D0646846

HEART DISEASE

A Textbook of Cardiovascular Medicine

5TH EDITION

HEART DISEASE

A Textbook of Cardiovascular Medicine

VOLUME 1

Edited by

EUGENE BRAUNWALD A.B., M.D., M.A. (hon.), M.D. (hon.), Sc.D. (hon.), F.R.C.P.

Vice President for Academic Programs, Partners HealthCare System; Distinguished Hersey Professor of Medicine, Faculty Dean for Academic Programs at Brigham and Women's Hospital and Massachusetts General Hospital, Harvard Medical School, Boston, Massachusetts

W.B. SAUNDERS COMPANY
A Division of Harcourt Brace & Company
PHILADELPHIA / LONDON / TORONTO / MONTREAL / SYDNEY / TOKYO

W.B. SAUNDERS COMPANY
A Division of Harcourt Brace & Company

The Curtis Center
Independence Square West
Philadelphia, Pennsylvania 19106

Library of Congress Cataloging-in-Publication Data

Heart disease: a textbook of cardiovascular medicine /
[edited by] Eugene Braunwald.—5th ed.

p. cm.

Includes bibliographical references and index.

ISBN 0–7216–5666–8 (single v.).—ISBN 0–7216–5663–3 (set).
ISBN 0–7216–5664–1 (v. 1).—ISBN 0–7216–5665–X (v. 2)

1. Heart—Diseases. 2. Cardiovascular system—Diseases.
I. Braunwald, Eugene
[DNLM: 1. Heart Diseases. WG 200 H4364 1997]

RC681.H362 1997 616.1′2—dc20

DNLM/DLC 95-24767

HEART DISEASE: A Textbook of
Cardiovascular Medicine, Fifth Edition

ISBN 0–7216–5666–8 (single vol.)
ISBN 0–7216–5663–3 (2-vol. set)
ISBN 0–7216–5664–1 (vol. 1)
ISBN 0–7216–5665–X (vol. 2)

Printed in the United States of America

Last digit is the print number: 9 8 7 6 5 4 3 2 1

Dedicated to

ELAINE

KAREN, ALLISON, JILL

DANA, ALEX, MARA, ELISE, CARI, *and* BENJAMIN

CONTRIBUTORS 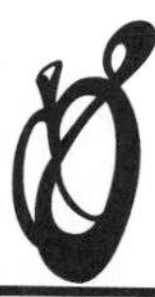

ELLIOTT M. ANTMAN, M.D.
Associate Professor of Medicine, Harvard Medical School. Director, Coronary Care Unit, Brigham and Women's Hospital, Boston, Massachusetts
Acute Myocardial Infarction; Medical Management of the Patient Undergoing Cardiac Surgery

S. SERGE BAROLD, M.D.
Professor of Medicine, University of Rochester School of Medicine and Dentistry. Chief, Cardiology Division, Department of Medicine, The Genesee Hospital, Rochester, New York
Cardiac Pacemakers and Antiarrhythmic Devices

JOHN A. BITTL, M.D.
Associate Professor of Medicine, Harvard Medical School. Director of Interventional Cardiology, Brigham and Women's Hospital, Boston, Massachusetts
Coronary Arteriography

ROBERT O. BONOW, M.D.
Goldberg Professor of Medicine and Chief, Division of Cardiology, Northwestern University Medical School. Chief, Division of Cardiology, Northwestern Memorial Hospital, Chicago, Illinois
Cardiac Catheterization

HARISIOS BOUDOULAS, M.D.
Professor of Medicine and Pharmacy, Ohio State University College of Medicine. Director, Overstreet Teaching and Research Laboratory (Division of Cardiology), Ohio State University Medical Center, Columbus, Ohio
Renal Disorders and Heart Disease

EUGENE BRAUNWALD, M.D.
Vice President for Academic Programs, Partners HealthCare System; Distinguished Hersey Professor of Medicine, Faculty Dean for Academic Programs at Brigham and Women's Hospital and Massachusetts General Hospital, Harvard Medical School, Boston, Massachusetts
The History; Physical Examination of the Heart and Circulation; Pathophysiology of Heart Failure; Assessment of Cardiac Function; Clinical Aspects of Heart Failure: High-Output Heart Failure; Pulmonary Edema; Management of Heart Failure; Pulmonary Hypertension; Valvular Heart Disease; Coronary Blood Flow and Myocardial Ischemia; Acute Myocardial Infarction; Chronic Coronary Artery Disease; The Cardiomyopathies and Myocarditides; Primary Tumors of the Heart; Traumatic Heart Disease; Hematological-Oncological Disorders and Heart Disease

BRUCE H. BRUNDAGE, M.D.
Professor of Medicine and Radiological Sciences, University of California, Los Angeles, School of Medicine, Los Angeles, California. Chief of Cardiology and Scientific Director, St. John's Cardiovascular Research Center, Harbor-UCLA Medical Center, Torrance, California
Relative Merits of Imaging Techniques

AGUSTIN CASTELLANOS, M.D.
Professor of Medicine, University of Miami School of Medicine. Director of Clinical Electrophysiology, Jackson Memorial Hospital, Miami, Florida
Cardiac Arrest and Sudden Cardiac Death

BERNARD R. CHAITMAN, M.D.
Professor of Medicine, St. Louis University School of Medicine. Chief of Cardiology, St. Louis University Health Sciences Center, St. Louis, Missouri
Exercise Stress Testing

KENNETH R. CHIEN, M.D., Ph.D.
Professor of Medicine and Member, Center for Molecular Genetics, University of California, San Diego, La Jolla, California. Attending Physician, University of California, San Diego, University Hospital, San Diego, California
Principles of Cardiovascular Molecular and Cellular Biology

JONATHAN S. COBLYN, M.D.
Assistant Professor of Medicine, Harvard Medical School. Associate Director, Robert B. Brigham Arthritis Center, Brigham and Women's Hospital, Boston, Massachusetts
Rheumatic Diseases and the Heart

PETER F. COHN, M.D.
Professor of Medicine and Chief, Cardiology Division, State University of New York Health Sciences Center, Stony Brook, New York
Traumatic Heart Disease

WILSON S. COLUCCI, M.D.
Professor of Medicine, Biochemistry and Physiology, Boston University School of Medicine. Associate Chief, Cardiovascular Division, and Director, Cardiomyopathy Program, Boston University Medical Center. Chief, Cardiology Section, Boston Veterans Affairs Medical Center, Boston, Massachusetts
Pathophysiology of Heart Failure; Clinical Aspects of Heart Failure: High-Output Heart Failure; Pulmonary Edema; Primary Tumors of the Heart

ADNAN S. DAJANI, M.D.
Professor of Pediatrics, Wayne State University School of Medicine. Director, Division of Infectious Diseases, Children's Hospital of Michigan, Detroit, Michigan
Rheumatic Fever

CHARLES J. DAVIDSON, M.D.
Associate Professor of Medicine, Northwestern University Medical School. Chief, Cardiac Catheterization Laboratories, Northwestern Memorial Hospital, Chicago, Illinois
Cardiac Catheterization

CHARLES DENNIS, M.D.
Chairman, Department of Cardiology, Deborah Heart and Lung Center, Browns Mills, New Jersey
Rehabilitation of Patients with Coronary Artery Disease

ROMAN W. DeSANCTIS, M.D.
Professor of Medicine, Harvard Medical School. Director of Clinical Cardiology and Physician, Massachusetts General Hospital, Boston, Massachusetts
Diseases of the Aorta

PAMELA S. DOUGLAS, M.D.

Associate Professor of Medicine, Harvard Medical School. Director, Noninvasive Cardiology, Beth Israel Hospital, Boston, Massachusetts

Coronary Artery Disease in Women

KIM A. EAGLE, M.D.

Associate Professor of Internal Medicine, University of Michigan School of Medicine. Director of Clinical Cardiology, University of Michigan Medical Center, Ann Arbor, Michigan

Diseases of the Aorta

URI ELKAYAM, M.D.

Professor of Medicine, Division of Cardiology, University of Southern California School of Medicine. Director, Heart Failure Program, and Director, High Risk Cardiology Perinatal Clinic, Los Angeles, California

Pregnancy and Cardiovascular Disease

JOHN A. FARMER, M.D.

Associate Professor of Medicine, Sections of Atherosclerosis and Cardiology, Baylor College of Medicine. Chief of Cardiology, Ben Taub General Hospital, Houston, Texas

Dyslipidemia and Other Risk Factors for Coronary Artery Disease

HARVEY FEIGENBAUM, M.D.

Distinguished Professor of Medicine, Indiana University School of Medicine. Senior Research Associate, Krannert Institute of Cardiology, Indianapolis, Indiana

Echocardiography

CHARLES FISCH, M.D.

Distinguished Professor Emeritus of Medicine, Indiana University School of Medicine, Indianapolis, Indiana

Electrocardiography

ROBERT F. FISHMAN, M.D.

Assistant Professor of Medicine, Northwestern University Medical School. Attending Physician, Northwestern Memorial Hospital, Chicago, Illinois

Cardiac Catheterization

WILLIAM F. FRIEDMAN, M.D.

J. H. Nicholson Professor of Pediatrics (Cardiology), Department of Pediatrics, and Senior Advisor, Clinical Affairs, to the Provost and Dean, University of California, Los Angeles, School of Medicine, Los Angeles, California

Congenital Heart Disease in Infancy and Childhood; Acquired Heart Disease in Infancy and Childhood

VALENTIN FUSTER, M.D., Ph.D.

Arthur M. and Hilda A. Master Professor of Medicine, Mount Sinai School of Medicine. Director, Cardiovascular Institute. Dean for Academic Affairs and Vice Chairman, Department of Medicine, Mount Sinai Medical Center, New York, New York

Hemostasis, Thrombosis, Fibrinolysis, and Cardiovascular Disease

PETER GANZ, M.D.

Associate Professor of Medicine, Harvard Medical School. Director of Research, Cardiac Catheterization Laboratory, Brigham and Women's Hospital, Boston, Massachusetts

Coronary Blood Flow and Myocardial Ischemia

BERNARD J. GERSH, M.B., D.Phil.

Professor of Medicine and Chief, Division of Cardiology, Georgetown University Medical Center, Washington, D.C.

Chronic Coronary Artery Disease

GARY GERSTENBLITH, M.D.

Professor of Medicine, Johns Hopkins University School of Medicine, Baltimore, Maryland

The Aging Heart: Structure, Function, and Disease

SAMUEL Z. GOLDHABER, M.D.

Associate Professor of Medicine, Harvard Medical School. Physician, Brigham and Women's Hospital, Boston, Massachusetts

Pulmonary Embolism

LEE GOLDMAN, M.D.

Julius Krevans Distinguished Professor and Chairman, Department of Medicine, and Associate Dean for Clinical Affairs, University of California, San Francisco, School of Medicine, San Francisco, California

Cost-Effective Strategies in Cardiology; General Anesthesia and Noncardiac Surgery in Patients with Heart Disease

ANTONIO M. GOTTO, Jr., M.D., D.Phil.

Distinguished Service Professor and Chairman, Department of Medicine, Baylor College of Medicine. Chief, Internal Medicine Service, Methodist Hospital, Houston, Texas

Dyslipidemia and Other Risk Factors for Coronary Artery Disease

ANDREW A. GRACE, Ph.D., M.R.C.P.

Senior Research Fellow, Departments of Medicine and Biochemistry, University of Cambridge, and Director, Cardiac Electrophysiology Service, Papworth Hospital, Cambridge, England. Visiting Scientist, Department of Medicine, University of California, San Diego, La Jolla, California.

Principles of Cardiovascular Molecular and Cellular Biology

WILLIAM GROSSMAN, M.D.

Adjunct Professor of Medicine, University of Pennsylvania School of Medicine, Philadelphia, Pennsylvania. Vice President, Clinical Research, Merck and Co., West Point, Pennsylvania

Clinical Aspects of Heart Failure: High-Output Heart Failure; Pulmonary Edema; Pulmonary Hypertension

CHARLES B. HIGGINS, M.D.

Professor and Vice-Chairman, Department of Radiology, University of California, San Francisco, San Francisco, California

Newer Cardiac Imaging Techniques: Magnetic Resonance Imaging and Computed Tomography

ERIC M. ISSELBACHER, M.D.

Instructor in Medicine, Harvard Medical School. Assistant in Medicine, Massachusetts General Hospital, Boston, Massachusetts

Diseases of the Aorta

NORMAN M. KAPLAN, M.D.

Professor of Internal Medicine and Head, Hypertension Division, University of Texas Southwestern Medical Center, Dallas, Texas

Systemic Hypertension: Mechanisms and Diagnosis; Systemic Hypertension: Therapy

WISHWA N. KAPOOR, M.D.

Falk Professor of Medicine, University of Pittsburgh. Chief, Division of Internal Medicine, Presbyterian-University Hospital, Pittsburgh, Pennsylvania

Syncope and Hypotension

ADOLF W. KARCHMER, M.D.

Professor of Medicine, Harvard Medical School. Chief, Division of Infectious Diseases, New England Deaconess Hospital, Boston, Massachusetts

Infective Endocarditis

RALPH A. KELLY, M.D.

Assistant Professor of Medicine, Harvard Medical School. Associate Physician, Division of Cardiology, Department of Medicine, Brigham and Women's Hospital, Boston, Massachusetts

Drugs Used in the Treatment of Heart Failure; Management of Heart Failure

EDWARD G. LAKATTA, M.D.

Professor of Medicine, Johns Hopkins School of Medicine. Professor of Physiology, University of Maryland School of Medicine. Chief, Laboratory of Cardiovascular Science, NIH/NIA/Gerontology Research Center, Baltimore, Maryland

The Aging Heart: Structure, Function, and Disease

THOMAS H. LEE, M.D., M.Sc.

Associate Professor of Medicine, Harvard Medical School and Brigham and Women's Hospital. Medical Director, Partners Community Health Care, Inc., Boston, Massachusetts

Practice Guidelines in Cardiovascular Medicine

CARL V. LEIER, M.D.

James W. Overstreet Professor of Medicine and Pharmacology, Ohio State University College of Medicine. Director, Division of Cardiology, and Director, Cardiac Transplantation Service, Ohio State University Medical Center, Columbus, Ohio

Renal Disorders and Heart Disease

DAVID C. LEVIN, M.D.

Professor of Radiology, Jefferson Medical College. Chairman, Department of Radiology, Thomas Jefferson University Hospital, Philadelphia, Pennsylvania

Radiology of the Heart; Coronary Arteriography

LEONARD S. LILLY, M.D.

Associate Professor of Medicine, Harvard Medical School. Associate Physician, Brigham and Women's Hospital, Boston, Massachusetts

The Heart in Endocrine and Nutritional Disorders

A. MICHAEL LINCOFF, M.D.

Assistant Professor of Medicine, Ohio State University. Director, Experimental Interventional Laboratory, Department of Cardiology, Center for Thrombosis and Vascular Biology, The Cleveland Clinic Foundation, Cleveland, Ohio

Interventional Catheterization Techniques

WILLIAM C. LITTLE, M.D.

Professor of Internal Medicine and Chief of Cardiology, Bowman-Gray School of Medicine of Wake Forest University. Chief of Cardiology and Associate Chief of Professional Services, North Carolina Baptist Hospital, Winston-Salem, North Carolina

Assessment of Cardiac Function

BEVERLY H. LORELL, M.D.

Associate Professor of Medicine, Harvard Medical School. Director, Hemodynamic Research Laboratory, and Associate Director, Cardiac Catheterization Laboratory, Beth Israel Hospital, Boston, Massachusetts

Pericardial Diseases

RICHARD A. MATTHAY, M.D.

Boehringer Ingelheim Professor of Medicine and Associate Director, Pulmonary and Critical Care Section, Department of Internal Medicine, Yale University School of Medicine, New Haven, Connecticut

Cor Pulmonale

ROBERT J. MYERBURG, M.D.

Professor of Medicine and Physiology and Director, Division of Cardiology, University of Miami School of Medicine. Chief of Cardiology, Jackson Memorial Medical Center, Miami, Florida

Cardiac Arrest and Sudden Cardiac Death

LIONEL H. OPIE, M.D., D.Phil., F.R.C.P.

Professor, Department of Medicine, University of Capetown. Director, Hypertension Clinic, Groote Schuur Hospital, Capetown, South Africa

Mechanisms of Cardiac Contraction and Relaxation

JOSEPH K. PERLOFF, M.D.

Streisand/American Heart Association Professor of Medicine and Pediatrics, University of California, Los Angeles, School of Medicine, Division of Cardiology, Departments of Medicine and Pediatrics, UCLA Center for the Health Sciences, Los Angeles, California

Physical Examination of the Heart and Circulation; Congenital Heart Disease in Adults; Neurological Disorders and Heart Disease

MARK G. PERLROTH, M.D.

Professor of Medicine, Division of Cardiovascular Medicine, Stanford University School of Medicine, Falk Cardiovascular Research Center. Professor of Medicine, Stanford University Medical Center and The Lucile Salter Packard Children's Hospital, Stanford, California. Consultant Cardiologist, Palo Alto Veterans Administration Medical Center, Palo Alto, California

Heart and Heart-Lung Transplantation

WILLIAM S. PIERCE, M.D.

Evan Pugh Professor of Surgery, Jane A. Fetter Professor of Surgery, and Chief, Division of Cardiothoracic Surgery, Department of Surgery, Pennsylvania State University College of Medicine, Hershey, Pennsylvania

Assisted Circulation and the Mechanical Heart

REED E. PYERITZ, M.D., Ph.D.

Chair, Department of Human Genetics, and Professor of Human Genetics, Medicine and Pediatrics, and Director, Institute for Medical Genetics, Medical College of Pennsylvania and Hahnemann University, Philadelphia and Pittsburgh, Pennsylvania. Director, Center for Medical Genetics, Allegheny General Hospital, Pittsburgh, Pennsylvania

Genetics and Cardiovascular Disease

BRUCE A. REITZ, M.D.
The Norman E. Shumway Professor and Chairman, Department of Cardiothoracic Surgery, Stanford University School of Medicine. Chief of the Cardiac Surgical Service, Stanford Health Services, Stanford, California. Chief of the Pediatric Cardiac Surgical Service, The Lucile Salter Packard Children's Hospital at Stanford, Palo Alto, California
Heart and Heart-Lung Transplantation

STUART RICH, M.D.
Professor of Medicine, University of Illinois, Chicago. Chief of Cardiology, University of Illinois, Chicago Medical Center, Chicago, Illinois
Pulmonary Hypertension

WAYNE E. RICHENBACHER, M.D.
Associate Professor, Division of Cardiothoracic Surgery, Department of Surgery, University of Iowa, Iowa City, Iowa
Assisted Circulation and the Mechanical Heart

DAVID S. ROSENTHAL, M.D.
Professor of Medicine, Harvard Medical School. Henry K. Oliver Professor of Hygiene, Harvard University. Physician, Brigham and Women's Hospital. Director and Physician, University Health Services, Harvard University, Cambridge, Massachusetts
Hematological-Oncological Disorders and Heart Disease

RUSSELL ROSS, Ph.D.
Professor, Department of Pathology, and Adjunct Professor, Department of Biochemistry, University of Washington School of Medicine, Seattle, Washington
The Pathogenesis of Atherosclerosis

JOHN D. RUTHERFORD, M.B., Ch.B., F.R.A.C.P.
Professor of Medicine, University of Texas, Gail Griffiths Hill Chair of Cardiology. Associate Director, Division of Cardiology, Southwestern Medical Center, Dallas, Texas
Chronic Coronary Artery Disease

HEINRICH R. SCHELBERT, M.D., Ph.D.
Professor of Pharmacology and Radiological Sciences and Vice Chairman, Department of Pharmacology, University of California, Los Angeles, School of Medicine, Los Angeles, California
Relative Merits of Imaging Techniques

FREDERICK J. SCHOEN, M.D., Ph.D.
Professor of Pathology, Harvard Medical School. Director, Cardiac Pathology, and Vice-Chairman, Department of Pathology, Brigham and Women's Hospital, Boston, Massachusetts
Primary Tumors of the Heart

ELLEN W. SEELY, M.D.
Assistant Professor of Medicine, Harvard Medical School. Director of Clinical Research, Endocrine-Hypertension Division, and Director, Ambulatory Clinical Research Center, Brigham and Women's Hospital, Boston, Massachusetts
The Heart in Endocrine and Nutritional Disorders

LAWRENCE N. SHULMAN, M.D.
Assistant Professor of Medicine, Harvard Medical School. Clinical Director, Hematology-Oncology Division, Brigham and Women's Hospital, Boston, Massachusetts
Hematological-Oncological Disorders and Heart Disease

DAVID J. SKORTON, M.D.

Professor of Medicine, College of Medicine, and Professor of Electrical and Computer Engineering, College of Engineering, University of Iowa. Co-Director, Adolescent and Adult Congenital Heart Disease Clinic. Staff Physician, University of Iowa Hospitals and Clinics. Consulting Physician, Department of Veterans Affairs Medical Center. Vice-President for Research, University of Iowa, Iowa City, Iowa

Relative Merits of Imaging Techniques

THOMAS W. SMITH, M.D.

Professor of Medicine, Harvard Medical School. Chief, Cardiovascular Division, and Senior Physician, Brigham and Women's Hospital, Boston, Massachusetts

Drugs Used in the Treatment of Heart Failure; Management of Heart Failure

ROBERT SOUFER, M.D.

Associate Professor of Diagnostic Radiology and Medicine (Cardiovascular Medicine), Yale University School of Medicine. Attending Physician, Internal Medicine, Yale-New Haven Hospital. Director, Positron Emission Tomography Center, Yale University-Veterans Administration PET Center, West Haven, Connecticut

Nuclear Cardiology

ROBERT M. STEINER, M.D.

Professor of Radiology and Medicine, Jefferson Medical College, Thomas Jefferson University Hospital, Philadelphia, Pennsylvania

Radiology of the Heart

LYNNE WARNER STEVENSON, M.D.

Associate Professor of Medicine, Harvard Medical School. Medical Director, Cardiomyopathy and Transplant Center, Brigham and Women's Hospital, Boston, Massachusetts

Management of Heart Failure

ERIC J. TOPOL, M.D.

Professor of Medicine, Cleveland Clinic Health Sciences Center, Ohio State University. Chairman, Department of Cardiology, and Director, Joseph J. Jacobs Center for Thrombosis and Vascular Biology, Cleveland Clinic Foundation, Cleveland, Ohio

Interventional Catheterization Techniques

MARC VERSTRAETE, M.D., Ph.D.

Professor of Medicine and Former Director, Center for Molecular and Vascular Biology, University of Leuven, Leuven, Belgium

Hemostasis, Thrombosis, Fibrinolysis and Cardiovascular Disease

FRANS J. TH. WACKERS, M.D.

Professor of Diagnostic Radiology and Medicine (Cardiology), Yale University School of Medicine. Director, Cardiovascular Nuclear Imaging and Exercise Laboratories, Yale-New Haven Hospital, New Haven, Connecticut

Nuclear Cardiology

HERBERT P. WEIDEMANN, M.D.

Chief, Pulmonary Department, The Cleveland Clinic Foundation, Cleveland, Ohio

Cor Pulmonale

MICHAEL E. WEINBLATT, M.D.

Associate Professor of Medicine, Harvard Medical School. Director of Clinical Rheumatology, Brigham and Women's Hospital, Boston, Massachusetts

Rheumatic Diseases and the Heart

MYRON L. WEISFELDT, M.D.

Samuel Bard Professor of Medicine and Chair, Department of Medicine, Columbia University College of Physicians and Surgeons. Director of the Medical Service and Attending Physician, Presbyterian Hospital, New York, New York

The Aging Heart: Structure, Function, and Disease

GORDON H. WILLIAMS, M.D.

Professor of Medicine, Harvard Medical School. Chief, Endocrine-Hypertension Division, and Director, Clinical Research Center, Brigham and Women's Hospital, Boston, Massachusetts

The Heart in Endocrine and Nutritional Disorders

GERALD L. WOLF, Ph.D., M.D.

Professor of Radiology, Harvard Medical School. Director, Center for Imaging and Pharmaceutical Research, Massachusetts General Hospital, Boston, Massachusetts

Relative Merits of Imaging Techniques

JOSHUA WYNNE, M.D.

Professor of Medicine and Chief, Division of Cardiology, Wayne State University. Chief, Section of Cardiology, Harper Hospital, Detroit Medical Center, Detroit, Michigan

The Cardiomyopathies and Myocarditides

BARRY L. ZARET, M.D.

Robert W. Berliner Professor of Medicine, Professor of Diagnostic Radiology, Chief, Section of Cardiovascular Medicine, and Associate Chair for Clinical Affairs, Department of Internal Medicine, Yale University School of Medicine. Chief of Cardiology, Yale-New Haven Hospital, New Haven, Connecticut

Nuclear Cardiology

DOUGLAS P. ZIPES, M.D.

Distinguished Professor of Medicine, Pharmacology, and Toxicology and Director, Division of Cardiology and Krannert Institute of Cardiology, Indiana University School of Medicine. Attending Physician, University Hospital, Wishard Memorial Hospital, and Roudebush Veterans Administration Hospital, Indianapolis, Indiana

Genesis of Cardiac Arrhythmias: Electrophysiological Considerations; Management of Cardiac Arrhythmias: Pharmacological, Electrical, and Surgical Techniques; Specific Arrhythmias: Diagnosis and Treatment; Cardiac Pacemakers and Antiarrhythmic Devices

PREFACE

As I complete the preparations of this new edition of *Heart Disease,* I am awed by the continued growth and progress in cardiovascular medicine. During my professional lifetime I have been privileged to observe the field's advance to a point at which the safe and accurate diagnosis and the effective treatment of most forms of heart disease is now feasible. While the overall population is aging and the total prevalence of heart disease rising, the age-adjusted mortality rate for cardiovascular disease in the United States has declined by approximately 1 per cent per year for the last 40 years, and this decline appears to be continuing.

The enormous advances in the field in the five years since the publication of the fourth edition have required the most extensive changes yet made in any revision of this text. Despite the need to include an enormous amount of new information, it was possible to retain the basic format of the previous edition of *Heart Disease.* The book is divided into five parts: Part I deals with the examination of the patient in the broadest sense, including clinical findings and the theory and application of modern noninvasive and invasive techniques to elicit information about the heart and circulation. Part II is concerned with the pathophysiology, diagnosis, and treatment of the principal abnormalities of circulatory function, including heart failure, arrhythmias, and abnormalities of arterial pressure. Part III, the longest in the book, consists of descriptions of the principal congenital and acquired diseases affecting the heart, pericardium, aorta, and pulmonary vascular bed in adults and children. Part IV deals with the interfaces between cardiology and broad fields such as genetics, aging, management of the postoperative cardiac patient, and the economics of cardiac care. Part V details the relationship between diseases of other organ systems and the circulation and vice versa.

Twenty-one new chapters—the most for any revision to date—have been added or substituted. Many other important new areas are covered in radically revised chapters.

A number of important areas are covered in this edition: The chapter on Physical Examination prepared with Perloff has been expanded and revised because the intelligent contemporary practice of cardiology requires careful integration of findings obtained from the clinical examination with those from the growing number of diagnostic modalities now available. The chapter on the Relative Merits of Imaging Techniques by Skorton and colleagues provides a rational approach to the intelligent selection among the several techniques now available to image the heart.

A new, and I believe unique, aspect of the fifth edition of *Heart Disease* is Lee's comprehensive chapter on Practice Guidelines in Cardiovascular Medicine. Increasingly, practice guidelines are influencing diagnosis and therapy and are rapidly becoming the basis for reimbursement of health care services. This new chapter provides a summary of the most important guidelines put together by authoritative groups—mostly key committees of the American Heart Association and the American College of Cardiology. In addition to a summary of the guidelines, Lee places them into the perspective of modern patient care. The chapter on Cost-Effective Strategies in Cardiology by Goldman explains how cost-conscious practice need not impair the quality of care.

Also of note is a new chapter on a subject that is attracting a great deal of interest—Coronary Artery Disease in Women—by Douglas, which complements the chapter on Aging in Cardiac Disease. This pair of chapters deals with two large groups of patients with special needs, problems, and issues, who together constitute an enormous percentage of the total population. Advances in interventional cardiology represent one of the most dramatic developments in the field and they are covered in an excellent new chapter by Lincoff and Topol. Cardiologists increasingly need an understanding of hemostasis, thrombosis, and fibrinolysis in their daily practice. Fuster and Verstraete have teamed up to provide a superb new chapter on this subject.

Because it is now clear that abnormalities of molecular processes may be the basis of many cardiovascular diseases and that genetic influences play critical roles in the development of these abnormalities, three new chapters have been included. Opie describes the basic mechanisms of cardiac contraction and relaxation. Chien and Grace present the impact of cell and molecular biology, while Pyeritz summarizes the genetics of cardiovascular disease. The important role played by genetics in cardiovascular disease is underscored by Figure 49–1, on pages 1652 and 1653, specially prepared for this book by Pyeritz, which shows the chromosomal location of 137 human genes whose mutations have been shown to produce deleterious effects on the cardiovascular system. This field is moving very swiftly indeed; undoubtedly many other genes will be identified and their chromosomal locations determined by the time the sixth edition of *Heart Disease* is published.

An important responsibility of an editor is to establish the boundaries of a book. In approaching this task, I have deliberately taken a broad approach—in the line with this book's subtitle "A Textbook of Cardiovascular Medicine." I believe that modern cardiologists will best serve their patients by being first broadly based physicians and second accomplished technical specialists. Cardiologists must remain the masters—not become the slaves—of the powerful new diagnostic and therapeutic tools now available. They must also understand the enormous influence that heart disease can exert on the function of other organ systems, as well as the equally important effect that disordered function of other organ systems can have on the circulation. Cardiologists must also be able to function effectively as a consultants to generalists, surgeons, and other specialists. The chapter on Pulmonary Embolism, and all of Part V (Heart Disease and Disorders of Other Organ Systems) explore the important interfaces between cardiology and other branches of medicine. The chapter by Antman on the medical management of the patient undergoing cardiac surgery should be helpful to the cardiologist and internist in what is a growing responsibility. Its companion chapter on noncardiac surgery in the patient with heart disease by Goldman provides an approach to an increasing challenge posed to the modern cardiologist and internist.

Considerable revisions have been made in both galley proofs and page proofs to include information about the most recent advances in the field. Particular emphasis has been placed on ensuring a comprehensive and up-to-date bibliography of more than 18,000 pertinent references, including hundreds to publications that appeared in 1996. Many of the 1,436 figures and 444 tables are new to this edition. The fifth edition of *Heart Disease* is approximately 15 per cent longer than the fourth. This has been accomplished with only a modest increase in the number of pages and bulk in the book through a more efficient page layout, the use of somewhat smaller illustrations, and the more liberal use of a special type face.

In order to allow the reader to keep pace with the enormous expansion of cardiovascular knowledge, the fifth edition is supplemented by a number of companion volumes. First, W.B. Saunders has just published the second edition of *Marcus Cardiac Imaging: A Companion to Braunwald's Heart Disease*, edited by Skorton, Schelbert, Wolf and Brundage, which provides an elegant analysis of the most important cardiovascular diagnostic imaging techniques now available. This companion book is especially useful given the profound advances in cardiovascular diagnosis made possible by modern imaging techniques. No area of cardiology has advanced more rapidly than therapeutics, and therefore it seems logical for the second companion to *Heart Disease* to be *Cardiovascular Therapeutics*. The editorial effort was ably led by my colleague at the Brigham, Thomas W. Smith, who enlisted the cooperation of a team of outstanding associate editors and authors.

Two other companions to *Heart Disease* are now in advanced stages of preparation—*Molecular Basis of Heart Disease*, edited by Chien, and *Clinical Trials in Cardiovascular Disease*, edited by Hennekens. In addition, a *Review and Assessment* book, prepared by Mendelsohn, will again accompany this edition of *Heart Disease*. It consists of 600 questions based on material discussed in the textbook and provides the answers as well as detailed explanations. This multipronged educational effort—*Heart Disease*, the growing number of companion volumes, as well as the *Review and Assessment* book, all appearing in print and electronic (CD-ROM) form—is designed to assist the reader with the awesome task of learning and remaining current in this dynamic field.

It is hoped that this textbook will prove useful to those who wish to broaden their knowledge of cardiovascular medicine. To the extent that it achieves this goal and thereby aids in the care of patients afflicted with heart disease, credit must be given to the many talented and dedicated persons involved in its preparation. My deepest appreciation goes to my fellow contributors for their professional expertise, knowledge and devoted scholarship, which are at the very "heart" of this book. At the W.B. Saunders Company, my editor, Richard Zorab, and the production team—Frank Polizzano, Edna Dick, Lorraine Kilmer, and Hazel Hacker—were enormously helpful. My editorial associate, Ms. Kathryn Saxon, rendered invaluable and devoted assistance.

This edition could not have become a reality were it not for the skillful and dedicated efforts of several other individuals. My responsibilities to the Harvard Medical School and the Brigham and Women's Hospital during the leave of absence that I required for much of my own writing were shouldered most effectively by my colleagues Drs. Dennis Kasper and Marshall Wolf, who provided the Department of Medicine with exemplary leadership. My administrative assistant, Ms. Diane Rioux, was enormously helpful in maintaining the orderly flow of activity essential to a busy Department of Medicine. I am especially indebted to Dr. Daniel C. Tosteson, Dean of the Harvard Medical School, and to Dr. H. Richard Nesson, President of the Partners HealthCare System and of the Brigham and Women's Hospital, for graciously allowing me the freedom to devote myself to this task. On a personal note, my wife, Elaine, provided the personal support, encouragement and understanding so essential for one who adds a task of this magnitude to an already full professional life.

EUGENE BRAUNWALD, 1996

Adapted from the PREFACE to the First Edition

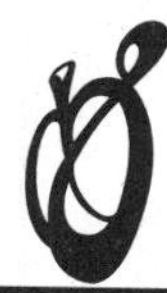

Cardiovascular disease is the greatest scourge afflicting the population of the industrialized nations. As with previous scourges—bubonic plague, yellow fever, and smallpox—cardiovascular disease not only strikes down a significant fraction of the population without warning but causes prolonged suffering and disability in an even larger number. In the United States alone, despite recent encouraging declines, cardiovascular disease is still responsible for almost one million fatalities each year and more than one half of all deaths; almost 5 million persons afflicted with cardiovascular disease are hospitalized each year. The cost of this disease in terms of human suffering and of material resources is almost incalculable.

Fortunately, research focusing on the causes, diagnosis, treatment, and prevention of heart disease is moving ahead rapidly. In the last 25 years in particular we have witnessed an explosive expansion of our understanding of the structure and function of the cardiovascular system—both normal and abnormal—and of our ability to evaluate it in the living patient, sometimes by means of techniques that require penetration of the skin but also, with increasing accuracy, by noninvasive methods. Simultaneously, remarkable progress has been made in preventing and treating cardiovascular disease by medical and surgical means. Indeed, in the United States, the aforementioned steady reduction in mortality from cardiovascular disease during the past decade suggests that the effective application of this increased knowledge is beginning to prolong the human life span—the most valued resource on earth.

An attempt to summarize our present understanding of heart disease in a comprehensive textbook for the serious student of this subject is a formidable undertaking. Following the untimely death of Dr. Charles K. Friedberg, whose masterful text served as a bible to me and to a whole generation of cardiologists during the 1950's and 1960's, the W.B. Saunders Company invited me to accept this responsibility. Younger colleagues, particularly cardiology fellows and medical residents at the Brigham, convinced me of the need for such a book.

In order to provide a comprehensive, authoritative text in a field that has become as broad and deep as cardiovascular medicine, I chose to enlist the aid of a number of able colleagues. However, I hoped that my personal involvement in the writing of about half of the book would make it possible to minimize the fragmentation, gaps, inconsistencies, organizational difficulties, and impersonal tone that sometimes plague multiauthored texts. I also sought a compromise between a book that is too long as a result of excessive repetition and one in which all duplication is eliminated, resulting in fragmented coverage of certain subjects. To help achieve this objective, extensive cross references have been provided within the text.

Since the early part of this century, clinical cardiology has had a particularly strong foundation in the basic sciences of physiology and pharmacology. More recently, the disciplines of molecular biology, genetics, developmental biology, biophysics, biochemistry, experimental pathology, and bioengineering have also begun to provide critically important information about cardiac function and malfunction. Although *Heart Disease: A Textbook of Cardiovascular Medicine* is primarily a clinical treatise and not a textbook of fundamental cardiovascular science, an effort has been made to explain, in some detail, the scientific basis of cardiovascular diseases.

EUGENE BRAUNWALD, 1980

COLOR PLATES 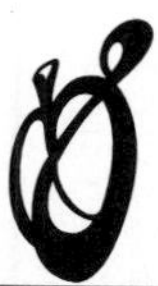

CONTENTS

PART I EXAMINATION OF THE PATIENT

PART II NORMAL AND ABNORMAL CIRCULATORY FUNCTION

PART III DISEASES OF THE HEART, PERICARDIUM, AORTA, AND PULMONARY VASCULAR BED

PART IV BROADER PERSPECTIVES ON HEART DISEASE AND CARDIOLOGIC PRACTICE

PART V HEART DISEASE AND DISORDERS OF OTHER ORGAN SYSTEMS

Part I
Examination of the Patient

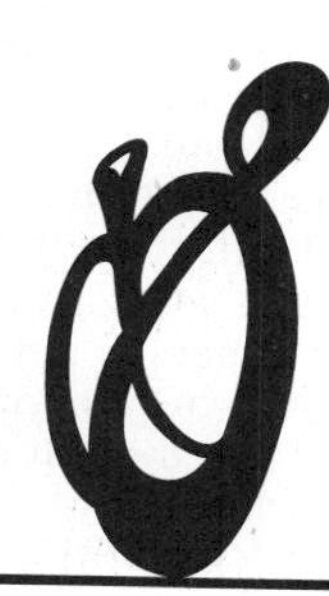

Chapter 1
The History

EUGENE BRAUNWALD

IMPORTANCE OF THE HISTORY

Specialized examinations of the cardiovascular system, presented in Chapters 3 to 11, provide a large portion of the data base required to establish a specific anatomical diagnosis of cardiac disease and to determine the extent of functional impairment of the heart. The development and application of these methods represent one of the triumphs of modern medicine. However, their appropriate use is to supplement but not to supplant a careful clinical examination. The latter remains the cornerstone of the assessment of the patient with known or suspected cardiovascular disease. There is a temptation in cardiology, as in many other areas of medicine, to carry out expensive, uncomfortable, and occasionally hazardous procedures to establish a diagnosis when a detailed and thoughtful history and physical examination are sufficient. Obviously, it is undesirable to subject patients to the unnecessary risks and expenses inherent in many specialized tests when a diagnosis can be made on the basis of an adequate clinical examination or when management will not be altered significantly as a result of these tests.[1] Intelligent selection of investigative procedures from the ever-increasing array of tests now available requires far more sophisticated decision-making than was necessary when the choices were limited to electrocardiography and chest roentgenography; some of the principles in such decision-making are dealt with in Chapters 11 and 53. The history and physical examination provide the critical information necessary for most of these decisions.

THE ROLE OF THE HISTORY. The overreliance on laboratory tests has increased as physicians attempt to utilize their time more efficiently by delegating responsibility for taking the history to a physician's assistant or nurse or even by limiting the history to a questionnaire—an approach that I consider to be an undesirable trend insofar as the patient with known or suspected heart disease is concerned.[2] First, it must be appreciated that the history remains the richest source of information concerning the patient's illness,[3,4] and any practice that might diminish the quality or quantity of information provided by the history is likely ultimately to impair the quality of care. Second, the physician's attentive and thoughtful taking of a history establishes a bond with the patient that may be valuable later in securing the patient's compliance in following a complex treatment plan, undergoing hospitalization for an intensive diagnostic work-up or a hazardous operation, and, in some instances, accepting that heart disease is not present at all.

Taking a history also permits the physician to evaluate the results of diagnostic tests that have strong subjective components, such as the determination of exercise capacity (Chap. 5). Perhaps most importantly, a careful history allows the physician to evaluate the impact of the disease, or the fear of the disease, on the various aspects of the patient's life and to assess the patient's personality, affect, and stability; often it provides a glimpse of the patient's responsibilities, fears, aspirations, and threshold for discomfort as well as the likelihood of compliance with one or another therapeutic regimen. Whenever possible, the physician should question not only the patient but also relatives or close friends to obtain a clearer understanding of the extent of the patient's disability and a broader perspective concerning the impact of the disease on both the patient and the family. (For example, the patient's spouse is much more likely than the patient to provide a history of Cheyne-Stokes [periodic] respiration.)

The combination of the widespread fear of cardiovascular disorders and the deep-seated emotional, symbolic, and sometimes even religious connotations surrounding the heart may, on the one hand, provoke symptoms that mimic those of organic heart disease in persons with normal cardiovascular systems. On the other, they cause so much fear that serious symptoms are repressed or denied by patients with established heart disease.

TECHNIQUE. Several approaches can be employed successfully in obtaining a medical history. I believe that patients should first be given the opportunity to relate their experiences and complaints in their own way. Although time-consuming and likely to include much seemingly irrelevant information, this technique has the advantage of providing considerable information concerning the patient's intelligence, emotional make-up, and attitude toward his or her complaints, as well as providing the patient with the satisfaction that he has been "heard" by the physician, rather than merely having had a few questions thrown at him and then been exposed to a battery of laboratory examinations. After the patient has given an account of the illness, the physician should direct the discussion and obtain information concerning the onset and chronology of symptoms; their location, quality, and intensity; the precipitating, aggravating, and alleviating factors, the setting in which the symptoms occur, and any associated symptoms; and the response to therapy.

Of course, a detailed general medical history including the personal past history, occupational history, nutritional history, and review of systems must be obtained. Of particular interest is a history of thyroid disease, recent dental extractions or manipulations, catheterization of the bladder, and earlier examinations that showed abnormalities of the cardiovascular system as reflected in restriction from physical activity at school and in rejection for life insurance, employment, or military service. Personal habits such as exercise, cigarette smoking, alcohol intake, and parenteral use of drugs—illicit and otherwise—should be ascertained. The exact nature of the patient's work, including the physical and emotional stresses, should be assessed. The increasing appreciation of the importance of genetic influences in many forms of heart disease (Chap. 49) underscores the importance of the family history.

A wide variety of disorders including, but not limited to, neurological (Chap. 60), endocrine (Chap. 61), and rheumatic (Chap. 56) may have important effects on the cardiovascular system; it is vital to ascertain the presence of these and other conditions that are not primarily cardiovascular. A history of the risk factors for ischemic heart disease—the history of cigarette smoking, hypertension, hypercholesterolemia, diabetes mellitus, artificial or early menopause, and long-term contraceptive pill ingestion, as well as the family history of ischemic heart disease (Chap. 35)—should always be sought.

Myocardial or coronary function that may be adequate at rest is often inadequate during exertion; therefore, specific attention should be directed to the influence of activity on the patient's symptoms. Thus, a history of chest discomfort and/or undue shortness of breath that appears only during activity is characteristic of heart disease, whereas the opposite pattern, i.e., the appearance of symptoms at rest and their remission during exertion, is almost never observed in patients with heart disease but is more characteristic of functional disorders. In attempting to assess the severity of functional impairment, both the *extent* of activity and the *rate* at which it is performed before symptoms develop should be determined and related to a detailed consideration of the therapeutic regimen. For example, the development of dyspnea after walking slowly up a flight of stairs in a patient receiving intensive treatment of heart failure denotes far more severe functional disability than does a similar symptom occurring in an untreated patient who has run up a flight of stairs.

As the patient relates the history, important nonverbal clues are often provided. The physician should observe the patient's attitude, reactions, and gestures while being questioned, as well as his or her choice of words or emphasis. Tumulty has aptly likened obtaining a meaningful clinical history to playing a game of chess:[5] "The patient makes a statement and based upon its content, and mode of expression, the physician asks a counter-question. One answer stimulates yet another question until the clinician is convinced that he understands precisely all of the circumstances of the patient's illness."

CARDINAL SYMPTOMS OF HEART DISEASE

The cardinal symptoms of heart disease include dyspnea, chest pain or discomfort, syncope, collapse, palpitation, edema, cough, hemoptysis, and excess fatigue. Cyanosis is more often a sign rather than a symptom, but it may be a key feature of the history, particularly in patients with congenital heart disease. Without doubt, history-taking is the most valuable technique available for determining whether or not these symptoms are caused by heart disease. Examples of the manner in which these symptoms may serve as a guide to diagnosis are given in the following pages, and reference is made to other portions of the book that contain more detailed information.

Dyspnea

(See also pp. 450 and 464)

Dyspnea is defined as an abnormally uncomfortable awareness of breathing; it is one of the principal symptoms of cardiac and pulmonary disease.[6] Since dyspnea is regularly caused by strenuous exertion in healthy, well-conditioned subjects and by only moderate exertion in those who are normal but unaccustomed to exercise, it should be regarded as abnormal only when it occurs at rest or at a level of physical activity not expected to cause this symptom. Dyspnea is associated with a wide variety of diseases of the heart and lungs, chest wall, and respiratory muscles as well as with anxiety[7–10]; the history is the most valuable means of establishing the etiology.[11,12] Table 1–1 provides a list of the various syndromes that may cause dyspnea and the primary pathophysiological mechanisms that are responsible.[13] Borg and Noble have developed a scale that is useful in quantitating the severity of dyspnea.[14]

The *sudden* development of dyspnea suggests pulmonary embolism, pneumothorax, acute pulmonary edema, pneumonia, or airway obstruction.[10] In contrast, in most forms of *chronic* heart failure, dyspnea progresses slowly over weeks or months. Such a protracted course may also occur in a variety of unrelated conditions, including obesity, pregnancy, and bilateral pleural effusion. *Inspiratory dyspnea* suggests obstruction of the upper airways, whereas *expiratory dyspnea* characterizes obstruction of the lower airways. Exertional dyspnea suggests the presence of organic diseases, such as left ventricular failure (Chap. 15) or chronic obstructive lung disease (Chap. 47), whereas dyspnea developing at rest may occur in pneumothorax, pulmonary embolism (Chap. 46), or pulmonary edema (Chap. 15), or it may be functional. Dyspnea that occurs only at rest and is absent on exertion is almost always functional. A *functional origin* is also suggested when dyspnea, or simply a heightened awareness of breathing, is accompanied by brief stabbing pain in the region of the cardiac apex or by prolonged (more than 2 hours) dull chest pain. It is often associated with difficulty in getting enough air into the lungs, claustrophobia, and sighing respirations that are relieved by exertion, by taking a few deep breaths, or by sedation. Dyspnea in patients with panic attacks is usually accompanied by hyperventilation. A history of relief of dyspnea by bronchodilators and corticosteroids suggests asthma as the etiology, whereas relief of dyspnea by rest, diuretics, and digitalis suggests left heart failure. Dyspnea accompanied by wheezing may be secondary to left ventricular failure (*cardiac* asthma) or primary bronchial constriction (*bronchial* asthma).

In patients with *chronic heart failure,* dyspnea is a clinical expression of pulmonary venous and capillary hyper-

TABLE 1-1 DISORDERS CAUSING DYSPNEA AND LIMITING EXERCISE PERFORMANCE; PATHOPHYSIOLOGY; AND DISCRIMINATING MEASUREMENTS

DISORDERS	PATHOPHYSIOLOGY	MEASUREMENTS THAT DEVIATE FROM NORMAL
Pulmonary		
Airflow limitation	Mechanical limitation to ventilation, mismatching of $\dot{V}_A/\dot{Q}$, hypoxic stimulation to breathing	$\dot{V}_E$ max/MVV, expiratory flow pattern, V_D, V_T; $\dot{V}O_2$ max, $\dot{V}_E/\dot{V}O_2$, $\dot{V}_E$ response to hyperoxia, (A − a)PO_2
Restrictive	Mismatching $\dot{V}_A/\dot{Q}$, hypoxic stimulation to breathing	
Chest wall	Mechanical limitation to ventilation	$\dot{V}_E$ max/MVV, P_ACO_2, $\dot{V}O_2$ max
Pulmonary circulation	Rise in physiological dead space as fraction of V_T, exercise hypoxemia	V_D/V_T, work-rate–related hypoxemia, VO_2 max, $\dot{V}_E/\dot{V}O_2$, (a − ET)PCO_2, O_2-pulse
Cardiac		
Coronary	Coronary insufficiency	ECG, $\dot{V}O_2$ max, anaerobic threshold $\dot{V}O_2$, $\dot{V}_E/\dot{V}O_2$, O_2-pulse, BP (systolic, diastolic, pulse)
Valvular	Cardiac output limitation (decreased effective stroke volume)	
Myocardial	Cardiac output limitation (decreased ejection fraction and stroke volume)	
Anemia	Reduced O_2-carrying capacity	O_2-pulse, anaerobic threshold $\dot{V}O_2$, $\dot{V}O_2$ max, $\dot{V}_E/\dot{V}O_2$
Peripheral circulation	Inadequate O_2 flow to metabolically active muscle	Anaerobic threshold $\dot{V}O_2$, $\dot{V}O_2$ max
Obesity	Increased work to move body; if severe, respiratory restriction and pulmonary insufficiency	$\dot{V}O_2$-work-rate relationship, P_AO_2, P_ACO_2, $\dot{V}O_2$ max
Psychogenic	Hyperventilation with precisely regular respiratory rate	Breathing pattern, PCO_2
Malingering	Hyperventilation and hypoventilation with irregular respiratory rate	Breathing pattern, PCO_2
Deconditioning	Inactivity or prolonged bed rest; loss of capability for effective redistribution of systemic blood flow	O_2-pulse, anaerobic threshold $\dot{V}O_2$, $\dot{V}O_2$ max

$\dot{V}_A$ = alveolar ventilation; $\dot{Q}$ = pulmonary blood flow; $\dot{V}_E$ = minute ventilation; MVV = maximum voluntary ventilation; V_D/V_T = physiological dead space/tidal volume ratio; O_2 = oxygen; VO_2 = O_2 consumption; (A − a)PO_2 = alveolar-arterial PO_2 difference; (a − ET)PCO_2 = arterial-end tidal PCO_2 difference.
Modified from Wasserman, D.: Dyspnea on exertion: Is it the heart or the lungs? JAMA *248*:2042, 1982. Copyright 1982 the American Medical Association.

tension (see p. 453). It occurs either during exertion or, in resting patients, in the recumbent position, and it is relieved promptly by sitting upright or standing *(orthopnea).* Patients with left ventricular failure soon learn to sleep on two or more pillows to avoid this symptom. In patients with heart failure, dyspnea is often accompanied by edema, upper abdominal pain (due to congestive hepatomegaly), and nocturia. The *sudden* occurrence of dyspnea in a patient with a history of mitral valve disease suggests the development of atrial fibrillation, rupture of chordae tendineae, or pulmonary embolism.

Paroxysmal nocturnal dyspnea is due to interstitial pulmonary edema and sometimes intraalveolar edema and is most commonly secondary to left ventricular failure (see p. 450). This condition, beginning usually 2 to 4 hours after the onset of sleep and often accompanied by cough, wheezing, and sweating, is quite frightening to the patient. Paroxysmal nocturnal dyspnea is often ameliorated by the patient's sitting on the side of the bed or getting out of bed; relief is not instantaneous but usually requires 15 to 30 minutes. Although paroxysmal nocturnal dyspnea secondary to left ventricular failure is usually accompanied by coughing, a careful history often discloses that the dyspnea *precedes* the cough, not vice versa. In contrast, patients with *chronic pulmonary disease* may also awaken at night, but cough and expectoration usually precede the dyspnea. These patients also often have a long history of smoking and a chronic cough with sputum production and wheezing and may be able to breathe more easily while leaning forward. Nocturnal dyspnea associated with pulmonary disease is usually relieved after the patient rids himself or herself of secretions rather than specifically by sitting up. Details of the value and limitations of the history of dyspnea in differentiating between primary diseases of the heart and lungs[15,16] are presented on page 451.

Patients with *pulmonary embolism* usually experience sudden dyspnea that may be associated with apprehension, palpitation, hemoptysis, or pleuritic chest pain (Chap. 46). The development or intensification of dyspnea, sometimes associated with a feeling of faintness, may be the only complaint of the patient with pulmonary emboli. *Pneumothorax* and *mediastinal emphysema* also cause dyspnea acutely, accompanied by sharp chest pain. Dyspnea accompanying thoracic pain occurs in *acute myocardial infarction.* Dyspnea is a common *"anginal equivalent"* (see p. 1290), i.e., a symptom secondary to myocardial ischemia that occurs in place of typical anginal discomfort.[16] This form of dyspnea may or may not be associated with a sensation of tightness in the chest, is present on exertion or emotional stress, is relieved by rest (more often in the sitting than in the recumbent position), is similar to angina in duration (i.e., 2 to 10 minutes), and is usually responsive to or prevented by nitroglycerin. The sudden development of severe dyspnea while sitting rather than lying, or whenever a particular position is assumed, suggests the possibility of a myxoma (see p. 1467) or ball-valve thrombus in the left atrium. When dyspnea is relieved by squatting, it is caused most commonly by tetralogy of Fallot or a variant thereof (see p. 929).

Chest Pain or Discomfort

(See also p. 1290)

Elucidation of the cause of chest pain is one of the key tasks of physicians, and this symptom is responsible for many cardiac consultations. The history remains the most important technique for distinguishing among the many causes of chest discomfort. Although chest pain or discomfort is one of the cardinal manifestations of cardiac disease, it is crucial to recognize that the pain may originate not only in the heart but also in (1) a variety of noncardiac intrathoracic structures, such as the aorta, pulmonary artery, bronchopulmonary tree, pleura, mediastinum, esophagus, and diaphragm; (2) the tissues of the neck or thoracic wall, including the skin, thoracic muscles, cervicodorsal spine, costochondral junctions, breasts, sensory nerves, and spinal cord; and (3) subdiaphragmatic organs such as the stomach, duodenum, pancreas, and gallbladder (Table 1–2). Pain of functional origin or factitious pain may also occur in the chest. Although a wide variety of laboratory tests is available to aid in the differential diagnosis of chest pain, without question the history remains the most valuable mode of examination. In obtaining the history of a patient with chest pain it is helpful to have a mental checklist and to ask the patient to describe the location, radiation, and character of the discomfort; what causes and relieves it; time relationships, including the duration, frequency, and pattern of recurrence of the discomfort; the setting in which it occurs; and associated symptoms. It is also particularly useful to observe the patient's gestures. Clenching the fist in front of the sternum while describing the sensation (Levine's sign) is a strong indication of an ischemic origin of the pain.

QUALITY. *Angina pectoris* may be defined as a discomfort in the chest and/or adjacent area associated with myocardial ischemia but without myocardial necrosis.[17–20] It is important to recognize that angina means *choking,* not pain. Thus, the discomfort of angina often is described not as pain at all but rather as an unpleasant sensation; "pressing," "squeezing," "strangling," "constricting," "bursting," and "burning" are some of the adjectives commonly used to describe this sensation (Table 1–3). "A band across the chest" and "a weight in the center of the chest" are other frequent descriptors. It is characteristic of angina that the intensity of effort required to incite it may vary from day to day and throughout the day in the same patient, but often a careful history will uncover explanations for this, such as meals ingested, weather, emotions, and the like. The anginal threshold is lower in the morning than at any other time of day; thus patients note frequently that activities that may cause angina in the morning or when first undertaken do not do so later in the day. When the threshold for angina is quite variable, defies any pattern, and is prominent at rest, the possibility that myocardial ischemia is caused by coronary spasm should be considered (see p. 1189). Thus, a careful history not only may indicate the cause of the pain (i.e., myocardial ischemia) but can also provide a clue to the mechanism of the ischemia (spasm vs. organic obstruction).

A history of prolonged, severe anginal chest discomfort accompanied by profound fatigue often signifies acute myocardial infarction.[21] There is some relationship between location of the chest pain and the site of coronary artery occlusion[22]; patients with ischemic heart disease who complain of substernal or left chest pain with radiation to the left arm often have heart disease involving the left coronary artery, while those with epigastric pain radiating to the neck or jaw may *not* have disease of the left anterior descending coronary artery.

When dyspnea is an "anginal equivalent," the patient may describe the midchest as the site of the shortness of breath, whereas true dyspnea is usually not well localized. Other anginal equivalents are discomfort limited to areas that are ordinarily sites of secondary radiation, such as the ulnar aspect of the left arm and forearm, lower jaw, teeth, neck, or shoulders, and the development of gas and belching, nausea, "indigestion," dizziness, and diaphoresis. Anginal equivalents above the mandible or below the umbilicus are quite uncommon. It is useful to determine whether the patient has symptoms or complications caused by atherosclerosis of other vascular beds, e.g., intermittent claudication, transient ischemic attacks, or stroke. In patients with suspected angina, a history of one of these manifestations of extracardiac atherosclerosis lends weight to the diagnosis of myocardial ischemia.

The chest discomfort of *pulmonary hypertension* (see p. 788) may be identical to that of typical angina[23,24]; it is caused by right ventricular ischemia or dilation of the pul-

TABLE 1–2 DIFFERENTIAL DIAGNOSIS OF EPISODIC CHEST PAIN RESEMBLING ANGINA PECTORIS

	DURATION	QUALITY	PROVOCATION	RELIEF	LOCATION	COMMENT
Effort angina	5–15 minutes	Visceral (pressure)	During effort or emotion	Rest, nitroglycerin	Substernal, radiates	First episode vivid
Rest angina	5–15 minutes	Visceral (pressure)	Spontaneous (? with exercise)	Nitroglycerin	Substernal, radiates	Often nocturnal
Mitral prolapse	Minutes to hours	Superficial (rarely visceral)	Spontaneous (no pattern)	Time	Left anterior	No pattern, variable character
Esophageal reflux	10 minutes to 1 hour	Visceral	Recumbency, lack of food	Food, antacid	Substernal, epigastric	Rarely radiates
Esophageal spasm	5–60 minutes	Visceral	Spontaneous, cold liquids, exercise	Nitroglycerin	Substernal, radiates	Mimics angina
Peptic ulcer	Hours	Visceral, burning	Lack of food, "acid" foods	Foods, antacids	Epigastric, substernal	
Biliary disease	Hours	Visceral (waxes and wanes)	Spontaneous, food	Time, analgesia	Epigastric, ? radiates	Colic
Cervical disc	Variable (gradually subsides)	Superficial	Head and neck movement, palpation	Time, analgesia	Arm, neck	Not relieved by rest
Hyperventilation	2–3 minutes	Visceral	Emotion, tachypnea	Stimulus removal	Substernal	Facial paresthesia
Musculoskeletal	Variable	Superficial	Movement, palpation	Time, analgesia	Multiple	Tenderness
Pulmonary	30 minutes +	Visceral (pressure)	Often spontaneous	Rest, time, bronchodilator	Substernal	Dyspneic

Reproduced with permission from Christie, L.G., Jr., and Conti, C.R.: Systematic approach to the evaluation of angina-like chest pain. Am. Heart J. *102*:897, 1981.

TABLE 1–3 SOME FEATURES DIFFERENTIATING CARDIAC FROM NONCARDIAC CHEST PAIN

FAVORING ISCHEMIC ORIGIN	AGAINST ISCHEMIC ORIGIN
Character of Pain	
Constricting Squeezing Burning "Heaviness," "heavy feeling"	Dull ache "Knife-like," sharp, stabbing "Jabs" aggravated by respiration
Location of Pain	
Substernal Across mid-thorax, anteriorly In both arms, shoulders In the neck, cheeks, teeth In the forearms, fingers In the interscapular region	In the left submammary area In the left hemithorax
Factors Provoking Pain	
Exercise Excitement Other forms of stress Cold weather After meals	Pain *after* completion of exercise Provoked by a specific body motion

From Selzer, A.: Principles and Practice of Clinical Cardiology. 2nd ed. Philadelphia, W.B. Saunders Company, 1983, p. 17.

monary arteries. The chest discomfort of *unstable angina* and *acute myocardial infarction* (see p. 1198) is similar in quality to that of angina pectoris in location and character; however, it usually radiates more widely than does angina, is more severe, and therefore is generally referred to by the patient as true *pain* rather than *discomfort*. This pain generally develops unrelated to unusual effort or emotional stress, often with the patient at rest or even sleeping. Usually nitroglycerin does not provide complete or lasting relief.

Acute pericarditis (see p. 1481) is frequently preceded by a history of a viral upper respiratory infection. The inflammation causes pain that is sharper than is anginal discomfort, is more left-sided than central, and is often referred to the neck. The pain of pericarditis lasts for hours and is little affected by effort but is often aggravated by breathing, turning in bed, swallowing, or twisting the body; unlike angina, the pain of acute pericarditis may lessen when the patient sits up and leans forward.

Aortic dissection (see p. 1554) is suggested by the sudden development of persistent, severe pain with radiation to the back and into the lumbar region in a patient with a history of hypertension. An expanding *thoracic aortic aneurysm* may erode the vertebral bodies and cause localized, severe, boring pain that may be worse at night. An aneurysmally enlarged left atrium in patients with mitral valve disease rarely causes chest pain; instead, patients commonly complain of discomfort in the back or right side of the chest that intensifies on exertion.

Chest-wall pain due to *costochondritis* or *myositis* is common in patients who present with fear of heart disease.[25] It is associated with both local costochondral and muscle tenderness, which may be aggravated by moving or coughing. Chest-wall pain[26] may also accompany chest injury, or *Tietze syndrome* (i.e., discomfort localized in swelling of the costochondral and costosternal joints, which are painful on palpation). When *herpes zoster* affects the left chest it may mimic myocardial infarction. However, its persistence, its localization to a dermatome, the extreme sensitivity of the skin to touch, and the appearance of the characteristic vesicles allow recognition of this condition. Pain in the chest wall is quite common following cardiac or thoracic surgery and may be confused with myocardial ischemia. Postsurgical pain is usually localized to the incision or the site of insertion of a chest tube.

The pain of *pulmonary embolism* (Ch. 46) usually commences suddenly, and, when it occurs at rest, is seen in patients at high risk for this condition (heart failure, venous disease, the postoperative state), and is accompanied by shortness of breath. It is typically described as tightness in the chest and is accompanied or followed by *pleuritic* chest pain, i.e., sharp pain in the side of the chest that is intensified by respiration or cough. Chest pain associated with *spontaneous pneumothorax* develops suddenly, is associated with acute dyspnea, and is located in the lateral area of the chest. The chest pain associated with *mediastinal emphysema* also commences suddenly and is accompanied by dyspnea, sometimes severe; it is located in the center of the chest.

Functional or *psychogenic chest* pain may be one feature of an anxiety state called Da Costa syndrome or neurocirculatory asthenia.[27–29] It is localized typically to the cardiac apex and consists of a dull, persistent ache that lasts for hours and is often accentuated by or alternates with attacks of sharp, lancinating stabs of inframammary pain of 1 or 2 seconds' duration. The condition may occur with emotional strain and fatigue, bears little relation to exertion, and may be accompanied by precordial tenderness. Attacks may be associated with palpitation, hyperventilation, numbness and tingling in the extremities, sighing, dizziness, dyspnea, generalized weakness, and a history of panic attacks and other signs of emotional instability or depression. The pain may not be completely relieved by any medication other than analgesics, but it is often attenuated by many types of interventions, including rest, exertion, tranquilizers, and placebos. Therefore, in contrast to ischemic discomfort, functional pain is more likely to show variable responses to interventions on different occasions. Since functional chest pain is often preceded by hyperventilation, which in turn may cause increased muscle tension and be responsible for diffuse chest tightness, some instances of so-called functional chest pain may, in fact, have an organic basis. Chest pain is common in patients with prolapse of the mitral valve (see p. 1029). The nature of the pain varies considerably among patients with this condition; it may be similar to that of classic angina pectoris or may resemble the chest pain of neurocirculatory asthenia described above.

LOCATION. Embryologically the heart is a midline viscus; thus, cardiac ischemia produces anginal symptoms that are characteristically felt substernally or across both sides of the chest (Figs. 1–1 and 1–2). Some patients complain of discomfort only to the left or less commonly only to the right of the midline. If the pain or discomfort can be localized to the skin or superficial structures and can be reproduced by localized pressure, it generally arises from the chest wall. If the patient can point directly to the site of discomfort, and if that site is quite small (<3 cm in diameter), it is usually not angina pectoris. Like other symptoms arising in deeper structures, angina tends to be diffuse and

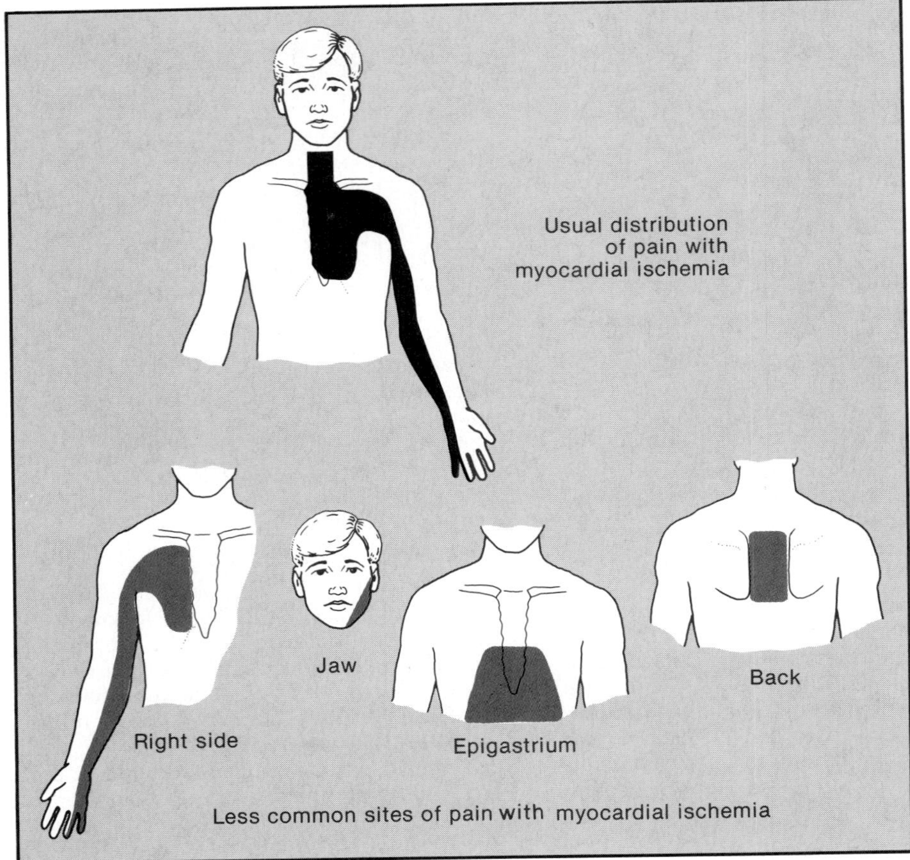

FIGURE 1–1. Pain patterns with myocardial ischemia. The usual distribution is referral to all or part of the sternal region, the left side of the chest, and the neck and down the ulnar side of the left forearm and hand. With severe ischemic pain, the right chest and right arm are often involved as well, although isolated involvement of these areas is rare. Other sites sometimes involved, either alone or together with other sites, are the jaw, epigastrium, and back. (From Horwitz, L. D.: Chest pain. *In* Horwitz, L. D., and Groves, B. M. [eds.]: Signs and Symptoms in Cardiology. Philadelphia, J. B. Lippincott, 1985, p. 9.)

eludes precise localization. Pain that is localized to the region of or under the left nipple or that radiates to the right lower chest[30] is usually noncardiac in origin and may be functional or due to osteoarthritis, gaseous distention of the stomach, or the splenic flexure syndrome. Although pain due to myocardial ischemia often radiates to the arm, especially the ulnar aspect of the left arm, wrist, epigastrium, or left shoulder, such radiation may also occur in pericarditis and disorders of the cervical spine. Radiation of pain from the chest to the neck and jaws is typical of myocardial infarction. Chest pain that radiates to the neck and jaw occurs in pericarditis as well as in myocardial ischemia. Dissection of the aorta or enlargement of an aortic aneurysm usually produces pain in the back in addition to the front of the chest.

DURATION. The duration of the pain is important in de-

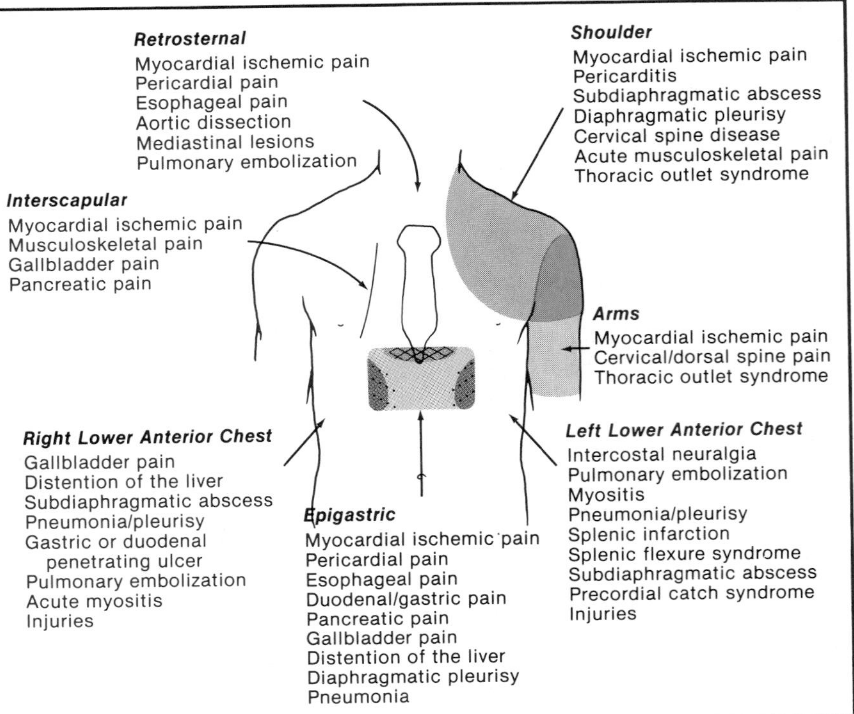

FIGURE 1–2. Differential diagnosis of chest pain according to location where pain starts. Serious intrathoracic or subdiaphragmatic diseases are usually associated with pains that begin in the left anterior chest, left shoulder, or upper arm, the interscapular region, or the epigastrium. The scheme is not all-inclusive; e.g., intercostal neuralgia occurs in locations other than the left, lower anterior chest area. (From Miller, A. J.: Diagnosis of Chest Pain. New York, Raven Press, 1988, p. 175.)

termining its etiology. Angina pectoris is relatively short, usually lasting from 2 to 10 minutes. However, if the pain is very brief, i.e., a momentary, lancinating, sharp pain, "stitch," or other discomfort that lasts less than 15 seconds, angina can usually be excluded; such a short duration points instead to musculoskeletal pain, pain due to hiatal hernia, or functional pain. Chest pain that is otherwise typical of angina but that lasts for more than 10 minutes or occurs at rest is typical of unstable angina. Chest pain lasting for hours may be seen with acute myocardial infarction, pericarditis, aortic dissection, musculoskeletal disease, herpes zoster, and anxiety.

PRECIPITATING AND AGGRAVATING FACTORS. Angina pectoris occurs characteristically on exertion, particularly when the patient is hurrying or walking up an incline. Thus, the development of chest discomfort or pain during walking, typically in the cold and against a wind, and after a heavy meal, is characteristic of angina pectoris. Angina may be precipitated by strong emotion or fright, by a nightmare, by working with the arms over the head, by cold exposure, or smoking a cigarette. Prinzmetal's (variant) angina characteristically occurs at rest (see p. 1340), and may or may not be affected by exertion; however, it must be remembered that (nonvariant) angina, although most often precipitated by effort, not uncommonly may be experienced at rest, as in unstable angina (see p. 1331); in these patients exertion intensifies the discomfort.

DIFFERENTIAL DIAGNOSIS. Chest pain that occurs after protracted vomiting may be due to the Mallory-Weiss syndrome, i.e., a tear in the lower portion of the esophagus. Pain that occurs while the patient is bending over is often radicular and may be associated with osteoarthritis of the cervical or upper thoracic spine. Chest pain occurring on moving the neck may be due to a herniated intervertebral disc.

Esophageal Pain. Substernal and epigastric discomfort during swallowing may be due to esophageal spasm or esophagitis, often with acid reflux, with or without a hiatal hernia. These conditions may also be associated with substernal or epigastric burning pain that is brought on by eating or lying down after meals and that may be relieved by antacids. Pain due to esophageal spasm has many of the features of and may be difficult to differentiate from angina pectoris.[30] Indeed, it is a common cause of chest pain considered atypical of angina pectoris.[31–34] A history of acid reflux into the mouth (water brash) and/or dysphagia[35] may be a useful diagnostic clue pointing to esophageal disease.[36] The chest discomfort secondary to esophageal reflux is most common after meals and occurs in the supine position or on bending. The difficulty in distinguishing angina from esophageal disease is compounded by the frequent coexistence of these two common conditions, by the observation that esophageal reflux lowers the threshold for the development of angina,[37] and by the observation that esophageal spasm may be precipitated by ergonovine and relieved by nitroglycerin. Esophageal pain radiates to the back more frequently than does angina pectoris.[32]

The discomfort produced by *peptic ulcer disease* is characteristically located in the midepigastrium. It may also resemble angina pectoris, but its characteristic relationship to food ingestion and its relief by antacids are important differentiating features. While the pain of *acute pancreatitis* may mimic acute myocardial infarction, with the former there is usually a history of alcoholism or biliary tract disease. The pain of pancreatitis, like that of myocardial infarction, may be predominant in the epigastrium. However, unlike the pain of myocardial infarction, it is usually transmitted to the back, is position-sensitive, and may be relieved in part by leaning forward.[30] Chest pain aggravated by coughing may be due to pericarditis, bronchitis, or pleurisy or may be of radicular origin. *Congenital absence of the pericardium* (see p. 1522) produces chest pain that is relieved by changing position in bed, is brought on by lying on the left side, and lasts a few seconds. Pain due to the *scalenus anticus (thoracic outlet) syndrome* may be confused with angina because it is often associated with paresthesias along the ulnar distribution of the arm and forearm. However, in contrast to angina, not only is it typically precipitated by abduction of the arm or lifting a weight, but it is not brought on by walking.

RELIEF OF PAIN. Rest and nitroglycerin characteristically relieve the discomfort of angina in approximately 1 to 5 minutes. If more than 10 minutes transpire before relief, the diagnosis of chronic stable angina becomes questionable and instead may be unstable angina, acute myocardial infarction, or pain not caused by myocardial ischemia at all. Although nitroglycerin commonly relieves the pain of angina pectoris, the discomfort of esophageal spasm and esophagitis may also be relieved by this drug. Angina pectoris is alleviated by quiet standing or sitting; sometimes resting in the recumbent position does not relieve angina. Chest pain secondary to *acute pericarditis* is characteristically relieved by leaning forward, whereas pain that is relieved by food or antacids may be due to *peptic ulcer disease* or esophagitis. Pain that is alleviated by holding the breath in deep expiration is commonly due to pleurisy. Some patients with upper gastrointestinal disease or anxiety report relief of symptoms after belching.

ACCOMPANYING SYMPTOMS. The physician should always be concerned about the patient who reports the presence of chest pain and profuse sweating. This combination of symptoms frequently signals a serious disorder, most often acute myocardial infarction, but also acute pulmonary embolism or aortic dissection. Severe chest pain accompanied by nausea and vomiting is also often due to myocardial infarction. The latter diagnosis, as well as pneumothorax, pulmonary embolism, or mediastinal emphysema, is suggested by pain associated with shortness of breath. Chest pain accompanied by palpitation may be due to the acute myocardial ischemia that results from a tachyarrhythmia-induced increase in myocardial oxygen consumption in the presence of coronary artery disease. Chest pain accompanied by hemoptysis suggests pulmonary embolism with infarction or lung tumor, whereas pain accompanied by fever occurs in pneumonia, pleurisy, and pericarditis. Functional pain is commonly accompanied by frequent sighing, anxiety, or depression.

Cyanosis

Cyanosis, both a symptom and a physical sign, is a bluish discoloration of the skin and mucous membranes resulting from an increased quantity of reduced hemoglobin or of abnormal hemoglobin pigments in the blood perfusing these areas[38,39] (see also pp. 885 and 891). There are two principal forms of cyanosis: (1) central cyanosis, characterized by decreased arterial oxygen saturation due to right-to-left shunting of blood or impaired pulmonary function, and (2) peripheral cyanosis, most commonly secondary to cutaneous vasoconstriction due to low cardiac output or exposure to cold air or water; if peripheral cyanosis is confined to an extremity, localized arterial or venous obstruction should be suspected. A history of cyanosis localized to the hands suggests Raynaud's phenomenon. Patients with central cyanosis due to congenital heart disease or pulmonary disease characteristically report that it worsens during exertion, whereas the resting peripheral cyanosis of congestive heart failure may be accentuated only slightly, if at all, during exertion.

Central cyanosis usually becomes apparent at a mean capillary concentration of 4 gm/dl reduced hemoglobin (or 0.5 gm/dl methemoglobin). In general, a history of cyanosis in light-skinned people is rarely elicited unless arterial saturation is 85 per cent or less; in pigmented races arterial saturation has to drop far lower before cyanosis is perceptible.

Although a history of cyanosis beginning in infancy suggests a congenital cardiac malformation with a right-to-left shunt, hereditary methemoglobinemia is another, albeit rare, cause of congenital cyanosis; the diagnosis of this condition is supported by a family history of cyanosis in the absence of heart disease.

A history of cyanosis limited to the neonatal period suggests the diagnosis of atrial septal defect with transient right-to-left shunting or, more commonly, pulmonary parenchymal disease or central nervous system depression. Cyanosis beginning at age 1 to 3 months may be reported when spontaneous closure of a patent ductus arteriosus causes a reduction of pulmonary blood flow in the presence of right-sided obstructive cardiac anomalies, most commonly tetralogy of Fallot. If cyanosis appears at age 6 months or later in childhood, it may be due to the development or progression of obstruction to right ventricular outflow in patients with ventricular septal defect. A history of the development of cyanosis in a patient with congenital heart disease between 5 and 20 years of age suggests an Eisenmenger reaction with right-to-left shunting as a consequence of a progressive increase in pulmonary vascular resistance (see p. 903). Cyanosis secondary to a pulmonary arteriovenous fistula also usually appears first in childhood.

Syncope

Syncope, which may be defined as a loss of consciousness (see also Chap. 28), results most commonly from reduced perfusion of the brain. The history is extremely valuable in the differential diagnosis of syncope (Table 1–4). Several daily attacks of loss of consciousness suggest (1) Stokes-Adams attacks, i.e., transient asystole or ventricular fibrillation in the presence of atrioventricular block; (2) other cardiac arrhythmias; or (3) a seizure disorder, i.e., petit mal epilepsy. These diagnoses are suggested when the loss of consciousness is abrupt and occurs over 1 or 2 seconds; a more gradual onset suggests vasodepressor syncope (i.e., the common faint) or syncope due to hyperventilation or, much less commonly, hypoglycemia.

CARDIAC SYNCOPE. This condition is usually of rapid onset without aura and is usually not associated with convulsive movements, urinary incontinence, and a postictal confusional state. Syncope in aortic stenosis[40,41] is usually precipitated by effort. Patients with epilepsy often have a prodromal aura preceding the seizure. Injury from falling is common, as are urinary incontinence and a postictal confusional state, associated with headache and drowsiness. Unconsciousness developing gradually and lasting for a few seconds suggests vasodepressor syncope or syncope secondary to postural hypotension, whereas a longer period suggests aortic stenosis or hyperventilation. Hysterical fainting is usually not accompanied by any untoward display of anxiety or change in pulse, blood pressure, or skin color, and there may be a question whether any true loss of consciousness occurred. It is often associated with paresthesias of the hands or face, hyperventilation, dyspnea, chest pain, and feelings of acute anxiety.

A history of syncope independent of body position suggests Stokes-Adams attacks, hyperventilation, or a convulsive disorder, whereas syncope of other etiology usually occurs in the upright position. Syncope occurring upon bending, leaning, or assuming a particular body position should raise the possibility of a left atrial myxoma (see p. 1467) or a ball-valve thrombus. Since syncope is an unusual feature of mitral stenosis, when it does occur in a patient thought to have this condition, the possibility of left atrial myxoma or ball-valve thrombus should be considered. A history of syncope occurring during or immediately following exertion suggests aortic stenosis, hypertrophic obstructive cardiomyopathy, or primary pulmonary hypertension. Syncope is rare in patients with angina pectoris unless the latter is secondary to one of the aforementioned conditions. Syncope following insulin administration suggests a hypoglycemic etiology; a history of syncope occurring several hours after eating is characteristic of reactive hypoglycemia. Loss of consciousness following an emotional stress suggests that it is vasodepressor syncope or secondary to hyperventilation.

Patients with vasodepressor syncope often have a history of recurrent fainting, commonly associated with emotional or painful stimuli. This, the most common form of syncope, may be precipitated by the sight or loss of blood or by physical or emotional stress; it can be averted by promptly lying down, and it is characteristically preceded by symptoms of autonomic hyperactivity such as dim vision, giddiness, yawning, sweating, and nausea. A history of syncope in the erect position may also be elicited in patients who have become hypovolemic as a consequence of overly vigorous diuresis. Syncope secondary to *cerebrovascular disturbance* is often preceded by aphasia, unilateral weakness, or confusion. A history of fainting following sudden movements of the head, shaving the neck, or wearing a tight collar suggests carotid sinus syncope. Syncope associated with chest pain may be secondary to massive acute myocardial infarction or infarction associated with arrhythmias; occasionally, following recovery of consciousness, the associated chest pain may be forgotten, and the infarction may be recognized only by the characteristic changes in serum enzymes and on the electrocardiogram. A history of syncope following chest pain may also occur in patients with *acute pulmonary embolism*.

REGAINING CONSCIOUSNESS. Consciousness is usually regained quite promptly in syncope of cardiovascular origin, but more slowly in patients with convulsive disorders. When consciousness is regained after vasodepressor syncope, the patient is often pale and diaphoretic with a slow heart rate, whereas after a Stokes-Adams attack, the face is often flushed and there may be cardiac acceleration. Patients who report an injury when falling during a fainting spell usually have epilepsy or occasionally syncope of cardiac origin, but patients who have unconsciousness related to emotional disturbance rarely sustain physical trauma.

DIFFERENTIAL DIAGNOSIS. A family history of syncope or near-syncope can often be elicited in patients with hypertrophic cardiomyopathy (see p. 1414) or ventricular tachyarrhythmias associated with Q-T

TABLE 1–4 CLUES FROM THE HISTORY IN ELUCIDATING THE CAUSE OF SYNCOPE

PRECEDING EVENTS	
Drugs:	Orthostatic hypotension (antihypertensives), hypoglycemia (insulin)
Severe pain, emotional stress:	Vasovagal syncope, hyperventilation
Movement of head and neck:	Carotid sinus hypersensitivity
Exertion:	Any form of obstruction to left ventricular outflow, Takayasu's arteritis
Upper extremity exertion:	Subclavian "steal"
TYPE OF ONSET	
Sudden:	Neurological (seizure disorder); arrhythmia (ventricular tachycardia or fibrillation, Stokes-Adams)
Rapid with premonition:	Vasovagal, neurological (aura)
Gradual:	Hyperventilation, hypoglycemia
POSITION AT ONSET	
Arising:	Orthostatic hypotension
Prolonged standing:	Vasovagal
Any position:	Arrhythmias, neurological, hypoglycemia, hyperventilation
POST-SYNCOPAL CLEARING OF SENSORIUM	
Slow:	Neurological
Rapid:	All others
ASSOCIATED EVENTS	
Incontinence, tongue biting, injury:	Neurological

Modified from Lindenfeld, J. A.: Syncope. *In* Horwitz, L. D., and Groves, B. M. (eds.): Signs and Symptoms in Cardiology. Philadelphia, J. B. Lippincott, 1985, 506 pp.

prolongation (see p. 685). A family history of epilepsy is positive in approximately 4 per cent of patients with convulsive disorders. A history of syncope associated with progressive intensification of cyanosis in an infant or child with cyanotic congenital heart disease is likely to be due to cerebral anoxia as a consequence of an increase in the right-to-left shunt, secondary to an increase in the obstruction to right ventricular outflow or a reduction in systemic vascular resistance (see p. 884). A history of syncope during childhood suggests the possibility of a cardiovascular anomaly obstructing left ventricular outflow—valvular, supravalvular, or subvalvular aortic stenosis. In patients with hypertrophic cardiomyopathy, syncope may be post-tussive and occurs characteristically in the erect position, when arising suddenly, after standing erect for long periods, and during or immediately after cessation of exertion.

Patients with syncope secondary to orthostatic hypotension may have a history of drug therapy for hypertension or of abnormalities of autonomic function, such as impotence, disturbances of sphincter function, peripheral neuropathy, and anhidrosis (see p. 865). When syncope is secondary to hypovolemia, there is often a history of melena, anemia, menorrhagia, or treatment with anticoagulants. Syncope due to cerebrovascular insufficiency is frequently associated with a history of unilateral blindness, weakness, paresthesias, or memory defects.

PALPITATION

This common symptom is defined as an unpleasant awareness of the forceful or rapid beating of the heart. It may be brought about by a variety of disorders involving changes in cardiac rhythm or rate, including all forms of tachycardia, ectopic beats, compensatory pauses, augmented stroke volume due to valvular regurgitation, hyperkinetic (high cardiac output) states, and the sudden onset of bradycardia. In the case of premature contractions the patient is more commonly aware of the postextrasystolic beat than of the premature beat itself, and it appears that it is the increased motion of the heart within the chest that is perceived. This explains why palpitation is not a characteristic feature of aortic or pulmonic stenosis or of severe systemic or pulmonary hypertension, conditions characterized by an increased force of cardiac contraction.

When episodes of palpitation last for an instant, they are described as "skipped beats" or a "flopping sensation" in the chest and most commonly are due to extrasystoles. On the other hand, the sensation that the heart has "stopped beating" often correlates with the compensatory pause following a premature contraction.

DIFFERENTIAL DIAGNOSIS. Palpitation characterized by a slow heart rate may be due to atrioventricular block or sinus node disease. When palpitation begins and ends abruptly, it is often due to a paroxysmal tachycardia such as paroxysmal atrial or junctional tachycardia, atrial flutter, or atrial fibrillation, whereas a gradual onset and cessation of the attack suggest sinus tachycardia and/or an anxiety state. A history of chaotic, rapid heart action suggests the diagnosis of atrial fibrillation; fleeting and repetitive palpitation suggests multiple ectopic beats. A history of multiple paroxysms of tachycardia followed by palpitation that occurs only with effort or excitement suggests paroxysmal atrial fibrillation that has become permanent—the palpitation being experienced only when the ventricular rate rises.

Some patients have taken their pulse during palpitation or have asked a companion to do so. A regular rate between 100 and 140 beats/min suggests sinus tachycardia, a regular rate of approximately 150 beats/min suggests atrial flutter, and a regular rate exceeding 160 beats/min suggests paroxysmal supraventricular tachycardia. As an adjunct to the history, it may be possible to ascertain the rhythm responsible for the palpitation by tapping the finger on the patient's chest in a variety of rhythms and asking the patient to identify the pattern that most closely resembles the abnormal feeling. Alternatively, patients can be asked to reproduce the arrhythmia by tapping their fingers on a tabletop at the rate and rhythm they perceived during palpitation. As described on p. 640, these maneuvers may provide important clues to the etiology of the responsible arrhythmia.

A history of palpitation during strenuous physical activity is normal, whereas palpitation during mild exertion suggests the presence of heart failure, atrial fibrillation, anemia, or thyrotoxicosis, or that the individual is severely "out of condition." A feeling of forceful heart action accompanied by throbbing in the neck suggests aortic regurgitation. When palpitation can be relieved suddenly by stooping, breath-holding, or induced gagging or vomiting, i.e., by vagal maneuvers, the diagnosis of paroxysmal supraventricular tachycardia is suggested. A history of syncope *following* an episode of palpitation suggests either asystole or severe bradycardia following the termination of a tachyarrhythmia or a Stokes-Adams attack. A history of palpitation associated with anxiety, a lump in the throat, dizziness, and tingling in the hands and face suggests sinus tachycardia accompanying an anxiety state with hyperventilation. Palpitation followed by angina suggests that myocardial ischemia has been precipitated by increased oxygen demands induced by the rapid heart rate.

A directed history is also useful (Table 1–5). Is there a history of cocaine or amphetamine abuse? Thyrotoxicosis? Anemia? Do the palpitations occur after heavy cigarette smoking or caffeine ingestion? Is there a family history of syncope, arrhythmia, or sudden death?

In many individuals no obvious cause for palpitation emerges despite careful work-up, including a correlation between episodes of palpitation with a simultaneously recorded ambulatory electrocardiogram (see p. 578) or an electrocardiogram recorded by transtelephonic transmission. Anxiety is responsible for the symptom in many such patients, some of whom are known to have heart disease and may be receiving a vasodilator for the treatment of hypertension or nifedipine for the treatment of myocardial ischemia. In these patients palpitation may be due to postural hypotension resulting in reflex cardiac acceleration.

Edema

LOCALIZATION. This is helpful in elucidating the etiology of edema.[42,43] Thus a history of edema of the legs that is most pronounced in the evening is characteristic of heart failure or bilateral chronic venous insufficiency. Inability to fit the feet into shoes is a common early complaint. In most patients any visible edema of both lower extremities is preceded by a weight gain of at least 7 to 10 lb. Cardiac edema is generally symmetrical. As it progresses, it usually ascends to involve the legs, thighs, genitalia, and abdominal wall. In patients with heart failure who are confined largely to bed, the edematous fluid localizes particularly in the sacral area. Edema affecting both the abdomen and the legs is observed in heart failure and hepatic cirrhosis. Edema may be generalized (anasarca) in the nephrotic syndrome, severe heart failure, and hepatic cirrhosis. A history of edema around the eyes and face is characteristic of the nephrotic syndrome, acute glomerulonephritis, angioneurotic edema, hypoproteinemia, and myxedema. A history of edema limited to the face, neck, and upper arms may be associated with obstruction of the superior vena cava, most commonly by carcinoma of the lung, lymphoma, or aneurysm of the aortic arch. A history of edema restricted to one extremity is usually due to venous thrombosis or lymphatic blockage of that extremity.

ACCOMPANYING SYMPTOMS. A history of dyspnea asso-

TABLE 1–5 ITEMS TO BE COVERED IN HISTORY OF PATIENT WITH PALPITATION

DOES THE PALPITATION OCCUR:	IF SO, SUSPECT:
As isolated "jumps" or "skips"?	Extrasystoles
In attacks, known to be of abrupt beginning, with a heart rate of 120 beats per minute or over, with regular or irregular rhythm?	Paroxysmal rapid heart action
Independent of exercise or excitement adequate to account for the symptom?	Atrial fibrillation, atrial flutter, thyrotoxicosis, anemia, febrile states, hypoglycemia, anxiety state
In attacks developing rapidly though not absolutely abruptly, unrelated to exertion or excitement?	Hemorrhage, hypoglycemia, tumor of the adrenal medulla
In conjunction with the taking of drugs?	Tobacco, coffee, tea, alcohol, epinephrine, ephedrine, aminophylline, atropine, thyroid extract, monoamine oxidase inhibitors
On standing?	Postural hypotension
In middle-aged women, in conjunction with flushes and sweats?	Menopausal syndrome
When the rate is known to be normal and the rhythm regular?	Anxiety state

From Goldman, L., and Braunwald, E.: Chest discomfort and palpitation. *In* Isselbacher, K. J., Braunwald, E., et al. (eds.): Harrison's Principles of Internal Medicine. 13th ed. New York, McGraw-Hill, 1994.

ciated with edema is most frequently due to heart failure, but may also be observed in patients with large bilateral pleural effusions, elevation of the diaphragm due to ascites, angioneurotic edema with laryngeal involvement, and pulmonary embolism. When dyspnea precedes edema, the underlying disorder is usually left ventricular dysfunction, mitral stenosis, or chronic lung disease with cor pulmonale. A history of jaundice suggests that edema may be of hepatic origin, whereas edema associated with a history of ulceration and pigmentation of the skin of the legs is most commonly due to chronic venous insufficiency or postphlebitic syndrome. When cardiac edema is not associated with orthopnea, it may be due to tricuspid stenosis or regurgitation or constrictive pericarditis; in these conditions edema is not always most prominent in the lower extremities but may be generalized and may even involve the face. A history of leg edema after prolonged sitting (particularly in the elderly in wheelchairs) may be due to stasis and not be associated with disease at all.

A history of ascites preceding edema suggests cirrhosis, whereas a history of ascites following edema suggests cardiac or renal disease. Angioneurotic edema occurs intermittently, particularly after emotional stress or eating certain foods. Idiopathic cyclic edema is associated with menstruation. A history of edema on prolonged standing is observed in patients with chronic venous insufficiency.

Cough

Cough, one of the most frequent of all cardiorespiratory symptoms, may be defined as an explosive expiration that provides a means of clearing the tracheobronchial tree of secretions and foreign bodies.[44–46] It can be caused by a variety of infectious, neoplastic, or allergic disorders of the lungs and tracheobronchial tree. Cardiovascular disorders most frequently responsible for cough include those that lead to pulmonary venous hypertension, interstitial and alveolar pulmonary edema, pulmonary infarction, and compression of the tracheobronchial tree (aortic aneurysm). Cough due to pulmonary venous hypertension secondary to left ventricular failure or mitral stenosis tends to be dry, irritating, spasmodic, and nocturnal. When cough accompanies exertional dyspnea, it suggests either chronic obstructive lung disease or heart failure, whereas in a patient with a history of allergy and/or wheezing, cough is often a concomitant of bronchial asthma. A history of cough associated with expectoration for months or years occurs in chronic obstructive lung disease and/or chronic bronchitis.

The character of the sputum may be helpful in the differential diagnosis. Thus, a cough producing frothy, pink-tinged sputum occurs in pulmonary edema; clear, white, mucoid sputum suggests viral infection or longstanding bronchial irritation; thick, yellowish sputum suggests an infectious cause; rusty sputum suggests pneumococcal pneumonia; blood-streaked sputum suggests tuberculosis, bronchiectasis, carcinoma of the lung, or pulmonary infarction.

A history of a combination of cough with hoarseness without upper respiratory disease may be due to pressure of a greatly enlarged left atrium on an enlarged pulmonary artery compressing the recurrent laryngeal nerve.

HEMOPTYSIS

The expectoration of blood or of sputum, either streaked or grossly contaminated with blood, may be due to (1) escape of red cells into the alveoli from congested vessels in the lungs (acute pulmonary edema); (2) rupture of dilated endobronchial vessels that form collateral channels between the pulmonary and bronchial venous systems (mitral stenosis); (3) necrosis and hemorrhage into the alveoli (pulmonary infarction); (4) ulceration of the bronchial mucosa or the slough of a caseous lesion (tuberculosis); minor damage to the tracheobronchial mucosa, produced by excessive coughing of any cause, can result in mild hemoptysis; (5) vascular invasion (carcinoma of the lung); or (6) necrosis of the mucosa with rupture of pulmonary-bronchial venous connections (bronchiectasis).

The history is often decisive in pinpointing the etiology of hemoptysis.[46] Recurrent episodes of minor bleeding are observed in patients with chronic bronchitis, bronchiectasis, tuberculosis, and mitral stenosis. Rarely, these conditions result in the expectoration of large quantities of blood, i.e., more than one-half cup. Massive hemoptysis may also be due to rupture of a pulmonary arteriovenous fistula; exsanguinating hemoptysis may occur with rupture of an aortic aneurysm into the bronchopulmonary tree.[47,48]

Hemoptysis associated with a history of expectoration of clear, gray sputum suggests chronic obstructive lung disease and of yellowish-green sputum, pulmonary infection. Hemoptysis associated with shortness of breath suggests mitral stenosis; in this condition the hemoptysis is often precipitated by sudden elevations in left atrial pressure during effort or pregnancy and is attributable to rupture of small pulmonary or bronchopulmonary anastomosing veins. Blood-tinged sputum in patients with mitral stenosis may also be due to transient pulmonary edema; in these circumstances it is usually associated with severe dyspnea.

A history of hemoptysis associated with acute pleuritic chest pain suggests pulmonary embolism with infarction. Recurrent hemoptysis in a young, otherwise asymptomatic woman favors the diagnosis of bronchial adenoma. Hemoptysis associated with congenital heart disease and cyanosis suggests Eisenmenger syndrome (see p. 799). A history of recurrent hemoptysis with chronic excessive sputum production suggests the diagnosis of bronchiectasis. Hemoptysis associated with the production of putrid sputum occurs in lung abscess, whereas hemoptysis associated with weight loss and anorexia in a male smoker suggests carcinoma of the lung. When blunt trauma to the chest is followed by hemoptysis, lung contusion is the probable cause.

A history of drug ingestion may be helpful in elucidating the etiology of hemoptysis; e.g., anticoagulants and immunosuppressive drugs can cause bleeding. A history of ingestion of contraceptive pills may be a risk factor for the development of deep vein thrombosis and subsequent pulmonary embolism and infarction.

FATIGUE AND OTHER SYMPTOMS

Cardiovascular disorders can cause symptoms emanating from every organ system. Several of these are mentioned here primarily to point out how detailed the history should be in providing a comprehensive evaluation of a patient suspected of having cardiovascular disease; fuller discussions are found elsewhere in this text.

FATIGUE. This is among the most common symptoms in patients with impaired cardiovascular function. However, it is also one of the most nonspecific of all symptoms in clinical medicine; in patients with impaired systemic circulation as a consequence of a depressed cardiac output, it may be associated with muscular weakness. In other patients with heart disease, fatigue may be caused by drugs, such as beta-adrenoceptor blocking agents. It may be the result of excessive blood pressure reduction in patients treated too vigorously for hypertension or heart failure. In patients with heart failure, fatigue may also be caused by excessive diuresis and by diuretic-induced hypokalemia. Extreme fatigue sometimes precedes or accompanies acute myocardial infarction.[20]

OTHER SYMPTOMS. *Nocturia* is a common early complaint in patients with congestive heart failure. *Anorexia,* abdominal fullness, right upper quadrant discomfort, weight loss, and cachexia are symptoms of advanced heart failure (see p. 452). Anorexia, *nausea, vomiting,* and *visual changes* are important signs of digitalis intoxication (see p. 484). Nausea and vomiting occur frequently in patients with acute myocardial infarction. Hoarseness may be caused by compression of the recurrent laryngeal nerve by an aortic aneurysm, a dilated pulmonary artery, or a greatly enlarged left atrium. A history of *fever* and *chills* is common in patients with infective endocarditis (see p. 1084).

The aforementioned symptoms are examples of the wide variety of symptoms that are not obviously associated with abnormalities of the cardiovascular system but that can be of critical importance in differential diagnosis when they are elicited in patients known to have or suspected of having heart disease. They serve to reemphasize that the physician whose responsibility it is to care for patients with heart disease must be first and foremost a broadly based clinician.

THE HISTORY IN SPECIFIC FORMS OF HEART DISEASE

Just as the history is of central importance in determining whether or not a specific symptom is caused by heart disease, it is equally valuable in elucidating the etiology of recognized heart disease. A few examples are given below; considerably greater detail is provided in later chapters that deal with each specific disease entity.

Heart Disease in Infancy and Childhood

The history is particularly helpful in establishing a diagnosis of congenital heart disease. In view of the familial incidence of certain congenital malformations (Chaps. 29 and 49), a history of congenital heart disease, cyanosis, or heart murmur in the family should be ascertained. Rubella in the first 2 months of pregnancy is associated with a number of congenital cardiac malformations (patent ductus arteriosus, atrial and ventricular septal defect, tetralogy of Fallot, and supravalvular aortic stenosis [see p. 919]). A maternal viral illness in the last trimester of pregnancy may be responsible for neonatal myocarditis. Syncope on exertion in a child with congenital heart disease suggests a lesion in which the cardiac output is fixed, such as aortic or pulmonic stenosis. Exertional angina in a child suggests severe aortic stenosis, pulmonary stenosis, primary pulmonary hypertension, or anomalous origin of the left coronary artery. A history of syncope or faintness with straining and associated with cyanosis suggests tetralogy of Fallot (see p. 929).

In infants or children with cardiac murmurs, it is important to ascertain as precisely as possible when the murmur was first detected. Murmurs due to either aortic or pulmonic stenosis are usually audible within the first 48 hours of life, whereas those produced by a ventricular septal defect are usually apparent a few days or weeks later. On the other hand, the murmur produced by an atrial septal defect often is not heard until age 2 to 3 months.

Frequent episodes of pneumonia early in infancy suggest a large left-to-right shunt, and a history of excessive diaphoresis occurs in left ventricular failure, most commonly due to ventricular septal defect in this age group. A history of squatting is most frequently associated with tetralogy of Fallot or tricuspid atresia (see p. 932). Dysphagia in early infancy suggests the presence of an aortic arch anomaly such as double aortic arch or an anomalous origin of the right subclavian artery passing behind the esophagus. A history of headaches, weakness of the legs, and intermittent claudication is compatible with the diagnosis of coarctation of the aorta (see p. 965). Weakness or lack of coordination in a child with heart disease suggests cardiomyopathy associated with Friedreich's ataxia or muscular dystrophy (Chap. 60). Recurrent bleeding from the nose, lips, or mouth, associated with dizziness and visual disturbances, and a family history of bleeding in a cyanotic child suggest hereditary hemorrhagic telangiectasia (Osler-Weber-Rendu disease) with pulmonary arteriovenous fistula(s) (see p. 461). A cerebrovascular accident in a cyanotic patient may be due to cerebral thrombosis or abscess or paradoxical embolization (see p. 885).

MYOCARDITIS AND CARDIOMYOPATHY

Rheumatic fever (Chap. 55) is suggested by a history of sore throat followed by symptoms including rash and chorea (St. Vitus dance). This is manifested as a period of twitching or clumsiness for a few months in childhood, as well as by frequent episodes of epistaxis and growing pains, i.e., nocturnal pains in the legs. In patients suspected of having myocarditis or cardiomyopathy, a history of Raynaud's phenomenon, dysphagia, or tight skin suggests scleroderma (see p. 1781). A history of dyspnea following an influenza-like illness with myalgia suggests acute myocarditis. Pain in the hip or lower back that awakens the patient in the morning and is followed by morning back stiffness suggests rheumatoid spondylitis, which is often associated with aortic valve disease (see p. 1780). *Carcinoid heart disease* is associated with a history of diarrhea, bronchospasm, and flushing of the upper chest and head (see p. 1434). A history of diabetes, particularly if resistant to insulin and associated with bronzing of the skin, suggests *hemochromatosis* (see p. 1790), which may be associated with heart failure due to cardiac infiltration. *Amyloid heart disease* (see p. 1427) is often associated with a history of postural hypotension and peripheral neuropathy. *Hypertrophic cardiomyopathy* (see p. 1414) is often associated with a family history of this condition and sometimes with a family history of sudden death. The characteristic symptoms are angina, dyspnea, and syncope, which are often intensified paradoxically by digitalis and which occur during or immediately after exercise.

HIGH-OUTPUT HEART FAILURE AND COR PULMONALE

Patients with symptoms of heart failure (breathlessness and excess fluid accumulation) with warm extremities often have *high-output heart failure* (see p. 460). They should be questioned about a history of anemia and of its common causes and accompaniments, such as menorrhagia, melena, peptic ulcer, hemorrhoids, sickle cell disease, and the neurological manifestations of vitamin B_{12} deficiency. Also, in such patients an attempt should be made to elicit a history of thyrotoxicosis (see pp. 461 and 1894) (weight loss, polyphagia, diarrhea, diaphoresis, heat intolerance, nervousness, breathlessness, muscle weakness, and goiter). Patients with beriberi heart disease responsible for high-output heart failure often have a history characteristic of peripheral neuritis, alcoholism, poor eating habits, fad diets, or upper gastrointestinal surgery.

Patients with chronic cor pulmonale (see Chap. 47) frequently have a history of smoking, chronic cough and sputum production, dyspnea, and wheezing relieved by bronchodilators. Alternatively, they may have a history of pulmonary emboli, phlebitis, and the sudden development of dyspnea at rest with palpitations, pleuritic chest pain, and, in the case of massive infarction, syncope.

PERICARDITIS AND ENDOCARDITIS

In patients in whom *pericarditis* or *cardiac tamponade* is suspected (Chap. 43), an attempt should be made to elicit a history of chest trauma, a recent viral infection, recent cardiac surgery, neoplastic disease of the chest with or without extensive radiation therapy, myxedema, scleroderma, tuberculosis, or contact with tuberculous patients. The *sequence of development* of abdominal swelling, ankle edema, and dyspnea should be determined, since in patients with chronic constrictive pericarditis, ascites often precedes edema, which in turn usually precedes exertional dyspnea. A history of joint symptoms with a face rash suggests the possibility of systemic lupus erythematosus (SLE), an important cause of pericarditis, and it should be recalled that procainamide, hydralazine, and isoniazid can produce an SLE-like syndrome (see p. 604).

The diagnosis of infective endocarditis is suggested by a history of fever, severe night sweats, anorexia, and weight loss and embolic phenomena expressed as hematuria, back pain, petechiae, tender finger pads, and a cerebrovascular accident (see p. 1084).

Drug-Induced Heart Disease

Since a wide variety of cardiac abnormalities can be induced by drugs,[49] a meticulous history of drug intake is of great importance. Table 1–6 summarizes the major drugs responsible for various cardiovascular manifestations.

Catecholamines, whether administered exogenously or secreted by a pheochromocytoma (see p. 1897), may produce myocarditis and arrhythmias. *Digitalis glycosides* can be responsible for a variety of tachyarrhythmias and bradyarrhythmias as well as gastrointestinal, visual, and central nervous system disturbances (see p. 499). *Quinidine* may cause Q-T prolongation, ventricular tachycardia of the torsades de pointes variety, syncope, and sudden death, presumably due to ventricular fibrillation (see p. 602). Paradoxically, the administration of antiarrhythmic drugs is one of the major causes of serious cardiac arrhythmias (see p. 600).

Disopyramide (see p. 604), *beta-adrenoceptor blockers* (see p. 610), and the calcium channel antagonists *diltiazem* and *verapamil* (see p. 616) may depress ventricular performance, and in patients with ventricular dysfunction these drugs may intensify heart failure. *Alcohol* is also a potent myocardial depressant and may be responsible for the development of cardiomyopathy (see p. 1412), arrhythmias, and sudden death. *Tricyclic antidepressants* may cause orthostatic hypotension and arrhythmias. *Lithium*, also used in the treatment of psychiatric disorders, can aggravate preexisting cardiac arrhythmias, particularly in patients with heart failure in whom the renal clearance of this ion is impaired. *Cocaine* can cause coronary spasm with resultant myocardial ischemia, myocardial infarction, and sudden death.[50,51]

The *anthracycline compounds* doxorubicin (Adriamycin) and daunorubicin, which are widely used because of their broad spectrum of activity against various tumors, may cause or intensify left ventricular failure, arrhythmias, myocarditis, and pericarditis (see p. 1800). *Cyclophosphamide*, an antineoplastic alkylating agent, may also cause

TABLE 1–6 CARDIOVASCULAR MANIFESTATIONS OF ADVERSE REACTIONS TO DRUGS

Acute Chest Pain (nonischemic)
- Bleomycin

Angina Exacerbation
- Alpha blockers
- Beta-blocker withdrawal
- Ergotamine
- Excessive thyroxine
- Hydralazine
- Methysergide
- Minoxidil
- Nifedipine
- Oxytocin
- Vasopressin

Arrhythmias
- Adriamycin
- Antiarrhythmic drugs
- Astemizole
- Atropine
- Anticholinesterases
- Beta blockers
- Daunorubicin
- Digitalis
- Emetine
- Erythromycin
- Guanethidine
- Lithium
- Papaverine
- Phenothiazines, particularly thioridazine
- Sympathomimetics
- Terfenadine
- Theophylline
- Thyroid hormone
- Tricyclic antidepressants
- Verapamil

AV Block
- Clonidine
- Methyldopa
- Verapamil

Cardiomyopathy
- Adriamycin
- Daunorubicin
- Emetine
- Lithium
- Phenothiazines
- Sulfonamides
- Sympathomimetics

Fluid Retention/Congestive Heart Failure/Edema
- Beta blockers
- Calcium blockers
- Carbenoxolone
- Diazoxide
- Estrogens
- Indomethacin
- Mannitol
- Minoxidil
- Phenylbutazone
- Steroids
- Verapamil

Hypotension (see also Arrhythmias)
- Amiodarone (perioperative)
- Calcium channel blockers, e.g., nifedipine
- Citrated blood
- Diuretics
- Interleukin-2
- Levodopa
- Morphine
- Nitroglycerin
- Phenothiazines
- Protamine
- Quinidine

Hypertension
- Clonidine withdrawal
- Corticotropin
- Cyclosporine
- Glucocorticoids
- Monoamine oxidase inhibitors with sympathomimetics
- NSAIDs (some)
- Oral contraceptives
- Sympathomimetics
- Tricyclic antidepressants with sympathomimetics

Pericarditis
- Emetine
- Hydralazine
- Methysergide
- Procainamide

Pericardial Effusion
- Minoxidil

Thromboembolism
- Oral contraceptives

From Wood, A. J.: Adverse reactions to drugs. *In* Isselbacher, K. J., Braunwald, E., et al. (eds.): Harrison's Principles of Internal Medicine. 13th ed. New York, McGraw-Hill, 1994.

TABLE 1–7 A COMPARISON OF THREE METHODS OF ASSESSING CARDIOVASCULAR DISABILITY

CLASS	NEW YORK HEART ASSOCIATION FUNCTIONAL CLASSIFICATION	CANADIAN CARDIOVASCULAR SOCIETY FUNCTIONAL CLASSIFICATION	SPECIFIC ACTIVITY SCALE
I	Patients with cardiac disease but without resulting limitations of physical activity. Ordinary physical activity does not cause undue fatigue, palpitation, dyspnea, or anginal pain.	Ordinary physical activity, such as walking and climbing stairs, does not cause angina. Angina with strenuous or rapid or prolonged exertion at work or recreation.	Patients can perform to completion any activity requiring ≤7 metabolic equivalents, e.g., can carry 24 lb up eight steps; carry objects that weigh 80 lb; do outdoor work (shovel snow, spade soil); do recreational activities (skiing, basketball, squash, handball, jog/walk 5 mph).
II	Patients with cardiac disease resulting in slight limitation of physical activity. They are comfortable at rest. Ordinary physical activity results in fatigue, palpitation, dyspnea, or anginal pain.	Slight limitation of ordinary activity. Walking or climbing stairs rapidly, walking uphill, walking or stair climbing after meals, in cold, in wind, or when under emotional stress, or only during the few hours after awakening. Walking more than two blocks on the level and climbing more than one flight of ordinary stairs at a normal pace and in normal conditions.	Patients can perform to completion any activity requiring ≤5 metabolic equivalents, e.g., have sexual intercourse without stopping, garden, rake, weed, roller skate, dance fox trot, walk at 4 mph on level ground, but cannot and do not perform to completion activities requiring ≥7 metabolic equivalents.
III	Patients with cardiac disease resulting in marked limitation of physical activity. They are comfortable at rest. Less than ordinary physical activity causes fatigue, palpitation, dyspnea, or anginal pain.	Marked limitation of ordinary physical activity. Walking one to two blocks on the level and climbing more than one flight in normal conditions.	Patients can perform to completion any activity requiring ≤2 metabolic equivalents, e.g., shower without stopping, strip and make bed, clean windows, walk 2.5 mph, bowl, play golf, dress without stopping, but cannot and do not perform to completion any activities requiring ≥5 metabolic equivalents.
IV	Patient with cardiac disease resulting in inability to carry on any physical activity without discomfort. Symptoms of cardiac insufficiency or of the anginal syndrome may be present even at rest. If any physical activity is undertaken, discomfort is increased.	Inability to carry on any physical activity without discomfort—anginal syndrome *may be* present at rest.	Patients cannot or do not perform to completion activities requiring ≥2 metabolic equivalents. *Cannot* carry out activities listed above (Specific Activity Scale, Class III).

Reproduced with permission from Goldman, L., Hashimoto, B., Cook, E. F., and Loscalzo, A.: Comparative reproducibility and validity of systems for assessing cardiovascular functional class: Advantages of a new specific activity scale. Circulation *64*:1227, 1981.

left ventricular dysfunction, while 5-fluorouracil and its derivatives (see p. 1803) may be responsible for angina secondary to coronary spasm (see p. 1189). Radiation therapy to the chest may cause acute and chronic pericarditis (see p. 1799), pancarditis, or coronary artery disease; further, it may enhance the aforementioned cardiotoxic effects of the anthracyclines.

Assessing Cardiovascular Disability

(Table 1–7)

One of the greatest values of the history is in categorizing the degree of cardiovascular disability, so that a patient's status can be followed over time, the effects of a therapeutic intervention assessed, and patients compared with one another. The Criteria Committee of the New York Heart Association has provided a widely used classification that relates functional activity to the ability to carry out "ordinary" activity.[52] The term "ordinary," of course, is subject to widely varying interpretation, as are terms such as "undue fatigue" that are used in this classification, and this has limited its accuracy and reproducibility. More recently, this Heart Association changed its evaluation from functional activity to a broader one, called Cardiac Status, which takes account of symptoms and other data gathered from the patient.[52] Cardiac status is classified as: (1) uncompromised, (2) slightly compromised, (3) moderately compromised, and (4) severely compromised.

Somewhat more detailed and specific criteria were provided by the Canadian Cardiovascular Society,[53] but this classification is limited to patients with angina pectoris. Goldman et al.[54] developed a specific activity scale in which classification is based on the estimated metabolic cost of various activities. This scale appears to be more reproducible and to be a better predictor of exercise tolerance than either the New York Heart Association Classification or the Canadian Cardiovascular Society Criteria.

A key element of the history is to determine whether the patient's disability is stable or progressive. A useful way to accomplish this is to inquire whether a specific task which now causes symptoms, e.g., dyspnea after climbing two flights of stairs, did so 3, 6, and 12 months previously. Precise questioning on this point is important since a gradual reduction of ordinary activity as heart disease progresses may lead to an underestimation of the apparent degree of disability.[55]

REFERENCES

IMPORTANCE OF THE HISTORY

1. Sandler, G.: The importance of the history in the medical clinic and the cost of unnecessary tests. Am. Heart J. *100*:928, 1980.
2. Hickman, D. H., Soc, H. C., Jr., and Soc, C. H.: Systematic bias in recording the history in patients with chest pain. J. Chronic Dis. *38*:91, 1985.
3. Sapira, J. D.: The history. *In* The Art and Science of Bedside Diagnosis. Baltimore, Urban Schwartzenberg, 1990, pp. 9–45.
4. Hampton, J. R., Harrison, M. J. G., Mitchell, J. R. A., et al.: Relative contributions of history-taking, physical examination, and laboratory investigation to diagnosis and management of medical outpatients. Br. Med. J. *2*:486, 1975.
5. Tumulty, P. A.: Obtaining the history. *In* The Effective Clinician. Philadelphia, W. B. Saunders Company, 1973, pp. 17–28.

CARDINAL SYMPTOMS OF HEART DISEASE

6. Szidon, J. P., and Fishman, A. P.: The first approach to the patient with respiratory signs and symptoms. *In* Fishman, A. P. (ed.): Pulmonary Diseases and Disorders. 2nd ed. New York, McGraw-Hill, 1988, pp. 313–367.
7. Weber, K. T., and Szidon, J. P.: Exertional dyspnea. *In* Weber, K. T., and Janick, J. S. (eds.): Cardiopulmonary Exercise Testing. Philadelphia, W. B. Saunders Company, 1986, pp. 290–301.
8. Cherniack, N. S.: Dyspnea. *In* Murray, J. F., and Nadel, J. A. (eds.): Textbook of Respiratory Medicine. 2nd ed. Philadelphia, W. B. Saunders Company, 1995, pp. 430–465.
9. Simon, P. M., Schwartzstein, R. M., Weiss, J. W., et al.: Distinguishable types of dyspnea in patients with shortness of breath. Am. Rev. Respir. Dis. *142*:1009, 1990.
10. Mahler, D. A.: Dyspnea: Diagnosis and management. Clin. Chest Med. *8*:215, 1987.
11. Elliott, M. W., Adams, I., Cockcroft, A., et al.: The language of breathlessness: Use of verbal descriptors by patients with cardiopulmonary diseases. Am. Rev. Respir. Dis. *144*:826, 1991.
12. Schwartzstein, R. M., et al.: Dyspnea: A sensory experience. Lung *169*:543, 1991.
13. Wasserman, K.: Dyspnea on exertion. Is it the heart or the lungs? JAMA *248*:2039, 1982.
14. Borg, G., and Noble, B.: Perceived exertion. *In* Wilmore, J. H. (ed.): Exercise and Sports. Science Reviews. New York, Academic Press, 1974, pp. 131–153.
15. Loke, J.: Distinguishing cardiac versus pulmonary limitation in exercise performance. Chest *83*:441, 1983.
16. Schmitt, B. P., Kushner, M. S., and Weiner, S. L.: The diagnostic usefulness of the history of the patient with dyspnea. J. Gen. Intern. Med. *1*:386, 1986.
17. Christie, L. G., and Conti, C. R.: Systematic approach to the evaluation of angina-like chest pain. Am. Heart J. *102*:897, 1981.
18. Constant, J.: The clinical diagnosis of nonanginal chest pain: The differentiation of angina from nonanginal chest pain by history. Clin. Cardiol. *6*:11, 1983.
19. Levine, H. J.: Difficult problems in the diagnosis of chest pain. Am. Heart J. *100*:108, 1980.
20. Matthews, M. B., and Julian, D. G.: Angina pectoris: Definition and description. *In* Julian, D. G. (ed.): Angina Pectoris. New York, Churchill Livingstone, 1985, p. 2.
21. Appels, A., and Mulder, P.: Excess fatigue as a precursor of myocardial infarction. Eur. Heart J. *9*:758, 1988.
22. Lichstein, E., Breitbart, S., Shani, J., et al.: Relationship between location of chest pain and site of coronary artery occlusion. Am. Heart J. *115*:564, 1988.
23. Ross, R. S., and Babe, B. M.: Right ventricular hypertension as a cause of angina. Circulation *22*:801, 1960.
24. Zimmerman, D., and Parker, B. M.: The pain of pulmonary hypertension: Fact or fancy? JAMA *246*:2345, 1981.
25. Cook, D. G., and Shaper, A. G.: Breathlessness, angina pectoris and coronary artery disease. Am. J. Cardiol. *63*:921, 1989.
26. Epstein, S. E., Gerber, L. N., and Boren, J. S.: Chest wall syndrome. A common cause of unexpected pain. JAMA *241*:279, 1979.
27. Bass, C., Chambers, J. B., Kiff, P., et al.: Panic anxiety and hyperventilation in patients with chest pain: A controlled study. Q. J. Med. *69*:260:949–959, 1988.
28. Beitman, B. D., Basha, I., Flaker, G. et al.: Atypical or nonanginal chest pain: Panic disorder or coronary artery disease? Arch. Intern. Med. *147*:1548, 1987.
29. Kane, F. J., Jr., Harper, R. G., and Wittels, E.: Angina as a symptom of a psychiatric illness. South. Med. J. *81*:1412, 1988.
30. Horwitz, L. D., and Groves, B. M. (eds.): Signs and Symptoms in Cardiology. Philadelphia, J. B. Lippincott, 1985, 506 pp.
31. Conte, M. R., Orzan, F., Magnacca, M., et al.: Atypical chest pain: Coronary or esophageal disease? Int. J. Cardiol. *13*:135, 1986.
32. Schofield, P. M., Whorwell, P. J., Jones, P. E., et al.: Differentiation of "esophageal" and "cardiac" chest pain. Am. J. Cardiol. *62*:315, 1988.
33. Hersh, T.: Gastrointestinal causes of chest discomfort. *In* Hurst, J. W. (ed.): The Heart, 7th ed. New York, McGraw-Hill, 1990, pp. 987–991.
34. Mellow, M. H.: A gastroenterologist's view of chest pain. Curr. Probl. Cardiol. *7*:36, 1983.
35. Patterson, D. R.: Diffuse esophageal spasm in patients with undiagnosed chest pain. J. Clin. Gastroenterol. *4*:415, 1982.
36. DeMeester, T. R., O'Sullivan, G. C., Bermudez, G. et al.: Esophageal function in patients with angina-type chest pain and normal coronary angiograms. Ann. Surg. *196*:488, 1982.
37. Davies, H. A., Rush, E. M., Lewis, M. J., et al.: Oesophageal stimulation lowers exertional angina threshold. Lancet *1*:1011, 1985.
38. Braunwald, E.: Cyanosis. *In* Isselbacher, K. J., Braunwald, E., et al. (eds.): Harrison's Principles of Internal Medicine. 13th ed. New York, McGraw-Hill, 1994, pp. 178–182.
39. Szidon, J. P., and Fishman, A. P.: Cyanosis and clubbing. *In* Fishman, A. (ed.): Pulmonary Diseases and Disorders. 2nd ed. Philadelphia, W. B. Saunders Company, 1988, p. 351.
40. Richards, A. M., et al.: Syncope in aortic valvular stenosis. Lancet *1*:1113, 1984.
41. Brooks, R., et al.: Evaluation of the patient with unexplained syncope. *In* Zipes, D. P., and Jalife, J. (eds.): Cardiac Electrophysiology. Philadelphia, W. B. Saunders Company, 1990.
42. Braunwald, E.: Edema. In Isselbacher, K. J., Braunwald, E., et al. (eds.): Harrison's Principles of Internal Medicine. 13th ed. New York, McGraw-Hill, 1994, pp. 183–187.
43. Rose, B. D.: Edematous states. *In* Clinical Physiology of Acid-Base and Electrolyte Disorders. New York, McGraw-Hill, 1989, pp. 416–463.
44. Irwin, R. S., et al.: Chronic cough: The spectrum and frequency of causes, key components of the diagnostic evaluation, and outcome of specific therapy. Am. Rev. Respir. Dis. *141*:640, 1990.
45. Poe, R. H., Harder, R. V., Israel, R. H., and Kallay, M. C.: Chronic persistent cough: Experience in diagnosis and outcome using an anatomic diagnostic protocol. Chest *95*:723, 1989.
46. Braunwald, E.: Cough and hemoptysis. *In* Isselbacher, K. J., Braunwald, E., et al. (eds.): Harrison's Principles of Internal Medicine. 13th ed. New York, McGraw-Hill, 1994, pp. 171–174.

47. Thompson, A. B., et al.: Pathogenesis, evaluation, and therapy for massive hemoptysis. Clin. Chest Med. *13*:69, 1992.
48. Jones, D. K., and Davies, R.: Massive hemoptysis. Br. Med. J. *300*:299, 1990.

THE HISTORY IN SPECIFIC FORMS OF HEART DISEASE

49. Bristow, M. R. (ed.): Drug-Induced Heart Disease. Amsterdam, Elsevier, 1980, 476 pp.
50. Virmani, R., Robinowitz, M., Smialek, J. E., and Smyth, D. F.: Cardiovascular effect of cocaine: An autopsy study of 40 patients. Am. Heart J. *115*:1068, 1988.
51. Isner, J. M., and Chokshi, S. K.: Cocaine and vasospasm. N. Engl. J. Med. *321*:1604, 1989.
52. The Criteria Committee of the New York Heart Association: Nomenclature and Criteria for Diagnosis. 9th ed. Boston, Little, Brown, 1994.
53. Campeau, L.: Grading of angina pectoris. Circulation *54*:522, 1975.
54. Goldman, L., Hashimoto, B., Cook, E. F., and Loscalzo, A.: Comparative reproducibility and validity of systems for assessing cardiovascular functional class: Advantages of a new specific activity scale. Circulation *64*:1227, 1981.
55. Goldman, L., Cook, E. F., Mitchell, N., et al.: Pitfalls in the serial assessment of cardiac functional status. How a reduction in "ordinary" activity may reduce the apparent degree of cardiac compromise and give a misleading impression of improvement. J. Chronic Dis. *35*:763, 1982.

GENERAL REFERENCES

Constant, J.: The evolving check list in history-taking. *In* Bedside Cardiology. 4th ed. Boston, Little, Brown, 1993, pp. 1–22.
Dressler, W.: Clinical Aids in Cardiac Diagnosis. New York, Grune and Stratton, 1970.
Fowler, N. O.: The history in cardiac diagnosis. *In* Fowler, N. O. (ed.): Cardiac Diagnosis and Treatment. 3rd ed. Hagerstown, Md., Harper and Row, 1980, pp. 23–29.
Hurst, J. W.: Cardiovascular Diagnosis: The Initial Examination. St. Louis, C. V. Mosby, 1993, 556 pp.
Kraytman, J.: Cardiorespiratory system. *In* The Complete Patient History. New York, McGraw-Hill, 1979, pp. 11–112.

Chapter 2
Physical Examination of the Heart and Circulation

JOSEPH K. PERLOFF, EUGENE BRAUNWALD

Two of the most common pitfalls in cardiovascular medicine are the failure by the cardiologist to recognize the effects of systemic illnesses on the cardiovascular system and the failure by the noncardiologist to recognize the cardiac manifestations of systemic illnesses that have major effects on other organ systems. In order to avoid these pitfalls, patients known to have or suspected of having heart disease require not only a detailed examination of the cardiovascular system but a meticulous general physical examination as well.

For example, the presence of coronary artery disease should prompt a careful search for frequent noncardiac concomitants such as atherosclerosis of the carotid arteries and of the arteries of the lower extremities and aorta. Conversely, the very high incidence (approximately 50 per cent) of coronary artery disease in patients with cerebrovascular disorders must be considered in dealing with patients with these conditions.

THE GENERAL PHYSICAL EXAMINATION

GENERAL APPEARANCE

An assessment of the patient's general appearance is usually begun with a detailed inspection at the time when the history is being obtained.[1–4] The general build and appearance of the patient, the skin color, and the presence of pallor or cyanosis should then be noted, as well as the presence of shortness of breath, orthopnea, periodic (Cheyne-Stokes) respiration (see p. 455), and distention of the neck veins. If the patient is in pain, is he or she sitting quietly (typical of angina pectoris); moving about, trying to find a more comfortable position (characteristic of acute myocardial infarction); or most comfortable sitting upright (heart failure) or leaning forward (pericarditis)? Simple inspection also reveals whether the patient's whole body shakes with each heartbeat and whether Corrigan's pulses (bounding arterial pulsations, as occur with the large stroke volume of severe aortic regurgitation, arteriovenous fistula, or complete atrioventricular [AV] block) are present in the head, neck, and upper extremities. Marked weight loss, malnutrition, and cachexia, which occur in severe chronic heart failure (see p. 455), may also be readily evident on inspection. The cold, sweaty palms and frequent sighing respirations typical of *neurocirculatory asthenia* may be detected, as well as the marked obesity, somnolence, and cyanosis reflecting the *Pickwickian syndrome* (see p. 801). Abdominally localized obesity (diameter of waist/diameter of hips > 0.85; normal = 0.7) is associated with adult onset diabetes and coronary artery disease and should also be looked for.

The distinctive general appearance of the *Marfan syndrome* (see p. 1837) is often apparent, i.e., long extremities with an arm span that exceeds the height; a longer lower segment (pubis to foot) than upper segment (head to pubis); and arachnodactyly (spider fingers). In *Cushing's syndrome*, a cause of secondary hypertension (see p. 1837), there is truncal obesity and rounding of the face, with disproportionately thin extremities.

HEAD AND FACE

Examination of the face often aids in the recognition of many disorders that can affect the cardiovascular system. For example, *myxedema* (see p. 1894) is characterized by a dull, expressionless face; periorbital puffiness; loss of the lateral eyebrows; a large tongue; and dry, sparse hair. An *earlobe crease* occurs more frequently in patients with coronary artery disease than in those without this condition.[5,6]

Bobbing of the head coincident with each heartbeat (de Musset's sign) is characteristic of severe aortic regurgitation. Facial edema may be present in patients with *tricuspid valve disease* or *constrictive pericarditis*.

The *muscular dystrophies*, the cardiac manifestations of which are described in Chapter 60, may also affect facial appearance profoundly. Patients with *myotonic dystrophy* exhibit a dull, expressionless face, with ptosis due to weakness of the levator muscles.

EYES

External ophthalmoplegia and ptosis due to muscular dystrophy of the extraocular muscles occur in the *Kearns-Sayre syndrome*, which may be associated with complete heart block (Fig. 60–16, p. 1876).

Exophthalmos and stare occur not only in hyperthyroidism, which can cause high-output cardiac failure (see p. 460), but also in advanced congestive heart failure, in which there is severe pulmonary venous hypertension and weight loss (see p. 455).[8] The stare is probably due to lid retraction caused by the increased adrenergic tone that accompanies heart failure. Severe tricuspid regurgitation can also cause pulsation of the eyeballs[9,10] (pulsatile exophthalmos), as well as of the earlobes.

Blue sclerae may be seen in patients with osteogenesis imperfecta[11] —a disorder that may be associated with aortic dilatation, regurgitation, and dissection and with prolapse of the mitral valve (Chap. 49).

FUNDI. Examination of the *fundi* allows classification of arteriolar disease in patients with hypertension (Fig. 2–1*A*), and may also be helpful in the recognition of arteriosclerosis. Beading of the retinal artery may be present in patients with hypercholesterolemia (Fig.

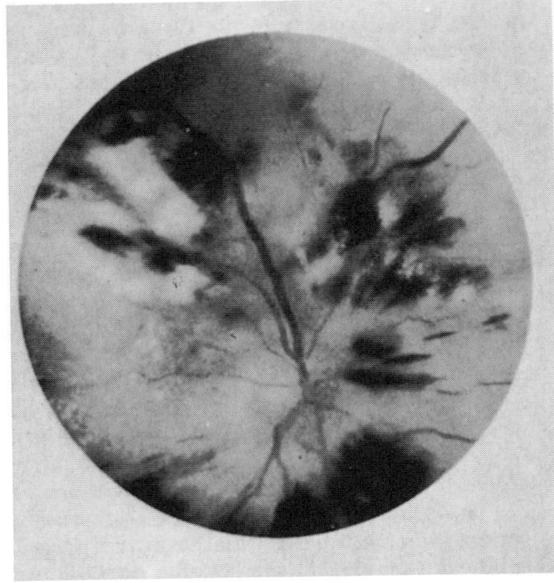

A

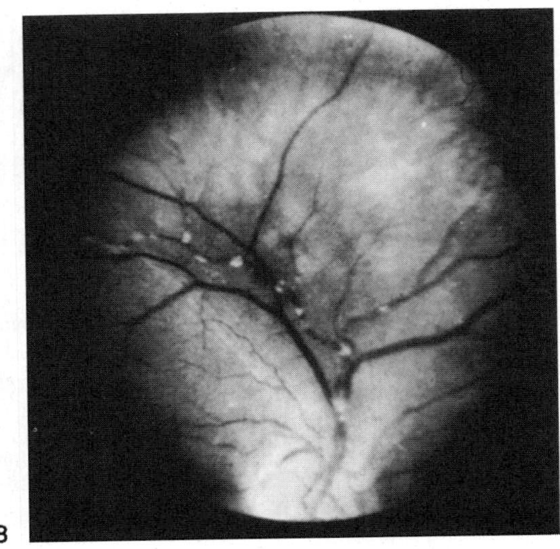

B

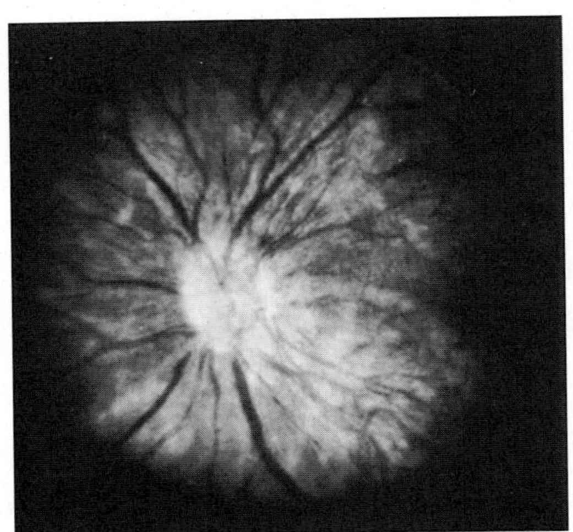

C

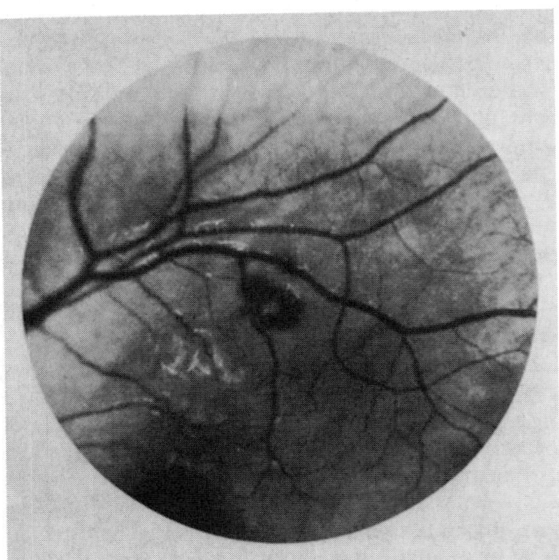

D

FIGURE 2–1. *A,* Severe hypertensive retinopathy. The patient was a 43-year-old man with the symptoms of malignant hypertension. He subsequently died of massive cerebral hemorrhage. *B,* Beading of the retinal artery in a patient with hypercholesterolemia. The patient was a 37-year-old man with a serum cholesterol level of 400 mg/100 ml. *C,* Proliferative retinopathy of Takayasu-Ohnishi disease. The patient was a 27-year-old Asian woman with postural amaurosis and hemiplegia. Brachial pulses were unobtainable. *D,* Roth spots (hemorrhage with white center) in a patient with subacute bacterial endocarditis. (From Cogan, D. G.: Ophthalmic Manifestations of Systemic Vascular Disease. Philadelphia, W. B. Saunders Company, 1974, p. 52.)

2–1*B*). Hemorrhages near the discs with white spots in the center (Roth's spots) occur in infective endocarditis (Fig. 33–7, p. 1085). Embolic retinal occlusions may occur in patients with rheumatic heart disease, left atrial myxoma, and atherosclerosis of the aorta or arch vessels. Papilledema may be present not only in patients with malignant hypertension (Chap. 26) but also in cor pulmonale with severe hypoxia.

SKIN AND MUCOUS MEMBRANES

Central cyanosis (due to intracardiac or intrapulmonary right-to-left shunting) involves the entire body, including warm, well-perfused sites such as the conjunctivae and the mucous membranes of the oral cavity, whereas peripheral cyanosis (due to reduction of peripheral blood flow, such as occurs in heart failure and peripheral vascular disease) is characteristically most prominent in cool, exposed areas that may not be well-perfused, such as the extremities, particularly the nailbeds and nose. Polycythemia can often be suspected from inspection of the conjunctivae, lips, and tongue, which in anemia are pale while in polycythemia are darkly congested.

Bronze pigmentation of the skin and loss of axillary and pubic hair occur in *hemochromatosis* (which may result in cardiomyopathy owing to iron deposits in the heart [see p. 1430]). Jaundice may be observed in patients following pulmonary infarction as well as in patients with congestive hepatomegaly or cardiac cirrhosis. *Lentigines,* i.e., small brown macular lesions on the neck and trunk that begin at about age 6 and do not increase in number with sunlight, are observed in patients with pulmonic stenosis and hypertrophic cardiomyopathy.[12]

Several types of *xanthomas,* i.e., cholesterol-filled nodules, are found either subcutaneously or over tendons in patients with hyperlipoproteinemia (Chap. 35). Premature atherosclerosis frequently develops in these individuals. *Tuberoeruptive xanthomas,* present subcutaneously or on the extensor surfaces of the extremities, and *xanthoma striatum palmare,* which produces yellowish, orange, or pink discoloration of the palmar and digital creases, occur most commonly in patients with Type III hyperlipoproteinemia. Patients with *xanthoma tendinosum* (Fig. 2–2), i.e., nodular swellings of the tendons, especially of the elbows, extensor surfaces of the hands, and Achilles' tendons, usually have Type II hyperlipoproteinemia (see p. 1143). *Eruptive xanthomas* are tiny yellowish nodules, 1 to 2 mm in diameter on an erythematous base, which may occur anywhere on the body and are associated with hyperchylomicronemia and are therefore often found in patients with Type I and Type V hyperlipoproteinemia.

Hereditary telangiectasias are multiple capillary hemangiomas occurring in the skin, lips (Fig. 2–3), nasal mucosa, and upper respiratory and gastrointestinal tracts and resemble the spider nevi seen in patients with liver disease. When present in the lung, they are associated with pulmonary arteriovenous fistulas and cause central cyanosis.

EXTREMITIES

A variety of congenital and acquired cardiac malformations are associated with characteristic changes in the extremities. Among the congenital lesions, short stature, cubitus valgus, and medial deviation of the extended forearm are characteristic of *Turner syndrome* (see p.

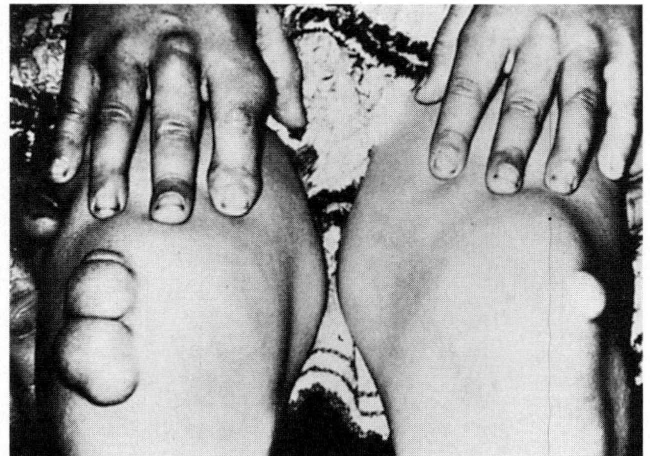

FIGURE 2–2. Tendinous xanthomas of the knees in a patient with familial hypercholesterolemia. The patient was a 10-year-old girl with a serum cholesterol level of 665 mg/100 ml. Several other members of the family had a similar syndrome. (From Cogan, D. G.: Ophthalmic Manifestations of Systemic Vascular Disease. Philadelphia, W. B. Saunders Company, 1974, pp. 14 and 15.)

1657). Patients with the *Holt-Oram syndrome*[13] (see p. 1661), i.e., atrial septal defect with skeletal deformities, often have a thumb with an extra phalanx, a so-called fingerized thumb, which lies in the same plane as the fingers, making it difficult to appose the thumb and fingers. In addition, they may exhibit deformities of the radius and ulna, causing difficulty in supination and pronation.

Arachnodactyly is characteristic of *Marfan syndrome* (p. 1669). Normally, when a fist is made over a clenched thumb, the latter does not extend beyond the ulnar side of the hand, but it usually does so in Marfan syndrome.

Systolic flushing of the nailbeds, which can be readily detected by pressing a flashlight against the terminal digits (Quincke's sign), is a sign of aortic regurgitation and of other conditions characterized by a greatly widened pulse pressure. *Differential cyanosis,* in which the hands and fingers (especially on the right side) are pink and the feet and toes are cyanotic, is indicative of patent ductus arteriosus with reversed shunt due to pulmonary hypertension (see p. 905); this finding can often be brought out by exercise. On the other hand, *reversed differential cyanosis,* in which cyanosis of the fingers exceeds that of the toes, suggests transposition of the great arteries, pulmonary hypertension, preductal narrowing of the aorta, and reversed flow through a patent ductus arteriosus.[14]

CLUBBING OF THE FINGERS AND TOES[15] (Fig. 2–4). Clubbing of the digits is characteristic of central cyanosis (cyanotic congenital heart disease or pulmonary disease with hypoxia). It may also appear within a few weeks of the development of infective endocarditis but usually develops after 2 or 3 years of central cyanosis. The earliest forms of clubbing are characterized by increased glossiness and cyanosis of the skin at the root of the nail.[16] Following obliteration of the normal angle between the base of the nail and the skin, the soft tissue of the pulp becomes hypertrophied, the nail root floats freely, and its loose proximal end can be palpated. In the more severe forms of clubbing, bony changes occur, i.e., *hypertrophic pulmonary osteoarthropathy;* these changes involve the terminal digits and in rare instances even the wrists, ankles, elbows, and knees. *Unilateral clubbing* of the fingers is rare but can occur when an aortic aneurysm interferes with the arterial supply to one arm.

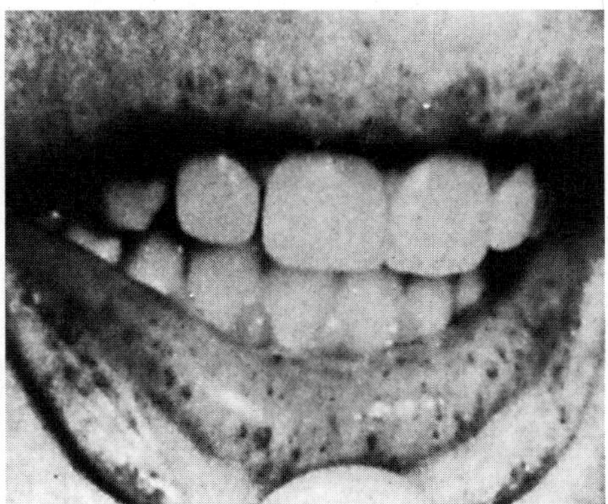

FIGURE 2–3. Hemorrhagic telangiectasia on the lips of a 25-year-old woman with pulmonary arteriovenous fistulas. (From Perloff, J. K.: The Clinical Recognition of Congenital Heart Disease. 4th ed. Philadelphia, W. B. Saunders Company, 1994, p. 719.)

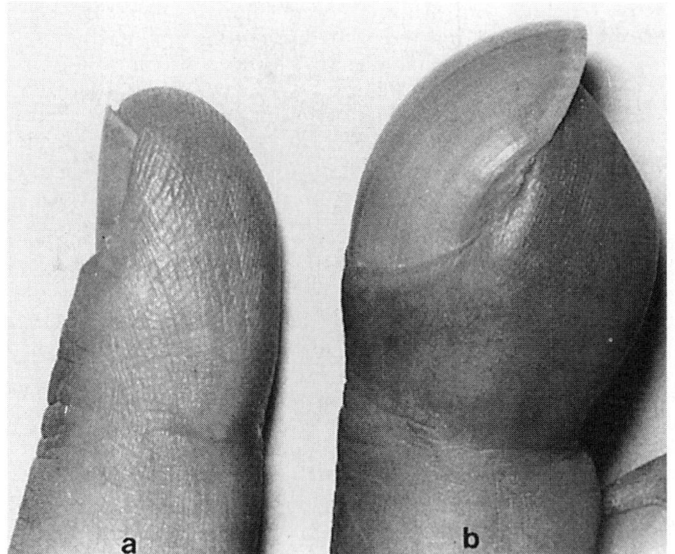

FIGURE 2–4. *A,* Normal finger. *B,* Advanced clubbing in a young cyanotic adult. (From Perloff, J. K.: The Clinical Recognition of Congenital Heart Disease. 4th ed. Philadelphia, W. B. Saunders Company, 1994, p. 7.)

Osler's nodes are small, tender, purplish erythematous skin lesions due to infected microemboli and occurring most frequently in the pads of the fingers or toes and in the palms of the hands or soles of the feet[17] (see p. 1085), whereas *Janeway lesions* are slightly raised, nontender hemorrhagic lesions in the palms of hands and soles of the feet; both these lesions as well as petechiae occur in infective endocarditis. When the latter occur under the nailbeds, they are termed *splinter hemorrhages.*

Edema of the lower extremities is a common finding in congestive heart failure; however, if it is present in only one leg, it is more likely due to obstructive venous or lymphatic disease than to heart failure. Firm pressure on the pretibial region for 10 to 20 seconds may be necessary for the detection of edema in ambulatory patients. In patients confined to bed, edema appears first in the sacral region. Edema may involve the face in children with heart failure of any etiology and in adults with heart failure associated with marked elevation of systemic venous pressure (e.g., constrictive pericarditis and tricuspid valve disease).

CHEST AND ABDOMEN

Examination of the thorax should begin with observations of the rate, effort, and regularity of respiration. The shape of the chest is important as well; thus, a barrel-shaped chest with low diaphragm suggests emphysema, bronchitis, and possibly cor pulmonale.

Inspection of the chest may reveal a bulging to the right of the upper sternum caused by an aortic aneurysm. This can also produce a venous collateral pattern caused by obstruction of the superior vena cava. *Kyphoscoliosis* of any etiology can cause cor pulmonale; this skeletal abnormality as well as pectus excavatum (funnel chest) and pectus carinatum (pigeon breast) is often present in Marfan syndrome.

Left ventricular failure and other causes of elevation of pulmonary venous pressure may cause pulmonary rales; wheezing is sometimes audible in pulmonary edema (cardiac asthma).

Painful enlargement of the *liver* may be due to venous congestion; the tenderness disappears in longstanding heart failure. Hepatic systolic expansile pulsations occur in patients with severe tricuspid regurgitation, and presystolic pulsations can be felt in patients with pure tricuspid stenosis and sinus rhythm. Patients with constrictive pericarditis also often have pulsatile hepatomegaly, the contour of the pulsations resembling those of the jugular venous pulse in this condition.[18,19] When firm pressure over the abdomen causes cervical venous distention, i.e., when there is *abdominojugular reflux,* right heart failure is usually present.[20] *Ascites* is also characteristic of heart failure, but is especially characteristic of tricuspid valve disease and chronic constrictive pericarditis.

Splenomegaly may occur in the presence of severe congestive hepatomegaly, most frequently in patients with constrictive pericarditis or tricuspid valve disease. The spleen may be enlarged and painful in infective endocarditis as well as following splenic embolization. Splenic infarction is frequently accompanied by an audible friction rub.

Both *kidneys* may be palpably enlarged in patients with hypertension secondary to polycystic disease. Auscultation of the abdomen should be carried out in all patients with hypertension; a systolic bruit secondary to renal artery stenosis may be audible near the umbilicus or in the flank.

Atherosclerotic aneurysms of the abdominal aorta are usually readily detected on palpation (see p. 1547), except in markedly obese patients. In patients with *coarctation of the aorta,* no abdominal pulsations are palpable despite the presence of prominent arterial pulses in the neck and upper extremities; arterial pulses in the lower extremities are reduced or absent.

JUGULAR VENOUS PULSE

Important information concerning the dynamics of the right side of the heart can be obtained by observation of the jugular venous pulse.[4,21,22,23] The *internal* jugular vein is ordinarily employed in the examination; the venous pulse can usually be analyzed more readily on the right than on the left side of the neck, because the right innominate and jugular veins extend in an almost straight line cephalad to the superior vena cava, thus favoring transmission of hemodynamic changes from the right atrium, while the left innominate vein is not in a straight line and may be kinked or compressed by a variety of normal structures, by a dilated aorta, or by an aneurysm.

The patient should be lying comfortably during the examination; clothing should be removed; although the head should rest on a pillow, it must not be at a sharp angle from the trunk. The jugular venous pulse may be examined effectively by shining a light tangentially across the neck. Most patients with heart disease are examined most effectively in the 45-degree position, but in patients in whom venous pressure is high, a greater inclination (60 or even 90 degrees) is required to obtain visible pulsations, while in those in whom jugular venous pressure is low, a lesser inclination (30 degrees) is desirable. In order to amplify the pulsations of the jugular veins, it may be helpful to place the patient in the supine position and try to increase venous return by elevating the patient's legs.

The internal jugular vein is located deep within the neck, where it is covered by the sternocleidomastoid muscle and is therefore not usually visible as a discrete structure, except in the presence of severe venous hypertension. However, its pulsations are transmitted to the skin of the neck, where they are usually easily visible. Sometimes difficulty may be experienced in differentiating between the carotid and jugular venous pulses in the neck, particularly when the latter exhibits prominent *v* waves, as occurs in patients with tricuspid regurgitation, in whom the valves in the internal jugular veins may be incompetent. However, there are several helpful clues[24]: (1) The arterial pulse is a sharply localized rapid movement that may not be readily visible but that strikes the palpating fingers with considerable force; in contrast, the venous pulse, while more readily visible, often disappears when the palpating finger is placed lightly on or below the pulsating area. (2) The arterial pulse usually exhibits a single upstroke while the venous pulse has two peaks and two troughs per cardiac cycle in sinus rhythm. (3) The arterial pulsations do not change when the patient is in the upright position or during respiration, whereas venous pulsations usually disappear or diminish greatly in the upright position and during inspiration, unless the venous pressure is greatly elevated. (4) Compression of the root of the neck does not affect the arterial pulse but usually abolishes venous pulsations, except in the presence of extreme venous hypertension.

Two principal observations can usually be made from examination of the neck veins: the level of venous pressure and the type of venous wave pattern. In order to estimate jugular venous pressure, the height of the oscillating top of the distended proximal portion of the internal jugular vein, which reflects right atrial pressure, should be determined. The upper limit of normal is 4 cm above the sternal angle, which corresponds to a central venous pressure of approximately 9 cm H_2O, since the right atrium is approximately 5 cm below the sternal angle. When the veins in the neck collapse in a subject breathing normally in the horizontal

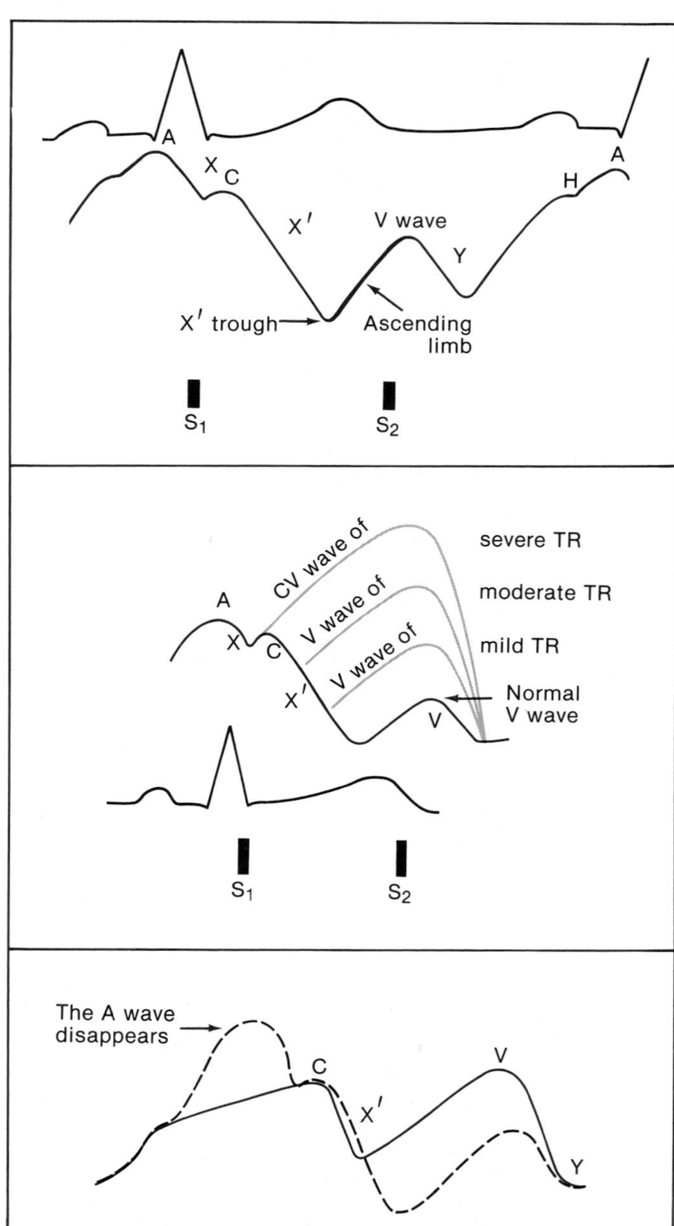

FIGURE 2–5. ***Top,*** **Normal jugular venous pulse: the jugular *v* wave is built up during systole, and its height reflects the rate of filling and the elasticity of the right atrium. Between the bottom of the *y* descent (*y* trough) and beginning of the *a* wave is the period of relatively slow filling of the "atrioventricle" or diastasis period. The wave built up during diastasis is the *H* wave. The *H* wave height also reflects the stiffness of the right atrium. S_1 and S_2 refer to the first and second heart sounds, respectively. *Center,* As the degree of tricuspid regurgitation (TR) increases, the *x′* descent is increasingly encroached upon. With severe TR, no *x′* descent is seen, and the jugular pulse wave is said to be "ventricularized." *Bottom,* Black broken line = normal jugular venous pulse and sinus rhythm; red continuous line = following development of atrial fibrillation. The dominant descent in atrial fibrillation is almost always the *y* descent; i.e., it has the superficial appearance of the pulse wave of TR. (From Constant, J.: Bedside Cardiology. 4th ed. Boston, Little, Brown & Co., 1994, pp. 81 and 89.)**

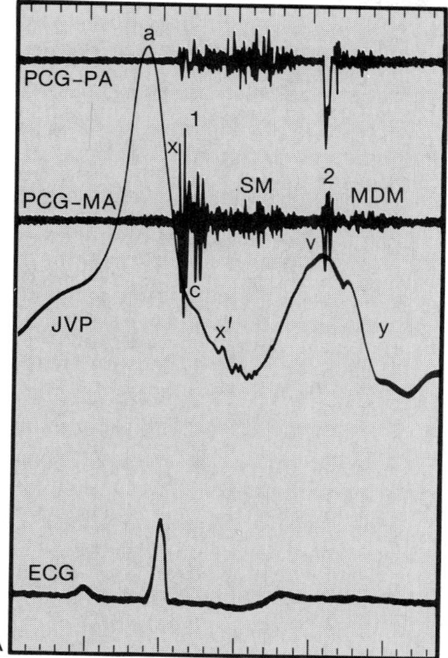

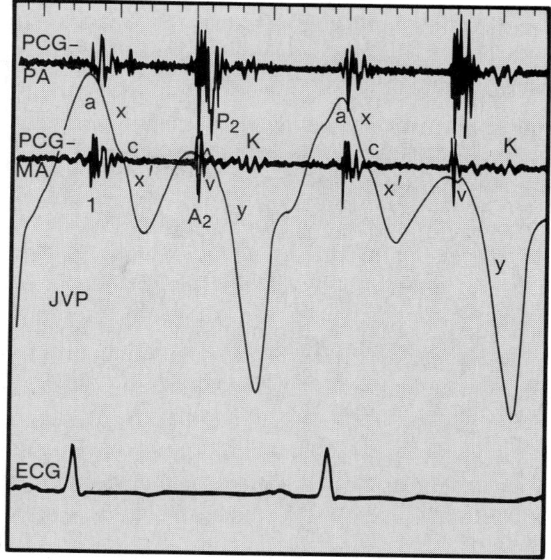

FIGURE 2–6. *A,* Jugular venous pressure (JVP) in mitral stenosis with pulmonary hypertension. The JVP is dominated by a very large *a* wave resulting from diminished compliance of the right ventricle associated with pulmonary hypertension. The peaked *a* wave represents a brief period of retrograde flow from right atrium to great veins. *B,* JVP in constrictive pericarditis. In this severe and longstanding case, the *x'* descent has become very shallow and the *y* descent is the principal feature, indicating that antegrade flow from the venous system to the right heart is now limited to early diastole. A pericardial knock (K) is seen at approximately the nadir of the *y* descent. (From Craige, E., and Smith, P.: Heart sounds. *In* Braunwald, E. [ed.]: Heart Disease: A Textbook of Cardiovascular Medicine. 3rd ed. Philadelphia, W. B. Saunders Company, 1988, pp. 61 and 62.)

position, it is likely that the central venous pressure is subnormal. When obstruction of veins in the lower extremities is responsible for edema, pressure in the neck veins is not elevated and the abdominal-jugular reflux is negative.

ABDOMINAL-JUGULAR REFLUX.[20,25] This can be tested by applying firm pressure to the periumbilical region for 10 to 30 seconds with the patient breathing quietly while the jugular veins are observed; increased respiratory excursions or straining should be avoided. In normal subjects, jugular venous pressure rises less than 3 cm H_2O and only transiently, while abdominal pressure is continued, whereas in right or left ventricular failure and/or tricuspid regurgitation the jugular venous pressure remains elevated. In the absence of these conditions a positive abdominal-jugular reflux suggests an elevated pulmonary artery wedge[21] or central venous pressure.[24]

PATTERN OF THE VENOUS PULSE. The events of the cardiac cycle, shown in Figure 12–22, p. 377, provide an explanation for the details of the jugular venous waveform (Fig. 2–5). The *a* wave in the venous pulse results from venous distention due to right atrial systole, while the *x* descent is due to atrial relaxation and descent of the floor of the right atrium during right ventricular systole; the latter, sometimes called the *x'* descent, interrupts the descent. The *c* wave, which occurs simultaneously with the carotid arterial pulse, is an inconstant wave in the jugular venous pulse and/or interruption of the descent following the peak of the *a* wave. (Many investigators refer to this wave as the *x* descent.) The *v* wave results from the rise in right atrial pressure when blood flows into the right atrium during ventricular systole when the tricuspid valve is shut, and the *y* descent, i.e., the downslope of the *v* wave, is related to the decline in right atrial pressure when the tricuspid valve reopens. Following the bottom of the *y* descent (the *y* trough) and beginning of the *a* wave is a period of relatively slow filling of the atrium or ventricle, the diastasis period, a wave termed the *H* wave.

While all or most of these events can usually be recorded, they may not be readily distinguishable on inspection. The descents or downward collapsing movements of the jugular veins are more rapid, produce larger excursions, and are therefore more prominent to the eye than are the ascents (Fig. 2–5). The normal dominant jugular venous descent, the *x'* descent, occurs just prior to the second heart sound, while the *y* descent ends after the second heart sound. With an increase in central venous pressure, the *v* wave becomes higher and the *y* collapse becomes more prominent. The *a* wave occurs just before the first sound or carotid pulse and has a sharp rise and fall. The *v* wave occurs just after the arterial pulse and has a slower, undulating pattern.

ALTERATIONS IN DISEASE. Elevation of jugular venous pressure reflects an increase in right atrial pressure and occurs in heart failure, reduced compliance of the right ventricle, pericardial disease, hypervolemia, obstruction of the tricuspid orifice, and obstruction of the superior vena cava. During inspiration, the jugular venous pressure normally declines but the *amplitude* of the pulsations increases. *Kussmaul's sign* is a paradoxical rise in the height of the jugular venous pressure during inspiration, which typically occurs in patients with chronic constrictive pericarditis and sometimes in congestive heart failure and tricuspid stenosis.

The *a* wave is particularly prominent in conditions in which the resistance to right atrial contraction is increased, such as right ventricular hypertrophy, pulmonary hypertension, and tricuspid stenosis (Fig. 2–6*A*). The *a* wave may also be tall in left ventricular hypertrophy when the thickened ventricular septum interferes with right ventricular filling. Tall *a* waves are present in patients with sinus rhythm and tricuspid stenosis or atresia, right atrial myxoma, or reduced compliance and/or marked hypertrophy of the right ventricle. Cannon (amplified) *a* waves are noted in patients with atrioventricular dissociation when the right atrium contracts against a closed tricuspid valve. In atrial fibrillation, the *a* wave and *x* descent disappear, and the x' descent becomes more prominent. In right ventricular failure and sinus rhythm, there may be increases in prominence of both the *a* and *v* waves. A steeply rising *H* wave is observed (or recorded) in restrictive cardiomyopathy, constrictive pericarditis, and right ventricular infarction. The *a* wave is absent in atrial fibrillation, accompanied by a diminished x' descent and a prominent *v* wave (Fig. 2–5, *Bottom*). The *x* descent may be prominent in patients with large *a* waves, as well as in patients with right ventricular volume overload (atrial septal defect).

Constrictive pericarditis (Fig. 2–6*B*) is characterized by a rapid and deep *y* descent followed by a rapid rise to a diastolic plateau (*H* wave) without a prominent *a* wave; occasionally, the x' descent is prominent in this condition as well, causing a "W"-shaped jugular venous pulse. However, it is in cardiac tamponade that the *x* descent is most prominent (Fig. 43–10, p. 1492). A prominent *v* wave or *c-v* wave, i.e., fusion of the *c* and *v* waves in the absence or attenuation of an x' descent, occurs in tricuspid regurgitation, sometimes causing a systolic movement of the ear lobe[29] (Figs. 2–5, *Center* and Fig. 32–46, p. 1058) and a right-to-left head movement with each ventricular systole. A prominent *v* wave and *y* descent are also seen in atrial septal defect; the *y* descent is gradual when right atrial emptying is impeded, as in tricuspid stenosis, and rapid when it is unimpeded, as in tricuspid regurgitation. A steep *y* descent is seen in any condition in which there is myocardial dysfunction, ventricular dilatation, and an elevated central venous pressure.

INDIRECT MEASUREMENT OF ARTERIAL PRESSURE

Systolic arterial pressure can be *estimated* without a sphygmomanometer cuff by gradually compressing the brachial artery while palpating the radial artery; the force required to obliterate the radial pulse represents the systolic blood pressure, and with practice, one can often estimate this level within 20 mm Hg. Ordinarily, however, a sphygmomanometer is used to obtain an indirect measurement of blood pressure.[26–28] The cuff should fit snugly around the arm, with its lower edge at least 1 inch above the antecubital space, and the diaphragm of the stethoscope should be placed close to or under the edge of the sphygmomanometer cuff. The width of the cuff selected should be at least 40 per cent of the circumference of the limb to be used.

The standard size, with a 5-inch-wide cuff, is designed for adults with an arm of average size. When this cuff is applied to a large upper arm or a normal adult thigh, arterial pressure is overestimated, leading to spurious hypertension in the obese (arm circumference >35 cm[3])[30,31]; when it is applied to a small arm, the pressure is underestimated. The cuff width should be approximately 1½ inches in infants and small children, 3 inches in young children (2 to 5 years), and 8 inches in obese adults. The rubber bag should be long enough to extend at least halfway around the limb (10 inches in adults). In patients with rigid, sclerotic arteries the systolic pressure may also be overestimated, by as much as 30 mm Hg. Mercury manometers are, in general, more accurate and reliable than the aneroid type; the latter should be calibrated at least once yearly.

BLOOD PRESSURE IN THE UPPER EXTREMITIES. In order to measure arterial pressure in an upper extremity,[32] the patient should be seated or lying comfortably and relaxed, the arm should be slightly flexed and at heart level, and the arm muscles should be relaxed. The cuff should be inflated rapidly to approximately 30 mm Hg above the anticipated systolic pressure.[33] These maneuvers, which diminish the volume of blood in the venous bed, decrease the tissue pressure distal to the cuff and thereby increase the flow into the occluded brachial artery. The cuff is then deflated slowly, no faster than 3 mm Hg/sec; the pressure at which the brachial pulse can be palpated is close to the systolic pressure.

The cuff should be deflated rapidly after the diastolic pressure is noted and a full minute allowed to elapse before pressure is remeasured in the same limb. Although excessive pressure on the stethoscope head does not affect systolic pressure, it does erroneously lower diastolic readings.[34] In one study, the anxiety associated with blood pressure measurement was shown to elevate arterial pressure by an average of 27/17 mm Hg[35]: ("white coat hypertension"). It is desirable for the patient to reduce anxiety and bladder distention and to avoid exercise, caffeine, eating, and smoking for a half hour preceding the screening. If doubt persists, a home blood pressure record should be obtained.

BLOOD PRESSURE IN THE LOWER EXTREMITIES. To measure pressure in the legs, the patient should lie on his or her abdomen, an 8-inch-wide cuff should be applied with the compression bag over the posterior aspect of the midthigh and should be rolled diagonally around the thigh to keep the edges snug against the skin, and auscultation should be carried out in the popliteal fossa. In order to measure pressure in the lower leg, an arm cuff is placed over the calf, and auscultation is carried out over the posterior tibial artery. Regardless of where the cuff is applied, care must be taken to avoid letting the rubber part of the balloon of the cuff extend beyond its covering and to avoid placing the cuff on so loosely that central ballooning occurs.

KOROTKOFF SOUNDS. There are five phases of Korotkoff sounds, i.e., sounds produced by the flow of blood as the constricting blood pressure cuff is gradually released. The first appearance of clear, tapping sound (phase I) represents the systolic pressure. These sounds are replaced by soft murmurs during phase II and by louder murmurs during phase III, as the volume of blood flowing through the constricted artery increases. The sounds suddenly become muffled in phase IV, when constriction of the brachial artery diminishes as arterial diastolic pressure is approached. Korotkoff sounds disappear in phase V, which is usually within 10 mm Hg of phase IV.

Diastolic pressure measured directly through an intraarterial needle and external manometer corresponds closely to phase V.[4] In severe aortic regurgitation, however, when the disappearance point is extremely low, sometimes 0 mm Hg, the sound of muffling (phase IV) is much closer to the intraarterial diastolic pressure than is the disappearance point (phase V). When there is a sizable difference between phases IV and V of the Korotkoff sounds (>10 mm Hg), both pressures should be recorded (e.g., 142/54/10 mm Hg).

Korotkoff sounds may be difficult to hear and arterial pressure difficult to measure when arterial pressure rises at a slow rate (as in severe aortic stenosis), when the arteries are markedly constricted (as in shock), and when the stroke volume is reduced (as in severe heart failure). Very soft or inaudible Korotkoff sounds can often be accentuated by dilating the blood vessels of the upper extremities simply by opening and closing the fist repeatedly. Sometimes in states of shock, the indirect method of measuring blood pressure is unreliable, and arterial pressure should be measured through an intraarterial needle.

The Auscultatory Gap. This is a silence that sometimes separates the first appearance of the Korotkoff sounds from their second appearance at a lower pressure. The phenomenon tends to occur when there is venous distention or reduced velocity of arterial flow into the arm. If the first muffling of sounds is considered to be the diastolic pressure, it will be overestimated. If the second appearance is taken as the systolic pressure, it will be underestimated. On the other hand, sounds transmitted through the arterial tree from prosthetic aortic valves may be responsible for falsely high readings.

BLOOD PRESSURE IN THE BASAL CONDITION. In order to determine arterial pressure in the basal condition, the patient should have rested in a quiet room for 15 minutes. It is desirable to record the arterial pressure in both arms at the time of the initial examination; differences in systolic pressure exceeding 10 mm Hg between the two arms when measurements are made simultaneously or in rapid sequence[36] suggest obstructive lesions involving the aorta or the origin of the innominate and subclavian arteries, or supravalvular aortic stenosis (in which pressure in the right arm exceeds that in the left). In patients with vertebral-basal artery insufficiency, a difference in pressure between the arms may signify that a subclavian "steal" is responsible for the cerebrovascular symptoms. In order to determine whether orthostatic hypotension is present, arterial pressure should be determined with the patient in both the supine and the erect positions. However, regardless of the patient's posture, the brachial artery should be at the level of the heart to avoid superimposition of the effects of gravity on the recorded pressure.

Normally, the systolic pressure in the legs is up to 20 mm Hg higher than in the arms, but the diastolic pressures are usually virtually identical. The recording of a higher diastolic pressure in the legs than in the arms suggests that the thigh cuff is too small. When systolic pressure in the popliteal artery exceeds that in the brachial artery by more than 20 mm Hg (Hill's sign), aortic regurgitation is usually present.[37] Blood pressure should be measured in the lower extremities in patients with hypertension to detect coarctation of the aorta or when obstructive disease of the aorta or its immediate branches is suspected.

To be *certain* from physical examination that the systolic pressure is different in the two arms or in the upper and lower extremities, two examiners should measure the pressures simultaneously, then switch extremities.[3]

ARTERIAL PULSE

The volume and contour of the arterial pulse are determined by a combination of factors, including the left ventricular stroke volume, the ejection velocity, the relative compliance and capacity of the arterial system, and the pressure waves that result from the antegrade flow of blood and reflections of the arterial pressure pulse returning from the peripheral circulation.[35] Bilateral palpation of the carotid, radial, brachial, femoral, popliteal, dorsalis pedis, and posterior tibial pulses should be part of the examina-

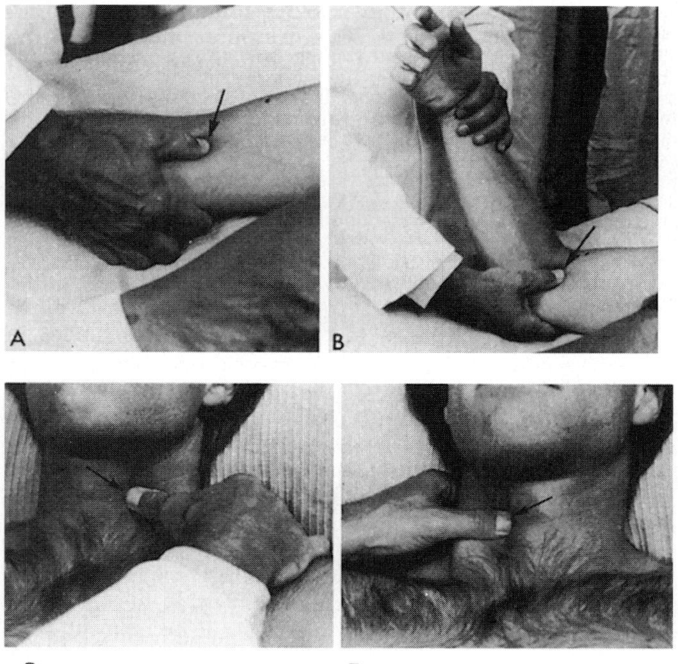

FIGURE 2–7. *A,* Palpation of the right brachial pulse with the thumb while the patient's arm lies at the side with the palm up. *B,* Palpation of the right brachial pulse with the patient's elbow resting in the palm of the examiner's hand. The thumb explores the antecubital fossa (arrow), while the patient's forearm is passively raised and lowered to achieve maximum relaxation of muscles around the elbow. *C* and *D,* Palpation of the carotid pulse. The examiner places the right thumb (arrow) on the patient's left carotid artery *(C).* The left thumb (arrow) is then applied separately to the right carotid *(D).* (From Perloff, J. K.: Physical Examination of the Heart and Circulation. Philadelphia, W. B. Saunders Company, 1990.)

tion of all cardiac patients, although caution should be exercised in bilateral carotid palpation, especially in the aged. The frequency, regularity, and shape of the pulse wave and the character of the arterial wall should be determined.[39] The carotid pulse (Fig. 2–7*C* and *D*) provides the most accurate representation of the central aortic pulse.[40] For palpation of the left carotid artery, the observer applies the right thumb to the patient's left carotid artery in the lower third of the neck[2] (Fig. 2–7*C*). The left femoral artery should be palpated with the right thumb. The patient should be supine with the head and chest at a 45-degree angle. The brachial artery is the vessel ordinarily most suitable for appreciating the rate of rise of the pulse and the contour, volume, and consistency of the peripheral vessels. This artery is located at the medial aspect of the elbow, and it may be helpful to flex the arm in order to improve palpation; palpation of the artery should be carried out with the thumb exerting pressure on the artery until its maximal movement is detected (Fig. 2–7*A* and *B*). A normal rate of rise of the arterial pulse suggests that there is no obstruction to left ventricular outflow, whereas a pulse wave of small amplitude with normal configuration suggests a reduced stroke volume.

THE NORMAL PULSE (Fig. 2–8). The pulse in the ascending aorta normally rises rapidly to a rounded dome; this initial rise reflects the peak velocity of blood ejected from the left ventricle. A slight anacrotic notch or pause is frequently recorded, but only occasionally felt, on the ascending limb of the pulse. The descending limb of the central aortic pulse is less steep than is the ascending limb, and it is interrupted by the incisura, a sharp downward deflection related to closure of the aortic valve. Immediately thereafter, the pulse wave rises slightly and then declines gradually throughout diastole. As the pulse wave is transmitted to the periphery, its upstroke becomes steeper, the systolic peak becomes higher, the anacrotic shoulder disappears, and the sharp incisura is replaced by a smoother, later dicrotic notch followed by a dicrotic wave.[41] Normally, the height of this dicrotic wave diminishes with age, hypertension, and arteriosclerosis. In the central arterial pulse (central aorta and innominate and carotid arteries), the rapidly transmitted impact of left ventricular ejection results in a peak in early systole, referred to as the *percussion wave;* a second, smaller peak, the *tidal wave,* presumed to represent a reflected wave from the periphery, can often be recorded but is not normally palpable. However, in older subjects, particularly those with increased peripheral resistance, as

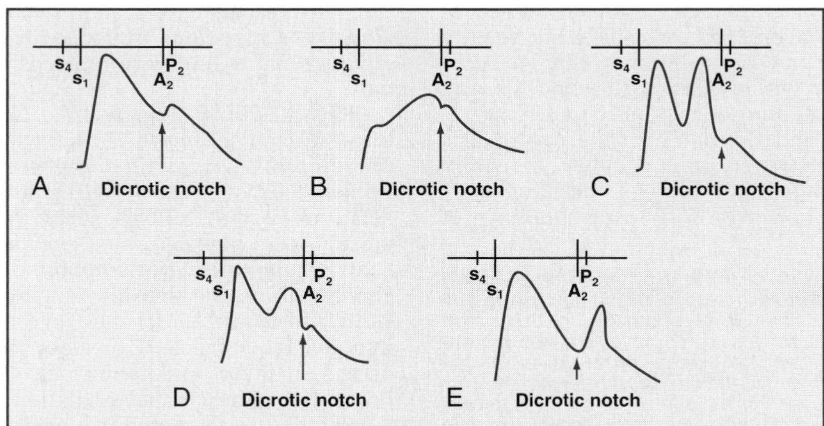

FIGURE 2–8. Schematic diagrams of the configurational changes in the carotid pulse and their differential diagnosis. Heart sounds are also illustrated. *A,* Normal. *B,* Anacrotic pulse with slow initial upstroke. The peak is close to the second heart sound. These features suggest fixed left ventricular outflow obstruction. *C,* Pulsus bisferiens with both percussion and tidal waves occurring during systole. This type of carotid pulse contour is most frequently observed in patients with hemodynamically significant aortic regurgitation or combined aortic stenosis and regurgitation with dominant regurgitation. It is rarely observed in mitral valve prolapse or in normal individuals. *D,* Pulsus bisferiens in hypertrophic obstructive cardiomyopathy. It is rarely appreciated at the bedside by palpation. *E,* Dicrotic pulse results from an accentuated dicrotic wave and tends to occur in sepsis, severe heart failure, hypovolemic shock, cardiac tamponade, and after aortic valve replacement. (S_4 = atrial sounds; S_1 = first heart sounds; A_2 = aortic component of the second heart sounds; P_2 = pulmonary component of the second heart sound). (From Chatterjee, K.: Bedside evaluation of the heart: The physical examination. *In* Chatterjee, K., et al. [eds.]: Cardiology: An Illustrated Text/Reference. Philadelphia, J. B. Lippincott, 1991, pp. 3.11–3.51.)

well as in patients with arteriosclerosis and diabetes, the tidal wave may be somewhat higher than the percussion wave; i.e., the pulse reaches a peak in late systole. In peripheral arteries, the pulse wave normally has a single sharp peak.

ABNORMAL PULSES. When peripheral vascular resistance and arterial stiffness are increased, as in hypertension or with the increased arterial stiffness that accompanies normal aging, there is an elevation in pulse wave velocity, and the pulse contour has a more rapid upstroke and greater amplitude. Reduced or unequal carotid arterial pulsations occur in patients with carotid atherosclerosis and with diseases of the aortic arch, including aortic dissection, aneurysm, and Takayasu's disease (see p. 1572). In *supravalvular aortic stenosis* there is a selective streaming of the jet toward the innominate artery, and the carotid and brachial arterial pulses are stronger and rise more rapidly on the right than on the left side, and pressures are higher in the right than in the left arm (see p. 919). The pulses of the upper extremities may be reduced or unequal in a variety of other conditions, including arterial embolus or thrombosis, anomalous origin or aberrant path of the major vessels, and cervical rib or scalenus anticus syndrome. Asymmetry of right and left popliteal pulses is characteristic of iliofemoral obstruction. Weakness or absence of radial, posterior tibial, or dorsalis pedis pulses on one side suggests arterial insufficiency. In *coarctation of the aorta* the carotid and brachial pulses are bounding, rise rapidly, and have large volumes, whereas in the lower extremities, the systolic and pulse pressures are reduced, their rate of rise is slow, and there is a late peak. This delay in the femoral arterial pulses can usually be readily detected by simultaneous palpation of the femoral and brachial arterial pulses.

In patients with fixed obstruction to left ventricular outflow (valvular aortic stenosis, and congenital fibrous subaortic stenosis), the carotid pulse rises slowly *(pulsus tardus)* (Fig. 2–8*B*); the upstroke is frequently characterized by a thrill (the *carotid shudder);* and the peak is reduced, occurs late in systole, and is sustained. There is a notch on the upstroke of the carotid pulse (anacrotic notch) that is so distinct that two separate waves can be palpated in what is termed an *anacrotic pulse. Pulsus parvus* is a pulse of small amplitude, usually because of a reduction of stroke volume. *Pulsus parvus et tardus* refers to a small pulse with a delayed systolic peak, which is characteristic of severe aortic stenosis. This type of pulse is more readily appreciated by palpating the carotid rather than a more peripheral artery. Patients with severe aortic stenosis and heart failure usually exhibit simply a reduced pulse amplitude, i.e., *pulsus parvus,* and the delay in the upstroke is not readily apparent. However, this delay is readily recorded. In elderly patients with inelastic peripheral arteries, the pulse may rise normally despite the presence of aortic stenosis.

The carotid arterial pulse may be prominent or exaggerated in any condition in which pulse pressure is increased, including anxiety, the hyperkinetic heart syndrome, anemia, fever, pregnancy, or other high cardiac output states (Chap. 15), as well as in bradycardia, and peripheral arteriosclerosis with reduction in arterial distensibility. In patients with *mitral regurgitation* or *ventricular septal defect,* the forward stroke volume (from the left ventricle into the aorta) is usually normal, but the fraction ejected during early systole is greater than normal; hence, the arterial pulse is of normal volume (the pulse pressure is normal), but the pulse may rise abnormally rapidly.[42] Exaggerated or bounding arterial pulses may be observed in patients with an elevated stroke volume, with sympathetic hyperactivity, and in patients with a rigid, sclerotic aorta. In *aortic regurgitation,* there is a very brisk rate of rise with an increased pulse pressure.

The *Corrigan* or *water-hammer pulse* of aortic regurgitation consists of an abrupt upstroke (percussion wave) followed by rapid collapse later in systole, but no dicrotic notch. Corrigan's pulse reflects a low resistance in the reservoir into which the left ventricle rapidly discharges an abnormally elevated stroke volume, and it can be exaggerated by raising the patient's arm. In *acute* aortic regurgitation, the left ventricle may not be significantly dilated, and premature closure of the mitral valve may occur and limit the volume of aortic reflux; therefore, the aortic diastolic pressure may *not* be very low, the arterial pulse *not* bounding, and the pulse pressure *not* widened despite a serious abnormality of valve function (see p. 1048).

Signs characteristic of severe chronic aortic regurgitation include "pistol-shot" sounds heard over the femoral artery when the stethoscope is placed on it *(Traube's sign);* a systolic murmur heard over the femoral artery when the artery is gradually compressed proximally; a diastolic murmur when the artery is compressed distally *(Duroziez's sign*[37,43]) and Quincke's sign (phasic blanching of the nail bed). Of these, Duroziez's sign is the most predictive. Bounding arterial pulses are also present in patients with patent ductus arteriosus or large arteriovenous fistulas; in hyperkinetic states such as thyrotoxicosis, pregnancy, fever, and anemia; in severe bradycardia; and in arteries proximal to coarctation of the aorta. In *Hill's sign* of aortic regurgitation (or any condition leading to an increased stroke volume, or the hyperkinetic circulatory state) the indirectly recorded systolic pressure in the lower extremities exceeds that in the arms by more than 20 mm Hg. Other signs of increased pulse pressure include *Becker's sign* (visible pulsations of the retinal arterioles) and *Mueller's sign* (pulsating uvula).

In the presence of AV dissociation, when atrial activity is irregularly transmitted to the ventricles, the strength of the peripheral arterial pulse depends on the time interval between atrial and ventricular contractions. In a patient with rapid heart action, the presence of such variations suggests ventricular tachycardia; with an equally rapid rate, an absence of variation of pulse strength suggests a supraventricular mechanism.

BISFERIENS PULSE (Fig. 2–8*C*). A bisferiens pulse is characterized by *two systolic peaks,* the percussion and tidal waves, separated by a distinct midsystolic dip; the peaks may be equal or either may be larger. This type of pulse is detected most readily by palpation of the carotid and less commonly of the brachial arteries. It occurs in conditions in which a large stroke volume is ejected rapidly from the left ventricle[44,45] and is observed most commonly in patients with pure aortic regurgitation or with a combination of aortic regurgitation and stenosis; it may disappear as heart failure supervenes.

A bisferiens pulse also occurs in patients with *hypertrophic obstructive cardiomyopathy,*[46,47] but the bifid nature may only be recorded, not palpated; on palpation there may merely be a rapid upstroke. In these patients the initial prominent percussion wave is associated with rapid ejection of blood into the aorta during early systole, followed by a rapid decline as obstruction becomes manifest in midsystole and by a tidal (reflected) wave. In some patients with hypertrophic cardiomyopathy with no or little obstruction to left ventricular outflow, the arterial pulse is normal or simply hyperkinetic in the basal state, but obstruction and a bisferiens pulse can be elicited by means of the Valsalva maneuver or inhalation of amyl nitrite. Occasionally, a bisferiens pulse is observed in hyperkinetic circulatory states, and very rarely it occurs in normal individuals.

DICROTIC PULSE (Fig. 2–8*E*). Not to be confused with a bisferiens pulse, in which both peaks occur in systole, is a dicrotic pulse, in which the second peak is in diastole immediately after the second heart sound.[39,40] The normally small wave that follows aortic valve closure (i.e., the dicrotic notch) is exaggerated and measures more than 50 per cent of the pulse pressure on direct pressure recordings and in which the dicrotic notch is low (i.e., near the diastolic pressure). A dicrotic wave may be present in normal hypotensive subjects with reduced peripheral resistance, as occurs in fever, and it may be elicited or exaggerated by inhalation alone or the inhalation of amyl nitrite. Rarely, a dicrotic pulse is noted in healthy adolescents or young adults, but it usually occurs in conditions such as cardiac tamponade, severe heart failure, and hypovolemic shock, in which a low stroke volume is ejected into a soft elastic aorta. In these conditions the dicrotic pulse is due to a reduction of the systolic wave with preservation of the incisura. A dicrotic pulse is rarely present when systolic pressure exceeds 130 mm Hg.

PULSUS ALTERNANS (alternating strong and weak pulses) (Fig. 2–9). Mechanical alternans is a sign of severe depression of myocardial function (see p. 455).[48] Although more readily recognized on sphygmomanometry, when the systolic pressure alternates by more than 20 mm Hg the

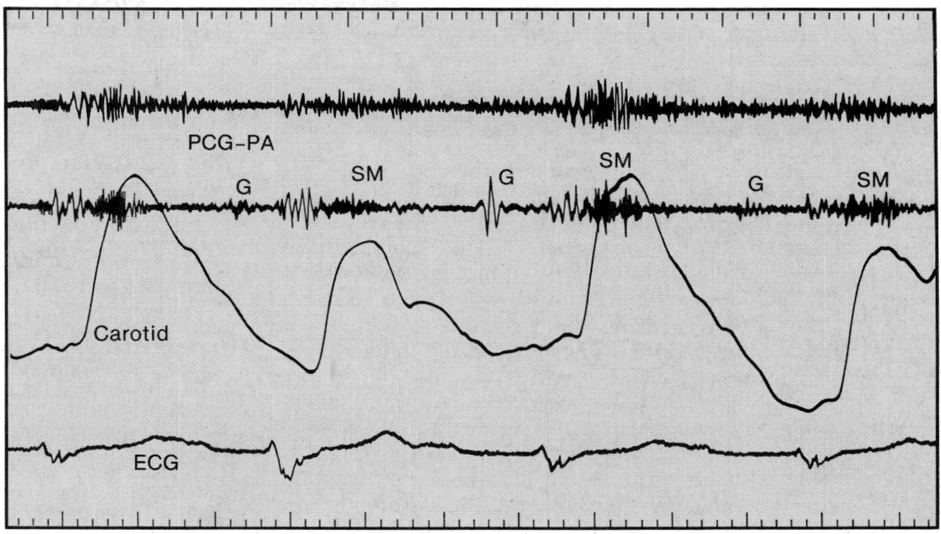

FIGURE 2–9. Pulsus alternans in a man with aortic stenosis and left ventricular failure. The first and third beats are of greater amplitude than the second and fourth beats. The stronger beats are also marked by a louder murmur (SM). The diastolic sound (G) is louder after the second (weak) beat. It is a summation sound caused by merging of S_3 and S_4, resulting from the combined effect of a rapid heart rate and a prolonged P-R interval. (From Craige, E., and Smith, D.: Heart sounds. *In* Braunwald, E. [ed.]: Heart Disease: A Textbook of Cardiovascular Medicine. 3rd ed. Philadelphia, W. B. Saunders Company, 1988, p. 57.)

alternans can be detected by palpation of a peripheral (femoral or brachial) pulse more frequently than by a more central pulse. Palpation should be carried out with light pressure and with the patient's breath held in midexpiration to avoid the superimposition of respiratory variation on the amplitude of the pulse. Pulsus alternans is generally accompanied by alternation in the intensity of the Korotkoff sounds and occasionally by alternation in intensity of the heart sounds. Rarely, pulsus alternans is so marked that the weak beat is not perceived at all. Aortic regurgitation, systemic hypertension, and reducing venous return by administration of nitroglycerin or by tilting the patient into the upright position all exaggerate pulsus alternans and assist in its detection. Pulsus alternans, which is frequently precipitated by a premature ventricular contraction, is characterized by a regular rhythm and must be distinguished from pulsus bigeminus (see below), which is usually irregular.

PULSUS BIGEMINUS. A bigeminal rhythm is caused by the occurrence of premature contractions, usually ventricular, after every other beat and results in alternation of the strength of the pulse, which can be confused with pulsus alternans. However, in contrast to the latter, in which the rhythm is regular, in pulsus bigeminus the weak beat always follows the shorter interval. In normal persons or in patients with fixed obstruction to left ventricular outflow, the compensatory pause following a premature beat is followed by a stronger-than-normal pulse. However, in patients with hypertrophic obstructive cardiomyopathy, the postpremature ventricular contraction beat is weaker than normal because of increased obstruction to left ventricular outflow[49] (see p. 1414).

PULSUS PARADOXUS (see p. 1489). This is an exaggerated reduction in the strength of the arterial pulse during normal inspiration or an exaggerated inspiratory fall in systolic pressure (more than 10 mm Hg during quiet breathing). When marked, i.e., an inspiratory reduction of pressure greater than 20 mm Hg, the paradoxical pulse can be detected by palpation of the brachial arterial pulse; in some instances there is inspiratory disappearance of the pulse. Milder degrees of a paradoxical pulse can be readily detected on sphygmomanometry: the cuff is inflated to suprasystolic levels and is deflated slowly at a rate of about 2 mm Hg per heartbeat; the peak systolic pressure during exhalation is noted. The cuff is then deflated even more slowly, and the pressure is again noted when Korotkoff sounds become audible throughout the respiratory cycle. Normally, the difference between the two pressures should not exceed 10 mm Hg during quiet respiration. (Pulsus alternans can also be detected by this maneuver by noting whether peak systolic pressure or the intensity of the Korotkoff sounds alternates when the breath is held.)

Pulsus paradoxus represents an exaggeration of the normal decline in systolic arterial pressure with inspiration. It results from the reduced left ventricular stroke volume and the transmission of negative intrathoracic pressure to the aorta. It is a frequent, indeed characteristic, finding in patients with cardiac tamponade (see p. 1486), occurs less frequently (in about half) in patients with chronic constrictive pericarditis (see p. 1496), and is also observed in patients with emphysema and bronchial asthma (who have wide respiratory swings of intrapleural pressure),[50] as well as in hypovolemic shock, pulmonary embolus, pregnancy, and extreme obesity. Aortic regurgitation tends to prevent the development of pulsus paradoxus despite the presence of cardiac tamponade. *Reversed* pulsus paradoxus (an inspiratory rise in arterial pressure) may occur in hypertrophic obstructive cardiomyopathy.[51]

THE ARTERIAL PULSE IN VASCULAR DISEASE. Examination of the arterial pulses is of critical importance in the diagnosis of extracardiac obstructive arterial disease. Systematic bilateral palpation of the common carotid, brachial, radial, femoral, popliteal, dorsalis pedis, and posterior tibial vessels, as well as palpation of the abdominal aorta (both above and below the umbilicus), should be part of every examination in patients suspected of having ischemic heart disease.[52] To diminish cold-induced vasoconstriction, peripheral pulses should be palpated after the patient has been in a warm room for at least 20 minutes.[53] Absent or weak peripheral pulses usually signify obstruction. However, the dorsalis pedis and posterior tibial arteries may be absent in approximately 2 per cent of normal persons because they pursue an abnormal course. Arterial bruits should be sought at specific anatomical sites. When the lumen diameter is reduced by approximately 50 per cent, a soft short systolic bruit is heard; as the obstruction becomes more severe, the bruit becomes high-pitched, louder, and longer. With approximately 80 per cent diameter reduction the murmur spills into early diastole, but disappears with very severe stenosis or complete occlusion. Arterial bruits are augmented by elevations of cardiac output (e.g., as occurs in anemia), by poor development of collaterals, and augmented arterial outflow (as occurs in regional exercise).

Auscultation over the spine in the interscapular region in patients with coarctation of the aorta may reveal a systolic or continuous murmur, and a systolic murmur may be heard over the lower abdomen in patients with aortic or iliofemoral obstructions.

INSPECTION

The cardiac examination proper should commence with inspection of the chest, which can best be accomplished with the examiner standing at the side or foot of the bed or examining table. Respirations—their frequency, regularity, and depth—as well as the relative effort required during inspiration and exhalation, should be noted. Simultaneously, one should search for cutaneous abnormalities, such as spider nevi (seen in hepatic cirrhosis and Osler-Weber-Rendu disease). Dilation of veins on the anterior chest wall with caudal flow suggests obstruction of the superior vena cava, whereas cranial flow occurs in patients with obstruction of the inferior vena cava. Precordial prominence is most striking if cardiac enlargement developed before puberty, but may also be present, although to a lesser extent, in patients in whom cardiomegaly developed in adult life, after the period of thoracic growth.[54,55]

A heavy muscular thorax, contrasting with less developed lower extremities, may occur in coarctation of the aorta, in which collateral arteries may be visible in the axillae and along the lateral chest wall. The upper portion of the thorax exhibits symmetrical bulging in children with stiff lungs in whom the inspiratory effort is increased. A "shield chest" is a broad chest in which the angle between the manubrium and the body of the sternum is greater than normal and is associated with widely separated nipples; shield chest is frequently observed in the Turner and Noonan syndromes. Careful note should be made of other deformities of the thoracic cage, such as *kyphoscoliosis*, which may be responsible for cor pulmonale (Chap. 47); *ankylosing spondylitis*, sometimes associated with aortic regurgitation (Chap. 56); and *pectus carinatum* (pigeon chest), which may be associated with Marfan syndrome but does not directly affect cardiovascular function.

Pectus excavatum, a condition in which the sternum is displaced posteriorly, is commonly observed in Marfan syndrome, homocystinuria, Ehlers-Danlos syndrome, Hunter-Hurler syndrome, and a small fraction of patients with mitral valve prolapse. This thoracic deformity rarely compresses the heart or elevates the systemic and pulmonary venous pressures, and the signs of heart disease are more often apparent rather than real. Displacement of the heart into the left thorax, prominence of the pulmonary artery, and a parasternal midsystolic murmur all may falsely suggest the presence of organic heart disease. Pectus excavatum may be associated with palpitations, tachycardia, fatigue, mild dyspnea, and some impairment of cardiac function.[56] Lack of normal thoracic kyphosis, i.e., the *straight back* syndrome,[1] is often associated with expiratory splitting of the second heart sound, a parasternal midsystolic murmur, and prominence of the pulmonary artery on radiography; less severe thoracic kyphosis is frequently associated with mitral valve prolapse.

CARDIOVASCULAR PULSATIONS. These should be looked for on the entire chest but specifically in the regions of the cardiac apex, the left parasternal region, and the third left and second right intercostal spaces. Prominent pulsations in these areas suggest enlargement of the left ventricle, right ventricle, pulmonary artery, and aorta, respectively. A thrusting apex exceeding 2 cm in diameter suggests left ventricular enlargement; systolic retraction of the apex may be visible in constrictive pericarditis. Normally, cardiac pulsations are not visible lateral to the midclavicular line; when present there, they signify cardiac enlargement unless there is thoracic deformity or congenital absence of the pericardium. Shaking of the entire precordium with each heartbeat may occur in patients with severe valvular regurgitation, large left-to-right shunts, especially patent ductus arteriosus, complete AV block, hypertrophic obstructive cardiomyopathy, and various hyperkinetic states (Chap. 15). Aortic aneurysms may produce visible pulsations of one of the sternoclavicular joints of the right anterior thoracic wall.

PALPATION

(Table 2–1)

Pulsations of the heart and great arteries that are transmitted to the chest wall are best appreciated when the examiner is positioned on the right side of a supine patient. In order to palpate the movements of the heart and great arteries, the examiner should use the fingertips or the area just proximal thereto. Precordial movements should be timed by using the simultaneously palpated carotid pulse or auscultated heart sounds.[58–60] The examination should be carried out with the chest completely exposed and ele-

TABLE 2–1 CHARACTERISTICS OF PRECORDIAL MOTION IN VARIOUS CARDIAC ABNORMALITIES

AORTIC REGURGITATION	ATRIAL SEPTAL DEFECT	CONGESTIVE CARDIOMYOPATHY	CORONARY ARTERY DISEASE
Apex impulse hyperdynamic in mild to moderate AR Severe AR: LV dilatation results in sustained impulse which is displaced laterally and downward (especially chronic AR) Systolic retraction medial to PMI Palpable *a* wave may be present	Hyperdynamic parasternal impulse PA impulse may be present RV impulse may be sustained if pulmonary hypertension is present and occasionally with large L to R shunt without elevated PA pressure	Sustained and displaced LV impulse, usually felt over 2 interspaces Palpable *a* wave (S_4) and S_3 common Parasternal lift, midsystolic bulge common	Usually normal at rest unless prior MI Palpable S_4 in left decubitus position Ectopic LV thrust if dyssynergy or LV aneurysm. May have transient abnormalities (e.g., bulge, heave) during acute infarction or attack of angina
HYPERTROPHIC CARDIOMYOPATHY	**MITRAL REGURGITATION**	**MITRAL STENOSIS**	**VALVULAR AORTIC STENOSIS**
Systolic thrill superior, medial to apex impulse Vigorous LV apical impulse, often sustained Large palpable *a* wave, especially in left decubitus position Occasional mid- or late systolic bulge—"triple ripple"	Apical systolic thrill in severe MR Apex impulse hyperdynamic Severe and/or chronic MR: apex is displaced laterally, sustained with amplitude Can have late parasternal impulse with severe MR without pulmonary hypertension Parasternal (RV) heave if significant pulmonary hypertension S_3 visible and palpable if severe MR S_4 palpable with acute onset MR	Small or impalpable apex impulse but S_1 typically palpable Opening snap palpable medial to apex Apical diastolic thrill in left decubitus position Parasternal lift is common; suggests pulmonary hypertension at rest or with effort	Systolic thrill—aortic area, 2 LICS. Or occasionally at apex Sustained and forceful LV apical impulse Little lateral (leftward) displacement of apex unless LV dilatation has occurred Palpable *a* wave (S_4) is common and indicates severe aortic obstruction

AR = aortic regurgitation; LV = left ventricular; PA = pulmonary artery; RV = right ventricular; MI = myocardial infarction; MR = mitral regurgitation; LICS = left intercostal space; L to R = left to right. Reproduced with permission from Abrams, J.: Examination of the precordium. Primary Cardiol. *8*:156–158, 1982.

vated to 30 degrees, both with the patient supine and in the partial left lateral decubitus positions; the latter increases the detection and evaluation of the left ventricular impulse.[2] Rotating the patient into the left lateral decubitus position with the left arm elevated over the head causes the heart to move laterally and increases the palpability of both normal and pathological thrusts of the left ventricle. Obese, muscular, emphysematous, and elderly persons may have weak or undetectable cardiac pulsations in the absence of cardiac abnormality, and thoracic deformities (e.g., kyphoscoliosis, pectus excavatum) can alter the pulsations transmitted to the chest wall. In the course of cardiac palpation, precordial tenderness may be detected; this important finding (see p. 1291) may result from costochondritis (Tzietse's syndrome) and may be an important indication that chest pain is not due to myocardial ischemia.

THE LEFT VENTRICLE. The *apex beat,* also referred to as the cardiac impulse and the apical thrust, is normally produced by left ventricular contraction and is the lowest and most lateral point on the chest at which the cardiac impulse can be appreciated and is normally above the anatomic apex (Fig. 2–10*B*). Although the apex beat may also be the point of maximal impulse (PMI), this is not necessarily the case, because the pulsations produced by other structures, e.g., an enlarged right ventricle, a dilated pulmonary artery, or an aneurysm of the aorta, may be more powerful than the apex beat. Normally the left ventricular impulse is medial and superior to the intersection of the left midclavicular line and the fifth intercostal space and is palpable as a single, brief outward motion. Although it may not be palpable in the supine position in as many as half of all normal subjects more than 50 years of age, the left ventricular impulse can usually be felt in the left lateral decubitus position. Displacement of the apex beat lateral to the midclavicular line or more than 10 cm lateral to the midsternal line is a sensitive but not specific indicator of left ventricular enlargement. However, when the patient is in the left lateral decubitus position a palpable apical impulse that has a diameter of more than 3 cm is an accurate sign of left ventricular enlargement.[61] Thoracic deformities —particularly scoliosis, straight back, and pectus excavatum—can result in the lateral displacement of a normal-sized heart.

The patient should be examined both supine and then in the left lateral decubitus position. The examination should be carried out with both the fingertips and the distal metacarpals. The subxiphoid region, which allows palpation of the right ventricle, should be examined with the tip of the index finger during held inspiration.

The apex cardiogram, which reflects the movement of the chest wall, represents the pulsation of the entire left ventricle. Its contour differs from what is perceived on palpation of the apex or what is recorded by the kinetocardiogram, a device in which the motion of specific points on the chest wall is recorded relative to a fixed point in space[62] and which therefore presents a more faithful graphic registration of the movements of the palpating finger on the chest wall.

SYSTOLIC MOTION. During isovolumetric contraction, the heart normally rotates counterclockwise (as one faces the patient), and the lower anterior portion of the left ventricle strikes the anterior chest wall, causing a brief outward motion followed by medial retraction of the adjacent chest wall during ejection (Fig. 2–11). The segment of the left ventricle responsible for the apex beat is usually medial to the actual cardiac apex identified on radiological or angiographic examination. For timing purposes it is useful to correlate pulsations while simultaneously listening to heart sounds; a convenient way to do this is to correlate the observed motion of the stethoscope, placed lightly at the apex, with the auscultatory events.

The peak outward motion of the left ventricular impulse is brief and occurs simultaneously with, or just after, aortic valve opening; then the left ventricular apex moves inward. In asthenic persons, in patients with mild left ventricular enlargement, and in subjects with a normal left ventricle but an augmented stroke volume, as occurs in anxiety and other hyperkinetic states, and in mitral or aortic regurgitation, the cardiac impulse may be overactive but with a normal contour; i.e., the outward thrust during systole is exaggerated in amplitude, but it is not sustained during ejection.

HYPERTROPHY AND DILATATION. With moderate or severe left ventricular concentric hypertrophy, the outward systolic thrust persists throughout ejection, often lasting up to the second heart sound (Fig. 2–11), and this motion is accompanied by retraction of the left parasternal region. This rocking motion can often be appreciated by placing the index finger of one hand on the apex beat and that of the other hand in the parasternal region and by observing the simultaneous outward motion of the former with retraction of the latter. The left ventricular heave or lift, which is more prominent in concentric hypertrophy than in left ventricular dilatation without volume overload, is characterized by a sustained outward movement of an area that is larger than the normal apex; i.e., it is more than 2 to 3 cm in diameter. In patients with left ventricular enlargement the systolic impulse is displaced laterally and downward into the sixth or seventh interspaces. In patients with ischemic heart disease a sustained apex beat is usually associated with a reduced ejection fraction.[63]

In patients with volume overload and/or sympathetic stimulation, the left ventricular impulse is *hyperkinetic,* i.e., it is brisker and larger than normal. It is hypokinetic in patients with reduced stroke volume, especially in acute myocardial infarction or dilated cardiomyopathy.

LEFT VENTRICULAR ANEURYSM. This produces a larger-than-normal area of pulsation of the left ventricular apex. Alternatively, it may produce a sustained systolic bulge several centimeters superior to the left ventricular impulse. In left ventricular pressure overload with normal ventricular function, the left ventricular impulse is prolonged and forceful. In patients with *left ventricular dyskinesia,* as occurs in acute myocardial ischemia following myocardial infarction, or left ventricular aneurysm, there may be two distinct impulses separated from each other by several centimeters; alternatively, a mid- or late systolic bulge may be palpated. In *mitral stenosis* there may be a brief prominent apical tap owing to an accentuated first sound, which must be distinguished from the apical thrust of the left ventricle.

OTHER CONDITIONS. A double systolic outward thrust of the left ventricle is characteristic of patients with hypertrophic obstructive cardiomyopathy (Fig. 2–12) who also often exhibit a typical presystolic cardiac expansion, thus resulting in three separate outward movements of the chest wall during each cardiac cycle.[46] In *aortic regurgitation* the apex exhibits a prominent outward thrust that may be followed by medial systolic retraction of the anterior chest wall as a consequence of the large stroke volume that evacuates the thorax during systole.

Constrictive pericarditis (as well as nonconstricting adherent pericarditis) is characterized by systolic retraction of the chest, particularly of the ribs in the left axilla (Broadbent's sign). This inward movement results from interference with the descent of the base of the heart and the compensatory exaggerated motion of the free wall of the left ventricle during ventricular ejection.[64] When left ventricular filling is very rapid during early diastole, outward movement of the chest wall may be particularly prominent and mistaken for systole, but it is usually accompanied by a third heart sound (see p. 35). A hypokinetic apical impulse is associated with a variety of low cardiac output states, including those secondary to hypovolemia, constrictive pericarditis, and pericardial effusion.

Diastolic Motion. The outward motion of the apex characteristic of rapid left ventricular diastolic filling is most readily palpated with the patient in the left lateral decubitus position and in full exhalation. The outward motion is accentuated when the inflow of blood into the left ventricle is accelerated, as occurs, for example, in mitral regurgitation, when the volume of the left ventricle is increased or its function is impaired.[55] This motion is the mechanical equivalent of and occurs simultaneously with a third heart sound. Prominent early diastolic left ventricular filling in constrictive pericarditis may be palpable.

When the atrial contribution to ventricular filling is augmented, as occurs in patients with reduced left ventricular compliance associated with concentric left ventricular hypertrophy, myocardial ischemia, and myocardial fibrosis, a presystolic pulsation (usually accompanying a fourth heart sound) is palpable, resulting in a double outward movement of the left ventricular impulse. This presystolic expansion is most readily discernible during exhalation, when the patient is in the left lateral decubitus position, and it can be confirmed by detecting the motion of the stethoscope placed over the left ventricular impulse or by observing the motion of an X mark over the left ventricular impulse. Presystolic expansion of the left ventricle can be enhanced by sustained handgrip, and is usually associated with marked elevation of left ventricular end-diastolic (rather than early diastolic) pressure. In contrast to prominence of early diastolic filling, in patients without ischemic

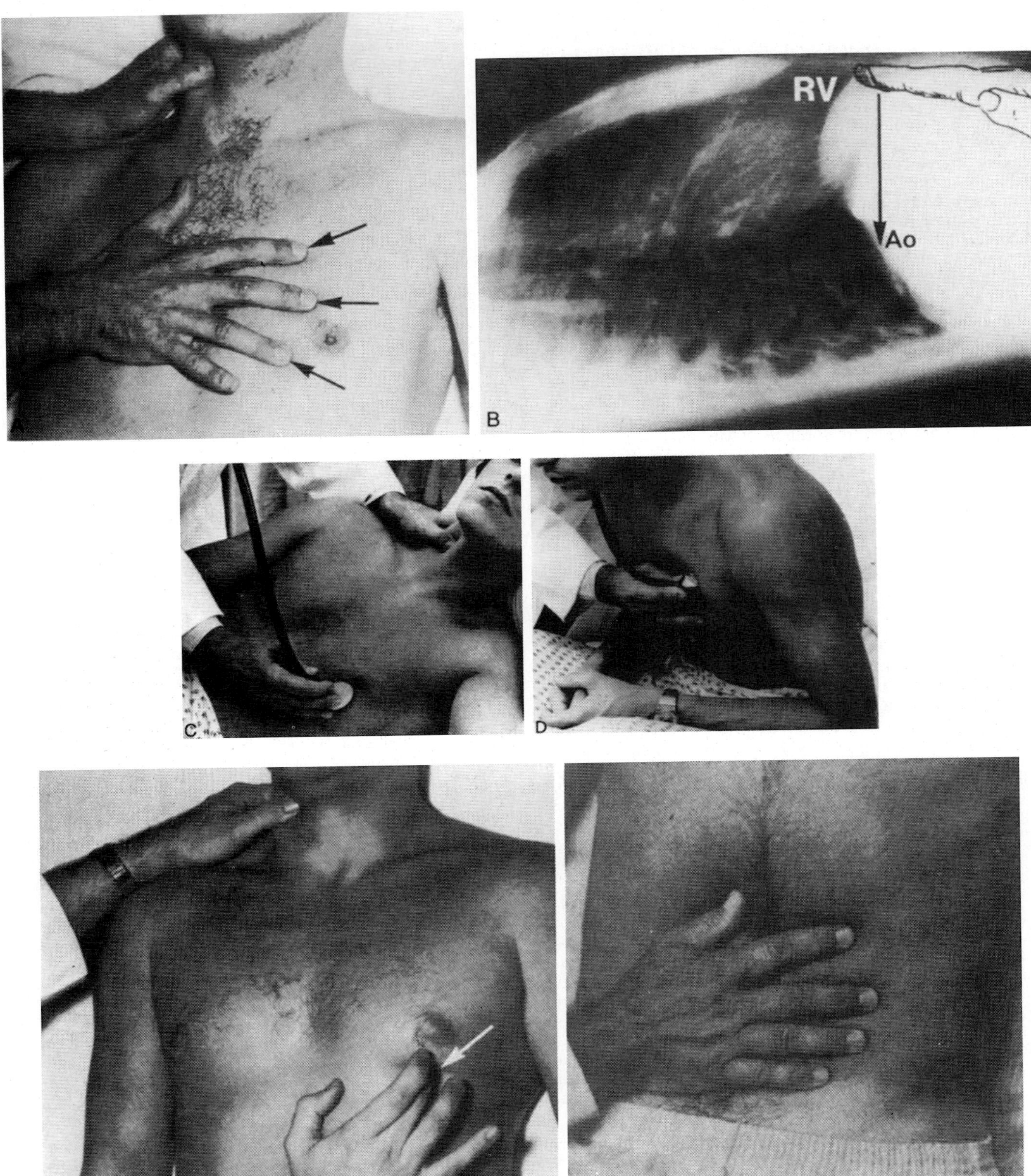

FIGURE 2–10. *A,* Palpation of the anterior wall of the right ventricle by applying the tips of three fingers in the third, fourth, and fifth interspaces, left sternal edge (arrows), during full held exhalation. Patient is supine with the trunk elevated 30 degrees. *B,* Subxiphoid palpation of the inferior wall of the right ventricle (RV) with the relative position of the abdominal aorta (Ao) shown by the arrow. *C,* The bell of the stethoscope is applied to the cardiac apex while the patient lies in a partial left lateral decubitus position. The thumb of the examiner's free left hand is used to palpate the carotid artery for timing purposes. *D,* The soft, high-frequency early diastolic murmur of aortic regurgitation or pulmonary hypertensive regurgitation is best elicited by applying the stethoscopic diaphragm very firmly to the mid-left sternal edge. The patient leans forward with breath held in full exhalation. *E,* Palpation of the left ventricular impulse with a fingertip (arrow). The patient's trunk is 30 degrees above the horizontal. The examiner's right thumb palpates the carotid pulse for timing purposes. *F,* Palpation of the liver. The patient is supine with knees flexed to relax the abdomen. The flat of the examiner's right hand is placed on the right upper quadrant just below the expected inferior margin of the liver; the left hand is applied diametrically opposite. (From Perloff, J. K.: Physical Examination of the Heart and Circulation. 2nd ed. Philadelphia, W. B. Saunders Company, 1990.)

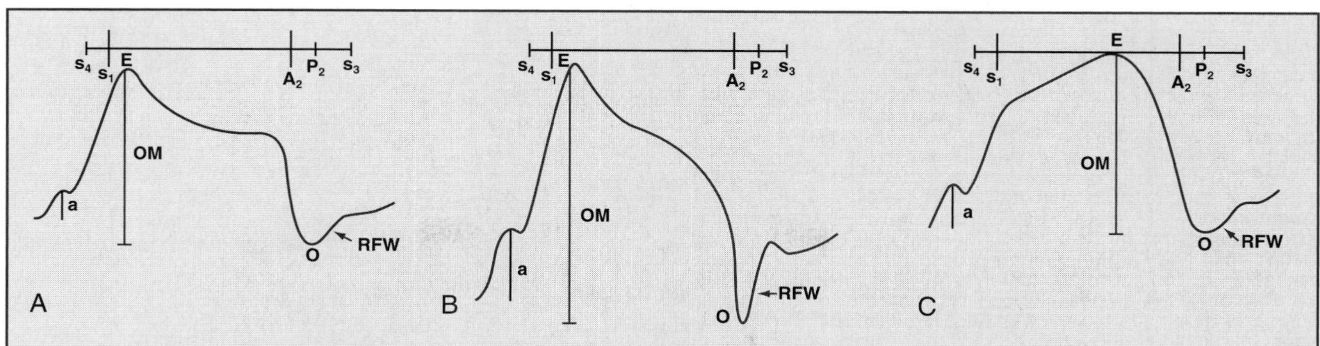

FIGURE 2–11. Schematic diagrams of normal hyperdynamic and sustained left ventricular impulse. Heart sounds are also illustrated. *A,* Normal apex cardiogram. The *a* wave, related to ventricular filling during atrial systole, usually does not exceed 15 per cent of the total height. E point usually coincides with the beginning of left ventricular ejection. Following E point, there is a gradual inward movement, explaining the brief duration of the normal left ventricular impulse. The O point approximately coincides with the mitral valve opening. *B,* Hyperdynamic left ventricular impulse is usually seen in left ventricular volume overloaded conditions such as primary mitral regurgitation and aortic regurgitation. Left ventricular ejection fraction is usually normal. Increased amplitude of *a* wave may be associated with palpable *a* waves, which are usually associated with increased left ventricular end-diastolic pressure. Accentuated rapid filling wave is frequently associated with audible S_3. *C,* Sustained left ventricular impulse (outward movement continued during ejection phase) is usually seen in the presence of decreased ejection fraction or when the left ventricle is markedly hypertrophied (S_4 = atrial sound; S_1 = first heart sound; A_2, = aortic component of the second heart sound; *a* = *a* wave; *E* = E point beginning of ejection; *OM* = outward movement; *O* = O point; *RFW* = rapid filling wave.) (From Chatterjee, K.: Bedside evaluation of the heart: The physical examination. *In* Chatterjee, K., et al. [eds.]: Cardiology: An Illustrated Text/Reference. Philadelphia, J. B. Lippincott, 1991, pp. 3.11–3.51.)

heart disease presystolic expansion is usually associated with normal or almost normal left ventricular function.[58] In patients with ischemic heart disease presystolic pulsation is usually associated with left ventricular dysfunction.[63] Presystolic expansion of the right ventricle occurs in right

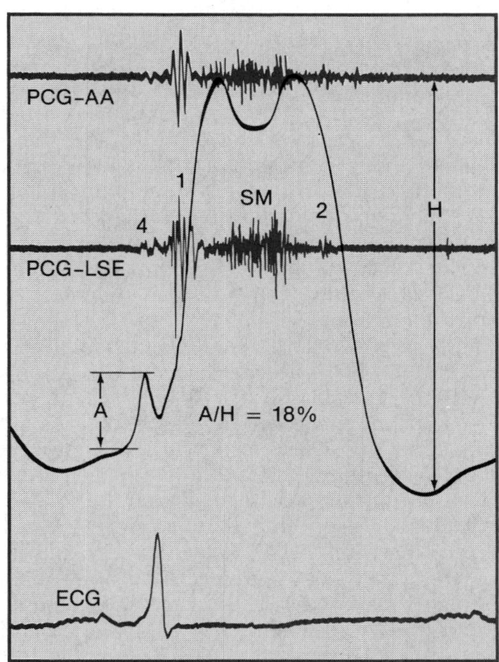

FIGURE 2–12. Apex cardiogram in hypertrophic obstructive cardiomyopathy. The *a* wave (A) is exaggerated in height, being 18 per cent of the entire amplitude of the apexcardiogram (H), and has an unusually rapid upstroke that culminates in a sharp peak, coinciding with the fourth heart sound (4). The systolic phase of the apexcardiogram has a bifid appearance with a prominent late systolic hump. The saddle-shaped decline in midsystole coincides in time with the systolic murmur and carotid pulse deformity, which, in turn, are related to the obstruction occasioned by the systolic anterior motion of the mitral valve. (From Craige, E., and Smith, D.: Heart sounds. *In* Braunwald, E. [ed.]: Heart Disease: A Textbook of Cardiovascular Medicine. 3rd ed. Philadelphia, W. B. Saunders Company, 1988, p. 59.)

ventricular hypertrophy and pulmonary hypertension and may be appreciated by subxiphoid palpation of the right ventricle during inspiration.

RIGHT VENTRICLE. Normally, neither this chamber, nor its motion, is palpable. A palpable anterior systolic movement (replacing systolic retraction) in the left parasternal region (Fig. 2–10*A*), best felt by the proximal palm or fingertips, and with the patient supine, usually represents *right ventricular enlargement* or hypertrophy.[65] In the absence of associated left ventricular enlargement, the right ventricular impulse is accompanied by reciprocal systolic retraction of the apex. In patients with pulmonary emphysema, even an enlarged right ventricle is not readily palpable at the left sternal edge but is better appreciated in the subxiphoid region. Exaggerated motion of the entire parasternal area, i.e., a hyperdynamic impulse with normal contour, usually reflects increased right ventricular contractility due to augmented stroke volume, as occurs in patients with atrial septal defect or tricuspid regurgitation, whereas a sustained left parasternal outward thrust reflects right ventricular hypertrophy due to pressure overload, as occurs in pulmonary hypertension or pulmonic stenosis. With marked right ventricular enlargement, this chamber occupies the apex because the left ventricle is displaced posteriorly.

When both ventricles are enlarged, both the left parasternal and the apical areas may rise with systole, but an area of systolic retraction between them can usually be appreciated. In patients with emphysema or obesity, an enlarged right ventricle is detected most readily in the subxiphoid region by palpating the epigastrium and pointing the fingers upward. With marked isolated right ventricular enlargement, the right ventricle may form the cardiac apex, and should not be confused with those of left or biventricular enlargement. When acute myocardial ischemia or myocardial infarction causes dyskinetic movement of the ventricular septum, there may be a transient left parasternal impulse not caused by right ventricular enlargement.

PULMONARY ARTERY. *Pulmonary hypertension* and/or increased pulmonary blood flow frequently produce a prominent systolic pulsation of the pulmonary trunk in the second intercostal space just to the left of the sternum. This pulsation is often associated with a prominent left parasternal impulse, reflecting right ventricular enlargement, or hypertrophy and a palpable shock synchronous with the second heart sound, reflecting forceful closure of the pulmonic valve.

LEFT ATRIUM. An enlarged left atrium or a large posterior left ventricular aneurysm can make right ventricular pulsations more prominent by displacing the right ventricle anteriorly against the left parasternal area, and in severe mitral regurgitation an expanding left atrium may be responsible for marked left parasternal movement, even in the absence of right ventricular hypertrophy. The systolic bulging of the left atrium, which is transmitted through the right ventricle, commences and terminates *after* the left ventricular thrust. Movement imparted by the systolic expansion of the left atrium can be appreciated by placing the index finger of one hand at the left ventricular apex and the index finger of the other in the left parasternal region in the third intercostal space; the movement of the latter finger begins and ends slightly later than that of the former. Although this difference in timing may be difficult to appreciate on palpation, particularly when the heart rate is rapid, recordings of chest wall motion in severe chronic mitral regurgitation demonstrate a delayed fall in the left lower precordium compared with the cardiac apex. Outward movement of the chest wall that is more marked to the right than to the left of the sternum is usually due to aneurysm of the aorta or to marked enlargement of the right atrium in the presence of tricuspid regurgitation. Occasionally, a giant left atrium is palpable in the right hemithorax. The left atrial appendage is sometimes visible and palpable in the third left intercostal space.

AORTA. Enlargement or aneurysm of the ascending aorta or aortic arch may cause visible or palpable systolic pulsations of the right or left sternoclavicular joint; and may also cause a systolic impulse in the suprasternal notch or the first or second right intercostal space.[1]

PALPABLE SOUNDS. Valve closure, if abnormally forceful or if normal in a patient with a thin chest wall, can be appreciated as a tapping sensation. A palpable sound occurs most prominently in the second left intercostal space in patients with pulmonary hypertension (pulmonic valve closure), in the second right intercostal space in patients with systemic hypertension (aortic valve closure), and at the cardiac apex in patients with mitral stenosis (mitral valve closure). Occasionally, in congenital aortic stenosis, aortic ejection sounds can be palpated at the cardiac apex; ejection sounds originating in a dilated aorta or pulmonary artery can sometimes be felt at the base of the heart.[61] Prominent third and fourth heart sounds are often palpable as diastolic movements at the cardiac apex. In patients with mitral stenosis an opening snap may be palpated at the apex.

THRILLS. The flat of the hand or the fingertips usually best appreciate thrills, vibratory sensations which are palpable manifestations of loud, harsh murmurs *having low-frequency to medium components.*[66] Because the vibrations must be quite intense before they are felt, far more information can be obtained from the auscultatory than from the palpatory features of heart murmurs. High-pitched murmurs such as those produced by valvular regurgitation, even when loud, are not usually associated with thrills.

PERCUSSION. Palpation is far more helpful than is percussion in determining cardiac size. However, in the absence of an apical beat, as in patients with pericardial effusion, or in some patients with dilated cardiomyopathy, heart failure, and marked displacement of a hypokinetic apical beat, the left border of the heart can be outlined by means of percussion. Also, percussion of dullness in the right lower parasternal area may, in some instances, aid in the detection of a greatly enlarged right atrium. Percussion aids materially in determining visceral situs, i.e., in ascertaining the side on which the heart, stomach, and liver are located. When the heart is in the right chest but the abdominal viscera are located normally, congenital heart disease is usually present. When both the heart and abdominal viscera are in the opposite side of the chest (situs inversus), congenital heart disease is uncommon.

CARDIAC AUSCULTATION

Principles and Technique

The modern binaural stethoscope is a well-crafted, airtight instrument with earpieces selected for comfort, with metal tubing joined to single flexible 12-inch-long, thick-walled rubber tubing (internal diameter of ⅛ inch) and with dual chest pieces—diaphragm for high frequencies, bell for low or lower frequencies—designed so that the examiner can readily switch from one chest piece to the other.[67,68] When the bell is applied with just enough pressure to form a skin seal, low frequencies are accentuated; when the bell is pressed firmly, the stretched skin becomes a diaphragm, damping low frequencies. Variable pressure with the bell provides a range of frequencies from low to medium.

Cardiac auscultation is best accomplished in a quiet room with the patient comfortable and the chest fully exposed.

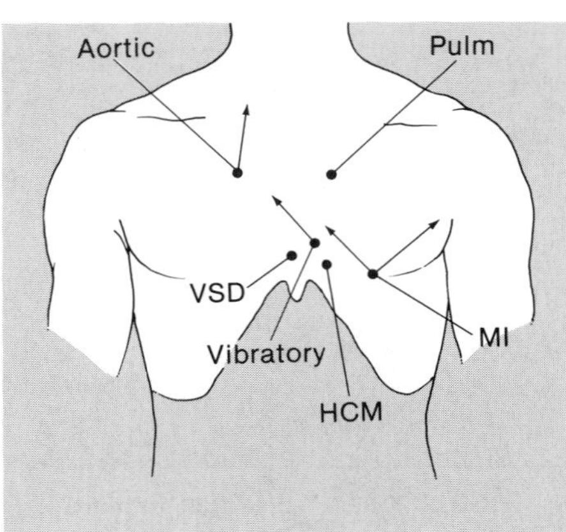

FIGURE 2–13. Maximal intensity and radiation of six isolated systolic murmurs. HCM = hypertrophic cardiomyopathy; MI = mitral incompetence; Pulm = pulmonary; VSD = ventricular septal defect. (From Barlow, J. B.: Perspectives on the Mitral Valve. Philadelphia, F. A. Davis, 1987, p. 140.)

Percussion should precede auscultation in order to establish visceral and cardiac situs, so that auscultation can be carried out with confidence in the topographic anatomy of the heart. Terms such as "mitral area," "tricuspid area," "pulmonary area," and "aortic area" should be avoided because they assume situs solitus without ventricular inversion and with normally related great arteries. The topographic areas for auscultation (Fig. 2–13), irrespective of cardiac situs, are best designated by descriptive terms—cardiac apex, left and right sternal borders interspace by interspace, and subxiphoid. For patients in situs solitus with a left thoracic heart, auscultation should begin at the cardiac apex (best identified in the left lateral decubitus) and contiguous lower left sternal edge (inflow), proceeding interspace by interspace up the left sternal border to the left base and then to the right base (outflow). This topographic sequence permits the examiner to think physiologically by using a pattern that conforms to the direction of blood flow—inflow/outflow. In addition to the routine sites described above, the stethoscope should be applied regularly to certain nonprecordial thoracic areas, especially the axillae, the back, the anterior chest on the opposite side, and above the clavicles. In patients with increased anteroposterior chest dimensions (emphysema), auscultation is often best achieved by applying the stethoscope in the epigastrium (subxiphoid).

Information derived from auscultation benefits not only from knowledge of the cardiac situs, but also from identification of palpable and visible movements of the ventricles. During auscultation, the examiner is generally on the patient's right; three positions are routinely employed: left lateral decubitus (assuming left thoracic heart), supine, and sitting. Auscultation should begin by applying the stethoscope to the cardiac apex with the patient in the left lateral decubitus position (Fig. 2–14). If tachycardia makes identification of the first heart sound difficult, timing can be established, with few exceptions, by simultaneous palpation of the carotid artery with the thumb of the free left hand (Fig. 2–14). Once the first heart sound is identified, analysis then proceeds by systematic, methodical, sequential attention to early, mid, and late systole, the second heart sound, then early, mid, and late diastole (presystole), returning to the first heart sound. When auscultation at the apex has been completed, the patient is turned into the supine position. Each topographic area—lower to upper left sternal edge interspace by interspace and then the right base—is interrogated using the same systematic sequence of analysis.

Assessment of pitch or frequency ranging from low to moderately high can be achieved by variable pressure of

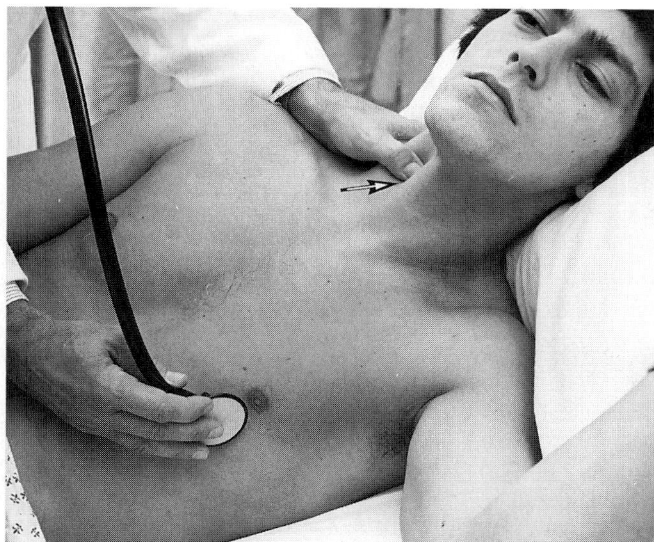

FIGURE 2–14. The bell of the stethoscope is applied to the cardiac apex while the patient lies in a left lateral decubitus position. The thumb of the examiner's free left hand palpates the carotid artery *(arrow)* for timing purposes.

the stethoscopic bell, whereas for high frequencies, the diaphragm should be employed. It is practical to begin by using the stethoscopic bell with varying pressure at the apex and lower left sternal edge, changing to the diaphragm when the base is reached. Low frequencies are best heard by applying the bell just lightly enough to achieve a skin seal. High frequency events are best elicited with firm pressure of the diaphragm, often with the patient sitting, leaning forward in full held exhalation.

The Heart Sounds

Heart sounds are relatively brief, discrete auditory vibrations of varying intensity (loudness), frequency (pitch), and quality (timbre). The first heart sound identifies the onset of ventricular systole, and the second heart sound identifies the onset of diastole. These two auscultatory events establish a framework within which other heart sounds and murmurs can be placed and timed.[1]

The basic heart sounds are the first, second, third, and fourth sounds (Fig. 2–15*A*). Each of these events can be normal or abnormal. Other heart sounds are, with few exceptions, abnormal, either intrinsically so or iatrogenic (e.g., prosthetic valve sounds, pacemaker sounds). A heart sound should first be characterized by a simple descriptive term that identifies where in the cardiac cycle the sound occurs. Accordingly, heart sounds within the framework established by the first and second sounds are designated as "early systolic, mid-systolic, late systolic," and "early diastolic, mid-diastolic, late diastolic (presystolic)" (Fig. 2–15*B*).[2] The next step is to draw conclusions based upon what a sound so identified represents. An *early systolic* sound might be an ejection sound (aortic or pulmonary) or an aortic prosthetic sound. Mid- and late systolic sounds are typified by the click(s) of mitral valve prolapse but occasionally are "remnants" of pericardial rubs. *Early diastolic* sounds are represented by opening snaps (usually mitral), early third heart sounds (constrictive pericarditis, less commonly mitral regurgitation), the opening of a mechanical inflow prosthesis, or the abrupt seating of a pedunculated mobile atrial myxoma ("tumor plop"). *Mid-diastolic* sounds are generally third heart sounds or summation sounds (synchronous occurrence of third and fourth heart sounds). *Late diastolic* or *presystolic* sounds are almost always fourth heart sounds, rarely pacemaker sounds.

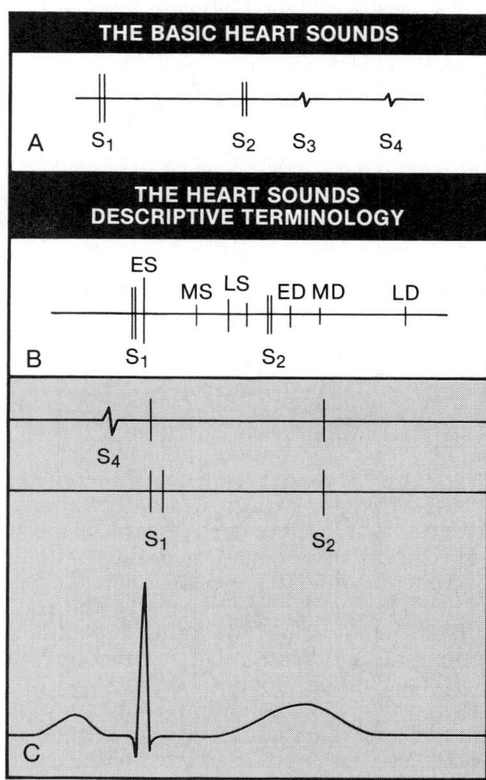

FIGURE 2–15. *A,* The basic heart sounds consist of the first heart sound (S_1), the second heart sound (S_2), the third heart sound (S_3), and the fourth heart sound (S_4). *B,* Heart sounds within the auscultatory framework established by the first heart sound (S_1) and the second heart sound (S_2). The additional heart sounds are designated descriptively as early systolic (ES), midsystolic (MS), late systolic (LS), early diastolic (ED), mid-diastolic (MD), and late diastolic (LD) or presystolic. *C,* Upper tracing illustrates a low-frequency fourth heart sound (S_4), and the lower tracing illustrates a split first heart sound (S_1), the two components of which are of the same quality.

The First Heart Sound

The first heart sound consists of two major components (Fig. 2–15*C*). The initial component is most prominent at the cardiac apex when the apex is occupied by the left ventricle.[69] The second component, if present, is normally confined to the lower left sternal edge, is less commonly heard at the apex, and is seldom heard at the base. The first major component is associated with closure of the mitral valve and coincides with abrupt arrest of leaflet motion when the cusps—especially the larger and more mobile anterior mitral cusp—reach their fully closed positions (maximal cephalad systolic excursion into the left atrium). The origin of the second major component of the first heart sound has been debated but is generally assigned to closure of the tricuspid valve based upon an analogous line of reasoning.[70] Opening of the semilunar valves with ejection of blood into the aortic root or pulmonary trunk usually produces no audible sound in the normal heart, although phonocardiograms sometimes record a low-amplitude sound following the mitral and tricuspid components and coinciding with the maximal opening excursion of the aortic cusps.[1] In complete right bundle branch block the first heart sound is widely split as a result of delay of the tricuspid component.[71] In complete left bundle branch block, the first heart sound is single as a result of delay of the mitral component.[72]

Because the two major audible components of the first heart sound are believed to originate in the closing movements of the atrioventricular valves, the quality of the two components (pitch) is similar (Fig. 2–15*C*). When the first heart sound is split, its first component is normally the

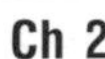

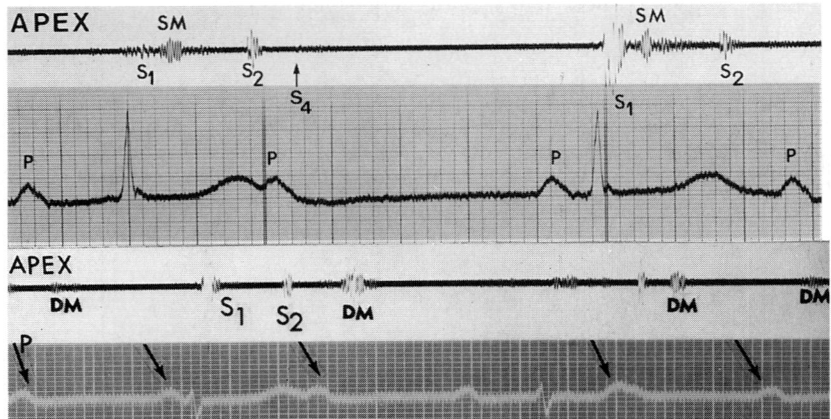

FIGURE 2–16. *Upper tracing,* Phonocardiogram and electrocardiogram (lead 2) from a 12-year-old girl with congenital complete heart block. The first heart sound (S_1) varies from soft (long P-R interval) to loud (short P-R interval). There is a grade 2/6 vibratory midsystolic murmur (SM). A soft fourth heart sound (arrow) follows the second P wave. *Lower tracing,* Phonocardiogram and electrocardiogram from a 15-year-old boy with congenital complete heart block. Arrows point to independent P waves. The first heart sound (S_1) varies from loud to soft depending upon the P-R interval. The short diastolic murmurs (DM) are especially prominent when atrial contraction (P wave) coincides with and reinforces the rapid filling phase (shortly after the T wave).

louder. The softer second component is confined to the lower left sternal edge but may also be heard at the apex. Only the louder first component is heard at the base. The intensity of the first heard sound, particularly its first major audible component, depends chiefly upon the position of the bellies of the mitral leaflets, especially the anterior leaflet, at the time the left ventricle begins to contract and less upon the rate of left ventricular contraction.[73] The first heart sound is therefore loudest when the onset of left ventricular systole finds the mitral leaflets maximally recessed into the left ventricular cavity, as in the presence of a rapid heart rate, a short P-R interval[74] (Fig. 2–16), short cycle lengths in atrial fibrillation, or mitral stenosis with a mobile anterior leaflet. In Ebstein's anomaly of the tricuspid valve, the first heart sound is widely split (delayed right ventricular activation), and the second component is loud provided the anterior tricuspid leaflet is large and mobile.[75]

Early Systolic Sounds

Aortic or pulmonary ejection sounds are the most common early systolic sounds.[76] "Ejection sound" is preferred to the term ejection "click," with the latter designation best reserved for the mid- to late systolic clicks of mitral valve prolapse (see p. 1032). Ejection sounds coincide with the fully opened position of the relevant semilunar valve, as in congenital aortic valve stenosis (Fig. 2–17*A*) or bicuspid aortic valve in the left side of the heart, or pulmonary valve stenosis (Fig. 2–18) in the right side of the heart.[75,77] Ejection sounds are relatively high frequency events, and depending upon intensity, have a pitch similar to that of the two major components of the first heart sound. An ejection sound originating in the aortic valve (congenital aortic stenosis or bicuspid aortic valve) or in the pulmonary valve (congenital pulmonary valve stenosis) indicates that the valve is mobile because the ejection sound is caused by abrupt cephalad doming (Fig. 2–17*B*).[77] Less certain is the origin of an ejection sound within a dilated arterial trunk that is guarded by a normal semilunar valve. Origin of the sound is assigned either to opening movement of the leaflets that resonate in the arterial trunk or to the wall of the dilated great artery. Aortic ejection sounds do not vary with respiration except those that originate in the large biventricular aorta of Fallot's tetralogy with pulmonary atresia or truncus arteriosus (Fig. 2–18).[75] The mechanism responsible for the respiratory variation in this setting is unclear.

Pulmonary ejection sounds often selectively and distinctively decrease in intensity during normal inspiration (Fig. 2–19*A*). The mechanism responsible for respiratory variation of a pulmonary ejection sound is most convincing in the setting of typical pulmonary valve stenosis.[78] An inspiratory increase in right atrial contractile force is transmitted into the right ventricle and onto the ventricular surface of the mobile stenotic valve, moving its cusps upward *before* the onset of ventricular contraction. Cephalad excursion of the valve during ventricular systole is therefore diminished, accounting for the inspiratory decrease in intensity of the ejection sound. This mechanism cannot apply to the respiratory variation of a pulmonary ejection sound asso-

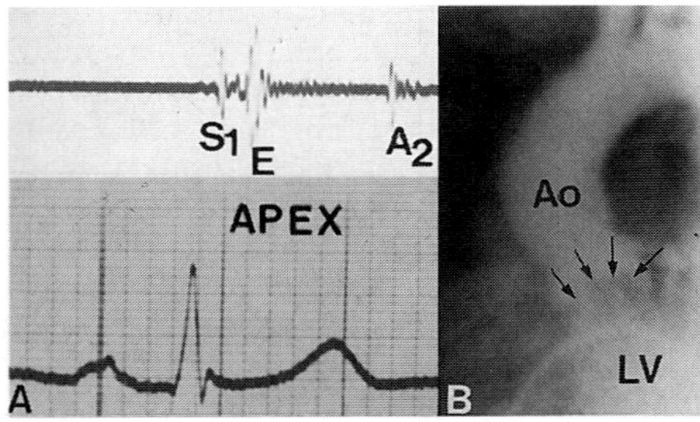

FIGURE 2–17. *A,* Phonocardiogram over the left ventricular impulse in a patient with mild congenital bicuspid aortic valve stenosis. The aortic ejection sound (E) is louder than the first heart sound (S_1). A_2 = Aortic component of the second heart sound. *B,* Left ventriculogram (LV) in another patient with congenital aortic valve stenosis. The cephalad systolic doming of the stenotic valve (arrows) produces the ejection sound.

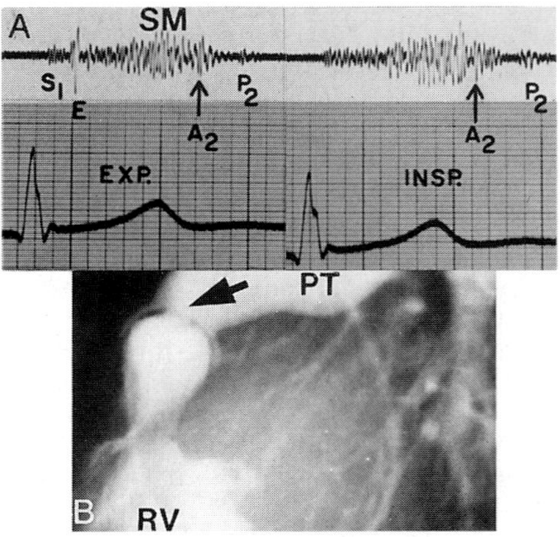

FIGURE 2–18. *A,* Phonocardiogram in the second left intercostal space of a patient with congenital pulmonary valve stenosis. The ejection sound (E) is obvious during exhalation (EXP) but disappears entirely during casual inhalation (INSP). The pulmonary component of the second heart sound (P_2) is delayed and soft. SM = Systolic murmur; S_1 = first heart sound. *B,* Right ventriculogram (RV) in another patient with pulmonary valve stenosis. The cephalad systolic doming of the mobile stenotic valve (arrow) produces the pulmonary ejection sound. There is post-stenotic dilatation of the pulmonary trunk (PT).

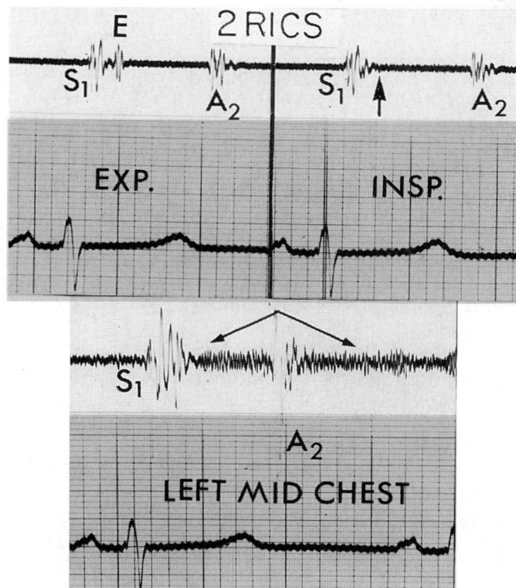

FIGURE 2–19. Phonocardiograms from an 11-year-girl with Fallot's tetralogy and pulmonary atresia. The upper tracing from the second right intercostal space (2RICS) shows an aortic ejection sound (E) that is prominent during exhalation (EXP) but absent during inspiration (INSP). The lower tracing from the left midchest shows a continuous murmur of aortopulmonary collaterals. The second heart sound is necessarily single and is represented by the aortic component (A_2). S_1 = First heart sound.

ciated with a dilated hypertensive pulmonary trunk (Fig. 2–20).[2,75]

Early systolic sounds accompany mechanical prostheses in the aortic location, especially the Starr-Edwards ball-in-cage valve, less so with a tilting disc valve such as the Björk-Shiley. Early systolic sounds do not occur with bioprosthetic valves (tissue valves) in either the aortic or pulmonary location.

Mid- to Late Systolic Sounds

Far and away the most common mid- to late systolic sound(s) are associated with mitral valve prolapse[2,79,80] (see p. 1029). The term "click" is appropriate because these mid- to late systolic sounds are of relatively high frequency and often, but not invariably, "clicking." Mid- to late systolic clicks of mitral valve prolapse coincide with maximal systolic excursion of a prolapsed leaflet (or scallop(s) of the posterior leaflet) into the left atrium and are ascribed to sudden tensing of the redundant leaflet(s) and elongated chordae tendinae. Variability epitomizes mitral systolic clicks, which from time-to-time may be replaced by a cluster of discrete late systolic "crackles." Physical or pharmacological interventions that *reduce* left ventricular volume, such as the Valsalva maneuver, or a change in position from squatting to standing (Fig. 2–21) causes the click(s) to occur earlier in systole.[79–82] Conversely, physical or pharmacological interventions that *increase* left ventricular volume, such as squatting (Fig. 2–21) or sustained hand grip, serve to delay the timing of the click(s). Multiple clicks are thought to arise from asynchronous tensing of different

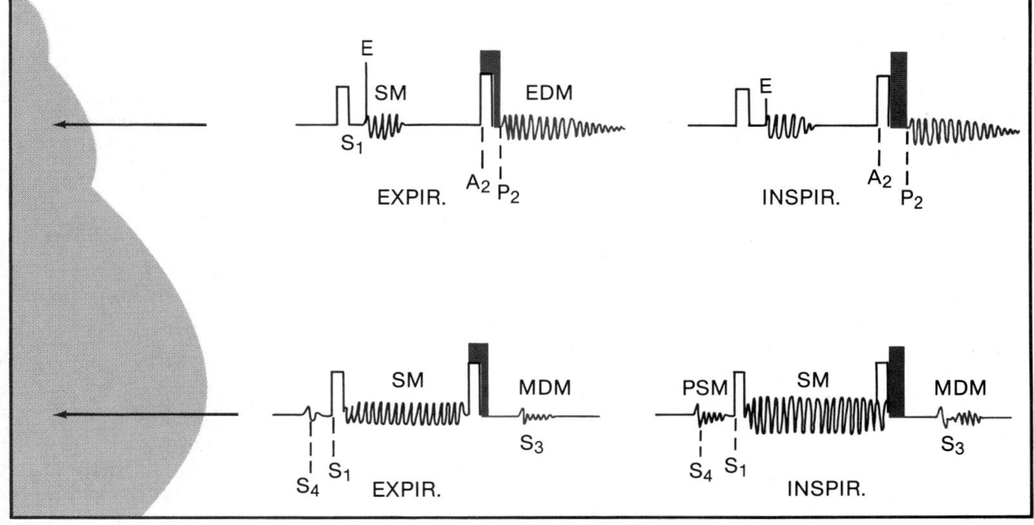

FIGURE 2–20. Composite of the principal auscultatory and phonocardiographic manifestations of pulmonary hypertension. (From Perloff, J. K.: Auscultatory and phonocardiographic manifestations of pulmonary hypertension. Prog. Cardiovasc. Dis. *9*:303, 1967.)

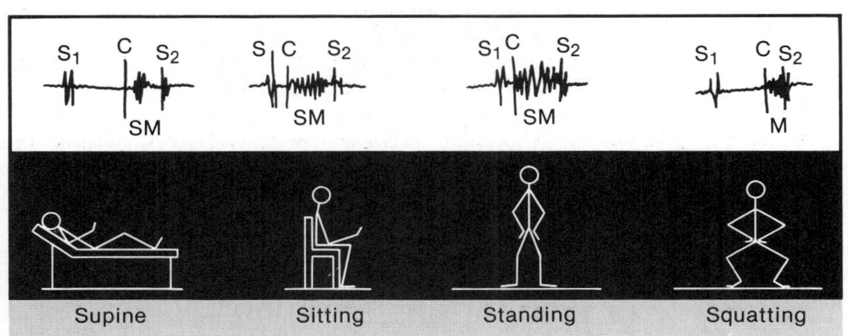

FIGURE 2–21. Postural maneuvers that affect the click(s) and late systolic murmur (SM) of mitral valve prolapse. A change from supine to sitting or standing causes the click to become earlier and the murmur longer although softer. Conversely, squatting delays the timing of the click, and the murmur becomes shorter but louder. (From Devereux, R., Perloff, J. K., Reichek, N., and Josephson, M.: Mitral valve prolapse. Circulation *54*:3, 1976, by permission of the American Heart Association.)

portions of redundant mitral leaflets, especially the triscalloped posterior leaflet.

On rare occasions, a pericardial friction rub leaves in its wake mid- to late systolic sounds—remnants of rubs—that persist after disappearance of the systolic phase of the rub. Carl Potain, in 1894, commented upon "small, short clicking sounds, well localized and such that one can scarcely attribute them to anything except the tensing of a pericardial adhesion."[83]

The Second Heart Sound

Respiratory splitting of the second heart sound was described by Potain in 1866,[84] and Leatham called the second heart sound the "key to auscultation of the heart."[85] The first component of the second heart sound is designated "aortic" and the second "pulmonary."[86,87] Each component coincides with the dicrotic incisura of its great arterial pressure pulse (Fig. 2–22).[69] Inspiratory splitting of the second heart sound is due chiefly to a delay in the pulmonary component, less to earlier timing of the aortic component.[88] During inspiration, the pulmonary arterial dicrotic incisura moves away from the descending limb of the right ventricular pressure pulse because of an inspiratory increase in capacitance of the pulmonary vascular bed, delaying the pulmonary component of the second heart sound.[89] Exhalation has the opposite effect. The earlier inspiratory timing of the aortic component of the second heart sound is attributed to a transient reduction in left ventricular volume coupled with unchanged impedance (capacitance) in the systemic vascular bed. Normal respiratory variations in the timing of the second heart sound are therefore ascribed principally to the variations in impedance characteristics (capacitance) of the pulmonary vascular bed, not to an inspiratory increase in right ventricular volume as originally proposed.[69,85] When an increase in capacitance of the pulmonary bed is lost because of a rise in pulmonary vascular resistance, inspiratory splitting of the second heart sound narrows and, if present at all, reflects an increase in right ventricular ejection time and/or earlier timing of the aortic component.[2]

The frequency compositions of the aortic and pulmonary components of the second heart sound are similar, but their normal amplitudes differ appreciably, reflecting the differences in systemic (aortic) and pulmonary arterial closing pressures. Splitting of the second heart sound is most readily identified in the second left intercostal space, because the softer pulmonary component is normally confined to that site, whereas the louder aortic component is heard at the base, sternal edge, and apex.[2,86]

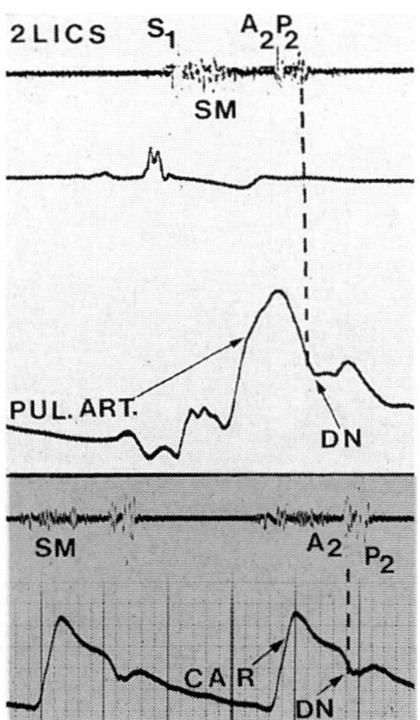

FIGURE 2–22. Tracings from a 28-year-old woman with an uncomplicated ostium secundum atrial septal defect. In the second left interspace (2LICS), the pulmonary component (P_2) of a widely split second heart sound is synchronous with the dicrotic notch (DN) of the pulmonary arterial pressure pulse. (S_1 = First heart sound; SM = midsystolic murmur). In the lower tracing, the aortic component (A_2) of the widely split second heart sound is synchronous with the dicrotic notch of the carotid arterial pulse (CAR).

TABLE 2–2 CAUSES OF SPLITTING OF THE SECOND HEART SOUND

NORMAL SPLITTING
DELAYED PULMONIC CLOSURE
Delayed electrical activation of the right ventricle
Complete RBBB (proximal type)
Left ventricular paced beats
Left ventricular ectopic beats
Prolonged right ventricular mechanical systole
Acute massive pulmonary embolus
Pulmonary hypertension with right heart failure
Pulmonic stenosis with intact septum (moderate to severe)
Decreased impedance of the pulmonary vascular bed (increased hang-out)
Normotensive atrial septal defect
Idiopathic dilatation of the pulmonary artery
Pulmonic stenosis (mild)
Atrial septal defect, postoperative (70%)
EARLY AORTIC CLOSURE
Shortened left ventricular mechanical systole (LVET)
Mitral regurgitation
Ventricular septal defect
REVERSED SPLITTING
DELAYED AORTIC CLOSURE
Delayed electrical activation of the left ventricle
Complete LBBB (proximal type)
Right ventricular paced beats
Right ventricular ectopic beats
Prolonged left ventricular mechanical systole
Complete LBBB (peripheral type)
Left ventricular outflow tract obstruction
Hypertensive cardiovascular disease
Arteriosclerotic heart disease
Chronic ischemic heart disease
Angina pectoris
Decreased impedance of the systemic vascular bed (increased hang-out)
Poststenotic dilatation of the aorta secondary to aortic stenosis or insufficiency
Patent ductus arteriosus
EARLY PULMONIC CLOSURE
Early electrical activation of the right ventricle
Wolff-Parkinson-White syndrome, type B

RBBB = right bundle-branch block; LVET = left ventricular ejection time; LBBB = left bundle-branch block.

Modified from Shaver, J. A., and O'Toole, J. D.: The second heart sound: Newer concepts. Parts 1 and 2. Mod. Concepts Cardiovasc. Dis. *46:*7 and 13, 1977.

ABNORMAL SPLITTING OF THE SECOND HEART SOUND. Three general categories of abnormal splitting are recognized: (1) persistently single, (2) persistently split (fixed or nonfixed), and (3) paradoxically split (reversed). When the second heart sound remains single throughout the respiratory cycle, one component is absent or the two components are persistently synchronous. The most common cause of a single second heart sound is inaudibility of the *pulmonary* component in older adults with increased anteroposterior chest dimensions. In the setting of congenital heart disease, a single second heart sound due to absence of the pulmonary component is a feature of pulmonary atresia (Fig. 2–18), severe pulmonary valve stenosis, dysplastic pulmonary valve or complete transposition of the great arteries (pulmonary component inaudible because of the posterior position of the pulmonary trunk).[75] Conversely, a single second heart sound due to inaudibility of the *aortic* component occurs when the aortic valve is immobile (severe calcific aortic stenosis) or atretic (aortic atresia). A single second sound due to persistent synchrony of its two components is a feature of Eisenmenger's complex, in which the aortic and pulmonary arterial dicrotic incisurae are virtually identical in timing.[75]

Both components of the second heart sound are sometimes inaudible at *all* precordial sites. This is likely to be so in older adults in whom fibrocalcific changes limit mobility of the aortic valve, whereas the pulmonary component is inaudible because of a large anteroposterior chest dimension (see above).

A single semilunar valve, as in truncus arteriosus, does not necessarily generate what is judged on auscultation to be a single second heart sound. Instead, the second sound may be perceived as "split" because of asynchronous closure of the unequal cusps of a quadricuspid valve.[75] In systemic or pulmonary hypertension, the duration of a single loud second heart sound may be sufficiently prolonged and slurred (reduplicated) to encourage the mistaken impression of splitting.

Persistent Splitting of the Second Heart Sound. This term applies when the two components remain audible (or recordable) during both inspiration and exhalation. Persistent splitting may be due to a delay in the pulmonary component, as in simple complete right bundle branch block[69] or to early timing of the aortic component, as occasionally occurs in mitral regurgitation.[90] Normal directional changes in the interval of the split (greater with inspiration, lesser with exhalation) in the presence of persistent audibility of both components defines the split as *persistent* but not *fixed.*

Fixed Splitting of the Second Heart Sound. This term applies when the interval between the aortic and pulmonary components is not only wide and persistent, but remains unchanged during the respiratory cycle.[69] Fixed splitting is an auscultatory hallmark of uncomplicated ostium secundum atrial septal defect. The aortic and pulmonary components are widely separated during exhalation and exhibit little or no change in the degree of splitting during inspiration or with the Valsalva maneuver. The *wide* splitting is caused by a delay in the pulmonary component because a marked increase in pulmonary vascular capacitance prolongs the interval between the descending limbs of the pulmonary arterial and right ventricular pressure pulses ("hangout"), and therefore delays the pulmonary incisura and the pulmonary component of the second heart sound (Fig. 2–22). The capacitance (impedance) of the pulmonary bed is appreciably increased, so there is little or no additional increase during inspiration and little or no inspiratory delay in the pulmonary component of the second sound. Phasic changes in systemic venous return during respiration in atrial septal defect are associated with reciprocal changes in the volume of the left-to-right shunt, minimizing respiratory variations in right ventricular filling. The net effect is the characteristic wide fixed splitting of the two components of the second heart sound.[75]

Paradoxical Splitting of the Second Heart Sound. This term refers to a reversed sequence of semilunar valve closure, the pulmonary component (P_2) preceding the aortic component (A_2).[69] Common causes of paradoxical splitting are complete left bundle branch block[91] or a right ventricular pacemaker, both of which are associated with initial activation of the right side of the ventricular septum, and delayed activation of the left ventricle owing to transseptal (right-to-left) depolarization.[92] When the second heart sound splits paradoxically, its two components separate during *exhalation* and become single (synchronous) during *inspiration.* Inspiratory synchrony is achieved as the two components fuse because of a delay in the pulmonary component, less to earlier timing of the aortic component.

Abnormal Loudness (Intensity) of the Two Components of the Second Heart Sound. Assessment of intensity requires that both components be compared when heard simultaneously at the same site. The relative softness of the normal pulmonary component is responsible for its localization in the second left intercostal space, whereas the relative loudness of the normal aortic component accounts for its audibility at all precordial sites (see earlier).[2] An increase in intensity of the *aortic* component of the second sound occurs with systemic hypertension. The intensity of the aortic component also increases when the aorta is closer to the anterior chest wall owing to root dilatation or transposition of the great arteries, or when an anterior pulmonary trunk is small or absent, as in pulmonary atresia (Fig. 2–18).[75]

A loud *pulmonary* component of the second heart sound (Figs. 2–20 and 2–23*A*) is a feature of pulmonary hypertension, and the loudness is enhanced by dilatation of a hypertensive pulmonary trunk. Graham Steell, in describing the auscultatory signs of pulmonary hypertension, remarked that ". . . extreme accentuation of the pulmonary second sound is always present, the closure of the pulmonary semilunar valve being generally perceptible to the hand placed over the pulmonary area, as a sharp thud."[93] An accentuated pulmonary component can be transmitted to the mid or lower left sternal edge, and when very loud, throughout the precordium to the apex and right base. A loud pulmonary component in the second left interspace may obscure a closely preceding aortic component. In this eventuality, auscultation at other precordial sites often identifies the transmitted but attenuated pulmonary component and allows detection of splitting. A moderate increase in loudness of the pulmonary component of the second heart sound sometimes occurs in the absence of pulmonary hypertension when the pulmonary trunk is dilated, as with idiopathic dilatation or ostium secundum atrial septal defect, or when there is a decrease in anteroposterior chest dimensions (loss of thoracic kyphosis) that places the pulmonary trunk closer to the chest wall.[94]

Early Diastolic Sounds

The opening snap of rheumatic mitral stenosis is the best known early diastolic sound (Fig. 2–23*B*). The term "snap" was introduced in 1908 by W. S. Thayer as the English equivalent to the "claquement d'ouverture" of Rouchès.[95] The diagnostic value derived from the pitch, loudness, and

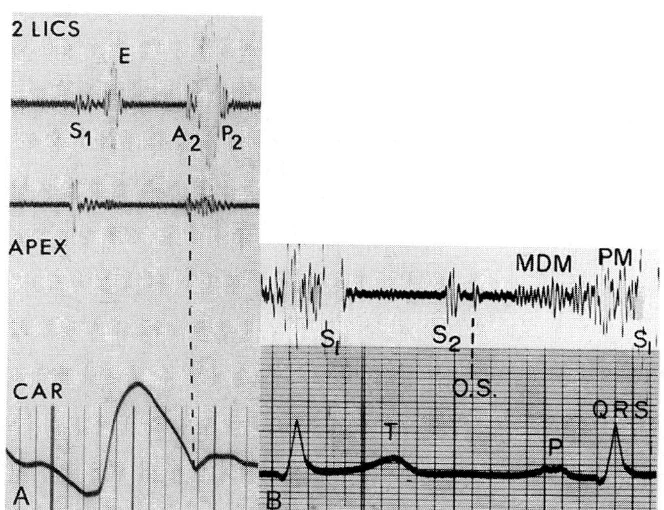

FIGURE 2–23. *A,* Tracings from a 32-year-old woman with an ostium secundum atrial septal defect, pulmonary hypertension, and a small right-to-left shunt. In the second left intercostal space (2LICS), the first heart sound is followed by a prominent pulmonary ejection sound (E). The second sound remains split. The pulmonary component (P_2) is very loud and is transmitted to the apex. (CAR = Carotid pulse). *B,* Phonocardiogram recorded in the left lateral decubitus position over the left ventricular impulse in a patient with pure rheumatic mitral stenosis. The first heart sound (S_1) is loud. The second heart sound (S_2) is followed by an opening snap (OS). There is a mid-diastolic murmur (MDM). The prominent presystolic murmur (PM) goes up to the subsequent loud first heart sound.

timing of the opening snap in the assessment of rheumatic mitral stenosis was established by Wood in his classic monograph, *An Appreciation of Mitral Stenosis*.[96] An audible opening snap indicates that the mitral valve is mobile, at least its longer anterior leaflet.[97] The snap is generated when superior systolic bowing of the anterior mitral leaflet is rapidly reversed toward the left ventricle in early diastole in response to high left atrial pressure. The mechanism of the opening snap is therefore a corollary to the loud first heart sound (Fig. 2–23*B*), which is generated by abrupt superior systolic displacement of a mobile anterior mitral leaflet that was recessed into the left ventricle during diastole by high left atrial pressure until the onset of left ventricular isovolumetric contraction (see earlier). The designation "snap" is appropriate because of the relatively high frequency of the sound.

The timing of the opening snap (OS) relative to the aortic component of the second heart sound (A_2) has important physiological meaning.[2] A short A_2-OS interval generally reflects the high left atrial pressure of *severe* mitral stenosis. However, in older subjects with systolic hypertension, mitral stenosis of appreciable severity can occur without a short A_2-OS interval because the elevated left ventricular systolic pressure takes longer to fall below the left atrial pressure. In the presence of atrial fibrillation, the A_2-OS interval varies inversely with cycle length, because (all else being equal) the higher the left atrial pressure (short cycle length), the earlier the stenotic valve opens and vice versa.

Early diastolic sounds are not confined to the opening snap of rheumatic mitral stenosis. In 1842, Dominic Corrigan, in a presentation to the Pathological Society of Dublin, described a "very loud bruit de frappement" in a patient with chronic constrictive pericarditis.[98] In French, "frapper" means "to knock," implying that Corrigan's "bruit de frappement" was what has come to be known as the pericardial "knock" of chronic constrictive pericarditis.[99] The term "knock" has also been applied to an early diastolic sound in pure severe mitral regurgitation with reduced left ventricular compliance. Both Corrigan's "pericardial knock" and the "knock" of mitral regurgitation are rapid filling sounds that are early and loud because a high-pressure atrium rapidly decompresses across an unobstructed AV valve into a recipient ventricle whose compliance is impaired.

Early diastolic sounds are sometimes caused by atrial myxomas.[100] The generation of such a sound, called a tumor "plop," requires a mobile myxoma attached to the atrial septum by a long stalk. The "plop" is believed to result from abrupt diastolic seating of the tumor within the right or left AV orifice.[100]

An early diastolic sound is generated by the opening movement of a mechanical prosthesis in the mitral location. This opening sound is especially prominent with a ball-in-cage prosthesis (Starr-Edwards) and less prominent with a tilting disc prosthesis (Björk-Shiley).

Mid-Diastolic and Late Diastolic (Presystolic) Sounds

Mid-diastolic sounds are, for all practical purposes, either normal or abnormal third heart sounds, and most if not all late diastolic or presystolic sounds are fourth heart sounds (Fig. 2–24). Each sound coincides with its relevant diastolic filling phase.[101] In sinus rhythm, the ventricles receive blood during two filling phases (Fig. 2–24). The first phase occurs when ventricular pressure drops sufficiently to allow the AV valve to open; blood then flows from atrium into ventricle. This flow coincides with the y descent of the atrial pressure pulse (Fig. 2–24) and is designated the "rapid filling phase," accounting for about 80 per cent of normal ventricular filling. The rapid filling phase is not a passive event in which the recipient ventricle merely expands in response to augmented inflow volume. Rather, ventricular relaxation is an active, complex, energy-dependent process.

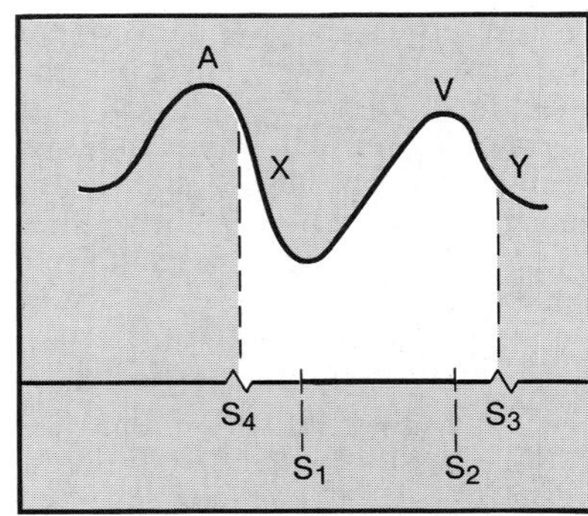

FIGURE 2–24. Atrial pressure pulse showing the *a* wave and *x* descent, and the *v* wave and *y* descent. The fourth heart sound (S_4) coincides with the phase of ventricular filling following atrial contraction. The third heart sound (S_3) coincides with the y descent (the phase of rapid ventricular filling). S_1 = First heart sound; S_2 = second heart sound.

The sound generated during the rapid filling phase is called the third heart sound (Fig. 2–24).[102] The second filling phase—diastasis—is variable in duration, usually accounting for less than 5 per cent of ventricular filling. The third phase of diastolic filling is in response to atrial contraction, which accounts for about 15 per cent of normal ventricular filling. The sound generated during the atrial filling phase is called the fourth heart sound (Fig. 2–24). Third and fourth heart sounds occur *within* the recipient ventricle as that chamber receives blood. Potain in 1876 attributed the third heart sound to sudden cessation of distention of the ventricle in early diastole, and he attributed the fourth heart sound to ". . . the abruptness with which the dilatation of the ventricle takes place during the presystolic period, a period which corresponds to the contraction of the auricle."[103] On both counts, he was not far from the mark.

The addition of either a third or a fourth heart sound to the cardiac cycle produces a *triple* rhythm. If both third *and* fourth heart sounds are present, a *quadruple* rhythm is produced. When diastole is short or the PR interval long, third and fourth heart sounds occur synchronously to form a summation sound.[2]

Children and young adults often have normal (physiological) *third* heart sounds but do not have normal fourth heart sounds.[104] Normal third heart sounds sometimes persist beyond age 40 years, especially in women.[105] After that age, however, especially in men, the third heart sound is likely to be abnormal.[106] Fourth heart sounds are sometimes heard in healthy older adults without clinical evidence of heart disease, particularly after exercise.[107] Such observations have led to the conclusion, still debated, that these fourth heart sounds are normal for age.

Because a fourth heart sound requires active atrial contribution to ventricular filling, the sound disappears when coordinated atrial contraction ceases, as in atrial fibrillation. When the atria and ventricles contract independently as in complete heart block (Fig. 2–16), fourth heart sounds or summation sounds occur randomly in diastole because the relationship between the P wave and the QRS of the electrocardiogram is random. Third and fourth heart sounds are events of ventricular filling, so obstruction of an AV valve, by impeding ventricular inflow, removes one of the prime preconditions for the generation of these filling sounds. Accordingly, the presence of a third or fourth heart sound implies an unobstructed (or relatively unobstructed) AV orifice on the side of the heart in which the sound originates. *Right ventricular* third or fourth heart sounds often respond selectively and distinctively to respiration, becoming more prominent during inspiration.[2] The inspiratory increase in right atrial flow is converted into an inspiratory augmentation of both mid-diastolic and presystolic filling.

Third and fourth heart sounds, either normal or abnormal, are relatively low-frequency events that vary considerably in intensity (loudness), that originate in either the left or right ventricle, and that are best elicited when the bell of the stethoscope is applied with just enough pressure to provide a skin seal. Left ventricular third and fourth heart sounds should be sought over the left ventricular impulse so identified with the patient in the left lateral decubitus position. Right ventricular third and fourth heart sounds should be sought over the right ventricular impulse (lower left sternal edge, occasionally subxiphoid) with the patient supine. An understanding of these simple principles sets the stage for bedside detection. The same principles can be used with advantage to distinguish a fourth heart sound preceding a single first heart sound from splitting of the two components of the first heart sound (Fig. 2–15*C*). The two components of the first heart sound are similar in frequency (pitch) although not in intensity (loudness), but differ in pitch from a preceding fourth heart sound. Selective pressure with the bell of the stethoscope enhances these distinctions.

Audibility of third heart sounds is improved by isotonic exercise that augments venous return and mid-diastolic AV flow. A few sit-ups usually suffice to produce the desired increase in venous return and acceleration in heart rate that increase the rate and volume of AV flow. Venous return can be increased by simple passive raising of both legs with the patient supine. The heart rate is also transiently increased by vigorous coughing. Left ventricular fourth heart sounds, especially in patients with ischemic heart disease, can be induced or augmented when resistance to left ventricular discharge is increased by sustained handgrip (isometric exercise, see later).

In the presence of sinus tachycardia, atrial contraction may coincide with the rapid filling phase, making it impossible to determine whether a given filling sound is a third heart sound, a fourth heart sound, or a summation sound. Carotid sinus massage transiently slows the heart rate, so the diastolic sound or sounds can be assigned their proper timing in the cardiac cycle.[2]

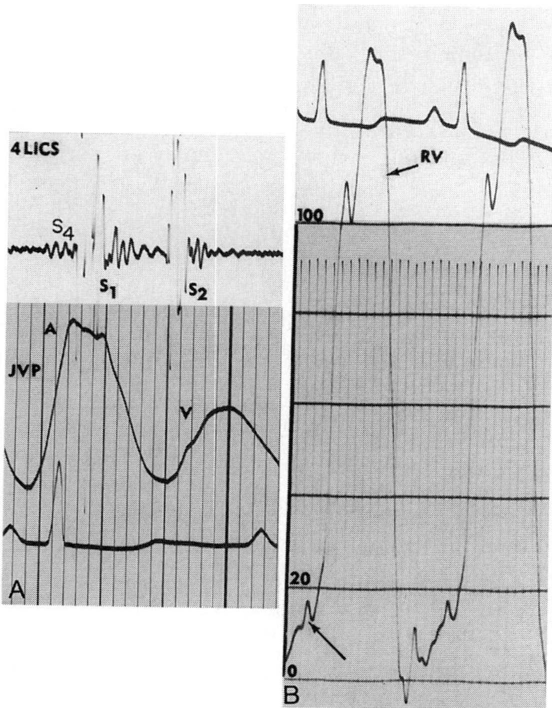

FIGURE 2–25. Tracings from an 18-year-old man with primary pulmonary hypertension. *A*, The phonocardiogram from the fourth left intercostal space (4LICS) shows a fourth heart sound (S_4). The jugular venous pulse (JVP) exhibits a prominent *a* wave. (S_1 = First heart sound; S_2 = second heart sound). *B*, The increased force of right atrial contraction, reflected in the large jugular venous *a* wave, results in presystolic distention (arrow) of the right ventricle (RV).

CAUSES OF THIRD AND FOURTH SOUNDS. The normal *third* heart sound is believed to be caused by sudden limitation of longitudinal expansion of the left ventricular wall during early diastolic filling.[108–111] The majority of *abnormal* third heart sounds are generated by altered physical properties of the recipient ventricle and/or an increase in the rate and volume of AV flow during the rapid filling phase of the cardiac cycle.[112] Abnormal *fourth* heart sounds occur when augmented atrial contraction generates presystolic ventricular distention (an increase in end-diastolic segment length) so that the recipient chamber can contract with greater force.[113,114] Typical substrates are the left ventricular hypertrophy of aortic stenosis or systemic hypertension in the left side of the heart,[115] or the right ventricular hypertrophy of pulmonary stenosis or pulmonary hypertension in the right side of the heart (Fig. 2–25).[113] Fourth heart sounds are also common in ischemic heart disease and are almost universal during angina pectoris or acute myocardial infarction because the atrial "booster pump" is needed to assist the relatively stiff ischemic ventricle.

A variation on the theme is the presystolic pacemaker sound.[116] A pacemaker electrode in the apex of the right ventricle may produce a presystolic sound that is relatively high-pitched and clicking and therefore different in pitch from a fourth heart sound. The presystolic pacemaker sound is believed to be extracardiac, resulting from contraction of chest wall muscle following spread of the electrical impulse from the pacemaker site.[116,117]

HEART MURMURS

According to O. H. Perry Pepper, *murmur* is a Latin word with probable onomatopoetic origins.[118] A cardiovascular murmur is a series of auditory vibrations that are more prolonged than a sound and are characterized according to intensity (loudness), frequency (pitch), configuration (shape), quality, duration, direction of radiation, and timing in the cardiac cycle. When these features are established, the stage is set for diagnostic conclusions that can be drawn from a murmur of a given description.

Intensity or loudness is graded from one to six, based upon the original recommendations of Samuel A. Levine in 1933.[119] A grade 1 murmur is so faint that it is heard only with special effort. A grade 2 is soft but readily detected; a grade 3 murmur is prominent but not loud; a grade 4 murmur is loud (and usually palpable); a grade 5 murmur is very loud. A grade 6 murmur is loud enough to be heard with the stethoscope just removed from contact with the chest wall. Frequency or pitch varies from high to low. The configuration or shape of a systolic murmur is best characterized as crescendo, decrescendo, crescendo-decrescendo (diamond-shaped), plateau (even), or variable (uneven). The duration of a murmur varies from short to long, with all gradations in between. A loud murmur radiates from its site of maximal intensity, and the direction of radiation is sometimes diagnostically useful. The timing of murmurs within the cardiac cycle is the basis for the following classification.

There are three categories of murmurs—systolic, diastolic, and continuous. A *systolic* murmur begins with or after the first heart sound and ends at or before the subsequent second heart sound on its side of origin. A *diastolic* murmur begins with or after the second heart sound and ends before the subsequent first heart sound. A *continuous* murmur begins in systole and continues without interruption through the timing of the second heart sound into all or part of diastole. The following classification of murmurs is based upon their timing relative to the first and second heart sounds.

Systolic Murmurs

Systolic murmurs are classified according to their time of onset and termination as midsystolic, holosystolic, early systolic, or late systolic (Fig. 2–26). A midsystolic murmur begins after the first heart sound and ends perceptibly before the second sound. The termination of a systolic murmur must be related to the relevant component of the second heart sound (Fig. 2–26). Accordingly, midsystolic murmurs originating in the *left* side of the heart end before the *aortic* component of the second heart sound; midsystolic murmurs originating in the *right* side of the heart end before the *pulmonary* component of the second sound. A *holosystolic* murmur begins with the first heart sound, occupies all of systole, and ends with the second heart sound on its side of origin. Holosystolic murmurs originating in the *left* side of the heart end with the *aortic* component of the second heart sound, and holosystolic murmurs originating in the *right* side of the heart end with the *pulmonary* component of the second sound.

The term "regurgitant systolic murmur," originally applied to murmurs that occupied all of systole,[69] has fallen out of use because "regurgitation" can be accompanied by holosystolic, midsystolic, early systolic, or late systolic murmurs.[2] Similarly, the term "ejection systolic murmur," originally applied to midsystolic murmurs, should be discarded, because midsystolic murmurs are not necessarily due to "ejection."[2]

MIDSYSTOLIC MURMURS. Midsystolic murmurs occur in five settings: (1) obstruction to ventricular outflow, (2) dilatation of the aortic root or pulmonary trunk, (3) accelerated systolic flow into the aorta or pulmonary trunk, (4) innocent (normal) midsystolic murmurs, and (5) some forms of mitral regurgitation. The physiological mechanism of *outflow* midsystolic murmurs reflects the pattern of phasic flow across the left or right ventricular outflow tract as originally described by Leatham (Fig. 2–27).[69] Isovolumetric contraction generates the first heart sound. Ventricular pressure rises, the semilunar valve opens, flow commences, and the murmur begins. As flow proceeds, the murmur increases in crescendo; as flow decreases, the murmur decreases in decrescendo. The murmur ends before ventricular pressure drops below the pressure in the central great artery, at which time the aortic and pulmonary valves close, generating the aortic and pulmonary components of the second heart sound.

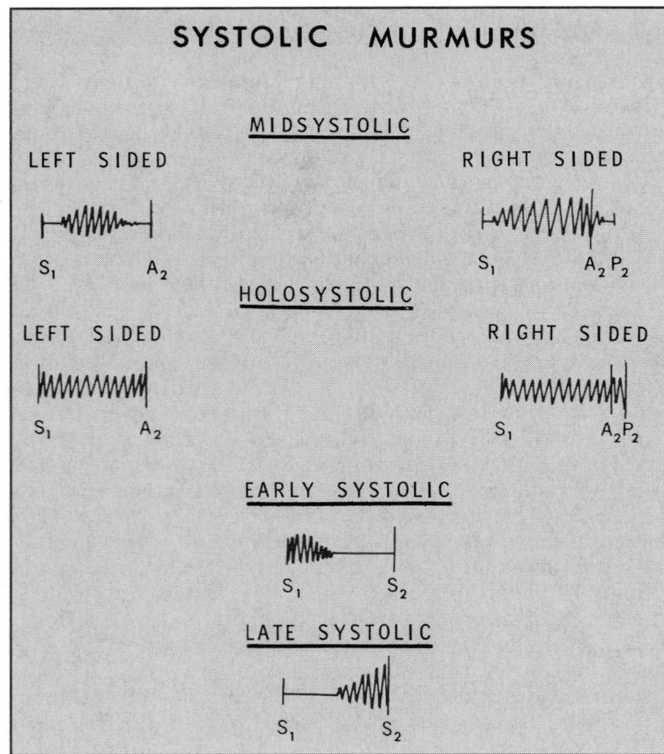

FIGURE 2–26. Systolic murmurs as illustrated here are descriptively classified according to their time of onset and termination as midsystolic, holosystolic, early systolic, and late systolic. The termination of the murmur must be related to the component of the second heart sound on its side of origin, that is, the aortic component (A_2) for systolic murmurs originating in the left side of the heart and the pulmonary component (P_2) for systolic murmurs originating in the right side of the heart.

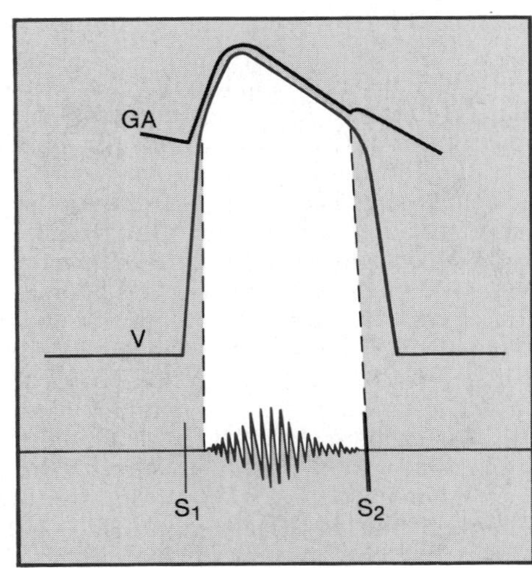

FIGURE 2–27. Illustration of the physiological mechanism of a midsystolic murmur generated by phasic flow into aortic root or pulmonary trunk. Ventricular (V) and great arterial (GA) pressure pulses are shown with phonocardiogram. The midsystolic murmur begins after the first heart sound (S_1), rises in crescendo to a peak as flow proceeds, then declines in decrescendo as flow diminishes, ending just before the second heart sound (S_2) as ventricular pressure falls below the pressure in the great artery.

Aortic valve stenosis is associated with a prototypical midsystolic murmur, which may have an early systolic peak and a short duration, a relatively late peak and a prolonged duration, or all gradations in between. Whether long or short, however, the murmur remains a symmetrical diamond beginning after the first heart sound (or with an aortic ejection sound), rising in crescendo to a systolic peak, and declining in decrescendo to end before the aortic component of the second heart sound. The high-velocity jet within the aortic root results in radiation of the murmur upward, to the right (second right intercostal space), and into the neck. An important variation occurs in older adults with previously normal trileaflet aortic valves rendered sclerotic or stenotic by fibrocalcific changes.[120] The accompanying murmur in the second right intercostal space is harsh, noisy, and impure, whereas the murmur over the left ventricular impulse is pure and often musical (Fig. 2–28). These two distinctive midsystolic murmurs—the noisy right basal and the musical apical—were described in 1925 by Gallavardin,[121] and the designation "Gallavardin dissociation" is still used. The impure right basal component of the murmur originates within the aortic root because of turbulence caused by the high-velocity jet. The pure musical component of the murmur heard over the left ventricular impulse originates from periodic high-frequency vibrations of the fibrocalcific aortic cusps (Fig. 2–29). The musical apical midsystolic murmur is sometimes dramatically loud. William Stokes (1855) reported that such a murmur was heard at a distance of 3 feet from the

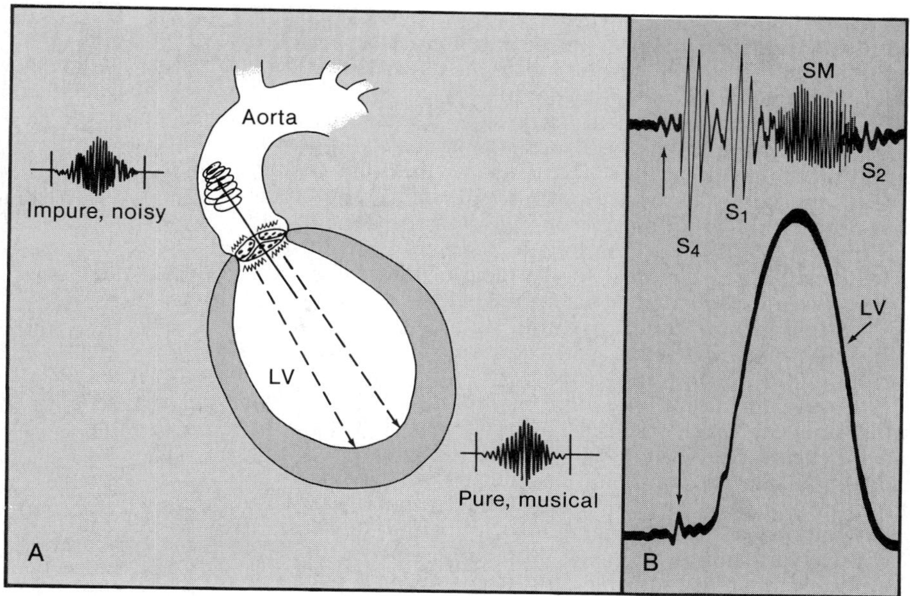

FIGURE 2–28. *A,* Illustration of "Gallavardin dissociation" of the basal and apical murmurs associated with a fibrocalcific trileaflet aortic valve in older adults. The impure, noisy midsystolic murmur at the right base originates within the aortic root because of turbulence caused by the high-velocity jet. The pure, musical midsystolic murmur at the apex results from high-frequency vibrations originating in the fibrocalcific but mobile aortic cusps and radiates selectively into the left ventricular cavity (LV). *B,* Left ventricular intracardiac phonocardiogram of an older adult with calcific aortic stenosis on a previously normal trileaflet valve. The pure, musical midsystolic murmur (SM) is recorded over the apex of the left ventricle (LV). A prominent fourth heart sound (S_4) coincides with presystolic distention of the left ventricle (lower vertical arrow). Upper vertical arrow identifies inaudible low-frequency vibrations preceding the fourth heart sound. S_1 = First heart sound; S_2 = second heart sound.

chest, and "this gentleman once observed to me that his entire body was one humming top."[122]

The high-frequency apical midsystolic murmur of aortic sclerosis or stenosis should be distinguished from the high-frequency apical murmur of mitral regurgitation, a distinction that may be difficult or impossible, especially if the aortic component of the second heart sound is soft or absent. However, when premature ventricular contractions are followed by pauses longer than the dominant cycle length, the apical midsystolic murmur of aortic stenosis or sclerosis increases in intensity in the beat following the premature contraction, whereas the intensity of the murmur of mitral regurgitation (whether midsystolic or holosystolic) remains relatively unchanged.[115] The same patterns hold following longer cycle lengths in atrial fibrillation. The validity of these observations assumes that aortic and mitral murmurs do not coexist at the apex.

The murmur of *pulmonary valve stenosis* is prototypical of a midsystolic murmur originating in the *right* side of the heart.[75] The murmur begins after the first heart sound or with a pulmonary ejection sound, rises in crescendo to a peak, then decreases in a slower decrescendo to end before a delayed or soft pulmonary component of the second heart sound (Fig. 2–19*A*). The length and configuration of the murmur are useful signs of the degree of obstruction.[75] The relative durations of right and left ventricular systole can be compared by relating the end of the pulmonary stenotic murmur (right-sided event) to the timing of the *aortic* component of the second heart sound (left-sided event) (Fig. 2–19*A*).

Short, soft midsystolic murmurs originate within a dilated aortic root or dilated pulmonary trunk. Midsystolic murmurs are also generated by rapid ejection into a *normal* aortic root or pulmonary trunk, as during pregnancy, fever, thyrotoxicosis, or anemia. The pulmonary midsystolic murmur of ostium secundum atrial septal defect results from *rapid* ejection into a *dilated* pulmonary trunk (Fig. 2–22). *Normal* (innocent) systolic murmurs are, except for the systolic mammary souffle, all midsystolic.[75]

The normal vibratory midsystolic murmur described by George Still in 1909[123] is short, buzzing, pure, and medium-frequency (Fig. 2–30) and is believed to be generated by low-frequency periodic vibrations of normal pulmonary leaflets at their attachments or periodic vibrations of a left ventricular false tendon. A second type of innocent midsystolic murmur occurs in children, adolescents, and young adults and represents an exaggeration of normal ejection vibrations within the pulmonary trunk. This normal pulmonary midsystolic murmur is relatively impure and is best heard in the second left intercostal space, in contrast to the vibratory midsystolic murmur of Still, which is typi-

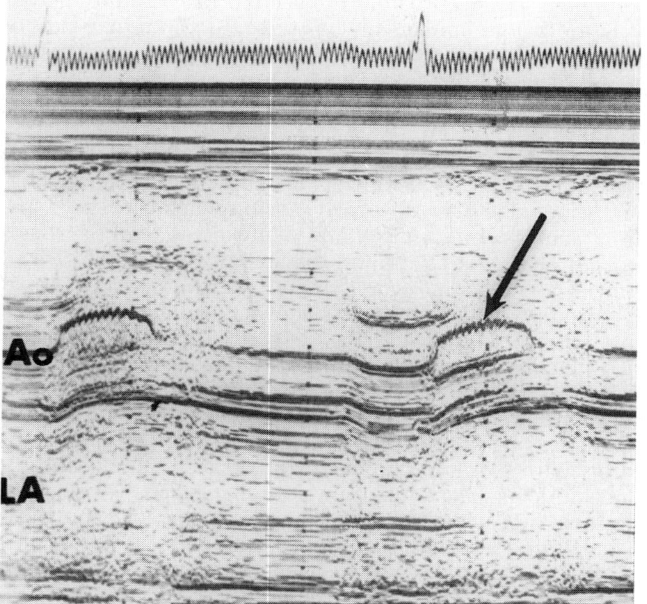

FIGURE 2–29. M-mode echocardiogram illustrating pure frequency vibrations of an open fibrocalcific mildly stenotic aortic valve (Ao) in a 64-year-old male with an apical musical midsystolic murmur of "Gallavardin dissociation" (see Fig. 2–28). LA = Left atrium.

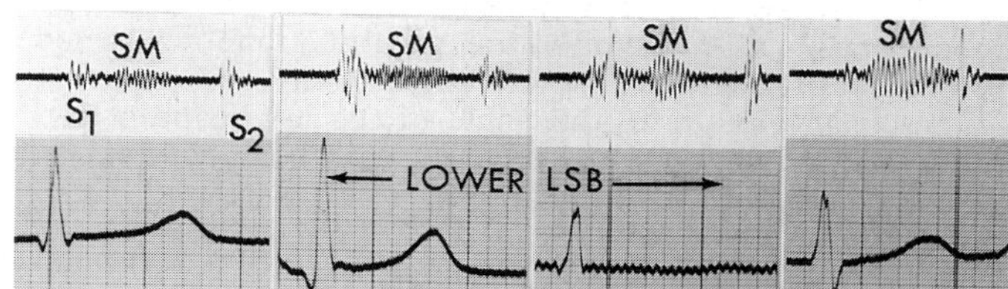

FIGURE 2–30. Four vibratory midsystolic murmurs (SM) from healthy children. These murmurs, designated "Still's murmur," are pure, medium frequency, relatively brief in duration, and maximal along the lower left sternal border (LSB). The last of the four murmurs was from a 5-year-old girl who was febrile. Following defervescence, the murmur decreased in loudness and duration.

cally heard between the lower left sternal edge and apex.[65] Normal pulmonary midsystolic murmurs are also heard in patients with diminished anteroposterior chest dimensions (loss of thoracic kyphosis, for example).[94]

The most common form of "innocent" midsystolic murmur in older adults has been designated the *"aortic sclerotic"* murmur (see above). The cause of this functionally benign murmur is fibrous or fibrocalcific thickening of the bases of otherwise normal aortic cusps as they insert into the sinuses of Valsalva.[75] As long as the fibrous or fibrocalcific thickening is confined to the *base* of the leaflets, the free edges remain mobile. No commissural fusion and no obstruction occurs. The Gallavardin dissociation phenomenon associated with such an aortic valve was described earlier.

It is not uncommon for *mitral regurgitation* to generate a midsystolic murmur.[90,124] The clinical setting is usually ischemic heart disease associated with left ventricular regional wall motion abnormalities. The physiological mechanism responsible for the midsystolic murmur of mitral regurgitation in this setting reflects impaired integrity of the muscular component of the mitral apparatus, with early systolic competence of the valve, midsystolic incompetence, followed by a late systolic decline in regurgitant flow. In any event, these midsystolic murmurs are unrelated to "ejection."

HOLOSYSTOLIC MURMURS. Just as the term "midsystolic" is preferable to "ejection" systolic, the term "holosystolic" is preferable to "regurgitant" because holosystolic murmurs are not necessarily due to regurgitant flow. A holosystolic murmur begins with the first heart sound and occupies all of systole (Gr. *holos* = entire) up to the second sound on its side of origin (Fig. 2–26).[69] Such murmurs are generated by flow from a vascular bed whose pressure or resistance throughout systole is higher than the pressure or resistance in the vascular bed receiving the flow. Holosystolic murmurs occur in the left side of the heart with mitral regurgitation, in the right side of the heart with high-pressure tricuspid regurgitation, between the ventricles through a restrictive ventricular septal defect, and between the great arteries through aortopulmonary connections.

The timing of holosystolic murmurs within the framework established by the first and second heart sounds reflects the physiological and anatomical mechanisms responsible for their genesis. Figure 2–31 illustrates the mechanism of the holosystolic murmur of mitral regurgitation or high-pressure tricuspid regurgitation. Ventricular pressure exceeds atrial pressure at the very onset of systole (isovolumetric contraction), so regurgitant flow begins with the first heart sound. The murmur persists up to or slightly beyond the relevant component of the second heart sound, provided that ventricular pressure at end-systole exceeds atrial pressure and provided that the AV valve remains incompetent.

Direction of radiation of the intraatrial jet of mitral regurgitation determines the chest wall distribution of the murmur.[90,125] When the direction of the intraatrial jet is forward and medial against the atrial septum near the origin of the aorta, the murmur radiates to the left sternal edge, to the base, and even into the neck (Fig. 2–32). When the flow generating the murmur of mitral regurgitation is directed posterolaterally within the left atrial cavity, the murmur radiates to the axilla, to the angle of the left scapula, and occasionally to the vertebral column, with bone conduction from the cervical to the lumbar spine (Fig. 2–32).

The *murmur of tricuspid regurgitation* is holosystolic when there is a substantial elevation of right ventricular systolic pressure, as schematically illustrated in Figure 2–31. A distinctive and diagnostically important feature of the tricuspid murmur is its selective inspiratory increase in loudness—Carvallo's sign (Fig. 2–20).[126] The tricuspid murmur is occasionally audible only during inspiration. The increase in intensity occurs because the inspiratory

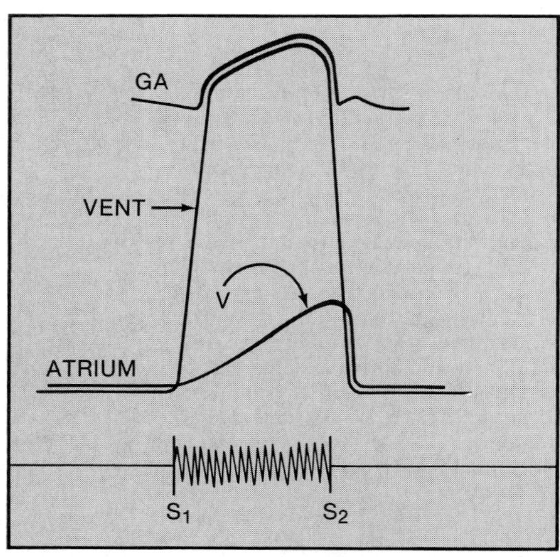

FIGURE 2–31. Illustration of great arterial (GA), ventricular (VENT), and atrial pressure pulses with phonocardiogram showing the physiological mechanism of a holosystolic murmur in some forms of mitral regurgitation and in high-pressure tricuspid regurgitation. Ventricular pressure exceeds atrial pressure at the very onset of systole, so regurgitant flow and murmur commence with the first heart sound (S_1). The murmur persists up to or slightly beyond the second heart sound (S_2) because regurgitation persists to the end of systole (ventricular pressure still exceeds atrial pressure). V = Atrial *v* wave.

augmentation in right ventricular volume is converted into an increase in stroke volume and in the velocity of regurgitant flow.[127] When the right ventricle fails, this capacity is lost, so Carvallo's sign vanishes.

The murmur of an uncomplicated restrictive ventricular septal defect is holosystolic because left ventricular systolic pressure and systemic resistance exceed right ventricular systolic pressure and pulmonary resistance from the onset to the end of systole. Holosystolic murmurs are perceived as such in patients with large aortopulmonary connections (aortopulmonary window, patent ductus arteriosus) when a rise in pulmonary vascular resistance abolishes the diastolic portion of the continuous murmur, leaving a murmur that is holosystolic or nearly so.[75]

EARLY SYSTOLIC MURMURS. Murmurs confined to early systole begin with the first heart sound, diminish in decrescendo, and end well before the second heart sound, generally at or before midsystole (Fig. 2–26). Certain types of mitral regurgitation, tricuspid regurgitation, or ventricular septal defects are the substrates.

Acute severe mitral regurgitation is accompanied by an early systolic murmur or a holosystolic murmur that is decrescendo, diminishing if not ending before the second heart sound (Fig. 2–33*A*).[128–130] The physiological mechanism responsible for this early systolic decrescendo murmur is acute severe regurgitation into a relatively normal-sized left atrium with limited distensibility. A steep rise in left atrial *v* wave approaches the left ventricular pressure at end-systole; a late systolic decline in left ventricular pressure favors this tendency (Fig. 2–33*B*). The stage is set for regurgitant flow that is maximal in early systole and minimal in late systole. The systolic murmur parallels this pattern, declining or vanishing before the second heart sound.

An early systolic murmur is a feature of tricuspid regurgitation with *normal* right ventricular systolic pressure.[131] An example is tricuspid regurgitation caused by infective endocarditis in drug abusers. The mechanisms responsible for the timing and configuration of the early systolic murmur of low-pressure tricuspid regurgitation are analogous to those just described for mitral regurgitation. The crest of the right atrial *v* wave reaches the level of normal right ventricular pressure in latter systole; the regurgitation and murmur are therefore chiefly, if not exclusively, *early* systolic. These murmurs are of medium frequency because

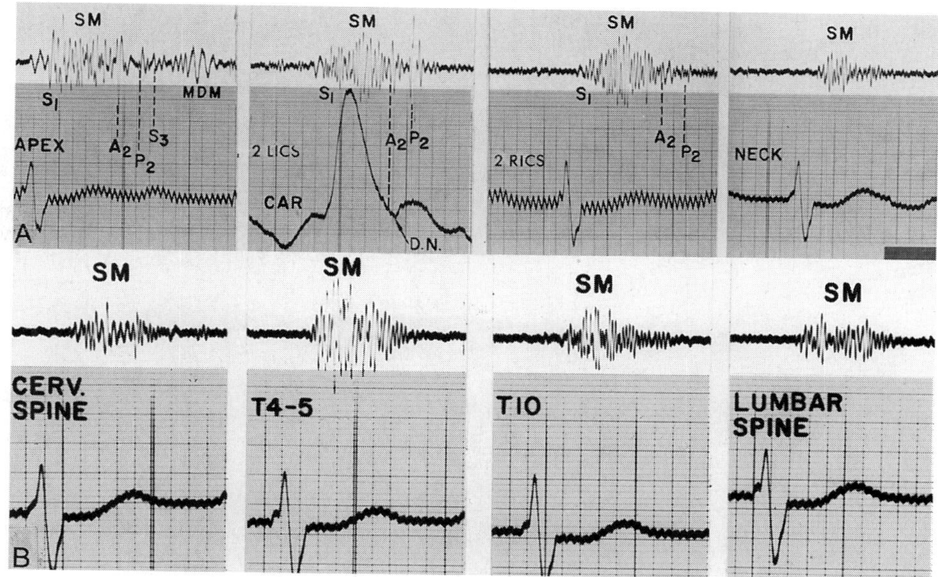

FIGURE 2–32. Phonocardiograms illustrating wide radiation of the murmur of mitral regurgitation. *A,* The holosystolic murmur (SM) radiates from the apex to the second left intercostal space (2LICS) to the second right intercostal space (2RICS) and into the neck. S_1 = First heart sound; A_2 = aortic component of the second sound; P_2 = pulmonary component of the second sound; S_3 = third heart sound; MDM = mid-diastolic murmur; CAR = carotid pulse; DN = dicrotic notch. *B,* The murmur of mitral regurgitation radiates to the cervical spine, down the thoracic spine (T4-5, T10) to the lumbar spine.

normal right ventricular systolic pressure generates comparatively low-velocity regurgitant flow in contrast to elevated right ventricular systolic pressure that generates a high-frequency holosystolic murmur (see earlier).

Early systolic murmurs also occur through ventricular septal defects, but under two widely divergent anatomical and physiological circumstances. A soft, pure, high-frequency, early systolic murmur localized to the mid- or lower left sternal edge is typical of a very small ventricular septal defect in which the shunt is confined to early systole.[75] A murmur of similar timing and configuration occurs through a nonrestrictive ventricular septal defect when an elevation in pulmonary vascular resistance decreases or abolishes late systolic shunting.[75]

LATE SYSTOLIC MURMURS. The term "late systolic" applies when a murmur begins in mid- to late systole and proceeds up to the second heart sound (Fig. 2–26). The late systolic murmur of *mitral valve prolapse* is prototypical (Fig. 2–33).[79,132] One or more mid- to late systolic clicks often introduce the murmur. The responses of the late systolic murmur and clicks to postural maneuvers (see earlier discussion) are illustrated in Figure 2–21. In response to a *diminution* in left ventricular volume, best achieved by prompt standing after squatting but also achieved by the Valsalva maneuver, the late systolic murmur becomes longer although softer.[79,82] In response to an *increase* in left ventricular volume associated with squatting or with sustained handgrip, the late systolic murmur becomes shorter but louder.[79,82] Pharmacological interventions that variably alter left ventricular volume, especially amyl nitrite (Fig. 2–34), produce analogous effects but are less practical at the bedside.

The late systolic murmur of mitral valve prolapse is occasionally replaced by an intermittent, striking, and sometimes disconcerting systolic whoop or honk, either spontaneously or in response to physical maneuvers.[79] The whoop is high-frequency, musical, widely transmitted, and

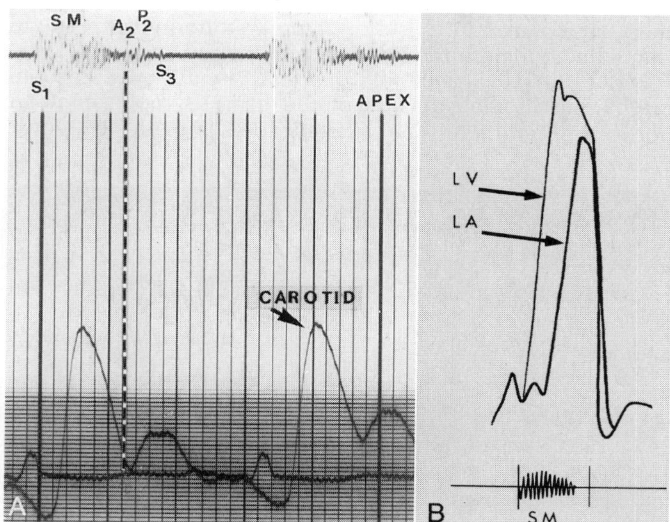

FIGURE 2–33. *A,* Phonocardiogram recorded from the cardiac apex of a patient with acute severe mitral regurgitation due to ruptured chordae tendineae. There is an early systolic decrescendo murmur (SM) diminishing if not ending before the aortic component (A_2) of the second heart sound. P_2 = Pulmonary component of the second heart sound; S_1 = first heart sound; S_3 = third heart sound. *B,* Left ventricular (LV) and left atrial (LA) pressure pulses with schematic illustration of the phonocardiogram showing the relationship between the decrescendo configuration of the early systolic murmur and late systolic approximation of the tall left atrial *v* wave and left ventricular end-systolic pressure. Regurgitant flow diminishes or ceases. The murmur therefore is early systolic and decrescendo, paralleling the hemodynamic pattern of regurgitation.

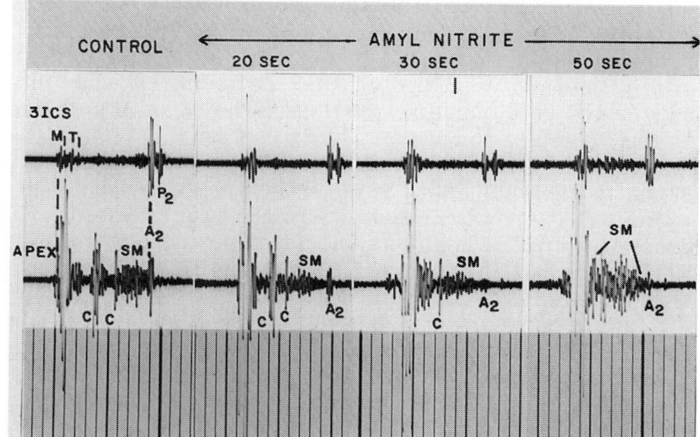

FIGURE 2–34. Phonocardiograms illustrating the response of the systolic clicks (C) and late systolic murmur (SM) of mitral valve prolapse to amyl nitrite inhalation. At 20 to 30 seconds, the clicks become earlier and the systolic murmur becomes longer but softer. At 50 seconds, the murmur is holosystolic and louder. M_1 = Mitral component of the first heart sound; T_1 = tricuspid component of the first heart sound; A_2 = aortic component of the second heart sound; P_2 = pulmonary component of the second sound.

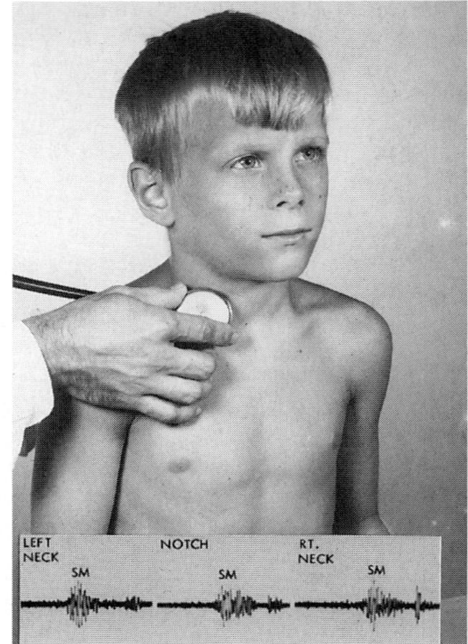

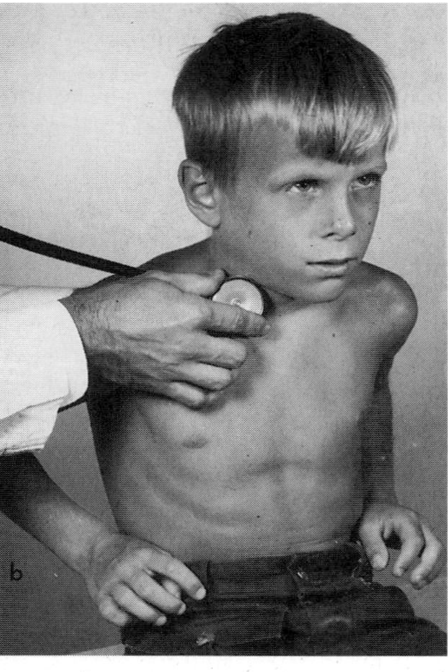

FIGURE 2–35. *Left,* Phonocardiogram showing a normal supraclavicular systolic arterial murmur maximal above the clavicles (left neck, right neck) and in the suprasternal notch. Auscultation is initially carried out while the patient sits with shoulders relaxed and arms resting in the lap. *Right,* When the elbows are brought well behind the back (hyperextension of the shoulders), the murmur markedly diminishes or disappears.

occasionally loud enough to be disturbing to the patient and sometimes to the physician.[133] The musical whoop is thought to arise from mitral leaflets and chordae tendineae set into high-frequency periodic vibration.

SYSTOLIC ARTERIAL MURMURS. Systolic murmurs can originate in anatomically normal arteries in the presence of normal or increased flow, or in abnormal arteries because of tortuosity or luminal narrowing. Detection of systolic arterial murmurs requires auscultation at nonprecordial sites. Timing with the first and second heart sounds is imprecise because the murmurs begin at variable distances from the heart. Nevertheless, the arterial murmurs dealt with here are essentially systolic and tend to have a crescendo-decrescendo configuration that reflects the rise and fall of pulsatile arterial flow.[2]

The "supraclavicular systolic murmur" (Fig. 2–35), often heard in children and adolescents, is believed to originate at the aortic origins of normal major brachiocephalic arteries.[75,134] The configuration of these murmurs is crescendo-decrescendo, the onset is abrupt, the duration is brief, and the intensity at times is surprisingly loud with radiation below the clavicles. Normal supraclavicular systolic murmurs decrease or vanish in response to hyperextension of the shoulders, which is achieved by bringing the elbows back until the shoulder girdle muscles are drawn taut (Fig. 2–35).[134]

In older adults, the most common cause of a systolic arterial murmur is atherosclerotic narrowing of a carotid, subclavian, or iliofemoral artery. A variation on this theme is the "compression artifact" that can be induced in the femoral artery in the presence of free aortic regurgitation. When the femoral artery is moderately compressed by the examiner's stethoscopic bell, a systolic arterial murmur is generated. Further compression causes the systolic murmur to continue into diastole, a sign described in 1861 by Duroziez.[75] The eponym is still in use.

A systolic "mammary souffle" is sometimes heard over the breasts because of increased flow through normal arteries during late pregnancy or more especially in the postpartum period in lactating women.[75,135] The murmur begins well after the first heart sound because of the interval between left ventricular ejection and arrival of flow at the artery of origin.

A systolic arterial murmur is present in the back between the scapulae over the site of coarctation of the aortic isthmus.[75] Transient systolic arterial murmurs originating in the pulmonary artery and its branches are occasionally heard in normal neonates because the angulation and disparity in size between the pulmonary trunk and its branches set the stage for turbulent systolic flow. These normal or innocent pulmonary arterial systolic murmurs disappear with maturation of the pulmonary bed, generally within the first few weeks or months of life.[75,136] Similar if not identical pulmonary arterial systolic murmurs are generated at sites of congenital stenosis of the pulmonary artery and its branches. Rarely, a pulmonary arterial systolic murmur is caused by luminal narrowing following a pulmonary embolus.[113]

Diastolic Murmurs

Diastolic murmurs are classified according to their time of *onset* as early diastolic, mid-diastolic, or late diastolic (presystolic) (Fig. 2–36). An *early* diastolic murmur begins with the aortic or pulmonary component of the second heart sound, depending upon its side of origin. A mid-diastolic murmur begins at a clear interval *after* the second heart sound. A late diastolic or presystolic murmur begins immediately before the first heart sound.

EARLY DIASTOLIC MURMURS. An early diastolic murmur originating in the left side of the heart is represented by *aortic regurgitation.* The murmur begins with the aortic

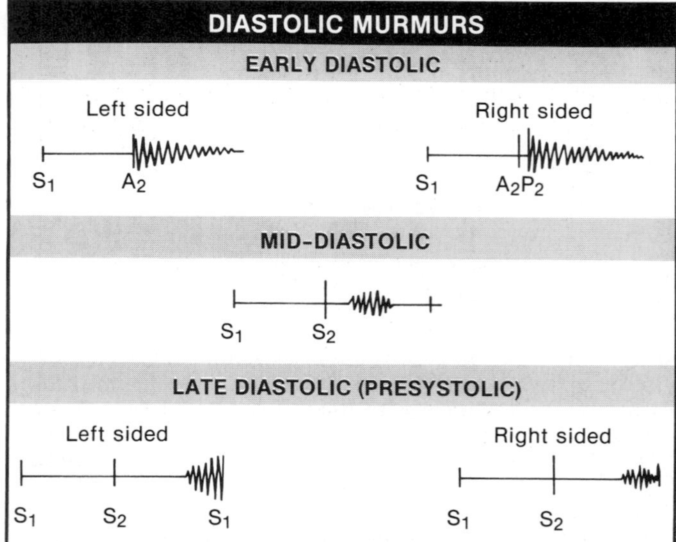

FIGURE 2–36. Diastolic murmurs are descriptively classified according to their time of *onset* as early diastolic, mid-diastolic, or late diastolic (presystolic). Diastolic murmurs originate in either the left or the right side of the heart.

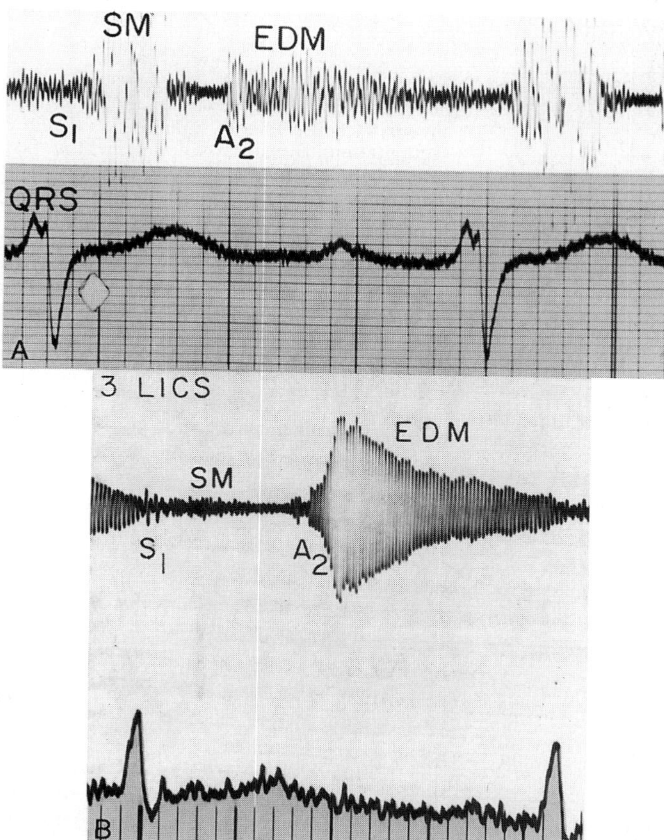

FIGURE 2–37. *A,* **Phonocardiogram recorded from the mid-left sternal edge of a patient with chronic pure severe aortic regurgitation. An early diastolic murmur (EDM) proceeds immediately from the aortic component (A_2) of the second heart sound. The murmur has an early crescendo followed by a late long decrescendo. There is a prominent midsystolic flow murmur (SM) across an unobstructed aortic valve. S_1 = First heart sound.** *B,* **Phonocardiogram in the third left intercostal space (3LICS) records a high-frequency, musical, early diastolic decrescendo murmur (EDM) caused by eversion of an aortic cusp. S_1 = First heart sound; SM = midsystolic murmur; A_2 = aortic component of the second sound.**

component of the second heart sound (Fig. 2–37*A*), i.e., as soon as left ventricular pressure falls below the aortic incisura. The configuration of the murmur tends to reflect the volume and rate of regurgitant flow. In chronic aortic regurgitation of moderate severity, the aortic diastolic pressure consistently and appreciably exceeds left ventricular diastolic pressure, so the decrescendo is subtle and the murmur is well heard throughout diastole. In chronic *severe* aortic regurgitation, the decrescendo is more obvious, paralleling the dramatic decline in aortic root diastolic pressure. Selective radiation of the murmur of aortic regurgitation to the *right* sternal edge implies aortic root dilatation, as in the Marfan syndrome. When an inverted cusp is set into high-frequency periodic vibration by aortic regurgitation, the accompanying murmur is musical, early diastolic, and decrescendo (Fig. 2–37*B*).

The diastolic murmur of *acute severe* aortic regurgitation differs importantly from the murmur of chronic severe aortic regurgitation as just described.[137] When regurgitant flow is both sudden *and* severe (bicuspid aortic valve infective endocarditis, aortic dissection), the diastolic murmur is relatively short because the aortic diastolic pressure rapidly equilibrates with the steeply rising diastolic pressure in the unprepared, nondilated left ventricle. The pitch of the murmur is likely to be medium rather than high because the velocity of regurgitant flow is less rapid than in chronic severe aortic regurgitation. This short, medium-frequency diastolic murmur of sudden severe aortic regurgitation may be disarmingly soft. These auscultatory features are in contrast to the long, pure, high-frequency, blowing early diastolic murmur of chronic severe aortic regurgitation (Fig. 2–37).

Early diastolic murmurs in the *right* side of the heart are represented by the Graham Steell murmur of pulmonary hypertensive pulmonary regurgitation described in 1888.[93] "I wish to plead for the admission among the recognized auscultatory signs of disease of a murmur due to . . . long-continuing excess blood pressure in the pulmonary artery. . . . When the second sound is reduplicated, the murmur proceeds from its latter part. That such a murmur as I have described does exist, there can, I think, be no doubt."[93]

The Graham Steell murmur begins with a loud *pulmonary* component of the second heart sound as Steell originally described (Fig. 2–20) because the elevated pressure exerted upon the incompetent pulmonary valve begins at the moment that right ventricular pressure drops below the pulmonary arterial incisura.[113] The high diastolic pressure generates high-velocity regurgitant flow and results in a high-frequency blowing murmur that may last throughout diastole. Because of the persistent and appreciable difference between pulmonary arterial and right ventricular diastolic pressures, the amplitude of the murmur is usually relatively uniform throughout most if not all of diastole.

MID-DIASTOLIC MURMURS. A mid-diastolic murmur begins at a clear interval after the second heart sound (Figs. 2–36 and 2–38). The majority of mid-diastolic murmurs originate across mitral or tricuspid valves during the rapid filling phase of the cardiac cycle (AV valve obstruction or abnormal patterns of AV flow) or across an incompetent pulmonary valve, provided that the pulmonary arterial pressure is not elevated.

The mid-diastolic murmur of rheumatic mitral stenosis is a prime example.[138,139] The murmur characteristically follows the mitral opening snap (Fig. 2–23*B*). Because the murmur originates within the left ventricular cavity, transmission to the chest wall is maximal over the left ventricular impulse. Care must be taken to place the bell of the stethoscope lightly against the skin precisely over the left ventricular impulse with the patient turned into the left lateral decubitus position (Fig. 2–14). Soft mid-diastolic murmurs are reinforced when the heart rate and mitral valve flow are transiently increased by vigorous voluntary coughs. In atrial fibrillation, the *duration* of the mid-diastolic murmur is a useful sign of the degree of obstruction at the mitral orifice (Fig. 2–38). A murmur that lasts up to the first heart sound even after long cycle lengths indicates that the stenosis is severe enough to generate a persistent gradient even at the end of long diastoles.

The mid-diastolic murmur of *tricuspid* stenosis occurs in the presence of atrial fibrillation. The tricuspid mid-diastolic murmur differs from the *mitral* mid-diastolic murmur in two important respects: (1) the loudness of the tricuspid murmur selectively and distinctively increases with inspiration; and (2) the tricuspid murmur is confined to a relatively localized area along the left lower sternal edge. The inspiratory increase in loudness occurs because inspiration is accompanied by an augmentation in right ventricular volume, by a fall in right ventricular diastolic pressure, and by an increase in gradient and flow rate across the stenotic tricuspid valve.[140] The murmur is localized to the lower left sternal edge because it originates within the inflow portion of the right ventricle and is transmitted to the overlying chest wall.

Mid-diastolic murmurs across *unobstructed* AV valves occur in the presence of augmented volume and velocity of flow. Examples in the left side of the heart are the mid-diastolic flow murmur of pure mitral regurgitation (Fig. 2–39) and the mid-diastolic mitral flow murmur that accompanies a large left-to-right shunt through a ventricular septal defect (Fig. 2–40*A*). Mid-diastolic murmurs due to augmented flow across unobstructed *tricuspid* valves are gen-

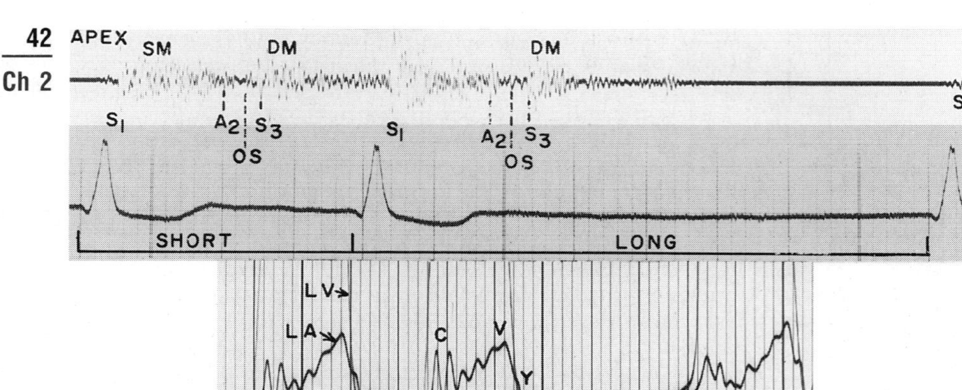

FIGURE 2–38. Tracings from a patient with rheumatic mitral stenosis, appreciable mitral regurgitation, and atrial fibrillation. The first heart sound (S_1) varies in intensity with cycle length. The aortic component of the second heart sound (A_2) is followed by a soft opening snap (OS), and a prominent third heart sound introduces a mid-diastolic murmur (DM). With a short cycle length, the murmur proceeds throughout diastole because there is an end-diastolic gradient between left atrium (LA) and left ventricle (LV). In the longer second cycle, the diastolic murmur ends, and the remainder of diastole is murmur-free, paralleling the equilibration of left atrial and left ventricular diastolic pressures (diastasis, D). C = c wave; V = v wave; Y = y descent.

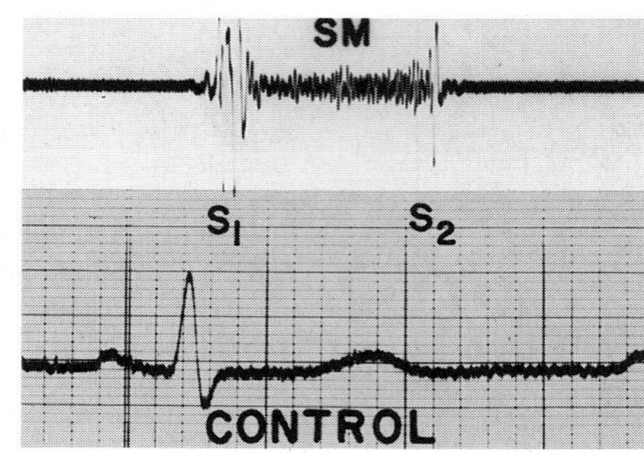

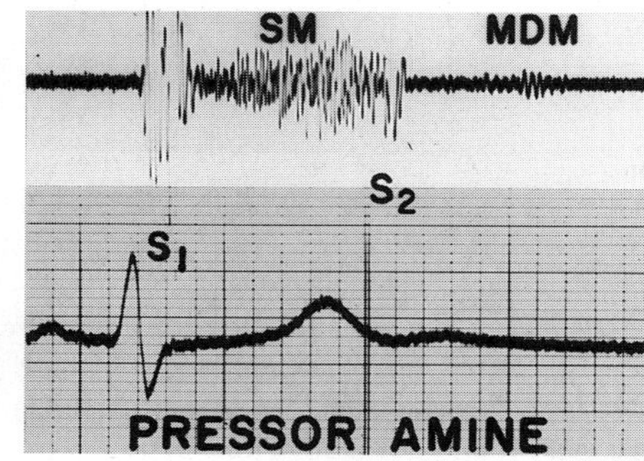

FIGURE 2–39. Phonocardiogram recorded over the left ventricular impulse of a patient with pure mitral regurgitation. When regurgitant flow is augmented in response to a pressor amine, the holosystolic crescendo murmur (SM) becomes more prominent, and a mid-diastolic flow murmur (MDM) appears.

erated by severe tricuspid regurgitation or by a large left-to-right shunt through an atrial septal defect (Fig. 2–40*B*). These mid-diastolic murmurs indicate appreciable AV valve incompetence or large left-to-right shunts and are often preceded by third heart sounds, especially in the presence of mitral or tricuspid regurgitation.

Short, mid-diastolic AV flow murmurs occur intermittently in complete heart block when atrial contraction coincides with the phase of rapid diastolic filling (Fig. 2–16). These murmurs are believed to result from antegrade flow across AV valves that are closing rapidly during filling of the recipient ventricle.[138] A similar mechanism is believed to be responsible for the Austin Flint murmur (Fig. 2–41), as Flint originally proposed (see below).[141–143]

A mid-diastolic murmur is a feature of pulmonary valve regurgitation, provided that the pulmonary arterial pressure is not elevated (Fig. 2–42*A*). The diastolic murmur typi-

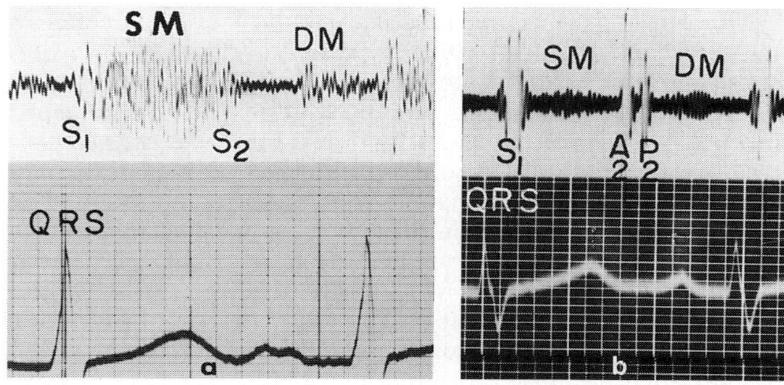

FIGURE 2–40. *a,* Phonocardiogram recorded at the apex of a patient with a moderately restrictive ventricular septal defect and increased pulmonary arterial blood flow. The mid-diastolic murmur (DM) results from augmented flow across the mitral valve. SM = Holosystolic murmur; S_1 = first heart sound; S_2 = second heart sound. *b,* Phonocardiogram at the lower left sternal edge of a patient with an ostium secundum atrial septal defect and increased pulmonary arterial blood flow. A mid-diastolic murmur (DM) resulted from augmented flow across the tricuspid valve. SM = Mid-systolic murmur; A_2 and P_2 = aortic and pulmonary components of a conspicuously split second heart sound.

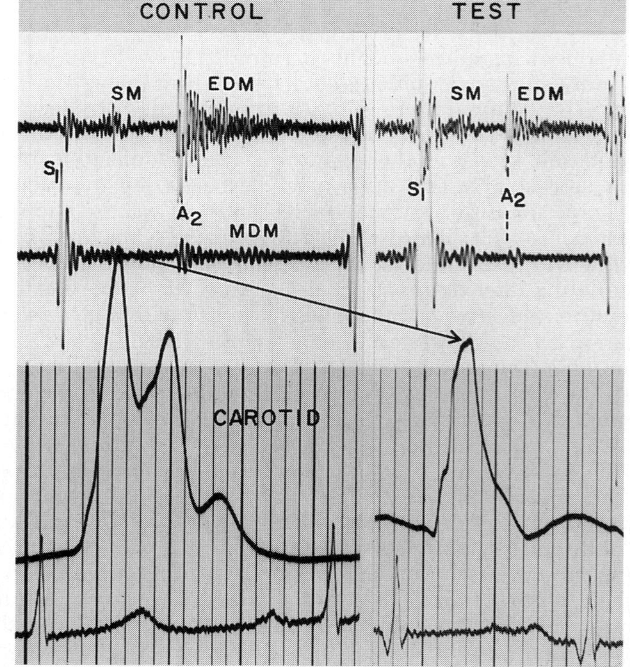

FIGURE 2–41. Phonocardiograms and simultaneous carotid pulse from a patient with chronic pure severe aortic regurgitation. Following amyl nitrite inhalation (test), the prominent early diastolic murmur (EDM) decreases, a mid-diastolic (MDM) Austin Flint murmur disappears, and the bisferiens carotid pulse becomes single-peaked.

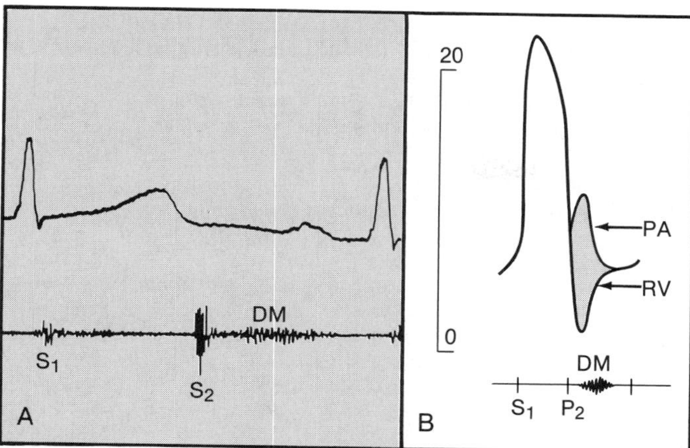

FIGURE 2–42. *A,* Phonocardiogram illustrating the mid-diastolic murmur (DM) of low-pressure pulmonary regurgitation in a heroin addict who had pulmonary valve infective endocarditis. The murmur begins well after the second heart sound (S_2), is medium-frequency and mid-diastolic, ending well before the subsequent first heart sound (S_1). *B,* Pressure pulses and phonocardiogram illustrate the physiological mechanism of the mid-diastolic murmur of low-pressure pulmonary regurgitation. Because the pressure exerted against the incompetent pulmonary valve is low, the murmur does not begin until well after the right ventricular (RV) and pulmonary arterial (PA) pressure pulses diverge. The murmur is maximal when the diastolic gradient *(cross-hatched area)* is greatest. Following an early diastolic dip in the RV pressure pulse, there is equilibration of the pulmonary arterial and right ventricular pressures in later diastole, so the regurgitant gradient is abolished and the murmur disappears.

cally begins at a perceptible interval after the pulmonary component of the second heart sound, is crescendo-decrescendo, ending well before the subsequent first heart sound.[75] The physiological mechanism responsible for the timing of this murmur is shown in Figure 2–42*B*. The diastolic pressure exerted upon the incompetent pulmonary valve is negligible at the inception of the pulmonary component of the second sound, so regurgitant flow is minimal. Regurgitation accelerates as right ventricular pressure dips below the diastolic pressure in the pulmonary trunk; at that point the murmur reaches its maximum (Fig. 2–42*B*). Late diastolic equilibration of pulmonary arterial and right ventricular pressures eliminates regurgitant flow and abolishes the murmur prior to the next first heart sound.

LATE DIASTOLIC OR PRESYSTOLIC MURMURS. A late diastolic murmur occurs immediately before the first heart sound, that is, in *presystole* (Fig. 2–26). With few exceptions, the late diastolic timing of the murmur coincides with the phase of ventricular filling that follows atrial systole and implies coordinated atrial contraction, generally sinus rhythm. Late diastolic or presystolic murmurs usually originate at the mitral or tricuspid orifice because of obstruction, but occasionally because of abnormal patterns of presystolic AV flow.

The best known presystolic murmur accompanies rheumatic mitral stenosis in sinus rhythm as AV flow is augmented in response to an increase in the force of left atrial contraction (Figs. 2–23*B* and 2–43*A*).[96] "Presystolic" accentuation of a mid-diastolic murmur is occasionally heard in mitral stenosis with atrial fibrillation, especially during short cycle lengths,[144,145] but the timing is actually early systolic, and the mechanism differs from the true presystolic murmur as described above and as shown in Figure 2–43*A*.

In *tricuspid* stenosis with sinus rhythm, a late diastolic or presystolic murmur typically occurs in the absence of a perceptible mid-diastolic murmur (Fig. 2–43*B*). This is so because the timing of tricuspid diastolic murmurs reflects the maximal acceleration of flow and gradient, which is usually negligible until powerful right atrial contraction.[140] The presystolic murmur of tricuspid stenosis is crescendo-decrescendo and relatively discrete, fading before the first heart sound (Fig. 2–43*B*). This is in contrast to the presystolic murmur of mitral stenosis, which tends to rise in crescendo that is interrupted by the first heart sound (Fig. 2–43*A*). The most valuable auscultatory sign of tricuspid stenosis in sinus rhythm is the effect of respiration on the intensity of the presystolic murmur (Figs. 2–43 and 2–44). Inspiration increases right atrial volume, provoking an increase in right atrial contractile force that coincides with a fall in right ventricular end-diastolic pressure. The result is an increase in the tricuspid gradient, in the velocity of tricuspid flow, and in the intensity of the tricuspid stenotic presystolic murmur (Fig. 2–44).[140]

Short, crescendo-decrescendo presystolic murmurs are occasionally heard in *complete heart block* when atrial contraction falls in late diastole. However, the murmur is usually mid-diastolic, as already described, occurring when atrial contraction coincides with and reinforces the rapid filling phase of the cardiac cycle (Fig. 2–16).

In 1862, Austin Flint described a presystolic murmur in patients with aortic regurgitation and proposed a mechanism that was astonishingly perceptive.[141–143,146,147] "Now in cases of considerable aortic insufficiency, the left ventricle is rapidly filled with blood flowing back from the aorta as well as from the auricle, before the auricular contraction takes place. The distention of the ventricle is such that the mitral curtains are brought into coaptation, and when the auricular contraction takes place, the mitral direct current passing between the curtains throws them into vibration and gives rise to the characteristic blubbering murmur."[141]

Continuous Murmurs

The term "continuous" appropriately applies to murmurs that begin in systole and *continue* without interruption through the second heart sound into all or part of diastole (Fig. 2–45). The presence of murmurs throughout both phases of the cardiac cycle (holosystolic followed by holodiastolic) (Fig. 2–45) is not the criterion for the designation "continuous." Conversely, a murmur that fades completely before the subsequent first heart sound *is* continuous, provided that the systolic portion of the murmur proceeds without interruption through the second heart sound (Fig. 2–45).

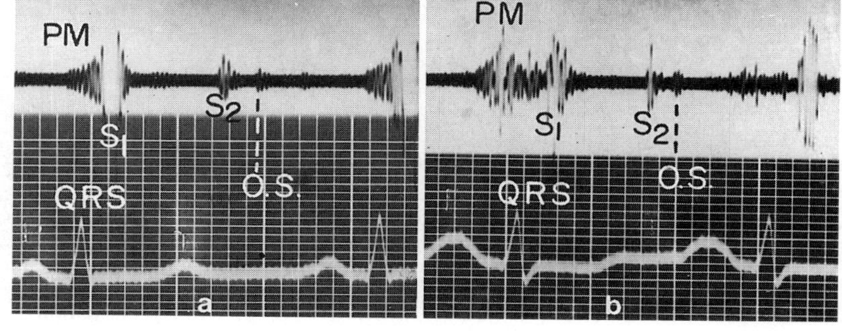

FIGURE 2–43. *a,* Phonocardiogram from the cardiac apex of a patient with pure rheumatic mitral stenosis. A presystolic murmur (PM) rises in a crescendo that is interrupted by a loud first heart sound (S_1). S_2 = Second heart sound; OS = mitral opening snap. *b,* Phonocardiogram from the lower left sternal edge of a patient with rheumatic tricuspid stenosis. The first cycle is during inspiration and is accompanied by a prominent presystolic murmur (PM) that is crescendo-decrescendo, decreasing before the first heart sound (S_1). During exhalation (second cycle), the presystolic murmur all but vanishes.

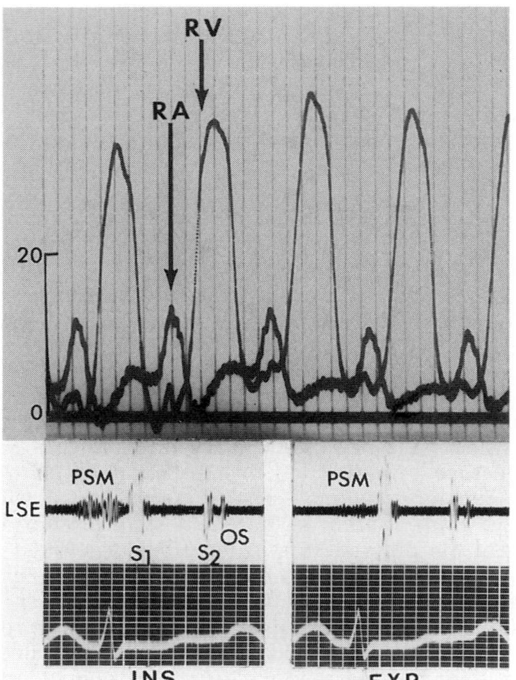

FIGURE 2–44. Pressure pulses and phonocardiogram illustrating the physiological mechanism of the respiratory variation in the presystolic murmur of tricuspid stenosis. During inhalation, a fall in intrathoracic pressure and an increase in systemic venous return result in an increase in the right atrial (RA) A wave and a decline in right ventricular (RV) end-diastolic pressure, so the presystolic murmur (PSM) increases in loudness. During exhalation, the right atrial A wave declines, the right ventricular diastolic pressure increases, the tricuspid gradient is at its minimum, and the presystolic murmur all but vanishes.

TABLE 2–3 DIFFERENTIAL DIAGNOSIS OF CONTINUOUS THORACIC MURMURS (IN ORDER OF FREQUENCY)

DIAGNOSIS	KEY FINDINGS
Cervical venous hum	Disappears on compression of the jugular vein
Hepatic venous hum	Often disappears with epigastric pressure
Mammary souffle	Disappears upon pressing hard with stethoscope
Patent ductus arteriosus	Loudest at 2nd left intercostal space
Coronary arteriovenous fistula	Loudest at lower sternal borders
Ruptured aneurysm of sinus of Valsalva	Loudest at upper right sternal border, sudden onset
Bronchial collaterals	Associated signs of congenital heart disease
High-grade coarctation	Brachial-pedal arterial pressure gradient
Anomalous left coronary artery arising from pulmonary artery	Electrocardiographic changes of myocardial infarction
Truncus arteriosus	
Pulmonary artery branch stenosis	Heard outside the area of cardiac dullness
Pulmonary AV fistula	Same as above
Atrial septal defect with mitral stenosis or atresia	Altered by the Valsalva maneuver
Aortic-atrial fistulas	

Adapted from Sapira, J. D.: The Art and Science of Bedside Diagnosis. Baltimore, Urban & Schwartzenberg, 1990.

Continuous murmurs are generated by uninterrupted flow from a vascular bed of higher pressure or resistance into a vascular bed of lower pressure or resistance without phasic interruption between systole and diastole. Such murmurs are due chiefly to (1) aortopulmonary connections, (2) arteriovenous connections, (3) disturbances of flow patterns in arteries, and (4) disturbances of flow patterns in veins.

The most celebrated continuous murmur is associated with the aortopulmonary connection of *patent ductus arteriosus* (Fig. 2–46). The murmur characteristically peaks just before and after the second heart sound which it envelops, decreases in late diastole—often appreciably, and may be soft or even absent before the subsequent first heart sound.[75] In 1847, the *London Medical Gazette* published the description of "a murmur accompanying the first heart sound . . . prolonged into the second sound so that there is no cessation of the murmur before the second sound had already commenced."[148] The author correctly assigned the cause of the murmur to patent ductus arteriosus and established the proper meaning of "continuous" as "no cessation of the murmur before the second sound had already commenced." George Gibson's description in 1900 was even more precise.[149] "It persists through the second sound

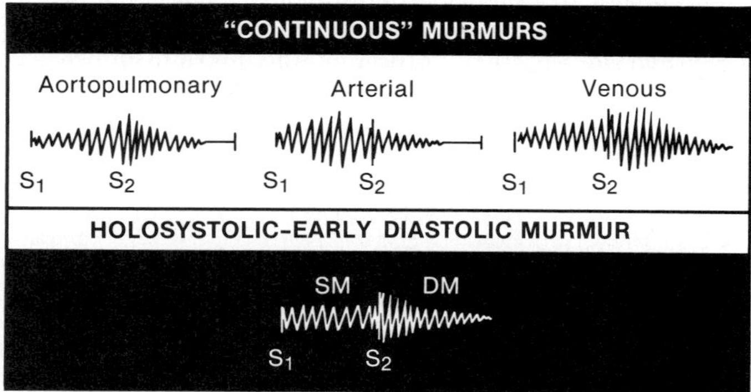

FIGURE 2–45. Continuous murmurs begin in systole and *continue* without interruption through the timing of second heart sound (S_2) into all or part of diastole. The continuous murmurs shown here are aortopulmonary, systemic arterial, and systemic venous. A holosystolic murmur (SM) followed by a holodiastolic murmur (DM) represents two separate murmurs, not one continuous murmur.

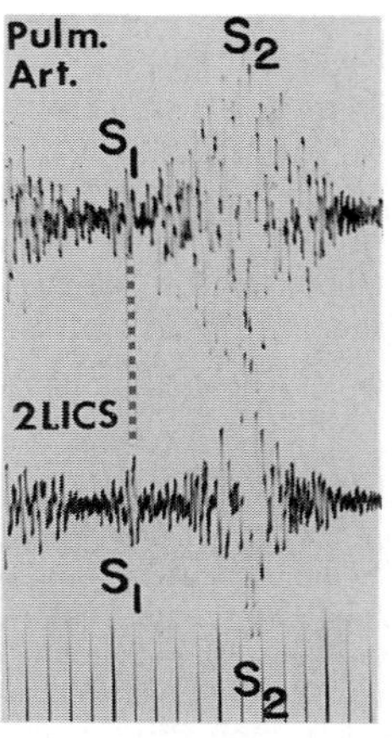

FIGURE 2–46. The classic continuous murmur of patent ductus arteriosus recorded from within the main pulmonary artery *(upper tracing)* and simultaneously on the chest wall at the second left intercostal space (2LICS). The murmur "begins softly and increases in intensity so as to reach its acme just about, or immediately after the incidence of the second sound, and from that point gradually wanes until its termination," as originally described by Gibson in 1900.[149]

and dies away gradually during the long pause. The murmur is rough and thrilling. It begins softly and increases in intensity so as to reach its acme just about, or immediately after, the incidence of the second sound, and from that point gradually wanes until its termination" (Fig. 2–46).

Arteriovenous continuous murmurs can be congenital or acquired and are represented in part by arteriovenous fistulas, coronary arterial fistulas, anomalous origin of the left coronary artery from the pulmonary trunk, and sinus of Valsalva–to–right heart communications.[75] The configuration, location, and intensity of arteriovenous continuous murmurs vary considerably among these different lesions. *Acquired* systemic arteriovenous fistulas are created surgically by forearm shunts for hemodialysis. *Congenital* arteriovenous continuous murmurs occur when a coronary arterial fistula enters the pulmonary trunk, right atrium, or right ventricle. At the latter site, the continuous murmur can be either softer or louder in systole, depending upon the degree of compression exerted on the fistulous coronary artery by right ventricular contraction.[75] Rupture of a congenital aortic sinus aneurysm into the right heart results in a continuous murmur that tends to be louder in either systole or diastole, sometimes creating a to-and-fro impression.[75]

Arterial continuous murmurs originate in either *constricted* or *nonconstricted* arteries. A common example of a continuous murmur arising in a constricted artery is carotid or femoral arterial atherosclerotic obstruction. Not surprisingly, these arterial continuous murmurs are characteristically louder in systole (Fig. 2–45) and more often than not are purely systolic.

Disturbances of flow patterns in *normal, nonconstricted* arteries sometimes produce continuous murmurs. The "mammary souffle" described earlier,[135] an innocent murmur heard during late pregnancy and the puerperium, is an arterial murmur which, when continuous, is typically louder in systole and maximal over either lactating breast. A distinct gap separates the first heart sound from the onset of the mammary souffle because of the relatively long interval that elapses before blood ejected from the left ventricle arrives at the artery of origin.[75] Light pressure with the stethoscope tends to augment the murmur and bring out its continuous features, whereas firm pressure with the stethoscope or by digital compression adjacent to the site of auscultation often abolishes the murmur.

Continuous murmurs in nonconstricted arteries originate in the large systemic-to-pulmonary arterial collaterals in certain types of cyanotic congenital heart disease, typically Fallot's tetralogy with pulmonary atresia (Fig. 2–19). These continuous murmurs are randomly located throughout the thorax because of the random location of the aortopulmonary collaterals.[75]

Continuous venous murmurs are well-represented by the innocent cervical venous hum (Fig. 2–47) described by Potain in 1867.[150] The hum is far and away the most common type of normal continuous murmur, universal in healthy children, and frequently present in healthy young adults, especially during pregnancy. Thyrotoxicosis and anemia, by augmenting cervical venous flow, initiate or reinforce the venous hum. The term "hum" does not necessarily characterize the quality of these cervical venous murmurs, which may be rough and noisy and are occasionally accompanied by a high-pitched whine.[75] The hum is truly continuous, although typically louder in diastole, as is generally the case with venous continuous murmurs (Fig. 2–47). The mechanism of the venous hum is unsettled. Silent laminar flow in the internal jugular vein may be disturbed by deformation of the vessel at the level of the transverse process of the atlas during head rotation designed to elicit the hum.[151]

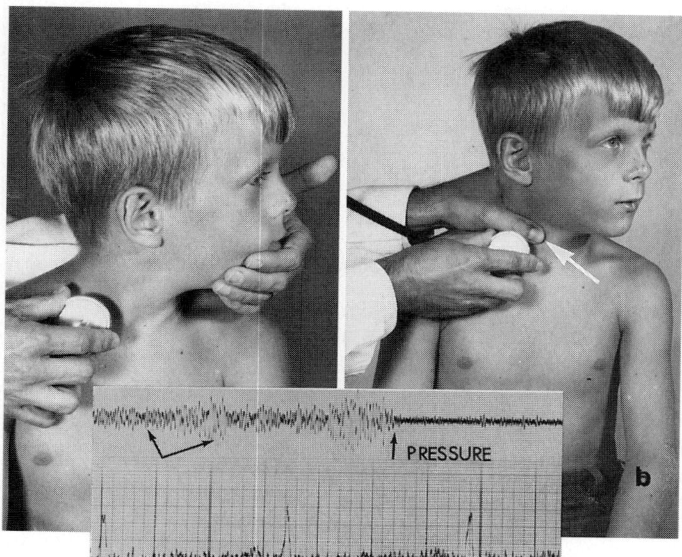

FIGURE 2–47. The phonocardiogram shows the continuous murmur of a normal venous hum. The *diastolic* component is louder (paired arrows). Digital pressure over the right internal jugular vein (vertical arrow) abolishes the murmur. The photographs show maneuvers used to elicit or abolish the venous hum. *Left,* The bell of the stethoscope is applied to the medial aspect of the right supraclavicular fossa as the examiner's left hand grasps the patient's chin from behind and pulls it tautly to the left and upward, stretching the neck. *Right,* The patient's head has returned to a more neutral position, and digital compression of the right internal jugular vein (arrow) abolishes the hum.

Pericardial Rubs

In sinus rhythm, the typical pericardial rub is triple-phased, that is, midsystolic, mid-diastolic, and presystolic.[152] Recognition is simplest when all three phases are present, and when the characteristic superficial scratchy, leathery quality is evident. The term "rub" is appropriate because the auscultatory sign is generated by abnormal visceral and parietal pericardial surfaces "rubbing" against each other. In the supine position, firm pressure with the stethoscopic diaphragm during full held exhalation reinforces visceral and parietal pericardial contact and accentuates the rub. Apposition of visceral and parietal pericardium can be even better achieved by examination while the patient rests on elbows and knees.

Of the three phases of the pericardial rub, the systolic phase is the most consistent, followed by the presystolic phase. In atrial fibrillation, the presystolic component necessarily disappears. The diagnosis of a pericardial rub is least secure, and often impossible, when only one phase remains, typically the midsystolic. The most common clinical setting in which pericardial rubs are heard is immediately after open heart surgery. However, auscultation often detects instead a "crunch" synchronous with the heart beat, especially in the left lateral decubitus position. This is not a pericardial rub, but is Hamman's sign caused by air in the mediastinum.[153]

THE CARDIORESPIRATORY MURMUR

Thoracic auscultation occasionally detects what has been called a "cardiorespiratory murmur." Richard Cabot was aware that "Cardiorespiratory murmurs may be produced without any adhesion of the lung to the pericardium under conditions not at present understood."[154] Cabot went on to say that: "Such murmurs may be heard under the left clavicle or below the angle of the left scapula, as well as near the apex of the heart—less than in other parts of the chest. . . . Cardiorespiratory murmurs may be either systolic or diastolic, but the vast majority of cases are systolic. The area over which they are audible is usually a very limited one. They are greatly affected by position and by respiration, and are heard most distinctly if not exclusively during inspiration, especially at the end of that act." The mechanism responsible for the cardiorespiratory murmur remains unclear, but the location, timing, and relation to respiration remain as Cabot described.[154]

DYNAMIC AUSCULTATION

This term refers to the technique of altering circulatory dynamics by means of respiration and a variety of physiological and pharmacological maneuvers and determining the effects of these maneuvers on heart sounds and murmurs.[155–158] The interventions most commonly employed in dynamic auscultation include respiration, postural changes, the Valsalva maneuver, premature ventricular contractions, isometric exercise, and one of the vasoactive agents—amyl nitrite, methoxamine, or phenylephrine. The clinical applications of dynamic auscultation are summarized in Table 2–4.

TABLE 2–4 RESPONSE OF MURMURS AND HEART SOUNDS TO PHYSIOLOGICAL AND PHARMACOLOGICAL INTERVENTIONS

CLINICAL DISORDER	INTERVENTION AND RESPONSE
SYSTOLIC MURMURS	
Aortic outflow obstruction	
Valvular aortic stenosis	Louder with passive leg-raising, with sudden squatting, with Valsalva release (after five to six beats), following a pause induced by a premature beat, or after amyl nitrite; fades during Valsalva strain and with isometric handgrip
Hypertrophic obstructive cardiomyopathy	Louder with standing, during Valsalva strain, or with amyl nitrite; fades with sudden squatting, recumbency, or isometric handgrip
Pulmonic stenosis	Midsystolic murmur increases with amyl nitrite except with marked right ventricular hypertrophy; also increases during first few beats after Valsalva release
Mitral regurgitation	
Rheumatic	Murmur louder with sudden squatting, isometric handgrip, or phenylephrine; softens with amyl nitrite
Mitral valve prolapse	Midsystolic click moves toward S_1 and late systolic murmur starts earlier with standing, Valsalva strain, and amyl nitrite; click may occur earlier on inspiration; murmur starts later and click moves toward S_2 during squatting, with recumbency, and often after pause induced by a premature beat
Papillary muscle dysfunction	Late systolic murmur generally softer after a pause induced by a premature beat; response to amyl nitrite variable, depending on acute or chronic nature of this disorder
Tricuspid regurgitation	Murmur increases during inspiration, with passive leg-raising, and with amyl nitrite
Ventricular septal defect	
Small defect with pulmonary hypertension	Fades with amyl nitrite; increases with isometric handgrip or phenylephrine
Large defect with hyperkinetic pulmonary hypertension	Louder with amyl nitrite; fades with phenylephrine
Large defect with severe pulmonary vascular disease	Little change with any of above interventions
Tetralogy of Fallot	Murmur softens with amyl nitrite
Supraclavicular bruit	Altered by compression of subclavian artery; may be eliminated by extension of ipsilateral shoulder
DIASTOLIC MURMURS	
Aortic regurgitation	
Blowing diastolic murmur	Increases with sudden squatting, isometric handgrip, or phenylephrine
Austin Flint murmur	Fades with amyl nitrite
Pulmonary regurgitation	
Congenital	Early or mid-diastolic rumble increases on inspiration and with amyl nitrite
Pulmonary hypertension	High-frequency blowing murmur not altered by above interventions
Mitral stenosis	Mid-diastolic and presystolic murmurs louder with exercise, left lateral position, coughing, isometric handgrip, or amyl nitrite; phenylephrine widens A_2-OS interval; inspiration produces sequence of A_2-P_2-OS
Tricuspid stenosis	Mid-diastolic and presystolic murmurs increase during inspiration, with passive leg-raising, and with amyl nitrite
CONTINUOUS MURMURS	
Patent ductus arteriosus	Diastolic phase amplified with isometric handgrip or phenylephrine; diastolic phase fades with amyl nitrite
Cervical venous hum	Obliterated by direct compression of jugular veins or by Valsalva strain
ADDED HEART SOUNDS	
Gallop rhythm	
Ventricular gallop (S_3) and atrial gallop (S_4)	Accentuated by lying flat with passive leg-raising; decreased by standing or during Valsalva; right-sided gallop sounds usually increase during inspiration; left-sided during expiration
Summation gallop	Separates into ventricular gallop (S_3) and atrial gallop (S_4) sounds when heart rate slowed by carotid sinus massage
Ejection sounds	Ejection sound in pulmonary stenosis fades and occurs closer to the first sound during inspiration

OS = opening snap of mitral valve
From Criscitiello, M. G.: Physiologic and pharmacologic aids in cardiac auscultation. *In* Fowler, N. O. (ed.): Cardiac Diagnosis and Treatment. Hagerstown, MD, Harper and Row, 1980.

RESPIRATION

SECOND HEART SOUND. The splitting of S_2 is best audible along the left sternal border and can usually be appreciated when A_2 and P_2 are separated by more than 0.02 sec. The effects of respiration on the splitting of the second heart sound are discussed on p. 32.

THIRD AND FOURTH SOUNDS AND EJECTION SOUNDS. When third and fourth sounds originate from the right ventricle, they are characteristically diminished during exhalation and augmented during inspiration, whereas they exhibit the opposite response when they originate from the left side of the heart. Like other left-sided events, the opening snap of the mitral valve may become softer during inspiration and louder during exhalation owing to respiratory alterations in venous return, whereas the opening snap of the tricuspid valve behaves in the opposite fashion. Inspiration also diminishes the intensity of ejection sounds in pulmonary valve stenosis because the elevation of right ventricular diastolic pressure causes partial presystolic opening of the pulmonary valve and therefore less upward motion of the valve during systole. On the other hand, respiration does not affect the intensity of aortic ejection sounds, except in Fallot's tetralogy with pulmonary atresias.

Murmurs

Respiration exerts more pronounced and consistent alterations on murmurs originating from the right than from the left side of the heart. During inspiration, the diastolic murmurs of tricuspid stenosis (Fig. 2–44) and low pressure pulmonary regurgitation, the systolic murmurs of tricuspid regurgitation[159] (Carvallo's sign) and the presystolic murmur of Ebstein's anomaly may all be accentuated. The inspiratory reduction in left ventricular size in patients with mitral valve prolapse increases the redundancy of the mitral valve and therefore the degree of valvular prolapse; consequently, the midsystolic click and the systolic murmurs occur earlier during systole and may become accentuated.[160]

THE VALSALVA MANEUVER. This maneuver was described in 1704 as a method for expelling pus from the middle ear by straining with the mouth and nose closed.[75] The Valsalva maneuver is readily performed at the bedside and consists of a relatively deep inspiration followed by forced exhalation against a closed glottis for 10 to 12 seconds. The patient should be instructed on how to perform the maneuver. Simulation by the examiner is a simple means of doing so. The examiner then places the flat of the hand upon the abdomen to provide the patient with a force against which to strain and to permit assessment of the degree and duration of the straining effort.[161–163] The normal response to the Valsalva maneuver consists of four phases. *Phase I* is associated with a transient rise in systemic blood pressure as straining commences. This phase cannot, as a rule, be identified at the bedside. *Phase II* is accompanied by a perceptible decrease in systemic venous return, blood pressure, and pulse pressure (small pulse) and is readily detectable by reflex tachycardia. *Phase III* begins promptly with cessation of straining, is associated with an abrupt, transient decrease in blood pressure and in systemic venous return, and is generally not perceived at the bedside. *Phase IV* is characterized by an overshoot of systemic arterial pressure and relatively obvious reflex bradycardia. During phase II, third and fourth heart sounds are attenuated and the A_2-P_2 interval narrows or is abolished (Fig. 2–48). As stroke volume and systemic arterial pressure fall, the systolic murmurs of aortic and pulmonary stenosis and of mitral and tricuspid regurgitation diminish, and the diastolic murmurs of aortic and pulmonary regurgitation and of tricuspid and mitral stenosis soften. As left ventricular volume is reduced, the systolic murmur of hypertrophic

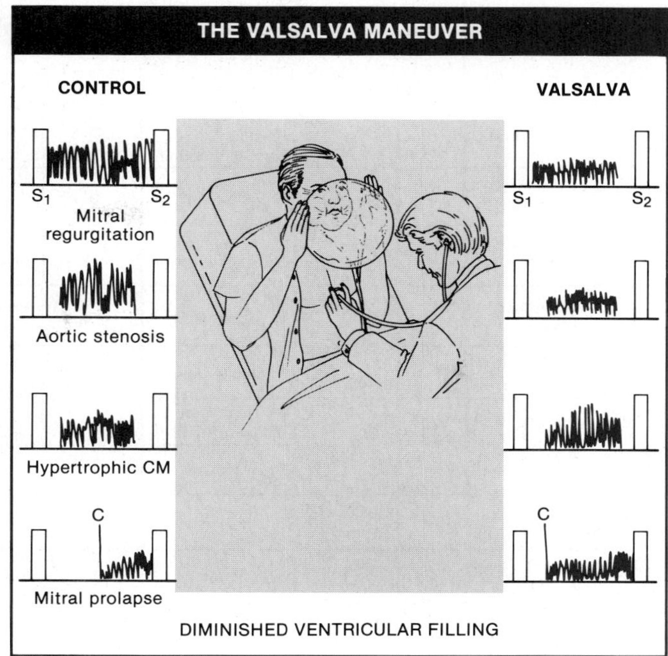

FIGURE 2–48. Changes in four left-sided systolic murmurs during the strain phase of the Valsalva maneuver. (From Grewe, K., Crawford, M. H., and O'Rourke, R. A.: Differentiation of cardiac murmurs by auscultation. Curr. Probl. Cardiol. *13*(10):669, 1988.)

obstructive cardiomyopathy amplifies, and the click and late systolic murmur of mitral valve prolapse begin earlier. In phase III, the sudden increase in systemic venous return is accompanied by wide splitting of the second heart sound and by augmentation of murmurs and filling sounds in the right side of the heart. Murmurs and filling sounds in the left side of the heart return to control levels and may transiently increase during the overshoot of phase IV.

In patients with atrial septal defect, mitral stenosis, or heart failure, the Valsalva maneuver provokes a "square wave" response, negating the four phases and their auscultatory equivalents. The Valsalva maneuver should not be performed in patients with ischemic heart disease because of the accompanying fall in coronary blood flow.

THE MÜLLER MANEUVER. This maneuver is the converse of the Valsalva maneuver but is less frequently employed because it is not as useful.[81] The maneuver is continued for about 10 seconds as the patient forcibly *inspires* while the nose is held closed and the mouth firmly sealed. The Müller maneuver exaggerates the inspiratory effort, widens the split second sound, and augments murmurs and filling sounds originating in the right side of the heart.

POSTURAL CHANGES AND EXERCISE

(Fig. 2–49)

Sudden assumption of the *lying* from the standing or sitting position or sudden passive elevation of both legs results in an increase in venous return, which augments first right ventricular and, several cardiac cycles later, left ventricular stroke volume. The principal auscultatory changes include widening of the splitting of S_2 in all phases of respiration and augmentations of right-sided S_3 and S_4 and, several cardiac cycles later, left-sided S_3 and S_4. The systolic murmurs of pulmonic valve stenosis and aortic stenosis, the systolic murmurs of mitral and tricuspid regurgitation and ventricular septal defect, and most functional systolic murmurs are augmented. On the other hand, because left ventricular end-diastolic volume is increased, the systolic murmur of hypertrophic obstructive

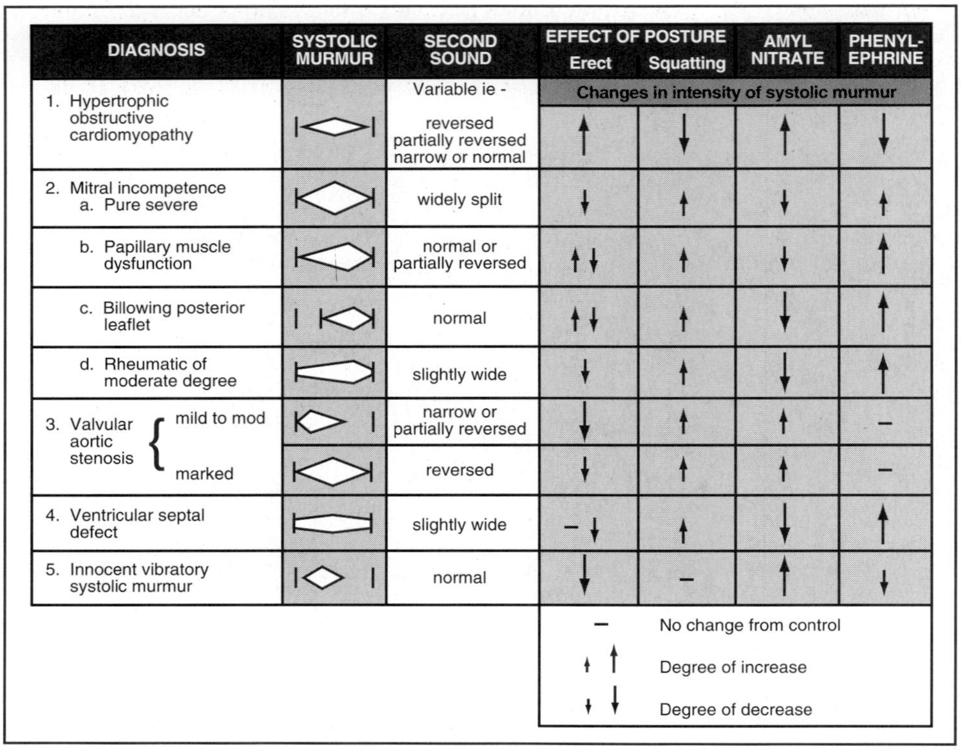

DIAGNOSIS	SYSTOLIC MURMUR	SECOND SOUND	EFFECT OF POSTURE Erect	EFFECT OF POSTURE Squatting	AMYL NITRATE	PHENYL-EPHRINE
			Changes in intensity of systolic murmur			
1. Hypertrophic obstructive cardiomyopathy		Variable ie - reversed partially reversed narrow or normal	↑	↓	↑	↓
2. Mitral incompetence a. Pure severe		widely split	↓	↑	↓	↑
b. Papillary muscle dysfunction		normal or partially reversed	↑↓	↑	↓	↑
c. Billowing posterior leaflet		normal	↑↓	↑	↓	↑
d. Rheumatic of moderate degree		slightly wide	↓	↑	↓	↑
3. Valvular aortic stenosis — mild to mod		narrow or partially reversed	↓	↑	↑	–
3. Valvular aortic stenosis — marked		reversed	↓	↑	↑	–
4. Ventricular septal defect		slightly wide	– ↓	↑	↓	↑
5. Innocent vibratory systolic murmur		normal	↓	–	↑	↓

– No change from control
↑ ↑ Degree of increase
↓ ↓ Degree of decrease

FIGURE 2–49. Diagrammatic representation of the character of the systolic murmur and of the second heart sound in five conditions. The effects of posture, amyl nitrite inhalation, and phenylephrine injection on the intensity of the murmur are shown. (Modified from Barlow, J. B.: Perspectives on the Mitral Valve. Philadelphia, F. A. Davis, 1987, p. 138.)

cardiomyopathy is diminished, and the midsystolic click and late systolic murmur associated with mitral valve prolapse are delayed and sometimes attenuated (see p. 31) (Fig. 2–21).

Rapid standing or sitting up from a lying position or rapid standing from a squatting posture has the opposite effect; in patients in whom there is relatively wide splitting of S_2 during exhalation—a finding that may be confused with fixed splitting—the width of the splitting is reduced, so that a normal pattern emerges during the respiratory cycle. No change in splitting occurs in patients with true fixed splitting. The decrease in venous return reduces stroke volume and innocent pulmonary flow murmurs as well as the murmurs of semilunar valve stenosis and of AV valve regurgitation. The auscultatory changes in hypertrophic cardiomyopathy and mitral valve prolapse are opposite to those on assumption of the lying posture described above.

SQUATTING. A sudden change from standing to squatting increases venous return and systemic resistance simultaneously. Stroke volume and arterial pressure rise, and the latter may induce a transient reflex bradycardia. The auscultatory features include augmentation of S_3 and S_4 (from both ventricles) and as a consequence of an increase in stroke volume, the systolic murmurs of pulmonary and aortic stenosis and the diastolic murmurs of tricuspid and mitral stenosis become louder, with right-sided events preceding left-sided events. Squatting may make audible a previously inaudible murmur of aortic regurgitation.

The elevation of arterial pressure increases blood flow through the right ventricular outflow tract of patients with tetralogy of Fallot and increases the volume of mitral regurgitation and of the left-to-right shunt through a ventricular septal defect, thereby increasing the intensity of the systolic murmur in these conditions. Also, the diastolic murmur of aortic regurgitation is augmented consequent to an increase in aortic reflux. The combination of elevated arterial pressure and increased venous return increases left ventricular size, which reduces the obstruction to outflow and thus the intensity of the systolic murmur of hypertrophic obstructive cardiomyopathy[2]; the midsystolic click and the late systolic murmur of mitral valve prolapse are delayed.

OTHER POSITIONAL CHANGES. *Assumption of the left lateral recumbent position* accentuates the intensity of S_1, S_3, and S_4 originating from the left side of the heart; the opening snap and the murmurs associated with mitral stenosis and regurgitation; the midsystolic click and late systolic murmur of mitral valve prolapse; and the Austin Flint murmur associated with aortic regurgitation. *Sitting up and leaning forward* make the diastolic murmurs of aortic and pulmonary regurgitation more readily audible.

Hyperextension of the shoulders is an important positional maneuver that assists in assessing supraclavicular systolic murmurs.[134] The mechanism responsible for diminution in the intensity of normal supraclavicular systolic murmurs with hyperextension of the shoulders is apparently related to the effect of the maneuver on the site of origin of the murmurs in the proximal brachiocephalic arteries as they leave the aortic arch. *Stretching the neck* to elicit a venous hum is illustrated in Figure 2–50.

Passive elevation of the legs with the patient supine transiently increases venous return and augments third heart sounds. Pericardial rubs may be more readily detected when the patient is on elbows and knees (Fig. 2–51), a physical maneuver designed to increase the contact of visceral and parietal pericardium (see above).

ISOMETRIC EXERCISE. This can be carried out simply and reproducibly using a calibrated handgrip device or hand ball. (It is useful to carry out isometric exercise bilaterally simultaneously.) Isometric exercise should be avoided in patients with ventricular arrhythmias and myocardial ischemia, both of which can be intensified by this activity. Handgrip should be sustained for 20 to 30 seconds, but a Valsalva maneuver during the handgrip must be avoided. Isometric exercise results in transient but significant increases in systemic vascular resistance, arterial pressure, heart rate, cardiac output, left ventricular filling pressure, and heart size. As a consequence, (1) S_3 and S_4 originating from the left side of the heart become accentuated, (2) the

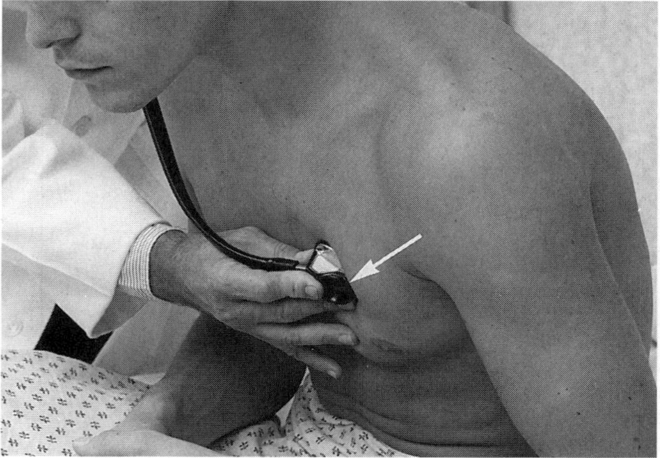

FIGURE 2–50. The soft, high-frequency early diastolic murmur of aortic regurgitation or pulmonary hypertensive regurgitation is best elicited by applying the diaphragm of the stethoscope very firmly to the mid-left sternal edge (arrow) as the patient sits and leans forward with breath held in full exhalation.

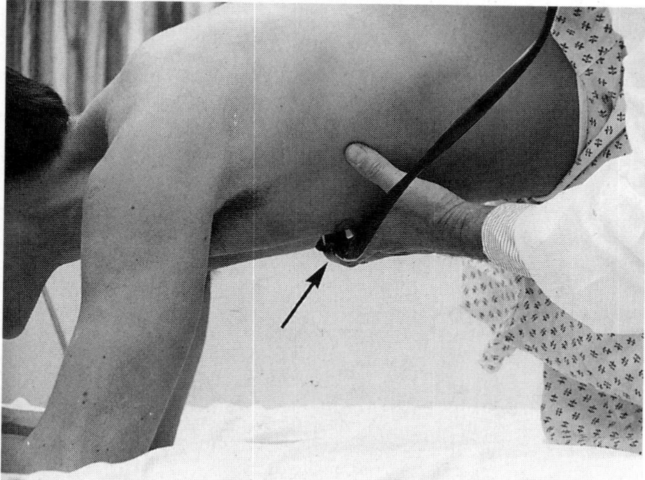

FIGURE 2–51. A technique for eliciting a pericardial rub. The diaphragm of the stethoscope is firmly applied to the precordium *(arrow)* while the patient rests on elbows and knees.

systolic murmur of aortic stenosis is diminished as a result of reduction of the pressure gradient across the aortic valve,[164,165] (3) the diastolic murmur of aortic regurgitation and the systolic murmurs of rheumatic mitral regurgitation and ventricular septal defect increase, (4) the diastolic murmur of mitral stenosis becomes louder consequent to the increase in cardiac output, and (5) the systolic murmur of hypertrophic obstructive cardiomyopathy diminishes and the systolic click and late systolic murmur of mitral valve prolapse are delayed because of the increased left ventricular volume.

PHARMACOLOGICAL AGENTS

(Fig. 2–49)

Inhalation of *amyl nitrite* is carried out by placing an ampule in gauze near the supine patient's nose and then crushing the ampule. The patient is asked to take three or four deep breaths over 10 to 15 seconds, after which the amyl nitrite is removed. The drug produces marked vasodilatation, resulting in the first 30 seconds in a reduction of systemic arterial pressure, and 30 to 60 seconds later in a reflex tachycardia, followed in turn by a reflex *increase* in cardiac output, velocity of blood flow, and heart rate.[2,155–158,166] The major auscultatory changes occur in the first 30 seconds following inhalation. S_1 is augmented and A_2 is diminished. The opening snaps of the mitral and tricuspid valves become louder, and as arterial pressure falls, the A_2-opening snap interval shortens. An S_3 originating in either ventricle is augmented, owing to greater rapidity of ventricular filling, but because mitral regurgitation is reduced, the S_3 associated with this lesion is diminished. The systolic murmurs of aortic valve stenosis, pulmonary stenosis, hypertrophic obstructive cardiomyopathy, tricuspid regurgitation, and functional systolic murmurs are all accentuated.

The reduction of arterial pressure increases the right-to-left shunt and decreases the blood flow from the right ventricle to the pulmonary artery and diminishes the midsystolic murmur in patients with tetralogy of Fallot. The increase in cardiac output augments the diastolic murmurs of mitral and tricuspid stenosis and of pulmonary regurgitation and the systolic murmur of tricuspid regurgitation. However, as a result of the fall in systemic arterial pressure, the systolic murmurs of mitral regurgitation and ventricular septal defect, the diastolic murmurs of aortic regurgitation (Fig. 2–41), and the Austin Flint murmur as well as the continuous murmurs of patent ductus arteriosus and of systemic arteriovenous fistula are all diminished.[164] The reduction of cardiac size results in an earlier appearance of the midsystolic click and late systolic murmur of mitral valve prolapse; the intensity of the systolic murmur exhibits a variable response.

The response to amyl nitrite is useful in distinguishing (1) the systolic murmur of aortic stenosis (which is augmented) from that of mitral regurgitation (which is diminished),[166] (2) the systolic murmur of tricuspid regurgitation (augmented) from that of mitral regurgitation (diminished), (3) the systolic murmur of isolated pulmonary stenosis (augmented) from that of tetralogy of Fallot (diminished), (4) the diastolic rumbling murmur of mitral stenosis (augmented) from the Austin Flint murmur of aortic regurgitation (diminished), and (5) the early blowing diastolic murmur of pulmonary regurgitation (augmented) from that of aortic regurgitation (diminished).

Methoxamine and *phenylephrine* increase systemic arterial pressure and exert an effect opposite to that of amyl nitrite. In general, methoxamine, 3 to 5 mg intravenously, elevates arterial pressure by 20 to 40 mm Hg for 10 to 20 minutes, but phenylephrine is preferred because of its shorter duration of action; 0.3 to 0.5 mg of phenylephrine administered intravenously elevates systolic pressure by approximately 30 mm Hg for only 3 to 5 minutes. Both drugs cause reflex bradycardia and decreased contractility and cardiac output. They should not be used in the presence of congestive heart failure and systemic hypertension.

After administration, the intensity of S_1 is usually reduced, and the A_2-mitral opening snap interval becomes prolonged. The responses of S_3 and S_4 are variable. As a result of the increased arterial pressure, the diastolic murmur of aortic regurgitation; the systolic murmurs of mitral regurgitation (Fig. 2–39), ventricular septal defect, and tetralogy of Fallot; and the continuous murmurs of patent ductus arteriosus and systemic arteriovenous fistula all become louder.[164] On the other hand, as a consequence of the increase in left ventricular size, the systolic murmur of hypertrophic obstructive cardiomyopathy becomes softer, and the click and late systolic murmur of mitral valve prolapse are delayed. The reduction in cardiac output diminishes the systolic murmur of aortic valve stenosis, functional systolic murmurs, and the diastolic murmur of mitral stenosis. The rumbling diastolic murmurs of mitral regurgitation and the Austin Flint murmur also diminish.

REFERENCES

THE GENERAL PHYSICAL EXAMINATION

1. Marriott, H. J. L.: Bedside Cardiac Diagnosis. Philadelphia, J. B. Lippincott Co., 1993.
2. Perloff, J. K.: Physical Examination of the Heart and Circulation. 2nd ed. Philadelphia, W. B. Saunders Company, 1990.
3. Sapira, J. D.: The Art and Science of Bedside Diagnosis. Baltimore, Urban & Schwartzenberg, 1990.
4. Constant, J.: Bedside Cardiology, 4th ed. Boston, Little, Brown & Co., 1993.
5. Brady, P. M., Zive, M. A., Goldberg, R. J., et al.: A new wrinkle to the earlobe crease. Arch. Intern. Med. *147*:65, 1987.
6. Kirkham, N., Murrels, T., Melcher, S. H., and Morrison, E. A.: Diagonal ear lobe creases and fatal cardiovascular disease: A necropsy study. Br. Heart J. *61*:361, 1989.
7. Roberts, N. K., Perloff, J. K., and Kark, R. A. P.: Cardiac conduction in the Kearns-Sayre syndrome (a neuromuscular disorder associated with progressive external ophthalmoplegia and pigmentary retinopathy). Am. J. Cardiol. *44*:1396, 1979.
8. Cogan, D. G.: Ophthalmic Manifestations of Systemic Vascular Disease. Philadelphia, W. B. Saunders Company, 1974.
9. Allen, S. J., and Naylor, D.: Pulsation of the eyeballs in tricuspid regurgitation. Can. Med. Assoc. J. *133*:119, 1985.
10. Byrd, M. D.: Lateral systolic pulsation of the earlobe: A sign of tricuspid regurgitation. Am. J. Cardiol. *54*:244, 1984.
11. Criscitiello, M. G., Ronan, J. A., Besterman, E. M., and Schoenwetter, W.: Cardiovascular abnormalities in osteogenesis imperfecta. Circulation *31*:255, 1965.
12. St. John Sutton, M. G., Tajik, A. J., Giuliani, E. R., et al.: Hypertrophic obstructive cardiomyopathy and lentiginosis: A little known neural ectodermal syndrome. Am. J. Cardiol. *47*:214, 1981.

13. Basson, C. T., Cowley, G. S., Solomon, S. D., et al.: The clinical and genetic spectrum of the Holt-Oram syndrome (heart-hand syndrome) N. Engl. J. Med. *330*:885, 1994; erratum, N. Engl. J. Med. *330*:1627, 1994.
14. Buckley, M. J., Mason, D. T., Ross, J., Jr., and Braunwald, E.: Reversed differential cyanosis with equal desaturation of the upper limbs. Syndrome of complete transposition of the great vessels with complete interruption of the aortic arch. Am. J. Cardiol. *15*:111, 1965.
15. Finger clubbing. Lancet *1*:1285, 1975.
16. Lanken, P. N., and Fishman, A. P.: Clubbing and hypertrophic osteoarthropathy. *In* Fishman, A. P. (ed.): Pulmonary Diseases and Disorders. New York, McGraw-Hill Book Co., 1980, pp. 84–91.
17. Yee, J., McAllister, C. K.: The utility of Osler's nodes in the diagnosis of infective endocarditis. Chest *92*:751, 1987.
18. Manga, P., Vythilingum, S., and Mitha, A. S.: Pulsatile hepatomegaly in constrictive pericarditis. Br. Heart J. *52*:465, 1984.
19. Coralli, R. J., and Crawley, I. S.: Hepatic pulsations in constrictive pericarditis. Am. J. Cardiol. *58*:370, 1986.
20. Ewy, G. A.: The abdominojugular test: Technique and hemodynamic correlates. Ann. Intern. Med. *109*:456, 1988.
21. Swartz, M. H.: Jugular venous pressure pulse: Its value in cardiac diagnosis. Primary Cardiol. *8*:197, 1982.
22. Stojnic, B. B., Brecker, S. J., Xiao, H. B., and Gibson, D. G.: Jugular venous "a" wave in pulmonary hypertension: New insights from a Doppler echocardiographic study. Br. Heart J. *68*:187, 1992.
23. Butman, S. M., Ewy, G. A., Standen, J. R., et al.: Bedside cardiovascular examination in patients with severe chronic heart failure: Importance of rest or inducible jugular venous distension. J. Am. Coll. Cardiol. *22*:968, 1993.
24. Ducas, J., Magder, S., and McGregor, M.: Validity of the hepatojugular reflux as a clinical test for congestive heart failure. Am. J. Cardiol. *52*:1299, 1983.
25. Sochowski, R. A., Dubbin, J. D., and Naqvi, S. Z.: Clinical and hemodynamic assessment of the hepatojugular reflux. Am. J. Cardiol. *66*:1002, 1990.
26. Petrie, J. C., et al.: Recommendations on blood pressure measurement. Br. Med. J. *293*:611, 1986.
27. Frohlich, E. D., et al.: Recommendations for human blood pressure determination by sphygmomanometers. Report of a special task force appointed by the steering committee, American Heart Association. Circulation *77*:501a, 1988.
28. O'Brien, E., et al.: Blood pressure measurement: Current practice and future trends. Br. Med. J. *290*:729, 1985.
29. Maisel, A. S., Atwood, J. E., Goldberger, A. L.: Hepatojugular reflux: Useful in the bedside diagnosis of tricuspid regurgitation. Ann. Intern. Med. *101*:781, 1984.
30. Linfors, E. W., Feussner, J. R., Blessing, C. L., et al.: Spurious hypertension in the obese patient. Effect of sphygmomanometer cuff size on prevalence of hypertension. Arch. Intern. Med. *144*:1482, 1984.
31. Manning, D. M., Kuchirka, C., and Kaminski, J.: Miscuffing: Inappropriate blood pressure cuff application. Circulation *68*:763, 1983.
32. Nelson, W. P., and Egbert, A. M.: How to measure blood pressure—accurately. Prim. Cardiol. *10*:14, 1984.
33. Kirkendall, W. M., Burton, A. C., Epstein, F. H., and Freis, E. D.: Recommendations for human blood pressure determination by sphygmomanometers. Circulation *36*:980, 1967.
34. Londe, S., and Klitzner, T. S.: Auscultatory blood pressure measurement—Effect of pressure on the head of the stethoscope. West. J. Med. *141*:193, 1984.
35. Mancia, G., Grassi, G., Pomidossi, G., et al.: Effects of blood-pressure measurement by the doctor on patient's blood pressure and heart rate. Lancet *2*:695, 1983.
36. Gould, B. A., Hornung, R. S., Kieso, H. A., et al.: Is the blood pressure the same in both arms? Clin. Cardiol. *8*:423, 1985.
37. Sapira, J. D.: Quincke, de Musset, Duroziez, and Hill: Some aortic regurgitations. South. Med. J. *74*:459, 1981.
38. Abrams, J.: The arterial pulse. Prim. Cardiol. *8*:138, 1982.
39. Schlant, R. C., and Feiner, J. M.: The arterial pulse—clinical manifestations. Curr. Probl. Cardiol. Vol. 1, No. 5, 1976, 50 pp.
40. Perloff, J. K.: The physiologic mechanisms of cardiac and vascular physical signs. J. Am. Coll. Cardiol. *1*:184, 1983.
41. Smith, D., and Craige, E.: Mechanism of the dicrotic pulse. Br. Heart J. *56*:531, 1986.
42. Elkins, R. C., Morrow, A. G., Vasko, J. S., and Braunwald, E.: The effects of mitral regurgitation on the pattern of instantaneous aortic blood flow. Clinical and experimental observations. Circulation *36*:45, 1967.
43. Rowe, G. G., Afonso, S., Castillo, C. A., and McKenna, D. H.: The mechanism of the production of Duroziez's murmur. N. Engl. J. Med. *272*:1207, 1965.
44. Fleming, P. R.: The mechanism of the pulsus bisferiens. Br. Heart J. *19*:519, 1957.
45. Talley, J. D.: Recognition, etiology, and clinical implications of pulsus bisferiens. Heart Dis. Stroke *3*:309, 1994.
46. Braunwald, E., Lambrew, C. T., Rockoff, S. D., et al.: Idiopathic hypertrophic subaortic stenosis. I. A description of the disease based upon an analysis of 64 patients. Circulation *30*(Suppl. 4):3, 1964.
47. Bartall, M., Auber, S., Desser, K. B., and Benchimol, A.: Normalization of the external carotid pulse tracing of hypertrophic subaortic stenosis during Müller's maneuver. Chest *74*:77, 1978.
48. Lab, M. J., and Seed, W. A.: Pulses alternans. Cardiovasc. Res. *27*:1407, 1993.
49. Brockenbrough, E. C., Braunwald, E., and Morrow, A. G.: A hemodynamic technic for the detection of hypertrophic subaortic stenosis. Circulation *23*:189, 1961.
50. Rebuck, A. S., and Pengelly, L. D.: Development of pulsus paradoxus in the presence of airways obstruction. N. Engl. J. Med. *288*:66, 1973.
51. Massumi, R. A., Mason, D. T., Zakauddin, V., et al.: Reversed pulsus paradoxus. N. Engl. J. Med. *289*:1272, 1973.
52. Kurtz, K. J.: Dynamic vascular auscultation. Am. J. Med. *76*:1066, 1984.
53. Linhart, J.: Bedside examination of peripheral vascular disease. Eur. Heart J. *4*:137, 1983.

THE CARDIAC EXAMINATION

54. Davies, H.: Chest deformities in congenital heart disease. Br. J. Dis. Chest *53*:151, 1959.
55. Perloff, J. K.: Diagnostic inferences drawn from observation and palpation of the precordium with special reference to congenital heart disease. Adv. Cardiopulm. Dis. *4*:13, 1969.
56. Beiser, G. D., Epstein, S. E., Stampfer, M., et al.: Impairment of cardiac function in patients with pectus excavatum. N. Engl. J. Med. *287*:267, 1972.
57. Ansari, A.: The "straight back" syndrome. Clin. Cardiol. *8*:290, 1985.
58. Abrams, J.: Precordial palpation. *In* Horwitz, L. D., and Groves, B. M. (eds.): Signs and Symptoms in Cardiology. Philadelphia, J. B. Lippincott, 1985, pp. 156–177.
59. O'Neill, T. W., Smith, M., Barry, M., and Graham, I. M.: Diagnostic value of the apex beat. Lancet *1*(8635):410, 1989.
60. Basta, I. L., and Bettinger, J. J.: The cardiac impulse: A new look at an old art. Am. Heart J. *97*:96, 1979.
61. Eilen, S. D., Crawford, M. H., and O'Rourke, R. A.: Accuracy of precordial palpation for detecting increased left ventricular volume. Ann. Intern. Med. *99*:628, 1983.
62. Bancroft, W. H., Jr., Eddleman, E. E., Jr., and Larkin, L. N.: Methods and physical characteristics of the kineto-cardiographic and apex cardiographic systems for recording low-frequency precordial motion. Am. Heart J. *73*:756, 1967.
63. Ranganathan, Juma, Z., and Sivaciyan, V.: The apical impulse in coronary heart disease. Clin. Cardiol. *8*:20, 1985.
64. Dressler, W.: Clinical Aids in Cardiac Diagnosis. New York, Grune and Stratton, 1970, 246 pp.
65. Gillam, P. M. S., et al.: The left parasternal impulse. Br. Heart J. *26*:726, 1964.
66. Counihan, T. B., Rappaport, M. B., and Sprague, H. B.: Physiologic and physical factors that govern the clinical appreciation of cardiac thrills. Circulation *4*:716, 1951.
67. Littmann, D.: An approach to the ideal stethoscope. JAMA *178*:504, 1961.
68. Kindig, J. R., Beeson, T. P., Campbell, R. W., et al.: Acoustical performance of the stethoscope: A comparative analysis. Am. Heart J. *104*:269, 1982.

HEART SOUNDS

69. Leatham, A.: Auscultation of the heart. Lancet *II*:703, 1958.
70. O'Toole, J. D., Reddy, P. S., Curtiss, E. L., et al.: The contribution of tricuspid valve closure to the first heart sound. An intracardiac micromanometer study. Circulation *53*:752, 1976.
71. Brooks, N., Leech, G., and Leatham, A.: Complete right bundle branch block: Echophonocardiographic study of the first heart sound and right ventricular contraction times. Br. Heart J. *41*:637, 1979.
72. Burggraf, G. W.: The first heart sound in left bundle branch block: An echophonocardiographic study. Circulation *63*:429, 1981.
73. Burggraf, G. W., and Craige E.: The first heart sound in complete heart block. Circulation *50*:17, 1974.
74. Leech, G., Brooks, N., Green-Wilkinson, A., and Leatham, A.: Mechanism of influence of PR interval on loudness of first heart sound. Br. Heart J. *43*:138, 1980.
75. Perloff, J. K.: The Clinical Recognition of Congenital Heart Disease, 4th ed. Philadelphia, W. B. Saunders Company, 1994.
76. Waider, W., and Craige, E.: The first heart sound and ejection sounds: Echophonocardiographic correlation with valvular events. Am. J. Cardiol. *35*:346, 1975.
77. Mills, P. G., Brodie, B., McLaurin, L., et al.: Echocardiographic and hemodynamic relationships of ejection sounds. Circulation *56*:430, 1977.
78. Hultgren, H. N., Reeve, R., Cohn, K., and McLeod, R.: The ejection click of valvular pulmonic stenosis. Circulation *40*:631, 1969.
79. Devereux, R., Perloff, J. K., Derchek, N., and Josephson, M.: Mitral valve prolapse. Circulation *54*:3, 1976.
80. Bank, A. J., Sharkey, S. W., Goldsmith, S. R., et al.: Atypical systolic clicks produced by prolapsing mitral valve masses. Am. J. Cardiol. *69*:1491, 1992.
81. Rothman, A., and Goldberger, A. L.: Aids to cardiac auscultation. Ann. Intern. Med. *99*:346, 1983.
82. Lembo, N. J., Dell'Italia, J. L., Crawford, M. H., and O'Rourke, R. A.: Bedside diagnosis of systolic murmurs. N. Engl. J. Med. *318*:1572, 1988.
83. Potain, P. C.: Clinique médicale de la Charité. Paris, Masson, 1894. *In* McKusick, V. A.: Cardiovascular Sound in Health and Disease. Baltimore, Williams and Wilkins Co., 1958.

84. Potain, P. C.: Note sur les dédoublements normaux des bruits du coeur. Bull. Mem. Soc. Med. Hop. Paris. 3:138, 1866.
85. Leatham, A.: The second heart sound. Key to auscultation of the heart. Acta Cardiol. 19:395, 1964.
86. Leatham, A.: Splitting of the first and second heart sounds. Lancet II:607, 1954.
87. Kupari, M.: Aortic valve closure and cardiac vibrations in the genesis of the second heart sound. Am. J. Cardiol. 52:152, 1983.
88. Curtiss, E. I., Matthews, D. G., and Shaver, J. A.: Mechanism of normal splitting of the second heart sound. Circulation 51:157, 1975.
89. Shaver, J. A., Nadolny, R. A., O'Toole, J. D., et al.: Sound-pressure correlates of the second heart sound. Circulation 49:316, 1974.
90. Perloff, J. K., and Harvey, W. P.: Auscultatory and phonocardiographic manifestations of pure mitral regurgitation. Prog. Cardiovasc. Dis. 5:172, 1962.
91. Xiao, H. B., Faiek, A. H., and Gibson, D. G.: Re-evaluation of normal splitting of the second heart sound in patients with classical left bundle branch block. Int. J. Cardiol. 45:163, 1994.
92. Hultgren, H. N., Craige, E., Nakamura, T., and Bilisoly, J.: Left bundle branch block and mechanical events of the cardiac cycle. Am. J. Cardiol. 52:755, 1985.
93. Steell, G.: The murmur of high pressure in the pulmonary artery. Med. Chron. (Manchester) 9:182, 1888–1889.
94. de Leon, A. C., Perloff, J. K., Twigg, H., and Moyd, M.: The straight back syndrome. Circulation 32:193, 1965.
95. Thayer, W. S.: On the early diastolic sound (the so-called third heart sound). Boston Med. Surg. J. 158:713, 1908.
96. Wood, P.: An appreciation of mitral stenosis. I. Clinical features. Br. Med. J. 1:1051, 1954; II. Investigations and results. 1:1113, 1954.
97. Joyner, C. R., Jr., and Dear, W. E.: The motion of the normal and abnormal mitral valve. A study of the opening snap. J. Clin. Invest. 45:1029, 1966.
98. Connolly, D. C., and Mann, R. J.: Dominic J. Corrigan (1802–1880) and his description of the pericardial knock. Mayo Clin. Proc. 55:771, 1980.
99. Tyberg, T. I., Goodyer, A. V. N., and Langou, R. A.: Genesis of the pericardial knock in constrictive pericarditis. Am. J. Cardiol. 46:570, 1980.
100. Bass, N. M., and Sharatt, G. J. P.: Left atrial myxoma diagnosed by echocardiography with observations on tumor movement. Br. Heart J. 35:1332, 1973.
101. Van de Werf, F., Minten, J., Carmeliet, P., et al.: Genesis of the third and fourth heart sounds. J. Clin. Invest. 73:1400, 1984.
102. Van de Werf, F., Boel, A., Geboers, J., et al.: Diastolic properties of the left ventricle in normal adults and in patients with third heart sounds. Circulation 69:1070, 1984.
103. Potain, P. C.: Concerning the cardiac rhythm called gallop rhythm. Bull. Men. Soc. Med. Hop. (Paris) 12:137, 1876.
104. Kupari, M., Koskinen, P., Virolainen, J., et al.: Prevalence and predictors of audible physiological third heart sound in a population sampled aged 36 to 37 years. Circulation 89:1189, 1994.
105. Van de Werf, F., Geboers, J., Math, L., et al.: The mechanism of disappearance of the physiologic third heart sound with age. Circulation 73:877, 1986.
106. Folland, E. D., Kriegel, B. J., Henderson, W. G., et al.: Implications of third heart sounds in patients with valvular heart disease. The Veterans Affairs Cooperative Study on Valvular Heart Disease. N. Engl. J. Med. 327:458, 1992.
107. Aronow, W. S., Papageorge's, N. P., Uyeyama, R. R., and Cassidy, J.: Maximal treadmill stress test correlated with postexercise phonocardiogram in normal subjects. Circulation 43:884, 1971.
108. Ozawa, Y., Smith D., and Craige, E.: Origin of the third heart sound. I. Studies in dogs. Circulation 67:393, 1983.
109. Ozawa, Y., Smith, D., and Craige, E.: Origin of the third heart sound. II. Studies in human subjects. Circulation 67:399, 1983.
110. Drzewiecki, G. M., Wasicko, M. J., and Li, J. K.: Diastolic mechanics and the origin of the third heart sound. Ann. Biomed. Engin. 19:651, 1991.
111. Downes, T. R., Dunson, W., Stewart, K., et al.: Mechanism of physiologic and pathologic S_3 gallop sounds. Am. Soc. Echocardiol. 5:211, 1992.
112. Ishimitsu, T., Smith, D., Berko, B., and Craige, E.: Origin of the third heart sound: Comparison of ventricular wall dynamics in hyperdynamic and hypodynamic types. J. Am. Coll. Cardiol. 5:268, 1985.
113. Perloff, J. K.: Auscultatory and phonocardiographic manifestations of pulmonary hypertension. Prog. Cardiovasc. Dis. 9:303, 1967.
114. Gibson, T. C., Madry, R., Grossman, W., et al.: The A wave of the apex cardiogram and left ventricular diastolic stiffness. Circulation 49:441, 1974.
115. Perloff, J. K.: Clinical recognition of aortic stenosis. Progr. Cardiovasc. Dis. 10:323, 1964.
116. Cheng, T. O., Ertem, G., and Vera, Z.: Heart sounds in patients with cardiac pacemakers. Chest 62:66, 1972.
117. Harris, A.: Pacemaker "heart sound." Br. Heart J. 29:608, 1967.

MURMURS

118. Pepper, O. H. P.: Medical Etymology. Philadelphia, W. B. Saunders Company, 1949.
119. Freeman, A. R., and Levine, S. A.: The clinical significance of the systolic murmur. A study of 1000 consecutive "non-cardiac" cases. Ann. Intern. Med. 6:1371, 1933.
120. Roberts, W. C., Perloff, J. K., and Costantino, T.: Severe valvular aortic stenosis in patients over 65 years of age. Am. J. Cardiol. 27:497, 1971.
121. Gallavardin, L., and Pauper-Ravault: Le souffle du rétré cissement aortique peut changer de timbre et devenir musical dans se propagation apexienne. Lyon Med. 1925, p. 523.
122. Stokes, W.: Diseases of the Heart in Aorta. Philadelphia, Lindsay and Blakiston, 1855.
123. Still, G. F.: Common Disorders and Diseases of Childhood. London, Henry Frowde, 1909.
124. Burch, G. E., DePasquale, N. P., and Phillips, J. H.: The syndrome of papillary muscle dysfunction. Am. Heart J. 75:399, 1968.
125. Perloff, J. K., and Roberts, W. C.: The mitral apparatus: Functional anatomy of mitral regurgitation. Circulation 46:227, 1972.
126. Rivero-Carvallo, J. M.: Sitno para el diagnostico de las insuficiencias tricuspideas. Arch. Inst. Cardiol. Mexico 16:531, 1946.
127. Leon, D. F., Leonard, J. J., Lancaster, J. F., et al.: Effect of respiration on pansystolic regurgitant murmurs as studied by biatrial intracardiac phonocardiography. Am. J. Med. 39:429, 1965.
128. Sanders, C. A., Scannell, J. G., Harthorne, J. W., and Austen, W. G.: Severe mitral regurgitation secondary to ruptured chordae tendineae. Circulation 31:506, 1965.
129. Sutton, G. C., and Craige, E.: Clinical signs of acute severe mitral regurgitation. Am. J. Cardiol. 20:141, 1967.
130. Ronan, J. A., Steelman, R. B., DeLeon, A. C., et al.: The clinical diagnosis of acute severe mitral insufficiency. Am. J. Cardiol. 27:284, 1971.
131. Rios, J. C., Massumi, R. A., Breesman, W. T., and Sarin, R. K.: Auscultatory features of acute tricuspid regurgitation. Am. J. Cardiol. 23:4, 1969.
132. Ronan, J. A., Perloff, J. K., and Harvey, W. P.: Systolic clicks and the late systolic murmur—intracardiac phonocardiographic evidence of their mitral valve origin. Am. Heart J. 70:319, 1965.
133. Osler, W.: On a remarkable heart murmur, heard at a distance from the chest wall. Med. Times Gaz. Lond. 2:432, 1980.
134. Nelson, W. P., and Hall, R. J.: The innocent supraclavicular arterial bruit—utility of shoulder maneuvers in its recognition. N. Engl. J. Med. 278:778, 1968.
135. Grant, R. P.: A precordial systolic murmur of extracardiac origin during pregnancy. Am. Heart J. 52:944, 1965.
136. Danilowicz, D. A., Rudolph, A. M., Hoffman, J. I. E., and Heyman, M.: Physiologic pressure differences between the main and branch pulmonary arteries in infants. Circulation 45:410, 1972.
137. Morganroth, J., Perloff, J. K., Zeldis, S. M., and Dunkman, W. B.: Acute severe aortic regurgitation: Pathophysiology, clinical recognition and management. Ann. Intern. Med. 87:223, 1977.
138. Fortuin, N. J., and Craige, E.: Echocardiographic studies of genesis of mitral diastolic murmurs. Br. Heart J. 35:75, 1973.
139. Ross, R. S., and Criley, J. M.: Cineangiocardiographic studies of the origin of cardiovascular physical signs. Circulation 30:255, 1964.
140. Perloff, J. K., and Harvey, W. P.: Clinical recognition of tricuspid stenosis. Circulation 22:346, 1960.
141. Flint, A.: On cardiac murmurs. Am. J. Med. Sci. 44:23, 1862.
142. Fortuin, N. J., and Craige, E.: On the mechanisms of the Austin Flint murmur. Circulation 45:558, 1972.
143. Landzberg, J. S., Tflugfelder, P. W., Cassidy, M. M., et al.: Etiology of the Austin Flint murmur. J. Am. Coll. Cardiol. 20:408, 1992.
144. Criley, J. M., and Hermer, H. A.: Crescendo pre-systolic murmur of mitral stenosis with atrial fibrillation. N. Engl. J. Med. 285:1284, 1971.
145. Criley, J. M., Feldman, J. M., and Meredith, T.: Mitral valve closure and the crescendo presystolic murmur. Am. J. Med. 51:456, 1971.
146. Reddy, P. S., Curtiss, E. L., and Salerni, R.: Sound-pressure correlates of the Austin Flint murmur: An intracardiac sound study. Circulation 53:210, 1976.
147. Berman, P.: Austin Flint—America's Laënnec revisited. Arch. Intern. Med. 148:2053, 1988.
148. Williams, X.: Comment in discussion of case of patent ductus arteriosus with aortic valve disease, coarctation of aorta and infective endocarditis reported by Babington. London Med. Gazette 4:822, 1847.
149. Gibson, G. A.: Persistence of the arterial duct and its diagnosis. Edinb. Med. J. 8:1, 1900.
150. Potain, P. C.: Des movements et de bruits qui se passent dans les veines jugulaires. Bull. Mem. Soc. Med. Hop. Paris 4:3, 1867.
151. Cutforth, R., Wideman, J., and Sutherland, R. D.: The genesis of the cervical venous hum. Am. Heart J. 80:488, 1970.
152. McGuire, J., Kotte, J. H., and Helm, R. A.: Acute pericarditis. Circulation 9:425, 1954.
153. Hamman, L.: Mediastinal emphysema. JAMA 128:1, 1945.
154. Cabot, R. C.: Physical Diagnosis. New York, William Wood and Co., 1915.

DYNAMIC AUSCULTATION

155. Grewe, K., Crawford, M. H., and O'Rourke, R. A.: Differentiation of cardiac murmurs by dynamic auscultation. Curr. Probl. Cardiol. 13:671, 1988.
156. Lembro, N. J., Dell'Italia, L. J., Crawford, M. H., and O'Rourke, R. A.: Bedside diagnosis of systolic murmurs. N. Engl. J. Med. 318:1572, 1988.
157. Baragan, J., Fernandez, F., and Thiron, J. M.: Dynamic Auscultation and Phonocardiography. Tavel, M. E., and Tavel, M. E. (eds.). Maryland, Charles Press, 1979.

158. Rothman, A., and Goldberger, A. L.: Aids to cardiac auscultation. Ann. Intern. Med. *99*:346, 1983.
159. Cha, S. D., and Gooch, A. S.: Diagnosis of tricuspid regurgitation. Arch. Intern. Med. *143*:1763, 1983.
160. Barlow, J. B.: Perspectives on the Mitral Valve, Philadelphia, F. A. Davis, 1987.
161. Vrewe, K., Crawford, M. H., and O'Rourke, R. A.: Differentiation of cardiac murmurs by dynamic auscultation. Curr. Probl. Cardiol. *13*:671, 1988.
162. Nishimura, R. A., and Tajik, A. J.: The Valsalva maneuver and response revisited. Mayo Clin. Proc. *61*:211, 1986.
163. Lembro, N. J., Dell'Italia, L. J., Crawford, M. H., and O'Rourke, R. A.: Bedside diagnosis of systolic murmurs. N. Engl. J. Med. *318*:1572, 1988.
164. Criscitiello, M.: Physiologic and pharmacologic aids in cardiac auscultation. *In* Fowler, N. O. (ed.): Cardiac Diagnosis and Treatment. 3rd ed. Hagerstown, Harper and Row, 1980, pp. 77–90.
165. McCraw, D. B., Siegel, W., Stonecipher, H. K., et al.: Response of the heart murmur intensity to isometric (handgrip) exercise. Br. Heart J. *34*:605, 1972.
166. Barlow, J., and Shillingford, J.: The use of amyl nitrite in differentiating mitral and aortic systolic murmurs. Br. Heart J. *20*:162, 1958.
167. Tavel, M. E.: Clinical Phonocardiography and External Pulse Recording. Chicago, Year Book Medical Publishers, 1985.

Chapter 3
Echocardiography

HARVEY FEIGENBAUM

PRINCIPLES OF ECHOCARDIOGRAPHY

CREATION OF IMAGES USING PULSED REFLECTED ULTRASOUND

The term *echocardiography* refers to a group of tests that utilize ultrasound to examine the heart and record information in the form of echoes, i.e., reflected sonic waves.[1-3] The upper limit for audible sound is 20,000 cycles/second, or 20 kiloHertz (kHz = 1000 cycles/second).[1] The sonic frequency used for echocardiography ranges from 1 to 10 million cycles/second, or 1 to 10 megaHertz (MHz).[2] In adults the frequencies commonly employed are 2.0 to 5.0 MHz, while in children they are usually higher, ranging from 3.5 to 10.0 MHz. The resolution of the recording, which is the ability to distinguish two objects that are spatially close together, varies directly with the frequency and inversely with the wavelength. High-frequency (short wavelength) ultrasound can identify separate objects that are less than 1 mm apart. Beams having lower frequencies and longer wavelengths have poorer resolution. However, the degree of penetration, which is the ability to transmit sufficient ultrasonic energy into the chest to provide a satisfactory recording, is inversely proportional to the frequency of the signal. Since a high-frequency ultrasonic beam (i.e., 5 or 10 MHz) is unable to penetrate a thick chest wall, lower frequency ultrasonic beams are used in adults. While this permits penetration through the chest wall, it partially sacrifices resolution; however, even with a transducer producing a beam of 2.50 MHz, which is commonly used in adult echocardiography, it is possible to resolve objects that are 1 to 2 mm apart.

Principles of Ultrasonic Imaging

The principles by which ultrasound creates an image are depicted in Figure 3–1. The transducer at the side of the beaker of water has a piezoelectric element that vibrates very rapidly and produces ultrasound when activated by an electrical field.[3] If a burst of electrical energy is imparted to the transducer, it will emit a burst of ultrasound, which travels through the beaker. As long as the medium through which the sound travels is homogeneous, the ultrasonic waves will travel in a straight line. When the ultrasound strikes an interface between two media that have different acoustical properties, the sound behaves according to the laws of reflection and refraction,[1,2] analogous to light. Whether or not ultrasound is reflected by an interface depends upon the difference in the acoustical impedances of the two media. Although acoustical impedance is the product of the density of the object and the velocity of sound through that object, for all practical purposes one can consider the acoustical impedance to be a function of density. Thus, if the interface is between a liquid and a solid, the ultrasonic wave will generally be reflected. If the interface is between two solids of different densities, the quantity of reflected ultrasound is usually less. Thus the quantity of energy reflected is directly proportional to the difference in the acoustical impedances (or densities) of the object and its surrounding media.

The left panel of Figure 3–1 shows diagrammatically an ultrasonic beam, which consists of individual bursts of ultrasound that leave the transducer, travel through the fluid, strike the far side of the beaker, are reflected by this interface, retrace their original path, and again strike the transducer. The piezoelectric element in the transducer not only converts electrical energy into ultrasonic impulses but also converts ultrasound back to electrical energy. Thus, when the reflected ultrasound (echo) strikes the piezoelectric element in the transducer, an electrical signal is produced. If the time it takes for (1) the ultrasound to leave the transducer and return and (2) the velocity of sound through the medium are both known, the distance between the transducer and the reflected interface can be calculated. By calibration of the echograph for a velocity of sound in the medium under examination the time that it takes for the ultrasound to leave and return as an echo can be automatically converted to distance. Thus, the far wall of the beaker is depicted on the oscilloscope as being 6 cm from the transducer.

If a rod is placed in the water so that it transects the ultrasonic beam, part of the energy will strike it and be reflected by the rod before the beam strikes the far side of the beaker. Thus, the returning ultrasonic energy or echo from the rod will strike the transducer sooner than that returning from the far side of the beaker, and the corresponding electrical signal produced by the echo from the rod will be closer to the transducer than will that from the beaker. Also, since some of the ultrasonic energy is reflected by the rod, less energy will remain to strike the far wall of the beaker, and the magnitude of the echo (Fig. 3–1, center panel) will be reduced. If the interface is a very strong reflector of sound, no energy may transverse the object and no images are obtained behind the object, i.e., acoustic shadowing. There are adjustments in ultrasonic instrumentation that provide depth compensation and thereby correct for the usually gradual loss of ultrasonic energy from distant or far objects. From examination of the A-mode echo ("A" refers to amplitude) in

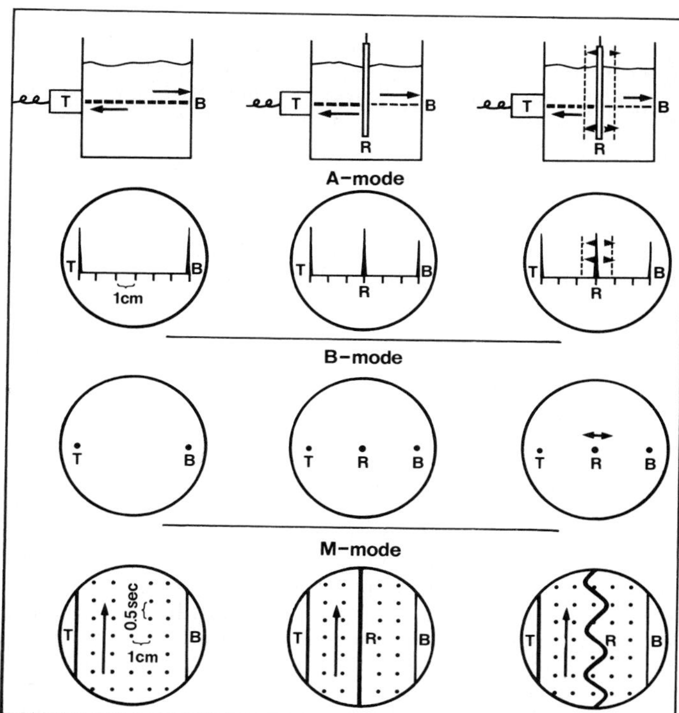

FIGURE 3–1. The principles of acoustic imaging using pulsed reflected ultrasound (see text for details). T = transducer; B = beaker; R = rod. (Modified from Feigenbaum, H., and Zaky, A.: Use of diagnostic ultrasound in clinical cardiology. J. Indiana State Med. Assoc. *59:*140, 1966.)

Figure 3–1 (center panel), one could deduce that the far wall of the beaker is 6 cm from the transducer and that an echo-reflecting object is present in the center of the beaker, 3 cm from the transducer.

Imaging a Moving Object

If the rod were moving back and forth as in the right panel of Figure 3–1, the ultrasonic examination would differ. The transducer functions as a transmitter of ultrasound for a very short time, just over 1 μsec in commercial echocardiographs. During the remaining time the transducer functions as a receiver, waiting for echoes to be converted into electrical signals. The rapidity of the repetition rate with which the transducer fires the 1 μsec impulses varies depending upon the design of the instrument. In most situations the transducer functions as a receiver for over 90 per cent of the time.

A-Mode, B-Mode, and M-Mode Presentations

In the left and center panels of Figure 3–1, the wall of the beaker and the rod are not moving. All the ultrasonic impulses firing at a rate of 1000/sec take the same time to leave the transducer and return as echoes. Therefore the signals or echoes seen on the oscilloscope are static. In the right panel, the object moves constantly, the time required for the ultrasound to leave the transducer and return as an echo varies correspondingly, and the echo signal on the oscilloscope moves. In the A-mode presentation the echo from the rod moves back and forth within the center of the beaker. To record the motion of the rod, one converts the amplitude of the echo to brightness, which changes the display from the A-mode to the B-mode ("B" refers to brightness), in which the returning echoes are displayed on the oscilloscope as dots rather than as spikes. Stronger signals are therefore taller on the A-mode and brighter on the B-mode presentation. On the M-mode presentation ("M" refers to motion), displayed in Figure 3–1, the oscilloscope sweeps from bottom to top. In the left and center panels the structures are fixed, and therefore the M-mode presentation shows simply a series of parallel lines. In the right panel the rod moves back and forth regularly, its echo inscribing a sinusoidal curve on the M-mode oscilloscope.

Thus, the M-mode presentation permits recording of amplitude and of the rate of motion of moving objects with great accuracy; the sampling rate is essentially 1000 pulses/sec, the repetition rate of the transducer. Because electrocardiograms and other cardiac parameters are conventionally displayed on the oscilloscope together with the echocardiographs, the oscilloscope usually sweeps from left to right rather than from bottom to top; therefore the transducer is generally displayed at the top of the oscilloscopic image rather than on the left side, as depicted in Figure 3–1.

M-Mode Echocardiography

TECHNIQUE. The ultrasonic transducer is ordinarily placed on the surface of the chest, usually along the left sternal border, and the ultrasonic beam is directed toward the part of the heart lobe examined. In Figure 3–2 the ultrasound is depicted as passing through a small portion of the right ventricle, the interventricular septum, and the cavity and posterior wall of the left ventricle. Structures such as the chest wall that do not move with cardiac activity are depicted as horizontal lines. Cardiac walls and valves that move with cardiac action inscribe wavy signals, while the blood-filled cavities are relatively echo free.

THE M-MODE TRACING. An M-mode recording is sometimes called a one-dimensional or an "ice pick" view of the heart. However, since time is the second dimension on M-mode tracings, this display is not truly one-dimensional. The information provided by an isolated M-mode view of the heart, as in Figure 3–2, can be augmented by changing the direction of the ultrasonic beam, as in an arc or sector. With the transducer placed along the left sternal border in approximately the third or fourth intercostal space, the ultrasonic beam can be swept in a sector between the apex and the base of the heart. When the transducer is pointed toward the apex of the heart. the ultrasonic beam traverses the left ventricular cavity at the level of the papillary muscles and passes through a small portion of the right ventricular cavity (Fig. 3–3, position 1). Tilting the transducer superiorly and medially causes the ultrasonic beam to traverse the left ventricular cavity at the level of the edges of the mitral valve leaflets or the chordae (position 2). The beam again passes through a small portion of the right

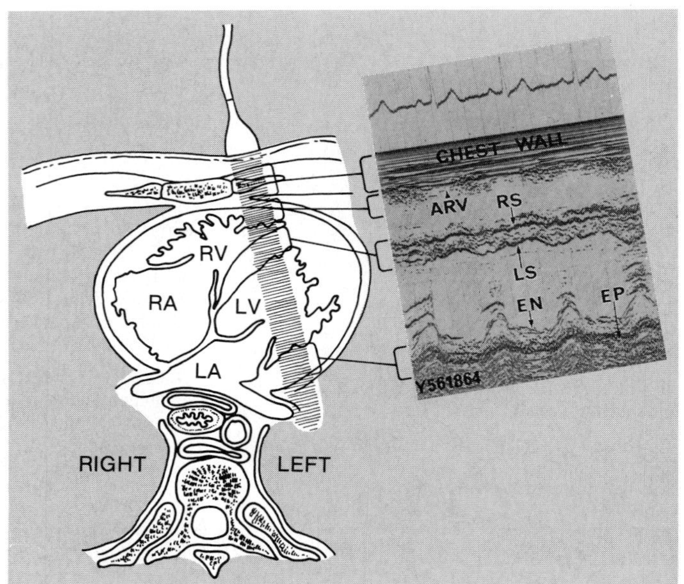

FIGURE 3–2. Cross-section of the heart and corresponding echocardiogram showing the cardiac structures transected by an ultrasonic beam directed toward the left ventricle. The ultrasound passes through the chest wall, the anterior right ventricular wall (ARV), a small portion of the right ventricular cavity, the interventricular septum, the cavity of the left ventricle, and the posterior left ventricular wall. RS = right side of the interventricular septum; LS = left side of interventricular septum; EN = posterior left ventricular endocardium; EP = posterior left ventricular epicardium. (Modified from Popp, R. L., et al.: Estimation of right and left ventricular size by ultrasound. A study of the echoes from the interventricular septum. Am. J. Cardiol. *24*:523, 1969.)

ventricle. By directing the transducer more superiorly and medially (position 3), more of the anterior leaflet of the mitral valve can be recorded and the beam may traverse part of the left atrial cavity. Further tilting of the transducer superiorly and medially (position 4) directs the beam through the root of the aorta, the leaflets of the aortic valve, and the body of the left atrium.

Figure 3–4 shows echoes from the aorta and aortic valve; by tilting the transducer medially from the aortic valve, it is possible to record the anterior leaflet of the tricuspid valve, which is similar in appearance to the recording from the anterior leaflet of the mitral valve. When the transducer is directed superiorly and laterally from the aortic valve, a posterior leaflet of the pulmonary valve can be recorded (Fig. 3–4).

Two-Dimensional Echocardiography

The principle of two-dimensional (2-D) echocardiography is depicted in Figure 3–5. The ultrasonic beam now moves in a sector so that a pie-shaped slice of the heart is interrogated. Most commercial 2-D echocardiographs move the ultrasonic beam so that approximately 30 slices/sec are obtained. The ultrasonic beam can be moved mechanically by oscillating a single transducer or by rotating a series of transducers. The ultrasound can also be steered electronically using the so-called phased array principles,[4] in which multiple ultrasonic elements are utilized to make up the beam and in which the firing sequence of the elements is controlled. A computer or microprocessor is necessary to control the firing of the elements and the direction of the beam. Figure 3–6 illustrates two individual frames representing stop-action sequences from a videotape recording of a normal heart in which the mitral and aortic valves and parts of the left ventricle, left atrium, and right ventricle are imaged.

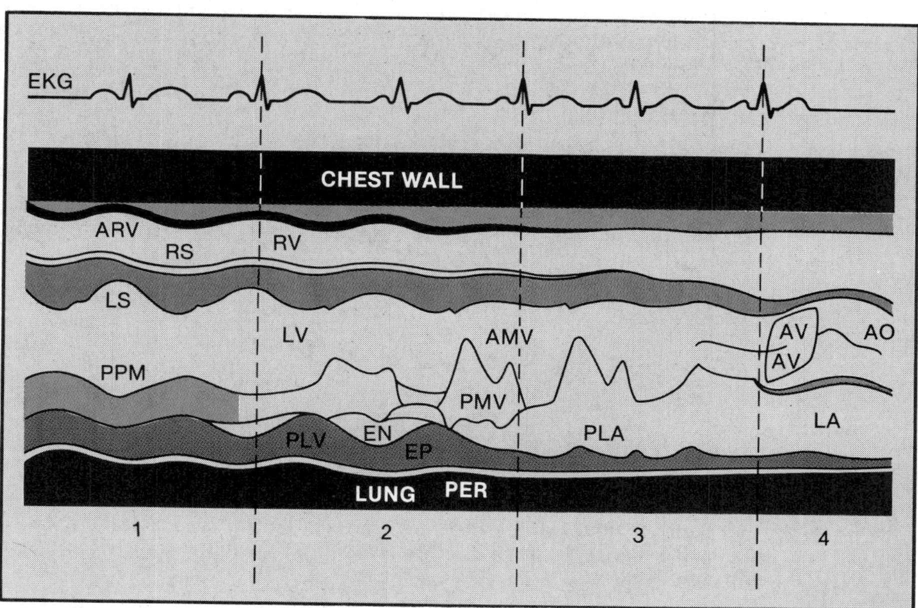

FIGURE 3–3. Presentation of an M-mode echocardiogram as the transducer is directed from the apex (position 1) to the base of the heart (position 4). Areas between the dotted lines correspond to the transducer position. EN = endocardium of the left ventricle; EP = epicardium of the left ventricle; PER = pericardium; PLA = posterior left atrial wall. (From Feigenbaum, H.: Clinical applications of echocardiography. Progr. Cardiovasc. Dis. *14*:531, 1972, by permission of Grune and Stratton.)

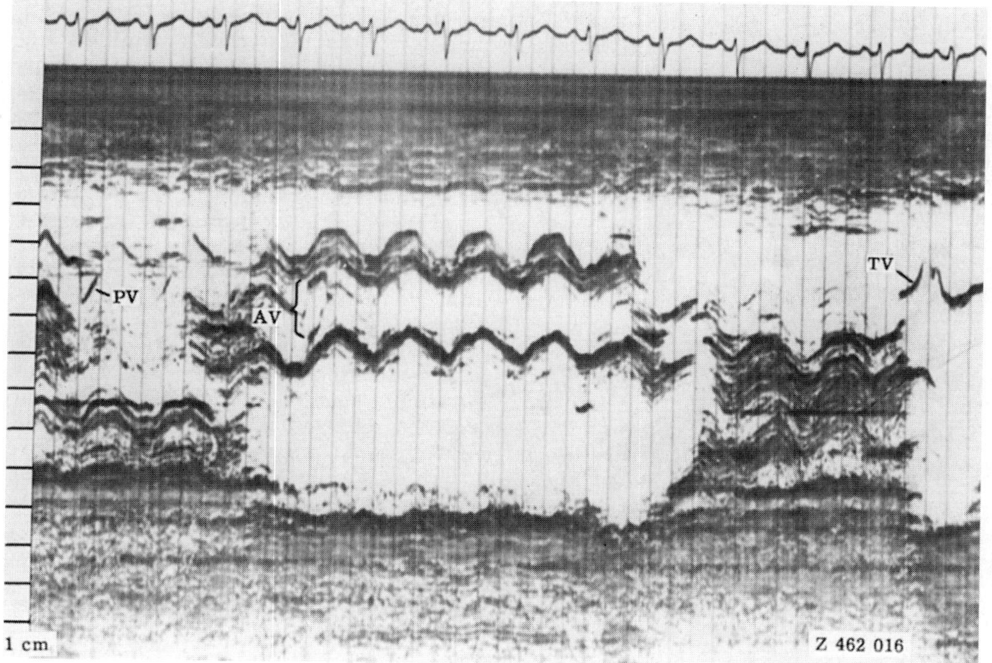

FIGURE 3–4. M-mode scan recording echoes from a pulmonic valve (PV), aortic valve (AV), and tricuspid valve (TV). (From Feigenbaum, H.: Echocardiography. 2nd ed. Philadelphia, Lea and Febiger, 1976.)

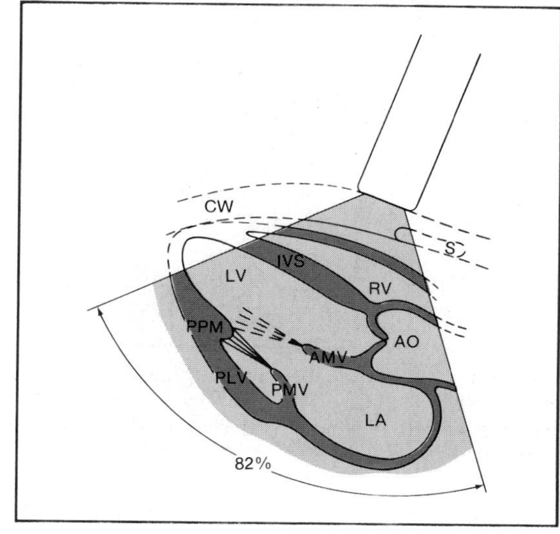

FIGURE 3–5. How to obtain a cross-sectional or 2-D image of the heart parallel to the long axis of the left ventricle. CW = chest wall.

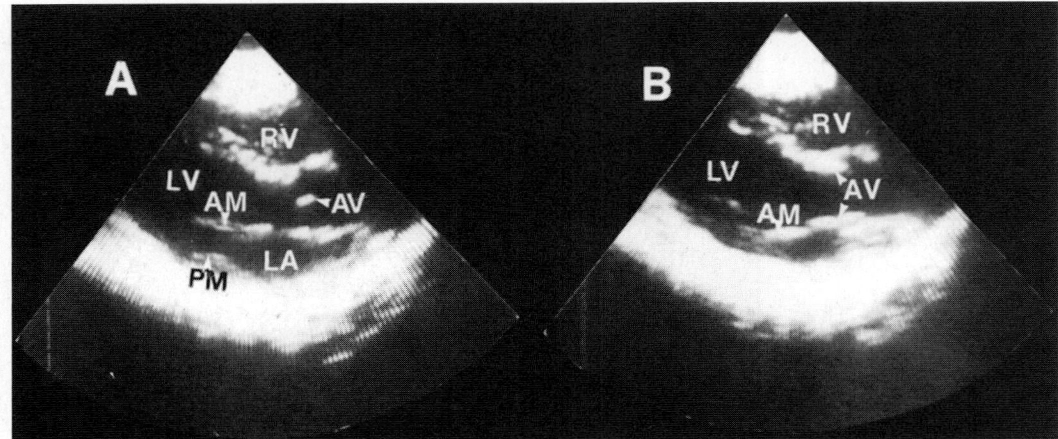

FIGURE 3–6. Long-axis 2-D echocardiographic images of the left ventricle (LV), right ventricle (RV), mitral valve, aortic valve, and left atrium (LA) during diastole *(A)* and systole *(B)*. During diastole the anterior (AM) and posterior (PM) mitral leaflets are apart and the aortic valve leaflets (AV) come together as a single echo in the midportion of the aorta *(A)*. With systole *(B)*, the mitral leaflets come together and the aortic valve leaflets separate.

Doppler Echocardiography

M-mode and 2-D echocardiography essentially create ultrasonic images of the heart. Doppler echocardiography utilizes ultrasound to record blood flow within the cardiovascular system. The principle of the Doppler effect is illustrated in Figure 3–7.[5,6] If the ultrasonic beam is reflected by a stationary object (Fig. 3–7), the transmitted frequency (f_t) and the reflected frequency (f_r) are equal. However, if the target reflecting the ultrasonic energy is moving toward the transducer (Fig. 3–7*B*), the reflected frequency is greater than the transmitted frequency. When the target is moving away from the transducer (Fig. 3–7*C*), the reflected frequency is less than the transmitted frequency. The difference between the reflected and transmitted frequencies represents the Doppler shift or Doppler frequency. By knowing the Doppler frequency it is possible to calculate the velocity of the moving target. Figure 3–8 shows the Doppler equations that relate Doppler frequency (f_d) and the velocity of the moving target (v). To determine the velocity of blood flow it is necessary to know the Doppler frequency, the angle (Θ) between the paths of the ultrasonic beam and moving target, and the velocity of sound in the medium being examined; in Doppler echocardiography the targets are the red blood cells.

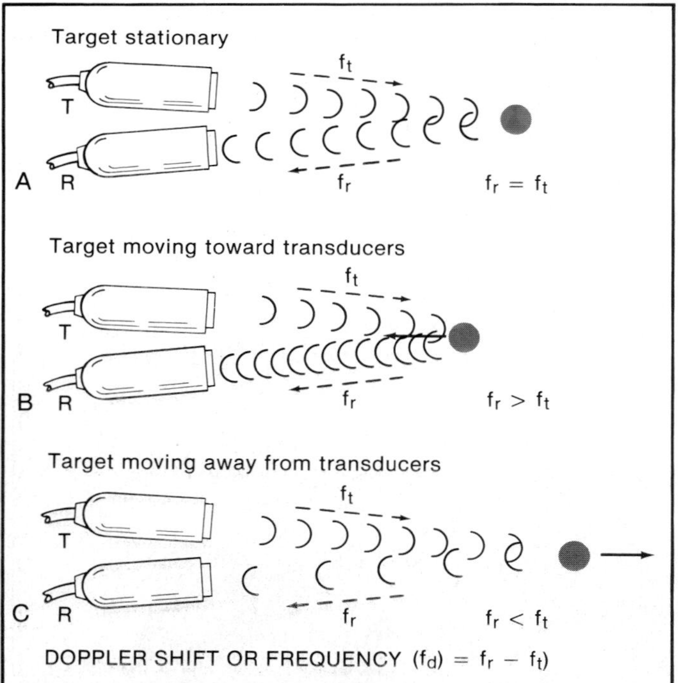

FIGURE 3–7. Demonstration of the Doppler effect using reflected sound from a target *(A)*. The reflected frequency (f_r) is greater than the transmitted frequency (f_t) when the target is moving toward the transducer *(B)*. The reflected frequency is smaller than the transmitted frequency when the target moves away from the transducer *(C)*. The Doppler shift or frequency (f_d) is the difference between the transmitted and reflected frequencies. (From Feigenbaum, H.: Echocardiography. 4th ed. Philadelphia, Lea and Febiger, 1986.)

Figure 3–7 illustrates the principles of continuous-wave Doppler. There are two transducers, one of which continuously transmits ultrasonic energy, and the other, which continuously records the reflected ultrasonic signals. One can also use pulsed ultrasound to obtain the Doppler information (Fig. 3–9). With pulsed Doppler only one transducer is needed. In addition, pulsed Doppler permits creation of a simultaneous M-mode or 2-D image.[7] To derive the Doppler frequency, the frequencies of the reflected and transmitted bursts of ultrasound are subtracted.

Significant differences exist between continuous wave and pulsed Doppler. The velocity that can be recorded using pulsed Doppler is limited by the pulse repetition

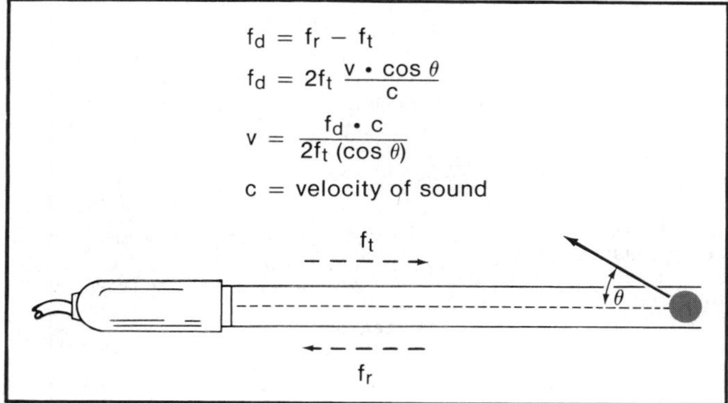

FIGURE 3–8. Doppler equations relating Doppler frequencies (f_d), received frequency (f_r), transmitted frequency (f_t), and the angle (θ) between the direction of the moving target and the path of the ultrasonic beam. (From Feigenbaum, H.: Echocardiography. 4th ed. Philadelphia, Lea and Febiger, 1986.)

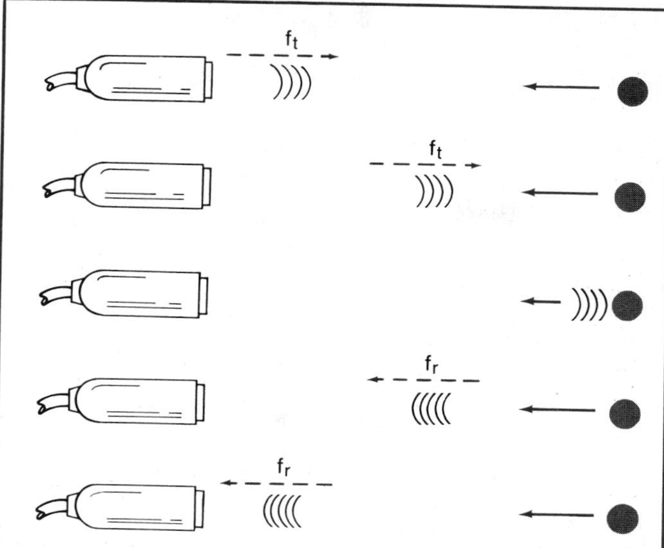

FIGURE 3–9. Demonstration of the principle of pulsed Doppler echocardiography. If the object reflecting the pulses with ultrasound is moving toward the transducer, the frequency of the received pulse (f_r) is greater than the transmitted frequency (f_t). (From Feigenbaum, H.: Echocardiography. 4th ed. Philadelphia, Lea and Febiger, 1986.)

frequency of the system. Thus, if the blood is moving very rapidly, as might occur when it is passing through a stenotic valve, then pulsed Doppler cannot sample rapidly enough to identify the Doppler frequency. This technical problem is known as *aliasing*.[8] As a result, continuous-wave Doppler is necessary for recording very high velocities within the cardiovascular system. An alternative way is to use a multiple pulsed or high pulse repetition frequency (high PRF) Doppler system. High PRF allows simultaneous imaging and recording of high flow rates; however, it is technically more difficult. The continuous wave approach is the more commonly used technique for recording high-frequency flows.[9]

The Doppler recording is a spectral display using fast Fourier analysis of the audible Doppler signal. The recording is usually on strip chart paper or videotape and is commonly referred to as *spectral Doppler*. The audio signal is helpful in interpreting the various types of flow and represents an important aspect of the Doppler examination.

COLOR DOPPLER. Doppler information from the cardiovascular system can also be recorded in a spatially correct format superimposed on an M-mode or 2-D echocardiogram. Doppler flow imaging is created by multiple Doppler gates that are spatially correct and display the moving blood within the 2-D or M-mode recording.[10] The direction of the blood is displayed in color as in Figure 3–10. With this particular instrument blood moving toward the transducer is depicted in shades of yellow and red, whereas blood moving away from the transducer is in shades of blue. Figure 3–11 shows an M-mode color Doppler or M/Q study of a patient with valvular disease. The tracing shows how turbulent flow can be displayed as green or as a mosaic of colors.[11]

Transesophageal Echocardiography

Although echocardiography is one of the most common noninvasive examinations, this ultrasonic examination need not be limited to merely placing the transducer on the surface of the chest. Transesophageal echocardiography has been available for many years. With the technical advances in placing a 2-D transducer at the end of a flexible endoscope, it is now possible to obtain high-quality 2-D images via the esophagus in multiple planes[12–14] (Figs. 3–12, 3–13). It is also possible to obtain Doppler information with this approach. Figure 3–14 demonstrates a transesophageal echocardiogram in a patient with mitral regurgitation. The regurgitant jet is multicolored instead of green.

FIGURE 3–10. See color plate 1.

FIGURE 3–11. See color plate 1.

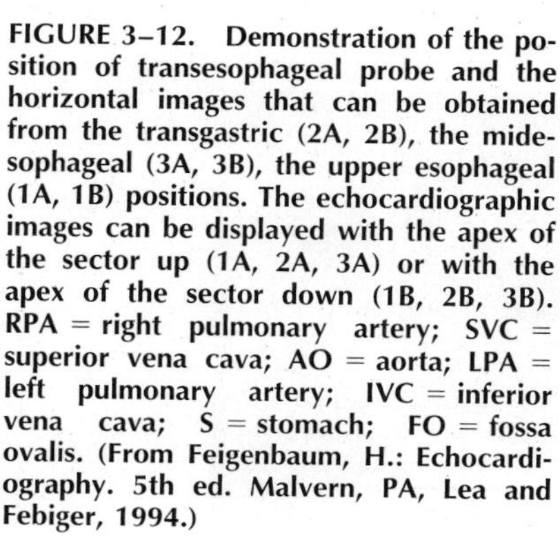

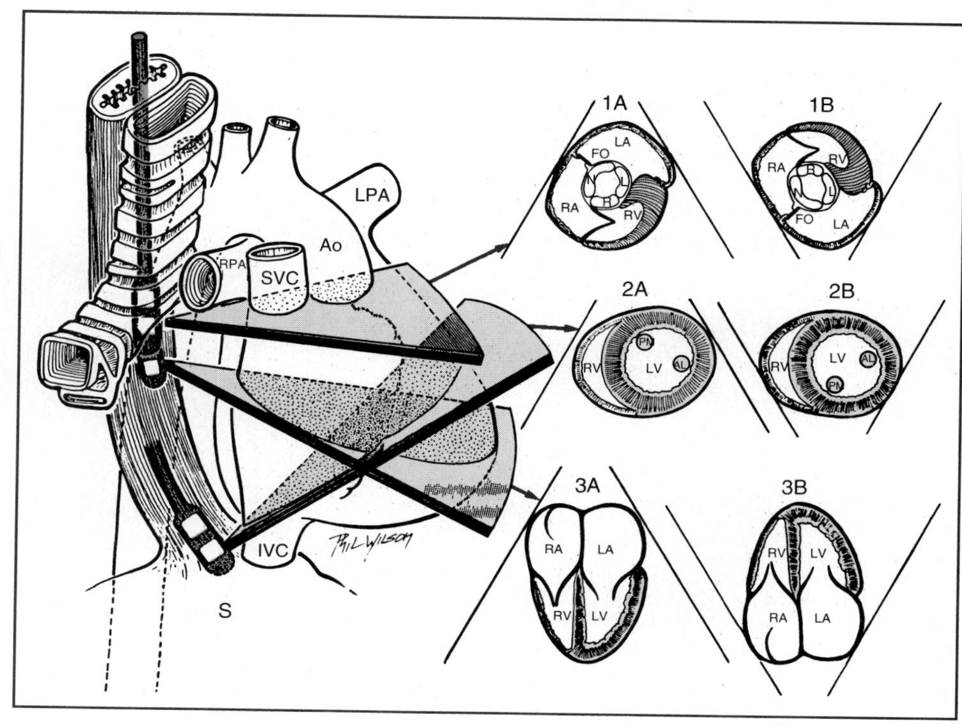

FIGURE 3–12. Demonstration of the position of transesophageal probe and the horizontal images that can be obtained from the transgastric (2A, 2B), the midesophageal (3A, 3B), the upper esophageal (1A, 1B) positions. The echocardiographic images can be displayed with the apex of the sector up (1A, 2A, 3A) or with the apex of the sector down (1B, 2B, 3B). RPA = right pulmonary artery; SVC = superior vena cava; AO = aorta; LPA = left pulmonary artery; IVC = inferior vena cava; S = stomach; FO = fossa ovalis. (From Feigenbaum, H.: Echocardiography. 5th ed. Malvern, PA, Lea and Febiger, 1994.)

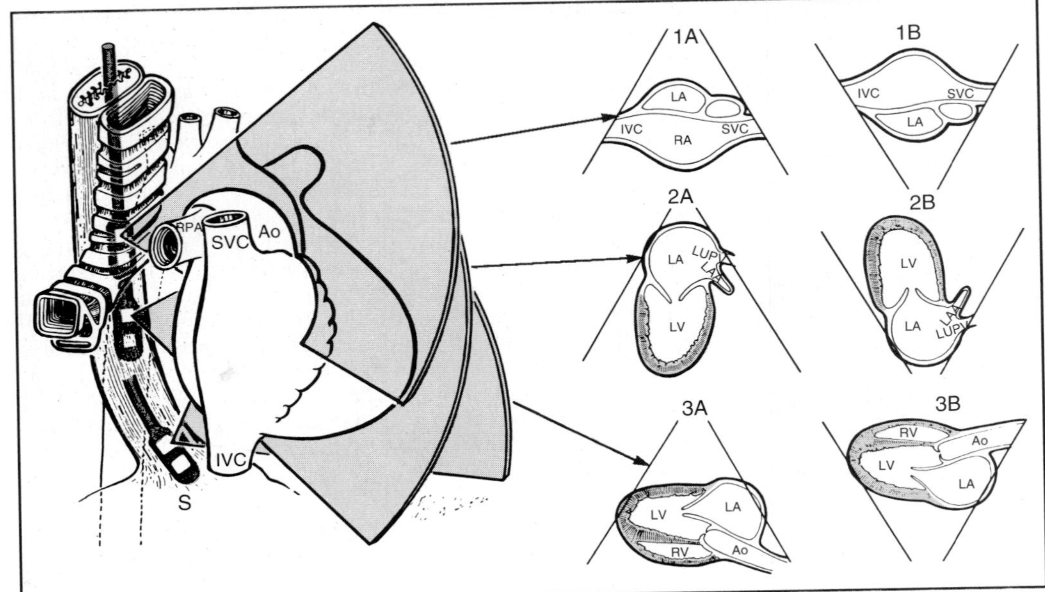

FIGURE 3–13. Views that can be obtained with the longitudinal transducer in the gastric (3A, 3B), midesophageal (2A, 2B), and upper esophageal (1A, 1B) positions. RPA = right pulmonary artery; SVC = superior vena cava; Ao = aorta; IVC = inferior vena cava; LA = left atrium; RA = right atrium; LUPV = left upper pulmonary vein; LAA = left atrial appendage; LV = left ventricle; RV = right ventricle. (From Feigenbaum, H.: Echocardiography. 5th ed. Malvern, PA, Lea and Febiger, 1994.)

Transesophageal echocardiography is useful in patients in whom the examination from the usual transthoracic approach is technically difficult or impossible.[15] This approach is particularly helpful in assessing prosthetic valves, vegetations, aortic disease, and intracardiac masses. Another major application for esophageal echocardiography is in the patient undergoing surgery. The esophageal ultrasonic probe can be used to monitor cardiac left ventricular function throughout the surgical procedure and into the postoperative state. Transesophageal echocardiography is being used in the operating room during open-heart surgery and to monitor myocardial ischemia during noncardiac surgery.[16] Cardiac surgeons are finding echocardiography helpful in assessing cardiac morphology and function before, during, and after surgical repair of valvular or congenital conditions.[17,18]

Echocardiography can also be used in conjunction with other invasive procedures such as pericardiocentesis[19] or diagnostic catheterization.[20] A similar type of monitoring has been useful to aid with endomyocardial biopsy.[21] Echocardiography may guide electrophysiological testing[22] and therapy.[23] Other therapeutic catheter techniques are also monitored effectively using echocardiography.[24–26]

INTRAVASCULAR ULTRASOUND. The ultrasonic transducer can be placed in a small catheter so that a vessel can be imaged via the lumen to provide an intravascular echocardiogram, a technique known as intravascular ultrasound. Several intravascular ultrasonic devices are currently being used.[27,28] The techniques utilize a rotating transducer, rotating ultrasonic mirror, or phased array multielement systems. These devices are generating considerable interest, especially for the ability to evaluate atherosclerosis from within the arteries (Fig. 3–15 and Figs. 39–12, p. 1381, and 39–13, p. 1383). Slightly larger intravascular ultrasonic devices are being used to visualize the heart from within the cardiac chambers.[29,30]

CONTRAST ECHOCARDIOGRAPHY. Ultrasound is an extremely sensitive detector of intravascular bubbles. The injection of almost any liquid into the intravascular spaces will introduce many microbubbles that appear as a cloud of echoes on the echocardiogram. Figure 3–16 demonstrates a transesophageal echocardiogram of a patient with an atrial septal aneurysm (arrows) (Fig. 3–16*A*). With the intravenous injection of saline agitated with a small amount of air, one sees the right atrium (RA) filled with echo-producing bubbles. Some of these bubbles (arrowheads) pass through the atrial septal aneurysm into the left atrium (Fig. 3–16*B*).

FIGURE 3–14. See color plate 1.

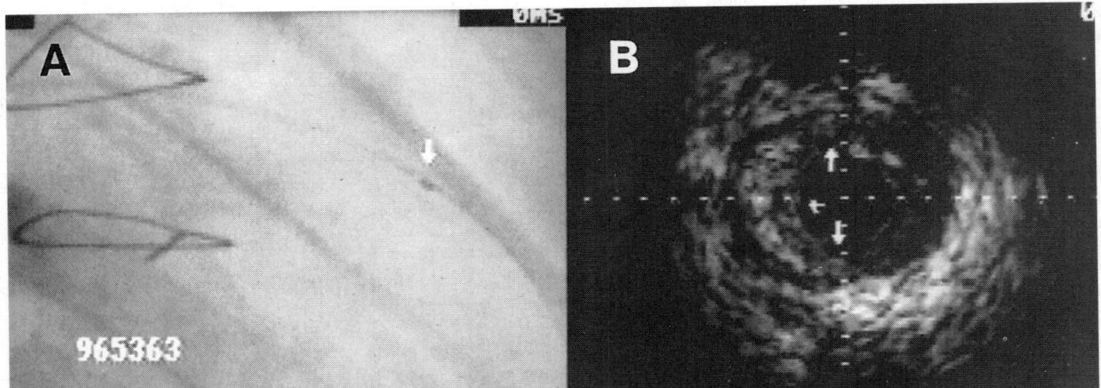

FIGURE 3–15. Intracoronary ultrasonic examination with the ultrasonic device within the left anterior descending coronary artery. The location of the transducer (arrow) can be seen in the angiogram *(A)*. The ultrasonic image *(B)* shows extensive atherosclerotic plaque (arrows) on the left side of the arterial wall. (From Feigenbaum, H.: Echocardiography. 5th ed. Malvern, PA, Lea & Febiger, 1994.)

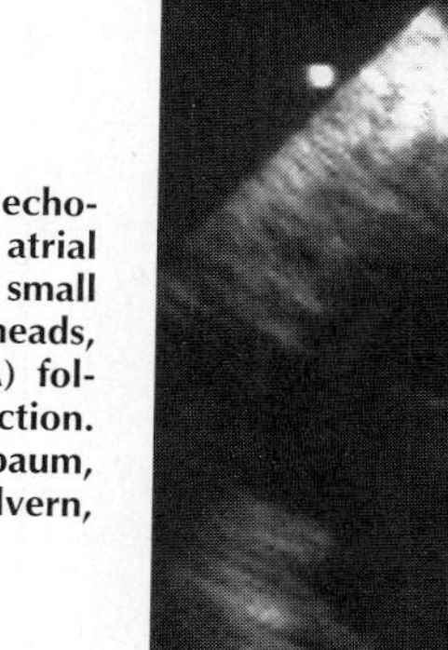
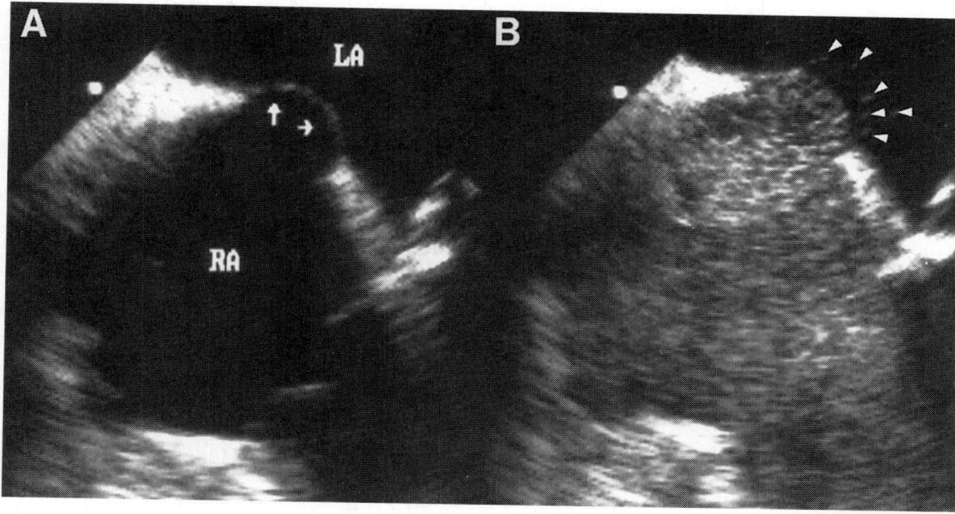

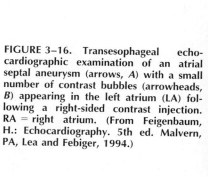

FIGURE 3–16. Transesophageal echocardiographic examination of an atrial septal aneurysm (arrows, *A*) with a small number of contrast bubbles (arrowheads, *B*) appearing in the left atrium (LA) following a right-sided contrast injection. RA = right atrium. (From Feigenbaum, H.: Echocardiography. 5th ed. Malvern, PA, Lea and Febiger, 1994.)

Contrast echocardiography is a very sensitive technique for detecting right-to-left shunts. The contrast agents that have been used include the patient's blood, saline, indocyanine green dye, agitated or sonicated angiographic contrast agents, and sonicated albumen. In all cases the contrast effect originates from suspended microbubbles in the fluid. Commercially manufactured microbubbles that traverse the pulmonary capillaries are now available.[31–33] The potential clinical uses for contrast echocardiography are numerous.[34–37]

FETAL ECHOCARDIOGRAPHY. Examination of the fetal heart in utero has become an important subspecialty of echocardiography. The examination is extremely demanding and requires great technical skill as well as an excellent understanding of fetal anatomy, physiology, and potential pathology.[38,39] The field is primarily in the hands of a few pediatric echocardiographers. Because of the highly specialized nature of this work it is beyond the scope of this particular discussion of echocardiography.

THREE-DIMENSIONAL ECHOCARDIOGRAPHY. A variety of approaches to recording echocardiograms that are oriented in three-dimensional (3-D) space have been proposed. One technique orients a 2-D transducer in 3-D space using spark gap sensors.[40–42] Most investigators are creating 3-D images of the heart using gated, reconstructed 2-D examinations.[43–45]

ADVANTAGES AND LIMITATIONS OF ECHOCARDIOGRAPHY. The advantages of echocardiography are numerous. The examination is painless, as best as can be determined it is virtually harmless,[46] and it is less costly than other sophisticated imaging techniques. However, some technical difficulties exist that require expertise on the part of the examiner and interpreter of the echocardiographic recordings. The principal problem is posed by the poor transmission of ultrasound through bony structures or air-containing lungs. The examiner must thus try to avoid these structures. A variety of techniques have been developed to circumvent this problem. The patient is commonly placed in the left recumbent position to move the heart from beneath the sternum. The subxiphoid or subcostal transducer position is frequently used in patients with hyperinflated lungs and a low diaphragm. Transesophageal echocardiography is available for the patient in whom the examination is extremely difficult. Thus, many examining techniques have been developed to minimize the technical difficulties in performing an echocardiographic examination.

EXAMINATION OF THE NORMAL HEART

TWO-DIMENSIONAL ECHOCARDIOGRAPHY. An infinite number of slices of the heart can theoretically be obtained using 2-D echocardiography. The American Society of Echocardiography has attempted to standardize and simplify the many 2-D examinations.[47] The Society thought that all views could be categorized into three orthogonal planes, as illustrated in Figure 3–17. These planes are the long-axis, short-axis, and four-chamber. The long-axis plane is the imaging plane that transects the heart perpendicular to the dorsal and ventral surfaces of the body and parallel to the long axis of the heart. The plane transecting the heart perpendicular to the dorsal and ventral surfaces of the body, but perpendicular to the long axis of the heart, is defined as the short-axis plane. The plane that transects the heart approximately parallel to the dorsal and ventral surfaces of the body is referred to as the four-chamber plan. It should be emphasized that these views or planes are with reference to the heart and not the thorax or body.

Transducer Locations. These ultrasonic planes or views can be obtained from more than one transducer location. Figure 3–18*A* demonstrates that the long-axis view can be obtained with the transducer in the apical position, in the parasternal position (left sternal border), or in the supra-

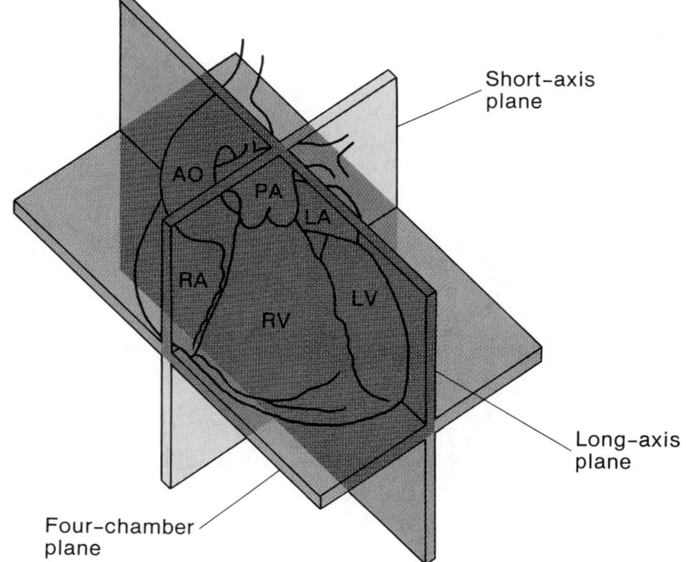

FIGURE 3–17. The three orthogonal planes for 2-D echocardiographic imaging. AO = aorta; PA = pulmonary artery; LA = left atrium; RA = right atrium; RV = right ventricle; LV = left ventricle. (Reproduced with permission from Henry, W. L., et al.: Report of the American Society of Echocardiography Nomenclature and Standards in Two-Dimensional Echocardiography. Circulation *62*:212, 1980. Copyright 1980 American Heart Association.)

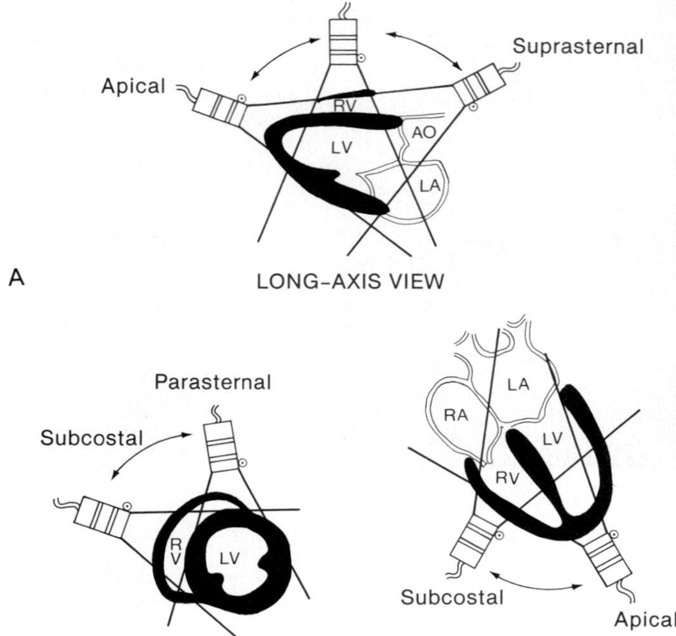

FIGURE 3–18. How the various orthogonal planes can be obtained from different transducer positions. (Reproduced with permission from Henry, W. L., et al.: Report of the American Society of Echocardiography Nomenclature and Standards in Two-Dimensional Echocardiography. Circulation *62:*212, 1980. Copyright 1980 American Heart Association.)

sternal notch. A short-axis view (Fig. 3–18*B*) cuts across the heart so that the left ventricle resembles a circle. The right ventricle can be seen curving around the left ventricle. Such an examination can be obtained with the transducer in the parasternal position or in the subcostal (subxiphoid) position. The four-chamber view is depicted in Figure 3–18*C*. Such a view permits the examination of all four cardiac chambers simultaneously. This type of examination can be obtained with the transducer over the cardiac apex or with the transducer in the subcostal position. Table 3–1 lists the various 2-D echocardiographic examinations categorized according to the location of the transducer, the plane of the examination, and the cardiac structure being examined.

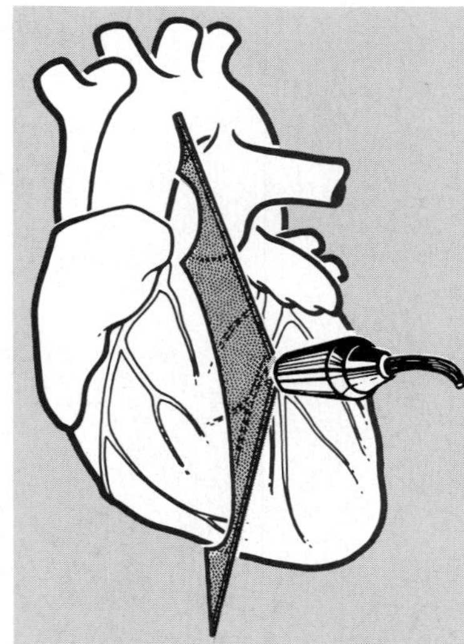

FIGURE 3–19. Transducer position for long-axis parasternal examination of the tricuspid valve, right atrium, and right ventricular inflow tract. (From Feigenbaum, H.: Echocardiography. 4th ed. Philadelphia, Lea and Febiger, 1986.)

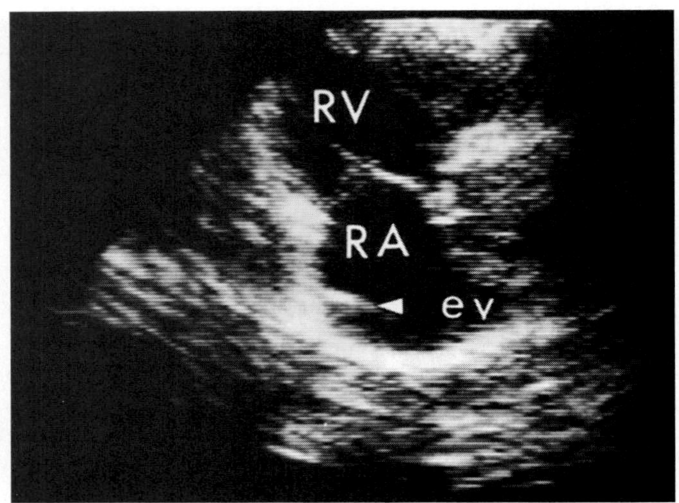

FIGURE 3–20. Two-dimensional echocardiogram of the right atrium (RA) and right ventricular inflow tract (RV). ev = eustachian valve. (From Feigenbaum, H.: Echocardiography. 4th ed. Philadelphia, Lea and Febiger, 1986.)

The right ventricle, right atrium, and tricuspid valve can be recorded with the transducer in the parasternal position (Fig. 3–19). The plane of the transducer does not exactly fit either the long axis or the short axis. However, the plane is closer to that of the long axis than that of the short axis and thus is categorized as a long-axis study. Figure 3–20 shows the right ventricular inflow tract and right atrium by way of such a parasternal examination.

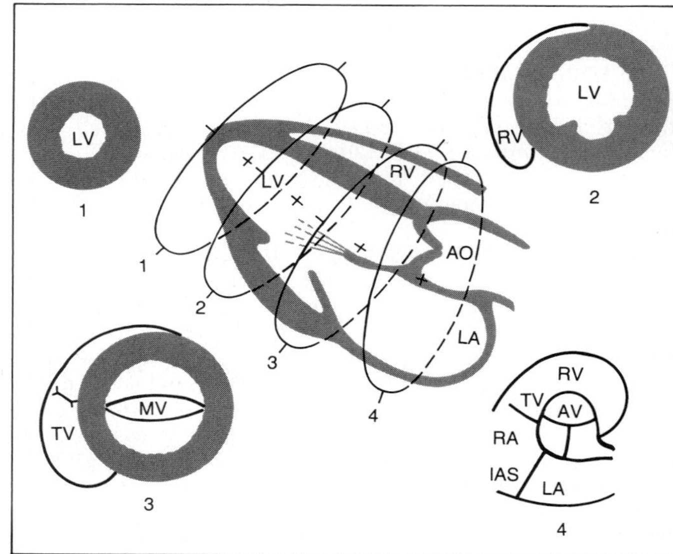

FIGURE 3–21. How short-axis echocardiographic cross-sectional images of the heart, which are perpendicular to the long axis of the left ventricle, are obtained. *Diagram 1* shows a short-axis left ventricular echocardiogram near the cardiac apex. *Diagram 2* demonstrates part of the right ventricle (RV) and the circular left ventricular cavity (LV) at the level of the papillary muscles, which can be seen to bulge into the LV cavity. *Diagram 3* is closer to the base of the heart and shows the left ventricle at the level of the mitral valve (MV). *Diagram 4* shows a short-axis cross-section of the base of the heart with the aorta, aortic valve (AV), left atrium (LA), interatrial septum (IAS), right atrium (RA), tricuspid valve (TV), and right ventricular outflow tract (RV). (From Feigenbaum, H.: Echocardiography. 4th ed. Philadelphia, Lea and Febiger, 1986.)

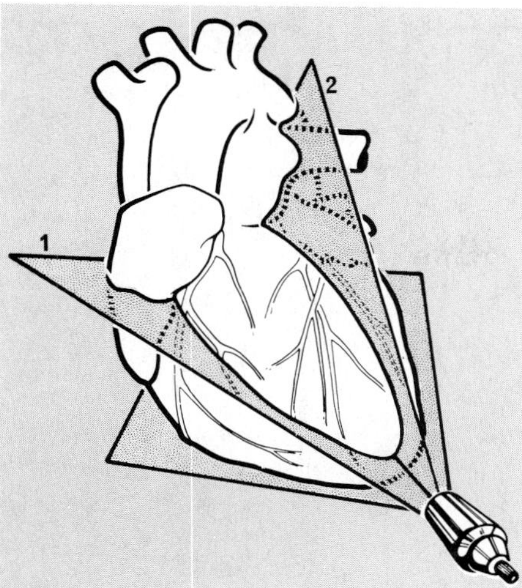

FIGURE 3–22. Transducer position and examining planes for apical 2-D echocardiograms. Plane 1 passes through the four-chamber plane of the heart. Plane 2 represents the path of the ultrasonic beam for the two-chamber apical examination. (From Feigenbaum, H.: Echocardiography. 4th ed. Philadelphia, Lea and Febiger, 1986.)

Various short-axis examinations are diagrammatically illustrated in Figure 3–21. The short-axis views are commonly obtained at the level of the apex, the papillary muscles, the mitral valve, and the base of the heart. With slight variation in angulation the short-axis examination of the base of the heart can also record the pulmonary valve and the pulmonary artery with its bifurcation. It is also possible to use this examination to record the origins of the coronary arteries and the left atrial appendage.

Figure 3–22 diagrammatically illustrates two commonly used 2-D echocardiographic views with the transducer placed at the cardiac apex. Plane 1 demonstrates an apical four-chamber view of the heart and plane 2 is a longitudinal slice through the left ventricle and atrium, the so-called two-chamber view. The two-chamber view does not exactly fit the three-plane scheme, since it is between the four-chamber and long-axis planes. Figure 3–23 shows four common 2-D echocardiographic views. The long-axis (LX) and short-axis (SX) echograms are with the transducer in the left parasternal position. The four chamber (4C) and two chamber (2C) views are obtained with the transducer at the apex.

TABLE 3–1 TWO-DIMENSIONAL ECHOCARDIOGRAPHIC EXAMINATION

PARASTERNAL APPROACH
Long-axis plane
Root of aorta–aortic valve, left atrium, left ventricular outflow tract
Body of left ventricle–mitral valve
Left ventricular apex
Right ventricular inflow tract–tricuspid valve
Short-axis plane
Root of the aorta–aortic valve, pulmonary valve, tricuspid valve, right ventricular outflow tract, left atrium, pulmonary artery, coronary arteries
Left ventricle–mitral valve
Left ventricle–papillary muscles
Left ventricle–apex
APICAL APPROACH
Four-chamber plane
Four chamber
Four chamber with aorta
Long-axis plane
Two chamber–left ventricle, left atrium
Two chamber with aorta
SUBCOSTAL APPROACH
Four-chamber plane–all four chambers and both septa
Short-axis plane
Left ventricle
Right ventricle
Inferior vena cava
SUPRASTERNAL APPROACH
Four-chamber plane
Arch of aorta–descending aorta
Long-axis plane
Arch of aorta–pulmonary artery, left atrium

The subcostal transducer location produces examinations roughly in the four-chamber and short-axis planes. The ultrasonic plane indicated in Figure 3–24*A* is similar to examining plane 1 in Figure 3–21. The resulting subcostal four-chamber echocardiogram appears in Figure 3–25*A*. Figures 3–24*B* and 3–25*B* show how the transducer can be rotated 90 degrees to provide a subcostal short-axis exami-

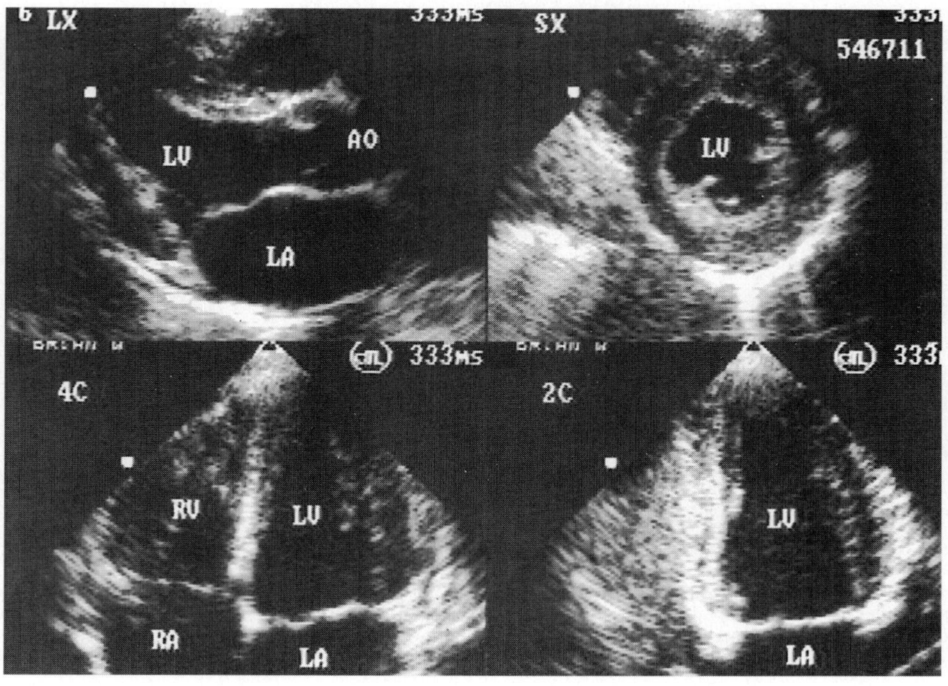

FIGURE 3–23. A quad screen display of four common 2-D echocardiographic views. LX = long axis; SX = short axis; 4C = four chamber; 2C = two chamber; LV = left ventricle; AO = aorta; LA = left atrium; RV = right ventricle; RA = right atrium. (From Feigenbaum, H.: Echocardiography. 5th ed. Malvern, PA, Lea and Febiger, 1994.)

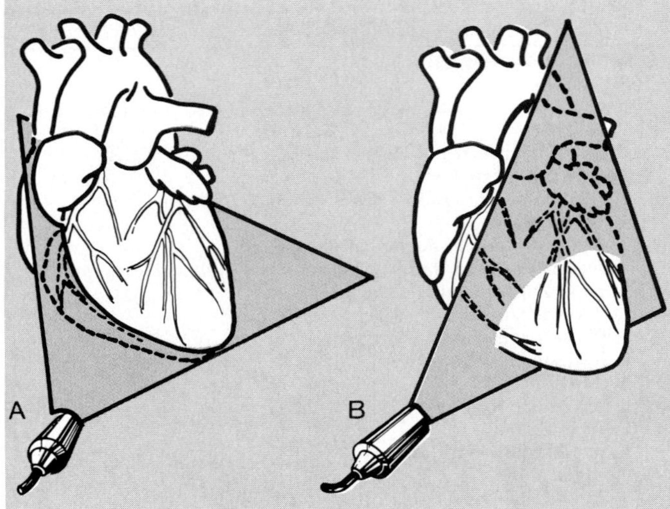

FIGURE 3–24. Transducer position and examining planes for a subcostal four-chamber examination *(A)* and a subcostal short-axis examination *(B)*. (From Feigenbaum, H.: Echocardiography. 4th ed. Philadelphia, Lea and Febiger, 1986.)

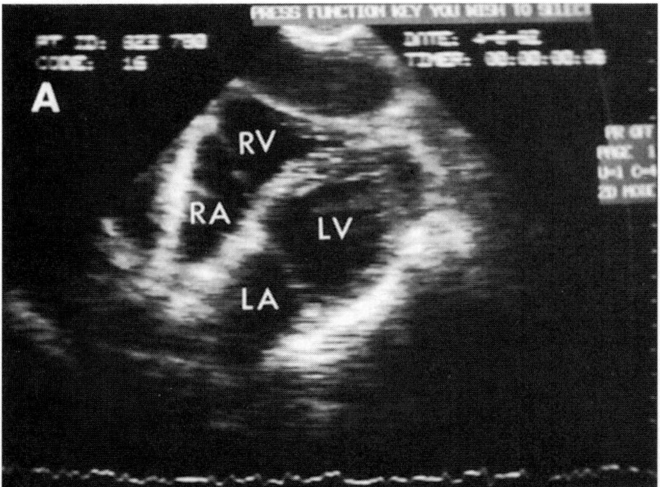

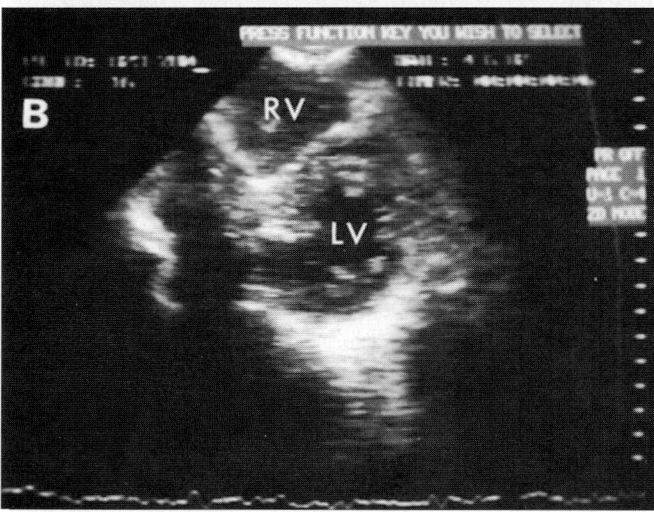

FIGURE 3–25. Two-dimensional echocardiograms obtained with the transducer in the subcostal position. Echocardiogram *A* represents a four-chamber view, and *B* is a short-axis examination. RV = right ventricle; RA = right atrium; LA = left atrium; LV = left ventricle.

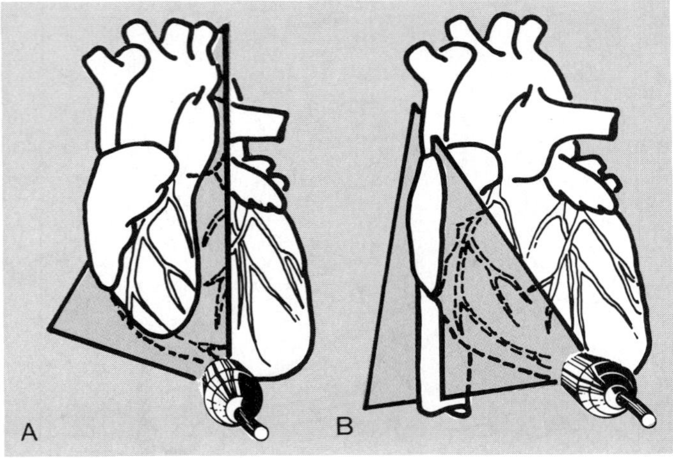

FIGURE 3–26. Examining planes and transducer positions for the subcostal examination of the right side of the heart *(A)* and the inferior vena cava *(B)*. (From Feigenbaum, H.: Echocardiography. 4th ed. Philadelphia, Lea and Febiger, 1986.)

nation of the heart. The subcostal four-chamber view is particularly helpful in examining the interatrial and interventricular septa. By directing the transducer in a slightly modified short-axis examination, one can obtain an excellent view of the right side of the heart. The subcostal location also permits an opportunity to direct the ultrasonic beam through the inferior vena cava and hepatic veins (Figs. 3–26*B* and 3–27).

The two examining planes with the transducer in the suprasternal notch are depicted in Figure 3–28. The ultra-

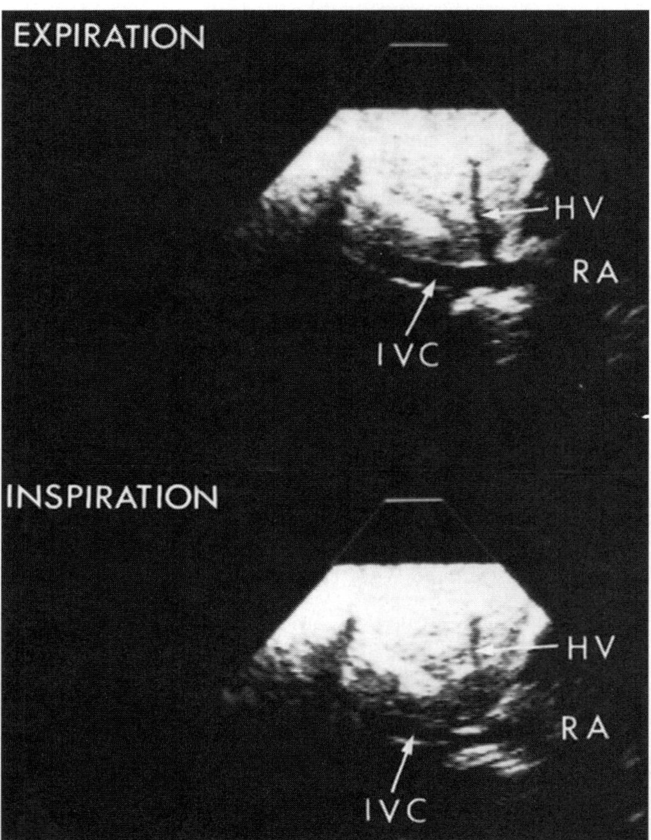

FIGURE 3–27. Subcostal 2-D echocardiograms of the inferior vena cava (IVC) and hepatic veins (HV). The inferior vena cava decreases in size with inspiration. RA = right atrium. (From Feigenbaum, H.: Echocardiography. 4th ed. Philadelphia, Lea and Febiger, 1986.)

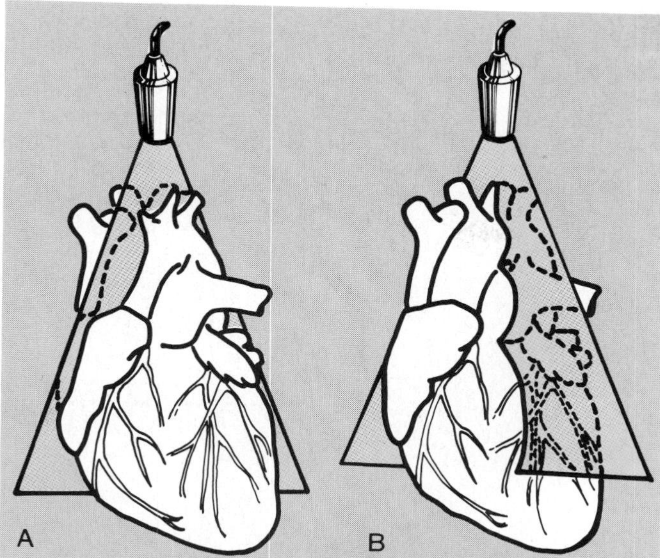

FIGURE 3–28. Transducer position in examining planes for the suprasternal examination parallel to the arch of the aorta *(A)* and perpendicular to the arch of the aorta *(B)*. (From Feigenbaum, H.: Echocardiography. 4th ed. Philadelphia, Lea and Febiger, 1986.)

sonic view in Figure 3–28*A* is roughly equivalent to that of a four-chamber plane, and the view in Figure 3–28*B* is somewhat comparable to that of the long-axis plane. However, it is probably best to orient the ultrasonic beam with regard to the arch of the aorta rather than to the heart, since one does not record much of the heart with the transducer in this position, especially in the adult. In addition, the planes are different from those with the transducer at the apex or subcostal region. Thus, better terminology with regard to the examining plane from the suprasternal location would be parallel or perpendicular to the arch of the aorta. Figure 3–29 shows a suprasternal examination parallel to the arch of the aorta.

M-MODE ECHOCARDIOGRAPHY. With the advent of 2-D echocardiography, and to some extent Doppler echocardiography, the M-mode examination now plays a lesser role in the ultrasonic examination of the heart.[48] The principal advantage of this examination is the high temporal resolution inherent in sampling cardiac motion at roughly 1000 times/second. One can utilize this examination to demonstrate subtle motion of cardiac structures. Figure 3–30 is an M-mode study of a normal mitral valve. One can appreciate the motion of the anterior and posterior leaflets with far greater detail than can be seen with a 2-D study that usually samples at 30 frames/sec. For example, the mid-diastolic reopening of the valve, which commonly is seen in normal persons, is rarely appreciated on a real-time 2-D examination. Figure 3–30 shows the usual labeling given to an M-mode mitral valve echogram.

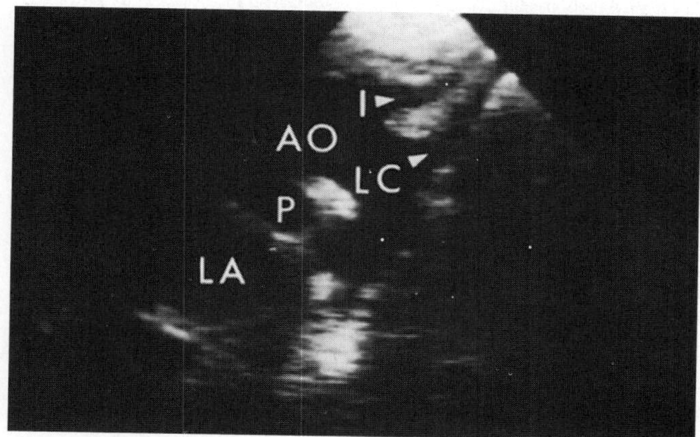

FIGURE 3–29. Suprasternal echocardiographic examination of the arch of the aorta (AO), pulmonary artery (P), and left atrium (LA). I = innominate artery; LC = left common carotid artery.

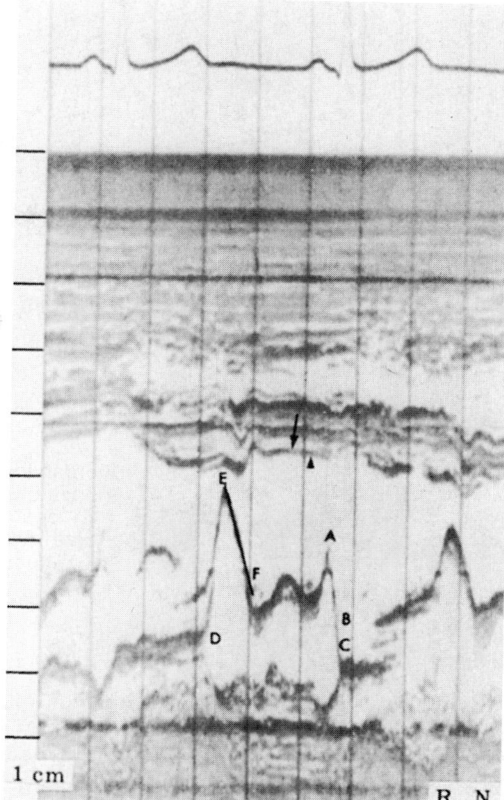

FIGURE 3–30. M-mode echocardiogram of a normal mitral valve. The letters A through F denote various portions of the anterior leaflet motion. The arrow indicates the leading edge of the echo from the left side of the interventricular septum; the arrowhead denotes the trailing edge of that echo. (From Feigenbaum, H.: Echocardiography. 2nd ed. Philadelphia, Lea and Febiger, 1976.)

One of the common uses of M-mode echocardiography is obtaining cardiac measurements. Figure 3–31 illustrates some of the M-mode measurements that are being used. The diastolic and systolic dimensions of the left ventricle can be used to calculate fractional shortening. One can also use an empirical formula to calculate volumes and provide ejection fraction. One can use M-mode dimensions for measuring septal and posterior wall thickness. These measurements can be combined to calculate left ventricular mass. Left atrial and aortic measurements are also commonly made with the M-mode examination. Table 3–2 shows some of the M-mode measurements and normal values for these determinations.[49]

DOPPLER ECHOCARDIOGRAPHY. Spectral Doppler echocardiographic recordings are basically of three types. There is the venous ventricular inflow and ventricular outflow pattern of Doppler flow (Fig. 3–32). Venous flow has both systolic and diastolic components. There will be some slight variation whether the recording is from systemic or pulmonary veins.[50] There is frequently reverse flow that moves downward or away from the transducer following atrial contraction.[51] Ventricular inflow is totally diastolic. There is an early component that peaks at the E wave and a late component following atrial contraction that peaks with an A wave. Ventricular outflow is entirely systolic in nature. Figure 3–33 shows the ventricular inflow or mitral flow pattern with the sample volume at the level of the mitral valve. One sees the early flow that peaks with the E

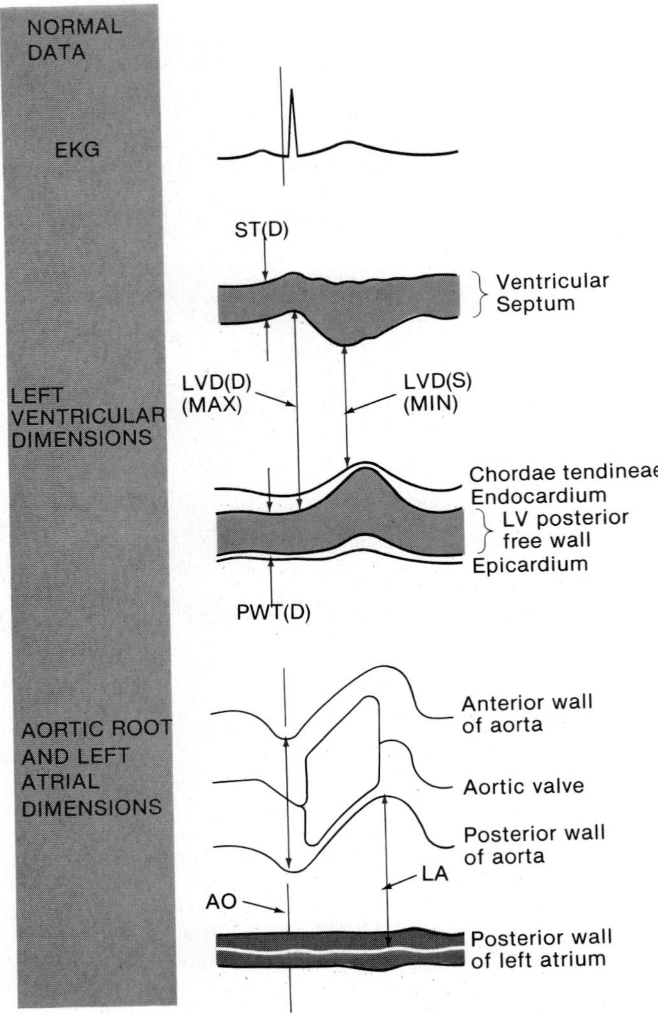

FIGURE 3–31. Methods for obtaining M-mode echocardiographic measurements. ST(D) = diastolic septal thickness; LVD (D) and LVD(S) = diastolic and systolic left ventricular diameters; PWT(D) = diastolic posterior wall thickness; AO = aorta; LA = left atrium. (Reproduced with permission from Henry, W. L., Gardin, J. M., and Ware, J. H.: Echocardiographic measurements in normal subjects from infancy to old age. Circulation *62*:1054, 1980. Copyright 1980 American Heart Association.)

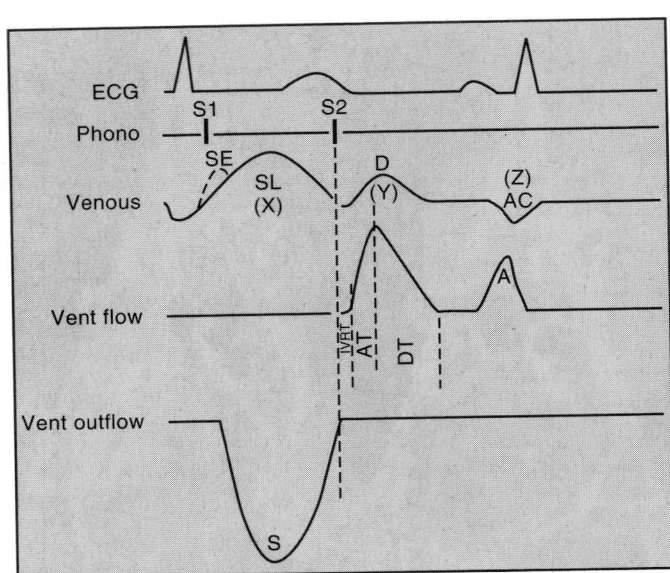

FIGURE 3–32. Relationship between the electrocardiogram (ECG), phonocardiogram (PHONO), venous, ventricular inflow, and ventricular outflow Doppler velocities. SE = early systole; SL = late systole; D = diastole; AC = atrial contraction; IVRT = isovolumic relaxation time; AT = acceleration time; DT = deceleration time. (From Feigenbaum, H.: Echocardiography. 5th ed. Malvern, PA, Lea and Febiger, 1994.)

wave and the late flow that peaks with the A wave. Figure 3–34 shows a pulsed Doppler recording of aortic flow taken with the transducer at the apex. With this "five-chamber" view one sees the systolic flow moving away from the transducer during systole. Doppler flow patterns on the right side of the heart are essentially the same except the velocities are lower. The peak mitral velocity in Figure 3–33 is about 100 cm/sec, and the aortic velocity in Figure 3–34 is about 120 cm/sec.

EVALUATION OF CARDIAC PERFORMANCE

M-MODE ECHOCARDIOGRAPHY. The ability to evaluate the function of the left ventricle by means of echocardiography has been one of the principal factors in the increasing ap-

TABLE 3–2 NORMAL VALUES OF M-MODE ECHOCARDIOGRAPHIC MEASUREMENTS IN ADULTS

	RANGE (CM)	MEAN (CM)	NUMBER OF SUBJECTS
Age (years)	13 to 54	26	134
Body surface area (M^2)	1.45 to 2.22	1.8	130
RVD—flat	0.7 to 2.3	1.5	84
RVD—left lateral	0.9 to 2.6	1.7	83
LVID—flat	3.7 to 5.6	4.7	82
LVID—left lateral	3.5 to 5.7	4.7	81
Posterior LV wall thickness	0.6 to 1.1	0.9	137
Posterior LV wall amplitude	0.9 to 1.4	1.2	48
IVS wall thickness	0.6 to 1.1	0.9	137
Mid IVS amplitude	0.3 to 0.8	0.5	10
Apical IVS amplitude	0.5 to 1.2	0.7	38
Left atrial dimension	1.9 to 4.0	2.9	133
Aortic root dimension	2.0 to 3.7	2.7	121
Aortic cusps' separation	1.5 to 2.6	2.9	93
Percentage of fractional shortening*	34% to 44%	36%	20%
Mean rate of circumferential shortening (Vcf)† or mean normalized shortening velocity	1.02 to 1.94 circ/sec	1.3 circ/sec	38

$$* \frac{\text{LVIDd} - \text{LVIDs}}{\text{LVIDd}}$$

$$\dagger \frac{\text{LVIDd} - \text{LVIDs}}{\text{LVIDd} \times \text{Ejection time}}$$

RVD = Right ventricular dimension
LVID = Left ventricular internal dimension; d = end diastole; s = end systole
LV = Left ventricle
IVS = Interventricular septum

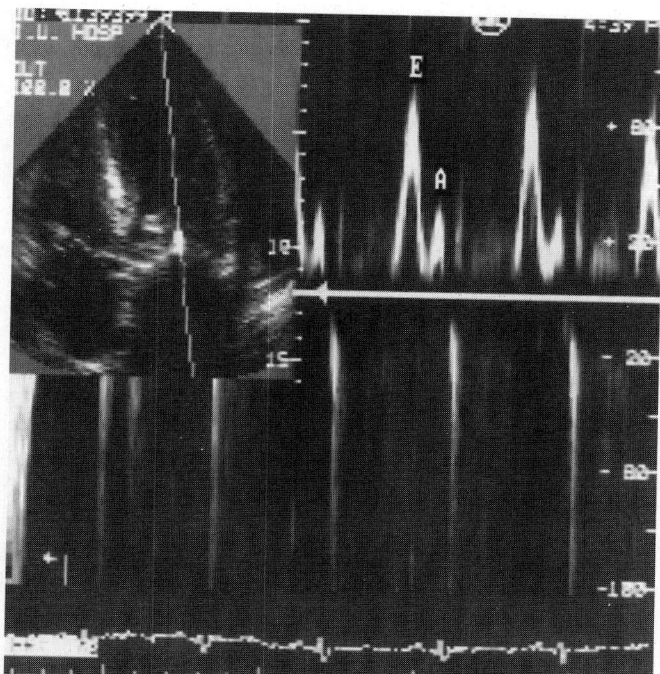

FIGURE 3–33. **Pulsed Doppler recording of mitral velocities showing the early diastolic flow (E) and late diastolic flow or velocity (A) following atrial systole.**

plication of this technique. The standard M-mode technique may be used to record a dimension of the left ventricle between the left side of the interventricular septum and the endocardial surface of the posterior left ventricular wall (Fig. 3–31).[52] This dimension may be measured in end diastole and end systole. Although these dimensions can be used to estimate ventricular volume, many errors can occur in such calculations,[53] since many assumptions that are not always valid are required to obtain the volume of a three-dimensional object from measurement of a single dimension. Irrespective of whether or not M-mode echocardiography can calculate true left ventricular volumes, simple dimensions of the left ventricle can provide an estimate of the overall size and performance of the left ventricle in many patients. Fractional shortening, i.e., the difference be tween the end-diastolic dimension, provides information about left ventricular systolic function. The quotient of fractional shortening and ejection time provides the mean fractional or circumferential shortening.[54] While these measurements are useful in judging left ventricular performance (Table 3–1), it must be appreciated that the ventricle must be contracting uniformly for them to reflect global function. These echocardiographic measurements assess the status of only the basal portion of the chamber and must be interpreted with caution in patients with segmentally diseased left ventricles,[55] with left bundle branch block, with a dilated right ventricle, or with a low echocardiographic window so that the M-mode measurement is closer to the major axis than the minor axis.

Another useful M-mode echocardiographic technique for assessing ventricular size is to measure the distance between the E point of mitral valve and the left side of the interventricular septum.[56] Normally the mitral E point and the left side of the septum are within a few millimeters of each other. The upper limits of normal of the mitral E point septal separation (EPSS) is approximately 8 mm. As the left ventricular ejection fraction decreases, the EPSS increases. As the left ventricle dilates, the septum moves anteriorly. The opening of the mitral valve is largely dependent upon the volume of blood passing through that orifice. As the mitral valve flow or left ventricular stroke volume decreases, the amplitude of the E point is decreased. Thus, with a decreased stroke volume and/or left ventricular dilatation, the septum and anterior mitral leaflet would move in opposite directions. Naturally, if there is valvular disease, such as mitral stenosis, then the excursion of the mitral valve is not a reliable indicator of flow through that orifice. In patients with aortic regurgitation, mitral valve flow is not an indicator of total left ventricular stroke volume, and one would not be able to provide an assessment of ejection fraction.

TWO-DIMENSIONAL ECHOCARDIOGRAPHY. The limited number of sampling sites for the M-mode dimensions and the lack of spatial orientation limit the clinical usefulness of these measurements. Thus, it is not surprising that 2-D echocardiography is being used to assess cardiac chambers. Hesitancy to use the 2-D approach and continued reliance on M-mode measurements are partially due to convenience and familiarity with M-mode measurements and the difficulty of making measurements from videotape recordings. However, with the widespread use of computer analysis of the 2-D images both on-line and off-line, this inconvenience is no longer a problem.

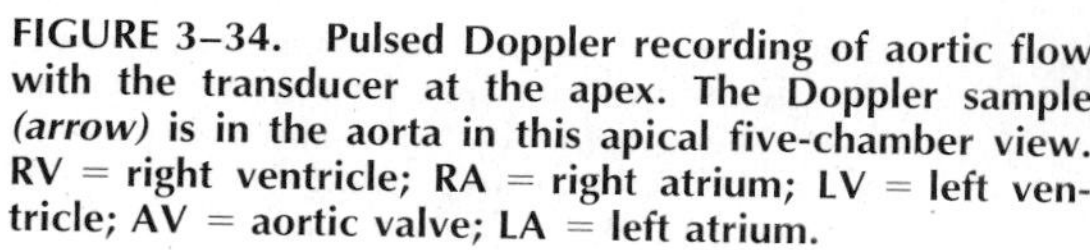

FIGURE 3–34. **Pulsed Doppler recording of aortic flow with the transducer at the apex. The Doppler sample** ***(arrow)*** **is in the aorta in this apical five-chamber view. RV = right ventricle; RA = right atrium; LV = left ventricle; AV = aortic valve; LA = left atrium.**

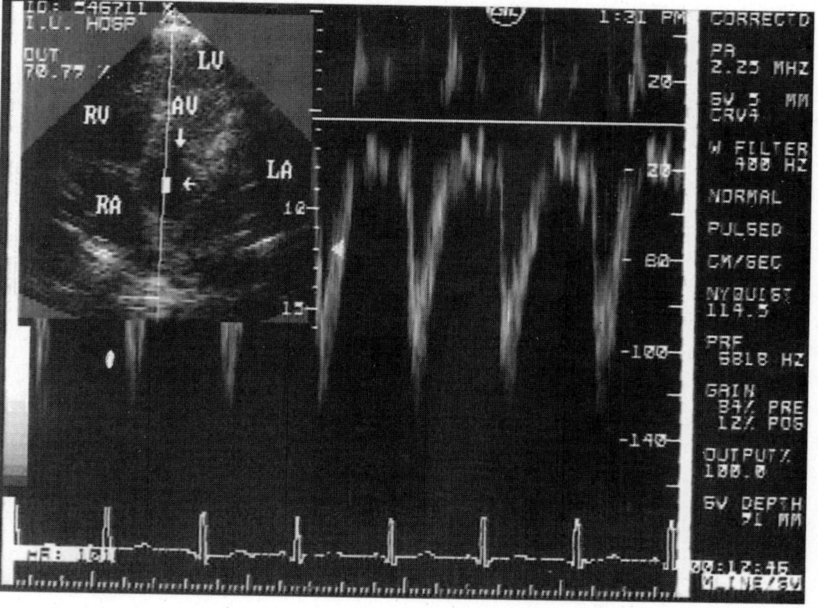

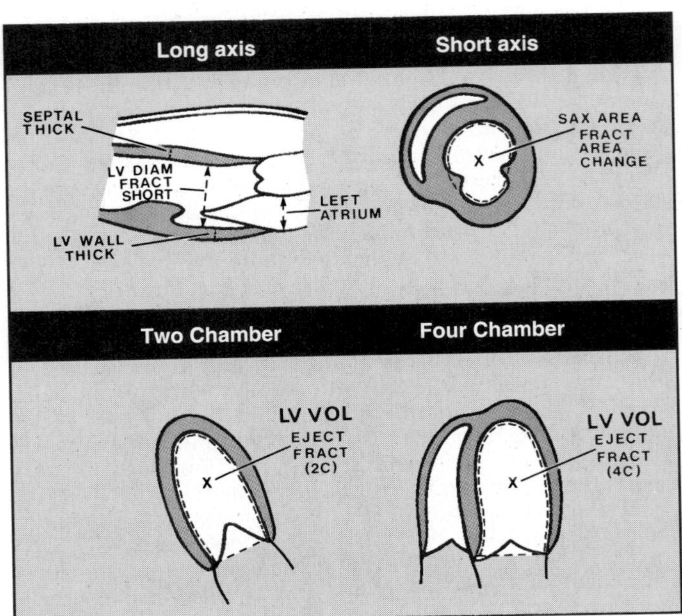

FIGURE 3–35. Some of the measurements that can be obtained from 2-D echocardiograms. The left ventricular diameter and fractional shortening provide an assessment of the size and systolic function of the base of the left ventricle. The short-axis (SAX) areas and fractional area change at the papillary muscle level give similar information for the midportion of the left ventricle. Left ventricular volumes (LV VOL) and ejection fraction can be determined from two-chamber and four-chamber echocardiograms using prolate ellipse or Simpson's rule formulas for calculating volumes. (From Feigenbaum, H.: Echocardiography. 5th ed. Malvern, PA, Lea and Febiger, 1994.)

Figure 3–35 shows some of the left ventricular measurements that are possible with 2-D echocardiography.[57] One can utilize the parasternal long-axis and short-axis views to obtain modified M-mode measurements. The long-axis examination permits measurements very similar to the M-mode measurements. The dimension between the interventricular septum and the posterior left ventricular wall provides an opportunity for calculating left ventricular dimensions and fractional shortening. It should be emphasized, however, that this dimension is not the same as the M-mode measurement. The M-mode dimension is usually not through the true minor dimension. The relationship of the M-mode measurement to the minor axis depends upon the available acoustic window. This window tends to be lower in older individuals. Thus the M-mode dimension changes with age. The dimensions from the long-axis view of the 2-D examination is truly through the minor dimension and is closer to the base of the heart. The 2-D fractional shortening essentially evaluates systolic function at the base of the left ventricle.[58] Septal thickness, posterior wall thickness, left atrial dimensions, and aortic dimensions are again possible using the long-axis 2-D examination as has been done with M-mode measurements. The short-axis view provides left ventricular area measurements and a systolic ejection index calculated as fractional area change.

To measure volumes the apical views are necessary. A variety of ways to calculate volumes have been proposed.[57] Probably the most accurate is to use a modified version of Simpson's rule because it minimizes the effect of geometric shape for calculating volumes. However, any of the angiographic techniques, such as the prolate ellipse or area-length methods, have also been used to calculate volumes using the apical 2-D echograms. A somewhat simplified formula for calculating volumes is the "bullet" formula, which takes five-sixths of the area in the short-axis view times the length of the left ventricle ($V = 5/6\ AL$). This formula is attractive because of its simplicity and because the area of the left ventricle and the length of the left ventricle can be easily obtained with 2-D echocardiography. It is also common practice for the physician interpreting echocardiograms to merely estimate the ejection fraction on the basis of visual inspection.[59] This approach is attractive because it avoids the necessity to make any measurements. However, the measurement is obviously qualitative and is highly subjective.

There are attempts to automate the quantitation of left ventricular function using 2-D echocardiography. Figure 3–36 shows a technique whereby the endocardial border is automatically detected. The instrument provides an instantaneous measure of the cross-sectional area of the left ventricle.[60] This technique has also been extrapolated to attempt to give volumes as well as area changes.[61] As with all quantitative measurements, this technique is very dependent upon the quality of the image and clear identification of endocardial borders.[62] As a general rule, apical

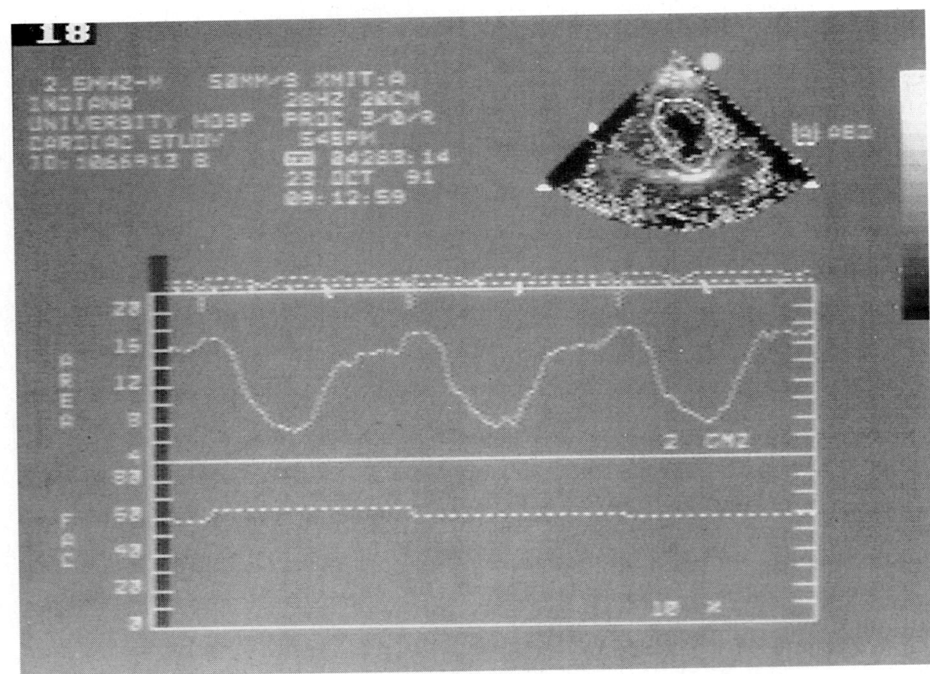

FIGURE 3–36. How a real-time edge detection device can produce a display of the cyclic variation in the area of the left ventricle. An area of interest is drawn around the left ventricular cavity, and an instrument automatically determines the area on a frame-to-frame basis. The graphic display shows change in area and fractional area change (FAC). (From Feigenbaum, H.: Echocardiography. 5th ed. Malvern, PA, Lea and Febiger, 1994.)

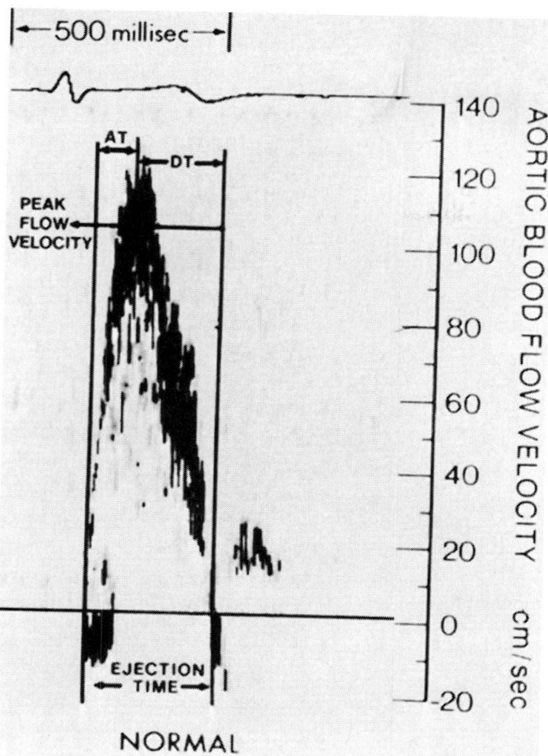

FIGURE 3–37. Pulsed Doppler recording of aortic blood flow velocity demonstrating how ejection time, peak flow velocity, acceleration time (AT), and deceleration time (DT) are measured. (From Gardin, J. M., et al.: Evaluation of blood flow velocity in the ascending aorta and main pulmonary artery of normal subjects by Doppler echocardiography. Am. Heart J. *107*:310, 1984.)

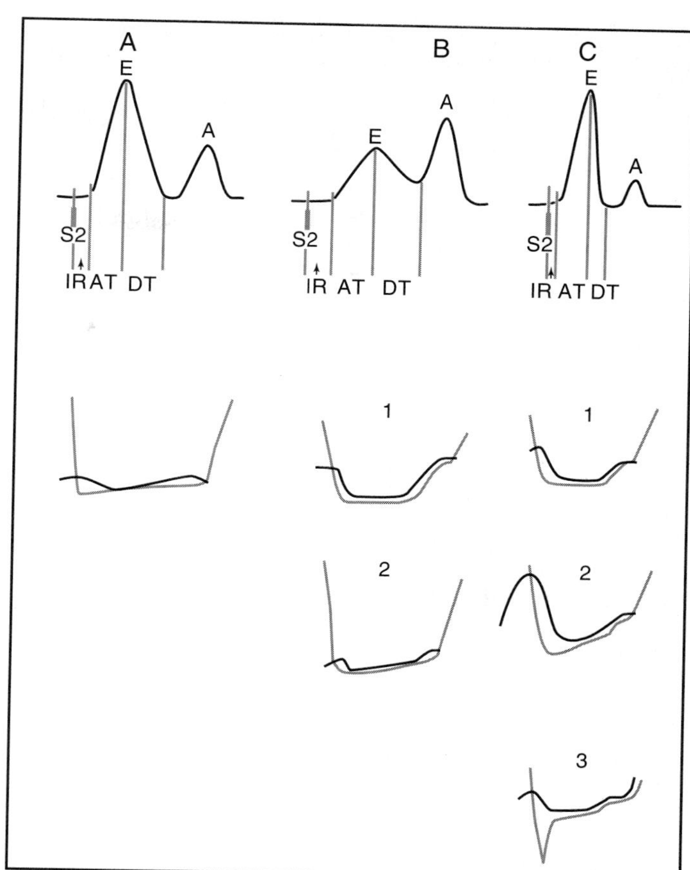

FIGURE 3–38. Relationship of mitral valve or left ventricular inflow Doppler velocities and left ventricular and left atrial pressures (see text for details). (From Feigenbaum, H.: Echocardiography. 5th ed. Malvern, PA, Lea and Febiger, 1994.)

views suffer more from loss of endocardial definition because the walls are parallel to the ultrasonic beam.

DOPPLER ECHOCARDIOGRAPHY. This technique can be used to evaluate left ventricular systolic function with a recording of flow in the ascending aorta. Acceleration time, from the onset of flow to the time of peak acceleration (Fig. 3–37), and peak acceleration have been shown to be related to global left ventricular systolic function.[63] The acceleration of the mitral regurgitant Doppler velocity may be an indicator of contractility.[64]

DIASTOLIC FUNCTION. Echocardiography has been used to evaluate left ventricular diastolic function. M-mode techniques have been used to record the rate of relaxation of the left ventricular cavity. This technique utilizes digitization of the borders of the left ventricular cavity, with the rapidity with which the left ventricular dimension increases in early diastole being noted.[66]

Doppler echocardiography currently is the primary technique used for evaluating left ventricular diastolic function.[67] Figure 3–38 shows the relationship between mitral flow and left ventricular and left atrial pressures.[68] With normal left-sided pressures the early diastolic mitral velocity (E) exceeds that following atrial systole (A). Under several conditions, one of which is normal aging,[69] the velocity in early diastole decreases and the late velocity increases (Fig. 3–38*B*). Among the pathologic states that produce this change are left ventricular hypertrophy and myocardial ischemia.[70] Both conditions produce abnormal relaxation and decreased early velocity into the left ventricle. This situation will commonly produce elevated left ventricular diastolic pressures (Fig. 3–38*B*-1). Unusually low filling pressures within the left atrium may also produce a similar pattern of flow (Fig. 3–38*B*-2).

If the left ventricular filling pressure is markedly elevated, as may occur with severe heart failure (Fig. 3–38*C*-1), then the left ventricular inflow velocity pattern changes dramatically.[71] Now there is a marked increase in the early diastolic velocity with an increase in the E velocity (Fig. 3–38*C*). The atrial velocity is now reduced. A similar pattern may also occur if one has severe mitral regurgitation with an elevated V wave in the left atrial pressure (Fig. 3–38*C*-2). This type of mitral flow may also occur if there is a restrictive pattern of filling of the left ventricle, as may occur with constrictive pericarditis or restrictive cardiomyopathy (Fig. 3–38*C*-3). It is apparent that with an abnormal left ventricle the flow pattern may change from normal (A) to abnormal relaxation (B) early in the disease. As the problem progresses and heart failure and/or mitral regurgitation develops, then the pattern may change to C.[72] Between *B* and *C* one can have "pseudonormalization" whereby an apparent normal pattern *(A)* is really a transition between *B* and *C*. Investigators are also measuring various time intervals such as isovolumetric relaxation time from Doppler recordings to assess left ventricular diastolic function.[73]

STRESS ECHOCARDIOGRAPHY. Although echocardiography has been used primarily for evaluating the cardiac chambers at rest, there is increasing interest in performing the ultrasonic examination during or immediately after some form of stress. These studies have utilized supine[74] or upright bicycle exercise,[75] immediate post-treadmill exercise,[76] pharmacological stress, and atrial pacing.[77] Many of the technical difficulties involved in recording an echocardiogram while the patient is hyperventilating following exercise have been overcome by using digital techniques that record a single cardiac cycle or continuous loop display.[78] This digital approach eliminates respiratory artifacts and permits the resting and exercise studies to be presented side by side for ease of interpretation. This type of examination is being done primarily for detecting exercise-induced regional wall motion abnormalities in patients with coronary artery disease. Exercise studies using Doppler measurements during exercise have also been used to assess global changes in left ventricular function and hemodynamics in patients with valvular heart disease[79,80] or congenital heart disease.[81]

WALL THICKNESS. Echocardiography may also be employed to measure the thickness of the walls of the ventricle[82] (Figs. 3–32 and 3–35). The absolute thickness of the ventricle is important in determining the presence of left ventricular hypertrophy, in estimating left ventricular mass,[83,84] and in calculating left ventricular end-systolic stress.[85,86] Echocardiography also permits measurement of changes in left ventricular thickness during the cardiac cycle.[87] Normally the left ventricular wall thickens during systole, but in pathological conditions this thickening decreases and actual systolic thinning has been noted in acute ischemia or myocardial infarction.[88]

OTHER CHAMBERS

Left Atrium. Echocardiography offers the opportunity to evaluate all four cardiac chambers and not just the left ventricle. Left atrial dilatation is readily recognized on the M-mode[89] (Fig. 3–31) or 2-D echocardiogram (Fig. 3–35).[90] A variety of quantitative measurements have been introduced. A simple anteroposterior dimension of the chamber is usually sufficient for identifying patients with dilated left atria. Such measurements can be done with either the M-mode or parasternal long-axis 2-D view. In patients in whom the left atrium does not uniformly expand or if there is distortion by a dilated aorta,[91] other views, including the apical 2-D views, can be used to assess the size of the left atrium.[92,93] Transesophageal echocardiography provides an excellent view of the left atrium, especially the atrial appendage. Since this site is a common location for clot formation, it has been studied extensively for function[94] as well as for clots.[95]

Right Ventricle and Atrium. The right ventricle is more difficult to evaluate quantitatively because of its unusual shape.[96] However, gross dilatation is easily assessed with M-mode[97] or 2-D examinations. Probably the most common technique is to use the relative size of the right and left ventricles in the apical four-chamber view. The thickness of the right ventricle walls can also be detected using either M-mode or 2-D echocardiography.[98] With right ventricular dilatation there is frequently distortion of the shape of the interventricular septum.[99] Whether this distortion occurs primarily during diastole or systole will indicate whether or not there is primarily a pressure or volume overload of the right ventricle.[100] With a diastolic overload the septum is flat in diastole and assumes a more normal curvature in systole. With a pressure overload the flattened interventricular septum is seen with systole.[101]

The right atrium can also be evaluated with 2-D echocardiography using the apical four-chamber or parasternal right ventricular inflow view. Transesophageal echocardiography provides excellent examination of the right atrium.

Hemodynamic Information

DOPPLER ECHOCARDIOGRAPHY. This is now the principal ultrasonic technique for obtaining hemodynamic information. By recording the velocity of intracardiac blood flow, one can obtain quantitative data concerning both blood flow and intracardiac pressures. The principle is illustrated in Figure 3–39. To calculate flow the mean velocity passing through an orifice or vessel and the cross-sectional area of the orifice or vessel must be known. The mean velocity is acquired by measuring the velocity time integral of the Doppler signal, which is the area under the recording. The cross-sectional area of the orifice through which the blood is flowing can be obtained directly with 2-D echocardiography; alternatively the diameter can be measured with either 2-D[102] or M-mode[103] echocardiography, and then the area can be calculated. Such flow determinations are feasible through any orifice or vessel.[104]

Blood flow in the ascending aorta is commonly used for cardiac output calculations.[105] The integrated velocity from the ascending aorta is combined with the calculated cross-sectional area determined at any of three locations: the aortic annulus, the separation of the aortic valve leaflets, or just past the sinus of Valsalva. All three approaches have been used with reasonable success. In a similar manner, pulmonary blood flow can be measured by taking Doppler pulmonary artery velocity and multiplying it by the cross-sectional area of the pulmonary artery. Flow through the mitral[106,107] and tricuspid valves[108] has also been calculated. Atrioventricular valve flow is somewhat more complicated because the flow is phasic, and early and late diastolic flow must be allowed for.[109] Although the measurements are more complex, they have been reasonably accurate.[110]

The effectiveness of Doppler echocardiography for measuring flow has been validated; however, there are many technical details in making such calculations. The biggest limitation is the calculation of the orifice or vessel area.[111] It is difficult to obtain an accurate cross-sectional area of the various orifices. Because the measured diameter must be squared in the calculation of blood flow, any error would also be squared. For example, in many adult patients it is difficult to obtain an accurate orifice measurement of the main pulmonary artery.

Although the Doppler technique for measuring blood flow is not routinely done in many laboratories, the potential clinical utility is readily apparent. It can be used to measure cardiac output or stroke volume.[12] The technique is particularly useful for following directional changes in these variables in a given patient.[113,114] By calculating flow through different orifices, regurgitant fraction[115] and shunt ratios can be quantified.[116,117] For example, pulmonary to systemic flow ratios can be obtained by measuring aortic and pulmonary artery flows. Mitral regurgitant fraction can be calculated by measuring aortic flow and mitral valve flow. With the increasing availability of computer analysis, the difficulties of making these determinations have been resolved. However, some limitations still exist.[118]

DOPPLER MEASUREMENT OF PRESSURE GRADIENTS. Possibly the most important development in Doppler echocardiography has been the utilization of a modified version of the Bernoulli equation to calculate the pressure drop or

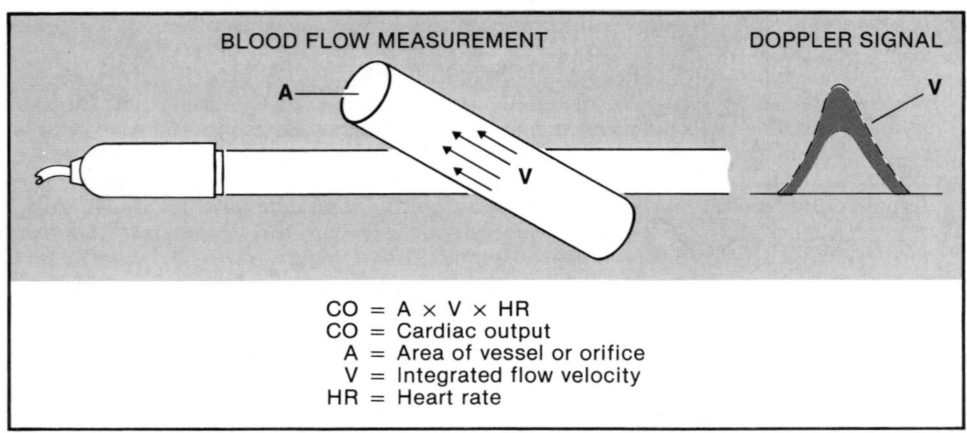

FIGURE 3–39. Principles of using Doppler echocardiography to measure blood flow. (From Feigenbaum, H.: Echocardiography. 4th ed. Philadelphia, Lea and Febiger, 1986.)

PLATE 1

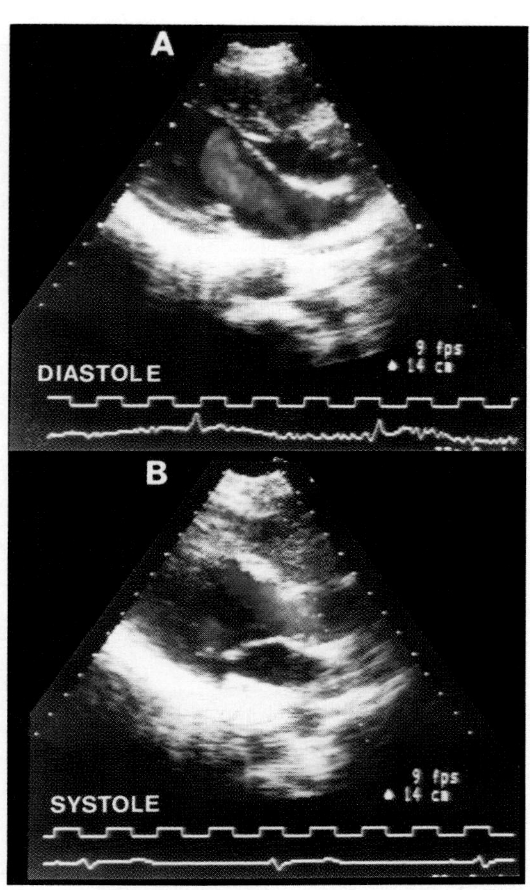

FIGURE 3–10. Two-dimensional color flow Doppler image of the left ventricular inflow *(A)* and outflow *(B)* in the parasternal long-axis view. The blood passing through the mitral valve during diastole *(A)* is moving toward the transducer and is encoded in red. During systole *(B)* the blood passes through the left ventricular outflow tract and is encoded in blue. As the velocity increases toward the aortic root, the intensity or brightness of the color increases.

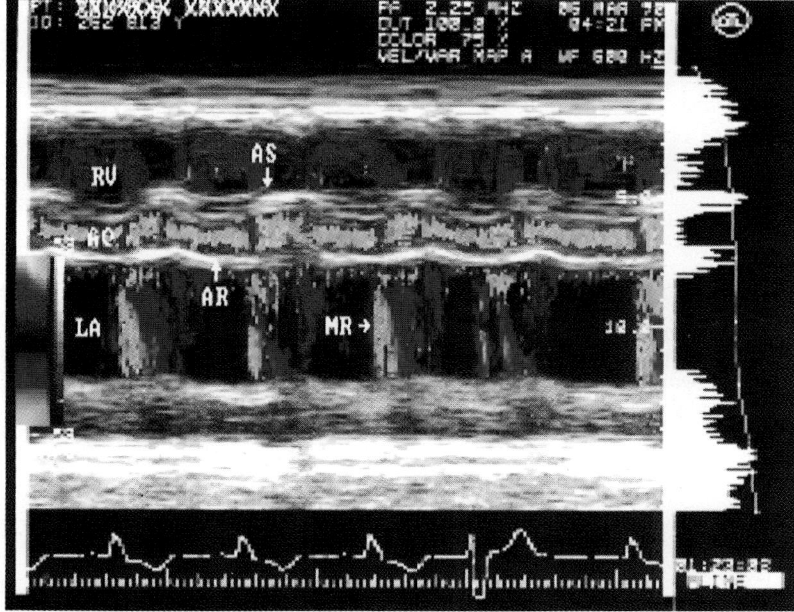

FIGURE 3–11. Color-encoded Doppler flow superimposed on an M-mode tracing in a patient with valvular heart disease. The high-velocity turbulent blood is encoded in green. Both the systolic aortic stenosis flow (AS) and the diastolic aortic regurgitation flow (AR) can be seen within the aorta (AO). The high-velocity mitral regurgitation jet (MR) is detected within the left atrium (LA) in systole. RV = right ventricle.

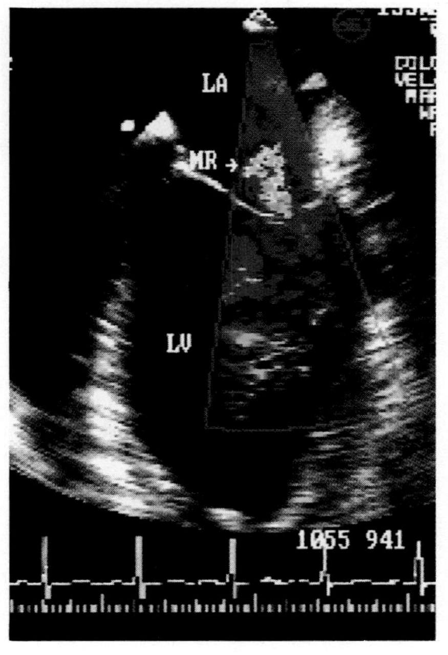

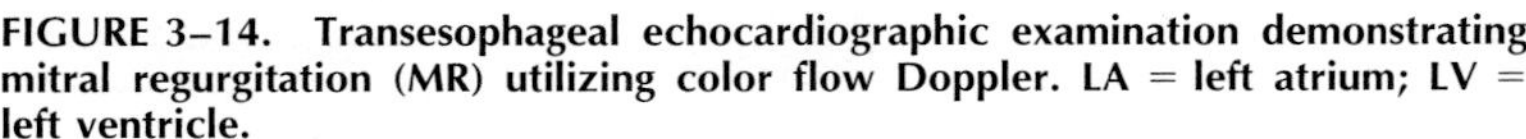

FIGURE 3–14. Transesophageal echocardiographic examination demonstrating mitral regurgitation (MR) utilizing color flow Doppler. LA = left atrium; LV = left ventricle.

PLATE 2

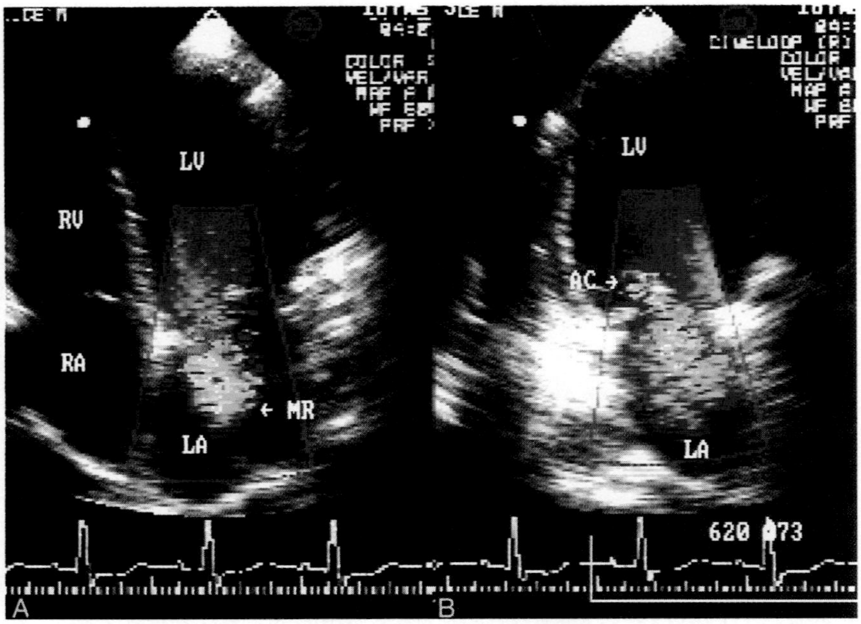

FIGURE 3–49. Color flow Doppler study of a patient with mitral regurgitation (MR) as viewed from the four-chamber *(A)* and two-chamber *(B)* views. There is acceleration of flow on the left ventricular side of the regurgitant mitral orifice (AC). LV = left ventricle; LA = left atrium; RV = right ventricle; RA = right atrium.

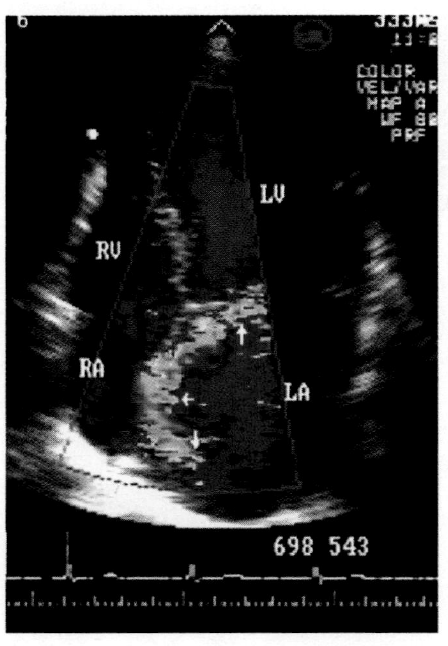

FIGURE 3–50. Color flow Doppler study of a patient with mitral regurgitation in whom the regurgitant jet (arrows) is eccentric and directed toward the interatrial septum. RV = right ventricle; LV = left ventricle; RA = right atrium; LA = left atrium.

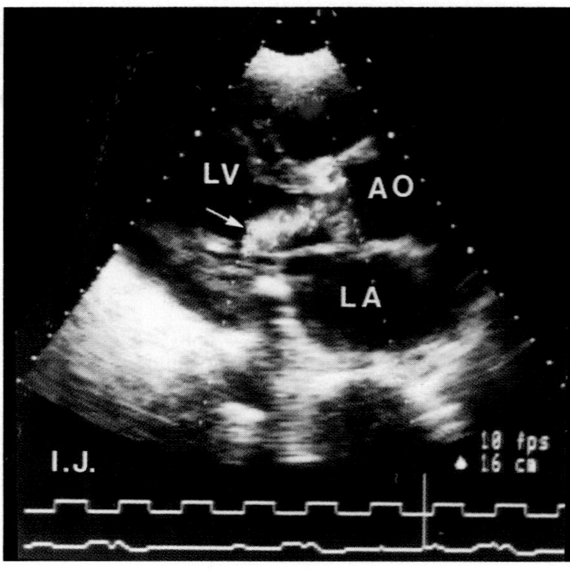

FIGURE 3–58. Color flow mapping in a patient with aortic regurgitation. The brightly colored, high-velocity jet can be seen passing from the aorta (AO) to the left ventricle (LV). The center of the jet is white, and the edges are shades of blue. Even though the velocity is extremely high, most of the jet is blue because the flow is almost perpendicular to the ultrasonic beam, and the velocities are registered as being lower than they actually are.

PLATE 3

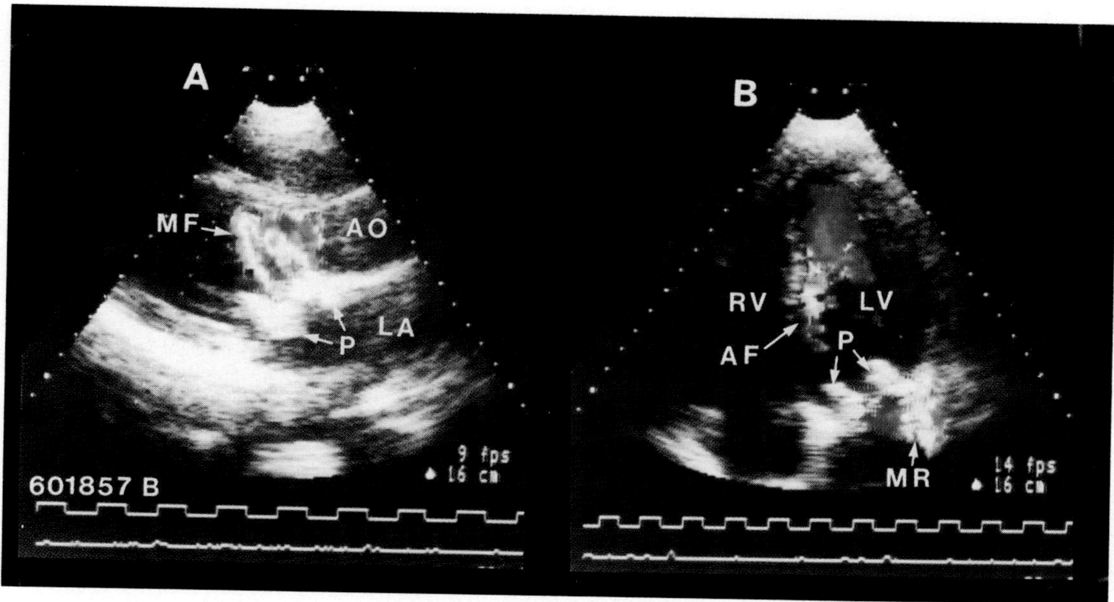

FIGURE 3–65. Color Doppler images in diastole *(A)* and systole *(B)* in a patient with a prosthetic mitral valve (P). During diastole *(A)*, turbulent multidirectional antegrade mitral flow (MF) is present. During systole *(B)*, a regurgitant jet (MR) is present within the left atrium along the lateral border of the prosthetic valve (P). Aortic flow (AF) exhibits aliasing in this patient who also had left ventricular outflow obstruction. The apical half of the left ventricular outflow tract is blue and the portion near the aorta is red. AO = aorta; LA = left atrium; RV = right ventricle; LV = left ventricle.

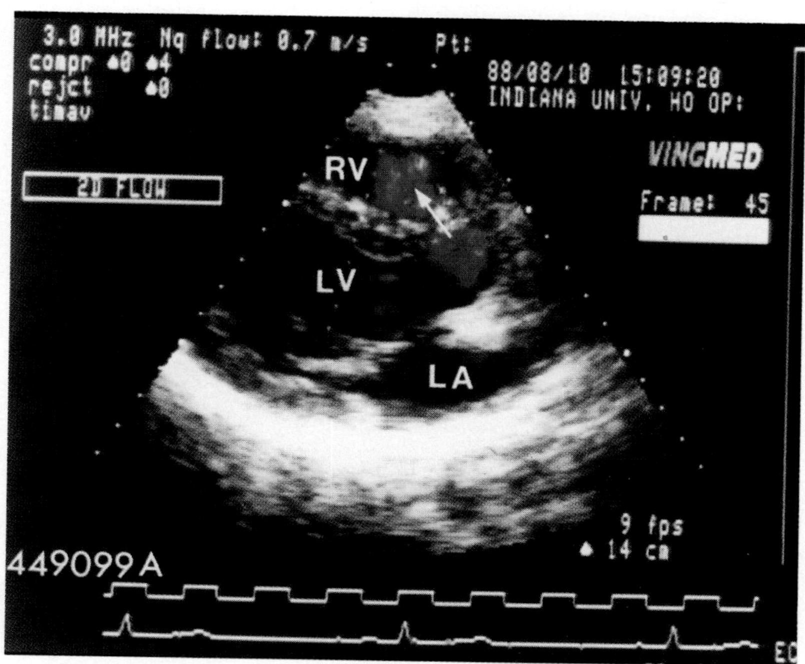

FIGURE 3–74. Color flow Doppler study of a patient with a membranous ventricular septal defect. The blood can be seen flowing toward the transducer and the right ventricle (RV) and is encoded in red (arrow). At the site of the defect the width of the jet is narrowed and the velocity is increased as noted by the multicolor nature of the flow map. LV = left ventricle; LA = left atrium.

PLATE 4

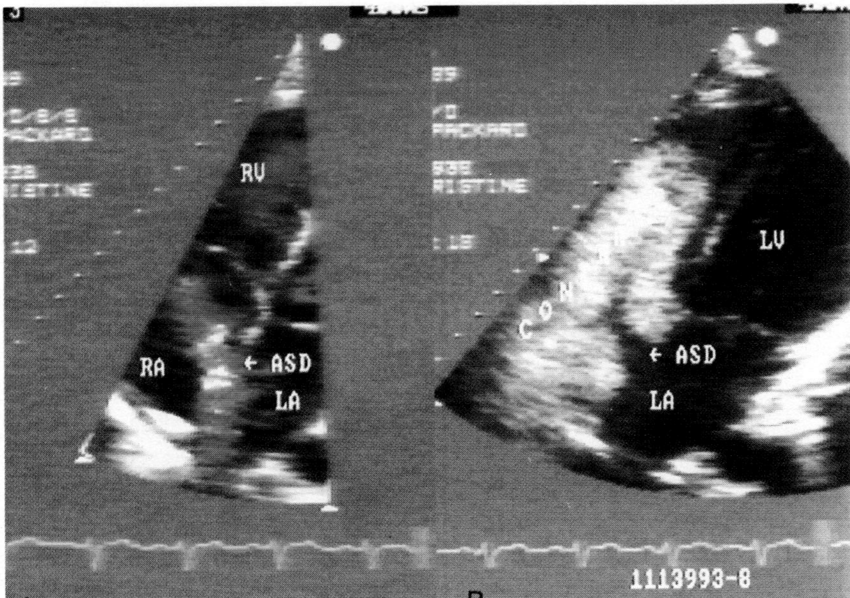

FIGURE 3–81. Color flow Doppler *(left)* and contrast echocardiogram *(right)* of a patient with a secundum atrial septal defect. The defect (ASD) is noted by red-encoded blood passing through the atrial septum on the color study and as a negative contrast with the contrast echocardiogram. RV = right ventricle; RA = right atrium; LA = left atrium; LV = left ventricle.

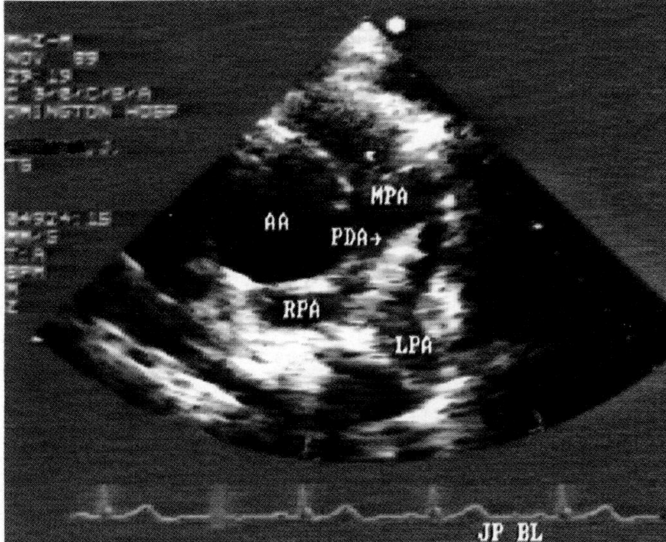

FIGURE 3–83. Color Doppler images in a patient with patent ductus arteriosus. The shunt flow passing from the aorta into the pulmonary artery can be seen as a blue jet (PDA) within the main pulmonary artery (MPA). RPA = right pulmonary artery; LPA = left pulmonary artery; AA = aorta.

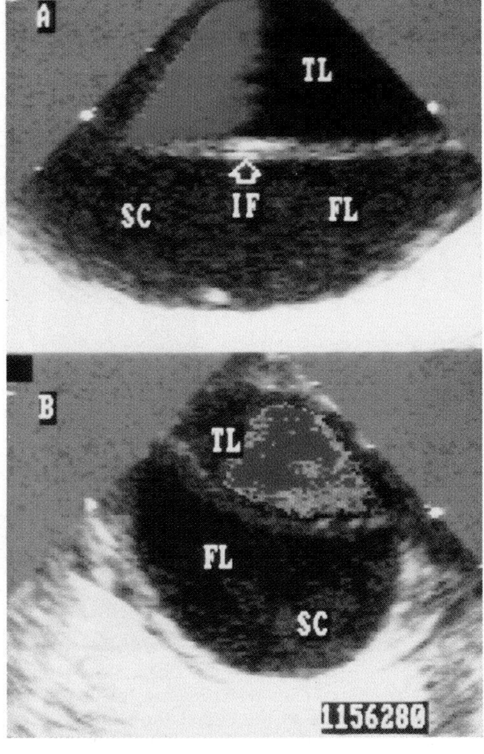

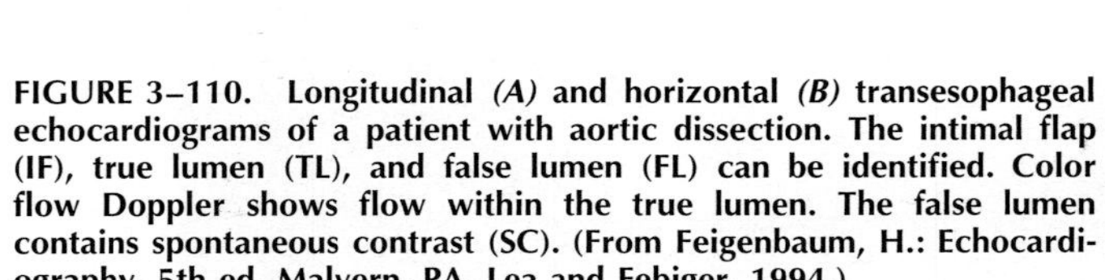

FIGURE 3–110. Longitudinal *(A)* and horizontal *(B)* transesophageal echocardiograms of a patient with aortic dissection. The intimal flap (IF), true lumen (TL), and false lumen (FL) can be identified. Color flow Doppler shows flow within the true lumen. The false lumen contains spontaneous contrast (SC). (From Feigenbaum, H.: Echocardiography. 5th ed. Malvern, PA, Lea and Febiger, 1994.)

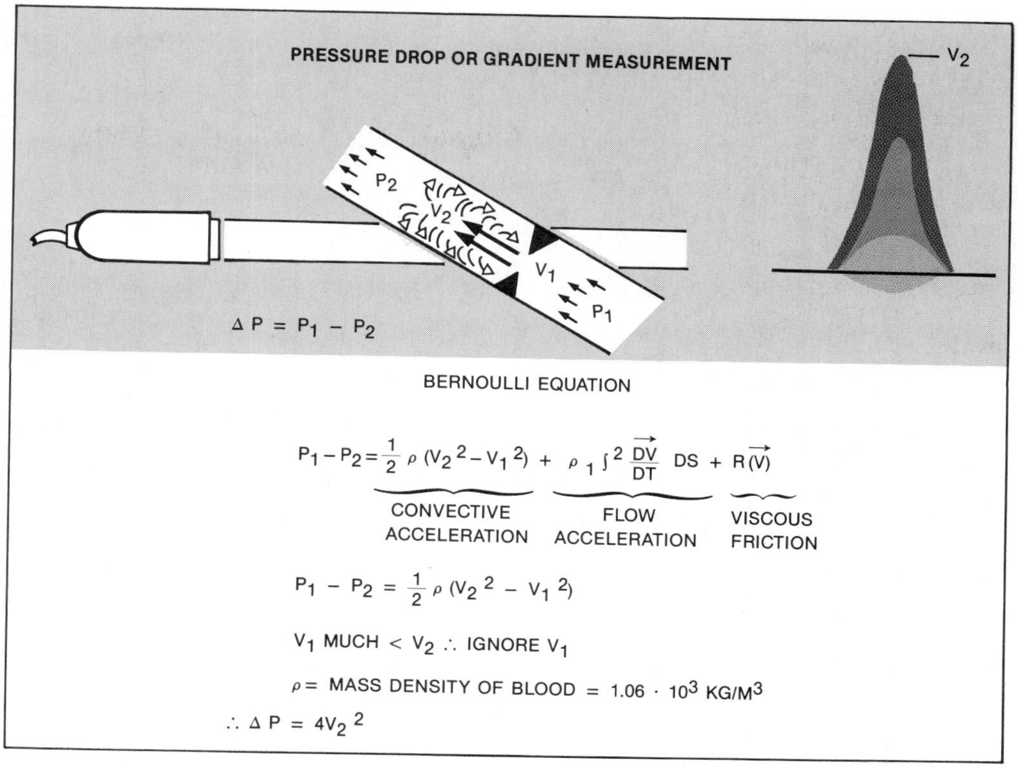

PRESSURE DROP OR GRADIENT MEASUREMENT

$\Delta P = P_1 - P_2$

BERNOULLI EQUATION

$$P_1 - P_2 = \frac{1}{2}\rho(V_2^2 - V_1^2) + \rho\int_1^2 \frac{\vec{DV}}{DT}DS + R(\vec{V})$$

CONVECTIVE ACCELERATION — FLOW ACCELERATION — VISCOUS FRICTION

$$P_1 - P_2 = \frac{1}{2}\rho(V_2^2 - V_1^2)$$

V_1 MUCH $< V_2 \therefore$ IGNORE V_1

$\rho =$ MASS DENSITY OF BLOOD $= 1.06 \cdot 10^3$ KG/M^3

$\therefore \Delta P = 4V_2^2$

FIGURE 3–40. Principles of using Doppler echocardiography to measure a pressure drop or gradient across an obstruction. P_2 = pressure distal to an obstruction; V_2 = blood velocity distal to an obstruction; V_1 = velocity proximal to an obstruction; P_1 = pressure proximal to an obstruction. (From Feigenbaum, H.: Echocardiography. 4th ed. Philadelphia, Lea and Febiger, 1986.)

gradient across a narrowed part of the cardiovascular system[5]; the principle is shown in Figure 3–40. Although the Bernoulli equation is fairly complex and involves convective acceleration, flow acceleration, and viscous friction, the equation can be limited to convective acceleration alone because flow acceleration and viscous friction are probably not relevant in the clinical setting. Essentially the equation relates the difference in pressure across a stenosis with the differences in velocities. As blood flows through a narrowed orifice, the velocity increases proportionally. With a few assumptions that seem to be clinically appropriate, a fairly complicated equation can be condensed to the difference in pressure (ΔP) equals 4 times the square of the velocity distal to the obstruction. The accuracy and validity of this approach have been confirmed in numerous laboratories.[119] This observation is now the basis for many clinical applications of Doppler echocardiography.

CLINICAL APPLICATIONS: THE ESTIMATION OF INTRACARDIAC PRESSURES. An early application of Doppler echocardiography was calculating a pressure gradient across a stenotic mitral valve.[120] The approach was then used with stenotic semilunar valves.[119] This same technique can be used to assess the difference in pressure across a regurgitant valve as well as a stenotic valve. For example, in the presence of tricuspid regurgitation the difference in pressure between the right ventricle and the right atrium in systole can be assessed by noting the peak velocity of the regurgitant jet (Fig. 3–41).[121] By knowing the pressure differential between the right ventricle and right atrium and adding an estimate of the right atrial pressure, one can calculate right ventricular systolic pressure. If there is no obstruction to right ventricular outflow, the pulmonary artery systolic pressure is also known. If the velocity of blood flow across a ventricular septal defect is measured, the difference in pressure between the left and right ventricles can also be calculated. By knowing the left ventricular systolic pressure and the gradient between this chamber and the right ventricle, one can calculate right ventricular systolic pressure.[122] A similar approach is possible with aortic-pulmonary shunts.[123] With the help of the modified Bernoulli equation, Doppler

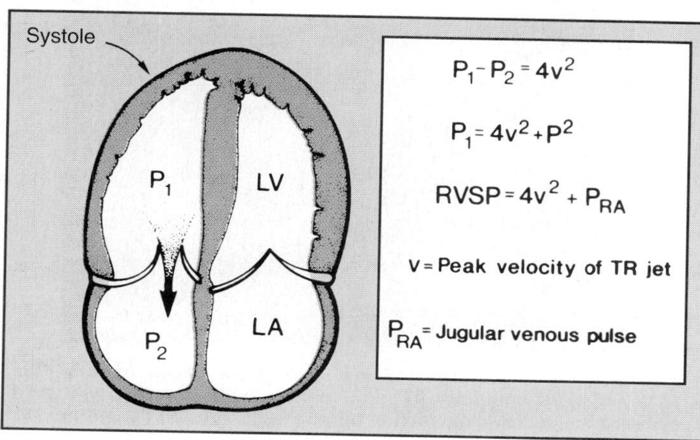

FIGURE 3–41. Measurement of right ventricular systolic pressure using Doppler recording of tricuspid regurgitation. Using the modified Bernoulli equation, one can calculate the pressure gradient across the regurgitant tricuspid valve ($P_1 - P_2$). The right ventricular systolic pressure of P_1 is equal to 4 times the square of the peak velocity of the tricuspid jet (v), plus the right atrial pressure (P_{RA}). (From Feigenbaum, H.: Echocardiography. 5th ed. Malvern, PA, Lea and Febiger, 1994.)

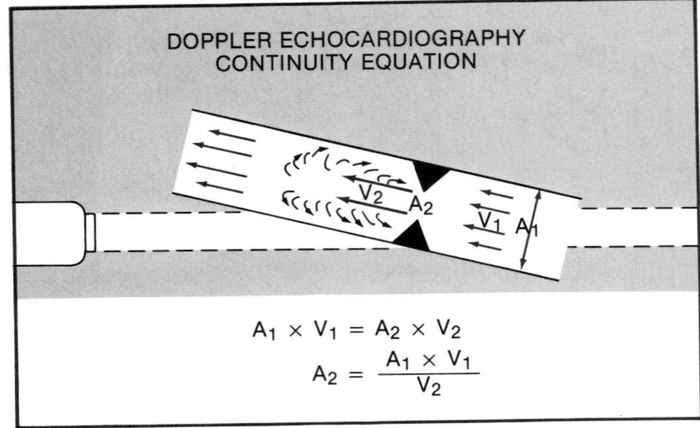

FIGURE 3–42. Principles of using Doppler echocardiography and the continuity equation for calculating the area of a stenotic orifice. A_1 = area proximal to the stenosis; A_2 = area of the stenosis; V_1 = velocity proximal to the stenosis; V_2 = velocity through the stenosis.

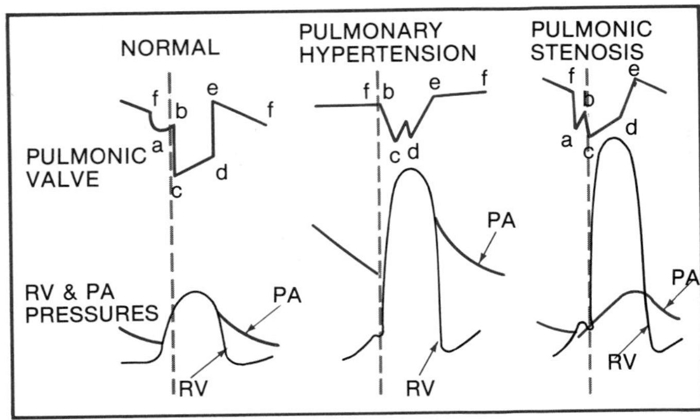

FIGURE 3–43. Relationship of the pulmonic valve echocardiogram and right-heart pressure in the normal state, with pulmonary hypertension and with pulmonic stenosis. PA = pulmonary artery pressure; RV = right ventricular pressure. (See text for details.) (From Feigenbaum, H.: Echocardiography. 2nd ed. Philadelphia, Lea and Febiger, 1976.)

echocardiography is playing an increasing role in estimating intracardiac pressures.

The pattern of the Doppler flow velocities can also provide hemodynamic information. Figure 3–38 shows the relationship between mitral flow and left-sided diastolic pressures. The flow pattern within the pulmonary artery can give clues to the presence of pulmonary hypertension.[124] However, this technique has been replaced by measurement of right ventricular systolic pressure.

DOPPLER MEASUREMENT OF VALVE AREA. Combining the Doppler principles for measuring blood flow and pressure gradient permits one to calculate a valve area utilizing the "continuity equation." Figure 3–42 shows the principle of how the area of a stenotic orifice can be calculated using a combination of Doppler and imaging ultrasound. From blood flow calculations (Fig. 3–39) stroke volume is a function of the product of the integrated velocity with the area. The continuity equation states that the blood flow proximal to the area of obstruction must equal the blood flow passing through the area of obstruction.[125] Thus, if the volume of blood proximal to an obstruction and the velocity of blood through the obstruction are known, the area of the stenotic orifice can be calculated (Fig. 3–42). In the case of aortic stenosis the velocity and the area of the left ventricular outflow tract must be measured to calculate blood flow proximal to a stenotic valve. Then by measuring the velocity of flow across the valve the aortic valve area can be calculated.

M-MODE VALVE RECORDINGS. M-mode recordings of the cardiac valves can also provide hemodynamic information. Abnormal closure of the mitral valve following atrial systole gives a qualitative assessment of elevated left atrial pressure. Normal valve motion between the A and C points (Fig. 3–30) is smooth and uninterrupted. If there is elevated left ventricular diastolic pressure secondary to a large increase with atrial systole, there will be interruption of this closure with a "B bump."[126,127] Premature closure of the mitral valve occurs with severe aortic regurgitation.[128] Analysis of the M-mode aortic valve recording is useful in patients with subaortic stenosis. With either dynamic or fixed obstruction one sees midsystolic closure of the aortic valve.[129] In patients with poor forward left ventricular stroke volume or severe mitral regurgitation there may be gradual closure of the aortic valve throughout systole. With severe aortic regurgitation and markedly elevated left ventricular diastolic pressure, the aortic valve may open before ventricular systole.[130]

Figure 3–43 diagrammatically shows the relationship of the M-mode pulmonary valve motion and right-sided pressures. Normally, atrial systole produces a slight downward motion of the pulmonary valve. With pulmonic stenosis, the right ventricular systolic and diastolic pressures rise without any similar elevation in pulmonary artery pressure. As a result, atrial contribution to right ventricular pressure is exaggerated and is usually sufficient to open the pulmonary valve prior to ventricular systole (Fig. 3–43).[131] In patients with elevated right ventricular diastolic pressures due to right ventricular failure, tricuspid regurgitation, constrictive pericarditis, or communication between the aorta and right ventricle, the elevated pressure in the right ventricle in early diastole may cause opening of the pulmonary valve even before the onset of atrial systole.[132] An increase in pulmonary artery pressure may change pulmonary valve motion in several ways (Fig. 3–43). One of the most consistent changes is the elimination of atrial systolic motion and the absence of the pulmonary valve A wave.[133] This A wave may reappear if right ventricular failure occurs with pulmonary hypertension. Another sign of pulmonary hypertension is midsystolic closure of the pulmonary valve.[134] These M-mode findings are now secondary to the Doppler measurement of right ventricular systolic pressure.[135]

EXAMINATION OF THE INFERIOR VENA CAVA. A 2-D echocardiographic examination of the inferior vena cava and hepatic vein gives information concerning right-sided hemodynamics (Fig. 3–44).[136] This examination can be helpful in assessing the central venous pressure. An increase in

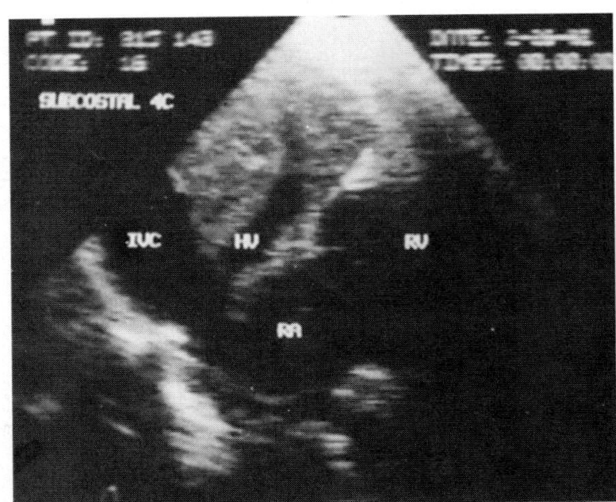

FIGURE 3–44. Subcostal 2-D echocardiogram of the right atrium (RA) and right ventricle (RV) in a patient with elevated right atrial pressure and a markedly dilated inferior vena cava (IVC) and hepatic vein (HV).

pressure dilates the veins[137] and eliminates the normal respiratory variation in the size of the inferior vena cava (Fig. 3–27).

ACQUIRED VALVULAR HEART DISEASE

(See also Chap. 32)

Mitral Stenosis

The detection of mitral stenosis (MS) was the first clinical application of echocardiography.[138] It remains an important technique in the evaluation of suspected mitral valve disease because echocardiography can allow visualization of the mitral valve in a manner not possible with any other procedure. The M-mode examination provides a sensitive assessment of the motion and thickness of the valve leaflets, while the 2-D technique provides a spatial image of the valve and allows direct measurement of the valve orifice.[139] Doppler echocardiography provides hemodynamic assessment of the stenotic orifice.

Figure 3–45 shows an M-mode echocardiogram of a patient with calcific MS. The motion of the mitral valve is considerably altered from the normal pattern seen in Figures 3–3 and 3–30; the normal M-shaped configuration during diastole is no longer present, since the presence of a holodiastolic atrioventricular pressure gradient (diastasis) prevents rapid closure of the valve in mid-diastole. Although sinus rhythm was present, there was no reopening of the valve with atrial contraction and no A wave. Thus, the M-mode echocardiographic hallmark of MS is the absence of valve closure in mid-diastole and of reopening in late diastole. Although this decreased (flat) diastolic (E-F) slope is characteristic of MS,[138] it is not specific. Other conditions such as decreased left ventricular compliance or low cardiac output may also reduce the diastolic slope of mitral valve motion.[140]

In addition to the change in motion of the valve, the number of echoes originating from the valve is increased when it is fibrotic or calcified, and another echocardiographic sign of MS is increased thickness of the valve leaflets. (Note that the quantity of echoes originating from the mitral valve in Figure 3–45 is considerably greater than in Figure 3–30.) Inadequate separation of the anterior and posterior leaflets of the valve occurs during diastole.[140] Normally the two leaflets move in opposite directions during diastole, but when fused, as in MS, they do not separate widely and may actually appear to move in the same direction (Fig. 3–45). The echocardiographic findings of reduced diastolic slope, increased thickness, and decreased separation of the valve leaflets provide a sensitive and accurate method for detection of MS.

The diagnosis of MS by 2-D echocardiography is made by noting thickening, doming, and restricted motion of the leaflets (Fig. 3–46). Doming of any valve on 2-D echocardiography is a characteristic sign of stenosis. This distortion in shape with opening of the valve indicates that the tips of the leaflets are restricted in their ability to open, whereas the bodies of the leaflets still wish to accommodate more blood flow; thus the leaflets are curved, or domed. The presence of doming distinguishes a valve that is truly stenotic from one that opens poorly because of low flow. Two-dimensional echocardiography provides an opportunity to visualize and measure the flow-restricting orifice of the stenotic mitral valve directly (Fig. 3–46*B*).[141]

Doppler echocardiography provides another means of quantitating the degree of MS.[142] Figure 3–47 shows a pulsed Doppler recording of a patient with MS and atrial fibrillation; there is no atrial contraction. The peak velocities are increased, and the fall in velocity in early diastole is decreased. The technique for quantitating the degree of MS depends on the rate of velocity decrease in early diastole. The time interval required for the peak velocity to reach half of its initial level is related directly to the severity of the obstruction of the mitral orifice.[143] This pressure half-time correlates reasonably well with the mitral valve area; however, there are some limitations to this technique.[144–146] The modified Bernoulli equation can also be used to calculate the mean gradient transmitral valve pressure gradient.[147] Mitral valve area can then be calculated using the Gorlin formula and a Doppler measurement for mitral blood flow.[148]

Echocardiography can help determine whether or not a stenotic valve is suitable for valvotomy by estimating its pliability and degree of calcification.[149] This ability is particularly valuable in evaluating patients for balloon valvuloplasty.[150,151] Two-dimensional echocardiography is the procedure of choice for assessing the fibrosis and pliability of the mitral valve apparatus, especially when subvalvular adhesions are present.[152] Secondary effects of mitral stenosis, such as left atrial dilatation and pulmonary hypertension, can be detected with various echocardiographic examinations.

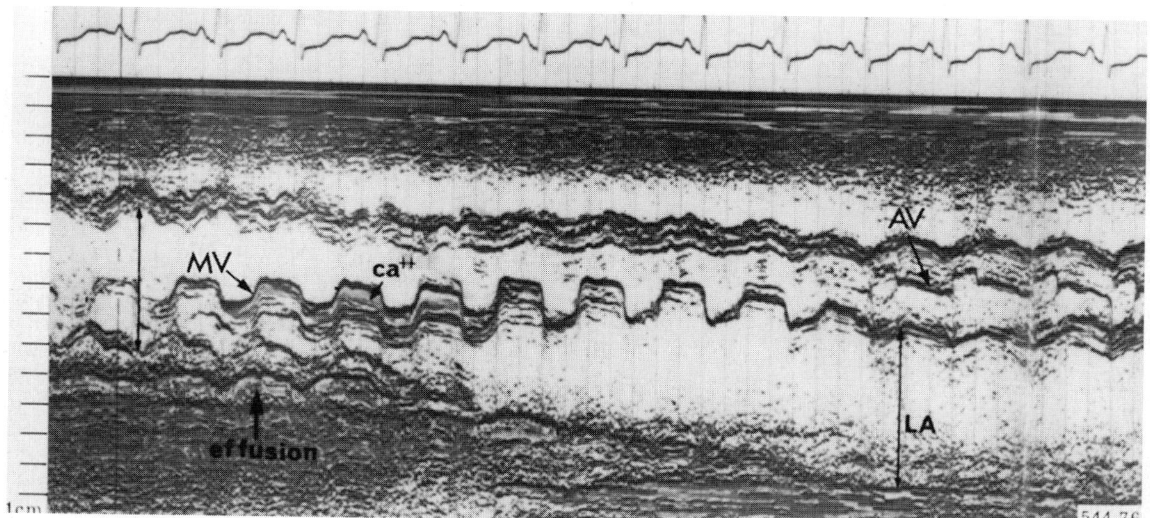

FIGURE 3–45. M-mode scan from a patient with mitral stenosis. The valve is calcified (Ca^{++}) and immobile. The left atrium (LA) is dilated, and there is moderate posterior pericardial effusion. AV = aortic valve. (From Chang, S.: M-Mode Echocardiographic Techniques and Pattern Recognition. Philadelphia, Lea and Febiger, 1976.)

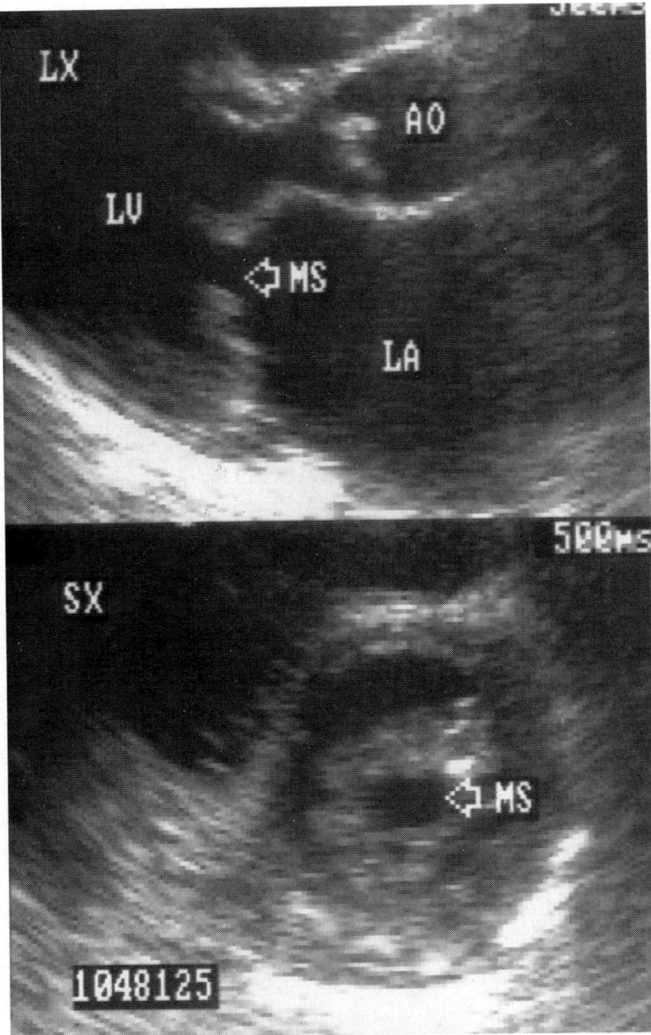

FIGURE 3–46. Long-axis (LX) and short-axis (SX) 2-D echocardiograms of a patient with mitral stenosis. The long-axis view shows typical doming of both leaflets with diminished separation (MS) between the anterior and posterior edges. The short-axis view shows the echo-free orifice in the center of the stenotic valve (MS). (From Feigenbaum, H.: Echocardiography. 5th ed. Malvern, PA, Lea and Febiger, 1994.)

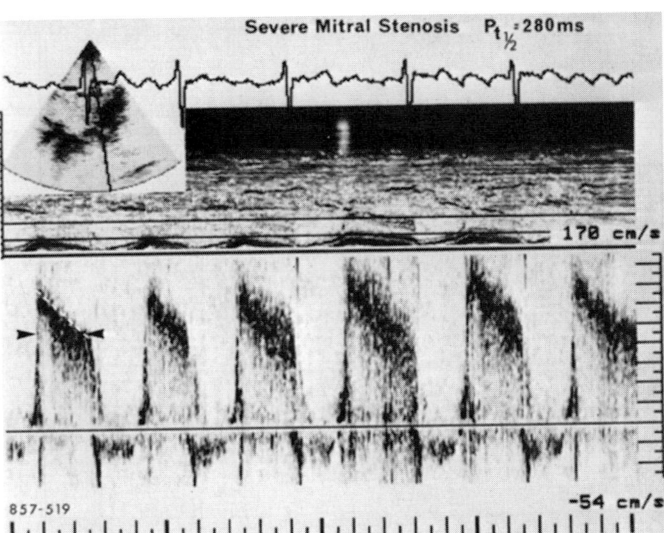

FIGURE 3–47. Pulsed Doppler echocardiogram of mitral flow in a patient with mitral stenosis, demonstrating how the pressure half-time ($P_{t_{1/2}}$) (arrowheads) is measured. (From Feigenbaum, H.: Echocardiography. 4th ed. Philadelphia, Lea and Febiger, 1986.)

Mitral Regurgitation

DOPPLER ECHOCARDIOGRAPHY. This is the ultrasonic procedure of choice for the detection of any valvular regurgitation.[153] Figure 3–48 shows a pulsed Doppler recording with the Doppler sample in the left atrium. With this type of examination, high-velocity flow which aliases is recorded during ventricular systole in the left atrium.

Color flow Doppler is the principal echocardiographic technique for assessing the presence and severity of mitral regurgitation (MR) (Fig. 3–49).[154] Transesophageal echocardiography is more sensitive in detecting MR than is the transthoracic approach.[155] The regurgitant blood flows into the left atrium during ventricular systole. The velocity is very high, and a mosaic, multicolored pattern is recorded because of aliasing. The location, direction, and size of the MR flow are readily depicted by the color flow system. There is a rough relationship between the size of the regurgitant jet and the extent of regurgitation,[156] but this relationship is influenced by many factors, such as the direction of the regurgant jet (Fig. 3–50). In Figure 3–49 the jet enters the center of the left atrium and fills much of the left

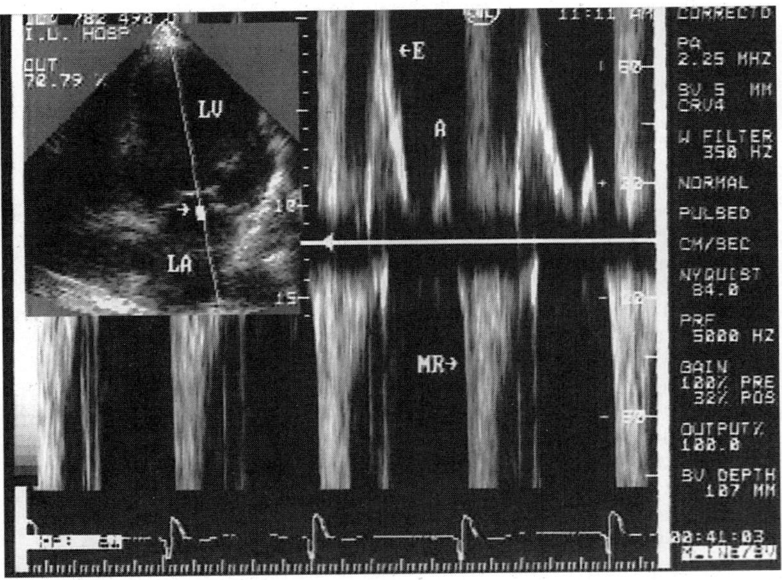

FIGURE 3–48. Pulsed Doppler examination of a patient with mitral regurgitation. The sample volume is within the left atrium (LA) and shows the high-velocity, aliasing mitral regurgitant jet (MR). LV = left ventricle. (From Feigenbaum, H.: Echocardiography. 5th ed. Malvern, PA, Lea and Febiger, 1994.)

FIGURE 3–49. See color plate 2.

FIGURE 3–50. See color plate 2.

atrium; it is known as a central jet. However, in Figure 3–50 the jet is directed toward the interatrial septum, and the flow curves around the atrial septum (arrows). Such Doppler flow is a wall jet.[157] The area of such a pattern underestimates the degree of regurgitation.

A useful sign when using color flow Doppler for valvular regurgitation is to look at the acceleration of flow proximal to the regurgitant orifice (AC) (Fig. 3–49). This acceleration is due to blood velocity increasing as it approaches the small regurgitant orifice.[158] This finding is usually indicative of significant blood flow or regurgitant flow. Techniques have been developed to use this proximal acceleration to calculate a proximal isovelocity area or PISA.[159] This area measurement has been used to quantitate the severity of MR.[160,161] Another technique is to record pulmonary venous Doppler velocities and noting systolic reverse flow.[162]

Unfortunately, all flow-mapping techniques with either color mapping or standard pulsed Doppler have only a limited relationship to the degree of MR.[163,164] Thus the quantitation of valvular regurgitation using Doppler flow mapping is at best semiquantitative. An alternative Doppler technique for quantifying MR is to calculate stroke volumes through two different orifices, one that reflects flow ejected from the left ventricle to the aorta and one measuring flow passing from the left atrium to the left ventricle.[165,166] The difference is the regurgitant volume, and regurgitant fraction can be calculated. This approach requires accurate stroke volume measurements and may not be possible in all patients.

Echocardiography is also helpful in assessing the hemodynamic consequences of the MR. The left atrium is invariably dilated, and left ventricular stroke volume increases with frequent left ventricular dilatation.[167] All of these findings are detectable on the echocardiogram. Possibly one of the most important uses of echocardiography is in identifying the etiology of the MR. Rheumatic MR almost always produces some thickening of the mitral valve and at least minimal echocardiographic evidence of MS. There are numerous other causes for MR, and echocardiography plays an important role in identifying these.

NONRHEUMATIC MITRAL REGURGITATION

Mitral Valve Prolapse (see p. 1029). Echocardiography is particularly useful in the diagnosis of this condition.[168] Figure 3–51 demonstrates the principal M-mode finding, a fairly abrupt posterior (downward) motion of the mitral valve apparatus in mid or late systole.[169] This motion often commences simultaneously with the mid or late systolic click (Fig. 3–51), a typical auscultatory and phonocardiographic finding in this condition (see p. 31). Although this mid or late systolic posterior motion of the mitral valve is a reasonably specific sign of mitral valve prolapse, it is not a very sensitive sign. Many patients with this lesion fail to show it, while in others the prolapse is a holosystolic event, i.e., there is posterior displacement of the valve throughout systole (Fig. 32–25, p. 1034).[170] Minor degrees of posterior displacement of the mitral valve can occur normally, and there is a troublesome "gray zone" in which it is difficult to determine whether the prolapse is normal or not.[171] Late or holosystolic prolapse, as in Figure 3–51, in which the leaflets move posteriorly by at least 5 mm, is generally accepted as abnormal. However, when

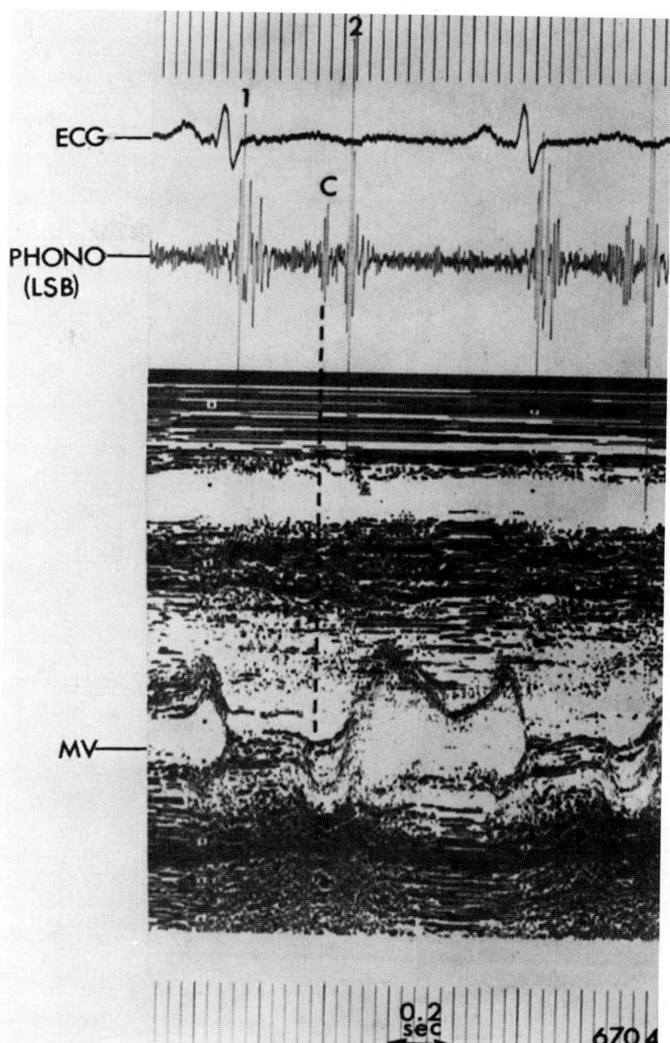

FIGURE 3–51. Phonocardiogram and M-mode echocardiogram from a patient with mitral valve prolapse. The late systolic click (C) on the phonocardiogram corresponds to late systolic posterior displacement of the mitral valve (MV). (From Tavel, M. E.: Clinical Phonocardiography and External Pulse Recordings. 3rd ed. Chicago, Year Book Medical Publishers, 1978.)

the holosystolic "hammocking" is less than 5 mm,[172] the diagnosis is not clear-cut.

Several findings on 2-D echocardiography have been suggested for the diagnosis of mitral valve prolapse,[173,174] including the recording of buckling of one or both mitral leaflets into the left atrium during systole. Figure 3–52 demonstrates a parasternal long-axis and a four-chamber examination of a patient with mitral valve prolapse. The posterior or mitral leaflet can be seen buckline or herniating into the left atrium in late systole. Unfortunately the amount of systolic prolapse noted on the 2-D echocardiograms also exhibits a continuum from normal to abnormal, and there may still be a problem in differentiating between prolapse and a normal variant with this technique.[175] The parasternal long-axis view is more specific for the diagnosis of prolapse[176] than is the four-chamber view.

Other echocardiographic findings in patients with mitral valve prolapse include excessive amplitude of motion of the valve during diastole that can be appreciated in both M-mode and 2-D examinations. Thickening of the leaflets is common and is presumably due to myxomatous degeneration.[177] The leaflets may also be redundant and seem to fold on themselves in diastole. When there is redundancy and thickening of the leaflets, the diagnosis of mitral valve

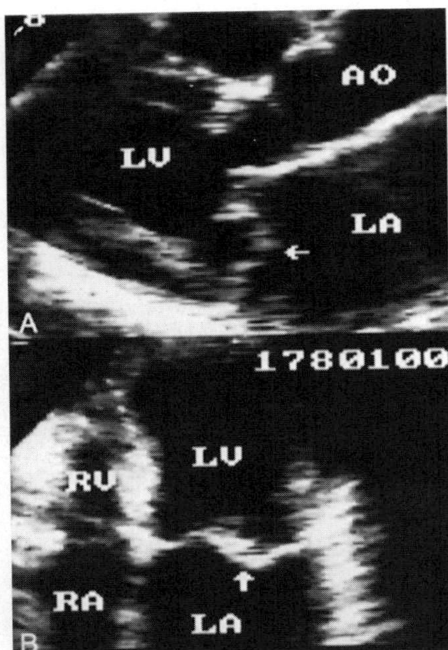

FIGURE 3–52. Two-dimensional echocardiogram in the parasternal long-axis *(A)* and apical four-chamber *(B)* views of a patient with mitral valve prolapse (arrows). LV = left ventricle; AO = aorta; LA = left atrium; RV = right ventricle; RA = right atrium.

prolapse is more secure than when the leaflets are seen to move into the left atrium only in systole.[178] It must be emphasized that although echocardiography can frequently be used to make a positive diagnosis of mitral valve prolapse, it is also difficult to distinguish minor degrees of prolapse from a normal variant.

Two-dimensional echocardiography is the examination of choice for establishing the presence of a flail mitral leaflet.[179] With this abnormality the leaflets are seen to protrude into the left atrium (Fig. 3–53).[180] The differentiation between a flail mitral leaflet and mitral valve prolapse depends on whether the tips of the leaflet point toward the left atrium (flail valve) or curve back and point toward the left ventricle (prolapse).[181] Color Doppler almost always reveals an eccentric jet with a flail mitral valve.[182] As would be expected, transesophageal echocardiography is excellent in detecting and evaluating a flail mitral valve.[183]

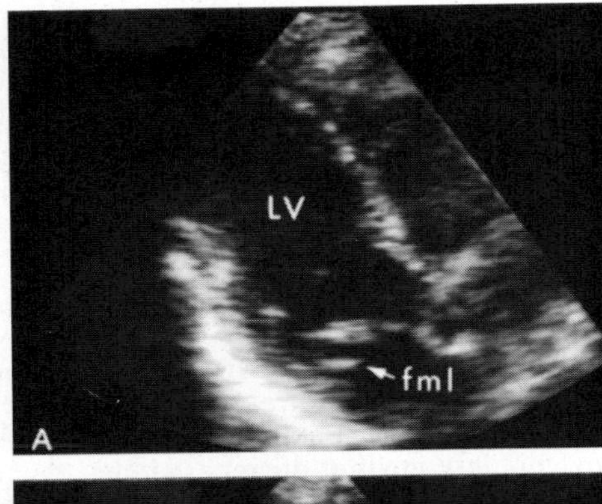

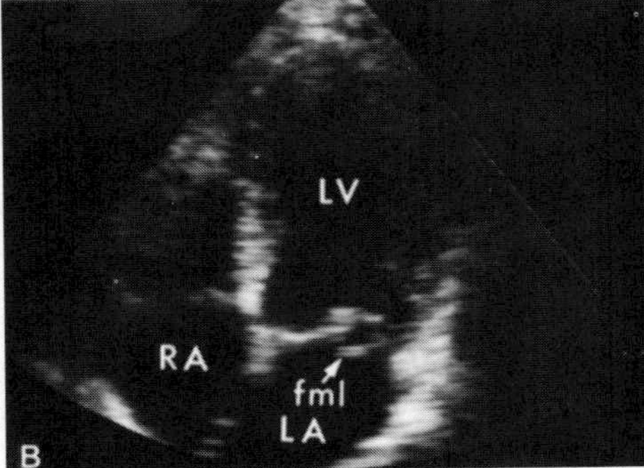

FIGURE 3–53. *A,* Apical two-chamber and *B,* four-chamber views of a patient with a flail mitral leaflet. The flail leaflet (fml) can be seen protruding into the left atrium (LA) during ventricular systole. LV = left ventricle; RA = right atrium. (From Feigenbaum, H.: Echocardiography. 4th ed. Philadelphia, Lea and Febiger, 1986.)

PAPILLARY MUSCLE DYSFUNCTION. Two-dimensional echocardiography provides an opportunity to detect incomplete closure of the mitral valve because of left ventricular dilatation or scarring of the papillary muscles. In this condition the leaflets in the four-chamber view fail to reach the level of the mitral annulus.[184]

Aortic Stenosis

Doppler echocardiography has revolutionized the role of echocardiography and indeed the management of patients with aortic stenosis (AS). M-mode and 2-D echocardiography have always provided an excellent qualitative diagnosis of AS. Doppler echocardiography now provides an opportunity for the quantitative diagnosis. The 2-D echocardiographic diagnosis of valvular aortic stenosis is doming, thickening, and restricted motion of the leaflets (Fig. 3–54).[185] The valve may be heavily calcified and immobile, in which case only distorted, echo-producing, immobile valve leaflets are apparent.[186] It is possible to make a semiquantitative assessment of AS with 2-D echocardiography by judging the mobility of the leaflets, especially in the short-axis view (Fig. 3–54). Although transthoracic 2-D echocardiography is rarely used to quantitate AS, there is renewed interest in using transesophageal echocardiography to measure the cross-sectional area of the aortic valve and thus quantitating AS.[187,188]

The best ultrasonic technique for quantifying AS utilizes continuous-wave Doppler.[119,189] Using the modified Bernoulli equation (Fig. 3–40), it is possible to measure the pressure gradient across the aortic valve. Figure 3–55 shows a composite of simultaneous Doppler recordings and intracardiac pressure measurements in four patients with AS; an increase in the Doppler velocity occurs as the gradient increases. There is an excellent relationship between the instantaneous gradient across the stenotic valve as measured by both catheterization and Doppler techniques.[189]

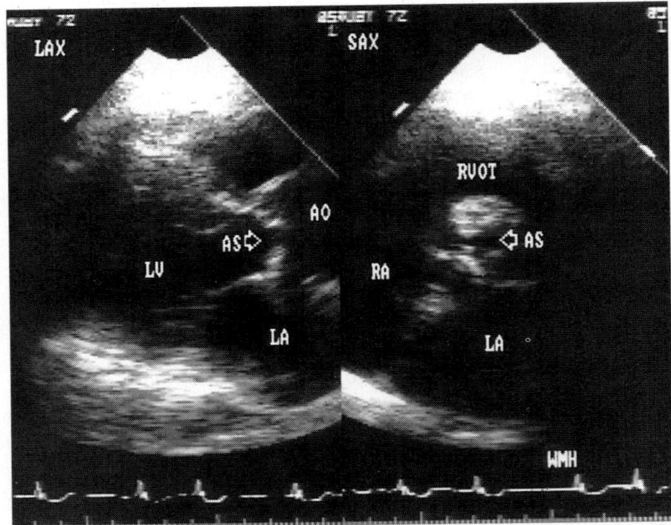

FIGURE 3–54. Long-axis (LAX) and short-axis (SAX) views from a patient with aortic stenosis (AS). The long-axis examination shows classic doming, restricted motion, and reduced separation of the leaflets. The elliptical orifice occasionally can be identified in the short-axis examination. LV = left ventricle; AO = aorta; LA = left atrium; RVOT = right ventricular outflow tract; RA = right atrium. (From Feigenbaum, H.: Echocardiography. 5th ed. Malvern, PA, Lea and Febiger, 1994).

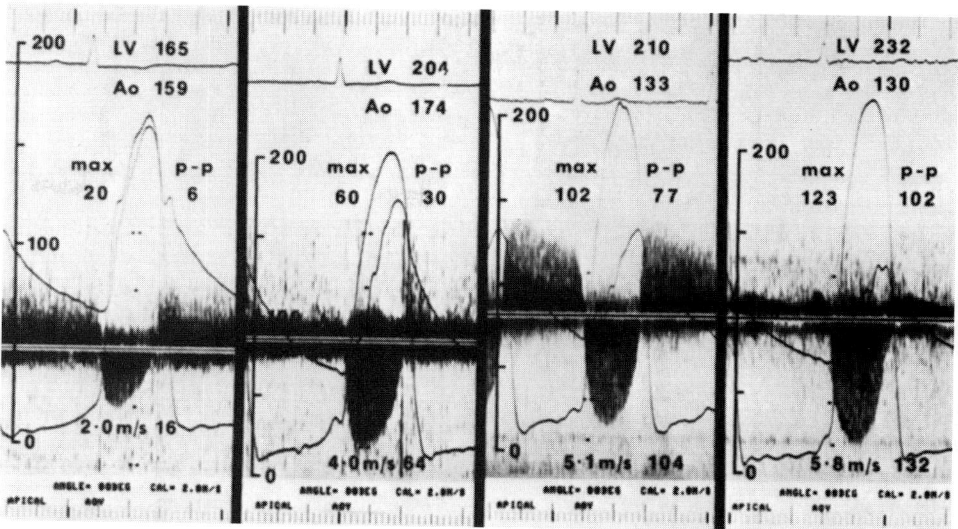

FIGURE 3–55. Simultaneous continuous wave Doppler and hemodynamic measurements in four different patients with valvular aortic stenosis. The peak velocity increases as the gradient between the left ventricular and aortic pressures increases. (Reproduced with permission from Currie, P. J., et al.: Continuous wave Doppler echocardiographic assessment of severity of calcific aortic stenosis: A simultaneous Doppler-catheter correlative study in 100 adult patients. Circulation *71*:1162, 1985. Copyright 1985 American Heart Association.)

In the cardiac catheterization laboratory it is customary to measure the aortic valve gradient as the difference between the peak left ventricular pressure and the peak aortic pressure (the "peak-to-peak" gradient) (Fig. 3–56). This gradient actually does not exist at any instant in time because the peak aortic pressure occurs later than the peak left ventricular pressure. The peak instantaneous pressure gradient measured by the Doppler technique is invariably larger. If one measures the more accurate mean gradients both in the catheterization laboratory and with the Doppler examination, then the measurements are quite similar.

The Doppler technique thus gives a good estimate of the gradient across the aortic valve. Obviously the gradient is dependent on both the aortic valve area and the flow across the valve. With reduced cardiac output one can have a small gradient in a patient with severe AS. Cardiac output could be measured with a right-heart catheter and thermodilution techniques[190] or by use of one of the Doppler stroke volume measurements through an orifice that does not have a diseased valve. Another Doppler approach for calculating aortic valve area uses the "continuity equation"[191] (Fig. 3–42). This technique has been used with reasonable accuracy to calculate the aortic valve orifice in patients with valvular AS. A modification of the continuity equation uses blood flow through the mitral orifice rather than the left ventricular outflow tract.[192]

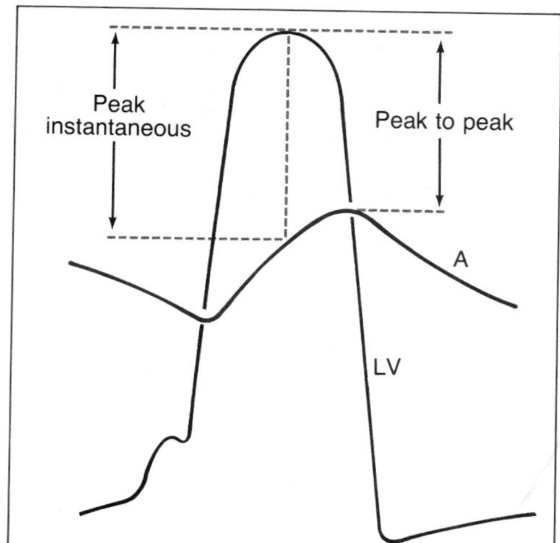

FIGURE 3–56. Left ventricular (LV) and aortic (A) pressures in aortic stenosis. The peak instantaneous pressure difference or gradient is greater than the peak-to-peak gradient because the peak aortic pressure occurs later than the peak left ventricular pressure. (From Feigenbaum, H.: Echocardiography. 4th ed. Philadelphia, Lea and Febiger, 1986.)

The theoretical basis for using Doppler echocardiography for calculating the valve gradient is well established. However, there are technical details that must be recognized.[193,194] It is crucial that the maximal velocity be recorded and that the ultrasonic beam be parallel to the aortic stenotic jet. This requirement can make the examination fairly lengthy. Various ultrasonic windows must be tried to make certain that the optimal jet is identified.

From a practical point of view, if a high-velocity jet (in excess of 4 m/sec) is identified, the probability of critical AS is extremely high and the patient's condition can be managed accordingly. On the other hand, if the velocity is within normal limits or mildly elevated, the possibility of significant AS can be excluded. When the velocity is in an intermediate zone, which would indicate a pressure gradient between 23 and 50 mm Hg, additional hemodynamic information may be necessary for proper management.[195]

There are secondary signs of AS that can be noted on the echocardiogram. Both M-mode and 2-D echocardiography can detect left ventricular hypertrophy with increased thickness of the left ventricular walls. Although the degree of left ventricular hypertrophy has been used to assess the severity of AS,[196] this technique is not nearly as reliable as the use of Doppler for valve gradients and valve area.

Aortic Regurgitation

As with all valvular regurgitation, Doppler echocardiography is the examination of choice for detecting the presence of aortic regurgitation (AR).[197,198] Figure 3–57 shows a Doppler sample in the left ventricular outflow tract and the recording of high-velocity flow during diastole. This type of examination is both sensitive and specific for the presence of AR. Color flow Doppler provides a 2-D display of the AR jet (Fig. 3–58). The accuracy of Doppler flow mapping for quantitating AR is at best semiquantitative.[199,200] The same limitations pertain to AR as were discussed with MR (see p. 72). The width of the aortic jet at the valve orifice as judged by color flow Doppler is used to judge the severity of AR,[13,200] and is clinically useful. The rate of decrease in velocity of the regurgitant blood as recorded in the left ventricular outflow tract using continuous-wave Doppler has been used as a reflection of severity of the AR (Fig. 3–59). Severe AR produces a faster fall in velocity as the pressure difference between the aorta and left ventricle falls rapidly.[201] AR can also be judged by the difference between aortic flow and pulmonary artery flow or mitral flow.[202] One can calculate a regurgitant orifice size using Doppler continuity equation.[203]

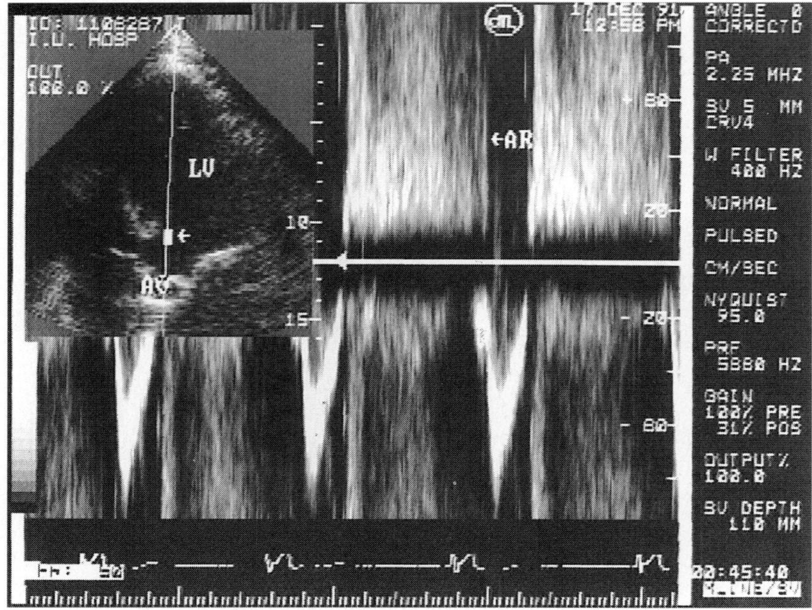

FIGURE 3–57. Pulsed Doppler echogram of a patient with aortic regurgitation. The Doppler sample *(arrow)* is within the left ventricular outflow tract, and the recording displays a high velocity, aliasing diastolic Doppler signal (AR). LV = left ventricle; AO = aorta. (From Feigenbaum, H.: Echocardiography. 5th ed. Malvern, PA, Lea and Febiger, 1994.)

FIGURE 3–58. See color plate 2.

One M-mode sign of AR that remains useful is premature closure of the mitral valve in the presence of severe, usually acute, AR[128] (see p. 1050). This premature mitral closure can also be noted on the Doppler recording.[204] With an elevated left ventricular diastolic pressure there may even be early opening of the aortic valve on the M-mode recording.[130] Both of these signs represent severe AR and markedly elevated left ventricular diastolic pressures. The secondary effects of AR on the left ventricle can be detected with both M-mode and 2-D echocardiographic examinations. Serial measurements of left ventricular size and systolic function are important in observing patients with chronic AR or judging the efficacy of surgery.[205] Deterioration in left ventricular systolic function is one criterion for valve replacement[206] (see p. 1052).

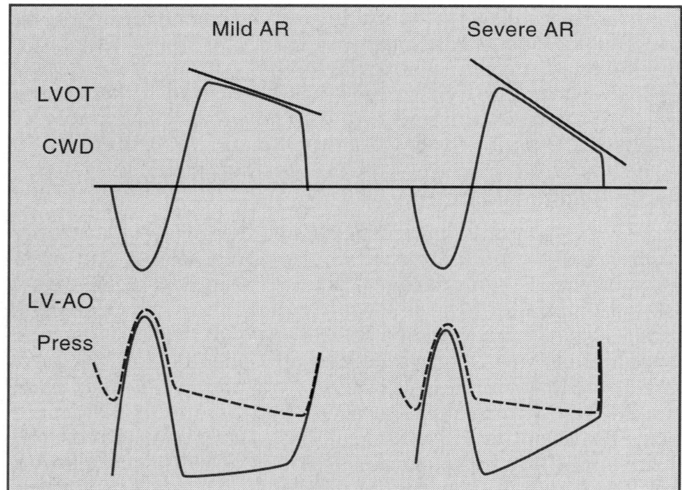

FIGURE 3–59. The principle of how the diastolic slope of the regurgitant jet can relate to the severity of aortic regurgitation (AR). The continuous-wave Doppler (CWD) signal is a function of the pressure difference between the left ventricle and the aorta (LV-AO). With relatively mild aortic regurgitation, the pressure difference gradually decreases as regurgitant blood is flowing into the left ventricle; however, with severe aortic regurgitation, the aortic pressure drops rapidly and the left ventricular pressure rises steeply as the large regurgitant volume increases the pressure. Thus the pressure differential decreases and the slope of the diastolic regurgitant jet increases. LVOT = left ventricular outflow tract. (From Feigenbaum, H.: Echocardiography. 5th ed. Malvern, PA, Lea and Febiger, 1994.)

Tricuspid Valve Disease

TRICUSPID STENOSIS. The echocardiographic findings of tricuspid stenosis and regurgitation are very similar to those for MS and MR. Two-dimensional and Doppler echocardiography are the procedures of choice for detecting tricuspid stenosis. Doming of the tricuspid valve on 2-D echocardiography is the hallmark of TS.[207] The Doppler findings of tricuspid stenosis are similar to those with MS.[208] The velocities passing through the orifice are increased, and the rate of diastolic decline in velocity is reduced. The pressure half-time can also be used to calculate the severity of the valvular obstruction.

TRICUSPID REGURGITATION. This abnormality is also best determined by pulsed, continuous wave, or color flow Doppler echocardiography.[209,210] As noted previously, the Doppler recording of tricuspid regurgitation can be used to estimate the pressure gradient across the tricuspid valve. This measurement provides an opportunity for estimating right ventricular systolic pressure by adding an estimate of right atrial pressure.

Two-dimensional echocardiography can help determine the etiology of tricuspid regurgitation. Rheumatic tricuspid regurgitation usually has an element of tricuspid stenosis and invariably exhibits MS. Pulmonary hypertension can be detected by estimating the right ventricular systolic pressure. Tricuspid valve prolapse gives an appearance similar to that of mitral valve prolapse (Fig. 3–60).[211] A flail tricuspid valve is indicated by the finding of parts of the tricuspid valve protruding into the right atrium in ventricular systole.[212] Carcinoid valve disease (see p. 1056) produces stiff immobile tricuspid leaflets that are continuously open.[213] Valve vegetations and Ebstein's anomaly are discussed on pp. 1083 and 934 respectively. As with all valvular disease, transesophageal echocardiography can provide higher quality images of tricuspid valve pathology.[214]

Secondary effects of tricuspid regurgitation can be noted on 2-D studies. Right ventricular and right atrial dilatation are invariably present. Abnormal diastolic motion of the interventricular septum indicates that right ventricular volume overload may be present.

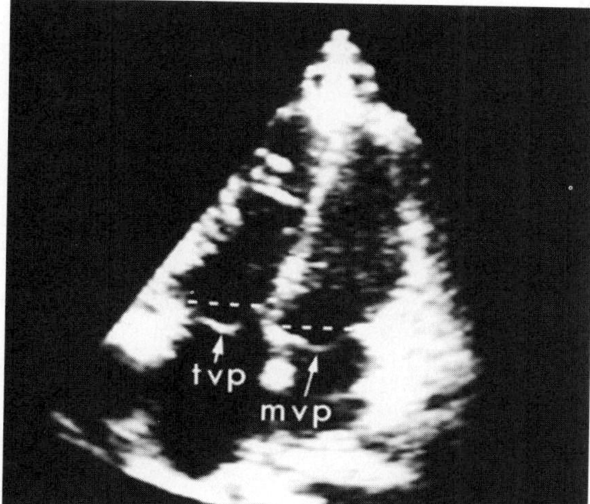

FIGURE 3–60. Apical four-chamber 2-D echocardiogram of a patient with tricuspid valve prolapse (tvp) and mitral valve prolapse (mvp). (From Feigenbaum, H.: Echocardiography. 4th ed. Philadelphia, Lea and Febiger, 1986.)

Infective Endocarditis

(See Chap. 33)

Echocardiography provides a means for visualizing the vegetations of infective valvular endocarditis, which appear as echo-producing masses attached to the infected valve (Fig. 3–61) (Fig. 33–4, p. 1084).[215] They are usually asymmetrical, commonly involving one leaflet more than another, but may be present on more than one valve. If the vegetation is associated with destruction of the valve or if it is on a long "stalk," it can be readily imaged; its excessive motion can be appreciated on both M-mode[216,217] and 2-D echocardiography.[218] Transesophageal echocardiography is proving to be much more sensitive than transthoracic echocardiography in detecting valvular vegetations.[219] Figure 3–62 shows a small vegetation on the aortic valve. This lesion was not seen on the routine transthoracic echocardiogram. (The greater sensitivity of transesophageal echocardiography for the detection of valvular vegetations may change our understanding as to why echocardiographic vegetations are frequently seen in patients with endocarditis and whether or not this ultrasonic technique can exclude the diagnosis.[220])

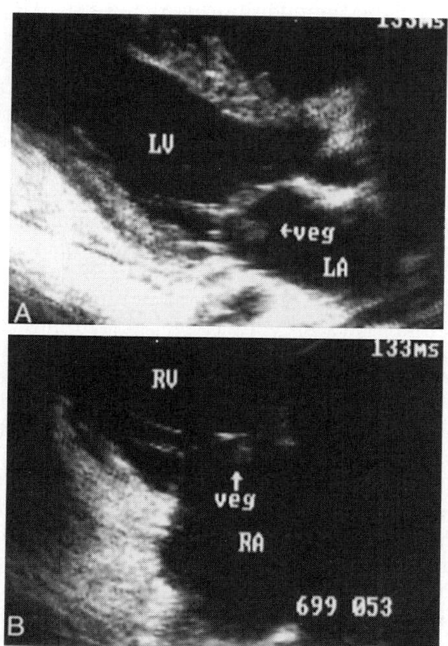

FIGURE 3–61. Two-dimensional echocardiograms of a patient with vegetation (veg) on the mitral *(A)* and tricuspid valves *(B)*. LV = left ventricle; LA = left atrium; RV = right ventricle; RA = right atrium.

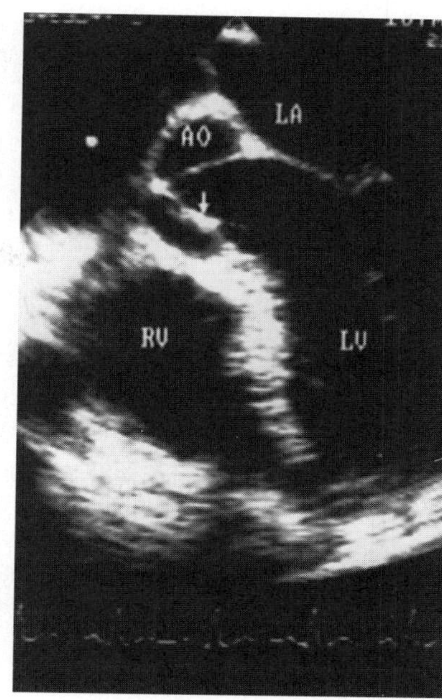

FIGURE 3–62. Transesophageal echocardiogram of a patient with a small vegetation (arrows) on the aortic valve. AO = aorta; LA = left atrium; RV = right ventricle; LV = left ventricle.

Vegetations visualized echocardiographically need not be bacterial[221,222] or even infected. Infected vegetations may be difficult to distinguish from myxomatous degeneration of the valve,[218] although this differentiation is usually readily accomplished clinically.

One of the major applications of echocardiography in patients with endocarditis is in the identification of complications. When the valve is damaged to the point that it is grossly incompetent, echocardiography can both detect and assess the hemodynamic importance of the valvular regurgitation. When the aortic valve is involved, premature closure of the mitral valve because of the very high left ventricular diastolic pressure may be evident. Another serious complication of aortic valve endocarditis is the development of an aortic root abscess (Fig. 3–63).[223] This prob-

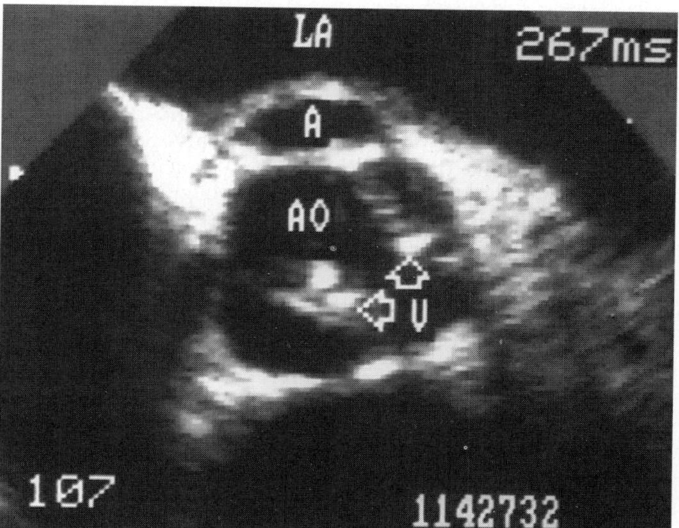

FIGURE 3–63. Transesophageal echocardiogram of a patient with vegetations (V) on the aortic valve and a periaortic abscess (A). LA = left atrium; AO = aorta. (From Feigenbaum, H.: Echocardiography. 5th ed. Malvern, PA, Lea and Febiger, 1994.)

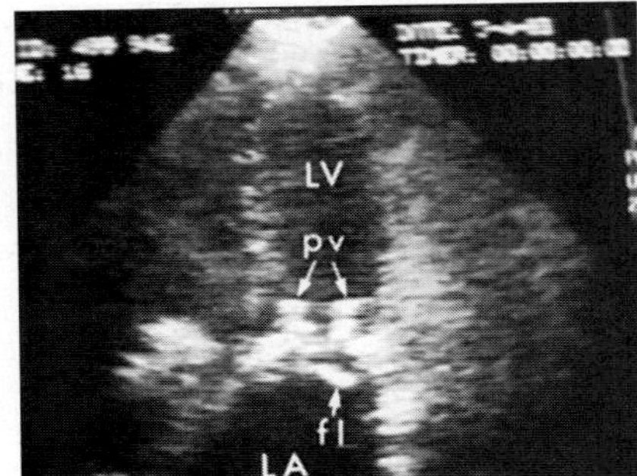

FIGURE 3–64. Apical four-chamber view in a patient with a degenerated flail porcine mitral prosthesis (pv). The flail leaflet (fl) can be seen protruding into the left atrium (LA) in systole. LV = left ventricle. (From Feigenbaum, H.: Echocardiography. 4th ed. Philadelphia, Lea and Febiger, 1986.)

lem is seen as a relatively echo-free space adjacent to the aortic root and is seen best with transesophageal echocardiography.[224] Mitral valve diverticulum can also be detected by means of esophageal echocardiography.[225]

Prosthetic Valves

There is a variety of echocardiographic signs of prosthetic valve malfunction. Most published reports of prosthetic valve malfunction represent isolated case studies.[226] Abnormal motion of a ball or disc usually results from a thrombus[227] or from ball variance.[226] A useful sign of a malfunctioning Björk-Shiley valve in the mitral position is a rounding of the E point on the M-mode echocardiogram.[229] An abnormal rocking motion of a prosthetic valve resulting from the sutures pulling loose from the annulus has been reported.[230] Thickening of the porcine valve leaflets is useful in judging deterioration of this valve.[231] A flail porcine valve, especially in the mitral position, can be easily identified with 2-D echocardiography (Fig. 3–64).[232]

DOPPLER ECHOCARDIOGRAPHY. This technique is very helpful in evaluating prosthetic valves.[233–235] Valvular regurgitation is detected readily with the Doppler technique. Color Doppler has the advantage of locating some of these unusually located valvular regurgitations (Fig. 3–65).[236] Doppler echocardiography can also assist in judging stenotic prosthetic valves. The technique is most effective with valves that have a central orifice, such as a tissue valve[237] or St. Jude mechanical valve.[238] Ball valves or tilting disc valves present more difficulties in judging the flow characteristics through the valve.

TRANSESOPHAGEAL ECHOCARDIOGRAPHY. This technique has made a major contribution to the detection of malfunctioning prosthetic valves, particularly in the mitral position.[239–241] Acoustic shadowing frequently prohibits the detection of MR involving a prosthetic valve when the examination is done through the chest. When the ultrasonic examination is performed via the esophagus, the view of the left atrium is unobstructed and the regurgitant jet is easily detected (Fig. 3–15).[242] In addition, the superior resolution inherent in the higher frequency transducer provides better visualization of the prosthetic valve, especially for the detection of minor abnormalities such as small thrombi or vegetations (Fig. 3–66).[243]

Calcified Mitral Annulus

(See p. 1017)

Calcification of a mitral annulus can be readily demonstrated by echocardiography.[244] The principal finding is a

FIGURE 3–65. See color plate 3.

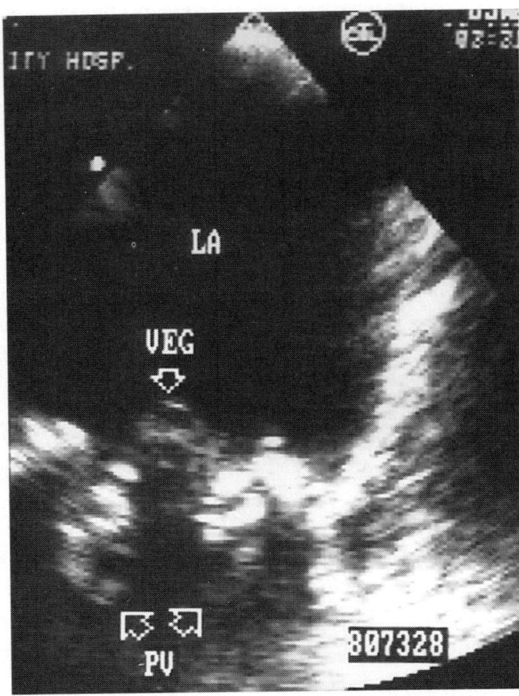

FIGURE 3–66. Transesophageal echocardiogram of a patient with a vegetation (VEG) on a porcine mitral valve (PV). LA = left atrium. (From Feigenbaum, H.: Echocardiography. 5th ed. Malvern, PA, Lea and Febiger, 1994.)

band of dense echoes between the mitral valve and the posterior left ventricular wall. Calcification can be extensive and involve the posterior mitral leaflet and much of the base of the heart.

CONGENITAL HEART DISEASE

(See also Chaps. 29 and 30)

Deductive Echocardiography

Echocardiography is an indispensable and frequently definitive examination for the evaluation of patients with known or suspected congenital heart disease. The availability of 2-D M-mode spectral Doppler, color Doppler, contrast and transesophageal echocardiography gives the clinician ample tools to decipher even the most complex congenital anomaly.[245] Echocardiography now can frequently obviate the need for more costly and dangerous invasive procedures.[246–248]

There are many ways in which echocardiography can be used to decipher the riddle of the congenitally malformed heart. The term *deductive echocardiography* refers to a technique by which an attempt is made to deduce the anatomy of the heart by systematically identifying the atria, atrioventricular valves, ventricles, semilunar valves, and great vessels. Several approaches can be used to identify the atria.[249,250] The right atrium contains the eustachian valve, has a different appearing appendage, and is not as round as the left atrium. Another technique is to identify the abdominal viscera and the venous drainage. Atrial and visceral situs are almost always concordant. The normal atrial relationship or atrial situs solitus can be determined by identifying a right-sided liver and left-sided stomach with an abdominal ultrasound examination from the subcostal position. The same examination can be used to identify the inferior vena cava, which almost invariably drains into the right atrium. One can also identify the pulmonary veins draining into the left atrium; however, this examination is technically more difficult, especially with the transthoracic examination.

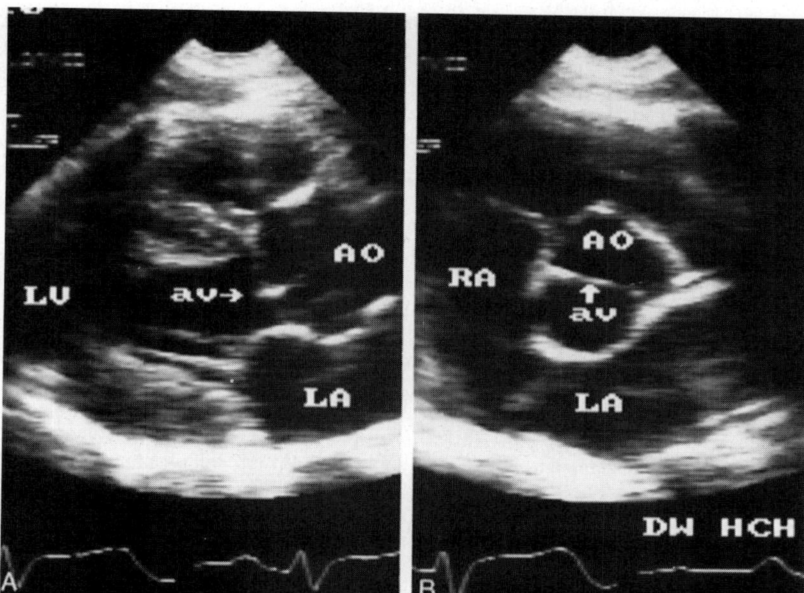

FIGURE 3–67. Long-axis *(A)* and short-axis *(B)* 2-D echocardiograms of a patient with a bicuspid aortic valve (av). LV = left ventricle; AO = aorta; LA = left atrium; RA = right atrium.

The ventricles are identified by the corresponding atrioventricular valve. The tricuspid valve is recognized by the fact that it inserts into the interventricular septum closer to the apex than does the mitral valve.[251] The right ventricle can also be identified by its trabeculations and the moderator band. The course of the great arteries and the bifurcation of the pulmonary artery help to distinguish the aorta from the pulmonary artery. The semilunar valves are always a part of the corresponding great vessel. This deductive approach can frequently unravel the mystery of even the most complex malformation.

Ventricular Inlet and Outlet Anomalies

VALVULAR STENOSIS. A bicuspid aortic valve (see p. 964) is probably the most common congenital cardiac anomaly. The best echocardiography criterion for making this diagnosis utilizes 2-D echocardiography. With this technique two cusps rather than the normal three cusps can be identified (Fig. 3–67). The diagnosis can be confusing, since occasionally a fused commissure may resemble a third leaflet echocardiographically. In addition, if the commissure is in an anterior-posterior direction, it is sometimes difficult to record echocardiographically.[252] The M-mode technique of identifying eccentric closure of the aortic valve within the aorta[253] is less reliable.

In aortic stenosis (see p. 1035), most echocardiographic findings are similar whether the valve is deformed on a congenital (see p. 914) or acquired basis. In the adult the valve is frequently heavily calcified, and the etiology is difficult to determine. The qualitative diagnosis is made by finding doming and/or restricted motion of the valve during systole. The quantitative diagnosis is now best obtained using continuous-wave Doppler (see p. 56).

A host of types of congenitally deformed mitral valves can be detected echocardiographically.[254] Congenital mitral stenosis is rare, but has been recognized by echocardiography. A parachute mitral valve has also a fairly characteristic echocardiographic appearance. Two-dimensional echocardiography can identify a double-orifice mitral valve.[255] The domed stenotic pulmonary valve resembles the congenitally stenotic aortic valve on 2-D echocardiography (Fig. 3–68*A*).[256] The M-mode recording of the pulmonary valve has an accentuated A wave (Fig. 3–43). The severity of congenital pulmonic stenosis may also be assessed by Doppler echocardiography.[257,258] If continuous-wave Doppler echocardiography and criteria similar to those for AS (see p. 74) are utilized, the gradient across the stenotic pulmonary valve can be estimated (Fig. 3–68*B*). A common abnormality associated with congenital pulmonic stenosis is pulmonic regurgitation. This abnormality is noted using Doppler recordings that reveal diastolic flow into the right ventricle.

EBSTEIN'S ANOMALY (see p. 934). The echocardiographic diagnosis of Ebstein's anomaly is based on the displacement of the tricuspid valve leaflets within the body of the right ventricle on the 2-D echocardiogram (Fig. 3–69).[259,260] Normally the tricuspid valve inserts on the interventricular septum slightly above the insertion of the mitral valve. However, with Ebstein's anomaly this displacement is marked, and much of the tricuspid valve lies within the body of the right ventricle. On M-mode echocardiography the diagnosis of Ebstein's anomaly is based on delayed closure of the tricuspid valve.[261] The 2-D echocardiogram is more specific and reliable for this diagnosis.

VALVULAR ATRESIA. Atresia of cardiac valves is generally associated with hypoplasia of the ipsilateral ventricle (Chap. 29). Thus, aortic or mitral atresia is associated with hypoplasia of the left ventricle.[262] Diminutive ventricles and the atretic valves have been imaged with both M-mode[263] and 2-D techniques (Fig. 3–70).[264,265]

SUBVALVULAR OBSTRUCTIONS. A variety of congenital subvalvular obstructions have been detected echocardiographically. Early systolic closure of the aortic valve has

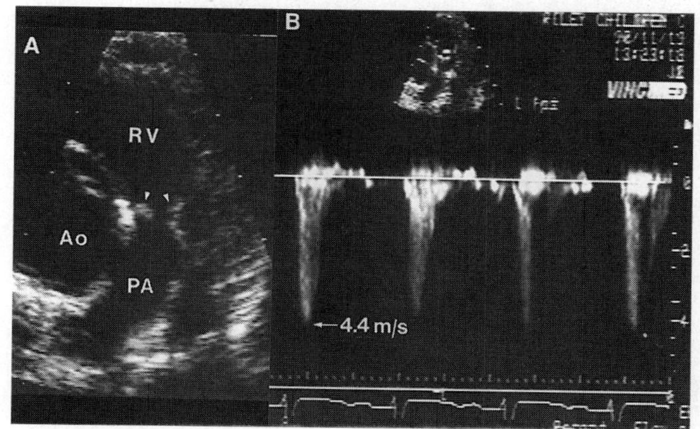

FIGURE 3–68. Two-dimensional *(A)* and continuous-wave Doppler *(B)* studies of a patient with valvular pulmonic stenosis. The 2-D study shows a thickened, domed pulmonary valve. The continuous-wave Doppler shows increased velocity that peaks at 4.4 M/sec, which is consistent with a systolic gradient of approximately 78 mm Hg. RV = right ventricle; Ao = aorta; PA = pulmonary artery. (From Feigenbaum, H.: Echocardiography. 5th ed. Malvern, PA, Lea and Febiger, 1994.)

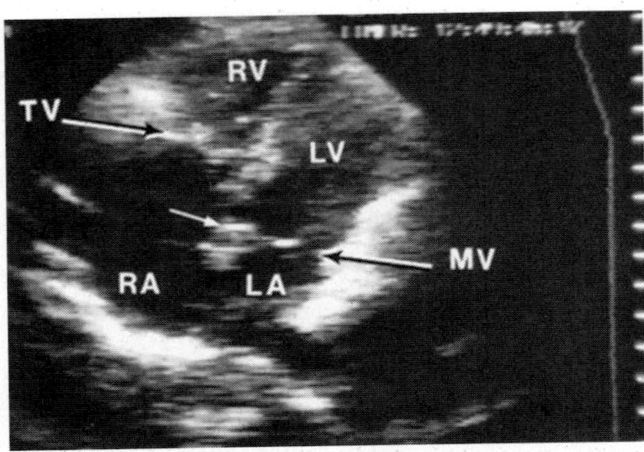

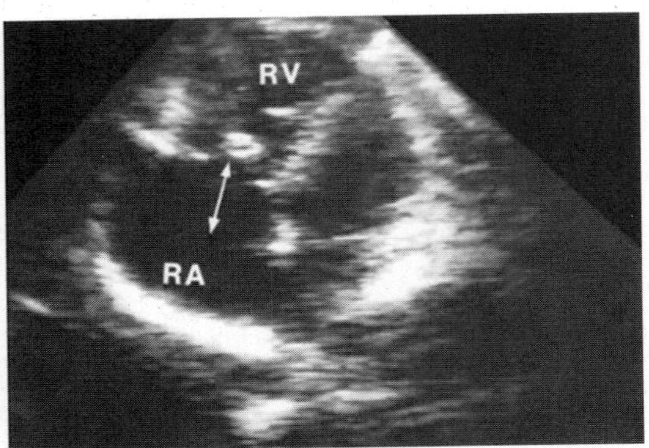

FIGURE 3–69. Apical four-chamber view in a patient with Ebstein's anomaly. The tricuspid valve (TV) is displaced from the tricuspid annulus (arrow). The effective right ventricular volume (RV) is decreased and the volume of the right atrium (RA) is increased. LV = left ventricle; LA = left atrium; MV = mitral valve. (From Feigenbaum, H.: Echocardiography. 4th ed. Philadelphia, Lea and Febiger, 1986.)

been observed in patients with both discrete (Fig. 3–71)[266] and hypertrophic obstructive cardiomyopathy (Fig. 41–17, p. 1418).[129] In addition, systolic fluttering of the aortic valve is often exaggerated, although some degree of aortic valve fluttering may be seen normally. Although midsystolic closure and fluttering of the aortic valve are not specific findings for subaortic stenosis, they can be very helpful in differentiating valvular from subvalvular obstruction, since they do not occur in the former condition.

Examination of the outflow tract is accomplished with transthoracic or transesophageal 2-D echocardiography, and the subvalvular obstruction can be identified directly by this technique (Fig. 3–72).[267,268] The 2-D technique also permits the classification of discrete obstruction into the discrete membranous and the diffuse types.[269] Distinguishing between them may be of considerable clinical importance, since their management may differ. The membranous form is frequently situated just below the aortic valve and may therefore be difficult to recognize at catheterization, since the short subvalvular chamber can be missed on a pull-out pressure recording. Indeed, the thin membrane can even be missed on the angiogram, so that its recognition by 2-D echocardiography can be very helpful. Doppler echocardiography can be used to assess the severity of subvalvular as well as valvular stenosis.[270]

In subpulmonic obstruction the M-mode tracing exhibits coarse fluttering of the pulmonary valve.[271] The actual subpulmonic obstruction can be detected, and its severity quantified in patients with tetralogy of Fallot by means of

FIGURE 3–70. Apical four-chamber view in a patient with tricuspid atresia. The atretic tricuspid annulus is indicated by arrowheads. A large atrial septal defect is present. The hypoplastic right ventricle (RV) is seen. RA = right atrium; LA = left atrium; LV = left ventricle. (From Feigenbaum, H.: Echocardiography. 5th ed. Malvern, PA, Lea & Febiger, 1994.)

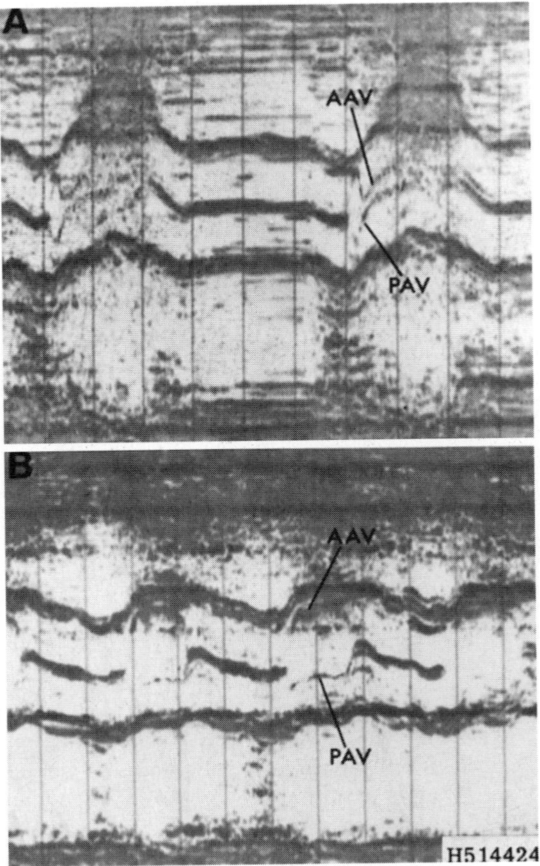

FIGURE 3–71. Aortic valve echocardiograms from a patient with discrete subaortic stenosis before *(A)* and *(B)* after surgery for the subaortic obstruction. Prior to surgery the aortic valve anterior (AAV) and posterior (PAV) leaflets come together shortly after the onset of ventricular ejection and remain essentially closed throughout systole. This systolic closure of the valve leaflets is no longer present after surgery. (From Davis, R. H., et al: Echocardiographic manifestation of discrete subaortic stenosis. Am. J. Cardiol. *33:*277, 1974.)

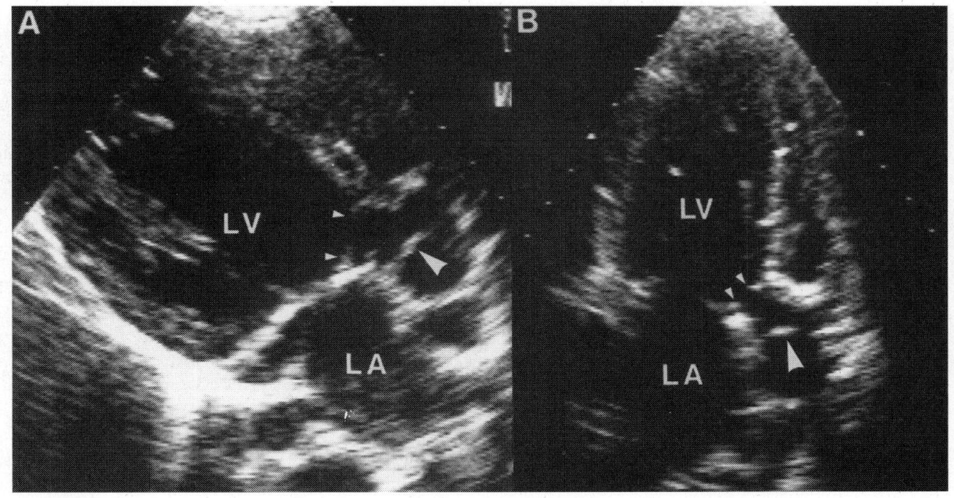

FIGURE 3–72. Parasternal *(A)* and apical *(B)* long-axis view from a patient with discrete, membranous subaortic stenosis. The aortic valve (large arrowhead) is thickened, but not stenotic. Immediately below the valve in the left ventricular outflow tract is a discrete membrane (small arrowheads). LA = left atrium; LV = left ventricle. (From Feigenbaum, H.: Echocardiography. 5th ed. Malvern, PA, Lea and Febiger, 1994.)

2-D examination of the right ventricular outflow tract and subpulmonic area.[272]

Subvalvular mitral obstruction can also occur. A fibrous membrane may be situated within the left atrial cavity (Fig. 3–73). Such a membrane obstructs flow and divides the left atrium into two chambers.[273] This anomaly is commonly known as *cor triatriatum* (see p. 923).[274] If the fibrous band is next to the mitral annulus, then the entity is known as a *supravalvular stenosing ring.*[275] Congenital stenoses of the pulmonary veins can also occur.

Cardiac Shunts

Echocardiography can be helpful in the diagnosis of cardiac shunts by detecting the actual defect between the two sides of the heart, by evaluating the hemodynamic consequences of the shunt, and by recording the shunted blood using color flow Doppler or contrast methods.

VENTRICULAR SEPTAL DEFECT (see also pp. 901 and 967). Pulsed Doppler is useful for detecting ventricular septal defects,[276] but color flow Doppler has become the technique of choice for visualizing these abnormalities[277,278] (Fig. 3–74). The examination is particularly helpful when multiple defects exist.[279] The defects can also be seen with 2-D echocardiography.[280] Figure 3–75 demonstrates a small membranous ventricular septal defect using 2-D echocardiography and contrast. Figure 3–76 demonstrates an apical four-chamber view in a patient with total absence of a ventricular septum or a single ventricle.[281] The continuous-wave Doppler velocity across the ventricular septal defect can reflect the pressure difference between the left and right ventricles during systole.[282] Subtracting the pressure gradient from the left ventricular systolic pressure provides an estimate of the right ventricular systolic pressure.

ATRIAL SEPTAL DEFECT (see also pp. 896 and 970). The 2-D echocardiographic examination, especially from the subcostal position, provides an opportunity for direct examination of the interarterial septum (Fig. 3–25*A*, p. 62).[283,284] Figure 3–77 demonstrates findings in a patient with an ostium secundum atrial septal defect. A remnant of the interatrial septum can be seen attached to the ventricular septum. In contrast, Figure 3–78 demonstrates an atrial septal defect in a patient with an ostium primum

FIGURE 3–74. See color plate 3.

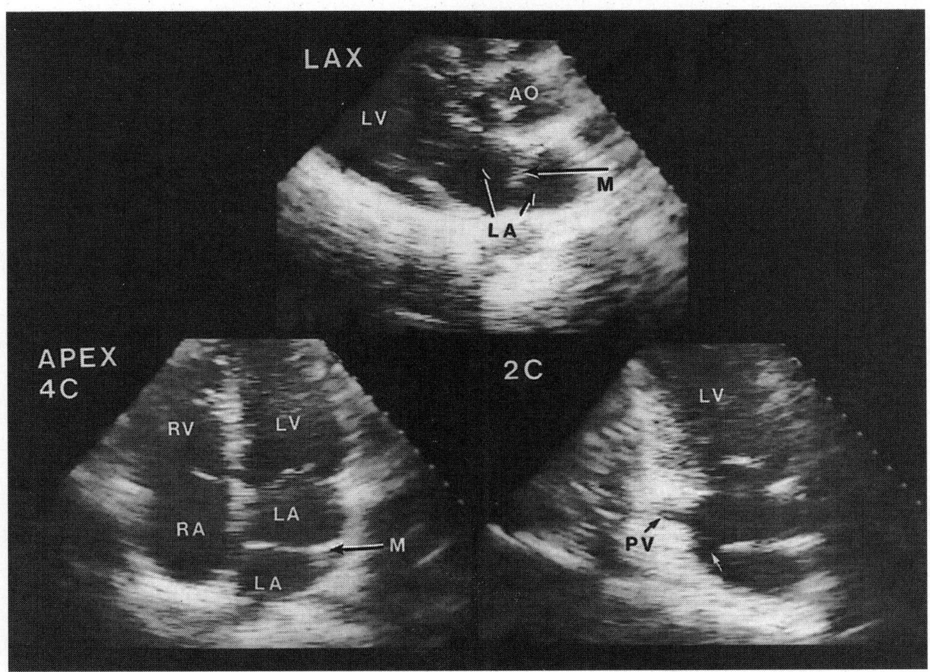

FIGURE 3–73. Parasternal long-axis and apical views from an asymptomatic patient with cor triatriatum. A linear echo courses posterior laterally within the left atrium, dividing it into two components. LA = left atrium; RA = right atrium; RV = right ventricle; LV = left ventricle; AO = aorta; M = left atrial membrane; PV = pulmonary vein. (From Feigenbaum, H.: Echocardiography. 5th ed. Malvern, PA, Lea and Febiger, 1994.)

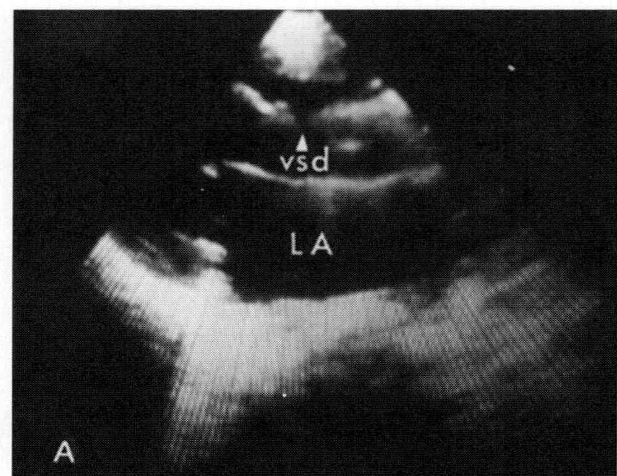

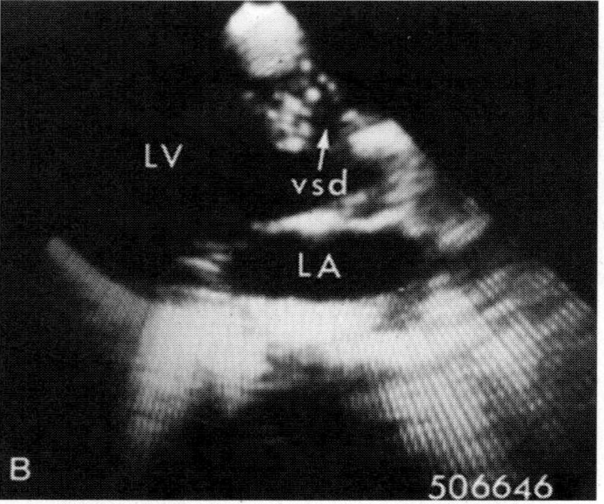

FIGURE 3–75. Two-dimensional long-axis echocardiograms of a patient with a membranous ventricular septal defect. *A,* The discontinuity of echoes from the ventricular septal defect (vsd) can be seen. *B,* A peripheral contrast injection fills the right ventricle, but an echo-free jet, i.e., negative contrast, can be seen anterior to the ventricular septal defect. LV = left ventricle; LA = left atrium. (From Feigenbaum, H.: Echocardiography. 4th ed. Philadelphia, Lea and Febiger, 1986.)

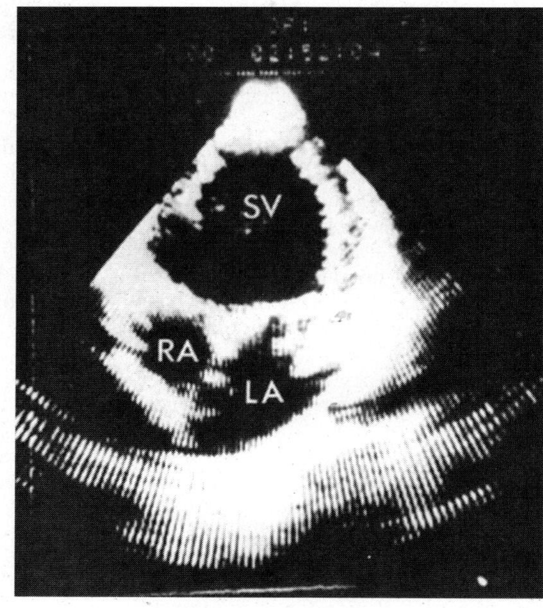

FIGURE 3–76. Cross-sectional echocardiogram of a patient with a single ventricle (SV). The ultrasonic probe is placed at the apex of the heart, and the plane of the scan transects the interatrial septum so that all chambers can be seen simultaneously. This view is particularly helpful in demonstrating the absence of the interventricular septum. RA = right atrium; LA = left atrium.

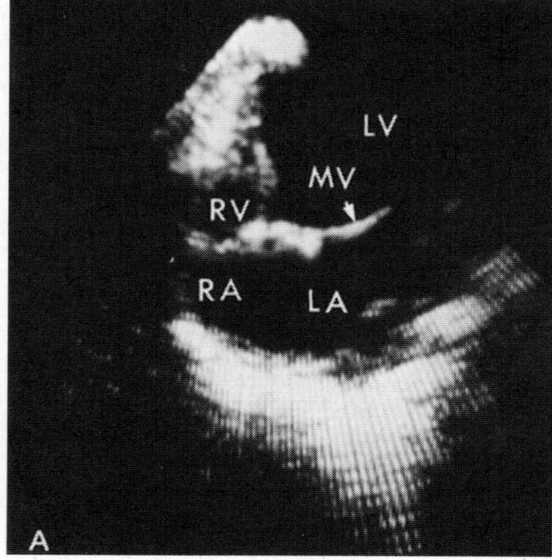

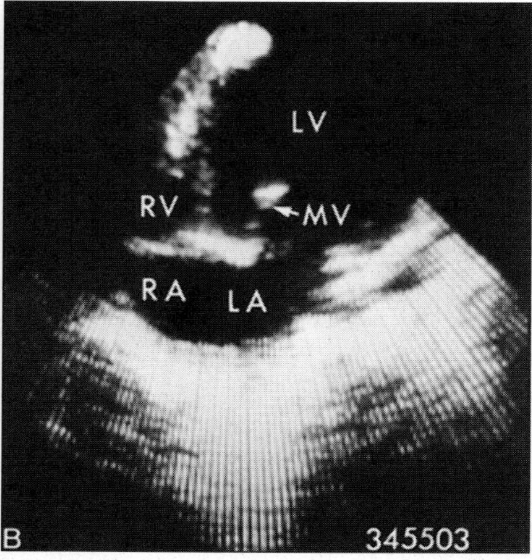

FIGURE 3–77. Subcostal 2-D echocardiogram of a patient with an ostium secundum atrial septal defect. Remnants of the interatrial septum are visible on both sides of the defect (ASD). RA = right atrium; LA = left atrium; LV = left ventricle. (From Feigenbaum, H.: Echocardiography. 3rd ed. Philadelphia, Lea and Febiger, 1981.)

defect. There is no residual septum attached to the ventricular septum. Thus, the 2-D technique not only helps to identify the presence of an atrial septal defect, but it is also an excellent means of differentiating a secundum from a primum type of abnormality. One can also identify more severe forms of an endocardial cushion defect with a coexistent ventricular septal defect (Fig. 3–79). A sinus venosus type of atrial septal defect is the most difficult type of atrial septal defect to detect with 2-D echocardiography[285] and is best seen with transesophageal echocardiography.[286] Actually, all atrial septal defects are better seen with the transesophageal approach[287] but such an examination is not always necessary.

Three-dimensional (3-D) echocardiography is an evolving technology that has great promise, especially in congenital heart disease.[288,289] Figure 3–80 shows a 3-D reconstructed echogram of a patient with both secundum and primum atrial septal defects. Figure 3–80*A* is equivalent to a 2-D four-chamber view cutting across the atrial septum. This 3-D examination permits one to appreciate the back walls

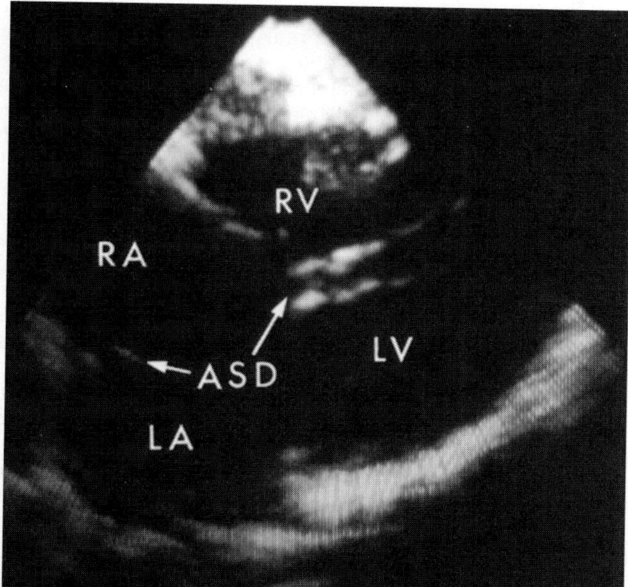

FIGURE 3–78. Subcostal 2-D echocardiogram of a patient with an ostium primum atrial septal defect. No residual septal tissue is apparent between the defect (ASD) and the interventricular septum. RA = right atrium; LA = left atrium; RV = right ventricle; LV = left ventricle. (From Feigenbaum, H.: Echocardiography. 3rd ed. Philadephia, Lea and Febiger, 1981.)

of the chambers as well as the cross-sectional appearance of the septa. By viewing the examination parallel to the septa (Fig. 3–80*B*), one now gains a new perspective of the atrial septum. Now as one examines the surface of the septum, what one sees is similar to what a surgeon might see in the operating room. With this approach one can appreciate the shape and size of the defects.

Color flow Doppler and contrast echocardiogram can both be used to demonstrate *atrial septal defects.* Figure 3–81 shows a color Doppler and a contrast echocardiogram in a patient with a secundum-type atrial septal defect.[290] With the Doppler study one can see the red-encoded blood passing from the left atrium to the right atrium through the defect. With the contrast examination one sees an echo-filled right atrium and right ventricle. The left atrium and left ventricle are echo free. As the non-contrast-containing left atrial blood passes through the atrial septal defect, a negative contrast effect within the right atrium (ASD) is

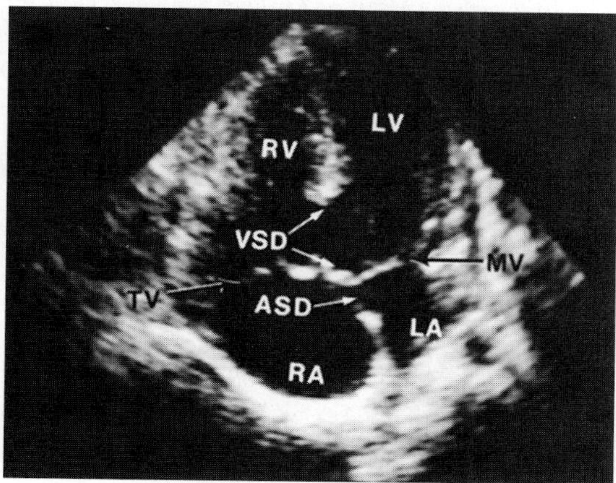

FIGURE 3–79. Apical four-chamber view in a patient with an endocardial cushion defect showing the perimembranous ventricular septal defect (VSD) and primum atrial septal defect (ASD). RA = right atrium; LA = left atrium; RV = right ventricle; LV = left ventricle; MV = mitral valve; TV = tricuspid valve. (From Feigenbaum, H.: Echocardiography. 4th ed. Philadelphia, Lea and Febiger, 1986.)

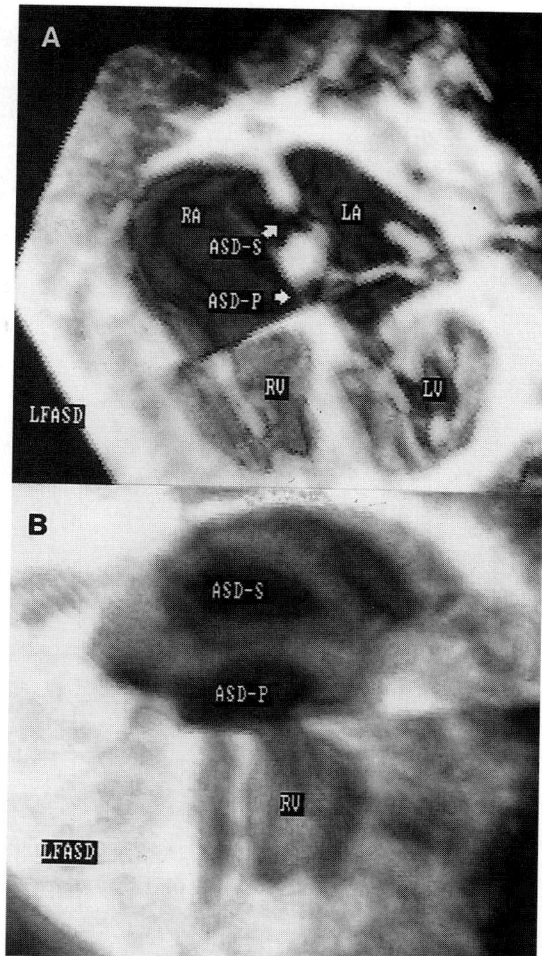

FIGURE 3–80. Three-dimensional reconstruction in an infant with a secundum (ASD-S) and primum (ASD-P) atrial septal defect. Figure *A* is comparable to a four-chamber view cutting through the atrial septal defects. The walls of the cardiac chambers are seen in the background. The 3-D view in *B* shows the surface of the atrial septa. Now one can better appreciate the size and shape of the two defects. RA = right atrium; LA = left atrium; RV = right ventricle; LV = left ventricle.

apparent.[291–293] If there were a right-to-left shunt, then contrast would be seen within the left atrium and left ventricle with such an injection.

In *total anomalous pulmonary venous return* all four pulmonary veins empty into a common pulmonary venous chamber behind the left atrium, which produces additional echoes posterior to the left atrium (Fig. 29–66, p. 944).[294,295]

Besides septal defects one can also record *septal aneurysms* frequently associated with septal defects. The aneurysm involving the membranous portion of the interventricular septum can be imaged on the right side of the septum.[296] Atrial septal aneurysms can also be detected by 2-D echocardiography and especially transesophageal echocardiography (Fig. 3–16).[297,298] These aneurysms are usually quite mobile and may be seen moving between the two atria throughout the cardiac cycle. These aneurysms frequently are fenestrated[299] and have been implicated in systemic emboli. Transesophageal echocardiography with contrast is proving to be a very sensitive way to identify a probe-patent foramen ovale.[300–302] (Fig. 3–16).

FIGURE 3–81. See color plate 4.

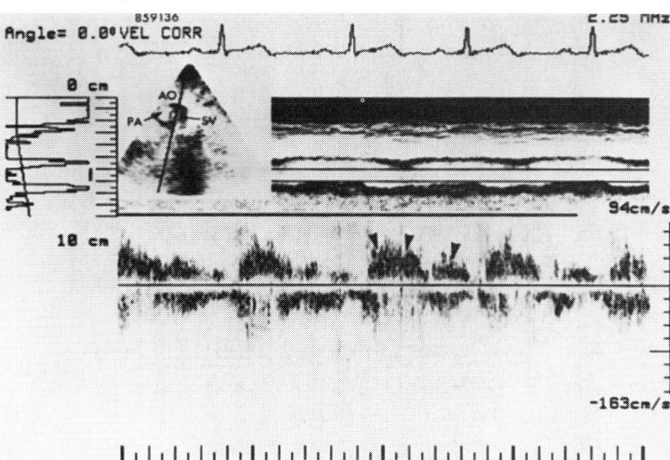

FIGURE 3–82. Pulsed Doppler examination with the sample volume (SV) placed in the wall of the pulmonary artery (PA) in the region of the presumed patent ductus. Note the presence of continuous flow in the region of the ductus *(arrowheads).* AO = aorta. (From Feigenbaum, H.: Echocardiography. 4th ed. Philadelphia, Lea and Febiger, 1986.)

FIGURE 3–83. See color plate 4.

ASSOCIATED LESIONS. Intracardiac shunts are frequently associated with other anomalies of the heart that can be recognized echocardiographically. For example, in patients with defects of the atrioventricular canal, anomalies of the mitral and/or tricuspid valves can be appreciated on the echocardiogram.[303] The mitral valve appears to be closer than normal to the interventricular septum, a finding consistent with abnormal insertion of the mitral leaflet in this anomaly. The cleft in the mitral valve commonly present with ostium primum atrial septal may be detected using 2-D echocardiography.[304]

Another valvular anomaly that may be associated with an intracardiac shunt is a tricuspid valve that overrides the ventricular septum, which can pose major problems in the repair of a ventricular septal defect and which is therefore important to recognize preoperatively. The echocardiographic findings in this condition resemble those in atrioventricular canal defects in that the tricuspid valve is recorded to the left of the interventricular septum.[305]

PATENT DUCTUS ARTERIOSUS (see also p. 905). Although 2-D echocardiography can occasionally visualize the patent ductus between the aorta and pulmonary artery, Doppler is more sensitive and reliable in detecting the abnormal communication.[306] Although continuous flow within the ductus itself has been detected, since the ductus is frequently perpendicular to the sample volume the Doppler signal can be somewhat difficult to record. It is actually easier to make the diagnosis by obtaining Doppler recording from the aorta and pulmonary artery. By placing the sampling volume in the pulmonary artery, flow into this vessel can be noted in both systole and diastole as the shunted blood comes from the aorta (Fig. 3–82). Figure 3–83 shows a color Doppler study of a patient with a patent ductus arteriosus. The abnormal flow within the pulmonary artery can be readily detected.[307]

Abnormalities of the Great Arteries

Supravalvular aortic stenosis (see p. 919) can be detected using 2-D echocardiography.[264,308] The method of examination is similar to that used for the detection of valvular aortic stenosis, except that the scanning is carried out superior to the aortic valve. *Coarctation of the aorta* (see p. 965) is detected with 2-D echocardiography by placing the probe in the suprasternal notch,[309] which allows imaging of both the narrowed segment of the aorta and the poststenotic dilation and detection of the excessive pulsation of the aorta proximal to the coarctation. Doppler echocardiography can be used to assess the hemodynamic obstruction across the coarctation.[310] Color flow Doppler is improving the ability to assess the severity of a coarctation.[311]

Tetralogy of Fallot (see p. 929) is detected echocardiographically by noting a membranous ventricular septal defect and a dilated aorta that overrides the interventricular septum (Fig. 3–84 and Fig. 29–48, p. 929). The short-axis view also demonstrates a narrowing of the right ventricular outflow tract, usually at the subpulmonic level.[272] *Double-outlet right ventricle* (see p. 941) is clinically similar to tetralogy of Fallot but can be differentiated echocardiographically from the more common anomaly when a mass of tissue can be noted betweeen the anterior mitral leaflet and the aorta.[312] This tissue indicates that the aorta is communicating directly with the right ventricle and cannot be repaired surgically as is possible in tetralogy of Fallot.

Two-dimensional echocardiography has greatly improved the ultrasonic detection of anomalies of the great arteries.[313] In the diagnosis of truncus arteriosus, 2-D echocardiography helps to establish the number of great arteries leaving the heart.[314] Normally, with a short-axis view of the great vessels, a circular aorta surrounded by a curved, tubular right ventricular outflow tract and pulmonary artery is recorded (Fig. 3–21, diagram 4); in truncus arteriosus only a single large circular vessel can be visualized. Actual recording of the branch of the truncus that supplies the lungs is more definitive in establishing the diagnosis of truncus arteriosus.

The 2-D technique for the detection of transposition of the great arteries (see p. 935) is based on determining the relationship between the two great arteries.[272,315] Normally the pulmonary artery twists around the aorta as the latter passes posteriorly. With transposition of the great arteries, on the other hand, the two arteries run parallel to each other, and with a 2-D view parallel to the arteries it is possible to appreciate how the transposed arteries do not twist around each other.[316] A perpendicular or short-axis view of the great vessels demonstrates two circular structures (Fig. 3–85) rather than the pulmonary artery normally wrapping around the circular aorta. Doppler examination

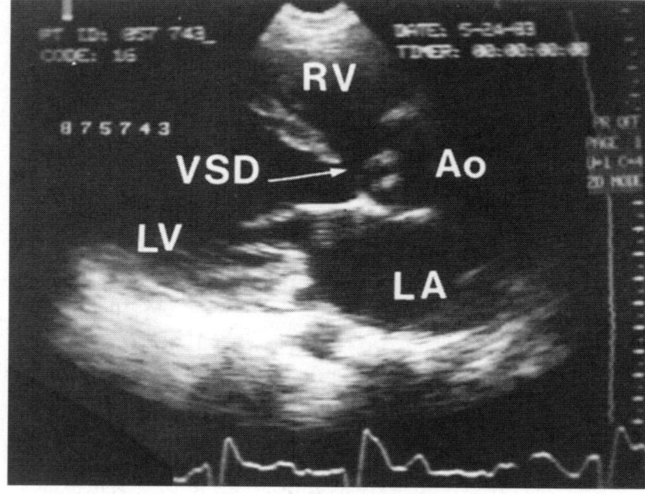

FIGURE 3–84. Parasternal long-axis examination in an adult with uncorrected tetralogy of Fallot. The ventricular septal defect (VSD) in the area of a membranous septum and overriding of the aorta (Ao) are apparent. LA = left atrium; LV = left ventricle; RV = right ventricle. (From Feigenbaum, H.: Echocardiography. 4th ed. Philadelphia, Lea and Febiger, 1986.)

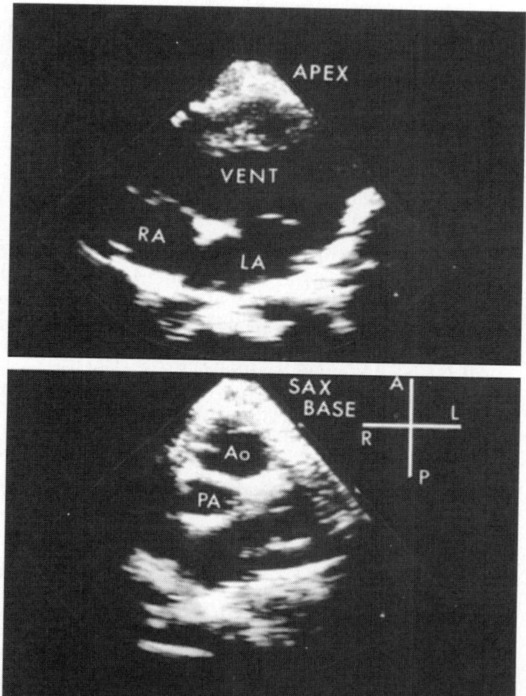

FIGURE 3–85. Apical four-chamber view *(top)* and short-axis (SAX) view *(bottom)* of the great vessels in a patient with a single ventricle and transposition of the great arteries. A single ventricular chamber (VENT) can be seen that received blood from both the right and left atria (RA, LA). In the short-axis view two great vessels oriented in a parallel direction can be seen. The aorta (Ao) is anterior and to the left of the pulmonary artery (PA). (From Feigenbaum, H.: Echocardiography. 4th ed. Philadelphia, Lea and Febiger, 1986.)

together with 2-D echocardiography helps in the recognition of corrected transposition.[317]

SURGICALLY CORRECTED CONGENITAL HEART DISEASE (see also p. 980). The adult cardiologist is increasingly being confronted with evaluating congenital anomalies that have been surgically repaired. In many ways these are far more difficult to evaluate than native congenital defects. It is frequently the role of echocardiography to try to evaluate the effectiveness and possible complications of the surgery.[318–320] The variety of procedures that are performed on these patients are too numerous to discuss in any detail at this time. Figure 3–86 gives one example of the type of challenge presented to the echocardiographer in examining surgically corrected congenital heart disease. In this illustration the patient had a Mustard procedure for *correction of transposition of the great arteries* (see p. 935). With this operation there are intra-atrial baffles diverting systemic venous flow into the left ventricle and pulmonary venous flow into the right ventricle. The echocardiogram in Figure 3–86 shows how an attempt has been made to trace the baffles, which creates the systemic venous atrium (SVA) and the pulmonary venous atrium (PVA) as they cross the deliver blood into the appropriate ventricles. The evaluation of such iatrogenic anomalies requires a great deal of experience in identifying the surgically produced structures and recognizing malfunction when it occurs. As these patients live longer and well into adult life, this type of evaluation is becoming the responsibility of adult and pediatric cardiologists working together in adult congenital heart clinics.

Ischemic Heart Disease

DETECTION OF MYOCARDIAL ISCHEMIA. Two-dimensional echocardiography can detect ischemic myocardium by evaluating the motion, thickening, and thickness of various segments of the heart.[321,322] Figure 3–87 shows diastolic and systolic frames in the long-axis and four-chamber views of a patient with ischemic heart disease. With systole the left ventricular cavity in both views becomes smaller. However, the smaller cavity is a function of hyperkinesis of the posterior wall in the long-axis view and the lateral wall in the four-chamber view. The anterior and medial septum and apex (arrows) fail to move from diastole to systole. This akinesis is a result of inadequate blood flow within the left anterior descending artery. One of the advantages of the 2-D examination in patients with coronary artery disease is that the various myocardial segments correlate fairly predictably to coronary artery perfusion. Figure 3–88 shows the relationship between four common 2-D echocardiographic views and the corresponding coronary artery perfusion. This diagram also shows the relationship between the short-axis view and the three longitudinal views (long-axis, two-chamber, and four-chamber). The recording of these four 2-D views can provide an excellent assessment of regional function in the setting of coronary artery disease.

Another advantage of 2-D echocardiography is that with chronic ischemia and scar formation there is frequently loss of myocardial tissue as well as increased intensity of the echoes from that segment. Figure 3–89 shows a patient with a scarred distal septum and apex. The chronically ischemic segments not only fail to move but also exhibit loss of diastolic wall thickness. Not all regional wall-motion abnormalities are due to coronary artery disease. Left bundle branch block,[323] right ventricular pacing, and open-heart surgery[325] can produce abnormal interventricular septal motion. It should also be emphasized that with acute ischemia the nonischemic myocardium is usually hyperkinetic.[326] This fact limits the usefulness of a global measurement such as ejection fraction.

Patients with coronary artery disease frequently have normal left ventricular function at rest. However, with stress there is inadequate blood flow, ischemia is produced,

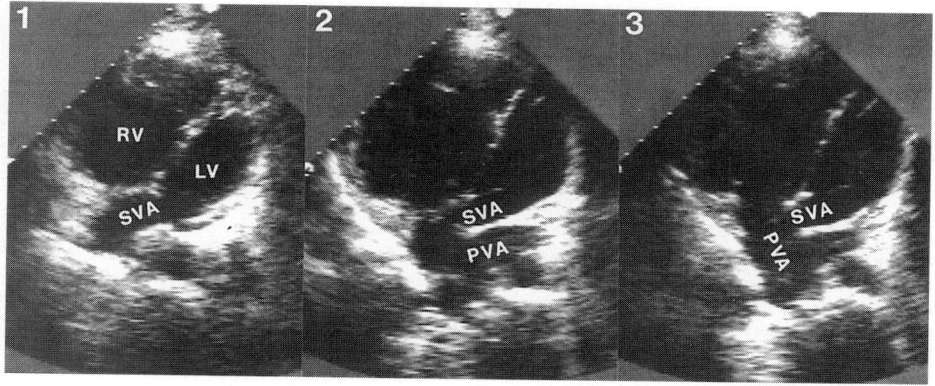

FIGURE 3–86. A series of three modified, four-chamber views from a patient following an intraatrial baffle procedure for transposition of the great arteries. By tilting the transducer at different angles, various limbs of the baffle can be visualized. In *panel 1,* the systemic venous atrium (SVA) is seen in continuity with the mitral valve and left ventricle (LV). In *panel 2,* both the systemic pulmonary venous atria (PVA) are seen. In *panel 3,* by tilting the transducer to a more anterior plane, continuity between the pulmonary venous atrium and the tricuspid valve and right ventricle is demonstrated. (From Feigenbaum, H.: Echocardiography. 5th ed. Malvern, PA, Lea and Febiger, 1994.)

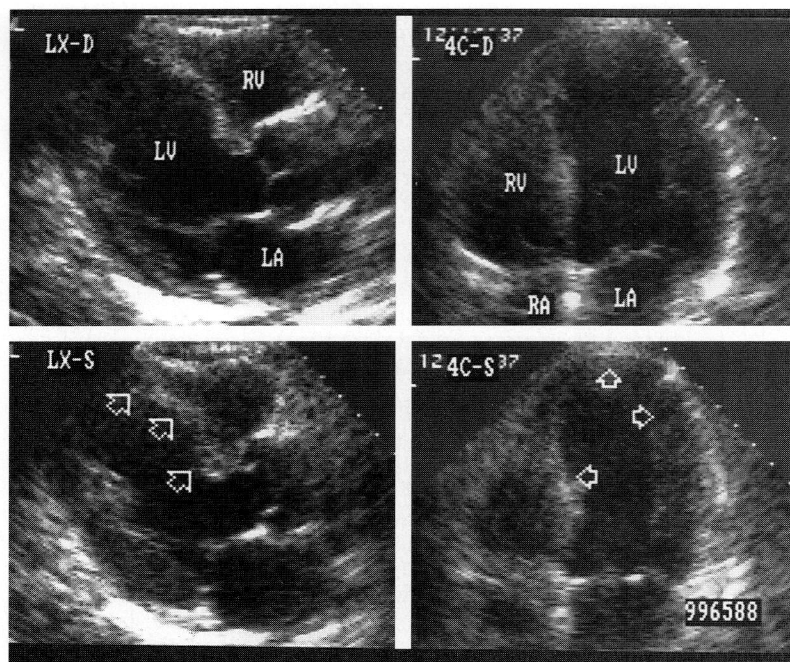

FIGURE 3–87. Long-axis (LX) and four-chamber 2-D echocardiogram of a patient with an anterior myocardial infarction secondary to occlusion of the left anterior descending artery. In systole there is akinesis (arrows) of the anterior system (LX-S) and distal septum, apex, and apical lateral wall (4C-S). LV = left ventricle; RV = right ventricle; LA = left atrium; RA = right atrium. (From Feigenbaum, H.: Echocardiography. 5th ed. Malvern, PA, Lea and Febiger, 1994.)

and the myocardium involved will stop moving. Figure 3–90 shows a patient before and immediately after exercise. At rest the long-axis and short-axis echocardiograms are normal at end-systole. Following exercise the septum stops moving (arrows) as noted in this end-systolic frame. A variety of stresses can be used with echocardiographic monitoring to identify stress-induced myocardial ischemia and regional dysfunction.[327–329] One can use immediate post-treadmill exercise,[330,331] supine[332] and upright[333] bicycle exercise, atrial pacing,[334] or a variety of pharmacological stresses.[335–338] The stress echocardiograms are frequently recorded digitally so that the resting and stress images are evaluated side by side on a computer screen.[339,340]

Not only is stress echocardiography being used for the detection and evaluation of coronary artery disease,[341,342] the examination is also valuable in establishing the prognosis following myocardial infarction,[343,344] for risk stratification of noncardiac surgery,[345,346] in establishing the prognosis in patients with high likelihood of coronary artery disease,[347–349] and in evaluating reperfusion procedures.[350,351]

ASSESSMENT OF LEFT VENTRICULAR PERFORMANCE. There are many echocardiographic techniques available for assessing left ventricular performance in patients with ischemic heart disease. Although the M-mode left ventricular dimensions are of limited value in patients with regional

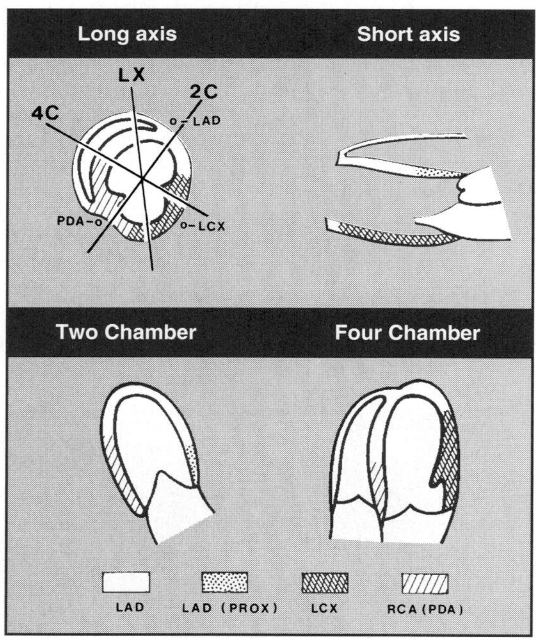

FIGURE 3–88. Relationship of 2-D echocardiographic views and coronary artery perfusion. 4C = four-chamber; LX = long-axis; 2C = two-chamber; LAD = left anterior descending; LCX = left circumflex artery; RCA = right coronary artery; PDA = posterior descending artery. (From Feigenbaum, H.: Echocardiography. 5th ed. Malvern, PA, Lea and Febiger, 1994).

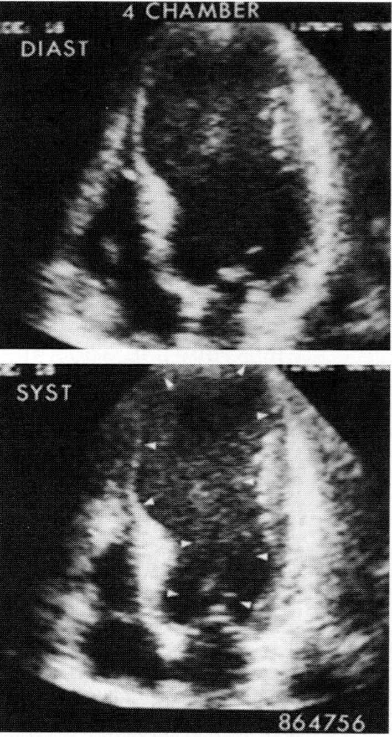

FIGURE 3–89. Apical four-chamber view in a patient with a scarred, dilated, aneurysmal apex and distal interventricular septum. The proximal half of the septum has normal thickness and contracts normally with systole. (From Feigenbaum, H.: Echocardiography. 4th ed. Philadelphia, Lea and Febiger, 1986.)

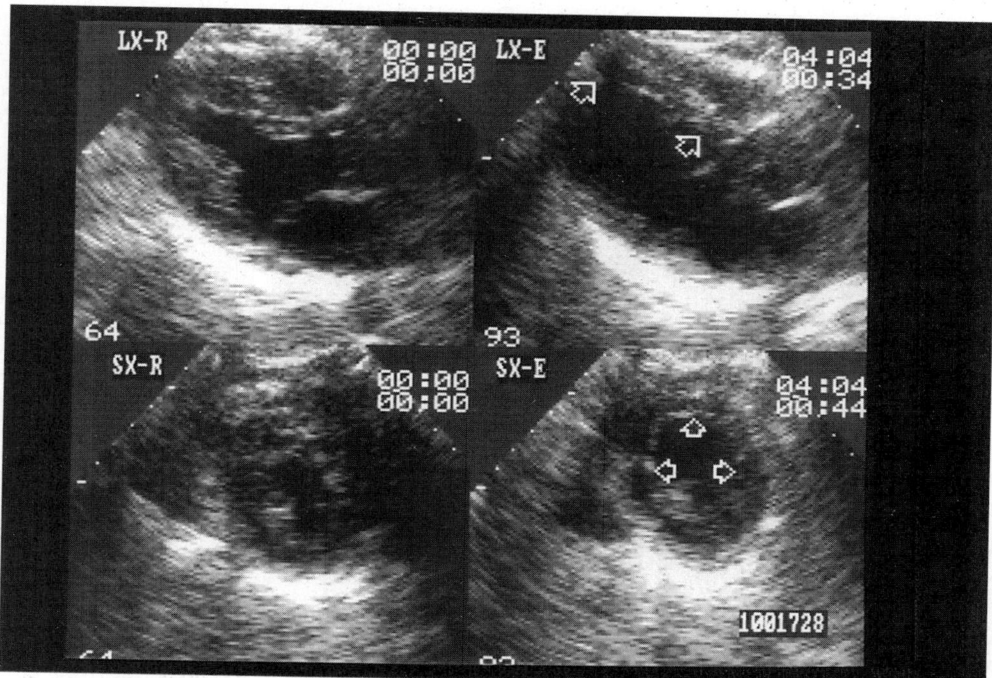

FIGURE 3–90. Exercise echocardiogram of a patient with an obstruction in the proximal left anterior descending coronary artery. The long-axis (LX-R) and short-axis (SX-R) resting images are normal. With exercise, however, the long-axis (LX-E) and short-axis (SX-E) examinations reveal that the septum and anterior wall (arrows) become akinetic. The heart rate is indicated in the left lower corner of each image; the numbers in the right upper corner indicate the exercise duration *(top)* and the postexercise duration *(bottom).* In this example, the long-axis examination was obtained at 34 seconds after exercise; the short-axis study was recorded 45 seconds after exercise. (From Feigenbaum, H.: Echocardiography. 5th ed. Malvern, PA, Lea and Febiger, 1994).

heart disease, measurements such as mitral valve E point–septal separation and abnormal closure of the mitral valve can give reasonable assessment of altered left ventricular function in patients with ischemic heart disease. The E point–septal separation increases when left ventricular ejection fraction decreases and abnormal closure of the mitral valve occurs in patients with elevated atrial components of left ventricular diastolic pressure. Doppler echocardiography can also be used to evaluate global left ventricular function. Acceleration and peak velocity are reduced as global left ventricular function deteriorates. Instantaneous mitral valve flow can reflect altered left ventricular filling.[352] With ischemia the early diastolic flow or E point is reduced and the velocity of flow with atrial systole (A point) is increased. As a result the E/A ratio changes from a normal positive value to a negative one[353] (Fig. 3–38*B*).

The best echocardiographic technique for evaluating regional left ventricular performance utilizes 2-D echocardiography and the assessment of regional wall motion.[354,355] The left ventricle is divided into a number of segments. Determining the motion of each segment provides a wall motion score for the entire chamber.[57,356] A number of schemes have been suggested in the literature. Any or all of these techniques provide reasonable assessment of both regional and global left ventricular function. Standard ejection fractions can also be calculated from the apical two-chamber or four-chamber views in patients with ischemic heart disease.[357,358] Because of the frequently distorted shape of the ventricle in these patients, Simpson's rule technique is preferred.[57] Minor axis measurements using parasternal long-axis or short-axis views can also be very helpful in patients with coronary artery disease by providing regional systolic function. Frequently the status of the base of the left ventricle is a better predictor of prognosis than is global ejection fraction, especially in patients with apical aneurysms.[359,360]

Myocardial Infarction

(See also Chap. 37)

COMPLICATIONS. All of the common complications of acute myocardial infarction (AMI) may be detected with echocardiographic techniques.[361] A common problem is the development of a left ventricular aneurysm.[360,362] Figure 3–89 shows the echocardiographic findings characteristic of aneurysm. There is a loss of myocardial thickness, scar formation, localized dilatation, and frequently dyskinesis. A pseudoaneurysm (see p. 1242) is a serious complication of MI, which represents rupture of the free wall. The blood leaving the cavity of the left ventricle is trapped in the pericardium, clot forms within the pericardial sac, and an aneurysmal wall consisting of clot and pericardium prevents exsanguination. The echocardiographic appearance of this complication is fairly characteristic, with the neck of the aneurysm being smaller than the body (Fig. 3–91).[363] Doppler flow patterns, especially color flow Doppler, within the aneurysm can help differentiate between a true and a false aneurysm.[364,365] Transesophageal echocardiography can assist with the diagnosis at times.[366] Indications for surgery are more urgent with a pseudoaneurysm; therefore the diagnosis is crucial. On rare occasion the initial rupture of the free wall can be detected echocardiographically.[367]

Aneurysmal dilatation and subsequent perforation of the ventricular septum (see p. 1243) are another complication of MI.[368] The septal aneurysm may be seen on the 2-D echocardiogram.[369] On rare occasions the actual perforation can be visualized.[370] The echocardiographic diagnosis, however, is best made with Doppler.[371] When the sample volume is put on the right ventricular side of the interventricular septum, the high-velocity systolic flow from the left

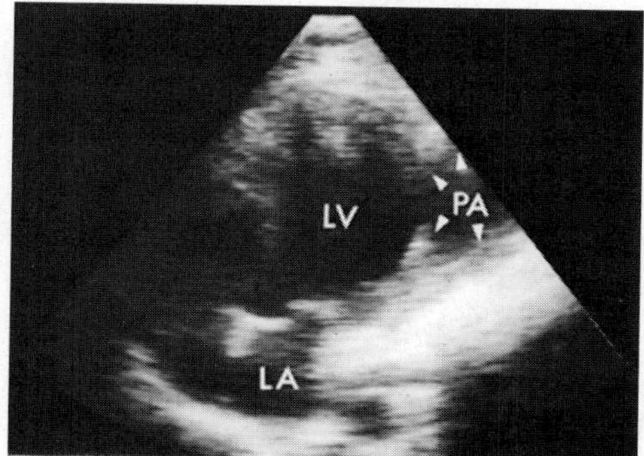

FIGURE 3–91. Four-chamber 2-D echocardiogram of a patient with a pseudoaneurysm (PA) adjacent to the posterior lateral free wall of the left ventricle (LV). LA = left atrium. (From Feigenbaum, H.: Echocardiography. 4th ed. Philadelphia, Lea and Febiger, 1986.)

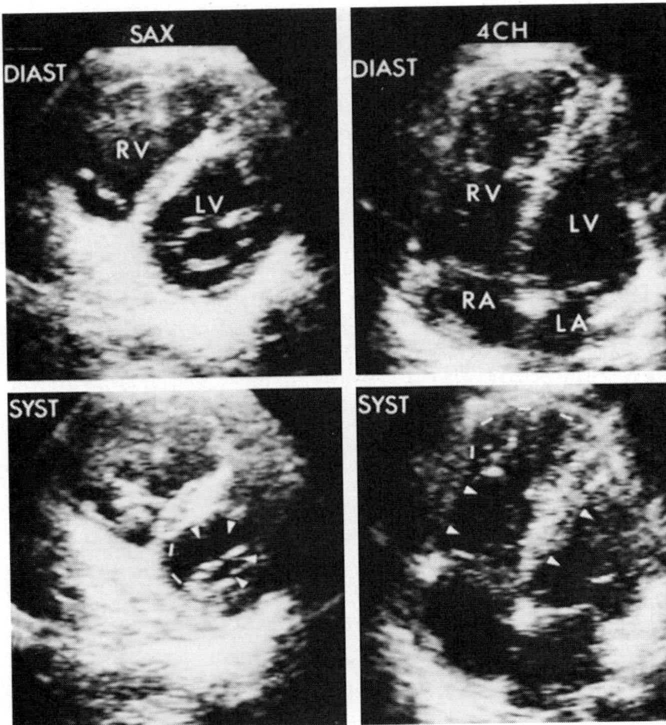

FIGURE 3–92. Short-axis (SAX) and four-chamber (4CH) 2-D echocardiograms of a patient with an inferior myocardial infarction complicated by right ventricular infarction. The posterior-inferior wall is akinetic (dashed line, SAX, SYST). In addition, the apical half of the right ventricular free wall is akinetic (dashed line, 4CH, SYST). The right ventricle (RV) is also dilated. RA = right atrium; LV = left ventricle; LA = left atrium. (From Feigenbaum, H.: Echocardiography. 4th ed. Philadelphia, Lea and Febiger, 1986.)

ventricle to the right ventricle through the ruptured septum can be recorded. Color flow Doppler recording of such a defect is the procedure of choice.[372,373] Transesophageal echocardiography may be useful in some patients.[374]

Right ventricular infarction (see p. 1192) is an increasingly recognized complication of MI and can have important clinical implications for management. Figure 3–92 shows the common echocardiographic findings with right ventricular infarction.[375,376] These patients usually have evidence of an inferior infarction. The inferior-posterior wall of the left ventricle is akinetic in systole (dashes) as noted in the short-axis view. The evidence for right ventricular infarction is right ventricular dilatation and right ventricular free wall motion akinesis (dashes) (Fig. 3–92). Premature pulmonary valve opening may occur with right ventricular infarction.[377] There may also be distortion of the interatrial septum so that it bulges toward the left atrium.[378]

Mural thrombus (see p. 1256) represents another common complication of AMI that can be detected with echocardiography.[379,380] These clots occur most often with aneurysms, especially those involving the anterior wall and apex. Figure 3–93 shows a variety of left ventricular clots. The thrombi may have various configurations. Those that protrude into the cavity and may be mobile, as in Figure 3–93*B* and *D*, are easier to detect echocardiographically and may have a greater likelihood of producing systemic emboli.[381–383] Other thrombi are layered along the wall and may not be as likely to break loose (Fig. 3–93*A*). Certain left ventricular echocardiographic flow patterns or spontaneous contrast may be precursors of thrombi.[384]

Other complications of AMI, such as mitral regurgitation[385–387] and pericardial effusion,[388] are easily detected echocardiographically.

NATURAL HISTORY AND PROGNOSIS. Echocardiography is ideal for serial studies in patients with MI.[389] Two-dimensional echocardiography carried out early in the course of an infarction is helpful in establishing the diagnosis.[390,391] and provides prognostic information as well.[392,393] This examination is useful in the assessment of the status of the myocardium not involved in the current infarction[394] because an unsuspected previous MI may be discovered. An early echocardiographic study also can serve as a baseline for detecting future ischemic events such as MI expansion[395,396] or other complications. The initial examination may even help identify the patients who are at high risk of experiencing complications.[397,398] A resting[399] or stress[400] 2-D echocardiogram before discharge can also provide long-term prognostic information.

Possibly one of the most important uses of echocardiography in patients with acute MI is to evaluate the efficacy of reperfusion therapy.[401,402] Figure 3–94 shows serial stud-

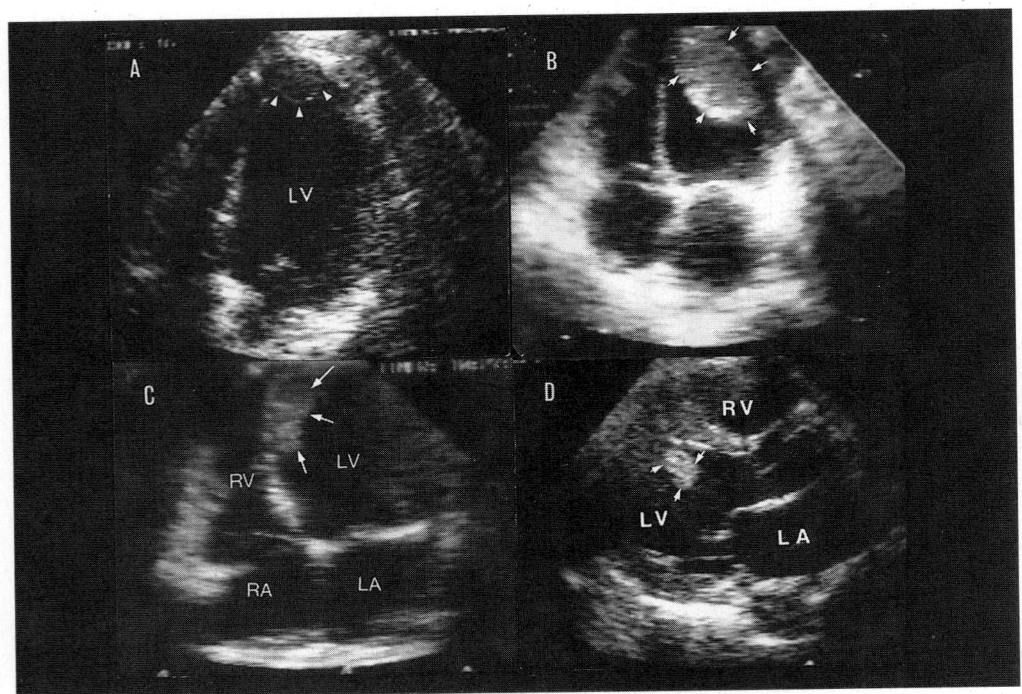

FIGURE 3–93. Echocardiograms demonstrating a variety of different left ventricular thrombi (arrows) that can be identified echocardiographically. The thrombi in *A* and *C* are relatively flat and adherent to the walls. The thrombus in *B* is large and protrudes into the cavity of the left ventricle. *D* demonstrates a relatively small (more mobile) thrombus attached to the interventricular septum. LV = left ventricle; RV = right ventricle; RA = right atrium; LA = left atrium. (From Feigenbaum, H.: Echocardiography. 5th ed. Malvern, PA, Lea and Febiger, 1994).

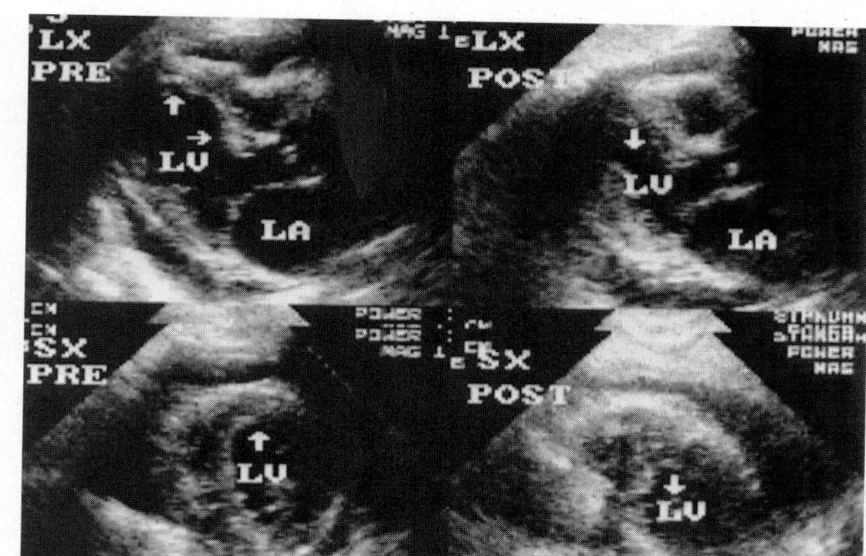

FIGURE 3–94. Long-axis (LX) and short-axis (SX) echocardiograms of a patient with an acute anterior myocardial infarction before (PRE) and after (POST) PTCA of the left anterior descending coronary artery. Before PTCA the anterior septum is dyskinetic (upward arrows). After successful PTCA the motion of the septum is normal (downward arrows).

ies of a patient who underwent angioplasty for an occluded left anterior descending coronary artery. During the acute infarction and before angioplasty the anterior septum was dyskinetic (reverse arrows). After successful reopening of the artery and recovery of the stunned myocardium, the septal motion returned to normal (arrows LX post, SX post).

STUNNED OR HIBERNATING MYOCARDIUM (see also p. 1176). Stunned or hibernating myocardium denotes viable but dysfunctional myocardial segments. It has been demonstrated that stressing the heart with dobutamine or dipyridamole can identify those segments that are viable and potentially functional by inducing them to contract, usually with low-dose pharmacologic agents.[403–405] With stunned myocardium the functional recovery will occur with time since the artery is already reopened. Reperfusion procedures are necessary to restore ventricular function with hibernating muscle.[406,407]

EXAMINATION OF THE CORONARY ARTERIES. Echocardiography is playing an increasing role in direct visualization of the coronary arteries. Ultrasonic transducers can be placed at the tip of an intracoronary catheter. These transducers are small enough to be inserted within the proximal coronary arteries (Fig. 3–15). The transducer then provides a cross-sectional picture of the artery.[408] This examination gives an excellent view of the arterial wall. The normal wall is very thin while atherosclerotic plaque has a thick crescent-shaped appearance (Fig. 3–15, arrows). Figure 3–95 illustrates the variety of coronary atherosclerotic lesions that can be detected with intravascular ultrasound. The ultrasonic technique has already changed our understanding of coronary artery disease.[409–413] The diffuse nature of this pathologic process is better appreciated with intracoronary ultrasound than is commonly noted with angiography.[414] This examination is being utilized with invasive angioplasty techniques.[415–417] Figure 3–96*A* illustrates two intracoronary echograms and accompanying diagrams of a patient with coronary atherosclerosis who underwent atherectomy for removal of the atherosclerotic plaque *(A)*. Following atherectomy much of the atherosclerotic material has been removed (arrowheads). In Figure 3–96*B* an intravascular echogram and diagram show the deployment of a

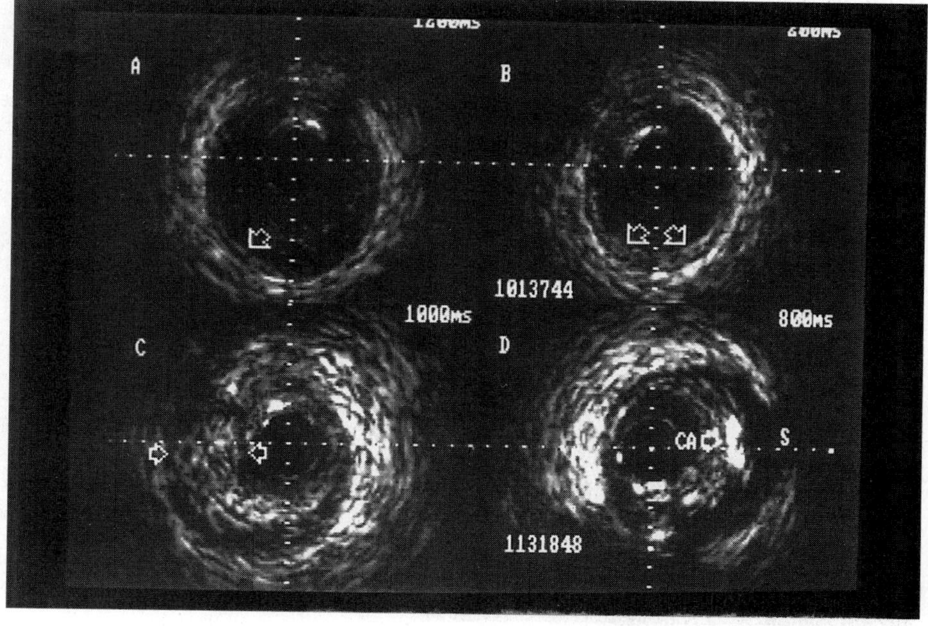

FIGURE 3–95. Intracoronary ultrasonic images demonstrating the different severity of coronary atherosclerosis: *A,* Small rim of thickened endothelium (arrow). *B,* Larger amount of eccentric endothelial thickening (arrows). *C,* Massive atherosclerotic plaque that is wider (arrows) than the residual lumen. *D,* Calcification in the plaque (CA) produces shadowing (S). (From Feigenbaum, H.: Echocardiography. 5th ed. Malvern, PA, Lea and Febiger, 1994).

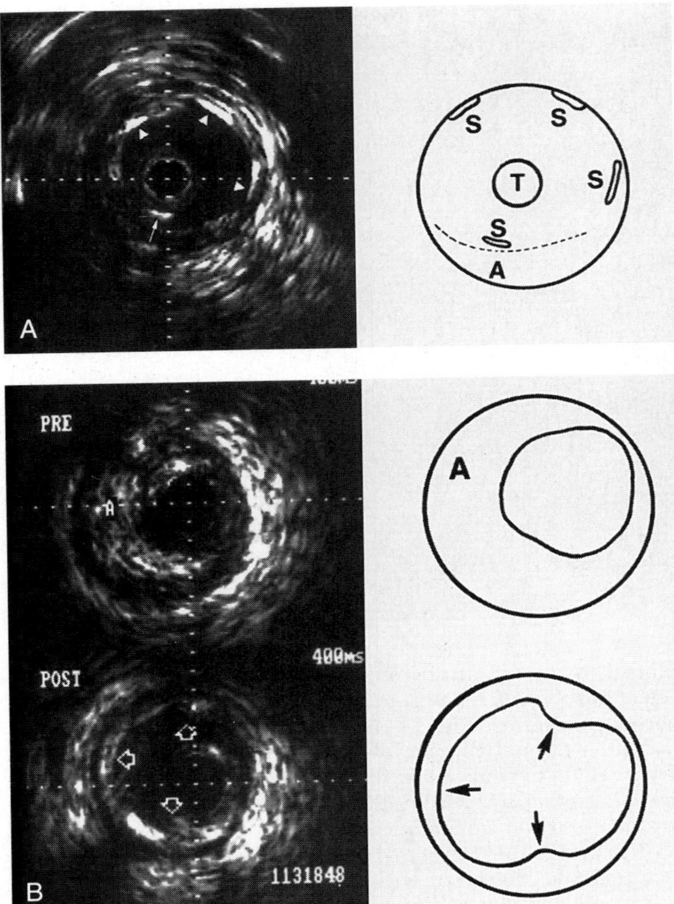

FIGURE 3–96. Intracoronary ultrasonic images and diagrams before (PRE) and after (POST) atherectomy and removal (arrows) of much of the preatherectomy atherosclerosis *(A).* (From Feigenbaum, H.: Echocardiography. 5th ed. Malvern, PA, Lea and Febiger, 1994.) *B,* Intracoronary echogram and diagram of a patient following elective placement of a Palmaz-Schatz stent. Although the proper angiographic deployment was observed, a single strut (arrow) did not demonstrate full apposition to the wall, whereas the other struts (arrowheads) are fully deployed. (Courtesy of R. L. Wilensky, M.D.)

Palmaz-Schatz stent (see p. 1380) in the vicinity of an atherosclerotic plaque. Three of the struts of the stent are in direct proximity to the arterial wall. However, one strut (arrow) abuts the atherosclerotic plaque but is not fully deployed against the arterial wall and may be prone to thrombose.

It is also possible to put a tiny Doppler transducer at the tip of an intracoronary catheter. In so doing one can record the blood velocities within the coronary arteries.[418,419] Using such a technique with a potent vasodilator provides an opportunity to record coronary flow reserve.[420,421] Normally there is a dramatic increase in the blood velocity with a vasodilator. In patients with reduced reserve this augmentation of flow is blunted.

Transesophageal and transthoracic echocardiography can also be used to examine the coronary arteries directly.[422,423] With the transesophageal approach one can record spatial Doppler velocities[424,425] and color flow imaging.[426] Both transthoracic and transesophageal imaging techniques can visualize the arterial walls. Figure 3–97 shows a transthoracic examination of a normal proximal left coronary artery. Atherosclerotic plaques within the proximal left coronary system can be identified as bright, segmental echoes that give an irregular appearance to the artery lumen.[427,428] Kawasaki's disease occurs in children and produces aneurysms of the coronary arteries.[429,430] These aneurysmal dilatations are identifiable with transthoracic echocardiography (Fig. 31–7, p. 996).[431] Congenital anomalies of the coronary arteries (pp. 909 and 966) can also be detected with both transthoracic and transesophageal 2-D, Doppler, and color Doppler echocardiography.[432–434] Coronary artery fistulas are also detected echocardiographically.[435]

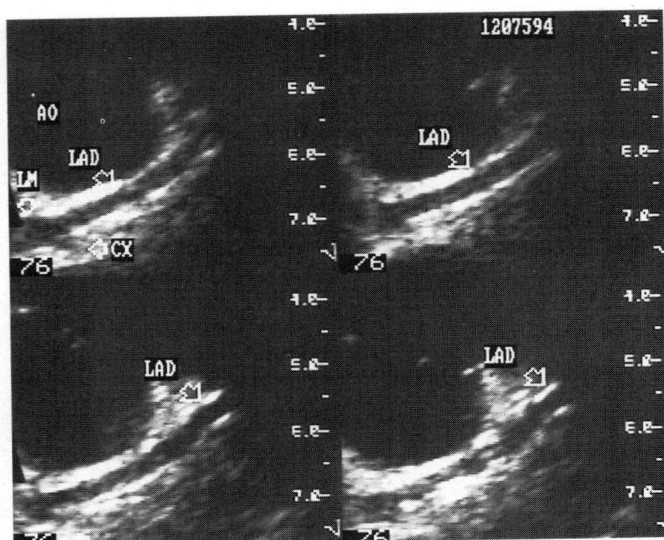

FIGURE 3–97. Left coronary artery examined with transthoracic echocardiography using a modified short-axis plane. LM = left main; AO = aorta; LAD = left anterior descending; CX = circumflex.

MYOCARDIAL PERFUSION USING CONTRAST ECHOCARDIOGRAPHY. Contrast echocardiography may also be employed to study myocardial perfusion.[436–438] If a fluid containing microbubbles is injected into the root of the aorta or directly into the coronary artery, the echogenicity of the myocardium will be increased (Fig. 3–98), provided that the blood supply is intact. When blood flow is impeded, the increase in echogenicity in that segment is reduced or absent. This examination has been done in a limited fashion in the catheterization laboratory or in the operating room. With the introduction of contrast agents that are visualized on the left side of the heart with intravenous injections, there is optimism for a less invasive recording of myocardial perfusion using this technique.[439,440]

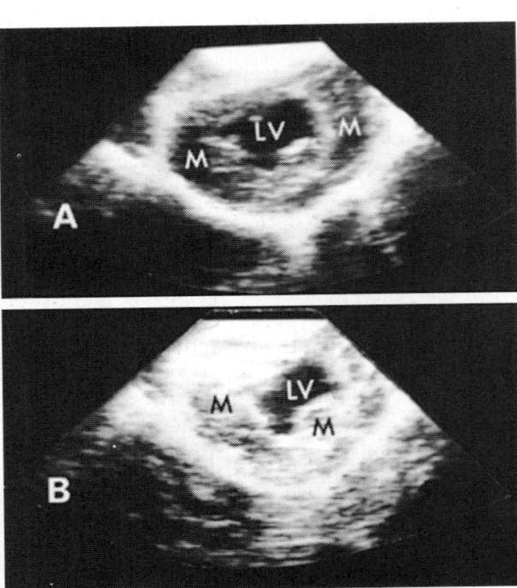

FIGURE 3–98. Short-axis 2-D echocardiogram of a dog before and after injection of contrast in the root of the aorta. Before contrast injection *(A)* the myocardium (M) is relatively echo free. Following the injection of fluid containing tiny microbubbles *(B)* the myocardium becomes uniformly echogenic.

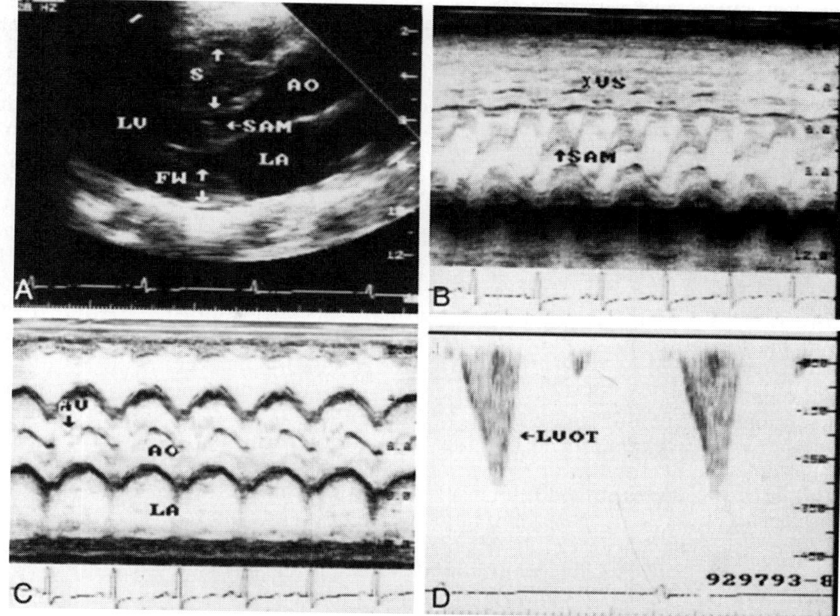

FIGURE 3–99. Two-dimensional, M-mode, and Doppler studies in a patient with hypertrophic obstructive cardiomyopathy. The 2-D long-axis study shows the thickened interventricular septum (S) and the systolic anterior motion of the mitral valve (SAM). The abnormal mitral motion and the thickened septum are also seen on the M-mode recording *(B)*. The M-mode recording of the aortic valve shows midsystolic closure (AV). The Doppler recording of the left ventricular outflow tract shows how the velocity within the outflow tract increases in the latter half of systole. LV = left ventricle; AO = aorta; FW = left ventricular free wall; LA = left atrium; IVS = interventricular septum; LVOT = left ventricular outflow tract.

CARDIOMYOPATHIES

(See also Chap. 41)

HYPERTROPHIC CARDIOMYOPATHY (HCM) (see also p. 1414). Echocardiography is an important diagnostic tool in patients with HCM and has enriched our understanding of this abnormality. An early echocardiographic abnormality to be noted was systolic anterior motion of the mitral valve (termed *SAM*) (Fig. 3–99*B*),[441] which appeared to be related to and was correlated with the presence of obstruction to left ventricular outflow.[442,443] The shorter the distance between the septum and the leaflet and the longer the duration of apposition between these two structures, the more severe the obstruction.[444] This echocardiographic finding also demonstrated the critical importance of involvement of the mitral valve apparatus in the obstruction in this condition.[445] More recently SAM has been noted in a variety of other patients, some of whom had no evidence of left ventricular hypertrophy.[446,447] It has been observed in patients with anemia and hypovolemia as well as in patients with a hyperdynamic left ventricle.[446] It is possible that SAM is a nonspecific sign that occurs whenever the left ventricular systolic volume is reduced, either because of hypertrophy, as in HCM, or in the presence of a hyperdynamic state.[448]

A second echocardiographic finding in patients with obstructive HCM is midsystolic closure of the aortic valve (Fig. 3–99*C*). However, as noted earlier, this sign is not specific for HCM and is also present in patients with discrete subaortic stenosis. While this finding is not sensitive, when present it usually indicates a significant amount of obstruction.

Hypertrophy of the septum with abnormal organization of myocardial cells may be one of the basic abnormalities of HCM[449] (p. 1416), and a key echocardiographic finding is disproportionate hypertrophy of the septum in relation to the posterior wall of the left ventricle, so that the ratio of thickness of the septum to the free wall exceeds 1.3:1.0 (Fig. 3–98)[450] and the motion of the hypertrophied septum is reduced.[451] It has also been shown that asymmetrical septal hypertrophy (ASH) is frequently transmitted as an autosomal dominant trait and that there are patients with asymmetrical septal hypertrophy who do not show SAM and therefore do not have obstruction to left ventricular outflow.[452] These patients may be considered to have HCM without obstruction. While the concept of recognizing ASH with or without obstruction to left ventricular outflow by echocardiography is an important one, there are limitations to echocardiographic diagnosis. First, the thickness of the septum may be difficult to measure precisely echocardiographically. (In Figure 3–99 the left side of the septum is clearly identified, but the right side is not as distinct.) Second, it must be appreciated that ASH is not pathognomonic for HCM and related myopathies and can occur in a variety of other disease states, including right ventricular hypertrophy. In addition, some patients with HCM may have concentric rather than asymmetrical hypertrophy, in which the septal and posterior left ventricular walls are equal in thickness (see p. 1415).

Two-dimensional echocardiography provides additional information by indicating the shape and location of the hypertrophied myocardium in patients with known or suspected HCM.[453,454] A variety of hypertrophied segments has been recorded by this technique. Figure 3–100 shows a hypertrophied septum limited to the basal two-thirds of the septum, while the apex is virtually free of muscular hyper-

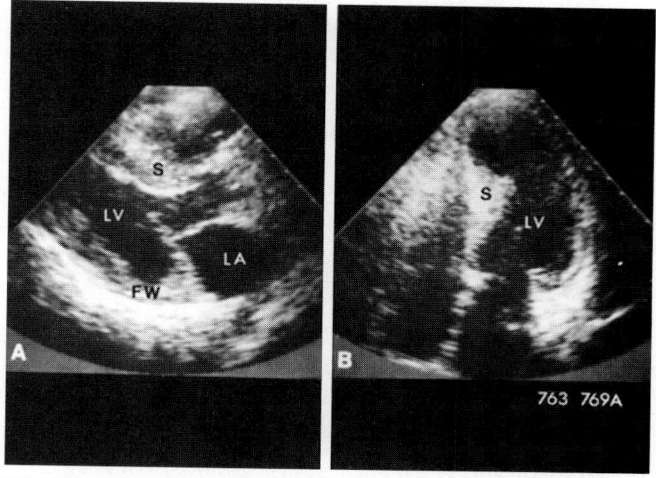

FIGURE 3–100. Long-axis *(A)* and apical four-chamber *(B)* echocardiograms of a patient with hypertrophic cardiomyopathy whose hypertrophy primarily involves the proximal two-thirds of the interventricular septum (S). The apex is spared from the hypertrophic process. LV = left ventricle; FW = left ventricular free wall; LA = left atrium. (From Feigenbaum, H.: Echocardiography. 4th ed. Philadelphia, Lea and Febiger, 1986.)

trophy. Other patients exhibit an apical form of hypertrophy with the proximal septum being relatively thin.[455,456] Concentric hypertrophy is also a fairly common form of hypertrophic myopathy (Fig. 3–101). Cavity obliteration with ventricular systole is almost always present with this type of disease. Two-dimensional echocardiography is useful in assessing the effectiveness of myotomy and myectomy. An intriguing observation is that the echoes from the diseased septum in HCM are more reflective or "speckled" than those from the free posterior wall.[457]

Doppler echocardiography may also be helpful in evaluating hypertrophic cardiomyopathy.[458,459] The Doppler recording of the left ventricular outflow may show an abnormal pattern with the abnormally high velocity occurring in late systole (Fig. 3–99*D*).[460] The systolic gradient can be estimated using the Doppler technique.[461] The left ventricular hypertrophy and reduced left ventricular compliance alter the Doppler recording of mitral valve flow. The early diastolic velocity or E point is reduced, and the late velocity with atrial systole is increased.[462] Color Doppler provides spatial visualization of the altered blood flow in patients with obstructive HCM.[463,464]

CONGESTIVE (DILATED) CARDIOMYOPATHY (see also p. 1407). The echocardiogram characteristically reveals a dilated poorly contracting left ventricle in patients with congestive cardiomyopathy.[465,466] Signs of reduced cardiac output include a poorly moving aorta, reduced opening of the mitral valve, and slow closure of the aortic valve. The left atrium is dilated, and the abnormal closure of the mitral valve indicative of elevated left diastolic pressure is frequently noted. Incomplete closure of the mitral valve or papillary muscle dysfunction and subsequent mitral regurgitation are common. Left ventricular filling on Doppler echograms changes as the disease progresses.[467,468] It must be appreciated that these findings are nonspecific and may also occur in patients with ischemic heart disease. However, at least one portion of the left ventricle continues to exhibit normal motion in most, although not all, patients with severe coronary artery disease.[465] In patients with cardiomyopathy the impairment of left ventricular wall motion is diffuse. If mitral regurgitation develops in patients with cardiomyopathy, septal motion may increase slightly in keeping with the left ventricular volume overload, although this increase in septal motion is certainly not as striking as that which occurs in primary mitral valve disease with secondary myocardial failure.

RESTRICTIVE (INFILTRATIVE) CARDIOMYOPATHY (see also p. 1426). The principal echocardiographic findings in patients with infiltrative cardiomyopathy are reduced wall motion and thickening of the left ventricular wall without dilatation.[469,470] These changes are usually uniform throughout the ventricle. There is also a characteristic left ventricular filling pattern with a tall E wave and short A wave on the mitral Doppler recording (Fig. 3–38*C*).[471] Obviously these findings are not specific for infiltrative cardiomyopathy, and like those obtained by means of electrocardiography, chest roentgenography, hemodynamics, and angiography, they must be interpreted in terms of the total clinical setting. In patients with amyloid heart disease (Fig. 3–102)[472] the echocardiographic findings are usually again nonspecific and show left ventricular hypertrophy. There are also frequently more specific findings in that the valves may be uniformly thickened in addition to the hypertrophy of the ventricular walls. The interatrial septum may also be unusually thick, and a peculiar speckled appearance of the myocardium may be noted, reflecting localized variations in echo density.[473] In the beginning course of amyloid heart disease early left ventricular filling is reduced. The Doppler mitral E wave is decreased and the A wave is

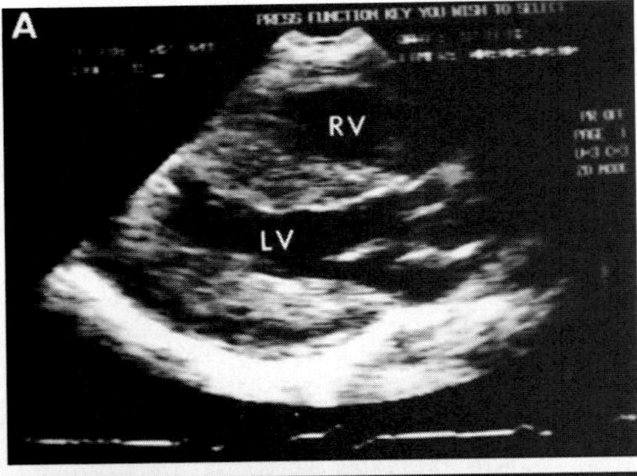

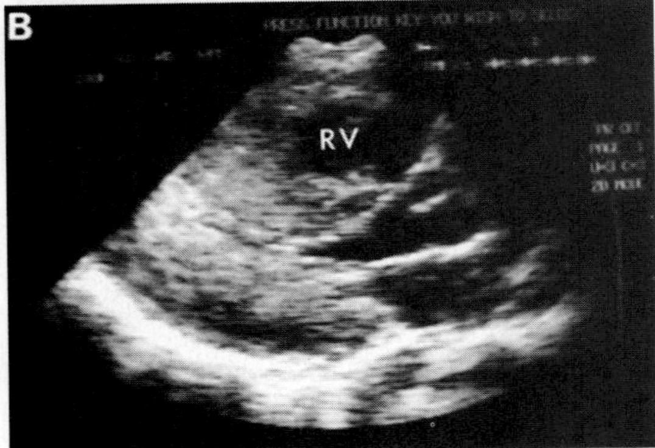

FIGURE 3–101. Long-axis 2-D echocardiogram of a patient with hypertrophic cardiomyopathy who exhibits uniform hypertrophy of the entire left ventricle (LV). RV = right ventricle; *A* = diastole; *B* = systole. (From Feigenbaum, H.: Echocardiography. 4th ed. Philadelphia, Lea and Febiger, 1986.)

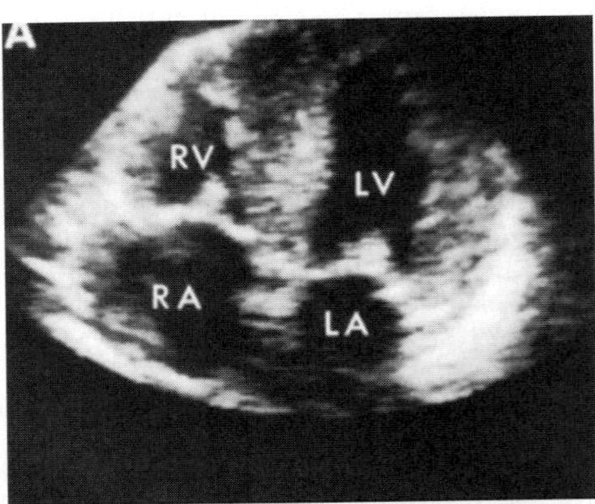

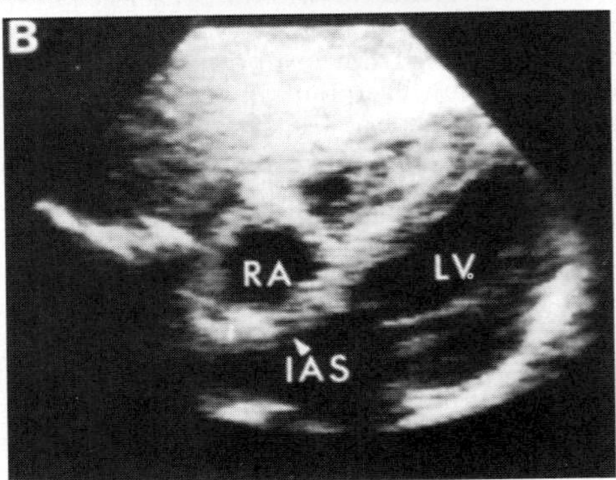

FIGURE 3–102. Four-chamber *(A)* and subcostal *(B)* 2-D echocardiograms of a patient with hereditary amyloidosis. The four-chamber view demonstrates markedly hypertrophied cardiac walls, especially the interventricular septum and free wall of the right ventricle. The tricuspid and mitral valve leaflets are also thickened. The left ventricle (LV) and right ventricle (RV) cavities are small. The subcostal examination demonstrates a thickened interatrial septum (IAS). RA = right atrium; LA = left atrium. (From Feigenbaum, H.: Echocardiography. 4th ed. Philadelphia, Lea and Febiger, 1986.)

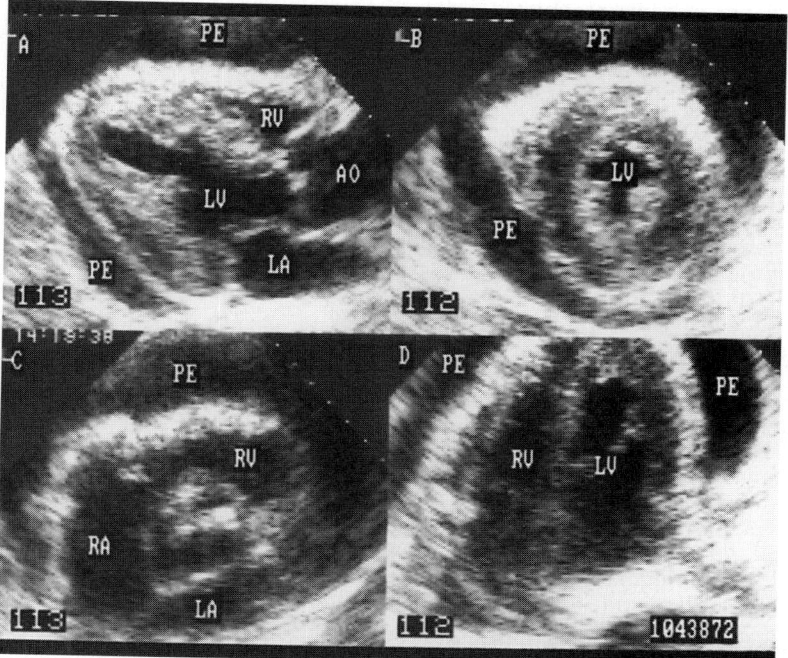

FIGURE 3–103. Long-axis *(A),* short-axis at the papillary muscle *(B),* short-axis at the base of the heart *(C),* and apical four-chamber *(D)* 2-D echocardiograms of a patient with a large pericardial effusion (PE). the relatively echo-free fluid can be seen surrounding the heart in all views. The visceral pericardium is echogenic and probably thickened. RV = right ventricle; LV = left ventricle; AO = aorta; LA = left atrium; RA = right atrium. (From Feigenbaum, H.: Echocardiography. 5th ed. Malvern, PA, Lea and Febiger, 1994.)

increased (Fig. 3–38*B*). Later, filling becomes more restrictive and the E and A waves are reversed (Fig. 3–38*C*), and in between there may be a pattern of "pseudonormalization."[474]

PERICARDIAL DISEASE

(See also Chap. 43)

PERICARDIAL EFFUSION (see also p. 1485). The theory underlying the use of ultrasound in the recognition of pericardial effusion is relatively simple; since the acoustic properties of fluid differ significantly from those of cardiac muscle, the effusion surrounding the heart is less echogenic than is the myocardium. Accordingly, the detection of effusion was one of the first and has remained one of the most useful applications of echocardiography.[475]

Figure 3–103 shows a 2-D echocardiographic examination of a patient with a large pericardial effusion (PE). One can see the echo-free space both anteriorly and posteriorly in the long-axis (A) and short-axis (B) views. The four-chamber view *(D)* shows the fluid on both the medial and lateral aspects of the heart. There is very little if any fluid posterior to the left atrium (*A* and *C*). The size of the effusion is estimated by the amount of echo-free space surrounding the heart. Frequently with small effusions one sees only a posterior echo-free space and very little fluid anteriorly. As the fluid increases it distributes both anteriorly and posteriorly. With large effusions, as in Figure 3–103, one usually sees more anterior fluid than posterior fluid as the heart tends to sink posteriorly.

There are several echocardiographic signs for cardiac tamponade.[476] One of the most frequent findings is collapse of the anterior right ventricular free wall.[477,478] Figure 3–104 shows the collapse of the right ventricular wall (arrow) in the long-axis view (LX). In the four-chamber view one notes collapse of the right atrial free wall (arrow). Right atrial collapse is slightly more sensitive but less specific than right ventricular collapse.[478a,479] Occasionally one may see collapse of the left atrium[480,481] and even on rare occasion the left ventricle.[482,483] Right ventricular collapse occurs in early diastole and may be better appreciated on an M-mode recording. Doppler echocardiography can also be used to identify cardiac tamponade.[484,485] Under this hemodynamic setting one can see a respiratory cyclical variation of both tricuspid and mitral flow.[486,487] With inspiration one finds an exaggerated increase in tricuspid flow and a decrease in mitral flow. The reverse occurs with expiration.

With very large effusions one can detect excessive motion of the heart within the pericardial sac. This excessive

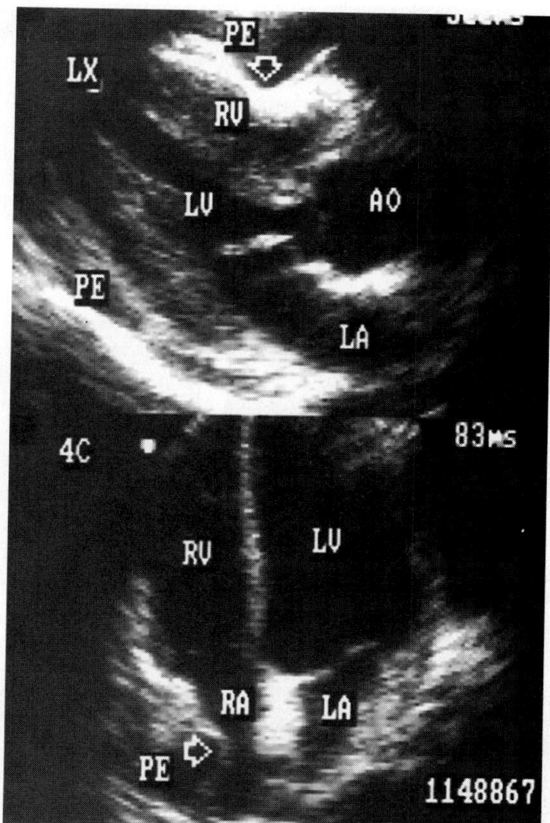

FIGURE 3–104. Long-axis (LX) and four-chamber (4C) 2-D echocardiographic views in a patient with pericardial effusion (PE) and cardiac tamponade. The long-axis view shows diastolic collapse of the right ventricular wall (arrow); the four-chamber view shows collapse of the right atrial free wall (arrow). RV = right ventricle; LV = left ventricle; AO = aorta; LA = left atrium; RA = right atrium. (From Feigenbaum, H.: Echocardiography. 5th ed. Malvern, PA, Lea and Febiger, 1994.)

motion has been noted as a "swinging heart."[488,489] If the motion is such that the heart does not resume its original position before the next electric depolarization occurs, then the axis of the QRS is altered and one notes electrical alternans on the electrocardiogram.

CONSTRICTIVE PERICARDITIS (see also p. 1496). Echocardiography is of some (albeit limited) value in the diagnosis of a thickened pericardium with constrictive pericarditis.[490,491] Although a thickened pericardium can be detected in many patients, particularly those who already have pericardial fluid (Fig. 3–103), this finding by itself does not imply the presence of constriction. The echocardiographic signs of constriction include lack of diastolic motion, i.e., a flat diastolic slope of the posterior left ventricular wall,[2,492,493] abnormal motion of the interventricular septum,[492] very short E to F slope of the mitral valve,[2] and a dilated inferior vena cava that does not get smaller with inspiration. Doppler studies of the tricuspid, mitral, pulmonary venous flow are probably the most useful current recordings for constriction.[494,495] One notes a typical restrictive filling pattern of the mitral valve flow with a tall E wave and very small A wave (Fig. 3–38*C*). In addition there is a respiratory variation that will distinguish this type of recording from restrictive cardiomyopathy.[496,497]

CONGENITAL ABSENCE OF THE PERICARDIUM (see p. 1522). On the M-mode echocardiogram, the right ventricle is usually dilated and there is paradoxical septal motion similar to a right ventricular volume overload. Two-dimensional echocardiography reveals bulging or displacement of part of the left ventricle or left atrium in a distorted manner that suggests absence of the pericardium.[498,499]

CARDIAC TUMORS AND THROMBI

(See also Chap. 42)

LEFT ATRIAL TUMORS. Left atrial myxoma (see p. 1467) is by far the most common cardiac tumor, and echocardiography has proved to be an extremely important diagnostic technique for its recognition.[500] Figure 3–105 demonstrates a 2-D echocardiogram of a patient with left atrial myxoma. The spatial orientation inherent in this examination provides additional useful information, and the size and shape of the mass are apparent. In addition, the site of attachment of the mass to the cardiac structure can frequently be detected. Transesophageal echocardiography provides an outstanding view of the left atrium[501,502] and has vastly improved our ability to detect all intracardiac masses.[503,504] Excellent definition of left atrial masses can be seen with this unobstructive view. Figure 3–106 shows four images of a small left atrial mass that is attached to the interatrial septum (IAS). Although this tumor was seen on a transthoracic 2-D echocardiogram, the clarity and detail were greater with the transesophageal examination[505] (Fig. 3–107).

LEFT ATRIAL THROMBI. Other space-occupying structures[506,507]—atrial thrombi—have been identified in the left atrium by means of echocardiography.[508] Since most are located near the left atrial appendage, transesophageal echocardiography is superior to conventional echocardiography in visualizing left atrial thrombi (Fig. 3–107). The transesophageal technique may detect spontaneous contrast in the left atrium, which is frequently associated with and may be a precursor of thrombus formation.[509,510]

RIGHT ATRIAL MASSES (see p. 1466). Right atrial myoma is not as common as the left atrial variety. Such tumors can also be detected echocardiographically.[511,512] They appear as a mass of echoes that are in the right atrium during systole and traverse the tricuspid valve during diastole. As on the left side of the heart, a large vegetation involving the tricuspid valve can simulate a right atrial myxoma. Bilateral atrial myxomas have been detected echocardiographically.[513] Right atrial thrombi that have the potential of producing massive pulmonary emboli have been detected with 2-D echocardiography.[514,515]

VENTRICULAR TUMORS. Myomas can occur in the ventricles as well as in the atria[516,517] (see p. 1466) and have been imaged in both ventricles. When the tumors are mobile, they can produce very dramatic echograms on both M-mode and 2-D examinations; they may move above the mitral valve into the left ventricular outflow tract during systole.[518] Pedunculated right ventricular masses can prolapse into the pulmonary artery[519] or simulate pulmonic stenosis.[520] Rhabdomyomas[521] and fibromas[522] can also in-

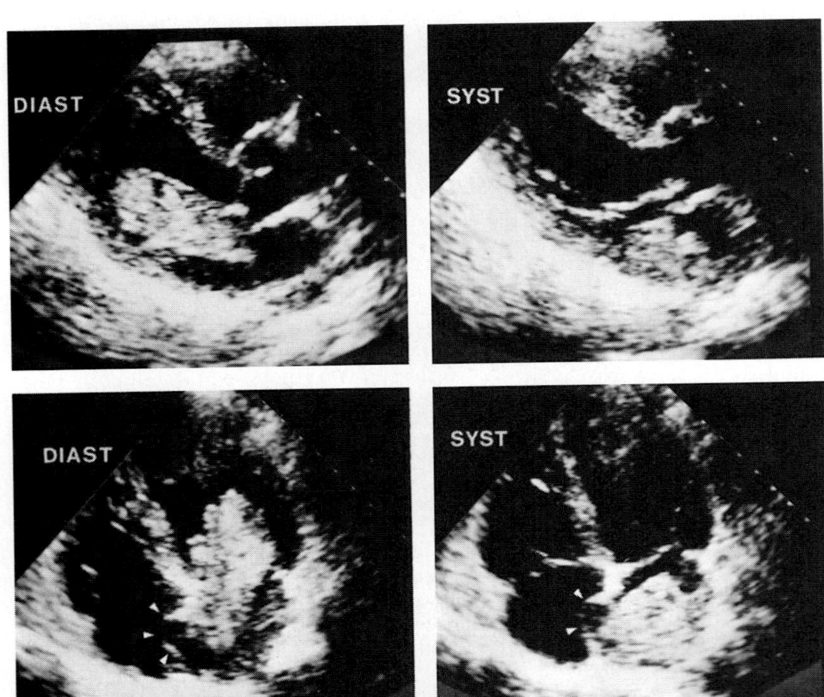

FIGURE 3–105. Long-axis *(top)* and apical four-chamber *(bottom)* 2-D echocardiograms in diastole and systole in a patient with a left atrial myxoma and an atrial septal aneurysm. The septal aneurysm (arrowheads) can be seen bulging toward the right atrium in both diastole and systole in the four-chamber view. (From Feigenbaum, H.: Echocardiography. 4th ed. Philadelphia, Lea and Febiger, 1986.)

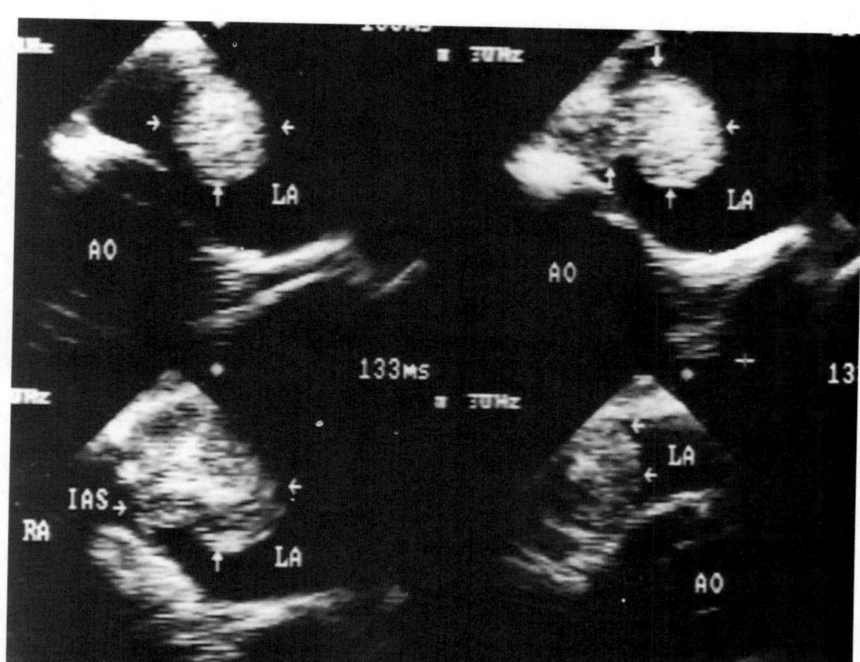

FIGURE 3–106. Transesophageal echocardiogram of a patient with a left atrial tumor (arrows). The tumor is attached to the interatrial septum (IAS). RA = right atrium; LA = left atrium; AO = aorta.

volve the ventricles; these two types of lesions have been imaged successfully.[523]

VALVULAR TUMORS. Neoplasms may involve the cardiac valves. Cardiac papillary fibroelastomas represent small tumors on the edges of the valve leaflets, primarily the mitral valve[524] and rarely the tricuspid valve.[525] Systemic emboli and stroke occur in patients with these neoplasms.[526] Other neoplasms, such as rhabdomyosarcoma, may also involve the mitral valve and can be detected echocardiographically.[527] Primary myxoma can also be attached to the mitral valve.[528]

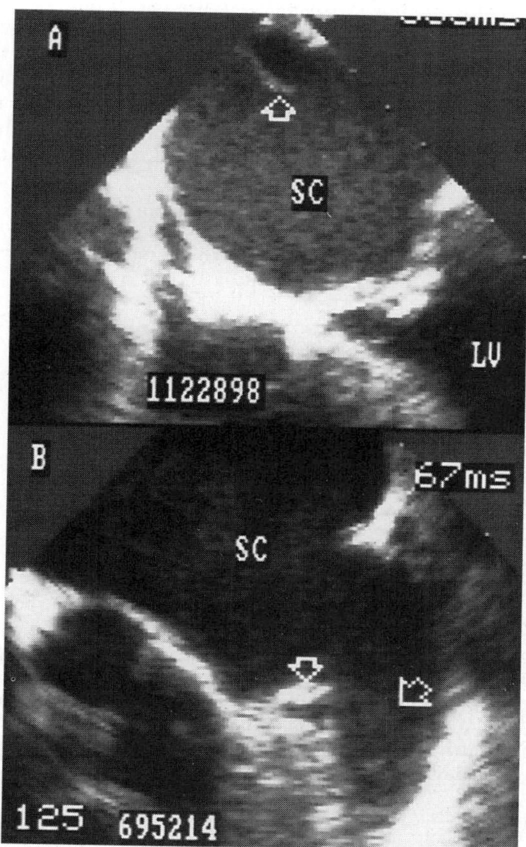

FIGURE 3–107. Transesophageal echocardiograms of two patients with spontaneous contrast (SC) and formed thrombi (arrows) in the left atrium. In *A* the thrombus is linear and immobile. In *B* a clot (small arrow) is attached to the junction of the left atrial appendage and the body of the left atrium. A less-dense echogenic mass (large arrow) is faintly seen within the left atrial appendage. LV = left ventricle. (From Feigenbaum, H.: Echocardiography. 5th ed. Malvern, PA, Lea and Febiger, 1994.)

OTHER INTRACARDIAC ECHOGENIC STRUCTURES. It should be kept in mind that not all echogenic structures in the heart are pathologic.[529] It is possible to detect various structures in the right atrium that are possibly normal variants. The so-called Chiari network may produce mobile echoes within the right atrium that may not be pathologic.[530,531] In addition, the eustachian valve may be prominent and simulate a pathologic mass.[532] Lipomatous hypertrophy of the interatrial septum may be striking but is benign.[533,534]

There are nonpathologic echo-producing structures on the left side of the heart as well.[535] Left ventricular bands or false tendons straddling the left ventricular chamber frequently can be imaged.[536] Moderator bands are routinely seen in the right ventricle. Iatrogenic masses, such as various catheters, are also easily detected on the 2-D echocardiogram. Occasionally this examination can help detect an incorrectly placed catheter or pacemaker catheter that may have perforated one of the cardiac walls.[537] Right atrial thrombi that have the potential of producing massive pulmonary emboli have been detected with 2-D echocardiography.[538,539]

INVASION AND METASTASIS TO THE HEART (see Ch. 57). Invasion of the wall of the heart[540,541] and compression of the heart[542] by neoplasms arising elsewhere have been imaged echocardiographically. Seeding of the pericardium with metastases and the production of pericardial effusion (see p. 1485) probably represent the most common types of cardiac involvement with malignant disease. Occasionally a massively thickened pericardium is produced. On echocardiography the position and configuration of the heart may be distorted by a large tumor mass in the mediastinum. Echocardiography has also been shown to be helpful in distinguishing between cystic and solid tumors involving the heart.[543] Transesophageal echocardiography can be very helpful in detecting paracardiac masses.[544]

PULMONARY ARTERY CLOTS. Transesophageal echocardiography now permits visualization of clots in the pulmonary arteries and is helpful in the diagnosis of pulmonary emboli.[545,546]

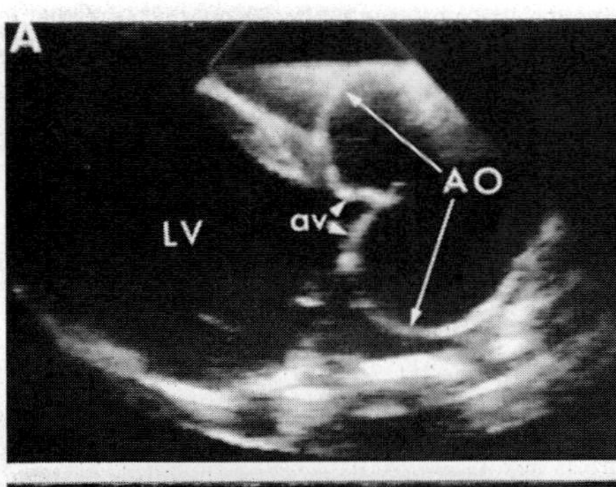

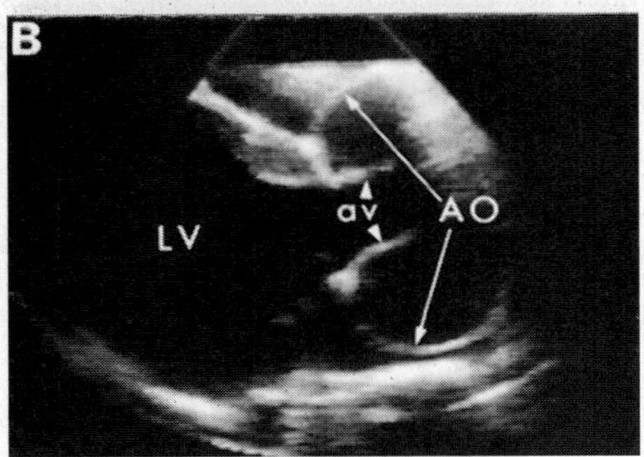

FIGURE 3–108. Diastolic *(A)* and systolic *(B)* long-axis, parasternal 2-D echocardiograms of a patient with Marfan syndrome. The aorta (AO) is markedly dilated. Note the marked discrepancy between the aortic valve (av) opening and the size of the aorta. LV = left ventricle. (From Feigenbaum, H.: Echocardiography. 3rd ed. Philadelphia, Lea and Febiger, 1981.)

DISEASES OF THE AORTA

(See also Chap. 45)

DILATATION AND ANEURYSM (see p. 1547). It is possible to examine almost the entire aorta using echocardiography.[547] The root of the aorta and proximal portion of the ascending aorta may be recorded with both M-mode and 2-D echocardiography. The 2-D technique utilizing the parasternal long-axis examination permits recording of the descending aorta posterior to the left atrium and left ventricle.[548] The suprasternal approach provides visualization of the arch of the aorta and the proximal portion of the descending aorta. The abdominal aorta can then be imaged with the transducer in the subcostal position or over the abdomen itself. Transesophageal echocardiography provides the most spectacular images of the aorta. Aside from a small section of the arch of the aorta, all of the aorta can be imaged very accurately with the transesophageal approach.

As might be expected, dilatation of the aorta, as occurs in the Marfan syndrome and cystic medial necrosis, is imaged relatively easily (Fig. 3–108).[549] The echocardiographic detection of coarctation of the aorta has already been discussed (see p. 84). Aneurysms of the abdominal aorta are routinely examined quite successfully by 2-D echocardiography.

AORTIC DISSECTION (see p. 1554). Two-dimensional echocardiography has been used extensively for the detection of aortic dissection (Fig. 3–109, p. 96).[550,551] In addition to the usual transducer position, the right parasternal position may be useful in detecting dissection with its true and false lumina and in indicating systolic fluttering of the intimal flap.[552] Transesophageal echocardiography is becoming the procedure of choice in the diagnosis of aortic dissection (Fig. 3–110, p. 96).[553–555] Doppler echocardiography has also been useful in the diagnosis of aortic dissection.[556] The flow characteristics in the false channel are distinctly different from those in the true channel. Color flow Doppler helps in establishing the correct diagnosis by indicating the difference between the false and true lumina (Fig. 3–111, p. 97) and helps to identify the entry point of the dissection.[557,558]

ANEURYSM OF THE SINUS OF VALSALVA. Because examination of the root of the aorta is possible, 2-D and transesophageal echocardiography have been used to image the sinus of Valsalva, allowing detection of aneurysms of these sinuses.[559,560] Bulging of the sinus, usually the anterior or

FIGURE 3–110. See color plate 4.

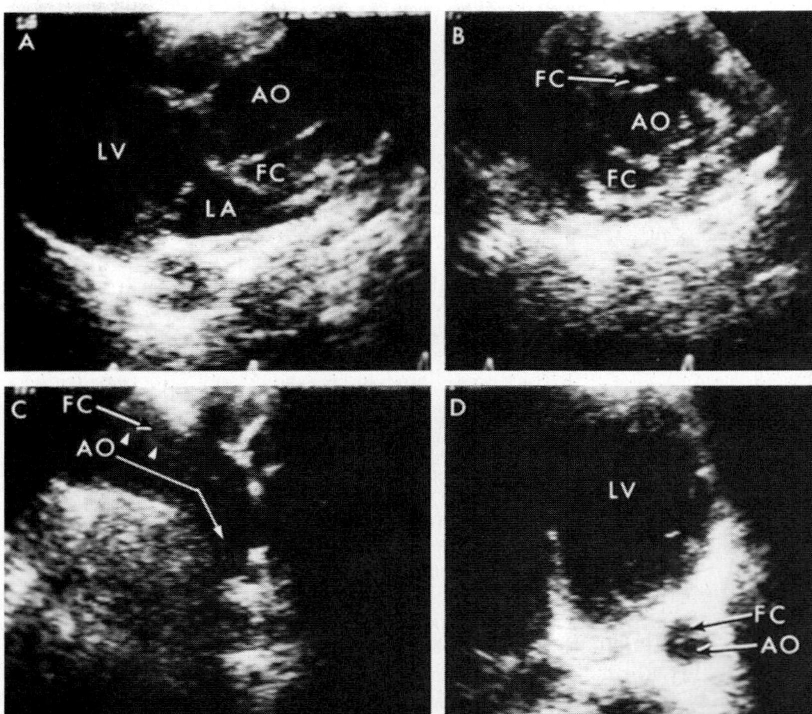

FIGURE 3–109. Parasternal long-axis *(A)*, short-axis *(B)*, suprasternal *(C)*, and apical *(D)* views in a patient with aortic dissection. The false channel (FC) can be seen in every view. The intimal flap (arrowheads) is only faintly seen in the suprasternal examination *(C)*. AO = true aortic lumen; LV = left ventricle; LA = left atrium. (From Feigenbaum, H.: Echocardiography. 4th ed. Philadelphia, Lea and Febiger, 1986.)

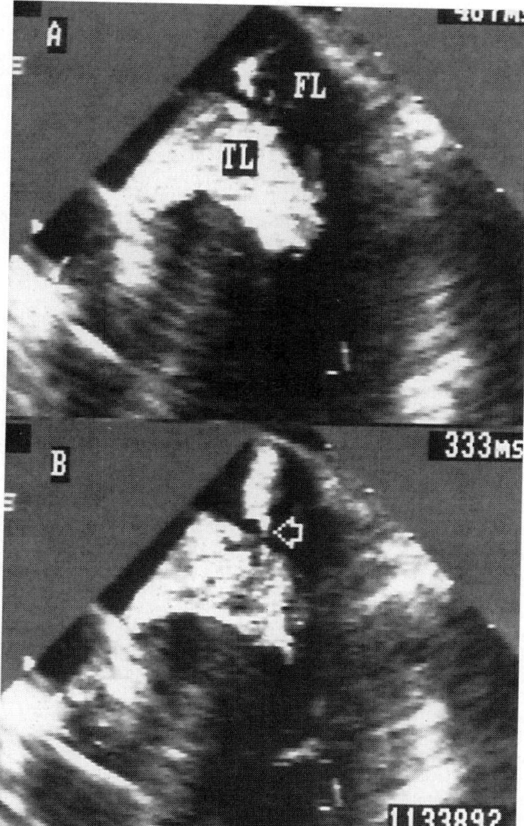

FIGURE 3–111. Doppler flow imaging in black and white showing an entry jet (arrow) passing from the true lumen (TL) into the false lumen (FL) of a patient with aortic dissection. (From Feigenbaum, H.: Echocardiography. 5th ed. Malvern, PA, Lea and Febiger, 1994.)

right coronary sinus, into the right ventricular outflow tract[561] or interventricular septum[562] has been recorded. With rupture there is discontinuity of the anterior wall of the sinus and mid-systolic closure and coarse fluttering of the right coronary cusp of the aortic valve.[563] With rupture of the sinus of Valsalva into the right side of the heart, fluttering of the tricuspid valve as well as premature opening of the pulmonary valve has been reported.[132] Doppler echocardiography, especially color flow, is the principal echocardiographic examination in the diagnosis of ruptured sinus of Valsalva aneurysms.[564] The abnormal jets of blood can be readily identified.

AORTIC ATHEROSCLEROSIS. Transesophageal echocardiography offers the opportunity to see atherosclerotic plaque within the thoracic aorta.[565,566] The masses vary in size and mobility[567] and may be responsible for systemic emboli.[568,569]

REFERENCES

PRINCIPLES OF ECHOCARDIOGRAPHY

1. Carlsen, E, N.: Ultrasound physics for the physician: A brief review. J. Clin. Ultrasound *3*:69, 1975.
2. Feigenbaum, H.: Echocardiography. 5th ed. Malvern, PA, Lea and Febiger, 1994.
3. Wells, P. N. T.: Ultrasonics in Clinical Diagnosis. 2nd ed. New York, Churchill Livingstone, 1977.
4. Von Ramm, O.T., and Thurstone, F. L.: Cardiac imaging using a phased array ultrasound system. Circulation *53*:258, 1976.
5. Hatle, L., and Angelsen, B.: Doppler ultrasound in cardiology: Physical principles and clinical applications. 2nd ed. Philadelphia, Lea and Febiger, 1984.
6. Goldberg, S. J., Allen, H. D., Marx, G. R., and Flinn, C. J.: Doppler Echocardiography. Philadelphia, Lea and Febiger, 1985.
7. Burns, P. N.: The physical principles of Doppler and spectral analysis. J. Clin. Ultrasound *15*:567, 1987.
8. Bom, K., deBoo, J., and Rijsterborgh, H.: On the aliasing problem in pulsed Doppler cardiac studies. J. Clin. Ultrasound. *12*:559, 1984.
9. Stewart, W. J., Galvin, K. A., Gillam, L. D., et al.: Comparison of high pulse repetition frequency and continuous wave Doppler echocardiography in the assessment of high flow velocity in patients with valvular stenosis and regurgitation. J. Am. Coll. Cardiol. *6*:565, 1985.
10. Stevenson, J. G.: Appearance and recognition of basic concepts in color flow imaging. Echocardiography *6*:451, 1989.
11. Ritter, S. B.: Red, green and blue: The flag of color flow mapping. Echocardiography *6*:369, 1989.
12. Seward, J. B., Khandheria, B. K., Oh, J. K., et al.: Transesophageal echocardiography: Technique, anatomic correlations, implementation, and clinical applications. Mayo Clin. Proc. *63*:649, 1988.
13. Tardif, J.-C., Schwartz, S. L., Vannan, M. A., et al.: Clinical usefulness of multiplane transesophageal echocardiography: Comparison to biplanar imaging. Am. Heart J. 128:156, 1994.
14. Seward, J. B., Khandheria, B. K., Edwards, W. D., et al.: Biplanar transesophageal echocardiography: Anatomic correlations, image orientation, and clinical applications. Mayo Clin Proc. *65*:1193, 1990.
15. Schiller, N. B., Maurer, G., Ritter, S. B., et al.: Transesophageal echocardiography. J. Am. Soc. Echocardiogr. *2*:354, 1989.
16. Eisenberg, M. J., London, M. J., Leung, J. M., et al.: Monitoring for myocardial ischemia during noncardiac surgery. A technology assessment of transesophageal echocardiography and 12-lead electrocardiography. The study of perioperative ischemia research group. JAMA *268*:210, 1992.
17. Tee, S. D. C., Shiota, T., Weintraub, R., et al.: Evaluation of ventricular septal defect by transesophageal echocardiography: Intraoperative assessment. Am. Heart J. *127*:585, 1994.
18. Cohen, G. I., Casale, P. N., Lytle, B. W., et al.: Transesophageal echocardiography guidance of closed mitral commissurotomy. J. Am. Soc. Echocardiogr. *6*:332, 1993.
19. Callahan, J. A., Seward, J. B., Nishimura, R. A., et al.: Two-dimensional echocardiographically guided pericardiocentesis: Experience in 117 consecutive patients. Am. J. Cardiol. *55*:476, 1985.
20. Koenig, P. R., Rossi, A., and Ritter, S. B.: Bedside cardiac catheterization using transesophageal echocardiographic guidance. Echocardiography *9*:637, 1992.
21. Pytlewski, G., Georgeson, S., Burke, J., et al.: Endomyocardial biopsy under transesophageal echocardiographic guidance can be safely performed in the critically ill cardiac transplant recipient. Am. J. Cardiol. *73*:1019, 1994.
22. Lee, M. S., Evans, S. J. L., Blumberg, S., et al.: Echocardiographically guided electrophysiologic testing in pregnancy. J. Am. Soc. Echocardiogr. *7*:182, 1994.
23. Chu, E., Fitzpatrick, A. P., Chin, M. C., et al.: Radiofrequency catheter ablation guided by intracardiac echocardiography. Circulation *89*:1301, 1994.
24. Thomas, M. R., Monaghan, M. J., Smyth, D. W., et al.: Comparative value of transthoracic and transesophageal echocardiography before balloon dilatation of the mitral valve. Br. Heart J. *68*:493, 1992.
25. Boutin, C., Dyck, J., Benson, L., et al.: Balloon atrial septostomy under transesophageal echocardiographic guidance. Pediatr. Cardiol. *13*:175, 1992.
26. VanDerVelde, M. E., Sanders, S. P., Keane, J. F., et al.: Transesophageal echocardiographic guidance of transcatheter ventricular septal defect closure. J. Am. Coll. Cardiol. *23*:1660, 1994.
27. Nissen, S. E., Grines, C. L., Gurley, J. C., et al.: Application of a new phased-array ultrasound imaging catheter in the assessment of vascular dimensions. Circulation *81*:660, 1990.
28. Pandian, N. G.: Intravascular and intracardiac ultrasound imaging. Circulation *80*:1091, 1989.
29. Chen, C., Guerrero, J. L., dePrada, J. A. V., et al.: Intracardiac ultrasound measurement of volumes and ejection fraction in normal, infarcted, and aneurysmal left ventricles using a 10-MHz ultrasound catheter. Circulation *90*:1481, 1994.
30. Chu, E., Kalman, J. M., Kwasman, M. A., et al.: Intracardiac echocardiography during radiofrequency catheter ablation of cardiac arrhythmias in humans. J. Am. Coll. Cardiol. *24*:1268, 1994.
31. Smith, M. D., Elion, J. L., McClure, R. R., et al.: Left heart opacification with peripheral venous injection of a new saccharide echo contrast agent in dogs. J. Am. Coll. Cardiol. *13*:1622, 1989.
32. Klein, A. L., Bailey, A. S., Moura, A., et al.: Reliability of echocardiographic measurements of myocardial perfusion using commercially produced sonicated serum albumin (Albunex). J. Am. Coll. Cardiol. *22*:1983, 1993.
33. Goldberg, B. B., Liu, J.-B., and Forsberg, F.: Ultrasound contrast agents: A review. Ultrasound Med. Biol. *20*:319, 1994.
34. Porter, T. R., Xie, F., Kricsfeld, A., et al.: Improved endocardial border resolution during dobutamine stress echocardiography with intravenous sonicated dextrose albumin. J. Am. Coll. Cardiol. *23*:1440, 1994.
35. Terasawa, A., Miyatake, K., Nakatani, S., et al.: Enhancement of Doppler flow signals in the left heart chambers by intravenous injection of sonicated albumin. J. Am. Coll. Cardiol. *21*:737, 1993.
36. Crouse, L. J., Cheirif, J., Hanly, D. E., et al.: Opacification and border delineation improvement in patients with suboptimal endocardial border definition in routine echocardiography. J. Am. Coll. Cardiol. *22*:1494, 1993.
37. Von Bibra, H., Becher, H., Firschke, C., et al.: Enhancement of mitral regurgitation and normal left atrial color Doppler flow signals with peripheral venous injection of a saccharide-based contrast agent. J. Am. Coll. Cardiol. *22*:521, 1993.

38. Martin, G. R., and Ruckman, R. N.: Fetal echocardiography: A large clinical experience and follow-up. J. Am. Soc. Echocardiogr 3:4, 1990.
39. Roberson, D. A., and Silverman, N. H.: Ebstein's anomaly: Echocardiographic and clinical features in the fetus and neonate. J. Am. Coll. Cardiol. 14:1300, 1989.
40. Sapin, P. M., Schroder, K. M., Gopal, A. S., et al.: Comparison of two- and three-dimensional echocardiography with cineventriculography for measurement of left ventricular volume in patients. J. Am. Coll. Cardiol. 24:1054, 1994.
41. Jiang, L., Vazquez de Prada, A., Handschumacher, M. D., et al.: Quantitative three-dimensional reconstruction of aneurysmal left ventricle. In vitro and in vivo validation. Circulation 91:222, 1995.
42. Handschumacher, M. D., Lethord, J.-P., Siu, S. C., et al.: A new integrated system for three-dimensional echocardiographic reconstruction: Development and validation for ventricular volume with application in human subjects. J. Am. Coll. Cardiol. 21:743, 1993.
43. Kupferwasser, I., Mohr-Kahaly, S., Erbel, R., et al.: Three-dimensional imaging of cardiac mass lesions by transesophageal echocardiographic computed tomography. J. Am. Soc. Endocardiogr. 7:561, 1994.
44. Roelandt, J. R. T. C., tenCate, F. J., Fletter, W. B., et al.: Ultrasonic dynamic three-dimensional visualization of the heart with a multiplane transesophageal imaging transducer. J. Am. Soc. Echocardiogr. 7:217, 1994.
45. Wang, X.-F., Li, Z.-A., Cheng, T. O., et al.: Clinical application of three-dimensional transesophageal echocardiography. Am. Heart J. 128:380, 1994.
46. Stewart, H. D., Stewart, H. F., Moore, R. M., and Garry, J.: Compilation of reported biological effects data and ultrasound exposure levels. J. Clin. Ultrasound 13:167, 1985.

EXAMINATION OF THE NORMAL HEART

47. Henry, W. L., DeMaria, A., Gramiak, R., et al.: Report of the American Society of Echocardiography Nomenclature and Standards in Two-Dimensional Echocardiography. Circulation 62:212, 1980.
48. Feigenbaum, H.: Current status of M-mode echocardiography. A.C.C. Current J. Review 3:58, 1994.
49. Huwez, F. U., Houston, A. B., Watson, J., et al.: Age and body surface area related normal upper and lower limits of M-mode echocardiographic measurements and left ventricular volume and mass from infancy to early adulthood. Br. Heart J. 72:276, 1994.
50. Kuecherer, H. F., Kusumoto, F., Muhiudeen, I. A., et al.: Pulmonary venous flow patterns by transesophageal pulsed Doppler echocardiography: Relation to parameters of left ventricular systolic and diastolic function. Am. Heart J. 122:1683, 1991.
51. Rossvoll, O., and Hatle, L. K.: Pulmonary venous flow velocities recorded by transthoracic Doppler ultrasound: Relation to left ventricular diastolic pressures. J. Am. Coll. Cardiol. 21:1687, 1993.

EVALUATION OF CARDIAC PERFORMANCE

52. Feigenbaum, H., Popp, R. L., Wolfe, S. B., et al.: Ultrasound measurements of the left ventricle: A correlative study with angiography. Arch. Intern. Med. 129:461, 1972.
53. Teichholz, L. E., Kreulen, T., Herman, M. V., et al.: Problems in echocardiographic volume determinations: Echocardiographic-angiographic correlations in the presence or absence of asynergy. Am. J. Cardiol. 37:7, 1976.
54. Quinones, M. A., Gaasch, W. H., and Alexander, J. K.: Echocardiographic assessment of left ventricular function: With special reference to normalized velocities. Circulation 50:42, 1974.
55. Feigenbaum, H.: Echocardiographic examination of the left ventricle. Circulation 51:1, 1975.
56. Ahmadpour, H., Shah, A. H., Allen, J. W., et al.: Mitral E point septal separation: A reliable index of left ventricular performance in coronary artery disease. Am. Heart J. 106:21, 1983.
57. Schiller, N. B., Shah, P. M., Crawford, M., et al.: Recommendations for qualitation of the left ventricle by two-dimensional echocardiography. J. Am. Soc. Echocardiogr. 5:362, 1989.
58. Ryan, T., Petrovic, O., Armstrong, W. F., et al.: Quantitative two-dimensional echocardiography assessment of patients undergoing left ventricular aneurysmectomy. Am. Heart J. 111:714, 1986.
59. Wong, M., Bruce, S., Joseph, D., et al.: Estimating left ventricular ejection fraction from two-dimensional echocardiograms: Visual and computer-processed interpretations. Echocardiography 8:1, 1991.
60. Waggoner, A. D., Miller, J. G., and Perez, J. E.: Two-dimensional echocardiographic automatic boundary detection for evaluation of left ventricular function in unselected adult patients. J. Am. Soc. Echocardiogr. 7:459, 1994.
61. Yvorchuk, K. J., Davies, R. A., and Chang, K.-L.: Measurement of left ventricular ejection fraction by acoustic quantification and comparison with radionuclide angiography. Am. J. Cardiol. 74:1052, 1994.
62. Katz, W. E., Gasior, T. A., and Reddy, S. C. B.: Utility and limitations of biplane transesophageal echocardiographic automated border detection for estimation of left ventricular stroke volume and cardiac output. Am. Heart J. 128:389, 1994.
63. Gardin, J. M.: Doppler measurements of aortic blood flow velocity and acceleration: Load-independent indexes of left ventricular performance? Am. J. Cardiol. 64:935, 1989.
64. Chen, C., Rodriguez, L., Lethord, J.-P., et al.: Continuous wave Doppler echocardiography for non-invasive assessment of left ventricular dP/dt and relaxation time constant from mitral regurgitant spectra in patients. J. Am. Coll. Cardiol. 23:970, 1994.
65. Kawai, H., Yokota, Y., and Yokoyama, M.: Noninvasive evaluation of contractile state by left ventricular dP/dtmax divided by end-diastolic volume using continuous-wave Doppler and M-mode echocardiography. Clin. Cardiol. 17:662, 1994.
66. Pandian, N. G., Nanda, N. C., Schwartz, S. L., et al.: Three-dimensional and four-dimensional transesophageal echocardiographic imaging of the heart and aorta in humans using a computed tomographic imaging probe. Echocardiography 9:677, 1992.
67. Taylor, R., and Waggoner, A. D.: Doppler assessment of left ventricular diastolic function. A review. J. Am. Soc. Echocardiogr. 5:603, 1992.
68. Thomas, J. D., and Weyman, A. E.: Echocardiographic Doppler evaluation of left ventricular diastolic function. Physics and physiology. Circulation 84:977, 1992.
69. Iwase, M., Nagata, K., Izawa, H., et al.: Age-related changes in left and right ventricular filling velocity profiles and their relationship in normal subjects. Am. Heart J. 126:419, 1993.
70. Pipilis, A., Meyer, T. E., Ormerdo, O., et al.: Early and late changes in left ventricular filling after acute myocardial infarction and the effect of infarct size. Am. J. Cardiol. 70:1397, 1992.
71. Ohno, M., Cheng, C.-P., and Little, W. C.: Mechanism of altered patterns of left ventricular filling during the development of congestive heart failure. Circulation 89:2241, 1994.
72. Oh, J. K., Ding, Z. P., Gersh, B. J., et al.: Restrictive left ventricular diastolic filling identifies patients with heart failure after acute myocardial infarction. J. Am. Soc. Echocardiogr. 5:497, 1992.
73. Thomas, J. D., Flachskampf, F. A., Chen, C., et al.: Isovolumic relaxation time varies predictably with its time constant and aortic and left atrial pressures: Implications for the noninvasive evaluation of ventricular relaxation. Am. Heart J. 124:1305, 1992.
74. Hecht, H. S., DeBord, L., Sotomayor, N., et al.: Truly silent ischemia and the relationship of chest pain and ST segment changes to the amount of ischemic myocardium: Evaluation of supine bicycle stress echocardiography. J. Am. Coll. Cardiol. 23:369, 1994.
75. Presti, C. F., Armstrong, W. F., and Feigenbaum, H.: Comparison of echocardiography at peak exercise and after bicycle exercise in evaluation of patients with known or suspected coronary artery disease. J. Am. Soc. Echocardiogr. 1:119, 1988.
76. Williams, M. J., Marwick, T. H., O'Gorman, D., et al.: Comparison of exercise echocardiography with an exercise score to diagnose coronary artery disease in women. Am. J. Cardiol. 74:435, 1994.
77. Iliceto, S., Sorino, M., D'Ambrosio, G., et al.: Detection of coronary artery disease by two-dimensional echocardiography and transesophageal atrial pacing. J. Am. Coll. Cardiol. 5:1188, 1985.
78. Feigenbaum, H.: Digital recording, display, and storage of echocardiograms. J. Am. Soc. Echocardiogr. 1:378, 1988.
79. Tischler, M. D., Battle, R. W., Saha, M., et al.: Observations suggesting a high incidence of exercise-induced severe mitral regurgitation in patients with mild rheumatic mitral valve disease at rest. J. Am. Coll. Cardiol. 25:128, 1995.
80. Otto, C. M., Pearlman, A. S., Kraft, C. D., et al.: Physiologic changes with maximal exercise in asymptomatic valvular aortic stenosis assessed by Doppler echocardiography. J. Am. Coll. Cardiol. 20:1160, 1992.
81. Kaplan, J. D., Foster, E., Redberg, R. F., et al.: Exercise Doppler echocardiography identifies abnormal hemodynamics in adults with congenital heart disease. Am. Heart J. 127:1572, 1994.
82. Feigenbaum, H., Popp, R. L., Chip, J. N., et al.: Left ventricular wall thickness measured by ultrasound. Arch. Intern. Med. 121:391, 1969.
83. Devereux, R. B., Alonso, D. R., Lutas, E. M., et al.: Echocardiographic assessment of left ventricular hypertrophy: Comparison to necropsy findings. Am. J. Cardiol. 57:450, 1986.
84. Byrd, B. F., Finkbeiner, W., Bouchard, A., et al.: Accuracy and reproducibility of clinically acquired two-dimensional echocardiographic mass measurements. Am. Heart J. 118:133, 1989.
85. Roman, M. J., Devereux, R. B., and Cody, R. J.: Ability of left ventricular stress-shortening relations, end-systolic stress/volume ratio and indirect indexes to detect severe contractile failure in ischemic or idiopathic dilated cardiomyopathy. Am. J. Cardiol. 64:1338, 1989.
86. Segar, D. S., Moran, M., Ryan, T., et al.: End-systolic regional wall stress-length and stress-shortening relations in an experimental model of normal, ischemic and reperfused myocardium. J. Am. Coll. Cardiol. 17:1651, 1991.
87. Goldberg, S. J.: Analysis and interpretation of thickening and thinning phases of left ventricular wall dynamics. Ultrasound Med. Biol. 10:797, 1984.
88. Corya, B. C., Rasmussen, S., Feigenbaum, H., et al.: Systolic thickening and thinning of the septum and posterior wall in patients with coronary artery disease, congestive cardiomyopathy, and atrial septal defect. Circulation 55:109, 1977.
89. Feigenbaum, H.: Estimation of left atrial size using ultrasound. Am. Heart J. 78:43, 1969.
90. Kircher, B., Abbott, J. A., Pau, S., et al.: Left atrial volume determination by biplane two-dimensional echocardiography: Validation by cine computed tomography. Am. Heart J. 121:864, 1991.
91. Lemire, F., Tajik, A. J., and Hagler, D. J.: Asymmetric left atrial enlargement: An echocardiographic observation. Chest 59:779, 1976.
92. Gehl, L. G., Mintz, G. S., Kotler, M. N., and Segal, B. L.: Left atrial volume overload in mitral regurgitation: A two-dimensional echocardiographic study. Am. J. Cardiol. 49:33, 1982.

93. Hiraishi, S., DiSessa, T. G., Jarmakani, J. M., et al.: Two-dimensional echocardiographic assessment of left atrial size in children. Am. J. Cardiol. *52*:1249, 1983.
94. Mugge, A., Kuhn, H., Nikutta, P., et al.: Assessment of left atrial appendage function by biplane transesophageal echocardiography in patients with nonrheumatic atrial fibrillation: Identification of a subgroup of patients at increased embolic risk. J. Am. Coll. Cardiol. *23*:599, 1994.
95. Salka, S., Saeian, K., and Sagar, K. B.: Cerebral thromboembolization after cardioversion of atrial fibrillation in patients without transesophageal echocardiographic findings of left atrial thrombus. Am. Heart J. *126*:722, 1993.
96. Gibson, T. C., Miller, S. W., Aretz, T., et al.: Method for estimating right ventricular volume by planes applicable to cross-sectional echocardiography. Correlation with angiographic formulas. Am. J. Cardiol. *55*:1584, 1985.
97. Popp, R. L., Wolfe, S. B., Hirata, T., et al.: Estimation of right and left ventricular size by ultrasound. A study of the echoes from the interventricular septum. Am. J. Cardiol. *24*:523, 1969.
98. Baker, B. J., Scovil, J. A., Kane, J. J., et al.: Echocardiographic detection of right ventricular hypertrophy. Am. Heart J. *105*:611, 1983.
99. King, M. E., Braun, H., Goldblatt, A., et al.: Interventricular septal configuration as a predictor of right ventricular systolic hypertension in children: A cross-sectional echocardiographic study. Circulation *68*:68, 1983.
100. Ryan, T., Petrovic, O., Dillon, J. C., et al.: An echocardiographic index for separation of right ventricular volume and pressure overload. J. Am. Coll. Cardiol. *5*:918, 1985.
101. Cheriex, E. C., Steeram, N., Eussen, Y. F. J. M., et al.: Cross-sectional Doppler echocardiography as the initial technique for the diagnosis of acute pulmonary embolism. Br. Heart J. *72*:52, 1994.
102. Robson, S. C., Murray, A., Peart, I., et al.: Reproducibility of cardiac output measurement by cross-sectional and Doppler echocardiography. Br. Heart J. *59*:680, 1988.
103. Bouchard, A., Blumlein, S., Schiller, N. B., et al.: Measurement of left ventricular stroke volume using continuous wave Doppler echocardiography of the ascending aorta and M-mode echocardiography of the aortic valve. J. Am. Coll. Cardiol. *9*:75, 1987.
104. Sahn, D. J.: Determination of cardiac output by echocardiographic Doppler methods: Relative accuracy of various sites for measurement. J. Am. Coll. Cardiol. *6*:663, 1985.
105. Moulinier, L., Venet, T., Schiller, N. B., et al.: Measurement of aortic blood flow by Doppler echocardiography: Day to day variability in normal subjects and applicability in clinical research. J. Am. Coll. Cardiol. *17*:1326, 1991.
106. Ascah, K. J., Stewart, W. J., Gillam, L. D., et al.: Calculation of transmitral flow by Doppler echocardiography: A comparison of methods in a canine model. Am. Heart J. *117*:402, 1989.
107. Shimamoto, H., Koto, H., Kawazoe, K., et al.: Transesophageal Doppler echocardiographic measurement of cardiac output by the mitral annulus method. Br. Heart J. *68*:510, 1992.
108. Meijboom, E. J., Horowitz, S., Valdes-Cruz, L. M., et al.: A Doppler echocardiographic method for calculating volume flow across the tricuspid valve: Correlative laboratory and clinical studies. Circulation *71*:551, 1985.
109. Valdes-Cruz, L. M., Horowitz, S., Goldberg, S. J., et al.: The mitral valve orifice method for noninvasive two-dimensional echo Doppler determinations of cardiac output. Circulation *67*:872, 1983.
110. Miller, W. E., Richards, K. L., and Crawford, M. H.: Accuracy of mitral Doppler echocardiographic output determinations in adults. Am. Heart J., *119*:620, 1990.
111. Lloyd, T. R., and Shirazi, F.: Nongeometric Doppler stroke volume determination is limited by aortic size. Am. J. Cardiol. *66*:883, 1990.
112. Nishimuta, R. A., Callahan, M. J., Schaff, H. V., et al.: Non-invasive measurement of cardiac output by continuous-wave Doppler echocardiography: Initial experience and review of the literature. Mayo Clin. Proc. *59*:484, 1984.
113. Ihlen, H., Myhre, E., Amlie, J. P., et al.: Changes in left ventricular stroke volume measured by Doppler echocardiography. Br. Heart J. *54*:378, 1985.
114. Gorcsan, J., III, Ball, D. P., and Hattler, B. G.: Intraoperative determination of cardiac output by transesophageal continuous wave Doppler. Am. Heart J. *123*:171, 1992.
115. Goldberg, S. J., and Allen, H. D.: Quantitative assessment by Doppler echocardiography of pulmonary or aortic regurgitation. Am. J. Cardiol. *56*:131, 1985.
116. Jenni, R., Ritter, M., Vieli, A., et al.: Determination of the ratio of pulmonary blood flow to systemic blood flow by derivation of amplitude weighted mean velocity from continuous wave Doppler spectra. Br. Heart J. *61*:167, 1989.
117. Jenni, R., Ritter, M., Vieli, A., et al.: Determination of the ratio of pulmonary blood flow to systemic blood flow by derivation of amplitude weighted mean velocity from continuous wave Doppler spectra. Br. Heart J. *61*:167, 1989.
118. Meijboom, E. J., Rijsterborgh, H., Bot, H., et al.: Limits of reproducibility of blood flow measurements by Doppler echocardiography. Am. J. Cardiol. *59*:133, 1987.
119. Stamm, R. B., and Martin, R. P.: Quantification of pressure gradients across stenotic valves by Doppler ultrasound. J. Am. Coll. Cardiol. *2*:707, 1983.
120. Hatle, L., Brubakk, A., Tromsdal, A., et al.: Noninvasive assessment of pressure drop in mitral stenosis by Doppler ultrasound. Br. Heart J. *40*:131, 1978.
121. Yock, P. G., and Popp, R. L.: Non-invasive estimation of right ventricular systolic pressure by Doppler ultrasound in patients with tricuspid regurgitation. Circulation *70*:657, 1984.
122. Silbert, D. R., Brunson, S. C., Schiff, R., and Diamant, S.: Determination of right ventricular pressure in the presence of a ventricular septal defect using continuous wave Doppler ultrasound. J. Am. Coll. Cardiol. *8*:379, 1986.
123. Marx, G. R., Allen, H. D., and Goldberg, S. J.: Doppler echocardiographic estimation of systolic pulmonary artery pressure in patients with aortic-pulmonary shunts. J. Am. Coll. Cardiol. *7*:880, 1986.
124. Isobe, M., Yazaki, Y., Takaku, F., et al.: Prediction of pulmonary arterial pressure in adults by pulsed Doppler echocardiography. Am. J. Cardiol. *57*:316, 1986.
125. Taylor, R.: Evaluation of the continuity equation in the Doppler echocardiographic assessment of the severity of valvular aortic stenosis. J. Am. Soc. Echocardiogr. *3*:326, 1990.
126. Konecke, L. L., Feigenbaum, H., Chang, S.: Abnormal mitral valve motion in patients with elevated left ventricular diastolic pressures. Circulation *47*:989, 1973.
127. Otsuji, Y., Toda, H., Ishigami, T., et al.: Mitral regurgitation during B bump of the mitral valve studied Doppler echocardiography. Am. J. Cardiol. *67*:778, 1991.
128. Botvinick, E. H., Schiller, N. B., Wickramasekaran, R., et al.: Echocardiographic demonstration of early mitral valve closure in severe aortic insufficiency. Its clinical implications. Circulation *51*:836, 1975.
129. Sabbah, H. N., and Stein, P. D.: Mechanism of early systolic closure of the aortic valve in discrete membranous subaortic stenosis. Circulation *65*:399, 1982.
130. Nathan, M. P. R., Arora, R., and Rubenstein, H.: Mid-diastolic aortic valve opening in bacterial endocarditis of aortic valve. Clin. Cardiol. *5*:294, 1982.
131. Weyman, A. E., Dillon, J. C., Feigenbaum, H., et al.: Echocardiographic patterns of pulmonic valve motion in pulmonic stenosis. Am. J. Cardiol. *34*:644, 1974.
132. Wann, L. S., Weyman, A. E., Dillon, J. C., et al.: Premature pulmonary valve opening. Circulation *55*:128, 1977.
133. Weyman, A. E., Dillon, J. C., Feigenbaum, H., et al.: Echocardiographic patterns of pulmonary valve motion with pulmonary hypertension. Circulation *50*:905, 1974.
134. Turkevich, D., Groves, B.M., Micco, A., et al.: Early partial systolic closure of the pulmonic valve relates to severity of pulmonary hypertension. Am. Heart J. *115*:409, 1988.
135. Stevenson, J. G.: Comparison of several noninvasive methods for estimation of pulmonary artery pressure. J. Am. Soc. Echocardiogr. *2*:157, 1989.
136. Moreno, F. L. L., Hagan, A. D., Holman, J. R., et al.: Evaluation of size and dynamics of the inferior vena cava as an index of right-sided cardiac function. Am. J. Cardiol. *53*:579, 1984.
137. Kircher, B. J., Himelman, R. B., Schiller, N. B.: Non-invasive estimation of right atrial pressure from the inspiratory collapse of the inferior vena cava. Am. J. Cardiol. *66*:493, 1990.

ACQUIRED VALVULAR HEART DISEASE

138. Edler, I.: Ultrasound cardiogram in mitral valve disease. Acta Chir. Scand. *111*:230, 1956.
139. Wann, L. S., Weyman, A. E., Dillon, J. C., et al.: Determination of mitral valve area by cross-sectional echocardiography. Ann. Intern. Med. *88*:337, 1978.
140. Duchak, J. M., Jr., Chang, S., and Feigenbaum, H.: The posterior mitral valve echo and the echocardiographic diagnosis of mitral stenosis. Am. J. Cardiol. *29*:628, 1972.
141. Riggs, T. W., Lapin, G. D., Paul, M. H., et al.: Measurement of mitral valve orifice area in infants and children by two-dimensional echocardiography. J. Am. Coll Cardiol. *1*:873, 1983.
142. Hatle, L., Brubakk, A., Tromsdal, A., et al.: Noninvasive assessment of pressure drop in mitral stenosis by Doppler ultrasound. Br. Heart J. *40*:131, 1978.
143. Smith, M. D., Handshoe, R., Handshoe, S., et al.: Comparative accuracy of two-dimensional echocardiography and Doppler pressure half-time methods in assessing severity of mitral stenosis in patients with and without prior commissurotomy. Circulation *73*:100, 1986.
144. Loyd, D., Ask, P., and Wranne, B.: Pressure half-time does not always predict mitral valve area correctly. J. Am. Soc. Echocardiogr. *1*:313, 1988.
145. Thomas, J. D., Wilkins, G. T., Choong, C. Y. P., et al.: Inaccuracy of mitral pressure half-time immediately after percutaneous mitral valvotomy. Circulation *78*:980, 1988.
146. Yoneda, Y., Suwa, M., Hanada, H., et al.: Noninvasive detection of left ventricular diastolic dysfunction using M-mode echocardiography to assess left ventricular posterior wall kinetics in hypertrophic cardiomyopathy. Am. J. Cardiol. *70*:1583, 1992.
147. Nishimura, R. A., Rihal, C. S., Tajik, A. J., et al.: Accurate measurement of the transmitral gradient in patient with mitral stenosis: A simultaneous catheterization and Doppler echocardiographic study. J. Am. Coll. Cardiol. *24*:152, 1994.
148. Fredman, C. S., Pearson, A. C., Labovitz, A. J., et al.: Comparison of hemodynamic pressure half-time method and Gorlin formula with Doppler and echocardiographic determination of mitral valve area in

patients with combined mitral stenosis and regurgitation. Am. Heart J. *119*:121, 1990.
149. Abascal, V. M., Wilkins, G. T., O'Shea, J. P., et al.: Prediction of successful outcome in 130 patients undergoing percutaneous balloon mitral valvotomy. Circulation *82*:448, 1990.
150. Chen, C., Wang, X., Wang, Y., et al.: Value of two-dimensional echocardiography in selecting patients and balloon sizes for percutaneous balloon mitral valvuloplasty. J. Am. Coll. Cardiol. *14*:1651, 1989.
151. Reid, C. L., Otto, C. M., Davis, K. B., et al.: Influence of mitral valve morphology on mitral balloon commissurotomy: Immediate and six-month results from the NHLBI balloon valvuloplasty register. Am. Heart J. *123*:657, 1992.
152. Zaretskii, V. V., Kuznetsoa, L. M., Bobkov, V. V., et al.: Diagnosis of subvalvular adhesions in mitral stenosis by 2-dimensional echocardiography. Kardiologiia *25*:68, 1985.
153. Patel, A. K., Rowe, G. G., Thomsen, J. H., et al.: Detection and estimation of rheumatic mitral regurgitation in the presence of mitral stenosis by pulsed Doppler echocardiography. Am. J. Cardiol. *51*:986, 1983.
154. Rivera, J. M., Vandervoort, P. M., Morris, E., et al.: Visual assessment of valvular regurgitation: Comparison with quantitative Doppler measurements. J. Am. Soc. Echocardiogr. *7*:480, 1994.
155. Castello, R., Fagan, L., Lenzen, P., et al.: Comparison of transthoracic and transesophageal echocardiography for assessment of left-sided valvular regurgitation. Am. J. Cardiol. *68*:1677, 1991.
156. Spain, M. B., Smith, M. D., Grayburn, P. A., et al.: Quantitative assessment of mitral regurgitation by Doppler color flow imaging: Angiographic and hemodynamic correlations. J. Am. Coll. Cardiol. *13*:585, 1989.
157. Enriquez-Sarano, M., Tajik, A. J., Bailey, K. R., et al.: Color flow imaging compared with quantitative Doppler assessment of severity of mitral regurgitation: Influence of eccentricity of jet and mechanism of regurgitation. J. Am. Coll. Cardiol. *21*:1211, 1993.
158. Appleton, C. P., Hatle, L. K., Nellesen, U., et al.: Flow velocity acceleration in the left ventricle: A useful Doppler echocardiographic sign of hemodynamically significant mitral regurgitation. J. Am. Soc. Echocardiogr. *3*:35, 1990.
159. Utsunomiya, T., Ogawa, T., Doshi, R., et al.: Doppler color flow: "Proximal isovelocity surface area" method for estimating volume flow rate: Effects of orifice shape and machine factors. J. Am. Coll. Cardiol. *17*:1103, 1991.
160. Shiota, T., Jones, M., Teien, D. E., et al.: Evaluation of mitral regurgitation using a digitally determined color Doppler flow convergence "centerline" acceleration method. Circulation *89*:2879, 1994.
161. Grayburn, P. A., Fehske, W., Omran, H., et al.: Multiplane transesophageal echocardiographic assessment of mitral regurgitation by Doppler color flow mapping of the vena contracta. Am. J. Cardiol. *74*:912, 1994.
162. Kamp, O., Huitink, H., vanEenige, M. J., et al.: Value of pulmonary venous flow characteristics in the assessment of severity of native mitral valve regurgitation: An angiographic correlated study. J. Am. Soc. Echocardiogr. *5*:239, 1992.
163. McCully, R. B., Enriquez-Sarano, M., Tajik, A. J., et al.: Overestimation of severity of ischemic/functional mitral regurgitation by color Doppler jet area. Am. J. Cardiol. *74*:790, 1994.
164. Rivera, J. M., Mele, D., Vendervoort, P. M., et al.: Physical factors determining mitral regurgitation jet area. Am. J. Cardiol. *74*:515, 1994.
165. Ascah, K. J., Stewart, W. J., Jiang, L., et al.: A Doppler two-dimensional echocardiographic method for quantitation of mitral regurgitation. Circulation *72*:377, 1985.
166. Tribouilloy, C., Shen, W. F., Slama, M. A., et al.: Non-invasive measurement of the regurgitant fraction by pulsed Doppler echocardiography in isolated pure mitral regurgitation. Br. Heart J. *66*:290, 1991.
167. Burwash, I. G., Blackmore, G. L., and Koilpillai, C. J.: Usefulness of left atrial and left ventricular chamber sizes as predictors of the severity of mitral regurgitation. Am. J. Cardiol. *70*:774, 1992.
168. Shah, P. M.: Echocardiographic diagnosis of mitral valve prolapse. J. Am. Soc. Echocardiogr. *7*:286, 1994.
169. Dillon, J. C., Haine, C. L., Chang, S., et al.: Use of echocardiography in patients with prolapsed mitral valve. Am. J. Cardiol. *43*:503, 1971.
170. DeMaria, A. N., King, J. F., Bogren, H. G., et al.: The variable spectrum of echocardiographic manifestations of the mitral valve prolapse syndrome. Circulation *50*:33, 1974.
171. Sahn, D. J., Wood, J., Allen, H. D., et al.: Echocardiographic spectrum of mitral valve motion in children with and without mitral valve prolapse. The nature of false positive diagnosis. Am. J. Cardiol. *39*:422, 1977.
172. Markiewicz, W., Stoner, J., London, E., et al.: Mitral valve prolapse in one hunderd presumably healthy young females. Circulation *53*:464, 1976.
173. Sahn, D. J., Allen, H. D., Goldberg, S. J., et al.: Mitral valve prolapse in children. A problem defined by real-time cross-sectional echocardiography. Circulation *53*:651, 1976.
174. Morganroth, J., Jones, R. H., Chen, C. C., et al.: Two dimensional echocardiography in mitral, aortic and tricuspid valve prolapse. The clinical problem, cardiac nuclear imaging considerations and a proposed standard for diagnosis. Am. J. Cardiol. *46*:1164, 1980.
175. Krivokapich, J., Child, J. S., Dadourian, B. J., et al.: Reassessment of echocardiographic criteria for diagnosis of mitral valve prolapse. Am. J. Cardiol. *61*:131, 1988.
176. Levine, R. A., Stathogiannis, E., Newell, J. B., et al.: Reconsideration of echocardiographic standards for mitral valve prolapse: Lack of association between leaflet displacement isolated to the apical four chamber view and independent echocardiographic evidence of abnormality. J. Am. Coll. Cardiol. *11*:1010, 1988.
177. Chun, P. K. C., and Sheehan, M. W.: Myxomatous degeneration of mitral valve M-mode and two-dimensional echocardiographic findings. Br. Heart J. *47*:404, 1982.
178. Ballester, M., Presbitero, P., Foale, R., et al.: Prolapse of the mitral valve in secundum atrial septal defect: A functional mechanism. Eur. Heart J. *4*:472, 1983.
179. Avgeropoulou, C. C., Rahko, P. S., and Patel, A. K.: Reliability of M-mode, two-dimensional, and Doppler echocardiography in diagnosing a flail mitral valve leaflet. J. Am. Soc. Echocardiogr. *2*:433, 1988.
180. Ballester, M., Foale, R., Presbitero, P., et al.: Cross-sectional echocardiographic features of ruptured chordae tendineae. Eur. Heart J. *4*:795, 1983.
181. Mintz, G. S., Kotler, M. N., Segal, B. L., et al.: Two-dimensional echocardiographic recognition of ruptured chordae tendineae. Circulation *57*:244, 1978.
182. Pearson, A. C., St. Vrain, J., Mrosek, A., et al.: Color Doppler echocardiographic evaluation of patients with a flail mitral leaflet. J. Am. Coll. Cardiol. *16*:232, 1990.
183. Shyu, K.-G., Lei, M.-H., Hwang, J.-J., et al.: Morphologic characterization and quantitative assessment of mitral regurgitation with ruptured chordae tendineae by transesophageal echocardiography. Am. J. Cardiol. *70*:1152, 1992.
184. Godley, R. W., Wann, L. S., Rogers, E. W., et al.: Incomplete mitral leaflet closure in patients with papillary muscle dysfunction. Circulation *63*:565, 1981.
185. Weyman, A. E., Feigenbaum, H., Dillon, J. C., et al.: Cross-sectional echocardiography in assessing the severity of valvular aortic stenosis. Circulation *52*:828, 1975.
186. Godley, R. W., Green, D., Dillon, J. C., et al.: Reliability of two-dimensional echocardiography in assessing the severity of valvular aortic stenosis. Chest *79*:657, 1981.
187. Tribouilloy, C., Shen, W. F., Peltier, M., et al.: Quantitation of aortic valve area in aortic stenosis with multiplane transesophageal echocardiography: Comparison with monoplane transesophageal approach. Am. Heart J. *128*:526, 1994.
188. Hoffmann, R., Flachskampf, F. A., and Hanrath, P.: Planimetry of orifice area in aortic stenosis using multiplane transesophageal echocardiography. J. Am. Coll. Cardiol. *22*:529, 1993.
189. Currie, P. J., Seward, J. B., Reeder, G. S., et al.: Continuous-wave Doppler echocardiographic assessment of severity of calcific aortic stenosis: A simultaneous Doppler-catheter correlative study in 100 adult patients. Circulation *71*:1162, 1985.
190. Warth, D. C., Stewart, W. J., Block, P. C., et al.: A new method to calculate aortic valve area without left heart catheterization. Circulation *70*:978, 1984.
191. Taylor, R.: Evolution of the continuity equation in the Doppler echocardiographic assessment of the severity of valvular aortic stenosis. J. Am. Soc. Echocardiogr. *3*:326, 1990.
192. Richards, K. L., Cannon, S. R., Miller, J. F., et al.: Calculation of aortic valve area by Doppler echocardiography: A direct application of the continuity equation. Circulation *73*:964, 1986.
193. Danielsen, R., Nordrehaug, J. E., and Vik-Mo, H.: Factors affecting Doppler echocardiographic valve area assessment in aortic stenosis. Am. J. Cardiol. *63*:1107, 1989.
194. Danielsen, R., Nordrehaug, J. E., Strangeland, L., et al.: Limitations in assessing the severity of aortic stenosis by Doppler gradients. Br. Heart J. *59*:551, 1988.
195. Yeager, M., Yock, P. G., and Popp, R. L.: Comparison of Doppler-derived pressure gradient to that determined at cardiac catheterization in adults with aortic valve stenosis: Implications of management. Am. J. Cardiol. *57*:644, 1986.
196. Reichek, N., and Devereux, R. B.: Reliable estimation of peak left ventricular systolic pressure by M-mode echographic-determined end-diastolic relative wall thickness: Identification of severe valvular aortic stenosis in adult patients. Am. Heart J. *103*:202, 1982.
197. Ciobanu, M., Abbasi, A. S., Allen, M., et al.: Pulsed Doppler echocardiography in the diagnosis and estimation of severity of aortic insufficiency. Am. J. Cardiol. *49*:339, 1982.
198. Grayburn, P. A., Smith, M. D., Handshoe, R., et al.: Detection of aortic insufficiency by standard echocardiography, pulsed Doppler echocardiography, and auscultation. Ann. Intern. Med. *104*:599, 1986.
199. Bouchard, A., Yock, P., Schiller, N. B., et al.: Value of color Doppler estimation of regurgitant volume in patients with chronic aortic insufficiency. Am. Heart J. *117*:1099, 1989.
200. Perry, G. J., Helmcke, F., Nanda, N. C., et al.: Evaluation of aortic insufficiency by Doppler color flow mapping. J. Am. Coll. Cardiol. *9*:952, 1987.
201. Samstad, S. O., Hegrenaes, L., Skjaerpe, T., et al.: Half time of the diastolic aortoventricular pressure difference by continuous wave Doppler ultrasound: A measure of the severity of aortic regurgitation? Br. Heart J. *61*:336, 1989.
202. Nishimura, R. A., Vonk, G. D., Rumberger, J. A., et al.: Semiquantitation of aortic regurgitation by different Doppler echocardiographic techniques and comparison with ultrafast computed tomography. Am. Heart J. *124*:995, 1992.
203. Yeung, A. C., Plappert, T., and St. John Sutton, M. G.: Calculation of aortic regurgitation orifice area by Doppler echocardiography: An application of the continuity equation. Br. Heart J. *68*:236, 1992.
204. Marcus, R. H., Neumann, A., Borow, M. K., et al.: Transmitral flow

velocity in symptomatic severe aortic regurgitation: Utility of Doppler for determination of preclosure of the mitral valve. Am. Heart J. *120*:449, 1990.
205. Fioretti, P., Roelandt, J., Sclavo, M., et al.: Postoperative regression of left ventricular dimensions in aortic insufficiency: A long-term echocardiographic study. J. Am. Coll. Cardiol. *5*:856, 1985.
206. Bonow, R. O., Rosing, D. R., Kent, K. M., et al.: Timing of operation for chronic aortic regurgitation. Am. J. Cardiol. *50*:325, 1982.
207. Guyer, D. E., Gillam, L. D., Foale, R. A., et al.: Comparison of the echocardiographic and hemodynamic diagnosis of rheumatic tricuspid stenosis. J. Am. Coll. Cardiol. *3*:1135, 1984.
208. Parris, T. M., Panidis, I. P., Ross, J., et al.: Doppler echocardiographic findings in rheumatic tricuspid stenosis. Am. J. Cardiol. *60*:1414, 1987.
209. Blanchard, D., Diebold, B., Guermonprez, J. L., et al.: Doppler echocardiographic diagnosis and evaluation of tricuspid regurgitation. Arch. Mal. Coeur. *75*:1357, 1982.
210. Mugge, A., Danile, W. G., Herrmann, G., et al.: Quantification of tricuspid regurgitant by Doppler color flow mapping after cardiac transplantation. Am. J. Cardiol. *66*:884, 1990.
211. Ogawa, S., Hayashi, J., Sasaki, H., et al.: Evaluation of combined valvular prolapse syndrome by two-dimensional echocardiography. Circulation *65*:174, 1982.
212. Eckfeldt, J. H., Weir, E. K., and Chesler, E.: Echocardiographic findings in ruptured chordae tendineae of the tricuspid valve. Am. Heart J. *105*:1033, 1983.
213. Forman, M. B., Byrd, B. F., Oates, J. A., et al.: Two-dimensional echocardiography in the diagnosis of carcinoid heart disease. Am. Heart J. *107*:492, 1984.
214. Winslow, T., Redberg, R., and Schiller, N. B.: Transesophageal echocardiography in the diagnosis of flail tricuspid valve. Am. Heart J. *123*:1682, 1992.
215. Yvorchuk, K. J., and Chan, K.-L.: Application of transthoracic and transesophageal echocardiography in the diagnosis and management of infective endocarditis. J. Am. Soc. Echocardiogr. *7*:294, 1994.
216. Dillon, J. C., Feigenbaum, H., Konecke, L. L., et al.: Echocardiographic manifestations of valvular vegetations. Am. Heart J. *86*:698, 1973.
217. Roy, P., Tajik, A. J., Giuliani, E. R., et al.: Spectrum of echocardiographic findings in bacterial endocarditis. Circulation *53*:474, 1976.
218. Gallis, H. A., Johnson, M. L., and Kisslo, J. A.: Two-dimensional echocardiographic assessment of vegetative endocarditis. Circulation *55*:346, 1977.
219. Lowry, R. W., Zoghbi, W. A., Baker, W. B., et al.: Clinical impact of transesophageal echocardiography in the diagnosis and management of infective endocarditis. Am. J. Cardiol. *73*:1089, 1994.
220. Sochowski, R. A., and Chan, K.-L.: Implication of negative results on a monoplane transesophageal echocardiographic study in patients with suspected infective endocarditis. J. Am. Coll. Cardiol. *21*:216, 1993.
221. Blanchard, D. G., Ross, R. S., and Dittrich, H. C.: Non-bacterial thrombotic endocarditis. Assessment by transesophageal echocardiography. Chest *102*:954, 1992.
222. Appelbe, A. F., Olson, D., Mixon, R., et al.: Libman-Sacks endocarditis mimicking intracardiac tumor. Am. J. Cardiol. *68*:817, 1991.
223. Pollak, S. J., and Felner, J. M.: Echocardiographic identification of an aortic valve ring abscess. J. Am. Coll. Cardiol. *7*:1167, 1986.
224. Leung, D. Y. C., Cranney, G. B., Hopkins, A. P., et al.: Role of transesophageal echocardiography in the diagnosis and management of aortic root abscess. Br. Heart J. *72*:175, 1994.
225. Teskey, R. J., Chan, K.-L., and Beanlands, D. S.: Diverticulum of the mitral valve complicating bacterial endocarditis: Diagnosis by transesophageal echocardiography. Am. Heart J. *118*:1063, 1989.
226. Wann, L. S., Pyhel, H. J., Judson, W. E., et al.: Ball variance in a Harken mitral prosthesis. Echocardiographic and phonocardiographic features. Chest *72*:785, 1977.
227. Pfeifer, J., Goldschlager, N., Sweatman, T., et al.: Malfunction of mitral ball valve prosthesis due to thrombus. Am. J. Cardiol. *29*:95, 1972.
229. Clements, S. D., and Perkins, J. V.: Malfunction of a Bjork-Shiley prosthetic heart valve in the mitral position producing an abnormal echocardiographic pattern. J. Clin. Ultrasound *6*:334, 1978.
230. Mehta, A., Kessler, K. M., Tamer, D., et al.: Two-dimensional echographic observations in major detachment of a prosthetic aortic valve. Am. Heart J. *101*:231, 1981.
231. Alam, M., Goldstein, S., and Lakier, J. B.: Echocardiographic changes in the thickness of porcine valves with time. Chest *79*:663, 1981.
232. Bansal, R. C., Morrison, D. L., and Jacobsen, J. G.: Echocardiography of porcine aortic prostheses with flail leaflets due to degeneration and calcification. Am. Heart J. *107*:591, 1984.
233. Burstow, D. J., Nishimura, R. A., Bailey, K. R., et al.: Continuous wave Doppler echocardiographic measurement of prosthetic valve gradients. Circulation *80*:504, 1989.
234. Ryan, T., Armstrong, W. F., Dillon, J. C., et al.: Doppler echocardiographic evaluation of patients with porcine mitral valves. Am. Heart J. *111*:237, 1986.
235. Ferrara, R. P., Labovitz, A. J., Wiens, R. D., et al.: Prosthetic mitral regurgitation detected by Doppler echocardiography. Am. J. Cardiol. *55*:229, 1985.
236. Chambers, J., Monaghan, M., and Jackson, G.: Colour Doppler mapping in the assessment of prosthetic valve regurgitation. Br. Heart J. *62*:1, 1989.
237. Rothbart, R. M., Castriz, J. L., Harding, L. V., et al.: Determination of aortic valve area by two-dimensional and Doppler echocardiography in patients with normal and stenotic bioprosthetic valves. J. Am. Coll. Cardiol. *15*:817, 1990.
238. Weinstein, I. R., Marbarger, J. P., and Perez, J. E.: Ultrasonic assessment of the St. Jude prosthetic valve: M-mode, two-dimensional and Doppler echocardiography. Circulation *68*:897, 1983.
239. Khandheria, B. K., Seward, J. B., Oh, J. K., et al.: Value and limitations of transesophageal echocardiography in assessment of mitral valve prostheses. Circulation *83*:1956, 1991.
240. Daniel, W. G., Mugge, A., Grote, J., et al.: Comparison of transthoracic and transesophageal echocardiography for detection of abnormalities of prosthetic and bioprosthetic valves in the mitral and aortic positions. Am. J. Cardiol. *71*:210, 1993.
241. Gueret, P., Vignon, P., Fournier, P., et al.: Transesophageal echocardiography for the diagnosis and management of nonobstructive thrombosis of mechanical mitral valve prosthesis. Circulation *91*:103, 1995.
242. Taams, M. A., Gussenhoven, E. J., Cahalan, M. K., et al.: Transesophageal Doppler color flow imaging in the detection of native and Bjork-Shiley mitral valve regurgitation. J. Am. Coll. Cardiol. *13*:95, 1989.
243. Alam, M., Rosman, H. S., and Sun, I.: Transesophageal echocardiographic evaluation of St. Jude Medical and bioprosthetic valve endocarditis. Am. Heart J. *123*:236, 1992.
244. Nair, C. K., Thomson, W., Ryschon, K., et al.: Long-term follow-up of patients with echocardiographically detected mitral annular calcium and comparison with age- and sex-matched control subjects. Am. J. Cardiol. *63*:465, 1989.

CONGENITAL HEART DISEASE

245. VanPraagh, R.: Diagnosis of complex congenital heart disease: Morphologic-anatomic method and terminology. Cardiovasc. Intervent. Radiol. *7*:115, 1984.
246. Lipshultz, S. E., Sanders, S. P., Mayer, J. E., et al.: Are routine preoperative cardiac catheterization and angiography necessary before repair of ostium primum atrial septal defect? J. Am. Coll. Cardiol. *11*:373, 1988.
247. Huhta, J. C., Glasow, P., Murphy, D. J., et al.: Surgery without catheterization for congenital heart defects: Management of 100 patients. J. Am. Coll. Cardiol. *9*:823, 1987.
248. Santoro, G., Marino, B., DiCarlo, D., et al.: Echocardiographically guided repair of tetralogy of Fallot. Am. J. Cardiol. *73*:808, 1994.
249. Foale, R., Stefanini, L., Rickards, A., et al.: Left and right ventricular morphology in complex congenital heart disease defined by two dimensional echocardiography. Am. J. Cardiol. *49*:93, 1982.
250. Silverman, N. H.: An ultrasonic approach to the diagnosis of cardiac situs, connections, and malpositions. Cardiol. Clin. *1*:473, 1983.
251. Hagler, D. J., Tajik, A. J., Seward, J. B., et al.: Atrioventricular and ventriculoarterial discordance (corrected transposition of the great arteries). Wide-angle two-dimensional echocardiographic assessment of ventricular morphology. Mayo Clin. Proc. *56*:591, 1981.
252. Lesbre, J. P., Scheuble, C., Kalisa, A., et al.: Echocardiography in the diagnosis of severe aortic valve stenosis in adults. Arch. Mal. Coeur. *76*:1, 1983.
253. Brandenburg, R. O., Jr., Tajik, A. J., Edwards, W. D., et al.: Accuracy of 2-dimensional echocardiographic diagnosis of congenitally bicuspid aortic valve: Echocardiographic-anatomic correlation in 115 patients. Am. J. Cardiol. *51*:1469, 1983.
254. Smallhorn, J., Tommasini, G., Deanfield, J., et al.: Congenital mitral stenosis. Anatomical and functional assessment by echocardiography. Br. Heart J. *45*:527, 1981.
255. Trowitzsch, E., Bano-Rodrigo, A., Burger, B. M., et al.: Two-dimensional echocardiographic findings in double orifice mitral valve. J. Am. Coll. Cardiol. *6*:383, 1985.
256. Weyman, A. E., Hurwitz, R. A., Girod, D. A., et al.: Cross-sectional echocardiographic visualization of the stenotic pulmonary valve. Circulation *56*:769, 1977.
257. Johnson, G. L., Kwan, O. L., Handshoe, S., et al.: Accuracy of combined two-dimensional echocardiography and continuous wave Doppler recordings in the estimation of pressure gradient in right ventricular outlet obstruction. J. Am. Coll. Cardiol. *3*:1013, 1984.
258. Hagler, D. J., Tajik, A. J., Seward, J. B., et al.: Noninvasive assessment of pulmonary valve stenosis, aortic valve stenosis, and coarctation of the aorta in critically ill neonates. Am. J. Cardiol. *57*:369, 1986.
259. Shiina, A., Seward, J. B., Edwards, W. D., et al.: Two-dimensional echocardiographic spectrum of Ebstein's anomaly: Detailed anatomic assessment. J. Am. Coll. Cardiol. *3*:356, 1984.
260. Radford, D. J., Graff, R. F., and Neilson, G. H.: Diagnosis and natural history of Ebstein's anomaly. Br. Heart J. *54*:517, 1985.
261. Milner, S., Meyer, R. A., Venables, A. W., et al.: Mitral and tricuspid valve closure in congenital heart disease. Circulation *53*:513, 1976.
262. Meyer, R. A., and Kaplan, S.: Echocardiography in the diagnosis of hypoplasia of the left or right ventricle in the neonate. Circulation *46*:55, 1972.
263. Lundstrom, N. R.: Ultrasound cardiographic studies of the mitral valve region in young infants with mitral atresia, mitral stenosis, hypoplasia of the left ventricle and cor triatriatum. Circulation *45*:324, 1972.
264. Weyman, A. E., Caldwell, R. L., Hurwitz, R. A., et al.: Cross-sectional echocardiographic characterization of aortic obstruction: I. Supravalvular aortic stenosis and aortic hypoplasia. Circulation *57*:491, 1978.
265. Cabrera, A., Pastor, E., and Lekuona, I.: Congenital aortic atresia with intact ventricular septum and normal left ventricle. Diagnosis by cross-sectional echocardiography. Int. J. Cardiol. *8*:339, 1985.

266. Davis, R. A., Feigenbaum, H., Chang, S., et al.: Echocardiographic manifestations of discrete subaortic stenosis. Am. J. Cardiol. *33*:277, 1974.
267. DiSessa, T. G., Hagan, A. D., Isabel-Jones, J. B., et al.: Two-dimensional echocardiographic evaluation of discrete subaortic stenosis from the apical long axis view. Am. Heart J. *101*:774, 1981.
268. Gnanapragasam, J. P., Houston, A. B., Doig, W. B., et al.: Transesophageal echocardiographic assessment of fixed subaortic obstruction in children. Br. Heart J. *66*:281, 1991.
269. Sreeram, N., Franks, R., and Walsh, K.: Aortic-ventricular tunnel in a neonate: Diagnosis and management based on cross sectional and colour Doppler ultrasonography. Br. Heart J. *65*:161, 1991.
270. Valdes-Cruz, L. M., Jones, M., Scagnelli, S., et al.: Prediction of gradients in fibrous subaortic stenosis by continous wave two-dimensional Doppler echocardiography: Animal studies. J. Am. Coll. Cardiol. *5*:1363, 1985.
271. Weyman, A. E., Dillon, J. C., Feigenbaum, H., et al.: Echocardiographic differentiation of infundibular from valvular pulmonary stenosis. Am. J. Cardiol. *36*:21, 1975.
272. Caldwell, R. L., Weyman, A. G., Hurwitz, R. A., et al.: Right ventricular outflow tract assessment by cross-sectional echocardiography in tetralogy of Fallot. Circulation *59*:395, 1979.
273. Horowitz, M. D., Zager, W., Bilsker, M., et al.: Cor triatriatum in adults. Am. Heart J. *126*:472, 1993.
274. Lengyel, M., Arvay, A., and Biro, V.: Two-dimensional echocardiographic diagnosis of cor triatriatum. *59*:484, 1987.
275. Sullivan, I. D., Robinson, P. J., DeLeval, M., et al.: Membranous supravalvular mitral stenosis: A treatable form of congenital heart disease. J. Am. Coll. Cardiol. *8*:159, 1986.
276. Magherini, A., Azzolina, G., Weichmann, V., et al.: Pulsed Doppler echocardiography for diagnosis of ventricular septal defects. Br. Heart J. *43*:143, 1980.
277. Helmcke, F., deSouza, A., Nanda, N. C., et al.: Two-dimensional and color Doppler assessment of ventricular septal defect of congenital origin. Am. J. Cardiol. *63*:1112, 1989.
278. Sommer, R. J., Golinko, R. J., and Ritter, S. B.: Intracardiac shunting in children with ventricular septal defect: Evaluation with Doppler color flow mapping. J. Am. Coll. Cardiol. *16*:1437, 1990.
279. Sutherland, G. S., Smyllie, J. H., Ogilvie, B. C., et al.: Colour flow imaging in the diagnosis of multiple ventricular septal defects. Br. Heart J. *62*:43, 1989.
280. Sharif, D. S., Huhta, J. C., Maranttz, P., et al.: Two-dimensional echocardiographic determination of ventricular septal defect size: Correlation with autopsy. Am. Heart J. *117*:1333, 1989.
281. Rigby, M. L., Anderson, R. H., Gibson, D., et al.: Two dimensional echocardiographic categorisation of the univentricular heart. Br. Heart J. *46*:603, 1981.
282. Houston, A. B., Lim, M. K., Doig, W. B., et al.: Doppler assessment of the interventricular pressure drop in patients with ventricular septal defects. Br. Heart J. *60*:50, 1988.
283. Shub, C., Dimopoulos, I. N., Seward, J. B., et al.: Sensitivity of two-dimensional echocardiography in the direct visualization of atrial septal defect utilizing the subcostal approach: Experience with 154 patients. J. Am. Coll. Cardiol. *2*:127, 1983.
284. Mehta, R. H., Helmcke, F., Nanda, N. C., et al.: Uses and limitations of transthoracic echocardiography in the assessment of atrial septal defect in the adult. Am. J. Cardiol. *67*:288, 1991.
285. Nasser, F. N., Tajik, A. J., Stewart, J. B., et al.: Diagnosis of sinus venosus atrial septal defect by two-dimensional echocardiography. Mayo Clin. Proc. *56*:568, 1981.
286. Sonoda, M., Wang, Y., Sakamoto, T., et al.: Visualization of sinus venosus-type atrial septal defect by biplane transesophageal echocardiography. J. Am. Soc. Echocardiogr. *7*:179, 1994.
287. Hausmann, D., Daniel, W. G., Mugge, A., et al.: Value of transesophageal color Doppler echocardiography for detection of different types of atrial septal defects in adults. J. Am. Soc. Echocardiogr. *5*:481, 1992.
288. Bartel, T., Muller, S., and Geibel, A.: Preoperative assessment of cor triatriatum in an adult by dynamic three dimensional echocardiography was more informative than transesophageal echocardiography or magnetic resonance imaging. Br. Heart J. *72*:4989, 1994.
289. Vogel, M., and Losch, S.: Dynamic three-dimensional echocardiography with a computed tomography imaging probe: Initial clinical experience with transthoracic application in infants and children with congenital heart defects. Br. Heart J. *71*:462, 1994.
290. Pollick, C., Sullivan, H., Cujec, B., et al.: Doppler color-flow imaging assessment of shunt size in atrial septal defect. Circulation *78*:522, 1988.
291. Weyman, A. E., Wann, L. S., Caldwell, R. L., et al.: Negative contrast echocardiography: A new method for detecting left-to-right shunts. Circulation *59*:498, 1979.
292. VanHare, G. G., and Silverman, N. H.: Contrast two-dimensional echocardiography in congenital heart disease: Techniques, indications and clinical utility. J. Am. Coll. Cardiol. *13*:673, 1989.
293. Konstantinides, S., Kasper, W., Geibel, A., et al.: Detection of left-to-right shunt in atrial septal defect by negative contrast echocardiography: A comparison of transthoracic and transesophageal approach. Am. Heart J. *126*:909, 1993.
294. Goswami, K. C., Shrivastava, S., Saxena, A., et al.: Echocardiographic diagnosis of total anomalous pulmonary venous connection. Am. Heart J. *126*:433, 1993.
295. Romero-Cardenas, A., Vargas-Barron, J., Rylaarsdam, M., et al.: Total anomalous pulmonary venous return: Diagnosis by transesophageal echocardiography. Am. Heart J. *121*:1831, 1991.
296. Barron, J. V., Sahn, D. J., Valdes-Cruz, L. M., et al.: Two-dimensional echocardiographic features of left ventricular septal aneurysm paradoxically bulging into the left ventricular outflow tract. Am. Heart J. *104*:156, 1982.
297. Schneider, B., Hofmann, T., Meinertz, T., et al.: Diagnostic value of transesophageal echocardiography in atrial septal aneurysm. Int. J. Cardiac Imaging *8*:143, 1992.
298. Wolf, W. J., Casta, A., and Sapire, D. W.: Atrial septal aneurysms in infants and children. Am. Heart J. *113*:1149, 1987.
299. Belkin, R. N., Waugh, R. A., and Kisslo, J.: Interatrial shunting in atrial septal aneurysm. Am. J. Cardiol. *57*:310, 1986.
300. Belkin, R. N., Pollack, B. D., Ruggiero, M. L., et al.: Comparison of transesophageal and transthoracic echocardiography with contrast and color flow Doppler in the detection of patent foramen ovale. Am. Heart J. *128*:520, 1994.
301. Stoddard, M. D., Keedy, D. L., Dawkins, P. R., et al.: The cough test is superior to the Valsalva maneuver, the delineation of right-to-left shunting through a patent foramen ovale during contrast transesophageal echocardiography. Am. Heart J. *125*:185, 1993.
302. Stollberger, C., Schneider, B., Abzieher, F., et al.: Diagnosis of patent foramen ovale by transesophageal contrast echocardiography. Am. J. Cardiol. *71*:604, 1993.
303. Beppu, S., Nimura, Y., Nagata, S., et al.: Diagnosis of endocardial cushion defect with cross-sectional and M-mode scanning of echocardiography. Differentiation from secundum atrial septal defect. Br. Heart J. *38*:911, 1976.
304. Beppu, S., Nimura, Y., Saka, H., et al.: Mitral cleft in ostium primum atrial septal defect assessed by cross-sectional echocardiography. Circulation *62*:1099, 1980.
305. Rice, M. J., Seward, J. B., Edwards, W. D., et al.: Straddling atrioventricular valve: Two-dimensional echocardiographic diagnosis, classification and surgical implications. Am. J. Cardiol. *55*:505, 1985.
306. Milne, M. J., Sung, R. Y. T., Fok, T. F., et al.: Doppler echocardiographic assessment of shunting via the ductus arteriosus in newborn infants. Am. J. Cardiol. *64*:102, 1989.
307. Liao, P.-K., Su, W.-J., and Hung, J.-S.: Doppler echocardiographic flow characteristics of isolated patent ductus arteriosus: Better delineation by Doppler color flow mapping. J. Am. Coll. Cardiol. *12*:1285, 1988.
308. Vogt, J., Rupprath, G., Grimm, T., et al.: Qualitative and quantitative evaluation of supravalvular aortic stenosis by cross-sectional echocardiography. Pediatr. Cardiol. *3*:13, 1982.
309. Snider, A. R., and Silverman, N. H.: Suprasternal notch echocardiography: A two-dimensional technique for evaluating congenital heart disease. Circulation *63*:165, 1981.
310. Rao, P. S., and Carey, P.: Doppler ultrasound in the prediction of pressure gradients across aortic coarctation. Am. Heart. J. *118*:299, 1989.
311. Simpson, I. A., Sahn, D. J., Valdes-Cruz, L. M., et al.: Color Doppler flow mapping in patients with coarctation of the aorta: New observations and improved evaluation with color flow diameter and proximal acceleration as predictors of severity. Circulation *77*:736, 1988.
312. Hagler, D. J., Tajik, A. J., Seward, J. B., et al.: Double-outlet right ventricle: Wide-angle two dimensional echocardiographic observations. Circulation *63*:419, 1981.
313. Daskalopoulos, D. A., Edwards, W. D., Driscoll, D. J., et al.: Correlation of two-dimensional echocardiographic and autopsy findings in complete transposition of the great arteries. J. Am. Coll. Cardiol. *2*:1151, 1983.
314. Marin-Garcia, J., and Tonkin, I. L. D.: Two-dimensional echocardiographic evaluation of persistent truncus arteriosus. Am. J. Cardiol. *50*:1376, 1982.
315. Marino, B., DeSimone, G., Pasquini, L., et al.: Complete transposition of the great arteries: Visualization of left and right outflow tract obstruction by oblique subcostal two-dimensional echocardiography. Am. J. Cardiol. *55*:1140, 1985.
316. Sahn, D. J., Terry, R., O'Rourke, R., et al.: Multiple crystal cross-sectional echocardiography in the diagnosis of cyanotic congenital heart disease. Circulation *50*:230, 1974.
317. Meissner, M. D., Panidis, I. P., Eshaghpour, E., et al.: Corrected transposition of the great arteries: Evaluation by two-dimensional and Doppler echocardiography. Am. Heart J. *111*:599, 1986.
318. Chin, A. J., Larsen, R. L., Seliem, M. A., et al.: Noninvasive imaging of intraatrial baffles in infants and children. J. Am. Soc. Echocardiogr. *6*:45, 1993.
319. Arisawa, J., Morimoto, S., Ikezoe, J., et al.: Pulsed Doppler echocardiographic assessment of portal venous flow patterns in patients after the Fontan operation. Br. Heart J. *69*:41, 1993.
320. Nascimento, R., Cunha, D. L., Bastos, P., et al.: Echo-Doppler study of right ventricular filling in asymptomatic patients with Senning operation for transposition of the great arteries. Am. J. Cardiol. *68*:693, 1991.

ISCHEMIC HEART DISEASE

321. Buda, A. J., Zotz, R. J., Pace, D. P., et al.: Comparison of two-dimensional echocardiographic wall motion and wall thickening abnormalities in relation to the myocardium at risk. Am. Heart J. *111*:587, 1986.
322. Heger, J. J., Weyman, A. E., Wann, L. S., et al.: Cross-sectional echocardiographic analysis of the extent of left ventricular asynergy in acute myocardial infarction. Circulation *61*:1113, 1980.

323. Xiao, H. B., Lee, C. H., and Gibson, D. G.: Effect of left bundle branch block on diastolic function in dilated cardiomyopathy. Br. Heart J. *66*:443, 1991.
325. Lehmann, K. G., Lee, F. A., McKenzie, W. B., et al.: Onset of altered interventricular septal motion during cardiac surgery. Circulation *82:* 1325, 1990.
326. Buda, A. J., Lefkowitz, C. A., and Gallagher, K. P.: Augmentation of regional function in nonischemic myocardium during coronary occlusion measured with two-dimensional echocardiography. J. Am. Coll. Cardiol. *16*:175, 1990.
327. Previtali, M., Lanzarini, L., Fetiveau, R., et al.: Comparison of dobutamine stress echocardiography, dipyridamole stress echocardiography and exercise stress testing for diagnosis of coronary artery disease. Am. J. Cardiol. *72*:865, 1993.
328. Beleslin, B. D., Ostojic, M., Stepanovic, J., et al.: Stress echocardiography in the detection of myocardial ischemia. Head-to-head comparison of exercise, dobutamine, and dipyridamole tests. Circulation *90*:1168, 1994.
329. Roger, V. L., Pellikka, P. A., Oh, J. K., et al.: Stress echocardiography: I. Exercise echocardiography: Techniques, implementation, clinical applications, and correlations. Mayo Clin. Proc. *70*:5, 1995.
330. Quinones, M. A., Verani, M. S., Haichin, R. M., et al.: Exercise echocardiography versus 201 T1 single photon emission computed tomography in evaluation of coronary artery disease. Circulation *85*:1026, 1992.
331. Rober, V. L., Pellikka, P. A., Oh, J. K., et al.: Identification of multivessel coronary artery disease by exercise echocardiography. J. Am. Coll. Cardiol. *24*:109, 1994.
332. Hecht, H. S., et al.: Digital supine bicycle stress echocardiography: A new technique for evaluating coronary artery disease. J. Am. Coll. Cardiol. *21*:950, 1993.
333. Ryan, T., Segar, D. S., Sawada, S. G., et al.: Detection of coronary artery disease with upright bicycle exercise echocardiography. J. Am. Soc. Echocardiogr. *6*:186, 1993.
334. Anselmi, M., Golia, G., Marino, P., et al.: Usefulness of transesophageal atrial pacing combined with two-dimensional echocardiography (echo-pacing) in predicting the presence and site of residual jeopardized myocardium after uncomplicated acute myocardial infarction. Am. J. Cardiol. *73*:534, 1994.
335. Pellikka, P. A., Roger, V. L., Oh, J. K., et al.: Stress echocardiography: II. Dobutamine stress echocardiography: Techniques, implementation, clinical applications, and correlations. Mayo Clin. Proc. *70*:16, 1995.
336. Takeishi, Y., Chiba, J., Abe, S., et al.: Adenosine-echocardiography for the detection of coronary artery disease. J. Cardiol. *24*:1, 1994.
337. Picano, E., Parodi, O., Lattanzi, F., et al.: Assessment of anatomic and physiological severity of single-vessel coronary artery lesions by dipyridamole echocardiography. Circulation *89*:753, 1994.
338. Segar, D. S., Brown, S. E., Sawada, S. G., et al.: Dobutamine stress echocardiography: Correlation with coronary lesion severity as determined by quantitative angiography. J. Am. Coll. Cardiol. *19*:1197, 1992.
339. Madu, E. C., Ahmar, W., Arthur, J., et al.: Clinical utility of digital dobutamine stress echocardiography in the noninvasive evaluation of coronary artery disease. Arch. Intern. Med. *154*:1065, 1994.
340. Marangelli, V., Iliceto, S., Piccinni, G., et al.: Detection of coronary artery disease by digital stress echocardiography: Comparison of exercise, transesophageal atrial pacing and dipyridamole echocardiography. J. Am. Coll. Cardiol. *24*:117, 1994.
341. Marcovitz, P. A., and Armstrong, W. F.: Accuracy of dobutamine stress echocardiography in detecting coronary artery disease. Am. J. Cardiol. *69*:1269, 1992.
342. Sawada, S. G., Segar, D. S., Ryan, T., et al.: Echocardiographic detection of coronary artery disease during dobutamine infusion. Circulation *83*:1605, 1991.
343. Camerieri, A., Picano, E., Landi, P., et al.: Prognostic value of dipyridamole echocardiography early after myocardial infarction in elderly patients. J. Am. Coll. Cardiol. *22*:1809, 1993.
344. Takeuchi, M., Araki, M., Nakashima, Y., et al.: The detection of residual ischemia and stenosis in patients with acute myocardial infarction with dobutamine stress echocardiography. J. Am. Soc. Echocardiogr. *7*:242, 1994.
345. Lalka, S. G., Sawada, S. G., Dalsing, M. C., et al.: Dobutamine stress echocardiography as a predictor of cardiac events associated with aortic surgery. J. Vasc. Surg. *15*:831, 1992.
346. Dávila-Román, V. G., Waggoner, A. D., Sicard, G. A., et al.: Dobutamine stress echocardiography predicts surgical outcome in patients with an aortic aneurysm and peripheral vascular disease. J. Am. Coll. Cardiol. *21*:957, 1993.
347. Sawada, S. G., Ryan, T., Conley, M. J., et al.: Prognostic value of a normal exercise echocardiogram. Am. Heart J. *120*:49, 1990.
348. Maseika, P. K., Nadazdin, A., and Oakley, C. M.: Prognostic value of dobutamine echocardiography in patients with high pretest likelihood of coronary artery disease. Am. J. Cardiol. *71*:33, 1993.
349. Krivokapich, J., Child, J. S., Gerber, R. S., et al.: Prognostic usefulness of positive or negative exercise stress echocardiography for predicting coronary events in ensuing twelve months. Am. J. Cardiol. *71*:646, 1993.
350. Akosah, K. O., Porter, T. R., Simon, R., et al.: Ischemia-induced regional wall motion abnormality is improved after coronary angioplasty: Demonstration by dobutamine stress echocardiography. J. Am. Coll. Cardiol. *21*:584, 1993.
351. Hecht, H. S., DeBord, L., Shaw, R., et al.: Usefulness of supine bicycle stress echocardiography for detection of restenosis after percutaneous transluminal coronary angioplasty. Am. J. Cardiol. *71*:293, 1993.
352. Stoddard, M. F., Pearson, A. C., Kern, M. J., et al.: Left ventricular diastolic function: Comparison of pulsed Doppler echocardiographic and hemodynamic indexes in subjects with and without coronary artery disease. J. Am. Coll. Cardiol. *13*:327, 1989.
353. Fujii, J., Yazaki, Y., Sawada, H., et al.: Noninvasive assessment of left and right ventricular filling in myocardial infarction with a two-dimensional Doppler echocardiographic method. J. Am. Coll. Cardiol. *5*:1155, 1985.
354. Erbel, R., Schweizer, P., Meyer, J., et al.: Sensitivity of cross-sectional echocardiography in detection of impaired global and regional left ventricular function: Prospective study. Int. J. Cardiol. *7*:375, 1985.
355. Ren, J-F., Kotler, M. N., Hakki, A-H., et al.: Quantitation of regional left ventricular function by two-dimensional echocardiography in normals and patients with coronary artery disease. Am. Heart J. *110*:552, 1985.
356. Shiina, A., Tajik, A. J., Smith, H. C., et al.: Prognostic significance of regional wall motion abnormality in patients with prior myocardial infarction: A prospective correlative study of two-dimensional echocardiography and angiography. Mayo Clin. Proc. *61*:254, 1986.
357. Van Reet, R. E., Quinones, M. A., Poliner, L. R., et al.: Comparison of two-dimensional echocardiography with gated radionuclide ventriculography in the evaluation of global and regional left ventricular function in acute myocardial infarction. J. Am. Coll. Cardiol. *3*:243, 1984.
358. Iliceto, S., Ricci, A., Sorino, M., et al.: Evaluation of the ejection fraction using two simplified echocardiographic methods in patients with ischemic heart disease and left ventricular asynergy. G. Ital. Cardiol. *15*:142, 1985.
359. Ryan, T., Petrovic, O., Armstrong, W. F., et al.: Quantitative two-dimensional echocardiographic assessment of patients undergoing left ventricular aneurysmectomy. Am. Heart J. *111*:714, 1986.
360. Visser, C. A., Kan, G., Meltzer, R. S., et al.: Assessment of left ventricular aneurysm resectability by two-dimensional echocardiography. Am. J. Cardiol. *56*:857, 1985.
361. Katz, A. S., Harrigan, P., and Parisi, A. F.: The value and promise of echocardiography in acute myocardial infarction and coronary artery disease. Clin. Cardiol. *15*:401, 1992.
362. Matsumoto, M., Watanabe, F., Goto, A., et al.: Left ventricular aneurysm and the prediction of left ventricular enlargement studied by two-dimensional echocardiography: Quantitative assessment of aneurysm size in relation to clinical course. Circulation *72*:280, 1985.
363. Hamilton, K., Ellenbogen, K., Lowe, J. E., et al.: Ultrasound diagnosis of pseudoaneurysm and contiguous ventricular septal defect complicating inferior myocardial infarction. J. Am. Coll. Cardiol. *6*:1160, 1985.
364. Sutherland, G. R., Smyllie, J. H., and Croelandt, J. R. T.: Advantages of colour flow imaging in the diagnosis of left ventricular pseudoaneurysm. Br. Heart J. *61*:59, 1989.
365. Bansal, R. C., Pai, R. G., Hauck, A. J., et al.: Biventricular apical rupture and formation of pseudoaneurysm: Unique flow patterns by Doppler and color flow imaging. Am. Heart J. *124*:497, 1992.
366. Burns, C. A., Paulsen, W., Arrowood, J. A., et al.: Improved identification of posterior left ventricular pseudoaneurysms by transesophageal echocardiography. Am. Heart J. *124*:796, 1992.
367. Deshmukh, H. G., Khosla, S., and Jefferson, K. K.: Direct visualization of left ventricular free wall rupture by transesophageal echocardiography in acute myocardial infarction. Am. Heart J. *126*:475, 1993.
368. Mascarenhas, D. A. N., Benotti, J. R., Daggett, W. M., et al.: Postinfarction septal aneurysm with delayed formation of left-to-right shunt. Am. Heart J. *122*:226, 1991.
369. Stephens, J. D., Giles, M. R., and Banim, S. O.: Ruptured postinfarction ventricular septal aneurysm causing chronic congestive cardiac failure. Detection by two-dimensional echocardiography. Br. Heart J. *46*:216, 1981.
370. Smith, G., Endresen, K., Sivertssen, E., and Semb, G.: Ventricular septal rupture diagnosed by simultaneous cross-sectional echocardiography and Doppler ultrasound. Eur. Heart J. *6*:631, 1985.
371. Panidis, I. P., Mintz, G. S., Goel, I., et al.: Acquired ventricular septal defect after myocardial infarction: Detection by combined two-dimensional and Doppler echocardiography. Am. Heart J. *111*:427, 1986.
372. Maurer, G., Czer, L. S. C., Shah, P. K., et al.: Assessment by Doppler color flow mapping of ventricular septal defect after acute myocardial infarction. Am. J. Cardiol. *64*:668, 1989.
373. Smyllie, J. H., Sutherland, G. R., Geuskins, R., et al.: Doppler color flow mapping in the diagnosis of ventricular septal rupture and acute mitral regurgitation after myocardial infarction. J. Am. Coll. Cardiol. *15*:1449, 1990.
374. Ballal, R. S., Sanyal, R. S., Nanda, N. C., et al.: Usefulness of transesophageal echocardiography in the diagnosis of ventricular septal rupture secondary to acute myocardial infarction. Am. J. Cardiol. *71*:367, 1993.
375. Jugdutt, B. I., Sussex, B. A., Sivaram, C. A., et al.: Right ventricular infarction: Two-dimensional echocardiographic evaluation. Am. Heart J. *107*:505, 1984.
376. Goldberger, J. J., Himelman, R. B., Wolfe, C. L., et al.: Right ventricular infarction: Recognition and assessment of its hemodynamic significance by two-dimensional echocardiography. J. Am. Soc. Echocardiogr. *4*:140, 1991.
377. Doyle, T., Troup, P. J., and Wann, L. S.: Mid-diastolic opening of the

pulmonary valve after right ventricular infarction. J. Am. Coll. Cardiol. *5*:366, 1985.

378. Lopez-Sendon, J., DeSa, E. L., Roldan, I., et al.: Inversion of the normal interatrial septum convexity in acute myocardial infarction: Incidence, clinical relevance and prognostic significance. J. Am. Coll. Cardiol. *15*:801, 1990.
379. Asinger, R. W., Mikell, F. L., Elsperger, J., et al.: Incidence of left-ventricular thrombosis after acute transmural myocardial infarction. Serial evaluation by two-dimensional echocardiography. N. Engl. J. Med. *305*:297, 1981.
380. Sharma, B., Carvalho, A., Wyeth, R., et al.: Left ventricular thrombi diagnosed by echocardiography in patients with acute myocardial infarction treated with intracoronary streptokinase followed by intravenous heparin. Am. J. Cardiol. *56*:422, 1985.
381. Keren, A., Goldberg, S., Gottlieb, S., et al.: Natural history of left ventricular thrombi: Their appearance and resolution in the posthospitalization period of acute myocardial infarction. J. Am. Coll. Cardiol. *15*:790, 1990.
382. Weintraub, W. S., and Ba'albaki, H. A.: Decision analysis concerning the application of echocardiography to the diagnosis and treatment of mural thrombi after anterior wall acute myocardial infarction. Am. J. Cardiol. *64*:708, 1989.
383. Jugdutt, B. I., Sivaram, C. A., Wortman, C., et al.: Prospective two-dimensional echocardiographic evaluation of left ventricular thrombus and embolism after acute myocardial infarction. J. Am. Coll. Cardiol. *13*:554, 1989.
384. Delemarre, B. J., Visser, C. A., Bot, H., et al.: Prediction of apical thrombus formation in acute myocardial infarction based on left ventricular spatial flow pattern. J. Am. Coll. Cardiol. *15*:355, 1990.
385. Barzilai, B., Gessler, C., Perez, J. E., et al.: Significance of Doppler-detected mitral regurgitation in acute myocardial infarction. Am. J. Cardiol. *61*:220, 1988.
386. Kono, T., Sabbah, H. N., Rosman, H., et al.: Mechanism of functional mitral regurgitation during acute myocardial ischemia. J. Am. Coll. Cardiol. *19*:1101, 1992.
387. Hanlon, J. T., et al.: Echocardiography recognition of partial papillary muscle rupture. J. Am. Soc. Echocardiogr. *6*:101, 1993.
388. Pierard, L. A., Albert, A., Henrard, L., et al.: Incidence and significance of pericardial effusion in acute myocardial infarction as determined by two-dimensional echocardiography. J. Am. Coll. Cardiol. *8*:517, 1986.
389. Berning, J., Launbjerg, J., and Appleyard, M.: Echocardiographic algorithms for admission and predischarge prediction of mortality in acute myocardial infarction. Am. J. Cardiol. *69*:1538, 1992.
390. Horowitz, R. S., Morganroth, J., Parrotto, C., et al.: Immediate diagnosis of acute myocardial infarction by two dimensional echocardiography. Circulation *65*:323, 1982.
391. Sabia, P., Abbott, R. D., Afrookiteh, A., et al.: Importance of two-dimensional echocardiographic assessment of left ventricular systolic function in patients presenting to the emergency room with cardiac-related symptoms. Circulation *84*:1615, 1991.
392. Kan, G., Visser, C. A., Koolen, J. J., et al.: Short and long term predictive value of admission wall motion score in acute myocardial infarction. Br. Heart J. *56*:422, 1986.
393. Abernethy, M., Sharpe, N., Smith, H., et al.: Echocardiographic prediction of left ventricular volume after myocardial infarction. J. Am. Coll. Cardiol. *17*:1527, 1991.
394. Ginzton, L. E., Conant, R., Rodrigues, D. M., et al.: Functional significance of hypertrophy of the noninfarcted myocardium after myocardial infarction in humans. Circulation *80*:816, 1989.
395. Weiss, J. L., Marino, P. N., and Shapiro, E. P.: Myocardial infarction expansion: Recognition, significance and pathology. Am. J. Cardiol. *68*:35D, 1991.
396. Jugdutt, B. I.: Identification of patients prone to infarct expansion by the degree of regional shape distortion on an early two-dimensional echocardiogram after myocardial infarction. Clin. Cardiol. *13*:28, 1990.
397. Nishimura, R. A., Tajik, A. J., Shib, C., et al.: Role of two-dimensional echocardiography in the prediction of in-hospital complications after acute myocardial infarction. J. Am. Coll. Cardiol. *4*:1080, 1984.
398. Abrams, D. S., Starling, M. R., Crawford, M. H., et al.: Value of noninvasive techniques for predicting early complications in patients with clinical class II acute myocardial infarction. J. Am. Coll. Cardiol. *2*:818, 1983.
399. Bhatnagar, S. K., and Al-Yusuf, A. R.: The role of prehospital discharge two-dimensional echocardiography in determining the prognosis of survivors of first myocardial infarction. Am. Heart J. *109*:472, 1985.
400. Ryan, T., Armstrong, W. F., O'Donnell, J. A., et al.: Risk stratification after acute myocardial infarction by means of exercise two-dimensional echocardiography. Am. Heart J. *114*:1305, 1987.
401. Bourdillon, P. D. V., Broderick, T. M., Williams, E. S., et al.: Early recovery of regional left ventricular function after reperfusion in acute myocardial infarction assessed by serial two-dimensional echocardiography. Am. J. Cardiol. *63*:641, 1989.
402. Otto, C. M., Stratton, J. R., Maynard, C., et al.: Echocardiographic evaluation of segmental wall motion early and late after thrombolytic therapy in acute myocardial infarction: The Western Washington tissue plasminogen activator emergency room trial. Am. J. Cardiol. *65*:132, 1990.
403. Smart, S. C., Sawada, S., Ryan, T., et al.: Low-dose dobutamine echocardiography detects reversible dysfunction after thrombolytic therapy of acute myocardial infarction. Circulation *88*:405, 1993.
404. Barilla, F., Gheorghiade, M., Alam, M., et al.: Low-dose dobutamine in patients with acute myocardial infarction identifies viable but not contractile myocardium and predicts the magnitude of improvement in wall motion abnormalities in response to coronary revascularization. Am. Heart J. *122*:1522, 1991.
405. Pierard, L. A., DeLandsheere, C. M., Berthe, C., et al.: Identification of viable myocardium by echocardiography during dobutamine infusion in patients with myocardial infarction after thrombolytic therapy: Comparison with positron emission tomography. J. Am. Coll. Cardiol. *15*:1021, 1990.
406. Charney, R., Schwinger, M. E., Chun, J., et al.: Dobutamine echocardiography and resting-redistribution thallium-201 scintigraphy predicts recovery of hibernating myocardium after coronary revascularization. Am. Heart J. *128*:864, 1994.
407. Cigarroa, C. G., deFilippi, C. R., Brickner, E., et al.: Dobutamine stress echocardiography identifies hibernating myocardium and predicts recovery of left ventricular function after coronary revascularization. Circulation *88*:430, 1993.
408. Hausmann, D., Lundkvist, A.-J.S., Friedrich, G. J., et al.: Intracoronary ultrasound imaging: Intraobserver and interobserver variability of morphometric measurements. Am. Heart J. *128*:674, 1994.
409. Hausmann, D., Lundkvist, A.-J. S., Friedrich, G., et al.: Lumen and plaque shape in atherosclerotic coronary arteries assessed by in vivo intracoronary ultrasound. Am. J. Cardiol. *74*:573, 1994.
410. Rasheed, Q., Nair, R., Sheehan, H., et al.: Correlation of intracoronary ultrasound plaque characteristics in atherosclerotic coronary artery disease in patients with clinical variables. Am. J. Cardiol. *73*:753, 1994.
411. Gerber, T. C., Erbel, R., Gorge, G., et al.: Extent of atherosclerosis and remodeling of the left main coronary artery determined by intravascular ultrasound. Am. J. Cardiol. *73*:666, 1994.
412. Pinto, F. J., Chenzbraum, A., Botas, J., et al.: Feasibility of serial intracoronary ultrasound imaging for assessment of progression of intimal proliferation in cardiac transplant recipients. Circulation *90*:348, 1994.
413. Yamagishi, M., Nissen, S. E., Booth, D. C., et al.: Coronary reactivity to nitroglycerin: Intravascular ultrasound evidence for the importance of plaque distribution. J. Am. Coll. Cardiol. *25*:224, 1995.
414. Ge, J., Erbel, R., Gerber, T., et al.: Intravascular ultrasound imaging of angiographically normal coronary arteries: A prospective study in vivo. Br. Heart J. *71*:572, 1994.
415. Nakamura, S., Colombo, A., Galione, A., et al.: Intracoronary ultrasound observations during stent implantation. Circulation *89*:2026, 1994.
416. Mintz, G. S., Potkin, B. N., Keren, G., et al.: Intravascular ultrasound evaluation of the effect of rotational atherectomy in obstructive atherosclerotic coronary artery disease. Circulation *86*:1383, 1992.
417. Hodgson, J. M., et al.: Intracoronary ultrasound imaging: Correlation of plaque morphology with angiography, clinical syndrome and procedural results in patients undergoing coronary angioplasty. J. Am. Coll. Cardiol. *21*:35, 1993.
418. Kern, M. J., Aguirre, F. V., Donohue, T. J., et al.: Continuous coronary flow velocity monitoring during coronary interventions: Velocity trend patterns associated with adverse events. Am. Heart J. *128*:426, 1994.
419. DiMario, C., Krams, R., Gil, R., et al.: Slope of the instantaneous hyperemic diastolic coronary flow velocity-pressure relation. A new index for assessment of the physiological significance of coronary stenosis in humans. Circulation *90*:1315, 1994.
420. Deychak, Y. A., Segal, J., Reiner, J. S., et al.: Doppler guide wire–derived coronary flow reserve distal to intermediate stenoses used in clinical decision making regarding interventional therapy. Am. Heart J. *128*:178, 1994.
421. Rossen, J. D., and Winniford, M. D.: Effect of increases in heart rate and arterial pressure on coronary flow reserve in humans. J. Am. Coll. Cardiol. *21*:343, 1993.
422. Tardif, J.-C., Vannan, M. A., Taylor, K., et al.: Delineation of extended lengths of coronary arteries by multiplane transesophageal echocardiography. J. Am. Coll. Cardiol. *24*:909, 1994.
423. Memmola, C., Iliceto, S., and Rizzon, P.: Detection of proximal stenosis of left coronary artery by digital transesophageal echocardiography: Feasibility, sensitivity, and specificity. J. Am. Soc. Echocardiogr. *6*:149, 1993.
424. Isaaz, K., Bruntz, J. F., Ethevenot, G., et al.: Abnormal coronary flow velocity pattern in patients with left ventricular hypertrophy, angina pectoris, and normal coronary arteries: A transesophagael Doppler echocardiographic study. Am. Heart J. *128*:500, 1994.
425. Isaaz, K., Bruntz, J. F., Ethevenot, G., et al.: Noninvasive assessment of coronary flow dynamics before and after coronary angioplasty using transesophageal Doppler. Am. J. Cardiol. *72*:1238, 1993.
426. Yamagishi, M., Yasu, T., Ohara, K., et al.: Detection of coronary blood flow associated with left main coronary artery stenosis by transesophageal Doppler color flow echocardiography. J. Am. Coll. Cardiol. *17*:87, 1991.
427. Faletra, F., Cipriani, M., Corno, R., et al.: Transthoracic high-frequency echocardiographic detection of atherosclerotic lesions in the descending portion of the left coronary artery. J. Am. Soc. Echocardiogr. *6*:290, 1993.
428. Sawada, S. G., Ryan, T., Segar, D., et al.: Distinguishing ischemic cardiomyopathy from nonischemic dilated cardiomyopathy with coronary echocardiography. Am. Heart J. *19*:1223, 1992.
429. Ching, K. J., Fulton, D. R., and Lapp, R.: One-year follow-up of cardiac and coronary artery disease in infants and children with Kawasaki disease. Am. Heart J. *115*:1263, 1988.

430. Eteedgui, J. A., Neches, W. H., and Pahl, E.: The role of cross-sectional echocardiography in Kawasaki disease. Cardiol. Young. *1*:221, 1991.
431. Capannari, T. E., Daniels, S. R., Meyer, R. A., et al.: Sensitivity, specificity, and predictive value of two-dimensional echocardiography in detecting coronary artery aneurysms in patients with Kawasaki disease. J. Am. Coll. Cardiol. *7*:355, 1986.
432. Sanders, S. P., Parness, I. A., and Colan, S. D.: Recognition of abnormal connections of coronary arteries with the use of Doppler color flow mapping. J. Am. Coll. Cardiol. *13*:922, 1989.
433. Oda, H., Kawada, Y., Toeda, T., et al.: Assessment of a coronary artery fistula to the pulmonary artery by transesophageal echocardiography. Am. Heart J. *125*:1460, 1993.
434. Maire, R., Gallino, A., and Jenni, R.: Initial detection in a teenager of anomalous left coronary artery from the pulmonary artery by color Doppler echocardiography. Am. Heart J. *125*:1803, 1993.
435. Thomas, M. R., Monaghan, M. J., Michalis, L. K., et al.: Aortoatrial fistulae diagnosed by transthoracic and transesophageal echocardiography: Advantages of the transesophageal approach. J. Am. Soc. Echocardiogr. *6*:21, 1993.
436. Agati L., Voci P., Bilotta F., et al.: Influence of residual perfusion within the infarct zone on the natural history of left ventricular dysfunction after acute myocardial infarction: A myocardial contrast echocardiographic study. J. Am. Coll. Cardiol. *24*:336, 1994.
437. Porter, T. R., D'Sa, A., Turner, C., et al.: Myocardial contrast echocardiography for the assessment of coronary blood flow reserve: Validation in humans. J. Am. Coll. Cardiol. *21*:349, 1993.
438. Ito, H., Tomooka, T., Sakai, N., et al.: Lack of myocardial perfusion immediately after successful thrombolysis. Circulation *85*:1699, 1992.
439. Voci, P., Bilotta, F., Merialdo, P., et al.: Myocardial contrast enhancement after intravenous injection of sonicated albumin microbubbles: A transesophageal echocardiography dipyridamole study. J. Am. Soc. Echocardiogr. *7*:337, 1994.
440. Skyba, D. M., Jayaweera, A. R., Goodman, N. C., et al.: Quantification of myocardial perfusion with myocardial contrast echocardiography during left atrial injection of contrast. Implications for venous injection. Circulation *90*:1513, 1994.

CARDIOMYOPATHIES

441. Shah, P. M., Taylor, R. D., and Wong, M.: Abnormal mitral valve coaptation in hypertrophic obstructive cardiomyopathy: Proposed role in systolic anterior motion of mitral valve. Am. J. Cardiol. *48*:258, 1981.
442. Henry, W. L., Clark, C. E., Glancy, D. L., et al.: Echocardiographic measurement of the left ventricular outflow gradient in idiopathic hypertrophic subaortic stenosis. N. Engl. J. Med *288*:989, 1973.
443. Panza, J. A., Maris, T. J., and Maron, B. J.: Development and determinants of dynamic obstruction to left ventricular outflow in young patients with hypertrophic cardiomyopathy. Circulation *85*:1398, 1992.
444. Pollick, C., Rakowski, H., and Wigle, E. D.: Muscular subaortic stenosis: The quantitative relationship between systolic anterior motion and the pressure gradient. Circulation *69*:43, 1984.
445. Henry, W. L., Clark, C. E., Griffith, J. M., et al.: Mechanism of left ventricular outflow obstruction in patients with obstructive aysmmetric septal hypertrophy (idiopathic hypertrophic subaortic stenosis). Am. J. Cardiol. *35*:337, 1975.
446. Mintz, G. S., Kotler, M. N., Segal, B. L., et al.: Systolic anterior motion of the mitral valve in the absence of asymmetric septal hypertrophy. Circulation *57*:256, 1978.
447. Maron, B. J., Epstein, S. E., Bonow, R. O., Wyngaarden, M. K., and Wesley, Y. E.: Obstructive hypertrophic cardiomyopathy associated with minimal left ventricular hypertrophy. Am. J. Cardiol. *53*:377, 1984.
448. Jiang, L., Levine, R. A., King, M. E., et al.: An integrated mechanism for systolic anterior motion of the mitral valve in hypertrophic cardiomyopathy based on echocardiographic observations. Am. Heart J. *113*:633, 1987.
449. Henry, W. L., Clark, C. E., Roberts, W. C., et al.: Difference in distributions of myocardial abnormalities in patients with obstructive and nonobstructive asymmetric septal hypertrophy (ASH): Echocardiographic and gross anatomic findings. Circulation *50*:447, 1974.
450. Henry, W. L., Clark, C. E., and Epstein, S. E.: Asymmetric septal hypertrophy (ASH). Echocardiographic identification of the pathognomonic anatomic abnormality of IHSS. Circulation *47*:225, 1973.
451. TenCate, F. J., Hugenholtz, P. G., and Roelandt, J.: Ultrasound study of dynamic behaviour of left ventricle in genetic asymmetric septal hypertrophy. Br. Heart J. *39*:627, 1977.
452. Clark, C. E., Henry, W. L., and Epstein, S. E.: Familial prevalence and genetic transmission of idiopathic hypertrophic subaortic stenosis. N. Engl. J. Med. *289*:709, 1973.
453. Lewis, J. F., and Maron, B. J.: Hypertrophic cardiomyopathy characterized by marked hypertrophy of the posterior left ventricular free wall: Significance and clinical implications. J. Am. Coll. Cardiol. *18*:421, 1991.
454. Maron, B. J., Gottdiener, J. S., and Epstein S. E.: Patterns and significance of distribution of left ventricular hypertrophy in hypertrophic cardiomyopathy. A wide angle, two-dimensional echocardiographic study of 125 patients. Am. J. Cardiol. *48*:418, 1981.
455. Webb, J. G., Sasson, Z., Rakowski, H., et al.: Apical hypertrophic cardiomyopathy: Clinical follow-up and diagnostic correlates. J. Am. Coll. Cardiol. *15*:83, 1990.
456. Ko, Y.-L., Lei, M.-H., Chiang, F.-T., et al.: Apical hypertrophic cardiomyopathy of the Japanese type: Occurrence with familial hypertrophic cardiomyopathy in a family. Am. Heart J. *124*:1626, 1992.
457. Lattanzi, F., Spirito, P., Picano, E., et al.: Quantitative assessment of ultrasonic myocardial reflectivity in hypertrophic cardiomyopathy. J. Am. Coll. Cardiol. *17*:1085, 1991.
458. Maron, B. J., Gottdiener, J. S., Arce, J., et al.: Dynamic subaortic obstruction in hypertrophic cardiomyopathy: Pulsed Doppler echocardiography. J. Am. Coll. Cardiol. *6*:1, 1985.
459. Zoghbi, W. A., Haichin, R. N., and Quinones, M. A.: Mid-cavity obstruction in apical hypertrophy: Doppler evidence of diastolic intraventricular gradient with higher apical pressure. Am. Heart J. *116*:1469, 1988.
460. Panza, J. A., Petrone, R. K., Fananapazir, L., et al.: Utility of continuous wave Doppler echocardiography in the noninvasive assessment of left ventricular outflow tract pressure gradient in patients with hypertrophic cardiomyopathy. J. Am. Coll. Cardiol. *19*:91, 1992.
461. Sasson, Z., Yock, P. G., Hatle, L. K., et al.: Doppler echocardiographic determination of the pressure gradient in hypertrophic cardiomyopathy. J. Am. Coll. Cardiol. *11*:752, 1988.
462. Spirito, P., and Maron, B. J.: Relation between extent of left ventricular hypertrophy and diastolic filling abnormalities in hypertrophic cardiomyopathy. J. Am. Coll. Cardiol. *15*:808, 1990.
463. Hoit, B. D., Penonen, E., Dalton, N., et al.: Doppler color flow mapping studies of jet formation and spatial orientation in obstructive hypertrophic cardiomyopathy. Am. Heart J. *117*:1119, 1989.
464. Schwammental, E., Block, M., Schwartzkopff, B., et al.: Prediction of the site and severity of obstruction in hypertrophic cardiomyopathy by flow mapping and continuous wave Doppler echocardiography. J. Am. Coll. Cardiol. *20*:964, 1992.
465. Douglas, P. S., Morrow, R., Ioli, A., et al.: Left ventricular shape, afterload and survival in idiopathic dilated cardiomyopathy. J. Am. Coll. Cardiol. *13*:311, 1989.
466. Goldberg, S. J., Valdes-Cruz, L. M., Sahn, D. J., et al.: Two dimensional echocardiographic evaluation of dilated cardiomyopathy in children. Am. J. Cardiol. *52*:1244, 1983.
467. Pinamonti, B., DiLenarda, A., Sinagra, G., et al.: Restrictive left ventricular filling pattern in dilated cardiomyopathy assessed by Doppler echocardiography: Clinical, echocardiographic and hemodynamic correlations and prognostic implications. J. Am. Coll. Cardiol. *22*:808, 1993.
468. Werner, G. S., Schaefer, C., Dirks, R., et al.: Doppler echocardiographic assessment of left ventricular filling in idiopathic dilated cardiomyopathy during one-year follow-up: Relation to the clinical course of disease. Am. Heart J. *126*:1408, 1993.
469. Siegel, R. J., Shah, P. K., and Fishbein, M. C.: Idiopathic restrictive cardiomyopathy. Circulation *70*:165, 1984.
470. Gross, D. M., Williams, J. C., Caprilio, C., et al.: Echocardiographic abnormalities in the mucopolysaccharide storage diseases. Am. J. Cardiol. *61*:170, 1988.
471. Spirito, P., Lupi, G., Melevendi, C., et al.: Restrictive diastolic abnormalities identified by Doppler echocardiography in patients with thalassemia major. Circulation *82*:88, 1990.
472. Simons, M., and Isner, J. M.: Assessment of relative sensitivities of noninvasive tests for cardiac amyloidosis in documented cardiac amyloidosis. Am. J. Cardiol. *69*:425, 1992.
473. Chandrasekaran, K., Aylward, P. E., Fleagle, S. R., et al.: Feasibility of identifying amyloid and hypertrophic cardiomyopathy with the use of computerized quantitative texture analysis of clinical echocardiographic data. J. Am. Coll. Cardiol. *13*:832, 1989.
474. Klein, A. L., Hatle, L. K., Taliercio, C. P., et al.: Prognostic significance of Doppler measures of diastolic function in cardiac amyloidosis. Circulation *83*:808, 1991.

PERICARDIAL DISEASE

475. Feigenbaum, H., Waldhausen, J. A., and Hyde, L. P.: Ultrasound diagnosis of pericardial effusion. JAMA *191*:107, 1965.
476. Levine, M. J., Lorell, B. H., Diver, D. J., et al.: Implications of echocardiographically assisted diagnosis of pericardial tamponade in contemporary medical patients: Detection before hemodynamic embarrassment. J. Am. Coll. Cardiol. *17*:59, 1991.
477. Armstrong, W. F., Schilt, B. F., Helper, D. J., et al.: Diastolic collapse of the right ventricle with cardiac tamponade: An echocardiographic study. Circulation *65*:1491, 1982.
478. Singh, S., Wann, L. S., Klopfenstein, H. S., et al.: Usefulness of right ventricular diastolic collapse in diagnosing cardiac tamponade and comparison to pulsus paradoxus. Am. J. Cardiol. *57*:652, 1986.
478a. Gillam, L. D., Guyer, D. E., Gibson, T. C., et al.: Hydrodynamic compression of the right atrium: A new echocardiographic sign of cardiac tamponade. Circulation *68*:294, 1983.
479. Kochar, G. S., Jacobs, L. E., and Kotler, M. N.: Right atrial compression in postoperative cardiac patients: Detection by transesophageal echocardiography. J. Am. Coll. Cardiol. *16*:511, 1990.
480. Torelli, J., Marwick, T. H., and Salcedo, E. E.: Left atrial tamponade: Diagnosis by transesophageal echocardiography. J. Am. Soc. Echocardiogr. *4*:413, 1991.
481. Brodyn, N. E., Rose, M. R., Prior, F. P., et al.: Left atrial diastolic compression in a patient with a large pericardial effusion and pulmonary hypertension. Am. J. Med. *88*:1, 1990.
482. Fusman, B., Schwinger, M. E., Charney, R., et al.: Isolated collapse of

left-sided heart chambers in cardiac tamponade: Demonstration by two-dimensional echocardiography. Am. Heart J. *121*:613, 1991.
483. Chuttani, K., Pandian, N. G., Mohanty, P. K., et al.: Left ventricular diastolic collapse. An echocardiographic sign of regional cardiac tamponade. Circulation *83*:1999, 1991.
484. Burstow, D. J., Oh, J. K., Bailey, K. R., et al.: Cardiac tamponade: Characteristic Doppler observations. Mayo Clin. Proc. *64*:312, 1989.
485. Schutzman, J. J., Obarski, T. P., Pearce, G. L., et al.: Comparison of Doppler and two-dimensional echocardiography for assessment of pericardial effusion. Am. J. Cardiol. *70*:1353, 1992.
486. Leeman, D. E., Levine, M. J., and Come, P. C.: Doppler echocardiography in cardiac tamponade: Exaggerated respiratory variation in transvalvular blood flow velocity integrals. J. Am. Coll. Cardiol. *11*:572, 1988.
487. Appleton, C. P., Hatle, L. K., and Popp, R. L.: Cardiac tamponade and pericardial effusion: Respiratory variation in transvalvular flow velocities studied by Doppler echocardiography. J. Am. Coll. Cardiol. *11*:1020, 1988.
488. Feigenbaum, H., Zaky, A., and Grabhorn, L.: Cardiac motion in patients with pericardial effusion: A study using ultrasound cardiography. Circulation *34*:611, 1966.
489. Kreuger, S. K., Zucker, R. P., Dzindzio, B. S., et al.: Swinging heart syndrome with predominant anterior pericardial effusion. J. Clin. Ultrasound *4*:113, 1976.
490. Lewis, B. S.: Real time two dimensional echocardiography in constrictive pericarditis. Am. J. Cardiol. *49*:1789, 1982.
491. Engel, P. J., Fowler, N. O., Tei, C., et al.: M-mode echocardiography in constrictive pericarditis. J. Am. Coll. Cardiol. *6*:471, 1985.
492. Morgan, J. M., Raposo, L., Clague, J. C., et al.: Restrictive cardiomyopathy and constrictive pericarditis: Non-invasive distinction by digitised M mode echocardiography. Br. Heart J. *61*:29, 1989.
493. Voelkel, A. G., Pietro, D. A., Folland, E. D., et al.: Echocardiographic features of constrictive pericarditis. Circulation *58*:871, 1978.
494. Oh, J. K., Hatle, L. K., Seward, J. B., et al.: Diagnostic role of Doppler echocardiography in constrictive pericarditis. J. Am. Coll. Cardiol. *23*:154, 1994.
495. Hatle, L. K., Appleton, C. P., and Popp, R.L.: Differentiation of constrictive pericarditis and restrictive cardiomyopathy by Doppler echocardiography. Circulation *80*:357, 1989.
496. Klein, A. L., Cohen, G. I., Pietrolungo, J. F., et al.: Differentiation of constrictive pericarditis from restrictive cardiomyopathy by Doppler transesophageal echocardiographic measurements of respiratory variations in pulmonary venous flow. J. Am. Coll. Cardiol. *22*:1935, 1993.
497. Vaitkus, P. T., and Kussmaul, W. G.: Constrictive pericarditis versus restrictive cardiomyopathy: A reappraisal and update of diagnostic criteria. Am. Heart J. *122*:1431, 1991.
498. Ruys, F., Paulus, W., Stevens, C., et al.: Expansion of the left atrial appendage is a distinctive cross-sectional echocardiographic feature of congenital defect of the pericardium. Eur. Heart J. *4*:738, 1983.
499. Kansal, S., Roitman, D., and Sheffield, L. T.: Two-dimensional echocardiography of congenital absence of pericardium. Am. Heart J., *109*:912, 1985.
500. Obeid, A. I., Marvasti, M., Parker, F., et al.: Comparison of transthoracic and transesophageal echocardiography in diagnosis of left atrial myxoma. Am. J. Cardiol. *63*:1006, 1989.
501. Tway, K. P., Shah, A. A., and Rahimtoola, S. H.: Multiple bilateral myxomas demonstrated by two-dimensional echocardiography. Am. J. Med. *71*:896, 1981.
502. Alam, M., and Sun, I.: Transesophagael echocardiographic evaluation of left atrial mass lesions. J. Am. Soc. Echocardiogr. *4*:323, 1991.
503. Reeder, G. S., Khandheria, B. K., Seward, J. B., et al.: Transesophageal echocardiography and cardiac masses. Mayo Clin. Proc. *66*:1101, 1991.
504. Pearson, A. C., Labovitz, A. J., Tatineni, S., et al.: Superiority of transesophageal echocardiography in detecting cardiac sources of embolism in patients with cerebral ischemia of uncertain etiology. J. Am. Coll. Cardiol. *17*:66, 1991.
505. Shyu, K.-G., Chen, J.-J., Cheng, J.-J., et al.: Comparison of transthoracic and transesophageal echocardiography in the diagnosis of intracardiac tumors in adults. J. Clin. Ultrasound *22*:381, 1994.
506. Saxon, L. A., Stevenson, W. G., Fonarow, G. C., et al.: Transesophageal echocardiography during radiofrequency catheter ablation of ventricular tachycardia. Am. J. Cardiol. *72*:658, 1993.
507. Brickner, M. E., Friedman, D. B., Cigarroa, C. G., et al.: Relation of thrombus in the left atrial appendage by transesophageal echocardiography to clinical risk factors for thrombus formation. Am. J. Cardiol. *74*:391, 1994.
508. Bansal, R. C., Heywood, J. T., Applegate, P. M., et al.: Detection of left atrial thrombi by two-dimensional echocardiography and surgical correlation in 148 patients with mitral valve disease. Am. J. Cardiol. *64*:243, 1989.
509. Hwang, J.-J., Kuan, P., Chen, J.-J., et al.: Significance of left atrial spontaneous echo contrast in rheumatic mitral valve disease as a predictor of systemic arterial embolization: A transesophageal echocardiographic study. Am. Heart J. *127*:880, 1994.
510. Fatkin, D., Kelly, R. P., and Feneley, M. P.: Relations between left atrial appendage blood flow velocity, spontaneous echocardiographic contrast and thromboembolic risk in vivo. J. Am. Coll. Cardiol. *23*:961, 1994.
511. Riggs, T., Paul, M. H., DeLeon, S., et al.: Two dimensional echocardiography in evaluation of right atrial masses: Five cases in pediatric patients. Am. J. Cardiol. *48*:961, 1981.
512. Sommariva, L., Auricchio, A., Polisca, P., et al.: Right atrial myxoma with atypical features of syndrome myxoma. Am. Heart J. *126*:256, 1993.
513. Dittmann, H., Voelker, W., Karsch, K. R., et al.: Bilateral atrial myxomas detected by transesophageal two-dimensional echocardiography. Am. Heart J. *118*:172, 1989.
514. Cameron, J., Pohlner, P. G., Stafford, E. G., et al.: Right heart thrombus: Recognition and management. J. Am. Coll. Cardiol. *5*:1239, 1985.
515. Sans, P., Provansal, D., Balansard, P., et al.: Large right intracardiac thrombus cause of recurrent pulmonary embolism. Arch. Mal. Coeur. *78*:650, 1985.
516. Meller, J., Teichholz, L. E., Pichard, A. O., et al.: Left ventricular myxoma. Echocardiographic diagnosis and review of the literature. Am. J. Med. *63*:816, 1977.
517. Roelandt, J., Bletter, W. B., Leuftink, E. W., et al.: Ultrasonic demonstration of right ventricular myxoma. J. Clin. Ultrasound *5*:191, 1977.
518. Levisman, J. A., MacAlpin, R. N., Abbasi, A. S., et al.: Echocardiographic diagnosis of a mobile, pedunculated tumor in the left ventricular cavity. Am. J. Cardiol. *36*:957, 1975.
519. Nanda, N. C., Barold, S. S., Gramiak, R., et al.: Echocardiographic features of right ventricular outflow tumor prolapsing into the pulmonary artery. Am. J. Cardiol. *40*:272, 1977.
520. Grantham, N.: Echocardiographic, angiocardiographic, and surgical correlations in right ventricular myxoma simulating valvular pulmonic stenosis. Circulation *55*:619, 1977.
521. Bass, J. L., Breningstall, G. N., and Swaiman, K. F.: Echocardiographic incidence of cardiac rhabdomyoma in tuberous sclerosis. Am. J. Cardiol. *55*:1379, 1985.
522. Yabek, S. M., Isabel-Jones, J., Gyepes, M. T., et al.: Cardiac fibroma in a neonate presenting with severe congestive heart failure. J. Pediatr. *91*:310, 1977.
523. Ports, T. A., Schiller, N. B., and Strunk, B. L.: Echocardiography of right ventricular tumors. Circulation *56*:439, 1977.
524. Topol, E. J., Biern, R. O., and Reitz, B. A.: Cardiac papillary fibroelastoma and stroke. Am. J. Med. *80*:129, 1986.
525. Schwinger, M. E., Katz, E. Rotterda, H., et al.: Right atrial papillary fibroelastoma: Diagnosis by transthoracic and transesophageal echocardiography and percutaneous transvenous biopsy. Am. Heart J. *118*:1047, 1989.
526. Fowles, R. E., Miller, D. C., Egbert, B. M., et al.: Systemic embolization from mitral valve papillary endocardial fibroma detected by two dimensional echocardiography. Am. Heart J. *102*:128, 1981.
527. Hajar, R., Roberts, W. C., and Folger, G. M.: Embryonal botryoid rhabdomyosarcoma of the mitral valve. Am. J. Cardiol. *57*:376, 1986.
528. Grosse, P., Herpin, D., Roudaut, R., et al.: Myxoma of the mitral valve diagnosed by echocardiography. Am. Heart J *111*:803, 1986.
529. Stoddard, M. F., Liddell, N. E., Longacker, R. A., et al.: Transesophageal echocardiography: Normal variants and mimickers. Am. Heart J. *124*:1587, 1992.
530. Cujec, B., Mycyk, T., and Khouri, M.: Identification of Chiari's network with transesophageal echocardiography. J. Am. Soc. Echocardiogr. *5*:96, 1992.
531. Cloez, J. L., Neimann, J. L., Chivoret, G., et al.: Echocardiographic rediscovery of an anatomical structure: The Chiari network. Apropos of 16 cases. Arch. Mal. Coeur *76*:1284, 1983.
532. Limacher, M. C., Gutgesell, H. P., Vick, G. W., et al.: Echocardiographic anatomy of the eustachian valve. Am. J. Cardiol. *57*:363, 1986.
533. Pochis, W. T., Saeian, K., and Sagar, K. B.: Usefulness of transesophageal echocardiography in diagnosing lipomatous hypertrophy of the atrial septum with comparison to transthoracic echocardiography. Am. J. Cardiol. *70*:396, 1992.
534. Cohen, I. S., and Raiker, K.: Atrial lipomatous hypertrophy: Lipomatous atrial hypertrophy with significant involvement of the right atrial wall. J. Am. Soc. Echocardiogr. *6*:30, 1993.
535. Keren, A., Billingham, M. E., and Popp, R. L.: Echocardiographic recognition and implications of ventricular hypertrophic trabeculations and aberrant bands. Circulation *70*:836, 1984.
536. Casta, A., and Wolf, W. J.: Left ventricular bands (false tendons): Echocardiographic and angiocardiographic delineation in children. Am. Heart J. *111*:321, 1986.
537. Chazal, R. A., and Feigenbaum, H.: Two-dimensional echocardiographic identification of epicardial pacemaker wire perforation. Am. Heart J. *107*:165, 1984.
538. Cameron, J., Pohlner, P. G., Stafford, E. G., et al.: Right heart thrombus: Recognition and management. J. Am. Coll. Cardiol. *51*:1239, 1985.
539. Sans, P., Provansal, D., Balansard, P., et al.: Large right intracardiac thrombus cause of recurrent pulmonary embolism. Arch. Mal. Coeur *78*:650, 1985.
540. Weg, I. L., Mehra, S., Azueta, V., et al.: Cardiac metastasis from adenocarcinoma of the lung. Am. J. Med. *80*:108, 1986.
541. Sobue, T., Iwase, M., Iwase, M., et al.: Solitary left ventricular metastasis of renal cell carcinoma. Am. Heart J. *125*:1801, 1993.
542. Cueto-Garcia, L., Shub, C., Sheps, S. G., et al.: Two-dimensional echocardiographic detection and mediastinal pheochromocytoma. Chest *87*:834, 1985.
543. Kruger, S. R., Michaud, J., and Cannom, D. S.: Spontaneous resolution of a pericardial cyst. Am. Heart J. *109*:1390, 1985.
544. Lestuzzi, C., Nicolosi, G. L., Mimo, R., et al.: Usefulness of transesophageal echocardiography in evaluation of paracardiac neoplastic masses. Am. J. Cardiol. *70*:247, 1992.
545. Torbicki, A., Tramarain, R., and Morpurgo, M.: Role of echo/Doppler in the diagnosis of pulmonary embolism. Clin. Cardiol. *15*:805, 1992.

546. Rittoo, D., Sutherland, G. R., Samuel, L., et al.: Role of transesophageal echocardiography in diagnosis and management of central pulmonary artery thromboembolism. Am. J. Cardiol. *71:*1115, 1993.
547. Goldstein, S. A., Mintz, G. S., and Lindsay, J., Jr.: Aorta: Comprehensive evaluation by echocardiography and transesophageal echocardiography. J. Am. Soc. Echocardiogr. *6:*634, 1993.
548. Come, P. C., Sacks, B., Vine, H., et al.: Ultrasonic visualization of the posterior thoracic aorta in long axis: Diagnosis of a saccular mycotic aneurysm. Chest *79:*470, 1981.
549. Simpson, I. A., deBelder, M. A., Treasure, T., et al.: Cardiovascular manifestations of Marfan's syndrome: Improved evaluation by transesophageal echocardiography. Br. Heart J. *69:*104, 1992.
550. Cigarroa, J. E., Isselbacher, E. M., DeSanctis, R. W., and Eagle, K. A.: Diagnostic imaging in the evaluation of suspected aortic dissection. Old standards and new directions. N. Engl. J. Med. *328:*35, 1993.
551. Granato, J. E., Dee, P., and Gibson, R. S.: Utility of two-dimensional echocardiography in suspected ascending aortic dissection. Am. J. Cardiol. *56:*123, 1985.
552. D'Cruz, I. A., Jain, M., Campbell, C., et al.: Ultrasound visualization of aortic dissection by right parasternal scanning, including systolic flutter of the intimal flap. Chest *80:*239, 1981.
553. Banning, A. P., Masani, N. D., Ikram, S., et al.: Transesophageal echocardiography as the sole diagnostic investigation in patients with suspected thoracic aortic dissection. Br. Heart J. *72:*461, 1994.
554. Chirillo, F., Cavallini, C., Longhini, C., et al.: Comparative diagnostic value of transesophageal echocardiography and retrograde aortography in the evaluation of thoracic aortic dissection. Am. J. Cardiol. *74:*590, 1994.
555. Duch, P. M., Chandrasekaran, K., Karalis, D. G., et al.: Improved diagnosis of coexisting types II and III aortic dissection with multiplane transesophageal echocardigraphy. Am. Heart J. *127:*699, 1994.
556. Hashimoto, S., Kumada, T., Osakada, G., et al.: Assessment of transesophageal Doppler echography in dissecting aortic aneurysm. J. Am. Coll. Cardiol. *14:*1252, 1989.
557. Iliceto, S., Nanda, N. C., Rizzon, P., et al.: Color Doppler evaluation of aortic dissection. Circulation *75:*748, 1987.
558. Chia, B. L., Yan, P. C., Ee, B. K., et al.: Two-dimensional echocardiography and Doppler color flow abnormalities in aortic root dissection. Am. Heart J. *116:*192, 1988.
559. Cabanes, L., Garcia, E., VanDamme, C., et al.: Aneurysm of the noncoronary sinus of Valsalva ruptured into the left atrium. Am. Heart J. *124:*1659, 1992.
560. Dev, V., Goswami, K. C., Shrivastava, S., et al.: Echocardiographic diagnosis of aneurysm of the sinus of Valsalva. Am. Heart J. *126:*930, 1993.
561. Kiefaber, R. W., Tabakin, B. S., Coffin, L. H., et al.: Unruptured sinus of Valsalva aneurysm with right ventricular outflow obstruction diagnosed by two-dimensional and Doppler echocardiography. J. Am. Coll. Cardiol. *7:*438, 1986.
562. Hands, M. E., Lloyd, B. L., and Hung, J.: Cross-sectional echocardiographic diagnosis of unruptured right sinus of Valsalva aneurysm dissecting into the interventricular septum. Int. J. Cardiol. *9:*380, 1985.
563. Terdjman, N., Bourdarias, J. P., Farcot, J. C., et al.: Aneurysms of sinus of Valsalva: Two-dimensional echocardiographic diagnosis and recognition of rupture into the right heart cavities. J. Am. Coll. Cardiol. *3:*1227, 1984.
564. Chia, B. L., Ee, B. K., Choo, M. H., et al.: Ruptured aneurysm of sinus of Valsalva: Recognition of Doppler color flow mapping. Am. Heart J. *115:*686, 1988.
565. Nihoyannopoulos, P., Jayshree, J., Athanasopoulos, G., et al.: Detection of atherosclerotic lesions in the aorta by transesophageal echocardiography. Am. J. Cardiol. *71:*1208, 1993.
566. Nishino, M., Masugata, H., Yamada, Y., et al.: Evaluation of thoracic aortic atherosclerosis by transesophageal echocardiography. Am. Heart J. *127:*336, 1994.
567. Dee, W., Geibel, A., Kasper, W., et al.: Mobile thrombi in atherosclerotic lesions of the thoracic aorta: The diagnostic impact of transesophageal echocardiography. Am. Heart J. *126:*707, 1993.
568. Horowitz, D. R., Tuhrim, S., Budd, J., et al.: Aortic plaque in patient with brain ischemia: Diagnosis by transesophageal echocardiography. Neurology *42:*1602, 1992.
569. Tunick, P. A., Rosenzweig, B. P., Katz, E. S., et al.: High risk for vascular events in patients with protruding aortic atheromas: A prospective study. J. Am. Coll. Cardiol. *23:*1085, 1994.

Chapter 4
Electrocardiography

CHARLES FISCH

The clinical electrocardiogram (ECG) records the changing potentials of the electrical field imparted by the heart. The ECG *does not record directly the electrical activity of the source itself.* Such activity is registered only when an electrode is in immediate contact with the tissue generating the current and at the moment when the electrode senses the edge of the wave of activation or recovery. In all other circumstances only potential differences in an electrical field are registered. It is important to appreciate that the ECG, while recording the changes of an electrical field, often provides only an *approximation of the actual* voltage generated by the heart. Efforts to predict surface potentials from the knowledge of behavior of the cardiac generator—the so-called electrocardiographic *forward problem*—or to predict the electrical behavior of the cardiac generator from the body surface potentials—the so-called electrocardiographic *inverse problem*—have to date been unsuccessful.[1]

Despite this basic limitation, the ECG has evolved into an extremely useful clinical laboratory tool and is the only practical means of recording the electrical behavior of the heart.[2] Its usefulness as a diagnostic method is the result of careful, often purely deductive analysis of innumerable patient records and of studies correlating the ECG with basic electrophysiological properties of the heart; with clinical and laboratory findings; and with anatomical, pathological, and experimental observations.[3] As a result, electrocardiography can be used, within limits, to identify anatomical, metabolic, ionic, and hemodynamic changes. It is often an independent marker of cardiac disease, occasionally the only indicator of a pathological process, and not infrequently a guide to therapy.[4–11]

Electrocardiography serves as a gold standard for the diagnosis of arrhythmias, which are discussed in detail in Chapters 20 to 24. Although arrhythmias have been studied by a variety of methods for centuries, none has approached the levels of sensitivity and specificity offered by the ECG.[12] Free of the assumptions required for interpreting the electrocardiographic waveforms, arrhythmias recorded from the surface of the body, with rare exceptions, accurately reflect intracardiac events. However, while most arrhythmias are due to disordered impulse formation or conduction (or both) of the specialized tissue, the ECG reflects the electrical behavior of the myocardium and not of the specialized tissue. This limitation, once appreciated as inherent in the ECG, rarely interferes with proper analysis of even the most complex arrhythmias.[11]

As with any other laboratory procedure, the sensitivity and specificity of the ECG and of its individual components are critical determinants of its clinical usefulness. This is far more complex for the ECG than for other laboratory techniques developed for any single purpose, since its multiple waveforms may be identically or differentially influenced by a wide spectrum of physiological, pathophysiological, or anatomical changes. Thus, it may be difficult—if not impossible—to identify a single cause for any given ECG abnormality.

THE NORMAL ELECTROCARDIOGRAM

Theoretical Considerations

Essential to an understanding of the derivation and interpretation of the clinical ECG is information about (1) the physical and electrophysiological events responsible for the electrical potential recorded as the transmembrane action potential and the spread of excitation, (2) the role of the volume conductor, and (3) the theoretical basis of the lead systems.

ELECTRICAL BASES AND THEORY

At any instant, the cardiac generator can be viewed as a dipole consisting of a positive and a negative charge separated by a small distance. Since the dipole generates a force that has magnitude and direction, it can be expressed as a vector. By convention, the arrowhead of the vector indicates the positive pole. When such a dipole is immersed in a volume conductor, an electrical field is generated.[13,14] In a homogeneous volume conductor, the field is symmetrically distributed. The lines of the electrical field are symmetrical in relation to a line that is perpendicular to and transects the dipole at its midpoint.

At any instant, the magnitude of the potential at a given point *(P)* in the volume conductor can be estimated using the solid-angle concept, or the concept relating the potential to an angle formed by a line drawn from *P* to the midpoint of the dipole axis and the dipole axis itself (Fig. 4–1).

The electrical surface with its boundary projected to P results in a cone and defines the solid angle subtended by the area in question. The segment of a sphere inscribed by a radius of unity drawn about point P, with P as the center of the sphere and its border delineated by the cone, is proportional to the area of electrical activity. With variables such as tissue resistance and geometry being constant, the voltage at P can be expressed as $Ep = \phi \cdot \Omega$, where ϕ is voltage per unit of the solid angle and Ω is the solid angle. An alternative and perhaps clinically more applicable approach to estimating Ep considers the distance (r) of P from the source, the strength of the source (m), and the cosine of the angle formed by a line drawn from P to the midpoint of the dipole axis and the dipole axis (Θ), with the magnitude of the angle estimated in reference to the positive pole of the dipole. This relationship can be expressed as

$$Ep = \frac{m \cos \Theta}{r^2}$$

According to this formula, when the angle is 90 degrees, the line drawn from *P* is perpendicular to the dipole axis, and the Ep is zero. In the ECG the inscription would be isoelectric or equiphasic. On the other hand, with the angle becoming smaller, the point P is closer to the positive pole of the dipole, and the voltage becomes greater.

Assuming that the volume conductor is homogeneous and infinite and has a uniform boundary and that the generator is located in the center of the volume conductor, both approaches for estimation of Ep at P are correct. Such assumptions, however, are not entirely valid in humans (see below).

The influence of polarity of the dipole, the distance of the electrode from the dipole, and the strength of the electrical field on waveform are important in analysis of the ECG. These relationships can be studied using a hypothetical dipole or tissue immersed in a homogeneous volume conductor. An electrode, located outside the electrical field, when moved into the negative field records a gradually increasing negativity. Halfway between the two poles, a sharp reversal of polarity is registered (intrinsic deflection), and the electrode enters the positive field. As the electrode is moved, positive voltage declines gradually until a potential difference is no longer registered. A similar sequence of events is registered with the electrode stationary and the electrical field moving relative to the electrode. When the positive field moves toward the electrode, a positive

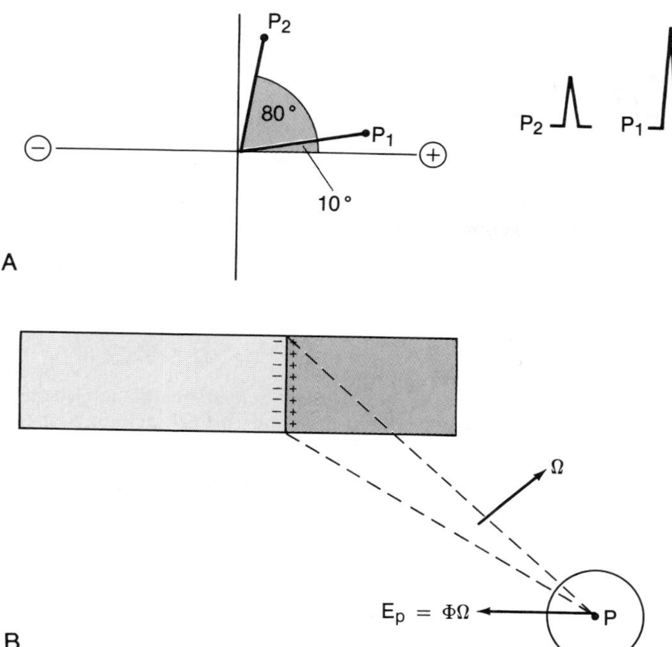

FIGURE 4–1. *A,* The potentials at points P_1 and P_2 are inversely proportional to the square of the distance from the source and proportional to the cosine of angle formed by a line drawn from point P to the midpoint of the dipole axis and the axis itself. *B,* The potential E is proportional to the solid angle Ω and the strength of the charged surface. (Modified from Wolff, L: Electrocardiography: Fundamentals and Clinical Application. 3rd ed. Philadelphia, W. B. Saunders Company, 1962, p. 15.)

potential is recorded; when the electrode finds itself in the negative field, a negative potential is recorded.

Transmembrane ionic fluxes are responsible for voltage differences between activated and resting tissue. These ionic fluxes are reflected as the transmembrane action potential, the cellular counterpart of the clinical ECG. The ECG counterparts of the phases 0, 1, 2, 3, and 4 of the transmembrane action potential are the QRS complex, the ST segment, the T wave, and the isoelectric baseline, respectively (see Chap. 20).

DEPOLARIZATION AND REPOLARIZATION. To progress logically toward an understanding of the ECG, we will review the effect of a muscle strip immersed in a homogenous volume conductor on the electrical field generated by the muscle strip and on the electrode immersed in the field.

A muscle strip, when uniformly positive on the outside, is in a resting or polarized state. Because it exhibits no difference of potential and fails to impart an electrical field, an electrode immersed in the volume conductor registers an isoelectric line. Stimulation of the muscle strip at any given point increases membrane permeability, and positive ions, largely sodium, enter the cell. The result is depolarized muscle whose external field is relatively negative in apposition to polarized muscle whose external field is relatively positive, with a potential difference across a boundary. In the surrounding medium the current flows from the positively (source) to the negatively (sink) charged muscle. The moving boundary between the polarized (positive) and the depolarized (negative) muscle can be represented by a dipole or vector. This dipole or vector moves along the muscle fiber from the point of excitation, leaving in its wake tissue that is electrically negative (depolarized) in relation to the still polarized (resting) muscle. When the wave of depolarization reaches the end of the muscle strip, the surface becomes uniformly negative, and the strip is now completely depolarized. Since a difference of potential no longer exists, an isoelectric baseline is inscribed. The most intense difference of potential exists at the boundary between depolarized and resting tissue, and the recorded voltage changes reflect the events taking place at this boundary.[13,14]

Restitution of membrane polarity, *repolarization,* can be viewed as a "wave" of positivity sweeping across the cells or tissue. As a result, the outside of the cell is again uniformly positive. Since the boundary moves in the direction of the depolarized, negative muscle, an electrode located at the point of origin of repolarization records a positive potential, while an electrode placed at the opposite end records a negative potential. In a preparation of *isolated myocardial tissue* (not the intact heart), the direction of repolarization is the same as that of depolarization but is preceded by the negative pole of the dipole. The repolarization inscribes an area equal to that inscribed by depolarization but of opposite polarity.

EFFECT OF THE BOUNDARY OF DEPOLARIZATION ON POLARITY OF THE RECORDED POTENTIAL. Three electrodes placed on a muscle strip will illustrate the effect of a boundary potential, which can be represented as a dipole or vector, on the recording electrode (Fig. 4–2). Electrode A is located at the point of excitation, electrode B at the midpoint of the muscle strip, and electrode C at the opposite end of the muscle strip. Immediately after excitation, electrode A is in the most intensively negative field. As the dipole moves away, the potential becomes less negative, and at the end of depolarization the inscription returns to the baseline. Thus, the electrode at point A inscribes a negative deflection. At the moment of excitation, electrode B is located in the positive field of the dipole, and as the dipole moves toward the recording electrode, the latter registers a gradually increasing positivity and records an upright deflection. When the dipole passes the electrode, there is a sudden reversal of polarity, termed the *intrinsic deflection,* and the electrode finds itself in a strongly negative field. A downward, negative deflection is recorded. With the dipole moving away, the electrode at point B registers a less negative potential, and finally, when the strip is completely depolar-

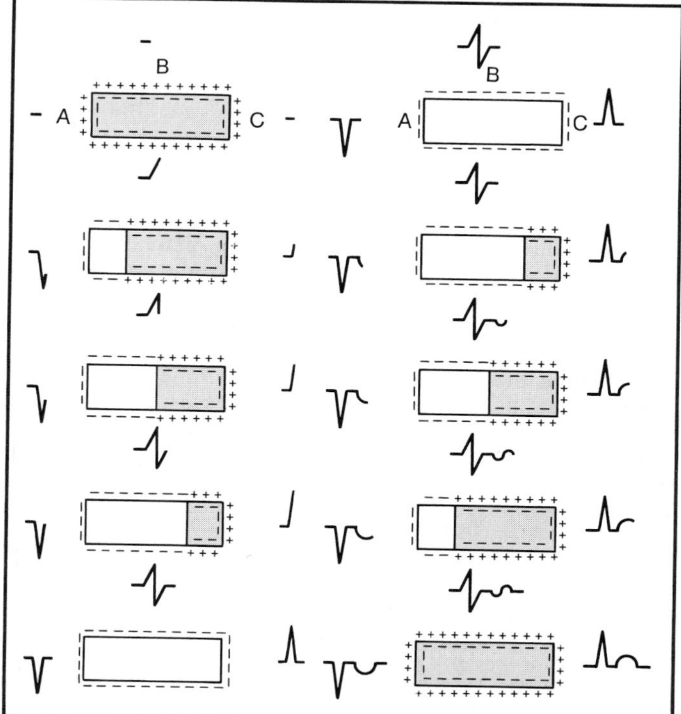

FIGURE 4–2. Potential generated during depolarization (left vertical sequence of panels) and repolarization (right vertical sequence of panels) recorded with an exploring electrode located at the endocardium (A), epicardium (C), and midway between the two (B). (Modified from Barker, J. M.: The Unipolar Electrocardiogram: A Clinical Interpretation. New York, Appleton-Century-Crofts, Inc., 1952.)

ized, an isoelectric baseline is recorded. Thus, the electrode at point B registers a positive-negative deflection. Electrode C is located in the positive field throughout the entire process of depolarization. As the dipole approaches the electrode, the field becomes more intensively positive, with the most intense positivity occurring at the moment immediately before completion of depolarization. Thus, the electrode at point C records an upright deflection.

SEQUENCE OF CARDIAC ACTIVATION. The sequence of cardiac activation has been studied in animals, primarily in the dog, and in the isolated perfused human heart.[15] The normal impulse originates in the sinoatrial (SA) node and traverses the atria in a wavelike front with a velocity of approximately 1000 mm/sec. The wave of atrial activation resembles a wavefront seen when a pebble is thrown into water. The sinoatrial node is located in the right atrium and initially activates the right atrium in a right and anterior direction, followed by excitation of the left atrium in a left and posterior direction. It has been suggested that preferential internodal pathways connect the SA node and the atrioventricular (AV) junctional tissue and that these specialized internodal pathways are capable of conducting an impulse in the presence of a quiescent atrium.

The impulse arrives at the AV node, where it is delayed, most probably because of decremental conduction (see p. 569). Study of the sequence of ventricular activation in the dog reveals an early (0 to 5 msec) and almost simultaneous activation of the central left side of the septum and the high anterior and apical posterior paraseptal areas of the left ventricle. At 5 to 10 msec after the onset of ventricular activation, the wave of activation envelops left and right ventricular walls and the remainder of the septum; the latter is completely activated at 12 msec. The earliest epicardial breakthrough occurs at the anterior right epicardial surface near the apex, followed by anterior and posterior paraseptal areas of the left ventricle. At 18 msec, activation of the central portion of the two ventricles is complete. Excitation continues along the lateral and basal aspects of the left ventricle, with the basal portion of the septum the last to become depolarized.

Studies of perfused human heart indicate that its path of activation closely follows that of the canine heart (Fig. 4–3).[15] The results obtained from the resuscitated human heart were validated by comparing the process of activation with that of a perfused and in situ dog heart. The only difference was that the activation proceeded more rapidly in the perfused dog preparation. Intracardiac mapping during surgery indicates that initial epicardial breakthrough occurs in the right ventricle followed by activation of the anterior and inferior left ventricle.

Human studies indicate that atrial repolarization follows approximately the same path as atrial depolarization, with the polarity of repolarization opposite to that of depolarization. Ventricular repolarization proceeds in a direction *opposite* to that of depolarization, and its polarity is therefore the *same* as that of depolarization. The process of repolarization in the intact ventricle begins at the epicardium—a sequence opposite to that observed in isolated muscle strip. The reason for the reversal in vivo of the order of repolarization is not entirely clear. The presence of a transmural pressure gradient may be an important factor, since it prolongs the duration of the excited state of the endocardium, and consequently, recovery begins at the epicardium.

VENTRICULAR GRADIENT. The ventricular gradient (G), introduced by Wilson, describes the relationships between depolarization (QRS) and repolarization (T).[16] In an isolated muscle strip, depolarization and repolarization are equal in duration and follow the same path. The net areas of the QRS complex (AQRS) and the T wave (AT) are equal but of opposite polarity so that their sum is zero and there is no gradient. In the intact heart, on the other hand, repolarization proceeds from the epicardium to endocardium, in a direction *opposite* to that of depolarization; the algebraic sum of their respective areas is no longer zero; and a gradient is said to exist. AQRS, AT, and G can be expressed as a vectorial quantity from any two of the three bipolar limb leads of the ECG. AQRS and AT are expressed in the form of vectors and are plotted using the Einthoven triangle or Bayley triaxial reference system. A parallelogram of the AQRS and the AT is constructed, with the resultant diagonal vector being the manifest AQRST vector or gradient (G). The G vector and the mean QRS vector are located in about the same plane. The G forms an angle of approximately 30 degrees with the mean spatial QRS vector.

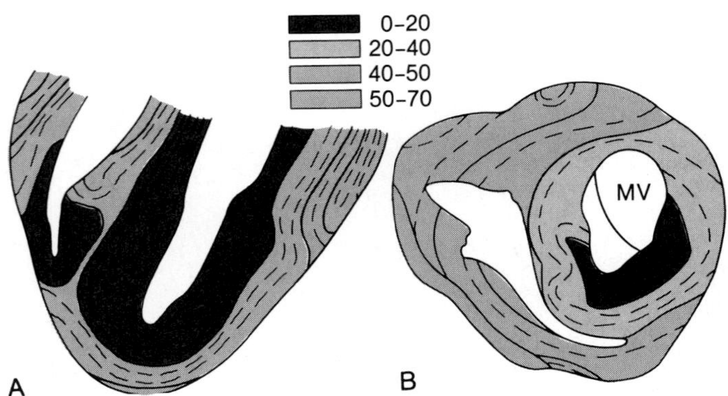

FIGURE 4–3. Sequence of ventricular activation of an isolated human heart. *A* and *B* represent sagittal and coronal sections, respectively. The dotted lines denote 5-msec sequences, while changes in pattern represent 20-msec intervals. (Reproduced with permission from Durrer, D., et al.: Total excitation of the isolated human heart. Circulation *41*:899, 1970. Copyright 1970 American Heart Association, Inc.)

THEORETICAL BASES OF SURFACE LEADS. At any instant the surface leads reflect projection of the electrical field of the equivalent or "net" dipole expressed as the mean instantaneous spatial vector. Orientation of a lead axis is defined as one that records a maximal voltage when its axis is parallel to that of the axis or vector of the equivalent dipole. The voltage registered in any lead, having magnitude and direction, can be expressed as a vector (lead vector), with the amplitude of deflection in any lead paralleling the magnitude of the vector. Since more than one dipole may exist at any instant, the net potential and consequently the resultant lead vector reflect the contribution of all such dipoles. Furthermore, because dipole vectors may vary in magnitude and direction, the equivalent or "net" dipole is an approximation of these forces, and consequently, its expression on a lead axis is also an approximation.

LEADS. *Bipolar limb leads,* introduced by Einthoven, register the direction, magnitude, and duration of voltage changes in the frontal plane. The three bipolar leads—I, II, and III—record the differences in potential between left arm (LA) and right arm (RA), left leg (LF) and RA, and LF and LA, respectively.

Unipolar limb leads are constructed by connecting all three extremities to a "central terminal" (Fig. 4–4*A*). Although in reality the central terminal registers a small voltage, for practical purposes it is considered to have a zero potential and serves as the *indifferent* or *reference electrode.* The potential differences recorded by the positive terminal, the *exploring electrode,* are dominated by local electrical events. When placed on the right arm, left arm, or left foot, the exploring electrode registers the potential from the respective limb. The letter *V* identifies a unipolar lead and the letters *r, l,* and *f* the respective extremities. If one disconnects the central terminal from the extremity from which the potential is being recorded, the amplitude registered by the respective unipolar limb lead is augmented, and the leads are designated as aV_r, aV_l, and aV_f.

Locations of the exploring electrode for the *precordial leads* are as follows: V_1—fourth interspace to the right of the sternum; V_2—fourth interspace to the left of the sternum; V_3—midway between leads V_2 and V_4; V_4—fifth interspace at the midclavicular line; V_5—anterior axillary line at the level of lead V_4; and V_6—midaxillary line at the level of lead V_4 (Fig. 4–4*A*).[17]

In the absence of major thoracic deformity or cardiac malposition, three pairs of precordial leads, i.e., leads V_1 and V_2, V_3 and V_4, and V_5 and V_6, face the right side of the septum, the septum itself, and the left side of the septum, respectively, and are referred to as *right ventricular, septal* or *transitional,* and *left ventricular leads,* respectively.

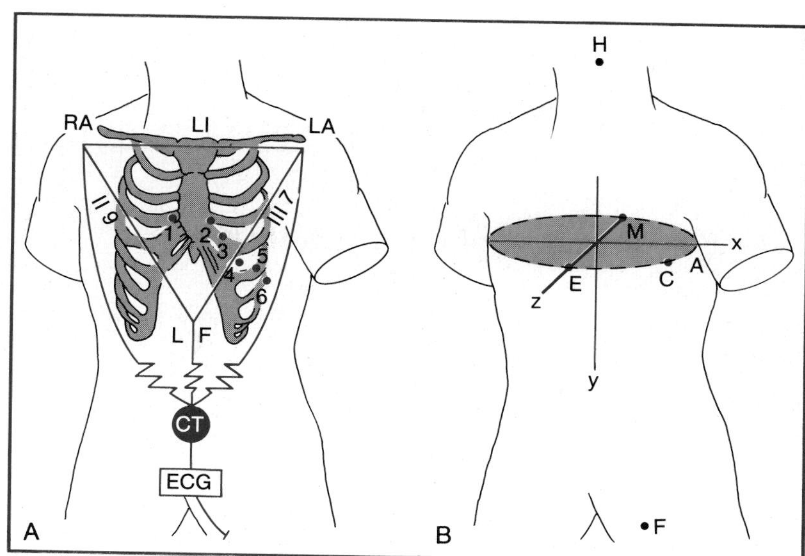

FIGURE 4–4. *A*, ECG lead system. Leads I, II, and III are formed by connecting RA-LA, RA-LF, and LA-LF, respectively. The indifferent electrode of the unipolar system is obtained by connecting RA, LA, and LF through 50,000-ohm resistance into a central terminal (CT). (For details about positioning of the exploring unipolar electrode, see discussion under Leads.) *B*, Frank electrode system. Five horizontal electrodes are placed at the level where the fifth intercostal space intersects the sternal line. Specific locations include fifth intercostal space and sternum (E), the midaxillary line (A,I) and the vertebral column (M). Electrode C is located halfway between points E and A, while electrodes H and F are on the back of the neck and left lower extremity, respectively.

Right precordial leads are of increasing interest because of their importance in the diagnosis of right ventricular infarction. The leads are recorded from the following positions on the right chest: V_3R—between V_1 and V_4R; V_4R—right midclavicular line in the fifth intercostal space; V_5R—right anterior axillary line in the same horizontal plane as V_4R; V_6R—right midaxillary line in the same horizontal plane as V_4R. Normally, an rS configuration is present in 98 per cent of V_3R leads. Secondary R wave (R′) increases in frequency and amplitude in the right lateral leads (for details see ref. 18).

The Standard 12-Lead Electrocardiogram

The P Wave

The cardiac impulse originating in the SA node activates the right and left atria in the general direction from right to left, inferiorly and posteriorly. Initial activation of the right atrium, an anterior chamber, is directed anteriorly and inferiorly and is followed by activation of the left or posterior atrium, directed to the left, posteriorly, and inferiorly.

The P wave is rounded with a notch corresponding to the separation between right and left atrial activation. Amplitude of the P wave is normally less than 0.20 mV (2.0 mm) with a duration less than 0.12 sec (Table 4–1). The P wave and the *Ta segment*, or atrial repolarization, define atrial electrical systole. The P vector varies from −50 to +60 degrees. In the precordial leads the P wave is positive except in lead V_1, where the P wave may be upright, biphasic, or negative.

The Ta segment may be inscribed during the P-R segment, the QRS complex, and the early part of the ST segment (Fig. 4–5). It is best seen in the presence of AV block. Duration of the Ta segment varies from 0.15 to 0.45 sec,

TABLE 4–1 P WAVE: AMPLITUDE AND DURATION IN NORMAL ADULTS

	LEAD I	LEAD II	LEAD III	LEAD V_1*
P Amplitude (mV)				
Mean	0.049	0.103	0.069	0.040
Range	0.02 to 0.10	0.03 to 0.20	0 to 0.20	0.005 to 0.080
P Duration (sec)				
Mean	0.08	0.09	0.16	0.05
Range	0.05 to 0.12	0.05 to 0.12	0.12 to 0.20	0 to 0.08
P-R Interval (sec)				
Mean	0.16	0.16		
Range	0.12 to 0.20	0.12 to 0.20		

AMPLITUDE OF Q, R, S, AND T WAVES IN SCALAR ELECTROCARDIOGRAM OF 100 NORMAL ADULTS†

	I	II	III	aV_r	aV_l	aV_f	V_1	V_5	V_6
Patients with Q Wave	38%	41%	50%	—	38%	40%	0%	60%	75%
Q Amplitude									
Mean	0.4	0.6	0.09	—	0.04	0.07	0	0.03	0.03
Range	0 to 0.1	0 to 0.16	0 to 0.23		0 to 0.11	0 to 0.17	0	0 to 0.18	0 to 0.18
R Amplitude									
Mean	0.56	0.89	0.45	0.13	0.34	0.6	0.19	1.2	1.0
Range	0.1 to 1.0	0.2 to 1.6	0.1 to 1.2	0 to 0.29	0 to 0.82	0 to 1.38	0.1 to 0.6	0.7 to 2.1	0.5 to 1.8
S Amplitude									
Mean	0.2	0.2	0.24	0.7	0.26	—	0.8	0.25	0.13
Range	0 to 0.5	0 to 0.37	0 to 0.64	0.22 to 1.18	0 to 0.58	—	0.3 to 1.3	0 to 0.5	0 to 0.2
T Amplitude									
Mean	0.19	0.23	0.1	—	0.03	0.17	0.1	0.33	0.1
Range	0.1 to 0.3	0.1 to 0.2	−0.2 to 0.2	—	−0.1 to 0.2	0 to 0.4	−0.2 to 0.2	0.2 to 0.7	0.1 to 0.4

* Twenty-five per cent of the series had a small terminal negative deflection of the P wave in lead V_1.
† Amplitude values are in millivolts (0.1 mV = 1 mm).
From Cooksey, J. D., et al.: Clinical Vectorcardiography and Electrocardiography. 2nd ed. Chicago, Year Book Medical Publishers, 1977.

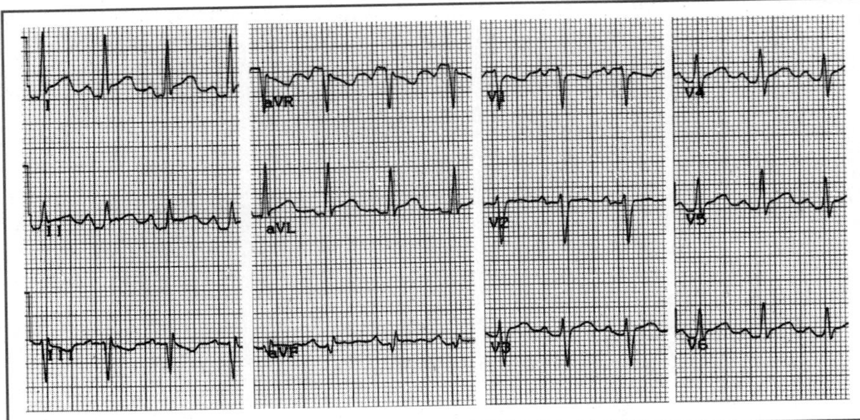

FIGURE 4–5. Acute pericarditis indicated by the diffuse ST-segment elevation without QRS or T-wave abnormality and with the highly diagnostic Ta segment depression in leads I, II, V_4, V_5, and V_6 and elevation in lead aV_r.

and its amplitude is low, reaching 0.08 mV. The magnitude of the Ta is directionally related to the area of the P wave. The orientation of the Ta segment is opposite to that of the P wave. The P wave and Ta areas are equal and opposite in direction, and the resultant gradient is zero. In the presence of atrial enlargement, the Ta segment may result in displacement of the ST segment.

P-R INTERVAL. The P-R interval includes the time for intraatrial, AV nodal, and His-Purkinje conduction, and its duration varies from 0.12 to 0.20 or 0.22 sec (Table 4–1; Chap. 20).

The QRS Complex

Ventricular activation proceeds chiefly symmetrically about the septum and from the endocardium to the epicardium. Consequently, much of its voltage is canceled; in fact, only 10 to 15 per cent of the potential generated by the heart is ultimately recorded on the surface ECG.

The normal QRS complex can be described by four vectors (Fig. 4–6): (1) initial septal activation from left to right, anteriorly, inferiorly, or superiorly, followed by further septal activation from left to right (0.01 sec); (2) an overlapping wave of excitation involving both ventricles, with the vector directed inferiorly and slightly to the left (0.02 sec); (3) unopposed activation of the apical and central portions of the left ventricle, the thin right ventricular wall having been depolarized, with a resultant vector directed posteriorly, inferiorly, and to the left (0.04 sec); and finally, (4) activation of the posterior basal portion of the left ventricle and septum, with a vector directed superiorly and posteriorly (0.06 sec).

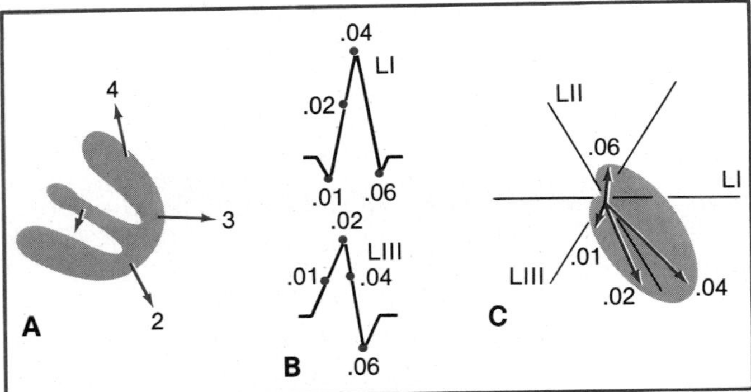

FIGURE 4–6. Correlation between the order of ventricular activation *(A)*, scalar ECG *(B)*, and vectorcardiogram *(C)*. *A*, The sequence of ventricular activation is represented by four instantaneous frontal plane vectors. *B*, The four vectors plotted on leads I and III at the appropriate time during inscription of the QRS. *C*, Using the method of construction of vectors described in Figure 4-7, one can derive each of the four vectors in the frontal plane. A line joining the ends of the vectors results in a frontal plane QRS loop. The same method can be used to derive the orthogonal X, Y, and Z leads from the frontal, transverse, or sagittal planes. (Times given are in seconds.)

Septal activation from left to right and anteriorly results, normally, in an initial Q wave in leads I, II, III, aV_l, V_5, and V_6 and an R wave in the right precordial and septal leads V_1 to V_4. Lead aV_f registers an R or Q wave depending on whether the septal vector is directed superiorly or inferiorly. The ventricular vector directed inferiorly and to the left is reflected by an R wave in leads II and III and in the transitional or septal leads V_3 and V_4. The third vector, that of the unopposed force directed to the left, posteriorly, and somewhat inferiorly, gives rise to an R wave in leads I, II, III, aV_l, aV_f, V_5, V_6, and occasionally V_4, with an S wave in leads aV_r, V_1, V_2, V_3, and at times V_4. The terminal force directed superiorly and posteriorly and perhaps to the right may result in a terminal S wave in leads I, V_5, and V_6. A lead positioned in the right fourth interspace in the midclavicular line (V_{4r}) may record a terminal R wave (R′), which also may occasionally be recorded in lead V_1.[17] The magnitudes of the Q, R, and S waves are given in Table 4–1.

One hundred msec is considered the upper limit of normal QRS duration. In a recent study of 1254 normal white males, however, a QRS complex of 100 to 120 msec in duration, some with R′ in leads V_1 and V_2, was present in 21 per cent of the group. This indicates that a QRS duration of 100 to 120 msec may be normal and does not necessarily indicate pathological intraventricular conduction defect.[19]

THE QRS AXIS, POSITION, AND ROTATION. The electrical position of the heart can be described by the QRS axis and the rotation of the heart on the anteroposterior and longitudinal (apex-to-base) axes. Because the *order* of activation can be viewed as a sequence of instantaneous dipoles or vectors, *total* cardiac activation can be presented as a mean QRS vector. When such a vector is placed within the triangle formed by leads I, II, and III, which define the frontal plane, and assuming that this triangle is equilateral, that the heart is located in its center, and that the thorax is a homogeneous volume conductor with a uniform boundary, projection of the vector on the respective leads permits an estimate of the magnitude of voltage recorded in each lead. Similarly, if the voltage in each of the leads is known, the mean QRS vector can be reconstructed and the axis of the QRS complex can be estimated (Fig. 4–7).

The preceding assumptions—the Einthoven postulates—are applicable in the experimental setting. In the human, however, the heart is a large organ; it is not a point generator nor is it centrally located, and the thorax is not a homogeneous conductor within a uniform boundary. Burger, using a model of a human torso, with nonhomogeneous conduction to reflect the nature of human organs and an eccentrically located generator, found that the triangle formed by the axes of leads I, II, and III is not equilateral

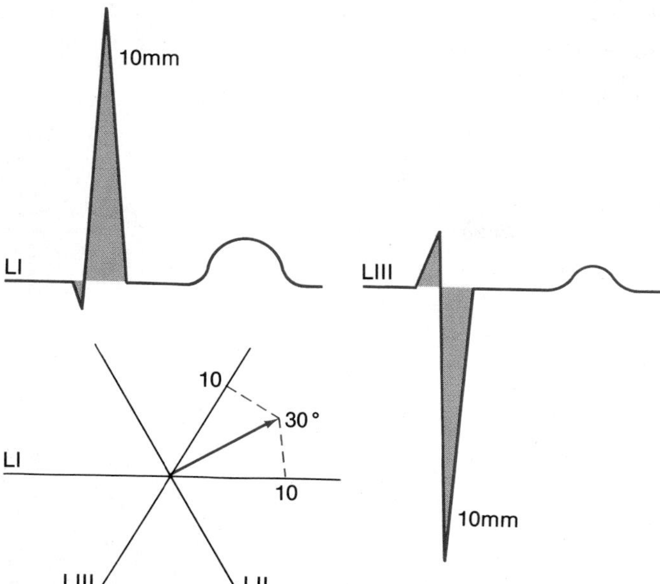

FIGURE 4–7. **Electrical axis plotted in leads I and II of the Einthoven triangle. Peak amplitudes of the R wave in lead I and of the S wave in lead III—in this instance each measuring 10 mm—are plotted on their respective leads. Perpendicular lines are dropped and the point at which these cross is identified. A line drawn from the point where leads I, II, and III cross to the point where the two "perpendicular" lines intersect identifies the electrical axis of the QRS (30 degrees). The same approach is used for plotting the P and T axes. When the P, QRS, or T wave area is plotted on the respective lead, the mean P, QRS, or T vector is identified. The latter represents the mean magnitude, direction, and polarity of the entire period of depolarization. This is a more accurate but impractical method of estimating the electrical axis. Although the direction of the QRS axis and of the mean QRS vector differ, as a rule both lie in the same quadrant.**

but is scalene, with lead I being shortest and lead III longest.[20] The scalene triangle configuration is more consistent with clinical electrocardiography.

The most accurate method for determining the QRS axis is based on estimation of the QRS area in each of the limb leads and a plot of these as vectors on the respective lead axis of a triaxial reference system. From the positive end of the vector, lines perpendicular to the lead axis are dropped. A vector is drawn from the center of the triaxial reference system to the point where the perpendicular lines cross. This vector defines the direction and magnitude of the mean QRS vector. The same method is used to estimate the T vector. Normally, the angle between the QRS and T vectors does not exceed 30 degrees. For practical purposes, however, the assumption that the magnitude of the force projected on a given lead axis is directionally related to the cosine of the angle subtended by the lead vector and lead axis allows a rapid and reasonably accurate estimate of the QRS axis. Thus, if the mean QRS vector is perpendicular to a given lead axis, the angle between the two is 90 degrees, the cosine of the angle is zero, and the QRS will be isoelectric, very small, or equiphasic. On the other hand, when the mean QRS vector is parallel to a lead axis, the angle between the two is zero, the cosine of the angle is one, and the amplitude of the QRS will be greatest in that lead.

Plotted on a hexaxial reference system, axes of −30 to +90 degrees, −30 to −90 degrees, +90 to 180 degrees, and −90 to 180 degrees are normal, left, right, and indeterminate, respectively (Fig. 4–8).[21]

An *anteroposterior axis* allows the apex to face either the left arm or the left foot or to assume a position between the two. Thus, when a QRS complex in aV_l resembles that in leads V_5 and V_6, the electrical position is said to be horizontal. On the other hand, when the QRS complex in aV_f reflects that in leads V_5 and V_6, the position is said to be vertical. Similarly, in the horizontal position the QRS complex in aV_f and in the vertical position the QRS complex in aV_r resemble the QRS complex in lead V_1. When the apex is approximately equidistant from the two extremities, both aV_l and V_f exhibit QRS complexes resembling those in leads V_5 and V_6, and the position is said to be intermediate. If the position shifts more toward the left arm or the left foot, the position is said to be semihorizontal and semivertical, respectively. In the semihorizontal position, the QRS complex in lead aV_l resembles that of leads V_5 and V_6, while the QRS complex in lead aV_f is small. In the semivertical position, the QRS complex in lead aV_f resembles that of leads V_5 and V_6, while the QRS complex in aV_l is small.

Clockwise and counterclockwise rotation along the *longitudinal, apex-to-base axis* can be recognized by analysis of the precordial leads. The direction of rotation is described by viewing the heart from the diaphragmatic surface. *Clockwise rotation* shifts the transitional zone (the position at which the rS complex changes to a qR complex) to the left, and consequently, the right ventricular QRS complex (rS) is displaced to the left and occasionally may be registered in all the precordial positions. *Counterclockwise rotation* results in a more anterior shift of the left ventricle and a more posterior displacement of the right ventricle. Consequently, the transitional zone is shifted to the right, and the left precordial QRS (qR) pattern may be registered, for example, in the V_3 position.

THE ST SEGMENT. The ST segment reflects phase 2 of the transmembrane action potential (see p. 109). Because there is little change in the potential during this phase, the ST segment is usually isoelectric in normal subjects.

THE T WAVE. The mechanism and sequence of ventricular repolarization were described on page 109. The right and left precordial T waves are upright in 75 and 50 per cent of newborns, respectively. Often, after about 8 hours, and invariably after 60 to 90 hours, the left precordial T waves become upright. The right precordial T waves usually become upright after the age of 16, but occasionally the negative T waves persist into early adulthood—a normal variant—termed the *juvenile* T wave.

In the adult, all the unipolar leads inscribe an upright T

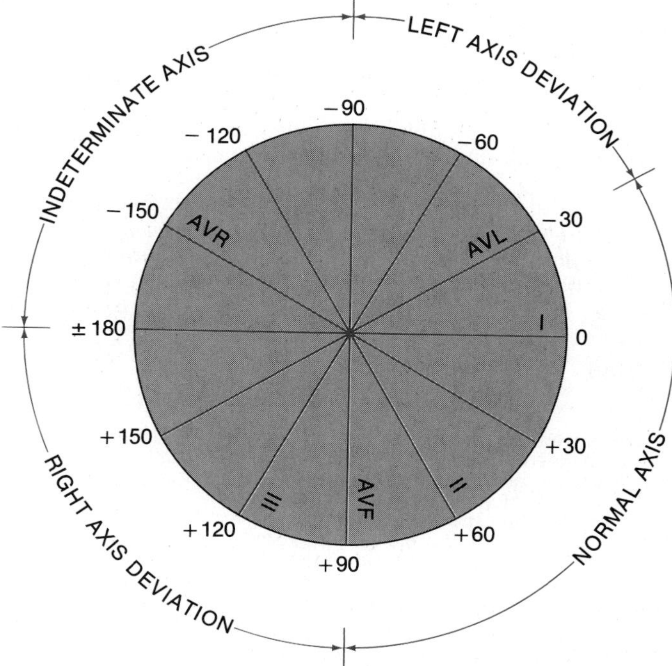

FIGURE 4–8. **The frontal plane hexaxial reference system and the respective ranges of axis deviation.**

wave except for aV_r and occasionally V_1. The amplitude of T waves is given in Table 4–1.

THE U WAVE. The genesis of the U wave, which follows the T wave, is not clear. It has been suggested that it represents a surface reflection of a negative afterpotential. The two prevailing concepts of the mechanism of the U wave include repolarization of the Purkinje fibers and a mechanical event, presumably ventricular relaxation.

The U wave is upright, and its amplitude is 5 to 50 per cent that of the T wave. The tallest U wave is recorded in leads V_2 and V_3, where its amplitude may reach 0.2 mV. Ordinarily the U and T waves are clearly separated. However, under conditions in which the U wave appears early, such as with abbreviated ventricular filling and ejection or when the Q-T interval is prolonged (as with hypocalcemia or after administration of drugs such as quinidine), the U wave may be difficult to separate from the T wave; on the other hand, when the Q-T interval is abbreviated, as with digitalis or hypercalcemia, the U wave is easily identifiable.

The Q-T Interval

The Q-T interval, measured from the beginning of the QRS complex to the end of the T wave, reflects, within limits, the duration of depolarization and repolarization. Importantly, the Q-T interval may not always accurately reflect the recovery time of the ventricles. In some portions of the ventricles repolarization is complete before the end of the Q-T interval, while in other areas repolarization may continue after the end of the Q-T interval, but because of the small magnitude of the potential or because of cancellation, it cannot be identified in the surface tracing. In addition, because the onset of the QRS complex or the end of the T wave or both may be difficult to define, one cannot always obtain an accurate measurement of the Q-T interval.[21a] The point at which the line of maximal downslope of the T wave crosses the baseline helps to identify the end of the T wave.

Duration of the Q-T interval varies with cycle length, and numerous formulas have been suggested to correct for heart rate. Bazett proposed a formula for estimating the Q-T interval corrected for heart rate,[22] or the *Q-T$_c$ interval:* Q-T/$\sqrt{\text{R-R}}$. The upper limit of the Q-T$_c$ interval is 0.39 sec for men and 0.44 sec for women. The earlier correction equations give conflicting results at low and high heart rates. This is especially true for the Bazett formula. An improved method for adjusting the Q-T interval for heart rate has been proposed using a linear regression model.[23] Similarly, a nomogram giving the number of milliseconds by which the Q-T interval should be corrected for the different heart rates results in an excellent adjustment of the Q-T for the heart rate.[24]

Because of the variability of measurements and potential influences other than heart rate, different ranges of normal are accepted by different investigators.[25] For practical purposes, therefore, minor deviations from the expected Q-T$_c$ interval should be disregarded as being of questionable clinical significance.

The Normal Vectorcardiogram

The concept of vectorcardiography, introduced in 1920 by Mann,[26] can be defined as registration of the time course of mean instantaneous spatial cardiac vectors. By plotting on a triaxial reference system a number of vectors derived simultaneously from leads I and III, and by connecting the ends of the derived vectors, Mann recorded a loop, which he termed a *monocardiogram* (Fig. 4–6C). The advent of the cathode-ray oscilloscope allowed for direct recording of the loop.

Vectorcardiogram (VCG) loops are recorded in three planes: frontal, transverse, and sagittal. Both right and left sagittal views are in use (Fig. 4–9). Any two of the three leads of the orthogonal system will define a plane and will inscribe a loop in a given plane. The combination of *X* and *Y*, *X* and *Z*, *Y* and *Z* will register the VCG loop in the frontal, transverse, or sagittal planes, respectively. To correct for nonuniformity of the conducting medium, eccentricity of the heart as a source, presence of a number of dipoles, and variation in vector-

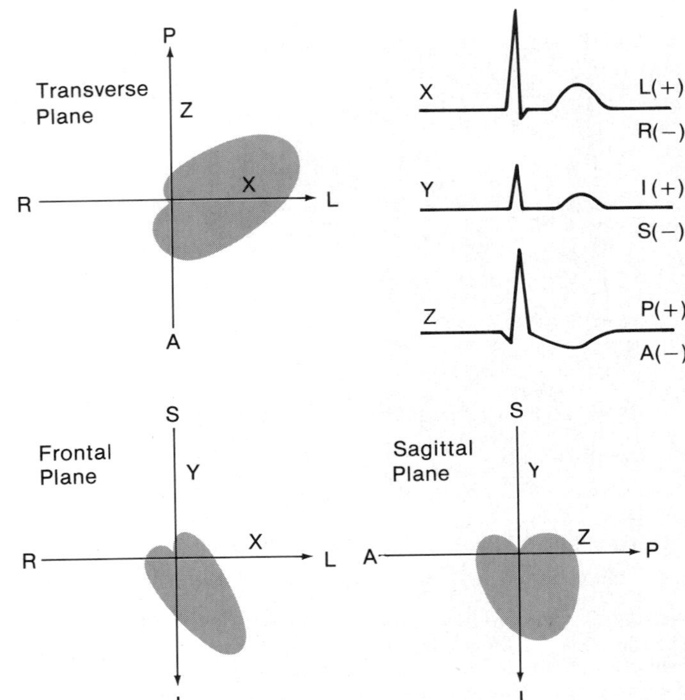

FIGURE 4–9. The transverse, frontal, and sagittal planes and the respective orthogonal leads XZ, XY, and YZ that define the planes. The arrow indicates the positive pole. Normal transverse, frontal, and right sagittal loops are diagrammed. The right upper panel diagrams the orthogonal X, Y, and Z leads. When the vector points to the left (L), inferiorly (I), or posteriorly (P), a positive or upright deflection is recorded. Similarly, if the current flows to the right (R), superiorly (S), or anteriorly (A), a negative or downward deflection is recorded. In this instance the mean vector is oriented to the left, inferiorly, and posteriorly.

ial expression of the magnitude of an electrical signal and to ensure that the three leads are perpendicular, a number of corrected orthogonal leads have been devised. Although none is ideal, the Frank system, because of its relative simplicity, is most widely used[27] (Fig. 4–4B).

The VCG differs from the ECG only in the method of display of the electrical field generated by the heart. *While the ECG reflects best the changes in time and amplitude, the VCG adds the important dimension of direction.* Despite the corrected nature of the orthogonal leads, the assumptions and limitations implicit in the ECG are also applicable to the VCG.

Whether because of the relative complexity of recording the VCG compared with the ECG or because of its failure to add significant information to that gained from the ECG, routine use of the VCG is no longer favored. The spatial VCG, however, is an excellent teaching tool, especially for the analysis of the QRS complex. It is for this reason that the QRS loop is discussed briefly in this chapter.

In a three-dimensional projection, the major portion of the normal QRS loop is located in the left, inferior, and posterior octant[27] (Fig. 4–9). In the frontal plane, the loop is narrow and elongated, and in about one-third of subjects the inscription is clockwise; in the remaining two-thirds the inscription is counterclockwise or a figure-of-eight. The loop is most frequently located in the left inferior quadrant. In the transverse plane, the loop is inscribed counterclockwise and is oval in appearance, and the major portion is located in the left posterior quadrant. In the right sagittal plane, the loop is inscribed clockwise and is located in the anterior and posterior quadrants.

Although the QRS loop is routinely inscribed in the three orthogonal planes, with few exceptions, the characteristic patterns can be recognized in the transverse plane. Patterns with a superior or inferior orientation require frontal projection for analysis. Of these, the most commonly encountered abnormalities include block of the divisions of the left bundle and inferior myocardial infarction. Normal values for the QRS loop are given in Table 4–2.

BODY SURFACE POTENTIAL MAPPING

Body surface potential mapping may contribute information not available from the 12-lead ECG or the VCG; i.e., it provides regional electrophysiological information that cannot be extracted using these methods. Analysis of surface potentials has been applied to the diagnosis of old inferior myocardial infarction, localization of the by-

TABLE 4–2 SOME CHARACTERISTICS OF THE NORMAL QRSsÊ LOOP

CHARACTERISTIC	TRANSVERSE PLANE Mean	TRANSVERSE PLANE 95% Range	RIGHT SAGITTAL PLANE Mean	RIGHT SAGITTAL PLANE 95% Range	FRONTAL PLANE Mean	FRONTAL PLANE 95% Range
Max QRS vector						
Direction (degrees)	−10	−80 to 20.0	100	50 to 165	35	10 to 65
Magnitude (mV)	1.30	0.85 to 1.95	1.00	0.3 to 1.9	1.50	0.9 to 2.2
0.02-sec vector						
Direction	55	0 to 120.0	15	−30 to 75	20	Widely scattered
Magnitude	0.40	0.15 to 0.75	0.30	0.10 to 0.55	0.25	0.05 to 0.7
0.04-sec vector						
Direction	−20	−90 to 25.0	110	60 to 170	35	−10 to 70
Magnitude	1.15	0.55 to 1.90	0.90	0.25 to 1.80	1.25	0.4 to 2.2
0.06-sec vector						
Direction	−90	−125 to −35	160	115 to 220	85	Widely scattered
Magnitude	0.45	0 to 0.9	0.55	0.1 to 1.0	0.25	0 to 0.6
Time of occurrence of max QRS vector (msec)	38	30 to 48	Same as transverse		Same as transverse	
Direction of inscription	Counterclockwise		Clockwise		Clockwise 65% Figure-of-eight 25% Counterclockwise 10%	

From Chou, T. C., et al.: Clinical Vectorcardiography. 2nd ed. New York, Grune and Stratton, 1974, p. 60.

pass pathway in the Wolff-Parkinson-White syndrome, recognition of ventricular hypertrophy, estimation of the size of a myocardial infarction, and the effects of different interventions designed to reduce infarct size. The limiting factor at present is the complexity of the recording and analysis, which requires 100 or more electrodes, sophisticated instrumentation, and dedicated personnel. Initial efforts toward reducing the number of electrodes without loss of pertinent information are promising. Once the technical obstacles are overcome, large numbers of patients can be studied, and the ultimate utility of this procedure can be evaluated.

THE ABNORMAL ELECTROCARDIOGRAM

Abnormal P Wave and the Ta Segment

Although an atrial abnormality often implies atrial enlargement or hypertrophy, P-wave changes may reflect altered intraatrial pressure, volume, or conduction. Furthermore, shift of the site of origin of the P wave with an intraatrial conduction disturbance may simulate a pathological state. *Right atrial enlargement* or preponderance is manifested by an atrial vector that is increased in magnitude and shifted to the right. The P wave is normal in duration, low or isoelectric in lead I, and tall—but more importantly, peaked or pointed—in leads II, III, and aV_f (Fig. 4–10*B*). P waves in leads V_{4r}, V_1, and V_2 may be upright and increased in amplitude. A P-wave axis of +90 degrees or greater, with an isoelectric P wave in lead I, is rarely, if ever, a normal finding. Using two-dimensional echocardiography as a reference, it appears that the most powerful predictor of right atrial enlargement is a P wave in lead V_2 greater than 1.5 mm, especially when associated with a QRS axis of +90 degrees and an R/S ratio greater than 1 in lead V_1. While P pulmonale alone detected only 6 per cent of patients with right atrial enlargement, the combined sensitivity of the three criteria was 49 per cent and the specificity was 100 per cent.[28]

In the adult the most common cause of right atrial abnormality is chronic obstructive lung disease (see p. 135). The predictive value of P wave amplitude for detecting right atrial enlargement diagnosed with two-dimensional echocardiography is low. P pulmonale pattern in the absence of right atrial enlargement, termed *pseudo–P pulmonale,* has been found in association with a variety of disorders of the left heart, including coronary artery disease with angina pectoris, and less often in the absence of heart disease. It has been suggested that in the presence of left heart disease, pseudo–P pulmonale reflects an increase of the left atrial component of the P waves.[29] This suggestion is supported by a recent observation that damage to the left atrium increases the right atrial vector and damage to the right atrium simulates left atrial enlargement.[30]

Left atrial enlargement is manifested by prolongation of the P wave, shortening or absence of the P-R segment, and a shift of the P vector to the left and posteriorly (Fig. 4–10*A*). The duration of the P wave is 0.12 sec or longer, the prolongation is at the expense of the P-R segment, the P wave is notched, and its axis is shifted to the left. Because the vector is increased in magnitude and oriented posteriorly, lead V_1 registers a prominent negative P wave. A negative P wave in lead V_1, 0.04 sec in duration and 0.1 mV in depth, is consistent with left atrial preponderance, the so-called *P mitrale.* In a study of 57 patients with

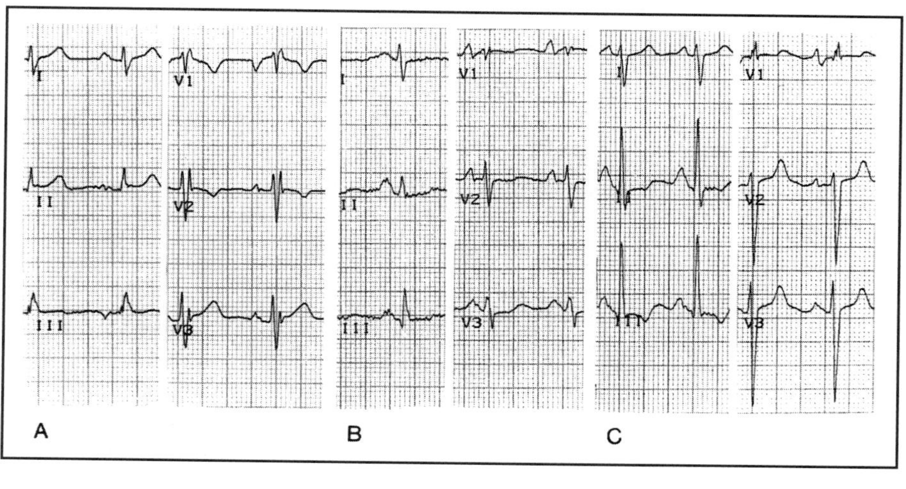

FIGURE 4–10. *A,* Left atrial enlargement manifest by prolonged notched P wave with left axis and the highly specific negative P wave in lead V_1. A common feature, not evident in this figure, is foreshortening or absence of the P-R segment. *B,* Right atrial enlargement with the diagnostic prominent positive P waves in leads V_1 and V_2. The other characteristic features of the P wave in the frontal plane, namely, right-axis deviation and prominent, pointed P waves in leads II and III, are shown in Figure 4–14. *C,* Biatrial enlargement manifest by a tall, broad P wave in lead II, a notched P wave in lead III, and a large biphasic P in lead V_1.

echocardiographically confirmed left atrial enlargement, the sensitivity of the various ECG criteria for left atrial enlargements varied from as low as 15 per cent for notched P wave with interpeak duration more than 0.04 sec to as high as 83 per cent for negative P wave of more than 0.04 sec in lead V_1. The specificity varied from 64 per cent for a foreshortened P-R segment to nearly 100 per cent for notched P wave with interpeak more than 0.04 sec.[31] Although P mitrale is common in mitral valve disease, the most frequent cause is left ventricular disease, with the increased left ventricular end-diastolic pressure reflected in the atrium.

In *biatrial* enlargement, both anterior and posterior forces are increased. The abnormality includes a prominent initial part of the P wave coupled with the left axis of the terminal portion of the P wave and a biphasic P wave in leads V_1 and occasionally in V_2 (Fig. 4–10*C*).

In the presence of atrial fibrillation, atrial disease can occasionally be suspected from an analysis of the QRS complex. With severe tricuspid regurgitation, right atrial enlargement displaces the tricuspid valve down and to the left. As a result, lead V_1 (and sometimes V_2), normally subtended by the right ventricle, now reflects the intracavitary (qR) right atrial potential as indicated by QR, qR, or qrS complexes in leads V_1 or V_1 and V_2 followed by a normal progression of R-wave amplitude from leads V_2 or V_3 to V_6 (Fig. 4–AE1, p. 146). Atrial enlargement also can be suspected when coarse, relatively large fibrillatory waves are present, especially in lead V_1. This is in contrast to atrial fibrillation complicating arteriosclerotic and hypertensive heart disease, in which the fibrillatory waves are fine and frequently unidentifiable.

Alteration of atrial repolarization (Ta), recognized by deviation from the T-P segment, can be either secondary or primary. Secondary changes appear in response to and are obligatory to atrial depolarization, while primary Ta changes are independent of atrial depolarization and indicate nonuniformity of atrial repolarization (Fig. 4–5). The usual pathological causes of secondary Ta-segment depression, which may exceed 1 mm (0.1 mV), include atrial dilation, hypertrophy, and intraatrial block. In chronic obstructive lung disease, for example, depression of the Ta segment may be exaggerated and mistaken for ST-segment displacement.

The usual causes of *primary* Ta-segment changes are pericarditis (Fig. 4–5), atrial infarction, and atrial injury due to penetrating wounds. *Pericarditis* exaggerates the normally negative Ta segment, and Ta-segment depression is recorded in all leads except aV_r, in which it is elevated. Occasionally, a Ta-segment abnormality may be the only convincing evidence of acute pericarditis.

The incidence of *atrial infarction* in myocardial infarction (see p. 1192) is difficult to estimate, and the reported numbers vary widely. In a study of 304 consecutive patients with Q-wave myocardial infarction, displacement of the Ta segment was noted in 10 per cent. However, in 12 patients the Ta depression was associated with a pericardial friction rub, making a differentiation of Ta abnormality due to infarction from that due to pericarditis difficult. A Ta depression suggested a larger infarct size and an increased in-hospital mortality.[32] Isolated atrial infarction in the absence of ventricular infarction is a most unlikely event. The manifestations of infarction may include elevation of the Ta segment in leads I, II, III, V_5, or V_6 or a depression that may exceed 0.15 mV in precordial leads and 0.1 mV in leads I, II, and III. Displacement of Ta segment in an opposite direction, a reciprocal change, may be recorded in "distal" leads, i.e., those facing noninfarcted areas of the atrium. Attempts to localize the site of atrial infarction by ECG have been unsuccessful. Supraventricular arrhythmias frequently accompany atrial infarction.

Penetrating injury of the atria due to gunshot wounds (see p. 1539) or perforation in the course of cardiac catheterization may be associated with diagnostic Ta-segment depression. Ta-segment displacement is also frequently observed following open heart surgery, and whether or not the displacement reflects mechanical injury, associated pericarditis, hemopericardium, or a combination of these factors is still unclear.

Ventricular Hypertrophy

Left Ventricular Hypertrophy (LVH)

ECG manifestations of LVH include an increase in voltage; shift of the mean QRS axis posteriorly, superiorly, and to the left; prolongation of depolarization (delayed intrinsicoid deflection); and gradual shift of the ST segment and T wave in a direction opposite to that of the QRS complex. The exact mechanism of the voltage increase is not clear.[33] In addition to the muscle mass, other factors may play a role, such as intracavitary blood volume, proximity to the chest wall, conducting properties of intrathoracic organs, location of the heart within the thorax, intraventricular and transmural pressures, and perhaps unopposed inscription of a portion of the QRS complex due to delayed activation.

The left superior and posterior orientation of the mean QRS vector in LVH is most likely related to hypertrophy of the basal portion of the left ventricle with delayed, and at times unopposed, activation. Variables that may be responsible for delayed depolarization include increased muscle mass, decreased Purkinje activation, and localized intraventricular conduction delays. Marked superior orientation is noted in association with left anterior divisional block.

Prolongation of the excited state through the myocardium and prolongation of activation result in a change in the order of repolarization, which proceeds from endocardium to epicardium, resulting in a reversal of T-wave polarity. Of the mechanisms responsible for this reversal of repolarization, increased muscle mass without a concomitant increase in the capillary bed, the so-called relative coronary insufficiency, may be an important factor. It is also possible that as the muscle mass outgrows the Purkinje fiber mass, more of the activation proceeds through the myocardium, and this can contribute to a change in the T-wave vector. ST-segment depression may be due to the onset of repolarization before the completion of depolarization.

The mean QRS vector, increased in magnitude and oriented toward the left, posteriorly and superiorly, results in a positive deflection in leads I, II, aV_l, V_5, and V_6 and a positive or negative deflection in leads III and aV_f. The precordial transitional zone is shifted to the left. Leads V_1 and V_2 record an rS pattern, but in some instances the initial R wave may be absent, most likely due to posterior rotation of the QRS loop (Fig. 4–11). Lack of the initial R wave may be erroneously interpreted as an anteroseptal myocardial infarction.

QRS voltage criteria for LVH include $R_I + S_{III} \geq 2.5$ mV, R in $aV_l > 1.2$ mV, R in $aV_f > 2.0$ mV, S in $V_1 \geq 2.4$ mV, R in V_5 or $V_6 > 2.6$ mV, and R in V_5 or V_6 + S in $V_1 >$ 3.5 mV.[34] The following point system for diagnosing LVH has been suggested. Amplitude of R or S wave in limb leads ≥ 2.0 mV *or* S wave in V_1 or V_2 ≥ 3.0 mV *or* R wave

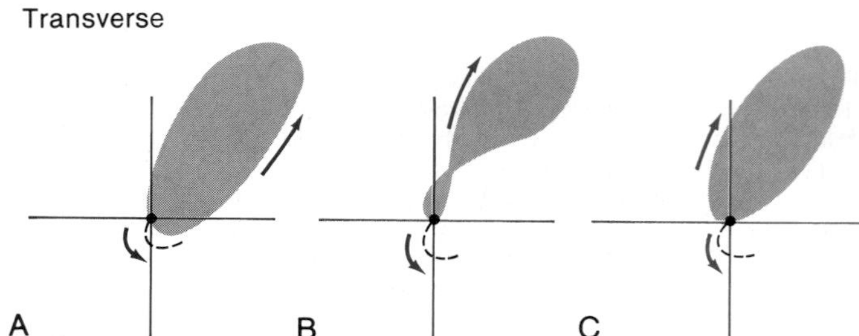

FIGURE 4–11. VCG loops in the transverse plane in left ventricular hypertrophy. The loops illustrate the occasional loss of the initial rightward force (*A*) and rightward and anterior forces (*B, C*) as a result of LVH. Such changes are reflected in the precordial ECG by diminution or loss of the initial R wave in right precordial leads, which could mistakenly suggest myocardial infarction. The dashed lines represent the initial normal forces.

in V_5 or $V_6 \geq 3.0$ mV = 3 points. ST segment changes with or without digitalis = 1 or 2 points, respectively. Left atrial enlargement = 3 points. Left-axis deviation of −30 degrees or more = 2 points. QRS duration ≥ 0.09 sec and intrinsicoid deflection in V_5 and $V_6 \geq 0.05$ sec = 1 point each. Left ventricular hypertrophy is considered to be likely if the points total 4 and to be present if the total is 5 or more. It also has been suggested that the strongest independent variables for LVH, when compared with the echocardiogram, include the S wave in lead V_3 and the R wave in aV_l. In men, the sum of R wave in aV_l and S wave in V_3 (the Cornell index) exceeding 35 mm indicates LVH.[35]

The diagnosis of LVH is strengthened by a delayed intrinsicoid deflection in lead V_5 or V_6, measuring more than 0.05 sec in the adult. The *intrinsicoid deflection*, based on the concept of intrinsic deflection (see p. 109) and applied to the indirect surface leads, is theoretically related to muscle mass. In the clinical ECG the time from the onset of the QRS to the peak of the R wave is an estimate of the intrinsicoid deflection. In the right (namely, V_1, V_2) and left (namely, V_5, V_6) precordial leads, the time from onset of the QRS to appearance of the intrinsicoid deflection is 0.035 and 0.055 sec or less, respectively. For practical purposes in the study of conduction delays, the term *R peak time* is preferred.[21]

The direction of the ST segment and T wave is opposite to that of the QRS complex in LVH. Characteristically, the T wave is negative and asymmetrical, its ascending limb being steeper with an occasional terminal positive inscription. The J point and the ST segment are depressed in leads I, aV_l, V_5, and V_6. The T-wave inversion is greater in lead V_6 than in V_4. In the presence of a vertical position, these changes are recorded in leads II, III, and aV_f. It has been suggested that depression of the J point, asymmetry of the T wave with a more rapid return to the baseline, terminal positivity of the T wave ("overshoot"), T-wave inversion in lead V_6 greater than 3 mm, and T-wave change greater in lead V_6 than V_4 support the diagnosis of LVH and help to distinguish LVH from coronary artery disease in the absence of voltage criteria for LVH.[36] Left atrial dilatation is common with LVH.

The limitations of the sensitivity of the ECG criteria for LVH are recognized. This is true for both the voltage criteria and the point system.[37] Anatomical and echocardiographic studies suggest a sensitivity of about 25 per cent for Sokolow-Lyons voltage criteria and approximately 50 per cent for Romhilt-Estes point score. The specificity is approximately 95 per cent for both. Sensitivity of the criteria for LVH varies depending on the etiology of the underlying heart disease, with the sensitivity lowest in the presence of coronary artery disease.

In a population with a true prevalence of LVH of less than 10 per cent, there are more false-positive than true-positive diagnoses. Similarly, autopsy data indicate that voltage changes consistent with LVH can be present in the absence of LVH.

The concept of *diastolic overload* may be useful clinically.[38] It may point to such lesions as patent ductus arteriosus, ventricular septal defect, or aortic or mitral valve regurgitation, in which there is volume overload. The ECG pattern is one of LVH but with a prominent Q wave in the leads facing the left side of the septum, namely, I, aV_l, V_5, and V_6, and a reciprocal, prominent R wave in the leads facing the right side of the septum, namely, V_1 and V_2. As a rule, the Q wave is narrow, measuring 0.025 sec or less, and its depth is 0.2 mV or greater (Figs. 4–AE2 and 4–AE3, p. 146). Systolic or "pressure" overload is characterized by high-amplitude R waves and ST-segment and T-wave changes in the left ventricular leads and may be present in disorders with an increased resistance to left ventricular outflow. However, the accuracy of the LVH pattern in predicting the hemodynamic abnormality is limited.

VECTORCARDIOGRAM. The VCG changes in LVH are due to an increase in and rotation of the forces farther to the left and posteriorly. These events are best reflected in the transverse plane. The VCG loop is increased in magnitude, elongated, inscribed counterclockwise as a rule, and shifted posteriorly. The occasional posterior orientation of the initial part of the loop simulates anteroseptal myocardial infarction (Fig. 4–11).

Right Ventricular Hypertrophy (RVH)

In contrast to LVH, RVH is not simply an exaggeration of the normal. For RVH to become manifested, the right ventricular mass must be sufficiently large to overcome the left ventricular forces (Fig. 4–12). For this reason, the specificity of the ECG pattern of RVH is much greater, but the sensitivity is relatively low, varying from 25 to 40 per cent depending on the criteria used.[33] While the ECG changes of RVH result largely from the chamber's anatomical dominance, the cause of the heart disease and associated hemodynamic alterations often contribute to the abnormal ECG pattern. At times, the etiology of the cardiac disorder and the severity of right ventricular pressure can be estimated from an analysis of the ECG.

In RVH the axis shifts to the right, the degree of axis deviation varying with the clinical disorder, and this is accompanied by vertical position and clockwise rotation. Based on the QRS pattern in lead V_1, RVH can generally be separated into three groups, namely, a dominant R wave (qR, rR, rsR') (Figs. 4–12 and 4–AE4, p. 146), RS complex (Rs, Rsr'), and rS or rsr' complex. The different QRS patterns may provide a clue to the degree of elevation in right ventricular pressure. In general, a qR complex, a prominent R wave with a slur on the upstroke, or an rsR' complex (incomplete right bundle branch block) suggests that right ventricular pressure exceeds (qR), is equal to (R or rR), or is lower than (rsR') left ventricular pressure, respectively. Ex-

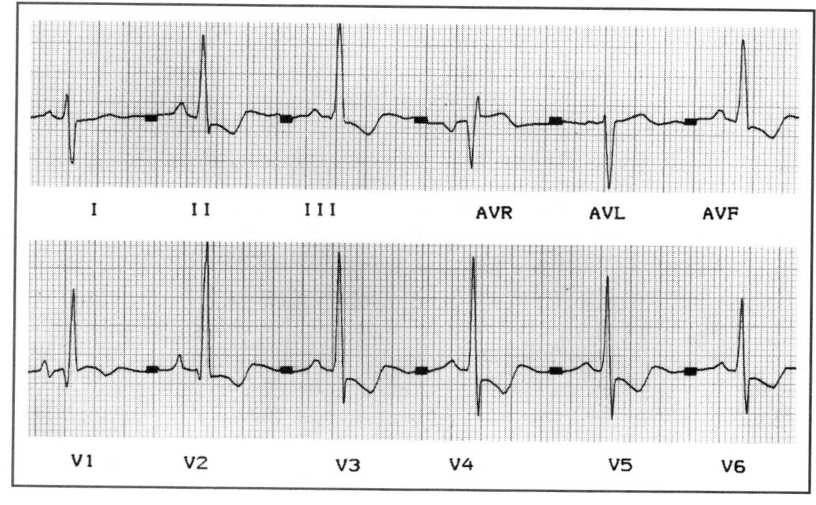

FIGURE 4–12. Right ventricular hypertrophy with marked right-axis deviation and vertical position of the QRS complex, a qR pattern in leads V_1 and V_2, and tall R wave in lead V_1. The qR pattern in leads V_1 and V_2 suggests that the right ventricular pressure exceeds the left ventricular pressure. Absence of the typical P wave changes in leads I, II, and III is compatible with pulmonary hypertension due to pulmonary fibrosis (see text). The ST-T changes are secondary to the right ventricular hypertrophy.

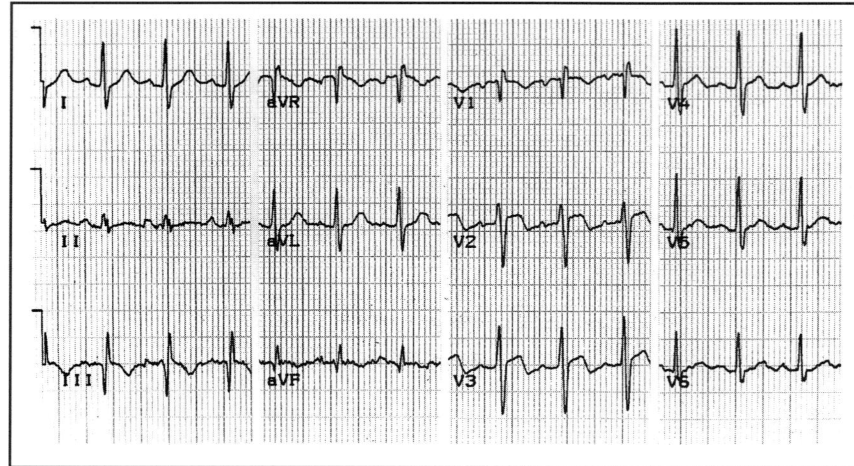

FIGURE 4–13. Acute massive pulmonary embolus with the characteristic S_1Q_3 pattern and the more common but nonspecific changes including incomplete right bundle branch block and ST segment elevation in leads V_1 to V_3 with terminal T wave inversion.

amples include severe pulmonary stenosis or primary pulmonary hypertension (qR), tetralogy of Fallot or Eisenmenger complex (R or rR), and atrial septal defect (rsR′), respectively. In the latter, hypertrophy of the outflow tract of the right ventricle is responsible for the R′ wave.

In the presence of RVH the delay of ventricular activation results in earlier recovery of the endocardium, and as in LVH, repolarization proceeds from endocardium to epicardium. The ST segment is thereby depressed and the T wave inverted in lead V_1 and occasionally in V_2. Significant ST-segment depression and T-wave inversion are, as a rule, indicative of moderate or severe right ventricular hypertension.

In the adult with acquired RVH the most commonly encountered ECG changes include right-axis deviation and an R/S ratio equal to or greater than 1 in V_1, with an R wave 0.5 mV or greater. Isolated right-axis deviation of +100 to −90 degrees is considered by some to be indicative of RVH, but this criterion alone is less sensitive (Fig. 4–AE5, p. 146). An R/S ratio greater than 1 in lead V_1 alone is not diagnostic of RVH, since it may be recorded in patients with a posterior infarction or occasionally in the absence of heart disease.

ACUTE PULMONARY EMBOLISM (ACUTE COR PULMONALE) (see Chap. 46). The most characteristic ECG feature of this disorder is probably the transient nature of the changes, and for this reason serial tracings are most helpful.[39] In 49 proven cases of acute pulmonary embolism, the ECG diagnosis was considered probable in 37 patients (76 per cent). This was based on the presence of three or more of the following ECG changes: (1) incomplete or complete RBBB ($n = 33$); associated with ST elevation ($n = 17$) and positive T wave in lead V_1 ($n = 3$); (2) S wave in leads I and aV_l of >1.5 mm ($n = 36$); (3) clockwise rotation ($n = 25$); (4) Q waves in leads III and aV_f but not in lead II ($n = 24$); (5) right-axis deviation >90 degrees ($n = 16$) or indeterminate axis ($n = 15$); (6) low-voltage QRS complex of <5 mm in limb leads ($n = 10$); and (7) T wave inversion in leads III and aV_f ($n = 16$) or leads V_1 to V_4 ($n = 13$) (Fig. 4–13). Of the 12 patients with normal ECG on admission, only 3 became positive on serial tracings.[40] The ECG changes are most likely related to acute pulmonary hypertension with right atrial and ventricular dilation, hypoxia, and perhaps myocardial ischemia. Acute atrial dilation coupled with myocardial ischemia is probably responsible for the frequent atrial arrhythmias. Despite the high incidence of abnormal tracings, the diagnosis is difficult because of the nonspecific nature of the ECG changes. While a single ECG is rarely helpful, a comparison with a tracing obtained before the acute episode and serial tracings after the episode increase significantly the sensitivity of the ECG.

CHRONIC OBSTRUCTIVE LUNG DISEASE (COLD) AND COR PULMONALE (see Chap. 47). The ECG pattern of COLD and COLD with pulmonary hypertension (cor pulmonale) can be ascribed to a combination of positional changes, increased lung volume, and RVH. ECG changes include right-axis deviation of the P wave, increased amplitude and "peaked" appearance of the P wave in the limb leads, and "peaked" and biphasic morphology wave in leads V_1 and V_2 (Figs. 4–10*B* and 4–14). A P-wave axis of +90 degrees is highly suggestive of COLD. The shift of the P-wave axis is most likely due to overinflation of the lungs. While right-axis deviation of the P wave is present in about 80 per cent of patients with obstructive lung disease, only 7 per cent of the patients with restrictive lung disease manifest right-axis deviation of the P wave. Similarly, 53 per cent of patients with restrictive lung disease manifest a horizontal P-wave axis as contrasted with only 8 per cent of the patients with obstructive lung disease.[41] Because of the large P-wave area, the Ta segment is exaggerated and occasionally interpreted as ST-segment depression. Right-

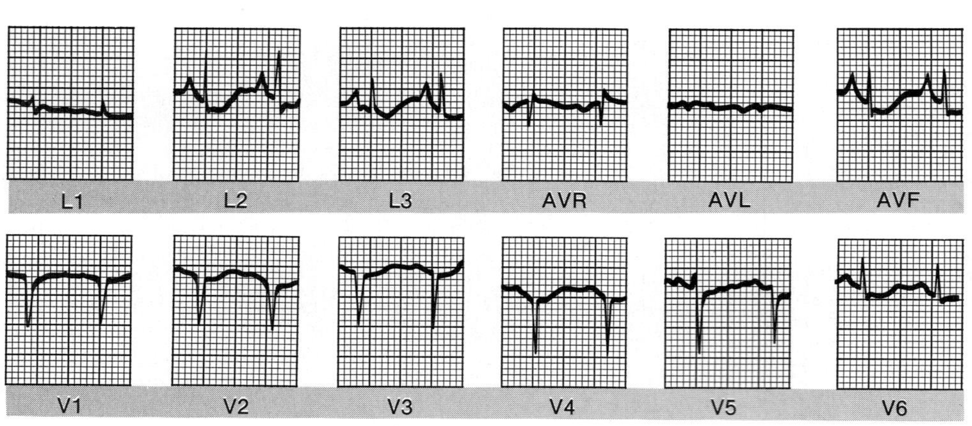

FIGURE 4–14. A case of chronic obstructive lung disease (COLD) simulating an anteroseptal myocardial infarction. The characteristic features of COLD include "pointed" tall P waves in leads 2, 3, AV_f with right-axis deviation (+90 degrees), tendency to right axis of the QRS, clockwise rotation, and "pseudo–ST segment" depression. The latter reflects atrial repolarization. The clockwise rotation simulates anteroseptal myocardial infarction.

axis deviation and clockwise rotation are characteristic findings. Occasionally, an $S_1S_2S_3$ pattern may be present.[42] Amplitude of the precordial R wave is reduced in leads V_5 and V_6, often measuring less than 0.7 mV. When the clockwise rotation is marked, absence of the R wave in precordial leads simulates an anterior myocardial infarction. With progression to pulmonary hypertension and RVH, prominent R waves may appear in leads V_1 and V_2. These changes are probably due to unopposed late activation of the crista terminalis and right ventricular free wall. Right atrial dilatation is probably responsible for the QR pattern in V_1, with the Q wave reflecting right atrial intracavitary potential (as occurs also in tricuspid regurgitation) (Fig. 4–AE1). As indicated, the sensitivity of the ECG for cor pulmonale is relatively low, the test being diagnostic in about 25 to 40 per cent of patients with confirmed RVH.

In *biventricular hypertrophy,* the LV forces are dominant and often obscure the RVH.

VECTORCARDIOGRAM. In RVH, the characteristic VCG changes of the QRS loop are recorded in the transverse plane, and these fall into three general types (Fig. 4–15). In type A, the configuration varies considerably. It may be oval, narrow, or figure-of-eight. The major segment of the loops is located anteriorly and to the right. The loop is inscribed clockwise or, as in the case of the figure-of-eight loop, initially counterclockwise with the latter component recorded clockwise. An oval loop is illustrated in Figure 4–15. In type B, the loop is inscribed clockwise or counterclockwise, is often figure-of-eight, and is located primarily in the left anterior and to a lesser extent in the left and right posterior quadrants. In type C, the loop is inscribed counterclockwise, with 50 per cent of the loop located in posterior left and right quadrants. Of the three, type A usually reflects severe RVH, while type B is most often encountered in patients with atrial septal defect and mitral stenosis. Type C can be recorded with chronic obstructive lung disease.

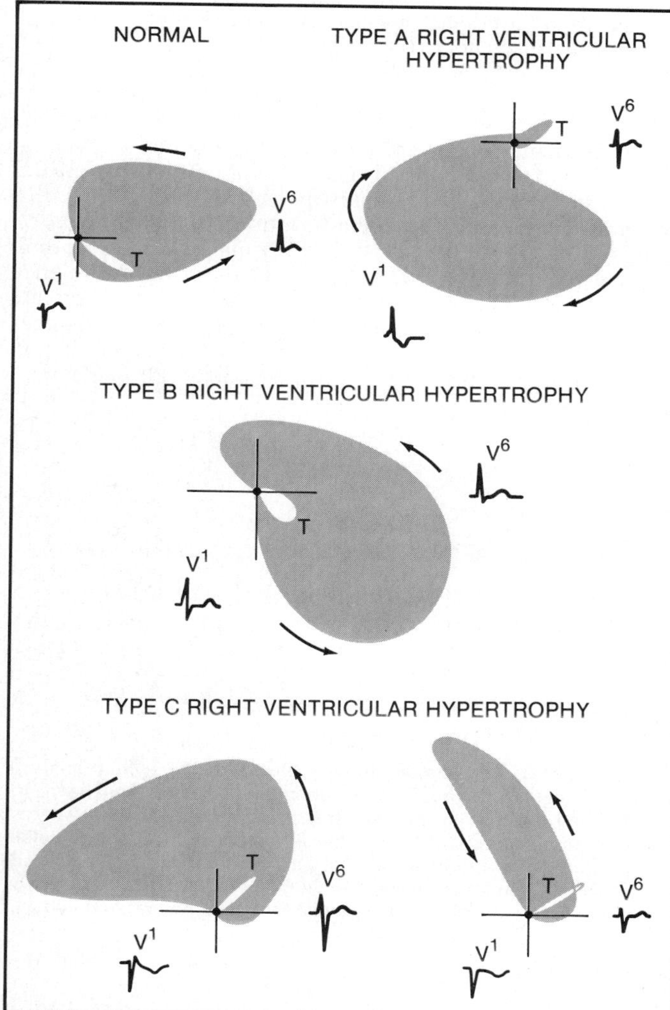

FIGURE 4–15. Diagrammatic representation of the three common, but not exclusive, VCG patterns of right ventricular hypertrophy recorded in the horizontal plane. When compared with the normal, the QRS loops are located in the right and left anterior quadrants in type A and in the left anterior and to a lesser extent left and right posterior quadrants in type B; a major portion of the loop is located in the left and right posterior quadrants in type C. (Modified from Chou, T. C., Helm, R. A., and Kaplan, S.: Clinical Vectorcardiography. 2nd ed. New York, Grune and Stratton, 1974, pp. 87, 99, 102.)

VENTRICULAR HYPERTROPHY IN THE PRESENCE OF CONDUCTION DEFECTS

The diagnosis of ventricular hypertrophy in the presence of intraventricular conduction defect is difficult, if not impossible, owing in part to the fact that a portion of cardiac activation may be unopposed for a period of time, resulting in misleading voltage changes[43] (Fig. 4–AE6, p. 146). It has been suggested that in the presence of right bundle branch block (RBBB), an R′ greater than 1.0 to 1.5 mV indicates associated RVH. However, it is not unusual to record preoperatively a normal QRS complex in lead V_1, only to register postoperatively an RBBB with an R′ wave greater than 1.0 or 1.5 mV, indicating that this criterion of RVH may not be valid in the presence of RBBB (Fig. 4–AE7, p. 147). Left bundle branch block (LBBB) makes a diagnosis of RVH and LVH essentially impossible. In the presence of RBBB, LVH may be suspected when the S wave in lead V_1 and the R wave in lead V_6 satisfy voltage criteria for LVH. However, such an interpretation is subject to the limitations imposed by the relatively low sensitivity and specificity of the voltage criteria. It also has been suggested that the QRS is significantly longer in LBBB with LVH than with isolated LBBB.

In a study of 50 patients with left anterior fascicular block, the sum of S in lead III and the maximal R + S in any precordial lead equal to or exceeding 3 mV (30 mm) showed a specificity of 87 per cent, a sensitivity of 96 per cent, a positive predictive value of 89 per cent, and a negative predictive value of 95 per cent for LVH.[44]

Intraventricular Conduction Defects

The bundle of His bifurcates into right and left bundles (see Fig. 20–5, p. 551). The ribbon-like right bundle descends subendocardially on the right side of the septum. At the base of the right ventricular anterior papillary muscle, it divides and supplies fibers to the free right ventricular wall and the right side of the septum. The left bundle divides into an anterior division (LAD) and posterior division (LPD), which supply the left ventricular wall and left side of the septum. Discrete anatomical lesions, asynchrony of conduction in the bundles or its branches, nonuniformity of refractoriness, changes in membrane responsiveness, and a decrease in the magnitude of phase 4 of the transmembrane action potential (see p. 109) may, singly or in combination, cause block of conduction in the bundle branches (BBB) and the divisions of the left bundle. However, most commonly BBB is due to an anatomical lesion. In transient BBB, the specific underlying electrophysiological mechanism may be difficult to define.

Left Bundle Branch Block (LBBB)

Interruption of the left bundle branch results in early activation of the right side of the septum and of the right ventricular myocardium. Transseptal activation from right to left is transmyocardial and thus slow, and probably a major cause of the prolonged ventricular activation. Initial activation of the ventricles proceeds from right to left, inferiorly, and more often anteriorly than posteriorly. This is followed by continued activation of the septum and of the adjacent free left ventricular wall, with the activation proceeding to the left, posteriorly, and inferiorly. This phase of activation is rapid, presumably because the impulse enters the Purkinje system below the site of the BBB. Last to be activated are the lateral wall and basal aspect of the left ventricle, with a vector oriented posteriorly, superiorly, and, less frequently, inferiorly.

In complete LBBB, the QRS complex is prolonged, measuring 0.12 to 0.18 sec (Fig. 4–16).[45] An upright notched or slurred R wave reflecting the right-to-left myocardial activation is recorded in leads I, aV_l, and V_6. A small R wave followed by an S wave is present in aV_f; the R wave and

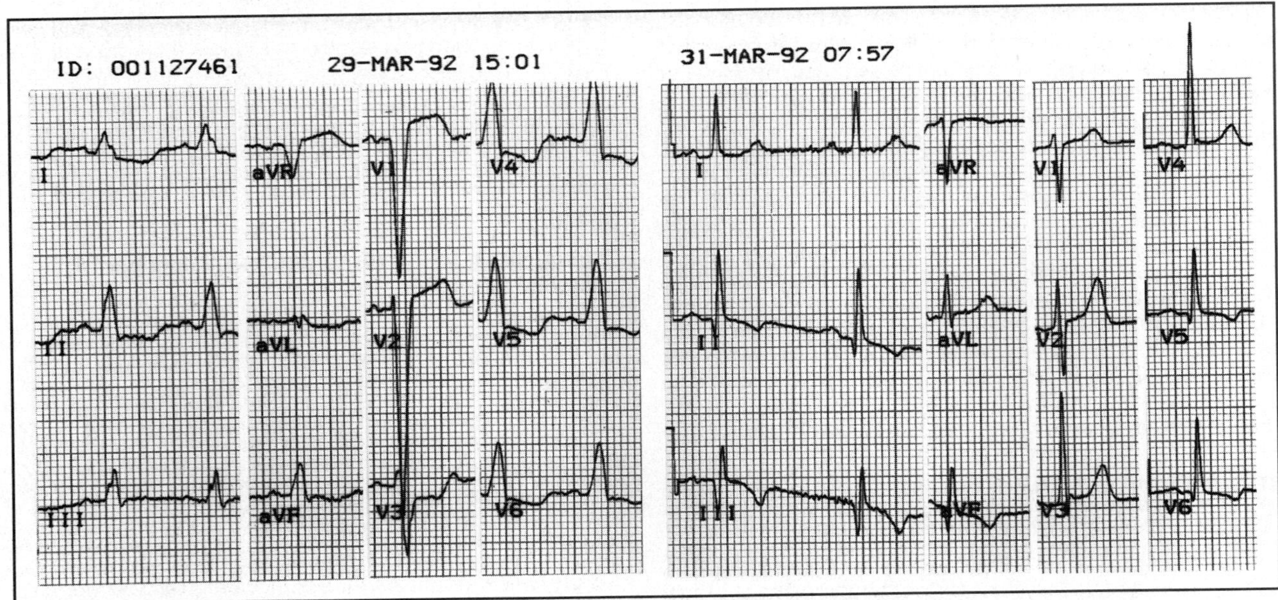

FIGURE 4–16. Left bundle branch block (LBBB) obscuring an inferior myocardial infarction. LBBB is present in the left panel at a heart rate of 100 beats/min. With slowing of the heart rate to 75 beats/min in the right panel, the intraventricular conduction normalizes with appearance of an inferior myocardial infarction and most likely ischemic T waves in leads V_5 and V_6. With LBBB, the septum depolarizes from right to left, and the left ventricular intracavitary potential is initially positive, thus in keeping with the "window" concept of ECG changes of myocardial infarction, precluding recording of a Q wave.

the S wave reflect, respectively, the initial septal activation directed inferiorly and the superior orientation of the final vector. An rS or a QS complex, depending on whether the initial activation is oriented anteriorly or posteriorly, is recorded in lead V_1, with the S wave reflecting activation of the left ventricle from right to left. An initial R wave in lead V_1 is present in about 45 per cent of cases of LBBB. The precordial leads V_1 to V_4 may exhibit a small R wave, with the R waves in the midprecordial leads occasionally lower in amplitude than those in the right precordial leads. One clinically important feature of LBBB is an absence of a septal Q, owing to the initial right-to-left septal activation. Similarly, a Q wave fails to register when either myocardial infarction complicates preexisting LBBB or when LBBB complicates an acute myocardial infarction (see p. 127) (Fig. 4–16). The frontal axis in LBBB may be either normal or directed to the left (−30 to −90 degrees), the prevalence of the two being about equal. Although it has been accepted that an abnormal left axis in excess of −45 degrees is nearly always due to a left anterior divisional block, LBBB per se also may result in pronounced left-axis deviation.

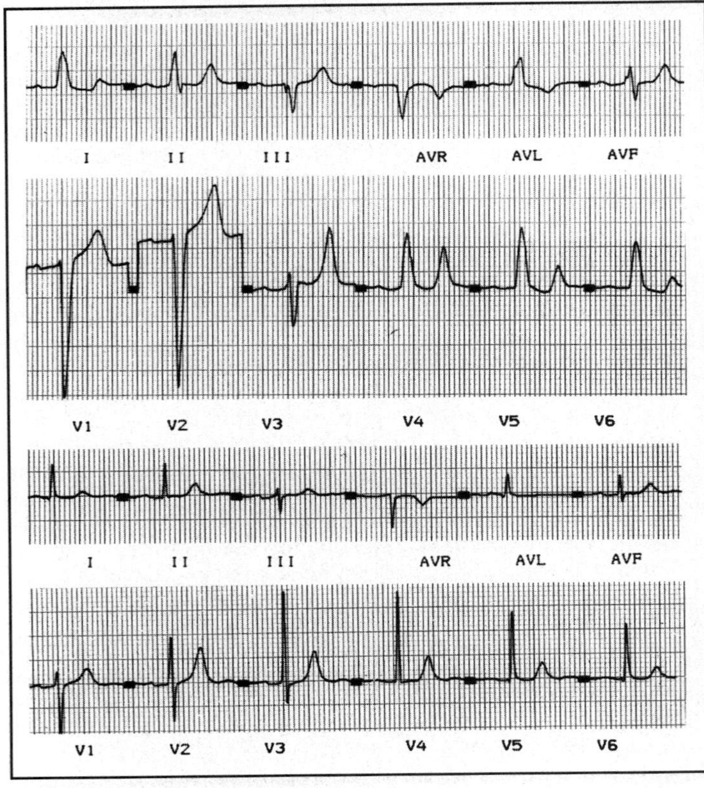

FIGURE 4–17. Left bundle branch block (LBBB) with primary T wave changes; i.e., the T waves are upright rather than being inverted and opposite to the QRS area. Such primary T waves suggest a primary myocardial disorder that is not secondary to the bundle branch block. In approximately 15 per cent, however, with normalization of the intraventricular conduction the electrocardiogram is normal *(lower panel)*. In this instance the LBBB was rate-related.

In LBBB, the direction of the ST-segment and T-wave vectors is opposite to that of the QRS vector. In the presence of an upright QRS complex in leads I, aV_l, and V_6, the ST segment is depressed and the T waves are inverted. The opposite is true in leads V_1, V_2, and V_3, in which a predominantly negative QRS complex is recorded. The ST-segment and T-wave changes are secondary to the conduction disturbance, and the magnitude of the change parallels the magnitude of the QRS aberration. Occasionally LBBB is associated with an isoelectric ST segment and a T-wave vector concordant with the QRS vector. Such primary T-wave changes suggest a myocardial abnormality independent of the LBBB, which may be due, for example, to accompanying myocardial ischemia. However, this is not always a reliable sign of a primary myocardial disorder (Fig. 4–17).

Incomplete LBBB implies a greater delay of conduction in the left than in the right bundle, with initial right-to-left septal activation and loss of the septal Q wave. In contrast to complete LBBB, the left bundle ultimately contributes to activation of the septum and left ventricular wall. ECG criteria for incomplete LBBB include a QRS complex of 0.10 to 0.12 sec, loss of the initial septal Q wave, slurring or notching, and often high voltage of the QRS complex.

In the transverse plane of the VCG, the QRS loop of LBBB is oriented to the left and posteriorly. The initial portion of the loop reflects septal activation and is inscribed slowly from right to left and anteriorly. The remainder of the loop is inscribed clockwise with slow inscription of the midportion, most likely reflecting slow intramyocardial conduction through the left ventricular wall. The T loop points in a direction opposite to that of the QRS.

Right Bundle Branch Block (RBBB)

In RBBB the septum is activated normally, from left to right. While the left ventricle is activated normally, right ventricular depolarization is delayed, the right ventricle being last to be activated, and this terminal activation is unopposed. Prolongation of the QRS complex is largely due to delayed activation of the right ventricular wall. The initial dominant septal force is directed from left to right, anteriorly and superiorly, followed by a vector dominated by the left ventricle, oriented to the left, inferiorly, and either somewhat anteriorly or posteriorly. The final vector representing activation of the right ventricle is directed to the right, anteriorly, and either superiorly, inferiorly, or horizontally.

The characteristic ECG changes of RBBB are recorded in lead V_1. The initial normal septal activation inscribes an R wave, followed by an S wave reflecting left ventricular activation and a final R′ wave due to depolarization of the right ventricle from left to right and anteriorly. The depth of the S wave in lead V_1 varies depending on whether the left ventricular activation generates a more posteriorly or anteriorly oriented vector. In the former, a prominent S wave separates the R wave from the R′ wave, while in the latter, the S wave may be shallow or a slur or, indeed, may be absent. Leads facing the left side of the septum, namely, I, aV_l, V_5, and V_6, record an initial Q wave followed by an R wave of normal duration and a prolonged, relatively shallow S wave. The latter reflects delayed activation of the right ventricle (Figs. 4–18 to 4–20). Because the initial septal activation is normal, namely, left to right, RBBB, in contrast to LBBB, does not obscure myocardial infarction.

The T wave is usually inverted in lead V_1 and occasionally in V_2, while it is upright in the remaining precordial and limb leads, a direction opposite to the *terminal* portion of the QRS complex.

Preliminary evidence suggests that patients with RBBB with a normal QT interval but persistent ST-segment elevation in leads V_1 to V_3 not explainable by electrolyte disturbances, ischemia, or structural heart disease are prone to rapid polymorphic ventricular tachycardia and sudden death.[46] Others propose that the terminal "delay" in the right precordial leads represents a J wave rather than delay due to RBBB. The mechanism of the J wave is unclear and may vary depending on the underlying clinical condition.[47]

The characteristic VCG feature is evident in the transverse plane and consists of a slowly inscribed terminal appendage directed to the right and anteriorly. The initial septal and left ventricular portion of the loop is normal.

Divisional (Fascicular) Blocks

The ventricular conduction system, including the right bundle branch and the two divisions of the left bundle, can be considered for purposes of clinical electrocardiography to consist of three divisions (fascicles) (Fig. 4–21). Divisional blocks are, with rare exception, acquired. Although the evidence for the existence of anatomically discrete divisions of the left bundle branch is not convincing, experimental data support a functional divisional conduction system.[48]

Furthermore, nearly simultaneous early endocardial activation at two sites—the middle anterior and posterior paraseptal areas—is consistent with the concept of functional divisions of the left bundle. This concept is also supported by distinctive and predictable ECG patterns. Thus, from the ECG standpoint, the concept of divisions of the left bundle is a useful one.[49]

BLOCK OF ANTERIOR DIVISION OF THE LEFT BUNDLE BRANCH (ANTERIOR FASCICULAR BLOCK). In the presence of left anterior divisional block, the initial septal activation proceeds inferiorly, anteriorly, to the right, and occasionally to the left. This is followed by activation of inferior and apical

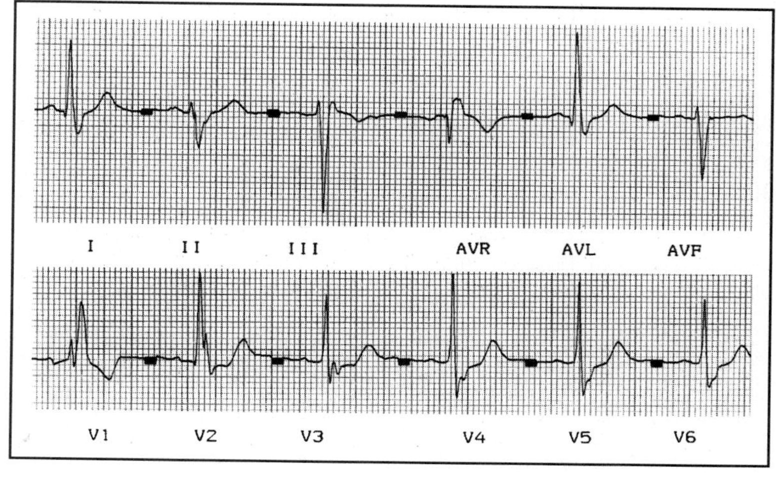

FIGURE 4–18. Right bundle branch block manifest by prominent S wave in leads I, aV_l, and the left ventricular precordial leads and an rsR pattern in lead V_1. The left anterior fascicular block is indicated by the marked left-axis deviation in the frontal leads.

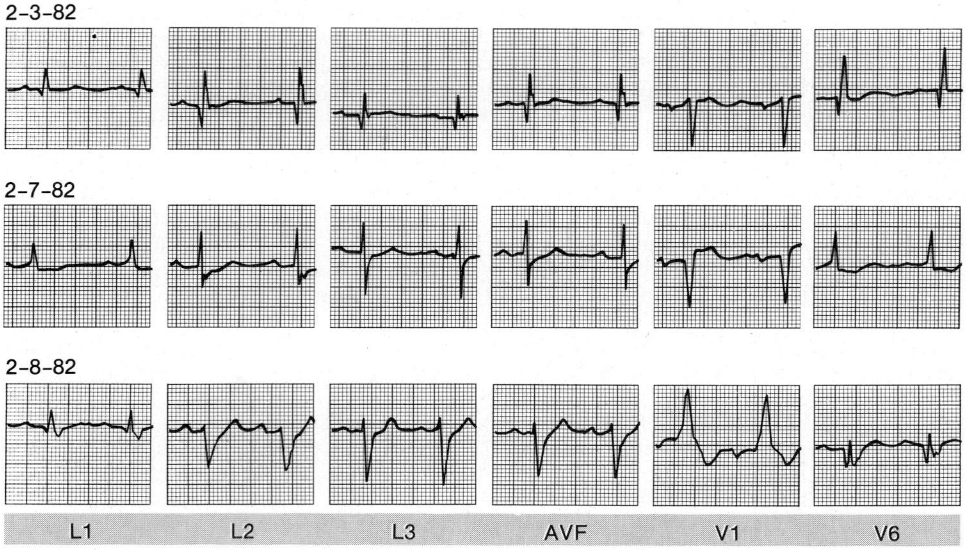

FIGURE 4–19. Masking of myocardial infarction Q waves by intraventricular conduction defects. Top trace (2-3-82) illustrates an inferolateral infarction manifested by Q waves in leads II, III, aV_f, and V_6. Incomplete LBBB and LAFB (left anterior fascicular block) in the middle trace (2-7-82) mask the inferior and lateral infarction. In the bottom trace (2-8-82), the LAFB masks the inferior infarction. The RBBB, in contrast to the incomplete LBBB in the middle trace, does not obscure the lateral infarction. (From Fisch, C.: Evolution of the clinical electrocardiogram. Reprinted with permission of the American College of Cardiology. J. Am. Coll. Cardiol. *14:*1127, 1989.)

areas with the vector oriented inferiorly, to the left, and anteriorly. Final activation is that of the anterolateral and posterobasal left ventricular wall, the vector oriented superiorly, posteriorly, and to the left (Fig. 4–AE8, p. 147).

The resultant ECG pattern is characteristic (Figs. 4–18 through 4–21). Lead I records a dominant R wave, with or without an initial Q wave. The criterion of a small Q wave in leads I and aV_l is the subject of continued controversy.[21] The presence or absence of a Q wave depends on whether the initial septal activation is directed to the right or to the left. Since the initial activation is directed inferiorly, leads II, III, and aV_f inscribe an R wave followed by a deep S wave reflecting activation of the anterolateral and posterobasal segments of the left ventricle. The QRS axis varies from −45 to −90 degrees. The duration of the QRS is less than 0.12 sec[21] (Figs. 4–18 and 4–20).

The precordial transitional zone is frequently displaced to the left. The amplitude of the R wave is diminished, with a prominent S wave in V_5 and V_6 reflecting the superior orientation of the mean left ventricular vector. The S wave is exaggerated when the final order of activation is directed to the right. Because of the inferior orientation of the initial vector, the right and midprecordial leads may register an initial Q wave. Such patterns could be mistaken for anteroseptal myocardial infarction were it not for the fact that an R wave is recorded when the leads are placed an interspace lower (Fig. 4–AE9, p. 147). The T waves are normally upright except in lead aV_r and occasionally in leads aV_l and V_1.

BLOCK OF POSTERIOR DIVISION OF THE LEFT BUNDLE BRANCH (POSTERIOR FASCICULAR BLOCK). Left posterior divisional block is a rare finding, and its pattern is nonspecific. It can be recorded in asthenic individuals and patients with emphysema, RVH, and extensive lateral infarction.[49] Diagnosis is secure only if a normal or a different ECG pattern is recorded before appearance of the block (Fig. 4–AE82, p. 147).

In the presence of left posterior divisional block, activation begins in the midseptal and paraseptal areas, with the vector directed to the left, anteriorly, and superiorly. This is followed by activation of the left ventricular anterior and anterolateral walls, with the vector directed to the left and anteriorly. Final activation is of the inferior and posterior walls with the vector directed inferiorly, posteriorly, and to the right. The QRS duration is less than 0.12 sec.[21] In the limb leads, the initial superior and left orientation of septal vectors is reflected as R waves in leads I and aV_l and a narrow, 0.025-msec Q wave in leads II, III, I, and aV_f. The

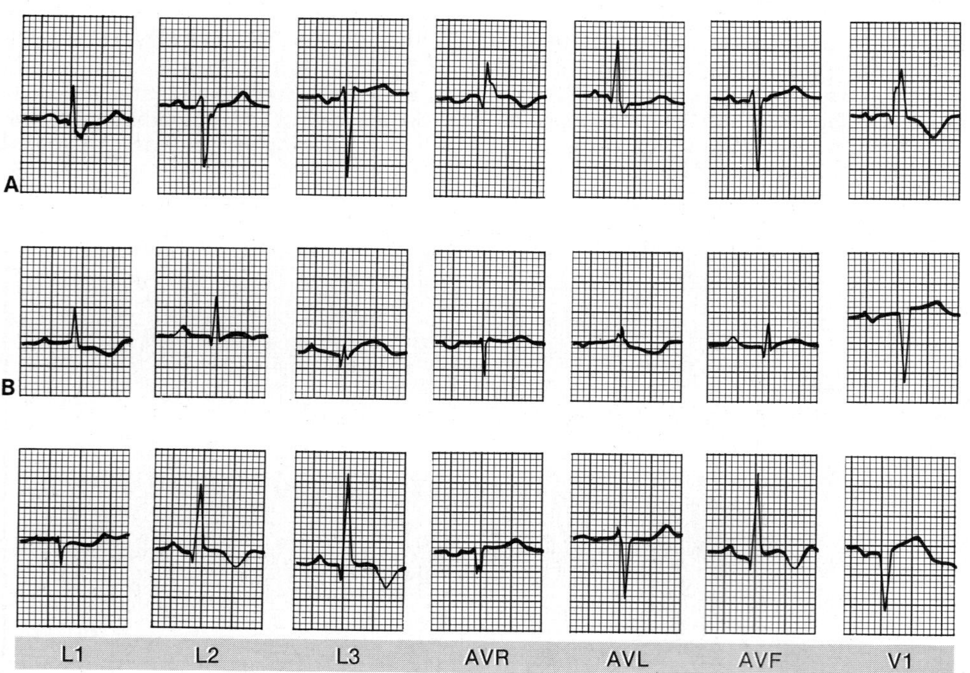

FIGURE 4–20. *A,* Right bundle branch block with left anterior divisional block. *B,* Upper trace, the control trace, illustrates an inferior myocardial infarction with a normal QRS axis. The bottom trace demonstrates left posterior divisional block (LPDB). Because the latter may be due to causes other than LPDB a diagnosis of LPDB requires evidence of normal conduction prior to appearance of LPDB such as illustrated in upper trace of panel B.

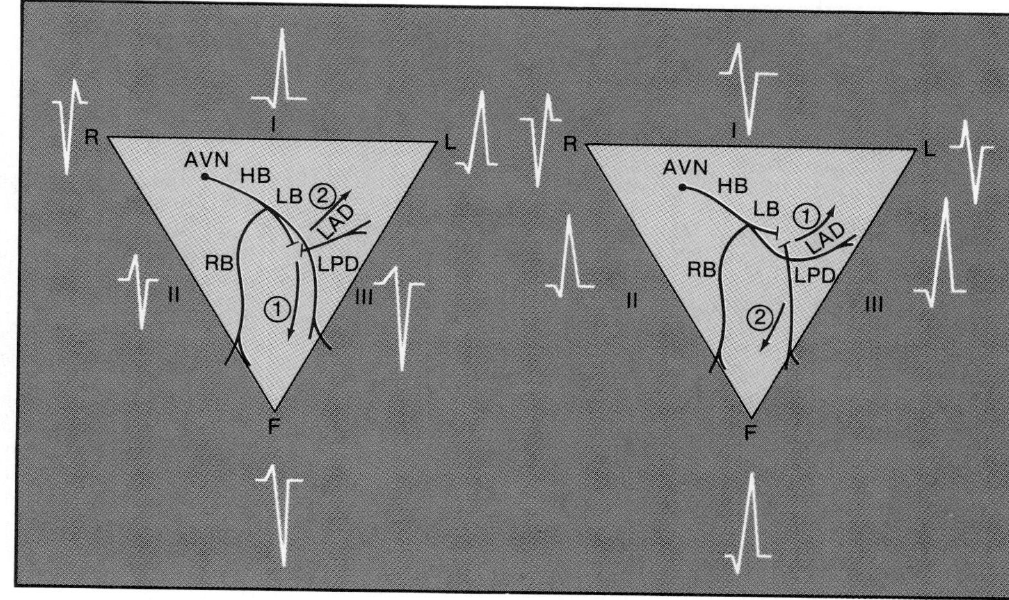

FIGURE 4–21. Diagrammatic representation of the conduction system. Interruption of the LAD *(left)* results in an initial inferior *(1)* followed by a dominant superior *(2)* direction of activation; interruption of the LPD *(right)* results in an initial superior *(1)* followed by a dominant inferior *(2)* direction of activation. AVN = atrioventricular node; HB = His bundle; LB = left bundle; RB = right bundle; LAD = left anterior division; LPD = left posterior division.

R waves in leads I and aV_l are small and followed by deep S waves reflecting the inferior, posterior, and right orientation of the wave of activation (Figs. 4–20 and 4–21). The initial superior force and final inferior force result in a QR complex in leads II, III, and aV_f. The amplitude of the R wave in lead III exceeds the R wave in lead II. The frontal axis varies from about +90 to +120 degrees, or perhaps +80 to +140 degrees. The T wave is usually normal.

RIGHT BUNDLE BRANCH BLOCK AND DIVISIONAL BLOCKS. RBBB with left anterior divisional block is the most common combination (Fig. 4–18). The activation during the first 0.08 sec determines the axis and identifies the left anterior divisional block. The delay of depolarization due to RBBB results in a final activation of the right ventricle to the right and anteriorly (Figs. 4–20 and 4–AE8, p. 147).

RBBB with left posterior divisional block is a rare combination. The initial 0.08 sec defines the axis and divisional block, while the final delayed activation, oriented to the right and anteriorly, reflects RBBB (Fig. 4–AE8).

Block of the right bundle and both divisions of the left bundle (trifascicular block) can occur in the presence of RBBB with alternating left anterior and posterior divisional blocks. Such patterns are usually associated with Mobitz (type II) AV block. It has been suggested that RBBB with either hemiblock and a prolonged P-R interval may be a manifestation of trifascicular block. Although the prolonged P-R interval may be due to delayed conduction in the remaining division, the delay also may reflect AV nodal delay.

NONSPECIFIC INTRAVENTRICULAR CONDUCTION DEFECT (IVCD). The QRS complex may be abnormally prolonged but without the characteristic pattern of either RBBB or LBBB. Such conduction delays are referred to as *nonspecific* IVCD. These often resemble LBBB or LBBB with an abnormal left-axis deviation, a combination suggesting left anterior hemiblock with peripheral conduction delay. Presence of a normal Q wave supports peripheral delay as the cause of QRS prolongation. Although such a nonspecific prolongation may be due to drugs or electrolyte abnormalities, it is most often due to organic heart disease. An interesting form of right ventricular conduction delay has been described in patients with arrhythmogenic ventricular dysplasia. The delayed activation is inscribed in the form of a sharp deflection after termination of the QRS, during the ST segment or upstroke of the T wave.[50]

MASQUERADING BUNDLE BRANCH BLOCK. This form of BBB is rare. It is manifest by RBBB, marked left-axis deviation, and absence of a significant S wave in leads I, aV_l, and V_6. In essence, it can be described as LBBB in the limb leads and RBBB in the chest leads. In contrast to the ordinary RBBB with left anterior fascicular block, or bifascicular block, the masquerading BBB is usually associated with significant heart disease and a relatively poor long-term prognosis. (Fig. 4–22).[51]

BILATERAL BUNDLE BRANCH BLOCK. This diagnosis can be considered when alternating RBBB and LBBB are present. Any other combination of conduction delays cannot be differentiated from block in the AV junction. For example, simultaneous block in both bundles results in complete AV block. Similarly, intermittent delay or block in one bundle and complete block of conduction in the contralateral bundle will manifest either as BBB with a prolonged P-R interval or intermittent AV block. In the presence of BBB, a superimposed AV block due to failure of conduction in the contralateral bundle branch cannot be differentiated from block in the AV junction (Fig. 4–23).

BUNDLE BRANCH BLOCK ALTERNANS. Bundle branch block (BBB) alternans is a rare finding and may be manifested as alternans of (1) RBBB or LBBB with a normal QRS, (2) RBBB and LBBB (see Bilateral BBB), or (3) complete and incomplete RBBB or LBBB.[52]

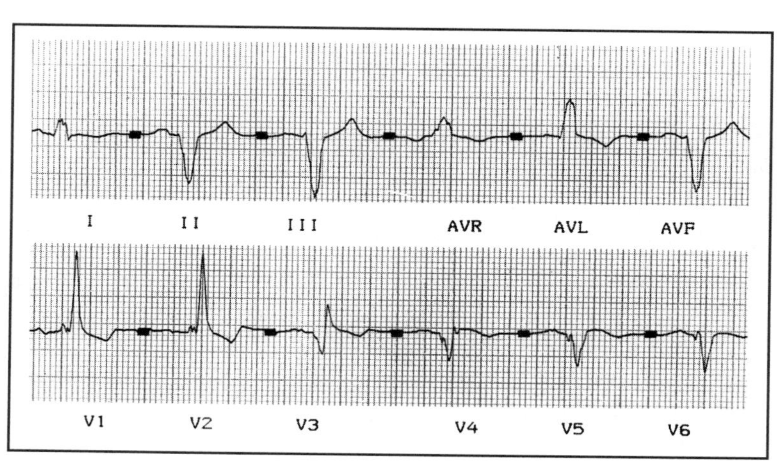

FIGURE 4–22. Anterolateral myocardial infarction with a "masquerading" bundle branch block. The latter is indicated by the right bundle branch block (RBBB)–like pattern in leads V_1 and V_2 but without the characteristic, diagnostic S wave in leads I and aV_l. The exact mechanism of this type of intraventricular conduction is unclear. It is possible that the changes in right precordial leads are not due to RBBB.

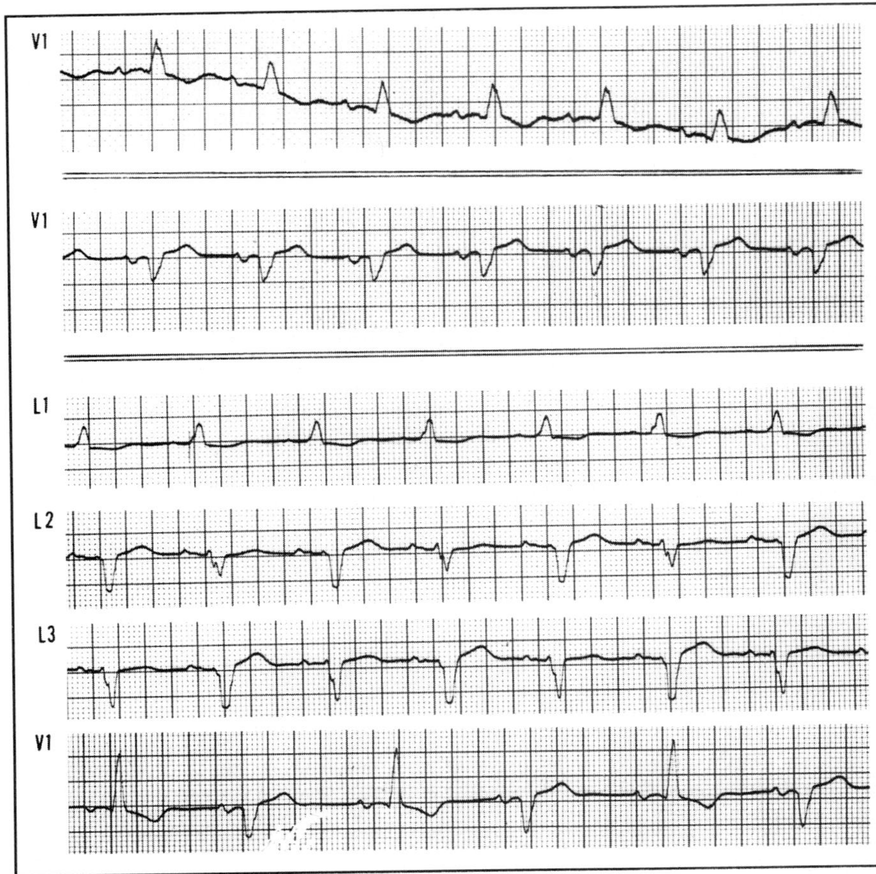

FIGURE 4–23. Alternating P-R interval and bundle branch block (BBB). *Top tracing,* V1 Right bundle branch block (RBBB) with a P-R interval of 280 msec. *Middle panel,* V1 Left bundle branch block (LBBB) with a P-R interval of 180 msec. *Lower panel,* RBBB alternating with LBBB with alternation of the P-R interval. Leads 1, 2, and 3 exhibit left anterior fascicular block. (From Fisch, C.: Electrocardiography of Arrhythmias. Philadelphia, Lea and Febiger, 1990, p. 433, with permission.)

Aberration

Intraventricular aberration describes a supraventricular impulse with abnormal, bizarre intraventricular conduction (Fig. 4–24).[53] It refers to intraventricular conduction abnormalities related to changing heart rate or other functional alterations in electrophysiological properties, anomalous AV conduction, metabolic and electrolyte abnormalities, and toxic effects of drugs. The term *aberration,* as used currently, does not include fixed organic conduction defects.

The mechanisms responsible for, or contributory to, aberration with changing cycle length include (1) excitation prior to completion of repolarization (i.e., in the presence of a reduced transmembrane potential), (2) unequal refractoriness of conducting tissue resulting in local delay or block of conduction, (3) prolongation of the action potential due to prolongation of the preceding cycle length, (4) failure of restitution of transmembrane electrolyte concentration during diastole, (5) failure of the refractory period to shorten in response to acceleration of the heart rate, (6) a reduced take-off potential secondary to diastole depolarization, (7) concealed transseptal conduction with delay or block of bundle branch conduction, and (8) diffuse depression of intraventricular conduction including that of specialized as well as myocardial tissue.

Aberration may result when any of these mechanisms alter conduction in the bundle branches or the divisions of the left bundle branch (or a combination of the two), the Purkinje fibers, or the myocardium. RBBB is the most common form of aberrancy and is frequently associated with left anterior divisional block. Aberrancy due to LBBB is much less common and in our experience often due to heart disease, although the heart disease may not be clinically evident. An abnormality of intraventricular conduction due to diffuse depression of conduction in the Purkinje system and in the myocardium should be suspected when both the initial and terminal portions of the QRS complex are abnormal.

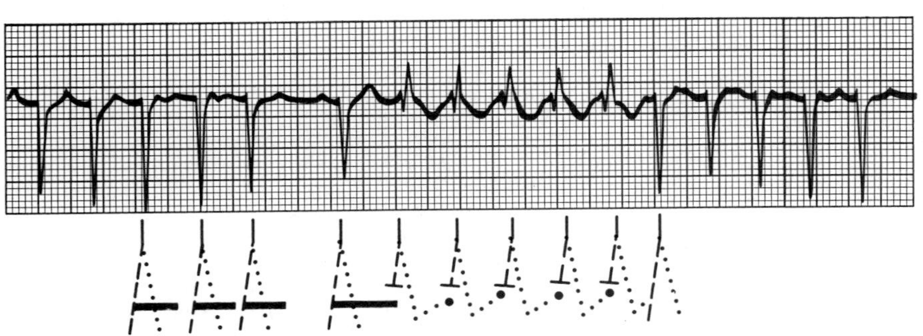

FIGURE 4–24. Atrial tachycardia with Wenckebach (type I) AV block, ventricular aberration due to the Ashman phenomenon, and probably concealed transseptal conduction. The long pause of the atrial tachycardia is followed by five QRS complexes with RBBB morphology. The RBBB of the first QRS reflects the Ashman phenomenon. The aberration is perpetuated by concealed transseptal activation from the left bundle into the right bundle with block of the anterograde conduction of the subsequent sinus impulse in the right bundle. Foreshortening of the R-R cycle, a manifestation of the Wenckebach structure, disturbs the relationship between transseptal and anterograde sinus conduction, and RBB conduction is normalized. In the ladder diagram below the tracing, the solid lines represent the His bundle, the dashes the RBB and the dots the LBB, while the solid horizontal bars denote the refractory period. Neither the P waves nor the AV node is identified in the diagram.

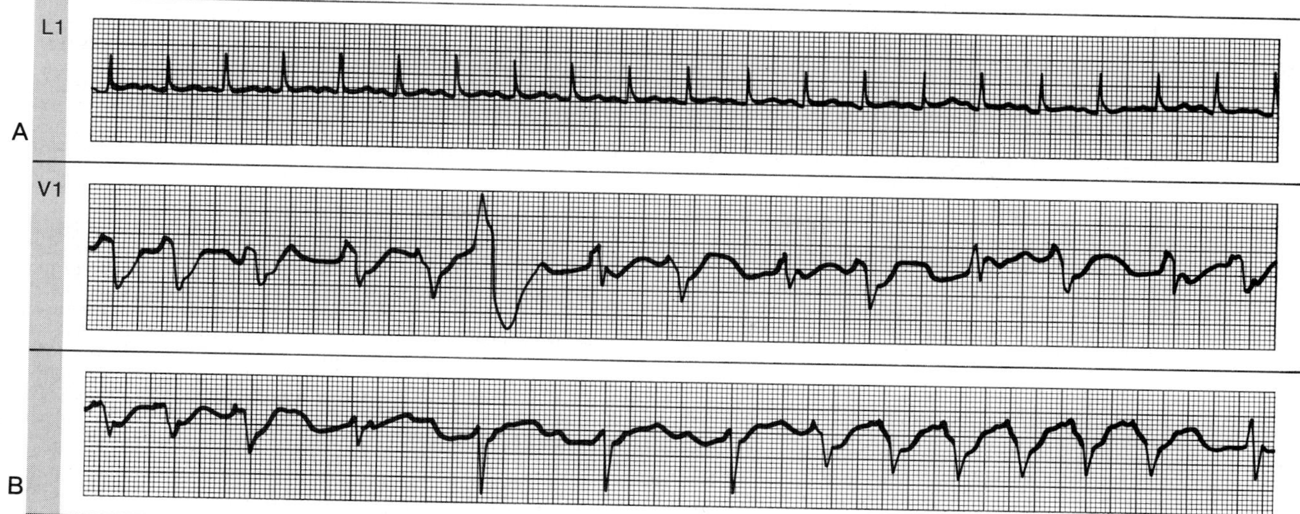

FIGURE 4–25. Intraventricular aberration due to quinidine and acceleration of the heart rate. In panel *A*, control tracing, the ECG is normal with a sinus rate of 130 beats/min. After administration of quinidine (panel *B*), the heart rate is 120 beats/min and the QRS widened to 0.20 sec with a 3:2 Wenckebach (type I) AV block interrrupted by one VPC. P wave duration is prolonged and the P-R interval is increased to 0.28 sec. The QRS complex which follows the longer pauses are narrower, probably owing to a longer period of recovery. In the bottom trace 1:1 AV conduction is interrupted by 2:1 AV conduction. P waves measure 0.20 sec in duration, the P-R interval is 0.40 sec, and the QRS complexes at onset of 2:1 AV block are foreshortened to 0.16 sec. The QRS prolongation to 0.16 sec is due to quinidine, while further widening of the QRS complexes to 0.20 sec in presence of 1:1 AV conduction reflects both the effect of quinidine and the accelerated heart rate.

Of the mechanisms and manifestations of aberration, seven will be considered in further detail: (1) premature excitation, (2) the Ashman phenomenon, (3) acceleration-dependent aberrancy, (4) deceleration-dependent aberrancy, (5) concealed conduction, (6) diffuse myocardial depression of conduction, and (7) postextrasystolic aberrancy.

PREMATURE EXCITATION. Conduction will fail or be delayed if the stimulus falls during the effective or the relative refractory period of recovery. When the impulse falls during the relative refractory period of a single bundle branch, the unilateral delay results in a bundle branch block. The duration of the refractory period may equal that of the transmembrane action potential, so-called voltage-dependent refractoriness, or it may exceed it, so-called time-dependent refractoriness. Duration of the refractory period depends to a great extent on the basic heart rate and on the duration of the immediately preceding cycle(s). Normally, the refractory period shortens with acceleration of the heart rate and lengthens with slowing of the heart rate. With all variables affecting conduction being constant, the degree of aberration is usually a function of prematurity of excitation.

The site of conduction depression and thus the morphology of the aberrant QRS complex is determined by the length of the refractory period of the AV node, the bundle of His, and the bundle system itself. Normally, at slow heart rates, the right bundle branch has the longest refractory period, with the left bundle and the AV node somewhat shorter and the bundle of His the shortest. Only at very rapid rates may the duration of the refractory period of the left bundle exceed that of the right bundle.

EFFECT OF CHANGING CYCLE LENGTH ON REFRACTORINESS (ASHMAN PHENOMENON). This form of aberrancy, also a function of premature excitation, differs from that due to early excitation just described in that the abnormal conduction is a function of an altered duration of the refractory period rather than of changing prematurity of stimulation. Since the duration of the refractory period is a function of the immediately preceding cycle length, the longer the preceding cycle, the longer the refractory period that follows. Consequently, with a relatively constant heart rate, sudden prolongation of the immediately preceding cycle length may result in aberration. This relationship of aberrancy to changes in the preceding cycle length is known as the *Ashman phenomenon.*[54] Aberrancy so initiated may persist for a number of cycles (Fig. 4–24), usually exhibits RBBB morphology, and may be associated with left anterior or rarely with left posterior divisional block.

In the presence of irregular supraventricular rhythms, such as atrial fibrillation, repetitive atrial tachycardia, or atrial tachycardia with Wenckebach (type 1) AV block (Fig. 4–24), aberration due to the Ashman phenomenon is suggested by the following: (1) a relatively long cycle immediately preceding the cycle terminated by the aberrant QRS complex, (2) RBBB aberrancy with normal orientation of the initial QRS vector, (3) irregular coupling of the aberrant QRS complex, and (4) lack of a compensatory pause following the aberrant QRS complex.

ACCELERATION-DEPENDENT ABERRATION (TACHYCARDIA-DEPENDENT ABERRANCY, PHASE 3 ABERRANCY). This form of aberration has been recognized since 1913.[55] At certain critical heart rates, impaired intraventricular conduction results in aberrancy (Figs. 4–25 and 4–26). This phenomenon has been described as tachycardia-dependent aberrancy or phase 3 aberrancy; however, the term *acceleration-dependent aberrancy* appears most appropriate. Aberration often appears at relatively slow rates, frequently below 75 beats/min; similarly, because of the slow rate at which the conduction fails, one would have to postulate an extremely long transmembrane action potential in order to accept excitation during phase 3 as the cause of the impaired conduction. Finally, conduction also will fail with excitation during phase 2 of the action potential.

The appearance and disappearance of aberration often depends on very small changes in cycle length, a change frequently difficult if not impossible to detect in the ECG. Assuming that a reasonably long recording is available, a comparison of the earliest available cycle length terminated by a normal QRS complex with the cycle length terminated by the first aberrant QRS complex will aid in the diagnosis

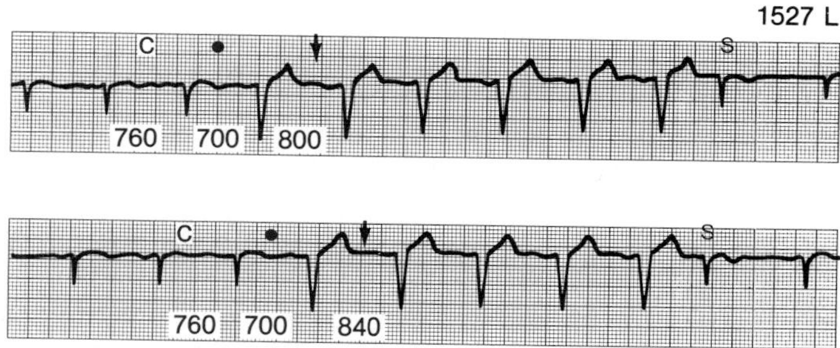

FIGURE 4–26. Acceleration-dependent QRS aberration with the paradox of persistence at a longer cycle and normalization at a shorter cycle than that which initiated the aberration. The duration of the basic cycle (C) is 760 msec. LBBB appears at a cycle length of 700 msec (·) and is perpetuated at cycle lengths of 800 (↓) and 840 (↓) msec; conduction normalizes after a cycle length of 600 msec. Perpetuation of LBBB at a cycle length of 800 and 840 (↓) msec is probably due to transseptal concealment, similar to that described in Figure 4–24. Unexpected normalization of the QRS (S) following the atrial premature contraction is probably due to equalization of conduction in the two bundles; however, supernormal conduction in the left bundle cannot be excluded. (Reproduced with permission from Fisch, C., et al.: Rate dependent aberrancy. Circulation *48:*714, 1973. Copyright 1973 American Heart Association.)

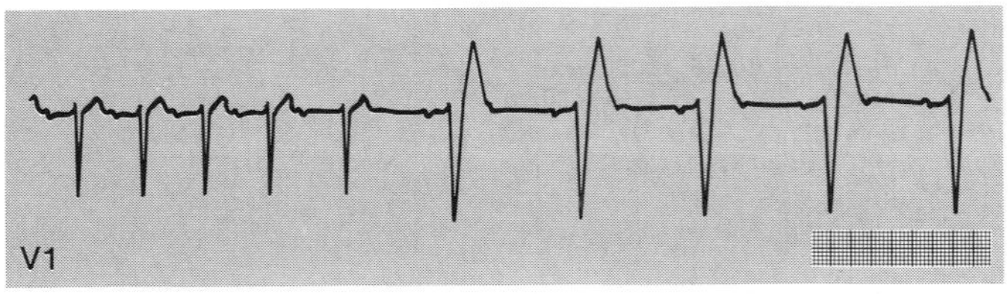

FIGURE 4–27. Deceleration-dependent aberration. The basic rhythm is sinus with Wenckebach (type I) AV block. With 1 : 1 AV conduction, the QRS complexes are normal in duration; with 2 : 1 AV block or after the longer pause of a Wenckebach sequence, LBBB appears. Slow diastolic depolarization (phase 4) of the transmembrane action potential during the prolonged cycle is implicated as the cause of the LBBB.

of acceleration-dependent aberrancy. The difference in the duration of two such cycles is often less than 0.04 sec.

Acceleration-dependent aberration differs from the physiological aberrancy observed in a normal heart. Differences include (1) appearance of aberrancy at relatively slow heart rates, (2) predominance of LBBB morphology, (3) independence from the immediately preceding cycle length, (4) occasional appearance without or with only a slight change in cycle length, and (5) association with heart disease.

QRS aberrancy may persist at an R-R interval considerably longer than the interval that initiated the aberrancy (Fig. 4–26). Three mechanisms have been suggested to explain this paradox: (1) concealed transseptal activation blocking conduction in the contralateral bundles, (2) "fatigue" of the bundle, and (3) concealed transseptal conduction coupled with suppression of conduction due to the increased heart rate, somewhat analogous to suppression of pacemakers by an ectopic tachycardia. A discrepancy of as much as 210 msec between the cycles initiating and terminating the aberration suggests that concealed transseptal conduction may not be the sole factor responsibile for the unexpected persistence of aberrancy at the longer cycle lengths. The difference cannot be explained solely on the basis of time consumed by conduction along the contralateral bundle and across the septum. Normal transseptal activation in the human heart is about 40 to 45 msec; in the diseased heart, it may be prolonged to 115 msec.[56–59] It is likely, therefore, that a combination of mechanisms is operative.

One mechanism that would explain the unexpected delay in normalization of intraventricular conduction is *fatigue,* a descriptive term that may reflect failure of restitution of transmembrane ionic gradients and lowering of the transmembrane resting potential and/or a shift of the membrane responsiveness to the right. The latter denotes a decrease in upstroke velocity of phase 0 for any given magnitude of transmembrane resting potential. A different mechanism, namely, concealed conduction, may explain the delayed normalization of bundle branch conduction in patients with atrial fibrillation. Concealed conduction of atrial fibrillatory impulses into the blocked bundle may result in a true bundle-to-bundle interval that is consistently shorter than the manifest QRS interval.

Occasionally, paradoxical normalization of the QRS complex without a change in heart rate—or, in fact, with acceleration of the heart rate—has been documented (Fig. 4–26). Mechanisms that may explain this phenomenon include physiological shortening of the refractory period in response to acceleration of the heart rate, equalization of conduction in the two bundles and conduction during the supernormal period, and the gap phenomenon.

DECELERATION-DEPENDENT ABERRANCY (BRADYCARDIA-DEPENDENT ABERRANCY, PHASE 4 ABERRANCY). A prolonged cycle may be terminated by an aberrant QRS and foreshortening of the cycle may normalize the QRS (Fig. 4–27).[60] It has been suggested that this form of aberrancy is due to a gradual loss of transmembrane resting potential during a prolonged diastole with excitation from a less negative take-off potential. Because a small change in resting potential may have a pronounced effect on the rate of rise of phase 0 of the action potential, deceleration aberrancy may be seen with a relatively small prolongation of the cycle length.

CONCEALED CONDUCTION. Conduction in the bundle branches may be impaired by concealed penetration of a supraventricular impulse or by transseptal activation from the contralateral bundle (Fig. 4–24). In atrial fibrillation, concealed conduction into a bundle branch can be considered when acceleration-dependent aberrancy persists at a QRS cycle that is longer than a cycle terminated by a normal QRS. Transseptal concealed conduction into a bundle branch from the contralateral bundle should be suspected if aberrancy, once initiated, persists at rates slower than the rate that initiated the aberrancy (Fig. 4–26).

MYOCARDIAL DEPRESSION. Drugs and metabolic and electrolyte disorders are frequent causes of QRS aberrancy (Fig. 4–25). The severity of depression of conduction varies, and the QRS may exhibit RBBB or LBBB, divisional block, or any combination. As indicated previously, aberrancy can be differentiated from ordinary BBB by the presence of distortion in the initial and terminal components of the QRS complex. The appearance of aberration is often rate related (Fig. 4–25).

POSTEXTRASYSTOLIC ABERRATION. Aberrant intraventricular conduction of a sinus impulse terminating a compensatory pause is rare and must be differentiated from an aberrant escape complex. The exact mechanism of the postpausal aberrancy is not clear. It may be due to slow diastolic depolarization, unequal recovery of conducting or myocardial tissue, or increased diastolic volume.

Wolff-Parkinson-White (WPW) Syndrome

(See pp. 574 and 667)

WPW, or preexcitation,[61] syndrome is an electrocardiographic syndrome characterized by a short P-R (≤ 0.12 sec) interval, prolonged QRS (≥ 0.12 sec) complex, a slur on the

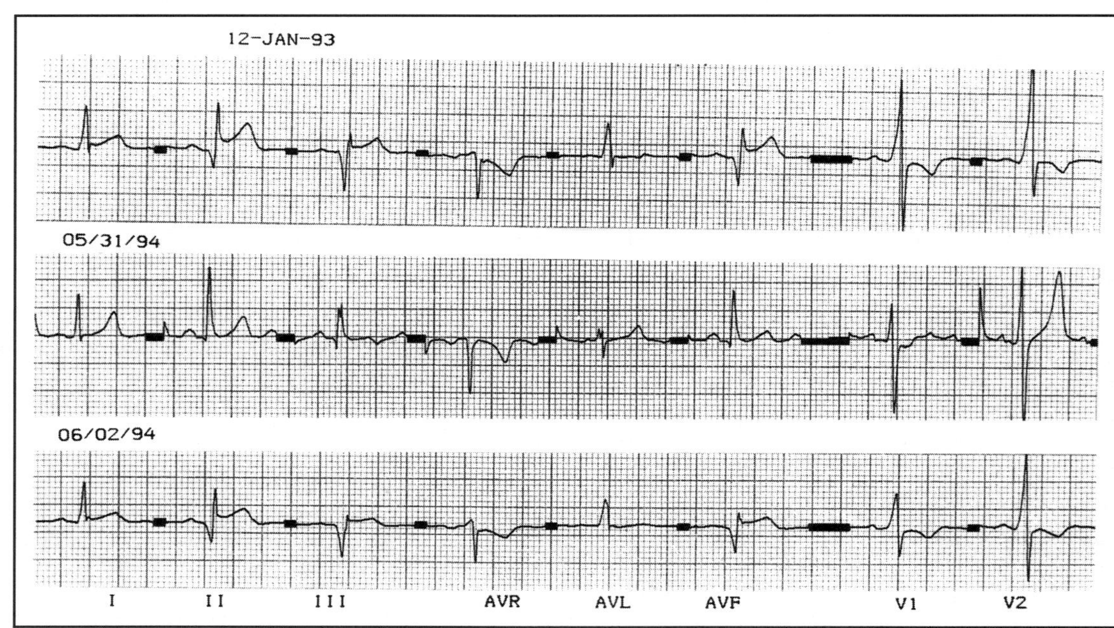

FIGURE 4–28. WPW syndrome simulating an inferior myocardial infarction. 1/12/93, WPW syndrome with negative delta wave suggestive of inferior infarction. 5/31/94, Normal AV conduction with normal QRS complexes. 6/2/94, Recurrence of WPW syndrome with negative delta wave, again simulating an inferior infarction. The normalization of the QRS in the recurrence of the pseudoinfarction Q wave on 6/2/94 rules out a myocardial infarction.

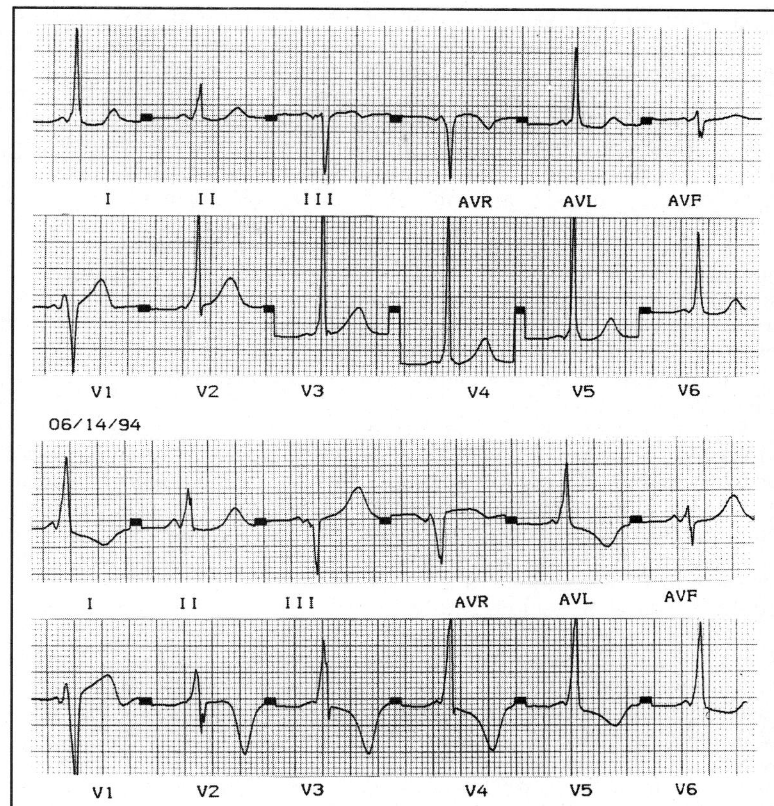

FIGURE 4–29. WPW syndrome and acute myocardial infarction. 1/12/93, WPW syndrome with a short P-R interval and a delta wave. The tracing of 6/14/94 was recorded during an acute myocardial infarction. The latter manifest by the negative T waves. Because of the conduction via the bypass toward the left ventricle, the left ventricular cavity is initially positive, thus precluding registration of the diagnostic Q wave (see Fig. 4–16).

upstroke of the QRS (delta wave), and (as a rule) a normal P-J interval (Figs. 4–28, 4–29, and 4–AE6). Secondary ST-segment and T-wave changes are nearly always present. Paroxysmal supraventricular tachycardia is recorded in about 50 per cent of patients with WPW. The characteristic pattern of WPW can be altered by abnormalities of AV and intraventricular conduction. The prevalence of WPW in the general population is approximately 3 per 1000.

Although Wilson is credited with the initial report of WPW[62] it was Cohn who brought the electrocardiograph to America and first described an ECG pattern to become known as WPW. His patient, described in 1913, exhibited the WPW pattern and supraventricular tachycardia.[63] In 1930, this pattern was recognized as a discrete ECG syndrome. Shortly thereafter the bypass concept of WPW was proposed, and this concept has stood the test of time.[64]

In WPW the QRS complex is a fusion between the impulse traversing the bypass and the normal AV junction. The bypass component of the QRS complex, or *delta wave,* varies depending on the size of the ventricular muscle mass activated through the bypass. In some instances, especially in the presence of AV conduction delay, the entire ventricular mass may be activated by the impulse propagated through the bypass, and the entire QRS complex becomes essentially a delta wave.

Traditionally, WPW has been classified into type A and type B. *Type A* is characterized by a prominent positive initial QRS deflection in leads V_1 and V_2 and *type B* by a predominantly negative deflection in leads V_1 and V_2.[65] In type A, the initial inscription of the QRS complex, the delta wave, reflects early activation of the posterior left ventricle and, in type B, early activation of the anterior superior right ventricle. *Type C WPW,* characterized by a negative delta wave in the left lateral leads, also has been described. Studies using surface potential mapping, epicardial mapping during surgery, and electrophysiological studies have identified a number of preexcitation sites.[66] Presence of more than one QRS pattern in an individual patient suggests the possibility of multiple bypass tracts. A short P-R interval with a normal QRS complex accompanied by paroxysmal supraventricular tachycardia has been suggested as a variant of WPW (see p. 667).

First-, second-, and third-degree AV block have been reported with WPW, as have right and left BBB. In the presence of a BBB, an ipsilateral bypass, by preexciting the ventricle normally activated by the blocked bundle branch, will obscure the BBB. Both supernormal and concealed conduction have been invoked to explain unexpected patterns of behavior of bypass conduction.

WPW often complicates ECG interpretation because it may obscure or simulate a variety of patterns. It may mask (Fig. 4–29) or simulate myocardial infarction (Fig. 4–28). When the QRS vector is directed toward the left ventricular cavity, the cavity becomes initially positive, and a Q wave will not be recorded. A diagnosis of ventricular hypertrophy in the presence of WPW (as in BBB) may be difficult if not impossible (Fig. 4–AE6). WPW has been mistaken for RBBB, LBBB, and RVH. Supraventricular arrhythmias with aberration, resulting from conduction through the bypass, have been mistaken for ventricular tachycardia. Aberration due to WPW should be suspected when the ventricular rate is rapid, often approaching 300 beats/min, or when the QRS morphology of the bizarre complexes is upright in leads V_1 and V_2 as well as in V_5 and V_6.

Myocardial Infarction

(See Chap. 37)

The ECG changes of myocardial infarction, first described in humans in 1920,[67] are those of ischemia, injury, and cellular death and are, within limits, reflected by T-wave changes, ST-segment displacement, and the appearance of Q waves, respectively. Such a clear-cut differentiation, although clinically useful, may be overly simplistic and artificial. For example, T-wave changes may be due to ischemia, injury, or death of muscle. Similarly, a Q wave may be due to impairment of transmembrane ionic fluxes and not necessarily cellular death. However, for the purpose of this discussion, T-wave changes, ST-segment displacement, and appearance of a Q wave are assumed to reflect ischemia, injury, and cell death, respectively.

ISCHEMIA. In the dog, the earliest change following ligation of a coronary artery is the almost immediate appearance of a primary, as a rule negative, T wave. After 60 or 90 seconds, there is a maximal shift of the ST segment. The T wave becomes positive and peaked, and the change is as a rule a primary change. The amplitude of the R wave decreases during the first 30 seconds after experimental occlusion. This is followed by an increase in the amplitude, which peaks 20 to 30 seconds after the maximal increase of the left ventricular volume. In humans, unless an ECG is recorded at the moment of occlusion, the initial T wave change is usually missed (Figs. 4–AE10 and 4–AE11, p. 147). Occasionally, a giant R wave is recorded early during the ischemic episode (Fig. 4–AE12, p. 147). Such changes in the QRS could contribute to the T-wave abnormality, and the abnormal T wave would reflect both primary and secondary changes of repolarization.

Normally the process of repolarization proceeds from the epicardium to the endocardium, and an upright T wave is recorded. Ischemia prolongs the regional duration of recovery, with the ischemic area being last to repolarize. If the ischemia is subendocardial, the direction of repolarization remains unchanged and the polarity of the T wave remains upright. In the presence of subepicardial ischemia, the duration of the excited state is longer in the epicardium; the normal order of repolarization is reversed, proceeding from endocardium to epicardium, and an inverted T wave is inscribed. Because of local prolongation of recovery, the late phase of repolarization may be unopposed, and a large and prolonged T wave may be registered.

INJURY. Two concepts based on systolic and diastolic phenomena have been suggested to explain the ST-segment displacement. One postulates local reduction or loss of resting potential, resulting in a *diastolic current of injury.* The second concept assumes an unopposed current flowing from the injured area during the isoelectric ST segment, resulting in a *systolic current of injury.* These systolic and diastolic phenomena cannot be differentiated with the ordinary clinical alternating-current (AC) electrocardiograph but can be recorded experimentally with direct-current (DC) equipment (Fig. 4–30).

The concept of the *diastolic current* of injury proposes that localized injury is associated with a flow of current from the uninjured to the injured area. As a result, the T-Q segment is displaced downward but is automatically shifted to control level by the capacitor-coupled amplifier of the ECG. When the entire heart (including the injured area) is depolarized, the ST segment is elevated with respect to the depressed but rectified (isoelectric) diastolic T-Q segment (Fig. 4–31).

The concept of the *systolic current* of injury proposes that during the ST segment, the normal heart is depolarized, but the injured area undergoes early repolarization. The result is a current flow from the more positive, injured area to a more negative, uninjured area. The result is true elevation of the ST segment. Similarly, if, rather than repolarizing early, the injured area fails to depolarize with the normal myocardium, a current of injury would exist and an elevated ST segment would be recorded (Fig. 4–31).

Earlier experimental studies indicate that during injury both systolic and diastolic currents are present,[68] and at times the systolic precedes the diastolic current of injury. Subsequent studies, however, indicate that the diastolic current predominates while the systolic current plays a lesser role and that the magnitude of the current is modified by the heart rate[69] (Fig. 4–30). As indicated, the clinical ECG does not differentiate between systolic and diastolic currents of injury. Furthermore, unless the onset of the injury is recorded, even a DC-coupled ECG would not identify the mechanism of the ST-segment shift.

An electrode facing subendocardial injury registers an elevated ST segment, while an epicardial electrode subtended by the normal myocardium registers ST-segment depression. Similarly, an electrode facing epicardial injury registers elevation of the ST segment, while the endocardial electrode inscribes ST-segment depression.

INFARCTION. The diagnostic feature of infarction (myocardial necrosis) is the *Q wave.* Two concepts have been invoked to explain the appearance of the Q wave. The theory of proximity, the "window" theory, suggests that the

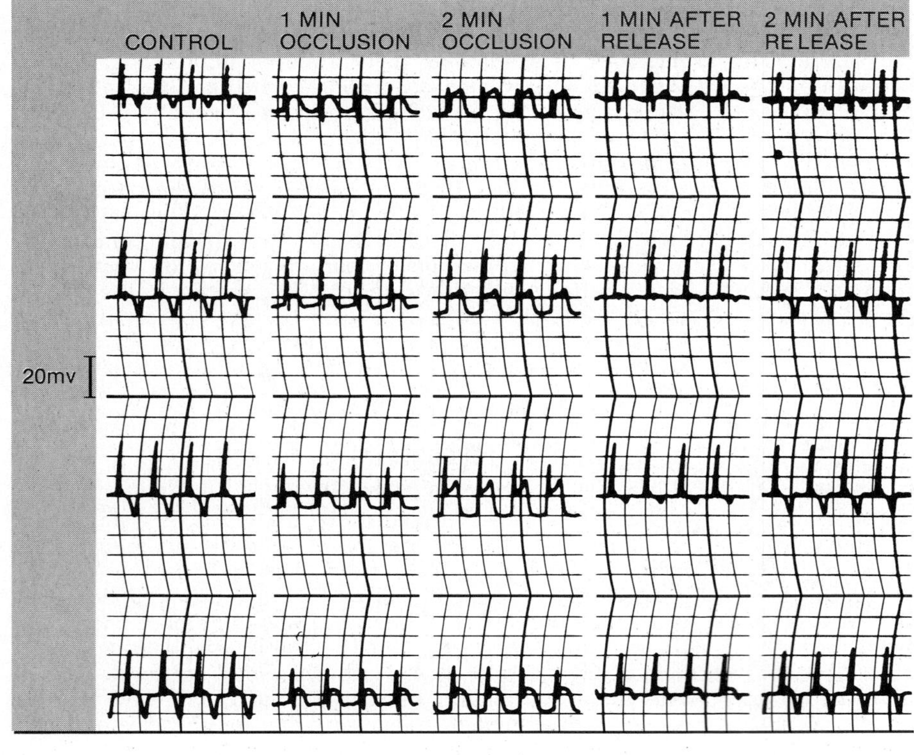

FIGURE 4–30. A series of simultaneous epicardial electrograms recorded from four sites. The electrodes were distributed randomly in the ischemic area, with some closer to the center of the ischemic area than others. After 1 minute of occlusion, TQ segment depression is apparent in all recordings. After 2 minutes of occlusion, TQ segment depression has increased. The ST segment take-off is slightly elevated or isoelectric in all recordings. The polarity of the T wave is changed from negative during the control period to positive. These recordings emphasize that major changes in action potential downstroke, shape, and timing can occur without significant alteration of phase 2 and of the action potential. Similarly, T wave changes can occur without a significant shift of the true ST segment. True TQ segment depression appears to be the major cause of ST segment displacement and the true ST segment shift of lesser magnitude and variable. T waveform is markedly altered with occlusion. (From Vincent, G. M., et al.: Mechanisms of ischemic ST-segment displacement. Circulation *56*:559, 1977, by permission of the American Heart Association, Inc.)

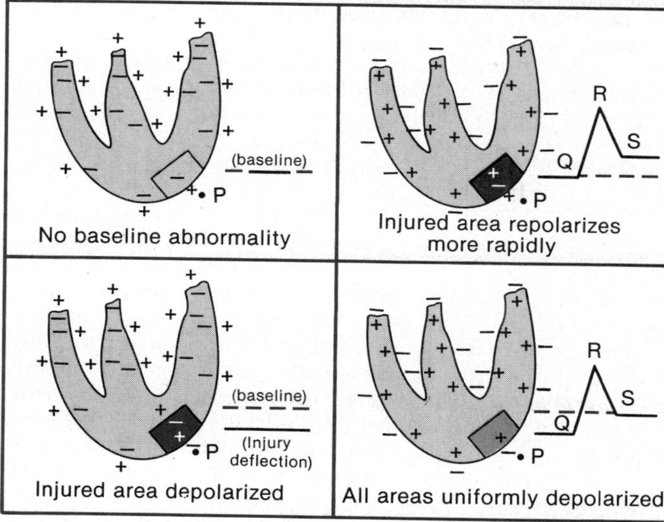

FIGURE 4–31. Systolic *(upper row)* and diastolic *(lower row)* currents of injury. *Upper row,* The ischemic area (pink) is electrically identical to the nonischemic heart at rest, and there is no shift of the baseline potential. During repolarization, however, the ischemic area (red) has repolarized early and is positive relative to the depolarized heart, the baseline is shifted upward (positive), and the ECG records an elevated ST segment. Similarly, if the ischemic area fails to depolarize with the remainder of the heart, it would be positive relative to the remainder of the heart and a positive ST segment would be recorded. This latter mechanism also may be operative. *Lower row,* The ischemic area (red) is depolarized at rest, thus negative relative to the remainder of the heart, and the baseline is shifted down (negative). This shift is not recognizable on ECG. However, with completion of depolarization the injured area is also depolarized; its potential becomes identical to that of the rest of the heart; and the ST segment, although isoelectric, is elevated relative to the depressed baseline; so that an elevated ST segment is registered. These two mechanisms cannot be differentiated with the ECG, and although both contribute to the current of injury, the systolic is thought to dominate (Fig. 4–30). (From Scher, A. M.: Electrocardiogram. *In* Ruch, I. C., and Patton, H. D. (eds.): Physiology and Biophysics. Philadelphia, W. B. Saunders Company, 1974, p. 94.)

electrically inert myocardium allows an electrode to record the intracavitary negativity. There is ample evidence, however, to suggest that a Q wave can be recorded in the absence of a transmural infarction. Heterogeneity of electrophysiological changes associated with the dynamic events of ischemic and subsequent healing, with intermingling of fibrous and viable tissue, has been suggested as an explanation.

According to the vectorial concept, the electrically inert myocardium fails to contribute to the normal electrical forces, and the result is a vector that points away from the area of infarction, reflected by a Q wave. Theoretically, the infarction vector represents the force that alters the normal vector. It is equal to but opposite in direction from the vector generated by the infarcted myocardium before infarction. If the net vector is directed normally but is reduced in magnitude, a Q wave will not be recorded, but the amplitude of the QRS complex will be reduced, indicating loss of myocardium. However, the specificity of such a change for infarction is low (Table 4–3).

Diagnosis

One of the most valuable contributions of the ECG is in the diagnosis of myocardial infarction. Usually it is the first laboratory test performed; the technique is reliable and reproducible, can be applied serially, and when properly interpreted is the cornerstone of the laboratory diagnosis of myocardial infarction and often dictates the initial therapy.[70]

THE INITIAL ECG. The initial ECG is "diagnostic" of acute infarction in approximately 50 per cent of patients, abnormal but not diagnostic in approximately 40 per cent, and normal in about 10 per cent. Serial tracings increase the sensitivity to near 95 per cent. A single ECG may never be "diagnostic." However, a pattern of ST-segment displacement, especially with associated Q-wave and T-wave changes, and a clinical history suggestive of ischemic heart disease is highly suggestive—if not diagnostic—of acute myocardial infarction.

CLASSIC PATTERN AND EVOLUTION OF INFARCTION. As in the experimental animal, if the ECG is inscribed at the

TABLE 4–3 SUMMARY OF VECTORCARDIOGRAPHIC CRITERIA FOR DIAGNOSIS OF MYOCARDIAL INFARCTION (MI)

Anteroseptal MI (1 and 2)*
1. Initial anterior QRS forces absent
2. 0.02-sec QRS vector directed posteriorly
Localized Anterior MI (1, 2, and 3)
1. Initial anterior septal forces present
2. 0.02-sec QRS vector directed posteriorly
3. Voltage criteria for left ventricular hypertrophy absent
Anterolateral MI (1, 2, and 3)
1. Initial anterior septal forces normal
2. Initial rightward QRS forces > 0.022 sec
3. Efferent limb of transverse plane QRS loop inscribed clockwise
4. Initial rightward QRS forces > 0.16 mV
5. Maximum frontal plane QRS vector > 40°, QRS loop inscribed counterclockwise
Extensive Anterior MI (1 and 2)
1. Initial anterior QRS forces absent
2. Transverse plane QRS loop inscribed clockwise
Inferior MI (1 or more)
1. Initial superior QRS forces > 0.025 sec
2. Initial superior QRS forces ≥ 0.020 sec, maximum left superior force ≥ 0.25 mV
3. Maximum frontal plane QRS vector < 10°, efferent limb of frontal QRS loop inscribed clockwise
4. Bites in afferent limb of frontal QRS loop
Inferolateral MI (1 and 2)
1. Initial rightward QRS forces > 0.022 sec
2. Initial superior QRS forces > 0.025 sec

* Numbers in parentheses after each type of infarction indicate the minimum requirements for the diagnosis.
From Chou, T. C., et al.: Clinical Vectorcardiography. 2nd ed. New York, Grune and Stratton, 1974, p. 229.

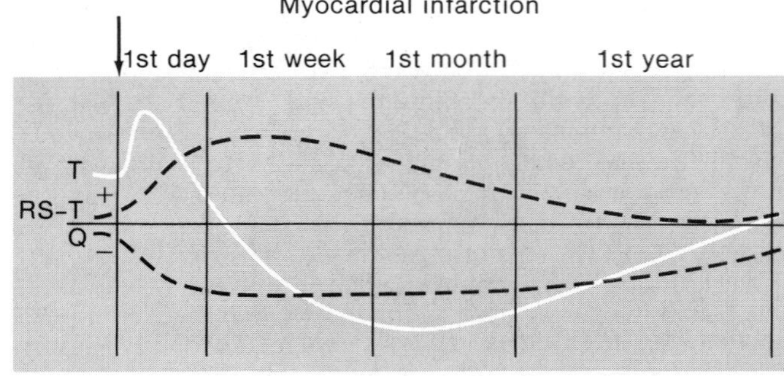

FIGURE 4–32. Evolution of the T wave, ST segment, and Q wave after myocardial infarction. (From Lepeschkin, E.: Modern Electrocardiography. Baltimore, Williams and Wilkins Co., 1951.)

onset of myocardial infarction, the characteristic early change—namely, an abnormal T wave—is often recorded (Figs. 4–AE10 and 4–AE11, p. 147). The T wave may be prolonged, increased in magnitude, and either upright or inverted. This is followed by ST segment elevation in leads facing the area of injury, with reciprocal depression in the "remote" opposite leads. The upright T wave may exhibit terminal inversion at a time when the ST segment is still elevated. A Q wave may be present in the first ECG or may not appear for hours or sometimes days.[70a] The amplitude of the QRS complex may diminish and may be replaced by a QS pattern. As the ST segment returns to the baseline, symmetrically inverted T waves evolve.[67] The time of appearance and the magnitude of the changes vary among patients (Fig. 4–32).

Occasionally, early in the course of evolution of acute infarction, a very tall R wave merging with an elevated ST segment with reduction or loss of the S wave may be present. The pattern resembles a monophasic action potential (Fig. 4–AE12, p. 147).[71]

The classic evolution of acute myocardial infarction is documented in approximately one-half to two-thirds of the patients (Fig. 4–33), while in those remaining the infarct is manifested by ST-segment, T-wave, and non-Q QRS changes (Fig. 4–34).

SUBTLE, ATYPICAL, NONSPECIFIC PATTERNS OF INFARCTION. Atypical features and characteristics of early infarction seen in about 40 to 50 per cent of the first ECG's include a normal ECG, subtle ST-segment and T-wave changes, isolated T-wave abnormality, transient normalization of the ST-segment, T-wave, or QRS complex, involvement of electrically "silent" areas (see Fig. 4–35 and 4–AE18), or the masking effect of conduction defects (Figs. 4–16, 4–19, and 4–29). Awareness and recognition of the early, nondiagnostic, "atypical" or subtle abnormalities will improve the diagnostic sensitivity of the ECG.

Although ECG changes can be documented within seconds after experimental coronary occlusion and in humans during angioplasty, such changes may be delayed. A normal initial ECG in a patient with evolving clinical acute myocardial infarction may be due to absence of ischemia at the time of the initial tracing, a delay in evolution of the characteristic pattern, an initially small infarct that produces diagnostic ECG changes only after extension, transient normalization of the ECG in the course of evolution of acute myocardial infarction, or infarction of an electrocardiographically "silent" area of the myocardium (Fig. 4–35).

Early changes of myocardial infarction may alter the terminal part of the QRS (Fig. 4–34). With an inferior infarction these may be manifested by an increase of the R wave amplitude in lead III and appearance of an S wave in aV_l. There also may be an associated increase in S wave amplitude in leads V_2 and V_3.[72] These changes are most likely due to conduction delays in the ischemic and injured

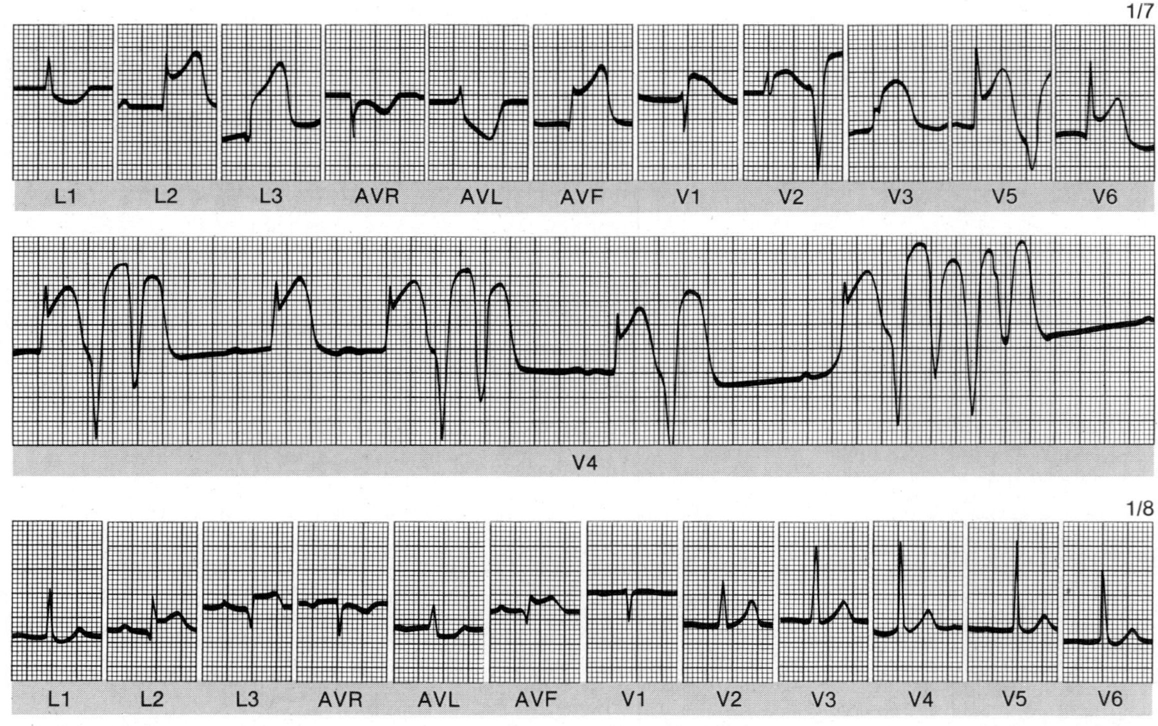

FIGURE 4–33. Acute inferior myocardial infarction and transient extensive anterior injury. Tracing made on 1/7 shows elevation of the ST segment in leads II, III, and aV_f, V_1 through V_6 with reciprocal depression of the ST segment in leads I and aV_l. In the second row the acute injury is accompanied by ventricular premature complexes (isolated and couplets) and a short run of ventricular tachycardia. In the tracing of 1/8, the anterior current of injury is no longer present, and the residual pattern is that of an acute inferior myocardial infarction manifest by a Q wave and ST segment elevation in leads II, III, and aV_f. The tall R in lead V_2 and upright right precordial R waves suggest an associated posterior infarction.

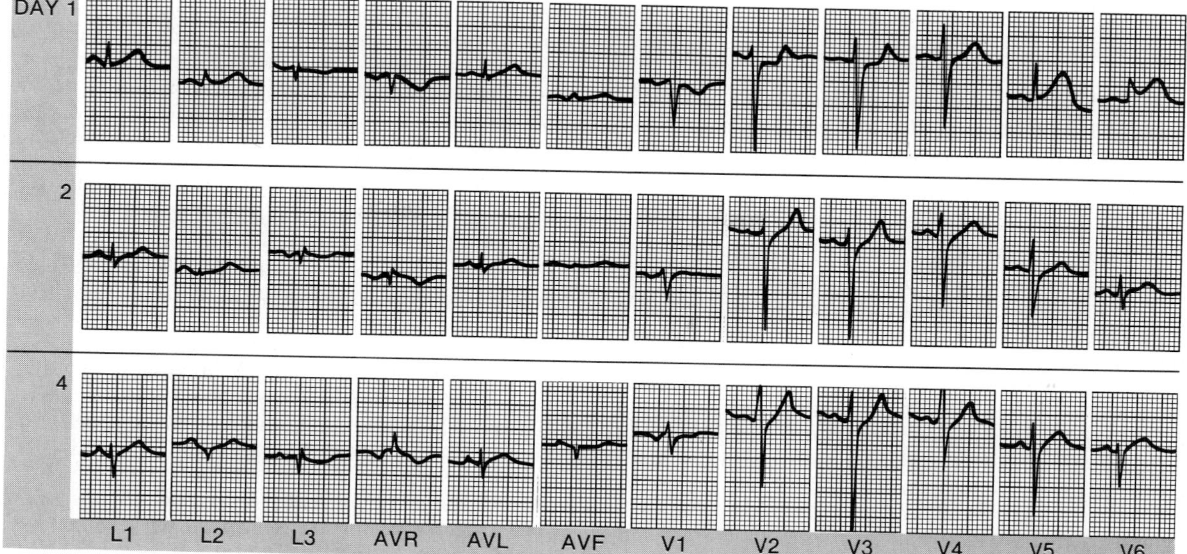

FIGURE 4–34. Acute myocardial infarction manifested by an altered sequence of ventricular activation. Tracing recorded on day 1 suggests a lateral infarction with reciprocal ST segment depression in leads V_1 to V_3. A shift of axis to right with prominent S waves in leads V_5 and V_6 is noted in the middle trace (Day 2). The Q waves in leads II, III, and aV_f with R waves of higher amplitude in leads V_1 and V_2 suggest that the infarct is inferior and probably posterior (Day 4). The marked right-axis duration and the prominent S waves in leads V_5 and V_6 indicate an inferior and posterior periinfarction block with the terminal ventricular excitation directed toward the infarction.

areas, in some way similar to periinfarction block (see p. 1251).

Evolution of the characteristic ST-segment and T-wave changes coupled with appearance of Q waves is highly specific for acute myocardial infarction. In the first ECG, the sensitivity and specificity of the ST-segment change alone, especially when marked, is high. With the passage of 4 to 12 hours, however, *evolving* changes in the ST segment need to be demonstrated, since conditions such as pericarditis, early repolarization, and ventricular aneurysm (Fig. 4–AE19) also may manifest ST-segment elevation, but it is usually persistent. Transient hyperkalemia (Fig. 4–45) and Prinzmetal's angina (see below) (Fig. 4–44), like acute myocardial infarction, also can cause transient ST-segment elevations. Although subtle, minor ST-segment elevation can be easily overlooked, it is a relatively common, isolated early finding.

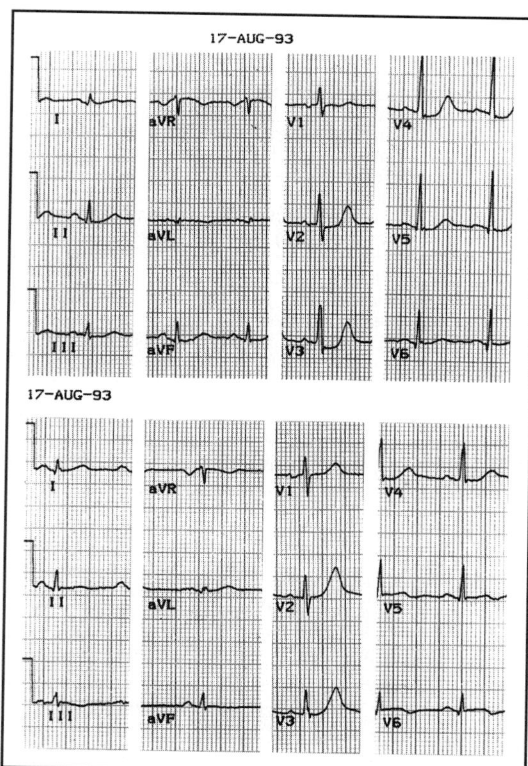

FIGURE 4–35. The top tracing illustrates what appears to be a "pure" posterior myocardial infarction manifest by tall R waves in leads V_1 and V_2 with ST segment depression in leads V_2 to V_4. The bottom tracing, however, discloses inferoapical changes. Pure posterior infarction without a concomitant inferior or lateral infarction or both is extremely rare (see Fig. 4–AE16, p. 149).

ST-segment depression may reflect subendocardial ischemia, infarction, or reciprocal changes secondary to infarction at a "remote" (opposite) site.[73–75] It also has been suggested that depression of the ST segment in leads V_1 to V_4 in the presence of an inferior infarction may indicate ischemia secondary to significant obstruction of the left anterior descending coronary artery. However, evidence indicates that the ST-segment depression is reciprocal to the inferior or posterolateral infarction and that the severity of the anterior wall ST-segment depression may be related to the severity and extent of the inferior ischemia rather than to anterior wall ischemia. There is evidence that inferior ST-segment depression noted with anterior ischemia is also a reciprocal phenomenon and does not reflect inferior ischemia.[76–80]

Minor, subtle ST-segment depression is a common early finding of acute myocardial infarction, especially non-Q wave infarction. However, since ST-segment depression is often a nonspecific change, it should be evaluated in light of other clinical and laboratory findings.

Tall, peaked T waves seen in experimental coronary occlusion are occasionally recorded in humans and are thought to reflect subendocardial ischemia (Fig. 4–AE10). More often, initially the T waves are isoelectric, negative (Fig. 4–AE11, p. 147), or biphasic. While subtle T-wave changes are often the earliest recorded signs of infarction, their value is limited because of nonspecificity. In about 20 to 30 percent of patients with myocardial infarction, a T-wave abnormality is the only sign of acute infarction.

In patients with ischemic heart disease, ST alternans is usually noted in limb leads and anterior precordial leads. It is characteristically associated with vasospastic angina

(Printzmetal's angina, p. 1340) but has been reported during acute infarction, during exercise tests, after subarachnoid hemorrhage, and rarely with other conditions.[52]

An *abnormal U wave* is a frequent marker of ischemic heart disease.[80a] Negative or biphasic U waves have been reported in up to 30 per cent of patients with chronic angina pectoris, either as a persistent finding or as a transient manifestation during an episode of angina. It is most often recorded in leads I, II, and V_4 to V_6. Appearance of a negative U wave during exercise-induced ischemia has been appreciated for some time and is highly specific for disease of the left anterior descending coronary artery.[81] When accompanying unstable angina or anterior myocardial infarction, the negative U wave frequently indicates multivessel disease with a severe lesion in the left anterior descending artery.[82] A negative U wave is seen in 10 to 60 per cent of patients with anterior infarction and in up to 30 per cent of patients with inferior infarction. When present in a setting of a previous myocardial infarction, the negative U waves are a sign of extensive infarction involving the apex and a marker of significant impairment of left ventricular function.[83] Appearance of a negative U wave may precede other ECG changes of infarction by several hours (Fig. 4–36), an observation supported by changes noted during PTCA.

An abnormal QRS complex, ST segment, and T wave may normalize transiently in the course of evolution of acute myocardial infarction. This may be due to reversible ischemia or injury or conduction defects, but it is also frequently observed in the normal evolution of acute myocardial infarction. Presence of an upright T wave longer than 48 hours after infarction or an early reversal of an inverted T wave to a positive deflection is indicative of postinfarction pericarditis with or without pericardial effusion and suggests the presence of transmural infarction.[84]

A premature ventricular complex with a qR or QR morphology even in the absence of ECG findings of infarction suggests the presence of myocardial infarction. This finding may prove particularly useful when the myocardial infarction is masked, for example, by LBBB or WPW. A recent study, however, questions the value of this finding in the absence of other ECG findings of myocardial infarction.

OLD INFARCTION. ECG diagnosis of old myocardial infarction is often difficult and frequently impossible without the availability of tracings documenting the acute episode. A definitive diagnosis of old infarction depends on the presence of a pathological Q wave. Only rarely can it be based on T-wave changes alone. While abnormal Q waves may be absent in transmural infarction and present in nontransmural infarction, the sensitivity and specificity of the ECG for diagnosis of an old myocardial infarction still depend on Q waves. The specificity of abnormal Q waves for myocardial infarction is relatively high; however, the sensitivity is quite low. Within 6 to 12 months after an acute myocardial infarction, about 30 per cent of the tracings, although abnormal, are no longer diagnostic of infarction, because the Q wave(s) are absent. Similarly, by the end of 10 years, or sooner, some 6 to 10 per cent of the cardiograms revert to normal. There is evidence to suggest that regression of Q waves following anterior myocardial infarction is associated with smaller areas of infarction.[85]

In a series of 1184 tracings correlating myocardial infarction with postmortem findings, the specificity and sensitivity of the Q wave were 89 and 61 per cent, respectively, and varied with location of the infarction. Anteriorly located Q waves (leads V_1 to V_4) and inferiorly located Q waves (leads II, III, and aV_f) were falsely positive in 46 per cent. Q waves longer than 0.03 sec in lateral leads (V_5 and V_6) or Q waves in more than one "electrocardiographic zone," i.e., inferior and lateral, were false positive in only 4 per cent. The sensitivity of the Q wave was lowest for infarction located in the lateral basal portion of the left ventricle.[86] This anatomical area is usually reflected in leads I and aV_l.[86a]

MYOCARDIAL INFARCTION AND CONDUCTION DELAYS. Conduction defects may not interfere with, may mask, or may falsely suggest the diagnosis of myocardial infarction. In RBBB, the initial order of activation is normal, and thus the pattern of infarction is unaltered. Rarely, the development of RBBB will unmask an anteroseptal infarction.[87] In LBBB the sequence of early activation is altered, with the initial septal vector directed from right to left. As a result, the earliest left ventricular intracavitary potential is positive. In keeping with the "window" concept of infarction, a Q wave cannot be registered except when there is extensive septal infarction. Restated in terms of the dipole or vector concept, since the free wall infarct is inscribed during the latter part of the QRS complex after the septal activation is complete, the direction of initial activation expressed as a dipole or vector is unaltered by the infarction, and the infarct is masked (Figs. 4–16 and 4–19).

LEFT BUNDLE BRANCH BLOCK. Numerous attempts at defining diagnostic criteria for myocardial infarction in the presence of LBBB have proven unsuccessful. The proposed criteria rarely correlate with autopsy findings. In a study of 52 patients with LBBB and autopsy findings of myocardial infarction, the following ECG findings were thought to correlate with myocardial infarction: (1) a Q wave 0.04 sec or greater in leads I, aV_l, V_5, or V_6; (2) rapid serial ST-segment and T-wave changes; (3) acute ST-segment elevation disproportionate to the area of the QRS complex; and (4) a Q wave of any size in lead V_6. Others suggest that a deep S wave in leads V_5 and V_6, a qRs complex with a slurred S wave in leads V_5 and V_6, loss of the R wave in the precordial leads, or a Q wave in leads II, III, and aV_f is consistent with myocardial infarction complicating LBBB. However, in another study of patients with LBBB, the significance of Q waves, broad R waves, notched middle and left precordial S waves, rsR′ complexes, ST-segment elevation, and T-wave changes was found to lack significant correlation with myocardial infarction.

In patients with LBBB, ischemia, and infarction, the following criteria were found highly specific and predictive for myocardial infarction in a range of 90 to 100 per cent: Q wave in at least two leads, leads I, aV_l, V_5, or V_6; R-wave regression from V_1 to V_4; notching on the upstroke of the S wave in at least two leads (leads V_3, V_4, or V_5), and primary ST-T changes in two or more adjacent leads (Fig. 4–17).[88] A somewhat better correlation was noted between an ECG sugges-

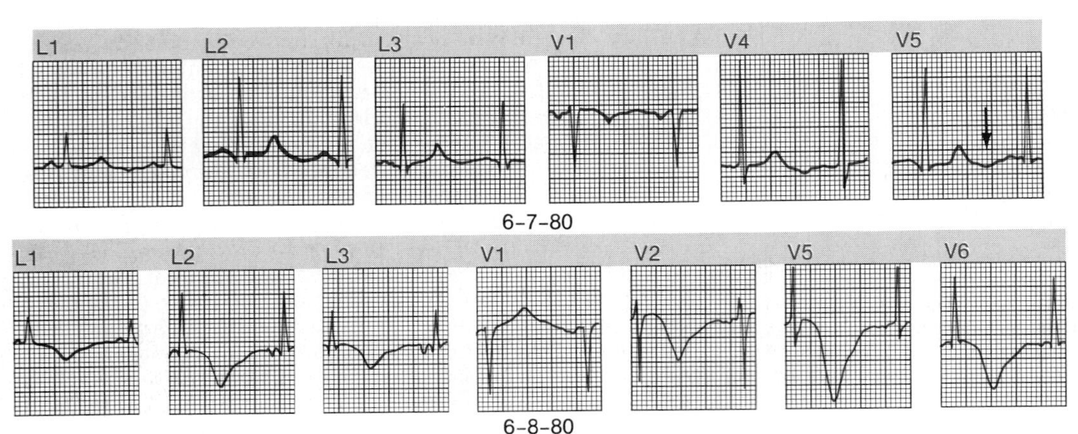

FIGURE 4–36. Negative U wave as the only marker of an acute ischemic episode. On 6/7/80 a negative U wave (↓) was recorded in leads I, V_4 and V_5, and an upright reciprocal U wave was present in lead V_1. In the tracing of 6/8/80 a prolonged Q-T interval and deeply inverted T waves are present in all the leads—evolutionary changes consistent with an acute myocardial infarction. At necropsy a subendocardial infarction was found.

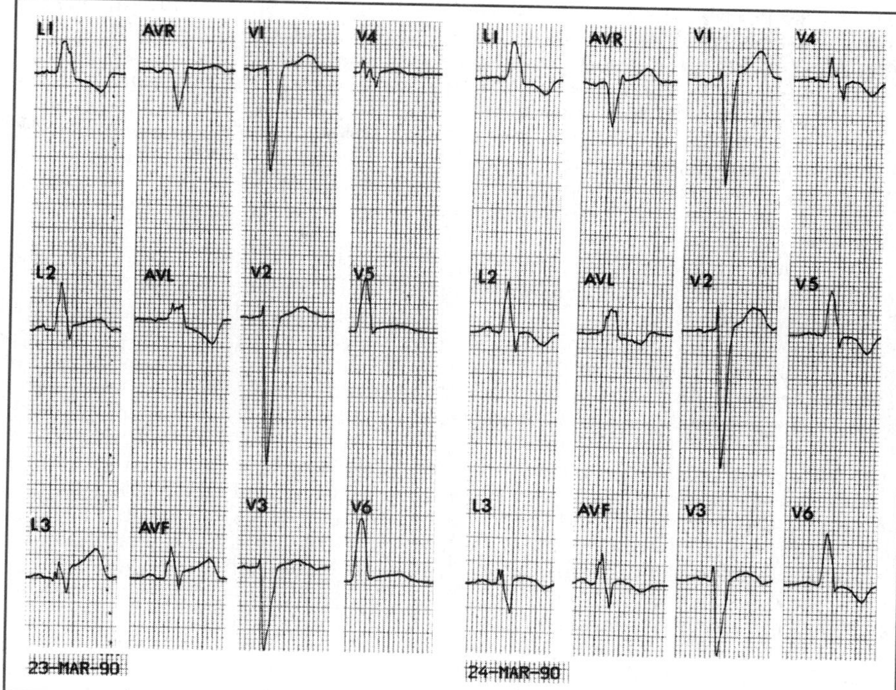

FIGURE 4–37. Acute myocardial infarction and LBBB. 3/23/90, The LBBB is accompanied by elevated ST segments in leads II, III, aV_f, and V_6 and depressed in leads I and aV_l. 3/24/90, Symmetrically inverted T waves are present in leads II, III, aV_f, V_4, V_5, and V_6. Although Q waves are not recorded, the evolution of the ST-T changes is consistent with the clinical history of acute myocardial infarction.

tive of acute inferior myocardial infarction and postmortem findings (Fig. 4–37). Observations made during angioplasty indicate that in the presence of LBBB with acute transmural ischemia, the ST segment becomes elevated over the area of the acute ischemia; this is a change similar to that observed with normal intraventricular conduction[89] (Fig. 4–AE13).

Studies of patients with intermittent LBBB and myocardial infarction provide additonal evidence that LBBB masks myocardial infarction (Fig. 4–16). It should be noted, however, that occasionally when acute infarction is evident during normal intraventricular conduction, acute changes are also recognizable in the presence of LBBB (Figs. 4–AE13, p. 148, and 4–37).

Block of the divisions of the LBBB may simulate or obscure myocardial infarction. Left anterior fascicular block (LAFB) may simulate an anterior infarction and obscure an inferior infarction (Fig. 4–19). In LAFB the R wave in lead aV_f is taller than in lead III and the R wave in lead II is taller than in lead aV_f (II > aV_f > III). A reversal of this progression, namely III > aV_f > II, is highly suggestive of a previous myocardial infarction.[90]

In WPW syndrome as in LBBB, the initial vector may be directed toward the left ventricular cavity, precluding the appearance of a Q wave (Fig. 4–29). The ECG pattern of infarction masked by WPW is recognizable in the presence of normal intraventricular conduction by ST-segment and T-wave changes.

PERIINFARCTION BLOCK. As originally defined, periinfarction block is a specific conduction abnormality due to myocardial infarction.[91–94] The ECG changes include a Q wave of 0.04 sec and a QRS complex in the limb leads of 0.10 sec, with a slurred prolonged terminal component facing the site of infarction. Peri-infarction block is not synonymous with left anterior divisional block. Peri-infarction block may be of help in the diagnosis of old inferior infarction when the characteristic changes are no longer evident. Presence of terminal, somewhat delayed activation facing leads II, III, or aV_f and a terminal negative wave in leads I, V_5, and V_6 (signs of peri-infarction block) strengthen the diagnosis of inferior myocardial infarction (Fig. 4–38).

In acute anterior infarction, slowing of conduction in the ischemic area is manifest by a decrease of the S wave in leads V_2 and V_3. In inferior infarction, the slowing of conduction is manifested by an increase in R wave in leads III and aV_f and S wave in lead aV_l.[95]

An RSR′ complex not related to RBBB but due to terminal conduction delay has been shown to be associated with severe segmental motion abnormality consistent with myocardial infarction scar tissue.[96]

THE ECG AND SITE OF CORONARY ARTERY OBSTRUCTION. The correlation of ECG pattern and site of obstruction early in the course of myocardial infarction was investigated arteriographically in 152 patients. The sensitivity, specificity, and predictive value for (1) ECG indicative of anterior infarction and occlusion of the left anterior descending coronary was 90, 95, and 96 per cent, respectively; (2) ECG indicative of inferior infarction and occlusion of the right coronary artery was 56, 97, and 80 per cent, respectively; (3) ECG indicative of posterior or lateral infarction and obstruction of the left circumflex coronary was 24, 98, and 75 per cent, respectively; (4) ECG indicative of inferior infarction and obstruction of the right or left circumflex coronary was 53, 98, and 94 per cent, respectively; and (5) ECG indicative of posterior or lateral infarction and obstruction of the right or left circumflex coronary was 53, 98, and 94 per cent, respectively.[97]

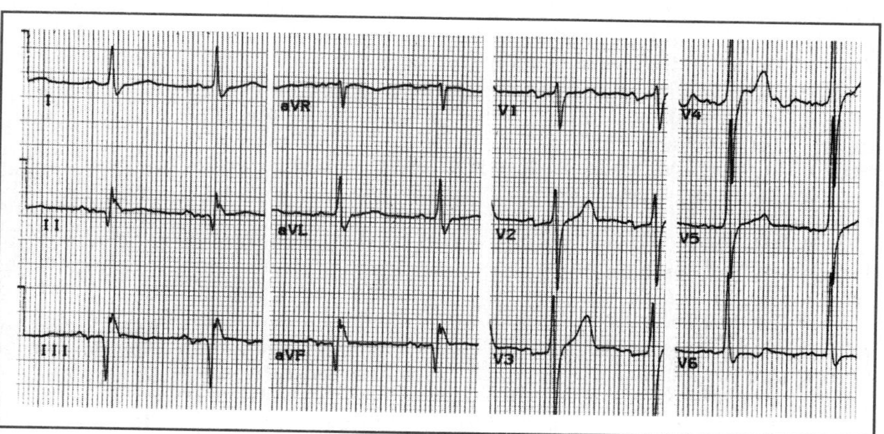

FIGURE 4–38. Inferior myocardial infarction and peri-infarction block. The inferior infarction is manifest by the Q waves in leads II, III, and aV_f. There is a terminal delay of depolarization toward the inferior infarction, as indicated by an S wave in leads I and aV_l and a terminal positive deflection of the QRS in leads III and aV_f. This terminal vector is due to an unopposed depolarization in the direction of the infarction. The delayed, slow depolarization is due to loss of the Purkinje fibers.

In acute inferior myocardial infarction, changes in the lateral leads (aV_l, V_5, and V_6) with an isoelectric or elevated ST in lead I identified obstruction of the circumflex coronary artery with a sensitivity, specificity, and predictive value of 83, 96, and 93, respectively. Changes in the lateral leads are rare, with inferior infarction resulting from obstruction of the right coronary artery.[98] There is evidence that lateral ECG abnormalities with an abnormal R wave in lead V_1 indicate a proximal left circumflex lesion.[99]

Two hundred and four consecutive patients with unstable angina manifesting abnormal ST-segment and terminal T-wave inversion in leads V_2 and V_3 without abnormal Q waves were found to have more than 50 per cent narrowing of proximal left anterior descending artery. Of this group, 33 had complete obstruction and 75 had collateral circulation to the affected vessel.[100] Others have made similar observations.

Presence of ST-segment elevation equal to or greater than 1 mm in lead V_4R has a sensitivity of 100 per cent and specificity of 87 per cent and a predictive accuracy of 92 per cent for occlusion of right coronary above the first right ventricular branch. The absence of ST-segment elevation of 1 mm excludes such lesions. Similarly, presence of ST-segment elevation in V_4R excluded isolated obstruction of left circumflex artery.[101]

THE ECG AND LOCATION OF INFARCTION. A precise anatomical location of anterior myocardial infarction based on ECG is not always possible.[101a] Accuracy of such localization is influenced, for example, by distance of the electrode from the heart, which varies considerably among individuals. The area subtending a given precordial electrode varies with the anteroposterior (AP) diameter of the chest and is greater in individuals with an increased diameter. Consequently, the same size anterior infarct would be recorded in more leads than in an individual with a normal AP diameter.

The diagnosis of transmural and nontransmural infarction when based on presence or absence of a Q wave shows a poor correlation with autopsy findings. Experimental and autopsy findings indicate that while nontransmural lesions may be accompanied by a Q wave, the Q wave may be absent in transmural infarction. It has been suggested that as many as 50 per cent of nontransmural myocardial infarctions manifest Q waves, making differentiation of nontransmural and transmural infarction based on the Q wave highly tenuous. It appears, therefore, that the terms Q and non-Q wave infarction (Fig. 4–36) may be preferable to transmural and nontransmural, unless necropsy findings are available.[102,103] Early elevation of the ST segment is a poor predictor of subsequent Q wave evolution.[104]

Septal Infarction. On the basis of the presence of Q waves, an infarct is considered septal when a Q wave is present in leads V_1 and V_2 (Fig. 4–AE14, p. 148); anterior when they are present in leads V_3 and V_4; anteroseptal if present in V_1 to V_4; lateral when present in leads I, aV_l, and V_6; anterolateral when present in leads I, aV_l, and V_3 to V_6; extensive anterior when present in leads I, aV_l, and V_1 to V_6, high lateral when present in leads I and aV_l (Fig. 4–AE15), and inferior when present in leads II, III, and aV_f (see Figs. 4–16, 4–33, and 4–34); and anteroinferior, or apical, when present in leads II, III, aV_l, and in one or more of the V_1 to V_4 leads. A posterior infarct is recognized by prominent R waves in lead V_1 or V_2 (Figs. 4–35 and 4–AE16 and 4–AE17, p. 149).

Loss of R waves in leads V_1 and V_2 indicates infarction of the septum and left anterior ventricular wall. Studies in isolated human hearts[18] suggest that the loss of the R wave is due to loss of the early excitation of the middle of the left side of the septum (Fig. 4–AE14).[105]

Isolated obstruction of the diagonal branch of the left anterior descending artery results in changes localized to leads I and aV_l and rarely involves the precordial leads.[106]

Right Ventricular Infarction. This is likely when an elevated ST segment in lead V_1 or V_2 complicates a Q-wave inferior left ventricular septal infarction (Fig. 4–39).[107] It has been suggested that simultaneous ST-segment elevation in lead V_1 and depression in lead V_2 is an important and specific sign for right ventricular infarction.[108] Although Q waves and ST elevation may appear in leads V_1 through V_3, their specificity is too low to be useful in the diagnosis of right ventricular infarction. Right ventricular infarction is more likely when the changes are recorded in right precordial leads, especially V_4R (Fig. 4–AE18, p. 149). The sensitivity and specificity of ST segment elevation in lead V_4R alone has been estimated between 82 to 100 and 68 to 77 per cent, respectively. ST-segment elevation equal to or greater than 1 mm in one or more leads V_4R to V_6R has been shown to have a sensitivity and specificity for infarction of the right ventricle of 90 and 91 per cent, respectively. It has been suggested that ST-segment elevation when greater in lead V_4R than in V_1, V_2, and V_3 reaches a specificity of 100 per cent, but its sensitivity is somewhat lower (78 per cent) than that of an elevated ST segment in V_4R alone.[109,110] During the acute phase of inferior infarction, ST segment elevation in right precordial leads V_4R to V_6R is a most reliable sign of right ventricular infarction. Q waves are superior to ST-segment elevation in patients admitted 12 hours or longer after onset of symptoms. Right ventricular infarction was recorded in 57 per cent of the 187 patients with inferior myocardial infarction.[111] Right ventricular conduction delay is a frequent finding in patients with right ventricular ischemia with an elevated ST segment.[112]

Posterior Left Ventricular Infarction. This is rarely detected. This area of the left ventricle, the last to be depolarized, is inscribed during the terminal 0.04 to 0.06 sec of the QRS complex. Theoretically, therefore, it cannot be expressed as an initial positive wave in leads V_1 and V_2. In keeping with the dipole concept, however, the S wave may become smaller, a sign that lacks any degree of specificity. In a small number of patients, posterior myocardial infarction may be suspected when there is ST-segment depression in lead V_1 or V_2 or both, an R wave in lead V_1 of 0.04 sec, and an R/S ratio greater than 1. The exact mechanism of the change in the initial QRS forces in leads V_1 and V_2 is not clear. Some have suggested that posterior myocardial infarction is not manifested in the ECG but that the find-

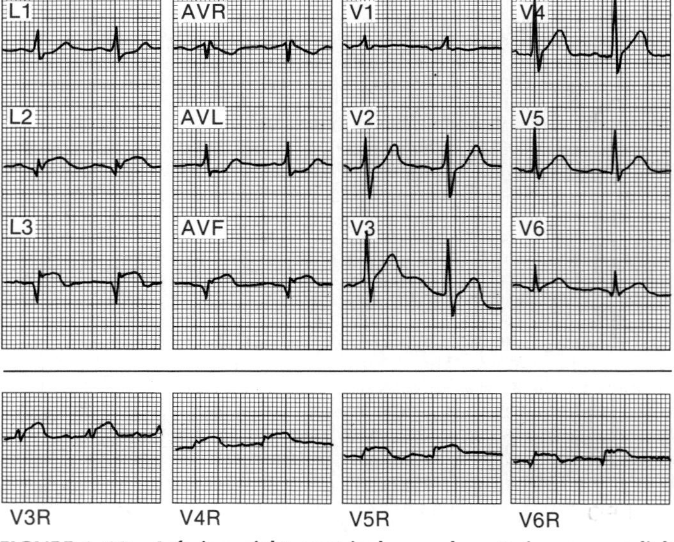

FIGURE 4–39. Inferior, right ventricular, and posterior myocardial infarction. The inferior infarct is manifested by Q waves and elevated ST segments in leads II, III, and aV_f, the posterior by the prominent R waves in leads V_1 and V_2, and the right ventricular by ST segment elevation in leads V_3R to V_6R.

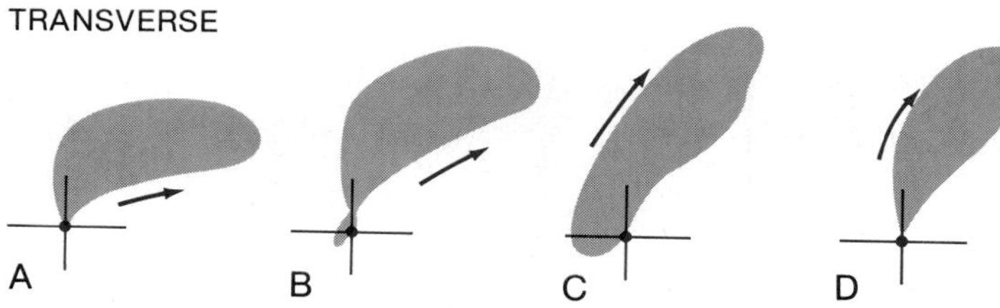

FIGURE 4–40. Vectorcardiogram (diagram) of anterior myocardial infarction. *A*, Anteroseptal; *B*, localized anterior; *C*, anterolateral; *D*, extensive anterior. (Modified from Chou, T. C., et al.: Clinical Vectorcardiography. 2nd ed. New York, Grune and Stratton, 1974, pp. 191, 196, 199.)

ings in lead V_1 or V_2 or both reflect an associated lateral infarction. In patients with an inferior or lateral myocardial infarction, an R wave of increased amplitude 0.04 sec in duration in leads V_1 and V_2 and an upright T wave in lead V_1 suggest concomitant posterior wall involvement (Figs. 4–35, 4–36, 4–AE16, and 4–AE17, p. 149). On occasion, ST-segment depression in leads V_2 and V_3 may be the early evidence of an evolving posterolateral myocardial infarction.[113]

In an effort to estimate the size of infarction, a QRS scoring system based on duration of the Q and R waves and loss of R-wave amplitude expressed in amplitude ratio of R/Q or R/S has been proposed.[114]

THE VCG IN MYOCARDIAL INFARCTION

The appearance of the vector loop in myocardial infarction depends on the site and size of the infarction. Deviation from normal reflects loss of forces normally generated by the infarcted area and resultant dominance of the noninfarcted myocardium. Anterior myocardial infarction is best visualized in the transverse plane, while inferior infarction is best displayed in the frontal or sagittal planes (Fig. 4–40 and 4–41).

Anteroseptal myocardial infarction is recognized in the transverse plane by loss of the first 10- to 20-msec forces, with the initial position of the loop oriented posteriorly and to the left. The entire loop is displaced posteriorly with loss of the anterior convexity. In the vast majority of cases, the loop is inscribed in a counterclockwise direction. The initial posterior and leftward orientation of the loop is reflected in the ECG as a QS complex in leads V_1 to V_4 (Fig. 4–40).

In *localized anterior infarction*, the transverse loop is similar in appearance to that present in anteroseptal myocardial infarction except for a normally inscribed initial force in a left and anterior direction. This initial inscription is displayed in the ECG as an R wave in lead V_1 and at times in V_2 (Fig. 4–40). In *extensive anterior infarction*, the transverse loop reflects loss of both the septal and free left ventricular walls. The initial normal anteriorly inscribed portion of the loop is lost, and the loop is shifted posteriorly and inscribed clockwise. The ECG shows a loss of R wave, at times, in all precordial leads.

Anterolateral infarction is inscribed clockwise or as a figure-of-eight in the transverse plane. The initial normal part of the loop is followed by posterior and somewhat rightward displacement, reflecting the more extensive loss of left ventricular wall. Loss of the lateral wall may result in an increase in magnitude of the initial left-to-right portion of the loop, reflected in the ECG as a tall R wave inscribed in the right precordial leads (Fig. 4–40).

Inferior myocardial infarction is best displayed in the frontal and sagittal planes (Fig. 4–41). In the frontal plane, the loop is most often inscribed in a clockwise direction. The initial portion is directed superiorly, the superior displacement exceeding 25 to 30 msec. The loop crosses the *X* axis to the left of the point of origin. It has been suggested that when the above diagnostic findings are absent, a shift to the left of the QRS loop combined with clockwise rotation is strongly indicative of an inferior infarction. Occasionally, when the inferior septum is spared, the initial loop may have a normal orientation, that is, to the right and inferiorly. This is followed by clockwise inscription and superior displacement of the remainder of the loop. In such instances the ECG will record small initial R waves in leads II, III, and aV_F.

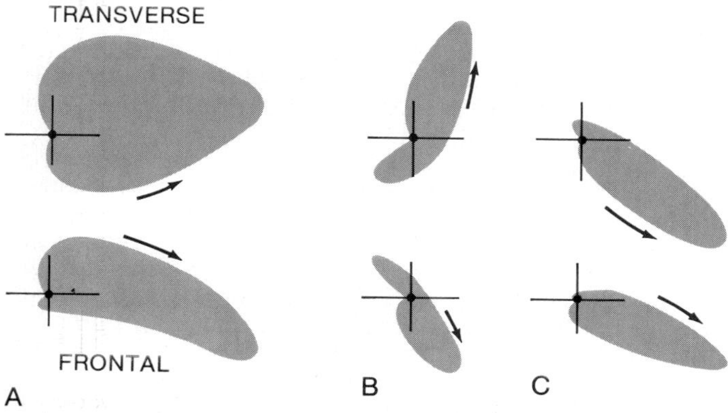

FIGURE 4–41. Vectorcardiogram of inferior and posterior myocardial infarction. *A*, Inferior; *B*, inferolateral; *C*, true posterior. (Modified from Chou, T. C., et al.: Clinical Vectorcardiography. 2nd ed. New York, Grune and Stratton, 1974, pp. 208, 220, 226.)

In *posterior myocardial infarction* the initial forces are normal in the transverse plane, but more than half the loop is ultimately displaced anteriorly. In the majority of cases, inscription of the loop is counterclockwise. The anterior displacement of the loop is reflected in the ECG by a prominent R wave in lead V_1 or V_2 that may exceed 0.04 sec in duration (Fig. 4–41).

A summary of VCG criteria for myocardial infarction is presented in Table 4–3 and Figures 4–40 and 4–41.

Noninfarction Q Waves

While the vast majority of abnormal Q waves are due to myocardial infarction, a significant number are due to other causes.

Noninfarction Q waves may be transient or permanent. Transient Q waves have been produced experimentally in animals and observed in patients during ischemic episodes.[115] Such Q waves have been explained by a transient loss of electrophysiological function, but without irreversible cellular damage, a phenomenon referred to by some as "myocardial concussion."[116,117] Q waves have been recorded with severe metabolic disturbances accompanying shock or pancreatitis. Similarly, transient Q waves have been noted during cardiac surgery and ascribed variously to transient ischemia and hypoxia, coronary spasm, localized metabolic and electrolyte disturbances, and possible hypothermia. Rarely a transient Q wave may result from tachycardia.

The largest group of noninfarction Q waves is due to myocardial disease, including myocarditis, AIDS (Fig. 4–AE19, p. 149), cardiac amyloidosis,[118] neuromuscular disorders such as progressive muscular dystrophy,[119] myotonia atrophica, Friedreich's ataxia, scleroderma, postpartum myopathy, myocardial replacement by tumor (Fig. 4–42), sarcoidosis, idiopathic cardiomyopathy, anomalous coronary artery, and coronary embolism.

Noninfarction Q waves are common in hypertrophic cardiomyopathy[120,121] and may simulate anterior or inferior myocardial infarction (Figs. 4–43 and 4–AE20, p. 149). Although the exact mechanism of the abnormal Q waves in this condition is unclear, increased septal mass or abnormal depolarization because of anomalous architecture of the septal myocardium, or both, have been proposed as the cause.

Abnormal Q waves can be associated with chronic obstructive lung disease (COLD) with or without cor pulmonale, pulmonary embolism, and pneumothorax. In COLD, findings in the precordial leads frequently simulate anterior myocardial infarction (Fig. 4–14). The mechanism responsible for the QS complex is clockwise rotation and downward displacement of the diaphragm and of the heart. As a result, the electrodes are located superior to the initial vector; when this vector is directed inferiorly, a QS pattern results. By placing the electrode one interspace lower, it is often possible to record an R wave and thus provide strong evidence against myocardial infarction. Occasionally in COLD the Q wave may simulate inferior myocardial infarction. The positional origin of the anterior or inferior Q

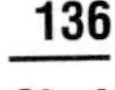

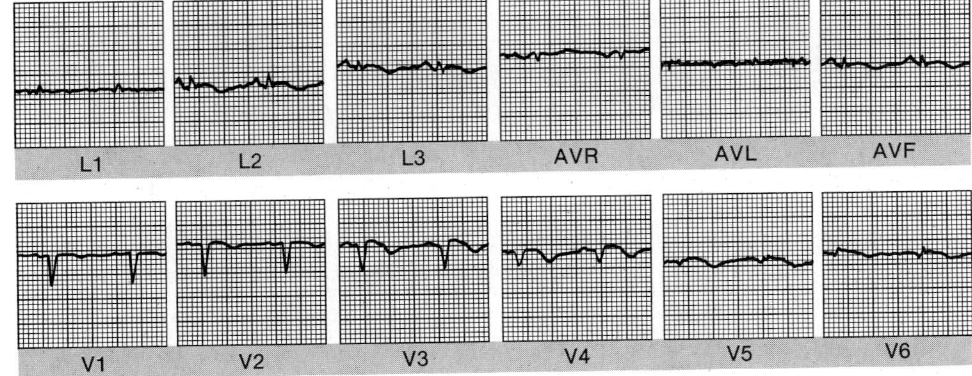

FIGURE 4–42. Extensive anterior and inferior myocardial infarction simulated by extensive myocardial metastasis of carcinoma of the breast.

waves may be suspected when the Q wave is accompanied by other ECG findings of COLD (see p. 115). However, since both COLD and myocardial infarction frequently coexist, differential diagnosis may at times be difficult or impossible.

Abnormal Q waves, especially in lead III and rarely in lead aV_f, with an S wave in lead I, can be recorded in acute cor pulmonale due to *pulmonary embolism* (Fig. 4–13). Clockwise rotation with superior orientation of the initial vector is most likely responsible for the Q waves in lead III. A Q wave in lead II is rarely recorded. Occasionally acute pulmonary embolus may simulate anterior myocardial infarction.

Spontaneous pneumothorax, particularly on the left, may result in a pattern simulating anterior myocardial infarction with occasional absence of the R wave in all the precordial leads.

In LBBB the initial forces are directed from right to left and either superiorly or inferiorly. When the inferiorly directed forces dominate, a QS complex may be recorded in the precordial leads, simulating an anterior myocardial infarction. If the initial vector is oriented to the left and superiorly, a QS complex may be registered in the inferior leads, suggesting inferior myocardial infarction.

With left anterior divisional block, the transitional zone is shifted to the left, and an initial Q wave may appear in the right precordial leads. Loss of the forces normally contributed by the left anterior division results in a vector directed inferiorly, posteriorly, and to the right. Consequently, right precordial leads may register a qrS complex suggestive of an anteroseptal infarction. By placement of the electrodes one interspace lower, an rS complex can be recorded attesting to the positional nature of the Q wave.

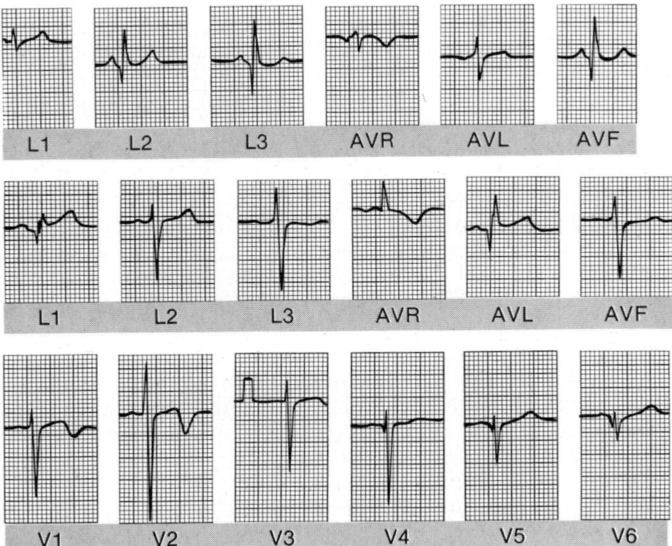

FIGURE 4–43. Hypertrophic cardiomyopathy simulating an inferior, high lateral (precordial leads, not shown, are normal) and anterolateral myocardial infarction in the upper, middle, and lower trace, respectively. (From Fisch, C.: Evolution of the clinical electrocardiogram. J. Am. Coll. Cardiol. *14*:1127, 1989. Reprinted by permission of the American College of Cardiology.)

Noninfarction Q waves are frequent in WPW (see p. 667). WPW type B, with the initial forces directed from right to left, registers a QS complex in the right precordial leads and may be mistaken for anteroseptal or anterior myocardial infarction. Rarely, preexcitation of the left lateral wall, with the vector oriented anteriorly and to the right, simulates lateral infarction. Most often, however, WPW simulates inferior infarction (Fig. 4–28). The Q waves recorded in leads II, III, and aV_f are due to superior orientation of the initial vector and may be seen with either type A or type B WPW.

In LVH, failure to record an R wave in leads V_1 to V_4 may suggest an anteroseptal myocardial infarction (Fig. 4–11). Similarly, reciprocal elevation of the ST segments in these leads may contribute to an erroneous diagnosis of myocardial infarction. The exact mechanism of the initial negative deflection of the QRS is not clear, but it may be related to posterior rotation or inferior orientation of the initial vector (Fig. 4–11).

ST-Segment and T-Wave Changes

ST-SEGMENT ELEVATION. In addition to the three most common organic causes of ST-segment elevations—acute myocardial infarction, pericarditis, and Prinzmetal's angina (Fig. 4–44)—ST-segment elevation is occasionally observed in acute cor pulmonale, hyperkalemia (Fig. 4–45), cerebrovascular accidents, LVH, LBBB, hypertrophic cardiomyopathy, invasion of the heart by neoplastic tissue, hypothermia, and cocaine abuse.[122] Elevation of the ST segment also may be an artifact caused by excessive inertia of the stylus of the electrocardiograph. In the normal heart the most common cause of ST-segment elevation is so-called *early repolarization*, a normal variant (Fig. 4–46).

T-WAVE ABNORMALITIES. A *primary T wave change* indicates a regional alteration in the duration of the depolarized state. Some common clinical conditions associated with primary T-wave changes include myocardial ischemia, ventricular aneurysm (Fig. 4–AE21), electrolyte abnormalities (Fig. 4–45), drugs, and a variety of primary myocardial and extracardiac disorders such as myocarditis and subarachnoid hemorrhage. A clinically important sequence of T-wave changes is one of abnormal baseline with normalization of the T wave during ischemia and return to the abnormal baseline after ischemia subsides. Lack of a control tracing could lead to an erroneous conclusion of non-Q wave infarction (Fig. 4–47).

Global, diffuse symmetrical T-wave inversion is a nonspecific finding[123] most often seen with patients with myocardial ischemia (Fig. 4–36), or infarction, following

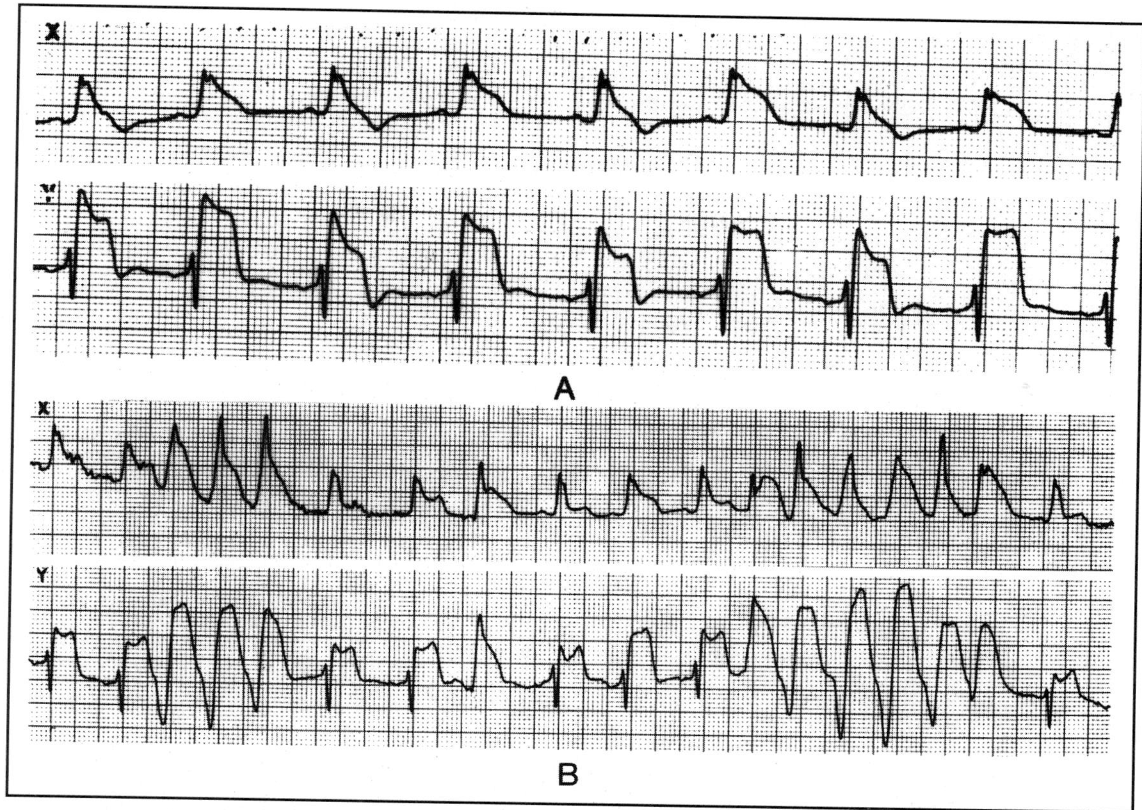

FIGURE 4–44. Printzmetal's angina with ST segment and T wave alternans in panel *A* and ST segment and T wave alternans and nonsustained VT in panel *B*.

cardiac resuscitation, cerebrovascular accidents, apical hypertrophic nonobstructive cardiomyopathy (Fig. 4–AE22, p. 150),[124,125] acute pulmonary embolism,[126] and rarely pheochromocytoma.[127] In a series of 29 patients, it was present in 6 individuals without evidence of organic heart disease. There is an unexplained female preponderance. This striking diffuse T-wave inversion does not in itself imply a poor prognosis. The prognosis is that of the disease.[123]

There is an interesting form of T-wave inversion ascribed to cardiac "memory." It was first noted following cardiac pacing, with the T-wave inversion persisting long after resumption of normal sinus rhythm.[128] Similar T-wave inversion has been recorded following radiofrequency ablation of the accessory pathway in WPW (Fig. 4–AE23, p. 150).[129,130]

Secondary T-wave changes result from alterations of the

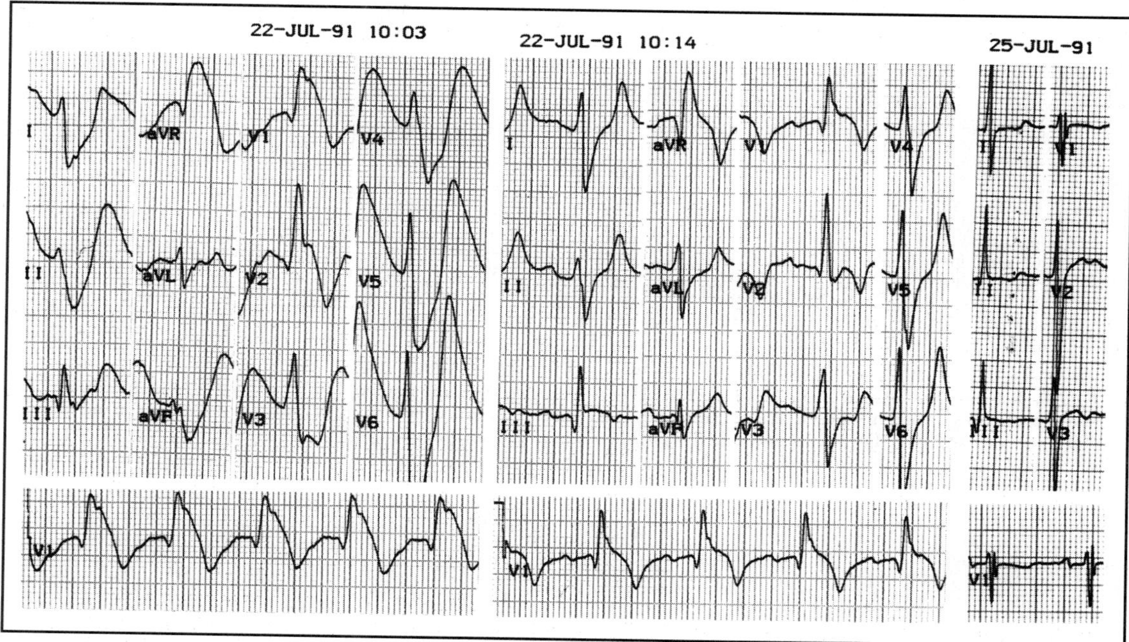

FIGURE 4–45. Severe hyperkalemia. 7/22/91, 10:03, P waves are absent, and there is a marked and diffused prolongation of the QRS with a "dialyzable" current of injury in leads V_1 and V_2. 7/22/91, 10:14, P waves are now present with a P-R interval of 0.24 sec. The QRS pattern is that of right bundle branch block with Q waves in leads V_1 and V_2 simulating a septal infarction. Elevation of the ST segment in lead V_1 is less pronounced. 7/25/91, The tracing is normal except for nonspecific ST-T changes in leads I, II, and III.

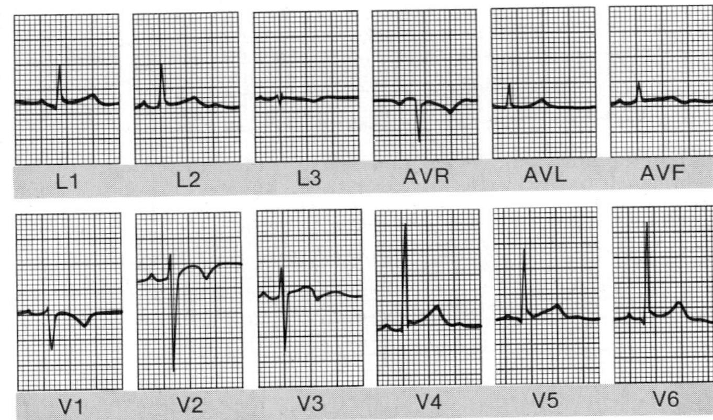

FIGURE 4–46. Normal tracing with juvenile T wave inversion in leads V_1, V_2, and V_3 and early repolarization manifested by ST-segment elevation in leads I, II, aV_f, V_4, V_5, and V_6.

timing or sequencing of depolarization or both, with an obligatory change of the order of repolarization. For example, in LBBB, left ventricular epicardial activation is delayed because of slow conduction through the ventricualr myocardium. As a result, repolarization begins in the subendocardium and an inverted T wave is recorded in precordial leads. The change in the area of the QRS complex and T waves is identical but opposite in direction. Occasionally LBBB is associated with an upright T wave in the left ventricular leads, suggesting that in addition to altered activation due to LBBB, regional abnormalities of repolarization contribute to the T-wave morphology (Fig. 4–17).

RATE-RELATED T-WAVE CHANGES. Postextrasystolic T-wave change was first described in 1915.[131] Since then, a number of mechanisms have been proposed to explain this observation, including an abnormal pathway of repolarization, prolonged diastolic filling time, and an abrupt change in the cycle length. Minor T-wave changes following an abrupt cycle change or after an interpolated ventricular premature complex may be recorded in normal tissue, while more pronounced T-wave alterations suggest an underlying myocardial disorder.

T-wave inversion is occasionally noted following supraventricular or ventricular tachycardia. The magnitude of the T-wave inversion varies, and when extreme, it may resemble the T-wave changes seen with cerebrovascular accidents or myocardial ischemia. The exact mechanism of the posttachycardia T wave is obscure.

T-WAVE ALTERNANS. Isolated T-wave alternans, i.e., without a change in either the QRS complex or the P wave, was first noted in the cat papillary muscle.[132] It is relatively rare and its mechanism not clear. Alternans of phases 2 and 3 of the action potential of the T wave has been recorded without any demonstrable change in phase 0, supporting the concept that isolated alternation of repolarization reflected in the T wave is possible. T-wave alternans of the type already mentioned is most often present during tachycardia or during a sudden change in cycle length. Isolated T-wave alternans, independent of tachycardia or premature systole, is nearly always associated with advanced heart disease or severe electrolyte disturbance (Fig. 4–48) following cardiac resuscitation, rarely with administration of amiodarone, acute pulmonary embolism, and idiopathic long Q-T syndrome. When T-wave alternans is associated with idiopathic pro-

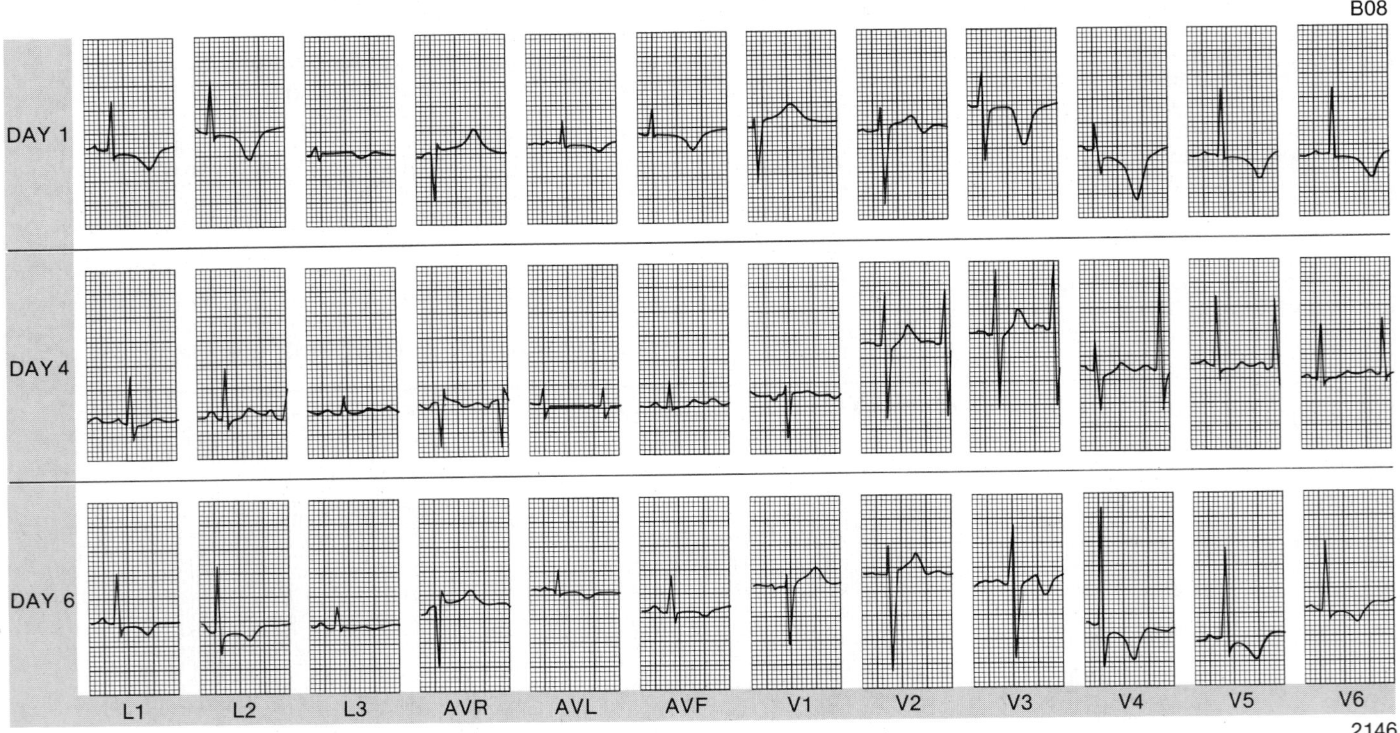

FIGURE 4–47. The top, control, trace recorded when the patient was asymptomatic illustrates symmetrical T wave inversion consistent with ischemic heart disease. During pain, on day 4, the T waves normalized, only to return to control after the pain subsided. If the top trace had been unavailable, the sequence of changes noted in the middle and lower traces coupled with the history could have been mistaken for a new non-Q-wave infarction.

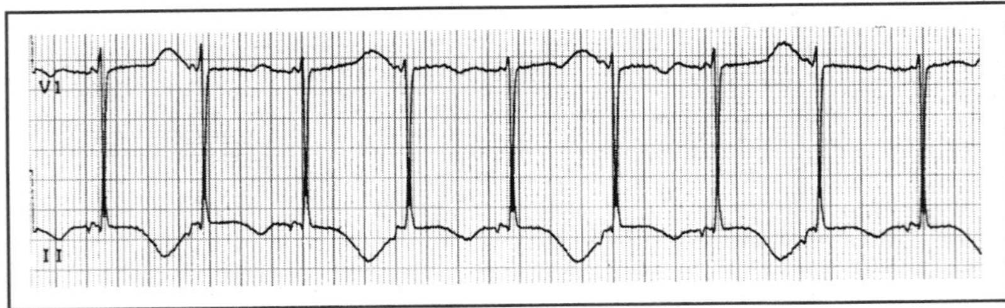

FIGURE 4–48. The QT interval is prolonged, measuring approximately 600 msec with T-wave alternans. The tracing was recorded in a patient with chronic renal disease shortly following dialysis.

longation of the Q-T interval, the risk is related to the prolonged Q-T interval rather than the T-wave alternans.[133–137]

NOTCHED, BIFID T WAVES. Notched, bifid T waves are relatively common in the absence of heart disease, especially in children. These waves also may be present in congenital organic heart disease, the prolonged Q-T syndrome, central nervous system disorders, alcoholic cardiomyopathy, and following the administration of drugs, especially the phenothiazines. The mechanism of bifid or notched T waves is unclear. It has been suggested that in some instances they are caused by nonuniform repolarization secondary to differential innervation of the anterior and posterior ventricular walls. It also has been proposed that in patients with left ventricular disease they may reflect regional delay of repolarization of the left ventricle. Notched or bifid T waves are much more common in association with a long Q-T interval and identify patients at higher risk for syncope or cardiac arrest.[138]

NONSPECIFIC ST-SEGMENT AND T-WAVE CHANGES. Although the ST segment and T wave represent different electrophysiological events and their respective changes may have different clinical connotations, the widespread practice among electrocardiographers is to refer to either one or both as *ST-T changes.* While it is more appropriate to discuss the two separately, it should be recognized that abnormalities of the ST segment and T wave frequently coexist.

Nondiagnostic ST-segment and T-wave changes are the most common ECG abnormality and account for about 50 per cent of the abnormal tracings recorded in a general hospital population and in 2.4 per cent of all cardiograms.[139] An abnormal T wave is extremely common because the wave is highly sensitive to physiological, pharmacological, and organic changes and therefore is least likely to suggest a specific diagnosis. This fact has been recognized since 1923, when Wilson first recorded inversion of the T wave following the ingestion of cold water.[140]

Although an abnormal T wave suggests the presence of an abnormal or, more appropriately, an altered state, it is recorded with relative frequency in the absence of any disorder (Fig. 4–45), as a reflection of physiological influences, e.g., in highly trained athletes,[141] or during paroxysmal supraventricular tachycardia.[142] For these reasons, an isolated T-wave change must be interpreted with caution and must *always* be correlated with all available clinical and laboratory information. Misinterpretation of the significance of a T-wave abnormality is the most common cause of "iatrogenic ECG heart disease." Attempts to identify the etiology of an abnormal ST segment, T wave, or ST-T segment in isolation from clinical and other laboratory findings often fail.

CLASSIC ST-T CHANGES. The specificity of the purported "classic" ST-T changes, such as those seen with LVH, digitalis administration, and ischemic heart disease, is relatively low. For example, a negative T wave reflecting persistence of a juvenile pattern cannot be differentiated from the symmetrically inverted T wave due to myocardial ischemia. The "classic" ST-T change of LVH also may be due to ischemic heart disease or digitalis, while the marked ST-segment depression due to ischemia or subendocardial infarction may be simulated by the administration of digitalis in the presence of moderate or severe disease. However, when correlated with clinical and other laboratory data, ST-T changes assume a greater predictive value. In a series of 410 abnormal tracings analyzed without regard to clinical data, 70 per cent could be interpreted only as "nonspecific ST-T change." This number was reduced to 10 per cent when such changes were correlated with available clinical information.[139]

The nonspecific and labile nature of the ST segment and the T wave, especially the latter, is expected. Repolarization is a much more diverse process than depolarization. Depolarization is rapid, with a reasonably uniform potential difference across the boundary of activation, and is reflected in the rate of rise of phase 0 and the amplitude of the action potential (see p. 555). Repolarization, displayed as the ST segment and T wave, reflects phases 2 and 3 of the action potential, is considerably longer, and is nonuniform, with many simultaneous boundaries and with differing potentials across various boundaries. It has been shown that shortening of the monophasic action potential by as little as 12 to 18 msec will alter the morphology of the T wave, and importantly, the change can be seen with involvement of 10 per cent or less of the myocardial mass.[143] The magnitude of the T-wave changes, unlike that of the QRS complex, is not related to the mass of the myocardium. The difference has been ascribed to cancellation of repolarization voltages and to uneven contributions from the different regions of repolarization to the genesis of the T wave. Such experimental findings explain, at least partially, the nonspecific character of ST-segment and T-wave changes.

A number of the clinical conditions that may alter the ST segment and T waves are listed in Table 4–4.

U WAVE ABNORMALITIES. An abnormal U wave may be increased in amplitude, inverted, or prolonged. A negative U wave is documented in about 1 per cent of cardiograms recorded in a general hospital. An exaggerated upright U wave may be due to hypokalemia, a variety of drugs (particularly digitalis), and some of the antiarrhythmic agents (e.g., amiodarone).

The most common causes of a *negative U wave* are hypertension (Fig. 4–AE24, p. 150), aortic and mitral valve disease, RVH, and myocardial ischemia (Fig. 4–36).[81,144] A negative U wave can occasionally be found in other metabolic or organic diseases. In hypertension, a negative U wave may be the earliest sign of myocardial involvement, appearing long before any change in the T wave, and has been reported in about 16 per cent of ECGs with an upright T wave and 45 per cent with negative T waves. It may revert to normal with control of the hypertension.[145] The majority of patients with aortic regurgitation and about 10 per cent of patients with aortic stenosis manifest negative U waves. Approximately 5 and 80 per cent of patients with systolic and diastolic overload of the right ventricle, respectively, manifest negative U waves in leads II, III, V_1, and V_2. While high-amplitude positive U waves are the usual finding in hypokalemia, on rare occasions profound hypokalemia may result in large negative U waves obscuring the hypokalemia.[146] In essence, a negative U wave, even as an isolated finding in an otherwise normal ECG, is strongly suggestive of a pathophysiological state.

Q-T INTERVAL ABNORMALITY (see also p. 114). *Shortening of the Q-T interval* may be recorded with hyperkalemia, digitalis, hypercalcemia, and acidosis. *Prolongation of the Q-T interval* may be primary and independent of the QRS, or it may reflect secondary changes of repolarization due to abnormal depolarization, or a combination of the two. Prolongation of the Q-T interval, independent of QRS duration, can be congenital (Figs. 4–49 and 4–AE25, p. 150) or acquired. Acquired disorders include ischemic heart disease, hypothermia, cardiomyopathy, mitral valve prolapse, complete heart block, the condition following cardiac resuscitation, electrolyte changes, and administration of drugs.[147–152] Q-T interval prolongation is a relatively frequent complication of acquired cerebral lesions, especially subarachnoid

TABLE 4–4 CAUSES OF ST-SEGMENT AND T WAVE CHANGES (SELECTED)

Physiological
Position, temperature, hyperventilation, anxiety, food (glucose), tachycardia, neurogenic influences, physical training
Pharmacological
Digitalis, antiarrhythmic and psychotropic drugs (phenothiazines, tricyclics, lithium)
Extracardiac Disorders
Electrolyte abnormalities, cerebrovascular accidents, shock, anemia, allergic reactions, infections, endocrine disorders, acute abdominal disorders, pulmonary embolism
Primary Myocardial Disease
Congestive, hypertrophic, postpartum cardiomyopathy, myocarditis
Secondary Myocardial Disease
Amyloidosis, hemochromatosis, neoplasm, sarcoidosis, connective tissue, neuromuscular disorders
Ischemic Heart Disease
Myocardial infarction

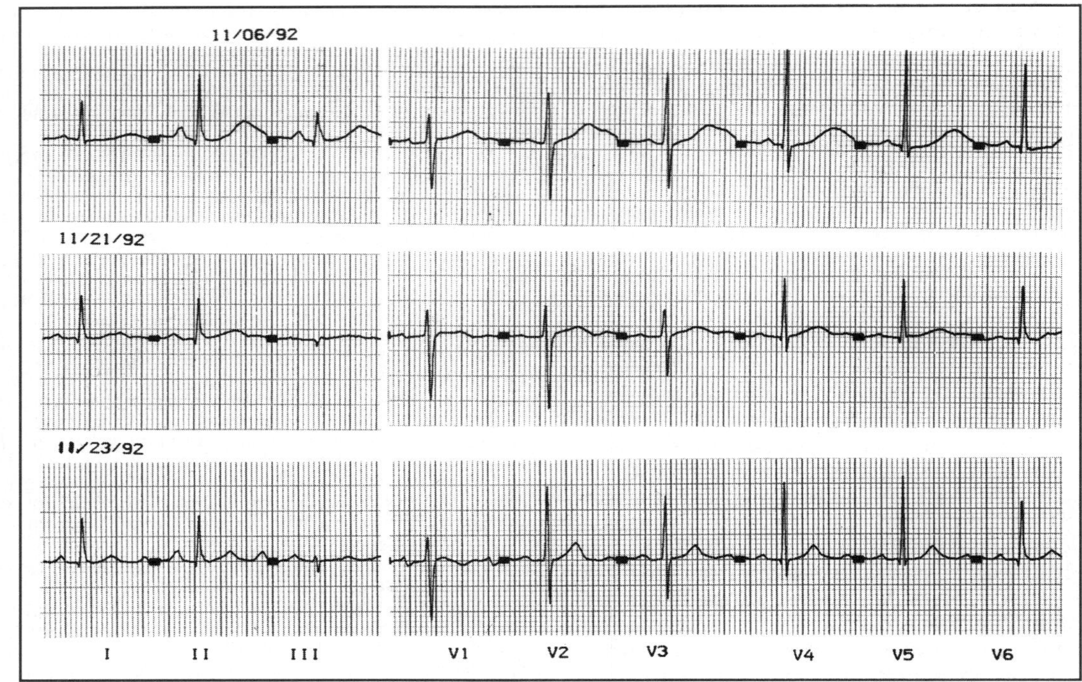

FIGURE 4–49. CVA with marked prolongation of the Q-T interval on 11/6/92. The Q-T interval is shorter but still prolonged on 11/21/92. On 11/23/92 the Q-T interval is normal.

hemorrhage, and also can be present during and following neurosurgical procedures.

ELECTRICAL ALTERNANS. Alternation of amplitude and direction of the QRS complex was noted in the experimental animal and humans as early as 1909 and 1910, respectively,[153] followed by documentation of alternation of the P wave, ST segment, and T wave[52] (Fig. 4–48). Isolated *alternation of the P wave* is seen frequently in the experimental setting but is rare in humans. Most often it accompanies alternation of the QRS complex and occasionally the QRS complex and the T wave. The latter is referred to as *total alternans* and suggests pericardial effusion, usually due to malignancy and frequently associated with tamponade or impending tamponade.

Although pericardial effusion is the most common cause of alternation of the QRS complex (see p. 112), *QRS alternans* is also seen with myocardial ischemia and myocardial disease due to other causes. Two mechanisms of QRS alternans have been proposed: positional oscillation and aberrancy of intraventricular conduction. The early suggestion that oscillation or alternation of position is the mechanism of alternans of the QRS complex was proved by means of echocardiography. The concept of oscillation also explains the fact that P-wave alternans is seen predominantly with massive pericardial effusion.

ST-segment alternans has been described in dogs after ligation of the coronary artery, in severely ill infants with congenital heart disease, and in patients with Prinzmetal's angina. *T-wave alternans* is discussed on page 137. *U-wave alternans* is least common and very difficult to recognize.

The mechanism of alternans in severe myocardial disorders but in the absence of pericardial effusion is obscure. It has been ascribed to uneven duration of the excited state or to two alternating foci of impulse formation. However, the fact that alternation of depolarization, activation, and repo-

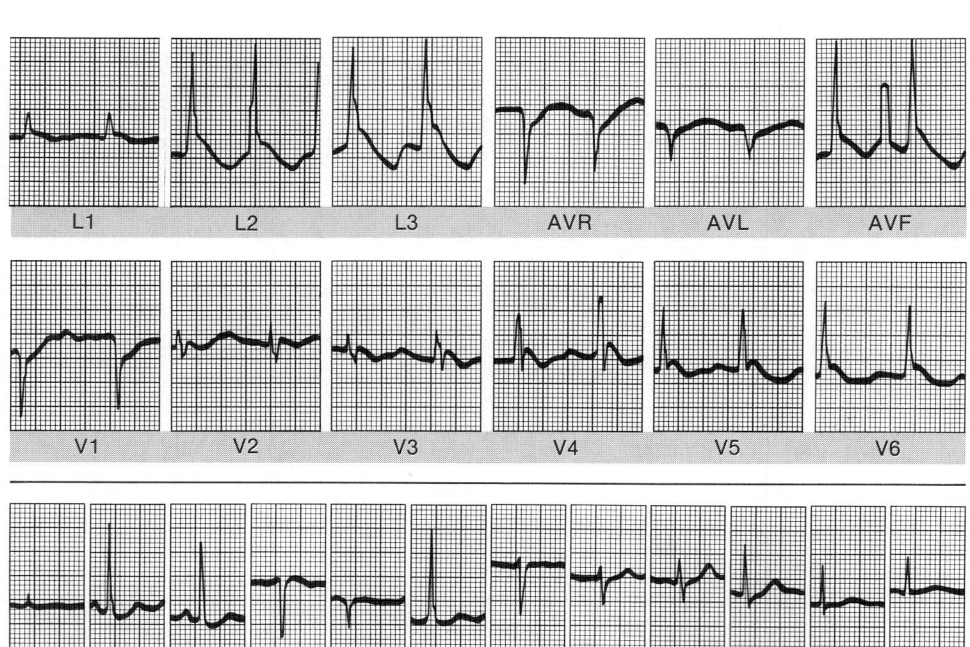

FIGURE 4–50. Osborne wave. Upper panel was recorded during hypothermia. The P-R interval is 0.28 sec; the QRS complex measures 0.10 sec and is followed by a wave (the Osborne wave) that merges with the ST segment: The T wave is inverted in leads I, II, III, aV_f, V_5, and V_6. It is difficult to separate the Osborne wave from the initial part of the ST segment. Bottom panel was recorded after the temperature returned to normal. The tracing is normal. The prolongation and increase in QRS amplitude noted during hypothermia, although within normal limits, are evident when compared with the normal ECG.

larization can be recorded in a single cell suggests that the mechanism is probably related to transmembrane ionic fluxes. Alternans of a human atrial monophasic action potential adds further credence to the primary role of transmembrane ionic events.[52]

THE OSBORNE WAVE. An Osborne wave, seen in hypothermia, is a deflection inscribed between the QRS complex and the beginning of the ST segment (Fig. 4–50).[154] It has been variously suggested that this wave reflects delay of depolarization, a current of injury, or early repolarization. In the left ventricular leads the polarity of the wave is positive and its amplitude is inversely related to body temperature. The electrophysiological mechanism of the Osborne wave remains unclear.

Abnormal ECG in Absence of Clinical Heart Disease

Abnormal ECGs may be recorded in patients with clinically normal hearts.[155,156] The abnormalities may be those of the QRS, ST segment, or T wave. Common abnormalities of the QRS include QS complexes in lead aV_l or QS or QR complexes in leads III and aV_f, a QS complex in leads V_1 and V_2, a tall R wave in leads V_1 and V_2, and high voltage of the R wave over the left ventricle. A frequent "normal" alteration of the ST segment is an elevation, the so-called early repolarization, which may be recorded in the inferior, left precordial, and rarely right precordial leads. Abnormal T waves include persistence of juvenile T-wave inversion over the right precordium (Fig. 4–45), isolated midprecordial T-wave inversion, and terminal T-wave inversion associated with ST-segment elevation due to early repolarization and right precordial T-wave inversion in middle-aged women. A variety of physiological influences alter the T wave of a normal heart (Table 4–4).

An abnormal ECG in the absence of clinical evidence of heart disease in the young should be evaluated carefully, because the prevalence of true heart disease in this setting is low and the chances are high that the tracing is false positive for disease.

Limb lead reversal is a relatively common error of technique and may result in an erroneous diagnosis of arrhythmias, myocardial ischemia or infarction, fascicular blocks, and ventricular hypertrophy. Lead reversal should be suspected when the limb leads exhibit significant changes while the precordial leads are normal and unchanged. The most common form of lead reversal is that of the right and left arms with a resultant "mirror image" of lead I. Right arm and right leg and left arm and right leg reversal should be suspected when lead II and III are isoelectric.[157] Not infrequently the sequence of leads V_1, V_2, and V_3 is reversed, and the computer will inevitably interpret the tracing as an anterior myocardial infarction (Fig. 4–AE25, p. 150). Such lead reversal is easily detected by analysis of the P wave. The inverted or biphasic P wave will identify lead V_1. However, when there is doubt, the cardiogram should be repeated.

The ECG and Electrolyte Abnormalities

HYPERKALEMIA. There is a good correlation between plasma K and the surface ECG in experimental hyperkalemia. The earliest ECG change, at a plasma level of about 5.7 mEq/liter, is a tall, peaked, most often symmetrical T wave with a narrow base and a normal or decreased $Q\text{-}T_c$ interval. The QRS complex widens uniformly at a level of 9 to 11 mEq/liter and an occasional acute current of injury resembling myocardial infarction may be present. Reduction in P-wave amplitude, intraatrial conduction delay, and P-R interval prolongation are recorded at a plasma level of about 7.0 mEq/liter. At plasma K levels of about 8.4 mEq/liter or higher, the P wave is no longer recognizable. When the plasma concentration exceeds 12 mEq/liter, either ventricular fibrillation or arrest follows. SA node fibers, being more resistant to the depressive action of K than is atrial myocardium, continue to generate impulses that are now delayed in their exit or may fail to propagate because of depressed intraatrial conduction. The result may be Wenckebach (type I) or Mobitz (type II) sinoatrial (SA) block (see p. 687). Junctional escape and junctional rhythm are relatively common in experimental hyperkalemia.

In clinical hyperkalemia, abnormalities of impulse information and conduction appear at K levels lower than those observed in the experimental animal, and the correlation between plasma K and the ECG is less reliable. A tall, peaked, symmetrical T wave with a narrow base, the so-called "tented" T wave, is the earliest ECG abnormality, usually best seen in leads II, III, V_2, V_3, and V_4. The pointed, symmetrical appearance and narrow base of the T wave help to differentiate the effect of hyperkalemia from other causes of tall T waves, including normal variants. The tented appearance and the narrow base are probably more characteristic of hyperkalemia than is the amplitude of the T wave. A decrease in amplitude of the R wave, appearance of a prominent S wave, widening of the QRS complex, depression of the ST segment, and an occasional elevation of the ST segment evolve as plasma K continues to rise and approaches 8 to 9 mEq/liter (Fig. 4–51). A decrease in amplitude and prolongation of the P wave and lengthening of the P-R interval followed by disappearance of the P wave often make recognition of arrhythmias in hyperkalemia difficult, if not impossible. At times hyperkalemia induces a current of injury called *dialyzable current of injury,* which may be mistaken for acute ischemia (Fig. 4–45).

With hyperkalemia, depression of intraventricular conduction is characteristically diffuse and fairly uniform and results in prolongation of both the initial and terminal parts of the QRS complex. The resulting pattern may resemble RBBB, LBBB, left anterior or posterior divisional block, or a combination of the four. When the ECG resembles RBBB, the initial phase of the QRS complex is prolonged, in contrast to the conventional RBBB, in which only the terminal portion of the QRS complex is delayed

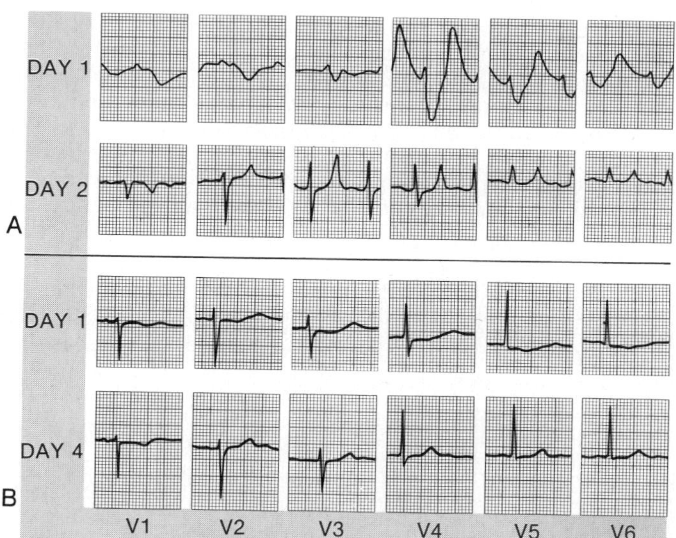

FIGURE 4–51. ECG changes in hyperkalemia *(A)* and hypokalemia *(B)*. Panel *A*, On day 1, at a K^+ level of 8.6 mEq/liter, the P wave is no longer recognizable and the QRS complex is diffusely prolonged. Initial and terminal QRS delay is characteristic of K^+-induced intraventricular conduction and is best illustrated in leads V_2 and V_6. On day 2, at a K^+ level of 5.8 mEq/liter, the P wave is recognizable with a P-R interval of 0.24 sec, the duration of the QRS complex is approximately 0.10 sec, and the T waves are characteristically "tented." Panel *B*, On day 1, at a K^+ level of 1.5 mEq/liter, the T and U waves are merged. The U wave is prominent and the Q-U interval prolonged. On day 4, at a K^+ level of 3.7 mEq/liter, the tracing is normal.

(Fig. 4–AE26, p. 150). Similarly, when the ECG simulates LBBB, an S wave indicates slowing of the terminal portion of the QRS (Fig. 4–51). In conventional LBBB, on the other hand, prolongation involves only the initial component of the QRS complex.

In humans, as in animals, SA block (see p. 687), either Wenckebach (type I) or Mobitz (type II), passive or accelerated junctional or ventricular escape rhythms may be present. Potassium may normalize physiologically or functionally inverted T waves, but as a rule it has no effect on T-wave inversion due to organic disorders or drugs.

HYPOKALEMIA. The ECG in *hypokalemia* is characterized by gradual depression of the ST segment, decrease of T-wave amplitude, occasionally inversion of the T wave, and a prominent U wave but without a significant change in the Q-T interval (Figs. 4–51 and 4–AE27, p. 151). In advanced hypokalemia the ST segment gradually fuses with the U wave, the latter greater in amplitude than the T wave. An increase in amplitude of the QRS complex may be present. There is reasonable correlation between ECG changes and K concentrations below 2.3 or 3.0 mEq/liter. Prominent U waves with ST-segment and T-wave changes are not specific for hypokalemia, however. Such abnormalities can be the result of administration of digitalis and other drugs, ventricular hypertrophy, and bradycardia.

CALCIUM. The effects of Ca on the ECG were recognized in 1922.[158] In general, the ECG changes due to alteration in Ca concentrations correlate with the effect of Ca ions on the transmembrane action potential. Changes in duration of phase 2 parallel the altered duration of the ST segment and the Q-T interval.

Hypocalcemia prolongs phase 2, reflected by prolongation of the ST segment and Q-T interval (Figs. 4–52 and 4–AE29). The Q-aT (Q to the apex of the T wave) and the Q-T intervals are prolonged, but the Q-T_c interval rarely exceeds 140 per cent of the normal. If longer, the U wave is likely to be included in the measurement. Hypocalcemia does not affect phase 3 of the action potential or the T wave. Hypocalcemia with hyperkalemia, most often seen in patients with chronic renal disease, results in a prolonged ST segment and a "tented" T wave. Hypocalcemia and hypokalemia exhibit a prolonged ST segment and a prominent terminal wave that includes both T and U waves.

Hypercalcemia shortens phase 2 of the action potential and the ST segment. The Q-T interval is shortened (Fig. 4–AE28, p. 151), the ST segment occasionally depressed, and the T wave inverted (Fig. 4–52).[159,160] A prominent J wave similar to that of hypothermia has been observed.

The correlation between the Q-T interval and serum Ca concentration is unpredictable, largely because the Q-T duration is affected by factors other than calcium levels, such as age, sex, heart rate, myocardial disease, drugs, and other electrolytes. It has been suggested that when factors known to alter the Q-T interval are eliminated, a reasonably good correlation is found between the ECG and calcium levels. This assumption is supported by the fact that Ca levels in pure hypocalcemia induced by EDTA show a reasonably good correlation with the Q-T interval. Of the three intervals—Q-T, Q-oT (Q to the onset of the T wave), and Q-aT (Q to the apex of the T wave)—the Q-aT interval can be measured with greatest accuracy and correlates best with the Ca level.

MAGNESIUM. Administration of magnesium may result in shortening of the Q-T interval and prolongation of the P-R interval, QRS complex, and intraatrial conduction. As a rule, however, abnormalities of the ST segment due to hypermagnesemia cannot be identified on the ECG because the changes are dominated by calcium.[161] Hypomagnesemia cannot be recognized on the ECG.

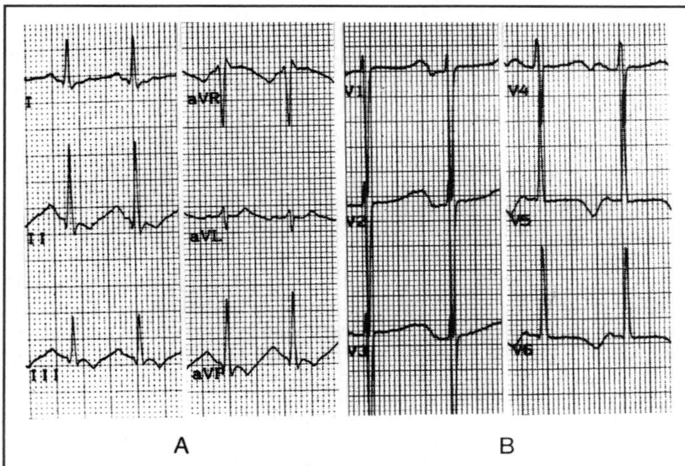

FIGURE 4–52. *A*, Hypercalcemia with a short Q-T interval (0.22 sec) and inverted T waves, the latter a rare manifestation of hypercalcemia. *B*, Hypocalcemia with a prolonged Q-T interval.

Effects of Drugs on the ECG

The effect of antiarrhythmic drugs on the ECG is considered in Chapter 21.

Digitalis

(See p. 664)

Alterations of the ST segment and the T wave are the earliest recognizable changes due to the digitalis glycosides. The T wave amplitude is lowered, and the ST segment is depressed and shortened, with occasional appearance of a prominent U wave.[162] While the "characteristic" digitalis-induced ST segment is described as sagging, it is often difficult if not impossible to differentiate it from ST-segment depresseion of other causes. When the ST segment is also shortened, digitalis is the likely cause of the depression. ST-segment displacement due to digitalis may be greatly exaggerated by myocardial disease, tachycardia, and high-amplitude QRS complexes. Rarely, digitalis causes symmetrical inversion of the T wave similar to that in pericarditis and ischemia, but there is usually associated shortening of the Q-T interval. A peaked, "tented" T wave, probably due to concomitant hyperkalemia, also can be present. Digitalis has no significant effect on depolarization of the atrium or ventricle. Consequently, prolongation of intraatrial and intraventricular conduction is rare.

DIGITALIS-INDUCED ARRHYTHMIAS. Digitalis has been known to induce nearly every known arrhythmia.[163,164]

1. Ectopic rhythms due to enhanced automaticity, reentry, or delayed diastolic afterdepolarizations: atrial tachycardia with block (Fig. 22-17, p. 657), atrial fibrillation and flutter, nonparoxysmal junctional tachycardia, ventricular premature contractions, ventricular tachycardia, ventricular flutter and fibrillation, multiple ectopic rhythms (Figs. 4–AE29 and AE30, p. 151), bidirectional ventricular tachycardia, or accelerated escape.
2. Depression of pacemaker: SA node arrest.
3. Depression of conduction: SA block, AV block, exit block, or reciprocation.
4. AV dissociation: Suppression of the dominant pacemaker with passive escape of the lower junctional focus or inappropriate acceleration of a subsidiary pacemaker, or, rarely, dissociation within the AV function (double junctional tachycardia).

Arrhythmias identical to those due to digitalis toxicity also can be caused by heart disease, drugs other than digitalis, and a variety of extracardiac factors.

THERAPEUTIC AND TOXIC EFFECTS (See p. 484). Appearance of ectopic rhythms in the course of digitalis administration is nearly always a sign of toxicity. On the other hand, depression of AV conduction may at times be a desirable therapeutic endpoint. Acknowledging that some degree of overlap is unavoidable and that the clinical significance of an arrhythmia may differ depending on the setting, the effects of digitalis on the ECG can be divided into three general groups—therapeutic, excessive and/or toxic, and unequivocally toxic.

The wide spectrum of arrhythmias induced by digitalis and the coexistence of a number of different arrhythmias in the same tracing can be explained by the interplay between digitalis and myocardial and extracardiac factors on the electrophysiological properties of cardiac tissues. The drug may have different effects on the same specialized tissue; i.e., it may depress conduction or enhance automaticity, or both. Also, digitalis may act directly on the specialized tissue or its action may be mediated through the sympathetic or parasympathetic system or both. In addition, the sensitivity of the tissues to digitalis may be altered by factors such as a changing acid-balance, plasma and intracellular electrolyte levels, oxygen tension, and mechanical stretch.

The arrhythmias most commonly caused by digitalis include atrial tachycardia with block, nonparoxysmal junctional tachycardia, ventricular tachyarrhythmias, AV dissociation, and AV conduction delay (see Ch.22).

ACCELERATED JUNCTIONAL ESCAPE. This arrhythmia is seen in the same clinical conditions as is nonparoxysmal junctional tachycardia, and its clinical significance is probably the same. Accelerated junctional escape follows the rules set for cardiac arrhythmias induced by delayed afterdepolarization and may be the clinical counterpart of the arrhythmias induced in the Purkinje fiber and the intact animal.

REFERENCES

1. Macfarlane, P. W., and Lawrie, V. T. D.: Comprehensive Electrocardiology. Vol. 1. New York, Pergamon Press, 1989.
2. Fye, W. B.: A history of the origin, evolution, and impact of electrocardiography. Am. J. Cardiol. *73*:937, 1994.
3. Horan, I. G.: Manifest orientation: The theoretical link between the anatomy of the heart and the clinical electrocardiogram. J. Am. Coll. Cardiol. *9*:1049, 1987.
4. Burch, G. E., and DePasquale, N. P.: A History of Electrocardiography. Chicago, Year Book Medical Publishers, 1964.
5. Fisch, C.: Evolution of the clinical electrocardiogram. J. Am. Coll. Cardiol. *14*:1127, 1989.
6. Waller, A. D.: A demonstration on man of electromotive changes accompanying the heart's beat. J. Physiol. *8*:229, 1887.
7. Einthoven, W.: Selected Papers on Electrocardiography. Snellen, A. (ed.). Leiden, University Press. 1977.
8. Lewis, T.: The Mechanism and Graphic Registration of the Heart Beat. London, Shaw and Sons, Ltd., 1920, p. 228.
9. Wilson, F. N.: Selected Papers of FD Johnston. Lepeschkin, F. D. E. (ed.). Ann Arbor, Edward Brothers, Inc., 1954.
10. Durrer, D.: Selected Papers. Meijler, F. L., and Burchell, H. B. (eds.). Amsterdam, North Holland Publishing Co., 1986.
11. Fisch, C.: Electrocardiography of Arrhythmias. Philadelphia, Lea and Febiger, 1989.
12. Fye, W. B.: Disorders of the Heartbeat: A historical overview from antiquity to mid-20th century. Am. J. Cardiol. *72*:1055, 1993.

THE NORMAL ELECTROCARDIOGRAM

13. Craib, W. H.: A study of the electrical field surrounding active heart muscle. Heart *14*:71, 1927.
14. Wilson, F. N., MacLeod, A. G., and Barker, P. S.: The distribution of the action currents produced by the heart muscle and other excitable tissues immersed in extensive conducting media. J. Gen. Physiol. *16*:423, 1933.
15. Durrer, D., VanDam, R. T., Freud, G. E., et al.: Total excitation of the isolated human heart. Circulation *41*:899, 1970.
16. Wilson, F. N., MacLeod, A. G., Barker, P. S., and Johnston, F. D.: The determination and the significance of the areas of the ventricular deflections of the electrocardiogram. Am. Heart J. *10*:46, 1934.
17. Wilson, F. N., Johnston, F. D., Rosenbaum, F. F., et al.: The precordial electrocardiogram. Am. Heart J. *27*:19, 1944.
18. Andersen, H. R., Nielsen, D., and Hansen, I. G.: The normal right chest electrocardiogram. J. Electrocardiol. *20*:27, 1987.
19. Selvester, R. H., Velasquez, D. W., Elko, P. P., and Cady, L. D.: Intraventricular conduction defect (IVCD), real or fancied, QRS duration in 1,254 normal adult white males by a multi-lead automated algorithm. J. Electrocardiol. *23*:118, 1990.
20. Burger, H. C., and Van Millaan, J. B.: Heart—Vector and leads. Br. Heart J. *9*:154, 1947.
21. Willems, J. L., Robles de Medina, E., Bernard, R., et al.: WHO task force on criteria for intraventricular conduction disturbances and pre-excitation. J. Am. Coll. Cardiol. *5*:1261, 1985.
21a. McLaughlin, N. B., Campbell, R. W. F., Murray, D.: Comparison of automatic QT measurement techniques in the normal 12 lead electrocardiogram. Br. Heart J. *74*:85, 1995.
22. Bazett, H. C.: An analysis of the time-relations of electrocardiograms. Heart *7*:353, 1920.
23. Sagie, A., Larson, M. G., Goldberg, R. J., et al.: An improved method for adjusting the QT interval for heart rate (the Framingham Heart Study). Am. J. Cardiol. *70*:797, 1992.
24. Karjalainen, J., Viitasalo, M., Manttari, M., and Manninen, V.: Relation between QT intervals and heart rates from 40 to 120 beats/min in rest electrocardiograms of men and a simple method to adjust QT interval values. J. Am. Coll. Cardiol. *23*:1547, 1994.
25. Schweitzer, P.: The values and limitations of the QT interval in clinical practice. Am. Heart J. *124*:1121, 1992.
26. Mann, H.: A method of analyzing the electrocardiogram. Arch. Intern. Med. *25*:283, 1920.
27. Frank, E.: An accurate, clinically practical system for spatial vectorcardiography. Circulation *13*:737, 1956.
28. Kaplan, J. D., Evans, G. T., Foster, E., et al.: Evaluation of electrocardiographic criteria for right atrial enlargement by quantitative two-dimensional echocardiography. J. Am. Coll. Cardiol. *23*:747, 1994.
29. Chou, T. C., and Helm, R. A.: The pseudo P pulmonale. Circulation *32*:96, 1965.
30. Medrano, G. A., De Micheli, A., and Osornio, S.: Interatrial conduction and STa in experimental atrial damage. J. Electrocardiol. *20*:357, 1987.
31. Munuswamy, K., Alpert, M. A., Martin, R. H., et al.: Sensitivity and specificity of commonly used electrocardiographic criteria for left atrial enlargement determined by M-mode echocardiography. Am. J. Cardiol. *53*:829, 1984.
32. Nagahama, Y., Sugiura, T., Takehana, K., et al.: Clinical significance of PQ segment depression in acute Q wave anterior wall myocardial infarction. J. Am. Coll. Cardiol. *23*:885, 1994.
33. Surawicz, B.: Electrocardiographic diagnosis of chamber enlargement. J. Am. Coll. Cardiol. *8*:714, 1986.
34. Sokolow, M., and Lyon, T. P.: The ventricular complex in left ventricular hypertrophy as obtained by unipolar precordial and limb leads. Am. Heart J. *37*:161, 1949.
35. Schillaci, G., Verdecchia, P., Borgioni, C., et al.: Improved electrocardiographic diagnosis of left ventricular hypertrophy. Am. J. Cardiol. *74*:714, 1994.
36. Huwez, F. U., Pringle, S. D., and Macfarlane, P. W.: Variable patterns of ST-T abnormalities in patients with left ventricular hypertrophy and normal coronary arteries. Br. Heart J. *67*:304, 1992.
37. Levy, D., Labib, S. B., Anderson, K. M., et al.: Determinants of sensitivity and specificity of electrocardiographic criteria for left ventricular hypertrophy. Circulation *81*:815, 1990.
38. Cabrera, E., and Gaxiola, A.: A critical reevaluation of systolic and diastolic overloading patterns. Prog. Cardiovasc. Dis. *2*:219, 1959.
39. Goldberger, A. L.: Myocardial Infarction. 3rd ed. St. Louis, C. V. Mosby Co., 1984.
40. Sreeram, N., Cheriex, E., Smeets, J. L. R. M., et al.: Value of the 12-lead electrocardiogram at hospital admission in the diagnosis of pulmonary embolism. Am. J. Cardiol. *73*:298, 1994.
41. Shah, N. S., Velury, S., Mascarenhas, D., and Spodick, D. H.: Electrocardiographic features of restrictive pulmonary disease, and comparison with those of obstructive pulmonary disease. Am. J. Cardiol. *70*:394, 1992.
42. Delise, P., Piccolo, E., O'Este, D., et al.: Electrogenesis of the S1S2S3 electrocardiographic pattern. J. Electrocardiol. *23*:23, 1990.
43. Xiao, H. B., Brecker, S. J. D., and Gibson, D. G.: Relative effects of left ventricular mass and conduction disturbance on activation in patients with pathological left ventricular hypertrophy. Br. Heart J. *71*:548, 1994.
44. Gertsch, M., Theier, A., and Foglia, E.: Electrocardiographic detection of left ventricular hypertrophy in the presence of left anterior fascicular block. Am. J. Cardiol. *61*:1098, 1988.
45. Flowers, N. C.: Left bundle branch block: A continuously evolving concept. J. Am. Coll. Cardiol. *9*:684, 1987.
46. Brugada, P., and Brugada, J.: Right bundle branch block, persistent ST segment elevation and sudden cardiac death: A distinct clinical and electrocardiographic syndrome. Am. Coll. Cardiol. *20*:1391, 1992.
47. Bjerregaard, P., Gussak, I., Kotar, S. L., et al.: Recurrent syncope in a patient with prominent J wave. Am. Heart J. *127*:1426, 1994.
48. Watt, T. B., Jr., Freud, G. E., Durrer, D., and Pruitt, R. D.: Left anterior arborization block combined with right bundle branch block in canine and primate hearts. An electrocardiographic study. Circ. Res. *22*:57, 1968.
49. Rosenbaum, M. B., Elizari, M. V., and Lazzari, J. O.: The Hemiblocks: New Concepts of Intraventricular Conduction Based on Human Anatomical Physiological, and Clinical Studies. Oldsmar, FL, Tampa Tracings, 1970.
50. Angelini, P., Springer, A., Sulbaran, T., and Livesay, W. R.: Right ventricular myopathy with an unusual intraventricular conduction defect (Epsilon potential). Am. Heart J. *101*:680, 1981.
51. Garcia-Moll, X. G., Guindo, J., Vinolas, X., et al.: Intermittent masked bifascicular block. Am. Heart J. *127*:214, 1994.
52. Surawicz, B., and Fisch, C.: Cardiac alternans: Diverse mechanisms and clinical manifestations. J. Am. Coll. Cardiol. *120*:483, 1992.
53. Lewis, T.: Observations upon disorders of the heart's action. Heart *3*:279, 1912.
54. Gouaux, J. L., and Ashman, R.: Auricular fibrillation with aberration simulating ventricular paroxysmal tachycardia. Am. Heart J. *34*:366, 1947.
55. Lewis, T.: Certain physical signs of myocardial involvement. Br. Med. J. *1*:484, 1913.
56. Katz, A., and Pick, A.: The transseptal conduction time in the human heart. Circulation *27*:1061, 1963.
57. Fisch, C., and Knoebel, S. B.: Vagaries of acceleration dependent aberration. Br. Heart J. *67*:16, 1992.
58. Moore, E. N., Spear, J. F., and Fisch, C.: "Supernormal" conduction and excitability. J. Cardiovasc. Electrophysiol. *4*:320, 1993.
59. Oreto, G., Smeets, J. L. R. M., Rodriguez, L. M., et al.: Supernormal conduction in the left bundle branch. J. Cardiovasc. Electrophysiol. *5*:345, 1994.
60. Dressler, W.: Transient bundle branch block occurring during slowing of the heart beat and following gagging. Am. Heart J. *58*:750, 1959.
61. Wolff, L., Parkinson, J., and White, P. D.: Bundle branch block with

short P-R interval in healthy young people prone to paroxysmal tachycardia. Am. Heart J. *5*:685, 1930.

62. Wilson, F. N.: A case in which the vagus influenced the form of the ventricular complex of the electrocardiogram. Arch. Intern. Med. *16*:1008, 1915.
63. Cohn, A. E., and Fraser, F. R.: Paroxysmal tachycardia and the effect of stimulation of the vagus nerves by pressure. Heart *5*:93, 1913.
64. Holzmann, N., and Scherf, D.: Ueber Elekrokardiogramme mit ver kuerzter Vornot-Kammer-Distanz und positiven P. Zacken Z Klin Med *121*:404, 1932.
65. Rosenbaum, F. F., Hecht, H. H., Wilson, F. N., and Johnston, F. D.: The potential variations of the thorax and the esophagus in anomalous atrioventricular excitation (Wolff-Parkinson-White syndrome). Am. Heart J. *29*:281, 1945.
66. Yuan, S., Iwa, T., Bando, T., and Bando, H.: Comparative study of eight sets of ECG criteria for the localization of the accessory pathway in Wolff-Parkinson-White syndrome. J. Electrocardiol. *25*:203, 1992.
67. Pardee, H. E. B.: An electrocardiographic sign of coronary artery obstruction. Arch. Intern. Med. *26*:244, 1920.
68. Samson, W. E., and Scher, A. N.: Mechanism of ST segment alteration during myocardial injury. Circ. Res. *8*:780, 1960.
69. Vincent, G. M., Abildskov, J. A., and Burgess, M. J.: Mechanisms of ischemic ST-segment displacement. Evaluation by direct current recordings. Circulation *56*:559, 1977.
70. Sharkey, S. W., Berger, C. R., Brunette, D. D., and Henry, T. D.: Impact of the electrocardiogram on the delivery of thrombolytic therapy for acute myocardial infarction. Am. J. Cardiol. *73*:550, 1994.
70a. Raitt, M. H., Maynard, C., Wagner, G. S., et al.: Appearance of abnormal Q waves early in the course of acute myocardial infarction: Implications for efficacy of thrombolytic therapy. J. Am. Coll. Cardiol. *25*:1084, 1995.
71. Madias, J. E.: The "Giant R Waves" ECG pattern of hyperacute phase of myocardial infarction. J. Electrocardiol. *26*:77, 1993.
72. Barnhill, J. E., III, Tendera, M., Cade, H., et al.: Depolarization changes early in the course of myocardial infarction: Significance of changes in the terminal portion of the QRS complex. J. Am. Coll. Cardiol. *14*:143, 1989.
73. Strasberg, B., Pinchas, A., Barbash, G. L., et al.: Importance of reciprocal ST segment depression in leads V5 and V6 as an indicator of disease of the left anterior descending coronary artery in acute inferior wall myocardial infarction. Br. Heart J. *63*:339, 1990.
74. Kracoff, O. S., Adelman, A. G., Marquis, J. F., et al.: Twelve-lead electrocardiogram recording during percutaneous transluminal coronary angioplasty. J. Electrocardiol. *23*:191, 1990.
75. Stevenson, R. N., Ranjadayalan, K., Umachandran, V., and Timmis, A. D.: Significance of reciprocal ST depression in acute myocardial infarction: A study of 258 patients treated by thrombolysis. Br. Heart J. *69*:211, 1993.
76. Sato, H., Kodama, K., Masuvama, T., et al.: Right coronary artery occlusion: Its role in the mechanism of precordial ST segment depression. J. Am. Coll. Cardiol. *14*:297, 1989.
77. Norell, M. S., Lyons, J. P., Gardener, J. E., et al.: Significance of "reciprocal" ST segment depression: Left ventriculographic observations during left anterior descending coronary angioplasty. J. Am. Coll. Cardiol. *13*:1270, 1989.
78. Edmunds, J. J., Gibbons, R. J., Bresnahan, J. F., and Clements, I. P.: Significance of anterior ST depression in inferior wall acute myocardial infarction. Am. J. Cardiol. *73*:143, 1994.
79. Kracoff, O. H., Adelman, A. G., Oettinger, M., et al.: Reciprocal changes as the presenting electrocardiographic manifestation of acute myocardial ischemia. Am. J. Cardiol. *71*:1359, 1993.
80. Birnbaum, Y., Solodky, A., Herz, I., et al.: Implications of inferior ST-segment depression in anterior acute myocardial infarction: Electrocardiographic and angiographic correlation. Am. Heart J. *127*:1467, 1994.
80a. Chikamori, T., Takata, J., Furuno, T., et al.: Usefulness of U wave analysis in detecting significant narrowing limited to a single coronary artery. Am. J. Cardiol. *75*:508, 1995.
81. Jain, A., Jenkins, M. G., and Gettes, L. S.: Lack of specificity of new negative U waves for anterior myocardial ischemia as evidenced by intracoronary electrogram during balloon angioplasty. J. Am. Coll. Cardiol. *15*:1007, 1990.
82. Gurick, A., Oral, D., Pamir, G., and Akyol, T.: Significance of resting U wave polarity in patients with atherosclerotic heart disease. J. Electrocardiol. *27*:157, 1994.
83. Kanemoto, N., Imaoka, C., and Suzuki, Y.: Significance of U wave polarities in previous anterior myocardial infarction. J. Electrocardiol. *24*:169, 1991.
84. Oliva, P. B., Hammill, S. C., and Talano, J. V.: T wave changes consistent with epicardial involvement in acute myocardial infarction. J. Am. Cardiol. *24*:1073, 1994.
85. Bergovec, M., Prpic, H., Zigman, M., et al.: Regression of ECG signs of myocardial infarction related to infarct size and left ventricular function. J. Electrocardiol. *26*:1, 1993.
86. Horan, L. G., Flowers, N. C., and Johnson, J. C.: Significance of the diagnostic Q wave of myocardial infarction. Circulation *43*:428, 1971.
86a. Parker, A. B. III, Waller, B. F., and Gering, L. E.: Usefulness of the 12-lead electrocardiogram in detection of myocardial infarction: Electrocardiographic-anatomic correlations—Part I. Clin. Cardiol. *19*:55, 1996.
87. Rosenbaum, M. B., Girotti, L. A., Lazzari, J. O., et al.: Abnormal Q waves in right sided chest leads provoked by onset of right bundle branch block in patients with anteroseptal infarction. Br. Heart J. *47*:227, 1982.
88. Hands, M. E., Cook, E. F., Stone, P. H., et al.: Electrocardiographic diagnosis of myocardial infarction in the presence of complete bundle branch block. Am. Heart J. *116*:23, 1988.
89. Cannon, A., Freedman, S. B., Bailey, B. P., and Bernstein, L.: ST-segment changes during transmural myocardial ischemia in chronic left bundle branch block. Am. J. Cardiol. *64*:1216, 1989.
90. Oreto, G., Saporito, F., Donato, G., et al.: The "Inverse" R wave progression in inferior leads in the presence of left anterior hemiblock: A clinical study. J. Electrocardiol. *24*:277, 1991.
91. First, S. R., Bayley, R. H., and Bedford, D. R.: Peri-infarction block electrocardiographic abnormality occasionally resembling bundle branch block and local ventricular block of other types. Circulation *2*:31, 1950.
92. Grant, R. P.: Peri-infarction block. Prog. Cardiovasc. Dis. *2*:237, 1959.
93. Babbitt, D. G., Binkley, P. F., and Schaal, S. F.: Clinical significance of terminal QRS abnormalities in the setting of inferior myocardial infarction. J. Electrocardiol. *24*:85, 1991.
94. Flowers, N. C., Horan, L. G., Wyids, A. C., et al.: Relation of peri-infarction block to ventricular late potentials in patients with inferior wall myocardial infarction. Am. J. Cardiol. *66*:568, 1990.
95. Barnhill, J. E., Tendera, M., Cade, H., et al.: Depolarization changes early in the course of myocardial infarction: Significance of changes in the terminal portion of the QRS complex. J. Am. Coll. Cardiol. *14*:143, 1989.
96. Varriale, P., and Chryssos, B. E.: The RSR′ complex not related to right bundle branch block: Diagnostic value as a sign of myocardial infarction scar. Am. Heart J. *123*:369, 1992.
97. Blanke, H., Cohen, M., Schlueter, G. V., et al.: Electrocardiographic and coronary arteriographic correlations during acute myocardial infarction. Am. J. Cardiol. *54*:249, 1984.
98. Hiasa, Y., Morimoto, S., Wada, T., et al.: Differentiation between left circumflex and right coronary artery occlusions: Studies on ST-segment deviation during percutaneous transluminal coronary angioplasty. Clin. Cardiol. *13*:783, 1990.
99. Shen, W. F., Tribouilloy, C., and Lesbre, J. P.: Relationship between electrocardiographic patterns and angiographic features in isolated left circumflex coronary artery disease. Clin. Cardiol. *14*:720, 1991.
100. de Zwaan, C., Bar, F. W., Janssen, J. J. A., et al.: Angiographic and clinical characteristics of patients with unstable angina showing an ECG pattern indicating critical narrowing of the proximal LAD coronary artery. Am. Heart J. *117*:557, 1989.
101. Braat, S. H., Brugada, P., Dulk, K., et al.: Value of lead V4R for recognition of the infarct coronary artery in acute inferior myocardial infarction. Am. J. Cardiol. *53*:1538, 1984.
101a. Shalev, Y., Fogelman, R., Oettinger, M., et al.: Does the electrocardiographic pattern of "anteroseptal" myocardial infarction correlate with anatomic location of myocardial surgery? Am. J. Cardiol. *75*:763, 1995.
102. Baer, M. F., Theissen, P., and Voth, E.: Morphologic correlate of pathologic Q waves as assessed by gradient-echo magnetic resonance imaging. Am. J. Cardiol. *74*:430, 1994.
103. Antaloczy, Z., Barcsak, J., and Magyar, E.: Correlation of electrocardiologic and pathologic findings in 100 cases of Q wave and non-Q wave myocardial infarction. J. Electrocardiol. *21*:331, 1988.
104. Boden, W. E., Gibson, R. S., Schechtman, K. B., et al.: ST segment shifts are poor predictors of subsequent Q wave evolution in acute myocardial infarction. Circulation *79*:537, 1989.
105. Tamura, A., Katooka, H., and Mikuriya, Y.: Electrocardiographic findings in a patient with pure septal infarction. Br. Heart J. *65*:166, 1991.
106. Iwasaki, K., Kusachi, S., Kita, T., and Taniguchi, G.: Prediction of isolated first diagonal branch occlusion by 12-lead electrocardiography: ST segment shift in leads I and aVL. J. Am. Coll. Cardiol. *23*:1557, 1994.
107. Kataoka, H., Kanzaki, K., and Mikuriva, Y.: Massive ST-segment elevation in precordial and inferior leads in right ventricular myocardial infarction. J. Electrocardiol. *21*:115, 1988.
108. Mak, K. H., Chia, B. L., Tan, A. T. H., and Johan, A.: Simultaneous ST segment elevation in lead V1 and depression in lead V2. A discordant ECG pattern indicating right ventricular infarction. J. Electrocardiol. *27*:203, 1994.
109. Andersen, H. R., Falk, E., and Nielsen, D.: Right ventricular infarction: Diagnostic accuracy of electrocardiographic right chest leads V3R to V7R investigated prospectively in 43 consecutive fatal cases from a coronary care unit. Br. Heart J. *62*:328, 1989.
110. Lopez-Sendon, J., Coma-Cannella, J., Alcasena, S., et al.: Electrocardiographic findings in acute right ventricular infarction: Sensitivity and specificity of electrocardiographic alterations in right precordial leads V_4R, V_3R, V_1, V_2 and V_3. J. Am. Coll. Cardiol. *8*:1273, 1985.
111. Zehender, M., Kasper, W., Kauder, E., et al.: Comparison of diagnostic accuracy, time dependency, and prognostic impact of abnormal Q waves, combined electrocardiographic criteria, and ST abnormalities in right ventricular infarction. Br. Heart J. *72*:119, 1994.
112. Kataoka, H., Tamura, A., Yano, S., and Kazaki, K.: Intraventricular conduction delay in acute right ventricular ischemia. Am. J. Cardiol. *64*:94, 1989.
113. Sclarovsky, S., Topaz, O., Rechavia, E., et al.: Ischemic ST segment depression in leads V_2–V_3 as the presenting electrocardiographic fea-

ture of posterolateral wall myocardial infarction. Am. Heart J. *113*:1085, 1987.
114. Bounous, E. P., Jr., Califf, R. M., Harrell, F. E., Jr., et al.: Prognostic value of the simplified Selvester QRS score in patients with coronary artery disease. J. Am. Coll. Cardiol. *11*:35, 1988.
115. Ascher, E. K., Stauffer, J. E., and Gaasch, W. H.: Coronary artery spasm, cardiac arrest, transient electrocardiographic Q waves and stunned myocardium in cocaine-associated acute myocardial infarction. Am. J. Cardiol. *61*:941, 939, 1988.
116. DePasquale, N. P., Burch, G. E., and Phillips, J. H.: Electrocardiograph alterations associated with electrically "silent" areas of myocardium. Am. Heart J. *68*:697, 1964.
117. Braunwald, E., and Kloner, R. A.: The stunned myocardium: Prolonged postischemic ventricular dysfunction. Circulation *66*:1146, 1982.
118. Hesse, A., Altland, K., Linke, R. P., et al.: Cardiac amyloidosis: A review and report of a new transthyretin (prealbumin) variant. Br. Heart J. *70*:111, 1993.
119. Yotsukura, M., Miyagawa, M., Tsuya, T., et al.: A 10-year follow-up study by orthogonal Frank lead ECG on patients with progressive muscular dystrophy of the Duchenne type. J. Electrocardiol. *25*:(4)345, 1992.
120. Lemery, R., Kleinebenne, A., Nihoyannopoulos, P., et al.: Q waves in hypertrophic cardiomyopathy in relation to the distribution and severity of right and left ventricular hypertrophy. J. Am. Coll. Cardiol. *16*:388, 1990.
121. Pelliccia, F., Clantrocca, C., Cristotani, R., et al.: Electrocardiographic findings in patients with hypertrophic cardiomyopathy. J. Electrocardiol. *23*:213, 1990.
122. Chakko, S., Sepulveda, S., Kessler, K. M., et al.: Frequency and type of electrocardiographic abnormalities in cocaine abusers. Am. J. Cardiol. *74*:710, 1994.
123. Walder, L. A., and Spodick, D. H.: Global T wave inversion: Long-term follow-up. J. Am. Coll. Cardiol. *21*:1652, 1993.
124. Usui, M., Inoue, H., Suzuki, J., et al.: Relationship between distribution of hypertrophy and electrocardiographic changes in hypertrophic cardiomyopathy. Am. Heart J. *126*:177, 1993.
125. Suzuki, J., Watanabe, F., Takenaka, K., et al.: New subtype of apical hypertrophic cardiomyopathy identified with nuclear magnetic resonance imaging as an underlying cause of markedly inverted T waves. J. Am. Coll. Cardiol. *22*:1175, 1993.
126. Lui, C. Y.: Acute pulmonary embolism as the cause of global T wave inversion and QT prolongation. J. Electrocardiol. *26*:91, 1993.
127. Trevethan, S., Castilla, R., Medrano, G., and Michelli, A.: Giant T waves simulating apical hypertrophic myocardiopathy that disappear with sodium nitroprusside administration. J. Electrocardiol. *24*:267, 1991.
128. Balzo, U., and Rosen, M. R.: T wave changes persisting after ventricular pacing in canine hearts are altered by 4-aminopyridine but not by lidocaine. Implications with respect to phenomenon of cardiac "memory." Circulation *85*:1464, 1992.
129. Wood, M. A., DiMarco, J. P., and Haines, D. E.: Electrocardiographic abnormalities after radiofrequency catheter ablation of accessory bypass tracts in the Wolff-Parkinson-White syndrome. Am. J. Cardiol. *70*:200, 1992.
130. Helguera, M. E., Pinski, S. L., Sterba, R., and Throman, R. G.: Memory T wave after radiofrequency catheter ablation of accessory atrioventricular connections in W-P-W syndrome. J. Electrocardiol. *27*:243, 1994.
131. White, P. D.: Alternation of the pulse: A common clinical condition. Am. J. Med. Sci. *150*:82, 1915.
132. Taussig, H. B.: Electrograms taken from isolated strips of mammalian ventricular cardiac muscle. Bull. Johns Hopkins Hosp. *43*:81, 1928.
133. Verrier, R. L., and Nearing, B. D.: Electrophysiologic basis for T wave alternans as an index of vulnerability to ventricular fibrillation. J. Cardiovasc. Electrophysiol. *5*:445, 1994.
134. Bardaji, A., Vidal, F., and Richart, C.: T wave alternans associated with amiodarone. J. Electrocardiol. *26*:155, 1993.
135. Tighe, D. A., Chung, E. K., and Park, C. H.: Electric alternans associated with acute pulmonary embolism. Am. Heart J. *128*:188, 1994.
136. Zareba, W., Moss, A. J., le Cessie, S., and Hall, W. J.: T wave alternans in idiopathic long QT syndrome. J. Am. Coll. Cardiol. *23*:1541, 1994.
137. Rosenbaum, D. S., Jackson, L. E., Smith, J. M., et al.: Electrical alternans and vulnerability to ventricular arrhythmias. N. Engl. J. Med. *330*:235, 1994.
138. Malfatto, G., Beria, G., Sala, S., et al.: Quantitative analysis of T wave abnormalities and their prognostic implications in the idiopathic long QT syndrome. Am. J. Cardiol. *23*:296, 1994.
139. Friedberg, C. K., and Zager, A.: "Nonspecific" ST and T-wave changes. Circulation *23*:655, 1961.
140. Wilson, F. N., and Finch, R.: The effect of drinking iced-water upon the form of the T deflection of the electrocardiogram. Heart *10*:275, 1923.
141. Balady, G. J., Cadigan, J. B., and Ryan, T. J.: Electrocardiogram of the athlete: An analysis of 289 professional football players. Am. J. Cardiol. *53*:1339, 1984.
142. Nelson, S. D., Kou, W. H., Annesiey, T., et al.: Significance of ST segment depression during paroxysmal supraventricular tachycardia. J. Am. Coll. Cardiol. *12*:383, 1988.
143. Autenrieth, G., Surawicz, B., Kuo, C. S., and Arita, M.: Primary T wave abnormalities caused by uniform and regional shortening of ventricular monophasic action potential in the dog. Circulation *51*:568, 1975.
144. Miwa, K., Miyagi, Y., Fujita, M., et al.: Transient terminal U wave inversion as a more specific marker for myocardial ischemia. Am. Heart J. *125*:981, 1993.
145. Twidale, N., Gallagher, A. W., and Tonkin, A. M.: Echocardiographic study of U wave inversion in the electrocardiograms of hypertensive patients. J. Electrocardiol. *22*:365, 1989.
146. Kanemoto, N., Nakayama, K., Ide, M., and Goto, Y.: Giant negative U waves in a patient with uncontrolled hypertension and severe hypokalemia. J. Electrocardiol. *25*:163, 1992.
147. Garson, A., Jr., Dick, M., 2d, Fournier, A., et al.: The long QT syndrome in children. An international study of 287 patients. Circulation *87*(6):1866, 1993.
148. Ward, O. C.: New familial cardiac syndrome in children. JAMA *54*:103, 1964.
149. Vincent, G. M., Timothy, K. W., Leppert, M., and Keating, M.: The spectrum of symptoms and QT intervals in carriers of the gene for the long QT syndrome. N. Engl. J. Med. *327*:846, 1992.
150. Martin, A. B., Garson, A., Jr., and Perry, J. C.: Prolonged QT interval in hypertrophic and dilated cardiomyopathy in children. Am. Heart J. *127*:64, 1994.
151. Schwartz, P. J., Moss, A. J., Vincent, G. M., et al.: Diagnostic criteria for the long QT syndrome. An update. Circulation *88*:782, 1993.
152. Surawicz, B., and Knoebel, S. B.: Long QT, good, bad or indifferent? J. Am. Coll. Cardiol. *4*:138, 1983.
153. Lewis, T.: Notes upon alternation of the heart. Q. J. Med. *4*:141, 1910.
154. Osborn, J. J.: Experimental hypothermia. Respiratory and blood pH changes in relation to cardiac function. Am. J. Physiol. *175*:389, 1953.
155. Fisch, C.: Abnormal ECG in clinically normal individuals. JAMA *250*:1321, 1983.
156. Zehender, M., Meinertz, T., Kaui, J., et al.: ECG variants and cardiac arrhythmias in athletes: Clinical relevance and prognostic importance. Am. Heart J. *119*:1378, 1990.
157. Haisty, W. K., Pahlm, O., Edenbrandt, L., and Newman, K.: Recognition of electrocardiographic electrode misplacements involving the ground (right leg) electrode. Am. J. Cardiol. *71*:1490, 1993.
158. Carter, E. P., and Andrus, E. C.: Q-T interval in human electrocardiogram in absence of cardiac disease. JAMA *78*:1922, 1922.
159. Ahmed, R., Yano, K., Mitsuoka, T., et al.: Changes in T wave morphology during hypercalcemia and its relations to the severity of hypercalcemia. J. Electrocardiol. *22*:125, 1989.
160. Lind, L., and Ljunghall, S.: Serum calcium and the ECG in patients with primary hyperparathyroidism. J. Electrocardiol. *27*:99, 1994.
161. Mosseri, M., Porath, A., Ovsyshcher, I., and Stone, D.: Electrocardiographic manifestations of combined hypercalcemia in hypermagnesemia. J. Electrocardiol. *23*:235, 1990.
162. Cohn, A. E., Fraser, F. R., and Jamieson, A.: The influence of digitalis on the T wave of the human electrocardiogram. J. Exp. Med. *21*:593, 1915.
163. Fisch, C., Knoebel, S. B.: Digitalis cardiotoxicity. J. Am. Coll. Cardiol. *5*:91A, 1985.
164. Smith, T. W., Antman, E. M., Friedman, P. L., et al.: Digitalis glycosides: Mechanisms and manifestations of toxicity. Prog. Cardiovasc. Dis. *26*:413, 1984.

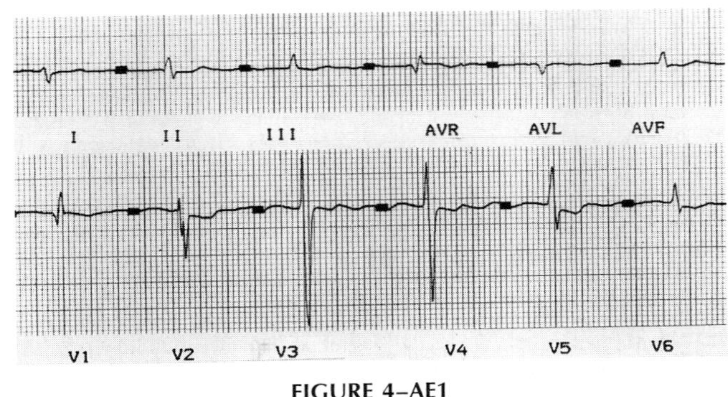

FIGURE 4–AE1

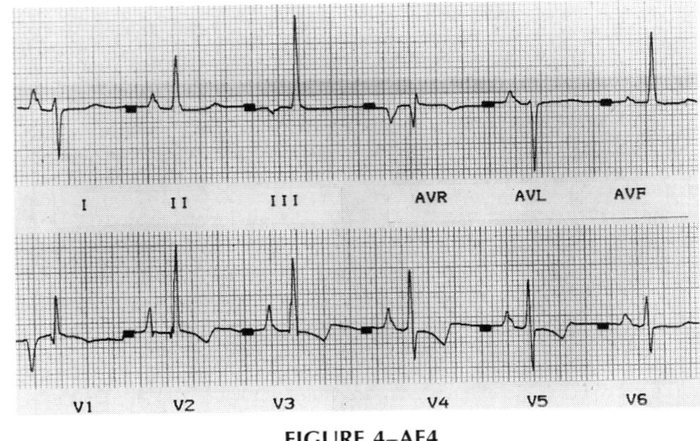

FIGURE 4–AE4

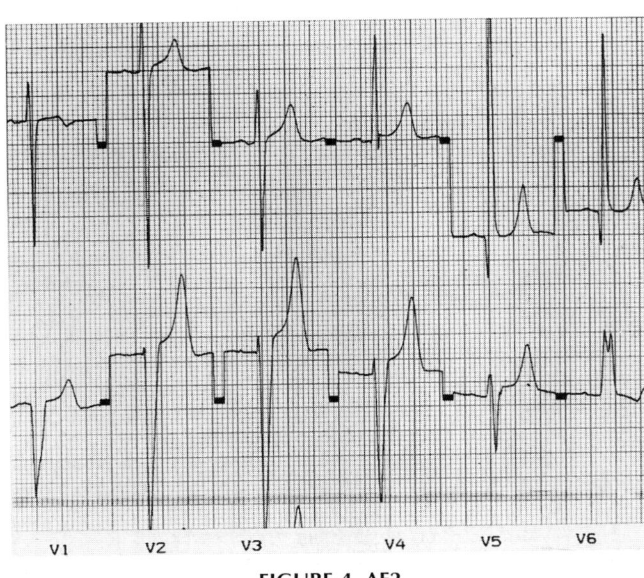

FIGURE 4–AE2

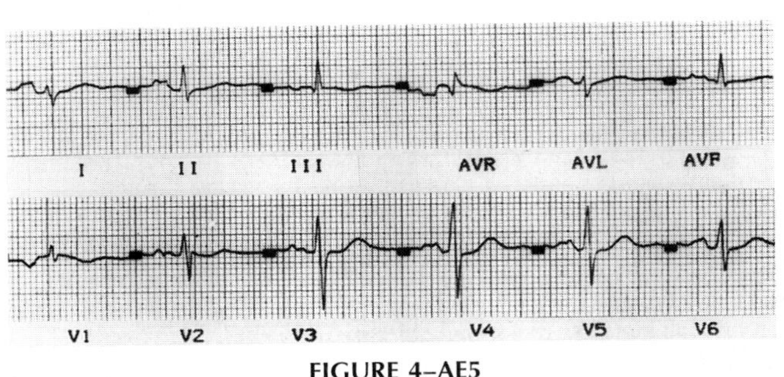

FIGURE 4–AE5

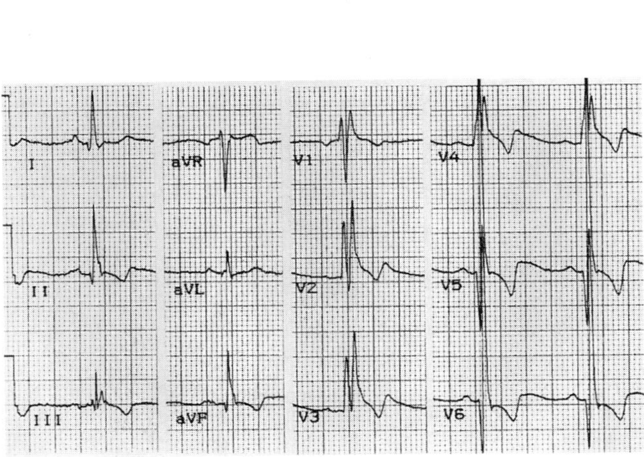

FIGURE 4–AE3

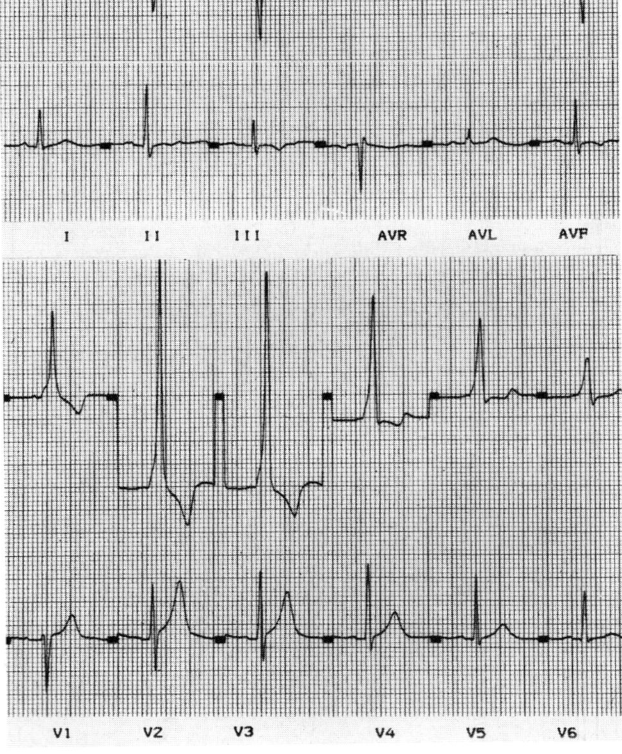

FIGURE 4–AE6

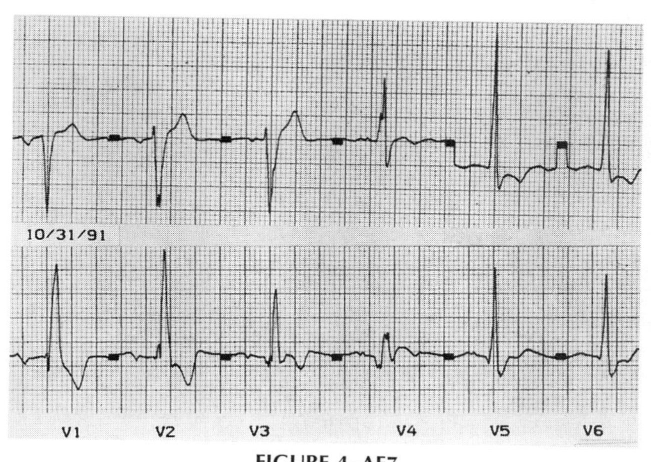

FIGURE 4–AE7

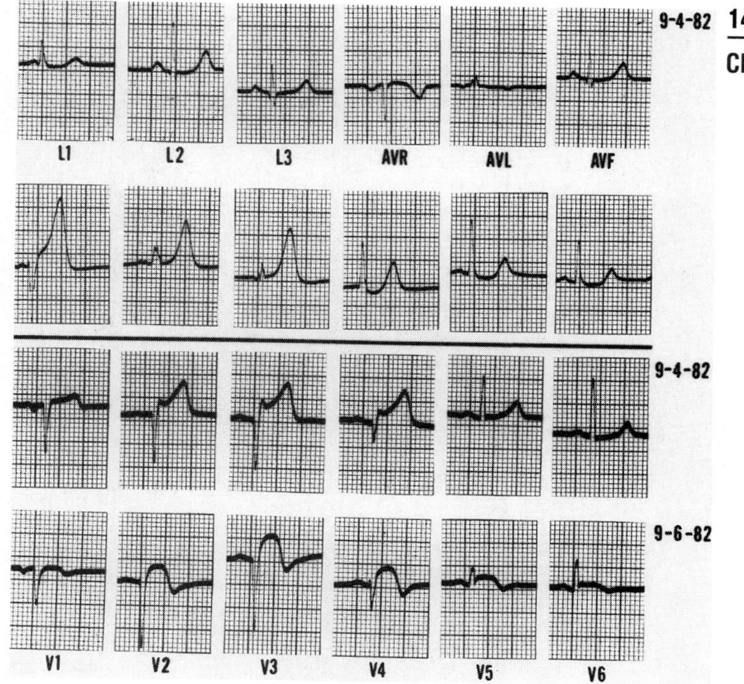

FIGURE 4–AE10

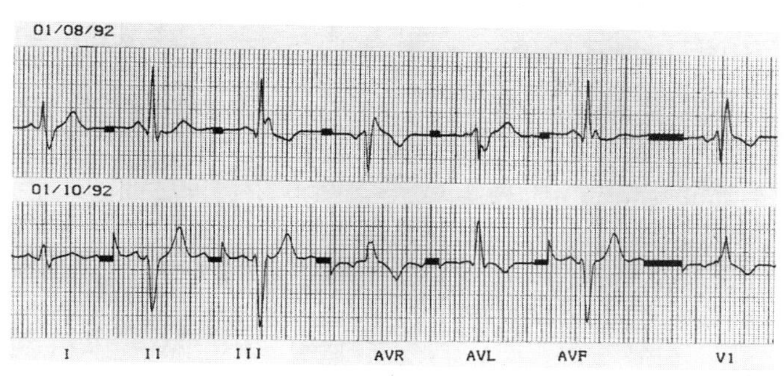

FIGURE 4–AE8

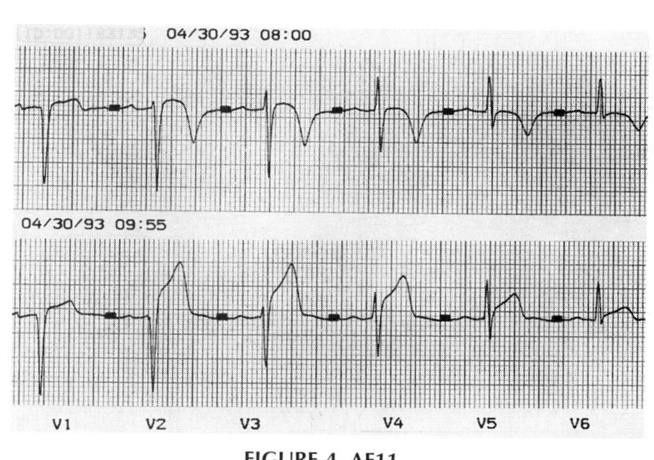

FIGURE 4–AE11

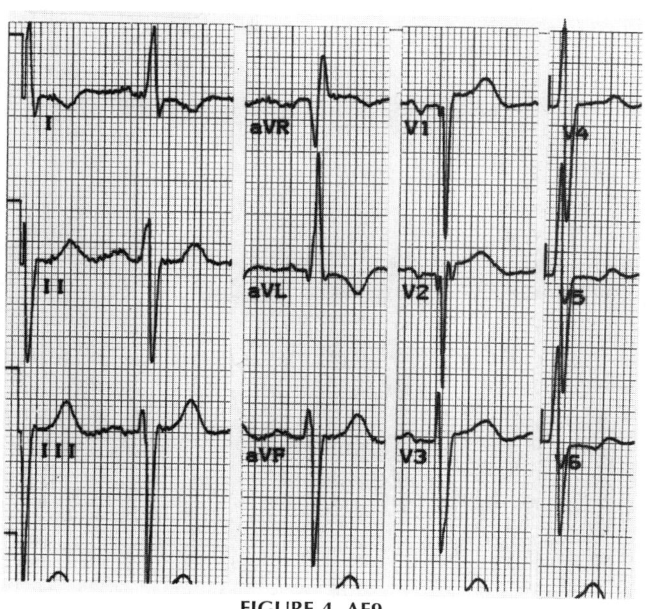

FIGURE 4–AE9

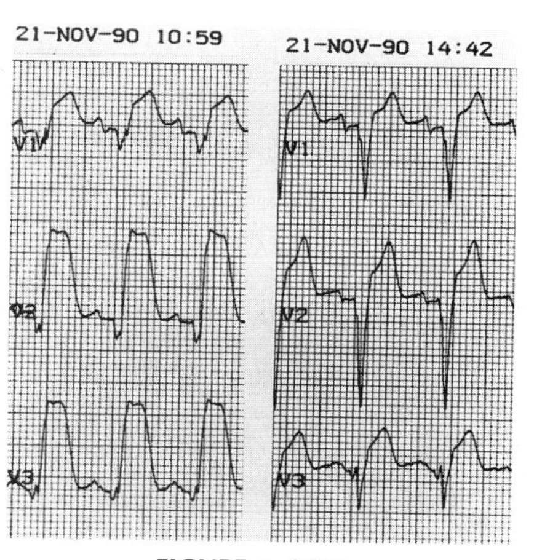

FIGURE 4–AE12

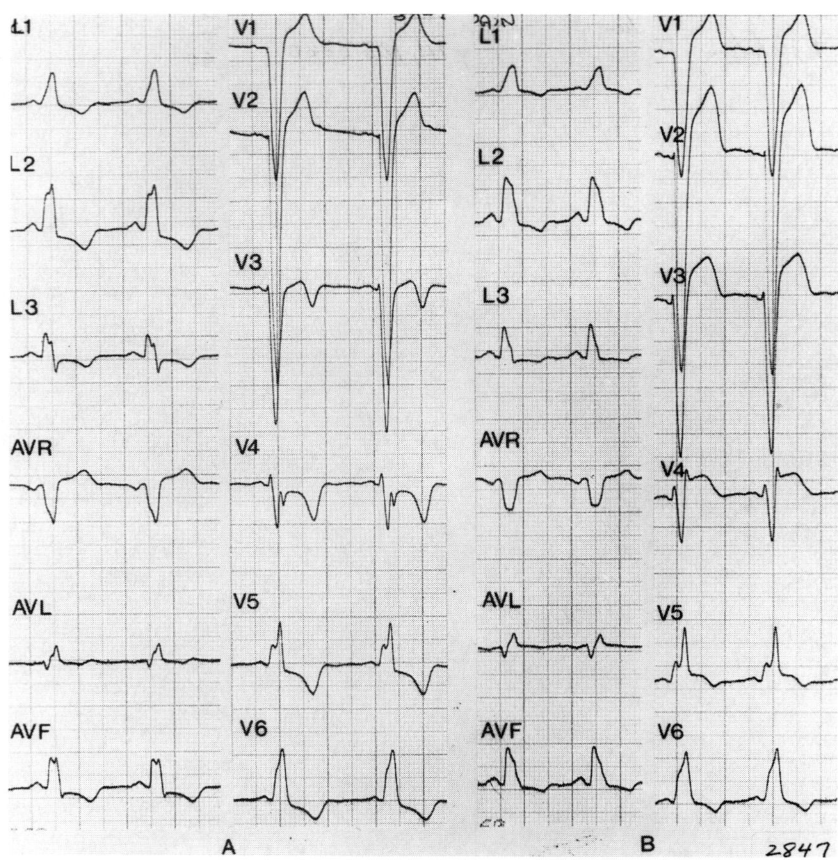

FIGURE 4–AE13

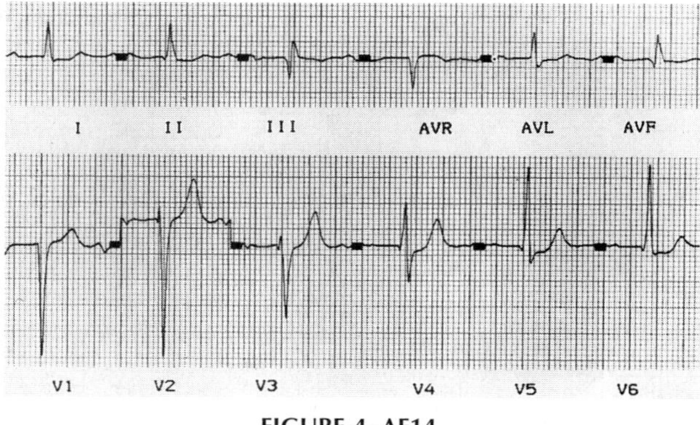

FIGURE 4–AE14

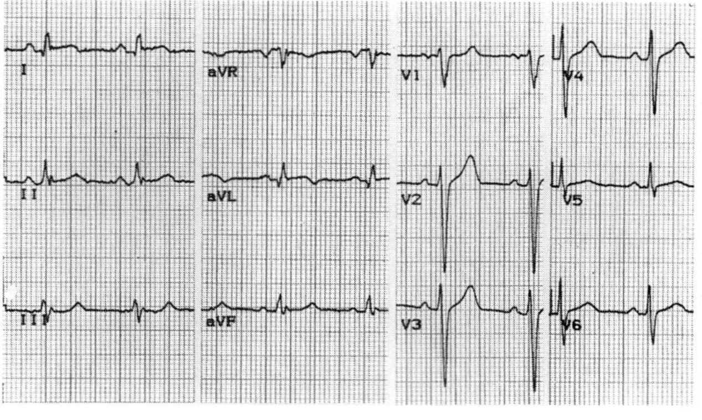

FIGURE 4–AE15

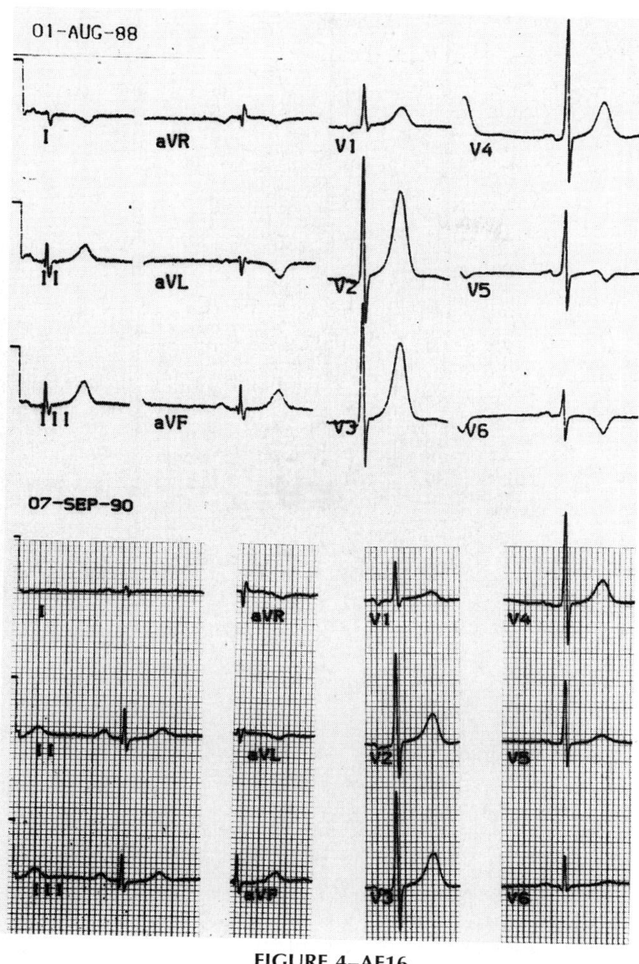

FIGURE 4–AE16

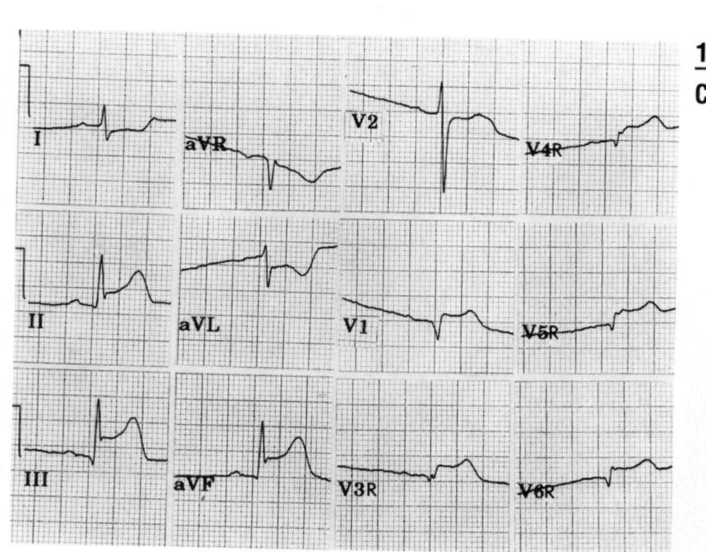

FIGURE 4–AE18

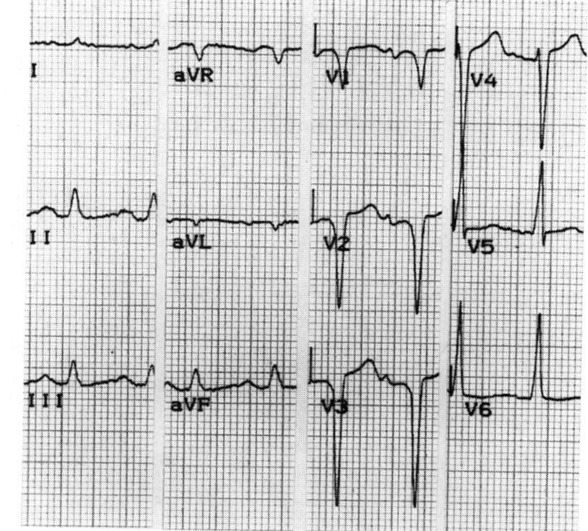

FIGURE 4–AE19

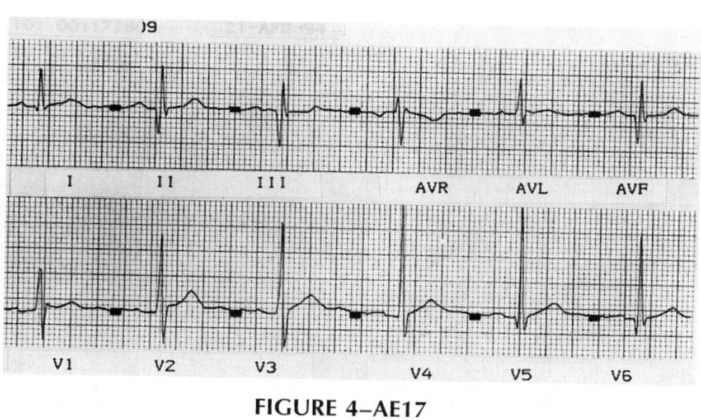

FIGURE 4–AE17

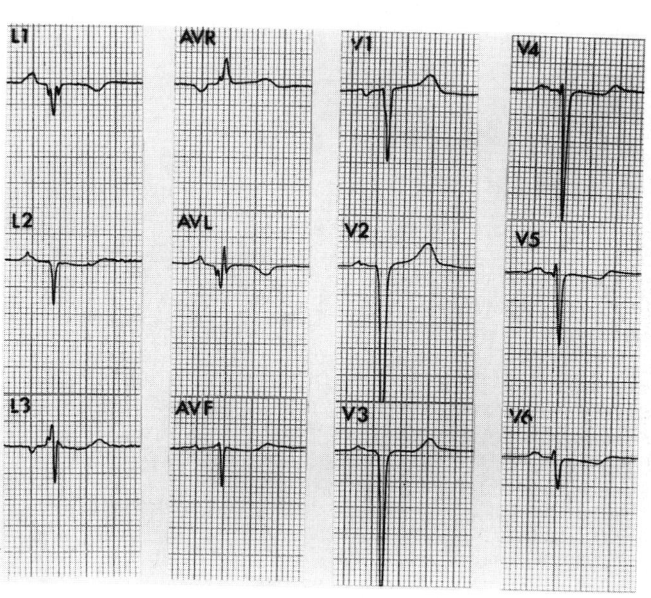

FIGURE 4–AE20

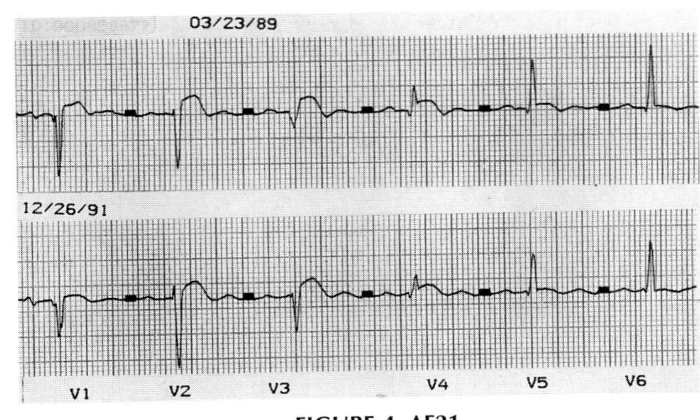

FIGURE 4–AE21

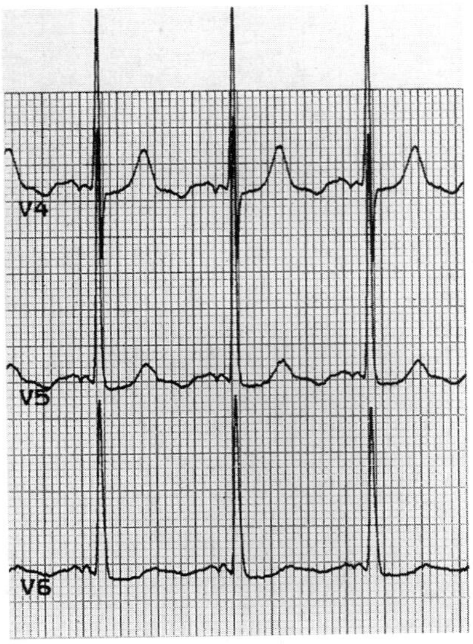

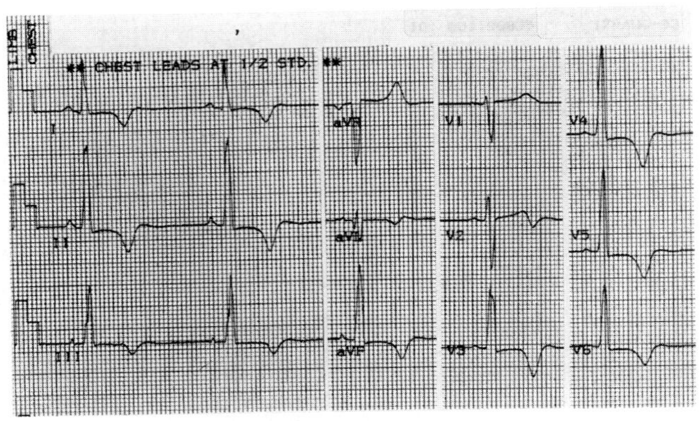

FIGURE 4–AE22

FIGURE 4–AE24

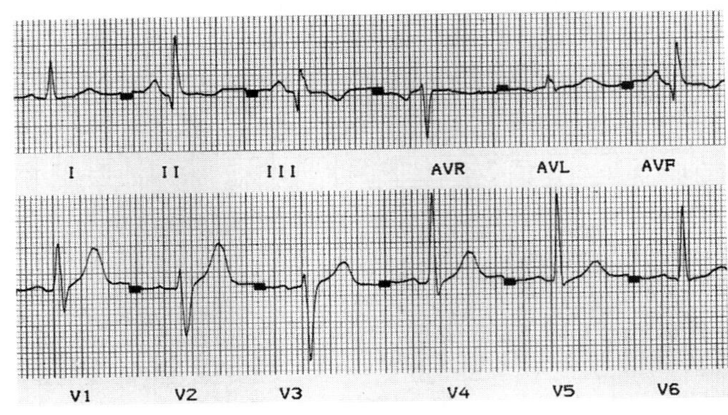

FIGURE 4–AE25

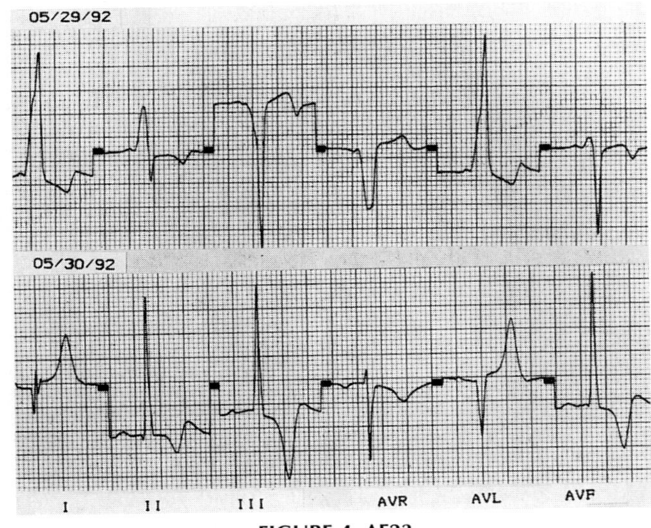

FIGURE 4–AE23

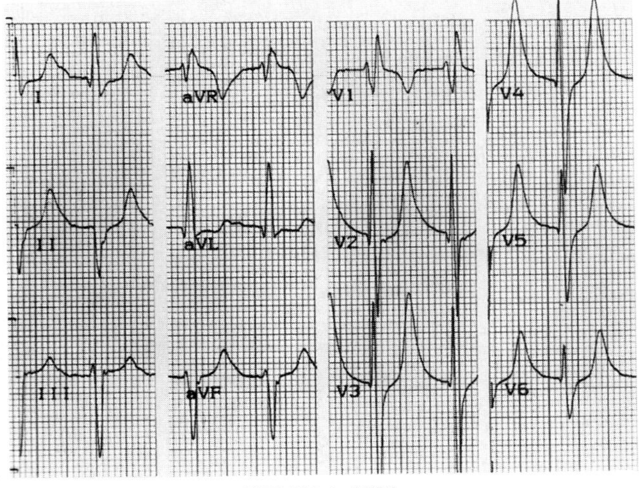

FIGURE 4–AE26

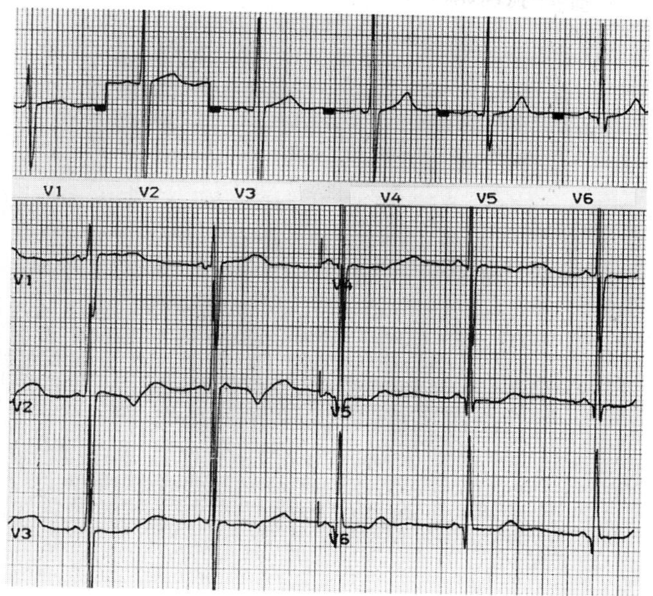

FIGURE 4–AE27

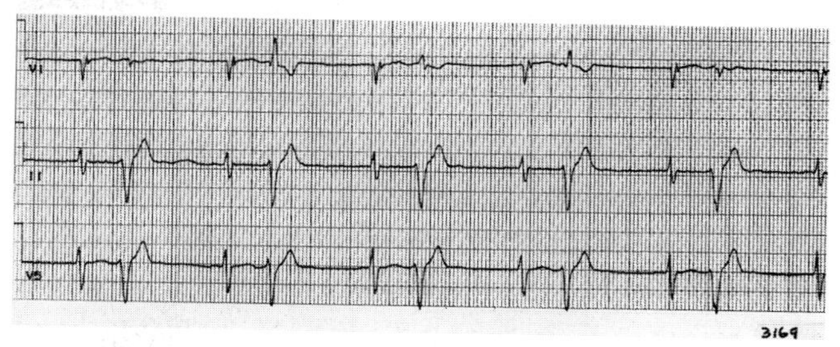

FIGURE 4–AE29

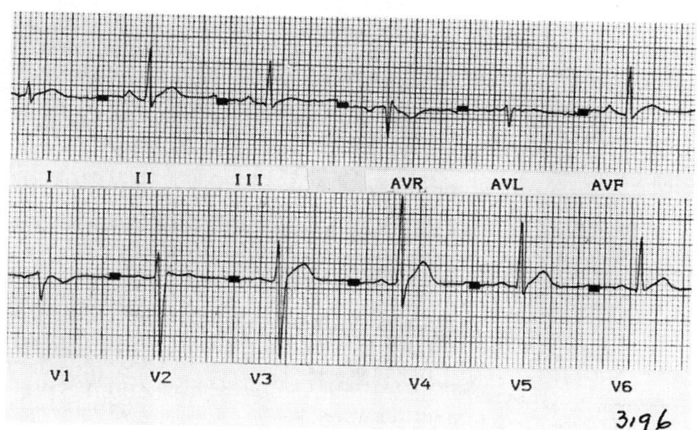

FIGURE 4–AE28

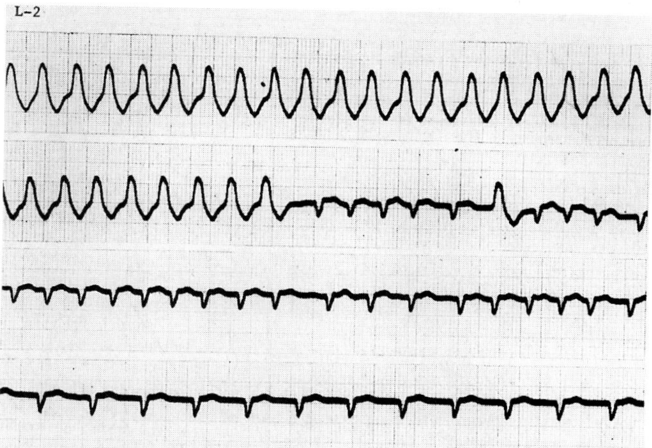

FIGURE 4–AE30

AF–Atrial fibrillation
LVH–Left ventricular hypertrophy
RVH–Right ventricular hypertrophy
LBBB–Left bundle branch block
RBBB–Right bundle branch block
IVCD–Intraventricular conduction delay
LAFB–Left anterior fascicular block
LPFB–Left posterior fascicular block
MI–Myocardial infarction

Figure 4–AE1
AF. The qR in lead V_1, in essence, a right atrial electrogram, is followed by a normal right-to-left R wave progression. The qR with a normal R wave progression beginning with lead V_2 is diagnostic of severe tricuspid insufficiency with a large right atrium subtending the V_1 electrode.

Figure 4–AE2
In the top tracing the large-amplitude QRS complexes with prominent Q waves in leads V_5 and V_6 indicates LVH due to a diastolic overload consistent with aortic regurgitation. In the lower tracing the LBBB obscures the Q waves and diminishes the R wave amplitude in leads V_4 to V_6. An IVCD, in this instance LBBB, makes a diagnosis of ventricular hypertrophy difficult if not impossible.

Figure 4–AE3
RBBB and LVH with a diastolic overload manifest by the high amplitude R waves, deep Q waves, and secondary ST-T changes recorded in a patient with a large patent ductus arteriosus.

Figure 4–AE4
Severe RVH. The q wave in V_1 suggests that the right ventricular pressure exceeds the left ventricular pressure. The left axis of the P wave and the prominent negative P wave in lead V_1 are unusual and most likely are due to a markedly enlarged right atrium projecting to the left and posteriorly. The prominent P waves in leads V_2 and V_3 are diagnostic of right atrial enlargement.

Figure 4–AE5
Mitral stenosis with pulmonary hypertension manifest by P mitrale, right-axis deviation, "squatty" QRS with a prominent R wave in V_1, and clockwise rotation.

Figure 4–AE6
Top row of each panel illustrates WPW with large-amplitude R waves in leads V_1 to V_4. In the lower row the AV conduction is normal with normal amplitude of the R waves. This tracing emphasizes the lack of specificity of QRS amplitude for ventricular hypertrophy in the presence of IVCD.

Figure 4–AE7
Top, IVCD with normal R wave amplitude in leads V_1, V_2, and V_3. 10/31/91 *(bottom)*. Postoperative RBBB with large-amplitude R waves in leads V_1, V_2, and V_3 stresses a lack of specificity of the tall R waves for RVH in presence of IVCD, in this instance RBBB. Q waves in leads V_3 and V_4 are consistent with an anterior MI.

Figure 4–AE8
1/8/92, RBBB with LPFB. 1/10/92, RBBB with LAFB. Both recorded from the same patient.

Figure 4–AE9
IVCD with LAFB simulating septal MI.

Figure 4–AE10
Prominent, tall, upright T waves in leads V_1 to V_4 recorded early during acute MI are illustrated in the top panel. Evolution of an acute anteroseptal MI is recorded in the lower panel.

Figure 4–AE11
The earliest tracing (8:00) recorded in the course of evolution of an acute MI illustrates T wave inversion due to ischemia. This is followed (9:55) by ST elevation and Q waves in leads V_1 and V_2 indicative of a current of injury and "death" of muscle respectively.

Figure 4–AE12
Acute MI with early high-amplitude R waves recorded at 10:59 and loss of R waves at 14:42.

Figure 4–AE13
A, LBBB with primary T waves in leads V_3 and V_4. *B*, LBBB with acute MI manifest by ST segment elevation in leads V_1 to V_5. While LBBB precludes recording of a Q wave, acute MI may occasionally be recognized by ST segment elevation.

Figure 4–AE14
Septal MI with the highly specific qrS pattern in lead V_2. The qrS pattern indicates reversal of septal activation, namely, from right to left, followed by right and left ventricular activation, respectively. Changes in leads III and aV_f are consistent with an inferior MI.

Figure 4–AE15
Isolated high lateral MI with changes confined to leads I and aV_l. The S waves in leads V_5 and V_6 are most likely due to peri-infarction block with the terminal activation directed toward the area of the MI.

Figure 4–AE16
Upper panel, Posterior and anterolateral MI manifest by the tall R waves in leads V_1 and V_2 and T wave changes in leads I, aV_l, V_5, and V_6. *Lower panel,* Suggests a pure posterior infarction were it not for the earlier evidence of the lateral infarction. Isolated posterior infarction is extremely rare.

Figure 4–AE17
Posterior MI manifest by delayed and large-amplitude R in leads V_1 and V_2 with an inferior MI, the latter manifest by Q waves in leads II, III, and aV_f.

Figure 4–AE18
Acute inferior and right ventricular MI. The latter is manifested by Q waves and elevated ST segments in leads V_1 to V_6R.

Figure 4–AE19
AIDS myocarditis simulating an anteroseptal MI.

Figure 4–AE20
Hypertrophic cardiomyopathy simulating an anteroseptal MI.

Figure 4–AE21
Anteroseptal myocardial infarction with persistence of ST segment elevation over a period of more than $2\frac{1}{2}$ years is characteristic of a ventricular aneurysm.

Figure 4–AE22
This tracing was recorded at $\frac{1}{2}$ standard and illustrates giant negative T waves occasionally present in patients with localized hypertrophic cardiomyopathy.

Figure 4–AE23
WPW recorded on 5/29/92. The tracing recorded on 5/30/92, after ablation of an accessory pathway illustrates inverted T waves in leads II, III, and aV_f. The latter is thought by some to reflect T wave "memory."

Figure 4–AE24
LVH with negative U waves. The latter are rarely, if ever, recorded in a normal heart.

Figure 4–AE25
Faulty technique with reversal of the order of recording of leads V_1, V_2, and V_3, invariably interpreted by the computer as an anterior MI. Analysis of the P wave leads to a correct diagnosis. Q waves in leads II, III, and aV_f indicate an inferior MI.

Figure 4–AE26
Hyperkalemia with a prolonged P-R interval best seen in lead I, depression of intraventricular conduction with the pattern of a RBBB with LAFB, and tall "tented" T waves.

Figure 4–AE27
Long Q-U interval due to hypokalemia. The prominent U waves are best seen in leads II, III, aV_f, V_2, and V_3. Although the T waves in hypokalemia are as a rule upright, on rare occasion the T wave may be inverted.

Figure 4–AE28
Hypercalcemia manifested by a short QT interval.

Figure 4–AE29
AF with a junctional rhythm and multiform VPC with fixed coupling. The presence of more than one ectopic rhythm and multiform VPC with fixed coupling is highly specific for digitalis intoxication.

Figure 4–AE30
AF treated with large doses of digitoxin which not only fails to slow the ventricular rate *(middle row)* but also induces a ventricular *(top row)* and junctional *(bottom row)* tachycardia. Recorded in a patient with pneumococcic pneumonia.

Chapter 5
Exercise Stress Testing

BERNARD R. CHAITMAN

Exercise testing is an important diagnostic and prognostic procedure in the assessment of patients with ischemic heart disease. The diagnostic utility of the electrocardiogram was recognized by Feil and Siegel as early as 1928, when ST- and T-wave changes following exercise were reported in three of four patients with chronic stable angina.[1] Master and Oppenheimer developed a standardized exercise protocol to assess functional capacity and hemodynamic response in 1929.[2] Continued research into causal mechanisms of ST-segment displacement, effect of lead position, refinement of exercise protocols, and determination of diagnostic and prognostic exercise variables in clinical patient subsets characterized the subsequent 30 years. Shortly after the advent of coronary angiography, the limitation of exercise-induced ST-segment depression as a diagnostic marker for obstructive coronary disease in patient populations with a low disease prevalence became apparent. The test is now most frequently used to estimate prognosis and to determine functional capacity, likelihood and extent of coronary disease, and effects of therapy.[3-10] Ancillary techniques such as metabolic gas analysis, radionuclide imaging, and echocardiography enhance the information content of exercise testing in selected patients.

EXERCISE PHYSIOLOGY

Anticipation of dynamic exercise results in an acceleration of ventricular rate due to vagal withdrawal, increase in alveolar ventilation, and increased venous return as a result of sympathetic vasoconstriction. In normal subjects, the net effect is to increase resting cardiac output before the start of exercise. The magnitude of hemodynamic response during exercise depends on the severity and amount of muscle mass involved. In the early phases of exercise in the upright position, cardiac output is increased by an augmentation in stroke volume mediated through the use of the Frank-Starling mechanism and heart rate; the increase in cardiac output in the latter phases of exercise is primarily due to an increase in ventricular rate (see p. 381). During strenuous exertion, sympathetic discharge is maximal and parasympathetic stimulation is withdrawn, resulting in vasoconstriction of most circulatory body systems, except for that in exercising muscle and in the cerebral and coronary circulations. Venous and arterial norepinephrine release from sympathetic postganglionic nerve endings is increased, and epinephrine levels are increased at peak exertion; this enhances ventricular contractility. As exercise progresses, skeletal muscle blood flow is increased, oxygen extraction increases by as much as threefold, total calculated peripheral resistance decreases, and systolic blood pressure, mean arterial pressure, and pulse pressure usually increase. Diastolic blood pressure is unchanged or may increase or decrease by approximately 10 mm Hg. The pulmonary vascular bed can accommodate as much as a sixfold increase in cardiac output with only modest increases in pulmonary artery pressure, pulmonary capillary wedge pressure, and right atrial pressure; in normal subjects, this is not a limiting determinant of peak exercise capacity.

Cardiac output increases by four- to sixfold above basal levels during strenuous exertion in the upright position, depending on genetic endowment and level of training.[3] The maximum heart rate and cardiac output are decreased in older individuals related in part to decreased beta-adrenergic responsivity[11] (see p. 1692). Maximum heart rate can be calculated from the formula 220 − age (years) with a standard deviation of 10 to 12 beats per minute.[6] The age-predicted maximum heart rate is a useful measurement for safety reasons. However, the wide standard deviation seen in the various regression equations used and the impact of drug therapy limit the usefulness of this parameter in arbitrary selection of limits of age-predicted maximum heart rate to define the adequacy of cardiac reserve in individual patients.

In the postexercise phase, hemodynamics return to baseline within minutes of termination. Vagal reactivation is an important cardiac deceleration mechanism after exercise and is accelerated in well-trained athletes but blunted in patients with chronic heart failure.[12] Intense physical work or important cardiorespiratory impairment may interfere with achievement of a steady state, and an oxygen deficit occurs during exercise. The total oxygen uptake in excess of the resting oxygen uptake during the recovery period is the oxygen debt.

PATIENT POSITION. At rest, the cardiac output and stroke volume are higher in the supine than in the upright position. With exercise in normal supine subjects, the elevation of cardiac output results almost entirely from an increase in heart rate with little augmentation of stroke volume. In the upright posture, the increase in cardiac output in normal subjects results from a combination of elevations in stroke volume and heart rate. A change from supine to upright posture causes decrease in venous return, left ventricular end-diastolic volume and pressure, stroke volume, and cardiac index. Renin and norepinephrine levels are increased. End-systolic volume and ejection fraction are not significantly changed. In normal individuals, end-systolic volume decreases and ejection fraction increases to a similar extent from rest to exercise in the supine and upright positions. The magnitude and direction of change in end-diastolic volume from rest to maximum exercise in both positions are small and may vary according to the patient population studied. The net effect on exercise performance is an approximate 10 per cent increase in exercise time, cardiac index, heart rate, and rate pressure product at peak exercise in the upright as compared with the supine position.

Cardiopulmonary Exercise Testing

Cardiopulmonary exercise testing involves measurements of respiratory oxygen uptake ($\dot{V}_{O_2}$), carbon dioxide production ($\dot{V}_{CO_2}$), and ventilatory parameters during a symptom-limited exercise test. During testing, the patient usually wears a nose clip and breathes through a nonrebreathing valve that separates expired air from room air. Important measurements of expired gas are O_2 tension, CO_2 tension, and airflow. A flowmeter is used to determine airflow. Ventilatory measurements include respiratory rate, tidal volume, and minute ventilation (VE). O_2 and CO_2 tension are sampled breath by breath or by use of a mixing chamber. The $\dot{V}_{O_2}$ and $\dot{V}_{CO_2}$ can be computed on-line from ventilatory volumes and differences between inspired and expired gases.[13] Under steady-state (equilibrium) conditions, $\dot{V}_{O_2}$ and $\dot{V}_{CO_2}$ measured at the mouth are equivalent to total-body oxygen consumption and CO_2 production. The relationship between work output, oxygen consumption, heart rate, and cardiac output during exercise is linear (Fig. 5–1). $\dot{V}_{O_2max}$ is the product of maximal arterial venous oxygen difference and cardiac output. In untrained persons, the arterial–mixed venous O_2 difference at peak exercise is relatively constant (14 to 17 vol per cent), and $\dot{V}_{O_2max}$ is an approximation of maximum cardiac output. $\dot{V}_{O_2max}$ does not reliably predict degree of systolic left ventricular dysfunction measured by ejection fraction.[14] Measured $\dot{V}_{O_2max}$ can be compared with predicted values from empirically derived formulas based on age, sex, weight, and height.[13,15,16] Peak exercise capacity is decreased when the ratio of measured to predicted $\dot{V}_{O_2max}$ is <85 to 90 per cent. Oximetry, determined noninvasively, can be used to monitor arterial oxygen saturation and normally does not decrease by more than 5 per cent during exercise. Estimates of oxygen saturation during strenuous exercise using pulse oximetry may be unreliable in some patients.[17]

ANAEROBIC THRESHOLD. *Anaerobic threshold* is a theoretical point during dynamic exercise when muscle tissue switches over to anaerobic metabolism as an additional energy source. All tissues do not shift simultaneously, and there is a brief interval during which exercising muscle tissue shifts from predominantly aerobic to anaerobic metabolism.[3,13,15,16,18] (Fig. 5–1). Lactic acid begins to accumulate when a healthy untrained subject reaches about 50 to 60 per cent of the maximal capacity for aerobic metabolism. The increase in lactic acid becomes greater as exercise becomes more intense, resulting in metabolic acidosis. As lactate is formed, it is buffered in the serum by the bicarbonate system, resulting in increased CO_2 excretion, which causes reflex hyperventilation. The gas exchange anaerobic threshold (AT_{ge}) is the point at which VE increases disproportionately relative to $\dot{V}_{O_2}$ and work; it occurs at 40 to 60 per cent of $\dot{V}_{O_2max}$ in normal, untrained individuals.[13] Below the anaerobic threshold, CO_2 production is proportional to oxygen consumption. Above the anaerobic threshold, CO_2 is produced in excess of oxygen consumption. There are several methods to determine AT_{ge}, which include (1) the V-slope method, the point at which the rate of increase in $\dot{V}_{CO_2}$ relative to $\dot{V}_{O_2}$ increases (Fig. 5–1), (2) the point at which the $\dot{V}_{O_2}$ and $\dot{V}_{CO_2}$ slopes intersect, and (3) the point at which the ratio of VE/$\dot{V}_{O_2}$ and end-tidal O_2 tension begins to increase systematically without an immediate increase in the VE/$\dot{V}_{O_2}$. The AT_{ge} is a useful parameter because work below AT_{ge} encompasses most activities of daily living. Anaerobic threshold is often reduced in patients with important cardiovascular disease. An increase in anaerobic threshold with training can greatly enhance an individual's capacity to perform sustained submaximal activities with consequent improvement in quality of life and daily living. Changes in anaerobic threshold with repeat testing can be used to assess disease progression, response to medical therapy, and improvement in cardiovascular fitness with training.

METABOLIC EQUIVALENT. The current usage of the term *MET* refers to the resting $\dot{V}_{O_2}$ for a 70-kg, 40-year-old male, and 1 MET is equivalent to 3.5 ml/min/kg of body weight. Work activities can be calculated in multiples of METs;

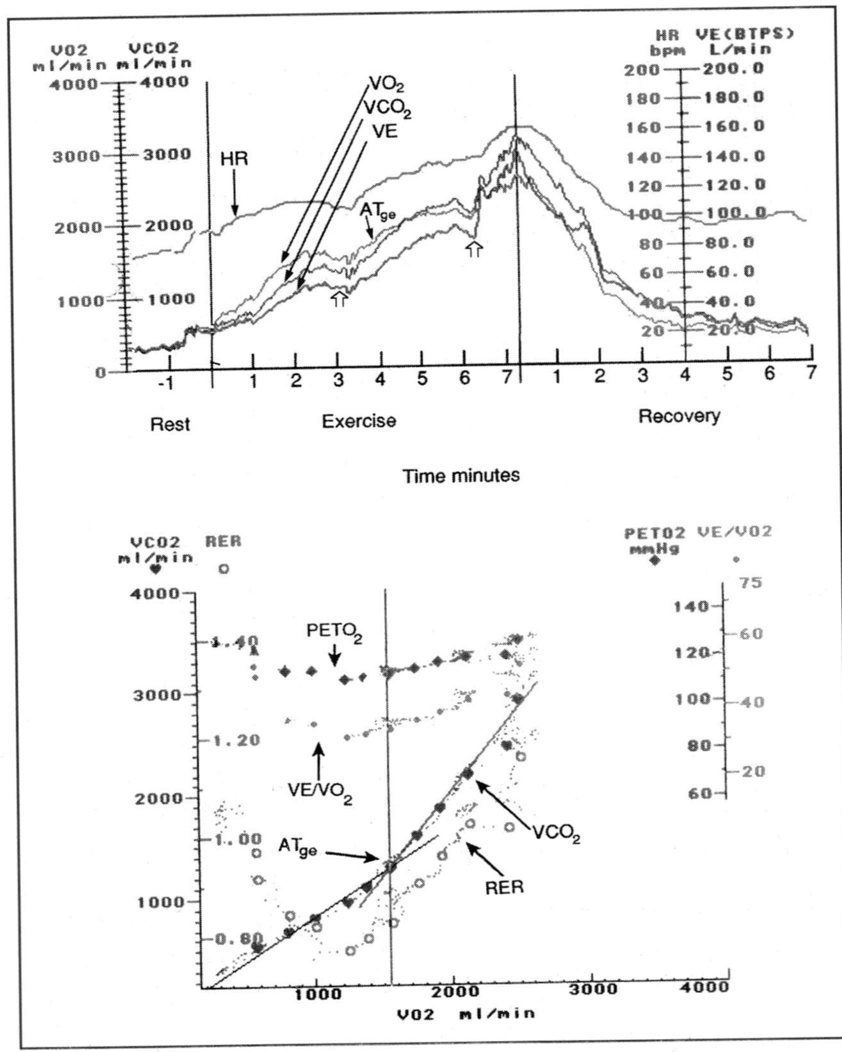

FIGURE 5–1. Cardiopulmonary exercise test in a 53-year-old, healthy man using the Bruce protocol. The progressive linear increase in work output, heart rate, and oxygen consumption ($\dot{V}_{O_2}$) is noted with steady-state conditions reached after 2 minutes in each of the first two stages *(top panel)*. Open arrows indicate the beginning of each new 3-minute stage. The subject completed 7 minutes and 10 seconds of exercise, and peak $\dot{V}_{O_2}$ was 3.08 liters/min. The anaerobic threshold (AT_{ge}), determined by the $\dot{V}$-slope method is the point at which the slope of the relative rate of increase in $\dot{V}_{CO_2}$ relative to $\dot{V}_{O_2}$ changes, and occurred at a $\dot{V}_{O_2}$ of 1.3 liters/min, or 42 per cent of peak $\dot{V}_{O_2}$, within predicted values for a normal sedentary population *(bottom panel)*. The AT_{ge} determined by the point at which the $\dot{V}_{O_2}$ and $\dot{V}_{CO_2}$ slopes intersect (1.8 liters/min) *(left panel)* is slightly greater than the AT_{ge} determined by the $\dot{V}$-slope method *(bottom panel)*. The $\dot{V}$-slope method usually provides a more reproducible estimate of AT_{ge}. PET_{O_2} = end-tidal pressure of oxygen; RER = respiratory exchange ratio; VE/$\dot{V}_{O_2}$ = ratio ventilation to oxygen uptake.

this measurement is useful to determine exercise prescriptions, assess disability, and standardize the reporting of submaximal and peak exercise workloads when different protocols are employed. An exercise workload of 3 to 5 METs is consistent with activities such as raking leaves, light carpentry, golf, and walking at 3 to 4 miles per hour. Workloads of 5 to 7 METs are consistent with exterior carpentry, singles tennis, and light backpacking. Workloads in excess of 9 METs are compatible with heavy labor, handball, squash, and running at 6 miles per hour (see p. 3004). Estimating $\dot{V}_{O_2}$ from work rate or treadmill time in individual patients may lead to misinterpretation of data if exercise equipment is not correctly calibrated or if the patient fails to achieve steady state, is obese, or has peripheral vascular disease, pulmonary vascular disease, or cardiac impairment. $\dot{V}_{O_2}$ does not increase linearly in some patients with cardiovascular or pulmonary disease as work rate is increased and may lead to overestimation of $\dot{V}_{O_2}$.[13] The measurements obtained with cardiopulmonary exercise testing are useful in understanding an individual patient's response to exercise and can be quite useful in the diagnostic evaluation of a patient with dyspnea.[19]

PATHOPHYSIOLOGY OF THE MYOCARDIAL ISCHEMIC RESPONSE

Myocardial oxygen consumption (M_{O_2}) is determined by heart rate, systolic blood pressure, left ventricular end-diastolic volume, wall thickness, and contractility.[6,10] The rate-pressure or double product (heart rate × systolic blood pressure) increases progressively with increasing work and can be used to estimate the myocardial perfusion requirement in normal subjects and in many patients with coronary artery disease. The heart is an aerobic organ with little capacity to generate energy through anaerobic metabolism. O_2 extraction in the coronary circulation is nearly maximal at rest. The only significant mechanism available to the heart to increase oxygen consumption is to increase perfusion, and there is a direct linear relationship between M_{O_2} consumption and coronary blood flow in normal individuals. The principal mechanism for increasing coronary blood flow during exercise is to decrease resistance at the coronary arteriolar level.[20] In patients with progressive atherosclerotic narrowing of the epicardial vessels, an ischemic threshold occurs beyond which exercise can produce abnormalities in diastolic and systolic ventricular function, electrocardiographic changes, and chest pain. The subendocardium is more susceptible to myocardial ischemia than the subepicardium because of increased wall tension, causing a relative increase in myocardial O_2 demand.

Dynamic changes in coronary artery tone at the site of an atherosclerotic plaque may result in diminished coronary flow during static or dynamic exercise; i.e., perfusion pressure distal to the stenotic plaque actually falls during exercise, resulting in reduced subendocardial blood flow[21] (see p. 404). Thus regional left ventricular myocardial ischemia may result not only from an increase in myocardial O_2 demand during exercise but also from a limitation of coronary flow as a result of coronary vasoconstriction and inability to vasodilate near the site of an atherosclerotic plaque.

EXERCISE PROTOCOLS

The main types of exercise are dynamic or isotonic exercise and static or isometric exercise. In daily living, a person frequently performs both types simultaneously. Dynamic protocols most frequently are used to assess cardiovascular reserve, and those suitable for clinical testing should include a low-intensity "warmup" phase. In general, 6 to 10 minutes of continuous progressive exercise during which the myocardial O_2 demand is elevated to the patient's maximal level is optimal for diagnostic and prognostic purposes. The protocol should include a suitable recovery or "cool-down" period. If the protocol is too strenuous for an individual patient, early test termination will result and will not allow an opportunity to observe clinically important responses. If the exercise protocol is too easy for an individual patient, the prolonged procedure will test endurance and not aerobic capacity. Thus exercise protocols should be individualized to accommodate the patient's limitations. Protocols may be set up at a fixed duration of exercise for a certain intensity to meet minimal qualifications for certain industrial tasks or sports programs.

STATIC EXERCISE. This form of isometric exercise generates force with little muscle shortening and produces a greater pressor response than with dynamic exercise. In a common form, the patient's maximal force on a hand dynamometer is recorded. The patient then sustains 25 to 33 per cent of maximal force for 3 to 5 minutes while ECG and blood pressures are recorded. The increase in myocardial $\dot{V}_{O_2}$ is often insufficient to initiate an ischemic response.

ARM ERGOMETRY. Arm crank ergometry protocols involve arm cranking at incremental workloads of 10 to 20 watts for 2 or 3 minute stages.[22] The heart rate and blood pressure responses to a given workload of arm exercise usually are greater than those for leg exercise. A bicycle ergometer with the axle placed at the level of the shoulders is used, and the subject sits or stands and cycles the peddles so that the arms are alternately fully extended. The most common frequency is 50 rpm's. In normal subjects, maximum $\dot{V}_{O_2}$ and VE for arm cycling approximates 50 to 70 per cent of leg cycling. Peak heart rate is approximately 70 per cent of that during leg testing.

BICYCLE ERGOMETRY. Bicycle protocols involve incremental workloads calibrated in watts or kilopond (KPD) meters/min. One watt is equivalent to 6 KPD meters/min in mechanically braked bicycles, work is determined by force and distance and requires a constant pedaling rate of 60 to 80 rpm, according to subject preference. Electronically braked bicycles provide a constant workload in spite of changes in pedaling rate and are less dependent on patient cooperation; although they are more costly than a mechanically braked bicycle, they are preferred for diagnostic and prognostic assessment. Most protocols begin at a workload of 25 watts and increase in 25-watt increments every 2 minutes. Younger subjects may start at 50 watts, with 50-watt increments every 2 minutes. A ramp protocol differs from the staged protocols in that the patient starts at 3 minutes of unloaded pedaling at a cycle speed of 60 rpm. Work rate is increased by a uniform amount each minute ranging from 5- to 30-watt increments depending on expected patient performance.[6,13] Exercise is terminated if the patient is unable to maintain a cycling frequency above 40 rpm. In the cardiac catheterization laboratory, hemodynamic measurements may be made during supine bicycle ergometry at rest and at one or two submaximal workloads.

In subjects unfamiliar with bicycle exercise, the muscles required for optimal performance are not as well developed as for treadmill exercise, and early fatigue may be a limiting factor. The bicycle ergometer is associated with a lower maximal $\dot{V}_{O_2}$ and anaerobic threshold than the treadmill, although maximal heart rate, maximal VE, and maximal lactate values are often similar. The metabolic requirements of ergometric workloads are inversely related to body mass, whereas the requirements of treadmill exercise are relatively independent of body mass. The bicycle ergometer has the advantage of requiring less space than a treadmill, is quieter, and permits sensitive precordial measurements without much motion artifact. However, in North America, treadmill protocols are more widely used in the assessment of patients with coronary disease.

TREADMILL PROTOCOL. The treadmill protocol should be consistent with the patient's physical capacity and the purpose of the test. In healthy individuals, the standard Bruce protocol is popular, and a large diagnostic and prognostic data base has been published.[6,10,23] In older individuals, or those whose exercise capacity is limited by cardiac disease, the Bruce protocol can be modified by two 3-minute warmup stages at 1.7 mph and 0 per cent grade and 1.7 mph and 5 per cent grade. The Bruce multistage maximal treadmill protocol has 3-minute periods to allow achievement of a steady state before workload is increased (Fig. 5–1). A limitation of the Bruce protocol is the relatively large increase in $\dot{V}_{O_2}$ between stages and the additional energy cost of running as compared with walking at stages in excess of Bruce stage III. The *Naughton* and *Weber protocols* use 1- to 2-minute stages with 1-MET increments between stages; these protocols may be more suitable for patients with limited exercise tolerance such as patients with congestive heart failure. The ACIP and modified ACIP (mACIP) protocols use 2-minute stages with 1.5-MET increments between stages after two 1-minute warmup stages with 1.0-MET increments. The ACIP protocols test patients with established coronary disease and result in a linear increase in heart rate and $\dot{V}_{O_2}$, permitting the time to occurrence of ST-segment depression over a wider range of heart rate and exercise time than protocols with more abrupt

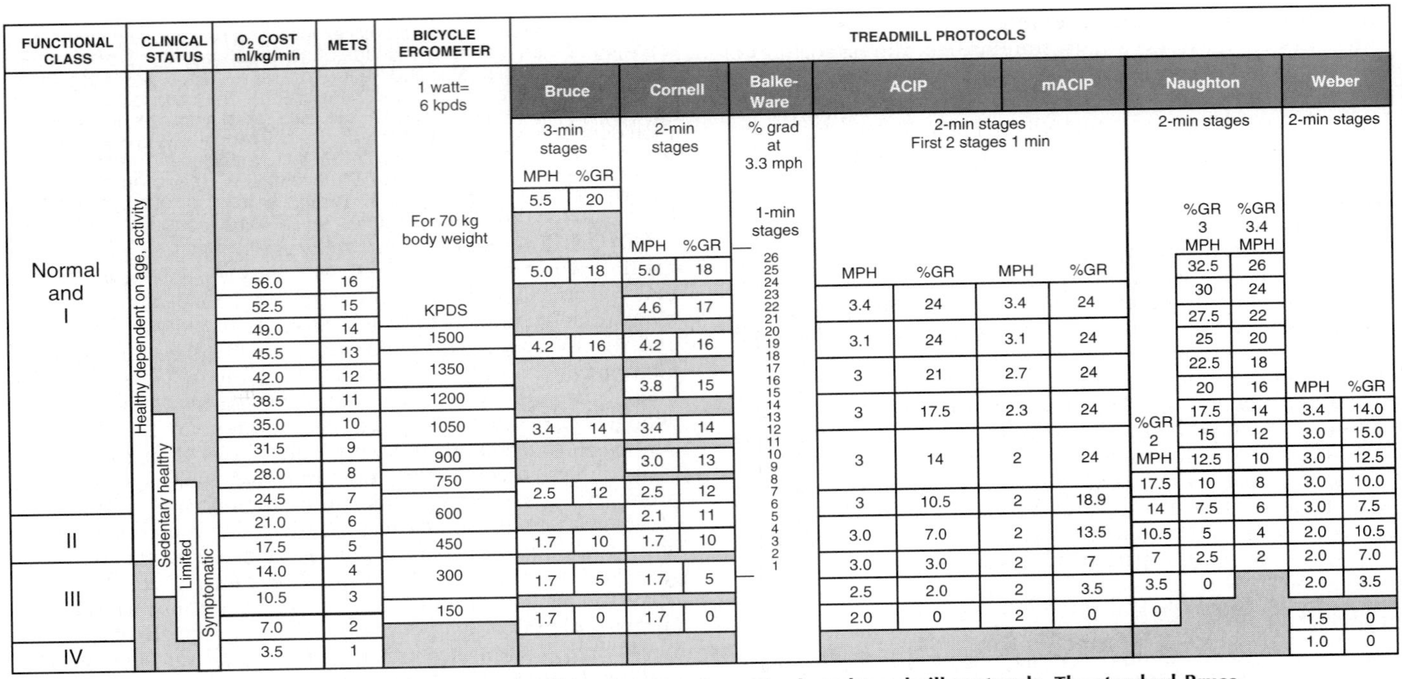

FUNCTIONAL CLASS	CLINICAL STATUS (Healthy dependent on age, activity; Sedentary healthy; Limited; Symptomatic)	O_2 COST ml/kg/min	METS
Normal and I		56.0	16
		52.5	15
		49.0	14
		45.5	13
		42.0	12
		38.5	11
		35.0	10
		31.5	9
		28.0	8
		24.5	7
II		21.0	6
		17.5	5
III		14.0	4
		10.5	3
		7.0	2
IV		3.5	1

BICYCLE ERGOMETER

1 watt= 6 kpds

For 70 kg body weight

KPDS
1500
1350
1200
1050
900
750
600
450
300
150

TREADMILL PROTOCOLS

Bruce — 3-min stages

MPH	%GR
5.5	20
5.0	18
4.2	16
3.4	14
2.5	12
1.7	10
1.7	5
1.7	0

Cornell — 2-min stages

MPH	%GR
5.0	18
4.6	17
4.2	16
3.8	15
3.4	14
3.0	13
2.5	12
2.1	11
1.7	10
1.7	5
1.7	0

Balke-Ware — % grad at 3.3 mph; 1-min stages

26, 25, 24, 23, 22, 21, 20, 19, 18, 17, 16, 15, 14, 13, 12, 11, 10, 9, 8, 7, 6, 5, 4, 3, 2, 1

ACIP and mACIP — 2-min stages; First 2 stages 1 min

ACIP MPH	ACIP %GR	mACIP MPH	mACIP %GR
3.4	24	3.4	24
3.1	24	3.1	24
3	21	2.7	24
3	17.5	2.3	24
3	14	2	24
3	10.5	2	18.9
3.0	7.0	2	13.5
3.0	3.0	2	7
2.5	2.0	2	3.5
2.0	0	2	0

Naughton — 2-min stages

%GR 2 MPH	%GR 3 MPH	%GR 3.4 MPH
	32.5	26
	30	24
	27.5	22
	25	20
	22.5	18
	20	16
	17.5	14
	15	12
	12.5	10
17.5	10	8
14	7.5	6
10.5	5	4
7	2.5	2
3.5	0	
0		

Weber — 2-min stages

MPH	%GR
3.4	14.0
3.0	15.0
3.0	12.5
3.0	10.0
3.0	7.5
2.0	10.5
2.0	7.0
2.0	3.5
1.5	0
1.0	0

FIGURE 5–2. Estimated oxygen cost of bicycle ergometer and selected treadmill protocols. The standard Bruce protocol starts at 1.7 mph and 10 per cent grade (5 METs) with a larger increment between stages than protocols such as the Naughton, ACIP, and Weber protocols, which start at less than 2 METs at 2 mph and increase by 1- to 1.5-MET increments between stages. The Bruce protocol can be modified by two 3-minute warmup stages at 1.7 mph and 0 per cent grade and 1.7 mph and 5 per cent grade. (Adapted with permission from Fletcher, G. F., Balady, G., Froelicher, V. F., et al: Exercise standards. A statement for healthcare professionals from the American Heart Association. Circulation *91*:580, 1995. Copyright 1995 American Heart Association.)

increments in workload between stages. The mACIP protocol produces a similar aerobic demand as the standard ACIP protocol for each minute of exercise and is well suited for short or elderly individuals who cannot keep up with a walking speed of 3 mph (Fig. 5–2).[24,25]

Ramp protocols start the patient at relatively slow treadmill speed, which is gradually increased until the patient has a good stride. The ramp angle of incline is progressively increased at fixed intervals (e.g., 10 to 60 seconds) starting at zero grade with the increase in grade calculated on the patient's estimated functional capacity such that the protocol will be complete at between 6 and 10 minutes.[6,10] In this type of protocol, the rate of work increase is continuous, and steady-state conditions are not reached. A limitation of ramp protocols is the requirement to estimate functional capacity from an activity scale; occasionally, under- or overestimation of functional capacity will result in an endurance test or premature cessation. One formula for estimating $\dot{V}_{O_2}$ from treadmill speed and grade is $\dot{V}_{O_2}$ (mlO_2/kg/min) = (mph × 2.68) + (1.8 × 26.82 × mph × grade ÷ 100) + 3.5.[26] $\dot{V}_{O_2}$ max is usually the same regardless of treadmill protocol used; the difference is the rate of time at which $\dot{V}_{O_2}$ is achieved.

It is important to encourage the patient not to grasp the handrails of the treadmill during exercise. Functional capacity can be overestimated by as much as 20 per cent in tests in which handrail support is permitted, and $\dot{V}_{O_2}$ is decreased. Since the degree of handrail support is difficult to quantify from one test to another, more consistent results can be obtained during serial testing when handrail support is not permitted.

The *6-minute walk test* can be used in patients with marked left ventricular dysfunction who cannot perform bicycle or treadmill exercise.[27] Patients are instructed to walk down a 100-foot corridor at their own pace, attempting to cover as much ground as possible in 6 minutes. At the end of the 6-minute interval, the total distance walked is determined and the symptoms experienced by the patient are recorded.

ELECTROCARDIOGRAPHIC MEASUREMENTS

LEAD SYSTEMS. The Mason-Likar modification of the standard 12-lead electrocardiogram requires that the extremity electrodes be moved to the torso to reduce motion artifact. The arm electrodes should be located in the lateral-most aspects of the infraclavicular fossae and the leg electrodes in a stable position above the anterior iliac crest and below the rib cage (Fig. 5–3). The Mason-Likar modification results in a right-axis shift and increased voltage in the inferior leads and may produce a loss of inferior Q waves and the development of new Q waves in lead aVl. Thus, the body torso limb lead positions cannot be used to interpret a diagnostic rest 12-lead ECG. The more cephalad the leg electrodes are placed, the greater is the degree of change and the greater is the augmentation of R-wave amplitude, potentiating exercise-induced ST-segment changes.

Bipolar lead groups place the negative or reference electrode over the manubrium (CM_5), right scapula (CB_5), RV_5 (CC_5), or on the forehead (CH_5), and the active electrode at V_5 or proximate location to optimize R-wave amplitude. In bipolar lead ML, which reflects inferior wall changes, the negative reference is at the manubrium and the active electrode in the left leg position. Bipolar lead groups may provide additional diagnostic information, and in some medical centers lead CM_5 is substituted for lead aV_r in the Mason-Likar modified lead system (Fig. 5–3). Bipolar leads are frequently used when only a limited ECG set is required (e.g., in cardiac rehabilitation programs). The use of more elaborate lead set systems is usually reserved for research purposes.

Types of ST Segment Displacement

In normal subjects, the P-R, QRS, and Q-T intervals shorten as heart rate increases. P amplitude increases and the P-R segment becomes progressively more downsloping in the inferior leads. J point, or junctional, depression is a normal finding during exercise (Fig. 5–4). However, in patients with myocardial ischemia, the ST segment usually becomes more horizontal (flattens) as the severity of the ischemic response worsens. With progressive exercise, the depth of ST-segment depression may increase, involving more ECG leads, and the patient may develop angina. In the immediate postrecovery phase, the ST-segment displacement may persist, with downsloping ST segments and T wave inversion, gradually returning to baseline after 5 to 10 minutes (Figs. 5–5 and 5–6). However, ischemic ST-segment displacement may be seen only during exercise, emphasizing the importance of adequate skin preparation and electrode placement to capture high-quality recordings during maximum exertion (Fig. 5–7). In about 10 per cent of patients, the ischemic response may appear only in the recovery phase.[27] The patient should not leave the exercise laboratory area until the postexercise ECG has returned to baseline. Figure 5–8 illustrates different ECG patterns seen during exercise testing.

MEASUREMENT OF ST-SEGMENT DISPLACEMENT. For purposes of interpretation, the PQ junction is usually chosen as the isoelectric point. The TP segment represents a true isoelectric point but is an impractical choice for most routine clinical measurements. The development of ≥0.10 mV (1 mm) of J point depression measured from the PQ junction, with a relatively flat ST-segment slope (<1 mV/sec), depressed ≥0.10 mV 60 to 80 msec after the J point in the three consecutive beats with a stable baseline is considered to be an abnormal response (Fig. 5–9). Occasionally, the ST segment at rest may be depressed. When this occurs, the J point and ST60 to ST80 measurements should be depressed an additional ≥0.10 mV to be considered abnormal. In patients with early repolarization and resting ST-segment elevation, return to the PQ junction is normal. Abnormal ST-segment depression in a patient with early repolarization should be measured from the PQ junction. A slow, upsloping ST segment is defined as J point depression with an upsloping ST segment (>1 mV/sec), depressed ≥0.15 mV at 60 to 80 msec after the J point, in three consecutive beats (Fig. 5–6).

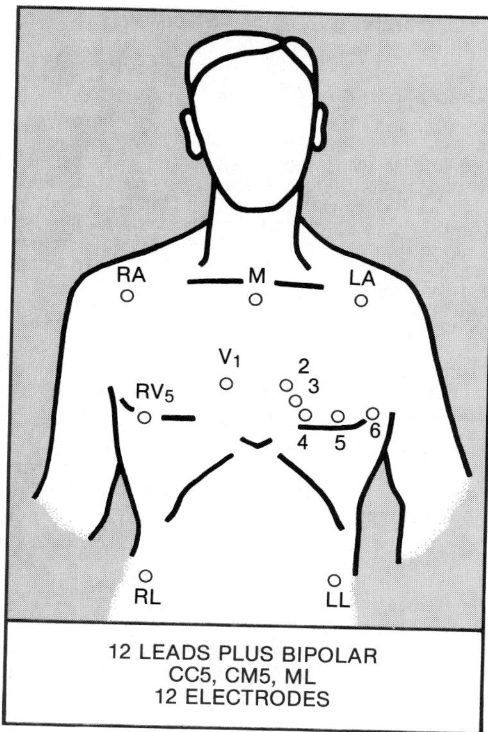

FIGURE 5–3. This lead group set reflects the Mason-Likar leads with the precordial electrodes in standard position and the arm and leg electrodes moved proximally to the subclavicular fossa and just above the anterior iliac crest. The position of the negative reference manubrial electrode and RV_5 electrode illustrates the position required for lead CM_5 and lead CC_5. In lead ML, the active electrode is in the left leg position.

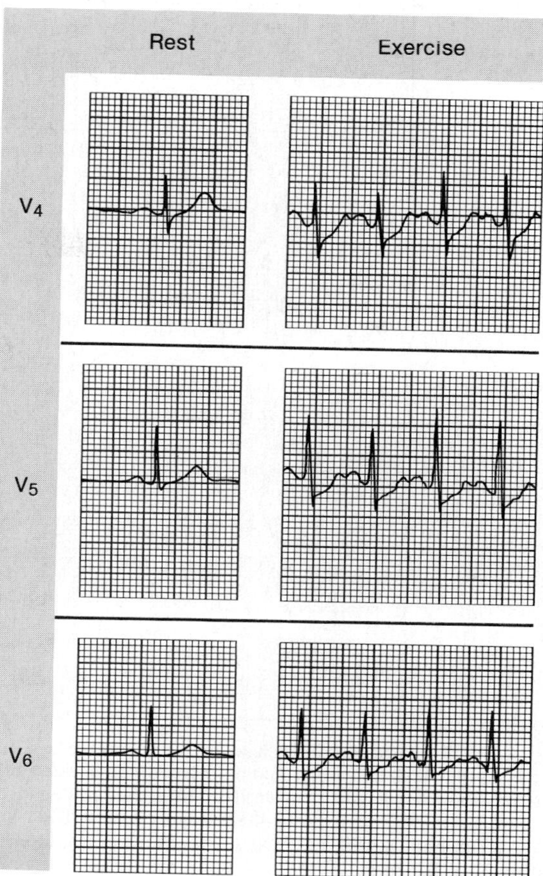

FIGURE 5–4. J point depression of 2 to 3 mm in leads V_4 to V_6 with rapid upsloping ST segments depressed approximately 1 mm 80 msec after the J point. The ST segment slope in leads V_4 and V_5 is ≥3.0 mV/sec. This response should not be considered abnormal.

Exercise-induced ST segment elevation may occur in Q wave or non-Q wave leads. The development of ≥0.10 mV (1 mm) of J point elevation, persistently elevated ≥0.10 mV at 60 to 80 msec after the J point in three consecutive beats, is considered an abnormal response (Figs. 5–8 and 5–10).

Exercise-induced ST segment depression does *not* localize the site of myocardial ischemia, *nor* does it provide a clue as to which coronary artery is involved.[29] For example, it is not unusual for patients with isolated right coronary disease to exhibit exercise-induced ST-segment depression only in leads V_4 to V_6, nor is it unusual for patients with disease of the left anterior descending coronary artery to exhibit exercise-induced ST-segment displacements in leads II, III, and aV_f. Exercise-induced ST-segment elevation is relatively specific for the territory of myocardial ischemia and the coronary artery involved.

T-WAVE CHANGES. The morphology of the T wave is influenced by body position, respiration, and hyperventilation. Occasionally, a patient may be referred for exercise testing who has T-wave inversion on the resting 12-lead ECG. Pseudonormalization of T waves (inverted at rest and becoming upright with exercise) is a nondiagnostic finding.[6] Although in rare instances this finding may be a marker for myocardial ischemia in a patient with docu-

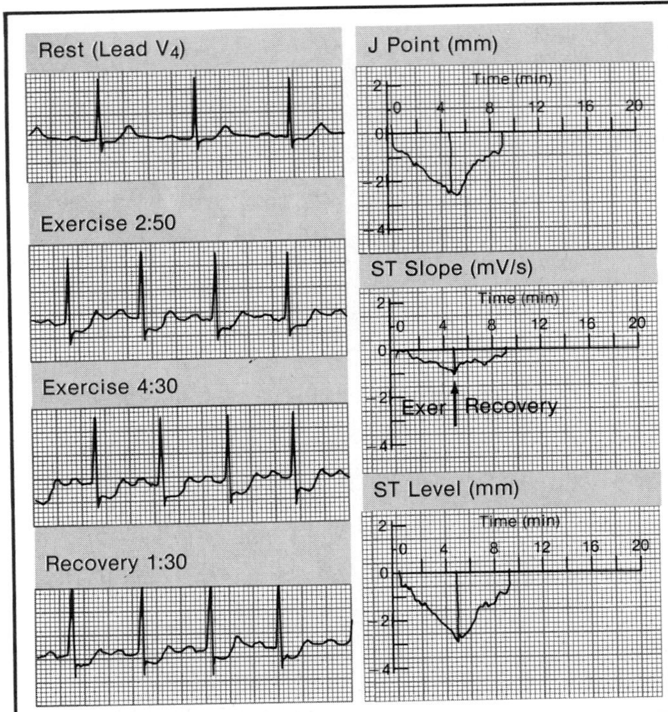

FIGURE 5–5. Bruce protocol. In lead V_4, the exercise ECG is abnormal early in the test, reaching 3 mm (0.3 mV) of horizontal ST-segment depression at the end of exercise. The ischemic changes persist for at least 1 min and 30 sec into the recovery phase. The right panel provides a continuous plot of the J point, ST slope, and ST-segment displacement at 80 msec after the J point (ST level) during exercise and in the recovery phase. Exercise ends at the vertical line at 4.5 min. The computer trends permit a more precise identification of initial onset and offset of ischemic ST-segment depression. This type of ECG pattern, with early onset of ischemic ST-segment depression, reaching more than 3 mm of horizontal ST-segment displacement, and persisting several minutes into the recovery phase, is consistent with a severe ischemic response.

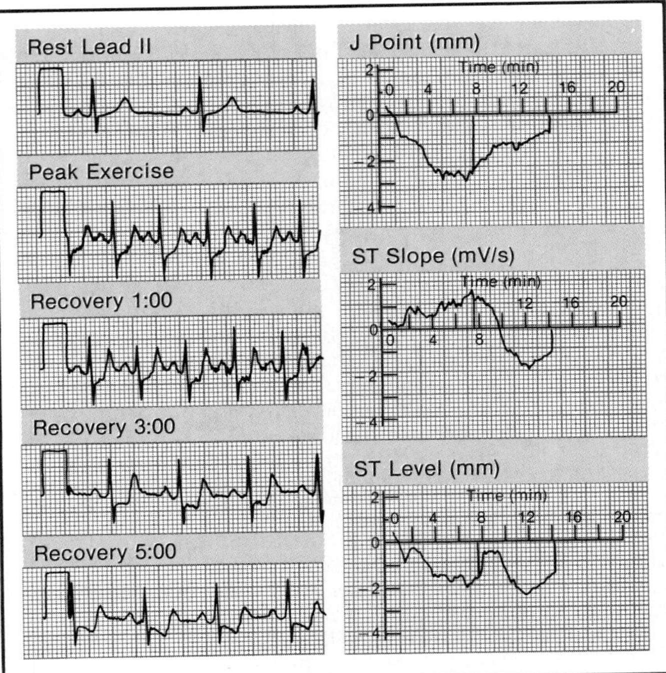

FIGURE 5–6. Bruce protocol. In this type of ischemic pattern, the J point at peak exertion is depressed 2.5 mm, the ST-segment slope is 1.5 mV/second, and the ST-segment level at 80 msec after the J point is depressed 1.6 mm. This "slow upsloping" ST segment at peak exercise indicates an ischemic pattern in patients with a high coronary disease prevalence pretest. A typical ischemic pattern is seen at 3 minutes of the recovery phase when the ST segment is horizontal and 5 minutes postexertion when the ST segment is downsloping. Exercise is discontinued at the vertical line in the right panels at 7.5 min.

mented coronary disease, it would need to be substantiated by an ancillary technique, such as the concomitant finding of a reversible thallium defect.

COMPUTER-ASSISTED ANALYSIS

The use of computers has facilitated the routine analysis and measurements required from exercise electrocardiography and can be performed on-line as well as off-line.[30] When the raw ECG data are high quality, the computer can filter and average or select median complexes from which the degree of J point displacement, ST-segment slope, and ST displacement 60 to 80 msec after the J point (ST60 to 80) can be measured. The selection of ST60 or ST80 depends on the heart rate response. At ventricular rates ≥ 130 beats/min, the ST80 measurement may fall on the upslope of the T wave, and the ST60 measurement should be employed instead. In some computerized systems, the PQ junction or isoelectric interval is detected by scanning before the R wave for the 10-msec interval with the least slope. J point, ST slope, and ST levels are determined, and the ST integral can be calculated from the area below the isoelectric line from the J point to ST60 to ST80. Computerized treatment of ECG complexes permits reduction of motion and myographic artifacts. However, the averaged or median beats occasionally may be erroneous because of ECG signal distortion caused by noise, baseline wander, or changes in conduction, and identification of the PQ junction and ST-segment onset may be imperfect. Therefore, it is crucial to ensure that the

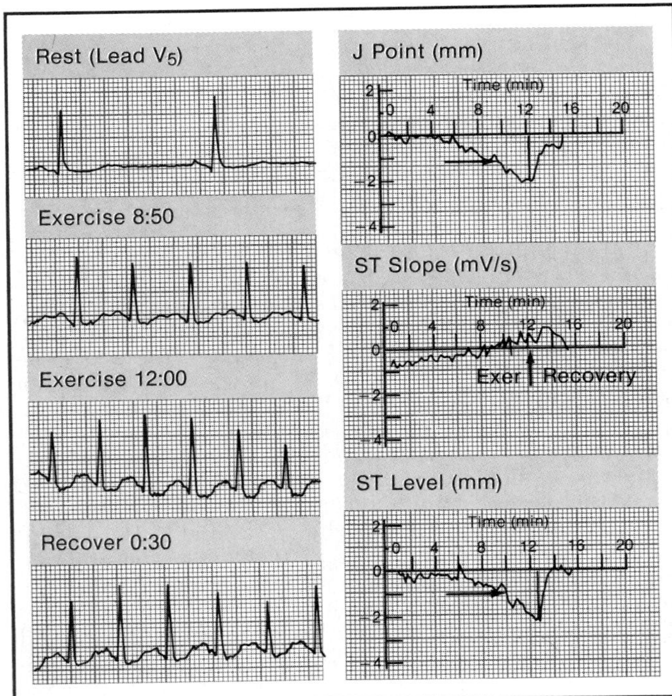

FIGURE 5–7. Bruce protocol. In lead V_4, the exercise ECG is abnormal early in the test, reaching 3 mm (0.3 mV) of horizontal ST-segment depression at the end of exercise. The ischemic changes persist for at least 1 min and 30 sec into the recovery phase. The right panel provides a continuous plot of the J point, ST slope, and ST-segment displacement at 80 msec after the J point (ST level) during exercise and in the recovery phase. Exercise ends at the vertical line at 4.5 min. The computer trends permit a more precise identification of initial onset and offset of ischemic ST-segment depression. This type of ECG pattern, with early onset of ischemic ST-segment depression, reaching $>$ 3 mm of horizontal ST-segment displacement, and persisting several minutes into the recovery phase, is consistent with a severe ischemic response.

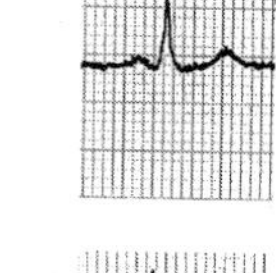
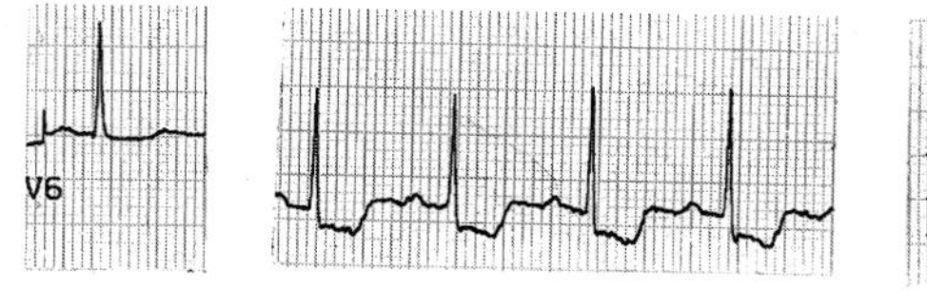
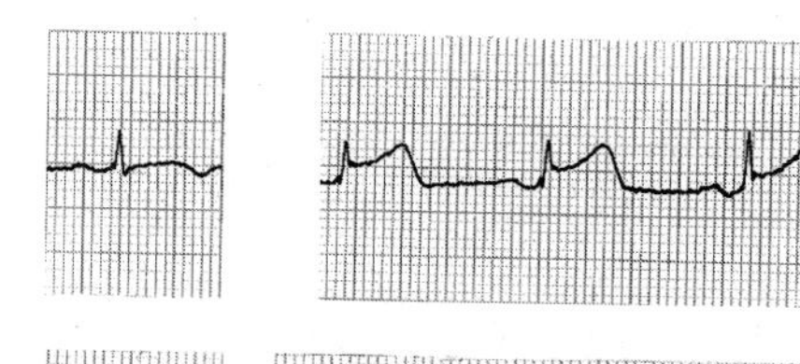

FIGURE 5–8. Illustration of typical exercise electrocardiographic patterns at rest and at peak exertion. The computer processed incrementally averaged beat corresponds with the raw data taken at the same time point during exercise and is illustrated in the last column. The patterns represent worsening ECG responses during exercise. In the column of computer-averaged beats, ST80 displacement (top number) indicates the magnitude of ST segment displacement 80 msec after the J point relative to the PQ junction or E point. ST segment slope measurement (bottom number) indicates the ST segment slope at a fixed time point after the J point to the ST80 measurement. At least three noncomputer average complexes with a stable baseline should meet criteria for abnormality before the exercise ECG can be considered abnormal (see Fig. 5–9). The normal and rapid upsloping ST segment responses are normal responses to exercise. J-point depression with rapid upsloping ST segments is a common response in an older, apparently healthy population. Minor ST depression can occur occasionally at submaximal workloads in patients with coronary disease; in this illustration, the ST segment is depressed 0.9 mm (0.09 mV) 80 ms after the J point. The slow upsloping ST segment pattern often demonstrates an ischemic response in patients with known coronary disease or those with a high pretest clinical risk of coronary disease. Criteria for slow upsloping ST segment depression include J-point and ST80 depression of 0.15 mV or more and ST segment slope of more than 1.0 mV/sec. Classic criteria for myocardial ischemia include horizontal ST-segment depression observed when both the J point and ST80 depression are 0.1 mV or more and ST segment slope is within the range of ± 1.0 mV/sec. Downsloping ST segment depression occurs when the J-point and ST80 depression are >0.1 mV and ST segment slope is > -1.0 mV/sec. ST segment elevation in a non–Q-wave, noninfarct lead occurs when the J point and ST60 are 1.0 mV or greater and represents a severe ischemic response. ST segment elevation in an infarct territory (Q-wave lead) indicates a severe wall motion abnormality and in most cases is not considered an ischemic response. (From Chaitman, B. R.: Exercise electrocardiographic stress testing. *In* Beller, G. A. (ed.): Chronic Ischemic Heart Disease. *In* Braunwald, E. (series ed.): Atlas of Heart Diseases. Vol. 5. Chronic Ischemic Heart Disease. Philadelphia, Current Medicine, 1995, pp 2.1–2.30.)

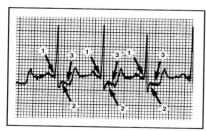

FIGURE 5–9. Magnified ischemic exercise-induced ECG pattern. Three consecutive complexes with a relatively stable baseline are selected. The PQ junction (1) and J point (2) are determined; the ST80 (3) is determined at 80 msec after the J point. In this example, average J point displacement is 2 mm (0.2 mV) and ST80 is 2.4 mm (0.24 mV). The average slope measurement from the J point to ST80 is -1.1 mV/sec.

computer-determined averages or median complexes reflect the raw ECG data, and physicians should program the computer to print out raw data during exercise and inspect the raw data to be certain that the QRS template is accurately reproduced before accepting the automatic measurements.

MECHANISM OF ST-SEGMENT DISPLACEMENT

The mechanism of exercise-induced ST-segment displacement is not completely understood (see also Fig. 4–30, p. 128). In normal persons, the action potential duration of the endocardial region is longer than that of the epicardial region, and ventricular repolarization is from epicardium to endocardium. The action potential duration is shortened in the presence of myocardial ischemia, and electrical gradients are created, resulting in ST-segment depression or elevation, depending on the surface ECG leads.[31] Increased myocardial oxygen demand associated with a failure to increase or an actual decrease in regional coronary blood flow will usually cause ST-segment depression; occasionally, ST-segment elevation may occur, depending on the severity of coronary flow reduction. ST-segment ele-

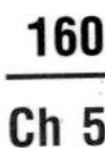

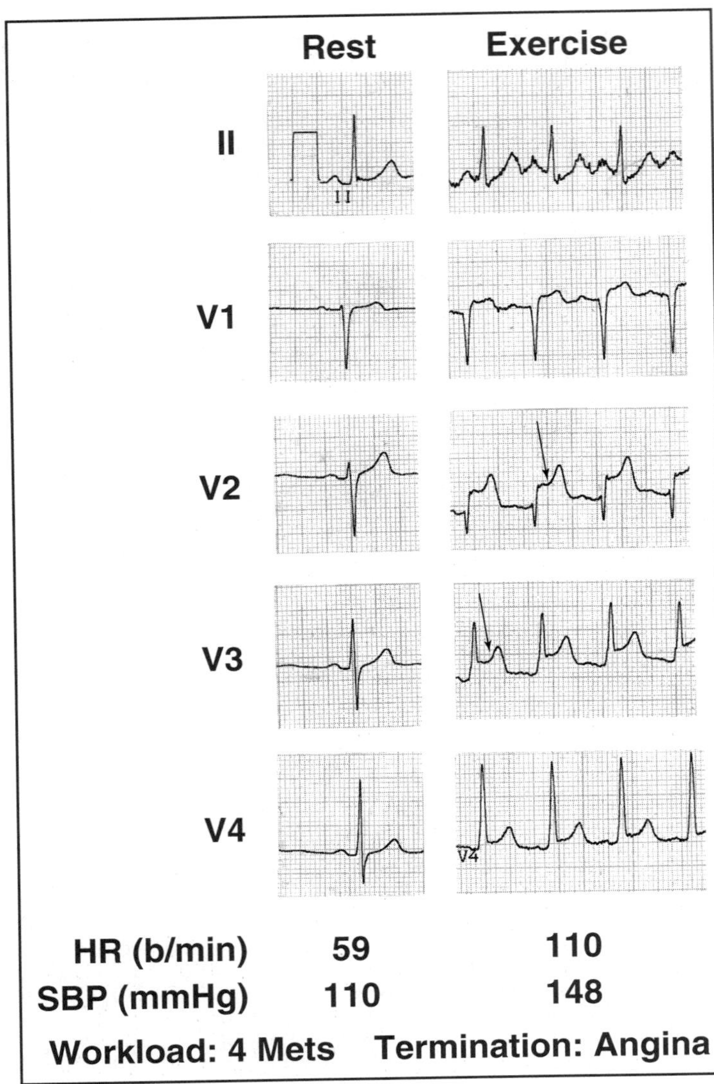

FIGURE 5–10. A 48-year-old man with several atherosclerotic risk factors and a normal rest ECG developed marked ST segment elevation (4 mm, [arrows]) in leads V_2 and V_3 with lesser degrees of ST-segment elevation in leads V_1 and V_4 and J point depression with upsloping ST segments in lead II, associated with angina. This type of ECG pattern is usually associated with a full-thickness, reversible myocardial perfusion defect in the corresponding left ventricular myocardial segments and high-grade intraluminal narrowing at coronary angiography. Rarely, coronary vasospasm will produce this result in the absence of significant intraluminal atherosclerotic narrowing. (From Chaitman, B. R.: Exercise electrocardiographic stress testing. *In* Beller, G. A., (ed.): Chronic Ischemic Heart Disease. *In* Braunwald, E. (series ed.): Atlas of Heart Diseases. Vol. 5. Chronic Ischemic Heart Disease. Philadelphia, Current Medicine, 1995, pp 2.1–2.30.)

vation in a non-Q wave lead is associated with a more severe degree of myocardial ischemia than is ST-segment depression.

EXERCISE TESTING

INDICATIONS. The most frequent indications for exercise testing are to aid in establishing the diagnosis of coronary artery disease in determining functional capacity and in estimating prognosis. The indications continue to evolve, with some that are uniformly accepted and others that are more controversial. The AHA and ACC Exercise Task Force determined several categories of test indications drawn from a large body of published literature on exercise testing[32] (Table 5–1). A class I indication indicates general agreement that exercise testing is justified; a class II indication indicates a condition for which exercise testing is frequently used but in which there is a divergence of opinion with respect to value and appropriateness; class III indicates general agreement that exercise testing is of little or no value or inappropriate. Exercise testing should not be used to screen very low-risk, asymptomatic individuals because the test has limited diagnostic and prognostic value in this situation, and the resultant undesirable consequences of a false-positive exercise test result in unnecessary follow-up, additional procedures, anxiety, and exercise restrictions.[7,8,32] Most asymptomatic subjects in an exercise screening program for coronary disease who die suddenly of cardiac causes have had a previous normal exercise test.

TECHNIQUES. The patient should be instructed not to eat, drink caffeinated beverages, or smoke for 3 hours prior to testing and to wear comfortable shoes and loose-fitting clothes. Unusual physical exertion should be avoided prior to testing. A brief history and physical examination should be performed, and the patient should be advised about the risks and benefits of the procedure. A written informed consent form is usually required. The indication for the test should be known. In many laboratories, the presence or absence of atherosclerotic risk factors is noted and cardioactive medication recorded. A 12-lead ECG should be obtained with the electrodes at the distal extremities.

Following recording of the standard 12-lead ECG, a torso ECG should be obtained in the supine position and in the sitting or standing position. Postural changes can bring out labile ST-T wave abnormalities. Hyperventilation is not recommended before exercise. If a false-positive test is suspected, hyperventilation should be performed after the test, and the hyperventilation tracing compared with the maximum ST segment abnormalities observed. The ECG and blood pressure should be recorded in both positions, and the patient should be instructed on how to perform the test.

Adequate skin preparation is essential for high-quality recordings, and the superficial layer of skin needs to be removed to augment signal-to-noise ratio. The areas of electrode application are rubbed with an alcohol-saturated pad to remove oil and rubbed with fine sandpaper or a rough material to reduce skin resistance to 5000 ohms or

TABLE 5–1 INDICATIONS FOR EXERCISE TESTING

CLASS 1 (CLEAR INDICATION)

Patients with suspected or proven coronary artery disease:

1. Diagnosis: patients with exercise related complaints of palpitations, dizziness, or syncope
2. Diagnosis: men with atypical symptoms
3. Prognostic assessment and functional capacity evaluation in patients with chronic stable angina or post-myocardial infarction
4. Symptomatic recurrent exercise-induced arrhythmias
5. Evaluation after revascularization procedure

CLASS 2 (TEST MAY BE INDICATED)

1. Diagnosis: women with typical or atypical angina pectoris
2. Functional capacity evaluation to monitor cardiovascular therapy in patients with CAD* or heart failure
3. Evaluation of patients with variant angina
4. Follow-up of patients with known CAD
5. Evaluation of asymptomatic men over 40 who are in special occupations (pilots, firefighters, police officers, bus or truck drivers, and railroad engineers), or who have two or more atherosclerotic risk factors or who plan to enter a vigorous exercise program

CLASS 3 (TEST PROBABLY NOT INDICATED)

1. Evaluation of patients with isolated premature ventricular beats and no evidence of CAD
2. Multiple serial testing during the course of cardiac rehab program
3. Diagnosis of CAD in patients, who have preexcitation syndrome or complete left bundle branch block or are on digitalis therapy
4. Evaluation of young or middle-aged asymptomatic men or women, who have no atherosclerotic risk factors or who have noncardiac chest discomfort

INDICATIONS FOR EXERCISE TESTING IN PATIENTS WITH VALVULAR HEART DISEASE OR HYPERTENSION

Test in common usage:

1. Evaluation of functional capacity in selected patients with valvular heart disease
2. Evaluation of blood pressure of hypertensive patients who wish to engage in vigorous dynamic or static exercise

* CAD = coronary artery disease

Data from ACC and AHA Subcommittee Report on Exercise Testing. Circulation *74*:653A, 1986.

less. Silver chloride electrodes with a fluid column to avoid direct metal-to-skin contact produce high-quality tracings; these electrodes have the lowest offset voltage.

Cables connecting the electrodes and recorders should be light, flexible, and properly shielded. In a small minority of patients, a fishnet jersey may be required over the electrodes and cables to reduce motion artifact. The electrode-skin interface can be verified by tapping on the electrode and examining the cathode-ray screen or by measuring skin impedance. Excessive noise indicates that the electrode needs to be replaced; replacement before the test rather than during exercise can save time. The ECG signal can be digitized systematically at the patient end of the cable by some systems, reducing powerline artifact. Exercise equipment should be calibrated regularly. Room temperature should be between 64 and 72°F (18 and 22°C) and humidity <60 per cent.

Treadmill walking should be demonstrated. The heart rate, blood pressure, and ECG should be recorded at the end of each stage of exercise, immediately before and immediately after stopping exercise, at the onset of an ischemic response, and for each minute for at least 5 to 10 minutes in the recovery phase. A minimum of three leads should be displayed continuously on the cathode-ray screen during the test. There is some controversy regarding optimal patient position in the recovery phase. In the sitting position, less space is required for a stretcher, and patients are more comfortable immediately after exertion. The supine position increases end-diastolic volume and has the potential to augment ST-segment changes.[33]

TABLE 5–2 TERMS USEFUL IN EVALUATION OF TEST RESULTS

True-positive (TP)	= abnormal test result in individual with disease
False-positive (FP)	= abnormal test result in individual without disease
True-negative (TN)	= normal test result in individual without disease
False-negative (FN)	= normal test result in individual with disease
Sensitivity:	percentage of patients with CAD who have an abnormal test = TP/(TP + FN)
Specificity:	percentage of patients without CAD who have a normal test = TN/(TN + FP)
Predictive value:	percentage of patients with abnormal test who have CAD = TP/(TP + FP)
Predictive value:	percentage of patients with normal test and of normal test without CAD = TN/(TN + FN)
Test accuracy:	percentage of true test results = (TP + TN)/total number tests performed
Likelihood ratio:	odds of a test result being true: of an abnormal test: sensitivity/(1 − specificity); of a normal test: specificity/(1 − sensitivity)
Relative risk:	$\frac{\text{disease rate in persons with a positive test result}}{\text{disease rate in persons with a negative test result}}$

DIAGNOSTIC USE OF EXERCISE TESTING

Appreciation of the exercise test literature requires an understanding of standard terminology such as sensitivity, specificity, and test accuracy (Table 5–2). The literature on the use of diagnostic exercise testing is extensive. The sensitivity of exercise ECG for single-vessel disease ranges from 25 to 71 per cent, with exercise-induced ST segment displacement most frequent in patients with left anterior descending coronary artery disease, followed by those with right coronary artery disease and those with isolated left circumflex coronary disease. An obstruction in an isolated left circumflex coronary artery has the tendency to exaggerate the depth of ST-segment depression when the ECG is abnormal, most likely related to the fact that the ischemic territory underlies the lateral precordial leads. Approximately 75 to 80 per cent of the diagnostic information on exercise-induced ST-segment depression is contained in leads V_4 to V_6. The ability to detect ECG changes in patients with right coronary disease can be augmented by recording lead V_5R.[34]

Gianrossi et al. performed an overview or meta-analysis of 147 consecutive published reports involving 24,074 patients who underwent both coronary angiography and exercise testing.[35] The mean sensitivity was 68 (range 23 to 100) per cent and mean specificity was 77 (range 17 to 100)

TABLE 5–3 NONCORONARY CAUSES OF ST-SEGMENT DEPRESSION

Severe aortic stenosis	Glucose load
Severe hypertension	Left ventricular hypertrophy
Cardiomyopathy	Hyperventilation
Anemia	Mitral valve prolapse
Hypokalemia	Intraventricular conduction disturbance
Severe hypoxia	Preexcitation syndrome
Digitalis	Severe volume overload (aortic, mitral regurgitation)
Sudden excessive exercise	Supraventricular tachyarrhythmias

per cent. In patients with multivessel coronary disease, the mean sensitivity was 81 (range 40 to 100) per cent and mean specificity was 66 (range 17 to 100) per cent.[36] The weighted mean sensitivity was 86 ± 11 per cent and mean specificity was 53 ± 24 per cent for left main or three-vessel coronary disease. The exercise ECG tends to be less sensitive in patients with extensive Q wave anterior wall myocardial infarction and when a limited-exercise ECG lead set is used.[37]

Selective referral of patients with a positive test for further study both decreases the rate of detection of true negative tests and increases the rate of detection of false-positive results, thus increasing sensitivity and decreasing specificity.[38] A positive exercise test cannot be considered false-positive for myocardial ischemia simply because angiography fails to reveal epicardial coronary disease. In patients with normal-appearing coronary arteries but abnormal coronary vasodilator reserve, ischemic ST-segment changes during exercise testing and abnormalities of left ventricular systolic and diastolic function during exercise have been reported (Table 5–3).[39]

SEVERITY OF ELECTROCARDIOGRAPHIC ISCHEMIC RESPONSE. The exercise ECG is more likely to be abnormal in patients with more severe coronary arterial obstruction, more extensive coronary disease, and after more strenuous levels of exercise. Early onset of angina, ischemic ST-segment depression, and fall in blood pressure at low exercise workloads are the most important exercise parameters associated with an adverse prognosis and multivessel coronary artery disease. Additional adverse markers include profound ST-segment displacement, ischemic changes in five or more ECG leads, and persistence of the changes late in the recovery phase of exercise (Table 5–4).

CORRELATION OF EXERCISE TEST RESULTS WITH CORONARY ANGIOGRAPHY. The traditional reference standard against which the exercise ECG has been measured is a qualitative assessment of the coronary angiogram using 50 to 70 per cent obstruction of the luminal diameter as the angiographic cutpoint. There are limitations of the angiographic classification of patients into one-, two-, and three-vessel coronary disease, and the length of the coronary artery narrowing and the impact of serial lesions are not accounted for in correlative studies comparing diagnostic exercise testing with coronary angiographic findings. Other approaches, including intracoronary Doppler flow studies and quantitative coronary angiography, have been proposed to assess coronary vascular reserve which may be more accurate than qualitative assessment of the angiogram.[40,41]

TABLE 5–4 EXERCISE PARAMETERS ASSOCIATED WITH AN ADVERSE PROGNOSIS AND MULTIVESSEL CORONARY ARTERY DISEASE

Duration of symptom-limiting exercise (<6 METs)
Failure to increase systolic blood pressure ≥ 120 mm Hg, or a sustained decrease ≥ 10 mm Hg, or below rest levels, during progressive exercise
ST segment depression ≥ 2 mm, downsloping ST segment, starting at <6 METs, involving ≥ 5 leads, persisting ≥ 5 minutes into recovery
Exercise-induced ST segment elevation (a V_r excluded)
Angina pectoris during exercise
Reproducible sustained (>30 sec) or symptomatic ventricular tachycardia

BAYESIAN THEORY (see also p. 1744). The depth of exercise-induced ST-segment depression and the extent of the myocardial ischemic response can be thought of as continuous variables. Cutpoints such as 1 mm of horizontal or downsloping ST-segment depression as compared with baseline cannot completely discriminate patients with disease from those without disease, and the requirement of more severe degrees of ST-segment depression to improve specificity will decrease sensitivity. Sensitivity and specificity are inversely related, and false-negative and false-positive results are to be expected when ECG or angiographic cutpoints are selected to optimize the diagnostic accuracy of the test.[38]

The use of Bayesian theory incorporates the pretest risk of disease and the sensitivity and specificity of the test (likelihood ratio) to calculate the posttest probability of coronary disease (Fig. 5–11). The results of the patient's clinical information and exercise test results are used to make a final estimate of the probability of coronary disease. The diagnostic power of the exercise test is maximal when the pretest probability of coronary artery disease is inter-

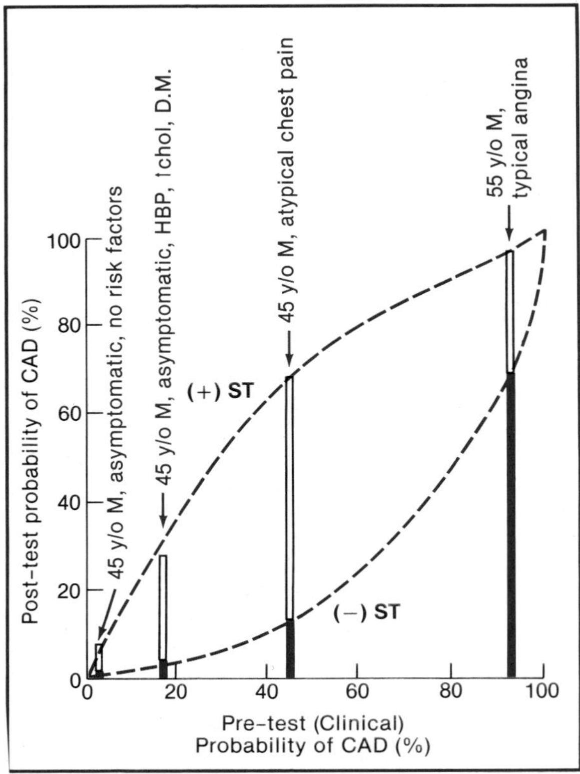

FIGURE 5–11. Use of Bayes theorem to calculate the probability of coronary artery disease (CAD). Four specific patient examples are shown by vertical bars where the height of the solid dark bar illustrates results for a negative exercise electrocardiogram (ECG) (−) ST, and a clear bar shows the results for a positive exercise ECG (+) ST. The posttest probability of coronary disease is optimal in patients with an intermediate coronary disease prevalence. (From Patterson, R. E., and Horowitz, S. F.: Importance of epidemiology and biostatistics in deciding clinical strategies for using diagnostic tests: A simplified approach using examples from coronary artery disease. Reprinted by permission of the American College of Cardiology. J. Am. Coll. Cardiol. *13*:1653, 1989.)

mediate (30 to 70 per cent). Exercise testing to diagnose coronary artery disease in young or middle-aged asymptomatic subjects without atherosclerotic risk factors is not useful, since the pretest risk is very low and a normal or abnormal exercise ECG result does not alter significantly the posttest risk of coronary artery disease[42] (Fig. 5–11).

MULTIVARIATE ANALYSIS. Multivariate analysis of exercise test variables to estimate posttest risk also can provide important diagnostic information. There is some controversy concerning whether to use Bayesian theory or multivariate analysis to estimate final posttest risk. Multivariate analysis offers the potential advantage that it does not require that the tests be independent of each other or that sensitivity and specificity remain constant over a wide range of disease prevalence rates. However, the multivariate technique depends critically on how patients are selected to establish the reference data base. Both Bayesian and multivariate techniques are acceptable.[43]

UPSLOPING SEGMENTS. Junctional or J point depression is a normal finding during maximum exercise, and a rapid upsloping ST segment (>1 mV/sec) depressed <1.5 mm (0.15 mV) after the J point should be considered to be normal. Occasionally, however, the ST segment will be depressed ≥1.5 mm (0.15 mV) at 80 msec after the J point. This type of "slow upsloping" ST segment may be the only ECG finding in patients with well-defined obstructive coronary disease and may depend on the lead set employed (Fig. 5–6). In patient subsets with a high disease prevalence, a slow upsloping ST segment depressed ≥1.5 mm at 80 msec after the J point should be considered to be abnormal. The importance of this finding in asymptomatic subjects or those with a low coronary disease prevalence is less certain. Increasing the degree of ST-segment depression at 80 msec after the J point to ≥2.0 mm (0.20 mV) in patients with a slow upsloping ST segment increases specificity but decreases sensitivity.[44]

ST-SEGMENT ELEVATION. Exercise-induced ST segment elevation in an infarct territory with abnormal Q waves is a marker for more severe left ventricular wall motion abnormalities and an adverse prognosis.[45] This finding occurs in approximately 30 per cent of patients with anterior myocardial infarctions and 15 per cent of those with inferior ones tested early (within 2 weeks) after the index event (Fig. 5–8) and decreases in frequency by 6 weeks. As a group, patients with exercise-induced ST-segment elevation have a lower ejection fraction than those without and greater severity of resting wall motion abnormalities. Exercise-induced ST-segment elevation in leads with abnormal Q waves is *not* a marker of more extensive coronary artery disease and rarely indicates myocardial ischemia. Occasionally, exercise-induced ST-segment elevation may occur in a patient who has regenerated R waves after an acute myocardial infarction; the clinical significance of this finding is similar to that observed when Q waves are present.

When ST-segment elevation develops during exercise in a non-Q wave lead in a patient without a previous myocardial infarction, the finding should be considered as likely evidence of transmural myocardial ischemia caused by coronary vasospasm or a high-grade coronary narrowing (Fig. 5–10). This finding is relatively uncommon, occurring in approximately 1 per cent of patients with obstructive coronary disease. The ECG site of ST-segment elevation is relatively specific for the coronary artery involved, and thallium scintigraphy will usually reveal a defect in the territory involved.

OTHER ELECTROCARDIOGRAPHIC MARKERS. Changes in R wave amplitude during exercise are relatively nonspecific and are related to the level of exercise performed. When the R wave amplitude meets voltage criteria for left ventricular hypertrophy, the ST-segment response *cannot* be used reliably to diagnose coronary disease, even in the absence of a left ventricular strain pattern. Loss of R wave amplitude, commonly seen after myocardial infarction, reduces the sensitivity of the ST-segment response in that lead to diagnose obstructive coronary artery disease. Occasionally, U wave inversion may be seen in the precordial leads at heart rates <120 beats/min. While this finding is relatively specific for coronary artery disease, it is relatively insensitive.[46]

ST/HEART RATE SLOPE MEASUREMENTS. Heart rate adjustment of ST-segment depression appears to improve the sensitivity of the exercise test, particularly the prediction of multivessel coronary disease.[47,48] The ST/heart rate slope depends on the type of exercise performed, number and location of monitoring electrodes, method of measuring ST-segment depression, and clinical characteristics of the study population. Calculation of maximal ST/heart rate slope in mV/beats/min is performed by linear regression analysis relating the measured amount of ST-segment depression in individual leads to the heart rate at the end of each stage of exercise, starting at end exercise. An ST/heart rate slope ≥2.4 mV/beats/min is considered abnormal, and values ≥6 mV/beats/min[47] are suggestive evidence of three-vessel coronary disease.[47] The use of this measurement requires modification of the exercise protocol such that increments in heart rate are gradual, as in the Cornell protocol, as opposed to more abrupt increases in heart rate between stages, as in the Bruce or Ellestad protocols, which limit the ability to calculate statistically valid ST-segment heart rate slopes. The measurement is not accurate in the early postinfarction phase. A modification of the ST-segment/heart rate slope method is the ΔST-segment/heart rate index calculation, which represents the average change of ST-segment depression with heart rate throughout the course of the exercise test. The ΔST/heart rate index measurements are less than the ST/heart rate slope measurements, and a ΔST/heart rate index ≥1.6 is defined as abnormal. The incremental additional prognostic content of ST-segment/heart rate slope measurements as compared with standard criteria is required before these measurements can be widely adopted for prognostic purposes.[49]

NONELECTROCARDIOGRAPHIC OBSERVATIONS

The ECG is only one part of the exercise response, and abnormal hemodynamics or functional capacity is just as important if not more so than ST-segment displacement.

BLOOD PRESSURE. The normal exercise response is to increase systolic blood pressure progressively with increasing workloads to a peak response ranging from 160 to 200 mm Hg, with the higher range of the scale seen in older patients with less compliant vascular systems.[6,10] As a group, black patients tend to have a higher systolic blood pressure response than do whites.[50] At high exercise workloads, it is sometimes difficult to obtain an accurate determination of systolic blood pressure.[51] In normal subjects the diastolic blood pressure does not change significantly, fluctuating ±10 mm Hg as compared with that at rest. Failure to increase systolic blood pressure ≥120 mm Hg, or a sustained decrease ≥10 mm Hg repeatable within 15 seconds, or a fall in systolic blood pressure below standing rest values is abnormal and reflects either inadequate elevation of cardiac output because of left ventricular systolic pump dysfunction or an excessive reduction in systemic vascular resistance.[52] The prevalence of exertional hypotension ranges from 2.7 to 9.3 per cent and is higher in patients with three-vessel or left main coronary disease. The finding of an abnormal systolic blood pressure response in patients with a high prevalence of coronary artery disease is associated with more extensive coronary disease and more extensive thallium defects. Conditions other than myocardial ischemia that have been associated with the failure to increase or an actual decrease in systolic blood pressure during progressive exercise are cardiomyopathy, cardiac arrhythmias, vasovagal reactions, left ventricular outflow tract obstruction, ingestion of antihypertensive drugs, hypovolemia, and prolonged vigorous exercise.[53]

It is important to make the distinction between a decline in blood pressure in the *postexercise* phase and a decrease or failure to increase systolic blood pressure *during* progressive exercise. The incidence of postexertional hypotension in asymptomatic subjects was 1.9 per cent in 781 asymptomatic volunteers in the Baltimore Longitudinal Study on Aging, with a 3.1 per cent incidence noted in subjects younger than age 55 and 0.3 per cent incidence in patients older than age 55.[54] In this series, most hypotensive episodes were symptomatic, and only two patients had hypotension associated with bradycardia and vagal symptoms. Although ST-segment abnormalities suggestive of ischemia occurred in one-third of the patients with hypotension, none of the patients had a cardiac event during 4 years of follow-up. Rarely, in young patients, vasovagal syncope can occur in the immediate postexercise phase, progressing through sinus bradycardia to several seconds of asystole and hypotension before reverting to sinus rhythm.

POSTEXERCISE SYSTOLIC BLOOD PRESSURE RATIOS. In the postexercise phase, there is a progressive decline in systolic and diastolic blood pressure. An abnormal postexercise systolic blood pressure response has been defined as a paradoxical increase in systolic blood pressure within minutes of stopping exercise. Some authors have reported a greater extent of exercise-induced myocardial ischemia, left ventricular dysfunction, and more extensive coronary disease with this finding.[55] Other investigators have not found this response to enhance diagnostic accuracy as compared with exercise-induced ST-segment depression alone.

MAXIMAL WORK CAPACITY. This variable is one of the most important prognostic measurements obtained from an exercise test.[56–60] Maximal work capacity in normal individuals is influenced by familiarization with the exercise test equipment, level of training, and environmental conditions at the time of testing. In patients with known or suspected coronary artery disease, a limited exercise capacity is associated with an increased risk of cardiac events, and in general, the more severe the limitation, the worse the coronary disease extent and prognosis. In estimating functional capacity, the amount of work performed (or exercise stage achieved) should be the parameter measured and not the number of minutes of exercise. Estimates of peak functional capacity for age and gender have been well established for most of the exercise protocols in common usage, subject to the limitations described in the section on cardiopulmonary testing.[61,62] Comparison of an individual's performance against normal standards provides an estimate of the degree of exercise impairment. There is a rough correlation between observed peak functional capacity during exercise treadmill testing and estimates derived from clinical data and specific activity questionnaires.[61]

Serial comparison of functional capacity in individual patients to assess significant interval change requires a careful examination of the exercise protocol used during both tests, of drug therapy and time of ingestion, of systemic blood pressure, and of other conditions that might influence test performance. All these variables need to be considered before attributing changes in functional capacity to progression of coronary artery disease or worsening of left ventricular function. Major reductions in exercise capacity usually indicate significant worsening of cardiovascular status; modest changes may not.

SUBMAXIMAL EXERCISE. The interpretation of an exercise test for diagnostic and prognostic purposes requires consideration of maximum work capacity. When a patient is unable to complete moderate levels of exercise or reach at least 85 to 90 per cent of age-predicted maximum, the level of exercise performed may be inadequate to test cardiac reserve. Thus, ischemic ECG, scintigraphic, or ventriculographic abnormalities may not be evoked and the test may be nondiagnostic.[63] Nondiagnostic tests are more common in patients with peripheral vascular disease, orthopedic limitation, or neurological impairment and in patients with poor motivation.

HEART RATE RESPONSE. The sinus rate increases progressively with exercise, mediated in part through sympathetic and parasympathetic innervation of the sinoatrial node and circulating catecholamines. In some patients who may be anxious about the exercise test, there may be an initial overreaction of heart rate and systolic blood pressure at the beginning of exercise with stabilization after approximately 30 to 60 seconds. Maximum heart rate during exercise is highest in childhood, decreases with age, and is slightly reduced in a trained athlete.

There are two types of abnormal heart rate responses to exercise. In patients with chronotropic incompetence, the heart rate increment per stage of exercise is less than normal and the heart rate may plateau at submaximal workloads.[12] This finding may indicate sinus node disease, may be present with drug therapy such as beta blockers, or may indicate a myocardial ischemic response. The second type of abnormal heart rate response is an inappropriate increase in heart rate of low exercise workloads. This response may occur in patients who are physically deconditioned, hypovolemic, or anemic or who have marginal left ventricular function and may persist for several minutes in the recovery phase.

RATE-PRESSURE PRODUCT. The heart rate–systolic blood pressure product, an indirect measure of myocardial oxygen demand (see p. 1162), increases progressively with exercise, and the peak rate pressure product can be used to characterize cardiovascular performance. Most normal subjects develop a peak rate pressure product of 20 to 35 mm Hg $\times$ beats/min $\times 10^{-3}$. In many patients with significant ischemic heart disease, rate-pressure products exceeding 25 mm Hg $\times$ beats/min $\times 10^{-3}$ are unusual. However, the cutpoint of 25 mm Hg $\times$ beats/min $\times 10^{-3}$ is not a useful diagnostic parameter; significant overlap exists between patients with disease and those without disease. Furthermore, cardioactive drug therapy will significantly influence this measurement.

CHEST DISCOMFORT. Characterization of chest discomfort during exercise can be a useful diagnostic finding, particularly when the symptom complex is compatible with typical angina pectoris. In some patients, the exercise level during the test may exceed that which the patient exhibits in day-to-day activities. Exercise-induced chest discomfort usually occurs after the onset of ischemic ST-segment abnormalities and may be associated with diastolic hypertension.[55,64] However, in some patients, chest discomfort may be the only marker that obstructive coronary artery disease is present. In patients with chronic stable angina, exercise-induced chest discomfort occurs less frequently than ischemic ST-segment depression. The severity of myocardial ischemia in a patient with exercise-induced angina and a normal ECG can often be assessed using thallium scintigraphy. The new development of an S_3 holosystolic apical murmur or basilar rates in the early recovery phase of exercise will enhance the diagnostic accuracy of the test.

EXERCISE TESTING IN DETERMINING PROGNOSIS

ASYMPTOMATIC POPULATION. The prevalence of an abnormal exercise electrocardiogram in middle-aged asymptomatic men ranges from 5 to 12 per cent.[64–69] The risk of developing a cardiac event such as angina, myocardial infarction, or death in men is 9 times greater when the test is abnormal as when it is normal; however, over 5 years of follow-up, only one in four such men will suffer a cardiac event, and this will most commonly be the development of angina. The risk is slightly greater when the test is strongly positive. In the LRC Prevention Trial, a strongly positive test was defined as one in which the ST response was ≥ 2 mm (0.2 mV) or occurred during the first 6 minutes of exercise or at heart rate at or below 163 $-$ 0.66 $\times$ age. Of 3806 middle-aged asymptomatic men who had a total cholesterol ≥ 265 mg/dl at entry, 3 per cent had a strongly positive test; the event rate was 2 per cent per year over an average of 4 years of follow-up.[66] A positive test was *not* significantly associated with nonfatal myocardial infarction; this indicates the difficulty in identifying patients destined to develop abrupt changes in plaque morphology.

In the Seattle Heart Watch, Bruce noted that an abnormal ST response to exercise in asymptomatic men did *not* increase the likelihood of developing cardiac events within 6 years in the absence of conventional risk factors. However, the likelihood of developing a cardiac event was increased when the patient had any conventional atherosclerotic risk factor (see Chap. 35) and two or more abnormal responses to exercise, with an abnormal exercise response defined as chest discomfort during the test, exercise duration <6 minutes or two stages, failure to achieve 90 per cent of age-predicted maximum heart rate, or ≥1 mm (0.1 mV) of horizontal or downsloping ST depression with exercise in early recovery. Only 1.1 per cent of the asymptomatic healthy men in this study were in a high-risk category.[68] The lead set and criteria for an abnormal ECG response were different in both studies. In the Baltimore Longitudinal Study on Aging, Fleg et al. performed maximal treadmill exercise electrocardiography and thallium scintigraphy in 407 asymptomatic volunteers whose mean age was 60 years. The only combination of test results predictive of subsequent cardiac events occurred in the 6 per cent of patients who had *both* an abnormal exercise ECG and thallium scan; 48 per cent had a cardiac event over an average 4-year follow-up.[69]

In asymptomatic middle-aged or older men with several atherosclerotic risk factors, a markedly abnormal exercise response is associated with a significant increased risk of subsequent cardiac events, particularly when there is additional supporting evidence for underlying coronary artery disease (e.g., coronary calcification, abnormal thallium scan, and the like).[69,70] Serial change of a negative exercise ECG to a positive one in an asymptomatic subject carries the same prognostic importance as an initially abnormal test.[71] However, when an asymptomatic subject with an initially abnormal test has significant worsening of the ECG abnormalities at lower exercise workloads, this finding may indicate significant coronary artery disease progression and warrants a more aggressive diagnostic workup.

The prevalence of an abnormal exercise ECG in middle-aged asymptomatic women ranges from 20 to 30 per cent.[6,23] In general, the prognostic value of an ST segment shift in women is less than in men. However, there are few prognostic data on large series of asymptomatic women stratified by age and atherosclerotic risk factors.

SYMPTOMATIC PATIENTS. Exercise testing should be routinely performed (unless this is not feasible or unless there are contraindications) before coronary angiography in patients with chronic ischemic heart disease. Patients who have excellent exercise tolerance (e.g., >10 METs) usually have an excellent prognosis regardless of the anatomical extent of coronary artery disease. The test provides an estimate of the functional significance of angiographically documented coronary artery stenoses. The impact of exercise testing in patients with proven or suspected coronary artery disease was studied by Weiner et al. in 4083 medically treated patients in the CASS study.[72] A high-risk patient subset was identified (12 per cent of the population) with an annual mortality ≥5 per cent a year when exercise workload was <Bruce stage I and the exercise ECG exhibited ≥1 mm (0.1 mV) ST-segment depression. A low-risk patient subset (34 per cent of the population) able to exercise into ≥Bruce stage III who had a normal exercise ECG had an annual mortality <1 per cent per year over 4 years of follow-up. Similar ECG and workload parameters were useful in risk stratifying patients with three-vessel coronary artery disease likely to benefit from coronary bypass grafting.[73]

Mark et al. developed a treadmill score based on 2842 consecutive patients in the Duke data bank with chest pain who had treadmill testing using the Bruce protocol and cardiac catheterization.[74] Patients with left bundle branch block or those with exercise-induced ST elevation in a Q wave lead were excluded. The treadmill score is calculated as follows: exercise time − (5 × ST deviation) − (4 × treadmill angina index). Angina index was assigned a value of 0 if angina was absent, 1 if typical angina occurred during exercise, and 2 if angina was the reason the patient stopped exercising. Exercise-induced ST deviation was defined as the largest net ST displacement in any lead. The 13 per cent of patients with a treadmill score ≤ − 11 had a 5-year survival of 72 per cent compared with 97 per cent in the 34 per cent of patients at low risk with a treadmill score ≥ + 5. The score added independent prognostic information to that provided by clinical data, coronary anatomy, and left ventricular ejection fraction. The stratified annual mortality rates predicted from the treadmill score were less in 613 outpatients referred for exercise testing from the same institution[75] (Fig. 5–12).

Morrow et al. developed a treadmill score based on 2546 male veterans who underwent exercise testing for prognostic purposes and were followed for 2.75 years. The scoring system uses a history of congestive heart failure or digoxin use and three exercise test variables (exercise-induced ST-segment depression, peak exercise capacity, and change in systolic blood pressure). The scoring system identified 77 per cent of patients at low risk (annual cardiac mortality rate <2 per cent), 18 per cent at moderate risk (annual cardiac mortality rate 7 per cent), and 6 per cent at high risk (annual cardiac mortality rate 15 per cent)[76,77] (Fig. 5–13).

Exercise scoring systems can be used to identify prognostic, intermediate–high-risk patients in whom coronary angiography would be indicated to define coronary anatomy. In patients with less extensive coronary disease (e.g., one to two vessels narrowed) and well-preserved left ventricular function, a similar degree of exercise-induced myocardial ischemia does not carry the same significant increased risk of cardiac events as in patients with more extensive disease (e.g., three vessels narrowed) or those with impaired left ventricular function.[60,78–80]

SILENT MYOCARDIAL ISCHEMIA (see p. 1344). In patients with documented coronary artery disease, the presence of exercise-induced ischemic ST-segment depression confers increased risk of subsequent cardiac events regardless of whether angina occurs during the test.[25,81–85] Exercise-induced chest pain tends to lose its apparent value as a clinical predictor when its analysis is restricted to coronary artery disease populations with a greater a priori likelihood of manifesting inducible ischemia.[83] The magnitude of the prognostic gradient in patients with an abnormal exercise ECG with or without angina varies considerably in the published literature, most likely a feature of patient selection.[84,85] In the CASS data bank, 7-year survival in patients with silent or symptomatic exercise-induced myocardial ischemia was similar in patients stratified by coronary anatomy and left ventricular function.[84] In the Asymptomatic Cardiac Ischemia Pilot (ACIP) trial, coronary revascularization was a more effective treatment strategy to reduce exercise-induced myocardial ischemia than medical therapy.[25]

UNSTABLE ANGINA (see p. 1331). The incidence of exercise-induced angina or ischemic ST-segment abnormalities in patients with unstable angina who undergo a predischarge low-level protocol ranges from 30 to 40 per cent. The finding of ischemic ST-segment changes or limiting chest pain is associated with a significantly increased risk of subsequent cardiac events. The *absence* of these findings identifies a low-risk patient subset.[86–88] Exercise testing should be considered in the outpatient evaluation of low-risk patients with unstable angina and should be performed in hospitalized low-to-intermediate-risk ambulatory patients who are free of angina or heart failure symptoms for at least 48 hours.[88]

MYOCARDIAL INFARCTION (see also Ch. 37). A low-level exercise test (achievement of 5 to 6 METs or 70 to 80 per cent of age-predicted maximum) is frequently performed before hospital discharge to establish the hemodynamic re-

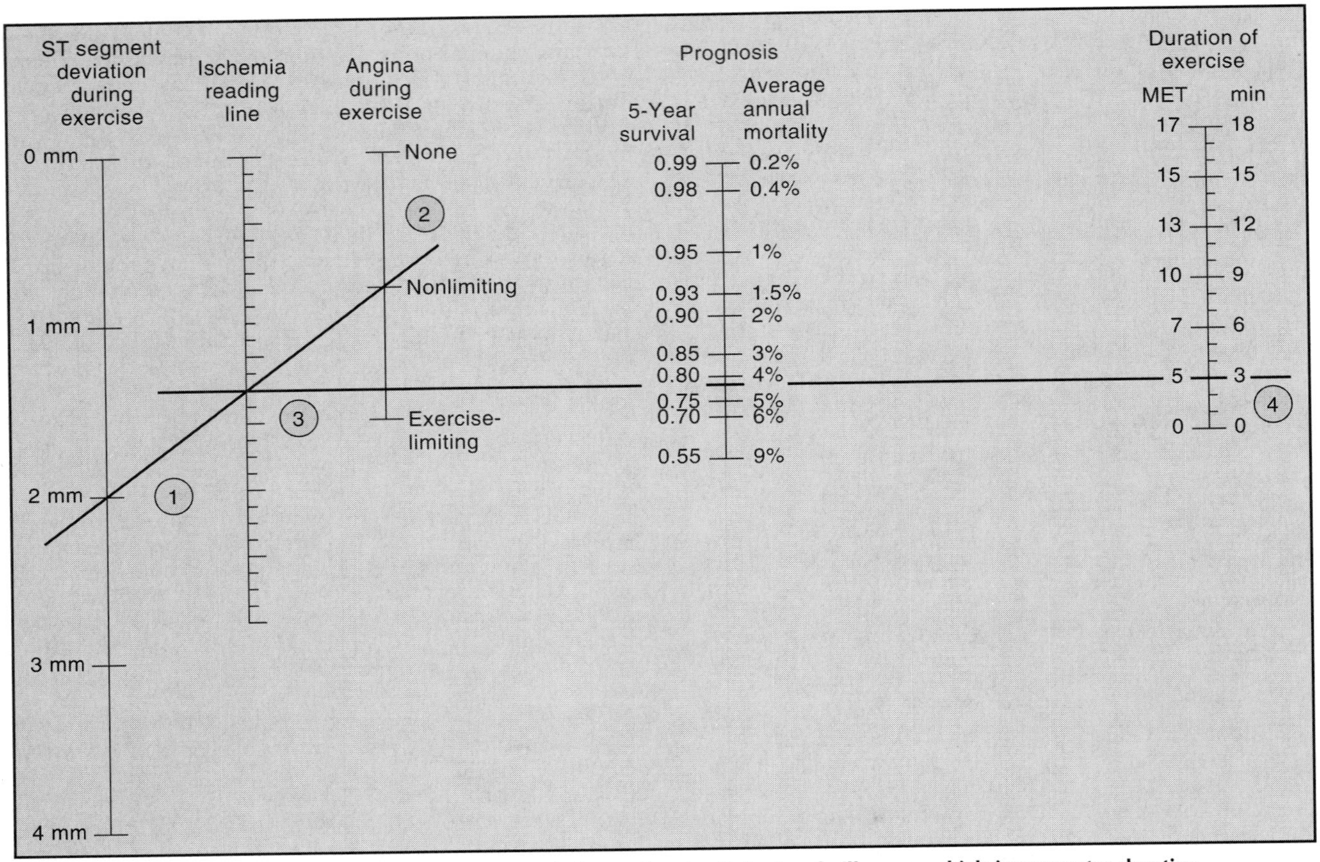

FIGURE 5–12. Nomogram of prognostic relations using the Duke treadmill score, which incorporates duration of exercise (in minutes) − (5 × maximal ST segment deviation during or after exercise) (in mm) − (4 × treadmill angina index). Treadmill angina index is 0 for no angina, 1 for nonlimiting angina, and 2 for exercise limiting angina. The nomogram can be used to assess the prognosis of ambulatory outpatients referred for exercise testing. In this example, the observed amount of exercise-induced ST-segment deviation (minus resting changes) is marked on the line for ST-segment deviation during exercise (1). The degree of angina during exercise is plotted (2), and the points are connected. The point of intersect on the ischemia reading line is noted (3). The number of METs (or minutes of exercise if the Bruce protocol is used) is marked on the exercise duration line (4). The marks on the ischemia reading line and duration of exercise line are connected, and the intersect on the prognosis line determines 5-year survival rate and average annual mortality for patients with these selected specific variables. In this example the 5-year prognosis is estimated at 78 per cent in this patient with exercise-induced 2-mm ST-depression, nonlimiting exercise angina, and peak exercise workload of 5 METs. (Adapted from Mark, D. B., et al.: Prognostic value of a treadmill exercise score in outpatients with suspected coronary artery disease. N. Engl. J. Med. *325*:849, 1991. Copyright Massachusetts Medical Society.)

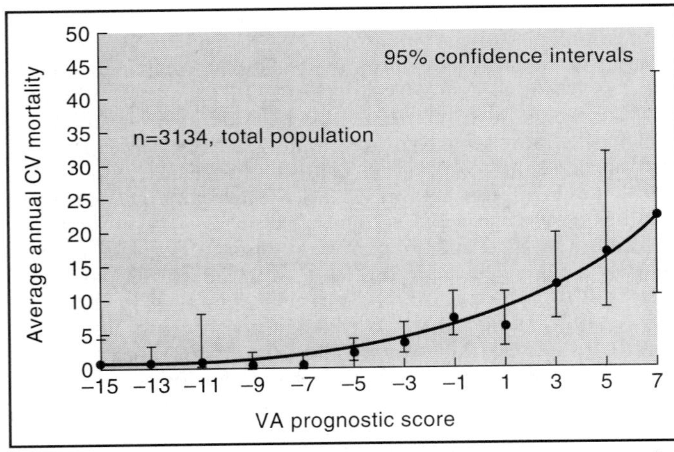

FIGURE 5–13. Plot of average cardiovascular mortality against the Veterans Affairs Prognostic Score including 95 per cent confidence intervals. A score of less than −2 is associated with an annual cardiac mortality rate of less than 2 per cent per year. (Reproduced with permission from Froelicher, V., et al.: Prediction of atherosclerotic cardiovascular death in men using a prognostic score. Am. J. Cardiol. *73*:133, 1994.)

sponse and functional capacity for exercise prescriptions, to identify serious ventricular arrhythmia, and to identify patients at increased risk of cardiac events.[37,89–95] The ability to complete 5 to 6 METs of exercise or 70 to 80 per cent of age-predicted maximum in the absence of abnormal ECG or blood pressure abnormalities is associated with a 1-year mortality of 1 to 2 per cent[6,37,60] (Fig. 5–14). Parameters associated with increased risk include inability to perform the low-level predischarge exercise test, poor exercise capacity, inability to increase or a decrease in exercise systolic blood pressure, and angina or exercise-induced ST-segment depression at low workloads.[37,60,90] The prognostic importance of painless ST-segment depression in postinfarct patients able to complete a low-level predischarge exercise test is less than in patients unable to complete the protocol.[91,93,95] The prognostic importance of exercise-induced ST-segment changes is influenced by the fact that many patients who have an abnormal test undergo coronary angiography and revascularization, which may alter the natural history of the disease process.[56] The performance of a predischarge maximum, symptom-limited test as opposed to a submaximal low-level test is gaining in popularity and is associated with an increased incidence of ischemic ST-segment depression and angina.[89] However, the

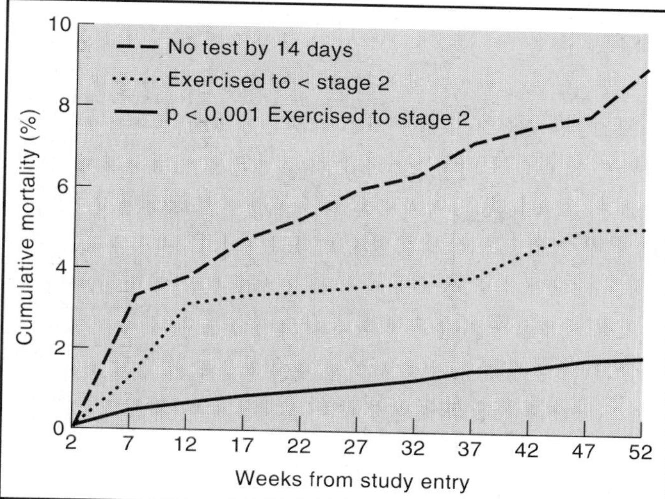

FIGURE 5–14. One-year mortality of patients assigned to the conservative strategy enrolled in the Thrombolysis in Myocardial Infarction (TIMI) II trial. All patients were treated with thrombolytic therapy within 4 hours of symptom onset. Patients unable to perform the exercise test were compared with individuals able to complete 200 kpm (< stage II) or 200 to 400 kpm (stage II) on a supine bicycle ergometry study performed within 2 weeks of the index event. Although the absolute mortality rates are less than patient series studied in the prethrombolytic era, a similar gradient of worsening prognosis is noted in patients unable to perform the low-level exercise test within 2 weeks of the index event, patients able to perform the test but unable to complete the protocol, and patients able to complete the low-level exercise test. (Reproduced with permission from Chaitman, B. R.: Impact of treatment strategy on predischarge exercise test in the Thrombolysis in Myocardial Infarction (TIMI) II trial. Am. J. Cardiol. *71*:131, 1993.)

safety and incremental increase in prognostic information in this approach require further study.

The relative prognostic value of a 6-week postdischarge exercise test is minimal once clinical variables and the results of the low-level predischarge test are adjusted for. For this reason, the timing of the exercise test after the infarct event favors predischarge exercise testing to allow implementation of a definitive treatment plan in patients in whom coronary anatomy is known as well as risk stratification of patients in whom coronary anatomy has not yet been determined.[37,92] A 6-week test is useful in clearing patients to return to work in occupations involving physical labor and to provide a better estimate of cardiovascular reserve at peak exercise performance.

The goals and basic principles of the predischarge evaluation have not been changed by the advent of reperfusion or direct PTCA therapy for acute infarction. The patient's clinical presentation and course during hospitalization are required to determine the indications for testing and to determine prognostic estimates.[37,95–98] After receiving intravenous thrombolytic therapy, uncomplicated myocardial infarct patients tend to exhibit exercise-induced angina and ST-segment depression less frequently than in consecutive postinfarct patients before thrombolysis was widely applied.[37] The indication to perform exercise testing in patients who have undergone coronary angiography or revascularization during hospital admission is to define the patient's functional status as part of the rehabilitation process and detect residual ischemia from incomplete revascularization or reocclusion of the infarct vessel. In the Primary Angioplasty Myocardial Infarct (PAMI) trial, a predischarge modified Bruce test was positive in 9 per cent of patients who received thrombolytic therapy versus 3 per cent of patients who received direct coronary angioplasty.[96]

Left ventricular ejection fraction is one of the most important prognostic determinants of mortality following acute myocardial infarction (see also pp. 1238 and 1260). The additional value of exercise testing in patients with a left ventricular ejection fraction <35 per cent by gated radionuclide scans 1 month after acute myocardial infarction was examined by Pilote et al.[97] Patients with an exercise capacity <4 METs have a 3.5-fold greater risk of dying than patients with an exercise capacity ≥7 METs.

CARDIAC ARRHYTHMIAS AND CONDUCTION DISTURBANCES

The genesis of cardiac arrhythmias includes reentry, delayed afterpotentials, and enhanced automaticity of ectopic foci (Chap. 20). Increased catecholamines during exercise accelerate impulse conduction velocity, shorten the myocardial refractory period, increase the amplitude of delayed afterpotentials, and increase the slope of phase 4 spontaneous depolarization of the action potential. Other potentiators of cardiac rhythm disturbance include metabolic acidosis and exercise-induced myocardial ischemia.[99] Ventricular premature beats occur frequently during exercise testing and increase with age.[100] Repetitive forms occur in 0 to 5 per cent of asymptomatic subjects without suspected cardiac disease and are not associated with an increased risk of cardiac death. Exercise-induced ventricular ectopic activity is not a useful diagnostic marker of ischemic heart disease in the absence of ischemic ST-segment depression. Suppression of ventricular ectopic activity during exercise is a nonspecific finding and may occur in patients with coronary artery disease as well as in normal subjects. The prognostic importance of ventricular arrhythmias in patients with chronic ischemic heart disease after adjustment for baseline, clinical, and left ventricular function characteristics is small.[101] Approximately 20 per cent of patients with known heart disease and 50 to 75 per cent of sudden cardiac death survivors have repetitive ventricular beats induced by exercise. In patients with a recent myocardial infarction, the presence of exercise-induced repetitive forms is associated with an increased risk of subsequent cardiac events.

Exercise-induced ventricular arrhythmias tend to be more frequent in the recovery phase of exercise because peripheral plasma norepinephrine levels continue to increase for several minutes after cessation of exercise and vagal tone is high in the immediate recovery phase. Beta-adrenergic blocking drugs may suppress exercise-induced ventricular arrhythmias. Continuous recording of the exercise test will enhance documentation of the cardiac arrhythmia.

EVALUATION OF VENTRICULAR ARRHYTHMIAS (see also Chap. 22). Exercise testing is useful in the assessment of patients with ventricular arrhythmias and has an important adjunctive role along with ambulatory monitoring and electrophysiological studies. Exercise testing provokes repetitive ventricular premature beats in most patients with a history of sustained ventricular tachyarrhythmia, and in approximately 10 to 15 per cent of such patients, spontaneously occurring arrhythmias are observed only during exercise testing (Fig. 5–15). The test is useful in the evaluation of the effects of antiarrhythmic drugs, the detection of supraventricular arrhythmias, the management of patients with chronic atrial fibrillation, and exposing possible drug toxicity in patients placed on antiarrhythmic drugs. Paradoxical prolongation of the QT_C interval ≥10 msec with exercise identifies patients likely to develop a proarrhythmic effect on type 1A antiarrhythmic drugs.[101] Exercise-induced widening of the QRS complex in patients using type 1C drugs may favor reentry induction of ventricular tachycardia.

SUPRAVENTRICULAR ARRHYTHMIAS. Supraventricular premature beats induced by exercise are observed in 4 to 10 per cent of normal subjects and up to 40 per cent of patients with underlying heart disease. Sustained supraven-

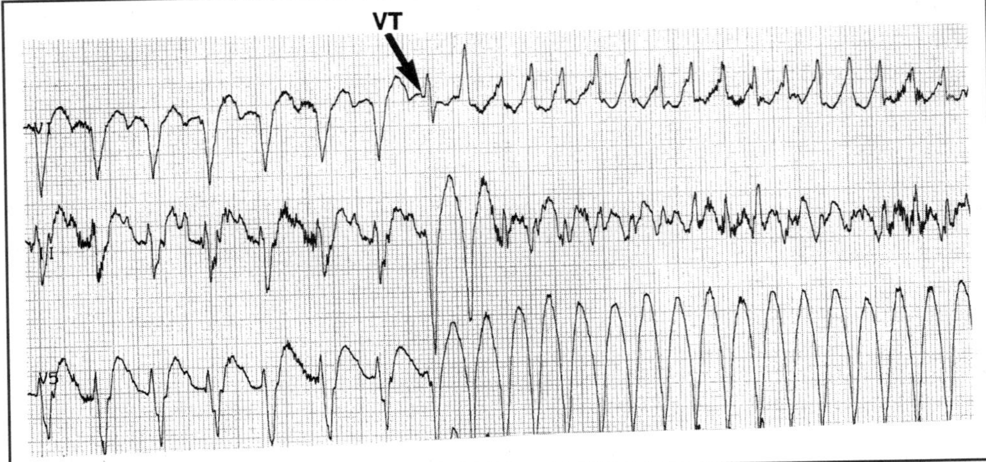

FIGURE 5–15. A 67-year-old man with ischemic cardiomyopathy referred for exercise testing had a left bundle branch block and first-degree AV block on the resting ECG. There was no worsening of the AV conduction disturbance immediately prior to ventricular tachycardia (VT) onset (arrow). At 4:55 minutes into the test, a 27-beat run of VT was noted, reproducing the patient's symptoms of dizziness and chest pounding. The exercise test proved useful in directing subsequent patient management to treatment of the ventricular arrhythmia.

tricular tachyarrhythmias occur in only 1 to 2 per cent of patients, although the frequency may approach as much as 10 to 15 per cent in patients referred for management of episodic supraventricular arrhythmias. The presence of supraventricular arrhythmias is not diagnostic for ischemic heart disease.

ATRIAL FIBRILLATION (see p. 654). Patients with chronic atrial fibrillation tend to have a rapid ventricular response in the initial stages of exercise and 60 to 70 per cent of the total change in heart rate usually occurs within the first few minutes of exercise (Fig. 5–16). The effect of digitalis preparations and beta-adrenergic and calcium antagonists on attenuating this rapid increase in heart rate for individual patients can be measured using exercise testing. Pharmacological control of the ventricular rate does not necessarily result in a significant increase in exercise capacity, which in many patients is related to the underlying cardiac disease process and not adequacy of control of the ventricular rate.

SICK SINUS SYNDROME (see p. 648). In general, patients with sick sinus syndrome have a lower heart rate at submaximal and maximal workloads compared with control subjects. However, as many as 40 to 50 per cent of patients will have a normal exercise heart rate response.

AV BLOCK. Exercise testing may help determine the need for AV sequential pacing in selected patients. In patients with congenital AV block, exercise-induced heart rates are low and some patients develop symptomatic rapid junctional rhythms which can be suppressed with DDD devices. In patients with acquired conduction disease, exercise can occasionally bring out advanced AV block.

LEFT BUNDLE BRANCH BLOCK (LBBB) (see also p. 119). Exercise-induced ST-segment depression is seen in most patients with LBBB and cannot be used as a diagnostic or prognostic indicator regardless of the degree of ST-segment abnormality. In patients referred to a tertiary center in whom exercise testing is carried out, the new development of exercise-induced transient left hemiblock is 0.3 per cent and left bundle branch block is 0.4 per cent, with a slightly greater incidence in older patients.[102] The development of ischemic ST-segment depression before the LBBB pattern appears or in the recovery phase after the LBBB has resolved does not attenuate the diagnostic yield of the ST-segment shift. The ventricular rate at which the LBBB appears and disappears can be significantly different (Fig. 5–17). In one series, permanent LBBB was reported in approximately half the patients who developed transient LBBB during exercise and who were followed for an average 6.6 years. High-grade AV block did not develop in any of the patients in this 15-patient series.[103]

RIGHT BUNDLE BRANCH BLOCK (RBBB). The resting ECG in RBBB is frequently associated with T wave and ST segment changes in the early anterior precordial leads (V_1 to V_3). Exercise-induced ST depression in leads V_1 to V_4 is a com-

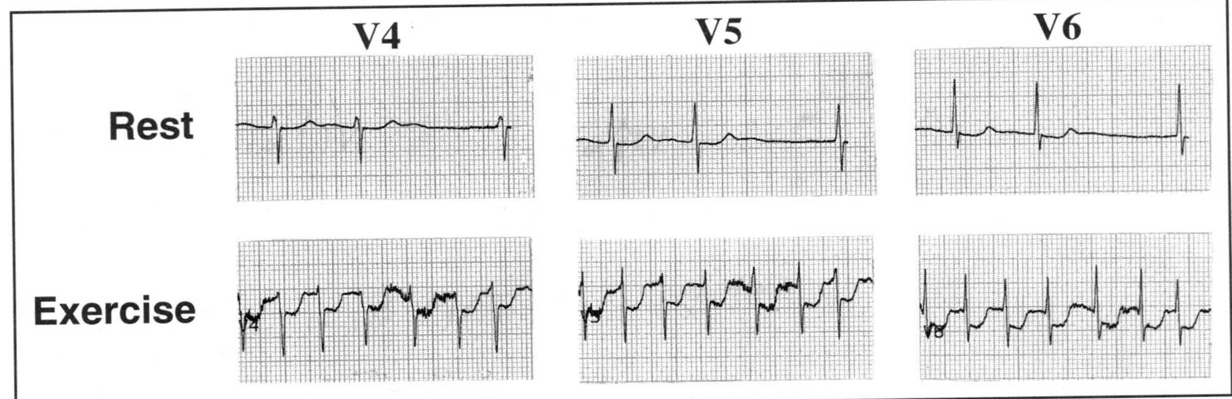

FIGURE 5–16. A 75-year-old woman with chronic atrial fibrillation and a 6-month history of atypical chest pain underwent mitral valve repair 1 year before testing, at which time nonobstructive coronary disease was noted. The patient exercised for 6 minutes, achieving a peak heart rate of 176 beats/min and peak blood pressure of 170/90 mm Hg. The resting ECG shows atrial fibrillation with a controlled ventricular response and minor ST-segment depression. At peak exertion, marked ST-segment depression is seen in the anterior leads, consistent with either digitalis effect or myocardial ischemia. In this type of patient, initial exercise testing with myocardial perfusion tracers or echocardiography would provide more useful diagnostic information than exercise testing alone.

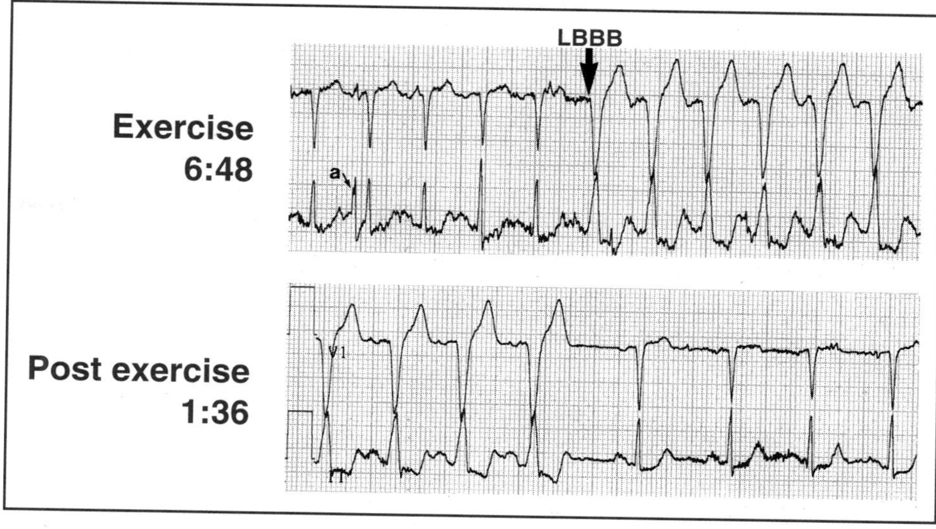

FIGURE 5–17. A 58-year-old hypertensive diabetic man with prior history of cigarette smoking was referred for evaluation of dyspnea and early fatigability during exercise. At 6:48 min into the test the patient developed a rate-related left bundle branch block (LBBB) at a heart rate of 133 beats/min which persisted during exercise and resolved at 1:36 min into the postexercise phase. The test was stopped because of dyspnea at a peak heart rate of 138 beats/min (85 per cent of predicted) and estimated workload of 6 METs. Peak blood pressure at end exercise was 174/94 mm Hg. Time to onset and offset of LBBB occurred at different ventricular rates related to fatigue in the left bundle, a common finding.

mon finding in patients with RBBB and is nondiagnostic. The new development of exercise-induced ST-segment depression in leads V_5 and V_6, reduced exercise capacity, and inability to adequately increase systolic blood pressure are useful in detecting patients with coronary artery disease who have a high clinical pretest risk of disease. The presence of RBBB decreases the sensitivity of the test.[104] The new development of exercise-induced RBBB is relatively uncommon, occurring in approximately 0.1 per cent of tests.

PREEXCITATION SYNDROME (see p. 693). The presence of WPW syndrome invalidates the use of ST-segment analysis as a diagnostic method for detecting coronary artery disease in preexcited as well as normally conducted beats; false-positive ischemic changes are frequently registered (Fig. 5–18). In patients with persistent preexcitation, exercise may normalize the QRS complex with disappearance of the delta wave in 20 to 50 per cent of cases dependent on the series studied.[105] Abrupt disappearance of the delta wave is presumptive evidence of a longer anterograde effective refractory period of the accessory pathway. Progressive disappearance of the delta wave is less reassuring and occurs when the improvement in AV node conduction is greater than in the accessory pathway; this finding does not exclude a possible significant or even critical shortening of the anterograde effective refractory period in the accessory pathway under the influence of sympathetic stimulation. Exercise-induced disappearance of the delta wave is more frequent with type A than type B WPW patterns. Although tachyarrhythmias appearing during an exercise test in patients with WPW are rare, when they do occur, they provide an opportunity to evaluate AV conduction velocity. The presence of WPW does not cause a limitation of physical work capacity.

SPECIFIC CLINICAL APPLICATIONS

WOMEN (see also Chap. 51). The specificity of exercise-induced ST-segment depression for obstructive coronary artery disease is less in women than in men. The decreased diagnostic accuracy results in part from a lower prevalence and extent of coronary artery disease in young and middle-aged women.[106] Women tend to have a greater release of catecholamines during exercise, which could potentiate coronary vasoconstriction and augment the incidence of abnormal exercise ECGs, and false-positive tests have been reported to be more common during menses or preovulation.[107]

The increased false-positive rate in women may potentiate gender differences in the use of follow-up diagnostic testing in women who have an initially abnormal noninvasive stress test result. In an 840-patient series evaluated for clinically suspect coronary disease using noninvasive tests, 62 per cent of women compared with only 38 per cent of men with an initial abnormal test result did not go on for additional diagnostic testing, even though the rates of initial abnormal test results were similar in both[108] (Fig. 5–19). Additional research to determine optimal diagnostic and prognostic algorithms for women is needed.[109]

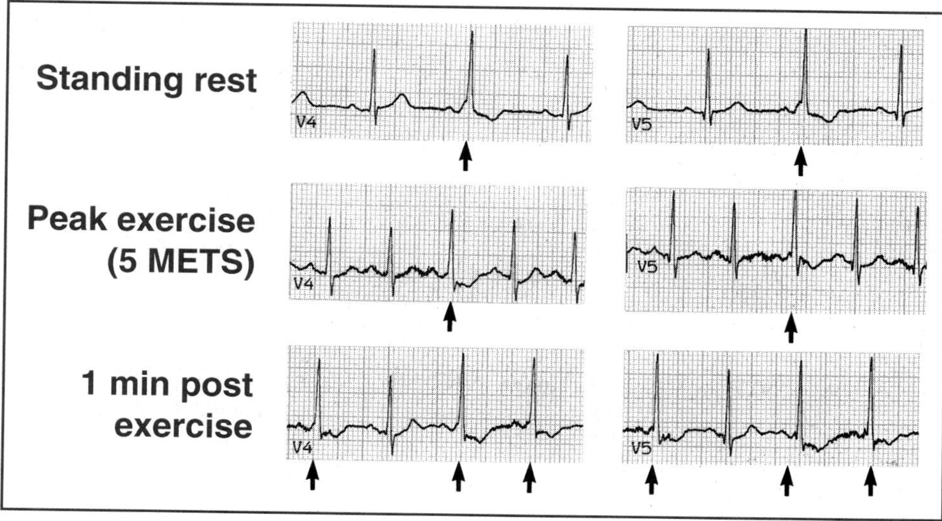

FIGURE 5–18. A 61-year-old man with atypical angina and a hiatal hernia was referred for diagnostic exercise testing. The test was stopped because of dyspnea. The standing rest ECG shows an intermittent WPW pattern (arrows). In the non-preexcited beats, ST-segment depression does not occur either at peak exercise or in the postexercise phase. However, in the preexcited beats (arrows) an additional 1.3 mm of downsloping ST-segment depression is noted as compared with baseline during and after exertion.

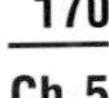

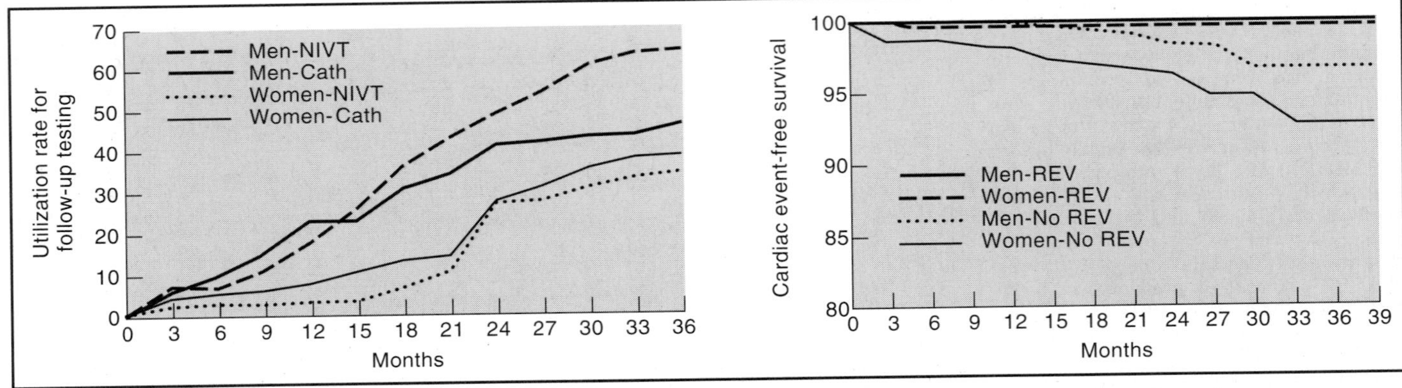

FIGURE 5–19. *Left panel,* A gender-based comparison of noninvasive test use rates over time. A greater percentage of men with initially abnormal test results received follow-up noninvasive testing (NIVT) compared with women ($p < 0.001$). Similarly, a comparison of use of coronary arteriography during the 2-year follow-up period showed that a greater percentage of men than women subsequently had catheterization (cath) ($p < 0.001$). *Right panel,* Cardiac events by gender. Patients who were revascularized (REV) had better cardiac event–free survival ($p < 0.001$). In patients with REV, cardiac events were more frequent in women. (From Shaw, L. J., et al.: Gender differences in the noninvasive evaluation and management of patients with suspected coronary artery disease. Ann. Intern. Med. *120*:559, 1994.)

HYPERTENSION. Exercise testing has been used in an attempt to identify patients with abnormal blood pressure response destined to subsequently develop hypertension. The optimal exercise protocol, and consensus on what constitutes an abnormal exercise response, requires additional study.[9] Different criteria may be required for blacks and whites, men and women, and younger versus older patients.[50] Severe systemic hypertension may interfere with subendocardial perfusion and cause exercise-induced ST-segment depression in the absence of atherosclerosis, even when the rest ECG does not show significant ST- or T-wave changes.[110] Beta and calcium channel blocking drugs decrease submaximal and peak systolic blood pressure in many hypertensive patients.

CONGESTIVE HEART FAILURE. Cardiac and peripheral compensatory mechanisms are activated in patients with chronic congestive heart failure to partly or fully restore impaired left ventricular performance.[108–112] There is a wide range of exercise capacity in patients who have a markedly reduced ejection fraction, with some patients having near-normal peak exercise capacity.[14] Symptoms in patients with congestive heart failure are related to an excessive increase in blood lactate during low exercise levels, reduction in quantity of oxygen consumed at peak exertion, and disproportionate increase in ventilation at submaximal and peak workloads. The increased ventilatory requirement assessed by the hyperventilatory response to exercise and increase in pulmonary dead space leads to rapid and shallow breathing during exercise. Fatigue may be related to altered skeletal muscle metabolism secondary to chronic physical deconditioning as well as impaired perfusion.[116] Dyspnea and fatigue are the usual reasons for exercise termination. Peak $\dot{V}_{O_2}$ measurements in patients with compensated congestive heart failure are useful in risk stratifying patients with congestive heart failure to determine subsequent incidence of cardiac events (Fig. 5–20). The ability to achieve a peak $\dot{V}_{O_2}$ of >20 ml/min/kg and AT_{ge} > 14 ml/min/kg is associated with a relatively good long-term prognosis and a maximum cardiac output >8 liters/min/m². Patients who are unable to achieve a peak $\dot{V}_{O_2}$ of 10 ml/min/kg and AT_{ge} of 8 ml/min/kg have a poor prognosis, and their maximum exercise cardiac output is usually <4 liters/min/m². Failure of $\dot{V}_{O_2}$ to decrease within 30 sec after peak exertion is associated with more severe reductions in left ventricular ejection fraction and moderate to severe impairment of pulmonary gas exchange. Inability to increase oxygen pulse is related to lack or minimal increase of stroke volume. A blunted heart rate response is not uncommon in patients with congestive heart failure caused by postsynaptic desensitization of beta-adrenergic receptors[12,111] (see p. 411).

Exercise protocols that limit exercise duration to 5 to 7 minutes are associated with the most reproducible peak $\dot{V}_{O_2}$ measurements in patients with heart failure. The interpretation of cardiopulmonary exercise tests in patients with heart failure can occasionally be difficult, because some patients hyperventilate during exercise, producing falsely low peak oxygen consumption, and it can be difficult to distinguish patients who are deconditioned from those who have impaired exercise performance and low peak $\dot{V}_{O_2}$ due to cardiac pathology. A 6-minute walk test also can be used to evaluate functional capacity in patients unable to exercise on a bicycle ergometer or treadmill.[27]

DRUGS. Digitalis glycosides can produce exertional ST segment depression even if the effect is not evident on the resting ECG and can accentuate ischemic exercise-induced ST segment changes (see p. 500). Absence of ST-segment deviation during an exercise test in a patient receiving a cardiac glycoside is considered a valid negative response. Hypokalemia in patients on long-term diuretic therapy may be associated with exercise-induced ST-segment depression. Antiischemic drug therapy with nitrates, beta-blocking drugs, or calcium channel blocking drugs will prolong the time to onset of ischemic ST-segment depression, increase exercise tolerance, and, in a small minority of patients (10 to 15 per cent), may normalize the exercise ECG response in patients with documented coronary artery disease.[6,23,25,117] The time and dose of drug ingestion may affect exercise performance. In some laboratories, cardioactive drug therapy is withheld for 3 to 5 half-lives and digitalis for 1 to 2 weeks before diagnostic testing. However, this is impractical in many cases. Heparin therapy may increase total exercise duration and ability to achieve a higher rate pressure product before the onset of angina, and at peak exertion.[118] The onset of ischemic ST-segment depression in patients with chronic ischemic heart disease occurs earlier in patients who are cold sensitive and who are exposed to low levels of carbon monoxide.[119,120] Amiodarone therapy increases the QRS duration during exercise by approximately 6 per cent in patients with a QRS duration <110 msec compared with 15 per cent in patients with a QRS duration >110 msec.[121]

CORONARY REVASCULARIZATION PROCEDURES. The degree of improvement in exercise-induced myocardial ischemia and aerobic capacity after coronary bypass grafting depends in part on the degree of revascularization achieved and left ventricular function.[25,59] Exercise-induced ischemic ST-seg-

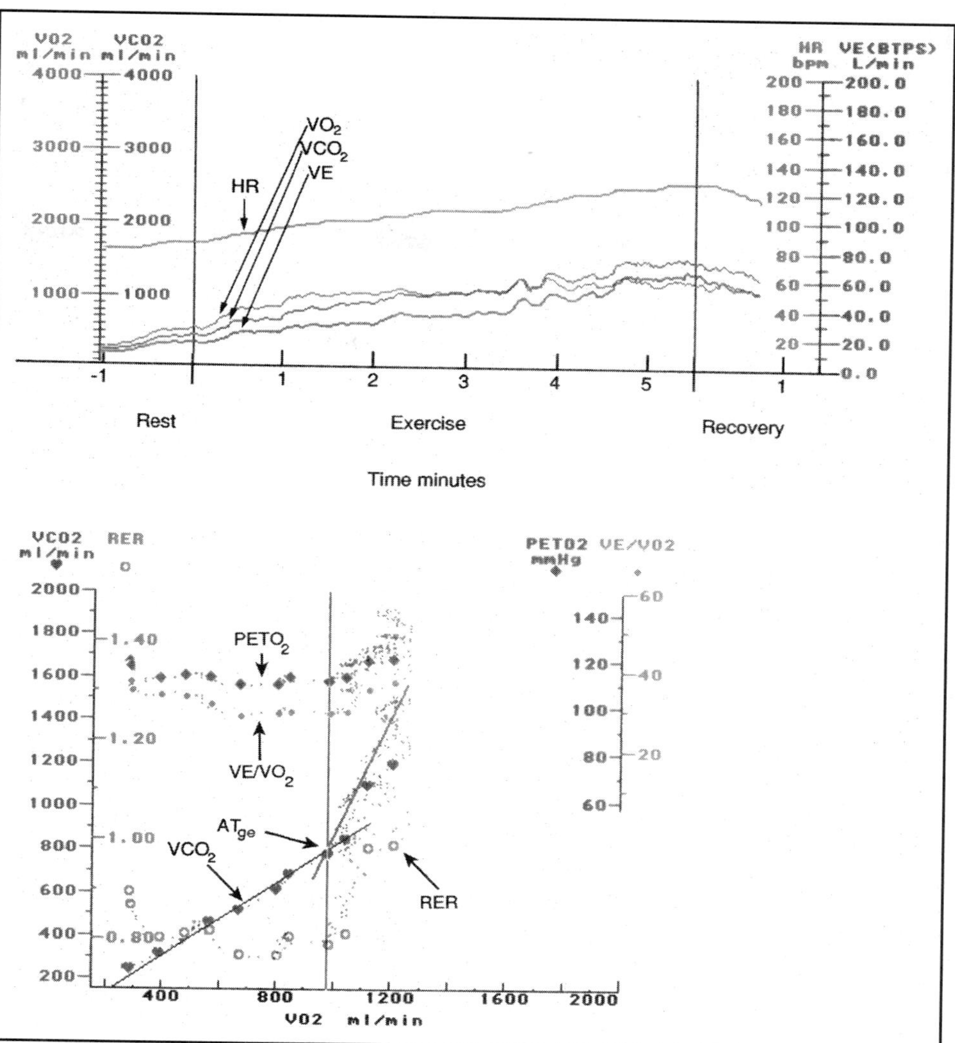

FIGURE 5–20. Cardiopulmonary exercise test in a 51-year-old man with cardiomyopathy in NYHA class III. A modified Bruce protocol was used. The patient reached a peak $\dot{V}_{O_2}$ of 14 ml/min/kg (4 METs), 44 per cent of predicted for age, size, and weight *(top panel)*. Anaerobic threshold (AT_{ge}) occurred at a $\dot{V}_{O_2}$ of 977 ml/min *(bottom panel)*. The blunted cardiopulmonary response is typical for a patient with severe cardiomyopathy and marked impairment of cardiac reserve. This patient was listed for cardiac transplantation.

ment depression may persist when incomplete revascularization is achieved, albeit at higher exercise workloads, and in approximately 5 per cent of patients in whom complete revascularization has been achieved.[122–124] It usually takes at least 6 weeks of convalescence before maximum exercise can be performed. The natural history of saphenous vein grafts and internal mammary artery conduits is different, and serial conversion from an initially normal to abnormal exercise ECG over time will depend in part on the type of conduit used and coronary disease progression in nongrafted vessels. The diagnostic and prognostic utility of exercise testing late after coronary revascularization (e.g., 5 to 10 years) is much greater than early (<1 year) testing, since a late abnormal exercise response is more likely to indicate graft occlusion, stenosis, or progression of coronary artery disease.

After coronary angioplasty (PTCA), restenosis occurs in approximately 20 to 40 per cent of patients, usually within the first 6 months, and is more common in patients with proximal LAD disease, long coronary artery narrowings, diabetic patients, patients with multivessel or multilesion dilation, and those in whom post PTCA luminal obstruction is >50 per cent. In the early post-PTCA phase (<1 month) an abnormal exercise ECG may be secondary to a suboptimal PTCA result, impaired coronary vascular reserve in a successfully dilated vessel, or incomplete revascularization.[125] The optimal time to perform an exercise test following PTCA depends in part on the success of the procedure and the degree of revascularization obtained. Exercise testing early after PTCA (within days) often can be used to help determine the need for a staged procedure and to provide a reference baseline for subsequent follow-up. In an otherwise asymptomatic patient, a 6-month postprocedure test allows a sufficient amount of time to document restenosis should it occur and allows the dilated vessel an opportunity to heal. In the absence of significant epicardial stenosis after PTCA, exercise-induced ST-segment depression may be associated with the presence of preprocedure regional left ventricular dysfunction that has recovered during follow-up.[126] Serial conversion of an initially normal exercise test post PTCA to an abnormal test in the initial 6 months after the procedure, particularly when it occurs at a lower exercise workload, is usually associated with restenosis. The use of thallium scintigraphy in selected patients enhances greatly the diagnostic content of the test and can help localize the territory of myocardial ischemia and guide indications for repeat coronary angiography in patients who have undergone multivessel/multilesion PTCA.

CARDIAC TRANSPLANTATION (see also Chap. 18). Cardiopulmonary exercise testing is useful in selecting patients with end-stage heart failure for cardiac transplantation. A peak oxygen uptake of less than 12 to 14 ml/kg/min or 40 to 50 per cent of predicted $\dot{V}_{O_2}$ is associated with 2-year survival rates of approximately 32 per cent. In patients awaiting heart transplantation, with initial poor exercise capacity, ability to increase peak oxygen uptake with increased peak oxygen pulse identifies a relatively lower-risk group in whom cardiac transplantation may be able to be deferred if the patient's clinical status is stable (Fig. 5–21).[129] Exercise performance in post-transplant recipients is influenced by the fact that the donor heart is surgically denervated without efferent parasympathetic or sympa-

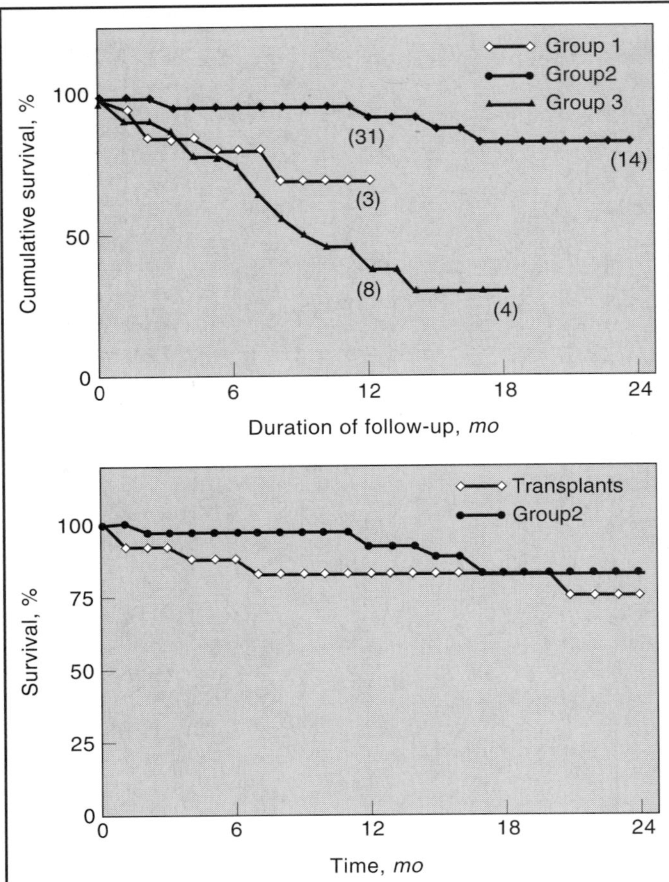

FIGURE 5–21. Cardiopulmonary exercise testing enhances the selection process for congestive heart failure patients considered for cardiac transplantation. The 2-year survival of 122 patients with an average ejection fraction of 19 per cent considered for heart transplantation was analyzed according to peak oxygen uptake ($\dot{V}_{O_2}$) and ability to reach anaerobic threshold *(top panel).* The survival of 35 patients accepted for cardiac transplantation with a peak $\dot{V}_{O_2}$ of 14 ml/kg/min or less (group 1) is compared with that of 52 patients for whom transplantation was considered unnecessary because of a peak $\dot{V}_{O_2} > 14$ ml/kg/min (group 2) and 27 patients with a peak $\dot{V}_{O_2}$ of 14 ml/kg/min or less rejected for transplantation because of noncardiac problems (group 3). *Bottom panel:* Group 2 patients had cumulative 1- to 2-year survival rates of 94 and 84 per cent, respectively, similar to survival levels after transplantation. Group 3 patients (not shown) had survival rates of only 47 and 32 per cent at 1 and 2 years, respectively. The data indicate that cardiac transplantation can be deferred safely in ambulatory patients with moderate-to-severe left ventricular dysfunction and a peak $\dot{V}_{O_2}$ of > 14 ml/kg/min. (Adapted with permission from Mancini, D. M.: Value of peak exercise oxygen consumption for optimal timing of cardiac transplantation in ambulatory patients with heart failure. Circulation *83:*778, 1991. Copyright 1991 American Heart Association.)

thetic innervation and by the occurrence of rejection and scar formation, donor-recipient size mismatch, systemic and pulmonary vascular resistance, and development of coronary atherosclerosis in the graft.[127,128] Maximum oxygen uptake and work capacity are reduced after cardiac transplantation compared with age-matched controls but are usually markedly improved compared with preoperative findings. Abnormalities of the ventricular rate response include a resting tachycardia due to parasympathetic denervation, a slow heart rate response during mild-to-moderate exercise, a more rapid response during more strenuous exercise, and a more prolonged time for the ventricular rate to return to baseline during recovery. The transplanted heart relies heavily on the Frank-Starling mechanism to increase cardiac output during mild-to-moderate exercise. Systemic vascular resistance may be increased because of cyclosporine therapy. The exercise electrocardiogram is relatively insensitive to detect coronary artery vasculopathy after cardiac transplantation.[130,131] However, the new development of an abnormal exercise ECG several years following cardiac transplantation may indicate focal intraluminal narrowing.

VALVULAR HEART DISEASE (see also Chap. 32). The hemodynamics of exercise provide an excellent opportunity to measure gradients across stenotic valves, to assess ventricular function in patients with primary valvular regurgitation or mixed lesions, and to assess pulmonary and systemic vascular resistance. The use of echocardiographic Doppler techniques is particularly valuable in evaluating patients whose symptoms are out of proportion to the degree of valvular disease observed and in assessing the results of valvulotomy or valve replacement.[132] Clinical and exercise noninvasive assessment of patients with valvular heart disease can provide very useful information on the timing of operative intervention and help achieve a more precise estimate of a patient's degree of incapacitation than can assessment of symptoms alone.[133]

CARDIAC PACEMAKERS (see also Chap. 23). The exercise protocol used to assess chronotropic responsiveness in patients before and after cardiac pacemaker insertion should adjust for the fact that many such patients are older individuals and may not tolerate high exercise workloads or abrupt and relatively large increments in work between stages of exercise. An optimal physiological cardiac pacemaker should normalize the heart rate response to exercise in proportion to oxygen uptake and increase heart rate 2 to 4 beats/min for an increase in $\dot{V}_{O_2}$ of 1 ml/min/kg, with a slightly steeper slope for patients with severe left ventricular function impairment.[134,135]

ELDERLY PATIENTS (see also Chap. 50). The exercise protocol in elderly patients should be selected according to estimated aerobic capacity. In patients with limited exercise tolerance, the test should be started at the slowest speed with a 0 per cent grade and adjusted according to the patient's ability. Older patients may need to grasp the handrails for support. Limited exercise tolerance is to be expected in many persons ≥ 80 years old. The frequency of abnormal exercise ECG patterns is greater in older than younger individuals, and the risk of cardiac events is significantly increased because of a concomitant increase in prevalence of more extensive coronary disease.[136,137]

Termination of Exercise

The use of standard test indications to terminate an exercise test will reduce risk (Table 5–5). Termination of exercise should be determined in part by the patient's recent activity level. The rate of perceived patient exertion can be estimated by the Borg scale (Table 40–2, p. 1396).[138] The

TABLE 5–5 INDICATIONS FOR TERMINATING EXERCISE TEST

Severe fatigue or dyspnea
Ataxia
Grade III/IV chest pain
Ischemic ST-segment depression ≥ 3.0 mm
Ischemic ST-segment elevation ≥ 1 mm in a non-Q wave lead
Unsuspected appearance of ventricular tachycardia
Ectopic supraventricular tachycardia
Progressive reproducible decrease in systolic blood pressure
Abnormal elevation of systolic blood pressure
Decreasing heart rate
Technical problems interfering with ECG or blood pressure interpretation

scale is linear with values of 7, very, very light; 9, very light; 11, fairly light; 13, somewhat hard; 15, hard; 17, very hard; and 19, very, very hard. Borg readings of 14 to 16 approximate anaerobic threshold, and readings ≥18 approximate a patient's maximum exercise capacity. Ataxia may indicate cerebral hypoxia. It is helpful to grade exercise-induced chest discomfort on a 1 to 4 scale, with 1 indicating the initial onset of chest discomfort and 4 the most severe chest pain the patient has ever experienced. The exercise technician should note the onset of grade 1 chest discomfort on the worksheet, and the test should be stopped when the patient reports grade 3 chest pain. In the absence of symptoms, it is prudent to stop exercise when a patient demonstrates ≥3 mm (0.3 mV) of ischemic ST-segment depression or ≥1 mm (0.1 mv) of ST-segment elevation in a lead without an abnormal Q wave. Significant worsening of ambient ventricular ectopy during exercise or the unsuspected appearance of ventricular tachycardia is an indication to terminate exercise. A progressive, reproducible decrease in systolic blood pressure of 10 mm Hg or more may indicate transient left ventricular dysfunction or an inappropriate decrease in systemic vascular resistance and is an indication to terminate exercise. The test should be stopped if the arterial blood pressure is ≥250 to 270/120–130 mm Hg.

A resuscitory cart and defibrillator should be available in the room where the test procedure is carried out and appropriate cardioactive medication available to treat cardiac arrhythmias, atrioventricular block, hypotension, and persistent chest pain. An intravenous line should be started in high-risk patients such as those being tested for adequacy of control of life-threatening ventricular arrhythmias. The equipment and supplies in the cart should be checked on a regular basis. A previously specified routine for cardiac emergencies needs to be determined which includes patient transfer and admission to a coronary care unit if necessary.

Clinical judgment is required to determine which patients can be tested safely in an office as opposed to a hospital-based setting. High-risk patients, such as those with evident left ventricular dysfunction, severe angina pectoris, history of cardiac syncope, and significant ambient ventricular ectopy on the pretest examination, should be tested in the hospital. Low-risk patients, such as asymptomatic subjects and those with a low pretest risk of disease, may be tested by specially trained nurses or physician assistants who have received ACLS certification, *with a physician in close proximity*.[139]

The exercise test report should contain basic demographic data, the indication for testing, a brief description of the patient profile, and exercise test results (Table 5–6).

TABLE 5–6 EXERCISE TEST REPORT INFORMATION

1. Demographic data: name, patient identifier, date of birth/age, gender, weight, height, test date
2. Indication(s) for test
3. Patient descriptors: atherosclerotic risk profile, drug usage, resting ECG findings
4. Exercise test results
   a. Protocol used
   b. Reason(s) for stopping exercise
   c. Hemodynamic data: rest and peak heart rate, rest and peak blood pressure, per cent maximum achieved heart rate, maximum rate of perceived exertion (Borg scale), peak workload, peak METs, total exercise duration in minutes
   d. Evidence for myocardial ischemia: time to onset and offset of ischemic ST-segment deviation or angina, maximum depth of ST-segment deviation, number of abnormal exercise ECG leads, abnormal systemic blood pressure response
5. General comments

TABLE 5–7 CONTRAINDICATIONS TO EXERCISE TESTING

- Unstable angina with recent rest pain
- Untreated life-threatening cardiac arrhythmias
- Uncompensated congestive heart failure
- Advanced atrioventricular block
- Acute myocarditis or pericarditis
- Critical aortic stenosis
- Severe hypertrophic obstructive cardiomyopathy
- Uncontrolled hypertension
- Acute systemic illness

Safety and Risks of Exercise Testing

Exercise testing has an excellent safety record. The risk is determined by the clinical characteristics of the patient referred for the procedure. In nonselected patient populations, the mortality is <0.01 per cent and morbidity <0.05 per cent.[140] The risk is greater when the test is performed soon after an acute ischemic event. In a survey of 151,941 tests conducted within 4 weeks of an acute myocardial infarction, mortality was 0.03 per cent, and 0.09 per cent of patients had either a nonfatal reinfarction or were resuscitated from cardiac arrest.[141] The relative risk of a major complication is about twice as great when a symptom-limited protocol is used as compared with a low-level protocol. Nevertheless, in the early postinfarction phase, the risk of a fatal complication during symptom-limited testing is only 0.03 per cent. The use of exercise testing as a screening procedure for low-risk patients who present to the emergency room with atypical angina or typical angina who have a normal ECG or minimal ST- and T-segment abnormalities at rest needs to be evaluated further in larger patient series. In a study of 93 patients who had a negative initial total CK and were considered clinically low risk, no complications of exercise testing were observed as a result of early exercise testing.[142] Exercise testing can be performed safely in patients with compensated congestive heart failure, with no major complications reported in 1286 tests in which a bicycle ergometer was used.[143] The risk of exercise testing in patients referred for life-threatening ventricular arrhythmias was examined by Young et al.[144] in a series of 263 patients who underwent 1377 tests; 2.2 per cent developed sustained ventricular tachyarrhythmias that required cardioversion, cardiopulmonary resuscitation, or antiarrhythmic drugs to restore sinus rhythm. The ventricular arrhythmias were more frequent in tests performed on antiarrhythmic drug therapy as compared with the baseline drug-free state.[144] In contrast to the high risk in the aforementioned patient subsets, the risk of complications in asymptomatic subjects is extremely low, with no fatalities reported in several series.[66,139]

The risk of incurring a major complication during exercise testing can be reduced by performing a careful history and physical examination before the test and observing the patient closely during exercise with monitoring of the electrocardiogram, arterial pressure, and symptoms. The standard 12-lead ECG should be verified before the test for any acute or recent change. There are well-defined contraindications to exercise testing (Table 5–7). After an episode of unstable angina, patients should be free of rest pain, of other evidence of ischemia, or of heart failure for at least 48 to 72 hours before testing. After an uncomplicated acute myocardial infarction, it is wise to wait at least 4 to 6 days before testing. Patients with critical obstruction to left ventricular outflow are at increased risk of cardiac events during exercise. In selected patients, low-level exercise can be quite useful in determining the severity of the left ventricular outflow tract gradient. The "cool-down" period should be prolonged to at least 2 minutes in patients with stenotic valves or those who have exertional hypotension, to avoid sudden pressure-volume shifts that occur in the immediate postexercise phase.

Uncontrolled systemic hypertension is a contraindication to exercise testing. Patients who present with systemic arterial pressure readings of ≥220/120 mm Hg should rest for 15 to 20 minutes and the blood pressure should be remeasured. If blood pressure remains at these levels, the test should be postponed until the hypertension is better controlled.

REFERENCES

EXERCISE TESTING FOR CARDIAC DISEASE

1. Feil, H., and Siegel, M. L.: Electrocardiographic changes during attacks of angina pectoris. Am. J. Med. Sci. *175*:255, 1928.
2. Master, A. M., and Oppenheimer, E. T.: A simple exercise tolerance test for circulatory efficiency with standard tables for normal individuals. Am. J. Med. Sci. *177*:223, 1929.
3. Guyton, A. C.: Textbook of Medical Physiology. 9th ed. Philadelphia, W. B. Saunders Company, 1995.
4. Pina, I. L., Balady, G. J., Hanson, P., et al: Guidelines for clinical exercise testing laboratories. A statement for healthcare professionals from the Committee on Exercise Cardiac Rehabilitation, American Heart Association. Circulation *91*:912, 1995.
5. Froelicher, V. F.: Manual of Exercise Testing. 2nd ed. St. Louis, Mosby–Year Book, 1994.
6. Froelicher, V. F., Myers, J., Follansbee, W. P., and Labovitz, A. J.: Exercise and the Heart. 3rd ed. St. Louis, Mosby–Year Book, 1993.
7. ESC Working Group on Exercise Physiology, Physiopathology and Electrocardiography: Guidelines for cardiac exercise testing. Eur. Heart J. *14*:969, 1993.
8. Gordon, N. F., Kohl, H. W., Scott, C. B., et al.: Reassessment of the guidelines for exercise testing. What alterations to current recommendations are required? Sports Med. *13*:293, 1992.
9. Washington, R. L., Bricker, J. T., Alpert, B. S., et al.: Guidelines for exercise testing in the pediatric age group. From the Committee on Atherosclerosis and Hypertension in Children, Council on Cardiovascular Disease in Young, the American Heart Association. Circulation *90*:2166, 1994.
10. Fletcher, G. F., Balady, G., Froelicher, V. F., et al.: Exercise standards. A statement for healthcare professionals from the American Heart Association. Circulation *91*:580, 1995.

EXERCISE PHYSIOLOGY

11. Fleg, J. L., Schulman, S., O'Connor, F., et al.: Effects of acute β-adrenergic receptor blockade on age-associated changes in cardiovascular performance during dynamic exercise. Circulation *90*:2333, 1994.
12. Imai, K., Sato, H., Hori, M., et al.: Vagally mediated heart rate recovery after exercise is accelerated in athletes but blunted in patients with chronic heart failure. J. Am. Coll. Cardiol. *24*:1529, 1994.
13. Wasserman, K., Hansen, J. E., Sue, D. Y., et al.: Principles of Exercise Testing and Interpretation. 2nd ed. Philadelphia, Lea and Febiger, 1994.
14. Smith, R. F., Johnson, G., Ziesche, S., et al.: Functional capacity in heart failure: Comparison of methods for assessment and their relation to other indexes of heart failure. The V-HeFT VA Cooperative Studies Group. Circulation *87*:VI88, 1993.
15. Weber, K. T., Janicki, J. S., McElroy, P. A., and Reddy, H. K.: Concepts and applications of cardiopulmonary exercise testing. Chest *93*:843, 1988.
16. Wasserman, K., Beaver, W. L., and Whipp, B. J.: Gas exchange theory and the lactic acidosis (anaerobic) threshold. Circulation *81*:II-14, 1990.
17. Norton, L. H., Squires, B., Craig, N. P., et al.: Accuracy of pulse oximetry during exercise stress testing. Int. J. Sports Med. *13*:523, 1992.
18. Cohen-Solal, A., Aupetit, J. F., Gueret, P., et al.: Can anaerobic threshold be used as an end-point for therapeutic trials in heart failure? Lessons from a multicentre randomized placebo-controlled trial. The $\dot{V}_{O_2}$ French Study Group. Eur. Heart J. *15*:236, 1994.
19. Eliasson, A. H., Phillips, Y. Y., Rajagopal, K. R., and Howard, R. S.: Sensitivity and specificity of bronchial provocation testing: An evaluation of four techniques in exercise-induced bronchospasm. Chest *102*:347, 1992.
20. Berdeaux, A., Ghaleh, B., Dubois-Rande, J. L., et al.: Role of vascular endothelium in exercise-induced dilation of large epicardial coronary arteries in conscious dogs. Circulation *89*:2799, 1994.
21. Kaufmann, P., Vassalli, G., Utzinger, U., and Hess, O. M.: Coronary vasomotion during dynamic exercise: Influence of intravenous and intracoronary nicardipine. J. Am. Coll. Cardiol. *26*:624, 1995.
22. Balady, G. J., Weiner, D. A., Rose, L., and Ryan, T. J.: Physiology responses to arm ergometry exercise relative to age and gender. J. Am. Coll. Cardiol. *16*:130, 1990.
23. Ellestad, M. H.: Stress Testing: Principles and Practice. 4th ed. Philadelphia, F. A. Davis Co., 1995.
24. Tamesis, B., Stelken, A., Byers, S., et al.: Comparison of the Asymptomatic Cardiac Ischemia Pilot and modified Asymptomatic Cardiac Ischemia Pilot versus Bruce and Cornell exercise protocols. Am. J. Cardiol. *72*:715, 1993.
25. Chaitman, B. R., Stone, P. H., Knatterud, G. L., et al.: Asymptomatic Cardiac Ischemia Pilot (ACIP) study: Impact of anti-ischemia therapy on 12-week rest ECG and exercise test outcomes. J. Am. Coll. Cardiol. *26*:585, 1995.
26. Blair, S. N., Gibbons, L. W., Painter, P., Pate, R. R., Taylor, C. B., and Will, J.: Guidelines for Exercise Testing and Prescriptions. 3rd ed. Phildelphia, Lea and Febiger, 1986.
27. Bittner, V., Weiner, D. H., Yusuf, S., et al.: Prediction of mortality and morbidity with a 6-minute walk test in patients with left ventricular dysfunction. JAMA *270*:1702, 1993.
28. Lachterman, B., Lehmann, K. G., Abrahamson, D., and Froelicher, V. F.: "Recovery only" ST-segment depression and the predictive accuracy of the exercise test. Ann. Intern. Med. *112*:11, 1990.

DIAGNOSTIC TESTING

29. Mark, D. B., Hlatky, M. A., Lee, K. L., Harrell, F. E., Califf, R. M., and Pryor, D. B.: Localizing coronary artery obstructions with the exercise treadmill test. Ann. Intern. Med. *106*:53, 1987.
30. Caralis, D. G., Shaw, L., Bilgere, B., et al.: Application of computerized exercise ECG digitization: Interpretation in large clinical trials. J. Electrocardogr. *25*:101, 1992.
31. Kubota, I., Yamaki, M., Shibata, T., et al.: Role of ATP-sensitive K^+ channel on ECG ST segment elevation during a bout of myocardial ischemia: A study on epicardial mapping in dogs. Circulation *88*:1845, 1993.
32. Schlant, R. C., Blonqvist, C. G., Brandenburg, R. O., et al.: Guidelines for exercise testing: A report of the Joint American College of Cardiology–American Heart Association Task Force on Assessment of Cardiovascular Procedures (Subcommittee on Exercise Testing). Circulation *74* (Suppl. III): 653a, 1986.
33. Shaw, L. J., Younis, L. T., Stocke, K. S., et al.: Effects of posture on metabolic and hemodynamic predischarge exercise response after acute myocardial infarction. Am J. Cardiol. *66*:134, 1990.
34. Couhan, L., Krone, R. J., Keller, A., and Eisenkramer, G.: Utility of lead V_4R in exercise testing for detection of coronary artery disease. Am. J. Cardiol. *64*:938, 1989.
35. Gianrossi, R., Detrano, R., Mulvihill, D., et al.: Exercise-induced ST depression in the diagnosis of coronary artery disease: A meta-analysis. Circulation *80*:87, 1989.
36. Detrano, R., Gianrossi, R., Mulvihill, D., et al.: Exercise-induced ST segment depression in the diagnosis of multivessel coronary disease: A metaanalysis. J. Am. Coll. Cardiol. *14*:1501, 1989.
37. Mark, D. B., and Froelicher, V. F.: Exercise treadmill testing and ambulatory monitoring. *In* Califf, R. M., Mark, D. B., and Wagner, G. S. (eds.): Acute Coronary Care. St. Louis, Mosby–Year Book, 1995, p. 767.
38. Patterson, R. E., and Horowitz, S. F.: Importance of epidemiology and biostatistics in deciding clinical strategies for using diagnostic tests: A simplified approach using examples from coronary artery disease: J. Am. Coll. Cardiol. *13*:1653, 1989.
39. Chauhan, A., Mullins, P. A., Petch, M. C., and Schofield, P. M.: Is coronary flow reserve in response to papaverine really normal in syndrome X? Circulation *89*:1998, 1994.
40. Folland, E. D., Vogel, R. A., Hartigan, P., et al.: Relation between coronary artery stenosis assessed by visual, caliper, and computer methods and exercise capacity in patients with single-vessel coronary artery disease. Circulation *89*:2005, 1994.
41. Kern, M. J., Donohue, T. J., Aguirre, F. V., et al.: Clinical outcome of deferring angioplasty in patients with normal translesional pressure-flow velocity measurements. J. Am. Coll. Cardiol. *25*:178, 1995.
42. Pryor, D. B., Shaw, L., McCants, C. B., et al.: Value of the history and physical in identifying patients at increased risk for coronary artery disease. Ann. Intern. Med. *118*:81, 1993.
43. Detrano, R., Leatherman, J., Salcedo, E. E., et al.: Bayesian analysis versus discriminant function analysis: Their relative utility in the diagnosis of coronary disease. Circulation *73*:970, 1986.
44. Chaitman, B. R.: The changing role of the exercise electrocardiogram as a diagnostic and prognostic test for chronic ischemic heart disease. J. Am. Coll. Cardiol. *8*:1195, 1986.
45. Bruce, R. A., Fisher, L. D., Pettinger, M., et al.: ST segment elevation with exercise: A marker for poor ventricular function and poor prognosis. Coronary Artery Surgery Study (CASS) confirmation of Seattle Heart Watch results. Circulation *77*:897, 1988.
46. Chikamori, T., Yamada, M., Takata, J., et al.: Exercise-induced prominent U waves as a marker of significant narrowing of the left circumflex or right coronary artery. Am. J. Cardiol. *74*:495, 1994.
47. Kligfield, P., Ameisen, O., and Okin, P. M.: Heart rate adjustment of ST segment depression for improved detection of coronary artery disease. Circulation *79*:245, 1989.
48. Kligfield, P., Okin, P. M., and Goldberg, H. L.: Value and limitations of heart rate–adjusted ST segment depression criteria for the identification of anatomically severe coronary obstruction: Test performance in relation to method of rate correction, definition of extent of disease, and β-blockade. Am. Heart J. *125*:1262, 1993.
49. Lachterman, B., Lehmann, K. G., Detrano, R., et al.: Comparison of ST segment/heart rate index to standard ST criteria for analysis of exercise electrocardiogram. Circulation *82*:44, 1990.
50. Ekelund, L. G., Suchindran, C. M., Karon, J. M., et al.: Black-white differences in exercise blood pressure. Circulation *31*:1568, 1990.
51. White, W. B., Lund-Johansen, P., and Omvik, P.: Assessment of four

ambulatory blood pressure monitors and measurements by clinicians versus intraarterial blood pressure at rest and during exercise. Am. J. Cardiol. *65:*60, 1990.
52. Lele, S. S., Scalia, G., Thomson, H., et al.: Mechanism of exercise hypotension in patients with ischemic heart disease: Role of neurocardiogenically mediated vasodilation. Circulation *90:*2701, 1994.
53. Derman, W. E., Sims, R., and Noakes, T. D.: The effects of antihypertensive medications on the physiological response to maximal exercise testing. J. Cardiovasc. Pharmacol. *19:*S122, 1992.
54. Fleg, J. L., and Lakatta, E. G.: Prevalence and significance of postexercise hypotension in apparently healthy subjects. Am. J. Cardiol. *57:*1380, 1986.
55. Hashimoto, M., Okamoto, M., Yamagata, T., et al.: Abnormal systolic blood pressure response during exercise recovery in patients with angina pectoris. J. Am. Coll. Cardiol. *22:*659, 1993.

EXERCISE TESTING DETERMINING PROGNOSIS

56. Chaitman, B. R., McMahon, R. P., Terrin, M., et al.: Impact of treatment strategy on predischarge exercise test in the Thrombolysis in Myocardial Infarction (TIMI) II trial. Am. J. Cardiol. *71:*131, 1993.
57. Morris, C. K., Ueshima, K., Kawaguchi, T., et al.: The prognostic value of exercise capacity: A review of the literature. Am. Heart J. *122:*1423, 1991.
58. Stevenson, L. W., Steimle, A. E., Fonarow, G., et al.: Improvement in exercise capacity of candidates awaiting heart transplantation. J. Am. Coll. Cardiol. *25:*163, 1995.
59. Vanhees, L., Fagard, R., Thijs, L., et al.: Prognostic significance of peak exercise capacity in patients with coronary artery disease. J. Am. Coll. Cardiol. *23:*358, 1994.
60. Younis, L. T., and Chaitman, B.R.: The prognostic value of exercise testing. Cardiol. Clin. *11:*229, 1993.
61. Myers, J., Do, D., Herbert, W., et al.: A nomogram to predict exercise capacity from a specific activity questionnaire and clinical data. Am. J. Cardiol. *73:*591, 1994.
62. Morris, C. K., Myers, J., Froelicher, V. F., et al.: Nomogram based on metabolic equivalents and age for assessing aerobic exercise capacity in men. J. Am. Coll. Cardiol. *22:*175, 1993.
63. Iskandrian, A. S., Heo, J., Kong, B., and Lyons, E.: Effect of exercise level on the ability of thallium-201 tomographic imaging in detecting coronary artery disease: analysis of 461 patients. J. Am. Coll. Cardiol. *14:*1477, 1989.
64. McCance, A. J., and Forfar, J. C.: Selective enhancement of the cardiac sympathetic response to exercise by anginal chest pain in humans. Circulation *80:*1642, 1989.
66. Ekelund, L. G., Suchindran, C. M., McMahon, R. P., et al.: Coronary heart disease morbidity and mortality in hypercholesterolemic men predicted from an exercise test: The Lipid Research Clinics Coronary Primary Prevention Trial. J. Am. Coll. Cardiol. *14:*556, 1989.
67. Rautaharju, P. M., Prineas, R. J., Eifler, W. J., et al.: Prognostic value of exercise electrocardiogram in men at high risk of future coronary heart disease: Multiple Risk Factor Intervention Trial experience. J. Am. Coll. Cardiol. *8:*1, 1986.
68. Bruce, R. A., and Fisher, L. D.: Exercise-enhanced assessment of risk factors for coronary heart disease in healthy men. J. Electrocardiol. (Suppl. October) *20:*162, 1987.
69. Fleg, J. L., Gerstenblith, G., Zonerman, A. B., et al.: Prevalence and prognostic significance of exercise-induced silent myocardial ischemia detected by thallium scintigraphy and electrocardiography in asymptomatic volunteers. Circulation *81:*428, 1990.
70. Fagan, L. F., Shaw, L., Kong, B. A., et al.: Prognostic value of exercise thallium scintigraphy in patients with good exercise tolerance and a normal or abnormal exercise electrocardiogram and suspected or confirmed coronary artery disease. Am. J. Cardiol. *69:*607, 1992.
71. Josephson, R. A., Shefrin, E., Lakatta, E. G., et al.: Can serial exercise testing improve the prediction of coronary events in asymptomatic individuals? Circulation *81:*20, 1990.
72. Weiner, D. A., Ryan, T. J., McCabe, C. H., et al.: Prognostic importance of a clinical profile and exercise test in medically treated patients with coronary artery disease. J. Am. Coll. Cardiol. *3:*772, 1984.
73. Weiner, D. A., Ryan, T. J., McCabe, C. H., et al.: Value of exercise testing in determining the risk classification and the response to coronary artery bypass grafting in three-vessel coronary artery disease: A report from the Coronary Artery Surgery Study (CASS) registry. Am. J. Cardiol. *60:*262, 1987.
74. Mark, D. B., Hlatky, M. A., Harrell, F. E., et al.: Exercise treadmill score for predicting prognosis in coronary artery disease. Ann. Intern. Med. *106:*793, 1987.
75. Mark, D. B., Shaw, L., Harrell, F. E. Jr., et al.: Prognostic value of a treadmill exercise score in outpatients with suspected coronary artery disease. N. Engl. J. Med. *325:*849, 1991.
76. Morrow, K., Morris, C. K., Froelicher, V. F., et al.: Prediction of cardiovascular death in men undergoing noninvasive evaluation for coronary artery disease. Ann. Intern. Med. *118:*689, 1993.
77. Froelicher, V., Morrow, K., Brown, M., et al.: Prediction of atherscolerotic cardiovascular death in men using a prognostic score. Am. J. Cardiol. *73:*133, 1994.
78. Chang, J., Atwood, J. E., and Froelicher, V.: Prognostic impact of myocardial ischemia. J. Am. Coll. Cardiol. *23:*225, 1994.
79. Miller, T. D., Christian, T. F., Taliercio, C. P., et al.: Severe exercise-induced ischemia does not identify high risk patients with normal left ventricular function and one- or two-vessel coronary artery disease. J. Am. Coll. Cardiol. *23:*219, 1994.
80. Quyyumi, A. A., Panza, J. A., Diodati, J. G., et al.: Prognostic implications of myocardial ischemia during daily life in low risk patients with coronary artery disease. J. Am. Coll. Cardiol. *21:*700, 1993.
81. Hecht, H. S., DeBord, L., Sotomayor, N., et al.: Truly silent ischemia and the relationship of chest pain and ST segment changes to the amount of ischemic myocardium: Evaluation by supine bicycle stress echocardiography. J. Am. Coll. Cardiol. *23:*369, 1994.
82. Benhorin, J., Pinsker, G., Moriel, M., et al.: Ischemic threshold during two exercise testing protocols and during ambulatory electrocardiographic monitoring. J. Am. Coll. Cardiol. *22:*671, 1993.
83. Klein, J., Chao, S. Y., Berman, D. S., and Rozanski, A.: Is "silent" myocardial ischemia really as severe as symptomatic ischemia? The analytical effect of patient selection biases. Circulation *89:*1958, 1994.
84. Weiner, D. A., Ryan, T. J., McCabe, C. H., et al.: Significance of silent myocardial ischemia during exercise testing in patients with coronary artery disease. Am. J. Cardiol. *59:*725, 1987.
85. Mark, D. B., Hlatky, M. A., Califf, R. M., et al.: Painless exercise ST deviation on the treadmill: Long-term prognosis. J. Am. Coll. Cardiol. *14:*885, 1989.
86. Nyman, I., Larsson, H., Areskog, J., et al. and the RISC Study Group: The predictive value of silent ischemia at an exercise test before discharge after an episode of unstable coronary artery disease. Am. Heart J. *123:*324, 1992.
87. Fruergaard, P., Launbjerg, J., Jacobsen, H. L., and Madsen, J. K.: Seven-year prognostic value of the electrocardiogram at rest and an exercise test in patients admitted for, but without, confirmed myocardial infarction. Eur. Heart J. *14:*499, 1993.
88. U.S. Department of Health and Human Services, Public Health Service Agency for Health Care Policy and Research, National Heart, Lung and Blood Institute: Clinical Practice Guideline. Unstable Angina: Diagnosis and Management. AHCPR Publication No. 94-0602, Number 10, March 1994.
89. Juneau, M., Colles, P., Theroux, P., et al.: Symptom-limited versus low level exercise testing before hospital discharge after myocardial infarction. J. Am. Coll. Cardiol. *20:*927, 1992.
90. Froelicher, E. S.: Usefulness of exercise testing shortly after acute myocardial infarction for predicting 10-year mortality. Am. J. Cardiol. *74:*318, 1994.
91. Khoury, Z., Keren, A., and Stern, S.: Correlation of exercise-induced ST depression in precordial electrocardiographic leads after inferior wall acute myocardial infarction with thallium-201 stress scintigraphy, coronary angiography and two-dimensional echocardiography. Am. J. Cardiol. *73:*868, 1994.
92. Morgan, C. D., Gent, M., Daly, P. A., et al.: Graded exercise testing following thrombolytic therapy for acute myocardial infarction: The importance of timing and infarct location. Can. J. Cardiol. *10:*897, 1994.
93. Moss, A. J., Goldstein, R. E., Hall, J., et al.: Detection and significance of myocardial ischemia in stable patients after recovery from an acute coronary event. J.A.M.A. *269:*2379, 1993.
94. Stevenson, R., Umachandran, V., Ranjadayalan, K., et al.: Reassessment of treadmill stress testing for risk stratification in patients with acute myocardial infarction treated by thrombolysis. Br. Heart J. *70:*415, 1993.
95. Arnold, A. E. R., Simoons, M. L., Detry, J. M. R., et al.: Prediction of mortality following hospital discharge after thrombolysis for acute myocardial infarction: Is there a need for coronary angiography? Eur. Heart J. *14:*306, 1993.
96. Grines, C. L., Browne, K. F., Marco, J., et al.: A comparison of immediate angioplasty with thrombolytic therapy for acute myocardial infarction: The Primary Angioplasty in Myocardial Infarction Study Group. N. Engl. J. Med. *328:*673, 1993.
97. Pilote, L., Silberberg, J., Lisbona, R., and Sniderman, A.: Prognosis in patients with low left ventricular ejection fraction after myocardial infarction. Circulation *80:*1636, 1989.
98. Aguirre, F. V., McMahon, R. P., Mueller, H., et al.: Impact of age on clinical outcome and postlytic management strategies in patients treated with intravenous thrombolytic therapy: Results from the TIMI II study. Circulation *90:*78, 1994.
99. Buckingham, T. A., and Chaitman, B. R.: Stress testing. *In* Zipes, D. P., and Rowlands, D. J. (eds.): Progress in Cardiology. Philadelphia, Lea and Febiger, 1988, p. 289.
100. Busby, M. J., Shefrin, E. A., and Fleg, J. L.: Prevalence and long-term significance of exercise-induced frequent or repetitive ventricular ectopic beats in apparently healthy volunteers. J. Am. Coll. Cardiol. *14:*1659, 1989.
101. Kadish, A. H., Weisman, H. F., Veltri, E. P., et al.: Paradoxical effects of exercise on the QT interval in patients with polymorphic ventricular tachycardia receiving type 1a antiarrhythmic agents. Circulation *81:*14, 1990.

CLINICAL APPLICATIONS

102. Williams, M. A., Esterbrooks, D. J., Nair, C. K., et al.: Clinical significance of exercise-induced bundle branch block. Am. J. Cardiol. *61:*346, 1988.
103. Heinsimer, J. A., Irwin, J. M., and Basnight, L. L.: Influence of underlying coronary artery disease on the natural history and prognosis of exercise-induced left bundle branch block. Am. J. Cardiol. *60:*1065, 1987.

104. Yen, R. S., Miranda, C., and Froelicher, V. F.: Diagnostic and prognostic accuracy of the exercise electrocardiogram in patients with preexisting right bundle branch block. Am. Heart J. *127:*1521, 1994.
105. Yamabe, H., Okumura, K., and Yasue, H.: Comparison of the effects of exercise and isoproterenol on the antegrade refractory period of the accessory pathway in patients with Wolff-Parkinson-White syndrome. Jpn. Circ. J. *58:*22, 1994.
106. Chaitman, B. R., Bourassa, M. G., Davis, K., et al.: Angiographic prevalence of high-risk coronary artery disease in patient subsets (CASS). Circulation *64:*360, 1981.
107. Clark, P. I., Glasser, S. P., Lyman, G. H., et al.: Relation of results of exercise tests in young women to phases of the menstrual cycle. Am. J. Cardiol. *61:*197, 1988.
108. Shaw, L. J., Miller, D. D., Romeis, J. C., et al.: Gender differences in the noninvasive evaluation and management of patients with suspected coronary artery disease. Ann. Intern. Med. *120:*559, 1994.
109. Mark, D. B., Shaw, L. K., DeLong, E. R., et al.: Absence of sex bias in the referral of patients for cardiac catheterization. N. Engl. J. Med. *330:*1101, 1994.
110. Otterstad, J. E., Davies, M., Ball, S. G., et al.: Left ventricular hypertrophy and myocardial ischaemia in hypertension: The THAMES study. Eur. Heart J. *14:*1622, 1993.
111. Colucci, W. S., Ribeiro, J. P., Rocco, M. B., et al.: Impaired chronotropic response to exercise in patients with congestive heart failure: Role of postsynaptic β-adrenergic desensitization. Circulation *80:*314, 1989.
112. Coats, A. J. S., Adamopoulos, S., Radaelli, A., et al.: Controlled trial of physical training in chronic heart failure: Exercise performance, hemodynamics, ventilation, and autonomic function. Circulation *85:*2119, 1992.
113. LeJemtel, T. H., Liang, C., Stewart, D. K., et al.: Reduced peak aerobic capacity in asymptomatic left ventricular systolic dysfunction: A substudy of the Studies of Left Ventricular Dysfunction (SOLVD). Circulation *90:*2757, 1994.
114. Myers, J., and Froelicher, V. F.: Hemodynamic determinants of exercise capacity in chronic heart failure. Ann. Intern. Med. *115:*377, 1991.
115. Waagstein, F., Bristow, M. R., Swedberg, K., et al.: Beneficial effects of metoprolol in idiopathic dilated cardiomyopathy: Metoprolol in Dilated Cardiomyopathy (MDC) Trial Study Group. Lancet *342:*1441, 1993.
116. Mancini, D. M., Walter, G., Reichek, N., et al.: Contribution of skeletal muscle atrophy to exercise intolerance and altered muscle metabolism in heart failure. Circulation *85:*1364, 1992.
117. Mahmarian, J. J., Fenimore, N. L., and Marks, G. F.: Transdermal nitroglycerin patch therapy reduces the extent of exercise-induced myocardial ischemia: Results of a double-blind, placebo-controlled trial using quantitative thallium-201 tomography. J. Am. Coll. Cardiol. *24:*25, 1994.
118. Melandri, G., Semprini, F., Cervi, V., et al.: Benefit of adding low molecular weight heparin to the conventional treatment of stable angina pectoris: A double-blind, randomized, placebo-controlled trial. Circulation *88:*2517, 1993.
119. Juneau, M., Johnstone, M., Dempsey, E., and Waters, D. D.: Exercise-induced myocardial ischemia in a cold environment: Effect of antianginal medications. Circulation *79:*1015, 1989.
120. Allred, E. N., Bleecker, E. R., Chaitman, B. R., et al.: Acute effects of carbon monoxide exposure on exercise performance in subjects with coronary artery disease. N. Engl. J. Med. *321:*1426, 1989.
121. Cascio, W. E., Woefel, A., Knisley, S. B., et al.: Use dependence of amiodarone during the sinus tachycardia of exercise in coronary artery disease. Am. J. Cardiol. *61:*1042, 1988.
122. Yli-Mayry, S., Huikuri, H. V., Airaksinen, K. E., et al.: Usefulness of a postoperative exercise test for predicting cardiac events after coronary artery bypass grafting. Am. J. Cardiol. *70:*56, 1992.
123. Parisi, A. F., Folland, E. D., and Hartigan, P.: A comparison of angioplasty with medical therapy in the treatment of single-vessel coronary artery disease: Veterans Affairs ACME Investigators. N. Engl. J. Med. *326:*10, 1992.
124. Weiner, D. A., Ryan, T. J., Parsons, L., et al.: Prevalence and prognostic significance of silent and symptomatic ischemia after coronary bypass surgery: A report from the Coronary Artery Surgery Study (CASS) randomization population. J. Am. Coll. Cardiol. *18:*343, 1991.
125. Uren, N. G., Crake, T., Lefroy, D. C., et al.: Delayed recovery of coronary resistive vessel function after coronary angioplasty. J. Am. Coll. Cardiol. *21:*612, 1993.
126. Beregi, J. P., Bauters, C., McFadden, E. P., et al.: Exercise-induced ST-segment depression in patients without restenosis after coronary angioplasty: Relation to preprocedural impaired left ventricular function. Circulation *90:*148, 1994.
127. Ehrman, J., Keteyian, S., Fedel, F., et al.: Cardiovascular responses of heart transplant recipients to graded exercise testing. J. Appl. Physiol. *73:*260, 1992.
128. Kao, A. C., Trigt, P. V., Shaeffer-McCall, G. S., et al.: Central and peripheral limitations to upright exercise in untrained cardiac transplant recipients. Circulation *89:*2605, 1994.
129. Mancini, D. M., Eisen, H., Kussmaul, W., et al.: Value of peak exercise oxygen consumption for optimal timing of cardiac transplantation in ambulatory patients with heart failure. Circulation *83:*778, 1991.
130. Smart, F. W., Ballantyne, C. M., Cocanougher, B., et al.: Insensitivity of noninvasive tests to detect coronary artery vasculopathy after heart transplant. Am. J. Cardiol. *67:*243, 1991.
131. Smart, F. W., Grinstead, W. C., Cocanougher, B., et al.: Detection of transplant arteriopathy: Does exercise thallium scintigraphy improve noninvasive diagnostic capabilities? Transplant. Proc. *23:*1189, 1991.
132. Burwash, I. G., Pearlman, A. S., Kraft, C. D., et al.: Flow dependence of measures of aortic stenosis severity during exercise. J. Am. Coll. Cardiol. *24:*1342, 1994.
133. Siemienczuk, D., Greenberg, B., Morris, C., et al.: Chronic aortic insufficiency: Factors associated with progression to aortic valve replacement. Ann. Intern. Med. *110:*587, 1989.
134. Hayes, D. L., Von Feldt, L., and Higano, S. T.: Standardized informal exercise testing for programming rate adaptive pacemakers. PACE *14;*1772, 1991.
135. McElroy, P. A., Janicki, J. S., and Weber, K. T.: Physiologic correlates of the heart rate response to upright isotonic exercise: relevance to rate-responsive pacemakers. J. Am. Coll. Cardiol. *11:*94, 1988.
136. Hilton, T. C., Shaw, L. J., Chaitman, B. R., et al.: Prognostic significance of exercise thallium-201 testing in patients aged greater than or equal to 70 years with known or suspected coronary artery disease. Am. J. Cardiol. *69:*45, 1992.
137. Ciaroni, S., Delonca, J., and Righetti, A.: Early exercise testing after acute myocardial infarction in the elderly: Clinical evaluation and prognostic significance. Am. Heart J. *126:*304, 1993.
138. Borg, G.: Perceived exertion as an indicator of somatic stress. Scand. J. Rehabil. Med. *2–3:*92, 1970.
139. Cahalin, L. P., Blessey, R. L., Kummer, D., and Simard, M.: The safety of exercise testing performed independently by physical therapists. J. Cardiopulmonary Rehabil. *7:*269, 1987.
140. Stuart, R. J., and Ellestad, M. H.: National survey of exercise stress testing facilities. Chest *77:*94, 1980.
141. Hamm, L. F., Crow, R. S., Stull, G. A., and Hannan, P.: Safety and characteristics of exercise testing early after acute myocardial infarction. Am. J. Cardiol. *63:*1193, 1989.
142. Lewis, W. R., and Amsterdam, E. A.: Utility and safety of immediate exercise testing of low-risk patients admitted to the hospital for suspected acute myocardial infarction. Am. J. Cardiol. *74:*987, 1994.
143. Tristani, F. E., Hughes, C. V., Archibald, D. G., et al.: Safety of graded symptom-limited exercise testing in patients with congestive heart failure. Circulation *76:*VI-54, 1987.
144. Young, D.Z., Lampert, S., Graboys, T. B., and Lown, B.: Safety of maximal exercise testing in patients at high risk for ventricular arrhythmia. Circulation *70:*184, 1984.

Chapter 6
Cardiac Catheterization

CHARLES J. DAVIDSON, ROBERT F. FISHMAN, ROBERT O. BONOW

HISTORICAL PERSPECTIVE

Procedures in the cardiac catheterization laboratory have evolved from purely diagnostic and research techniques to potentially life-saving interventional procedures. In 1733, Stephen Hales described the mechanics of blood circulation and went on to directly measure blood pressure and its response to various physiological conditions in animals and humans. Almost 200 years later, in 1929, Werner Forssmann performed the first human cardiac catheterization. During his training as a surgeon in Eberswalde, Germany, he used fluoroscopic guidance to advance a urethral catheter through his own left antecubital vein into the right atrium. In an attempt to develop a technique for direct delivery of drugs into the heart, he performed right heart catheterizations on himself on at least six occasions. He tried to opacify the heart with contrast medium injection into the right atrium, but because of poor fluoroscopic imaging, he was unable to visualize the heart structures. Although intense criticism eventually caused him to abandon this pursuit and to undertake a career as a urologist, he was awarded the Nobel prize in medicine in 1956 for his pioneering work. It was not until 1941 that right heart catheterization was routinely undertaken in humans to study cardiac physiology. Right heart catheterization was facilitated in 1970 when balloon-tipped flow-directed catheters that could be inserted without fluoroscopy were introduced by Swan and Ganz.[1]

Zimmerman and coworkers[2] undertook the first retrograde left heart catheterization in 1950 using a No. 6 French catheter inserted through the ulnar artery. The technique was facilitated greatly when Seldinger in 1953 described the method of percutaneous needle puncture and catheter exchange over a guidewire. In 1945, Radner visualized coronary arteries by nonselective injection of radiopaque contrast medium into the ascending aorta, but it was not until 1958 that the first selective injection of contrast medium into the coronary arteries was performed by Sones.[3] The following year, transseptal heart catheterization with interatrial puncture of the septum was described by Ross and by Cope.[4,5] Various retrograde percutaneous femoral artery coronary angiographic techniques were developed by Ricketts and Abrams,[6] Amplatz and colleagues,[7] and Judkins.[8] The catheter created by Judkins permits relatively easy and safe selective coronary arteriography. One of Judkins' favorite phrases was that the left coronary catheter will seek the lumen of the coronary artery unless thwarted by the operator.[9] The percutaneous femoral technique introduced by Judkins and the brachial arteriotomy technique pioneered by Sones are the most widely used today. Each method has its own set of advantages and disadvantages, which will be discussed later in greater detail.

Dotter and Judkins developed the technique of transluminal angioplasty in 1964. In 1977, Andreas Gruentzig performed the first percutaneous balloon coronary angioplasty in humans. Percutaneous revascularization strategies have evolved to include the use of intracoronary stents, various atherectomy methods, and laser technology. Technology is advancing to the point that genetic manipulation may be feasible in the catheterization laboratory.

INDICATIONS FOR DIAGNOSTIC CARDIAC CATHETERIZATION

As with any procedure, the decision to recommend cardiac catheterization is based on an appropriate risk-benefit ratio. In general, diagnostic cardiac catheterization is recommended whenever it is clinically important to define the presence or severity of a suspected cardiac lesion that cannot be adequately evaluated by noninvasive techniques. Intracardiac pressure measurements and coronary arteriography are procedures that can be performed only by catheterization as of this writing, although some intracardiac pressures and rudimentary coronary artery anatomy can be evaluated with echocardiography and magnetic resonance imaging, respectively. Since the mortality from cardiac catheterization is approximately 0.1 per cent in most laboratories, there are few patients who cannot be studied safely in an active laboratory.

The guidelines for diagnostic coronary angiography have been reported by a joint task force of the American College of Cardiology and the American Heart Association[10] (see p. 3012). These guidelines describe a three-tiered priority classification for specific disease states. Class I applications exist for those conditions in which there is general agreement that coronary angiography is justified, although this may not be the only appropriate diagnostic procedure. Class II indications apply to those conditions in which coronary angiography is frequently performed, but there is divergence of opinion with respect to justification of the value and appropriateness of the procedure. Class III conditions are those in which there is general agreement that cardiac catheterization is not ordinarily justified. Diseases are grouped under several categories: known or suspected coronary heart disease, atypical chest pain, acute myocardial infarction, valvular heart disease, congenital heart disease, and other conditions. Table 6–1 summarizes the recommendations of the task force.

The indications for cardiac catheterization are changing and are likely to continue to evolve. The trend during the last 10 years in the United States has been in two divergent directions. At the one extreme, many critically ill and hemodynamically unstable patients are being studied during acute myocardial ischemia. At the other end of the spectrum, an increasing number of studies are being performed in an outpatient setting. The result has been the expansion of traditional indications for cardiac catheterization to include both seriously ill patients and ambulatory patients.

Cardiac catheterization should be considered to be a diagnostic test for use in combination with other complementary noninvasive tests in cardiology. For example, cardiac catheterization in valvular or congenital heart disease is best done with full knowledge of the echocardiographic and any other functional information. Then, catheterization can be directed and simplified without obtaining redundant anatomical information.

Identification of coronary artery disease and assessment of its extent and severity are the most common indications for cardiac catheterization in adults. The information obtained by catheterization is crucial to optimize the care of patients with various chest pain syndromes. In addition, the presence of dynamic coronary vascular lesions, such as spasm or thrombosis, may be identified. The consequences of coronary heart disease, such as ischemic mitral regurgi-

TABLE 6–1 INDICATIONS FOR CORONARY ANGIOGRAPHY

KNOWN OR SUSPECTED CORONARY DISEASE (Known: previous myocardial infarction, or coronary bypass surgery or PTCA. Suspected: rest- or exercise-induced ECG abnormalities suggesting silent ischemia.)

ASYMPTOMATIC PATIENTS

Class I indications

1. Evidence for high risk on noninvasive testing
2. Individuals in high-risk occupations (airline pilots, bus drivers)
3. Following successful resuscitation from cardiac arrest

Class II indications

1. Positive noninvasive test in non–high-risk patient
2. Multiple risk factors for coronary artery disease
3. Prior MI with positive noninvasive testing
4. Following cardiac transplantation
5. After CABG or PTCA with positive ischemia
6. Before noncardiac surgery with positive noninvasive test

SYMPTOMATIC PATIENTS

Class I indications

1. Inadequate response to medical treatment
2. Unstable angina
3. Printzmetal's or variant angina
4. Canadian Cardiovascular Society functional Class I or II angina associated with the following:
   - a. Positive exercise test
   - b. History of MI or hypertension with ECG changes
   - c. Side effects of medical therapy
   - d. Occupational or lifestyle "need to know"
   - e. Episodic pulmonary edema
5. Before major vascular surgery if angina present or noninvasive positive test results
6. After resuscitation from cardiac arrest

Class II indications

1. Any angina in the following groups:
   - a. Female patients <40 yr of age with positive noninvasive testing
   - b. Male patients <40
   - c. Patients <40 with prior MI
   - d. Patients requiring major nonvascular surgery
2. Class 3 or 4 angina that improves on medical therapy
3. Patients who cannot be risk-stratified by other techniques

ATYPICAL CHEST PAIN OF UNCERTAIN ORIGIN

Class I indications

1. When noninvasive stress test reveals high risk for coronary disease
2. Suspected coronary artery
3. Associated symptoms or signs of abnormal LV function or failure

Class II indications

1. Patients in whom coronary disease cannot be excluded by noninvasive studies
2. Severe symptoms despite negative noninvasive tests

ACUTE MYOCARDIAL INFARCTION

Acute, Evolving MI

Class I indications

1. None*

Class II indications

1. Within the first 6 hr in candidates for revascularization therapy
2. After IV thrombolytic therapy when PTCA contemplated (see text)

Completed Myocardial Infarction (after 6 hr and before discharge evaluation)

Class I indications

1. Recurrent episodes of ischemic chest pain
2. Suspected ruptured septum or acute mitral regurgitation with CHF
3. Suspected left ventricular pseudoaneurysm

Class II indications

1. Thrombolytic therapy during evolving MI period
2. CHF and/or hypotension during intensive medical therapy
3. Recurrent VT and/or VF
4. Cardiogenic shock
5. MI due to coronary embolism

Convalescent Myocardial Infarction (predischarge to 8 wks)

Class I indications

1. Angina at rest or with minimal activity
2. CHF, recurrent ischemia, or ventricular arrhythmias
3. Positive noninvasive study
4. Non-Q-wave infarction

Class II indications

1. Mild angina
2. Asymptomatic and younger than 50
3. Need to return to unusually active or vigorous activity
4. Previous history of MI or angina for >6 mo before the current MI
5. Thrombolytic therapy given during evolving phase

VALVULAR HEART DISEASE

Class I indications

1. Before valve surgery in an adult with chest discomfort and/or ECG changes
2. Before valve surgery in a male patient ≥35
3. Before valve surgery in postmenopausal women

Class II indications

1. During left heart catheterization in men <35 or women >40 when aortic or mitral valve surgery is being considered
2. Multiple risk factors for coronary disease
3. Reoperation for valve surgery when angiography >1 year
4. In infective endocarditis when coronary embolization occurs

CONGENITAL HEART DISEASE

Class I indications

1. Signs or symptoms of angina
2. Suspected congestive coronary anomaly
3. Male patient >40 or postmenopausal woman

Class II indications

1. Presence of a congenital lesion with high frequency of coronary anomalies

MISCELLANEOUS

Class I indications

1. Disease of the aorta in which the presence or extent of coronary disease will affect management
2. LV failure without obvious cause
3. Angina associated with hypertrophic cardiomyopathy in patients ≥35 or postmenopausal women with angina

Class II indications

1. Dilated cardiomyopathy
2. Recent blunt chest trauma
3. Male patients >35 or postmenopausal women to undergo other cardiac surgery
4. Prospective transplant donors
5. Kawasaki's disease (coronary aneurysms)

Data from Ross J, Brandenburg RO, Dinsmore RE, and members of the subcommittee task force on coronary angiography of the AHA/ACC. J Am Coll Cardiol *10*:935, 1987.

* Revised ACC/AHA task force guidelines indicate a clinical role (Class I) for PTCA during acute myocardial infarction (Circulation *88*:2987, 1993). See text for details.

tation or left ventricular dysfunction and aneurysm, can be defined. In the current era of acute catheter intervention for coronary artery disease, patients may be studied during myocardial infarction or in the early period after acute myocardial injury. The aggressiveness of individual centers in approaching such patients depends on local facilities and treatment philosophies as well as the availability of appropriate therapy and surgical support.

According to the ACC/AHA task force recommendations, coronary angiography has no indications during the acute phase of myocardial infarction. However, several recent prospective randomized trials have demonstrated that immediate cardiac catheterization with direct percutaneous transluminal coronary angiography (PTCA) of the infarct-related artery produces clinical outcomes that are equivalent to and possibly superior to thrombolytic therapy[11] (see p. 1313). In certain patient subgroups, particularly those not at low risk, PTCA appears to be safer and more effective than thrombolytic therapy. The task force guidelines also suggest that coronary angiography is desirable during the evolving phase of acute myocardial infarction after thrombolytic therapy has been administered. Data from several large randomized prospective trials indicate that emergent catheterization should not be routinely performed after successful thrombolytic therapy.[12,13] Thus, the recommendations of the 1987 task force for cardiac catheterization during acute evolving myocardial infarction may be outdated based on the current literature.

The 1993 ACC/AHA task force recommendations regarding the use of PTCA in the setting of acute myocardial infarction and acute ischemic syndromes more accurately reflect current practice guidelines[14] (see p. 1221). These recommendations acknowledge that acute cardiac catheterization and PTCA are appropriately indicated (i.e., Class I) for evolving acute myocardial infarction and after acute myocardial infarction during initial hospitalization.

In patients with myocardial disease, cardiac catheterization may provide crucial information. It can exclude coronary artery disease as the cause of symptoms and evaluate left ventricular dysfunction in patients with cardiomyopathy. Cardiac catheterization also permits quantification of the severity of both diastolic and systolic dysfunction, differentiation of myocardial restriction from pericardial constriction, assessment of the extent of valvular regurgitation, detection of active myocarditis by endomyocardial biopsy, and observation of the cardiovascular response to acute pharmacological intervention.

In patients with valvular heart disease, cardiac catheterization provides both confirmatory and complementary data to noninvasive echocardiography and nuclear studies. Roberts[15] and Rahimtoola[16] have emphasized that the risk-benefit ratio of preoperative cardiac catheterization is weighted heavily in favor of the cardiac catheterization. Catheterization may be unnecessary in some preoperative situations, such as in patients with an atrial myxoma or young patients with endocarditis or acute mitral or acute aortic regurgitation. Nevertheless, additional confirmation of the severity of the valvular lesion, identification of associated coronary disease, quantification of the hemodynamic consequences of the valvular lesions (such as pulmonary hypertension), and occasionally the acute hemodynamic response to pharmacological therapy all provide useful preoperative information that fully defines the operative risk and permits a more directed surgical approach.

The current role of cardiac catheterization in certain congenital disease states is less well defined, as echocardiography, Doppler techniques, and cardiac magnetic resonance imaging have improved in accuracy and image quality. Because gross cardiac anatomy can generally be well defined by these methods, catheterization is required only if certain hemodynamic information (e.g., shunt size or pulmonary vascular resistance) is important in determining the indications for surgical procedures, if catheter interventional methods are contemplated, or if coronary anomalies are suspected.

COMPLICATIONS ASSOCIATED WITH CARDIAC CATHETERIZATION

(Table 6–2)

Cardiac catheterization is a relatively safe procedure but has a well-defined risk of morbidity and mortality.[17–22] The potential risk of major complications during cardiac catheterization may be difficult to ascertain due to the confounding aspects of comorbid disease and disparities in methodology used to collect complication data. Recent advances including the use of nonionic contrast media, lower profile diagnostic catheters, and extensive operator experience all serve to reduce further the incidence of complications. Several large trials including the American Heart Association's Cooperative Study on cardiac catheterization,[17] the Society for Cardiac Angiography's Registry,[18] and others[19,21,22] permit insight into the incidence of major events and delineate patient cohorts that are at increased risk. Two studies evaluating the specific risk of coronary angiography are also available—a survey of 46,904 patients[23] and the report from the Collaborative Study of Coronary Artery Surgery that included 7553 patients who were studied prospectively.[20]

TABLE 6–2 RISK GROUPS FOR CARDIAC CATHETERIZATION

	MORTALITY RATE (%)
Overall mortality	0.14
Age-related mortality	
Less than 1 year	1.75
More than 60 years	0.25
Coronary artery disease	
One-vessel disease	0.03
Three-vessel disease	0.16
Left main disease	0.86
Coronary heart failure	
NYHA functional Class I or II	0.02
NYHA functional Class III	0.12
NYHA functional Class IV	0.67
Valvular heart disease	0.28
PATIENTS AT HIGHEST RISK FOR COMPLICATIONS AND UNSUITABLE FOR CATHETERIZATION IN AN AMBULATORY SETTING	
Coronary artery disease	
Unstable or progressive angina	
Recent myocardial infarction (<7 days)	
Pulmonary edema thought due to ischemia	
High risk for left main disease by noninvasive testing	
Congestive heart failure	
NYHA functional Class III or IV	
Severe right heart failure	
Valvular heart disease	
Suspected severe AS	
Suspected severe AI (pulse pressure ≥80 mm Hg)	
Congenital heart disease	
Suspected severe pulmonary hypertension	
Severe right heart failure	
PATIENTS WHO REQUIRE PROLONGED MONITORING AFTER CARDIAC CATHETERIZATION AND MAY BE UNSUITABLE FOR AMBULATORY CARDIAC CATHETERIZATION	
Severe peripheral vascular disease	
General debility, mental confusion, or cachexia	
Need for continuous anticoagulation or a bleeding diathesis	
Uncontrolled systemic hypertension	
Poorly controlled diabetes mellitus	
Recent stroke (<1 month)	
Renal insufficiency (creatinine ≥2 mg/dl)	

Modified from Bashore, TM: Traditional and nontraditional cardiac catheterization laboratory settings. *In* Pepine, C. J., Hill, J. A., and Lambert, C. R.: Diagnostic and Therapeutic Cardiac Catheterization. 2nd ed. Baltimore, Williams and Wilkins, 1994, pp. 18, 19.

* Adapted from ACC/AHA Ad Hoc Task Force on Cardiac Catheterization. Guidelines for cardiac catheterization and cardiac catheterization laboratories. J Am Coll Cardiol 1991; 84:2213–2247.

Death from diagnostic cardiac catheterization occurs in 0.14 to 0.75 per cent of patients, depending on the population studied. Data from the Society for Cardiac Angiography identified subsets of patients with an increased mortality rate.[19] These include patients with >50 per cent stenosis of the left coronary artery (0.94 per cent), left ventricular ejection fraction <30 per cent (0.54 per cent), New York Heart Association (NYHA) functional class III or IV heart failure (0.24 per cent), age greater than 60 years (0.23 per cent), aortic valvular disease (0.23 per cent), and three-vessel coronary artery disease (0.13 per cent).[18] In an analysis of 58,332 patients studied in 1990, multivariate predictors of significant complications were moribund status, advanced NYHA functional class, hypertension, shock, aortic valve disease, renal insufficiency, unstable angina, mitral valve disease, acute myocardial infarction within 24 hours, congestive heart failure, and cardiomyopathy.[21] The risk of cardiac catheterization appears to be further increased in octogenarians,[24] in whom overall mortality is approximately 0.8 per cent and the risk of nonfatal major complications, which are primarily peripheral vascular, is about 5 per cent.

The risk of myocardial infarction varies from 0.07 to 0.6 per cent, cerebrovascular accidents from 0.03 to 0.2 per cent, and significant brady- or tachyarrhythmias from 0.56 to 1.3 per cent. Reports of the incidence of major vascular complications have varied widely, with most series suggesting a slightly higher frequency when the brachial approach is used. Recent data suggest the incidence of major vascular complications to be approximately 0.40 per cent.[21] Major vascular complications include occlusion requiring arterial repair or thrombectomy, retroperitoneal bleeding, hematoma formation, pseudoaneurysm, arteriovenous fistula formation, and infection. The risk of requiring surgical repair for vascular injury is related to advanced age, congestive heart failure, and larger body surface area.[25]

Systemic complications can vary from mild vasovagal responses to severe vagal reactions that lead to cardiac arrest. Prolonged hypotension during the procedure may also occur as a result of various mechanisms that include the vasodepressor vagal response, contrast medium–induced vasodilation or osmotic diuresis, cardiac tamponade due to myocardial perforation or coronary laceration, myocardial infarction, and an acute anaphylactoid reaction to the contrast media. Minor complications occur in approximately 4 per cent of patients undergoing routine cardiac catheterization.[26] The most common untoward effects are transient hypotension and brief episodes of angina lasting less than 10 minutes. However, with the use of low osmolar contrast media, bradycardia is infrequent and usually responds to cough. Rarely, administration of intravenous atropine is necessary.

After the procedure, diuresis from the radiographic contrast load and subsequent hypotension can be common. Intravenous hydration given before and after the procedure can usually restore the intravascular volume to compensate for the anticipated diuresis. A recent prospective trial evaluated the effects of saline, mannitol, and furosemide in preventing acute decreases in renal function due to contrast media–induced nephrotoxicity.[27] The authors concluded that saline alone was most effective in reducing the acute increase in serum creatinine. The incidence of acute renal dysfunction in patients with baseline renal insufficiency was 28 and 40 per cent with mannitol and furosemide, respectively, compared with 11 per cent with saline hydration alone.

Controversy exists regarding the use of low osmolar nonionic or hemionic versus high osmolar ionic contrast media for routine cardiac catheterization and angiography. Consensus is growing regarding the types of patients in whom use of low osmolar contrast agents should be considered (Table 6–3). Several reviews have suggested that contrast media–related toxicity occurs in 1.4 to 2.3 per cent of patients receiving ionic contrast media.[28,29] High osmolar ionic contrast media produce various adverse hemodynamic and electrophysiologic effects during coronary angiography. Most of these adverse events are clearly related to the osmolality, sodium content, and calcium binding characteristics of the ionic contrast solutions. In addition, myocardial depression, peripheral vasodilation, and increased coronary blood flow occur.[30] Nonionic low osmolar contrast agents clearly reduce acute adverse hemodynamic and electrophysiological reactions[31,32] and may reduce nephrotoxicity in patients at highest risk. They appear to release less histamine from mast cells and potentially reduce allergic reactions.[33] Clinical studies suggest no advantage of low osmolar contrast over ionic contrast media in the prevention of nephrotoxicity in patients with normal renal function.[26,34] However, other data indicate that the risk of contrast media–induced nephropathy may be reduced in patients with baseline renal insufficiency if nonionic contrast medium is utilized.[35]

TABLE 6–3 INDICATIONS FOR USE OF LOW OSMOLAR CONTRAST AGENTS

Unstable ischemic syndromes
Congestive heart failure
Diabetes mellitus
Renal insufficiency
Hypotension
Severe bradycardia
History of contrast allergy
Severe valvular heart disease
Internal mammary artery injection

From Hill JA, Lambert CR, Pepine CJ: Radiographic contrast agents. *In* Pepine CJ, Hill JA, and Lambert CR: Diagnostic and Therapeutic Cardiac Catheterization. 2nd ed. Baltimore, Williams and Wilkins, 1994, p. 192.

Baseline renal insufficiency has been consistently shown to be an independent predictor of subsequent contrast nephrotoxicity.[26] Contrast media–induced renal dysfunction can be minimized if the dosage of contrast medium is kept below 30 ml for the entire study.[36] The question of some inherent thrombogenicity of nonionic agents has also been raised,[37] and this possibility may relate to the formation of "thin" fibrin in the thrombus.[38] Because a substantial difference in costs exists between ionic and nonionic media, the controversy regarding the exclusive use of nonionic contrast media for routine cardiac catheterization is unresolved.

TECHNICAL ASPECTS OF CARDIAC CATHETERIZATION

CATHETERIZATION LABORATORY FACILITIES

Cardiac catheterization facilities have evolved to include traditional hospital-based laboratories with in-house cardiothoracic surgical programs, hospital-based laboratories without on-site surgical programs, free-standing laboratories, and mobile laboratories. The relative merits of each type of facility have been discussed in detail by a task force of the American Heart Association and the American College of Cardiology,[39] and guidelines for development of a mobile facility have been outlined by the Society for Cardiac Angiography and Interventions.[40] The goals of the free-standing and mobile cardiac catheterization facilities are to reduce cost while offering services in a convenient location for low-risk patients. In one study evaluating the safety of mobile catheterization involving 1001 low-risk patients, no patient died, 0.9 per cent required urgent referral for clinical instability, 0.6 per cent had major complications, and 27 per cent required further referral to a tertiary site for additional diagnostic or therapeutic procedures.[41] The issue of cost-saving potential of mobile and free-standing laboratories, as well as quality of patient care and ethical issues, remains unresolved. Because the majority of patients in the United States live within 30 to 60 minutes of a hospital-based facility,[39] it is generally recommended that catheterization be performed in traditional settings.

Because of cost containment considerations and the documented safety of diagnostic cardiac catheterization, there has been increasing pressure to perform catheterization on an ambulatory outpatient basis.[42,43] Criteria for ambulatory catheterization have been reported.[39,44] In general, patients who are not appropriate candidates for ambulatory catheterization include those with severe peripheral vascular disease, mechanical prosthetic valves, severe congestive heart failure, bleeding disorders, severe ischemia during stress testing, ischemia at rest, known or highly suspected severe left main or proximal three-vessel disease, critical aortic stenosis, and severe comorbid disease. Despite careful screening for low-risk patients, 12 per cent of patients may require hospitalization.[45]

PERSONNEL

Personnel in the catheterization laboratory include the director, physicians, nurses, and radiologic technologists. All members should be trained in cardiopulmonary resuscitation and preferably in advanced cardiac life support. It is desirable for facilities to be associated with a cardiothoracic surgical program. In general, high-risk diagnostic studies and all elective percutaneous interventions should be performed in laboratories with on-site surgical facilities. The re-

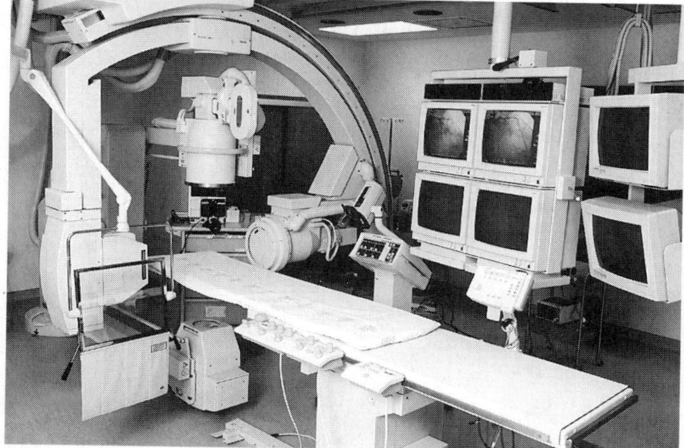

FIGURE 6–1. Cardiac catheterization laboratory at Northwestern University, Northwestern Memorial Hospital. Biplane radiographic equipment including x-ray tube and image intensifier assembly, hemodynamic physiological monitors, power injector, and emergency cart are shown.

cent American Heart Association/American College of Cardiology task force assessment of diagnostic and therapeutic cardiovascular procedures suggests that PTCA of high-risk patients with acute myocardial infarction may be performed by trained physicians without on-site surgical backup if the patient cannot be transferred to a more traditional setting without additional risk.[14]

In order to maintain proficiency, laboratories for adult studies should perform a minimum of 300 procedures per year, and physicians performing diagnostic catheterization should perform a minimum of 150 procedures per year.[39,46] Regular evaluation of laboratory and physician performance is also mandatory.[47]

EQUIPMENT

The physical requirements for the catheterization facility have been described in detail elsewhere.[39] Necessary equipment includes the radiographic system, physiological data monitoring and acquisition instrumentation, sterile supplies, and an emergency cart. Also included are support equipment consisting of a power injector, cineangiographic film or digital archiving, film processors, and viewing equipment (Fig. 6–1).

RADIOGRAPHIC EQUIPMENT. High-resolution x-ray imaging is required for optimal performance of catheterization procedures. The necessary equipment includes a generator, x-ray tube, image intensifier, video system, and usually a cinecamera.[48] While most facilities continue to use traditional film-based cineangiography, many laboratories have made the transition to using digital technology, thus becoming "cinefilm-less" laboratories.[49,50] The advantages of digital acquisition and archiving include the ability to have on-line review, quantitative computer analysis of high-quality images, image manipulation capabilities, and flicker-free images at very low frame rates thereby minimizing radiation exposure. Using these technologies, transfer of images between cardiac catheterization laboratories, hospitals, and physician offices could be accomplished using a common network. In order for this goal to be achieved, however, the digital archiving systems must be compatible.[51]

PHYSIOLOGICAL MONITORS. Continuous monitoring of blood pressure and the electrocardiogram (ECG) is required during cardiac catheterization. Systemic, pulmonary, and intracardiac pressures are generally recorded using fluid-filled catheters connected to strain-gauge pressure transducers and then transmitted to a monitor. Equipment for determination of cardiac output and blood gas determination, as well as a standard 12-lead ECG machine, are necessary.

RADIATION SAFETY

The patient and catheterization laboratory personnel must be protected from the harmful effects of radiation. Installing and maintaining optimal x-ray imaging equipment will reduce unnecessary radiation exposure. The amount of radiation exposure to the patient can be reduced by limiting fluoroscopic and image acquisition time, collimation of the beam to the anatomical region of interest, using low-intensity fluoroscopy, acquiring images at lower frame rates (i.e., 15 frames/sec), maintaining a minimum distance between the image intensifier and the x-ray tube, and using lead shielding when appropriate. Personnel in the laboratory can limit radiation exposure by minimizing acquisition and fluoroscopy times and by using low-dose fluoroscopy and 15 frames/sec acquisition rates. The most important factors are maximizing distance from the source of x-rays and using appropriate shielding (lead aprons, lead thyroid collars, lead eyeglasses, and moveable leaded glass barriers). A method for measuring radiation exposure for personnel is required. The maximum allowable radiation dose per year for those working with radiation is 5 roentgen-equivalents–man (rem). A full discussion of radiation safety has been presented by the Society for Cardiac Angiography and Interventions and others.[39,52,53]

Catheterization Laboratory Protocol

PREPARATION OF THE PATIENT FOR CARDIAC CATHETERIZATION. Before arrival in the catheterization laboratory, the cardiologist responsible for the procedure should fully explain the procedure including its risk and benefits to the patient and answer questions that the patient and/or family may have. Precatheterization evaluation includes a patient history, physical examination, laboratory evaluation (complete blood count, platelet count, blood urea nitrogen, serum creatinine, serum electrolytes, blood glucose, prothrombin time, and partial thromboplastin time), chest x-ray, and ECG. Important components of the history that need to be addressed include possible insulin-dependent diabetes mellitus, renal insufficiency, chronic anticoagulation, and peripheral vascular disease as well as previous contrast media reactions. A full knowledge of any prior procedures, including prior cardiac catheterizations, percutaneous interventions, and cardiac surgery, are necessary before the procedure. The patient should be fasting and an intravenous line should be established. Usually, oral or intravenous sedation should be administered (e.g., benzodizepine). Many laboratories routinely premedicate patients with antihistamines such as diphenhydramine (25 mg intravenous push) to decrease allergic reactions and prolong mild sedation.

CATHETERIZATION PROTOCOL. Each physician should develop an individual routine for performing diagnostic catheterization to ensure efficient acquisition of all pertinent data. The particular technical approach and necessary procedures should be individualized for each patient so that the specific clinical questions can be addressed (Table 6–4). In general, hemodynamic measurements and cardiac output determination should be made before angiography to most accurately reflect basal conditions and to guide angiography. When angiography is performed, the vessel or chamber with most clinical importance should be visualized first, in case an untoward reaction to the contrast media or another complication of the procedure should occur.

Controversy exists regarding whether right heart catheterization should be performed in *all* patients undergoing routine coronary angiography. Some physicians believe that right heart catheterization including screening oximetric analysis, measurement of right heart pressures, and determination of cardiac output should be performed in every patient because the risks are limited and potential benefits exist (uncovering an unsuspected problem). A prospective study evaluated 200 patients undergoing left heart catheterization for suspected coronary artery disease in whom data from right heart catheterization were not considered necessary for clinical management before the procedure.[54] The right heart catheterization took approximately 6 additional minutes of procedure time and 86 seconds of fluoroscopy time. Management was altered in only 1.5 per cent of patients as a result of the data obtained by right heart catheterization. While routine right heart catheterization does not appear necessary for patients undergoing routine coronary angiography, it is clearly indicated when the clinical question cannot be answered by isolated left heart catheterization or when there is left ventricular dysfunction, congestive heart failure, complicated acute myocardial infarction, valvular disease, suspected pulmonary hypertension, congenital anomaly, or pericardial disease.[39]

While the use of a temporary pacemaker is not indicated for routine cardiac catheterization, operators should understand the techniques for proper insertion and setting of the pacemaker if needed (Chap. 24). Even in patients with isolated left bundle branch block, right heart catheterization

TABLE 6–4 CATHETERIZATION PROTOCOL

CLINICAL ISSUE	LHC	RHC	CORO	LV	AO	RV	PA	BX	PROVO	IABP	PTCA
Known or suspected coronary artery disease											
stable angina	✓		✓	✓							
positive stress test	✓		✓	✓							
preoperative evaluation	✓		✓	✓							
atypical chest pain	✓		✓	✓					±		
unstable or new-onset angina	✓		✓	✓							±
acute myocardial infarction	✓	✓	✓	±						±	±
failed thrombolysis	✓	✓	✓	±						±	±
post-infarction angina	✓		✓	±						±	±
cardiogenic shock	✓	✓	✓	±						±	±
mechanical complications	✓	✓	✓	✓						±	±
sudden cardiac death	✓	✓	✓	✓							
Valvular heart disease	✓	✓	✓	✓	✓						
Myocardial disease	✓	✓	✓	✓	✓			±			
Pericardial disease	✓	✓	✓	✓							
Congenital heart disease	✓	✓	✓	✓	±	±	±				
Aortic dissection	✓	±	✓	±	✓						
Pulmonary disease	✓	✓	✓	✓		±	±				

AO, aortogram; BX, biopsy; CORO, coronary angiography; IABP, intra-aortic balloon pump; LHC, left heart catheterization, including measurement of left ventricular end-diastolic pressure and aortic valve gradient; LV, left ventriculography; PA, pulmonary angiography or wedge pulmonary angiography; PROVO, provocative challenge (i.e., ergot alkaloids, acetylcholine); PTCA, percutaneous transluminal coronary angioplasty; RHC, right heart catheterization including pressure measurement, determination of cardiac output, oximetric analysis; RV, right ventriculography; ✓, appropriate; ±, may be appropriate in certain clinical circumstances.

can generally be performed safely with balloon flotation catheters without causing additional conduction disturbance.

CATHETERS AND ASSOCIATED EQUIPMENT. Physicians performing cardiac catheterization should be familiar with technical aspects of the equipment used during the procedure.[55] Catheters used for cardiac catheterization come in various lengths, sizes, and shapes. Typical catheter lengths vary between 50 and 125 centimeters, with 100 centimeters being the most commonly used length for adult left heart catheterization via the femoral approach. The outer diameter of the catheter is specified using French units where one French unit (F) = 0.33 mm. The inner diameter of the catheter is smaller than the outside diameter due to the thickness of the catheter material. Guidewires used during the procedure must be small enough to pass through the inner diameter of both the introducer needle and the catheter. Guidewires are described by their length in centimeters, diameter in inches, and tip conformation. A commonly used wire is a 150-cm, 0.035-inch J-tipped wire. The introducer sheaths are specified by the French number of the largest catheter that will pass freely through the inner diameter of the sheath, rather than its outer diameter. Therefore, a No. 7F introducer sheath will accept a 7F catheter but will have an outer diameter of more than 7F or 2.31 mm.

The choice of the size of the catheters to be used is made by balancing the need to opacify the coronary arteries and cardiac chambers adequately, to have adequate catheter manipulation, to limit vascular complications, and to permit early ambulation. While the larger catheters (7F and 8F) allow greater catheter manipulation and excellent visualization, the smaller catheters (5F and 6F) permit earlier ambulation after catheterization. Catheter technology has advanced such that 5 French systems may be used for routine angiography without significant compromise of angiographic quality.[56] Use of the smaller-sized catheters requires greater technical skill of manipulation in order to achieve adequate angiography and thus may be less appropriate for the training of students of catheterization. The 6F diagnostic catheter is most widely used for routine angiography as this size catheter appears to most appropriately balance the needs outlined above. The relationship between sheath size and vascular complications is not clear. Rather, anticoagulation status and operator experience are more important factors related to vascular complications.[57]

Techniques

Right Heart Catheterization

Right heart catheterization allows for measurement and analysis of right heart, pulmonary artery, and pulmonary capillary wedge pressures, measurement of cardiac output by thermodilution, screening for intracardiac shunts, temporary ventricular pacing, assessment of arrhythmias, and pulmonary wedge angiography.[58] Right heart catheterization is performed antegrade through either the inferior or superior vena cava. Percutaneous entry is achieved via the femoral, subclavian, jugular, or antecubital vein. The anatomy of the major arteries and veins used for cardiac catheterization are shown in Figures 6–2 and 6–3. In the cardiac catheterization laboratory, the femoral venous access is used most often because the Judkins technique of left heart catheterization is performed concurrently. Balloon flotation catheters are the simplest and most widely employed. If thermodilution cardiac outputs are necessary, catheters that contain thermistors, such as Swan-Ganz catheters, should be used. These catheters have balloon tips, proximal and distal ports, and thermistors. Therefore, intracardiac pressures and oxygen saturation to evaluate intracardiac shunts can be obtained. Screening blood samples for oximetric analysis should be obtained from the superior vena cava and the pulmonary artery to evaluate for intracardiac shunts. Cardiac output can also be determined by thermodilution techniques. These catheters are both flexible and flow-directed, but when the femoral approach is employed, fluoroscopic guidance is almost always necessary to cannulate the pulmonary artery and to obtain pulmonary capillary wedge position. While most right heart catheters have a J-shaped curvature distally to facilitate passage from the superior vena cava to the pulmonary artery, a catheter with an S-shaped distal end has been designed for femoral insertion. Although manipulation is limited, the balloon flotation catheters are the safest and most rapid method to obtain right heart pressures and blood samples. Other balloon flotation end hole catheters that are stiffer and therefore allow better manipulation are available for right heart

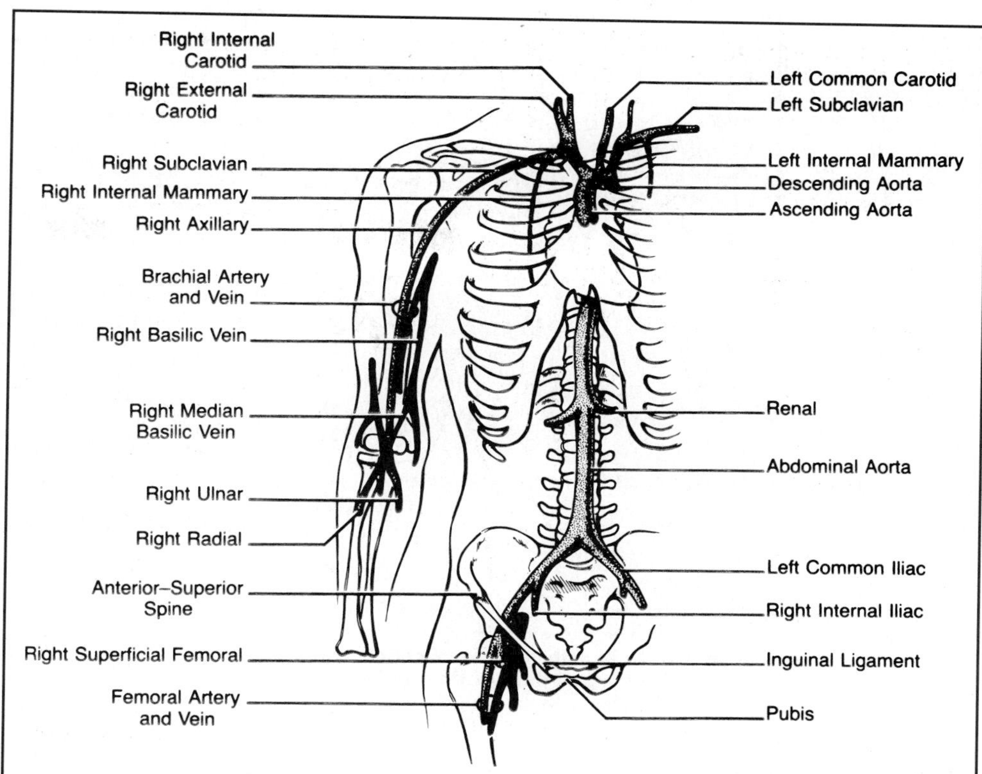

FIGURE 6–2. Principal arteries used for access during cardiac catheterization. Only the superficial veins are shown on the forearm. (Modified from Anthony, C. P.: Textbook of Anatomy and Physiology. 11th ed. St. Louis, C. V. Mosby, 1983. *In* Kern M. J.: The Cardiac Catheterization Handbook. 2nd ed. St. Louis, C. V. Mosby, 1995.)

catheterization. These lack the ability to obtain thermodilution cardiac outputs but yield better pressure fidelity, due to less catheter whip artifact and a larger end hole.

There are two methods to advance a balloon flotation catheter from the femoral vein. On many occasions, the catheter can be advanced directly through the right atrium and across the tricuspid valve. Once in the right ventricle, the catheter is manipulated to point superiorly and directly into the right ventricular outflow tract. This can usually be achieved while the catheter is advanced with slight clockwise rotation. Once in the outflow tract, the balloon tip should allow flotation into the pulmonary artery and wedge positions. When necessary, deep inspiration or cough can facilitate this maneuver and assist in crossing the pulmonic valve. If the catheter continues to point inferiorly toward the right ventricular apex, another technique should be employed, because further advancement can risk perforation of the right ventricular apex.

One such additional technique for performing right heart catheterization with a balloon flotation catheter is shown in Figure 6–4. A loop is formed in the right atrium with the catheter tip directed laterally. The loop can be created by hooking the catheter tip on the hepatic vein or by advancing the catheter while it is directed laterally in the right atrium. Once the loop is formed, the catheter should be advanced further; this will direct the tip inferiorly and then medially across the tricuspid valve. Antegrade blood flow should then direct the catheter into the pulmonary artery. After the catheter is placed into the wedge position, the redundant loop should be removed by slow withdrawal.

When an end hole catheter that does not have a balloon tip is used, the technique for cannulating the pulmonary artery is markedly different. Manipulation and torquing of the nonflotation catheter are necessary to advance into the pulmonary artery. The catheter should be directed inferiorly across the tricuspid valve and then superiorly into the right ventricular outflow tract. It is generally recommended to attempt to form a loop in the right atrium before advancement into the right ventricle in order to lessen the risk of perforation. These stiffer catheters can often prolapse into the left atrium with mild pressure against the interatrial septum in patients with a probe-patent foramen ovale. Left atrial position can be verified by the pressure

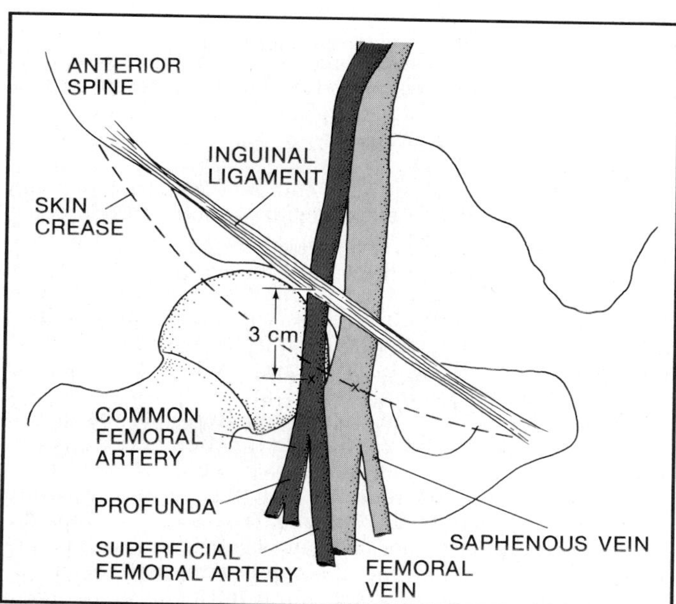

FIGURE 6–3. Anatomy relevant to percutaneous catheterization of femoral artery and vein: the right femoral artery and vein run underneath the inguinal ligament, which connects the anterior-superior iliac spine and pubic tubercle. The arterial skin nick (indicated by X) should be placed approximately 1½ to 2 fingerbreadths (3 cm) below the inguinal ligament and directly over the femoral artery pulsation. The venous skin nick should be placed at the same level, but approximately 1 fingerbreadth medial. (From Baim, D. S., and Grossman, W.: Percutaneous approach. *In* Grossman, W., and Baim, D. S. [eds.]: Cardiac Catheterization, Angiography, and Intervention. 4th ed. Philadelphia, Lea and Febiger, 1991.)

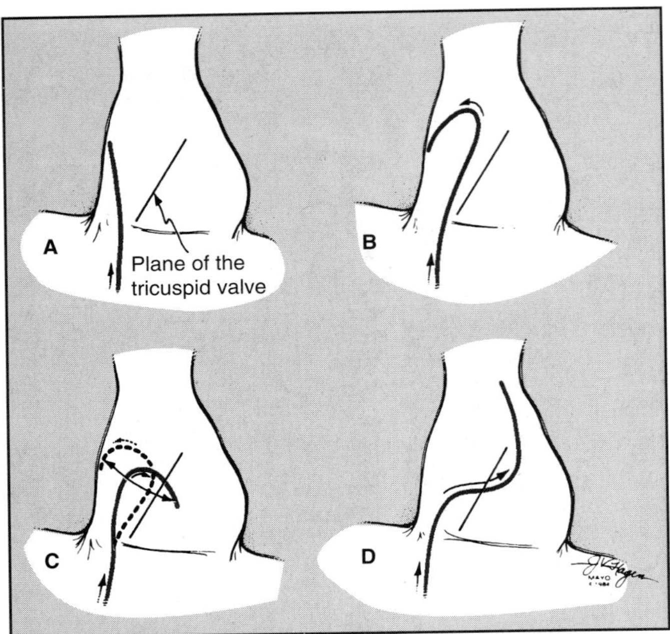

FIGURE 6–4. Technique of right heart catheterization from the femoral approach. *A*, The catheter is advanced through the inferior vena cava. *B*, A loop is created in the catheter by hooking on the hepatic vein or lateral right arterial wall. *C*, Clockwise rotation and advancement of catheter cross the tricuspid valve. *D*, Additional rotation and withdrawal straightens the catheter and directs it superiorly so that it may be advanced through the right ventricular outflow tract. (From Schwartz, R. S., et al.: Cardiac catheterization and angiography. *In* Giuliani, E. R., Fuster, V., Gersh, B. J., McGoon, M. D., and McGoon, D. C. [eds.]: Cardiology Fundamentals and Practice. 2nd ed. St. Louis, C. V. Mosby, 1991. By permission of Mayo Foundation.)

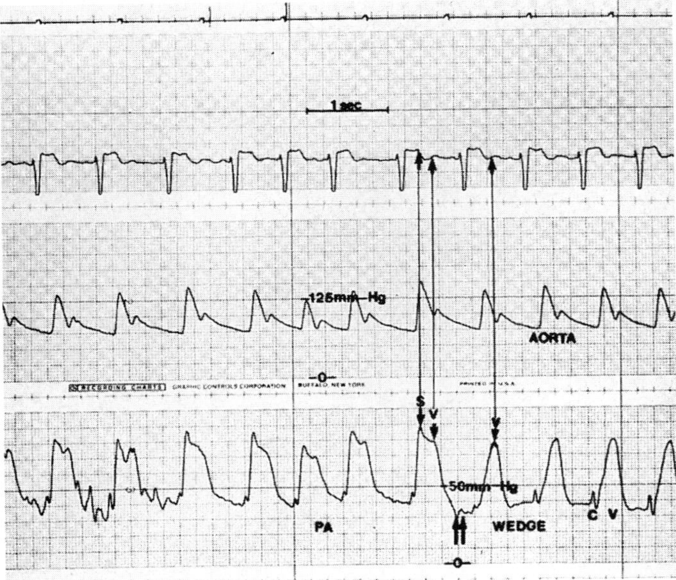

FIGURE 6–5. Arterial, pulmonary artery (PA) and pulmonary capillary wedge waveforms in a patient with acute mitral regurgitation. A prominent *v* wave is present in both the pulmonary artery and wedge tracings. The *v* wave occurs after the ECG T wave. Inflation of the balloon of the right heart catheter (double arrows) obliterates the pulmonary artery systolic (*s*) wave when the catheter wedges. The large *v* wave can cause the wedge to be mistaken for the PA tracing if the difference in timing between the *s* and *v* waves is not noticed. (From Sharkey, S. W.: Beyond the wedge: Clinical physiology and the Swan-Ganz catheter. Am. J. Med. *83:*115, 1987.)

waveform, by blood samples demonstrating arterial saturation, or by hand contrast injection.

The most common complications of right heart catheterization are nonsustained atrial and ventricular arrhythmias. Major complications associated with right heart catheterization are infrequent. These include pulmonary infarction, pulmonary artery or right ventricular perforation, and infection. Pulmonary artery rupture can be avoided by the combined use of fluoroscopic guidance and constant evaluation of the pressure waveform. Confusion as to the location of the distal end of the catheter may arise in the setting of large *v* waves in the pulmonary capillary wedge pressure tracing, which the operator may mistake for a pulmonary artery waveform. Careful attention to the timing of the peak pulmonary artery systolic pressure and the *v* wave with respect to the ECG along with the use of fluoroscopy will prevent inadvertent inflation of the balloon in the wedged position, which can cause pulmonary artery rupture (Fig. 6–5).

Left Heart Catheterization and Coronary Arteriography

THE JUDKINS TECHNIQUE. Because of its relative ease, speed, reliability, and low complication rate,[20] the Judkins technique[8] has become the most widely used method of left heart catheterization and coronary arteriography in the United States. After local anesthesia with 1 per cent lidocaine (Xylocaine), percutaneous entry of the femoral artery is achieved by puncturing the vessel 1 to 3 cm (or 1 to 2 fingerbreadths) below the inguinal ligament. The ligament can be palpated as it courses from the anterior superior iliac spine to the superior pubic ramus. It should be used as the landmark and not the inguinal crease; use of this crease is misleading. A transverse skin incision is made over the femoral artery with a scapel. Using a modified Seldinger technique (Fig. 6–6), an 18-gauge thin-walled needle (Fig. 6–7) is inserted at a 30- to 45-degree angle into the femoral artery, and a 0.035- or 0.038-inch J-tip Teflon-coated guidewire is advanced through the needle into the artery. The wire should pass freely up the aorta. After obtaining arterial access, a sheath at least equal in size to the coronary catheter is usually inserted into the femoral artery. It is generally recommended that the patient receive 3000 to 5000 units of heparin after access is obtained. The technique of coronary arteriography using this approach is described on p. 249.

Left ventricular systolic and end-diastolic pressures can be obtained by advancing a pigtail catheter into the left ventricle (Fig. 6–8). In assessing valvular aortic stenosis, left ventricular and aortic pressures should be recorded simultaneously. In suspected mitral stenosis, left ventricular and wedge or left atrial pressures should be obtained simultaneously. Left ventriculography is performed in the 30-degree RAO and 45- to 50-degree LAO views. A pigtail catheter is most commonly used for this purpose. Power injection of 30 to 50 ml of contrast medium into the ventricle is used to assess left ventricular function and the severity of mitral regurgitation. After ventriculography, pressure measurements may be repeated and the systolic pressure should be recorded as the catheter is withdrawn from the left ventricle into the aorta. If an aortic transvalvular gradient is present, recording these pressures will detect it. For measurement of suspected intraventricular gradients, a multipurpose catheter with an end hole is desirable to localize the gradient in the left ventricle. Pigtail catheters contain side holes, which will obscure the capacity to define whether the gradient is intraventricular or transvalvular.

After coronary arteriography and left heart catheterization have been completed, the catheters are removed and firm pressure is applied to the femoral area for 15 to 20 minutes, either by hand or by a mechanical clamp. The patient should be instructed to lie in bed for several hours, with the leg remaining straight to prevent hematoma formation.

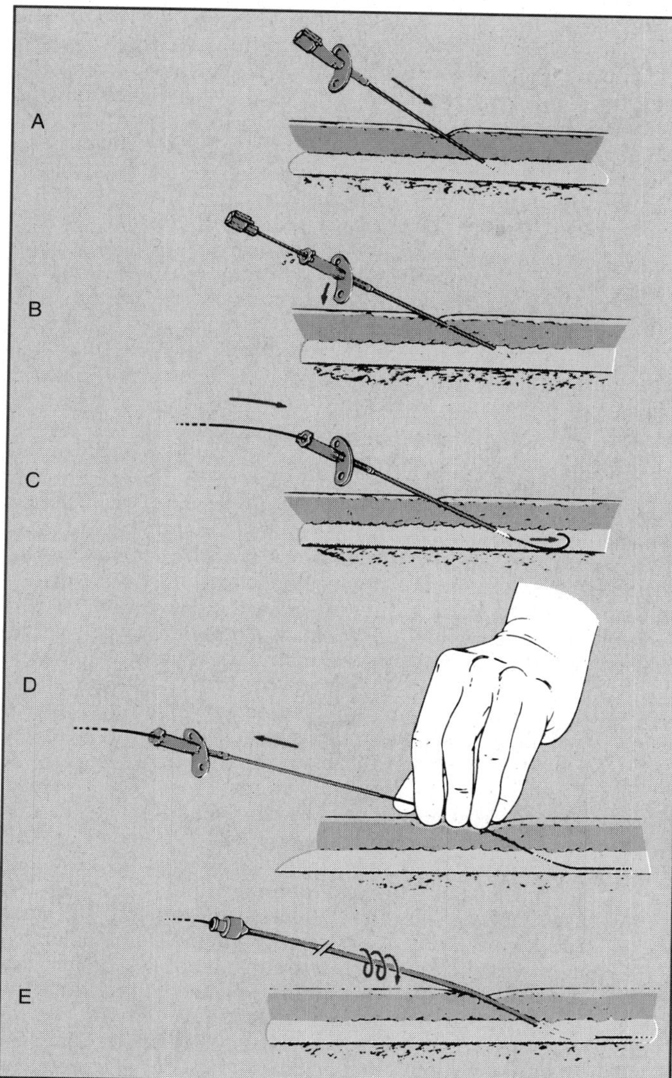

FIGURE 6–6. Basic procedure for the Seldinger technique. *A,* The vessel is punctured with the needle at a 30- to 40-degree angle. *B,* The stylet is removed and free blood flow is observed; the angle of the needle is then reduced. *C,* The flexible tip of the guidewire is passed through the needle into the vessel. *D,* The needle is removed over the wire while firm pressure is applied at the site. *E,* The tip of the catheter is passed over the wire and advanced into the vessel with a rotating motion. (From Tilkian, A. G., and Dailey, E. K.: Cardiovascular Procedures: Diagnostic Techniques and Therapeutic Procedures. St. Louis, C. V. Mosby, 1986.)

With No. 5F catheters, 2 hours of bed rest is usually sufficient, whereas use of 6F catheters usually involves at least 3 to 4 hours.

The main advantage of the Judkins technique is the speed and ease of selective catheterization. However, these attributes do not preclude the importance of extensive operator experience to ensure quality studies with acceptable safety. The main disadvantage of this technique is its use in patients with ileofemoral atherosclerotic disease in whom retrograde passage of catheters through areas of extreme narrowing or tortuosity may be difficult or impossible.

BRACHIAL ARTERY TECHNIQUE—SONES TECHNIQUE. Sones and colleagues[3] introduced the first technique for coronary artery catheterization by means of a brachial artery cutdown. The Sones technique is still popular in many centers and is described on p. 244.

PERCUTANEOUS BRACHIAL ARTERY TECHNIQUE

A modification of Sones technique is the percutaneous brachial artery technique utilizing pre-formed Judkins catheters. This technique uses the Seldinger method of percutaneous brachial artery entry. A No. 5F or 6F sheath is placed into the brachial artery, and 5000 units of heparin are infused into the side port. A guidewire is then advanced to the ascending aorta under fluoroscopic control. A No. 5F or 6F left, right, and pigtail catheters are passed over the guidewire for routine arteriography and ventriculography. Occasionally the guidewire may be necessary to direct the left coronary catheter into the left sinus of Valsalva and the ostium of the left main coronary artery.

The main advantage of the percutaneous brachial technique is that it avoids a brachial artery cutdown and repair. The main disadvantage is that manipulation of catheters can be difficult. When this tech-

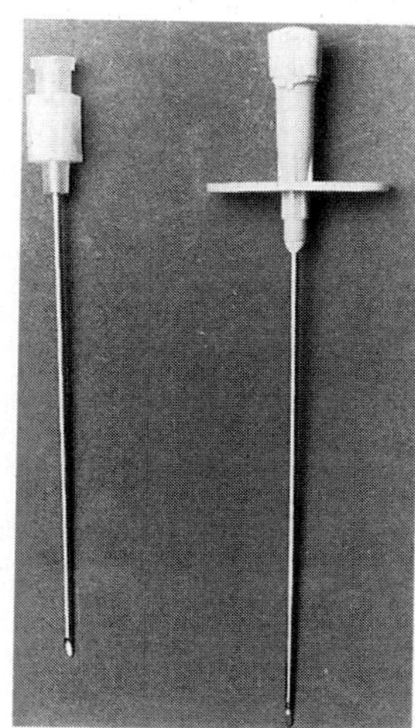

FIGURE 6–7. Two most commonly used needle types for vascular access. On the left, a single-piece, thin-walled "frontwall needle"; on the right, a two-component, thin-walled Seldinger needle. (From MacDonald, R. G.: Catheters, sheaths, guidewires, needles and related equipment. *In* Pepine, C. J., Hill, J. A., and Lambert, C. R. [eds.]: Diagnostic and Therapeutic Cardiac Catheterization. 2nd ed. Baltimore, Williams and Wilkins, 1994, p. 112.)

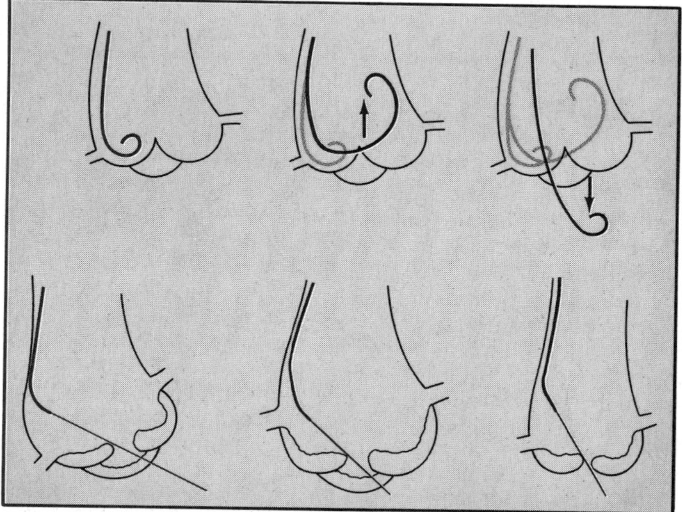

FIGURE 6–8. Technique for retrograde crossing of an aortic valve using a pigtail catheter. The upper row shows the technique for crossing a normal aortic valve. In the bottom row, the use of a straight guidewire and pigtail catheter in combination is shown. Increasing the length of protruding guidewire straightens the catheter curve and causes the wire to point more toward the right coronary ostium; reducing the length of protruding wire restores the pigtail contour and deflects the guidewire tip toward the left coronary artery. Once the correct length of wire and the correct rotational orientation of the catheter have been found, repeated advancement and withdrawal of catheter and guidewire together will allow retrograde passage across the valve. In a dilated aortic root, the angled pigtail catheter is preferable. In a small aortic root (bottom row, right) a right coronary Judkins catheter may have advantages. (From Baim, D. S., and Grossman, W.: Percutaneous approach. *In* Grossman, W., and Baim, D. S. [eds.]: Cardiac Catheterization, Angiography, and Intervention. 4th ed. Philadelphia, Lea and Febiger, 1991.)

nique was compared with the femoral technique, patient comfort, hemostasis time, and time to ambulation favor the brachial technique, while procedural efficiency, time of radiation exposure, and diagnostic film quality were more favorable with the femoral approach.[59] Complication rates appear similar.

PERCUTANEOUS RADIAL ARTERY TECHNIQUE

Left heart catheterization via the radial artery approach was developed as an alternative to the percutaneous transbrachial approach in an attempt to limit vascular complications.[60] The inherent advantages of the transradial approach are that the hand has a dual arterial supply connected via the palmar arches and that there are no nerves or veins at the site of puncture. In addition, prolonged bedrest is unnecessary after the procedure, thus allowing for more efficient outpatient angiography.

The procedure requires a normal Allen test: Following manual compression of both the radial and ulnar arteries during fist clenching, normal color returns to the opened hand within 10 seconds after releasing pressure over the ulnar artery, and significant reactive hyperemia is absent upon releasing pressure over the radial artery.[61] The arm is abducted and the wrist hyperextended over a gauze roll. Routine skin anesthesia is used, a small incision is made just proximal to the styloid process of the radius, and the subcutaneous tissue is tunneled using a forceps. An 18-gauge needle is introduced at a 45-degree angle and an exchange-length 0.035- or 0.038-inch J-tip guidewire is inserted. A 23-cm long 5F sheath is then introduced. Heparin, 5000 units, is administered through the side arm of the sheath. No. 5F coronary catheters are then advanced over the exchange wire into the ascending aorta. The left coronary artery is intubated using a left 4-cm tip Judkins (JL 4.0), a left Amplatz, or a brachial Castillo type II catheter. The right coronary artery is intubated using a 4-cm right Judkins (JR 4.0), a left Amplatz, or a multipurpose catheter. Left ventriculography can be performed using a multipurpose catheter with side holes or a pigtail catheter. Exchanges are best performed over the guidewire. Hemostasis is obtained at the end of the procedure after sheath removal using digital pressure. It is recommended that the arterial puncture site be allowed to bleed for several beats before maintaining digital pressure. The radial pulse should be monitored regularly for several hours after the procedure.

The potential limitations of this procedure include the inability to cannulate the radial artery owing to its smaller size and propensity to develop spasm, poor visualization of the coronary arteries resulting from the small-caliber catheters with limited manipulation potential, and risk of arterial occlusion caused by dissection or thrombus formation. In addition, when right heart catheterization is required, other approaches are necessary. While there is little debate that the femoral approach is the simplest and probably the safest technique for left heart catheterization, the transradial approach for left heart catheterization could gain in popularity with refinements in technique and equipment.

Transseptal Catheterization

Transseptal left-sided heart catheterization has received renewed interest recently with the growth of percutaneous balloon mitral commissurotomy as a viable option to surgical commissurotomy and with increasing utilization of disc valves in the aortic position. These mechanical prosthetic valves cannot be crossed safely and prohibit retrograde left heart catheterization.

The original technique of transseptal heart catheterization has been well described[4,5,62] and various techniques currently exist. The transseptal catheter is a short, curved catheter with a tapered tip and side holes. One approach is to place a 0.032-inch guidewire via the femoral vein through the right atrium and into the superior vena cava. A Mullins transseptal sheath and dilator are then advanced over the wire into the superior vena cava. The guidewire is removed and replaced with a Brokenbrough needle, and the distal port is connected to a pressure manifold. With the needle tip just proximal to the Mullins sheath tip, the entire catheter system is withdrawn. The catheter is simultaneously rotated from a 12 o'clock to 5 o'clock position. The operator experiences two abrupt rightward movements. The first occurs as the catheter descends from the superior vena cava to the right atrium. The second occurs as the Mullins dilator tip passes over the limbic edge into the fossa ovalis. The curve of the sheath and needle should be oriented slightly anteriorly. The dilator and needle can then be advanced as a unit. Steady pressure often is adequate to advance the system into the left atrium. If not, the needle should be advanced sharply across the interatrial septum, while holding the Mullins sheath.

Left atrial position can be confirmed by the increase in pressure with left atrial *a* and *v* waveforms, hand injection of contrast medium, or measurement of arterial oxygen saturation. Once position is confirmed, the dilator and sheath can be safely advanced 2 to 3 cm into the left atrium. The sheath is held firmly and the dilator and needle are removed. Left atrial pressure measurements may then be repeated. If measurement of left ventricular pressure and/or left ventriculography is necessary, the catheter can usually be advanced easily into the left ventricle after slight counterclockwise rotation. The risk of major morbidity with skilled operators should be less than 2 per cent.[63] The major risk of transseptal catheterization lies in inadvertent puncture of atrial structures, such as the atrial free wall or coronary sinus, or entry into the aortic root or pulmonary artery.

Direct Transthoracic Left Ventricular Puncture

The sole indication for direct left ventricular puncture is to measure left ventricular pressure and to perform ventriculography in patients with mechanical prosthetic valves in both the mitral and aortic positions, thus preventing retrograde arterial and transseptal catheterization. Crossing tilting disc valves with catheters should be avoided as this may result in catheter entrapment, occlusion of the valve, or possible dislodgment of the disc with embolization. The procedure is performed after localizing the left ventricular apex via palpation or preferably using echocardiography.[64] After local anesthesia is administered, a 3½-inch-long 18-gauge needle is inserted at the upper rib margin and directed slightly posteriorly and toward the right shoulder. An 0.035-inch J-tip guidewire is introduced into the ventricle under fluoroscopic guidance, followed by a No. 4F dilator and then a 4F pigtail catheter.[65] The risks of this procedure include cardiac tamponade, hemothorax, pneumothorax, laceration of the left anterior descending coronary artery, embolism of left ventricular thrombus, vagal reactions, and ventricular arrhythmias. The risk of pericardial tamponade, however, is limited in patients who have undergone prior cardiac surgery because mediastinal fibrosis will be present. With the advent of transesophageal echocardiography, this procedure is now infrequently performed.

Endomyocardial Biopsy

Endomyocardial biopsy can be performed using a variety of bioptomes (Fig. 6–9). The most common devices in use as of this writing include the stiff-shaft Caves-Schulz Stanford bioptome[66,67] and the floppy-shaft King's bioptome.[68,69] Right ventricular biopsy may be performed using the internal jugular vein,[67,70] the subclavian vein,[71] or the femoral vein.[72] Left ventricular biopsy may be performed using the femoral arterial approach.[69]

For performing right ventricular biopsy via the right internal jugular vein, a No. 7–9F sheath is introduced using the usual Seldinger technique. A No. 7–9F bioptome is advanced under fluoroscopic guidance to the lateral wall of the right atrium. Using counterclockwise rotation, the device is advanced across the tricuspid valve and toward the interventricular septum. Position of the bioptome against the interventricular septum is confirmed using 30-degree right anterior oblique and 60-degree left anterior oblique fluoroscopic projections. Alternatively, two-dimensional echocardiography has been used to guide the position of the bioptome with good results.[73] Contact with the myocardium is confirmed by the presence of premature ventricular contractions, lack of further advancement, and transmission of ventricular impulse to the operator. The bioptome is then withdrawn from the septum slightly, the forceps jaws are opened, the bioptome is readvanced to contact the myocardium, and the forceps is closed. A slight tug is felt upon removal of the device. Approximately four to six samples of myocardium are required

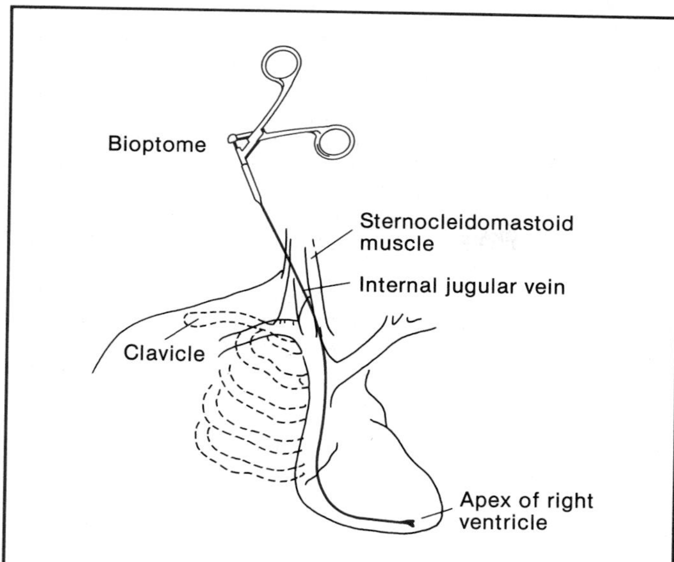

FIGURE 6–9. Endomyocardial biopsy. The bioptome is introduced by way of the right internal jugular vein and is passed across the tricuspid valve into the right ventricle. With the bioptome, a small segment of right ventricular endocardium is removed from the interventricular septum for microscopic examination. (From Mason, J. W., et al.: Myocardial biopsy. *In* Willerson, J. T., and Sanders, C. A. [eds.]: Clinical Cardiology. New York, Grune and Stratton, 1977.)

for adequate pathological analysis. Consultation with a pathologist should be obtained to ensure appropriate specimen collection and processing.

Right or left ventricular biopsy from the femoral vein or artery requires insertion of a long No. 6F or 7F sheath directed toward the portion of the ventricle to be sampled. The sheath used for right ventricular biopsy has a 45-degree angle on its distal end to allow for easier access to the right ventricle. An angled pigtail catheter and long guidewire system are used to enter the right ventricle. The sheath is then advanced over the pigtail catheter into the right ventricle, the catheter is withdrawn, the sheath is flushed, and pressure is measured. The bioptome is advanced through the sheath as flush solution is being continuously infused through the sheath. Samples of myocardium are taken in a manner similar to that described above. If left ventricular biopsy is to be performed, the biopsy sheath is generally positioned over a multipurpose or pigtail catheter which has been positioned in the ventricle. The sheath is advanced below the mitral apparatus and away from the posterobasal wall. The catheter is then withdrawn and either a long King's bioptome or the Stanford left ventricular bioptome is inserted. Care must be taken when left ventricular biopsy is performed to prevent air embolism while introducing the bioptome into the sheath. A constant infusion of flush solution through the sheath minimizes the risk of air or thrombus embolism.

Complications of endomyocardial biopsy include cardiac perforation with cardiac tamponade, emboli (air, tissue, or thromboembolus), arrhythmias, electrical conduction disturbances, injury to heart valves, vasovagal reactions, and pneumothorax.[74] The overall complication rate is between 1 and 2 per cent, with the risk of cardiac perforation with tamponade generally reported in less than 0.05 per cent.[75] Systemic embolization and ventricular arrhythmias are more common with left ventricular biopsy. Left ventricular biopsy should generally be avoided in patients with right bundle branch block because of the potential for developing complete atrioventricular block, and in patients with known left ventricular thrombus.

The indications for endomyocardial biopsy remain controversial.[76–78] Generally, there is agreement that endomyocardial biopsy is indicated to monitor cardiac allograft rejection and may also be useful to monitor for anthracycline cardiotoxicity.[76] However, considerable controversy persists regarding endomyocardial biopsy to evaluate the cause of dilated cardiomopathy.[78,79] Other possible indications for endomyocardial biopsy include differentiation between restrictive and constrictive myopathies,[80,81] determination of whether myocarditis is the cause of ventricular arrhythmias,[76,78] and assessment of patients with left ventricular dysfunction associated with human immunodeficiency virus infection.[82–84]

Percutaneous Intraaortic Balloon Pump Insertion

The intraaortic balloon counterpulsation devices available for adult usage are positioned in the descending thoracic aorta. They have a balloon volume of 30 to 50 ml, use helium as the inflation gas, and are timed to inflate during diastole and deflate during systole. Details of the technique of balloon insertion have been well described.[85] Briefly, the device is inserted via the femoral artery using the standard Seldinger technique. The device is placed such that the tip is just below the level of the left subclavian artery. Optimal positioning requires fluoroscopic guidance. Timing of the balloon is adjusted during 1:2 pumping such that inflation of the balloon will occur at the aortic dicrotic notch and deflation will occur immediately before systole to ensure maximal augmentation of diastolic flow and maximal systolic unloading.

Favorable hemodynamic effects include reduction in left ventricular afterload and improvement in myocardial oxygenation.[86,87] Therefore, intraaortic balloon pump (IABP) insertion is indicated for patients with angina refractory to medical therapy, cardiogenic shock, mechanical complications of myocardial infarction (including severe mitral regurgitation, ventricular septal defect), or those with severe left main coronary artery stenosis who will be undergoing cardiac surgery. IABP may also be valuable in patients undergoing high-risk angioplasty and after primary angioplasty in the setting of acute myocardial infarction.[88–90] IABP insertion is contraindicated in patients with moderate or severe aortic insufficiency, aortic dissection, aortic aneurysm, patent ductus arteriosus, severe peripheral vascular disease, bleeding disorders, or sepsis.

Complications of IABP insertion include limb ischemia requiring early balloon removal or vascular surgery, balloon rupture, balloon entrapment, hematomas, and sepsis.[91–93] The incidence of vascular complications ranges from 12 per cent[92] to over 40 per cent.[91] Most patients who develop limb ischemia after insertion of a balloon pump device have resolution of the ischemia upon balloon removal and do not require surgical intervention (thrombectomy, vascular repair, fasciotomy, or amputation). The risk of limb ischemia is heightened in patients with diabetes or peripheral vascular disease, in women, and in patients with a postinsertion ankle-brachial index of less than 0.8.[91] With the development of smaller size catheters (No. 8.5F to 9.5F) and the advent of the sheathless insertion techniques, vascular complications have been reduced.[93,94]

HEMODYNAMIC DATA

The hemodynamic component of the cardiac catheterization procedure focuses on pressure measurements, the measurement of flow (cardiac output, shunt flows, flow across a stenotic orifice, regurgitant flows, coronary blood flow, and so on), and the determination of vascular resistances. Simply stated, flow through a blood vessel is determined by the pressure difference within the vessel and the vascular resistance as described by Ohm's law: $Q = \Delta P/R$.

Pressure Measurements

The accurate recording of pressure waveforms and the correct interpretation of physiological data derived from these waveforms is a major goal of cardiac catheterization. A pressure wave is the cyclical force generated by cardiac muscle contraction, and its amplitude and duration are influenced by various mechanical and physiological parameters. The pressure waveform from a particular cardiac chamber is influenced by the force of the contracting chamber and its surrounding structures including the contiguous chambers of the heart, the pericardium, the lungs, and the vasculature. Physiological variables of heart rate and the respiratory cycle also influence the pressure waveform. An understanding of the various components of the cardiac cycle is essential to the correct interpretation of hemodynamic data obtained in the catheterization laboratory (Fig. 12–22).

PRESSURE MEASUREMENT SYSTEMS. Intravascular pressures are typically measured using a fluid-filled catheter that is attached to a pressure transducer. The pressure wave is transmitted from the catheter tip to the transducer by the fluid column within the catheter. The majority of pressure transducers used currently are disposable electrical strain-gauges. The pressure wave distorts the diaphragm or wire within the transducer. This energy is then converted to an electric signal proportional to the pressure being applied using the principle of the Wheatstone bridge. This signal is then amplified and recorded as an analog signal.[95]

There are a number of sources of error when pressures are measured using a fluid-filled catheter/transducer system.[96] Distortion of the output signal occurs as a result of the frequency response characteristics and damping characteristics of the system. The frequency response of the system is the ratio of the output amplitude to input amplitude over a range of frequencies of the input pressure wave. The natural frequency is the frequency that the system oscillates when it is shock-excited in the absence of friction. If the energy of the system is dissipated, such as by friction, this is called *damping.* In order to ensure a high-frequency response range, the pressure measurement system should have the highest possible natural frequency and optimal damping. Optimal damping dissipates the energy gradually, thus maintaining the frequency response curve as close to an output/input ratio of 1 as it approaches the system's natural frequency. This is achieved by using a short wide-bore, noncompliant catheter/tubing system that is directly connected to the transducer using a low-density liquid from which all air bubbles have been removed.[95]

The pressure transducer must be calibrated against a known pressure, and the establishment of a zero reference must be undertaken at the start of the catheterization procedure. In order to "zero" the transducer, the tranducer is placed at the level of the heart, which is approximately midchest. If the transducer is attached to the manifold and is therefore at variable positions during the procedure, a second fluid-filled catheter system should be attached to the transducer and positioned at the level of the heart. All transducers being used during the procedure should be zeroed and calibrated simultaneously.

Other sources of error include catheter whip artifact (motion of the tip of the catheter within the measured chamber), end pressure artifact (an end hole catheter measures an artificially elevated pressure on account of streaming or high velocity of the pressure wave), catheter impact artifact (when the catheter is impacted by the walls or valves of the cardiac chambers), and catheter tip obstruction within small vessels or valvular orifices occurring because of the size of the catheter itself. The operator must be aware of the many sources of potential error, and when there is a discrepancy between the observed data and the clinical scenario, the system should be examined for errors or artifacts.

Use of micromanometer catheters, which have the pressure transducer mounted at their catheter tip, greatly reduces many of these errors in measurement. However, their utility is limited by the additional cost and time to properly calibrate and utilize the system. These catheters have higher natural frequencies and more optimal damping characteristics because the interposing fluid column is eliminated. In addition, there is a decrease in catheter whip artifact. The pressure waveform is less distorted and is without the 30- to 40-millisecond delay seen in the fluid-filled catheter/transducer system. Commercially available high-fidelity micromanometer systems (Millar Instruments, Houston, TX) have both an end hole and side holes to allow for an over-the-wire insertion into the circulation while also permitting angiography. Catheters that have two transducers separated by a short distance are useful for accurate measurement of gradients across valvular structures and within ventricular chambers. The micromanometer system has been used for research purposes to measure the rate of ventricular pressure rise (dP/dt), wall stress, the rate of ventricular pressure decay (− dP/dt), and the time constant of relaxation, and to determine ventricular pressure-volume relationships.[97]

There are several disadvantages of the micromanometer catheter systems including their expense and fragility and the need for sterilization between usage. In addition, the zero level of these systems may drift after the pressure is zeroed to the fluid-filled lumen within the catheter.

Normal Pressure Waveforms

An understanding of the normal pressure waveform morphologies is necessary to comprehend the abnormalities that characterize certain pathological conditions. Normal pressures in the cardiac chambers and great vessels are given in Table 6–5. Simply stated, whenever fluid is added

TABLE 6–5 NORMAL PRESSURES AND VASCULAR RESISTANCES

PRESSURES	AVERAGE (mm Hg)	RANGE (mm Hg)
Right atrium		
a wave	6	2–7
v wave	5	2–7
mean	3	1–5
Right ventricle		
peak systolic	25	15–30
end-diastolic	4	1–7
Pulmonary artery		
peak systolic	25	15–30
end-diastolic	9	4–12
mean	15	9–19
Pulmonary capillary wedge		
mean	9	4–12
Left atrium		
a wave	10	4–16
v wave	12	6–21
mean	8	2–12
Left ventricle		
peak systolic	130	90–140
end-diastolic	8	5–12
Central aorta		
peak systolic	130	90–140
end-diastolic	70	60–90
mean	85	70–105
VASCULAR RESISTANCES	**MEAN ($dyne\text{-}sec\text{-}cm^{-5}$)**	**RANGE ($dyne\text{-}sec\text{-}cm^{-5}$)**
Systemic vascular resistance	1100	700–1600
Total pulmonary resistance	200	100–300
Pulmonary vascular resistance	70	20–130

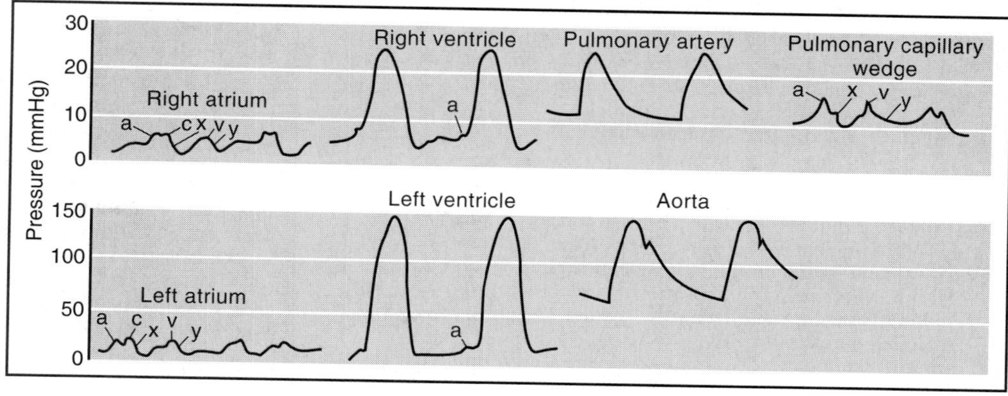

FIGURE 6–10. Normal right and left heart pressures recorded from fluid-filled catheter systems in a human. (From Pepine, C.: Diagnostic and Therapeutic Cardiac Catheterization. Baltimore, Williams and Wilkins, 1989.)

to a chamber or compressed within a chamber, the pressure usually rises; conversely, whenever fluid exits from a chamber or the chamber relaxes, the pressure usually falls. One exception to this rule is the early phase of ventricular diastolic filling when ventricular volume increases after mitral valve opening but ventricular pressure continues to decrease because of active relaxation.[98] Examples of normal pressure waveforms are given in Figure 6–10.

ATRIAL PRESSURE. The *right atrial pressure waveform* has three positive deflections, the *a*, *c*, and *v* waves. The *a* wave is due to atrial systole and follows the P wave of the ECG. The height of the *a* wave depends on atrial contractility and the resistance to right ventricle filling. The *x* descent follows the *a* wave and represents relaxation of the atrium and the downward pulling of the tricuspid annulus by right ventricular contraction. The *x* descent is interrupted by the *c* wave, which is a small positive deflection due to protrusion of the closed tricuspid valve into the right atrium. Pressure in the atrium rises after the *x* descent owing to passive atrial filling. The atrial pressure then peaks as the *v* wave, which represents right ventricular systole. The height of the *v* wave is related to atrial compliance and the amount of blood returning to the atrium from the periphery. The right atrial *v* wave is generally smaller than the *a* wave. The *y* descent occurs after the *v* wave and reflects tricuspid valve opening and right atrial emptying into the right ventricle. During spontaneous respiration, there is a decline in right atrial pressure during inhalation as intrathoracic pressure falls. Right atrial pressure rises during exhalation as intrathoracic pressures increase. The opposite effect is seen when patients are mechanically ventilated.

The *left atrial pressure waveform* is similar to that of the right atrium, although normal left atrial pressure is higher, reflecting the high pressure system of the left side of the heart. In the left atrium, as opposed to the right atrium, the *v* wave is generally higher than the *a* wave. This occurs because the left atrium is constrained posteriorly by the pulmonary veins, while the right atrium can easily decompress throughout the inferior and superior venae cavae. The height of the left atrial *v* wave most accurately reflects left atrial compliance.

PULMONARY CAPILLARY WEDGE PRESSURE. The pulmonary capillary wedge pressure waveform is similar to the left atrial pressure waveform but is slightly damped and delayed as a result of transmission through the lungs. The *a* and *v* waves with both *x* and *y* descents are visible, but *c* waves may not be seen. In the normal state, the pulmonary artery diastolic pressure is similar to the mean pulmonary capillary wedge pressure because the pulmonary circulation has low resistance. In certain disease states that are associated with an elevated pulmonary vascular resistance (hypoxemia, pulmonary embolism, and chronic pulmonary hypertension), and occasionally after mitral valve surgery, the pulmonary capillary wedge pressure may not accurately reflect left atrial pressure. Pulmonary capillary wedge may overestimate true left atrial pressure in this circumstance. Thus, accurate measurement of mitral valve gradient may require obtaining direct left atrial pressure.

VENTRICULAR PRESSURE. Right and left ventricular waveforms are similar in morphology. They differ mainly with respect to their magnitudes, with left ventricular systolic and diastolic pressures being higher. The duration of systole and isovolumic contraction and relaxation are longer, and the ejection period shorter in the left than in the right ventricle. There may be a small ($\leq$5 mm Hg) systolic gradient between the right ventricle and the pulmonary artery. Ventricular diastolic pressure is characterized by an early rapid filling wave during which most of the ventricle fills, a slow-filling phase and the *a* wave denoting atrial systolic activity. End-diastolic pressure is generally measured at the *c* point, which is the rise in ventricular pressure at the onset of isovolumic contraction (Fig. 12–22). When the *c* point is not well seen, a line is drawn from the R wave on the simultaneous ECG to the ventricular pressure waveform, and this is used as the end-diastolic pressure.

GREAT VESSEL PRESSURES. The contour of the *central aortic pressure* and the *pulmonary artery pressure* tracing consists of a systolic wave, the incisura (indicating closure of the semilunar valves), and a gradual decline in pressure until the following systole. The pulse pressure reflects the stroke volume and compliance of the arterial system. The mean aortic pressure more accurately reflects peripheral resistance. As the systemic pressure wave is transmitted through the length of the aorta, the systolic wave increases in amplitude and becomes more triangular in shape, while the diastolic wave decreases until it reaches the midthoracic aorta and then increases. The mean aortic pressures, however, are usually similar, with the mean *peripheral arterial pressure* typically $\leq$5 mm Hg lower than the mean central aortic pressure. The difference in systolic pressures between the central aorta and the periphery (femoral, brachial, or radial arteries) is greatest in younger patients due to their increased vascular compliance. These potential differences between proximal aorta and peripheral artery must be considered in order to measure and interpret the peak systolic pressure gradient between the left ventricle and systemic arterial system in patients with suspected aortic stenosis.

ABNORMAL PRESSURE CHARACTERISTICS. Abnormal pressure waveforms may be diagnostic of specific pathological conditions. Although these conditions are discussed in greater detail elsewhere in this book, Table 6–6 summarizes the more commonly encountered waveforms.

Cardiac Output Measurements

There is no totally accurate method to measure cardiac output, but it can be estimated on the basis of various assumptions. The two most commonly used methods are the Fick method and thermodilution method. For comparison among patients, cardiac output is often corrected for the patient's size based on the body surface area and expressed as cardiac index.

TABLE 6–6 PATHOLOGICAL WAVEFORMS

I. RIGHT ATRIAL PRESSURE WAVEFORMS

A. Low mean atrial pressure
   1. Hypovolemia
   2. Improper zeroing of the transducer
B. Elevated mean atrial pressure
   1. Intravascular volume overload states
   2. Right ventricular failure due to valvular disease (tricuspid or pulmonic stenosis or regurgitation)
   3. Right ventricular failure due to myocardial disease (right ventricular ischemia, cardiomyopathy)
   4. Right ventricular failure due to left heart failure (mitral stenosis/regurgitation, aortic stenosis/regurgitation, cardiomyopathy, ischemia)
   5. Right ventricular failure due to increased pulmonary vascular resistance (pulmonary embolism, chronic obstructive pulmonary disease, primary pulmonary hypertension)
   6. Pericardial effusion with tamponade physiology
   7. Obstructive atrial myxoma
C. Elevated *a* wave (any increase to ventricular filling)
   1. Tricuspid stenosis
   2. Decreased ventricular compliance due to ventricular failure, pulmonic valve stenosis, or pulmonary hypertension
D. Cannon *a* wave
   1. Atrial-ventricular asynchrony (atria contract against a closed tricuspid valve, as during complete heart block, following premature ventricular contraction, during ventricular tachycardia, with ventricular pacemaker)
E. Absent *a* wave
   1. Atrial fibrillation or atrial standstill
   2. Atrial flutter
F. Elevated *v* wave
   1. Tricuspid regurgitation
   2. Right ventricular heart failure
   3. Reduced atrial compliance (restrictive myopathy)
G. *a* wave equal to *v* wave
   1. Tamponade
   2. Constrictive pericardial disease
   3. Hypervolemia
H. Prominent *x* descent
   1. Tamponade
   2. Subacute constriction and possibly chronic constriction
   3. Right ventricular ischemia with preservation of atrial contractility
I. Prominent *y* descent
   1. Constrictive pericarditis
   2. Restrictive myopathies
   3. Tricuspid regurgitation
J. Blunted *x* descent
   1. Atrial fibrillation
   2. Right atrial ischemia
K. Blunted *y* descent
   1. Tamponade
   2. Right ventricular ischemia
   3. Tricuspid stenosis
L. Miscellaneous abnormalities
   1. Kussmaul's sign (inspiratory rise or lack of decline in right atrial pressure): constrictive pericarditis, right ventricular ischemia
   2. Equalization (≤ 5 mm Hg) of mean right atrial, right ventricular diastolic, pulmonary artery diastolic, pulmonary capillary wedge, and pericardial pressures in tamponade
   3. M or W patterns: right ventricular ischemia, pericardial constriction, congestive heart failure
   4 Ventricularization of the right atrial pressure: severe tricuspid regurgitation
   5. Saw tooth pattern: atrial flutter
   6. Dissociation between pressure recording and intracardiac ECG: Ebstein's anomaly

II. LEFT ATRIAL PRESSURE/PULMONARY CAPILLARY WEDGE PRESSURE WAVEFORMS

A. Low mean pressure
   1. Hypovolemia
   2. Improper zeroing of the transducer
B. Elevated mean pressure
   1. Intravascular volume overload states
   2. Left ventricular failure due to valvular disease (mitral or aortic stenosis or regurgitation)
   3. Left ventricular failure due to myocardial disease (ischemia or cardiomyopathy)
   4. Left ventricular failure due to systemic hypertension
   5. Pericardial effusion with tamponade physiology
   6. Obstructive atrial myxoma
C. Elevated *a* wave (any increase to ventricular filling)
   1. Mitral stenosis
   2. Decreased ventricular compliance due to ventricular failure, aortic valve stenosis, or systemic hypertension
D. Cannon *a* wave
   1. Atrial-ventricular asynchrony (atria contract against a closed mitral valve, as during complete heart block, following premature ventricular contraction, during ventricular tachycardia, with ventricular pacemaker)
E. Absent *a* wave
   1. Atrial fibrillation or atrial standstill
   2. Atrial flutter
F. Elevated *v* wave
   1. Mitral regurgitation
   2. Left ventricular heart failure
   3. Ventricular septal defect
G. *a* wave equal to *v* wave
   1. Tamponade
   2. Constrictive pericardial disease
   3. Hypervolemia
H. Prominent *x* descent
   1. Tamponade
   2. Subacute constriction and possibly chronic constriction
I. Prominent *y* descent
   1. Constrictive pericarditis
   2. Restrictive myopathies
   3. Mitral regurgitation
J. Blunted *x* descent
   1. Atrial fibrillation
   2. Atrial ischemia
K. Blunted *y* descent
   1. Tamponade
   2. Ventricular ischemia
   3. Mitral stenosis
L. Pulmonary capillary wedge pressure not equal to left ventricular end-diastolic pressure
   1. Mitral stenosis
   2. Left atrial myxoma
   3. Cor triatriatum
   4. Pulmonary venous obstruction
   5. Decreased ventricular compliance
   6. Increased pleural pressure
   7. Placement of catheter in a nondependent zone of lung

III. PULMONARY ARTERY PRESSURE WAVEFORMS

A. Elevated systolic pressure
   1. Primary pulmonary hypertension
   2. Mitral stenosis or regurgitation
   3. Congestive heart failure
   4. Restrictive myopathies
   5. Significant left to right shunt
   6. Pulmonary disease (pulmonary embolism, hypoxemia, chronic obstructive pulmonary disease)
B. Reduced systolic pressure
   1. Hypovolemia
   2. Pulmonary artery stenosis
   3. Sub- or supravalvular stenosis
   4. Ebstein's anomaly
   5. Tricuspid stenosis
   6. Tricuspid atresia
C. Reduced pulse pressure
   1. Right heart ischemia
   2. Right ventricular infarction
   3. Pulmonary embolism
   4. Tamponade
D. Bifid pulmonary artery waveform
   1. Large left atrial *v* wave transmitted backward (i.e., MR)
E. Pulmonary artery diastolic pressure greater than pulmonary capillary wedge pressure
   1. Pulmonary disease
   2. Pulmonary embolus
   3. Tachycardia

TABLE 6–6 PATHOLOGICAL WAVEFORMS—Continued

IV. VENTRICULAR PRESSURE WAVEFORMS
A. Systolic pressure elevated
1. Pulmonary or systemic hypertension
2. Pulmonary valve or aortic valve stenosis
3. Ventricular outflow tract obstruction
4. Supravalvular obstruction
5. Right ventricular pressure elevation with significant:
a. Atrial septal defect
b. Ventricular septal defect
6. Right ventricular pressure elevation due to factors that increase pulmonary vascular resistance (see factors that increase right atrial pressure)
B. Systolic pressure reduced
1. Hypovolemia
2. Cardiogenic shock
3. Tamponade
C. End-diastolic pressure elevated
1. Hypervolemia
2. Congestive heart failure
3. Diminished compliance
4. Hypertrophy
5. Tamponade
6. Regurgitant valvular disease
7. Pericardial constriction
D. End-diastolic pressure reduced
1. Hypovolemia
2. Tricuspid or mitral stenosis
E. Diminished or absent *a* wave
1. Atrial fibrillation or flutter
2. Tricuspid or mitral stenosis
3. Tricuspid or mitral regurgitation when ventricular compliance is increased
F. Dip and plateau in diastolic pressure wave
1. Constrictive pericarditis
2. Restrictive myopathies
3. Right ventricular ischemia
4. Acute dilatation associated with:
a. Tricuspid regurgitation
b. Mitral regurgitation
G. Left ventricular end-diastolic pressure > right ventricular end-diastolic pressure
1. Restrictive myopathies
V. AORTIC PRESSURE WAVEFORMS
A. Systolic pressure elevated
1. Systemic hypertension
2. Arteriosclerosis
3. Aortic insufficiency
B. Systolic pressure reduced
1. Aortic stenosis
2. Heart failure
3. Hypovolemia
C. Widened pulse pressure
1. Systemic hypertension
2. Aortic insufficiency
3. Significant patent ductus arteriosus
4. Significant ruptures sinus of Valsalva aneurysm
D. Reduced pulse pressure
1. Tamponade
2. Congestive heart failure
3. Cardiogenic shock
4. Aortic stenosis
E. Pulsus bisferiens
1. Aortic insufficiency
2. Obstructive hypertrophic cardiomyopathy
F. Pulsus paradoxus
1. Tamponade
2. Chronic obstructive airway disease
3. Pulmonary embolism
G. Pulsus alternans
1. Congestive heart failure
2. Cardiomyopathy
H. Pulsus parvus et tardus
1. Aortic stenosis
I. Spike and dome configuration
1. Obstructive hypertrophic cardiomyopathy

INDICATOR-DILUTION TECHNIQUES. The indicator-dilution method has been used to measure cardiac output since its introduction by Stewart in 1897 and subsequent modification by Hamilton and associates in 1932. The basic equation, commonly referred to as the Stewart-Hamilton equation, is shown below:

$$\text{Cardiac output (1/min)} = \frac{\text{amount of indicator injected (mg)} \times 60 \text{ sec/min}}{\text{mean indicator concentration (mg/ml)} \times \text{curve duration}}$$

The assumption is made that after the injection of a certain quantity of an indicator into the circulation, the indicator appears and disappears from any downstream point in a manner commensurate with the cardiac output. For example, if the indicator rapidly appears at a specific location downstream and then washes out quickly, the assumption is that the cardiac output is high. Although variation can occur, the site of injection is usually a systemic vein or the right side of the heart, and the sampling site is generally a systemic artery. The normal curve itself has an initial rapid upstroke followed by a slower downstroke and eventual appearance of recirculation of the tracer. In practice, this recirculation creates some uncertainty on the tail of the curve, and assumptions are required to correct for this distortion. Because the indicator concentration declines exponentially in the absence of recirculation, the initial data points from the descending limb are used to extrapolate the remainder of the descending limb. The area under both the ascending and descending limbs is then determined along with the total curve duration. The area of the curve is assumed to be a function of the mean indicator concentration. Both variables can be substituted in the Stewart-Hamilton equation to calculate the cardiac output.

There are several sources of error in this determination. Because the dye is unstable over time and can be affected by light, fresh preparations of indocyanine green dye are necessary. The exact amount of dye must be accurately measured, as it is crucial to the performance of the study. It is generally administered through a tuberculin syringe and injected rapidly as a single bolus. After injection, the indicator must mix well before reaching the sampling site, and the dilution curve must have an exponential decay over time so that extrapolation can be performed. If, for example, there is severe valvular regurgitation or a low cardiac output state in which the washout of the indicator is prolonged and recirculation begins well before an adequate decline in the indicator curve occurs, determinations will be erroneous. Intracardiac shunts may also greatly affect the shape of the curve.

THERMODILUTION TECHNIQUES. Because of the rather tedious and time-consuming nature of the indicator-dilution method, it has been replaced by thermodilution techniques in many laboratories. The development of balloon flotation (e.g., Swan-Ganz) catheters with a proximal port and distal thermistor has greatly expanded the ability to obtain thermodilution cardiac outputs in many clinical settings.

The thermodilution procedure requires the injection of a bolus of liquid (saline or dextrose) into the proximal port of the catheter. The resultant change in temperature in the liquid is measured by a thermistor mounted in the distal end of the catheter. The change in temperature versus time can be plotted in a manner similar to the dye-dilution method described above (in which the indicator is now the cooler liquid). The cardiac output is then calculated using an equation that considers the temperature and specific gravity of the injectate and the temperature and specific gravity of the blood, along with the injectate volume. A calibration factor is also used. The cardiac output is inversely related to the area under a thermodilution curve, plotted as a function of temperature versus time, with a smaller area indicative of a higher cardiac output.

The thermodilution method has several advantages. It obviates the need for withdrawal of blood from an arterial site and is less affected by recirculation. Perhaps its greatest advantage is the rapid display of results using computerized methods. Computers use the washout rate represented by the downslope of the curve to obtain a decay constant to correct the descending limb and compute the cardiac output.

Thermodilution cardiac outputs are susceptible to pitfalls similar to those encountered with indicator-dilution methods using indocyanine green. Because the data represent right-sided heart output, tricuspid regurgitation can be a particular problem as the bolus of saline is subsequently broken up. The thermodilution method tends to overestimate cardiac output in low-output states, because the dissipation of the cooler temperature to the surrounding cardiac structures results in reduction in the total area under the curve, causing a falsely elevated cardiac output value. Other difficulties include fluctuations in blood temperature during respiratory or cardiac cycles and the warming of the temperature of the injectate before its injection into the catheter. Because of these possible limitations, the general practice is to calculate the average of several (usually 3 to 5) cardiac output determinations.

From a practical viewpoint, thermodilution cardiac outputs have become standard practice. Their variability can be relatively large; thus small changes should not be overinterpreted. Practically, cardiac output data can be defined only to within a 15 per cent range.[99]

FICK TECHNIQUE. The Fick principle was first described by Adolph Fick in 1870. It assumes that the rate in which oxygen is consumed is a function of the rate of blood flow times the rate of oxygen pickup by the red blood cells. The basic assumption is that the flow of blood in a given period of time is equal to the amount of substance entering the stream of flow in the same period of time divided by the difference between the concentrations of the substance in the blood upstream and downstream from its point of entry into the circulation[100] (Fig. 6–11). The same number of red blood cells that enter the lung must leave the lung, if no intracardiac shunt is present. Thus, if certain parameters were known (the number of oxygen molecules that were attached to the red blood cells entering the lung, the number of oxygen molecules that were attached to the red blood cells leaving the lung, and the number of oxygen molecules consumed during travel through the lung), then the rate of flow of these red blood cells as they pass through the lung could be determined. This can be expressed in the following terms:

$$\text{Cardiac output (L/min)} = \frac{O_2 \text{ consumption (ml/min)}}{A - VO_2 \text{ difference (vol \%)} \times 10}$$

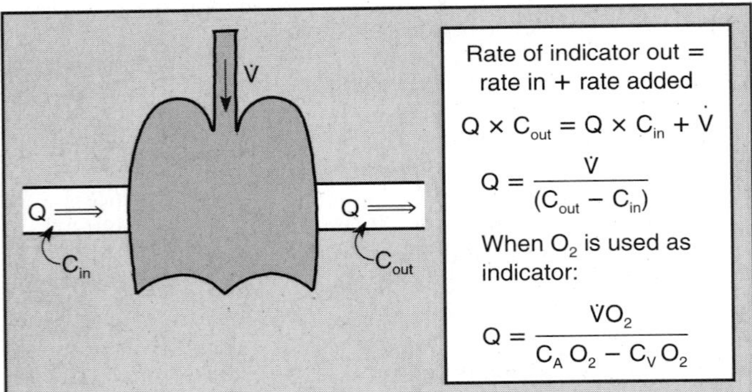

FIGURE 6–11. Schematic illustration of flow measurement using the Fick principle. Fluid containing a known concentration of an indicator (C_{in}) enters a system at flow rate, Q. As the fluid passes through the system, indicator is continuously added at rate $\dot{V}$, raising the concentration in the outflow to C_{out}. In a steady state, the rate of indicator leaving the system (QC_{out}) must equal the rate at which it enters (QC_{in}) plus the rate at which it is added ($\dot{V}$). When oxygen is used as the indicator, cardiac output can be determined by measuring oxygen consumption ($\dot{V}O_2$), arterial oxygen content (C_AO_2), and mixed venous oxygen content (C_VO_2). (From Winniford, M. D., and Lambert, C. R. [eds.]: Blood flow measurement. *In* Pepine, C. J., Hill, J. A., and Lambert, C. R. [eds.]: Diagnostic and Therapeutic Cardiac Catheterization. 2nd ed. Baltimore, Williams and Wilkins, 1994, p. 322.)

Measurements must be done in steady state. Automated methods can accurately determine the oxygen content within the blood samples. Thus, the greatest source of measurement variability is that of the oxygen consumption. Traditional Fick determinations used Van Slyke's method, in which expiratory gas samples were collected in a large bag over a specified period of time. By measuring the oxygen consumption within the bag and by knowing the concentration of oxygen in room air, the quantity of oxygen consumed over time could be determined. Newer techniques now allow for the measurement of oxygen consumption by a polargraphic method in which expired oxygen can be quantified by calculating the change in electrical current between a gold cathode and silver anode embedded in a potassium chloride gel. These devices can be connected to the patient by use of a plastic hood or by a mouthpiece and tubing.

The Fick method suffers primarily from the difficulty in obtaining accurate oxygen consumption measurements and the inability to obtain a steady state under certain conditions. Since the method assumes mean flow over a period of time, it is not suitable during rapid change in flow. It requires considerable time and effort on the part of the catheterization laboratory to obtain the appropriate data. Many laboratories use an "assumed" Fick method in which oxygen consumption index is assumed on the basis of the patient's age, gender, and body surface area or an estimate made (125 ml/m^2) on the basis of body surface area. The advantage of the Fick method is that it is the most accurate method in patients with low cardiac output and thus is preferred over the thermodilution method in these circumstances. It is also independent of the factors that affect curve shape and cause errors in thermodilution cardiac output. The inaccuracy of oxygen consumption measurements results in up to 10 per cent variability in the calculated cardiac output, which may be even greater when assumed oxygen consumption, rather than measured oxygen consumption, is used.

ANGIOGRAPHIC CARDIAC OUTPUT. Angiographic stroke volume can be calculated from tracing the end-diastolic and end-systolic images. Stroke volume is the amount of blood ejected with each beat. End-diastolic volume is the maximum left ventricular volume and occurs immediately before the onset of systole. This occurs immediately after atrial contraction in patients in sinus rhythm. End-systolic volume is the minimum volume during the cardiac cycle. Calibration of the images with calibrated grids or ventricular phantoms is necessary to obtain accurate ventricular volumes. Angiographic cardiac output and stroke volume are derived from the equation:

$$\text{Stroke volume} = \text{EDV} - \text{ESV}$$

$$\text{Cardiac output} = (\text{EDV} - \text{ESV}) \times \text{heart rate}$$

where EDV = end-diastolic volume and ESV = end-systolic volume. The inherent inaccuracies of calibrating angiographic volumes often make this method of measurement unreliable. In cases of valvular regurgitation or atrial fibrillation, angiographic cardiac output will not accurately measure true systemic outputs. However, the angiographic cardiac output is preferred over the Fick or thermodilution outputs for calculation of stenotic valve areas in patients with significant aortic or mitral regurgitation.

DETERMINATION OF VASCULAR RESISTANCE. Vascular resistance calculations are based on hydraulic principles of fluid flow, in which resistance is defined as the ratio of the decrease in pressure between two points in a vascular segment and the blood flow through the segment. Although this straightforward analogy to Ohm's law represents an oversimplification of the complex behavior of pulsatile flow in dynamic and diverse vascular beds, the calculation of vascular resistance based on these principles has proven to be of value in a number of clinical settings.

The determination of the resistance in a vascular bed requires measurement of the mean pressure of the proximal and distal ends of the vascular bed and accurate measurement of cardiac output. For this purpose, measurement of cardiac output by the Fick, the indicator-dilution, or the thermodilution method is preferred. Vascular resistance (R) is usually defined in absolute units (dynes-sec-cm^{-5}) and is defined as R = [mean pressure gradient (dyne/cm^2)]/[mean flow (cm^3/sec)]. Hybrid units (Wood units) are less often used.[101]

Systemic vascular resistance in absolute units is calculated using the equation:

$$SVR = \frac{80(Ao_m - RA_m)}{Q_s}$$

where Ao_m and RA_m are the mean pressures (in mm Hg) in the aorta and right atrium, respectively, and Q_s is the systemic cardiac output (in liters/min). The constant 80 is used to convert units from mm Hg/liters/min (Wood units) to the absolute resistance units dynes-sec-cm^{-5}. If the right atrial pressure is not known, the term RA_m can be dropped, and the resulting value is called the *total peripheral resistance* (TPR).

$$TPR = \frac{80(Ao_m)}{Q_s}$$

Similarly, the pulmonary vascular resistance is derived from the equation:

$$PVR = \frac{80(PA_m - LA_m)}{Q_p}$$

where PA_m and LA_m are the pulmonary artery and left atrial pressures, respectively, and Q_p is the pulmonary blood flow. Mean pulmonary capillary wedge pressure is commonly substituted for mean left atrial pressure if the latter has not been measured directly.[102–104] In the absence of an intracardiac shunt, Q_p is equal to the systemic cardiac output.

Elevated resistances in the systemic and pulmonary circuits may represent reversible abnormalities or may be fixed owing to irreversible anatomical changes. In several clinical situations, such as congestive heart failure, valvular heart disease, primary pulmonary hypertension, and congenital heart disease with intracardiac shunting, determination of whether elevated systemic or pulmonary vascular resistance can be lowered transiently in the catheterization laboratory may provide important insights into potential management strategies. Interventions that may be used in the laboratory for this purpose include the administration of vasodilating drugs (e.g., nifedipine, sodium nitroprusside), exercise, and (in patients with pulmonary hypertension) oxygen inhalation.

Vascular impedance measurements account for blood viscosity, pulsatile flow, reflected waves, and arterial compliance. Hence, vascular impedance has the potential to describe the dynamic relation between pressure and flow more comprehensively than is possible using the simpler calculations of vascular resistance. However, because the simultaneous pressure and flow data required for the calculation of impedance are complex and difficult to obtain, the concept of impedance has failed to gain widespread acceptance, and vascular impedance has not been adopted as a routine clinical index in most laboratories.

Evaluation of Valvular Stenosis

(See also Chap. 32)

Determining the severity of valvular stenosis based on the pressure gradient and flow across the valve is one of the most important aspects of evaluation in the catheterization laboratory of patients with valvular heart disease. In most patients, the magnitude of the pressure gradient alone is sufficient to distinguish clinically significant from insignificant valvular stenosis.

DETERMINATION OF PRESSURE GRADIENTS. In patients with *aortic stenosis* (see p. 1035), the transvalvular pressure gradient should be measured, whenever possible, with a catheter in the left ventricle and another in the proximal aorta. Although it is convenient to measure the gradient between the left ventricle and the femoral artery, downstream augmentation of the pressure signal and delay in pressure transmission between the proximal aorta and femoral artery may alter the pressure waveform substantially and introduce errors into the measured gradient.[105]

Left ventricular–femoral artery pressure gradients may suffice in many patients as an estimate of the severity of aortic stenosis to confirm the presence of a severely stenotic valve. If the side port of the arterial introducing sheath is used to monitor femoral pressure, the inner diameter of the sheath should be 1F size larger than the outer diameter of the catheter being used. The left ventricular–femoral artery gradient should not be relied on in the calculation of valve orifice area in patients with equivocal valve gradients. Thus, measurements obtained with two catheters, one positioned in the body of the left ventricle and the other in the proximal aorta, or in a careful single catheter pullback from left ventricle to aorta, are preferable to simultaneous measurement of left ventricular and femoral artery pressures. Alternatively, a single catheter with distal and proximal lumens, or a micromanometer catheter with distal and proximal transducers, may be used for simultaneous measurement of left ventricular pressure and central aortic pressure.

In patients with very severe aortic stenosis, the left ventricular catheter itself may reduce the effective orifice area, resulting in an artifactual increase in the measured pressure gradient.[106] This overestimation of the severity of aortic stenosis is rarely an important issue, as the diagnosis of severe aortic stenosis is usually already apparent in such patients.

The mean pressure gradient across the aortic valve is determined by planimetry of the area separating the left ventricular and aortic pressures using multiple beats (Fig. 6–12), and it is this gradient that is applied to calculation of the valve orifice area. The peak-to-peak gradient, measured as the difference between peak left ventricular pressure and peak aortic pressure, is commonly used to quantify the valve gradient, because this measurement is rapidly obtained and can be estimated visually. However, there is no physiological basis for the peak-to-peak gradient, since the maximum left ventricular and aortic pressures rarely occur simultaneously. The peak-to-peak gradient measured in the catheterization laboratory is generally lower than the peak instantaneous gradient measured in the echocardiography laboratory. This is because the peak instantaneous gradient represents the maximum pressure difference between the left ventricle and aorta when measured simultaneously. This occurs on the upslope of the aortic pressure tracing (Fig. 6–12). Therefore, apparent disparities between cardiac catheterization and echocardiographic measures of peak gradient occur because cardiac catheterization uses peak-to-peak gradient determinations, whereas Doppler echocardiography reports peak instantaneous gradient. Mean aortic transvalvular gradient and aortic valve area are well correlated with both techniques (r = 0.86 – 0.90 and r = 0.88 – 0.95, respectively).[107]

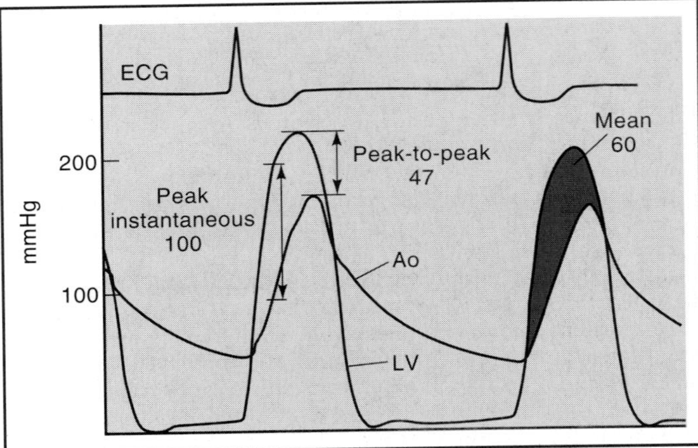

FIGURE 6–12. Various methods of describing an aortic transvalvular gradient. The peak-to-peak gradient (47 mm Hg) is the difference between the maximal pressure in the aorta (Ao) and the maximal left ventricle (LV) pressure. The peak instantaneous gradient (100 mm Hg) is the maximal pressure difference between the Ao and LV when the pressures are measured in the same moment (usually during early systole). The mean gradient *(shaded area)* is the integral of the pressure difference between the LV and Ao during systole (60 mm Hg). (From Bashore, T. M.: Invasive Cardiology: Principles and Techniques. Philadelphia, B. C. Decker Inc., 1990.)

In patients with *mitral stenosis* (see p. 1007), the most accurate means of determining mitral valve gradient is the measurement of left atrial pressure using the transseptal technique with simultaneous measurement of left ventricular pressure and with planimetry of the area bounded by the left ventricular and left atrial pressures in diastole using multiple cardiac cycles (Fig. 6–13). In most laboratories, the pulmonary capillary wedge pressure is substituted for the left atrial pressure, as the pulmonary wedge pressure is more readily obtained. The pulmonary wedge pressure tracing must be realigned with the left ventricular tracing for accurate mean gradient determination. Although it has been generally accepted that pulmonary capillary wedge pressure is a satisfactory estimate of left atrial pressure,[102–104] other studies indicate that the pulmonary wedge pressure may systematically overestimate the left atrial pressure by 2 to 3 mm Hg (up to 53 per cent), thereby increasing the measured mitral valve gradient.[108,109] In addition, accurate wedge tracings may be difficult to obtain in patients with mitral stenosis because of pulmonary hypertension or dilated right-sided heart chambers. Improperly wedged catheters, resulting in damped pulmonary artery pressure recordings, will further overestimate the severity of mitral stenosis. If there is doubt about the accurate position of the catheter in the wedge position, the position can be confirmed by slow withdrawal of blood for oximetric analysis. An oxygen saturation equal to that of the systemic circulation confirms the wedge position.

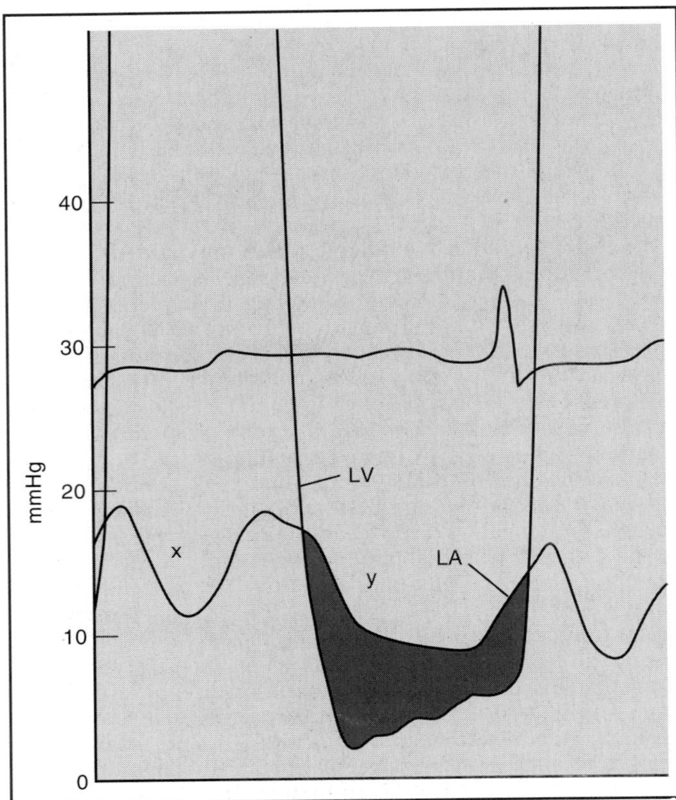

FIGURE 6–13. Pressure gradient in a patient with mitral stenosis. The pressure in the left atrium (LA) exceeds the pressure in the left ventricle (LV) during diastole, producing a diastolic pressure gradient *(shaded area).* (From Bashore, T. M.: Invasive Cardiology: Principles and Techniques. Philadelphia, B. C. Decker Inc., 1990.)

In *pulmonic stenosis,* the valve gradient is usually obtained by a catheter pullback from the pulmonary artery to the right ventricle, although multilumen catheters are available for simultaneous pressure recordings. Tricuspid valve gradients should be assessed with simultaneous recording of right atrial and right ventricular pressures.

CALCULATION OF STENOTIC VALVE ORIFICE AREAS. The stenotic orifice area is determined from the pressure gradient and cardiac output using the formula developed by Gorlin and Gorlin from the fundamental hydraulic relationships linking the area of an orifice to the flow and pressure drop across the orifice.[110] Flow (F) and orifice area (A) are related by the fundamental formula $F = cAV$, where V is velocity of flow and c is a constant accounting for central streaming of fluid through an orifice which tends to reduce the effective orifice size. Hence,

$$A = F/cV$$

Velocity is related to the pressure gradient through the relation $V = k\sqrt{2g\Delta P}$, where k is a constant accounting for frictional energy loss, g is the acceleration due to gravity (980 cm/s^2), and ΔP is the mean pressure gradient (mm Hg). Substituting for V in the orifice area equation and combining c and k into one constant C:

$$A = \frac{F}{C\sqrt{1960\Delta P}} = \frac{F}{44.3C\sqrt{\Delta P}}$$

Gorlin and Gorlin determined the value of the constant C by comparing the calculated valve area to actual valve area measured at autopsy or at surgery in 11 mitral valves. The maximal discrepancy between the actual mitral valve area and calculated values was only 0.2 cm^2 when the constant 0.85 was used. No data were obtained for aortic valves, a limitation noted by the Gorlins, and a constant of 1.0 was assumed. Because flow across the aortic valve occurs only in systole, the flow value for calculating aortic valve area (cm^2) is the cardiac output in ml/minute divided by the systolic ejection period (SEP) in seconds/beat times the heart rate (HR) in beats/min. The systolic ejection period is defined from aortic valve opening to closure. Hence, the aortic valve area is calculated from the Gorlin formula using the equation:

$$\text{Aortic valve area} = \frac{\text{cardiac output}}{44.3(\text{SEP})(\text{HR})\sqrt{\text{mean gradient}}}$$

Similarly, as mitral flow occurs only in diastole, the cardiac output is corrected for the diastolic filling period (DFP) in seconds/beat in the equation for mitral valve area, where the diastolic filling period is defined from mitral valve opening to mitral valve closure:

$$\text{Mitral valve area} = \frac{\text{cardiac output}}{37.7(\text{DFP})(\text{HR})\sqrt{\text{mean gradient}}}$$

The normal aortic valve area is 2.6 to 3.5 cm^2 in adults. Valve areas of 0.8 cm^2 or less represent severe aortic stenosis. The normal mitral valve area is 4 to 6 cm^2, and severe mitral stenosis is present with valve areas less than 1.0 to 1.5 cm^2.

The calculated valve area often is crucial in management decisions in patients with aortic stenosis or mitral stenosis. Hence, it is essential that accurate and simultaneous pressure gradient and cardiac output determinations be made, especially in patients with borderline or low pressure gradients. As the square root of the mean gradient is used in the Gorlin formula, the valve area calculation is more strongly influenced by errors in the cardiac output measurement than by errors in the pressure gradient. Thus, errors in measuring cardiac output may have profound effects on the calculated valve area, particularly in patients with low cardiac outputs in whom the calculated valve area is often of greatest importance.

The Fick method of determining cardiac output is the most accurate for assessing cardiac output, especially in low-output states. As noted previously, both the dye-dilution technique and the thermodilution technique may provide inaccurate cardiac output data when cardiac output is reduced or when concomitant aortic, mitral, or tricuspid regurgitation is present. In patients with mixed valvular disease (stenosis and regurgitation) of the same valve, the use of forward flow as determined by the Fick method or thermodilution technique will overestimate the severity of the valvular stenosis. This is because the Gorlin formula depends on total forward flow across the stenotic valve, not net forward flow. If valvular regurgitation is present, the angiographic cardiac output is the most appropriate measure of flow. If both aortic and mitral regurgitation are present, flow across a single valve cannot be determined and neither aortic valve area nor mitral valve area can be assessed accurately.

There are other potential errors and limitations in the use of the Gorlin formula,[111,112] related both to inaccuracies in measurement of valve gradients and to more fundamental issues regarding the validity of the assumptions underlying the formula. In low-output states the Gorlin formula may systematically predict smaller valve areas than are actually present. Several lines of evidence indicate that the aortic valve area by the Gorlin formula increases with increases in cardiac output.[113–116] Although this may represent an actual greater opening of stenotic valves by the higher proximal opening pressures that result from increases in transvalvular flow, the flow dependence of the calculated valve area may also reflect inherent errors in the assumptions underlying the Gorlin formula, particularly with respect to the aortic valve.[111,117]

Cannon et al.[115] demonstrated in valves of fixed orifice size that the constant in the Gorlin formula is actually not constant but varies with the square root of the mean pressure gradient ($C = k\sqrt{\text{mean gradient}}$). This concept would transform the Gorlin formula such that the square root disappears and the valve area varies inversely with the mean gradient:

$$\text{Valve area} = \frac{\text{Flow}}{44.3C\sqrt{\Delta P}} = \frac{\text{Flow}}{44.3(k\sqrt{\Delta P})\sqrt{\Delta P}} = \frac{\text{Flow}}{K\Delta P} + h$$

This concept has particular implications in aortic stenosis, in which the higher valve gradients have a greater effect on the Gorlin constant than the considerably smaller gradients encountered in mitral stenosis. The constant h was added to correct for a small offset between predicted and measured valve areas. The values of the new constants K and h have not been fully determined or validated, and the complete independence of these constants from transvalvular flow has not been fully investigated.

Other alternative formulas for determining valve areas have been proposed. Hakki[118] observed empirically that the effects of the systolic ejection period and the diastolic filling period were relatively constant at normal heart rates and proposed eliminating this term from the equation. This assumes that $(HR \times SEP \times 44.3) \approx 1000$ in most circumstances. In this modified and simplified approach, the aortic valve area would be determined by the formula:

$$\text{Aortic valve area} = \frac{\text{cardiac output (L/min)}}{\sqrt{\text{mean gradient (mm Hg)}}}$$

Angel et al.[119] tested this approach at various heart rates and proposed adding an empiric constant for heart rates less than 75 beats/min for mitral stenosis and more than 90 beats/min for aortic stenosis. As is the case with the Cannon modification of the Gorlin formula, this alternate approach to determining valve area has not been fully validated.

To surmount the limitations of the Gorlin formula in low-flow states, a number of investigators have advocated maneuvers in the cardiac catheterization laboratory to increase cardiac output and calculate valve area at the higher output and valve gradient. However, definitive data are lacking to indicate that this is a valid approach that actually yields more accurate valve area calculations. A second approach to the patient with a low aortic transvalvular gradient and low cardiac output is to calculate the aortic valve resistance using the formula:

$$\text{Aortic valve resistance} = \frac{\text{mean gradient}}{\text{flow}} = \frac{1.33\ \text{(mean gradient)(HR)(SEP)}}{\text{cardiac output}}$$

where HR is heart rate, SEP is systolic ejection period, and valve resistance is expressed in dynes-sec-cm^{-5}.[116,120] The limited data available using aortic valve resistance suggest that this measure may be a helpful adjunct in distinguishing those patients with borderline aortic valve areas (0.6 to 0.8 cm^2) who have severe from those with mild aortic stenosis.

Measurement of Intraventricular Pressure Gradients

The demonstration of an intracavitary pressure gradient is among the most interesting and challenging aspects of diagnostic catheterization. Simultaneous pressure measurements are usually obtained in the central aorta and from within the ventricular cavity. Pullback of the catheter from the ventricular apex to a posterior position just beneath the aortic valve will demonstrate an intracavitary gradient. An erroneous intracavitary gradient may be seen if the catheter becomes entrapped by the myocardium.

The intracavitary gradient is distinguished from aortic valvular stenosis due to the loss of the aortic–left ventricular gradient when the catheter is still within the left ventricle yet proximal to the myocardial obstruction. In addition, careful analysis of the upstroke of the aortic pressure waveform will distinguish a valvular from a subvalvular stenosis, as the aortic pressure waveform demonstrates a slow upstroke in aortic stenosis. Other methods to localize intracavitary gradients include the use of a dual-lumen catheter or a double-sensor micromanometer catheter, or placement of an end hole catheter in the left ventricular outflow tract while a transseptal catheter is advanced into the left ventricle, with pressure measured simultaneously. An intracavitary gradient may be increased by various provocative maneuvers including the Valsalva maneuver, inhalation of amyl nitrate, introduction of a premature ventricular beat, or isoproterenol infusion (see section on physiological maneuvers).

Assessment of Valvular Regurgitation

The severity of valvular regurgitation is generally graded by visual assessment, although calculation of the regurgitant fraction is used occasionally. A full description of the techniques of left ventriculography and aortography can be found elsewhere in this textbook (see Chap. 7).

VISUAL ASSESSMENT OF REGURGITATION. Valvular regurgitation may be assessed visually by determining the relative amount of radiographic contrast medium that opacifies the chamber proximal to its injection. The estimation of regurgitation depends on the regurgitant volume as well as the size and contractility of the proximal chamber. The original classification scheme devised by Sellers remains the standard in most catheterization laboratories:[121]

+	Minimal regurgitant jet seen. Clears rapidly from proximal chamber with each beat.
++	Moderate opacification of proximal chamber, clearing with subsequent beats.
+++	Intense opacification of proximal chamber, becoming equal to that of the distal chamber.
++++	Intense opacification of proximal chamber, becoming more dense than that of the distal chamber. Opacification often persists over the entire series of images obtained.

REGURGITANT FRACTION. A gross estimate of the degree of valvular regurgitation may be obtained by determining the regurgitant fraction. The difference between the angiographic stroke volume and the forward stroke volume can be defined as the regurgitant stroke volume. The regurgitant fraction (RF) is that portion of the angiographic stroke volume that does not contribute to the net cardiac output.

$$\text{Regurgitant stroke volume} = \text{angiographic stroke volume} - \text{forward stroke volume}$$

$$\text{RF} = \frac{\text{angiographic stroke volume} - \text{forward stroke volume}}{\text{angiographic stroke volume}}$$

Forward stroke volume is the cardiac output determined by the Fick or thermodilution method divided by the heart rate. Thermodilution cardiac output cannot be used if there is significant concomitant tricuspid regurgitation.

An RF of ≤ 20 per cent is roughly equivalent to 1+ regurgitation as detected visually; an RF of 21 to 40 per cent is equivalent to 2+ regurgitation; an RF of 41 to 60 per cent is equivalent to 3+ regurgitation; and an RF of 60 per cent or more is equivalent to 4+ regurgitation. The assumption underlying regurgitation fraction determination is that the angiographic and forward cardiac outputs are accurate and comparable, a state requiring similar heart rates, stable hemodynamic states between measurements, and only a single regurgitant valve. Given these conditions, the equation yields only a gross approximation of regurgitant flow.

Shunt Determinations

Normally, pulmonary blood flow and systemic blood flow are equal. When there is an abnormal communication between intracardiac chambers or great vessels, blood flow is shunted either from the systemic circulation to the pulmonary circulation (left-to-right shunt), from the pulmonary circulation to the systemic circulation (right-to-left shunt), or in both directions (bidirectional shunt). While many shunts are suspected before cardiac catheterization, physicians performing the procedure should be vigilant in determining the cause of unexpected findings. For example, an unexplained pulmonary artery oxygen saturation exceeding 80 per cent should raise the operator's suspicion of a left-to-right shunt, whereas unexplained arterial desaturation (<95 per cent) may indicate a right-to-left shunt.[122] Arterial desaturation commonly results from alveolar hypoventilation and associated "physiological shunting," the causes of which include oversedation from premedication, pulmonary disease, pulmonary venous congestion, pulmonary edema, and cardiogenic shock. If arterial desaturation persists after the patient takes several deep breaths or coughs, or following administration of 100 per cent oxygen, a right-to-left shunt must be highly suspected.

Several noninvasive and invasive methods are available for detection of intracardiac shunts. Noninvasive methods include echocardiographic, radionuclide, and magnetic resonance imaging techniques. The most commonly used method in the cardiac catheterization laboratory is the oximetric method.

OXIMETRIC METHOD. The oximetric method is based on blood sampling from various cardiac chambers for oxygen saturation determination. A left-to-right shunt is detected when there is a significant increase in blood oxygen saturation between two right-sided vessels or chambers.[123,124]

A screening oxygen saturation measurement for any left-to-right shunt should be performed with every right heart catheterization by sampling blood in the superior vena cava (SVC) and the pulmonary artery. If the difference in oxygen saturation between these samples is 8 per cent or more, a left-to-right shunt may be present, and a full oximetry "run" should be performed.[122] This includes obtaining blood samples from all right-sided locations including the superior vena cava (SVC), inferior vena cava (IVC), right atrium, right ventricle, and pulmonary artery. In cases of interatrial or interventricular shunts, it may be helpful to obtain multiple samples from the high, middle, and low right atrium or the right ventricular inflow tract, apex, and outflow tract in order to localize the level of the shunt. One may miss a small left-to-right shunt using the right atrium for screening purposes rather than the SVC because of incomplete mixing of blood in the right atrium, which receives blood from the IVC, SVC, and coronary sinus. Oxygen saturation in the IVC is higher than in the SVC because the kidneys use less oxygen relative to their blood flow than do other organs, while coronary sinus blood has very low oxygen saturation. Mixed venous saturation is most accurately measured in the pulmonary artery after complete mixing has occurred.

A full saturation run involves obtaining samples from the high and low IVC; high and low SVC; high, mid, and low right atrium; right ventricular inflow, outflow tracts, and mid-cavity; main pulmonary artery; left or right pulmonary artery; pulmonary vein and left atrium if possible; left ventricle; and distal aorta. When a right-to-left shunt must be localized, oxygen saturation samples must be taken from the pulmonary veins, left atrium, left ventricle, and aorta. While the major weakness of the oxygen step-up method is its lack of sensitivity, clinically significant shunts are generally detected by this technique. Another method of oximetric determination of intracardiac shunts uses a balloon-tipped fiberoptic catheter that allows for continuous registration of oxygen saturation as it is withdrawn from the pulmonary artery through the right heart chambers into the SVC and IVC.

SHUNT QUANTIFICATION. The principles used to determine Fick cardiac output are used to quantify intracardiac shunts. To determine the size of a left-to-right shunt, pulmonary blood flow and systemic blood flow determinations are required. Pulmonary blood flow (PBF) is simply oxygen consumption divided by the difference in oxygen content across the pulmonary bed, while systemic blood flow (SBF) is oxygen consumption divided by the difference in oxygen content across the systemic bed. The effective blood flow (EBF) is the fraction of mixed venous return received by the lungs without contamination by the shunt flow. In the *absence* of a shunt, PBF, SBF, and EBF are all equal. These equations are shown below:

$$PBF = \frac{O_2 \text{ consumption (ml/min)}}{(PV\ O_2 - PA\ O_2)}$$

$$SBF = \frac{O_2 \text{ consumption (ml/min)}}{(SA\ O_2 - MV\ O_2)}$$

$$EBF = \frac{O_2 \text{ consumption (ml/min)}}{(PV\ O_2 - MV\ O_2}$$

where PV O_2, PA O_2, SA O_2, and MV O_2 are the oxygen contents (in milliliters of oxygen per liter of blood) of pulmonary venous, pulmonary arterial, systemic arterial, and mixed venous bloods, respectively. The oxygen content is determined as outlined in the section on Fick cardiac output.

If a pulmonary vein is not sampled, systemic arterial oxygen content may be substituted, assuming systemic arterial saturation is 95 per cent or more. As discussed above, if systemic arterial saturation is less than 95 per cent, a right-to-left shunt may be present. If arterial desaturation is present but not secondary to a right-to-left shunt, systemic arterial oxygen content is used. If a right-to-left shunt is present, pulmonary venous oxygen content is calculated as 98 per cent of the oxygen capacity.

The mixed venous oxygen content is the average oxygen content of the blood in the chamber proximal to the shunt. When assessing a left-to-right shunt at the level of the right atrium, one must calculate mixed venous oxygen content on the basis of the contributing blood flow from the IVC, SVC, and coronary sinus. The most common formula used is the Flamm formula:[125]

Mixed venous oxygen content

$$= \frac{3(\text{SVC } O_2 \text{ content}) + 1(\text{IVC } O_2 \text{ content})}{4}$$

Assuming conservation of mass, the size of a left-to-right shunt, when there is no associated right-to-left shunt, is simply:

$$L \rightarrow R \text{ shunt} = PBF - SBF$$

When there is evidence of a right-to-left shunt in addition to a left-to-right shunt, the approximate left to right shunt size is:

$$L \rightarrow R \text{ shunt} = PBF - EBF$$

while the approximate right-to-left shunt size is:

$$R \rightarrow L \text{ shunt} = SBF - EBF$$

The flow ratio PBF/SBF (or QP/QS) is used clinically to determine the significance of the shunt. A ratio of less than 1.5 indicates a small left-to-right shunt. A ratio of 2.0 or more indicates a large left-to-right shunt and generally requires repair in order to prevent future pulmonary and/or right ventricular complications. A flow ratio of less than 1.0 indicates a net right-to-left shunt. If oxygen consumption is not measured, the flow ratio may be calculated as follows:

$$\frac{PBF}{SBF} = \frac{(SA\ O_2 - MV\ O_2)}{(PV\ O_2 - PA\ O_2)}$$

where SA O_2, MV O_2, PV O_2, and PA O_2 are systemic arterial, mixed venous, pulmonary venous, and pulmonary arterial blood oxygen saturations, respectively.

Indicator-Dilution Method

While the indicator-dilution method is more sensitive than the oximetric method in detection of small shunts, it cannot be used to localize the level of a left-to-right shunt (Fig. 6–14). An indicator such as indocyanine green dye is injected into a proximal chamber while a sample is taken from a distal chamber using a densitometer and the density of dye is displayed over time. In order to detect a left-to-right shunt, dye is injected into the pulmonary artery and sampling is performed in a systemic artery. Presence of a shunt is indicated by early recirculation of the dye on the *downslope* of the curve.[126] The presence of aortic or mitral regurgitation may distort the downslope of the curve, thereby yielding a false positive result. In adults, the indocyanine green method provides estimates of shunt magnitude that are somewhat smaller than those of the oximetric method, although they are in general agreement with one another concerning the QP/QS.[127,128] In order to detect a right-to-left shunt, dye is injected into the right heart proximal to the presumed shunt and sampling is performed in a systemic artery. If there is a right-to-left shunt, a distinctive early peak is seen on the *upslope* of the curve.[129] The level of the right-to-left shunt may be localized by injecting more distally until the early peak disappears. Shunts may also be quantified using this technique.

Miscellaneous Techniques

A sensitive method for detection and localization of a left-to-right shunt is to check systematically within the various right heart chambers for the early appearance of an indicator that is injected distal to the presumed shunt. Indicators that have been used for this

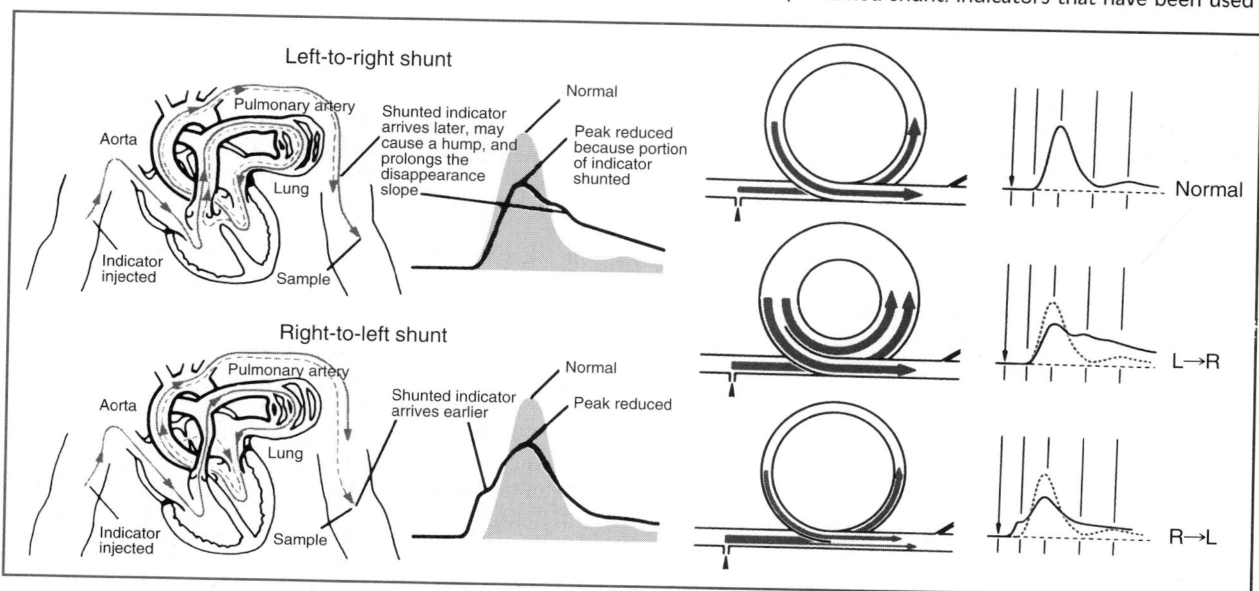

FIGURE 6–14. Left-to-right shunt (increased pulmonic flow). Indicator is not cleared rapidly but recirculates through central circulation via defect. Based on magnitude of shunt, a constant fraction leaves the central pool with each circulation. Maximal deflection is reduced and the disappearance is prolonged as a result of slow clearance. Right-to-left shunt (decreased pulmonic flow). A portion of the indicator passes directly to the arterial circulation via the defect without passing through the lungs and arrives at the arterial sampling site before the portion that did traverse the pulmonary circulation. (From Kern, M. J., Deligonul, U., Donohue, T., et al.: Hemodynamic data. *In* Kern, M. J.: The Cardiac Catheterization Handbook. 2nd ed. St. Louis, Mosby–Year Book, 1995, p. 142.)

purpose include indocyanine green dye, inhaled hydrogen, hydrogen dissolved in saline, and ascorbic acid. Platinum-tipped electrodes are used for detection when hydrogen and ascorbic acid are used. These techniques may also be used to detect small right-to-left shunts by altering of the sites of injection and sampling.

Selective injection of radiographic contrast (angiocardiography) can detect both left-to-right and right-to-left shunts, although these cannot be quantified. Angiocardiography is a useful adjunct to transesophageal echocardiography as part of a preoperative evaluation. It is also very useful in detecting pulmonary arteriovenous fistulas that may not be detected by other methods.

Physiological and Pharmacological Maneuvers

Potentially significant cardiac abnormalities may be silent in the resting condition. Abnormal hemodynamics may not be shown without physiological stresses in valvular, myocardial, and coronary disease states. Therefore, if the physician performing a cardiac catheterization procedure cannot elucidate the cause of the patient's symptoms at rest, various physiological and pharmacological maneuvers can be considered.

DYNAMIC EXERCISE. Dynamic exercise in the catheterization laboratory is most commonly performed using supine bicycle ergometry, although straight leg raises or arm or upright bicycle exercise may be used. Upright treadmill exercise may also be performed outside the catheterization laboratory, using a balloon flotation catheter inserted through an antecubital vein to measure pulmonary artery and wedge pressure and cardiac output. The associated changes in the heart rate, cardiac output, oxygen consumption, and intracardiac pressures are monitored at steady state during progressive stages of exercise. Normally, the increased oxygen requirements of exercise are met by an increase in cardiac output and an increase in oxygen extraction from arterial blood.[130] Patients with cardiac dysfunction are unable to increase their cardiac output appropriately in response to exercise and must meet the demands of the exercising muscle groups by increasing the extraction of oxygen from arterial blood, thereby increasing the arteriovenous oxygen difference. Dexter and colleagues found that the relationship between cardiac output and oxygen consumption was linear and that a regression formula may be used to calculate the predicted cardiac index at a given level of oxygen consumption.[131] The actual cardiac index divided by the predicted cardiac index is defined as the *exercise index.* A value of 0.8 or more indicates a normal cardiac output response to exercise.[130] The *exercise factor* is another method of describing the same relationship between the cardiac output and oxygen consumption. The exercise factor is the increase in cardiac output divided by the increase in oxygen consumption. Normally, for every 100 ml/min increase in oxygen consumption with exercise, the cardiac output should increase by at least 600 ml/min. Therefore, a normal exercise factor should be 0.6 or more.[130]

Supine exercise will normally cause a rise in mean arterial and pulmonary pressures. There will be a proportionally greater decrease in systemic vascular resistance compared with pulmonary vascular resistance and an increase in heart rate. Myocardial contractility increases owing to both the increase in heart rate and increased sympathetic tone. Left ventricular ejection fraction rises. During early levels of exercise, increased venous return augments left ventricular end-diastolic volume, leading to an increase in stroke volume.[132] At progressively higher levels of exercise, both left ventricular end-systolic and end-diastolic volumes decrease such that there is a negligible rise in stroke volume. Thus, the augmentation in cardiac output during peak supine exercise in the catheterization laboratory is generally caused by an increase in heart rate. For this reason, all agents that may impair the chronotropic response should be discontinued before catheterization if exercise is contemplated during the procedure.

Exercise may provoke symptoms in a patient who had been diagnosed as having valvular disease of borderline significance in the resting state. Exercise increases the gradient across the mitral valve in mitral stenosis and may provoke symptoms not experienced at rest. The hemodynamic response to exercise is also useful in evaluating regurgitant valvular lesions. Clinically significant valvular regurgitation exists if an increase occurs in left ventricular end-diastolic pressure, pulmonary capillary wedge pressure, and systemic vascular resistance, in conjunction with a reduced exercise index and abnormal exercise factor. Simultaneous echocardiographic data may also be useful in equivocal cases. Patients with myocardial disease, ischemic or otherwise, may have pronounced increases in left ventricular end-diastolic pressure with exercise.[133]

ISOMETRIC EXERCISE. Isometric handgrip exercise causes an increase in heart rate, mean arterial pressure, and cardiac output. Since the systemic vascular resistance does not rise, the elevation in arterial pressure is due to the rise in cardiac output rather than a vasoconstrictor response. Patients with left ventricular dysfunction respond abnormally to isometric exercise (i.e., significant increase in left ventricular end-diastolic pressure, a failure to increase stroke work appropriately, and a blunted rise in left ventricular peak dP/dT).[130]

PACING TACHYCARDIA. Rapid atrial or ventricular pacing increases myocardial oxygen consumption and myocardial blood flow.[134] In distinction from dynamic or isometric exercise, left ventricular end-diastolic volume decreases with pacing and there is little change in cardiac output.[135] This method may be used to determine the significance of coronary artery disease or valvular abnormalities. For example, the gradient across the mitral valve increases with rapid atrial pacing owing to the increase in heart rate. Pacing has the advantage of allowing for greater control and rapid termination of the induced stress.

PHYSIOLOGICAL STRESS. The *Valsalva maneuver* (forcible expiration against a closed glottis) should increase the systolic subaortic pressure gradient in patients with obstructive hypertrophic cardiomyopathy in the strain phase, during which there is a decrease in venous return and decreased left ventricular volume (see p. 1420). This maneuver is often abnormal in patients with heart failure.[136] The *Mueller maneuver* (forced inspiration against a closed glottis) causes the opposite effect on the systolic pressure gradient in patients with obstructive hypertrophic cardiomyopathy. Another useful maneuver in patients with hypertrophic obstructive cardiomyopathy is the introduction of a *premature ventricular beat* (Brockenbrough maneuver). Premature ventricular contractions normally increase the pulse pressure of the subsequent ventricular beat. In obstructive hypertrophic cardiomyopathy, the outflow gradient is increased during the postpremature beat with a decrease in the pulse pressure of the aortic contour. A premature ventricular beat may also accentuate the spike-and-dome configuration of the aortic pressure waveform. *Rapid volume loading* may reveal occult pericardial constriction, when atrial and ventricular filling pressures are relatively normal under baseline conditions owing to hypovolemia,[137] and may help distinguish pericardial constriction from myocardial restriction. *Kussmaul's sign* occurs in pericardial constriction (see p. 1497). This is demonstrated when, with inspiration, right atrial pressure fails to decrease or actually increases related to impaired right ventricular filling. *Cold pressor testing,* whereby the forearm of the patient is exposed to ice water, may induce coronary vasoconstriction in patients with coronary artery disease.[138]

PHARMACOLOGICAL MANEUVERS. *Isoproterenol infusion* may be used to simulate supine dynamic exercise, although untoward side effects may limit its applicability. This drug's positive inotropic and chronotropic effects may increase the gradients in obstructive hypertrophic cardiomyopathy and mitral stenosis. *Nitroglycerin* and *amyl nitrate* decrease preload and accentuate the systolic gradient in patients with obstructive hypertrophic cardiomyopathy. Amyl nitrate is generally inhaled and its onset of action is very rapid. Agents that increase systemic vascular resistance, such as *phenylephrine,* reduce the gradient in obstructive hypertrophic cardiomyopathy. Infusion of *sodium nitroprusside* may improve the cardiac output and filling pressures in patients with dilated cardiomyopathies and in patients with mitral regurgitation by lowering systemic and pulmonary vascular resistances. A favorable response to sodium nitroprusside infusion may predict a good clinical outcome. The use of *ergonovine* for provocation of coronary spasm as a diagnostic tool is limited by its lack of specificity.[139] In addition, production of this drug has recently been halted because of limited use.

Coronary Blood Flow Determinations

Four methods are generally used to measure human coronary blood flow in the cardiac catheterization laboratory: thermodilution, digital subtraction angiography, and the use of electromagnetic flow meters, and of Doppler velocity probes. Although most current methods measure relative changes in coronary blood flow, useful information regarding the physiological significance of stenosis,[140] cardiac hypertrophy,[141] and pharmacological interventions[142] can be obtained from these measurements.

Ganz and colleagues[143] introduced thermodilution methods for measuring coronary sinus flow in humans (Fig. 6–15). This inexpensive, widely available technique is the most frequently applied method for measuring global coronary blood flow in humans.[144] By injecting iced saline in the distal end of the catheter placed in the coronary sinus and measuring the temperature change from a proximal thermistor, the rate of change in temperature can be used to define coronary flow. The frequency response of this system is sufficient to measure flow changes that occur in 2 to 3 seconds and are greater than 30 per cent.[143] This technique has several serious limitations, however.[144] Although the method has been validated in vitro with the thermodilution catheter attached to the coronary sinus,[143] weaker correlations have been shown when the thermodilution catheter is allowed to move within the coronary sinus.[145] Meanwhile, no studies have clearly demonstrated the accuracy of this method in patients with severe coronary artery disease or myocardial infarction. Other fundamental limitations include the fact that (1) rapid changes in flow cannot be assessed because of the slow time constant of the technique, (2) right atrial and ventricular perfusion cannot be evaluated because the venous drainage does not occur by means of the coronary sinus, and (3) regional function and specifically transmural coronary flow cannot be assessed.

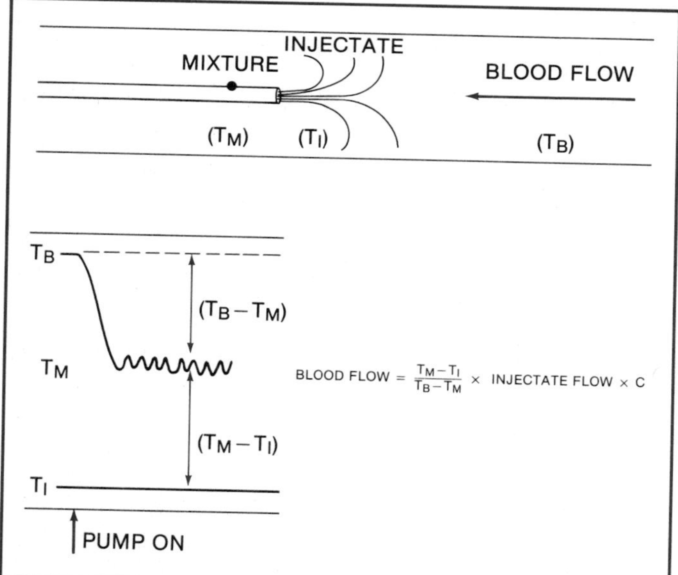

FIGURE 6–15. Schematic illustration of venous thermodilution method for measurement of coronary blood flow. The thermal indicator (injectate) at temperature T_I is infused at a constant rate (e.g., 15 ml/min). Turbulence causes mixing of the injectate with coronary venous blood at temperature T_B, resulting in a blood-injectate mixture at temperature T_M. The catheter tip thermistor monitors T_B and T_M, while an internal thermistor monitors T_I, and these are recorded continuously on a uniform temperature scale *(lower left).* Because heat loss by blood is gained by injectate, coronary venous flow is calculated using the measured temperatures, the rate of indicator injection, and the constant derived from the specific heats of blood and injectate. (From Bradley, A. B., and Baim, D. S.: Measurement of coronary blood flow in man. Methods and implications for clinical practice. Cardiovasc. Clin. *14*:67, 1984.)

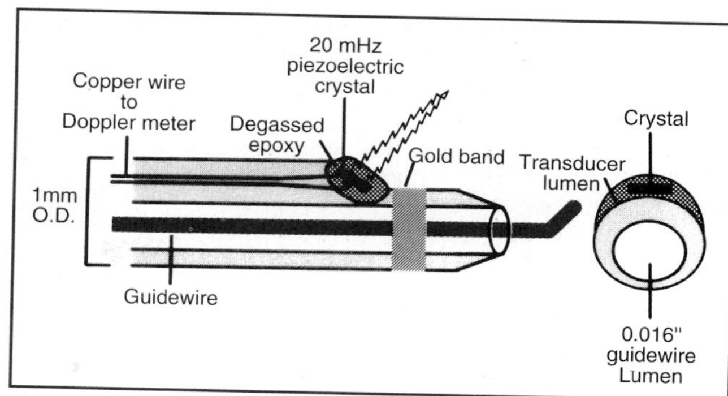

FIGURE 6–16. Schematic diagram of the distal portion of a 3F intracoronary Doppler catheter with side-mounted piezoelectric crystal. The copper wires attached to the crystal exit from the proximal end of the catheter and are connected to a 20 mHz pulsed Doppler velocimeter. The catheter is advanced into the coronary artery over an 0.014-inch angioplasty guidewire. O.D., outer diameter. (Modified from Wilson, R. F., Laughlin, D. E., and Ackell, P. H., et al.: Transluminal, subselective measurement of coronary artery blood flow velocity and vasodilator reserve in man. Circulation *72*:82, 1985. Copyright 1985 American Heart Association.)

To measure coronary flow with digital subtraction angiography, contrast medium is power injected into a coronary artery at a rate sufficient to replace blood within the artery completely. It is assumed that the contrast bolus is undiluted until the peak concentration has been imaged distally in the arterial segment. Regional flow reserve can be calculated in a number of ways, including the use of downstream appearance time and maximal contrast concentration before and during reactive hyperemia.[146] The assumption is that transit time within a region is inversely proportional to coronary blood flow in that region. This is true if the volume of distribution is constant. The technique is limited by a slow time constant and the inability to measure absolute flow. Evaluation of coronary flow reserve has been validated for this method in dogs by comparing digital flow ratio estimates with electromagnetic flow ratio measurements.[147,148] In humans, flow reserve has been shown to be abnormal in stenosed coronary arteries and bypass grafts and after coronary angioplasty.[149] Further human validation is necessary.

The electromagnetic flow meter is based on Faraday's induction law, which states that a conductor moving in an electric field produces current. A major advantage of electromagnetic flow meters is the high-frequency response.[141] Although these flow meters have been used to measure aortic blood flow velocity in humans,[150] they have not been developed to the point at which they are useful for measuring coronary blood flow at catheterization, in part because most methods require placement directly around the coronary artery. Electromagnetic flow meters are still in occasional use intraoperatively to evaluate flow in aortocoronary bypass grafts.

The Doppler flow meter is based on the principle of the Doppler effect (Fig. 6–16). It is the most widely applied technique for measurement of coronary flow in humans. High-frequency sound waves are reflected from moving red blood cells and undergo a shift in sound frequency that is proportional to the velocity of the blood flow. In pulsed-wave Doppler methods, a single piezoelectric crystal can both transmit and receive high-frequency sound waves. These methods have been applied successfully in humans by using miniaturized crystals fixed to the tip of catheters. Recent developments in technology have further miniaturized steerable 12-mHz Doppler guidewires to 0.014 inch in diameter. Therefore, flow can be assessed distal and proximal to a stenosis. The Doppler guidewire measures phasic flow velocity patterns and tracks linearly with flow rates in small, straight coronary arteries.[151] It has been advocated for use in determining the severity of intermediate stenosis (40 to 60 per cent) and in evaluating whether normal blood flow has been restored after PTCA. Validation studies have been performed that compare Doppler flow probes with labeled microspheres[152] and electromagnetic flow probes.[153] The use of this technique in 200 patients in the cardiac catheterization laboratory has been reported.[154] It has the advantage of permitting repeated sampling and at high frequency, thus allowing measurements after physiological or pharmacological interventions. The use of smaller Doppler catheters allows selective coronary artery flow velocity to be measured. By noting the increase in flow velocity following a strong coronary vasodilator, such as papaverine, the coronary flow reserve can be defined. Coronary flow reserve (CFR) provides an index of the functional significance of coronary lesions that obviates some of the ambiguity of anatomical description.[154]

Animal data indicate that stenosis exceeding 50 per cent is associated with a reduction in absolute flow reserve. It has been suggested that stenosis flow reserve (SFR) is a more reliable method of functional severity.[155] For a fixed arterial dimension and stenosis geometry, directly measured arterial CFR can be zero if no aortic perfusion is present or may change with other physiological conditions. Thus, CFR can be broken into its component parts of SFR, i.e., the flow reserve of the proximal arterial stenosis, and myocardial perfusion reserve (MPR), the flow reserve of the distal vascular bed. SFR is defined by geometric quantitative coronary dimensions using standard physiological conditions. MPR is directly or indirectly measured and is affected by geometric as well as physiological variables. The equation relating pressure change across a lesion and flow is:

$$\Delta P = Pa - Pc = A(Q/Qrest) + B(Q/Qrest)^2$$

where ΔP is the translesional gradient, Pc is distal coronary pressure, Pa is aortic pressure, Q and Qrest are flow and rest flow, and A and B are related to lesion geometry. A and B are defined by lesion length, minimal cross-sectional area of the lesion and reference segment, and blood viscosity.

The limitation of the current Doppler probe method is that only changes in flow velocity, rather than absolute velocity or volumetric flow, are measurable. The change in flow velocity is directly proportional to changes in volumetric flow only when vessel dimensions are constant at the site of the sample volume. Furthermore, there is concern that changes in luminal diameter and arterial cross-sectional area during interventions are not reflected in measurements of flow velocity, thus potentially causing underestimation of the true volume flow.[146]

REFERENCES

HISTORICAL PERSPECTIVE

1. Swan, H. J. C., Ganz, W., Forrester, J. S., et al.: Catheterization of the heart in man with use of a flow-directed balloon-tipped catheter. N. Engl. J. Med. *283*:447, 1970.
2. Zimmerman, H. A., Scott, R. W., and Becker, N. O.: Catheterization of the left side of the heart in man. Circulation *1*:357, 1950.
3. Sones, F. M., Jr., Shivey, E. K., Proudfit, W. L., and Westcott, R. N.: Cinecoronary arteriography (Abstract). Circulation *20*:773, 1959.
4. Ross, J., Jr.: Transseptal left heart catheterization: A new method of left atrial puncture. Ann. Surg. *1949*:395, 1959.
5. Cope, C.: Technique for transseptal catheterization of the left atrium: Preliminary report. J. Thorac. Surg. *37*:482, 1959.
6. Ricketts, H. J., and Abrams, H. L.: Percutaneous selective coronary cine arteriography. JAMA *181*:140, 1962.
7. Amplatz, K., Formonek G., Stranger, P., and Wilson, W.: Mechanics of selective coronary artery catheterization via the femoral approach. Radiology *89*:1040, 1967.
8. Judkins, M. P.: Selective coronary arteriography. I: A percutaneous transfemoral technique. Radiology *89*:815, 1967.
9. Acierno, L. J.: The History of Cardiology. 1st ed. Pearl River, NY, The Parthenon Publishing Group Inc., 1994.

INDICATIONS FOR DIAGNOSTIC CARDIAC CATHETERIZATION

10. Ross, J., Jr., Pepine, C. J., Brandenburg, R. O., et al.: Guidelines for coronary angiography. A report of the American College of Cardiology/American Heart Association Task Force on Assessment of Diagnostic and Therapeutic Cardiovascular Procedures (Subcommittee on Coronary Angiography). J. Am. Coll. Cardiol. *10*:935, 1987.
11. Grines, C. L., Browne, K. F., Marco, J., et al.: A comparison of immediate angioplasty with thrombolytic therapy for acute myocardial infarction. N. Engl. J. Med. *328*:673, 1993.
12. Topol, E. J., Califf, R. M., George, B. S., et al.: A randomized prospective trial of immediate versus delayed elective angioplasty after intravenous tissue plasminogen activator in acute myocardial infarction. N. Engl. J. Med. *317*:581, 1987.
13. The TIMI Study Group: Comparison of invasive and conservative strategies after treatment with intravenous tissue plasminogen activatorin acute myocardial infarction: Results of the Thrombolysis in Acute Myocardial Infarction (TIMI) Phase II Trial. N. Engl. J. Med. *320*:618, 1989.
14. Ryan, T. J., Bauman, W. B., Kennedy, J. W., et al.: Guidelines and indications for percutaneous transluminal coronary angioplasty. A report of the American College of Cardiology/American Heart Association Task Force on Assessment of Diagnostic and Therapeutic Cardiovascular Procedures (Subcommittee on Percutaneous Transluminal Coronary Angioplasty). Circulation *88*:2987, 1993.
15. Roberts, W. C.: Reasons for cardiac catheterization before cardiac valve replacement. N. Engl. J. Med. *306*:1291, 1982.
16. Rahimtoola, S. H.: The need for cardiac catheterization and angiography in valvular heart disease is not disproven. Ann. Intern. Med. *97*:433, 1982.

COMPLICATIONS ASSOCIATED WITH CARDIAC CATHETERIZATION

17. Braunwald, E., and Swan, H. J. C.: Cooperative study on cardiac catheterization. Circulation *37*(Suppl.III):1, 1968.
18. Kennedy, J. W.: Complication associated with cardiac catheterization and angiography. Cathet. Cardiovasc. Diagn. *8*:13, 1982.
19. Johnson, L. W., Lozner, E. C., Johnson, S., et al.: Coronary arteriography 1984–1987: A report of the Registry of the Society for Cardiac Angiography and Interventions. Results and complications. Cathet. Cardiovasc. Diagn. *17*:5, 1989.
20. Davis, K., Kennedy, J. W., Kemp, H. G., et al.: Complications of coronary arteriography from the collaborative study of coronary artery surgery (CASS). Circulation *59*:1105, 1979.
21. Laskey, W., Boyle, J., Johnson, L. W., and the Registry Committee of the Society for Cardiac Angiography and Interventions: Multivariable model for prediction of risk of significant complication during diagnostic cardiac catheterization. Cathet. Cardiovasc. Diagn. *30*:185, 1993.
22. Davidson, C. J., Mark, D. B., Pieper, K. S., et al.: Thrombotic and cardiovascular complications related to nonionic contrast media during cardiac catheterization. Analysis of 8517 patients. Am. J. Cardiol. *65*:1481, 1990.
23. Adams, D. F., Fraser, D. B., and Abrams, H. L.: The complications of coronary arteriography. Circulation *48*:609, 1973.
24. Clark, V. L., and Khaja, F.: Risk of cardiac catheterization in patients aged >80 years without previous cardiac surgery. Am. J. Cardiol. *74*:1076, 1994.
25. McCann, R. L., Schwartz, L. B., Pieper, K. S.: Vascular complications of cardiac catheterization. J. Vasc. Surg. *14*:375, 1991.
26. Davidson, C. J., Hlatky, M., Morris, G. G., et al.: Cardiovascular and renal toxicity of a nonionic radiographic contrast agent after cardiac catheterization. Ann. Intern. Med. *110*:119, 1989.
27. Solomon, R., Werner, C., Mann, D., D'Elia, J., and Silva, P.: Effects of saline, mannitol, and furosemide on acute decreases in renal function induced by radiocontrast agents. N. Engl. J. Med. *331*:1416, 1994.
28. Fareed, J., Moncada, R., Messmore, H. L., et al.: Molecular markers of contrast media–induced adverse reactors. Semin. Thromb. Hemost. *10*:306, 1984.
29. Shehadi, W. H.: Contrast media adverse reactions: Occurrence, recurrence and distribution patterns. Radiology *143*:11, 1982.
30. Fischer, H. W., and Thomson, K. R.: Contrast media in coronary arteriography: A review. Invest. Radiol. *13*:450, 1978.
31. Bashore, T. M., Davidson, C. J., Mark, D. B., et al.: Iopamidol use in the cardiac catheterization laboratory: A retrospective analysis of 3,313 patients. Cardiology *5*(Suppl.):6, 1988.
32. Higgins, C. B., Sovak, M., Schmidt, W. S., et al.: Direct myocardial effects of intracoronary administration of new contrast agents with low osmolality. Invest. Radiol. *15*:39, 1980.

33. Salem, D. N., Findlay, S. R., Isner, J. M., et al.: Comparison of histamine release effects of ionic and nonionic radiographic contrast media. Am. J. Med. *80*:382, 1986.
34. Schwab, S., Hlatky, M. A., Pieper, K. S., et al.: Contrast nephrotoxicity: A randomized study of the nephrotoxicity of ionic versus nonionic contrast following cardiac catheterization. N. Engl. J. Med. *320*:149, 1989.
35. Hill, J. A., Winniford, M., Van Fossen, D. B., et al.: Nephrotoxicity following cardiac angiography: A randomized double blind multicenter trial of ionic and nonionic contrast media in 1194 patients. Circulation *84*:II-333, 1991.
36. Manske, C. L., Sprafka, J. M., Strony, J. T., Wang, Y.: Contrast nephrotoxicity in an azotemic diabetic patient undergoing coronary angiography. Am. J. Med. *89*:615, 1990.
37. Grollman, J. H., Liu, C. K., Astone, R. A., and Lurie, M. D.: Thromboembolic complications in coronary angiography associated with the use of nonionic contrast medium. Cathet. Cardiovasc. Diagn. *14*:159, 1988.
38. Granger, C. B., Gabriel, D. A., Reece, N. S., et al.: Fibrin modification by ionic and non-ionic contrast media during cardiac catheterization. Am. J. Cardiol. *69*:8217, 1992.

TECHNICAL ASPECTS OF CARDIAC CATHETERIZATION

39. Pepine, C. J., Allen, H. D., Bashore, T. M., et al.: ACC/AHA guidelines for cardiac catheterization and cardiac catheterization laboratories. J. Am. Coll. Cardiol. *18*:1149, 1991.
40. Goss, J. E., and Cameron, A., for the Society for Cardiac Angiography and Interventions Laboratory Performance Standards Committee: Mobile cardiac catheterization laboratories. Cathet. Cardiovasc. Diagn. *26*:71, 1992.
41. Bersin, R. M., Elliott, C. M., Fedor, J. M., et al.: Mobile cardiac catheterization registry: Report of the first 1,001 patients. Cathet. Cardiovasc. Diagn. *31*:1, 1994.
42. Lee, J. C., Bengtson, J. R., Lipscomb, J., et al.: Feasibility and cost-saving potential of outpatient cardiac catheterization. J. Am. Coll. Cardiol. *15*:378, 1990.
43. Clements, S. D., Jr., and Gatlin, S.: Outpatient cardiac catheterization: A report of 3,000 cases. Clin. Cardiol. *14*:477, 1991.
44. Clark, D. A., Moscovich, M. D., Vetrovec, G. W., and Wexler, L.: Guidelines for the performance of outpatient catheterization and angiographic procedures. Cathet. Cardiovasc. Diagn. *27*:5, 1992.
45. Block, P., Ockene, I., Goldberg, R. J., et al.: A prospective randomized trial of outpatient versus inpatient cardiac catheterization. N. Engl. J. Med. *319*:1252, 1988.
46. Cameron, A., for the Society for Cardiac Angiography and Interventions Laboratory Performance Standards Committee: Guidelines for professional staff privileges in the cardiac catheterization laboratory. Cathet. Cardiovasc. Diagn. *21*:203, 1990.
47. Heupler, F. A., Al-Hani, A. J., Dear, W. E., and Members of the Laboratory and Performance Standards Committee of the Society for Cardiac Angiography and Interventions: Guidelines for continuous quality improvement in the cardiac catheterization laboratory. Cathet. Cardiovasc. Diagn. *30*:191, 1993.
48. Holmes, D. R., Jr., Wondrow, M. S., and Tulsrud, P. R.: Radiographic techniques used in cardiac catheterization. *In* Pepine, C. J., Hill, J. A., and Lambert, C. R. (eds.): Diagnostic and Therapeutic Cardiac Catheterization. 2nd ed. Baltimore, Williams and Wilkins, 1994, p. 141.
49. Tobis, J. M.: The future of digital angiography. Cathet. Cardiovasc. Diagn. *27*:14, 1992.
50. Nissen, S. E.: Principles and applications of digital imaging in cardiac and coronary angiography. *In* Pepine, C. J., Hill, J. A., and Lambert, C. R. (eds.): Diagnostic and Therapeutic Cardiac Catheterization. 2nd ed. Baltimore, Williams and Wilkins, 1994, p. 162.
51. Nissen, S. E., Pepine, C. J., Bashore, T. M., et al.: Cardiac angiography without cine film: Erecting a "Tower of Babel" in the cardiac catheterization laboratory. J. Am. Coll. Cardiol. *24*:834, 1994.
52. Balter, S., and Members of the Laboratory and Performance Standards Committee of the Society for Cardiac Angiography and Interventions: Guidelines for personnel radiation monitoring in the cardiac catheterization laboratory. Cathet. Cardiovasc. Diagn. *30*:277, 1993.
53. Johnson, L. W., Moore, R. J., and Balter, S.: Review of radiation safety in the cardiac catheterization laboratory. Cathet. Cardiovasc. Diagn. *25*:186, 1992.
54. Hill, J. A., Miranda, A. A., Keim, S. G., et al.: Value of right-sided cardiac catheterization in patients undergoing left-sided cardiac catheterization for evaluation of coronary artery disease. Am. J. Cardiol. *65*:590, 1990.
55. MacDonald, R. G.: Catheters, sheaths, guidewires, needles and related equipment. *In* Pepine, C. J., Hill, J. A., and Lambert, C. R. (eds.): Diagnostic and Therapeutic Cardiac Catheterization. 2nd ed. Baltimore, Williams and Wilkins, 1994, p. 111.
56. Kern, M. J., Cohen, M., Talley, J. D., et al.: Early ambulation after 5 French diagnostic cardiac catheterization: Results of a multicenter trial. J. Am. Coll. Cardiol. *15*:1475, 1990.
57. Popma, J. J., Satler, L. F., Pichard, A. D., et al.: Vascular complications after balloon and new device angioplasty. Circulation *88*(part I):1569, 1993.
58. Sharkey, S. W.: Beyond the wedge: Clinical physiology and the Swan-Ganz catheter. Am. J. Med. *83*:111, 1987.
59. Bush, C. A., Van Fossen, D. B., Kolibash, A. J., et al.: Cardiac catheterization and coronary angiography using 5F preformed (Judkins) catheters from the percutaneous right brachial approach. Cathet. Cardiovasc. Diagn. *29*:267, 1993.
60. Campeau, L.: Percutaneous radial artery approach for coronary angiography. Cathet. Cardiovasc. Diagn. *16*:3, 1989.
61. Kieffer, R. W., and Dean, R. H.: Complications of intra-arterial monitoring. Problems Gen. Surg. *2*:116, 1985.
62. Braunwald, E.: A new technique for left ventricular angiography and transseptal left heart catheterization. Am. J. Cardiol. *6*:1062, 1960.
63. Clugston, R., Lau, F. Y. K., and Ruiz, C.: Transseptal catheterization update 1992. Cathet. Cardiovasc. Diagn. *26*:266, 1992.
64. Vignola, P. A., Swaye, P. S., and Gosselin, A. J.: Safe transthoracic left ventricular puncture performed with echocardiographic guidance. Cathet. Cardiovasc. Diagn. *6*:317, 1980.
65. Baim, D. S., and Grossman, W.: Percutaneous approach, including transseptal catheterization and apical left ventricular puncture. *In* Grossman, W. and Baim, D. S. (eds.): Cardiac Catheterization, Angiography, and Intervention. 4th ed. Philadelphia, Lea and Febiger, 1991, p. 62.
66. Caves, P. K., Schulz, W. P., and Dong, E., Jr.: New instrument for transvenous cardiac biopsy. Am. J. Cardiol. *33*:264, 1974.
67. Mason, J. W.: Techniques for right and left ventricular endomyocardial biopsy. Am. J. Cardiol. *41*:887, 1978.
68. Richardson, P. J.: King's endomyocardial bioptome. Lancet *1*:660, 1974.
69. Brooksby, I. A. B., Jenkins, B. S., Coltast, D. J., et al.: Left ventricular endomyocardial biopsy. Lancet *2*:1222, 1974.
70. Hauptman, P. J., Selwyn, A. P., and Cooper, C. J.: Use of the left internal jugular vein approach in endomyocardial biopsy. Cathet. Cardiovasc. Diagn. *32*:42, 1994.
71. Corley, D. D., and Strickman, N.: Alternative approaches to right ventricular endomyocardial biopsy. Cathet. Cardiovasc. Diagn. *31*:236, 1994.
72. Anderson, J. L. and Marshall, H. W.: The femoral venous approach to endomyocardial biopsy: Comparison with internal jugular and transarterial approaches. Am. J. Cardiol. *53*:833, 1984.
73. Miller, L. W., Labovitz, A. J., McBride, L. A., et al.: Echocardiography-guided endomyocardial biopsy: A 5-year experience. Circulation 78(suppl III):III-99, 1988.
74. Sekiguchi, M., and Take, M.: World survey of catheter biopsy of the heart. *In* Sekiguchi, M., and Olsen, E. G. J. (eds.): Cardiomyopathy. Clinical, Pathological, and Theoretical Aspects. Baltimore, University Park Press, 1980, p. 217.
75. Fowler, R. E., and Mason, J. W.: Role of cardiac biopsy in the diagnosis and management of cardiac disease. Prog. Cardiovasc. Dis. *27*:153, 1984.
76. Mason, J. W., and O'Connell, J. B.: Clinical merit of endomyocardial biopsy. Circulation *79*:971, 1989.
77. Abelmann, W. H., Baim, D. S., and Schnitt, S. J.: Endomyocardial biopsy: Is it of clinical value? Postgrad. Med. J. *68*(suppl. 1):S44, 1992.
78. Mason, J. W.: Endomyocardial biopsy and the causes of dilated cardiomyopathy. J. Am. Coll. Cardiol. *23*:591, 1994.
79. Kasper, E. K., Agema, W. R. P., Hutchins, G. M., et al.: The causes of dilated cardiomyopathy: A clinicopathologic review of 673 consecutive patients. J. Am. Coll. Cardiol. *23*:586, 1994.
80. Schoenfeld, M. H., Supple, E. W., Dec, G. W., et al.: Restrictive cardiomyopathy versus constrictive pericarditis: Role of endomyocardial biopsy in avoiding unnecessary thoracotomy. Circulation *75*:1012, 1987.
81. Vaitkus, P. T., and Kussmaul, W. G.: Constrictive pericarditis versus restrictive cardiomyopathy: A reappraisal and update of diagnostic criteria. Am. Heart J. *122*:1431, 1991.
82. Hershkowitz, A., Vlahov, D., Willoughby, S. B., et al.: Prevalence and incidence of left ventricular dysfunction in patients with human immunodeficiency syndrome. Am. J. Cardiol. *71*:955, 1993.
83. Cohen, I. S., Anderson, D. W., Virmani, R., et al.: Congestive cardiomyopathy in association with the acquired immunodeficiency syndrome. N. Engl. J. Med. *315*:628, 1986.
84. Beschorner, W. E., Baughman, K., Turnicky, R. P., et al.: HIV-associated myocarditis, pathology and immunopathology. Am. J. Pathol. *137*:1365, 1990.
85. Nanas, J. N., and Moulopoulos, S. D.: Counterpulsation: Historical background, technical improvements, hemodynamic and metabolic effects. Cardiology *84*:156, 1994.
86. Weber, K. T., and Janick, J. S.: Intraaortic balloon counterpulsation: a review of physiologic principles, clinical results, and device safety. Ann. Thorac. Surg. *17*:602, 1974.
87. Kern, M. J., Aguirre, F. V., Jatineni, S., et al.: Enhanced coronary blood flow velocity during intraaortic balloon counterpulsation in critically ill patients. J. Am. Coll. Cardiol. *21*:359, 1993.
88. Aguire, F. V., Kern, M. J., Bach, R., et al.: Intraaortic balloon pump support during high-risk coronary angioplasty. Cardiology *84*:175, 1994.
89. Mueller, H. S.: Role of intra-aortic counterpulsation in cardiogenic shock and acute myocardial infarction. Cardiology *84*:186, 1994.
90. Ohman, E. M., George, B. S., White, C. J., et al.: Use of aortic counterpulsation to improve sustained coronary artery patency during acute myocardial infarction: Results of a randomized trial. Circulation *90*:792, 1994.
91. Alderman, J. D., Gabliani, G. I., McCabe, C. H., et al.: Incidence and management of limb ischemia with percutaneous wire guided intraaortic balloon catheters. J. Am. Coll. Cardiol. *9*:524, 1987.
92. Barnett, M. G., Swartz, M. T., Peterson, G. J., et al.: Vascular complications from intraaortic balloons: Risk analysis. J. Vasc. Surg. *19*:81, 1994.

93. Eitchaninoff, H., Dimas, A. P., and Whitlow, P. L.: Complications associated with percutaneous placement and use of intraaortic balloon counterpulsation. Am. J. Cardiol. *71*:328, 1993.
94. Nash, I. S., Lorell, B. H., Fishman, R. F., et al.: A new technique for sheathless percutaneous intraaortic balloon catheter insertion. Cathet. Cardiovasc. Diagn. *23*:57, 1991.

HEMODYNAMIC DATA

95. Grossman, W.: Pressure measurement. *In* Grossman, W., and Baim, D. S. (eds.): Cardiac Catheterization, Angiography, and Intervention. 4th ed. Philadelphia, Lea and Febiger, 1991, p. 123.
96. Milnor, W. R.: Hemodynamics. Baltimore, Williams and Wilkins, 1982.
97. Gersh, B. J., Hahn, C. E. W., and Prys-Roberts, C.: Physical criteria for measurement of left ventricular pressure and its first derivative. Cardiovasc. Res. *5*:32, 1971.
98. Bonow, R. O., and Udelson, J. E.: Left ventricular diastolic dysfunction as a cause of congestive heart failure: Mechanisms and management. Ann. Intern. Med. *117*:502, 1992.
99. Grondelle, A. van, Ditchey, R. V., Groves, B. M., et al.: Thermodilution method overestimates low cardiac low output in humans. Am. J. Physiol. *245*:H690, 1983.
100. Fargard, R., and Conway, J.: Measurement of cardiac output: Fick principle using catheterization. Eur. Heart J. *11*:1, 1990.
101. Nichols, W. W., and O'Rourke, M. F. (eds.): McDonald's Blood Flow in Arteries. 3rd ed. Philadelphia, Lea and Febiger, 1990.
102. Werko, L., Varnauskas, E., Eliasch, H., et al.: Further evidence that the pulmonary capillary wedge pressure pulse in man reflects cyclic pressure changes in the left atrium. Circ. Res. *1*:337, 1953.
103. Luchsinger, P. C., Seipp, H. W., and Patel, D. J.: Relationship of pulmonary artery-wedge pressure to left atrial pressure in man. Circ. Res. *11*:315, 1962.
104. Lange, R. A., Moore, D. M., Jr., Cigarroa, R. G., and Hillis, L. D.: Use of pulmonary capillary wedge pressure to assess severity of mitral stenosis. Is true left atrial pressure needed in this condition? J. Am. Coll. Cardiol. *13*:825, 1989.
105. McDonald, D. A., and Taylor, M. G.: The hydrodynamics of the arterial circulation. Prog. Biophys. Chem. *9*:107, 1959.
106. Carabello, B. A., Barry, W. H., and Grossman, W.: Changes in arterial pressure during left heart pullback in patients with aortic stenosis: A sign of severe aortic stenosis. Am. J. Cardiol. *44*:424, 1979.
107. Otto, C. M.: Echo-Doppler evaluation of aortic stenosis and the effect of percutaneous balloon aortic valvuloplasty. *In* Bashore, T. M. and Davidson, C. J. (eds.): Percutaneous Balloon Valvuloplasty and Related Techniques. Baltimore, Williams and Wilkins, 1991, p. 67.
108. Schoenfield, M. H., Palacios, I. F., Hutter, A. M., Jr., et al.: Underestimation of prosthetic mitral valve areas: Role of transseptal catheterization in avoiding unnecessary repeat mitral valve surgery. J. Am. Coll. Cardiol. *5*:1387, 1985.
109. Nishimura, R. A., Rihal, C. S., Tajik, A. J., and Holmes, D. R.: Accurate measurement of the transmitral gradient in patients with mitral stenosis: A simultaneous catheterization and Doppler echocardiographic study. J. Am. Coll. Cardiol. *24*:152, 1994.
110. Gorlin, R., and Gorlin, S. G.: Hydraulic formula for calculation of the area of the stenotic mitral valve, other cardiac valves, and central circulatory shunts. Am. Heart J. *41*:1, 1951.
111. Gorlin, R.: Calculations of cardiac valve stenosis: Restoring an old concept for advanced applications. J. Am. Coll. Cardiol. *19*:920, 1987.
112. Kass, D.: Hemodynamic assessment of valvular stenosis. *In* Bashore, T. M. and Davidson, C. J. (eds.): Percutaneous Balloon Valvuloplasty and Related Techniques. Baltimore, Williams and Wilkins, 1991, p. 37.
113. Bache, R. J., Wang, Y., and Jorgensen, C. R.: Hemodynamic effects of exercise in isolated valvular aortic stenosis. Circulation *44*:1003, 1971.
114. Ubago, J. L., Figueroa, A., Colman, T., et al.: Hemodynamic factors that affect calculated orifice areas in the mitral Hancock xenograft valve. Circulation *61*:388, 1980.
115. Cannon, S. R., Richards, K. L., and Crawford, M.: Hydraulic estimation of stenotic orifice area: A correction of the Gorlin formula. Circulation *71*:1170, 1985.
116. Cannon, J. D., Zile, M. R., Crawford, F. A., and Carabello, B. A.: Aortic valve resistance as an adjunct to the Gorlin formula in assessing the severity of aortic stenosis in symptomatic patients. J. Am. Coll. Cardiol. *20*:1517, 1992.
117. Carabello, B. A.: Advances in the hemodynamic assessment of stenotic cardiac valves. J. Am. Coll. Cardiol. *10*:912, 1987.
118. Hakki, A. H.: A simplified valve formula for the calculation of stenotic cardiac valve areas. Circulation *63*:1050, 1981.
119. Angel, J., Soler-Soler, J., Anivarro, I., and Domingo, E.: Hemodynamic evaluation of stenotic cardiac valves. II: Modification of the simplified formula for mitral and aortic valve calculation. Cathet. Cardiovasc. Diagn. *11*:127, 1985.
120. Ford, L. E., Feldman, T., Chiu, Y. C., and Carroll, J. D.: Hemodynamic resistance as a measure of functional impairment in aortic valvular stenosis. Circ. Res. *66*:1, 1990.
121. Sellers, R. D., Levy, M. J., Amplatz, K., and Lillehei, C. W.: Left retrograde cardioangiography in acquired cardiac disease: Technique, indications and interpretations in 700 cases. Am. J. Cardiol. *14*:437, 1964.
122. Grossman, W.: Shunt detection and measurement. *In* Grossman, W. and Baim, D. S. (eds.): Cardiac Catheterization, Angiography, and Intervention. 4th ed. Philadelphia, Lea and Febiger, 1991, p. 166.
123. Dexter, L., Haynes, F. W., Burwell, C. S., et al.: Studies of congenital heart disease. II. The pressure and oxygen content of blood in the right auricle, right ventricle, and pulmonary artery in control patients, with observations on the oxygen saturation and source of pulmonary capillary blood. J. Clin. Invest. *26*:554, 1947.
124. Antman, E. M., Marsh, J. D., Green, L. H., and Grossman, W.: Blood oxygen measurements in the assessment of intracardiac left to right shunts: A critical appraisal of methodology. Am. J. Cardiol. *46*:265, 1980.
125. Flamm, M. D., Cohn, K. E., and Hancock, E. W.: Measurement of systemic cardiac output at rest and exercise in patients with atrial septal defect. Am. J. Cardiol. *23*:258, 1969.
126. Swan, H. J. C., and Wood, E. H.: Localization of cardiac defects by dye-dilution curves recorded after injection of T-1824 at multiple sites in the heart and great vessels during cardiac catheterization. Proc. Staff Meet. Mayo Clin. *28*:95, 1953.
127. Daniel, W. C., Lange, R. A., Willard, J. E., et al.: Oximetric versus indicator dilution techniques for quantitating intracardiac left-to-right shunting in adults. Am. J. Cardiol. *75*:199, 1995.
128. Dehmer, G. J., and Rutala, W. A.: Current use of green dye curves. Am. J. Cardiol. *75*:170, 1995.
129. Castillo, C. A., Kyle, J. C., Gilson, W. E., and Rowe, G. G.: Simulated shunt curves. Am. J. Cardiol. *17*:691, 1966.
130. Lorell, B. H., and Grossman, W.: Dynamic and isometric exercise during cardiac catheterization. *In* Grossman, W. and Baim, D. S. (eds.): Cardiac Catheterization, Angiography, and Intervention. 4th ed. Philadelphia, Lea and Febiger, 1991, p. 267.
131. Dexter, L., Whittenberger, F. W., Haynes, W. T., et al.: Effects of exercise on circulatory dynamics of normal individuals. J. Appl. Physiol. *3*:439, 1951.
132. Bonow, R. O.: Left ventricular response to exercise. *In* Fletcher, G. F. (ed.): Cardiovascular Response to Exercise. American Heart Association Monograph Series. Mount Kisco, NY, Futura Publishing Co., 1993, p. 31.
133. Carroll, J. D., Hess, O. M., and Krayenbuehl, H. P.: Diastolic function during exercise-induced ischemia in man. *In* Grossman, W., and Lorell, B. H. (eds.): Diastolic Relaxation of the Heart. Boston, Martinus Nijhoff, 1986, p. 217.
134. Forrester, J. S., Helfart, R. H., Pasternac, A., et al.: Atrial pacing in coronary heart disease. Effects on hemodynamics, metabolism, and coronary circulation. Am. J. Cardiol. *27*:237, 1971.
135. Udelson, J. E., Bacharach, S. L., Cannon, R. O., and Bonow, R. O.: Minimum left ventricular pressure during beta-adrenergic stimulation in human subjects: Evidence for elastic recoil and diastolic "suction" in the normal heart. Circulation *82*:1174, 1990.
136. Gorlin, R., Knowles, J. H., and Storey, C. F.: The Valsalva maneuver as a test of cardiac function. Pathologic physiology and clinical significance. Am. J. Med. *22*:197, 1957.
137. Buch, C. A., Stang, J. M., Wooley C. F., and Kilman, J. W.: Occult constrictive pericardial disease: Diagnosis by rapid volume expansion and correction by pericardiectomy. Circulation *56*:924, 1977.
138. Mudge, G. H., Grossman, W., Mills, R. M., Jr., et al.: Reflex increase in coronary vascular resistance in patients with ischemic heart disease. N. Engl. J. Med. *295*:1333, 1976.
139. Harding, M. B., Leithe, M. E., Mark, D. B., et al.: Ergonovine maleate testing during cardiac catheterization: A 10-year perspective in 3447 patients without significant coronary artery disease or Prinzmetal's variant angina. J. Am. Coll. Cardiol. *20*:107, 1992.
140. Wilson, R. F., Marcus, M. L., and White, C. W.: Prediction of the physiologic significance of coronary artery lesions by quantitative lesion geometry in patients with limited coronary artery disease. Circulation *75*:723, 1987.
141. Marcus, M. L.: Effects of cardiac hypertrophy on the coronary circulation. *In* Marcus, M. L. (ed.): The Coronary Circulation in Health and Disease. New York, McGraw-Hill Book Company, 1983, p. 285.
142. Klocke, F. J., Ellisa, K., and Canty, J. M., Jr.: Interpretation of changes in coronary flow that accompany pharmacologic interventions. Circulation *75*(suppl. V):34, 1987.
143. Ganz, W., Tamura, K., Marcus, H. S., et al.: Measurement of coronary sinus blood flow by continuous thermodilution in man. Circulation *44*:181, 1971.
144. Marcus, M. L., Wilson, R. F., and White, C. W.: Methods of measurement of myocardial blood flow in patients: A critical review. Circulation *76*:245, 1987.
145. Mathey, D. G., Chatterjee, K., Tyberg, J. V., et al.: Coronary sinus reflux: A source of error in the measurement of thermodilution coronary sinus flow. Circulation *57*:778, 1978.
146. Klocke, F. J.: Measurement of coronary flow reserve: Defining pathophysiology versus making decisions about patient care. Circulation *76*:1183, 1987.
147. Cusma, J. T., Toggart, E. J., Folts, J. D., et al.: Digital subtraction angiographic imaging of coronary flow reserve. Circulation *75*:461, 1987.
148. Hodgson, J. M., LeGrand, V., Bates, E. R., et al.: Validation in dogs of a rapid digital angiographic technique to measure relative coronary blood flow during routine cardiac catheterization. Am. J. Cardiol. *55*:188, 1985.
149. Vogel, R. A.: Digital radiographic assessment of coronary flow reserve. *In* Buda, A. J., and Delp, E. J. (eds.): Digital Cardiac Imaging. Boston, Martinus Nijhoff, 1985, p. 106.
150. Klinke, W. P., Christie, L. G., Nichols, W. W., et al.: Use of catheter-tip

velocity-pressure transducer to evaluate left ventricular function in man: Effects of intravenous propranolol. Circulation *61*:946, 1980.
151. Doucette, J. W., Cori, P. D., Payne, H. M., et al.: Validation of a Doppler guidewire for intravascular measurement of coronary artery flow velocity. Circulation *85*:1899, 1992.
152. Wangler, R. D., Peters, K. G., Laughlin, D. E., et al.: A method for continuously assessing coronary velocity in the rat. Am. J. Physiol. *10*:H816, 1981.
153. Marcus, M., Wright, C., Doty, D., et al.: Measurement of coronary velocity and reactive hyperemia in the coronary circulation in humans. Circ. Res. *49*:877, 1981.
154. Wilson, R. F., and White, C. W.: Measurement of maximal coronary flow reserve: A technique for assessing the physiologic significance of coronary arterial lesions in humans. Herz *12*:163, 1987.
155. Dehmer, L., Gould, K. L., and Kirkeeide, R.: Assessing stenosis severity, coronary flow reserve, collateral function, quantitative coronary arteriography, position imaging, and digital subtraction angiography. A review and analysis. Prog. Cardiovasc. Dis. *30*:307, 1988.

Chapter 7
Radiology of the Heart

ROBERT M. STEINER, DAVID C. LEVIN

HISTORICAL PERSPECTIVE

The history of cardiac imaging is almost as old as radiology itself. Within one year of Roentgen's discovery, Francis H. Williams of Boston published two articles on cardiac imaging.[1] He reported, "I found that the outline of the heart as seen . . . through the fluoroscope corresponded to the outline drawn on the skin with percussion as a guide." Williams was a true pioneer. Using fluoroscopy, he was the first to describe the difference in pulsations between pericardial effusion and an enlarged heart.[2] By 1899 Williams concluded that radiography was the best method of determining heart size based on a comparison of radiographic findings, digital percussion, and autopsy specimens in 546 patients.[2]

During the decades that followed, dramatic developments in imaging technology occurred, highlighted by the Coolidge hot cathode ray tube in 1913, kymography in the 1920's, angiocardiography in the early 1930's, and the image intensifier in 1952.[3] Since the 1950's, a number of new modalities including radioisotope scanning, ultrasound, computed tomography (CT) and magnetic resonance imaging (MRI) have revolutionized cardiac imaging, allowing real-time anatomically detailed examination of the heart not possible with plain film techniques. In spite of these advances, the plain chest radiograph continues to yield unique and valuable information about the structure and function of the heart and the great vessels. As a screening examination patients undergo on entering the hospital or at an outpatient office for a wide variety of cardiopulmonary as well as other disorders, the chest radiograph presents an opportunity to identify subtle or overlooked cardiac pathology, including significant vascular calcification, chamber enlargement, and evidence of pulmonary arterial or venous hypertension. Adult-onset congenital heart disease, which may be overlooked clinically, is often identified by plain film chest radiography. The chest film frequently helps to confirm a clinical impression of valvular heart disease, acute or chronic pericarditis, ischemic heart disease, left ventricular failure, or pulmonary edema.

The former mainstay of cardiac diagnosis, the four-view heart series with a barium esophagram and cardiac fluoroscopy, has been supplanted by more sensitive and specific imaging modalities such as angiography,[4,5] CT (Chap. 10),[4,6–10] nuclear cardiology (Chap. 9),[11–12] MRI (Chap. 10),[6,11,13–18a] and echocardiography (Chap. 3).[19–21]

In recent years, the bedside portable chest roentgenogram has gained special importance in the evaluation and monitoring of patients with cardiac disease in the intensive care unit, including the postoperative cardiac patient.[5,22,23]

In this chapter we discuss the role of plain film chest radiology, emphasizing cardiovascular anatomy and alterations of that anatomy in a variety of pathological disorders. Correlation with cross-sectional imaging is used to clarify important anatomical questions.

NORMAL CARDIAC ANATOMY

Plain Chest Radiography

There is excellent contrast between the air-filled lung and the adjacent soft tissue structures in the normal chest radiograph. As a result, the pulmonary arteries and veins and the interlobar fissures are visualized in great detail. For this reason, the chest film remains the study of first choice for the evaluation of pulmonary parenchymal and vascular disease. On the other hand, the heart and other mediastinal structures appear as a featureless, opaque silhouette. Blood, myocardium, pericardium, coronary arteries and great vessels, valves, and mediastinal fat cannot be separated because they have similar radiographic attenuation characteristics, so that there is little or no contrast available to differentiate these structures. However, the cardiac borders are clearly outlined, and deviation from the normal configuration does suggest disease. Thus, knowledge of the appearance of the normal and pathological cardiac silhouettes is essential for the initial evaluation of the cardiac patient.

FRONTAL VIEW. In a well-positioned posteroanterior (PA) or frontal chest roentgenogram, the normal cardiac and other vascular structures are predictably outlined against the lung as a series of indentations and bulges along the right and left mediastinal borders (Fig. 7–1).

Left Subclavian Artery. The left subclavian artery is the border-forming structure along the upper left mediastinum above the aortic arch. Although the left innominate vein is actually lateral in position to the left subclavian artery, it is adjacent to the anterior chest wall so that there is no available contrast in the frontal view to single out the left innominate vein as a distinct structure. The left subclavian artery usually forms a concave border with the lung, extending from the clavicle to the aortic arch. The left subclavian artery may bulge laterally when there is increased blood flow through the vessel, as in postductal coarctation of the aorta or when the vessel is tortuous due to atherosclerosis or hypertension. A straight or a convex left supraaortic border is found in patients with persistent left superior vena cava (Fig. 7–2).

Aortic Arch. The aortic arch or "knob" forms a sharply marginated convex border immediately below the left subclavian artery. It is usually small in the young patient, with a diameter of 2.0 ± 1.0 cm, and represents the left posterior-lateral portion of the aortic arch. The trachea is displaced slightly to the right at the level of the aortic arch. When a right aortic arch is present, the trachea is displaced slightly to the left, a clear indication of that anomaly. A small bump or "nipple" measuring about 2 to 3 mm in diameter, representing the left superior intercostal vein, can be seen along the aortic arch in a minority of individuals (4 to 10 per cent) (Fig. 7–3).[23,24] When enlarged, the left superior intercostal vein has the same significance as a dilated azygos vein; i.e., it is due to increased central venous pressure or increased blood flow resulting from diversion from other major venous structures, as may occur in superior vena cava syndrome, inferior vena caval obstruction, or deep mediastinal venous obstruction.

The aortic arch is prominent on the frontal view in older individuals with pronounced aortic regurgitation, systemic hypertension, or atherosclerosis (Fig. 7–4). It is wider and higher than in the normal aorta and may even reach the level of the clavicle. The ascending aorta protrudes farther to the right side. The descending aorta assumes a tortuous or serpentine configuration (Fig. 7–4*A*). Aortic dissection (Fig. 7–4*B*) and aneurysm of the aortic arch (Fig. 7–4*C*) are evident on the frontal view. The brachiocephalic vessels also dilate and become tortuous. At times, a dilated right brachiocephalic artery may mimic the appearance of a substernal thyroid or other superior mediastinal mass and may require CT or MRI for diagnosis. In one of 1500 patients there is a right-sided aortic arch related to either an

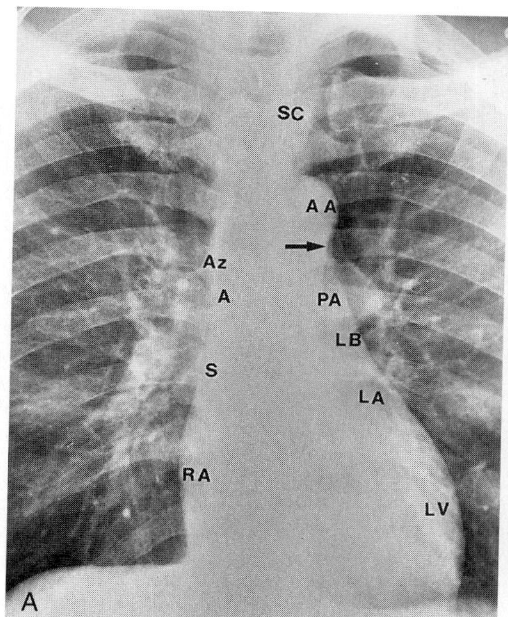

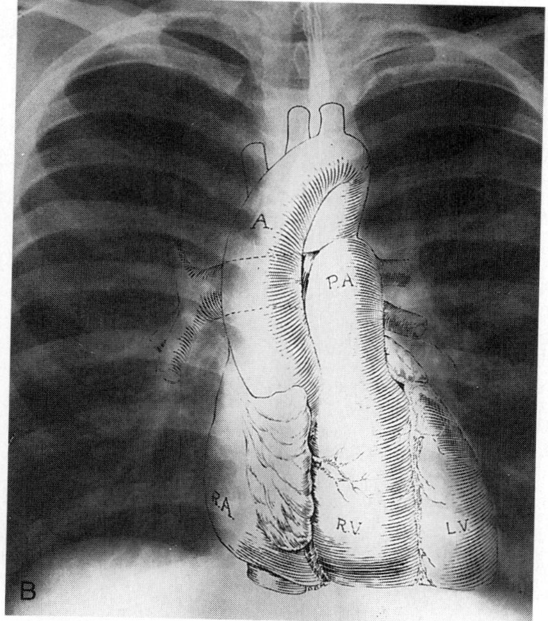

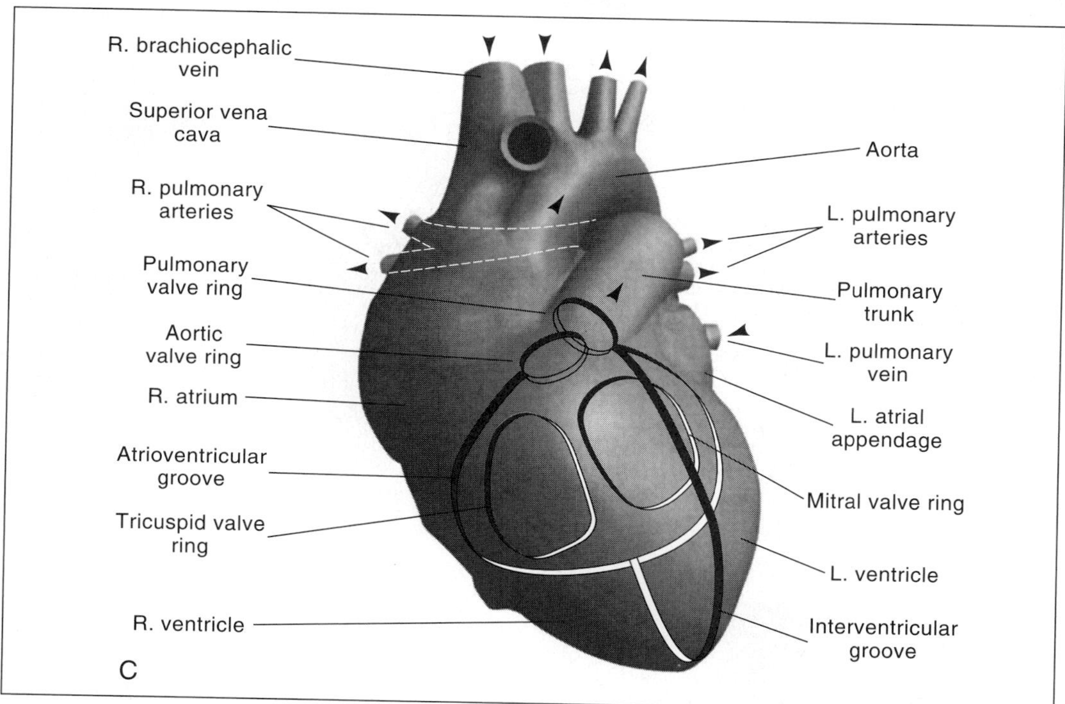

FIGURE 7–1. **Frontal projection of the heart and great vessels.** ***A,*** **Left and right heart borders in the frontal projection. SC = left subclavian artery; A = ascending aorta; LV = left ventricle; B = left bronchus; LA = left atrial appendage; PA = main pulmonary artery; RA = right atrium; S = superior vena cava; AA = aortic arch; Az = azygos vein; arrow = aorticopulmonary window.** ***B,*** **Superimposed line drawing demonstrates the position of the heart and great vessels. PA = pulmonary artery; RV = right ventricle; A = aorta; LV = left ventricle; RA = right atrium. (*A* and *B* from Van Houten, F. X., et al.: Radiology of valvular heart disease.** ***In*** **Sonnenblick, E., and Lesch, M. [eds.]: Valvular Heart Disease. New York, Grune and Stratton, 1974.)** ***C,*** **Line drawing in the frontal projection demonstrates the relationship of the cardiac valves, rings, and sulci to the cardiac silhouette.**

aberrent left subclavian artery or a mirror image arch. When no aortic knob is visible on the left side, displacement of the trachea to the left and an aortic arch on the right should lead to the diagnosis of right aortic arch[25,26] (Fig. 7–5).

The left mediastinal border immediately below the aortic arch is characterized by a variable-sized indentation of the lung into the mediastinum. This indentation is the aorticopulmonary window (Fig. 7–6). It is bordered superiorly by the inferior margin of the aortic arch and inferiorly by the upper margin of the left pulmonary artery. This small space contains, in addition to fat and soft tissue, several important anatomical structures. These include the left recurrent laryngeal nerve, the ligamentum or ductus arteriosus, and the ductus node. Lymphadenopathy or a ductus diverticulum may cause a convex bulge in the normally concave mediastinal reflection of the aorticopulmonary window.[27,28] Encroachment on the recurrent laryngeal nerve within the aorticopulmonary window by a neoplasm, a ductus diverticulum, or an enlarged lymph node or extrinsic pressure on the nerve from an aortic aneurysm or large left atrium can cause paralysis of the left vocal cord.

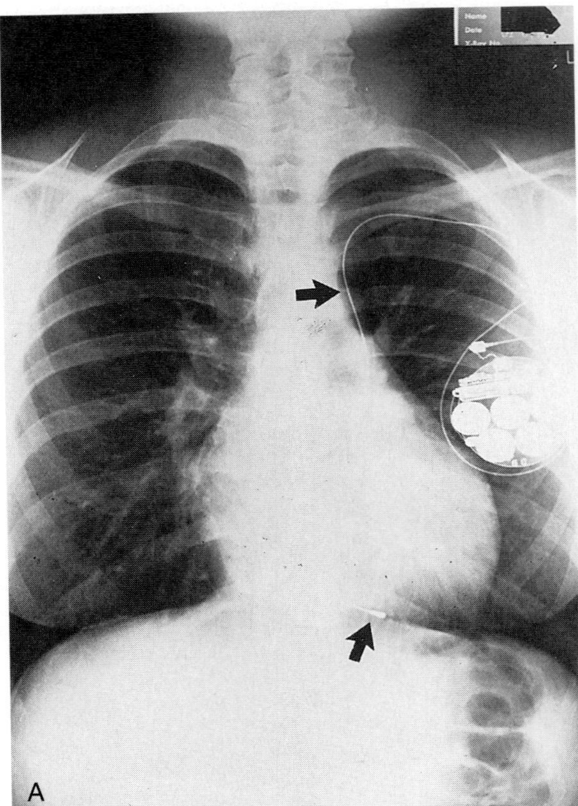

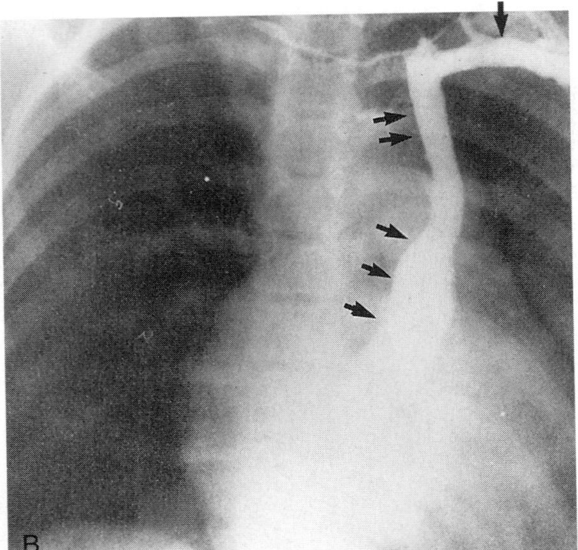

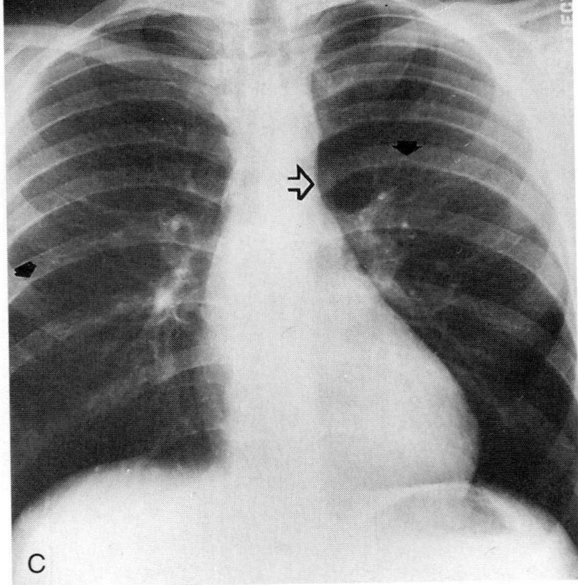

FIGURE 7–2. Persistent left superior vena cava (LSVC). *A,* PA chest film in a man with a normally functioning intravenous cardiac pacemaker. The course of the lead is as follows: LSVC (upper arrow) to coronary sinus, to right atrium and right ventricular apex (lower arrow). *B,* Left subclavian venogram illustrates the course of the LSVC: the subclavian vein (one arrow), the LSVC (two arrows), and the coronary sinus (three arrows). *C,* The left subclavian artery is prominent (open arrow) in this patient with coarction of the aorta. Rib notching is present (arrows).

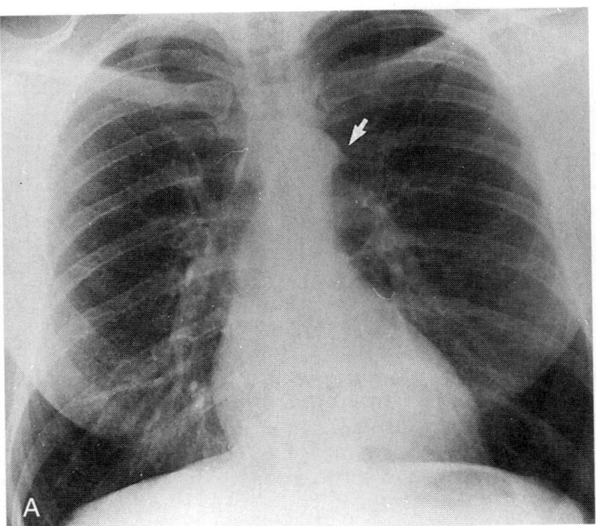

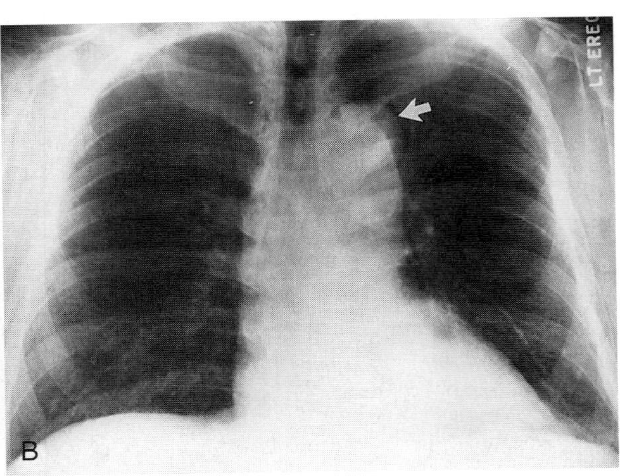

FIGURE 7–3. Left superior intercostal vein (LSIV). A small nipple or bulge is visible on the aortic knob. The LSIV normally measures 2 to 3 mm in diameter. Enlargement may be due to deep venous obstruction or altered hemodynamics. *A,* PA projection in a young woman. LSIV is a beak-like bulge that extends to the left at the aortic knob (arrow). *B,* A larger convex "mass" than that shown in *A* overlying the aortic knob (arrow).

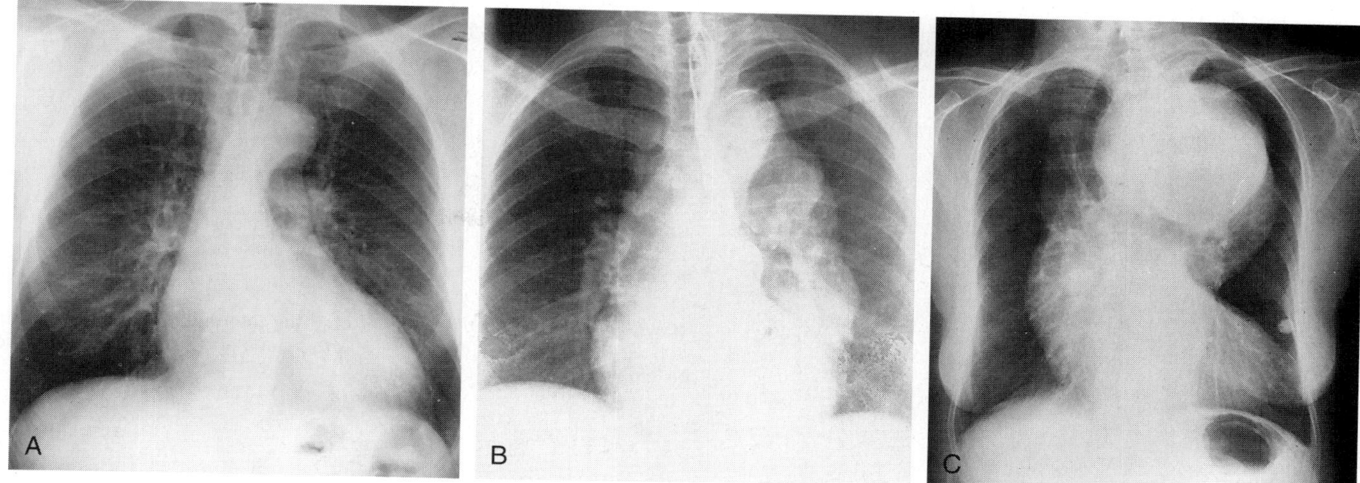

FIGURE 7–4. *A,* Aortic enlargement. A 63-year-old man with longstanding systemic hypertension and aortic regurgitation. There is marked dilatation and uncoiling of the aortic arch and descending aorta. *B,* Chronic aortic dissection. Marked dilation and elongation of the arch and descending aorta. The barium-filled esophagus follows the aorta and cannot be used to evaluate left atrial size. *C,* Giant aneurysm of the aortic arch with marked displacement of the trachea to the right.

Main Pulmonary Artery. The origin of the left main pulmonary artery is located immediately below the aorticopulmonary window and is border-forming with the left lung (Fig. 7–1*A, B*). It is identified as a small to moderate-sized, smoothly marginated arc at the level where the left pulmonary artery branches. Another indication of the location of the main pulmonary artery is the position of the left main stem bronchus. The left pulmonary artery arches over the left main stem bronchus, unlike the right pulmonary artery, which is located between the right upper lobe and right middle lobe bronchus. When enlarged, the normally slightly convex main pulmonary artery will form a prominent convex bulge. Enlargement of the main pulmonary artery is caused by increased flow, as in patients with anemia or a left-to-right shunt. A large main pulmonary artery may also be related to turbulent blood flow, as in pulmonary valvular stenosis, or to increased pressure related to Eisenmenger physiology, pulmonary hypertension associated with scleroderma, or primary pulmonary hypertension. Finally, a large main pulmonary artery may be found in disorders of vascular wall collagen such as Marfan syndrome or "idiopathic pulmonary artery dilatation." On the other hand, the main pulmonary artery border may be flat or not seen at all in patients with transposition of the great vessels, truncus arteriosus, tetralogy of Fallot, or pulmonary atresia (Fig. 7–7).

Left Atrium. The left atrial appendage or auricle lies immediately below the left main stem bronchus in the frontal projection. The left atrial appendage normally forms a smooth and slightly concave segment of the left heart border. When the left atrial border is straightened or bulges laterally, atrial enlargement should be suspected. Nonvascular pathology may simulate enlargement of the left atrial appendage. For example, a pericardial fibroma or cyst, lymphoma, or other mediastinal or pleural neoplasms may present as a convexity of the upper left mediastinal border. Congenital absence of the pericardium also causes bulging of the left atrial appendage. An important sign of left atrial

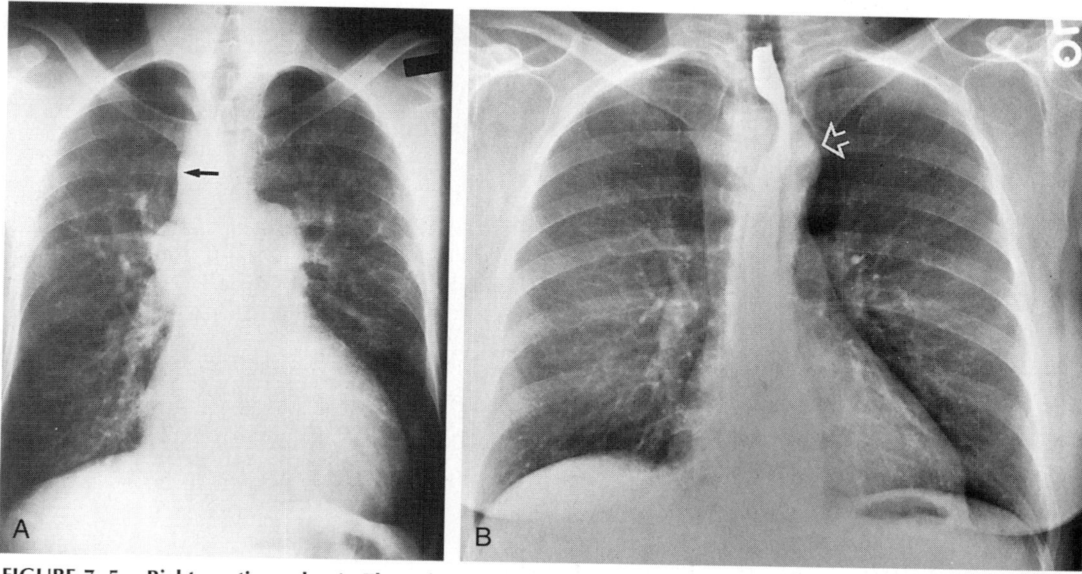

FIGURE 7–5. Right aortic arch. *A,* There is no evidence of a left-sided aortic knob in this patient with a right-sided arch (arrow). The pulmonary arteries are enlarged in this cyanotic 25-year-old man with truncus arteriosus type I. *B,* Frontal view of the chest in an adult female. The barium column is displaced to the left by the right aortic arch. The bulge on the left is due to the wide origin of the aberrant left subclavian artery (the diverticulum of Kommerall) (arrow).

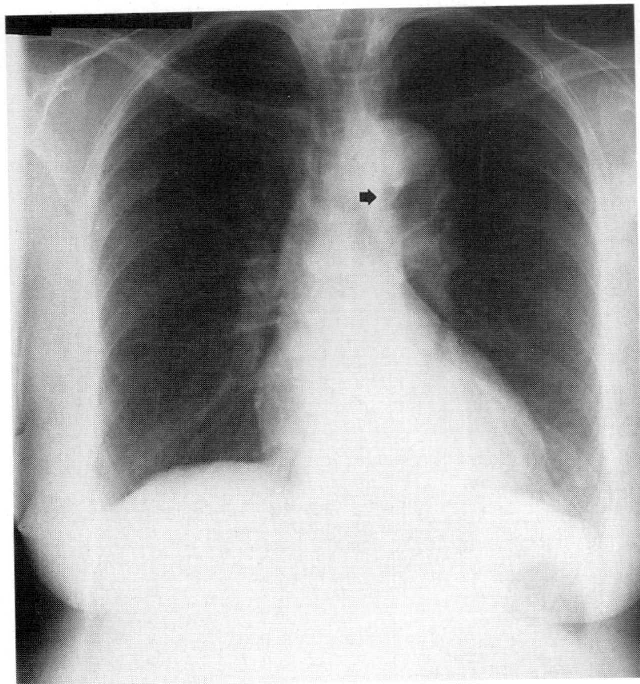

FIGURE 7–6. The deep recess between the inferior margin of the aortic arch and the superior edge of the left pulmonary artery represents the aorticopulmonary window (arrow).

enlargement in the frontal projection is elevation of the main stem bronchus so that the carinal angle is greater than the normal value of up to 75 degrees[29,30] (Figs. 7–8, 7–9).

Left Ventricle. The left ventricular border seamlessly blends with the left atrial border (Fig. 7–1*A*) without a specific landmark to differentiate between the two chambers. The left ventricular border is mildly convex extending to the diaphragm. It may be rounded and the apex elevated with hypertrophy due to aortic stenosis or hypertrophic cardiomyopathy. When the left ventricle is enlarged because of dilatation, as may occur with aortic regurgitation or aneurysm, the apex is displaced downward and laterally. Much of the downward displaced apex may be obscured by the overlying left diaphragmatic dome (Fig. 7–10).

With dilatation of the left ventricle due to volume overload as occurs, for example, in mitral regurgitation, the dimensions of the chamber increase markedly and the heart assumes a globular appearance. The left ventricular border extends to the left and may even reach the rib convexities. As the left ventricle enlarges, it obscures the left atrial border. The left anterior oblique projection helps to separate the two chambers so that their relative sizes can be discerned. The ability to separate the left heart chambers assumes importance when the differential diagnosis lies between ischemic cardiomyopathy (in which case the left ventricle is larger than the left atrium) and mitral regurgitation (in which case the left atrium may be larger than the left ventricle).

Right Atrium. The right atrial border forms a gentle convex interface with the adjacent right middle lobe. In the frontal projection, the inferior vena caval border below the right atrium is usually straight, and in a good inspiratory film it can be separated from the convex right atrial border.[30] The outline of the normal left atrium is seen deep to the right atrial border as an additional convex density.

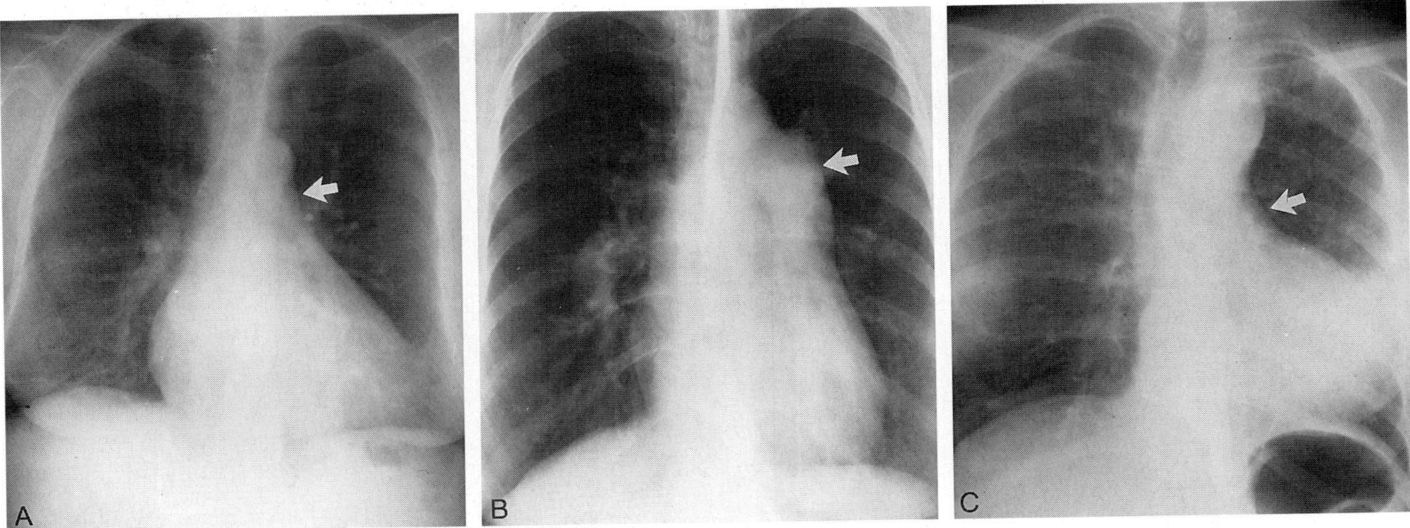

FIGURE 7–7. The pulmonary artery contour. *A*, Normal pulmonary artery segment in a 36-year-old woman with sickle cell anemia and moderate cardiomegaly (arrow). *B*, The main pulmonary artery is grossly enlarged in this patient with primary pulmonary hypertension (arrow). *C*, The pulmonary artery contour is small in this 16-year-old with tetralogy of Fallot and moderate pulmonary infundibular stenosis (arrow).

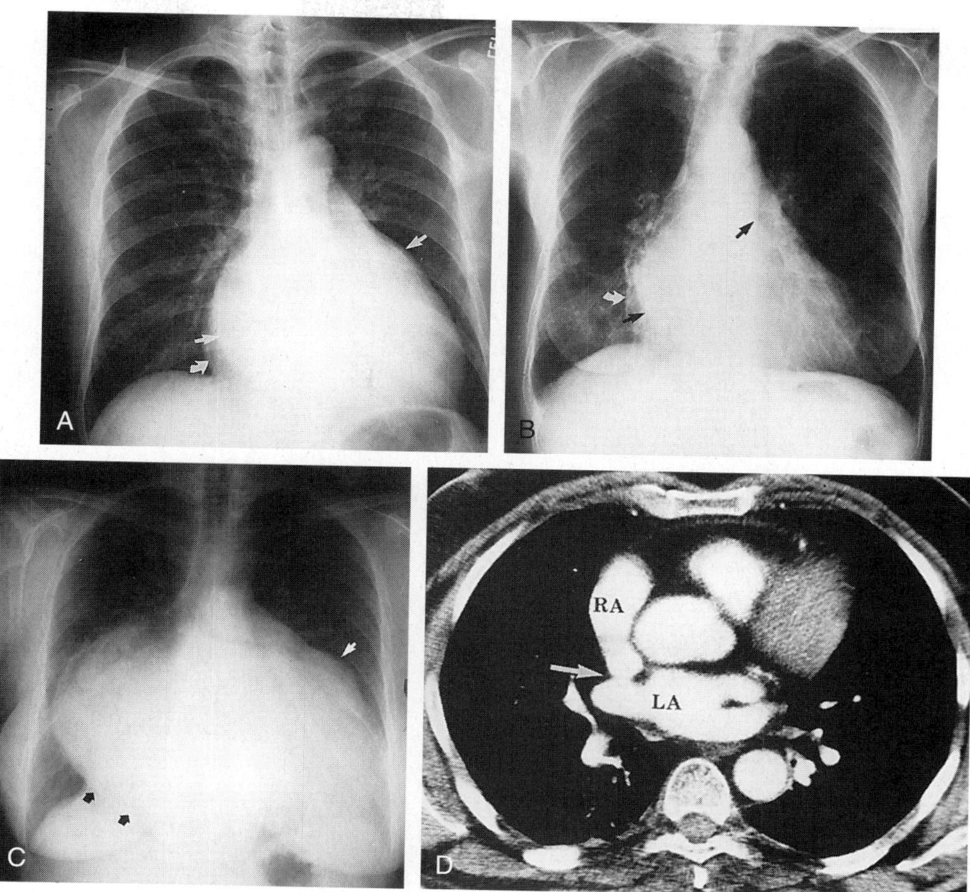

FIGURE 7–8. Prominent left atrial (LA) contour. *A,* The left atrial appendage bulges laterally to the left in this patient with multivalvular rheumatic heart disease (arrow). The double convex contour of enlarged right (curved arrow) and left (arrow) atria is present along the right atrial border (arrow). *B,* A 40-year-old woman with mitral stenosis. There is left atrial enlargement with a double right-sided heart border (white arrow = right atrium; black arrow = left atrial border). The left main stem bronchus is elevated (black arrow). *C,* Left atrial (LA) enlargement. A large convex bulge is seen in the area of the LA appendage (white arrow). The LA is grossly enlarged and is border-forming on the right side after traversing the smaller right atrium. The inferior border of the left atrium is visualized (black arrows) as it extends back toward the midline. If this were the right atrial border instead, it would have blended imperceptibly with the right hemidiaphragm and inferior vena cava. *D,* Enhanced CT demonstrates the anatomical relationship between the anterior RA and the posterior LA. The indentation of lung and fat between the atria (arrow) permits separation of the right-sided borders of both atria as seen in the PA chest radiograph.

The confluence of the right pulmonary veins is directed toward the epicenter of this bulge. The left atrium is clearly visualized within the right atrial shadow because of an interface of lung between the posteriorly positioned left atrium and the more anteriorly positioned right atrium. If the left atrium is markedly enlarged, the left atrial border may actually be lateral to the right atrium (Fig. 7–8). The borders of the right and left atria can be differentiated because the inferior border of the right atrium blends with the inferior vena cava while the left atrial shadow crosses the midline toward the left side of the heart. The upper right atrial border blends superiorly with the superior vena cava, which forms a straight interface with the adjacent lung as it continues toward the neck (Fig. 7–1). The right

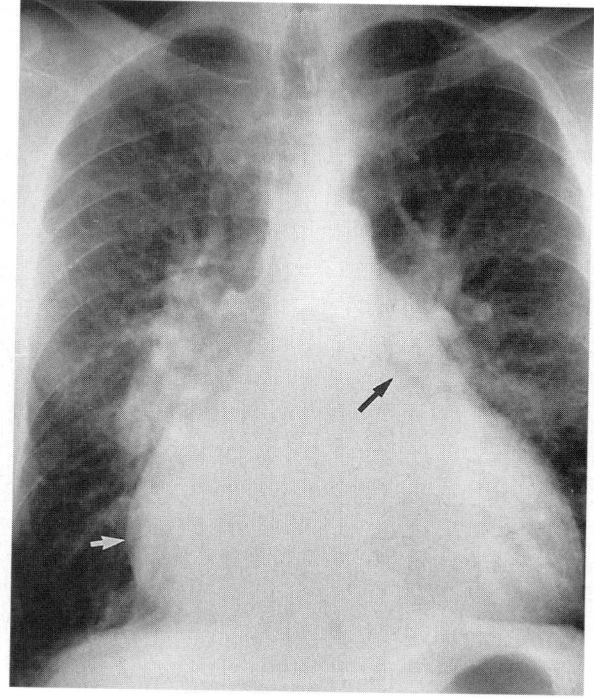

FIGURE 7–9. Prominent right atrial contour (white arrow). The RA border is prominent and convex (white arrow). There is cephalization of the pulmonary vasculature. The left atrium is deep to the enlarged right atrium. The left main stem bronchus is elevated (black arrow) in this patient with a dilated cardiomyopathy with mitral and tricuspid regurgitation.

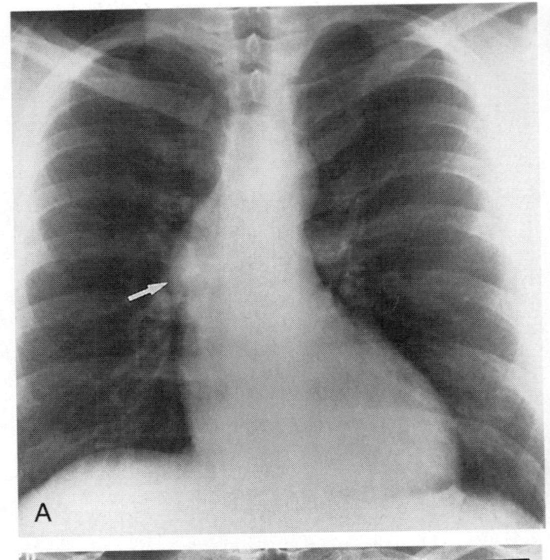

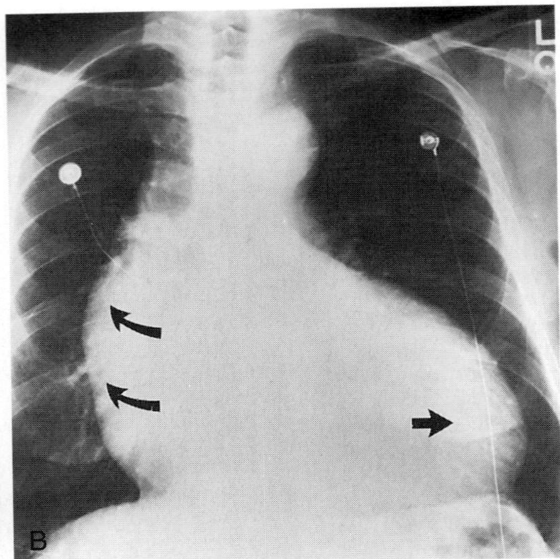

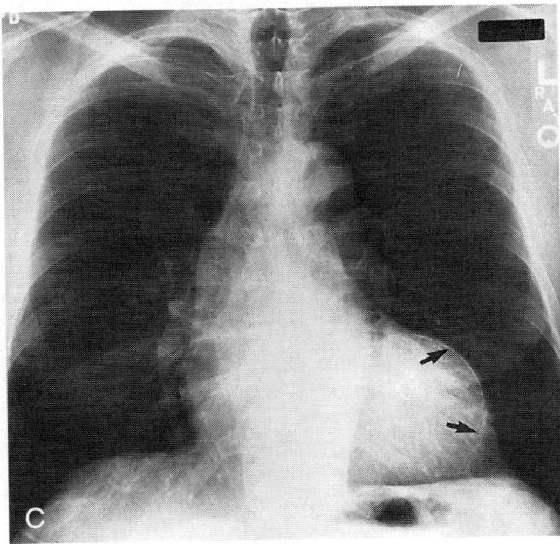

FIGURE 7–10. *A,* Aortic stenosis. The left ventricular border is rounded and prominent due to left ventricular hypertrophy. The proximal ascending aorta is prominent due to poststenotic dilatation (arrow). *B,* Aortic regurgitation in a patient with Marfan syndrome. Prominent left ventricular border (arrow). The LV chamber is dilated due to aortic regurgitation and the ascending aorta is convex (curved arrows). The descending aorta is dilated. *C,* The ascending aorta is enlarged, and there is a thin mural calcification within the left ventricle due to a large aneurysm (arrows).

atrial border is considered enlarged when it bulges more than 5.5 cm to the right of the midline[8] (Fig. 7–9).

Right Ventricle. The right ventricle is not border-forming in the frontal projection and cannot be directly viewed (Fig. 7–11; see also Fig. 7–1). As the right ventricle dilates, the left ventricle is displaced posteriorly and to the left, causing widening of the cardiac shadow. In selected cases such as tetralogy of Fallot, the enlarged right ventricle displaces the left ventricle laterally and superiorly, creating a high round left ventricular border.

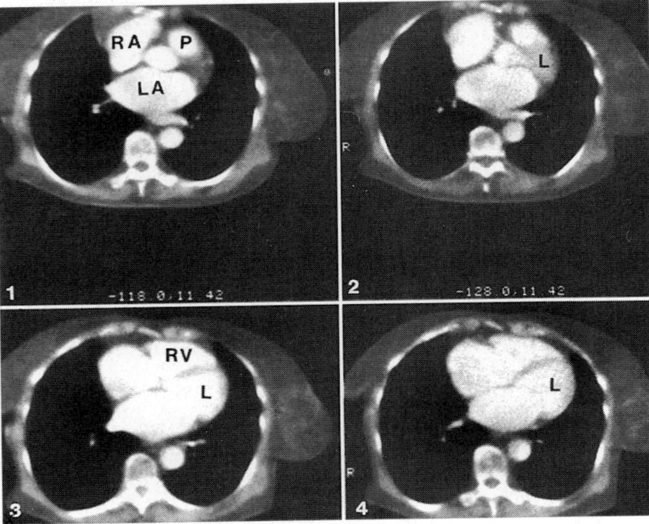

FIGURE 7–11. Enhanced ultrafast CT shows the anatomic relationships of the right ventricle. *Frame 1,* The main pulmonary artery is border-forming on the left and the right atrium is border-forming on the right. *Frame 2,* The left ventricle borders the left side of the heart. *Frames 3 and 4,* The right ventricle is border-forming anteriorly but not border-forming laterally or posteriorly. (RA = right atrium; LA = left atrium; P = pulmonary artery; L = left ventricle; RV = right ventricle.)

Ascending Aorta. This structure is superimposed on the superior vena cava and forms a convex border above the right atrium (Fig. 7–1). The aortic valve and annulus, the proximal ascending aorta, and the coronary arteries are not visible on plain films unless they are calcified, since their attenuation characteristics are similar to those of the rest of the heart. Enlargement of the aorta is shown in Figure 7–4.

Azygos Vein. The azygos vein is an elliptical structure at the right tracheobronchial angle. The azygos vein ascends in the right paravertebral sulcus and arches forward over the right main stem bronchus to enter the back of the superior vena cava (Fig. 7–12). The azygos vein and its left-sided equivalent, the hemiazygos vein, receive intercostal veins and act as an important collateral pathway when the deep mediastinal veins are obstructed.[30] Normally measuring 0.7 to 1 cm in the erect and 1 to 1.3 cm in the supine anteroposterior position, the azygos vein is a good indicator of changing cardiovascular dynamics. It is enlarged in superior vena caval and inferior vena caval obstruction, in the absence of the intrahepatic portion of the inferior vena cava, in portal vein obstruction, and in both left- and right-sided cardiac failure.[31] A change in diameter of the azygos vein will parallel changes in pulmonary venous pressure, making it a useful guide to the development of congestive heart failure on plain film x-rays. There is an azygos fissure in 3 per cent of the population. When this occurs the azygos vein is displaced laterally and superiorly and will dilate for the same reasons as a normally positioned azygos vein.[30]

LATERAL VIEW (Fig. 7–13). Proper positioning of the patient in the lateral projection is critical for accurate identification of cardiac structures.[32] The need for accurate positioning is exemplified by the right atrium. The normal right atrium is not border-forming in this projection, but if the patient is rotated backward the right atrium will form part of the lower posterior cardiac border, simulating enlargement.[30] The right ventricle is border-forming in the subxyphoid area and usually extends superiorly to a point about one-third of the distance between the diaphragm and the thoracic apex. As the right ventricle dilates, it encroaches further upon the retrosternal space.[33] The relationship between the size of the right ventricle and the extent of retrosternal encroachment is affected by body habitus and lung volume. For example, in the patient with emphysema, right ventricular enlargement may coexist with an expanded retrosternal space (Fig. 7–14*A*). In a patient with a small anterior-posterior (AP) diameter and/or a pectus excavatum deformity, the retrosternal space may be obliterated despite the absence of right ventricular enlargement (Fig. 7–14*B*). CT and MRI as well as echocardiography, unlike the chest film, portray relationships of the right ventricle to nearby structures with great accuracy and permit a clear analysis of right ventricular volume and function.[8,33,34]

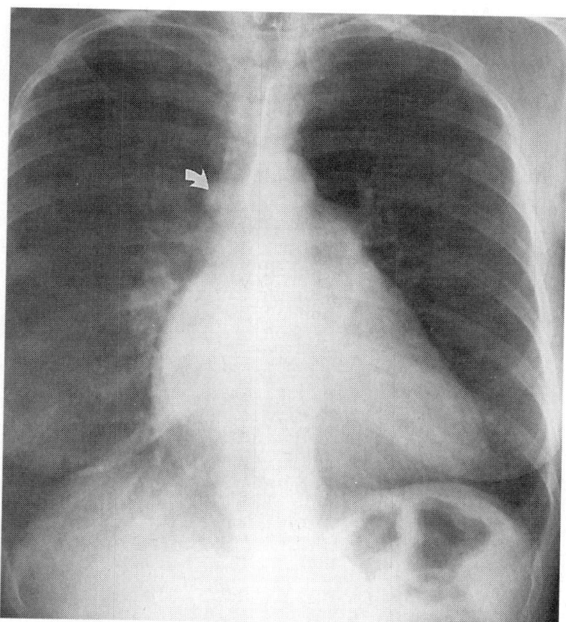

FIGURE 7–12. **The azygos vein forms an elliptical opacity at the junction of the trachea and right main stem bronchus. It is enlarged in this patient with mitral and tricuspid regurgitation (arrow).**

The anterior margin of the pulmonary artery and the ascending aorta lie above the right ventricle; however, because of abundant mediastinal fat, neither structure is visualized clearly in the normal patient. In patients with severe emphysema, however, the increased lung volume permits the main pulmonary artery and the ascending aorta to be well outlined. The arch of the aorta is usually clearly seen except at the level where the superior vena cava crosses the aorta and where the brachiocephalic arteries enter the aorta. The inferior margin of the posterior aortic arch is often visible because of the indentation of the lung into the aorticopulmonary window. The semilunar lucency of the aorticopulmonary window also outlines the superior margin of the left pulmonary artery. The descending aorta is usually not clearly discernible in the normal individual because it lies adjacent to the spine and the posterior mediastinal fat. However, in patients with hyperaeration or those with a tortuous or calcified aorta, the descending aorta is better seen.

The normal *left atrium* forms a shallow convex bulge at the upper aspect of the posterior border of the heart on the lateral view. It may be easily identified because the posterior border of the left atrium lies immediately anterior to the pulmonary venous confluence.

The normal *left ventricle* forms a long convexity at the posterior inferior heart border just above the diaphragm. Enlargement of the left ventricle is suggested by the use of the Hoffman-Rigler sign—a measurement determined by drawing a 2-cm line upward along the inferior vena cava from the point where the left ventricle and inferior vena cava cross in the lateral projection. At this point a second line is drawn parallel to the vertebral bodies. The distance between the left ventricle and the inferior vena cava should not exceed 1.8 cm. If it does, left ventricular enlargement is suggested. Although this sign is helpful, it is far from accurate because a poor positioning for a lateral chest film or backward displacement of the left ventricle due to right ventricular enlargement may influence this measurement.[32,35]

The *esophagus* lies immediately behind the left atrium and, when filled with contrast medium, can be used to locate the posterior border of the left atrial chamber. Normally the left atrium does not displace the esophagus, but when the left atrium is enlarged, posterior displacement of the esophagus from the area of the left main stem bronchus to the level of the left ventricle will occur (Fig. 7–14*C*). The normal left ventricle usually does not displace the esophagus but extends posterior and lateral to the esophagus. When both the left atrium and left ventricle are enlarged, the barium-filled esophagus may be pushed backward in one long curve.[36] Sometimes the left atrium enlarges without displacing the barium-filled esophagus because the esophagus may slide off the back of the left atrium to the left or right. When the aorta is tortuous and dilated (Fig. 7–4*B*) or when there is a scoliosis, the esophagus parallels the spinal curvature and cannot be used to evaluate left atrial size.

RIGHT ANTERIOR OBLIQUE (RAO) PROJECTION (Fig. 7–15). Chest radiography in this projection is performed with the patient in a 45-degree right anterior oblique relationship to the film cassette (right shoulder toward the cassette). In this view there is elongation of the ventricles; the long axes

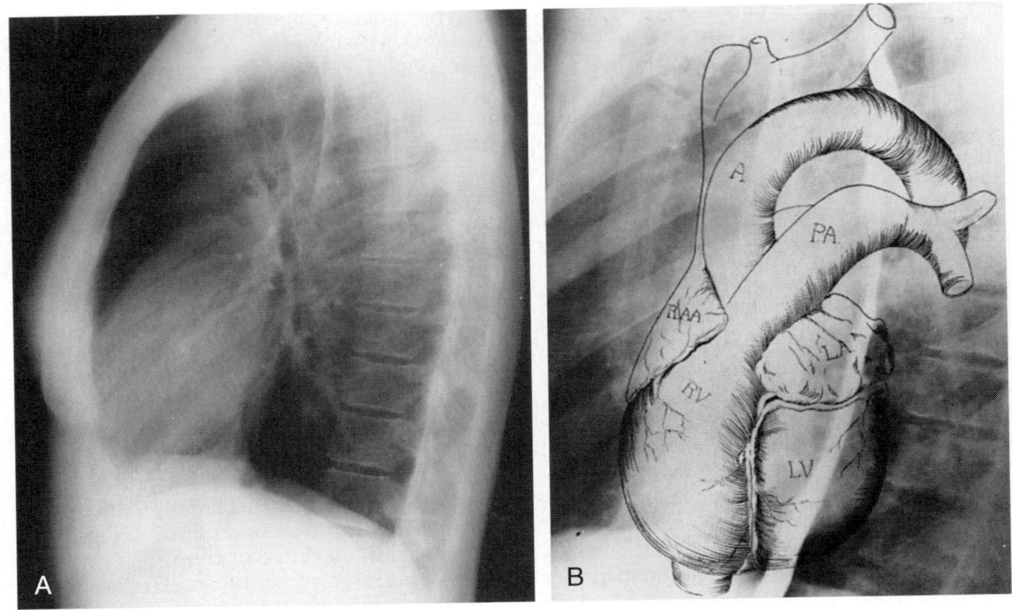

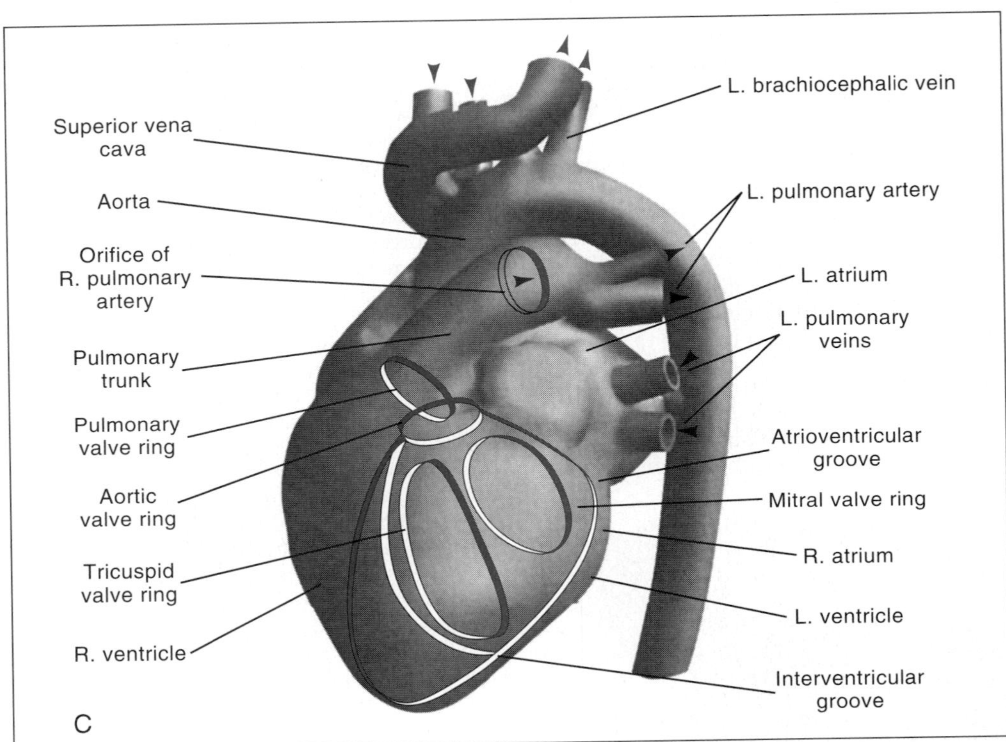

FIGURE 7–13. *A,* **Lateral chest film.** *B,* **Superimposed anatomical drawing of the cardiac chambers and great vessels. (***A, B* **from Van Houten, F. X., et al: Radiology of valvular heart disease.** *In* **Sonnenblick, E., and Lesch, M. [eds.]: Valvular Heart Disease. New York, Grune and Stratton, 1974.)** *C,* **Lateral projection of the heart showing position of valve rings.**

of the ventricles are in view and the atrioventricular groove is in profile. This position permits optimal visualization of a calcified mitral or tricuspid valve. The right anterior oblique view is used by angiographers to determine the presence of left atrial enlargement, a common feature in mitral stenosis (Fig. 7–16). It is also helpful to the fluoroscopist when studying the function of a mechanical mitral valve prosthesis. The aortic arch is foreshortened in this view, so that the arch and proximal descending aorta are often superimposed and obscured. The anterior border of the heart consists of the sinus portion of the right ventricle inferiorly and the right ventricular outflow tract and the main pulmonary artery superiorly. The right-sided or posterior heart border consists of the right atrium superiorly and the left atrium inferiorly.[36,37]

LEFT ANTERIOR OBLIQUE (LAO) PROJECTION (Fig. 7–17). The left anterior oblique projection is performed with the patient in a 60-degree oblique relationhip to the cassette. This is a useful angiographic view to diagnose the presence of left ventricular enlargement. Since the ventricular septum is in profile in the LAO projection, septal defects, dyskinesia, and displacement, due to right heart enlargement, can be identified. In this projection the aortic and pulmonary valves are in profile, so that aortic valve calcifi-

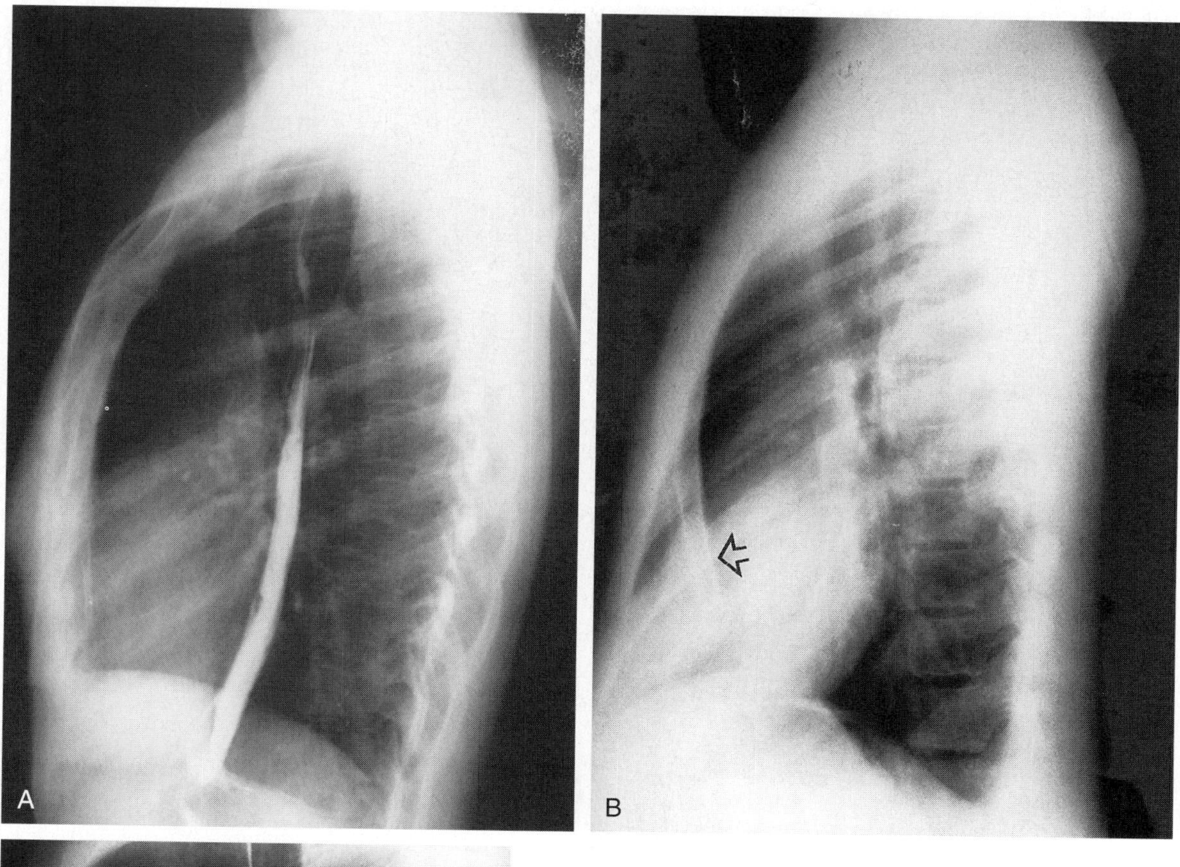

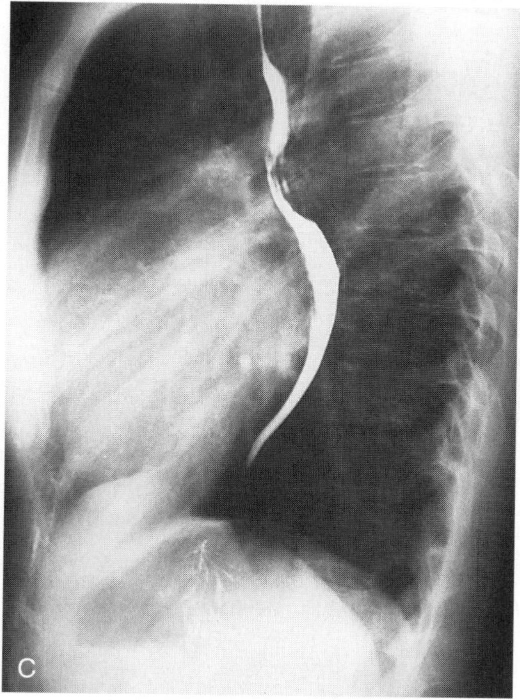

FIGURE 7–14. *A,* The extent of right ventricular encroachment on the retrosternal space is reduced by the hyperinflated lung due to emphysema. *B,* Severe pectus excavatum in patient with prolapsed mitral valve (arrow). The deformity exaggerates the extent of retrosternal encroachment. *C,* There is discrete posterior displacement of the barium column due to left atrial enlargement in a patient with mitral stenosis.

cations can be clearly visualized and aortic or pulmonary stenosis and regurgitation can be assessed.[32,37,38] The aortic arch is also in profile in the LAO projection so that abnormalities of the arch including dissection, contained rupture, aortitis, aneurysm, and coarctation can be detected with aortography or cross-sectional imaging.[30,39,40] The anterior (right) heart border consists of the right atrium above and right ventricle below. Along the left posterior heart border, the left atrium is border-forming superiorly and the left ventricle inferiorly.[41] The LAO projection is superior to other projections for detecting right ventricular enlargement, characterized by an increase in the convexity of the anterior border of the cardiac silhouette. An enlarged right atrium may cause bulging of the upper anterior border of the cardiac shadow, producing a shelf-like configuration.[30]

Fluoroscopy of the Heart

Fluoroscopy is performed to study cardiac motion and to identify cardiac and other mediastinal calcifications.[42]

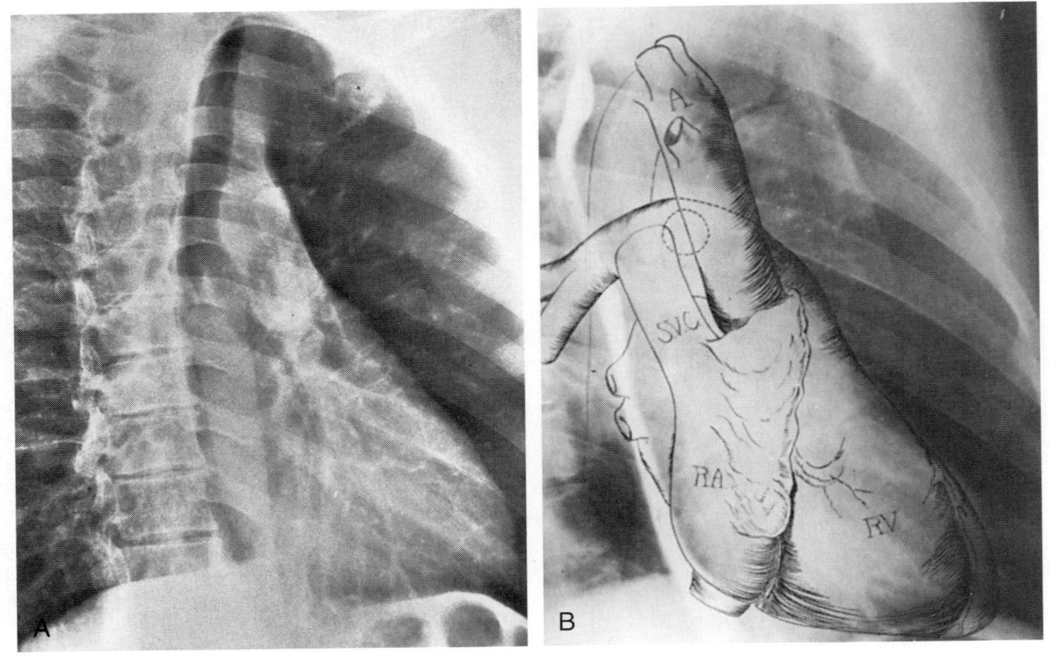

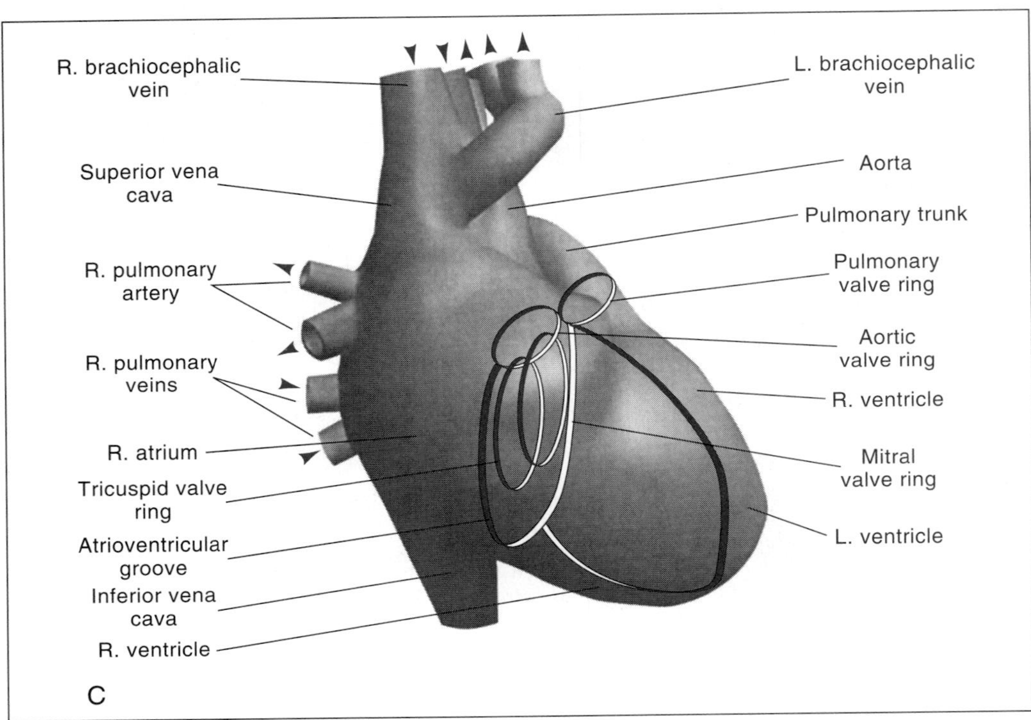

FIGURE 7–15. Right anterior oblique (45-degree) projection. ***A,*** **Chest radiograph.** ***B,*** **Line drawing shows position of cardiac chambers. (*A, B* from Van Houten, F. X., et al.: Radiology of valvular heart disease. *In* Sonnenblick, E., and Lesch, M. [eds.]: Valvular Heart Disease. New York, Grune and Stratton, 1974.)** ***C,*** **Drawing shows position of valve rings.**

Today, cardiac fluoroscopy is no longer performed routinely but is used largely to solve specific clinical questions. Because fluoroscopy potentially causes significant radiation risk to the patient, it should be used selectively, with careful beam collimation. Exposure time should be kept to a minimum, preferably not more than 5 minutes.[43] Perhaps the most important applications of fluoroscopy today are to evaluate prosthetic valve function and to detect coronary artery, valvular, and pericardial calcifications.[44–53]

Cardiac fluoroscopy is usually performed with the patient in the upright position at 68 to 75 kVp to enhance contrast and reduce mottle. The patient's position is determined by the structure to be studied. For example, if the presence or absence of aortic valve calcification is to be determined, positioning for a LAO projection is optimal. If the function of a mitral valve prosthesis is in question, or if the presence of mitral calcification is suspected, the RAO projection is most suitable. Coronary calcifications are best studied in the left and right oblique projections. In the 60-degree LAO projection, the right coronary artery, left circumflex, and left main coronary artery are seen to advantage. In the lateral and RAO projections, calcification of the left anterior descending artery is easily discernible.[49]

Although large calcifications may be seen on the chest film, small calcifications are often obscured because of mo-

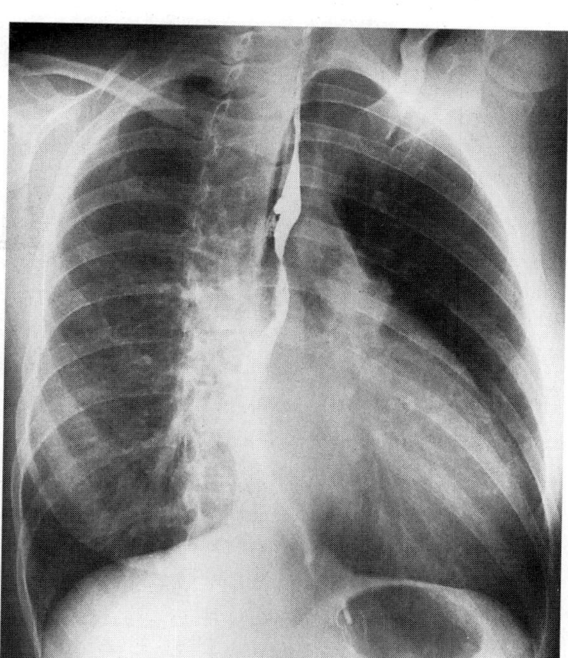

FIGURE 7–16. Right anterior oblique view. There is posterior displacement of the barium column by an enlarged LA in this patient with mitral stenosis.

tion. On the other hand, motion is an advantage with fluoroscopy and even small coronary artery calcifications are seen clearly as opaque tracks of calcification moving perpendicular to their long axes in a "to and fro" motion. The right main and circumflex coronary arteries move more vigorously than the anterior and posterior descending arteries. Subepicardial fat represents an important landmark for the identification of vascular and valvular anatomy and is best seen with fluoroscopy. Fat surrounding the coronary arteries and within the atrioventricular groove is well visualized so that the location of the mitral and tricuspid valves, the coronary sinus, and circumflex and right coronary arteries can be determined.

Fluoroscopy with videotape recording is useful in analyzing the integrity of the radiopaque components of prosthetic valves.[45,46] Excursion of the sewing ring exceeding 9 to 12 degrees between systole and diastole is associated with significant dehiscence (Fig. 7–18). Limitation of poppet or disc occluder motion suggests the presence of thrombus or vegetation. The results of fluoroscopic analysis of mechanical components compare favorably with echocardiography and phonocardiography but do not yield useful information about the degree of valvular regurgitation as will Doppler echocardiography, MRI, and angiography.[45,54,55]

Measuring Cardiac Size

Measurement of the size of the heart with plain film radiography has been de-emphasized in recent years because more accurate analyses of cardiac chamber dimensions and volume are available with echocardiography, radioisotope scanning, CT, and MRI. However, since an enlarged heart is abnormal, estimation of the cardiothoracic ratio remains a valuable yardstick to gain an impression of cardiac size and particularly serial changes in heart size coinciding with cardiac events. This may be done subjectively by estimating whether a heart is normal in size, enlarged, or grossly enlarged on the basis of an average cardiothoracic ratio of ≤0.50 with a range of 0.39 to 0.55.[37,56] Using more objective criteria, the cardiothoracic ratio may be expressed as the ratio between the maximum transverse diameter of the heart divided by the maximum width of the thorax. To obtain these diameters, a vertical line is drawn on the radiograph through the midpoint of the spine from the sternum to the diaphragm. The maximum transverse diameter of the heart is obtained by adding the widest distance of the heart border from the midline on the right and the left side (Fig. 7–19*A*). This value is then divided by the maximum transverse diameter of the thorax.[57,58] The normal range of the transverse diameter of the heart is 10 cm in a small, thin individual to 16.5 cm in a tall, heavy person. A measurement 10 per cent beyond these values represents the upper limits of normal.[59] Normal differences of transverse cardiac diameter in systole and diastole of 0.3 to 0.9 cm must be taken into account when analyzing cardiac size.[58] While the cardiothoracic ratio is helpful, it serves only as a guide. The normal heart may appear large in the frontal projection because of a small AP diameter of the thorax caused by pectus excavatum deformity or straight back. A large heart may appear smaller than it really is because of a downwardly displaced cardiac apex in patients with aortic regurgitation. The heart will be truly small in patients with Addison's disease, or anorexia nervosa due to the absence of brown fat (Fig. 7–19*B*).

Because of cardiac magnification on AP films (including portable radiographs), a visual correction must be made in order to avoid overdiagnosis of heart enlargement.[60] A correction of 10 to 12.5 per cent, depending on the anode-to-tube distance, will amend this discrepancy. High-kilovoltage PA airgap films also magnify the mediastinum approximately 6.6 per cent when compared with low-kV films in which an airgap is not used.[61] For the most part, calculated cardiothoracic ratios are of historical or research interest. In practice, these calculations are seldom performed because they are time consuming, and more accurate estimations of cardiac volume and size may be obtained with other imaging techniques.[13,14,62]

THE PULMONARY VASCULATURE

Normal Radiographic Anatomy

The pulmonary blood flow mirrors the hemodynamics of the heart itself. Because the pulmonary blood vessels are clearly visualized on the chest film, both normal and abnormal patterns of pulmonary blood flow can be identified. Increased, decreased, redistributed, or asymmetrical flow can be identified and correlated with other indications of

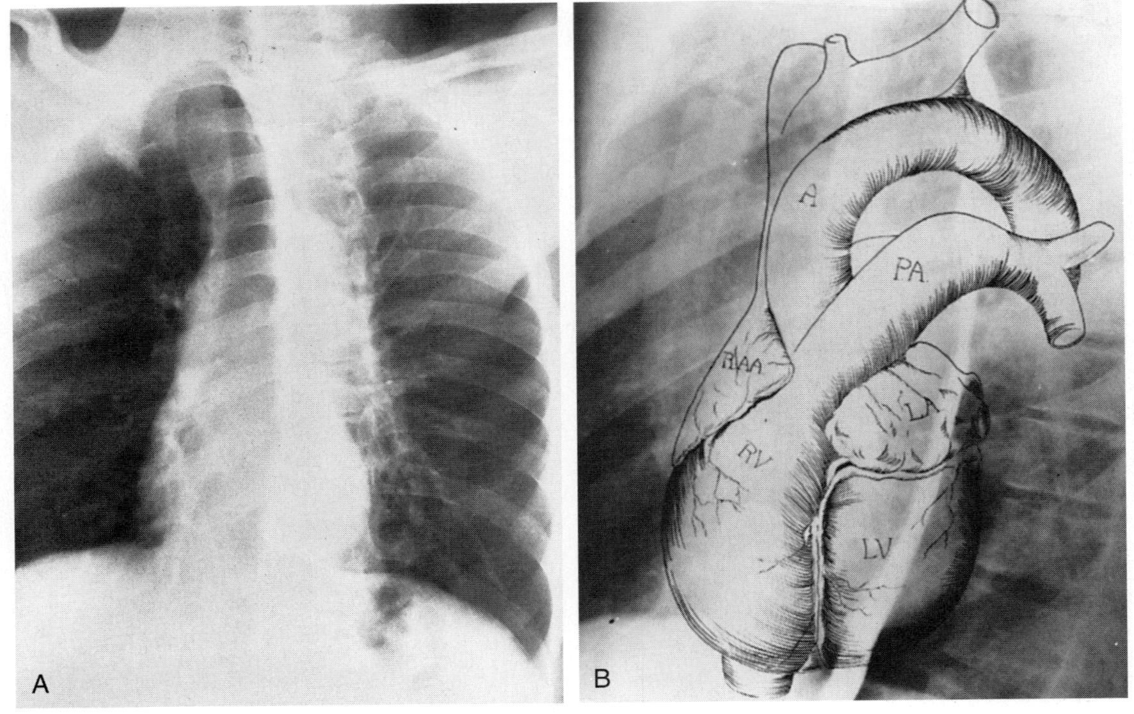

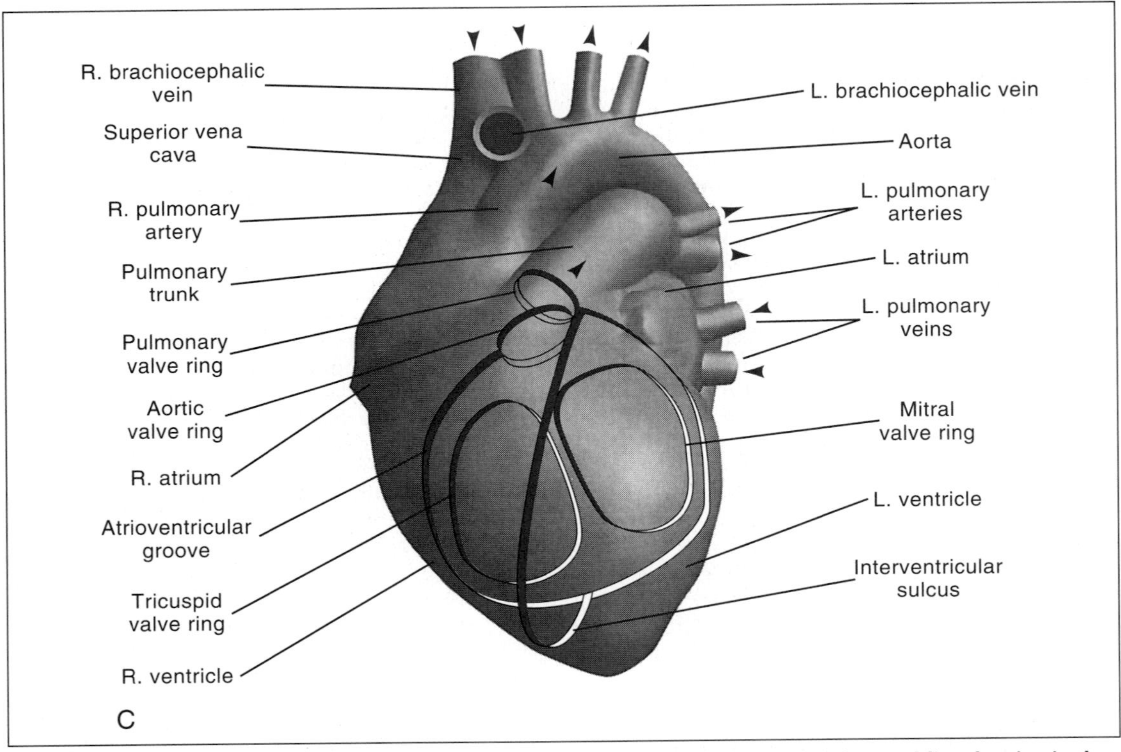

FIGURE 7–17. Sixty-degree left anterior oblique projection. *A,* Chest film. *B,* Superimposed line drawing in the same patient. (*A* and *B* from Van Houten, F. X., et al: Radiology of valvular heart disease. *In* Sonnenblick, E., and Lesch, M. [eds.]: Valvular Heart Disease. New York, Grune and Stratton, 1974.) *C,* Diagram in the left anterior oblique projection showing valves, rings, and sulci.

disease. The main pulmonary artery bifurcates within the mediastinum. The left pulmonary artery then courses to the left and backward, and its borders are visible just above the center of the left hilum (Fig. 7–1). In the lateral view, the left pulmonary artery passes over the left main stem bronchus paralleling the aortic arch (Fig. 7–13). The right pulmonary artery follows a horizontal course within the mediastinum, forming a round or elliptical opacity anterior to the right main stem bronchus on the lateral view. The right pulmonary artery divides within the mediastinum proximal to the right hilum. The intrapulmonary branches parallel the bronchi, divide in an orderly manner, and gradually taper toward the periphery of the lung. The arteries and bronchi subtending the same segment are of ap-

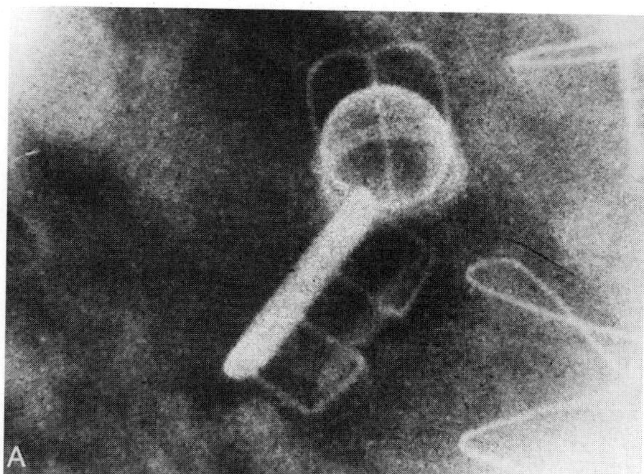

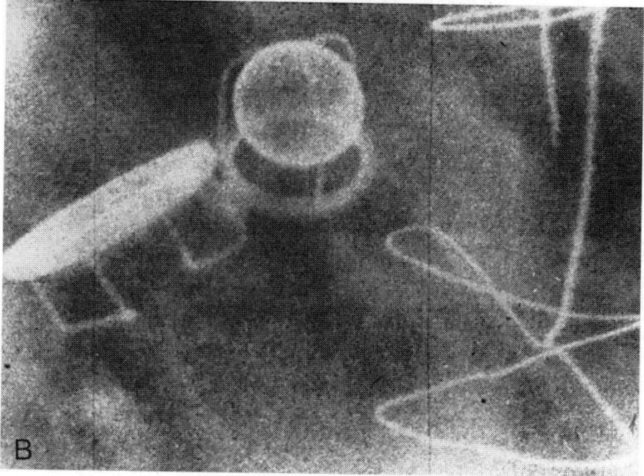

FIGURE 7–18. Abnormal excursion of a Beall mitral valve prosthesis due to partial dehiscence at the sewing ring. *A,* Diastole; *B,* systole.

proximately the same diameter at any particular level, with a ratio of 1.2:1.0. This relationship assumes importance when objective criteria are needed to support the impression of increased or redistributed blood flow (Fig. 7–20).

In the erect position, blood flow is greater to the lower lobes than to the upper lobes, partly because of the effects of gravity.[63,64] Another contributing factor affecting the normal distribution of pulmonary blood flow is differential intraalveolar pressures, as described by West.[63] In the supine and prone chest films, blood flow appears equal in both the upper and lower lung zones. Actually, flow is greatest in the dependent position or posterior third of each lung in the recumbent position, best appreciated with axial CT images.

In normal individuals, the pulmonary arteries and veins in the outer third of the lung are too small to be seen clearly on chest roentgenograms. The central pulmonary veins usually can be distinguished from pulmonary arteries because they follow different pathways. Pulmonary veins course centrally in the interlobular septa, converging in the left atrium 2 to 3 cm below the hila. The pulmonary arteries radiate from the hila several centimeters above the pulmonary venous confluences. The veins of the upper lobes are usually lateral to or superimposed on their companion pulmonary arteries, and for the most part, the veins are larger and branch less frequently than arteries. In practice, because the venous drainage and arterial supply to the upper lobes are so variable, it is often difficult to distinguish vein from artery.

Abnormal Pulmonary Blood Flow

INCREASED PULMONARY FLOW. The size of the pulmonary arteries is proportional to the volume of pulmonary blood flow so that if there is an increase in right-sided cardiac output the vessels will enlarge as long as the reserve of the

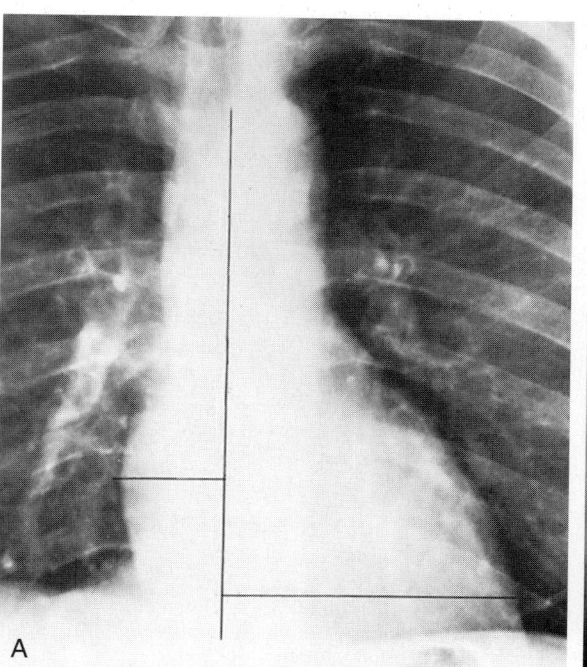

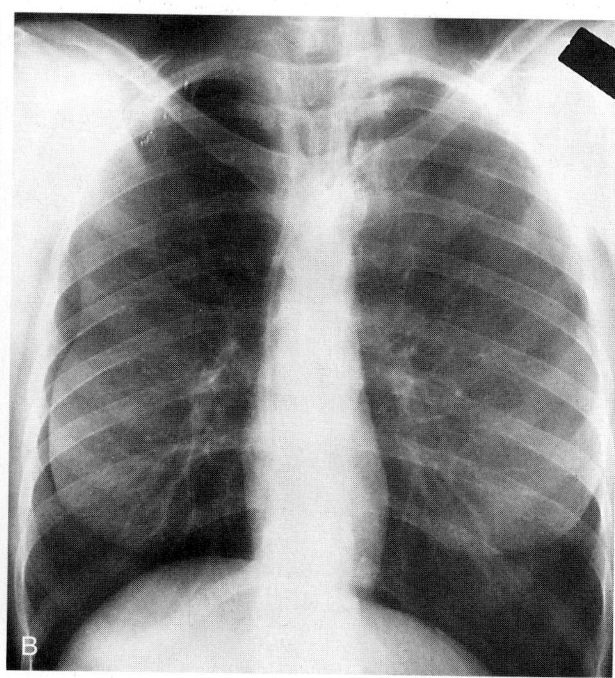

FIGURE 7–19. *A,* Measurement of the transverse cardiac diameter. A vertical reference line is drawn through the spinous processes of the vertebrae. The greatest distance from this line to the right and left margins of the cardiac shadow are then measured. The sum is the transverse cardiac diameter. *B,* The heart is unusually small in this young woman with anorexia nervosa.

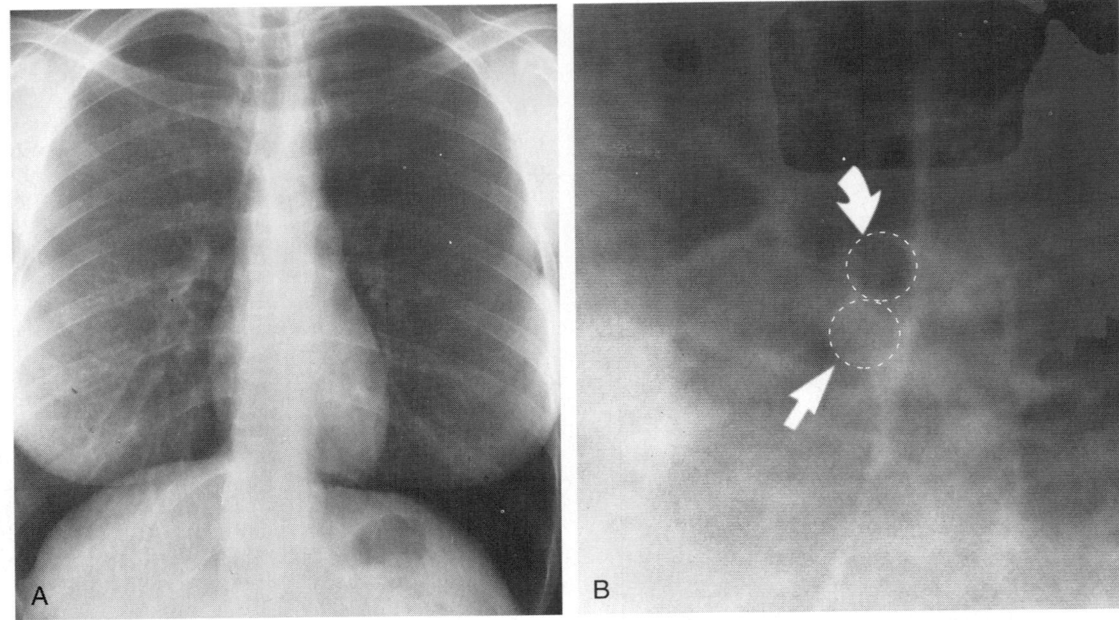

FIGURE 7–20. *A,* Normal pulmonary blood flow. The lower lobe vessels are two to three times greater in diameter than upper lobe vessels due to gravity and relative lung volumes. *B,* Magnification of paired anterior segment right upper lobe bronchus and pulmonary artery in a normal erect patient. The bronchus *(top)* and vessel *(bottom)* are of approximately the same size. This arterial-bronchial ratio is helpful in analyzing alterations in pulmonary vasculature.

pulmonary vascular bed (8 times normal flow) is not exceeded. When the reserve volume is overwhelmed or reduced because of vascular disease, the size of the vessels will be related to both blood flow and blood pressure or to pressure alone[37] (Fig. 7–21). The pulmonary veins also enlarge as pulmonary arterial blood flow rises. Enlarged pulmonary branches are found in a variety of conditions including left-to-right shunt, admixture lesions such as transposition of the great arteries, and conditions that produce an increase in cardiac output, such as chronic anemia, hyperthyroidism, arteriovenous fistula, and pregnancy. As pulmonary artery flow increases, radiographs demonstrate enlarged pulmonary arteries clearly seen to the edge of the lung. In a small left-to-right shunt, the increase may appear confined to the lower lobes, but in larger shunts there is recruitment of the upper lobe vessels as well, so that the differential flow between the upper and lower lobe vessels is lost. In left-to-right shunts smaller than 1.8/1, pulmonary vascular abnormalities may not be detected at all.

The size of the pulmonary vessels can be measured objectively by determining the transverse diameter of the right descending pulmonary artery immediately above the origin of the right middle lobe branch. The normal transverse diameter of this vessel is 10 to 15 mm in males and 9 to 14 mm in females. A variation of ±1.0 mm beyond these limits is abnormal.[65]

PULMONARY ARTERIAL HYPERTENSION. As the pulmonary vascular reserve is fully recruited by increased blood flow

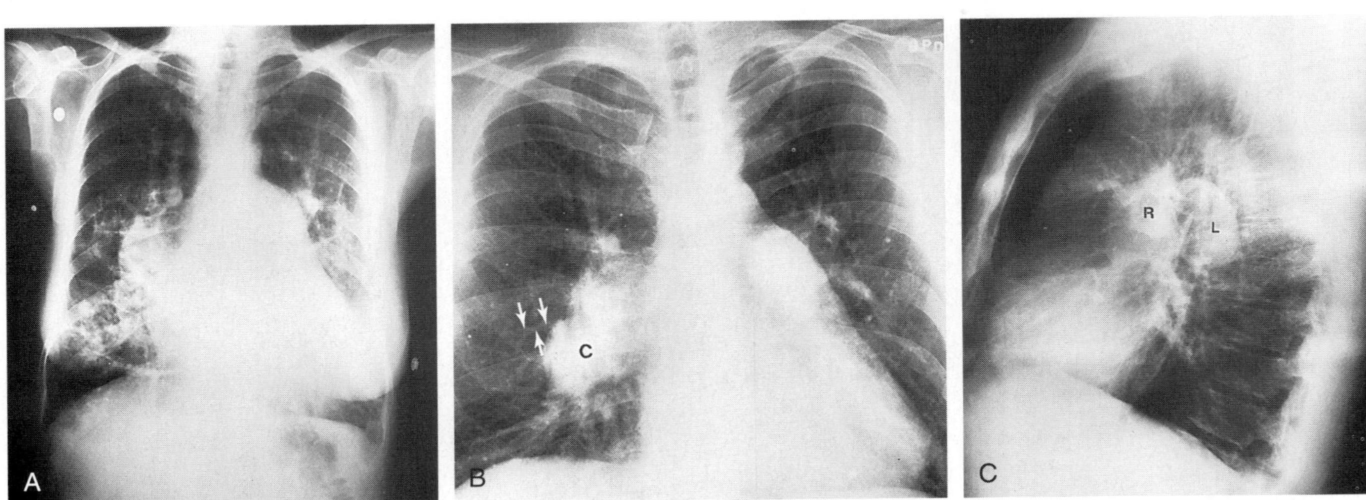

FIGURE 7–21. *A,* Increased pulmonary blood flow. This 41-year-old woman has an atrial septal defect, ostium primum type, with a pulmonary to systemic flow ratio of 5:1. There is secondary mitral regurgitation due to a cleft aortic leaflet of the mitral valve. There is moderate pulmonary hypertension with disparity between central and peripheral arterial branches. The right atrial border, the main pulmonary artery, and the upper and lower lobe vessels are enlarged and their branches are visible in the outer third of both lungs. *B,* There is a disparity between large central and smaller peripheral vessels in this patient with ventricular septal defect and pulmonary arterial hypertension (Eisenmenger physiology). C = central pulmonary arteries. Arrows indicate peripheral pulmonary artery. *C,* In the same patient as in *B,* the large pulmonary arteries are clearly seen on the lateral view. (L = left pulmonary artery; R = right pulmonary artery.)

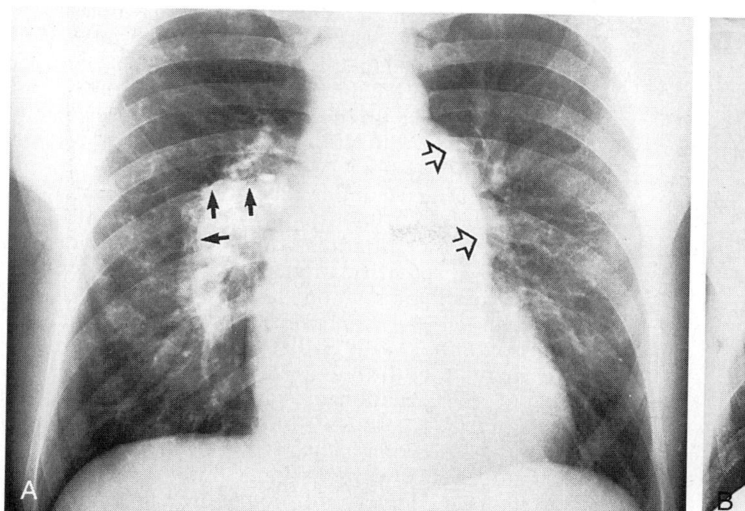
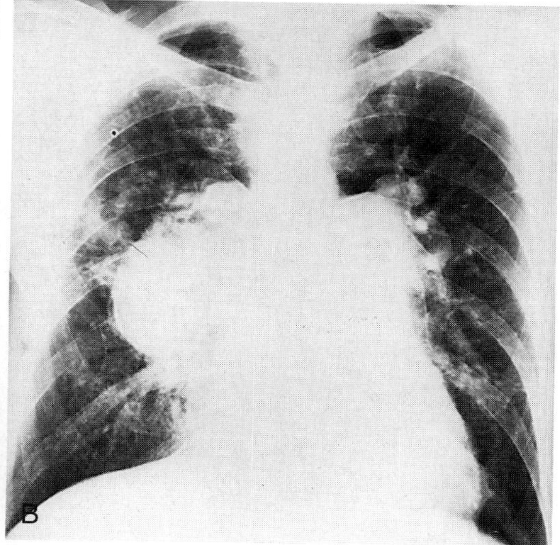

FIGURE 7–22. Pulmonary arterial hypertension. *A*, PA projection of chest of a 50-year-old male with a known membranous ventricular septal defect and cyanosis. There is calcification of the large right central pulmonary artery (arrows). The main pulmonary artery is enlarged in this patient with pulmonary hypertension and Eisenmenger physiology (open arrows). *B*, Severe longstanding pulmonary hypertension in a 64-year-old patient with an atrial septal defect and Eisenmenger physiology. The pulmonary arteries are calcified and aneurysmal.

or reduced by pulmonary arteritis or emphysema, pulmonary arterial pressure rises. The vascular engorgement that characterizes increased pressure is accompanied by vasospasm, peripheral vasoconstriction, and vessel wall thickening. Eventually, there is a decrease in peripheral blood flow, and the outer one-third of the lungs appears more lucent radiographically. The central elastic vessels enlarge, including the main pulmonary artery, the right and left pulmonary arteries, and second-order branching vessels. Calcification of the main pulmonary artery and the proximal branches may develop in longstanding and severe pulmonary arterial hypertension[66] (Fig. 7–22). Pulmonary arterial hypertension may be primary, particularly in women in the childbearing age group. It may also be secondary to chronic recurrent pulmonary thromboembolic disease, a longstanding left-to-right shunt, or pulmonary venous hypertension.[25,67,68]

PULMONARY VENOUS HYPERTENSION. Left ventricular failure, mitral stenosis, and other causes of vascular obstruction distal to the pulmonary arterial bed cause an increase in pulmonary venous pressure above the normal range of 8 to 12 mm Hg. As pressure rises to between 12 mm Hg and 18 mm Hg, pulmonary blood flow is directed into the upper lobes in the erect position and anteriorly in the supine position so that there is reversal of the normal difference in size between the small upper lobe and larger lower lobe vessels. With further elevation of pulmonary venous pressure above 18 mm Hg, pulmonary interstitial edema occurs. With pressure above 25 mm Hg, alveolar edema is seen (Fig. 7–23).

Radiographically, "cephalization" or redistribution of pulmonary venous and arterial flow to the upper lobes is the earliest sign of pulmonary venous hypertension (Fig. 7–24). A clue to the recognition of pulmonary venous hypertension is the diameter of vessels in the first anterior interspace. Normally, they do not measure more than 3 mm in diameter. If they are larger, increased or redirected flow should be considered.

Although the exact mechanism of vascular redistribution remains unresolved, one explanation has been proposed by several authors.[36,37,69–71] With an increase in pulmonary venous pressure, there is leakage of fluid from the pulmonary veins into the interlobular spaces, occurring first in the lower lobes because of gravitational effects. Fluid accumulation in the interlobular spaces decreases pulmonary compliance and increases interstitial pressure. These two

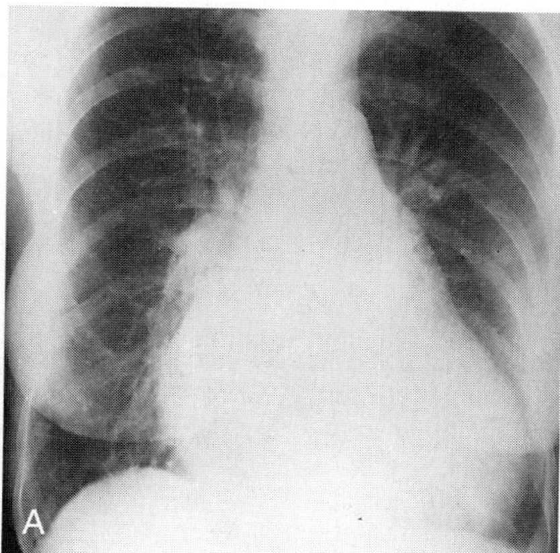
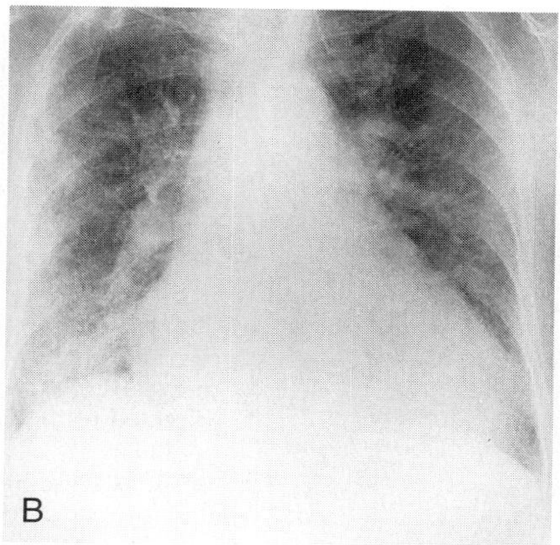
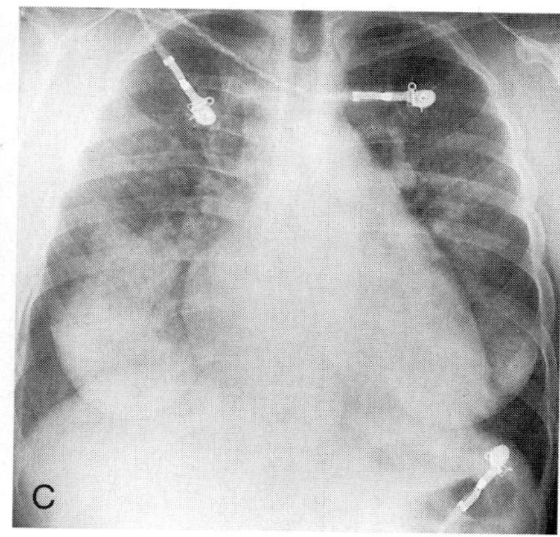

FIGURE 7–23. *A*, Pulmonary blood flow redistribution. Enlargement of the upper lobe vessels in this patient with ischemic cardiomyopathy and elevated pulmonary venous pressure. *B*, Pulmonary interstitial edema. The vessels are indistinct and enlarged. There is peribronchial cuffing. *C*, Pulmonary alveolar edema in a patient with congestive cardiomyopathy. The central parahilar distribution of edema, termed "bat wing" edema, is typical of cardiovascular or fluid overload (uremic) pulmonary alveolar edema.

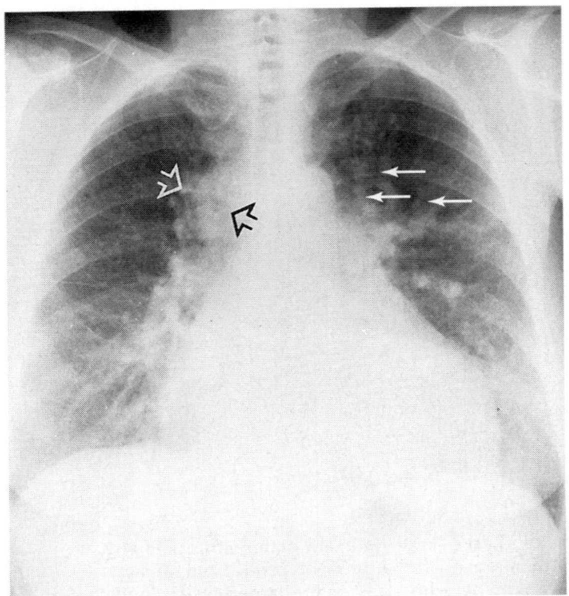

FIGURE 7–24. Congestive heart failure. There is vascular redistribution to the upper lung zones. The vessels in the lung at the first anterior interspaces are enlarged (small arrows) due to "cephalization." The prominent bulge at the right tracheobronchial angle is a dilated azygous vein (open arrows).

phenomena restrict flow to the lower lobes. Arterial spasm may also be a factor. Since these processes first develop in the lower lobes, redistribution of blood flow to the upper lobes follows.

DECREASED PULMONARY BLOOD FLOW. When blood flow is reduced, usually because of pulmonary outflow tract obstruction or an intracardiac right-to-left shunt, the pulmonary arteries and veins are reduced in size. The central vessels narrow and the peripheral vessels are not visible. Reduced pulmonary blood flow may be generalized, as in tetralogy of Fallot, or may be regional as a result of pulmonary embolus, emphysema, and narrowing of vessels due to tumor invasion or to the reduced perfusion of arteritis. When pulmonary perfusion is reduced, as in pulmonary atresia with ventricular septal defect or chronic pulmonary thromboembolism, there is an increase in bronchial and other collateral arterial circulation. Radiographically, bronchial vessels are tortuous, small, and nontapered, and because they emanate from the aorta they do not radiate from the hilum. Otherwise normal but small pulmonary arteries and veins also contribute to pulmonary opacity in lungs with significant bronchial circulation because pulmonary arteries and bronchial arteries interconnect, and preferential flow from the higher pressure systemic bronchial arteries to the lower pressure pulmonary arteries occurs.[66,72]

ASYMMETRICAL PULMONARY BLOOD FLOW. Asymmetrical pulmonary blood flow is due to the presence of vessels in one lung that are smaller than those in the other lung. As already indicated, these patterns of differential flow may be localized, as in pulmonary embolism, chronic obstructive pulmonary disease, or arteritis. Unilateral decrease or absence of pulmonary blood flow may also occur in patients with pulmonary artery branch atresia, hemitruncus, and tetralogy of Fallot with unilateral pulmonary artery branch narrowing. In addition, asymmetrical increased flow may be found after creation of a Blalock-Taussig, Waterston, or Potts shunt. Sometimes, the differences in blood flow in congenital heart disease are caused by orientation of the pulmonary outflow tract. For example, in pulmonary valvular stenosis, the flow of blood through the stenotic valve may be directed toward the left pulmonary artery[73] (Fig. 7–25). In patent ductus arteriosus, the preferential flow is often toward the left because the ductus is oriented toward the left pulmonary artery.

PULMONARY EDEMA (Fig. 7–23*C*). In the normal individual, there is continuous passage of fluid from the pulmonary veins into adjacent interlobular lymphatics that return the fluid to the central mediastinal veins. If the lymphatic reserve is overcome by increased transudate as a result of elevated pulmonary venous pressure, the interlobular septa are thickened and become visible radiographically. Redistribution of blood flow to the upper lung zone, or "cephalization," will occur following reduction in compliance or vasoconstriction in the lower lobes roughly paralleling the increase in pulmonary venous pressure.[67,69,74,75] Interlobular septal lines, or Kerley B lines, are visible as thin horizontal lines present at both lung bases perpendicular to the lateral pleural surface on the frontal chest film.[74,75] Prominent interstitial linear opacities throughout the lung reflect additional thickened septal lines. If the origin of the pulmonary interstitial edema is related to the cardiovascular system, the heart may be normal or enlarged, depending upon the chronicity of cardiac failure. In addition to cardiac failure, prominent interstitial lines may occur in a wide variety of noncardiac diseases including sarcoidosis, lymphatic spread of tumor, interstitial pneumonia, and asbestosis. When pulmonary interstitial edema is present, the lungs may be clear to auscultation—a clue that the extravascular fluid is confined to the interstitium. With further increases in pulmonary venous pressure above 25 mm Hg, there is

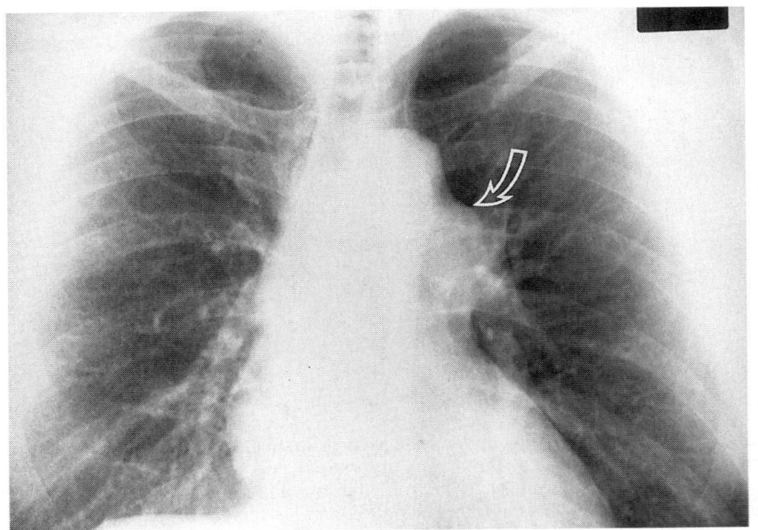

FIGURE 7–25. Asymmetrical pulmonary blood flow in a 51-year-old male with pulmonary valvular stenosis. The left pulmonary artery is larger than the right because the jet of blood is directed to the left pulmonary artery (arrow).

leakage of fluid into the pulmonary air spaces leading to alveolar edema.

Radiographically, pulmonary alveolar edema typically involves the inner two-thirds of the lung, producing a "butterfly" or "bat wing" appearance (Fig. 7–23*C*). An explanation for this pattern is that the outer third of the lung or cortex has better aeration, better compliance, and more efficient lymphatic drainage than the inner two-thirds, and for this reason fluid concentrates in the central portion of the lung.[69,73] Distinguishing pulmonary edema caused by congestive heart failure from that caused by increased "capillary permeability" or "overhydration" pulmonary edema is often difficult. Recent studies have attempted to separate cardiovascular pulmonary edema from the other forms by definable characteristics such as change in heart size, width of the pulmonary vascular pedicle, blood flow distribution, interstitial thickening, and regional distribution of pulmonary edema. In these studies, cardiovascular pulmonary edema is characteristically associated with a large heart, vascular redistribution, diffuse distribution of pulmonary edema fluid, a widened vascular pedicle, and increased pulmonary blood volumes, septal lines, and pleural effusions. Overhydration pulmonary edema is characterized by a balanced blood flow and perihilar pulmonary edema. In capillary permeability pulmonary edema, there is no cardiac enlargement, the vascular pedicle is normal or reduced in size, no septal lines are found, and the pulmonary edema has a peripheral rather than central pattern.[76,77]

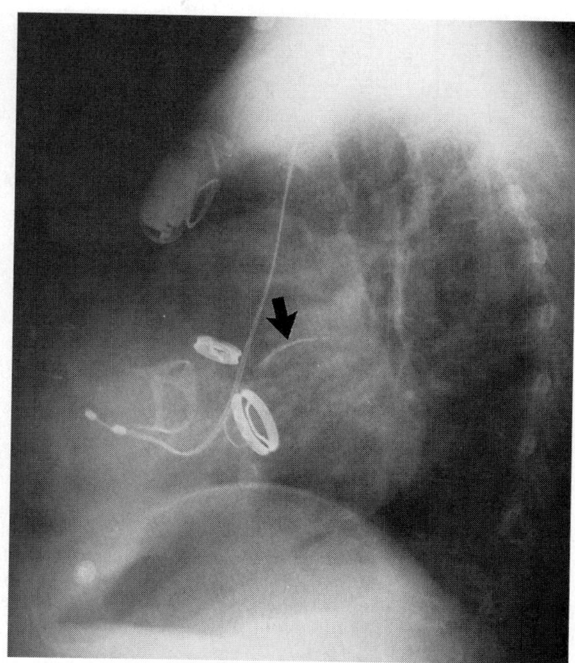

FIGURE 7–26. Left atrial calcification. A thin curvilinear calcification (arrow) is present in the superior and anterior wall of the left atrium in this patient with multivalvular rheumatic heart disease and atrial fibrillation. Prosthetic valves are seen in the tricuspid, mitral, and aortic areas.

CARDIAC CALCIFICATION

MYOCARDIAL CALCIFICATION. Dystrophic calcification of the heart is usually caused by a large myocardial infarction and is reported to occur in 8 per cent of infarcts more than 6 years old.[37,44] It has also been described following cardiac trauma, particularly in the anterior wall of the right ventricle.[78] The deposition of calcium is related to the slow production of carbon dioxide in slowly metabolizing tissue. Consequently, there is development of relative alkalinity and reduced solubility of calcium.[79] Myocardial calcification occurs most frequently in a left ventricular aneurysm and in the apical and anterior lateral aspects of the left ventricular wall. The calcium deposits are usually curvilinear in shape within the periphery of the infarct or aneurysm and occasionally may be homogeneous when an entire infarcted area calcifies.

Calcification may also occur within the left atrium and left atrial appendage, particularly in patients with rheumatic heart disease associated with mitral stenosis or regurgitation. Left atrial calcification is most often found in the endo- or subendocardial layers and is seen less often within an organized thrombus adherent to the chamber wall. Left atrial calcification is usually thin-walled and curvilinear, forming a shell around the circumference of the left atrial chamber or confined to the left atrial appendage[37,44,80,81] (Fig. 7–26).

VALVULAR CALCIFICATION. The radiographic presence of calcification within a cardiac valve suggests the presence of hemodynamically significant stenosis.[45,82] In the mitral valve, calcification appears clump-like or linear, usually measuring about 2 to 4 cm in diameter, and is most often caused by rheumatic heart disease.[44,83,84] Isolated aortic valve calcification in patients under age 40 generally signifies marked aortic stenosis related to a bicuspid valve (Fig. 7–27). In patients over 65 years of age, aortic valve calcification can be due to sclerosis with degeneration of normal valve leaflets or may be a manifestation of hemodynamically significant aortic stenosis.[54,82,82a]

The radiographic appearance of the calcification may help to determine the origin of the valvular deformity. For example, a thick, irregular semilunar ring pattern with a central bar or knob is typical of stenotic bicuspid valve and is found in 65 per cent of patients with congenital aortic stenosis[25,48,85] (Fig. 7–27). This pattern is due to calcification of the valve ring and the dividing ridge or raphe of one of the two cusps or the conjoint leaflet. The abundance of calcification in this entity is thought to be due to constant wear and tear from the abnormal tension-producing motion of the bicuspid valve leaflets. Occasionally three-leaflet aortic valves will mimic bicuspid valves because of fusion of two of the three leaflets. In these patients, three sinuses of Valsalva are present.[36] Calcification of the pulmonary valve occurs occasionally in pulmonary valvular stenosis with gradients in excess of 80 mm Hg or in longstanding severe pulmonary hypertension. Calcification of the tricuspid valve is unusual and is caused most frequently by rheumatic disease.[86]

ANNULAR CALCIFICATION. Annular calcification is found in the valve rings or fibroskeleton of the heart. It is a degenerative process occurring with aging and is found most often in individuals above the age of 40 years and especially in women.[83,86,87] Mitral annular calcification (see p. 1017) presents radiographically as a wavy O-, J-, or C-shaped opacity[87] (Fig. 7–28). When calcification is limited to the posterior-medial portion of the annulus at the base of the posterior leaflet there are usually no complications.[83] When the calcification is more extensive it may involve the valve leaflets and cause limitation of motion leading to regurgitation or, occasionally, an obstructive gradient during diastole.[84,87,88] Aortic annular calcification may also extend into the ascending aorta and down into the interventricular septum (Fig. 7–28*B*, *C*). Atrial fibrillation, conduction abnormalities, endocarditis, and mitral valve incompetence are associated findings.[83] Tricuspid annular calcification is rare, usually occurring in patients with longstanding pulmonary valvular stenosis, atrial septal defect, and/or right ventricular hypertension.[86]

Several methods have been suggested to identify the location of valvular calcification on plain films. A line drawn on the lateral chest film from the junction of the anterior chest wall and the diaphragm through the hilum to the lung apex will separate anterior superior aortic calcifica-

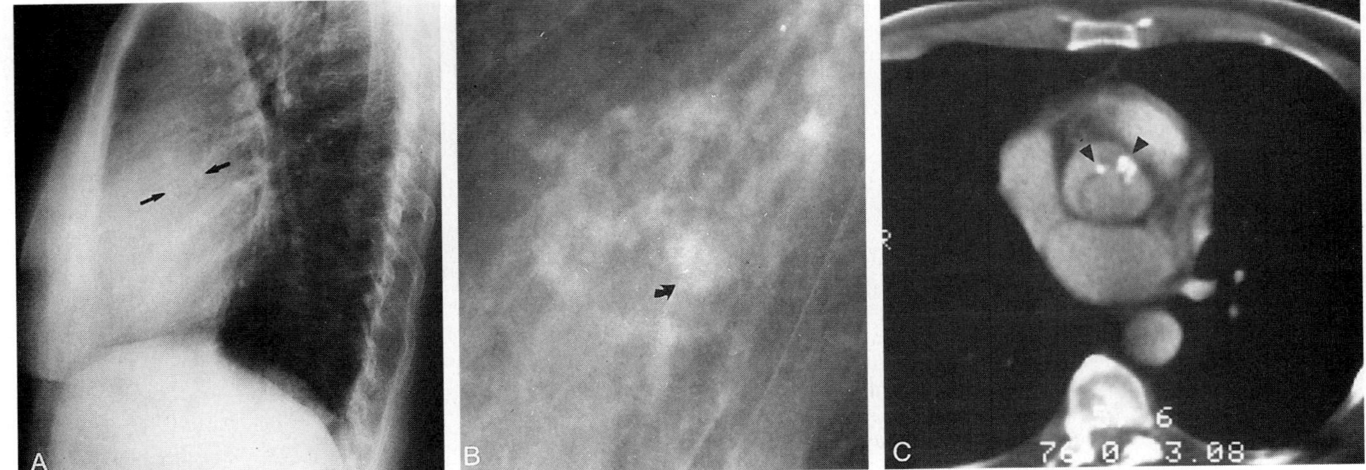

FIGURE 7–27. Aortic valve calcification. *A,* Lateral projection shows the typical pattern of calcification of congenital bicuspid aortic valve in a 60-year-old woman with secondary aortic regurgitation (arrows). *B,* A fluoroscopic spot film shows the calcified valve to better advantage (curved arrow indicates calcified raphe). *C,* Cine CT demonstrates calcification of the aortic valve leaflets in a different patient with congenital bicuspid aortic valve (arrowheads). (Courtesy of Stephanie Flicker, M.D.)

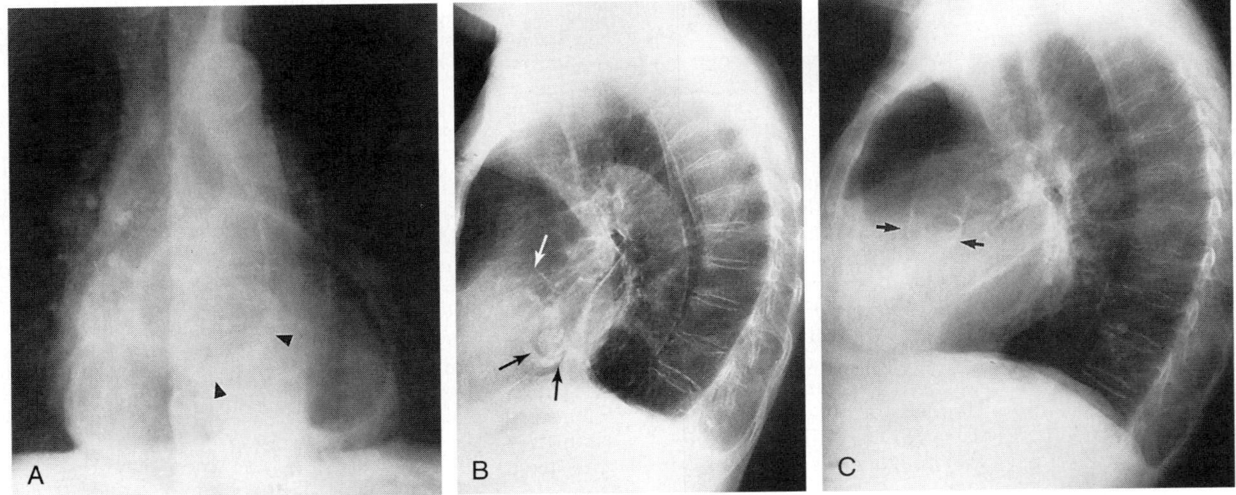

FIGURE 7–28. *A,* Calcified aortic and mitral annulus in an elderly woman. The air in a large hiatal hernia permits excellent visualization of the mitral annulus (arrowheads) in the PA projection. *B,* In the lateral projection, calcification can be seen in both the aortic (white arrow) and mitral (black arrows) annuli. *C,* Aortic annular calcification (arrows) in an elderly patient without signs or symptoms of aortic stenosis.

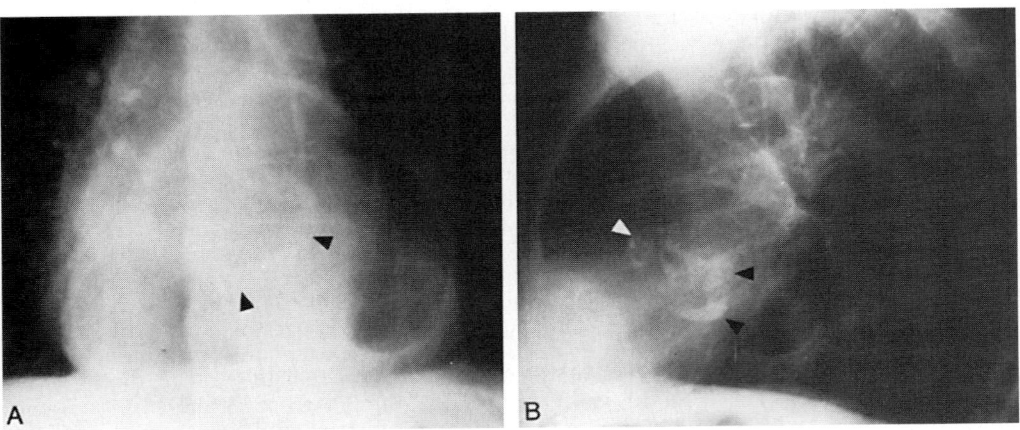

FIGURE 7–29. Mitral valve calcification. In the lateral projection, *(B),* the valve calcification (black arrows) lies below the line drawn from the left main bronchus to the anterior costophrenic sulcus, localizing it to the mitral valve. The aortic valve in this projection lies more anteriorly and above the line (open arrows).

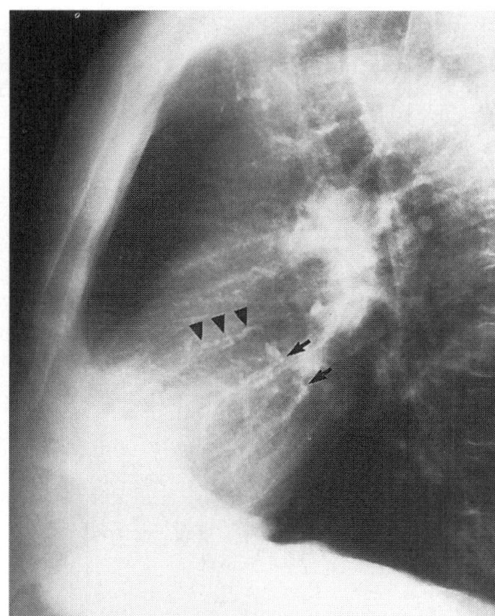

FIGURE 7–30. Lateral projection demonstrates the "tram track" pattern of coronary artery calcifications involving the left anterior descending (arrowheads) and circumflex coronary arteries (arrows).

tions from posterior inferior mitral calcifications (Fig. 7–29). Another approach is to divide the heart on the lateral view into six sections; this will permit identification of the aortic valve in the upper row middle section and mitral calcification in the lower row posterior section.

CORONARY ARTERY CALCIFICATION. Calcium is deposited early in the formation of an atherosclerotic plaque in the coronary arteries, and calcification can be used to monitor the evolution of the atherosclerotic process. Coronary artery calcification can be detected by a number of imaging modalities including plain radiography, fluoroscopy, ultrafast CT, and ultrasonography[89–93] (Fig. 7–30). Of these modalities, fluoroscopy has been studied most intensively.[89]

A number of studies have compared the efficacy of fluoroscopy with arteriography and exercise testing for the identification of significant coronary artery disease.[4,49,53,89] As a result of these studies, a direct relationship between fluoroscopically identified coronary calcification and the frequency and severity of stenotic lesions has been established. In one study of 360 patients undergoing arteriography for coronary artery disease who also underwent cardiac fluoroscopy, 97 per cent of those with calcified coronary arteries on fluoroscopy had significant (≥70 per cent occlusion) coronary artery stenosis of at least one major vessel on arteriography. Of those with significant coronary disease on arteriography, 56 per cent had calcification at fluoroscopy.[53] Another study was performed in asymptomatic patients with type II hyperlipidemia who were under the age of 55 years. Of those with both positive exercise tests and coronary calcification on fluoroscopy, 92 per cent had angiographically determined coronary artery disease. Fluoroscopy had an 82 per cent accuracy in the detection of significant (≥50 per cent occlusion) coronary artery disease.[89] In yet a third study in a randomly selected group of 108 asymptomatic men who underwent cardiac fluoroscopy and exercise testing, 81 per cent of those with a positive exercise test had coronary calcifications, and 35 per cent of these had a positive exercise test. Only 4 per cent of those without calcified coronary arteries had a positive exercise test. Finally, in this same series 92 per cent had at least one stenosed (≥50 per cent occlusion) coronary artery diagnosed by angiography.[51] Bartel et al. showed that approximately 90 per cent of patients with fluoroscopically detectable coronary calcifications had significant coronary disease.[53]

Since exercise tests alone yield 10 to 20 per cent positive results in an asymptomatic middle-aged male population without coronary artery disease (false-positives), fluoroscopy has been suggested as an effective additional screening test for identification of patients with critical coronary artery disease. Fluoroscopy is most valuable when there is atypical chest pain or cardiomyopathy or for screening asymptomatic patients. Those at particular risk are cigarette smokers, have hyperlipidemia, or have other positive prognostic indicators.

Coronary calcifications in the proximal left coronary artery may be identified with plain chest radiography or fluoroscopy in the frontal projection medial to the left atrial appendage. In the lateral view, calcification of the left anterior descending artery is often seen vividly as a double line of calcification extending along the anterior border of the cardiac silhouette (Fig. 7–30). Circumflex and right coronary artery calcification may also be identified by means of chest radiography, particularly oblique views.

CT is superior to fluoroscopy for the detection of coronary calcification.[4,52,90] In fact, approximately twice as many patients will be found to have calcified coronary arteries with CT than with fluoroscopy.[91–93] There is a similar detection yield of critical coronary artery disease when compared with those obtained by fluoroscopy. Although CT has been considered impractical as a screening test because of cost and limited availability, recent studies with cine CT have emphasized its value as a highly sensitive screening procedure in three selected populations.[90,93] Since CT is performed routinely for other disease indications, it is important to make note of coronary calcifications and their distribution on CT to alert the clinician to their significance.

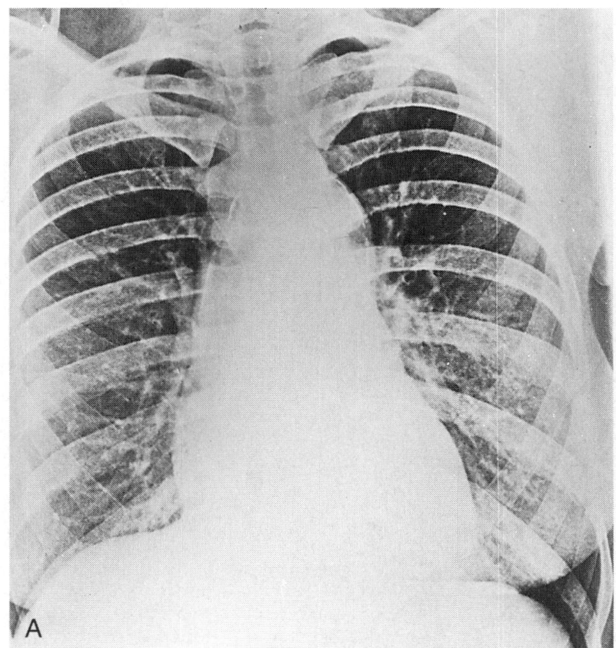

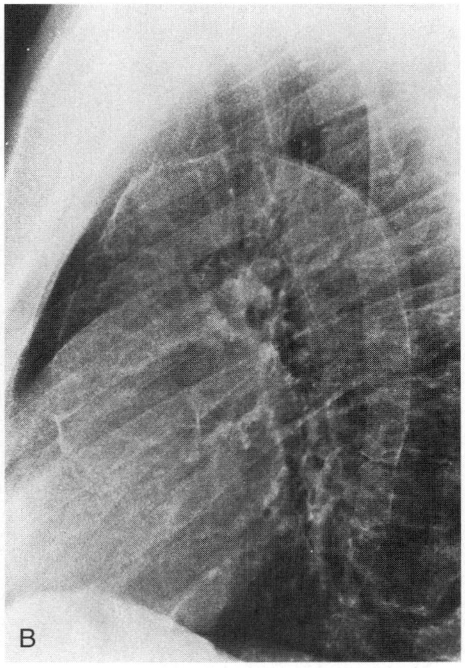

FIGURE 7–31. ***A,*** **PA projection.** ***B,*** **Lateral projection. Abundant thin line calcification extending from the aortic root to the distal descending thoracic aorta in a 30-year-old woman. Biopsy demonstrated Takayasu's arteritis.**

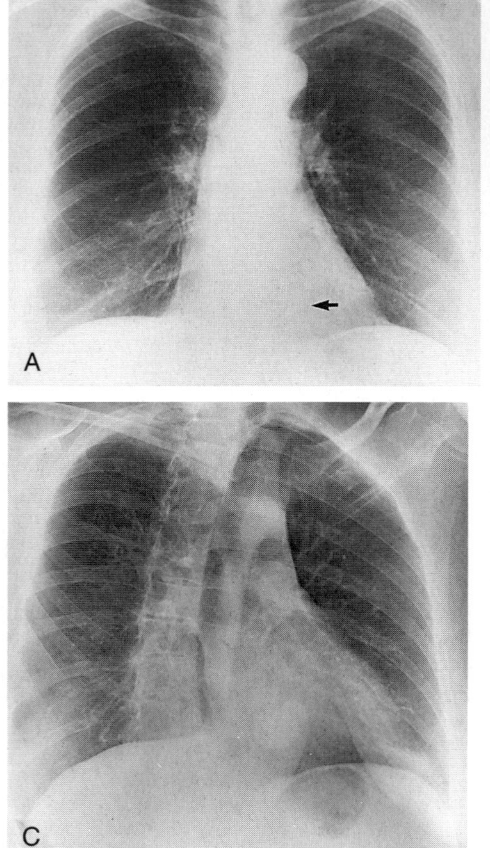
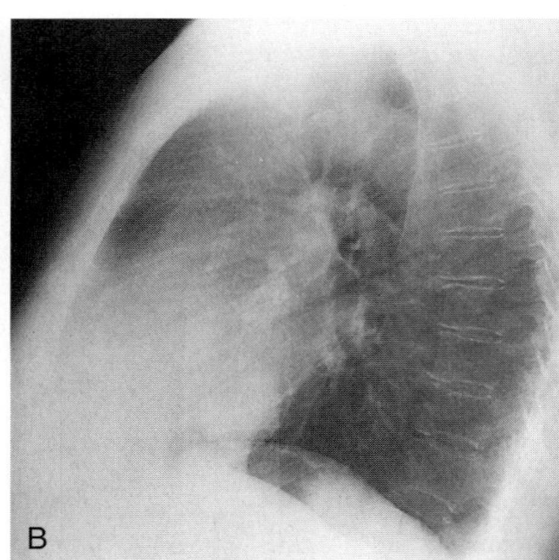

FIGURE 7–32. Tumor calcification. *A,* A large clump of calcification is present in the left atrium, faintly seen on the PA projection (arrow) and well demonstrated on the *(B)* lateral and *(C)* RAO projections of the chest. A myxoma was found at surgery.

CALCIFICATION OF THE GREAT VESSELS. Aortic calcification, particularly in the region of the arch, is almost ubiquitous in individuals over the age of 50. It is usually noted on chest radiographs as a thin curvilinear opacity near the lateral border of the arch. When the calcification is located deep to the aortic border, dissection may be present. Other causes of aortic calcification are syphilis (usually involving the ascending aorta), sinus of Valsalva aneurysm, and Takayasu's arteritis[86,94] (Fig. 7–31). The main pulmonary artery occasionally calcifies following right ventricular out-

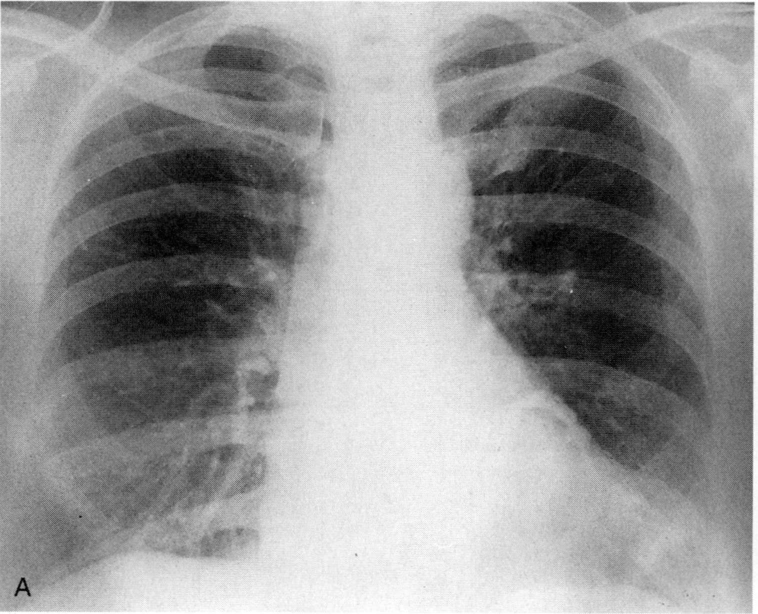
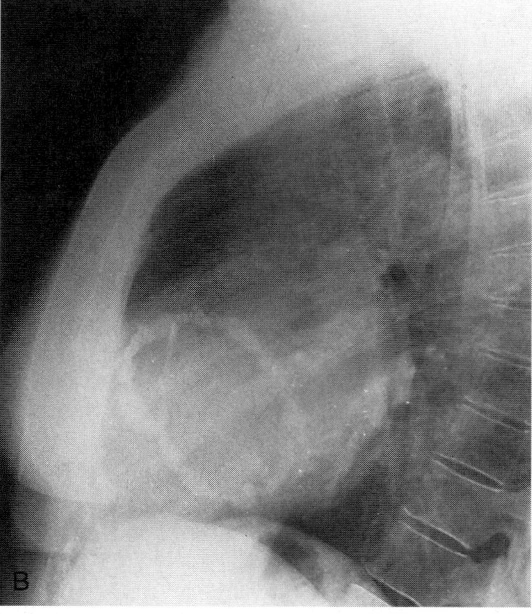

FIGURE 7–33. Pericardial calcification. *A,* PA projection. *B,* Lateral projection. Both show extensive calcification of the pericardium in the atrioventricular groove in a patient with a history of rheumatic heart disease. (From Moncada, R., et al.: Multimodality approach to pericardial imaging. *In* Kotler, M. N., and Steiner, R. M. (eds.): Cardiac Imaging: New Technologies and Clinical Applications. Philadelphia, F. A. Davis, 1986.)

flow tract surgery for total correction of tetralogy of Fallot. Calcification of the main pulmonary artery also occurs in severe longstanding pulmonary hypertension.

TUMOR CALCIFICATION. The most common primary tumor of the heart is myxoma (see p. 1467), a polypoid mass occurring most frequently in the left atrium (Fig. 7–32). About 10 per cent of myxomas calcify sufficiently to be seen radiographically.[95,96] Calcifications in cardiac tumors vary from a speckled pattern to a round clump of calcium mimicking mitral annular or valve calcification. Calcification may be visible on plain film or may be seen only with fluoroscopy or CT. With fluoroscopy or cine CT, a calcified atrial tumor may be seen to prolapse through the atrioventricular valve during diastole and cause obstructive symptoms. Echocardiography and cine MRI will demonstrate prolapse of a noncalcified myxoma.[96,96a]

PERICARDIAL CALCIFICATION (see also Chap. 43). Pericardial calcification occurs most often in association with previous acute pericarditis or trauma.[78,97] The most common causes are viral illness, especially Coxsackie or influenza A and B virus infection, granulomatous disease including tuberculosis and histoplasmosis, hemopericardium following trauma, and autoimmune disease—particularly systemic lupus erythematosus and rheumatic heart disease[98] (Fig. 7–33).

Occasionally, pericardial tumors (among them intrapericardial teratomas and cysts) calcify.[98] Calcification is present in up to 50 per cent of patients with constrictive pericarditis. On the other hand, extensive calcification may be present without the signs and symptoms of pericardial constriction.[99,100] Pericardial and myocardial calcifications are frequently confused with each other.[79] However, pericardial calcifications can be distinguished from myocardial calcification by differences in their distribution. Pericardial calcifications are most abundant along the right atrial and ventricular borders and in the area of the atrioventricular groove. The pericardium adjacent to the left ventricle is usually free of calcification, probably because of its vigorous pulsations, and calcification rarely occurs in the left atrial pericardium because of the absence of pericardium behind the left atrium.[80] On the other hand, myocardial calcification is usually localized to the left ventricle and is rare in the right atrium or ventricle.[79] Pericardial calcification is often obscured on a frontal chest film because of underexposure of the mediastinum. Overpenetrated films or fluoroscopy studies are helpful for localizing mediastinal calcifications, and CT may demonstrate calcium not seen on plain chest films.

ACQUIRED HEART DISEASE

The diagnosis and assessment of the severity of acquired heart disease is assisted by a combination of imaging studies including plain chest radiography.[54] The chest film is particularly useful to assess cardiac size and pulmonary vascularity. At the same time it offers important clues to the enlargement of individual cardiac chambers, although cineangiography, echocardiography, and other cross-sectional imaging techniques are more reliable.[101–104] Nevertheless, the plain film remains a useful first examination in the work-up of the cardiac patient.[51]

Valvular Heart Disease

AORTIC STENOSIS (see also p. 1035). In critical aortic stenosis the size of the aortic valve orifice is reduced from a normal cross-sectional area of 2.5 to 3.5 cm^2 to a cross-sectional area of less than 0.7 cm.[2,25] With mild to moderate constriction of the aortic valve orifice, there is compensatory concentric hypertrophy of the left ventricle (Fig. 7–10). With further increases in the severity of the stenosis, cardiac output and left ventricular contractility decrease, resulting in left ventricular dilatation, elevated left ventricular end-diastolic pressure, and pulmonary venous hypertension together with the signs and symptoms of congestive heart failure.

The typical radiographic changes of mild to moderate aortic stenosis include a normal-sized heart with rounding of the left ventricular border or an elongated cardiac silhouette with downward displacement of the cardiac apex due to concentric left ventricular hypertrophy[38,82] (Fig. 7–10). There is a characteristic discrete bulge on the right side of the ascending aorta just above the sinus of Valsalva due to poststenotic dilatation best visualized in the LAO or PA projection.[37] In pure aortic stenosis, the aortic arch and descending aorta remain normal in size and aortic valve calcification is frequent. It increases with the severity of stenosis and the age of the patient so that by the age of 40 years, more than 90 per cent of patients with aortic stenosis have visible aortic calcification (Fig. 7–27). Aortic valvular calcification has also been associated with a peak systolic gradient at the aortic valve of greater than 30 mm Hg in 97 per cent of patients.[37]

With severe aortic stenosis, the left atrium and ventricle will decompensate and enlarge.[79] The degree of enlargement of both chambers is correlated with the severity of aortic stenosis and with mitral regurgitation due to left ventricular dilatation or to associated intrinsic mitral valve disease. Isolated aortic stenosis is usually nonrheumatic in origin and is most often due to degeneration, scarring, and fusion of a congenital bicuspid valve (see p. 1036). Additional causes of left ventricular outflow tract narrowing, causing left ventricular enlargement without valvular calcification, are hypertrophic cardiomyopathy and supravalvular and subvalvular aortic stenosis.

Congenital aortic stenosis may take two principal forms. The more common is a bicuspid valve with congenital commissural fusion and a central or eccentric orifice. The second form is a bicuspid valve that is initially nonobstructive but undergoes commissural fusion with time. Turbulent blood flow traumatizes the valve and causes irregular nodular scarring of both leaflets, which subsequently undergo gradual fusion and calcification[48,82a] (Fig. 7–27). With time, these valves may also become insufficient due either to incomplete closure of the deformed valve leaflets or to infective endocarditis.

Degenerative and rheumatic aortic valvular stenosis may be found in normally tricuspid valves. On the chest film, linear or clumped calcifications may be found in the area of the aortic valve leaflets or annulus. In patients with rheumatic aortic stenosis, mitral calcifications also are frequently present.[37,105]

Both the obstructive and nonobstructive forms of hypertrophic cardiomyopathy and membranous subaortic stenosis are characterized radiographically by left ventricular enlargement alone.[19,101] Although the plain film findings are suggestive, a specific diagnosis of hypertrophic cardiomyopathy can be established with MRI, echocardiography, and/or radionuclide studies[19] (see p. 1421). Since the aortic leaflets are uninvolved, blood flow is normal during ventricular systole, and as a result, the ascending aorta does not dilate and the aortic valve does not calcify. Left atrial enlargement, when present, is usually associated with mitral regurgitation.[101,105]

AORTIC REGURGITATION (see also p. 1045). Aortic regurgitation may result from a stenotic bicuspid valve that developed insufficiency due to endocarditis or degeneration (Fig. 7–10*B*). *Rheuma*tic valvulitis and infective endocarditis are other important primary causes. A secondary cause of aortic regurgitation is dilatation of the aortic annulus in diseases preferentially affecting the ascending aorta, such as ankylosing spondylitis, annuloaortic ectasia, Marfan syndrome, Reiter syndrome, psoriatic arthritis, and others (Chap. 45).[106] The aortic regurgitation due to rheumatic heart disease is commonly associated with mitral disease

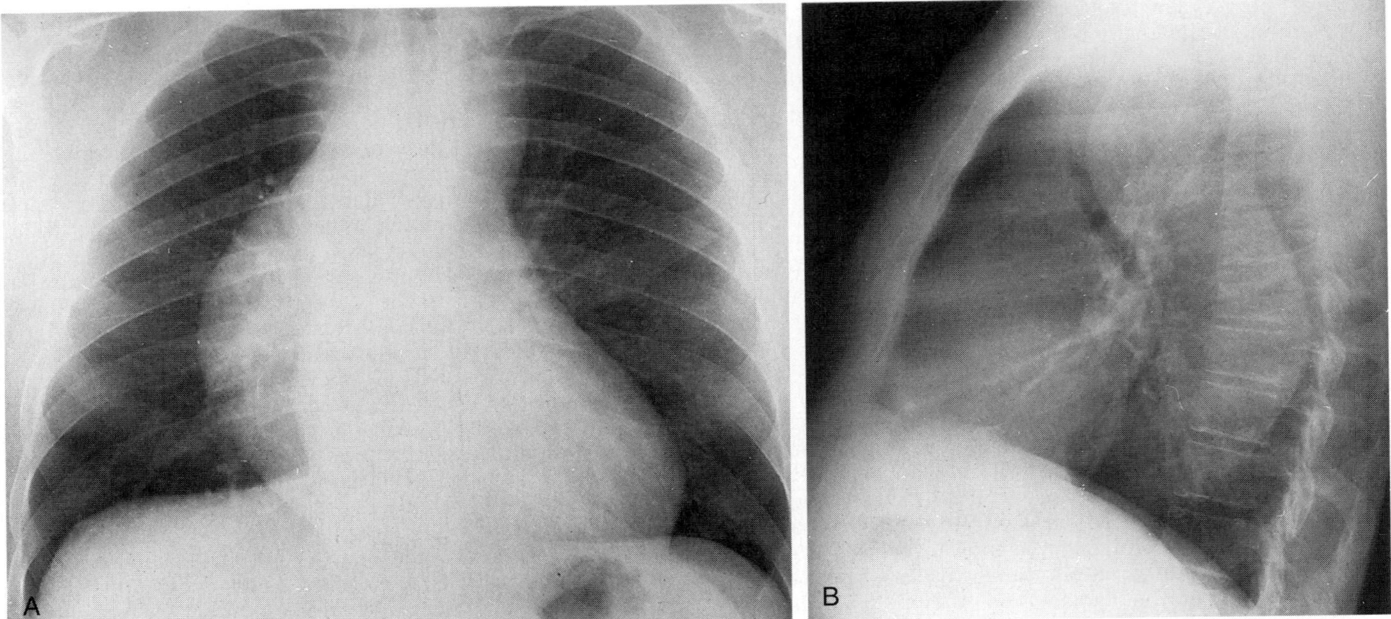

FIGURE 7–34. Aortic regurgitation. There is massive aortic dilatation in this man with severe aortic regurgitation related to annuloaortic ectasia. *A,* PA projection. *B,* Lateral projection.

alone or may involve all four cardiac valves (see p. 1045). Aortic regurgitation may also be due to trauma or may accompany dissection of the ascending aorta.[106]

In mild aortic regurgitation, the aorta is radiographically normal or mildly enlarged and the left ventricle remains normal in size. With moderate or severe regurgitation, there is increased dilatation of the left ventricle, and the cardiothoracic ratio usually exceeds 0.55. The aorta is diffusely and often massively dilated, unlike in aortic stenosis, in which only the ascending aorta is involved (Fig. 7–34). If the sinus portion of the ascending aorta is the only portion selectively dilated, Marfan syndrome (annuloaortic ectasia) is the most likely diagnosis. If the ascending aorta is also calcified, syphilis or, occasionally, Takayusu's aortitis is the likely diagnostic possibility. If the valve itself is calcified, aortic regurgitation secondary to a congenital bicuspid aortic valve or rheumatic disease should be considered.[105] If the mitral valve is also regurgitant, the left atrium may be markedly enlarged visually, obscuring the enlarged left ventricle. When aortic regurgitation occurs acutely due to infective endocarditis, trauma, or dissection, the left ventricle remains normal in size, but because end-diastolic pressure is dramatically increased, the pulmonary venous pressure rises and pulmonary interstitial and/or alveolar edema may be observed. In chronic compensated aortic regurgitation, progressive volume overload occurs with left ventricular dilatation and increase in overall cardiac size but with normal-appearing lungs.[106]

As is true of aortic stenosis, aortic regurgitation is best diagnosed by Doppler echocardiography (see p. 1051) or cine MRI (see p. 1051). In selected cases, however, analysis of the plain chest radiograph will often establish the diagnosis or reveal specific findings that support the diagnosis of this abnormality.

MITRAL STENOSIS (see also p. 1007). Rheumatic carditis is the most common cause of mitral stenosis. Left atrial

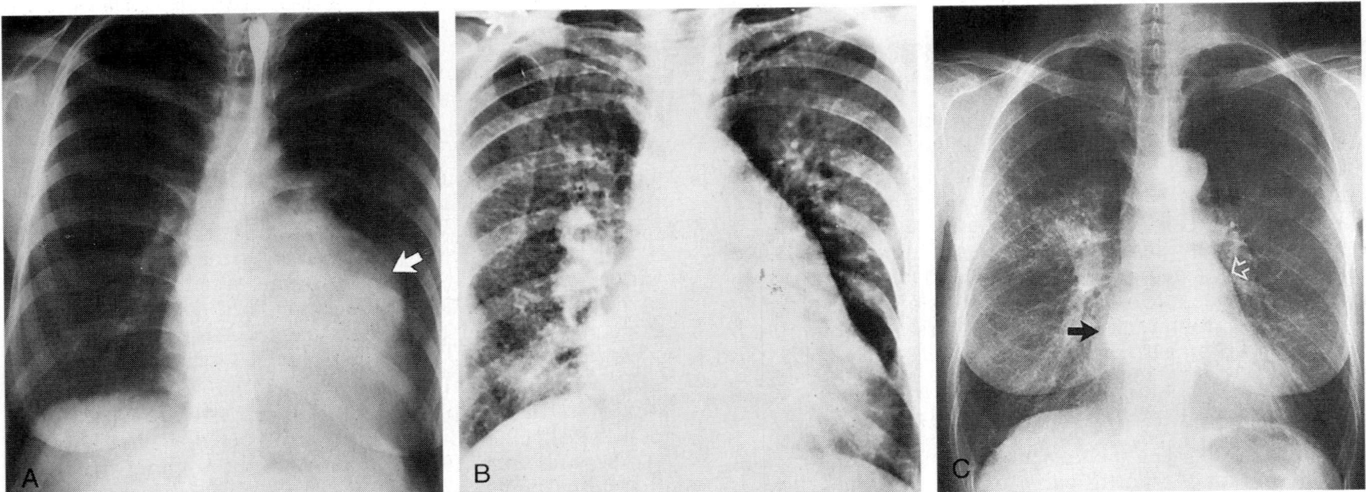

FIGURE 7–35. Mitral stenosis. *A,* The left atrial border is prominently convex. The aorta is small in this 19-year-old patient with mitral stenosis (arrow). *B,* In another patient, the lungs are studded with small nodules of moderate radiodensity due to hemosiderosis. The left atrium and left ventricle are enlarged. Kerley B lines are present in the lateral basal portions of the lungs. *C,* There is a subtle convex bulge at the level of the left atrial appendage (open arrow). A double atrial shadow is present on the right atrial border (black arrow). The heart is not enlarged in this 54-year-old woman with mitral stenosis.

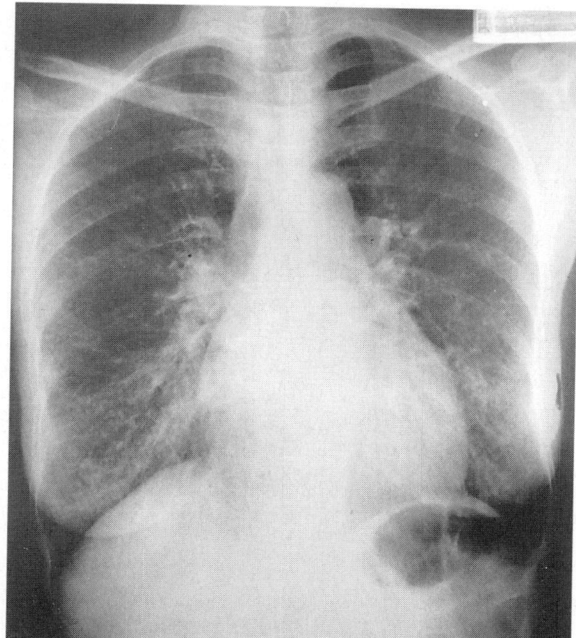

FIGURE 7–36. Mitral stenosis. There is chronic interstitial pulmonary edema with small punctate opacities representing small islands of ossification within the alveoli.

myxoma and, rarely, congenital mitral stenosis are also causes of mitral valve obstruction. The early roentgenographic signs of mitral stenosis are often subtle and include mild left atrial enlargement and posterior or posterior-lateral displacement of the barium-filled esophagus on the lateral chest. In most patients with mitral stenosis, the left ventricle and the pulmonary vessels are normal in appearance.

With more severe mitral stenosis, the left atrium usually increases further in size; however, in any given patient there is poor correlation between the severity of mitral stenosis and the size of the left atrial chamber[69,107] (Fig. 7–35). The left atrial appendage can be disproportionately enlarged, but the shape of the appendage appears to bear no relationship to the presence or absence of thrombosis.[81,108,109] The left main stem bronchus may be displaced upward by the enlarged left atrium. The right atrium is displaced to the right, and there is evidence of vascular redistribution of pulmonary blood flow to the upper lobes. The main pulmonary artery is enlarged, the left ventricle and aorta are usually normal or small, and the mitral valve is often calcified. In addition, calcification of the left atrial wall (often associated with atrial fibrillation) may be seen. The enlarged left atrium displaces the barium-filled esophagus posteriorly (Fig. 7–16). Left atrial wall calcification is most common in the posterior portion of the left atrial chamber as well as the appendage in patients with rheumatic heart disease (Fig. 7–26). There is evidence of pulmonary interstitial edema, characterized by "hilar haze" or central vascular indistinctness, Kerley B lines at the lung bases, and cephalization as pulmonary venous pressure rises to the range of 25 mm Hg.[70,107]

Interlobular effusions are also seen and are described as Kerley C lines or a reticular pattern representing superimposed Kerley B lines. Kerley A lines are best observed in the lateral projection as long, opaque lines merging into the hila, representing thickened perivascular connective tissue planes.[74,75] Hemosiderosis, due to recurrent small hemorrhages related to chronically elevated capillary pressure, is often associated with chronic mitral stenosis (Fig. 7–35*B*). The radiographic appearance in hemosiderosis is that of interstitial or miliary lung disease most prominent in the mid and lower lung zones.[36] With chronic pulmonary interstitial edema, small punctate pulmonary opacities may be found which represent small islands of bone within the alveoli and are visible as dense nodules on the chest radiograph (Fig. 7–36).

MITRAL REGURGITATION (see also p. 1017). Acute mitral regurgitation may be related to ruptured chordae tendineae, rupture of the papillary muscles, ischemic dysfunction, or infective endocarditis. While the heart may not be enlarged in acute mitral regurgitation, severe pulmonary edema is frequently present as a result of left-sided cardiac failure (Fig. 7–37). Although pulmonary edema secondary to mitral regurgitation[110,111] is usually symmetrical, selective right upper lobe pulmonary edema has been described in as many as 9 per cent of patients with acute or chronic mitral regurgitation. It is probably due to selective retrograde flow from the mitral valve to the right upper lobe pulmonary veins[110,112] (Fig. 7–38). Chronic mitral regurgitation may be secondary to rheumatic heart disease, mitral prolapse due to myxomatous degeneration, infective endocarditis, ischemic cardiomyopathy, hypertrophic cardiomyopathy, extensive mitral annulus calcification, Marfan syndrome, and other causes (see p. 1669).

Radiographically, in chronic mitral regurgitation, the left atrium as well as the left ventricle is enlarged and may be massive in size because of volume overload and increased

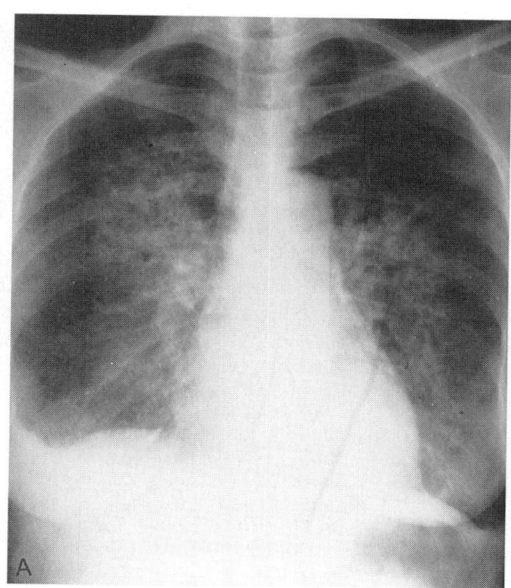

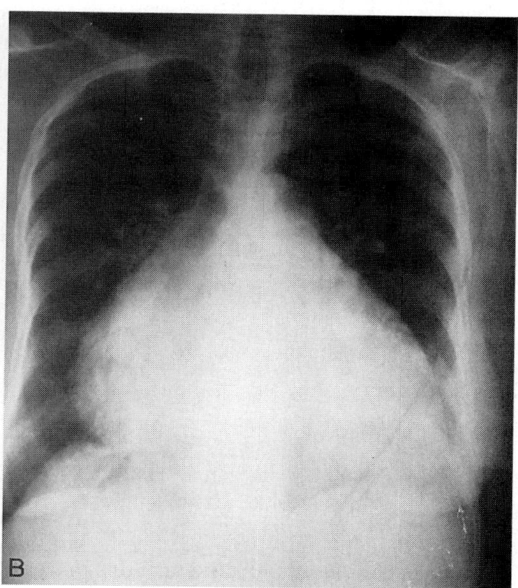

FIGURE 7–37. *A,* Acute post–myocardial infarction papillary muscle dysfunction. Acute pulmonary interstitial edema is present but there is no cardiac enlargement. *B,* Dilated cardiomyopathy. There is diffuse dilatation of the heart in this woman with systemic lupus erythematosus.

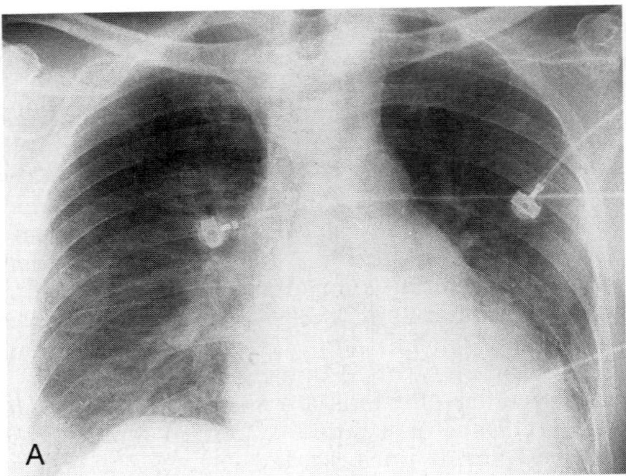

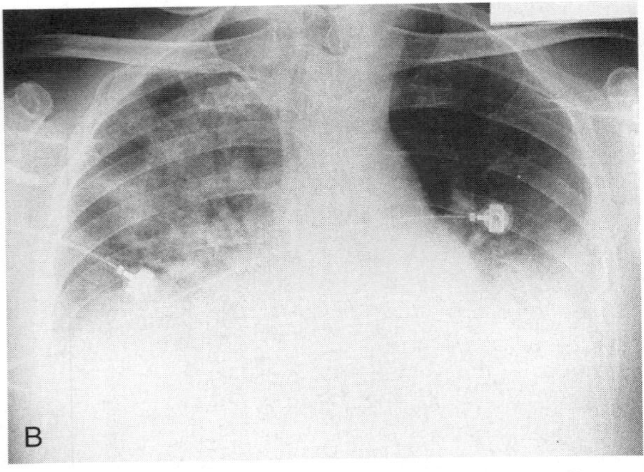

FIGURE 7–38. Mitral regurgitation. This 53-year-old patient developed mitral regurgitation secondary to dilated cardiomyopathy. He was admitted in congestive failure. There is localized development of alveolar edema in the right upper lobe. This phenomenon is due to preferential regurgitant flow toward the right upper lobe pulmonary vein. *A,* Portable AP chest film on admission. *B,* Three days later, patient is clinically in congestive heart failure.

pressure.[113] When the left atrium is enlarged, it may extend toward the right side and may be observed as a double shadow along the right atrial border. In the LAO projection, the large atrium causes upward displacement of the left main stem bronchus. Coexistent pulmonary arterial hypertension or tricuspid regurgitation may cause dilatation of the right atrium and ventricle and enlargement of the pulmonary arteries.[8,114,115] MRI and echocardiography can demonstrate the abnormality of the valve apparatus and evaluate the amount of regurgitant flow.

Ischemic Heart Disease

Many imaging modalities contribute to the diagnosis of ischemic heart disease, including coronary arteriography, radionuclide scintigraphy, echocardiography, CT, and MRI.[115,116] In ischemic cardiomyopathy, the chest roentgenogram can be entirely normal, even in patients with advanced disease; however, left ventricular enlargement and/or aneurysm are often present. Following infarction of 25 per cent or more of left ventricular muscle mass, pulmonary edema may occur, even in patients with a normal-sized heart.[116] When congestive heart failure persists in spite of treatment, complications of myocardial infarction, such as aneurysm, pseudoaneurysm, ventricular wall or papillary muscle rupture, and interventricular septal defect must be excluded.[10,115–120]

MYOCARDIAL INFARCTION (Chap. 37). An interventricular septal defect occurs in 0.5 to 1.0 per cent of patients with recent septal infarction and is characterized by cardiomegaly, pulmonary edema, and poor myocardial contractility (see p. 1243). On the plain film radiograph, the typical shunt pattern may not be appreciated because of pulmonary edema but can emerge months later if the patient survives. Such defects usually involve the muscular septum and occur within 7 to 12 days after myocardial infarction. The radiographic picture of post–myocardial infarction syndrome (Dressler syndrome) is that of an enlarged heart due to pericardial effusion. Unilateral or, less often, bilateral pleural effusions are common, and lower lobe consolidation, particularly on the left side, occurs in fewer than 20 per cent of patients. It generally occurs 2 to 6 weeks following myocardial infarction and is analogous to the postpericardiotomy syndrome.[116]

Aneurysm of the left ventricle is an abnormal bulge or outpouching of the myocardial wall that develops in 12 to 15 per cent of patients following myocardial infarction[115] (see p. 1256). It occurs most commonly at the cardiac apex or along the anterior free wall of the left ventricle. The chest film shows a localized bulge along the ventricular wall near the apex, with or without a thin rim of calcification. Angiography, CT, MRI, and echocardiography will also demonstrate the filling defect of a mural thrombus (if one is present) in the aneurysm. The differential diagnosis of left ventricular aneurysm includes pericardial cyst, mediastinal or pleural tumor, thymoma, and other mediastinal masses.

Cardiac rupture usually occurs in patients who have had an acute transmural infarction[119–121] (see p. 1241). Most die immediately, but in a minority of patients the rupture is contained or enclosed by the surrounding extracardiac soft tissues and a pseudoaneurysm is formed. Radiographically, a paracardiac mass is present, with sharply marginated edges free of calcification. The mass is usually posterior on the lateral projection, unlike the more anterior position of a true aneurysm.[121] A firm diagnosis is made by echocardiography, MRI, or contrast ventriculography. Coronary arteriography will show a complete absence of vessels in the wall of the pseudoaneurysm, unlike a true aneurysm, which may have a rim of mural vessels.[120]

Papillary muscle rupture following myocardial infarction occurs in approximately 1 per cent of patients (Fig. 7–37*A*) (see p. 1243). Plain film radiographic findings vary from a normal chest to gross cardiomegaly with left atrial and ventricular enlargement and pulmonary edema. Left ventriculography, MRI, or Doppler echocardiography will demonstrate the flail mitral valve leaflets and estimate the degree of mitral regurgitation.[45]

THE CARDIOMYOPATHIES (Chap. 41). The term cardiomyopathy describes a spectrum of myocardial disorders of varying etiology and pathophysiology. They are classified as dilated or congestive, infiltrative, restrictive, hypertrophic, and ischemic cardiomyopathies.[36,122]

In congestive, dilated, and ischemic cardiomyopathy, the left ventricular ejection fraction is reduced, often severely. Chest radiographs exhibit a wide spectrum of findings from a normal heart to diffuse nonspecific enlargement, which may resemble a large pericardial effusion (Fig. 7–37*B*). Echocardiography will demonstrate decreased ventricular contraction and enlargement of the left atrium and ventricle. With time, the right atrium and ventricle also enlarge. Doppler echocardiography or MRI may reveal mitral or tricuspid regurgitation caused by dilatation of the valve annulus.[123] Left-sided and later biventricular failure occur in most patients, an important predictive indicator of shortened survival time.

The radiographic appearance of *hypertrophic cardiomyopathy* (see p. 1414) is variable. Chest roentgenograms may demonstrate a normal heart or enlargement of the left ventricle, which can be focal or diffuse. If mitral regurgitation is present, the left atrium is also enlarged. Unlike in aortic valvular stenosis, no ascending aortic dilatation is present unless the patient has coincidental systemic hypertension or atherosclerotic uncoiling of the aorta.[82] The diagnosis is usually established by echocardiography, and cardiac catheterization with angiography is reserved for those cases in which noninvasive techniques are technically inadequate, coronary disease is suspected, or surgery is contemplated.[19] Angiography demonstrates, during systole, a narrow slitlike left ventricular chamber, marked wall thickening, and hyperdynamic contractions. CT and MRI are less invasive alternatives to angiography (Chap. 10).[19,123–126]

Restrictive cardiomyopathy (see p. 1426) is characterized by marked myocardial rigidity with poor left ventricular diastolic relaxation.[127] Radiographically, there are no consistent features of restrictive cardiomyopathy. The heart is normal in size or may be moderately or, more rarely, even markedly enlarged. The left atrium may also be enlarged when mitral regurgitation is present. Pulmonary congestion occurs in most patients, and calcification of the right or left ventricular wall may be seen. Contrast ventriculography (and radionuclide angiography) demonstrates rapid relaxation during early diastole followed by "plateauing" and absence of an "atrial kick".

POSTOPERATIVE CARDIAC RADIOLOGY

(See also Chap. 52)

With the unrelenting growth of coronary bypass graft surgery and the increased frequency of other cardiac surgical procedures during the last three decades, the postoperative supine portable chest roentgenogram has become one of the most frequently ordered examinations. In the Department of Radiology at Thomas Jefferson University Hospital, over 50 per cent of inpatient chest roentgenograms are performed at the bedside, usually in the intensive care unit. About one-third of these studies are of postsurgical cardiac patients. In order to interpret properly the postoperative chest film, special attention must be given to optimization of technique.[128–130] Adequate complementary film-screen combinations as well as careful patient positioning are needed to overcome the effects of low-capacity portable equipment and motion artifacts. Knowledge of the appearance of the preoperative film often aids in clarifying abnormalities seen on the postoperative portable roentgenogram. When the pre- and postoperative films are compared, the differences in vascularity, cardiac size, and degree of inspiration between the preoperative erect PA and the postoperative supine AP films must be taken into account.[131] For example, an 11 per cent increase in cardiac diameter, a 9 per cent increase in cardiothoracic ratio, and a 15 per cent increase in mediastinal width when an inspiratory PA film is compared with an inspiratory AP chest film have been described. For this reason, many surgeons and radiologists recommend that a preoperative supine AP film be taken prior to operation to guarantee the availability of a comparative film.[132]

Most cardiac surgery is performed through an extrapleural median sternotomy with the use of cardiopulmonary bypass. Except for specific problems related to the patient's preexisting cardiac disorder or to the specific surgical procedure, alterations found in the postoperative chest film are common to all cardiac surgical procedures.[133–136]

Immediately after operation, the lungs appear normal or there are varying degrees of subsegmental left lower lobe atelectasis related to incomplete reexpansion of the lungs after cardiopulmonary bypass. There may be mediastinal widening due to intraoperative edema or hemorrhage, and a small pneumomediastinum may also be present.

A number of tubes, wires, and catheters are present in or overlie the postoperative chest[23,133–137] (Fig. 7–39). These include an endotracheal tube, which should be positioned 5 to 7 cm above the carina to allow excursion in both flexion and extension of the neck. If the endotracheal tube is too close to the carina, flexion of the head or neck may force the distal end of the tube into the right or, less often, the left main stem bronchus, causing varying degrees of atelectasis of the opposite lung and barotrauma if assisted ventilation is used.[128] If the tube is too high, the patient may run the risk of aspiration, and dead space is increased.[134,135]

The central venous pressure catheter is ideally placed in the superior vena cava. However, its distal tip is often found in the right atrium, in which case pressure measurements remain accurate, but there is an increased risk of cardiac perforation when the catheter is placed in the thin-walled right atrium.[23] In addition to malposition, compression or "pinch-off" of the catheter by the clavicle and first rib may produce narrowing or kinking of the catheter. Pinch-off occurs in 1 per cent of catheter placements.[138] When pinch-off occurs, the catheter should be removed and replaced with a more rigid catheter, one that is oval rather than round in cross section.

A Swan-Ganz catheter is usually placed in either major pulmonary artery (ideally with the tip lying within a dependent branch) to monitor pulmonary artery or pulmonary capillary wedge pressure and to obtain mixed venous blood samples. If the catheter is too peripheral in position, the inflated balloon near the tip of the catheter may

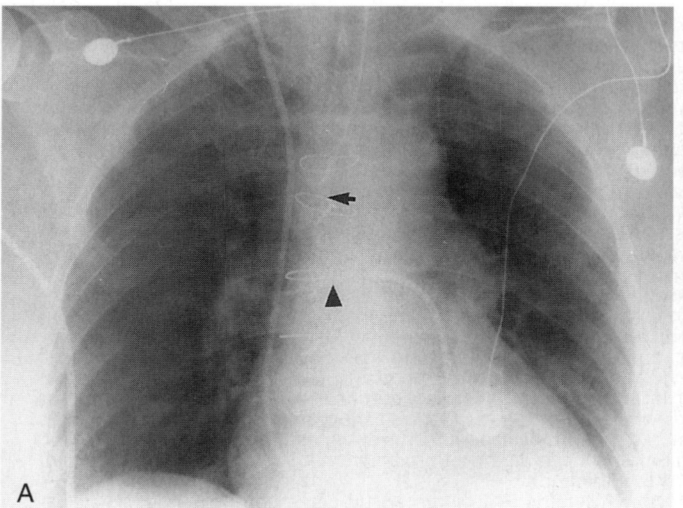

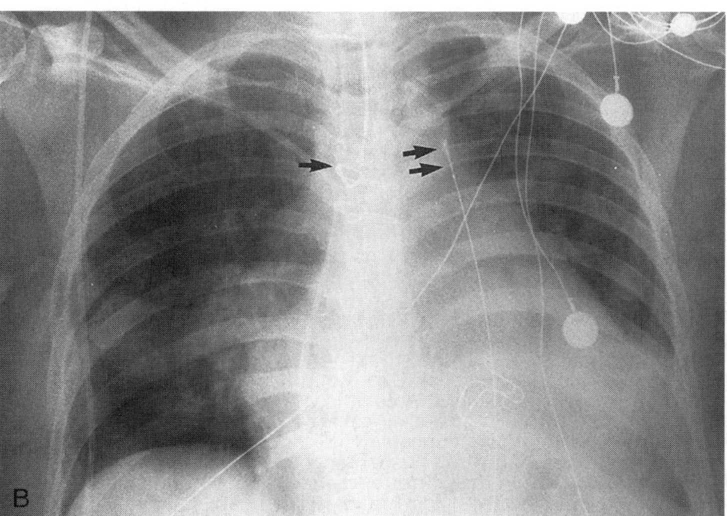

FIGURE 7–39. ***A,*** **An early postoperative chest radiograph. There is a Swan-Ganz catheter in the right pulmonary artery (arrowhead). The endotracheal tube lies 2 cm above the carina (arrow). It should be repositioned proximally to prevent selective bronchial placement.** ***B,*** **This 60-year-old man developed a massive myocardial infarction. The endotracheal tube lies just above the carina (left arrow). The intraaortic balloon catheter is located at the top of the arch near the orifice of the left subclavian artery (double arrows on right) and required at least 2 cm of retraction.**

damage the pulmonary artery wall and cause a perforation leading to a pseudoaneurysm.[137] The tip should lie in a large central branch from which it can float distally to a wedged position, whereupon the balloon is inflated.

Anterior mediastinal drainage catheters are located in the parasternal area, and posterior mediastinal drainage catheters usually lie on the left side behind the heart. Epicardial pacing wires or pacemaker wires project over the heart and lungs.[135,136] When circulatory assistance is needed, an intraaortic counterpulsation balloon catheter may be positioned with its tip just below the level of the left subclavian artery within the proximal descending aorta[136] (Fig. 7–39*B*). Pacemaker leads,[23,133] prosthetic valves,[46] and implantable cardioverter-defibrillators[139] require careful observation for lead or component malposition, pouch infection, or fracture.[133] A nasogastric tube is also usually present. It may be inadvertently placed in a bronchus and pass into the lung or even the pleura. If malposition of a nasogastric tube is unrecognized, aspiration of fluid may occur, causing a chemical pulmonary edema or pneumonia. Early recognition of the normal and abnormal positions of the large number of catheters, wires, and tubes found on the postoperative chest radiograph requires rapid interpretation by a physician thoroughly familiar with both the appearance of the postoperative chest and the possible complications that may frequently occur.

EARLY POSTOPERATIVE FILM. The first postoperative chest film usually demonstrates varying degrees of lower lobe atelectasis, mediastinal widening, pulmonary edema, and pleural effusion.[130,140] Unilateral or bilateral lower lobe atelectasis, usually accompanied by small pleural effusions, is the source of lower lung zone opacities found in almost all cardiac surgery patients.[135] Elevation of the involved hemidiaphragm is also present.[141] The lower lobe opacities usually appear within 8 hours after surgery and clear within 5 to 7 days. Although pneumonia can occur as a complication, it is unusual. These changes occur most commonly on the left side. The mechanisms for preferential left lower lobe atelectasis include paralysis of the phrenic nerve caused by cardioplegic solutions or crushed ice administered for myocardial preservation or retained secretions.[141] Decreased diaphragmatic motion may persist for many weeks after operation but will eventually resolve in most patients.

Pleural Effusion. Radiographically, pleural effusions manifested by blunting of the costophrenic angle, loss of sharpness of the diaphragmatic contour, and increased opacity behind the diaphragmatic dome are seen. Postoperative effusions are probably related to pericardial fluid that leaks into the pleural space through the surgically created pericardial window or to irritation of the pleura during operation. Postpericardiotomy syndrome and congestive heart failure are the sources of pleural effusion in some patients.[142] Increasingly larger or persistent pleural effusions may be due to hemomediastinum, with blood escaping into the pleural space through a pleural tear. Large pleural effusions are more common after left internal mammary bypass surgery because the pleural space is entered in that procedure.

Pulmonary Consolidation. Patchy or occasionally diffuse consolidation in both lungs following cardiac surgery is usually caused by pulmonary edema. Pulmonary edema due to increased capillary permeability or adult respiratory distress syndrome is common after cardiac surgery because of vasoactive substances released during cardiopulmonary bypass, which affect capillary permeability. Pulmonary edema usually occurs within 2 days of surgery and is reversible with supportive therapy including diuretics.[135] Post-perfusion pulmonary edema occurs after cardiopulmonary bypass, which causes a marked increase in fluid in the extravascular space. The mechanism for post-perfusion pulmonary edema is thought to be related to the contact of circulating blood with foreign surfaces during bypass.[131] Congestive heart failure following cardiac bypass surgery occurs in patients with poor cardiac output. Typically, vascular redistribution to the upper lobes, Kerley B lines, small bilateral pleural effusions, and the patchy opacities due to pulmonary edema are present.

Other early complications of cardiac surgery identified by plain film chest radiography include sternal dehiscence, pneumothorax, pneumomediastinum, mediastinal hematoma, pneumopericardium, subcutaneous emphysema, and the findings of pulmonary embolism[143–145] (Fig. 7–40). Rib fractures occur in 2 to 4 per cent of patients and are usually identified by plain films. Their importance lies in the possible misdiagnosis of chest pain of another cause, including angina or aortic dissection.

Pneumothorax is often difficult to identify in the supine patient.[129] It is characterized radiographically as a poorly defined radiolucency overlying the lower lung zones. Decubitus views are helpful in clearly defining the presence of a pleural air collection. Pneumomediastinum may occur when the mediastinum is entered during surgery. In most cases the mediastinal air resolves spontaneously within several days. A radiolucency overlying the center of the sternum following median sternotomy is due to a small gap in the sternum and soft tissues at the surgical site; this occurs in approximately one-third of patients. There is no proven correlation between this thin radiolucency and sternal dehiscence.[143]

Mediastinal Hemorrhage. This complication is common after cardiac surgery but is seldom serious enough to require reoperation. In the typical postoperative patient the mediastinum is widened by up to 35 per cent compared with preoperative PA chest films. Katzberg et al. found that if the mediastinum is widened more than 70 per cent compared with the baseline radiograph, surgery is usually required to remove the hematoma.[130] However, considerable bleeding may be present without visible mediastinal widening, especially if the patient is receiving positive end-expiratory pressure support, which may compress the mediastinum. Moreover, some patients may have a wide mediastinum but are hemodynamically stable, have no significant bloody drainage, and do not require reoperation.

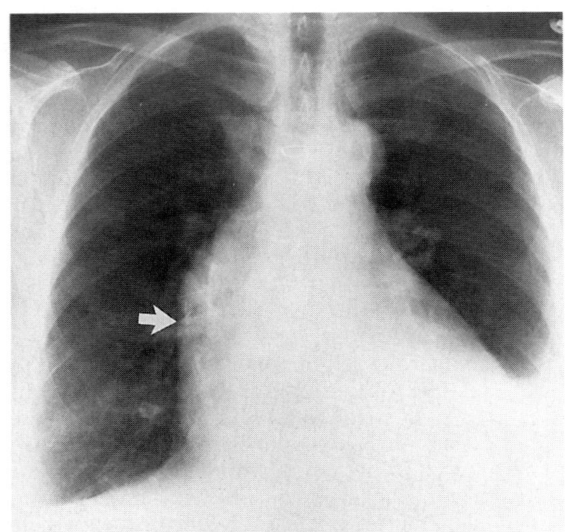

FIGURE 7–40. Mediastinal hemorrhage. There is marked widening of the right side of the mediastinum in the area of the ascending aorta (arrow). A large left pleural effusion is also present. Three days after CABG surgery.

Both CT and echocardiography can be helpful in establishing the diagnosis of intrapericardial hematoma. With echocardiography the hematoma has an echo-free center and a refractile margin. CT, with and without contrast enhancement, is also useful to differentiate hematoma from other masses. On nonenhanced CT the hematoma is denser than other soft tissues and the pericardium is visualized alongside the collection.[131,146]

Enlargement of the cardiac silhouette occurring during the early postoperative period may be due to cardiac failure with or without myocardial infarction or to a mediastinal or pericardial fluid collection. In some patients, pericardial tamponade occurs from bleeding of small arteries in the area of the sternal incision. Equalization of diastolic pressures and elevation of the pulmonary capillary wedge pressure without pulmonary redistribution or edema, together with diffuse enlargement of the cardiac silhouette, suggest pericardial tamponade. Although the chest roentgenogram is suggestive, both CT and echocardiography will clearly reveal the presence of pericardial fluid, while CT is the procedure of choice to detect a mediastinal fluid collection.[145]

LATE COMPLICATIONS OF CARDIAC SURGERY. Postpericardiotomy Syndrome (see p. 1520). This common late complication of cardiac surgery is characterized by pleuritis, pericarditis, and fever. It is believed to be the result of an immune response to the necrotic epicardium. It generally occurs several weeks after operation and is self-limited.[142] Occasionally, cardiac tamponade or constrictive pericarditis occurs as a complication of the postpericardiotomy syndrome. Radiographically, unilateral or bilateral pleural effusions, diffuse enlargement of the cardiac silhouette caused by pericardial effusion, and small basilar pulmonary opacities are found. Echocardiography or CT will identify the pleural or pericardial fluid collections.[142,145] Other late postoperative complications of cardiac surgery include sternal osteomyelitis, especially after internal mammary artery surgery,[147] dehiscence,[143] mediastinitis, and cardiac rupture.[119]

Pseudoaneurysm of the Thoracic Aorta (Fig. 7–41). This complication is associated with sternal and mediastinal inflammation following median sternotomy.[148–150] Pseudoaneurysm is a rare but serious complication of cardiac surgery and may occur at the site of an aortic cannulation or vent, the aortic clamp line, or the saphenous graft-aortic anastomosis.[150] Cardiac pseudoaneurysms can also occur at sites where full-thickness cardiac incisions were made. Although plain film radiographs will demonstrate a mass in the cardiac or aortic region, enhanced CT or MRI is diagnostic and should be performed before reoperation.[148,150]

Aortic Dissection. Although aortic dissection rarely occurs in patients who have undergone surgery of the aorta and aortic valve replacement, it should be considered in the differential diagnosis of mediastinal widening or anterior mediastinal mass. A dissection may appear immediately after operation but is more likely to occur weeks to months later. Although aortography is diagnostic, contrast-enhanced CT is helpful to distinguish between dissection on the one hand, and hematoma, abscess, tumor, or prominent mediastinal fat on the other.[148]

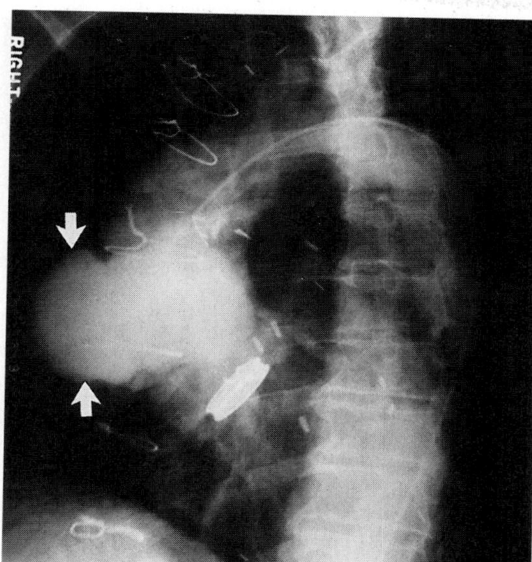

FIGURE 7–41. Pseudoaneurysm of the ascending aorta. This saccular pseudoaneurysm (arrows) developed 5 months after valve replacement at the aortotomy site in a 78-year-old man. (From Sullivan, K. L., et al.: Pseudoaneurysm of the ascending aorta following cardiac surgery. Chest *93*:138, 1988.)

PROSTHETIC VALVE SURGERY (see also p. 1065). The chest roentgenogram is helpful in following patients for the potential complications of valve implantation. Identification of the site of the prosthetic valve is not as simple as that of calcified native cardiac valves because only an AP film may be available during the early postoperative period and the prosthetic valves vary in position and often overlap each other.[151] If the patient fails to improve clinically after valve replacement or if there is pulmonary edema after a brief period of improvement, malfunction of the prosthetic valve may be the cause. Major malfunctions result from sewing ring dehiscence, strut fracture, tissue encroachment into the ring orifice, disc- or poppet-induced thrombosis, and infective endocarditis.[45,46] Plain chest film may show enlargement of the adjacent cardiac chambers or pulmonary edema. Calcification of a heterograft or homograft valve may be seen and is usually caused by tissue degeneration. Fracture and separation of radiopaque components and their distal migration may be identified by fluoroscopy or on radiographs of the chest and abdomen.[47,55]

Fluoroscopy documents prosthetic valve motion, the integrity of the mechanical components, and the presence of calcification. If there is more than 12 degrees of rocking of the mitral or aortic sewing ring in systole and diastole, prosthesis dehiscence at the ring should be considered.[54] Reduced or absent excursion of the valve occluder suggests thrombus, tissue intrusion, or vegetation. Doppler echocardiography will document regurgitant blood flow proximal to the valve. Enhanced cine CT and cine MRI are complementary studies to diagnose valvular regurgitation.

CORONARY ARTERY SURGERY (Chap. 30). The early plain film radiographic findings after coronary bypass surgery are nonspecific and are similar to those of other cardiac surgical procedures.[62,130,152] Radiographic evaluation of coronary bypass grafts utilizing ultrafast CT or MRI sometimes aids in distinguishing graft occlusion from other causes of postoperative chest pain.[132,153,154] MRI has an accuracy of 91 per cent for determination of patency and is 72 per cent accurate for determination of occlusion[154] (Fig. 10–10, p. 323). In comparison, CT exhibits 85 to 95 per cent accuracy in demonstrating occlusions and up to 100 per cent accuracy in demonstrating patency (Fig. 10–36, p. 338).[152] A drawback to these noninvasive techniques is that they neither exclude nonocclusive stenosis of the grafts nor document progression of disease in native vessels. Moreover, they do not eliminate the need to perform cardiac catheterization in patients in whom reoperation is contemplated.

CARDIAC TRANSPLANTATION (Chap. 18). Most transplant candidates have a history of end-stage cardiac failure caused by ischemic heart disease or cardiomyopathy. The heart is invariably enlarged, and pulmonary vascular redistribution or edema is generally present. In orthotopic cardiac transplantation, the recipient heart is removed and the donor heart, with intact aorta and pulmonary arteries, is attached to a cuff of native left atrium containing the pulmonary veins. Following transplant surgery, typical radiographic changes associated with median sternotomy are found, including a widened mediastinum, pleural effusion, left lower lobe consolidation, and atelectasis. Within 2 months after transplantation, the heart becomes smaller and reaches stability 6 months after surgery. Persistent cardiomegaly most likely is caused by pericardial effusion, which may result from cyclosporine therapy or placement of a small donor heart in a large pericardial sac. Following transplantation the radiograph often has a double density in the vicinity of the right atrial border because of the overlapping donor and recipient atria. MRI or CT can clearly depict postoperative transplantation anatomy as well as the presence of pericardial effusion and lymphadenopathy.[155]

If graft rejection occurs, the heart enlarges, but pulmonary edema does not usually develop. The diagnosis of rejection, made by endomyocardial biopsy, demonstrates lymphocytic infiltration and myocytic necrosis.[156] MRI can demonstrate alterations in signal intensity in moderate and severe rejection.[157] Accelerated coronary atherosclerosis can lead to myocardial infarction and left ventricular enlargement. Pulmonary infection due to immunosuppressive therapy is common and may be bacterial, viral, or protozoan in origin.

Heart-lung transplantation is usually performed in patients with a history of primary pulmonary hypertension, end-stage chronic pulmonary disease with right ventricular decompensation, or Eisenmenger physiology. Early complications in this group of patients include cytomegalovirus and bacterial pneumonia. Long-term sequelae include accelerated coronary atherosclerosis and bronchiolitis obliterans with or without organizing pneumonia. Radiographically, the parenchymal pattern of bronchiolitis obliterans is characterized by coarse, asymmetrical nodular or reticular-nodular densities throughout the lungs with relative sparing of the upper lobes.[158–160]

CONGENITAL HEART DISEASE IN THE ADULT

Adults with congenital cardiac disorders (see Chap. 30) fall into three different clinical groups: those whose cardiac disorder was recognized in childhood and surgically treated, those whose cardiac abnormalities were recognized but did not undergo surgery and were followed medically, and those patients who survived into adulthood with unrecognized or misdiagnosed congenital cardiac disease.

The radiographic findings in adult congenital heart disease can be classified in a number of ways, based on the frequency of the disorder or a combination of the hallmarks of disease including the state of the pulmonary vasculature, the position of the aortic arch, cardiac size, and abdominal situs. Combining the radiographic findings with a history of the presence or absence of cyanosis, the time of onset of the cardiac murmur, and the clinical state of the patient should narrow the diagnostic choices. Several of the more common congenital cardiovascular disorders found with some frequency in adults are discussed below.

Coarctation of the Aorta

Coarctation of the aorta (see p. 965) is a common anomaly, accounting for 8 per cent of congenital heart defects in children and about 6 per cent of adult congenital heart disease.[25] In the adult patient, localized postductal narrowing of the aorta is most common. It represents a deformity in the aortic media that narrows the lumen by a curtain-like unfolding of the vessel wall.[161,162] The clinical presentation is highly variable and ranges from left ventricular failure in infancy to hypertension in otherwise asymptomatic adult patients, depending on the site and severity of the coarctation and the presence of associated abnormalities.[163,164] The most common associated anomaly is bicuspid aortic valve, which occurs in as many as 85 per

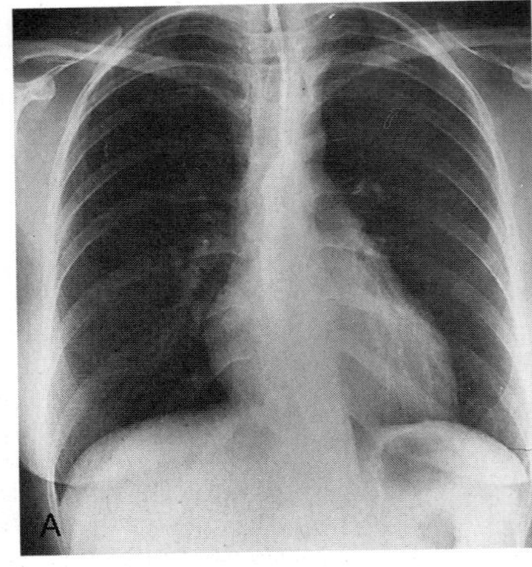

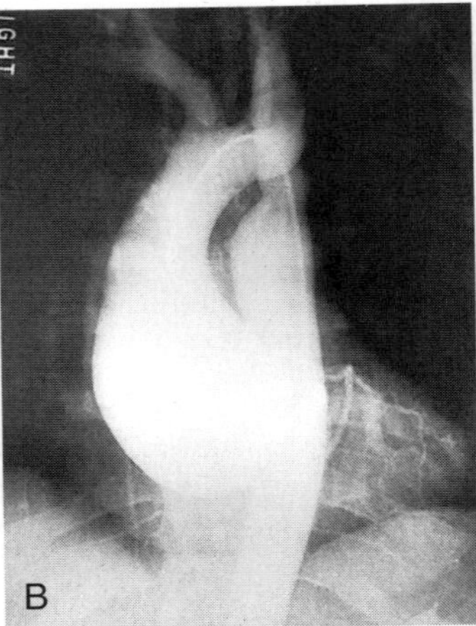

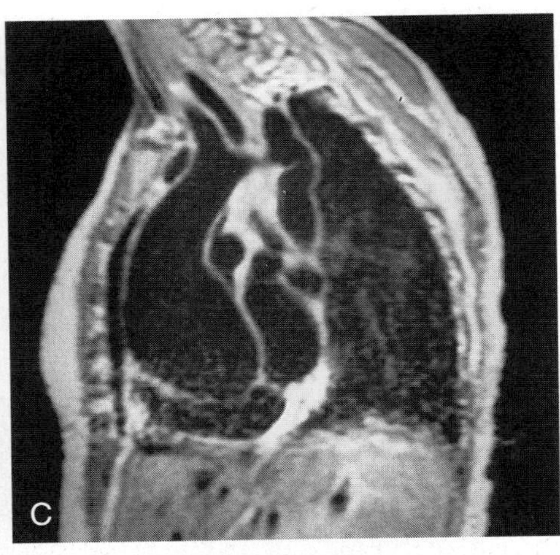

FIGURE 7–42. Coarctation of the aorta. *A,* There is displacement of the barium column to the right above and below the coarctation. *B,* Thoracic aortography. The luminal narrowing at the isthmus and enlargement of the LSCA are characteristic of coarctation. It may be described as a "3" sign or "E" sign becaue of the precoarctation bulge of the LSCA, the coarctation itself, and postcoarctation aortic dilatation. The dilatation of the ascending aorta is due to a regurgitant bicuspid aortic valve. *C,* Sagittal T1-weighted MRI in the same patient shows the same findings as the aortogram but without contrast media, radiation, or catheterization.

cent of patients with coarctation of the aorta.[25] Other associated congenital anomalies include ventricular septal defect, stenosis or atresia of the left subclavian artery, patent ductus arteriosus, Turner syndrome, or mitral valve prolapse.[165]

ROENTGENOGRAPHIC FINDINGS. The diagnosis of coarctation of the aorta can be established from the PA chest film alone in up to 92 per cent of patients.[161] The most useful radiographic sign is an abnormal contour of the aortic arch, which may appear as a double bulge above and below the usual site of the aortic knob.[166] This pattern has been described as a "figure 3" sign. The upper arc of the "3" is the dilated arch proximal to the coarctation and/or a dilated left subclavian artery (Fig. 7–42). The lower arc or bulge is the poststenotic dilatation of the aorta immediately below the coarctation. The indentation between the two bulges is the coarctation itself. When the esophagus is filled with barium, a reverse "3" or "E" sign is often seen, representing a mirror image of the areas of pre- and poststenotic dilatation. The "3" sign is variable in that the upper arc may be small and the lower arc large or vice versa (Fig. 7–42). Superior mediastinal widening due to large internal mammary collateral arteries is visible in some patients.[167] The aortic arch may also be obscured in the frontal view due to overlapping of the aorta by an enlarged left subclavian artery.[166] Left ventricular enlargement usually occurs with coarctation, particularly when there is an associated bicuspid aortic valve and aortic stenosis.

Bilateral symmetrical rib notching, readily appreciated on the chest film, is diagnostic of aortic coarctation. It is due to obstruction to blood flow at the narrowed aortic segment with collateral blood flow through the intercostal vessels. Rib notching is unusual in infancy, but it becomes more prominent with increased age and is present in 75 per cent of adults with coarctation. Rib notching occurs along the inferior margin of the third to the eighth ribs due to the pulsations of the dilated intercostal arteries. The major pathways of collateral flow include (1) subclavian artery to internal mammary artery to intercostal arteries, (2) subclavian artery to the costovertebral trunk to the intercostal arteries, and (3) transverse cervical and suprascapular arteries to the intercostal arteries. Dilatation of the internal mammary arteries acting as a collateral pathway may cause scallop-edged retrosternal notching.[167]

Cardiac catheterization and angiography are diagnostic, demonstrating both the site of the coarctation and associated anomalies, including aortic valvular disease (Fig. 7–42*B*). Cross-sectional imaging modalities yield important diagnostic information. Echocardiography, for example, demonstrates the presence or absence of bicuspid aortic and mitral valve deformities. MRI is useful in demonstrating both the coarctation itself and restenosis of the aorta following surgery or angioplasty[164,165,168,169] (Fig. 7–42*C*).

Left-to-Right Shunts

OSTIUM SECUNDUM ATRIAL SEPTAL DEFECT (ASD) (see also p. 966). This is the most common left-to-right shunt diagnosed in adult life, accounting for over 40 per cent of adult congenital heart defects.[170–171a] Although the chest radiograph may be normal in a patient with a small shunt, typically the main pulmonary artery, the peripheral pulmonary branches, the right atrium, and right ventricu-

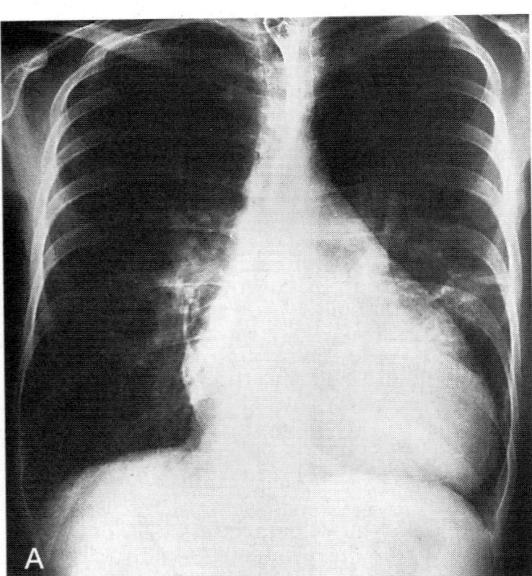

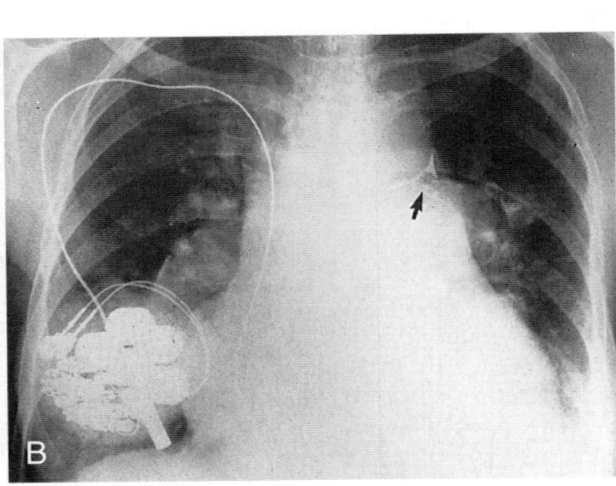

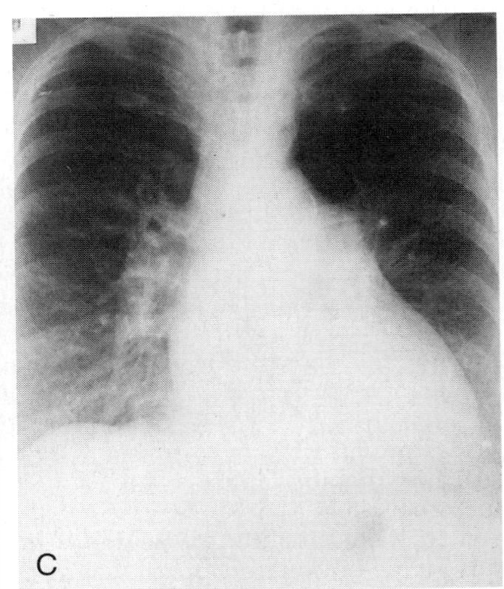

FIGURE 7–43. *A,* Atrial septal defect. A 45-year-old woman with an ostium secundum defect. The pulmonary artery is enlarged and there is prominence of the right atrial border. The enlargement of the right ventricle causes rounding of the left heart border. *B,* Patent ductus arteriosus in a patient with a cardiac pacemaker. An inverted "Y" calcification is present above an enlarged pulmonary artery (arrow). *C,* Ventricular septal defect. There is an increase in the size of the central pulmonary arteries in this patient with VSD and Eisenmenger physiology.

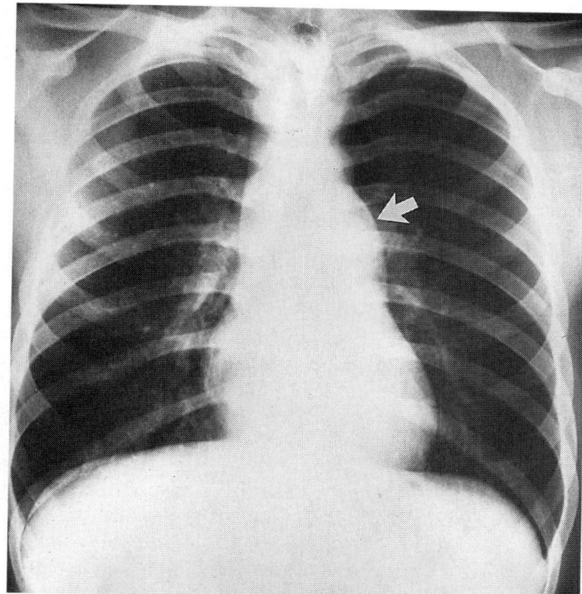

FIGURE 7–44. Pulmonary valvular stenosis. Pulmonary blood flow and cardiac size are normal, but the main pulmonary artery is enlarged (arrow) in this young woman with pulmonary valvular stenosis.

lar borders are enlarged (Fig. 7–21*A*). Differentiation from other left-to-right shunts is often possible. There is usually less pulmonary artery dilatation in patent ductus arteriosus (PDA) than in ASD, and both PDA and ventricular septal defect (VSD) are associated with enlarged left-sided cardiac chambers. In the adult over the age of 50 years, the radiographic findings of ASD are often atypical and may include left atrial enlargement, evidence of pulmonary venous hypertension, and pulmonary edema (Fig. 7–43*A*). These changes are associated with smaller shunts and a higher prevalence of left ventricular dysfunction and pulmonary arterial hypertension.[172] Echocardiography is diagnostic in ASD (Fig. 3–77, p. 82); right ventricular chamber dilation and paradoxical anterior systolic motion of the interventricular septum are seen. The size and the location of the ASD can often be visualized, as well as associated abnormalities including mitral valve prolapse. Cine CT and MRI also demonstrate the defect of the atrial septum.[169]

VENTRICULAR SEPTAL DEFECT (see also p. 967). VSD accounts for 30 per cent of cardiac malformations in the newborn but comprises only 10 per cent of adult-onset congenital heart defects. The relatively small incidence in adults is due to spontaneous closure of the defect in childhood or surgical repair.[173] If the VSD is small, the chest film is normal. However, if there is a large left-to-right shunt or secondary pulmonary hypertension, the pulmonary arteries are enlarged, as are both ventricles and the left atrium (Fig. 7–43*C*). The ascending aorta is small or normal in size, whereas the aorta is enlarged in PDA. Cine CT, MRI, and echocardiography will demonstrate the site of the defect.[162,164,173]

PULMONARY VALVULAR STENOSIS (see also p. 968). Pulmonary valvular stenosis in adults is usually an isolated anomaly.[174] Most patients are asymptomatic even with severe obstruction. There is mild to moderate enlargement of the main pulmonary artery due to post-stenotic dilatation resulting from the jet effect of blood flow through the narrowed pulmonary valve orifice (Fig. 7–44). Since the jet is directed toward the left, the left pulmonary artery is often preferentially enlarged. Calcification of the pulmonary valve is rare in this condition. The differential diagnosis of pulmonary valvular stenosis includes primary and secondary pulmonary hypertension and idiopathic pulmonary artery dilatation.

CONGENITAL CORRECTED TRANSPOSITION OF THE GREAT ARTERIES (see also p. 966). In this condition ventricular inversion and transposition of the pulmonary artery and aorta result from formation of a left (levo or l) rather than a right (dextro or d) bulboventricular loop. The systemic venous flow is transmitted to the lungs by way of a right-sided anatomical left ventricle and the transposed pulmonary artery. Pulmonary venous flow traverses the left atrium and a left-sided anatomical right ventricle en route to the aorta.

Radiographically, the ascending aorta is positioned to the left, forming a long continuous shadow along the left cardiac border from the ventricular apex to the aortic arch[175] (Fig. 7–45*A,B*). The main pulmonary artery lies behind and to the right of the aorta and is not border-forming with the lung in the PA view. A left-to-right shunt may or may not be present, and left atrioventricular valve regurgitation and conduction abnormalities leading to heart block are fairly common. The heart is normal to enlarged in size, depending on the degree of atrioventricular valve regurgitation. Cross-sectional imaging supports the plain film diagnosis, showing an anterior left-sided aorta and a pulmonary artery lying behind and medial to the aorta.[176,177]

Cyanotic Congenital Heart Disease in the Adult

TETRALOGY OF FALLOT (see also p. 968). This is the most common cyanotic congenital cardiac lesion in adults as well as in children. Most adults with tetralogy of Fallot demonstrate mild to moderate pulmonary hypovascularity. Those with mild infundibular pulmonary stenosis have normal pulmonary blood flow (Fig. 7–7*C*). Small tortuous bronchial arteries are found in both lungs when severe pulmonary outflow tract stenosis or atresia is present. There is a right aortic arch in 25 per cent of patients.[178] The combination of right aortic arch and cyanosis should always suggest the diagnosis of tetralogy of Fallot, although the same combination of findings can also be seen in the rare examples of truncus arteriosus or double-outlet right ventricle in the adult patient. Echocardiography often demonstrates a high and large ventricular septal defect, overriding of the ventricular septum by the aorta, and right ventricular hypertrophy. Cine CT and MRI can demonstrate the septal defect and the large ascending aorta, as well a right aortic arch.[164,169] Plain films show a boot-shaped heart in some adult patients, but this is less common than in children because those who survive into adulthood are less likely to have severe right ventricular outflow tract stenosis.

EBSTEIN'S ANOMALY (see also p. 969). In this condition the tricuspid valve is malformed and partially fused to the walls of the right ventricle. This results in downward displacement of the tricuspid orifice, and regurgitation ensues. There is a right-to-left shunt at the atrial

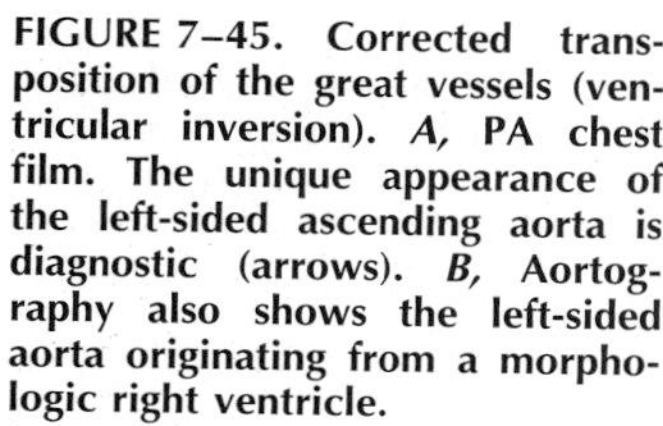

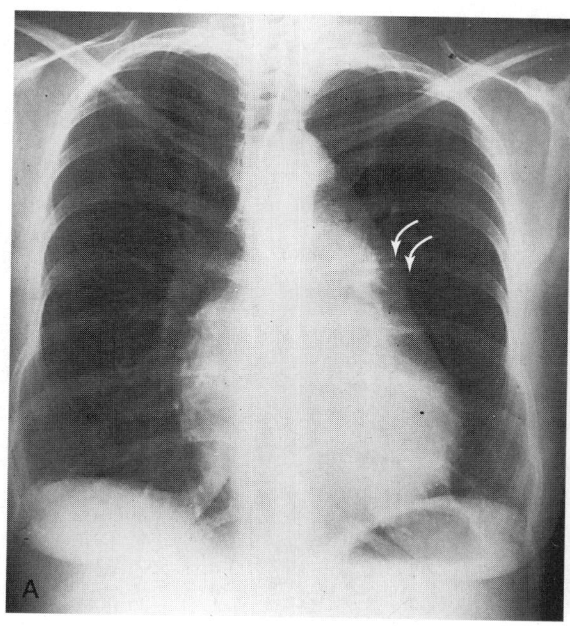

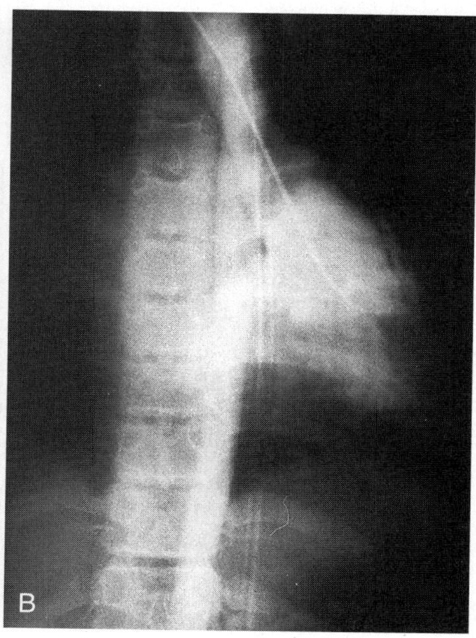

FIGURE 7–45. Corrected transposition of the great vessels (ventricular inversion). *A,* PA chest film. The unique appearance of the left-sided ascending aorta is diagnostic (arrows). *B,* Aortography also shows the left-sided aorta originating from a morphologic right ventricle.

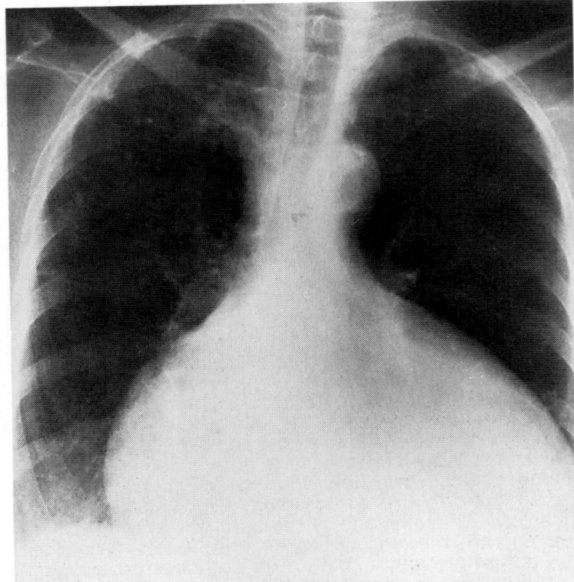

FIGURE 7–46. Ebstein's anomaly. There is globular cardiac enlargement due to severe tricuspid regurgitation and right heart enlargement. The pulmonary blood flow is reduced.

level, causing cyanosis. The right heart chambers are enlarged, often markedly, as a manifestation of the tricuspid regurgitation. The typical roentgenographical findings are those of a large rounded or triangular heart with a narrow vascular pedicle.[179,180] The pulmonary vasculature is reduced, depending on the degree of right-to-left shunting. The greater the shunt, the more diminished the vascularity. Echocardiography shows the abnormal placement of the tricuspid valve with downward displacement of the septal and posterior leaflets. Tricuspid regurgitation can be evaluated by two-dimensional and Doppler echocardiography. MRI and CT also demonstrate the downward displacement of the valve and enlargement of the right atrium[169,179,180] (Fig. 7–46).

THE PERICARDIUM

(See also Chap. 43)

The incidence of pericardial disease in the patient with cardiac disease parallels the frequency of cardiac surgery, multisystem inflammatory disease, thoracic irradiation, and the use of an array of therapeutic agents that affect the pericardium. There is also increasing recognition of the presence of pericardial disease because of modalities, such as echocardiography, which portray pericardial disease with great accuracy.

NORMAL PERICARDIUM. The normal pericardium is frequently identified on lateral plain film projections of the chest as a thin linear opacity separating the anterior subxiphoid mediastinal fat from the subepicardial fat[181–183] (Fig. 7–47*B*). The pericardium may also be visualized in the frontal projection paralleling the left heart border. The extent of the normal and abnormal pericardium is best appreciated with CT and MRI in most patients because of the superior contrast resolution of both techniques.[183,184] With both CT and MRI, the anterior, lateral, and posterior pericardium are clearly separated from mediastinal fat, and subtle discontinuous areas of mild pericardial thickening and loculated effusions may be clearly seen.[185–187] One disadvantage of MRI and CT is that while the pericardial recesses are clearly defined, they may on occasion mimic an aortic dissection or mediastinal lymphadenopathy.[186]

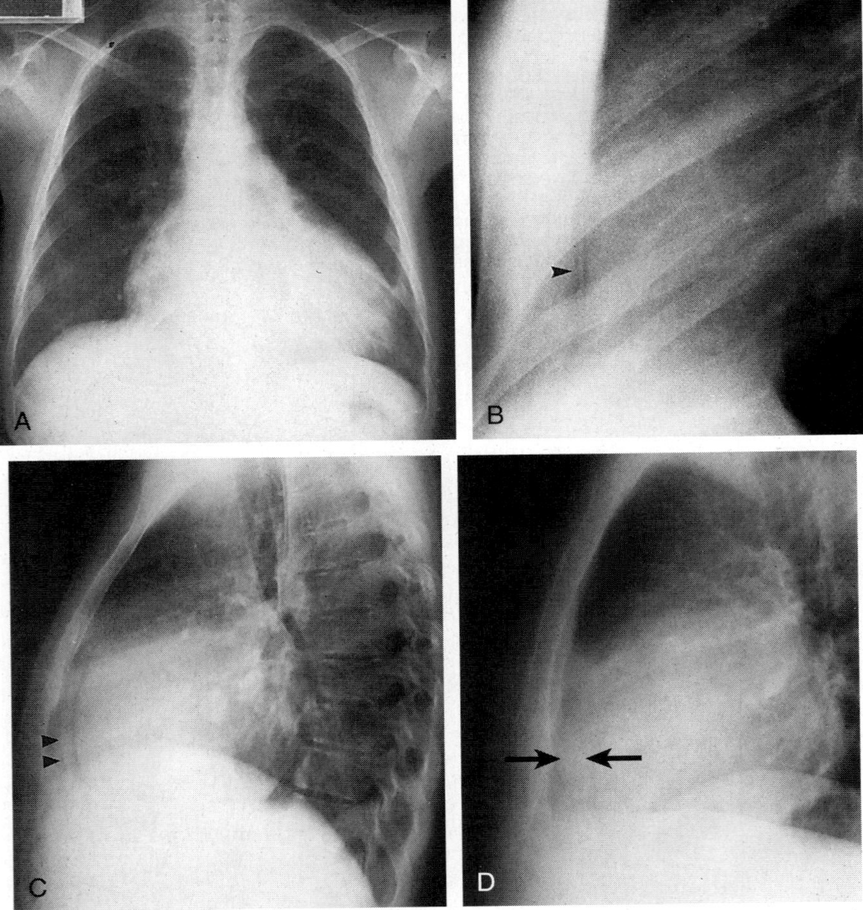

FIGURE 7–47. Pericardial effusion. *A,* The heart assumes a globular rounded shape following development of a pericardial effusion. The normal indentations along the heart borders are effaced so that the cardiac silhouette is smooth and featureless. *B,* The subepicardial radiolucent fat stripe is separated from the subxiphoid fat by the thin, higher density stripe of pericardial fluid (arrowhead). *C,* The pericardial stripe (arrowheads) is wider than in *B* because of a small pericardial effusion. *D,* A large pericardial effusion is present (arrows).

Echocardiography is probably the most sensitive technique for the diagnosis of small pericardial effusions. It is most often the imaging study of choice when pericardial effusion is clinically suspected or is considered as a possibility by plain film radiograph.[186]

PERICARDIAL EFFUSION (see also p. 1485). The effusion may be a transudate or exudate, hemorrhagic, gaseous, or chylous and may be due to a wide variety of causes.[37,186,187] When fluid accumulates in the pericardial space, the cardiac silhouette develops a "flask-like," triangular, or "globular" silhouette (Fig. 7–47). The normal indentations and prominences along both the left and right heart borders are effaced so that the shape of the cardiac silhouette becomes smooth and featureless. Since the pericardium extends up to the pulmonary bifurcation, when a large pericardial effusion is present, the hilar structures are draped and obscured by the distended pericardial cavity. This radiographic appearance should help to distinguish a large pericardial effusion from massive cardiomegaly, which will not obscure the hilar vessels.

In the lateral chest radiograph in the patient with pericardial effusion, the retrosternal space is typically narrowed or obliterated by the expanding cardiac silhouette. Normally the low-density subepicardial fat merges imperceptibly with the mediastinal fat since the two fat planes are separated only by the 2-mm-thick stripe of the pericardium.[182] When pericardial effusion is present the subepicardial fat is displaced posteriorly by the higher-density fluid, which may be visible as a wide opaque vertical band between the anterior border of the heart and the mediastinum (Fig. 7–47). This "epicardial fat pad sign" is visualized best on the lateral projection and is highly specific for pericardial effusion.[182,183,185]

Echocardiography is the most efficient method for the detection of simple pericardial effusion and/or thickening[188] (Fig. 3–104, p. 93). A major advantage of echocardiography is that the ultrasound apparatus can be transported to the bedside to examine critically ill patients. The technique is noninvasive and is diagnostically sensitive to fluid-filled structures. When the pericardial fluid volume is small, it appears as an elliptical hypoechoic region behind the left ventricle. When the effusion is large, the pericardial hypoechoic zone expands to surround the right ventricular apex. In some cases echocardiography may fail to identify pericardial thickening when constrictive pericarditis, neoplasm, or hemorrhage is present.

If echocardiography is inconclusive, CT can be helpful in detecting pericardial thickening, diffuse or loculated effusion, calcification, and adjacent mediastinal and pulmonary disease, as well as neoplasm[145,185,189] (Fig. 10–40, p. 340). The nature of the fluid may be identified by an analysis of CT density numbers. For example, there are higher CT density values in hemopericardium than in serous effusions. Chylous pericardial effusions may have a lower attenuation value than normal pericardial fluid.[185]

MRI and CT can clearly detect pericardial effusion.[190] On T1-weighted images, MRI will show the pericardial cavity as a dark signal void because of the motion of the fluid in the pericardial sac. On the other hand, the pericardial effusion is bright on a gradient echo sequence.[185] Pericardial fibrosis will present with a medium-intensity signal on T1-weighted or dark signal on T2-weighted images. Intrapericardial masses, cysts, and diffuse thickening are well demonstrated with MRI.[189] Furthermore, MRI can clearly define pericardial recesses, mediastinal fat, and other anatomical landmarks that may present pitfalls for the echocardiographer.[189–191a]

PERICARDIAL CONSTRICTION (see also p. 1496). Pericardial constriction may complicate viral or tuberculous pericarditis, hemopericardium, pericarditis associated with radiation, and postpericardiotomy syndrome.[186,187] In patients with chronic pericardial constriction, the overall heart size is large when the pericardium is thickened to 2 cm or more; otherwise the cardiac silhouette remains normal or small. The right atrial border is flattened, and there may be pulmonary vascular redistribution.[182,191]

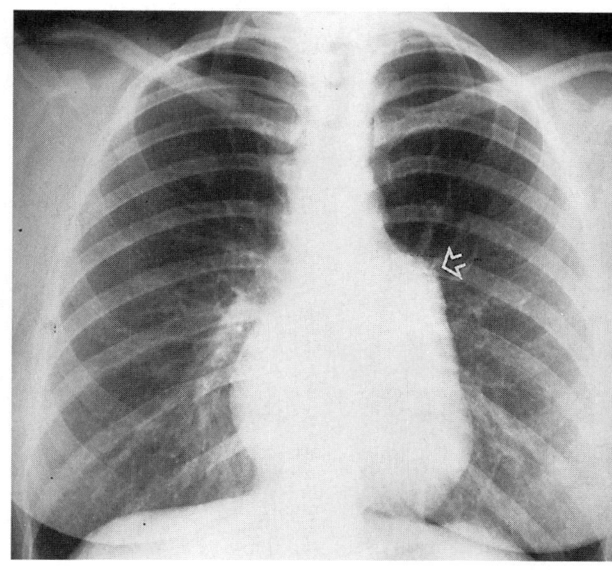

FIGURE 7–48. Partial absence of the pericardium: There is a convex bulge (open arrow) along the left atrial border due to herniation of the left atrial appendage through the pericardial defect.

Small to large pleural effusions are found in 60 per cent of patients with pericardial constriction, and enlargement of the azygos vein and left atrium occurs in 20 per cent of patients. In the past, tuberculous pericarditis was a frequent cause of pericardial calcification and constriction. But today tuberculosis is relatively uncommon. As a result, pericardial calcification occurs in fewer than 20 per cent of patients with chronic pericardial constriction[145] (Fig. 7–33). Pericardial calcification is best appreciated along the anterior and inferior cardiac borders or in the atrioventricular groove. While it is important to appreciate that the presence of pericardial calcification indicates chronic pericarditis, it does not in itself establish a diagnosis of pericardial constriction.

Pericardial constriction is often confused with restrictive cardiomyopathy, and MRI and CT are particularly helpful in differentiating between these entities (see p. 1501). The pericardium in patients with restrictive cardiomyopathy is normal in thickness and no calcification is present. In addition, there is diffuse limitation of global cardiac excursion in systole and diastole together with myocardial thickening in hearts with restrictive cardiomyopathy.[187]

CONGENITAL ANOMALIES (see also p. 1522). Congenital absence of the pericardium may be partial or complete. Complete absence is less common than partial absence and is usually left-sided.[192,193] Partial absence most frequently occurs along the upper border of the pericardium on either side.[183] If the left-sided defect is small, herniation of the left atrial appendage and/or the pulmonary trunk may occur. On the frontal chest film, herniation through a pericardial defect may resemble the appearance of pulmonary stenosis, mitral stenosis, or a mediastinal tumor (Fig. 7–48). When there is complete absence of the left pericardium, the aortic knob remains in its usual position, but the remainder of the cardiac silhouette shifts to the left and rotates toward the right, so that the right ventricle may become border-forming and the pulmonary artery and left atrial appendage become prominent.[192,193]

In patients with absence of the left pericardium, the plain film shows the lung interposed between the medial border of the pulmonary artery and the thoracic aorta outlining the pulmonary artery on both its medial and lateral sides, so that the lung may be visible between the heart and the diaphragm.[192] CT and MRI demonstrate to best

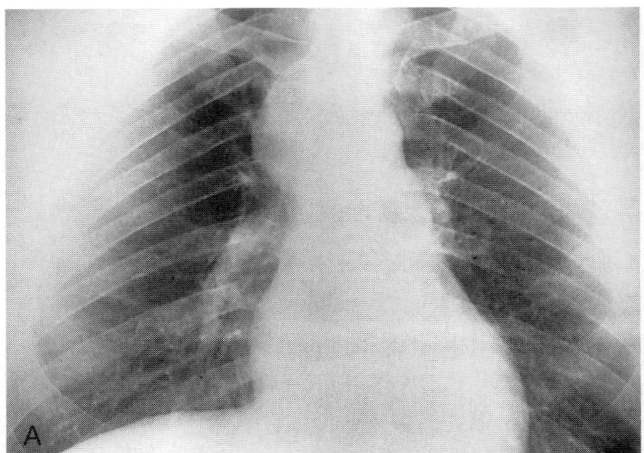

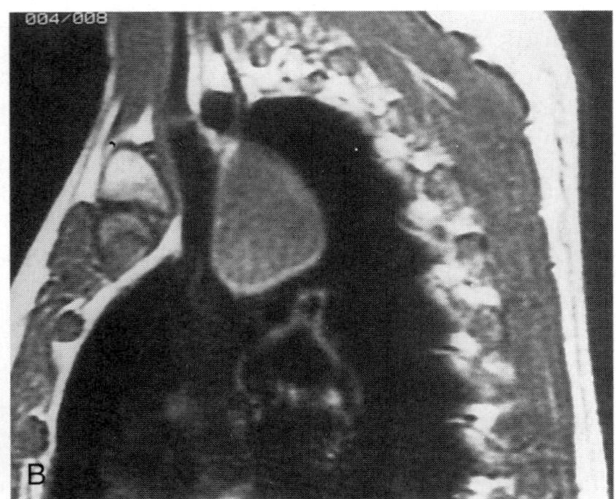

FIGURE 7–49. Pericardial recess cyst. *A,* PA chest film shows a mediastinal bulge along the right paratracheal line. *B,* MRI in sagittal plane shows the cyst as a homogeneous-intensity structure.

advantage the absence of the left anterior pericardium between ascending aorta and the main pulmonary artery. Displacement of the main pulmonary artery laterally and anteriorly is often a clue to the diagnosis.

PERICARDIAL CYST. A pericardial cyst generally appears as a smooth convex bulge along the middle or lower right heart border near the cardiophrenic sulcus. However, 20 per cent of pericardial cysts lie along the left heart border, sometimes mimicking a prominent left atrial appendage or left ventricular aneurysm.[194] Occasionally, pericardial recess cysts present as a soft tissue mass along the right superior mediastinal border in the area of the superior vena cava[194] (Fig. 7–49). While pericardial cysts are usually asymptomatic, chest pain has been described due to torsion or rapid increase in pericardial cyst volume due to intracystic bleeding.[195] Pericardial cysts rarely calcify and do not communicate with the pericardial space. Their clinical importance lies in the need to differentiate pericardial cysts from other masses with a similar appearance, such as fibroma, lymphoma, postoperative hematoma,[146,196] bronchogenic cyst, and cardiac neoplasm. Pericardial cysts are best diagnosed by echocardiography, CT, or MRI as smoothly marginated, fluid-filled structures adjacent to the right heart border.[194,195]

PERICARDIAL NEOPLASM. Pericardial tumors are demonstrated best by CT, MRI, or echocardiography[183] (Fig. 43–23, p. 1514). They generally do not cause a discrete bulge on the plain chest radiograph, but rather infiltrate the heart. When there is associated pericardial effusion, the cardiac silhouette will globally enlarge. CT can clearly identify associated pleural and parenchymal disease including metastatic lesions in the pleural space.

Metastatic neoplasm of the pericardium is far more common than primary tumor. The most common sources of pericardial metastases are the lung, breast, lymphoma, leukemia, and melanoma. Benign masses are unusual and include teratomas, bronchogenic cysts, lipomas, and fibromas.[98,189,195] The principal primary pericardial malignancy is mesothelioma, a rare pericardial tumor without a clear relationship to asbestos exposure (p. 1514). The tumor may be a single mass, multicentric, or diffuse with extensive encasement. Typically, pericardial mesothelioma is manifested by a clinical picture of pericardial constriction.[185]

REFERENCES

HISTORICAL PERSPECTIVE

1. Williams, F. H.: Notes on x-rays in medicine. Trans. Assoc. Am. Physicians *11*:375, 1896.
2. Williams, F. H.: A method for more fully determining the outline of the heart by means of a fluoroscope together with other uses of this instrument in medicine. Boston Med. Surg. J. *135*:335, 1896.
3. Eisenberg, R. L.: Radiology: An Illustrated History. St. Louis, Mosby-Year Book, 1992.
4. Schultz, K. W., Thorsen, M. K., Gurney, J. W., et al.: Comparison of fluoroscopy, angiography and CT in coronary artery calcification. Appl. Radiol. *6*:38, 1989.
5. Henry, D. A., Jolles, H., Berberich, J. J., and Schmelzer, V.: The post-cardiac surgery chest radiograph: A clinically integrated approach. J. Thorac. Imaging *4*:20, 1989.
6. Bank, E. R., and Hernandez, R. J.: CT and MR of congenital heart disease. Radiol. Clin. North Am. *26*:241, 1988.
7. Thompson, B. H., and Stanford, W.: Evaluation of cardiac function with ultrafast computed tomography. Radiol. Clin. North Am. *32*:537, 1994.
8. Stanford, W., and Galvin, J. R.: The radiology of right heart dysfunction: Chest roentgenogram and computed tomography. J. Thorac. Imaging *4*:7, 1989.
9. Holt, W. W., Wong, E., and Lipton, M. J.: Conventional and ultra-fast cine-computed tomography in cardiac imaging. Curr. Opin. Radiol. *1*:159, 1989.
10. Budoff, M. J., Georgiou, D., Brody, A., et al.: Number of calcified coronary vessels by ultrafast computed tomography as a mediator of angiographic coronary artery disease in a symptomatic population. Am. J. Card. Imaging *8*(51):6, 1994.
11. Ahmad, M., Johnson, R. F., Jr., Fawcett, H. D., et al.: Left ventricular aneurysm in short axis: A comparison of magnetic resonance, ultrasound and thallium-201 SPECT images. Magn. Reson. Imaging *5*:293, 1987.
12. Brown, K. A., Altland, E., and Rowen, M.: Prognostic value of normal technetium 99m-sestamibi cardiac imaging. J. Nucl. Med. *35*:554, 1994.
13. Utz, J. A., Herfkens, R. J., Heinsimer, J. A., et al.: Cine MR determination of left ventricular ejection fraction. A.J.R. *148*:839, 1987.
14. Sechtem, U., Pflugfelder, P. W., Gould, R. G., et al.: Measurement of right and left ventricular volumes in healthy individuals with cine MR imaging. Radiology *163*:697, 1987.
15. Kersting-Sommerhoff, B. A., Diethelm, L., Stanger, P., et al.: Evaluation of complex congenital ventricular anomalies with magnetic resonance imaging. Am. Heart J. *120*:133, 1990.
16. Mitchell, L., Jenklins, J. P. R., Watson, Y., et al.: Diagnosis and assessment of mitral and aortic valve disease by cine-flow magnetic resonance imaging. Magn. Reson. Med. *12*:181, 1989.
17. Higgins, C. B., and Caputo, G. R.: Role of MR imaging in acquired and congenital cardiovascular disease. A.J.R. *161*:13, 1993.
18. Davis, C. P., McKinnow, G. C., Debatin, J. F., et al.: Normal heart: Evaluation with echo-planar MR imaging. Radiology *191*:691, 1994.
18a. Wetter, D. R., McKinnow, G. C., Debatin, J. F., and Von Schulthess, G. K.: Cardiac echo-planar MR imaging: Comparison of single and multiple shot techniques. Radiology *194*:765, 1995.
19. Needleman, L., Gardiner, G. A., Jr., and Levin, D. C.: Hypertrophic cardiomyopathy: Changing concepts over the last two decades. A.J.R. *150*:1219, 1988.
20. Gordon, S., and Butler, M.: Echocardiography in cardiac tamponade. J. Clin. Ultrasound *17*:428, 1989.
21. Hartnell, G. G.: Developments in echocardiography. Radiol. Clin. North Am. *32*:461, 1994.
22. Wandtke, J. C.: Bedside chest radiography. Radiology *190*:1, 1994.
23. Wechsler, R. J., Steiner, R. M., and Kinori, I.: Monitoring the monitors: The radiology of thoracic catheters, wires and tubes. Semin. Roentgenol. *23*:61, 1988.

NORMAL CARDIAC ANATOMY

24. Ball, J. B., and Proto, A. V.: The variable appearance of the left superior intercostal vein. Radiology *144*:445, 1982.
25. Steiner, R. M., Gross, G., Flicker, S., et al.: Congenital heart disease in the adult patient. J. Thorac. Imaging *10*:1, 1995.

26. Benedikt, R. A., Jellnec, J. S., Schaefer, P. S., et al.: Right-side aortic arch with aneurysm of aberrant left subclavicular artery: MR imaging appearance. J. Magn. Reson. Imaging *1*:485, 1991.
27. Danza, F. M., Fusco, A., Breda, M., et al.: Ductus arteriosus aneurysm in an adult. A.J.R. *143*:131, 1984.
28. Salomonowitz, E., Edwards, J. E., Hunter, D. W., et al.: The three types of aortic diverticula. A.J.R. *142*:673, 1984.
29. Carlsson, E., Gross, R., and Hold, R. G.: The radiological diagnosis of cardiac valvar insufficiencies. Circulation *55*:921, 1977.
30. Jefferson, K., and Rees, S.: Clinical Cardiac Radiology. 2nd ed. London, Butterworths, 1980.
31. Berdon, W. E., and Baker, D. H.: Plain film findings in azygos continuation of the inferior vena cava. A.J.R. *104*:452, 1968.
32. Bachman, D. M., Ellis, K., and Austin, J. H. M.: The effect of minor degrees of obliquity on the lateral chest radiograph. Radiol. Clin. North Am. *16*:465, 1978.
33. Murphy, M. L., Blue, L. R., Ferris, E. J., et al.: Sensitivity and specificity of chest roentgenogram criteria for right ventricular hypertrophy. Invest. Radiol. *23*:853, 1988.
34. Marzullo, P., L'Abbate, A. L., and Marcus, M.: Patterns of global and regional systolic and diastolic function in the normal right ventricle assessed by ultrafast computed tomography. J. Am. Coll. Cardiol. *17*:1318, 1991.
35. Hoffman, R. B., and Rigler, L. G.: Evaluation of left ventricular enlargement in the lateral projection of the chest. Radiology *85*:93, 1965.
36. Baron, M. G.: Radiological and angiographic examination of the heart. *In* Braunwald, E. (ed.): Heart Disease: A Textbook of Cardiovascular Medicine. 3rd ed. Philadelphia, W. B. Saunders Co., 1988, p. 140.
37. Chen, J. T. T.: Essentials of Cardiac Roentgenology. Boston, Little Brown, 1987.
38. Van Houten, F. X., Adams, D. F., and Abrams, H. L.: Radiology of valvular heart disease. *In* Sonnenblick, E., and Lesch, M. (eds.): Valvular Heart Disease. New York, Grune and Stratton, 1974.
39. Mandalam, K. R., Subramanyan, R., Joseph, S., et al.: Natural history of aortoarteritis: Angiographic study in 26 survivors. Clin. Radiol. *49*:38, 1994.
40. Morgan, P. W., Goodman, L. R., Aprahamian, C., et al.: Evaluation of traumatic aortic injury: Does dynamic contrast enhanced CT play a role? Radiology *182*:661, 1992.
41. Baron, M.: Left anterior oblique view for evaluation of left atrial size. Circulation *44*:926, 1971.
42. Sos, T. A., Levin, D. C., Sniderman, K. W., et al.: Cinefluoroscopy in evaluating left ventricular contractility and aneurysms. Circulation *56* (Suppl. III):18, 1977.
43. Benson, J. S.: Patient and physician radiation during fluoroscopy. Radiology *182*:286, 1992.
44. Freundlich, L. M., and Lind, T. A.: Calcification of the heart and great vessels. C.R.C. Crit. Rev. Clin. Radiol. Nucl. Med. *6*:171, 1975.
45. Kotler, M. N., Mintz, G. S., Panidis, I., et al.: Noninvasive evaluation of normal and abnormal prosthetic valve function. J. Am. Coll. Cardiol. *2*:151, 1983.
46. Steiner, R. M., Mintz, G., Morse, D., et al.: Radiology of cardiac valve prosthesis. Radiographics *8*:277, 1988.
47. Guit, G. L., Van Voorthuisen, A. E., and Steiner, R. M.: Outlet strut fracture of the Björk-Shiley mitral prosthesis. Radiology *154*:298, 1985.
48. Spindola-Franco, H., Fish, B. G., Dachman, A., et al.: Recognition of bicuspid aortic valve by plain film calcification. A.J.R. *139*:867, 1982.
49. Green, C. E., and Kelley, M. J.: A renewed role for fluoroscopy in the evaluation of cardiac disease. Radiol. Clin. North Am. *18*:345, 1980.
50. Schultz, K. W., Thorsen, M. K., Gurney, J. W., et al.: Comparison of fluoroscopy, angiography and CT in coronary artery calcification. Appl. Radiol. *19*:38, 1989.
51. Kelley, M. J., Huang, E. K., and Langou, R. A.: Correlations of fluoroscopically detected coronary artery calcification with exercise stress testing in asymptomatic men. Radiology *729*:1, 1978.
52. Stanford, W., Thompson, B. H., Weiss, R. M., and Galvin, J. R.: Coronary artery visualization using ultrafast computed tomography. Am. J. Card. Imaging *7*:243, 1993.
53. Bartel, A. G., Chen, J. T. T., Peter, R. H., et al.: The significance of coronary calcification detected by fluoroscopy: A report of 360 patients. Circulation *49*:1247, 1974.
54. Duerinckx, A. J., and Higgins, C. B.: Valvular heart disease. Radiol. Clin. North Am. *32*:613, 1994.
55. Bordlee, R. P.: Cardiac valve reconstruction and replacement: A brief review. Radiographics *12*:659, 1992.
56. Van der Jagt, E. J., and Smits, H. J.: Cardiac size in the supine chest film. Eur. J. Radiol. *14*:173, 1992.
57. Kabala, J. E., and Wilde, P.: Measurement of heart size in the anteroposterior chest radiograph. Br. J. Radiol. *60*:981, 1987.
58. Gammill, S. L., Krebs, C., Meyers, P., et al.: Cardiac measurements in systole and diastole. Radiology *94*:115, 1970.
59. Glover, L., Baxley, W. A., and Dodge, H. T.: A quantitative evaluation of heart size measurements from chest roentgenograms. Circulation *47*:1289, 1973.
60. Milne, E. N. C., Burnett, K., Aufrichtig, D., et al.: Assessment of cardiac size on portable chest films. J. Thorac. Imaging *3*:64, 1988.
61. Peerry, M. M., Irfan, A. Y., Simmons, S. P., et al.: Heart size in high-kilovoltage chest radiography. Clin. Radiol. *36*:335, 1985.
62. Righetti, A., Crawford, M. H., O'Rourke, R. A., et al.: Echocardiographic and roentgenographic determination of left ventricular size after coronary arterial bypass graft surgery. Chest *72*:455, 1977.
63. West, J. B.: Regional differences in gas exchange in the lung in erect man. J. Appl. Physiol. *17*:893, 1963.
64. Milne, E. N. C.: A physiological approach to reading critical care unit films. J. Thorac. Imaging *1*:60, 1986.
65. Chang, C. H.: The normal roentgenographic measurement of the right descending artery in 1085 cases. A.J.R. *87*:929, 1962.
66. Gutierrez, F. R., Moran, C. J., Ludbrook, P. A., et al.: Pulmonary arterial calcification with reversible pulmonary hypertension. A.J.R. *135*:177, 1980.
67. Harrison, M. O., Conte, P. J., and Heitzman, E. R.: Radiological detection of clinically occult cardiac failure following myocardial infarction. Br. J. Radiol. *44*:265, 1971.
68. Auger, W. R., Fedullo, P. F., Moser, K. M., et al.: Chronic major vessel thromboembolic pulmonary artery obstruction appearance at angiography. Radiology *182*:393, 1992.
69. Milne, E. N. C., Pistolesi, M., Miniati, M., et al.: The radiologic distinction of cardiogenic and noncardiogenic edema. A.J.R. *144*:879, 1985.
70. Chen, J. T. T., Behar, V. S., Morris, J. J., Jr., et al.: Correlation of roentgen findings with hemodynamic data in pure mitral stenosis. A.J.R. *102*:280, 1968.
71. Herman, P. C., Khan, A., Kallman, C. E., et al.: Limited correlation of left ventricular end-diastolic pressure with radiographic assessment of pulmonary hemodynamics. Radiology *174*:721, 1990.
72. Tanaka, F., Hayakawa, R., Satol, Y., et al.: Evaluating bronchial drainage in patients with lung disease using digital subtraction and angiography. Invest. Radiol. *28*:434, 1993.
73. Chen, J. T. T., Robinson, A. E., Goodrich, F. K., et al.: Uneven distribution of pulmonary blood flow between left and right lungs in isolated valvular pulmonary stenosis. A.J.R. *107*:343, 1969.
74. Grainger, R. G.: Interstitial pulmonary oedema and its radiological diagnosis. A sign of pulmonary venous and capillary hypertension. Br. J. Radiol. *31*:201, 1958.
75. Kerley, P. J.: Radiology in heart disease. Br. Med. J. *2*:594, 1933.
76. Milne, E. N. C., Pistolesi, M., Miniati, M., et al.: The vascular pedicle of the heart and the vena azygos. I: The normal subject. Radiology *152*:1, 1984.
77. Pistoles, M., Milne, E. N. C., Miniati, M., et al.: The vascular pedicle and the vena azygos. II: Acquired heart disease. Radiology *152*:9, 1984.

CARDIAC CALCIFICATION

78. Soulen, R. L., and Freeman, E.: Radiologic evaluation of traumatic heart disease. Radiol. Clin. North Am. *9*:285, 1971.
79. Lasser, A.: Calcification of the myocardium. Hum. Pathol. *14*:824, 1983.
80. Leonard, J. J., Katz, S., and Nelson, D.: Calcification of the left atrium: Its anatomic location, diagnostic significance, and roentgenologic demonstration. N. Engl. J. Med. *256*:629, 1957.
81. Matsuyama, S., Watabe, T., Kuribayashi, S., et al.: Plain film diagnosis of thrombosis of left atrial appendage in mitral valve disease. Radiology *146*:15, 1983.
82. Rodan, B. A., Chen, J. T. T., Halber, M. D., et al.: Chest roentgenographic evaluation of the severity of aortic stenosis. Invest. Radiol. *17*:453, 1982.
82a. Lippert, J. A., White, C. S., Mason, A. C., and Plotnick, G. D.: Calcification of aortic valve detected incidentally on CT scans: prevalence and clinical significance. A.J.R. *164*:73, 1995.
83. Pounder, D. J.: Calcification of the mitral annulus and its complications. Am. J. Forensic Med. Pathol. *3*:109, 1982.
84. Osterberger, L. E., Goldstein, S., Khaja, F., and Lakier, J. B.: Functional mitral stenosis in patients with massive annular calcification. Circulation *64*:472, 1981.
85. Spindola-Franco, H., and Fish, B. G.: Radiology of the Heart. New York, Springer-Verlag, 1985, p. 259.
86. Rogers, J. V., Chandler, N. W., and Franch, R. H.: Calcification of the tricuspid annulus. A.J.R. *106*:550, 1969.
87. Roberts, W. C., and Waller, B. F.: Mitral valve "anular" calcium forming a complete circle or "O" configuration. Clinical and necropsy observations. Am. Heart J. *101*:619, 1981.
88. Fulkerson, P. K., Beaver, B. M., Auseon, J. C., et al.: Calcification of the mitral annulus: Etiology, clinical associations, complications, and therapy. Am. J. Med. *66*:967, 1979.
89. Aldrich, R. F., Brensike, J. F., Battaglini, J. W., et al.: Coronary calcification in the detection of coronary artery disease and comparison with electrocardiographic exercise testing. Circulation *59*:113, 1979.
90. Stanford, W., Rooholamini, M., Rumberger, J., et al.: Evaluation of coronary bypass graft patency by ultrafast computed tomography. J. Thorac. Imaging *3*(2):52, 1988.
91. Stanford, W., Thompson, B. H., and Weiss, R. M.: Coronary artery calcification: Clinical significance and current methods of detection. A.J.R. *161*:1139, 1993.
92. Shemesh, J., Tenenbaum, A., Fisman, E. Z., et al.: Coronary calcium as a reliable tool for differentiating ischemic from nonischemic cardiomyopathy. Am. J. Cardiol. *77*:191, 1996.
93. Moore, E. H., Greenberg, R. W., Merrick, S. H., et al.: Coronary artery calcifications: Significance of incidental detection on CT scans. Radiology *172*:711, 1989.
94. Sharma, S., Rajani, M., and Talwar, K. K.: Angiographic morphology in

nonspecific aortoarteritis (Takayasu's arteritis). Cardiovasc. Intervent. Radiol. *15*:160, 1992.
95. Nomeir, A. M., Watts, L. E., Seagle, R., et al.: Intracardiac myxomas: Twenty-year echocardiographic experience with review of the literature. J. Am. Soc. Echocardiogr. *2*:139, 1989.
96. Pucillo, A. L., Schechter, A. G., Kay, R. H., et al.: Identification of calcified intracardiac lesions using gradient echo MR imaging. J. Comput. Assist. Tomogr. *14*:743, 1990.
96a. Masui, T., Takahashi, M., Miura, K., et al. Cardiac myxoma: Identification of intratumoral hemorrhage and calcification on MR images. A.J.R. *164*:850, 1995.
97. McComb, B. L., and Steiner, R. M.: Pericardial disease. *In* Goodman, L., and Putman, C. (eds.): Critical Care Imaging. 3rd. ed. Philadelphia, W.B. Saunders Co., 1992.
98. Moncada, R., Baker, M., Salinas, M., et al.: Diagnostic role of computed tomography in pericardial heart disease: Congenital defects, thickening, neoplasms and effusions. Am. Heart J. *103*:263, 1982.
99. Crawley, I. S.: Noninvasive diagnosis of pericardial disease. *In* Miller, D. D., Burns, R. J., Gill, J. B., Ruddy, T. D. (eds.): Clinical Cardiac Imaging. New York, McGraw-Hill, 1988, p. 521.
100. Doppman, J. L., Rienmuller, R., Lissner, J., et al.: Computed tomography in constrictive pericardial disease. J. Comput. Assist. Tomogr. *5*:1, 1981.

ACQUIRED HEART DISEASE

101. Braunwald, E., Morrow, A. G., Cornell, W. P., et al.: Idiopathic hypertrophic subaortic stenosis: Clinical, hemodynamic and angiographic manifestations. Am. J. Med. *29*:924, 1960.
102. Lipton, M. J.: Quantitation of cardiac function by cine CT. Radiol. Clin. North Am. *23*:613, 1985.
103. de Roos, A., Reichek, N., Axel, L., et al.: Cine MR imaging in aortic stenosis. J. Comput. Assist. Tomogr. *13*:421, 1989.
104. Utz, J. A., Herfkens, R. J., Heinsimer, J. A., et al.: Valvular regurgitation: Dynamic MR imaging. Radiology *168*:91, 1988.
105. Raphael, M. J.: Acquired valvular heart disease. *In* Grainger, R. G., and Allison, J. (eds.): Diagnostic Radiology. 2nd ed. London, Churchill Livingstone, 1992.
106. Follman, D. F.: Aortic regurgitation. Postgrad. Med. *93*:1, 1993.
107. Probst, P., Goldschlager, N., and Selzer, A.: Left atrial size and atrial fibrillation in mitral stenosis: Factors influencing their relationship. Circulation *48*:1282, 1973.
108. Green, C. E., Kelley, M. J., and Higgins, C. B.: Etiologic significance of enlargement of the left atrial appendage in adults. Radiology *142*:21, 1982.
109. Sharma, S., Kumar, M. V., Aggarwal, S., et al.: Chest radiographs are unreliable in predicting thrombi in the left atrium or its appendage in rheumatic mitral stenosis. Clin. Radiol. *43*:337, 1991.
110. Gurney, J. W., and Goodman, L. R.: Pulmonary edema localized to the right upper lobe accompanying mitral regurgitation. Radiology *171*:397, 1989.
111. Raphael, M. J., Steiner, R. E., and Raftery, E. B.: Acute mitral incompetence. Clin. Radiol. *18*:126, 1967.
112. Schnyder, P., Sarraj, A. M., Duvoisin, B. E., et al.: Pulmonary edema associated with mitral regurgitation. A.J.R. *161*:33, 1993.
113. Rubin, S. A., Hightower, C. W., and Flicker, S.: Giant right atrium after mitral valve replacement: Plain film findings in 15 patients. A.J.R. *149*:257, 1987.
114. Gal, R. A., Shalev, Y., and Schmidt, D. H.: Mitral regurgitation: Parameters that affect the correlation between Doppler echocardiography and contrast ventriculography. Int. J. Cardiol. *28*:87, 1990.
115. Higgins, C. B., and Lipton, M. J.: Radiography of acute myocardial infarction. Radiol. Clin. North Am. *18*:359, 1980.
116. Watanabe, A. M.: Ischemic heart disease. *In* Kelly, N. W. (ed.): Essentials of Internal Medicine. Philadelphia, J. B. Lippincott, 1994.
117. Revel, D., and Higgins, C. B.: Magnetic resonance imaging of ischemic heart disease. Radiol. Clin. North Am. *23*:719, 1985.
118. Björk, L.: Radiology in diagnosis of mitral valve prolapse. Ann. Radiol. *245*:327, 1981.
119. Oliva, P. B., Hammill, S. C., and Edwards, W. D.: Cardiac rupture, a clinically predictable complication of acute myocardial infarction: Report of 70 cases with clinicopathologic correlations. J. Am. Coll. Cardiol. *22*:720, 1993.
120. Topaz, O., DiSciascio, G., and Vetrovec, G. W.: Acute ventricular septal rupture: Perspectives on the current role of ventriculography and coronary arteriography and their implication for surgical repair. Am. Heart J. *120*:412, 1990.
121. Higgins, C. B., Lipton, M. J., Johnson, A. D., et al.: False aneurysms of the left ventricle. Radiology *127*:21, 1978.
122. Johnson, R. A., and Palacios, I.: Dilated cardiomyopathies of the adult. N. Engl. J. Med. *307*:1051, 1119, 1982.
123. Sardenelli, F., Molinari, G., Petillo, A., et al.: MRI in hypertrophic cardiomyopathy: Morphofunctional study. J. Comput. Assist. Tomogr. *17*:862, 1993.
124. Higgins, C. B., Byrd, B. F., III, and Stark, D.: Magnetic resonance imaging in hypertrophic cardiomyopathy. Am. J. Cardiol. *55*:1121, 1985.
125. Wojtowicz, J., Pawlak, B., Lehman, Z., et al.: Cardiac chambers and their walls in cardiomyopathies as evaluated with CT. Eur. J. Radiol. *4*:93, 1984.
126. Bisset, G. S., III, and Meyer, R. A.: Obstructive left heart lesions. Semin. Roentgenol. *20*:244, 1985.
127. Chiles, C., Adams, G. W., and Ravin, C. E.: Radiographic manifestations of cardiac sarcoid. A.J.R. *145*:711, 1985.

POSTOPERATIVE CARDIAC RADIOLOGY

128. Goodman, L. R.: Postoperative chest radiograph: II. Alterations after major intrathoracic surgery. A.J.R. *134*:803, 1980.
129. Tocino, I. M., Miller, M. H., and Fairfax, W. R.: Distribution of pneumothorax in the supine and semi-recumbent critically ill adult. A.J.R. *144*:901, 1985.
130. Katzberg, R. W., Whitehouse, G. H., and deWeese, J. A.: The early radiologic findings in the adult chest after cardiopulmonary bypass surgery. Cardiovasc. Radiol. *1*:205, 1978.
131. Henry, D. A., Jolles, H., Berberich, J. J., and Schmelzer, V.: The post-cardiac surgery chest radiograph: A clinically integrated approach. J. Thorac. Imaging *4*:20, 1989.
132. Harris, R. S.: The preoperative chest film in relation to postoperative management—some effects of different projection, posture and lung inflation. Br. J. Radiol. *53*:96, 1950.
133. Steiner, R. M., Tegtmeyer, C. J., Morse, D., et al.: Radiology of cardiac pacemakers. Radiographics *6*:373, 1986.
134. Goodman, L. R., Conrardy, P. A., Laing, F., et al.: Radiologic evaluation of endotracheal tube position. A.J.R. *127*:433, 1976.
135. Thorsen, M. K., and Goodman, L. R.: Extracardiac complications of cardiac surgery. Semin. Roentgenol. *23*:32, 1988.
136. Landay, M. J., Mootz, A. R., and Estrera, A. S.: Apparatus seen on chest radiographs after cardiac surgery in adults. Radiology *174*:477, 1990.
137. Dieden, J. D., Friloux, L. A., and Renner, J. W.: Pulmonary artery false aneurysms secondary to Swan-Ganz pulmonary artery catheters. A.J.R. *149*:901, 1987.
138. Ramsen, W. H., Coehn, A. T., and Blanshard, K. S.: Case report: Central venous catheter fracture due to compression between the clavicle and first rib. Clin. Radiol. *50*:59, 1995.
139. Anderson, M. H., Ward, D. E., Camm, A. J., and Wilson, A.: Radiological appearance of implantable defibrillator systems. Clin. Radiol. *50*:29, 1995.
140. Peng, M-J., Vargas, F. S., Cukier, A., et al.: Postoperative pleural changes after coronary revascularization. Chest *10*:32, 1992.
141. Wheeler, W. E., Rubis, L. J., and Jones, C. W.: Etiology and prevention of topical cardiac hypothermia-induced phrenic nerve injury and left lower lobe atelectasis during cardiac surgery. Chest *88*:680, 1985.
142. Kaminsky, M. E., Rodan, B. A., Osborne, D. R., et al.: Postpericardiotomy syndrome. A.J.R. *138*:503, 1982.
143. Ziter, F. M.: Major thoracic dehiscence: Radiographic considerations. Radiology *122*:587, 1977.
144. Josa, M., Siouffi, S. Y., Silverman, A. B., et al.: Pulmonary embolism after cardiac surgery. J. Am. Coll. Cardiol. *21*:990, 1993.
145. Moncada, R., Kotler, M. N., Churchill, R. J., et al.: Multimodality approach to pericardial imaging. *In* Kotler, M. N., and Steiner, R. M. (eds.): Cardiac Imaging: New Technologies and Clinical Applications. Philadelphia, F. A. Davis, 1986, p. 409.
146. Fyke, F. E., Tancredi, R. G., Shub, C., et al.: Detection of intrapericardial hematoma after open heart surgery: The role of echocardiography. J. Am Coll. Cardiol. *5*:1496, 1985.
147. Grossi, E. A., Esposito, R., Harris, L. J., et al.: Sternal wound infections and the use of internal mammary artery grafts. J. Thorac. Cardiovasc. Surg. *102*(3):342, 1991.
148. Goodwin, J. D.: Conventional CT of the aorta. J. Thorac. Imaging *5*:18, 1990.
149. Thorsen, M. K., Goodman, L. R., Sagel, S. S., et al.: Ascending aorta complications of cardiac surgery: CT evaluation. J. Comput. Assist. Tomogr. *10*:219, 1986.
150. Sullivan, K. L., Steiner, R. M., Smullens, S. N., et al.: Pseudoaneurysm of the ascending aorta following cardiac surgery. Chest *93*:138, 1988.
151. Gross, B. H., Shirazi, K. K., and Slater, A. D.: Differentiation of aortic and mitral valve prosthesis based on postoperative frontal chest radiographs. Radiology *149*:389, 1983.
152. Goodwin, J. D., Califf, R. M., Korobkin, M., et al.: Clinical value of coronary bypass graft evaluation with CT. A.J.R. *140*:649, 1983.
153. Sherry, C. S., and Harms, S. E.: MR imaging of pseudoaneurysms in aorticocoronary bypass graft. J. Comput. Assist. Tomogr. *13*(3):426, 1989.
154. White, R., Caputo, G., Mark, A., et al.: Coronary bypass graft patency: Noninvasive evaluation with MR imaging. Radiology *164*:681, 1987.
155. Henry, D. A., Corcoran, H. L., Lewis, T. D., et al.: Orthotopic cardiac transplantation: Evaluation with CT. Radiology *170*:343, 1988.
156. Florence, S. H., Hutton, L. C., McKenzie, F. N., et al.: Cardiac transplantation: Postoperative chest radiographs. J. Can. Assoc. Radiol. *39*:115, 1989.
157. Aherne, T., Tscholakoff, D., Finkbeiner, W., et al.: Magnetic resonance imaging of cardiac transplants: The evaluation of rejection of cardiac allografts with and without immunosuppression. Circulation *74*(1):145, 1986.
158. Griffith, J. P., Hardesty, R. L., Trento, A., et al.: Heart-lung transplantation: Lessons learned and future hopes. Ann. Thorac. Surg. *43*:6, 1987.
159. Bonser, R. S., Fragomeni, L. S. U., and Jamieson, S. W.: Heart-lung transplantation. Invest. Radiol. *24*:310, 1989.
160. Holland, S. A., Hutton, L. C., and McKenzie, F. N.: Radiologic findings in heart-lung transplantation: A preliminary experience. J. Can. Assoc. Radiol. *40*:94, 1989.
161. Martin, E. C., Stratford, M. A., and Gersony, W. M.: Initial detection of

coarctation of the aorta: An opportunity for the radiologist. A.J.R. *127*:1015, 1981.
162. Gross, G. W., and Steiner, R. M.: Radiologic manifestations of congenital heart disease in the adult patient. Radiol. Clin. North Am. *29*:293, 1991.
163. Perloff, J. K., and Child, J. S.: Congenital Heart Disease in Adults. Philadelphia, W. B. Saunders Co., 1991.
164. Perloff, J. K.: Congenital heart disease in the adult: Clinical approach. J. Thorac. Imaging *9*:260, 1994.
165. Greenberg, B., Balsara, R. K., and Faerber, E. N.: Coarctation of the aorta: Diagnostic imaging after corrective surgery. J. Thorac. Imaging *10*:36, 1995.
166. Chen, J. T. T., Khoury, M., and Kirks, D. R.: Obscured aortic arch on the lateral view as a sign of coarctation. Radiology *153*:595, 1984.
167. Woodring, J. H., and Rhodes, R. A.: Posterior superior mediastinal widening in aortic coarctation. A.J.R. *144*:23, 1985.
168. Gomes, A. S.: MR imaging of congenital anomalies of the thoracic aorta and pulmonary arteries. Radiol. Clin. North Am. *27*:1171, 1989.
169. Wexler, L., Higgins, C. B., and Herfkens, R. J.: Magnetic resonance imaging in adult congenital heart disease. J. Thorac. Imaging *9*:219, 1994.
170. Whittemore, R., Wells, J. A., and Castellsague, X.: A second-generation study of 427 probands with congenital heart disease and their 837 children. J. Am. Coll. Cardiol. *23*:1459, 1994.
171. Green, C. E., Gottdiener, J. S., and Goldstein, H. A.: Atrial septal defect. Semin. Roentgenol. *20*:214, 1985.
171a. Eichhorn, P., Vogt, P., Ritter, M., et al.: Malformations of the interatrial septum: Recognition, prevalence and clinical relevance in adults. Schweiz. Med. Wochenschr. *125*:1336, 1995.
172. Sanders, C., Bittner, V., Nath, P. H., et al.: Atrial septal defects in older adults: Atypical radiographic appearances. Radiology *167*:123, 1988.
173. Soto, B., Bergeron, L. M., Jr., and Dethlein, E.: Ventricular septal defect. Semin. Roentgenol. *20*:200, 1985.
174. Hoeffel, J. C., Dally, P., Legras, B., et al.: Roentgen aspects of isolated pulmonary valvular stenosis. Radiology *26*:248, 1986.
175. Guit, G. L., Kroon, H. M., Van Voorthuisen, A., et al.: Congenitally corrected transposition in adults with left atrioventricular valve incompetence. Radiology *155*:567, 1985.
176. Takasugi, J. E., Godwin, J. D., and Chen, J. T. T.: CT in congenitally corrected transposition of the great vessels. Comput. Radiol. *11*:215, 1987.
177. Soulen, R. L., Donner, R. M., and Capitanio, M.: Postoperative evaluation of complex congenital heart disease by magnetic resonance imaging. Radiographics *7*:975, 1987.
178. Greenberg, B., Faerber, E. N., and Balsara, R. K.: Tetralogy of Fallot: Diagnostic imaging after palliative and corrective surgery. J. Thorac. Imaging *10*:26, 1995.
179. Deutsch, V., Wexler, L., Blieden, L. C., et al.: Ebstein's anomaly of tricuspid valve: Critical review of roentgenological features and additional angiographic signs. A.J.R. *125*:395, 1985.
180. Mu-sheng, T., Partridge, J., and Radford, D.: The plain film chest radiograph in uncomplicated Ebstein's disease. Clin. Radiol. *37*:551, 1986.

THE PERICARDIUM

181. Levy-Ravetch, M., Auh, Y. H., Rubenstein, W. A., et al.: CT of the pericardial recesses. A.J.R. *144*:707, 1985.
182. Carsky, E. W., Mauceri, R. A., and Azimi, R.: The epicardial fat pad sign. Radiology *137*:303, 1980.
183. Steiner, R. M., and Rao, V. M.: Radiology of the pericardium. *In* Grainger, R. G., and Allison, J. (eds.): Diagnostic Radiology. London, Churchill Livingstone, 1991.
184. Olson, M. C., Posniak, H. V., McDonald, V., et al.: Computed tomography and magnetic resonance imaging of the pericardium. Radiographics *9*:633, 1989.
185. Miller, S. W.: Imaging pericardial disease. Radiol. Clin. North Am. *27*:1113, 1989.
186. Boxt, L. M., and Katz, J.: Effect of drugs on the radiographic appearance of the heart. J. Thorac. Imaging *6*(1):76, 1991.
187. Vaitkus, P. T., and Kussmaul, W. G.: Constrictive pericarditis versus restrictive cardomyopathy: A reappraisal and update of diagnostic criteria. Am. Heart J. *122*:1431, 1991.
188. Engel, P. J.: Echocardiography in pericardial disease. Cardiovasc. Clin. *13*(2):181, 1993.
189. Brown, J. J., Barakos, J. A., and Higgins, C. B.: Magnetic resonance imaging of cardiac and paracardiac masses. J. Thorac. Imaging *4*(2):58, 1989.
190. Sechtem, U., Tscholakoff, D., and Higgins, C. B.: MRI of the abnormal pericardium. A.J.R. *147*:245, 1986.
191. Sutton, F. J., Whitley, N. O., and Applefield, M. M.: The role of echocardiography and computed tomography in the evaluation of constrictive pericarditis. Am. Heart J. *109*:350, 1985.
191a. Protopapas, Z., and Westcott, J. L.: Left pulmonic recess of the pericardium: Findings at CT and MR imaging. Radiology *196*:85, 1995.
192. Gutierrez, F. R., Shackelford, G. D., McKnight, R. C., et al.: Diagnosis of congenital absence of left pericardium by MR imaging. J. Comput. Assist. Tomogr. *9*:551, 1985.
193. Decanay, S., Hsieh, A. M., Fitzgerald, S. W., et al.: Diagnosis of congenital absence of the left pericardium. Am. J. Card. Imaging *6*:267, 1992.
194. Vinee, P., Stover, B., Sigmund, G., et al.: MR imaging of the pericardial cyst. J. Magn. Reson. Imaging *2*:593, 1992.
195. Feigin, D. S., Fenoglio, J. J., McAllister, H. A., et al.: Pericardial cysts. A radiologic-pathologic correlation and review. Radiology *125*:15, 1977.
196. Ellis, K., Malm, J. R., Bowman, F. O., Jr., and King, D. L.: Roentgenographic findings after pericardial surgery. *9*:327, 1971.

Chapter 8
Coronary Arteriography

JOHN A. BITTL, DAVID C. LEVIN

Coronary arteriography is the imaging method of choice for establishing the presence or absence of coronary artery disease and for providing the most reliable information for making critical decisions about the need for medical therapy, angioplasty, or bypass surgery. First performed by Sones in 1959,[1] coronary arteriography has become one of the most widely performed and accurate tests in cardiovascular medicine. Almost one million coronary arteriograms are performed every year in the United States[2] in 1537 of the 6044 acute care hospitals (25 per cent).[3] The growing use of coronary arteriography over the past 35 years has increased the need for universal standards to ensure optimal utilization and performance of this procedure.[4] Although the original purpose of coronary arteriography was limited to defining the presence or absence of significant narrowings in the epicardial coronary arteries, newer interventional cardiovascular therapies have increased the importance of precise anatomical assessment of lesion characteristics before and after interventional cardiovascular procedures, thus placing greater demands on the angiographer for ensuring high-quality imaging with optimal spatial and contrast resolution. The physician performing coronary arteriography should thus be an expert in angiography and in cardiovascular medicine and must consult carefully with the referring physician before carrying out the procedure. The aims of this chapter are to provide the serious angiographer with a discussion of the indications and techniques of coronary arteriography with emphasis on interventional arteriography, to present a detailed review of normal and pathological coronary anatomy, and to highlight the relations between coronary arteriographic anatomy and clinical outcome.

INDICATIONS FOR CORONARY ARTERIOGRAPHY

The primary indications for coronary arteriography are to establish the presence or absence of coronary artery disease, define therapeutic options, and determine prognosis (see Table 63–6, p. 3012). Coronary arteriography is thus recommended for patients with a history of stable angina refractory to medical management. Patients with a history of angina and an exercise treadmill test showing high-risk features such as hypotension, more than 2 mm of ST-segment depression associated with decreased exercise capacity,[5] or myocardial perfusion scanning showing increased lung uptake or multiple perfusion defects ordinarily should undergo coronary arteriography.[6] Coronary arteriography is also recommended for middle-aged and older patients scheduled to undergo surgery for valvular heart disease or congenital heart disease. Patients with a history of angina or provocable ischemia who are scheduled for vascular surgery should undergo coronary arteriography.

Coronary arteriography is important in certain patients who present with chest pain of unclear etiology. In patients with cardiac risk factors and chest pain atypical for angina, the finding of angiographically normal coronary arteries provides important information about therapy and prognosis. The diagnosis of coronary artery spasm relies on the clinical presentation, but coronary arteriography remains useful in patients with clinical evidence of coronary spasm to exclude the presence of fixed atherosclerotic lesions (see p. 264). Provocative testing for coronary artery spasm with ergonovine has recently been reintroduced in the United States. Provocative testing with other agents such as acetylcholine is too sensitive, because coronary artery spasm can be provoked in almost all patients with coronary atherosclerosis.[7]

Patients with unstable angina often require urgent coronary arteriography (see p. 288). Recurrent symptoms after initial medical management are an indication of refractory unstable angina and should initiate the referral for urgent coronary arteriography. Coronary arteriography should be carried out in most patients judged to be at high risk for complications of unstable angina, including those with prolonged chest pain lasting more than 20 minutes, pulmonary edema, new mitral regurgitation, dynamic ST-segment changes, S_3 or rales, hypotension, impaired left ventricular function with an ejection fraction of less than 50 per cent, or significant ventricular arrhythmias or atrioventricular block.[8] The rationale for using coronary arteriography in patients with unstable angina is supported by the Thrombolysis in Myocardial Ischemia (TIMI) IIIB study.[9] Although major complications of death or myocardial infarction, or positive exercise tests occurred with similar frequencies in patients randomized to early coronary arteriography and in patients managed conservatively, fewer postdischarge procedures and hospitalizations were required in the patients who underwent early coronary arteriography (7.8 versus 14.1 per cent; $P < 0.001$).[9] Thus patients managed with early diagnostic coronary arteriography and revascularization techniques had greater relief of angina without increasing the risk of major complications. Coronary arteriography also should be carried out in most patients with unstable angina if they have had prior angioplasty or bypass surgery.

Coronary arteriography is performed increasingly in the setting of acute myocardial infarction without antecedent thrombolytic therapy as a prelude to direct angioplasty because of reports that direct angioplasty results in a greater reduction in the incidence of death or nonfatal reinfarction at 6 weeks as compared with thrombolytic therapy[10] (see p. 1221). Coronary arteriography is also performed increasingly as a prelude to "rescue" angioplasty in patients who have received thrombolytic therapy but show no evidence of reperfusion[11] (see p. 1221). Coronary arteriography should be performed in many patients with non-Q-wave myocardial infarction or when myocardial infarction is complicated by congestive heart failure, cardiac arrest, mitral regurgitation, or ventricular septal rupture. Patients with angina or provocable ischemia after myocardial infarction also benefit from coronary arteriography, because revascularization may reduce the high risk of reinfarction in this group of patients.[5]

Coronary arteriography is commonly performed annually in patients after cardiac transplantation in the absence of clinical symptoms because of the diffuse nature of graft atherosclerosis[12] (see p. 525). Coronary arteriography is useful in potential donors for cardiac transplantation whose age or cardiac risk profile increases the likelihood of coronary artery disease. Coronary arteriography often provides important diagnostic information about the presence of coronary artery disease in patients with intractable arrhythmias who are scheduled to undergo electrophysiological testing. Coronary arteriography is also useful for establishing the presence of coronary artery disease associated with ischemic cardiomyopathy in patients with dilated cardiomyopathy of unknown etiology. Patients with severe coronary artery disease and impaired left ventricular function may benefit from revascularization.

Contraindications to coronary arteriography include unexplained fever, untreated infection, severe anemia with hemoglobin less than 8 gm/dl, severe electrolyte imbalance, severe active bleeding, uncontrolled systemic hypertension, digitalis toxicity, previous contrast material allergy but no pretreatment with glucocorticoids, and active stroke. Risk factors for significant complications after catheterization include advanced age, as well as several general medical, vascular, and cardiac characteristics (Table 8–1). Patients with these characteristics should be monitored closely after coronary arteriography for a minimum of 18 to 24 hours.

TABLE 8–1 PATIENTS AT INCREASED RISK FOR COMPLICATIONS AFTER CORONARY ARTERIOGRAPHY

INCREASED GENERAL MEDICAL RISK
Age >70 years
Complex congenital heart disease
Morbid obesity
General debility or cachexia
Uncontrolled glucose intolerance
Arterial oxygen desaturation
Severe chronic obstructive lung disease
Renal insufficiency with creatinine greater than 1.5 mg/dl
INCREASED CARDIAC RISK
Three-vessel coronary artery disease
Left main coronary artery disease
Functional class IV
Significant mitral or aortic valve disease or mechanical prosthesis
Low ejection fraction less than 35 per cent
High-risk exercise treadmill test results (hypotension or severe ischemia)
Pulmonary hypertension
Pulmonary artery wedge pressure greater than 25 mm Hg
INCREASED VASCULAR RISK
Anticoagulation or bleeding diathesis
Uncontrolled systemic hypertension
Severe peripheral vascular disease
Recent stroke
Severe aortic insufficiency

PREPARATION OF THE PATIENT

The optimal timing of coronary arteriography is one of the most important features of the diagnostic management of patients with coronary artery disease. The study should be performed at a time when problems such as congestive heart failure, renal failure, or mental status changes are stable or improving. Otherwise, the risk of complications increases. Under many circumstances, however, coronary arteriography must be performed under emergency conditions with increased risk of complications. The study should be performed after careful consultation between the referring physician and the angiographer so that all important information can be obtained from the procedure. Under all circumstances, the physician performing the study must review the history, physical examination, and laboratory data and then obtain informed consent from the patient after describing the procedure and explaining its benefits and potential complications.

A baseline electrocardiogram, measurement of serum electrolytes and creatinine, complete blood count, and coagulation parameters must be obtained and reviewed, ideally within 24 hours before the procedure. All cardiac medications, including aspirin, should be continued before the procedure. Warfarin sodium should be discontinued 2 days before elective coronary arteriography is performed. Elective studies can be undertaken safely when the international normalized ratio (INR) is less than 2.0. For patients at increased risk for systemic thromboembolism upon withdrawal of warfarin sodium, such as those with atrial fibrillation and mitral stenosis or those with a prior history of systemic thromboembolism, admission to the hospital 1 day before the procedure for full heparinization is necessary.

Coronary arteriography is often performed along with other invasive procedures such as right-heart catheterization or left ventriculography at the time of cardiac catheterization. The sequence of procedures depends on priority. For patients in whom the diagnosis or treatment of coronary artery disease is the primary indication for cardiac catheterization, coronary arteriography should be performed before left ventriculography. For patients with valvular or congenital heart disease, on the other hand, hemodynamic measurements, oximetric determinations, and left ventriculography or aortography should be performed before coronary arteriography.

TECHNIQUE OF CORONARY ARTERIOGRAPHY

Equipment for Coronary Arteriography

JUDKINS CATHETERS. The Judkins catheters are shaped specifically to aid entry into the coronary ostia (Fig. 8–1). The catheters are constructed of polyethylene or polyurethane with a fine wire braid within the wall to allow advancement and directional control (torque ability) and yet prevent kinking. The size of the catheters ranges from No. 4 French (4F) to 8F (each French number = 0.33 mm in diameter), but 6F catheters are used most commonly. Diagnostic catheter dimensions are given by the outer diameter. Most diagnostic catheters have a 0.45-inch inner lumen diameter.

The shape or configuration of the catheters varies (Fig. 8–2). Selection of catheter shape is based on the body habitus of the patient and size of the aortic root. Whereas the left coronary artery is easily intubated with the Judkins left

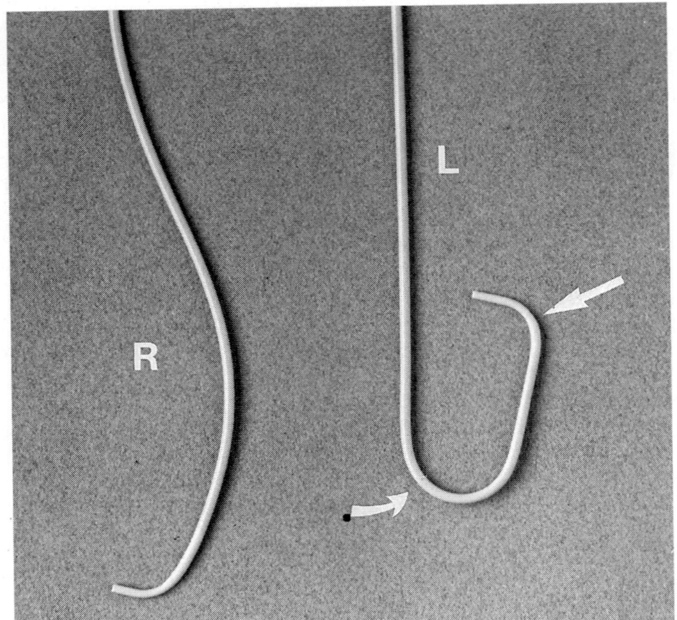

FIGURE 8–1. Judkins catheters. The right (R) and left (L) Judkins are shown. The primary (straight arrow) and secondary (curved arrow) curves of the left Judkins catheter are shown. (Photograph courtesy of Cordis Corporation.)

4.0 catheter in most patients, patients with a dilated ascending aorta (e.g., in the setting of congenital aortic stenosis and poststenotic dilatation) may require the use of a Judkins left 5.0 or 6.0 catheter, and the patient with an ascending aortic aneurysm may require catheterization with shapes modified by use of a sterile metal guide and steam to achieve a Judkins left 7.0 to 10.0 shape. Use of a Judkins shape that is too small for the ascending aorta often leads to folding or re-forming of the catheter. The best technique for removing a re-formed Judkins left catheter from the body involves withdrawing the reshaped catheter into the descending aorta and advancing a guidewire anterograde in the contralateral common iliac artery. Upon withdrawal of the catheter and guidewire together, the catheter will straighten and can be removed safely from the body without disrupting the arterial access site.

AMPLATZ CATHETERS. Amplatz catheters[13] can be used for the femoral or brachial approach to coronary arteriography (Fig. 8–3). Although the Amplatz catheters are used less commonly than the Judkins catheters, they are an excellent alternative in cases in which the Judkins catheter is not appropriately shaped to enter the coronary arteries.

MULTIPURPOSE CATHETERS. A single catheter that can be used for selective left and right coronary arteriography, as well as for left ventriculography, via the femoral approach was originally described by Schoonmaker and King.[14] The catheter shape is similar to that of the Sones catheter, but the tip is shorter (Fig. 8–4). The maneuvers required are also similar to those for the Sones catheter via the brachial approach.

MANIFOLD. The coronary catheter is attached to a three-way manifold, which enables the angiographer to switch among pressure measurement, saline flushing, and contrast injection all in a closed system that allows for speed and maintenance of sterility. In addition to the three side ports, the manifold has a rotating adapter for attachment to the catheter itself, while the other end has a locking fitting to which a fingertip-control syringe is attached for contrast or saline injection.

FEMORAL SHEATH. The Judkins catheters are usually inserted into the femoral artery through a side arm sheath (Fig. 8–5). The sheath is inserted into the femoral artery over a polyethylene dilator, which has been advanced over a guidewire previously inserted in the femoral artery through the entry needle. The sheath is constructed of Teflon and contains a hemostatic valve at its external end. It

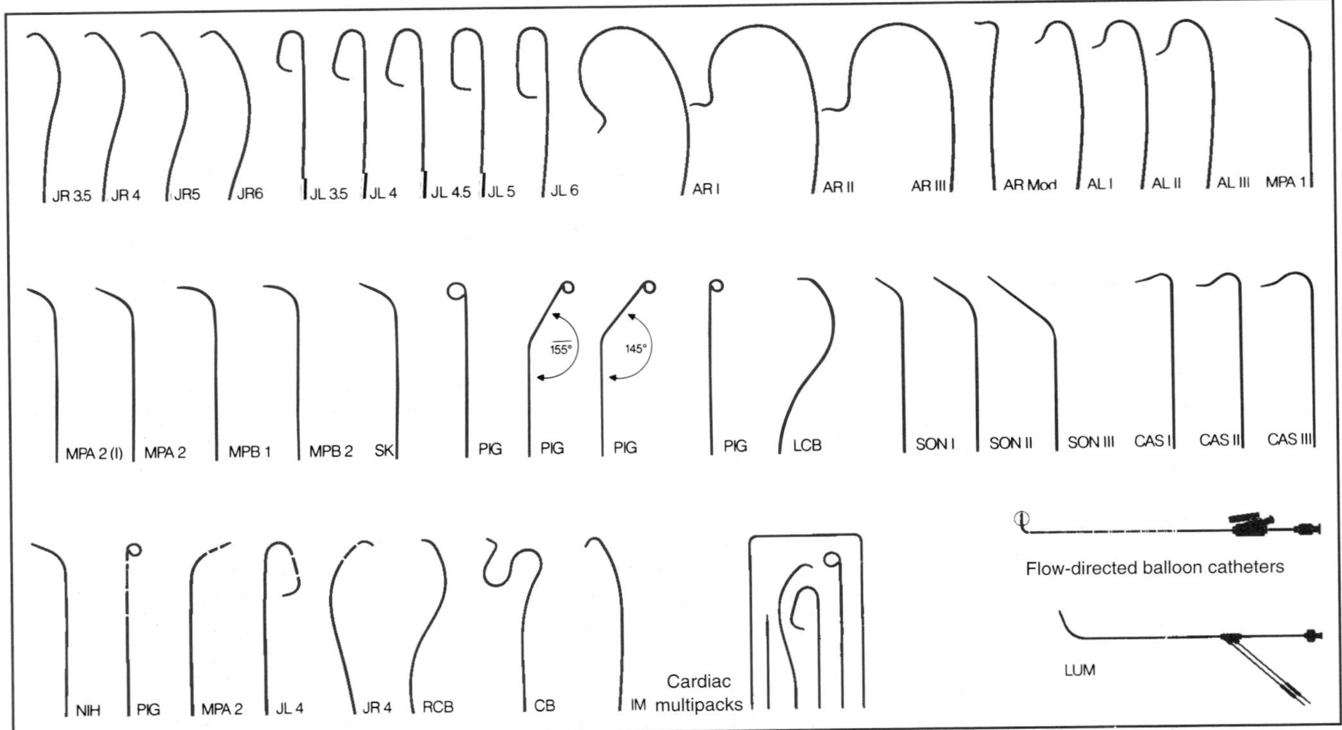

FIGURE 8–2. Coronary catheters. The tip configurations for several catheters useful in coronary arteriography are shown. JR = Judkins right; JL = Judkins left; AR = Amplatz right; Mod = modified; AL = Amplatz left; MP = multipurpose; PIG = pigtail; LCB = left coronary bypass graft; SON = Sones; CAS = Castillo; NIH = National Institutes of Health; RCB = right coronary bypass graft; CB = coronary bypass catheter; IM = internal mammary; LUM = lumen. (Photograph courtesy of Cordis Corporation.)

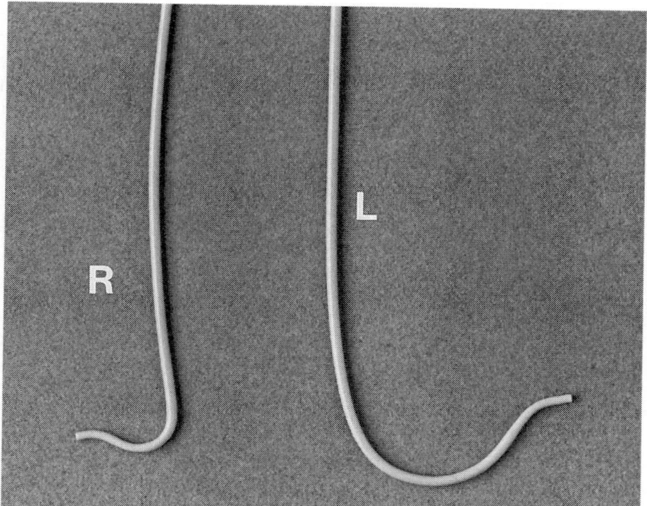

FIGURE 8–3. Amplatz catheters. The right (R) and left (L) Amplatz catheters are shown. (Photograph courtesy of Cordis Corporation.)

also has a side arm through which femoral artery pressure can be measured. The advantage of the sheath is that it permits multiple catheter exchanges without femoral site compression. The inner diameter of the sheath must permit easy passage of the diagnostic catheter, so the outer diameter of the sheath is approximately 1.5F larger than the sheath itself (i.e., a 6F sheath has an outer diameter of approximately 7.5F). Although the sheath requires a larger arteriotomy, the protection provided by the sheath minimizes arterial injury from multiple catheter exchanges and manipulations and reduces patient discomfort from manual compression during catheter exchange.

After the procedure, the sheath can be removed if the patient has not been treated with heparin. Compression of the femoral puncture site manually or with a compression device usually results in stable hemostasis after 20 minutes. Patients can sit up approximately 6 to 8 hours after coronary arteriography if no hematoma or bleeding has developed at the puncture site.

GUIDEWIRES. The standard guidewire for coronary arteriography is the 180-cm, 0.035-inch diameter, Teflon-coated guidewire with a 3-mm J-tip. The J configuration allows the guidewire to be advanced atraumatically through most iliac and brachial arteries. Occasionally, a 0.15-mm J-tip is required for advancement through small brachial arteries. In the presence of atherosclerotic disease in the iliac or subclavian arteries, other wire configurations such as those containing either a 15-mm J-tip, a long floppy distal segment, or a hydrophilic coating are required for successful passage.

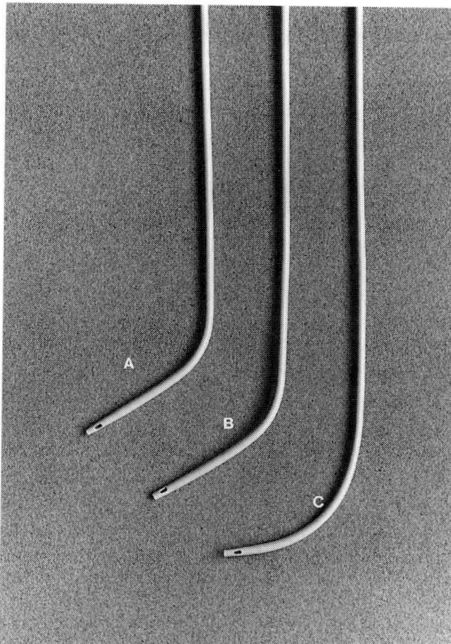

FIGURE 8–4. Multipurpose catheters. The multipurpose A, B, and C type catheters are shown. (Photograph courtesy of Cordis Corporation.)

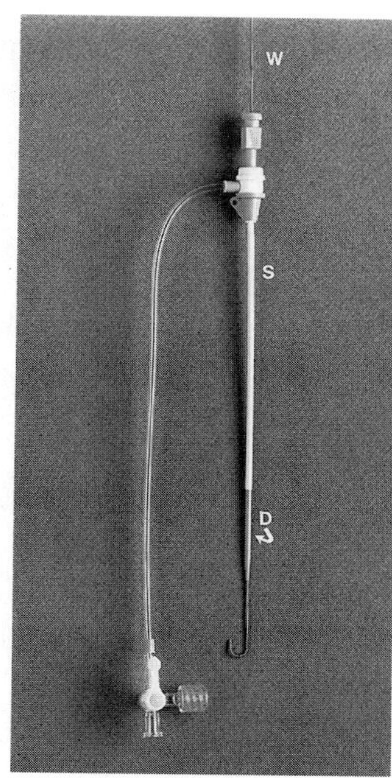

FIGURE 8–5. Side arm sheath. The side arm sheath (S) consists of a dilator (D) for entry into the artery over a guidewire (W). (Photograph courtesy of Cordis Corporation.)

Catheterization of the Coronary Arteries

FEMORAL APPROACH. A combination of physical and radiographic landmarks is used to identify the common femoral artery for arterial puncture. The common femoral artery should be punctured several centimeters below the inguinal ligament at the point of maximal impulse by palpation (Fig. 6–3, p. 183). This is usually located approximately 1 to 2 cm below the inguinal crease, which has a variable relation with the inguinal ligament. To confirm the location of the common femoral artery, the radiographic landmark of the femoral head is very useful. With 1 to 2 seconds of fluoroscopy, the course of the common femoral artery across the junction between the middle and medial thirds of the femoral head can be ascertained. If the puncture site is proximal to the inguinal ligament, hemostasis after the procedure may be impossible to achieve with manual compression, and retroperitoneal hemorrhage may ensue. If the puncture site is at the bifurcation of the common femoral artery, a pseudoaneurysm may appear.

After infiltration of the skin, subcutaneous tissue, and perivascular space surrounding and deep to the common femoral artery with 1 per cent lidocaine, the common femoral artery is entered either upon withdrawal of the Seldinger needle (Fig. 6–6, p. 185) or advancement of an 18-gauge thin-walled needle puncturing only the anterior wall of the artery. The guidewire is then passed through the needle into the aorta. The needle is removed over the guidewire, and the sheath and its dilator are advanced into the vessel with slight rotating motion and firm axial support to prevent buckling. Once the sheath is positioned correctly in the artery, the guidewire and dilator are quickly removed, and the side arm is connected to a two-

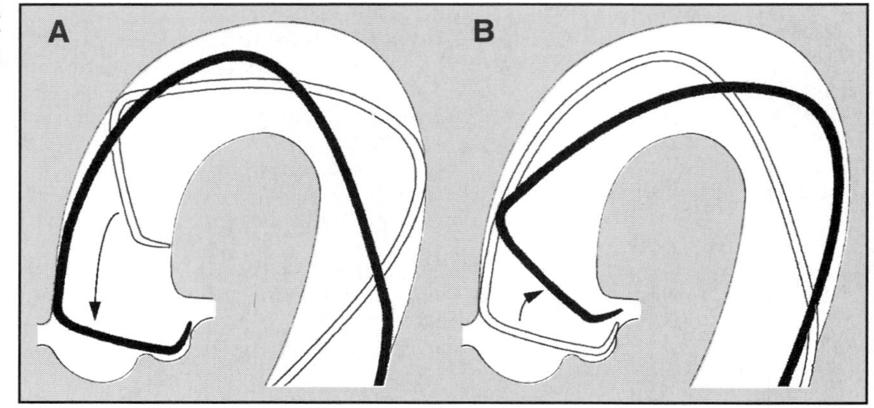

FIGURE 8–6. The push-pull technique for catheterizing the left coronary artery with the Judkins left catheter. In the left anterior oblique view, the coronary catheter is positioned in the ascending aorta over a guidewire, and the guidewire is removed. The catheter is advanced so that the tip enters the left sinus of Valsalva. If the catheter does not selectively enter the ostium of the left coronary artery, further slow advancement forces the tip deep into the left sinus of Valsalva and imparts a temporary acute angle at the catheter tip *(A)*. Prompt withdrawal of the catheter over a short distance allows easy entry into the ostium of the left coronary artery *(B)*.

way manifold for pressure monitoring and flushing of the system with saline.

The guidewire is then loaded into the Judkins coronary catheter so that the flexible tip of the wire protrudes beyond the tip of the catheter. The guidewire is barely retracted into the catheter, and both are inserted together through the femoral sheath. The guidewire is then advanced from the femoral sheath into the aorta under fluoroscopic guidance, and both the guidewire and catheter are advanced together to the ascending aorta. After the guidewire has been advanced to the aortic valve, its position is fixed while the catheter tip is advanced to a position approximately 10 cm above the aortic valve in the ascending aorta. The guidewire is removed, blood is aspirated from the catheter and discarded, and the catheter is connected to the three-way manifold and flushed with saline to remove all traces of blood or air bubbles.

To catheterize either coronary artery, the angiographer should position the image intensifier so that the patient's heart is viewed in the left anterior oblique (LAO) view. Viewed in this position, the left main coronary artery (LMCA) originates from the left sinus of Valsalva, while the right coronary artery (RCA) originates from the right side of the aorta (Fig. 8–6). From a true anatomical point of view, the LMCA originates from the left posterolateral aspect of the aorta, while the RCA originates from its anterior part inferior to the origin of the LMCA (for abbreviations, see Table 8–2).

Other Approaches to Coronary Arteriography

BRACHIAL TECHNIQUE

The brachial artery can be approached by cutdown with blunt dissection or by percutaneous entry. If cutdown is used, the brachial pulsation is identified 1 cm proximal to the antecubital crease, and the skin, subcutaneous tissue, and perivascular tissue are infiltrated carefully with 1 per cent lidocaine to avoid injection of the median nerve or brachial artery itself. The artery is identified, isolated with Silastic tubing, and entered after a small transverse nick is made with a No. 11 blade. A sheath can be inserted into the artery to prevent injury to the vessel during catheter manipulation or exchanges, or the procedure can be carried out without a sheath.

The technique most commonly used from the right brachial artery involves use of the Sones catheter, the multipurpose catheter, or preformed Amplatz catheters. From the left brachial artery, preformed Judkins catheters can be used. The Sones and the multipurpose catheters have an end hole and two to four small side holes near the catheter tip (Fig. 8–4). The multipurpose catheter forms an open loop on the right aortic cusp so that the shaft of the catheter and its tip form a 45-degree angle directed toward the left aortic cusp. Rapid advancement and withdrawal of the catheter will permit entry into the left sinus of Valsalva, and slow advancement with gentle catheter rotation will permit selective engagement of the left coronary ostium.

In some cases, slight withdrawal of the catheter results in deep engagement of the left main coronary artery, which can be detected by observing catheter advancement and the presence of an abnormal pressure recording at the tip of the catheter, and by practicing deep intubation during test injections with small amounts of contrast medium. If deep engagement is detected, the catheter should be withdrawn, and selective arteriography of the left coronary artery may be performed. After left coronary arteriography, the catheter tip is withdrawn into the left sinus of Valsalva. A slightly smaller open loop is formed, and the catheter is rotated clockwise to enter the right sinus of Valsalva anteriorly. Advancement and further rotation will allow the catheter to enter the right coronary artery.

Catheterization of bypass grafts via the brachial artery is straightforward and involves the same catheters used for the femoral approach. Catheterization of the internal mammary artery, however, is most easily performed from the ipsilateral brachial artery. Contralateral catheterization of the left internal mammary artery from the right brachial artery is technically more challenging and may require the use of an H1H or "headhunter" catheter for selective entry into the left subclavian artery.

RADIAL TECHNIQUE. Coronary arteriography can be performed via the radial artery with 5F and 6F catheters in adults. Before the procedure is performed, the Allen test should be carried out to ensure that the ulnar artery is patent.

TABLE 8–2 ABBREVIATIONS

ABBREVIATION	DEFINITION
Vessels	
LCA	Left coronary artery
LMCA	Left main coronary artery
LAD	Left anterior descending artery
LCx	Left circumflex coronary artery
RCA	Right coronary artery
IMA	Internal mammary artery
SVG	Saphenous vein bypass graft
Angiographic projections	
LAO	Left anterior oblique
AP	Anteroposterior
RAO	Right anterior oblique

Drugs Used During Coronary Arteriography

Adequate *premedication* of the patient is important for safe and comfortable coronary arteriography. The goal of premedication is to achieve a state of *conscious sedation*, defined as a "minimally depressed level of consciousness that allows a patient to respond appropriately to verbal commands and to maintain a patent airway."[15] The minimum number of personnel required to evaluate the patient during conscious sedation is two: the cardiologist performing the procedure and a clinical monitor trained to evaluate appropriate physiological variables and to provide support if resuscitation is required. Several different sedation regimens are recommended, but most involve the use of diazepam in doses of 2.5 to 10 mg orally and diphenhydramine in doses of 25 to 50 mg orally 1 hour before the procedure. For the elderly or frail patient, one or both premedications may be used in lower doses or skipped altogether. During the procedure, midazolam in doses of 1 to 2 mg can be given intravenously, but respiratory failure and arrest have been reported, especially when this agent is administered concurrently with a narcotic.[16] If midazolam is not used, conscious sedation may be achieved safely with the combination of fentanyl 25 μg and promethazine 12.5 mg, both given intravenously and repeated if necessary.

HEPARIN. The need for *heparin* for coronary arteriography performed via the femoral artery is controversial. Data from the Coronary Artery Surgery Study (CASS) Registry suggested that this was not beneficial.[17] For patients at increased risk for thromboembolic complications, however, 5000 units of heparin should be administered after the catheters have entered the central circulation. Patients at increased risk for thromboembolic complications include those who have severe, progressive peripheral arterial disease, arterial atheroembolic disease, or a need for prolonged use of guidewires in the central circulation for catheterization of the internal mammary arteries, bypass grafts, or the stenotic aortic valve. For catheter manipulation in the central circulation not requiring guidewires, frequent flushing of the catheter with contrast medium or heparinized saline approximately every 30 to 60 seconds avoids the formation of microthrombi within the catheter tip and reduces the risk of thromboembolism. It should be emphasized that prolonged use of guidewires in the central circulation (greater than 1 minute of uninterrupted guidewire use) should be accompanied by systemic anticoagulation with approximately 5000 units of heparin administered intravenously to reduce the risk of systemic thromboembolism. After heparin has been administered, guidewires should not remain in the central circulation for more than 2 minutes without removal and catheter flushing. For patients undergoing cardiac catheterization and coronary arteriography via the brachial or radial artery, 5000 units of heparin is administered before the arteriotomy is performed.

After the procedure, the anticoagulant effect of heparin can be reversed with *protamine,* in a dose of approximately 1 mg for every 100 units of heparin. It should be noted, however, that the use of protamine is associated with a risk of anaphylaxis or serious hypotensive episodes in approximately 2 per cent of patients. The risk of protamine reactions is increased in patients with prior exposure to neutral protamine H (NPH) insulin. Thus, protamine should not be administered to patients with prior exposure to NPH insulin. Protamine should not be used in patients with a history of unstable angina, those with high-risk coronary anatomy such as left main coronary artery disease, or those who have undergone coronary arteriography via the brachial or radial artery. If heparin is not reversed with protamine, femoral sheaths can be removed after the anticoagulant effect of heparin has dissipated, as evidenced by an activated clotting time of less than 180 seconds.

Although *atropine* frequently was recommended in the past to prevent vagal reactions and heart rate slowing during radiographic contrast injection, skillful technique and selective use of radiographic contrast agents have decreased the consequences of heart rate slowing during coronary arteriography. Atropine is used now only for circumstances of persistent bradycardia and hypotension and is not recommended as a prophylactic agent because of the risk of exacerbating unstable angina in patients with severe coronary disease.

Nitroglycerin diminishes the tone of the epicardial coronary arteries. For patients with adequate blood pressure greater than 100 mm Hg, this drug can be administered at a dose of 0.4 mg sublingually, 50 to 200 μg intracoronary, or 25 μg/min in a constant intravenous infusion.

Beta blockers frequently are required during coronary arteriography in patients with unstable angina and severe coronary artery disease. For patients with heart rates greater than 80 beats per minute and no contraindication to beta blockers such as bronchospastic disease or left ventricular dysfunction, an agent such as metoprolol can be administered in a dose of 5 mg intravenously over 1 minute.

Prednisone in a dose of 60 mg should be administered approximately 12 hours before coronary arteriography in any patient with a history of contrast allergy.[18]

Mechanical ventilation before coronary arteriography is required for all patients with respiratory failure, refractory pulmonary edema, or inability to protect the airway.

Intraaortic balloon counterpulsation is a useful adjunct for performing coronary arteriography in patients with cardiogenic shock or refractory pulmonary edema. The capability for this treatment must exist in any laboratory performing coronary arteriography.

Support equipment for coronary arteriography includes hemodynamic and electrocardiographic monitoring, oxygen and suction ports, general anesthesia cart, intraaortic balloon console, resuscitation cart, activated clotting time analyzer, blood gas analyzer or hemoglobin-oxygen saturation analyzer, and close proximity of Doppler echocardiography capability and expertise.

Continuous electrocardiographic, pressure, and oximetric monitoring is required for the safe performance of coronary arteriography.[4] Electrocardiographic monitoring involves the continuous display of standard limb lead I or II. Physiological measurements of blood pressure must be calibrated against a mercury manometer in every case. Transcutaneous monitoring of arterial hemoglobin-oxygen saturation with pulse oximetry should be used to ensure adequate oxygenation.

RADIOGRAPHIC CONTRAST AGENTS. These agents may produce a number of adverse hemodynamic, electrophysiological, and renal effects consequent to coronary arteriography. The monomeric ionic contrast agents that have been used in coronary arteriography for many years are high-osmolar methylglucamine and sodium salts of diatrizoic acid. These substances dissociate into cations and iodine-containing anions,[19] resulting in aqueous solutions of 1940 mOsmol/kg, as compared with the osmolality of human plasma of 300 mOsmol/kg. The hypertonicity of these compounds produces sinus bradycardia, heart block, Q-T interval and QRS prolongation, ST-segment depression, giant T-wave inversion, decreased left ventricular contractility, decreased systolic pressure, and increased left ventricular end-diastolic pressure. One cause of these hemodynamic and electrocardiographic effects is the presence of calcium-chelating properties of some of these agents. If the contrast agents are injected into a damped coronary catheter with ventricular pressure tracing or given too rapidly in too great a volume (e.g., more than approximately 5 ml for opacification of the right coronary artery), ventricular tachycardia or fibrillation may ensue.

Non-ionic agents such as iohexol and iopamidol also are available. Because they go into solution as single neutral molecules, their osmolality is substantially reduced (<850 mOsmol/kg). They also do not contain calcium-chelating agents. The standard ionic contrast agents have an inhibitory effect on clot formation when mixed with blood, whereas non-ionic agents exhibit less of this inhibitory effect. Because contrast agents and blood are in direct contact in syringes and tubing for varying time intervals during arteriography, clots are more likely to form when non-ionic agents are used. Serious thromboembolic complications have been reported anecdotally. The risk of such complications may be reduced, however, with careful attention to catheter technique.

The low-osmolality ionic dimer methylglucamine–sodium ioxaglate is another alternative to the high-osmolar agents. Ioxaglate retains most of the anticoagulant properties of diatrizoate sodium[20–22] and may have advantages in the unstable patient with hemodynamic compromise.

Radiographic contrast agents can lead to worsening azotemia. Patients with preexisting renal impairment or diabetes mellitus are at increased risk for developing radiocontrast-induced renal failure.[23] Other risk factors for radiocontrast-induced renal failure include advanced age, intravascular volume depletion, congestive heart failure, and the volume of contrast media administered.[24] In patients with renal insufficiency who undergo coronary arteriography, hydration with intravenous saline provides better protection against radiocontrast-induced renal failure than does mannitol or furosemide.[25]

Contrast agents produce several syndromes characterized as allergic. The incidence of anaphylaxis (bronchospasm, angioedema, urticaria, and hypotension) is approximately 0.15 per cent in individuals given intraarterial contrast agents.[24] In patients with a prior allergic reaction, pretreatment with steroids 12 and 2 hours before repeat challenge reduced the likelihood of allergic reaction.[18]

STANDARD VERSUS LOW-OSMOLAR AGENTS. The major drawback of the low-osmolar, low-ionic and non-ionic contrast agents is their 20-fold increase in cost relative to ionic agents. Although some laboratories routinely use low-osmolar agents, it appears that most have avoided doing so because of the associated high costs and lack of clear benefit. A rational and cost-effective policy is to use the standard ionic agents for most elective procedures. The use of low-osmolar, low-ionic, or non-ionic agents should be reserved for patients with resting heart rates of less than 55 to 60 beats per minute, unstable angina, acute myocardial infarction, renal failure, age older than 65 to 70, congestive heart failure, or a previous reaction to contrast agents. When ionic agents are selected, additional precautions are needed to avoid complications. Patients should be "coached" about coughing before the first selective coronary arteriogram is performed, and use of the minimal amount of contrast agent to fill the entire coronary artery for two cardiac cycles and allow brief reflux of contrast into the aortic root is needed. Often, only 4 to 5 ml of contrast agent for the left coronary artery and 1 to 2 ml for the right coronary artery is needed for optimal yet safe selective coronary arteriography.

Cineangiographic Equipment

ANGIOGRAPHIC EQUIPMENT. Cineangiographic equipment is composed of several components (Fig. 8–7): (1) An x-ray generator with an output of 80 to 100 kW with the potential applied preferably by a technique known as "secondary switching" is used in order to reduce preexposure and postexposure radiation release from stored radiation in the capacitance of high-voltage cables. A cine pulse system with exposure settings in the range of 5 to 8 msec is needed to optimize image quality. Longer exposures are associated with motion artifact, whereas shorter exposures may require increased voltage, which results in decreased image resolution. Automatic exposure control sets the brightness level of the image intensifier by varying voltage, current, and exposure duration. (2) An x-ray tube for the conversion of electrical energy to x-radiation is usually mounted in a **C**-arm configuration for multiaxial projection. Radiographic carbon fiber grids are commonly used to improve contrast by decreasing the scatter of radiation. (3) A dual- or triple-mode cesium iodide image intensifier with a resolution capability of approximately 5 line pairs per millimeter, a contrast ratio of greater than 15:1, and a conversion factor of greater than 50 for the small mode is recommended for coronary arteriography. The intensifier should have at least two modes, the large mode approximating 9 inches to be able to image large ventricles and a small mode (magnified mode) of 6 inches or less. (4) An optical system consisting of an objective lens, an image-distributing mirror, and a cine camera lens should be engineered to maximize image quality. The focal length of the camera lens should allow the proper degree of overframing. A diaphragm should be interposed in front of the cine camera lens, and ideally, the entire system should be set up so that the lens can operate at two f-stops above maximum aperture. (5) A cine camera capable of operating at either 30 or 60 frames per second with low vibration levels is required to record coronary arteriography with the optimal recording medium. (6) Cinefilm with a speed and average gradient appropriate for the system should be chosen carefully. (7) A cinefilm processor should be selected that can maintain highly stable developer temperature and immersion time; it also must provide adequate replenishment of chemical solutions, proper agitation, and recirculation. (8) A television system must be used that has excellent image clarity and minimal lag. A high-quality television camera and 525- or 1023-line monitor with a signal/noise ratio of at least 45 dB are suggested.[4] The 1023-line television system results in reduced raster line artifact.

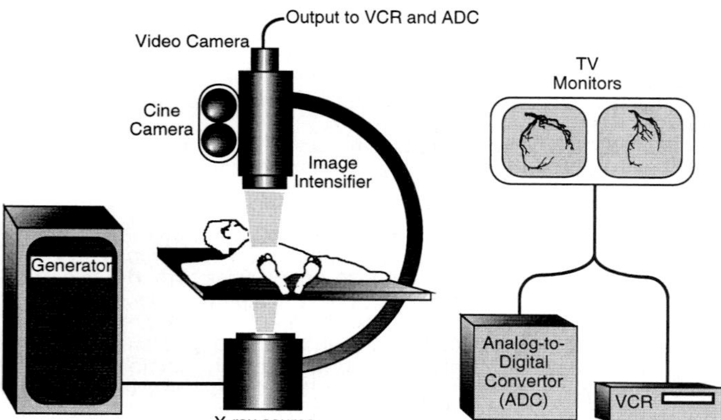

FIGURE 8–7. Cineangiographic equipment. The major components include a generator, x-ray tube, image intensifier attached to a positioner such as a C-arm, optical system, cine camera, video camera, videocassette recorder (VCR), analog-to-digital convertor, and television monitors. The x-ray tube is the source of the x-ray beam, which passes superiorly through the patient.

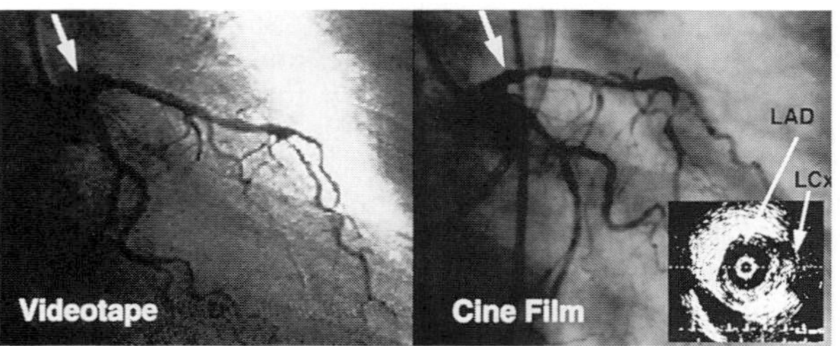

FIGURE 8–8. Comparison of analog videotape with 35-mm cinefilm. Nearly simultaneous recordings of the left coronary artery of an 82-year-old patient were made with both analog videotape and 35-mm cinefilm. Although both images were transferred using identical image-processing parameters such as line resolution, gray-scale range, and gamma curves, the videotape image has significant degradation in image quality as compared with cinefilm. An artifact representing a possible stenosis at the origin of the left anterior descending artery (*A*, arrow) was found to be a minor stenosis on cinefilm (*B*, arrow) and confirmed by intravascular ultrasound (*inset*).

IMAGE RECORDING AND STORAGE

The medium of choice for recording and storage of coronary arteriograms is 35-mm cinefilm. Despite its relative expense, 35-mm cinefilm currently meets the desirable criteria of exchangeability, adherence to a standard format, high quality of resolution, a permanent record format, and suitability for quantitative analysis. So long as quality control in film development is adequate, no other recording medium can compete with the spatial resolution or the dynamic contrast range of 35-mm cinefilm. Optimal radiographic imaging is crucial to the success of coronary arteriography. Under ideal circumstances, modern radiographic imaging techniques provide spatial resolution of 5 line pairs per millimeter, a level of resolution that must be considered of borderline adequacy for imaging coronary vessels as small as 1 mm.

Despite being the industry standard, use of 35-mm cinefilm has certain drawbacks, including high cost, delay in access, and inability for processing of data directly on film. Therefore, several other modalities, including analog videotape, digital tape, and optical discs, are currently being developed as possible replacements for cinefilm.[26] A few laboratories have already replaced cinefilm storage with analog videotape using super-VHS videotapes as the storage medium. Unfortunately, much of the spatial resolution is lost in the transfer of digital images to analog tape, which is caused by the poor signal/noise ratio and limited bandwidth of videotape.[27] The corresponding deterioration in image quality strongly interferes with decision-making regarding the need for revascularization (Fig. 8–8). Thus, analog videotape cannot be recommended as a replacement for cinefilm at the current time.[28]

Another alternative to cinefilm is digital tape or optical disc recording. Although these media may overcome most of the limitations of image degradation seen with analog videotape, requirements for storage (1 to 2.5 gigabytes per study) and difficulties with later retrieval are shortcomings.[29] In addition, no set of uniform standards exists for digital formats, so a digital arteriogram recorded in one laboratory may not be interpretable in another. Despite the current limitations of digital formats, further development of uniform standards can be expected eventually to identify a recording medium that may ultimately supplant 35-mm cinefilm.

Quantitative Coronary Arteriography

The role of quantitative coronary arteriography in judging the severity of coronary artery stenoses is one of the most controversial subjects in the field of invasive cardiology. It

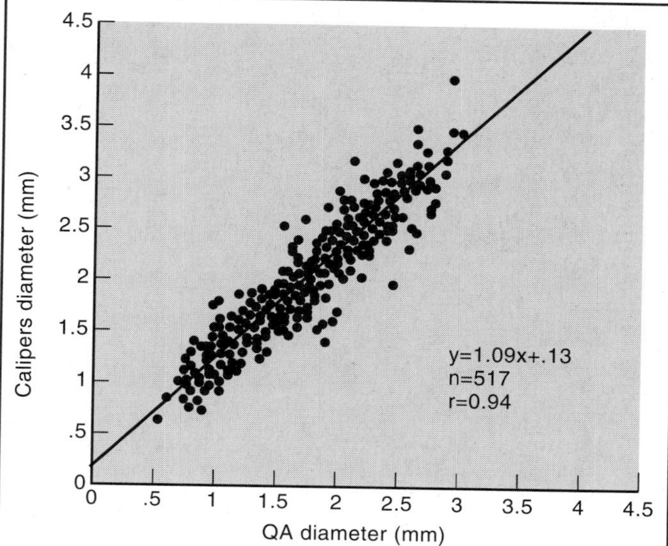

FIGURE 8–9. Coronary artery lumen diameter. The relationship between coronary artery lumen diameter measured with electronic digital calipers as compared with that measured with computerized quantitative coronary angiography (QA) shows excellent correlation and agreement. (Reproduced with permission from Uehata, A., Matsugushi, T., Bittl, J. A., et al.: The accuracy of electronic digital calipers compared with quantitative angiography in measuring arterial diameters. Circulation *88*:1724, 1993. Copyright 1993 American Heart Association.)

has been suggested that no technique in invasive cardiology is discussed more but utilized less than quantitative coronary arteriography.[30] Despite the development of several computer-assisted approaches to quantitative coronary arteriography, the standard method for interpreting the presence and severity of stenoses in the epicardial coronary arteries continues to be visual assessment. Several studies have suggested, however, that visual assessment of lesion severity suffers from a suboptimal degree of interobserver variability and accuracy.[31–34] Therefore, several computer-assisted systems have been promoted, but lack of uniform standards and unclear relation between quantitative measures of stenosis severity and clinical outcome have made recommendations difficult.

Quantitative angiography defines the edge of the vessel at the points of maximal rate of change of density of contrast, whereas visual assessment defines the minimal lumen diameter at the point where any gradient is detected. An approach that benefits from excellent interobserver variability and yet maintains the ability of the angiographer to integrate the visual information from several frames relies on the use of hand-held electronic digital calipers, which have been found to have acceptable agreement with computer-assisted methods (Fig. 8–9).[36]

CORONARY ARTERY ANATOMY

Coronary arteriography visualizes only a small portion of the coronary circulation: the major epicardial branches and their second-, third-, and perhaps fourth-order branches. The myriad small intramyocardial branches are not visualized because of their small size, cardiac motion, and limitations in resolution of cine imaging systems. Although these small "resistance" vessels play a major role in regulation of coronary blood flow, they are thought to play a small role in human coronary artery disease, limiting blood flow and contributing to ischemia in patients with left ventricular hypertrophy or systemic hypertension in the absence of epicardial coronary artery stenosis.

Because the heart is oriented obliquely in the thoracic cavity, the direct frontal and lateral views are not commonly used during coronary arteriography. Instead, the coronary circulation is imaged in the right anterior oblique (RAO) and left anterior oblique (LAO) views (Figs. 8–10 and 8–11). The major coronary arteries traverse the atrioventricular and interventicular grooves, which in turn are aligned with the long and short axes of the heart. Thus, the best angiographic projections to visualize these vessels in profile are the oblique views. Because the straight RAO and LAO views of the heart have serious shortcomings caused by foreshortening and superimposition of branches,[37,38] the rotation of the x-ray beam about the patient in the transverse plane for RAO and LAO projections is almost always accompanied by rotation of the x-ray beam about the patient in the sagittal plane for cranial and caudal angulation.

General recommendations about routine views, however, can be made for most patients, and tailored views are required to accommodate possible variations. During coronary arteriography, the anteroposterior (AP) view with shallow caudal angulation is often performed first to evaluate the possibility of left main coronary artery disease. Other important views include the LAO view with cranial angulation to evaluate the left anterior descending artery. This view should have sufficient leftward positioning of the image intensifier to prevent overlap between the left anterior descending artery (LAD) and the spine. This is followed by the LAO caudal view to evaluate the proximal segment of the left circumflex coronary artery (LCx), RAO view with caudal angulation to assess the LCx and marginal branches in full profile, and shallow RAO or AP cranial view to evaluate the midportion of the LAD. Although the foregoing sequence of views is recommended for the minimal assessment of the left coronary artery (LCA), a rigid sequence of views is not mandated. Instead, the views must be selected based on the rotation of the heart and the presence of lesions that may be targeted for revascularization techniques.

TERMINOLOGY OF VIEWS. The terminology originally proposed to describe these views was somewhat confusing, because several different terms were introduced by different authors. A simple nomenclature has evolved that defines the cineangiographic projection as the relation between the image intensifier and the patient. In most cardiac catheterization laboratories, the x-ray tube is under the patient table, and the image intensifier, with its coupled video and cinecameras, is over the patient table (Fig. 8–7). If the over-table image intensifier is tilted up toward the head of the patient, the resulting projection is referred to as the "cranial" view. The images recorded in this view appear as if the angiographer were looking down at the heart from the patient's head. Conversely, if the image intensifier is tilted down toward the feet of the patient, this is referred to as the "caudal" view and provides images as if the angiographer were looking up at the heart from the patient's feet. Cranial and caudal angulations have become a standard part of coronary arteriography and are used routinely in most laboratories that have the necessary **U**- or **C**-arm mounting units for their cine systems.

It is difficult to predict which angulated views will be most useful in any given patient. The usefulness of the angiographic projections depends largely on body habitus, variations in the coronary anatomy, and location of lesions. For this reason, it is recommended that coronary angiographers routinely use both cranial and caudal angulation views in both the LAO and RAO projections of the left coronary system. These views also can be helpful on occasion during examination of the right coronary system, especially in visualizing the origin of the posterior descending artery in the LAO cranial projection.

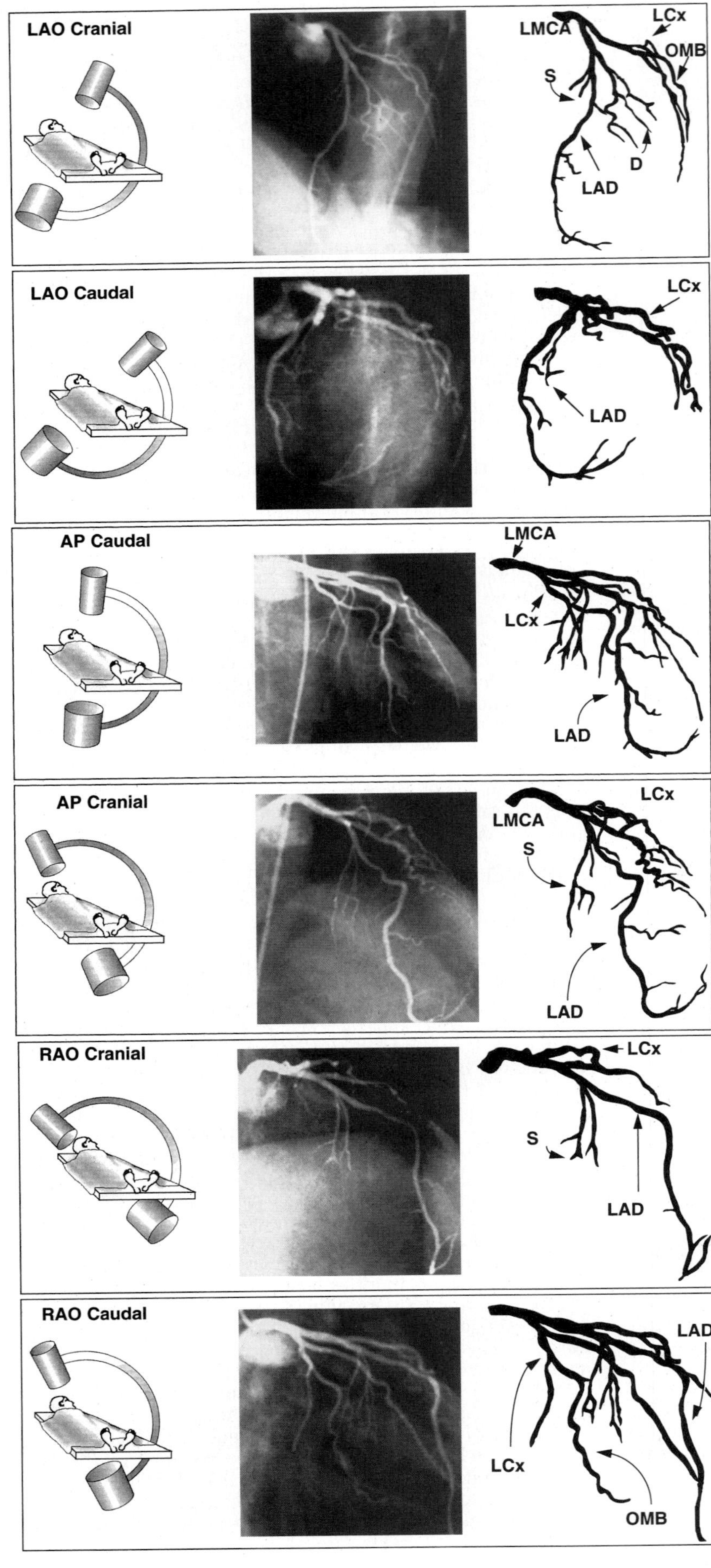

FIGURE 8–10. Angiographic views of the left coronary artery. The approximate positions of the x-ray tube and image intensifier are shown for each of the commonly used angiographic views. The 60-degree left anterior oblique view with 20 degrees of cranial angulation (LAO cranial) shows the ostium and occasionally the distal portion of the LMCA, the middle and distal portions of the LAD, septal perforators (S), diagonal branches (D), the proximal LCx and superimposed obtuse marginal branch (OMB). The 60-degree left anterior oblique view with 25 degrees of caudal angulation (LAO caudal) shows the proximal LMCA and the proximal segments of the LAD and LCx. The anteroposterior projection with 20 degrees of caudal angulation (AP caudal) shows the distal LMCA and proximal segment of the LAD and LCx. The proximal segment of the LCx is characterized by a 75- to 90-degree angle, but the midportion of the LCx and septal branches are superimposed. The anteroposterior projection with 20 degrees of cranial angulation (AP cranial) displays the midportion of the LAD and its septal (S) and diagonal branches. The 30-degree right anterior oblique projection with 20 degrees of cranial angulation (RAO cranial) shows the course of the LAD and its diagonal branches. The 30-degree right anterior oblique projection with 25 degrees of caudal angulation (RAO caudal) shows the LCx and marginal branches.

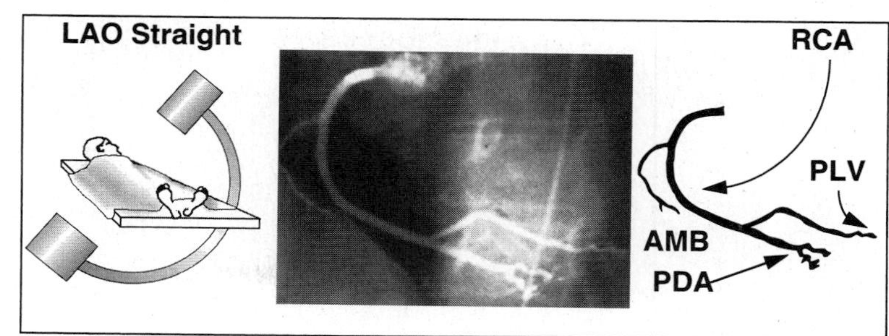

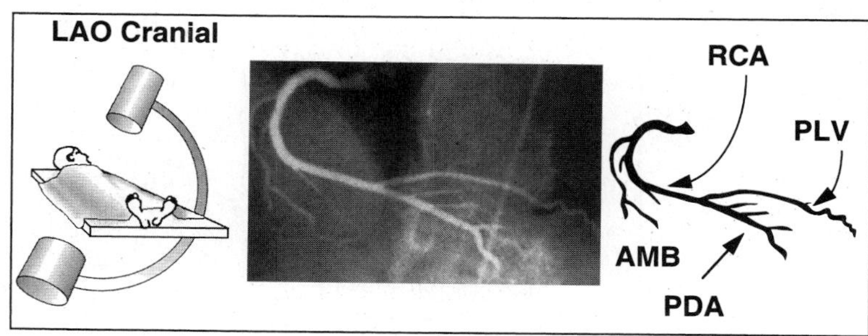

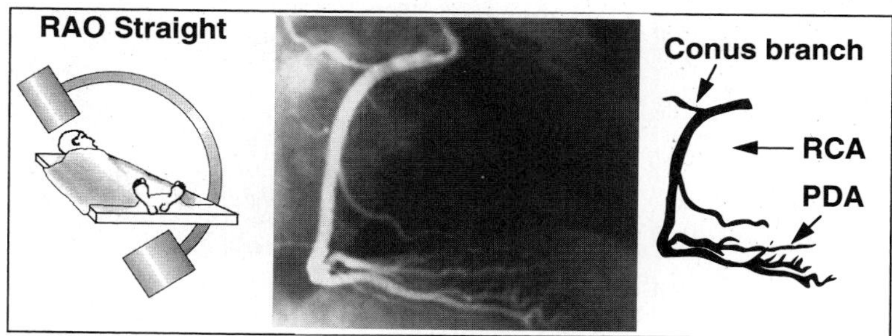

FIGURE 8–11. Angiographic views of the right coronary artery. The approximate positions of the x-ray tube and image intensifier are shown for each of the commonly used angiographic views. The 60-degree left anterior oblique view (LAO straight) shows the proximal and midportions of the right coronary artery (RCA), as well as the acute marginal branch (AMB). The 60-degree left anterior oblique view with 25-degree cranial angulation (LAO cranial) shows the midportion of the RCA and the origin and course of the PDA. The 30-degree right anterior oblique view (RAO straight) shows the conus branch, the midportion of the RCA, and the course of the PDA.

Dominance

The term "dominance" often is used to describe coronary artery anatomy. With this nomenclature, the dominant vessel is the one that supplies the posterior diaphragmatic portion of the interventricular septum and the diaphragmatic surface of the left ventricle (Figs. 8–12, 8–13, and 8–14). The right coronary artery (RCA) is dominant in about 85 per cent of humans. Use of the term dominance is somewhat misleading because it implies that the RCA is the more important vessel in 85 per cent of patients. Because human coronary artery disease (CAD) is primarily the result of interruption of blood supply to the left ventricular myocardium, a nondominant left coronary artery (LCA) is almost always more important than the dominant RCA. With this understanding, the term dominance nevertheless is used because it is a commonly accepted anatomical concept. Dominance is most easily assessed in the LAO cranial view.

Left Coronary Artery Catheterization Technique

The technique for catheterizing the left main coronary artery involves advancing the Judkins left coronary catheter toward the left coronary ostium (Fig. 8–6). If the catheter begins to turn out of profile (so that one or both curves of the catheter are no longer visualized en face), it can be rotated very slightly and advanced slowly to enter the left sinus of Valsalva. Overrotation of the left Judkins catheter "will only thwart attempts" to enter the left coronary ostium.[39] Further slow advancement will permit the catheter tip to engage the ostium of the left coronary artery. In conditions of a large ascending aorta, advancement of the Judkins left coronary catheter is associated with formation of an acute secondary angle. Further advancement should be avoided, because this would re-form the catheter shape and prevent catheterization of the left coronary artery. In the presence of a mildly dilated ascending aorta, the guidewire can be temporarily reinserted into the catheter to straighten the secondary bend and permit the catheter to be advanced to the left sinus of Valsalva.

If the ascending aorta is significantly dilated, however, the catheter should be exchanged for a larger size (e.g., Judkins left 5.0 or 6.0). If the tip of the Judkins left catheter advances beyond the ostium of the left coronary artery without engagement, the primary bend of the catheter can be reshaped within the patient's body by further careful advancement and prompt withdrawal of the catheter, allowing the tip to "pop" into the ostium of the left coronary artery. This maneuver, along with gentle clockwise or counterclockwise rotation, frequently permits selective engagement of the left coronary artery when the initial attempt has failed. It is imperative, however, to ensure that the catheter tip has not entered the left main coronary artery before further advancement is made.

To catheterize the left main coronary artery with the Amplatz catheter, the broad secondary curve of the appropriately sized left Amplatz catheter is positioned so that it rests on the right aortic cusp with its tip pointing toward the left aortic cusp. Alternating advancement and retraction of the catheter with slight clockwise or counterclockwise rotation allows the catheter tip to enter the left coronary ostium. Once the tip enters the ostium, the position of the catheter usually can be stabilized with slight retraction.

After the left coronary ostium is entered, the pressure at the tip of the catheter should be checked immediately to ensure that it matches femoral artery pressure. If this is the case, the catheter tip is most likely aligned coaxially with the origin of the coronary artery and free within its lumen. This can be verified by the gentle injection of a small amount of contrast medium. If a damped or ventricularized pressure tracing is obtained, the catheter should be removed immediately from the left coronary artery, and an attempt at repositioning should be made. If abnormal pressure recordings persist, it is reasonable to withdraw the catheter slightly from the coronary artery and perform a nonselective injection of contrast medium into the left coronary artery in the anteroposterior view to evaluate the possibility of left main coronary artery disease. If the pressure measured at the catheter tip is normal and a small test injection of contrast medium suggests the absence of left main coronary artery disease, left coronary arteriography is then performed using multiple projections.

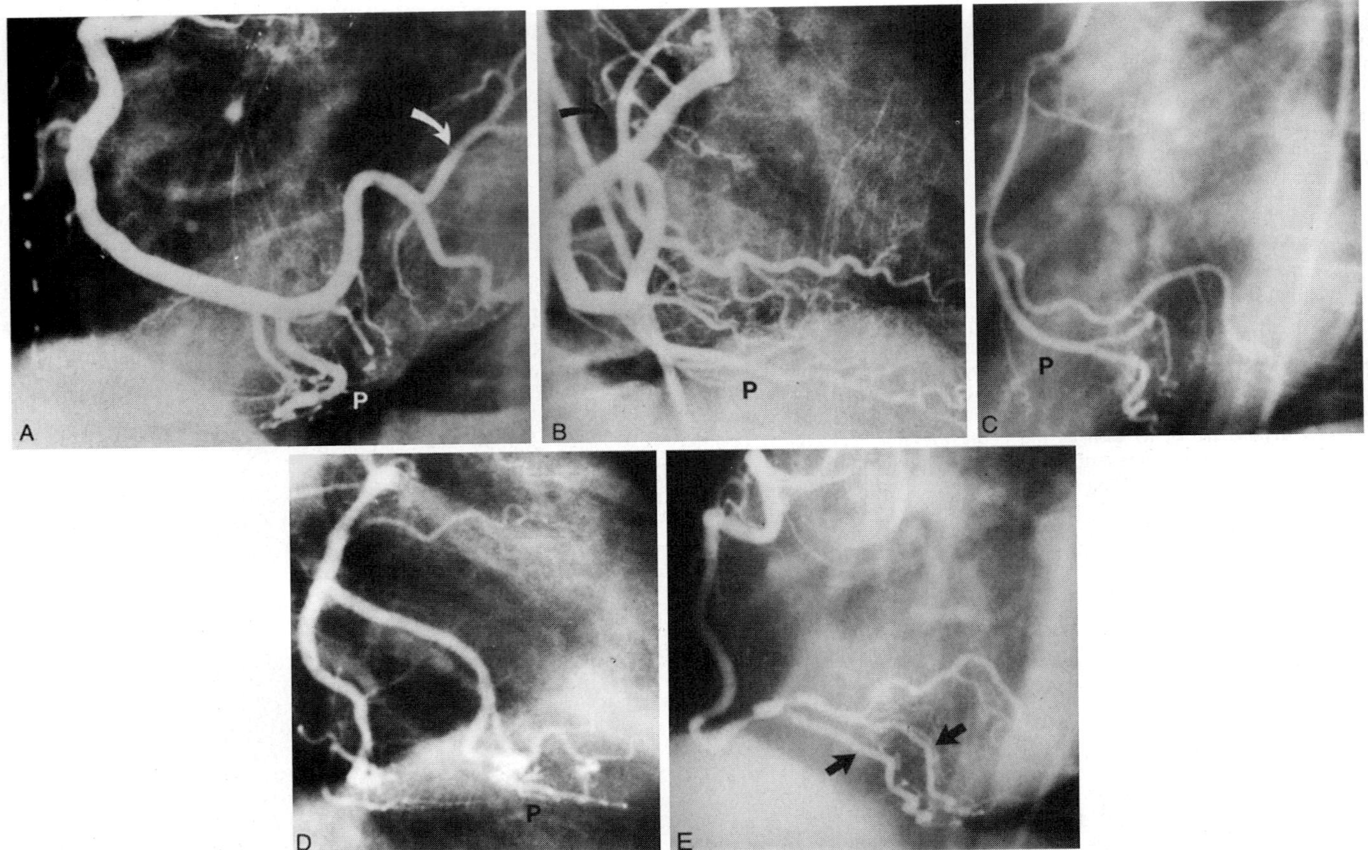

FIGURE 8–12. Strongly dominant right coronary artery. *A* and *B,* LAO and RAO views of the RCA show that the distal segment (arrows) extends to the left atrioventricular groove. After giving rise to the posterior descending artery, the RCA gives rise to multiple posterior left ventricular and obtuse marginal branches. *C,* A variation in the origin of the posterior descending artery, which originates early from the RCA, runs parallel to it, and enters the posterior interventricular groove. (From Levin, D. C., and Baltaxe, H. A.: Angiographic demonstration of important anatomic variations of the posterior descending artery. A. J. R. *116:*41, 1972, with permission). *D,* RAO right coronary arteriogram showing the posterior descending artery arising from a right ventricular branch of the RCA. *E,* LAO right coronary arteriogram showing duplicated posterior descending arteries (arrows). (From Levin, D. C., and Baltaxe, H. A.: Angiographic demonstration of important anatomic variations of the posterior descending artery. A. J. R. *116:*41, 1972, copyright 1972, American Roentgen Ray Society.)

Left Coronary Artery Anatomy

Left Main Coronary Artery (LMCA)

The LMCA arises from the upper portion of the left aortic sinus, just below the sinotubular ridge of the aorta, which defines the border separating the left sinus of Valsalva from the smooth (tubular) portion of the aorta. The diameter of the LMCA ranges from 3 to 6 mm. Quantitative analysis has shown that the diameter of the LMCA is greater for patients with entirely normal coronary arteries (4.5 ± 0.5 mm [± S.D.]) than in those with disease in the distal LCA (4.0 ± 0.3 mm) or disease in the adjacent segment of the LCA (3.8 ± 0.3 mm).[40] The LMCA passes behind the right ventricular outflow tract and may extend for 0 to 10 mm. It usually then bifurcates into the LAD and LCx branches.

Left Anterior Descending Artery (LAD)

The LAD passes down the anterior interventicular groove toward the cardiac apex. In the RAO projection, it extends toward the anterior aspect of the heart. In the LAO projection, it passes down the cardiac midline, between the right and left ventricles (Fig. 8–10). Its major branches are the septal and diagonal branches.

The septal branches emanate from the LAD at approximately 90-degree angles and pass into the interventricular septum. They vary in size, number, and distribution. In some cases there is a large first septal branch, which is vertically oriented and divides into a number of secondary branches that ramify throughout the septum. In other cases a more horizontally oriented, large first septal branch is present, which passes parallel to and below the LAD itself. In still other cases a number of septal arteries are roughly comparable in size. These septal branches interconnect with similar septal branches passing upward from the posterior descending branch of the RCA to produce a network of potential collateral channels. The interventicular septum is the most densely vascularized area of the heart, and the first septal branch is its most important potential collateral channel.

The diagonal branches of the LAD pass over the anterolateral aspect of the heart. Although virtually all patients have a single LAD in the anterior interventicular groove, there is wide variability in the number and size of diagonal branches. More than 90 per cent have one to three such branches.[41] Because less than 1 per cent of patients have no diagonal branches, the angiographer should suspect the presence of acquired atherosclerotic occlusion of the diagonal branch(es) if none are seen. This is particularly true in cases in which there are unexplained contraction abnormalities of the anterolateral left ventricle. Visualization of the origin of the diagonal branches often requires very

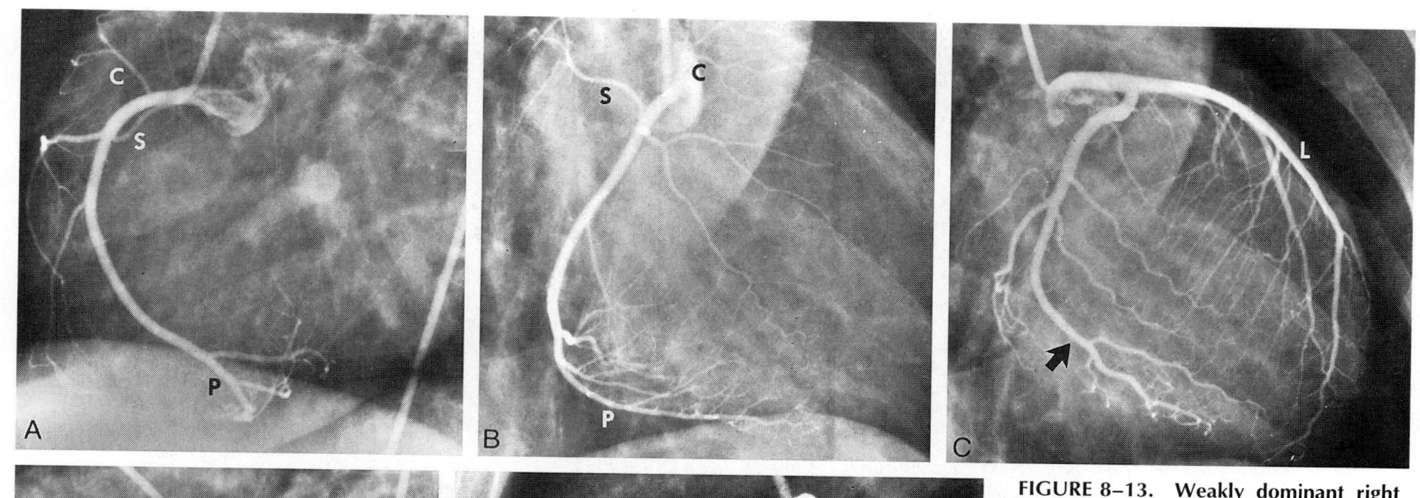

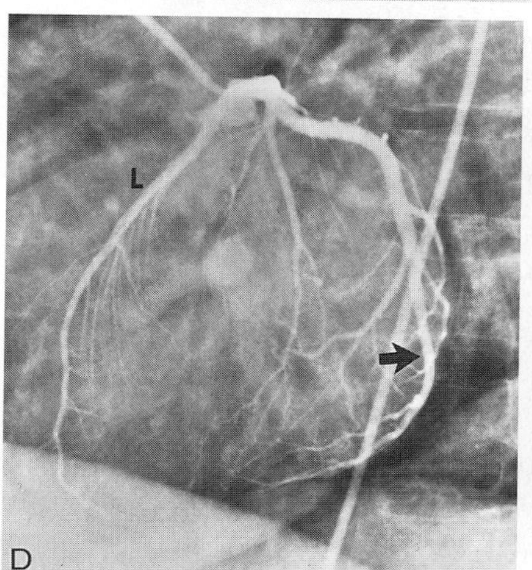

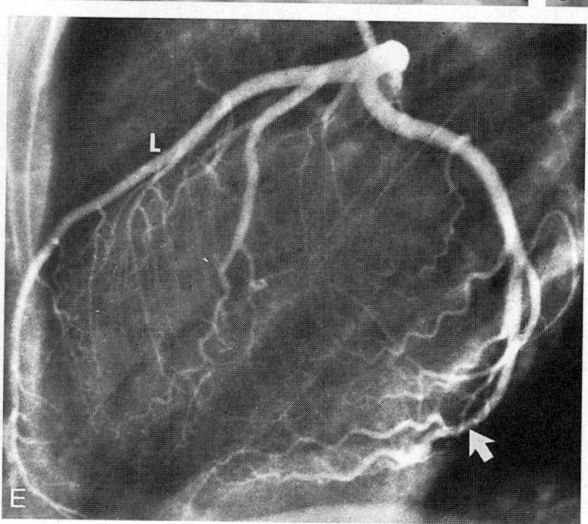

FIGURE 8–13. Weakly dominant right coronary artery. *A* and *B,* LAO and RAO views of the RCA. Both the conus and sinoatrial node artery arise from the RCA. The distal portion of the RCA beyond the origin of the posterior descending artery is short and gives rise to a single small posterior left ventricular branch. *C, D,* and *E,* LCA in the RAO, LAO, and left lateral projections, respectively. Note that the circumflex artery gives rise to four obtuse marginal branches, the most distal of which *(arrow)* supplies some of the diaphragmatic surface of the left ventricle. The LAD gives rise to two small and one medium-sized diagonal branches. C = conus branch; L = left anterior descending artery; P = posterior descending artery; S = sinoatrial nodal artery.

steep LAO cranial views involving as much as 80 degrees of leftward angulation and 20 to 40 degrees of cranial skew for optimal projection. The origin of the diagonal branches often can be brought into relief with less severely angulated RAO cranial or caudal projections.

In 37 per cent of patients, the LMCA trifurcates into the LAD, LCx, and *ramus medianus*.[41] In these cases, the ramus arises between the LAD and LCx arteries. This vessel is analogous to a diagonal branch and usually supplies the free wall along the lateral aspect of the left ventricle.

In 78 per cent of patients, the LAD courses beyond the left ventricular apex and terminates along the diaphragmatic aspect of the left ventricle. In 22 per cent of patients, however, the LAD fails to reach the diaphragmatic surface, terminating instead either at or before the cardiac apex.[42] In these latter cases, the posterior descending branch of the RCA is larger and longer than usual, supplies the apex, and may be informally termed "superdominant." In these patients, the LAD does not supply the cardiac apex, and its distal segment is smaller and shorter than usual. Early attenuation and a distal narrow segment in these cases do not necessarily signify LAD disease if some or all of the cardiac apex is supplied by the posterior descending artery.

The LAD requires carefully constructed projections to assess the ostium of the vessel and to separate it from its multiple septal and diagonal side branches. The best angiographic projections for viewing the course of the LAD are the cranially angulated views. The LAO caudal view (Fig. 8–10), however, will display the origin of the LAD in a horizontally oriented heart, and the AP caudal or shallow RAO caudal view also will project the proximal LAD well. The LAO cranial view displays the midportion of the LAD and origins of the diagonal branches but superimposes the LAD and the septal branches. The RAO cranial view displays the proximal, middle, and distal segments of the LAD but often superimposes the midportion of the LAD and the diagonal branches. The left lateral view often shows the midportion of the LAD only. Views designed to assess the origin of the diagonal branches and define ostial lesions of these branches are often tailored LAO cranial or RAO cranial views. Lastly, variations of the AP view requiring 20 to 40 degrees of cranial skew often will project the midportion of the LAD in best relief, separating the vessel from its diagonal branches.

In some patients, no LMCA is present. In these cases, separate ostia for the LAD and LCx are present, which can be separately engaged for selective arteriography. In general, the LAD has a more anterior origin than the LCx. The LAD can be engaged with the left Judkins catheter in this setting with paradoxical counterclockwise rotation, which rotates the secondary bend of the catheter to a posterior position in the aorta and turns the primary bend and tip of the catheter to an anterior position. The opposite maneuver may be used to engage the LCx selectively in the setting of separate LAD and LCx ostia. On the other hand, a Judkins catheter such as the Judkins left 5.0 with a larger curve will selectively engage the downward-coursing left circumflex, and a catheter with a shorter curve such as the Judkins left 3.5 will tend to engage selectively the more anterior and superior left anterior descending coronary artery.

Left Circumflex Artery (LCx)

The left circumflex artery originates at the bifurcation (or trifurcation) of the LMCA and passes down the left atrioventricular groove (Fig. 8–10). In about 85 per cent of human hearts, the LCx artery is the nondominant vessel and varies in size and length, depending on the actual degree of right coronary dominance. The LCx usually gives

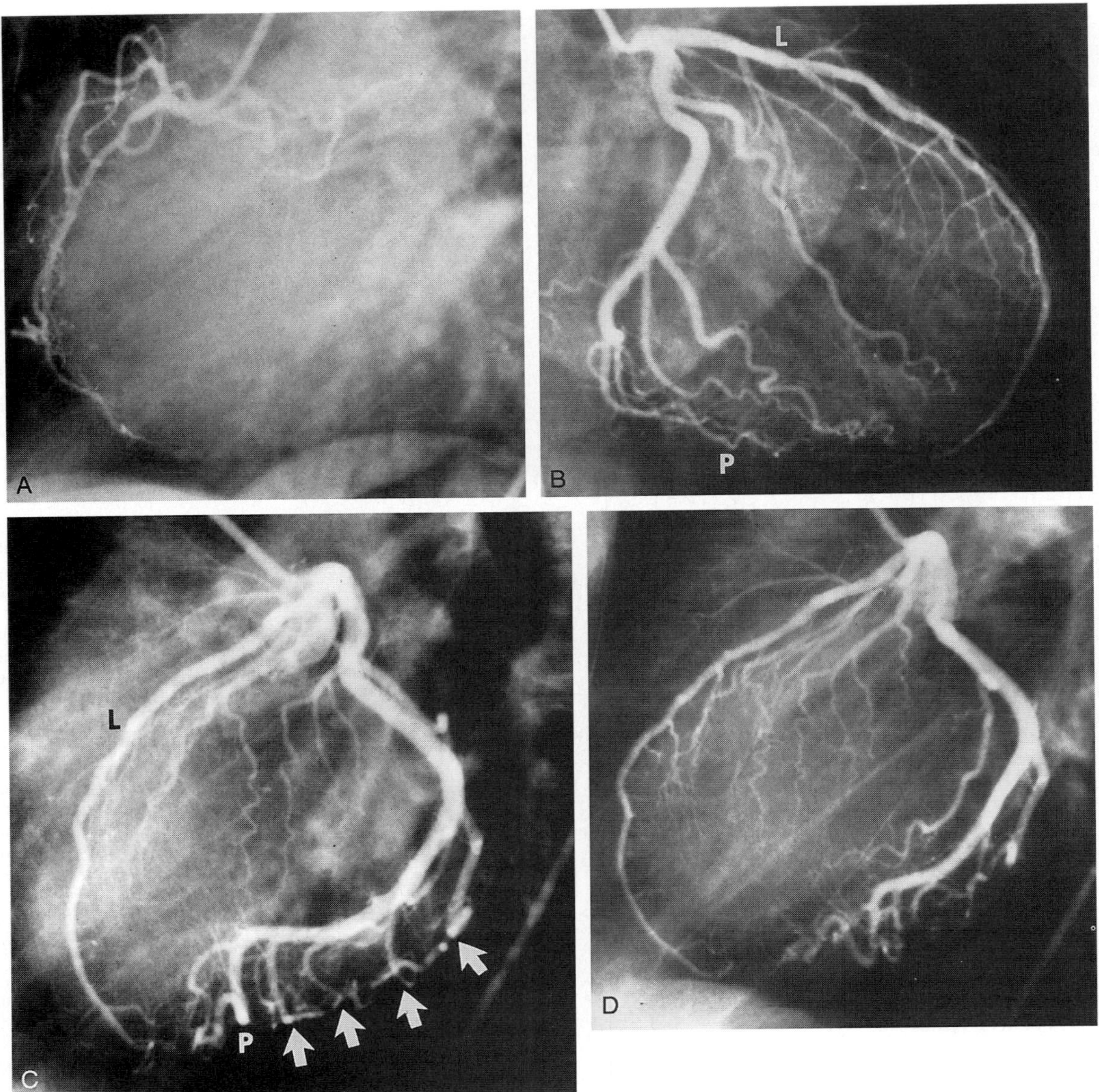

FIGURE 8–14. Dominant left coronary system. *A,* **The LAO projection shows that the RCA is small and terminates before reaching the crux.** *B, C,* **and** *D.* **The RAO, LAO, and left lateral projections show that the LCx is large and gives rise to the posterior descending artery at the crux of the heart, and to several posterior descending arteries.**

off one to three large *obtuse marginal branches* (OMBs) as it passes down the atrioventricular groove. These are the principal branches of the LCx, since they supply the free wall of the left ventricle along its lateral aspect. Beyond the origins of the obtuse marginal branches, the distal LCx tends to be small. The actual position of the LCx can be determined on the late phase of a left coronary injection, when the coronary sinus becomes opacified with diluted contrast material. The position of the coronary sinus identifies the position of the left atrioventricular groove and the proper LCx artery, which runs along the left ventricular side of the coronary sinus. The optimal projections for viewing the LCx and obtuse marginal branches usually involve caudal angulation to project the posteriorly and inferiorly coursing LCx into the plane of the angiographic film. The ostium of the LCx often requires the LAO caudal or RAO caudal view. The midportion of the LCx and the origins of the obtuse marginal branches are often best viewed in the AP caudal views or RAO caudal view with only 5 to 15 degrees of rightward angulation. More severe rightward angulation often superimposes the origins of the obtuse marginal branches on the LCx. If the LCA is dominant, the optimal projection for the posterior descending artery is the LAO cranial view.

The LCx also gives rise to one or two left atrial circumflex branches. These branches supply the lateral and posterior aspects of the left atrium.

Right Coronary Artery Catheterization Technique

Catheterization of the RCA is also performed in the LAO position, but this requires different maneuvers than catheterization of the LMCA. Whereas the left Judkins catheter naturally seeks the ostium of the LMCA, the right coronary catheter must be rotated by the angiographer to engage the vessel. This usually is accomplished by first passing the catheter to a point just above the aortic valve in the left sinus of Valsalva and then rotating the catheter clockwise, which forces the tip to move anteriorly from the left sinus of Valsalva to the right sinus of Valsalva. Entry into the right coronary ostium is signified by a sudden rightward and downward movement of the catheter tip. If the ostium of the RCA is not easily located, the most common reason is that the ostium has a higher and more anterior origin than anticipated. Repeat attempts to engage the RCA should be made at a level slightly more distal to the aortic valve. Nonselective contrast medium injections in the right sinus of Valsalva may reveal the site of origin of the RCA. Positioning an Amplatz catheter in the ostium of the RCA requires a catheterization technique similar to that used with the right Judkins catheter. If a gentle attempt to withdraw the Amplatz catheter results in paradoxical deep entry into the coronary artery, removal of the catheter can be achieved by clockwise or counterclockwise rotation and advancement to prolapse the catheter into the aortic sinus.

The catheter-tip pressure should be checked to ensure that damping or ventricularization has not occurred. An abnormal pressure tracing may suggest the presence of an ostial stenosis or spasm, selective engagement of the conus branch, or deep intubation of the RCA. If an abnormal pressure tracing has been encountered, the catheter tip should be rotated gently counterclockwise and withdrawn slightly in an effort to free the tip of the catheter. If persistent damping occurs, a very small amount of contrast medium (<1 ml) can be injected carefully and the catheter immediately withdrawn in a "shoot-and-run" maneuver, which may allow the cause of damping to be identified.

If the pressure tracing is normal on entry into the RCA, the vessel should be imaged in at least two projections. The initial injection should be gentle, because of the possibility that forceful injection through a catheter whose tip is immediately adjacent to the vessel wall may lead to dissection. The standard LAO and RAO projections usually will suffice, but on occasion cranial angulation should be added to view the origin and course of the posterior descending artery.

The ideal angiographic projections for evaluating the right coronary artery are the standard LAO and RAO views. The ostium of the RCA is best evaluated in the LAO view, with or without cranial angulation. If the standard Judkins catheter encounters a lesion at the ostium, this catheter should be replaced by a right Amplatz catheter or a short-tipped Judkins catheter to decrease the likelihood of vessel dissection. The origin of the posterior descending artery (PDA) is evaluated in the LAO cranial view, whereas the midportion of the RCA occasionally requires the left lateral view.

Right Coronary Artery Anatomy

The RCA originates from the right aortic sinus at a point somewhat lower than the origin of the LCA from the left aortic sinus (Fig. 8–11). It passes down the right atrioventricular groove toward the crux (a point on the diaphragmatic surface of the heart where the right atrioventricular groove, the left atrioventricular groove, and the posterior interventricular groove come together).

The first branch of the RCA is considered to be the *conus artery.* In about 50 per cent of hearts, this vessel arises at the right coronary ostium or within the first few millimeters of the RCA. It passes anteriorly and upward over the right ventricular outflow tract toward the LAD. The Judkins right coronary catheter frequently engages the conus artery subselectively, and this almost always produces a damped or ventricularized pressure tracing. Gentle withdrawal and further clockwise rotation may allow the catheter to enter the proper RCA. The primary importance of the conus artery is to serve as a source of collateral circulation in patients with LAD occlusion. In the other 50 per cent of hearts, the conus artery is not actually a branch of the RCA but arises from a separate ostium in the right aortic sinus just above the right coronary ostium.[43] In this group of patients, subselective conus branch arteriography may fail to opacify the RCA proper unless sufficient reflux of contrast medium occurs to fill the separate ostium.

The second branch of the RCA usually is the *sinoatrial node artery.* It has been found that this vessel arises from the RCA in 59 per cent, from the LCx in 38 per cent, and from both arteries with a dual blood supply in 3 per cent.[44] When it originates from the RCA, it passes obliquely backward through the upper portion of the atrial septum and the anteromedial wall of the right atrium. It sends branches to the sinus node and usually also to the right atrium or both atria. When the sinoatrial node artery originates from the LCx, it may pass backward in the atrial septum or around the posterolateral wall of the left atrium to reach the area of the sinus node.

The midportion of the RCA usually gives rise to one or more medium-sized acute marginal branches. These branches supply the anterior wall of the right ventricle and are relatively unimportant, except insofar as they also may serve as sources of collateral circulation in patients with LAD occlusion.

The next important branch of the RCA is the *posterior descending artery* (PDA) (Fig. 8–11). When the RCA is dominant, as it is in about 85 per cent of patients, the PDA originates at or shortly before the crux and passes forward in the posterior interventricular groove. During its course along this groove, it gives rise to a number of small inferior septal branches which pass upward to supply the lower portion of the interventricular septum and interdigitate with superior septal branches passing down from the LAD. After giving rise to the PDA, a dominant RCA continues beyond the crux and begins to pass upward along the distal portion of the left atrioventricular groove. Here it usually terminates by giving rise to one or several posterior left ventricular (PLV) branches, which supply the diaphragmatic surface of the left ventricle.

About 15 per cent of patients do not have RCA dominance; about half these patients have LCA dominance. With this anatomical pattern, the LCx artery is large and continues down to the diaphragmatic surface of the left ventricle, where it gives rise to the PLV branches and then reaches the crux and turns forward to become the PDA. In these cases, the RCA is very small, terminating before reaching the crux, and therefore does not supply any blood to the left ventricular myocardium. The other half of patients without RCA dominance have a mixed or "balanced" circulation, wherein the RCA gives rise to the PDA, while the LCx gives rise to the PLV branches.

At or near the crux, the dominant artery gives rise to a small atrioventricular node artery, which passes upward to supply the node.

In about 25 per cent of patients with RCA dominance, there are significant anatomical variations in the origin of the PDA. These variations include partial supply of the PDA territory by acute marginal branches, double PDA, and early origin of the PDA proximal to the crux.

Coronary Bypass Angiography

Angiography after coronary bypass is commonly performed to evaluate the cause of recurrent angina in surgically treated patients. It is estimated that more than 300,000 bypass operations are performed each year in the United States.[2] Although bypass surgery may achieve 99 per cent revascularization of target segments initially,[45] only 87 per cent of saphenous vein grafts (SVGs) remain open at 6 months,[46] and only 75 per cent of target segments remain revascularized 3 years after surgery.[45] The short- and long-term patency rates for SVGs have been reported in several large clinical studies (see p. 1319). In the CASS trial, patency of SVGs was 90 per cent within 60 days of surgery, 82 per cent at 18 months, and about 80 per cent at 3 years.[47] Similar results were seen in the European Coronary Surgery Study, in which SVGs were found to have a 77 per cent patency rate 9 to 18 months after surgery.[48] In patients at the Montreal Heart Institute, SVG patency at 1 year was about 80 per cent, and there was no further reduction in patency between 1 and 6 years after operation.[47] By the time 10 to 12 years had elapsed after surgery, the patency rate of SVGs had dropped to 63 per cent. Moreover, almost half the grafts still patent showed significant atherosclerotic changes. In 161 patients undergoing bypass surgery in the German Angioplasty Bypass Surgery Investigation (GABI),[46] 92 per cent were discharged from the hospital angina-free, but this proportion decreased to 84 per cent at 3 months and to 74 per cent at 6 months.

The patency of SVGs and internal mammary artery (IMA) grafts has been compared (see p. 1318). After a mean follow-up period of 36 months, the patency rate for IMA grafts was 96 per cent, whereas the patency rate for SVGs at a mean follow-up period of 39 months was 77 per cent.[49] At 6 months after bypass surgery, 93 per cent of IMA grafts were functioning.[46] At 7 to 10 years after surgery, IMA graft patency was in the range of 85 to 95 per cent.

The right gastroepiploic artery (GEA) has been used increasingly as a conduit for coronary artery bypass surgery. The right GEA has a slightly greater tendency to develop atherosclerosis than the IMA, with moderate to severe atherosclerosis seen in 12 per cent of right GEAs versus 0 per cent of IMAs at pathological examination.[50] Late GEA graft patency has been documented in 94 per cent of patients 2 to 5 years after surgery.[51]

Several mechanisms lead to failure of bypass grafts. The development of symptoms in the immediate postoperative period after bypass surgery may be due to incomplete revascularization, spasm of the internal mammary artery, or early thrombotic graft occlusion of saphenous vein grafts. The development of symptoms within 1 year of bypass surgery may be due to fibrointimal hyperplasia of saphenous vein grafts.[52] Symptoms in patients more than 1 year after bypass surgery may be due to development of atherosclerosis[52] in the bypass grafts[53] or progression of native vessel disease.[53]

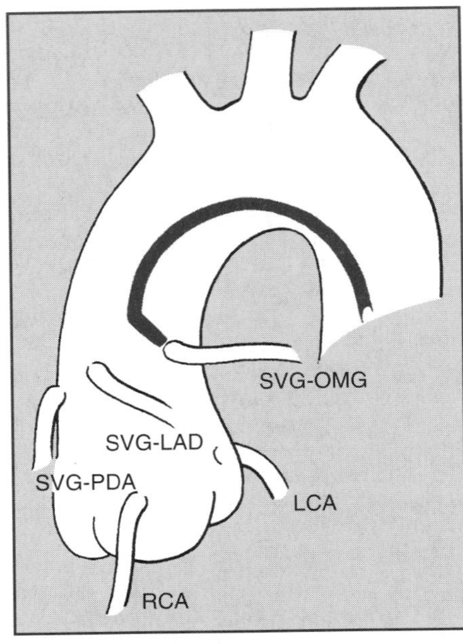

FIGURE 8–15. Catheterization of saphenous vein bypass grafts. In the LAO projection, saphenous vein bypass grafts to the native coronary arteries are positioned and oriented in a predictable manner. Bypass grafts anastomosing to the obtuse marginal branches (SVG-OMB) are characteristically the most leftward and superior of the grafts, those anastomosing primarily with posterior descending artery (SVG-PDA) are the most rightward and inferior, and those to the left anterior descending artery (SVG-LAD) are intermediate in position and orientation. (From Judkins, M. W.: Coronary arteriography. *In* Douglas, J. S., Jr., King, S. B., III [eds.]: Coronary Arteriography and Intervention. New York, McGraw-Hill, 1985, p. 229, with permission.)

Coronary Bypass Graft Catheterization Technique

Selective catheterization of coronary bypass grafts may be more difficult than catheterization of the native coronary arteries because the locations of graft ostia are more variable, even when surgical clips or ostia markers are used. The experienced angiographer, however, can easily locate graft ostia because the sites of origin for grafts leading to each coronary artery are very predictable. It is therefore crucial for the angiographer to review the operative note describing the number, course, and types of bypass grafts before performing graft arteriography.

Saphenous vein grafts (SVGs) from the aorta to the distal right coronary artery or posterior descending artery originate from the right anterolateral aspect of the aorta approximately 2 cm above the origin of the sinotubular ridge, whereas SVGs to the LAD originate from the anterior portion of the aorta about 4 cm above the sinotubular ridge, and SVGs to the obtuse marginal branches arise from the left anterolateral aspect of the aorta about 5 to 6 cm above the sinotubular ridge (Fig. 8–15). In most patients, all SVGs can be engaged with a single catheter. Use of the Amplatz right 2.0 catheter results in a very high rate of successful SVG catheterizations. Other catheters useful for engaging bypass grafts include the right and left bypass graft catheters (Fig. 8–2).

The eye-hand coordination of the angiographer contributes to the success of graft angiography. Viewed in the LAO projection, the Amplatz catheter will rotate anteriorly from the leftward position as the angiographer turns the catheter in a clockwise direction at the femoral artery. The relation between movement of the catheter shaft at the femoral artery, and the response of the catheter tip on fluoroscopy immediately informs the angiographer whether the catheter tip is positioned anteriorly in the aorta and thus likely to enter a graft ostium or positioned posteriorly and thus unlikely to engage an SVG. Steady advancement and withdrawal of the catheter tip proximal and distal in the ascending aorta, approximately 2 to 6 cm above the sinotubular ridge, with varying degrees of rotation usually results in entry into the graft.

Entry into the graft is associated with abrupt outward motion of the tip of the catheter. When this occurs, a small test injection of contrast material verifies that the catheter is in the SVG. Even if the graft is occluded, a well-circumscribed "stump" is almost always present. Each graft or stump must be viewed in nearly orthogonal views. The relation between the origin of the grafts and surgical clips confirms whether all targeted SVGs have been visualized. If neither a patent graft nor a stump can be located, it may be necessary to perform an ascending aortogram (preferably in biplane) in an attempt to visualize all SVGs.

GOAL OF BYPASS GRAFT ANGIOGRAPHY. This is to provide an assessment of the ostium of the graft, its entire course, and the distal insertion site at the anastomosis between the bypass graft and the native coronary vessel. The ostium of a bypass graft must be evaluated by achieving a parallel relation between the tip of the catheter and the origin of the graft. The midportion (body) of the graft must be evaluated in the absence of contrast streaming, because inadequate opacification produces an angiographic artifact suggestive of friable filling defects. It is critical to assess the graft insertion site in full profile without any overlap of the distal graft or the native vessel. Angiographic assessment of the native vessels beyond graft anastomotic sites requires views that are conventionally used for the native segments themselves but modified to avoid overlap with the graft itself.

INTERNAL MAMMARY ARTERY CATHETERIZATION

The left IMA arises inferiorly from the left subclavian artery approximately 10 cm from its origin. Catheterization of the left IMA is easily performed (Fig. 8–16) with a specially designed J-tip catheter, referred to as the "IM catheter" (Fig. 8–2). Advancement of the catheter into the aortic arch distal to the origin of the left subclavian artery in the LAO projection, counterclockwise rotation of the catheter, and gentle withdrawal of the catheter with the tip pointing in a cranial direction will easily allow entry into the left subclavian artery, which is usually located immediately under the head of the clavicle. If a small injection of contrast material or guidewire position confirms catheter position in the left subclavian artery, the guidewire is advanced to the left subclavian artery under the distal third of the clavicle. The artery is then viewed "down the barrel" in the RAO projection as the catheter is withdrawn and rotated slightly anteriorly and inferiorly (counterclockwise), tip down, to selectively engage the left IMA.

CATHETERIZATION OF THE RIGHT IMA. This also involves use of the IM catheter. The innominate artery is entered in the LAO projection. The guidewire must be advanced cautiously because of easy entry into the right common carotid artery. Once the guidewire is advanced to the distal right subclavian artery, the catheter is advanced to a point distal to the expected origin of the right IMA. The catheter is withdrawn in the LAO view, while the angiographer looks "down the barrel" of the right IMA.

Often, selective catheterization of the IMAs is compromised by tortuosity of the subclavian arteries. Another catheter that may be use-

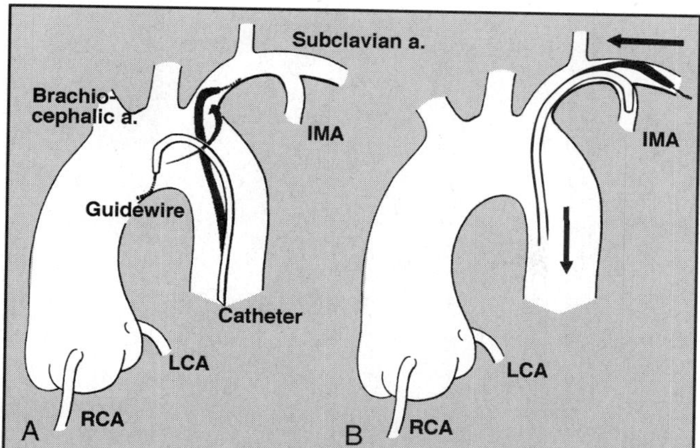

FIGURE 8–16. Catheterization of the left internal mammary artery. The internal mammary catheter is positioned in the aortic arch and visualized in the LAO position. The catheter tip is rotated so that it engages the origin of the left subclavian artery immediately subjacent to the head of the left clavicle *(A)*. This is followed by gentle advancement of the guidewire into subclavian artery to a point distal to the origin of the left internal mammary artery. After the guidewire is removed, the left subclavian is visualized in the RAO projection, the catheter is gently withdrawn, and the catheter tip engages the ostium of the left internal mammary artery selectively *(B)*. (From Judkins, M. W.: Coronary arteriography. *In* Douglas, J. S., Jr., King, S. B., III [eds.]: Coronary Arteriography and Intervention. New York, McGraw-Hill, 1985, p. 231, with permission.)

ful to enter the left subclavian or the innominate artery is the Headhunter catheter. The ability to advance the guidewire and catheter through the subclavian system also may be compromised by tortuosity and require the use of floppy-tip or hydrophilic-coated guidewire.

As the IMA has been used increasingly because of its superiority as a bypass conduit, the need for selective IMA arteriography also has increased. The IMA itself is rarely affected by atherosclerosis, which may be attributable to superior endothelial properties of anticoagulation, vasodilatation, and growth inhibition as compared with SVGs and native coronary arteries.[54] The distal insertion site, however, is subject to focal stenosis. Thus angiographic studies of the IMAs must assess not only the patency of the graft itself but also the distal anastomosis, where most of IMA graft compromise occurs.[47]

The LAO cranial view is often disappointing in projecting the anastomosis of the IMA with the LAD because of overlap, but the straight LAO and LAO caudal views are often helpful. The risk of catheter-induced dissection of the origin of the IMA can be reduced by careful manipulation of the catheter tip and avoidance of forceful advancement without the protection of the guidewire. If the IMA cannot be selectively engaged because of tortuosity of the subclavian artery, nonselective arteriography can be enhanced by placing a blood pressure cuff on the ipsilateral arm and inflating it to a pressure above systolic arterial pressure. The occurrence of IMA spasm can be treated with 50 to 200 μg of intraarterial nitroglycerin or 50 to 100 μg of intraarterial verapamil.

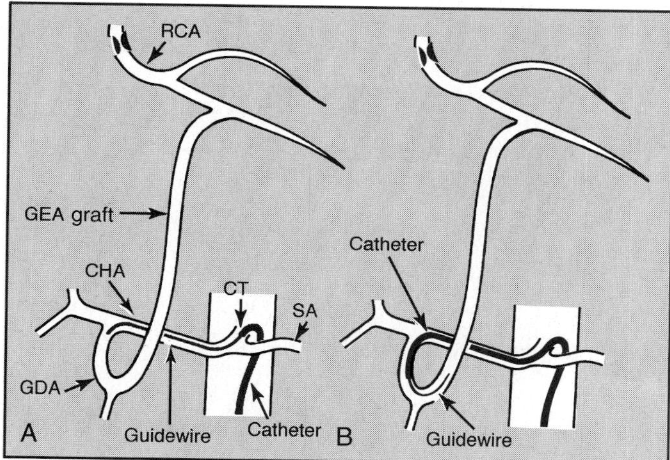

FIGURE 8–17. Catheterization of the right gastroepiploic artery graft. The celiac trunk (CT) is selectively engaged with a cobra catheter, and a torquable, hydrophilic-coated guidewire is gently advanced to the gastroduodenal artery (GDA) and the GEA (gastroepiploic) artery *(A)*. The catheter is advanced over the guidewire for selective arteriography of the GEA graft *(B)*. CHA = common hepatic artery; RCA = right coronary artery; SA = splenic artery. (From Isshiki, T., Yamaguchi, T., Tamura, T., et al.: Percutaneous angiography of stenosed gastroepiploic artery grafts. J. Am. Coll. Cardiol. *21:*727, 1993. Reprinted with permission from the American College of Cardiology.)

GASTROEPIPLOIC ARTERY CATHETERIZATION

The right gastroepiploic artery (GEA) is the largest terminal artery of the gastroduodenal artery. The other terminal branch of the gastroduodenal artery is the superior pancreaticoduodenal artery. The gastroduodenal artery arises from the common hepatic artery in 75 per cent of cases, but it also may arise from the right or left hepatic artery or the celiac trunk. Catheterization of the right GEA is carried out by first entering the common hepatic artery with a cobra catheter (Fig. 8–17). The angiographer then gently advances a torquable, hydrophilic-coated guidewire to the gastroduodenal artery and then to the right GEA. Exchange of the cobra for a multipurpose or Judkins right coronary catheter will then permit selective arteriography of the right GEA.

Pitfalls of Coronary Arteriography

GENERAL PRINCIPLES OF ARTERIOGRAPHIC INTERPRETATION. A systematic approach based on a few common sense principles is needed to avoid pitfalls in the performance and interpretation of coronary arteriography. It should be recalled that the normal coronary artery tapers gradually from proximal to distal and has smooth walls completely free of irregularities. Although it is tempting in some cases to invoke the diagnosis of an anatomical variant to account for a particular arteriographic finding, it must be emphasized that the prevalence of acquired coronary artery disease is several orders of magnitude greater than the rare occurrence of congenital variants. Thus, attention to the following three rules of congenital variations[55] is needed: (1) acquired atherosclerotic coronary artery disease is far more frequent than are the unusual anatomical variations; (2) there are thousands of collaterals for any one anomalous vessel; and (3) before an unusual vessel is accepted as a variant, an occlusion or large collateral channel should be suspected.

LEFT MAIN CORONARY ARTERY STENOSIS. The left main coronary artery should be viewed in several projections with the vessel off the spine. Catheter pressure damping and the absence of reflux suggest the presence of LMCA disease (Figs. 8–18 and 8–19). Unrecognized LMCA stenosis often results in inappropriate referral of patients for coronary intervention.[56]

INADEQUATE OPACIFICATION. Inadequate filling of the coronary artery with contrast medium may result in streaming of contrast medium and give the impression of ostial stenoses, missing side branches, or thrombus. Similarly, superselective injection of contrast medium into the left circumflex artery through a short left main coronary artery may give the impression of total occlusion of the left anterior descending coronary artery. Adequate filling of the coronary arteries and bypass grafts is required to overcome the native flow of unopacified blood and produce high-quality coronary arteriograms. Stenoses may be under- or overassessed if incomplete filling is achieved. The causes of incomplete filling include competition from increased native coronary blood flow in the setting of left ventricular hypertrophy associated with aortic insufficiency or anemia and inadequate placement of the diagnostic catheter with subselective injection. The problem of underfilling can be overcome by more forceful contrast material injection as long as the catheter-tip position and pressure recording confirm the safety of such a maneuver. Under some conditions, switching to an angioplasty guiding catheter with a soft, short tip and a larger lumen than a diagnostic catheter

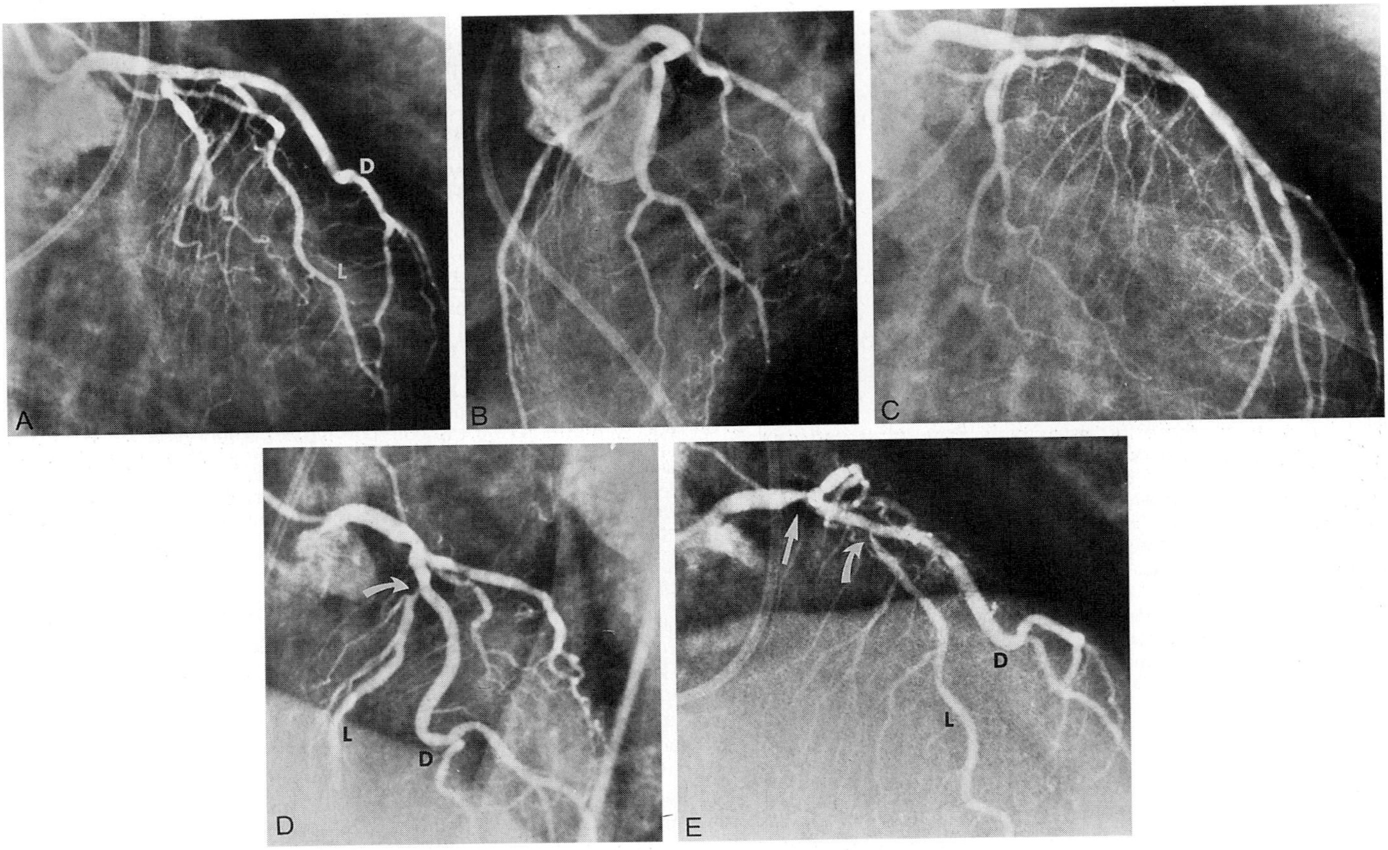

FIGURE 8–18. Missed left main coronary artery stenosis. *A–C,* left coronary arteriography in the standard RAO, LAO, and RAO caudal views fails to demonstrate significant stenoses of the LMCA or LAD. *D,* LAO cranial view shows severe stenosis (curved arrow) of the LAD (L) immediately beyond the origin of the diagonal branch (D). *E,* RAO cranial view shows the LAD stenosis (curved arrow) but also shows a severe stenosis of the LMCA (straight arrow) at its bifurcation.

may allow for more complete opacification of the target coronary artery or bypass graft.

ECCENTRIC STENOSES. Coronary atherosclerosis more often leads to eccentric or slit-like atherosclerotic narrowings than to concentric narrowings. If, in such cases, the long axis of the eccentric lumen is projected, the vessel may appear to have a normal or near-normal caliber. Only if the short axis of the stenotic lumen is projected will the narrowing be visible (Fig. 8–20). For this reason, coronary arteries must be viewed in at least two projections approximately 90 degrees apart.

A related problem is that of the band-like or membranous

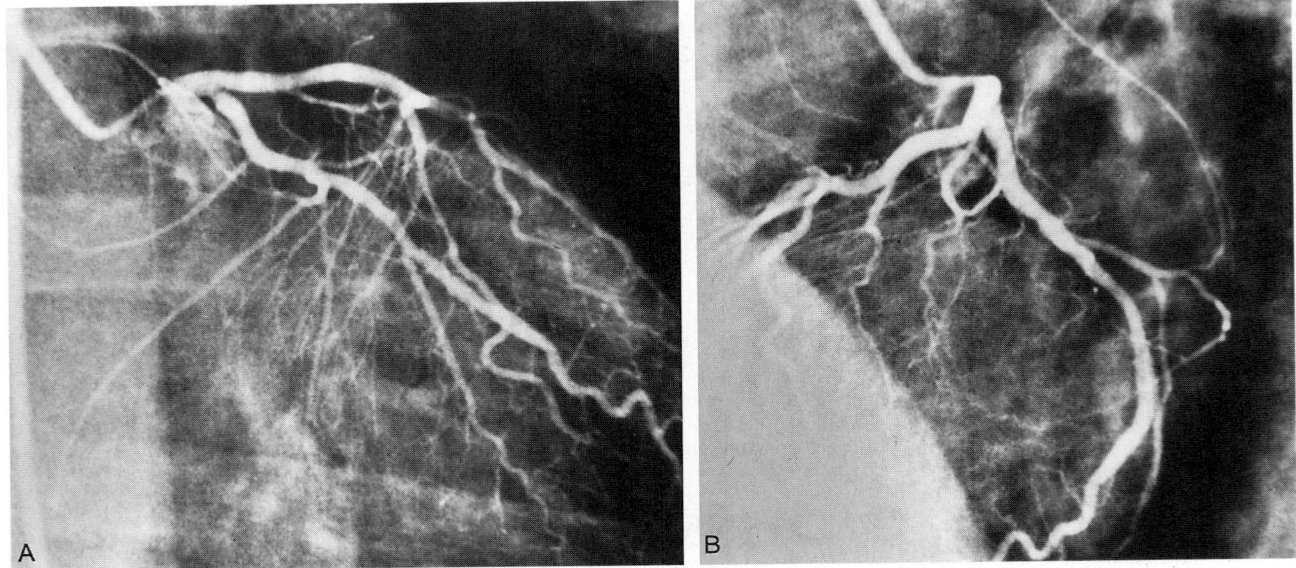

FIGURE 8–19. Difficulty in detecting ostial left main coronary artery stenosis. *A,* Shallow RAO views of the LAD with the catheter not well seated in the vessel result in poor visualization of the ostial stenosis of the LMCA. *B,* LAO cranial view shows the catheter tip selectively positioned in the LMCA without reflux of contrast around the tip.

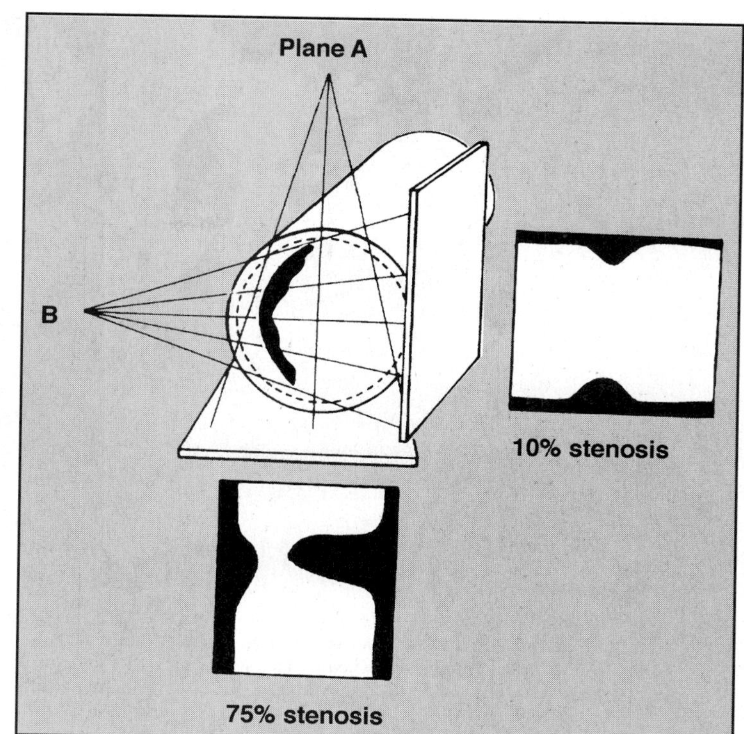

FIGURE 8–20. Importance of orthogonal projections. Each vascular segment of the coronary artery must be recorded in two orthogonal or nearly orthogonal views to avoid missing important diagnostic information about eccentric stenoses. In plane A the image is associated with a 75 per cent stenosis, but in plane B the image results in 10 per cent stenosis. (From Miller, S. W.: Coronary artery disease. *In* Miller, S. W. [ed.]: Cardiac Angiography. Boston, Little, Brown, 1984, p. 87, with permission.)

stenosis. Lesions such as this may be exceedingly difficult to detect. It is not clear whether these peculiar lesions represent pure atherosclerotic stenosis or are caused in some instances by congenital membranous bands.[57] Aside from the difficulty in detecting these lesions, it is difficult to ascertain their hemodynamic significance. Measurement of the pressure gradient across the lesion through a small inner catheter inserted through the angiographic catheter may be useful in this regard. The use of intravascular ultrasound also may be very helpful.

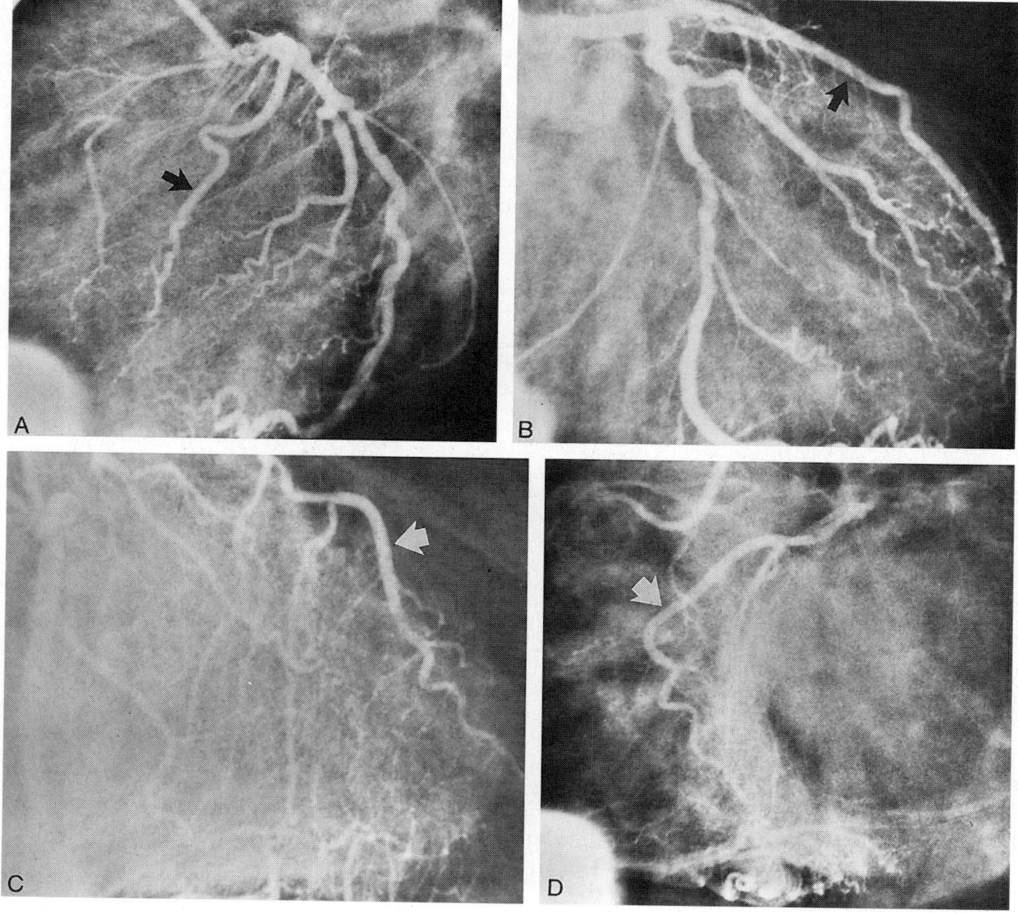

FIGURE 8–21. Superimposition of branches. *A, B,* LAO and RAO views of the left coronary arteriogram show that the LAD is totally occluded, although the point of occlusion is not visualized. There is a large diagonal branch (black arrows) that closely parallels the LAD in both projections and could be mistaken for the LAD. Late-phase frames from an RAO *(C)* and LAD *(D)* right coronary arteriogram show filling of the LAD (white arrows) via septal collaterals.

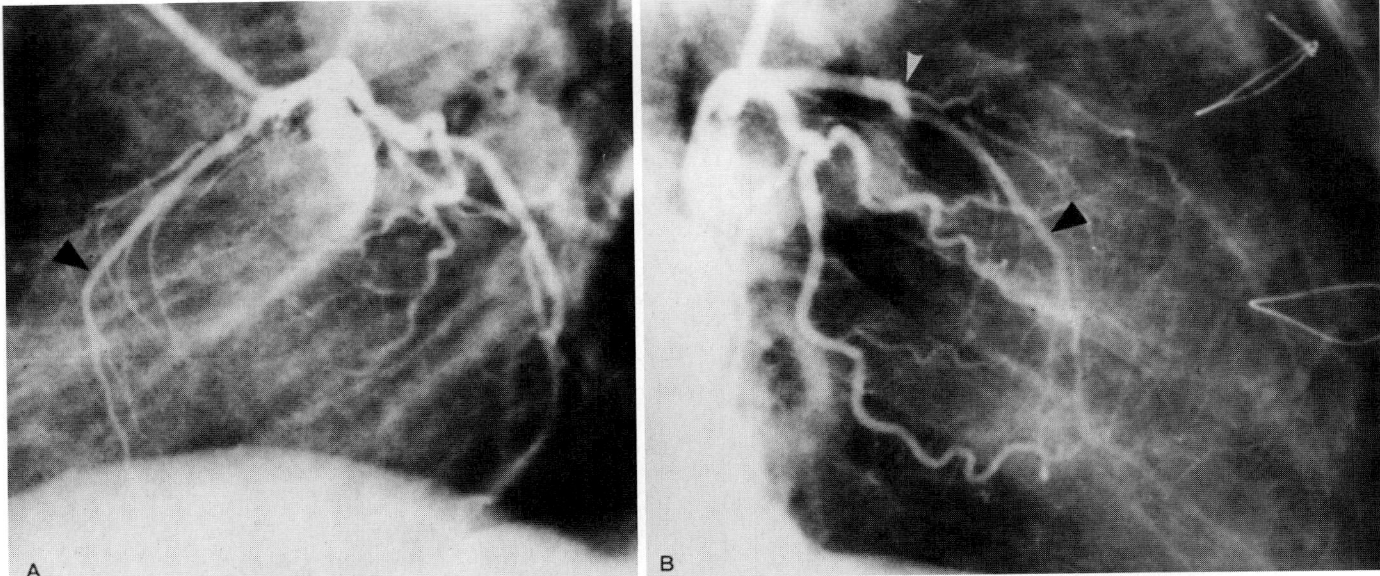

FIGURE 8–22. Septal branch mimicking the LAD. *A*, LAO left coronary arteriogram shows an enlarged septal branch (arrowhead) occupying the expected course of the LAD. *B*, The RAO view shows that the LAD is totally occluded (white arrowhead). The septal branch (black arrowhead) runs in a course approximately parallel to the LAD but below it and within the interventricular septum. (From Levin, D. C., Baltaxe, H. A., and Sos, T. A.: Potential sources of error in coronary arteriography. II. Interpretation of the study. A. J. R. *124*:386, 1975, copyright 1975 American Roentgen Ray Society.)

UNRECOGNIZED OCCLUSIONS. Flow disturbances associated with branch points predispose to the development of atherosclerosis and total occlusions of major arteries at these locations.[58,59] Because of this fact and the variability in the number and distribution of side branches in the normal coronary circulation, it is possible for occlusions at branch origins to escape detection. In some cases, occlusion of a branch can be recognized only by late filling of the distal segment of this branch by means of collateral circulation (Fig. 8–21).

SUPERIMPOSITION OF BRANCHES. Superimposition of major branches of the left coronary tree in the LAO and RAO projections can result in failure to detect stenoses or total occlusions of these branches. Although this problem most commonly affects the LAD and parallel diagonal branches (Fig. 8–19), it is alleviated by the use of cranial and caudal angulation. It should be noted that septal branches may mimic the LAD in the LAO cranial projection (Fig. 8–22). When the LAD is occluded beyond the origin of the first septal branch, this branch often enlarges in an attempt to provide collateral circulation to the vascular bed of the distal LAD.

MYOCARDIAL BRIDGING. The major coronary arteries pass over the epicardial surface of the heart. In some cases, however, short segments descend into the myocardium for a variable distance. This occurs in 5 to 12 per cent of humans and is almost always confined to the LAD.[60] Because a "bridge" of myocardial fibers passes over the involved segment of the LAD, each systolic contraction of these fibers can cause narrowing of the artery. Myocardial bridging has a characteristic appearance on cineangiography (Fig. 8–23). The bridged segment is of normal caliber during diastole but abruptly narrows with each systole. Systolic narrowing caused by myocardial bridging should not be confused with an atherosclerotic plaque. Although bridging is not thought to have any hemodynamic significance in most cases, some have suggested that when it produces severe systolic narrowing, ischemia or infarction

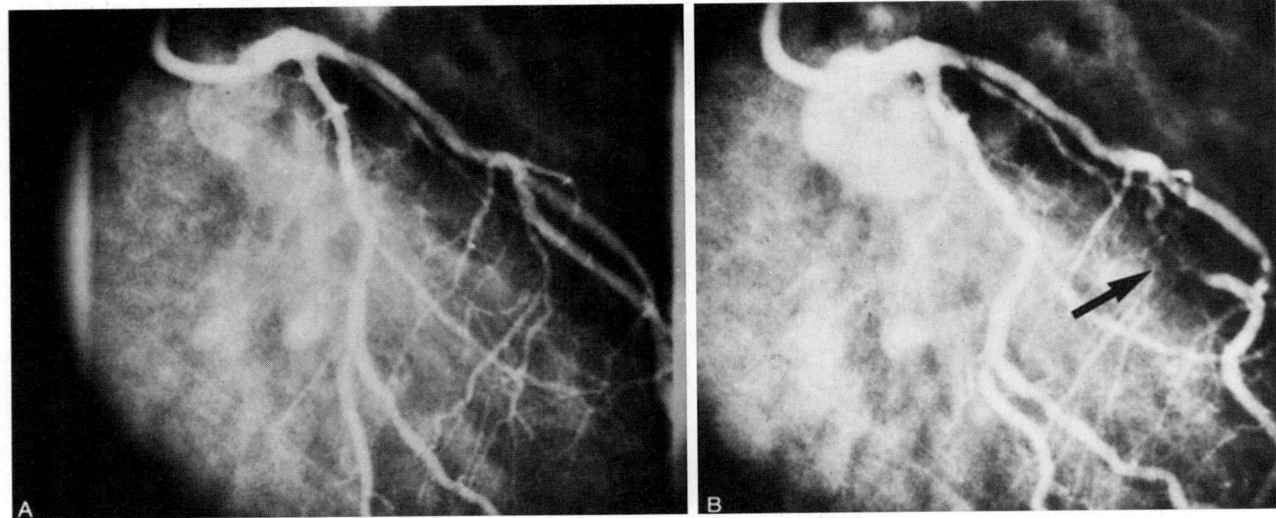

FIGURE 8–23. Myocardial bridging. *A*, RAO left coronary arteriogram shows a normal LAD during diastole. *B*, During systole, there is pronounced narrowing of the LAD (arrow).

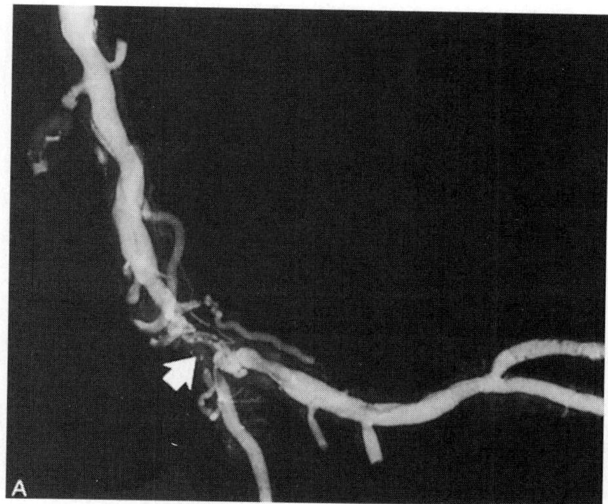

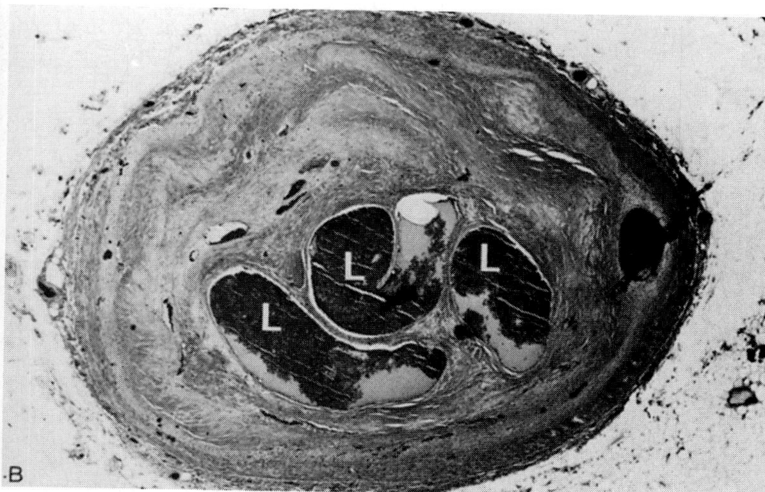

FIGURE 8–24. Recanalization of a total occlusion. *A,* Postmortem injection specimen. The RCA was injected with barium-gelatin mixture and then dissected from the epicardial surface of the heart. The recanalized segment (arrow) demonstrates several irregular channels. It is likely that angiography of such a segment in a living patient would not have sufficient resolution to demonstrate these channels. The angiographic appearance would likely be a total occlusion. *B,* Histologic section of the recanalized segment. L = recanalized lumina filled with the barium-gelatin mixture.

may result. The presence of myocardial bridging has important implications for interventional cardiovascular therapy because bridges do not respond to angioplasty.

RECANALIZATION. Although a narrowed segment of a coronary artery seen on arteriography usually is considered a "stenosis," such lesions may actually be segments which were once totally occluded but have recanalized. Pathological studies suggest that approximately one-third of totally occluded coronary arteries ultimately recanalize.[61] The arteriographic appearances of stenosis and recanalization may be indistinguishable. Recanalization usually results in the development of multiple tortuous channels, which are quite small and close to one another, creating an impression on cineangiography of a single, slightly irregular channel (Fig. 8–24). The spatial resolution of cineangiography is insufficient to demonstrate this degree of detail in most patients with recanalized total occlusions, but this has important implications for interventional cardiovascular treatments, because they are unlikely to be successful in the setting of multiple small channels.

COMPLICATIONS

The incidence of complications of coronary arteriography has been given in several large, multicenter reports. Data on complications for coronary arteriography for the 13 institutions participating in the CASS Registry involved a total of 7553 consecutive procedures.[17] The complications in 1087 patients undergoing coronary arteriography via the brachial approach were compared with those in 6328 patients undergoing the femoral approach. Death occurred in 0.51 per cent of the brachial patients and in 0.14 per cent of the femoral patients. Cerebral ischemia occurred in 0.17 per cent of the brachial patients and in 0.08 per cent of the femoral patients. Local vascular complications such as thrombosis occurred in 1.85 per cent of the brachial patients and in 0.24 per cent of the femoral patients.

The complications of outpatient coronary arteriography via the femoral approach have been reported.[62] In 3071 consecutive patients, death occurred in 0.13 per cent, nonfatal myocardial infarction in 0.07 per cent, neurological complications in 0.14 per cent, and local vascular complications in 0.35 per cent. The most extensive analysis of complications of coronary arteriography is the report of the Registry of the Society for Cardiac Angiography and Interventions.[63] Among 222,553 patients entered into this registry between 1984 and 1987, death occurred in 0.10 per cent, myocardial infarction in 0.06 per cent, stroke in 0.07 per cent, vascular complications in 0.46 per cent, and contrast reactions in 0.23 per cent. Major complications (death, myocardial infarction, and stroke) occurred with similar frequencies using the femoral and brachial approaches, but vascular complications were increased fourfold with the brachial approach. The incidence of death was increased in the presence of left main coronary artery disease (0.55 per cent), with ejection fraction less than 30 per cent (0.30 per cent), and in NYHA functional class IV (0.29 per cent). More recent registries have identified equivalent complication rates despite increasing age and acuity of illness in the patients undergoing coronary arteriography.[64]

The risk of clinically significant coronary air embolus during diagnostic coronary arteriography is low, probably occurring in less than 0.1 per cent of cases. If the syndrome of coronary air embolus and air lock does occur, 100 per cent O_2 should be administered to encourage rapid resorption of N_2, morphine sulfate is given for pain relief, and ventricular arrhythmias are anticipated and treated with lidocaine and direct-current (DC) cardioversion. Small amounts of air are usually resorbed within 2 to 4 minutes on 100 per cent oxygen.

ABNORMALITIES OF THE CORONARY CIRCULATION

Congenital Anomalies That Cause Myocardial Ischemia

(See also Chap. 29)

CORONARY ARTERY FISTULAS (see p. 908). A review of a large series of patients with congenital anomalies of the coronary arteries revealed that coronary artery fistula is by far the most common.[65] Although about half the patients with large fistulas remain asymptomatic, the other half develop congestive heart failure, infective endocarditis, myocardial ischemia, or rupture of an aneurysmal fistula. About half these fistulas arise from the RCA or its branches, slightly fewer than half arise from the LAD or LCx artery or their branches, and in the remaining cases there are multiple origins (Fig. 8–25). Drainage occurs into the right ventricle in 41 per cent, into the right atrium in 26 per cent, into the pulmonary artery in 17 per cent, into the left ven-

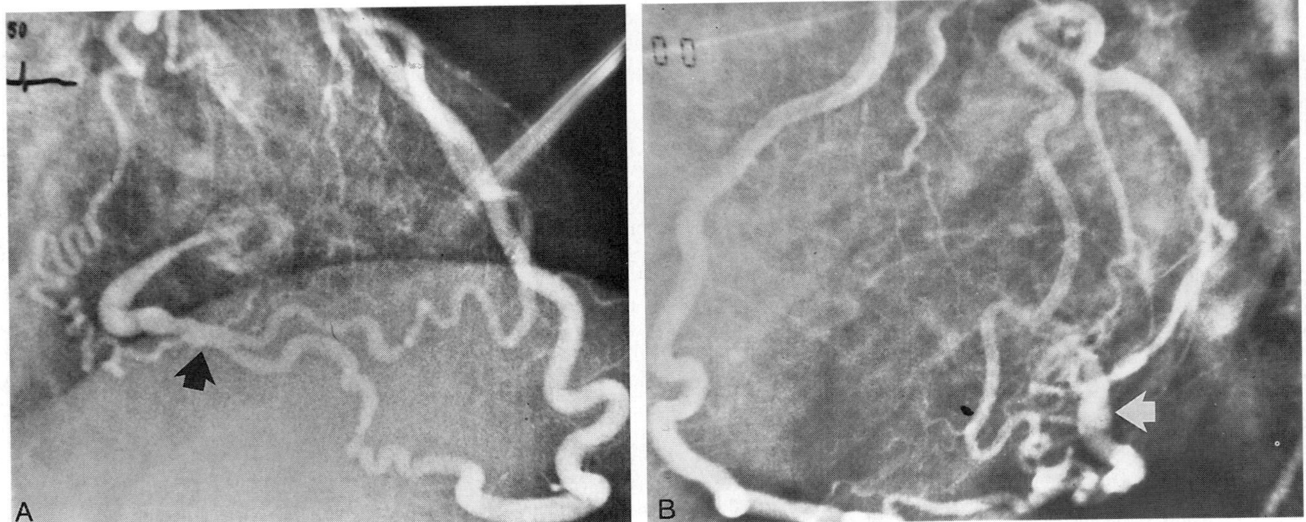

FIGURE 8–25. Congenital fistula. *A,* RAO cranial view of the left coronary arteriogram shows a congenital fistula (arrow) arising from branches of both the LAD and LCx and draining into the left ventricle. *B,* LAO view of the left coronary arteriogram shows the fistula (arrow).

tricle in 3 per cent, and into the superior vena cava in 1 per cent.[65] Thus a left-to-right shunt exists in more than 90 per cent of cases. Selective coronary arteriography is the only way to demonstrate the origin of these fistulas.

ORIGIN OF THE LEFT CORONARY ARTERY FROM THE PULMONARY ARTERY. Most patients with origin of the LCA from the main pulmonary artery develop myocardial ischemia early in life. About 25 per cent survive to adolescence or adulthood but frequently experience mitral regurgitation, angina, or congestive heart failure.[66] Aortography typically shows a large RCA with absence of a left coronary ostium in the left aortic sinus. During the late phase of the aortogram, patulous LAD and LCx branches fill by means of collateral circulation from RCA branches. Still later in the filming sequence, retrograde flow from the LAD and LCx opacifies the main LCA and its origin from the main pulmonary artery (Fig. 8–26). The clinical course of the patient tends to be more favorable if extensive collateral circulation exists. In rare instances, the RCA rather than the LCA may arise from the pulmonary artery.

CONGENITAL CORONARY STENOSIS OR ATRESIA. Congenital stenosis or atresia of a coronary artery can occur as an isolated lesion or in association with other congenital diseases such as calcific coronary sclerosis, supravalvular aortic stenosis, homocystinuria, Friedreich's ataxia, Hurler's syndrome, progeria, and rubella syndrome.[65] In these latter cases, the atretic vessel usually fills by means of collateral circulation from the contralateral side.

ANOMALOUS ORIGIN OF EITHER CORONARY ARTERY FROM THE CONTRALATERAL SINUS. Origin of the LCA from the proximal RCA or the right aortic sinus with subsequent passage between the aorta and the right ventricular outflow tract has been associated with sudden death during or shortly after exercise in young persons.[67–71] After its aberrant origin, the LCA takes an abrupt leftward turn and tunnels between the aorta and the right ventricular outflow tract. Sudden death is thought to result from transient occlusion of the anomalous LCA caused by an increase in blood flow through the aorta and pulmonary artery that occurs during exercise and creates either a kink at the sharp leftward bend or a pinchcock mechanism in the tunnel. Origin of the RCA from the LCA or left aortic sinus with passage between the aorta and the right ventricular outflow tract is somewhat less dangerous. This anomaly, however, also has been associated with myocardial ischemia or sudden death, presumably through the same mechanism.[69,71,72] In rare cases of anomalous origin of the LCA from the right aortic sinus, myocardial ischemia may occur even if the LCA passes anterior to the right ventricular outflow tract

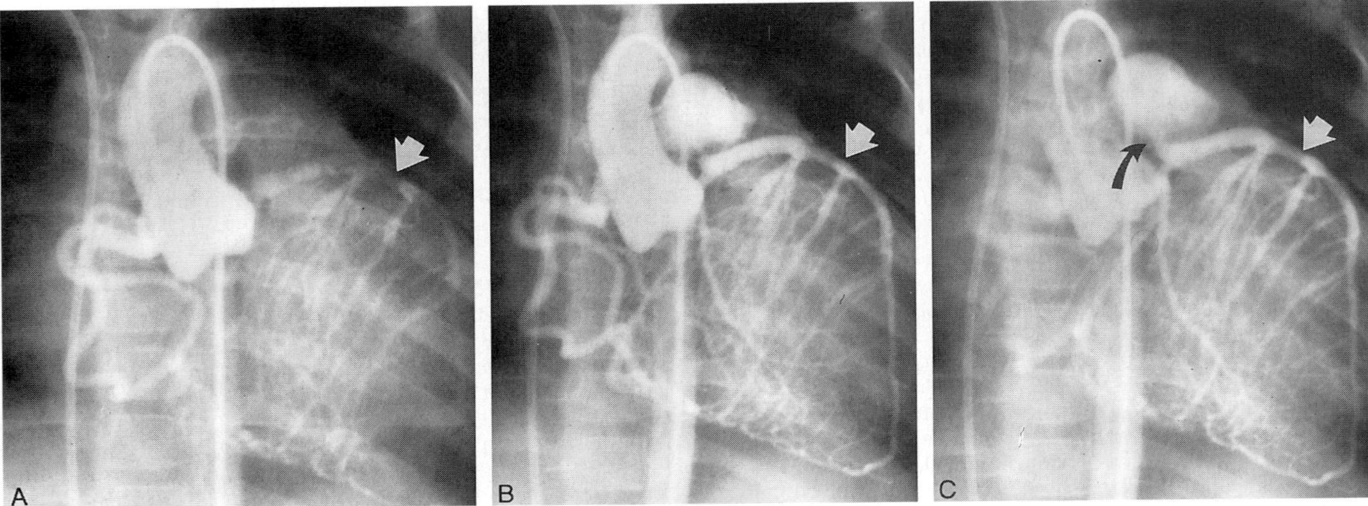

FIGURE 8–26. Anomalous origin of the LCA from the pulmonary artery. *A, B,* and *C,* The thoracic aortogram shows a large RCA and no antegrade filling of the LCA. The LCA fills primarily through extensive collaterals from the RCA to the LAD (white arrows). The anomalous origin of the LCA from the pulmonary artery is demonstrated in late phases of the aortogram (*C,* curved arrow).

or posterior to the aorta (i.e., not through a tunnel between the two great vessels),[73] but the cause of the defect is not clear.

The course of the anomalous coronary arteries is easily assessed by angiography in the RAO view (Fig. 8–27). There are four common courses for the anomalously arising LCA from the right sinus of Valsalva, one common course for the anomalous RCA arising from the left sinus of Valsalva, and one common course for the anomalous LCx arising from the right sinus of Valsalva. The anomalous LCA arising from the right sinus of Valsalva may take either a septal, anterior, interarterial, or posterior course (Fig. 8–27).[74] The posterior course of the anomalous LCA arising from the left sinus of Valsalva is similar to the almost unvarying course of the anomalous LCx arising from the right sinus of Valsalva, whereas the common interarterial course of the anomalous RCA from the left sinus of Valsalva (Fig. 8–28) is by symmetry similar to the interarterial course of the anomalous LCA arising from the right sinus of Valsalva.

When either the LCA or the LAD arises anomalously from the right aortic sinus, an alternative angiographic method to identify the course of the anomalous vessel is first to pass a catheter into the main pulmonary artery and then to perform an arteriogram of the aberrant coronary artery in the steep AP caudal projection. This places the aberrant coronary artery, the rightward and anterior pulmonary valve, and the leftward and posterior aortic valve all in one plane (see Fig. 8–27). From this "laid-back arteriogram," which can be used even in mapping the course of anomalous coronary arteries in transposition of the great vessels, it is usually possible to confirm whether the course of the aberrant coronary artery is between the great vessels.

Although angiography is useful for establishing the presence of anomalous coronary arteries, transesophageal echocardiography may be an important adjunctive diagnostic tool for defining the course of the vessels.[75]

CONGENITAL CORONARY ANOMALIES NOT CAUSING MYOCARDIAL ISCHEMIA

In this category of anomalies, the coronary arteries originate from the aorta, but their origins are in unusual locations. Although myocardial perfusion is normal, the angiographer may have trouble locating the arteries. These anomalies occur in about 0.5 to 1.0 per cent of adult patients undergoing coronary arteriography.[76]

ORIGIN OF THE LEFT CIRCUMFLEX ARTERY FROM THE RIGHT AORTIC SINUS. Anomalous origin of the LCx from the right aortic sinus is the most common of these anomalies (Fig. 8–29). In a series of almost

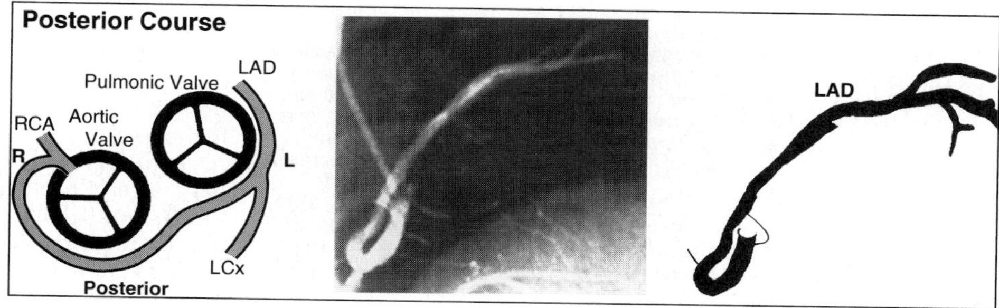

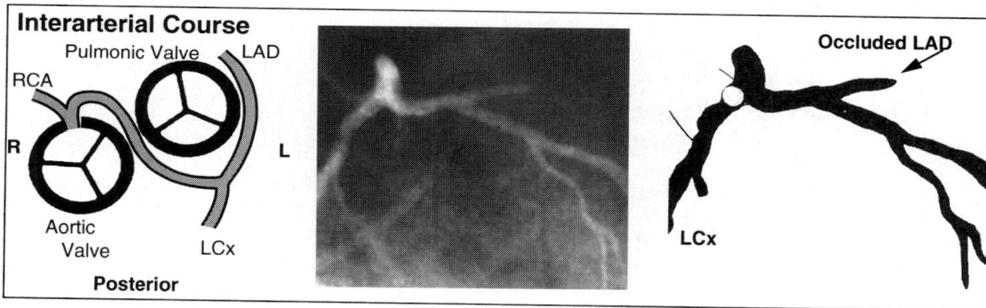

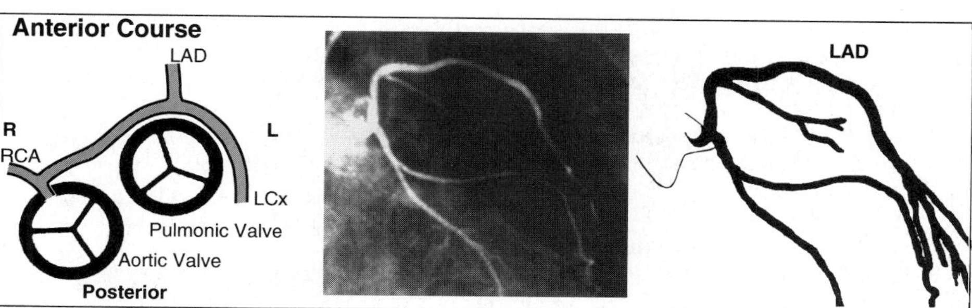

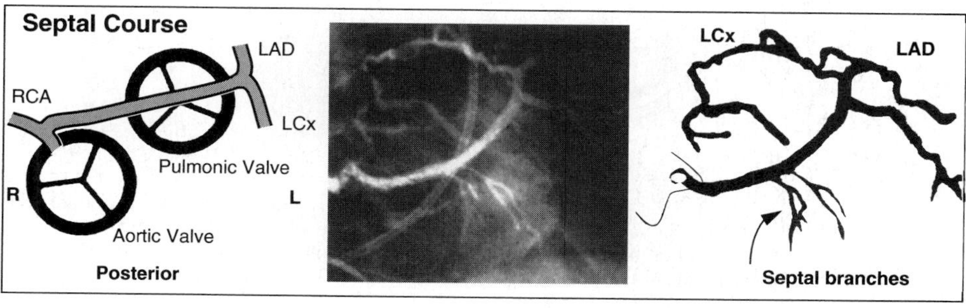

FIGURE 8–27. Anomalous origin of the left coronary artery from the right sinus of Valsalva. Each panel includes a caudo-cranial cross-sectional schematic representation at the level of the semilunar valves, showing the course of the anomalous coronary. The RAO angiograms and bitmaps show examples of each of four most common courses of the anomalous left coronary artery aberrantly arising from the right sinus of Valsalva: posterior (retroaortic), interarterial, anterior, and septal (subpulmonic) courses.

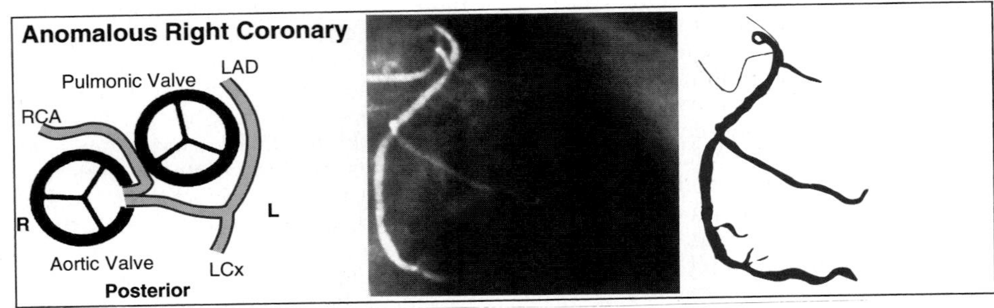

FIGURE 8–28. Anomalous origin of the right coronary artery. RAO coronary arteriogram shows an anomalous RCA arising from left sinus of Valsalva. The origin of the aberrantly arising artery, which is engaged with a left Judkins catheter, arises immediately anterior to the origin of the left coronary artery (not shown in the arteriogram). The anomalous right coronary follows an interarterial course opposite but analogous to that for the anomalous LCA arising from the right sinus of Valsalva (see Fig. 8–27).

3000 patients, this anomaly was found in 0.67 per cent.[77] In virtually every case, the anomalous LCx arises posterior to the right coronary artery and courses inferiorly and posteriorly to the aorta to enter the left atrioventricular groove. An interarterial course for an anomalously arising LCx from the right sinus of Valsalva would be almost unprecedented.

SINGLE CORONARY ARTERY. Although there are numerous variations of this anomaly,[78] it assumes hemodynamic significance when a major branch passes between the aorta and the right ventricular outflow tract, as described earlier.

ORIGIN OF ALL THREE CORONARY ARTERIES FROM EITHER THE RIGHT OR LEFT AORTIC SINUS VIA MULTIPLE SEPARATE OSTIA. This rare anomaly is similar to single coronary artery. There is absence of a coronary ostium in either the left or right aortic sinus. The missing vessels arise in the contralateral aortic sinus, but instead of arising as a single coronary artery, they arise through two or even three separate ostia.

HIGH ANTERIOR ORIGIN OF THE RIGHT CORONARY ARTERY. This anomaly is commonly encountered but of no hemodynamic significance. The inability to engage the ostium of the RCA selectively from conventional catheter manipulation raises the question of superior origin of the RCA above the sinotubular ridge. Forceful, nonselective injection of contrast medium into the right sinus of Valsalva may reveal the anomalous takeoff of the RCA, which can then be selectively engaged with a Judkins right 5.0 catheter or an Amplatz left 1.0 or 1.5 catheter.

Angiographic Assessment of Myocardial Blood Flow

Angiographic evidence of coronary artery perfusion can be based on the flow grades first proposed by the Thrombolysis in Myocardial Infarction (TIMI) study group.[79] With this scheme, coronary perfusion is classified as follows:

Grade 0: No perfusion. No anterograde flow of contrast medium is detected beyond the point of occlusion.

Grade 1: Penetration without perfusion. Contrast medium passes through the point of obstruction, but anterograde flow fails to opacify the distal portion of the vessel at any time.

Grade 2: Partial perfusion. Contrast material penetrates through the point of obstruction but enters the distal vessel at a rate slower than that for nonobstructed arteries in the same patient.

Grade 3: Complete perfusion. Anterograde flow into the distal coronary bed is rapid and complete.

The rate of coronary flow as assessed by the TIMI flow grade is determined by two major factors: the severity of the stenosis in the vessel and the status of the microvasculature. The clinical outcome after thrombolysis for acute myocardial infarction is related to TIMI flow grade. After receiving thrombolytic therapy for acute myocardial infarction, patients with TIMI grade 3 flow at 90 minutes had lower mortality rates than those with TIMI grade 2 flow.[80] A method for quantifying the angiographic rates of coronary artery perfusion has been proposed using the TIMI frame count. With this method, the number of cinefilm frames required for opacification of the involved vessel is counted by means of an automated frame counter, which is present on most cineprojectors. The quantitative frame count method offers the advantages of being more objective, more reproducible, and more strongly correlated with clinical outcomes than conventional methods.[81]

Coronary Collateral Circulation

(See also p. 1174)

In the normal human heart, myriad tiny anastomotic branches interconnect the major coronary arteries.[82] Most of these anatomical vessels are less than 200 μm in diameter, and they are the precursors of the collateral circulation. In coronary arteriograms of patients with normal or mildly diseased coronary arteries, they cannot be visualized because they carry only minimal flow and their small caliber is well beyond the spatial resolution capabilities of cine imaging systems. If, however, obstruction of a major coronary artery occurs, a pressure gradient is created in the anastomotic vessels connecting the distal segment of the involved artery with either its proximal segment or the

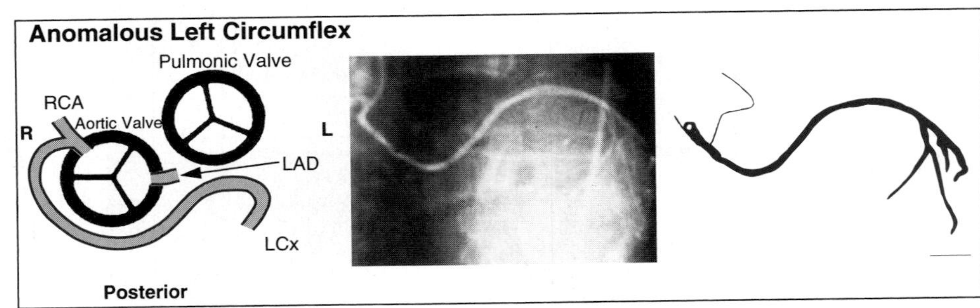

FIGURE 8–29. Anomalous origin of the left circumflex. The caudo-cranial cross-sectional view at the level of the semilunar valves shows the common course of the left circumflex coronary artery aberrantly arising from the right sinus of Valsalva. The LCx passes behind the aortic root and runs to the left atrioventricular groove following an initial course identical to that for the anomalous LCA arising from the right sinus of Valsalva that follows a posterior, retroaortic course (see Fig. 8–27).

nearby segments of other vessels. With the creation of this gradient, an increased volume of blood is propelled through the anastomotic vessels, which progressively dilate and eventually become visible angiographically as collateral channels. The reason this process seems to occur effectively in some patients and ineffectively in others is not entirely clear, but it may involve the rate at which obstruction develops. The most favorable clinical circumstance is gradual development of the obstruction, thereby allowing collateral channels to enlarge and become functional before the native vessel becomes totally occluded.

Other factors that affect collateral development are patency of the feeding arteries and the size and vascular resistance of the postobstructive segment.[83] Some interesting observations on the temporal sequence of collateral development resulted from an angiographic study of patients who showed persistent occlusion of the infarct artery after acute myocardial infarction.[84] Among patients studied within 6 hours of infarction, about half demonstrated angiographically visible collaterals. Among those studied more than 24 hours after infarction, virtually all had visible collaterals. This suggests that collateral flow may develop more quickly than previously thought, perhaps within hours after total occlusion. In any event, collateral circulation does not represent the formation of new vessels but rather the utilization of vessels that already exist but carry little blood flow until the need arises. Collaterals usually cannot be demonstrated at coronary arteriography unless the recipient vessel has developed at least 90 per cent diameter stenosis by visual estimates.[82,85]

A large number of collateral pathways exist in patients with severe coronary artery disease (Figs. 8–30 to 8–32). The functional role of coronary collateral circulation has been debated for many years. In patients with total occlusions, regional left ventricular contraction was significantly better in segments supplied by adequate collateral circulation than in those segments supplied by inadequate or no collateral circulation.[82] In another study, patients with acute myocardial infarction undergoing emergency coronary arteriography without antecedent thrombolytic therapy were divided into those with adequate collateral circulation to the infarct-related vessel and those with inadequate or no collateral circulation to the infarct vessel.[86] The group with adequate collaterals had significantly lower left ventricular end-diastolic pressures, higher cardiac index, higher ejection fraction, and lower percentage of area dyssynergy. None of the patients with adequate collaterals died, whereas the majority with inadequate or no collaterals died. Patients with severe coronary obstruction without collateral circulation were found to have a significantly higher incidence of thallium-201 myocardial perfusion defects than those with collateral circulation.[87] This suggests that collaterals may improve myocardial perfusion in the ischemic zone.

The advent of percutaneous transluminal coronary angioplasty (PTCA, see Chap. 39) has provided opportunities to study hemodynamic aspects and angiographic patterns of the coronary collateral circulation, since balloon inflation during PTCA simulates abrupt occlusion of a previously stenotic vessel. Using bilateral coronary angiography, Rentrop and Cohen[88] developed a grading system of 0 to 3 for collateral filling classified as follows:

Grade 0: No collaterals present

Grade 1: Barely detectable collateral flow. Contrast medium passes through collateral channels but fails to opacify the epicardial vessel at any time.

Grade 2: Partial collateral flow. Contrast material enters but fails to opacify the target epicardial vessel completely.

Grade 3: Complete perfusion. Contrast material enters and completely opacifies the target epicardial vessel.

With balloon inflation during PTCA, patients with well-developed collaterals experienced less pain, less left ventricular dyssynergy, and less summed ST-segment elevation than those with poorly developed collaterals.[88] Distal coronary perfusion pressure during balloon inflation is higher in patients with well-developed collaterals than in those with poorly developed collateral circulation.[89–91]

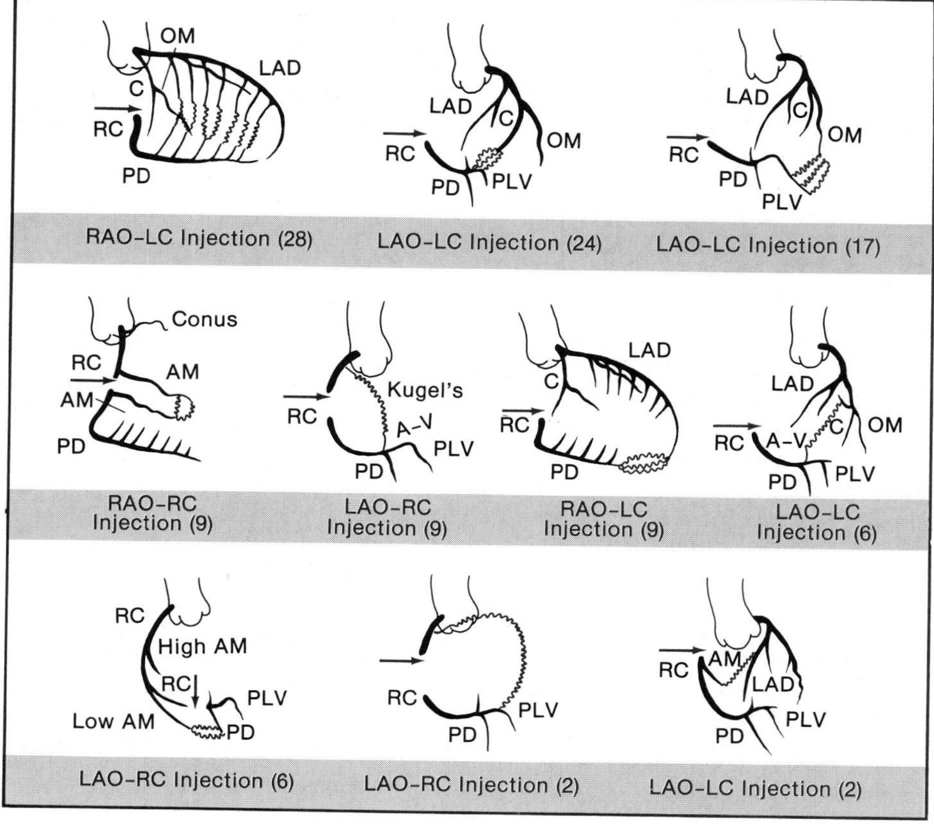

FIGURE 8–30. Coronary collaterals seen with RCA occlusion. Common collateral pathways seen with RCA occlusion. The arrows point to the site of obstruction. The small tortuous channels represent the collateral connections. Numbers in parentheses refer to the frequency with which each pathway was visualized in a series of 200 patients with significant coronary disease. RC = right coronary artery, C = circumflex artery, OM = obtuse marginal branch of the circumflex artery, PD = posterior descending branch of the right coronary artery, PLV = posterior left ventricular branch of the right coronary artery, AM = acute marginal branch of the right coronary artery, A-V = artery to the atrioventricular node. (Reproduced with permission from Levin, D. C.: Pathways and functional significance of the coronary collateral circulation. Circulation *50*:831, 1974, Copyright 1974 American Heart Association.)

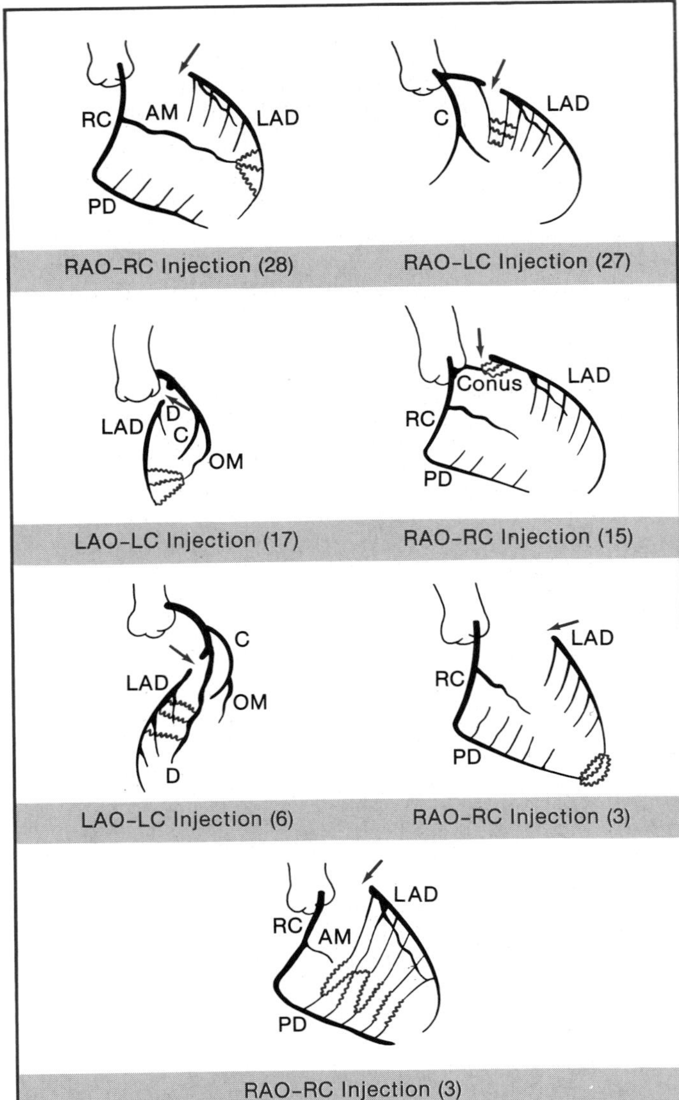

FIGURE 8–31. Common collateral pathways seen with LAD occlusion. (See Fig. 8–30 legend for abbreviations.) (From Levin, D. C.: Pathways and functional significance of the coronary collateral circulation. Circulation *50*:831, 1974. Copyright 1974 American Heart Association.)

Coronary Artery Spasm

(See also p. 1340)

Almost four decades have elapsed since Prinzmetal and coworkers[92] described an unusual or variant form of angina in which the onset of chest pain was not provoked by the usual factors, such as exercise, emotional upset, cold, or ingestion of a meal. According to currently accepted theories, patients considered to have variant angina are those in whom chest pain commences at rest or occurs both at rest and during exertion.[93] The pain often occurs in a cyclical pattern at the same time every day, generally in the morning, and usually is accompanied by ST-segment elevation if an electrocardiogram is recorded. Symptoms may occur many times daily, cease for weeks or months, and then recur. Although the ST-segment elevation often is striking, it rapidly reverts to normal when the pain disappears spontaneously or is terminated by the administration of nitroglycerin. Ischemic episodes may be accompanies by atrioventricular block, ventricular ectopic activity, ventricular tachycardia, or ventricular fibrillation. Although the original description of this syndrome emphasized its transient nature and its onset at rest, it has become apparent through further studies that coronary spasm also can play a role in exercise-induced angina, unstable angina, acute myocardial infarction, and sudden death.[92]

The mechanisms of coronary vasospasm are varied. Current evidence suggests that the presence of coronary atherosclerosis interferes with the normal ability of the endothelium to reduce resting tone of the coronary artery. The normal endothelium releases nitric oxide and prostacyclin (PGI_2), which relax the underlying smooth muscle cells and produce vasodilatation. Aggregating platelets release vasoconstrictor substances such as thromboxane A_2 and serotonin (5-hydroxytryptamine). Atherosclerosis interferes with the synthesis and action of the vasoactive substances produced by the endothelium. Thrombin has antithrombotic properties in intact endothelium. It is able to release enough nitric oxide and prostacyclin to overcome platelet-induced contraction resulting from the direct activation of platelets by thrombin.[54]

Coronary arteriography has played an important role in understanding the pathophysiology and clinical consequences of coronary artery spasm. In the early 1970's, several angiographic studies demonstrated spasm in patients with clinical variant angina.[94] These studies showed that although spasm usually was superimposed on areas of fixed stenosis, in some cases it occurred in segments of coronary arteries that appeared angiographically normal. Postmortem studies, however, have essentially confirmed the relation between spasm and coronary atherosclerosis, with only one case serving as an exception to the general rule that coronary artery spasm is associated with coronary atherosclerosis. In the late 1970's, intravenous ergonovine maleate was used to provoke spasm in patients with suspected variant angina who were undergoing coronary arteriography.[95] A comprehensive angiographic study of the frequency of coronary spasm was carried out by Bertrand

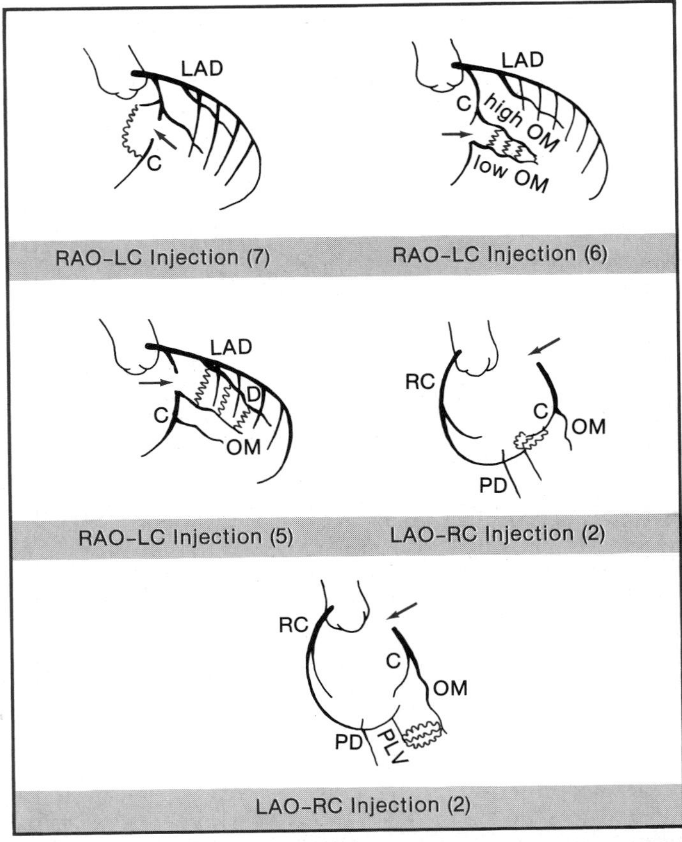

FIGURE 8–32. Common collateral pathways seen with LCx occlusion. (See Fig. 8–30 legend for abbreviations.) (From Levin, D. C.: Pathways and functional significance of the coronary collateral circulation. Circulation *50*:831, 1974. Copyright 1974 American Heart Association.)

and coworkers[96] in 1089 consecutive patients undergoing coronary arteriography for chest pain. Patients with left main coronary artery disease, severe three-vessel disease, NYHA functional class III or IV symptoms, or spontaneously occurring spasm were excluded. Of the 1089 patients, 134 exhibited spasm after ergonovine; in 59 per cent of these patients spasm was associated with angiographic evidence of a coronary stenosis, whereas in 41 per cent it occurred in an angiographically normal segment. Although ergonovine-induced spasm occurred rarely (less than 5 per cent) in patients with atypical chest pain or exertional angina, it occurred in 14 per cent of patients with symptoms of both exertional and resting angina. Ergonovine-induced coronary spasm was seen in 85 per cent of patients with primarily rest angina who were observed to have episodes of ST-segment elevation. In patients with recent myocardial infarction (less than 6 weeks), ergonovine-induced spasm was noted in 20 per cent.

Serious complications, including irreversible occlusion,[97] occur on rare occasions during ergonovine testing. The use of acetylcholine for diagnosing spasm is limited by the increased sensitivity and lack of specificity of the test; almost all patients with coronary atherosclerosis show evidence of at least mild constriction upon treatment with acetylcholine.[7] The diagnosis of coronary artery spasm must be supported by clinical features and response to treatment with nitrate compounds and calcium channel blockers.

INTERVENTIONAL CORONARY ARTERIOGRAPHY

(See also Chap. 39)

The introduction of balloon angioplasty by Grüntzig and coworkers[98] in 1977 and the subsequent development of atherectomy, coronary stenting, and laser angioplasty for specific lesion types have placed new demands on coronary arteriography for accurate characterization of lesion morphology. The angiographer must identify projections that show each target lesion clearly without foreshortening. In addition, the approach to the target lesion must be clearly delineated. For most cardiologists, this is probably a natural goal of the arteriographic procedure because approximately two-thirds of angiographers also perform angioplasty.[99] Several recommendations for interventional coronary arteriography can thus be made:

1. Before an intervention is planned, disease in the unprotected LMCA must be excluded. If pressure damping with a diagnostic catheter is detected, this probably reflects significant narrowing of the LMCA and predicts the likelihood of significant pressure damping when larger coronary guide catheters are used.
2. The course to the target lesion must be displayed conspicuously.
3. The target lesion itself should be projected in at least two views before interventional therapy.
4. The morphology of the lesion should be plainly defined by the angiographic procedure.
5. The lesion after angioplasty must be viewed in multiple projections after all intracoronary guidewires are retracted to assess adequacy of treatment, residual thrombus, and vessel dissection.

Lesion Morphology

In the American College of Cardiology/American Heart Association classification for coronary angioplasty,[100] lesion types are defined as simple (Type A), moderately complex (Type B), and complex (Type C) (Table 39–3, p. 1370). In a recent series of patients undergoing conventional balloon angioplasty,[101] most lesions were found to be moderately complex (Table 8–3).

TABLE 8–3 LESION CHARACTERISTICS OF PATIENTS UNDERGOING ANGIOPLASTY

N	733 (%)
Lesion complexity (ACC-AHA score)*	
A	227 (31)
B	314 (43)
C	192 (26)
Specific lesion types	
Saphenous vein graft lesion	517 (70)
Eccentric stenosis	169 (23)
Tubular lesion (10–20 mm)	121 (17)
Diffuse disease (>20 mm)	56 (7.6)
Total occlusion	60 (8.2)
Ostial stenosis	10 (1.4)
Bifurcation lesion	31 (4.2)
Ulcerated lesion	56 (7.6)
Thrombus present	21 (2.9)
Lesion in bend >45 degrees	16 (2.2)
Lesion in bend >90 degrees	4 (0.5)
Severely calcified stenosis	9 (1.2)

*ACC-AHA = American College of Cardiology/American Heart Association Task Force on PTCA.[100]

Wolfe, M. W., Roubin, G. S., Schweiger, M., et al.: Length of hospital stay and complications after percutaneous transluminal coronary angioplasty: Clinical and procedural predictors. Circulation *92*:311, 1995. Copyright 1995 American Heart Association.

Lesion eccentricity is assessed in a nonforeshortened projection and is evident by asymmetry. Although a quantitative assessment of the eccentricity index as the percentage deviation of the stenosis centerline from the vessel centerline has been used in some studies,[102] it is more common to use qualitative assessment.

Lesion angulation also must be assessed in a nonforeshortened end-diastolic projection. Visual assessment is frequently used but is less accurate than the semiquantitative method, in which the angle between 20-mm arterial centerlines originating at the stenosis is calculated to define the angle between the proximal and distal segments.[103] Although a hand-held protractor may be useful to measure the angle,[104] some angiographers measure the angle of the noninflated balloon catheter positioned across the stenosis.[104] Lesions associated with bends of 45 degrees or more are simply classified as "angulated," and lesions with bends of 90 degrees or more are commonly classified as "severely angulated."

CORONARY THROMBUS. Because coronary angiography provides a silhouette of lesion edges, it has limited ability to identify intracoronary thrombus as compared with other imaging modalities such as angioscopy.[105] Despite its limitations, the angiographic detection of complex lesions or thrombus in unstable angina has important prognostic and therapeutic implications. Angiographic-pathological correlations have suggested that an eccentric stenosis with a narrow neck, overhanging edge, or scalloped border corresponds to plaque rupture or hemorrhage, with superimposed partially occlusive or recanalized thrombus.[106] The most specific angiographic hallmark of intracoronary thrombus, however, is the presence of a globular filling defect, completely surrounded by contrast material and usually located distal to the point of most severe stenosis (Figs. 8–33 and 8–34). When an eccentric lesion is associated with contrast retention, thrombolytic intervention is often unsuccessful, suggesting that these lesions may actually represent areas of microvascular channels and not thrombus.[107]

The angiographic detection of thrombus varies from 6 to 17 per cent in angioplasty series and from 16 to 57 per cent in angiographic series.[107–116] The variation in the reporting of coronary thrombus in angiography is attributed to the type of study performed, the patient population studied, and definitions used. Patients in angioplasty series have a lower incidence of intracoronary thrombus than those in

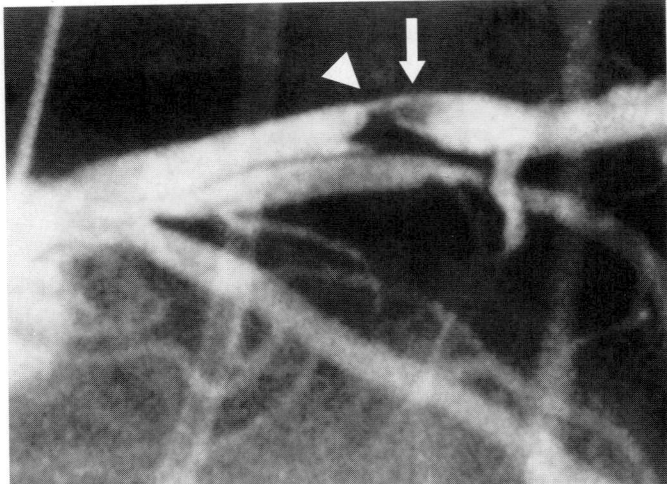

FIGURE 8–33. Intracoronary thrombus in acute myocardial infarction. In the setting of acute myocardial infarction, this RAO caudal left coronary arteriogram shows an eccentric lesion (arrowhead) in the proximal left anterior descending artery, immediately followed by a globular filling defect (arrow) surrounded by contrast medium on all sides.

angiographic series because angioplasty is often postponed when thrombus is detected.[104,110,113–118] Patients with rest angina or postinfarction angina have been found to have a higher likelihood of intracoronary thrombus than those with crescendo angina.[108,110] Angiographic detection of complex or ulcerated lesions in unstable angina is associated with an increased likelihood of thrombosis and an increased risk of adverse cardiac events.[119]

CORONARY DISSECTION. Interventional cardiovascular treatments occasionally are associated with the formation of vessel dissection, and rarely the performance of diagnostic coronary arteriography may be associated with vessel dissection. Thus, the angiographer must be familiar with the angiographic patterns of vessel dissection. Patients with severe dissections associated with contrast retention or propagation are more likely to experience complications outside the cardiac catheterization laboratory than those with mild dissections[120] (Fig. 8–35). The National Heart, Lung, and Blood Institute (NHLBI) Registry scoring system for vessel dissection has been modified to provide a uniform scale for rating dissections[120,121]:

Grade A: A radiolucent area, often linear, within the coronary lumen during contrast injection with minimal or no persistence of contrast after the dye has cleared.

Grade B: Parallel tracts or double lumen separated by a

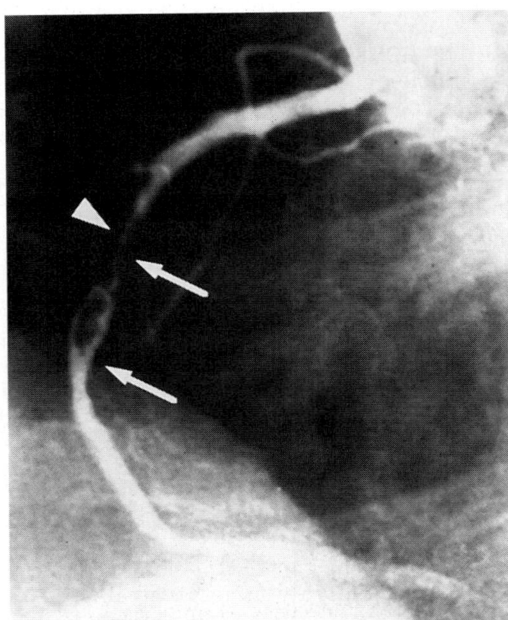

FIGURE 8–34. Intracoronary thrombus in unstable angina. This LAO right coronary arteriogram shows a severe stenosis in the mid-portion of the RCA (arrowhead), followed by a large filling defect surrounded by contrast medium on all sides (arrows).

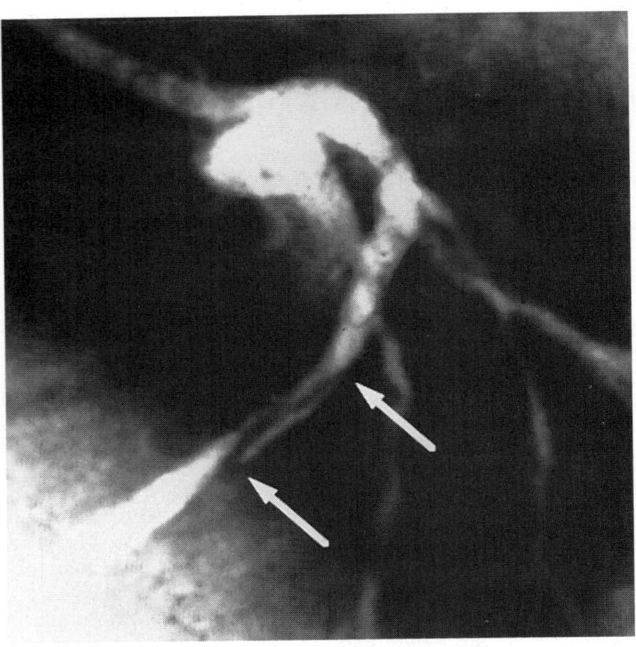

FIGURE 8–35. Moderately severe coronary dissection. This LAO cranial left coronary arteriogram shows a large intramural collection of contrast medium (arrows) at the site of angioplasty in the proximal LAD. Although contrast medium cleared rapidly from LAD itself, contrast medium persisted within the dissection itself, thus meeting criteria for a Grade C dissection (see text discussion).[120,121]

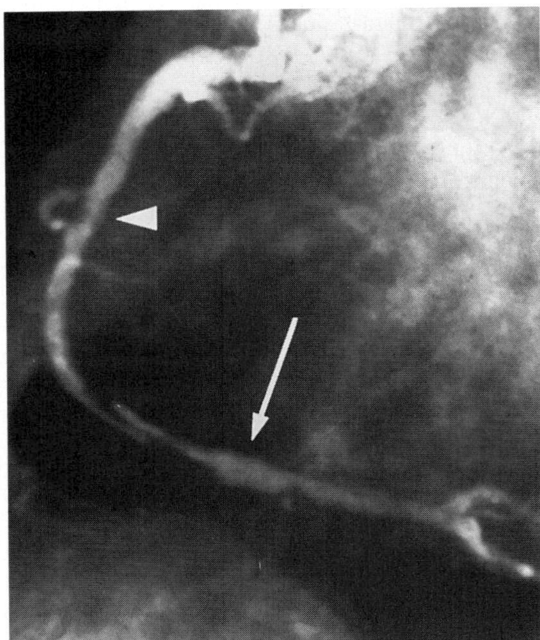

FIGURE 8–36. Spiral dissection. This LAO right coronary arteriogram shows evidence of a vessel dissection emanating from the site of angioplasty in the midportion of the RCA (arrowhead) and extending to the distal RCA (arrow), thus meeting criteria for a severe Grade D dissection.[120,121]

radiolucent area during contrast injection with minimal or no persistence after dye clearance.

Grade C: Contrast material immediately outside the coronary lumen but within the vessel wall with persistence of contrast material in the area after clearance of dye from the coronary lumen.

Grade D: Spiral luminal filling defects, frequently with extensive contrast material staining of the vessel (Fig. 8–36).

Dissection is more commonly detected than thrombus by angiography and by angioscopy in patients experiencing abrupt vessel closure. In 109 patients with abrupt vessel closure, 39 (34 per cent) had angiographic evidence of dissection, but 30 had evidence of thrombus (27 per cent).[122] In 65 patients with abrupt vessel closure, 31 (48 per cent) had dissection, but 27 (42 per cent) had evidence of thrombus.[101] In an angioscopic evaluation of abrupt vessel closure, 14 of 17 patients had evidence of dissection or extruded atheromatous plaque, but only 3 of 17 patients had evidence of thrombus.[123]

TOTAL OCCLUSIONS. Angiography of total occlusions requires detailed assessment of the anatomy at the site of the occlusion, the extent of collateral development, and the length of the totally occluded segment. The morphology at the point of total occlusion influences the likelihood of success with interventional cardiovascular procedures. Total occlusions associated with a blunt occlusion (Fig. 8–37) are less likely to result in successful angioplasty than those with a tapering funnel[124] (Fig. 8–38). The vascular segment distal to the obstruction occasionally requires visualization via contralateral collaterals.

PSEUDOLESIONS. When a tortuous coronary artery is straightened with an angioplasty wire, the redundant intimal tissue may compress via a "concertina effect" to produce coronary "pseudonarrowings"[125] or intimal intussusception (Fig. 8–39). These narrowings are not responsive to nitroglycerin and usually are resistant to balloon angioplasty. The characteristic appearance of sharply angulated protrusions of tissue into the lumen in a staircase pattern is a clue to the presence of coronary pseudonarrowings. Removal of the guidewire abolishes this angiographic finding.

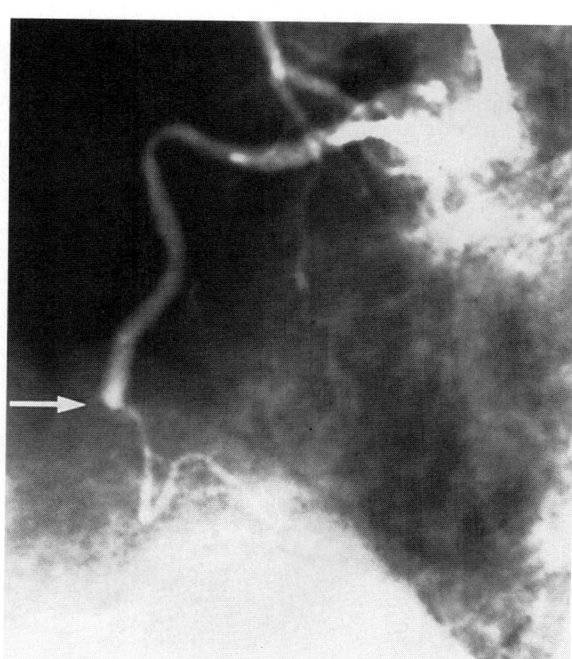

FIGURE 8–37. Total occlusion with blunt appearance. The LAO right coronary arteriogram shows a blunt total occlusion (arrow) of the midportion of the right coronary artery associated with a side branch. The blunt appearance and the presence of the side branch are characteristics that suggest that angioplasty may be unsuccessful.

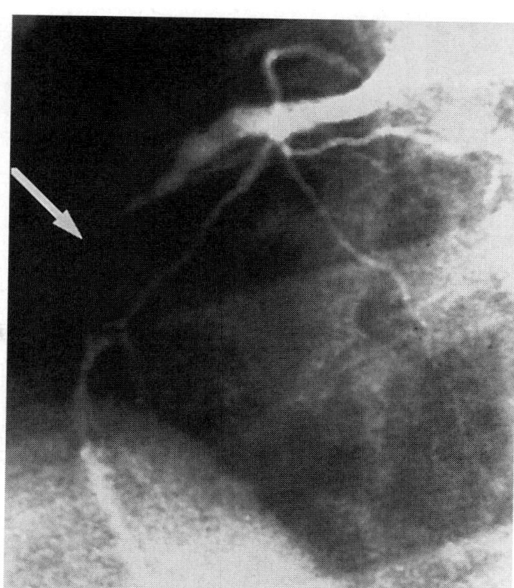

FIGURE 8–38. Total occlusion with taper. The LAO right coronary arteriogram shows a total occlusion (arrow) of the midportion of the RCA, but the smoothly tapering appearance of the site of total occlusion suggests that attempts with angioplasty may be successful.

RELATION BETWEEN ARTERIOGRAPHIC FINDINGS AND CLINICAL OUTCOME

Numerous studies have determined that the strongest predictors of survival in patients with coronary artery disease are (1) extent of coronary artery disease, (2) left ventricular function, and (3) exercise tolerance measured as time on the treadmill test (Chap. 38).

In the CASS Registry, the 7-year survival rate was 96 per cent among patients with completely smooth coronary arteries and 92 per cent among patients with luminal irregularities associated with less than 50 per cent stenosis of one or more coronary segments.[126] Among 1977 patients followed in the Duke University Cardiovascular Disease Databank, those with completely normal vessels had an infarct-free 10-year survival rate of 98 per cent, whereas those with less than a 75 per cent stenosis of any coronary artery

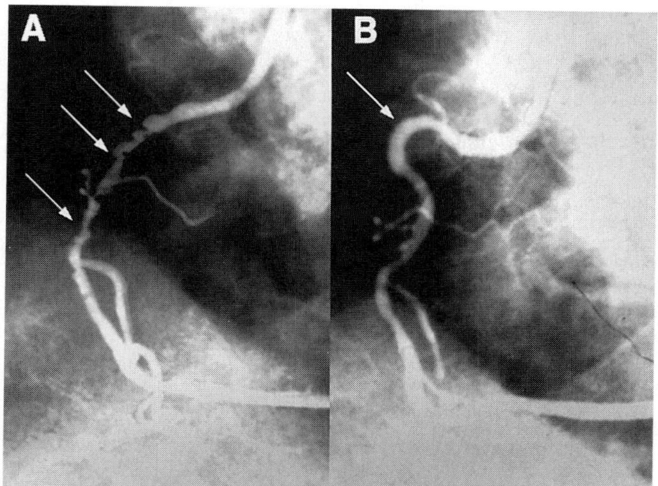

FIGURE 8–39. Coronary pseudolesions. The LAO coronary arteriogram shows evidence of multiple, sharply angulated narrowings (arrows) in the proximal RCA when an angioplasty guidewire is present with its tip in the distal RCA *(A)*. These areas were unresponsive to intracoronary nitroglycerin but immediately resolved upon removal of the guidewire *(B)*, revealing a very tortuous RCA with a prominent shepherd's crook (arrow) in the proximal segment.

TABLE 8–4 RELATION BETWEEN 4-YEAR SURVIVAL (%) AND EXTENT OF CORONARY ARTERY DISEASE AND LEFT VENTRICULAR DYSFUNCTION

EXTENT OF CAD	EF > 50%	EF 35 – 49%	EF < 35%
One-vessel CAD	95	91	74
Two-vessel CAD	93	83	57
Three-vessel CAD	82	71	50

Reproduced from Mock, M. B., Ringqvist, I., Fisher, L.D., et al.: Survival of medically treated patients in the Coronary Artery Surgery Study (CASS) registry. Circulation *66*:562, 1982. Copyright 1982 American Heart Association.

had an infarct-free 10-year survival rate of 90 per cent.[127] Patients with significant left main coronary artery disease are at increased risk. The cumulative survival among a group of medically treated patients with more than 70 per cent stenosis of the left main coronary artery was 72 per cent at 1 year and 41 per cent at 3 years.[128] For patients with left main coronary artery stenosis between 50 and 70 per cent, the prognosis was more favorable, with 91 per cent survival at 1 year and 66 per cent survival at 3 years. For patients with at least 75 per cent left main coronary artery stenosis on medical therapy, 42-month survival was 48 per cent for medically treated patients and 75 per cent for patients undergoing coronary artery bypass surgery.[129] Thus left main coronary artery disease is an indication for bypass surgery (see p. 1322).

The relations among survival, coronary artery disease, and left ventricular function have been assessed in the CASS Registry in 20,088 patients.[130] The 4-year survival rate for patients with more than 70 per cent diameter stenosis of one coronary artery was 92 per cent, for two coronary arteries 84 per cent, and for three coronary arteries 68 per cent. Left ventricular ejection fraction (EF), however, was found to be a more important predictor of survival (Table 8–4). Four-year survival was 95 per cent for patients with one-vessel disease and an EF greater than 50 per cent, 91 per cent for patients with an EF in the range of 35 to 49 per cent, and 74 per cent for patients with an EF of less than 35 per cent. Similar relations between survival and left ventricular dysfunction were seen for patients with two-vessel and three-vessel disease as well.

Relation Between Coronary Lesion Morphology and Clinical Presentation

It has been accepted from angiographic,[106,108,109,119,131] angioscopic,[105,132,133] and histological[134–139] observations that plaque inflammation, rupture, and nonocclusive thrombus formation precipitate unstable angina (see p. 1333). However, there is wide variability in the detection of these pathogenic events with angiographic and angioscopic methods. For example, only 10 to 26 per cent of patients with unstable angina have angiographic evidence of thrombus,[9,107–110,119,131] whereas the majority of such patients show angioscopic findings of intracoronary thrombus.[105,132,133] New information from the examination of atherectomy specimens[112,138] confirms the role of coronary thrombus formation in a significant proportion of patients with unstable angina but raises important questions about pathophysiology in the remaining patients. Although many episodes of unstable angina are undoubtedly caused by plaque rupture and thrombus formation, other mechanisms that alter the balance between myocardial oxygen supply and demand must be considered. For example, vasoconstriction may occur in the absence of deep arterial injury if endothelial function is abnormal.[140]

Several studies have suggested that angiographic plaque morphology is correlated with the clinical status and prognosis of the patient. In a study of 110 patients with stable or unstable angina, Ambrose and coworkers[131] classified lesions into four categories: concentric stenoses with smooth borders, eccentric stenoses with smooth borders, eccentric stenoses with complex borders (narrow base or neck caused by overhanging edges, or scalloped borders), and lesions with multiple irregularities. Among patients with stable angina, complex angiographic stenoses were present in 18 per cent of coronary arteries. Among the patients with unstable angina, complex lesions were seen in 56 per cent. These data show that in patients with unstable angina, lesions characterized by overhanging edges, scalloped or irregular borders, or multiple irregularities were more than three times as common than in patients with stable angina.

UNSTABLE ANGINA **(see also p. 1331)**. Because a broad spectrum of patients with myocardial ischemia varying widely in cause, prognosis, and responsiveness to therapy are lumped together under the single diagnosis of "unstable angina pectoris," a new clinical classification that depends on the timing of rest pain and its relation to previous myocardial infarction has been proposed.[141] The new classification is based on the acuity of presentation (presence and timing of rest pain) and the clinical presentation. In 246 consecutive patients with unstable angina and 50 patients with stable angina, the severity of angina was based on a score derived from the clinical circumstances (0 = stable angina, 1 = unstable angina secondary to a noncardiac condition such as anemia, 2 = unstable angina de novo, and 3 = postinfarction angina) and the acuity of presentation (0 = stable angina, 1 = no rest pain, 2 = rest pain occurring more than 48 hours before evaluation, and 3 = rest pain occurring 48 hours or less before evaluation).

Angiographic findings varied widely.[108] Depending on both the acuity and clinical circumstances of presentation, the probability of minimal obstruction (<50 per cent stenosis) ranged from 2.1 to 20.0 per cent, and the incidence of intracoronary filling defects varied from 0.0 to 22.2 per cent. The unstable angina score was identified as the most important predictor of presence of intracoronary filling defects. Multiple regression analysis showed that the unstable angina score also predicted lesion complexity in the ischemia-related vessel ($P = 0.001$). The multiple regression model, which included unstable angina score and quantitative measurements of lesion severity such as minimal lumen diameter and flow, may account for about 55 per cent of the variability in lesion complexity ($r^2 = 0.55$, $P = 10^{-6}$). Thus, unstable angina pectoris is a heterogeneous syndrome with a wide range of clinical presentations and underlying coronary morphology. The classification of unstable angina[141] predicts underlying angiographic anatomy and may thus aid in the decision regarding diagnostic procedures as well as provide a sound basis for evaluating the response to therapy in patients with unstable angina.

Relation Between Stenosis Severity and Clinical Outcome

(See also Chap. 38)

It was long assumed that the risk posed to the patient with a given coronary artery stenosis is related to the severity of the obstruction: The greater the degree of narrowing, the greater is the degree of risk of myocardial infarction and death. Conversely, mild or moderate stenoses (less than 50 per cent) were assumed to cause less risk. Investigations using sequential coronary arteriograms with or without lipid-lowering interventions have disproved this notion.

Angiographic studies of cholesterol reduction have provided additional insights into the relation between lesion severity and clinical events. In the National Heart, Lung, and Blood Institute Type II Coronary Intervention Study,[142] a total of 116 men with elevated low-density lipoprotein (LDL) cholesterol levels were randomly assigned to treatment with dietary modification alone or dietary modification plus cholestyramine. Coronary arteriography was performed at baseline and at 5 years. Although cholestyramine resulted in a 17 per cent reduction in cholesterol levels, coronary artery disease progressed in 32 per cent of cholestyramine patients versus 49 per cent of control patients.[142]

In the Familial Atherosclerosis Treatment Study (FATS),[143] 120 men with coronary artery disease were given dietary counseling and randomly assigned to treatment with lovastatin plus colestipol, niacin plus colestipol, or placebo. After 2.5 years of treatment, total cholesterol levels were reduced by 34 per cent in the group receiving lovastatin plus colestipol, by 23 per cent in the group receiving niacin plus colestipol, and by 4 per cent in the control group. Progression of coronary artery disease was detected in 21 per cent in the group receiving lovastatin plus colestipol, 25 per cent in the group receiving niacin plus colestipol, and 46 per cent in the control group. Regression of disease was detected in 32 per cent in the group receiving lovastatin plus colestipol, 39 per cent in the group receiving niacin plus colestipol, and 11 per cent in the control group. Although stenosis severity was reduced by a modest 0.3 and 1.1 per cent in the two groups with active treatment, there was a striking difference in clinical events: fatal or nonfatal myocardial infarction occurred in 4 per cent in the group receiving lovastatin plus colestipol, 6 per cent in the group receiving niacin plus colestipol, but in 19 per cent in the control group.[143]

A similar relation between quantitative angiography and clinical events after cholesterol reduction has been observed in several other studies. In the St. Thomas' Atherosclerosis Regression Study (STARS),[144] cholestyramine and dietary modification reduced stenosis severity by 1.5 per cent. This was associated with a substantial reduction in death and cardiovascular events.[144] Thus, cholesterol-lowering therapy results in modest reductions in stenosis severity but striking reductions in the incidence of cardiovascular events. One possible explanation for this apparent discrepancy may relate to endothelial function and the propensity for plaque rupture.[145,146]

The relation between stenosis severity and the likelihood of myocardial infarction has been evaluated in several studies. Ambrose and colleagues[147] compared the degree of baseline coronary stenoses in 38 patients who underwent two separate coronary arteriograms and had experienced either myocardial infarction or new total occlusion without infarction during the interval. In the infarct group, only 22 per cent of the culprit lesions were initially greater than 70 per cent, whereas in the noninfarct group, 61 per cent of the lesions that subsequently progressed to total occlusion were initially greater than 70 per cent. The lesions responsible for Q-wave myocardial infarction were characterized by a mean stenosis of only 34 per cent.

In another similar study of the progression of coronary artery disease, it was found that only 15 per cent of lesions that produced myocardial infarctions were severe (greater than 75 per cent) and half were mild (less than 50 per cent) on the initial angiogram.[148] Most patients who developed new total occlusion did not experience infarcts; 48 per cent of these stenoses were greater than 75 per cent on the initial coronary arteriograms. Little and colleagues[149] in a separate report reviewed coronary arteriograms in 42 consecutive patients who had been studied both before and shortly after acute myocardial infarction. In 29 patients a new total occlusion was observed on the second arteriogram. Among these 29 patients, 66 per cent of the culprit stenoses had been less than 50 per cent on the initial arteriogram, and almost all of them had been less than 70 per cent.

These observations are inconsistent with the simplistic notion that the severity of obstruction is proportional to an increased risk of myocardial infarction and cardiac death. Rather, the angiographic evidence of the presence of coronary artery disease provides more clinical information than the severity of the obstruction itself. This lack of correlation may be related to the inability of angiography to identify unstable plaques that are at high risk of rupture and to distinguish them from critically obstructive stenoses that are stable.

REFERENCES

1. Sones, F. M., and Shirey, E. K.: Cine coronary arteriography. Med. Concepts Cardiovasc. Dis. *31*:735, 1962.
2. Graves, E. J.: Vital and Health Statistics: National Hospital Discharge Survey: Annual Summary 1991. Hyattsville, Md., National Center for Health Statistics, 1993.
3. American Hospital Association guide to the health care field. Chicago, American Hospital Association, 1993.
4. Pepine, C. J., Allen, H. D., Bashore, T. M., et al.: ACC/AHA guidelines for cardiac catheterization and cardiac catheterization laboratories: American College of Cardiology/American Heart Association Ad Hoc Task Force on Cardiac Catheterization. Circulation *84*:2213, 1991.

INDICATIONS FOR CORONARY ARTERIOGRAPHY

5. Fletcher, G. F., Balady, G., Froelicher, V. F., et al.: Exercise standards: A statement for healthcare professionals from the American Heart Association. Circulation *91*:580, 1995.
6. Travin, M. I., Boucher, C. A., Newell, J. B., et al.: Variables associated with a poor prognosis in patients with an ischemic thallium-201 exercise test. Am. Heart J. *125*:335, 1993.
7. Ludmer, P. L., Selwyn, A. P., Shook, T. L., et al.: Paradoxical vasoconstriction induced by acetylcholine in atherosclerotic coronary arteries. N. Engl. J. Med. *315*:1046, 1986.
8. Braunwald, E., Jones, R. H., Mark, D. B., et al.: Diagnosing and managing unstable angina. Circulation *90*:613, 1994.
9. The TIMI IIIB Investigators: Effects of tissue plasminogen activator and a comparison of early invasive and conservative strategies in unstable angina and non–Q-wave myocardial infarction. Circulation *89*:1545, 1994.
10. Michels, K. B., and Yusuf, S.: Does PTCA in acute myocardial infarction affect mortality and reinfarction rates? A quantitative overview (meta-analysis) of the randomized clinical trials. Circulation *91*:476, 1995.
11. Ellis, S. G., Ribeiro da Silva, E., Heyndrickx, G., et al.: Randomized comparison of rescue angioplasty with conservative management of patients with early failure of thrombolysis for acute anterior myocardial infarction. Circulation *90*:2280, 1994.
12. Fish, R. D., Nabel, E. G., Selwyn, A. P., et al.: Responses of coronary arteries of cardiac transplant patients to acetylcholine. J. Clin. Invest. *81*:21, 1988.
13. Amplatz, K., Formanek, G., Stanger, P., and Wilson, W.: Mechanics of selective coronary artery catheterization via femoral approach. Radiology *89*:1040, 1967.
14. Schoonmaker, F. W., and King, S. B., III: Coronary arteriography by the single catheter percutaneous femoral technique. Circulation *50*:735, 1974.
15. Holzman, R. S., Cullen, D. J., Eichhorn, J. H., and Philip, J. H.: Guidelines for sedation by nonanesthesiologists during diagnostic and therapeutic procedures. J. Clin. Anesthesiol. *6*:265, 1994.
16. Bailey, P. L., Pace, N. L., Ashburn, M. A., et al.: Frequent hypoxemia and apnea after sedation with midazolam and fentanyl. Anesthesiology *73*:826, 1990.
17. Davis, K., Kennedy, J. W., Kemp, H. G., Jr., et al.: Complications of coronary arteriography. Circulation *59*:1105, 1979.
18. Lasser, E. D., Berry, C. C., Talner, L. B., et al.: Pretreatment with corticosteroids to alleviate reactions to intravenous contrast material. N. Engl. J. Med. *317*:845, 1987.
19. Bettmann, M. A.: Radiographic contrast agents—A perspective. N. Engl. J. Med. *317*:891, 1987.
20. Levi, M., Pascucci, C., Agnelli, G., et al.: Effect on thrombus growth and thrombolysis of two types of osmolar contrast media in rabbits. Invest. Radiol. *25*:533, 1990.
21. Ing, J. J., Smith, D. C., and Bull, B. S.: Differing mechanisms of clotting inhibition by ionic and nonionic contrast agents. Radiology *172*:345, 1989.
22. Rasuli, P., McLeish, W. A., and Hammond, D. I.: Anticoagulant effects of contrast materials: In vitro study of iohexol, ioxaglate, and diatrizoate. A.J.R. *152*:309, 1989.
23. Taliercio, C. P., McCallister, B. H., Holmes, D. R., Jr., et al.: Nephrotoxicity of nonionic contrast media after cardiac angiography. Am. J. Cardiol. *64*:815, 1989.
24. Brogan, W. C., III, Hillis, L. D., and Lange, R. A.: Contrast agents for cardiac catheterization: Conceptions and misconceptions. Am. Heart J. *122*:1129, 1991.
25. Solomon, R., Werner, C., Mann, D., et al.: Effects of saline, mannitol, and furosemide to prevent acute decreases in renal function induced by radiocontrast agents. N. Engl. J. Med. *331*:1416, 1994.
26. Holmes, D. R., Jr., Wondrow, M. A., and Julsrud, P. R.: Radiographic techniques used in cardiac catheterization. *In* Pepine, C. J., Hill, J. A., Lambert, C. R. (eds.): Diagnostic and Therapeutic Cardiac Catheterization. Baltimore, Williams and Wilkins, 1994, p. 141.
27. Gurley, J. C., Nissen, S. E., Booth, D. C., et al.: Comparison of simultaneously performed digital and film-based angiography in the assessment of coronary artery disease. Circulation *78*:1411, 1988.
28. Nissen, S. E.: Principles and applications of digital imaging in cardiac and coronary angiography. *In* Pepine, C. J., Hill, J.A., Lambert, C. R. (eds.): Diagnostic and Therapeutic Cardiac Catheterization. Baltimore, Williams and Wilkins, 1994, p. 162.
29. Nissen, S. E.: Principles of Radiographic Imaging. *In* Roubin, G. S., Califf, R. M., O'Neill, W. W., et al. (eds.): Interventional Cardiovascular Medicine. New York, Churchill Livingstone, 1994, p. 409.
30. King, S. B., III: Foreword. *In* Serruys, P. W., Foley, D. P., and De Feyter, P. J. (eds.): Quantitative Coronary Angiography in Clinical Practice. Boston, Kluwer Academic Publishers, 1994, p. xvii.
31. Folland, E. D., Vogel, R. A., Hartigan, P., et al.: Relation between coronary artery stenosis assessed by visual, caliper, and computer methods and exercise capacity in patients with single-vessel coronary artery disease. Circulation *89*:2005, 1994.
32. Beauman, G. J., and Vogel, R. A.: Accuracy of individual and panel visual interpretations of coronary arteriograms: Implications for clinical decisions. J. Am. Coll. Cardiol. *16*:108, 1990.
33. Kalbfleisch, S. J., McGillem, M. J., Pinto, I. M. F., et al.: Comparison of automated quantitative coronary angiography with caliper measurements of percent diameter stenosis. Am. J. Cardiol. *65*:1181, 1990.
34. White, C. W., Wright, C. B., Doty, D. B., et al.: Does the visual interpretation of the coronary arteriogram predict the physiologic significance of a coronary stenosis? N. Engl. J. Med. *310*:819, 1984.
35. Stadius, M. L., and Alderman, A. L.: Coronary artery revascularization: Critical need for, and consequences of, objective angiographic assessment of lesion severity. Circulation *82*:2231, 1990.
36. Uehata, A., Matsugushi, T., Bittl, J. A., et al.: The accuracy of electronic digital calipers compared with quantitative angiography in measuring arterial diameters. Circulation *88*:1724, 1993.

37. Bunnell, I. L., Greene, D. G., Tandon, R. N., and Arani, D. T.: The half axial projection: A new look at the proximal left coronary artery. Circulation *48*:151, 1973.
38. Arani, D. T., Bunnell, I. L., and Greene, D. G.: Lordotic right posterior oblique projection of the left coronary artery: A special view for special anatomy. Circulation *52*:504, 1975.
39. Judkins, M. W.: Coronary arteriography. *In* Douglas, J. S., Jr., and King, S. B., III (eds.): Coronary Arteriography and Intervention. New York, McGraw-Hill, 1985.
40. Leung, W.-H., Alderman, E. L., Lee, T. C., and Stadius, M. L.: Quantitative arteriography of apparently normal coronary segments with nearby or distant disease suggests the presence of occult, nonvisualized atherosclerosis. J. Am. Coll. Cardiol. *25*:311, 1995.
41. Levin, D. C., Harrington, D. P., Bettmann, M. A., et al.: Anatomic variations of the left coronary arteries supplying the anterolateral aspect of the left ventricle: Possible explanation for the "unexplained" left ventricular aneurysm. Invest. Radiol. *17*:458, 1982.
42. Perlmutt, L. M., Jay, M. E., and Levin, D. C.: Variations in the blood supply of the left ventricular apex. Invest. Radiol. *18*:138, 1983.
43. Levin, D. C., Bechmann, C. F., Garnic, J. D., et al.: Frequency and clinical significance of failure to visualize the conus artery during coronary arteriography. Circulation *63*:833, 1981.
44. Kyriakidis, M. K., Kouraouklis, C. B., Papaioannou, J. T., et al.: Sinus node coronary arteries studied with angiography. Am. J. Cardiol. *51*:749, 1983.
45. King, S. B., III, Lembo, N. J., Weintraub, W. S., et al.: A randomized trial comparing coronary angioplasty with coronary bypass surgery. N. Engl. J. Med. *331*:1044, 1994.
46. Hamm, C. W., Reimers, J., Ischinger, T., et al.: A randomized study of coronary angioplasty compared with bypass surgery in patients with symptomatic multivessel coronary disease. N. Engl. J. Med. *331*:1037, 1994.
47. Bourassa, M. G., Fisher, L. D., Campeua, L., et al.: Long-term fate of bypass grafts: The Coronary Artery Surgery Study (CASS) and the Montreal Heart Institute experiences. Circulation *72* (Suppl. V):V-71, 1985.
48. European Coronary Surgery Study Group: Long-term results of prospective randomized study of coronary artery bypass surgery in stable angina pectoris. Lancet *2*:1173, 1982.
49. Loop, F. D., Lytle, B. W., Cosgrove, D. M., et al.: Influence of the internal-mammary-artery graft on 10-year survival and other cardiac events. N. Engl. J. Med. *314*:1, 1986.
50. Suma, H., and Takanashi, R.: Arteriosclerosis of the gastroepiploic and internal thoracic arteries. Ann. Thorac. Surg. *50*:413, 1990.
51. Suma, H., Wanibuchi, Y., and Terada, Y.: The right gastroepiploic artery graft: Clinical and angiographic mid-term results in 200 patients. J. Thorac. Cardiovasc. Surg. *105*:615, 1993.
52. de Feyter, P. J., van Suylen, R.-J., de Jaegere, P. P. T., et al.: Balloon angioplasty for the treatment of lesions in saphenous vein bypass grafts. J. Am. Coll. Cardiol. *21*:1539, 1993.
53. Hwang, M. H., Meadows, W. R., Palac, R. T., et al.: Progression of native coronary artery disease at 10 years: Insight from a randomized study of medical versus surgical therapy for angina. J. Am. Coll. Cardiol. *16*:1066, 1990.
54. Luscher, T. F., Diederich, D., Siebenmann, R., et al.: Difference between endothelium-dependent relaxation in arterial and in venous coronary bypass grafts. N. Engl. J. Med. *319*:462, 1988.
55. Gensini, G. G.: Coronary arteriography. *In* Braunwald, E. (ed.): Heart Disease: A Textbook of Cardiovascular Medicine. Philadelphia, W. B. Saunders Company, 1984, p. 337.
56. Hermiller, J. B., Buller, C. E., Taneglia, A. N., et al.: Unrecognized left main coronary artery disease in patients undergoing interventional procedures. Am. J. Cardiol. *71*:173, 1993.
57. Haraphongse, M., and Rossall, R. E.: Diaphragmatic coronary lesion mimics significant coronary stenosis: Report of 4 cases. Cathet. Cardiovasc. Diagn. *11*:173, 1985.
58. Zarins, C. K., Giddens, D. P., Bharadvaj, B. K., et al.: Carotid bifurcation atherosclerosis: Quantitative correlation of plaque localization with flow velocity profiles and wall shear stress. Circ. Res. *53*:502, 1983.
59. Fuster, V., Badimon, J. J., and Badimon, L.: Clinical-pathological correlations of coronary disease progression and regression. Circulation *86* (Suppl. III):III-1, 1992.
60. Kramer, J. R., Kitazume, H., Proudfit, W. L., and Sones, F. M., Jr.: Clinical significance of isolated coronary bridges: Benign and frequent condition involving the left anterior descending artery. Am. Heart J. *103*:282, 1982.
61. Friedman, M.: The coronary canalized thrombus: Provenance, structure, function and relationship to death due to coronary artery disease. Br. J. Exp. Pathol. *48*:556, 1967.
62. Klinke, W. P., Kubac, G., Talibi, T., and Lee, S. J. K.: Safety of outpatient catheterizations. Am. J. Cardiol. *56*:639, 1985.
63. Johnson, L. W., Lozner, E. C., Johnson, S., et al.: Coronary arteriography 1984–1987: A report of the Registry of the Society for Cardiac Angiography and Interventions: I. Results and complications. Cathet. Cardiovasc. Diagn. *17*:5, 1989.
64. Johnson, L. W., and Krone, R.: Cardiac catheterization 1991: A report of the Registry of the Society for Cardiac Angiography and Interventions. Cathet. Cardiovasc. Diagn. *28*:219, 1993.
65. Levin, D. C., Fellows, K. E., and Abrams, H. L.: Hemodynamically significant primary anomalies of the coronary arteries: Angiographic aspects. Circulation *58*:25, 1978.
66. Wilson, C. L., Dlabal, P. W., Holeyfield, R. W., et al.: Anomalous origin of left coronary artery from pulmonary artery: Case reports and review of literature concerning teenagers and adults. J. Thorac. Cardiovasc. Surg. *73*:887, 1977.
67. Cheitlin, M. D., Decastro, D. M., and McAllister, H. A.: Sudden death as a complication of anomalous left coronary origin from the anterior sinus of Valsalva. Circulation *50*:780, 1974.
68. Liberthson, R. R., Dinsmore, R. E., and Fallon, J. T.: Aberrant coronary artery origin from the aorta: Report of 18, review of literature and delineation of natural history and management. Circulation *59*:748, 1979.
69. Roberts, W. C.: Major anomalies of coronary artery origin seen in adulthood. Am. Heart J. *111*:941, 1986.
70. Roberts, W. C., Siegel, R. J., and Zipes, D. P.: Origin of the right coronary artery from the left sinus of Valsalva and its functional consequences: Analysis of 10 necropsy patients. Am. Heart J. *49*:863, 1982.
71. Kragel, A. H., and Roberts, W. C.: Anomalous origin of either the right or left main coronary artery from the aorta with subsequent coursing between aorta and pulmonary trunk: Analysis of 32 necropsy cases. Am. J. Cardiol. *62*:771, 1988.
72. Brandt, B., III, Martins, J. B., and Marcus, M. L.: Anomalous origin of the right coronary artery form the left sinus of Valsalva. N. Engl. J. Med. *309*:596, 1983.
73. Kimbiris, D., Iskandrian, A. S., Segal, B. L., and Bemis, C. E.: Anomalous aortic origin of coronary arteries. Circulation *58*:606, 1978.
74. Serota, H., Barth, C. W., III, Seuc, C. A., et al.: Rapid identification of the course of anomalous coronary arteries in adults: The "dot and eye" method. Am. J. Cardiol. *65*:891, 1990.
75. Fernandes, F., Alam, M., Smith, S., and Khaja, F.: The role of transesophageal echocardiography identifying anomalous coronary arteries. Circulation *88*:2532, 1993.
76. Click, R. L., Holmes, D. R., Jr., Vlietstra, R. E., et al.: Anomalous coronary arteries: Location, degree of atherosclerosis and effect on survival—A report from the Coronary Artery Surgery Study. J. Am. Coll. Cardiol. *12*:531, 1989.
77. Page, H. L., Jr., Engel, H. J., Campbell, W. B., and Thomas, C. S., Jr.: Anomalous origin of the left circumflex coronary artery: Recognition, angiographic demonstration and clinical significance. Circulation *50*:768, 1974.
78. Lipton, M. J., Barry, W. H., Obrez, I., et al.: Isolated single coronary artery: Diagnosis, angiographic classification, and clinical significance. Radiology *130*:39, 1979.
79. TIMI Study Group: The Thrombolysis in Myocardial Infarction (TIMI) trial: Phase I findings. N. Engl. J. Med. *312*:932, 1985.
80. The GUSTO Angiographic Investigators: The effects of tissue plasminogen activator, streptokinase, or both on coronary artery patency, ventricular function, and survival after acute myocardial infarction. N. Engl. J. Med. *329*:1615, 1993.
81. Gibson C. M.: TIMI frame count: A new standardization of infarct-related artery flow grade, and its relationship to clinical outcomes in the TIMI-4 trial. Circulation *90* (Abs.):I-220, 1994.
82. Levin, D. C.: Pathways and functional significance of the coronary collateral circulation. Circulation *50*:831, 1974.
83. Newman, P. E.: Coronary collateral circulation: Determinants and functional significance in ischemic heart disease. Am. Heart J. *102*:431, 1981.
84. Schwartz, H., Leiboff, R. H., and Bren, G. B.: Temporal evolution of the human coronary collateral circulation following acute myocardial infarction. J. Am. Coll. Cardiol. *4*:1088, 1984.
85. Freedman, S. B., Dunn, R. F., Bernstein, L., et al.: Influence of coronary collateral blood flow on the development of exertional ischemia and Q wave infarction in patients with severe single-vessel disease. Circulation *71*:681, 1985.
86. Williams, D. O., Amsterdam, E. A., Miller, R. R., and Mason, D. T.: Functional significance of coronary collateral vessels in patients with acute myocardial infarction: Relation to pump performance, cardiogenic shock, and survival. Am. J. Cardiol. *37*:345, 1976.
87. Tubau, J. F., Chaitman, B. R., Bourassa, M. G., et al.: Importance of coronary collateral circulation in interpreting exercise test results. Am. J. Cardiol. *47*:27, 1981.
88. Cohen, M., and Rentrop, P.: Limitation of myocardial ischemia by collateral circulation during sudden controlled coronary artery occlusion in human subjects. Circulation *74*:469, 1986.
89. Mizuno, K., Horiuchi, K., Matui, H., et al.: Role of coronary collateral vessels during transient coronary occlusion during angioplasty assessed by hemodynamic, electrocardiographic, and metabolic changes. J. Am. Coll. Cardiol. *12*:624, 1988.
90. Meier, B., Luethy, P., Fincy, L., et al.: Coronary wedge pressure in relation to spontaneously visible and recruitable collaterals. Circulation *75*:906, 1987.
91. Probst, P., Zangl, W., and Pachinger, O.: Relation of coronary arterial occlusion pressure during percutaneous transluminal coronary angiolasty to presence of collaterals. Am. J. Cardiol. *55*:1264, 1985.
92. Prinzmetal, M., Kennamer, R., Merliss, R., et al.: Angina pectoris: I. Variant form of angina pectoris. Am. J. Med. *27*:375, 1959.

93. Braunwald, E.: Coronary artery spasm: Mechanisms and clinical relevance. JAMA *256:*1957, 1981.
94. Olivas, P. B., Potts, D. E., and Pluss, R. G.: Coronary arterial spasm in Prinzmetal angina: Documentation by coronary arteriography. N. Engl. J. Med. *288:*745, 1973.
95. Curry, R. C., Jr., Pepine, C. J., Varnell, J. H., et al.: Clinical usefulness and safety of the ergonovine test in patients with chest pain. Am. J. Cardiol. *41:*369, 1978.
96. Bertrand, M. E., LaBlanche, J. M., Tilmant, P. Y., et al.: Frequency of provoked coronary arterial spasm in 1089 consecutive patients undergoing coronary arteriography. Circulation *65:*1299, 1982.
97. Crevey, B. J., Owen, S. F., and Pitt, B.: Irreversible coronary occlusion related to administration of ergonovine. Circulation *66:*252, 1982.

INTERVENTIONAL CORONARY ARTERIOGRAPHY

98. Grüntzig, A. R., Senning, A., and Siegenthaler, W. E.: Nonoperative dilatation for coronary artery stenosis—Percutaneous transluminal coronary angioplasty. N. Engl. J. Med. *301:*61, 1979.
99. Ritchie, J. L., Phillips, K. A., and Luft, H. S.: Coronary angiopasty: Statewide experience in California. Circulation *88:*2735, 1993.
100. Ryan, T. J., Bauman, W. B., Kennedy, J. W., et al.: Guidelines for percutaneous transluminal coronary angioplasty: A report of the American Heart Association/American College of Cardiology Task Force on Assessment of Diagnostic and Therapeutic Cardiovascular Procedures (Subcommittee on Percutaneous Transluminal Coronary Angioplasty). Circulation *88:*2987, 1993.
101. Wolfe, M. W., Roubin, G. S., Schweiger, M., et al.: Length of hospital stay and complications after percutaneous transluminal coronary angioplasty: Clinical and procedural predictors. Circulation *92:*311, 1995.
102. Ghazzal, Z. M. B., Hearn, J., Litvack, F., et al.: Morphological predictors of acute complications after percutaneous excimer laser coronary angioplasty. Results of a comprehensive angiographic analysis: Importance of the eccentricity index. Circulation *86:*820, 1992.
103. Ellis, S. G., and Topol, E. J.: Results of percutaneous transluminal coronary angioplasty of high-risk angulated stenoses. Am. J. Cardiol. *66:*932, 1990.
104. Ellis, S. G., Roubin, G. S., King, S. B., III, et al.: Angiographic and clinical predictors of acute closure after native vessel coronary angioplasty. Circulation *77:*372, 1988.
105. Sherman, C. T., Litvack, F., Grundfest, W., et al.: Coronary angioscopy in patients with unstable angina pectoris. N. Engl. J. Med. *315:*913, 1986.
106. Holmes, D. R., Hartzler, G. O., Smith, H. C., and Fuster, V.: Coronary artery thrombosis in patients with unstable angina. Br. Heart J. *45:*411, 1981.
107. The TIMI IIIA Investigators: Early effects of tissue-type plasminogen activator added to conventional therapy on the culprit coronary lesion in patients presenting with ischemia cardiac pain at rest: Results of the Thrombolysis in Myocardial Ischemia (TIMI IIIA) trial. Circulation *87:*38, 1993.
108. Ahmed, W. H., Bittl, J. A., and Braunwald, E.: Relation between clinical presentation and angiographic findings in unstable angina pectoris, and comparison with that in stable angina. Am. J. Cardiol. *72:*544, 1993.
109. Gotoh, K., Minamino, T., Katoh, O., et al.: The role of intracoronary thrombus in unstable angina: Angiographic assessment and thrombolytic therapy during ongoing anginal attacks. Circulation *77:*526, 1988.
110. Bentivoglio, L. G., Detre, K., Yeh, W., et al.: Outcome of percutaneous transluminal coronary angioplasty in subsets of unstable angina pectoris: A report of the 1985–1986 National Heart, Lung, and Blood Institute Percutaneous Transluminal Coronary Angioplasty Registry. J. Am. Coll. Cardiol. *24:*1195, 1994.
111. Ellis, S. G., Topol, E. J., Gallison, L., et al.: Predictors of success for coronary angioplasty performed for acute myocardial infarction. J. Am. Coll. Cardiol. *12:*1407, 1988.
112. Sullivan, E., Kearney, M., Isner, J. M., et al.: Pathology of unstable angina: Analysis of biopsies obtained by directional coronary atherectomy. J. Thromb. Thrombol. *1:*63, 1994.
113. Sutton, J. M., Ellis, S. G., Roubin, G. S., et al.: Major clinical events after coronary stenting: The multicenter registry of acute and elective Gianturco-Roubin stent placement. Circulation *89:*1126, 1994.
114. Popma, J. J., Leon, M. B., Mintz, G. S., et al.: Results of coronary angioplasty using the transluminal extraction catheter. Am. J. Cardiol. *70:*1526, 1992.
115. Safian, R. D., Grines, C. L., May, M. A., et al.: Clinical and angiographic results of transluminal extraction coronary atherectomy in saphenous vein bypass grafts. Circulation *89:*302, 1994.
116. Mabin, T. A., Holmes, D. R., Jr., Smith, H. C., et al.: Intracoronary thrombus: Role in coronary occlusion complicating percutaneous transluminal coronary angioplasty. J. Am. Coll. Cardiol. *5:*198, 1985.
117. Grassman, E. D., Leya, F., Johnson, S. A., et al.: Percutaneous transluminal coronary angioplasty for unstable angina: Predictors of outcome in a multicenter study. J. Thromb. Thrombol. *1:*73, 1994.
118. Estella, P., Ryan, T. J., Jr., Landzberg, J. S., and Bittl, J. A.: Excimer laser-assisted angioplasty for lesions containing thrombus. J. Am. Coll. Cardiol. *21:*1550, 1993.
119. Freeman, M. R., Williams, A. E., Chisholm, R. J., and Armstrong, P. W.: Intracoronary thrombus and complex morphology in unstable angina: Relation of timing of angiography and in-hospital cardiac events. Circulation *80:*17, 1989.
120. Huber, M. S., Mooney, J. F., Madison, J., and Mooney, M. R.: Use of a morphologic classification to predict clinical outcome after dissection from coronary angioplasty. Am. J. Cardiol. *68:*467, 1991.
121. Dorros, G., Cowley, M. J., Simpson, J., et al.: Percutaneous transluminal coronary angioplasty: Report of complications from the National Heart, Lung, and Blood Institute PTCA Registry. Circulation *67:*723, 1983.
122. Lincoff, A. M., Popma, J. J., Ellis, S. G., et al.: Abrupt vessel closure complicating coronary angioplasty: Clinical, angiographic and therapeutic profile. J. Am. Coll. Cardiol. *19:*926, 1992.
123. White, C. J., Ramee, S. R., Collins, T. J., et al.: Coronary angioscopy of abrupt occlusion after angioplasty. J. Am. Coll. Cardiol. *25:*1681, 1995.
124. Stone, G. W., Rutherford, B. D., McConahay, D. R., et al.: Procedural outcome of angioplasty for total coronary artery occlusion: An analysis of 971 lesions in 905 patients. J. Am. Coll. Cardiol. *15:*849, 1990.
125. Tenaglia, A. N., Tcheng, J. E., Phillips, H. R., III, and Stack, R. S.: Creation of a pseudonarrowing during coronary angioplasty. Am. J. Cardiol. *67:*658, 1991.

RELATION BETWEEN ARTERIOGRAPHIC FINDINGS AND CLINICAL OUTCOME

126. Kemp, H. G., Kronmal, R. A., Vlietstra, R. E., et al.: Seven-year survival of patients with normal or near normal coronary arteriograms: A CASS Registry study. J. Am. Coll. Cardiol. *7:*479, 1986.
127. Papanicolaou, M. N., Califf, R. M., Hlatky, M. A., et al.: Prognostic implications of angiographically normal and insignificantly narrowed coronary arteries. Am. J. Cardiol. *58:*1181, 1986.
128. Conley, M. J., Ely, R. L., Kisslo, J., et al.: The prognostic spectrum of left main stenosis. Circulation *57:*947, 1978.
129. Takaro, T., Peduzzi, P., Detre, K. M., et al.: Survival in subgroups of patients with left main coronary artery disease: Veterans Administration Cooperative Study of Surgery for Coronary Arterial Occlusive Disease. Circulation *66:*14, 1982.
130. Mock, M. B., Ringqvist, I., Fisher, L. D., et al.: Survival of medically treated patients in the Coronary Artery Surgery Study (CASS) Registry. Circulation *66:*562, 1982.
131. Ambrose, J. A., Winters, S. L., Stern, A., et al.: Angiographic morphology and the pathogenesis of unstable angina pectoris. J. Am. Coll. Cardiol. *5:*609, 1985.
132. Mizuno, K., Satomura, K., Miyamoto, A., et al.: Angioscopic evaluation of coronary-artery thrombi in acute coronary syndromes. N. Engl. J. Med. *326:*287, 1992.
133. Forrester, J. S., Litvack, F., Grundfest, W., and Hickey, A.: A perspective of coronary disease seen through the arteries of living man. Circulation *75:*505, 1986.
134. Falk, E.: Unstable angina with fatal outcome: Dynamic coronary thrombosis leading to infarction and/or sudden death. Circulation *71:*699, 1983.
135. Davies, M. J., and Thomas, A. C.: Plaque-fissuring: The cause of acute myocardial infarction, sudden ischaemic death, and crescendo angina. Br. Heart J. *53:*363, 1985.
136. Davies, M. J., Thomas, A. C., Knapman, P. A., and Hangartner, J. R.: Intramyocardial platelet aggregation in patients with unstable angina suffering ischemic cardiac death. Circulation *73:*418, 1986.
137. Lendon, C. L., Davies, M. J., Born, G. V., and Richardson, P. D.: Atherosclerotic plaque caps are locally weakened when macrophage density is increased. Atherosclerosis *87:*87, 1991.
138. Flugelman, M. Y., Virmani, R., Correa, R., et al.: Smooth muscle cell abundance and fibroblast growth factors in coronary lesions of patients with nonfatal unstable angina. Circulation *88:*2493, 1993.
139. van der Wal, A. C., Becker, A. E., van der Loos, C. M., and Das, P. K.: Site of intimal rupture or erosion of thrombosed coronary atherosclerotic plaques is characterized by an inflammatory process irrespective of the dominant plaque morphology. Circulation *89:*36, 1994.
140. Fuster, V., Badimon, L., Badimon, J. J., and Chesebro, J. H.: The pathophysiology of coronary artery disease and the acute coronary syndromes. N. Engl. J. Med. *326:*242, 1992.
141. Braunwald, E.: Unstable angina: A classification. Circulation *80:*410, 1989.
142. Brensike, J. F., Levy, R. I., Kelsey, S. F., et al.: Effects of therapy with cholestyramine on progression of coronary arteriosclerosis: Results of the NHLBI Type II Coronary Intervention Study. Circulation *69:*313, 1984.
143. Brown, G., Albers, J. J., Fisher, L. D., et al.: Regression of coronary artery disease as a result of intensive lipid-lowering therapy in men with high levels of apolipoprotein B. N. Engl. J. Med. *323:*1289, 1990.
144. Watts, G. F., Lewis, B., Brunt, J. N. H., et al.: Effects on coronary artery disease of lipid-lowering diet, or diet plus cholestyramine, in the St. Thomas' Atherosclerosis Regression Study (STARS). Lancet *339:*563, 1992.
145. Treasure, C. B., Klein, J. L., Weintraub, W. S., et al.: Beneficial effects of cholesterol-lowering therapy on the coronary endothelium in patients with coronary artery disease. N. Engl. J. Med. *332:*481, 1995.
146. Anderson, T. J., Meredith, I. T., Yeung, A. C., et al.: The effect of cholesterol-lowering and antioxidant therapy on endothelium-dependent coronary vasomotion. N. Engl. J. Med. *332:*488, 1995.
147. Ambrose, J. A., Tannenbaum, M. A., and Alexopoulos, D.: Angiographic

progression of coronary artery disease and the development of myocardial infarction. J. Am. Coll. Cardiol. *12*:56, 1988.
148. Webster, M. W., Chesebro, J. H., Smith, H. C., et al.: Myocardial infarction and coronary artery occlusion: A prospective 5-year angiographic study. J. Am. Coll. Cardiol. *15*(Abs.):218A, 1990.
149. Little, W. C., Constantinescu, M., Applegate, R. J., et al.: Can coronary angiography predict the site of a subsequent myocardial infarction in patients with mild-to-moderate coronary artery disease? Circulation *78*:1157, 1988.
150. Bär, F. W., Raynaud, P., Renkin, J. P., et al.: Coronary angiographic findings do not predict clinical outcome in patients with unstable angina. J. Am. Coll. Cardiol. *24*:1453, 1994.
151. Isshiki, T., Yamaguchi, T., Tamura, T., et al.: Percutaneous angioplasty of stenosed gastroepiploic artery grafts. J. Am. Coll. Cardiol. *21*:727, 1993.
152. Miller, S. W.: Coronary artery disease. *In* Miller, S. W. (ed.): Cardiac Angiography. Boston, Little, Brown, 1984, p. 87.

Chapter 9
Nuclear Cardiology

FRANS J. TH. WACKERS, ROBERT SOUFER, BARRY L. ZARET

Nuclear cardiology has been an active clinical discipline for more than two decades. Since the initial evolution from investigative studies to clinical studies, new techniques have evolved progressively. Major advances have occurred in both instrumentation and radiopharmaceutical development. In a parallel fashion, studies have actively pursued issues relating to clinical relevance, efficacy, and outcomes. The discipline has moved from the primary diagnostic sphere to an equally intense involvement in the functional categorization of patients with known disease. This has provided numerous insights into risk stratification and prognosis. In this chapter, following an introduction of some principles of instrumentation, the major techniques of nuclear cardiology are discussed. In each section, relevant technical issues necessary for adequate test performance are presented together with the clinical and investigative impact of the derived data.

INSTRUMENTATION

The acquisition and display of a nuclear image depend on the detection of radiation emitted from the patient following the administration of a radionuclide. In radionuclide cardiac imaging, the radionuclides are either extracted by the myocardium or remain in the cardiac blood pool. Several components are required to acquire gamma rays and to produce an image. These include a scintillation device such as the sodium iodide (NaI) crystal, which absorbs the gamma rays and generates photons that are converted to an electrical signal by photomultiplier tubes. The electrical signal then is amplified and accelerated such that the energy of the gamma ray initially absorbed by the crystal is directly proportional to the height of the generated electrical pulse. Different radionuclides emit at different energies. This allows discrimination between photons from the target and scatter.

THE SCINTILLATION (GAMMA) CAMERA

Nuclear cardiology studies are performed with a scintillation camera interfaced with a computer. Radionuclide images are the result of gamma rays passing through several principal camera components: a collimator, a large NaI crystal, and a hexagonal array of 37 to 91 photomultiplier tubes. The gamma camera provides an image of the location and intensity of a radiopharmaceutical in the body. The image is the result of the interaction between gamma rays and the camera crystal, which converts part of this energy into light (scintillation).

The photomultiplier tubes translate these scintillations into voltage pulses; these are measured as an electrical signal that defines the position at which gamma ray and crystal interact. This is accomplished by electronic circuits that compute x and y coordinates of crystal interaction and display this interaction in a two-dimensional matrix anatomically analogous to the site of occurrence within the patient. A multichannel analyzer defines the appropriate energy of the event; thus, low-energy (Compton) scatter events are not accepted.

COLLIMATION. Collimation is important for radionuclide imaging. It can be thought of as comparable to a focusing lens on a photographic camera. A collimator is composed of lead channels designed in either a parallel or diverging manner. Gamma rays must pass through the collimator before reaching the crystal. The purpose of the collimator is to approximate the origin of the photon emission within the patient to an analogous location within the crystal. Parallel-hole collimators are of either the high-resolution or the high-sensitivity variety. The high-resolution collimator permits better spatial resolution (the ability of the detector source to discriminate between neighboring sources of activity and visually resolve various components within the field of view), but with a loss of count sensitivity (the number of counts acquired per unit time).

Alternatively, a high-sensitivity collimator maximizes count sensitivity at the expense of spatial resolution. A compromise between the two types of collimators is the low-energy all-purpose or general all-purpose collimator, which is intermediate with respect to sensitivity and resolution. The thickness of the crystal and the type of collimation determine the sensitivity of a gamma camera. The type of collimation used for a particular study is based on these simple concepts. For instance, a parallel-hole high-sensitivity is appropriate for rapidly acquired studies such as first-pass blood pool studies.

Characteristics that influence the overall performance of the gamma camera are intrinsic and partial resolution, field uniformity, and count rate linearity. Most scintillation cameras have a spatial resolution of 10 to 12 mm, with a count rate linearity of approximately 75,000 counts per second and a flood of uniformity of ± 5 per cent.

COMPUTING. The computer is a principal component of all nuclear imaging systems. These data processing systems are interfaced with the gamma camera. The routine use of computers makes radionuclide imaging intrinsically quantitative. The computers have software containing algorithms for quantification of both static and dynamic digital images. The principal hardware components of the computer include analog digital convertor, central processing unit, image memory, mass storage, an array processor, and a display monitor. The scintigraphic matrix is generally 64×64 or 128×128 pixels (picture elements).

SINGLE-PHOTON EMISSION COMPUTED TOMOGRAPHY (SPECT)

Over the past several years SPECT acquisition has been used more commonly in cardiovascular nuclear medicine imaging. With SPECT, a series of planar images is obtained over a 180-degree arc around the patient's thorax. Transaxial images are recreated using a technique called filtered backprojection. These transaxial images are reconstructed into short axis and horizontal and vertical long axis orientations relative to the anatomical axis of the heart. The overall result is an improvement in anatomical resolution and contrast. Alternatively, SPECT imaging requires more attention to detail with regard to the parameters set for acquisition and more stringent quality control measures.

TECHNICAL ADVANCES. Conventional gamma cameras have one detector head. In planar imaging the detector head remains in position and acquires the projection of radioactivity in one plane. For SPECT imaging the detector head rotates around the patient while acquiring multiple projection images. From these planar projection images a three-dimensional image is constructed by backprojection. Recently, gamma cameras with multiple detector heads have been developed. These systems have improved electronics and count sensitivities, which improve image resolution and decrease SPECT imaging time. The optimal detector configuration is two camera crystal heads separated by 90 degrees. Because two camera heads are used simultaneously, the full 180-degree orbit may be required, with only a 90-degree motion resulting in half the acquisition time. Optimal 360-degree acquisition may be performed with triple head systems, in which each head is separated by 120-degrees. The increased count sensitivity of these detectors allows high-resolution collimation and improved image quality and quantification.

FUTURE DEVELOPMENTS. A significant limitation of traditional single-photon imaging is inhomogeneous attenuation of radiation by soft tissue. Attenuation artifacts are most commonly located in the anterior wall owing to breast or chest wall attenuation or in the inferior wall owing to diaphragmatic attenuation. Attenuation correction systems currently are under clinical investigation. Another problem with SPECT imaging is patient motion. Motion correction software has been developed but as yet is not widely used clinically. Finally, scatter photons are a major source of degraded image quality. Scatter correction signifies a major improvement of radionuclide image quality. A more detailed discussion of instrumentation used in cardiovascular nuclear medicine is beyond the scope of this chapter and may be found elsewhere.[1,2]

MYOCARDIAL PERFUSION IMAGING

The regional distribution of myocardial perfusion can be visualized using radiopharmaceuticals that accumulate proportional to regional myocardial blood flow. The first scintigraphic images of myocardial perfusion were acquired in 1964 by Carr et al.[3] using cesium-131. Exercise-induced myocardial ischemia was initially visualized with potassium-43 in 1973 by Zaret et al.[4] Thallium-201 (^{201}Tl), a potassium analog, became available in 1974 and has since been employed successfully.[5–8] Recently, new technetium-99m (^{99m}Tc)–labeled compounds with better imaging characteristics and novel biological properties have been introduced for visualization of myocardial perfusion.[10–16] Employing any of these imaging agents, the *relative* distribution of myocardial blood flow can be visualized. *Absolute* quantification of myocardial blood flow is not feasible using single-photon emitting radioisotopes but can be achieved with positron emission tomography.

The most important clinical application of myocardial perfusion imaging is in conjunction with stress testing for evaluation of ischemic heart disease. Numerous investigators have shown the diagnostic usefulness of exercise myocardial perfusion imaging[8,9] using either ^{201}Tl or the ^{99m}Tc-labeled imaging agents.[10–16] Generally good agreement is found between the results of stress myocardial perfusion imaging and findings on contrast coronary angiography. More importantly, it has been demonstrated that findings on stress myocardial perfusion images reflect the hemodynamic and functional significance of coronary artery stenoses and thus provide important prognostic information. Finally, the information derived from radionuclide myocardial perfusion imaging has independent and incremental value over that derived by other diagnostic methods.

RADIOPHARMACEUTICALS

THALLIUM-201. Thallium-201 is cyclotron-produced and emits mercury x-rays at 69 to 83 keV (88 per cent) and gamma rays at 135, 165, and 167 keV (12 per cent). Its physical half-life is 74 hours; however, its biological half-life is approximately 58 hours. The estimated absorbed radiation dose to the whole body is 0.21 rad/mCi, to the kidney 0.24 rad/mCi, and to the large intestine 0.54 rad/mCi. Because of the relatively long half-life of ^{201}Tl, only a relatively small amount of radioactivity can be administered. For planar imaging, usually 2 to 2.5 mCi is administered, whereas for tomographic imaging is 3.5 to 4.0 mCi is given. The first-pass myocardial extraction fraction of ^{201}Tl of 85 per cent is relatively high.[17] The initial myocardial accumulation of ^{201}Tl is proportional to myocardial blood flow. Once ^{201}Tl has entered the myocyte, a continuous exchange of ^{201}Tl takes place across the cell membrane. This process involves the Na^+, K^+-ATPase pump. The intrinsic half-life of ^{201}Tl within the myocardial cell is approximately 85 minutes. However, because of continued cellular reaccumulation of ^{201}Tl, the effective half-life of ^{201}Tl in the heart is 7.5 hours. A unique aspect of ^{201}Tl studies is that images obtained *early* and *late* after injection provide different pathophysiologic information:

1. Images immediately after injection reflect the flow-dependent initial distribution and thus regional myocardial blood flow.
2. Images taken after a delay of 2 to 24 hours reflect the distribution of the potassium pool and hence myocardial viability.

TECHNETIUM-99m–LABELED COMPOUNDS. A number of ^{99m}Tc-labeled compounds have been introduced in recent years for myocardial imaging. The first to be approved by the Food and Drug Administration and the most widely used compound in this class is ^{99m}Tc-sestamibi,[10,11] a lipophilic monovalent cation. Technetium-99m–tetrofosmin[14,15] and ^{99m}Tc-furifosmin[16] have at the time of this writing been tested in phase-two and phase-three clinical trials but have not yet been approved for routine clinical use. The ^{99m}Tc label emits gamma rays at 140 keV and has a physical half-life of 6 hours. Because of the slow body clearance, the biological half-life of sestamibi, tetrofosmin, and furifosmin is approximately the same. The whole-body absorbed radiation dose for these agents is approximately 0.02 rad/mCi. The target organ is the gallbladder, which receives approximately 0.29 rad/mCi.

Because of favorable dosimetry of the ^{99m}Tc-labeled compounds compared with ^{201}Tl, up to 30 mCi of these agents can be administered per day (see imaging protocols). The initial myocardial distribution of ^{99m}Tc-labeled agents is similar to that of ^{201}Tl and is proportional to regional distribution of myocardial blood flow. However, in contrast to ^{201}Tl, simultaneous rapid accumulation in the liver and subsequent clearance into the biliary tract occur. Myocardial extraction of ^{99m}Tc-sestamibi with an extraction fraction of 65 per cent, is substantially less efficient than that of ^{201}Tl. Sestamibi enters the myocyte by passive diffusion and binds stably to intracellular membranes. Because of intracellular retention and additional subsequent myocardial uptake during recirculation, the *absolute net retention* of ^{99m}Tc agents at several minutes after administration is comparable to that of ^{201}Tl.[18] Because myocardial distribution of ^{99m}Tc agents remains relatively fixed over time and no significant redistribution occurs, the distribution of myocardial blood flow *at the time of injection* is "frozen" over time and can be imaged for several hours. In addition, two separate injections are required to evaluate myocardial uptake at rest and exercise.

Technetium-99m–Teboroxime. Another recently developed ^{99m}Tc-labeled myocardial perfusion imaging agent with markedly different physiological characteristics is teboroxime. Technetium-99m–teboroxime is a neutral cation and a boronic acid adduct of technetium oxime (BATO). In contrast to the other ^{99m}Tc-labeled compounds, this imaging agent has both the rapid and efficient myocardial extraction (80 to 90 per cent myocardial extraction fraction) and subsequent rapid washout from the heart.[12] In addition, intense early hepatic activity may hinder complete evaluation of myocardial uptake, particularly of the inferior wall.

TABLE 9–1 COMPARATIVE CHARACTERISTICS OF VARIOUS MYOCARDIAL PERFUSION IMAGING AGENTS

	^{201}Tl	^{99m}Tc-SESTAMIBI ^{99m}Tc-TETROFOSMIN ^{99m}Tc-FURIFOSMIN	^{99m}Tc-TEBOROXIME
Energy emissions	69–83 keV (x-rays) 135, 165, 167 keV	140 keV	140 keV
Physical half-life	74 hr	6 hr	6 hr
Biological half-life	58 hr	6 hr	<6 hr
Heart half-life	3–4 hr	6–7 hr	<10 min
Dose	2–4.0 mCi	30 mCi	30 mCi
Radiation dose			
Whole body	0.21 rad/mCi	0.02 rad/mCi	0.02 rad/mCi
Intestines	0.54 rad/mCi	0.18 rad/mCi	0.11 rad/mCi
Myocardial EF	85%	65%	80–90%
% ID heart	4%	1.5%	?
Visualizes			
Blood flow	+	+	+
Viability	+ (delayed image)	+	–
Redistribution	+	Minimal	–
LVEF (first pass)	–	+	+
ECG gating	–	+	–
Imaging time/views			
Planar	10 min	5 min	1–2 min
Tomography	21 min	11 min	1 min

Abbreviations: EF = Extraction fraction; % ID = Per cent of injected dose; LVEF = Left ventricular ejection fraction

Myocardial washout of teboroxime is biexponential: At 5 minutes after injection only 25 per cent of the initial activity remains in the heart. The estimated whole-body absorbed radiation dose is 0.02 rad/mCi. The target organs are liver and large intestine, which receive 0.12 rad/mCi and 0.11 rad/mCi, respectively. This imaging agent requires rapid serial imaging during the 5 minutes immediately following injection.[13] The main characteristics of the various imaging agents are summarized in Table 9–1.

Technical Considerations

GAMMA CAMERA. For planar imaging, a camera with 10-inch diameter detector and a ¼-inch thick crystal is preferred. Low-energy photons of ^{201}Tl do not adequately penetrate thicker crystals, resulting in images of inadequate count density. Tomographic cameras with large field of view (20-inch diameter) generally have a ⅜-inch thick crystal and are thus not ideally suited for ^{201}Tl imaging but are ideally suited for imaging of ^{99m}Tc-labeled agents.

COLLIMATION. For both planar and SPECT imaging with ^{201}Tl, a general all-purpose parallel-hole collimator is preferred to ensure adequate count density. Owing to the higher photon flux with ^{99m}Tc-labeled imaging agents, good-quality images are obtained with a high-resolution parallel-hole collimator.

ENERGY WINDOW. For ^{201}Tl imaging, a dual window is preferred: 25 per cent window over the 80-keV mercury x-ray peak and 20 per cent window over the 167-keV gamma-ray peak. The latter window accounts for approximately 10 per cent additional counts. For ^{99m}Tc-labeled imaging agents, a 20 per cent window is placed over the 140-keV peak.

COMPUTER ACQUISITION. Radionuclide images are acquired on computer and stored on computer disk or magnetic tape for data processing. For planar myocardial perfusion imaging, acquisition in 128 × 128 matrix is preferred, whereas for SPECT imaging a 64 × 64 matrix is commonly used.

IMAGING PROTOCOLS

Because of the introduction of new imaging agents and new insights in ^{201}Tl biokinetics, imaging protocols have recently been modified considerably. Figure 9–1 provides a schematic representation of the most frequently used imaging protocols at the time of this writing. For a more detailed discussion of various imaging protocols, see a recent review by Wackers.[19]

For *Tl-201 stress imaging* (Fig. 9–1*A*), one single dose of ^{201}Tl is injected at peak exercise. Initial stress imaging should be started *within 5 minutes* of the injection. Delayed or redistribution imaging is performed *2 to 4 hours later* (timing of delayed imaging should be standardized in each laboratory). For complete assessment of viable myocardium, a second injection of ^{201}Tl is administered at rest in selected patients. The repeat rest injection can be given either following redistribution imaging or on a different day (see p. 294).

For imaging with *^{99m}Tc-labeled perfusion imaging agents* (Fig. 9–1*B, C*) two separate injections are given: one during exercise and a second at rest. Employing ^{99m}Tc-sestamibi, imaging is started approximately *15 minutes after injection during exercise and 60 minutes after injection at rest.* Because ^{99m}Tc-tetrofosmin and ^{99m}Tc-furifosmin clear more rapidly from the liver after rest injection, rest imaging with these compounds can be started relatively early *(15 minutes after injection)*. Thus, with these latter agents both rest and exercise imaging is started at 15 minutes after injection.

With ^{99m}Tc-teboroxime the patient should be imaged rapidly, starting at *1 minute after injection.* After 5 to 10 minutes not enough teboroxime remains in the heart to allow adequate quality imaging.

DUAL ISOTOPE IMAGING (Fig. 9–1*D*). This is a "hybrid" imaging protocol, designed to overcome the disadvantage of a relatively lengthy imaging protocol using two injections of sestamibi.[20] Using the dual-isotope protocol a rest injection of ^{201}Tl (3.5 mCi) is given first, followed by rest ^{201}Tl imaging. The patient is then stressed and injected

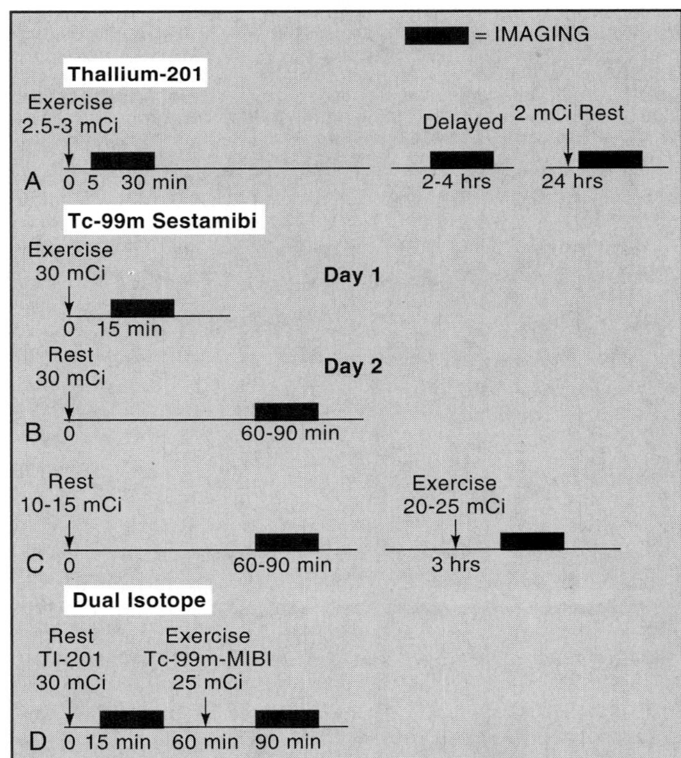

FIGURE 9–1. Schematic representation of preferred myocardial perfusion imaging protocols using either ^{201}Tl, ^{99m}Tc-sestamibi, or dual isotope imaging (see text).

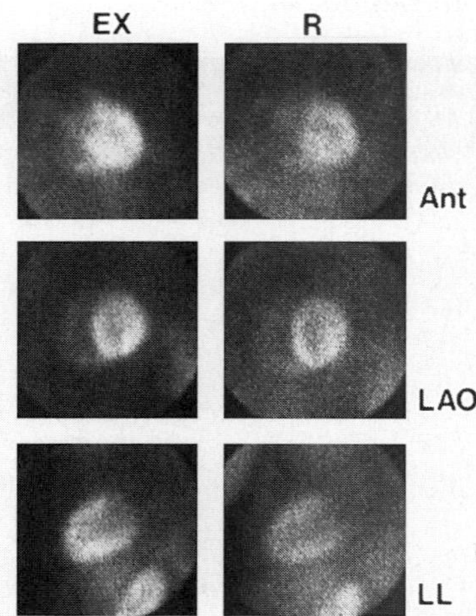

FIGURE 9–2. Normal planar exercise (EX) and redistribution (R) planar ^{201}Tl images. Ant = Anterior view; LAO = left anterior oblique view; LL = left lateral view.

with 25 to 30 mCi of sestamibi at peak stress, followed after 15 minutes by sestamibi imaging. This imaging protocol can be completed in 1½ to 2 hours.

Imaging Techniques

PLANAR IMAGING. Although SPECT imaging at the present time is the predominant imaging technique used in clinical nuclear cardiology, the technical basis for good-quality SPECT imaging remains the ability to perform good-quality planar imaging. To acquire optimal planar myocardial perfusion images, some basic requirements should be met.[21,22] The most frequent reasons for suboptimal quality images are (1) insufficient count density within the heart, (2) inconsistent *patient positioning and repositioning,* (3) the use of *too large a zoom factor,* and (4) inadequate display of images.

ADEQUATE COUNT DENSITY. Images should have at least 600,000 counts in the field of view. However, when extracardiac activity is present, such as in lungs or subdiaphragmatic organs, the count density in the field of view does not reflect the count density in the heart. Longer imaging time is needed to obtain adequate counts from the heart. Therefore, it is recommended to acquire images for a certain *preset time.* For planar ^{201}Tl imaging, 8- to 10-minute acquisitions per view usually results in adequate count density imaging. Using ^{99m}Tc-labeled imaging agents, adequate count density is readily achieved because 20 to 30 mCi is administered. Employing the latter agents, 1.5 to 2 million counts per field of view can be obtained with 5-minute acquisitions per view.

PATIENT POSITIONING. Planar imaging is routinely performed in three positions. The *left anterior oblique* (LAO) view usually is obtained with the patient lying supine. An optimal LAO is the projection that shows best separation of right and left ventricular cavities with the septum straight and vertical. This angulation should be used as a reference angle for the other views. The *anterior view* is obtained with the patient lying supine, 45 degrees to the right of the LAO view. For the *left lateral view* the patient should be turned on his *right side,* with the camera head in the same position as for the anterior view. The detector head should be angled in such a way that it is as close as possible to the patient's chest wall.

On all views the heart should be in the *center* of the field of view. *Repositioning* of the patient at delayed imaging should be performed with great care. The position of heart on the exercise images should be reproduced as close as possible.

ZOOM FACTOR. When a large field of view camera is used, the *zoom factor* (magnification) should not exceed 1.2 times. On an optimal image, the heart is approximately one-third to one-fourth of the diameter of the field of view.

PLANAR IMAGE DISPLAY. The *display* of myocardial perfusion images is important for reproducible and consistent interpretation. Color display of *planar* images should be discouraged. "White on black" display using a linear gray scale is preferred (Fig. 9–2). On these images the heart is white (radioactivity). When interpretation is performed from a computer screen, standardization of display is important. Arbitrarily changing contrast intensity and gray scales should be limited to a minimum. We recommend use of the test pattern designed by the Society for Motion Picture and Television Engineers (SMPTE) for quality control. The linear gray scale should be normalized to the "hottest pixel" within the heart (Fig. 9–3). In this manner the gray scale is fully utilized in the representation of the heart. This is particularly important for display of images acquired with ^{99m}Tc-labeled agents. Exercise and rest/delayed images should be displayed side by side for comparison.

TOMOGRAPHIC (SPECT) IMAGING. Careful attention to technical details is even more important for SPECT imaging than for planar imaging. Energy settings are the same as for planar imaging. Usually a general all-purpose collimator is used. For imaging with ^{99m}Tc-labeled myocardial perfusion agents, a high-resolution parallel-hole collimator is preferred because of higher count rate.[23] During cardiac SPECT imaging, the gamma camera rotates thorough a 180-degree arc with 32 stops. For imaging with ^{201}Tl, the duration of each stop is 40 seconds. Employing ^{99m}Tc-sestamibi, the time for each stop can be shortened to 25 seconds for a high-dose (22 to 25 mCi) study. For the low-dose (8 to 10 mCi) study, 40 seconds per stop is recommended.

The basic principle of tomographic reconstruction involves the acquisition of multiple planar projection images around an object and the reconstruction of the three-dimensional object by "filtered backprojection."[24] For cardiac SPECT, because the heart lies eccentrically in the chest, 180-degree image acquisition may be used. The pos-

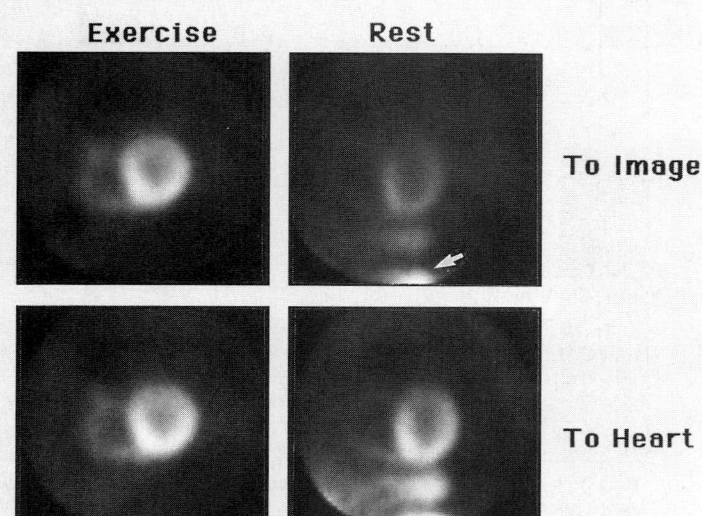

FIGURE 9–3. Normalization of exercise/rest ^{99m}Tc-sestamibi images. Intense subdiaphragmatic activity (arrow) may cause problems with adequate display of the image of the heart. Radionuclide images are usually normalized to the "hottest" area in the field of view. On the exercise sestamibi images the heart is the hottest organ. However, on the rest image the gastrointestinal tract is the hottest area (arrow). Consequently, when the rest image is normalized to subdiaphragmatic activity, the heart is only faintly visualized *(top).* Using ^{99m}Tc-labeled myocardial perfusion imaging agents, images should be normalized to the heart, as shown in the bottom panel, for adequate visualization of the heart. (From Wackers, F. J. Th.: Myocardial perfusion imaging. *In* Sandler, M. P., Coleman, R. E., Wackers, F. J. Th., et al.: Diagnostic Nuclear Medicine. 3rd ed. Baltimore, Williams and Wilkins, 1995.)

terior 180-degree arch is not used with ^{201}Tl because it contains low count data as a result of greater distance from the heart and substantial attenuation. Using ^{99m}Tc-labeled radiotracers that are better suited for gamma camera imaging and the new multihead gamma cameras, data acquired over a 360-degree orbit can be used for reconstruction. After backprojection, filtering techniques are used to correct for reconstruction artifacts and enhance the image quality. Tomographic slices are generated perpendicular to the anatomical axis of the heart, rather than those of the body.

PATIENT POSITIONING

Patient positioning and patient preparation are extremely important for optimal SPECT imaging. Patient motion is a common cause for artifacts on SPECT imaging.[30] *Motion* may involve movement of the patient's upper body but may also result from a change in position of the heart within the chest. Immediately after exercise, because of deeper breathing, the heart may be in a vertical position. While the patient recovers from exercise, the heart may move into a horizontal position. This phenomenon of "upward creep" can cause artifactual inferior wall defects on reconstructed slices.[25] This can be avoided by delaying the start of SPECT imaging after termination of exercise for approximately 10 minutes. This allows for acquisition of one *planar* image immediately after exercise, which is useful for evaluation of increased lung uptake. Because SPECT imaging with ^{99m}Tc-labeled agents is not started before 15 minutes after exercise, upward creep is not an issue using these radiotracers.

Adequate count density is a frequently ignored aspect of tomographic perfusion imaging. As mentioned above, gamma cameras used for SPECT imaging have a ¾-inch thick crystal, which is not optimal for ^{201}Tl imaging. Therefore, a relatively high dose of at least 3.5 mCi (129.5 MBq) of ^{201}Tl should be administered. Using ^{99m}Tc-labeled compounds, 10 to 30 mCi (370 to 1110 MBq) is administered. Consequently, count densities are usually adequate for good-quality SPECT images. Unfortunately, most commercially available computer software does not provide information on count density of unprocessed planar projection images. Poor count density on reconstructed and filtered SPECT images should be suspected when the distribution of radiopharmaceutical appears to occur in multiple "patches" of apparent higher and lower activity, a pattern that does not match the usual anatomy of coronary artery disease.

SPECT ORBIT. Many cameras provide a choice of various acquisition orbits. The camera may rotate around the patient in a perfect *circle*, or may follow the *body contour* of the patient. A body-contour orbit may cause artifacts because of varying gamma camera resolution with varying distance of the detector head from the target organ. These artifacts are characteristic and consist of small 180-degree diametrical defects on the short-axis slices.[26] High-resolution collimation reduces the effect of varying spatial resolution and resulting artifacts. Therefore, a circular orbit is preferred for cardiac SPECT imaging.

SPECT IMAGE DISPLAY. The display of reconstructed SPECT slices has been standardized (Fig. 9–4).[27] Images should be displayed "white on black" using a linear gray scale (Fig. 9–5). Three sets of slices are reconstructed: short-axis slices, horizontal long-axis slices, and vertical long-axis slices. The exercise and rest (or delayed) images are displayed side by side to facilitate comparison. Because of the multitude of images, it is useful to "condense" all information into one color-coded polar map, or "bull's-eye" image[28] (see Figs. 9–17*B* and 9–18*B*, p. 284).

Normal Planar Myocardial Perfusion Images

In planar imaging, perfusion is visualized as the projection of myocardial radioactivity on a plane parallel to the crystal surface of the gamma camera. The "left ventricular cavity" as it appears on planar images is in part an optical illusion.[21] The familiar horseshoe appearance of the left ventricle on ^{201}Tl images is a result of attenuation of radiation from the distant myocardial wall by ventricular blood pool and the relatively greater myocardial mass of the walls perpendicular to the plane of view. The "facing" myocardial wall contains relatively less radiopharmaceutical, which creates the illusion of visualization of the ventricular cavity.

Because of overprojection of myocardial regions in one plane, it is necessary to obtain multiple planar images from different angles to visualize all segments of left ventricular myocardium. The anatomy of the heart as projected on various planar views and the various coronary artery territories are shown in Figure 9–6.

NORMAL VARIATIONS OF PLANAR MYOCARDIAL PERFUSION IMAGES. The interpretation of myocardial perfusion images may be difficult at times because of normal variations in the pattern of radiotracer uptake.[21]

Apex. A well-recognized area of normally decreased tracer activity is at the apex of the left ventricle. In patients with a vertical position of the heart, this may be a prominent feature. An apical variant appears as a narrow slit or cleft-like area, aligned with the long axis of the left ventricle.

Aortic Valve Plane. On the LAO view the membranous septum and aortic valve plane are projected at the open end of the horseshoe, at times causing an apparent high septal defect. This may be seen prominently in patients with a horizontal position of the heart.

Mitral Valve Plane. The mitral valve plane is seen as the open end of the horseshoe in all three views.

ARTIFACTS ON PLANAR IMAGES

ANTERIOR VIEW. In most normal subjects the intensity of radiotracer uptake in the inferoseptal wall on the planar anterior view is approximately equal to that of the anterolateral wall. However, in a patient with enlargement of the right ventricle (e.g., in chronic obstructive pulmonary disease), the right ventricular blood pool may attenuate inferoseptal activity and produce an apparent defect. Such artifacts can be unmasked by imaging the patient in the upright position, thereby changing the position of the right ventricle in the chest.

LEFT ANTERIOR OBLIQUE VIEW. The appearance of the heart in the planar LAO view depends on both the position of the heart in the chest and the size of the heart. Patients with left ventricular dilatation may have clockwise rotation. In the latter situation a routine 45-degree LAO view may display an image similar to that usually seen in the anterior projection. The (normal) open end of the horseshoe could be misinterpreted as a septal defect. A steeper (60-degree)

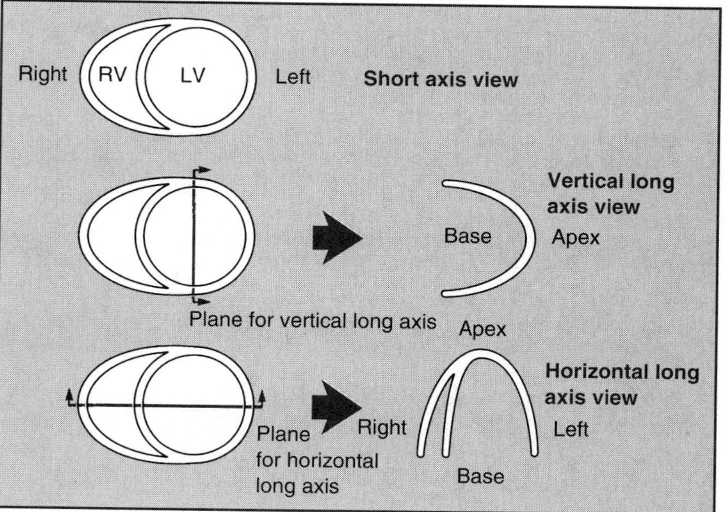

FIGURE 9–4. Standardized display of SPECT myocardial perfusion images. The short-axis slices are displayed with the right ventricle left and the left ventricle right. The short-axis slices are displayed as a horizontal row of images, starting with the apical slice on the left and the basal slices on the right. The vertical long-axis slices are cut from the septum toward the lateral wall, displaying the septal slices on the left and the lateral slices on the right. The horizontal long-axis slices are cut from the inferior wall toward the anterior wall, displaying the inferior wall slices on the left and the anterior wall slices on the right. (From the Cardiovascular Imaging Committee, American College of Cardiology; the Committee on Advanced Cardiac Imaging and Technology, Council of Clinical Cardiology, American Heart Association; and the Board of Directors, Cardiovascular Council Society of Nuclear Medicine: ACC/AHA/SNM Policy Statement: Standardization of cardiac tomographic imaging. J. Nucl. Cardiol. *1*:117, 1994.)

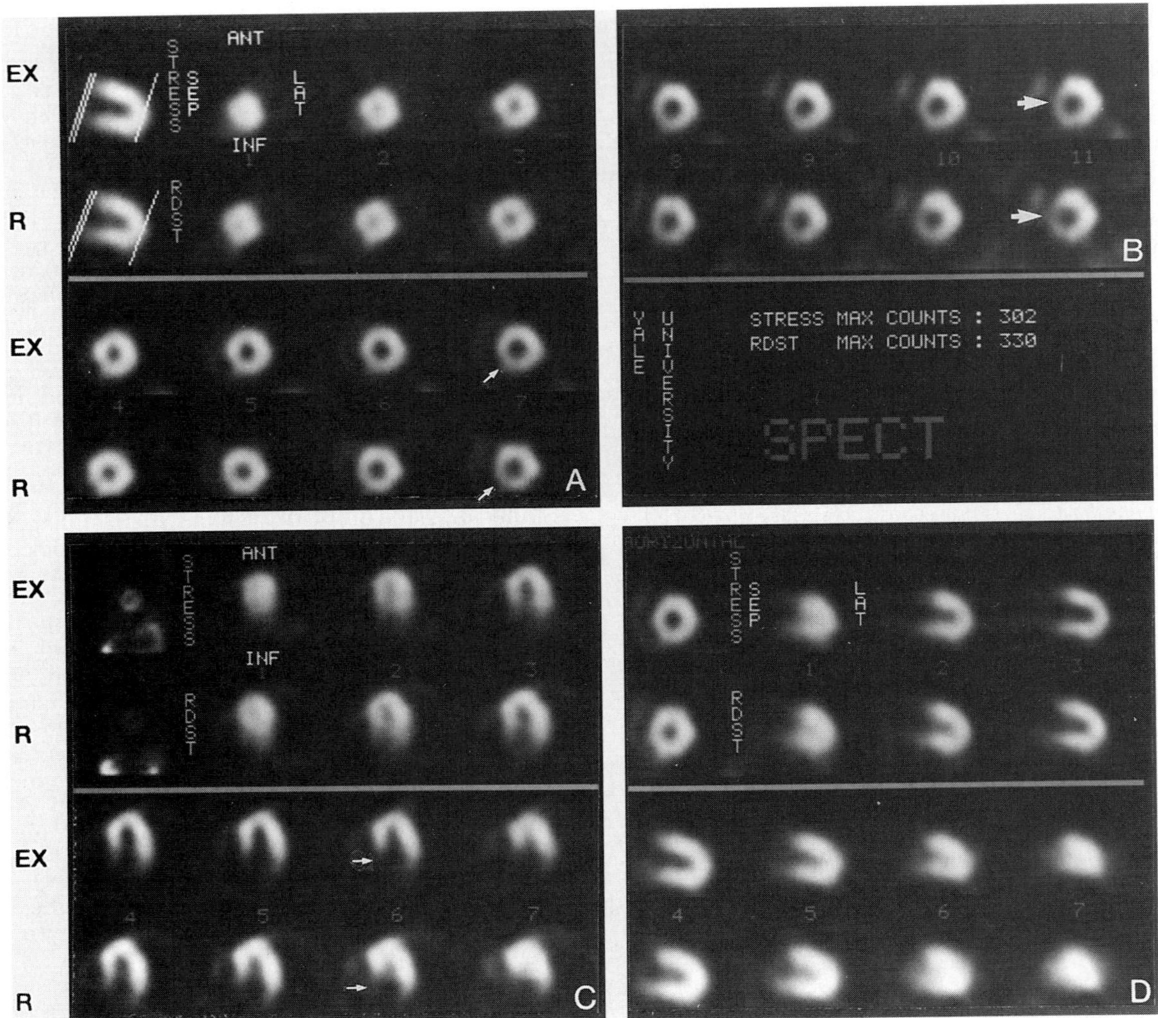

FIGURE 9–5. SPECT ^{99m}Tc-sestamibi myocardial images after exercise and at rest in a normal subject, showing normal variations of radiopharmaceutical distribution. On the midventricular short-axis slices *(A)* the inferior septal areas (small arrows) have slightly less activity than the lateral wall. This is a normal variation. The hottest area is in the lateral wall. On the basal slices *(B)* an apparent septal defect is present (large arrow). This is the membranous portion of the septum. This "septal defect" and normal variation are also seen in the horizontal long-axis slices *(C)*, where the septum is shorter (arrows) than the lateral wall. Vertical long-axis slices are shown in *D*. (From Wackers, F. J. Th.: Artifacts in planar and SPECT myocardial perfusion imaging. Am. J. Cardiac Imaging 6:42, 1992.)

angulation may project the left ventricle correctly along the long axis, thereby restoring the "typical" doughnut-shaped configuration.

LEFT LATERAL VIEW. Acquisition of a steep LAO or left lateral image with the patient *supine* may cause artifactual inferior wall defects. This artifact is seen in approximately one-fourth of the patients imaged in the supine position.[29] This artifact is caused by attenuation of the inferior wall activity by the left hemidiaphragm. Turning the patient on his or her right side causes the heart to shift into a vertical position (Fig. 9–7). Moreover, in this position of the left hemidiaphragm makes larger excursions. This results in less attenuation and improved projection of the inferoposterior wall.

OBESE PATIENTS/LARGE BREASTS. In extremely obese patients or in women with large breasts, attenuation of radiation may cause apparent defects. These artifactual defects often appear as anterior defects on the anterior and left lateral views, whereas the location of artifacts is less predictable on the LAO view. We find it useful to employ radioactive string markers to outline the breasts and thus define the relationship between the breasts and cardiac defects (Fig. 9–8). Superimposition of breast tissue over the heart may also result in linear areas of relatively *increased* activity. This linear artifact is believed to be caused by a small-angle scatter from the breast tissue fold. Breast artifacts are the most frequent cause of false-positive ^{201}Tl studies. The use of breast markers is an important aid in correctly interpreting ^{201}Tl images.[21,22,30]

NORMAL PLANAR IMAGES WITH TECHNETIUM-99m–LABELED AGENTS. Images with ^{99m}Tc-labeled myocardial perfusion imaging agents are generally of better quality than ^{201}Tl images. Compared with ^{201}Tl, these images have substantially less low-radiation background scatter and are therefore clearer than ^{201}Tl images. The normal variants and artifacts described above can also be observed on images with ^{99m}Tc-labeled compounds. The most important difference from ^{201}Tl is the amount of subdiaphragmatic uptake, such as in liver, gallbladder, and large intestine (Fig. 9–9). The liver clearance of sestamibi, tetrofosmin, and furifosmin after exercise is relatively rapid. Postexercise imaging can be started at 15 minutes after injection. However, there is a difference in liver clearance *after rest injection* between various ^{99m}Tc-labeled compounds. The clearance of sestamibi is slow and rest imaging often has to be postponed until 60 to 90 minutes after injection.[10] In contrast, tetrofosmin and furifosmin clear relatively rapidly after rest injection, and rest imaging can be started at 15 minutes after injection.

Because of significant extracardiac activity, images with ^{99m}Tc-labeled compounds should be displayed with the gray scale normalized to the "hottest" pixel within the heart (Fig. 9–3). Nevertheless, planar images with ^{99m}Tc-labeled compound may be difficult to interpret, particularly the inferior wall in the left lateral view, owing to intense subdiaphragmatic activity.

Technetium-99m-Teboroxime. Images with this radiopharmaceutical are characterized by rapid initial accumulation of the radiotracer within the heart and subsequent fast

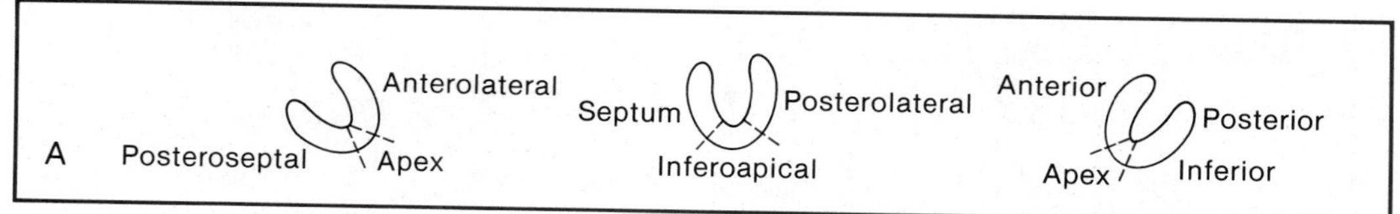

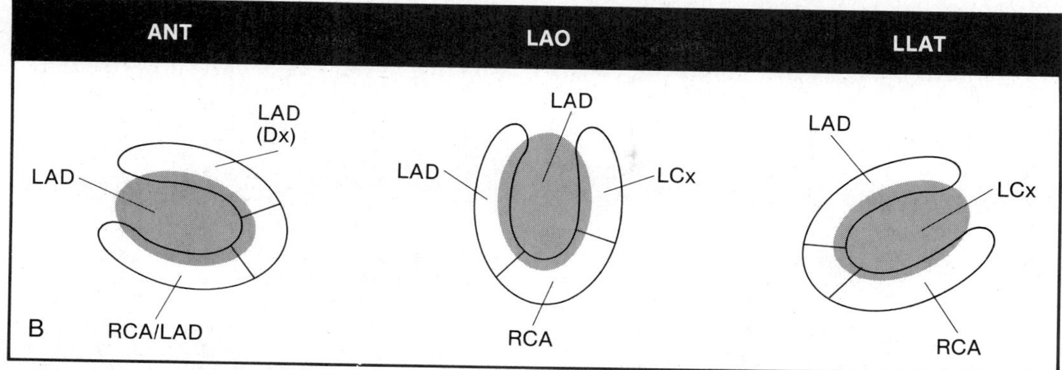

FIGURE 9–6. *A*, Anatomy of the heart as projected on planar views. *B*, Coronary artery territories on three planar views. The shaded area indicates the facing myocardium overlying the left ventricular cavity. LAD = Left anterior descending coronary artery; RCA = right coronary artery; Dx = diagonal artery; LCx = left circumflex artery; ANT = anteroposterior; LAO = left anterior oblique; LLAT = left lateral.

clearance (within 2 to 3 minutes) from the heart and intensive accumulation (within 2 to 3 minutes) in the liver.[12] Consequently, the heart can be imaged only for a few minutes after administration of the radiopharmaceutical (Fig. 9–10). The appearance of the heart is very similar in quality to that with ^{201}Tl. The intense subdiaphragmatic activity also may interfere with analysis of the inferior wall.

Characteristics of Normal SPECT Myocardial Perfusion Images

SPECT images are reconstructed as multiple slices oriented along the anatomical axis of the left ventricle. For interpretation of the short-axis slices it is convenient to divide the slices into three groups: apical slices, midventricular slices, and basal slices. To avoid apical artifacts by partial volume effect, only apical slices that clearly show the ventricular cavity should by analyzed. When interpreting basal slices, slices showing that membranous septum are excluded. SPECT anatomy and coronary territories are shown in Figure 9–11.

NORMAL VARIATIONS OF SPECT MYOCARDIAL PERFUSION IMAGES. A useful practical rule for interpreting a SPECT study is that a perfusion defect should be seen on at least three consecutive slices in order to be considered a true abnormality.

The *vertical long-axis slices* and the *horizontal long-axis* slices contain the same information shown on the short-axis slices. However, the apex and base of the heart can be analyzed in these views without partial volume artifacts. Only slices that clearly show the left ventricular cavity should be analyzed.

Slightly less inferoseptal uptake can be noted in male patients as a normal variant (Fig. 9–5). In females radiotracer distribution is usually more homogeneous. The basal short-axis slices usually show a septal defect. This is a normal finding and represents the membranous portion of the septum.

ARTIFACTS ON SPECT IMAGES

Motion artifacts and how to avoid them have been discussed above (Patient Positioning). Although computer software has been developed to correct for patient motion, this is not widely used in clinical practice.

Other common artifacts are caused by *attenuation.* The supine position of the patient may cause inferior wall defects by attenuation by the left hemidiaphragm (Figs. 9–7 and 9–12). To avoid such artifacts, alternative patient positioning has been proposed. For instance, the patient can be imaged prone (lying on the stomach),[31,32] turned on the right side,[33] or sitting in an upright position.[34]

Attenuation by breast tissue can cause artifacts on SPECT imaging as well. Breast artifacts are in general easier to recognize on planar images than on reconstructed SPECT images.[35] It is important to be alert to the potential presence of artifact *before* the interpretation of images. For SPECT imaging, images with breast markers cannot be obtained as is done for planar imaging. For SPECT imaging careful

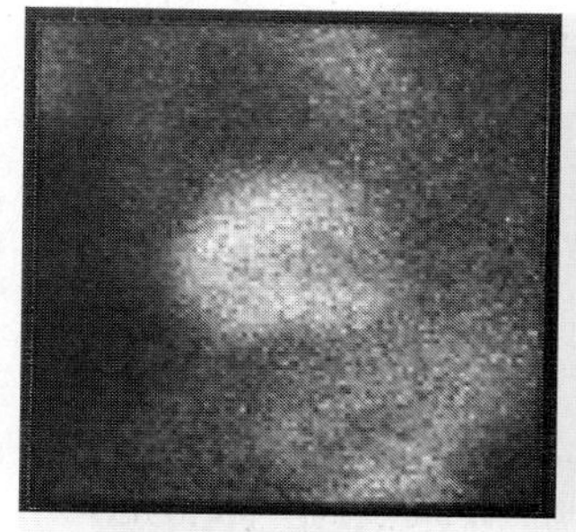

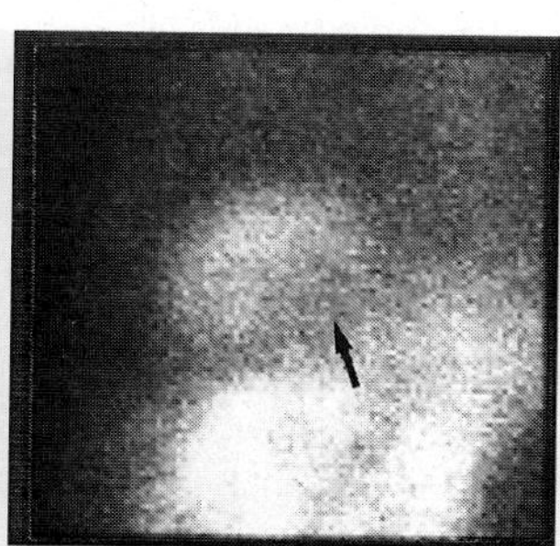

FIGURE 9–7. Artifactual inferoposterior defect in the supine position. ^{201}Tl images following exercise in a patient with angiographically normal coronary arteries. A definite inferoposterior myocardial perfusion defect (arrow) is seen on the left lateral (LL) supine projection. A LL view obtained with the patient lying on his right side demonstrates a normal inferoposterior wall. The two left lateral images were acquired immediately after each other. (From Wackers, F. J. Th.: Artifacts in planar and SPECT myocardial perfusion imaging. Am. J. Cardiac Imaging *6*:42, 1992.)

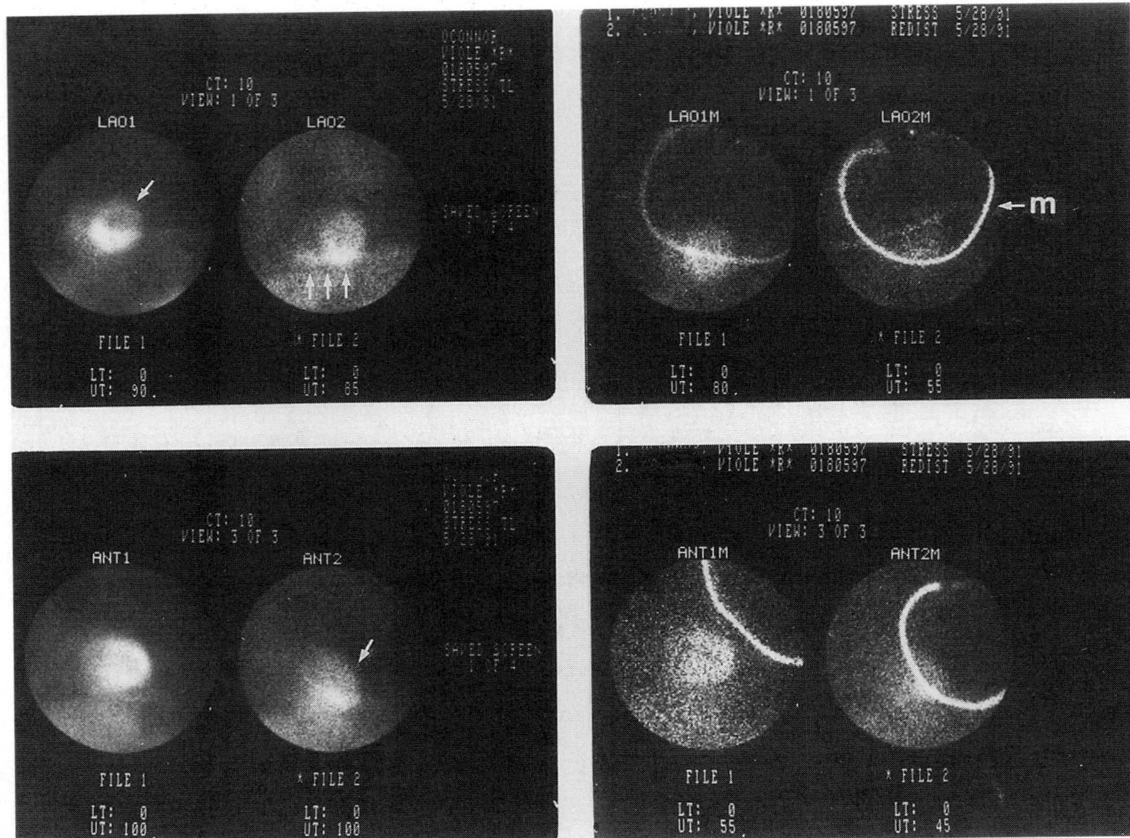

FIGURE 9–8. Planar ^{201}Tl left anterior oblique (LAO) and anterior (ANT) images in a woman with large breasts (LAO1, ANT1 = exercise images; LAO2, ANT2 = delayed images). The breasts are marked with radioactive line markers (m) in the images on the right. On the LAO exercise images *(top)*, a definite attenuation artifact is present (arrow). At delayed imaging, the breast contour is lower and is visualized as a linear area (arrow) with increased activity due to "small-angle scatter." The exercise anterior view *(bottom)* is normal because the breast did not cover the heart. However, at delayed imaging, the contour of the breast is across the heart, causing an attenuation artifact (arrow). This is an example of how breast attenuation artifacts can vary in the same view owing to different breast positions. Note that on the delayed LAO image, unequal attenuation mimics an image with increased lung uptake of ^{201}Tl. (From Wackers, F. J. Th.: Artifacts in planar and SPECT myocardial perfusion imaging. Am. J. Cardiac Imaging *6*:42, 1992.)

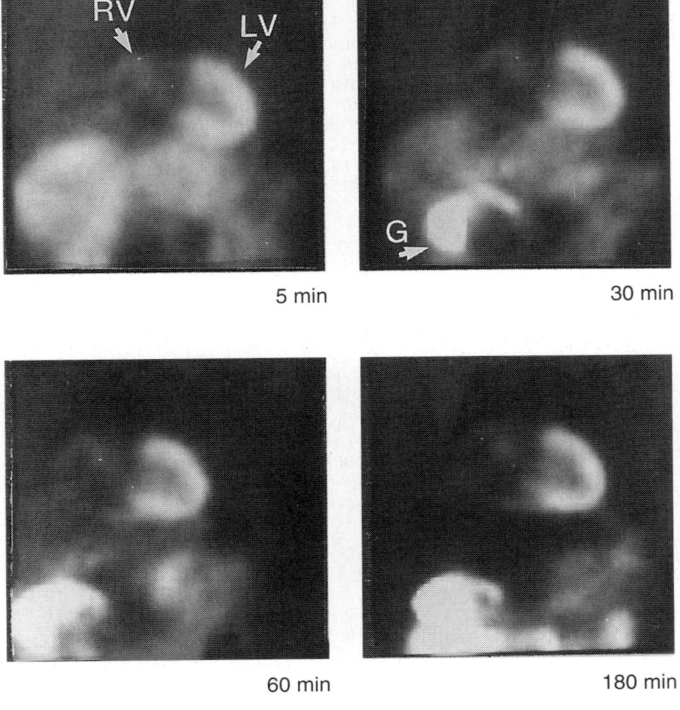

FIGURE 9–9. Planar myocardial perfusion images with ^{99m}Tc-sestamibi. Images of normal volunteer after exercise. The images are taken with a large field-of-view camera. Both the right *(RV)* and left *(LV)* ventricles are well visualized. The imaging agent initially accumulated in the liver and cleared into the gallbladder *(G)*. After 30 minutes there is no significant liver accumulation. Solid-colored line, 10 to 19 per cent; broken line, <10 per cent; p = 0.0032; white line, >20 per cent. (Reprinted by permission of the Society of Nuclear Medicine from Wackers, F. J. Th., Berman, D. S., Maddahi, J., et al.: Technetium-99m Hexakis 2-methoxyisobutyl isonitrile: Human biodistribution, dosimetry, safety and preliminary comparison to thallium-201 for myocardial perfusion imaging. J. Nucl. Med. *30*:301, 1989.)

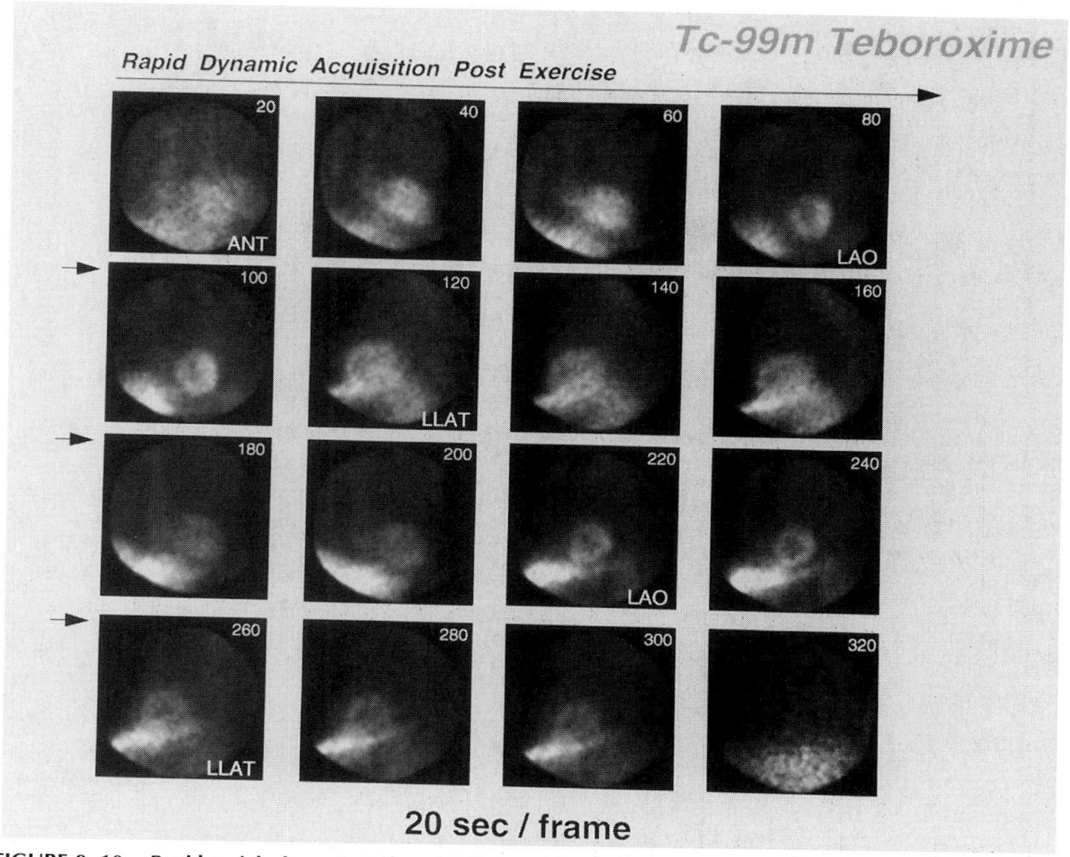

FIGURE 9–10. Rapid serial planar imaging with ^{99m}Tc-teboroxime. Each planar image is taken for 20 seconds, starting in the anterior (ANT) position immediately after termination of exercise. The patient was seated upright on a swivel chair and rotated from the anterior to the left anterior oblique (LAO) and left lateral (LLAT) position and again ANT, LAO, and LLAT. Note the rapid disappearance of ^{99m}Tc-teboroxime from the heart in 260 seconds and intensive liver uptake. (From Wackers, F. J. Th.: Artifacts in planar and SPECT myocardial perfusion imaging. Am. J. Cardiac Imaging *6*:42, 1992.)

inspection of the *cine display of unprocessed projection images* may help to anticipate a potential attenuation problem. The breast can often be recognized as a shadow moving over the heart in certain projections and therefore may cause attenuation artifacts. Attenuation artifacts are the most common source of error in SPECT imaging. Attenuation correction software is currently being developed but as yet has not been clinically validated.

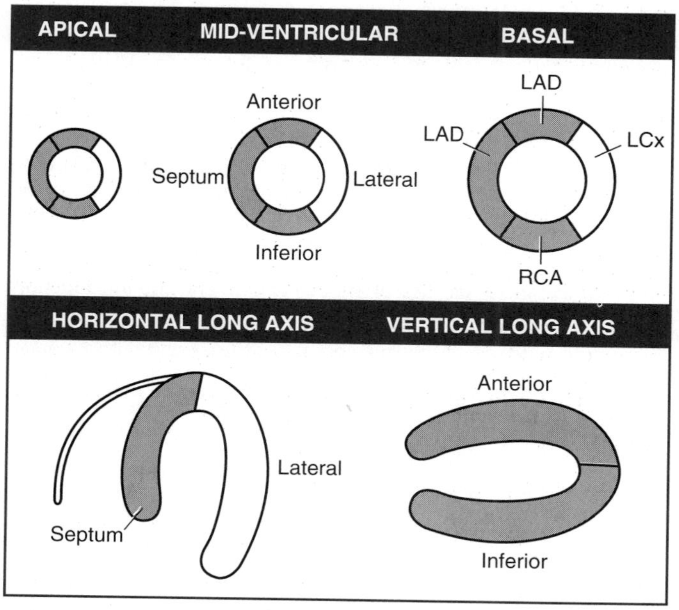

FIGURE 9–11. Left ventricular anatomy and coronary artery territories on SPECT slices.

Quality control should be performed systematically as a part of the interpretation of a SPECT study and should involve the following:

1. Inspection of cine display of 32 planar projection images to assess motion of the patient or of the heart and identify the presence of a breast shadow. The cine display also allows one to evaluate whether the heart is in the center of rotation.
2. A check for adequate count density—*at least 100 counts* within the "hottest" pixel of the heart in one of the unprocessed anterior projection images.
3. Assessment of the presence of diaphragmatic attenuation of the inferoposterior wall. This can be done readily by comparing a planar left lateral supine view with a planar left lateral right side down view (Figs. 9–7 and 9–12).

Image Interpretation

Planar and SPECT images are interpreted qualitatively by visual analysis, often aided by computer quantification. Image interpretation can be described as follows (Fig. 9–13):

NORMAL. Homogeneous uptake of the radiopharmaceutical throughout the myocardium.

DEFECT. A localized myocardial area with a relative decrease in radiotracer uptake. Defects may vary in intensity, from slightly reduced activity to almost absent activity.

REVERSIBLE DEFECT. A defect present on the initial stress images is no longer present or is present to a lesser degree on the resting or delayed images. This pattern indicates myocardial ischemia. Improvement over time on ^{201}Tl imaging is referred to as *redistribution*. It is not appropriate to use this terminology for ^{99m}Tc-labeled agents.

Fixed Defect. A defect is unchanged and present on both exercise and rest (delayed) images. This pattern generally indicates infarction and scar tissue. However, in some patients with fixed ^{201}Tl defects on 2- to 4-hour delayed

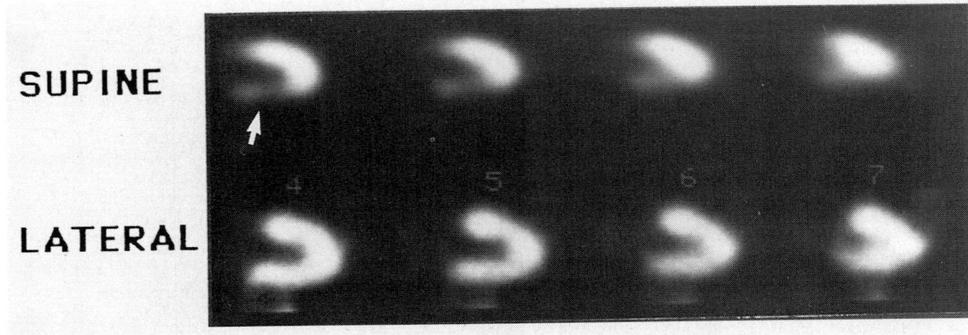

FIGURE 9–12. Vertical long-axis ^{201}Tl SPECT images of the patient shown in Figure 9–7. Images acquired with the patient lying on his back *(supine)* are shown in the top panel. An inferior wall myocardial perfusion defect is present (arrow). The patient was turned on the right side *(lateral)* and SPECT imaging was repeated. This time the vertical long-axis images are normal. The erroneous inferior wall defect on supine imaging is caused by attenuation by the left hemidiaphragm. Turning the patient on the right side diminishes diaphragmatic attenuation. (From Wackers, F. J. Th.: Artifacts in planar and SPECT myocardial perfusion imaging. Am. J. Cardiac Imaging *6*:42, 1992.)

imaging, improved uptake can be noted on 24-hour redistribution imaging or after a new resting injection (see below).[36,37] It is controversial at the time of this writing whether a fixed defect with ^{99m}Tc-labeled agents (which involves a rest injection) at times may underestimate myocardial viability.

REVERSE REDISTRIBUTION. This pattern occurs only with ^{201}Tl imaging. The initial stress images either are normal or show a defect, whereas the delayed images show a new or a more severe defect.[38] This pattern is frequently observed in patients with infarction who have undergone thrombolytic therapy or percutaneous coronary angioplasty. The phenomenon is thought to be caused by initial *excess* of tracer uptake in a reperfused area with a mixture of scar tissue and viable myocytes. Initial accumulation is followed by rapid clearance from scar tissue. Although the significance of this finding is controversial, it does *not* represent evidence of exercise-induced ischemia. With positron emission tomography with F18-deoxyglucose, the presence of residual viable myocardium has been demonstrated within areas with reverse redistribution.[39]

RADIOTRACER LUNG UPTAKE. Normally very little or no radiotracer is noted in the lung fields on postexercise images. Increased lung uptake can be quantitated as lung/heart ratio (normal < 0.5 for ^{201}Tl) or as lung washout (normal < 42 per cent for ^{201}Tl). This abnormal pattern has been well documented for ^{201}Tl and indicates exercise-induced left ventricular dysfunction.[40] Increased lung uptake has also been noted in occasional patients with ^{99m}Tc-labeled agents,[41] but less frequently than with ^{201}Tl. At the time of this writing it is still unclear whether increased lung uptake of ^{99m}Tc-labeled compounds has the same significance as noted for ^{201}Tl.

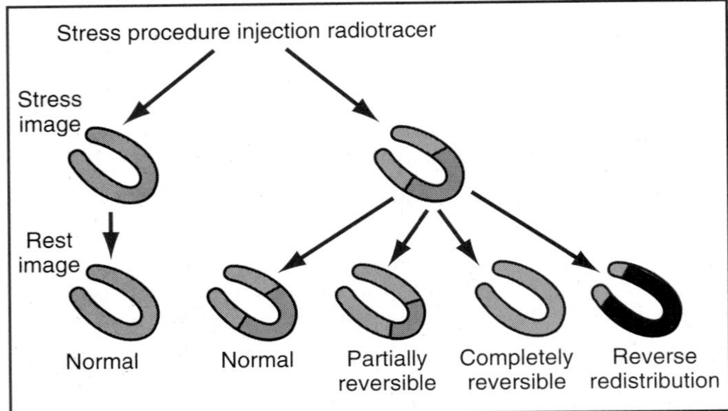

FIGURE 9–13. Schematic representation of interpretation of myocardial perfusion images. The shaded areas indicate myocardial perfusion defects.

TRANSIENT LEFT VENTRICULAR DILATION. Occasionally the left ventricle is noted to be larger following exercise than on the rest or delayed image. This pattern indicates exercise-induced left ventricular dysfunction.[42]

Image Quantification

Myocardial perfusion images are relatively difficult to interpret. As with visual interpretation of any data set, considerable intraobserver and interobserver variability exists for subjective interpretation, even among experienced readers.[43] Reproducibility of interpretation is related to a number of factors: (1) overall quality of raw data, (2) quality of image display, (3) degree of abnormality, (4) degree of change between exercise and rest images, and (5) familiarity with normal variations.

Computer quantification of myocardial perfusion images provides an important means of improving consistency of image interpretation and decreasing reader variability.[43] Several approaches to image quantification have been described. Irrespective of planar or SPECT imaging, the output of computer quantification generally consists of the following: (1) graphic or polar map display of relative myocardial distribution of radiotracer, (2) quantitative comparison of relative radiotracer distribution with a normal reference data base, (3) quantitative comparison of stress defect size with rest (delayed) defect size and quantification of defect reversibility, and (4) quantification of myocardial kinetics (applicable only for ^{201}Tl).

MYOCARDIAL KINETICS OF THALLIUM-201. Quantitative analysis of ^{201}Tl kinetics has become of decreasing importance over the last few years with the increased use of SPECT imaging and the introduction of ^{99m}Tc-labeled radiopharmaceuticals that show no significant redistribution. After injection at peak exercise, ^{201}Tl accumulates rapidly in myocardium supplied by normal coronary arteries and subsequently clears slowly from the myocardium (Fig. 9–14). In normal patients washout at 2 hours after injection is approximately 30 per cent, and at 4 hours 35 per cent. The rate of ^{201}Tl washout is related to peak exercise heart rate, exercise duration, and ^{201}Tl blood level. The kinetics of ^{201}Tl in *ischemic myocardium* is variable.[44]

When a significant coronary artery stenosis is present, the initial uptake of ^{201}Tl during exercise is lower than in normal myocardium. Subsequently, the washout of ^{201}Tl from ischemic tissue is lower than normal, and accumulation of ^{201}Tl may even occur over time. The initial uptake of ^{201}Tl in infarcted or scarred myocardium is considerably lower than in normal myocardium. On planar images ^{201}Tl clearance from an infarct parallels that of normal myocardium. This is very likely explained by overlap of normal myocardium on planar images.

MYOCARDIAL KINETICS OF TECHNETIUM-99m–LABELED AGENTS. During the first 3 hours after injection, approximately 30 per cent of a

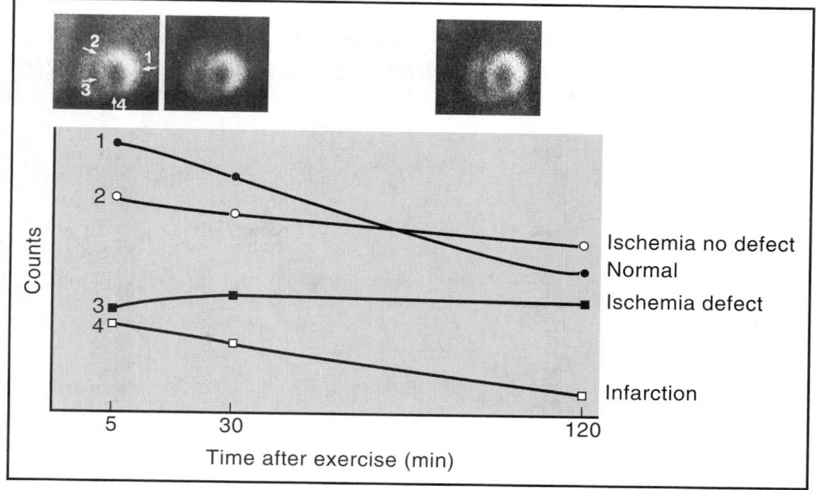

FIGURE 9–14. ^{201}Tl time activity curves after exercise in normal myocardium (1), transiently ischemic myocardium without visual defect (2), transiently ischemic myocardium with a visible defect (3), and old myocardial infarction (4). Normal myocardium (1) shows a gradual decrease of ^{201}Tl activity over time. After transient ischemia, ^{201}Tl clearance is slower than normal (2), or ^{201}Tl uptake may increase (3) in the myocardium over time. An old infarct area (4) without exercise-induced myocardial ischemia shows gradual decrease in ^{201}Tl activity over time similar to that in normal myocardium. The images show an example of a septal defect that gradually fills in over time, except at the apex where an old scar is present (4).

^{99m}Tc-labeled myocardial perfusion imaging agent clears from the heart (Fig. 9–15). Although redistribution of sestaMIBI in ischemic defects has been demonstrated in experimental animals[45] and in selected patients, the degree of redistribution in humans is minimal and does not have clinical significance. For practical clinical imaging, two separate injections are required to assess reversibility of stress-induced defects.

QUANTIFICATION OF PLANAR IMAGES

Planar exercises and rest images usually show marked differences in background radiotracer activity.[21] Accordingly, before quantification, interpolative background correction is performed.[46] After background correction, the relative distribution of radiopharmaceutical in the myocardium can be displayed in several ways: either as traverse count profiles or as circumferential count profiles.[47–49]

For the transverse count profile method, usually four profiles are generated across the left ventricle in each planar view. The count profiles are normalized to the pixel with maximal activity and compared with the lower limit of normal radiotracer distribution. In addition, myocardial clearance can be assessed by measuring the change in absolute myocardial count density over time.

With circumferential count profiles (Fig. 9–16), the mean regional distribution of radiopharmaceutical is displayed, sampling the entire left ventricle in 36 or more segments. Exercise and rest circumferential profiles are normalized to the segment with highest tracer activity, and the patient's profiles are compared with those of a normal data base. A normal data base is usually not derived from patients with normal angiographic coronary arteries but rather from subjects with a low (<3 per cent) likelihood of coronary artery disease.

In a normal image, all data points of either transverse or circumferential profiles are above the lower limit of normal. In a patient with a myocardial perfusion defect, the count profile is below the lower limit of normal in the anatomical location corresponding to the visually perceived defect. With circumferential profiles, a defect can be quantified as a *defect integral*, that is, the area below the lower limit of normal curve proportional to the total potentially visualized normal myocardium (Fig. 9–16). The reproducibility of these methods has been well established.[50]

QUANTIFICATION OF SPECT IMAGING

In SPECT imaging a multitude of reconstructed images are available for analysis. A typical SPECT study consists of approximately 32 paired (stress and rest) images in short-axis, vertical long-axis, and horizontal long-axis slices (Figs. 9–17*A* and 9–18*A*). Computer quantification is usually performed on reconstructed short-axis slices.

THE POLAR MAP (BULL'S EYE DISPLAY). The most widely used and commercially available approach is that of polar map or bull's-eye display (Figs. 9–17*B* and 9–18*B*). The purpose of a polar map is to generate one single image that encompasses the relative radiopharmaceutical distribution in the entire heart.[28] Relative radiopharmaceutical uptake on short-axis images is compressed to color-coded concentric rings, with the apical slice in the center and the basal slices on the periphery of the polar map.

It is important to understand that *a polar map is not a true image* but a simplified color-coded derivative of analog images. The bull's-eye image can be compared with a normal reference polar map. As mentioned above, a normal data base is usually derived from subjects with a low likelihood of coronary artery disease. Considerable variation exists with regard to the generation of a SPECT normal data base. In some software packages, the lower limit is a uniform mean minus two standard deviations. In other approaches, different criteria are applied for each coronary artery territory. Gender-specific data bases also have been recommended.[28]

Areas with a significant myocardial perfusion defect (i.e., relative count distribution below the lower limit of normal) can be highlighted on a polar map as a "black-out area" (Fig. 9–18*C*). By comparing stress and rest polar maps and image subtraction, the amount of defect reversibility can be visualized and quantified.[51] Although several commercially available software packages exist for generation of polar maps, manufacturers often do not supply a normal data base. Consequently, in many laboratories, SPECT polar maps are inter-

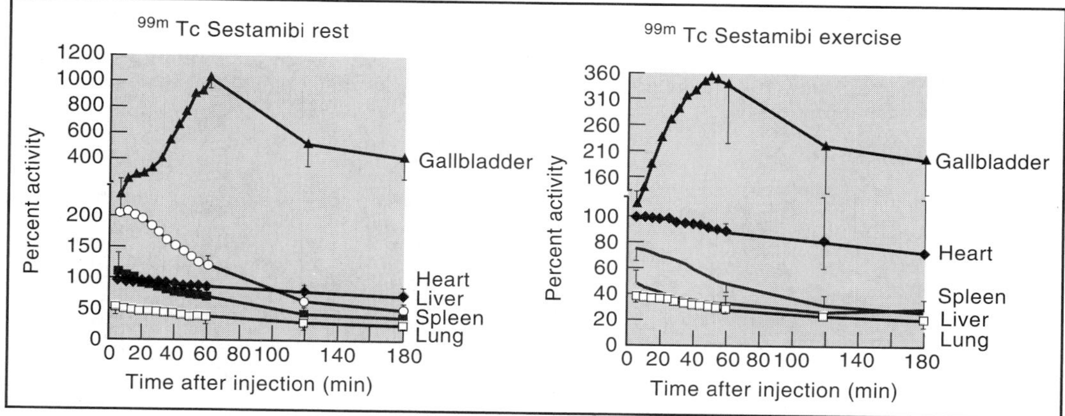

FIGURE 9–15. ^{99m}Tc-sestamibi organ time activity curves after injection at rest and after exercise in 5 normal volunteers (mean ± standard deviation). The data are normalized at cardiac activity at 5 minutes after injection. For clarity, standard deviations are shown only at 5, 60, 120, and 180 minutes. ^{99m}Tc-hexamibi is obsolete nomenclature for ^{99m}Tc-sestamibi. (Reprinted by permission of the Society of Nuclear Medicine from Wackers, F. J. Th., Berman, D. S., Maddahi, J., et al.: Technetium-99m Hexakis 2-methoxyisobutyl isonitrile: Human biodistribution, dosimetry, safety and preliminary comparison to Thallium-201 for myocardial perfusion imaging. J. Nucl. Med. *30*:301, 1989.)

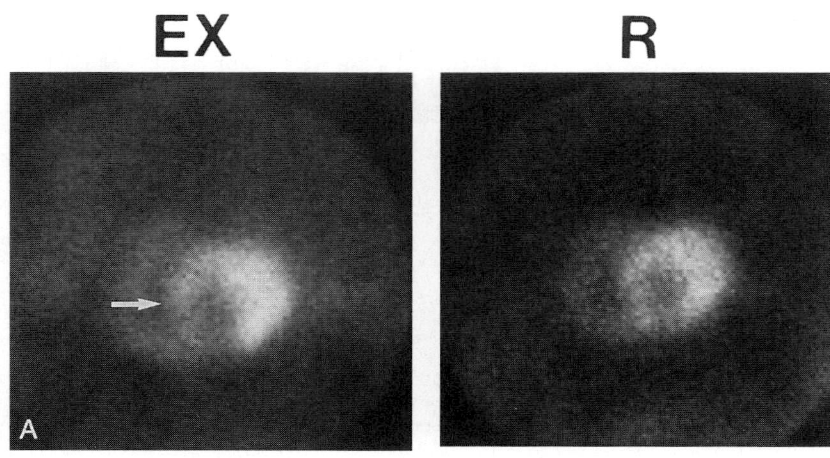

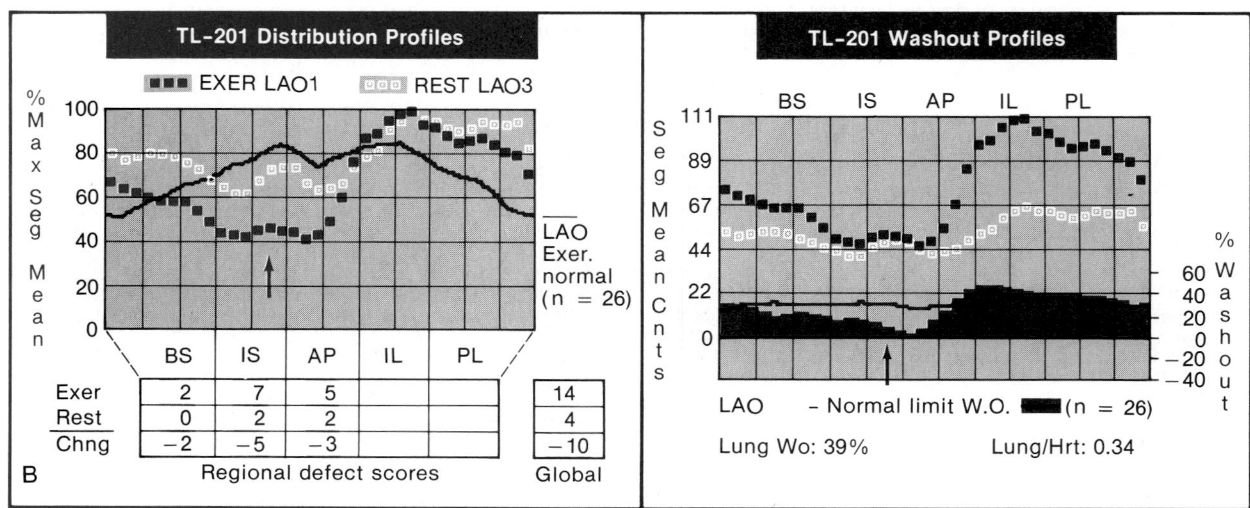

FIGURE 9–16. Left anterior oblique (LAO) images after exercise (EX) and at redistribution (R) imaging, and circumferential count distribution and washout profiles generated from these images. *A,* The analog images show a reversible exercise-induced inferoseptal defect (arrow). *B, Left,* Circumferential count distribution profiles display myocardial activity from basal septum (BS) to posterolateral (PL) wall. The continuous black line indicates the lower-limit-of-normal ^{201}Tl distribution (mean − 2 deviations). The exercise (colored dots) and delayed (white dots) profiles are normalized to the area with maximal counts (i.e., PL wall). The exercise profile is below the lower limit of normal in the basal septal (BS), inferoseptal (IS), and apical septal (AP) segments. This exercise defect (arrow) is quantified as an integral of 14. The delayed profile shows the graphic representation of a reversible defect (closer to the lower limit of normal). The defect on the delayed images is 4. The change in defect size (reversibility) is 10. *Right,* The washout (WO) profiles show thallium distribution as absolute counts. In the (normal) inferolateral and posterolateral area absolute counts decreased over time, with a measured washout of approximately 40 per cent. This is shown as the colored histogram on the bottom. The continuous black line indicates the lower limit of normal washout. In the ischemic BS, IS, and AP areas there is no change in absolute counts. In these areas the washout is below the lower-limit-of-normal curve (arrow). The patient's lung washout is normal at 39 per cent, and the lung/heart ratio is normal at 0.34.

FIGURE 9–17. See color plate 5.

FIGURE 9–18. See color plates 6 and 7.

preted visually without normal reference file and without quantification.

CIRCUMFERENTIAL PROFILES. An alternative approach to the polar map display for quantification of SPECT images is the use of circumferential profiles (Fig. 9–17*C*), similar to that described for planar images. Multiple circumferential profiles are generated over each of the short-axis slices and compared with those of a normal reference data base.[52] In a normal image, all data points of circumferential profiles are above the lower limit of normal. In a patient with a myocardial perfusion defect (Fig. 9–18*C*), the count profile is below the lower limit of normal in the areas corresponding to visually perceived defect. With circumferential profiles, a defect can be quantified as an integral, i.e., the area below the lower limit of a normal curve proportional to the total potentially visualized normal myocardium.

The total size of a myocardial perfusion defect can be expressed as a percentage of the entire left ventricle. The computed defect size is adjusted for slice thickness and varying diameter of each short-axis slice from base to apex. This approach provides quantification of total exercise defect size, rest defect size, and per cent defect reversibility.

Regardless of the quantitative approach used, the advantage of computer quantification is in providing a graphic display of the relative distribution of radiopharmaceutical uptake in the myocardium and the degree of perfusion abnormality compared with a normal reference data base.

Clinical Use of Quantification of Myocardial Perfusion Imaging

Computer quantification of myocardial perfusion imaging enhances the overall accuracy of the detection of coronary artery disease and also enhances reproducibility of interpretation. However, quantification should be used astutely. In general, from a standpoint of diagnostic interpretation, quantification should confirm the impression derived from visual analysis of analog images. If quantitative information appears to be discordant, one should inspect the analog images again. Frequently, one may recognize that quantification was correct. However, sometimes artifacts cause abnormal quantitative results. The process of integrating analog and quantitative information can be referred to as "quantitative analysis with visual overread." It is important to realize that artifacts, such as those caused by attenuation due to overlying soft tissue or diaphragm or resulting from patient motion, often have an unpredictable effect on the appearance of reconstructed slices. Although a normal data base, to a certain extent, incorporates normal variations, computer quantification per se should not be expected to distinguish between true perfusion defects and artifacts.

Electrocardiograph (ECG)-Gated Myocardial Perfusion Imaging

The high photon flux of ^{99m}Tc-sestamibi and of other ^{99m}Tc-labeled compounds makes it feasible to acquire myocardial perfusion images in ECG-gated mode.[53] ECG-gated myocardial perfusion images can be displayed as an endless-loop cine, similar to that commonly used for ECG-gated equilibrium radionuclide angiocardiography. The interpretation of ECG-gated *planar* images is not always unequivocal because of confluence of "endocardial edges" due to thickening of the facing myocardial wall.[53] However, interpretation of ECG-gated *SPECT* images is usually easier.[54] ECG-gated SPECT images allow assessment of regional wall motion and regional wall thickening. ECG gating is usually applied to the study in which the agent is injected during stress. However, because the acquisition is performed at rest, it is possible to evaluate *resting* wall motion and *resting* wall thickening in areas with exercise-induced myocardial perfusion defects (Figs. 9–17*D* and 9–18*D*). Combined interpretation of perfusion and function of ECG-gated images substantially increases confidence of interpretation. ECG-gated images are also useful for the recognition of artifactual defects due to attenuation (breast and diaphragm). Several investigators have demonstrated the feasibility of determining left ventricular ejection fraction ventricular volumes and regional wall thickening from ECG-gated SPECT slices.[55,56]

CLINICAL APPLICATIONS OF MYOCARDIAL PERFUSION IMAGING

Acute Myocardial Infarction

(See also Chap. 37)

DETECTION. Myocardial perfusion imaging with either ^{201}Tl or ^{99m}Tc-labeled compounds is an extremely sensitive and reliable means for early visualization of acute myocardial infarction (Figs. 9–19 and 9–20*A* and *B*). The timing of imaging after the onset of acute chest pain is relevant for the results of imaging. Images obtained during the first 6 hours after the onset of myocardial infarction show perfusion abnormalities at the anatomical location of infarction almost without exception.[57] However, as the time interval after onset of chest pain increases, some patients may have normal perfusion images. Serial imaging in patients with acute myocardial infarction revealed that in some patients the size of myocardial perfusion defect may decrease over time. These observations, initially made in 1974 with ^{201}Tl, are currently better understood. In approximately 20 per cent of patients with acute infarction, spontaneous throm-

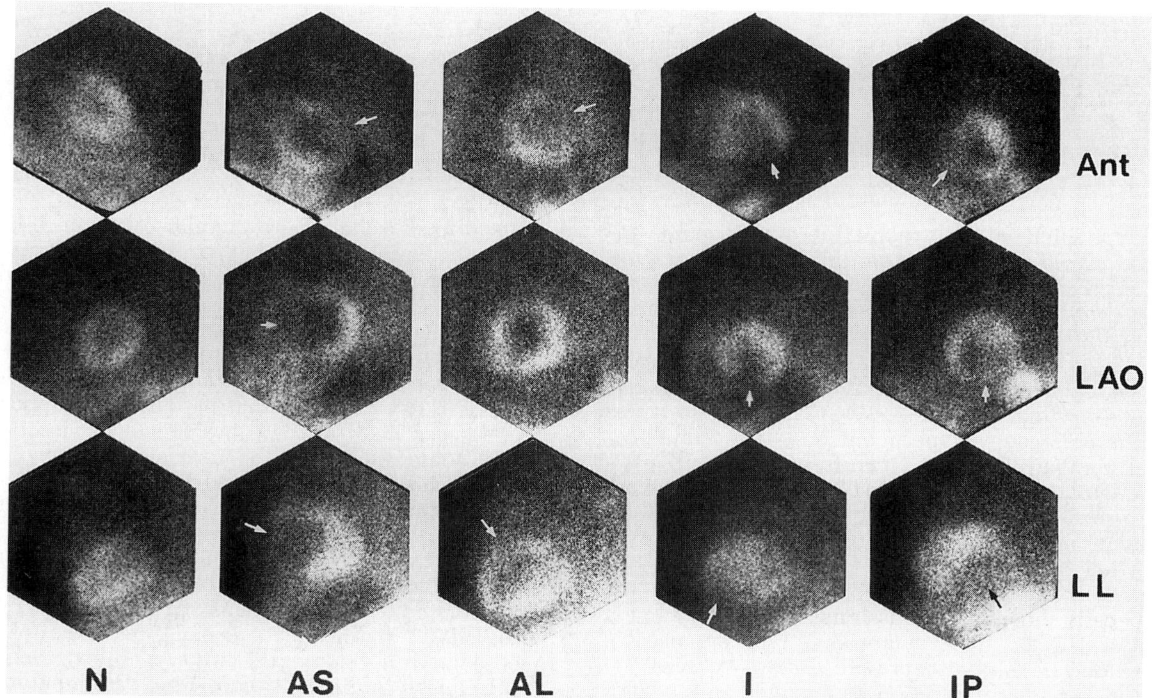

FIGURE 9–19. Planar ^{201}Tl images in acute myocardial infarction. Typical images of acute myocardial infarction in three projections. The first column shows normal ^{201}Tl images (N), the second to fourth columns show typical images of acute myocardial infarcts at anteroseptal (AS), anterolateral (AL), inferior (I), and inferoposterior (IP) locations. The defects are marked by arrows. (From Wackers, F. J. Th., Busemann Sokole, E., Samson, G., et al.: Value and limitations of thallium-201 scintigraphy in the acute phase of myocardial infarction. N. Engl. J. Med. *295*:1, 1976. Copyright Massachusetts Medical Society.)

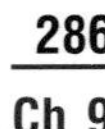

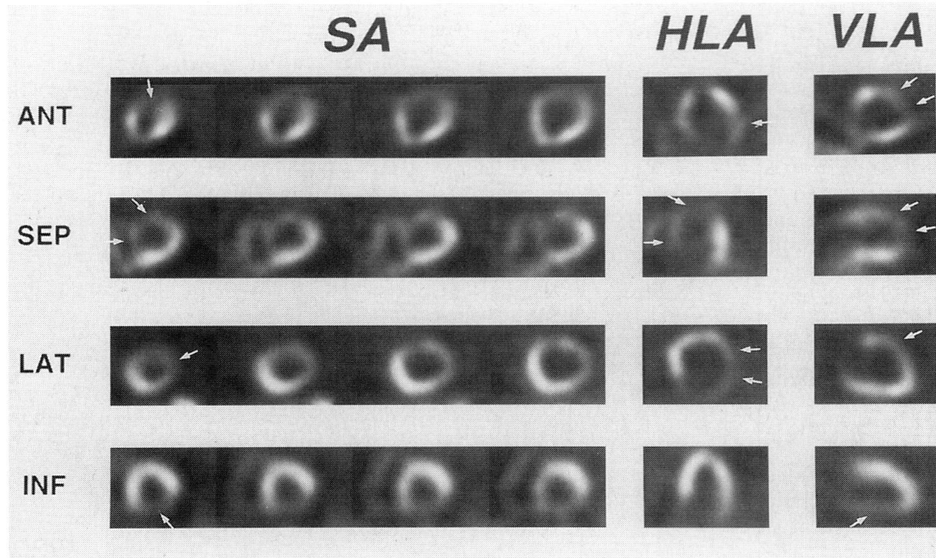

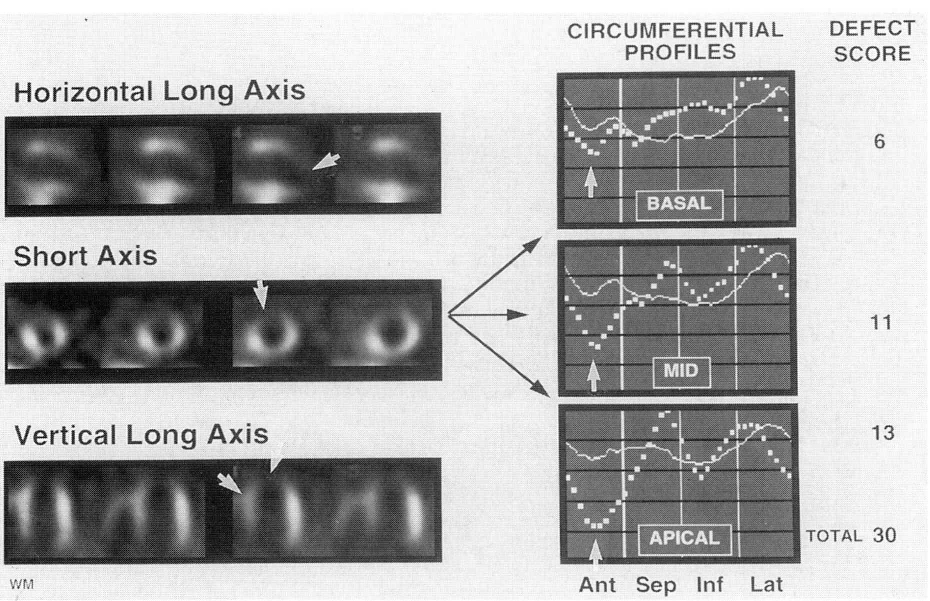

FIGURE 9–20. *Top,* SPECT ^{99m}Tc-sestamibi images of acute myocardial infarction. Typical ^{99m}Tc-sestamibi SPECT images of acute myocardial infarction in short-axis (SA), horizontal long-axis (HLA), and vertical long-axis (VLA) slices. From top to bottom: anterior (ANT), anteroseptal (SEP), lateral (LAT), and inferior (INF) infarctions. Defects are indicated by arrows. (From Wackers, F. J. Th.: Myocardial perfusion imaging. *In* Sandler, M. P., Coleman, R. E., Wackers, F. J. Th. (eds.): Diagnostic Nuclear Medicine. Baltimore, Williams & Wilkins, 1995.) *Bottom,* Quantification of infarct size on SPECT myocardial perfusion images. ^{99m}Tc-sestamibi images in a patient with anteroseptal myocardial infarction are shown. The images on the left show horizontal long-axis, short-axis, and vertical long-axis slices. An anterior apical myocardial perfusion defect (arrow) is present. On the right, circumferential profiles count distribution. The thin line represents the lower-limit-of-normal distribution of sestamibi. The white data points represent patient's circumferential profile. The circumferential profile is below the lower limit of normal in the anteroseptal and lateral areas. The defect is quantified as 30 per cent of the total left ventricle.

bolysis occurs, which could explain the spontaneous improvement of myocardial perfusion images. The location and size of myocardial perfusion defects in acute myocardial infarction correlate well with findings at postmortem.[58]

MYOCARDIAL PERFUSION IMAGING IN THE EMERGENCY DEPARTMENT. Because acute regional myocardial hypoperfusion can be visualized almost instantaneously with myocardial perfusion imaging, potential use as a means to triage patients in the emergency department has been evaluated. A substantial number of patients seen in emergency departments with complaints of acute chest pain have a nondiagnostic electrocardiogram. These patients are often admitted to rule out acute myocardial infarction. However, in only a small proportion of these patients (15 to 20 per cent) can acute coronary disease be confirmed. The majority of patients have costly hospital admissions without having a true cardiac cause for their symptoms. Wackers et al.[59] showed that none of the patients with normal "acute ^{201}Tl images" had either acute infarction or unstable angina after further clinical evaluation. In contrast, more than 80 per cent of patients who later were proven to have either acute infarction or unstable angina had abnormal ^{201}Tl perfusion images on admission in the emergency room.[59]

The new ^{99m}Tc-labeled myocardial perfusion imaging agents are better suited than ^{201}Tl for imaging patients with chest pain in the emergency department. Because these agents do not redistribute significantly, imaging does not have to be performed immediately, and myocardial perfusion during chest pain can be imaged at a convenient time. Moreover, SPECT imaging can be performed, which allows more detailed evaluation of various coronary vascular territories. Varetto et al.[60] and Hilton et al.[61] injected sestamibi in patients with chest pain and nondiagnostic electrocardiograms. They observed that patients with abnormal sestamibi images had a high incidence of coronary events (death, acute infarction, or revascularization) during follow-up, whereas patients with normal acute myocardial perfusion images in general had a favorable outcome. If these observations are confirmed in larger series of patients, myocardial perfusion imaging in the emergency department could become an important and cost-effective means for the triage of patients with acute chest pain.[62]

THROMBOLYTIC THERAPY. During the early hours of acute myocardial infarction, evaluation of myocardial perfusion is of interest in patients who have thrombolytic therapy. Serial myocardial perfusion imaging can demonstrate a decrease in myocardial perfusion defect size over time in patients who had successful reperfusion. Imaging with ^{201}Tl is not practical in this setting. Because of ^{201}Tl redistribution, myocardial imaging has to be performed *before* initiation of therapy. This would cause a clinically unacceptable delay in treatment. A more practical approach is the use of

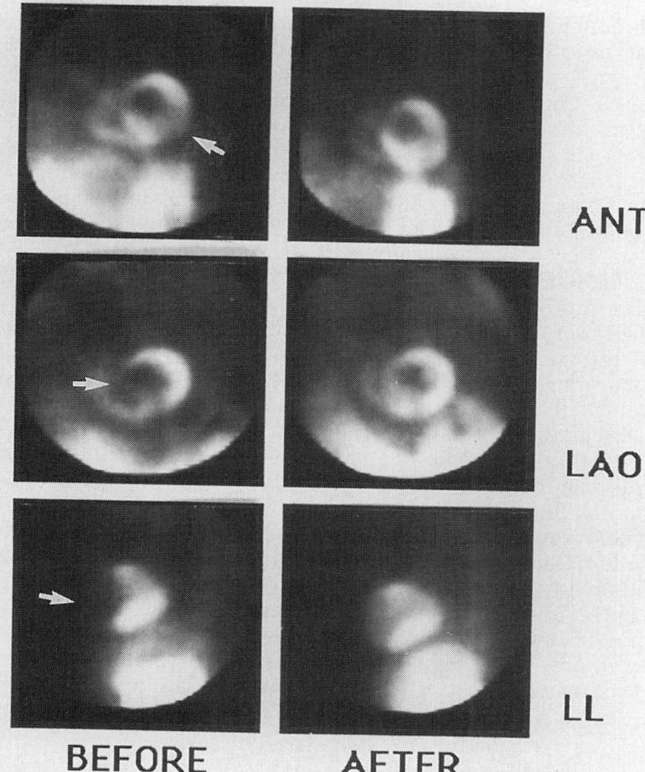

FIGURE 9–21. Planar myocardial perfusion imaging with ^{99m}Tc-sestamibi before and after thrombolytic therapy in a patient with an acute anteroseptal myocardial infarct. ^{99m}Tc-sestamibi was injected immediately before initiation of thrombolytic therapy and imaging was performed 2 hours later. Because of the lack of significant redistribution of ^{99m}Tc-sestamibi, the distribution of myocardial blood flow at the time of injection is "frozen" in time. The images before thrombolytic therapy show an anteroseptal myocardial perfusion defect (arrows) that was quantified as 53. The patient was reinjected with ^{99m}Tc-sestamibi when thrombolytic therapy was completed. These images show improved perfusion of the anteroseptal segments, indicating successful reperfusion of the infarcted artery. The perfusion defect size after thrombolytic therapy was 35. Therefore, 33 per cent of myocardium was salvaged by thrombolytic therapy in this patient. (From Wackers, F. J. Th., Gibbons, R. J., Verani, M. S., et al.: Serial quantitative planar technetium-99m-isonitrile imaging in acute myocardial infarction: Efficacy for noninvasive assessment of thrombolytic therapy. Reprinted with permission from the American College of Cardiology. J. Am. Coll. Cardiol. *14*:861, 1989.)

^{99m}Tc-sestamibi. Because of the lack of significant redistribution, this imaging agent can be injected *before* initiation of thrombolytic therapy, and imaging of myocardial perfusion can be performed later using either planar imaging at the bedside or SPECT imaging in the nuclear cardiology laboratory.[63–68] Gibbons et al.[63] and Wackers et al.[64] showed that successful thrombolysis of the infarct artery can be predicted by a decrease of the size of myocardial perfusion defects on serial ^{99m}Tc-sestamibi imaging (Fig. 9–21).

The noninvasive demonstration of successful myocardial reperfusion by thrombolysis could be useful in defining management of individual patients. For example, patients who apparently had failure of thrombolytic therapy (i.e., no change in myocardial perfusion defect) may be candidates for a more aggressive and invasive approach, whereas patients who had apparently successful reperfusion, as demonstrated by improvement of myocardial perfusion, may be more appropriate candidates for conservative management. With the use of a "split-dose" technique (i.e., a small dose initially followed by a larger dose later), it is feasible to obtain the same information on risk area and salvage within a few hours after the patient's arrival in the emergency room.

Serial myocardial perfusion imaging with sestamibi has provided new insights on the pathophysiology of acute human myocardial infarction. Gibbons et al. conducted a series of important clinical studies with sestamibi in patients with acute infarction. Their experience can be summarized as follows.

The myocardial area at risk varies greatly in individual patients.[63,64] Little correlation exists between extent of the risk area as demonstrated with sestamibi imaging and the anatomic site of occlusion of the infarct artery, i.e., distal or proximal.[69] The area at risk in acute anterior myocardial infarction is usually larger than that in acute inferior infarction.[71] Patients with collateral coronary circulation to the infarct artery have smaller ultimate infarct size than patients without collateral vessels.[71]

A decrease in myocardial perfusion defect size on serial imaging before and after thrombolytic therapy is a reliable predictor of reperfusion on the infarct artery and subsequent improvement of left ventricular regional wall motion.[72] Serial myocardial perfusion imaging has further shown that in many patients (approximately 40 per cent) myocardial perfusion defect size continues to decrease during the days after thrombolytic therapy was administered.[64] Others have confirmed this observation.[73,74]

Marcassa et al.[75] observed the same phenomenon of continued decreasing resting defect size in stable patients late (7 months) after anterior wall infarction. This may cause an apparent increase of stress-induced ischemia. The pathophysiological basis of this phenomenon remains unclear. Ito et al.[76] demonstrated delayed recovery from microvascular damage after acute infarction. This could be a potential explanation for late improvement in defect size.

Serial myocardial perfusion imaging with ^{99m}Tc-labeled myocardial perfusion imaging agents is now recognized as a potentially useful clinical research tool to assess the efficacy of various thrombolytic strategies in acute myocardial infarction.[77] The patient serves as his own control, and fewer patients needed to be recruited for a clinical trial. In a comparative trial of primary angioplasty versus thrombolysis for acute myocardial infarction, Gibbons et al.[78] demonstrated with acute sestamibi imaging that the area at risk in both patient groups was the same.

EARLY ASSESSMENT OF PROGNOSIS AFTER ACUTE INFARCTION. The size of myocardial perfusion defects in stable patients after acute myocardial infarction has been shown to be of prognostic significance. Silverman et al.[79] showed that patients with large resting myocardial perfusion defects had a significantly poorer prognosis and survival than patients with small myocardial perfusion defects. This outcome appeared to be independent of other clinical parameters. Similar prognostic information on the size of SPECT myocardial perfusion defect was reported by Cerqueira et al.[80] after thrombolytic therapy (Fig. 9–22).

Visualization of the right ventricle at rest[81] and increased ^{201}Tl uptake in the lung at rest in patients with recent infarction[82] have been reported as additional indicators of an unfavorable course after myocardial infarction.

Brown et al.[83] evaluated the potential of pharmacological vasodilation and myocardial perfusion imaging for early (first to fourth day) risk stratification in patients with recent acute myocardial infarction. Patients who had evi-

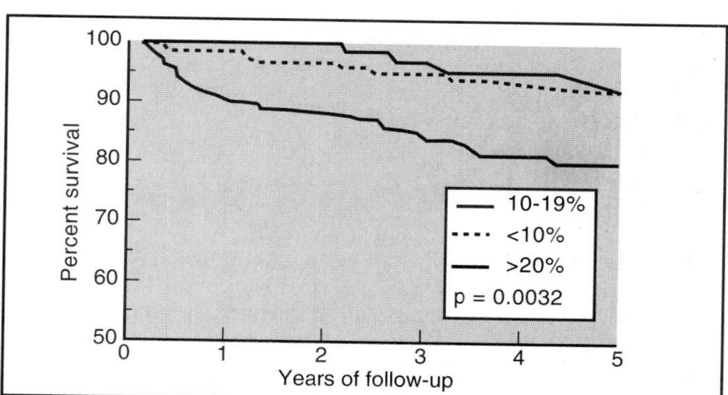

FIGURE 9–22. ^{201}Tl SPECT infarct size and per cent survival during follow-up after thrombolytic therapy for acute myocardial infarction. Patients with large (>20 per cent of left ventricle) myocardium perfusion defects after thrombolytic therapy for myocardial infarction had significantly poorer prognosis than patients with a small (<10 per cent) or moderate (10 to 19 per cent) sized myocardial perfusion defect. (From Cerqueira, M. D., Maynard, C., Ritchie, J. L., et al.: Long-term survival in 618 patients from the Western Washington streptokinase in myocardial infarction trials. Reprinted with permission from the American College of Cardiology. J. Am. Coll. Cardiol. *20*:1452, 1992.)

dence of residual jeopardized myocardium (i.e., partially reversible defects) had a significantly higher in-hospital complication rate than patients who had fixed myocardial perfusion defects.

UNSTABLE ANGINA (see p. 1331). In patients with unstable angina without prior myocardial infarction, rest myocardial perfusion defects have been demonstrated. These perfusion defects are demonstrable not only when the radiopharmaceutical is injected *during* chest pain but also for considerable time *after* the angina has subsided.[84–86] Resting ^{201}Tl defects in patients with unstable angina are invariably reversible, indicating transient hypoperfusion of viable myocardium.

Technetium-99m–labeled myocardial perfusion imaging agents that do not redistribute have a particular advantage in patients with unstable angina. The lack of redistribution makes it possible to inject the radiotracer during pain and acquire images at a later time when the patient is pain free and stable. Bilodeau et al.[86] reported similar observations in patients with unstable angina using sestamibi SPECT imaging as described above with ^{201}Tl. Patients with abnormal electrocardiographic findings during pain had larger myocardial perfusion defects than those who did not. The observations with myocardial perfusion imaging in patients with unstable angina indicate that impaired regional myocardial blood flow persists longer than can be judged from the clinical status or electrocardiogram. Patients with reversible resting myocardial perfusion defects usually have severe multivessel coronary artery disease. Resting myocardial perfusion imaging during pain was more sensitive and more specific for significant coronary artery disease than the resting electrocardiogram.

Resting imaging in patients with recurrent chest pain after infarction or with unstable angina is useful for objectively demonstrating the presence of transient myocardial hypoperfusion and viable myocardium. This information can be very helpful when myocardial revascularization is considered. In patients with unstable angina who have been stabilized, subsequent exercise myocardial perfusion defect size has been shown to be a reliable predictor of the extent of coronary artery disease.[87]

DETECTION OF OLD MYOCARDIAL INFARCTION. Myocardial perfusion imaging does not differentiate between acute myocardial infarction, acute ischemia, or old scar. A substantial number of patients with small or old myocardial infarction may have normal perfusion images. Frequently, prior myocardial infarction can be recognized only as "thinner" myocardial segments. In approximately one-half of patients with old infarction, planar myocardial perfusion images may become normal. This occurs particularly in patients with old inferior wall myocardial infarcts. SPECT imaging appears to be more sensitive in detecting such small myocardial scars.

Chronic Coronary Artery Disease

(See also Chap. 38)

In patients with chronic stable coronary artery disease who are capable of physical exercise, myocardial perfusion imaging is used in conjunction with exercise testing. Physical exercise can be performed either on a treadmill, which is most popular in the United States, or on an upright bicycle, which is frequently used in Europe and other countries. Physical exercise has the advantage of providing additional useful clinical and physiological parameters, such as duration of exercise, total workload, maximum heart rate, exercise-induced symptoms, electrocardiographic changes, and blood pressure response. However, a substantial number of patients referred for evaluation cannot physically exercise because of orthopedic, neurological, or peripheral vascular problems. In the latter group of patients pharmacological vasodilatation with dipyridamole or adenosine or pharmacological stress with dobutamine provides useful alternative approaches.

The basic principle of using various modes of stress in conjunction with radionuclide myocardial perfusion imaging is to create *heterogeneity of myocardial blood flow* between vascular territories supplied by normal coronary arteries and that supplied by an artery with significant obstructive coronary artery stenosis (Fig. 9–23). Heterogeneity of regional myocardial blood flow can be visualized with radionuclide myocardial perfusion agents. Heterogeneity of regional myocardial blood flow is a requirement for abnormal images. However, regional hypoperfusion does not necessarily imply myocardial ischemia.

PHYSICAL EXERCISE. Several standardized treadmill exercise protocols exist. The most widely used protocol was designed by Bruce. Nonimaging endpoints are reproduction of the patient's symptoms, exhaustion, hypotension or decrease in systolic blood pressure of 20 mm Hg or more, ventricular arrhythmias, and electrocardiographic severe ST-segment depression on electrocardiography. An intravenous line should be in place in a large antecubital vein for injection of the radiopharmaceutical agent. When the endpoint of exercise is reached, the radiopharmaceutical is injected rapidly in the intravenous line and flushed with saline. The patient is then encouraged to exercise for another 1 to 2 minutes at the same level of exercise. This continuation of exercise after injection of the radiotracer is crucial for diagnostic stress imaging. It is important to maintain heart rate, and thus myocardial blood flow, at peak exercise level to allow for accumulation of the radio-

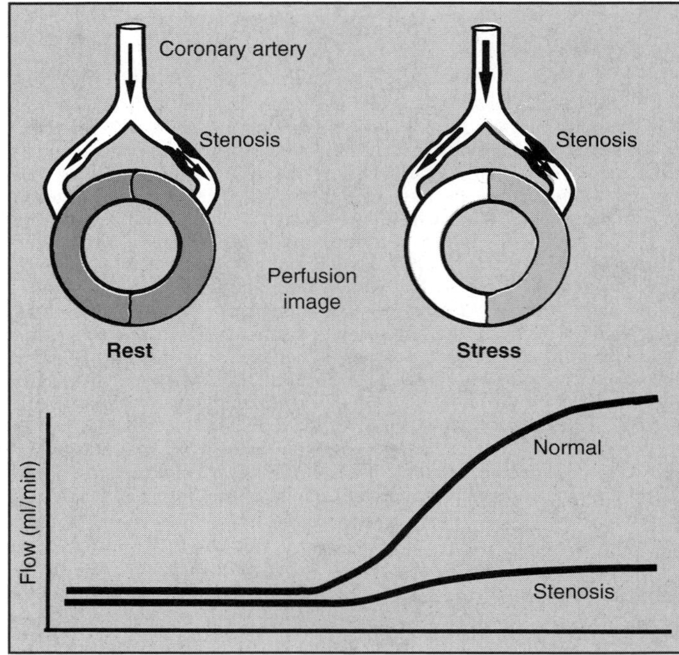

FIGURE 9–23. Schematic representation of the principle of rest/stress myocardial perfusion imaging. *Top,* Two branches of a coronary artery are schematically shown; the left branch is normal, and the right branch has a significant stenosis *(middle).* Myocardial perfusion images of the territories supplied by two branches. *Bottom,* Schematic representation of coronary blood flow in the branches at rest and during stress. At rest, myocardial blood flow is similar in both coronary artery branches. When a myocardial perfusion imaging agent is injected at rest, myocardial uptake is homogeneous (normal image). During stress, coronary blood flow increases 2.0 to 2.5 times in the normal branch, but not to the same extent in the stenosed branch, resulting in heterogeneous distribution of blood flow. This heterogeneity of blood flow can be visualized with ^{201}Tl or ^{99m}Tc-sestamibi as an area with relatively decreased radiotracer uptake (myocardial perfusion defect). (Reprinted by permission of the Society of Nuclear Medicine from Wackers, F. J. Th.: Exercise myocardial perfusion imaging. J. Nucl. Med. *35*:726, 1994.)

tracer during a "steady ischemic state." If the patient is unable to continue exercising at the same level, the speed and grade of the treadmill can be decreased to a lower level.

For bicycle exercise a similar graded exercise protocol is used. Usually the patient starts at 25 kpm, and the resistance is increased every 3 minutes until an exercise end-point is reached.

The purpose of exercise is to increase cardiac metabolic demands and to test the ability of the coronary circulation to meet these demands with an appropriate increase of myocardial blood flow. Consequently, myocardial ischemia is frequently provoked with physical exercise.

PHARMACOLOGICAL VASODILATION. Patients with orthopedic, neurological, or peripheral vascular problems are incapable of exercising adequately on a treadmill or bicycle. These patients can be evaluated for the presence of significant coronary artery disease by use of pharmacological vasodilation in combination with radionuclide myocardial perfusion imaging. Furthermore patients on beta-blocking medication who are unable to increase their heart rate adequately by physical exercise have been studied successfully with pharmacological coronary vasodilation. In addition, patients with complete left bundle branch block are preferably studied with dipyridamole to avoid artifactual perfusion defects.

Intravenous infusion of *dipyridamole* blocks the cellular reabsorption of adenosine and thus increases the concentrations of adenosine, an endogenous vasodilator that activates specific receptors. Coronary blood flow is autoregulated by adenosine to meet myocardial metabolic demands.[88] In patients without coronary artery disease dipyridamole infusion creates vasodilatation and increases coronary blood flow three to five times above baseline levels. In patients with significant coronary artery disease the resistance vessels distal to a stenosis are already dilated, often maximally, in order to maintain normal resting flow. In these patients, infusion of dipyridamole does not cause further significant vasodilatation in the diseased vascular bed. However, in the adjacent myocardium supplied by normal coronary arteries, a substantial increase in myocardial blood flow occurs. In this manner, *heterogeneity of regional myocardial blood flow is created:* Territories supplied by diseased arteries are relatively hypoperfused compared with normal regions (Fig. 9–23). Pharmacological vasodilation by dipyridamole or adenosine infusion usually does not provoke myocardial ischemia.

DIPYRIDAMOLE INFUSION PROTOCOL. Dipyridamole is infused over a 4-minute period (0.142 mg/kg/min).[88] At approximately 4 minutes after completion of the infusion, maximal dilatory effect is achieved. At this time the radiotracer is injected intravenously. Maximal vasodilatory effect is usually associated with a modest increase in heart rate (10 beats per minute) and slight decrease (10 mm Hg) in systolic blood pressure. In some laboratories dipyridamole infusion is combined with low-level exercise. This appears to decrease the incidence of side effects, which occur in about 50 per cent of patients during infusion of dipyridamole.[89] Approximately 10 per cent may have electrocardiographic changes, and 20 per cent may experience angina, although most frequent complaints are headache, flushing, and nausea (Table 9–2).[90,91]

Ischemia may be caused by "coronary steal." In this situation, the marked increase in blood flow in the *normal* myocardial zones "steals" blood away via collaterals from the vascular bed supplied by significantly diseased coronary arteries. This and other undesirable side effects can usually be reversed quickly by blocking adenosine receptor sites with intravenous aminophylline.

ADENOSINE INFUSION. Clinical experience of direct intravenous infusion of adenosine (maximal 140 μg/kg/min) has been comparable to that reported for dipyridamole.[92,93] The coronary vasodilatory effect of adenosine appears to be more potent and more consistent than that of dipyridamole.[94] However, side effects are more common, occurring in about 75 per cent of patients (Table 9–2). Approximately 50 per cent of patients may have chest pain, and many have headache, nausea, and flushing. Atrioventricular conduction abnormalities have been reported occasionally in patients using adenosine infusion. This has been of some concern. However, because of the short half-life of adenosine, side effects can be reversed almost instantaneously by termination infusion of adenosine. Samuels et al.[95] observed that adenosine-SPECT imaging was well tolerated by patients with moderate to severe aortic valvular stenosis who were evaluated for coexisting coronary artery disease.

DOBUTAMINE STRESS. For patients who have contraindications to dipyridamole or adenosine infusion, such as those with bronchospastic pulmonary disease, or for patients who are on xanthine derivatives or who have consumed caffeine, dobutamine infusion offers an alternative diagnostic approach.[96,97] Dobutamine increases myocardial oxygen demand by increasing myocardial contractility, heart rate, and blood pressure. The increase in coronary blood flow is comparable to that during physical exercise (two- to three-fold) but less than that with adenosine or dipyridamole.

Nevertheless dobutamine infusion should not be considered equivalent to physical exercise. Useful clinical information such as duration of exercise, exercise capacity, and reproduction of symptoms is not obtained. The increase in heart rate is usually lower than with exercise. Thus, dobutamine pharmacological stress should be considered

TABLE 9–2 REPORTED SIDE EFFECTS (% OF PATIENTS) OF INTRAVENOUS DIPYRIDAMOLE, ADENOSINE, AND DOBUTAMINE MYOCARDIAL PERFUSION IMAGING

	DIPYRIDAMOLE (RANHOSKY AND RAWSON[90])	ADENOSINE (VERANI et al.[92])	DOBUTAMINE (HAYS et al.[97])
Cardiac			
Fatal myocardial infarction	0.05	0	0
Nonfatal myocardial infarction	0.05	0	0
Chest pain	19.7	57	31
ST-T changes on ECG	7.5	12	50
Ventricular ectopy	5.2	?	43
Tachycardia	3.2	?	1.4
Hypotension	4.6	?	0
Blood pressure lability	1.6	?	?
Hypertension	1.5	?	1.4
Atrioventricular block	0	10	0.6
Noncardiac			
Headache	12.2	35	14
Dizziness	11.8	?	4
Nausea	4.6	?	9
Flushing	3.4	29	14
Pain (nonspecific)	2.6	?	7
Dyspnea	2.6	15	14
Paresthesia	1.3	?	12
Fatigue	1.2	?	?
Dyspepsia	1.0	?	?
Acute bronchospasm	0.15	0*	?

*Patients with history of bronchospasm excluded
? = Not reported

TABLE 9–3 SENSITIVITY AND SPECIFICITY FOR DETECTION OF CORONARY ARTERY DISEASE BY QUANTITATIVE PLANAR ^{201}Tl SCINTIGRAPHY

AUTHOR	NUMBER OF PATIENTS	SENSITIVITY (%)	SPECIFICITY (%)
Berger et al. 1981[99]	140	91	90
Maddahi et al. 1981[100]	67	93	91
Wackers et al. 1985[49]	150	89	95
Kaul et al. 1986[102]	325	90	80
van Train et al. 1986[101]	157	84	88
TOTAL	839	89	89

a last resort in patients who cannot exercise, rather than a substitute for exercise.

Dobutamine Infusion Protocol. Infusion of dobutamine is started with a low dose of 5 μg/kg/min. The dose is increased each 3 minutes, if tolerated, to a maximal dose of 40 μg/kg/min. The radiopharmaceutical is injected during infusion of maximal dose, and infusion is continued for 2 to 3 minutes. Table 9–2 shows the incidence of side effects during dobutamine infusion.[97] A similar infusion protocol is used for dobutamine stress echocardiography. In a recent review of 2942 patients who had dobutamine-atropine stress echocardiography, nine patients (0.3 per cent) had serious cardiac side effects, including two nonfatal infarctions, two instances of ventricular fibrillation, two instances of sustained ventricular tachycardia, two cases of sustained severe hypotension, and one case of prolonged severe myocardial ischemia.[98]

Clinical Results of Exercise Testing and Myocardial Perfusion Imaging

Each year more than 2.5 million patients undergo stress myocardial perfusion imaging in the United States. Currently, approximately 70 per cent of all studies are performed with ^{201}Tl, and the remaining studies are obtained with ^{99m}Tc-sestamibi. About 60 to 70 per cent of studies are performed in conjunction with physical exercise and 30 per cent with pharmacological vasodilation. Eighty per cent of all studies in the United States use SPECT imaging.

Over the last 20 years the clinical usefulness of stress myocardial perfusion imaging has been well established. Although the majority of data in the literature are based on planar ^{201}Tl imaging, recent published reports indicate that similar results are obtained with SPECT imaging and ^{99m}Tc-labeled agents.

The introduction of computer processing and quantification of *planar* myocardial perfusion images improved overall detection of coronary artery disease substantially (Table 9–3). For instance, the detection of single-vessel disease with ^{201}Tl improved from 55 per cent by visual analysis to 84 per cent by quantitative analysis. Almost all patients with double- or triple-vessel coronary artery disease are detected by quantitative myocardial perfusion imaging.[49,99–102]

ASSESSMENT OF MYOCARDIAL PERFUSION. In 1994 the American Medical Association performed a Diagnostic And Therapeutic Technology Assessment (DATTA) of SPECT myocardial perfusion imaging.[103] This extensive review of the literature revealed sensitivities for planar imaging ranging from 67 to 96 per cent and sensitivities for SPECT imaging ranging from 83 to 98 per cent. The range of specificities for planar imaging varied from 40 to 100 per cent and from 53 to 100 per cent for SPECT imaging. The report did not address the potential contribution of image quantification on improvement of diagnostic accuracy. The DATTA panel of experts considered ^{201}Tl SPECT myocardial perfusion imaging a well-established and proven technology. Representative results of qualitative and quantitative SPECT imaging are shown in Table 9–4.[104–112]

The ability to accurately predict coronary disease in specific individual vessels has been consistently suboptimal by planar imaging and reflects an inherent limitation of planar technology. Using SPECT imaging, detection of coronary artery disease in individual vessels, in particular the left circumflex coronary artery, is significantly improved.[105] Consequently, SPECT stress myocardial perfusion imaging is particularly useful in following patients who had coronary angioplasty (see below).

VALUE OF TECHNETIUM-99m RADIOPHARMACEUTICALS. Since the introduction of ^{99m}Tc-sestamibi in 1989, thousands of patients have been evaluated with this new myocardial perfusion agent. Several comparative studies, both by planar and SPECT technique, have shown that the detection of coronary artery disease with ^{99m}Tc-sestamibi is comparable to that with ^{201}Tl.[10,11,113–116] Similar results have been reported recently for ^{99m}Tc-tetrofosmin[15,117,118] and ^{99m}Tc-furifosmin.[119,120]

The relatively high dose of ^{99m}Tc administered makes it feasible to acquire images in ECG-gated mode and to perform first-pass angiocardiography in combination with myocardial perfusion imaging.[54,114] The feasibility of acquiring simultaneous myocardial perfusion and myocardial contraction data (*"one-stop shop"*) using the same radiopharmaceutical injection is one of the major advantages of the ^{99m}Tc-labeled compounds over ^{201}Tl (Fig. 9–24). Combined analysis of "still" slices and perfusion wall motion images further improves accuracy and confidence of interpretation. The clinical importance of acquiring both resting and peak exercise left ventricular ejection fraction is discussed elsewhere in this chapter.

Technetium-99m–Teboroxime. The clinical experience with ^{99m}Tc-teboroxime is still limited to a relatively small number of patients (Fig. 9–10). The diagnostic yield of this agent to detect coronary artery disease appears to be comparable to that of ^{201}Tl.[12,13,121,122] This imaging agent is of

TABLE 9–4 SENSITIVITY AND SPECIFICITY FOR DETECTION OF CORONARY ARTERY DISEASE BY ^{201}Tl SINGLE-PHOTON EMISSION COMPUTERIZED TOMOGRAPHY

AUTHOR	NUMBER OF PATIENTS	SENSITIVITY (%)	SPECIFICITY (%)	NORMALCY RATE
Tamaki et al. 1984[109]	104	91	92	
De Pasquale et al. 1988[105]	210	95	71	
Borges-Neto et al. 1988[112]	100	92	69	
Maddahi et al. 1989[104]	110	96	56	86
Fintel et al. 1989[106]	112	91	90	
Iskandrian et al. 1989[110]	164	88	62	93
Go et al. 1990[108]	202	76	80	
Mahmarian et al. 1990[107]	360	93	87	
van Train et al. 1990[111]	242	95	56	
TOTAL	1901	91	73	90

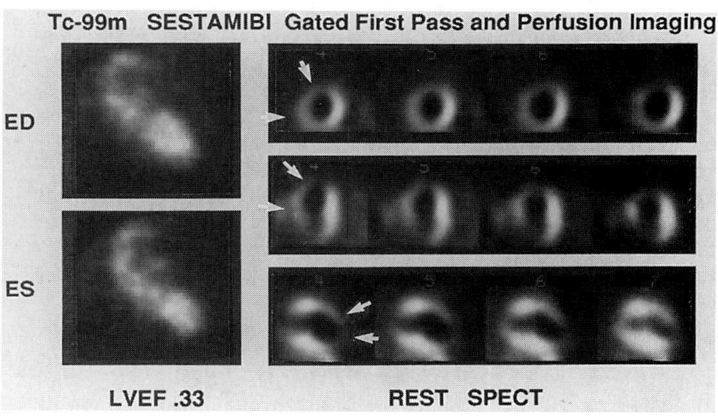

FIGURE 9–24. Simultaneous assessment of myocardial perfusion and function. ^{99m}Tc-sestamibi imaging in acute myocardial infarction allows assessment of both function and perfusion. In this patient with large anteroseptal infarction, the resting injection of sestamibi was used for first-pass radionuclide angiography *(left)*. The end-diastolic and systolic frames are shown. Global left ventricular ejection fraction was severely depressed at 0.33. On the right are resting SPECT sestamibi images in short-axis and vertical and horizontal long-axis slices. A large anteroseptal myocardial perfusion defect is present (arrows).

particular interest because the relatively short residence time in the heart allows for multiple injections and repeat simultaneous assessment of left ventricular function by first-pass radionuclide angiocardiography and myocardial perfusion. Preliminary data suggest that it may be feasible to derive pathophysiological information with regard to the presence of significant coronary artery disease by analysis of regional differences in myocardial washout of ^{99m}Tc-teboroxime.[123,124] The sensitivities and specificities to detect coronary artery disease using pharmacological vasodilation with various myocardial perfusion imaging agents have been reported to be similar to those used for physical exercise.[125,131]

REFERRAL BIAS. As mentioned above, many investigators report a relatively low specificity of stress SPECT myocardial perfusion imaging. The reported specificities range from 53 to 100 per cent. This lack of specificity has been explained by "referral bias."[132] That is, since stress myocardial imaging has become accepted in the clinical practice of cardiology, patients with normal stress radionuclide images are no longer referred for cardiac catheterization. Thus, the occasional patient who has normal coronary arteries on angiography almost always is referred because of abnormal stress myocardial perfusion images. The true specificity of stress SPECT imaging therefore can no longer be assessed in patients undergoing coronary angiography because of this referral bias.

Specificity should, however, be tested in patients with low likelihood of coronary artery disease. In such patients the "normalcy rate" is determined. The normalcy rate of planar imaging using ^{201}Tl and ^{99m}Tc-labeled compounds is generally over 95 per cent. With SPECT imaging, normalcy rate ranges from 85 per cent for ^{201}Tl to 95 to 100 per cent for ^{99m}Tc-labeled agents.

DETECTION OF HIGH-RISK CORONARY ARTERY DISEASE. The greater the functional severity of coronary artery disease, the more abnormal exercise myocardial perfusion images are likely to be. Most patients (approximately 95 per cent) with left main coronary disease have abnormal stress myocardial perfusion images.[133] However, the expected typical left main pattern, i.e., defects in the anteroseptal and posterolateral walls, is found in only a minority (approximately 14 per cent) of patients with left main coronary artery disease.[133–135] The majority (approximately 75 per cent) of patients have multiple perfusion defects and frequently abnormally increased lung uptake of ^{201}Tl.[136]

Although most patients with triple-vessel disease have abnormal stress images, approximately 60 per cent have multiple defects in two or more vascular regions. Most frequently, disease in the left circumflex coronary artery is not detected on planar stress myocardial perfusion images.

High-risk myocardial perfusion images (Figs. 9–18 and 9–25) can be characterized by (1) multiple reversible defects in two or more coronary artery territories[137]; (2) quantitatively large myocardial perfusion defects[138–142]; (3) increased pulmonary radiotracer uptake after exercise[40,41]; and (4) transient dilatation of the left ventricle immediately after exercise.[42]

This high-risk pattern is highly specific (approximately 95 per cent) for multivessel coronary artery disease; however, the sensitivity is only about 70 per cent. Therefore, in the absence of the above-mentioned scintigraphic characteristics, the presence of multivessel disease cannot be ruled out.

SEVERITY OF MYOCARDIAL PERFUSION DEFECTS. Myocardial perfusion defects vary in intensity. A defect can be very dense (severe), i.e., almost without any radiotracer uptake. On the other hand, some residual activity may still be present within the defect. The severity of perfusion defects is often assessed using a semiquantitative visual scoring system: 0 = normal, 1 = mildly reduced or equivocal, 2 = moderately reduced, and 3 = severely reduced. Computer quantification of circumferential count distribution profiles provides a means of quantifying precisely the extent (the number of angles below the lower limit) and severity (area below the lower limit) of a perfusion defect. This measurement can be expressed as an integrated defect score.[50–52]

Stress Myocardial Perfusion Imaging and Prognosis

The detection of coronary artery disease is only one aspect of the clinical value of stress myocardial perfusion imaging. An important additional feature is the ability to

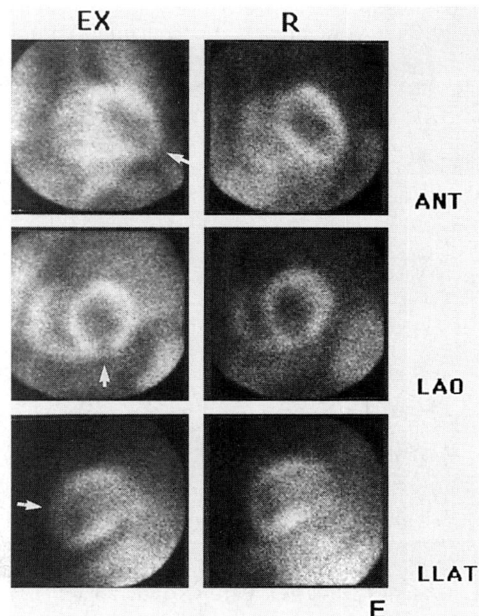

FIGURE 9–25. High risk ^{201}Tl images. After exercise the heart is enlarged and there is increased lung uptake of ^{201}Tl. Furthermore, there is a partially reversible anteroapical myocardial perfusion defect (arrows).

predict prognosis and to identify high- and low-risk patients. The first critical finding on myocardial perfusion images is the presence or absence of defect reversibility, i.e., ischemia.[141] Patients with evidence of transient ischemia on planar ^{201}Tl images have been shown to have a higher incidence of future cardiac events than patients with fixed defects. In patients with suspected or known chronic coronary artery disease, semiquantitative and quantitative assessment of the number or extent of myocardial perfusion defects and the magnitude of defect reversibility are predictive of cardiac events during follow-up (Figs. 9–26 and 9–27).[138,143]

Gibson et al.[137] evaluated patients who had uncomplicated myocardial infarction at the time of hospital discharge by planar quantitative ^{201}Tl stress imaging. Patients with a fixed single ^{201}Tl stress defect and without washout abnormalities (i.e., normal clearance of ^{201}Tl from the heart) at hospital discharge had only a 6 per cent cardiac event rate (death, recurrent infarction, or unstable angina), whereas patients who had high-risk findings on predischarge ^{201}Tl stress images (multiple defects in more than one vascular region, abnormal washout, or increased lung uptake) had a 51 per cent cardiac event rate. Numerous other investigators have since reported similar prognostic value of stress myocardial perfusion imaging after myocardial infarction using either physical or pharmacological stress.[144–147] Brown et al.[145] reported that patients with recurrent chest pain *after myocardial infarction* frequently had ischemia *within* the infarct region (75 per cent of patients), whereas only 25 per cent of patients had ischemia at distance. Patients with evidence of reversibility had a substantially poorer prognosis and higher incidence of revascularization procedures than patients who did not have demonstrable defect reversibility. Evidence of transient left ventricular dysfunction during stress (i.e., transient postexercise dilatation and/or increased radiotracer lung uptake) constitutes an important additional scintigraphic marker of adverse outcome.[148]

Bateman et al.[149] showed that categorization of results of SPECT imaging in high- and low-risk subsets is an effective strategy to select appropriate patients for coronary angiography, as well as to avoid unnecessary cardiac catheterization. Recently Nallamother et al.[149a] reported similar results, suggesting a future role for SPECT imaging as a "gatekeeper" for coronary angiography.

Alternatively, the presence of *quantitatively normal planar or SPECT stress myocardial perfusion images,* even

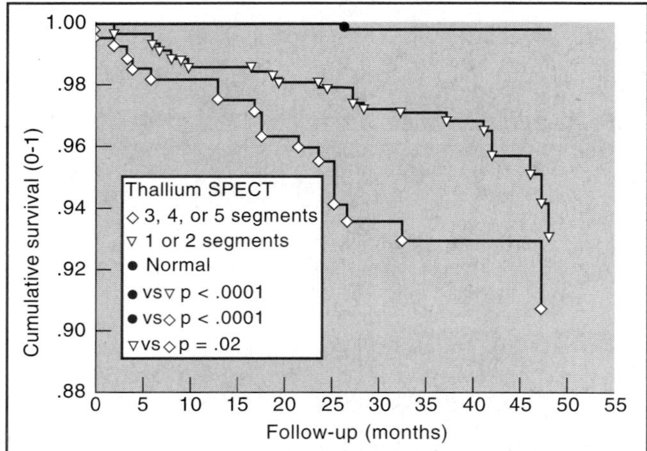

FIGURE 9–26. Cardiovascular cumulative survival and number of abnormal segments on SPECT ^{201}Tl stress scintigraphy. (From Manchecourt, J., Longere, P., Fagret, D., et al.: Prognostic value of thallium-201 single-photon emission computed tomographic myocardial perfusion imaging according to extent of myocardial defect. Reprinted with permission from the American College of Cardiology. J. Am. Coll. Cardiol. *23:*1096, 1994.)

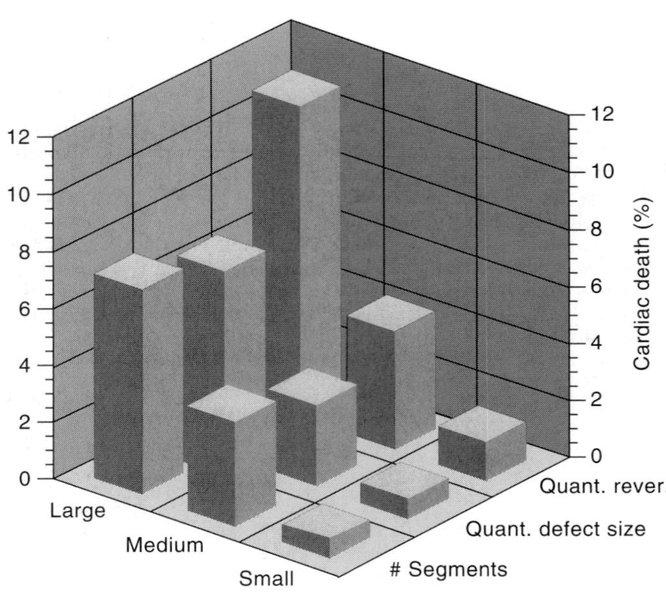

FIGURE 9–27. Prognostic importance of size and type of myocardial perfusion abnormality. Data are from 816 patients with stable coronary artery disease enrolled in the Multicenter Study on Silent Myocardial Ischemia (MSSMI). The patients had 26 months follow-up. All patients had quantitative planar ^{201}Tl stress imaging. The graph relates the size of exercise defects, defect reversibility, and number of abnormal segments to cardiac death rate during follow-up. The highest cardiac death rate occurred in patients with most abnormal images. In particular, patients with greatest defect reversibility had highest cardiac death rate. (Modified from Bodenheimer, M. M., Wackers, F. J. Th., Schwartz, R. G., et al.: Prognostic significance of a fixed thallium defect one to six months after onset of acute myocardial infarction or unstable angina. Am. J. Cardiol. *74:*1196, 1994.)

when coronary artery stenosis is angiographically documented, indicates favorable prognosis with low subsequent cardiac event rate.[150–156] Patients with quantitatively normal myocardial perfusion images have a yearly nonfatal myocardial infarction rate of 0.6 per cent and a mortality rate of 0.5 per cent per year.

These data on abnormal and normal stress myocardial perfusion images indicate that the extent of myocardial perfusion defects, or the lack thereof, provide significant physiological and prognostic information that surpassess the anatomical information obtained from coronary angiograms. Recent data in the literature suggest that the prognostic predictive value of stress myocardial perfusion imaging is independent of the imaging technique applied (planar or SPECT) or the radiopharmaceutical used (^{201}Tl or ^{99m}Tc-sestamibi).[157,158]

INDEPENDENT INCREMENTAL VALUE OF STRESS MYOCARDIAL PERFUSION IMAGING. In clinical practice diagnostic tests are usually used in conjunction with each other. The clinician usually has other clinical and diagnostic information available. The pathophysiological prognostic value of stress myocardial perfusion imaging as outlined above is important. However, if similar information can be derived from other less costly and readily available tests, it may not be cost-effective to perform radionuclide myocardial perfusion imaging. The incremental prognostic value of various diagnostic data obtained in succession (clinical data, exercise ECG, planar ^{201}Tl stress imaging, and coronary angiography) was assessed by Pollock et al.[159] and Melin et al.[160] The combination of clinical and exercise ^{201}Tl variables provide greater prognostic information than the combination of clinical and angiographic data. Iskandrian et al.[161] observed similar independent and incremental prognostic information using SPECT ^{201}Tl stress imaging, even when cardiac catheterization data are available (Fig. 9–28).

Bodenheimer et al.[140] reported that the extent of myocardial perfusion abnormality on quantitative SPECT was the

PLATE 5

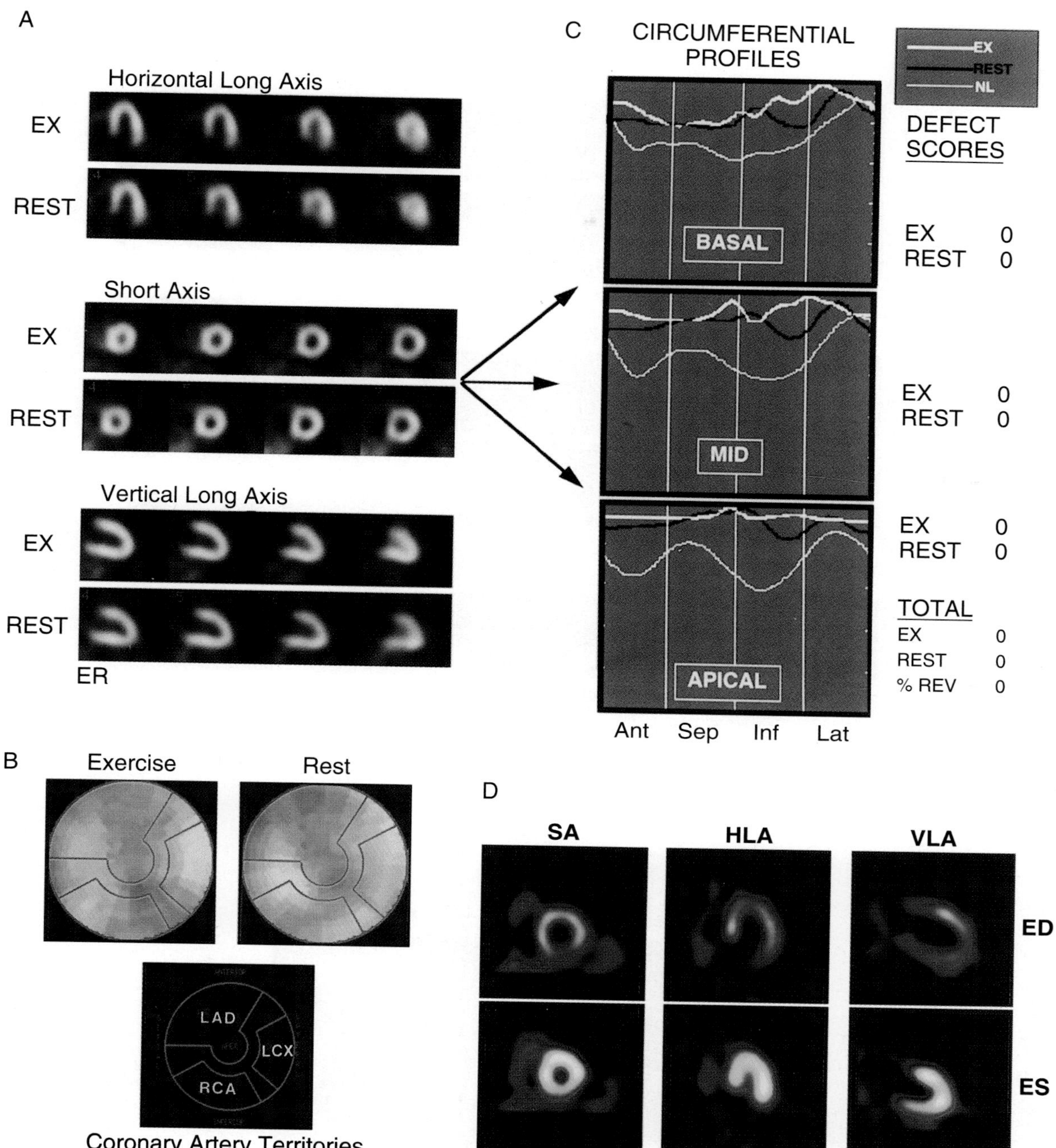

FIGURE 9–17. Exercise and rest SPECT myocardial perfusion imaging with ^{99m}Tc-sestamibi in a normal subject.

A, Horizontal long-axis, short-axis, and vertical long-axis slices. Normal distribution of ^{99m}Tc-sestamibi is noted.

B, Exercise and rest polar maps (bull's-eye display) of tomographic slices in *A.* On both the exercise and rest polar map, distribution of radiopharmaceutical is approximately homogeneous. Color scale: White represents the area with highest activity; yellow, orange, red, violet blue, and black indicate gradually decreasing count activity. The coronary artery territories of the LAD (left anterior coronary artery), LCX (left circumflex coronary artery), and RCA (right coronary artery) are indicated. The yellow, white, and orange colors represent normal perfusion.

C, Circumferential count profiles. Relative activity of sestamibi on the exercise images is displayed as a white line. The relative activity of sestamibi of the rest images is displayed as a black line. The lower-limit-of-normal sestamibi distribution is indicated as the thin white line. The relative radiotracer activity in the anterior (ANT), septum (SEP), interior (INF), and lateral (LAT) walls is shown in representative basal, midventricular, and apical short-axis slices. In this normal subject the relative distribution of sestamibi is above the lower-limit-of-normal distribution, indicating absence of perfusion defects and thus normal images.

D, ECG-gated exercise myocardial perfusion images of the same patient. End-diastolic and end-systolic frames of the short-axis slices (SA), horizontal long-axis slices (HLA), and vertical long-axis slices (VLA) are shown. The color coding is the same as in *B.* Comparison of the end-diastolic and end-systolic frames allow assessment of regional wall motion and regional wall thickening. In this normal subject wall motion and thickening are homogeneous: The color in the anterior wall, septum, and lateral wall changes from yellow to white; in the inferior wall color changes from orange to yellow. The relatively lesser activity in the inferior wall is due to diaphragmatic attenuation.

PLATE 6

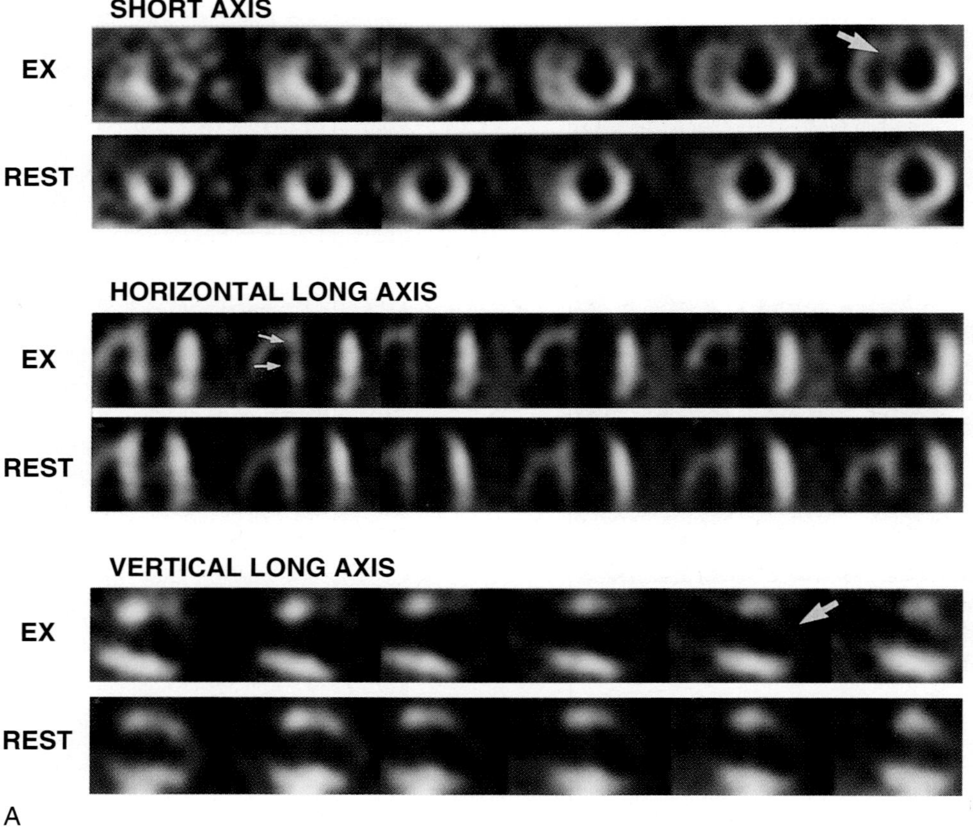

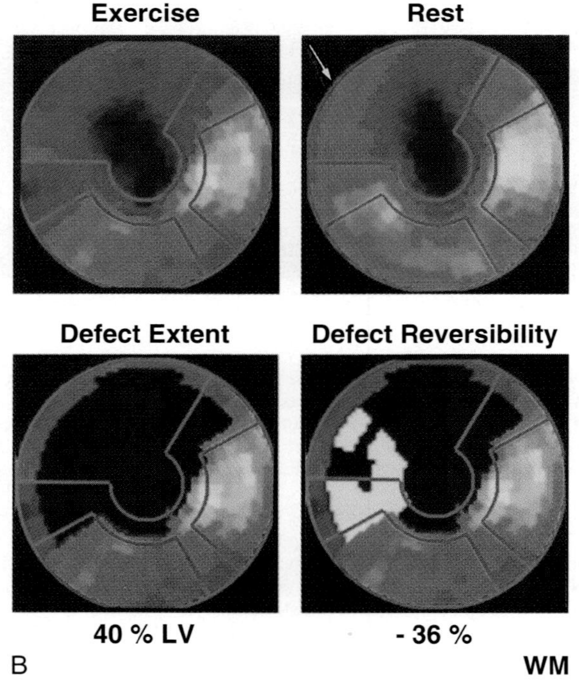

Legend on opposite page

PLATE 7

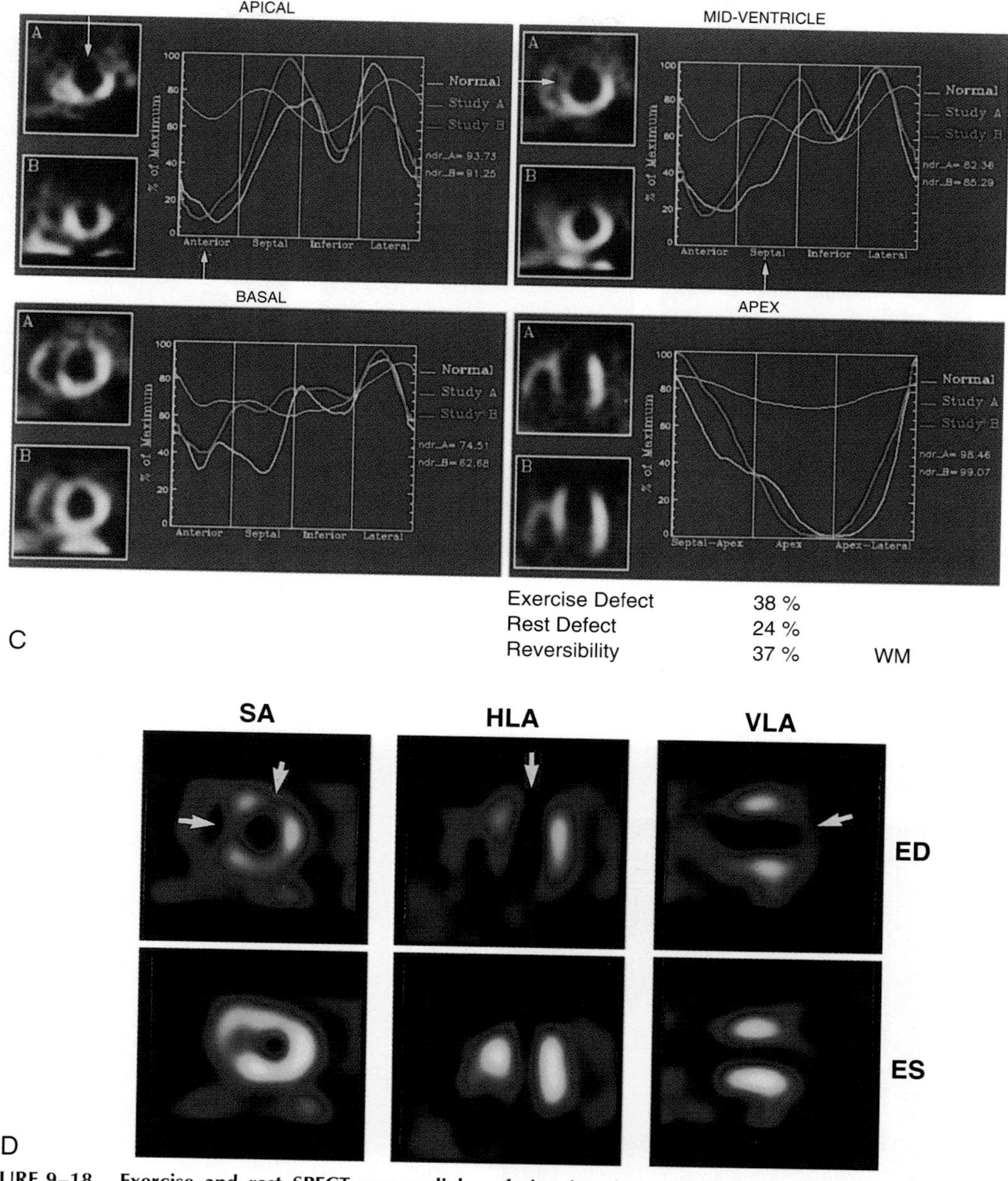

FIGURE 9–18. Exercise and rest SPECT myocardial perfusion imaging with ^{99m}Tc-sestamibi in a patient with anterior infarction and extensive triple-vessel coronary artery disease.

A, Reconstructed short-axis, horizontal long-axis, and vertical long-axis slices. On the exercise (EX) short-axis images an extensive anteroseptal myocardial perfusion defect (arrow) is present, which is partially reversible on the basal rest images. On the horizontal long-axis slices, a fixed apical defect is present with some reversibility in the septal area (arrows). On the vertical long-axis slices an extensive anteroapical myocardial perfusion defect is present which shows only minimal reversibility at rest.

B, Polar map display of short-axis slices in *A.* The color coding is the same as in Figure 9–17. On the exercise polar map an extensive anteroseptal myocardial perfusion defect is present. On the rest polar map, improvement in the septum (arrow) can be appreciated. On the bottom polar map, defect extent is compared with a normal data base. The abnormal area is black. The extent of the defect is calculated as 40 per cent of the left ventricle. On the reversibility polar map defect (white), reversibility is quantified as 36 per cent of the exercise defect.

C, Circumferential profiles analysis. The relative distribution of radiopharmaceutical is displayed for representative apical, midventricular, and basal short-axis slices. The yellow line represents the exercise study, the orange line the rest study, and the thin white line the lower-limit-of-normal distribution. The apical slice *(top left)* shows no significant improvement on the resting study. In contrast, the septal defect reversibility is demonstrated in the midventricular slice *(top right)* and the basal slice *(bottom left).* The apical defect *(bottom right)* is fixed. Total exercise myocardial perfusion defect size is quantified as 38 per cent of total left ventricle. The rest defect is 24 per cent. Defect reversibility is 34 per cent.

D, ECG-gated exercise SPECT images. End-diastolic and end-systolic frames are shown for the short-axis slices (SA), horizontal long-axis slices (HLA), and vertical long-axis slices (VLA). On the end-diastolic frames an extensive anteroapical and septal myocardial perfusion defect (arrow) is present. Analysis of wall motion shows absence of thickening in the anteroapical segment on the vertical long-axis and horizontal long-axis slices. On the short-axis slice and horizontal long-axis slice, in spite of the presence of an exercise-induced anteroseptal myocardial perfusion defect, thickening (change from orange and blue to yellow) of the anteroseptal segment can be appreciated.

PLATE 8

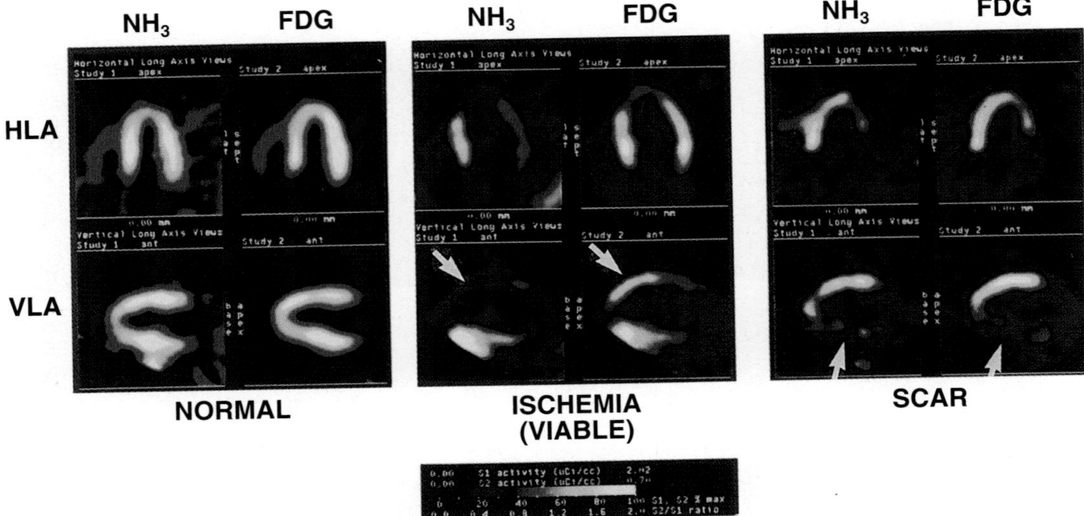

FIGURE 9–40. Three PET scintigraphic presentations are shown. On each panel, perfusion is represented by NH_3 and glucose metabolism by FDG. The left panel shows normal homogeneous uptake of NH_3 and FDG. In the middle panel, the arrows point to markedly reduced blood flow with preserved glucose uptake in a patient with myocardial viability in an area of an old anterior wall myocardial infarction. On the right, the arrows point to concordant reduction of blood flow and FDG in a patient with remote inferior wall myocardial infarction. (From Zaret, B. L., and Wackers, F. T.: Nuclear Cardiology (I). N. Engl. J. Med. *329*:775, 1993. Copyright 1993 Massachusetts Medical Society.)

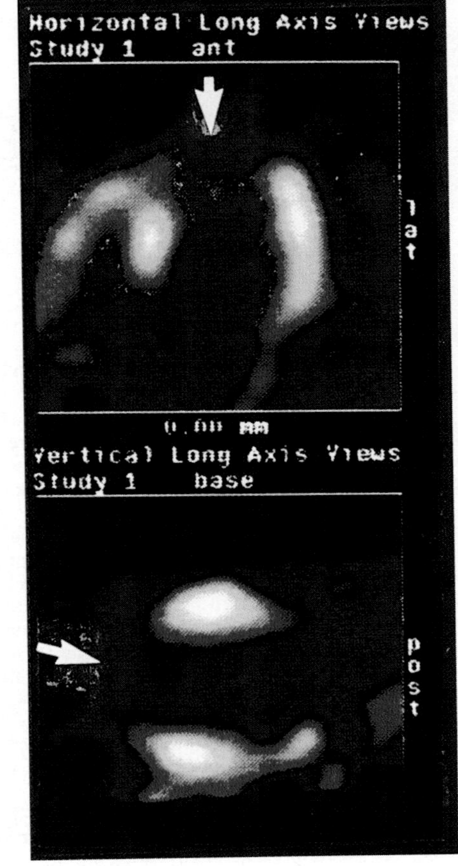

FIGURE 9–41. Static ^{11}C acetate images in a patient within one week of an anterior wall myocardial infarction are shown. The white arrows point to marked decrease of ^{11}C acetate in the anteroapical region. Serial data acquisition over time revealed marked decrease of ^{11}C acetate washout in these regions.

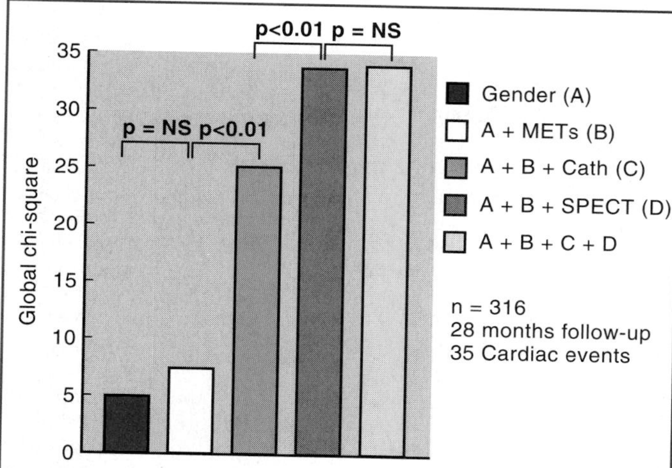

FIGURE 9–28. Independent and incremental prognostic power of clinical, exercise, catheterization, and quantitative ^{201}Tl SPECT variables. Data shown represent the global chi-square statistics of various clinical and diagnostic variables. SPECT imaging provides independent and incremental information to identify high-risk patients. Note that angiography (Cath) has less incremental value over clinical variables than ^{201}Tl-SPECT imaging. (From Iskandrian, A. S., Chae, S. C., Heo, J., et al.: Independent and incremental prognostic value of exercise single-photon emission computed tomographic (SPECT) thallium imaging in coronary artery disease. Reprinted with permission from the American College of Cardiology. J. Am. Coll. Cardiol. *22:*665, 1993.)

single most important prognostic predictor. Petretta et al.[162] and Fagan et al.[163] noted that the exercise ECG should be taken into consideration when the exercise ECG is normal and the additive prognostic value of stress myocardial perfusion imaging is less than when the exercise ECG is abnormal or nondiagnostic.

STRESS MYOCARDIAL PERFUSION IMAGING AFTER THROMBOLYIS. Several investigators[164,165] reported apparent diminished sensitivity of stress myocardial perfusion imaging for predicting multivessel coronary artery disease and cardiac events after treatment with thrombolysis for acute myocardial infarction. There may be several potential explanations for this observation. It is well recognized that patients eligible for thrombolytic therapy constitute a patient cohort at relatively low risk. These patients are generally younger and have fewer prior myocardial infarctions, fewer non-Q-wave infarctions, and less multivessel coronary artery disease than patients with acute infarction in the prethrombolytic era.

Because of the favorable outcome and low mortality in these patients, one would predict, based on Bayesian principles, diminished predictive value for stress myocardial perfusion imaging. Another confounding factor is that patients with abnormal stress perfusion images after acute myocardial infarction are generally referred for coronary angiography and revascularization if coronary anatomy is suitable. Accordingly, Gimple and Beller[166] have suggested that "the excellent outcome in patients treated with thrombolytic therapy and risk stratified with exercise testing provides strong empiric support for the continued use of noninvasive testing of patients without complication after thrombolytic therapy." Dakik et al.[167] reported that quantitative predischarge SPECT ^{201}Tl imaging in patients who had thrombolytic therapy for acute infarction provided a reliable means of identifying patients at high, intermediate, and low risk for future adverse events.

DETECTION OF CORONARY ARTERY DISEASE IN WOMEN (see also p. 1705). Exercise electrocardiography has been reported to be less accurate in women than in men to detect coronary artery disease. This can be explained in part by differences in disease prevalence in men and women.[168] Moreover, women more often have an abnormal baseline electrocardiogram, which affects accuracy of interpretation of the exercise electrocardiograms. Although breast attenuation artifacts may make the interpretation of stress myocardial perfusion images in women more difficult, Desmarais et al.[169] demonstrated that experienced interpreters usually recognize artifacts and can avoid false-positive interpretations.

Several investigators have examined the performance of stress myocardial perfusion imaging in women. Although women in general achieve lower exercise workload, the detection of significant coronary artery disease using radionuclide stress perfusion imaging[170–172] is similar to that in men. Moreover, Chae et al. and others showed that low- and high-risk patients are identified without gender differences.[155,171,173] Hendel et al.[174] reported that long-term outcome for vascular surgery patients also can be predicted by dipyridamole ^{201}Tl imaging irrespective of gender.

Syndrome X (typical exertional angina pectoris, positive ECG response to exercise, and angiographically normal coronary arteries (see p. 1343), occurs predominantly in postmenopausal women.[175] These patients, who have a good prognosis, generally have normal myocardial perfusion images, although myocardial perfusion abnormalities have been noted in an occasional patient.

PATIENTS WITH LEFT BUNDLE BRANCH BLOCK. In patients with complete left bundle branch block, the conduction abnormality precludes the use of conventional electrocardiographic criteria for the diagnosis of infarction or exercise-induced ischemia. It was expected that myocardial distribution of myocardial perfusion imaging agents would be unaffected by the electrocardiographic abnormality.[176] Indeed, in patients with left bundle branch block without prior myocardial infarction, *resting* myocardial perfusion images are generally normal. However, the septum is frequently thin and in older patients the left ventricle is often dilated.

A number of investigators have reported exercise-induced myocardial perfusion defects in anteroapical and anteroseptal areas in patients with complete left bundle branch block and angiographic normal coronary arteries.[177,178] In some patients partial or complete reversibility of these defects have been observed. Hirzel et al.[179] proposed, based upon experimental animal data with right ventricular pacing, that diminished septal myocardial blood flow during abnormal sequence of electrical ventricular depolarization caused septal defects. Shefcyk et al.[180] compared regional myocardial uptake of ^{201}Tl during rapid atrial pacing (normal conduction) with that during rapid right ventricular pacing (left bundle branch block). These investigators found no significant quantitative difference in regional ^{201}Tl uptake. Thus, it appears that the altered sequence of ventricular depolarization *itself* is not a principal cause of myocardial perfusion defects in left bundle branch block.

We noted a relationship between the presence of exercise-induced myocardial perfusion defects in left bundle branch block and degree of *left ventricular dilatation* at rest. Patients with left bundle branch block often have clinically unexpected cardiomyopathy with ventricular dilation and depressed left ventricular ejection fraction. Thus, altered geometry and partial volume effect may be other plausible explanations for observed defects. The use of pharmacological vasodilation with dipyridamole has been shown to reduce the incidence of artifactual perfusion defects in left bundle branch block.[181] We recommend that patients with electrocardiographic left bundle branch block be studied with pharmacologic vasodilation with dipyridamole or adenosine rather than with physical exercise to avoid false-positive results.

THALLIUM-201 STRESS IMAGING IN NONCORONARY ARTERY DISEASE. Thallium-201 imaging has been used in a number of clinical conditions that may be present with symptoms of chest pain but angiographically normal epicardial arteries.[182,183] In a number of these patients abnormal and "false-positive" ^{201}Tl images have been observed. LeGrand et al.[184] demonstrated that in patients with syndrome X, abnormal coronary reserve also could be demonstrated. Cannon et al.[185] found that these patients also had abnormal global and regional systolic and diastolic function. At least some of the so-called false-positive ^{201}Tl images in patients with angiographic normal coronary arteries may in fact reveal true abnormalities in myocardial microcirculation.[185a] In patients with mitral valve prolapse and atypical chest pain, several investigators have demonstrated normal ^{201}Tl stress images.

MYOCARDIAL PERFUSION IMAGING FOR PREOPERATIVE SCREENING (see also p. 1759). An important clinical application of myocardial perfusion imaging is the preoperative evaluation of patients undergoing noncardiac surgery. This has had its most meaningful application in the study of patients prior to revascularization surgery involving the descending aorta and the lower extremities. This group of patients has a strong likelihood coexisting coronary artery disease. Boucher et al.[186] were the first to show that dipyridamole thallium imaging is predictive of subsequent perioperative cardiac events in this patient's subgroup. The findings of reversibility on the dipyridamole thallium study were the single most important prognostic indicator.

Subsequent studies have indicated that the total cohort of patients can be stratified prior to perfusion scintigraphy based upon clinical variables. Eagle et al.[187] demonstrated that, based upon simple clinical assessment of specified risk factors, those with high risk of coronary disease and those with very low risk of coronary disease did not require perfusion studies for appropriate risk stratification. However, the majority of patients fell into an intermediate clinical group who were categorized quite effectively by perfusion studies. Further studies in this area have also demonstrated that the simple qualitative characterization of a perfusion study as either positive or negative for ischemia may be insufficient. However, appropriate categorization can be obtained using quantitative techniques that allow definition of a large potential ischemic burden as well as the identification of specific "high-risk" findings.[188,191] It has also recently been shown that dipyridamole thallium scintigraphy is of value in predicting long-range outcomes, beyond the perioperative period, in this group of patients.[191]

The predictive value of dipyridamole thallium imaging in preoperative assessment has been questioned in two recent studies.[192,193] However, it should be noted that both studies had potential for significant selection bias in the populations studied. It should also be noted that at the present time further prospective analysis of efficacy may be somewhat difficult because clinicians use the results of perfusion studies in routine preoperative management.[191] Consequently, those with substantial abnormalities are often evaluated further with preoperative coronary angiography which, if found to be abnormal, often lead to additional procedures such as coronary angioplasty or bypass surgery prior to vascular surgery.

MYOCARDIAL PERFUSION IMAGING BEFORE AND AFTER REVASCULARIZATION. A main purpose for performing stress myocardial perfusion imaging is not only to detect significant coronary artery disease, but also to aid in patient management decisions. Patients with markedly abnormal and high-risk stress myocardial perfusion images are usually considered candidates for coronary revascularization, either by coronary bypass surgery or percutaneous transluminal coronary angioplasty. Myocardial perfusion imaging is not routinely performed after coronary bypass surgery and is indicated only when symptoms recur. Because many patients have nonspecific ST-T segment changes on the baseline electrocardiogram after surgery, myocardial perfusion imaging is preferred over the exercise electrocardiography in the evaluation of these patients.

Coronary Angioplasty. Stress myocardial perfusion imaging is particularly useful after coronary angioplasty because often only one vessel is dilated and its vascular territory can be evaluated readily with SPECT imaging. The optimal timing of imaging after angioplasty is controversial. Some investigators[194] reported a high incidence of false-positive myocardial perfusion abnormalities early after angioplasty, presumably because of delayed return of coronary reserve. This is not a general experience. Most patients have normal myocardial perfusion images within the first week of successful angioplasty. At approximately 4 weeks after coronary angioplasty, a good correlation has been demonstrated between stress-induced myocardial perfusion abnormalities and the presence or absence of restenosis, independent of clinical symptoms.[195–197] In our own laboratory we perform electrocardiographic treadmill stress testing shortly after angioplasty to assess functional status and exercise-induced symptoms. Stress myocardial perfusion imaging is performed in patients who develop symptoms supportive of restenosis, or at 6 months in those who are asymptomatic.[190]

SPECT imaging is particularly useful in patients with known coronary artery disease. Tomographic localization of perfusion abnormalities allows us to determine whether clinical ischemia is likely to be caused by coronary graft closure, restenosis at the site of angioplasty, or progression of disease in other coronary arteries.

ASSESSMENT OF MYOCARDIAL VIABILITY (see also p. 1296). In patients with recurrent angina, known previous infarction(s), and left ventricular dysfunction, a reliable method for assessing the presence, extent, and location of viable myocardium is of considerable clinical importance when therapeutic decisions on revascularization procedures are made.

It is now well established that, using the conventional ^{201}Tl imaging protocol with 2- to 4-hour delayed imaging, myocardial viability occasionally may be underestimated in patients who appear to have "scintigraphic scar," i.e., a fixed perfusion defect.[36,37] Apparently fixed defects may improve after coronary bypass surgery or coronary angioplasty. Depending on patient selection, approximately 30 to 50 per cent of patients with a fixed ^{201}Tl stress defect on 2- to 4-hour delayed imaging may show "late filling-in" on either 24-hour redistribution imaging or after reinjection at rest (Fig. 9–29).[199–201] Because 24-hour redistribution images are generally of suboptimal quality, reinjection of ^{201}Tl at rest is preferred. Reinjection of ^{201}Tl can be done either *on the same day* of the stress test by administration of a new dose (1 mCi) of ^{201}Tl immediately after completion of the 2- to 4-hour delayed images or *on a different day* by injection of a new dose (2 mCi) of ^{201}Tl at rest (Fig. 9–1). In some laboratories, delayed ^{201}Tl imaging has been abolished and 1 mCi of ^{201}Tl is reinjected at rest as soon as stress imaging is completed. Rest imaging is then performed 3 hours later.

The phenomenon of "rest filling-in" with ^{201}Tl cannot be predicted readily by clinical parameters such as the presence of prior infarction, the presence of angina, or electrocardiographic signs of ischemia. Rest filling-in correlates in selected patients with improvement of wall motion after revascularization and shows substantial concordance with the demonstration of metabolically viable myocardium on positron F18-deoxyglucose imaging.[202] Although in most laboratories rest ^{201}Tl imaging is performed at approximately 15 to 45 minutes after injection, the highest yield for detection of myocardial viability is probably obtained by 3- to 4-hour rest-delayed imaging.[203]

Comparison with PET imaging showed further that ^{201}Tl defect intensity was predictive of the presence of viable myocardium.[204] Mild to moderate fixed defects (on 2- to 4-hour delayed imaging) with greater than 50 per cent of normal ^{201}Tl uptake showed evidence of viability on PET imaging in more than 95 per cent of cases. In contrast, only one-half of defects with less than 50 per cent of normal uptake had evidence of viable myocardium. However, on rest reinjection of ^{201}Tl in patients with fixed defects with

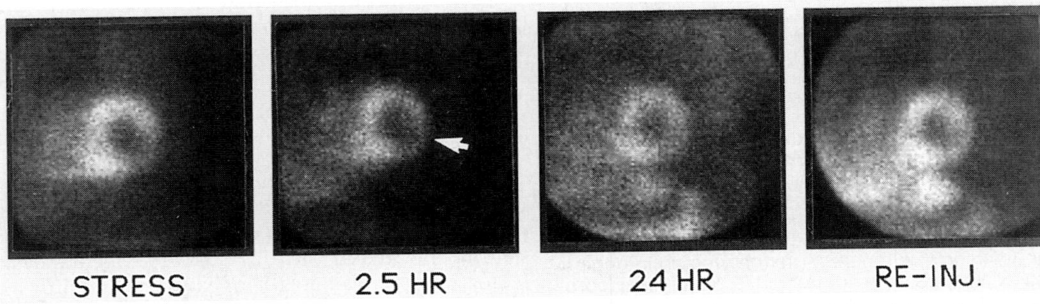

FIGURE 9–29. ^{201}Tl images after exercise (stress), 2.5-hr delayed imaging, 24-hr delayed imaging, and a reinjection of ^{201}Tl at rest. This patient has an apparently fixed defect (arrow) at 2.5-hr delayed imaging. However, on 24-hr redistribution imaging, filling-in of the defect can be appreciated. After reinjection of ^{201}Tl at rest, further normalization of the image can be appreciated.

less than 50 per cent of normal uptake, concordance of "filling-in" and "no filling-in" with PET evidence of metabolic activity was 88 per cent. Zimmerman et al.[205] demonstrated that the level of residual ^{201}Tl activity in defects after reinjection is significantly related to the mass of preserved viable myocytes in myocardial biopsies.

Thus, for assessment of myocardial viability on myocardial perfusion images one should consider two aspects: (1) the quantitative reduction in radiotracer uptake relative to normal myocardium and (2) the presence of defect reversibility. Thallium-201 uptake greater than 50 per cent of normal and/or defect reversibility (complete or partial) suggests viable myocardium. When clinical decisions on revascularization are to be made, the extent of viable myocardium that can be revascularized should be taken into account[206] (see p. 1313). Revascularization of only small quantities of viable myocardium cannot be expected to result in substantial improvement of global ventricular function, although ischemia may be abolished. At the time of this writing, no well-defined quantitative imaging criteria have been developed to guide such clinical decisions on revascularization.

There is considerable (and, at the time of this writing, inconclusive) debate in the literature whether *resting ^{99m}Tc-sestamibi imaging* is comparable to resting ^{201}Tl imaging for detecting myocardial viability. Experimental studies have shown that only viable myocardial cells with preserved membrane integrity accumulate and retain sestamibi.[207] However, the delivery of sestamibi is primarily flow dependent and only minimal redistribution occurs.[45] Other confounding factors are the physical and imaging differences between the two radiotracers.[208] Thus far, comparative studies involve only a relatively small number of patients. Although differences in uptake between ^{201}Tl and sestamibi are noted, the predictive accuracy of sestamibi uptake for improved wall motion after revascularization is similar to that of ^{201}Tl.[199–201] Udelson et al.[212] reported similar quantitative uptake of the two radiotracers in patients with unstable angina and left ventricular dysfunction. Dilsizian et al.[213] stressed the potential importance of 4-hour rest-redistribution sestamibi images. Because of known differences in tracer kinetics, one should probably use different tracer uptake threshold values when evaluating myocardial viability. Several investigators[214,215] have suggested resting sestamibi imaging in conjunction with nitrate administration as an improved means to predict accurately myocardial viability. In summary, the role of sestamibi and other ^{99m}Tc-labeled radiotracers for evaluating myocardial viability has not been as yet fully elucidated. More properly designed studies using an appropriate adequate gold standard for myocardial viability are needed.[216]

Selection of Patients for Myocardial Perfusion Stress Imaging

Although the sensitivity and specificity of myocardial perfusion imaging for detection of coronary artery disease is better than that of electrocardiographic stress testing, false-negative and false-positive results occur. According to Bayes' theorem, the significance of test results relates not only to the sensitivity and specificity of a test but also to the prevalence of disease in the population under study.[217,218] Quantitative planar ^{201}Tl and ^{99m}Tc-sestamibi stress imaging has a reported sensitivity of approximately 90 per cent and a specificity of approximately 95 per cent.

A positive result obtained in a population with a very low prevalence of coronary disease (e.g., less than 3 per cent) has a predictive value of only 36 per cent because, compared with expected true-positive results, a relatively large absolute number of false positives can be anticipated. However, in a patient population with a high prevalence of coronary disease, e.g., 90 per cent, a positive result has a predictive value of 99 per cent. In this setting, relative to the true-positive results, only a few false-positive results are obtained. On the other hand, in a population with a high prevalence of disease, a relatively large number of false-negative results are also obtained, and the predictive value of the negative test for absence of coronary disease is only 51 per cent.

Thus, in a population with a low prevalence of coronary disease (such as young asymptomatic subjects) a positive test is of little predictive value, whereas in a population with a high prevalence of coronary artery disease (50- to 60-year-old males with typical angina pectoris), a negative test is of little practical diagnostic value. The difference between pretest probability of disease (determined by the patient's age, symptoms, and stress ECG) and post-test probability (determined by the results of myocardial perfusion stress imaging) indicates the practical value of the test. Stress myocardial perfusion imaging has optimal discriminative value in a patient population with a pretest probability of coronary artery disease ranging from about 40 to 70 per cent. This population includes patients with atypical chest pain, asymptomatic patients with major risk factors, or asymptomatic patients with a positive stress electrocardiogram.[219]

When ordering a stress test for diagnostic purposes, the baseline electrocardiogram should be considered. In patients with normal baseline electrocardiograms, the ST-T segment response to maximal exercise is of diagnostic value. We and others[220,221] observed that patients with a normal ST-segment response to maximal exercise almost without exception also had normal exercise myocardial perfusion images. Thus, *myocardial perfusion imaging did not provide additional new information*. However, of patients with positive or equivocal exercise electrocardiograms, a substantial number had normal exercise myocardial perfusion images. Thus, in certain patient populations it may be cost-effective to perform exercise electrocardiography as a first test in patients with normal baseline electrocardiograms and repeat the exercise test with added myocardial perfusion imaging only in patients with abnormal exercise electrocardiograms. However, Nallamothu et al.[222] showed that in patients with an intermediate to high likelihood of coronary artery disease and normal baseline ECG, SPECT is superior to the electrocardiographic response in detecting coronary artery disease.

UNIQUE VALUE OF RADIONUCLIDE IMAGING COMPARED WITH OTHER DIAGNOSTIC MODALITIES. Compared with other diagnostic modalities, radionuclide imaging has certain unique characteristics: (1) Radionuclide imaging provides information regarding the physiological significance of disease that surpasses anatomical information. (2) Radionuclide imaging provides information that has independent and incremental prognostic value over other clinical and diagnostic information, including the contrast coronary angiogram. (3) Radionuclide images are digital count-based images that can be quantified readily. (4) Quantitative radionuclide imaging has been shown to be highly reproducible. (5) Diagnostic quality radionuclide images can be acquired in almost all patients, regardless of body habitus or patient cooperation. The above attributes are uniquely related to the use of radiotracers for imaging.

From the early days of nuclear cardiology, myocardial infarction was visualized either as a "cold spot" (perfusion defect) or as a "hot spot." Cold-spot imaging has been extensively discussed above. When a radiopharmaceutical localizes specifically in an area of recent infarction, the infarct is visualized as a "hot spot." The advantage of hot-spot imaging is that it is generally easier to image the presence of a tracer than its absence. The clinical usefulness of infarct imaging still requires clear definition. The diagnosis of acute myocardial infarction in the majority of patients can readily be made on the basis of simple and inexpensive tests, such as electrocardiography and cardiac enzyme analysis.

TECHNETIUM-99m-Sn–PYROPHOSPHATE

The first clinically useful hot spot imaging of acute infarction was performed using ^{99m}Tc-Sn-pyrophosphate (Fig. 9–30). This imaging agent was very sensitive for detecting acute myocardial infarction from 24 hours to 5 days after the onset of chest pain.[223] However, small and nontransmural infarcts were often not detected. Although as a rule scintigraphy was negative very early after infarction, some infarcts were positive within a few hours after onset of chest pain. Based upon present knowledge, it seems likely that spontaneous reperfusion occurred in these patients.[224] On the other hand, some very large acute infarcts remained scintigraphically negative, apparently because of absence of residual flow to the infarct region. The intensity and pattern of ^{99m}Tc-Sn-pyrophosphate uptake were found to be of prognostic significance. At the present time ^{99m}Tc-pyrophosphate infarct imaging is mainly of historic interest and is performed infrequently in most laboratories. In occasional patients who are suspected of having sustained an acute infarction 2 to 3 days prior to the hospital admission ^{99m}Tc-pyrophosphate imaging may be useful to establish the diagnosis at a time when plasma enzyme levels have returned to normal. SPECT imaging appears to be more sensitive than planar imaging.

Technetium-99m–pyrophosphate is also a specific but not very sensitive imaging agent to detect cardiac amyloidosis.[225]

INDIUM-111 LEUKOCYTES. Another approach to hot-spot infarction imaging, which has never come to routine clinical application, involves the use of ^{111}In-labeled leukocytes.[226] The patient's own white blood cells are labeled in vitro with ^{111}In and then reinjected. On the second or third day after acute infarction, migration of white cells occurs into the infarct area and can be visualized by imaging with ^{111}In.

INDIUM-111–ANTIMYOSIN. More recently, imaging with a monoclonal antibody specific for intracellular myosin has shown promising clinical results. Indium-111 murine monoclonal antimyosin binds selectively to irreversibly damaged myocytes.[227] Imaging is performed after administration of approximately 2 mCi of ^{111}In-antimyosin. Planar or SPECT imaging is performed 24 hours after antibody injection. The gamma camera is peaked on both photopeaks (171 and 245 keV) of ^{111}In. A medium-energy collimator is used. Either the conventional three planar views—anterior, LAO, and left lateral—or 360-degree SPECT is obtained.

Typical ^{111}In-antimyosin images of an acute infarct demonstrate discrete uptake in the myocardium. In addition, substantial liver and spleen uptake may be seen. Initial clinical duties have been encouraging. Indium-111–labeled antimyosin appears highly specific (100 per cent) and sensitive (92 per cent) for the detection of acute myocardial necrosis.[228] In addition to positive images in patients with acute myocardial infarction, uptake of ^{111}In-antimyosin has been noted in patients with unstable angina. The intensity and extent of ^{111}In-antimyosin accumulation appears to be of prognostic significance, both in patients with acute infarction and in those with unstable angina. Patients with extensive antimyosin uptake, i.e., greater than 50 per cent of the myocardium, had a four- to nine-fold increased risk for future cardiac events (cardiac death and nonfatal myocardial infarction) than patients with less or no uptake. The positive uptake seen in patients with unstable angina probably should be interpreted as the noninvasive demonstration of small, clinically undetectable focal areas of necrosis.

The potential prognostic significance of the extent of antimyosin uptake is important and has to be investigated in a larger number of patients. It has been proposed that simultaneous dual tracer imaging (^{201}Tl and ^{111}In-antimyosin) may have a role in the assessment of myocardial salvage after thrombolytic therapy (Fig. 9–31).

In addition to imaging of acute myocardial infarction, ^{111}In-antimyosin imaging may have a role in cardiac transplant patients for detection of cardiac rejection.[229] Furthermore, in patients with active myocarditis, diffuse ^{111}In-antimyosin uptake has been observed.[230] More patients (55 per cent) had abnormal ^{111}In-antimyosin images than abnormal endomyocardial biopsies (22 per cent). Nearly all patients with abnormal myocardial biopsies had abnormal ^{111}In-antimyosin images. More than half of the patients with positive antimyosin images

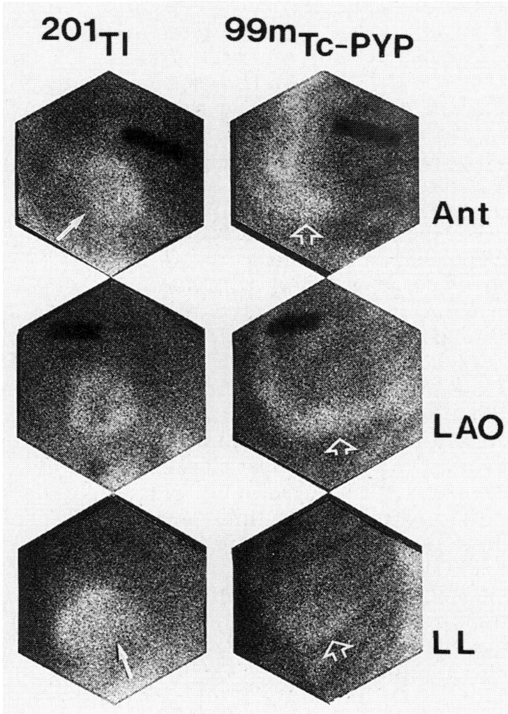

FIGURE 9–30. *Left,* ^{201}**Tl images in a patient with acute inferior wall myocardial infarction. An inferior** ^{201}**Tl myocardial perfusion defect can be seen (arrow). Right,** ^{99m}**Tc-Sn-pyrophosphate (PYP) imaging in the same patient. Uptake of** ^{99m}**Tc-pyrophosphate occurred in matching area (open arrow). On the LAO view, intense uptake of** ^{99m}**Tc-pyrophosphate is present in the inferior wall and extends into the right ventricle. This patient had, in addition to left ventricular infarction, right ventricular involvement.**

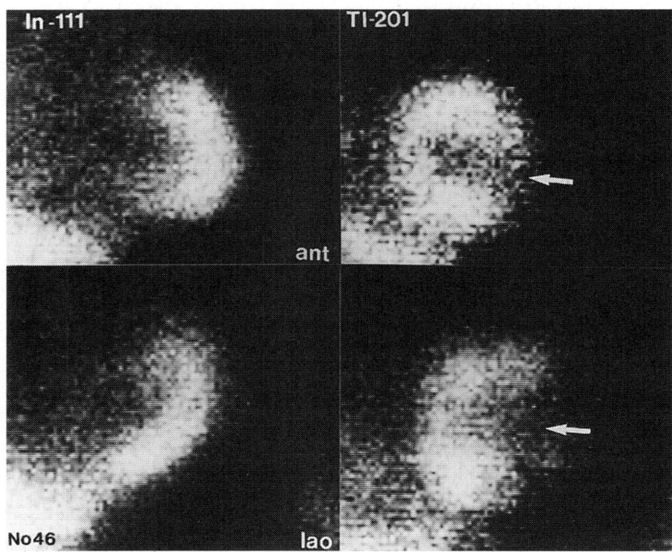

FIGURE 9–31. ^{111}**In-antimyosin** *(left)* **and** ^{201}**Tl imaging in a patient with acute anterolateral infarction. The** ^{201}**Tl defects (arrow) correspond with areas of** ^{111}**In-antimyosin accumulation. (From Lahiri, A., and Jain, D.: New radionuclide imaging in cardiovascular disease. Curr. Opin. Cardiol.** ***2:*****1070, 1986.)**

showed improvement of left ventricular function over time, whereas only 18 per cent of patients with normal scans improved. This clinical course was independent of biopsy results. These observations suggest that imaging with ^{111}In-antimyosin provides independent important clinical information in myocarditis. Further studies are needed to define the usefulness of ^{111}In-antimyosin imaging in acute ischemic syndromes and other cardiac diseases associated with cellular necrosis.[231]

ASSESSMENT OF CARDIAC PERFORMANCE

Cardiac performance can be assessed with radionuclide techniques by either of two generic approaches. The first involves analysis of the first transit of a radionuclide bolus through the central circulation (first-pass radionuclide angiocardiogram). The second, more widely applied method involves analysis following equilibrium intravascular labeling, which allows repeat imaging over several hours (equilibrium radionuclide angiocardiogram).

Variations of each technique involve assessment of the right and left ventricles, diastolic as well as systolic function, regional or global performance, ventricular volumes, and adaptations for longer term or ambulatory monitoring. Although the radionuclide approach for the evaluation of ventricular function has been challenged recently by echocardiography, these techniques continue to play an important role in the quantitative assessment of cardiac performance. These specific approaches, their clinical implications, and applications are discussed below.

EQUILIBRIUM RADIONUCLIDE ANGIOCARDIOGRAPHY

The concept of utilizing a physiological signal such as the electrocardiogram to "gate," or physiologically control, the otherwise static imaging of the cardiac blood pool was initially proposed in 1971.[232,233] The ERNA utilizes electrocardiographic events to define the temporal relationship between the acquisition of nuclear data and the volumetric components of the cardiac cycle. Sampling is performed repetitively over several hundred heartbeats with physiological segregation of nuclear data according to occurrence within the cardiac cycle (Fig. 9–32). Data are accumulated until radioactivity count density is sufficient for statistically meaningful analysis. The electrocardiogram provides a reasonably sensitive and easily defined physiological signal with which to link the static imaging technique. Data are quantified and displayed in an endless loop cine format for additional qualitative visual interpretation and analysis.

TECHNICAL CONSIDERATIONS. Because analysis involves the summation of several hundred cardiac cycles, a number of factors must be considered for the study to be deemed adequate. First, the patient must be able to remain relatively still beneath the detector during the period of data acquisition. In general, studies should be obtained in multiple views for interpretation to be complete. These include the standard anterior and LAO views, as well as the left lateral and/or left posterior oblique views (Figs. 9–33 and 9–34).

The need for multiple views is inherent in this form of imaging because overlying radioactivity in multiple cardiac and noncardiac structures can obscure a given ventricular region in any one view. In addition, specific abnormalities in regional left ventricular performance, such as ventricular aneurysms or akinesis of the posterobasal segment, may be appreciated only in lateral or posterior oblique views.[234] It is also assumed that cardiac performance remains relatively stable during the entire period of acquisition. This obviously is not the case in the presence of substantial arrhythmia such as atrial fibrillation or frequent premature beats.

The presence of major arrhythmia must be accounted for in interpretation; otherwise, the potential exists for substantially underestimating ventricular performance. Some currently available programs routinely exclude premature beats. Finally, the radionuclide label also must remain stable during the period of analysis, and the interval of data acquisition (framing interval) must be sufficiently short to allow adequate temporal resolution for definition of both systolic and diastolic performance parameters.

PERFORMANCE. Equilibrium blood pool labeling is achieved using ^{99m}Tc. The intravascular label is established with the patient's own red blood cells, using an in vitro or modified in vitro technique. Unlabeled stannous pyrophosphate is used to facilitate this reaction. The labeling techniques are now well standardized and quality control can be assured.[235] Following a single labeling procedure, serial studies can be readily obtained for periods ranging from 4 to 6 hours. If necessary, additional labeling can be achieved and the duration of observation extended.

Conventional Anger scintillation cameras are employed for these studies. Equipment is sufficiently portable to be brought to the bed-

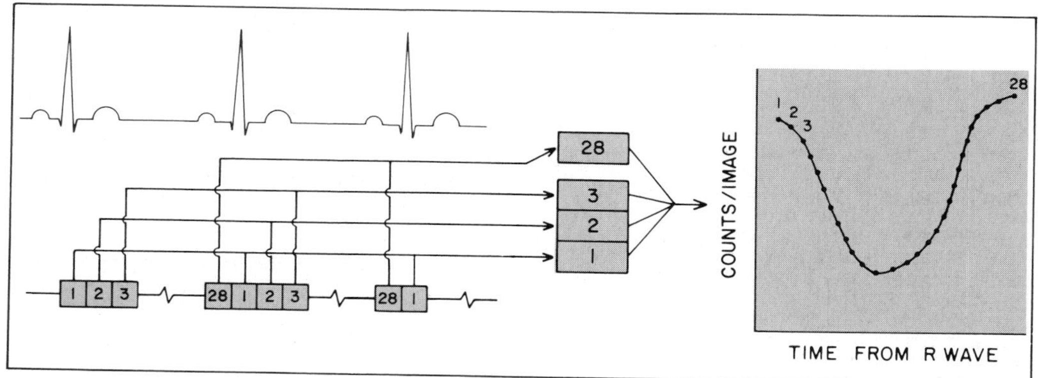

FIGURE 9–32. Diagrammatic representation of the technique for equilibrium radionuclide angiocardiography. Each cardiac cycle is divided into 28 equal segments. For each heartbeat, data are accumulated and then stored in a separate file. To the right, these data for the 28 portions of the cycle are displayed as a single summed ventricular volume curve. The numbers 1 to 28 refer to the temporal sequence within the cardiac cycle. (From Zaret, B. L., and Berger, H. J.: Nuclear cardiology. *In* Hurst, J. W. (ed.): The Heart, Arteries and Veins. 7th ed. New York, McGraw-Hill Book Co., 1990, p. 1899.)

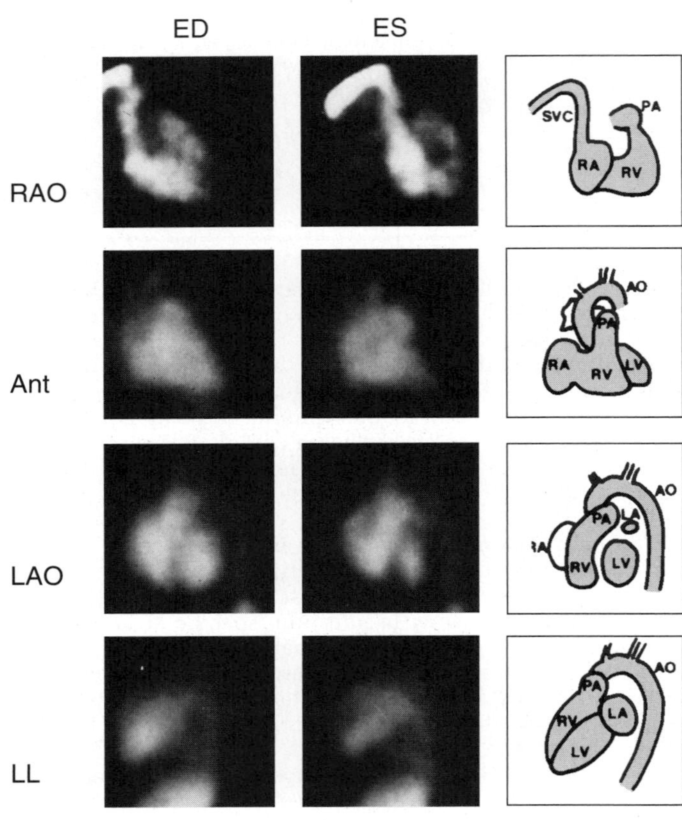

FIGURE 9–33. End-diastolic (ED) and end-systolic (ES) images obtained from a gated first-pass and equilibrium radionuclide angiocardiogram study. The anatomical configuration is shown diagrammatically to the right. In the upper panel, a gated first-pass study for evaluating the right ventricle is shown in the right anterior oblique (RAO) view. In the lower three panels (the equilibrium radionuclide angiocardiogram), images are shown for the anterior (Ant), left anterior oblique (LAO), and left lateral (LL) views. Note a normal contraction pattern in each view. (AO = aorta, LA = left atrium, LV = left ventricle, PA = pulmonary artery, RA = right atrium, RV = right ventricle, SVC = superior vena cava.)

side of acutely ill patients. Data are analyzed by computer, generally with some operator interaction. Analysis may be obtained in either the "frame" or "list" mode.[235] Radionuclide data are collected and segregated temporally. In the frame mode, which is employed most frequently, the R-R interval of electrocardiogram is divided into 20- to 50-msec portions, depending upon the patient's intrinsic heart rate and the conditions of the study, i.e., rest or exercise. If one is interested in defining diastolic filling events, a relatively short framing interval is required. The process generally requires 3 to 10 minutes for completion of each view. Following data acquisition, the data from the several hundred individual beats are summed, processed, and displayed as a single "representative cardiac cycle."

Data from the LAO view also are utilized for qualitative analysis of global left ventricular function. In this view, there is minimal overlap of the two ventricles. Using a count-based approach, left ventricular ejection fraction as well as other indices of filling and ejection are calculated from the left ventricular radioactivity present at various points throughout the cardiac cycle (Fig. 9–35). Measurements obtained in this manner correlate well with other defined standards, such as contrast left ventricular angiography.

BACKGROUND ACTIVITY. Because radioactivity is present within the entire intravascular space, it is necessary to correct for contribution of activity in adjacent intravascular structures to the overall measured left ventricular radioactivity. Major contributions to this "background" come from lungs and left atrium. Because the left atrium is posterior to the left ventricle in the LAO view, its background contribution is attenuated substantially by the more anterior left ventricular blood pool. Semiautomated methods are now routine for determining regions of interest as well as background zones. With the equilibrium technique, a variable region of interest is used for determining the left ventricular blood pool for each frame of the cardiac cycle. This is necessary because using a so-called fixed or single region of interest throughout the cardiac cycle introduces error and results in an underestimation of ejection fraction.

INTERPRETATION. Interpretation of ERNA requires both visual and

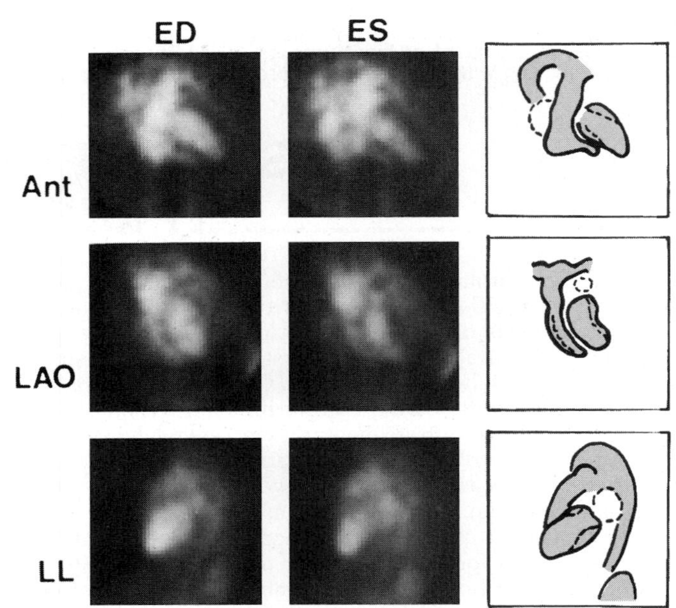

FIGURE 9–34. Equilibrium radionuclide angiocardiogram demonstrating anterior, apical, and septal akinesis in a patient with left ventricular ejection fraction of 33 per cent. End-diastolic (ED) and end-systolic (ES) frames are shown for the anterior (Ant), left anterior oblique (LAO), and left lateral (LL) views. A diagrammatic representation of superimposed end-diastolic and end-systolic contours are shown to the right of each image pair.

quantitative analysis. The approximate 45-degree LAO view provides data for the quantitative count-based assessment of left ventricular function. In the equilibrium study, quantitative analysis of right ventricular function is difficult because of contamination from overlying anterior right atrial activity. For this reason, right ventricular function is best evaluated by first-pass techniques. The degree of left anterior obliquity must be individualized based upon specific patient anatomy and cardiac orientation within the thorax. The degree of obliquity is determined in a manner providing optimal separation of right and left ventricles ("best septal view"). This is a relatively straightforward approach that can be used by the technologist without physician interaction. The LAO view also provides qualitative information concerning contraction of the septal, inferoapical, and lateral walls. The anterior view provides data concerning regional motion of the anterior and apical segments. The left lateral or left posterior oblique views provide optimal qualitative information concerning contraction of the inferior wall and posterobasal segment.

Ventricular aneurysm can be assessed best in the lateral views as

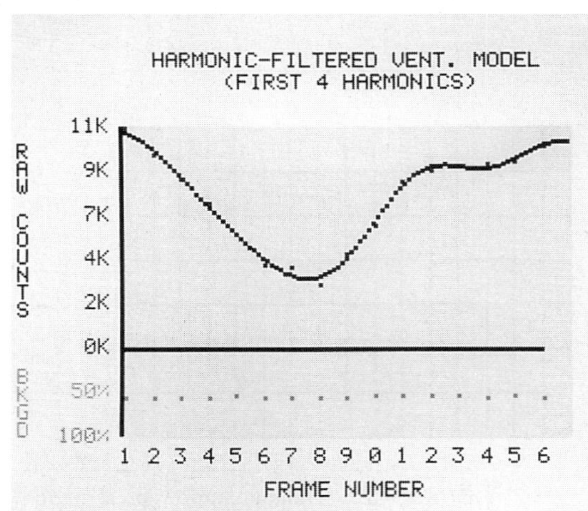

FIGURE 9–35. Ventricular volume curve derived from an equilibrium radionuclide angiocardiographic study. The raw data have been smoothed using a Fourier filter technique to four harmonics. Note the discrimination of the period of rapid diastolic filling as well as the atrial contribution to diastolic filling.

well. Analysis of only the anterior and LAO views may give the false impression of an enlarged, diffusely hypokinetic ventricle, when in fact there are additional obscured zones of normally contracting myocardium. In addition to a purely visual assessment, a point scoring system can be utilized for assessing regional function. This is generally done with a 5-point score for each segment, with specific numerical grades assigned for dyskinesis, akinesis, mild and severe hypokinesis, and normal function.[236]

An advantage of labeling the entire intravascular blood pool involves visualization of all cardiac and vascular structures. Such a visual assessment can provide information concerning relative cardiac chamber sizes and the relative adequacy of contraction of each chamber. In addition, the size, orientation, and pathology of the great vessels can be defined. The relative thickness of the interventricular septum can be appreciated, as can the presence of filling defects representing intracardiac masses such as left atrial myxoma or intraventricular thrombus.

The ERNA can easily be combined with additional physiological stress testing or provocation. This may be in the form of either physiological stress such as exercise, pharmacological stress with positive ionotropic agents such as dobutamine or isoproterenol, or psychological stress.[237] Because equilibrium labeling is stable for the short term, studies can be repeated, allowing for multiple stress and control measurements.

VENTRICULAR VOLUMES. Ventricular volume also can be determined by count-based methods.[238,239] Because radioactivity at equilibrium is directly proportional to volume, it is straightforward to establish a relationship between volume of a chamber and counts emanating from a region of interest representing that chamber in the two-dimensional display. The study also requires a blood sample to serve as a calibration standard. In addition, radiation attenuation must be accounted for.[238] Attenuation measurement represents the major source of error of the technique. However, volumes measured in this manner correlate well with other analyses. Because analysis is count-based, data are independent of the constraints and errors associated with fitting a deformed left ventricle to a geometrically ideal shape. There are now available new count-based approaches to measuring volume that do not involve attenuation correction.[239] This innovative new approach simplifies substantially current volumetric analyses.

The ability to measure ventricular volumes is quite important, because volumetric changes may be critical for analysis of patients with heart failure and severely depressed systolic function. In such individuals, therapeutic benefit may be documented by a reduction in ventricular size while ejection fraction does not change. Measurement of volume is also key to understanding the process of ventricular remodeling. Furthermore, linking volumetric analysis to concomitantly obtained pressure measurements can provide important insights into ventricular pressure–volume relations during both systole and diastole. This particular approach has been employed using both nonimaging nuclear probes and gamma camera equilibrium studies in the cardiac catheterization laboratory in which direct intracavitary pressure measurements are available.[240]

Marmor et al. have utilized equilibrium blood pool studies in conjunction with a noninvasive Doppler technique for accurately measuring central aortic systolic pressure from peripheral signals. With this procedure, an assessment of systolic pressure-volume relationships as well as a measure of ventricular power can be obtained noninvasively. Ventricular power is a measurement that is relatively independent of afterload and appears suitable for following patients with depressed ventricular function receiving a variety of interventions.[242]

QUANTIFICATION OF REGIONAL FUNCTION. The equilibrium technique has been adapted for quantitative measurement of regional left ventricular function. In the LAO view, this is best done using a regional ejection fraction technique.[242,243] This technique is based upon the same principles utilized for measuring global ejection fraction. However, when regional function is assessed, the left ventricular blood pool is divided into several discrete regions with well-established anatomical correlates. The best

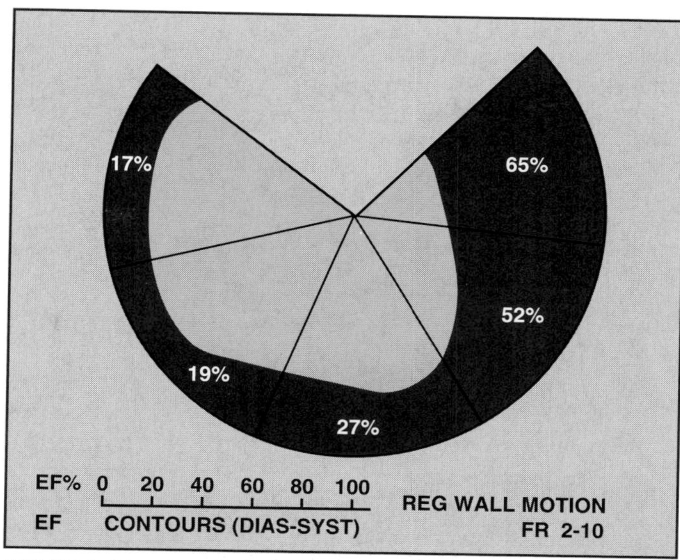

FIGURE 9–36. A typical regional ejection fraction display obtained from a left anterior oblique equilibrium study. The left ventricle is divided into five sectors. An upper sector involving the valve planes is excluded. These sectors, from upper left to upper right counterclockwise, involve upper septum, lower septum, apex, and inferolateral and posterolateral segments. In this particular study, there is a decrease of regional ejection fraction in the upper and lower septum as well as the apex, with maintained contraction of the two lateral segments.

approach involves division of the left ventricular blood pool into five regions of equal size (Fig. 9–36). These are upper and lower septal regions and inferoapical, inferolateral, and posterolateral regions. An upper zone involving the valve planes is excluded. This particular technique has been utilized in the TIMI multicenter trial and has provided meaningful insights into regional left ventricular function at rest and exercise following thrombolytic therapy.[243]

PHASE ANALYSIS OF CONTRACTION. Regional function can also be assessed from phase analysis based upon the onset, timing, and extent of contraction.[244] The phase and amplitude images also can be used for specific localization of bypass tracts in Wolff-Parkinson-White syndrome, as well as for definition of the site of sustained ventricular ectopy or tachycardia.[245]

OTHER CIRCULATORY BEDS. With the same study in which an ERNA is obtained, it is also possible to gather quantitative data concerning circulatory beds other than the heart. Since counts are proportional to volume, relative change in counts provides information concerning alterations in volume of various capacitance beds. This approach has been utilized to assess the effects of exercise and of drugs.[246,247]

Nonimaging Probe Studies

A variation of the equilibrium technique involves application of nonimaging probes for longer term (several hours) ventricular function monitoring.[248] The probes employed initially were high-sensitivity devices that provided beat-by-beat analysis as well as equilibrium analysis. High temporal resolution also allowed relatively easy assessment of diastolic filling.[249] The nonimaging probe has been utilized in a number of clinical studies; one example involved evaluation of graded infusions of intravenous nitroglycerin in patients with unstable angina.[250] The principle of monitoring ventricular function in unstable intensive care unit patients is appealing. The initial nonimaging probe called the "nuclear stethoscope" is no longer commercially available. However, new miniaturized devices have been developed.[251] This device can be affixed easily to the patient's chest and allows for serial monitoring in the intensive care unit environment. Preliminary data indicate that ejection fraction measured in this manner correlates well with that measured with conventional gamma cameras.

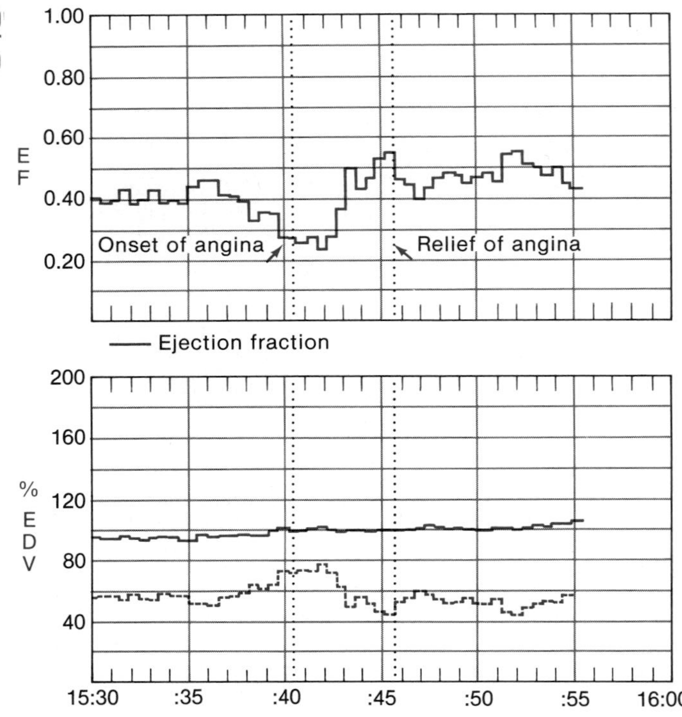

FIGURE 9–37. Trended data obtained with the VEST in a patient developing postmyocardial infarction ischemia. Data for ejection fraction are shown in the upper panel and data for relative end-diastolic volume and end-systolic volume are shown in the lower panel. Continuous data are shown for a 25-minute period. The times of onset and relief of angina are indicated. The fall in ejection fraction precedes the clinical occurrence of angina. This fall is associated predominantly with a rise in end-systolic volume, with minimal change in end-diastolic volume. (From Kayden, D. S., Wackers, F. J., and Zaret, B. L.: Silent left ventricular dysfunction during routine activity after thrombolytic therapy for acute myocardial infarction. Reprinted by permission of the American College of Cardiology. J. Am. Coll. Cardiol. *15:*1500, 1990.)

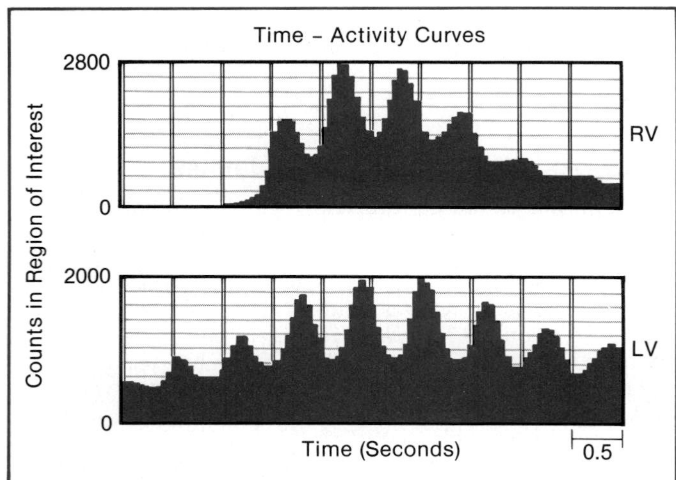

FIGURE 9–38. Radionuclide time activity curves obtained from a right ventricular (RV) and left ventricular (LV) region of interest during a first-pass radionuclide angiocardiogram. Each peak and valley represents a single cardiac cycle. Data from this study are summed to provide right and left ventricular ejection fractions. (From Zaret, B. L., and Berger, H. J.: Nuclear Cardiology. *In* Hurst, J. W. (ed.): The Heart, Arteries and Veins. 7th ed. New York, McGraw-Hill Book Co., 1990, p. 1899.)

Ambulatory Monitoring

Further application of the technique of equilibrium angiocardiography relates to utilization of miniaturized equipment suitable for monitoring patients during routine activities. A newly developed instrument, called the VEST, allows for monitoring over several hours following blood pool labeling.[252] It again employs the basic principles of ERNA. The device is worn by patients so that they are fully ambulatory (Fig. 9–37). Radionuclide and electrocardiographic data are stored on tape in a manner comparable to that of the Holter monitor employed for arrhythmia detection. Offline analysis provides trended data concerning ventricular function (Fig. 9–38). This instrumentation has been validated and standardized in several laboratories and is ready for broader clinical application. Initial studies suggest a potential major role for this device in the assessment of silent myocardial ischemia and mental stress.[253–255]

SPECT Studies

The equilibrium radionuclide technique may also be suitable for application to SPECT studies. At this time, work in this area is still relatively early and experimental.[256] However, tomographic studies may provide optimal radionuclide three-dimensional assessment of global and regional function.[257]

FIRST-PASS RADIONUCLIDE ANGIOCARDIOGRAPHY

First-pass radionuclide angiocardiography was the first radionuclide technique applied to the study of cardiac physiology. The initial reports of Blumgart and Weiss occurred in 1927.[258] However, it was not until the early 1970's that the clinical and investigative impact of the measurement was appreciated.[259] The first-pass approach remains a viable alternative to equilibrium studies. At present, it is performed much less frequently than ERNA. However, with the recent availability and use of technetium-labeled myocardial perfusion agents (see p. 274), the first-pass technique may take on new significance because ventricular function can be assessed by first-pass methods at the time of injection of the perfusion agent before subsequent static perfusion imaging.

TECHNICAL CONSIDERATIONS

The FPRNA technique involves sampling for only seconds during the initial transit of the bolus through the central circulation. The high-frequency components of this radioactive passage are recorded and analyzed quantitatively.[234] It is assumed that there is sufficient mixing of the indicator with blood such that changes in count rates are proportional to volumetric changes. During the initial passage, there should be temporal and anatomical separation of radioactivity within each ventricle. Because of this, it is possible to analyze right and left ventricular function independently during this brief transit. Regional function also can be assessed from generated outlines of ventricular silhouettes.

THE SCINTILLATION CAMERA. In contrast to the equilibrium study, the choice of scintillation camera for the first-pass study is critical. Instrumentation must be utilized that provides high sensitivity with respect to count rate acquisition. If system linearity is lacking and there are major dead time losses, then data are inaccurate. For this reason the multicrystal scintillation camera was initially developed. This instrument has since been replaced by second- and third-generation digital cameras that are suitable for rapid acquisition of the high count rate data necessary for first-pass studies.

Several technical issues are relevant to performance of first-pass studies. First, the injection technique must be impeccable; it is necessary to have a compact radionuclide bolus without streaming. Injections can be made from either the jugular or the antecubital venous systems. Injections at more peripheral sites are not suitable. The presence of major arrhythmia during the evaluation invalidates the data. Because analysis is based upon at most 8 to 10 cardiac cycles, the presence of rhythmic irregularity or premature beats negates the validity of the study.

RADIOPHARMACEUTICALS. ^{99m}Tc radiopharmaceuticals are used for first-pass studies; for the most part, in the past technetium pertechnetate or technetium complexed to either DTPA or sulfur colloid was used. Thus, based on the clearance of individual tracers, multiple injections can be made during a single study. Again, with the advent of technetium-labeled perfusion agents, it is now possible also to utilize these perfusion agents for several purposes including first-pass functional evaluation. In the past, attempts were made to develop additional radiopharmaceuticals suitable for first-pass techniques. However, these short-lived generator systems have been purely investigational and have been employed for the most part only in individual laboratories with a specific research interest in their use.

PROCESSING OF FIRST-PASS STUDIES. The first-pass study is computer-processed in frame mode. Regions of interest are selected over either the right or left ventricle; generally, a fixed region of interest is used. Activity is analyzed only when the initial bolus passes through the specific chamber of interest. This temporal segregation of radioactivity compensates for the potential problem of overlapping regions of interest. Background corrections are necessary for which a variety of approaches have been described. The same approach utilized for the equilibrium study can be applied to the first-pass technique. In such a manner, global and regional left ventricular performance can be assessed. The first-pass technique is the radionuclide modality of choice for assessing *right* ventricular function.[260] This can be carried out in concert with left ventricular analysis as part of a total first-pass evaluation.

GATED FIRST-PASS TECHNIQUE. Alternatively, a gated first-pass technique can be employed at the time of tracer injection for a subsequent equilibrium study. With this latter technique, first-pass data are acquired synchronously with the electrocardiogram. They are stored temporally and several beats are subsequently summed, forming a representative cardiac cycle obtained during the right heart phase. This particular approach provides higher count rate data than could be obtained with simple bolus injection and conventional Anger camera acquisition. The data from this study also can be viewed in endless loop cine format. Unlike the case for the left ventricle, poor contrast angiographic standards exist with which right ventricular radionuclide data can be compared. For this reason, normal values for right ventricular ejection fraction have been established independently and the technique standardized.[260] Right ventricular ejection fraction is a highly afterload-dependent measure. The finding of abnormal right ventricular ejection in the absence of intrinsic right ventricular disease is excellent evidence of acquired pulmonary hypertension.[260]

Shunt Studies

The first-pass study also can be used to detect and quantify intracardiac shunts.[261] With this particular approach, a region of interest is selected over the lung field. A pulmonary time-activity curve from the region is analyzed. Normally, there is a sharp rise and subsequent fall-off of radioactivity as it enters and leaves the pulmonary vasculature. A second, lower amplitude peak occurs as a result of normal recirculation of the bolus. In the presence of a significant left-to-right shunt, persistent activity remains in the lungs and there is relatively slow washout. Techniques have been developed for applying this approach to quantification of the degree of shunting. By deconvolution of the pulmonary time-activity curve using a gamma-variate fit, the magnitude of shunting can be determined. This correlates extremely well with oximetry measures of left-to-right shunting. From right-to-left shunting, qualitative assessment demonstrating early appearance of activity in the aorta is often sufficient. Quantitative approaches also exist for defining the degree of right-to-left shunts.

Comparison of First-Pass and Equilibrium Techniques

Both the ERNA and FPRNA techniques have advantages and limitations. In addition, any one laboratory should perform that study with which it is most familiar and for which its equipment is optimal. The ERNA has several distinct advantages: (1) multiple studies can be performed following a single radionuclide injection; (2) regional assessment can be done in as many views as are relevant for analysis; (3) sequential and serial data can be obtained during a variety of control, physiological, and/or pharmacological states; (4) the statistical reliability of high count rate equilibrium studies is superior to that of the first-pass technique; (5) the entire cardiovascular blood pool may be viewed at equilibrium; and (6) the equilibrium study is less prone to invalidation because of transient arrhythmia than is the first-pass study. On the other hand, additional activity from adjacent or overlying tissues can hinder optimal visualization of a specific ventricular segment in the ERNA. Evaluation of right ventricular performance, as well as shunt detection, is better achieved with the first-pass than the equilibrium technique. While equipment necessary for performing first-pass studies is more complex, as already stated, first-pass techniques will likely achieve resurgent popularity when combined with perfusion studies involving technetium-labeled agents.

CLINICAL ASSESSMENT OF CARDIAC PERFORMANCE

Diastolic Function

Diastolic function of the ventricles (see pp. 385 and 448) can be evaluated from either the equilibrium or first-pass study, although the former has been more frequently used. A number of indices have been described for assessing diastolic function. The most widely employed are the peak filling rate and the time-to-peak filling rate.[262] Filling fraction also has been recently studied.[263] High temporal resolution is necessary for performing these studies. Equilibrium studies have often been obtained in list mode so that ectopic or irregular beats can be eliminated from analysis. It is crucial that there be high temporal resolution and reliability of the diastolic filling phase if accurate data are to be obtained. Fourier filtering techniques, in conjunction with polynomial mathematical algorithms, have been applied to volume curves obtained by frame mode equilibrium studies of lower temporal resolution in a manner that provides accurate data. High temporal resolution nuclear probe studies also provide excellent analyses of diastole.[249]

Assessment of diastolic function has achieved increasing importance with clinical recognition of the entity of congestive heart failure associated with normal systolic and abnormal diastolic function (see p. 448). This has been most commonly observed in left ventricular hypertrophy and coronary artery disease,[262,264] as well as in restrictive cardiomyopathies. Abnormal peak filling rates have been noted in a majority of patients with coronary disease, even in the presence of normal systolic function.[262] Improvement in filling parameters has been noted following successful coronary angioplasty or after the institution of antianginal therapy. Abnormal diastolic function has been estimated to occur in as many as 30 to 40 per cent of patients hospitalized with congestive heart failure.[265]

A group of 54 such patients was described. The majority of patients with unequivocal heart failure and intact systolic performance had hypertensive or coronary disease, alone or in combination.[249] Follow-up of these patients over a 5-year period has indicated substantial cardiovascular morbidity and mortality that is not dissimilar to that of individuals manifesting systolic dysfunction alone.[266] Treatment with verapamil has been shown to improve objective and clinical parameters of heart failure as well as left ventricular filling in such patients.[267] Measurement of diastolic function is an important dimension in the assessment of ventricular performance in patients with heart failure. However, it must be noted that parameters of diastolic filling are age-dependent. Abnormal filling is noted, proportional to age, in the absence of disease.[268]

RESTING VENTRICULAR PERFORMANCE. Measurement of right and left ventricular performance at rest is clearly of value in the evaluation of patients with congestive heart failure. In the simplest assessment, this particular study can be utilized to distinguish cardiac from pulmonary or other noncardiac causes of the symptom complex. Resting function is valuable in assessing preoperative surgical risk.[269] The cause of heart failure may be inferred from the involvement of the right and/or the left ventricle as well as the presence of diffuse left ventricular dysfunction as opposed to regional dysfunction.[235] Systolic versus diastolic heart failure may be differentiated by this study. Relative chamber size may also provide important insights concerning the occurrence of concomitant or primary valvular disease.

Coronary Artery Disease

Perhaps the widest clinical and investigative application of resting radionuclide ventricular function studies has been in the assessment of patients with myocardial infarction. Several reports have documented the importance of prognostic stratification on the basis of global ventricular function as measured by ejection fraction. Ejection fraction, certainly in the prethrombolytic era, was a key factor in defining prognosis (see also p. 425).[270–274] In the thrombolytic era, ejection fraction at rest still remains an important prognostic index; however, for any level of ejection fraction, mortality is substantially lower than noted in the prethrombolytic period (Fig. 9–39).[270a] The CASS trial has also shown the importance of prognostic stratification based upon ejection fraction in patients with multivessel disease when survival was compared in patients assigned to surgical as opposed to medical therapy.[275] In patients who have survived out-of-hospital cardiac arrest, the single best prognostic factor also has been the degree of impairment in global function as measured by ejection fraction.[276]

In addition, the finding of a postinfarction functional left ventricular aneurysm carries further prognostic significance. In one study involving patients with an anterior wall infarction, the finding of aneurysm formation, as defined by nuclear data, provided relevant prognostic information not available from the ejection fraction alone.[277] In the setting of acute infarction, radionuclide studies at rest also are of major value in distinguishing true aneurysm from pseudoaneurysm and in distinguishing right from left ventricular infarction.

EXERCISE STUDIES. Ventricular performance during exercise can be assessed with either equilibrium or first-pass techniques. In general, exercise may be performed in the supine, semisupine, or nearly upright position. A normal exercise response is generally defined by an increment of at least 5 per cent (in absolute terms) in global ejection fraction of both right and left ventricles. In patients with coronary artery disease, abnormal ventricular reserve is manifested by failure of such augmentation. The finding of a major fall (>5 per cent) in ejection fraction from rest to exercise carries with it a poor prognosis.[278] Lee and colleagues have defined the prognostic impact of exercise ejection fraction data.[279] They have noted that the exercise ejection fraction itself as an absolute number provides the most relevant prognostic information. The ventricular response to exercise in patients with abnormal resting function may have greater prognostic significance than the extent of coronary disease.[280] The exercise response may also be used effectively to monitor the prognostic effects of medical therapy.[281]

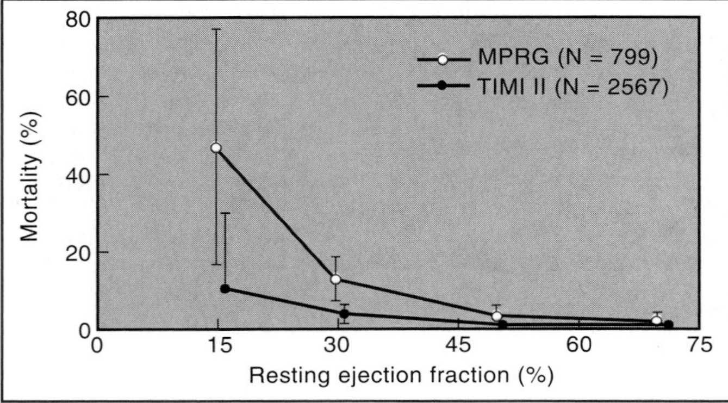

FIGURE 9–39. Relationship of rest ejection fraction to cardiac mortality in the TIMI II study *(black circles)* and MPRG (Multicenter Post Infarction Research Group Study *(open circles)*. Note the comparable shape of both mortality curves and the significantly lower mortality noted in the TIMI II study of the lower ejection fraction levels. (From Zaret, B. L., Wackers, F. J., Terrin, M. L., et al.: Value of radionuclide rest and exercise left ventricular ejection fraction to assess survival of patients following thrombolytic therapy for acute myocardial infarction: Results of the Thrombolysis in Myocardial Infarction (TIMI) Phase II study. Reprinted with permission of the American College of Cardiology. J. Am. Coll. Cardiol. *26*:73, 1995.

SILENT MYOCARDIAL ISCHEMIA (see also p. 1344). The prognosis associated with ischemia appears not to be affected by the presence or absence of a concomitant pain syndrome.[282] Because it is recognized that radionuclide exercise studies generally add to the sensitivity and specificity of the exercise ECG, it is not surprising that the study of left ventricular function during rest and exercise provides additional information concerning prognosis in silent ischemia.[283] The ability to detect silent myocardial ischemia during routine activities (as opposed to exercise in the laboratory) is of additional importance. It is within this context that ambulatory ventricular function monitoring has achieved prominence (Fig. 9–38). Transient abnormalities in global left ventricular function during routine activity frequently occur silently.[254] Abnormal VEST responses have also been noted in the absence of symptoms during balloon occlusion at the time of coronary angioplasty, a situation producing transient transmural ischemia.[284]

Silent ventricular dysfunction also is relatively common under conditions of mental stress. This phenomenon has been demonstrated in studies using the gamma camera or nuclear probe during several forms of induced mental stress.[237,255] Regional wall motion abnormalities were readily demonstrated during mental stress in patients with coronary artery disease, with or without an associated abnormal global ejection fraction response. These responses occurred in the absence of major increments in heart rate; this suggests that altered myocardial oxygen supply is the major mechanism. Jain et al. recently demonstrated the independent prognostic significance of mental stress–induced ventricular dysfunction.[285]

Congestive Heart Failure

Analysis of left ventricular function is cardinal for the assessment of patients with known or presumed congestive heart failure. Radionuclide studies provide systolic and diastolic data of relevance. The finding of diastolic dysfunction as the primary pathophysiological abnormality may necessitate use of a different therapeutic regimen (see p. 507) from that used when systolic dysfunction alone is noted. The radionuclide study also can provide insight into the presence of valvular problems complicating or mimicking heart failure. Serial radionuclide studies provide a basis for monitoring the effects of therapy. In the presence of unexplained congestive heart failure, the demonstration of intact right ventricular function with abnormal left ventricular function speaks against primary cardiomyopathy as a cause. Generally, the most likely culprits in such a circumstance are coronary artery disease (ischemic cardiomyopathy), hypertensive heart disease, or aortic valvular disease. However, it should be noted that the converse is not necessarily true; patients with advanced left ventricular dysfunction may develop secondary pulmonary hypertension and, with this, secondary right ventricular dysfunction.

DOXORUBICIN CARDIOTOXICITY (see also p. 1800). A major role for serial radionuclide left ventricular function studies involves the moni-

TABLE 9–5 GUIDELINES FOR MONITORING PATIENTS RECEIVING DOXORUBICIN

Perform baseline radionuclide angiocardiography at rest for LVEF prior to administration of 100 mg/m² doxorubicin. Subsequent studies at least 3 weeks after the indicated total cumulative doses have been given, but before next dose.

A. PATIENTS WITH NORMAL BASELINE LVEF (≥50%)
Perform the second study after 250 to 300 mg/m²
Repeat study after 400 mg/m² in patients with known heart disease, radiation exposure, abnormal electrocardiogram, or cyclophosphamide therapy; or after 450 mg/m² in the absence of any of these risk factors
Perform sequential studies thereafter before each dose
Discontinue doxorubicin if absolute decrease in LVEF ≥10% (EF units) with a decline to a level ≤50% (EF units)

B. PATIENTS WITH ABNORMAL BASELINE LVEF (<50%)
Doxorubicin therapy should not be initiated with baseline LVEF ≤30%
In patients with LVEF >30% and <50%, sequential studies should be obtained before each dose
Discontinue doxorubicin if absolute decrease in LVEF ≥10% (EF units) and/or final LVEF ≤30%

Modified from Schwartz, R. G., McKenzie, W. B., Alexander, J., et al.: Congestive heart failure and left ventricular dysfunction complicating doxorubicin therapy: Seven-year experience using serial radionuclide myocardiography. Am. J. Med. *82*:1109, 1987.

toring of patients with neoplastic disease for drug-induced cardiotoxicity. Doxorubicin, a commonly employed antineoplastic agent, may be associated with development of a severe cardiomyopathy that is often both irreversible and ultimately fatal. Radionuclide ventriculography has become established as a means of detecting presymptomatic cardiotoxicity.[286-288]

Guidelines for patient management with doxorubicin based upon resting ejection fraction data have been developed and are now currently employed (Table 9–5). Retrospective analysis noted marked differences in outcome between individuals who were managed with adherence to the radionuclide guidelines and those who were not.

It appears that resting ejection fraction provides an optimal means of assessing patients receiving cardiotoxic medication. The addition of exercise stress does not appear to add significantly to this prognostic assessment.

VALVULAR HEART DISEASE (see also Chap. 32). Rest and exercise ventricular performance studies have been employed in the study of valvular heart disease. It has been suggested that exercise left ventricular responses are of value in patients with aortic regurgitation with respect to defining the indications for aortic valve replacement, even in the asymptomatic state.[289] At the present time, this general approach is not popular. Resting studies of ventricular performance clearly play a role in the assessment of patients with suspected or known valvular disease in whom surgery is being contemplated. In the context of the mitral regurgitation, such an evaluation may be particularly relevant clinically with respect to the definition of operability.

CHRONIC OBSTRUCTIVE PULMONARY DISEASE (see also Chap. 47). Patients with chronic obstructive pulmonary disease were studied intensively when radionuclide techniques for assessing the right ventricle were developed initially.[260] It is recognized that the right ventricle is an extremely afterload-dependent structure. The presence of abnormal right ventricular ejection fraction in such patients strongly suggests the presence of significant pulmonary hypertension. Abnormalities in right ventricular performance also can be related to the degree of ventilatory and physiological impairment.[260] Right ventricular performance, as measured by ejection fraction, is responsive to agents that both augment inotropic performance as well as serve as pulmonary vasodilators.

The impact of positive end-expiratory pressure (PEEP) upon right ventricular function has also been evaluated.[290] Therapy involving PEEP is now routine in patients with severe respiratory insufficiency. Patients with normal baseline right ventricular function have no change in right ventricular volumetric status or contractile performance with PEEP. In contrast, those with depressed baseline right ventricular function manifest abnormal right ventricular hemodynamic responses to PEEP. On the basis of such data, a baseline evaluation of right ventricular performance before the institution of PEEP therapy seems reasonable. In addition, the impact of right coronary flow upon right ventricular responses to PEEP has been studied. Abnormal right ventricular performance during PEEP frequently occurs under conditions of coronary stenosis or obstruction.[290] This also has been confirmed in experimental animal preparations.[291]

SPECIAL IMAGING TECHNIQUES

ASSESSMENT OF MYOCARDIAL FATTY ACID METABOLISM BY SPECT

Long-chain fatty acids are important substrates for myocardial oxidative metabolism. Approximately 60 to 80 per cent of ATP produced derives from fatty acid oxidation.[292] In the presence of myocardial ischemia, oxidation of fatty acids is generally suppressed, with a more active role played by glucose metabolism. The study of fatty acid metabolism involves radioactive iodine labeling of free fatty acids and has been an area of active research since the early 1970's. Initially research in this area was limited by problems with loss of the radioiodine label and the subsequent introduction of substantial artifact. Recently a number of ^{123}I-labeled fatty acids have been introduced for imaging.[293]

There are two general groups of iodinated fatty acid compounds utilized: straight-chain fatty acids and branched-chain fatty acids. The straight-chain fatty acids are metabolized via beta-oxidation and released from the myocardium. Therefore fatty acid utilization can be assessed directly by evaluation of the washout kinetics of the radioactive tracer. This requires rapid dynamic acquisition. In the presence of ischemia, washout is slowed substantially. Consequently, by evaluating the initial degree of uptake and the subsequent washout, one can assess metabolism. The prototype straight-chain fatty acid used for imaging is ^{123}I phenyl pentadecanoic acid (IPPA).[293]

In order to measure absolute regional uptake of the fatty acid and quantify the initial distribution in the most precise manner, the regional uptake of the tracer must be maintained for a substantial period of time. In order to do this, the fatty acid compound can be modified with the introduction of a branched chain. This leads to metabolic trapping and allows for the acquisition of metabolic images of high quality without change in distribution during the imaging period. The methyl branching of the fatty acid chain protects the compounds from metabolism via beta-oxidation while retaining some of the physiological properties such as uptake and turnover rate in the triglyceride pool.

Currently, there are two iodinated branched chain fatty acids with which one can effectively image uptake distribution patterns: ^{123}I-methyl-pentadecanoic acid (BMIBP) and ^{123}I-dimethyl-pentadecanoic acid (DMIBP).[294]

Initial studies using both types of fatty acids have demonstrated potential for assessing myocardial viability in the presence of left ventricular dysfunction as well as myocardial ischemia in association with stress. Combined imaging with a perfusion agent allows for appropriate assessment of regional metabolism and regional perfusion in a manner comparable to that performed with PET.[294]

IODINE-123-LABELED METAIODOBENZYLGUANIDINE IMAGING

Metaiodobenzylguanidine (MIBG) may be labeled with ^{125}I, ^{131}I, or ^{123}I. The analog participates in the same uptake and storage mechanisms as norepinephrine.[295] It is not metabolized by catechol-O-methyltransferase or monoamine oxidase. MIBG uptake for imaging involves mainly the specific uptake-1 path by which norepinephrine is stored in presynaptic vesicles. Imaging of this uptake consequently provides evidence of the intactness of sympathetic cardiac innervation as assessed by the uptake-1 pathway.[296] Doses of 4 to 10 mCi of ^{123}I MIBG are used for either planar or SPECT modes. Cardiac uptake can be quantified on both a global and regional basis.[296] Decreased MIBG uptake has been noted in congestive heart failure. This is consistent with the pathophysiological observations involving depletion of cardiac stores of norepinephrine in association with this condition (see p. 409).

Scintigraphic measurements of cardiac MIBG uptake have been used to evaluate patients with idiopathic cardiomyopathy. Scintigraphically determined ^{123}I MIBG activity correlates with that measured from endomyocardial biopsy samples.[297] Diminished MIBG uptake has been repeatedly related to various indices of left ventricular dysfunction, including left ventricular ejection fraction, cardiac index, and intraventricular pressures. In a study of 90 patients with heart failure, MIBG uptake was related inversely to prognosis. Uptake, measured as a heart/mediastinum activity ratio, had a high predictive value for survival. Multivariate analysis showed that MIBG cardiac uptake was an independent predictor.[298]

Abnormalities of regional MIBG uptake have been noted in the presence of acute ischemia, both in experimental animals and in humans.[296] Iodine-123 MIBG has been used to delineate the denervated area after myocardial infarction. Studies have demonstrated the zone of denervation to be larger than the comparable perfusion defect associated with the infarct. Altered MIBG uptake may also play a significant role in the assessment of arrhythmogenic potential in patients with heart disease as well as cardiomyopathy.

Currently, the most commonly used radiotracers reflect physiological or biochemical processes that respond to changes in cellular viability and integrity. Because oxygen supply to the heart is fundamental for cardiac function, an assessment of tissue oxygen content by tracers extracted readily by and retained significantly in the myocardium in direct response to tissue oxygen levels may provide a means of imaging hypoxic myocardium.

A class of compounds with high electron affinity, the radiolabeled nitroimidazoles, is under active evaluation for this purpose. These lipophilic compounds diffuse across the cell membrane and undergo reduction in the cytoplasm to form a radical.[299-301] When oxygen is abundant in the cell, nitroimidazol reacts with the radical anion formed to yield superoxide and noncharged nitroimidazole that then diffuses out of the cell. When intracellular hypoxia is present, the nitroimidazole radical anion is reduced further to form nitrous compounds that combine covalently with cytosolic macromolecules and are trapped intracellularly.

Enhanced retention of nitroimidazoles in hypoxic cells has been demonstrated in intact dogs[302,303] and perfused hearts[304] using [^{18}F]fluoromisonidazole and in isolated adult rat myocytes[305] and dogs[306] using [^{3}H]fluoromisonidazole. In order to have wider clinical applications, ^{99m}Tc-nitroimidazole (BMS-181321) has been developed recently to be used as a potential hypoxic marker in SPECT. Preliminary studies in dogs,[307,308] perfused hearts,[309] and isolated myocytes[309] indicate that ^{99m}Tc-nitroimidazole (BMS-181321) may serve as a sensitive marker for hypoxic myocardium. Ng et al. evaluated myocardial kinetics of ^{99m}Tc-nitroimidazole. They confirmed that tissue retention of nitroimidazol was inversely proportional to perfusate oxygen level. This report found the threshold for myocellular binding to be 60 per cent or less of the perfusate oxygen level.[310] In the future, hypoxic compounds that are more lipophilic and thus have greater myocardial retention will be developed.

POSITRON EMISSION TOMOGRAPHY

Positron emission tomography (PET), long viewed as primarily a research imaging modality, is currently becoming a clinically important technique.[311] The uniqueness of PET imaging lies in its ability to image and quantify metabolic processes, receptor occupancy, and blood flow. The main advantages of positron imaging are the ability to label and thus image biologically active compounds and drugs. A major result of these advantages is the ability to derive absolute quantitative measurements with the appropriate kinetic model.

TECHNICAL CONSIDERATIONS

Conventional single-photon emitters such as ^{99m}Tc, ^{123}I, ^{201}Tl, and ^{111}In have several limitations. These isotopes decay with the emission of a single photon traveling in a random direction. The percentage of photons reaching the detector depends upon scatter attenuation and the distance between photon source and detector. These factors result in loss of relevant physiological information, which precludes accurate quantification of volumes, blood flow, and metabolism. Positron-emitting isotopes overcome these limitations. Positron-emitting radionuclides are characterized by excess protons. This unstable structure results in the conversion of an excess proton to a neutron; in the process, a positron (antielectron) is emitted. The positron travels a few millimeters in tissue; when it encounters an electron, an annihilation ensues. This results in the release of a photon pair with characteristic energy of 511 keV. These photon gamma rays travel at 180 degrees from each other. Using detectors that are paired and aligned, the photon pairs emitted from the positron annihilation can be detected by coincidence counting.

Images are obtained in a tomographic manner similar to SPECT imaging. However, in SPECT studies a single or several camera head(s) (each containing NaI crystal) are used, which rotate on a gantry. In contrast, PET imaging utilizes 1200 to 1500 small stationary crystal/detectors arranged in a circle, allowing photons to be detected in coincidence. This principle provides for correction for body attenuation and for the ability of this technology to electronically, not structurally, collimate data. These factors result in better count statistics and the ability to quantify various metabolic processes. With present technology, up to 21 simultaneous tomographic slices may be obtained, with reconstruction along cardiac planes similar to those displayed in cardiac SPECT imaging.

PROCEDURES. Current PET imaging protocols depend on both the positron emitter and detector source. Briefly, the heart must be localized by either fluoroscopy or various transmission scan programs. The patient is positioned with arms above the head or at the sides so that the heart is within the 12-cm detector range. After the patient is made comfortable, a 10- to 30-minute attenuation scan (depending on the ring source) is acquired. This allows subtraction of activity in noncardiac structures from the overall field of view, thereby providing an isolated image of only cardiac activity. The positron-emitting radionuclide then is injected. Allowance must be made for individual variation in the time needed for accumulation and subsequent acquisition of each radiopharmaceutical. For example, metabolic imaging with ^{18}FDG (fluorodeoxyglucose) requires injection of 5 to 10 mCi. Then 30 to 40 minutes must elapse before FDG image acquisition is initiated for an additional 20 to 30 minutes.

RADIOPHARMACEUTICALS. Many positron emitters are unique because their naturally occurring counterparts (hydrogen, carbon, nitrogen, and oxygen) are predominant constituents of natural compounds. Positron-emitting isotopes of carbon, nitrogen, and oxygen may replace stable counterparts in the synthesis of metabolic substrate, receptor ligands, drugs, and other biologically active compounds without disrupting biochemical properties or activity. Fluorine-18 is also a suitable substitute for naturally occurring hydrogen because of its strong carbon-fluorine bond and stearic effect similar to that of hydrogen. Positron-emitting tracers generally have shorter physical half-lives than most single-photon emitters. This property allows for repeat injections as a means of observing rapidly changing events over time. Table 9–6 summarizes the PET radioisotopes, half-lives, and synthesized radiopharmaceuticals suitable for use in cardiovascular medicine.

Clinical Indications

PET studies are recommended for the identification of myocardial viability in patients with established coronary

TABLE 9–6 POSITRON EMITTERS IN CARDIOVASCULAR IMAGING

ISOTOPE	HALF-LIFE	LABELED COMPOUND	APPLICATION
^{18}F	109 min	^{18}F Fluoro-2-deoxyglucose (^{18}FDG)	Carbohydrate metabolism
		^{18}F Fluorodopamine	Adrenergic neuronal imaging
		^{18}F-6 Fluorometaraminol	Adrenergic neuronal imaging
		^{18}F Misonidazole	Tissue hypoxia
^{13}N	10 min	^{13}N Ammonia	Perfusion
		^{13}N Amino acids (glutamate, alanine, leucine, aspartate)	Amino acid metabolism
^{11}C	20 min	^{11}C Amino acids (alanine, leucine, tryptophan)	Amino acid metabolism
		^{11}C Palmitate	Fatty acid metabolism
		^{11}C Acetate	Myocardial oxygen consumption
		^{11}C Butanol	Perfusion
		^{11}C Hydroxyephedrine	Adrenergic neuronal imaging
		^{11}C CGP 12177	Muscarinic receptor density
		^{11}C Carazolol	Beta-receptor imaging
^{15}O	2 min	^{15}O Oxygen	Oxygen utilization
		^{15}O Water	Blood flow quantification
^{82}Rb	75 sec	^{82}Rb Chloride	Perfusion
^{68}Ga	68 min	^{68}Ga Platelets	Thrombus formation

artery disease and regional or global left ventricular dysfunction[311,312] and for the noninvasive diagnosis of coronary artery disease. Other readily available imaging alternatives have limited PET application for these indications. These include conventional perfusion imaging, reinjection thallium imaging, and the development of new classes of ^{99m}Tc-perfusion agents.[313] Although ^{201}Tl and PET both have high accuracies for predicting recovery of regional and global left ventricular dysfunction after revascularization, PET has a higher positive and negative predictive accuracy for improvement in left ventricular function and is considered the gold standard for detection of viability.[314] Specific comparisons between various modalities are discussed below.

Assessment of Myocardial Viability

An accurate assessment of the presence and extent of viable yet poorly contractile myocardium and its discrimination from purely infarcted tissue are of clinical importance.[315] Myocardial viability is particularly relevant to current cardiology practice because revascularization and reperfusion can be established by surgery or by a variety of catheter-based techniques (see p. 286). An assessment of viability is important with respect to establishing the appropriateness of these procedures as well as their ultimate efficacy. Available imaging techniques must be able to differentiate "stunned" or "hibernating" myocardium from true infarcted tissue.

For institutions without PET facilities, myocardial viability is generally assessed with ^{201}Tl scintigraphy (see p. 294). The assessment of myocardial viability with ^{99m}Tc-sestaMIBI still is under active investigation, and results are variable with regard to the positive and negative predictive accuracies for reversal of wall motion abnormalities after revascularization or to direct comparison with thallium scintigraphy.[209,316–318] Although modified single-photon imaging protocols for detecting viable myocardium have been performed, the results are still suboptimal. PET imaging generally is regarded as the gold standard and final arbiter in decisions regarding viability. Viable but dysfunctional myocardium can be assessed by metabolic PET imaging with ^{18}F-FDG as a marker of glucose utilization, ^{11}C-acetate as a marker of oxidative metabolism, and $^{15}O\text{-}H_2O$ (water-perfusable tissue index) to assess the rate of water exchange.

FLUORINE-18 DEOXYGLUCOSE. Assessment of myocardial viability by PET imaging involves comparison of regional myocardial perfusion with regional glucose utilization. Myocardial perfusion can be visualized and quantified with flow tracers such as ^{82}Rb, ^{13}N ammonia, and ^{15}O water. Regional myocardial metabolism is visualized with ^{18}F-fluorodeoxyglucose (FDG). Experimental studies have demonstrated that glucose utilization is *augmented* in segments that are hypoperfused and ischemic but nevertheless viable. During ischemia energy production shifts from the oxidation of free fatty acids to that of glucose. Under normal conditions, glycolysis (glucose utilization) predominantly results in CO_2 production with minimal lactate generation. However, during ischemia, lactate production is increased relative to CO_2 production; glucose may contribute up to 70 per cent of the total energy production during ischemia.[319]

Metabolism as assessed with ^{18}F-FDG, traces exogenous glucose utilization. When FDG exchanges across the cellular membrane in proportion to glucose exchange, it competes for the enzyme hexokinase. The phosphorylated glucose analog, FDG-6-phosphate, unlike the native glucose-6-phosphate, is a poor substrate for glycolysis, glycogen synthesis, or the fructose-pentose shunt. It also is relatively impermeable to cell membranes, because the enzyme that catalyzes the reverse reaction, glucose-6-phosphatase, is absent or present in only negligible quantities. Therefore, the tracer becomes trapped in the myocardium and its persistent activity reflects regional rates of exogenous glucose uptake and utilization.[320] In myocardial segments with irreversible injury, tissue glucose utilization declines linearly with blood flow. Thus, in patients with ischemic heart disease, PET imaging with ^{18}F deoxyglucose has been useful in discriminating hypoperfused but viable tissue from regions with irreversible injury.[321–325]

Cross-sectional left ventricular images are acquired 2 to 5 minutes following intravenous injection of a flow tracer. Then, 5 to 15 mCi of FDG are injected and metabolic images obtained 30 to 50 minutes after injection. These images can be analyzed by circumferential activity profile analysis similar to that employed in SPECT thallium image processing.[326]

Three basic patterns of comparative blood flow and metabolism activity distribution are demonstrable (Fig. 9–40). First, there may be a match between flow and metabolic activity with homogeneous myocardial distribution of each tracer (normal). Second, regional blood flow may be decreased while glucose utilization in the same area is normal or increased relative to normally perfused myocardium or to the regions with reduced blood flow. This pattern of blood flow–metabolism mismatch is the PET scintigraphic signature of myocardial viability in the presence of ventricular dysfunction. Third, regional myocardial blood flow and glucose utilization may be concordantly decreased. This pattern is the marker of myocardial scar and irreversible damage.

CLINICAL APPLICATIONS. There have been several clinical investigations demonstrating that blood flow–metabolism mismatch on PET images is representative of hypoperfused but viable myocardium. These studies are based on the demonstration of improvement in regional wall motion after revascularization in regions demonstrating flow-metabolism mismatch (diminished flow, increased glucose uptake).[202,325,327,328]

Tillisch and colleagues evaluated 17 patients with a total of 73 regions with abnormal resting wall motion.[202] Those myocardial segments that showed preserved glucose uptake in regions of abnormal wall motion predicted reversibility of wall motion abnormalities following bypass surgery. In contrast, abnormal motion in regions with depressed glucose uptake did not improve following revascularization. Abnormal contraction in 35 of 41 segments was correctly predicted to be reversible (85 per cent predictive accuracy). Abnormal contraction in 24 of 26 regions was correctly predicted to be irreversible (92 per cent predictive accuracy). In the 17 patients, left ventricular ejection fraction averaged 32 ± 14 per cent before and 41 ± 15 per cent after revascularization. This improvement was more marked in 11 patients with two or more regions that were either normal or revealed glucose activity in hypoperfused segments. Left ventricular ejection fraction increased in these patients from 30 ± 11 per cent to 45 ± 14 per cent ($P < 0.05$), compared with no improvement in the remaining 6 patients with only one or no mismatched FDG/blood flow regions.

In a comparable study, Tamaki et al. performed PET myocardial perfusion and FDG metabolic imaging before and 5 to 7 weeks after coronary artery bypass surgery in 22 patients.[325] Postoperative improvement in wall motion abnormalities was observed more often in the metabolically active segments (78 per cent) than in the metabolically inactive segments (22 per cent) ($P < 0.001$). Thus, the persistence of metabolic activity with FDG identifies viable, dysfunctional myocardium. An alternative approach using postexercise FDG PET imaging was used by Marwick et al. to determine the spectrum of metabolic responses of hibernating myocardium, as well as to predict improvement in exercise capacity after revascularization.[327,328]

These studies reinforce the concept that metabolic imaging with PET is a useful tool to predict the reversal of preoperative wall motion abnormalities after successful revascularization. These studies also point out that although a subgroup shows improvement in wall motion and perfusion after revascularization, myocardial metabolism may remain abnormal. The latter occurred in segments with extensive perfusion and metabolic changes preoperatively.[328] In a separate study by the same author, postexercise FDG uptake in patients with previous myocardial infarction predicted improvement in regional systolic function as well as in exercise tolerance after revascularization.[327] Studies addressing the ability of modified SPECT camera systems to accept 511-keV photons, specifically ^{18}FDG, have been performed.[329,330] These preliminary studies suggest that ^{18}FDG SPECT

FIGURE 9–40. **See color plate 8.**

TABLE 9–7 POSITRON IMAGING PATTERNS AND MORTALITY IN CORONARY ARTERY DISEASE AND LEFT VENTRICULAR DYSFUNCTION

STUDY	NUMBER OF PATIENTS	VIABLE		NONVIABLE	
		Medical	Revascularization	Medical	Revascularization
Eitzman et al.[331]	83	6/18	1/26	2/24	0/14
DiCarli et al.[332]	93	7/17	3/26	3/33	1/17
Lee et al.[333]	137	10/21	4/49	2/40	2/19
TOTAL	313	23/56	8/101	7/97	3/50
% mortality		41%	8%	7%	6%

imaging may be a clinical and cost-effective means for the metabolic assessment of left ventricular myocardial viability.

PROGNOSIS AND PET IMAGING FOR MYOCARDIAL VIABILITY. Prognostic stratification of patients with coronary artery disease and left ventricular dysfunction recently has been addressed with metabolic PET imaging. There are three reports (one retrospective, two prospective) that address this issue using paired perfusion-FDG metabolic PET studies (Table 9–7).[331–333] In each of these studies patients were characterized as FDG viable or nonviable and then according to treatment with medical therapy or revascularization. Both studies then looked at mortality among four subgroups. The mortality rate was significantly lower in patients with a PET mismatch pattern who were revascularized. When these three studies are combined in a total of 313 patients, patients with a PET scintigraphic marker of viability had significantly lower mortality following revascularization compared with medical therapy (8 per cent versus 41 per cent). The patients were followed for approximately 1 year in two studies[331,332] and for a mean of 18 months in the remaining study.[333]

Another study also determined the prognostic value of PET in patients who underwent either revascularization or medical therapy.[334] This study was based on infarct size and viability measured by rubidium PET. The extent of scar and the presence of viable myocardium by PET in vascular areas at risk in patients with myocardial infarction were highly predictive of 3-year mortality. This study differed from the others discussed above because it included patients with a normal ejection fraction.[334] In a study by Tamaki et al., 158 patients with myocardial infarction were referred for FDG PET and stress thallium imaging.[335] Eighty-four patients were followed for a mean interval of 23 months. This study confirmed that an increase in FDG uptake was the best predictor of future cardiac events when compared with clinical, angiographic, and radionuclide variables. An increase in FDG uptake was also predictive even when a stress thallium-201 scan did not show redistribution.

COMPARISON OF PET FDG WITH THALLIUM-201-REDISTRIBUTION/REINJECTION SCINTIGRAPHY. Studies directly comparing ^{201}Tl redistribution scintigraphy and PET have been performed.[336–339] As detailed above, standard ^{201}Tl redistribution imaging underestimates the amount of viable myocardium compared with reinjection imaging. Thus, although these studies indicate that PET metabolic imaging is superior to standard thallium scintigraphy without reinjection in the delineation of viable myocardium, they currently are not particularly relevant.

Two reports have compared thallium reinjection and PET FDG imaging.[204,340] In the study by Bonow et al., PET FDG scintigraphic findings correlated a high percentage of the time with ^{201}Tl reinjection scintigraphy in severe irreversible defects that had less than 50 per cent of maximum counts on the initial post-stress image. However, moderate and mild irreversible thallium defects, when imaged with PET FDG and subsequent thallium reinjection, showed a greater discordance.[204] This was confirmed in a study by Tamaki et al., in which the thallium reinjection defect scores were not segregated according to the magnitude of the defect, and an overall discordance rate of 25 per cent was noted.[340]

COMPARISON OF PET FDG WITH SESTAMIBI SCINTIGRAPHY. Several studies have been performed comparing FDG and MIBI in the assessment of myocardial viability in patients with chronic coronary artery disease.[213,316–318, 341, 342] Some authors found FDG uptake in 23 per cent of the resting perfusion defects as assessed with sestamibi.[317] FDG is most helpful in distinguishing viability in those MIBI defects that were 31 to 50 per cent of peak normalized counts, clinically considered to be severe defects.

The potential for sestamibi to underestimate viability has been addressed by two additional studies.[318,342] In the study by Sawada et al., FDG evidence of viability was present in 50 per cent of segments with ^{99m}Tc-sestamibi activity less than 40 per cent. Moderate defects (50 to 59 per cent of peak activity) were viable as assessed by FDG.[342] These results were reinforced by another study, which revealed that a major portion of the discordance was contributed by the inferior wall myocardial segments.[318] The latter suggests that inferior wall attenuation artifact on sestamibi SPECT imaging may contribute significantly to the underestimation of viability by sestamibi.

A study by Dilsizian et al. showed that same-day rest/stress sestaMIBI imaging incorrectly identified 36 per cent of myocardial regions as irreversibly impaired and nonviable compared with both thallium redistribution/reinjection and PET FDG imaging.[213]

OTHER CONSIDERATIONS. Several aspects of FDG metabolic imaging require resolution. The dietary state of patients undergoing metabolic imaging is to be standardized. Some investigators studied patients with FDG in the fasting state and others after feeding and glucose loading. We recommend PET imaging using ^{13}N-ammonia and ^{18}FDG in the glucose-loaded state.[343] It also is not clear how accurate PET assessments of viability will be when tomography is performed early in the postinfarct period. Most studies to date have been performed late after the acute event. Other issues concern the accuracy of this technique in patients with diabetes and the lack of data concerning interobserver and intraobserver variability.

ADDITIONAL PET MARKERS OF MYOCARDIAL METABOLISM

The study of flow/FDG relationships is only one approach for the assessment of myocardial metabolism in ischemic conditions. Metabolic perturbation may occur on a cellular level as a result of acute or chronic ischemia and not be detected by flow/FDG relationships. Cardiac work depends on the availability of high-energy phosphate production, which is derived normally from the oxidation of long-chain fatty acids.[319] Only when fatty acid levels are low and glucose levels are high (as in the postprandial state) does the heart utilize glucose oxidation as a major source of energy. Therefore, it is relevant to evaluate other markers of myocardial metabolism in patients with coronary artery disease.[344–348]

^{11}C-ACETATE. Dynamic PET studies of ^{11}C-acetate kinetics provide a noninvasive measurement of regional myocardial oxygen consumption.[349] Furthermore, myocardial blood flow may be quantified using the same tracer injection. Clearance of ^{11}C-acetate from the myocardium is bi-exponential.[350] The decay constant of the initial component of the clearance curve is linearly related to myocardial oxygen consumption. Analysis of ^{11}C kinetics is thought to accurately reflect myocardial oxygen consumption and thus mitochondrial oxidative flux in human subjects.[351]

Gropler et al. quantified myocardial oxidative metabolism by analysis of the rate of myocardial clearance of ^{11}C-acetate in 35 patients with ischemic myocardial dysfunction who were undergoing coronary revascularization. Glucose metabolism was assessed preoperatively and by analysis of FDG uptake. The predictive value for recovery of regional function based on measurements of oxidative and glucose metabolism was compared. In myocardial segments with initially severe dysfunction, ^{11}C-acetate clearance appeared to have better positive and negative predictive values than FDG, although the difference did not reach statistical significance.[352] The complementary role of ^{11}C-acetate in PET myocardial viability imaging may be its ability to distinguish viable from nonviable myocardium in acute infarction (Fig. 9–41). In this setting where myocardial stunning may be predominant, an index of overall oxidative metabolism may be more accurate than FDG.[320] Additionally, because ^{11}C-acetate is not influenced by substrate availability, it may be more useful than FDG imaging in diabetic patients with chronic coronary artery disease. Imaging with ^{11}C-acetate in this setting would make unnecessary the titration of serum insulin levels with an insulin clamp and/or serial serum glucose measurements titrated by insulin administration.[353]

RUBIDIUM-82. Myocardial viability also can be assessed by dynamic measurements of resting myocardial kinetics of ^{82}Rb. ^{82}Rb is extracted

FIGURE 9–41. See color plate 8.

and retained by viable and normal myocardium, whereas it clears rapidly from necrotic myocardium, resulting in a defect.[354] Further studies addressing the functional outcome after revascularization are needed to establish the clinical usefulness of ^{82}Rb as a marker of myocardial viability.

WATER-PERFUSABLE TISSUE INDEX. The water-perfusable tissue index assesses myocardial viability based on the principle that normal or viable myocardium, and not scar, exchanges water rapidly.[355] Preliminary data by DeSilva et al. in patients with chronic coronary artery disease and previous myocardial infarction who underwent revascularization show that the perfusable tissue index accurately predicted contractile recovery after revascularization, and that there was good agreement with FDG in this regard. This study should be considered preliminary until performed in a larger group of patients.[356]

ASSESSMENT OF MYOCARDIAL BLOOD FLOW

The assessment of myocardial blood flow with PET can be performed with either ^{82}Rb, ^{13}N ammonia, ^{15}O-labeled water, or copper pyruvaldehyde bis (N^4-methylthiosemicarbazonate) (PTSM). ^{82}Rb and ^{13}N ammonia are transiently trapped in the myocardium proportional to regional distribution of blood flow.[357–359] ^{15}O water is an inert diffusible tracer that accumulates in and clears from the myocardium as a function of blood flow.[358] Rubidium is a potassium analog that in part requires the sodium-potassium transport pump for uptake and thus utilizes energy for its myocardial trapping.[360,361] Its first-pass extraction fraction is 65 per cent.[359] ^{82}Rb is a unique and convenient radiopharmaceutical to use because it is generator-produced and does not depend upon a cyclotron for production. Because its half-life is only 76 seconds, repeated measurements may be performed to assess the effects of rapid physiological interventions.[359]

Copper PTSM is another noncyclotron, generator-produced tracer with a high single pass extraction, and it may prove to be another alternative for measuring blood flow with PET.[362,363] ^{13}N ammonia has a first-pass extraction fraction of 80 per cent and requires energy for myocardial trapping.[357] ^{13}N ammonia is converted to ^{13}N glutamine by the glutamine synthetase reaction.[326] Myocardial uptake of ^{13}N is linear over a wide range of myocardial blood flow (44 and 200 ml/min/100 g). However, at flows higher than 200 ml/min/100 g, uptake is not linear and flow measurement is inaccurate in this range. Similar lack of linearity at high blood flow has been observed for ^{82}Rb.[360] This characteristic is true for all myocardial perfusion agents, including ^{201}Tl, sestaMIBI, and tetrofosmin.

It has not been firmly established that flow measurements with either of these positron emitters are totally independent of metabolic conditions. Accumulation of these tracers depends upon some level of tissue viability following the ischemic insult.[323,364,365] Therefore, absolute quantification of blood flow with these two tracers may be limited by the nonlinear uptake at high flow rates and the extent to which metabolic factors affect the myocardial retention of these tracers. In contrast, water labeled with ^{15}O (half-life = 2.1 minutes) is a diffusible tracer of myocardial blood flow. Its extraction fraction is independent of the metabolic state of the myocardium.[366] Accurate measurements of absolute myocardial blood flow may be performed across a wide spectrum of flow values[367]; however, measurements with this tracer may be more technically challenging.

CORONARY BLOOD FLOW. The noninvasive absolute quantification of myocardial blood flow in vivo is a major advantage of positron imaging. The relationship between myocardial blood flow and the severity of coronary artery stenosis has been measured by positron emission tomography with ^{15}O-labeled water at rest and during hyperemia induced with intravenous adenosine.[368] Absolute quantitative basal myocardial blood flow remained constant regardless of the severity of coronary artery stenosis. In contrast, during hyperemia there was a progressive decrease in flow reserve when the degree of stenosis was 40 per cent or more. This study supports the high degree of sensitivity for PET to detect the functional significance of subcritical stenosis during pharmacological intervention.

The augmentation of myocardial perfusion reserve after coronary angioplasty has been quantified by PET H_2 ^{15}O studies.[369] The high concentration of ^{15}O water in the intracavitary blood pool occurs concomitantly with myocardial activity. This necessitates subtraction of the blood pool activity in order to obtain an accurate assessment of myocardial perfusion.[370,371]

Diagnosis of Coronary Artery Narrowing

The anatomical delineation of coronary artery luminal narrowing by coronary angiography may not accurately reflect the functional significance of coronary artery disease.[372] PET imaging with $^{13}NH_3$ and ^{82}Rb has identified abnormal flow reserve in patients with coronary artery disease. The term "flow reserve" is meaningful to the extent that absolute measurement before and after pharmacological intervention is measured. Absolute flow reserve reflects the cumulative effects of physiological factors such as vasomotor tone, workload, hypertrophy, and stenosis. Relative flow reserve measurement reflects more specifically coronary stenosis independent of these other physiological variables and thus is comparable (with regard to mechanism) to reversible/nonreversible SPECT flow tracers for the assessment of CAD. PET myocardial perfusion imaging using either ^{82}Rb, ^{13}N ammonia, or ^{15}O-labeled water has identified abnormal perfusion reserve in patients with coronary artery disease with high sensitivity and specificity[108,373–382] (Table 9–8). Cardiac PET detects coronary artery disease with similar accuracy in asymptomatic as well as symptomatic subjects[375] and is equal to or better than arteriography for following changes in stenosis severity.[359]

TABLE 9–8 DIAGNOSTIC ASSESSMENT OF CORONARY ARTERY DISEASE WITH POSITRON EMISSION TOMOGRAPHY

STUDY	NUMBER OF PATIENTS	SENSITIVITY (%)	SPECIFICITY (%)
Gupta[377]	48	94	95
Stewart et al.[381]	81	84	88
Williams[378]	208	98	93
Go et al.[108]	132	95	82
Stewart[379]	60	87	82
Demer et al.[376]	193	94	95
Tamaki et al.[375]	51	88	90
Yonekura et al.[382]	60	97	100
Gould et al.[374]	50	95	100
Schelbert et al.[373]	32	97	100
TOTAL	915	93%	93%

In another study, 50 patients were studied with either ^{82}Rb or ^{13}N ammonia after intravenous dipyridamole and isometric handgrip stress. Quantitative coronary arteriography was obtained to determine coronary flow reserve. Those patients with a coronary flow reserve of less than 3 were identified accurately by PET imaging.[374]

Limited coronary artery perfusion reserve can also be delineated with ^{15}O-labeled water. Abnormalities in myocardial perfusion reserve have been reported in relative and absolute terms.[358,369,380] In one study, perfusion distal to a coronary stenosis after dipyridamole increased to only 64 per cent of that in normal anatomical areas. However, as quantified with PET, areas with successfully dilated arteries had postdipyridamole perfusion similar to areas supplied by nonstenotic vessels.[371]

COMPARISON WITH THALLIUM-201 SCINTIGRAPHY. The higher-energy photons released from positron-emitting tracers in conjunction with attenuation correction and higher resolution overcome to a major extent the photon attenuation problems commonly encountered with thallium studies. Three studies directly compared ^{201}Tl stress scintigraphy and PET perfusion studies in the same patient.[375,379,381]

Tamaki and colleagues studied 51 patients (48 with coronary artery disease) with exercise thallium SPECT and PET employing dipyridamole and ^{13}N ammonia. Both qualitative and semiquantitative image interpretation and qualitative analysis of the coronary arteriogram were employed. Of the 48 coronary artery disease patients, SPECT showed abnormal perfusion in 46 (96 per cent), and PET detected abnormalities in 47 (98 per cent). The sensitivity for detecting disease in individual coronary arteries ($>$50 per cent stenosis) was similar for SPECT (81 per cent) and PET (88 per cent). However, preliminary data in 60 patients who underwent ^{82}Rb PET and Tl-SPECT imaging within a 4-week interval recorded a higher specificity for PET.[381]

GATED PET PERFUSION STUDIES. Gated myocardial PET also has been performed, quantified, and compared with magnetic resonance imaging in controls and with left ventriculography in patients with coronary artery disease.[383] In controls, percentage of wall thickening showed a good correlation with percentage of count increase. In coronary artery disease patients, count increase decreased significantly as wall motion worsened. This investigational technique could eventually provide assessment of left ventricular regional function at the time of PET perfusion imaging.

NEUROCARDIOLOGIC POSITRON EMISSION TOMOGRAPHIC IMAGING

Several reports utilizing single-photon imaging with radioiodinated *M*-iodobenzylguanidine (MIBG) have underscored the usefulness of evaluating presynaptic adrenergic neuronal function.[384–386] However, this agent defines activity only in the presynaptic system and requires several hours for detection and resolution of MIBG-derived radioactivity in cardiac tissue compared with that in blood.[387] Thus, conventional MIBG imaging is not suited for kinetic analysis and quantification of sympathetic function.

PET neurocardiac studies may develop into a new approach focusing on sympathetic and parasympathetic interactions, neural regulation of the coronary circulation, adrenergic mechanisms in the genesis of arrhythmias, cardiac reflexes, and sympathetic innervation in the failing heart. Currently, PET imaging may assess preganglionic and postganglionic neurochemistry, providing the opportunity to gain insights in cardiovascular neurohormonal interactions. ^{18}F-fluorodopamine can be used to visualize sympathetic innervation and function in vivo.[388] ^{18}F-fluorodopamine is converted to ^{18}F-fluoronorepinephrine in synaptic adrenergic vesicles. Imaging with this agent allows depiction of tissue sites of uptake, retention, and excretion for 3 hours after injection. The homogeneous uptake of the tracer occurs within 2 to 5 minutes after injection and is independent of blood flow because displacement with reserpine and desipramine inhibit uptake and retention of the tracer.

Visualization of the cardiac sympathetic nervous system has also been performed with ^{11}C hydroxyephedrine (^{11}C HED), an analog of norepinephrine.[389] Comparative studies were performed in six normal volunteers and five cardiac transplant patients, the latter representing a model of global cardiac denervation. The normal volunteers showed homogeneous uptake of ^{11}C HED and of ^{82}Rb. However, the transplant patients, while demonstrating normal blood flow with ^{82}Rb, had a markedly reduced uptake of ^{11}C HED.

Other cardiac neuronal agents such as [^{18}F] 6-fluorometaraminol are under investigation.[390] Furthermore, true postganglionic receptor imaging may be possible with the ongoing development of muscarinic and beta-receptor ligands. In a recent study by Valette et al., PET was used serially in dogs to assess changes in ventricular muscarinic and beta-adrenergic densities following chemical and surgical denervation with the ligand CGP 12177. Their results showed an up-regulation of beta-adrenergic receptor densities following chemical or surgical denervation without any serial changes in muscarinic receptor density.[391] Adrenergic receptor imaging has direct clinical applicability in patients with left ventricular dysfunction, heart failure, and painful or silent myocardial ischemia. In patients with heart failure, quantification of specific beta-adrenergic receptor binding may provide a useful index for beta-blocker therapy in congestive heart failure.[392]

The reason for the lack of pain perception in silent myocardial ischemia is unclear. Although peripheral levels of circulating endorphins correlate with pain threshold, recent observations indirectly measuring central nervous system modulation of opiate receptor outflow challenge the contribution of opiate pathways in silent myocardial ischemia.[393,394] The quantification of regional opiate receptors with tracers such as ^{11}C diprenorphine may deliver important insights into silent myocardial ischemia and the central nervous system modulation of specific cardiovascular presentations.[395]

NONINVASIVE ASSESSMENT OF CHOLESTEROL LOWERING

Evidence supports the benefits of aggressive cholesterol lowering in secondary prevention studies, which results in a decrease in coronary events.[396–399] Longitudinal noninvasive management with dipyridamole PET has been shown to demonstrate a decrease in the size and severity of perfusion abnormalities in patients with successful vigorous cholesterol lowering during a 90-day intensive lowering treatment plan.[400] These same patients had a final control period off their lipid-lowering regimens, with repeat rest-dipyridamole PET which showed significant increases (worsening) in the size and severity of perfusion abnormalities. The pathophysiological mechanisms that may account for improved perfusion defects over such a short period of cholesterol lowering are not likely explained by anatomical regression of atherosclerosis but may be more consistent with restoration of endothelium-dependent vasodilatation by a reduction and/or pharmacological manipulation of serum lipids.[401] These provocative observations provide a basis for future studies with larger populations that would address absolute serial changes in perfusion.

Future of Clinical Cardiovascular PET Imaging

The initial capital costs and maintenance of PET technology have limited its availability. In those institutions where both PET and SPECT are available, established referral patterns suggest that PET is used in situations where conventional modalities render equivocal results (for example, attenuation artifacts on SPECT imaging or questions about the presence of viable myocardium). The higher spatial resolution and attenuation correction may justify direct PET referrals when the pretest likelihood of coronary artery disease is low.[402] Socioeconomic changes have influenced institutions with PET capability to offer PET imaging at competitive cost compared with SPECT and conventional nuclear cardiology studies. In institutions where SPECT and PET are both available, for reasons stated above PET viability studies frequently are a final resort for making difficult clinical decisions in high-risk coronary artery disease patients after conventional myocardial perfusion imaging, echocardiography, and coronary angiography have been performed.[318,322,323,332]

In the future, the clinical indications for cardiac PET may be more widely used if the prices of PET studies decline, and regional distribution of PET radiopharmaceuticals or generator-produced radiopharmaceuticals becomes available. These trends already are in place in some locales and may play an important role in the wider future use of PET in clinical cardiology. Patterson et al. addressed economic aspects of a multimodality approach to the diagnosis of coronary artery disease with a comparison of stress PET, SPECT, coronary angiography, and stress ECG.[403] Their analysis suggested that stress PET is most economical with lowest cost per use in patients with a less than 70 per cent pretest likelihood of coronary artery disease. Two future diagnostic indications may provide an expanded role for PET in clinical cardiology. These include absolute quantification of regional myocardial blood flow and the assessment of adrenergic neuronal integrity.

To the extent that endothelial dysfunction represents the results of lipid deposition and is expressed clinically by altered vasomotor control, the absolute quantification of myocardial blood flow with interventions designed to detect early coronary artery disease with PET may emerge.[404,405] In addition, the interaction between flow and mechanical left ventricular function may be addressed in various clinical situations such as ventricular remodeling and in those instances in which mechanical dysfunction exceeds the extent of coronary artery disease.

Adrenergic receptor density in the myocardium may be of increasing importance in the future. Given the neurohormonal contribution to presentations such as congestive heart failure,[406] acute myocardial infarction,[407] long Q-T syndrome,[408] and sudden death,[409] PET may play an important role in identifying, stratifying, and monitoring therapy in these patients.

REFERENCES

INSTRUMENTATION

1. Garcia, E. V.: Quantitative myocardial perfusion single-photon emission computed tomographic imaging: Quo vadis? (Where do we go from here?) J. Nucl. Cardiol. *1*:83, 1994.
2. Rullo, F., and Patton, J. A.: Instrumentation and information portrayal. *In* Freeman, L. M. (eds.): Freeman and Johnson's Clinical Radionuclide Imaging. Orlando, Grune & Stratton, 1988, p. 203.

MYOCARDIAL PERFUSION IMAGING

3. Carr, E. A., Gleason, G., Shaw, J., et al.: The direct diagnosis of myocardial infarction by photoscanning after administration of cesium-131. Am. Heart J. *68*:627, 1964.
4. Zaret, B. L., Strauss, H. W., Martin, N. D., et al.: Noninvasive regional myocardial perfusion with radioactive potassium. N. Engl. J. Med. *288*:809, 1973.
5. Bradley-Moore, P. R., Lebowitz, E., Greene, M. W., et al.: Thallium-201 for medical use. II: Biologic behavior. J. Nucl. Med. *16*:156, 1975.
6. Strauss, H. W., Harrison, K., Langan, J. K., et al.: Thallium-201 for myocardial imaging. Relation of thallium-201 to regional myocardial perfusion. Circulation *51*:641, 1975.
7. Wackers, F. J. Th., van der Schoot, J. B., Busemann Sokole, E., et al.: Noninvasive visualization of acute myocardial infarction in man with thallium-201. Br. Heart J. *37*:741, 1975.
8. Kaul, S.: A look at 15 years of planar thallium-201 imaging. Am. Heart J. *118*:581, 1989.
9. Brown, K. A.: Prognostic value of thallium-201 myocardial perfusion imaging: A diagnostic tool comes of age. Circulation *83*:363, 1991.
10. Wackers, F. J. Th., Berman D. S., Maddahi, J., et al.: Technetium-99m Hexakis 2-methyoxyisobutyl isonitrile: Human biodistribution, dosimetry, safety and preliminary comparison to thallium-201 for myocardial perfusion imaging. J. Nucl. Med. *30*:301, 1989.
11. Kiat, H., Maddahi, J., Roy, L. T., et al.: Comparison of technetium-99m-methyoxy isobutyl isonitrile and thallium-201 for evaluation of coronary artery disease by planar and tomographic methods. Am. Heart J. *117*:1, 1989.
12. Seldin, D. W., Johnson, L. L., Blood, D. K., et al.: Myocardial perfusion imaging with technetium-99m SQ30217: Comparison with thallium-201 and coronary anatomy. J. Nucl. Med. *30*:312, 1989.

13. Hendel, R. C., McSherry, B., Karimeddini, M., et al.: Diagnostic value of a new myocardial perfusion agent, teboroxime (SQ30,217), utilizing a rapid planar imaging protocol: Preliminary results. J. Am. Coll. Cardiol. *16*:855, 1990.
14. Jain, D., Wackers, F. J. Th., Mattera, J., et al.: Biokinetics of ^{99m}Tc-tetrofosmin, a new myocardial perfusion imaging agent: Implications for a one day imaging protocol. J. Nucl. Med. *34*:1254, 1993.
15. Zaret, B. L., Rigo, P., Wackers, F. J. Th., et al.: The Tetrofosmine International Trial Study Group: Myocardial perfusion imaging with ^{99m}Tc-tetrofosmin. Comparison to ^{201}Tl imaging and coronary angiography in a phase III multicenter trial. Circulation *91*:313, 1995.
16. Gerson, M. C., Millard, R. W., Roszell, N. J., et al.: Kinetic properties of ^{99m}Tc-Q12 in canine myocardium. Circulation *89*:1291, 1994.
17. Weich, H. F., Strauss, H. W., and Pitt, B.: The extraction of thallium-201 by the myocardium. Circulation *56*:188, 1977.
18. Marshall, R. C., Leidholdt, E. M., Zhang, D. Y., et al.: Technetium-99m hexakis 2-methoxy-2-isobutyl isonitrile and thallium-201 extraction, washout, and retention at varying coronary flow rates in rabbit heart. Circulation *82*:998, 1990.
19. Wackers, F. J. Th.: The maze of myocardial perfusion imaging protocols anno 1994. J. Nucl. Cardiol. *1*:180, 1994.
20. Berman, D. S., Kiat, H., Friedman, J. D., et al.: Separate acquisitions rest thallium–201/stress technetium–99m sestamibi dual-isotope myocardial perfusion single-photon emission computed tomography: A clinical validation study. J. Am. Coll. Cardiol. *22*:1455, 1993.
21. Wackers, F. J. Th.: Myocardial perfusion imaging. *In* Sandler, M. P., Coleman, R. E., Wackers, F. J. Th., et al. (eds.): Diagnostic Nuclear Medicine. 3rd ed. Baltimore, Williams & Wilkins, 1995.
22. Wackers, F. J. Th., and Mattera, J. A.: Optimizing planar Tl-201 imaging: Computer quantification. Cardiology *7*:103, 1990.
23. Berman, D. S., Kiat, H. S., Van Train, K. F., et al.: Myocardial perfusion imaging with technetium-99m sestamibi: Comparative analysis of available imaging protocols. J. Nucl. Med. *35*:681, 1994.
24. DePuey, E. G., Berman, D. S., and Garcia, E. V.: Cardiac SPECT Imaging. New York, Raven Press, 1995.
25. Friedman, J., Van Train, K., Maddahi, J., et al.: "Upward creep" of the heart: A frequent source of false positive reversible defects during thallium-201 stress-distribution SPECT. J. Nucl. Med. *30*:1718, 1989.
26. Maniawski, P. J., Morgan, H. T., Wackers, F. J. Th.: Orbit related variation in spatial resolution as a source of artifactual defects in Tl201 SPECT. J. Nucl. Med. *32*:871, 1991.
27. The Cardiovascular Imaging Committee, American College of Cardiology; The Committee on Advanced Cardiac Imaging and Technology, Council of Clinical Cardiology, American Heart Association; and the Board of Directors, Cardiovascular Council, Society of Nuclear Medicine: ACC/AHA/SNM Policy Statement: Standardization of cardiac tomographic imaging. J. Nucl. Cardiol. *1*:117, 1994.
28. Eisner, R. I., Tammas, M. J., Colinger, K., et al.: Normal SPECT thallium-201 bull's eye display: Gender differences. J. Nucl. Med. *29*:1901, 1988.
29. Johnstone, D. E., Wackers, F. J. Th., Berger, H. J., et al.: Effect of patient positioning on left lateral thallium-201 myocardial images. J. Nucl. Med. *20*:183, 1979.
30. Wackers, F. J. Th.: Artifacts in planar and SPECT myocardial perfusion imaging. Am. J. Cardiac Imaging *6*:42, 1992.
31. Segal, G. M., and Davis, M. J.: Prone versus supine thallium myocardial SPECT: A method to decrease artifactual inferior wall defects. J. Nucl. Med. *30*:548, 1989.
32. Esquerre, J. P., Coca, F. J., Martinez, S. J., et al.: Prone decubitus: A solution to inferior wall attenuation in thallium-201 myocardial tomography. J. Nucl. Med. *30*:398, 1989.
33. Suzki, A., Muto, S., Oshima, M., et al.: A new scanning method for thallium-201 myocardial SPECT: Semi-decubital position method. Clin. Nucl. Med. *14*:736, 1989.
34. Barr, S. A., Shen, M. Y. H., Sinusas, A. J., et al.: Reduced inferior attenuation on rest SPECT myocardial perfusion imaging in the upright position using a rotating chair: Comparison with standard supine SPECT imaging. J. Nucl. Med. *35*:91P, 1994.
35. DePuey, E. G., and Garcia, E. V.: Optimal specificity of thallium-201 SPECT through recognition of imaging artifacts. J. Nucl. Med. *30*:441, 1989.
36. Cloninger, K. G., DePuey, E. G., Garcia, E. V., et al.: Incomplete redistribution of delayed thallium-201 single photon emission computed tomographic (SPECT) images: An overestimation of myocardial scarring. J. Am. Coll. Cardiol. *12*:955, 1988.
37. Kiat, H. K., Berman, D. S., Maddahi, J., et al.: Late reversibility of tomographic myocardial thallium-201 defects: An accurate marker of myocardial viability. J. Am. Coll. Cardiol. *12*:1456, 1988.
38. Weiss, A. T., Maddahi, J., Lew, A. S., et al.: Reverse redistribution of thallium-201: A sign of nontransmural myocardial infarction with patency of the infarct-related coronary artery. J. Am. Coll. Cardiol. *7*:61, 1986.
39. Soufer, R., Dey, H. M., Lawson, A. J., et al.: Relationship between reverse redistribution on planar thallium scintigraphy and regional myocardial viability: A correlative PET study. J. Nucl. Med. *36*:180, 1995.
40. Gill, J. B., Ruddy, T. D., Newell, J. B., et al.: Prognostic importance of thallium uptake by the lungs during exercise in coronary artery disease. N. Engl. J. Med. *317*:1485, 1987.
41. Giubbini, R., Campini, R., Milan, E., et al.: Evaluation of technetium-99m-sestamibi lung uptake: Correlation with left ventricular function. J. Nucl. Med. *36*:58, 1995.
42. Weiss, A. T., Berman, D. S., Lew, A. S., et al.: Transient ischemic dilation of the left ventricle on stress thallium-201 scintigraphy: A marker of severe and extensive coronary artery disease. J. Am. Coll. Cardiol. *9*:752, 1987.
43. Wackers, F. J. Th., Bodenheimer, M., Fleiss, J. L., et al.: Factors affecting uniformity in interpretation of planar Tl-201 imaging in a multicenter trial. J. Am. Coll. Cardiol. *21*:1064, 1993.
44. Beller, G. A., Watson, D. D., and Pohost, G. M.: Kinetics of thallium distribution and redistribution: Clinical applications in sequential myocardial imaging. *In* Strauss, H. W., and Pitt, B. (eds.): Cardiovascular Nuclear Medicine, 2nd ed. St. Louis, C. V. Mosby Co., 1979.
45. Sinusas, A. J., Bergin, J. D., Edwards, N. C., et al.: Redistribution of ^{99m}Tc-Sestamibi and ^{201}Tl in presence of a severe coronary artery stenosis. Circulation *89*:2332, 1994.
46. Goris, M. L., Daspit, S. G., McLaughlin, P., et al.: Interpolative background subtraction. J. Nucl. Med. *17*:744, 1976.
47. Watson, D. D., Campbell, N. P., Read, E. K., et al.: Spatial and temporal quantitation of plane thallium myocardial images. J. Nucl. Med. *22*:577, 1981.
48. Garcia, E., Maddahi, J., Berman, D. S., et al.: Space/time quantitation of thallium-201 myocardial scintigraphy. J. Nucl. Med. *22*:309, 1981.
49. Wackers, F. J. Th., Fetterman, R. C., Mattera, J. A., et al.: Quantitative planar thallium-201 stress scintigraphy: A critical evaluation of the method. Semin. Nucl. Med. *15*:46, 1985.
50. Sigal, S. L., Soufer, R., Fetterman, R. C., et al.: Reproducibility of quantitative planar thallium-201 scintigraphy. Quantitative criteria for reversibility of myocardial perfusion defects. J. Nucl. Med. *32*:759, 1991.
51. Klein, J. L., Garcia, E. V., DePuey, G., et al.: Reversibility bulls-eye: A new polar bulls-eye may quantify reversibility of stress-induced SPECT thallium-201 myocardial perfusion defects. J. Nucl. Med. *31*:1240, 1990.
52. Wackers, F. J. Th.: Science, art and artifacts: How important is quantification for the practicing physician interpreting myocardial perfusion studies. J. Nucl. Cardiol. *1*:S109, 1994.
53. Wackers, F. J. Th., Maniawski, P., and Sinusas, A. J.: Evaluation of left ventricular wall function by ECG-gated Tc-99m-Sestambi imaging. *In* Beller, G. A., and Zaret, B. L. (eds.): Nuclear Cardiology: State of the Art and Future Direction. St. Louis, C. V. Mosby Co., 1993, p. 85.
54. Chua, T., Kiat, H., Germano, G., et al.: Gated technetium-99m sestamibi for simultaneous assessment of stress myocardial perfusion, postexercise regional ventricular function and myocardial viability. J. Am. Coll. Cardiol. *23*:1107, 1994.
55. Germano, G., Kavanaugh, P. B., Kiat, H., et al.: Automated analysis of gated myocardial SPECT: Development and initial validation of a method. J. Nucl. Med. *35*:816, 1994.
56. DePuey, E. G., Nichols, K., and Dobrinsky, C.: Left ventricular ejection fraction assessed from gated technetium-99m-sestamibi SPECT. J. Nucl. Med. *34*:1871, 1993.

CLINICAL APPLICATIONS OF MYOCARDIAL PERFUSION IMAGING

57. Wackers, F. J. Th., Busemann Sokole, E., Samson, G., et al.: Value and limitations of thallium-201 scintigraphy in the acute phase of myocardial infarction. N. Engl. J. Med. *295*:1, 1976.
58. Wackers, F. J. Th., Becker, A. E., Samson, G., et al.: Location and size of acute transmural myocardial infarction estimated from thallium-201 scintiscans. Circulation *56*:71, 1977.
59. Wackers, F. J. Th., Lie, K. I., Liem, K. I., et al.: Potential value of thallium-201 scintigraphy as a means of selecting patients for the coronary care unit. Br. Heart J. *41*:111, 1979.
60. Varetto, T., Cantalupi, D., Altiero, A., et al.: Emergency room technetium-99m-sestamibi imaging to rule out acute myocardial ischemic events in patients with nondiagnostic electrocardiograms. J. Am. Coll. Cardiol. *22*:1804, 1993.
61. Hilton, T. C., Thompson, R. C., Williams, H. J., et al.: Technetium-99-sestamibi myocardial perfusion imaging in the emergency room evaluation of chest pain. J. Am. Coll. Cardiol. *23*:1016, 1994.
62. Radensky, P. W., Stowers, S. A., Hilton, T. C., et al.: Cost-effectiveness of acute myocardial perfusion imaging with Tc-99m-sestamibi for risk stratification of emergency room patients with acute chest pain. Circulation *90*(Abs.):528, 1994.
63. Gibbons, R. J., Verani, M. S., Behrenbeck, T., et al.: Feasibility of tomographic ^{99m}Tc-hexakis-2-methoxy-2-methylpropyl-isonitrile imaging for the assessment of myocardial area at risk and the effect of treatment in acute myocardial infarction. Circulation *80*:177, 1989.
64. Wackers, F. J. Th., Gibbons, R. J., Verani, M. S., et al.: Serial quantitative planar technetium-99m-isonitrile imaging in acute myocardial infarction: Efficacy for noninvasive assessment of thrombolytic therapy. J. Am. Coll. Cardiol. *14*:861, 1989.
65. Santoro, G. M., Bisi, G., Sciagra, R., et al.: Single photon emission computed tomography with technetium-99m-hexakis 2-methoxy isobutyl isonitrile in acute myocardial infarction before and after thrombolytic treatment: Assessment of salvaged myocardium and prediction of late functional recovery. J. Am. Coll. Cardiol. *15*:301, 1990.
66. Decoster, P. M., Wijns, W., Cauwe, F., et al.: Area-at-risk determination by technetium-99m-hexakis-2-methoxyisobutyl isonitrile in experimental reperfused myocardial infarction. Circulation *82*:2152, 1990.
67. Bisi, G., Sciagra, R., Santoro, G. M., et al.: Comparison of tomography and planar imaging for the evaluation of thrombolytic therapy in acute myocardial infarction using pre- and post-treatment myocardial scintigraphy with technetium-99m sestamibi. Am. Heart J. *122*:13, 1991.

68. Faraggi, M., Assayag, P., Messian, O., et al.: Early isonitrile SPECT in acute myocardial infarction: Feasibility and results before and after fibrinolysis. Nucl. Med. Communications *10*:539, 1989.
69. Gibbons, R. J.: Perfusion imaging with ^{99m}Tc-sestamibi for the assessment of myocardial area at risk and the efficacy of acute treatment in myocardial infarction. Circulation *84*(Suppl I.):1, 1991.
70. Christian, T. F., Gibbons, R. J., and Gersh, B. J.: Effect of infarct location on myocardial salvage assessed by technetium-99m isonitrile. J. Am. Coll. Cardiol. *17*:1303, 1991.
71. Christian, T. F., Schwartz, R. S., and Gibbons, R. J.: Determinants of infarct size in reperfusion therapy for acute myocardial infarction. Circulation *86*:81, 1992.
72. Christian, T. F., Behrenbeck, T., Pellikka, P. A., et al.: Mismatch of left ventricular function and infarct size demonstrated by technetium-99m isonitrile imaging after reperfusion therapy for acute myocardial infarction: Identification of myocardial stunning and hyperkinesia. J. Am. Coll. Cardiol. *16*:1632, 1990.
73. Pellikka, P. A., Behrenbeck, R., Verani, M. S., et al.: Serial changes in myocardial perfusion using tomographic technetium-99m-hexakis-2-methoxy-2-methylpropyl-isonitrile imaging following reperfusion therapy of myocardial infarction. J. Nucl. Med. *31*:1269, 1990.
74. Gibbons, R. J.: Technetium-99m sestamibi in the assessment of acute myocardial infarction. Semin. Nucl. Med. *21*:213, 1991.
75. Marcassa, C., Galli, M., Luigi, P., et al.: Technetium-99m-sestamibi tomographic evaluation of residual ischemia after anterior myocardial infarction. J. Am. Coll. Cardiol. *25*:590, 1995.
76. Ito, H., Iwakura, K., Oh, H., et al.: Temporal changes in myocardial perfusion patterns in patients with reperfused anterior wall myocardial infarction. Their relation to myocardial viability. Circulation *91*:656, 1995.
77. Gibbons, R. J., Christian, T. F., Hopfenspringer, M., et al.: Myocardium at risk and infarct size after thrombolytic therapy for acute myocardial infarction: Implications for the design of randomized trials of acute intervention. J. Am. Coll. Cardiol. *24*:616, 1994.
78. Gibbons, R. J., Holmes, D. R., Reeder, G. S., et al.: Immediate angioplasty compared with the administration of a thrombolytic agent followed by conservative treatment for myocardial infarction. N. Engl. J. Med. *328*:685, 1993.
79. Silverman, K. J., Becker, L. C., Bulkley, B. H., et al.: Value of early thallium-201 scintigraphy for predicting mortality in patients with acute myocardial infarction. Circulation *61*:996, 1980.
80. Cerqueira, M. D., Maynard, C., Ritchie, J. L., et al.: Long-term survival in 618 patients from the Western Washington streptokinase in myocardial infarction trials. J. Am. Coll. Cardiol. *20*:1452, 1992.
81. Nestico, P. E., Hakki, A., Felsher, J., et al.: Implications of abnormal right ventricular thallium uptake in acute myocardial infarction. Am. J. Cardiol. *58*:230, 1986.
82. Jain, D., Lahiri, A., Raftery, E. B., et al.: Clinical and prognostic significance of lung thallium uptake on rest imaging in acute myocardial infarction. Am. J. Cardiol. *65*:154, 1990.
83. Brown, K. A., O'Meara, J., Chambers, C. E., et al.: Ability of dipyridamole-thallium-201 imaging one to four days after acute myocardial infarction to predict in-hospital and late recurrent myocardial ischemic events. Am. J. Cardiol. *65*:160, 1990.
84. Wackers, F. J. Th., Lie, K. I., Liem, K. L., et al.: Thallium-201 scintigraphy in unstable angina pectoris. Circulation *57*:738, 1978.
85. Berger, B. C., Watson, D. D., Burwell, L. R., et al.: Redistribution of thallium at rest in patients with stable and unstable angina and the effect of coronary artery bypass surgery. Circulation *60*:1114, 1979.
86. Bilodeau, L., Theroux, P., Gregoire, J., et al.: Technetium-99m sestamibi tomography in patients with spontaneous chest pain: Correlations with clinical, electrocardiographic and angiographic findings. J. Am. Coll. Cardiol. *18*:1684, 1991.
87. Freeman, M. R., Chisholm, R. J., and Armstrong, P. W.: Usefulness of exercise electrocardiography and thallium scintigraphy in unstable angina pectoris in predicting the extent and severity of coronary artery disease. Am. J. Cardiol. *62*:1164, 1988.
88. Gould, K. L.: Noninvasive assessment of coronary stenoses by myocardial perfusion imaging during pharmacologic coronary vasodilatation. I. Physiologic basis and experimental validation. Am. J. Cardiol. *41*:267, 1978.
89. Casale, P. N., Guiney, T. E., Strauss, H. W., et al.: Simultaneous low level treadmill exercise and intravenous dipyridamole stress thallium imaging. Am. J. Cardiol. *62*:799, 1988.
90. Ranhosky, A., and Rawson, J.: The safety of intravenous dipyridamole thallium myocardial perfusion imaging. Circulation *81*:1205, 1990.
91. Lette, J., Tatum, J. L., Fraser, S., et al.: Safety of dipyridamole testing in 73,806 patients: The multicenter dipyridamole safety study. J. Nucl. Cardiol. *2*:3, 1995.
92. Verani, M. S., Mahmarian, J. J., Hixson, J. B., et al.: Diagnosis of coronary artery disease by controlled coronary vasodilation with adenosine and thallium-201 scintigraphy in patients unable to exercise. Circulation *82*:80, 1990.
93. Nguyen, T., Heo, J., Ogilby, J. D., et al.: Single photon emission computed tomography with thallium-201 during adenosine-induced coronary hyperemia: Correlation with coronary arteriography, exercise thallium imaging and two-dimensional echocardiography. J. Am. Coll. Cardiol. *16*:1375, 1990.
94. Wilson, R. F., Wyche, K., Christensen, B. V., et al.: Effects of adenosine on human coronary arterial circulation. Circulation *82*:1595, 1990.
95. Samuels, B., Kiat, H., Friedman, J. D., et al.: Adenosine pharmacologic stress myocardial perfusion tomographic imaging in patients with significant aortic stenosis. Diagnostic efficacy and comparison of clinical, hemodynamic and electrocardiographic variables with 100 age-matched control subjects. J. Am. Coll. Cardiol. *25*:99, 1995.
96. Pennell, D. J., Underwood, R., Swanton, R. H., et al.: Dobutamine thallium myocardial perfusion tomography. J. Am. Coll. Cardiol. *18*:147, 1991.
97. Hays, J. T., Mahmarian, J. J., Cochran, A. J., et al.: Dobutamine thallium-201 tomography for evaluating patients with suspected coronary artery disease unable to undergo exercise or vasodilator pharmacologic stress testing. J. Am. Coll. Cardiol. *21*:1583, 1993.
98. Picano, E., Mathias, W., Pingitore, A., et al.: Safety and tolerability of dobutamine-atropine stress echocardiography: A prospective, multicentre study. Lancet *344*:1190, 1994.
99. Berger, B. C., Watson, D. D., Taylor, G. J., et al.: Quantitative thallium-201 exercise scintigraphy for detection of coronary artery disease. J. Nucl. Med. *22*:585, 1981.
100. Maddahi, J., Garcia, E. V., Berman, D. S., et al.: Improved noninvasive assessment of coronary artery disease by quantitative analysis of regional stress myocardial distribution and washout of thallium-201. Circulation *64*:924, 1981.
101. van Train, K. F., Berman, D. S., Garcia, E. V., et al.: Quantitative analysis of stress thallium-201 myocardial scintigrams: A multicenter trial. J. Nucl. Med. *27*:17, 1986.
102. Kaul, S., Boucher, C. A., Newell, J. B., et al.: Determination of the quantitative thallium imaging variables that optimize detection of coronary artery disease. J. Am. Coll. Cardiol. *7*:527, 1986.
103. Henkin, R. E., Kalousdian, S., Kikkawa, R. M., et al.: Diagnostic and therapeutic technology assessment (DATTA) myocardial perfusion imaging utilizing single-photon emission-computed tomography (SPECT). Washington Manual of Therapeutic Technology, 1994, p. 2850.
104. Maddahi, J., van Train, K., Prigent, F., et al.: Quantitative single photon emission computed thallium-201 tomography for detection and localization of coronary artery disease: Optimization and prospective validation of a new technique. J. Am. Coll. Cardiol. *14*:1689, 1989.
105. DePasquale, E. E., Nody, A. C., DePuey, E. G., et al.: Quantitative rotational thallium-201 tomography for identifying and localizing coronary artery disease. Circulation *77*:316, 1988.
106. Fintel, D. J., Links, J. M., Brinker, J. A., et al.: Improved diagnostic performance of exercise thallium-201 single photon emission computed tomography over planar imaging in the diagnosis of coronary artery disease: A receiver operating characteristic analysis. J. Am. Coll. Cardiol. *13*:600, 1989.
107. Mahmarian, J. J., Boyce, T. M., Goldberg, R. K., et al.: Quantitative exercise thallium-201 single photo emission computed tomography for the enhanced diagnosis of ischemic heart disease. J. Am. Coll. Cardiol. *15*:318, 1990.
108. Go, R. T., Marwick, T. H., MacIntyre, W. J., et al.: A prospective comparison of rubidium-82 PET and thallium-201 SPECT myocardial perfusion imaging utilizing a single dipyridamole stress in the diagnosis of coronary artery disease. J. Nucl. Med. *31*:1899, 1990.
109. Tamaki, N., Yonekura, Y., Mukai, T., et al.: Stress thallium-201 transaxial emission computed tomography: Quantitative versus qualitative analysis for evaluation of coronary artery disease. J. Am. Coll. Cardiol. *4*:1213, 1984.
110. Iskandrian, A. S., Heo, J., Kong, B., et al.: Effect of exercise level on the ability of thallium-201 tomographic imaging in detecting coronary artery disease: Analysis of 461 patients. J. Am. Coll. Cardiol. *14*:1477, 1989.
111. van Train, K. F., Maddahi, J., Berman, D. S., et al.: Quantitative analysis of tomographic stress thallium-201 myocardial scintigrams: A multicenter trial. J. Nucl. Med. *31*:1168, 1990.
112. Borges-Neto, S., Mahmarian, J. J., Jain, A., et al.: Quantitative thallium-201 single photon emission computed tomography after oral dipyridamole for assessing the presence, anatomic location and severity of coronary artery disease. J. Am. Coll. Cardiol. *11*:962, 1988.
113. Taillefer, R., Lambert, R., Dupras, G., et al.: Clinical comparison between thallium-201 and Tc-99m-methoxyisobutyl isonitrile (hexamibi) myocardial perfusion imaging for the detection of coronary artery disease. Eur. J. Nucl. Med. *15*:280, 1989.
114. Iskandrian, A., Heo, J., Kong, B., et al.: Use of technetium-99m isonitrile (RP-30A) in assessing left ventricular perfusion and function at rest and during exercise in coronary artery disease, and comparison with coronary arteriography and exercise thallium-201 SPECT imaging. Am. J. Cardiol. *64*:270, 1989.
115. Maddahi, J., Kiat, H., Friedman, J. D., et al.: Technetium-99m-sestamibi myocardial perfusion imaging for evaluation of coronary artery disease. *In* Zaret, B. L., and Beller, G. A. (eds.): Nuclear Cardiology. St. Louis, C. V. Mosby Co., 1993, p. 191.
116. van Train, K. F., Garcia, E. V., Maddahi, J., et al.: Multicenter trial validation of quantitative analysis of same-day rest stress technetium-99m-sestamibi myocardial tomograms. J. Nucl. Med. *35*:609, 1994.
117. Rigo, P., Leclercq, B., Itti, R., et al.: Technetium-99m-tetrofosmin myocardial imaging: A comparison with thallium-201 and angiography. J. Nucl. Med. *35*:587, 1994.
118. Heo, J., Cave, V., Wasserleben, V., et al.: Planar and tomographic imaging with technetium 99m-labeled tetrofosmin: Correlation with thallium 201 and coronary angiography. J. Nucl. Cardiol. *1*:317, 1994.
119. Gerson, M. C., Lukes, J., Deutsh, E., et al.: Comparison of technetium 99m Q12 and thallium-201 for detection of angiographically docu-

mented coronary artery disease in humans. J. Nucl. Cardiol. *1*:499, 1994.
120. Hendel, R. C., Gerson, M. C., Verani, M. S., et al.: Perfusion imaging with Tc-99m furisfosmin (Q12): Multicenter phase III trial to evaluate safety and comparative efficacy. Circulation *90*(Abs.):449, 1994.
121. Iskandrian, A. S., Heo, J., Nguyen, T., et al.: Tomographic myocardial perfusion imaging with technetium-99m teboroxime during adenosine-induced coronary hyperemia: Correlation with thallium-201 imaging. J. Am. Coll. Cardiol. *19*:307, 1992.
122. Serafini, A. N., Topchik, S., Jiminez, H., et al.: Clinical comparison of technetium-99m-teboroxime and thallium-201 utilizing a continuous SPECT imaging protocol. J. Nucl. Med. *33*:1304, 1992.
123. Henzlova, M. J., and Machac, J.: Clinical utility of technetium-99m-teboroxime myocardial washout imaging. J. Nucl. Med. *35*:575, 1994.
124. Stewart, R. E., Heyl, B., O'Rourke, R. A., et al.: Demonstration of differential post-stenoic myocardial technetium-99m-teboroxime clearance kinetics after experimental ischemia and hyperemic stress. J. Nucl. Med. *32*:2000, 1991.
125. Albro, P. C., Gould, K. L., Westcott, R. J., et al.: Noninvasive assessment of coronary stenoses by myocardial imaging during pharmacologic coronary vasodilatation. III. Clinical trial. Am. J. Cardiol. *42*:751, 1978.
126. Sochor, H., Pachinger, O., Ogris, E., et al.: Radionuclide imaging after coronary vasodilation: Myocardial scintigraphy with thallium-201 and radionuclide angiography after administration of dipyridamole. Eur. Heart J. *5*:400, 1984.
127. Francisco, D. A., Collins, S. M., Go, R. T., et al.: Tomographic thallium-201 myocardial perfusion scintigrams after maximal coronary artery vasodilation with intravenous dipyridamole: Comparison of qualitative and quantitative approaches. Circulation 66:370, 1982.
128. Kong, B. A., Shaw, L., Miller, D. D., et al.: Comparison of accuracy for detecting coronary artery disease and side-effect profile of dipyridamole thallium-201 myocardial perfusion imaging in women versus men. Am. J. Cardiol. *70*:168, 1992.
129. Verani, M. S., Mahmarian, J. J., Hixson, J. B., et al.: Diagnosis of coronary artery disease by controlled coronary vasodilation with adenosine and thallium-201 scintigraphy in patients unable to exercise. Circulation *82*:80, 1990.
130. Iskandrian, A. S., Heo, J., Nguyen, T., et al: Assessment of coronary artery disease using single photon emission computed tomography with thallium-201 during adenosine induced coronary hyperemia. Am. J. Cardiol. *67*:1190, 1991.
131. Santos-O'Campos, C. D., Herman, S. D., Travin, M. I., et al.: Comparison of exercise, dipyridamole, and adenosine by use of technetium 99m sestamibi tomographic imaging. J. Nucl. Cardiol. *1*:57, 1994.
132. Rozanski, A., Diamond, G., Forrester, J. S., et al.: Declining specificity of exercise radionuclide ventriculography. N. Engl. J. Med. *309*:518, 1983.
133. Maddahi, J., Abdulla, A., Garcia, E. V., et al.: Noninvasive identification of left main and triple vessel coronary artery disease: Improved accuracy using quantitative analysis of regional myocardial stress distribution and washout of thallium-201. J. Am. Coll. Cardiol. *7*:53, 1986.
134. Dash, H., Massie, B. M., Botvinick, E. H., et al.: The noninvasive identification of left main and three-vessel coronary artery disease by myocardial stress perfusion scintigraphy and treadmill exercise electrocardiography. Circulation *60*:276, 1979.
135. Nygaard, T. W., Gibson, R. S., Ryan, J. M., et al.: Prevalance of high-risk thallium-201 scintigraphic findings in left main coronary artery stenosis: Comparison with patients with multiple and single-vessel coronary artery disease. Am. J. Cardiol. *53*:462, 1984.
136. Kushner, F. G., Okada, R. D., Kirshenbaum, H. D., et al.: Lung thallium-201 uptake after stress testing in patients with coronary artery disease. Circulation *63*:341, 1981.
137. Gibson, R. S., Watson, D. D., Craddock, G. B., et al.: Prediction of cardiac events after uncomplicated myocardial infarction: A prospective study comparing predischarge exercise thallium-201 scintigraphy and coronary angiography. Circulation *68*:321, 1983.
138. Brown, K. A., Boucher, C. A., Okada, R. D., et al.: Prognostic value of exercise thallium-201 imaging in patients presenting for evaluation of chest pain. J. Am. Coll. Cardiol. *1*:994, 1983.
139. Abraham, R. D., Freedman, S. B., Dunn, R. F., et al.: Prediction of multivessel coronary artery disease and prognosis early after acute myocardial infarction by exercise electrocardiography and thallium-201 myocardial perfusion scanning. Am. J. Cardiol. *58*:423, 1986.
140. Bodenheimer, M. M., Wackers, F. J. Th., Schwartz, R. G., et al.: Prognostic significance of a fixed thallium defect one to six months after onset of acute myocardial infarction or unstable angina. Am. J. Cardiol. *74*:1196, 1994.
141. Kaul, S., Finkelstein, D. M., Homma, S., et al.: Superiority of quantitative exercise thallium-201 variables in determining long-term prognosis in ambulatory patients with chest pain: A comparison with cardiac catheterization. J. Am. Coll. Cardiol. *12*:25, 1988.
142. Manchecourt, J., Longere, P., Fagret, D., et al.: Prognostic value of thallium-201 single-photon emission computed tomographic myocardial perfusion imaging according to extent of myocardial defect. J. Am. Coll. Cardiol. *23*:1096, 1994.
143. Miller, D. D., Stratmann, H. G., Shaw, L., et al.: Dipyridamole technetium 99m sestamibi myocardial tomography as an independent predictor of cardiac event-free survival after acute ischemic events. J. Nucl. Cardiol. *1*:172, 1994.
144. Leppo, J. A., O'Brien, J., Rothendler, J. A., et al.: Dipyridamole-thallium-201 scintigraphy in the prediction of future cardiac events after acute myocardial infarction. N. Engl. J. Med. *310*:1014, 1984.
145. Brown, K. A., Weiss, R. M., Clements, J. P., et al.: Usefulness of residual ischemic myocardium within prior infarct zone for identifying patients at high risk late after acute myocardial infarction. Am. J. Cardiol. *60*:15, 1987.
146. Kamal, A., Fattah, A. A., Pancholy, S., et al.: Prognostic value of adenosine single-photon emission computed tomographic thallium imaging in medically treated patients with angiographic evidence of coronary artery disease. J. Nucl. Cardiol. *1*:254, 1994.
147. Olona, M., Candell-Riera, J., Permanyer-Miralda, G., et al.: Strategies for prognostic assessment of uncomplicated first myocardial infarction: 5 year follow-up study. J. Am. Coll. Cardiol. *25*:815, 1995.
148. Krawczynska, E. G., Weintraub, W. S., Garcia, E. V., et al.: Left ventricular dilation and multivessel coronary artery disease on thallium-201 SPECT are important prognostic indicators in patients with large defects in the left anterior descending distribution. Am. J. Cardiol. *74*:1233, 1994.
149. Bateman, T. M., O'Keefe, J. H., Dong, V. M., et al.: Coronary angiography rates following stress SPECT scintigraphy. J. Nucl. Cardiol. *2*:217, 1995.
149a. Nallamothu, N., Pancholy, S. B., Lee, K., et al.: Impact of exercise single-photon emission computed tomographic thallium imaging on patient management and outcome. J. Nucl. Cardiol. *2*:334, 1995.
150. Wackers, F. J. Th., Russo, D. J., Russo, D., et al.: Prognostic significance of normal quantitative planar thallium-201 stress scintigraphy in patients with chest pain. J. Am. Coll. Cardiol. *6*:27, 1985.
151. Pamelia, F. X., Gibson, R. S., Watson, D. D., et al.: Prognosis with chest pain and normal thallium-201 exercise scintigrams. Am. J. Cardiol. *55*:920, 1985.
152. Wahl, J., Hakki, A. H., and Iskandrian, A. S.: Prognostic implications of normal exercise thallium-201 images. Arch. Intern. Med. *145*:253, 1985.
153. Staniloff, H. M., Forrester, J. S., Berman, D. S., et al.: Prediction of death, myocardial infarction, and worsening chest pain using thallium scintigraphy and exercise electrocardiography. J. Nucl. Med. *27*:1842, 1986.
154. Brown, K. A., Altland, E., and Rowen, M.: Prognostic value of normal Tc-99m sestamibi cardiac imaging. J. Nucl. Med. *35*:554, 1994.
155. Raiker, K., Sinusas, A. J., Zaret, B. L., et al.: One year prognosis of patients with normal Tc-99m-sestamibi stress imaging. J. Nucl. Cardiol. *1*:449, 1994.
156. Berman, D. S., Kiat, H., Cohen, J., et al.: Prognosis of 1044 patients with normal exercise Tc-99m sestamibi myocardial perfusion SPECT. J. Am. Coll. Cardiol. *1A*:63A, 1994.
157. Miller, D. D., Stratmann, H. G., Shaw, L., et al.: Dipyridamole technetium-99m-sestamibi myocardial tomography as an independent predictor of cardiac event-free survival after acute ischemic events. J. Nucl. Cardiol. *1*:172, 1994.
158. Stratmann, H. G., Williams, G. A., Wittry, M. D., et al.: Exercise technetium-99m sestamibi tomography for cardiac risk stratification of patients with stable chest pain. Circulation *89*:615, 1994.
159. Pollock, S. G., Abbott, R. D., Boucher, C. A., et al.: Independent and incremental prognostic value of tests performed in hierarchical order to evaluate patients with suspected coronary artery disease. Circulation *85*:237, 1992.
160. Melin, J. A., Robert, A., Luwaert, R., et al.: Additional prognostic value of exercise testing and thallium-201 scintigraphy in catheterized patients without previous myocardial infarction. Int. J. Cardiol. *27*:235, 1990.
161. Iskandrian, A. S., Chae, S. C., Heo, J., et al.: Independent and incremental prognostic value of exercise single-photon emission computed tomographic (SPECT) thallium imaging in coronary artery disease. J. Am. Coll. Cardiol. *22*:665, 1993.
162. Petretta, M., Cuocolo, A., Carpinelli, A., et al.: Prognostic value of myocardial hypoperfusion indexes in patients with suspected or known coronary artery disease. J. Nucl. Cardiol. *1*:325, 1994.
163. Fagan, L. F., Shaw, L., Kong, B. A., et al.: Prognostic value of exercise thallium scintigraphy in patients with good exercise tolerance and a normal or abnormal exercise electrocardiogram and suspected or confirmed coronary artery disease. Am. J. Cardiol. *69*:607, 1992.
164. Tilkemeier, P. L., Guiney, T. E., LaRaia, P. J., et al.: Prognostic value of predischarge low-level exercise thallium testing after thrombolytic treatment of acute myocardial infarction. Am. J. Cardiol. *66*:1203, 1990.
165. Sutton, J. M., Topol, E. J.: Significance of a negative exercise thallium test in the presence of a critical residual stenosis after thrombolysis for acute myocardial infarction. Circulation *83*:1278, 1991.
166. Gimple, L. W., and Beller, G. A.: Assessing prognosis after acute myocardial infarction in the thrombolytic era. J. Nucl. Cardiol. *1*:198, 1994.
167. Dakik, H. A., Kimball, K. T., Koutelou, M., et al.: Prognostic value of exercise thallium-201 tomography after myocardial infarction in the thrombolytic era. Circulation *88*(Abs.):487, 1993.
168. Weiner, D. A., Ryan, T. J., McCabe, C. H., et al.: Correlations among history of angina, ST-segment response and prevalence of coronary artery disease in the coronary artery surgery study (CASS). N. Engl. J. Med. *301*:230, 1979.
169. Desmarais, R. L., Kaul, S., Watson, D. D., et al.: Do false positive thallium-201 scans lead to unnecessary catheterization? Outcome of patients with perfusion defects on quantitative planar thallium-201 scintigraphy. J. Am. Coll. Cardiol. *21*:1058, 1993.
170. Kong, B. A., Shaw, L., Miller, D. D., et al.: Comparison of accuracy for detecting coronary artery disease and side-effect profile of dipyrida-

mole thallium-201 myocardial perfusion imaging in women versus men. Am. J. Cardiol. *70*:168, 1992.
171. Chae, S. C., Heo, J., Iskandrian, A. S., et al.: Identification of extensive coronary artery disease in women by exercise single-photon emission computed tomographic (SPECT) thallium imaging. J. Am. Coll. Cardiol. *21*:1305, 1993.
172. Shaw, L. J., Miller, D. D., Romeis, J. C., et al.: Gender differences in the noninvasive evaluation and management of patients with suspected coronary artery disease. Ann. Intern. Med. *120*:559, 1994.
173. Travin, M. I., Rama, P. R., Arthur, A. L., et al.: The relationship of gender to the use and prognostic value of stress technetium-99m sestamibi myocardial SPECT scintigraphy. J. Nucl. Med. *35*:60P, 1994.
174. Hendel, R. C., Chen, M. H., L'Italien, G. J., et al.: Sex differences in perioperative and long term cardiac event-free survival in vascular surgery patients. An analysis of clinical and scintrigraphic variables. Circulation *91*:1044, 1995.
175. Kaski, J. C., Rosano, G. M. C., Collins, P., et al.: Cardiac syndrome X: Clinical characteristics and left ventricular function. J. Am. Coll. Cardiol. *25*:807, 1995.
176. Wackers, F. J. Th.: Complete left bundle branch block: Is the diagnosis of myocardial infarction possible? Int. J. Cardiol. *2*:521, 1983.
177. McGowan, R. L., Welch, T. G., Zaret, B. L., et al.: Noninvasive myocardial imaging with potassium-43 and rubidium-81 in patients with left bundle branch block. Am. J. Cardiol. *38*:422, 1976.
178. DePuey, E. G., Guertler-Krawczynska, E., and Robbins, W. L.: Thallium-201 SPECT in coronary artery disease patients with left bundle branch block. J. Nucl. Med. *29*:1479, 1988.
179. Hirzel, H. O., Senn, M., Neusch, K., et al.: Thallium-201 scintigraphy in complete left bundle branch block. Am. J. Cardiol. *53*:764, 1984.
180. Shefcyk, D. I., Gingrich, S., Nino, A. F., et al.: Altered left ventricular depolarization sequences in left bundle branch block is not a cause for false-positive thallium-201. J. Am. Coll. Cardiol. *17*:II-78A, 1991.
181. Burns, R. J., Galligan, L., Wright, L. M., et al.: Improved specificity of myocardial thallium-201 single-photon emission computed tomography in patients with left bundle branch block by dipyridamole. Am. J. Cardiol. *68*:504, 1991.
182. Berger, H. J., Sands, M. J., Davies, R. A., et al.: Exercise left ventricular performance in patients with chest pain, ischemic-appearing exercise electrocardiograms, and angiographically normal coronary arteries. Ann. Intern. Med. *94*:186, 1981.
183. Berger, B. C., Abramowitz, R., Park, C. H., et al.: Abnormal thallium-201 scans in patients with chest pain and angiographically normal coronary arteries. Am. J. Cardiol. *52*:365, 1983.
184. Legrand, V., Hodgson, J. M., Bates, E. R., et al.: Abnormal coronary flow reserve and abnormal radionuclide exercise test results in patients with normal coronary angiograms. J. Am. Coll. Cardiol. *6*:1245, 1985.
185. Cannon, R. O., Bonow, R. O., Bacharach, S. L., et al.: Left ventricular dysfunction in patients with angina pectoris, normal epicardial coronary arteries, and abnormal vasodilator reserve. Circulation *71*:218, 1985.
185a. Zeiher, A. M., Krause, T., Schächinger, V., et al.: Impaired endothelium-dependent vasodilation of coronary resistance vessels is associated with exercise-induced myocardial ischemia. Circulation *91*:2345, 1995.
186. Boucher, C. A., Brewster, D. C., Darling, R. C., et al.: Determination of cardiac risk by dipyridamole-thallium imaging before peripheral vascular surgery. N. Engl. J. Med. *312*:389, 1985.
187. Eagle, K. A., Singer, D. E., Brewster, D. C., et al.: Dipyridamole thallium scanning in patients undergoing vascular surgery. Optimizing preoperative evaluation of cardiac risk. JAMA *257*:2185, 1987.
188. Lane, S. E., Lewis, S. M., Pippin, J. J., et al.: Predictive value of quantitative dipyridamole thallium scintigraphy and assessing cardiovascular risk after vascular surgery in diabetes mellitus. Am. J. Cardiol. *64*:1275, 1989.
189. Lette, J., Waters, D., Bernier, H., et al.: Preoperative and long term risk cardiac assessment. Predictive value of 23 clinical descriptors, 7 multivariates scoring systems and quantitative dipyridamole imaging in 360 patients. Ann. Surg. *216*:192, 1992.
190. Levinson, J. R., Boucher, C. A., Coley, C. M., et al.: Usefulness of semiquantitative analysis of dipyridamole thallium-201 redistribution from proving risk stratification before vascular surgery. Am. J. Cardiol. *66*:406, 1990.
191. Fleisher, L. A., Rosenbaum, S. H., Nelson, A. H., et al.: Preoperative dipyridamole thallium imaging and ambulatory electrocardiographic monitoring as a predictor of perioperative cardiac events and long term outcome. Anesthesiology *83*:906, 1995.
192. Mangano, D. T., London, M. J., Tubau, J. F., et al.: Dipyridamole thallium-201 scintigraphy as a preoperative screening test. A re-examination of its predictive potential. Circulation *84*:493, 1991.
193. Baron, J. F., Mundler, O., Bertran, D., et al.: Dipyridamole thallium scintigraphy and gated radionuclide angiography to assess cardiac risk before abdominal aortic surgery. N. Engl. J. Med. *330*:663, 1994.
194. Manyari, D. E., Knudson, M., Kloiber, R., et al.: Sequential thallium-201 myocardial perfusion studies after successful percutaneous transluminal coronary artery angioplasty: Delayed resolution of exercise-induced scintigraphic abnormalities. Circulation *77*:86, 1988.
195. Hecht, H. S., Shaw, R. E., Bruce, T. R., et al.: Usefulness of tomographic thallium-201 imaging for detection of restenosis after percutaneous transluminal coronary angioplasty. Am. J. Cardiol. *66*:1314, 1990.
196. Jain, A., Mahmarian, J. J., Borges-Neto, S., et al.: Clinical significance of perfusion defects by thallium-201 single photon emission tomography following oral dipyridamole early after coronary angioplasty. J. Am. Coll. Cardiol. *11*:970, 1988.
197. Miller, D. D., Liu, P., Strauss, H. W., et al.: Prognostic value of computer-quantitated exercise thallium imaging early after percutaneous transluminal coronary angioplasty. J. Am. Coll. Cardiol. *10*:275, 1987.
198. Miller, D. D., and Verani, M. S.: Current status of myocardial perfusion imaging after percutaneous transluminal coronary angioplasty. J. Am. Coll. Cardiol. *24*:260, 1994.
199. Dilsizian, V., Rocco, T. P., Freedman, N. M. T., et al.: Enhanced detection of ischemic but viable myocardium by the reinjection of thallium after stress-redistribution imaging. N. Engl. J. Med. *323*:141, 1990.
200. Rocco, T. P., Dilsizian, V., McKusick, K. A., et al.: Comparison of thallium redistribution with rest "reinjection" imaging for the detection of viable myocardium. Am. J. Cardiol. *66*:158, 1990.
201. Kayden, D. S., Zaret, B. L., Wackers, F. J. Th., et al.: 24 hour planar thallium-201 delayed imaging: Is reinjection necessary? Circulation *80*(Abs.):376, 1989.
202. Tillisch, J., Brunken, R., Marshall, R., et al.: Reversibility of cardiac wall-motion abnormalities predicted by positron tomography. N. Engl. J. Med. *314*:884, 1986.
203. Favaro, L., Masini, F., Serra, W., et al.: Thallium-201 for detection of viable myocardium: Comparison of different reinjection protocols. J. Nucl. Cardiol. *1*:515, 1994.
204. Bonow, R. O., Dilsizian, V., Cuocolo, A., et al.: Identification of viable myocardium in patients with chronic coronary artery disease and left ventricular dysfunction and PET imaging with ^{18}F-fluorodeoxyglucose. Circulation *83*:26, 1991.
205. Zimmerman, R., Mall, G., Rauch, B., et al.: Residual ^{201}Tl activity in irreversible defects as a marker of myocardial viability. Clinicopathological study. Circulation *91*:1016, 1995.
206. Ragosta, M., Beller, G. A., Watson, D. D., et al.: Quantitative planar rest-redistribution ^{201}Tl imaging in detection of myocardial viability and prediction of improvement in left ventricular function after coronary bypass surgery in patients with severely depressed left ventricular function. Circulation *87*:1630, 1993.
207. Piwnica-Worms, D., Chiu, M. L., and Kronauge, J. F.: Divergent kinetics of ^{201}Tl and ^{99m}Tc-sestamibi in cultured chick ventricular myocytes during ATP depletion. Circulation *85*:1531, 1992.
208. Weinstein, H., King, M. A., Reinhardt, C. P., et al.: A method of simultaneous dual-radionuclide cardiac imaging with technetium-99m and thallium-201. I: Analysis of interradionuclide crossover and validation in phantoms. J. Nucl. Cardiol. *1*:39, 1994.
209. Cuocolo, A., Pace, L., Ricciardell, B., et al.: Identification of viable myocardium in patients with chronic coronary artery disease: Comparison of thallium 201 scintigraphy with reinjection and technetium-99m-methoxyisobutyl isonitrile. J. Nucl. Med. *33*:505, 1992.
210. Maurea, S., Cuocolo, A., Pace, L., et al.: Left ventricular dysfunction in coronary artery disease: Comparison between rest-redistribution thallium-201 and resting technetium 99m methoxyisobutyl isonitrile cardiac imaging. J. Nucl. Cardiol. *1*:165, 1994.
211. Marzullo, P., Sambuceti, G., and Parodi, O.: The role of sestamibi scintigraphy in the radioisotopic assessment of myocardial viability. J. Nucl. Med. *33*:1925, 1992.
212. Udelson, J. E., Coleman, P. S., Metherall, J., et al.: Predicting recovery of severe regional ventricular dysfunction: Comparison of resting scintigraphy with ^{201}Tl and ^{99m}Tc-sestamibi. Circulation *89*:2552, 1994.
213. Dilsizian, V., Arrighi, J. A., Diodati, J. G., et al.: Myocardial viability in patients with chronic coronary artery disease. Comparison of ^{99m}Tc-sestamibi with thallium reinjection and [^{18F}]Fluorodeoxyglucose. Circulation *89*:578, 1994.
214. Galli, M., Marcassa, C., Imparato, A., et al.: Effects of nitroglycerin by technetium-99m sestamibi tomoscintigraphy of resting regional myocardial hypoperfusion in stable patients with healed myocardial infarction. Am. J. Cardiol. *74*:843, 1994.
215. Bisi, G., Sciagra, R., Santoro, G. M., et al.: Rest technetium-99m sestamibi tomography in combination with short-term administration of nitrates: Feasibility and reliability for prediction of postrevascularization outcome of asynergic territories. J. Am. Coll. Cardiol. *24*:1282, 1994.
216. Udelson, J. E.: Can technetium-99m-labeled sestamibi track myocardial viability? J. Nucl. Cardiol. *1*:571, 1994.
217. Diamond, G. A., and Forrester, J. S.: Analysis of probability as an aid in the clinical diagnosis of coronary artery disease. N. Engl. J. Med. *300*:1350, 1979.
218. Epstein, S. E.: Implications of probability analysis on the strategy used for noninvasive detection of coronary artery disease. Role of single or combined use of exercise electrocardiographic testing, radionuclide cineangiography and myocardial perfusion imaging. Am. J. Cardiol. *46*:491, 1980.
219. Hamilton, G. W., Trobaugh, G. B., Ritchie, J. C., et al.: Myocardial imaging with ^{201}Thallium: An analysis of clinical usefulness based on Bayes' theorem. Semin. Nucl. Med. *8*:358, 1978.
220. Arain, S. A., Mattera, J. A., Sinusas, A. J., et al.: Is myocardial perfusion imaging necessary in patients with normal baseline ECG referred for stress testing? J. Nucl. Med. *36*(Abs.):110P, 1995.
221. Christian, T. F., Miller, T. D., Bailey, K. R., et al.: Exercise tomographic thallium-201 imaging in patients with severe coronary artery disease and normal electrocardiograms. Ann. Intern. Med. *121*:825, 1994.
222. Nallamothu, N., Ghods, M., Heo, J., et al.: Comparison of thallium-201 single photon emission computed tomography and electrocardiographic

response during exercise in patients with normal rest electrocardiographic results. J. Am. Coll. Cardiol. *25*:830, 1995.

INFARCT IMAGING

223. Rude, R. E., Parkey, R. W., Bonte, F. J., et al.: Clinical implications of the technetium-99 stannous pyrophosphate myocardial scintigraphic "doughnut" pattern in patients with acute myocardial infarcts. Circulation *59*:721, 1979.
224. Schofer, J., Spielmann, R. P., Bromel, T., et al.: Thallium-201/technetium-99m pyrophosphate overlap in patients with acute myocardial infarction after thrombolysis: Prediction of depressed wall motion despite thallium uptake. Am. Heart J. *112*:291, 1986.
225. Gertz, M. A., Brown, M. L., Hauser, M. F., et al.: Utility of technetium-99m pyrophosphate bone scanning in cardiac amyloidosis. Arch. Intern. Med. *147*:1039, 1987.
226. Davies, A. D., Thakur, M. L., Berger, H. J., et al.: Imaging the inflammatory response to acute myocardial infarction in man using Indium-111 labeled autologous leukocytes. Circulation *63*:826, 1981.
227. Narula, J., Torchilin, V. P., Petrov, A. N., et al.: In vivo targeting of acute myocardial infarction with negative-charge, polymer-modified antimyosin antibody: Use of different cross-linkers. J. Nucl. Cardiol. *2*:26, 1995.
228. Johnson, L. L., Seldin, D. W., Becker, L. C., et al.: Antimyosin imaging in acute transmural myocardial infarctions: Results of a multicenter clinical trial. J. Am. Coll. Cardiol. *13*:27, 1989.
229. Carrio, I., Bernia, L., Ballester, M., et al.: Indium-111 antimyosin scintigraphy to assess myocardial damage in patients with suspected myocarditis and cardiac rejection. J. Nucl. Med. *29*:1900, 1988.
230. Dec, G. W., Palacios, I., Yasuda, T., et al.: Antimyosin antibody cardiac imaging: Its role in the diagnosis of myocarditis. J. Am. Coll. Cardiol. *16*:97, 1990.
231. Lahiri, A., Jain, D.: New radionuclide imaging in cardiovascular disease. Curr. Opin. Cardiol. *2*:1070, 1987.

ASSESSMENT OF CARDIAC PERFORMANCE

232. Zaret, B. L., Strauss, H. W., Hurley, P. J., et al.: A noninvasive scintiphotographic method for detecting regional ventricular dysfunction in man. N. Engl. J. Med. *284*:1165, 1971.
233. Strauss, H. W., Zaret, B. L., Hurley, P. J., et al.: A scintiphotographic method for measuring left ventricular ejection fraction in man without cardiac catheterization. Am. J. Cardiol. *28*:575, 1971.
234. Berger, H. J., and Zaret, B. L.: Radionuclide assessment of cardiovascular performance. *In* Freeman, L. M. (ed.): Freeman and Johnson's Clinical Radionuclide Imaging. 3rd ed. New York, Grune and Stratton, 1984, p. 364.
235. Zaret, B. L., and Berger, H. J.: Nuclear cardiology. *In* Hurst, J. W. (ed.): The Heart, Arteries and Veins. 7th ed. New York, McGraw-Hill Book Co., 1990, p. 1899.
236. Kimchi, A., Rozanski, A., Fletcher, C., et al.: Reversal of rest myocardial asynergy during exercise: A radionuclide scintigraphic study. J. Am. Coll. Cardiol. *6*:1004, 1985.
237. Rozanski, A., Bairey, C. N., Krantz, D. S., et al.: Mental stress and the induction of silent myocardial ischemia in patients with coronary artery disease. N. Engl. J. Med. *318*:1005, 1988.
238. Links, J. M., Becker, L. C., Shindledecker, J. G., et al.: Measurement of absolute left ventricular volume from gated blood pool studies. Circulation *65*:82, 1982.
239. Massardo, T., Gal, R. A., Grenier, R. P., et al.: Left ventricular volume calculation using a count-based ratio method applied to multigated radionuclide angiography. J. Nucl. Med. *31*:450, 1990.
240. Gerson, M. C.: Radionuclide ventriculography: Left ventricular volumes and pressure-volume relations. *In* Gerson M. C. (ed.): Cardiac Nuclear Medicine. New York, McGraw-Hill Book Co., 1991, p. 81.
241. Marmor, A., Jain, D., Cohen, L. S., et al.: Left ventricular peak power during exercise: A noninvasive approach for assessment of contractile reserve. J. Nucl. Med. *34*:1877, 1993.
242. Marmor, A., Jain, D., and Zaret, B. L.: Beyond ejection fraction. J. Nucl. Med. *1*:477, 1994.
243. Zaret, B. L., Wackers, F. J., Terrin, M., et al.: Assessment of global and regional left ventricular performance at rest and during exercise after thrombolytic therapy for acute myocardial infarction: Results of the Thrombolysis in Myocardial Infarction (TIMI II) study. Am. J. Cardiol. *69*:1, 1992.
244. Starling, M. R., Walsh, R. Z., Lasher, J. C., et al.: Quantification of left ventricular regional dyssynergy by radionuclide angiography. J. Nucl. Med. *28*:1725, 1987.
245. Botvinick, E. H., Dae, M. W., O'Connell, J. W., et al.: First harmonic Fourier (phase) analysis of blood pool scintigrams for the evaluation of cardiac contraction and conduction. *In* Gerson, M. D. (ed.): Cardiac Nuclear Medicine. New York, McGraw-Hill Book Co., 1991, p. 81.
246. Robinson, V. J. B., Smiseth, O. A., Scott-Douglas, N. W., et al.: Assessment of splanchnic vascular capacity and capacitance using quantitative equilibrium blood pool scintigraphy. J. Nucl. Med. *31*:154, 1990.
247. Flamm, S. D., Taki, J., Moore, R., et al.: Redistribution of regional and organ blood volume and effect on cardiac function in relation to upright exercise intensity in healthy human subjects. Circulation *81*:1550, 1990.
248. Zaret, B. L., and Jain, D.: Continuous monitoring left ventricular function with miniaturized nonimaging detectors. *In* Zaret, B. L., and Beller, G. A. (eds.): Nuclear Cardiology: State-of-the-Art and Future Directions. St. Louis, C. V. Mosby Co., 1993, p. 136.
249. Soufer, R., Wohlgelernter, D., Vita, N. A., et al.: Intact systolic left ventricular function in clinical congestive heart failure. Am. J. Cardiol. *55*:1032, 1985.
250. Breisblatt, W. M., Vita, N. A., Armuchastegui, M., et al.: Usefulness of serial radionuclide monitoring during graded nitroglycerin infusion for unstable angina pectoris for determining left ventricular function and individualized therapeutic dose. Am. J. Cardiol. *61*:685, 1988.
251. Broadhurst, P., Cashman, P., Crawley, J., et al.: Clinical validation of a miniature nuclear probe system for continuous on-line monitoring of cardiac function and ST-segment. J. Nucl. Med. *32*:37, 1991.
252. Tamaki, N., Yasuda, T., Moore, R., et al.: Continuous monitoring of left ventricular function by an ambulatory radionuclide detector in patients with coronary artery disease. J. Am. Coll. Cardiol. *12*:669, 1988.
253. Kayden, D. S., Wackers, F. J., and Zaret, B. L.: Silent left ventricular dysfunction during routine activity after thrombolytic therapy for acute myocardial infarction. J. Am. Coll. Cardiol. *15*:1500, 1990.
254. Zaret, B. L., and Kayden, D. S.: Ambulatory monitoring of left ventricular function: A new modality for assessing silent myocardial ischemia. *In* Kellerman, J. J., and Braunwald, E. (eds.): Silent Myocardial Ischemia: A Critical Appraisal. Basel, Karger, 1990, p. 105.
255. Berg, M. M., Jain, D., Soufer, R., et al.: Role of behavioral and psychological factors in mental stress induced silent left ventricular dysfunction in coronary artery disease. J. Am. Coll. Cardiol. *22*:440, 1993.
256. Corbett, J. R.: Tomographic radionuclide ventriculography: Opportunity ignored? J. Nucl. Cardiol. *1*:567, 1994.
257. Lu, P., Liu, X, Shi, R., et al.: Comparison of tomographic and planar radionuclide ventriculography in the assessment of regional left ventricular function in patients with left ventricular aneurysm before and after surgery. J. Nucl. Cardiol. *1*:537, 1994.

FIRST-PASS RADIONUCLIDE ANGIOCARDIOGRAPHY

258. Blumgart, H. L., and Weiss, S.: Studies on the velocity of blood flow. VII. The pulmonary circulation time in normal resting individuals. J. Clin. Invest. *4*:399, 1927.
259. Van Dyke, D. C., Anger, H. O., Sullivan, R. W., et al.: Cardiac evaluation for radioisotope dynamics. J. Nucl. Med. *13*:585, 1972.
260. Zaret, B. L., and Wackers, F. J.: Measurement of right ventricular function. *In* Gerson, M. C. (ed.): Cardiac Nuclear Medicine. New York, McGraw-Hill Book Co., 1991, p. 183.
261. Gelfand, M. J., and Hannon, D. W.: Pediatric Nuclear Cardiology. *In* Gerson, M. C. (ed.): Cardiac Nuclear Medicine. New York, McGraw-Hill Book Co., 1991, p. 551.
262. Bonow, R. O., Bacharach, S. L., Green, M. V., et al.: Impaired left ventricular diastolic filling in patients with coronary artery disease: Assessment with radionuclide angiography. Circulation *64*:315, 1981.
263. Bashore, T. M., Leithe, M. E., and Shaffer, P.: Diastolic function. *In* Gerson, M. C. (ed.): Cardiac Nuclear Medicine. New York, McGraw-Hill Book Co., 1991, p. 195.
264. Fouad, F. M., Slominski, J. M., and Tarazi, R. C.: Left ventricular diastolic function in hypertension: Relation to left ventricular mass and function. J. Am. Coll. Cardiol. *3*:1500, 1984.
265. Cohn, J. N., Johnson, G., and the Veterans Administration Cooperative Study Group: Heart failure with normal ejection fraction. Circulation *82*(Suppl. III):4A, 1990.
266. Setaro, J., Soufer, R., Remetz, M. S., et al.: Long term outcome in patients with congestive heart failure and intact systolic left ventricular performance. Am. J. Cardiol. *69*:1212, 1992.
267. Setaro, J. F., Zaret, B. L., Schulman, D. S., et al.: Usefulness of verapamil for congestive heart failure, abnormal diastolic filling and normal left ventricular systolic performance. Am. J. Cardiol. *66*:981, 1990.
268. Iskandrian, A. S., and Hakki, A.: Age-related changes in left ventricular diastolic performance. Am. Heart J. *112*:75, 1986.

CLINICAL APPLICATIONS OF CARDIAC PERFORMANCE STUDIES

269. Kazmers, A., Cerqueira, M. D., and Zierler, R. E.: The role of preoperative radionuclide ejection fraction in direct abdominal aortic aneurysm repair. J. Vasc. Surg. *8*:128, 1988.
270. The Multicenter Postinfarction Research Group: Risk stratification and survival after myocardial infarction. N. Engl. J. Med. *309*:331, 1983.
270a. Zaret, B. L., Wackers, F. J., Terrin, M. L., et al.: Value of radionuclide rest and exercise left ventricular ejection fraction to assess survival of patients following thrombolytic therapy for acute myocardial infarction: Results of the Thrombolysis in Myocardial Infarction (TIMI) Phase II study. J. Am. Coll. Cardiol. *26*:73, 1995.
271. Abraham, R. D., Harris, P. G., Rubin, G. S., et al.: Usefulness of ejection fraction response to exercise one month after acute myocardial infarction in predicting coronary anatomy and prognosis. Am. J. Cardiol. *60*:225, 1987.
272. Ahnve, S., Gilpin, E., Henning, H., et al.: Limitations and advantages of the ejection fraction for defining high risk after acute myocardial infarction. Am. J. Cardiol. *58*:872, 1986.
273. Kuchard, L., Frund, J., Yates, M., et al.: Enhanced prediction of major cardiac events after myocardial infarction using exercise radionuclide ventriculography. Aust. N.Z. J. Med. *17*:228, 1987.
274. Mazzotta, G., Camerini, A., Scopinaro, G., et al.: Predicting cardiac mortality after uncomplicated myocardial infarction by exercise radio-

nuclide ventriculography and exercise-induced ST-segment elevation. Eur. Heart J. *13*:330, 1992.
275. CASS Principal Investigators: Coronary artery surgery study (CASS): A randomized trial of coronary bypass surgery. Survival data. Circulation *68*:939, 1983.
276. Ritchie, J. L., Hallstrom, A. P., Troubaugh, C. B., et al.: Out-of-hospital sudden coronary death: Rest and exercise left ventricular function in survivors. Am. J. Cardiol. *55*:645, 1985.
277. Meizlish, J., Berger, H. J., Plankey, R. T., et al.: Functional left ventricular aneurysm formation following acute anterior transmural myocardial infarction: Incidence, natural history and prognostic implications. N. Engl. J. Med. *311*:101, 1984.
278. Bonow, R. O., Kent, K. M., Rosing, D. R., et al.: Exercise-induced ischemia in mildly symptomatic patients with coronary artery disease and preserved left ventricular function: Identification of subgroups at risk of death during medical therapy. N. Engl. J. Med. *311*:1339, 1984.
279. Lee, K. L., Pryor, D. B., Pieper, K. S., et al.: Prognostic value of radionuclide angiography in medically treated patients with coronary artery disease: A comparison with clinical and catheterization variables. Circulation *82*:1705, 1990.
280. Mazzotta, G., Pace, L., and Bonow, R. O.: Risk stratification of patients with coronary artery disease and left ventricular dysfunction by exercise radionuclide angiography and exercise electrocardiography. J. Nucl. Cardiol. *1*:529, 1994.
281. Lim, R., Dyke, L., and Dymond, D. S.: Objective assessment of "cardioprotective" efficacy as a prognostic guide in the management of mildly symptomatic revascularisible coronary artery disease. J. Am. Coll. Cardiol. 1995 *(in press)*.
282. Schlant, R. C.: The prognosis of individuals with silent myocardial ischemia. *In* Kellerman, N. J. J., and Braunwald, E. (eds.): Silent Myocardial Ischemia: A Critical Appraisal. Vol. 37. Basel, Karger, 1990, p. 187.
283. Breitenbucher, A., Pfisterer, M., Hoffman, A., et al.: Long-term follow-up of patients with silent ischemia during exercise radionuclide angiography. J. Am. Coll. Cardiol. *15*:999, 1990.
284. Kayden, D. S., Remetz, M. S., Cabin, H. S., et al.: Validation of continuous radionuclide left ventricular function monitoring in detecting myocardial ischemia during balloon angioplasty of the left anterior descending artery. Am. J. Cardiol. *67*:1339, 1991.
285. Jain, D., Burg, M., Soufer, R., et al.: Prognostic implications of mental stress induced silent left ventricular dysfunction of patients with stable angina pectoris. Am. J. Cardiol. *76*:31, 1995.
286. Alexander, J., Dainiak, N., Berger, H. J., et al.: Serial assessment of doxorubicin cardiotoxicity with quantitative radionuclide angiocardiography. N. Engl. J. Med. *300*:278, 1979.
287. Schwartz, R. G., McKenzie, W. B., Alexander, J., et al.: Congestive heart failure and left ventricular dysfunction complicating doxorubicin therapy: Seven-year-experience using serial radionuclide angiocardiography. Am. J. Med. *82*:1109, 1987.
288. Schwartz, R. G., and Zaret, B. L.: The diagnosis and treatment of drug-induced myocardial disease. *In:* Muggia, F. M., Green, M. D., and Speyer, J. L. (eds.): Cancer Treatment and the Heart. Baltimore, John Hopkins University Press, 1992, p. 173.
289. Borer, J. S., Bacharach, S. L., Green, M. V., et al.: Exercise-induced left ventricular dysfunction in symptomatic and asymptomatic patients with aortic regurgitation: Assessment by radionuclide cineangiography. Am. J. Cardiol. *42*:351, 1978.
290. Schulman, D. S., Biondi, J. W., Matthay, R. A., et al.: Differing responses in ventricular filling, loading, and volumes during positive and expiratory pressure in man. Am. J. Cardiol. *64*:772, 1989.
291. Schulman, D. S., Biondi, J. W., Zohgbi, S., et al.: Coronary flow limits right ventricular performance during positive and exploratory pressure. Am. Rev. Respir. Dis. *141*:1531, 1990.

OTHER SPECIAL IMAGING STUDIES

292. Tamaki, N., Fujibayas, H. I. Y., Magata, Y., et al.: Radionuclide assessment of myocardial fatty acid metabolism by PET and SPECT. J. Nucl. Cardiol. *2*:256, 1995.
293. Iskandrian, A. S., Powers, J., Cave, E. V., et al.: Assessment of myocardial viability by dynamic tomographic I-123 iodophenyl pentadecanoic acid imaging: Comparison to rest-redistribution thallium-201 imaging. J. Nucl. Cardiol. *2*:101, 1995.
294. Nishimura, T., Uehara, T., Shimonagata, T., et al.: Clinical results with beta-methyl iodolphenylpentadecanoic acid single photon emission computer tomography in cardiac disease. J. Nucl. Cardiol. *1*:S65, 1994.
295. Dae, M. W., O'Connell, J. W., and Botvinick, E. H.: Scintigraphic assessment of regional cardiac adrenergic innervation. Circulation *79*:634, 1989.
296. Merlet, P. T., Valette, H., DuBois-Rande, J. L., et al.: Iodine 123-labeled metaiodobenzylguanidine imaging in heart disease. J. Nucl. Cardiol. *1*:S79, 1994.
297. Schofer, J., Spielmann, R., Schubert, A., et al.: Iodine-123 metaiodobenzylguanidine scintigraphy: A non-invasive method to demonstrate myocardial adrenergic system disintegrity in patients with idiopathic dilated cardiomyopathy. J. Am. Coll. Cardiol. *12*:1252, 1988.
298. Merlet, P., Vailette, H., DuBois-Rande, J. L., et al.: Prognostic value of cardiac MIBG imaging in patients with congestive heart failure. J. Nucl. Med. *33*:471, 1992.

HYPOXIA IMAGING

299. Chapman, J. D.: Hypoxic sensitizers: Implications for radiation therapy. N. Engl. J. Med. *301*:1429, 1979.
300. Frank, A. J., Chapman, J. D., and Doch, C. J.: Binding of misonidazole to EMT6 and V79 spheroids. Int. J. Radiat. Oncol. Biol. Phys. *8*:737, 1982.
301. Miller, G. G., Ngan-Lee, J., and Chapman, J. D.: Intracellular localization of radioactivity labeled misonidazole in EMT-6 tumor cells in vitro. Int. J. Radiat. Oncol. Biol. Phys. *8*:741, 1982.
302. Martin, G. V., Caldwell, J. H., Graham, M. M., et al.: Noninvasive detection of hypoxic myocardium using fluorine-18-fluoromisonidazole and positron emission tomography. J. Nucl. Med. *33*:2202, 1992.
303. Shelton, M. E., Dence, C. S., Hwang, D. R., et al.: In vivo delineation of myocardial hypoxia during coronary occlusion using fluorin-18-fluoromisonidazole and positron emission tomography: A potential approach for identification of jeopardized myocardium. J. Am. Coll. Cardiol. *16*:477, 1990.
304. Shelton, M. E., Dence, C. S., Hwang, D. R., et al.: Myocardial kinetics of fluorine-18 misonidazole: A marker for hypoxic myocardium. J. Nucl. Med. *30*:351, 1989.
305. Martin, G. V., Cerqueira, M. D., Caldwell, J. H., et al.: Fluoromisonidazole a metabolic marker for myocyte hypoxia. Circ. Res. *67*:240, 1990.
306. Martin, G. V., Caldwell, J. H., Rasey, J. S., et al.: Enhanced binding of the hypoxic cell marker [^{3}H]Fluoromisonidazole in ischemic myocardium. J. Nucl. Med. *30*:194, 1989.
307. Rumsey, W. L., Patel, B., Kuczynski, B., et al.: Planar and SPECT imaging of ischemic canine myocardium using a novel ^{99m}Tc-nitroimidazole. J. Nucl. Med. *34*(Abs.):(5):15P, 1993.
308. Shi, W., Dione, D. P., Singer, M. J., et al.: Technetium-99m nitroimidazole: A positive imaging agent for the detection of myocardial ischemia. Circulation *88*(Abs.)(4):1, 1993.
309. Rumsey, W. L., Cyr, J. E., Raju, N., et al.: A novel [99m]technetium-labeled nitroheterocycle capable of identification of hypoxia in heart. Biochem. Biophys. Res. Comm. *193*:1239, 1993.
310. Ng, C. K., Sinusas, A. J., Zaret, B. L., et al.: Kinetic analysis of technetium-99m labeled nitroimidazole (BMS-181321) as a tracer of myocardial hypoxia. Circulation *92*:1261, 1995.

POSITRON EMISSION TOMOGRAPHY

311. Schelbert, H., Bonow, R. O., Geltman, E., et al.: Position statement: Clinical use of cardiac positron emission tomography. Position paper of the Cardiovascular Council of the Society of Nuclear Medicine. J. Nucl. Med. *34*:1385, 1993.
312. ACC/AHA Task Force Report: Guidelines for clinical use of cardiac radionuclide imaging. Report of the ACC/AHA task force on assessment of diagnostic and therapeutic procedures (committee on radionuclide imaging), developed in collaboration with the American Society of Nuclear Cardiology. J. Am. Coll. Cardiol. *25*:521, 1995.
313. Bonow, R. O., Berman, D. S., Gibbons, R. J., et al.: Cardiac positron emission tomography. A report for health professionals from the committee on advanced cardiac imaging and technology of the Council on Clinical Cardiology, American Heart Association. Circulation *84*:447, 1991.
314. Maddahi, J., Schelbert, H., Brunken, R., et al.: Role of thallium-201 and PET imaging in evaluation of myocardial viability and management of patients with coronary artery disease and left ventricular dysfunction. J. Nucl. Med. *35*:707, 1994.
315. Mody, F. V., Brunken, R. C., Stevenson, L. W., et al.: Differentiating cardiomyopathy of coronary artery disease from nonischemic dilated cardiomyopathy utilizing positron emission tomography. J. Am. Coll. Cardiol. *17*:373, 1991.
316. vom Dahl, J., Altehoefer, C., Biedermann, M., et al.: Technetium-99m methoxy-isobutyl-isonitrile as a tracer of myocardial viability? A quantitative comparison with F-18 FDG in 100 patients with coronary artery disease. J. Am. Coll. Cardiol. *21*(Suppl A):283A, 1993.
317. Altehoefer, C., Hans-Jurgen, K., Dorr, R., et al.: Fluorine-18 deoxyglucose PET for assessment of viable myocardium in perfusion defects in Tc-99m MIBI SPECT: A comparative study in patients with coronary artery disease. Eur. J. Nucl. Med. *19*:334, 1992.
318. Soufer, R., Dey, H. M., Ng, C. K., et al.: Comparison of sestamibi single photon emission computed tomography to positron emission tomography for estimating left ventricular myocardial viability. Am. J. Cardiol. *75*:1214, 1995.
319. Camici, P., Ferrannini, E., and Opie, L. H.: Myocardial metabolism in ischemic heart disease: Basic principles and application to imaging by positron emission tomography. Prog. Cardiovasc. Dis. *32*:217, 1989.
320. Bergmann, S. R.: Use and limitations of metabolic tracers labeled with positron-emitting radionuclides in the identification of viable myocardium. J. Nucl. Med. *35*(Suppl):15S, 1994.
321. Marshall, R. C., Tillisch, J. H., Phelps, M. E., et al.: Identification and differentiation of resting myocardial ischemia and infarction in man with positron computed tomography, ^{18}F-labeled fluorodeoxyglucose and N-13 ammonia. Circulation *67*:766, 1983.
322. Brunken, R., Tillisch, J., Schwaiger, M., et al.: Regional perfusion, glucose metabolism and wall motion in patients with chronic electrocardiographic Q wave infarctions: Evidence for persistence of viable tissue in some infarct regions by positron emission tomography. Circulation *73*:951, 1986.

323. Schelbert, H. R., and Buxton, D.: Insights into coronary artery disease gained from metabolic imaging. Circulation *78*:496, 1988.
324. Fudo, T., Kambara, H, Hashimoto, T., et al.: F-18 deoxyglucose and stress N-13 ammonia positron emission tomography in anterior wall healed myocardial infarction. Am. J. Cardiol. *61*:1191, 1988.
325. Tamaki, N., Yonekura, Y., Yamashita, K., et al.: Positron emission tomography using F-18 deoxyglucose in evaluation of coronary artery bypass grafting. Am. J. Cardiol. *64*:860, 1989.
326. Brunken, R. C., and Schelbert, H. R.: Positron emission tomography in clinical cardiology. Cardiol. Clin. *7*:607, 1989.
327. Marwick, T. H., Nemec, J. J., Lafont, A., et al.: Prediction by post exercise fluoro-18-deoxyglucose positron emission tomography of improvement in exercise capacity after revascularization. Am. J. Cardiol. *69*:854, 1992.
328. Marwick, T. H., MacIntyre, W. J., Lafont, A., et al.: Metabolic responses of hibernating and infarcted myocardium to revascularization: A follow-up study of regional perfusion, function, and metabolism. Circulation *85*:1347, 1992.
329. Burt, R. W., Perkins, O. W., Oppenheim, B. E., et al.: Direct comparison of fluorine-18-FDG SPECT, fluorine-18-FDG PET and rest thallium-201 SPECT for detection of myocardial viability. J. Nucl. Med. *36*:176, 1995.
330. Bax, J. J., Visser, F. C., van Lingen, A., et al.: Feasibility of assessing regional myocardial uptake of 18F-fluorodeoxyglucose using single photon emission computed tomography. Eur. Heart J. *14*:1675, 1993.
331. Eitzman, D., Al-Aouar, Z., Kanter, H. L., et al.: Clinical outcome of patients with advanced coronary artery disease after viability studies with positron emission tomography. J. Am. Coll. Cardiol. *20*:559, 1992.
332. DiCarli, M. F., Davidson, M., Little, R., et al.: Value of metabolic imaging with positron emission tomography for evaluating prognosis in patients with coronary artery disease and left ventricular dysfunction. Am. J. Cardiol. *73*:527, 1994.
333. Lee, K. S., Marwick, T. H., Cook, S. A., et al.: Prognosis of patients with left ventricular dysfunction, with and without viable myocardium after myocardial infarction: Relative efficacy of medical therapy and revascularization. Circulation *90*:2687, 1994.
334. Yoshida, K., and Gould, K. L.: Quantitative relation of myocardial infarct size and myocardial viability by positron emission tomography to left ventricular ejection fraction and 3-year mortality with and without revascularization. J. Am. Coll. Cardiol. *22*:984, 1993.
335. Tamaki, N., Kawamoto, M., Takahashi, N., et al.: Prognostic value of an increase in fluorine-18-deoxyglucose uptake in patients with myocardial infarction: Comparison with stress thallium imaging. J. Am. Coll. Cardiol. *22*:1621, 1993.
336. Brunken, R., Schwaiger, M., Grover-McKay, M., et al.: Positron emission tomography detects tissue metabolic activity in myocardial segments with persistent thallium perfusion defects. J. Am. Coll. Cardiol. *10*:557, 1987.
337. Brunken, R. C., Kottou, S., Nienabar, C. A., et al.: PET detection of viable tissue in myocardial segments with persistent defects at Tl-201 SPECT. Radiology *172*:65, 1989.
338. Tamaki, N., Yonekura, Y., Yamashita, K., et al.: Relation of left ventricular perfusion and wall motion with metabolic activity in persistent defects on thallium-201 tomography in healed myocardial infarction. Am. J. Cardiol. *62*:202, 1988.
339. Tamaki, N., Yonekura, Y., Yamashita, K., et al.: SPECT thallium-201 tomography and positron tomography using N-13 ammonia and F-18 fluorodeoxyglucose in coronary artery disease. Am. J. Cardiac Imag. *3*:3, 1989.
340. Tamaki, N., Ohtani, H., Yamashita, K., et al.: Metabolic activity in the areas of new fill-in after thallium-201 reinjection: Comparison with positron emission tomography using fluorine-18-deoxyglucose. J. Nucl. Med. *32*:673, 1991.
341. Altehoefer, C., vom Dahl, J., Biedermann, M., et al.: Significance of defect severity in technetium-99m-MIBI SPECT at rest to assess myocardial viability: Comparison with fluorine-18-FDG PET. J. Nucl. Med. *35*:569, 1994.
342. Sawada, S. G., Allman, K. C., Muzik, O., et al.: Positron emission tomography detects evidence of viability in rest technetium-99m sestamibi defects. J. Am. Coll. Cardiol. *23*:92, 1994.
343. Berry, J. J., Baker, J. A., Pieper, K. S., et al.: The effect of metabolic milieu on cardiac PET imaging using fluorine-18-deoxyglucose and nitrogen-13-ammonia in normal volunteers. J. Nucl. Med. *32*:1518, 1991.
344. Schwaiger, M., Schelbert, H. R., Ellison, D., et al.: Sustained regional abnormalities in cardiac metabolism after transient ischemia in the chronic dog model. J. Am. Coll. Cardiol. *6*:336, 1985.
345. Sobel, B. E., Geltman, E. M., Tiefenbrunn, A. J., et al.: Improvement of regional myocardial metabolism after coronary thrombolysis induced with tissue-type plasminogen activator or streptokinase. Circulation *69*:983, 1984.
346. Schwaiger, M., Schelbert, H. R., Keen, R., et al.: Retention and clearance of C-11 palmitic acid in ischemic and reperfused canine myocardium. J. Am. Coll. Cardiol. *6*:310, 1985.
347. Grover-McKay, M., Schelbert, H. R., Schwaiger, M., et al.: Identification of impaired metabolic reserve in patients with significant coronary artery stenosis by atrial pacing. Circulation *74*:281, 1986.
348. Rosamond, T. L., Abendschein, D. R., Sobel, B. E., et al.: Metabolic fate of radiolabeled palmitate in ischemic canine myocardium: Implications for positron emission tomography. J. Nucl. Med. *28*:1322, 1987.
349. Armbrecht, J. J., Buxton, D. B., Brunken, R. C., et al.: Regional myocardial oxygen consumption determined noninvasively in humans with [1-^{11}C] acetate and dynamic positron tomography. Circulation *80*:863, 1989.
350. Buxton, D. B., Nienaber, C. A., Luxen, A., et al.: Noninvasive quantitation of regional myocardial oxygen consumption in vivo with [1-11C]acetate and dynamic positron emission tomography. Circulation *79*:134, 1989.
351. Ng, C. K., Huang, S. C., Schelbert, H. R., et al.: Validation of a model for [1-^{11}C]acetate as a tracer of cardiac oxidative metabolism. Am. J. Physiol. *255*:H1304, 1994.
352. Gropler, R. J., Geltman, E. M., Sampathkumaran, K., et al.: Comparison of carbon-11-acetate with fluorine-18-fluorodeoxyglucose for delineating viable myocardium by positron emission tomography. J. Am. Coll. Cardiol. *22*:1587, 1993.
353. Vom Dahl, J., Herman, W. H., Hicks, R. J., et al.: Myocardial glucose uptake in patients with insulin-dependent diabetes mellitus assessed quantitatively by dynamic positron emission tomography. Circulation *88*:395, 1993.
354. Gould, L., Yoshida, K., Hess, M., et al.: Myocardial metabolism of fluorodeoxyglucose compared to cell membrane integrity for the potassium analogue rubidium-82 for assessing infarct size in man by PET. J. Nucl. Med. *32*:1, 1991.
355. Yamamoto, Y., deSilva, R., Rhodes, C., et al.: A new strategy for the assessment of viable myocardium and regional myocardial blood flow using ^{15}O-water and dynamic positron emission tomography. Circulation *86*:167, 1992.
356. DeSilva, R., Yamamoto, Y., Rhodes, C., et al.: Detection of hibernating myocardium using $H_2{}^{15}O$ and positron emission tomography (PET). Circulation *86*:1738, 1992.
357. Shah, A., Schelbert, H. R., Schwaiger, M., et al.: Measurement of regional myocardial blood flow with N-13 ammonia and positron emission tomography in intact dogs. J. Am. Coll. Cardiol. *5*:92, 1985.
358. Bergmann, S. R., Herrero, P., Markham, J., et al.: Noninvasive quantitation of myocardial blood flow in human subjects with oxygen-15-labeled water and positron emission tomography. J. Am. Coll. Cardiol. *14*:639, 1989.
359. Gould, K. L.: PET perfusion imaging and nuclear cardiology. J. Nucl. Med. *32*:579, 1991.
360. Goldstein, R. A., Mullani, N. A., Marani, S. K., et al.: Myocardial perfusion with rubidium-82. II. Effects and pharmacologic intervention. J. Nucl. Med. *24*:907, 1983.
361. Mullani, N. A., Goldstein, R. A., Gould, K. L., et al.: Myocardial perfusion with rubidium-82. I. Measurement of extraction fraction and flow with external detectors. J. Nucl. Med. *24*:898, 1983.
362. Shelton, M. E., Green, M. A., Mathias, C. J., et al.: Kinetics of copper-PTSM in isolated hearts: A novel tracer for measuring blood flow with positron emission tomography. J. Nucl. Med. *30*:1843, 1989.
363. Shelton, M. E., Green, M. A., Mathias, C. J., et al.: Assessment of regional myocardial and renal blood flow with copper-PTSM and positron emission tomography. Circulation *82*:990, 1990.
364. Goldstein, R. A.: Kinetics of rubidium-82 after coronary occlusion and reperfusion: Assessment of patency and viability in open-chested dogs. J. Clin. Invest. *75*:1131, 1985.
365. Goldstein, R. A.: Rubidium-82 kinetics after coronary occlusion: Temporal relation of net myocardial accumulation and viability in open-chested dogs. J. Nucl. Med. *27*:1456, 1986.
366. Bergmann, S. T., Hack, S., Tweson, T., et al.: Dependence of accumulation of $^{13}NH_3$ by myocardium on metabolic factors and its implications for the quantitative assessment of perfusion. Circulation *61*:34, 1980.
367. Bergmann, S. R., Fox, K. A. A., Rand, A. L., et al.: Quantification of regional myocardial blood flow in vivo with $H_2{}^{15}O$. Circulation *70*:724, 1984.
368. Uren, N. G., Melin, J. A., DeBruyne, B., et al.: Relation between myocardial blood flow and the severity of coronary artery stenosis. N. Engl. J. Med. *330*:1782, 1994.
369. Walsh, M. N., Geltman, E. M., Steele, R. L., et al.: Augmented myocardial perfusion reserve after coronary angioplasty quantified by positron emission tomography with $H_2{}^{15}O$. J. Am. Coll. Cardiol. *15*:119, 1990.
370. Soufer, R., and Zaret, B. L.: Positron emission tomography and the quantitative assessment of regional myocardial blood flow (editorial). J. Am. Coll. Cardiol. *15*:128, 1990.
371. Huang, S. C., Schwaiger, M., Carson, R. E., et al.: Quantitative measurement of myocardial blood flow with oxygen-15 water and positron computed tomography: An assessment of potential and problems. J. Nucl. Med. *26*:616, 1985.
372. Gould, K. L.: Percent coronary stenosis: Battered gold standard, pernicious relic or clinical practicality. J. Am. Coll. Cardiol. *11*:886, 1988.
373. Schelbert, H. R., Wisenberg, C., Phelps, M. E., et al.: Noninvasive assessment of coronary stenosis by myocardial imaging during pharmacologic coronary vasodilation. VI. Detection of coronary artery disease in human beings with intravenous N-13 ammonia and positron computed tomography. Am. J. Cardiol. *49*:1197, 1982.
374. Gould, K. L., Goldstein, R. A., Mullani, N. A., et al.: Noninvasive assessment of coronary stenosis by myocardial perfusion imaging during pharmacologic coronary vasodilation. VIII. Clinical feasibility of positron cardiac imaging without a cyclotron using generator-produced rubidium-82. J. Am. Coll. Cardiol. *7*:775, 1986.
375. Tamaki, N., Yonekura, Y., Senda, M., et al.: Value and limitation of stress thallium-201 single photon emission computed tomography:

Comparison with nitrogen-13 positron tomography. J. Nucl. Med. *29:*1181, 1988.
376. Demer, L. L., Gould, K. L., Goldstein, R. A., et al.: Assessment of coronary artery disease severity by positron emission tomography. Comparison with quantitative arteriography in 193 patients. Circulation *79:*825, 1989.
377. Gupta, N. C.: Adenosine in myocardial perfusion imaging using positron emission tomography. Am. Heart J. *122:*293, 1991.
378. Williams, B. R.: Positron emission tomography for the assessment of ischemia and myocardial viability. J. Myocard. Ischemia *2*(4):38, 1990.
379. Stewart, R.: Comparison of rubidium-82 positron emission tomography and thallium-201 SPECT imaging for detection of coronary artery disease. Am. J. Cardiol. *67:*1303, 1991.
380. Walsh, M. N., Bergmann, S. R., Steele, R. L., et al.: Delineation of impaired regional myocardial perfusion by positron emission tomography with $H_2{}^{15}O$. Circulation *78:*620, 1988.
381. Stewart, R., Kalus, M., Molina, E., et al.: Rubidium-82 PET versus thallium-201 SPECT for the diagnosis of regional coronary artery disease. Circulation *80:*209, 1989.
382. Yonekura, Y., Tamaki, N., Senda, M., et al.: Detection of coronary artery disease with N-13 ammonia and high-resolution positron emission computed tomography. Am. Heart J. *113:*645, 1987.
383. Yamashita, K., Tamaki, N., Yonekura, Y., et al.: Quantitative analysis of regional wall motion by gated myocardial positron emission tomography: Validation and comparison with left ventriculography. J. Nucl. Med. *30:*1775, 1989.
384. Sisson, J. C., and Wieland, D. M.: Radiolabeled meta-iodobenzylguanidine: Pharmacology and clinical studies. Am. J. Physiol. Imaging *1:*96, 1986.
385. Glowniak, J. V., Turner, F. E., Gray, L. L., et al.: Iodine-123-metaiodobenzylguanidine imaging of the heart in idiopathic congestive cardiomyopathy and cardiac transplants. J. Nucl. Med. *30:*1182, 1989.
386. Fagret, D., Wolf, J. E., Vanzetto, G., et al.: Myocardial uptake of metaiodobenzylguanidine in patients with left ventricular hypertrophy secondary to valvular aortic stenosis. J. Nucl. Med. *34:*57, 1993.
387. Dae, M. W., O'Connell, J. W., Botvinick, E. H., et al.: Scintigraphic assessment of regional cardiac innervation. Circulation *79:*634, 1989.
388. Goldstein, D. S., Chang, P. C., Eisenhofer, G., et al.: Positron emission tomographic imaging of cardiac sympathetic innervation and function. Circulation *81:*1606, 1990.
389. Schwaiger, M., Kalff, V., Rosenspire, K., et al.: Noninvasive evaluation of sympathetic nervous system in human heart by positron emission tomography. Circulation *82:*457, 1990.
390. Rosenspire, K. C., Gildersleeve, D. L., Massin, C. C., et al.: Metabolic fate of the heart agent [18F]6-Fluorometaraminol. Nucl. Med. Biol. *16:*735, 1989.
391. Valette, H., Deleuze, P., Syrota, A., et al.: Canine myocardial beta-adrenergic, muscarinic receptor densities after denervation: A PET study. J. Nucl. Med. *36:*140, 1995.
392. Berridge, M. S., Nelson, A. D., Zhen, L., et al.: Specific beta-adrenergic receptor binding of carazolol measured with PET. J. Nucl. Med. *35:*1665, 1994.
393. Droste, C., and Roskamm, H.: Pain perception and endogenous pain modulation in angina pectoris. Adv. Cardiol. *37:*142, 1990.
394. Marchant, B., Umachandran, V., Wilkinson, P., et al.: Reexamination of the role of endogenous opiates in silent myocardial ischemia. J. Am. Coll. Cardiol. *23:*645, 1994.
395. Johes, A. K. P., Luthra, S. K., Maziere, B., et al.: Regional cerebral opioid receptor studies with [^{11}C]diprenorphine in normal volunteers. J. Neurosci. Methods *23:*121, 1988.
396. Haskell, W. L., Alderman, E. L., Fair, J. M., et al.: Effects of intensive multiple risk factor reduction on coronary atherosclerosis and clinical cardiac events in men and women with coronary artery disease: The Standard Coronary Risk Intervention Project (SCRIP). Circulation *89:*975, 1994.
397. National Cholesterol Education Program: Second report of the expert panel on detection, evaluation and treatment of high blood cholesterol in adults (adult treatment panel II). Circulation *89:*1329, 1994.
398. Buchwald, H., Matts, J. P., Fitch, L. L., et al.: Changes in sequential coronary arteriograms and subsequent coronary events: Program on the Surgical Control of the Hyperlipidemias (POSCH) Group. JAMA *268:*1429, 1992.
399. Superko, H. R., and Drauss, R. M.: Coronary artery disease regression: Convincing evidence for the benefit of aggressive lipoprotein management. Circulation *90:*1056, 1994.
400. Gould, K. L., Martucci, J. P., Goldberg, D. I., et al.: Short-term cholesterol lowering decreases size and severity of perfusion abnormalities by positron emission tomography after dipyridamole in patients with coronary artery disease: A potential noninvasive marker of healing coronary endothelium. Circulation *89:*1530, 1994.
401. Harrison, D. G., Armstrong, M. L., Frieman, P. C., et al.: Restoration of endothelium-dependent relaxation by dietary treatment of atherosclerosis. J. Clin. Invest. *80:*1801, 1987.
402. Schelbert, H. R., and Maddahi, J.: Clinical cardiac PET: Quo vadis? J. Nucl. Cardiol. *1:*576, 1994.
403. Patterson, R. E., Eisner, R. L., and Horowitz, S. F.: Comparison of cost-effectiveness and utility of exercise ECG, single photon emission computed tomography, positron emission tomography and coronary angiography for diagnosis of coronary artery disease. Circulation *91:*54, 1995.
404. Zeiher, A., Drexler, H., Wollschlager, H., et al.: Endothelial dysfunction of the coronary microvasculature is associated with impaired coronary blood flow regulation in patients with early atherosclerosis. Circulation *84:*1984, 1991.
405. Grambow, D., Dayanikli, F., Muzik, O., et al.: Assessment of endothelial function with PET cold pressure test in patients with various degrees of coronary atherosclerosis. J. Nucl. Med. *34:*P36, 1993.
406. Packer, M.: The neurohormonal hypothesis: A theory to explain the mechanism of disease progression in heart failure (editorial). J. Am. Coll. Cardiol. *20:*248, 1992.
407. Allman, K., Wieland, D., Muzik, O., et al.: Carbon-11 hydroxyephedrine with positron emission tomography for serial assessment of cardiac adrenergic neuronal function after acute myocardial infarction in humans. J. Am. Coll. Cardiol. *22:*368, 1993.
408. Calkins, H., Lehmann, M. H., Allman, K., et al.: Scintigraphic pattern of regional cardiac sympathetic innervation in patients with familial long QT syndrome using positron emission tomography. Circulation *87:*1616, 1993.
409. Calkins, H., Allman, K., Bolling, S., et al.: Correlation between scintigraphic evidence of regional sympathetic neuronal dysfunction and ventricular refractoriness in the human heart. Circulation *88:*172, 1993.

Chapter 10
Newer Cardiac Imaging Techniques: Magnetic Resonance Imaging and Computed Tomography

CHARLES B. HIGGINS

MAGNETIC RESONANCE IMAGING OF THE HEART

Magnetic resonance imaging (MRI) has several important attributes that make it intrinsically advantageous for cardiovascular diagnosis. First, a high natural contrast exists between the blood pool and the cardiovascular structures because of the lack of signal from flowing blood with the spin-echo MRI technique or the bright signal from blood with the gradient-echo (cine MRI) technique. When the spin-echo technique is used, blood appears black on images; therefore, internal structures of the heart can be visualized within the signal void of the cardiac chambers. Using the gradient-echo technique, the blood pool appears white and has substantially higher signal than the myocardium, again providing good edge definition of the endocardial margin. Consequently, contrast medium is not required for discrimination of the blood pool, as MRI is an entirely noninvasive imaging technique. Second, a wide range of soft tissue contrast provides the potential for the characterization of myocardial tissue. This contrast among tissues depends on proton (hydrogen nuclei) density, magnetic relaxation times of the protons, and magnetic susceptibility effects. Third, imaging can be done in any plane, including those parallel and perpendicular to the major axis of the ventricles.

MAGNETIC RESONANCE GLOSSARY

Brief descriptions of the MRI process, general imaging techniques, and specific imaging techniques for the heart are given below, along with some useful terminology for MRI. A more detailed description of the principles underlying MRI is available elsewhere.

ECHOPLANAR IMAGING. A method for obtaining MR images in 30 to 50 msecs. Data for all points in the image matrix are obtained with a single pulse repetition (single TR). In echoplanar imaging, a very rapid series of echoes is generated by rapidly switching a strong phase-encoding gradient in the presence of a weaker read gradient.

FREE INDUCTION DECAY. The signal produced by the release of energy absorbed by the nuclei from a previously applied radiofrequency (RF) pulse. The free induction decay is the signal analyzed in MRI and spectroscopy.

GRADIENT-ECHO IMAGING SEQUENCE. A method by which images are acquired more rapidly than with spin-echo imaging by substantially reducing the repetition time (TR). The technique uses a flip angle of 90 degrees or less and a short TR. This reduction is achieved by switching the read gradient to focus the signal rather than by a time-consuming refocusing RF pulse. Contrast on these images is very different from that for spin-echo images. A major difference is that flow blood produces strong signal and appears bright.

HYDROGEN DENSITY (SPIN DENSITY, PROTON DENSITY). Density of protons at a site in a sample which are resonating as part of the magnetic resonance process. From the point of view of quantum mechanics, these are the protons making transitions from high-energy states to lower ones and vice versa, when energy just equal to the difference between these two states is applied.

MAGNETIC MOMENT. Intensity and direction of the net magnetic field of spinning nuclei. In a magnetic field, nuclei align to produce a net magnetic moment parallel to the field.

MAGNETIC RESONANCE IMAGING (MRI). Spatial two- or three-dimensional map of nuclei resonating at a characteristic frequency when placed in a magnetic field and subjected to intermittently applied RF pulses.

PROTON MRI. Imaging dependent on the concentration and relaxation time of hydrogen nuclei.

MULTINUCLEAR MRI. Imaging using nuclei other than hydrogen, such as sodium-23 and phosphorus-31.

MAGNETIC RESONANCE SIGNAL. During relaxation after cessation of an RF pulse, energy absorbed from this pulse is released and provides an RF signal.

RELAXATION. Return of nuclei to the original state of alignment with a magnetic field after having been tilted by an RF pulse.

MAGNETIC RESONANCE SPECTROSCOPY. Spectrum of resonant frequencies of a specific nucleus contained within a sample. This spectrum results from the chemical shift of a nucleus caused by the influence of the local chemical environment. Consequently, the resonant frequency of phosphorus in the inorganic state is slightly different from its frequency in creatine phosphate. Magnetic resonance spectroscopy detects and maps these chemical shifts of a nucleus.

PROTON SPECTROSCOPY. Spectrum of resonant frequencies of hydrogen nuclei (protons) in relation to the chemical environment. Proton spectroscopy can define chemical peaks representative of substances such as fats, water, lactic acid, choline, and carnitine.

PARAMAGNETIC SUBSTANCES. Substances that alter the natural relaxation times of nuclei undergoing the magnetic resonance process. These are usually molecules with unpaired electrons which reduce the relaxation times of resonating nuclei. These substances are being used and developed as contrast media for magnetic resonance imaging.

RELAXATION TIMES. Relaxation of nuclei undergoing the magnetic resonance process has two components called T1 and T2 relaxation times. These relaxation times are time-constant, measured as the magnetization vector processes into alignment with the magnetic field after perturbation by an RF pulse.

RESONANT FREQUENCY. Each nucleus that is sensitive to the magnetic resonance process must be tilted in the magnetic field by a specific frequency (resonant frequency) in order to induce resonance. When this frequency is applied, the nucleus is rotated away from its equilibrium alignment with the magnetic field. When the RF pulse ceases, the nucleus realigns with the magnetic field through a process of magnetic relaxation.

SPIN-ECHO IMAGING SEQUENCE. Images are produced by sampling signal after an initial 90-degree RF pulse, followed by one or more 180-degree pulses. The 180-degree pulse refocuses spins and thereby enhances the signal from them. Signal is sampled some time after the 180-degree pulse.

SURFACE COILS. RF receiver coils placed upon the surface of the subject or upon an organ of interest in order to detect the magnetic resonance signal. These coils increase the efficiency and signal strength for both MRI and spectroscopy.

T1 RELAXATION TIME. Also called spin-lattice or longitudinal relaxation time. T1 relaxation is a measure of the exponential rate of growth of the magnetization vector along the direction of the external magnetic field after the nuclei have been tilted (flipped) by an RF pulse.

T1-WEIGHTED IMAGE. Image in which the intensity of image voxels depends greatly on the T1 relaxation time of tissues. For the spin-echo technique, this is done with a short TR and TE.

T2 RELAXATION TIME. Also called spin-spin or transverse relaxation time. Immediately after cessation of a 90-degree RF pulse, the nuclei process in phase, resulting in a magnetization vector in the transverse plane. There is gradual dephasing of nuclei, leading to cancellation of the magnetization vector in the transverse plane.

T2-WEIGHTED IMAGE. Image in which the intensity of image voxels depends heavily upon the T2 relaxation time of tissues. For the spin-echo technique, this is done with a long TR and TE.

TE. Echo delay time. Time between the initiation of a pulse sequence (90-degree pulse) and the sampling of the spin-echo signal. For the spin-echo sequence, this sampling is done after the 180-degree pulse. For example, the first spin-echo signal is sampled at a time that is twice the duration between the initial 90-degree pulse and the 180-degree refocusing pulse.

Technical Aspects

Atomic nuclei with a net charge have a magnetic moment. A net charge exists when a nucleus contains unpaired (an odd number) of protons, neutrons, or both. The hydrogen nucleus contains only a proton; it is positively charged and has a strong magnetic moment. The magnetic properties of nuclei are expressed when they are placed in an external magnetic field. When protons or other nuclei with magnetic moment lie within a magnetic field and are then exposed to electromagnetic radiation (RF waves), energy is absorbed and subsequently emitted. This absorption and release of energy causes resonance—nuclear magnetic resonance. The RF necessary to induce resonance has to be proportional to the local magnetic field (H_L) and a constant (magnetogyric ratio) related to the specific nucleus involved. The relationship between frequency (f) and magnetic field is expressed by the following equation:

$$f = \delta H_L / 2\pi$$

When nuclei at equilibrium in a magnetic field are irradiated at the resonant frequency, they attain a higher energy state. When they return to equilibrium, they emit energy at the same frequency if the magnetic field remains constant. If the magnetic field changes between the time of excitation and emission, then the emission occurs at a frequency corresponding to the new field strength as expressed by this equation.

Localization of Magnetic Resonance Signal

MRI depends on the reception of the emitted RF signal from resonating nuclei and on the capability of locating these nuclei in space. Location of the resonating nuclei can be achieved by spatially varying the field strength in a known manner. Because resonance frequency of a nucleus at a specific site is related to local field strength, the emitted frequency characterizes the spatial location of the nucleus when a magnetic gradient exists in one or more planes.

Selection of a transverse section for imaging is done by applying a magnetic gradient along the Z axis (long axis of the body). In such a gradient, each transverse plane (XY plane) has a specific and different resonant frequency. If the body is irradiated with a 90-degree RF pulse consisting of a narrow range of frequencies corresponding to the resonance frequency of a single plane, only the nuclei in that plane resonate *selective irradiation,* and the image plane is delineated.

Once a plane is excited by selective irradiation, spatial localization is attained in that plane by another gradient oriented parallel to that plane. After the selective 90-degree RF pulse is applied, a magnetic field gradient is produced in the X or Y direction. Nuclei at the stronger end of the field gradient resonate at a higher frequency than those at the weaker end of the gradient. This provides spatial localization within the selected plane.

The magnetic signal from a sample undergoing MRI is detected by an RF receiver coil. The intensity of the signal at foci in the imaging plane depends on the concentration of resonating nuclei at the site and the magnetic relaxation times of the nuclei. The relaxation times are measures of the interaction of the resonating protons with the static magnetic field and the intermittently applied RF pulses.

The net magnetic moment of nuclei at any site can be expressed as a vector with length (intensity) and direction. At equilibrium, the vector points along the main static magnetic field. The vector can be tipped 90 degrees by the application of an RF pulse. The component of the net magnetic moment that points along the main magnetic field is called *longitudinal magnetization.* The component at 90 degrees to the main field is the *transverse magnetization.* The component at 90 degrees to the main field is fully aligned with the magnetic field (equilibrium); the vector varies continuously between longitudinal and transverse magnetization and gradually approaches full longitudinal magnetization.

MAGNETIC RELAXATION TIMES

After the application of a 90-degree RF pulse, net magnetization is rotated from the longitudinal direction (ZY plane) into the transverse direction (XY plane). At this instant, transverse magnetization is maximum and longitudinal magnetization is zero. Immediately after this, longitudinal magnetization gradually recovers toward its equilibrium value. This exponential growth has a time constant called *T1.* Likewise, after the 90-degree pulse, transverse magnetization exponentially decays; the time constant is called *T2.* In tissues, T2 is much shorter than T1. These relaxation times are related to several characteristics of tissues, including temperature. Tissues have different relaxation times, and these differences contribute to contrast among tissues during imaging. Contrast between two tissues can be accentuated by sampling signal at an instant when the difference between the relaxation times of the two tissues is maximal.

IMAGING, TR, AND TE. The MR image is produced by applying the sets of RF pulses many times over several minutes; generally, 128 to 512 pulse sequences are used. The time between application of sets of RF pulses is called the *repetition time* (TR). Depending on the technique employed for imaging, each set consists of one or more RF pulses. The time between the initial pulse in a sequence and the instant when signal is acquired from the sample is called the *echo delay time* (TE). It is possible to alter the pulse sequences in such a way that differences in T1 and T2 relaxation times among the tissues can be accentuated to produce contrast among these tissues. This is referred to as *T1* or *T2 weighting of the images.* T1-weighted images have short TR and TE intervals, while T2-weighted images have long TR and TE intervals when using the spin-echo technique. T1 and T2 weighting for new fast-imaging techniques is achieved to some extent by variations in the flip angles induced in the nuclei by the initial RF pulses.

EFFECTS OF MOVING BLOOD. During an imaging sequence, the motion of nuclei through the region that is being imaged greatly influences signal intensity. Although the influence of blood flow on MR images is complex, motion of the excited nuclei causes either a loss or increase of signal intensity, depending upon the RF pulse sequence employed. For the spin-echo sequence, moving blood in the lumina of vessels appears dark (no signal), providing considerable natural contrast for visualization of the internal surfaces of the blood vessels and walls of the cardiac chambers (Fig. 10–1). Because contrast medium is not required to mark the blood pool, MRI is a totally noninvasive technique for cardiovascular diagnosis. When blood veloc-

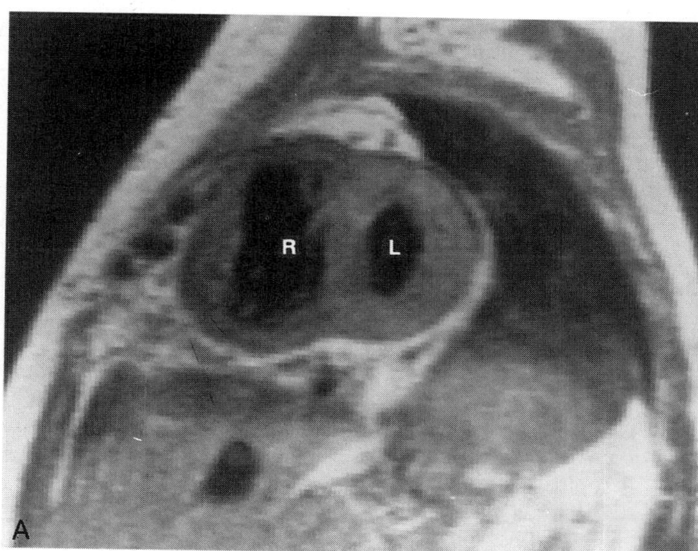

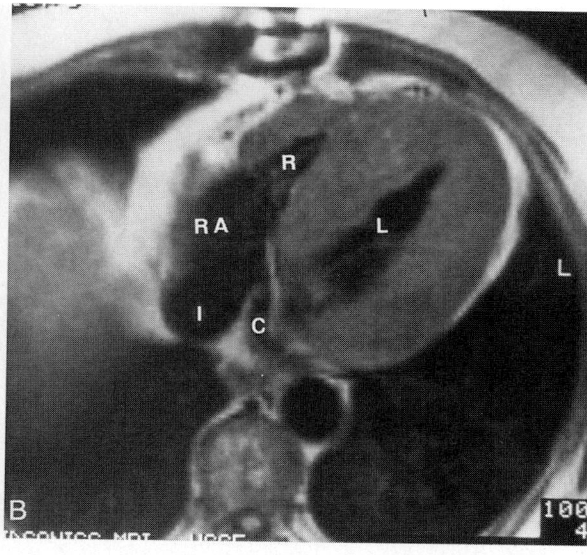

FIGURE 10–1. *A,* ECG-gated spin-echo MR image acquired in the short-axis plane through the middle of the ventricles. On this type of image the moving blood within the chambers of the heart produces little or no signal, resulting in high contrast between the blood pool and myocardial walls. The right ventricular wall is thickened in this patient. L = left ventricle; R = right ventricle. *B,* ECG-gated spin-echo image acquired in the transverse plane. The endocardial border is sharply demarcated owing to the contrast between the blood pool and the myocardium. There is severe left ventricular hypertrophy. I = inferior vena cava; L = left ventricle; RA = right atrium; R = right ventricle; C = coronary sinus. Note that the cardiac short-axis image transects the heart perpendicular to the long axis of the heart while the transverse plane sections the ventricles obliquely.

ity is such that protons move through the thickness of the tomogram (usually 5 to 10 mm) in the time between the 90-degree and 180-degree pulses of the spin-echo sequence, signal is lost from the blood. Using standard spin-echo sequences, this time (TE/2) is usually 7 to 15 msec for the first such image. For the gradient-echo pulse sequence, signal is received from blood flowing at normal velocities in the cardiac chambers and all blood vessels. The signal of flowing blood increases in proportion to the rate of flow (velocity) over a moderate range of velocities until a plateau of nearly constant signal is reached. In this circumstance, blood appears substantially brighter (white) than the cardiac walls (Fig. 10–2). With jet flow at very high velocities, signal is lost. This loss of signal from high-velocity disturbed flow in jets can be minimized by the use of short TE (<5 msec). High-velocity jets produced by flow across stenotic or regurgitant valves can be recognized as a signal void within the signal-filled cardiac chambers.

Techniques for MRI of the Heart

Cardiac imaging requires some form of physiological gating of the imaging sequence. Acquisition of MR signals of the thorax without gating results in poor cardiac images owing to loss of the signal from moving structures and to the variable position of the cardiac structure relative to imaging pixels when data are acquired indiscriminantly throughout the cardiac cycle.

GATING WITH MRI. This is associated with unique problems. Sensors, wire leads, and transducers are usually composed of ferromagnetic materials, which can generate noise or may grossly distort the images within the RF-shielded room containing the MRI device. Consequently, gating with MRI requires the use of a nonferromagnetic physiological signal-sensing circuit. An electronically isolated electrocardiogram (ECG) electrode-lead circuit containing very little metal has been used for repetitive synchronization, i.e., ECG gating, of pulse sequences to fixed segments of the cardiac cycle.

MULTISLICE TECHNIQUES. Several imaging strategies have been used, depending upon the information desired. For anatomical diagnosis, the *ECG-gated multislice technique* is used. This technique is economical in time, requiring less than 10 minutes for the acquisition of tomograms (0.3 to 1.0 cm in thickness) at multiple, usually 10 to 12, anatomical levels, which encompasses the entire heart and root of the great vessels. A difference of about 30 to 50 msec exists between each adjacent level, so the images are obtained at different phases of the cardiac cycle. Images can be obtained at multiple anatomical levels during a single imaging sequence because the time required to complete a set of RF pulses and sample the emitted signal for each line on that image is usually 15 to 30 msec (TE interval) for T1-weighted images, while the time between the application of repetitive sets of pulses is approximately 500 to 1000 msec (TR interval). Consequently, the inactive time for each cycle is long, frequently greater than 90 per cent of the cycle. Efficiency is improved by applying the set of spin-echo pulses at other levels during the magnetization recovery period. For example, upon completion of a 50-msec duty cycle at one level, the full set of pulses is selectively applied at the next adjacent tomographic level and then the next, and so forth. With this multislice technique, the total number of tomographic levels that can be imaged is approximately TR/TE. As indicated earlier, TR equals the length of the cardiac cycle (R-R interval) when using ECG gating.

The *multiphasic multislice technique* can be used for the evaluation of cardiac dimensions and function. With this technique, each anatomical section is imaged at 5 to 10 phases of the cardiac cycle. From end-diastolic and end (late)-systolic images of each anatomical level, measurement can be made of diastolic and systolic volumes, stroke volume, ejection fraction, myocardial mass, and extent of left ventricular regional wall thickening. With this technique, wall thickening dynamics have been measured for various regions of the left ventricle in normal subjects and patients with global and regional myocardial dysfunction and in patients with focal and generalized hypertrophy.

CINE MRI. This can be accomplished by ECG referencing of gradient-echo sequences. This approach can produce a set of images corresponding to multiple evenly spaced phases of the cardiac cycle. The temporal window for each phasic image is usually 20 to 30 msec for acquisition at a single anatomical level, but double or triple the time if acquisitions are done simultaneously at two or three levels. Acquisitions are usually done at two levels simultaneously, and 16 phasic images are produced at each level. These images are laced together in a cinematic display so that wall motion of the ventricles, valve motion, and blood flow patterns in the heart and great vessels can be visualized.

FAST GRADIENT-ECHO MRI. These fast gradient-echo imaging techniques are important for MRI of the heart. For conventional spin-echo and gradient-echo techniques, one line of the imaging matrix (usually 128 to 256 lines compose an imaging matrix) is acquired for each TR interval (R-R interval for gated acquisitions). With fast gradient-echo imaging, multiple lines (usually eight) are acquired for each TR interval. This reduces the acquisition time by a factor of 8 (number of lines acquired), so that a cine acquisition can be done in a breath hold period of about 12 to 14 seconds (breath-hold cine MR imaging).[1] Because multiple lines or a segment of the image matrix (K space) is acquired rather than a single line, this technique is sometimes called segmented fast gradient-echo imaging. Because the respiration is suspended during the acquisition, cine MR images are produced which are free of motion artifacts associated with breathing.

Another fast imaging method uses very short TR and TE intervals for gradient-echo acquisition with a course matrix (64 to 128 lines) to produce low spatial resolution images in about 600 to 2000 msec. These are sometimes called fast gradient-echo or turbo gradient-

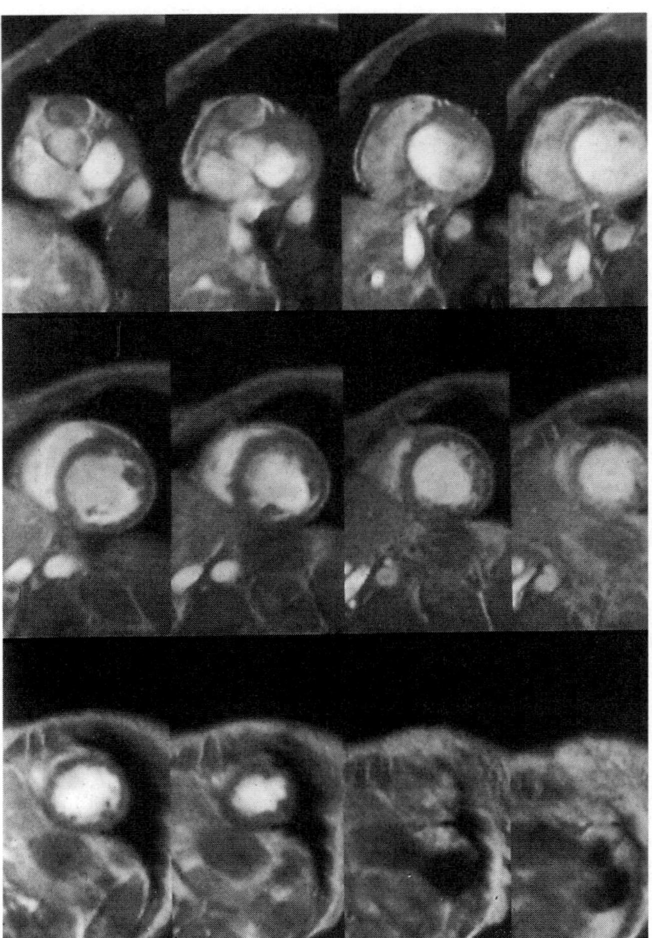

FIGURE 10–2. Series of cine MR images extending from base *(upper left)* to apex *(lower right)* of the heart. Images are acquired at the same phase of the cardiac cycle. From such a set of images acquired at end-diastole and end-systole, direct measurements of right and left ventricular volumes and mass can be done. With this type of imaging sequence (gradient-echo), the blood pool produces higher signal than the myocardium, resulting in substantial contrast between the two, and sharp delineation of the endocardial margin.

echo images. These can be weighted for T1 or T2 contrast by applying a preparation pulse before the imaging sequence, such as an inversion recovery (180-degree) pulse before the image sequence. These sequences have been initially applied to provide 1- to 2-second monitoring of the initial passage of injected contrast medium through the central circulation and myocardium in order to evaluate regional myocardial perfusion.[2,3]

Echo planar imaging (EPI) is the fastest MRI technique.[4] It can provide an image in an acquisition time of 40 to 50 msec. The acquisition can be done so that all lines in the image matrix or K space are acquired in a single TR interval (single-shot EPI) or in a few (usually two to four) sequential TR intervals (multishot or interleaved EPI).[5] Echoplanar imaging sequences can be either spin-echo EPI or gradient-echo EPI. In addition, preparatory pulses can be used to increase the T1 weighting of the imaging; inversion recovery EPI is very sensitive to T1 contrast effects such as those produced by low doses of MR contrast medium.[6]

EVALUATION OF SPECIFIC CARDIAC DISEASES

The clinical use of MRI has been primarily for the demonstration of pathological anatomy. However, in the past few years cine MRI has been used for the quantification of global and regional function of the right and left ventricles, for the quantification of valvular heart disease, for the measurement of blood flow in the heart and great arteries, and for the assessment of myocardial perfusion and even coronary blood flow. Precise demonstration of anatomical abnormalities has been useful for the evaluation of patients with ischemic heart disease, cardiomyopathies, pericardial disease, neoplastic disease, congenital heart disease, and thoracic aortic disease.

Ischemic Heart Disease

The role of MRI in ischemic heart disease has been quite minor up to the current time. However, recent advances in technology provide capabilities by which MRI could evolve as a comprehensive imaging technique for ischemic heart disease.[7] In this regard, morphology can be assessed with the ECG-gated spin-echo and cine MRI techniques, permitting determination of the extent of wall thinning caused by previous infarctions and depiction of complications of infarctions, such as true and false aneurysms. Segmental myocardial function can be quantified by measuring the extent of regional wall thickening or wall motion on standard or breath-hold cine MRI. Moreover, regional myocardial ischemia can be demonstrated by analysis of regional myocardial wall thickening in the basal state and during pharmacological stress induced by dipyridamole or dobutamine.[8,9] Using breath-hold cine MRI, images of the major coronary arteries can be produced.[10,11] Breath-hold velocity-encoded techniques can be applied for measuring coronary blood flow or velocity at rest and during interventions intended to test coronary flow reserve.[12,13] Finally, contrast-prepared fast gradient-echo imaging can be used to evaluate myocardial perfusion in the basal and vasodilated states to identify myocardium jeopardized by coronary arterial stenosis.[14,15]

MORPHOLOGY. MRI provides direct visualization of the myocardium with excellent delineation of the epicardial and endocardial interfaces. Consequently, it can define accurately segmental wall thinning that is indicative of previous myocardial infarction.[16–18] In some patients with a history of transmural infarction, residual myocardium can be demonstrated at the site of the infarction. In others, MRI shows virtually complete absence of remnant muscle. Direct visualization of the myocardium can be used to determine whether there is sufficient residual myocardium in the region jeopardized by a coronary arterial lesion to warrant a bypass graft (Fig. 10–3). Regional wall thickening can also be assessed.[19] It has been shown that a wall thickness of less than 6 mm at end-diastole and wall thickening of less than 1 mm are indicative of myocardial scar when

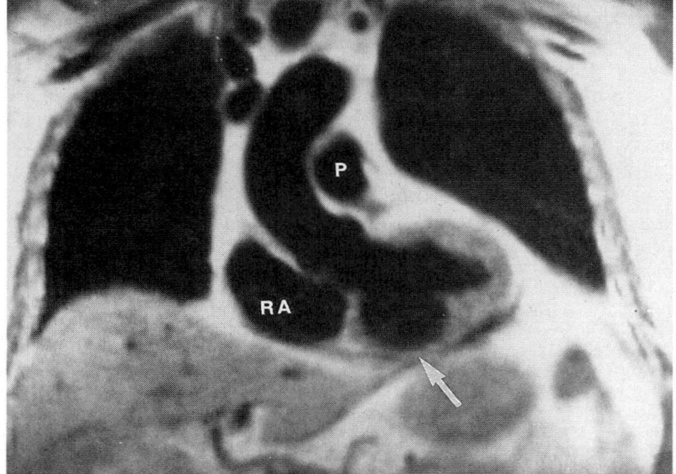

FIGURE 10–3. ECG-gated spin-echo image in the coronal plane displays a chronic transmural myocardial infarction (arrow) of the diaphragmatic wall of the left ventricle, which has caused severe wall thinning and aneurysmal bulging. P = pulmonary artery; RA = right atrium.

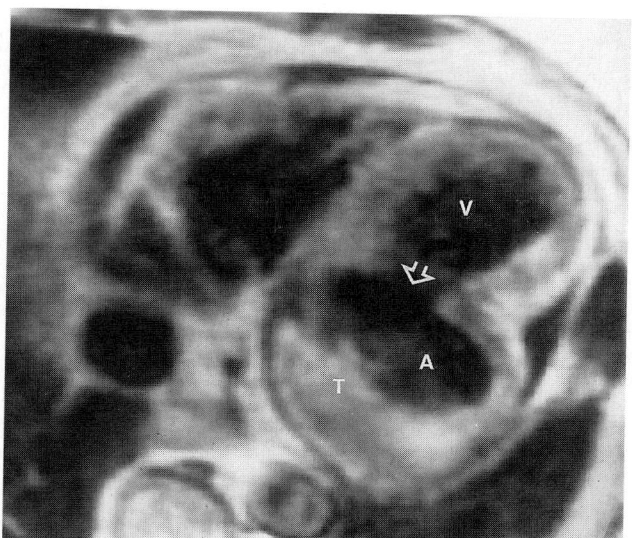

FIGURE 10–4. ECG-gated spin-echo image of a false aneurysm of the left ventricle. There is a narrow ostium (open arrow) connecting the large posterior aneurysm (A) to the ventricular (V) chamber. There is thrombus (T) in the aneurysm.

compared with uptake of ^{99m}Tc-sestamibi single-photon emission tomography.

The recognition of decreased signal intensity of the myocardial wall at the site of old myocardial infarction suggests that MRI can identify the replacement of myocardium by fibrous scar.[17] Gated MRI has also demonstrated complications of myocardial infarctions, such as left ventricular thrombus and aneurysms[16,17] (Fig. 10–4). Transverse or short-axis tomography facilitates the recognition of the small ostium connecting the left ventricular chamber and the false aneurysm (Fig. 10–4); this is a distinguishing feature of the false compared with the true left ventricular aneurysm.

Acute myocardial infarctions have been demonstrated by gated MRI. The region of ischemically damaged myocardium displays increased signal intensity compared with normal myocardium.[21–25] Contrast between infarcted and normal myocardium increases on images with greater T2 contribution to signal intensity. Because cardiac pulsations and respiration can cause high-intensity artifacts projected over the myocardial region, caution must be used in the interpretation of this finding.[25] Comparison of changes in contrast among images with increasing TE value and estimation of T2 relaxation times can alleviate this problem.[22] Administration of MR contrast medium (gadolinium chelates) with T1-weighted spin-echo images causes greater enhancement of infarcted than of normal myocardium (Fig. 10–5).

Regional Contraction Abnormalities. The major role of noninvasive imaging techniques in ischemic heart disease is the detection of ischemic myocardium and other features indicative of the presence of obstructive coronary arterial disease. Ischemic myocardium can be demonstrated directly or indirectly by MRI. Indirectly, it is shown by demonstrating a regional contraction abnormality, usually by wall thickening measurement, at rest or during pharmacological stress. Cine MRI in the basal state and during pharmacological intervention with dobutamine or dipyridamole has correlated closely with nuclear perfusion imaging and/or coronary arteriography for demonstrating potentially ischemic myocardial segments.[7–9] Directly, the monitoring of the first-pass distribution of MR contrast medium with T1-sensitive fast GRE imaging in basal and vasodilated states has shown regions of decreased myocardial perfusion in association with coronary arterial stenosis[14,15] (Fig. 10–6).

Visualization of Coronary Arteries. The unique information provided by MRI relevant to ischemic heart disease is visualization of the major coronary arteries using newly developed MR angiographic techniques[10,11] (Fig. 10–7). One report has shown approximately 90 per cent correlation between coronary MRA and coronary x-ray angiography for identifying hemodynamically significant coronary arterial stenoses or occlusions.[26] Equally intriguing is the possibility of measuring volume or velocity of flow in the major coronary arteries using breath-hold gradient-echo or echo planar velocity-encoded techniques[12,13] (Figs. 10–8 and 10–9). These techniques have already been used in human subjects to document an increase in volume flow or flow velocity in response to vasodilators; the exclusion or confirmation of coronary arterial disease by the noninvasive assessment of coronary flow may be an important future application of MRI in ischemic heart disease.

CORONARY ARTERY BYPASS GRAFTS. Gated MRI has been used to evaluate the patency of bypass grafts. Because blood usually flows rapidly through the grafts, they appear

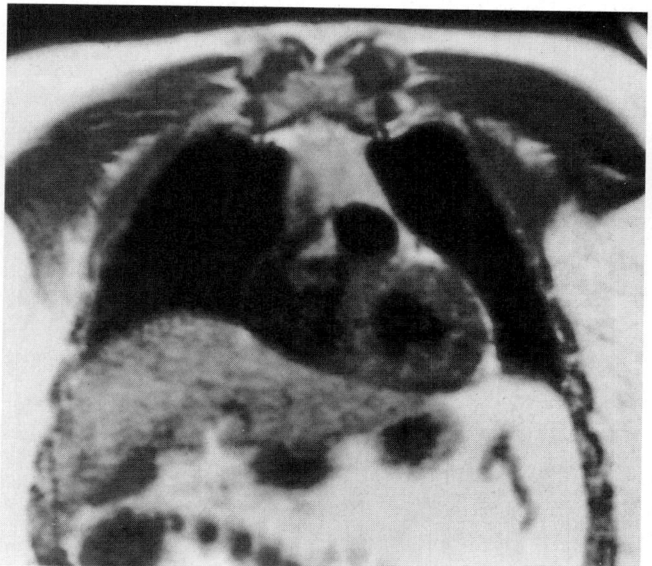

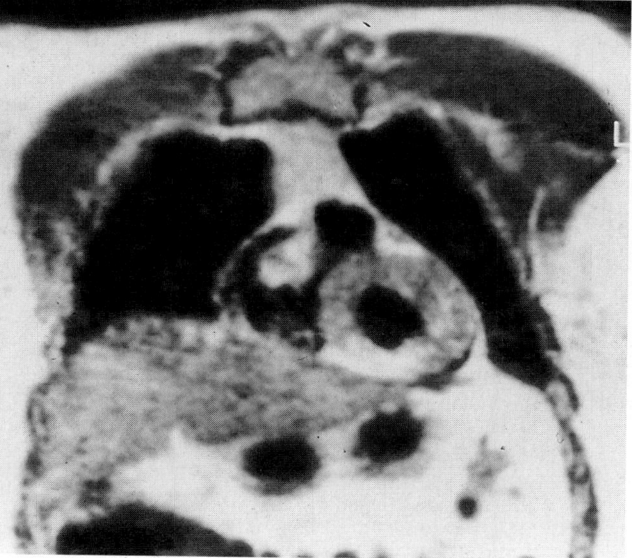

FIGURE 10–5. ECG-gated spin-echo image in the coronal plane before *(left)* and after *(right)* the administration of MR contrast medium (gadolinium chelate). The contrast medium causes greater enhancement of the infarcted area and demarcates it on the postcontrast image.

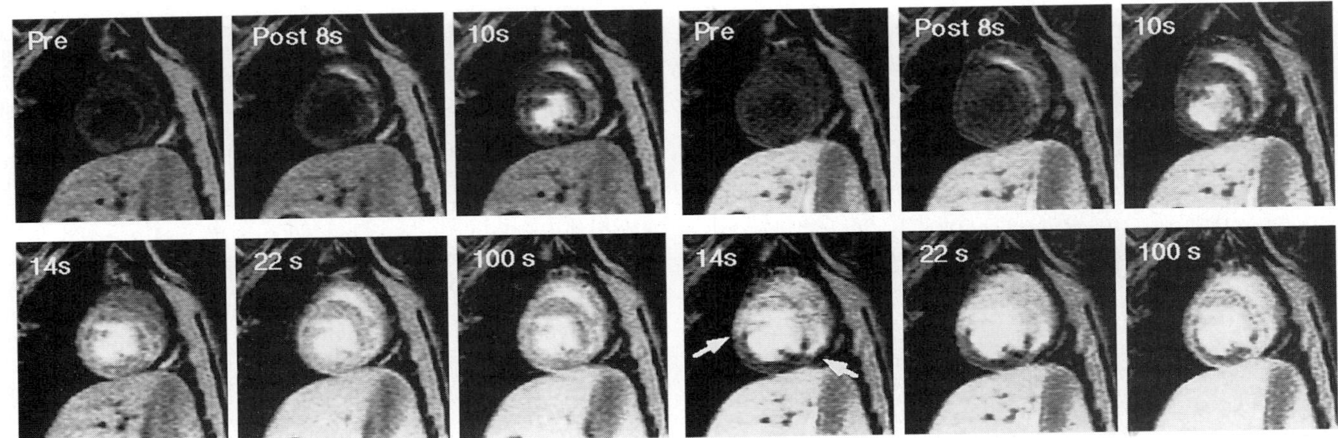

FIGURE 10–6. Sequential inversion recovery fast gradient-echo images acquired during the first passage of MR contrast medium (gadolinium chelate) through the heart. The series of images was performed in the basal *(left)* and vasodilated *(right)* states. In this animal model of a nonocclusive coronary arterial stenosis, the potentially ischemic region is not evident in the basal state. After dipyridamole the ischemic region is demarcated as a low-intensity zone (arrows) compared with normal myocardium.

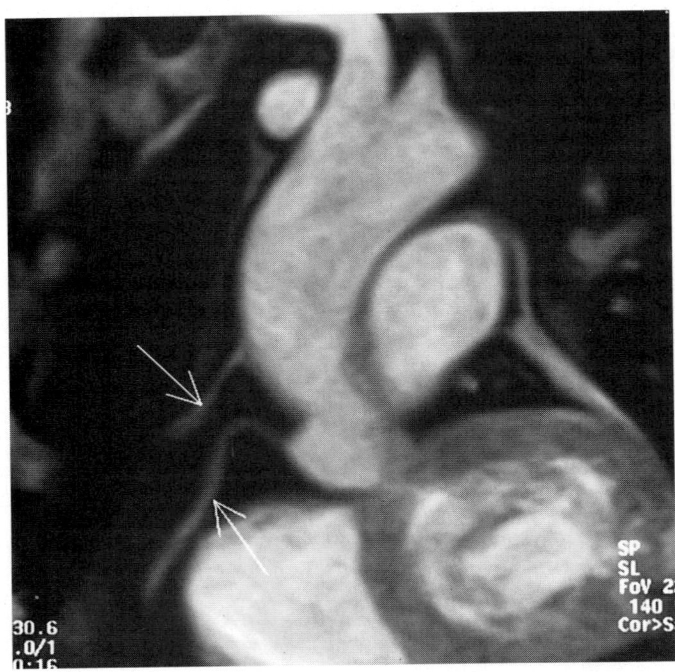

FIGURE 10–7. Breath-hold cine MR image demonstrates the proximal portion of the right coronary artery (arrow) and a bypass graft (arrow) to the right coronary artery. (Courtesy of Robert Edelman, M.D.)

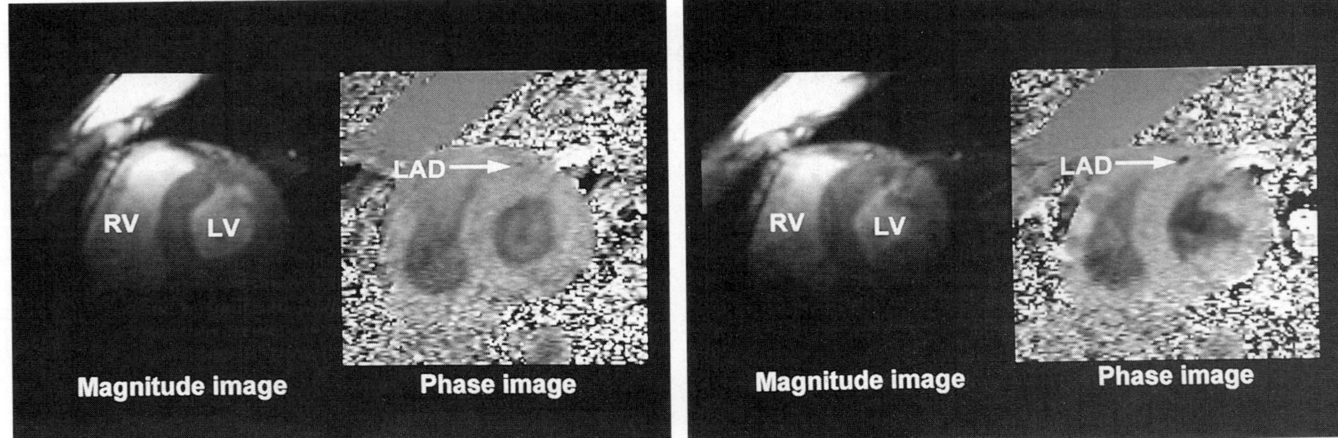

FIGURE 10–8. Magnitude and phase images in the short-axis planes display the left anterior descending coronary artery (LAD, arrow) in the basal *(left)* and vasodilated *(right)* states. Signal of the artery is increased in the vasodilated state due to increased flow induced by dipyridamole. These images were derived from breath-hold velocity-encoded MR sequences.

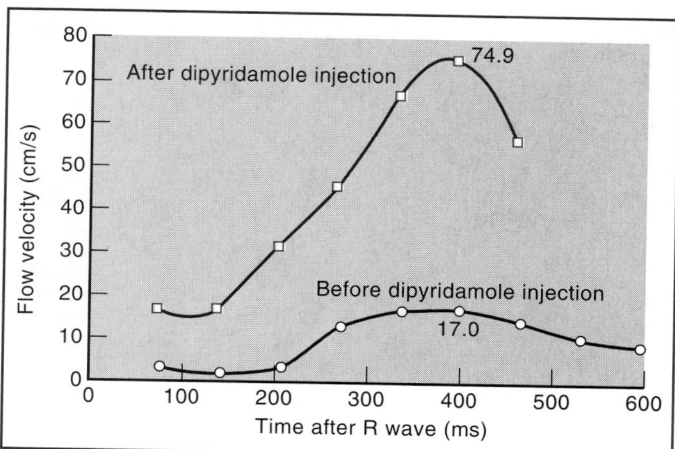

FIGURE 10–9. Graph showing left anterior descending coronary flow velocity in basal and vasodilated states.

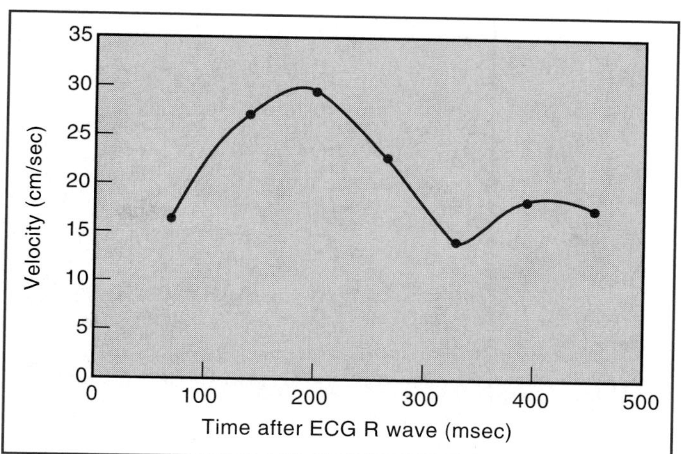

FIGURE 10–11. Plot of the flow velocity versus time curve from an internal mammary artery bypass conduit.

as small circular structures with absence of a luminal signal. For visualization of grafts, ECG-gated images are acquired in order to minimize the effect of motion of the grafts. Generally, images are acquired at each anatomical level during multiple phases of the cardiac cycle to ensure that an image is acquired at a phase when the rate of flow through the graft is rapid. High flow rate in the graft produces a flow void in the lumen of the graft using spin-echo MRI and thus indicates patency of the graft. With the cine (gradient-echo) MRI and MR angiographic techniques, flowing blood causes bright signal intensity; therefore, bright signal rather than flow void indicates graft patency with this technique (Fig. 10–10). MRI has an accuracy of 80 to 90 per cent for defining graft patency.[27–31] Phase-contrast gradient-echo techniques have been used to demonstrate flow and to estimate flow velocity in coronary bypass conduits[32,33] (Fig. 10–11).

Cardiomyopathies

(See also Chap. 41)

HYPERTROPHIC CARDIOMYOPATHIES (see also p. 1414). MRI has been used to define the presence, distribution, and severity of hypertrophic cardiomyopathies.[34,35] It has displayed the extent of septal involvement (Fig. 10–12) and has been particularly useful for identifying the unusual distribution of hypertrophy in the variant forms of hypertrophic cardiomyopathy. Left ventricular[36,37] and right ventricular[37,38] mass and wall thickness have been quantified using spin-echo and cine MRI. Substantial right ventricular hypertrophy has been shown by MRI measurements in patients with hypertrophic cardiomyopathy.[37,38] Cine MRI has also been used to assess ventricular diastolic parameters by constructing volume-time curves during the cardiac cycle; reduced filling rate and time to peak filling have been demonstrated in patients with hypertrophic cardiomyopathy.[38]

DILATED CARDIOMYOPATHY (see also p. 1407). MRI has depicted the morphologic[39] and functional[40] alterations in congestive (dilated) cardiomyopathy. It has been used to quantify left ventricular volume and systolic wall stress in patients with congestive cardiomyopathies.[41,42] Cine MRI has also been performed sequentially in order to monitor the effect of drug therapy in patients with congestive cardiomyopathy; it has demonstrated significant decreases in left ventricular volume, mass, and systolic wall stress during 3 months of treatment with an angiotensin-converting enzyme inhibitor.[42] Because MRI provides excellent discrimination of the edges of the myocardium, it can also be used to assess myocardial mass and wall thickness in patients with cardiomyopathies; several studies have indicated the accuracy of MRI for quantifying myocardial mass in both normally and abnormally shaped left ventricles.[43,44] Cine MRI has also been found to be highly reproducible in measuring left ventricular mass and volumes between two studies in the same subject.[43,44] The interstudy variability of mass measurements is less than 5 per cent. Cine MRI has demonstrated considerable increase in left ventricular mass and markedly elevated end-systolic wall stress in patients with dilated cardiomyopathy.[41,42,44] Cine MRI has demonstrated both a decrease in the extent of wall thickening and a change in the regional pattern of wall thickening

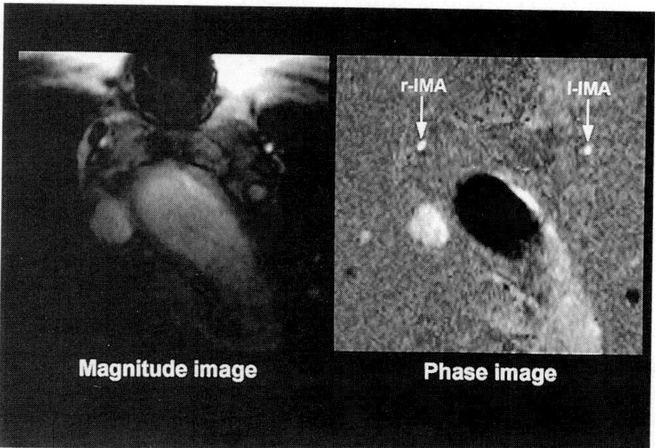

FIGURE 10–10. Magnitude and phase images of right (R-IMA) and left (L-IMA) internal mammary bypass grafts.

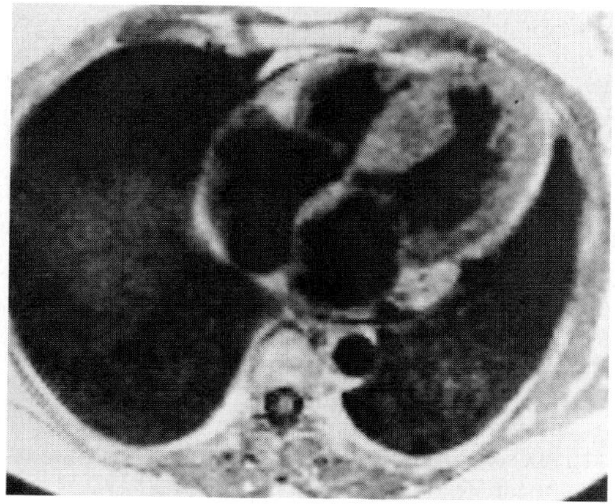

FIGURE 10–12. Hypertrophic cardiomyopathy. MRI displays severe hypertrophy of the entire septum and normal thickness of the lateral wall.

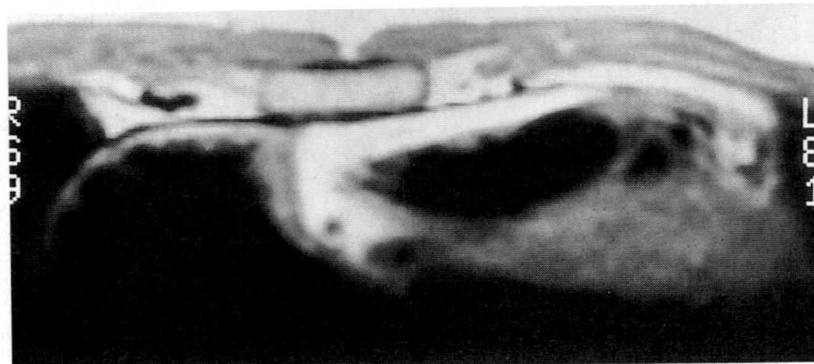

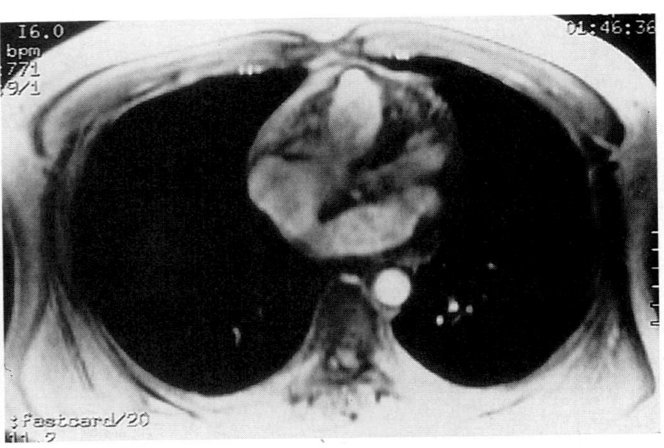

FIGURE 10–13. Spin-echo image *(left)* in a patient with right ventricular dysplasia shows transmural fat in the right ventricular free wall. Cine MR image *(right)* shows wall thinning and aneurysmal bulging of the right ventricular free wall in another patient with right ventricular dysplasia.

in patients with dilated cardiomyopathy compared with normal subjects.[40]

RESTRICTIVE CARDIOMYOPATHY (see also p. 1426). ECG-gated spin-echo MRI has displayed features considered to be characteristic for restrictive cardiomyopathy.[45] There is substantial enlargement of the atria and the inferior vena cava, with usually less prominent ventricular enlargement. Because of resistance caused by the noncompliant ventricles to atrial emptying during diastole, prominent signal is observed in the atrial blood. Such intra-atrial signal originates from slowly moving blood on spin-echo MR images. The major contribution of MRI to establishing the diagnosis of restrictive cardiomyopathy is the demonstration of normal pericardial thickness, which essentially excludes the alternate diagnosis of constrictive pericarditis. In *amyloid heart disease,* MRI has demonstrated thickened myocardial walls and diminished wall thickening during the cardiac cycle.[46,47] Cine MRI indicates apparent hypertrophy of the left ventricle with normal or decreased left ventricular contraction rather than hypercontractile left ventricle expected in left ventricular hypertrophy. MRI has also demonstrated infiltration of the myocardium by tumorous and inflammatory processes[48]; detection of such myocardial infiltrates can be useful for the diagnosis of specific forms of restrictive myocardial diseases.

The MRI findings in cardiomyopathies have thus far been limited to *anatomical* and *functional* abnormalities. No consistent changes in MRI relaxation times have been found for the myocardium in hypertrophic or congestive cardiomyopathies or in amyloid heart disease.

RIGHT VENTRICULAR DYSPLASIA (see also p. 749). Right ventricular dysplasia is represented pathologically by variable replacement or infiltration of right ventricular myocardium by fatty or fibrous tissue. Aside from suggestive clinical and electrophysiological features, the diagnosis has been definitively established by tissue examination after endomyocardial biopsy. The major differential diagnoses for ventricular arrhythmias of right ventricular origin in the presence of a grossly normal right ventricle are right ventricular dysplasia and right ventricular outflow tract tachycardia. ECG-gated spin-echo MRI has been used to identify transmural or focal fat in the right ventricular free wall in order to establish the diagnosis of right ventricular dysplasia[49] (Fig. 10–13). Focal or generalized wall thinning of the right ventricle also is consistent with this diagnosis[49] (Fig. 10–13). Focal wall thinning and focal bulging (aneurysm) of the right ventricular outflow tract has been shown also on MRI in right ventricular outflow tract tachycardia.[50] One report has shown that MRI actually demonstrates fat in the right ventricular free wall in less than half of patients with right ventricular dysplasia, but a regional contractile abnormality is demonstrated by cine MRI in a majority.[51]

Pericardial Disease

(See also Chap. 43)

Gated MRI provides direct visualization of the pericardium.[52] It has been effective for the assessment of patients with suspected pericardial disease. Normal pericardium is composed primarily of fibrous tissue and has low MRI signal intensity. The thickness of pericardial line measured in normal subjects was 1.5 ± 0.4 mm (S.D.) with a range from 0.8 to 2.6 mm.[52] A variation of thickness of the low-intensity line has been observed during the cardiac cycle in normal subjects. These latter observations, along with information from postmortem studies, indicate that the normal pericardium measures less than 3.0 mm and suggest that the low-intensity pericardial line consists of pericardium and some adherent pericardial fluid. A thickness of 4 mm or greater is abnormal (Fig. 10–14). This is probably responsible for the pericardial line observed on CT as well because normal CT measurements of pericardial thickness are similar to MRI measurements. On spin-echo MR images, pericardial effusion causes a low signal intensity space separating the heart and pericardium (Fig. 10–15). The distinction between the pericardium itself and pericardial fluid can also be achieved on cine MR images, on which the fluid has bright signal and the pericardium is a dark line (Fig. 10–15). MRI has been used to establish the diagnosis of congenital absence of the left pericardium.[53] Pericardial thickening and effusions are characteristic features of acute pericarditis.

Gated MRI has been useful for demonstrating pericardial thickness in patients with suspected constrictive pericarditis.[52,54,55] The signal intensity of the thickened pericardium is variable. The purely fibrous or calcified pericardium in chronic constrictive pericardial disease has low signal intensity. However, in subacute forms of constrictive pericarditis caused by irradiation, surgical trauma, or uremia, the thickened pericardium has moderate to high intensity on spin-echo images.[52] The effusive-constrictive form of pericardial disease has thickened pericardium and pericardial effusion. One study[55] has demonstrated a diagnostic accuracy of 93 per cent for MRI in distinguishing between constrictive pericarditis and restrictive cardiomyopathy by demonstrating thickened pericardium (≥4 mm) in the former disease.

MRI demonstrates even the small amount of pericardial fluid present in normal subjects. Fluid in the superior pericardial recesses is commonly seen even when fluid is not evident posterior to the left ventricle. The appearance of pericardial fluid is different on spin-echo and cine MRI (gradient-echo) images (Fig. 10–15). Nonhemorrhagic fluid shows low intensity on short-TR, short-TE sequences (T1-weighted) and has high intensity on long-TR, long-TE se-

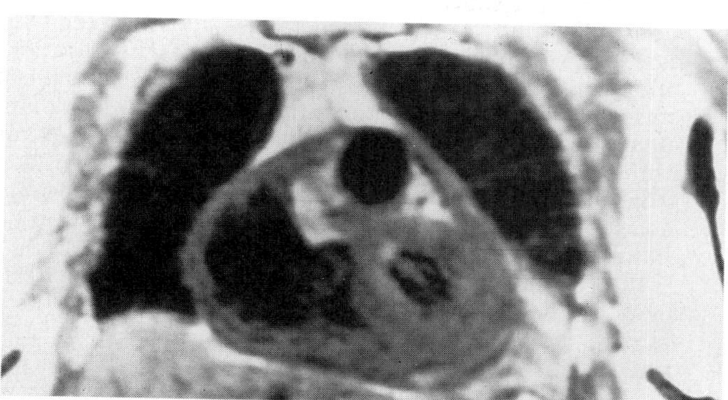

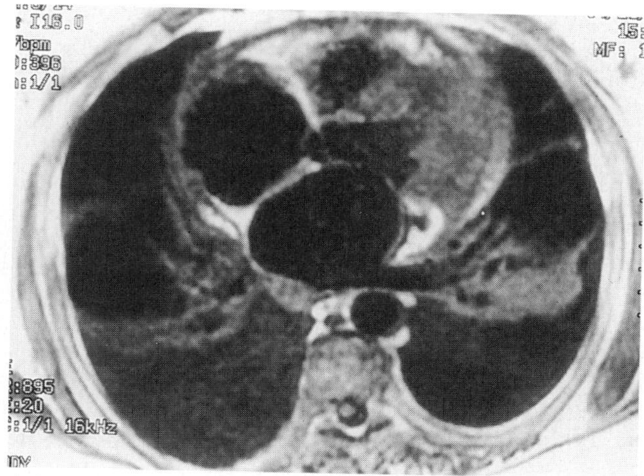

FIGURE 10–14. ECG-gated spin-echo images in coronal *(left)* and transverse *(right)* planes of a patient with constrictive pericarditis. The pericardium is substantially thickened. Thick pericardium can be visualized extending over the pulmonary artery on the coronal image.

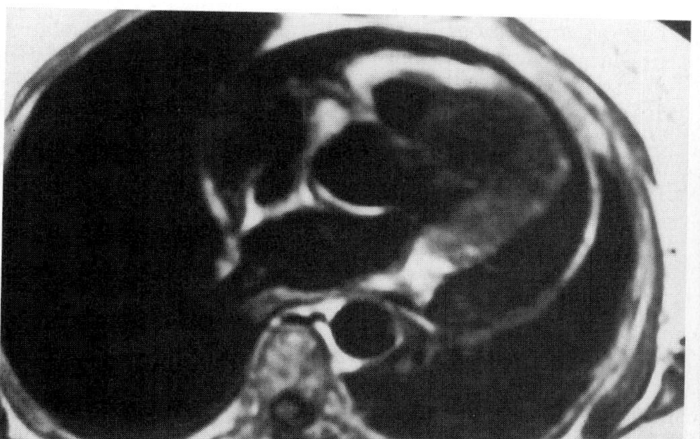

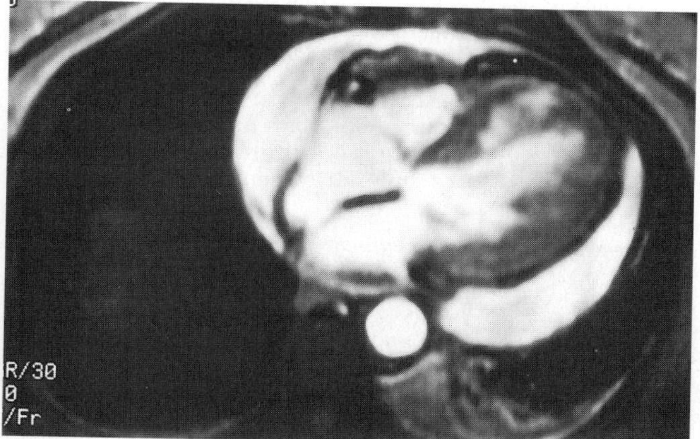

FIGURE 10–15. Spin-echo *(left)* and gradient-echo (cine MR) *(right)* images of a patient with a large pericardial effusion.

quences (T2-weighted). On the other hand, pericardial hematoma has high intensity on T1-weighted images (Fig. 10–16) and may have high intensity on T2-weighted images, depending on the age of the hematoma and the magnetic field strength of the imager. On cine MRI, the nonhemorrhagic effusion is bright and the hemorrhagic one may be low intensity.

In pericardial disease the role of MRI must be considered in the light of the established effectiveness of echocardiography. An advantage of MRI over echocardiography is the capability to differentiate pericardial hematoma from other types of effusions. Because of the wide field of view, MRI seems to be useful in locating loculated effusions. Determination of pericardial thickening seems to be a clear indication for the use of MRI.

Neoplastic Disease

(See also Chaps. 42 and 57)

Several reports have documented the clinical utility of gated MRI for the evaluation of intracardiac and paracardiac masses.[56–60] Because of the unequivocal delineation of the pericardium, myocardial walls, and chambers of the heart on MR images, the precise relationship of tumors to cardiovascular structures can be defined. Tumors within the myocardial wall may be identified by virtue of a difference in signal intensity (usually higher) compared with the myocardium. In this regard, MR contrast media can be used in an attempt to accentuate differences in signal intensity between tumor and myocardium.[61]

Secondary cardiac involvement by tumors (see p. 1794) is about 40 times more frequent than primary tumors (see p. 1464). Secondary involvement occurs by three routes: direct extension from the mediastinum and lungs (Fig. 10–

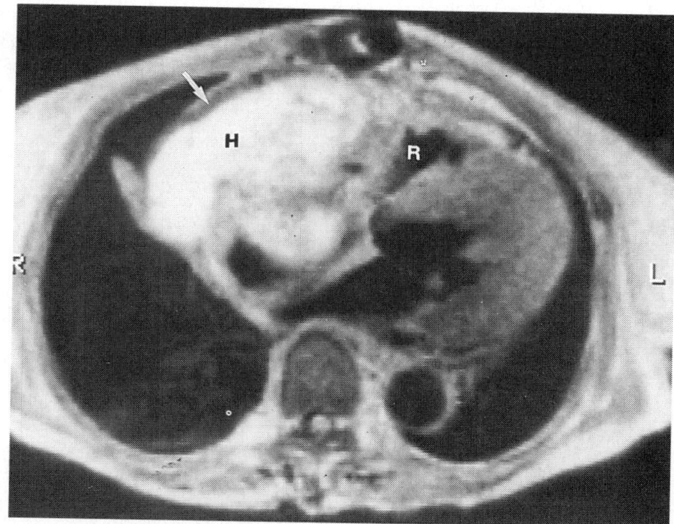

FIGURE 10–16. ECG-gated spin-echo images show a pericardial hematoma (H). The hemorrhagic pericardial effusion causes bright signal intensity on the T1-weighted (TE = 30 msec) image. The right atrium and right ventricle are compressed by the hematoma. Pericardium (arrow) is thickened. R = right ventricle.

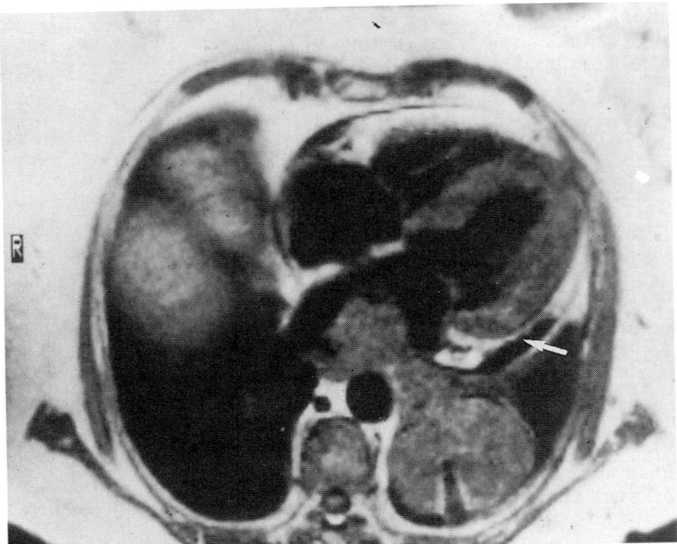

FIGURE 10–17. ECG-gated spin-echo image shows a lung tumor extending through the pericardium and into the left atrial chamber. The MR image clearly displays the extracardiac and intracardiac parts of the mass and a small pericardial effusion (arrow).

17, metastases to the pericardium or cardiac chambers, and direct extension of upper abdominal tumors through the inferior vena cava or lung tumors through the pulmonary veins. MRI appears to be superior to computed tomography (CT) for assessing the extent and effect of mediastinal masses adjacent to cardiovascular structures.[60,62] Gated MRI is the imaging procedure of choice for identifying paracardiac masses, defining their nature, and determining invasion of the pericardium. The intensity on spin-echo images can be used to differentiate such masses from innocuous lipomas, the pericardial fat pad, pericardial cysts, loculated pericardial effusions, and unusual enlargement or displacement of cardiac chambers. Gated MRI has been extremely useful for demonstrating invasion of cardiac chambers by pulmonary and mediastinal malignancies (Fig. 10–17). Metastases to the pericardium and the accompanying pericardial effusion can be readily depicted by gated MRI.

Intracardiac tumors can be clearly identified within the signal void of the cardiac blood pool. Because of its wide field of view, MRI is ideal for defining both the intracardiac and extracardiac extent of masses (Figs. 10–17 to 10–19). For the evaluation of intracardiac masses, it is advisable to acquire spin-echo and gradient-echo MR images and to obtain images with at least two planes perpendicular to each other. A recent investigation has suggested that intracardiac or intravascular tumors can be distinguished from thrombus using cine MRI in most instances[63] (Fig. 10–19). Tumors are represented by medium signal (higher signal or similar signal compared with myocardium), whereas thrombus produces very low signal (less than myocardium). This low signal is due to elements in the thrombus (e.g., hemosiderin, deoxyhemoglobin) that induce a magnetic susceptibility effect and vitiate signal from the region. The cine MRI sequence is very sensitive to this effect.

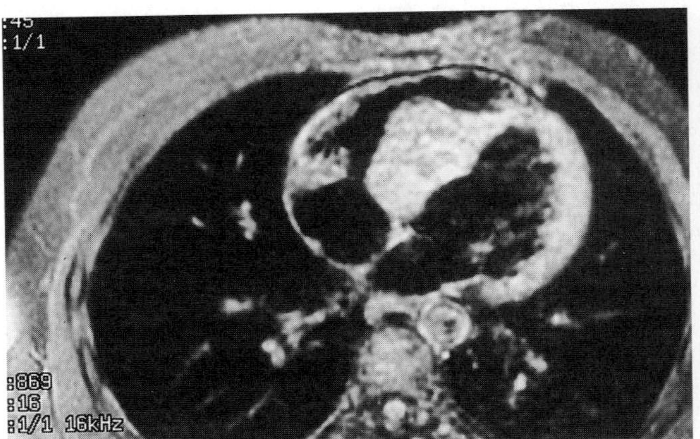

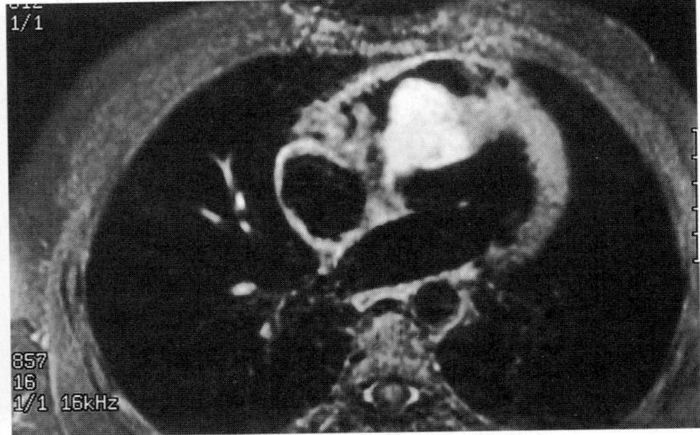

FIGURE 10–18. ECG-gated spin-echo images before *(left)* and after *(right)* injection of gadolinium chelate in a patient with a sarcoma of the ventricular septum. A fat saturation technique was used after contrast medium in order to accentuate the effect of the contrast medium. The tumor is contrast-enhanced to a greater degree than myocardium.

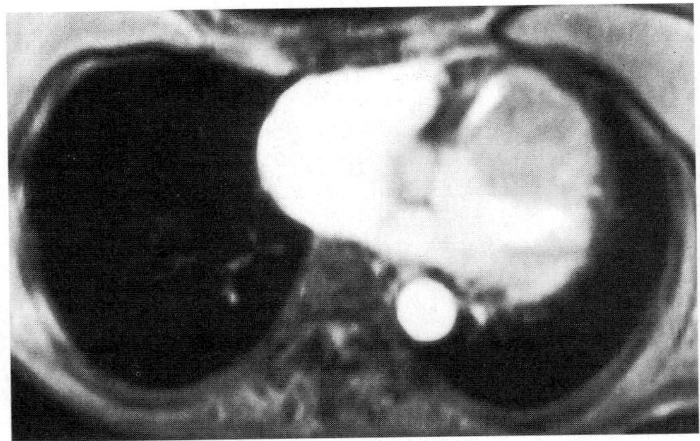

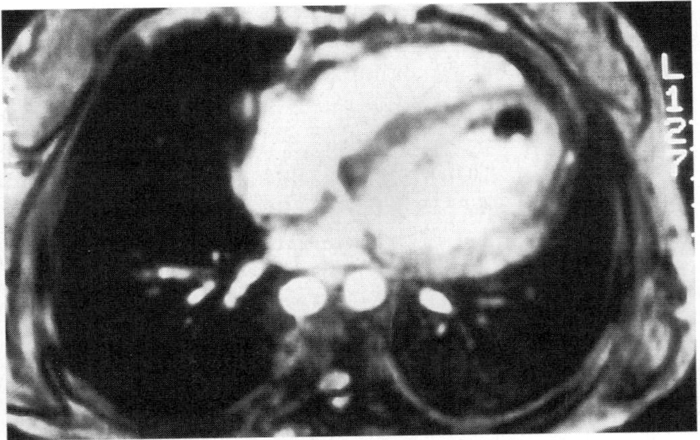

FIGURE 10–19. Gradient-echo (cine MR) images in two patients with intracardiac masses. *Left,* Metastatic tumor in the right ventricle has medium intensity. *Right,* Thrombus at the left ventricular apex has low intensity. (From Higgins, C. B., Hricak, H., and Helms, C. A.: MRI of the Body, 2nd ed. New York, Raven Press, 1992.)

Some myxomas contain a considerable amount of iron and can show the same effect, so confident distinction between myxoma and clot may not always be possible. Differentiation between tumor and thrombus has not been possible using the ECG-gated spin-echo sequence. Differentiation between tumor and blood clots can also be done using MR contrast media. The contrast media enhances the signal of tumor but not that of clots.[61]

Congenital Heart Disease

(See also Chaps. 29 and 30)

MRI has multiple capabilities for the evaluation of congenital heart disease. Morphological information is provided by ECG-gated spin-echo and cine MRI. Ventricular volumes, mass, and function can be obtained using cine MRI. The volumes of shunts, valvular function, and pressure gradients across valves and conduits can be estimated using velocity-encoded cine MRI (velocity-flow mapping). However, the clinical use of these capabilities is influenced by the widespread application of echocardiography and Doppler techniques for many of these same purposes. Consequently, the current clinical role of MRI is to supplement the information acquired by echocardiography.

Reports from several centers indicate encouraging results with MRI for the evaluation of patients with congenital heart disease.[64–82] In several studies in which the results of MRI were corroborated by angiography and/or two-dimensional echocardiography, accurate anatomical diagnosis of anomalies was achieved by MRI in more than 90 per cent of patients.[66,70,72]

Visceroatrial situs, the type of ventricular loop, and the relationship of the great vessels could be identified in all patients in whom studies encompassing the entire heart were done.[72] The diagnostic accuracy of MRI exceeded 90 per cent for abnormalities of arterioventricular connections; great vessel anomalies such as coarctation and vascular rings; ventricular and atrial septal defects, and abnormalities of venous connections.[72] Likewise, determination of visceroatrial situs and type of ventricular loop reached an accuracy of nearly 100 per cent with MRI.[72] The major limitation of spin-echo MRI was the determination of stenosis and regurgitation of the semilunar and atrioventricular valves; however, valvular atresia was accurately defined. The limitation of spin-echo MRI for valvular disease can be overcome with the use of cine MRI.

In another report,[70] blinded analysis of MR images has shown a sensitivity and specificity of over 90 per cent for the identification of atrial level abnormalities, including ostia secundum and primum atrial septal defects as well as anomalous pulmonary venous connection. However, it is recognized that a thin fossa ovalis can be confused with an atrial septal defect on static MR images. It may be possible to avoid this misinterpretation by using cine MRI techniques.

Much of the diagnostic information provided by MRI can also be shown by two-dimensional echocardiography (see p. 78). The role of MRI must therefore be considered in respect to the established role of echocardiography. The unique capabilities of MRI in congenital heart disease are visualization of the central pulmonary arteries in cases of pulmonary atresia[76] (Fig. 10–20) and assessment of anomalies of the thoracic aorta[65,68] (Fig. 10–21): complete definition of complex anomalies involving both the great vessels and ventricles[69,73] and the postoperative evaluation of patients who have undergone complicated supracardiac operations for cyanotic congenital heart disease.[74,75,77–80] MRI has been shown to be reliable for both preoperative and postoperative evaluation of coarctation of the aorta[65,68]; angiography can be obviated in most patients (Fig. 10–21). Several reports[74–80] have shown the effectiveness of MRI for the postoperative evaluation of the Fontan, Rastelli, Norwood, Damus, Glenn, and Jatene procedures. MRI has been used to quantitatively monitor the size of the pulmonary arteries after surgical procedures that either involve the pulmonary arteries or are intended to increase their size by altering pulmonary blood flow.[79,81] A comparative study between echocardiography and MRI for the evaluation of the pulmonary arteries after surgery showed that MRI was superior for the evaluation of right and left pulmonary stenoses and dimensions.[81] MRI has been used to monitor pulmonary arteries through multiple staged surgeries such as the Fontan[79] and Norwood[77] procedures. Velocity-encoded MRI has been effective for estimating and monitoring the gradient across Rastelli conduits.[80]

Therefore, the major indications for MRI in patients with congenital heart disease are evaluation of thoracic aortic anomalies such as coarctation and aortic arch anomalies, determination of pulmonary arterial size in patients with

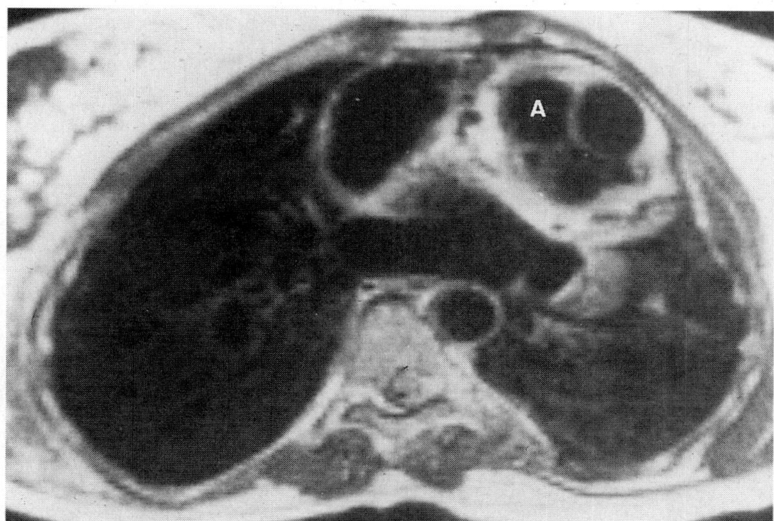

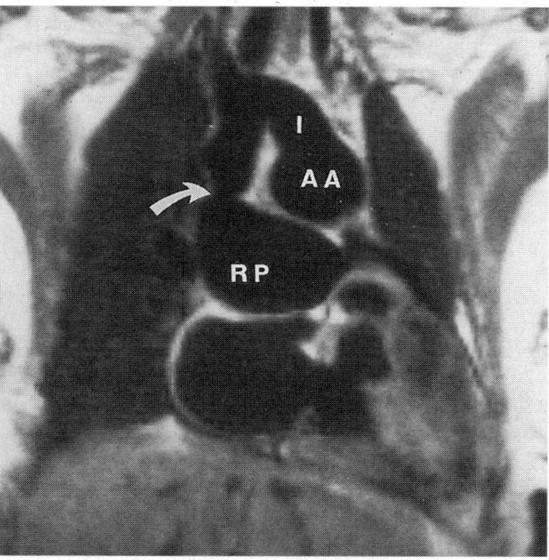

FIGURE 10–20. Transverse *(left)* and coronal *(right)* spin-echo images of a patient with transposition of the great arteries, pulmonary atresia, and ventricular septal defect. The transverse image acquired at the base of the heart shows only the aortic valve (A). Coronal image shows the right subclavian to pulmonary arterial anastomosis (curved arrow). The right pulmonary artery is aneurysmal while the left pulmonary artery is absent. The heart is shifted to the left owing to decreased size of the left lung. AA = aortic arch; I = innominate artery; RP = right pulmonary artery.

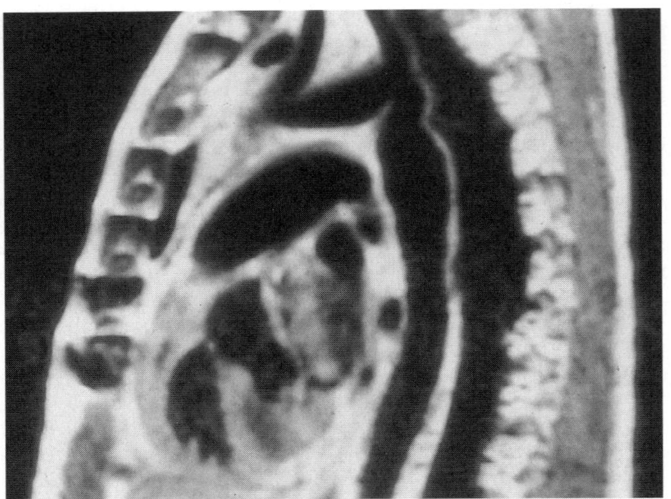

FIGURE 10–21. ECG-gated spin-echo image in oblique sagittal plane in a patient with re-coarctation of the aorta. Three-millimeter slice thickness was used for this image.

pulmonary atresia or severe obstruction, definition of complex cyanotic lesions in which precise definition of septal size and chamber size are needed, and assessment of the status of surgically created shunts, anastomoses, and conduits. MRI more completely depicts the segmental anatomy of the heart and great vessels in patients with complex cyanotic anomalies than is possible with angiography.[73] Likewise, a comparative study also showed that MRI was at least as effective as angiography for demonstrating the anatomy and complications associated with surgical procedures involving supracardiac structures.[74] Because echocardiography is limited for the demonstration of supracardiac anatomy, MRI may be the most effective technique for the monitoring of patients after various operations such as the Rastelli, Damus, Fontan, Jatene, and Norwood procedures.

The role of MRI in the evaluation of congenital heart disease is evolving rapidly. Experience at many institutions in large numbers of patients has not been achieved, so widespread familiarity with the technique and its attributes, limitations, and indications does not exist. As reliance upon angiography as the definitive diagnostic procedure for congenital heart disease wanes, it seems likely that echocardiography and MRI will be used increasingly for this purpose and will eventually obviate angiography, both for preoperative analysis and for postoperative monitoring of the morphology of congenital heart disease. Because the tomographic thickness can be reduced to 2 to 3 mm, MRI can be used to display morphology of the heart of infants. However, limitations exist for its use in critically ill neonates because of lack of portability and difficulties in management of such patients in the MR environment.

The capability of MRI in congenital heart disease has been extended by cine MRI and velocity-encoded cine MRI. The former technique can provide multiple images per cardiac cycle so that ventricular function can be evaluated, whereas the latter technique permits measurement of blood flow and velocity in the aorta and pulmonary artery and across valves and conduits. High-velocity flow causes a signal void within the blood pool on cine MRI images; this enables the recognition of flow through sites of stenosis,[80] as well as depiction of valvular regurgitant flow. Functional evaluation of congenital heart disease using MR techniques is discussed below.

Diseases of the Thoracic Aorta

(See also Chap. 45)

A number of reports attest to the effectiveness of MRI for the evaluation of aortic dissection, true and false aneurysms, periaortic abscess and hematoma, aortic arch anomalies, and coarctation of the aorta.[83–93] In aortic dissection, MRI can depict the intimal flap and the proximal extent of the dissection, and it can distinguish true from false channels (Fig. 10–22). On spin-echo MR images, intraluminal signal is usually seen in the false channel as a result of thrombus, slow blood flow, or both. Differentiation between slow flow and thrombus is evident on cine MRI (gradient-echo) images because the former produces high or moderate intraluminal signal whereas thrombus causes low signal on this type of image (Fig. 10–22). Velocity-encoded cine MRI provides a measurement of the differential flow velocity in the true and false channels.[90] Using multiple images per cardiac cycle, a velocity-time curve can be generated to display the disparate flow pattern in the two channels.

The recent availability of *breath-hold cine MRI* (segmental fast gradient-echo imaging) can provide multiple evenly spaced images through the cardiac cycle at a single anatomical level in a period of about 14 seconds.[11] The patient usually suspends respiration during this rapid acquisition. Because the entire thoracic aorta can be imaged in less than 5 minutes with this technique, it is attractive for providing a rapid evaluation of the thoracic aorta in patients with suspected aortic dissection[91] (Fig. 10–23).

A recent report[93] has shown high sensitivity for transesophageal echocardiography, CT, and MRI for the diagnosis of *aortic dissection*. However, the specificity of CT and MRI was significantly better than that of transesophageal echocardiography. The wide field of view of CT and MRI is

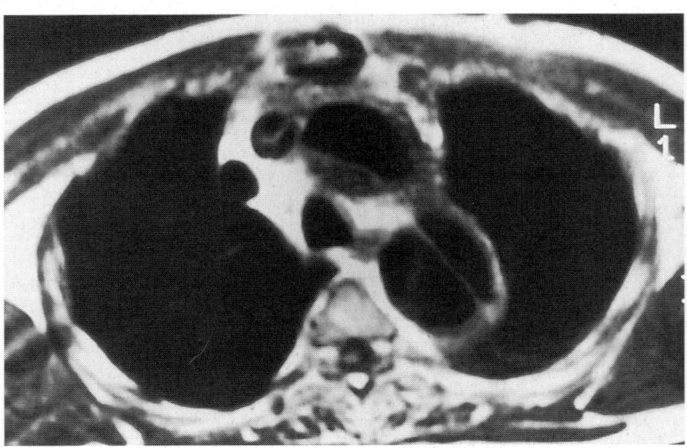

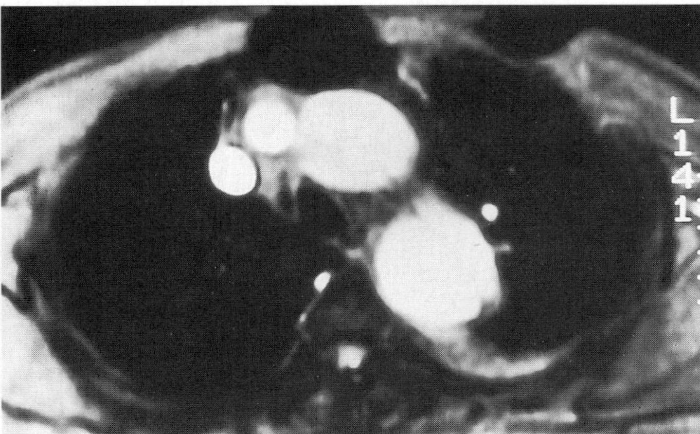

FIGURE 10–22. Spin-echo *(left)* and gradient-echo (cine MR) *(right)* images in a patient with type A aortic dissection.

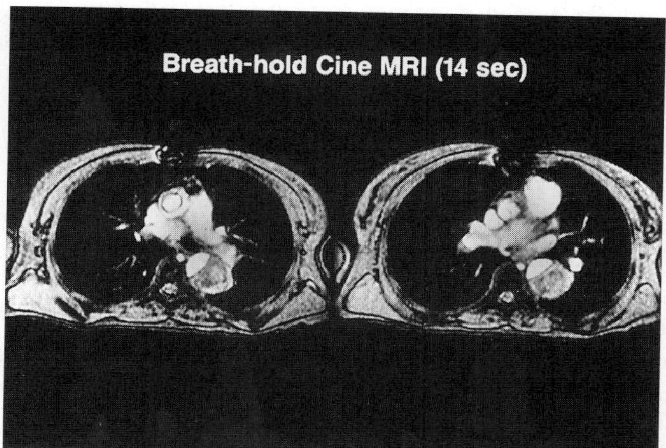

FIGURE 10–23. Breath-hold cine MR images of a patient after repair of type A aortic dissection. Images are taken from a series of cine MR images acquired during a 14-second breath-hold period.

an additional advantage for showing the extent of the dissection. On the other hand, transesophageal echocardiography has the important advantage of portability.

MRI has been used to monitor the size of the thoracic aorta in patients with the *Marfan syndrome* and to exclude the presence of an occult dissection.[88] Dimensions at various segments of the thoracic aorta have been defined for normal subjects and patients with aneurysmal dilatation due to Marfan syndrome and other causes. Because MRI is a completely noninvasive technique, it is ideal for monitoring patients with aortic diseases and patients who have undergone surgical or medical treatment of aortic dissection.[89] MRI is also the most logical technique for the study of patients whose chest roentgenogram suggests a substantial increase in the size of the thoracic aorta.

MRI has been used to detect periaortic abscess complicating bacterial endocarditis.[92] The three-dimensional tomographic nature of the technique permits precise localization of these abscesses. MRI can also demonstrate the presence of intramural[93] or periaortic hematoma. Using T1-weighted spin-echo images, mediastinal intramural or pericardial blood has high intensity.

Evaluation of Cardiovascular Function

(See also Chap. 14)

A variety of MRI techniques has been employed for the evaluation of several aspects of cardiovascular function. These include standard cine MRI for the quantitation of global and regional contraction of the left and right ventricles.[94,95] The cine MRI technique usually produces gradient-echo images at 16 to 30 evenly spaced intervals through the cardiac cycle (Fig. 10–24). With standard cine MRI, the data acquisition period occupies 256 cardiac cycles. A fast version can be performed in only 16 cardiac cycles and has been called breath-hold cine MRI or segmental fast cine gradient-echo imaging.[1]

Blood flow volume and flow velocity can be quantified using velocity-encoded cine MRI (velocity flow mapping).[96–99] This technique provides a velocity image (velocity map, phase image) at evenly spaced intervals, usually 16, throughout the cardiac cycle. Analysis of the velocity image can be done to measure peak velocity or average velocity in any selected region of interest in the flow channel. Velocity-encoded sequences can be coupled with either standard cine MRI or breath-hold cine MRI. Using the multiple phase images collected over the cardiac cycle, flow or velocity versus time curve can be made.[98,99]

ECHOPLANAR IMAGING. The most attractive technique for evaluating cardiovascular function is *echoplanar imaging* (EPI), which essentially constitutes real-time MRI. It can be used in "single shot" or "multishot" modes.[5,100,101] The "single-shot" mode acquires the entire image in about a 40- to 80-msec interval of a single heart beat. The "multishot" mode acquires the image in 20- to 40-msec intervals of two to four consecutive heart beats. Thus, a cine version of EPI can be done during a single cardiac cycle or acquired over two to four cardiac cycles. Velocity-encoded EPI can also be done. Thereby, analysis of contractile function of the ventricles and blood flow quantification are possible in essentially real time and on a nearly beat-to-beat basis using cine and velocity-encoded cine versions of EPI.

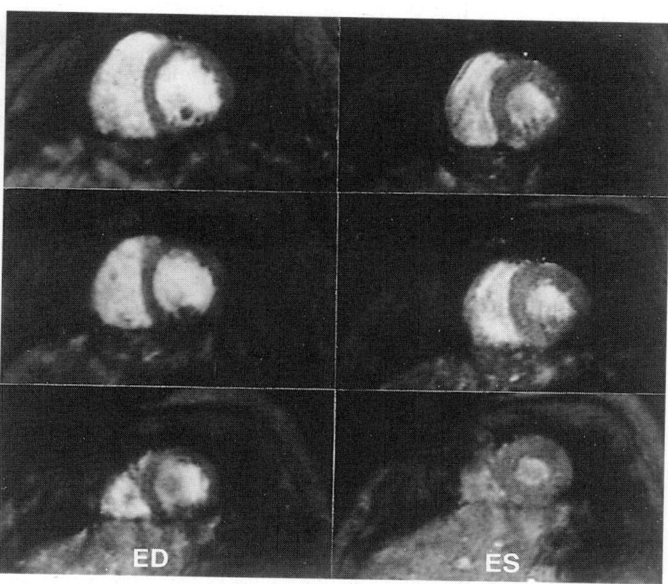

FIGURE 10–24. Cine MR images in the short-axis plane acquired at end-diastole (ED) and end-systole (ES) near the base *(upper panels)*, middle *(middle panels)*, and apex *(lower panels)* of the left ventricle. These images demonstrate symmetrical wall thickening of the left ventricle. From such images encompassing the length of both ventricles, measurement of ventricular volume and global function can be made.

Because MRI is a three-dimensional imaging technique, it can provide direct measurements upon which the clinical evaluation of global left ventricular function has been based. Using sets of images encompassing the left ventricle, it is possible to calculate end-diastolic, end-systolic, and stroke volumes, and ejection fraction (Fig. 10–24). This can be done directly and does not depend upon the geometric assumptions used for such measurements from echocardiograms and x-ray angiograms. Moreover, MRI provides a three-dimensional direct visualization of the myocardium with excellent mural edge discrimination, thereby allowing quantitation of left ventricular mass.[1,43,44,102,103] MRI measurements have correlated closely with postmortem measurements of left ventricular mass.[102,103] Measurements of volumes and mass using a single MR image acquired in the long-axis plane of the left ventricle or in two perpendicular long- or short-axis planes, assuming various geometrical models, have been validated.[104–106]

RIGHT VENTRICULAR FUNCTION. Because MRI also defines the right ventricular myocardium, it may serve as the preferred technique for the accurate determination of right ventricular mass.[107] Reasonable accuracy has been shown for the measurement of right ventricular end-diastolic, end-systolic, and stroke volumes as well as ejection fraction.[107–109] Moreover, comparison of right and left ventricular stroke volumes has been used to estimate the regurgitant fraction in patients with aortic and mitral regurgitation.[109]

REGIONAL LEFT VENTRICULAR FUNCTION. Acquisition of MR images at various phases of the cardiac cycle provides a noninvasive method of assessing regional myocardial function.[46,110] Using various MR techniques, the extent of regional wall thickening in normal subjects has been defined.[46,110] Diminished regional wall thickening has been demonstrated in patients with acute myocardial infarction,[46,110] and generalized wall-thickening abnormalities have been demonstrated in patients with congestive cardiomyopathy and concentric left ventricular hypertrophy.[46]

Regional function is usually assessed with standard or breath-hold cine MRI because of the ability to segment the cardiac cycle into multiple frames (usually 16 to 30 per cycle) (Fig. 10–24). A study in normal individuals and patients with prior myocardial infarction demonstrated that cine MRI readily distinguished the site of previous injury by a diminution or absence of wall thickening during systole.[110] Systolic wall thickening of less than 2 mm was found in 31 of 40 abnormal segments (shown to be abnormal by angiography or echocardiography) and was found in only 3 of 78 segments of normal subjects. In addition, dyskinetic segments showed significantly thinned walls at end-diastole compared with normal values, whereas hypokinetic and akinetic segments did not show such severe wall thinning. Therefore, residual systolic wall thickening and nearly normal wall thickness at end diastole may indicate the presence of residual viable myocardium in a previously infarcted region. Infarcted segments as defined by ^{99m}Tc-sestamibi single-photon emission tomography have generally correlated with the cine MRI characteristics of wall thickness less than 6 mm and wall thickening of 1 mm or less.[20] Pharmacological stress has been successfully applied with cine MRI to provoke regional wall thickening abnormalities in patients with hemodynamically significant coronary arterial stenosis.[8,9]

Wall Thickening. For accurate measurements of wall thickness, imaging planes perpendicular to the long axis of the left ventricular wall (cardiac short-axis plane) are used (Fig. 10–24). These cardiac imaging planes (short- or long-axis) can minimize the problem of overestimation of wall thickness caused by oblique sectioning of the heart using the standard transverse planes. However, because of the ellipsoid shape of the left ventricle, some obliquity is unavoidable even when using planes oriented to the intrinsic axes of the left ventricle. This may be even more pronounced during systole because of shortening of the left ventricle along its long axis, resulting in possible overestimation of wall thickening at the apical level. A study with cine MRI acquired in short-axis planes showed a gradient of wall thickening increasing progressively from the base to the apex.[40] The influence of the imaging plane on this finding is not clear, but a similar gradient in the extent of regional myocardial shortening has been observed using sonomicrometer measurements in dogs.[111]

Although cine MRI provides an accurate means to quantify wall thickening, the major limiting factor to its widespread clinical implementation will be the time required to manually create the ventricular epicardial and endocardial contours. With the future development of a computerized automated contour-detection algorithm, time efficient, accurate, and reproducible analysis of ventricular volumes and wall thickening dynamics by cine MRI can be implemented clinically.

MYOCARDIAL TAGGING. Recently, myocardial tagging, a new method for quantitation of myocardial motion with MRI, has been developed.[112,113] Specified regions of the myocardium can be labeled by restricted localized RF pulses; these are placed perpendicular to the myocardial wall. These RF pulses are followed by a conventional imaging sequence after a short, specified delay. The labeled or "tagged" myocardial regions can be tracked precisely during systolic contraction. Myocardial motion occurring between RF excitation of the tag and image formation can be expressed as the displacement and distortion of the tagged regions, which appear as dark stripes (Fig. 10–25). The extent of the displacement of the tagged myocardium can be measured as the distance between a given tag and its original position at end-diastole. Heterogeneous myocardial motion among various segments of the left ventricle has been shown in normal subjects.[112] The longitudinal displacement of the tag during systole is significantly greater at the basal layer than at the mid or apical layers of the left ventricle. Short-axis images with tagging showed heterogeneous rotation of the wall with an increasing degree of counterclockwise rotation from the base to the apex. This technique has been used to characterize abnormal contraction and twisting of various myocardial regions in hypertrophic cardiomyopathy.[114] It has also demonstrated tethering and compensatory regional contraction of normal myocardial segments after acute myocardial infarction.[115] This technique may provide the first noninvasive method for quantitating the complex multidirectional motion of myocardial segments.

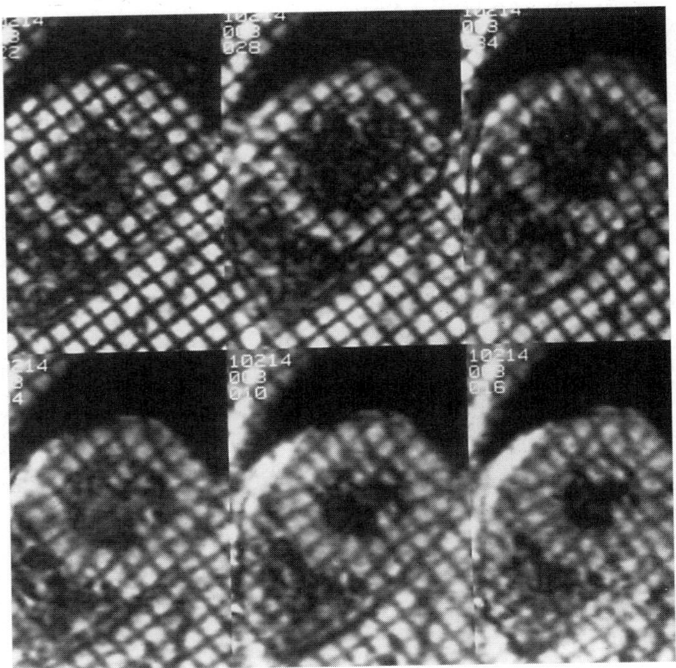

FIGURE 10–25. Composite of six short-axis views of the left ventricle (LV) from end-diastole *(upper left)* to end-systole *(lower right)* in a patient with left ventricular hypertrophy. The pattern of diagonal lines is a magnetic grid created in the tissue with spatial modulation of magnetization (SPAMM). Initially the grid moves with the underlying tissue, enabling analysis of regional wall motion within separate delineated elements of the wall. (Courtesy of Leon Axel, M.D., University of Pennsylvania Medical School.)

Quantification of Valvular Regurgitation

(See also Chap. 32)

Accurate determination of the severity of valvular regurgitation is important for the evaluation of medical therapy and timing of surgical interventions. Among various methods, Doppler echocardiography has been used as the main diagnostic tool to detect valvular regurgitation because of its high sensitivity and specificity. However, quantification of severity has been less successful. Mapping of the spatial extent of the disturbed flow in the regurgitant chamber with pulse Doppler or color Doppler is useful for routine serial evaluation but provides only a semiquantitative estimate of the severity of valvular regurgitation. In this regard, cine MRI provides several methods for quantifying the extent of valvular regurgitation, including measurement of signal void on cine MRI and determination of the difference in stroke volumes of the two ventricles. In addition, velocity-encoded cine MRI can be used to measure the volume of retrograde flow in the ascending aorta or pulmonary artery in aortic and pulmonary regurgitation, respectively.

THE SIGNAL VOID IN REGURGITATION. The high-velocity jet caused by regurgitation can be readily identified on cine MR images because it produces a signal void in the recipient cardiac chamber[116–123] (Fig. 10–26). Mitral regurgitation causes a systolic signal void extending from the incompetent mitral valve into the left atrium, whereas aortic regurgitation causes a diastolic signal void extending from the

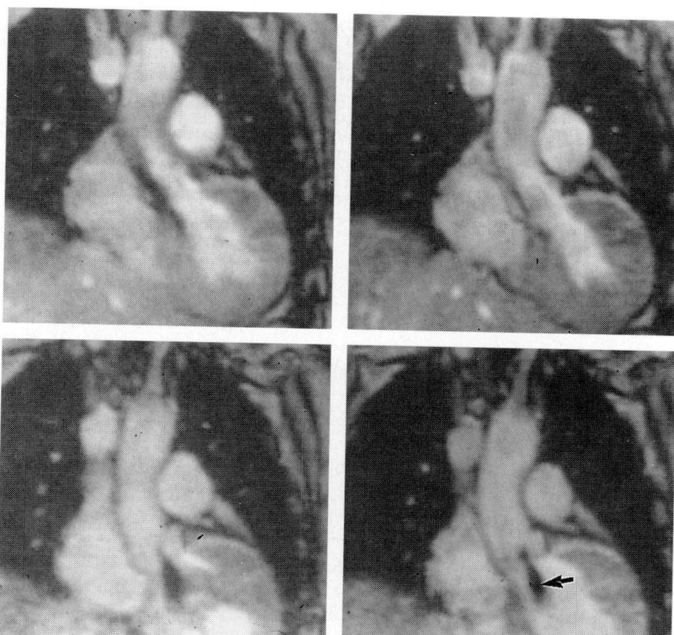

FIGURE 10–26. Series of cine MR images obtained in the coronal plane. Images in upper panels are from systole and those in the lower panels are from diastole. A signal void (arrow) originates from the closed aortic valve during diastole, indicating aortic regurgitation.

aortic valve *into* the left ventricle. Measurements of the signal void have been used to provide a semiquantitative estimation of the severity of mitral or aortic regurgitation.[117,119,121,123] The area of signal loss roughly corresponds to the extent of turbulent retrograde flow and has been correlated with the severity of regurgitation established by angiography, echocardiography,[117,119] or regurgitant volumes calculated as the difference between right and left ventricular stroke volumes using cine MRI.[119]

Some possible pitfalls should be considered in measuring signal void on cine MRI. The size of the flow void can be affected by the velocity of the jet flow and the relationship between the direction of regurgitant flow and orientation of the imaging plane. The signal void is influenced also by the size of the aperture in the closed valve and pressure differential between the two chambers or artery. In addition, the size of the void varies relative to the echo delay time (TE) used for imaging. With shortening of the TE, the size of the void is reduced. Therefore, serial quantification of valvular regurgitation or direct comparison of results among groups may be possible only if identical imaging parameters are used.

STROKE VOLUME RATIO AND REGURGITANT VOLUME. The difference between end-diastolic and end-systolic volume for a ventricle with a regurgitant valve includes both the forward stroke volume and the regurgitant volume. Because the forward or net stroke volume is equal to the volume ejected from normal ventricle, the difference in stroke volumes between a regurgitant ventricle (e.g., left ventricle with aortic and mitral regurgitation) and normal ventricle (e.g., right ventricle) is the regurgitant volume. The sum of the forward and regurgitant volume is called total stroke volume of the regurgitant ventricle.

Several reports have verified that ventricular volume can be accurately measured from cine MRI images.[40,108] In the absence of regurgitation, the stroke volumes of the right and left ventricle are nearly equal.[108] However, in patients with aortic and/or mitral regurgitation, the stroke volume of the left ventricle exceeds that of the right ventricle by a value equivalent to the regurgitant volume. The regurgitant fraction can be calculated as the regurgitant volume divided by the total stroke volume of the regurgitant ventricle. The stroke volume ratio can also be calculated from the stroke volumes of the two ventricles. These measurements derived from cine MRI have distinguished patients with mild, moderate, and severe left-sided regurgitant lesions, as shown by independent imaging techniques.[109]

The major limitation of utilizing stroke volume difference for quantification of regurgitation is in the presence of multiple valve disease. If both aortic and mitral regurgitation are present, the calculation determines only the total volume of regurgitation. If regurgitation coexists on both sides of the heart, this calculation is not meaningful.

VELOCITY-ENCODED CINE MRI. The most effective MR technique for quantifying valvular function is velocity-encoded cine MRI or velocity-flow mapping. It has been used to quantify the volumes of aortic[124] and mitral[125] regurgitation and to estimate the pressure gradients in aortic[126,127] and mitral[127,128] stenosis. The methodology, validation, and applications of velocities accorded cine MRI are discussed below.

Quantification of *aortic regurgitation* by velocity-encoded cine MRI has been accomplished in two ways. Measurement of blood flow in the ascending aorta and main pulmonary artery provides stroke volume for the left and right ventricles, respectively. The difference between the two stroke volumes is the aortic regurgitant volume. Moreover, because retrograde as well as antegrade flow can be determined from the instantaneous flow changes throughout the cardiac cycle using velocity-encoded cine MRI, the volume of aortic regurgitation or pulmonary regurgitation can be measured directly by the time integration of diastolic regurgitant flow[124] (Fig. 10–27).

Mitral regurgitation has been quantified by measuring diastolic inflow to the left ventricle by a velocity-encoded cine MR acquisition in a short-axis plane positioned at the level of the mitral annulus, and systolic outflow by a velocity-encoded cine MR acquisition positioned at the level of the proximal ascending aorta. The difference between the two volumes is the volume of mitral regurgitation.[125]

Measurement of Blood Flow

Measurement of blood flow velocity with MRI has been achieved in several laboratories using a technique originally proposed by Moran[129] and introduced clinically by Underwood and associates.[130] The version used in the laboratory of the author is called "velocity-encoded cine MRI." This method is principally based on the phase shifts of moving spins in the magnetic field gradient.[131,132] The extent of phase shifts of moving spins is proportional to velocity along the velocity-encoding direction. Velocity encoding is performed by using bipolar gradient pulses. The direction of velocity encoding can be done in any orthogonal or oblique axis of the body.

Velocity encoding of blood flow in each pixel provides two-dimensional quantitative velocity mapping of the vascular system (Figs. 10–27 to 10–29). The instantaneous flow in the ascending aorta can be determined by the product of the cross-sectional area and mean velocity of the blood within the aorta. The integration of the instantaneous flow at the base of the aorta through the cardiac cycle provides a measure of left ventricular stroke volume and the same done at the proximal pulmonary artery is a measure of right ventricular stroke volume (Fig. 10–29). The stroke volumes measured in this manner have correlated well with ventricular stroke volumes measured by planimetry of the multiple adjacent cine MR images.[97]

VELOCITY-ENCODED CINE MRI. Measurement of flow by velocity-encoded cine MRI should be very accurate provided that the flowing blood generates enough signal to calculate phase; the velocity phase-encoding gradients are accurately calibrated; and the correct range of velocity in the vessels being interrogated has been selected. The calculation of blood flow in the main pulmonary artery by the velocity-encoded cine MRI technique has shown nearly equivalent values to the sum of the flow in the right and left pulmonary arteries.[133] A distinctly different flow pattern in the pulmonary artery has been observed in patients with pulmonary hypertension than in normal subjects using this technique.[134,135]

Velocity-encoded cine MRI has been tested for an array of applications, including measurement of stroke volume of both ventricles,[97] quantification of valvular regurgitation[124,125] (Figs. 10–27 and 10–28), estimation of the gradient across valvular and vascular stenoses,[126–128] and the measurement of the volume of left-to-right shunts[136] (Fig. 10–29). Velocity encoding can be used with the breath-hold cine MRI sequence[12,13] (Fig. 10–8) and with EPI. Some pitfalls accompany the

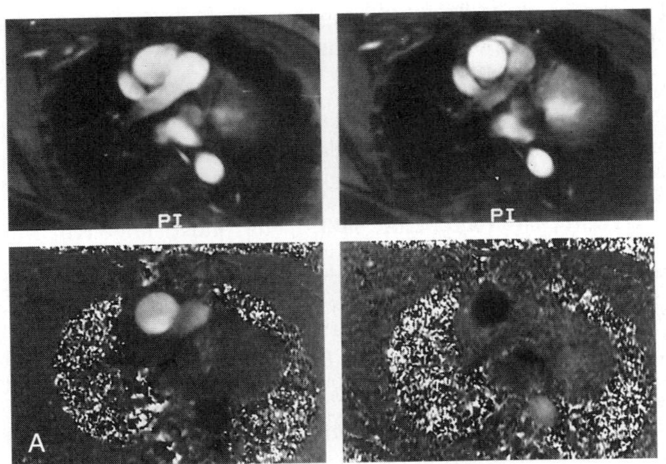

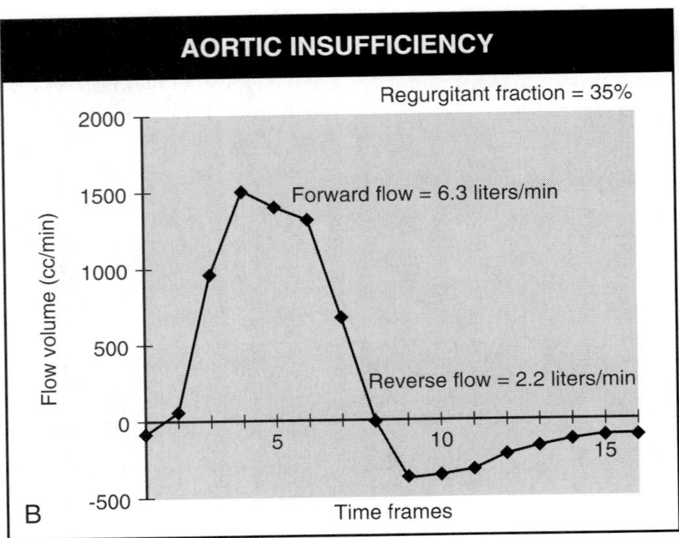

FIGURE 10–27. *A,* magnitude *(above)* and phase *(below)* images in systole *(left)* and diastole *(right)* of a patient with aortic regurgitation on phase images. Bright signal in the ascending aorta in systole represents antegrade flow. In diastole, dark signal in the ascending aorta represents retrograde flow due to aortic regurgitation. *B,* Flow versus time curve in a patient with aortic regurgitation. Reverse flow in diastole represents aortic insufficiency. The area under this curve provides a direct measurement of the volume of aortic regurgitation. (From Higgins, C. B., and Caputo, G. R.: MRI of valvular heart disease. *In* Pohost, G. M., (ed.): Cardiovascular Applications of Magnetic Resonance. Mt. Kisco, NY, Futura Publishing, 1993.)

use of the velocity-encoded cine MRI technique for measuring blood flow. These include aliasing due to setting of the maximum velocity range to less than the actual velocity. The finite slice thickness also results in volume averaging, causing underestimation of peak velocity. Furthermore, orientation may not provide optimal interrogation of the jet, so that velocity is underestimated.

ESTIMATION OF PRESSURE GRADIENTS AND SHUNTS. Doppler echocardiography has been found to be effective for measuring peak velocity across valvular stenoses and for estimating the pressure gradient with the modified Bernoulli equation (peak pressure gradient = 4 × peak velocity^2; $\Delta P = 4V^2$) (see Fig. 3–41, p. 69). By the same principle, velocity-encoded cine MRI can provide estimates of the gradients of aortic and mitral stenoses. The velocity-encoded cine estimates have correlated with measurements obtained via catheterization and/or echocardiography.[126–128]

Velocity-encoded cine MRI can be used to measure flow in the ascending aorta and pulmonary artery simultaneously in order to quantify the volume of some left-to-right shunts and to calculate the pulmonary-to-systemic flow ratio (Qp/Qs) of cardiovascular shunts (Fig. 10–29). The MR measurement of Qp/Qs has correlated closely with that derived from oximetric data acquired during cardiac catheterization in patients with atrial septal defects.[136] Measurement of blood flow separately in the right and left pulmonary arteries can be used to quantify the distribution of pulmonary blood flow in lesions causing unequal flow. This technique can also be applied to estimate the gradient across pulmonary vascular stenosis, stenosis of branches of the pulmonary artery, coarctation of the aorta, and Rastelli conduits.[80]

Recently, velocity-encoded cine MRI has been used to provide an estimate of the collateral circulation in coarctation.[137] In healthy subjects the total flow in the distal part of the descending aorta is slightly decreased compared with the flow in the proximal part of the descending aorta because of runoff through the intercostal arteries. In patients with hemodynamically significant coarctation, the MR measurements have revealed a substantial increase in flow in the distal compared with the proximal part of the descending aorta. This increase in flow is presumably due to retrograde flow in the branches of the descending aorta.

CORONARY FLOW VELOCITY. Velocity-encoded cine MR images can also be acquired during a single breath hold and have been used to measure coronary flow velocity in humans[12,13] (Fig. 10–8). Volume flow and flow velocity in the coronary circulation can be augmented severalfold in response to increased oxygen demands caused by exercise or in response to vasodilators. Coronary vasodilator reserve is ablated or attenuated in the presence of a hemodynamically significant stenosis of the coronary arteries. Breath-hold velocity-encoded MRI has shown an increase in coronary flow velocity in response to the vasodilator adenosine[12] and dipyridamole.[13] Thus, MRI has the potential to provide noninvasive imaging of the major coronary arteries and, additionally, to test the physiological integrity of the coronary circulation by quantifying coronary vasodilator reserve. Breath-hold velocity-encoded MRI can also be used to determine the adequacy of flow in internal mammary arterial and saphenous venous bypass grafts. The normal flow pattern in grafts and in native coronary arteries has a characteristic biphasic pattern with substantial flow velocity in diastole (Figs. 10–9 and 10–10). Loss of the phasic pattern and/or loss of vasodilator reserve may indicate failing coronary bypass conduits.

Characterization of Myocardial Tissue

Characterization of myocardial tissue depends on estimation of signal intensity on images with varying TR and TE values, hydrogen density, and T1 and T2 relaxation times. The measurements of relaxation times from gated images are approximations rendered inexact by cardiac and respiratory motion.[138] Despite these limitations, the T2 relaxation times have been found to discriminate between normal and pathological myocardium of the in situ beating heart.

Ex vivo measurements have revealed that several myocardial diseases, including ischemic myocardial injury[139,140] and cardiac transplant rejection[141] produce significant alteration of relaxation time. Increases in signal intensity and T2 relaxation times have been found in experimental animals[21,142,143] with acute myocardial infarction and in humans with acute and subacute infarction.[22,23] The utility of MR for myocardial tissue characterization is not clear, and little attention has been focused on this topic in recent years.

MRI CONTRAST MEDIA FOR MYOCARDIAL ENHANCEMENT. ECG-gated spin-echo MRI can demonstrate the presence of acute myocardial infarction without the use of contrast agents. However, this ability to detect acute infarction depends on the prolongation of T1 and T2 relaxation times, which is caused by increased tissue water content and does not reach a detectable level until several hours after coronary artery occlusion. Therefore, acute ischemia is not visible until the onset of myocardial edema. Consequently, contrast agents seem to be necessary for identifying acute ischemia. Moreover, contrast agents may be useful to enhance the contrast between myocardial infarction and normal myocardium by differently altering the relaxation times of the two regions. The current status of myocardial contrast media has been reviewed recently.[144]

Contrast agents currently used can be classified by the mechanisms of action.[144] The first class of MRI contrast agents are *relaxivity agents,* which affect signal by enhancing relaxation of neighboring protons. In this class, paramagnetic compounds mainly decrease T1 relaxation time

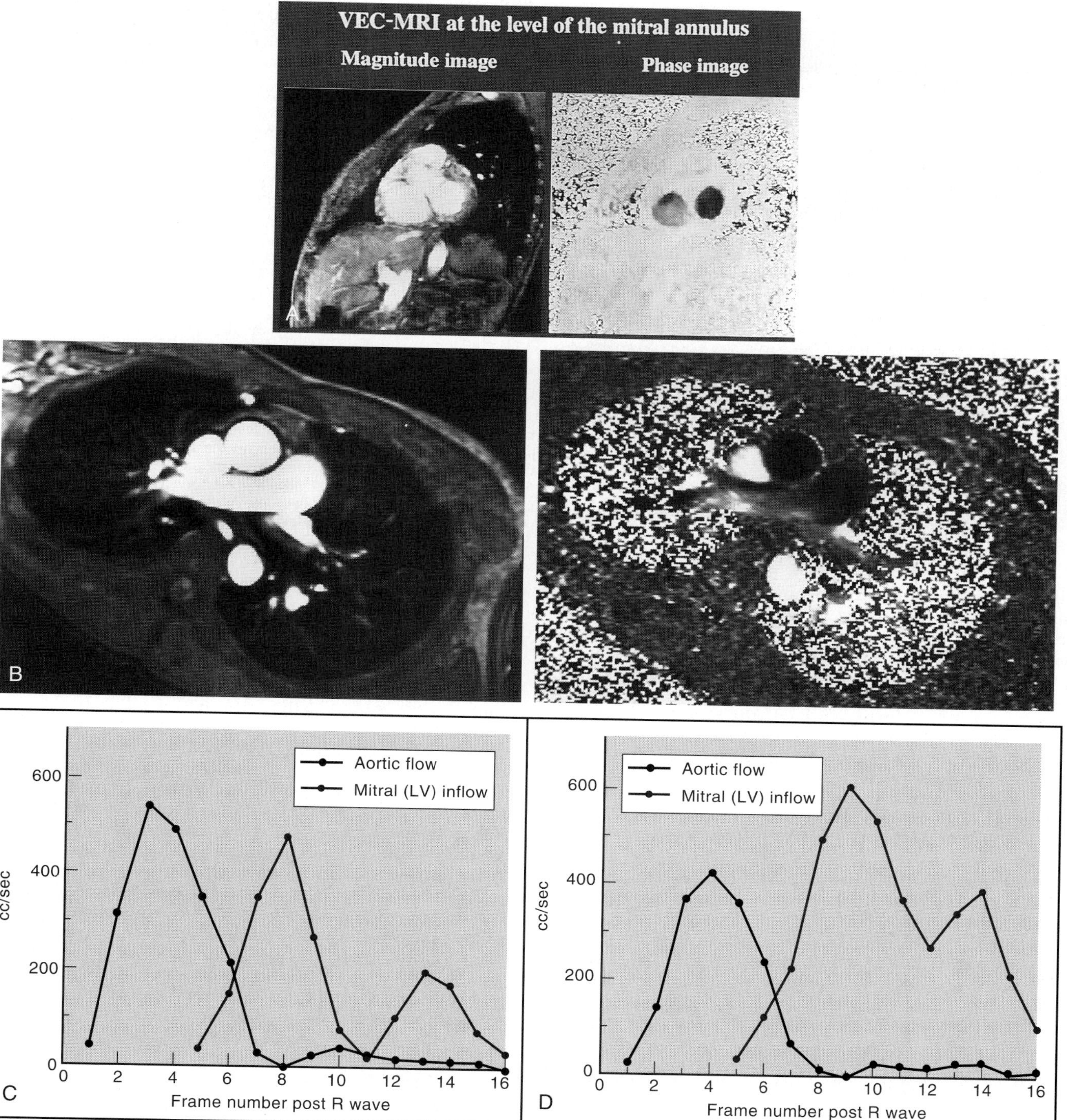

FIGURE 10–28. *A,* Magnitude and phase images at the level of the mitral annulus. The phase image is used to measure mitral inflow. *B,* Magnitude *(left)* and phase *(right)* images at the level of the proximal aorta. *C,* Flow versus time curve for mitral inflow and aortic outflow in a normal subject. *D,* Flow versus time curve in a patient with mitral regurgitation. Using phase images, flow is calculated as the spatial average velocity in the region of interest (i.e., aorta) and the cross-sectional area of the region of interest. The areas under the two curves in *C* are nearly equal. In *D,* the area under the mitral inflow curve is considerably greater than the area of the aortic outflow curve. The difference between the two areas is the volume of mitral regurgitation. (From Fujita, N., Chazouilleres, A. F., Hartiala, J. J., et al.: Quantification of mitral regurgitation by velocity-encoded cine magnetic resonance imaging. J. Am. Coll. Cardiol. *23:*951–958, 1994.)

and thereby enhance the regional intensity of tissues. The effect is maximal on T1-weighted images (Fig. 10–6). Examples of relaxivity agents are gadolinium chelates. The second class of MRI contrast media are *magnetic susceptibility agents;* these agents cause inhomogeneity in the local magnetic field within tissues and by this mechanism decrease signal intensity. The effect of this agent is maximal on T2-weighted images. Examples of susceptibility agents are dysprosium chelates[145] and iron oxide particles.

PARAMAGNETIC AGENTS. Most MR contrast agents used to date for myocardial imaging have been predominantly paramagnetic agents. They are soluble, aqueous substances much like x-ray contrast media. The magnitude of relaxation enhancement is influenced by magnetic field strength

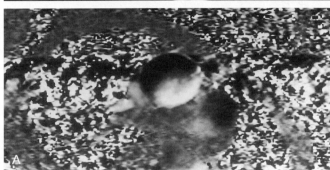

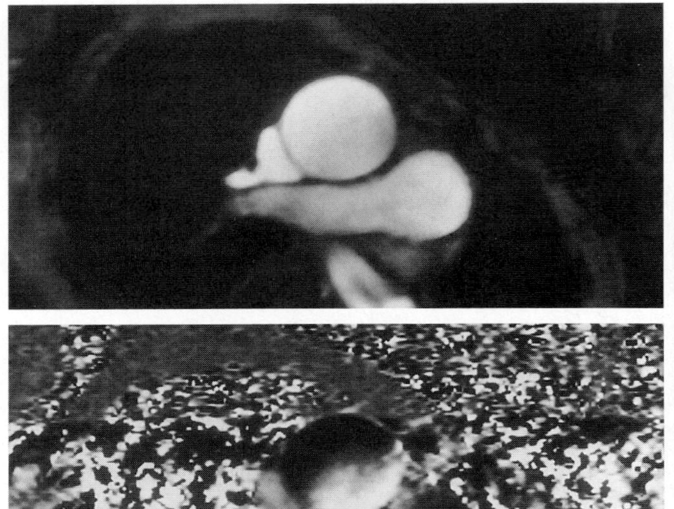

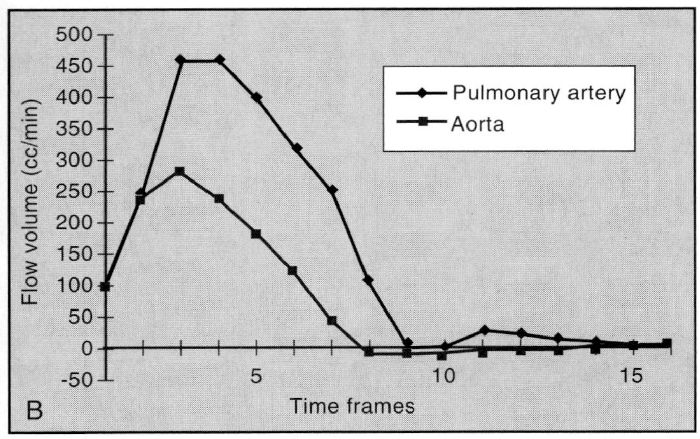

FIGURE 10–29. *A,* Phase image at level of ascending aorta and main pulmonary artery. Flow is calculated on the spatial average velocity of the vessel and the cross-sectional area of the vessel. *B,* Flow versus time curves for the aorta and pulmonary artery. The difference in area under the two curves is the volume of the left-to-right shunt in a patient with an atrial septal defect.

and the concentration of the paramagnetic agents. Although they can cause shortening of both T1 and T2 relaxation times, T1 shortening predominates at lower doses and T2 effects are dominant at higher doses. Myocardial intensity after administration of a paramagnetic agent depends upon myocardial perfusion as well as other factors, including diffusion of the agent through the capillaries, affinity of the agent for myocardial cells, volume of the interstitial space, and rate of elimination of the agent from myocardial tissue and bloodstream. The currently used paramagnetic MR contrast media are ionic or nonionic chelates of gadolinium (Gd) such as Gd DTPA (Magnevist, Schering AG, Berlin), and Gd DTPA-BMA (Omniscan Nycomed, Oslo).

Paramagnetic contrast media have been used to improve demarcation between infarcted and normal myocardium; the infarcted myocardium is enhanced to a greater degree than normal myocardium on images acquired during the steady-state distribution of the media[144,146,147] (Fig. 10–5). This has been observed both in animals[144,146] and in humans.[147–149] These media have also shown a different intensity enhancement pattern for reperfused compared with occlusive myocardial infarctions in experimental animals using spin-echo imaging[150] and a different early distribution pattern using EPI.[151]

Regional myocardial perfusion has been assessed using T1-sensitive fast gradient-echo imaging (images acquired at the rate of one every 1 or 2 seconds) after the bolus injection of gadolinium chelates in the basal state and in a vasodilated state induced by dipyridamole[15] (Fig. 10–6).

MAGNETIC SUSCEPTIBILITY AGENTS. These MR contrast media cause a decrease in signal intensity of the tissues to which they are distributed because they induce local differences in the magnetic field of the tissues. Acute myocardial ischemia is demarcated as a region of high signal in the myocardium owing to greater reduction of signal of the normal myocardium.[145]

The recent experience with MRI contrast media in animal models of ischemic heart disease indicates that these agents expand the capability of MRI for characterizing various tissue alterations caused by ischemia. The potential role of MRI contrast media in ischemic heart disease includes distinguishing between normal and acutely ischemic myocardium; demonstration of reperfusion of myocardial

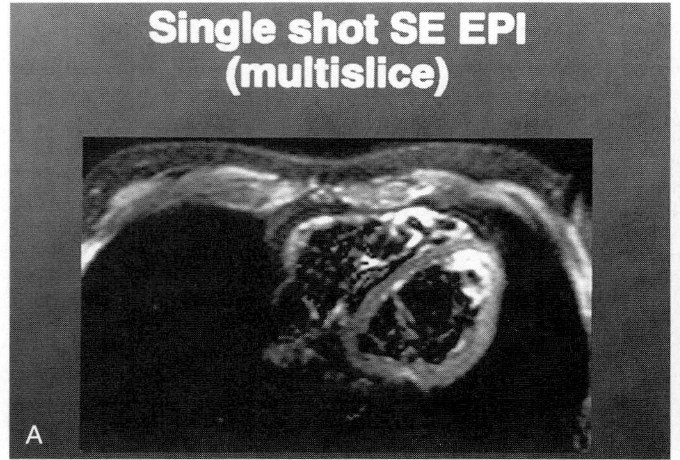

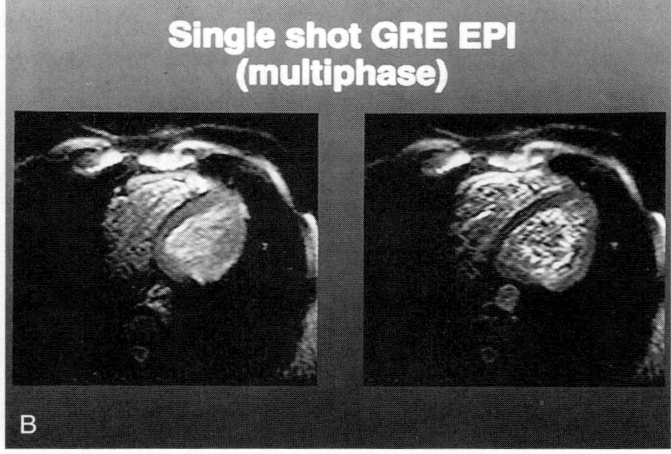

FIGURE 10–30. Single-shot echoplanar images. Each image was acquired in approximately 50 msec. *A,* Spin-echo pulse sequence. *B,* Gradient-echo pulse sequence.

infarctions; and possibly differentiation between reperfused reversibly injured and irreversibly injured myocardium. It is reasonable to expect considerable progress in this area of research in the next few years.

ECHOPLANAR IMAGING. In the past 2 years MR imagers capable of producing MR images in approximately 50 msec (Fig. 10–30) have been put into operation at a few centers around the world. The EPI technique provides the possibility of imaging the entire heart in a single heart beat. Moreover, it can be used to assess myocardial perfusion of the entire left ventricle at a temporal resolution of 1 second during the first passage of MR contrast media. It can be applied to measure blood flow on a beat-to-beat basis. Consequently, this technique is expected to have an important impact on the cardiovascular applications of MRI.

COMPUTED TOMOGRAPHY

Technical Aspects

Computed tomographic (CT) scanning of the heart usually requires modification of the standard CT techniques used for investigating other parts of the body. For some purposes, such as evaluation of thoracic aortic disease, pericardial disease, paracardiac and intracardiac tumors, and patency of coronary arterial bypass grafts, newer standard CT scanners with exposure times of less than 2 seconds are usually adequate.[152–155] Continuously rotating (spiral) CT scanners have an exposure time of 1 second for each image with no interscan delay between images at sequential anatomical levels, producing images of the entire heart in approximately 12 to 20 seconds. Although adequate anatomical depiction of cardiovascular anatomy is attained with spiral CT, scans corresponding to precise phases of the cardiac cycle cannot be obtained. For the assessment of cardiac dimensions and function in addition to morphology, millisecond CT scanners are required.[156,157] The evolution of CT scanning of the heart in the early stages also involved ECG gating of CT data acquisition. However, such gating techniques proved to be cumbersome and never received clinical acceptance. This approach has been discarded.

SPIRAL CT SCANNER. CT scans at multiple adjacent anatomical levels are obtained during a breath-hold period. Each CT scan is acquired in approximately 1 second. This is accomplished by multiple rotations of the CT scanner gantry while the table is continuously incremented through the gantry. This permits multiple transaxial scans, 4 mm to 10 mm in thickness, of most or the entire thorax during a single breath-hold period at the time of peak contrast enhancement of the cardiovascular structures. Approximately 80 to 100 ml of contrast medium at a rate of 2 to 3 ml/sec is injected intravenously, and CT acquisition is started at 20 to 30 seconds after the start of the injection (circulation time).

ULTRAFAST (CINE, ELECTRON BEAM) CT SCANNER. The ultrafast CT scanner employs a scanning focused x-ray beam, which provides complete cardiac imaging in 50 msec without the need for ECG gating (Fig. 10–31). This CT scanner is not limited by the inertia associated with moving mechanical parts. It uses a focused electron beam that is successively swept across four cadmium tungstate target arcs at the speed of light. Each of the four targets generates a fan beam of photons that pass from beneath the patient to a bank of photon detectors arranged in a semicircle above the patient.

The ultrafast CT scanner can be operated in three different modes: (1) the *cine mode* is used to assess global and regional myocardial function. The scans are obtained at an exposure time of 50 msec and at a rate of 17 scans per second[153] (Fig. 10–32). The *triggered mode*, used for flow analysis, employs a series of 20 to 40 successive scans in which each 50-msec exposure is triggered at a specific phase of the cardiac cycle of successive heart beats or every other heart beat. From such a series of scans, time-density curves can be constructed for specific regions of interest in the cardiac chamber or myocardium, providing an estimate of transit time, perfusion, or blood flow.[154] The *volume mode* provides eight scans by the use of all four target arcs in an imaging period of approximately 200 msec. These eight transverse scans can sometimes encompass the entire left ventricular chamber and thereby provide an estimate of left ventricular volume and mass. Usually 10 to 12 tomographic levels are needed to entirely encompass the heart.

Because multiple images can be acquired at multiple levels, ultrafast CT permits the acquisition of images at end-diastole and endsystole because both are approximately 60 msec in duration. Real-time sequential imaging is accomplished within a single heart beat at multiple levels, and these images can then be displayed in a close-loop cine format (cine CT display).

CONTRAST ENHANCEMENT. For nearly all purposes, intravenous injection of iodinated contrast medium is used to delineate the blood pool on CT scans. The contrast medium can be given as an intravenous bolus injection or a rapid infusion. For evaluation of the heart and great vessels, contrast medium is usually delivered in a bolus over several seconds and in a volume of approximately 30 to 60 ml. Scans are exposed at the estimated time of peak enhancement of the structure of interest. In order to identify the time of arrival of contrast medium in the left-sided cardiac chamber and aorta, a preliminary bolus injection of indocyanine dye can be given in order to define circulation time. This time is then used to specify the time of acquisition of the series of ultrafast CT scans. Scans are sometimes obtained without contrast medium in order to identify calcification of cardiac structures.

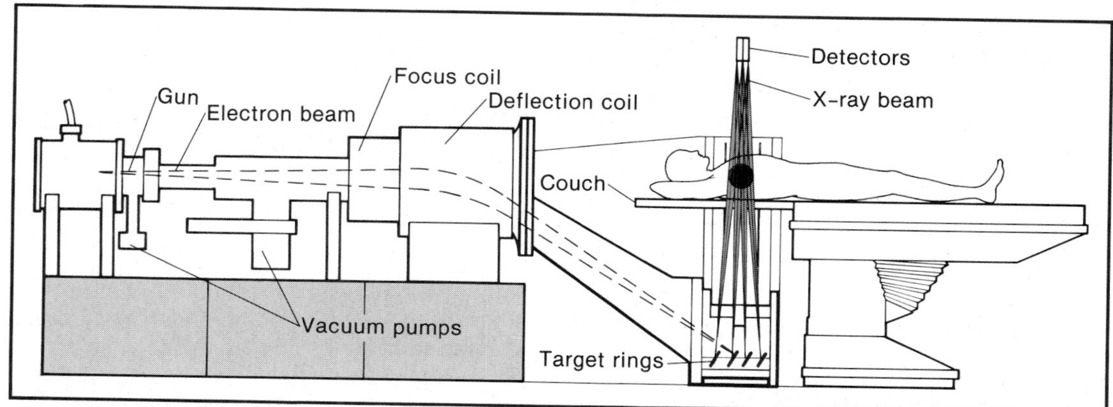

FIGURE 10–31. Diagram of cine CT scanner. Electron gun produces a stream of electrons that are magnetically focused and directed onto four tungsten target rings. Each target ring emits two fan beams of x-ray. Transmission of x-rays through the subject is registered by detectors arranged over a 180-degree arc.

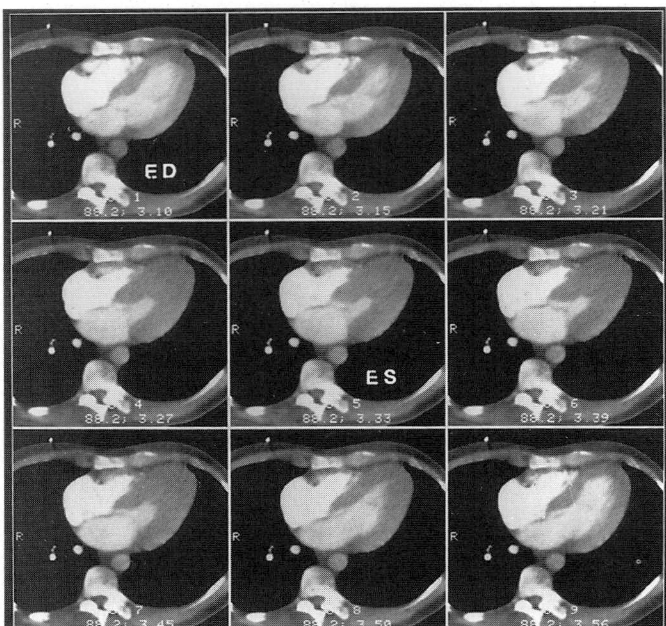

FIGURE 10–32. Series of CT scans of the same anatomical level acquired every 50 msec during a single cardiac cycle in a patient with hypertrophic cardiomyopathy. These are 9 of 17 scans acquired in approximately one cardiac cycle. Frame at upper left is near end-diastole (ED) and middle frame is near end-systole (ES). Note the change in ventricular volumes during the cardiac cycle and wall thickening during systole. (Courtesy of J. Rumberger, Ph.D., M.D., Mayo Clinic.)

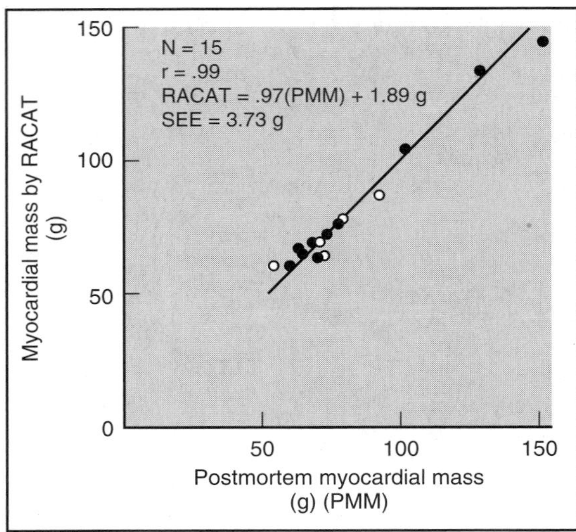

FIGURE 10–33. Graph plots mass determined by rapid-acquisition computer-assisted tomography (RACAT) versus postmortem measurement of left ventricular mass (PMM). RACAT is another denotation for cine CT. This study was done in anesthetized dogs. (Reproduced with permission from Feiring, A., et al.: Determination of left ventricular mass in dogs with rapid-acquisition cardiac CT scanning. Circulation *72:*1355, 1985. Copyright 1985 American Heart Association.)

Evaluation of Cardiac Dimensions and Function

CT scans have the capability of identifying not only the inner endocardial wall but also the epicardial surface. Wall thickness and myocardial mass have been estimated accurately with ultrafast CT[162] (Fig. 10–33). A close correlation has been found between CT measurements and postmortem anatomical measurements of wall thickness and mass[158,159] (Fig. 10–33). It has also been employed to estimate right ventricular mass by measuring the mass of the free wall.[160,161] Right ventricular mass was demonstrated to be substantially increased in patients with pulmonary arterial hypertension compared with measurements in normal subjects.[161]

CT scanning can be used in the assessment of the dynamics of *regional myocardial wall-thickening.*[162–164] A series of tomograms in a short-axis plane acquired during multiple phases of the cardiac cycle provides the capability to measure area ejection fraction and wall thickening at various levels of the left ventricle, extending from the base to the apex. In normal human subjects, a variation in both regional ejection fraction and extent of wall thickening has been defined; a gradient in both area ejection fraction and extent of wall thickening increases progressively from basal to apical layers.[164] Cine CT has demonstrated dysfunction of wall thickening and wall motion in global and regional myocardial abnormalities.[165–167]

Left ventricular volumes and *ejection fraction* can be estimated by contrast angiography, echocardiography, and gated blood pool nuclear images. While the quantitation of ventricular volumes and ejection fraction by cine CT is not a unique capability, the accuracy of CT can potentially exceed that of the other techniques. Other cardiac imaging techniques such as echocardiography and LV angiography estimate left ventricular volume, making geometric assumptions from measurements performed in one or two planes. These assumptions lead to inaccuracies of volume measurement in the presence of left ventricular conformational abnormalities. Ultrafast CT directly measures chamber volumes by planimetry of the cardiac blood pool on each tomogram, allowing precise volume determination. It has been demonstrated that left ventricular volume, ejection fraction, and stroke volume can be acquired by ultrafast CT with high accuracy and close reproducibility among observers and among studies on different occasions in the same subject.[168,169] In normal subjects the stroke volumes of the right and left ventricle as measured by ultrafast CT were equal.[169]

Ultrafast CT provides a measurement of total ventricular *stroke volume.* If an independent technique is used for the measurement of forward (effective) stroke volume, then these measurements can be combined to estimate regurgitant volume; regurgitant volume is the difference between total stroke volume and forward stroke volume. Ultrafast CT can also be applied for the simultaneous quantification of the right and left ventricular stroke volumes.[169,170] The difference in the stroke volume between the ventricles is equal to the total regurgitant volume of valves on one side of the heart. This method has been shown to be highly accurate for measuring the regurgitant volume in an animal model of acute aortic regurgitation.[170] The method is not relevant for circumstances in which valvular regurgitation is present in both the right and left ventricles.

EVALUATION OF SPECIFIC CARDIAC DISEASES

Ischemic Heart Disease

After myocardial infarction, CT can be used to demonstrate regional wall thinning[171–174] and complications of infarction, such as left ventricular aneurysm (Figs. 10–34 and 10–35) and mural thrombus. Gated CT and ultrafast CT have demonstrated reduced wall thickening and wall motion as evidence of left ventricular segmental dysfunction in ischemic heart disease. In one large series in which ECG-gated CT was compared with left ventricular cineangiography, a sensitivity of 94 per cent and a specificity of 87 per cent were shown for the detection of a regional wall

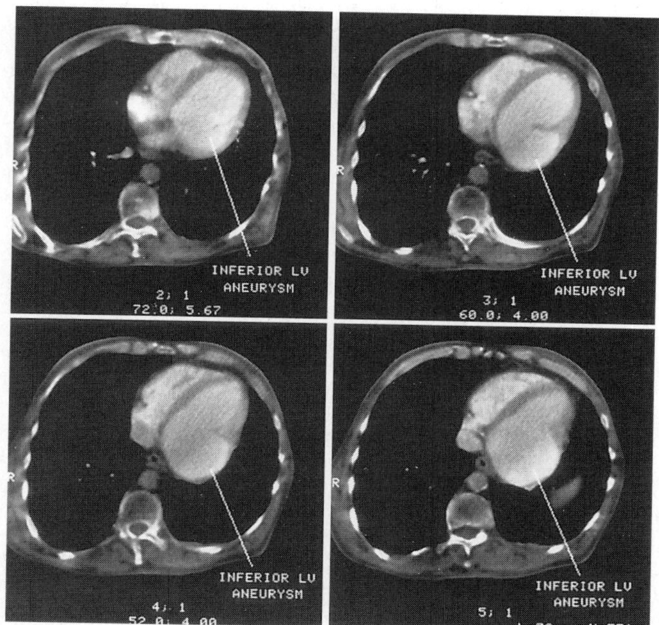

FIGURE 10–34. Cine (ultrafast) CT images at four adjacent anatomical levels (*upper left,* cranial to *lower right,* caudal) in a patient with inferior left ventricular aneurysm. The CT images demonstrate the location and extent of the aneurysm. (Courtesy of Imatron, Inc.)

abnormality.[171] The accuracy of detecting the anatomical and functional sequelae of infarction was substantially better for the anterior wall than for the posterior and diaphragmatic walls of the left ventricle because of the orientation of the heart in relation to the fixed transverse imaging. The ability of present-day methodology to acquire images in a plane approximating the cardiac short axis by elevating and tilting the table has considerably alleviated this limitation.

CT provides unequivocal spatial separation between various regions of the left ventricle, enabling better localization and estimation of the extent of wall thinning after infarction compared with projectional techniques such as left ventriculography and most scintigraphic techniques. Likewise, the site and extent of anterior (Fig. 10–35) and posterior aneurysms of the left ventricle can be well demonstrated. The differentiation by CT between true aneurysm and pseudoaneurysm depends on the identification of the small ostium connecting the left ventricular cavity and the aneurysm. False aneurysms are usually substantially larger than true aneurysms and frequently arise from the posterior or inferior wall of the left ventricle.

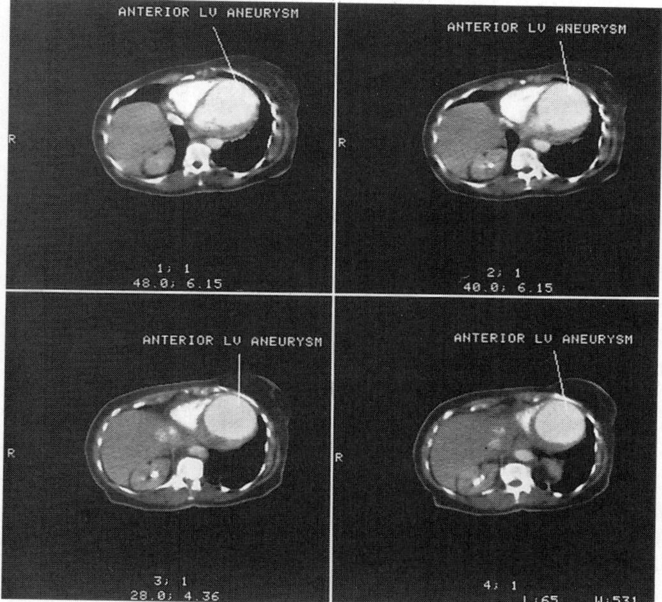

FIGURE 10–35. Cine (ultrafast) CT images at four adjacent anatomical levels (*upper left,* cranial to *lower right,* caudal) demonstrate an anterior left ventricular aneurysm. There is severe thinning of the anteroseptal and anterior walls and bulging of the left ventricle anteriorly. (Courtesy of Imatron, Inc.)

CT has been found to be as accurate as two-dimensional echocardiography for identifying left ventricular *mural thrombus.*[175,176] Moreover, comparative studies have shown greater accuracy of CT compared with two-dimensional echocardiography in demonstration of thrombus in the left atrium.[177] The comparative accuracy of CT and transesophageal echocardiography has not been established.

REGIONAL WALL MOTION. For the evaluation of regional myocardial function, the cine mode of the ultrafast CT scanner is used to acquire images at 17 scans per second at the time of peak opacification of the left ventricle (Fig. 10–34). Quantitation of systolic myocardial wall thickening appears to be a particularly useful technique for evaluating regional myocardial contractile function in patients with ischemic heart disease. Ultrafast CT has been effective in identifying the region of ischemia by demonstrating loss of regional wall thickening during acute coronary occlusion in a canine experimental model.[165] Using ultrafast CT scanning with contrast enhancement for demonstrating regional contraction abnormalities in patients with prior infarctions, a 91 per cent correlation with left ventriculography for identifying abnormal myocardial segments has been reported.[173] Regional wall thickening and inward motion were used as the parameters of regional function on CT scans; they correlated well with wall motion abnormalities demonstrated on left ventriculography and critical coronary stenoses shown by coronary angiography.[174]

MYOCARDIAL PERFUSION. Ultrafast CT may also be able to provide an indication of *regional myocardial perfusion.*[178–181] Estimates of myocardial perfusion are obtained by drawing regions of interest over various sites of the myocardium displayed on the transverse CT scans. The density of the myocardial regions is measured on sequential 50-msec scans acquired during an appropriate duration of the myocardial contrast-enhancement phase. From these measurements, time-density curves are constructed; analyses of these curves in regard to contrast appearance and wash-out are used to estimate regional myocardial perfusion. Thus, fast CT has the potential of providing both regional function and perfusion in a single study. Experiments have shown that flow can be reliably estimated under variable physiological (vasodilatation) and pathological (stenosis) states in comparison to radiolabeled microspheres.[179,181] Measurements of regional flow in response to a vasodilator could be used to test coronary flow reserve in various regions and to identify a region served by an artery with a critical stenosis by failure of flow to rise in response to a vasodilator.

MYOCARDIAL INFARCTION. CT with contrast enhancement provides direct visualization of the infarction because of differences between normal and infarcted myocardium in the distribution kinetics of iodinated contrast media.[182] After intravenous administration of contrast material, temporally distinct phases of enhancement of normal and ischemically damaged myocardium have been depicted on CT. During the perfusion phase, normal myocardium is maximally enhanced (maximum increase in x-ray attenuation value), whereas the area of damage is nonenhanced or minimally enhanced. Several minutes after administration of contrast material, enhancement of normal myocardium has declined and the damaged myocardium is nearly maximally enhanced. In the perfusion phase, the ischemically damaged area appears as a low-density defect within the myocardium, whereas in the later phase it appears as a high-density region.

In animal studies quantitation of infarct volume or mass from a series of transverse CT scans encompassing the full extent of the left ventricle has been found to correlate closely with postmortem measurements.[182,183] In a canine model, sequential CT scans have been utilized to monitor the mass of the infarct and of the remaining normal myocardium during the initial month after coronary occlusion.[182] The noninfarcted myocardial mass in animals with infarcts was found to increase during the initial month after occlusion, presumably representing compensatory hypertrophy. CT scans have also been used to document the beneficial effects of reperfusion 2 hours after occlusion in the dog.[183]

CORONARY ARTERY BYPASS GRAFTS. The patency of coronary artery bypass grafts can be assessed by sequential CT scans during the transit of intravenously administered contrast medium through the arterial side of the circulation. An early study[152] showed 93 per cent sensitivity and 95 per cent specificity for defining graft patency using coronary angiography as the standard of reference. Subsequent reports in larger numbers of patients have shown somewhat lower diagnostic accuracy of standard CT in defining graft patency.[153,154] Although all reports show high diagnostic accuracy for evaluation of grafts to the left anterior descending coronary artery system, the accuracy for assessing grafts to the circumflex and right coronary arterial systems is poorer.[152–154] Another limitation of the technique is the inability to identify grafts with significant stenoses.[184] Several reports have indicated high accuracy of ultrafast CT for defining the patency of coronary artery bypass grafts.[185–187] The diagnostic accuracy of ultrafast CT for defining the patency of saphenous grafts and internal mammary bypasses has been shown to be greater than 90 per cent in amulticenter study.[185] High accuracy was shown for defining patency of grafts to the left anterior descending, circumflex branches, and right coronary arterial branches. CT scanning has been used to assess graft patency within the first several days after bypass surgery with a view to reoperation in the event of documented early occlusion.[188,189]

The site of the bypass graft on contrast-enhanced CT scans can be related to a clock. The grafts to the right coronary artery are situated between 9 and 11 o'clock; grafts to the left anterior descending artery system are situated at 12 to 2 o'clock, and the graft to the circumflex coronary system is located at 2 to 4 o'clock (Fig. 10–36). Diagnostic confidence is enhanced by visualizing the grafts at two adjacent anatomical levels and by showing contrast enhancement of the graft simultaneously with aortic opacification.

CORONARY ARTERIAL CALCIFICATION. Calcification in the coronary arteries usually indicates the presence of atherosclerosis (p. 1298). Although the early stages of atherosclerosis exist without calcification and calcification can exist in the coronary arteries in the absence of hemodynamically significant arterial obstruction, the detection of calcification increases the likelihood of significant coronary arterial obstructive disease in a specified population of patients. Older studies[190–192] have revealed that in patients being studied by coronary arteriography, the absence of fluoroscopically detectable coronary arterial calcification is usually associated with no significant arterial stenoses and the presence of calcification with significant stenoses (>50 per cent reduction in luminal diameter). Because the population of patients used in these studies contained a preponderance of patients with symptomatic disease, the role of detection of calcium as an indicator of occult disease was an unresolved question. Hamby et al.[190] demonstrated in a large group of patients that fluoroscopically detectable calcification increased the likelihood of significant coronary arterial disease by severalfold in patients less than 60 years of age. The positive predictive value was highest in younger subjects and in women. In comparison with exercise electrocardiography, fluoroscopic detection of calcification has been shown to be more sensitive for defining the presence of some degree of atherosclerotic disease but less specific than exercise electrocardiography for identifying patients with hemodynamically significant lesions.[192]

Ultrafast CT has been used in the past few years for the detection of calcification in the coronary arteries. It can be performed more rapidly than can fluoroscopy, without the presence of a physician, which potentially makes it feasible as a low-cost screening test. It is more sensitive than fluoroscopy in detecting calcification, with excellent intra- and interobserver and interstudy reproducibility.[193,194] Several studies using excised hearts or excised coronary arteries have shown a nearly one-to-one correlation between sites of coronary calcification depicted by ultrafast CT and postmortem histomorphometry.[195–198]

A close correlation has been found between the total mass of calcium in the coronary arteries as reflected in the calcium score (area of calcium on scan × density of calcium as expressed by the range of CT density numbers) and the total mass of atherosclerotic plaques, numbers of arterial segments with stenosis, and numbers of arteries and segments with greater than 75 per cent reduction in luminal diameter.[195–198] In one postmortem study, greater than 97 per cent of arterial segments without calcification were free of hemodynamically significant stenosis (<75 per cent area stenosis), and no hemodynamically significant stenosis was shown in any vessel without calcification in any segment.[195] Thus, ultrafast CT examination of postmortem specimens shows that the technique detects coronary calcification when it is present and can accurately quantify the mass of calcium in the coronary arteries. The mass of the calcium as mea-

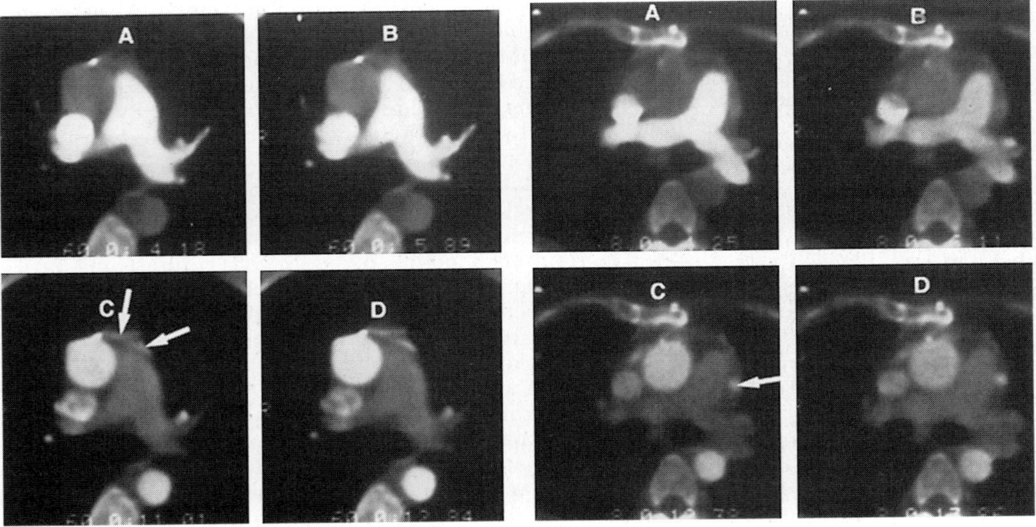

FIGURE 10–36. *Left,* Sequential cine CT scans show patent bypass grafts (arrows) to the left anterior descending artery and acute diagonal. *Right,* Graft to the obtuse marginal branch of the circumflex artery (arrow). Note that the grafts opacify simultaneously with the ascending aorta. Each set of four images was obtained at the same anatomical level. The images were done with the passage of contrast medium through the central circulation. Early images *(A,B)* show contrast in the pulmonary artery and later images *(C,D)* show contrast in the aorta and bypass grafts.

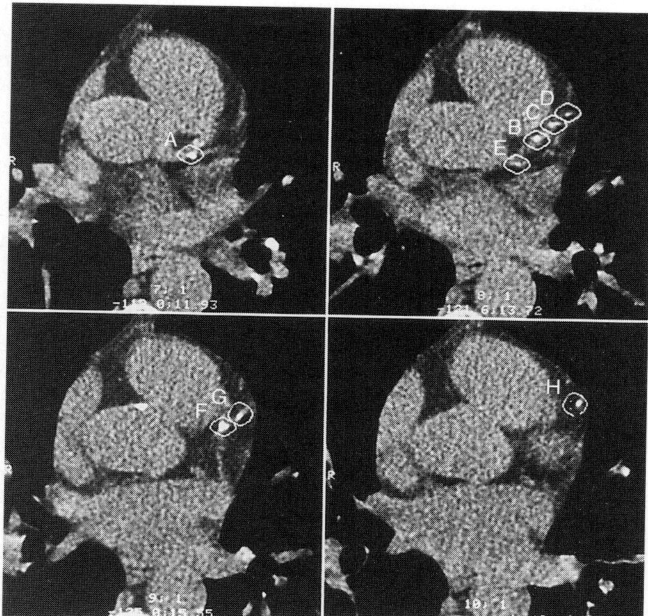

FIGURE 10–37. Cine CT scans obtained without contrast medium used to detect the presence, severity, and extent of coronary arterial calcification. Adjacent images extending from cranial *(upper left)* to caudal *(lower right)*. Sites of calcification are labeled A to H. There are multiple sites of calcification in the proximal and mid left anterior descending artery.

sured by ultrafast CT is closely related to the number of arterial segments and number of arteries containing nonobstructive and obstructive atherosclerotic plaques and the total atherosclerotic burden of the coronary arterial system.

PREDICTION OF PRESENCE OF CORONARY STENOSIS. The presence of coronary arterial calcification, the number of coronary arteries with calcification, and the total mass of coronary calcification in the coronary circulation have been used to predict the presence of any degree of coronary arterial stenosis and hemodynamically significant stenosis compared with coronary arteriography.[199–201] The sensitivity for predicting any degree of stenosis or hemodynamically significant stenosis has been high, usually exceeding 90 per cent, but the specificity is only fair. The mass of calcium is quantified by calculating the calcium score (total area of calcium × density weighting) (Fig. 10–37).[193]

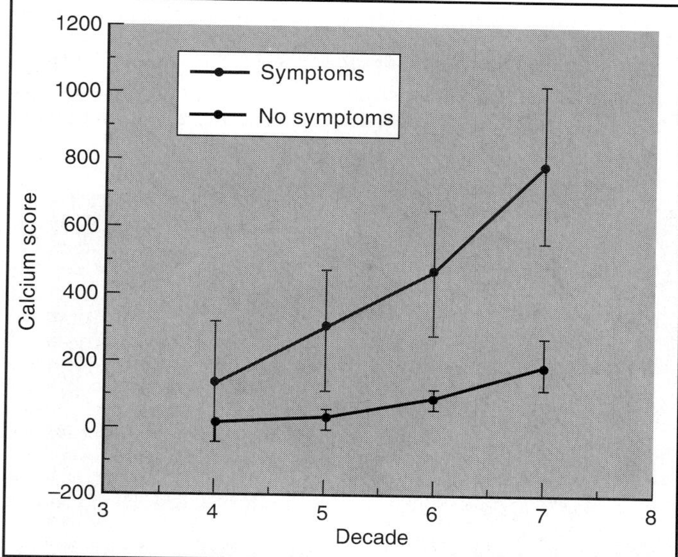

FIGURE 10–38. Plot of coronary arterial calcium score versus decade of age for groups of patients with and without known (symptomatic) coronary disease. (From Agatston, A. S., Janowitz, W. R., Hildner, E. J., et al.: Quantification of coronary artery calcium using ultrafast computed tomography. Reprinted with permission of the American College of Cardiology. J. Am. Coll. Cardiol. *15*:827, 1990.)

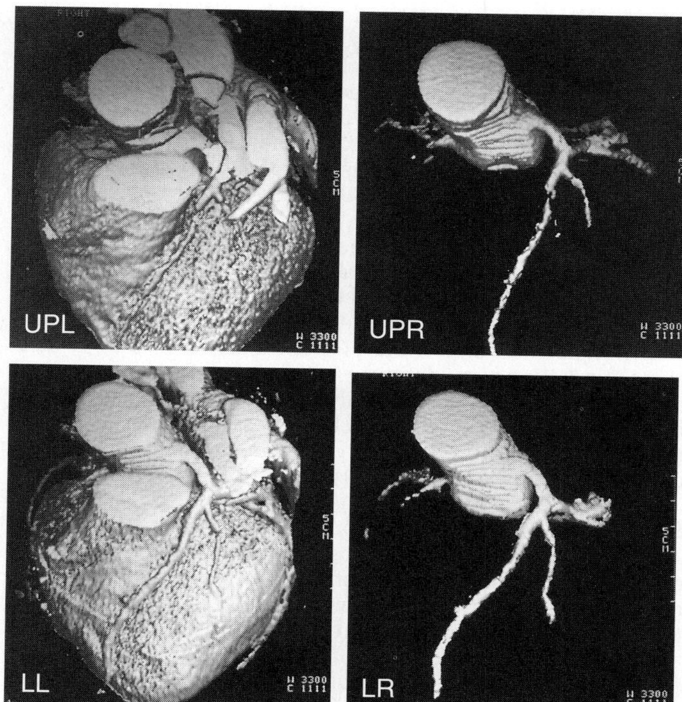

FIGURE 10–39. Reconstructed image of the left anterior ascending coronary artery produced from contiguous ultrafast CT scans acquired in diastole. Postprocessing of data shows three-dimensional reconstructions *(left)* of the images and isolated projectional images *(right)* of the artery before *(above)* and after angioplasty *(below)*. (Courtesy of Imatron, Inc., and Werner Moshage, M.D., University of Erlangen.)

The prevalence of coronary arterial calcification detected by ultrafast CT in women is half that of men until the age of 60; the distribution of calcium scores of men between the ages 40 and 69 years was nearly identical to that of women between ages 50 and 79.[201] Because the presence of coronary calcification and the calcium score increase with age,[193] the usefulness of ultrafast CT for identifying patients at a higher risk for significant coronary arterial disease decreases with increasing age (Fig. 10–38). Although the sensitivity remains high even in patients under 50 years, the specificity for predicting significant stenosis is still only fair.[202]

The role of ultrafast CT in identifying patients at higher risk for the development of symptomatic coronary arterial disease, cardiac morbidity, and death remains somewhat controversial. As a potential screening test, it does have high sensitivity and can be performed rapidly, inexpensively, and noninvasively. Perhaps its role at the current time is to indicate patients with some degree of atherosclerotic coronary arterial disease who should enter strict risk-reduction programs. The absence of coronary arterial calcification by ultrafast CT makes the presence of significant coronary arterial disease very unlikely. However, it does not totally exclude such disease.[202]

CORONARY ANGIOGRAPHY. Recently, ultrafast CT has been used to image the coronary arteries. This is done by acquiring contiguous or overlapping thin CT scans at the same phase of diastole during breath holding. From this three-dimensional data set, projectional images are produced which display the major coronary arterial branches (Fig. 10–39). Postprocessing of the data set can be done to subtract the heart from the image and thereby provide an isolated projectional image of the coronary arteries (Fig. 10–39).

Pericardial Disease

(See also Chap. 43)

Computed tomography provides distinct visualization of the pericardium in most patients. Discrimination of the pericardial line from the myocardium depends upon the presence of some epicardial and pericardial fat; it has been reported to be visible on CT scans of 95 per cent of normal subjects.[203] Although visible over the right atrium and ventricle in most subjects, it is frequently not detectable on the lateral and posterior walls of the left ventricle. The mean width of the line in normal subjects is 2.2 mm at its thinnest portion and is always less than 4 mm. Pericardial thickness is usually normal near its diaphragmatic attachments. CT also frequently demonstrates the superior recesses of the pericardium extending over the ascending aorta and lateral to the main pulmonary artery. These recesses may be distended in the presence of a pericardial effusion.

Two-dimensional echocardiography is an extremely effective technique for the diagnosis of pericardial abnormalities and is the primary modality for evaluation of suspected pericardial disease (p. 93). Although it is extremely sensitive for the detection of pericardial effusion, it has some limitations in defining loculated effusions, hemorrhagic effusions, and especially pericardial thickening. CT is especially effective in depicting these entities.[204,205] Consequently, it is complementary to echocardiography in the diagnosis and assessment of pericardial disease.

CONGENITAL ABNORMALITIES AND CYSTS OF THE PERICARDIUM (see also p. 1522). Congenital abnormalities, such as absence of the pericardium[206] and pericardial cyst[204,205,207,208] can be well demonstrated by CT. Pericardial defect (usually partial or complete absence of left-sided pericardium) is recognized on CT by the discontinuity of the pericardial line over the left aspect of the heart, with shift of the heart leftward or bulging of the left atrial appendage through the defect. CT demonstrates interposition of a tongue of lung tissue between the proximal ascending aorta and main pulmonary artery at the base of the heart in the absence of the left-sided pericardium.

A pericardial cyst appears as a paracardiac mass with a thin capsule that is occasionally partially or completely calcified and has a homogeneous internal density nearly equivalent to that of water. However, rarely the cyst contains mucoid material, causing the density to be higher than water; such a cyst usually cannot be reliably distinguished from a solid mass. *Thymic* and *bronchogenic cysts,* which may be adjacent to the pericardium, also may show homogeneous water density on CT densitometry and may be indistinguishable from pericardial cysts.

PERICARDIAL FLUID (see also p. 1485). Fluid in the pericardial space may be reliably detected by CT.[204,209] This technique can also provide an accurate estimate of the volume of this fluid.[209] Although two-dimensional echocardiography is sufficient and, for economic and logistic reasons, more clinically efficacious for the primary evaluation of most pericardial effusions, CT is indicated in some special situations. Loculated effusions (especially anterior loculations), which may pose difficulty for echocardiography, are readily demonstrated on CT[205] because of the wide field of view provided and the potentially three-dimensional nature of the technique. CT can be effective not only for diagnosing loculated effusions but also for guiding pericardiocentesis.[210] CT density measurements provide some degree of characterization of pericardial fluid.[204,205,209] Density numbers (Hounsfield numbers) exceeding water density (water density = 0 to 12 units) are suggestive of hemopericardium, purulent exudate, or effusions associated with hypothyroidism. Low-density pericardial effusions have been reported in the presence of chylopericardium.[209]

CONSTRICTIVE PERICARDITIS (see also p. 1501). The establishment of the diagnosis of constrictive pericarditis can be substantially aided by CT. Because CT shows the pericardium, it can document pericardial thickening, defined as thickness greater than 4 mm. Focal plaques of thickening or the greater thickness of the pericardium near the diaphragm should not be confused with the more extensive pericardial thickening associated with constrictive pericarditis. However, the pericardial thickening may be limited to the right side of the heart, a form that appears to be more prevalent in patients who have undergone coronary arterial bypass surgery.

The documentation of pericardial thickening is the major discriminatory feature between constrictive pericarditis and restrictive cardiomyopathy (Fig. 10–40). However, thickened pericardium per se is not indicative of constrictive disease. Pericardial thickening without constriction is frequently observed in the early postoperative period and may persist for several months following operation in patients with the postpericardiotomy syndrome.[204] Thickened pericardium without constriction has also been observed in association with inflammation of the pericardium caused by a variety of conditions, including uremia, rheumatic heart disease, rheumatoid arthritis, sarcoidosis, and postmediastinal irradiation. Pericardial thickening may also be caused by metastatic carcinoma, thymoma,[211] and lymphoma[204] and mesothelioma. These conditions are usually associated with effusion. Likewise, primary sarcoma of the heart and mediastinal and lung malignant tumors extending to the pericardium produce local or diffuse pericardial thickening and loculated or generalized pericardial effusion. Moreover, thickened pericardium is to be expected in many patients for several weeks after cardiac surgery. It may be present for a prolonged period in patients afflicted by the postpericardiotomy syndrome (Dressler's syndrome).

EFFUSIVE-CONSTRICTIVE PERICARDITIS (see also p. 1505). This condition is demonstrated by an effusion in association with thickened pericardium; however, it may not

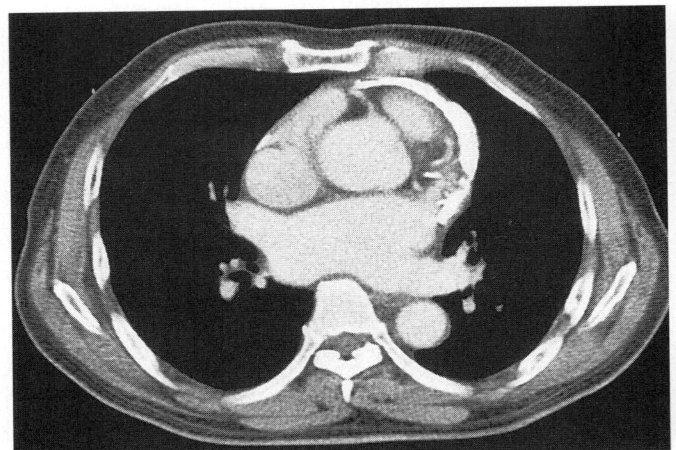
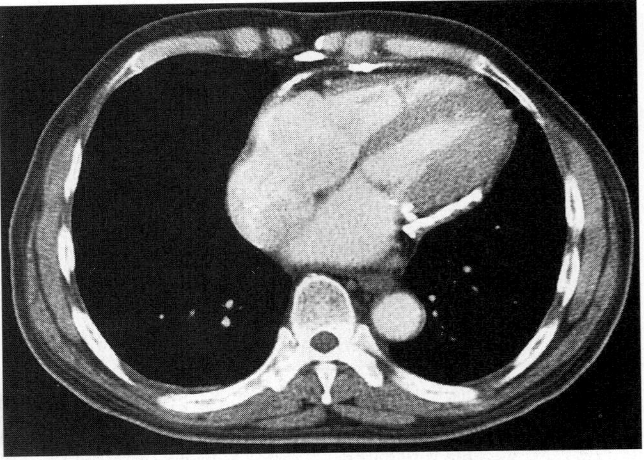

FIGURE 10–40. Calcific constrictive pericarditis. Cine CT scans at the base of the heart *(left)* and at mid ventricular level *(right).* Note the heavy calcification at multiple sites of the pericardium and extending into the posterior atrioventricular grove. (Courtesy of Imatron, Inc.)

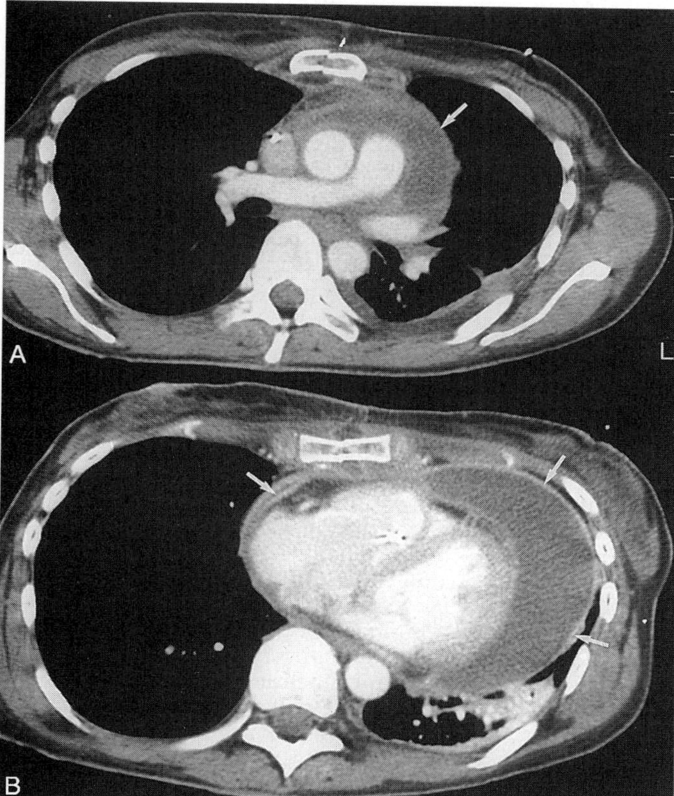

FIGURE 10–41. Cine CT scans at the levels of the right pulmonary artery *(A)* and at the ventricles *(B)* in a patient with a pericardial inflammation and large effusion (outlined by the arrows). The effusion extends over the pulmonary artery as well as the ventricles. There is contrast enhancement of the pericardium, suggesting pericardial inflammation. (Courtesy of Imatron, Inc.)

always be possible to distinguish a small effusion from thickened pericardium.[204] Pericardial thickening alone usually measures between 5 and 20 mm, while greater thickening generally indicates associated effusion or effusion alone. Contrast enhancement of the thickened pericardium is indicative of pericardial inflammation[212] (Fig. 10–41). Additional CT findings in constrictive pericarditis often reflect the anatomical and physiological consequences of the thickened pericardium on the cardiac chambers.[213,214] CT shows substantial dilatation of the inferior vena cava and some enlargement of the atria, especially the right atrium (Fig. 10–40). The ventricles tend to have a small volume and a narrow tubular configuration.[213] In some cases, a sigmoid-shaped ventricular septum or prominent leftward convexity of the septum has been observed. Unusual contours, such as straightening or focal indentation of the free wall of either the right or left ventricle, have been noted on CT scans.[213]

The density resolution of CT makes it the most sensitive technique for identifying pericardial calcification. Pericardial calcific deposits are usually residuals of pericardial inflammation and are most commonly found in the visceral layer along the atrioventricular and interventricular grooves. Extensive calcification of the pericardium suggests but does not prove the presence of cardiac constriction.

Paracardiac, Pericardial, and Cardiac Masses

(See also Chaps. 42 and 57)

CT is useful for the evaluation of pericardial and paracardiac masses. CT and more recently MRI have emerged as the preferential techniques for defining the site and extent of such masses and in some cases even indicate their nature.[204,205,207,208,215,216] CT may show the water density of pericardial cysts; this is an especially useful finding when the cyst is located in an unusual mediastinal location[209] or when it protrudes inwardly, displacing the atrial wall.[217] In one series CT detected eight of eight intrapericardial masses compared with echocardiography, which identified only one.[216] CT and MRI are currently the best techniques for defining the extension of mediastinal neoplasms (including lymphoma) and of carcinoma of the lung into the pericardium. Metastatic involvement of the pericardium is suggested by the CT findings of effusion with an irregularly thickened pericardium or the actual demonstration of a mass involving the pericardium.[204,205,216] An effusion with high CT density (hemopericardium) along with pericardial thickening also suggests metastatic pericardial involvement.[205]

CT sometimes provides insight into the nature of the mass by demonstrating the shape, defining the density measurements, or showing multiple masses. The CT demonstration of multiple pericardial nodules suggests metastatic tumor or, rarely, multicentric mesothelioma. Pericardial cysts have water density, whereas lipomas have a very low density value (− 55 or fewer Hounsfield units). Demonstration of calcium or bone and fat in a paracardiac mass by CT suggests teratoma.

Intracardiac masses can be detected very well by echocardiography (Fig. 3–105, p. 94) and angiography. However, CT not only can detect masses within the cardiac chambers but also can define fully their extent (Fig. 10–42). CT can demonstrate components of the mass within the myocardial wall and extending outside of the heart. The contrast resolution of CT may provide some insight

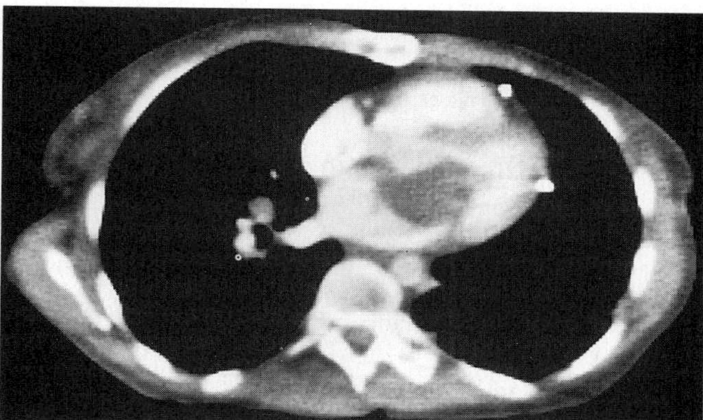

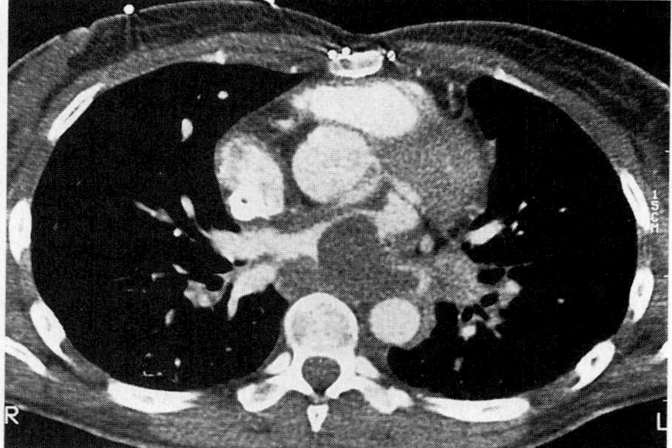

FIGURE 10–42. *Left,* Cine CT scans of left atrial myxoma. The attachment of the myxoma to the atrial septum and prolapsing across the mitral valve are shown. *Right,* Malignant tumor invading the left atrium.

into the composition of the mass, such as demonstrating the presence of fat or calcium. CT has detected simple intracardiac masses such as atrial myxoma[171,218,219] and complex masses involving the myocardial wall with extracardiac extension.[171] Finally, by defining clearly the myocardial wall, CT allows distinguishing of the extracardiac location of tumors which produce compression and invagination of cardiac walls, simulating an intracardiac origin.[217]

INTRACARDIAC THROMBUS. The most frequent intracardiac mass is a thrombus. Intracardiac thrombi are usually located in the left atrium in patients with mitral valve disease or patients with atrial fibrillation from any cause; and in the left ventricle in patients with recent myocardial infarction or patients with dilated (congestive) cardiomyopathy. Although transthoracic echocardiography is usually the initial study used to detect intracardiac thrombi or an intracardiac source of peripheral embolism, recent studies have revealed that CT is as sensitive but more specific for identifying ventricular thrombus[176] and more sensitive for defining left atrial thrombus.[177] Thrombi in the left atrial appendage and lateral wall of the atrium are more readily detected with MRI and CT than with transthoracic echocardiography. MRI and CT are very effective techniques for the detection of intracardiac thrombus; however, their accuracy compared with transesophageal echocardiography has yet to be systematically evaluated.

Congenital Heart Disease

(See also Chaps. 28 and 29)

Standard CT, ultrafast CT (cine CT), and MRI are useful noninvasive techniques for the visualization of cardiovascular anatomy in patients with congenital heart disease (CHD). Ultrafast CT and MRI can also provide assessment of cardiovascular function in these patients. MRI appears to be the most suitable of these techniques for assessing congenital heart disease. The x-ray exposure, contrast media requirement, and inability to image in multiple plane are limitations of CT for the evaluation of CHD.

STANDARD CT. This technique has been found to be useful for evaluation of suspected *anomalies of the aortic arch*.[220–222] Contrast-enhanced CT is usually required to show the vascular tissue surrounding the trachea in the presence of double aortic arch and the retroesophageal vascular structure indicating anomalous origin of the subclavian artery. Double arch is also suggested by the presence of four paratracheal vessels arranged symmetrically at the cervicothoracic junction.[220]

Although many cardiac anomalies such as septal defects, tetralogy of Fallot, Ebstein's anomaly, abnormal arterioventricular connections, and others have been demonstrated by CT,[221,223,224] the technique has not found widespread use owing to the ease and the usual diagnostic superiority of two-dimensional echocardiography and more recently MRI. An exception is the definitive demonstration of systemic veins, liver, and spleen possible with CT; this is important for complete evaluation of situs-splenic syndromes.[223]

ULTRAFAST CT. At a few centers ultrafast CT has also been tested for its potential for the evaluation of congenital heart disease.[223–225] Ultrafast CT has been found to be accurate in defining systemic and pulmonary venous connections. Likewise, it has demonstrated atrial and ventricular septal defects. Transverse tomograms provide clear spatial separation of the inflow and outflow portions of the ventricular septum. This permits localization of defects and facilitates the detection of multiple ventricular septal defects.[223,224] In addition, an assessment of the hemodynamic effects of septal defects (and of other lesions) can be made by evaluation of chamber dimension and wall thickness. Because of the absence of overlying structures defined on CT scans and the three-dimensional nature of ultrafast CT acquisition, the size of the ventricles can be measured.

Normal and abnormal atrioventricular valves can be demonstrated by ultrafast CT,[223,224] which can be used to diagnose both tricuspid and mitral atresia. It can also demonstrate the size of the atrium above the atretic valve.

Ultrafast CT has been effective for demonstrating abnormal arterioventricular connections, including transposition complexes and double-outlet right ventricle.[223,224] Abnormalities of the pulmonary arteries, such as congenital absence, peripheral coarctations, and hypoplasia, have been demonstrated by this technique.[224] However, cine CT is not recommended for this purpose because multiplanar MRI has been shown in recent years to be the most effective technique for assessing pulmonary arterial anomalies.

Congenital anomalies of the coronary arteries (see p. 967) have been demonstrated very well using ultrafast CT scans positioned at the base of the heart.[226] Ectopic origin of coronary arteries and coronary arteriovenous fistulae have been effectively demonstrated by this technique.[226] Contrast-enhanced ultrafast CT is probably the noninvasive procedure of choice for the diagnosis and exclusion of major or minor anomalies of origin and course of the coronary arteries.

EVALUATION OF CARDIAC FUNCTION IN CONGENITAL HEART DISEASE. This can be accomplished in patients with congenital heart disease by ultrafast CT which, along with cine MRI, may be the best technique for quantitating right ventricular volumes and ejection fraction. In addition, ultrafast CT can be used to estimate the volume of shunts; its accuracy has been documented in an experimental right-to-left shunt model in the dog.[225] This is accomplished by measuring density of contrast medium within a cardiac chamber receiving shunt flow on sequential CT scans obtained during passage of contrast medium through the central circulation. A density-versus-time curve can be generated for such a region of interest. The normal curve is unimodal as contrast medium enters and leaves a cardiac chamber. A bimodal time-density curve may be generated from the region-of-interest cursor placed over any chamber involved in a shunt. Using a gamma variate fit method, the areas under the primary and secondary portions of the curve can be measured in order to calculate pulmonary-to-systemic flow ratios. A close correlation has been found for the measurement of pulmonary-to-systemic flow ratio by cine CT and oximetry in experimental animals[225] and in patients.[224]

Another method for calculating the net shunt is to compare the difference in stroke volume between the two ventricles. For a left-to-right shunt at the ventricular level, the difference between the larger left ventricular stroke volume and right ventricular stroke volume indicates the net shunt value. Such an approach can be used also to calculate net volume and fraction of regurgitant lesions.

Cine CT appears to be an excellent technique for the evaluation of both right and left ventricular function in surgically corrected congenital heart disease. Because volumes[164,168,169] and mass[159,160] of both ventricles can be measured accurately by CT, this technique can be used to evaluate the expected regression of ventricular dilatation and hypertrophy after corrective procedures.

Disease of the Thoracic Aorta

(See also Chap. 45)

CT has been shown to be extremely accurate for the diagnosis of thoracic aortic aneurysm and dissection.[227–231]

AORTIC DISSECTION. In one prospective study in 26 patients with suspected aortic dissection there were no false-negative or false-positive CT scans for this diagnosis.[229] In this study CT correctly indicated the true extent of dissection in some patients in whom it was underestimated by angiography. In general, CT has an accuracy of greater than 90 per cent and is equivalent to MRI and better than x-ray

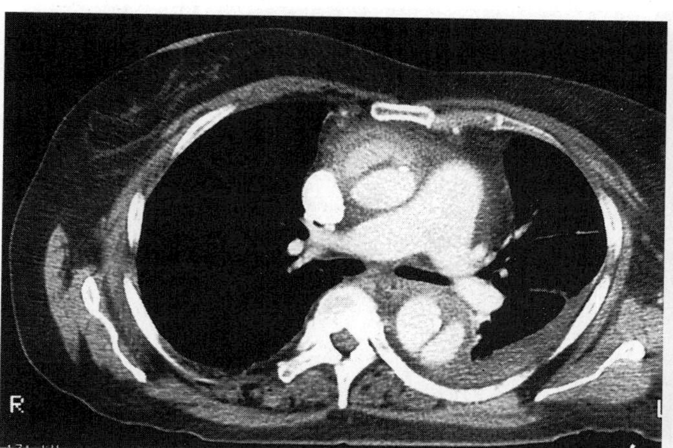

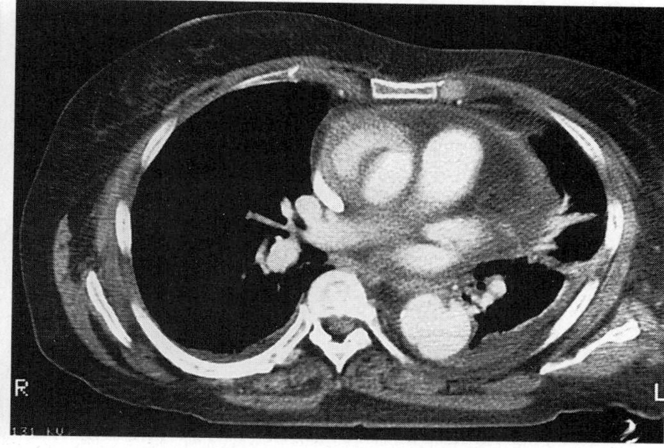

FIGURE 10–43. Type A aortic dissection, cine CT scans at level of right pulmonary artery *(left)* and 1 cm caudal *(right)* demonstrate intimal flap in ascending and descending aorta. Note also the pericardial effusion, indicating probable leakage from the false channel. (Courtesy of Imatron, Inc.)

angiography for the diagnosis of a variety of diseases of the thoracic aorta.[230,232] A recent study comparing CT, MRI, and transesophageal and transthoracic echocardiography has shown greater diagnostic accuracy of CT and MRI than of the echocardiographic techniques.[232] However, some instances of false-negative CT examination in aortic dissection have been reported.[227,230] Diagnosis of dissection requires the demonstration of the intimal flap, appearing as a lucency within the lumen of the contrast-enhanced aortic lumen on CT scans (Fig. 10–43). Intramural hematoma has been reported as a feature of aortic dissection without entry into the lumen of the aorta.[233] This has been reported in approximately 30 per cent of patients with dissection in a report from Japan.[232] It is likely that this is an early stage of some acute dissections, but not all intramural hematomas progress to the typical feature of acute dissection. Supportive findings for the diagnosis of aortic dissection are differential temporal enhancement of the true and false aortic channels or compression of the opacified true lumen by a thrombosed false channel. Inward displacement of calcium in the aortic wall is also a sign of aortic dissection. CT can distinguish between dissections that involve the ascending aorta and those that are limited to the descending aorta. In the former, the intimal flap can be demonstrated in the ascending aorta. It may be difficult to differentiate a dissection with thrombus of the false channel from an aortic aneurysm with mural thrombus. A dissection is more likely when CT scans at multiple levels show the thrombus extending for more than 10 cm longitudinally. Also, dissection usually results in a compressed true aortic lumen whereas aneurysm has a normal or increased lumen.

CT also may be used for following the course of thoracic aortic dissections after initial treatment.[234–237] After surgical placement of an ascending aortic graft, the false channel beyond the distal anastomosis of the graft frequently remains patent. Sequential CT studies have also revealed persistent patency of the false channel after medical as well as surgical therapy: Eventual thrombosis of the false channel or even its disappearance is seen in some patients.[236,237] CT has also been used to follow the alterations in the false channel of untreated type B dissections; in a minority of patients the aorta reverts to a normal appearance after months to years.[235]

AORTIC ANEURYSM. This is characterized by an increase in aortic diameter and by outward displacement of calcium of the aortic wall (Fig. 10–44). CT is an effective method for defining the maximum diameter of the aneurysm and monitoring the diameter over time. A diameter exceeding 4 cm is considered aneurysmal and one exceeding 6 cm is usually an indication for surgery of thoracic aortic aneurysm.

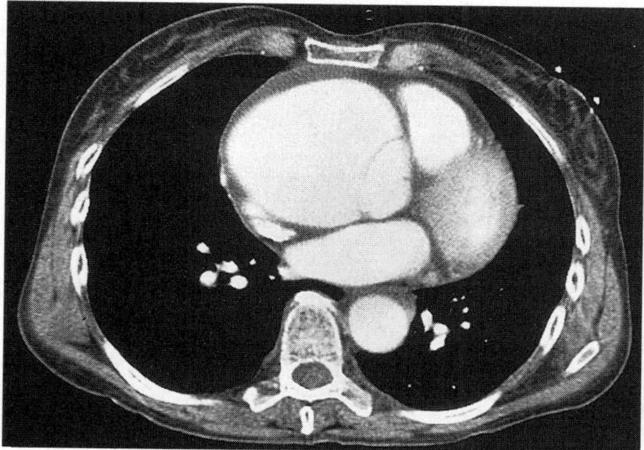

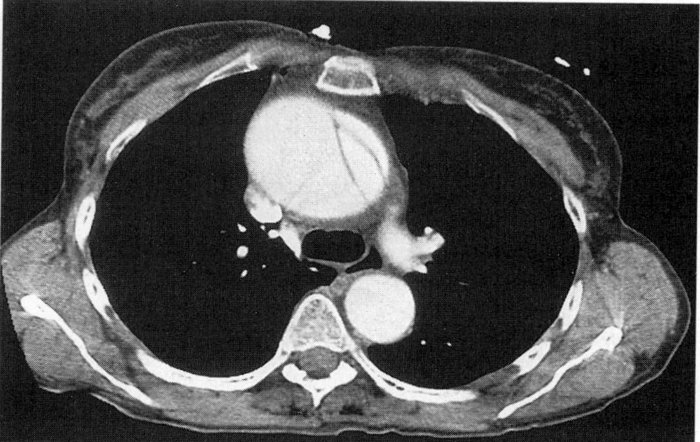

FIGURE 10–44. Thoracic aortic aneurysm and type A dissection, cine CT scans at the level of the sinus of Valsalva *(left)* and distal ascending aorta *(right)*. There is aneurysmal dilatation of the sinuses of Valsalva and ascending aorta. Note also the intimal flap in the ascending aorta. There is no dissection of the descending aorta. (Courtesy of Imatron, Inc.)

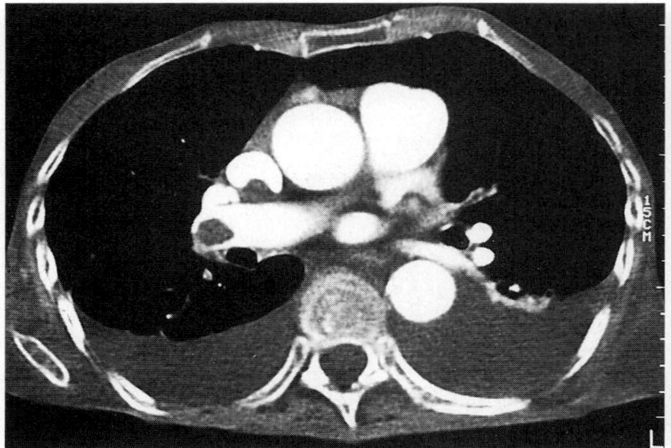

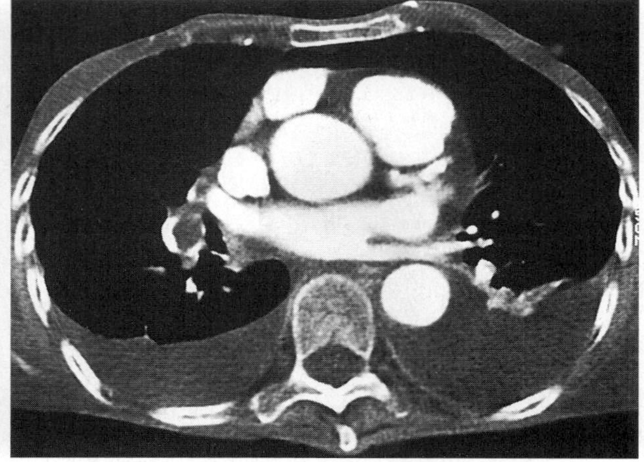

FIGURE 10–45. Ultrafast CT scans of pulmonary arteries demonstrate a thrombus in the central right pulmonary artery *(left)* and extending into the descending branch of the right pulmonary artery *(right)*. (Courtesy of Imatron, Inc.).

PULMONARY EMBOLISM. Ultrafast[238] and spiral[239] CT have been used in recent years for establishing or excluding the diagnosis of pulmonary embolism (Fig. 10–45). Both techniques have been shown to provide high diagnostic accuracy for this purpose. It has been proposed that CT scanning be used to confirm the diagnosis of pulmonary embolism in patients with intermediate likelihood of the diagnosis by nuclear pulmonary perfusion scans. At some centers, ultrafast or spiral CT has substantially replaced x-ray angiography for the definitive diagnosis of pulmonary embolism.

REFERENCES

MAGNETIC RESONANCE IMAGING

1. Sakuma, H., Fujita, N., Foo, T. K., et al.: Evaluation of LV volume and mass with breath hold cine MR imaging. Radiology *188*:377, 1993.
2. Atkinson, D. J., Burstein, D., and Edelman, R. R.: First pass cardiac perfusion: Evaluation with ultrafast MR imaging. Radiology *174*:757, 1990.
3. Saeed, M., Wendland, M. F., Lauerma, K., et al.: First pass contrast-enhanced inversion recovery and driven equilibrium fast GRE imaging studies: Detection of acute myocardial ischemia. J. Magn. Reson. Imag. *5*:515, 1995.
4. Mansfield, P.: Real time echo planar imaging by NMR. Br. Med. Bull. *40*:187, 1984.
5. McKinnon, G. C.: Ultrafast interleaved gradient echoplanar imaging on a standard scanner. Magn. Reson. Med. *30*:609, 1993.
6. Wendland, M. F., Saeed, M., Masui, T., et al.: Echoplanar MR imaging of normal and ischemic myocardium with gadodiamide injection. Radiology *186*:535, 1993.

EVALUATION OF SPECIFIC CARDIAC DISEASES

7. Steffens, J. C., Bourne, M. W., Sakuma, H., et al.: MR imaging of ischemic heart disease. Am Heart J. *(in press)*.
8. Pennell, D. J., Underwood, S. R., and Langmore, D. B.: Detection of coronary artery disease using MR imaging with dipyridamole. J. Comput. Assist. Tomogr. *14*:167, 1990.
9. Baer, F. M., Smolarz, K., Jungebulsing, M., et al.: Feasibility of high dose dipyridamole-magnetic resonance imaging for the detection of coronary disease and comparison with coronary angiography. Am. J. Cardiol. *69*:51, 1992.
10. Edelman, R. R., Manning, W. J., Burstein, D., et al.: Coronary arteries: Breath hold MR angiography. Radiology *181*:641, 1991.
11. Sakuma, H., Caputo, G. R., Steffens, J. C., et al.: Breath-hold MR cine angiography of coronary arteries in healthy volunteers: Value of multiangle oblique imaging planes. A.J.R. *163*:533, 1994.
12. Edelman, R. R., Manning, W. L., Gervino, E., et al.: Flow velocity quantification in human coronary arteries with breath hold MR angiography. J. Magn. Reson. Imag. *3*:699, 1993.
13. Sakuma, H., Blake L. M., Amidon, T. M., et al.: Noninvasive measurement of coronary flow reserve in humans using breath-hold velocity encoded cine MR imaging. Radiology. *(submitted for publication)*.
14. Wilke, N., Simm, C., Zhong, J., et al.: Contrast enhanced first pass myocardial perfusion imaging: Correlation between myocardial blood flow in dogs at rest and during hyperemia. Magn. Reson. Med. *29*:485, 1993.
15. Saeed, M., Wendland, M. F., Sakuma, H., et al.: Coronary artery stenosis: Detection with contrast-enhanced MR imaging in dogs. Radiology *196*:79, 1995.
16. Higgins, C. B., Lanzer, P., Stark, D., et al.: Imaging by nuclear magnetic resonance in patients with chronic ischemic heart disease. Circulation *69*:523, 1984.
17. McNamara, M. T., and Higgins, C. B.: Magnetic resonance imaging of chronic myocardial infarctions in man. A.J.R. *146*:315, 1986.
18. Akins, E. W., Hill, J. A., Sievers, K. W., et al.: Assessment of left ventricular wall thickness in healed myocardial infarction by magnetic resonance imaging. Am. J. Cardiol. *59*:24, 1987.
19. Sechtem, U., Sommerhoff, B. A., Markiewicz, W., et al.: Assessment of regional left ventricular wall thickening by magnetic resonance imaging: Evaluation in normal persons and patients with global and regional dysfunction. Am. J. Cardiol. *59*:145, 1987.
20. Sechtem, U., Voth, E., Schneider, C., et al.: Assessment of myocardial viability in patients with myocardial infarction using magnetic resonance imaging. Int. J. Card. Imaging. *9*:31, 1993.
21. Wesbey, G., Higgins, C. B., Lanzer, P., et al.: In vivo imaging and characterization of acute myocardial infarction using gated nuclear magnetic resonance. Circulation *69*:125, 1984.
22. McNamara, M. T., Higgins, C. B., Schechtmann, N., et al.: Detection and characterization of acute myocardial infarctions in man using gated magnetic resonance imaging. Circulation *71*:717, 1985.
23. Wisenberg, G., Finnie, K., Jablonsky, G., et al.: Nuclear magnetic resonance and radionuclide angiographic assessment of acute myocardial infarction in a randomized trial of intravenous streptokinase. Am. J. Cardiol. *62*:1011, 1988.
24. Wisenberg, G., Proto, F. S., Carrol, S. E., et al.: Serial NMR imaging of acute myocardial infarction with and without reperfusion. Am. Heart. J. *115*:510, 1988.
25. Filipchuk, N. G., Peshock, R. M., Malloy, C. R., et al.: Detection and localization of recent myocardial infarction by MRI. Am. J. Cardiol. *58*:214, 1986.
26. Manning, W. J., Lil, W., and Edelman, R. R.: A preliminary report comparing magnetic resonance coronary angiography with conventional angiography. N. Engl. J. Med. *328*:828, 1993.
27. White, R. D., Caputo, G. R., Mark, A. S., et al.: Noninvasive evaluation of coronary artery bypass graft patency using magnetic resonance imaging. Radiology *164*:681, 1987.
28. White, R. D., Pflugfelder, P. W., Lipton, M. J., et al.: Coronary artery bypass grafts: Evaluation of patency with cine MR imaging. A.J.R. *150*:1271, 1988.
29. Gomes, A. S., Lois, J. F., Drinkwater, D. C., et al.: Coronary artery bypass grafts: Visualization with MR imaging. Radiology *162*:175, 1987.
30. Frija, G., Schouman-Clays, E., Lacombe, P., et al.: A study of coronary artery bypass graft patency using MR imaging. J. Comput. Assist. Tomogr. *13*:226, 1989.
31. Aurigemma, G. R., Reichek, N., Axel, L., et al.: Noninvasive determination of coronary artery bypass graft patency by cine magnetic resonance imaging. Circulation *80*:1595, 1989.
32. Underwood, S. R., Firmin, D. W., Klipstein, R. H., et al.: The assessment of coronary artery bypass grafts using MRI with velocity mapping. Br. Heart. J. *57*:93, 1982.
33. Debatin, J. F., Strong, J. A., Sostman, H. D., et al.: MR characterization of blood flow in native and grafted internal mammary arteries. J. Magn. Resn. Imag. *3*:443, 1993.
34. Higgins, C. B., Byrd, B. F., McNamara, M. T., et al.: Magnetic resonance imaging of the heart: A review of the experience in 172 subjects. Radiology *155*:671, 1985.
35. Higgins, C. B., Byrd, B. F., and Stark, D.: Magnetic resonance imaging of hypertrophic cardiomyopathy. Am. J. Cardiol. *55*:1121, 1985.

36. Wagner, S., Chew, W. M., Semelka, R., et al.: Integrative analysis of cardiac function and metabolism in patients with idiopathic hypertrophic cardiomyopathy with cine MR imaging and P-31 spectroscopy. Radiology *173*:238, 1989.
37. Suzuki, J-I., Chang, J-M., Caputo, G. R., et al.: Evaluation of right ventricular early diastolic filling by cine nuclear magnetic resonance imaging in patients with hypertrophic cardiomyopathy. J. Am. Coll. Cardiol. *18*:809, 1991.
38. Suzuki, J. I., Sakamoto, T., Takenaka, K., et al.: Assessment of the thickness of the right ventricular free wall by MRI in patients with hypertrophic cardiomyopathy. Br. Heart J. *60*:440, 1988.
39. Byrd, B. F., Schiller, N. B., Botvinick, E. H., et al.: Magnetic resonance imaging and 2D echocardiography in dilated cardiomyopathy. Circulation *72*(Suppl III):III22, 1985.
40. Buser, P. T., Auffermann, W., Holt, W. W., et al.: Noninvasive evaluation of the global left ventricular function using cine MR imaging. J. Am. Coll. Cardiol. *13*:1294, 1989.
41. Wagner, S., Auffermann, W., Buser, P., et al.: Functional description of the left ventricle in patients with volume overload, pressure overload and myocardial disease using cine nuclear magnetic resonance imaging (NMRI). Am. J. Cardiac. Imaging *5*:87, 1991.
42. Doherty, N. E. III, Seelos, K. C., Suzuki, J-I., et al.: Application of cine NMR imaging for sequential evaluation of response to angiotensin converting enzyme inhibitor therapy in dilated cardiomyopathy. J. Am. Coll. Cardiol. *19*:1294, 1992.
43. Semelka, R. C., Tomei, E., Wagner, S., et al.: Normal left ventricular dimensions and function: Interstudy reproducibility of measurements with cine MR imaging. Radiology *174*:763, 1990.
44. Semelka, R. C., Tomei, E., Wagner, S., et al.: Interstudy reproducibility of dimensional and functional measurements between cine magnetic resonance studies in the morphologically abnormal left ventricle. Am. Heart J. *119*:1367, 1990.
45. Sechtem, U., Higgins, C. B., Sommerhoff, B. A., et al.: Magnetic resonance imaging of restrictive cardiomyopathy: A report of 3 cases. Am. J. Cardiol. *59*:480, 1987.
46. Sechtem, U., Sommerhoff, B. A., Markiewicz, W., et al.: Assessment of regional left ventricular wall thickening by MRI. Am. J. Cardiol. *59*:149, 1987.
47. O'Donnell, J. K., Go, R. T., Bolt-Silverman, C., et al.: Cardiac amyloidosis: Comparison of MR imaging and echocardiography. Radiology *153*(Abs.):261, 1984.
48. Riedy, K., Fisher, M., Belic, N., et al.: MR imaging of myocardial sarcoidosis. A.J.R. *151*:915, 1988.
49. Blake, L. M., Scheinman, M. M., and Higgins, C. B.: MR features of arrhythmogenic right ventricular dysplasia. A.J.R. *162*:809, 1994.
50. Carlson, M. D., White, R. D., Trohman, R. G., et al.: Right ventricular outflow tract tachycardia: Detection of previously unrecognized abnormalities using cine MRI. J. Am. Coll. Cardiol. *24*:720, 1994.
51. Auffermann, W., Wichter, T., Bretthardt, G., et al.: Arrhythmogenic right ventricular disease: MR imaging vs angiography. A.J.R. *161*:549, 1993.
52. Sechtem, U., Tscholakoff, D., and Higgins, C. B.: Pericardial disease: Diagnosis by MRI. A.J.R. *147*:245, 1986.
53. Guttierrez, F. R., Shackleford, G. D., McKnight, R. L., et al.: Diagnosis of congenital absence of left pericardium by MR imaging. J. Comput. Assist. Tomogr. *9*:551, 1985.
54. Soulen, R. L., Stark, D. D., and Higgins, C. B.: Magnetic resonance imaging of constrictive pericardial disease. Am. J. Cardiol. *55*:480, 1985.
55. Masui, T., Finck, S., and Higgins, C. B.: Constrictive pericarditis and restrictive cardiomyopathy: Evaluation with MR imaging. Radiology *182*:369, 1992.
56. Amparo, E. G., Higgins, C. B., Farmer, D., et al.: Gated MRI of cardiac and paracardiac masses: Initial experiment. A.J.R. *143*:1151, 1984.
57. Go, R. T., O'Donnell, J. K., Underwood, D. A., et al.: Comparison of gated cardiac MRI and 2D echocardiography of intracardiac neoplasms. A.J.R. *145*:21, 1985.
58. Conces, D. J., Vox, V. A., and Klatte, E. C.: Gated MR imaging of left atrial myxomas. Radiology *156*:445, 1985.
59. Fujita, N., Caputo, G. R., and Higgins, C. B.: Diagnosis and characterization of intracardiac masses by magnetic resonance imaging. Am. J. Cardiac Imaging *8*:69, 1994.
60. Barakos, J. A., Brown, J. J., and Higgins, C. B.: Magnetic resonance imaging of secondary cardiac and paracardiac masses. A.J.R. *153*:48, 1989.
61. Funari, M., Fujita, N., Peck, W. W., et al.: Cardiac tumors: Assessment with Gd-DTPA enhanced MR imaging. J. Comput. Assist. Tomogr. *15*:953, 1992.
62. von Schulthess, G. K., McMurdo, K., Tscholakoff, D., et al.: Mediastinal masses: MR imaging. Radiology *158*:289, 1986.
63. Seelos, K., Caputo, G. R., Carrol, C. L., et al.: Cine gradient refocused (GRE) echo imaging of intravascular masses: Differentiation between tumor and nontumor thrombus. J. Comput. Assist. Tomogr. *16*:169, 1992.
64. Higgins, C. B., Byrd, B. F. III, Farmer, D., et al.: Magnetic resonance imaging in patients with congenital heart disease. Circulation *70*:851, 1984.
65. Rees, S., Sommerville, J., Ward, C., et al.: Coarctation of the aorta: MR imaging in late postoperative assessment. Radiology *173*:499, 1989.
66. Didier, D., Higgins, C. B., Fisher, M. R., et al.: Congenital heart disease in 72 patients. Radiology *158*:227, 1986.
67. Didier, D., and Higgins, C. B.: Identification and localization of ventricular septal defects by gated magnetic resonance imaging. Am. J. Coll. Cardiol. *57*:1363, 1986.
68. von Schulthess, G. K., Higashino, S. M., Higgins, S. S., et al.: Coarctation of the aorta: MR imaging. Radiology *158*:474, 1986.
69. Peshock, R. M., Parrish, M., Fixler, D., et al.: MR imaging in the evaluation of single ventricle. Radiology *158*:474, 1986.
70. Diethelm, L., Dery, R., Lipton, M. J., et al.: Atrial level shunts: Sensitivity and specificity of MR diagnosis. Radiology *162*:181, 1987.
71. Hirsch, R., Kilner, P. J., Connelly, M. S., et al.: Diagnosis in adolescents and adults with congenital heart disease: Prospective of individual and combined roles of MRI and TEE. Circulation *90*:2937, 1994.
72. Kersting-Sommerhoff, B. A., Diethelm, L., Teitel, D. F., et al.: Magnetic resonance imaging of congenital heart disease: Sensitivity and specificity using receiver operating characteristic curve analysis. Am. Heart. J. *118*:155, 1989.
73. Kersting-Sommerhoff, B. A., Diethelm, L., Stanger, P., et al.: Evaluation of complex congenital ventricular anomalies with magnetic resonance imaging. Am. Heart J. *120*:133, 1990.
74. Kersting-Sommerhoff, B. A., Seelos, K. C., Hardy, C., et al.: Evaluation of surgical procedures for cyanotic congenital heart disease using MR imaging. A.J.R. *155*:259, 1990.
75. Julsrud, P. P., Ehman, R. L., Hagler, D. J., et al.: Extracardiac vasculature in candidates for Fontan surgery: MR imaging. Radiology *173*:503, 1989.
76. Sommerhoff, B. K., Sechtem, U. P., and Higgins, C. B.: Evaluation of pulmonary blood supply by nuclear magnetic resonance imaging in patients with pulmonary atresia. J. Am. Coll. Cardiol. *11*:166, 1988.
77. Kondo, C., Hardy, C., Higgins, S. S., et al.: MR imaging of the palliative operation for hypoplastic left heart syndrome. J. Am. Coll. Cardiol. *18*:809, 1991.
78. Blankenberg, F., Rhee, J., Hardy, C., et al.: MRI vs echocardiography in the evaluation of the Jatene procedure. J. Comput. Assist. Tomogr. *18*:749, 1994.
79. Fogel, M. A., Donofrio, M. T., Romaciotti, C., et al.: Magnetic resonance and echocardiographic imaging of pulmonary artery size throughout stages of Fontan reconstruction. Circulation *90*:2927, 1994.
80. Martinez, J. E., Mohiaddin, R. H., Kilner, P. J., et al.: Obstruction in extracardiac ventriculopulmonary conduits: Value of NMR imaging with velocity mapping and Doppler echocardiography. J. Am. Coll. Cardiol. *20*:338, 1992.
81. Duerinckx, A. J., Wexler, L., Banerjee, A., et al.: Postoperative evaluation of pulmonary arteries in congenital heart surgery by MR imaging: Comparison with echocardiography. Am. Heart J. *128*:1139, 1994.
82. Sechtem, U., Pflugfelder, P., Cassidy, M. C., et al.: Ventricular septal defect: Visualization of shunt flow and determination of shunt size by cine magnetic resonance imaging. A.J.R. *149*:689, 1987.
83. Amparo, E. G., Higgins, C. B., Hricak, H., et al.: Aortic dissection: Magnetic resonance imaging. Radiology *155*:399, 1985.
84. White, R. C., Dooms, G. C., and Higgins, C. B.: Advances in imaging thoracic aortic disease. Invest. Radiol. *21*:761, 1986.
85. Dinsmore, R. E., Liberthson, R. R., Wismer, G. L., et al.: Magnetic resonance imaging of thoracic aortic aneurysms. A.J.R. *146*:309, 1986.
86. Kersting-Sommerhoff, B. A., Higgins, C. B., White, R. D., et al.: Aortic dissection: Sensitivity and specificity of MR imaging. Radiology *3*:651, 1988.
87. Laissy, J-P., Blanc, F., Soyer, P., et al.: Thoracic aortic dissection: Diagnosis with transesophageal echocardiography vs MR imaging. Radiology *194*:331, 1995.
88. Sommerhoff, B. A., Sechtem, U. P., Schiller, N. B., et al.: MRI of thoracic aorta in Marfan patients. J. Comput. Assist. Tomogr. *11*:633, 1987.
89. White, R. D., Ullyot, D. J., and Higgins, C. B.: MR imaging of the aorta after surgery for aortic dissection. A.J.R. *150*:87, 1988.
90. Chang, J-M., Friese, K., Caputo, G. R., et al.: MR measurement of blood flow in the true and false channel in chronic aortic dissection. J. Comput. Assist. Tomogr. *15*:418, 1991.
91. Sakuma, H., Globits, S., O'Sullivan, M., et al.: Flow velocity measurements in native internal mammary arteries and coronary artery bypass grafts with breath-held velocity encoded cine MR imaging. J. Magn. Reson. Imaging *(in press)*.
92. Winkler, M. L., and Higgins, C. B.: Magnetic resonance imaging of perivalvular infectious pseudoaneurysms. A.J.R. *147*:153, 1986.
93. Nienaber, C. A., Spielmann, R. P., Von Kodolitsch, Y., et al.: Diagnosis of thoracic aortic dissection: Magnetic resonance imaging vs transesophageal echocardiography. Circulation *85*:434, 1992.
94. Higgins, C. B., and Caputo, G. R.: Role of MR imaging in acquired and congenital cardiovascular disease. A.J.R. *161*:13, 1993.
95. Szolar, D., Sakuma, H., and Higgins, C. B.: Cardiovascular application of magnetic resonance flow and velocity measurements. J. Magn. Reson. Imaging *(in press)*.
96. Firmin, D. N., Naigler, G. L., Klipstein, R. H., et al.: In vivo validation of MR velocity mapping. J. Comput. Assist. Tomogr. *11*:751, 1987.
97. Kondo, C., Caputo, G. R., Semelka, R., et al.: Right and left ventricular stroke volume measurements with velocity encoded cine NMR imaging: In vitro and in vivo validation. A.J.R. *157*:9, 1991.
98. Mostbeck, G. H., Caputo, G. R., and Higgins, C. B.: MR measurement of blood flow in the cardiovascular system. A.J.R. *159*:453, 1992.
99. Mohiaddin, R. H., and Longmore, D. B.: Functional aspects of cardio-

vascular nuclear magnetic resonance imaging. Circulation *88:*264, 1993.

100. Wetter, D. R., McKinnon, G. C., Debatin, J. F., and von Schulthess, G. K.: Cardiac echo-planar MR imaging: Comparison of single- and multiple-shot techniques. Radiology *194:*765, 1995.
101. Untermerger, M., Debatin, J. F., Leung, D. A., et al.: Cardiac volumetry: Comparison of echoplanar and conventional cine MR data acquisition strategies. Invest. Radiol. *29:*994, 1994.
102. Caputo, G. R., Tscholakoff, D., Sechtem, U., et al.: Measurement of canine left ventricular mass using gated magnetic resonance imaging. A.J.R. *148:*33, 1987.
103. Maddahi, J., Crues, J., Berman, D. S., et al.: Noninvasive quantitation of left ventricular mass by gated proton NMR imaging. J. Am. Coll. Cardiol. *10:*682, 1987.
104. Underwood, S. R., Firmin, D. N., Klipstein, H., et al.: Rapid measurement of left ventricular volume from single oblique MR images. Radiology *157:*309, 1986.
105. Cranney, G. B., Lotan, C. S., Dean, L., et al.: Left ventricular volume measurement using cardiac axis NMR imaging. Circulation *82:*154, 1990.
106. Dulce, M-C., Mostbeck, G. H., Friese, K. K., et al.: Quantification of the left ventricular volumes and function with cine MRI: Comparison of geometric models with three-dimensional data. Radiology *188:*371, 1993.
107. Doherty, N. E., Fujita, N., Caputo, G. R., et al.: Measurement of right ventricular mass in normal and dilated cardiomyopathic ventricles using cine MRI. Am. J. Cardiol. *69:*1225, 1992.
108. Sechtem, U., Pflugfelder, P., Gould, R., et al.: Measurement of right and left ventricular volumes in healthy individuals with cine MR imaging. Radiology *163:*697, 1987.
109. Sechtem, U., Pflugfelder, P. W., Cassidy, M. M., et al.: Mitral or aortic regurgitation: Quantification of regurgitant volumes with cine MR imaging. Radiology *167:*425, 1988.
110. Pflugfelder, P. W., Sechtem, U. P., White, R. D., et al.: Quantification of regional myocardial function by rapid (cine) magnetic resonance imaging. A.J.R. *150:*523, 1988.
111. LeWinter, M. M., Kent, R. S., Kroener, J. M., et al.: Regional differences in myocardial performance in the left ventricle of the dog. Circ. Res. *37:*191, 1975.
112. Zerhouni, E. A., Parish, D. M., Roger, W. J., et al.: Human heart: Tagging with MR imaging—a method for noninvasive assessment of myocardial motion. Radiology *169:*59, 1988.
113. Axel, L., and Dougherty, L.: MR imaging of motion with spatial modulation of magnetization. Radiology *171:*841, 1989.
114. Maier, S. E., Fischer, S. E., McKinnon, G. C., et al.: Evaluation of left ventricular segmental wall motion in hypertrophic cardiomyopathy with myocardial tagging. Circulation *86:*1919, 1992.
115. Lima, J. A. C., Jeremy, R., Guier, W., et al.: Accurate systolic wall thickening by MRI with tissue tagging: Correlation with sonomicrometers in normal and ischemic myocardium. J. Am. Coll. Cardiol. *21:*1741, 1993.
116. Sechtem, U., Pflugfelder, P. W., White, R. D., et al.: Cine MRI: Potential for the evaluation of cardiovascular function. A.J.R. *148:*239, 1987.
117. Pflugfelder, P. W., Sechtem, U. P., White, R. D., et al.: Noninvasive evaluation of mitral regurgitation by analysis of left atrial signal loss in cine magnetic resonance. Am. Heart J. *117:*1113, 1989.
118. Pflugfelder, P. W., Landzberg, J. S., Cassidy, M. M., et al.: Comparison of cine MR imaging with Doppler echocardiography for the evaluation of aortic regurgitation. A.J.R. *152:*729, 1989.
119. Wagner, S., Auffermann, W., Buser, P., et al.: Diagnostic accuracy and estimation of the severity of valvular regurgitation from the signal void on cine magnetic resonance images. Am. Heart J. *118:*760, 1989.
120. Underwood, S. R., Klipstein, P. H., Firmin, D. N., et al.: Magnetic resonance assessment of aortic and mitral regurgitation. Br. Heart J. *56:*455, 1986.
121. Higgins, C. B., Wagner, S., Kondo, C., et al.: Evaluation of valvular heart disease using cine GRE magnetic resonance imaging. Circulation (Suppl.) *84*(3):I-198, 1991.
122. Cranney, G. B., Lotan, C. S., and Pohost, G. M.: Nuclear magnetic resonance imaging for assessment and follow up of patients with valve disease. Circulation (Suppl.) *84:*216, 1991.
123. Globits, S., and Higgins, C. B.: Assessment of valvular heart disease using magnetic resonance imaging. Am. Heart J. *129:*369, 1995.
124. Dulce, M-C., Mostbeck, G., O'Sullivan, M. M., et al.: Severity of aortic regurgitation: Interstudy reproducibility of measurements with velocity-encoded cine MR imaging. Radiology *185:*235, 1992.
125. Fujita, N., Chazouilleres, A. F., Hartiala, J. J., et al.: Quantification of mitral regurgitation by velocity-encoded cine magnetic resonance imaging. J. Am. Coll. Cardiol. *23:*951, 1994.
126. Eichenberger, A. C., Jenni, R., and von Schulthess, G. K.: Aortic valve pressure gradients in patients with aortic valve stenosis: Quantification with velocity encoded cine MRI. A.J.R. *160:*971, 1992.
127. Kilner, P. J., Firmin, D. N., Rees, R. S. O., et al.: Valve and great vessel stenosis: Assessment with MR jet velocity mapping. Radiology *178:*229, 1991.
128. Hendenreich, P. A., Steffens, J. C., Fujita, N., et al.: The evaluation of mitral stenosis with velocity-encoded cine magnetic resonance imaging. Am. J. Cardiol. *75:*365, 1995.
129. Moran, P. R.: A flow zeugomatographic interface for NMR imaging in humans. Magn. Reson. Imaging *1:*197, 1982.
130. Underwood, S. R., Firmin, D. N., Klipstein, R. H., et al.: Magnetic resonance velocity mapping: Clinical application of a new technique. Br. Heart J. *57:*404, 1987.
131. Meier, D., Meier, S., and Böseger, P.: Quantitative flow measurements on phantoms and on blood vessels with MR. Magn. Reson. Med. *8:*25, 1988.
132. Moran, P. R., Moran, R. A., and Karstaedt, N. K.: Verification and evaluation of internal flow and motion. Radiology *154:*433, 1985.
133. Caputo, G. R., Kondo, C., Masui, T., et al.: Right and left lung perfusion: In vitro and in vivo validation with oblique-angle, velocity-encoded cine MR imaging. Radiology *180:*693, 1991.
134. Bogren, H. G., Klipstein, R. H., Mohiaddin, R. H., et al.: Pulmonary artery distensibility and blood flow patterns: A magnetic resonance study of normal subjects and of patients with pulmonary arterial hypertension. Am. Heart J. *118:*990, 1989.
135. Kondo, C., Caputo, G. R., Masui, T., et al.: Pulmonary hypertension: Pulmonary flow quantification and flow profile analysis with velocity-encoded cine MR imaging. Radiology *183:*751, 1992.
136. Brenner, L. D., Caputo, G. R., Mostbeck, G., et al.: Quantification of left to right atrial shunts with velocity encoded cine nuclear magnetic resonance imaging. J. Am. Coll. Cardiol. *20:*1246, 1992.
137. Steffens, J. C., Bourne, M. W., Sakuma, H., et al.: Quantification of collateral blood flow in coarctation of the aorta by velocity encoded cine MRI. Circulation *90:*937, 1994.
138. Ehman, R. L., McNamara, M. T., Brasch, R. C., et al.: Influence of physiologic motion on the appearance of tissue in MR images. Radiology *159:*777, 1986.
139. Higgins, C. B., Herfkens, R., Lipton, M. J., et al.: Nuclear magnetic resonance imaging of acute myocardial infarction in dogs: Alterations in magnetic relaxation times. Am. J. Cardiol. *52:*184, 1983.
140. Johnston, D. L., Brady, T. J., Ratner, A. V., et al.: Assessment of myocardial ischemia with proton magnetic resonance: Effects of a three hour coronary occlusion with and without perfusion. Circulation *71:*595, 1985.
141. Tscholakoff, D., Aherne, T., Yee, E. S., et al.: Cardiac transplantation in dogs: Evaluation with MRI. Radiology *157:*697, 1985.
142. Tscholakoff, D., Higgins, C. B., McNamara, M. T., et al.: Early phase myocardial infarction: Evaluation by magnetic resonance imaging. Radiology *159:*667, 1986.
143. Pflugfelder, P. W., Wisenberg, G., Prato, F. S., et al.: Early detection of canine myocardial infarction by magnetic resonance imaging in vivo. Circulation *71:*587, 1985.
144. Saeed, M., Wendland, M. F., and Higgins, C. B.: Contrast media for MR imaging of the heart. J. Magn. Reson. Imag. *4:*269, 1994.
145. Saeed, M., Wendland, M. F., and Tomei, E.: Demarcation of myocardial ischemia: Magnetic susceptibility effect of contrast medium in MR imaging. Radiology *173:*763, 1989.
146. Saeed, M., Wendland, M. F., Yu, K. K., et al.: Dual effects of gadodiamide injection in depiction of the region of myocardial ischemia. J. Magn. Reson. Imag. *3:*21, 1993.
147. Dulce, M-C., Duerinckx, A. J., Hartiala, J., et al.: MR imaging of the myocardium using nonionic contrast medium: Signal intensity changes in patients with subacute myocardial infarction. A.J.R. *160:*1, 1993.
148. Eichstaedt, H. W., Felix, R., Dougherty, F. C., et al.: Magnetic resonance imaging (MRI) in different stages of myocardial infarction using the contrast agent gadolinium-DTPA. Clin. Cardiol. *9:*527, 1986.
149. de Roos, A., van Rossum, A. C., van der Wall, E., et al.: Reperfused and nonreperfused myocardial infarction: Diagnostic potential of Gd-DTPA-enhanced MR imaging. Radiology *172:*717, 1989.
150. Saeed, M., Wendland, M. F., Takehara, Y., et al.: Reperfusion and irreversible myocardial injury: Identification with a nonionic MR imaging contrast medium. Radiology *182:*675, 1991.
151. Wendland, M. F., Saeed, M., Masui, T., et al.: Echo-planar MR imaging of normal and ischemic myocardium with gadodiamide injection. Radiology *186:*535, 1993.

COMPUTED TOMOGRAPHY

152. Brundage, B., Lipton, M. J., Herfkens, R. J., et al.: Detection of patent coronary artery bypass grafts by computed tomography: A preliminary report. Circulation *61:*826, 1980.
153. Moncada, R., Salinas, M., Churchill, R., et al.: Patency of saphenous aortocoronary grafts demonstrated by computed tomography. N. Engl. J. Med. *303:*503, 1980.
154. Kohl, F. C., Wolfman, N. T., and Watts, L. E.: Evaluation of aortocoronary bypass graft status by computed tomography. Am. J. Cardiol. *48:*304, 1981.
155. Higgins, C. B., Carlsson, E., and Lipton, M. J. (eds.): CT of the Heart and Great Vessels. Mt. Kisco, N.Y., Futura Publishing Co., 1983, p. 167.
156. Lipton, M. J., Higgins, C. B., Farmer, D., et al.: Cardiac imaging with a high-speed cine-CT scanner: Preliminary results. Radiology *152:*579, 1983.
157. Sinak, L. F., and Ritman, E. L.: Dynamic spatial reconstructor. *In* CT of the Heart and Great Vessels. Mt. Kisco, N.Y., Futura Publishing Co., 1983, p. 61.
158. Rumberger, J. A., Feiring, A. J., Reiter, S. J., et al.: Ultrafast computed tomography: Evaluation of global left ventricular anatomy and function. *In* Pohost, G. M., Higgins, C. B., Morganroth, J., et al. (eds.): New Con-

cepts in Cardiac Imaging. Chicago, Year Book Medical Publishers, 1988, p. 195.
159. Feiring, A., Rumberger, J. A., Reiter, S. J., et al.: Determination of left ventricular mass in dogs with rapid-acquisition cardiac CT scanning. Circulation *72*:1355, 1985.
160. Hajkuczok, Z. D., Weiss, R. M., Stanford, W., et al.: Determination of right ventricular mass in humans and dogs with ultrafast cardiac computed tomography. Circulation *82*:202, 1990.
161. Himelman, R. B., Abbott, J. A., Lipton, M. J., et al.: Cine CT compared with echocardiography in the evaluation of cardiac function in emphysema. Am. J. Cardiac Imaging *2*:283, 1988.
162. Lanzer, P., Garrett, J., Lipton, M. J., et al.: Quantitation of regional myocardial function by cine computed tomography: Pharmacologic changes in wall thickness. J. Am. Coll. Cardiol. *8*:682, 1986.
163. Caputo, G. R., and Lipton, M. J.: Evaluation of regional left ventricular function using ultrafast CT. *In* Pohost, G. L., Higgins, C. B., Morganroth, J., et al. (eds.): New Concepts in Cardiac Imaging. Chicago, Year Book Medical Publishers, 1988, p. 231.
164. Feiring, A. J., Rumberger, J. A., Reiter, S. J., et al.: Sectional and segmental variability of left ventricular function: Experimental and clinical studies using ultrafast computed tomography. J. Am. Coll. Cardiol. *12*:415, 1988.
165. Farmer, D. W., Lipton, M. J., Higgins, C. B., et al.: In vivo assessment of left ventricular wall and chamber dynamics during transient myocardial ischemia using cine CT. Am. J. Cardiol. *55*:560, 1985.
166. Marcus, M. L., and Weiss, R. M.: Evaluation of cardiac structures and function with ultrafast computed tomography. *In* Marcus, M. L., Schelbert, H. R., Skorton, D. J., et al. (eds.): Cardiac Imaging. Philadelphia, W.B. Saunders Company, 1991, p. 669.
167. Roig, E., Chomka, E. V., Costaner, A., et al.: Exercise ultrafast computed tomography for the detection of coronary artery disease. J. Am. Coll. Cardiol. *13*:1073, 1989.
168. McMillan, R. M., and Rees, M. R.: Determinants of left ventricular ejection fraction by ultrafast CT. Angiology *39*:203, 1988.
169. Reiter, S. J., Rumberger, J. A., Feiring, A. J., et al.: Precision of right and left ventricular stroke volume measurements by rapid acquisition cine CT. Circulation *74*:890, 1986.
170. Reiter, S. J., Rumberger, J. A., Stanford, W., et al.: Quantitative determination of aortic regurgitant volumes in dogs by ultrafast computed tomography. Circulation *76*:728, 1987.

EVALUATION OF SPECIFIC CARDIAC DISEASES

171. Lackner, K., and Thurn, P.: Computed tomography of the heart: ECG gated and continuous scans. Radiology *140*:413, 1981.
172. Kramer, P., Goldstein, J., Herfkens, R., et al.: Imaging of acute myocardial infarction in man with contrast enhanced computed transmission tomography. Am. Heart J. *108*:1514, 1984.
173. Lipton, M. J., Farmer, D. W., Killebrew, E. J., et al.: Regional myocardial dysfunction: Evaluation of patients with prior myocardial infarction with fast CT. Radiology *157*:735, 1985.
174. Lackner, K.: Clinical application of CTT for evaluation of ischemic heart disease—comparison with other imaging methods. *In* Higgins, C. B. (ed.): CTT of the Heart and Great Vessels. Mt. Kisco, N.Y., Futura Publishing Co., 1982, p. 267.
175. Tomoda, H., Hoshiai, M., Furuya, H., et al.: Evaluation of intracardiac thrombus with computed tomography. Am. J. Cardiol. *51*:843, 1983.
176. Tomoda, H., Hoshiai, M., Furuya, H., et al.: Evaluation of left ventricular thrombus with computed tomography. Am. J. Cardiol. *48*:573, 1981.
177. Tomoda, H., Hoshiai, M., Tozawa, R., et al.: Evaluation of left atrial thrombus with computed tomography. Am. Heart J. *100*:306, 1980.
178. Rumberger, J. A., Feiring, A. J., Lipton, M. J., et al.: Use of ultrafast computed tomography to quantitate regional myocardial perfusion: A preliminary report. J. Am. Coll. Cardiol. *9*:59, 1987.
179. Gould, R. G., Lipton, M. J., McNamara, M. T., et al.: Measurement of regional myocardial flow in dogs using ultrafast CT. Invest. Radiol. *23*:348, 1988.
180. Wolfkiel, C. J., Ferguson, J. L., Chomka, E. V., et al.: Measurement of myocardial blood flow by ultrafast computed tomography. Circulation *76*:1262, 1987.
181. Rumberger, J. A., Bell, M. R., Feiring, A. J., et al.: Measurement of myocardial perfusion using fast computed tomography. *In* Marcus, M. L., Schelbert, H. R., Skorton, D. J., et al. (eds.): Cardiac Imaging. Philadelphia, W.B. Saunders Company, 1991, p. 688.
182. Peck, W. A., Mancini, G. B. J., Mattrey, R. F., et al.: In vivo assessment by CT of natural progression of infarct size, left ventricular mass, and function after myocardial infarction in the dog. Am. J. Cardiol. *53*:929, 1984.
183. Mancini, G. B. J., Peck, W. W., Ross, J., Jr., et al.: Use of computerized tomography to assess myocardial infarct size and ventricular function in dogs during acute coronary occlusion and reperfusion. Am. J. Cardiol. *53*:282, 1984.
184. Daniel, W. G., Doring, W., Stender, H. S., et al.: Value and limitations of computed tomography in assessing aortocoronary bypass graft patency. Circulation *67*:983, 1983.
185. Stanford, W., Brundage, B. H., MacMillan, R., et al.: Sensitivity and specificity of assessing coronary bypass graft patency with ultrafast computed tomography: Results of a multicenter study. J. Am. Coll. Cardiol. *12*:1, 1988.
186. Bateman, T. M., Gray, R. J., Whiting, J. S., et al.: Ultrafast computed tomographic evaluation of aortocoronary bypass graft patency. J. Am. Coll. Cardiol. *8*:693, 1986.
187. Bateman, T. M., Gray, R. J., Whiting, J. S., et al.: Prospective evaluation of ultrafast CT for determination of coronary bypass graft patency. Circulation *75*:1018, 1987.
188. Ullyot, D. J., Turley, K., McKay, C. R., et al.: Assessment of saphenous vein graft patency by contrast enhanced computed tomography. J. Thorac. Cardiovasc. Surg. *83*:512, 1982.
189. McKay, C. R., Brundage, B. H., Ullyot, D. J., et al.: Evaluation of early postoperative coronary artery bypass graft patency by contrast enhanced computed tomography. J. Am. Coll. Cardiol. *2*:312, 1983.
190. Hamby, R. I., Tabrah, F., Wisoff, B. G., et al.: Coronary artery calcification: Clinical implications and angiographic correlates. Am. Heart J. *87*:565, 1974.
191. Bartel, A. G., Chen, J. T., Peter, R. H., et al.: The significance of coronary arterial calcification detected by fluoroscopy. Circulation *49*:1247, 1974.
192. Aldrich, R. F., Brensike, J. F., Battaglini, J. W., et al.: Coronary calcification in the detection of coronary artery disease and comparison with electrocardiographic exercise testing. Circulation *59*:113, 1979.
193. Agatston, A. S., Janowitz, W. R., Hildner, F. J., et al.: Quantification of coronary artery calcium using ultrafast computed tomography. J. Am. Coll. Cardiol. *15*:827, 1990.
194. Kaufman, R. B., Sheedy, P. F., Breen, J. F., et al.: Detection of heart calcification with electron beam CT: Interobserver and intraobserver reliability for scoring quantification. Radiology *190*:347, 1994.
195. Simon, D. B., Schwartz, R. S., Edwards, W. O., et al.: Noninvasive detection of anatomic coronary artery disease by ultrafast tomographic scanning: A quantitative pathologic comparison study. J. Am. Coll. Cardiol. *20*:1118, 1992.
196. Mautner, S., Mautner, G., Frolich, J., et al.: Coronary artery disease: Prediction with in vitro electron beam CT. Radiology *192*:625, 1994.
197. Mautner, G., Mautner, S. L., Frolich, J., et al.: Coronary artery calcification: Assessment with electron beam CT and histomorphometric correlation. Radiology *192*:619, 1994.
198. Rumberger, J. A., Schwartz, R. S., Simons, D. B., et al.: Relation of coronary calcium determined by electron beam computed tomography and lumen narrowing by autopsy. Am. J. Cardiol. *74*:1169, 1994.
199. Breen, J. F., Sheedy, P. F., Schwartz, R. S., et al.: Coronary artery calcification detected by ultrafast CT as an indication of coronary artery disease. Radiology *185*:435, 1992.
200. Agatson, A. S., Janowitz, W. R., Kaplan, G., et al.: Ultrafast computed tomography detected coronary calcium reflects the angiographic extent of coronary arterial stenosis. Am. J. Cardiol. *74*:1272, 1994.
201. Janowitz, W. R., Agathson, A. S., Kaplan, G., et al.: Differences in prevalence and extent of coronary artery calcium detected by ultrafast computed tomography in asymptomatic men and women. Am. J. Cardiol. *72*:247, 1993.
202. Fallavolleta, J. A., Brody, A. S., Bannell, I., et al.: Fast detection of coronary calcification in the diagnosis of coronary artery disease. Circulation *72*:247, 1993.
203. Silverman, P. M., and Harell, G. S.: Computed tomography of the normal pericardium. Invest. Radiol. *18*:141, 1983.
204. Moncada, R., Baker, M., Salinas, M., et al.: Diagnostic role of computed tomography in pericardial heart disease: Congenital defects, thickening, neoplasms and effusions. Am. Heart J. *103*:263, 1981.
205. Isner, J. M., Carter, B. L., Bankoff, M. S., et al.: Computed tomography in the diagnosis of pericardial heart disease. Ann. Intern. Med. *97*:473, 1982.
206. Baim, R. S., MacDonald, I. L., Wise, D. J., et al.: Computed tomography of absent left pericardium. Radiology *135*:127, 1980.
207. Roger, C. I., Seymour, Q., and Brock, G. I.: Atypical pericardial cysts location: The value of computed tomography. J. Comput. Assist. Tomogr. *4*:583, 1980.
208. Pugatch, R. D., Braver, J. H., Robbins, A. H., et al.: CT diagnosis of pericardial cysts. A.J.R. *131*:515, 1978.
209. Tomoda, H., Hoshiai, M., Furuya, H., et al.: Evaluation of pericardial effusion with computed tomography. Am. Heart J. *99*:701, 1980.
210. Higgins, C. B., Mattrey, R. F., and Shea, P.: CT localization and aspiration of postoperative pericardial fluid collection. J. Comput. Assist. Tomogr. *7*:734, 1983.
211. Zerhouni, E. A., Scott, W. W., Baker, R. R., et al.: Invasive thymomas: Diagnosis and evaluation by computed tomography. J. Comput. Assist. Tomogr. *6*:92, 1982.
212. Hackney, D., Mattrey, R., Peck, W. W., et al.: Experimental pericardial inflammation evaluated by computed tomography. Radiology *151*:145, 1984.
213. Doppman, J. C., Reinmuller, R., Lissner, J., et al.: Computed tomography in constrictive pericardial disease. J. Comput. Assist. Tomogr. *5*:1, 1981.
214. Isner, J. M., Carter, B. L., Bankoff, M. S., et al.: Differentiation of constrictive pericarditis from restrictive cardiomyopathy by computed tomographic imaging. Am. Heart J. *105*:1019, 1983.
215. Handler, J. B., Higgins, C. B., Warrent, S. E., et al.: Computerized tomographic diagnosis of paracardiac masses. West. J. Med. *135*:271, 1981.
216. Glazer, G. M., Gross, B. H., Oringer, M. B., et al.: Computed tomography of pericardial masses. J. Comput. Assist. Tomogr. *8*:895, 1984.
217. Patel, B. K., Markivee, C. R., and George, E. A.: Pericardial cyst simulating intracardiac mass. A.J.R. *141*:292, 1983.

218. Norlindh, T., Lilja, B., Nyman, U., et al.: Left atrial myxoma demonstrated by CT. A.J.R. *137:*153, 1981.
219. Huggins, T. J., Huggins, M. J., Schnopf, D. J., et al.: Left atrial myxoma: Computed tomography as a diagnostic modality. Invest. Radiol. *12:*559, 1977.
220. Baron, R. L., Guitterez, F. R., and McKnight, R. C.: Computed tomographic evaluation of the great arteries and aortic arch anomalies. *In* Freedman, W. F., and Higgins, C. B. (eds.): Pediatric Cardiac Imaging. Philadelphia, W.B. Saunders Company, 1984, pp. 135–156.
221. Farmer, D. W., Lipton, M. J., Webb, W. R., et al.: Computed tomography in congenital heart disease. J. Comput. Assist. Tomogr. *8:*677, 1984.
222. Webb, W. R., Gamsu, G., Speckman, G., et al.: CT demonstration of mediastinal aortic arch anomalies. J. Comput. Assist. Tomogr. *6:*445, 1982.
223. Eldridge, W. J.: Comprehensive evaluation of congenital heart disease using ultrafast computed tomography. *In* Marcus, M. L., Schelbert, H. R., Skorton, D. J., et al. (eds.): Cardiac Imaging. Philadelphia, W.B. Saunders Company, 1991, p. 714.
224. Eldridge, W. J., Flicker, S., and Steiner, R. M.: Cine CT in the anatomical evaluation of congenital heart disease. *In* Pohost, G., Higgins, C. B., Morgenroth, J., et al. (eds.): New Concepts in Cardiac Imaging. Vol. 3. Chicago, Year Book Medical Publishers, 1987, p. 265.
225. Garrett, J. S., Jaschke, W., Aherne, T., et al.: Quantitation of intracardiac shunts by cine CT. J. Comput. Assist. Tomogr. *12:*82, 1988.
226. MacMillan, R. M., Shakriari, A., Sumithisena, F., et al.: Contrast enhanced cine computed tomography for the diagnosis of right coronary to coronary sinus arteriovenous fistulae. Am. J. Cardiol. *56:*997, 1985.
227. Helberg, E., Wolverson, M., Sundaram, M., et al.: CT finding in thoracic aortic dissection. A.J.R. *136:*13, 1981.
228. Thorsten, M. K., San Drelto, M. A., Lawson, T. L., et al.: Dissecting aortic aneurysms: Accuracy of computed tomographic diagnosis. Radiology *148:*773, 1983.
229. Dudkerk, M., Overbosch, E., and Dee, P.: CT recognition of acute aortic dissection. A.J.R. *141:*671, 1983.
230. White, R. C., Lipton, M. J., Higgins, C. B., et al.: Noninvasive evaluation of suspected thoracic aortic disease by contrast-enhanced computed tomography. Am. J. Cardiol. *57:*282, 1986.
231. Cizarros, J. E., Isselbacher, E. M., DeSanctis, R. W., et al.: Diagnostic imaging in the evaluation of suspected aortic dissection: Old standards and new directions. N. Engl. J. Med. *328:*35, 1993.
232. Nienaber, C. A., Von Kodolitsch, Y., Nichols, V., et al.: The diagnosis of thoracic aortic dissection by noninvasive imaging procedures. N. Engl. J. Med. *328:*1, 1993.
233. Yamada, T., Toda, S., and Harada, J.: Aortic dissection without intimal rupture: Diagnosis with MR imaging and CT. Radiology *168:*347, 1988.
234. Guthaner, D. F., Miller, D. C., Silverman, J. F., et al.: Fate of the false lumen following surgical repair of aortic dissection: An angiographic study. Radiology *133:*1, 1979.
235. Yamaguchi, T., Naito, H., Ohta, M., et al.: False lumens in type III aortic dissection: Progress in CT study. Radiology *156:*757, 1985.
236. Yamaguchi, T., Guthaner, D. F., and Wexler, L.: Natural history of the false channel of type A aortic dissection after surgical repair: CT study. Radiology *170:*743, 1989.
237. Mathieu, D., Keita, K., Loisance, D., et al.: Postoperative CT follow-up of aortic dissection. J. Comput. Assist. Tomogr. *10:*216, 1986.
238. Teigen, C. L., Maus, T. P., Sheedy, P. F., et al.: Pulmonary embolism: Diagnosis with contrast enhanced electron beam CT and comparison with pulmonary angiography. Radiology *194:*313, 1995.
239. Remy-Jardin, M., Remy, J., Wattinne, L., et al.: Central pulmonary thromboembolism: Diagnosis with spiral volumetric CT with single breath hold technique—comparison with pulmonary angiography. Radiology *185:*381, 1992.

Chapter 11
Relative Merits of Imaging Techniques

DAVID J. SKORTON, BRUCE H. BRUNDAGE, HEINRICH R. SCHELBERT, GERALD L. WOLF

Evaluation of the patient with known or suspected cardiovascular disease is becoming both more accurate and more precise due to the availability of an already broad and still growing array of diagnostic methods (described in the first 10 chapters of this book). The process of diagnosis in the mid-1990's still begins with a careful and thorough history (Chap. 1) and physical examination (Chap. 2). Often, these are followed by a resting 12-lead electrocardiogram (Chap. 4) and chest roentgenogram (Chap. 7). At this point in the diagnostic process, the clinician usually forms presumptive diagnostic hypotheses. To confirm or refute these hypotheses, the clinician can turn to a range of laboratory examinations, including measurements made on blood and urine, exercise electrocardiographic testing (Chap. 5), electrophysiological monitoring or testing, and a large number of sophisticated imaging techniques. With the exception of evaluating arrhythmias and conduction disturbances, methods of imaging the heart are the predominant laboratory diagnostic methods in cardiology.[1,2] Thus, the clinician needs to be conversant with the several methods of imaging the heart and circulation. However, because of the wealth of sometimes redundant information offered by these methods, in the interest of efficient and cost-effective diagnosis, the clinician also needs to be aware of the relative strengths and weaknesses of these techniques under particular clinical circumstances. In Chapters 3 and 7 through 10, details regarding the use and interpretation of each of the individual imaging techniques are presented. It is the purpose of this chapter to offer some insights into the relative advantages and disadvantages of these several modalities.

SCOPE OF CARDIAC IMAGING

The several available and developing methods of cardiac imaging may be categorized in various ways; we choose to divide them, somewhat arbitrarily, into "standard" and "evolving" methods (Table 11–1). The basis of this distinction is the general availability of and clinical experience with the methods. Only a few investigative centers have all these methods available for routine clinical use. In general, those we classify as standard are widely available and thus are methods with which most clinicians have at least some experience. The modalities classified as evolving are relatively new or not widely employed, so most clinicians have relatively little direct experience with them.

Projection versus Tomographic Imaging

The distinction between *projection* and *tomographic* imaging is of theoretical and practical importance. The standard chest roentgenogram is a good example of a projection imaging method. The patient is placed between an x-ray source and an x-ray detector (a film-screen system). The x-rays are launched; they pass through the patient and are then received and detected on film. Thus, the imaging energy is *projected* through the patient so that attenuation of x-rays occurs not only due to the structure of interest (e.g., the heart) but also due to other structures interposed along the path taken by the x-rays (such as chest wall and lung). Because of this projection phenomenon, x-ray shadows in the resulting roentgenogram represent a superimposition of wanted and unwanted information. Plain-film

TABLE 11–1 STANDARD AND EVOLVING METHODS OF CARDIAC IMAGING

STANDARD METHODS
Chest roentgenography
Echocardiography
Radionuclide methods
Planar and single-photon emission computed tomography
Myocardial perfusion scintigraphy (thallium-201 and technetium-99m agents)
Radionuclide ventriculography (technetium-99m-labeled red blood cells)
Infarct-avid imaging (technetium-99m pyrophosphate or indium-111 antimyosin antibody)
Selective angiography
Ventriculography/aortography
Pulmonary angiography
Coronary angiography
EVOLVING METHODS
Computer-assisted echocardiography
Perfusion (contrast) studies
Ultrasound tissue characterization
Three-dimensional reconstructions
Radionuclide methods
Newer imaging tracers
Positron emission tomography
Digital angiography
Fast computed tomography
Electron beam
Slip-ring
Magnetic resonance methods
Magnetic resonance imaging
Magnetic resonance spectroscopy

roentgenography, fluoroscopy, and angiography are all examples of projection imaging methods.

Projection radionuclide images are usually referred to as *planar.* In the case of planar radionuclide images (see p. 276), the basic data consist of photons emitted by the injected radionuclide; these photons are detected externally by a gamma camera. The resulting images may be degraded by interactions of the photons with other tissues interposed along the paths taken by the photons as they travel from the tissue of interest to the gamma camera.

The other basic approach to imaging is the selective depiction of a slice, or *tomogram,* through the patient. For example, in the case of x-ray computed tomography (CT) (Chap. 10), the production of a tomogram is accomplished by acquiring x-ray attenuation measurements from many different angles around the patient within a selected plane. At each angle, x-rays are sent from an x-ray source through the patient and are then received by a detector on the opposite side of the patient. This process is repeated for many angles around the patient, yielding a set of x-ray attenuation profiles. By computer reconstruction methods,[3] these many x-ray attenuation profiles are combined to produce an image depicting the two-dimensional distribution of x-ray attenuation data for a slice, or tomogram, through the patient. Since the resulting data selectively represent x-ray attenuation only in the "slice" under study, the problem of superimposition found in projection methods does not occur. Thus, the tomographic imaging techniques permit clearer delineation of physical characteristics and anatomical features of selected body regions than is possible with nontomographic, projection methods. Two-dimensional echocardiography, single-photon emission radionuclide CT, x-ray CT, and magnetic resonance imaging (MRI) are all examples of tomographic imaging methods. Tomographic imaging methods virtually all depend on digital computer image processing methods for image generation, display, and analysis.

Standard Imaging Methods

Standard widely available imaging methods include chest roentgenography, fluoroscopy, echocardiography, myocardial perfusion scintigraphy employing thallium-201 (^{201}Tl) or agents labeled with technetium-99m (^{99m}Tc) (including both planar scintigraphy and single-photon emission computed tomography [SPECT]), radionuclide ventriculography, infarct scans, and selective angiocardiography. The information content of these several imaging methods varies widely, because the method of image formation is different in each type of technique. Each imaging method represents the use of a particular energy source to produce an image containing anatomical and/or physiological information. As the energy sources vary, so do the types of information that may be extracted by application of the different methods. Table 11–2 lists the basic energy forms used to produce medical image data with an indication of some of the biophysical bases of image formation by each technique. Standard radiographic techniques (including chest roentgenography, fluoroscopy, and selective angiocardiography) are based on differential attenuation of x-rays by tissues of varying density. In angiography, attenuation of x-rays by blood is increased selectively by the infusion of iodinated contrast media. Ultrasonographic imaging is based on differential reflection and absorption of ultrasound (mechanical) energy by structures of varying density and elasticity. Radionuclide image data depend on both the radioisotope used as a label and the biologically relevant compound to which the label is attached. The regional image intensity reflects the regional distribution of that particular radiotracer in the body or the organ under study at the time of imaging.

TABLE 11–2 SOME DETERMINANTS OF IMAGE INTENSITY

ENERGY FORM	IMAGE INTENSITY DETERMINANTS
X-ray based methods	**Density of tissue**
Plain-film radiography	**Local contrast (iodine) concentration**
Angiography	
Computed tomography	
Ultrasound	**Acoustic velocity**
	Density of tissue
	Tissue elasticity
	Contrast agent
Radionuclides	**Tracer concentration (depends on biological activity of ligand)**
	Photon energy
Magnetic resonance methods	**Proton (spin) density (i.e., water content)**
	Nuclear magnetic resonance relaxation times
	Chemical shift
	Blood flow
	Contrast agent effect

Evolving Imaging Methods

Evolving and/or less commonly used imaging methods include newer, computer-assisted ultrasound applications (including contrast-based perfusion imaging,[4] tissue characterization,[5] and three-dimensional reconstruction[6]), positron emission tomography (PET)[7] (Chap. 9), digital angiography,[8], magnetic resonance methods[9] (both imaging [MRI][10] and spectroscopy[11] [Chap. 10]), and fast x-ray computed tomography (fast CT).[12] (We use the term "fast CT" to include at least two methods of rapid acquisition CT: slipring methods and electron beam CT [the latter previously referred to as "ultrafast CT"].) As discussed already for standard imaging methods, the information content of the evolving methods also varies widely and is based on the energy form used to produce the image. The newer computer-assisted ultrasound applications depend on standard ultrasound interactions with tissue and therefore share the determinants of image intensity noted for standard echocardiography, but they employ new image data acquisition and processing methods. Similarly, PET image data are related to unique radionuclides and biologically relevant ligands. CT and digital angiography remain x-ray–based techniques in which image intensity is related to tissue density, but signal detection and image formation allow new capabilities. Image intensity in MRI (for proton images, the only widely available type) is a complex function of several variables, including regional water content, flow, motion, so-called nuclear magnetic resonance (NMR) relaxation times (both spin-lattice, or T_1, and spin-spin, or T_2, relaxation times), chemical shift and possibly other factors not fully understood[13] (Chap. 10). To summarize, the evolving and standard imaging methods are based on production of pictures using a wide variety of energy forms and biophysical determinants. Thus, these methods should be considered potentially complementary in the information they may offer.

A final general point to be emphasized is that the evolving imaging methods depend to a greater degree than do the standard methods on digital computer image processing technology for data acquisition, image production, display, storage, and analysis.[14,15] For example, chest roentgenography and selective angiocardiography may be performed without the aid of computer storage or manipulation of image data, although digital applications are becoming more common in these two modalities. However, computed tomographic techniques (including x-ray CT, SPECT, and PET) depend completely on computer technology for acquisition of basic image data, reconstruction of these data into tomographic images, and display, enhancement, and storage of the resulting images. Similarly, modern echocardiographic and MRI systems depend on computer methods for

TABLE 11–3 RELATIVE USEFULNESS OF CONVENTIONAL IMAGING TECHNIQUES IN ACHIEVING DIAGNOSTIC GOALS*

DIAGNOSTIC GOAL	CXR	ANGIO†	ECHO	RADIONUCLIDE VENTRICULOGRAPHY	MYOCARDIAL SCINTIGRAPHY
CARDIAC ANATOMY					
Chamber size	+	+++	+++	++	+
Myocardial mass	0	+	+++	0	+
Intracardiac masses	0	+++	++++	+	0
Valvular anatomy	0	++	++++	0	0
Pericardial disease	+	++	+++	0	0
Coronary anatomy	0	++++	+	0	0
Graft patency	0	++++	+	0	0
CARDIAC PHYSIOLOGY					
Ventricular systolic function	+	+++	+++	++	+
Ventricular diastolic function	0	++++	+++	++	0
Valvular stenosis/insufficiency	+	++++	+++	+	0
Intracardiac shunt	+	++++	+++	++	0
Myocardial blood flow	0	+	+	0	+++
Tissue characterization	0	0	+	0	0
Myocardial metabolism	0	0	0	0	+

* 0, no information; ++++, maximum information; angio, angiography; CXR, chest roentgenogram; echo, echocardiography.
† Angio includes both imaging and hemodynamic evaluation.
Modified and updated from Grover-McKay, M., and Skorton D. J.: Comparative aspects of modern imaging techniques. *In* Zipes, D. P., and Rowlands, D. J. (eds.): Progress in Cardiology. Philadelphia, Lea and Febiger, 1990, p. 3.

image generation and display. Once images are produced, digital computer technology is feasible for quantitative image analyses.

MEETING THE GOALS OF CARDIAC IMAGING

The complete assessment of a patient with known or suspected heart disease ideally should include information on cardiac anatomy (including the detailed anatomy of the coronary arteries), the function of the heart chambers and valves, myocardial perfusion and metabolism and their responses to exercise stress and/or pharmacologic agents, and tissue characteristics such as the replacement of normal myocardium by scar or infiltration by abnormal substances. Standard imaging methods give very useful information on cardiovascular anatomy and on chamber and valvular function (Table 11–3). In addition, information on relative regional deficits in myocardial perfusion is offered by myocardial perfusion scintigraphy employing thallium-201 or agents labeled with technetium-99m. However, none of the standard imaging methods offers information on the *absolute* level of regional myocardial perfusion, the details of regional myocardial metabolism, or the definition of tissue characteristics. Thus, development of the evolving imaging methods has been based in part on the perceived need to realize all the goals of cardiac imaging in clinical practice (Table 11–4). No single standard or evolving imaging modality is likely to be capable of optimal achievement of all the goals of cardiac imaging. Conversely, several techniques permit assessment of cardiac anatomy and function; there-

TABLE 11–4 RELATIVE USEFULNESS OF EVOLVING IMAGING TECHNIQUES IN ACHIEVING DIAGNOSTIC GOALS*

DIAGNOSTIC GOAL	DIGITAL ANGIO†	COMPUTER-ASSISTED ECHO	MRI	MRS	FCT	PET
CARDIAC ANATOMY						
Chamber size	+++	+++	++++	0	++++	++
Myocardial mass	+	+++	++++	0	++++	++
Intracardiac masses	+++	++++	++++	0	++++	0
Valvular anatomy	++	++++	+++	0	+++	0
Pericardial disease	++	+++	++++	0	++++	0
Coronary anatomy	++++	++	++	0	++	0
Graft patency	++++	+	++	0	+++	++
CARDIAC PHYSIOLOGY						
Ventricular systolic function	+++	+++	++++	0	++++	++
Ventricular diastolic function	++++	+++	++	0	++	0
Valvular stenosis/insufficiency	++++	+++	+++	0	++	0
Intracardiac shunt	++++	+++	+++	0	+++	0
Myocardial blood flow	++	++	+	0	++	++++
Tissue characterization	0	++	++	+++	+	+++
Myocardial metabolism	0	0	0	++++	0	++++

* 0, no information; ++++, maximum information; angio, angiography; echo, echocardiography; MRI, magnetic resonance imaging; MRS, magnetic resonance spectroscopy; PET, positron emission tomography; FCT, fast computed tomography.
† Angio includes both imaging and hemodynamic evaluation.
Modified and updated from Grover-McKay, M., and Skorton D. J.: Comparative aspects of modern imaging techniques. *In* Zipes, D. P., and Rowlands, D. J. (eds.): Progress in Cardiology. Philadelphia, Lea and Febiger, 1990, p. 3.

fore, redundant information will be obtained if these techniques are used additively without consideration of their relative strengths in the attainment of all imaging goals.

Assessment of Anatomy

Cardiac chamber and great vessel anatomy can be evaluated accurately with the use of any of several imaging techniques, including echocardiography, selective angiocardiography, CT, and MRI. An estimate of chamber size and shape also can be obtained from radionuclide ventriculograms. However, because of relatively coarse spatial resolution (on the order of several millimeters to 1 cm), the radionuclide techniques are not the methods of choice for assessing the detailed aspects of cardiac morphology. Selective angiocardiography has been the traditional standard for chamber volume against which other techniques have been judged. Tomographic methods, however, are superior in assessment of cardiac size and shape because of their ability to delineate wall thickness clearly, because of their relative freedom from problems caused by superimposition, and because their use in assessing chamber volume or mass does not require simplified geometric assumptions. Thus, echocardiography, CT, and MRI are the best methods for determining chamber and great vessel morphology. Fast CT permits enormously accurate and precise determination of cardiac anatomy.[16] However, CT has the disadvantages of not being portable and of having the problems associated with the need for iodinated contrast medium and radiation exposure. In the patient who can lie relatively still for several minutes, MRI can produce exquisitely detailed images of cardiac anatomy.[17] More recent, rapid methods of MRI image acquisition are increasing the utility of MRI in assessment of cardiac anatomy.[18] However, like CT, MRI is not portable. Because of these considerations, echocardiography is often considered the initial procedure of choice for assessment of chamber and great vessel morphology in patients in whom studies of diagnostic quality can be achieved. Particularly with the advent of transesophageal echocardiography (see p. 57), it is possible to assess accurately cardiac chamber and great vessel anatomy in the vast majority of patients by using ultrasound methods.

Determination of the detailed anatomy of the coronary arteries in routine clinical practice continues to be the domain of selective coronary arteriography (Chap. 8). Whether recorded on 35-mm cine film or in digital format, selective coronary angiograms exhibit the high spatial and temporal resolution necessary to image the coronary arteries sufficiently accurately to plan and evaluate catheter and/or surgical interventions. This is true particularly for the distal portions of the coronary vasculature or severely diseased vessels in which arterial lumen diameters may be 1 mm or smaller. CT shows potential for visualization of selected portions of the coronary arteries.[19] Both transesophageal echocardiography[20] and MRI[21] also may be used to visualize portions of the coronary tree and to assess flow within the vessels. However, it is unlikely that any technique other than selective coronary angiography will be capable within the next few years of defining the details of coronary anatomy throughout the epicardial coronary tree in the great majority of patients. The one exception to this statement may be intravascular ultrasound imaging (see p. 58), which offers unique information on not only luminal but also vessel wall anatomy.

Delineation of the anatomy of coronary bypass grafts (whether of internal mammary or saphenous vein origin) is also best done using angiography with selective graft injections (Fig. 8–17, p. 255). However, CT[22] (Fig. 10–36, p. 338) and MRI[23] (Fig. 10–10, p. 323) have substantial utility in identification of bypass graft patency.

Evaluation of Chamber and Valvular Function

LEFT VENTRICULAR FUNCTION. Global systolic and diastolic function of the left ventricle can be assessed with echocardiography, radionuclide ventriculography, selective angiocardiography, CT, and MRI. Because of its portability, safety, and high patient acceptance, echocardiography (including both imaging and Doppler approaches) is commonly used as the initial tool to assess left ventricular global and regional function. Echocardiography permits accurate assessment of left ventricular function[24] when studies of adequate quality are obtained; with the widespread availability of transesophageal echocardiography, this includes most patients. However, clinicians may not wish to undertake transesophageal echocardiography strictly for the assessment of left ventricular function. Echocardiograms of sufficient quality for at least semiquantitative analysis of left ventricular function can be obtained by the transthoracic approach in most patients. However, echocardiography has some inherent problems that limit its ability to define precisely left ventricular volume, mass, and ejection fraction. Among these problems is the fact that echocardiographic images are not acquired in mutually parallel or perpendicular orientations but are obtained at somewhat arbitrary angles, dictated by the constraints of the intercostal spaces and other aspects of thoracic anatomy. As opposed to these problems of echocardiography, CT and MRI permit the acquisition of multiple parallel, high-resolution tomograms from the apex to the base of the left ventricle, yielding quite precise and accurate assessment of chamber volume,[25–27] mass,[16,25,28] and function[29,30] (Figs. 10–34 and 10–35, p. 337). Whether the additional precision and accuracy afforded by CT and MRI justify the additional expense of these techniques and the biological hazards of CT (contrast media and small radiation exposure) remains to be proved. Nonetheless, in terms of theoretical and practical experience, the newer tomographic methods should be considered the most precise and accurate in this application.

Radionuclide methods, while not extremely precise for the calculation of left ventricular mass or volume, nonetheless offer acceptable accuracy for the determination of left ventricular systolic and diastolic performance[31] (see p. 434). Radionuclide determinations of left ventricular function are achieved without the necessity of the geometrical assumptions common to echocardiography and without the requirements for detailed definition of endocardial and epicardial contours (by hand or computer tracing) that are characteristic of echocardiographic, CT, and MRI methods.

Echocardiographic or radionuclide techniques can be used at the bedside and thus are the techniques of choice in the assessment of left ventricular function in the critical care unit or the emergency department. Overall, radionuclide techniques appear to offer a good balance of accuracy, ease of use, portability, and cost-effectiveness for the quantitative determination of left ventricular function. In situations in which extremely precise determinations of left ventricular mass or volume are desired, the use of CT or MRI may be justified (Fig. 10–2, p. 320).

RIGHT VENTRICULAR FUNCTION. Assessment of the function of the right ventricle is more difficult than that of the left ventricle because of the complex shape of the right ventricle, which defies easy representation by simple geometrical models. Although echocardiographic methods of quantitatively assessing right ventricular function have been developed,[32] there has not been widespread use of these techniques. Fast CT is extremely precise and accurate in the derivation of right ventricular volumes[33] and stroke volumes,[34] and MRI methods also appear to have impressive accuracy for assessment of right ventricular function[27,35] and mass.[35,36] First-pass radionuclide ventriculography[37] (see p. 300) is a relatively inexpensive and simple method that can determine right ventricular ejection fraction accurately at the bedside or in the clinical imaging area.

VALVULAR FUNCTION. A complete assessment of valvular function requires determining the anatomical and physiological characteristics of the valve itself (such as the degree of stenosis or regurgitation) as well as defining the effect of the valvular abnormality on ventricular or atrial anatomy and performance. For the determination of valvular anatomy, transvalvular gradient, and the severity of valvular regurgitation, echocardiographic methods (including imaging and Doppler approaches) are the current procedures of choice.[38] Particularly with the wide availability of high-quality pulsed, continuous-wave, and color flow Doppler systems, coupled with transesophageal echocardiography in selected patients, the assessment of valvular heart disease in general falls within the domain of echocardiography (Figs. 3–55, p. 75, and 3–63, p. 77). With regard to determining the effect of the valvular abnormality on chamber size and function, the previous comments concerning the relative precision and accuracy of radionuclide, ultrasound, CT, and MRI methods apply.

Assessment of Myocardial Perfusion

At present, the only approach widely used clinically to identify regional deficits in perfusion is radionuclide imaging with thallium-201 or with the more recently developed technetium-99m–labeled perfusion agents, performed at rest and with exercise stress or pharmacological vasodilation (Figs. 9–19, p. 285, and 9–20, p. 286). Unfortunately, these techniques have shortcomings in terms of both the physics of the imaging agents and the inability of conventional radionuclide imaging to estimate *absolute* values of regional myocardial perfusion. Therefore, several additional methods of determining perfusion are being developed. As shown in Figure 11–1, the various methods of assessing perfusion or indices related to perfusion can be considered systematically on the basis of the anatomical level at which data are acquired, beginning at the level of the epicardial coronary arteries. Clinicians commonly interpret the severity of narrowing of a particular coronary artery on the cineangiogram as an indicator of the likelihood of hypoperfusion distal to that stenosis. Thus arterial stenoses in excess of 50 to 75 per cent diameter narrowing are commonly assumed to represent hydraulically significant stenoses, capable of limiting flow at high rates.[39] Unfortunately, percentage diameter stenosis is an imperfect estimator of the functional significance of individual coronary lesions.[40] Further, this approach gives no information on *absolute* levels of regional perfusion. Videodensitometric techniques evaluate transit time or other measures of flow rate through an epicardial coronary artery based on angiograms and showed some potential in early studies.[41,42] However, due in part to the relative complexity of the measurements, quantitative assessment of coronary angiographic transit time has not gained widespread acceptance. Doppler ultrasound devices, either mounted on intracoronary catheters or placed directly on the epicardial coronary arteries in the operating room, have been used to measure velocity of coronary flow.[43] These devices may be used to estimate relative coronary flow at rest and after a hyperemic stimulus, giving a measure of coronary flow reserve. Once again, these methods do not yield absolute measures of myocardial perfusion or regional perfusion data and are not widely employed in routine clinical practice.

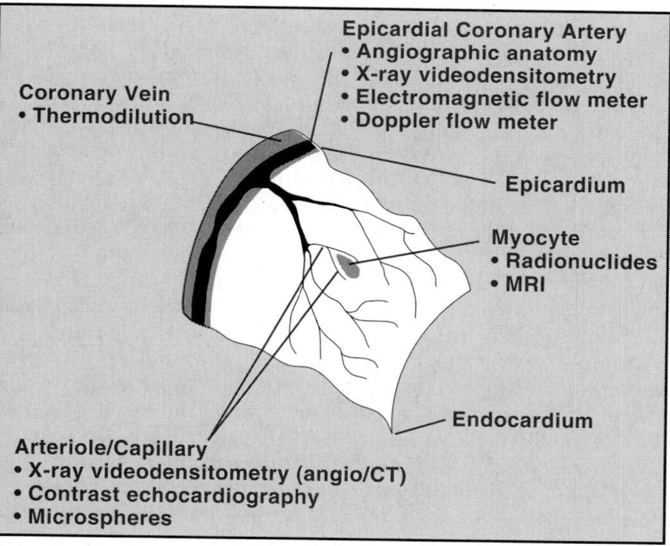

FIGURE 11–1. Current and evolving approaches to the assessment of coronary artery flow and myocardial perfusion. A schematic cross section of the left ventricular wall is shown, along with an indication of the anatomical levels at which various methods are used to evaluate perfusion. At the level of the epicardial coronary arteries, angiographic anatomy is commonly used to identify hydraulically significant stenoses, thereby inferring the potential for hypoperfusion with stress. X-ray videodensitometry and electromagnetic and Doppler flowmeters also may be used to assess perfusion at the level of the coronary arteries. (Some of these methods can be used only with an open chest.) Coronary venous thermodilution methods offer some insight into global or regional perfusion. At the arteriolar/capillary level, x-ray videodensitometry, contrast echocardiography, and microspheres may be employed. Finally, radionuclide and magnetic resonance imaging (MRI) methods attempt to assess perfusion at the level of the myocyte. Angio, angiography; CT, computed tomography.

The next anatomical level to consider is that of the coronary microvasculature. Several densitometric methods use various indicators and the principles of indicator-dilution theory to assess myocardial perfusion. Thus the kinetics of indicator entry into and washout from the myocardium may be assessed utilizing angiography[44] or CT[45] (in which an iodinated contrast medium is the indicator) or echocardiography[4,46] (in which "microbubbles" or other echogenic material is used as the indicator) (Fig. 3–98, p. 90). Perhaps most relevant to the clinician and physiologist would be the determination of nutrient flow at the level of the myocyte, utilizing indicators that are taken up by normally perfused cells. Thus radionuclides such as thallium-201[47] or technetium-99m–labeled perfusion agents[48] are used for the qualitative assessment of regional perfusion because of their relatively avid uptake by myocardial cells.

The most promising radionuclide approach to quantitative myocardial perfusion imaging is PET (see p. 304). The combination of the high-energy photons released during positron annihilation (511 keV) and the method of coincidence detection for image formation permits high-resolution depiction of the distribution of a perfusion tracer. The high temporal resolution, together with a quantitative imaging capability, combined with the use of multicompartment tracer kinetic models permits accurate estimates of absolute levels of myocardial perfusion.[49–52]

MRI methods, coupled with paramagnetic contrast agents, also show promise for the delineation of myocardial perfusion (Fig. 10–6, p. 322). For example, regional myocardial concentration of manganese has been shown to correlate with microsphere-determined blood flow.[53] Recent studies using gadolinium-based MRI contrast agents or other substances also appear promising for the assessment of myocardial perfusion.[54–56]

As of this writing, PET and fast CT appear to be the methods most capable of accurate, absolute measurements of regional myocardial perfusion at rest and with stress.

Assessment of Myocardial Metabolism

Two general approaches to the assessment of myocardial metabolism appear to be possible through imaging techniques: PET and MR spectroscopy. These two methods should be viewed as complementary,[57] since they offer different insights into the biochemistry of the myocardium. PET offers a wide range of metabolic information. Chief among these are studies of the uptake of fuel substrates such as glucose[58] and fatty acids.[59] Further, oxidative metabolism may be assessed quantitatively using PET.[60] Measurements of receptor density and function[61] and of other aspects of intermediary metabolism also may be performed utilizing PET (Fig. 9–40, Color plate 7).

MR spectroscopy of the myocardium is still in its infancy compared with PET. Nonetheless, MR spectroscopy shows promise and potentially can be performed using a variety of nuclei including protons (hydrogen nuclei), phosphorus-31, carbon-13, fluorine-19, and sodium-23.[62–64] Currently, whole-body spectroscopy seems most feasible with phosphorus-31 or proton methods. Phosphorus-31 spectroscopy allows quantitation of the relative amounts of myocardial high-energy phosphates, including phosphocreatine, inorganic phosphate, and adenosine triphosphate.[62,63,65] In addition to a "snapshot" assessment of the relative amounts of various high-energy phosphate compounds at a given point in time, magnetization transfer techniques show promise for the assessment of enzyme kinetics in vivo.[66] Finally, phosphorus-31 spectroscopy offers the potential of assessing intracellular pH, and MR spectroscopy using carbon-13 or protons offers insights into aspects of intermediary metabolism.

Delineation of Tissue Characteristics

In selected patients, clinicians will wish to have information on the physical characteristics or composition of the myocardium. For example, identification of the amount of scar tissue versus viable myocardium present after myocardial infarction is of great clinical interest. Similarly, knowledge of the degree of myocardial fibrosis attendant to long-standing volume overload in aortic regurgitation likely would be of use in the timing of valve replacement. The two techniques that appear to be most promising in the assessment of tissue characteristics are ultrasonography and MRI.

Myocardial reflection or absorption of ultrasound depends in part on tissue composition. Thus, acoustic characteristics of injured tissue may differ from those of normal myocardium. For example, edema related to acute ischemia and infarction, necrosis attendant to acute infarction, collagen deposition in chronic infarction, and atherosclerosis in vessel walls have all been identified using acoustic ultrasonographic analyses.[67] Further, diffuse cardiomyopathies, such as amyloidosis (Fig. 41–21, p. 1428) and hypertrophic cardiomyopathy, have been identified and differentiated from each other and from hypertensive left ventricular hypertrophy utilizing ultrasonographic tissue characterization methods.[68] Although many technical problems related to the acquisition of ultrasound data remain to be solved before these methods will be widely useful clinically, the general approach appears promising.

MRI techniques also may identify alterations in tissue composition based on differing image brightness in appropriately weighted images or on measurement of tissue NMR relaxation times. For example, alterations in image intensity, in myocardial T_1 and T_2 relaxation times, or in proton spectra have been demonstrated in infarction,[69–71] scar,[72] and "stunned" myocardium.[73] Paramagnetic contrast agents such as gadolinium appear to accentuate the image intensity and relaxation time differences and thus improve identification of myocardial abnormalities with MRI.[74]

EVALUATING SPECIFIC CATEGORIES OF CARDIAC DISEASE WITH IMAGING METHODS

In Table 11–5 and the following paragraphs is a summary of our opinions on the relative current utility of the various imaging methods in specific patient groups.

Ischemic Heart Disease

(See also Chaps. 37 and 38)

CORONARY ATHEROSCLEROSIS. The presence and extent of coronary atherosclerosis can be characterized most definitively utilizing selective coronary angiography. Particularly in the present era of aggressive interventional techniques to reduce the severity of coronary atherosclerotic narrowing, a large percentage of patients with ischemic heart disease will continue to be candidates for selective coronary angiography. As sophisticated methods of analyzing coronary arteriograms are further developed and validated, some advantages may accrue to the acquisition of coronary arteriographic data in digital format so that the newer computer analysis algorithms may be easily applied.[75]

Two other imaging approaches also make contributions to the diagnosis of coronary atherosclerosis. Intravascular ultrasound (see p. 58) permits extremely high resolution imaging of coronary lumen and adjacent wall thickness and composition (e.g., the presence of calcified plaque).[76,77] Recent intravascular ultrasound studies have demonstrated atherosclerosis in regions of coronary arteries judged normal on angiography.[76] CT also can contribute to the diagnosis of coronary atherosclerosis by the identification of coronary calcification[78,79] (Fig. 10–37, p. 339).

ACUTE FLOW DISTURBANCE AND TRANSIENT ISCHEMIA. In many patients with ischemic heart disease, coronary angiography is not indicated, particularly upon initial presentation. Thus, methods of identifying reduced coronary flow reserve or transient ischemia, particularly with exercise stress or pharmacological coronary vasodilation, are of great interest to clinicians. Thallium-201 scintigraphy (employing exercise stress or pharmacological vasodilation[47]) remains a useful procedure for the identification of regional myocardial ischemia, including the approximate severity of ischemia (Fig. 9–29, p. 294) and, in some patients, the identification of multivessel disease. The newer ^{99m}Tc-based myocardial perfusion tracers (Fig. 9–1, p. 275) and PET will ensure a continued important role for radionuclide methods in the assessment of transient ischemia.

Exercise or pharmacological stress radionuclide ventriculography and echocardiography offer an indirect but especially useful marker for acute ischemia: the appearance of new regional wall motion disturbances resulting from acute hypoperfusion of the myocardium. Although it does not give direct information on myocardial perfusion, the delineation of new regional wall motion disturbances (particu-

TABLE 11–5 RELATIVE USEFULNESS OF CARDIAC IMAGING METHODS IN SPECIFIC PATIENT GROUPS*

DISORDER	CXR	ECHO/DOPPLER	ANGIO†	RADIONUCLIDES	FCT	MRI
Ischemic	+	++	++++	+++	++	++
Valvular	++	++++	++++	++	+++	+++
Congenital	++	++++	++++	++	++++	++++
Traumatic	++	+++	+++	++	++	++
Cardiomyopathy	+	++++	+++	++	+++	+++
Pericardial	+	+++	++	0	++++	++++
Endocarditis	+	++++	++	0	++	+++
Masses	0	++++	+++	+	++++	++++

* 0, no information; ++++, maximum information; CXR, chest x-ray; echo, echocardiography; angio, angiography; FCT, fast computed tomography; MRI, magnetic resonance imaging.

† Angio includes both imaging and hemodynamic evaluation.

larly systolic ventricular wall thinning) will likely make stress echocardiography a more widely used technique in the future[80] (Fig. 3–90, p. 87). CT methods are much less widely used in the identification of transient ischemia because of the relatively small number of installed systems capable of performing high-speed CT imaging with pharmacologic stress. MRI may prove useful in the diagnosis of ischemia if paramagnetic contrast agents are found to be efficacious in identifying regional deficits in perfusion[81] or if spectroscopy becomes widely available.[82] However, because of the widespread availability of radionuclide methods and echocardiography, MRI probably will *not* be a first-line method for assessing acute or transient ischemia in the near future.

INFARCTION/REPERFUSION (see Chap. 37). The only clinically available imaging methods capable of directly identifying acutely necrotic myocardium are ^{99m}Tc pyrophosphate scintigraphy and labeled monoclonal antimyosin-specific antibody[83] scintigraphy (Fig. 9–19, p. 285). Although these methods permit the identification of acute necrosis, their clinical applicability is somewhat limited by their poor spatial resolution, which precludes detailed assessment of the size of myocardial infarction. Nonetheless, infarct-avid scintigraphy is, in selected patients, a useful method of infarct identification. Metabolic imaging with PET (see p. 306) shows great promise in the identification and quantitation of acute myocardial infarction.[84] MR spectroscopy using ^{31}P also may prove to be useful in identifying infarction.[65]

Analysis of regional wall motion is also a useful method of indirectly identifying acute myocardial infarction. If a patient is known to have had normal wall motion in a particular region before an infarction, echocardiographic delineation of regional wall motion disturbances in that region permit some assessment of the size of infarction, as do similar wall motion analyses utilizing radionuclide, CT, or MRI techniques. However, the assessment of regional wall motion abnormalities is plagued by the inherent biological heterogeneity of contraction in normal subjects,[85] by the fact that regional wall motion patterns appear to be load-dependent,[86] and by the nonspecificity of regional wall motion abnormalities. Acute ischemia, infarction, and scar may all be associated with similar wall motion abnormalities. Thus, in the future, these indirect techniques may have a lesser place in the identification of infarction than more direct methods.

Discrimination among reperfused, nonreperfused but viable, and irreversibly injured tissue is important, particularly with the availability of potent thrombolytic agents and other interventional procedures. The reversal of a regional wall motion disturbance identified by echocardiography, radionuclide ventriculography, CT, or MRI is a good marker for reperfusion of viable myocardium. Wall motion may not immediately return to normal, however, because the myocardium may be "stunned" (see p. 388) or "hibernating" (see p. 388). Echocardiography performed before and after pharmacological stimulation of the myocardium (e.g., with dobutamine) (see p. 289) may reveal an increase in regional contraction after stimulation. This approach is showing promise as a method of determining myocardial viability.[87] The most direct method available to help the clinician negotiate the quandary of assessing myocardial viability is metabolic imaging with PET. For example, the combination of PET scans of fuel substrate uptake and perfusion offers a unique strategy to differentiate viable from irreversibly injured myocardium (Fig. 9–41, Color plate 8). Fatty acids are the preferred substrate for normal myocardium; nonetheless, normal myocardium does take up glucose. Ischemic but viable myocardium may take up increased amounts of glucose as it operates in an oxygen-limited environment. Thus, the combination of PET scans showing preserved or *increased* glucose uptake in a region of *decreased* perfusion (a "mismatch") suggests that the region is, in fact, potentially viable. A concordant decrement in perfusion and fuel substrate uptake identifies irreversibly injured myocardium.[88]

The assessment of high-energy phosphate stores by MR spectroscopy also offers the potential for identification of the presence and extent of irreversibly injured myocardial tissue, although this approach remains investigative.

CHRONIC INFARCTION/SCAR FORMATION (see Chap. 38). As already described, the combination of lack of perfusion and lack of fuel substrate uptake on PET identifies a region as infarcted, although scar tissue from earlier infarction may produce the same pattern (Fig. 9–40, Color plate 8). Fibrosis may be identified directly in the future by the use of echocardiographic[89] or MRI tissue characterization[90] techniques or by PET as the fraction of tissue unable to exchange water rapidly.[91] As of this writing, however, no widely available imaging method is capable of identifying directly the presence and extent of myocardial fibrosis in the clinical setting. Thus, clinicians must depend on persistent abnormalities of regional contraction and decreased wall thickness (as delineated by echocardiography, radionuclide ventriculography, CT, or MRI) to identify chronic infarction.

Valvular Heart Disease

(See also Chap. 32)

Echocardiography remains the procedure of choice for the initial assessment of patients with valvular heart disease. Frequently, decisions regarding medical and surgical management are based on echocardiography without the need for invasive evaluation. In selected patients, angiography and cardiac catheterization are still quite useful, particularly in the identification of concomitant coronary artery disease and when ultrasound examinations yield equivocal results. CT and MRI methods offer the ability to determine left ventricular mass more precisely than does echocardiography. Regurgitant volume also can be determined accurately with CT[34] (see p. 336). This may prove useful in selected patients with valvular heart disease.

Congenital Heart Disease

(See also Chaps. 29 and 30)

Clinicians caring for patients with congenital heart disease require accurate information on cardiac morphology, often in settings of extremely complex spatial relationships among atria, ventricles, and great vessels. Methods capable of high-resolution anatomical assessment are of paramount importance in congenital heart disease. Currently, echocardiography is the initial method of choice in evaluating the anatomy of the heart and great vessels, whether in fetus, newborn, child, adolescent, or adult with established or suspected congenital heart disease. In addition to echocardiography, first-pass radionuclide angiography also offers information of use in congenital heart disease by permitting accurate noninvasive quantitation of cardiac shunts.[92] CT[93] and MRI[94] also permit shunt identification and quantitation.

Echocardiographic methods (including Doppler techniques) frequently yield diagnostic information of sufficient reliability to obviate the need for cardiac catheterization in relatively simple abnormalities, such as atrial septal defects in patients younger than 40 years of age. Invasive angiographic, oximetric, and hemodynamic studies will be needed, however, in many complex anomalies before surgical intervention. For abnormalities of the great vessels, particularly disorders of the aorta and pulmonary arteries, CT (Fig. 10–41, p. 341) and MRI (Fig. 10–20, p. 327) offer extremely useful information in selected patients. Finally, assessment of patients who have undergone complex repairs, particularly those involving the placement of conduits or baffles, is greatly aided by CT and especially MRI studies. The three-dimensional imaging characteristics of

MRI and the ability to assess intracardiac, great vessel, and conduit flow may make MRI of increasing importance in these patients.[95–97]

Traumatic Heart Disease and Aortic Disease

(See also Chaps. 44 and 45)

Assessment of the trauma patient with suspected cardiovascular sequelae generally involves a search for myocardial contusion, deceleration injuries (e.g., chordal rupture, aortic dissection), and, in the case of penetrating wounds, a wide variety of problems (including hemopericardium, tricuspid valve damage, and coronary artery laceration). While echocardiography is of use in the identification of acute valvular disruption, it may be difficult to perform after major thoracic trauma. Transesophageal echocardiography,[98] CT,[99] and MRI[100] are useful in identifying acute aortic dissection or rupture; of these three methods, only echocardiography can be performed at the bedside (Fig. 45–15, p. 1562).

Echocardiography, CT, or MRI may be used to identify abnormalities of regional ventricular contraction that indirectly suggest myocardial contusion. Technetium-99m pyrophospate scintigraphy identifies myocardial contusion directly (Fig. 44–7, p. 1541) but has a temporal limitation: the need to wait at least 24 hours after injury for acceptable scan sensitivity.

Cardiac catheterization may be required to assess the condition of selected patients after trauma, particularly those with suspected coronary injuries. Most, however, will be evaluated adequately using echocardiography, CT, and/or MRI.

Cardiomyopathies

(See also Chap. 41)

Although echocardiography is capable of differentiating among dilated, hypertrophic, and restrictive cardiomyopathies in most patients, it offers limited insight into the specific causes of these disorders. Observations of unusual echocardiographic textural appearance of the myocardium in amyloidosis (Fig. 3–102, p. 92) and hypertrophic cardiomyopathy have led to investigative quantitative approaches to discrimination among these disorders with ultrasound tissue characterization methods.[68] Although as of this writing these are not clinically applicable, tissue characterization may become available in the future. Perhaps more promising in selected disorders will be metabolic studies with PET and MR spectroscopy. As of this writing, invasive studies, including hemodynamic evaluation and sometimes endomyocardial biopsy, also are required in selected cases for complete characterization of the type and severity of cardiomyopathy.

Pericardial Disease

(See also Chap. 43)

Echocardiographic methods can ascertain the presence of pericardial effusion as well as give some indication of the existence of tamponade; therefore, echocardiography is the initial procedure of choice in investigating the patient with suspected pericardial effusion (Fig. 3–104, p. 93). In selected cases, echocardiography may be supplemented by CT or MRI. Due to the wider field of view of these latter methods, in some patients a better appreciation of the quantity and anatomical distribution of the effusion may be gained (Figs. 10–15, p. 325, and 10–41, p. 341). However, echocardiography, CT, and MRI give limited information on the cause of the effusion. Positron emission tomography and MRI may eventually offer assistance in this regard.

Echocardiographic images are of only limited value in identifying pericardial thickening and delineating the physiology of constrictive pericarditis. CT[101] and MRI[102] offer excellent visualization of the pericardium (Fig. 10–14, p. 325, and 10–40, p. 340) and are probably more useful than echocardiography in precise measurement of the thickness of the pericardium. Recent investigations with Doppler echocardiography,[103] CT,[104] and MRI[105] suggest that these noninvasive techniques may give information relevant to the diagnosis of constrictive pericarditis. Thus noninvasive assessment of diastolic filling may offer some help in the diagnosis of constrictive pericarditis, but these methods are still not as well established as hemodynamic data obtained at cardiac catheterization (see p. 187).

Infective Endocarditis

(See also Chap. 33)

The presence of vegetations may be established in the majority of patients using echocardiography (Fig. 3–61, p. 77). The advent of transesophageal echocardiography has substantially improved the sensitivity of ultrasonic identification of vegetations.[106] Thus, ultrasound is the initial imaging technique of choice in the patient suspected of having infective endocarditis. It should be emphasized, however, that failure to identify a vegetation by echocardiography should not be used to exclude definitively a diagnosis of endocarditis, since false-negative examination results do occur, even with transesophageal echocardiography.

The complications of endocarditis, including valve disruption and abscess formation, often can be identified with echocardiography (Fig. 3–63, p. 77), and likely with CT or MRI as well. Catheterization and angiocardiography are rarely necessary to identify either the presence of endocarditis or its attendant complications.

Intracardiac Masses

(See also Chaps. 42 and 57)

In addition to vegetations, clinicians will encounter other varieties of intracardiac mass lesions, including thrombi, myxomata, and metastatic tumors. Once again, echocardiography is quite useful in assessment of these patients (Fig. 3–105, p. 94). Transesophageal echocardiography has proved particularly helpful in identifying thrombi in areas that are difficult to image by other methods, such as the left atrial appendage in patients with a suspected cardiogenic source of cerebral emboli.[107] CT and MRI are also excellent methods of identifying intracardiac masses (Figs. 10–18, p. 326, and 10–42, p. 341) and should be considered when the results of echocardiography are equivocal. The determination of the nature of an intracardiac mass is best made currently by indirect evidence, such as the anatomical position and attachment of the mass, but such methods as characterization of the tissue by ultrasonography or MRI may prove helpful in this regard in the future.

COST CONSIDERATIONS IN CARDIAC IMAGING

A major, global change is occurring in the practice of medicine, wherein the intellectual challenge is framed less by what we *can* do and more by what we *should* do. Increasingly, the physician is faced with the dilemma that the best possible care for the patient is not necessarily aligned with the optimal use of resources for society. Even when imaging is likely to be beneficial, recommendations can be expected to differ between a managed care organization concerned with "covered lives" and a physician who has responsibility for an individual patient. The clinician strives to do the right thing for a patient even when outcomes data, cost-effectiveness information, and practice guidelines are of dubious relevance to the individual case. Only the personal physician can be aware of the diverse factors impacting the patient's care at any given time.

The several methods of imaging the heart and circulation vary widely in their costs. In considering these variations, several types of expenses should be considered (Table 11–6). These include the initial purchase price of the system

TABLE 11–6 SOME COSTS ASSOCIATED WITH CARDIAC IMAGING METHODS

Purchase price of system
Site preparation
Power, water, and environmental costs
Personnel
Physicians
Nurses
Technicians
Support personnel (physicists, engineers, pharmacists, others)

and any necessary expenditures for site preparation. Once the system is installed, consideration must be given to power and environmental costs. Personnel costs to be considered include the physicians, technicians, and nurses who deal with the day-to-day operation of the system, as well as support personnel for maintenance and quality control testing. Overall, in terms of establishing and operating a particular imaging system, excluding chest roentgenography, echocardiography falls at the least expensive end of the spectrum, although a complete modern echocardiographic system costs about $250,000. At the other end of the spectrum are CT, MRI, and PET, all of which cost in excess of $1 million. Conventional radionuclide imaging falls between these extremes of the cost spectrum.

Currently evolving changes in the health care reimbursement system, however, may render some of these cost comparisons less relevant. The total cost of a complete diagnostic evaluation for a particular disorder will likely become the factor of key interest. Thus a relatively more expensive technique that eliminates other tests may reduce the overall cost of an individual patient workup. An a priori expensive test may become, thereby, a rather cost-effective test. This approach, however, will necessitate discipline on the part of the responsible clinician to choose only those imaging tests which add unique information that will significantly impact patient management decisions.

SUMMARY AND CONCLUSION

A large, at times bewildering set of choices in diagnostic imaging methods confronts clinicians evaluating patients with known or suspected cardiovascular disease. The varying biophysical bases of the several available imaging approaches suggest their complementarity in patient evaluation. We have offered our consensus opinions on the relative merits of available and evolving imaging methods in general and for specific patient groups. In the individual practice setting, availability and local expertise are additional, critical factors to be considered.

REFERENCES

SCOPE OF CARDIAC IMAGING

1. Skorton, D. J., Schelbert, H. R., Wolf, G. L., and Brundage, B. H. (eds.): Marcus Cardiac Imaging. 2nd ed. (A companion to E. Braunwald, Heart Disease.) Philadelphia, W. B. Saunders Company, 1996.
2. Pohost, G. M., and O'Rourke, R. A.: Principles and Practice of Cardiovascular Imaging. Boston, Little, Brown, 1991.
3. Hounsfield, G. N.: Computed medical imaging (Nobel lecture, December 8, 1979). J. Comput. Assist. Tomogr. *4*:665, 1980.
4. Jayaweera, A. R., and Kaul, S.: Quantifying myocardial blood flow with contrast echocardiography. Am. J. Cardiac Imaging *7*:317, 1993.
5. Wickline, S. A., Verdonk, E. D., Wong, A. K., et al.: Structural remodeling of human myocardial tissue after infarction: Quantification with ultrasonic backscatter. Circulation *85*:259, 1992.
6. Siu, S. C., Rivera, J. M., Guerrero, J. L., et al.: Three-dimensional echocardiography: In vivo validation for left ventricular volume and function. Circulation *88* (Part 1):1715, 1993.
7. Schelbert, H. R.: Blood flow and metabolism by PET. *In* Verani, M. S. (ed.): Cardiology Clinics, Nuclear Cardiology: State of the Art. Vol. 12. Philadelphia, W.B. Saunders Company, 1994, p. 303.
8. Koning, G., Brandvanden, M., Zorn, I., et al.: Usefulness of digital angiography in the assessment of left ventricular ejection fraction. Cathet. Cardiovasc. Diagn. *21*:185, 1990.
9. Edelman, R. R., and Warach, S.: Magnetic resonance imaging. N. Engl. J. Med. *328*:708, 1993.
10. Mohiaddin, R. H., and Longmore, D. B.: Functional aspects of cardiovascular nuclear magnetic resonance imaging: Techniques and application. Circulation *88*:264, 1993.
11. Weiss, R. G., Bottomley, P. A., Hardy, C. J., and Gerstenblith, G.: Regional myocardial metabolism of high-energy phosphates during isometric exercise in patients with coronary artery disease. N. Engl. J. Med. *323*:1593, 1990.
12. Brundage, B. H.: Myocardial imaging with ultrafast computed tomography. *In* Zoreb, B. L., Kaufman, L., Berson, A. S., and Dunn, R. A. (eds.): Frontiers in Cardiovascular Imaging. New York, Raven Press, 1993, p. 35.
13. Jones, J. P.: Physics of the MR image: From the basic principles to image intensity and contrast. *In* Partain, C. L., Price, R. R., Patton, J. A., et al. (eds.): Magnetic Resonance Imaging. 2nd ed. Vol. 2: Physical Principles and Instrumentation. Philadelphia, W.B. Saunders Company, 1988, p. 1003.
14. Collins, S. M., and Skorton, D. J. (eds.): Cardiac Imaging and Image Processing. New York, McGraw-Hill Book Co., 1986.
15. Buda, A. J., and Delp, E. J.: Digital Cardiac Imaging. Boston, Martinus Nijhoff, 1985.

MEETING THE GOALS OF CARDIAC IMAGING

16. Feiring, A. J., Rumberger, J. A., Reiter, S. J., et al.: Determination of left ventricular mass in dogs with rapid-acquisition cardiac computed tomographic scanning. Circulation *72*:1355, 1985.
17. Pattynama, P. M. T., de Roos, A., van der Wall, E. E., and van der Voorthuisen, A. D. E.: Evaluation of cardiac function with magnetic resonance imaging. Am. Heart J. *128*:595, 1994.
18. Pearlman, J. D., and Edelman, R. R.: Ultrafast magnetic resonance imaging: Segmented turboflash, echo-planar, and real-time nuclear magnetic resonance. Radiol. Clin. North Am. *32*:593, 1994.
19. Napel, S., Rutt, B. K., and Pflugfelder, P.: Three-dimensional images of the coronary arteries from ultrafast computed tomography: Method and comparison with two-dimensional arteriography. Am. J. Cardiac Imaging *3*:237, 1989.
20. Iliceto, S., Marangelli, V., Memmola, C., and Rizzon, P.: Transesophageal Doppler echocardiography evaluation of coronary blood flow velocity in baseline conditions and during dipyridamole-induced coronary vasodilation. Circulation *83*:61, 1991.
21. Manning, W. J., Li, W., and Edelman, R. R.: A preliminary report comparing magnetic resonance coronary angiography with conventional angiography. N. Engl. J. Med. *328*:828, 1993.
22. Stanford, W., Brundage, B. H., MacMillan, R., et al.: Sensitivity and specificity of assessing coronary bypass graft patency with ultrafast computed tomography: Results of a multicenter study. J. Am. Coll. Cardiol. *12*:1, 1988.
23. Stanford, W., Galvin, J. R., Thompson, B. H., Grover-McKay, M., and Skorton, D. J.: Nonangiographic assessment of coronary artery bypass graft patency. Int. J. Cardiac Imaging *9*:77, 1993.
24. Schiller, N. B., Shah, P. M., Crawford, M., DeMaria, A., et al.: American Society of Echocardiography Committee on Standards, Subcommittee on Quantitation of Two-Dimensional Echocardiograms: Recommendations for quantitation of the left ventricle by two-dimensional echocardiography. J. Am. Soc. Echocardiogr. *2*:358, 1989.
25. Roig, E., Georgiou, D., Chomka, E. V., Wolfkiel, C., LoGalbo-Zak, C., Rich, S., and Brundage, B. H.: Reproducibility of left ventricular myocardial volume and mass measurement by ultrafast computed tomography. J. Am. Coll. Cardiol. *18*:990, 1991.
26. Hunter, G. J., Hamberg, L. M., Weisskoff, R. M., Halpern, E. F., and Brady, T. J.: Measurement of stroke volume and cardiac output within a single breath hold with echo-planar MR imaging. J. Magn. Reson. Imaging *4*:51, 1994.
27. Kondo, C., Caputo, G. R., Semelka, R., et al.: Right and left ventricular stroke volume measurements with velocity-encoded cine MR imaging: In vitro and in vivo validation. A.J.R. *157*:9, 1991.
28. Florentine, M. S., Grosskreutz, C. L., Chang, W., et al.: Measurement of left ventricular mass in vivo using gated nuclear magnetic resonance imaging. J. Am. Coll. Cardiol. *8*:107, 1986.
29. Rumberger, J. A., Weiss, R. M., Feiring, A. J., et al.: Patterns of regional diastolic function in the normal human left ventricle: An ultrafast computed tomography study. J. Am. Coll. Cardiol. *14*:119, 1989.
30. Beache, G. M., Wedeen, V. J., and Dinsmore, R. E.: Magnetic resonance imaging evaluation of left ventricular dimensions and function and pericardial and myocardial disease. Coronary Artery Dis. *4*:328, 1993.
31. Gibbons, R. J.: Equilibrium radionuclide angiography. *In* Skorton, D. J., Schelbert, H. R., Wolf, G. L., and Brundage, B. H. (eds.): Marcus Cardiac Imaging. 2nd ed. (A companion to E. Braunwald, Heart Disease.) Philadelphia, W. B. Saunders Company, 1996.
32. Aebischer, N. M., and Czegledy, F.: Determination of right ventricular volume by two-dimensional echocardiography with a crescentic model. J. Am. Soc. Echocardiogr. *2*:110, 1989.
33. Mahoney, L. T., Smith, W., Noel, M. P., et al.: Measurement of right ventricular volume using cine computed tomography. Invest. Radiol. *22*:451, 1987.
34. Reiter, S. J., Rumberger, J. A., Feiring, A. J., et al.: Precision of measurements of right and left ventricular volume by cine computed tomography. Circulation *74*:890, 1986.
35. Pattynama, P. M. T., Lamb, H. J., Van der Geest, R., et al.: Reproducibil-

ity of MRI-derived measurements of right ventricular volumes and myocardial mass. J. Magn. Reson. Imaging *13*:53, 1995.
36. Doherty, N. E., Fujita, N., Caputo, G. R., and Higgins, C. B.: Measurement of right ventricular mass in normal and dilated cardiomyopathic ventricles using cine magnetic resonance imaging. Am. J. Cardiol. *69*:1223, 1992.
37. Rezai, K., Weiss, R., Stanford, W., et al.: Relative accuracy of three scintigraphic methods for determination of right ventricular ejection fraction: A correlative study with ultrafast CT. J. Nucl. Med. *32*:429, 1991.
38. van den Brink, R. B., Verheul, H. A., Hoedemaker, G., et al.: The value of Doppler echocardiography in the management of patients with valvular heart disease: analysis of one year of clinical practice. J. Am. Soc. Echocardiogr. *4*:109, 1991.
39. Gould, K. L., and Lipscomb, K.: Effects of coronary stenoses on coronary flow reserve and resistance. Am. J. Cardiol. *34*:48, 1974.
40. White, C. W., Wright, C. B., Doty, D. B., et al.: Does the visual interpretation of the coronary arteriogram predict the physiological importance of a coronary stenosis? N. Engl. J. Med. *310*:819, 1984.
41. Rutishauser, W., Noseda, G., Bussman, W. D., and Preter, B.: Blood flow measurements through single coronary arteries by roentgen densitometry: II. Right coronary artery flow in conscious man. A.J.R. *109*:21, 1970.
42. Smith, H. C., Sturm, R. E., and Wood, E. H.: Videodensitometric system for measurement of vessel blood flow, particularly in the coronary arteries, in man. Am. J. Cardiol. *32*:144, 1973.
43. Wilson, R. F., Laughlin, D. E., Ackell, P. H., et al.: Transluminal subselective measurement of coronary artery blood flow velocity and vasodilator reserve in man. Circulation *72*:82, 1985.
44. Hodgson, J. M., LeGrand, V., Bates, E. R., et al.: Validation in dogs of a rapid digital angiographic technique to measure relative coronary blood flow during routine cardiac catheterization. Am. J. Cardiol. *5*:188, 1985.
45. Wolfkiel, C. J., and Brundage, B. H.: Measurement of myocardial blood flow by UFCT: Towards clinical applicability. Int. J. Cardiac Imaging *7*:89, 1991.
46. Feinstein, S. B., Lang, R. M., Dick, C., et al.: Contrast echocardiography during coronary arteriography in humans: Perfusion and anatomic studies. J. Am. Coll. Cardiol. *11*:59, 1988.
47. Beller, G.: Myocardial perfusion imaging with thallium-201. J. Nucl. Med. *35*:674, 1994.
48. van Train, K.: Multicenter trial validation for quantitative analysis of same-day rest-stress technetium-99m-sestamibi myocardial tomograms. J. Nucl. Med. *35*:609, 1994.
49. Kuhle, W., Porenta, G., Huang, S. C., et al.: Quantification of regional myocardial blood flow using ^{13}N-ammonia and reoriented dynamic positron emission tomographic imaging. Circulation *86*:1004, 1992.
50. Bergmann, S. R., Herrero, P., Markham, J., et al.: Noninvasive quantitation of myocardial blood flow in human subjects with oxygen-15–labeled water and positron emission tomography. J. Am. Coll. Cardiol. *14*:639, 1989.
51. Krivokapich, J., Smith, G. T., Huang, S. C., et al.: N-13 ammonia myocardial imaging at rest and with exercise in normal volunteers: Quantification of absolute myocardial perfusion with dynamic positron emission tomography. Circulation *80*:1328, 1989.
52. Czernin, J., Müller, P., Chan, S., et al.: Influence of age and hemodynamics on myocardial blood flow and flow reserve. Circulation *88*:62, 1993.
53. Schaefer, S., Lange, R. A., Kulkarni, P. V., et al.: In vivo nuclear magnetic resonance imaging of myocardial perfusion using the paramagnetic contrast agent manganese gluconate. J. Am. Coll. Cardiol. *14*:472, 1989.
54. Edelman, R. R., and Li, W.: Contrast-enhanced echo-planar MR imaging of myocardial perfusion: Preliminary study in humans. Radiology *190*:771, 1994.
55. Wendland, M. F., Saeed, M., Masui, T., Derugin, N., and Higgins, C. B.: First pass of an MR susceptibility contrast agent through normal and ischemic heart: Gradient-recalled echo-planar imaging. J. Magn. Reson. Imaging *3*:755, 1993.
56. Saeed, M., Wendland, M. F., Masui, T., et al.: Dual mechanisms for change in myocardial signal intensity by means of a single MR contrast medium: Dependence on concentration and pulse sequence. Radiology *186*:175, 1993.
57. Syrota, A., and Jehenson, P.: Complementarity of magnetic resonance spectroscopy, positron emission tomography and single photon emission tomography for the in vivo investigation of human cardiac metabolism and neurotransmission. Eur. J. Nucl. Med. *18*:897, 1991.
58. Choi, Y., Brunken, R., Hawkins, R., et al.: Factors affecting myocardial 2-[F-18]fluoro-2-deoxy-D-glucose uptake in positron emission tomography studies of normal humans. Eur. J. Nucl. Med. *20*:308, 1993.
59. Schelbert, H. R., Henze, E., Sochor, H., et al.: Effects of substrate availability on myocardial C-11 palmitate kinetics by positron emission tomography in normal subjects and patients with ventricular dysfunction. Am. Heart J. *111*:1055, 1986.
60. Armbrecht, J. J., Buxton, D. B., Brunken, R. C., et al.: Regional myocardial oxygen consumption determined noninvasively in humans with [1-^{11}C]acetate and dynamic positron tomography. Circulation *80*:863, 1989.
61. Merlet, P., Delforge, J., Syrota, A., et al.: Positron emission tomography with ^{11}C CGP-12177 to assess β-adrenergic receptor concentration in idiopathic dilated cardiomyopathy. Circulation *87*:1169, 1993.
62. Bottomley, P. A.: Noninvasive study of high-energy phosphate metabolism in human heart by depth-resolved P-31 NMR spectroscopy. Science *229*:769, 1985.
63. Bottomley, P. A., Hardy, C. J., and Roemer, P. B.: Phosphate metabolite imaging and concentration measurements in human heart by nuclear magnetic resonance. Magn. Reson. Med. *14*:425, 1990.
64. Jelicks, L. A., and Gupta, R. K.: Nuclear magnetic resonance measurement of intracellular sodium in the perfused normotensive and spontaneously hypertensive rat heart. Am. J. Hypertens. *7*:429, 1994.
65. Scholz, T. D., Grover-McKay, M., Fleagle, S. R., and Skorton, D. J.: Quantitation of the extent of acute myocardial infarction by phosphorus-31 nuclear magnetic resonance spectroscopy. J. Am. Coll. Cardiol. *18*:1380, 1991.
66. Zahler, R., and Ingwall, J. S.: Estimation of heart mitochondrial creatine kinase flux using magnetization transfer NMR spectroscopy. Am. J. Physiol. *262*:H1022, 1992.
67. Pérez, J. E., and Miller, J. G.: Ultrasonic backscatter tissue characterization in cardiac diagnosis. Clin. Cardiol. *14* (Suppl V):V-4, 1991.
68. Chandrasekaran, K., Aylward, P. E., Fleagle, S. R., et al.: Feasibility of identifying amyloid and hypertrophic cardiomyopathy with the use of computerized quantitative texture analysis of clinical echocardiographic data. J. Am. Coll. Cardiol. *13*:832, 1989.
69. Johnston, D. L.: Myocardial tissue characterization with magnetic resonance imaging techniques. Am. J. Cardiac Imaging *8*:140, 1994.
70. de Roos, A., van der Wall, E. E., Bruschke, A. V. G., and van Voorthuisen, A. E.: Magnetic resonance imaging in the diagnosis and evaluation of myocardial infarction. Magn. Reson. Q. *7*:191, 1991.
71. Saeed, M., Wendland, M. R., Yu, K. K., et al.: Identification of myocardial reperfusion with echo planar magnetic resonance imaging: Discrimination between occlusive and reperfused infarctions. Circulation *90*:1492, 1994.
72. Wisenberg, G., Prato, F. S., Carroll, S. E., et al.: Serial nuclear magnetic resonance imaging of acute myocardial infarction with and without reperfusion. Am. Heart J. *115*:510, 1988.
73. Reeves, R. C., Evanochko, W. T., Canby, R. C., et al.: Demonstration of increased myocardial lipid with postischemic dysfunction ("myocardial stunning") by proton nuclear magnetic resonance spectroscopy. J. Am. Coll. Cardiol. *13*:739, 1989.
74. Saeed, M., Wendland, M. F., and Higgins, C. B.: Contrast media for MR imaging of the heart. J. Magn. Reson. Imaging *4*:269, 1994.

EVALUATING SPECIFIC CATEGORIES OF CARDIAC DISEASE

75. Rensing, B. J., Hermans, W. R. M., Deckers, J. W., et al.: Lumen narrowing after percutaneous transluminal coronary balloon angioplasty follows a near gaussian distribution: A quantitative angiographic studyin 1445 successfully dilated lesions. J. Am. Coll. Cardiol. *19*:939, 1992.
76. St.Goar, F. G., Pinto, F. J., Alderman, E. L., et al.: Intracoronary ultrasound in cardiac transplant recipients: In vivo evidence of "angiographically silent" intimal thickening. Circulation *85*:979, 1992.
77. Linker, D. T., Kleven, A., Grønningsaether, Å., et al.: Tissue characterization with intra-arterial ultrasound: Special promise and problems. Int. J. Cardiac Imaging *6*:255, 1991.
78. Agatston, A. S., Janowitz, W. R., Hildner, F. J., Zusmer, N. R., Viamonte, M., and Detrano, R.: Quantification of coronary artery calcium using ultrafast computed tomography. J. Am. Coll. Cardiol. *15*:827, 1990.
79. Mautner, S. L., Mautner, G. L., Froelich, J., Feurstein, I. M., Proschan, M. A., Roberts, W. C., and Doppman, J. L.: Predicting coronary artery disease by electron beam tomography. Radiology *192*:625, 1994.
80. Ryan, T., Segar, D. S., Sawada, S. G., et al.: Detection of coronary artery disease using upright bicycle exercise echocardiography. J. Am. Soc. Echocardiogr. *6*:186, 1993.
81. Wendland, M. F., Saeed, M., Masui, T., Derugin, N., Moseley, M. E., and Higgins, C. B.: Echo-planar MR imaging of normal and ischemic myocardium with gadodiamide injection. Radiology *186*:535, 1993.
82. Yabe, T., Mitsunami, K., Okada, M., Morikawa, S., Inubushi, T., and Kinoshita, M.: Detection of myocardial ischemia by ^{31}P magnetic resonance spectroscopy during handgrip exercise. Circulation *89*:1709, 1994.
83. Maddahi, J.: Clinical applications of antimyosin monoclonal antibody imaging. Am. J. Cardiac Imaging *8*:249, 1994.
84. Hicks, R., Melon, P., Kalff, V., et al.: Metabolic imaging by positron emission tomography early after myocardial infarction as a predictor of recovery of myocardial function after reperfusion. J. Nucl. Cardiol. *1*:124, 1994.
85. Pandian, N. G., Skorton, D. J., Collins, S. M., et al.: Heterogeneity of left ventricular segmental wall thickening and excursion in two-dimensional echocardiograms of normal human subjects. Am. J. Cardiol. *51*:1667, 1983.
86. Weiss, R. M., Shonka, M. D., Kinzey, J. E., et al.: Effects of loading alterations on the pattern of heterogeneity of regional left ventricular function (Abs.). FASEB J *2*:1494A, 1988.
87. LaCanna, G., Alfieri, O., Giubbini, R., et al.: Echocardiography during infusion of dobutamine for identification of reversible dysfunction in patients with chronic coronary artery disease. J. Am. Coll. Cardiol. *23*:617, 1994.
88. Tillisch, J., Brunken, R., Marshall, R., et al.: Reversibility of cardiac wall-motion abnormalities predicted by positron tomography. N. Engl. J. Med. *314*:884, 1986.
89. Hoyt, R. H., Collins, S. M., Skorton, D. J., et al.: Assessment of fibrosis

in infarcted human hearts by analysis of ultrasonic backscatter. Circulation *71:*740, 1985.
90. Hsu, J. C. M., Johnson, G. A., and Smith, W. M.: Magnetic resonance imaging of chronic myocardial infarcts in formalin-fixed human autopsy hearts. Circulation *89:*2133, 1994.
91. Yamamoto, Y., De Silva, R., Rhodes, C., et al.: A new strategy for the assessment of viable myocardium and regional myocardial blood flow using ^{15}O-water and dynamic positron emission tomography. Circulation *86:*167, 1992.
92. Alazraki, N.: Nuclear imaging of valvular disease, left atrial myxoma, and shunts. *In* Elliott, L. P. (ed.): Cardiac Imaging in Infants, Children and Adults. Philadelphia, J. B. Lippincott Co., 1991, p. 796.
93. Garrett, J., Jaschke, W., Aherue, T., et al.: Quantitation of intracardiac shunts by cine-CT. J. Comput. Asst. Tomogr. *12:*82, 1988.
94. Sieverding, L., Jung, W. I., Klose, U., and Apitz, J.: Noninvasive blood flow measurement and quantification of shunt volume by cine magnetic resonance in congenital heart disease: Preliminary results. Pediatr. Radiol. *22:*48, 1992.
95. Link, K. M., and Lesko, N. M.: Magnetic resonance imaging in the evaluation of congenital heart disease. Magn. Reson. Q. *7:*173, 1991.
96. Fellows, K. E., Weinberg, P. M., Baffa, J. M., and Hoffman, E. A.: Evaluation of congenital heart disease with MR imaging: Current and coming attractions. A.J.R. *159:*925, 1992.
97. White, R. D.: Magnetic resonance imaging of congenital heart disease. *In* Pohost, G. M. (ed.): Cardiovascular Applications of Magnetic Resonance. Mount Kisco, N.Y., Futura, 1993, p. 59.
98. Smith, M. D., Cassidy, J. M., Souther, S., et al.: Transesophageal echocardiography in the diagnosis of traumatic rupture of the aorta. N. Engl. J. Med. *332:*356, 1995.
99. Stanford, W., Rooholamini, S. A., and Galvin, J. R.: Ultrafast computed tomography in the diagnosis of aortic aneurysms and dissections. J. Thoracic Imaging *5:*32, 1990.
100. Link, K. M., and Lesko, N. M.: The role of MR imaging in the evaluation of acquired disease of the thoracic aorta. A.J.R. *158:*1115, 1992.
101. Grover-McKay, M., Burke, S., Thompson, S. A., et al.: Measurement of pericardial thickness by cine computed tomography. Am. J. Cardiac Imaging *5:*98, 1991.
102. Didier, D., Terrier, R., and Grossholz, M.: Imaging of the pericardium using magnetic resonance (German). Radiologe *33:*87, 1993.
103. Oh, J. K., Hatle, L. K., Seward, J. B., et al.: Diagnostic role of Doppler echocardiography in constrictive pericarditis. J. Am. Coll. Cardiol. *23:*154, 1994.
104. Oren, R. M., Grover-McKay, M., Stanford, W., and Weiss, R. M.: Accurate preoperative diagnosis of pericardial constriction using cine computed tomography. J. Am. Coll. Cardiol. *22:*832, 1993.
105. Masui, T., Finck, S., and Higgins, C. B.: Constrictive pericarditis and restrictive cardiomyopathy: Evaluation with MR imaging. Radiology *182:*369, 1992.
106. Erbel, R., Rohmann, S., Drexler, M., et al.: Improved diagnostic value of echocardiography in patients with infective endocarditis by transesophageal approach: A prospective study. Eur. Heart J. *9:*43, 1988.
107. Pearson, A. C., Labovitz, A. J., Tatineni S., and Gomez, C. R.: Superiority of transesophageal echocardiography in detecting cardiac source of embolism in patients with cerebral ischemia of uncertain etiology. J. Am. Coll. Cardiol. *17:*66, 1991.

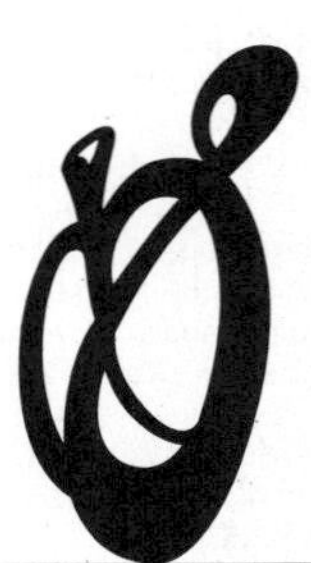

Part II
Normal and Abnormal Circulatory Function

Chapter 12
Mechanisms of Cardiac Contraction and Relaxation

LIONEL H. OPIE

MICROANATOMY OF CONTRACTILE CELLS AND PROTEINS

Ultrastructure of Contractile Cells

The contractile proteins of the heart lie within the muscle cells *(cardiomyocytes)*, which constitute about 75 per cent of the total volume of the myocardium, although only about one-third in number of all the cells.[1] About half of each ventricular myocyte is occupied by myofibrils and about one-quarter to one-third by mitochondria (Table 12–1).[2] A *myofiber* is a group of myocytes (Fig. 12–1) held together by surrounding collagen connective tissue. Further strands of collagen connect myofibers to each other,[3] and excess collagen, as in left ventricular (LV) hypertrophy, may cause LV diastolic dysfunction.[1]

The individual cardiomyocytes that account for more than half of the heart's weight are roughly cylindrical in shape (Fig. 12–1). Those in the atrium are quite small, less than 10 microns in diameter and about 20 microns in length. Relative to atrial cells, human ventricular myocytes are large, measuring about 17 to 25 microns in diameter and 60 to 140 microns in length (Table 12–1).

When examined under the light microscope, the atrial and ventricular muscle cells have cross-striations and are branched.[2] Each cell is bounded by a complex cell membrane, the *sarcolemma* (*sarco* = flesh; *lemma* = thin husk), and is filled with rodlike bundles of *myofibrils* (Fig. 12–1). The latter are the contractile elements. The sarcolemma of the myocyte invaginates to form an extensive tubular network *(T tubules)* that extends the extracellular space into the interior of the cell (Figs. 12–1 and 12–2). The nucleus, which contains almost all of the cell's genetic information, is often centrally located. Some myocytes have several nuclei. Interspersed between the myofibrils and immediately beneath the sarcolemma are many *mitochondria,* the main function of which is to generate the energy in the form of adenosine triphosphate (ATP) needed to maintain the heart's contractile function and the associated ion gradients. Of the other organelles, the *sarcoplasmic reticulum* (SR), is most important (Fig. 12–3).

Anatomically, the SR is a fine network spreading throughout the myocytes, demarcated by its lipid bilayer which is rather similar to that of the sarcolemma. Parts of the SR lie in very close apposition to the T tubules.[2] Here the tubules of the SR expand into bulbous swellings, still hollow, which lie along the inner surface of the sarcolemma or are wrapped around the T tubules (Fig. 12–1). These expanded areas of the SR have several names: *subsarcolemmal cisternae* (baskets, Latin) or *junctional SR.* Sometimes the cisternae occur in pairs *(dyads)* lying astride the T tubule, the whole having the appearance of *triads.* Their function is to release calcium from the *calcium release channel* (also called the ryanodine receptor) to initiate the contractile cycle (Fig. 12–3 and Fig. 16–5, p. 481).

The second part of the SR, the *longitudinal* or *network SR,* consists of ramifying tubules (Fig. 12–1) and is concerned with the uptake of calcium that initiates relaxation. This uptake is achieved by the ATP-requiring calcium pump, also called SERCA (sarcoendoplasmic reticulum Ca^{++}-ATPase), that increases its activity in response to beta-adrenergic stimulation (see p. 405). Calcium taken up

TABLE 12–1 CHARACTERISTICS OF CARDIAC CELLS, ORGANELLES, AND CONTRACTILE PROTEINS

MICROANATOMY OF HEART CELLS

	Ventricular Myocyte	Atrial Myocyte	Purkinje Cells
Shape	Long and narrow	Elliptical	Long and broad
Length (microns)	60–140	About 20	150–200
Diameter (microns)	About 20	5–6	35–40
Volume (microns^3)	15–45,000	About 500	135,000–250,000
T tubules	Plentiful	Rare or none	Absent
Intercalated disc	Prominent end-to-end transmission	Side-to-side as well as end-to-end transmission	Very prominent; abundant gap junctions. Fast end-to-end transmission
General appearance	Mitochondria and sarcomeres very abundant Rectangular branching bundles with little interstitial collagen	Bundles of atrial tissue separated by wide areas of collagen	Fewer sarcomeres, paler

COMPOSITION AND FUNCTION OF VENTRICULAR CELL

Organelle	Percentage of Cell Volume	Function
Myofibril	About 50–60	Interaction of thick and thin filaments during contraction cycle
Mitochondria	16 in neonate 33 in adult rat 23 in adult man	Provide ATP chiefly for contraction
T system	About 1	Transmission of electrical signal from sarcolemma to cell interior
Sarcoplasmic reticulum (SR)	33 in neonate 2 in adult	Takes up and releases Ca^{++} during contraction cycle
Terminal cisternae of SR	0.33 in adult	Site of calcium storage and release
Rest of network of SR	Rest of volume	Site of calcium uptake en route to cisternae
Sarcolemma	Very low	Control of ionic gradients; channels for ions (action potential); maintenance of cell integrity; receptors for drugs and hormones
Nucleus	About 5	Protein synthesis
Lysosomes	Very low	Intracellular digestion and proteolysis
Sarcoplasm (= cytoplasm) (+ nuclei + other structures)	About 12 in adult rat, 18 in humans	Provides cytosol in which rise and fall of ionized calcium occurs; contains other ions and small molecules

is then stored at high concentration in a number of storage proteins, including *calsequestrin,* before being released again.

The *cytoplasm* is the intracellular fluid and proteins therein, contained within the sarcolemma but excluding the contents of organelles such as mitochondria and the SR. The fluid component of the cytoplasm, minus the proteins, is called the *cytosol.* It is in the cytosol that the concentrations of calcium ions rise and fall to cause cardiac contraction and relaxation. The proteins of the sarcoplasm include many specialized molecules, the *enzymes,* that act to accelerate the conversion of one chemical form to another, thereby eventually producing energy.

Contractile Proteins

The major function of myocardial myocytes lies in the contraction-relaxation cycle. The major molecules involved include the two chief contractile proteins, the thin *actin* filament and the thick *myosin* filament. The molecular structure of the myosin head is now well understood (Fig. 12–4). Of note is the concept that it is the elongated basal part of the head that changes configuration during the contractile cycle, and not flexion and extension at the head-tail junction, as previously thought. Calcium ions interact with troponin-C at binding sites now identified to relieve the inhibition otherwise exerted by troponin-I (Fig. 12–4). *Titin* is a newly discovered large elastic molecule that supports myosin. During contraction, the filaments slide over each other without the individual molecules of actin or myosin actually shortening. As they slide, they pull together the two ends of the fundamental contractile unit called the *sarcomere.* On electron microscopy, the sarcomere is limited on either side by the *Z line* (Z, abbreviation for German *Zückung,* contraction), to which the actin filaments are attached (Fig. 12–2). Conversely, the myosin filaments extend from the center of the sarcomere in either direction toward but not actually reaching the Z lines (Fig. 12–1).

The myosin heads interact with actin filaments when sufficient calcium is present (Fig. 12–5). The process is called *crossbridge cycling.* As the actin filaments move inward toward the center of the sarcomere, drawing the Z lines closer together, the sarcomere shortens. The energy for this shortening is provided by the breakdown of ATP, chiefly made in the mitochondria.

Titin (also called *connectin*), the largest protein molecule yet described, is an extraordinarily long, flexible, and slender myofibrillar protein.[4] It acts as a third filament and provides elasticity.[5] Between 0.6 and 1.2 μm in length, the titin molecule extends from the Z line, stopping just short of the M line (Fig. 12–1). It has two distinct segments: an inextensible segment that interacts with myosin and an extensible segment that stretches as sarcomere length increases.[6] Titin has two functions: It tethers the myosin molecule to the Z line, and as it stretches its elasticity explains the stress-strain elastic relation of striated muscle, without having to postulate a major role for nonmyofibrillar structures such as extracellular connective tissue.[6]

ACTIN AND TROPONIN-C. To understand the indispensable role of calcium ions in providing a crucial switch-on signal to the crossbridge cycle requires a brief outline of the molecular structure of the actin filament. Thin filaments are composed of *two actin units,* which intertwine in a helical pattern, both being carried on a heavier tropomyosin molecule that functions as a "backbone" (Fig. 12–4). At regular intervals of 38.5 nm along this twisting structure is a closely bound group of three regulatory proteins called the *troponin complex.*[7] Of these three, it is troponin-C that

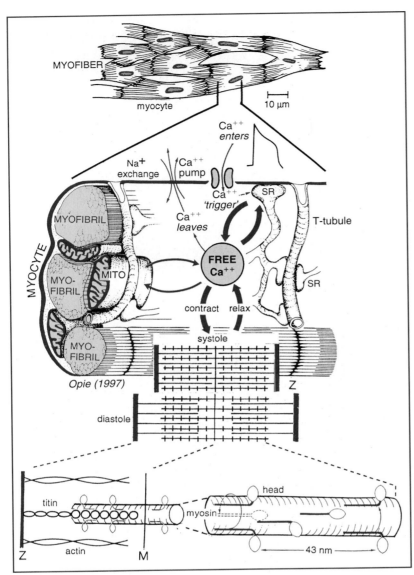

FIGURE 12–1. The crux of the contractile process lies in the changing concentrations of Ca^{++} ions in the myocardial cytosol. Ca^{++} ions are schematically shown as entering via the calcium channel, which opens in response to the wave of depolarization that travels along the sarcolemma. These Ca^{++} ions "trigger" the release of more calcium from the sarcoplasmic reticulum (SR) and thereby initiate a contraction-relaxation cycle. Eventually the small amount of calcium that has entered the cell leaves, predominantly by a Na^{+}/Ca^{++} exchanger with a lesser role for the sarcolemmal calcium pump. The varying actin-myosin overlap is shown for systole and diastole. The myosin heads, attached to the thick filaments, interact with the thin actin filaments, as shown in Figure 12–6. For role of titin, see Figure 12–4. (Upper panel reproduced with permission from Braunwald E., et al.: Mechanisms of Contraction of the Normal and Failing Heart. 2nd ed. Boston, Little, Brown, & Co., 1976; middle and lower panels reprinted with permission. Copyright ©1997 L. H. Opie.)

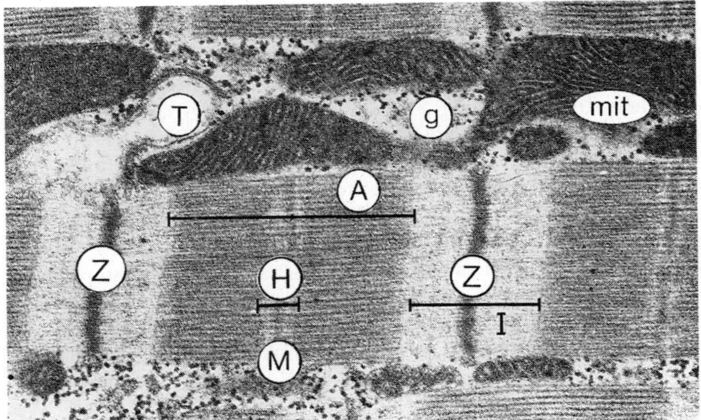

FIGURE 12–2. The sarcomere is the distance between the two Z lines. Note the presence of numerous mitochondria (mit) sandwiched between the myofibrils, and the presence of T tubules (T), which penetrate into the muscle at the level of the Z lines. This two-dimensional picture should not disguise the fact that the Z line is really a "Z disc," as is the M line (M). H = Central clear zone containing only myosin filament bodies and the M line; A = band of actin-myosin overlap; I = band of actin filaments, titin, and Z line; g = glycogen granules. ×32,000 rat papillary muscle. (Courtesy of Dr. J. Moravec, Dijon, France.)

responds to the calcium ions that are released in large amounts from the SR to start the crossbridge cycle.

Schematically, when the cytosolic calcium level is low, the *tropomyosin* molecule is twisted in such a way that the myosin heads cannot interact with actin (Fig. 12–5). When more calcium ions arrive at the start of the contractile cycle and interact with troponin-C, then the activated troponin-C binds tightly to the inhibitory molecule, *troponin-I.* This process repositions troponin-M (tropomyosin) on the thin filament,[8] which removes the inhibition exerted by tropomyosin on the actin-myosin interaction. Thus, the crossbridge cycle is initiated. When troponin-I is phosphorylated by beta-adrenergic stimulation, then the rate of relaxation is enhanced.[9]

STRONG AND WEAK BINDING STATES. Although at a molecular level the events underlying the crossbridge cycle are exceedingly complex, one simple current hypothesis is a revival of a two-state model first proposed by Huxley.[10] According to this proposal, the crossbridges exist in either a strong or a weak binding state (Fig. 12–5).[8] The arrival of calcium ions at the contractile proteins is a crucial link in the series of events known as *excitation-contraction coupling.* The ensuing interaction of calcium with troponin-C and the deinhibition of troponin-I puts the crossbridges in the strong binding state. As long as enough calcium ions are present, the strong binding state potentially dominates (Fig. 12–5). If, however, the strong binding state were con-

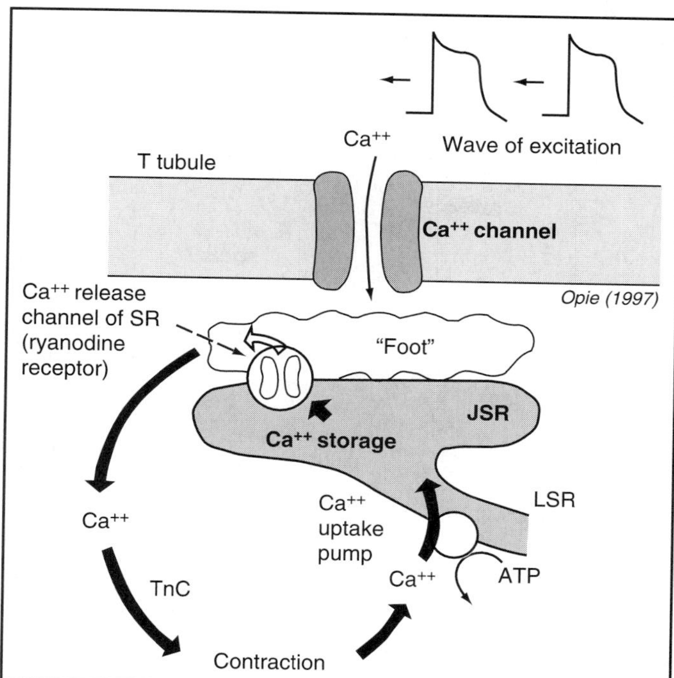

FIGURE 12–3. The sarcoplasmic reticulum (SR) plays an essential role in the contraction-relaxation cycle. When the wave of excitation opens the Ca^{++} channel of the T tubule, the Ca^{++} ions thus entering release much more Ca^{++} from the SR. The function of the "foot" is shown in Figure 12–10. This Ca^{++} is released from the ryanodine receptor located in the junctional SR (JSR), and is also called the Ca^{++} release channel of the SR. The Ca^{++} thus released into the cytosol interacts with troponin-C to trigger the contractile process (Figs. 12–4 to 12–7). Ca^{++} ions are then taken up from troponin-C into the longitudinal SR (L-SR) to be stored at high concentrations in the JSR in association with calsequestrin and other storage proteins. Then the Ca^{++} ions can once again be released when more Ca^{++} triggers the process during the next wave of excitation. (Reprinted with permission. Copyright ©1997 L. H. Opie.)

tinuously present, then the contractile proteins could never relax. Thus, the proposal is that the binding of ATP to the myosin head puts the crossbridges into a weak binding state even when the calcium concentration is high.[8] Conversely, when ATP is hydrolyzed to ADP and P_i, the strong binding state again predominates. Thus, the ATP-induced changes in the molecular configuration of the myosin head result in corresponding variations in the physical properties (a similar concept is common in metabolic regulation).

When cystosolic calcium levels fall at the start of diastole, a master switch is turned off as the calcium ions leave troponin-C and tropomyosin again assumes the inhibitory configuration. The weak binding state now predominates.

MODEL FOR MOLECULAR BASIS OF MUSCULAR CONTRACTION. Each myosin head is the terminal part of a heavy chain. The bodies of two of these chains intertwine, and each terminates in a short "neck" that carries the elongated myosin head (Fig. 12–4). It is the base of the head, also sometimes called the neck, that changes configuration in the contractile cycle. Together with the "bodies" of all the other heads, the myosin thick filament is formed. Each lobe of the bilobed head has an *ATP-binding pocket* (also called nucleotide-pocket) and a narrow cleft that extends from the base of this pocket to the actin-binding face.[11] ATP and its breakdown products ADP and P_i bind to the nucleotide pocket, which has in close proximity the myosin ATPase activity that breaks down ATP to its products (Fig. 12–6). According to the revised Rayment model,[12] the narrow cleft that splits the central 50-kDA segment of the myosin head responds to the binding of ATP or its breakdown products to the nucleotide pocket in such a way that the conformational changes necessary for movement of the head are produced. Starting with the rigor state (Fig. 12–6*A*), the binding of ATP to its pocket changes the molecular configuration of the myosin head so that the head detaches from actin to terminate the rigor state (Fig. 12–6*B*). Next, the ATPase activity of the myosin head splits ATP into ADP and P_i and the head flexes (Fig. 12–6*C*). As ATP is hydrolyzed, the cleft extending from the nucleotide pocket to the actin-binding face starts to close, and, once it is closed, the myosin head transiently binds weakly to an actin unit. Then P_i is released from the head, the cleft finally closes, and there is strong binding of the myosin head to actin (Fig. 12–6*D*). Next, the head extends, i.e., straightens. A power stroke takes place, the actin molecule moves by 5 to 10 nm,[11,13] and the myosin head is now in the rigor state. The pocket then releases ADP, ready for acceptance of ATP, and repetition of the cycle. A major point of emphasis is that it is straightening and not flexion of the light chain region of the head (i.e., the "neck") that produces the power stroke; however, the angle between the straightened head and the myosin body does decrease to give the appearance of flexion of head on the body.

Myosin ATPase activity normally responds to calcium in such a way that an increase of calcium ion concentration from 10^{-7} M to 5×10^{-5} M results in a fivefold increase in activity.[14] Similar calcium concentrations are associated with contraction in the whole heart (Fig. 12–7).

Myosin heavy chain isoforms help regulate myosin ATPase activity. Each myosin filament consists of two heavy chains, the bodies of which are intertwined and each ending in one head, and four light chains, two in apposition to each head. The heavy chains, containing the myosin ATPase activity on the heads, occur in two isoforms, alpha and beta of the same molecular weight, but with substantially different ATPase activities. The beta-heavy chain (β-MHC) isoform has lower ATPase activity and is the predominant form in the adult human. In small animals, the faster α-MHC form changes to a predominant β-MHC pattern in experimental heart failure. A mutant gene for β-MHC is thought to be responsible for some kindreds of patients with human hypertrophic cardiomyopathy (see p. 1664).[15] Less commonly, mutants for tropomyosin or troponin-T are responsible[15] (see p. 1664).

Two *myosin light chains* surround the elongated base of each myosin head (four per bilobed head). The *essential myosin light chain* (MLC-1), an integral part of the structure of the myosin head, appears to inhibit the contractile process by a newly described interaction with actin.[16] The other *regulatory myosin light chain* (MLC-2) is a potential site for phosphorylation, for example in response to beta-adrenergic stimulation. Such phosphorylation (i.e., the gaining of a phosphate grouping) promotes crossbridge cycling by increasing the affinity of myosin for actin.[8] In vascular smooth muscle, a similar phosphorylation occurs under the influence of the enzyme, myosin light chain kinase (MLCK), and is an obligatory step in the initiation of the contractile process.

Effects of Increased Cytosolic Calcium Levels on Crossbridge Cycle

Calcium ions stimulate the contractile process at multiple control sites.[8,17,18] Their interaction with troponin-C is essential for crossbridge cycling.[7] Two major models are proposed to account for increased force development at greater calcium ion concentrations (Figs. 12–7 and 12–8). First, it has been held that calcium acts as an on-off switch, and, therefore, the enhanced force development in the presence of calcium ions must be due to recruitment of additional crossbridge sites.[19] The alternate point of view is that the crossbridges react to calcium in a graded manner.[18,20]

The cellular mechanisms in the "graded model" may involve (1) a graded response of troponin-C to calcium ions,

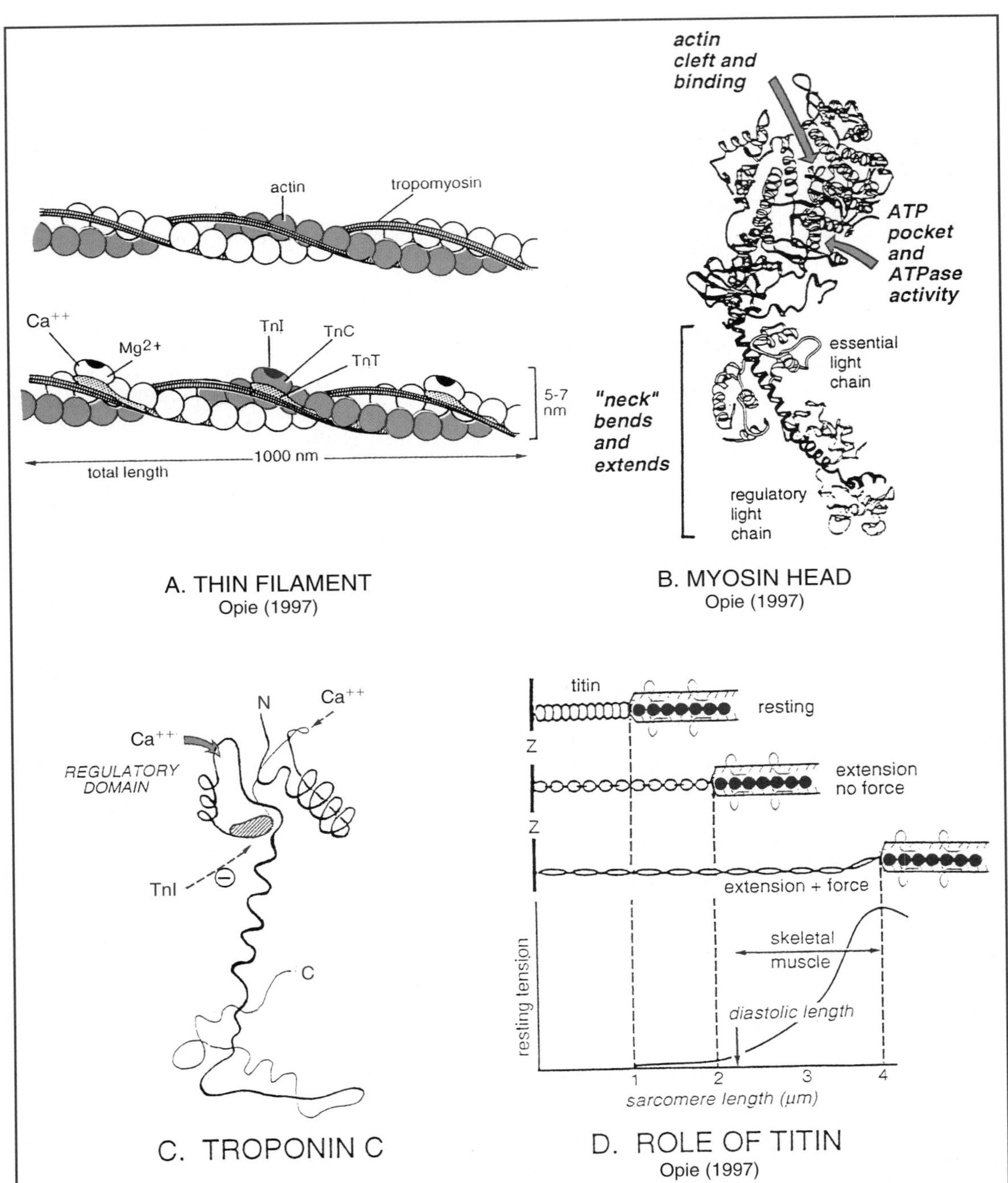

FIGURE 12–4. The major molecules of the contractile system. The thin actin filament *(A)* interacts with the myosin head *(B)* when Ca^{++} ions arrive at troponin-C *(C)*. The giant molecule titin *(D)* provides structural support by linking myosin to the Z line. The molecular aspects are as follows: The thin actin filament *(A)* contains troponin-C (TnC) and its Ca^{++} binding sites. When TnC is not activated by Ca^{++}, then troponin-I (TnI) inhibits the actin-myosin interaction. The role of troponin-T (TnT) is less well defined. *B,* Myosin head molecular structure, based on Rayment et al.,[11] is composed of heavy and light chains. The heavy head chain in turn has two major domains: one of 70 kDA (i.e., 70,000 molecular weight) that interacts with actin at the actin cleft and has an ATP-binding pocket. The other domain of 20 kDA is elongated, extends and bends, and has two light chains attached to it. The essential light chain (ELC) is part of the structure. The other regulatory light chain (RLC) influences the extent of the actin-myosin interaction. *C,* TnC with sites in the regulatory domain for activation by calcium and for interaction with TnI. *D,* Titin, the very large elongated protein with elasticity that binds myosin to the Z line. (Modified from Wang, K., McCarter, R., Wright, J., et al.: Regulation of skeletal muscle stiffness and elasticity by titin isoforms: A test of the segmental extension model of resting tension. Proc. Natl. Acad. Sci. *88:*7101–7105, 1991; with permission.) As the sarcomere is stretched to its maximum diastolic length of 2.2 microns (Fig. 12–24), titin is increasingly stretched and contributes to the elastic properties of the sarcomere. For differences between cardiac and skeletal titin, see reference 6. (Reprinted with permission. Copyright ©1997 L. H. Opie.)

which is unlikely in view of the very steep relationship between force development; (2) a graded response of myosin ATPase to calcium[14] (Fig. 12–7); and/or (3) increased myosin light chain phosphorylation—this is still speculative. Additional possibilities are, first, that there could be "near neighbor" self-activation whereby actin-myosin interaction activates additional crossbridges even in the absence of binding of calcium to the troponin-C of those cross-

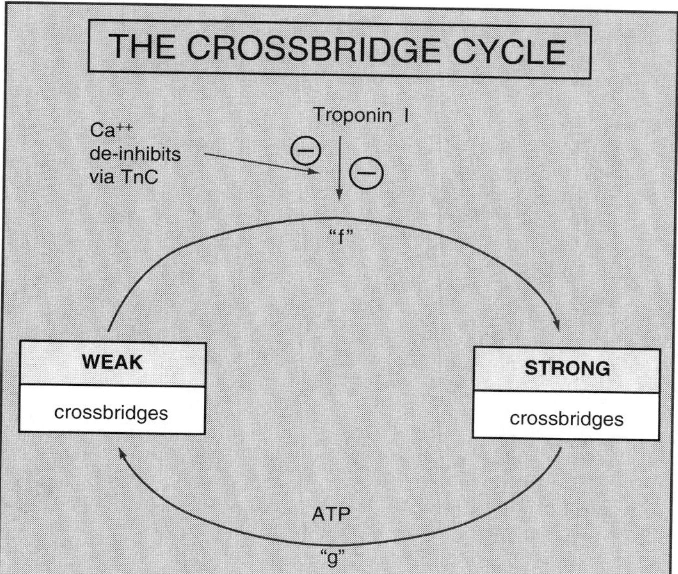

FIGURE 12–5. Hypothesis for crossbridge cycle based on concepts of Brenner.[20] Strong crossbridges are required for the power stroke (Fig. 12–6). The probability of such crossbridges forming is decreased by troponin-I. When Ca^{++} interacts with troponin-C (TnC), de-inhibition occurs and the strong crossbridges form more easily. ATP, when attached to the myosin head, causes the strong binding state to change to the weak state and, therefore, inhibits rigor formation (Fig. 12–6). During force generation, the molecular force-generators (myosin crossbridges) cycle between weak and strong states with apparent rate constants, f and g. According to Brenner,[20] calcium, by activating TnC, increases the probability of forming strong, force-generating crossbridges. The responsiveness to calcium depends on the relative values of f and g, as well as on the calcium affinity of TnC. For original concepts, see Rüegg.[24]

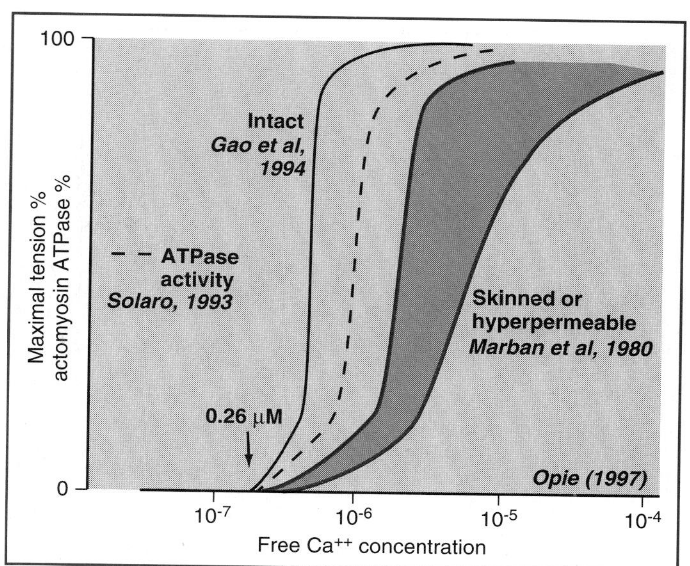

FIGURE 12–7. Relation of free ionized Ca^{++} to tension development in (1) intact rat trabeculae, at fixed diastolic fiber lengths of 2.2 μm, shown on left, and taken from Gao et al.[17] and (2) a variety of skinned and hyperpermeable preparations from Gao et al.[17] and Marban et al.,[25] shown in slashes. The dashed line indicates the effect of $[Ca^{++}]_i$ on actomyosin ATPase activity from Solaro et al.[14] Note the steep curve of activation of intact fibers and of actomyosin ATPase activity. Also note that the myofibrils of intact preparations are much more sensitive to calcium than those of skinned preparations. (Reprinted with permission. Copyright ©1997 L. H. Opie.)

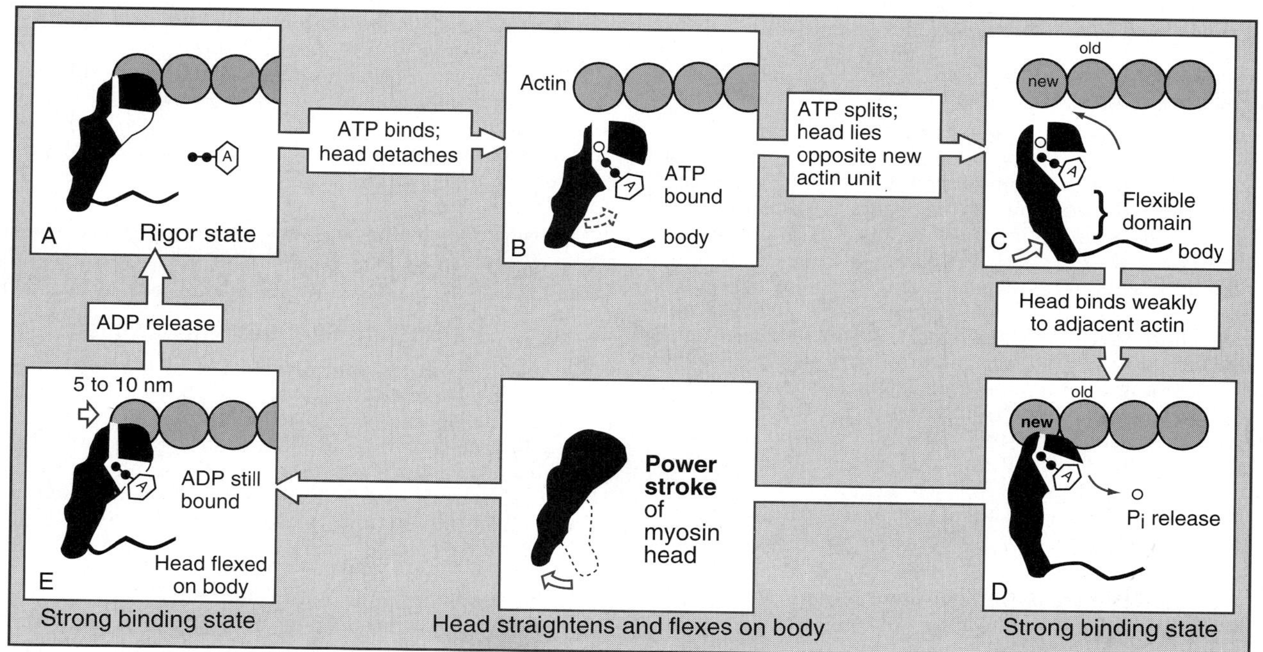

FIGURE 12–6. Schema modified from the Rayment[11] five-step model for interaction between the myosin head and the actin filament, taking into account revisions[12] and additional changes proposed by the present author. The cycle starts with the rigor state *(A)*, in which the myosin head is still attached to actin at the end of the power stroke. ATP binds to the ATP-binding pocket to cause the head to assume the same molecular configuration as before the power stroke. Binding of the head to an adjacent actin monomer occurs first weakly and then strongly. Myosin ATPase activity splits the ATP into ADP (adenosine diphosphate) and P_i (inorganic phosphate). As P_i is released, the power stroke occurs, and the actin filament is moved by 5 to 10 nm. The actin monomer with which the myosin head is interacting is dotted. (Professor J. C. Rüegg of Heidelberg University, Germany, is thanked for comments.)

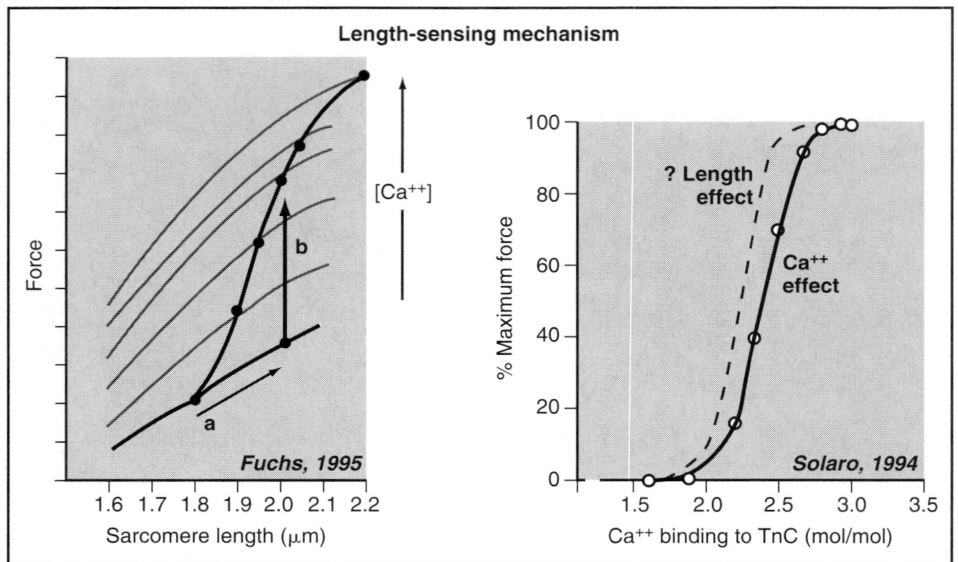

FIGURE 12–8. The proposed explanation for the Starling effect, whereby a greater end-diastolic fiber length develops a greater force. The left panel shows how the steep ascending limb of the cardiac force-length curve is explained by an interaction between sarcomere length and calcium ions. Light lines show a family of hypothetical force-length curves for increasing free Ca^{++} concentrations, each drawn on the assumption that the shape of the curve is determined solely by the degree of overlap of thin and thick filaments (Fig. 12–1). It is postulated that a change in end-diastolic fiber length (a) at any given free Ca^{++} concentration would increase force by the Starling effect and would, in addition, cause cooperative interactions within the thin filament, the latter leading to a greater binding of Ca^{++} to the thin filament. Hence there would be a greater force (b) than would be expected simply on the basis of the change in filament overlap (a). The right panel proposes that the effects of Ca^{++} and length can be explained by the properties of troponin-C (TnC) and the binding of calcium to TnC. As more Ca^{++} ions bind to TnC in a skinned fiber preparation, more force is developed. There is a steep relation, similar to that shown in the left panel. When the fiber is stretched and the sarcomere length increased, it is postulated that for any given number of Ca^{++} ions binding to TnC there is a greater force development, so that TnC has become sensitized to Ca^{++}. (Modified from Fuchs, F.: Mechanical modulation of the Ca^{2+} regulatory protein complex in cardiac muscle. NIPS *10*:6–12, 1995; and Solaro, R. J., Wolska, B. M., and Westfall, M.: Regulatory proteins and diastolic relaxation. *In* Lorell, B. H., and Grossman, W. (eds.): Diastolic Relaxation of the Heart. Norwell, MA, Kluwer Academic Publishers, 1994, pp. 43–53.)

bridges.[14] Second, once crossbridge attachment has occurred, the affinity of troponin-C for calcium may increase.[21,22]

Length-Dependent Activation

The other major factor influencing the strength of contraction is the length of the muscle fiber at the end of diastole, just before the onset of systole. Starling observed that the greater the volume of the heart in diastole, the more forceful the contraction (see p. 464). The increased volume translates into an increased muscle length, which acts by a length-sensing mechanism (Fig. 12–8). Previously this relation was ascribed to a more optimal overlap between actin and myosin. The current view is that a complex interplay occurs between anatomical and regulatory factors,[23] including the concept that an increased sarcomere length leads to greater sensitivity of the contractile apparatus to the prevailing cytosolic calcium,[8] thereby explaining length-dependent activation. The mechanism for this regulatory change, although not yet clarified, may hypothetically involve increased sensitivity of the calcium-binding domain of troponin-C to calcium (Fig. 12–8).[8]

Crossbridge Cycling Versus Cardiac Contraction-Relaxation Cycle

The crossbridge and the cardiac cycles must be distinguished. The former cycle is the repetitive interaction between myosin heads and actin, according to the five-step model (Fig. 12–6). So long as enough calcium ions are bound to troponin-C, many repetitive cycles of this nature occur. Thus, at any given moment, some myosin heads are flexing or have flexed, some are extending or have extended, some are attached to actin, and some are detached from actin. Numerous such crossbridge cycles, each lasting only a few microseconds, actively move the thin actin filaments toward the central bare area of the thick myosin filaments, thereby shortening the sarcomere. The sum total of all the shortening sarcomeres leads to systole, which is the contraction phase of the cardiac cycle. When calcium ions depart from their binding sites on troponin-C, crossbridge cycling cannot occur, and the diastolic phase of the cardiac cycle sets in.

CALCIUM ION FLUXES IN CARDIAC CONTRACTION-RELAXATION CYCLE

Pattern of Calcium Movements

Despite the critical role of calcium in regulating the contraction and relaxation phases of the cardiac cycle, the exact details of the associated calcium ion fluxes that link contraction to the wave of excitation are not yet fully clarified, although a working model can be conceptualized (Fig. 12–9). A generally accepted hypothesis is based on the critical role of calcium release from the SR.[26] Relatively small amounts of calcium ions actually enter and leave the cell during each cardiac cycle, whereas much larger amounts move in and out of the SR. The theory of *calcium-induced calcium release*[27] explains most of the current available data.[26] The basic proposal is that the SR releases relatively large amounts of calcium ions into the cytosol in response to the much smaller amounts entering the cardiac myocyte with each wave of depolarization.[28] This process elevates by about tenfold the concentration of calcium ions in the cytosol.[27] The result is the increasing interaction of calcium ions with troponin-C to trigger the contractile process. This theory, also called the *chemical synapse theory*,[29] has recently received strong support from

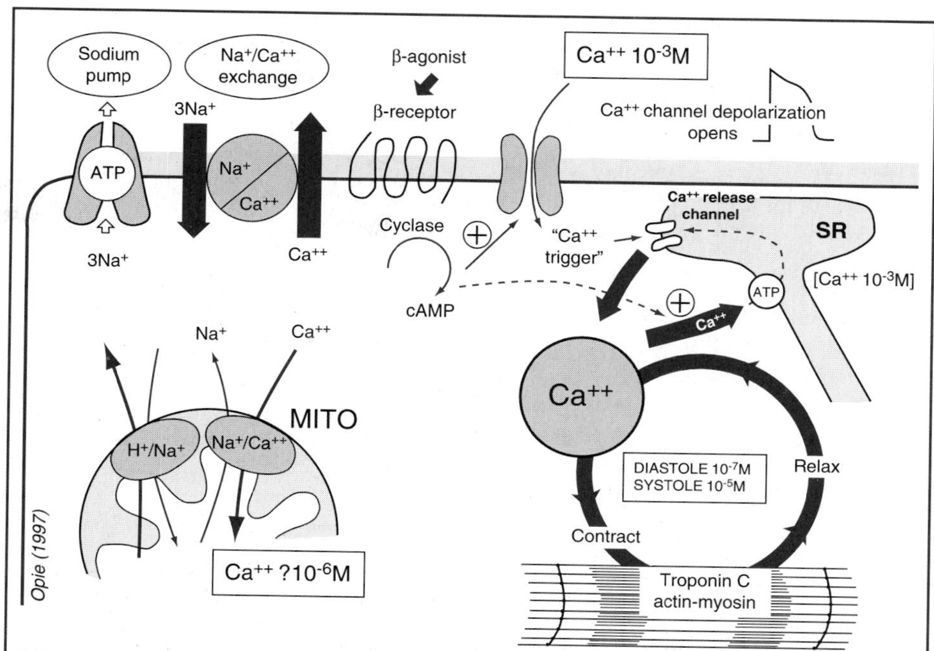

FIGURE 12–9. Calcium fluxes in the myocardium. Crucial features are (1) entry of Ca^{++} ions via the voltage-sensitive Ca^{++} channel, acting as a trigger to the release of Ca^{++} ions from the sarcoplasmic reticulum (SR) as shown in Figure 12–3; (2) the effect of beta-adrenergic stimulation with adenylate cyclase forming cyclic AMP, the latter both helping to open the Ca^{++} channel and to increase the rate of uptake of Ca^{++} into the SR; and (3) exit of Ca^{++} ions chiefly via the Na^{+}/Ca^{++} exchange, with the sodium pump thereafter extruding the Na^{+} ions thus gained. The latter process requires ATP. Note the much higher extracellular (10^{-3} M) than intracellular values (Fig. 12–7) and a hypothetical mitochondrial value of about 10^{-6} M. The mitochondria can act as a buffer against excessive changes in the free cytosolic calcium concentration. MITO = Mitochondria. (Reprinted with permission. Copyright ©1997 L. H. Opie.)

the molecular characterization of the receptor on the SR that releases calcium[30] from the anatomical proximity of the junctional SR to the sarcolemma of the T tubule (Fig. 12–10), and from electrophysiological evidence closely linking the duration of the action potential with the extent of Ca^{++} release.[28]

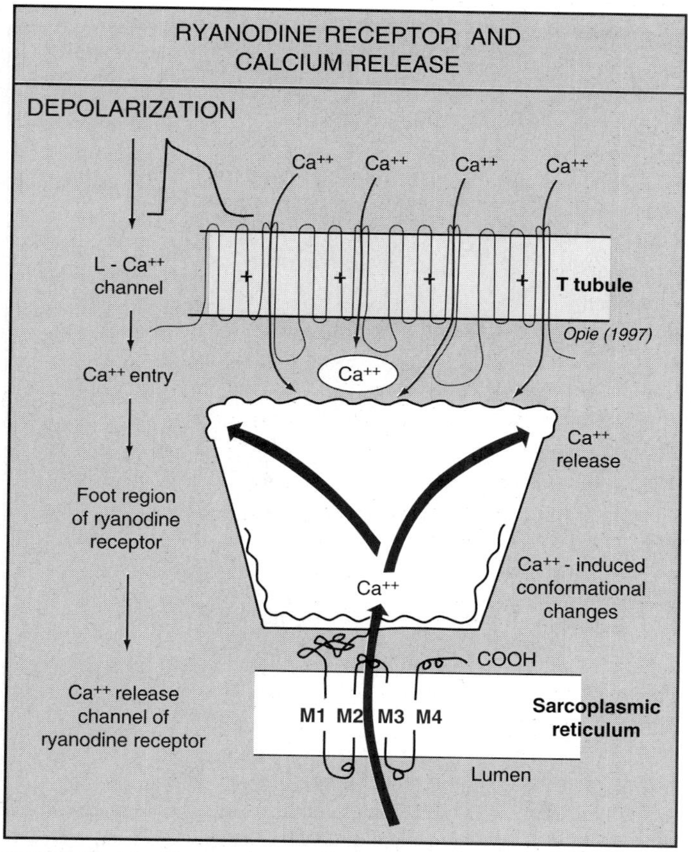

The rise of cytosolic calcium concentration comes to an end as the wave of excitation passes, no more calcium ions enter, and the release of calcium from the SR ceases. The latter event could be explained by one or more of several proposals, namely (1) that the cytosolic calcium ion concentration has risen high enough to inhibit the process of calcium-induced calcium release[27]; (2) the release of calcium from the SR is tightly linked to opening of the calcium channel, so that when the latter closes the release of calcium from the SR ceases[31]; (3) the rising cytosolic calcium ion concentration can activate the calcium uptake pump of the SR[32]; or (4) calcium release from the SR continues only for the duration of action potential duration.[28] The overall effect of these mechanisms is that the cytosolic calcium ion concentration starts to fall and relaxation is initiated. As the cytosolic calcium decreases, tropomyosin again starts to inhibit the interaction between actin and myosin, and relaxation proceeds.

To balance the small amount of calcium ions entering the heart cell with each depolarization, a similar quantity must leave the cell by one of two processes. First, calcium can be exchanged for sodium ions entering by the Na^{+}/Ca^{++} exchange, and, second, an ATP-consuming sarcolemmal calcium pump can transfer calcium into the extracellular space against a concentration gradient.

FIGURE 12–10. Proposed crucial role of T tubule, the feet and calcium release channel of the sarcoplasmic reticulum (SR) in excitation-contraction coupling. Depolarization stimulates the L-type calcium channel of the T tubule to allow calcium ion entry, which interacts with the "foot" region of the ryanodine receptor to cause molecular conformational changes that eventually result in calcium release from the calcium-release channel of the ryanodine receptor of the SR. For molecular structure of the foot, see Wagenknecht et al.[34] (Reprinted with permission. Copyright ©1997 L. H. Opie.)

Calcium Release Channel of the Sarcoplasmic Reticulum

Each sarcolemmal voltage-operated calcium channel is thought to control a cluster of SR release channels[31,33] by virtue of close anatomical proximity of the sarcolemmal calcium channels, situated on the T tubules, to the calcium release channels, situated on the SR. The calcium release channel is part of the complex structure known as the *ryanodine receptor*, so called because it coincidentally binds the potent insecticide ryanodine.[32] Part of this receptor extends from the membrane of the SR toward the T tubule to constitute the *foot structure* or *junctional channel complex* that bridges the gap between the SR and the T tubule.[34] After the wave of depolarization has reached the T tubule and induced the voltage-operated calcium channels to open, the calcium ions enter the cardiac myocyte to reach the foot regions of the ryanodine receptors (Fig. 12–10). The result is a change in the molecular configuration

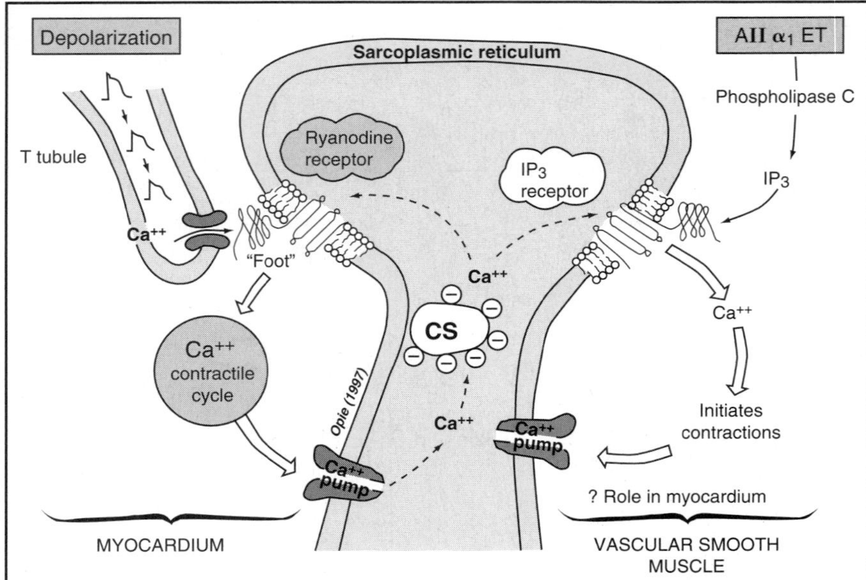

FIGURE 12–11. In the *myocardium* (left side of figure), calcium is released from the sarcoplasmic reticulum (SR) via the calcium release channel (part of the ryanodine receptor), chiefly in response to calcium that has entered during voltage depolarization. Calcium is taken up again by the calcium pump of the longitudinal SR, to interact with the storage protein calsequestrin (CS), thence to be released again. In contrast, in *vascular smooth muscle,* stimulation of vasoconstrictor receptors, such as angiotensin II (AII), alpha$_1$-adrenergic (α_1), and endothelin (ET), leads to release of inositol trisphosphate (IP_3) that acts on its receptor to release calcium from the SR. The role of IP_3 as a signal in the myocardium is still under evaluation. (Reprinted with permission. Copyright ©1997 L. H. Opie.)

of the ryanodine receptor that opens the calcium release channel of the SR to discharge calcium ions, probably into the subsarcolemmal space between the foot and the T tubule[34] and thence into the cytosol.

From the molecular point of view, the calcium release channel of the SR has been analyzed by cloning and sequencing the complementary DNA.[35] The predicted structure is that of a large protein comprising over 5000 amino acids, with two major components. The larger part is the foot, which links the T tubules and the SR, and the smaller structure is the C-terminal region, which constitutes the actual pore-containing channel of the SR.[34,35] The density of this channel, as measured by ryanodine binding, is very high with nearly 800 receptors per μm^2 of the junctional SR.[36]

IP_3-Induced Release of Calcium from Sarcoplasmic Reticulum

A totally different calcium release signal system may also be involved. In addition to the ryanodine receptor on the SR, there is a second receptor, that for inositol trisphosphate (IP_3) (Fig. 12–11). This IP_3 receptor has a high degree of molecular homology with the ryanodine receptor, although only about half its size. IP_3 is one of the messengers of the phosphatidylinositol pathway, responding to certain agonists with vasoconstriction as their major physiological role, namely alpha$_1$-adrenergic stimulation, angiotensin II, and endothelin.[30] Calcium released from the SR by IP_3 may stimulate Na^+/Ca^{++} exchange directly.[37] In vascular smooth muscle, this IP_3 messenger system is of fundamental importance in regulating the release of calcium from the SR. In cardiac muscle, the role of IP_3 is still sufficiently controversial to question its role in the inotropic response.[38] An attractive possibility is that in human heart failure, the IP_3 receptor becomes upregulated in relation to the ryanodine receptor, perhaps to help maintain release of calcium from the SR.[39]

Calcium Uptake by the Calcium ATPase of the Sarcoplasmic Reticulum

Calcium ions are taken up into the SR by the activity of the calcium pump, that is, the *calcium-pumping ATPase* of the SR (also called SERCA), that constitutes nearly 90 per cent of the protein component of the SR.[40,41] Its molecular weight is about 115 kDA, and it straddles the SR membrane in such a way that part of it actually protrudes into the cytosol.[42] It exists in several isoforms.[40] For each mole of ATP hydrolyzed by this enzyme, two calcium ions are taken up to accumulate within the SR (Fig. 12–12).

Phospholamban, which means "phosphate receiver," is the major regulator of this calcium pump.[32] Phospholamban is a pentamer protein, consisting of five subunits, each with a molecular weight of 6 kDA, found in a 1:1 molar ratio to the ATPase of the calcium pump. The activity of phospholamban is governed by its state of phosphorylation, a process that alters the molecular configuration of the calcium pump in such a way that the normal inhibition exerted by unphosphorylated phospholamban on the calcium uptake pump is removed (Fig. 12–12). Each of the five

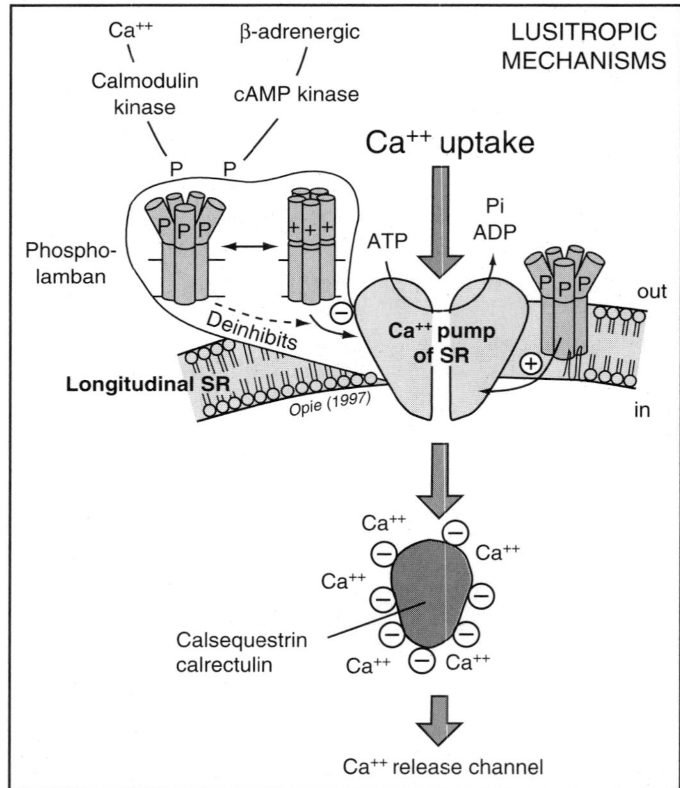

FIGURE 12–12. Calcium uptake by the energy-requiring calcium pump into the sarcoplasmic reticulum (SR). Phospholamban can be phosphorylated (P) to remove the inhibition exerted by its unphosphorylated form (positive charges) on the calcium pump. Calcium uptake is thereby increased either in response to an enhanced cytosolic calcium or in response to beta-adrenergic stimulation. Thus, two phosphorylations activate phospholamban at distinct sites and their effects are additive. An increased rate of uptake of calcium into the SR enhances the rate of relaxation (lusitropic effect). (Reprinted with permission. Copyright ©1997 L. H. Opie.)

subunits of phospholamban can be phosphorylated at two different sites[43] by at least two and possibly three protein kinases.[41] Of specific interest is that one of the two major protein kinases involved, the one activated by cyclic AMP, responds to beta-adrenergic stimulation of the cardiac myocyte by enhancing the uptake of calcium into the SR to increase the rate of relaxation.[41] The further proposal is that the increased store of calcium in the SR is then released by the subsequent waves of depolarization with an increased rate and force of contraction. This sequence is strongly supported by the transgenic mouse model, totally deficient in phospholamban, in which rates of contraction and relaxation are maximal and do not vary in response to beta-adrenergic stimulation by isoproterenol.[41]

The calcium taken up into the SR by the calcium pump is stored prior to further release. The highly charged storage protein, *calsequestrin,* is found in that part of the SR that lies near the T tubules.[44] Calcium stored with calsequestrin is thought to become available for the release process as calsequestrin discharges calcium ions into the inner mouth of the calcium release channel. This process replaces those calcium ions liberated from the outer mouth into the cytosol. *Calrectulin* is another Ca^{++}-storing protein, very similar in structure to calsequestrin, and probably similar in function.[32]

Role of Sarcoplasmic Reticulum in Heart Failure

(See also p. 405)

In heart failure, the force of cardiac contraction is reduced and there is an abnormal delayed pattern of cardiac relaxation. Because the SR is so intimately concerned in both of these phases of the cardiac contractile cycle, it is not surprising that abnormalities of the SR are thought to play a fundamental role in heart failure. The calcium release channel of the SR of the failing heart is diminished in activity and markedly less sensitive to caffeine.[45] Furthermore, the levels of the messenger RNAs of the proteins regulating calcium uptake and release are decreased in end-stage human heart failure. The mRNAs for the ryanodine receptor, the calcium uptake pump, and phospholamban are all abnormally deficient.[46] One hypothesis currently favored is that abnormal calcium handling by the SR of the failing myocardium is due to impaired expression of the genes encoding these specific SR proteins. These proposals tie in with the downgraded state of the ryanodine receptor in SR from patients in severe heart failure.[39]

SARCOLEMMAL CONTROL OF CALCIUM AND OTHER IONS

Ion Channels

(See also Chap. 20)

All current models of excitation-contraction coupling ascribe a crucial role to the voltage-induced opening of the sarcolemmal L-type calcium channels in the initiation of the contractile process.[28] Channels are pore-forming macromolecular proteins that span the sarcolemmal lipid bilayer to allow a highly selective pathway for ion transfer into the heart cell when the channel changes from a closed to an open state.[47,48] Ion channels have two major properties: gating and permeation. Guarding each channel are two or more hypothetical gates that control its opening. Ions can permeate through the channel only when both gates are open. In the case of the sodium and calcium channels, which are best understood, the activation gate is shut at the normal resting membrane potential and the inactivation gate is open, so that the channels are *voltage-gated.* Depolarization opens the activation gate.

MOLECULAR STRUCTURE OF L-TYPE CALCIUM CHANNELS. There is a striking molecular similarity between the sodium and calcium channels.[48] "This finding shows a conservation of structure probably among all the voltage-gated ion channels and suggests a common gene family."[49] Both channels contain a major alpha-subunit with four transmembrane subunits or domains, very similar to each other in structure. In addition, both sodium and calcium channels include in their overall structure a number of other subunits whose function is less well understood, such as the beta-subunit. Each of the four transmembrane domains of the alpha-subunit is made up of six helices. In each domain, one specific helical segment, called S4, is rich in amino acids, is highly positively charged, and is the proposed site of the voltage sensor (Fig. 12–13).

Activation is now understood in molecular terms as the change in charge on the fourth transmembrane segment, S4, called the *voltage sensor,* of each of the four subunits of the sodium or calcium channel.[50] *Inactivation* is the process whereby the current initially elicited by depolarization decreases with time despite continuation of the original stimulus.[50] For the Na^+ channel and hypothetically also for the calcium channel, it is the intracellular linker region between subunits 3 and 4 that inactivates (Fig. 12–13). This linker chain is the proposed molecular explanation for the

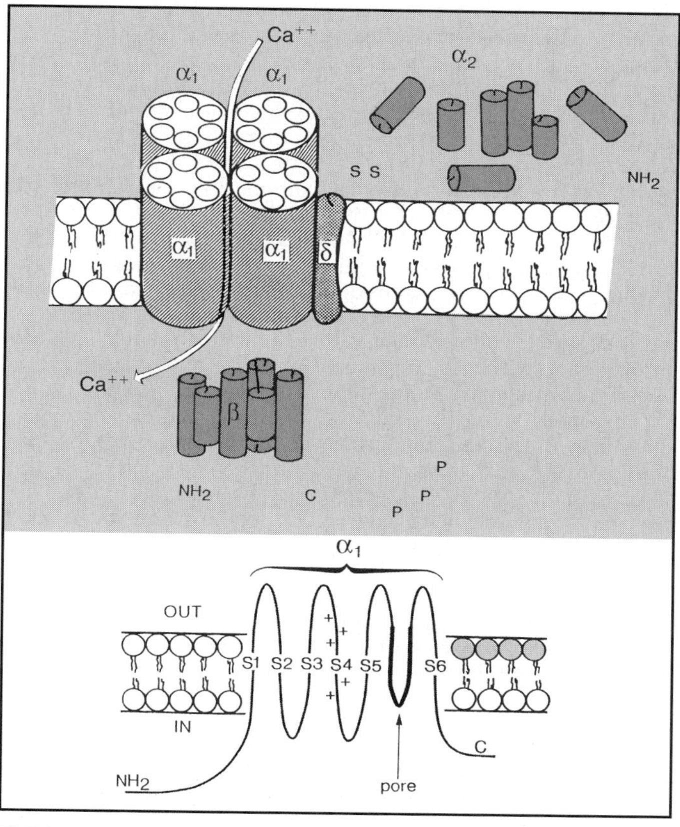

FIGURE 12–13. Simplified model of Ca^{++} channel showing the alpha$_1$-subunit (α_1) forming the central pore, the regulatory beta-subunit (β), and α_2 and delta-subunits of unknown function. Beta-adrenergic stimulation, via cyclic AMP, promotes phosphorylation (P) and the opening probability of the Ca^{++} channel. The proposal is that four domains, each similar to that shown in the righthand panel and composed of six spanning segments, combine to form the α_1-subunit. Segment S_4 is thought to respond to voltage depolarization (+ = positive charges) by altering the molecular configuration of the loop between S_5 and S_6 (part of the pore), so that there is a greater probability of Ca^{++} ions entering (channel opens). For more details, see Heinemann and Stuhmer.[50] (Upper panel modified from Varadi, G., et al.: Molecular determinants of Ca^{2+} channel function and drug action. Trends Pharmacol. Sci. *16*:43–49, 1995, with permission of the authors and Elsevier Science Ltd. Lower panel modified from Tomaselli, G. F., et al.: Molecular basis of permeation in voltage-gated ion channels. Circ. Res. *72*:491–496, 1993. Copyright 1993 American Heart Association.)

previous concept of the internal inactivation gate (f). The actual channel pore is probably contained in the alpha$_1$-subunit, lying between helices S5 and S6, where calcium ions are potentially admitted. Each of the four domains of the alpha$_1$-subunit appears to be folded in on itself, so that the four S5-S6 spans structurally combine to form the single functioning pore of each calcium channel. The beta-subunit acts to enhance the calcium current flow through the alpha-subunit pores.[51] The amino acid structure of the channel pores has critical properties. For example, the presence of the glutamate residue helps determine the presence of high-affinity calcium binding and therefore the calcium ion specificity of the pore.[52]

Channels are not simply open or closed. Rather, the open state is the last of a sequence of many molecular states, varying from a fully closed to a fully open configuration. Therefore, it is more correct to speak of the *probability of channel opening.*

CALCIUM CHANNEL PHOSPHORYLATION. The alpha$_1$-subunit (the organ-specific subunit) of the sarcolemmal calcium channel can be phosphorylated at several sites, especially in the C-terminal tail.[53] During beta-adrenergic stimulation, cyclic AMP increases within the cell and phosphate groups are transferred from ATP to the alpha$_1$-subunit. Thereby, the electrical charges near the inner mouth of the nearby pores are altered to induce changes in the molecular conformation of the pores, so that there is an increased probability of opening of the calcium channel.[48] Either the time that the channel remains in the open state is increased so that more calcium ions flow with the same degree of voltage activation, or phosphorylation activates calcium channels that were otherwise inactive.

T- AND L-TYPE CALCIUM CHANNELS. There are two major subpopulations of sarcolemmal calcium channels relevant to the cardiovascular system, namely the T channels and the L channels.[53,54] The T (transient) channels open at a more negative voltage, have short bursts of opening and do not interact with conventional calcium antagonist drugs.[53] The T channels presumably account for the earlier phase of the opening of the calcium channel, which may also give them a special role in the early electrical depolarization of the sinoatrial node, and hence of initiation of the heart beat. Although T channels are found in atrial cells,[54] their existence in normal ventricular cells is controversial.

The sarcolemmal L (longlasting) channels are the standard calcium channels found in the myocardium and are involved in calcium-induced calcium release. The L channels have two patterns in which their gates work (modes of gating). Mode 1 has short bursts of opening, and mode 2 has longer periods of opening. The sites to which the calcium channel antagonist drugs bind are located in those transmembrane-spanning helices that are close to the pores, mostly on segment S6.[53]

Ion Exchangers

Sodium-Calcium Exchanger

During relaxation, the sarcoplasmic calcium uptake pump and the Na^+/Ca^{++} exchanger compete for the removal of cytosolic calcium, with the SR pump normally being dominant.[55] Restitution of calcium balance takes place by the activity of a series of transsarcolemmal exchangers, the chief of which is the Na^+/Ca^{++} exchanger[56] (Fig. 12–14). The exchanger (molecular weight of 108 kDA) consists of 970 amino acids[57] and does not have substantial homology to any other known protein.[56] A specific inhibitory peptide (XIP = exchange inhibitor peptide) has been identified.[58] The direction of ion exchange is responsive to the membrane potential and to the concentrations of sodium and calcium ions on either side of the sarcolemma. Because sodium and calcium ions can exchange either inward or outward in response to the membrane potential, there must be a specific membrane potential, called the reversal or equilibrium potential, at which the ions are so distributed that they can move as easily one way as the other.[56] The reversal potential may lie about halfway between the resting membrane potential and the potential of the fully depolarized state.[59] Changing the membrane potential from the resting value of, say, −85 mV to +20 mV in the phase of rapid depolarization of the action potential may therefore briefly affect the direction of Na^+/Ca^{++} exchange.[56] During depolarization the charge on the inner side of the sarcolemma becomes positive, which tends to hinder the entrance of sodium ions with their positive charge. Thus, the sodium ions that have just entered during the opening of the sodium channel tend to leave, and calcium ions tend to enter. This process, still controversial, is termed "reverse mode Na^+/Ca^{++} exchange"[60] to distinguish it from the standard "forward mode" (Na^+ in, Ca^{++} out) (compare Figs. 12–14 and 12–15).

A major unsolved problem in relation to the activity of the Na^+/Ca^{++} exchanger is the true value of the internal sodium or calcium ion concentrations, which may differ in the subsarcolemmal "fuzzy space" from the bulk cytosol (Fig. 12–15). Using a sophisticated computer model, very different patterns for the operation of this exchanger during the action potential can be obtained.[61] In particular, if the subsarcolemmal sodium ion concentration is low enough, then the early "reversed mode" exchange with outward movement of sodium ions does not occur, and the exchanger does not contribute to the action potential plateau.

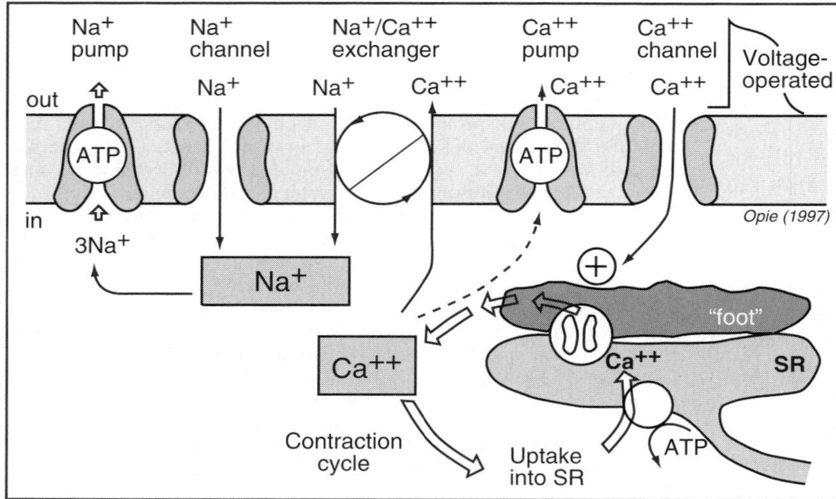

FIGURE 12–14. Regulation of Ca^{++} balance within myocardial cell, showing role of sarcoplasmic reticulum (SR) in contraction-relaxation cycle, as in Figure 12–3. There is a balance between the Ca^{++} ions entering upon depolarization *(right)* and those leaving the cell by the Na^+/Ca^{++} exchange mechanism. A smaller number of Ca^{++} ions leave by an ATP-dependent sarcolemmal Ca^{++} pump. Ion gradients for Na^+ and K^+ are maintained by the operation of the sodium pump (Na^+/K^+-ATPase). An increased internal Ca^{++} following Ca^{++} release from the SR is reduced by competition among one of three routes: uptake into the sarcoplasmic reticulum (SR), Na^+/Ca^{++} exchange, and outward pumping by the membrane Ca^{++}-ATPase. The dominant uptake mechanism is into the SR, followed by the exchanger, followed by the membrane pump. (Reprinted with permission. Copyright ©1997 L. H. Opie.)

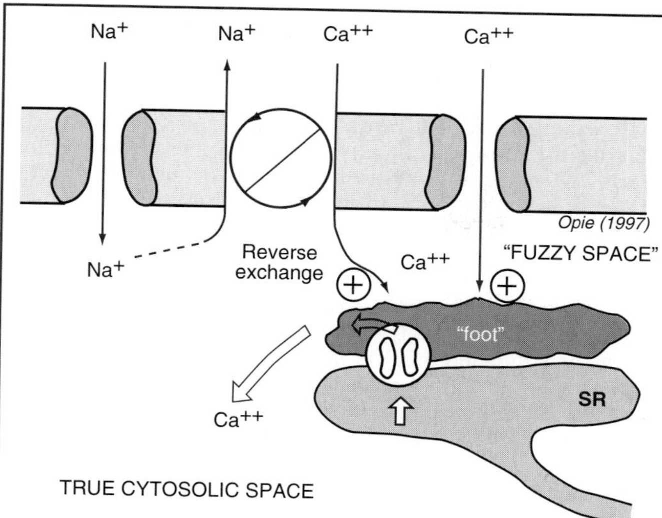

FIGURE 12–15. Proposal for "reverse mode" Na^+/Ca^{++} exchange in the direction of calcium entry following accumulation of sodium ions in the "fuzzy space."[71] According to this proposal, the Na^+/Ca^{++} exchange may play a role in the liberation of calcium involved in the cardiac contractile cycle. For criticism of proposal, see Johnson and Lemieux.[72] (Reprinted with permission. Copyright ©1997 L. H. Opie.)

PHYSIOLOGICAL SIGNIFICANCE OF SODIUM-CALCIUM EXCHANGER. First, transsarcolemmal calcium entry during reversed mode exchange may participate in calcium-induced calcium release.[37,62,63] Second, the exchanger participates in the restitution of ionic balances.[56] Third, this exchanger may participate in the force-frequency relationship (Treppe or Bowditch phenomenon).[62] According to the "sodium pump lag" hypothesis, the rapid accumulation of calcium ions during rapid stimulation of the myocardium outstrips the ability of the Na^+/Ca^{++} exchanger and the sodium pump to achieve return to ionic normality. The result is an accumulation of calcium ions within the SR and an increased force of contraction.[64]

Sodium-Proton Exchange and Acid-Base Homeostasis

The internal pH, pH_i, is more alkaline than can be expected if protons (H^+) were passively distributed across the cardiac cell membrane. To achieve transport of protons out of the myocyte, the electroneutral 1-for-1 exchange of Na^+ and H^+ is driven by the gradient of Na^+ ions, much higher outside than inside the myocyte (Fig. 12–16). The exchanger can be inhibited by the diuretic amiloride and its more specific derivatives, and also by the novel highly specific inhibitor HOE 694.

Physiologically, Na^+/H^+ exchange is thought to play a role in the regulation of protein synthesis, because cytoplasmic alkalinization, for example by insulin, may regulate certain crucial steps in protein synthesis. Alkalinization may also explain why angiotensin II opens Ca^{++} channels in rabbit myocardium.[65]

This exchanger also corrects an acid load during ischemia and acidosis, or during early *postischemic reperfusion,* by transporting protons (H^+) out of the cell while transporting Na^+ into the cell. The resultant increase of internal Na^+ can be dealt with either by the operation of the Na^+/Ca^{++} exchanger or by Na^+/K^+ pump or by sodium-bicarbonate cotransport or by Na^+/K^+ cotransport. Alternatively, the exchanger could operate in the reverse direction to extrude Na^+ from the cells at the expense of a gain of protons that in turn could be dealt with by decreasing the activity of the bicarbonate-chloride exchanger.

The *sodium/bicarbonate cotransporter* helps the Na^+/H^+ exchanger to correct acidosis by the inward transport of bicarbonate, at the cost, however, of a simultaneous gain of Na^+ ions.[66] Such Na^+ gain must be offset by the activity of the Na^+/K^+ pump at the cost of ATP.

The *bicarbonate/chloride exchanger* acidifies by outward movement of the bicarbonate ion, leaving behind protons.[66] In contrast, the Na^+/H^+ exchanger acts chiefly as an alkalinizing mechanism. When acidification is required, the bicarbonate-chloride exchanger transports HCO_3^- outward, leaving H^+ behind. The steady-state pH of cardiac cells is, therefore, controlled at about 7.0 to 7.2 by a balance between the alkalinizing and acidifying exchangers and the metabolic production of acids.[67] Recently, the bicarbonate-chloride exchanger has been cloned from the human heart.[67] Beta-adrenergic stimulation causes acidification by increasing the activity of this exchanger.[68]

Sodium Pump

The sarcolemma becomes highly permeable to Na^+ only during the opening of the Na^+ channel during early depolarization, and Na^+ also enters during the exit of Ca^{++} by Na^+/Ca^{++} exchange. Most of this influx of Na^+ across the sarcolemma must be corrected by the activity of the Na^+/K^+ pump, also called the Na^+/K^+-ATPase or simply the Na^+ pump.[69] The pump is activated by internal Na^+ or external K^+.[69] One ATP molecule is used per transport cycle. The ions are first secluded within the pump protein and then extruded to either side. Although there has been some dispute about the exact ratio of Na^+ to K^+ that are pumped, a generally accepted model is that for every three Na^+ ex-

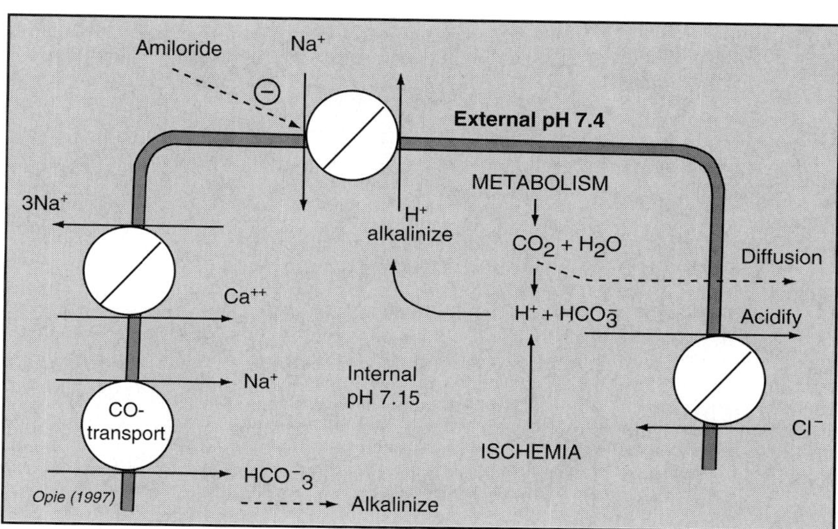

FIGURE 12–16. The difference between extracellular pH (7.40) and intracellular pH (7.15) is maintained by the activity of a series of exchanges and transporters. Intracellular pH is lower because of the generation of CO_2 and H_2O by metabolism, and hence formation of H^+ and HCO_3^-. Note the crucial role of H^+ extrusion by Na^+/H^+ exchange with subsequent activity of the Na^+/Ca^{++} exchanger to transport outward the Na^+ ions gained from Na^+/H^+ exchange. Further adjustments are possible by varying the rates of bicarbonate entry *(bottom left)* and exit *(bottom right).* During intracellular acidosis as in ischemia, the necessity to extrude H^+ means that there is a gain of Na^+ and hence indirectly of Ca^{++}. (Reprinted with permission. Copyright ©1997 L. H. Opie.)

ported, two K^+ are imported.[70] During this process, one positive charge must leave the cell. Hence, the pump is electrogenic and is also called the electrogenic Na^+ pump.[69] The current induced by sustained activity of the pump may contribute about −10 mV to the resting membrane potential.[69] Because the pump must extrude Na^+ ions entering by either Na^+/Ca^{++} exchange or by the Na^+ channel, its sustained activity is essential for the maintenance of normal ion balance (Fig. 12–14).

RECEPTORS AND SIGNAL SYSTEMS

The autonomic nervous system can initiate signal systems that profoundly alter the fluxes of calcium and other ions. Thus, adrenergic or cholinergic stimulation of the sarcolemmal receptors inaugurates the activity of a complex system of sarcolemmal and cytosolic messengers.[73] Occupancy of the beta-adrenergic receptor is coupled by a G-protein complex (Fig. 12–17) to activation of a sarcolemmal enzyme, adenylate cyclase.[74,75] The G-protein complex involved, being stimulatory, is called G_s.[75] Situated in the

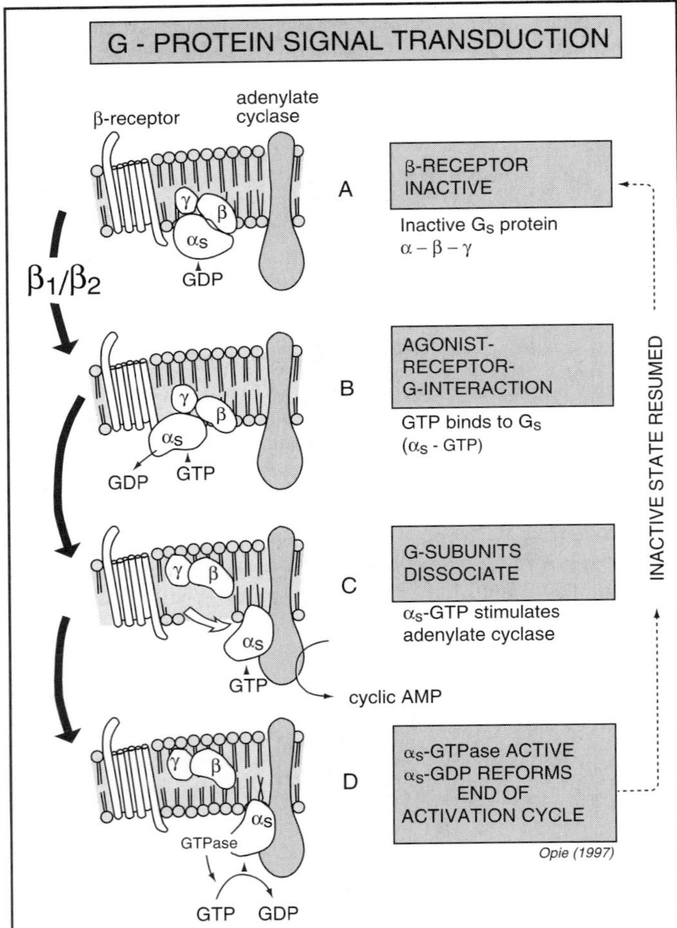

FIGURE 12–17. G proteins and their role in signal transduction in response to beta-adrenergic stimulation. Steps in G_S protein cycle: *(A)* inactive beta-receptor, inactive G_S protein ($\alpha + \beta + \gamma$); *(B)* beta-receptor occupancy, GTP binds to alpha-subunit of $G_S(\alpha_S)$ to displace GDP; *(C)* the G-subunits dissociate. Affinity of receptor for agonist decreases. α_S-GTP stimulates activity of adenylate cyclase with formation of cyclic AMP; *(D)* GTPase becomes active; converts GTP to GDP, α_S-GDP reforms. End of activation cycle. Inactive state resumed. α_S = stimulatory alpha-subunit of G protein; β = beta-subunit of G protein; γ = gamma-subunit of G protein; GDP = guanine diphosphate; G_S = stimulatory G-protein; GTP = guanine triphosphate. (Reprinted with permission. Copyright ©1997 L. H. Opie.)

sarcolemma, G_s passes on the signal from the beta-receptor to adenylate cyclase.[74,76] In the sinus node, a similar messenger system increases the heart rate. Adenylate cyclase, stimulated by G_s, produces the second messenger, cyclic AMP, which then acts through a further series of intracellular signals and specifically the third messenger protein kinase A, to increase cytosolic calcium transients. In contrast, cholinergic stimulation exerts inhibitory influences, largely on the heart rate, but also on atrial contraction, acting at least in part by decreasing the rate of formation of cyclic AMP.[73]

Other cardiac receptors, such as the alpha-adrenergic receptor, have an alternate dual messenger system involving inositol trisphosphate (IP_3) and diacylglycerol, with the latter activating protein kinase C.[30,77] Such signals are of established importance in controlling calcium flux in vascular smooth muscle, thereby regulating vascular tone and indirectly the blood pressure. In the case of cardiac myocytes, it is now appreciated that receptors coupled to protein kinase C, such as angiotensin II, may play a major role in the regulation of cardiac myocyte growth[78] and sometimes have inotropic effects.

Yet other messenger systems exist to convey different signals. For example, in blood vessels, nitric oxide formed in the inner endothelial layer stimulates the formation of cyclic GMP in the smooth muscle layer, thereby causing relaxation (vasodilation).

The sum total of these processes converting an extracellular hormonal or neural stimulus to an intracellular physiological change is called *signal transduction,* which typically starts with the agonist binding to a receptor site.[30,75]

Beta-Adrenergic Receptors and G Proteins

Cardiac beta-adrenergic receptors are chiefly the beta$_1$-subtype, whereas most noncardiac receptors are beta$_2$. There are also beta$_2$-receptors in the human heart, about 20 per cent of the total beta-receptor population in the left ventricle and about twice as high a percentage in the atria.[79] These beta$_2$-receptors appear to have greater efficacy in their capacity to activate the G-protein–adenylate cyclase system than do the beta$_1$-receptors.[80]

The receptor site is highly stereospecific, the best fit among catecholamines being obtained with the synthetic agent isoproterenol (ISO) rather than with the naturally occurring catecholamines, norepinephrine (NE), and epinephrine (E). In the case of beta$_1$-receptors, the order of agonist activity is ISO > E = NE, whereas in the case of beta$_2$-receptors, the order is ISO > E > NE.[81] The structure of the beta$_2$-receptor has been particularly well studied. The transmembrane domains are held to be the site of agonist and antagonist binding, whereas the cytoplasmic domains interact with G proteins. One of the phosphorylation sites lies on the terminal COOH tail and may be involved in the process of desensitization (see next section).

THE STIMULATORY G PROTEIN. G proteins are a superfamily of proteins that bind guanine triphosphate (GTP) and other guanine nucleotides, a process that is crucial in linking the effect of the first messenger on the receptor to the activity of the membrane-bound enzyme system that produces the second messenger (Fig. 12–17).[74] The triple combination of the beta-receptor, the G-protein complex, and adenylate cyclase is termed the *beta-adrenergic system.*[82] The G protein itself is a heterotrimer composed of G_α, G_β, and G_γ, which upon receptor stimulation splits into the alpha-subunit that is bound to GTP, and the beta-gamma-subunit.[83] Either of these subunits may regulate differing effectors such as adenylate cyclase, phospholipase C, and ion channels. The activity of adenylate cyclase is controlled by two different G-protein complexes, namely G_s which stimulates and G_i which inhibits.[84] The alpha-subunit of G_s (α_s) combines with GTP and then separates from the other two subunits to enhance activity of adenylate cyclase. The beta- and gamma-subunits appear to be linked structurally and in function.

THE INHIBITORY G PROTEIN. In contrast, a second trimeric GTP-binding protein, G_i, is responsible for inhibition of adenylate cyclase.[83] During cholinergic signaling, the muscarinic receptor is stimulated and GTP binds to the inhibitory alpha-subunit, α_i.[75] The latter then dissociates from the other two components of the G-protein complex, which are, as in the case of G_s, the combined beta-gamma-subunits. Whereas the role of α_i is not clear, the beta-gamma-subunits act as follows. By stimulating the enzyme GTPase,[85] they break down the active alpha$_s$-subunit (α_s-GTP), so that the activation of adenylate cyclase in response to beta-stimulation becomes less. Furthermore, the beta-gamma-subunit activates the K_{ACh} channel[86] that, in turn, can inhibit the sinoatrial node to contribute to the bradycardic effect of cholinergic stimulation. The alpha$_i$-subunit activates another potassium channel (K_{ATP})[86] whose physiological function is still under discussion.

A third G protein, G_q, is involved in linking myocardial alpha-adrenergic receptors to another membrane-associated enzyme, phospholipase C (see p. 375). G_q has at least four isoforms, of which two have been found in the heart. This G protein, unlike G_i, is not susceptible to inhibition by the pertussis toxin.[75]

Role of Cyclic Adenosine Monophosphate (Cyclic AMP)

Adenylate cyclase is the only enzyme system producing cyclic AMP and specifically requires low concentrations of ATP (and magnesium) as substrate. Surprisingly, the proposed molecular structure resembles certain channel proteins, such as that of the calcium channel. Most of the protein is located on the cytoplasmic side,[87] the presumed site of interaction with the G protein.

Cyclic AMP acts as the second messenger of beta-adrenergic receptor activity (Fig. 12–18), while another cyclic nucleotide, cyclic GMP, acts as a second messenger for some aspects of vagal activity (Fig. 12–19). In vascular smooth muscle, cyclic GMP is the second messenger of the nitric oxide messenger system. These messenger chemicals are present in the heart cell in minute concentrations, that of cyclic AMP being roughly about 10^{-9} M and that of cyclic GMP about 10^{-11} M.[88] Cyclic AMP has a very rapid turnover as a result of a constant dynamic balance between its formation by adenylate cyclase and removal by another enzyme, phosphodiesterase. In general, directional changes in the tissue content of cyclic AMP can be related to directional changes in cardiac contractile activity (Table 7–3[89]). For example, beta-adrenergic stimulation increases both, whereas beta-blockade inhibits the increases induced by beta-agonists. *Forskolin,* a direct stimulator of adenylate cy-

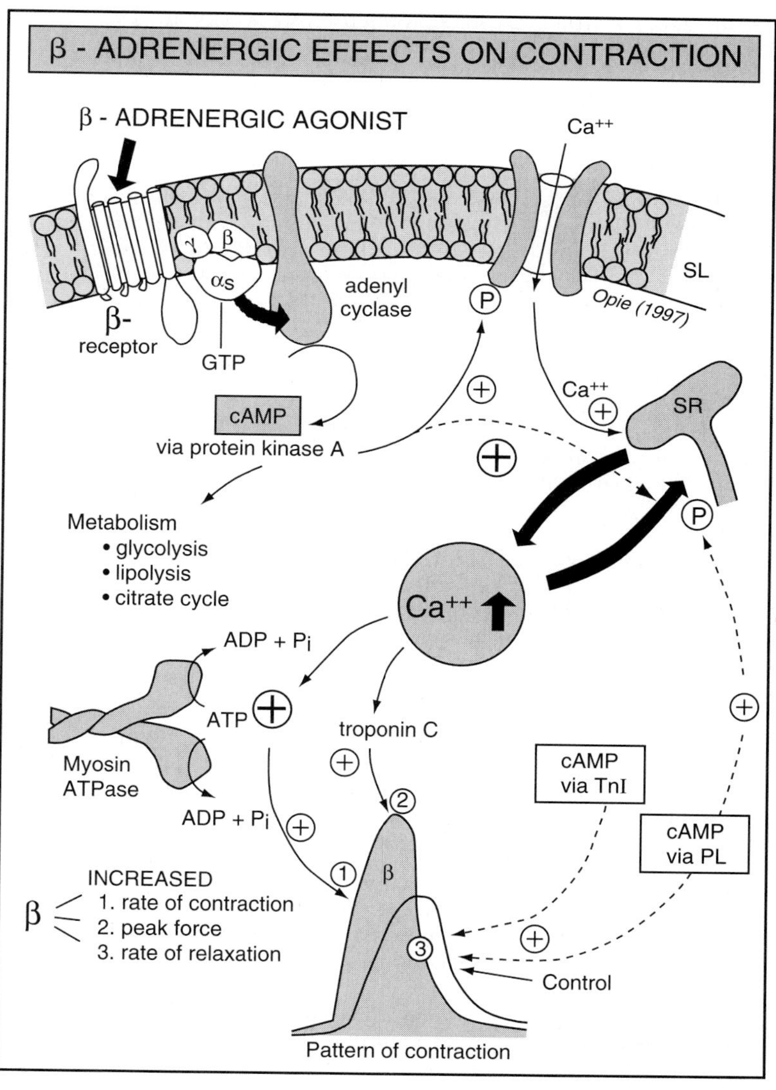

FIGURE 12–18. Signal systems involved in positive inotropic and lusitropic (enhanced relaxation) effects of beta-adrenergic stimulation. When the beta-adrenergic agonist interacts with the beta-receptor, a series of G protein–mediated changes (Fig. 12–17) lead to activation of adenylate cyclase and formation of cyclic AMP (cAMP). The latter acts via protein kinase A to stimulate metabolism *(left)* and to phosphorylate the calcium channel protein (Fig. 12–13). The result is an enhanced opening probability of the calcium channel, thereby increasing the inward movement of Ca^{++} ions through the sarcolemma (SL) of the T tubule. These Ca^{++} ions release more calcium from the sarcoplasmic reticulum (SR) (Fig. 12–3) to increase cytosolic calcium and to activate troponin-C. Calcium ions also increase the rate of breakdown of ATP to ADP and inorganic phosphate (P_i). Enhanced myosin ATPase activity explains the increased rate of contraction, with increased activation of troponin-C explaining increased peak force development. An increased rate of relaxation is explained because cyclic AMP also activates the protein phospholamban, situated on the membrane of the SR, that controls the rate of uptake of calcium into the SR (Fig. 12–12). The latter effect explains enhanced relaxation (lusitropic effect). P = phosphorylation; PL = phospholamban; SL = sarcolemma; SR = sarcoplasmic reticulum. (Reprinted with permission.)

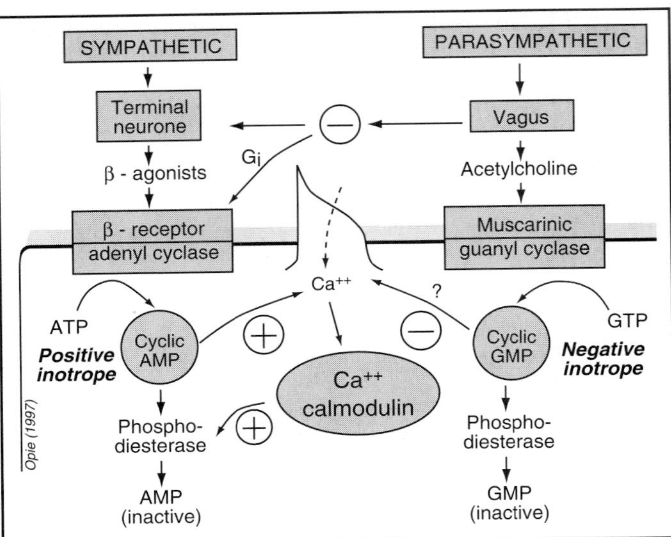

FIGURE 12–19. Interaction between parasympathetic and sympathetic systems at a cellular level may involve two opposing cyclic nucleotides, cyclic AMP and cyclic GMP. Many effects of vagal stimulation could best be explained by the inhibitory effect on the formation of cyclic AMP, including formation of inhibitory G protein, G_i, in response to M_2-receptor stimulation (Fig. 12–21). (Reprinted with permission. Copyright ©1997 L. H. Opie.)

clase, increases cyclic AMP and contractile activity. Adenosine, acting through A_1-receptors, inhibits adenylate cyclase, decreases cyclic AMP, and lessens contractile activity.

A number of hormones can couple to myocardial adenylate cyclase independently of the beta-adrenergic receptor. These are glucagon, thyroid hormone, prostacyclin (PGI_2), and the calcitonin gene-related peptide.

INHIBITION OF CYCLIC AMP FORMATION. The major physiological stimulus to G_s is thought to be vagal muscarinic receptor stimulation (Fig. 12–19). There are two additional inhibitory agonists. First, adenosine, interacting with A_1-receptors, couples to G_i to inhibit contraction and heart rate.[90] The adenosine A_2-receptor, also found in the heart, paradoxically increases cyclic AMP. The latter effect is thought to be of major importance in vascular smooth muscle but of only ancillary significance in the heart.[90] Second, endothelin may also inhibit cyclic AMP formation through a G_s-linked receptor[91] to have a potentially negative inotropic effect, in contrast to the possible positive effect generated by the coupling of the endothelin receptor to phospholipase C.

CYCLIC AMP–DEPENDENT PROTEIN KINASES. It is now clear that most if not all of the effects of cyclic AMP are ultimately mediated by the protein kinases that phosphorylate various important proteins and enzymes.[92,93] *Phosphorylation* is the donation of a phosphate group to the enzyme concerned, acting as a fundamental metabolic switch that can extensively amplify the signal.

Each protein kinase is composed of two subunits, regulatory (R) and catalytic (C). When cyclic AMP interacts with the inactive protein kinase, it binds to the R-subunit to liberate the active kinase, which is the C-subunit:

$$(R_2 + C_2) + 2\ cAMP \rightarrow 2\ RcAMP + 2\ C$$

At a molecular level, this active kinase catalyzes the transfer of the terminal phosphate of ATP to serine and threonine residues of the protein substrates, leading to phosphorylation and modification of the properties of the proteins concerned, thereby leading to further key reactions. Protein kinase A occurs in different cells in two isoforms: *protein kinase II* predominates in cardiac cells.[93] The proposed anchorage of this kinase to specific organelles could help explain the phenomenon of *cyclic AMP compartmentation*.[94] In addition, the G-protein system may not be evenly spread throughout the sarcolemma but localized to certain focal areas.[83] Thus, it is very likely that there is a specific compartment of cyclic AMP available to increase contractile activity.[95,96]

Physiological Beta-Adrenergic Effects

The probable sequence of events describing the positive inotropic effects of catecholamines is shown in Figure 12–18 and is as follows[89]:

Catecholamine stimulation → beta-receptor → molecular changes → binding of GTP to alpha$_s$-subunit of G protein → GTP-alpha$_s$-subunit stimulates adenylate cyclase → formation of cyclic AMP from ATP → activation of cyclic AMP–dependent protein kinase (PKA) → phosphorylation of a sarcolemmal protein p27 → increased entry of calcium ion through increased opening of the voltage-dependent L-type calcium channels → greater calcium-induced calcium release via ryanodine receptor of sarcoplasmic reticulum → more rise of intracellular free calcium ion concentration → increased calcium–troponin-C interaction with deinhibition of tropomyosin effect on actin-myosin interaction → increased rate and number of crossbridges interacting with increased myosin ATPase activity → increased rate and peak force development.

The increased lusitropic (relaxant) effect is the consequence of increased protein kinase A–mediated phosphorylation of phospholamban (Fig. 12–18).

Cholinergic Receptors

In the case of the parasympathetic system, signaling is again an extracellular first messenger (acetylcholine), a receptor system (the muscarinic receptor), and a sarcolemmal signaling system (the G-protein system). The myocardial *muscarinic receptor (M_2)* is associated specifically with the activity of the vagal nerve endings. Receptor stimulation produces a negative chronotropic response that is inhibited by atropine.

Regarding the *negative inotropic effect of vagal stimulation* (Fig. 12–19), the mechanism is multiple, including (1) heart rate slowing (negative Treppe phenomenon); (2) an inhibition of the formation of cyclic AMP; and (3) a direct negative inotropic effect mediated by cyclic GMP.[97] It should be noted that ventricular tissue is much less responsive to muscarinic agonists than atrial tissue, although the receptor populations are similar in density.[73] Thus, there must be postreceptor differences between atrial and ventricular tissue, probably in the degree of G-protein coupling. In general, the negative inotropic effect has been best observed in the presence of beta-stimulation (Table 12–2) when vagal effects counteract those of prior beta-stimulation.[73,98] The proposal is that muscarinic stimulation inhibits the G_s activation that results from beta-receptor occupation.

Cyclic GMP may act as a second messenger to vagal stimulation just as cyclic AMP does to beta-adrenergic stimulation. Thus, the vagus may have a dual effect on second messengers, inhibiting the formation of cyclic AMP and increasing that of cyclic GMP.[97] Cyclic GMP may in turn inhibit the activity of the L-calcium channel by a cyclic GMP–dependent kinase (G kinase).[99,100] Favoring this view is the finding that cell-permeable analogs of cyclic GMP have antiadrenergic effects. The problem with this hypothesis is the inconstant increase in ventricular cyclic GMP in response to vagal stimulation. The explanation could lie in cell compartmentation of cyclic GMP, as postulated for cyclic AMP. Also the effects of cyclic GMP on contractility may be more subtle than changes in the pattern of peak force development. Rather, there may be decreased sensitivity of the myofilaments to Ca^{++} and earlier relaxation.[101]

Yet another mechanism for parasympathetic-sympathetic interaction lies at the level of the sympathetic terminal

TABLE 12–2 IONIC EFFECTS OF ADRENERGIC AND CHOLINERGIC STIMULATION: RELATION TO HEART RATE AND CONTRACTILE ACTIVITY

AGONIST	IONIC CURRENT	EFFECT
Beta-adrenergic stimulation[1,2]	I_{Ca} increased I_k increased I_{to} increased I_f increased I_{Na} increased	+ inotropic − inotropic − inotropic Heart rate + Contraction + Conduction +
ACh during beta-stimulation[1,3]	I_{Ca} decreased I_{Na} decreased I_f decreased	− inotropic − dromotropic − chronotropic
ACh direct effect on K^+ currents[4]	I_{kACh} and I_{kATP} increased	Heart rate decreased
Alpha$_1$-adrenergic stimulation[5]	I_{to} decreased I_k decreased I_{kACh} decreased	+ inotropic + inotropic Atrial current, effects not clear

− = negative; + = positive
[1] Matsuda et al.[98]
[2] Matsuda et al.[130]
[3] Chang and Cohen[131]
[4] Kurachi[86]
[5] Fedida[108]

neuronse, where a *presynaptic muscarinic M_2 receptor* inhibits the release of norepinephrine.[73]

Additionally, both adrenergic and cholinergic stimuli exert complex and potentially important effects on ion channels that can be translated into opposing effects on cardiac function (Table 12–2). The presence of such multiple mechanisms for the inhibitory effects of vagal stimulation on the heart rate and inotropic state suggest that "braking" of beta-adrenergic stimulation is desirable. Otherwise, the risk may be that intense beta-adrenergic stimulation would excessively increase the heart rate or inotropic state.

Receptors Linked to Phospholipase C

There is an important group of receptors previously thought to act chiefly on the myocardium at the presynaptic level to enhance release of norepinephrine, and on postsynaptic vascular receptors to cause vasoconstriction. Such receptors include those for alpha$_1$-adrenergic catecholamines, angiotensin II, and endothelin. They are all linked to phospholipase C by a G protein, G_q (Fig. 12–20). Currently, two aspects of their action are under intense focus. First, the signaling system involved is clearly different from that involved in beta-adrenergic effects.[30] Second, these receptors have been identified in ventricular myocytes, posing the question of their physiological role—a problem that is still not fully clarified.[77]

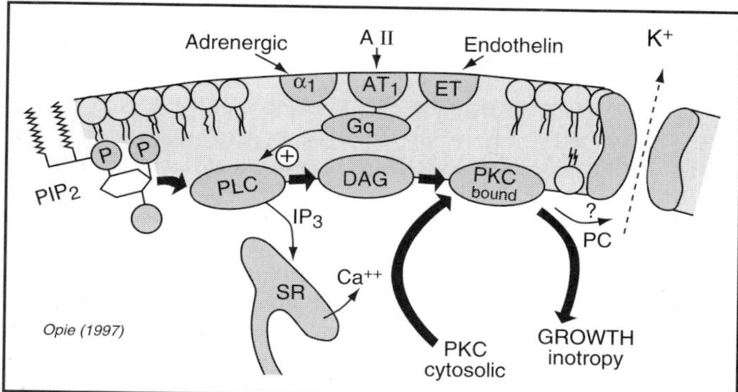

FIGURE 12–20. Phospholipase C (PLC) signaling system in myocardium, coupled to alpha$_1$-adrenergic, angiotensin AT_1, and endothelin (ET) receptors by G proteins G_q. PLC splits phosphatidylinositol bisphosphate (PIP_2) to inositol trisphosphate (IP_3) and diacylglycerol (DAG), the latter being membrane-bound. IP_3 (and IP_4) release Ca^{++} from the sarcoplasmic reticulum (SR) to activate protein kinase C (PKC) by translocating it from a cytosolic to a membrane-bound situation. PKC plays a role in growth regulation and possibly in inotropy and ion channel control. Hypothetically, PKC is an effector of preconditioning (PC) and activates potassium channels. (Reprinted with permission. Copyright ©1997 L. H. Opie.)

PHOSPHATIDYLINOSITOL SYSTEM. When any of these agonists occupies its receptor, then the link to phospholipase C is by one of the G-protein family, namely G_q. The exact steps involved are not as well understood as is the coupling of the beta-receptor to adenylate cyclase, but similar components of the G-protein complex appear to be involved.[102] First, G_q activates phospholipase C to split the compound phosphatidylinositol bisphosphate (PIP_2), part of the membrane phospholipid system, into two second messengers, *inositol trisphosphate* (IP_3) and 1,2-diacylglycerol (DAG). IP_3, in turn, stimulates the slow release of calcium from the SR and increases calcium oscillations.[103] This calcium acts on the next messenger in the system, protein kinase C, by promoting the translocation of this enzyme from cytosol to sarcolemma.[104] Once translocated, protein kinase C becomes activated by DAG, the other second messenger of phospholipase C activity. DAG, being highly lipophilic, stays in the cell membrane and, together with a resident serine component of the membrane lipids, stimulates protein kinase C into activity by reducing the calcium requirement of the protein kinase C to micromolar values.[93]

PROTEIN KINASE C. Protein kinase C has at least nine isoforms, the functions of which are poorly understood.[105] Some of the isoforms may hypothetically be associated with enhanced growth via proto-oncogenes.[106] Other isoforms may be concerned with inotropy.[107] The involvement of different isoforms may be concerned with inotropy.[107] The involvement of different isoforms may explain variable effects on contraction, mostly positive with some negatives.[73,108,109] Hypothetically, protein kinase C is an effector of preconditioning,[110] perhaps activating potassium channels (Fig. 12–20).[111]

Other Signals

Nitric Oxide as Messenger with Cyclic GMP as Target

In the myocardium, the proposal is that cyclic GMP can, by stimulation of the appropriate protein G kinases (PKG), result in a decreased heart rate and in a negative inotropic effect.[100] Formation of cyclic GMP, under the influence of guanylate cyclase, is thought to occur in response to (1) cholinergic stimulation, as already discussed, and (2) the nitric oxide signaling path.

In vascular smooth muscle, soluble guanylate cyclase responds to stimulation by nitric oxide, released by the vascular endothelium, by formation of cyclic GMP.[112] The latter vasodilates through a mechanism not fully understood but thought to involve G kinase and a decrease of cytosolic calcium. Until recently it was thought that nitric oxide played no role in the regulation of myocardial cell function. Yet, in ventricular myocytes, production of nitric oxide enhances the negative inotropic effect of acetylcholine and decreases the positive inotropic effects of beta-stimulation.[113] Therefore, the nitric oxide system, it is proposed, may have a negative modulatory role on the cardiac effects of autonomic stimulation in keeping with the proposed formation of cyclic GMP. Nonetheless, in cardiac muscle not undergoing beta-adrenergic stimulation, physiological concentrations of nitric oxide do not appear to alter cardiac contractile behavior.[114] Thus, the physiological role of the nitric oxide messenger system in the myocardium remains controversial.

Adenosine Signaling

Adenosine, like nitric oxide, is a physiological vasodilator. It is formed from the breakdown of ATP both physiologically (as during an increased heart load) and pathologically (as in ischemia). Adenosine can diffuse from myocardial cells to act on coronary arterial smooth muscle to cause vasodilation (see p. 386). The mechanism of the latter effect is reasonably well understood and involves the stimulation of vascular adenylate cyclase and cyclic AMP formation. A_2-Receptors mediate such vasodilation. Although A_2-receptors have also been identified in cardiomyocytes, stimulation of such receptors does not appear to have functional consequences.[115] Therefore only the A_1-receptors coupled to adenylate cyclase by the inhibitory G protein (alpha$_i$-subunit) are functional in the myocardium.

Other signal systems are also involved.[116] First, A_1-receptors couple to the acetycholine-sensitive potassium channel (current I_{kACh}) to stimulate channel opening and thereby to exert inhibitory effects on the sinus and AV nodes, the latter inhibition being the basis for the use of adenosine in the treatment of supraventricular nodal reentry arrhythmias (see p. 618). Second, A_1-receptors may in some circumstances couple to phospholipase C, which hypothetically explains their role in preconditioning.

Stretch Receptors

Both myocardial and vascular cells can respond to stretch by activation of a group of poorly understood mechanoreceptors, also called stretch receptors. Activation of these receptors is linked to a series of phosphorylations, including those of two crucial enzymes in the growth cascade, namely MAP (mitogen-activated protein) kinase and S6 kinase.[117] Stretch may initiate a series of conformational changes in ion channels or receptors to allow increased entry of a specific ion, such as sodium, which could then be converted to a calcium signal by Na^+/Ca^{++} exchange. Another example of a mechanoreceptor is the response of the ATP-sensitive potassium channel of atrial muscle.[118] Of considerable interest is the concept that an early event in the sequence leading from muscle stretch to hypertrophy is release of angiotensin II from the stretched muscle.[78] The mechanism of this stretch-induced release of angiotensin II is not known but may include stimulation of formation of the cardiac mRNA for renin.[119]

Signaling Systems in Heart Failure

(See also Chap. 13)

In congestive heart failure (Fig. 12–21), changes to the beta-adrenergic–cyclic AMP system include (1) major beta$_1$-receptor downregulation[79,120]; (2) beta$_2$-receptor uncoupling from adenylate cyclase[120]; (3) decreased adenylate cyclase activity[120,121]; and (4) increased levels of inhibitory G_i proteins.[122] In combination, these changes may explain the poorly developed and low-amplitude calcium transients in human tissue from severe heart failure subjects.[123] There is a major (50 to 70 per cent) *downregulation* of the beta$_1$-receptor with decreased receptor density, especially when the heart failure is caused by idiopathic cardiomyopathy.[120] Of the beta-receptor subtypes in the human ventricle, the normal ratio of the beta$_1$ to beta$_2$ of about 80:20 is changed to a ratio of about 60:40,[79,124] so that beta$_2$-mediated inotropic effects may become relatively more important. The previous proposal that the beta$_1$-receptor downregulation occurs in response to the excess level of circulating catecholamines seems not valid.[120] Rather, a poorly understood local mechanism translates into a decrease of the mRNA for the beta$_1$-receptor.[120,125] In addition, both Beta$_1$- and beta$_2$-receptors become moderately uncoupled from their signaling systems, so that even beta$_2$-stimulation is less positively inotropic than expected.[79,120] In this context, although it might be anticipated that alpha$_1$-mediated positive inotropic effects would become more prominent as a compensatory mechanism, nonetheless the response to alpha$_1$-stimulation in heart failure is much diminished.[124]

Uncoupling of the beta-receptor from the signaling system may be explained as follows.[125,126] Sustained beta-agonist stimulation rapidly induces the activity of the beta-agonist receptor kinase (βARK) that is involved in the transfer of the phosphate group to the phosphorylation site on the terminal COOH tail of the receptor, which of itself does not markedly affect the signaling properties. Rather, βARK increases the affinity of the beta-receptor for another protein family, the *arrestins*,[125,127] that cause the uncoupling. Hypothetically, the molecular configuration of the receptor is changed in such a way that the G proteins cannot interact optimally with it. Resensitization of the receptor occurs if the phosphate group is split off by a phosphatase and the receptor may then more readily be linked to G_s.[81]

Physiologically, the βARK-arrestin mechanism causes a very rapid desensitization of beta-receptor within minutes to seconds, yet this mechanism also plays a role in long-term desensitization as in heart failure.[125,127]

Also causing physiological (but not pathological) desensitization is phosphorylation of the beta-receptor by protein kinase A,[127] occurring within minutes and acting as a feedback mechanism to prevent adverse effects of excess cyclic AMP elevation and protein kinase activation such as severe arrhythmias.[128] Long-term desensitization may be associated with receptor internalization, sequestration,[127] and even lysosomal degradation.[129]

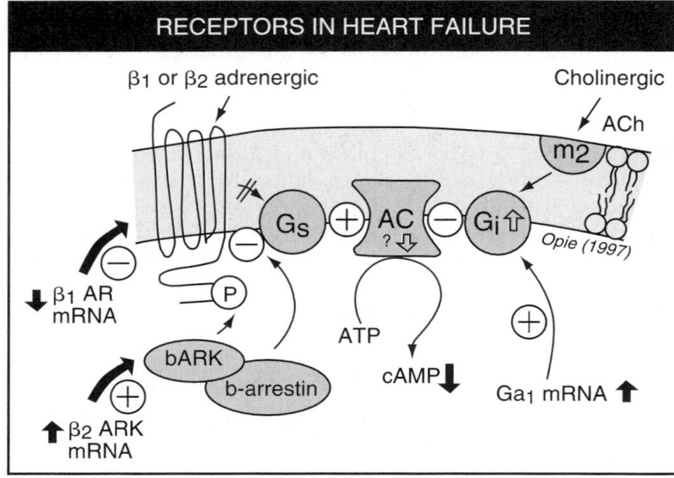

FIGURE 12–21. Proposed changes in beta-adrenergic receptor signal system in severe congestive heart failure (CHF). For concepts, see Lohse.[125] AC = Adenylate cyclase; β_1AR = beta$_1$-adrenergic receptor; β_2AR = beta$_2$-adrenergic receptor; βARK = beta-adrenergic receptor kinase; M_2 = muscarinic receptor; ACh = acetylcholine; G_i = inhibitory G protein; G_s = stimulatory G protein. (Reprinted with permission. Copyright ©1997 L. H. Opie.)

CONTRACTILE PERFORMANCE OF THE INTACT HEART

There are three main determinants of myocardial mechanical performance, namely the Frank-Starling mechanism, the contractile state, and the heart rate. This section describes the cardiac cycle and then the determinants of left ventricular (LV) function.

The Cardiac Cycle

The cardiac cycle, fully assembled by Lewis[132] but first conceived by Wiggers,[133] yields important information on the temporal sequence of events in the cardiac cycle. The three basic events are (1) LV contraction, (2) LV relaxation, and (3) LV filling (Table 12–3). Although similar mechanical events occur in the right side of the heart, those on the left side are the focus.

LV CONTRACTION. LV pressure starts to build up when the arrival of calcium ions at the contractile proteins starts to trigger actin-myosin interaction. On the electrocardio-

TABLE 12–3 THE CARDIAC CYCLE

LV CONTRACTION
Isovolumic contraction (b)
Maximal ejection (c)
LV RELAXATION
Start of relaxation and reduced ejection (d)
Isovolumic relaxation (e)
LV filling: rapid phase (f)
Slow LV filling (diastasis) (g)
Atrial systole or booster (a)

The letters a to g refer to the phases of the cardiac cycle shown in Wiggers' diagram (Fig. 12–22). These letters are arbitrarily allocated so that atrial systole (a) coincides with the A wave and (c) with the C wave of the jugular venous pressure.

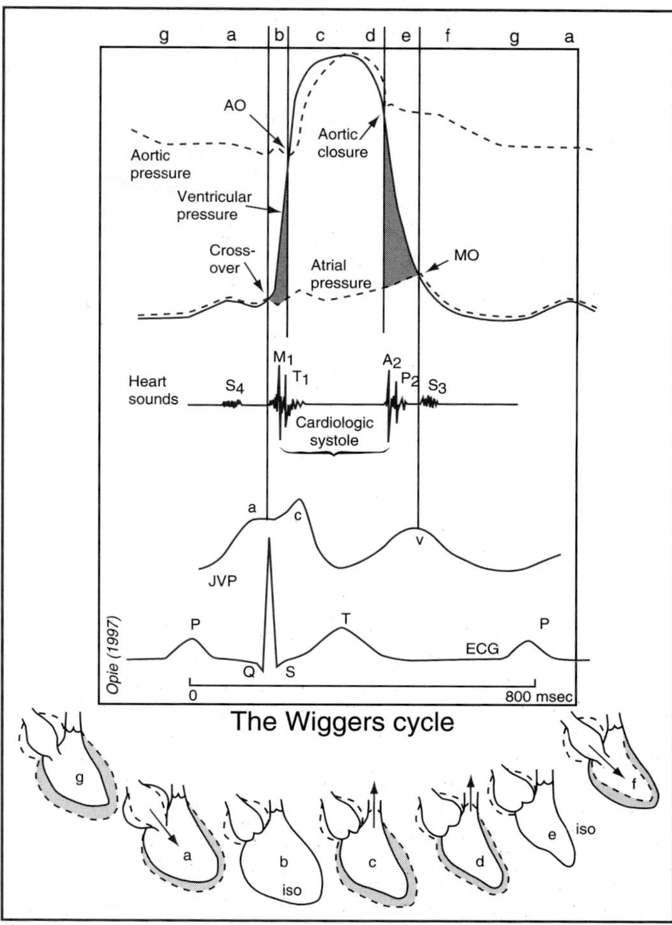

FIGURE 12–22. The mechanical events in the cardiac cycle, first assembled by Lewis in 1920 but first conceived by Wiggers in 1915.[133] Note that mitral valve closure occurs *after* the crossover point of atrial and ventricular pressures at the start of systole. (Visual phases of the ventricular cycle in bottom panel are modified from Shepherd J. T., and Vanhoutte P. M.: The Human Cardiovascular System. New York, Raven Press, 1979, p. 68.) For explanation of phases a to g, see Table 12–3. ECG = Electrocardiogram; JVP = jugular venous pressure; M_1 = mitral component of first sound at time of mitral valve closure; T_1 = tricuspid valve closure, second component of first heart sound; AO = aortic valve opening, normally inaudible; A_2 = aortic valve closure, aortic component of second sound; P_2 = pulmonary component of second sound, pulmonary valve closure; MO = mitral valve opening, may be audible in mitral stenosis as the opening snap; S_3 = third heart sound; S_4 = fourth heart sound; a = wave produced by right atrial contraction; c = carotid wave artifact during rapid LV ejection phase; v = venous return wave which causes pressure to rise while tricuspid valve is closed. Cycle length of 800 msec for 75 beats per minute. (Copyright ©1997 L. H. Opie.)

gram (ECG), the advance of the wave of depolarization is indicated by the peak of the R wave (Fig. 12–22). Soon after LV pressure in the early contraction phase builds up and exceeds that in the left atrium (normally 10 to 15 mm Hg), followed about 20 msec later by M_1, the mitral component of the first sound. The exact relation of M_1 to mitral valve closure is open to debate.[134,135] Although mitral valve closure is often thought to coincide with the crossover point at which the LV pressure starts to exceed the left atrial pressure,[132,133,136] in reality mitral valve closure is delayed because the valve is kept open by the inertia of the blood flow.[135,137] Shortly thereafter, pressure changes in the right ventricle, similar in pattern but lesser in magnitude to those in the left ventricle, cause the tricuspid valve to close, thereby creating T_1, which is the second component of the first heart sound.

During this phase of contraction between mitral valve and aortic valve opening, the LV volume is fixed *(isovolumic contraction),* because both aortic and mitral valves are shut. As more and more myofibers enter the contracted state, pressure development in the left ventricle proceeds. The interaction of actin and myosin increases, and cross-bridge cycling augments. When the pressure in the left ventricle exceeds that in the aorta, the aortic valve opens. Opening of the aortic valve is followed by the phase of *rapid ejection,* determined not only by the pressure gradient across the aortic valve, but also by the elastic properties of the aorta and the arterial tree, which undergoes systolic expansion. LV pressure rises to a peak and then starts to fall.

LV RELAXATION. As the cytosolic calcium ion concentration starts to decline because of uptake of calcium into the SR under the influence of phospholamban, more and more myofibers enter the state of relaxation and the rate of ejection of blood from the left ventricle into the aorta falls (phase of *reduced ejection*). During this phase, blood flow from the LV to the aorta rapidly diminishes but is maintained by aortic distensibility—the Windkessel effect.[138] The pressure in the aorta exceeds the falling pressure in the LV. The aortic valve closes, creating the first component of the second sound, A_2 (the second component, P_2, results from closure of the pulmonary valve as the pulmonary artery pressure exceeds that in the right ventricle). Thereafter, the ventricle continues to relax. Because the mitral valve is closed during this phase, the LV volume does not change *(isovolumic relaxation).* When the LV pressure falls to below that in the left atrium, the mitral valve opens and the filling phase of the cardiac cycle starts (Fig. 12–22). Mitral valve opening is normally silent, but in mitral stenosis there may be an audible opening snap.

LV FILLING. As LV pressure drops below that in the left atrium, just after mitral valve opening, the *phase of rapid or early filling* occurs to account for most of ventricular filling.[139] Active diastolic relaxation of the ventricle may also contribute to early filling (see section on Ventricular Suction). Such rapid filling may cause the physiological third heart sound (S_3), particularly when there is a hyperkinetic circulation.[140] As pressures in the atrium and ventricle equalize, LV filling partially stops (*diastasis,* separation). Renewed filling requires that the pressure gradient from the atrium to the ventricle should increase. This is achieved by *atrial systole* (or the *left atrial booster*), which is especially important when a high cardiac output is required as during exercise, or when the LV fails to relax normally as in LV hypertrophy.[139]

DEFINITIONS OF SYSTOLE AND DIASTOLE. *Systole* means contraction in Greek, and *diastole* is derived from two Greek words, *to send* and *apart.* For the physiologist, systole lasts from the start of isovolumic contraction (where LV pressure crosses over atrial pressure, Fig. 12–22) to the peak of the ejection phase, so that physiological diastole commences as the LV pressure starts to fall (Table 12–4). In contrast, *cardiological* systole is demarcated by the heart sounds and extends from the first heart sound (M_1) to the closure of the aortic valve (A_2), with the rest of the cardiac cycle being defined as cardiological diastole. Mitral valve

TABLE 12–4 PHYSIOLOGICAL VERSUS CARDIOLOGICAL SYSTOLE AND DIASTOLE

PHYSIOLOGICAL SYSTOLE	CARDIOLOGICAL SYSTOLE
Isovolumic contraction Maximal ejection	From M_1 to A_2 Only part of isovolumic contraction* Maximal ejection Reduced ejection
PHYSIOLOGICAL DIASTOLE	**CARDIOLOGICAL DIASTOLE**
Reduced ejection Isovolumic relaxation Filling phases	A_2-M_1 interval (Filling phases included)

* Note that M_1 occurs with a definite delay after the start of LV contraction.

closure (M_1) actually occurs about 20 msec after the onset of physiological systole at the crossover point of pressure.[135] The term *protodiastolic* (early diastole) for the physiologist is the early part of the relaxation phase—from when aortic flow begins to fall until the aortic valve shuts. For the cardiologist, protodiastole is the early phase of rapid filling, the time when the third heart sound (S_3) can be heard. This sound probably reflects ventricular wall vibrations during rapid filling and becomes audible with an increase in LV diastolic pressure or wall stiffness or rate of filling.

Frank-Starling Relationship

PRELOAD. The preload, literally the load before contraction has started, is provided by the venous return that fills the left atrium, which in turn empties into the LV during diastole.[141] When the preload increases, the LV distends, the LV pressure development becomes more rapid and rises to a higher peak pressure,[142] and the stroke volume augments. Because the heart rate also increases (see later in this section), the cardiac output rises as the venous pressure rises, as originally described by Starling. An example of such increases in the venous return are the increased cardiac output of exercise or of volume expansion as during an infusion of excess intravenous fluids. The preload is physiologically determined by the *venous return,* which in turn is influenced by venous compliance. There is also a lesser effect of a hemodynamically inactive "venous storage" component, also called the "unstressed volume," which is increased in size by venodilators.[143]

AFTERLOAD. During systole, the LV contracts against the afterload (the load *after* the onset of contraction, against which the LV contracts during LV ejection). It is less well known that Starling also studied the effect of an acute increase in afterload on LV performance. He and his coworkers abruptly increased the blood pressure of the heart-lung preparation and found that LV performance increased to overcome the greater peripheral resistance. Both systolic and diastolic LV volumes rose, indicating that the left ventricle did not empty completely. The increased diastolic volume acted in a manner similar to an increased preload to prevent the stroke volume from falling as the afterload increased. Such an afterload-dependent myocardium was probably the result of experimental conditions in which the left ventricle was in a state of incipient failure. In experimental preparations and in normal humans, a sudden increase in blood pressure is compensated for by an increased force of contraction (see Anrep effect) and by a reflex decrease of the peripheral vascular resistance mediated by the baroreflexes.

FORCE-LENGTH RELATIONSHIPS IN CALCIUM TRANSIENTS. The temptation is to link "optimal sarcomere length" with Starling's law and the force-length relationship, by supposing that ventricular stretch gives rise to such optimal overlap of actin and myosin. Whereas the overlap theory explains the force-length relationship in skeletal muscle, in cardiac muscle the situation is different (Fig. 12–23). In the case of skeletal muscle, the argument is as follows: "Because each actin filament projects about 1 micron from each side of the Z-disc, active force would decline when the sarcomere length was less than the sum of the lengths of the individual actin filaments, i.e., less than 2.0–2.2 microns."[23] In cardiac muscle, however, even at 80 per cent of the optimal length, only 10 per cent or less of the maximal force is developed (Fig. 12–23). Thus, it can be predicted that cardiac sarcomeres must function near the upper limit of their maximal length (L_{max}). Rodriguez et al.[144] have tested this prediction by relating sarcomere length changes to volume changes of the intact heart. By implanting small radiopaque beads in only about 1 cm^3 of the LV free wall and using biplane cineradiography, the motion of the markers can be tracked through various cardiac cycles with allowances made for local myocardial deformation. Thus, the change in sarcomere length from approximately 85 per cent of L_{max} to L_{max} itself is able to effect physiological LV volume changes (Fig. 12–24).

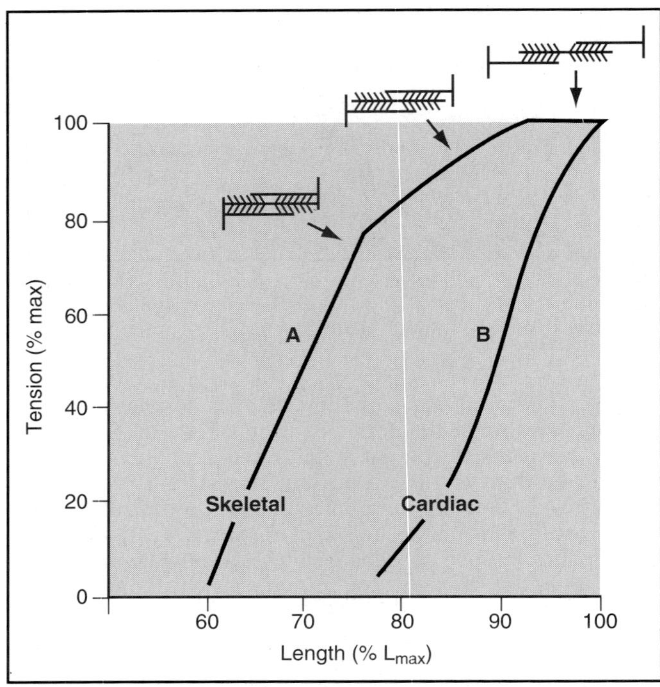

FIGURE 12–23. Schematic drawing illustrating general shape of ascending limb of *force-length relationship* in skeletal (A) and cardiac (B) muscle. Normalized force is plotted as a function of normalized length, i.e., length relative to length at which maximum force is generated (L_{max}). Also shown is approximate disposition of thick and thin filaments at different points along the physiologically relevant portion of the ascending limb. The maximum length (L_{max} 100 per cent) corresponds to the situation at maximum sarcomere lengths (2.2 microns, Fig. 12–24) or 2.15 microns (Fig. 12–25). (From Fuchs, F.: Mechanical modulation of the Ca^{2+} regulatory protein complex in cardiac muscle. NIPS *10:*6–12, 1995.)

The favored explanation for the steep length-tension relation of cardiac muscles is *length-dependent activation,* whereby an increase in calcium sensitivity is the major factor explaining the steep increase of force development as the initial sarcomere length increases.[8,145] At a molecular level, it is supposed that an increased length sensitizes troponin-C to the prevailing cytosolic calcium transient.[23] Proof that there is no increase in the calcium transient as the sarcomere length increases is provided by direct measurements (Fig. 12–25).

It should be noted that Starling did not relate sarcomere length nor LV end-diastolic pressure nor the pulmonary capillary wedge pressure but rather the *LV volume* to cardiac output. The relation between LV end-diastolic volume and LV end-diastolic pressure is curvilinear depending on the LV compliance.

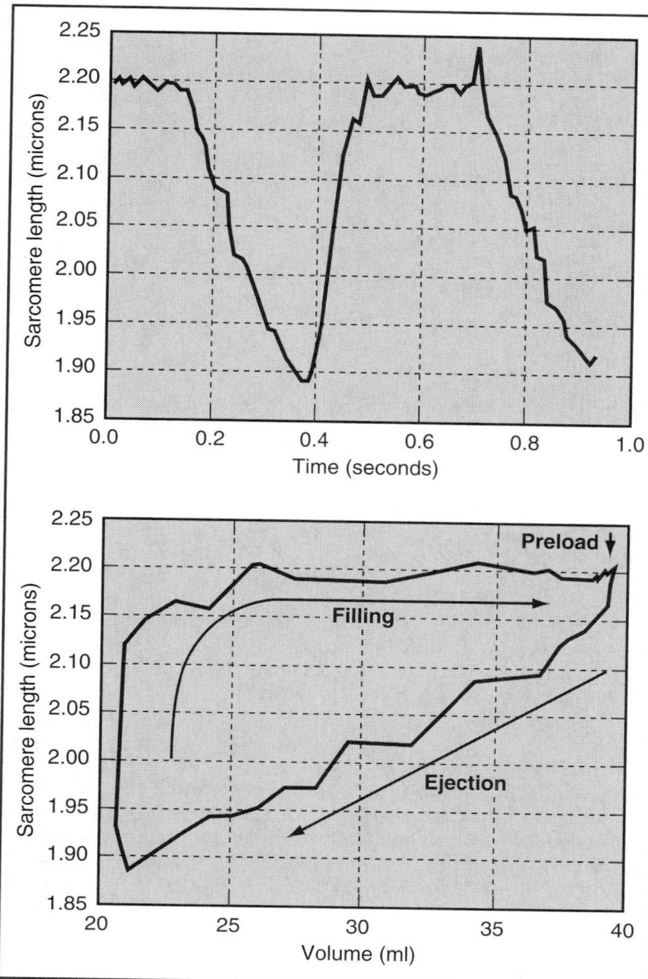

FIGURE 12–24. Changes in sarcomere length during a typical cardiac contraction-relaxation cycle in the intact dog heart. Top panel shows that during diastole the sarcomere length is 2.2 microns, reducing to 1.90 microns during systole. Bottom panel relates sarcomere length to LV volume. Starting at the top right, the preload is the maximum sarcomere length just before the onset of contraction. Then ejection decreases the LV volume, in this case by about half. Sarcomere length falls from 2.20 to 1.90 microns. Then, during the rapid phase of filling (Fig. 12–32), the sarcomere length increases from 1.90 to 2.15 microns, to be followed by the phase of constant sarcomere length (diastasis). (Modified from Rodriguez, E. K., Hunter, W. C., Royce, M. J., et al.: A method to reconstruct sarcomere lengths and orientations at transmural sites in beating canine hearts. Am J. Physiol. *263:*H293–H306, 1992.)

ANREP EFFECT: ABRUPT INCREASE IN AFTERLOAD. When the aortic pressure is elevated abruptly, a positive inotropic effect follows within 1 or 2 minutes. This was called *homeometric* autoregulation (*homeo* = the same; *metric* = length) because it was apparently independent of muscle length and by definition a true inotropic effect. A reasonable speculation would be that increased LV wall tension could act on myocardial stretch receptors to increase cytosolic sodium[146] and then, by Na^+/Ca^{++} exchange, cytosolic calcium. Thus, this effect would differ from that of an increase in preload (which acts by length-activation).

Wall Stress

Stress develops when tension is applied to a cross-sectional area, and the units are force per unit area (Fig. 14–6, p. 426). According to the *Laplace law* (Fig. 12–26):

$$\text{Wall stress} = \frac{\text{pressure} \times \text{radius}}{2 \times \text{wall thickness}}$$

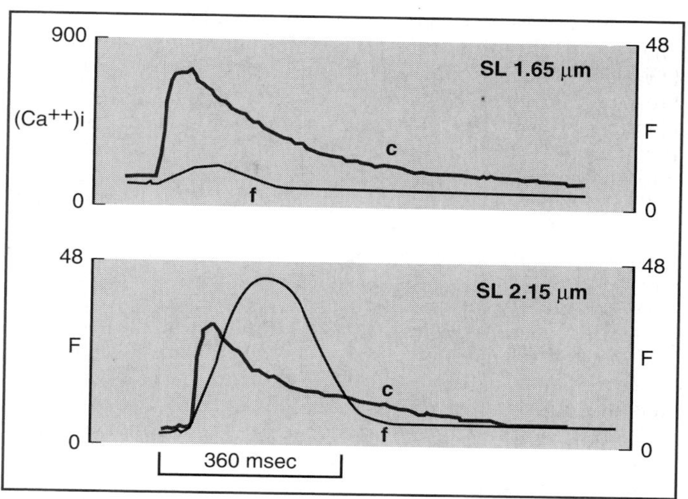

FIGURE 12–25. Length-sensitization of the sarcomere. *Top,* the sarcomere length (SL) is 1.65 microns, which gives very little force (f) development (Fig. 12–8). *Bottom,* at a near maximum sarcomere length (Figs. 12–8 and 12–24), the same $[Ca^{2+}]$ transient (c) with the same peak value and overall pattern causes a much greater force development. Therefore, there has been length-induced calcium sensitization. (Modified from Backx, P. H., and ter Keurs, H. E. D. J.: Fluorescent properties of rat cardiac trabeculae microinjected with fura-2 salt. Am. J. Physiol. *264:*H1098–H1110, 1993.)

This equation, although an oversimplification, emphasizes two points. First, the bigger the left ventricle and the greater its radius, the greater the wall stress. Second, at any given radius (LV size), the greater the pressure developed by the LV, the greater the wall stress. An increase in wall stress achieved by either of these two mechanisms (LV size or intraventricular pressure) increases myocardial oxygen uptake. This is because a greater rate of ATP use is required, as the myofibrils develop greater tension. (For more details and formulas for circumferential and meridional wall stress, see Chapter 14, pp. 426 and 427).

In cardiac hypertrophy, Laplace's law explains the effects of changes in wall thickness on wall stress (Fig. 12–26). The increased wall thickness due to hypertrophy balances

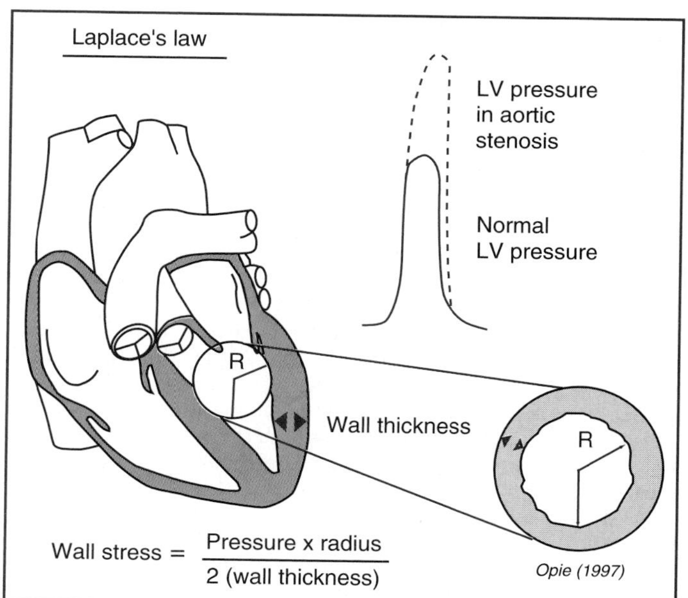

FIGURE 12–26. Wall stress increases as the afterload increases. The formula shown is derived from the Laplace law. The increased LV pressure in aortic stenosis is compensated for by LV wall hypertrophy, which decreases the denominator on the right side of the equation, thereby maintaining wall stress at control levels. (Reprinted with permission. Copyright ©1997 L. H. Opie.)

the increased pressure, and the wall stress remains unchanged during the phase of compensatory hypertrophy. In congestive heart failure, the heart dilates so that the increased radius elevates wall stress. Furthermore, because ejection of blood is inadequate, the radius stays too large throughout the contractile cycle, and both end-diastolic and end-systolic tensions are higher.

WALL STRESS, PRELOAD, AND AFTERLOAD. *Preload* can now be defined more exactly as the wall stress at the end of diastole and therefore at the maximal resting length of the sarcomere (Fig. 12–24). Measurement of wall stress in vivo is difficult because the radius of the left ventricle (see preceding sections) neglects the confounding influence of the complex anatomy of the left ventricle.[147] Surrogate measurements of the indices of preload include LV end-diastolic pressure or dimensions (the latter being the major and minor axes of the heart in a two-dimensional echocardiographic view). The *afterload,* being the load on the contracting myocardium, is also the wall stress during LV ejection. Increased afterload means that an increased intraventricular pressure has to be generated first to open the aortic valve and then during the ejection phase. These increases translate themselves into an increased myocardial wall stress, which can be measured either as an average value or at a given phase of systole, such as end-systole. Systolic wall stress reflects the two major components of the afterload, namely the arterial blood pressure and the arterial compliance. Decreased arterial compliance and increased afterload can be anticipated when there is aortic dilation as in severe systemic hypertension or in the elderly. Generally, in clinical practice, it is a sufficient approximation to take the arterial blood pressure as a measure of the afterload, provided that there is no significant aortic stenosis nor change in arterial compliance.

The *aortic impedance,* also termed the arterial input impedance, gives another accurate measure of the afterload. The aortic impedance is the aortic pressure divided by the aortic flow at that instance, so that this index of the afterload varies at each stage of the contraction cycle. Factors reducing aortic flow, such as high arterial blood pressure or aortic stenosis or loss of aortic compliance, increase impedance and hence the afterload. During systole, when the aortic valve is open, an increased afterload communicates itself to the ventricles by increasing wall stress. In LV failure, aortic impedance is augmented not only by peripheral vasoconstriction but by decreases in aortic compliance.[148] The problem with the clinical measurement of aortic impedance is that invasive instrumentation is required. An approximation can be found by using transesophageal echocardiography to determine aortic blood flow at, for example, the time of maximal increase of aortic flow just after aortic valve opening.

Heart Rate and Force-Frequency Relation

TREPPE OR BOWDITCH EFFECT. An increased heart rate progressively increases the force of ventricular contraction, even in an isolated papillary muscle preparation (Bowditch staircase phenomenon[149]). Alternative names are the *treppe* (steps, German) phenomenon or positive inotropic effect of activation or force-frequency relation (Figs. 12–27 and 12–28). Conversely, a decreased heart rate has a negative staircase effect. When stimulation becomes too rapid, force decreases.[150] The proposal is that during rapid stimulation, more sodium and calcium ions enter the myocardial cell than can be handled by the sodium pump and the mechanisms for calcium exit. Opposing the force-frequency effect is the negative contractile influence of the decreased duration of ventricular filling at high heart rates. The longer the filling interval, the better the ventricular filling and the stronger the subsequent contraction. This phenomenon can be shown in patients with mitral stenosis and atrial fibrillation with a variable filling interval.

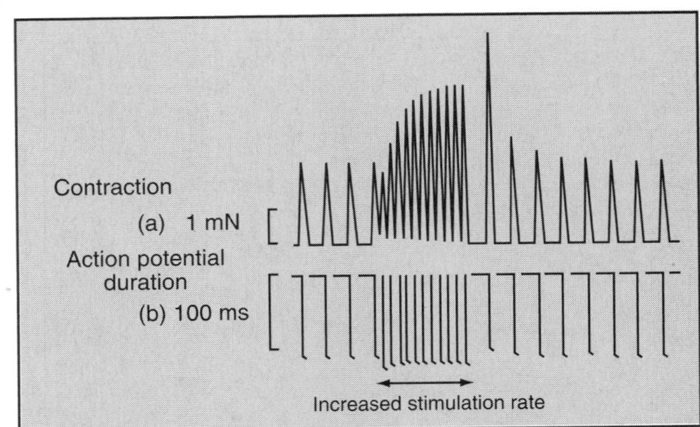

FIGURE 12–27. The Bowditch or *treppe* phenomenon, whereby a faster stimulation rate *(bottom panel)* increases the force of contraction *(top panel).* The stimulus rate is shown as the action potential duration on an analog analyzer (ms = milliseconds). The tension developed by papillary muscle contraction is shown in milliNewtons (mN) in the top panel. On cessation of rapid stimulation, the contraction force gradually declines. Hypothetically, the explanation for the increased contraction during the increased stimulation is repetitive Ca^{++} entry with each depolarization and, hence, an accumulation of cytosolic calcium. (From Noble, M. I. M.: Excitation-contraction coupling. *In* Drake-Holland, A. J., and Noble, M. I. M. (eds.): Cardiac Metabolism. Chichester, John Wiley, 1983, pp. 49–71.)

Post-extrasystolic potentiation and the inotropic effect of *paired pacing* can be explained by the same model,[151] again assuming an enhanced contractile state after the prolonged interval between beats. Nonetheless, the exact cellular mechanism remains to be clarified.[152]

FORCE-FREQUENCY RELATIONSHIP IN HUMANS. Muscle strips prepared from patients with mitral regurgitation behave very differently from normal muscle in response to an increased stimulation of frequency (Fig. 12–28). Normally, peak contractile force at a fixed muscle length (isometric contraction) is reached at about 150 to 180 stimuli per minute.[150] This is the human counterpart of the *treppe*

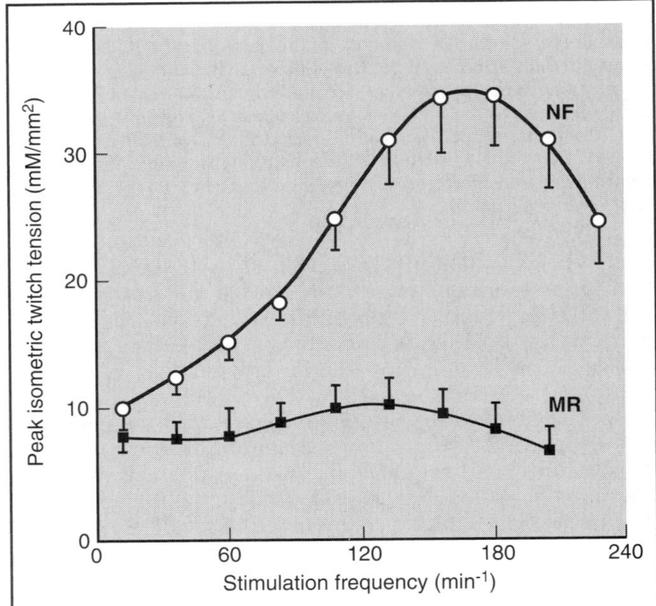

FIGURE 12–28. Plot of average steady-state isometric twitch tension versus stimulation frequency. Each point represents the mean ± SEM of eight nonfailing, control preparations (NF) and eight failing, mitral regurgitation preparations (MR). Temperature 37°C. (Data from Mulieri, L. A., et al.: Myocardial force-frequency defect in mitral regurgitation heart failure is reversed by forskolin. Circulation *88:*2700, 1993. Copyright 1993 American Heart Association.)

phenomenon. In severe mitral regurgitation there is hardly any response to an increased stimulation frequency. In another study on muscle strips from normal hearts, optimal force development was reached at rates of about 120 to 150 beats per minute,[153] whereas in patients with cardiomyopathy, an increased heart rate produced a decreased twitch tension.

HEART RATE IN SITU. In situ, the optimal heart rate is not only the rate that would give maximal mechanical performance of an isolated muscle strip, but is also determined by the need for adequate time for diastolic filling. In normal humans, it is not possible to attach exact values to the heart rate required to decrease rather than increase cardiac output or to keep it steady. Pacing rates of up to 150 per minute can be tolerated whereas higher rates cannot because of the development of AV block. In contrast, during exercise, indices of LV function still increase up to a maximum heart rate of about 170 beats per minute, presumably because of enhanced contractility and peripheral vasodilation.[154] It is presumed that the increased heart rate during exercise produces an increase in contractile force in keeping with the *treppe* phenomenon and in response to (1) adrenergic discharge and (2) activation of mechanoreceptors in the left atrium.

Myocardial Oxygen Uptake

The myocardial oxygen demand can be increased by heart rate, preload, or afterload (Fig. 12–29), factors that can all precipitate myocardial ischemia in those with coronary artery disease. A less commonly known but equally important concept is that the oxygen uptake can be augmented by increased contractility as during beta-adrenergic stimulation.[155]

Because myocardial oxygen uptake ultimately reflects the rate of mitochondrial metabolism and of ATP production, any increase of ATP requirement is reflected in an increased oxygen uptake. In general, factors increasing wall stress increase the oxygen uptake. An increased afterload causes an increased systolic wall stress, which needs a greater oxygen uptake. An increased diastolic wall stress, resulting from an increased preload, also requires more oxygen because the greater stroke volume must be ejected against the afterload. In states of enhanced contractility, the rate of change of wall stress is increased. Thus, thinking in terms of wall stress provides a comprehensive approach to the problem of myocardial oxygen uptake. Because the systolic blood pressure is an important determinant of the afterload, a practical index of the oxygen uptake is systolic blood pressure × heart rate, the *double-product*.[156] In addition, there may be a metabolic component to the oxygen uptake which is usually small but may be prominent in certain special conditions, such as the "oxygen wastage" found during abnormally high circulating free fatty acid values.[157,158] The concept of wall stress in relation to oxygen uptake also explains why heart size is such an important determinant of the myocardial oxygen uptake (because the larger radius increases wall stress).

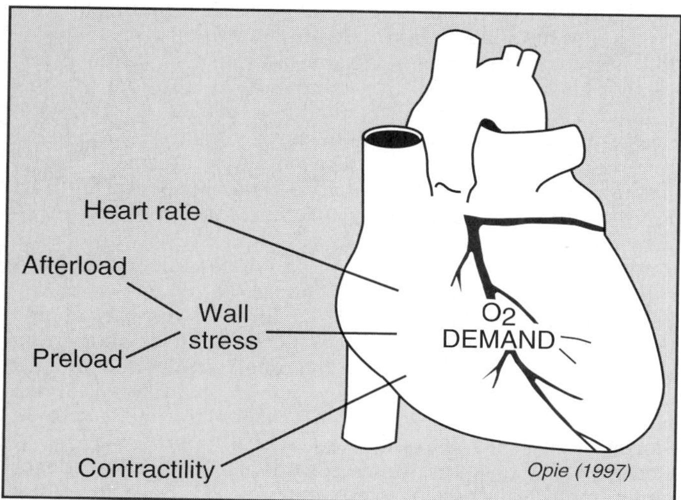

FIGURE 12–29. Major determinants of the oxygen demand of the normal heart are heart rate, wall stress, and contractility. For use of pressure-volume area as index of oxygen uptake, see Figure 12–33. (Reprinted with permission. Copyright ©1997 L. H. Opie.)

WORK OF THE HEART. External work is done when, for example, a mass is lifted a certain distance. In terms of the heart, the cardiac output is the mass moved, and the resistance against which it is moved is the blood pressure. Because volume work needs less oxygen than pressure work,[151,159] it might be supposed that external work is not an important determinant of the myocardial oxygen uptake. However, three determinants of the myocardial oxygen uptake are involved: preload (because this helps determine the stroke volume), afterload (in part determined by the blood pressure), and heart rate, as can be seen from the following formula:

$$\text{Minute work} = \text{SBP} \times \text{SV} \times \text{heart rate}$$

where SBP = systolic blood pressure and SV = stroke volume. Thus, it is not surprising that heart work is related to oxygen uptake.[156] The *pressure-work index* takes into account both the double-product (SBP × HR) and the HR × stroke volume, i.e., cardiac output.[156] The *pressure-volume area* is another index of myocardial oxygen uptake, requiring invasive monitoring for accurate measurements.[151] External cardiac work can account for up to 40 per cent of the total myocardial oxygen uptake.[156]

In strict terms, the work performed *(power production)* needs to take into account not only pressure but kinetic components.[160] It is the pressure work that has been discussed (product of cardiac output and peak systolic pressure). The kinetic work is the component required to move the blood against the afterload. Normally kinetic work is less than 1 per cent of the total. In aortic stenosis, kinetic work increases sharply as the cross-sectional area of the aorta narrows, whereas pressure work increases as the gradient across the aortic valve rises. Currently, noninvasive measures of peak power production are being assessed as indices of cardiac contractility.[161]

Efficiency of work is the relation between the work performed and the myocardial oxygen uptake.[151] Exercise increases the efficiency of external work, an improvement that offsets any metabolic cost of the increased contractility.[162] Certain pharmacological agents, such as dobutamine, also improve efficiency in the failing heart.[163] The subcellular basis for changes in efficiency of work are not fully understood. Because as little as 12 to 14 per cent of the oxygen uptake may be converted to external work,[162] it is probably the "internal work" that becomes less demanding. Internal ion fluxes ($Na^+/K^+/Ca^{++}$) account for about 20 to 30 per cent of the ATP requirement of the heart,[89] so that most ATP is spent on actin-myosin interaction, and much of that on generation of heat rather than on external work. An increased initial muscle length is known to sensitize the contractile apparatus to calcium, thereby theoretically increasing the efficiency of contraction by diminishing the amount of calcium flux required. In addition, muscle shortening in itself appears to increase efficiency, again by an unknown mechanism.[164]

Contractility or the Inotropic State

Although difficult to define with precision, increased contractility results in a greater velocity of contraction, which reaches a greater peak force or pressure when other factors influencing the myocardial oxygen uptake, such as the heart rate, the preload, and the afterload, are kept constant. An alternate name for contractility is the *inotropic state* (*ino* = fiber; *tropos* = to move). Contractility is one of the major determinants of the myocardial oxygen uptake (Fig. 12–29). Factors that increase contractility include adrenergic stimulation (exercise, emotion), digitalis, and other inotropic agents. *A useful hypothesis is that the factor common to all situations with an increased inotropic state is enhanced interaction between calcium ions and the contractile proteins.* Such interaction could result from either an increased systolic rate of rise and peak of the cytosolic calcium ion concentration or from sensitization of the contractile proteins to a given level of cytosolic calcium, as during the action of certain positively inotropic drugs acting through this mechanism.[165] Some experimental data suggest that sensitization may be a physiological mechanism for the increase in contractility in response, for example, to alpha-adrenergic stimulation.[108]

Conversely, contractility is decreased whenever calcium transients are depressed, as when beta-adrenergic blockade decreases calcium entry through the L-type calcium channel, when the ATP required for the activity of the calcium uptake pump of the SR is impaired as during anoxia or ischemia, or when there are abnormalities of the SR as in congestive heart failure.

The concept of contractility has at least two serious defects, including (1) the absence of any potential index that can be measured in situ and is free of significant criticism and, in particular, the absence of any acceptable noninvasive index; and (2) the impossibility of separating the cellular mechanisms of contractility changes from those of load or heart rate. Thus, an increased heart rate through the sodium pump lag mechanism gives rise to an increased cytosolic calcium, which is thought to explain the *treppe* phenomenon. An increased preload involves increased fiber stretch, which in turn causes length activation, explicable by sensitization of the contractile proteins to the prevailing cytosolic calcium concentration. An increased afterload may increase cytosolic calcium through stretch-sensitive channels. Thus, there is a clear overlap between contractility, which should be independent of load or heart rate, and the effects of load and heart rate on the cellular mechanisms. Hence, the traditional separation of inotropic state from load/heart rate effects as two independent regulators of cardiac muscle performance is no longer simple now that the underlying cellular mechanisms have been uncovered.[166] In clinical terms, it nonetheless remains important to separate the effects of a primary increase of load or heart rate from a primary increase in contractility (Fig. 14–2, p. 422). This distinction is especially relevant when attempting to dissect the multiple abnormalities found in congestive heart failure, where a decreased contractility could indirectly or directly result in increased afterload, preload, and heart rate, all of which factors then predispose to a further decrease in myocardial performance. Thus, decreased contractility is eventually self-augmenting.

FORCE-VELOCITY RELATIONSHIP AND MAXIMUM CONTRACTILITY IN MUSCLE MODELS. If the concept of contractility is truly independent of the load and the heart rate, then unloaded heart muscle stimulated at a fixed rate should have a maximum value of contractility for any given magnitude of the cytosolic calcium transient. This value, the V_{max} of muscle contraction, is defined as the *maximal velocity of contraction* when there is no load on the isolated muscle or no afterload to prevent maximal rates of cardiac ejection (Fig. 12–30). Beta-adrenergic stimulation increases V_{max}, and converse changes are found in the failing myocardium. V_{max} is also termed V_0 (the maximum velocity at zero load). The problem with this relatively simple concept is that V_{max} cannot be measured directly but is extrapolated from the peak rates of force development in unloaded muscle obtained from the intercept on the velocity axis.[167] In another extreme condition, there is no muscle shortening at all (zero shortening), and all the energy goes into development of pressure (P_0) or force (F_0). This situation is an example of *isometric shortening* (*iso* = the same; *metric* = length). Because the peak velocity is obtained at zero load when there is no external force development, the relationship is usually termed the *force-velocity relationship*.

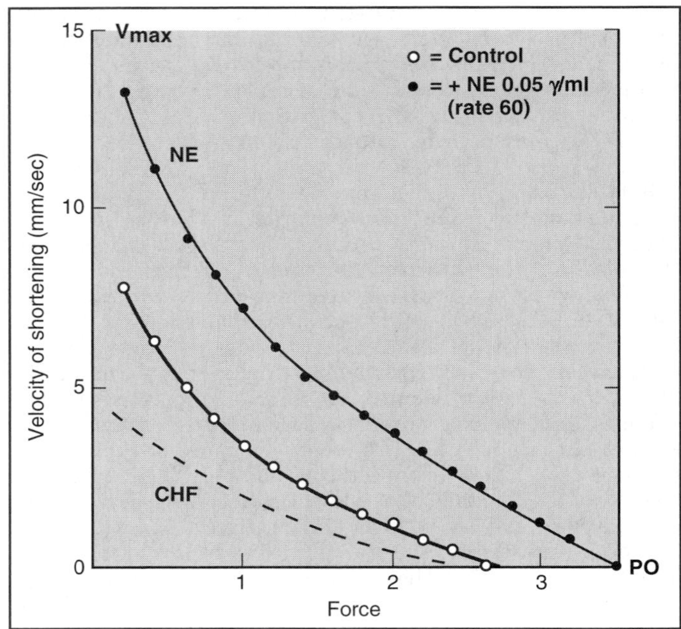

FIGURE 12–30. Effects of the addition of norepinephrine (NE) on the force-velocity relation of the cat papillary muscle. NE induces an increase in the velocity of shortening at any load, in the force of isometric contraction (P_0) and in the maximum velocity of zero-load shortening (V_{max}). The dashed line adds hypothetical data from congestive heart failure (CHF). (Modified from Braunwald, E., Sonnenblick, E. H., and Ross, J.: Normal and abnormal circulatory function. *In* Braunwald, E. (ed.): Heart Disease: A Textbook of Cardiovascular Medicine. 4th ed. Philadelphia, W. B. Saunders Company, 1992, pp. 351–392.)

The concept of V_{max} has been subject to much debate over many years, chiefly because of the technical difficulties in obtaining truly unloaded conditions. Braunwald et al.[168] used cat papillary muscle to define a hyperbolic force-velocity curve, with V_{max} relatively independent of the initial muscle length, but increased by the addition of norepinephrine (Fig. 12–30).

Another preparation used to examine force-velocity relations uses single cardiac myocytes isolated by enzymatic digestion of the rat myocardium and then permeabilized with a staphylococcal toxin. Again, the force-velocity relation is hyperbolic, suggesting the existence of intracellular *passive elastic elements* that contribute to the load on the isolated myocyte.[169] In fact, the more hyperbolic and increased curvilinear nature of the force-velocity relationship in isolated myocytes than in the papillary muscle suggests that internal passive forces such as those generated by titin (Fig. 12–4) are greater than expected in the isolated myocytes. In the intact heart, the noncontractile components contribute relatively little to overall mechanical behavior, at least in physiological circumstances.[170]

Do similar relations hold at the level of the sarcomere? Ter Keurs[171] carefully measured the velocity of shortening of the central sarcomeres in a maximally unloaded muscle and found that V_{max} was the same at sarcomere lengths between 1.85 and 2.35 microns, although decreasing at shorter lengths to become zero at 1.6 microns. Thus, it seems as if V_{max} is truly length-independent at the longer and more physiological sarcomere lengths. Both the work on papillary muscle and that on sarcomeres suggest that in unloaded conditions the intrinsic contractility as assessed by V_{max} does not change with initial fiber or sarcomere length.

MECHANISM OF BETA-ADRENERGIC EFFECTS ON FORCE-VELOCITY RELATIONSHIP. The data on papillary muscles showing that norepinephrine can increase V_{max} could be explained by either an effect of beta-adrenergic stimulation on enhancing calcium ion entry or a direct effect on the contractile proteins, or both. Strang et al.[172] showed that either isoproterenol (beta-stimulant) or protein kinase A (intracellular messenger) increased V_{max} by about 40 per cent, concurrently with phosphorylation of troponin-I and C protein in an isolated ventricular myocyte preparation. Hypothetically, such phosphorylations increase the rate of crossbridge cycling, possibly by promoting release of ADP from myosin, or else by increasing myosin ATPase activity.[169] In contrast, de Tombe and ter Keurs[173] emphasize the dominant role of calcium ion entry, because they could find the expected increase V_{max} with beta-stimulation only when the external calcium ion concentration of their preparation was suboptimal.

The overall concept is that beta-adrenergic stimulation mediates the major component of its inotropic effect through increasing the cytosolic calcium transient and the factors controlling it, such as the rate of entry of calcium ions through the sarcolemmal L-type channels, the rate of calcium uptake under the influence of phospholamban into the SR, and the rate of calcium release from the ryanodine receptor in response to calcium entry in association with depolarization. Of all these factors, phosphorylation of phospholamban may be most important (see p. 368).

ISOMETRIC VERSUS ISOTONIC CONTRACTION. Despite the similarities in the force-velocity patterns between the data obtained on papillary muscle and isolated myocytes, it should be considered that a number of different types of muscular contraction may be involved. For example, data for P_0 are obtained under isometric conditions (length unchanged). When muscle is allowed to shorten against a steady load, the conditions are *isotonic* (*iso* = same; *tonic* = contractile force). Yet measurements of V_{max} have to be under totally unloaded conditions, both in the papillary muscles and in permeabilized myocytes.[167] Thus, the force-velocity curve may be a combination of initial isometric conditions followed by isotonic contraction and then may follow abrupt and total unloading to measure V_{max}. Although isometric conditions can be found in the whole heart as an approximation during isovolumic contraction, isotonic conditions cannot prevail because the load is constantly changing during the ejection period, and complete unloading is impossible. Therefore, the application of force-velocity relations to the heart in vivo is limited.

PRESSURE-VOLUME LOOPS. Accordingly, measurements of pressure-volume loops are among the best of the current approaches to the assessment of the contractile behavior of the intact heart (Figs. 14–1 and 14–2, p. 422). Major criticisms arise when it is assumed that the slope of the pressure-volume relationship (E_S) is necessarily linear (it may be curvilinear[174]) or when E_S is used as an index of "absolute" contractility (for E_S, see Fig. 12–31). Also in clinical practice, the need to change the loading conditions and the requirement for invasive monitoring lessen the usefulness of this index.[175] Invasive measurements of the LV pressure are required for the full loop, which is an indirect measure of the Starling relationship between the force (as measured by the pressure) and the muscle length (measured indirectly by volume). Measuring LV volume adequately and continuously throughout the cardiac cycle is not easy.

During a positive inotropic intervention, the pressure-volume loop reflects a smaller end-systolic volume and a higher end-systolic pressure, so that E_s has moved upward and to the left (Fig. 12–31). When the positive inotropic intervention is by beta-adrenergic stimulation, then enhanced relaxation (lusitropic effect) results in a lower pressure-volume curve during ventricular filling than in controls.

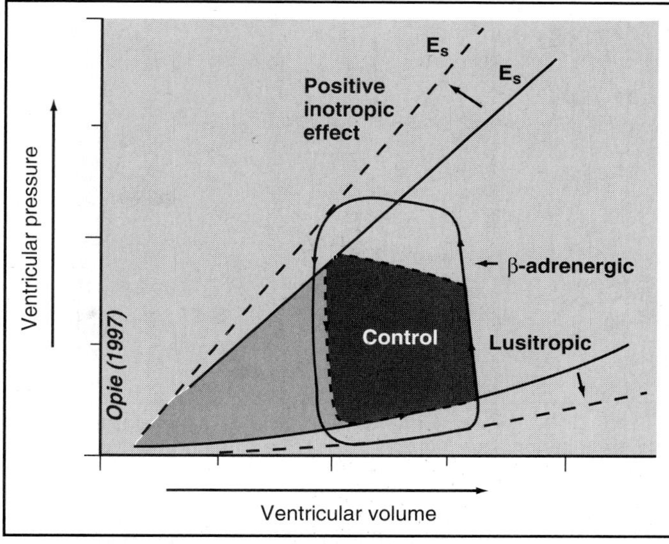

FIGURE 12–31. Note the effects of beta-adrenergic catecholamines with both positive inotropic (increased slope of line E_s) and increased lusitropic (relaxant) effects. E_s = Slope of pressure-volume relationship. The total pressure-volume area (sum of slashed and dotted areas for control) is closely related to the myocardial oxygen uptake.[151] (Reprinted with permission. Copyright ©1997 L. H. Opie.)

Ventricular Relaxation and Diastolic Dysfunction

(See also p. 402)

Among the many complex cellular factors influencing relaxation, four are of chief interest. First, the cytosolic calcium level must fall to cause the relaxation phase, a process requiring ATP and phosphorylation of phospholamban for uptake of calcium into the SR. Second, the inherent viscoelastic properties of the myocardium are important. In the hypertrophied heart, relaxation occurs more slowly. Third, increased phosphorylation of troponin-I enhances the rate of relaxation.[9] Fourth, relaxation is influenced by the systolic load. The history of contraction affects crossbridge relaxation.[176,177] Within limits, the greater the systolic load, the faster the rate of relaxation.

This complex relationship has been explored in detail by Brutsaert and Sys[178] and Brutsaert et al.[179] but could perhaps be simplified as follows. When the workload is high, peak cytosolic calcium is also thought to be high. A high end-systolic cytosolic calcium means that the rate of fall of calcium also can be greater, provided that the uptake mechanisms are functioning effectively. In this way a systolic pressure load and the rate of diastolic relaxation can be related. Furthermore, a greater muscle length (when the workload is high) at the end of systole should produce a more rapid rate of relaxation by the opposite of length-dependent sensitization, so that there is a more marked response to the rate of decline of calcium in early diastole. Yet, when the systolic load exceeds a certain limit, the rate of relaxation is delayed,[177] perhaps because of too great a mechanical stress on the individual crossbridges. Thus, in congestive heart failure caused by an excess systolic load, relaxation becomes increasingly afterload-dependent, so that therapeutic reduction of the systolic load should improve LV relaxation.[180]

IMPAIRED RELAXATION AND CYTOSOLIC CALCIUM. Hemodynamically, diastole can be divided into four phases (Fig. 12–32). For these purposes, this chapter has used the clincial definition of diastole according to which diastole extends from aortic valve closure to the start of the first heart sound. The first phase of diastole is the isovolumic phase, which, by definition, does not contribute to ventricular filling. The second phase of rapid filling provides most of

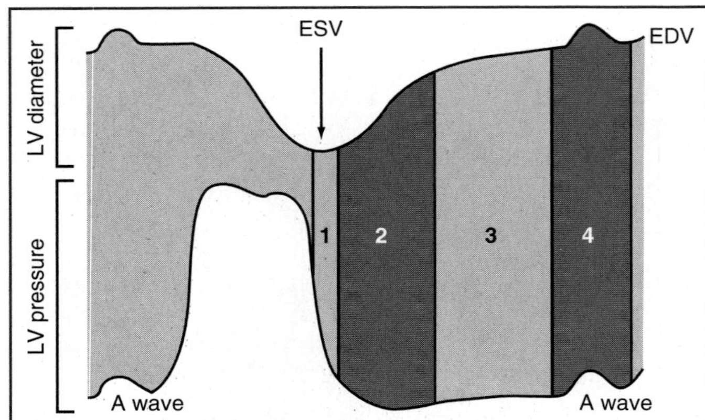

FIGURE 12–32. Phases of left ventricular (LV) diastole. 1, Isovolumic relaxation period, from aortic valve closure to mitral valve opening. 2, Rapid filling period, from mitral valve opening to onset of plateau (diastasis) of LV volume curve. 3, Diastasis, from onset of plateau on volume curve to atrial systole. 4, Atrial systole with end-diastolic volume. Arrow, end-systolic volume. (Modified from Harizi, R. C., Bianco, J. A., and Alpert, J. S.: Diastolic function of the heart in clinical cardiology. Arch. Intern. Med. *148:*99–109, 1988.) For A wave, see Figure 12–22. For further details, see Figure 14–22.

ventricular filling. The third phase of slow filling or diastasis accounts for only 5 per cent of the total filling. The final atrial booster phase accounts for the remaining 15 per cent. The first phase of isovolumic relaxation is energy-dependent.

ISOVOLUMIC RELAXATION. This phase of the cardiac cycle is energy-dependent, requiring ATP for the uptake of calcium ions by the SR (Fig. 12–33) which is an active, not a passive, process. Impaired relaxation is an early event in angina pectoris. A proposed metabolic explanation is that there is impaired generation of energy, which diminishes the supply of ATP required for the early diastolic uptake of calcium by the SR. The result is that the cytosolic calcium level, at a peak in systole, delays its return to normal in the early diastolic period. In other conditions, too, there is a relationship between the rate of diastolic decay of the calcium transient and diastolic relaxation, with a relation to impaired function of the SR.[181] When the rate of relaxation is prolonged by hypothyroidism, the rate of return of the systolic calcium elevation is likewised delayed, whereas opposite changes occur in hyperthyroidism.[182] In congestive heart failure, diastolic relaxation also is delayed and irregular, as is the rate of decay of the cytosolic calcium elevation.[182] Most patients with coronary artery disease have a variety of abnormalities of diastolic filling, probably related to those also found in angina pectoris. Theoretically, such abnormalities of relaxation are potentially reversible because they depend on changes in patterns of calcium ion movement. Indices of the isovolumic phase and other indices of diastolic function are shown in Table 12–5. Of interest is the echocardiographic determination in patients with regurgitant valve disease of $-dP/dt_{max}$[183] and of *tau*, the time constant of relaxation.[184]

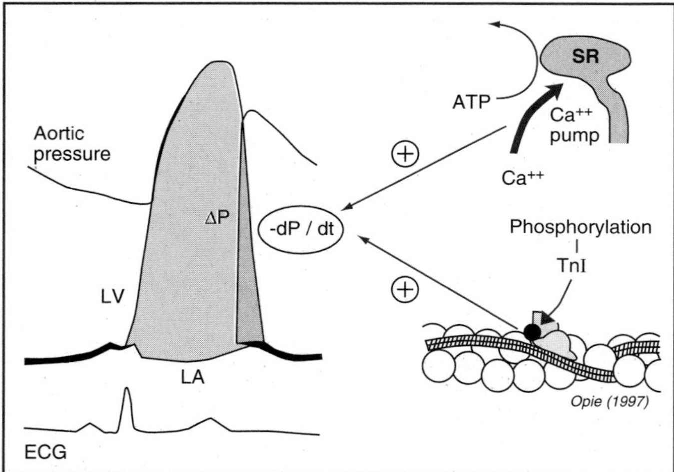

FIGURE 12–33. Factors governing the isovolumic relaxation phase of the cardiac cycle (see Fig. 12–32). This period of the cycle extends from the aortic second sound (A_2) (Fig. 12–22) to the crossover point between the left ventricular and left atrial pressures. The maximum negative rate of pressure development ($-dP/dt_{max}$), which gives the isovolumic relaxation rate, is measured either invasively or by a continuous wave Doppler velocity spectrum in aortic regurgitation.[183] Isovolumic relaxation is increased (+ sign) when the rate of calcium uptake into the sarcoplasmic reticulum (SR) is enhanced, for example during beta-adrenergic stimulation (Fig. 12–18). Isovolumic relaxation is also enhanced when phosphorylation of troponin I (TnI), as in response to beta-adrenergic stimulation, decreases the affinity of the contractile system for calcium. Copyright ©1997 L. H. Opie.)

DOES THE LEFT VENTRICLE "SUCK" DURING EARLY FILLING? Whether the LV suction by active relaxation could increase the pressure gradient from left atrium to LV during the early filling phase remains controversial, although well supported by the data. An LV suction effect can be found by carefully comparing LV and left atrial pressures, and it occurs especially in the early diastolic phase of rapid filling. The sucking effect may be of most importance in mitral stenosis, when the mitral valve does not open as it otherwise should in response to diastolic suction. During catecholamine stimulation, the rate of relaxation may increase to enhance the sucking effect[185] and to prolong the period of filling. The proposed mechanism of sucking is as follows.[186] When the end-systolic volume is less than the equilibrium volume, the shortened muscle fibers and collagen matrix may act as a compressed spring, to generate recoil forces in diastole.

ATRIAL FUNCTION. The left atrium, besides its well-known function as a blood-receiving chamber, also acts as follows: First, by presystolic contraction and its booster function, it helps to complete LV filling.[187] Second, it is the volume sensor of the heart, releasing atrial natriuretic peptide (ANP) in response to intermittent stretch and several other stimuli, including angiotensin II[188] and endothelin.[189] Third, the atrium contains receptors for the afferent arms of various reflexes, including mechanoreceptors that increase sinus discharge rate, thereby contributing to the tachycardia of exercise as the venous return increases (Bainbridge reflex).

The atria have a number of differences in structure and function from the ventricles, having smaller myocytes with a shorter action potential duration as well as a more fetal type of myosin (both in heavy and light chains). Furthermore, the atria are more reliant on the phosphatidylinositol signal transduction pathway,[190] which may explain the relatively greater positive inotropic effect in the atria than in

TABLE 12–5 SOME INDICES OF DIASTOLIC FUNCTION

ISOVOLUMIC RELAXATION
(−) dP/dt_{max} (Fig. 12–33)
Aortic closing–mitral opening interval
Peak rate of LV wall thinning
Time constant of relaxation, *tau**
EARLY DIASTOLIC FILLING
Relaxation kinetics on ERNA (rate of volume increase)
Early filling phase (E phase) on Doppler transmitral velocity trace
DIASTASIS
Pressure-volume relation indicates compliance
ATRIAL CONTRACTION
Invasive measurement of atrial and ventricular pressures
Doppler transmitral pattern (E to A ratio)

* For noninvasive measurements by continuous-wave Doppler velocity profile in mitral regurgitation, see Chen et al.[184]
ERNA = Equilibrated radionuclide angiography

the ventricles in response to angiotensin II.[191] The more rapid atrial repolarization is thought to be due to increased outward potassium currents, such as I_{to} and I_{kACh}.[192,193] In addition, some atrial cells have the capacity for spontaneous depolarization.[194] In general, these histological and physiological changes can be related to the decreased need for the atria to generate high intrachamber pressures, rather than being sensitive to volume changes, while retaining enough contractile action to help with LV filling and to respond to inotropic stimuli.[187]

MEASUREMENT OF DIASTOLIC FUNCTION (see also p. 434). The rate of isovolumic relaxation can be measured by negative dP/dt_{max} at invasive catheterization. *Tau*, the time constant of relaxation, describes the rate of fall of LV pressure during isovolumic relaxation and also requires invasive techniques for precise determination.[184] *Tau* is increased as the systolic LV pressure rises.[177] Another index of relaxation can be obtained echocardiographically from the peak rate of wall thinning.[195] The isovolumic relaxation time lies between aortic valve closure and mitral valve opening measured by signals of valve movements taken by Doppler echocardiography.[196] In mitral regurgitation, the Doppler velocity profile can be used to calculate *tau*.[184] In each case, precise measurement is difficult, and the range of normality is large.

DIASTOLIC DYSFUNCTION IN HYPERTROPHIC MYOCARDIUM. In hypertrophic hearts, as in chronic hypertension or severe aortic stenosis,[197] abnormalities of diastole are common and may precede systolic failure. The mechanism is not clear, although it is thought to be related to the extent of ventricular hypertrophy or indirectly to a stiff left atrium.[198] Conceptually, impaired relaxation must be distinguished from prolonged systolic contraction with delayed onset of normal relaxation.[179] Experimentally, there are several defects in early hypertensive hypertrophy, including decreased rates of contraction and relaxation, and decreased peak force development.[181] Of specific interest is the concept that the loss of the load-sensitive component of relaxation is due to impaired activity of the SR. Impaired relaxation is associated with an increase of the late (atrial) filling phase, so that E/A ratio on the mitral Doppler pattern declines. In time, with both increased hypertrophy and the development of fibrosis, chamber compliance decreases (Fig. 14–20, p. 435). Such multiple abnormalities are difficult to detect in the transmitral flow pattern (Fig. 14–23, p. 437).

Vascular Compliance

Because vascular compliance is one of the two major factors influencing the afterload (the other being arterial blood pressure), increasing attention is being paid to its changes in disease states and during drug therapy. For example, severe hypertension decreases arterial compliance while nitrates increase large arterial diameter, thereby showing that compliance has increased.[199] Some workers distinguish between the distensibility of the arteries, taken as a measure of the elastic properties, and the compliance, a measure of the buffering capacity.[199]

Aortic-Ventricular Coupling

The interaction between physical properties of the arterial tree and the mechanical function of the left ventricle is influenced by numerous factors, including distensibility of the ascending aorta.[200] The latter can be measured noninvasively by the change in aortic diameter in relation to the pulse pressure using echocardiography[200] or magnetic resonance imaging.[201]

From the conceptual point of view, the aorta functions as a Windkessel, i.e., as a pressure chamber, which provides compliance to act as a buffer.[202] If aortic pressure oscillations can be measured, then aortic flow can be calculated and hence the cardiac output measured noninvasively. In practice, models and extrapolations from the radial pulse pressure patterns can be used to estimate aortic pressure pulsations.[202]

Ventricular Interaction

Thus far, LV function has been discussed as if the left ventricle were working in isolation. In reality, its function is intimately linked to that of the right ventricle, both functionally and anatomically. The cardiac output of the left ventricle must equal that of the right ventricle unless there is a state of imbalance, as in conditions of acute LV failure when blood may accumulate in the lungs to cause pulmonary edema. In general, the right ventricle is working against a low resistance circuit, and afterload is not a major problem in physiological conditions. What the right ventricle receives by means of its filling pressure in the venous system, it empties in response to the Starling effect. The amount of pressure work generated by the right ventricle is relatively low, which explains the thinner right ventricular wall and the dominance of LV function in calculations of pressure work or of myocardial oxygen uptake.

Anatomically, the two ventricles are interlinked. They share a common septum. That septum constitutes part of the load against which each ventricle must work. In LV hypertrophy, which includes the septum, the right ventricle must, therefore, work harder and tends to become hypertrophied. This is *systolic ventricular interaction*. One type of diastolic ventricular interaction is the *Bernheim effect*, whereby a large left ventricle compresses the right ventricle, the volume on the left side being so great that the right side is unable to fill properly. A converse ventricular interaction can occur in severe heart failure, when the dilated right ventricle may impinge on the left. When the right ventricle is unloaded by the venodilator agent nitroglycerin, it can decrease in size and allow the LV function to improve. Similarly, following surgical thromboendarterectomy for chronic thromboembolic pulmonary hypertension, LV diastolic function improved as the interventricular septum changed position.[203]

When there is a physical impairment of the mechanical function of one ventricle on the other as a result of volume overloading with blood, the result is *diastolic ventricular interference*.[204]

Pericardium

(See also Chap. 43)

The normal pericardium has an important restraining effect on the diastolic properties of the ventricles, especially the right ventricle.[205] Without the pericardium, the right ventricle would dilate by about 40 per cent and the right atrium by about 70 per cent. Therefore, the physical properties of the pericardium help to determine ventricular pressure-volume relations and, indirectly, the compliance. Normally LV diastolic pressure is greater than that in the other chambers by the amount of its transmural pressure (5 to 10 mm Hg), the low pericardial pressure being equally applied to all chambers. During pericardial disease with cardiac tamponade, the pressure within the pericardial cavity rises as the volume increases, especially with a volume above 200 ml,[206] so that the intrapericardial pressure equals or exceeds the normal diastolic filling pressure. When this happens, diastole is interrupted and ventricular diastolic collapse can be seen on echocardiography.[207]

Endocardium

The vascular and endocardial endothelium constitute "one continuous sheet of tissue."[208] A current proposal is that there is intracavity autoregulation by endocardial endothelial cells. Release of an endothelin-like agent, endocardin, from the stretched endocardium could, it is proposed, increase the duration of contraction.[209] The dilated failing left ventricle could thereby generate an autoregulating inotropic stimulus. Yet there is thought to be a defect in the endocardial endothelium in heart failure causing, for example, a decreased response to alpha$_2$-adrenergic inotropic stimulation.[208] What is thus far not explained is how, if the properties of endocardin resemble those of endothelin, a preferential positive inotropic effect rather than vasoconstriction could be achieved unless endocardin preferentially stimulates adjacent endocardial papillary muscle cells.

EFFECTS OF ISCHEMIA AND REPERFUSION ON CONTRACTION AND RELAXATION

Contractile Impairment in Ischemia

(See p. 1162)

Despite experimental differences, there is now widespread agreement that early contractile failure (Fig. 12–34) can occur even when *calcium transients* are normal or near normal,[212–214] and, therefore, a metabolic cause must be sought. The latter could be either decreased sensitivity of the contractile proteins to calcium, as for example caused by acidosis, or inhibition of the crossbridge cycle, as for example from the early rise in inorganic phosphate. As creatine phosphate falls, the activity of the creatine phosphate shuttle decreases so that "local" ATP, required for calcium movements in the contractile cycle, falls.[215] In addition, the free energy of hydrolysis of ATP decreases during ischemia.[216,216a] The large increase in P_i, as a result of creatine phosphate breakdown, decreases free energy of hydrolysis, as do the smaller decreases in ATP and increases in ADP. Creatine phosphate fall can also indirectly inhibit contractility by accumulation of inorganic phosphate, which decreases the contractile effects of any given cytosolic calcium level.[217] Inorganic phosphate may act by promotion of formation of weak rather than strong crossbridges.

Accumulation of neutral lactate can promote mitochondrial damage, decrease the action potential duration, and inhibit glyceraldehyde-3-phosphate dehydrogenase.[218] The mechanism of these lactate effects is not clarified and may include extracellular acidosis with Na^+/H^+ exchange, a subsequent gain in cell Na^+, and then Na^+/Ca^{++} exchange with gain of harmful Ca^{++}.[219]

Potassium Efflux. The mechanism of early potassium efflux in ischemia is not well understood, and there are three major theories. First, the ATP-inhibited potassium channel (K_{ATP}) may open as a result of cytosolic ATP deficiency (Fig. 12–35).[220] Not all potassium loss can be blocked by sulfonylureas,[221] so that other potassium channels such as those activated by sodium or by fatty acids may play a role. Second, inhibition of the sodium-potassium pump has long been suspected, but the onset of such inhibition is probably too late to explain early potassium egress, although probably contributing to the later phase of potassium loss. Third, co-ionic loss of potassium with negatively charged lactate and phosphate ions has often been proposed, but the evidence is scanty.[222] For example, inhibition of lactate transport by alpha-cyanohydroxycinnamic acid does not change extracellular potassium accumulation in ischemia.[220] The importance of potassium loss is that because the action potential duration is shortened, calcium influx may be diminished.[28]

Adenosine. This substance is formed during ischemia from the breakdown of ATP. It is potentially recyclable as a building block of ATP during resynthesis. Besides being the probable origin of the ischemic anginal pain,[223] adenosine has complex cardioprotective qualities. In response to stimulation of the A_1-receptor,[115] adenosine increases the inhibitory G protein G_i, which, in turn, lessens the activity of adenylate cyclase and increases the opening probability of two types of potassium channels. The consequences include negative inotropic, chronotropic, and dromotropic effects, as well as coronary vasodilation. Adenosine may also play an important role in preconditioning.[224]

SUPPLY VERSUS DEMAND ISCHEMIA. Apstein and Grossman[225] proposed that ischemia has different effects on the systolic and diastolic properties of the left ventricle, depending on how ischemia is produced. In *supply ischemia*, with a decreased oxygen supply as the dominant metabolic change, there is an early increase in diastolic distensibility (compliance increases, ischemic area bulges). The proposed mechanism is lack of washout of ischemic metabolites that impair the interaction of the increased cytosolic calcium with the myofilaments. In contrast, when *demand ischemia* is precipitated, for example by rapid atrial pacing in the presence of experimental coronary stenosis, the diastolic distensibility acutely decreases, so that there is stiffening and the failure of the ischemic tissue to relax, with a rise in LV end-diastolic pressure. The proposed metabolic explanation is that intracellular calcium is thought to increase without a significant acidosis so that ischemia-induced loss of compliance takes place and the myocardium stiffens.

In reality, these distinctions between supply and demand ischemia are not absolute. The real differences may lie more in the severity of ischemia than in the mode of its

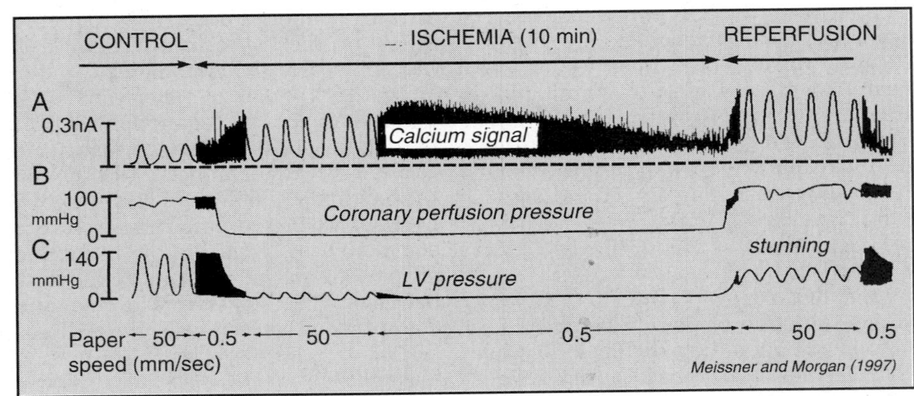

FIGURE 12–34. Can LV mechanical failure during severe ischemia be explained by changes in the cytosolic calcium? These data show that when there is abrupt ischemic LV failure (LV pressure falls to zero in *C*), the calcium signal *(A)* increases before it falls. Ischemia is designated by the abrupt fall of coronary perfusion pressure to zero in this isolated rat heart preparation. During reperfusion there is also a dissociation between the cytosolic calcium oscillations, which are augmented (righthand panel of A) in contrast to LV contraction which is decreased (righthand aspect of bottom panel), so that there is mechanical stunning. It is thought that excess calcium oscillations damage the contractile proteins (Fig. 12–38). (From Meissner, A., and Morgan, J. P.: Contractile dysfunction and abnormal Ca^{2+} modulation during postischemic reperfusion in rat heart. Am. J. Physiol. *268:*H100–H111, 1995.)

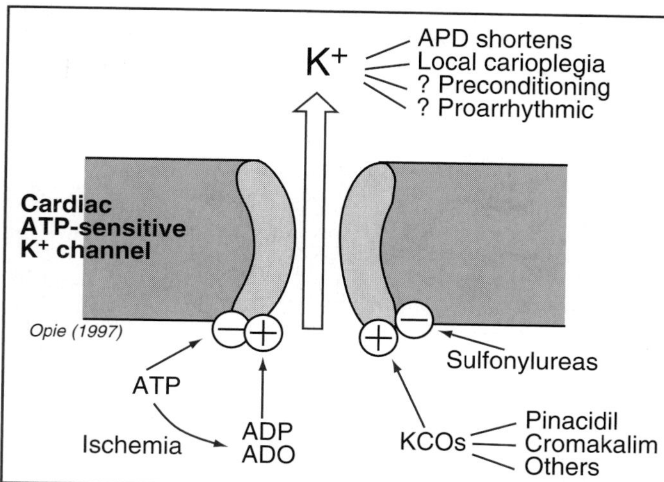

FIGURE 12–35. Proposed role of ATP-sensitive potassium channel in promotion of potassium loss in early ischemia. As ATP decreases and breaks down in ischemia to ADP and adenosine (ADO), the probability is greater that this potassium channel is open. The consequences include shortening of the action potential duration (APD), low cardioplegia, and possibly preconditioning and proarrhythmic effects. The potassium channel openers (KCOs) act on a site integral to the channel pore to promote the probability of channel opening, whereas the sulfonylureas act on a site not integral to the pore, to inhibit the potassium channel opening. For further details, see Edwards and Weston.[265] (Reprinted with permission. Copyright ©1997 L. H. Opie.)

production.[226] Thus, balloon occlusion in angioplasty is more likely to produce severe ischemia and increased distensibility than is pacing ischemia in the same patient.[227,228]

ISCHEMIC CONTRACTURE. After 5 to 20 minutes of severe ischemia, but depending on variable metabolic circumstances, including the cardiac glycogen reserve,[229] there is the gradual onset of ischemic contracture with a rise in diastolic pressure virtually without systolic activity. In general, even complete reperfusion never fully relieves ischemic contracture. The mechanisms for contracture include ATP depletion and a rise in cytosolic calcium (Fig. 12–36). Of interest is the proposal that continued glycolysis and production of glycolytic ATP have roles in the maintenance of intracellular calcium homeostasis, probably acting indirectly by maintaining activity of the sodium pump.[230] As glycolysis is inhibited, diastolic tension increases.[231]

INTERMITTENT ISCHEMIA AND PRECONDITIONING. Whereas many repetitive episodes of ischemia should produce cumulative damage, relatively few episodes or even one burst of short-lived severe ischemia followed by complete reperfusion causes preconditioning. The latter is a condition in which the myocardium is protected against a greater subsequent ischemic insult, with less threat of infarction.[232,233] The mechanism of the protective effect of preconditioning is still speculative. Of note is the important proposal that G_i is upregulated (Fig. 12–37) so that activation of receptors coupled to it, such as adenosine A_1- and muscarinic M_2-receptors, leads to greater inhibition of adenylate cyclase and hence to an indirect antiadrenergic effect.[234–236] In addition, G_i may mediate other potentially protective mechanisms, such as direct inhibition of L-calcium channels and activation of the ATP-sensitive potassium channels in the ventricles.[224] An alternate hypothesis is that adenosine formed during the preconditioning ischemic period activates protein kinase C, which mediates the subsequent protection by an unknown mechanism (Fig. 12–20).[110,237]

Preconditioning is an important phenomenon, probably with clinical implications, because repetitive anginal episodes in patients may develop into full-fledged infarction. Patients with preinfarction angina may suffer from a less

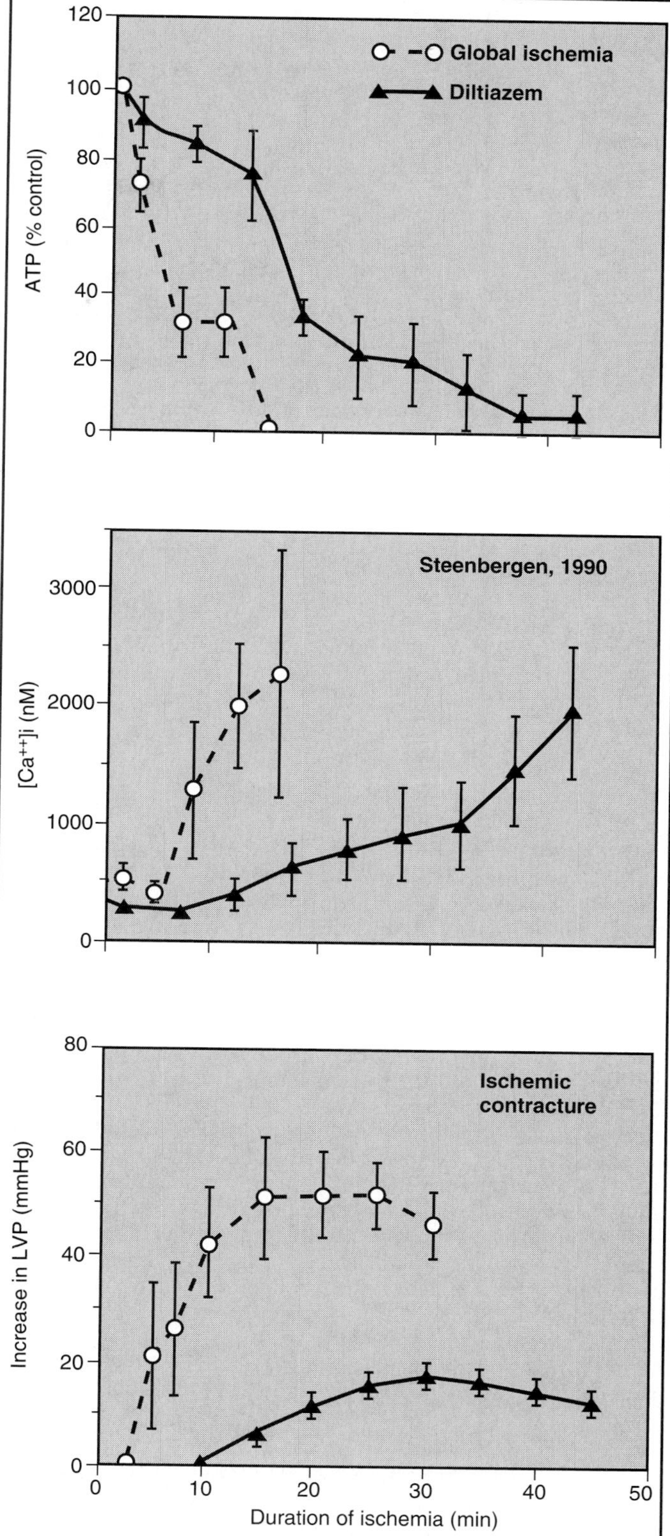

FIGURE 12–36. Ischemic contracture in isolated rat hearts under control conditions and in the presence of diltiazem (0.9 μm). In control hearts, note rapid fall of ATP followed by rise of internal Ca^{++} at time of onset of ischemic contracture. Diltiazem (and K^+ cardioplegia, not shown) reduced the rate of fall of ATP and delayed the onset of rise in $[Ca^{++}]_i$ and in ischemic contracture. Preservation of ATP and in particular glycolytically generated ATP delays ischemic contracture. (Data from Figures 2 and 7 of Steenbergen, C., et al.: Correlation between cytosolic free calcium, contracture, ATP, and irreversible ischemic injury in perfused rat heart. Circ. Res. *66*:135–146, 1990. Copyright 1990 American Heart Association.)

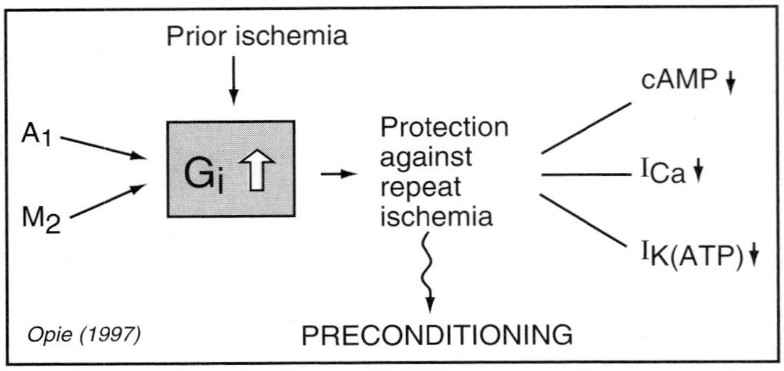

Prior ischemia

A1 → Gi ⇧ ← M2 → Protection against repeat ischemia → cAMP↓, ICa↓, IK(ATP)↓

PRECONDITIONING

Opie (1997)

FIGURE 12–37. Proposed role of inhibitory G protein, G_i, in mediating effects of preconditioning.[234] The proposal is that prior ischemia (preconditioning episode) upregulates G_i according to Niroomand et al.[236] G_i, by inhibiting formation of cyclic AMP, lessens L-type calcium channel activity and promotes opening of the ATP-dependent K^+ channel. Thus, when ischemia is repeated, there is relative protection. A_1 = Subtype 1 of adenosine receptor; M_2 = subtype 2 of muscarinic receptor; I_{Ca} = L-type calcium current; $I_{k(ATP)}$ = ATP-dependent potassium current. (Reprinted with permission. Copyright ©1997 L. H. Opie.)

severe infarct than those thought to undergo sudden coronary occlusion without the opportunity for preconditioning.[238,239] In contrast, patients with multiple short-lived attacks of ischemia might become tolerant to the development of protective preconditioning, according to animal data.[240]

Hibernating Heart

(See also pp. 89 and 1176)

The hibernating myocardium, like the hibernating animal, is temporarily asleep and can wake up to function normally when the blood supply is fully restored (Table 12–6). The proposal is that the fall of myocardial function to a lower level copes with the reduced myocardial oxygen supply and leads to self-preservation, the so-called smart heart.[241] However, a greater flow reduction should lead to true ischemia. When the myocardium is blood-perfused, the exact limit to hibernation is not so clearly defined but could be only about 70 to 80 per cent of normal coronary flow, judging from human data.[242] Hibernation is a complex clinical situation without a good animal model. When ischemia in patients is delineated echocardiographically as depressed regional wall motion, the hypocontractile segments that still have a sustained glucose extraction, as shown by positron emission tomography (PET), have a high chance of recovery after coronary artery bypass surgery. In contrast, those segments with a decreased glucose extraction almost uniformly fail to recover.[243]

An alternative point of view, gaining ground, is that hibernation can occur even when the resting coronary flow is normal despite the presence of coronary disease. The proposed mechanism is that recurrent episodes of ischemia leave behind stunned myocardium, so that hibernation is the sum of repetitive and cumulative stunning.[244,245]

Stunning

(See also pp. 89 and 1176)

The first observation was that the recovery of mechanical function following transient coronary occlusion was not instant but delayed.[246] Thereafter, Braunwald and Kloner[247] defined the "stunned myocardium" as one characterized by prolonged postischemic myocardial dysfunction with eventual return of normal contractile activity. In addition, the "diagnosis of reversible impairment of contractility requires simultaneous measurements of regional myocardial function and flow."[248] Thus, either coronary angiography or some other measurement of flow, such as PET, would need to be performed. In practice, myocardial stunning is often inferred from circumstantial evidence. By such criteria, stunning is thought to occur in several clinical situations, including delayed recovery from effort angina, unstable angina, after thrombolytic reperfusion, and following ischemic cardioplegia. The two chief explanations for stunning are an increased cytosolic calcium[249–251] and formation of free radicals upon reperfusion.[248,252]

MECHANISM OF INCREASED CYTOSOLIC CALCIUM DURING EARLY REPERFUSION. In view of the excess cytosolic calcium found in prolonged severe ischemia,[214,253] the $[Ca^{++}]_i$ is high at the start of reperfusion. Thus, restoration of energy with reperfusion induces excess oscillations (Fig. 12–38). Second, opening of the voltage-sensitive calcium channels during early reperfusion may also be important.[254] The highly specific L-calcium channel antagonist, nisoldipine, when given only at the time of reperfusion, lessens stunning, as do the nonorganic ions, magnesium and manganese.[254] Third, release of calcium from the SR is also likely,[255,256] probably in response to free radicals.[257,258] Fourth, considerable evidence indicates that calcium may enter the reperfused cells via the process of Na^+/Ca^{++} exchange, consequent on Na^+/H^+ exchange.[254,259] Fifth, it may be predicted that all agents stimulating the phosphatidylinositol cycle and increasing inositol trisphosphate[103] at the time of reperfusion should worsen stunning. These would include angiotensin II, endothelin,[260] and alpha$_1$-adrenergic stimulation.[261] Increased calcium transients may also explain reperfusion arrhythmias.[103,251,262] Decreased systolic force generation may be linked to a calcium-induced abnormality in the thin filaments.[251]

CHRONIC STUNNING. Although experimental stunning typically lasts for hours, full mechanical recovery can sometimes take much longer. Full recovery from thrombolytic reperfusion in patients with acute myocardial infarction may be delayed over weeks. To explain this finding, a current proposal is that there is a condition of late or chronic stunning,[263] hypothetically the end-result changes

TABLE 12–6 CHARACTERISTICS OF STUNNING, HIBERNATION, AND ISCHEMIA

PARAMETER	STUNNING	HIBERNATION	TRUE ISCHEMIA
Myocardial function	Reduced	Reduced	Reduced
Coronary blood flow	Normal/high	Modestly reduced	Most severely reduced
Myocardial energy metabolism	Normal or excessive	Reduced; in steady state	Reduced; increasingly severe as ischemia proceeds
Duration	Hours to days	Days to hours to months	Minutes to hours
Outcome	Full recovery	Recovery if blood flow restored	Infarction if severe ischemia persists
Proposed change in metabolic regulation of calcium	Cytosolic overload of calcium in early reperfusion	Possibly just enough glycolytic ATP to prevent contracture	Insufficient glycolytic ATP to prevent ischemic contracture and irreversibility

Modified from Opie, L. H.: Stunning, Hibernation and Calcium in Myocardial Ischemia and Reperfusion. Norwell, MA, Kluwer Academic Publishers, 1992.

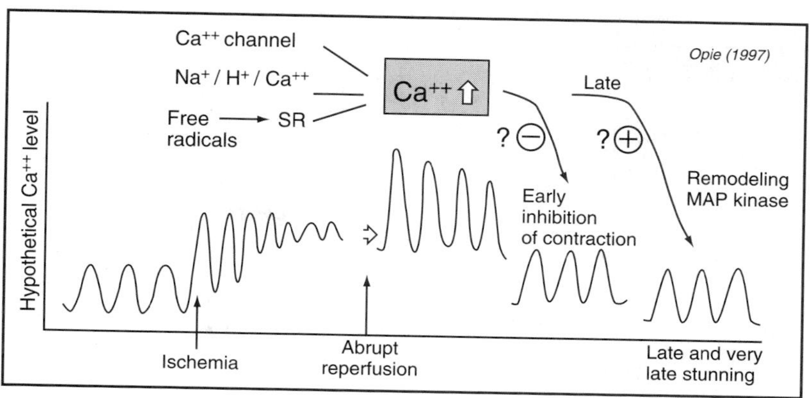

FIGURE 12–38. Proposed role of increased cytosolic calcium in causing early stunning after reperfusion and in hypothetically playing a role in late remodeling by stimulation of protein synthesis, possibly at the level of MAP kinase (mitogen-actived protein kinase). $Na^+/H^+/Ca^{++}$ = Sodium/proton and sodium/calcium exchange mechanisms; SR = sarcoplasmic reticulum. (Reprinted with permission. Copyright ©1997 L. H. Opie.)

in cytosolic calcium, perhaps acting as a trigger to complex changes in protein synthesis and degradation.[264] Chronic stunning may be the explanation for some aspects of hibernation. For example, repetitive ischemia precipitated by excitement in pigs with severe coronary stenosis can cause depressed mechanical function even in the absence of any measurable reduction of coronary blood flow at rest.[245]

REFERENCES

MICROANATOMY OF CONTRACTILE PROTEINS

1. Brilla, C. G., Janicki, J. S., and Weber, K. T.: Impaired diastolic function and coronary reserve in genetic hypertension. Role of interstitial fibrosis and medial thickening of intramyocardial coronary arteries. Circ. Res. *69*:107–115, 1991.
2. Forbes, M. S., and Sperelakis, N.: Ultrastructure of mammalian cardiac muscle. *In* Sperelakis, N. (ed.): Physiology and Pathophysiology of the Heart. 3rd ed. Boston, Kluwer Academic Publishers, 1995, pp. 1–35.
3. Weber, K. T., Sun, Y., Tyagi, S. C., and Cleutjens, J. P. M.: Collagen network of the myocardium: Function, structural remodeling and regulatory mechanisms. J. Mol. Cell. Cardiol. *26*:279–292, 1994.
4. Wang, K., Ramirez-Mitchell, R., and Palter, D.: Titin is an extraordinarily long, flexible, and slender myofibrillar protein. Proc. Natl. Acad. Sci. *81*:3685–3689, 1984.
5. Hein, S., Scholz, D., Fujitani, N., et al.: Altered expression of titin and contractile proteins in failing human myocardium. J. Mol. Cell Cardiol. *26*:1291–1306, 1994.
6. Trombitas, K., Jin, J.-P., and Granzier, H.: The mechanically active domain of titin in cardiac muscle. Circ. Res. *77*:856–861, 1995.
7. Perry, S. V.: The regulation of contractile activity in muscle. Biochem. Soc. Trans. *7*:593–617, 1979.
8. Solaro, R. J., Wolska, B. M., and Westfall, M.: Regulatory proteins and diastolic relaxation. *In* Lorell, B. H., and Grossman, W. (eds.): Diastolic Relaxation of the Heart. Boston, Kluwer Academic Publishers, 1994, pp. 43–53.
9. Zhang, R., Zhao, J., Mandveno, A., and Potter, J. D.: Cardiac troponin-I phosphorylation increases the rate of cardiac muscle relaxation. Circ. Res. *76*:1028–1035, 1995.
10. Huxley, A. F.: Muscle structure and theories of contraction. Prog. Biophys. Chem. *7*:255–318, 1957.
11. Rayment, I., Holden, H. M., Whittaker, M., et al.: Structure of the actin-myosin complex and its implications for muscle contraction. Science *261*:58–65, 1993.
12. Fisher, A. J., Smith, C. A., Thoden, J., et al.: Structural studies of myosin: Nucleotide complexes: A revised model for the molecular basis of muscle contraction. Biophys. J. *68*:19s–28s, 1995.
13. Irving, M., Lombardi, V., Piazzesi, G., and Ferenczi, M. A.: Myosin head movements are synchronous with the elementary force-generating process in muscle. Nature *357*:156–158, 1992.
14. Solaro, R. J., Powers, F. M., Gao, L., and Gwathmey, J. K.: Control of myofilament activation in heart failure. Circulation *87*(Suppl VII): 38–43, 1993.
15. Watkins, H., McKenna, W. J., Thierfelder, L., et al.: Mutations in the genes for cardiac troponin-T and alpha-tropomyosin in hypertrophic cardiomyopathy. N. Engl. J. Med. *332*:1058–1064, 1995.
16. Morano, I., Ritter, O., Bonz, A., et al.: Myosin light chain–actin interaction regulates cardiac contractility. Circ. Res. *76*:720–725, 1995.
17. Gao, W. D., Backx, P. H., Azan-Backx, M., and Marban, E.: Myofilament Ca^{2+} sensitivity in intact versus skinned rat ventricular muscle. Circ. Res. *74*:408–415, 1994.
18. Wolff, M. R., McDonald, K. S., and Moss, R. L.: Rate of tension development in cardiac muscle varies with level of activator calcium. Circ. Res. *76*:154–160, 1995.
19. Hancock, W. O., Martyn, D. A., and Huntsman, L. L.: Ca^{2+} and segment length dependence of isometric force kinetics in intact ferret cardiac muscle. Circ. Res. *73*:603–611, 1993.
20. Brenner, B.: Effect of Ca^{2+} on crossbridge turnover kinetics in skinned rabbit psoas fibers. Proc. Natl. Acad. Sci. U.S.A. *85*:3265–3269, 1988.
21. Hofmann, P. A., and Fuchs, F.: Evidence for a force-dependent component of calcium binding to cardiac troponin-C. Am. J. Physiol. *253*:C541–C546, 1987.
22. Hannon, J. D., Martyn, D. A., and Gordon, A. M.: Effects of cycling and rigor crossbridges on the conformation of cardiac troponin-C. Circ. Res. *71*:984–991, 1992.
23. Fuchs, F.: Mechanical modulation of the Ca^{2+} regulatory protein complex in cardiac muscle. News Physiol. Sci. *10*:6–12, 1995.
24. Rüegg, J. C.: Towards a molecular understanding of contractility. Cardioscience *1*:163–167, 1990.
25. Marban, E., Rink, T. J., Tsien, R. W., and Tsien, R. Y.: Free calcium in heart muscle at rest and during contraction measured with Ca^{2+}-sensitive microelectrodes. Nature *286*:845–850, 1980.

CALCIUM ION FLUXES IN CARDIAC CONTRACTION-RELAXATION CYCLE

26. Gibbons, W. R., and Zygmunt, A. C.: Excitation-contraction coupling in heart. *In* Fozzard, H. A., et al. (eds.): The Heart and Cardiovascular System. 2nd ed. New York, Raven Press, 1992, pp. 1249–1279.
27. Fabiato, A.: Calcium-induced release of calcium from the cardiac sarcoplasmic reticulum. Am. J. Physiol. *245*:C1–C14, 1983.
28. Bouchard, R. A., Clark, R. B., and Giles, W. R.: Effects of action potential duration on excitation-contraction coupling in rat ventricular myocytes. Action potential voltage-clamp measurements. Circ. Res. *76*:790–801, 1995.
29. Kohmoto, O., Levi, A. J., and Bridge, J. H. B.: Relation between reverse sodium-calcium exchange and sarcoplasmic reticulum calcium release in guinea pig ventricular cells. Circ. Res. *74*:550–554, 1994.
30. Berridge, M. J.: Inositol trisphosphate and calcium signalling. Nature *361*:315–325, 1993.
31. Wier, W. G., Egan, T. M., Lopez-Lopez, J. R., and Balke, C. W.: Local control of excitation-contraction coupling in rat heart cells. J. Physiol. *474*:463–471, 1994.
32. Lytton, J., and MacLennan, D. H.: Sarcoplasmic reticulum. *In* Fozzard, H. A., et al. (eds.): The Heart and Cardiovascular System. 2nd ed. New York, Raven Press, 1992, pp. 1203–1222.
33. Sipido, K. R., Callewaert, G., and Carmeliet, E.: Inhibition and rapid recovery of Ca^{2+} current during Ca^{2+}-release from sarcoplasmic reticulum in guinea pig ventricular myocytes. Circ. Res. *76*:102–109, 1995.
34. Wagenknecht, T., Grassucci, R., Frank, J., et al.: Three-dimensional architecture of the calcium channel/foot structure of sarcoplasmic reticulum. Nature *338*:167–170, 1989.
35. Takeshima, H., Nishimura, S., Matsumoto, T., et al.: Primary structure and expression from complementary DNA of skeletal muscle ryanodine receptor. Nature *339*:439–445, 1989.
36. Wibo, M., Bravo, G., and Godraind, T.: Postnatal maturation of excitation-contraction coupling in rat ventricle in relation to the subcellular localization and surface density of 1,4-dihydropyridine and ryanodine receptors. Circ. Res. *68*:662–673, 1991.
37. Gilbert, J. C., Shirayama, T., and Pappano, A. J.: Inositol trisphosphate promotes Na-Ca exchange current by releasing calcium from sarcoplasmic reticulum in cardiac myocytes. Circ. Res. *69*:1632–1639, 1991.
38. Brown, J. H., and Martinson, E. A.: Phosphoinositide-generated second messengers in cardiac signal transduction. Trends Cardiovasc. Med. *2*:209–214, 1992.
39. Go, L. O., Moschella, M. C., Handa, K. K., et al.: Differential regulation of two types of intracellular calcium-release channels during end-stage human heart failure. Circulation *90*(Abs.):I-L, 1994.
40. Arai, M., Matsui, H., and Periasamy, M.: Sarcoplasmic reticulum gene expression in cardiac hypertrophy and heart failure. Circ. Res. *74*:555–564, 1994.
41. Luo, W., Grupp, I. L., Harrer, J., et al.: Targeted ablation of the phospholamban gene is associated with markedly enhanced myocardial contractility and loss of beta-agonist stimulation. Circ. Res. *75*:401–409, 1994.

42. Tada, M., and Katz, A. M.: Phosphorylation of the sarcoplasmic reticulum and sarcolemma. Ann. Rev. Physiol. *44*:401–423, 1982.
43. Gasser, J., Paganetti, P., Carafoli, E., and Chiesi, M.: Heterogeneous distribution of calmodulin- and cAMP-dependent regulation of Ca^{2+} uptake in cardiac sarcoplasmic reticulum subfractions. Eur. J. Biochem. *176*:535–541, 1988.
44. McLeod, A. G., Shen, A. C. Y., Campbell, K. P., et al.: Frog cardiac calsequestrin. Identification, characterization, and subcellular distribution in two structurally distinct regions of peripheral sarcoplasmic reticulum in frog ventricular myocardium. Circ. Res. *69*:344–359, 1991.
45. D'Agnolo, A., Luciani, G. B., Mazzucco, A., et al.: Contractile properties and Ca^{2+} release activity of the sarcoplasmic reticulum in dilated cardiomyopathy. Circulation *85*:518–525, 1992.
46. Arai, M., Alpert, N. R., MacLennan, D. H., et al.: Alterations in sarcoplasmic reticulum gene expression in human heart failure. A possible mechanism for alterations in systolic and diastolic properties of the failing myocardium. Circ. Res. *72*:463–469, 1993.

SARCOLEMMAL CONTROL OF CALCIUM AND OTHER IONS

47. Katz, A. M.: Cardiac ion channels. N. Engl. J. Med. *328*:1244–1251, 1993.
48. Tomaselli, G. F., Backx, P. H., and Marban, E.: Molecular basis of permeation in voltage-gated ion channels. Circ. Res. *72*:491–496, 1993.
49. Schwartz, A.: Calcium antagonists: Review and perspective on mechanism of action. Am. J. Cardiol. *64*(Suppl.):3I–9I, 1989.
50. Heinemann, S. H., Stuhmer, W.: Molecular structure of potassium and sodium channels and their structure-function correlation. *In* Sperelakis, N. (ed.): Physiology and Pathophysiology of the Heart. 3rd ed. Boston, Kluwer Academic Publishers, 1995, pp. 101–114.
51. Pragnell, M., De Waard, M., Mori, Y., et al.: Calcium channel beta-subunit binds to a conserved motif in the I-II cytoplasmic linker of the $alpha_1$-subunit. Nature *368*:67–70, 1994.
52. Yatani, A., Bahinski, A., Mikala, G., et al.: Single amino acid substitutions within the ion permeation pathway alter single-channel conductance of the human L-type cardiac Ca^{2+} channel. Circ. Res. *75*:315–323, 1994.
53. Flockerzi, V., and Hofmann, F.: Molecular structure of the cardiac calcium channel. *In* Sperelakis, E. (ed.): Physiology and Pathophysiology of the Heart. 3rd ed. Boston, Kluwer Academic Publishers, 1995, pp. 91–99.
54. Bean, B. P.: Two kinds of calcium channels in canine atrial cells. Differences in kinetics, selectivity and pharmacology. J. Gen. Physiol. *86*:1–30, 1985.
55. Bers, D. M., Bassani, J. W. M., and Bassani, R. A.: Competition and redistribution among calcium transport systems in rabbit cardiac myocytes. Cardiovasc. Res. *27*:1772–1777, 1993.
56. Reeves, J. P.: Cardiac sodium-calcium exchange sytstem. *In* Sperelakis, N. (ed.): Physiology and Pathophysiology of the Heart. 3rd ed. Boston, Kluwer Academic Publishers, 1995, pp. 309–318.
57. Nicoll, D. A., Longoni, S., and Philipson, K. D.: Molecular cloning and functional expression of the cardiac sarcolemmal Na^+–Ca^{2+} exchanger. Science *250*:562–565, 1990.
58. Chin, T. K., Spitzer, K. W., Philipson, K. D., and Bridge, J. H. B.: The effect of exchanger inhibitory peptide (XIP) on sodium-calcium exchange current in guinea-pig ventricular cells. Circ. Res. *72*:497–503, 1993.
59. Bers, D. M.: Excitation-Contraction Coupling and Cardiac Contractile Force. Boston, Kluwer Academic Publishers, 1991.
60. Leblanc, N., and Hume, J. R.: Sodium current-induced release of calcium from cardiac sarcoplasmic reticulum. Science *248*:372–376, 1990.
61. Noble, D., Noble, S. J., Bett, C. L., et al.: The role of sodium-calcium exchange during the cardiac action potential. Ann. N. Y. Acad. Sci. *639*:334–353, 1991.
62. Sheu, S.-S., and Blaustein, M. P.: Sodium/calcium exchange and control of cell calcium and contractility in cardiac and vascular smooth muscles. *In* Fozzard, H. A., et al. (eds.): The Heart and Cardiovascular System. 2nd ed. New York, Raven Press, 1992, pp. 903–943.
63. Levi, A. J., Brooksby, P., and Hancox, J. C.: A role for depolarisation-induced calcium entry on the Na-Ca exchange in triggering intracellular calcium release and contraction in rat ventricular myocytes. Cardiovasc. Res. *27*:1677–1690, 1993.
64. Han, S., Schiefer, A., and Isenberg, G.: Ca^{2+} load of guinea-pig ventricular myocytes determines efficacy of brief Ca^{2+} currents as trigger for Ca^{2+} release. J. Physiol. *480*:411–421, 1994.
65. Kaibara, M., Mitarai, S., Yano, K., and Kameyama, M.: Involvement of Na^+/H^+ antiporter in regulation of L-type Ca^{2+} channel current by angiotensin-II in rabbit ventricular myocytes. Circ. Res. *75*:1121–1125, 1994.
66. Vandenberg, J. I., Metcalfe, J. C., Grace, A. A.: Mechanisms of pH_i recovery after global ischemia in the perfused heart. Circ. Res. *72*:993–1003, 1993.
67. Yanoukakos, D., Stuart-Tilley, A., Fernandez, H. A., et al.: Molecular cloning, expression, and chromosomal localization of two isoforms of the AE3 anion exchanger from human heart. Circ. Res. *75*:603–614, 1994.
68. Desilets, M., Puceat, M., and Vassort, G.: Chloride dependence of pH modulation by beta-adrenergic agonist in rat cardiomyocytes. Circ. Res. *75*:862–869, 1994.
69. Eisner, D. A., and Smith, T. W.: The Na-K pump and its effectors in cardiac muscle. *In* Fozzard, H. A., et al. (eds.): The Heart and Cardiovascular System. 2nd ed. New York, Raven Press, 1992, pp. 863–902.
70. Lelievre, L., and Charlemagne, D.: The myocyte sarcolemma in cardiac hypertrophy: Na^+/K^+-ATPase, Ca^{2+}-ATPase, Na^+/Ca^{2+} exchange and phospholipids. *In* Swynghedauw, B. (ed.): Research in Cardiac Hypertrophy and Failure. INSERM/John Libbey Eurotext, London, 1990, pp. 171–184.
71. Carmeliet, E.: A fuzzy subsarcolemmal space for intracellular Na^+ in cardiac cells? Cardiovasc. Res. *26*:433–442, 1992.
72. Johnson, E. A., and Lemieux, R. D.: Sodium-calcium exchange. Science *251*:1370, 1991.

RECEPTORS AND SIGNAL SYSTEMS

73. Lindemann, J. P., and Watanabe, A. M.: Mechanisms of adrenergic and cholinergic regulation of myocardial contractility. *In* Sperelakis, N. (ed.): Physiology and Pathophysiology of the Heart. 3rd ed. Boston, Kluwer Academic Publishers, 1995, pp. 467–494.
74. Fleming, J. W., Wisler, P. L., and Watanabe, A. M.: Signal transduction by G-proteins in cardiac tissues. Circulation *85*:420–433, 1992.
75. Neer, E. J., and Clapham, D. E.: Signal transduction through G-proteins in the cardiac myocyte. Trends Cardiovasc. Med. *2*:6–11, 1992.
76. Lefkowitz, R. J.: Clinical implications of basic research. N. Engl. J. Med. *332*:186–187, 1995.
77. De Jonge, H. W., Van Heugten, H. A. A., and Lamers, J. M. J.: Signal transduction by the phosphatidylinositol cycle in myocardium. J. Mol. Cell Cardiol. *27*:93–106, 1995.
78. Sadoshima, J., Xu, Y., Slayter, H. S., and Izumo, S.: Autocrine release of angiotensin-II mediates stretch-induced hypertrophy of cardiac myocytes in vitro. Cell *75*:977–984, 1993.
79. Bristow, M. R., Hershberger, R. E., Port, J. D., and Rasmussen, R.: $Beta_1$ and $beta_2$ adrenergic receptor–mediated adenylate cyclase stimulation in nonfailing and failing human ventricular myocardium. Mol. Pharmacol. *35*:295, 1989.
80. Levy, F. O., Zhu, X., Kaumann, A. J., and Birnbaumer, L.: Efficacy of β_1-adrenergic receptors is lower than that of β_2-adrenergic receptors. Proc. Natl. Acad. Sci. *90*:10798–10802, 1993.
81. Raymond, J. R., Hantowich, M., Lefkowitz, R. J., and Caron, M. G.: Adrenergic receptors. Models for regulation of signal transduction processes. Hypertension *15*:119–131, 1990.
82. Spinale, F. G., Tempel, G. E., Mukherjee, R., et al.: Cellular and molecular alterations in the β-adrenergic system with cardiomyopathy induced by tachycardia. Cardiovasc. Res. *28*:1243–1250, 1994.
83. Neubig, R. R.: Membrane organization in G-protein mechanisms. FASEB J. *8*:939–946, 1994.
84. Port, J. D., and Malbon, C. C.: Integration of transmembrane signaling. Cross-talk among G-protein–linked receptors and other signal transduction pathways. Trends Cardiovasc. Med. *3*:85–92, 1993.
85. Coleman, D. E., Berghuis, A. M., Lee, E., et al.: Structures of active conformations of $G_{i\alpha1}$ and the mechanism of GTP hydrolysis. Science *265*:1405–1412, 1994.
86. Kurachi, Y.: G-protein control of cardiac potassium channels. Trends Cardiovasc. Med. *4*:64–69, 1994.
87. Schofield, P. R., and Abbott, A.: Molecular pharmacology and drug action: Structural information casts light on ligand binding. TIPS *10*:207–212, 1989.
88. Kumar, R., Joyner, R. W., Hartzell, H. C., et al.: Postnatal changes in the G-proteins, cyclic nucleotides and adenylyl cyclase activity in rabbit heart cells. J. Mol. Cell Cardiol. *26*:1537–1550, 1994.
89. Opie, L. H.: The Heart: Physiology and Metabolism. 2nd ed. New York, Raven Press, 1991, pp. 67–126, 147–175.
90. Liang, B. T., and Haltiwanger, B.: Adenosine A_{2a} and A_{2b} receptors in cultured fetal chick heart cells. High- and low-affinity coupling to stimulation of myocyte contractility and cAMP accumulation. Circ. Res. *76*:242–251, 1995.
91. Ono, K., Eto, K., Sakamoto, A., et al.: Negative chronotropic effect of endothelin 1 mediated through ET_A receptors in guinea pig atria. Circ. Res. *76*:284–292, 1995.
92. Shabb, J. B., and Corbin, J. D.: Protein phosphorylation in the heart. *In* Fozzard, H. A., et al.: The Heart and Cardiovascular System. 2nd ed. New York, Raven Press, 1992, pp. 1539–1562.
93. Walsh, D. A., and Van Patten, S. M.: Multiple pathway signal transduction by the cAMP-dependent protein kinase. FASEB J. *8*:1227–1236, 1994.
94. Scott, J. D., and Carr, D. W.: Subcellular localization of the Type II cAMP-dependent protein kinase. NIPS *7*:143–148, 1992.
95. Hohl, C. M., and Li, Q.: Compartmentation of cAMP in adult canine ventricular myocytes. Relation to single cell free Ca^{2+} transients. Circ. Res. *69*:1369–1379, 1991.
96. Worthington, M., and Opie, L. H.: Contrasting effects of cyclic AMP increase caused by beta-adrenergic stimulation or by adenylate cyclase activation on ventricular fibrillation threshold of isolated rat heart. J. Cardiovasc. Pharmacol. *20*:595–600, 1992.
97. Bartel, S., Karczewski, P., and Krause, E.-G.: Protein phosphorylation and cardiac function: Cholinergic-adrenergic interaction. Cardiovasc. Res. *27*:1948–1953, 1993.
98. Matsuda, J. J., Lee, H. C., and Shibata, E. F.: Acetylcholine reversal of isoproterenol-stimulated sodium currents in rabbit ventricular myocytes. Circ. Res. *72*:517–525, 1993.
99. Sumii, K., and Sperelakis, N.: cGMP-dependent protein kinase regula-

tion of the L-type Ca^{2+} current in rat ventricular myocytes. Circ. Res. *77*:803–812, 1995.
100. Lohmann, S. M., Fischmeister, R., and Walter, U.: Signal transduction by cGMP in heart. Basic Res. Cardiol. *86*:503–514, 1991.
101. Shah, A. M., Spurgeon, H. A., Sollott, S. J., et al.: 8-Bromo-cGMP reduces the myofilament response to Ca^{2+} in intact cardiac myocytes. Circ. Res. *74*:970–978, 1994.
102. Deckmyn, H., Ven Geet, C., and Vermylen, J.: Dual regulation of phospholipase C activity by G-proteins. NIPS *8*:61–63, 1993.
103. Du, X.-J., Anderson, K.E., Jacobsen, A., et al.: Suppression of ventricular arrhythmias during ischemia-reperfusion by agents inhibiting Ins(1, 4,5)P_3 release. Circulation *91*:2712–2716, 1995.
104. Rogers, T. B., and Lokuta, A. J.: Angiotensin-II signal transduction pathways in the cardiovascular system. Trends Cardiovasc. Med. *4*:110–116, 1994.
105. Hug, H., and Sarre, T. F.: Protein kinase C isoenzymes: Divergence in signal transduction? Biochem. J. *291*:329–343, 1993.
106. Gu, X., and Bishop, S. P.: Increased protein kinase C and isozyme redistribution in pressure-overload cardiac hypertrophy in the rat. Circ. Res. *75*:926–931, 1994.
107. Johnson, J. A., and Mochly-Rosen, D.: Inhibition of the spontaneous rate of contraction of neonatal cardiac myocytes by protein kinase C isozymes. Circ. Res. *76*:654–663, 1995.
108. Fedida, D.: Modulation of cardiac contractility by α_1-adrenoceptors. Cardiovasc. Res. *27*:1735–1742, 1993.
109. Steinberg, S. F., Goldberg, M., and Rybin, V. O.: Protein kinase C isoform diversity in the heart. J. Mol. Cell Cardiol. *27*:141–153, 1995.
110. Mitchell, M. B., Meng, X., Brown, J. M., et al.: Preconditioning of isolated rat heart is mediated by protein kinase C. Circ. Res. *76*:73–81, 1995.
111. Tomai, F., Crea, F., Gaspardone, A., et al.: Ischemic preconditioning during coronary angioplasty is prevented by glibenclamide, a selective ATP-sensitive K^+ channel blocker. Circulation *90*:700–705, 1994.
112. Forstermann, U., Pollock, J. S., and Nakane, M.: Nitric oxide synthases in the cardiovascular system. Trends Cardiovasc. Med. *3*:104–110, 1993.
113. Balligand, J.-L., Kelly, R. A., Marsden, P. A., et al.: Control of cardiac muscle cell function by an endogenous nitric oxide signaling system. Proc. Natl. Acad. Sci. *90*:347–351, 1993.
114. Weyrich, A. S., Ma, X., Buerke, M., et al.: Physiological concentrations of nitric oxide do not elicit an acute negative inotropic effect in unstimulated cardiac muscle. Circ. Res. *75*:692–700, 1994.
115. Shryock, J., Song, Y., Wang, D., et al.: Selective A_2-adenosine receptor agonists do not alter action potential duration, twitch shortening, or cAMP accumulation in guinea pig, rat, or rabbit isolated ventricular myocytes. Circ. Res. *72*:194–205, 1993.
116. Stiles, G. L.: Adenosine receptors. J. Biol. Chem. *267*:6451–6454, 1992.
117. Komuro, I., and Yazaki, Y.: Intracellular signaling pathways in cardiac myocytes induced by mechanical stress. Trends Cardiovasc. Med. *4*:117–121, 1994.
118. Van Wagoner, D. R.: Mechanosensitive gating of atrial ATP-sensitive potassium channels. Circ. Res. *72*:973–983, 1993.
119. Boer, P. H. Ruzicka, M., Lear, W., et al.: Stretch-mediated activation of the cardiac renin gene. Am. J. Physiol. *267*:H1630–H1636, 1994.
120. Bristow, M. R., Anderson, F. L., Port, D., et al.: Differences in beta-adrenergic neuroeffector mechanisms in ischemic versus idiopathic dilated cardiomyopathy. Circlation *84*:1024–1039, 1991.
121. Böhm, M., Reiger, B., Schwinger, R. H. G., and Erdmann, E.: cAMP concentrations, cAMP dependent protein kinase activity, and phospholamban in non-failing and failing myocardium. Cardiovasc. Res. *28*:1713–1719, 1994.
122. Böhm, M., Eschenhagen, T., Gierschik, P., et al.: Radioimmunochemical quantification of Giα in right and left ventricles from patients with ischaemic and dilated cardiomyopathy and predominant left ventricular failure. J. Mol. Cell Cardiol. *26*:133–149, 1994.
123. Beuckelmann, D. J., Nabauer, M., and Erdmann, E.: Intracellular calcium handling in isolated ventricular myocytes from patients with terminal heart failure. Circulation *85*:1046–1055, 1992.
124. Steinfath, M., Danielsen, W., von der Leyen, H., et al.: Reduced α_1- and β_2-adrenoceptor-mediated positive inotropic effects in human end-stage heart failure. Br. J. Pharmacol. *105*:463–469, 1992.
125. Lohse, M. J.: G-protein-coupled receptor kinases and the heart. Trends Cardiovasc. Med. *5*:63–68, 1995.
126. Hausdorff, W. P., Caron, M. G., and Lefkowitz, R. J.: Turning off the signal: Desensitization of beta-adrenergic receptor function. FASEB J. *4*:2881–2889, 1990.
127. Ungerer, M., Böhm, M., Elce, J. S., et al.: Altered expression of β-adrenergic receptor kinase and β_1-adrenergic receptors in the failing human heart. Circulation *87*:454–463, 1993.
128. Lubbe, W. F., Podzuweit, T., and Opie, L. H.: Potential arrhythmogenic role of cyclic AMP and cytosolic calcium overload: Implications for prophylactic effects of beta-blockers and proarrhythmic effects of phosphodiesterase inhibitors. J. Am. Coll. Cardiol. *19*:1622–1633, 1992.
129. Muntz, K. H., Zhao, M., and Miller, J. C.: Downregulation of myocardial β-adrenergic receptors. Receptor subtype selectivity. Circ. Res. *74*:369–375, 1994.
130. Matsuda, J. J., Lee, H., and Shibata, E. F.: Enhancement of rabbit cardiac sodium channels by β-adrenergic stimulation. Circ. Res. *70*:199–207, 1992.
131. Chang, F., and Cohen, I. S.: Mechanism of acetylcholine action on pacemaker current (I_f) in canine Purkinje fibers. Pflugers Arch. *420*:389–392, 1992.

CONTRACTILE PERFORMANCE OF THE INTACT HEART

132. Lewis, T.: The Mechanism and Graphic Registration of the Heart Beat. London, Shaw and Sons, 1920, p. 24.
133. Wiggers, C. J.: Modern Aspects of the Circulation in Health and Disease. Philadelphia, Lea and Febiger, 1915, p. 98.
134. Laniado, S., Yellin, E. L., Miller, H., and Frater, R. W. M.: Temporal relation of the first heart sound to closure of the mitral valve. Circulation *47*:1006–1014, 1973.
135. Parisi, A. F., and Milton, B. G.: Relation of mitral valve closure to the first heart sound in man. Echocardiographic and phonocardiographic assessment. Am. J. Cardiol. *32*:779–782, 1973.
136. Rhodes, J., Udelson, J. E., Marx, G. R., et al.: A new noninvasive method for the estimation of peak dP/dt. Circulation *88*:2693–2699, 1993.
137. Hirschfeld, S., Meyer, R., Korfhagen, J., et al.: The isovolumic contraction time of the left ventricle. An echographic study. Circulation *54*:751–756, 1976.
138. Belz, G. G.: Elastic properties and Windkessel function of the human aorta. Cardiovasc. Drugs Ther. *9*:73–83, 1995.
139. Ohno, M., Cheng, C.-P., and Little, W. C.: Mechanism of altered patterns of left ventricular filling during the development of congestive heart failure. Circulation *89*:2241–2250, 1994.
140. Glower, D. D., Murrah, R. L., Olsen, C. O., et al.: Mechanical correlates of the third heart sound. J. Am. Coll. Cardiol. *19*:450–457, 1992.
141. Starling, E. H.: The Linacre Lecture on the Law of the Heart. London, Longmans, Green and Co., 1918.
142. Frank, O.: Zur Dynamik des Herzmuskels. Z. Biol. *32*:370–447, 1895. Translated in Am. Heart J. *58*:282–317, 467–478, 1958.
143. Greenway, C. V., and Wayne Lautt, W.: Blood volume, the venous system, preload and cardiac output. Can. J. Physiol. Pharmacol. *64*:383–387, 1986.
144. Rodriguez, E. K., Hunter, W. C., Royce, M. J., et al.: A method to reconstruct myocardial sarcomere lengths and orientations at transmural sites in beating canine hearts. Am. J. Physiol. *263*:H293–H306, 1992.
145. Backx, P. H., ter Keurs, H. E. D. J.: Fluorescent properties of rat cardiac trabeculae microinjected with fura-2 salt. Am J. Physiol. *264*:H1098–H1110, 1993.
146. Kent, R. L., Hoober, K., and Cooper, G.: Load responsiveness of protein synthesis in adult mammalian myocardium: Role of cardiac deformation linked to sodium influx. Circ. Res. *64*:74–85, 1989.
147. Borow, K. M.: Clinical assessment of contractility in the symmetrically contracting left ventricle: Part I. Mod. Concepts Cardiovasc. Dis. *57*:29–34, 1988.
148. Eaton, G. M., Cody, R. J., and Binkley, P. F.: Increased aortic impedance precedes peripheral vasoconstriction at the early stage of ventricular failure in the paced canine model. Circulation *88*:2714–2721, 1993.
149. Bowditch, H.: Uber die Eigenthumlickkeiten der Reizbarkeit, welche die Muskelfasern des Herzens Zeigen. Arb. Physiol. Inst. Lpz. *6*:139, 1871.
150. Mulieri, L. A., Leavitt, B. J., Martin, B. J., et al.: Myocardial force-frequency defect in mitral regurgitation heart failure is reversed by forskolin. Circulation *88*:2700–2704, 1993.
151. Suga, H.: Ventricular energetics. Physiol. Rev. *70*:247–277, 1990.
152. Cooper, M. W.: Postextrasystolic potentiation. Do we really know what it means and how to use it? Circulation *88*:2962–2971, 1993.
153. Hasenfuss, G., Reinecke, H., Studer, R., et al.: Relation between myocardial function and expression of sarcoplasmic reticulum Ca^{2+}-ATPase in failing and nonfailing human myocardium. Circ. Res. *75*:434–442, 1994.
154. Pierard, L. A., Serruys, P. W., Roelandt, J., and Meltzer, R. S.: Left ventricular function at similar heart rates during tachycardia induced by exercise and atrial pacing: An echocardiographic study. Br. Heart J. *57*:154–160, 1987.
155. Braunwald, E., and Sobel, B. E.: Coronary blood flow and myocardial ischemia. *In* Braunwald, E. (ed.): Heart Disease. A Textbook of Cardiovascular Medicine. 4th ed. Philadelphia, W. B. Saunders Company, 1992, pp. 1161–1199.
156. Rooke, G. A., and Feigl, E. O.: Work as a correlate of canine left ventricular oxygen consumption, and the problem of catecholamine oxygen wasting. Circ. Res. *50*:273–286, 1982.
157. Simonsen, S., and Kjekshus, J. K.: The effect of free fatty acids on myocardial oxygen consumption during atrial pacing and catecholamine infusion in man. Circulation *58*:484–491, 1978.
158. Burkhoff, D., Weiss, R. G., Schulman, S. P., et al.: Influence of metabolic substrate on rat heart function and metabolism at different coronary flows. Am. J. Physiol. *261*:H741–H750, 1991.
159. Braunwald, E.: Control of myocardial oxygen consumption. Physiologic and clinical considerations. Am. J. Cardiol. *27*:416–432, 1971.
160. Kannengiesser, G. J., Opie, L. H., and van der Werff, T. J.: Impaired cardiac work and oxygen uptake after reperfusion of ischaemic myocardium. J. Mol. Cell Cardiol. *11*:197–207, 1979.
161. Kass, D. A., and Beyar, R.: Evaluation of contractile state by maximal ventricular power divided by the square of end-diastolic volume. Circulation *84*:1698–1708, 1991.

162. Nozawa, T., Cheng, C.-P., Noda, T., and Little, W. C.: Effect of exercise on left ventricular mechanical efficiency in conscious dogs. Circulation *90:*3047–3054, 1994.
163. Beanlands, R. S. B., Bach, D. S., Raylman, R., et al.: Acute effects of dobutamine on myocardial oxygen consumption and cardiac efficiency measured using carbon-11 acetate kinetics in patients with dilated cardiomyopathy. J. Am. Coll. Cardiol. *22:*1389–1398, 1993.
164. Burkhoff, D., de Tombe, P. P., Hunter, W. C., and Kass, D. A.: Contractile strength and mechanical efficiency of left ventricle are enhanced by physiological afterload. Am. J. Physiol. *260:*H569–H578, 1991.
165. Opie, L. H.: Regulation of myocardial contractility. J. Cardiovasc. Pharmacol. *26*(Suppl. 1):S1–S9, 1995.
166. Lakatta, E. G.: Starling's Law of the heart is explained by an intimate interaction of muscle length and myofilament calcium activation. J. Am. Coll. Cardiol. *10:*1157–1164, 1987.
167. Schlant, R. C., and Sonnenblick, E. H.: Normal physiology of the cardiovascular system. *In* Schlant, R. C., and Alexander, R. W. (eds.): The Heart, Arteries and Veins. New York, McGill Inc., 1994, pp. 113–151.
168. Braunwald, E., Sonnenblick, E. H., and Ross, J.: Normal and abnormal circulatory function. *In* Braunwald, E. (ed.): Heart Disease. A textbook of Cardiovascular Medicine. 4th ed. Philadelphia, W. B. Saunders Company, 1992, pp. 351–392.
169. Sweitzer, N. K., and Moss, R. L.: Determinants of loaded shortening velocity in single cardiac myocytes permeabilized with alpha-hemolysin. Circ. Res. *73:*1150–1162, 1993.
170. Campbell, K. B., Kirkpatrick, R. D., Tobias, A. H., et al.: Series coupled non-contractile elements are functionally unimportant in the isolated heart. Cardiovasc. Res. *28:*242–251, 1994.
171. Ter Keurs, H. E. D. J.: Calcium and contractility. *In* Drake-Holland, A. J., and Noble, M. I. M. (eds.): Cardiac Metabolism. Chicester, John Wiley, 1983, pp. 73–99.
172. Strang, K. T., Sweitzer, N. K., Greaser, M. L., and Moss, R. L.: Beta-adrenergic receptor stimulation increases unloaded shortening velocity of skinned single ventricular myocytes from rats. Circ. Res. *74:*542–549, 1994.
173. de Tombe, P. P., and ter Keurs, H. E. D. J.: Lack of effect of isoproterenol on unloaded velocity of sarcomere shortening in rat cardiac trabeculae. Circ. Res. *68:*382–391, 1991.
174. Kass, D. A., Beyar, R., Lankford, E., et al.: Influence of contractile state on curvilinearity of in situ end-systolic pressure-volume relations. Circulation *79:*167–178, 1989.
175. Carabello, B. A.: The role of end-systolic pressure-volume analysis in clinical assessment of ventricular function. Trends Cardiovasc. Med. *1:*337–341, 1991.
176. Hori, M., Kitakaze, M., Ishida, Y., et al.: Delayed end ejection increases isovolumic ventricular relaxation rate in isolated perfused canine hearts. Circ. Res. *68:*300–308, 1991.
177. Leite-Moreira, A. F., and Gillebert, T. C.: Nonuniform course of left ventricular pressure fall and its regulation by load and contractile state. Circulation *90:*2481–2491, 1994.
178. Brutsaert, D. L., and Sys, S. U.: Relaxation and diastole of the heart. Physiol. Rev. *69:*1228–1315, 1989.
179. Brutsaert, D. L., Sys, S. U., and Gillebert, T. C.: Diastolic failure: Pathophysiology and therapeutic implications. J. Am. Coll. Cardiol. *22:*318–325, 1993.
180. Eichhorn, E. J., Willard, J. E., Alvarez, L., et al.: Are contraction and relaxation coupled in patients with and without congestive heart failure? Circulation *85:*2132–2139, 1992.
181. Cory, C. R., Grange, R. W., and Houston, M. E.: Role of sarcoplasmic reticulum in loss of load-sensitive relaxation in pressure overload cardiac hypertrophy. Am. J. Physiol. *266:*H68–H78, 1994.
182. Morgan, J. P., and Morgan, K. G.: Intracellular calcium and cardiovascular function in heart failure: Effects of pharmacologic agents. Cardiovasc. Drugs Ther. *3:*959–970, 1989.
183. Yamamoto, K., Masuyama, T., Doi, Y., et al.: Noninvasive assessment of left ventricular relaxation using continuous wave Doppler aortic regurgitant velocity curve. Its comparative value to the mitral regurgitation method. Circulation *91:*192–200, 1995.
184. Chen, C., Rodriguez, L., Levine, R. A., et al.: Noninvasive measurement of the time constant of left ventricular relaxation using the continuous-wave Doppler velocity profile of mitral regurgitation. Circulation *86:*272–278, 1992.
185. Udelson, J. E., Bacharach, S. L., Cannon, R. O., and Bonow, R. O.: Minimum left ventricular pressure during beta-adrenergic stimulation in human subjects. Circulation *82:*1174–1182, 1990.
186. Gilbert, J. C., and Glantz, S. A.: Determinants of left ventricular filling and of the diastolic pressure-volume relation. Circ. Res. *64:*827–852, 1989.
187. Hoit, B. D., Shao, Y., Gabel, M., and Walsh, R. A.: In vivo assessment of left atrial contractile performance in normal and pathological conditions using a time-varying elastance model. Circulation *89:*1829–1838, 1994.
188. Focaccio, A., Volpe, M., Ambrosio, G., et al.: Angiotensin-II directly stimulates release of atrial natriuretic factor in isolated rabbit hearts. Circulation *87:*192–198, 1993.
189. Fyrhquist, F., Sirvio, M.-L., Helin, K., et al.: Endothelin antiserum decreases volume-stimulated and basal plasma concentration of atrial natriuretic peptide. Circulation *88:*1172–1176, 1993.
190. Mouton, R., Lochner, J. De V., and Lochner, A.: New emphasis on atrial cardiology. S. Afr. Med. J. *82:*222–223, 1992.
191. Holubarsch, C., Hasenfuss, G., Schmidt-Schweda, S., et al.: Angiotensin-I and II exert inotropic effects in atrial but not in ventricular human myocardium. An in vitro study under physiological experimental conditions. Circulation *88:*1228–1237, 1993.
192. Wang, Z., Fermini, B., and Nattel, S.: Delayed rectifier outward current and repolarization in human atrial myocytes. Circ. Res. *73:*276–285, 1993.
193. Koumi, S.-I., and Wasserstrom, J. A.: Acetylcholine-sensitive muscarinic K^+ channels in mammalian ventricular myocytes. Am. J. Physiol. *266:*H1812–H1821, 1994.
194. Rozanski, G. J., Lipsius, S. L., and Randall, W. C.: Functional characteristics of sinoatrial and subsidiary pacemaker activity in the canine right atrium. Circulation *67:*1378–1387, 1983.
195. Douglas, P. S., Berko, B., Lesh, M., and Reichek, N.: Alterations in diastolic function in response to progressive left ventricular hypertrophy. J. Am. Coll. Cardiol. *13:*461–467, 1989.
196. Myreng, Y., and Smiseth, O. A.: Assessment of ventricular relaxation by Doppler echocardiography. Comparison of isovolumic relaxation time and transmitral flow velocities with time constant of isovolumic relaxation. Circulation *81:*260–266, 1990.
197. Villari, B., Vassalli, G., Monrad, E. S., et al.: Normalization of diastolic dysfunction in aortic stenosis late after valve replacement. Circulation *91:*2353–2358, 1995.
198. Mehta, S., Charbonneau, F., Fitchett, D. H., et al.: The clinical consequences of a stiff left atrium. Am. Heart J. *122:*1184–1191, 1991.
199. Kool, M. J., Spek, J. J., Struyker Boudier, H. A., et al.: Acute and subacute effects of nicorandil and isosorbide dinitrate on vessel wall properties of large arteries and hemodynamics in healthy volunteers. Cardiovasc. Drugs Ther. *9:*331–337, 1995.
200. Stefanadis, C., Stratos, C., Boudoulas, H., et al.: Distensibility of the ascending aorta: Comparison of invasive and non-invasive techniques in healthy men and in men with coronary artery disease. Eur. Heart J. *11:*990–996, 1990.
201. Adams, J. N., Brooks, M., Redpath, T. W., et al.: Aortic distensibility and stiffness index measure by magnetic resonance imaging in patients with Marfan's syndrome. Br. Heart J. *73:*265–269, 1995.
202. Wesseling, K. H., Jansen, J. R. C., Settels, J. J., and Schreuder, J. J.: Computation of aortic flow from pressure in humans using a nonlinear, three-element model. J. Appl. Physiol. *74:*2566–2573, 1993.
203. Dittrich, H. C., Chow, L. C., and Nicod, P. H.: Early improvement in left ventricular diastolic function after relief of chronic right ventricular pressure overload. Circulation *80:*823–830, 1989.
204. Feneley, M. P., Olsen, C. O., Glower, D. D., and Rankin, J. S.: Effect of acutely increased right ventricular afterload on work output from the left ventricle in conscious dogs. Systolic ventricular interaction. Circ. Res. *65:*135–145, 1989.
205. Hamilton, D. R., Dani, R. S., Semlacher, R. A., et al.: Right atrial and right ventricular transmural pressures in dogs and humans. Effects of the pericardium. Circulation *90:*2492–2500, 1994.
206. Refsum, H., Junemann, M., Lipton, M. J., et al.: Ventricular diastolic pressure-volume relations and the pericardium. Effects of changes in blood volume and pericardial effusion in dogs. Circulation *64:*997–1004, 1981.
207. Chuttani, K., Pandian, N. G., Mohanty, P. K., et al.: Left ventricular diastolic collapse. An echocardiographic sign of regional cardiac tamponade. Circulation *83:*1999–2006, 1991.
208. Li, K., Rouleau, J. L., Calderone, A., et al.: Endocardial function in pacing-induced heart failure in the dog. J. Mol. Cell Cardiol. *25:*529–540, 1993.
209. Brutsaert, D. L., and Andries, L. J.: The endocardial endothelium. Am. J. Physiol. *263:*H985–H1002, 1992.
210. Noble, M. I. M.: Excitation-contraction coupling. *In* Drake-Holland, A. J., and Noble, M. I. M. (eds.): Cardiac Metabolism. New York, John Wiley, 1983, pp. 49–71.
211. Harizi, R. C., Bianco, J. A., and Alpert, J. S.: Diastolic function of the heart in clinical cardiology. Arch. Intern. Med. *148:*99–109, 1988.

EFFECTS OF ISCHEMIA AND REPERFUSION ON CONTRACTION AND RELAXATION

212. Figueredo, V., Brandes, R., Weiner, M. W., et al.: Endocardial versus epicardial differences of intracellular free calcium under normal and ischemic conditions in perfused rat hearts. Circ. Res. *72:*1082–1090, 1993.
213. Urthaler, F., Harris, K., Walker, A. A., et al.: Beat to beat $[Ca^{2+}]_i$ and left ventricular function during brief bouts of ischemia in rats. J. Am. Coll. Cardiol. 22(Abs.):317A, 1994.
214. Meissner, A., and Morgan, J. P.: Contractile dysfunction and abnormal Ca^{2+} modulation during postischemic reperfusion in rat heart. Am. J. Physiol. *268:*H100–H111, 1995.
215. Korge, P., Byrd, S. K., and Campbell, K. B.: Functional coupling between sarcoplasmic reticulum-bound creatine kinase and Ca^{2+}-ATPase. Eur. J. Biochem. *213:*973–980, 1993.
216. Cross, H. R., Clarke, K., Opie, L. H., and Radda, G. K.: Is lactate-induced myocardial ischaemic injury mediated by decreased pH or increased intracellular lactate? J. Mol. Cell Cardiol. *27:*1369–1381, 1995.
216a. Sata, M., Sugiura, S., Yamashita, H., et al.: Coupling between myosin ATPase cycle and creatine kinase cycle facilitates cardiac actomyosin

sliding in vitro. A clue to mechanical dysfunction during myocardial ischemia. Circulation *93*:310, 1996.
217. Kentish, J. C.: The effects of inorganic phosphate and creatine phosphate on force production in skinned muscles from rat ventricle. J. Physiol. *370*:585–604, 1986.
218. Opie, L. H.: Myocardial metabolism in ischemia. *In* Heusch, G. (ed.): Pathophysiology and Rational Therapy of Myocardial Ischemia. Darmstadt, Steinkopff Verlag, 1990, pp. 37–57.
219. Turvey, S. E., and Allen, D. G.: Changes in myoplasmic sodium concentration during exposure to lactate in perfused rat heart. Cardiovasc. Res. *28*:987–993, 1994.
220. Gasser, R. N. A., and Klein, W.: Contractile failure in early myocardial ischemia: Models and mechanisms. Cardiovasc. Drugs Ther. *8*:813–822, 1994.
221. Kantor, P., Coetzee, W. A., Carmeliet, E., et al.: Reduction of ischemic K^+ loss and arrhythmias in rat hearts. Effects of glibenclamide, a sulfonylurea. Circ. Res. *66*:478–485, 1990.
222. Weiss, J. N., and Shieh, R.-C.: Potassium loss during myocardial ischaemia and hypoxia: Does lactate efflux play a role? Cardiovasc. Res. *28*:1125–1132, 1994.
223. Sylven, C.: Mechanisms of pain in angina pectoris—A critical review of the adenosine hypothesis. Cardiovasc. Drugs Ther. *7*:745–759, 1993.
224. Yao, Z., and Gross, G. J.: A comparison of adenosine-induced cardioprotection and ischemic preconditioning in dogs. Efficacy, time course, and role of K_{ATP} channels. Circulation *89*:1229–1236, 1994.
225. Apstein, C. S., and Grossman, W.: Opposite initial effects of supply and demand ischemia on left ventricular diastolic compliance: The ischemic-diastolic paradox. J. Mol. Cell Cardiol. *19*:119–128, 1987.
226. Applegate, R. J., Walsh, R. A., and O'Rourke, R. A.: Comparative effects of pacing-induced and flow-limited ischemia on left ventricular function. Circulation *81*:1380–1392, 1990.
227. De Bruyne, B., Bronzwaer, J. G. F., Heyndrickx, G. R., and Paulus, W. J.: Comparative effects of ischemia and hypoxemia on left ventricular systolic and diastolic function in humans. Circulation *88*:461–471, 1993.
228. Takano, H., and Glantz, S. A.: Left ventricular contractility predicts how the end-diastolic pressure-volume relation shifts during pacing-induced ischemia in dogs. Circulation *91*:2423–2434, 1995.
229. King, L. M., Boucher, F., and Opie, L. H.: Coronary flow rate and glucose delivery as determinants of contracture in the ischaemic myocardium. J. Mol. Cell Cardiol. *27*:701–720, 1995.
230. Cross, H. R., Radda, G. K., and Clarke, K.: The role of Na^+/K^+ ATPase activity during low flow ischemia in preventing myocardial injury: A ^{31}P, ^{23}Na and ^{87}Rb NMR spectroscopic study. Mag. Res. Med. *in press*.
231. Owen, P., Dennis, S., and Opie, L. H.: Glucose flux rate regulates onset of ischemic contracture in globally underperfused rat hearts. Circ. Res. *66*:344–354, 1990.
232. Murry, C. E., Jennings, R. B., and Reimer, K. A.: Preconditioning with ischemia: A delay of lethal cell injury in ischemic myocardium. Circulation *74*:1124–1136, 1986.
233. Schott, R. J., Rohmann, S., Braun, E. R., and Schaper, W.: Ischemic preconditioning reduces infarct size in swine myocardium. Circ. Res. *66*:1133–1142, 1990.
234. Thornton, J. D., Liu, G. S., and Downey, J. M.: Pretreatment with pertussis toxin blocks the protective effects of preconditioning: Evidence for a G-protein mechanism. J. Mol. Cell Cardiol. *25*:311–320, 1993.
235. Ashraf, M., Suleiman, J., and Ahmad, M.: Ca^{2+} preconditioning elicits a unique protection against the Ca^{2+} paradox injury in rat heart. Role of adenosine. Circ. Res. *74*:360–367, 1994.
236. Niroomand, F., Weinbrenner, C., Weis, A., et al.: Impaired function of inhibitory G proteins during acute myocardial ischemia of canine hearts and its reversal during reperfusion and a second period of ischemia. Possible implications for the protective mechanism of ischemic preconditioning. Circ. Res. *76*:861–870, 1995.
237. Ytrehus, K., Liu, Y., and Downey, J.: Preconditioning protects ischemic rabbit heart by protein kinase C activation. Am. J. Physiol. *266*:H1145–H1152, 1994.
238. Ottani, F., Galvani, M., Ferrini, D., et al.: Prodromal angina limits infarct size. A role for ischemic preconditioning. Circulation *91*:291–297, 1995.
239. Kloner, R. A., Shook, T., Przyklenk, K., and TIMI-4 Investigators: Previous angina alters in-hospital outcome in TIMI-4. A clinical correlate to preconditioning? Circulation *91*:37–45, 1995.
240. Cohen, M. V., Yang, X.-M., and Downey, J. M.: Conscious rabbits become tolerant to multiple episodes of ischemic preconditioning. Circ. Res. *74*:998–1004, 1994.
241. Rahimtoola, S. H.: The hibernating myocardium. Am. Heart J. *117*:211–221, 1989.
242. Maes, A., Flameng, W., Nuyts, J., et al.: Histological alterations in chronically hypoperfused myocardium. Correlation with PET findings. Circulation *90*:735–745, 1994.
243. vom Dahl, J., Eitzman, D. T., Al-Aouar, Z. R., et al.: Relation of regional function, perfusion, and metabolism in patients with advanced coronary artery disease undergoing surgical revascularization. Circulation *90*:2356–2366, 1994.
244. Vanoverschelde, J.-L., Wijns, W., Depre, C., et al.: Mechanisms of chronic regional post-ischemic dysfunction in humans. New insights from the study of noninfarcted collateral-dependent myocardium. Circulation *87*:1513–1523, 1993.
245. Shen, Y.-T., and Vatner, S. F.: Mechanism of impaired myocardial function during progressive coronary stenosis in conscious pigs. Hibernation versus stunning? Circ. Res. *76*:479–488, 1995.
246. Heyndrickx, G. R., Baig, H., Nellens, P., et al.: Depression of regional blood flow and wall thickening after brief coronary occlusions. Am. J. Physiol. *234*:H653–H659, 1978.
247. Braunwald, F., and Kloner, R. A.: The stunned myocardium: Prolonged, postischemic ventricular dysfunction. Circulation *66*:1146–1149, 1982.
248. Bolli, R., Hartley, C. J., and Rabinovitz, R. S.: Clinical relevance of myocardial "stunning." *In* Opie, L. H. (ed.): Stunning, Hibernation, and Calcium in Myocardial Ischemia and Reperfusion. Boston, Kluwer Academic Publishers, 1992, pp. 56–82.
249. Opie, L. H.: Reperfusion injury and its pharmacological modification. Circulation *80*:1049–1062, 1989.
250. Kusuoka, H., and Marban, E.: Cellular mechanism of myocardial stunning. Annu. Rev. Physiol. *54*:243–256, 1992.
251. Gao, W. D., Atar, D., Backx, P. H., and Marban, E.: Relationship between intracellular calcium and contractile force in stunned myocardium. Direct evidence for decreased myofilament Ca^{2+} responsiveness and altered diastolic function in intact ventricular muscle. Circ. Res. *76*:1036–1048, 1995.
252. Hearse, D. J.: Stunning: A radical re-view. Cardiovasc. Drugs Ther. *5*:853–876, 1991.
253. Lee, J. A., and Allen, D. G.: Mechanisms of acute ischemic contractile failure of the heart. Role of the intracellular calcium. J. Clin. Invest. *88*:361–367, 1991.
254. Du Toit, E. F., and Opie, L. H.: Modulation of severity of reperfusion stunning in the isolated rat heart by agents altering calcium flux at onset of reperfusion. Circ. Res. *70*:960–967, 1992.
255. Du Toit, E. F., and Opie, L. H.: Role for the Na^+/H^+ exchanger in reperfusion stunning in isolated perfused rat heart. J. Cardiovasc. Pharmacol. *22*:877–883, 1993.
256. Smart, S., Schultz, J., Sagar, K., and Warltier, D.: Intracoronary doxorubicin, but not intracoronary verapamil, improves recovery of postischemic function. J. Am. Coll. Cardiol. *21*(Abs.):164A, 1993.
257. Matsuura, H., and Shattock, M. J.: Membrane potential fluctuations and transient inward currents induced by reactive oxygen intermediates in isolated rabbit ventricular cells. Circ. Res. *68*:319–329, 1991.
258. Jabr, R. I., and Cole, W. C.: Alterations in electrical activity and membrane currents induced by intracellular oxygen-derived free radical stress in guinea pig ventricular myocytes. Circ. Res. *72*:1229–1244, 1993.
259. Kusuoka, H., Camilion de Hurtado, M. C., and Marban, E.: Role of sodium-calcium exchange in the mechanism of myocardial stunning: Protective effect of reperfusion with high sodium solution. J. Am. Coll. Cardiol. *21*:240–248, 1993.
260. Brunner, F., Du Toit, E. F., and Opie, L. H.: Endothelin release during ischaemia and reperfusion of isolated perfused rat hearts. J. Mol. Cell Cardiol. *24*:1291–1305, 1993.
261. Mouton, R., Genade, S., Huisamen, B., et al.: The effect of ischaemia-reperfusion on [3H]inositol phosphates and Ins(1,4,5)P3 levels in cardiac atria and ventricles—a comparative study. Mol. Cell Biochem. *115*:195–202, 1992.
262. Du Toit, E. F., and Opie, L. H.: Antiarrhythmic properties of specific inhibitors of sarcoplasmic reticulum calcium ATPase in the isolated perfused rat heart after coronary artery litigation. J. Am. Coll. Cardiol. *23*:1505–1510, 1994.
263. Opie, L. H.: Chronic stunning: The new switch in thought. Invited Comment. Basic Res. Cardiol. *90*:303–304, 1995.
264. Sadoshima, J., Qiu, Z., Morgan, J. P., and Izumo, S.: Angiotensin-II and other hypertrophic stimuli mediated by G protein–coupled receptors activate tyrosine kinase, mitogen-activated protein kinase, and 90-kD S6 kinase in cardiac myocytes. The critical role of Ca^{2+}-dependent signaling. Circ. Res. *76*:1–15, 1995.
265. Edwards, G., and Weston, A. H.: Pharmacology of the potassium channel openers. Cardiovasc. Drugs Ther. *9*:185–193, 1995.
266. Opie, L. H.: Stunning, Hibernation, and Calcium in Myocardial Ischemia and Reperfusion. Boston, Kluwer Academic Publishers, 1992.

Chapter 13
Pathophysiology of Heart Failure

WILSON S. COLUCCI, EUGENE BRAUNWALD

Heart (or cardiac) failure is the pathophysiological state in which the heart is unable to pump blood at a rate commensurate with the requirements of the metabolizing tissues or can do so only from an elevated filling pressure. It is usually, but not always, caused by a defect in myocardial contraction, i.e., by *myocardial failure*. However, in some patients with heart failure, a similar clinical syndrome is present, but there is no detectable abnormality of *myocardial* function. In many such cases heart failure is caused by conditions in which the normal heart is suddenly presented with a load that exceeds its capacity or in which ventricular filling is impaired.[1] *Heart failure* should be distinguished from *circulatory failure*, in which an abnormality of some component of the circulation—the heart, the blood volume, the concentration of oxygenated hemoglobin in the arterial blood, or the vascular bed—is responsible for the inadequate cardiac output.

Thus, the terms myocardial failure, heart failure, and circulatory failure are not synonymous, but refer to progressively more inclusive entities. Myocardial failure, when sufficiently severe, always causes heart failure, but the converse is not necessarily the case, because a number of conditions in which the heart is suddenly overloaded (e.g., acute aortic regurgitation secondary to acute infective endocarditis) can cause heart failure in the presence of normal myocardial function, at least early in the course of the illness. Also, conditions such as tricuspid stenosis and constrictive pericarditis, which interfere with cardiac filling, can cause heart failure without myocardial failure. Heart failure, in turn, always causes circulatory failure, but again the converse is not necessarily the case, because a variety of noncardiac conditions, e.g., hypovolemic shock, can produce circulatory failure at a time when cardiac function is normal or only modestly impaired.

The hemodynamic, contractile, and wall motion disorders in heart failure are discussed in the chapters on echocardiography (Chap. 3), cardiac catheterization (Chap. 6), radionuclide imaging (Chap. 9), and assessment of cardiac function (Chap. 14). In this chapter, the focus is on the physiological, neurohumoral, biochemical, and cellular changes characteristic of heart failure.

ADAPTIVE MECHANISMS

In the presence of a primary disturbance in myocardial contractility or an excessive hemodynamic burden placed on the ventricle, or both, the heart depends on a number of adaptive mechanisms for maintenance of its pumping function[2,3] (Table 13–1). Most important among these are (1) the Frank-Starling mechanism, in which an increased preload helps to sustain cardiac performance (see p. 378); (2) myocardial hypertrophy with or without cardiac chamber dilatation, in which the mass of contractile tissue is augmented (see p. 399); and (3) activation of neurohumoral systems, especially the release of the neurotransmitter norepinephrine (NE) by adrenergic cardiac nerves (see p. 408), which augments myocardial contractility and the activation of the renin-angiotensin-aldosterone system (see p. 446), and other neurohumoral adjustments (see p. 414) that act to maintain arterial pressure and perfusion of vital organs. In acute heart failure, these adaptive mechanisms may be adequate to maintain the overall pumping performance of the heart at relatively normal levels. However, the capacity of each of these mechanisms to sustain cardiac performance in the face of hemodynamic overload relative to myocardial contractility is finite and, when chronically maintained, becomes maladaptive (Fig. 13–1).

Cardiac output is often depressed and the arterial–mixed venous oxygen difference is widened in the basal state in patients with the common forms of heart failure secondary to ischemic heart disease, hypertension, primary myocardial disease, valvular disease, and pericardial disease (so-called low-output heart failure).[4,5] In cases of mild heart failure, the cardiac output may be normal at rest but fails to rise normally during exercise (see p. 451).[5] When the volume of blood delivered into the systemic arterial bed is chronically reduced, and/or when one or both ventricles has an elevated filling pressure, a complex sequence of adjustments occurs that ultimately results in the retention of sodium and water in the intravascular and interstitial compartments (see Chap. 62).[6] Many of the clinical manifestations of heart failure such as dyspnea and edema are secondary to this excessive retention of fluid (see Chap. 15).

Interactions Between Frank-Starling Mechanism and Adrenergic Nervous System in Heart Failure

It may be useful to consider the function of the normal and failing heart within the framework of the Frank-Starling mechanism, in which an increase in preload, reflected in an elevation of end-diastolic volume, augments ventricular performance. The normal relationship between ventricular end-diastolic volume and performance is shown in Figure 13–2, curve 1. During exercise and other stresses, the increases in adrenergic nerve impulses to the myocardium, the concentration of circulating catecholamines (see p. 374), and tachycardia all augment myocardial contractil-

TABLE 13–1 SHORT-TERM AND LONG-TERM RESPONSES TO IMPAIRED CARDIAC PERFORMANCE

RESPONSE	SHORT-TERM EFFECTS*	LONG-TERM EFFECTS†
Salt and water retention	Augments preload	Causes pulmonary congestion, anasarca
Vasoconstriction	Maintains blood pressure for perfusion of vital organs (brain, heart)	Exacerbates pump dysfunction (afterload mismatch); increases cardiac energy expenditure
Sympathetic stimulation	Increases heart rate and ejection	Increases energy expenditure
Sympathetic desensitization	—	Spares energy
Hypertrophy	Unloads individual muscle fibers	Leads to deterioration and death of cardiac cells; cardiomyopathy of overload
Capillary deficit	—	Leads to energy starvation
Mitochondrial density	Increase in density helps meet energy demands	Decrease in density leads to energy starvation
Appearance of slow myosin	—	Increases force, decreases shortening velocity and contractility; is energy-sparing
Prolonged action potential	—	Increases contractility and energy expenditure
Decreased density of sarcoplasmic reticulum calcium-pump sites	—	Slows relaxation; may be energy-sparing
Increased collagen	May reduce dilatation	Impairs relaxation

* Short-term effects are mainly adaptive and occur after hemorrhage and in acute heart failure.
† Long-term effects are mainly deleterious and occur in chronic heart failure.
Reprinted by permission from Katz, A. M.: Cardiomyopathy of overload: A major determinant of prognosis in congestive heart failure. N. Engl. J. Med. *322*:100, 1990. Copyright Massachuetts Medical Society.

ity with a shift from curve 1 to curve 2. Ventricular performance, as reflected in stroke work or cardiac output, increases with little change in end-diastolic pressure and volume. This is represented by a shift from point A to point B in Figure 13–2. Vasodilation occurs in the exercising muscles, reducing peripheral vascular resistance and aortic impedance. This ultimately allows achievement of a greatly elevated cardiac output during exercise, at an arterial pressure only slightly greater than in the resting state. During intense exercise, cardiac output can rise to a maximal level if use is made of the Frank-Starling mechanism, as reflected in modest increases in the left ventricular end-diastolic volume and pressure (point B to point C).

In moderately severe systolic heart failure, as represented by curve 3, cardiac output and external ventricular performance at rest are within normal limits but are maintained at these levels only because the end-diastolic fiber

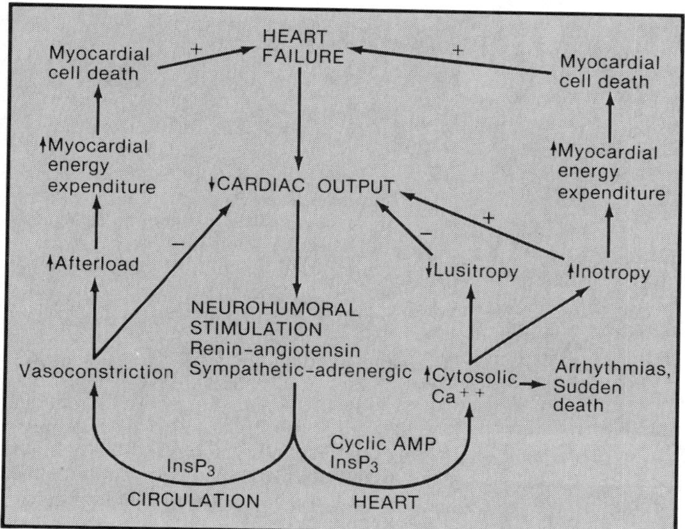

FIGURE 13–1. The low-output state can accelerate the rate of cell death in the failing heart by stimulating the renin-angiotensin and sympathetic-adrenergic systems, which act on both the circulation and the heart. Vasoconstriction increases afterload, which further decreases cardiac output; the increased afterload may also accelerate the rate of myocardial cell death by increasing the work of the heart. In the heart, increased concentrations of cyclic AMP and inositol-1,4,5-tris phosphate ($InsP_3$) promote calcium entry, augmenting contractility; along with a chronotropic response (not shown), this inotropic response increases cardiac output and is thus compensatory. However, the increased amount of calcium that enters the cytosol can overload the systems that pump this ion out of the cell during diastole, thus impairing relaxation. Calcium overload may also induce arrhythmias and lead to sudden death. Because the inotropic and chronotropic responses to sympathetic-adrenergic stimulation increase myocardial energy expenditure, they may also accelerate the rate of cell death in the failing heart. Thus, when the initial adaptive responses of both the circulation and the heart to a chronic low-output state become sustained, they can have deleterious long-term effects in patients with congestive heart failure. (Reprinted with permission from Katz, A. M.: Cardiomyopathy of overload: A major determinant of prognosis in congestive heart failure. N. Engl. J. Med. *322*:100, 1990. Copyright Massachusetts Medical Society.)

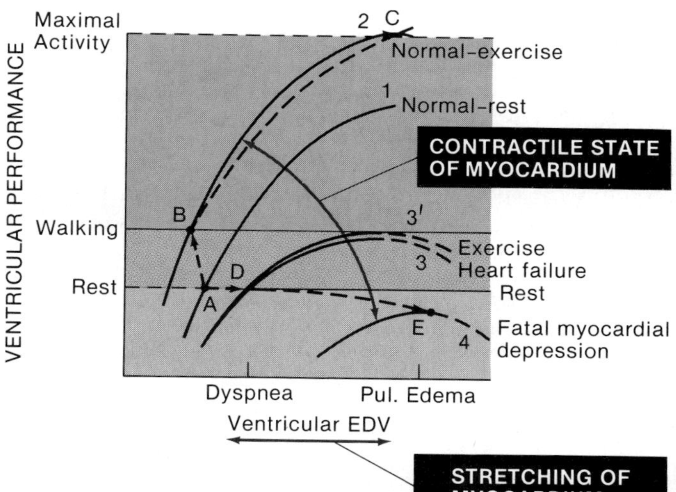

FIGURE 13–2. Diagram showing the interrelationship of influences on ventricular end-diastolic volume (EDV) through stretching of the myocardium and the contractile state of the myocardium. Levels of ventricular EDV associated with filling pressures that result in dyspnea and pulmonary edema are shown on the abscissa. Levels of ventricular performance required during rest, walking, and maximal activity are designated on the ordinate. The dotted lines are the descending limbs of the ventricular performance curves, which are rarely seen during life but which show what the level of ventricular performance would be if end-diastolic volume could be elevated to very high levels. (Modified from Braunwald, E., Ross, J., Jr., and Sonnenblick, E. H.: Mechanisms of Contraction of the Normal and Failing Heart. Boston, Little, Brown and Co., 1968.)

length and the ventricular end-diastolic volume (ventricular preload) are elevated, i.e., through the operation of the Frank-Starling mechanism. The elevations of left ventricular diastolic pressure are associated with abnormally high levels of pulmonary capillary pressure, contributing to the dyspnea experienced by patients with heart failure, sometimes even at rest (point D).

Heart failure is frequently accompanied by reductions in NE stores and myocardial beta-adrenoceptor density (see p. 410) and therefore in the inotropic response to impulses in the cardiac adrenergic nerves. As a consequence, ventricular function (performance) curves cannot be elevated to normal levels by the adrenergic nervous system, and the normal improvement of contractility that takes places during exercise is attenuated (curves 3 and 3′). The factors that tend to augment ventricular filling during exercise push the failing ventricle even farther along its flattened, depressed function curve, and there is an inordinate elevation of ventricular end-diastolic volume and pressure and therefore of pulmonary capillary pressure.[7] The elevation of the latter intensifies dyspnea and plays an important role in limiting the intensity of exercise that the patient can perform. According to this formulation, left ventricular failure becomes fatal when the left ventricular function curve becomes depressed (curve 4) to the point at which either cardiac output is insufficient to satisfy the requirements of the peripheral tissue at rest or the left ventricular end-diastolic and pulmonary capillary pressures are elevated to levels that result in pulmonary edema, or both (point E).

REDISTRIBUTION OF LEFT VENTRICULAR OUTPUT. Heart failure is characterized by generalized adrenergic activation (see p. 412) and parasympathetic withdrawal[8] (see p. 413), as illustrated in Figure 13–3. This leads to tachycardia, sodium retention, renin release, and generalized systemic vasoconstriction. Maintenance of arterial pressure in the presence of a reduced cardiac output is a primitive but effective compensatory mechanism. In hypovolemia and heart failure, this important mechanism is brought into play in order to allow the limited cardiac output to be most useful for survival. Vasoconstriction, mediated in part by the adrenergic nervous system, plays an important role in

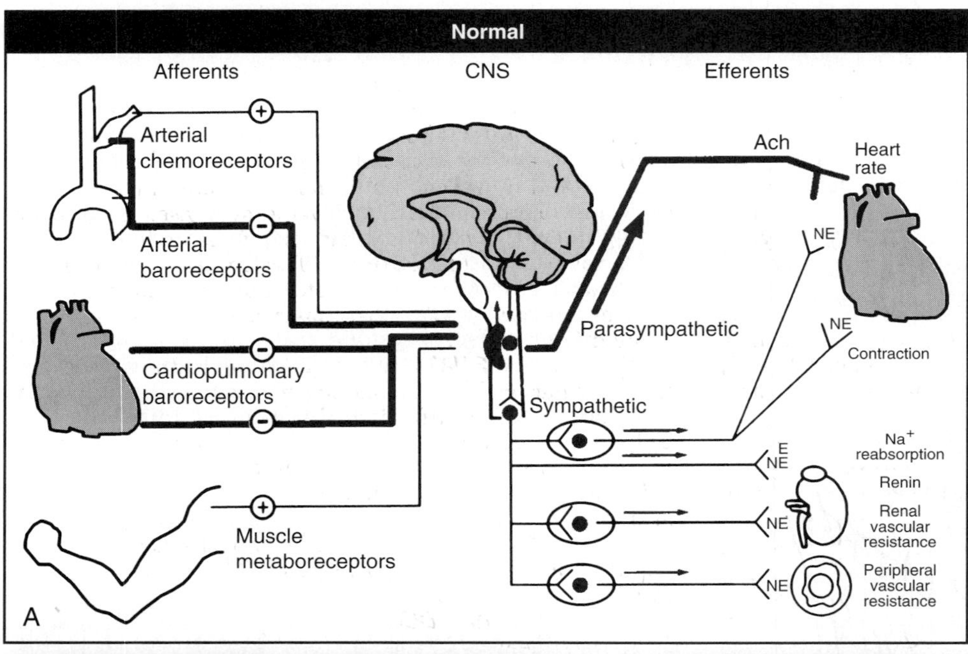

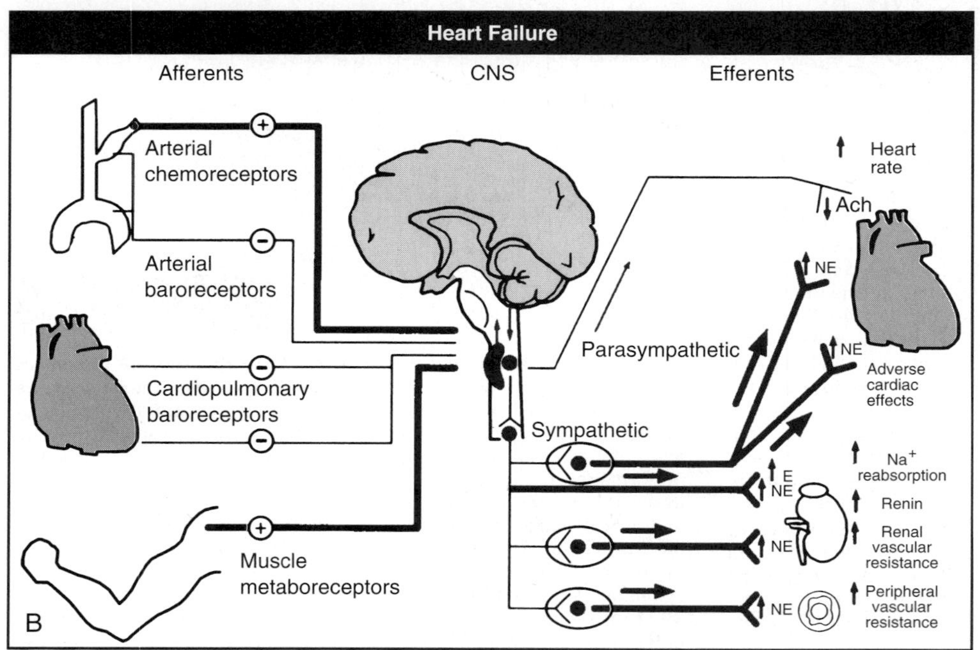

FIGURE 13–3. Mechanisms for generalized sympathetic activation and parasympathetic withdrawal in heart failure. *A,* Under normal conditions, inhibitory (−) inputs from arterial and cardiopulmonary baroreceptor afferent nerves are the principal influence on sympathetic outflow. Parasympathetic control of heart rate is also under potent arterial baroreflex control. Efferent sympathetic traffic and arterial catecholamines are low and heart rate variability high. *B,* As heart failure progresses, inhibitory input from arterial and cardiopulmonary receptors decreases and excitatory (+) input increases. The net response to this altered balance includes a generalized increase in sympathetic nerve traffic, blunted parasympathetic and sympathetic control of heart rate, and impairment of the reflex sympathetic regulation of vascular resistance. Anterior wall ischemia has additional excitatory effects on efferent sympathetic nerve traffic. See text for details. Ach = acetylcholine; CNS = central nervous system; E = epinephrine; Na^+ = sodium; NE = norepinephrine. (From Floras, J. S.: Clinical aspects of sympathetic activation and parasympathetic withdrawal in heart failure. Reprinted with permission from the American College of Cardiology. J. Am. Coll. Cardiol. *22:*72A, 1993.)

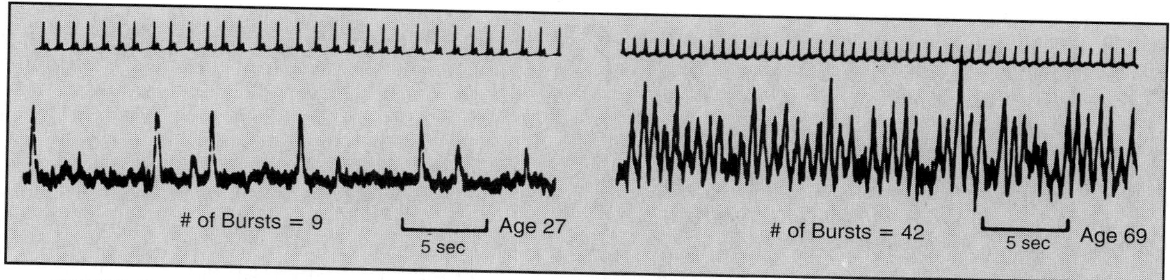

FIGURE 13–4. Representative tracings of the electrocardiograms *(upper tracings)* and mean voltage neurograms of muscle sympathetic nerve activity *(lower tracings)* in a normal subject *(left)* and a patient with heart failure *(right)*. (Reproduced by permission from Leimbach, W. N., Walling, B. G., Victor, R. G., et al.: Direct evidence from intraneural recordings for increased central sympathetic outflow in patients with heart failure. Circulation *73*:913, 1986. Copyright 1986 American Heart Association.)

this redistribution of peripheral blood flow. Neurograms obtained from adrenergic nerves to the limbs display an increased traffic in heart failure (Fig. 13–4).[9] In patients with moderately severe heart failure, in whom the cardiac output at rest is normal, abnormal vasoconstriction occurs when an additional burden (such as exercise, fever, or anemia) is imposed on the circulation and the cardiac output does not rise normally to meet the peripheral demands. As cardiac performance declines, left ventricular output is ultimately redistributed, even at rest.[10–13] This redistribution maintains the delivery of oxygen to vital organs such as the brain and heart, while blood flow to less crucial areas, such as the skin, skeletal muscle, and kidney, is reduced.[14,15] This underperfusion of skeletal muscle leads to anaerobic metabolism,[16] lactic acidosis, an excess oxygen debt, weakness, and fatigue. Occasionally, serious complications can result from the redistribution of cardiac output and the resulting regional reductions of blood flow. These include marked sodium and nitrogen retention as a consequence of diminished renal perfusion (see Chap. 62) and, very rarely, gangrene of the tips of the phalanges and mesenteric infarction.

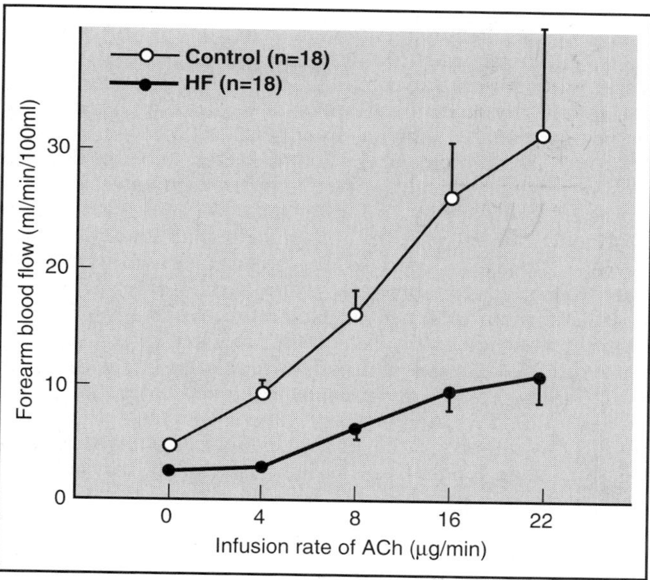

FIGURE 13–5. Responses of forearm blood flow (FBF) to acetylcholine in patients with heart failure (HF) (●) and in control subjects (○). The FBF at rest and during infusion of acetylcholine (ACh) was less in patients with heart failure than in control subjects. The magnitudes of the increases in FBF in response to ACh were less in patients with heart failure than in control subjects. In contrast, the responses to sodium nitroprusside were comparable. (Reproduced by permission from Hirooka, Y., Imaizumi, T., Tagawa, T., et al.: Effects of L-arginine on impaired acetylcholine-induced and ischemic vasodilation of the forearm in patients with heart failure. Circulation *90*:658, 1994. Copyright 1994 American Heart Association.)

ENDOTHELIAL DYSFUNCTION. Both ischemia and exercise-induced vasodilation in the extremities are attenuated in patients with heart failure.[17] This attenuation is related in part to endothelial dysfunction (see p. 1166). The response of blood flow to infused acetylcholine and methacholine, endothelium-dependent vasodilators, is reduced in heart failure (Fig. 13–5). The vasodilator response can be restored by the administration of L-arginine, a precursor of endothelium-derived nitric oxide.[18,19] These findings suggest that defective endothelial function contributes to the impaired vasodilator capacity in heart failure. The mechanisms potentially responsible include impaired endothelial cell receptor function, deficiency of L-arginine substrate, abnormal expression of nitric oxide synthase, and the impaired release or rapid degradation of the endothelium-derived relaxing factor, nitric oxide.[19] In addition to abnormalities in endothelial vasodilator function, the release by the endothelium of the vasoconstrictor endothelin is augmented (see p. 415).

CHANGES IN THE VASCULAR WALL. The sodium content of the vascular wall is increased in heart failure, and this contributes to the stiffening, thickening, and compression of blood vessel walls, which raises vascular resistance and also prevents normal vasodilation during exercise.[12] The veins in the extremities of patients with heart failure are also constricted by the activity of the adrenergic nervous system as well as by circulating venoconstrictors (norepinephrine and angiotensin II). This venoconstriction results in displacement of blood to the heart and lungs.

2,3-DIPHOSPHOGLYCERATE. A progressive decline in the affinity of hemoglobin for oxygen due to an increase in 2,3-diphosphoglycerate (DPG) also occurs in heart failure.[20] The rightward shift in the oxygen-hemoglobin dissociation curve represents a compensatory mechanism that facilitates oxygen transport; the increased DPG, tissue acidosis, and the slowed circulation characteristic of heart failure act synergistically to maintain the delivery of oxygen to the metabolizing tissues in the face of a reduced cardiac output.

CONTRACTILITY OF HYPERTROPHIED AND FAILING MYOCARDIUM

When an excessive pressure or volume load is imposed on the ventricle, myocardial hypertrophy develops, providing one of the aforementioned key compensatory mechanisms that permits the ventricle to sustain an increased load.[2,4,21] However, as described below, a ventricle subjected to an abnormally elevated load for a prolonged period may fail to maintain compensation despite the presence of ventricular hypertrophy, and pump failure may ultimately occur.

ISOLATED MUSCLE. Cardiac muscle isolated from animals in which the heart had been subjected to a controlled stress has been studied by many investigators. One convenient

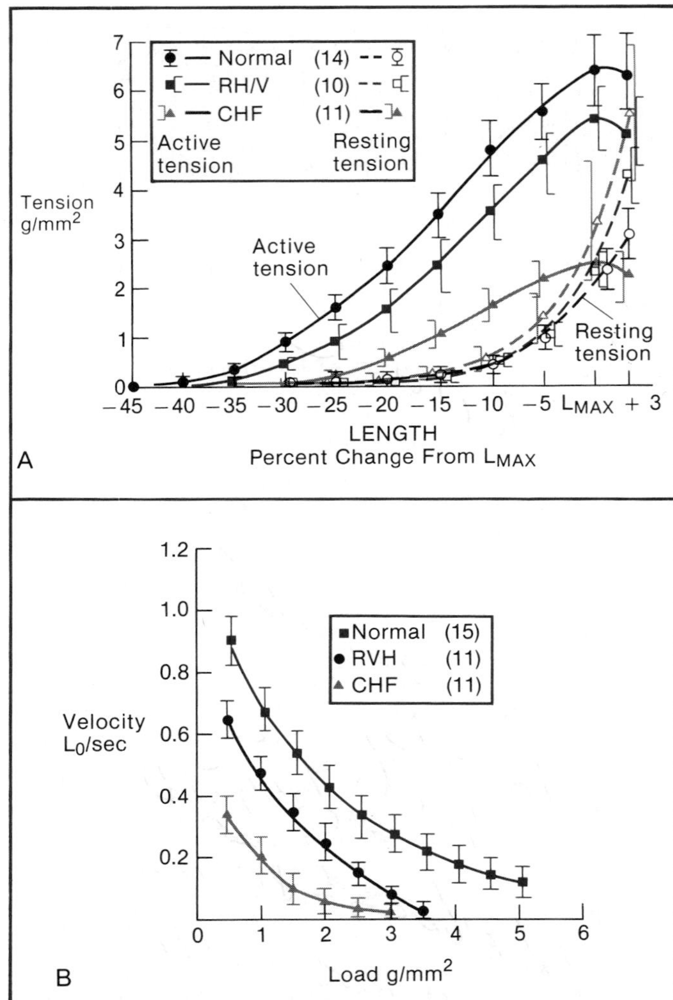

FIGURE 13–6. *A,* **Relation between muscle length and tension of papillary muscles from normal (circles), hypertrophied (squares), and failing (triangles) right ventricles. Open symbols = resting tension; filled symbols = actively developed tension. Tension is corrected for cross-sectional area (g/mm²). Numbers in parentheses = number of animals.** *B,* **Force-velocity relations of the three groups of cat papillary muscles. Average values ± SEM are given for each point. Velocity has been corrected to muscle lengths per second (L_0/sec). (Reproduced by permission from Spann, J. F., Jr., Buccino, R. A., Sonnenblick, E. H., and Braunwald, E.: Contractile state of cardiac muscle obtained from cats with experimentally produced ventricular hypertrophy and heart failure. Circ. Res.** ***21*****:341, 1967. Copyright 1967 American Heart Association.)**

experimental model of ventricular pressure overload is the cat (or ferret) with pulmonary artery constriction. Papillary muscles are then removed from the right ventricles in which either hypertrophy or overt failure has developed, and the excised muscles are studied in vitro.[22,23] Both right ventricular hypertrophy and failure reduce the maximum velocity of (unloaded) shortening ($\dot{V}_{max}$) of excised muscle below the values observed in muscles obtained from normal cats. These changes are more marked in animals in which heart failure has been present than in those with hypertrophy alone (Fig. 13–6). Because the depression of myocardial contractility is evident in vitro, when the muscle's physical and chemical milieu is controlled, it is considered to be *intrinsic,* and not the result of any humoral or neural stimuli or abnormal loading conditions that are often present in vivo. The depression of contractility in hypertrophied myocardium is less marked or even absent when the stress is imposed slowly and when the measurements are made during a stable phase of the ventricular response to overload.[24]

The findings summarized above are, in general, consonant with those of a number of other investigations on cardiac muscle isolated from animals with experimentally produced pressure overload. For example, the trabeculae carnae or papillary muscles removed from the left ventricles of rats with left ventricular hypertrophy secondary to aortic constriction or renovascular hypertension also exhibit depression of the velocity of isotonic shortening and prolongation of duration of the action potential, of isometric contraction, and of the time-to-peak tension, even when the development of isometric tension is normal.[25] The force and rate of force development are also depressed in isometrically contracting myocardium obtained from hearts with totally different forms of heart failure (e.g., Syrian hamsters with hereditary cardiomyopathy), as well as papillary muscles removed from the left ventricles of patients with heart failure due to chronic valvular disease.[26] In contrast to the depressed performance of cardiac muscle removed from pressure-overloaded hearts, contractility has been found to be normal in papillary muscles removed from cats with a volume overload resulting from an experimentally produced atrial septal defect.[27]

In nonfailing myocardium, the force of contraction and rate of tension development rise with increased stimulation frequency, the so-called *positive force-frequency relationship* (Fig. 12–28, p. 380). However, there is evidence of an abnormal (negative) force-frequency relationship in failing human myocardium.[28] Gwathmey et al. showed in myocardium obtained from failing human hearts that pacing-induced tachycardia results in calcium accumulation.[29] These observations provide a potential explanation for the further deterioration of cardiac function that occurs with tachycardia in patients with heart failure and possibly for the beneficial effects of slowing the heart rate with beta blockade (see p. 486) or digitalis.

Structural Changes. There are a number of structural features of hypertrophied human myocytes (Fig. 13–7).[30] These include abnormal Z-band patterns, multiple intercalated discs, and prominent collagen fibrils connecting adjacent myocardial cells. Nuclei are enlarged and lobulated and contain well-developed nucleoli; there is an abundance of ribosomes, presumably reflecting enhanced protein synthesis. However, electron microscopic studies of myocardium removed from overloaded, dilated hearts fixed at the elevated filling pressures that existed during life have revealed sarcomere lengths averaging 2.2 μm—no longer than those at the apex of the length/active tension curve of normal cardiac muscle.[31] This finding indicates that the depressed contractility of failing heart muscle is *not* due to the disengagement of actin and myosin filaments.

INTACT HEARTS. Changes in performance of the intact heart subjected to abnormal hemodynamic loads are, in general, similar to those in isolated cardiac tissue. Thus, the right ventricles of cats with pulmonary artery constriction exhibit a marked depression paralleling that observed in the isolated papillary muscles removed from these ventricles.[32] When compared with normal values, the active tension developed by the right ventricle at equivalent end-diastolic fiber lengths is markedly reduced in cats with heart failure produced by pressure overload.

Immediately following the imposition of a volume overload (such as the opening of a large arteriovenous fistula), the contractility of the ventricle—as reflected in the end-systolic stress-circumference relationship—may actually increase, perhaps as a consequence of adrenergic stimulation. However, it then declines, while overall hemodynamic performance, i.e., cardiac work, is sustained.[33] Later in the course of a large volume overload, overt clinical heart failure develops, accompanied by increases in left ventricular end-diastolic volume and in the ratio of left ventricular weight to body weight and by depressed indices of left ventricular contractility[34,35] (see Chap. 14). As the ventricle fails, it moves to the right along a depressed performance (function) curve, so that it requires an abnormally elevated end-diastolic volume (and often an elevation of end-diastolic pressure as well) to generate a level of tension equal to that achieved by the normal heart at a normal end-diastolic volume (Fig. 13–1).

MYOCARDIAL HYPERTROPHY

PATTERNS OF VENTRICULAR HYPERTROPHY. The development of ventricular hypertrophy constitutes one of the principal mechanisms by which the heart compensates for an increased load.[36] One of the early cellular changes that occurs after a stimulus for hypertrophy is applied is the synthesis of mitochondria; presumably the expanded mitochondrial mass provides the high-energy phosphates required to meet the increased energy demands of the hypertrophied cell. This is accompanied by an expansion of the myofibrillar mass (Fig. 13–7). Myocytes isolated from patients with heart failure are longer than normal myocytes[37,38] (Fig. 13–8). After the neonatal period, the increase in myocardial mass is associated with a proportional increase in the size of individual cells, i.e., hypertrophy, without any increase in the number of cells (or a minimal increase), i.e., without hyperplasia.[2] These changes within the myocyte are accompanied by the laying down of interstitial collagen.[39]

There is evidence that hemodynamic overload reactivates growth factors present in the embryonic heart but dormant in the normal adult heart (Fig. 13–9). These reactivated growth factors accelerate protein synthesis.[3] Current understanding of the fundamental mechanisms responsible for hypertrophy is described on pages 747 to 748.

Grossman et al. examined systolic and diastolic wall stresses in normal subjects and in patients with chronic pressure- and volume-overloaded left ventricles who were compensated and not in heart failure.[40] Left ventricular mass was increased approximately equally in both the pressure- and volume-overloaded groups. There was a substantial increase in wall thickness in the pressure-overloaded ventricles but only a mild increase in wall thickness in the volume-overloaded ventricles (Fig. 13–10). The latter was just sufficient to counterbalance the increased radius, so that the ratio of wall thickness to radius remained normal for the patients with volume-overload hypertrophy. This ratio was substantially increased in patients with pressure-overload hypertrophy, in whom there was disproportionate thickening of the ventricular wall. These observations are consistent with those of other investigators, who have indicated that myocardial hypertrophy develops in a manner that maintains systolic stress within normal limits.[41–43] Thus, when the primary stimulus to hypertrophy is pressure overload, the resultant acute increase in systolic wall stress leads to parallel replication of myofibrils, thickening of individual myocytes,[44] and concentric hypertrophy. The wall thickening is usually sufficient to maintain a normal level of systolic stress (Fig. 13–11). When the primary stimulus is ventricular volume overload, increased diastolic wall stress leads to replication of sarcomeres in series, elongation of myocytes, and ventricular dilatation. This, in turn, results in a modest increase in systolic stress[45] (by the Laplace relationship), which causes proportional wall thickening that returns systolic stress toward normal. Thus, in compensated subjects, both volume and pressure overload alter ventricular geometry and wall thickness, so that systolic stress does not change greatly.

Left ventricular wall thickness is a crucial determinant of ventricular performance in patients with pressure-overload hypertrophy due to aortic stenosis or hypertension. Impaired performance in such patients may be secondary to inadequate hypertrophy leading to increased wall stress (afterload), which in turn may be responsible for inadequate muscle shortening. This condition has been termed "afterload-mismatch" by Ross.[46] His group found that when the aorta in conscious dogs was suddenly constricted, left ventricular systolic pressure rose, the left ventricle dilated, and the left ventricular wall thinned; this was associated with a large increase in wall stress and a reciprocal reduction in the extent and velocity of shortening.[47] During the next few weeks the left ventricle became hypertrophied and left ventricular wall stress and shortening both returned toward

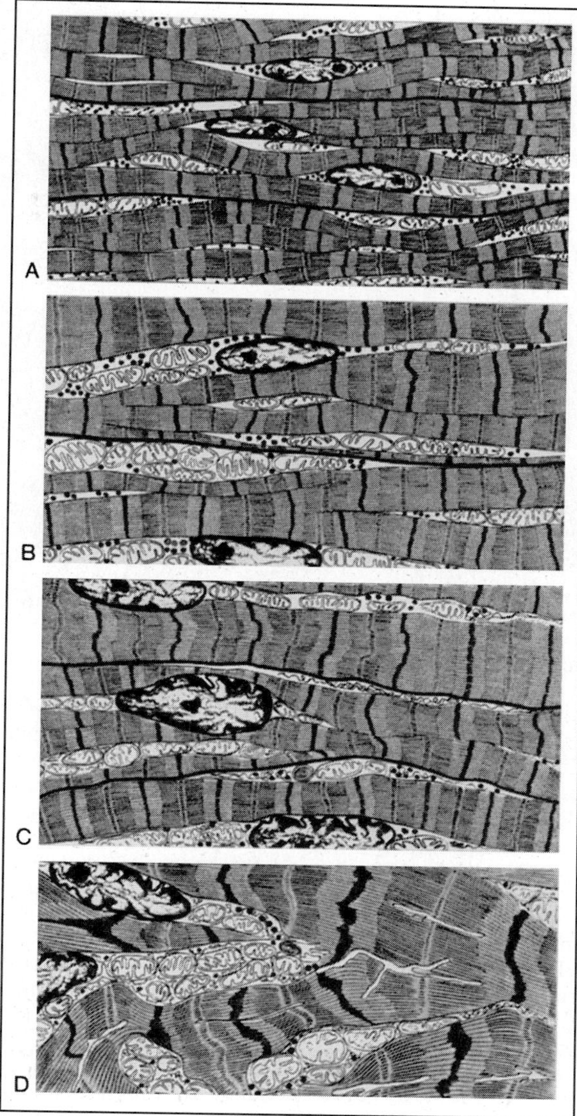

FIGURE 13–7. The early stage of cardiac hypertrophy *(A)* is characterized morphologically by increases in the number of myofibrils and mitochondria as well as enlargement of mitochondria and nuclei. Muscle cells are larger than normal, but cellular organization is largely preserved. At a more advanced stage of hypertrophy *(B)*, preferential increases in the size or number of specific organelles, such as mitochondria, as well as irregular addition of new contractile elements in localized areas of the cell, result in subtle abnormalities of cellular organization and contour. Adjacent cells may vary in their degree of enlargement. Cells subjected to longstanding hypertrophy *(C)* show more obvious disruptions in cellular organization, such as markedly enlarged nuclei with highly lobulated membranes, which displace adjacent myofibrils and cause breakdown of normal Z-band registration. The early preferential increase in mitochondria is supplanted by a predominance by volume of myofibrils. The late stage of hypertrophy *(D)* is characterized by loss of contractile elements with marked disruption of Z bands, severe disruption of the normal parallel arrangement of the sarcomeres, deposition of fibrous tissue, and dilation and increased tortuosity of T tubules. (From Ferrans, V. J.: Morphology of the heart in hypertrophy. Hosp. Pract. *18*:69, 1983. © 1983 The McGraw-Hill Companies, Inc.)

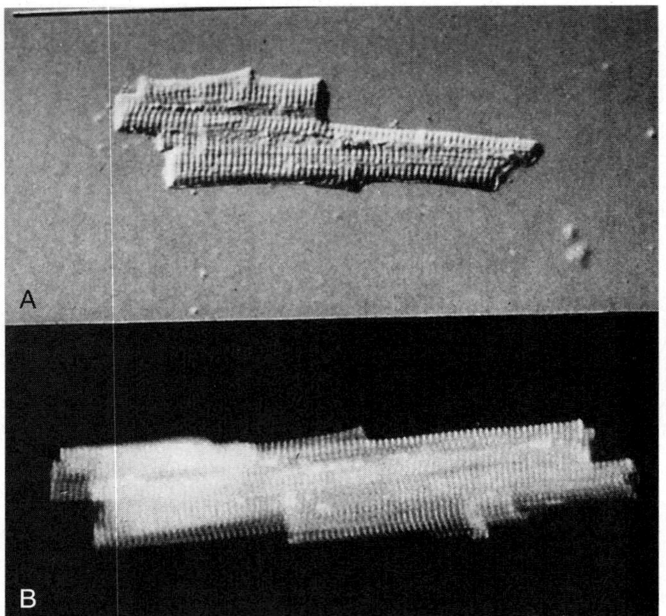

FIGURE 13–8. Isolated cardiac myocytes obtained from human left ventricular myocardium. *A,* Myocyte from a normal heart (bar = 100 μm). *B,* A hypertrophied myocyte from the left ventricle of a patient with ischemic cardiomyopathy, viewed at the same magnification as in *A.* This myocyte is longer than the normal myocyte. The myocytes have been stained with rhodamine-phalloidin for visualization of the sarcomere structure. In the myocyte from the failing heart, there has been addition of sarcomeres. These are otherwise organized in a normal pattern. (Modified by permission from Gerdes, A. M., et al.: Structural remodeling of cardiac myocytes in patients with ischemic cardiomyopathy. Circulation *86*:426, 1992. Copyright 1992 American Heart Association.)

normal. When the constriction was suddenly released, wall stress declined and shortening became supernormal.

Prolonged athletic training causes a moderate increase in myocardial mass.[48] Isotonic exercise, such as long-distance running or swimming, resembles volume overload and causes an increase in left ventricular diastolic volume, with only mild thickening of the wall. Isometric exercise, such as weightlifting or wrestling, resembles pressure overload and causes an increase in wall thickness. Neither form of hypertrophy appears to be deleterious in the absence of heart disease and rapidly disappears when training is discontinued.

DEVELOPMENT OF HEART FAILURE. When the ventricle is stressed, by either a pressure or a volume overload, the initial response is an increase in sarcomere length, so that the overlap between myofilaments becomes optimal, i.e., approximately 2.2 μm (see p. 360). This is followed by an increase in the total muscle mass, although, as already noted, the pattern of hypertrophy differs depending on whether the stress is a pressure load or a volume load (see p. 399).

When the hemodynamic overload is severe, myocardial contractility becomes depressed. In its mildest form, this depression is manifested by a reduction in the velocity of shortening of unloaded myocardium ($\dot{V}_{max}$) (Fig. 13–6) or by a reduction in the rate of force development during isometric contraction,[22] but by little if any reduction in the development of maximal isometric force or in the extent of shortening of afterloaded isotonic contractions. As myocardial contractility becomes further depressed, a more extensive reduction in $\dot{V}_{max}$ occurs, now accompanied by a decline in isometric force development and shortening. At this point, circulatory compensation may still be provided by cardiac dilation and an increase in muscle mass, which tend to maintain wall stress at normal levels. Although cardiac output and stroke volume remain normal in the

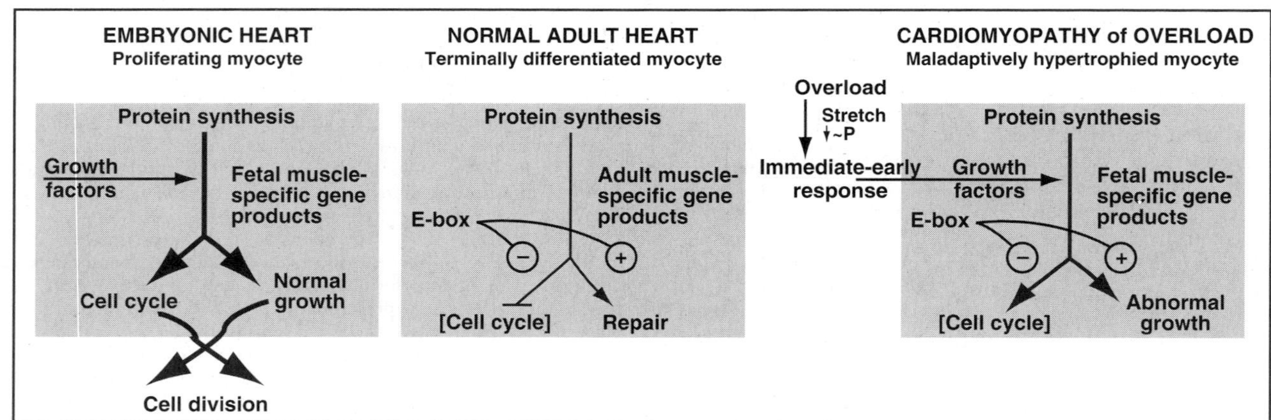

FIGURE 13–9. Overall growth pattern in the proliferating myocytes of the embryonic heart, the terminally differentiated myocytes of the normal adult heart, and the maladaptively hypertrophied myocytes of the failing heart. *Left,* In the embryonic heart, growth factors stimulate synthesis of fetal-specific gene products that, because protein synthesis is matched to active cell cycling, lead to normal cell division. *Center,* Withdrawal of growth factors and binding of myogenic factors to the E box (a DNA sequence found in muscle-specific genes) in the terminally differentiated cells of the normal adult heart slows protein synthesis, inhibits the cell cycle, and favors the synthesis of adult muscle-specific gene products. *Right,* Overloading of the adult heart initiates an immediate-early gene response that reactivates growth factor stimulation; this, in turn, accelerates protein synthesis and favors the expression of fetal muscle-specific gene products. However, because the cell cycle remains blocked, the overloaded heart undergoes an unnatural growth response which may lead to myocardial cell death. (From Katz, A. M.: The cardiomyopathy of overload: An unnatural growth response in the hypertrophied heart. Ann. Intern. Med. *121*:363, 1994.)

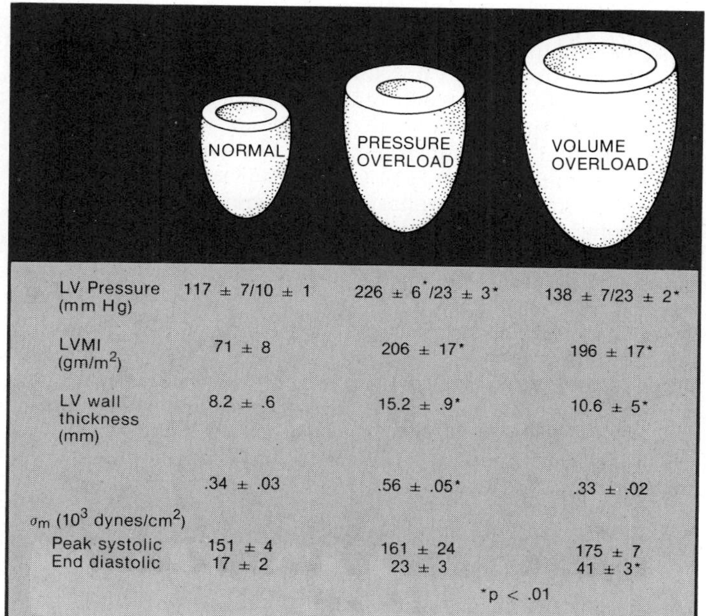

NORMAL
PRESSURE OVERLOAD
VOLUME OVERLOAD
LV Pressure (mm Hg) 117 ± 7/10 ± 1 226 ± 6*/23 ± 3* 138 ± 7/23 ± 2*
LVMI (gm/m2) 71 ± 8 206 ± 17* 196 ± 17*
LV wall thickness (mm) 8.2 ± .6 15.2 ± .9* 10.6 ± 5*
.34 ± .03 .56 ± .05* .33 ± .02
σm (10^3 dynes/cm^2)
Peak systolic 151 ± 4 161 ± 24 175 ± 7
End diastolic 17 ± 2 23 ± 3 41 ± 3*
*p < .01

FIGURE 13–10. Mean values for left ventricular (LV) pressure, mass index (LVMI), left ventricular wall thickness, the ratio of wall thickness to radius (h/R), and peak systolic and end-diastolic meridional wall stress in patients with normal (6 subjects), pressure-overloaded (6 subjects), and volume-overloaded (18 subjects) ventricles. Although mass is increased similarly in both pressure- and volume-overloaded groups, the increase is accomplished primarily by wall thickening in the pressure-overloaded group. The h/R ratio is normal in volume-overload hypertrophy, indicating a "magnification" type of growth. In pressure overload, concentric hypertrophy is quantified by the increase in h/R. Patients were compensated with respect to heart failure, and peak systolic tension (σ_m) was not statistically different from normal. However, end-diastolic stress was consistently elevated in the volume-overloaded group. See text for details. (Reproduced from Grossman, W., et al.: Wall stress and patterns of hypertrophy in the human left ventricle. J. Clin. Invest. *56*:56, 1975, by copyright permission of the American Society for Clinical Investigation.)

resting state, the ejection fraction at rest, as well as the maximal cardiac output that can be attained during stress, decline. As contractility falls further, overt congestive heart failure, reflected in a depression of cardiac output and work and/or an elevation of ventricular end-diastolic volume and pressure at rest, supervenes.

TRANSITION FROM HYPERTROPHY TO HEART FAILURE. As described by Meerson[49] (Table 13–2), immediately upon imposition of a large pressure load, the increase in work performed by the ventricle exceeds the augmentation of cardiac mass and the heart dilates. As a consequence, a

TABLE 13–2 THREE STAGES IN THE RESPONSE TO A SUDDEN HEMODYNAMIC OVERLOAD

Stage 1: (Days) Transient breakdown	
Circulatory:	Acute heart failure; pulmonary congestion, low output
Cardiac:	Acute left ventricular dilatation, early hypertrophy
Myocardial:	Increased content of mitochondria relative to myofibrils
Stage 2: (Weeks) Stable hyperfunction	
Circulatory:	Improved pulmonary congestion and cardiac output
Cardiac:	Established hypertrophy
Myocardial:	Increased content of myofibrils relative to mitochondria
Stage 3: (Months) Exhaustion and progressive cardiosclerosis	
Circulatory:	Progressive left ventricular failure
Cardiac:	Further hypertrophy with progressive fibrosis
Myocardial:	Cell death

From Katz, A. M.: Energy requirements of contraction and relaxation: Implications of inotropic stimulation of the failing heart. *In* Just, H., Holubarsch, C., and Scholz, H. (eds.): Inotropic Stimulation and Myocardial Energetics. New York, Springer-Verlag, 1989, p. 49.

compensatory phase sets in as the ventricle hypertrophies, and the contractile function returns to approximately normal levels. Mitochondria proliferate, and myofibrils are laid down in parallel and sarcomeres in series so that both the length and cross-sectional diameter of myocytes is increased[44] (Fig. 13–7). Later, alterations in cellular organization take place. In what Meerson has termed the "exhaustion" phase several events take place: (1) there is lysis of myofibrils, (2) lysosomes increase in number (presumably to digest worn-out cell constituents), (3) the sarcoplasmic reticulum becomes distorted,[30] (4) the surface densities of the key tubular system are reduced, and (5) fibrous tissue takes the place of cardiac cells.[50] In addition, capillary density and coronary reserve, as reflected in the increase in coronary blood flow during adenosine infusion (see p. 289), become reduced.[51] The resulting ischemia, most severe in the subendocardium (Fig. 36–15, p. 1170), may contribute further to the impairment of cardiac function. Myocyte function then deteriorates (see p. 1179), and overt heart failure occurs.

MYOCYTE NECROSIS. This is an important component of the transition to heart failure. Myocyte necrosis may be localized, as in myocardial infarction, which affects the ventricle in a manner analogous to a volume overload, with an increase both in diameter and length of the remaining cells. Necrosis may be diffuse, as in ischemic cardiomyopathy[36] or idiopathic dilated cardiomyopathy, or as in myocardium damaged by toxic agents such as daunorubicin (see p. 1800) or by myocarditis. Regardless of the cause of

FIGURE 13–11. The normal (N) relationship between LV wall thickness (h) and chamber radius (r) is shown *(first panel)*. An acute increase in systolic pressure (acute load) causes an increase in systolic wall stress, which can be approximated by the equation P × r/h, where P is LV systolic pressure. Diastolic wall stress is also increased when there is chamber dilatation or when diastolic pressure is elevated *(second panel)*. If sufficient compensatory hypertrophy occurs, the increase in ventricular wall thickness may normalize the systolic and diastolic wall stresses *(third panel)*. However, if additional chamber dilatation occurs or the increase in wall thickness is insufficient, systolic and diastolic wall stresses remain abnormally elevated. In this situation, further chamber dilatation may occur in association with hemodynamic failure *(fourth panel)*. (From Thaik, C. M., and Colucci, W. S.: Molecular and cellular events in myocardial hypertrophy and failure. *In* Colucci, W. S. (ed.): Heart Failure: Cardiac Function and Dysfunction, Atlas of Heart Diseases. Vol. 4. St. Louis, Mosby-Year Book, 1995, pp. 4.1–4.15.)

	Normal	Acute load	Compensatory hypertrophy	Cardiac failure
LV systolic pressure	N	+	+	+
LV radius	N	+	+	+
LV wall thickness	N	N	+	+
LV diastolic volume	N	+	+/–	++
Systolic wall stress	N	+	N	+
Diastolic wall stress	N	+	N	+

myocyte death, the load on the remaining cells rises and leads to reactive hypertrophy, which may impair further the function of these myocytes. This may be responsible for a vicious circle.

Drop-out of individual myocytes has been observed in the senescent rat[52] and human heart (Chap. 50). Olivetti et al. reported a loss of an average of 38 million nuclei per year in aging people without cardiovascular disease. This loss in myocyte number was accompanied by a reciprocal increase in myocyte cell volume per nucleus, averaging 110 μm^3 per year, thereby preserving ventricular wall thickness.[53] This process may contribute to the development of cardiac dysfunction and, when there is an additional stress such as hypertension, to heart failure in the elderly (see Chap. 50).

Myocardial overload, regardless of cause, can lead to heart failure as a consequence of afterload mismatch, i.e., inadequate hypertrophy. A marked increase in wall stress (afterload) may cause ventricular dilatation, which causes a further increased wall stress, in turn reducing myocardial fiber shortening, leading to further dilatation, and creating a vicious circle.[54] However, excess afterload may also cause *intrinsic* myocardial contractility to decline. Thus, Aoyagi et al.[55] studied an animal model of pressure overload hypertrophy produced by gradually tightening a hydraulic constrictor around the ascending aorta. A depression of myocardial contractility, as assessed by *load-independent* contractility indices, occurred (Fig. 13–12). They concluded that the cardiac dysfunction in this model was not due to insufficient hypertrophy causing afterload mismatch but to a depression of the myocardium's *intrinsic* contractility. Impaired myocardial contractility has also been observed in patients with hypertension and fully compensatory ventricular hypertrophy, normal myocardial stress, and apparently normal pump function. Such patients have displayed reduction of intramural myocardial shortening, as determined by spatial modulation of magnetization, using magnetic resonance imaging techniques[56]; this reduction indicates a depression of myocardial contractility in the presence of apparently normal loading conditions.

The transition from pressure overload hypertrophy to heart failure in the rat with aortic stenosis can be delayed by means of inhibition of angiotensin-converting enzyme, indicating that the renin-angiotensin system contributes to this transition (see p. 413).[57] There is experimental evidence that impaired coronary reserve and inadequate subendocardial blood flow contribute to the transition as well. Thus, Vatner et al. have demonstrated a diminished response of endocardial blood flow to adenosine and exercise-induced vasodilation in dogs with pressure overload hypertrophy.[58] This is caused in part by hypertrophy and in part by an exercise-induced increase in left ventricular subendocardial wall stress. The reduced subendocardial perfusion in turn may cause subendocardial ischemic injury and replacement fibrosis, which impair both systolic and diastolic function, accelerating the development of heart failure (Fig. 36–15, p. 1170).

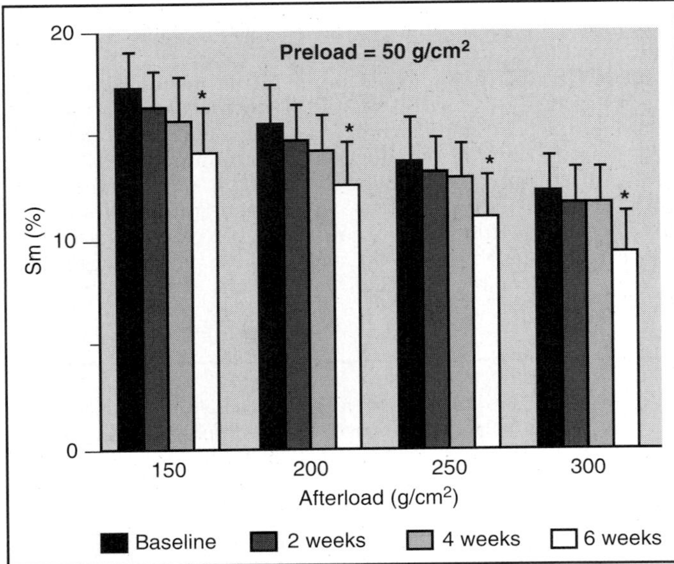

FIGURE 13–12. Time course of myocardial contractility following gradual imposition of a pressure load. Sm indicates midwall shortening at common preload of 50 g/cm² and various afterloads. Significant depression of myocardial contractility was detected (*P < .05) at the sixth week of the aortic constriction. (Reproduced by permission from Aoyagi, T., Fujii, A. M., Flanagan, M. F., et al.: Transition from compensated hypertrophy to intrinsic myocardial dysfunction during development of left ventricular pressure-overload hypertrophy in conscious sheep. Systolic dysfunction precedes diastolic dysfunction. Circulation *88*:2415, 1993. Copyright 1993 American Heart Association.)

PATHOPHYSIOLOGY OF DIASTOLIC HEART FAILURE

(See also pp. 447 and 503)

Alterations in Diastolic Properties

Approximately one-third of patients with congestive heart failure have dominant diastolic heart failure, which may be defined as pulmonary (or systemic) venous congestion, and the symptoms consequent thereto, in the presence of normal or almost normal systolic function.[59–61] Another third have impairment of both systolic and diastolic function, and the remainder primarily disordered systolic function.

ALTERED VENTRICULAR RELAXATION. While two aspects of the heart's diastolic characteristics, i.e., relaxation and wall stiffness, are often considered together, they actually describe two different properties. Relaxation (inactivation of contraction) is a dynamic process that begins at the termination of contraction and occurs during isovolumetric relaxation and early ventricular filling (Fig. 13–13*A*; see also

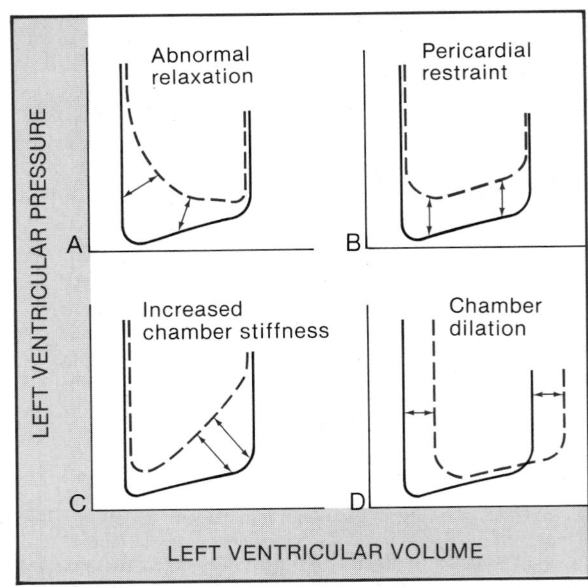

FIGURE 13–13. Mechanisms that cause diastolic dysfunction. Only the bottom half of the pressure-volume loop is depicted. Solid lines represent normal subjects; dashed lines represent patients with diastolic dysfunction. (Reproduced by permission from Zile, M. R.: Diastolic dysfunction: Detection, consequences, and treatment. Part 2: Diagnosis and treatment of diastolic function. Mod. Concepts Cardiovasc. Dis. *59*:1, 1990. Copyright 1990 American Heart Association.)

TABLE 13–3 CALCIUM HOMEOSTASIS IN FAILING HUMAN MYOCARDIUM

INTRACELLULAR CALCIUM LEVELS
Basal (diastolic) ↑
Peak (systolic) ↑
Rate of fall with diastole ↓
CALCIUM-HANDLING PROTEINS AND/OR mRNA LEVELS
SR Ca^{++}-ATPase ↓
Phospholamban ↓
Ca^{++} release channel ↓
Voltage-dependent Ca^{++} channels ↓
Na^{+}/Ca^{++} exchanger ↑
Calsequestrin ↔

Fig. 12–32, p. 384). The rate of ventricular relaxation is controlled primarily by the uptake of Ca^{++} by the sarcoplasmic reticulum, but also by the efflux of Ca^{++} from the myocyte. These processes are regulated by the sarcoplasmic reticulum calcium ATPase, as well as by sarcolemmal calcium pumps (pp. 369 and 405, Table 13–3). Because these Ca^{++} movements are against concentration gradients, they are energy-consuming. Therefore, ischemia-induced ATP depletion interferes with these processes and slows myocardial relaxation. On the other hand, beta-adrenergic receptor stimulation, by increasing cyclic AMP and cyclic AMP–dependent protein kinase activity, causes the phosphorylation of phospholamban (see p. 368), which accelerates Ca^{++} uptake by the sarcoplasmic reticulum and thereby enhances relaxation.

An acute increase in ventricular afterload has also been shown to slow myocardial relaxation.[62] Thus, when pressure overload is applied (before compensatory hypertrophy has normalized afterload), ventricular relaxation is slowed. Myocardium isolated from patients with hypertrophic cardiomyopathy[63] and from ferrets with pressure-overload hypertrophy[64] exhibits a prolonged calcium transient (i.e., a prolonged elevation of myoplasmic Ca^{++}), associated with a prolonged tension decay, findings consistent with delayed uptake of Ca^{++} by the sarcoplasmic reticulum.

ALTERED VENTRICULAR FILLING. During early ventricular filling the myocardium normally lengthens rapidly and homogeneously. Regional variation in the onset, rate, and extent of myocardial lengthening is referred to as *ventricular heterogeneity,* or *diastolic asynergy;* temporal dispersion of relaxation, with some fibers commencing to lengthen later than others, is referred to as *asynchrony.*[65,66] Both diastolic asynergy and asynchrony interfere with early diastolic filling. In contrast to these early diastolic events, myocardial *elasticity,* i.e., the change in muscle length for a change in force, ventricular *compliance,* i.e., the change in ventricular volume for a given change in pressure, and ventricular *stiffness,* the inverse of compliance, are generally measured in the relaxed ventricle at end-diastole.

These diastolic properties of the ventricle are described by its curvilinear pressure-volume relation (Figs. 12–32, p. 384; 13–13; and 14–1, p. 422). The slope of a tangent to this curvilinear relation (dP/dv) defines the chamber compliance at any level of filling pressure. An increase in chamber stiffness may occur secondary to any one or a combination of these three mechanisms: (1) A rise in filling pressure,[67] i.e., movement of the ventricle up along its pressure-volume (stress-strain) curve to a steeper portion (Fig. 14–20, p. 435). This may occur in conditions such as volume overload secondary to acute valvular regurgitation and in acute left ventricular failure due to myocarditis. (2) A shift to a steeper ventricular pressure-volume (Fig. 13–13*C*) or stress-strain curve. This results most commonly from an increase in ventricular mass and wall thickness. Thus, while hypertrophy constitutes a principal compensatory mechanism to sustain systolic emptying of the overloaded ventricle, it may simultaneously interfere with the ventricle's diastolic properties and impair ventricular filling. This shift to a steeper pressure-volume curve can also be caused by an increase in *intrinsic* myocardial stiffness (the stiffness of a unit of the cardiac wall regardless of the total mass or thickness of the myocardium), as occurs with disorders in which there is myocardial infiltration (e.g., amyloidosis), endomyocardial fibrosis, or myocardial ischemia (Fig. 13–14). (3) A parallel upward displacement of the diastolic pressure-volume curve, generally referred to as a *decrease in ventricular distensibility,* usually caused by extrinsic compression of the ventricles (Fig. 13–13*B*).

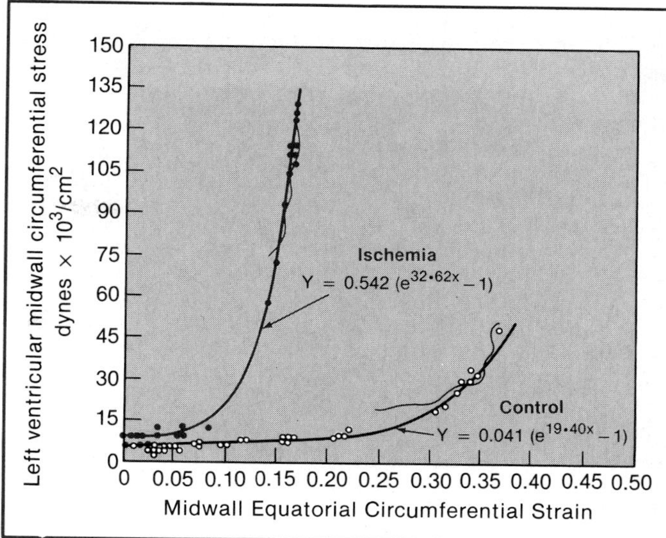

FIGURE 13–14. Diastolic pressure-strain and stress-strain relationships constructed from observations during control period and during ischemia. (Reproduced by permission from Visner, M. S., et al.: Effects of global ischemia on the diastolic properties of the left ventricle in the conscious dog. Circulation *71*:616, 1985. Copyright 1985 American Heart Association.)

Chronic Changes in Ventricular Diastolic Pressure-Volume Relationships

The compliance of the left ventricle, reflected in the end-diastolic pressure-volume relationship, is altered in a variety of cardiac disorders (p. 447). Substantial shifts in the diastolic pressure-volume curve of the left ventricle can be demonstrated during sustained volume overload.[68] For example, dogs with large chronic arteriovenous fistulas exhibit a rightward displacement of the entire diastolic pressure-volume curve, whereby ventricular volume is greater at any end-diastolic pressure but the slope of this curve is steeper, indicating increased chamber stiffness.[69] Patients with severe volume overloading due to chronic aortic and/or mitral regurgitation demonstrate similar shifts of the diastolic left ventricular pressure-volume relationship. Similar changes frequently occur in patients with dilated or ischemic cardiomyopathy or following large transmural myocardial infarction (see below).

In contrast, concentric left ventricular hypertrophy, as occurs in aortic stenosis, hypertension, and hypertrophic cardiomyopathy, shifts the pressure-volume relation of the ventricle to the left along its volume axis so that at any diastolic volume ventricular diastolic pressure is abnormally elevated[70–72] (Figs. 13–13*C* and 15–1, p. 447). In contrast to the changes in the diastolic properties of the ventricular *chamber,* the stiffness of *each unit of myocardium* may or may not be altered in the presence of myocardial hypertrophy secondary to pressure overload.[73]

In the presence of concentric left ventricular hypertrophy, there is an inverse relationship between the thickness of the posterior wall of the ventricle and its peak

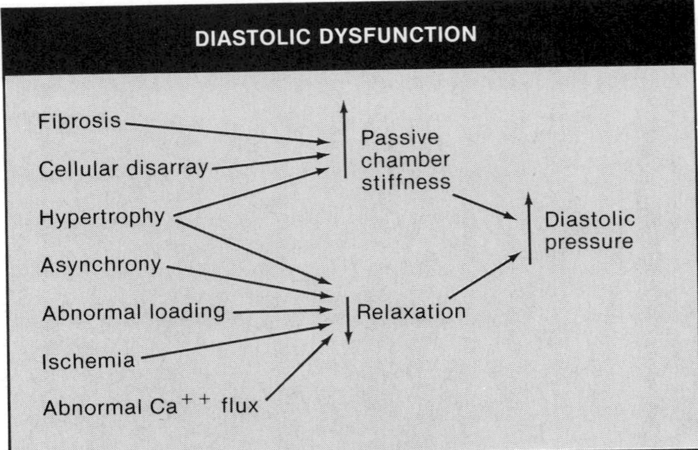

FIGURE 13–15. Factors responsible for diastolic dysfunction and increased left ventricular diastolic pressure. (From Gaasch, W. H., and Izzi, G.: Clinical diagnosis and management of left ventricular diastolic dysfunction. *In* Hori, M., Suga, H., Baan, J., and Yellin, E. L. [eds.]: Cardiac Mechanics and Function in the Normal and Diseased Heart. New York, Springer-Verlag, 1989, p. 296.)

thinning rate during early diastole[74]; a higher-than-normal diastolic ventricular pressure is required to fill the hypertrophied ventricle. Patients with hypertension have demonstrated slowing of ventricular filling by radionuclide angiography[75] and echocardiography, even when systolic function is normal.[76]

ISCHEMIC HEART DISEASE. Marked changes in the diastolic properties of the left ventricle can occur in the presence of ischemic heart disease (see p. 1194). First, as already pointed out, acute myocardial ischemia slows ventricular relaxation (Fig. 13–13*A*) and increases myocardial wall stiffness[77,78] (Figs. 13–14 and 13–15). Myocardial infarction causes more complex changes in ventricular pressure-volume relationships, depending on the size of the infarct and the time following infarction at which the measurements are made. Infarcted muscle tested very early exhibits reduced stiffness.[79–81] Subsequently, the development of myocardial contracture, interstitial edema, fibrocellular infiltration, and scar contribute to stiffening of the necrotic tissue and thereby to increased chamber stiffness, with a steeper ventricular pressure-volume curve (a greater increase in pressure for any increase in volume).[82] Later still, in the case of large infarcts, left ventricular remodeling and dilatation cause a rightward displacement of the pressure-volume curve,[83] resembling that observed in volume overload. The subendocardial ischemia that is characteristic of severe concentric hypertrophy (even in the presence of a normal coronary circulation) intensifies the failure of relaxation,[58,84] and when coronary artery obstruction accompanies severe hypertrophy, this abnormality may be particularly severe.[83] Tachycardia, by reducing the duration of diastole and thereby intensifying ischemia, exaggerates this diastolic abnormality and may raise ventricular diastolic pressure even while reducing diastolic ventricular volume, whereas bradycardia has the opposite effect. Successful treatment of ischemia improves diastolic relaxation and lowers ventricular diastolic and pulmonary venous pressures, thereby reducing dyspnea.

CARDIOMYOPATHY AND PERICARDIAL DISEASE. The restrictive cardiomyopathies, especially those such as amyloid heart disease with intracardiac infiltration (see p. 1427), the transplanted heart during rejection, and endomyocardial fibrosis (see p. 1433), all are characterized by upward and leftward displacement of the diastolic pressure-volume relation, with a higher pressure at any volume and a greater increase in diastolic pressure for any increase in volume. Pericardial tamponade and constrictive pericarditis also change the apparent diastolic properties of the heart. Early filling is unimpaired because the myocardium is normal. However, filling is abruptly halted in mid-diastole by the constricted or tamponading pericardium, which imposes its mechanical properties on those of the ventricle in the latter half of diastole (Fig. 13–13*B*; Fig. 43–20, p. 1503).

ROLE OF COLLAGEN. The diastolic properties of the ventricle are determined not only by its myocytes but also by the coronary vessels, nerves, and interstitial connective tissue, consisting of fibroblasts, and types I and III fibrillar collagen.[39,85,86] The latter provide struts along which the myocytes are aligned. Branches of collagen fibers course at right angles to connect and align muscle bundles. Weber has pointed out that the diastolic properties of the ventricle are influenced profoundly by the quantity of collagen relative to myocytes, as well as by its elastic properties and its physical disposition.[85] The messenger RNA for types I and III collagen that is present in fibroblasts increases markedly after aortic banding in experimental animals,[87] and the left ventricular concentration of collagen is increased in experimentally induced chronic pressure overload hypertrophy,[39] as well as in patients with hypertension. Less information is available on the role of collagen in volume overload hypertrophy; however, the increase in diastolic stiffness sometimes seen in this condition has been associated with increased cross-linking of types I and III collagens.[88]

CELLULAR AND MOLECULAR MECHANISMS OF MYOCARDIAL DYSFUNCTION

Important changes at the cellular and molecular levels have been identified in hypertrophied and failing myocardium. Functional abnormalities in excitation-contraction coupling, contractile protein function, and energetics have been identified in failing animal and human myocardium, and at the molecular level alterations have been observed in the expression of several proteins that are central to normal myocardial structure and function.[89] There is strong evidence from in vitro and animal studies to suggest that these molecular and cellular events are secondary to both mechanical forces and a variety of neuronal, endocrine, and autocrine/paracrine mediators that act on the myocardium. Some of the responses are adaptive and sustain cardiac function. Others are maladaptive. It is not clear which or whether any of these are *responsible* for the impaired myocardial function of heart failure, or play contributory roles, or simply accompany the heart failure state as "epiphenomena."[90]

Excitation-Contraction Coupling and the Role of Ca^{++}

(See also p. 366 and Table 13–3, p. 403)

Ca^{++} plays a central role in the regulation of myocardial contraction and relaxation.[91] Hypocalcemia, secondary to hypoparathyroidism and a variety of other conditions, can cause heart failure that is responsive to the infusion of calcium.[92,93] Elevation of serum ionized Ca^{++} has been shown to augment contractility in patients with renal failure undergoing dialysis[94] and in patients with severe heart failure secondary to cardiomyopathy who have downregulation of beta-adrenergic receptors.[95]

Myocardium obtained at the time of cardiac transplantation from patients with end-stage heart failure exhibits abnormal prolongation of the action potential and developed force, and impaired relaxation.[29] Observations using the Ca^{++} indicator aequorin in whole myocardium have shown that these alterations in electrical and contractile properties are associated with a prolonged elevation of the intracellular Ca^{++} transient during relaxation.[29] Likewise, in myocytes obtained from patients with end-stage heart failure, the action potential is prolonged. The intracellular Ca^{++}

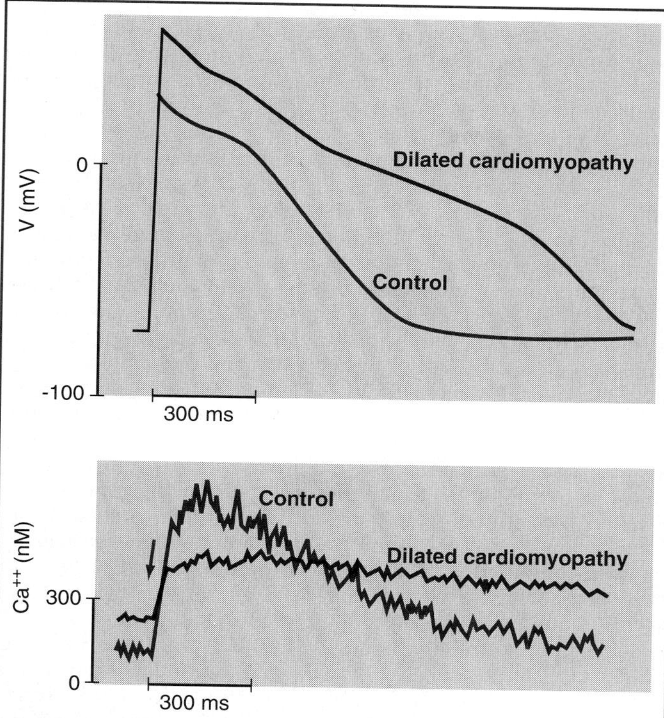

FIGURE 13–16. Abnormal action potential and intracellular calcium transient in failing cardiac myocytes. ***Top panel,*** **The action potential recorded in a myocyte isolated from the heart of a patient with dilated cardiomyopathy is markedly prolonged, as compared to that in a myocyte from a normal heart (control). Such abnormalities could contribute to both the generation of arrhythmias and abnormal diastolic relaxation.** ***Bottom panel,*** **The intracellular calcium transient measured with the fluorescent calcium indicator fura-2 are also markedly abnormal in myocytes isolated from the myocardium of patients with dilated cardiomyopathy. As compared to a normal myocyte (control), the myocyte from a patient with dilated cardiomyopathy shows an attenuated rise with depolarization** ***(arrow)*** **and a markedly delayed return to baseline. These abnormalities reflect the altered expression or function of key calcium handling proteins (e.g., Ca++-ATPase) and likely contribute to the abnormal action potential illustrated in Panel A. (Modified by permission from Beuckelmann, D. J., Nabauer, M., and Erdmann, E.: Intracellular calcium handling in isolated ventricular myocytes from patients with terminal heart failure. Circulation** ***85:*****1046, 1992. Copyright 1992 American Heart Association.)**

transient, as assessed by the fluorescent indicator fura-2, demonstrates a blunted rise with depolarization reflecting a slower delivery of Ca^{++} to the contractile apparatus (causing slower activation) and a slowed rate of fall during repolarization (causing slowed relaxation) (Fig. 13–16).[96] These two abnormalities can explain both systolic and diastolic dysfunction.

Additional evidence of abnormal myocardial Ca^{++} handling is provided by the observation that there is a reduction in the amount of tension-independent heat produced in myocardium from patients with heart failure.[97] Tension-independent heat, which is believed to reflect the energy expended for Ca^{++} transport, can be used to estimate the amount of Ca^{++} cycled per heartbeat.[98] With this approach, it was shown that Ca^{++} cycling is reduced by approximately 50 per cent in failing human myocardium.[97]

Excitation-contraction coupling can also be assessed by examination of the force-frequency response. As already pointed out (see p. 398), in normal myocardium, contractile force increases with increasing rates of stimulation, whereas in myocardium obtained from patients with end-stage heart failure the force-frequency response is markedly attenuated.[99] A similar phenomenon is observed in patients with heart failure studied at the time of catheterization.[99a] In patients with normal ventricular function, left ventricular contractility (as measured by +dP/dt or the end-systolic pressure-volume ratio) increases progressively as heart rate is increased by atrial pacing. By comparison, in patients with severe heart failure there is little or no increase in either contractile index.

The intracellular concentration of Ca^{++} is regulated by several enzymes and channels that are located in the sarcolemma, sarcoplasmic reticulum (SR), and mitochondria[91] (Chap. 12). Evidence is accumulating that the expression and/or function of a number of these proteins may be altered in hypertrophied and failing myocardium[100] (Table 13–3).

SARCOPLASMIC RETICULUM Ca^{++}-ATPase. Ca^{++} reuptake by the SR is mediated primarily by the ATP-dependent enzyme Ca^{++}-ATPase (SERCA2).[100] The activity of SERCA2 is inhibited by the associated protein, phospholamban,[100–102] and this inhibition is relieved by cyclic AMP–mediated phosphorylation of phospholamban (e.g., by beta-adrenergic receptor stimulation) thereby resulting in increased Ca^{++} reuptake into the SR and the acceleration of diastolic relaxation. The reuptake of Ca^{++} by the SR is also important for normal systolic function, which requires that ample SR Ca^{++} be available for release during systole to mediate contraction.[100]

Although these observations remain controversial, reports have indicated that the levels of SERCA2[103–105] and phospholamban[104–106] mRNA and SERCA2 protein[105] are reduced in myocardium obtained from patients with end-stage heart failure. In one study, the decrease in the level of SERCA2 mRNA was inversely related to the level of atrial natriuretic factor mRNA (Fig. 13–17), suggesting that the reduced expression of this adult muscle-specific protein is coupled to the reexpression of a fetal gene program.[104] These observations are consistent with several studies that have demonstrated a reduction in SR Ca^{++} reuptake in animal models of heart failure[107–109] and some[110] but not all[111] studies in patients with heart failure. In mice deficient in phospholamban due to targeted gene ablation, there is a marked increase in basal myocardial contractility and a loss of both the contractile and relaxant effects of beta-adrenergic stimulation.[102] It is therefore possible that a decrease in phospholamban activity is an adaptive response to the decrease in SERCA2 activity.

THE Ca^{++} RELEASE CHANNEL. The Ca^{++} release channel (CRC), located on the SR, mediates the release of Ca^{++} from the SR into the myoplasm during systole.[91] Studies in failing human myocardium have shown decreases in the

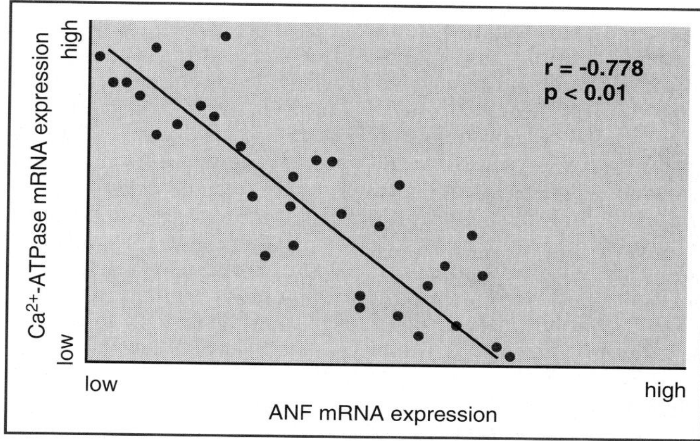

FIGURE 13–17. Inverse relationship between the mRNA levels for the fetal gene atrial natriuretic factor (ANF) and the adult muscle-specific gene encoding Ca++-ATPase in ventricular myocardium obtained from patients with various degrees of myocardial failure. The reexpression of a fetal gene program is typical of hypertrophied and failing myocardium. (Modified by permission from Arai, M., Matsui, H., and Periasamy, M.: Sarcoplasmic reticulum gene expression in cardiac hypertrophy and heart failure. Circ. Res. ***74:*****555, 1994. Copyright 1994 American Heart Association.)**

mRNA level for the CRC. In one study, the mRNA level for CRC was reduced in patients with ischemic cardiomyopathy but not those with dilated cardiomyopathy.[112] In another study, the level of CRC mRNA was decreased in patients with heart failure of both causes.[104]

VOLTAGE-DEPENDENT Ca^{++} CHANNEL. The mRNA and protein levels of the voltage-dependent Ca^{++} channel also have been shown to be decreased in failing human myocardium obtained from patients with both ischemic heart disease and dilated cardiomyopathy.[113]

Na^{+}/Ca^{++} EXCHANGER. The Na^{+}/Ca^{++} exchanger is the major route by which Ca^{++} is removed from the cardiac myocyte and can account for approximately 20 per cent of the removal of Ca^{++} from the cytoplasm during diastole.[105] The mRNA and protein levels of the Na^{+}/Ca^{++} exchanger were found to be increased in myocardium obtained from patients with heart failure due to both ischemic and idiopathic dilated cardiomyopathy, and correlated inversely with the decrease in SERCA2 mRNA levels.[105] This augmentation in Na^{+}/Ca^{++} exchange activity might be a compensatory response to the reduction in Ca^{++} reuptake caused by a decrease in SERCA2. Although this would facilitate diastolic Ca^{++} removal, it might do so at the expense of increased arrhythmogenicity, because this Ca^{++} efflux is associated with an influx of Na^{+} that can prolong depolarization and cause afterdepolarizations.

CALSEQUESTRIN. This is the major protein in the SR that binds Ca^{++} and thereby serves a storage function. Several studies have found calsequestrin mRNA levels to be unchanged in failing human myocardium.[104,111,113]

Contractile Apparatus

The fraction of cell volume composed of myofibrils is initially increased in animal models of pressure-induced hypertrophy.[34,114] Patients with aortic stenosis without heart failure exhibit a normal fraction of myofibrils per cell, whereas those with left ventricular failure show a significant reduction in cell volume occupied by myofibrils, suggesting that this reduction in the quantity of the contractile machinery may play a role in the development of cardiac decompensation.[115] In end-stage heart failure in the human, electron microscopic observations likewise show a reduction of ventricular myofibrillar protein.[116]

REDUCTION OF MYOSIN ATPase. Considerable data suggest that qualitative, as well as quantitative, alterations of contractile proteins occur in heart failure. First, the finding that the reduced velocity of contraction of failing myocardium occurs in chemically skinned ventricular fibers suggests that this change reflects intrinsic alterations in the contractile apparatus. Early studies showed that the activity of myofibrillar ATPase is reduced in the hearts of patients who died of heart failure[117,118] and in dogs with naturally occurring heart failure.[119] Furthermore, reductions in the activities of myofibrillar ATPase, actomyosin ATPase, or myosin ATPase have been demonstrated in heart failure induced in cats by pulmonary artery constriction,[120] in guinea pigs with constriction of the ascending aorta,[121] in dogs with constriction of the pulmonary artery or aorta,[122] and in rats with renovascular hypertension.[123] These depressions of enzymatic activity could occur if an altered subunit of the myosin molecule, i.e., the portion of the molecule responsible for the ATPase activity, were produced in the overloaded heart and reduced contractility by lowering the rate of interaction between actin and myosin filaments. A reduction in the Mg^{++}-ATPase activity (which expresses the response of myofibrils to Ca^{++}) has been demonstrated in myofibrils obtained from patients with end-stage heart failure at the time of transplantation and in less sick patients undergoing valve replacement.[124]

MYOSIN ISOFORM CHANGES. Animal studies have indicated that when the adult heart hypertrophies, fetal and neonatal forms of contractile proteins (termed isoforms) and other proteins (such as atrial natriuretic peptide) reappear, signifying reexpression of the genes for these fetal and neonatal isoforms. Thus, hemodynamic overload leads to enhanced overall protein synthesis,[3] but it alters the proteins qualitatively, i.e., it leads to the synthesis of protein isoforms that were present during fetal and neonatal life when protein synthesis in the heart was also rapid.[124a] Altered isoforms of cardiac proteins may arise from the expression of different members of a multigene family or from the assembly of the same gene in a different pattern. In rodents the predominant myosin heavy chain (MHC) is the "fast" V_1 isoform (high ATPase activity, encoded by the alpha-MHC gene). With pressure-induced hypertrophy or myocardial failure following myocardial infarction in the rat, there is the reexpression of the "slow" V_3 isoform (low ATPase activity, encoded by the beta-MHC gene), and deinduction of the V_1 isoform.[125–129]

Although a shift in MHC isoforms would provide an attractive explanation for the reduction in myofibrillar ATPase activity observed in failing human myocardium, the predominant MHC isoform in humans is the slower V_3 isoform (encoded by the beta-MHC gene). In failing human myocardium, as in normal myocardium, alpha-MHC mRNA is not detectable; beta MHC and alpha cardiac actin are reduced and correlate inversely with the increase in atrial natriuretic factor mRNA level; and alpha-skeletal actin mRNA, which is expressed in normal human myocardium, is unchanged.[104] These observations are consistent with a general decrease in contractile protein-expression; however, they make it unlikely that a shift in myosin isoforms is responsible for the observed decrease in myosin ATPase activity. It remains possible that functional alterations in myosin and/or actin may be present, and it has been reported that there is a reduction in the number of cells containing alpha-MHC in failing human myocardium.[130]

ALTERED REGULATORY PROTEINS. Another possible cause of a decrease in contractile protein function is an alteration in the expression and/or activity of regulatory proteins. In animals with experimental heart failure, there are changes in the myosin light chain and the troponin-tropomyosin complex.[131,132] Changes in myosin light-chain isoforms have been observed in the atria and ventricles of patients sub-

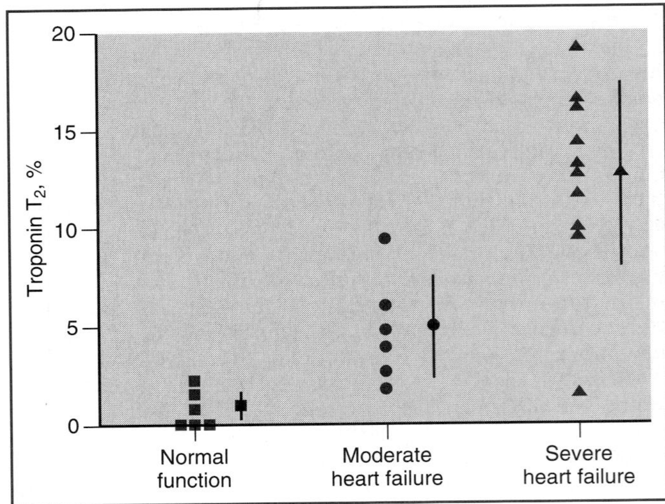

FIGURE 13–18. Increased expression in failing human myocardium of the troponin-T_2 isoform of troponin-T, a component of the tropomyosin complex which regulates the interaction of actin and myosin. Changes in the expression of troponin-T, or other regulatory proteins (e.g., myosin light chains), could contribute to altered contractile protein function in such patients. (Modified from Anderson, P. A. W., Malouf, N. N., Oakeley, A. E., et al.: Troponin T isoform expression in the normal and failing human left ventricle: A correlation with myofibrillar ATPase activity. Basic Res. Cardiol. *87*:175, 1992.)

jected to increased mechanical stress,[133] and the expression of troponin-T, a component of the troponin complex that regulates the interaction of myosin and actin, was found to be altered in failing human myocardium.[134] In normal myocardium, troponin-T is expressed as a single isoform (T_1), which accounts for approximately 98 per cent of the troponin-T. In myocardium from patients with end-stage heart failure, a second isoform (T_2) was expressed at increased levels, and its level of expression was related to the severity of heart failure (Fig. 13–18).[134] The functional significance of these changes in the expression of regulatory proteins is not known. However, these observations suggest that changes in myosin activity could be due to changes in regulatory proteins and need not reflect alterations in the contractile proteins themselves.

Myocardial Energetics

Heart failure frequently occurs in the presence of adequate myocardial perfusion, oxygen, and substrate. In early studies, measurement of coronary blood flow utilizing coronary sinus catheterization, both in humans and in dogs with chronic heart failure, showed that the coronary blood flow per gram of myocardium did not differ significantly from normal.[135] Several preparations of failing heart muscle were shown to require less oxygen than does normal muscle. When contractility is acutely depressed, myocardial oxygen consumption of the intact ventricle also declines.[136] Similarly, patients with chronic impairment of left ventricular performance and reduction of the velocity of myocardial fiber shortening exhibit reduction of coronary blood flow and myocardial oxygen consumption per unit of muscle.[137] Marked reductions in myocardial oxygen consumption have been described in the Syrian hamster with hereditary cardiomyopathy.[138] Papillary muscles removed from cats with pressure overload–induced right ventricular hypertrophy exhibit a depression of both contractility and oxygen consumption per unit of tension development.[23] These lowered energy needs of the failing heart may serve a protective function, reducing the likelihood of the exacerbation of heart failure by an imbalance between energy supply and demand.

MYOCARDIAL ENERGY PRODUCTION. Considerable dispute has centered on the question of whether or not mitochondrial oxidative phosphorylation, i.e., energy production, is abnormal in heart failure. Early studies indicated that electron transport and the tightness of respiratory control are normal in mitochondria obtained from failing human hearts[139] and cat hearts with experimental heart failure produced by pressure overload.[140] On the other hand, in one study in which mitochondria from the hearts of patients with end-stage dilated cardiomyopathy were studied, a reduction in cytochrome-a content and in cytochrome-dependent enzyme activity was reported.[141] The cytochromes are located in the inner mitochondrial membrane and are constituents of the respiratory chain that couples oxidation to the synthesis of chemical energy. Mitochondria obtained from failing human cardiac muscle have also shown reduced oxygen consumption during active phosphorylation and reduced rates of NADH-linked respiratory activity.[141] These and other observations have led to the thesis that myocardial failure in the setting of hemodynamic overload may be related to an inability of the energy-producing system, i.e., the mitochondria, to keep pace with the needs of the contractile apparatus.

The nucleotide-transporting protein located on the inner mitochondrial membrane, the so-called ADP-ATP carrier, has been identified as an autoantigen in viral myocarditis and dilated cardiomyopathy. In guinea pigs immunized to this carrier protein, both myocardial oxygen consumption and cardiac work fell.[142] These findings are compatible with the hypothesis that the impaired cardiac performance in some cases of myocarditis (and dilated cardiomyopathy) may be secondary to an imbalance between energy delivery and demand.

MYOCARDIAL ENERGY RESERVES. In compensated hypertrophy, observations on myocardial ATP concentration have shown no consistent change.[143] However, in myocardium from dogs with myocardial failure due to rapid pacing or chronic ischemia and from humans with end-stage cardiomyopathy, total creatine kinase activity and the concentrations of phosphocreatine and creatine are decreased.[143–145] These observations have led to the hypothesis that myocardial failure may be the consequence of a decreased energy reserve.[143] The measurement of creatine kinase flux provides a sensitive measure of myocardial energy reserves and may detect abnormalities in the absence of changes in ATP and phosphocreatine concentrations. By studying high-energy flux in vivo using nuclear magnetic resonance technology, it was demonstrated that creatine kinase activity is markedly reduced in the myopathic Syrian hamster.[146] This abnormality was almost completely corrected by treatment with the converting enzyme inhibitor enalapril. The mechanism responsible for a decrease in creatine kinase activity is not understood but is associated with alterations in the isoform of creatine kinase. In failing myocardium, there is a decrease in the adult (MM) isoform and an increase or no change in the fetal isoform (MB).[143]

One unusual form of heart failure that is primarily related to a reduction of myocardial energy stores is that due to phosphate deficiency. Chronic hypophosphatemia induced by dietary means is associated with reversible depression of myocardial performance in isolated muscle as well as in the intact heart of animals and humans, presumably as a consequence of reduced ATP stores.[147,148]

NEUROHORMONAL, AUTOCRINE, AND PARACRINE ADJUSTMENTS

A complex series of neurohormonal changes takes place consequent to the two principal hemodynamic alterations in heart failure: reduction of cardiac output and atrial hypertension (Fig. 13–19). Many of these neurohormonal changes occur in response to the inadequate arterial volume characteristic of systolic heart failure. In the early stages of acute systolic failure, these changes—heightened adrenergic drive, activation of the renin-angiotensin-aldosterone axis, and the augmented release of vasopressin and endothelin—are truly compensatory and act to maintain perfusion to vital organs and to expand the inadequate arterial blood volume. However, each of these mechanisms may be thought of as a "double-edged sword." As heart failure becomes chronic, several of these compensatory mechanisms can cause undesirable effects such as excessive vasoconstriction, increased afterload, excessive retention of salt and water, electrolyte abnormalities, and arrhythmias (Table 13–1). In contrast, other responses, such as the release of atrial natriuretic peptide (ANP) in response to atrial distention, may oppose these adverse effects by causing vasodilation and increased excretion of salt and water.

A variety of mediators are involved in control of the cardiovascular system in heart failure. Some are circulating hormones (endocrine effect). Some act on neighboring cells of another type (paracrine effect) or on the cell of origin (autocrine effect).[149] These include peptides that primarily act locally in the vicinity of their production, such as endothelin, peptide growth factors (e.g., transforming growth factor-alpha), and inflammatory cytokines (e.g., interleukin-1 beta and tumor necrosis factor-alpha). These and other local mediators act in concert with the autonomic nervous system and circulating hormones to modulate cardiovascular organ function. In addition, many if not all of these mediators have effects on the growth of cardiovascular tis-

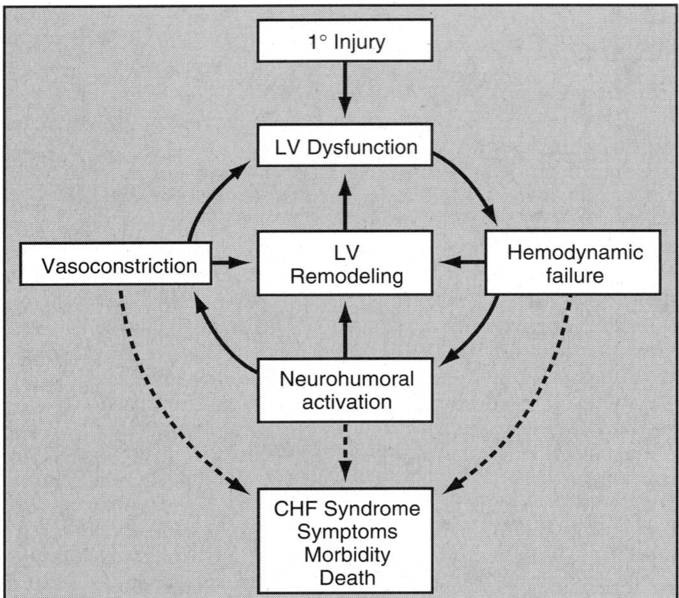

FIGURE 13–19. Schematic illustrating the proposed relationship between primary myocardial injury and secondary events which contribute to the clinical syndrome of heart failure and progression of the underlying myocardial disease. According to this thesis, hemodynamic and neurohormonal consequences of the initial myocardial injury result in both acute impairment of ventricular function due to increased ventricular afterload and chronic progression of disease due to ventricular remodeling.

sues and may thereby play an important role in the "remodeling" of myocardium and vasculature.

Autonomic Nervous System

INCREASED SYMPATHETIC ACTIVITY (see Fig. 13–2, p. 395). Measurements of the concentration of the adrenergic norepinephrine (NE) in arterial blood provide an index of the activity of this system, which is crucial to the normal regulation of cardiac performance. At rest, in patients with advanced heart failure, the circulating NE concentration is much higher, generally two to three times the level found in normal subjects,[150–153] and is accompanied by elevation of circulating dopamine and sometimes by epinephrine as well; the latter reflects increased adrenomedullary activity. Measurement of 24-hour urinary NE excretion also reveals marked elevations in patients with heart failure.[152] In the prevention arm of the SOLVD study (see p. 495), plasma NE was significantly elevated, even in asymptomatic patients, and was further elevated in patients with symptomatic heart failure (Fig. 13–20).[154] During comparable levels of exercise, much greater elevations in circulating NE occur in patients with heart failure than in normal subjects, presumably reflecting greater activation of the adrenergic nervous system during exercise in these patients.[155–157]

Elevation of Circulating Norepinephrine. The elevation of circulating NE may result from a combination of increased release of NE from adrenergic nerve endings and its consequent "spillover" into plasma,[158,159] as well as reduced uptake of NE by adrenergic nerve endings.[160] Patients with heart failure demonstrate increased adrenergic

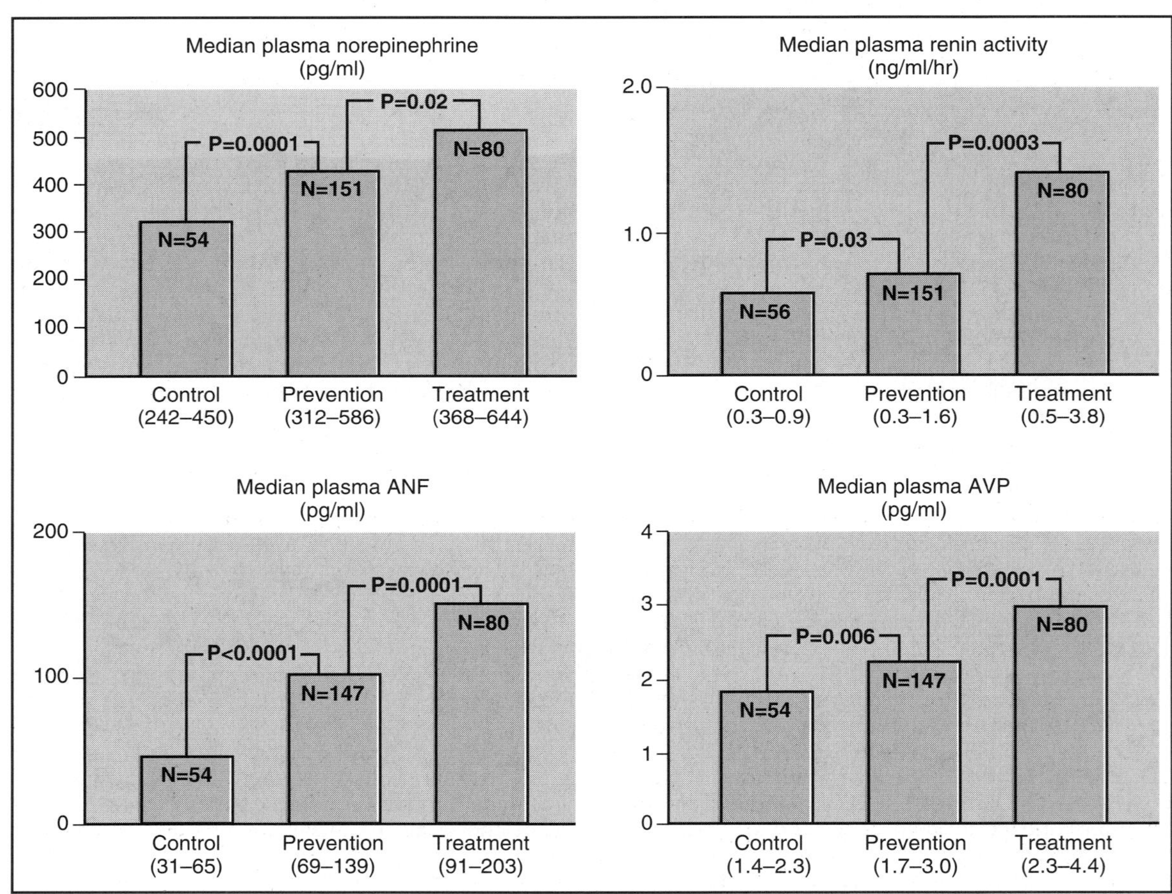

FIGURE 13–20. Activation of neurohormonal systems in patients with heart failure. In patients studied in the SOLVD trials, plasma norepinephrine, renin activity, atrial natriuretic factor (ANF), and arginine vasopressin (AVP) were elevated in patients with symptomatic heart failure enrolled in the treatment trial, and also, albeit to a lesser degree, in asymptomatic patients enrolled in the prevention trial. (Modified by permission from Francis, G. S., Benedict, C., Johnstone, D. E., et al.: Comparison of neuroendocrine activation in patients with left ventricular dysfunction with and without congestive heart failure. A substudy of the studies of left ventricular dysfunction (SOLVD). Circulation *82*:1724, 1990. Copyright 1990 American Heart Association.)

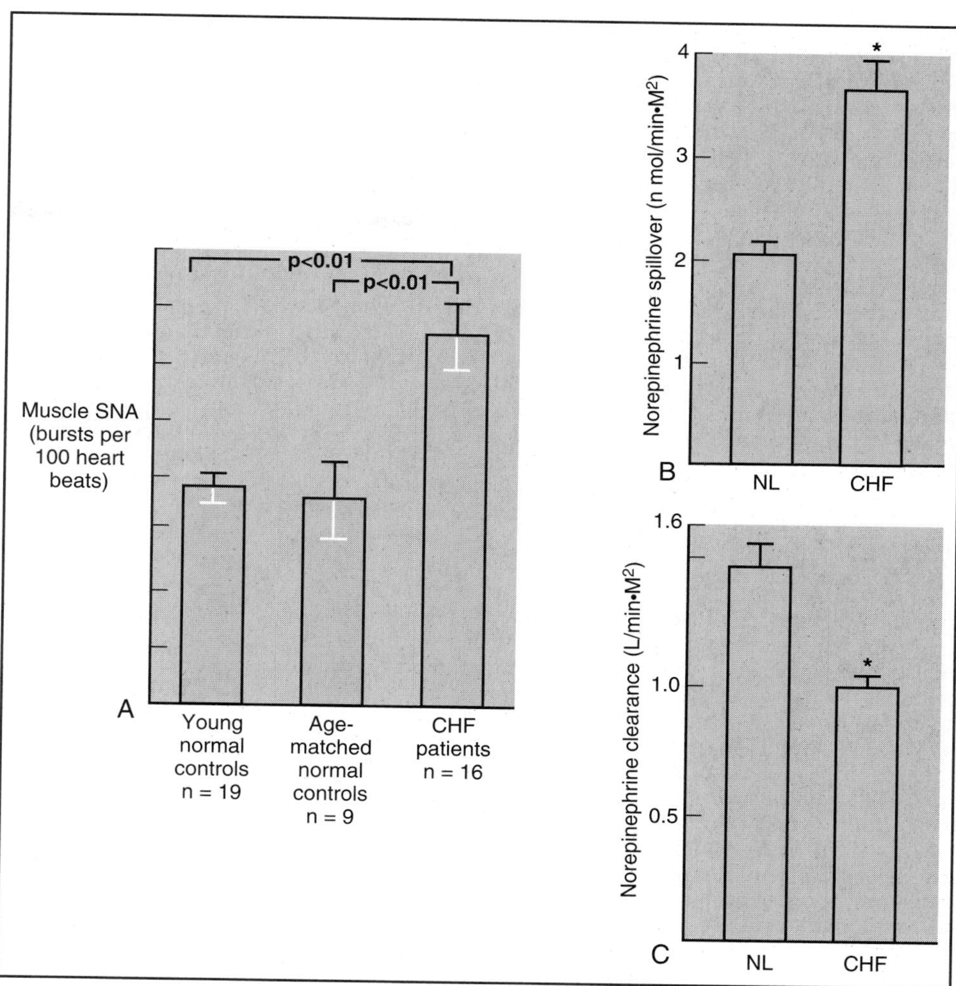

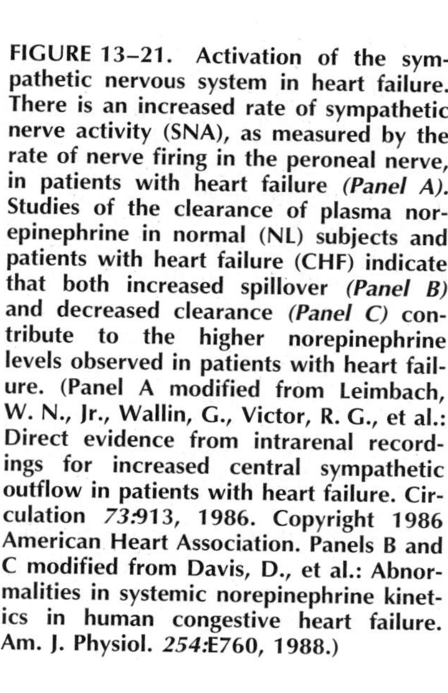

FIGURE 13–21. Activation of the sympathetic nervous system in heart failure. There is an increased rate of sympathetic nerve activity (SNA), as measured by the rate of nerve firing in the peroneal nerve, in patients with heart failure *(Panel A)*. Studies of the clearance of plasma norepinephrine in normal (NL) subjects and patients with heart failure (CHF) indicate that both increased spillover *(Panel B)* and decreased clearance *(Panel C)* contribute to the higher norepinephrine levels observed in patients with heart failure. (Panel A modified from Leimbach, W. N., Jr., Wallin, G., Victor, R. G., et al.: Direct evidence from intrarenal recordings for increased central sympathetic outflow in patients with heart failure. Circulation *73:*913, 1986. Copyright 1986 American Heart Association. Panels B and C modified from Davis, D., et al.: Abnormalities in systemic norepinephrine kinetics in human congestive heart failure. Am. J. Physiol. *254:*E760, 1988.)

nerve outflow, as measured by microneurography of the peroneal nerve (Fig. 13–4), and the level of nerve activity correlates with the concentration of plasma NE (Fig. 13–21).[161] The level of adrenergic nerve activity also correlates directly with the levels of left and right ventricular filling pressures.[161] While the normal heart usually extracts NE, in patients with heart failure the coronary sinus NE level exceeds the arterial level, indicating increased adrenergic activation of the heart.[158] Drugs such as the alpha$_2$-agonist guanabenz (which reduces adrenergic nerve impulse traffic) and bromocriptine (a presynaptic dopamine-2 agonist[162]) reduce plasma NE, indicating that presynaptic control of adrenergic nervous activity is intact in patients with heart failure.[151] It has been suggested that treatment with such agents might be useful in interrupting the vicious circle already referred to.[162]

The extent of elevation of plasma NE concentration that occurs in patients with heart failure correlates directly with the severity of the left ventricular dysfunction,[150] as reflected in the height of the pulmonary capillary wedge pressure and depression of the cardiac index,[151,153] and with cardiac mortality.[163] The augmented adrenergic outflow from the central nervous system in patients with heart failure may trigger ventricular tachycardia or even sudden cardiac death, particularly in the presence of myocardial ischemia. However, it is not clear whether the elevated levels of circulating NE in patients who subsequently die of heart failure are causally related to death as a consequence of their vasoconstrictor, arrhythmogenic, or other actions or whether they represent an "epiphenomenon" that merely reflects the severity of the underlying heart failure.

In addition to activation of beta-adrenergic receptors in the heart, the heightened activity of the adrenergic nervous system leads to stimulation of myocardial alpha$_1$-adrenergic receptors, which elicits a modest positive inotropic effect.[164] Stimulation of myocardial alpha$_1$-adrenergic receptors may also cause myocyte hypertrophy, changes in phenotype characterized by the reexpression of a fetal gene program,[165] and the induction of peptide growth factors.[166] Alpha$_1$-adrenergic receptors are of low density in the human heart; however, in contrast to beta$_1$-adrenergic receptors, which are downregulated, alpha$_1$-adrenergic receptors appear to be unchanged in number in failing human myocardium.[167]

CARDIAC NOREPINEPHRINE DEPLETION. The concentration of NE in atrial[152] and ventricular tissue[26] removed at operation from patients with heart failure is extremely low. In patients, it has been reported that cardiac NE content determined from endomyocardial biopsies correlates directly with the ejection fraction and inversely with plasma epinephrine concentration.[168] NE concentrations are also markedly depressed in the ventricles of dogs with right ventricular failure produced by the creation of pulmonary stenosis and tricuspid regurgitation.[170] Local cardiac NE stores do not appear to play any role in the *intrinsic* contractile state of cardiac muscle. Thus, no differences were found in the length-tension or force-velocity relationships displayed by papillary muscles removed from normal cats and from cats with NE depletion produced by chronic cardiac denervation or reserpine pretreatment.[170] However, the reduction in cardiac NE stores represents a depletion of the adrenergic neurotransmitter in adrenergic nerve endings, and as a consequence the response to activation of the sympathetic nervous system is blunted[171] (Fig. 13–2, p. 395).

The mechanism responsible for cardiac NE depletion in severe heart failure is not clear; it may be an "exhaustion" phenomenon from the prolonged adrenergic activation of the cardiac adrenergic nerves in heart failure. Reductions in the activity of tyrosine hydroxylase,[172] which catalyzes the rate-limiting step in the biosynthesis of NE, and in the rate at which noradrenergic vesicles can take up dopamine[173] have also been incriminated. In patients with cardiomyopathy, [^{131}I]-labeled metaiodobenzylguanidine (MTBG), a radiopharmaceutical that is taken up by adrenergic nerve endings, is not taken up normally.[174] The technique based on this observation may provide a noninvasive approach to assessing disturbances in adrenergic function in heart failure.

ABNORMAL BAROREFLEX CONTROL IN HEART FAILURE. Increased adrenergic activity in heart failure is due, in part, to abnormal baroreflex control of adrenergic outflow from the central nervous system (Fig. 13–3). In dogs with experimental heart failure, carotid occlusion elicits a blunted reflex response of heart rate, arterial pressure, and vascular resistance.[175,176] The possibility of defective adrenergic control of heart rate in patients with heart failure has been studied by observing the reflex hemodynamic responses to stimuli such as upright tilt and vasodilator-induced hypotension.[177–181]

An inappropriately depressed increase in heart rate in humans with heart failure was observed when arterial pressure was reduced through administration of vasodilators.[182] While the changes in mean arterial pressure observed in response to the vasodilators were similar in patients with heart failure and in control subjects, the changes in heart rate after vasodilators correlated significantly with the changes in concentration of circulating NE and with the sum of circulating NE and epinephrine. In normal individuals, both heart rate and catecholamine concentrations rose, whereas in patients with heart failure, in whom resting catecholamine levels were already increased, cardiac acceleration was blunted, and catecholamine concentration failed to rise normally. Similarly, during upright tilt there is a blunting of the normal increases in plasma NE, forearm vascular resistance, and hepatic vascular resistance in patients with heart failure.[117,178] Some patients with heart failure exhibit a major reduction in arterial pressure during tilting, analogous to what is observed in idiopathic orthostatic hypotension.[179] In such patients, not surprisingly, exercise capacity in the upright position is markedly reduced.[183] Further evidence for impairment of baroreflex control of the systemic circulation comes from investigations in which lower body negative pressure fails to cause normal reflex augmentation of forearm vascular resistance.[180]

Atrial Stretch Receptors. Abnormal baroreflex control also contributes to the reduced ability of patients with heart failure to excrete salt and water. Under normal circumstances, elevated left atrial pressure stimulates atrial stretch receptors. The increased activity of both myelinated and nonmyelinated (C-fiber) afferents[184] inhibits the release of ADH, thereby increasing water excretion, which in turn reduces plasma volume and would act to restore left atrial pressure to normal. In addition, enhanced left atrial stretch receptor activation depresses renal efferent sympathetic nerve activity and increases renal blood flow and glomerular filtration rate, thereby enhancing the ability of the kidney to reduce plasma volume.

With continued stimulation as occurs in heart failure, there is desensitization of atrial (and arterial) baroreceptors. Zucker et al. observed that the decreased sensitivity of left atrial stretch receptors in dogs with heart failure is the result of cardiac dilatation and alterations in atrial compliance and is reversible following reversal of heart failure.[185,186] This resetting of atrial receptors may be responsible for the inappropriately high plasma ADH levels in heart failure[187] and may contribute to the renal vasoconstriction, peripheral edema, ascites, and hyponatremia characteristic of chronic severe heart failure. With chronic heart failure and its attendant cardiac distention and decreased sensitivity of cardiac receptors, the reflex inhibition of adrenergic activity disappears. The adrenergic drive to the peripheral vascular bed and the adrenal medulla is enhanced, contributing to the sodium retention, tachycardia, and the vasoconstricted state characteristic of heart failure.

There is evidence that abnormal baroreflex control is associated with increased activity of Na^+, K^+-ATPase in the baroreceptors.[188] Digitalis glycosides can partially correct the blunted baroreceptor responsiveness in patients with heart failure.[180] This effect of digitalis is apparently due to a direct action on one or more components of the baroreflex pathway rather than to an improvement in hemodynamic function, because a similar effect is not seen when hemodynamic function is acutely improved by infusion of the beta-adrenergic agonist dobutamine.[180] This thesis is also supported by the observation that, in dogs with pacing-induced heart failure, the selective perfusion of the carotid sinus with ouabain corrected abnormal baroreflex function.[188] This ability of digitalis to correct baroreflex function and thereby suppress adrenergic nerve activity may play a significant role in its clinical efficacy (see Chap. 16). The abnormal baroreflex response in patients with heart failure is usually corrected by cardiac transplantation,[189] indicating that it is a secondary manifestation (not a cause) of heart failure.

ADRENERGIC CONTROL OF THE SPLANCHNIC AND RENAL CIRCULATIONS. Substantial changes also occur in heart failure in the function of the adrenergic nerves that innervate splanchnic and renal vessels.[190,191] Adrenergically mediated vasoconstriction normally occurs in the vessels supplying the splanchnic viscera and kidneys during exercise. However, it has been shown that exercise induces a much more marked reduction in mesenteric blood flow and elevation of mesenteric vascular resistance in dogs with heart failure produced experimentally by inducing tricuspid regurgitation and constriction of the pulmonary artery than in normal dogs.[192] Similar changes during exercise were observed in other major visceral vascular beds, such as the renal bed. Evidence that this intense vasoconstriction during exercise is mediated by the adrenergic nervous system is provided by observations on dogs with experimentally produced heart failure in which one kidney was denervated. Blood flow through the normal kidney declined precipitously during exercise, and calculated renal vascular resistance increased markedly. In contrast, little change in renal blood flow and calculated renal vascular resistance occurred in the denervated kidney.[192] This intensive visceral vasoconstriction during exercise helps to divert the limited cardiac output to exercising muscle but, conversely, may contribute to hypoperfusion of the gut and kidneys.

Beta-Adrenergic Receptor–G Protein–Adenylate Cyclase Pathway

BETA-ADRENERGIC RECEPTORS. Ventricles obtained from patients with heart failure demonstrate a marked reduction in beta-adrenergic receptor density, isoproterenol-mediated adenylate cyclase stimulation, and the contractile response to beta-adrenergic agonists (Table 13–4).[193] It is generally believed that the downregulation of beta-adrenergic receptors is mediated by increased levels of NE in the vicinity of the receptor. In patients with right ventricular failure secondary to primary pulmonary hypertension, beta$_1$-adrenergic receptors are downregulated in the right ventricle but not in the normally functioning left ventricle,[194] suggesting that beta-adrenergic receptor downregulation is due to a local chamber-specific mechanism, presumably an increase in local NE concentrations. In patients with dilated cardiomyopathy, this reduction in receptor density is proportional to the severity of heart failure[195] and involves primarily beta$_1$, but not beta$_2$, receptors, thus reducing the ratio of beta$_1$ to beta$_2$ receptors (Fig. 13–22*A*).[196] The beta$_2$ receptor, although not downregulated, becomes partially

TABLE 13–4 ALTERATIONS IN THE BETA-ADRENERGIC RECEPTOR PATHWAY IN FAILING HUMAN MYOCARDIUM

CONTRACTILE RESPONSES TO VARIOUS AGONISTS (COMPARED WITH NORMAL MYOCARDIUM)
Calcium ↔
Forskolin ↔
β_2-adrenergic agonist ↔/↓
β_1-adrenergic agonist ↓↓
COMPONENTS OF THE β-AR/ADENYLATE CYCLASE PATHWAY (COMPARED WITH NORMAL MYOCARDIUM)
Number of β_1-AR/mRNA ↓↓/↓↓
Number of β_2-AR/mRNA ↔/↔
G_i activity/mRNA ↑/↔
G_s activity/mRNA ↔/↔
βARK activity/mRNA ↑↑/↑↑

↔ = no change.

"uncoupled" from its effector enzyme (adenylate cyclase),[197] producing a similar effect.

The relative roles of beta-adrenergic receptor downregulation versus receptor uncoupling may depend on the cause of heart failure. In myocardium obtained from patients with heart failure secondary to ischemic heart disease, there is a relatively greater degree of receptor desensitization than in myocardium from patients with ischemic cardiomyopathy.[198] This observation, together with apparent differences in the regulation of G-protein function (discussed below), has led to the suggestion that there are differences in the behavior of the beta-adrenergic receptor G-protein complex in these forms of heart failure. The beneficial hemodynamic effects of chronic therapy with the beta-adrenergic antagonist bucindolol were significantly better in patients with idiopathic rather than ischemic cardiomyopathy,[199] suggesting that such differences in pathophysiology may also have therapeutic implications.

In myocardium from patients with heart failure the level of beta$_1$-adrenergic receptor mRNA is decreased, indicating that downregulation of beta$_1$-adrenergic receptors is mediated, at least in part, by a decrease in receptor synthesis, whereas the level of beta$_2$-adrenergic receptor mRNA is unchanged (Fig. 13–22*A*).[202] In addition, there are increases in the expression of beta-adrenergic receptor kinase (BARK) and its mRNA level in failing human myocardium (Fig. 13–22*B*).[203] BARK is an enzyme that phosphorylates both beta$_1$- and beta$_2$-adrenergic receptors and thereby plays a central role in uncoupling of the receptor from its G protein.[203] Increased BARK activity may therefore contribute to the uncoupling of both beta$_1$- and beta$_2$-adrenergic receptors in patients with heart failure.

Downregulation of beta$_1$ receptors in patients with heart failure may be reversed by the administration of metoprolol, a relatively specific beta$_1$ antagonist. The long-term clinical benefit of beta blockade in heart failure (see p. 486) has been reported to be associated with both a restoration of myocardial beta receptor density and the contractile response to administered catecholamines.[204]

G PROTEINS AND ADENYLATE CYCLASE. G proteins play a crucial role in coupling receptors, including beta-adrenergic

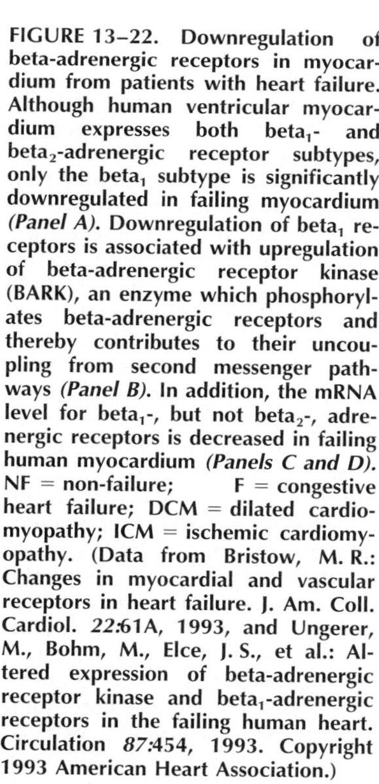

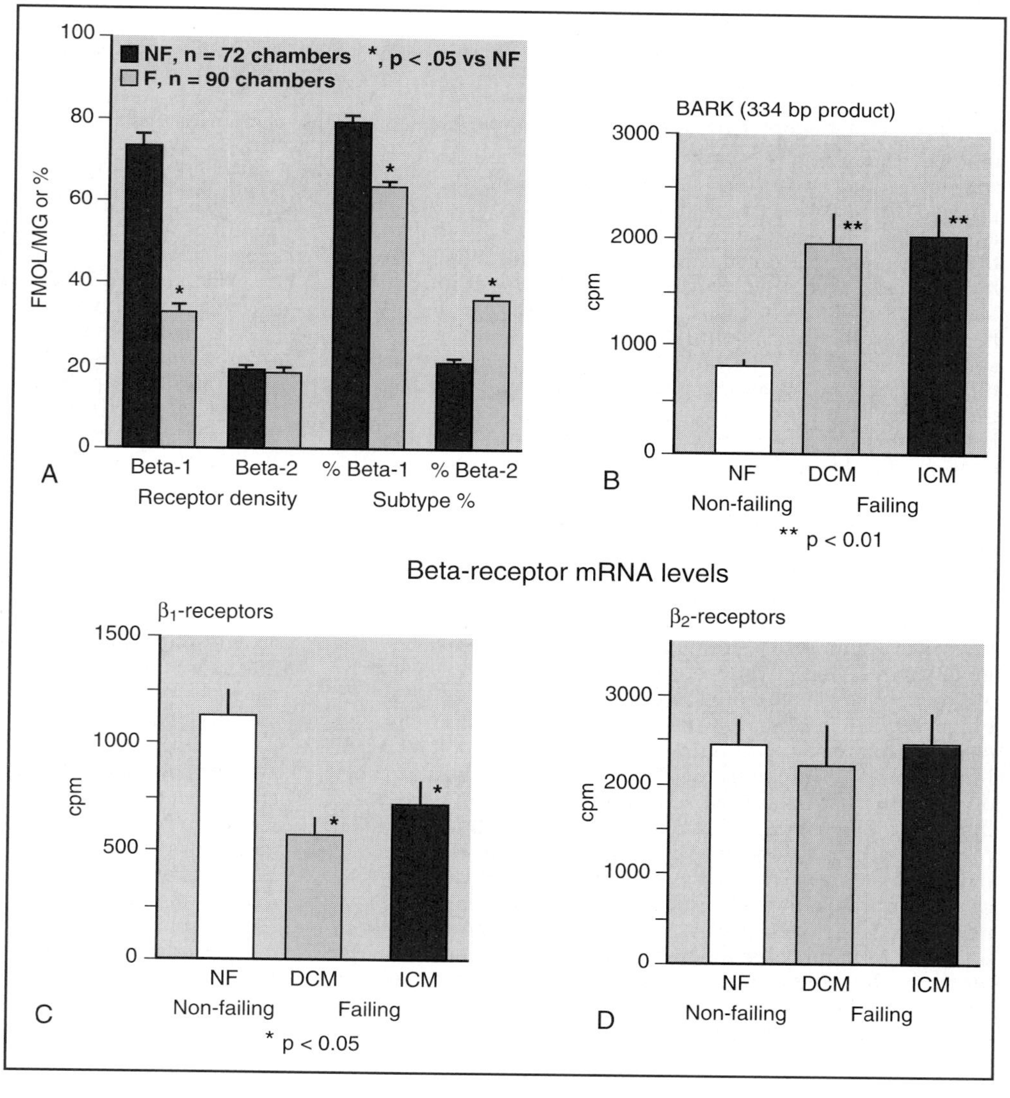

FIGURE 13–22. Downregulation of beta-adrenergic receptors in myocardium from patients with heart failure. Although human ventricular myocardium expresses both beta$_1$- and beta$_2$-adrenergic receptor subtypes, only the beta$_1$ subtype is significantly downregulated in failing myocardium *(Panel A)*. Downregulation of beta$_1$ receptors is associated with upregulation of beta-adrenergic receptor kinase (BARK), an enzyme which phosphorylates beta-adrenergic receptors and thereby contributes to their uncoupling from second messenger pathways *(Panel B)*. In addition, the mRNA level for beta$_1$-, but not beta$_2$-, adrenergic receptors is decreased in failing human myocardium *(Panels C and D)*. NF = non-failure; F = congestive heart failure; DCM = dilated cardiomyopathy; ICM = ischemic cardiomyopathy. (Data from Bristow, M. R.: Changes in myocardial and vascular receptors in heart failure. J. Am. Coll. Cardiol. *22*:61A, 1993, and Ungerer, M., Bohm, M., Elce, J. S., et al.: Altered expression of beta-adrenergic receptor kinase and beta$_1$-adrenergic receptors in the failing human heart. Circulation *87*:454, 1993. Copyright 1993 American Heart Association.)

receptors, to effector enzymes such as adenylate cyclase (see p. 376). Cardiac cells contain at least two types of G proteins: (1) G_s, which mediates the stimulation of adenylate cyclase (and thereby causes a rise in intracellular cyclic AMP, which in turn stimulates Ca^{++} influx into the myocyte through Ca^{++} channels in the sarcolemma and accelerates the uptake of Ca^{++} by the sarcoplasmic reticulum); and (2) G_i, which mediates the inhibition of adenylate cyclase and has the opposite effect on the movements of Ca^{++}.

Heart failure caused by dilated cardiomyopathy is associated with an increase in G_i activity and protein level in heart muscle,[205,206] which may be accompanied by a reduction in the activity of adenylate cyclase.[207] The mechanism responsible for the increase in G_i activity is not known. The level of G_i assessed by Western blotting is increased in myocardium from patients with idiopathic dilated cardiomyopathy but not from those with ischemic heart disease, suggesting that alterations in G protein function are related to the cause of heart failure.[208] The mRNA levels of G_i are not increased in myocardium of patients with heart failure,[209] further suggesting that the increase in G_i activity reflects events at the post-transcriptional level. A reduction in the function of G_s has been reported in the Syrian hamster with dilated cardiomyopathy,[210] but G_s appears normal in failing human myocardium.[205] Overall, heart failure is characterized by an increase in the ratio of $G_i:G_s$.[206,209]

The functional consequences of an increase in G_i activity remain to be established. Although an increase in G_i activity could suppress adenylate cyclase activity and thereby depress basal and beta-adrenergic receptor–stimulated responses, the responses to muscarinic agonists and adenosine, which act via G_i to inhibit adenylate cyclase, are not altered in myocardium from patients with dilated cardiomyopathy.[208]

ADRENERGIC SUPPORT OF THE FAILING HEART. The importance of the adrenergic nervous system in maintaining ventricular contractility when myocardial function is depressed in heart failure is demonstrated by the effects of adrenergic blockade. Acute pharmacological blockade of the adrenergic nervous system may cause intensification of heart failure as well as sodium and water retention.[202,211,212] The acute administration of beta blockers to patients with heart failure results in reductions in both systolic and diastolic myocardial function[213] associated with falls in cardiac output and arterial pressure, and increased filling pressures.[214] Despite the long-term salutary effects of beta-blocker therapy in patients with heart failure (see p. 486), caution should be exercised in using these agents, particularly at the initiation of therapy.

Because of the depletion of cardiac NE stores and the changes in the postsynaptic beta-adrenoceptor pathway, the capacity of the myocardium to produce cyclic AMP is diminished, sometimes profoundly, in patients with heart failure.[193,215] As a consequence, the failing heart loses an important compensatory mechanism. In patients with heart failure, downregulation of postsynaptic beta-adrenoceptors in the sinoatrial node contributes to the attenuated chronotropic response to exercise.[157] Likewise, the positive inotropic response to an intracoronary infusion of the beta-adrenergic agonist dobutamine is markedly reduced in patients with heart failure.[216] The degree of attenuation of both the chronotropic and positive inotropic responses to adrenergic stimulation are correlated with the level of baseline adrenergic activation as reflected by the concentration of plasma norepinephrine (Fig. 13–23).[157,216] An important therapeutic consequence of the alterations of the beta-adrenergic pathway described above is that the positive inotropic response to beta-adrenoceptor agonists, and to a lesser extent to phosphodiesterase inhibitors, is markedly reduced in myocardium obtained from patients with end-stage heart failure.[215]

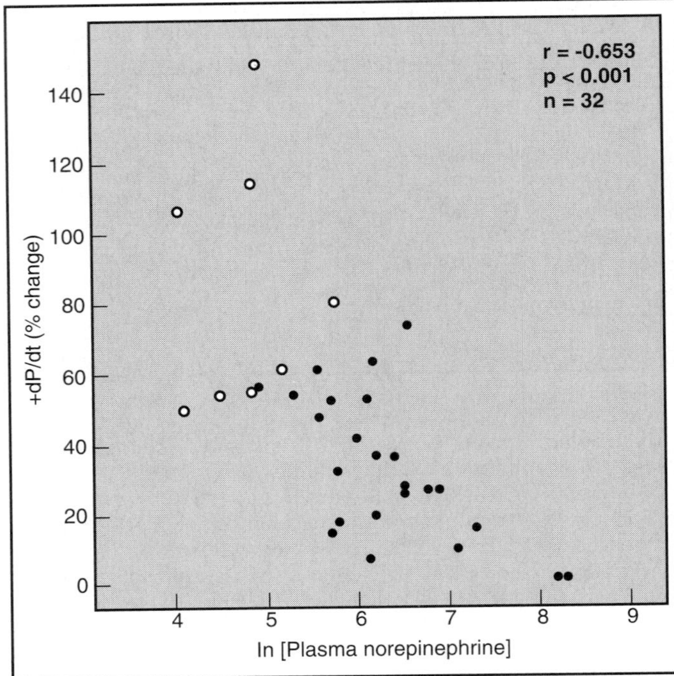

FIGURE 13–23. Relationship between plasma norepinephrine concentration and myocardial beta-adrenergic responsiveness. The positive inotropic response to an intracoronary infusion of the beta-adrenergic agonist dobutamine, as measured by an increase in +dP/dt, was inversely related to the resting level of the logarithm (ln) plasma norepinephrine in patients with heart failure *(solid circles)* or normal ventricular function *(open circles)*. (Reproduced from Colucci, W. S., Denniss, A. R., Leatherman, G. F., et al.: Intracoronary infusion of dobutamine to patients with and without severe congestive heart failure. Dose-response relationships, correlation with circulating catecholamines, and effect of phosphodiesterase inhibition. J. Clin. Invest. *81*:1103, 1988, by copyright permission of the American Society for Clinical Investigation.)

ADVERSE EFFECTS OF ADRENERGIC STIMULATION. Although increased adrenergic activity may play a compensatory role over the short term, chronic adrenergic activation may be deleterious by increasing afterload, precipitating cardiac arrhythmias, and perhaps by exerting toxic and direct receptor-mediated effects on the failing myocardium. Thus, it has been postulated that in heart failure there may be a positive feedback loop causing a vicious circle (Fig. 13–19). According to this concept, heart failure activates the adrenergic nervous system (as well as activating the renin-angiotensin system and stimulating the release of vasopressin and endothelin); this causes increases in preload and afterload that intensify heart failure.

Increased adrenergic nerve activity may also affect the growth and phenotype of the myocardium due to the direct effects of NE on alpha- and beta-adrenergic receptors located on several cell types, including cardiac myocytes, vascular smooth muscle cells, endothelial cells, and fibroblasts. NE, acting on $alpha_1$-adrenergic receptors, induces growth of both cardiac myocytes[165,217,218] and vascular smooth muscle cells.[219] In cardiac myocytes, this effect is associated with the reappearance of fetal genes and fetal isoforms of proteins involved in the development of contractile force, the regulation of myocardial energetics, and excitation-contraction coupling.[89] In addition, NE, acting on both $alpha_1$-adrenergic and beta-adrenergic receptors located on cardiac myocytes and fibroblasts,[166,220] can induce the expression of a variety of peptide growth factors that have been shown to have important effects on the growth and phenotype of myocytes and fibroblasts.[221]

Parasympathetic Function in Heart Failure

Cardiac enlargement, with or without heart failure, is associated with marked disturbances of parasympathetic as well as sympathetic function.[222] The parasympathetic restraint on sinoatrial node automaticity is markedly reduced in patients with heart failure (Fig. 13–3), who exhibit less heart rate slowing for any given elevation of systemic arterial pressure than do normal subjects. The sensitivity of the baroreceptor reflex to an increase in pressure has also been shown to be significantly reduced in dogs with heart failure.[175] Measurements of heart rate variability, which indirectly reflect autonomic nervous system function, indicate that parasympathetic activity in patients with heart failure is abnormal both at rest and in response to exercise.[223]

Abnormal parasympathetic function may also be altered at the level of the peripheral nerve and the postsynaptic receptor. Cardiomyopathic hamster hearts display a reduction in the activity of choline acetyltransferase, an enzyme that provides an estimate of the density of parasympathetic innervation,[224] and there is evidence that the density of high-affinity muscarinic receptors is reduced in the hearts of dogs with experimental heart failure.[225]

Renin-Angiotensin System

(See also pp. 819–820)

In low cardiac output states, there is activation of the renin-angiotensin system (RAS), which operates in concert with the activated adrenergic nervous–adrenal medullary system to maintain arterial pressure. These two compensatory systems are clearly coupled; stimulation of beta$_1$-adrenoceptors in the juxtaglomerular apparatus of the kidneys as a consequence of heightened adrenergic drive is a principal mechanism responsible for the release of renin in acute heart failure. Activation of the baroreceptors in the renal vascular bed by a reduction of renal blood flow is also responsible for the release of renin, and in patients with severe chronic heart failure following salt restriction and diuretic treatment, reduction of the sodium presented to the macula densa contributes to the release of renin. Elevated plasma renin activity is a common, although not universal, finding in heart failure.[151,154,226,227] In the SOLVD study, plasma angiotensin II was significantly elevated even in asymptomatic patients and was further elevated in patients with symptomatic heart failure (Fig. 13–20).[154]

Angiotensin II is a potent peripheral vasoconstrictor and contributes, along with increased adrenergic activity, to the excessive elevation of systemic vascular resistance and the vicious circle already referred to (see p. 402) in patients with heart failure. Angiotensin II also enhances the adrenergic nervous system's release of NE. Aldosterone has potent sodium-retaining properties. Therefore, it is not surprising that interruption of the renin-angiotensin-aldosterone axis by means of an angiotensin-converting enzyme inhibitor reduces system vascular resistance, diminishes afterload, and thereby elevates cardiac output in heart failure. In some patients, these compounds also exert a mild diuretic action, presumably by lowering the angiotensin II-stimulated production of aldosterone.

TISSUE RENIN ANGIOTENSIN SYSTEM (RAS). The major portion (90 to 99 per cent) of angiotensin-converting enzyme (ACE) in the body is found in tissues, and only 1 to 10 per cent is found in the circulation.[228,229] All of the necessary components of the RAS (Fig. 13–24) are likewise present in several organs and tissues, including the vasculature, heart, and kidneys. In myocardium from animals with experimental myocardial hypertrophy or failure, there is increased expression of ACE[230,231] and angiotensinogen,[232] the substrate for angiotensin I production by renin. It has been suggested that the tissue RAS may be activated during compensated heart failure at a time when activity of the circulating system can be relatively normal (Fig. 13–25),[228]

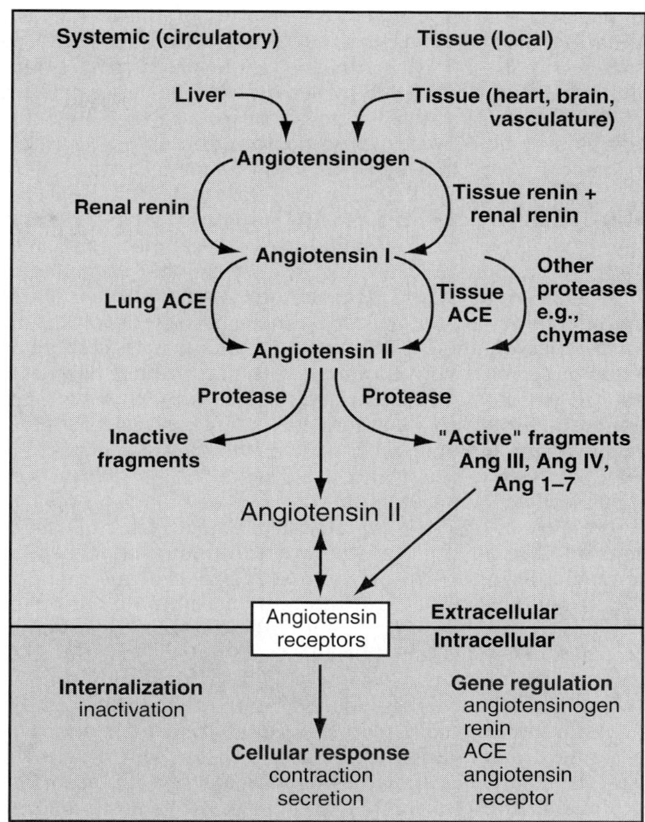

FIGURE 13–24. The systemic and tissue components of the renin-angiotensin system. Several tissues, including myocardium, vasculature, kidney, and brain, have the capacity to generate angiotensin II independent of the circulating renin-angiotensin system. Angiotensin II produced at the tissue level may play an important role in the pathophysiology of heart failure. (Modified from Timmermans, P. B., Wong, P. C., Chiu, A. T., et al.: Angiotensin II receptors and angiotensin II receptor antagonists. Pharmacol. Rev. *45:*205, 1993.)

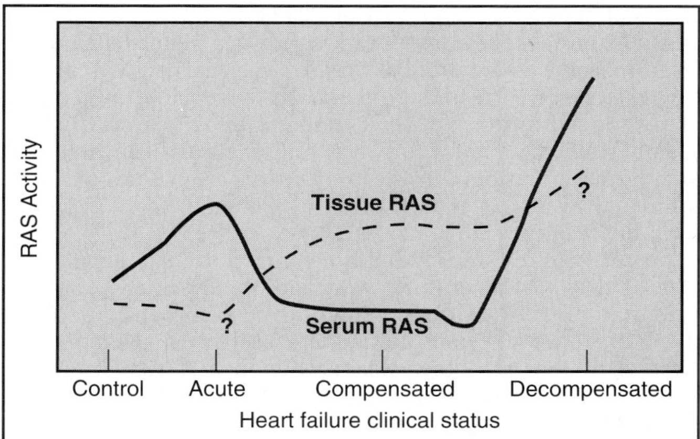

FIGURE 13–25. Relative roles of the circulating and tissue renin-angiotensin systems postulated in patients with heart failure. The tissue system may have alternative pathways for the production of angiotensin II that do not depend on converting enzyme (e.g., chymase), and which therefore are not suppressed by converting enzyme inhibitors. It has been proposed that activation of the tissue renin-angiotensin system may follow a different time course than that of the circulating system, particularly during the compensated phase of heart failure when the circulating renin-angiotensin system may be relatively quiescent and during treatment with converting enzyme inhibitors which may increase the activity of the tissue system by elevating circulating renin levels. (Modified from Dzau, V. J.: Tissue renin-angiotensin system in myocardial hypertrophy and failure. Arch. Intern. Med. *153:*937, 1993.)

and there is evidence that the activities of the tissue and circulating RAS systems can be regulated differentially in animals with heart failure.[233] The tissue production of angiotensin II may also occur by a pathway not dependent on ACE (the chymase pathway). It has been suggested that this pathway may be of major importance in the myocardium,[234] particularly when the levels of renin and angiotensin I are increased by the use of ACE inhibitors.

ANGIOTENSIN RECEPTORS. The predominant angiotensin receptor subtype in the vasculature is the angiotensin$_1$ subtype.[235] In human myocardium it appears that both angiotensin$_1$ and angiotensin$_2$ receptor subtypes are present, and the angiotensin$_2$ receptor predominates in a ratio of 2:1.[236] The number of angiotensin$_1$ and angiotensin$_2$ receptors is normal in patients with moderate heart failure but downregulated in patients with end-stage heart failure.[237] Downregulation of angiotensin receptors has been observed in myocardium from patients with both ischemic and idiopathic dilated cardiomyopathy and associated with a decrease in the mRNA level for the receptor.

Several observations suggest that a direct effect of angiotensin on cardiac angiotensin receptors may play a central role in modifying the structure and function of the myocardium in patients with heart failure by acting on a variety of cell types to promote cell growth and alter gene expression. In cardiac myocytes and fibroblasts obtained from the neonatal rat, angiotensin caused myocyte hypertrophy and fibroblast proliferation associated with the induction of mRNA for several early response genes (c-*fos*, c-*jun*, *jun B*, *Egr-1*, and c-*myc*), angiotensinogen and the peptide growth factor, transforming growth factor-beta$_1$.[238,239] In addition, angiotensin induced mRNA for the fetal genes encoding atrial natriuretic factor and alpha-skeletal actin in myocytes.[238] Because these observations were made in cultured cells, they indicate that angiotensin can exert important effects on the growth and phenotype of cardiac cells, independent of changes in loading conditions on the heart.

Arginine Vasopressin

Arginine vasopressin (AVP) is a pituitary hormone that plays a central role in the regulation of free water clearance and plasma osmolality. Circulating AVP is elevated in many patients with heart failure,[240] even after correction for plasma osmolality. Patients with acute heart failure secondary to massive myocardial infarction may have particularly elevated levels,[241] which are usually associated with elevated concentrations of catecholamines and renin. The plasma AVP concentration was significantly elevated in asymptomatic patients in the prevention arm of the SOLVD study and was elevated further in patients with symptomatic heart failure (Fig. 13–20).[154]

Control of circulating AVP concentration is abnormal in patients with heart failure who fail to show the normal reduction of AVP with a reduction of osmolality.[242] This may contribute to their inadequate ability to excrete free water and hence to the plasma hypoosmolarity in some patients with heart failure. Decreased sensitivity of atrial stretch receptors, which normally inhibit AVP release with atrial distention, may contribute to the elevation of circulating AVP.[243] In addition, patients with heart failure exhibit failure of the normal suppression of AVP following administration of ethanol[244] as well as failure of the normal augmentation of circulating AVP in response to orthostatic stress.[245]

Two types of AVP receptors (V_1 and V_2) have been identified in a variety of tissues. In dogs with pacing-induced heart failure, the selective inhibition of V_1 receptors increased cardiac output without affecting electrolytes or hormone levels.[245] In contrast, inhibition of V_2 receptors increased serum sodium concentration, plasma renin activity, and plasma AVP levels but did not affect hemodynamics. When the two inhibitors were combined, the hemodynamic effects were potentiated. These results suggest that, in addition to regulating free water clearance through the V_2 receptor, in heart failure AVP may contribute to systemic vasoconstriction through the V_1 receptor.

Natriuretic Peptides

Three natriuretic peptides—atrial natriuretic peptide (ANP), brain natriuretic peptide (BNP), and C-natriuretic peptide (CNP)—have been identified in humans.[246] ANP is stored mainly in the right atrium and released in response to an increase in atrial distending pressure. This peptide causes vasodilation and natriuresis and counteracts the water-retaining effects of the adrenergic, renin-angiotensin, and AVP systems. BNP is stored mainly in cardiac ventricular myocardium and may be responsive—albeit less so than ANP—to changes in ventricular filling pressures.[247] BNP has a high level of homology with ANP at the structural level and, like ANP, causes natriuresis and vasodilation. CNP is located primarily in the vasculature. Although the physiological role of CNP is not yet clarified, it appears that it may play an important regulatory role in juxtaposition to the RAS system. At least three receptors for natriuretic peptides (A, B, and C) have been identified.[246] The A and B receptors mediate the vasodilatory and natriuretic effects of the peptides. The C type receptor appears to act primarily as a clearance receptor, which along with neutral endopeptidase, regulates available levels of the peptides.

Circulating levels of both ANP and BNP are elevated in the plasma of patients with heart failure.[248,249] In normal human hearts, ANP predominates in the atria, where there is also a low level of expression of BNP and CNP. In patients with heart failure, the atrial content of ANP is unchanged, and the contents of BNP and CNP increase 10-fold and 2- to 3-fold, respectively.[249] In the SOLVD study, the level of plasma ANP was elevated even in asymptomatic patients and was further elevated in patients with symptoms (Fig. 13–20).[154] Although the atrial peptides are present only in very low levels in normal ventricular myocardium, in patients with heart failure all three peptides are markedly elevated,[249] and ventricular production contributes significantly to the circulating levels.[250] The secretion of ANP and BNP appears to be regulated mainly by wall tension. The N-terminal of the ANP free-hormone (N-terminal pro-ANP) has a longer half-life and greater stability than ANP and has been shown to be a powerful and independent predictor of cardiovascular mortality and the development of heart failure.[251] ANP levels normalize following cardiac transplantation.[252]

The hemodynamic and natriuretic responses to an infusion of ANP are attenuated in patients and experimental animals with heart failure.[253,254] However, studies using an ANP receptor antagonist in dogs with pacing-induced heart failure showed that, despite attenuated hemodynamic and renal effects, the peptide continues to exert an important suppressive effect on the activity of the RAS and NE levels.[255]

One approach that attempts to capitalize on the beneficial effects of the natriuretic peptides is to inhibit their degradation through the use of neutral endopeptidase inhibitors. The infusion of the endopeptidase inhibitor candoxatrilat into patients with heart failure mimics the action of infused ANP; it causes a reduction in left and right heart filling pressures associated with suppression of plasma NE levels and a transient reduction in plasma vasopressin, aldosterone, and renin activity.[256] In addition to the beneficial effect of natriuretic peptides on neurohormones, renal function, and hemodynamics, there is evidence that the natriuretic peptides may directly inhibit myocyte and vascular smooth muscle hypertrophy and interstitial fibrosis.[257–259]

Endothelin

Endothelin is a potent peptide vasoconstrictor released by endothelial cells throughout the circulation.[260] Three endothelin peptides (endothelin-1, endothelin-2, and endothelin-3) have been identified, all of which are potent constrictors. At least two subtypes of endothelin receptors (types A and B) have been recognized. The release of endothelin from endothelial cells in vitro can be enhanced by several vasoactive agents (e.g., NE, angiotensin II, thrombin) and cytokines (e.g., transforming growth factor-beta and interleukin-1 beta).

Several reports have documented an increase in circulating levels of endothelin-1 in patients with heart failure.[261–264] Plasma endothelin correlates directly with pulmonary artery pressures and, in particular, the pulmonary vascular resistance and the resistance ratio of pulmonary vascular resistance to systemic resistance. This has led to the suggestion that endothelin plays a pathophysiological role in mediating pulmonary hypertension in patients with heart failure.[261,263]

In normal subjects, plasma endothelin levels increase with orthostatic stress. However, in heart failure patients, endothelin levels are already elevated and show no further increase with orthostatic stress, similar to the pattern of response seen with a variety of other vasoconstrictor substances, including angiotensin and NE.[262] Plasma endothelin levels have been shown to be increased in patients with acute myocardial infarction and to correlate with the Killip class in these patients.[264]

Antagonists of endothelin receptors are available and have been used to demonstrate the physiological effects of endothelin. When administered to rats with heart failure following myocardial infarction, the endothelin antagonist bosentan, which blocks both endothelin$_A$ and endothelin$_B$ receptors, significantly decreased arterial pressure and had an additive effect to that of an ACE inhibitor.[265] In cultured cardiac myocytes, endothelin induces cellular hypertrophy associated with the induction of fetal genes.[266,267] In rats with pressure overload–induced hypertrophy caused by aortic banding, administration of the endothelin$_A$ receptor antagonist BQ123 transiently inhibited myocyte hypertrophy and prevented fetal gene induction.[268] These observations suggest that endothelin receptor antagonists may be of value in both the acute and chronic treatment of patients with heart failure.

Cytokines

Several peptide mediators, including peptide growth factors and inflammatory cytokines, can have important effects on the myocardium and vasculature and appear to be involved in heart failure. Peptide growth factors can induce growth and modulate gene expression in cardiac myocytes, vascular smooth muscle cells, endothelial cells, and fibroblasts.[228] Several peptide growth factors have been shown to cause hypertrophy associated with the expression of fetal genes.[228] Peptide growth factors can be expressed by several cell types in the heart, including cardiac myocytes[166] and fibroblasts,[227] and there is increased expression of peptide growth factors in response to hemodynamic overload and NE. Increased levels of transforming growth factor-beta$_1$ have been observed in the myocardium in response to myocardial infarction in the rat.[269] These observations suggest that peptide growth factors may play a central role in mediating the changes in myocardial structure and function that occur in heart failure.

The circulating levels of the inflammatory cytokine, tumor necrosis factor-alpha (TNF-alpha) are increased in patients with heart failure.[270,271] TNF-alpha can induce immediate myocardial dysfunction and has been shown to attenuate intracellular calcium transients in vitro.[272–274] The

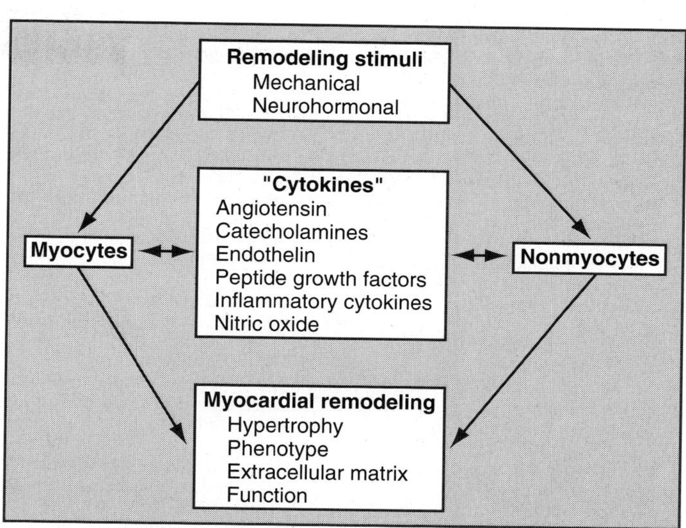

FIGURE 13–26. Central role of cell-to-cell interactions in myocardial remodeling. Both myocytes and nonmyocytes (e.g., fibroblasts, endothelial cells, vascular smooth muscle cells) in the myocardium produce a number of intercellular mediators, many of which are cytokines, that may act on neighboring cells in an autocrine or paracrine manner and thereby play a central role in modulating changes in the structure and function of the myocardium.

inflammatory cytokine, interleukin-1 beta, has been shown to induce myocyte hypertrophy in vitro,[275,276] and can induce the expression of nitric oxide synthase (NOS), resulting in increased levels of nitric oxide.[277] Nitric oxide has been shown to attenuate the positive inotropic response to a beta-adrenergic agonist in cardiac myocytes.[278,279] In normal subjects, the intracoronary infusion of nitroprusside, a nitric oxide donor, improved left ventricular distensibility,[280] whereas inhibition of nitric oxide synthesis by the intracoronary infusion of an NOS inhibitor potentiated the positive inotropic response to dobutamine in patients with left ventricular dysfunction.[281]

The role of inflammatory cytokines and nitric oxide in the pathophysiology of heart failure remains to be determined. The inflammatory cytokines may contribute to the myocardial depression that occurs in patients with inflammatory processes such as myocarditis, sepsis, and transplantation rejection. However, it also appears that inflammatory cytokines may play a role in patients without obvious inflammatory processes, such as those with ischemic and idiopathic dilated cardiomyopathy.[272] Cytokines may exert long-term effects on the remodeling of myocardial and vascular tissue and thereby contribute to the pathophysiology of chronic heart failure (Fig. 13–26). It is of interest that vesnarinone, an oral agent that appears to improve survival in patients with heart failure (see p. 485), has been shown to decrease the plasma levels of inflammatory cytokines.[282]

REFERENCES

ADAPTIVE MECHANISMS

1. Braunwald, E., Mock, M. B., and Watson, J. (eds.): Congestive Heart Failure: Current Research and Clinical Applications. New York, Grune and Stratton, 1982, 384 pp.
2. Katz, A. M.: Cardiomyopathy of overload: A major determinant of prognosis in congestive heart failure. N. Engl. J. Med. *322*:100, 1990.
3. Katz, A. M.: The cardiomyopathy of overload: An unnatural growth response in the hypertrophied heart. Ann. Int. Med. *121*:363, 1994.
4. Braunwald, E., Ross, J., Jr., and Sonnenblick, E. H.: Mechanisms of Contraction of the Normal and Failing Heart. 2nd ed. Boston, Little, Brown and Co., 1976, 417 pp.
5. Jennings, G. L., and Esler, M. D.: Circulatory regulation at rest and exercise and the functional assessment of patients with congestive heart failure. Circulation *81*(Suppl II):5, 1990.
6. Anand, I. S., Ferrari, R., Kalra, G. S., et al.: Studies of body water and sodium, renal function, hemodynamic indexes, and plasma hormones in untreated congestive heart failure. Circulation *80*:299, 1989.

7. Ross, J., Jr., and Braunwald, E.: Studies on Starling's law of the heart. IX. The effects of impeding venous return on performance of the normal and failing human left ventricle. Circulation *30:*719, 1964.
8. Floras, J. S.: Clinical aspects of sympathetic activation and parasympathetic withdrawal in heart failure. J. Am. Coll. Cardiol. *22:*72A, 1993.
9. Leimbach, W. N., Wallin, B. G., Victor, R. G., et al.: Direct evidence from intraneural recordings for increased central sympathetic outflow in patients with heart failure. Circulation *73:*913, 1986.
10. Vanhoutte, P. M.: Adjustments in the peripheral circulation in chronic heart failure. Eur. Heart J. *4*(Suppl. A):67, 1983.
11. Higgins, C. B., Vatner, S. F., Braunwald, E., et al.: Alterations in regional hemodynamics in experimental heart failure in conscious dogs. Trans. Assoc. Am. Physicians *85:*267, 1972.
12. Zelis, R., Mason, D. T., and Braunwald, E.: A comparison of the effects of vasodilator stimuli on peripheral resistance vessels in normal subjects and in patients with congestive heart failure. J. Clin. Invest. *47:*960, 1968.
13. Zelis, R., Mason, D. T., and Braunwald, E.: Partition of blood flow to the cutaneous and muscular beds of the forearm at rest and during leg exercise in normal subjects and in patients with heart failure. Circ. Res. *24:*799, 1969.
14. Zelis, R., Sinoway, L. I., Musch, T. I., et al.: Regional blood flow in congestive heart failure. Concept of compensatory mechanisms with short and long term constants. Am. J. Cardiol. *62:*2E, 1988.
15. Wilson, J. R., Mancini, D. M., McCully, K., et al.: Noninvasive detection of skeletal muscle underperfusion with near-infrared spectroscopy in patients with heart failure. Circulation *80:*1668, 1989.
16. Mancini, D. M., Coyle, E., Coggan, A., et al.: Contribution of intrinsic skeletal muscle changes to 31P NMR skeletal muscle metabolic abnormalities in patients with chronic heart failure. Circulation *80:*1338, 1989.
17. Wilson, J. R., and Mancini, D. M.: Factors contributing to the exercise limitation of heart failure. J. Am. Coll. Cardiol. *22*(Suppl. A):93a, 1993.
18. Kubo, S. H., Rector, T. S., Bank, A. J., et al.: Endothelium-dependent vasodilatation is attenuated in patients with heart failure. Circulation *84:*1589, 1991.
19. Hirooka, Y., Imaizumi, T., Tagawa, T., et al.: Effects of L-arginine on impaired acetylcholine-induced and ischemic vasodilation of the forearm in patients with heart failure. Circulation *90:*658, 1994.
20. Woodson, R. D., Torrance, J. D., Shappell, S. D., and Lenfant, C.: The effect of cardiac diseases on hemoglobin-oxygen binding. J. Clin. Invest. *49:*1349, 1970.

CONTRACTILITY OF HYPERTROPHIED AND FAILING MYOCARDIUM

21. Krayenbuehl, H. P., Hess, O. M., Schneider, J., and Turina, M.: Physiologic or pathologic hypertrophy. Eur. Heart J. *4*(Suppl. A):29, 1983.
22. Spann, J. F., Jr., Buccino, R. A., Sonnenblick, E. H., and Braunwald, E.: Contractile state of cardiac muscle obtained from cats with experimentally produced ventricular hypertrophy and heart failure. Circ. Res. *21:*341, 1967.
23. Cooper, G., IV, Tomanek, R. J., Ehrhardt, J. D., and Marcus, M. L.: Chronic progressive pressure overload of the cat right ventricle. Circ. Res. *48:*488, 1981.
24. Crozatier, B., and Hittinger, L.: Mechanical adaptation to chronic pressure overload. Eur. Heart J. *9:*E-7, 1988.
25. Capasso, J. M., Aronson, R. S., and Sonnenblick, E. H.: Reversible alterations in excitation-contraction coupling during myocardial hypertrophy in rat papillary muscle. Circ. Res. *51:*189, 1982.
26. Chidsey, C. A., Sonnenblick, E. H., Morrow, A. G., and Braunwald, E.: Norepinephrine stores and contractile force of papillary muscle from the failing human heart. Circulation *33:*43, 1966.
27. Cooper, G., IV, Puga, F., Zujko, K. J., et al.: Normal myocardial function and energetics in volume-overload hypertrophy in the cat. Circ. Res. *32:*140, 1973.
28. Schwinger, R. H., Boh, M., Muller-Ehrnsen, J., et al.: Effect of inotropic stimulation on the negative force-frequency relationship in the failing human heart. Circulation *88:*2267, 1993.
29. Gwathmey, J. K., Copelas, L., MacKinnon, R., et al.: Abnormal intracellular calcium handling in myocardium from patients with end-stage heart failure. Circ. Res. *61:*70, 1987.
30. Dalen, H., Saetersdal, T., and Odegarden, S.: Some ultrastructural features of the myocardial cells in the hypertrophied human papillary muscle. Virchows Arch. A. *410:*281, 1987.
31. Ross, J., Jr., Sonnenblick, E. H., Taylor, R. R., and Covell, J. W.: Diastolic geometry and sarcomere length in the chronically dilated canine left ventricle. Circ. Res. *28:*49, 1971.
32. Spann, J. F., Jr., Covell, J. W., Eckberg, D. L., et al.: Contractile performance of the hypertrophied and chronically failing cat ventricle. Am. J. Physiol. *223:*1150, 1972.
33. Alyono, D., Ring, W. S., Anderson, M. R., and Anderson, R. W.: Left ventricular adaptation to volume overload from large aortocaval fistula. Surgery *96:*360, 1984.
34. Legault, D., Rouleau, J. L., Juneau, C., et al.: Functional and morphological characteristics of compensated and decompensated cardiac hypertrophy in dogs with chronic infrarenal aortocaval fistulas. Circ. Res. *66:*846, 1990.
35. Carabello, B. A., Nakano, K., Corin, W., et al.: Left ventricular function in experimental volume overload hypertrophy. Am. J. Physiol. *256:*H974, 1989.

MYOCARDIAL HYPERTROPHY

36. Cohn, J. N.: Structural basis for heart failure. Ventricular remodeling and its pharmacological inhibition. Circulation *91:*2504, 1995.
37. Beltrami, C. A., Finato, N., Rocco, M., et al.: Structural basis of end-stage failure in ischemic cardiomyopathy in humans. Circulation *89:*151, 1994.
38. Zak, R.: Cardiac hypertrophy: Biochemical and cellular relationships. Hosp. Pract. *18:*85, 1983.
39. Weber, K. T., Nanicki, J. S., Schroff, S. G., Pick, R., et al.: Collagen remodeling of the pressure-overloaded, hypertrophied nonhuman primate myocardium. Circ. Res. *62:*757, 1988.
40. Grossman, W., Jones, D., and McLaurin, L. P.: Wall stress and patterns of hypertrophy in the human left ventricle. J. Clin. Invest. *56:*56, 1975.
41. Gunther, S., and Grossman, W.: Determinants of ventricular function in pressure overload hypertrophy in man. Circulation *59:*679, 1979.
42. Donner, R., Carabello, B. A., Black, I., and Spann, J. F.: Left ventricular wall stress in compensated aortic stenosis in children. Am. J. Cardiol. *51:*946, 1983.
43. Spann, J. F., Bove, A. A., Natarajean, G., and Kreulen, T.: Ventricular performance, pump function and compensatory mechanisms in patients with aortic stenosis. Circulation *82:*2075, 1990.
44. Anversa, P., Ricci, R., and Olivetti, G.: Quantitative structural analyses of the myocardium during physiologic growth and induced cardiac hypertrophy: A review. J. Am. Coll. Cardiol. *7:*1140, 1986.
45. Hayashida, W., Kumada, T., Nohara, R., et al.: Left ventricular regional wall stress in dilated cardiomyopathy. Circulation *82:*2075, 1990.
46. Ross, J., Jr.: Afterload mismatch and preload reserve: A conceptual framework for the analysis of ventricular function. Prog. Cardiovasc. Dis. *18:*255, 1976.
47. Sasayama, S., Ross, J., Jr., Franklin, D., et al.: Adaptations of the left ventricle to chronic pressure overload. Circ. Res. *38:*172, 1976.
48. Pelliccia, A., Maron, B. J., Spataro, A., et al.: The upper limit of physiologic cardiac hypertrophy in highly trained elite athletes. N. Engl. J. Med. *324:*295, 1991.
49. Meerson, F. Z.: The myocardium in hyperfunction, hypertrophy, and heart failure. Circ. Res. *25*(Suppl. 2):1, 1969.
50. Ferrans, V. J.: Morphology of the heart in hypertrophy. Hosp. Pract. *18:*67, 1983.
51. Breisch, E. A., White, F. C., and Bloor, C. M.: Myocardial characteristics of pressure overload hypertrophy: A structural and functional study. Lab. Invest. *51:*333, 1984.
52. Anversa, P., Palackal, T., Sonnenblick, E. H., et al.: Myocyte cell loss and myocyte cellular hyperplasia in the hypertrophied aging rat heart. Circ. Res. *67:*871, 1990.
53. Olivetti, G., Melissari, M., Capasso, J. M., and Anversa, B.: Cardiomyopathy of the aging human heart: Myocyte loss and reactive cellular hypertrophy. Circ. Res. *68:*1560, 1991.
54. Pouleur, H. G., Konstam, M. A., Udelson, J. E., and Rousseau, M. F.: Changes in ventricular volume wall thickness and wall stress during progression of left ventricular dysfunction. J. Am. Coll. Cardiol. *224*(Suppl. 4A):43a, 1993.
55. Aoyagi, T., Fujii, A. M., Flanagan, M. F., et al.: Transition from compensated hypertrophy to intrinsic myocardial dysfunction during development of left ventricular pressure-overload hypertrophy in conscious sheep. Systolic dysfunction precedes diastolic dysfunction. Circulation *88:*2415, 1993.
56. Palmon, L. C., Reichek, N., Yeon, S. B., et al.: Intramural myocardial shortening in hypertensive left ventricular hypertrophy with normal pump function. Circulation *89:*122, 1994.
57. Weinberg, E. O., Schoen, F. J., George, D., et al.: Angiotensin-converting enzyme inhibition prolongs survival and modifies the transition to heart failure in rats with pressure overload hypertrophy due to ascending aortic stenosis. Circulation *90:*1410, 1994.
58. Vatner, S. F., and Hittinger, L.: Coronary vascular mechanisms involved in decompensation from hypertrophy to heart failure. J. Am. Coll. Cardiol. *224*(Suppl. 4A):34a, 1993.

PATHOPHYSIOLOGY OF DIASTOLIC HEART FAILURE

59. Lenihan, D. J., Gerson, M. C., Hoit, B. D., et al.: Mechanisms, diagnosis and treatment of diastolic heart failure. Am. Heart J. *130:*153, 1995.
60. Soufer, R., Wohlgelernter, D., Vita, N. A., et al.: Intact systolic left ventricular function in clinical congestive heart failure. Am. J. Cardiol. *55:*1032, 1985.
61. Grossman, W.: Diastolic dysfunction in congestive heart failure. N. Engl. J. Med. *325:*1557, 1991.
62. Brutsaert, D. L., Rademakers, F. E., and Sys, S. U.: Triple control of relaxation: Implications in cardiac disease. Circulation *69:*190, 1984.
63. Gwathmey, J. K., Warren, S. E., Briggs, G. M., et al.: Diastolic dysfunction in hypertrophic cardiomyopathy; effect on active force generation during systole. J. Clin. Invest. *87:*1023, 1991.
64. Gwathmey, J. K., and Morgan, J. P.: Altered calcium handling in experimental pressure-overload hypertrophy in the ferret. Circ. Res. *57:*836, 1985.
65. Heyndrickx, G. R., and Paulus, W. J.: Effect of asynchrony on left ventricular relaxation. Circulation *81*(Suppl. III):41, 1990.
66. Bonow, R. O.: Regional left ventricular nonuniformity: Effects of left ventricular diastolic function in ischemic heart disease, hypertrophic cardiomyopathy, and the normal heart. Circulation *81*(Suppl. III):54, 1990.

67. Gaasch, W. H., Levine, H. J., Quinnes, M. A., and Alexander, J. K.: Left ventricular compliance: Mechanisms and clinical implications. Am. J. Cardiol. *38:*645, 1976.
68. Corin, W. J., Murakami, T., Monrad, E. S., et al.: Left ventricular passive diastolic properties in chronic mitral regurgitation. Circulation *83:*797, 1991.
69. McCullagh, W. H., Covell, J. W., and Ross, J., Jr.: Left ventricular dilatation and diastolic compliance changes during chronic volume overloading. Circulation *45:*943, 1972.
70. Lecarpentier, Y., Waldenstrom, A., Clergue, M., et al.: Major alterations in relaxation during cardiac hypertrophy induced by aortic stenosis in guinea pig. Circ. Res. *61:*107, 1987.
71. Warren, S. E., Coh, L. H., Schoen, F. J., et al.: Advanced diastolic heart failure in familial hypertrophic cardiomyopathy managed with cardiac transplantation. J. Appl. Cardiol. *3:*415, 1988.
72. Douglas, P. S., Berko, B., Lesh, M., and Reichek, N.: Alterations in diastolic function in response to progressive left ventricular hypertrophy. J. Am. Coll. Cardiol. *13:*461, 1989.
73. Williams, J. F., Jr., Potter, R. D., Hern, D. L., et al.: Hydroxyproline and passive stiffness of pressure-induced hypertrophied kitten myocardium. J. Clin. Invest. *89:*309, 1982.
74. Fifer, M. A., Borow, K. M., Colan, S. D., and Lorell, B. H.: Early diastolic left ventricular function in children and adults with aortic stenosis. J. Am. Coll. Cardiol. *5:*1147, 1985.
75. Smith, V. E., Schulman, P., Karimeddini, M. K., et al.: Rapid ventricular filling in left ventricular hypertrophy. II. Pathologic hypertrophy. J. Am. Coll. Cardiol. *5:*869, 1985.
76. Papademetriou, V., Gottdiener, J. S., Fletcher, R. D., and Freis, E. D.: Echocardiographic assessment by computer-assisted analysis of diastolic left ventricular function and hypertrophy in borderline or mild systemic hypertension. Am. J. Cardiol. *56:*546, 1985.
77. Serizawa, T., Carabello, B. A., and Grossman, W.: Effect of pacing induced ischemia on left ventricular diastolic pressure-volume relations in dogs with coronary stenosis. Circ. Res. *46:*430, 1980.
78. Hess, O. M., Osakada, G., Lavelle, J. F., et al.: Diastolic myocardial wall stiffness and ventricular relaxation during partial and complete coronary occlusions in the conscious dog. Circ. Res. *52:*387, 1983.
79. Forrester, J., Diamond, C., Parmley, W. W., and Swan, H. J. C.: Early increase in left ventricular compliance following myocardial infarction. J. Clin. Invest. *51:*598, 1972.
80. Pirzada, F. A., Ekong, E. A., Vokonas, P. S., et al.: Experimental myocardial infarction. XIII. Sequential changes in left ventricular pressure-length relations in the acute phase. Circulation *53:*970, 1976.
81. Farhi, E. R., Canty, J. J., and Klocke, F. J.: Effects of graded reductions in coronary perfusion pressure on the diastolic pressure-segment length relation and the rate of isovolumic relaxation in the resulting conscious dog. Circulation *80:*1458, 1989.
82. Diamond, C., and Forrester, J. S.: Effect of coronary artery disease and acute myocardial infarction on left ventricular compliance in man. Circulation *45:*11, 1972.
83. Fletcher, P. J., Pfeffer, J. M., Pfeffer, M. A., and Braunwald, E.: Left ventricular diastolic pressure-volume relations in rats with healed myocardial infarction. Effects on systolic function. Circ. Res. *49:*618, 1981.
84. Vatner, S. F., Shannon, R., and Hittinger, L.: Reduced subendocardial coronary reserve: A potential mechanism for impaired diastolic function in the hypertrophied and failing heart. Circulation *81*(Suppl. III):8, 1990.
85. Weber, K. T., Jalil, J. E., Janicki, J. S., and Pick, R.: Myocardial collagen remodeling in pressure overload hypertrophy. Am. J. Hypertens. *2:*931, 1989.
86. Weber, K. T., Pick, R., Silver, M. A., et al.: Fibrillar collagen and remodeling of dilated canine left ventricle. Circulation *82:*1387, 1990.
87. Iimoto, D. S., Covell, J. W., and Harper, E.: Increase in cross-linking of Type I and Type III collagens associated with volume-overloaded hypertrophy. Circ. Res. *63:*399, 1988.
88. Chapman, D., Weber, K. T., and Eghbali, M.: Regulation of fibrillar collagen Types I and III and basement membrane Type IV collagen gene expression in pressure-overloaded rat myocardium. Circ. Res. *67:*787, 1990.

CELLULAR AND MOLECULAR MECHANISMS OF MYOCARDIAL DYSFUNCTION

89. Thaik, C. M., and Colucci, W. S.: Molecular and cellular events in myocardial hypertrophy and failure. *In* Braunwald, E. (ed.): Atlas of Heart Diseases. Heart Failure: Cardiac Function and Dysfunction. Vol. IV. Colucci, W. S. (volume ed.). St. Louis, Mosby-Year Book, 1995, p 4.2.
90. Mann, D. L., Urabe, Y., Kent, R. L., et al.: Cellular versus myocardial basis for the contractile dysfunction of hypertrophied myocardium. Circ. Res. *68:*402, 1991.
91. Morgan, J. P.: Abnormal intracellular modulation of calcium as a major cause of cardiac contractile dysfunction. N. Engl. J. Med. *325:*625, 1991.
92. Connor, T. B., Rosen, B. L., Blaustein, M. P., et al.: Hypocalcemia precipitating congestive heart failure. N. Engl. J. Med. *307:*869, 1982.
93. Levine, S. N., and Rheams, C. N.: Hypocalcemic heart failure. Am. J. Med. *78:*1033, 1985.
94. Henrich, W. L., Hunt, J. M., and Nixon, J. V.: Increased ionized calcium and left ventricular contractility during hemodialysis. N. Engl. J. Med. *310:*19, 1984.
95. Ginsburg, R., Esserman, L. J., and Bristow, M. R.: Myocardial performance and extracellular ionized calcium in a severely failing human heart. Ann. Intern. Med. *98:*603, 1983.
96. Beuckelmann, D. J., Nabauer, M., and Erdmann, E.: Intracellular calcium handling in isolated ventricular myocytes from patients with terminal heart failure. Circulation *85:*1046, 1992.
97. Hasenfuss, G., Mulieri, L. A., Leavitt, B. J., et al.: Alteration of contractile function and excitation-contraction coupling in dilated cardiomyopathy. Circ. Res. *70:*1225, 1992.
98. Hasenfuss, G., Mulieri, L. A., Blanchard, E. M., et al.: Energetics of isometric force development in control and volume-overload human myocardium: Comparison with animal species. Circ. Res. *68:*836, 1991.
99. Mulieri, L. A., Hasenfuss, G., Leavitt, B., Allen, P. D., and Alpert, N. R.: Altered myocardial force–frequency relation in human heart failure. Circulation *85:*1743, 1992.
99a. Feldman, M. D., Alderman, J. D., Aroesty, J. M., et al.: Depression of systolic and diastolic myocardial reserve during atrial pacing tachycardia in patients with dilated cardiomyopathy. J. Clin. Invest. *82:*1661, 1988.
100. Arai, M., Matsui, H., and Periasamy, M.: Sarcoplasmic reticulum gene expression in cardiac hypertrophy and heart failure. Circ. Res. *74:*555, 1994.
101. Sham, J. S. K., Jones, L. R., and Morad, M.: Phospholamban mediates the beta adrenergic–enhanced Ca^{2+} uptake in mammalian ventricular myocytes. Am. J. Physiol. *261:*H1344, 1991.
102. Luo, W., Grupp, I. L., Harrer, J., et al.: Targeted ablation of the phospholamban gene is associated with markedly enhanced myocardial contractility and loss of beta-agonist stimulation. Circ. Res. *75:*401, 1994.
103. Mercadier, J.-J., Lompre, A.-M., Duc, P., et al.: Altered sarcoplasmic reticulum Ca^{2+}-ATPase gene expression in the human ventricle during end-stage heart failure. J. Clin. Invest. *85:*305, 1990.
104. Arai, M., Alpert, N. R., MacLennan, D. H., et al.: Alterations in sarcoplasmic reticulum gene expression in human heart failure. A possible mechanism for alterations in systolic and diastolic properties of the failing myocardium. Circ. Res. *72:*463, 1993.
105. Studer, R., Reinecke, H., Bilger, J., et al.: Gene expression of the cardiac Na^{+}-Ca^{2+} exchanger in end-stage human heart failure. Circ. Res. *75:*443, 1994.
106. Feldman, A. M., Ray, P. E., Silan, C. M., et al.: Selective gene expression in failing human heart. Quantification of steady-state levels of messenger RNA in endomyocardial biopsies using the polymerase chain reaction. Circulation *83:*1866, 1991.
107. Sordahl, L. A., McCollum, W. B., Wood, W. G., and Schwartz, A.: Mitochondria and sarcoplasmic reticulum function in cardiac hypertrophy and failure. Am. J. Physiol. *224:*497, 1973.
108. Ito, Y., Suko, J., and Chidsey, A. A.: Intracellular calcium and myocardial contractility: V. Calcium uptake of sarcoplasmic reticulum fractions in hypertrophied and failing rabbit hearts. J. Mol. Cell. Cardiol. *6:*237, 1974.
109. Whitmer, J. T., Kumar, P., and Solaro, R. J.: Calcium transport properties of cardiac sarcoplasmic reticulum from cardiomyopathic Syrian hamsters (BIO 53.58 and 14.6): Evidence for a quantitative defect in dilated myopathic hearts not evident in hypertrophic hearts. Circ. Res. *62:*81, 1988.
110. Limas, C. J., Olivari, M.-T., Goldenberg, I. F., et al.: Calcium uptake by cardiac sarcoplasmic reticulum in human dilated cardiomyopathy. Cardiovasc. Res. *21:*601, 1987.
111. Movsesian, M. A., Karimi, M., Green, K., and Jones, L. R.: Ca^{2+}-transporting ATPase, phospholamban, and calsequestrin levels in nonfailing and failing human myocardium. Circulation *90:*653, 1994.
112. Brillantes, A.-M., Allen, P., Takahasi, T., et al.: Differences in cardiac calcium release channel (ryanodine receptor) expression in myocardium from patients with end-stage heart failure caused by ischemic versus dilated cardiomyopathy. Circ. Res. *71:*18, 1992.
113. Takahashi, T., Allen, P. D., Lacro, R. V., et al.: Expression of dihydropyridine receptor (Ca^{2+} channel) and calsequestrin genes in the myocardium of patients with end-stage heart failure. J. Clin. Invest. *90:*927, 1992.
114. Page, E., and McCallister, L. P.: Quantitative electron microscopic description of heart muscle cells. Application to normal, hypertrophied and thyroxin-stimulated hearts. Am. J. Cardiol. *31:*172, 1973.
115. Schwarz, F., Schaper, J., Kittstein, D., et al.: Reduced volume fraction of myofibrils in myocardium of patients with decompensated pressure overload. Circulation *63:*1299, 1981.
116. Hammond, E. H., Anderson, J. L., and Menlove, R. L.: Prognostic significance of myofilament loss in patients with idiopathic cardiomyopathy determined by electron microscopy. J. Am. Coll. Cardiol. *7:*204A, 1986.
117. Alpert, N. R., and Gordon, M. S.: Myofibrillar adenosine triphosphate activity in congestive failure. Am. J. Physiol. *202:*940, 1962.
118. Gordon, M. S., and Brown, A. L.: Myofibrillar adenosine triphosphate activity of human heart tissue and congestive failure: Effects of ouabain and calcium. Circ. Res. *19:*534, 1966.
119. Luchi, R. J., Dritcher, E. M., and Thyrum, P. T.: Reduced cardiac myosin adenosine triphosphate activity in dogs with spontaneously occurring heart failure. Circ. Res. *24:*513, 1969.
120. Chandler, B. M., Sonnenblick, E. H., Spann, J. R., Jr., and Pool, P. E.: Association of depressed myofibrillar adenosine triphosphatase and reduced contractility in experimental heart failure. Circ. Res. *21:*717, 1967.

121. Draper, M., Taylor, N., and Alpert, N. R.: Alteration in contractile protein in hypertrophied guinea pig hearts. *In* Alpert, N. (ed.): Cardiac Hypertrophy. New York, Academic Press, 1971, p. 315.
122. Wikman–Coffelt, J., Kamiyama, T., Salel, A. F., and Mason, D. T.: Differential responses of canine myosin ATPase activity and tissue gases in the pressure-overloaded ventricle dependent upon degree of obstruction—mild versus severe pulmonic and aortic stenosis. *In* Kobayashi, T., Yoshio, I., and Rona, G. (eds.): Recent Advances in Studies on Cardiac Structure and Metabolism. Vol. 12. Cardiac Adaption. Baltimore, University Park Press, 1978, p. 367.
123. Scheuer, J., Malhotra, A., Hirsch, C., et al.: Physiologic cardiac hypertrophy corrects contractile protein abnormalities associated with pathologic hypertrophy in rats. J. Clin. Invest. *70:*1300, 1983.
124. Solaro, R. J., Powers, F. M., Gao, L., and Gwathmey, J. K.: Control of myofilament activation in heart failure. Circulation *87:*VII–38, 1993.
124a. Kitsis, R. N., and Scheuer, J.: Functional significance of alterations in cardiac contractile protein isoforms. Clin. Cardiol. *19:*9, 1996.
125. Walsh, R. A., Henkel, R., and Robbins, J.: Cardiac myosin heavy- and light-chain gene expression in hypertrophy and heart failure. Heart Failure *6:*238, 1991.
126. Gorza, L., Pauletto, P., Pessina, A. C., et al.: Isomyosin distribution in normal and pressure-overloaded rat ventricular myocardium. An immunohistochemical study. Circ. Res. *49:*1003, 1981.
127. Geenen, D. L., Malhotra, A., Scheuer, J.: Ventricular function and contractile proteins in the infarcted rat heart exposed to chronic pressure overload. Am. J. Physiol. *256:*H745, 1989.
128. Scheuer, J.: Cardiac contractile proteins and congestive heart failure. J. Appl. Cardiol. *4:*407, 1989.
129. Bugaisky, L. B., Anderson, P. G., Hall, R. S., and Bishop, S. P.: Differences in myosin isoform expression in the subepicardial and subendocardial myocardium during cardiac hypertrophy in the rat. Circ. Res. *66:*1127, 1990.
130. Bouvagnet, P., Mairhofer, H., Leger, J. O. C., et al.: Distribution of pattern of and myosin in normal and diseased human ventricular myocardium. Basic Res. Cardiol. *84:*91, 1989.
131. Malhotra, A., and Scheuer, J.: Troponin-tropomyosin dysfunction in cardiomyopathy. Circulation *78:*179, 1988.
132. Malhotra, A.: Regulatory proteins in hamster cardiomyopathy. Circ. Res. *66:*1302, 1990.
133. Walsh, R. A., Henkel, R., and Robbins, J.: Cardiac myosin heavy- and light-chain gene expression in hypertrophy and heart disease. Heart Failure *6:*238, 1991.
134. Anderson, P. A. W., Malouf, N. N., Oakeley, A. E., et al.: Troponin T isoform expression in the normal and failing human left ventricle: A correlation with myofibrillar ATPase activity. Basic Res. Cardiol. *87:*175, 1992.
135. Bing, R. L.: The biochemical basis of myocardial failure. Hosp. Pract. *18:*93, 1983.
136. Graham, T. P., Jr., Ross, J., Jr., and Covell, J. W.: Myocardial oxygen consumption in acute experimental cardiac depression. Circ. Res. *21:*123, 1967.
137. Henry, P. D., Eckberg, D., Gault, J. H., and Ross, J., Jr.: Depressed inotropic state and reduced myocardial oxygen consumption in the human heart. Am. J. Cardiol. *31:*300, 1973.
138. Sievers, R., Parmley, W. W., James, T., and Coffelt-Wilman, J.: Energy levels at systole vs. diastole in normal hamster hearts vs. myopathic hamster hearts. Circ. Res. *53:*759, 1983.
139. Chidsey, C. A., Weinbach, E. C., Pool, P. E., and Morrow, A. G.: Biochemical studies of energy production in the failing human heart. J. Clin. Invest. *45:*40, 1966.
140. Sobel, B. E., Spann, J. F., Jr., Pool, P. E., et al.: Normal oxidative phosphorylation in mitochondria from the failing heart. Circ. Res. *21:*355, 1967.
141. Buchwald, A., Till, H., Unterberg, C., et al.: Alterations of the mitochondrial respiratory chain in human dilated cardiomyopathy. Eur. Heart J. *11:*509, 1990.
142. Schulze, K., Becker, B. F., Schauer, R., and Schultheiss, H. P.: Antibodies to ADP-ATP carrier—an autoantigen in myocarditis and dilated cardiomyopathy—impair cardiac function. Circulation *81:*959, 1990.
143. Ingwall, J. S.: Is cardiac failure a consequence of decreased energy reserve? Circulation *87:*VII–58, 1993.
144. Conway, M. A., Allis, J., Ouwerkerk, R., et al.: Detection of low phosphocreatine to ATP ratio in failing hypertrophied human myocardium by ^{31}P magnetic resonance spectroscopy. Lancet *338:*973, 1991.
145. Hardy, C. J., Weiss, R. G., Bottomley, P. A., and Gerstenblith, G.: Altered myocardial high-energy phosphate metabolites in patients with dilated cardiomyopathy. Am. Heart J. *122:*795, 1991.
146. Nascimben, L., Friedrich, J., Liao, R., et al.: Enalapril treatment increases cardiac performance and energy reserve via the creatine kinase reaction in myocardium of Syrian myopathic hamsters with advanced heart failure. Circulation *91:*1824, 1995.
147. Capasso, J. M., Aronson, R. S., Strobeck, J. E., and Sonnenblick, E. H.: Effects of experimental phosphate deficiency on action potential characteristics and contractile performance of rat myocardium. Cardiovasc. Res. *16:*71, 1982.
148. Davis, S. V., Olichwier, K. K., and Chakko, S. C.: Reversible depression of myocardial performance in hypophosphatemia. Am. J. Med. Sci. *295:*183, 1988.

NEUROHORMONAL, AUTOCRINE, AND PARACRINE ADJUSTMENTS

149. Dzau, V. J.: Autocrine and paracrine mechanisms in the pathophysiology of heart failure. Am. J. Cardiol. *70:*4C, 1992.
150. Thomas, J. A., and Marks, B. H.: Plasma norepinephrine in congestive heart failure. Am. J. Cardiol. *41:*233, 1978.
151. Francis, G. S., Goldsmith, S. R., Levine, T. B., et al.: The neurohumoral axis in congestive heart failure. Ann. Intern. Med. *101:*370, 1984.
152. Chidsey, C. A., Braunwald, E., and Morrow, A. G.: Catecholamine excretion and cardiac stores of norepinephrine in congestive heart failure. Am. J. Med. *39:*442, 1965.
153. Viquerat, C. E., Daly, P., Swedberg, K., et al.: Endogenous catecholamine levels in chronic heart failure: Relation to the severity of hemodynamic abnormalities. Am. J. Med. *78:*455, 1985.
154. Francis, G. S., Benedict, C., Johnstone, D. E., et al.: Comparison of neuroendocrine activation in patients with left ventricular dysfunction with and without congestive heart failure. A substudy of the studies of left ventricular dysfunction (SOLVD). Circulation *82:*1724, 1990.
155. Chidsey, C. A., Harrison, D. C., and Braunwald, E.: Augmentation of plasma norepinephrine response to exercise in patients with congestive heart failure. N. Engl. J. Med. *267:*650, 1962.
156. Francis, G. S., Goldsmith, S. R., Ziesche, S., et al.: Relative attenuation of sympathetic drive during exercise in patients with congestive heart failure. J. Am. Coll. Cardiol. *5:*832, 1985.
157. Colucci, W. S., Ribeiro, J. P., Rocco, M. B., et al.: Impaired chronotropic response to exercise in patients with congestive heart failure. Role of postsynaptic beta-adrenergic desensitization. Circulation *80:*314, 1989.
158. Rose, C. P., Burgess, J. H., and Cousineau, D.: Tracer norepinephrine kinetics in coronary circulation of patients with heart failure secondary to chronic pressure and volume overload. J. Clin. Invest. *76:*1740, 1985.
159. Hasking, G. J., Esler, M. D., Jennings, G. L., et al.: Norepinephrine spillover to plasma in patients with congestive heart failure: Evidence of increased overall and cardiorenal sympathetic nervous activity. Circulation *73:*615, 1986.
160. Liang, C.-S., Fan, T.-H. M., Sullebarger, J. T., and Sakamoto, S.: Decreased adrenergic neuronal uptake activity in experimental right heart failure. A chamber-specific contributor to beta-adrenoceptor downregulation. J. Clin. Invest. *84:*1267, 1989.
161. Leimbach, W. N., Jr., Wallin, G., Victor, R. G., et al.: Direct evidence from intrarenal recordings for increased central sympathetic outflow in patients with heart failure. Circulation *73:*913, 1986.
162. Francis, G. S., Parks, R., and Cohn, J. N.: The effects of bromocriptine in patients with congestive heart failure. Am. Heart J. *106:*100, 1983.
163. Cohn, J. N., Levine, T. B., Olivari, M. T., et al.: Plasma norepinephrine as a guide to prognosis in patients with chronic congestive heart failure. N. Engl. J. Med. *311:*819, 1984.
164. Landzberg, J. S., Parker, J. D., Gauthier, D. F., and Colucci, W. S.: Effects of myocardial alpha$_1$-adrenergic receptor stimulation and blockade on contractility in humans. Circulation *84:*1608, 1991.
165. Bisphoric, N. H., Simpson, P. C., and Ordahl, C. P.: Induction of the skeletal alpha-actin gene in alpha$_1$-adrenoreceptor-mediated hypertrophy of rat cardiac myocytes. J. Clin. Invest. *80:*1194, 1987.
166. Takahashi, N., Calderone, A., Izzo, N. J., Jr., et al.: Hypertrophic stimuli induce transforming growth factor-beta$_1$ expression in rat ventricular myocytes. J. Clin. Invest. *94:*1470, 1994.
167. Bristow, M. R., Minobe, W., Rasmussen, R., et al.: Alpha$_1$ adrenergic receptors in the nonfailing and failing human heart. J. Pharmacol. Exp. Ther. *247:*1039, 1988.
168. Schoffer, J., Tews, A., Langes, K., et al.: Relationship between myocardial norepinephrine content and left ventricular function—an endomyocardial biopsy study. Eur. Heart J. *8:*748, 1987.
169. Chidsey, C. A., Kaiser, G. A., Sonnenblick, E. H., and Braunwald, E.: Cardiac norepinephrine stores in experimental heart failure. J. Clin. Invest. *43:*2386, 1964.
170. Spann, J. F., Jr., Sonnenblick, E. H., Cooper, T., and Braunwald, E.: Cardiac norepinephrine stores and the contractile state of heart muscle. Circ. Res. *19:*317, 1966.
171. Covell, J. W., Chidsey, C. A., and Braunwald, E.: Reduction of the cardiac response to postganglionic sympathetic nerve stimulation in experimental heart failure. Circ. Res. *19:*51, 1966.
172. Pool, P. E., Covell, J. W., Levitt, M., et al.: Reduction of cardiac tyrosine hydroxylase activity in experimental congestive heart failure. Its role in depletion of cardiac norepinephrine stores. Circ. Res. *20:*349, 1967.
173. Sole, M. J.: Alterations in sympathetic and parasympathetic neurotransmitter activity: *In* Braunwald, E., Mock, M. B., and Watson, J. (eds.): Congestive Heart Failure: Current Research and Clinical Applications. New York, Grune and Stratton, 1982, p. 101.
174. Henderson, E. B., Kahn, J. K., Dorbett, J. R., et al.: Abnormal I-123 Metaoidobenzylguanidine myocardial washout and distribution may reflect myocardial adrenergic derangement in patients with congestive cardiomyopathy. Circulation *78:*1192, 1988.
175. Higgins, C. B., Vatner, S. F., Eckberg, D. L., and Braunwald, E.: Alterations in the baroreceptor reflex in conscious dogs with heart failure. J. Clin. Invest. *51:*715, 1972.
176. White, C. W.: Reversibility of abnormal arterial baroreflex control of heart rate in heart failure. Am. J. Physiol. *241:*H778, 1981.
177. Levine, T. B., Francis, G. S., Goldsmith, S. R., and Cohn, J. N.: The neurohumoral and hemodynamic response to orthostatic tilt in patients with congestive heart failure. Circulation *67:*1070, 1983.

178. Goldsmith, S. R., Francis, G. S., Levine, T. B., and Cohn, J. N.: Regional blood flow response to orthostasis in patients with congestive heart failure. J. Am. Coll. Cardiol. *1*:1391, 1983.
179. Kubo, S. H., and Cody, R. J.: Circulatory autoregulation in chronic congestive heart failure: Responses to head-up tilt in 41 patients. Am. J. Cardiol. *52*:512, 1983.
180. Ferguson, D. W., Abboud, F. M., and Mark, A. L.: Selective impairment of baroreflex-mediated vasoconstrictor responses in patients with ventricular dysfunction. Circulation *69*:451, 1984.
181. Marin-Neto, J. A., Pintya, A. O., Gallo, L., Jr., and Maciel, B. C.: Abnormal baroreflex control of heart rate in decompensated congestive heart failure and reversal after compensation. Am. J. Cardiol. *67*:604, 1991.
182. Levine, T. B., Olivari, T., and Cohn, J. N.: Dissociation of the responses of the renin-angiotensin system and sympathetic nervous system to a vasodilator stimulus in congestive heart failure. Int. J. Cardiol. *12*:165, 1986.
183. Stone, G. W., Kubo, S. H., and Cody, R. J.: Adverse influence of baroreceptor dysfunction on upright exercise in congestive heart failure. Am. J. Med. *80*:799, 1986.
184. Thoren, P., and Ricksten, S.-E.: Cardiac C-fiber endings in cardiovascular control under normal and pathophysiological conditions. *In* Abboud, F. M., Fozzard, H. A., Gilmore, J. P., and Reis, D. J. (eds.): Disturbances in Neurogenic Control of the Circulation. Bethesda, MD, Am. Physiol. Soc., 1981, p. 17.
185. Zucker, I. H., Earle, A. M., and Gilmore, J. P.: The mechanism of adaptation of left atrial stretch receptors in dogs with chronic congestive heart failure. J. Clin. Invest. *60*:323, 1977.
186. Zucker, I. H., Earle, A. M., and Gilmore, J. P.: Changes in the sensitivity of left atrial receptors following reversal of heart failure. Am. J. Physiol. *237*:H555, 1979.
187. Riegger, G. A. J., Leibau, G., and Kocksiek, K.: Antidiuretic hormone in congestive heart failure. Am. J. Med. *72*:49, 1982.
188. Wang, W., Chen, J.-S., and Zucker, I. H.: Carotid sinus baroreceptor sensitivity in experimental heart failure. Circulation *81*:1959, 1990.
189. Ellenbogen, K. A., Mohanty, P. K., Szentpetery, S., and Thames, M. D.: Arterial baroreflex abnormalities in heart failure. Reversal after orthotopic cardiac transplantation. Circulation *79*:51, 1989.
190. Leier, C. V., Binkley, P. F., and Cody, R. J.: Alpha-adrenergic component of the sympathetic nervous system in congestive heart failure. Circulation *82*:168, 1990.
191. Kubo, S. H., Rector, T. S., Heifets, S. M., and Cohn, J. N.: Alpha$_2$-receptor–mediated vasoconstriction in patients with congestive heart failure. Circulation *80*:1660, 1989.
192. Higgins, C. B., Vatner, S. F., Millard, R. W., et al.: Alterations in regional hemodynamics in experimental heart failure in conscious dogs. Trans. Assoc. Am. Physicians *85*:267, 1972.
193. Bristow, M. R.: Changes in myocardial and vascular receptors in heart failure. J. Am. Coll. Cardiol. *22*:61A, 1993.
194. Bristow, M. R., Minobe, W., Rasmussen, R., et al.: Beta-adrenergic neuroeffector abnormalities in the failing human heart are produced by local rather than systemic mechanisms. J. Clin. Invest. *89*:803, 1992.
195. Fowler, M. B., Laser, J. A., Hopkins, G. L., et al.: Assessment of the beta-adrenergic receptor pathway in the intact failing human heart. Circulation *74*:1290, 1986.
196. Bristow, M. R., Ginsburg, R., Umans, V., et al.: Beta$_1$- and beta$_2$-adrenergic–receptor subpopulations in nonfailing and failing human ventricular myocardium: Coupling of both receptor subtypes to muscle contraction and selective beta$_1$-receptor downregulation in heart failure. Circ. Res. *59*:297, 1986.
197. Bristow, M. R., Hershberger, R. E., Port, J. D., and Rasmussen, R.: Beta$_1$- and beta$_2$-adrenergic receptor–mediated adenylate cyclase stimulation in nonfailing and failing human ventricular myocardium. Mol. Pharmacol. *35*:295, 1989.
198. Bristow, M. R., Anderson, F. L., Port, J. D., et al.: Differences in beta-adrenergic neuroeffector mechanisms in ischemic versus idiopathic dilated cardiomyopathy. Circulation *84*:1024, 1991.
199. Woodley, S. L., Gilbert, E. M., Anderson, J. L., et al.: Beta-blockade with bucindolol in heart failure caused by ischemic versus idiopathic dilated cardiomyopathy. Circulation *84*:2426, 1991.
200. Ungerer, M., Bohm, M., Elce, J. S., et al.: Altered expression of beta-adrenergic receptor kinase and beta$_1$-adrenergic receptors in the failing human heart. Circulation *87*:454, 1993.
201. Bristow, M. R., Minobe, W. A., Raynolds, M. V., et al.: Reduced beta-1 receptor messenger RNA abundance in the failing human heart. J. Clin. Invest. *92*:2737, 1993.
202. Gaffney, T. E., and Braunwald, E.: Importance of the adrenergic nervous system in the support of circulatory function in patients with congestive heart failure. Am. J. Med. *34*:320, 1963.
203. Hausdorff, W. P., Caron, M. G., and Lefkowitz, R. J.: Turning off the signal: Desensitization of beta-adrenergic receptor function. FASEB J. *4*:2881, 1990.
204. Heilbrunn, S. M., Shah, P., Bristow, M. R., et al.: Increased beta-receptor density and improved hemodynamic response to catecholamine stimulation during long-term metoprolol therapy in heart failure from dilated cardiomyopathy. Circulation *79*:483, 1989.
205. Feldman, A. M., Gates, A. E., Veazey, W. B., et al.: Increase of the 40,000-mol wt pertussis toxin substrate (G protein) in the failing human heart. J. Clin. Invest. *82*:189, 1988.
206. Neumann, J., Schmitz, W., Scholz, H., et al.: Increase in myocardial G$_1$ proteins in heart failure. Lancet *22*:936, 1988.
207. Denniss, A. R., Marsh, J. D., Quigg, R. J., et al.: Beta-adrenergic receptor number and adenylate cyclase function in denervated transplanted and cardiomyopathic human hearts. Circulation *79*:1028, 1989.
208. Böhm, M., Gierschik, P., Jakobs, K.-H., et al.: Increase of G$_i$ in human hearts with dilated but not ischemic cardiomyopathy. Circulation *82*:1249, 1990.
209. Feldman, A. M., Ray, P. E., and Bristow, M. R.: Expression of alpha-subunits of G proteins in failing human heart: A reappraisal utilizing quantitative polymerase chain reaction. J. Mol. Cell. Cardiol. *23*:1355, 1991.
210. Feldman, A. M., Tena, R. G., Kessler, P. D., et al.: Diminished beta-adrenergic responsiveness and cardiac dilatation in hearts of myopathic Syrian hamsters (BIO 53,58) are associated with a function abnormality of the G stimulatory protein. Circulation *81*:1341, 1990.
211. Epstein, S. E., and Braunwald, E.: The effect of beta-adrenergic blockade on patterns of urinary sodium excretion: Studies in normal subjects and in patients with heart disease. Ann. Intern. Med. *75*:20, 1966.
212. Vogel, J. H. K., and Chidsey, C. A.: Cardiac adrenergic activity in experimental heart failure assessed with beta-receptor blockade. Am. J. Cardiol. *24*:198, 1969.
213. Haber, H. L., Simek, C. L., Gimple, L. W., et al.: Why do patients with congestive heart failure tolerate the initiation of beta blocker therapy? Circulation *88*:1610, 1993.
214. Hjalmarson, A., and Waagstein, F.: Use of beta blockers in the treatment of dilated cardiomyopathy. *In* Gwathmey, J. D., Briggs, G. M., and Allen, P. D. (eds.): Heart Failure. Basic Science and Clinical Aspects. Marcel Dekker, New York, 1993, p. 223.
215. Feldman, M. D., Copelas, L., Gwathmey, J. K., et al.: Deficient production of cyclic AMP: Pharmacologic evidence of an important cause of contractile dysfunction in patients with end-stage heart failure. Circulation *75*:331, 1987.
216. Colucci, W. S., Denniss, A. R., Leatherman, G. F., et al.: Intracoronary infusion of dobutamine to patients with and without severe congestive heart failure. Dose-response relationships, correlation with circulating catecholamines, and effect of phosphodiesterase inhibition. J. Clin. Invest. *81*:1103, 1988.
217. Simpson, P., and McGrath, A.: Norepinephrine-stimulated hypertrophy of cultured rat myocardial cells is an alpha$_1$-adrenergic response. J. Clin. Invest. *72*:732, 1983.
218. Iwaki, K., Sukhatme, V. P., Shubeita, H. E., and Chien, K. R.: α- and β-adrenergic stimulation induces distinct patterns of immediate early gene expression in neonatal rat myocardial cells. J. Biol. Chem. *265*:13809, 1990.
219. Nakaki, T., Nakayama, M., Yamamoto, S., and Kato, R.: α_1-Adrenergic stimulation and beta$_2$-adrenergic inhibition of DNA synthesis in vascular smooth muscle cells. Molec. Pharmacol. *37*:30, 1990.
220. Long, C. S., Hartogensis, W. E., and Simpson, P. C.: Beta-adrenergic stimulation of cardiac non-myocytes augments the growth-promoting activity of non-myocyte conditioned medium. J. Mol. Cell. Cardiol. *25*:915, 1993.
221. Schneider, M. D., and Parker, T. G.: Cardiac myocytes as targets for the action of peptide growth factors. Circulation *81*:1443, 1990.
222. Eckberg, D. L., Drabinsky, M., and Braunwald, E.: Defective cardiac parasympathetic control in patients with heart disease. N. Engl. J. Med. *285*:877, 1971.
223. Arai, Y., Saul, J. P., Albrecht, P., et al.: Modulation of cardiac autonomic activity during and immediately after exercise. Am. J. Physiol. *256*:H132, 1989.
224. Roskoski, R., Jr., Schmid, P. G., Mayer, H. E., and Abboud, F. M.: In vitro acetylcholine biosynthesis in normal and failing guinea pig hearts. Circ. Res. *36*:547, 1975.
225. Vatner, D. E., Lee, D. L., Schwarz, K. R., et al.: Impaired cardiac muscarinic receptor function in dogs with heart failure. J. Clin. Invest. *81*:1836, 1988.
226. Levine, T. B., Francis, G. S., Goldsmith, S. R., et al.: Activity of the sympathetic nervous system and renin-angiotensin system assessed by plasma hormone levels and their relation to hemodynamic abnormalities in congestive heart failure. Am. J. Cardiol. *49*:1659, 1982.
227. Kluger, J., Cody, R. J., and Laragh, J. H.: The contributions of sympathetic tone and the renin-angiotensin system to severe chronic congestive heart failure. Response to specific inhibitors (prazosin and captopril). Am. J. Cardiol. *49*:1667, 1982.
228. Dzau, V. J.: Tissue renin-angiotensin system in myocardial hypertrophy and failure. Arch. Int. Med. *153*:937, 1993.
229. Dzau, V. J., and Re, R.: Tissue angiotensin system in cardiovascular medicine. A paradigm shift? Circulation *89*:493, 1994.
230. Hirsch, A. T., Talsness, C. E., Schunkert, H., et al.: Tissue-specific activation of cardiac angiotensin converting enzyme in experimental heart failure. Circ. Res. *69*:475, 1991.
231. Schunkert, H., Dzau, V. J., Tang, S. S., et al.: Increased rat cardiac angiotensin converting enzyme activity and mRNA expression in pressure overload left ventricular hypertrophy. Effects on coronary resistance, contractility, and relaxation. J. Clin. Invest. *86*:1913, 1990.
232. Lindpaintner, K., Lu, W., Niedermajer, N., et al.: Selective activation of cardiac angiotensinogen gene expression in post-infarction ventricular remodeling in the rat. J. Mol. Cell. Cardiol. *25*:133, 1993.
233. Huang, H., Arnal, J.-F., Llorens-Cortes, C., et al.: Discrepancy between plasma and lung angiotensin-converting enzyme activity in experimental congestive heart failure. A novel aspect of endothelium dysfunction. Circ. Res. *75*:454, 1994.

234. Urata, H., Healy, B., Stewart, R. W., et al.: Angiotensin II-forming pathways in normal and failing human hearts. Circ. Res. *66*:883, 1990.
235. Timmermans, P. B., Wong, P. C., Chiu, A. T., et al.: Angiotensin II receptors and angiotensin II receptor antagonists. Pharmacol. Rev. *45*:205, 1993.
236. Regitz-Zagrosek, V., Friedel, N., Heymann, A., et al.: Regulation, chamber localization, and subtype distribution of angiotensin II receptors in human hearts. Circulation *91*:1461, 1995.
237. Nozawa, Y., Haruno, A., Oda, N., et al.: Angiotensin II receptor subtypes in bovine and human ventricular myocardium. J. Pharmacol. Exp. Ther. *270*:566, 1994.
238. Sadoshima, J.-I., and Izumo, S.: Molecular characterization of angiotensin II-induced hypertrophy of cardiac myocytes and hyperplasia of cardiac fibroblasts. Critical role of the AT_1 receptor subtype. Circ. Res. *73*:413, 1993.
239. Crawford, D. C., Chobanian, A. V., and Brecher, P.: Angiotensin II induces fibronectin expression associated with cardiac fibrosis in the rat. Circ. Res. *74*:727, 1994.
240. Goldsmith, S. R., Francis, G. S., and Cowley, A. W.: Arginine vasopressin and the renal response to water loading in congestive heart failure. Am. J. Cardiol. *58*:295, 1986.
241. Schaller, M.-D., Nussberger, J., Feihl, F., et al.: Clinical and hemodynamic correlates of elevated plasma arginine vasopressin after acute myocardial infarction. Am. J. Cardiol. *60*:1178, 1987.
242. Goldsmith, S. R.: Control of arginine vasopressin and congestive heart failure. Am. J. Cardiol. *71*:629, 1993.
243. Greenberg, T. T., Richmond, W. H., Stocking, R. A., et al.: Impaired atrial receptor responses in dogs with heart failure due to tricuspid insufficiency and pulmonary artery stenosis. Circ. Res. *32*:424, 1973.
244. Goldsmith, S. R., and Dodge, D.: Response of plasma vasopressin to ethanol in congestive heart failure. Am. J. Cardiol. *55*:1354, 1985.
245. Naitoh, M., Suzuki, H., Murakami, M., et al.: Effects of oral AVP receptor antagonists OPC-21268 and OPC-31260 on congestive heart failure in conscious dogs. Am. J. Physiol. *267*:H2245, 1994.
246. Struthers, A. D.: Ten years of natriuretic peptide research: A new dawn for their diagnostic and therapeutic use? Br. Med. J. *308*:1615, 1994.
247. Moe, G. W., Grima, E. A., Wong, N. L., et al.: Dual natriuretic peptide system in experimental heart failure. J. Am. Coll. Cardiol. *22*:891, 1993.
248. Yoshimura, M., Yasue, H., Okumura, K., et al.: Different secretion patterns of atrial natriuretic peptide and brain natriuretic peptide in patients with congestive heart failure. Circulation *87*:464, 1993.
249. Wei, C. M., Heublein, D. M., Perrella, M. A., et al.: Natriuretic peptide system in human heart failure. Circulation *88*:1004, 1993.
250. Yasue, H., Yoshimura, M., Sumida, H., et al.: Localization and mechanism of secretion of B-type natriuretic peptide in comparison with those of A-type natriuretic peptide in normal subjects and patients with heart failure. Circulation *90*:195, 1994.
251. Hall, C., Rouleau, J. L., Moye, L., et al.: N-terminal proatrial natriuretic factor. An independent predictor of long-term prognosis after myocardial infarction. Circulation *89*:1934, 1994.
252. Weston, M. W., Cintron, G. B., Giordano, A. T., and Vesely, D. L.: Normalization of circulating atrial natriuretic peptides in cardiac transplant recipients. Am. Heart J. *127*:129, 1994.
253. Cody, R. J., Atlas, S. A., Laragh, J. H., et al.: Atrial natriuretic factor in normal subjects and heart failure patients: Plasma levels and renal, hormonal, and hemodynamic responses to peptide infusion. J. Clin. Invest. *78*:1362, 1986.
254. Kohzuki, M., Hodsman, G. P., and Johnston, C. I.: Attenuated response to atrial natriuretic peptide in rats with myocardial infarction. Am. J. Physiol. *256*:H533, 1989.
255. Wada, A., Tsutamoto, T., Matsuda, Y., and Kinoshita, M.: Cardiorenal and neurohumoral effects of endogenous atrial natriuretic peptide in dogs with severe congestive heart failure using a specific antagonist for guanylate cyclase-coupled receptors. Circulation *89*:2232, 1994.
256. Münzel, T., Kurz, S., Holtz, J., et al.: Neurohormonal inhibition and hemodynamic unloading during prolonged inhibition of ANF degradation in patients with severe chronic heart failure. Circulation *86*:1089, 1992.
257. Calderone, A., Takahashi, N., Thaik, C. M., and Colucci, W. S.: Atrial natriuretic factor and cyclic guanosine monophosphate modulate cardiac myocyte growth and phenotype. Circulation *90*(Suppl. I):I-317, 1994.
258. Itoh, H., Pratt, R. E., and Dzau, V. J.: Atrial natriuretic polypeptide inhibits hypertrophy of vascular smooth cells. J. Clin. Invest. *86*:1690, 1990.
259. Cao, L., and Gardner, D. G.: Natriuretic peptides inhibit DNA synthesis in cardiac fibroblasts. Hypertension *25*:227, 1995.
260. Yanagisawa, M., Kurihara, H., Kimura, S., et al.: A novel potent vasoconstrictor peptide produced by vascular endothelial cells. Nature *332*:411, 1988.
261. Cody, R. J., Haas, G. J., Binkley, P. F., Capers, Q., and Kelley, R.: Plasma endothelin correlates with the extent of pulmonary hypertension in patients with chronic congestive heart failure. Circulation *85*:504, 1992.
262. Stewart, D. J., Cernacek, P., Costello, K. B., and Rouleau, J. L.: Elevated endothelin-1 in heart failure and loss of normal response to postural change. Circulation *85*:510, 1992.
263. Tsutamoto, T., Wada, A., Maeda, Y., et al.: Relation between endothelin-1 spillover in the lungs and pulmonary vascular resistance in patients with chronic heart failure. J. Am. Coll. Cardiol. *23*:1427, 1994.
264. Tomoda, H.: Plasma endothelin-1 in acute myocardial infarction with heart failure. Am. Heart J. *125*:667, 1993.
265. Teerlink, J. R., Loffler, B. M., Hess, P., et al.: Role of endothelin in the maintenance of blood pressure in conscious rats with chronic heart failure. Acute effects of the endothelin receptor antagonist Ro 47-0203 (bosentan). Circulation *90*:2510, 1994.
266. Shubeita, H. E., McDonough, P. M., Harris, A. N., et al.: Endothelin induction of inositol phospholipid hydrolysis, sarcomere assembly, and cardiac gene expression in ventricular myocytes. A paracrine mechanism for myocardial cell hypertrophy. J. Biol. Chem. *265*:20555, 1990.
267. Ito, H., Hirata, Y., Hiroe, M., et al.: Endothelin-1 induces hypertrophy with enhanced expression of muscle-specific genes in cultured neonatal rat cardiomyocytes. Circ. Res. *69*:209, 1991.
268. Ito, H., Hiroe, M., Hirata, Y., et al.: Endothelin ET_A receptor antagonist blocks cardiac hypertrophy provoked by hemodynamic overload. Circulation *89*:2198, 1994.
269. Casscells, W., Bazoberry, F., Speir, E., et al.: Transforming growth factor-beta1 in normal heart and in myocardial infarction. Ann. NY Acad. Sci. *593*:148, 1990.
270. Levine, B., Kalman, J., Mayer, L., Fillit, H. M., and Packer, M.: Elevated circulating levels of tumor necrosis factor in severe chronic heart failure. N. Engl. J. Med. *323*:236, 1990.
271. McMurray, J., Abdullah, I., Dargie, H. J., and Shapiro, D.: Increased concentrations of tumor necrosis factor in "cachectic" patients with severe chronic heart failure. Br. Heart J. *66*:356, 1991.
272. Mann, D. L., and Young, J. B.: Basic mechanisms in congestive heart failure. Recognizing the role of proinflammatory cytokines. Chest *105*:897, 1994.
273. Finkel, M. S., Oddis, C. V., Jacob, T. D., et al.: Negative inotropic effects of cytokines on the heart mediated by nitric oxide. Science *257*:387, 1992.
274. Yokoyama, T., Vaca, L., Rossen, R. D., et al.: Cellular basis for the negative inotropic effects of tumor necrosis factor-alpha in the adult mammalian heart. J. Clin. Invest. *92*:2303, 1993.
275. Thaik, C. M., Calderone, A., Takahashi, N., and Colucci, W. S.: Interleuken-1 beta modulates the growth and phenotype of neonatal rat cardiac myocytes. J. Clin. Invest. *96*:1093, 1995.
276. Palmer, J. N., Hartogensis, W. E., Patten, M., Fortuin, F. D., and Long, C. S.: Interleuken-1 beta induces cardiac myocyte growth but inhibits cardiac fibroblast proliferation in culture. J. Clin. Invest. *95*:2555, 1995.
277. Tsujino, M., Hirata, Y., Imai, T., et al.: Induction of nitric oxide synthase gene by interleukin-1 beta in cultured rat cardiocytes. Circulation *90*:375, 1994.
278. Balligand, J.-L., Kelly, R. A., Marsden, P. A., Smith, T. W., and Michel, T.: Control of cardiac muscle cell function by an endogenous nitric oxide signaling system. Proc. Natl. Acad. Sci. *90*:347, 1993.
279. Hare, J. M., and Colucci, W. S.: Role of nitric oxide in the regulation of myocardial function. Prog. Cardiovasc. Dis. *38*:1, 1995.
280. Paulus, W. J., Vantrimpont, P. J., and Shah, A. M.: Acute effects of nitric oxide on left ventricular relaxation and diastolic distensibility in humans. Assessment by bicoronary sodium nitroprusside infusion. Circulation *89*:2070, 1994.
281. Hare, J. M., Loh, E., Creager, M. A., and Colucci, W. S.: Nitric oxide inhibits the positive inotropic response to beta-adrenergic stimulation in humans with left ventricular dysfunction. Circulation *92*:2198, 1995.
282. Matsumori, A., Shioi, T., Yamada, T., et al.: Vesnarinone, a new inotropic agent, inhibits cytokine production by stimulated human blood from patients with heart failure. Circulation *89*:955, 1994.

Chapter 14
Assessment of Cardiac Function

WILLIAM C. LITTLE, EUGENE BRAUNWALD

THEORETICAL CONSIDERATIONS

Reasons to Focus on Left Ventricle

The cardiovascular system supplies the tissues with oxygen and metabolic substrates and removes carbon dioxide and other products of metabolism. This requires the integration of all of its components (venous circulation, right heart, pulmonary vascular system, left heart, arterial circulation, and blood). Most (but not all) circulatory dysfunction of cardiac origin in adults is due to abnormalities of the left heart. Thus the clinical evaluation of cardiac function predominantly involves assessment of the performance of the left ventricle.

Levels of Integration: Myocardium, Pump, Cardiac Output

The performance of the left ventricle as a pump depends on the contraction of the sarcomeres in the myocardium as well as the configuration of the left ventricular chamber and loading conditions. Ultimately the interaction of the left ventricle, the other cardiac chambers, and the arterial, pulmonary, and venous circulations results in the cardiac output. Thus, cardiac function can be evaluated at several levels of integration: (1) myocardial function, (2) chamber (usually left ventricular) pump performance, and (3) integrated cardiac output. It is important to recognize at which level of integration cardiac function is being evaluated. For example, changes in cardiac output or the level of left ventricular pump function can result from many factors and do not merely reflect myocardial contractility.[1] Thus, measurement of cardiac output alone provides a limited and insensitive assessment of ventricular function or of myocardial contractility. Furthermore, evaluation of left ventricular pump function alone cannot assess the adequacy of cardiac output or the level of myocardial contractility.

Factors Controlling Myocardial Function

As described in Chapter 13, myocardial shortening is determined by four factors: (1) preload, (2) afterload, (3) contractility, (4) and heart rate and cardiac rhythm. *Preload* is proportional to the stretch of the myocardium prior to stimulation and reflects the initial sarcomere length. Within the physiological range, the greater the preload the stronger the contraction and the greater the extent of shortening. *Afterload* is the load that the myocardium must bear to contract; the greater the afterload the less the amount of shortening. *Myocardial contractility* refers to a fundamental property of cardiac tissue reflecting the level of activation, and the formation and cycling of the cross bridges between actin and myosin filaments (Fig. 12–5, p. 365). At constant preload and afterload, increased contractility results in a greater extent and velocity of shortening. The final determinants of cardiac function are the *heart rate* and *rhythm*. Within wide limits, with increasing rate there is enhancement of contractility (positive force-frequency relation). These factors (preload, afterload, contractility, rate, and rhythm) represent a simplification of the fundamental processes, since at the level of the sarcomere, load, contractility, and frequency are interrelated.[2,3]

Left Ventricle in Pressure-Volume Plane: Transformation of Myocardial to Pump Function

The transformation of myocardial function to left ventricular pump function can be understood by plotting the cardiac cycle in the pressure-volume plane.

LEFT VENTRICULAR PRESSURE-VOLUME LOOP. The relationship between left ventricular pressure and volume in a normal ejecting beat is shown in Figure 14–1. Contraction of the left ventricular myocardium begins at end diastole. The energy of the contraction is first utilized to increase ventricular pressure to the level of aortic diastolic pressure without a change in volume as the aortic and mitral valves are closed. When left ventricular pressure exceeds aortic pressure, the aortic valve opens. Myocardial fibers shorten as blood is ejected through the open aortic valve, and ventricular volume decreases. After the contraction reaches its peak at end systole, the myocardial fibers begin to relax, and when left ventricular pressure falls below aortic pressure, the aortic valve closes and cardiac ejection stops. Then, as the ventricle relaxes, ventricular pressure declines rapidly. With opening of the mitral valve, left ventricular filling begins, and the left ventricular pressure-volume loop is completed.

When cardiac ejection is prevented in an experimental preparation, peak isovolumetric left ventricular pressure increases as diastolic pressure increases, describing a straight line in the physiological range.[4,5] This is the end-systolic pressure-volume relation (ESPVR). Similarly, the upper left corner of the pressure-volume loops of variably loaded beats, denoted as end systole in Figure 14–1, fall close to isovolumetric ESPVR. The slope of this line, end-systolic elastance, termed E_{ES}, has units of pressure per volume and denotes the maximum stiffness or *elastance* of the left ventricle. The slope and position of the ESPVR respond to changes in myocardial contractile state. An increase in contractility increases the slope of the ESPVR, shifting the line toward the left in the physiological range. Conversely, the ESPVR flattens and shifts to the right when there is depressed myocardial contractile function. Thus the position and slope of the ESPVR can be used to measure contractile state (see below).

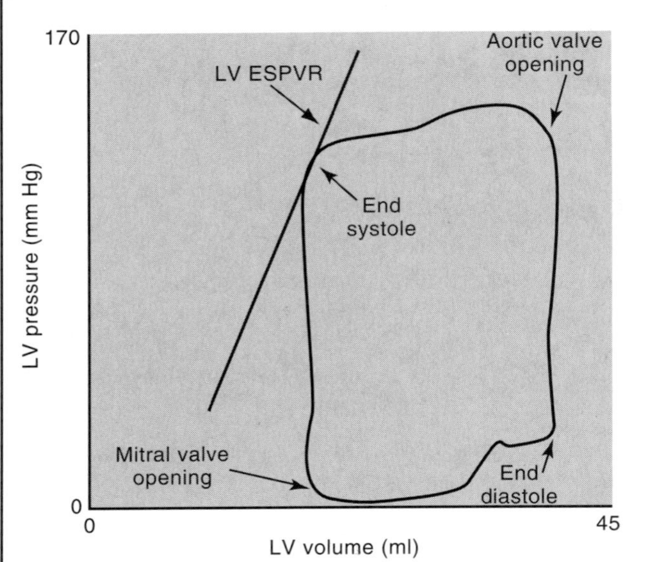

FIGURE 14–1. A left ventricular (LV) pressure-volume loop describing one cardiac cycle. At end diastole the mitral valve closes. The left ventricle is a closed chamber as the pressure increases without a change in volume during isovolumetric contraction. When left ventricular pressure exceeds aortic pressure, the aortic valve opens. During left ventricular ejection, left ventricular volume falls. Aortic valve closure occurs near the time of end systole. Following aortic valve closure, left ventricular pressure falls without a change in left ventricular volume until left ventricular pressure falls below left atrial pressure and mitral valve opening occurs. During diastole left ventricular volume increases, completing the cardiac cycle. End systole falls on the left ventricular end-systolic pressure-volume relation (ESPVR). (Data from Little, W. C., and Cheng, C. P.: Left ventricular-arterial coupling in conscious dogs. Am. J. Physiol. *261*:H70, 1991.)

The effects on left ventricular performance of altering preload, afterload, and contractility are readily described in the left ventricular pressure-volume plane. In the intact circulation, alteration of any of these three determinants of left ventricular performance elicits a prompt compensatory response that modifies the other two factors and heart rate. However, it is useful to analyze the effect of a change in each of these parameters, assuming for illustrative purposes that the other two factors remain constant.

An acute increase in afterload results in a greater proportion of the contractile energy being utilized to develop pressure so there is less myocardial shortening (Fig. 14–2). As a consequence, emptying is impaired, causing reduced stroke volume and decreased ejection fraction. Thus, increased afterload can decrease left ventricular systolic emptying in the absence of any depression of myocardial contractility. An increase in preload (increased end-diastolic volume), if it occurs without a change in end-systolic pressure, results in a larger stroke volume as the ventricle ejects to a similar end-systolic volume. A primary increase in myocardial contractility effects a steeper ESPVR. If preload and afterload remain constant, this brings about an increase in stroke volume.

MEASUREMENT OF KEY VARIABLES

Pressures

The intracardiac, arterial, and venous pressures are important variables used in assessing cardiac function. These pressures have been traditionally measured using fluid-filled catheters (see p. 423). Arterial pressure can be obtained noninvasively by sphygmomanometry. Recently, Doppler echocardiographic techniques have allowed noninvasive estimation of some intracardiac pressures.

TECHNICAL CONSIDERATIONS. Intracardiac pressures can be measured through a fluid-filled catheter connected to a strain-gauge manometer. If the system is carefully flushed to eliminate air bubbles, it has a flat frequency response from 0 to about 10 Hz.[6,7] These fluid-filled systems typically have a resonant frequency of approximately 15 Hz. Thus, catheter systems can accurately measure pressures when the waveform is not rapidly varying (Fig. 14–3). For example, venous pressures and late diastolic and late systolic ventricular and aortic pressures can be accurately measured. However, a fluid-filled catheter system cannot accurately determine rapidly changing pressures as occur during left ventricular isovolumetric contraction and relaxation. During a rapid change in pressure, the fluid-filled system initially lags behind the true pressure. After the transient, the fluid-filled system overshoots and may resonate. These effects can be minimized, but not entirely prevented, by optimal damping. Therefore the time derivative of left ventricular pressure (dP/dt) or the time constant of the isovolumetric fall in left ventricular pressure cannot be accurately determined from a fluid-filled catheter system.

Catheters tipped with a micromanometer provide a flat frequency response to above 100 Hz. Thus a micromanometer can accurately measure cardiac pressures throughout the cardiac cycle. Micromanometers are required to measure left ventricle dP/dt and determine the time constant of the isovolumetric decline in left ventricular pressure. Accurate pressure measurement with a micromanometer requires careful attention to calibration, drift, zeroing, and hydrostatic pressure gradients.[7a]

NONINVASIVE PRESSURE MEASUREMENT. Cuff sphygmomanometry (see p. 20) accurately measures arterial systolic and diastolic pressures. The combination of computer-controlled cuff inflation gated by the electrocardiogram with

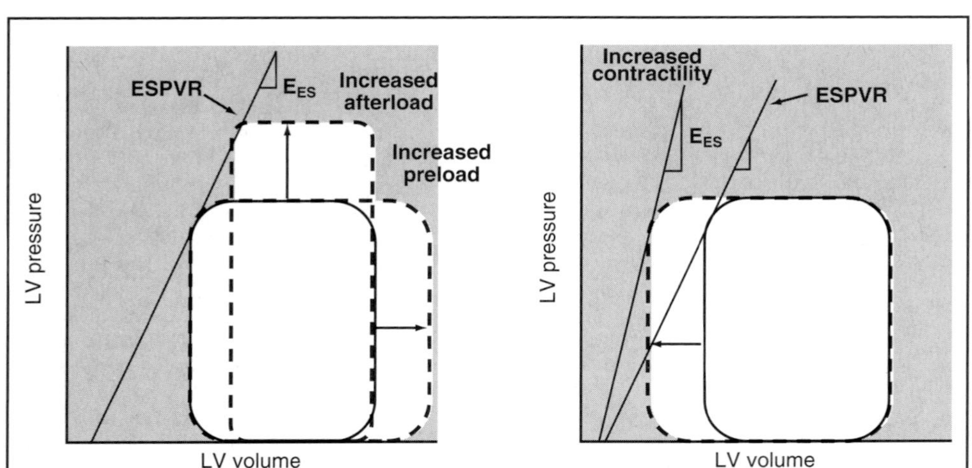

FIGURE 14–2. The responses of the left ventricle to increased afterload, increased preload, and increased contractility are shown in the pressure-volume plane. ESPVR = end-systolic pressure-volume relation; E_{ES} = the slope of the end-systolic pressure-volume relation. See text for discussion.

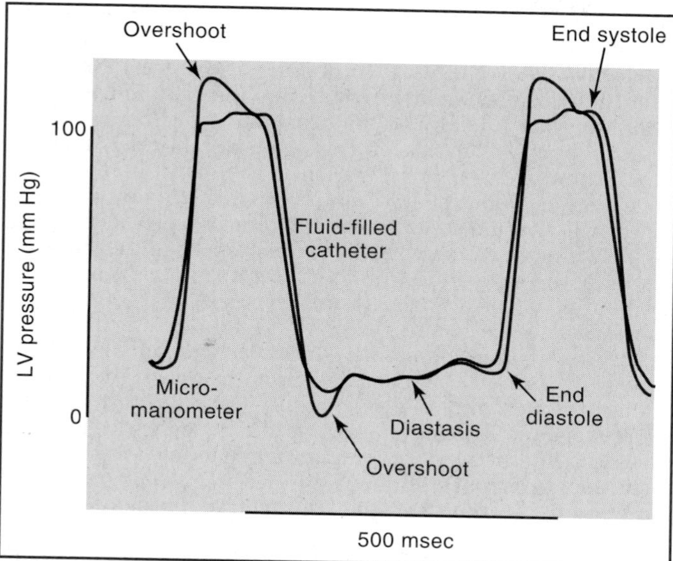

FIGURE 14–3. Recording of left ventricular pressure from a fluid-filled catheter and a micromanometer catheter. The recording with the fluid-filled catheter is delayed slightly relative to the recording with the micromanometer. During portions of the cardiac cycle when left ventricular pressure is not rapidly changing (diastasis, end diastole, end systole) the pressures recorded through the two systems are nearly identical. When pressure is rapidly increasing or decreasing, the pressure recorded through the fluid-filled catheter initially lags behind the micromanometer pressure and then overshoots. (Recording courtesy of Dr. Che-Ping Cheng, Bowman Gray School of Medicine of Wake Forest University.)

Doppler measurements of brachial arterial flow provides a quantitative measure of the entire arterial waveform.[8]

Doppler echocardiography can determine the velocity (v) of systolic regurgitant jet across the tricuspid, mitral, or aortic valves (see p. 56). Using the modified Bernoulli equation ($\Delta P = 4v^2$), the pressure gradient (ΔP) responsible for the regurgitant jet can be calculated. This can be used to estimate the time course of right and left ventricular systolic pressures.[9–11]

PULMONARY CAPILLARY WEDGE PRESSURE. The diastolic pressure that distends the left ventricle and determines left ventricular preload is the left ventricular end-diastolic pressure. This is measured at the relative nadir of left ventricular pressure that occurs after the *a* wave produced by atrial contraction. In the absence of mitral stenosis, left atrial and left ventricular pressures are equal during the mid-diastolic period (diastasis) and at end diastole. Because the pulmonary venous pressure approximates left atrial pressure in most circumstances, the mean pulmonary capillary wedge pressure provides a clinically useful estimate of mean left atrial pressure and the left ventricular filling pressure (see p. 421). The waveform of the pulmonary capillary wedge pressure also approximates the phasic left atrial wave pressure. However, the peak *a* and *v* waves in the pulmonary capillary wedge pressure are damped and delayed relative to the left atrial pressure.[12] Accurate recording of pulmonary wedge pressures requires correct positioning of the catheter tip in the true wedge position to avoid recording a damped pulmonary arterial pressure.[13] Failure to correct for the phase delay or mistaking a damped pulmonary arterial pressure for the wedge pressure may result in overestimating left atrial pressure.[14]

Ventricular Volume

Angiographic techniques, described below, provide the most widely accepted means of measuring ventricular chamber volumes and segmental wall motion. They allow calculation of the extent and velocity of wall shortening and assessment of regional wall motion. When they are combined with measurements of intraventricular pressure and wall thickness, wall tension can be calculated and both ventricular systolic and diastolic stiffness can be determined. Although noninvasive techniques are now widely used in the assessment of ventricular dimensions and volumes, their application to the assessment of cardiac function is based on the earlier work using ventricular angiography, which remains a benchmark for these measurements.

QUANTITATIVE ANGIOCARDIOGRAPHY. The left ventricle is outlined most clearly by direct injection of contrast material into the ventricular cavity. In patients with severe aortic regurgitation the contrast material may be injected into the aorta, with the resultant reflux outlining the left ventricular cavity. Digital subtraction angiography utilizing injections into a peripheral vein, pulmonary artery, or left ventricle also may be used to define the left ventricle.[15,16]

Unless the effects of premature contractions and of the resultant postextrasystolic potentiation (see p. 380) are to be examined, ventricular irritability should be avoided during injection of the contrast material. Contact should be avoided between the tip of the catheter and the myocardium and a multiholed catheter used to diminish the impact of the jet of contrast agent striking the endocardium. If premature contractions are induced, the premature contraction itself and the postpremature beats may exhibit marked changes in cardiac function. The premature ventricular contraction also may induce mitral and/or tricuspid regurgitation. However, because the contrast material usually is injected within 3 or 4 sec and filming is carried out for 5 to 8 sec, one or two cardiac cycles usually are available for analysis, even if a single premature contraction occurs at the beginning of the injection.

Injection of the contrast agent does not begin to produce hemodynamic changes (except for premature beats) until about the sixth beat after injection.[17] The hyperosmolarity produced by the contrast agent increases the blood volume, which begins to increase preload and heart rate within 30 sec of the injection, an effect that may persist for as long as 2 hours. Regular contrast agents (so-called ionic agents, such as meglumine diatrizoate [see p. 245]) depress contractility directly. However, newer nonionic agents minimize these adverse effects and may be safer for patients with marked elevations of left ventricular end-diastolic pressures (>25 mm Hg) or depressed cardiac function.[18] Digital subtraction techniques also are useful, since they allow the injection of much smaller quantities of contrast agent and still provide excellent resolution.[15]

In calculation of ventricular volumes or dimensions from angiograms, it is essential to take into account and apply appropriate correction factors for magnification as well as for distortion resulting from nonparallel X-ray beams (pincushion distortion).[19,20] To apply these correction factors, care must be exercised to determine with accuracy the tube-to-patient and tube-to-film distances.

THE CONDUCTANCE CATHETER

The conductance technique provides a useful method to measure left ventricular volume on-line in the cardiac catheterization laboratory, avoiding the problems associated with multiple injections of contrast agent.[21] In this technique, a multielectrode catheter is passed across the aortic valve, and the tip is advanced to the apex of the left ventricle. An electric field is generated (20 kHz, 0.03 mA RMS current) in the left ventricle between electrodes positioned at the top of the catheter in the apex and just above the aortic valve (Fig. 14–4). Sensing electrodes that are evenly distributed along the catheter are used to measure the potential produced by the current.

From these measurements, the *resistance* (and its inverse—*conductance*) between electrode pairs spanning the long axis of the left ventricle is calculated. The conductances from the electrode pairs are summed and converted to volume using a signal conditioner, assuming that all the current flows through blood in the left ventricular chamber. An uncorrected volume of the ventricle (V_M) at any time (t) is proportional to the sum of the measured conductances (G_M) and calculated as:

$$V_M(t) = L^2 \rho G_M(t)$$

where L is the distance between sensing electrodes, and ρ is the resistivity of blood, which is inversely related to conductivity.[21]

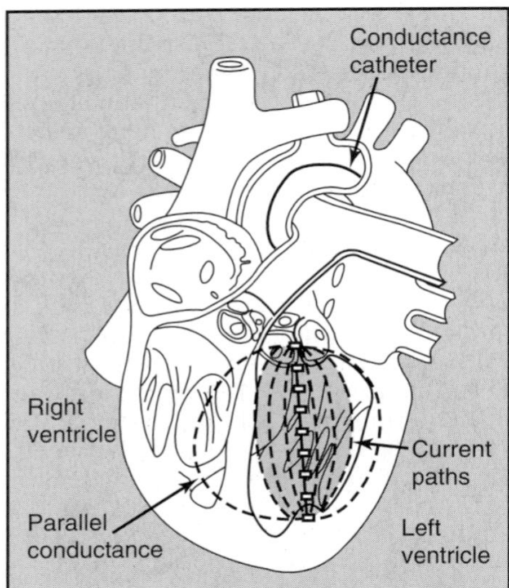

FIGURE 14–4. Measurement of left ventricular volume using a conductance catheter. A multielectrode catheter is passed retrograde across the aortic valve and positioned along the long axis of the left ventricle with the tip in the apex. A current is induced between the electrode in the tip of the left ventricle and an electrode positioned in the aorta above the aortic valve. Most of the current travels within the left ventricle. Thus the conductance of current between electrode pairs is proportional to the volume of blood in that portion of the ventricle. Some current may also travel through the right ventricle and left ventricular walls. These current paths outside the left ventricle contribute to the parallel conductance.

Most of the induced current flows through the blood in the left ventricular cavity. However, some current travels through the left ventricular wall, the right ventricle, and the pericardium. These other paths contribute to the total measured conductance. This is termed the *parallel conductance*, G_P, and produces a volume offset, V_C, equal to:

$$V_C = (L^2\rho)G_P$$

Thus the left ventricular volume corrected for parallel conductance is given by:

$$V(t) = (1/\alpha)(V_M(t) - \alpha V_C)$$

where α is a unitless constant, V is left ventricular volume corrected for parallel conductance volume, and αV_C is the volume correction because of parallel conductance. Usually α is assumed to be 1.0. Baan et al.[21] developed a technique to calculate V_C by transiently altering blood conductivity within the left ventricle without actually changing left ventricular volume or ejection fraction. In this technique, hypertonic saline (5 ml 20% NaCl) is injected into the pulmonary artery, causing a transient increase in measured volume, V_M.

The calculation of parallel conductance by the saline method assumes that V_C remains constant and that ejection fraction does not change. The line characterizing the relation between the end-diastolic (ED) and end-systolic (ES) V_M is computed. This line is extrapolated to the point where end-diastolic and end-systolic V_M are equal. This point is equal to V_C because any V_M arising from parallel conductance is outside the left ventricle. Baan et al.,[21] Burkhoff et al.,[22] and Kass et al.[23] have evaluated this approach in the isolated heart and open-chest anesthetized dogs and have found that the saline method accurately measured parallel conductance (V_C). An alternate method to determine V_C is to subtract absolute left ventricular volume measured by quantitative angiography from the uncorrected volume measured by conductance.

The conductance catheter can be used to determine stroke volume accurately over a wide range of physiological values.[21,24,25] Determination of absolute left ventricular volumes under steady-state conditions, when α and V_C are nearly constant, is also feasible using the conductance catheter and the saline method of calculating parallel conductance volume. However, because of volume-dependent changes in α and V_C, the conductance catheter may not provide absolute volume measurements when volume varies over a wide range.[26,27] Particularly, analysis of ESPVRs over a range of volumes using the conductance catheter may underestimate the absolute slope because of volume-dependent changes in α and V_C. However, the direction and magnitude of changes in inotropic state are accurately measured by the conductance catheter.[27] In addition, the effect of maneuvers or pharmacological interventions on the ESPVR measured over similar volume ranges can be accurately compared in a single subject.[28] However, comparisons over markedly different volume ranges in a subject may be inaccurate. The recent development of a dual-field stimulation technique may help minimize these technical problems with the conductance catheter.[29]

NONINVASIVE METHODS. Cardiac catheterization and quantitative selective angiography are the standard tools for evaluating the function of the heart, but these invasive procedures have some risk and are not suitable for repeated application in the same patient. Therefore investigators have searched for reliable noninvasive methods of assessing cardiac volume. Such methods are needed particularly for detecting serial changes in cardiac function and in evaluating both acute and chronic effects of interventions such as pharmacological agents and cardiac operations. Discussed elsewhere in this book are the four principal noninvasive methods for assessing cardiac performance: echocardiography (see p. 64), radionuclide angiography (see p. 300), ultrafast computed tomography (CT) (see p. 336), and gated magnetic resonance imaging (MRI) (see p. 329). All of these are alternatives to contrast angiography for measurement of ventricular volumes and/or dimensions and therefore permit the noninvasive estimation of ejection phase indices (see below). Other than in patients with obstruction to left ventricular outflow, wall stress (afterload) can be estimated from a combination of systemic arterial pressure, ventricular radius, and wall thickness. All four noninvasive imaging methods allow estimation of ventricular systolic and diastolic volumes and both global and regional ejection fractions (EFs).

LEFT VENTRICULAR VOLUME. The area-length method developed by Dodge and Sheehan is the most accepted technique for calculating left ventricular volume (Fig. 14–5).[20] In each of two orthogonal projections, the longest length (L) of the ventricular chamber, i.e., from the apex to the root of the aortic valve, is measured, and the diameter (D) of the ventricle is calculated from the formula D = 4A/L, where A = area of left ventricular cavity determined by planimetry. Ordinarily this calculation is made for images exposed in both 30-degree right anterior oblique (RAO) and 60-degree left anterior oblique (LAO) projections. The shape of the left ventricle usually resembles a prolate ellipsoid with one major and two minor diameters.[20,30] With use of this assumption, left ventricular volume is calculated from the formula:

$$V = \frac{8}{3\pi} \cdot \frac{A_{RAO} - A_{LAO}}{L_{min}}$$

where L_{min} is the shorter L in the RAO or LAO projection.

The actual ventricular volume is determined from the calculated volume using a regression formula that takes into account the volume occupied by the papillary muscles and chordae tendineae within the ventricular chamber as well as corrections for distortion of X-ray beams. Studies based on human autopsy specimens as well as on models and ventricular casts have proved the accuracy of this approach.[31]

Biplane angiographic methods are superior to single-plane methods for the calculation of left ventricular volumes. However, in patients without serious regional wall motion disorders, ventricular aneurysm, or distortion of the ventricular cavity, ventricular volume can be obtained by utilizing the RAO projection. Assuming that the two diameters (D) of the left ventricle are equal, ventricular volume is calculated from the formula:

$$V = L \cdot D^2 \cdot CF^3 \cdot \pi/6$$

where CF represents a one-dimensional correction factor.[31] Standardization of the degree of obliquity—usually 30-degree RAO and 60-degree LAO—is required for application of any particular correction factor in the calculation of ventricular volume. A close correlation has been found between left ventricular volume determined in the RAO projection and true cardiac volume; however, the overestimation of true volume is greater than with the biplane oblique volume method, and appropriate corrections must be made.[32,33]

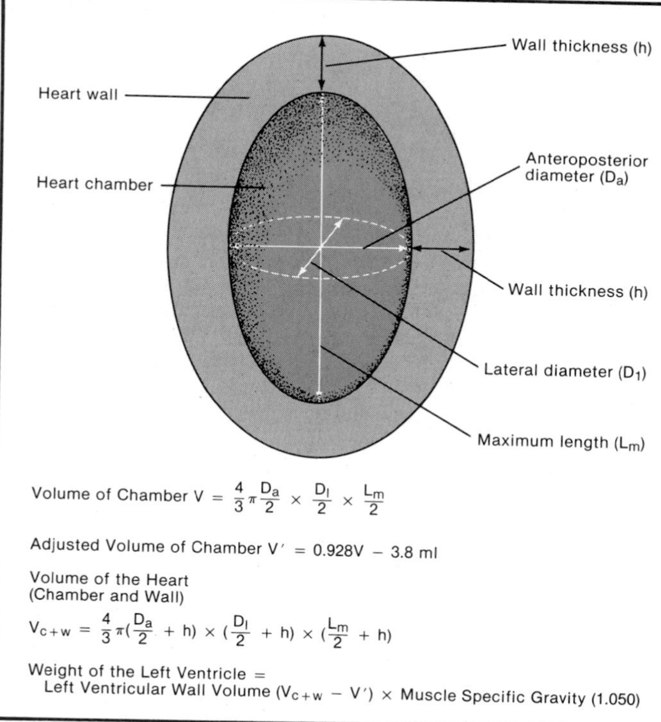

FIGURE 14–5. A method to calculate left ventricular volume by means of quantitative angiocardiography. Margins of the projected image of the left ventricular chamber are traced, and maximum length is measured in the anteroposterior and lateral views. Minor axes are derived from the planimetered areas of the chamber in both views; all dimensions are corrected to allow for distortion caused by nonparallel X-rays. Left ventricular volumes are calculated using the formula for the volume of an ellipsoid, since (with regression-equation adjustment) this has given results that tally closely with directly measured ventricular volume. To determine left ventricular mass, volume of the ventricular chamber is subtracted from volume of chamber plus wall; multiplying wall volume by the specific gravity of cardiac muscle converts volume to heart weight or mass. (From Dodge, H. T.: Hemodynamic aspects of cardiac failure. *In* Braunwald, E. [ed.]: The Myocardium: Failure and Infarction. New York, HP Publishing Co., 1974, p. 70. Reproduced by permission of the McGraw-Hill Co. Illustration by Bunji Tagawa.)

The normal left ventricular end-diastolic volume averages 70 ± 20 (SD) ml/m² (Table 14–1).[33,34] Left ventricular performance ordinarily is considered to be depressed when ventricular end-diastolic volume is clearly elevated (i.e., >110 ml/m², or >2 SDs above the normal mean) and total stroke volume and/or cardiac index and work are either reduced or within normal limits, while heart rate and arterial pressure are normal.

Left ventricular stroke volume (SV) is the quantity of blood ejected with each beat and is the difference between end-diastolic volume (EDV) and end-systolic volume (ESV). The normal SV is 45 ± 13 ml/m² (Table 14–1). The cardiac output is equal to the product of the SV and heart rate. In the absence of valvular regurgitation or intracardiac shunt, the angiographic SV should correlate closely with an independent measurement of SV (cardiac output/heart rate) using the Fick or thermodilution method. In the presence of valvular regurgitation or a shunt, the total SV determined by angiocardiography is greater than the effective forward SV determined by the Fick or indicator dilution method. The difference between the two represents the regurgitant (or shunt) flow per cardiac cycle.

Ejection Fraction (EF). This is the ratio between SV and EDV (SV/EDV). In the presence of valvular regurgitation, the total SV ejected by the ventricle, i.e., the sum of forward and regurgitant volumes, is used in this calculation. The regurgitant fraction (RF) is the ratio of regurgitant flow per beat to the total left ventricular SV:

$$RF = \frac{\text{SV total} - \text{SV forward}}{\text{SV total}},$$

where SV total is determined by angiography and SV forward by the Fick or indicator dilution method. When mitral and aortic regurgitation coexist, the regurgitant fraction reflects the sum of the two regurgitant volumes and does not distinguish between them. It is important to recognize that there are errors in measuring both total SV and forward SV. These errors may summate in the calculation of the regurgitant volume and the regurgitant fraction. Thus it is difficult to determine these parameters with accuracy.

LEFT VENTRICULAR MASS. Although left ventricular mass is usually calculated using echocardiography, it also can be determined by angiocardiography. Wall thickness, h, measured along the free lateral wall of the left ventricle just below the equator at end diastole (best measured on the AP or RAO projection), is added to the major and minor semiaxis to obtain the sum of volumes of the chamber and wall. This volume minus the chamber volume equals the volume of the wall. The product of wall volume and the specific gravity of heart muscle (1.050) equals left ventricular mass.[34] A simplifying assumption in this method, which introduces some inaccuracy, is that left ventricular wall thickness is uniform around the entire left ventricular cavity. However, this method has been validated by postmortem studies comparing actual and projected left ventricular weights.[33]

Left ventricular mass can be determined by two-dimensional echocardiography using several techniques.[35,36] In

TABLE 14–1 LEFT VENTRICULAR VOLUME DATA

GROUP	NO. OF PATIENTS	END-DIASTOLIC VOLUME (ml/m²)	STROKE VOLUME (ml/m²)	MASS (gm/m²)	EJECTION FRACTION
Normal*	—	70 ± 20.0	45 ± 13.0	92 ± 16.0	0.67 ± 0.08
AS	14	84 ± 22.9	44 ± 10.1	172 ± 32.7	0.56 ± 0.17
AR	22	193 ± 55.4	92 ± 30.9	223 ± 73.0	0.56 ± 0.13
AS and AR	13	138 ± 36.5	75 ± 19.1	231 ± 56.9	0.53 ± 0.10
MS	37	83 ± 21.2	43 ± 11.9	98 ± 24.1	0.57 ± 0.14
MR	29	160 ± 53.1	87 ± 21.3	166 ± 49.9	0.47 ± 0.10
MS and MR	29	106 ± 34.4	58 ± 14.7	119 ± 27.8	0.57 ± 0.12
A and M combined	45	130 ± 55.8	69 ± 25.5	156 ± 55.9	0.55 ± 0.12
Myocardial disease	15	199 ± 75.7	44 ± 14.5	145 ± 27.6	0.25 ± 0.09

From Dodge, H. T., and Baxley, W. A.: Left ventricular volume and mass and their significance in heart disease. Am. J. Cardiol. 23:528, 1969.

* Normal values from Kennedy, J. W., et al.: Quantitative angiocardiography. The normal left ventricle in man. Circulation 34:272, 1966.

AS = aortic valve stenosis with peak systolic pressure gradient >30 mm Hg; AR = aortic valve insufficiency with regurgitant flow >30 ml/beat; MS = mitral valve area <1.5 sq cm; MR = mitral valve regurgitant flow >20 ml/beat; A and M combined = combined aortic and mitral valve disease; Myocardial disease = primary cardiomyopathy or myocardial disease secondary to coronary atherosclerosis.

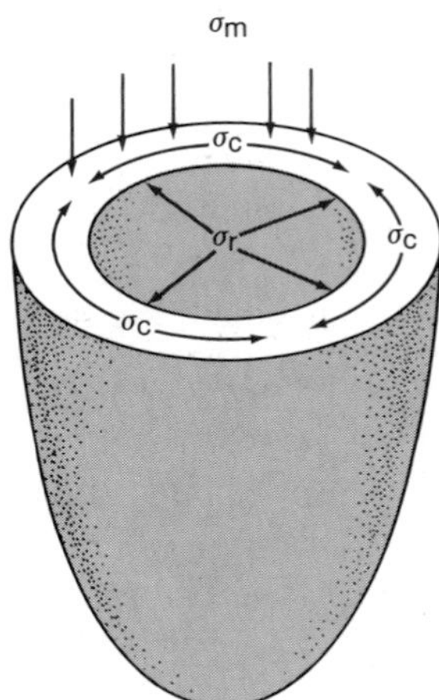

FIGURE 14–6. Circumferential (σ_c), meridional (σ_m), and radial (σ_r) components of left ventricular wall stress from an ellipsoid model. The three components of wall stress are mutually perpendicular. (From Fifer, M.A., and Grossman, W.: Measurement of ventricular volumes, ejection fraction, mass, and wall stress. *In* Grossman, W. [ed.]: Cardiac Catheterization and Angiography. 3rd ed. Philadelphia, Lea and Febiger, 1986, p. 293. Reproduced by permission.)

one of these, left ventricular mass is calculated as the difference between total ventricular volume (estimated from the product of the epicardial left ventricular length and the area of the left ventricle in the short axis) and the volume of the left ventricular cavity. This method has been validated against directly measured ventricular mass.[37] Echocardiographically determined left ventricular mass is an important prognostic factor.[38–40] Computed tomography and magnetic resonance imaging also are useful methods to measure left ventricular mass accurately.

Left ventricular wall thickness normally averages 10.9 ± 2.0 (SD) mm and left ventricular mass, 92 ± 16 gm/m^2 (Table 14–1).[31,34] Chronic cardiac dilatation secondary to volume overload or primary myocardial disease increases left ventricular mass, as does chronic pressure overload. Hypertrophy caused by pressure overload (such as aortic stenosis) is characterized by increased muscle mass resulting from augmentation of wall thickness with little change in ventricular chamber volume (concentric hypertrophy) (Table 14–1). In contrast, hypertrophy caused by volume overload or by primary myocardial disease is characterized by increased muscle mass resulting from ventricular dilatation, with only a slight increase in wall thickness (eccentric hypertrophy) (Table 14–1).

LEFT VENTRICULAR FORCES. The forces acting on the myocardial fibers within the ventricular wall can be calculated from the dimensions of the left ventricular cavity, wall thickness, and intraventricular pressure. Tension (force/cm) is defined as the force acting on a hypothetical slit in the ventricular wall that would tend to pull its edges apart. According to Laplace's law, tension is the product of the intraventricular pressure and radius. *Wall stress* (σ) is the force or tension per unit of cross-sectional area of the ventricular wall. Wall stress may be considered to act in three directions—circumferential, meridional, and radial (Fig. 14–6). The calculation of stress requires assumptions concerning the shape and configuration of the ventricle.[41,42] Circumferential wall stress, the strongest force generated within the ventricular wall, can be approximated as:

$$\text{CWS} = \frac{(\text{P} \cdot \text{b})}{\text{h}}\left(1 - \frac{\text{h}}{2\text{b}}\right)\left(1 - \frac{\text{hb}}{2\text{a}^2}\right)$$

where CWS = circumferential wall stress in dynes per square centimeter $\times 10^3$; P = left ventricular pressure in dynes per square centimeter; a and b are major and minor semiaxes (i.e., half the longest lengths), respectively, in centimeters; and h = left ventricular wall thickness in square centimeters.[7] *Meridional wall stress* (MWS) can be approximated as:

$$\text{MWS} = \frac{\text{P} \cdot \text{r}}{2\text{h}(1 + \text{h}/2\text{r})}$$

where r is the internal radius of the ventricle in centimeters.[43]

Simultaneous recording of left ventricular dimensions (by angiography) and intraventricular pressure recorded with a high-fidelity micromanometer allows calculation of left ventricular tension and stress throughout the cardiac cycle (Fig. 14–7). A simpler method of analyzing the instantaneous left ventricular tension throughout the cardiac cycle consists of recording left ventricular pressure simultaneously with left ventricular diameter across the minor axis of the left ventricle determined by echocardiography. This combination of measurements provides the data necessary to calculate ventricular circumferential fiber shortening (at either the endocardium or the midwall) and midwall circumferential stress, using minor modifications of the equations presented above.[44] However, the use of echocardiography—especially M-mode—for these calculations is based on the assumption of uniform wall motion. This assumption is reasonable only in conditions that affect left ventricular function relatively uniformly, such as dilated cardiomyopathy or aortic or mitral regurgitation. These assumptions are not correct when there is regional left ventricular dysfunction.

During isovolumetric contraction, left ventricular wall

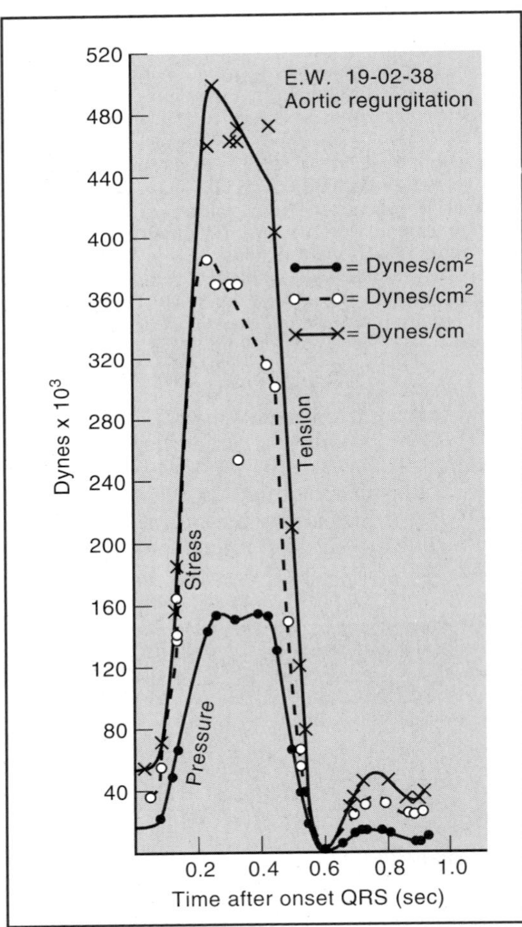

FIGURE 14–7. Sequential changes in left ventricular tension, stress, and pressure are shown throughout the cardiac cycle in a patient with aortic regurgitation. Note that tension and stress decline during ejection, although left ventricular pressure is maintained. (Reproduced with permission from Rackley, C. E.: Quantitative evaluation of left ventricular function by radiographic techniques. Circulation *54*:862, 1976. Copyright 1976 the American Heart Association.)

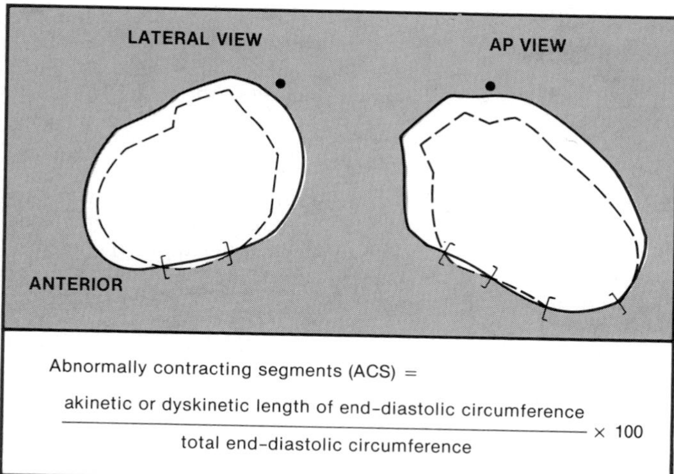

FIGURE 14–8. Systolic *(dashed)* and diastolic *(solid)* lateral and anteroposterior (AP) contrast left ventriculograms are superimposed with a central marker as a reference point. The abnormally contracting segments are enclosed by the brackets on the diastolic silhouette. (Reproduced with permission from Rackley, C. E.: Quantitative evaluation of left ventricular function by radiographic techniques. Circulation *54*:862, 1976. Copyright 1976 the American Heart Association.)

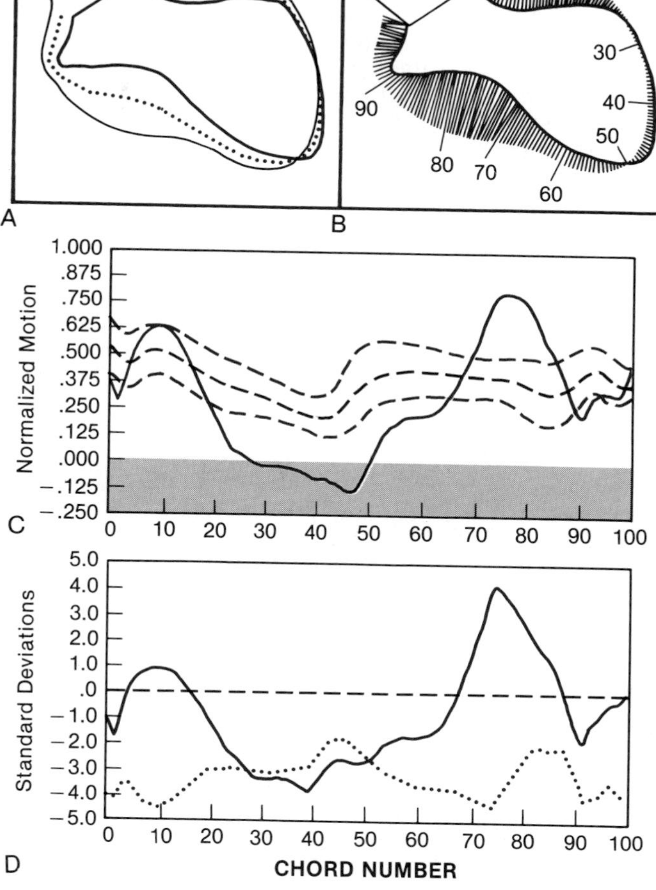

FIGURE 14–9. Center line method of left ventricular regional wall motion analysis. *A,* A center line is constructed midway between the end-diastolic and end-systolic endocardial contours. *B,* Motion is measured along 100 chords constructed perpendicular to the center line. *C,* Motion at each chord is normalized by the end-diastolic perimeter length to yield a shortening fraction. The contraction pattern ± SD measured in a normal population is plotted with a dashed line. *D,* The patient's wall motion is plotted in units of standard deviation (SD) from the normal mean *(dotted line).* Wall motion abnormality in the central infarct region, peripheral infarct region, and noninfarct region is calculated by averaging the motion of chords lying within these regions. (From Kennedy, J. W., and Sheehan, F. H.: Ventriculography. *In* Pepine, C. J., Hill, J. A., and Lambert, C. R. [eds.]: Diagnostic and Therapeutic Cardiac Catheterization. Baltimore, Williams and Wilkins, 1989, p. 171. Reproduced by permission.)

tension and stress rise rapidly as the ventricle contracts without decreasing the chamber volume. During ejection, as the left ventricular cavity decreases in size and wall thickness increases, the stress and tension decline even though pressure is maintained (Fig. 14–7).

REGIONAL VENTRICULAR WALL MOTION. Ischemic heart disease may produce focal, regional abnormalities of contraction. Hyperkinesis of normal areas may compensate for impaired function of an abnormal region, leaving global left ventricular function normal or only minimally depressed. Thus, assessment of regional wall motion is more sensitive in detecting ventricular dysfunction in such patients than analysis of global ventricular function.

Regional wall motion can be assessed with a variety of methods, including contrast angiography.[45] Marked focal abnormalities of contraction can be appreciated by visual inspection of cineventriculograms; segments of abnormal ventricular contraction can be localized by superimposing end-diastolic and end-systolic outlines of the left ventricular cavity. Akinesis is present when a portion of each of the two silhouettes shares a common line; dyskinesis is present when the end-systolic silhouette extends outside the end-diastolic silhouette. The abnormally contracting segments (both akinetic and dyskinetic) may be expressed simply as percentages of the total end-diastolic circumference (Fig. 14–8). Hypokinesis (focal decreases in the extent of contraction) as well as asynchrony (abnormalities of timing of contraction) are less severe disturbances of contraction. Analysis of wall motion from multiple cineframes and automated border detection may be necessary for the detection of these more subtle abnormalities.[46] By use of such techniques it is apparent that focal hypokinesis and abnormalities of timing of segmental wall motion cannot be readily detected by visual inspection of cineangiograms, and that they are relatively common disturbances, especially in ischemic heart disease.

The Center Line Method. Sheehan et al.[47,48] developed a technique in which end-diastolic and end-systolic endocardial contours are traced from a normal sinus beat (Fig. 14–9). A center line is drawn midway between the end-systolic and end-diastolic silhouettes (Fig. 14–9); 100 chords are then constructed perpendicular to this center line. The length of each chord is determined, and after appropriate corrections for ventricular size, it is then compared with that for a group of normal subjects expressed in units of standard deviation from the normal mean.

RIGHT VENTRICULAR AND ATRIAL VOLUME. The shape of the right ventricle is much more complex than the shape of the left ventricle. Thus the prolate ellipsoid that is a useful model to calculate left ventricular volume is not appropriate for the right ventricle.[49] One method is to consider the right ventricle as a pyramid with a triangular base.[50] An alternate approach is to calculate right ventricular volume using Simpson's rule.

The shapes of the atria are less complex than those of the right ventricle. Thus, the atrial volumes can be calculated assuming an ellipsoidal geometry.[51]

ASSESSMENT OF LEFT VENTRICULAR MYOCARDIAL FUNCTION

The factors that determine myocardial function (preload, afterload, contractility, heart rate, and rhythm) can be estimated from left ventricular pressure and volume.

Preload

Left ventricular preload can be assessed from the left ventricular filling pressure, the left ventricular end-diastolic volume, or left ventricular end-diastolic stress.[52,53] The pressure distending the ventricle immediately prior to contraction is the end-diastolic pressure. In the absence of disease of the mitral valve this is equivalent to the pressure in the left atrium at this time (the post *a*-wave or *z*-point pressure). When there is a vigorous atrial contraction, the end-diastolic pressure is substantially higher than the mean left atrial pressure. It is important to recognize that the amount of pulmonary congestion is related to the mean pulmonary capillary (or left atrial) pressure, while the end-diastolic volume is determined by the left ventricular end-diastolic pressure.[52] In the absence of pulmonary vascular disease, mean pulmonary capillary wedge pressure approximates the pulmonary artery diastolic pressure. In the presence of a tall *v* wave, the mean atrial pressure (and mean pulmonary capillary edge pressure) may exceed the ventricular end-diastolic pressure.[54,55]

The left ventricular preload depends on the end-diastolic volume produced by the distending pressure of the ventricle. Since interventions that alter end-diastolic pressure may also alter the relation between end-diastolic volume and pressure, changes in end-diastolic pressure do not always represent changes in end-diastolic volume or changes in end-diastolic fiber stretch.[56,57]

Afterload

Following aortic valve opening the ventricle ejects into the arterial circulation. Thus, in the simplest sense the systolic pressure represents the afterload opposing left ventricular ejection. However, arterial systolic pressure is not a pure measure of left ventricular afterload.[58] The tension in the ventricular wall that the sarcomeres must overcome to shorten is related not only to the systolic pressure but also to the cavity size through the Laplace relation. Thus, at similar systolic pressures a larger ventricle will have greater wall tension than a smaller ventricle. Furthermore, the arterial systolic pressure depends not only on the characteristics of the arterial circulation but also on the pumping performance of the left ventricle. The more vigorous the left ventricular contraction, the greater the volume ejected and the higher the systolic pressure. Thus, left ventricular systolic function and left ventricular afterload are interrelated.

The steady-state arterial load opposing left ventricular ejection can be quantified as the peripheral vascular resistance.[59] This is calculated as the cardiac output divided by the mean arterial pressure minus the mean venous pressure (see p. 439). Because mean venous pressure is very low relative to mean arterial pressure, it is frequently neglected in this calculation. The peripheral vascular resistance provides only steady-state information concerning the relation between flow and pressure in the arterial system. In fact, the left ventricular ejection is pulsatile and there are pulsatile elements to the arterial load that increase in importance with tachycardia, aging, and peripheral vascular disease.[60,61]

The full relation between flow and arterial pressure can be evaluated in the frequency domain as the *arterial input impedance*.[62–64] Calculation of the input impedance spectrum requires the high-fidelity measurement of aortic pressure and flow at the same point. The impedance spectrum consists of a magnitude and phase at each frequency. The magnitude of the impedance at a given frequency is the ratio of a sinusoidally varying pressure and related flow at that frequency. Since arterial pressure and flow do not vary sinusoidally, the Fourier transformation is used to mathematically describe the aortic pressure and flow as a combination of a fundamental sine wave (at the heart rate) and a series of harmonic waves. The impedance spectrum is then calculated as the ratio of the pressure to flow at each frequency. Figure 14–10 provides an example of such an impedance spectrum. Although the impedance spectrum contains all the information concerning the relation between pulsatile flow and pressure in the arterial circulation, its clinical usefulness is limited by the difficulty in obtaining the appropriate measurement and the calculations.

Evaluation of the interaction of the left ventricle and the arterial system requires that they be described in similar terms. Description of the arterial system in the frequency domain does not easily allow this coupling to be assessed because the left ventricle is difficult to describe in these terms. Because the left ventricle can be evaluated in the pressure-volume plane, Sunagawa et al.[65] proposed that the arterial system be evaluated in an analogous manner. In this analysis, the arterial system is described by the relation between the stroke volume and end-systolic pressure (Fig. 14–11). The higher the stroke volume, the greater the end-systolic pressure. The slope of this relation represents the effective arterial end-systolic elastance (E_A). If it is assumed that this relation passes through the origin, then E_A can be calculated as the ratio of end-systolic pressure to stroke volume. As shown in Figure 14–11, this can be plotted on the left ventricular pressure-volume loop. End systole occurs at the intersection of the arterial and ventricular relations. The production of stroke work is maximum when the E_{ES} and E_A are approximately equal.[66]

Under usual conditions, E_A, the slope of the arterial end-systolic pressure stroke volume relation, can be approximated by the product of the peripheral vascular resistance and the heart rate.[67] In older hypertensive patients, E_A may exceed peripheral vascular resistance times heart rate. However, E_A can be accurately estimated over a wide range

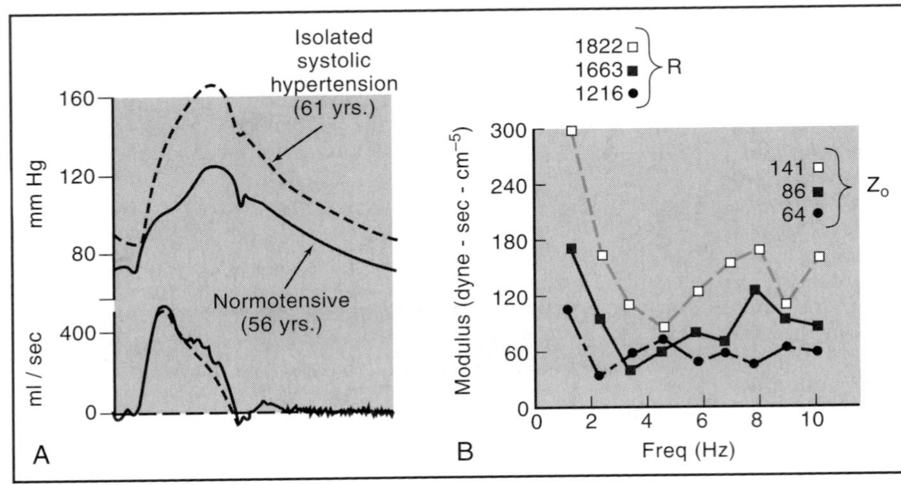

FIGURE 14–10. *A,* Recordings of ascending aortic pressure and flow, and *B,* the resulting aortic input impedance spectra from a 56-year-old normotensive subject *(solid colored lines/closed boxes)* and a 61-year-old subject with isolated systolic hypertension *(broken lines/open boxes),* with an impedance spectrum from a young (28 years) normotensive subject *(solid dots),* shown for comparison. Peripheral vascular resistance (R), impedance moduli of the first harmonic, and characteristic impedance (Z_0) were all higher in the subject with isolated systolic hypertension. Also, the impedance moduli minimum was shifted to a higher frequency in the subject with isolated systolic hypertension. Freq = frequency. (From Nichols, W. W., Nicolini, F. A., and Pepine, C. J.: Determinants of isolated systolic hypertension in the elderly. J. Hypertension *10*[Suppl. 6]:S73, 1992. Reproduced by permission of Current Science Ltd.)

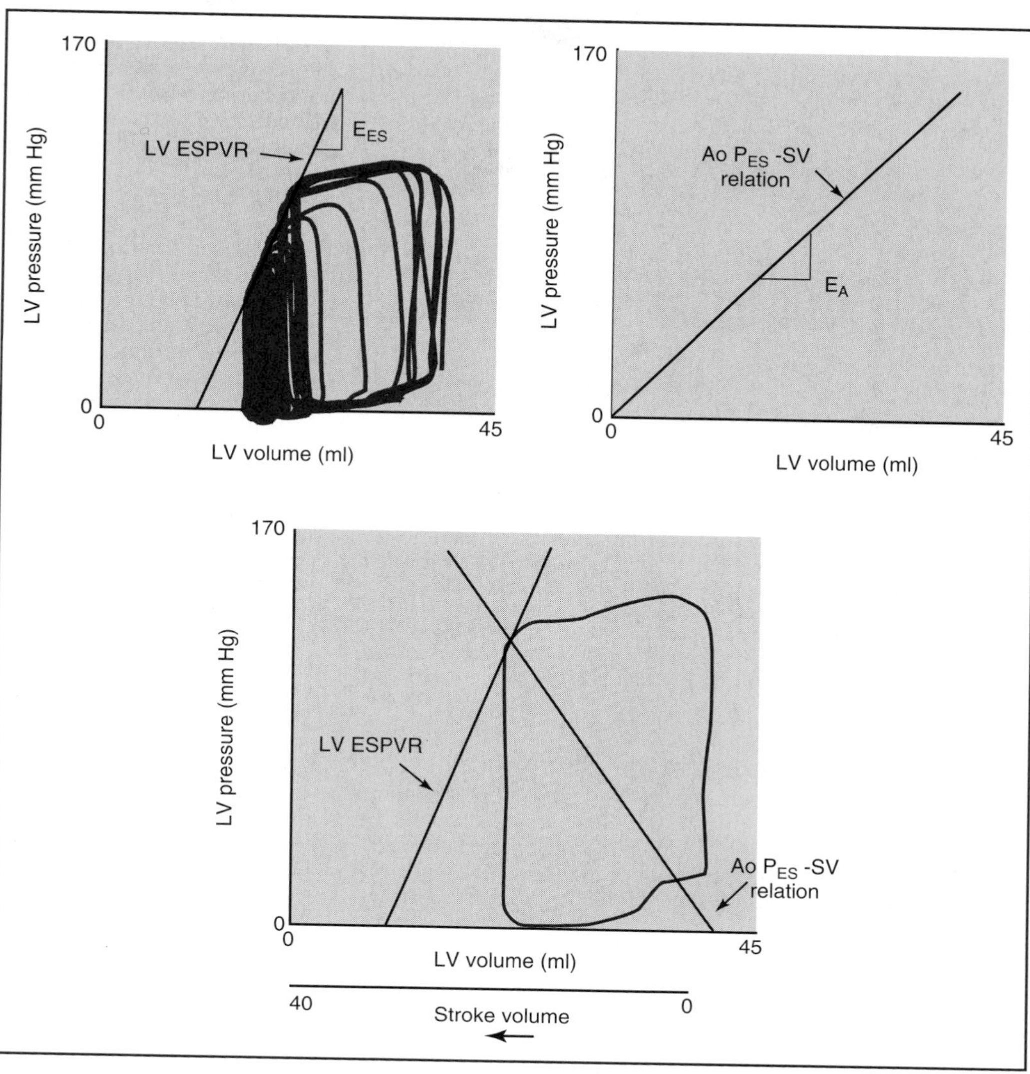

FIGURE 14–11. Left ventricular–arterial coupling assessed in the pressure-volume plane. The left ventricular (LV) end-systolic pressure-volume relation (ESPVR) is used to describe left ventricular systolic performance. In the upper left panel, pressure-volume loops for variably loaded beats are shown with the upper left corner of each beat falling on the end-systolic pressure-volume relation. In the upper right panel, the arterial circulation is described as a relation between stroke volume (SV) and end-systolic pressure. The slope of this relation represents the effective end-systolic arterial elastance (E_A). In the lower panel, the left ventricular ESPVR and the aortic end-systolic pressure-volume relation (A_OP_{ES}-V_{SV}) are plotted on the same axis. End systole occurs at the intersection of the two relations. Thus, description of the arterial circulation in terms of the aortic P_{ES}-SV relation allows understanding of the coupling between the left ventricle and arterial circulation. (Redrawn from Little, W. C., and Cheng, C. P.: Left ventricular–arterial coupling in conscious dogs. Am. J. Physiol. *261*:H70, 1991. Reproduced by permission of the American Physiological Society.)

of conditions from arterial systolic (P_{SYS}) and diastolic pressures (P_{diast}) as: $(2 \cdot P_{SYS} + P_{dias})/3$ divided by the SV.[67]

Contractility

In isolated cardiac muscle or in the isolated heart, loading can be readily controlled and the effects of an intervention on the strength, extent, and velocity of muscle shortening indicate its effect on contractility (Fig. 12–8, p. 366). It is more difficult to make analogous measurements in patients in whom preload, afterload, or both may be abnormal and cannot be readily controlled. Many drugs that affect myocardial contractility also act on the arterial and/or venous beds, thereby altering cardiac loading. Furthermore, in patients with valvular heart disease, it is necessary to evaluate the level of myocardial contractility despite the marked alterations in loading conditions. These considerations have led to the search for methods of evaluating cardiac function that go beyond analysis of the pumping function of the ventricle and provide an assessment of contractility. A number of indices of contractility have been proposed and investigated empirically. Unfortunately, there is no absolute measure of myocardial contractility, i.e., there is no gold standard with which these indices can be compared. Furthermore, at the sarcomere level, contractility and load are interrelated and thus not independent variables.[2,3]

Many indices have been proposed as measures of left ventricular contractile function[23,68] (Table 14–2). These can be divided into isovolumetric phase indices, ejection phase indices, and measures derived from left ventricular pressure-volume relations.

TABLE 14–2 EVALUATION OF LEFT VENTRICULAR SYSTOLIC PERFORMANCE: NORMAL VALUES FOR SOME ISOVOLUMETRIC AND EJECTION PHASE INDICES

CONTRACTILITY INDICES		NORMAL VALUES (MEAN ± S.D.)
ISOVOLUMETRIC PHASE INDICES		
Maximum dP/dt		1610 ± 290 mm Hg/sec
		1670 ± 320 mm Hg/sec
		1661 ± 323 mm Hg/sec
Maximum (dP/dt)/P)		44 ± 8.4 sec^{-1}
VPM or peak $\left[\frac{dP/dt}{28P}\right]$		1.47 ± 0.19 ML/sec
dP/dt/DP at DP = 40 mm Hg		37.6 ± 12.2 sec^{-1}
EJECTION PHASE INDICES		
LVSW		81 ± 23 gm-m
LVSWI		53 ± 22 gm-m/M^2
		41 ± 12 gm-m/M^2
EF	angio:	0.72 ± 0.08
MNSER	angio:	3.32 ± 0.84 EDV/sec
	echo:	2.29 ± 0.30 EDV/sec
Mean V_{CF}	angio:	1.83 ± 0.56 ED circ/sec
		1.50 ± 0.27 ED circ/sec
	echo:	1.09 ± 0.12 ED circ/sec

From Grossman, W.: Evaluation of systolic and diastolic function of the myocardium. *In* Grossman, W., and Baim, D. S. (eds.): Cardiac Catheterization, Angiography and Intervention. Philadelphia, Lea and Febiger, 1991, p. 326.

dP/dt = rate of rise of left ventricular (LV) pressure; DP = developed LV pressure; EF = ejection fraction; MNSER = mean normalized systolic ejection rate; ML = muscle lengths; ED = end-diastolic; V = volume; circ = circumference.

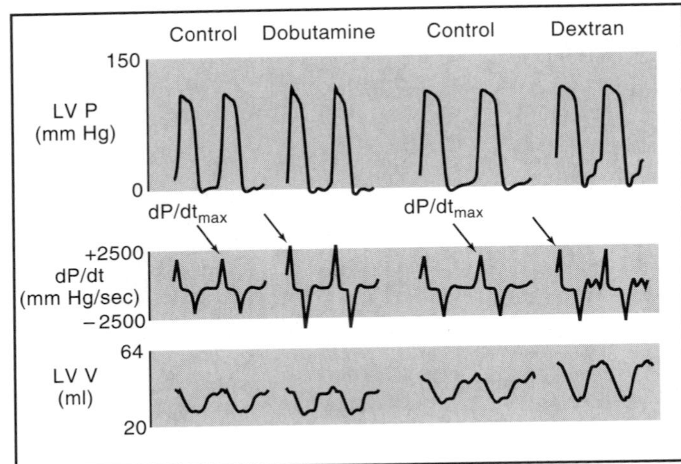

FIGURE 14–12. Recording of left ventricular pressure (LVP), the rate of change of left ventricular pressure (dp/dt), and left ventricular volume (LV V). The maximum value of dP/dt (dP/dt_{max}) increases in response to dobutamine; however, dP/dt_{max} also increases when left ventricular end-diastolic volume is increased by infusing dextran. This demonstrates the sensitivity of dP/dt_{max} to both contractility and left ventricular end-diastolic volume (preload). (Data from Little, W. C.: The left ventricular dP/dt_{max}-end-diastolic volume relation in closed chest dogs. Circ. Res. *56*:808, 1985. Copyright 1985 American Heart Association.)

ISOVOLUMETRIC PHASE INDICES OF CONTRACTILITY. Ventricular dP/dt. The maximum rate of rise of ventricular pressure (dP/dt_{max}) is highly sensitive to acute changes in contractility (Fig. 14–12).[69–71] Under normal conditions dP/dt_{max} occurs before aortic valve opening; thus it is not affected by steady-state alterations in aortic pressure.[72] However, dP/dt_{max} may be delayed until after aortic valve opening in patients with severe left ventricular depression or marked arterial vasodilation with very low aortic diastolic pressures. In the absence of these conditions, dP/dt_{max} can be considered to be relatively independent of afterload. However, dP/dt_{max} is very sensitive to changes in preload.[69,71] This preload sensitivity is greater in ventricles with enhanced contractility and reduced in depressed ventricles.[71] A change in dP/dt_{max} without a change in preload or with an opposite change in preload indicates an alteration in contractility. Another difficulty with the use of dP/dt_{max} as an index of contractility is that it can be altered by ventricular hypertrophy. This difficulty can be surmounted, however, by calculating the peak rate of stress development ($d\sigma/dt$).[73]

Although dP/dt_{max} correlates with contractility, the wide variation between individuals and the marked preload dependence decrease its usefulness for assessing *basal* contractility. Instead, dP/dt_{max} is more useful in assessing *directional* changes in contractility during acute interventions when used in combination with a measure of left ventricular preload. For example, dP/dt_{max} increases during exercise,[73] with tachycardia,[74] and after administration of inotropic agents.[75]

V_{max}. V_{max} is the maximum velocity of shortening of the unloaded contractile elements (CEs). It was originally proposed as a measure of myocardial contractility that is independent of preload or afterload. However, there are theoretical and practical limitations to the calculation of CE V_{max} in isolated muscle, and even more so in the intact heart.[76] Because of the theoretical problems and practical difficulties in calculating V_{max}, it is no longer used as a clinical measure of contractility.

Relation Between dP/dt and Developed Pressure. Some of the difficulties involving the calculation of V_{max} can be partially avoided by the selection of certain points on the curve relating dP/dt to DP, the developed left ventricular pressure (i.e., left ventricular pressure minus end-diastolic pressure). The dP/dt at a DP of 40 mm Hg, a level of pressure that almost always occurs before the opening of the aortic valve, is commonly used. dP/dt at a DP of 40 mm Hg and the maximum dP/dt/DP are useful for assessing directional changes in contractility, since it is unaffected by changes in afterload and less sensitive to changes in preload than dP/dt_{max}.[77–79]

EJECTION PHASE INDICES. The extent of left ventricular ejection can be measured as the stroke volume, ejection fraction, or fractional shortening, and the rate of ejection quantified as the mean and peak velocity of shortening (V_{CF}). All of these measurements are influenced by both contractility and load.[80] The marked preload dependence of the stroke volume is minimized by dividing by the end-diastolic volume producing the EF. However, the EF remains highly sensitive to changes in afterload, so it is best to consider it a measure of systolic performance and not a pure measure of contractility (see below).

The afterload dependence of the ejection fraction or measures of the left ventricular shortening can be minimized using concepts derived from the myocardial force-velocity relation of isolated cardiac muscle (Fig. 14–13). For example, the relation between fractional myocardial fiber shortening (determined noninvasively) and left ventricular end-systolic stress (obtained in the basal state), sometimes supplemented by the measurements made during a pharmacologically altered afterload, provides a useful and practical framework for assessing the basal level of ventricular contractility.[81–86] Similarly, the relation between end-systolic stress and mean V_{CF} at various levels of wall stress is relatively preload independent and incorporates afterload. Thus, changes in the relation between the extent (or velocity) of myocardial wall shortening and the simultaneous ventricular wall stress reflect acute changes in contractility. For example, augmentation of (V_{CF}) at a constant wall stress signifies improvement of contractility. The relation between end-systolic wall stress and left ventricular fractional shortening of V_{CF} can also provide assessment of the basal level of contractility. This relation is particularly

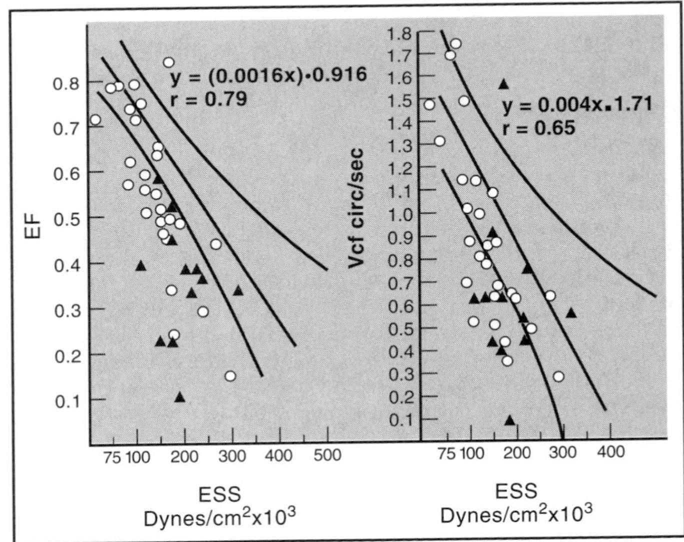

FIGURE 14–13. The ejection fraction (EF)–end-systolic stress (ESS) relationship is shown on the *left* and the mean velocity of circumferential fiber shortening (Vcf)–end-systolic stress relationship is shown on the *right*. In this example, data from patients with valvular heart disease are compared to observations from normal subjects (95 per cent confidence limits are shown for the normal relation). Those patients who fell down and to the left of the normal limits demonstrated reduced ejection performance for any given level of afterload suggesting impaired contractility. (From Carabello, B. A., Williams, H., Gash, A. K., et al.: Hemodynamic predictors of outcome in patients undergoing valve replacement. Circulation *74*:1309, 1986. Copyright 1986 American Heart Association.)

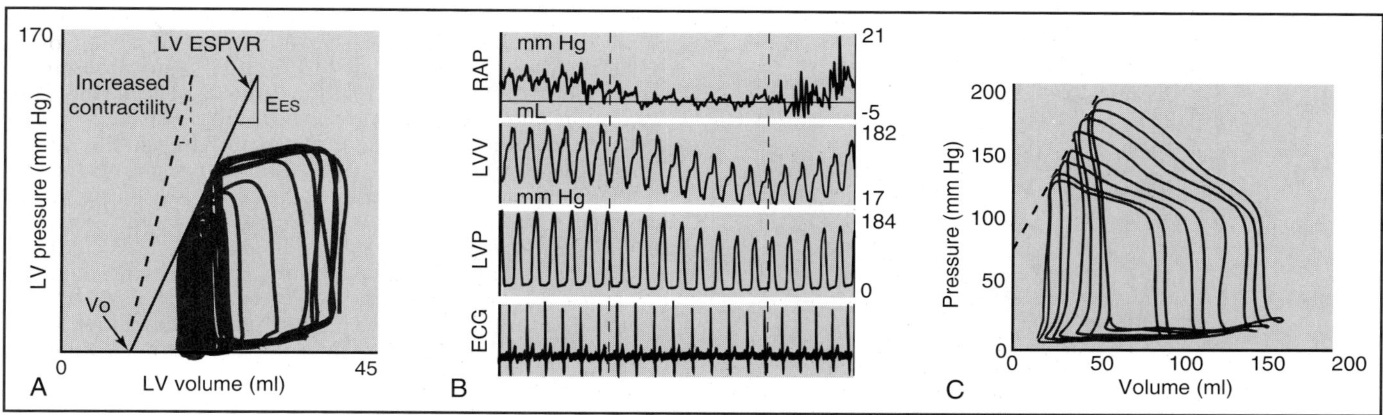

FIGURE 14–14. *A,* **Variably loaded pressure-volume loops produced by caval occlusion in a conscious experimental animal. End systole occurs at the upper left corner of the pressure-volume loops. The end-systolic points of the variably loaded beats fall along a single relation, the left ventricular end-systolic pressure-volume relation (LV ESPVR). Within the physiological range, this relation is approximated by a straight line. The line can be described in terms of its slope (E_{ES}) and volume axis intercept (V_0). Note that the volume axis intercept results from extrapolation of the line outside the range of end-systolic pressures in which data can be acquired.**

An increase in contractile state, produced by infusing dobutamine, shifts the left ventricular end-systolic pressure-volume relation toward the left while increasing the slope (E_{ES}). (Data from Little, W. C., Cheng, C. P., Mumma, M., et al.: Comparison of measures of left ventricular contractile performance derived from pressure-volume loops in conscious dogs. Circulation *80:*1378, 1989. Reproduced by permission of the American Heart Association, Inc.)

B, **Recording of right atrial pressure (RAP), left ventricular volume (LVV) measured with the conductance catheter, and left ventricular pressure (LVP) in a patient during transient balloon occlusion of the inferior vena cava. These variably loaded beats are shown in the pressure-volume plane on the right *(C).* The upper left corner of these loops defines the left ventricular end-systolic pressure-volume relation *(dotted line).* (From Kass, D. A.: Clinical ventricular pathophysiology: A pressure-volume view. *In* Waltier, D. C.: Ventricular Function. Baltimore, Williams and Wilkins, 1995, p. 111. Reproduced by permission of the Society of Cardiovascular Anesthesiologists.)**

useful in patients who have a reduced EF, because it distinguishes between reduced myocardial shortening due to excessive afterload and that due to depressed myocardial contractility.[87]

Because the $V_{CF} - \sigma_{ES}$ relation during a single beat is not defined by parallel straight lines, it may not be accurately defined from measurements made at a single loading condition.[88]

PRESSURE-VOLUME RELATIONS. As discussed above, consideration of the left ventricle in the pressure-volume plane provides a powerful method to understand left ventricular performance.[5,89–91] The generation of variably loaded beats allows determination of several relations that provide information concerning left ventricular contractility and systolic performance. The variably loaded beats can be produced by transient balloon occlusion of the inferior vena cava.[23,91,92] An alternate approach is to generate a range of loading conditions using graded infusions of vasoactive agents, such as methoxamine and nitroprusside.[93,94]

Left Ventricular ESPVR. The upper left corner of variably loaded pressure-volume loops defines the left ventricular end-systolic pressure-volume relation (Fig. 14–14). In the physiological range, this relation can be approximated as a straight line and can therefore be described with a slope (E_{ES}) and volume axis intercept (V_0), i.e., $P_{ES} = E_{ES}(V_{ES} - V_0)$.[89,95] E_{ES} has dimensions of pressure/volume (units of mm Hg/ml). This represents the end-systolic stiffness of the left ventricle and indicates how sensitive ejection is to increases in afterload (as reflected in the end-systolic pressure). With enhanced contractility, E_{ES} increases. The volume axis intercept (V_0) of the ESPVR has been referred to as the *dead volume* of the ventricle. This is the volume at which the left ventricle would generate no pressure. This volume intercept cannot be directly measured clinically. Instead it must be determined by extrapolation and thus is subject to significant errors.[89,95,96] In many clinical studies the extrapolated V_0 is negative, which is a physiological impossibility. This indicates the difficulties involved in accurately determining V_0 in clinical studies.[89]

The position of the ESPVR on the volume axis at the operating pressure (e.g., the end-systolic volume associated with an end-systolic pressure of 100 mm Hg) indicates the extent of contraction. Global increases in contractility, such as the infusion of dobutamine, both increase E_{ES} and shift the ESPVR to the left in the physiological range.[89,95] Thus, at a constant afterload (i.e., constant left ventricular end-systolic pressure) the left ventricle with enhanced contractility ejects to a lower volume and is less sensitive to changes in systolic pressure. Global decreases in contractility produce the opposite effect. Thus, E_{ES} and the position of the ESPVR in the physiological range provide load-insensitive measures of contractility.[89,95]

Regional left ventricular dysfunction resulting from coronary artery occlusion produces a nearly parallel rightward shift of the left ventricular ESPVR in the physiological range with little change in the E_{ES}[97,98] (Fig. 14–15). A similar parallel shift of the ESPVR occurs when the normal activation sequence of the left ventricle is altered by pacing.[99]

An echocardiographically determined left ventricular end-systolic dimension or cross-sectional area can be used as a surrogate for left ventricular volume in the left ventricular end-systolic pressure-volume relation provided that there is no segmental wall motion abnormality.[100] Automated echocardiographic border detection makes it possible to determine pressure-area relations on-line.[101]

There are practical and theoretical difficulties in using the ESPVR as a clinical measure of left ventricular contractility. First, to define accurately the ESPVR, a wide range of loading conditions must be obtained. Such alterations in load may induce reflexly mediated changes in heart rate and left ventricular contractility. In addition, arterial vasoconstriction and vasodilation produce parallel shifts of the left ventricular ESPVR.[102,103] Thus, the interventions required to define the ESPVR accurately may themselves

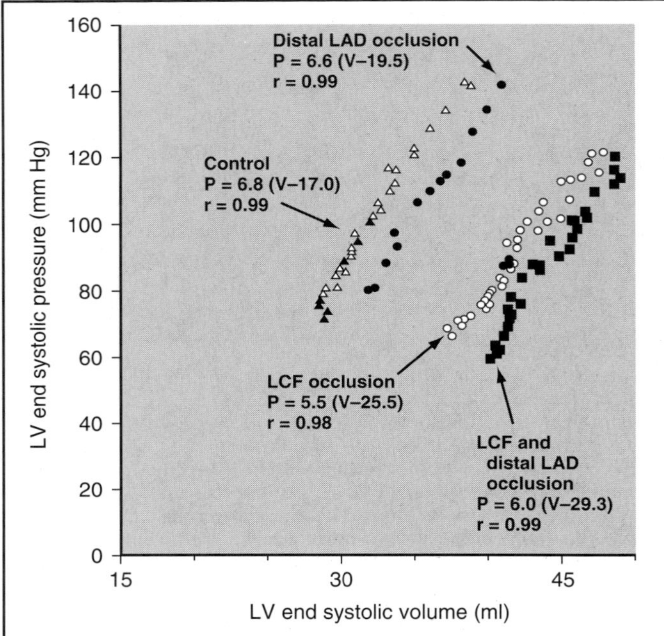

FIGURE 14–15. Left ventricular (LV) end-systolic pressure-volume (P-V) relations from a conscious experimental animal during a control period and after occlusion of the distal left anterior descending coronary artery (LAD), the proximal left circumflex coronary artery (LCF), and both the distal left anterior descending coronary artery and proximal left circumflex coronary artery. Progressively larger amounts of regional ischemia produce greater parallel leftward shifts of the end-systolic pressure-volume relations. (From Little, W. C., and O'Rourke, R. A.: Effect of regional ischemia on the left ventricular end-systolic pressure-volume relation in chronically instrumented dogs. Reproduced by permission of the American College of Cardiology.) J. Am. Coll. Cardiol. *5*:297, 1985.

alter the relation, confounding the ability to define the ESPVR with precision in clinical studies.

A second difficulty in evaluating the ESPVR is the determination of the timing of end systole, defined as the upper left corner of the pressure-volume loop. This may not correspond exactly to aortic valve closure or the time of maximum ventricular elastance. This difference may be accentuated when there is reduced impedance to left ventricular ejection, as occurs in mitral regurgitation.[104]

A third difficulty is that because the slope of the ESPVR depends on the size of the ventricle, it is not possible to define a normal range for E_{ES}. Attempts to correct for ventricular size have not been uniformly successful. However, this does not prevent E_{ES} from differentiating patients with normal from those with abnormal left ventricular contractile function.[105] One method of correcting for differences in LV size is to evaluate the LV in the stress-strain plane.[106] In this analysis the LV end-systolic stress-strain relation is analogous to the ESPVR except that it has been normalized for wall thickness and chamber size and configuration.

If V_0 is assumed to be small, E_{ES} can be approximated by the ratio of LV systolic pressure to end-systolic volume (P_{ES}/V_{ES}).[89,107] This approach has the advantage of avoiding the need to evaluate multiply loaded beats and can be performed noninvasively. However, the P_{ES}/V_{ES} ratio is subject to significant errors in estimating E_{ES} when V_0 is large, and is not a sensitive measure of contractile performance.

Despite the theoretical and practical limitations to the clinical evaluation of contractility using the ESPVR, left ventricular pressure-volume analysis provides a powerful tool to help understand the interaction of contractile state and load to produce ventricular performance (Fig. 14–16).

Other Pressure-Volume Relations. Two other relations can be derived from variably loaded pressure-volume loops: the dP/dt_{max}–end-diastolic volume (V_{ED}) relation and the SW-V_{ED} relation (Fig. 14–17).

During caval occlusion, dP/dt_{max} and V_{ED} are linearly related.[71] The slope of the relation (dE/dt_{max}) represents the maximum rate of change of left ventricular elastance during contraction and is very sensitive to contractile state.[71] Thus, this resting $dP/dt_{max} - V_{ED}$ relation accounts for the preload dependence of dP/dt_{max}, which increases when contractile state is augmented. Although it is very sensitive to changes in contractile state, the $dP/dt_{max} - V_{ED}$ relation has several limitations. First, dP/dt_{max} is more variable than P_{ES}, and this relation is less stable than the ESPVR.[108] Second, the $dP/dt_{max} - V_{ED}$ relation saturates at volumes only slightly above the operating point.[109] Thus this relation can be defined only by preload reduction and not by pharmacologically produced increases in load.

Stroke work (SW) is the external work performed by the left ventricle and is calculated as the area of the pressure-volume loop. It can be approximated as the product of stroke volume and mean arterial pressure. Thus, SW integrates the two determinants of tissue perfusion: flow and pressure.[65] During caval occlusions, SW and V_{ED} are linearly related. SW is insensitive to arterial load in the physiological range; thus the SW-V_{ED} relation is afterload independent under these conditions.[66,110,111] In response to an increase in contractile state the slope of this relation, termed *preload recruitable stroke work* (PRSW), increases. Thus, PRSW has been proposed as a load-independent measure of contractile state.[112] However, the SW-V_{ED} relation is not only determined by contractile state, it also can be altered by changes in the diastolic left ventricular pressure-volume relation.[108] For example, the diastolic pressure-volume relation can be altered under some circumstances without a change in the ESPVR.[113] This would alter the LV SW-V_{ED} relation and PRSW. Although importantly influenced by contractility, the SW-V_{ED} relation is best considered as a measure of integrated pump function (see below).

The SW-V_{ED} relation has several important advantages.[108] First, because SW integrates pressure and volume throughout the cardiac cycle, it is free of noise and is remarkably stable. Second, during reductions in preload as produced by caval occlusion, both determinants of SW (stroke volume and end-systolic pressure) decline, producing a wide range of SW values. This wide range of data increases the statistical precision with which the SW-V_{ED} relation can be defined. Finally, because the slope (PRSW) has dimensions of pressure, it therefore is independent of left ventricle cavity size.

PRELOAD ADJUSTED POWER. The power generated by the left ventricle can be calculated as the product of aortic flow and pressure. The maximum power (PWR_{max}) responds to changes in contractile state, is insensitive to changes in the arterial circulation, and is linearly related to the square of V_{ED} (V_{ED}^2) in the physiological range.[114] Thus, PWR_{max}/V_{ED}^2 may provide a preload-independent measure of contractility. PWR_{max}/V_{ED}^2 can be determined noninvasively using nuclear techniques or Doppler echocardiography to determine aortic flow, and measuring arterial pressure using indirect means.[115]

LEFT VENTRICULAR PUMP FUNCTION

The contraction of individual sarcomeres is integrated into the myocardial shortening that ultimately is expressed as the pumping function of the left ventricle. The left heart can be analyzed as a pump with an input (the pulmonary venous or mean left atrial pressure) and an output (which in simplest terms is the cardiac output = stroke volume × heart rate). The relationship between the input and output is the ventricular function curve or the Frank-Starling rela-

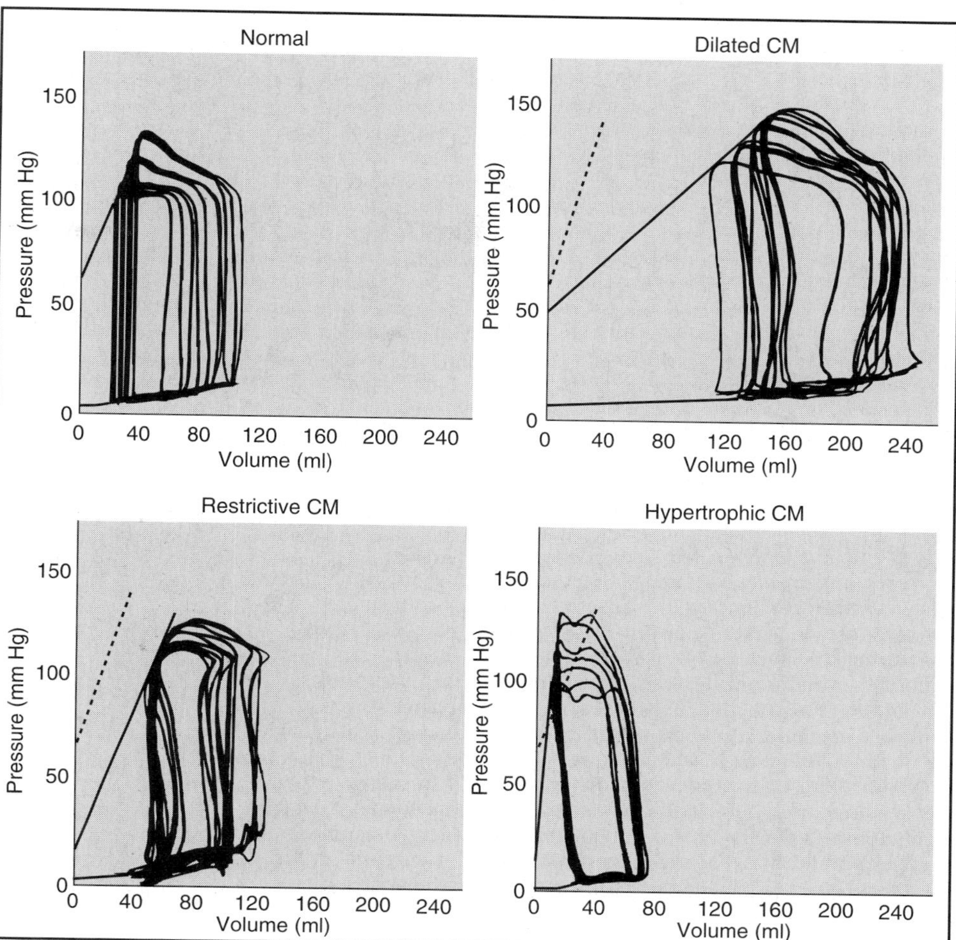

FIGURE 14–16. Variably loaded pressure-volume loops used to define the left ventricular end-systolic pressure-volume relations in four patients: *A,* normal ventricle; *B,* dilated cardiomyopathy (CM); *C,* restrictive heart disease; *D,* hypertrophic cardiomyopathy. (From Kass, D. A.: Clinical ventricular pathophysiology: A pressure-volume view. *In* Warltier, D. C.: Ventricular Function. Baltimore, Williams and Wilkins, 1995, p. 111. Reproduced by permission of the Society of Cardiovascular Anesthesiologists.)

tionship[116,117] (Figs. 14–18 and 14–19). In this relationship the output can be considered to be the SV, cardiac output, or the SW.

A family of Frank-Starling curves reflects the response of the pump performance of the ventricle to a spectrum of contractile states, and the position of a given curve provides a description of ventricular contractility. Movement along a single curve represents the operation of the Frank-Starling principle, which indicates that SV, cardiac output, or SW varies with preload. By contrast, upward or downward displacement of the curve represents a positive or negative inotropic effect, i.e., augmentation or depression of contractility, respectively (Fig. 14–18). However, it is important to recognize that in an intact patient or animal the standard ventricular function curve represents a complex interaction of preload, afterload, and contractility.

The pump performance of the left ventricle depends on its ability to fill (diastolic performance) and to empty (systolic performance) (Fig. 14–19). The SV is equal to the product of the end-diastolic volume and the effective ejection fraction. Thus the generation of stroke volume depends on the conversion of the filling pressure to end-diastolic volume (diastolic performance) and on the effective ejection fraction (systolic performance).[53]

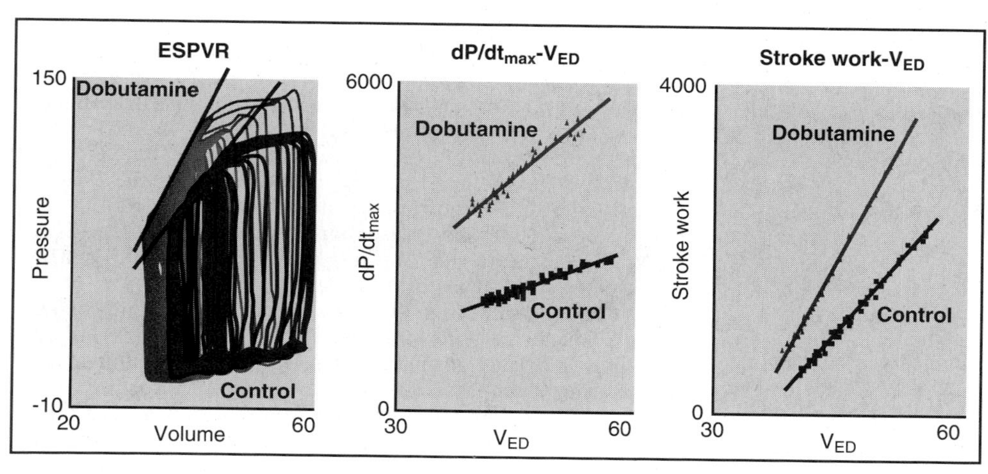

FIGURE 14–17. Three relations describing left ventricular contractile performance derived from variably loaded pressure-volume loops: the left ventricular end-systolic pressure-volume relation (ESPVR); the relation between dP/dt_{max} and end-diastolic volume (V_{ED}); and the relation between stroke work and V_{ED}. All three relations can be approximated by a straight line within the range of data generated by transient caval occlusion. Each relation is shifted toward the left with an increase in slope in response to increase in contractile state produced by dobutamine. (Reproduced with permission from Little, W. C., Cheng, C. P., Mumma, M., et al.: Comparison of measures of left ventricular contractile performance derived from pressure-volume loops in conscious dogs. Circulation *80*:1378, 1989. Copyright 1989 the American Heart Association.)

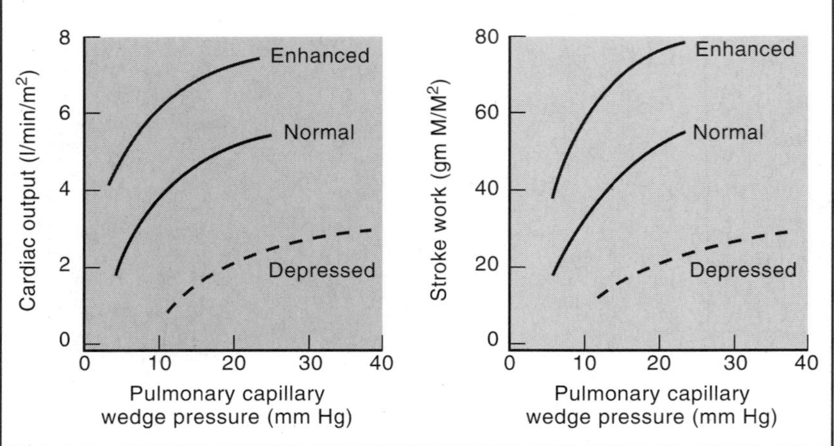

FIGURE 14–18. The Starling relationship. With increasing left ventricular filling pressure measured by the pulmonary capillary wedge pressure (reflecting the pulmonary venous pressure), there is an increase in cardiac output and stroke work. The positions of the curves are influenced by the contractile state of the left ventricle. An enhancement of contractile state shifts the curves upward while a depression produces a downward shift.

Systolic Performance

Left ventricular systolic performance is the ability of the left ventricle to empty. Because myocardial contractility is an important determinant of the left ventricle's systolic performance, systolic performance and contractility are frequently considered to be interchangeable. However, they are not the same because the systolic performance of the left ventricle is also importantly influenced by load and ventricular configuration. Thus it is possible to have abnormal systolic performance despite normal contractility when left ventricular afterload is excessive. Alternatively, left ventricular systolic performance may be nearly normal despite decreased myocardial contractility if left ventricular afterload is low, as occurs in some patients with mitral regurgitation.

Left ventricular systolic performance can be quantified as the left ventricular emptying fraction or ejection fraction (EF). In the presence of a left-sided valvular regurgitant lesion (mitral regurgitation or aortic regurgitation), or left-to-right shunt (ventricular septal defect or patent ductus arteriosus), the left ventricular stroke volume may be high, while the forward stroke volume (stroke volume minus regurgitant volume or shunt volume), which contributes to useful cardiac output, is lower. Accordingly, we define the *effective ejection fraction* as the forward stroke volume divided by end-diastolic volume.[53,118] The effective EF is a useful means to quantify systolic function because it represents the functional emptying of the left ventricle and is relatively independent of left ventricular end-diastolic volume over the clinically relevant range. An operational definition of systolic dysfunction is an effective EF of less than 50 per cent.[27,118] When defined in this manner, systolic left ventricular dysfunction may result from impaired myocardial function, increased left ventricular afterload, and/or structural abnormalities of the left heart.

The forward SV is equal to the product of the effective ejection fraction and the end-diastolic volume (Fig. 14–19). If left ventricular contractile state and arterial properties remain constant as end-diastolic volume increases, the EF stays constant or increases slightly.[80] Thus an increase in the end-diastolic volume will allow for a normal forward SV despite a reduced effective EF.

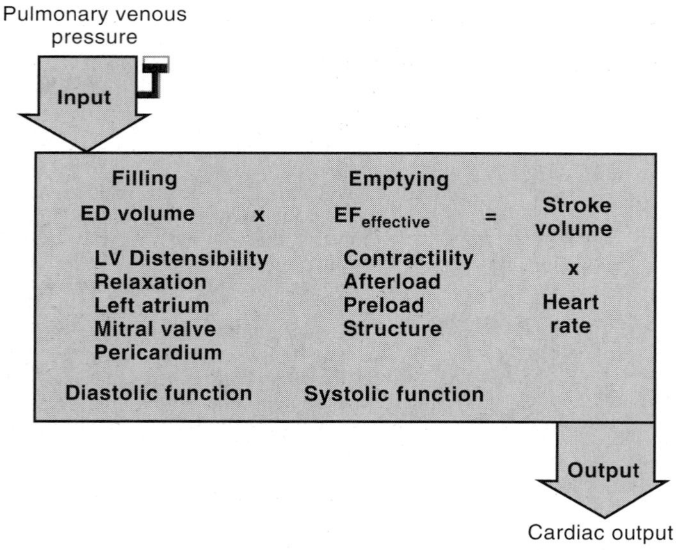

FIGURE 14–19. Left ventricular pump performance. The input is considered to be the pulmonary venous pressure and the output the cardiac output. The stroke volume is equal to the product of the end-diastolic volume (ED) and the effective left ventricular ejection fraction (EF). Thus, the generation of the stroke volume depends on the conversion of the filling pressure to end-diastolic volume (diastolic perfomance) and on the effective ejection fraction (systolic performance).

Diastolic Performance (See also p. 383)

For the left ventricle to function as a pump, it must not only empty but also fill. The left atrial (and pulmonary venous) pressure is the source pressure for left ventricular filling. Thus, normal left ventricular diastolic function can be defined as filling of the left ventricle sufficient to produce a cardiac output commensurate with the body's needs with a normal mean pulmonary venous pressure that does not exceed 12 mm Hg.[52]

A patient with systolic dysfunction (reduced effective ejection fraction) requires a larger end-diastolic volume to produce an adequate stroke volume and cardiac output. The achievement of a higher left ventricular end-diastolic volume without abnormally high pulmonary venous pressure, secondary to rightward displacement of the left ventricular diastolic pressure-volume curve (from curve B to curve A in Figure 14–20), can compensate for impaired systolic performance. However, more often the greater end-diastolic volume requires elevation of left ventricular diastolic, left atrial, and pulmonary venous pressures. Thus, systolic dysfunction is the most common cause of elevation of left ventricular diastolic pressure.

Diastolic dysfunction also occurs in the absence of systolic dysfunction and may be due to obstruction of left ventricular filling, impaired left ventricular distensibility, or external compression of the left ventricle.[53,119–122] A common cause of such primary diastolic dysfunction is altered diastolic distensibility. In the pressure-volume plane, this is represented by a leftward and upward shift of the end-diastolic pressure-volume relation (EDPVR) (Fig. 14–20). When this occurs, significantly higher pressures

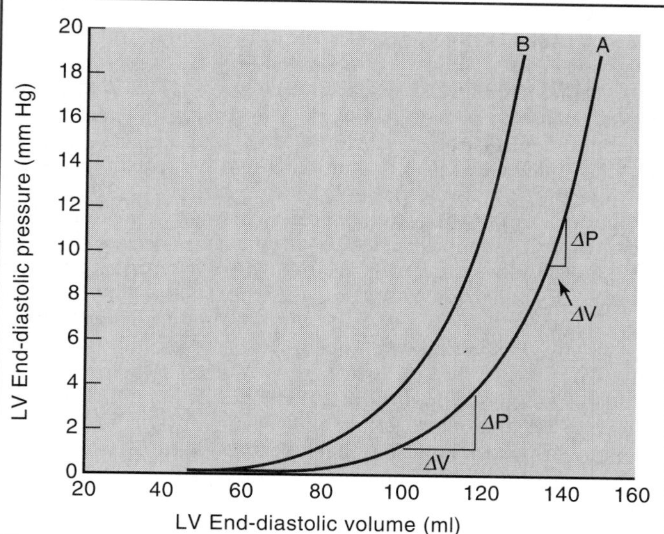

FIGURE 14–20. The slope of the LV end-diastolic pressure-volume relation indicates the passive chamber stiffness. Since the relation is exponential in shape, the slope (ΔP/ΔV) increases as the end-diastolic pressure increases. A shift of the curve from A to B indicates that a higher LV pressure will be required to distend the LV to a similar volume, indicating that the ventricle is less distensible. (From Little, W. C., and Downes, T. R.: Clinical evaluation of left ventricular diastolic performance. Prog. Cardiovasc. Dis. *32*(4):273, 1990. Reproduced by permission.)

are required to distend the left ventricle to achieve the same end-diastolic volume. If the shift in the EDPVR is severe enough, filling of the left ventricle to the level sufficient to produce a normal stroke volume can be achieved only with elevated pulmonary venous pressure that will be associated with pulmonary congestion. Thus, an alteration in diastolic distensibility may produce pulmonary congestion and congestive heart failure in the absence of systolic dysfunction.[119,120,122,123]

Evaluation of Diastolic Performance

The indices of diastolic function can be organized into three groups: measures of isovolumetric relaxation, indices of passive left ventricular characteristics derived from the diastolic left ventricular pressure-volume relations, and measurements of the pattern of left ventricular diastolic filling, which are obtained from Doppler echocardiography or radionuclide angiography.[52,124,125]

ISOVOLUMETRIC RELAXATION. Isovolumetric relaxation can be quantified by measuring its duration or by describing the time course of the fall in left ventricular pressure. The duration of isovolumetric relaxation, or the time from aortic valve closure to mitral valve opening, can be measured by M-mode echocardiography. A similar interval, the time from aortic valve closure to the onset of mitral valve flow, can be measured by combining phonocardiography and Doppler echocardiography. Unfortunately, the duration of isovolumetric relaxation depends not only on the rate of left ventricular relaxation but also on the difference in pressures between the aorta at the time of aortic valve closure and the left atrium at mitral valve opening.[126] Thus, the duration of isovolumetric relaxation can be increased by an elevation of aortic pressure or decreased by an elevation of left atrial pressure. The time from minimum left ventricular volume to peak left ventricular filling rate can be measured using radionuclear angiography.[125] Because this time interval spans both isovolumetric relaxation and part of early filling, the interpretation is even more complicated than the duration of isovolumetric relaxation alone.

The time course of isovolumetric pressure decline has been quantitatively described by the peak rate of pressure fall (dP/dt_{min}) and the time constant of an exponential fit of the time course of isovolumetric pressure decline. Each of these requires the measurement of left ventricular pressure using a micromanometer. dP/dt_{min} is strongly influenced by the pressure at the time of aortic valve closure and is not a good measure of the rate of isovolumetric relaxation.

After aortic valve closure, left ventricular pressure declines in an exponential manner during isovolumetric relaxation[127] (Fig. 14–21). The rate of pressure decline can be quantified by the time constant of the exponential decline. The time constant (τ) is increased by processes such as ischemia or other causes of myocardial depression that slow ventricular relaxation.[128,129] It is shortened by acceleration of the rate of active relaxation, as caused by an increase in heart rate or sympathetic stimulation. The time constant of isovolumetric pressure decline can also be altered by changes in loading conditions. An increase in arterial pressure or end-diastolic volume can increase the time constant, although changes in the preload at a constant arterial pressure may have less effect.[129,130]

Calculation of the time constant of left ventricular isovolumetric pressure decline has several technical limitations. Data are analyzed from the time of minimum dP/dt to a pressure 5 or 10 mm Hg above end-diastolic pressure. Even if pressure is measured every 2 msec, there are only a limited number of data points. This contributes to a large beat-to-beat variability of τ.[131]

If mitral in-flow is prevented, left ventricular pressure will decline to subatmospheric levels. Thus, it has been suggested that the data should be fit to an exponential function with an asymptote (P_B):

$$P(t) = P_o e^{-t/\tau} + P_B.$$

This is usually done by differentiating both sides and then using the linear least squares technique to fit the equation:

$$dP(t)/dt = -(1/\tau)(P - P_B)$$

The normal range of values of τ calculated using this method is 37 to 67 msec.[132]

The use of an asymptote to calculate τ is particularly important when the external pressure of the left ventricle may be changing.[133] However, τ determined from a nonfilling beat in an experimental animal in which the full

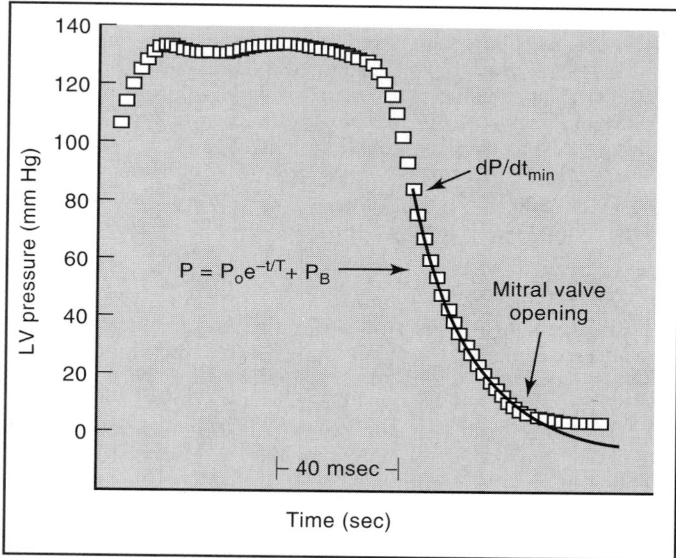

FIGURE 14–21. LV pressure measured at 2-msec intervals using a micromanometer. The LV pressure from the time of minimum dP/dt (dP/dt_{min}) to mitral valve opening is described by an exponential relation *(solid line)*. After mitral valve opening, LV pressure deviates from the exponential line. $P_o + P_b$ = pressure (P) at dP/dt_{max}; t = time; T = time constant of relaxation; P_B = baseline pressure. (From Little, W. C., and Downes, T. R.: Clinical evaluation of left ventricular diastolic performance. Prog. Cardiovasc. Dis. *32*(4):273, 1990. Reproduced by permission.)

time course of left ventricular relaxation is available correlates most closely with τ calculated from a normal beat without the use of an asymptote (i.e., $P = P_o e^{-t/\tau}$).[134] To avoid the computational properties of nonlinear fitting in the calculation on τ without an asymptote, the relation is linearized using a natural logarithm transformation to result in:

$$\ln P = \ln P_o - t/\tau$$

The data are then fit to this equation using the linear least squares technique to determine τ. When calculated using this method, the normal range of values for τ is 28 to 45 msec.[132]

Recently, the time course of LV pressure during isovolumetric relaxation has been characterized using noninvasive Doppler measurement of the velocity of a regurgitant jet across the mitral or aortic valve.[10,11,135] In this method the modified Bernoulli equation is used to approximate LV pressure during isovolumetric relaxation allowing calculation of the maximum rate of left ventricular pressure decline and the exponential time constant.

PASSIVE DIASTOLIC CHARACTERISTICS OF THE LEFT VENTRICLE. The passive characteristics of the left ventricle can be described as the diastolic pressure-volume relation.[119,120,129] Optimally the passive left ventricular diastolic pressure-volume relation should be constructed from points that are obtained after relaxation is complete and at slow filling rates, so that viscous effects are not present.[129,136] Practically, this can be approximated using points obtained late in diastole, when relaxation is assumed to be complete, or from variously loaded beats at end diastole. However, it is important to correct for the effect of respiratory changes in intrathoracic pressure.

The slope of the end-diastolic pressure-volume relation is the *chamber stiffness.* Since the pressure-volume relation is nonlinear, the chamber stiffness depends on the point on the curve in which it is measured; stiffness increases with increasing volume (Fig. 14–20). Several techniques have been proposed to correct for this effect by normalizing chamber stiffness. One approach is to approximate the pressure-volume relation by an exponential function.[137] Another technique is to compare the chamber stiffness at a common pressure or volume. However, the analysis of chamber stiffness does not account for shifts in the pressure-volume relation that can occur from the alteration of load, diseases, or pharmacological agents.[56,57,129,136] The position of the diastolic pressure-volume relation indicates the distensibility of the left ventricle, an upward shift indicating a less distensible ventricle.[119]

The *diastolic pressure-volume* relation represents the net passive characteristics of the left ventricular chamber. To derive information concerning the properties of the myocardium alone, the effects of wall thickness, ventricular configuration, size, and external pressure must be removed.[138] This can be accomplished by deriving the myocardial stress-strain relation from the chamber transmural pressure-volume relation. In contrast to the slope of the pressure-volume relation that assesses the amount of ventricular chamber distention under pressure, the stress-strain relation represents the resistance of the myocardium to stretch when subjected to stress. Thus, it should not be influenced by the configuration of the left ventricle. However, calculation of stress requires the use of a geometrical model of the left ventricle, and calculation of strain requires assumption of the unstressed left ventricular volume. In addition to these potential theoretical limitations, these calculations require accurate measurements over a wide range of left ventricular pressures and volumes. Measurements made during rapid filling may be inappropriately influenced by active myocardial relaxation and viscoelastic effects. Observations during diastasis and atrial systole do not have this problem, but they may not supply a wide enough range of data points. The theoretical problems and the technical difficulties in determining myocardial stress-strain relations have limited their clinical application.

PATTERNS OF LEFT VENTRICULAR DIASTOLIC FILLING. Recently there has been interest in assessing quantified diastolic left ventricular performance by analyzing the pattern of left ventricular filling. Such information can be obtained by determining the left ventricular volume or dimension throughout the cardiac cycle, using contrast or radionuclide angiography, M-mode or two-dimensional echocardiography, or by measuring the left ventricular in-flow velocity using a Doppler determination of mitral valve flow velocities. The most widely used methods today are radionuclide angiography[125] and Doppler mitral valve flow-velocity determination[52,124,139–142] (see Fig. 4–37, p. 72).

Mechanisms of Diastolic Filling. To understand the significance of the patterns of left ventricular filling, it is important to consider the mechanisms of normal left ventricular filling.[142,143] The events surrounding normal left ventricular filling are shown in Figure 14–22. From the time of aortic valve closure until mitral valve opening, the left ventricle is normally a closed chamber with a constant volume. Myocardial relaxation begins in the latter part of systole and causes a steep, exponential fall in intraventricular pressure as elastic elements of the left ventricle that compressed and twisted during ejection are allowed to recoil. Although no filling occurs during isovolumetric relax-

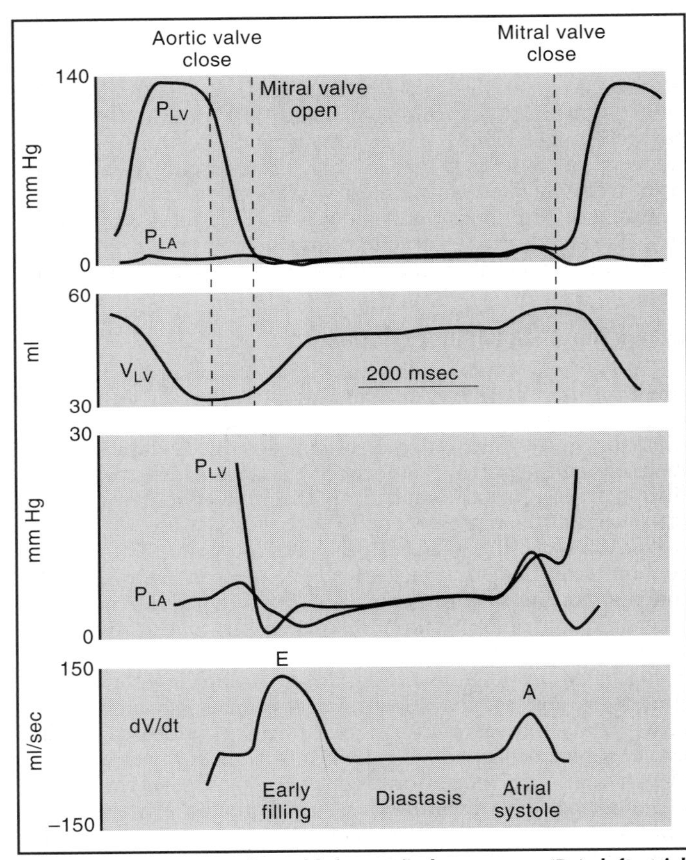

FIGURE 14–22. Recording of left ventricular pressure (P_{LV}), left atrial pressure (P_{LA}), left ventricular volume (V_{LV}), and the rate of change of left ventricular volume (dV/dt), which indicates the rate of left ventricular filling. Left ventricular filling occurs early in diastole and during atrial systole in response to pressure gradient from the left atrium to the left ventricle. The early diastolic pressure gradient is generated as left ventricular pressure falls below left atrial pressure and the late diastolic gradient is generated as atrial contraction increases left atrial pressure above left ventricular pressure. (Data from Cheng, C. P., Freeman, G. L., Santamore, W. P., et al.: Effect of loading conditions, contractile state and heart rate on early diastolic left ventricular filling in conscious dogs. Circ. Res. *66*:814, 1990. Copyright 1990 American Heart Association.)

ation, the processes that determine the rate of decline of the isovolumetric pressure influence ventricular filling following opening of the mitral valve.[134,144] For the first 30 to 40 msec after mitral valve opening, decline of left ventricular wall tension is normally rapid enough to cause left ventricular pressure to fall, despite a substantial increase in left ventricular volume.[143] This fall in left ventricular pressure produces a pressure gradient that accelerates blood from the left atrium into the left ventricle, resulting in rapid early diastolic filling. The rate of early left ventricular filling is determined by the mitral valve pressure gradient (left atrial pressure–left ventricular pressure).[134,143,145] Although peak filling occurs after the peak pressure gradient, the two are closely related. Two major factors (myocardial relaxation and LA pressure) determine the early diastolic mitral valve pressure gradient and the rate of left ventricular filling. Under normal circumstances more than two-thirds of the stroke volume enters the left ventricle during early diastole.

After filling of the left ventricle begins, the mitral valve pressure gradient decreases and then transiently reverses. This occurs because left ventricular relaxation is nearing completion and the flow of blood from the left atrium fills the left ventricle, raising the left ventricular pressure while lowering the left atrial pressure. This reversed mitral valve pressure gradient decelerates and then stops the rapid flow of blood into the left ventricle early in diastole. The pressures in the left atrium and left ventricle equilibrate as mitral flow nearly ceases; thus, little left ventricular filling occurs during the midportion of diastole, termed *diastasis.*

Atrial contraction increases atrial pressure late in diastole producing a left atrium–to–left ventricle pressure gradient that again propels blood into the left ventricle. Following atrial systole, as the LA relaxes, its pressure decreases below left ventricular pressure, causing the mitral valve to begin closing.[146] The onset of ventricular systole produces a rapid increase in left ventricular pressure that seals the mitral valve and ends diastole.

Normal Pattern of Left Ventricular Filling. The normal pattern of left ventricular filling is characterized by rapid filling early in diastole with some additional filling during atrial contraction. This normal filling pattern can be quantified by measuring the peak early diastolic filling rate or mitral flow velocity (E), the integral of the early diastole filling or flow velocity, and the peak filling rate or mitral flow velocity during atrial contraction (A).[52,134,139–142] The relative contribution of early and late (atrial) filling is commonly expressed as the E/A ratio. Normally the E/A ratio is greater than 1. The time required for deceleration of the early diastolic flow (t_{dec}) and the rate of this deceleration (E/t_{dec}) are two other important parameters of the filling pattern. A variety of other measures have also been proposed. Table 14–3 contains a list of the ranges of normal values for these measures of left ventricular filling. The wide range of normal values is probably caused by variations in the technique of performing the observations, which are both operator and equipment sensitive. Furthermore, the measures can be altered by many physiological factors.

Abnormal Patterns of Left Ventricular Filling. The normal pattern of left ventricular filling is altered in many patients with cardiac disease.[52,124,139–141,147–149] By means of Doppler mitral flow velocity, three abnormal patterns (in the absence of mitral stenosis) have been identified indicating progressively greater impairment of diastolic function (Fig. 14–23).

The first abnormal pattern of filling has been termed *delayed relaxation.*[140,150] In this pattern there is reduced peak rate and amount of early left ventricular filling, and the relative importance of atrial filling is enhanced. This results in a reversed E/A ratio of less than 1 (i.e., E < A). The reduced peak rate of early filling is due to a decreased early diastolic left atrial–to–left ventricular pressure gradient, resulting from a slowed rate of left ventricular relaxation[151] (Fig. 14–24). A delayed relaxation pattern can be seen in patients with left ventricular hypertrophy, arterial hypertension, and coronary artery disease and in normal elderly subjects. In many of these patients, mean left atrial pressure is within the normal range at rest and the patients are asymptomatic.[52] In this situation the vigorous atrial contraction compensates for the reduced early filling due to impaired left ventricular relaxation while maintaining a normal mean left atrial pressure.

TABLE 14–3 PARAMETERS OF LEFT VENTRICULAR DIASTOLIC FILLING MEASURED BY DOPPLER ECHOCARDIOGRAPHY

Peak E	79 ± 26 cm/sec
Peak A	48 ± 22 cm/sec
E/A	1.7 ± 0.6
E Deceleration time	184 ± 24 msec
E Deceleration rate	5.6 ± 2.7 m/sec²
Isovolumetric relaxation time	74 ± 26 msec
Peak pulmonary venous AR wave	19 ± 4 cm/sec

Adapted from Little, W. C., and Downes, T. R.: Clinical evaluation of left ventricular diastolic performance. Prog. Cardiovasc. Dis. *32*(4):273, 1990.

A second pattern of abnormal filling has been termed *pseudonormalized.*[140] This pattern, in which the E/A ratio is greater than 1 (as occurs in normal persons), is seen in patients with more severe impairment of diastolic performance than the pattern of delayed relaxation. The pseudonormalized pattern is due to restoration of the normal early diastolic left ventricular pressure gradient due to an increase in left atrial pressure that compensates for the slowed rate of left ventricular relaxation[151] (Fig. 14–24). The pseudonormalized pattern of filling is distinguished from normal by a more rapid rate of early diastolic flow deceleration and faster deceleration time (<150 msec). The deceleration time is proportional to the inverse of the square root of the left ventricular chamber stiffness.[151,152] Thus, the faster deceleration time indicates increased left ventricular diastolic chamber stiffness.

A third abnormal pattern of left ventricular filling indicating a severe diastolic abnormality has been termed the *restrictive pattern.*[140,150] In this pattern the early filling is increased above the control level and greatly exceeds the filling that occurs during atrial contraction, and the E/A ratio is usually greater than 2. In fact, there may be little or

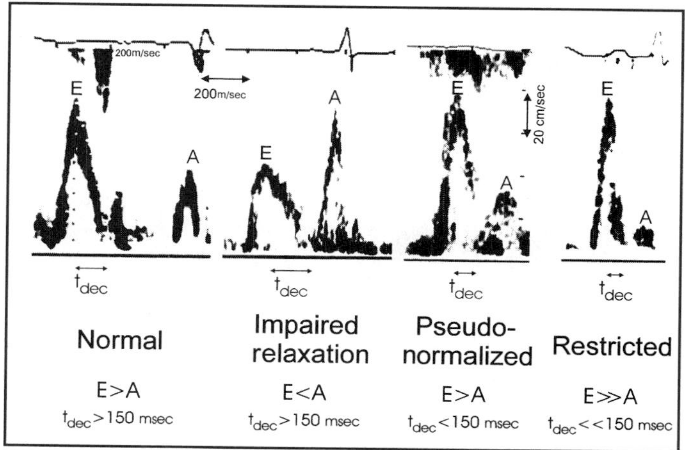

FIGURE 14–23. Patterns of left ventricular filling as recorded by diastolic Doppler mitral flow velocities. In the normal pattern there is a large E wave and a small A wave. There are three abnormal patterns of mitral filling representing progressively worsening left ventricular diastolic performance. With "delayed relaxation" the E wave is less than the A wave. The left ventricular deceleration (t_{dec}) is normal or prolonged. In the "pseudonormalized" pattern the E wave is larger than the A wave; however, t_{dec} is shortened. In the restricted filling pattern E is much larger than A with a very short t_{dec}.

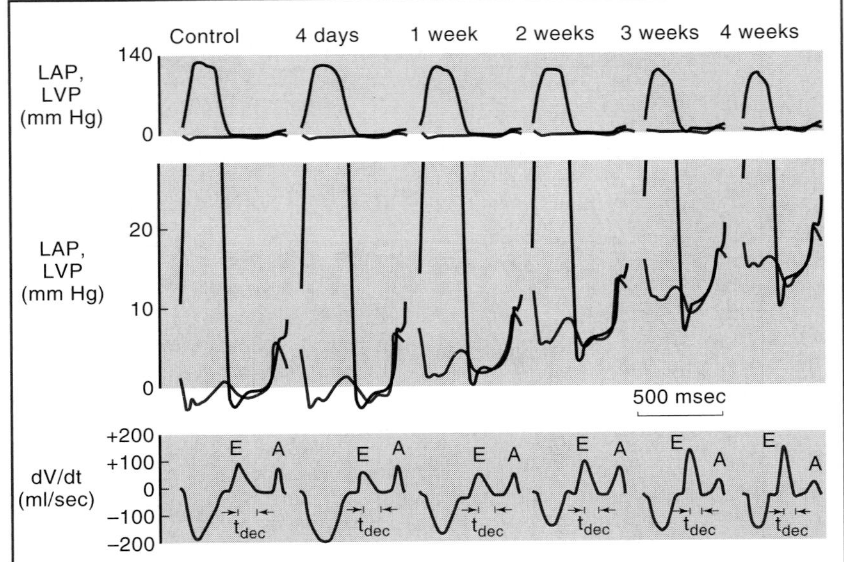

FIGURE 14–24. Recordings of left ventricular (LVP) and left atrial pressures (LAP) and the rate of change of left ventricular volume (dV/dt) during control and serially during the development of pacing-induced heart failure in an experimental animal. During control there is a normal filling pattern with E (early diastolic filling) larger than A (diastolic filling during atrial systole). At 4 days a pattern of "delayed relaxation" has developed with a small E and large A. This occurs in response to a slowing of the rate of left ventricular relaxation and a smaller pressure gradient from the left atrium to the left ventricle early in diastole. As heart failure subsequently worsened, left atrial pressure increased. This ultimately resulted in a pattern of "pseudonormalization" at 2 to 3 weeks and a pattern of "restricted filling" at 4 weeks. The increased early filling (E) occurring during these patterns was associated with increases in the early diastolic left atrial to left ventricular pressure gradient produced by the marked increase in left atrial pressure. (From Ohno, M., Cheng, C. P., and Little, W. C.: Mechanism of altered patterns of left ventricular filling during the development of congestive heart failure. Circulation *89*:2241, 1994. Copyright 1994 American Heart Association.)

no filling during atrial contraction. The deceleration time is much less than 150 msec. This pattern is seen in patients with severe diastolic dysfunction and pulmonary congestion. The enhanced early filling in the restrictive pattern results from markedly elevated LA pressure that more than offsets the slowing of left ventricular relaxation.[151] In this situation, in which left ventricular stiffness is increased, the early flow deceleration time is very short, and the deceleration rate of early flow is rapid. The restrictive filling pattern is seen in patients with severe pulmonary congestion,[153] constrictive pericarditis,[154] and restrictive cardiomyopathies such as cardiac amyloidosis.[155]

The three abnormal patterns of left ventricular filling represent a continuum of increasing severity of diastolic abnormalities. The pattern of delayed relaxation may be observed in asymptomatic patients with only impaired diastolic reserve, while the pseudonormalized and restrictive patterns occur in patients with progressively more severe diastolic dysfunction who almost always have pulmonary congestion.

Pulmonary Venous Flow Patterns. The pattern of blood flow in the pulmonary veins provides additional information on diastolic filling.[124,150,156,157] The velocity of pulmonary venous flow can be measured by transthoracic Doppler in some patients and by transesophageal Doppler in most patients. The pulmonary venous flow velocity has three waves (Fig. 14–25): (1) the S wave, indicating antegrade flow into the left atrium during ventricular systole, (2) the D wave, indicating antegrade flow early in diastole just following the peak of the E wave mitral valve flow, and (3) the AR wave of retrograde flow out of the left atrium during atrial systole. The S and D waves correspond to the *x* and *y* descents in the left atrial pressure, while the pulmonary venous AR wave corresponds to the left atrial *a* wave. When left ventricular end-diastolic stiffness is increased, the AR wave is augmented and prolonged, unless atrial systolic failure or atrial fibrillation is present. Thus, pseudonormalized and restricted mitral flow patterns are associated with large, prolonged AR waves with a peak flow velocity >35 cm/sec.[150]

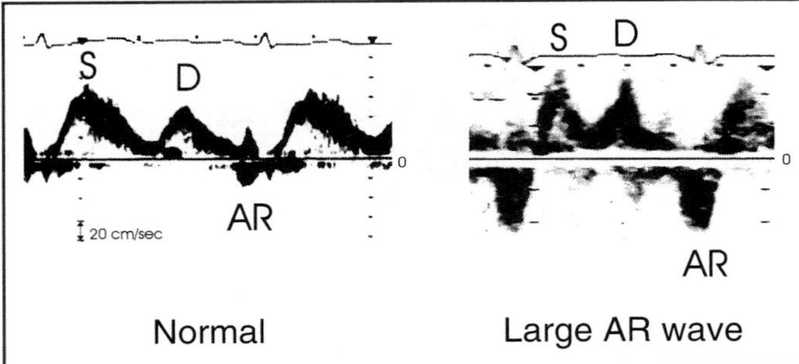

FIGURE 14–25. On the left is a normal pulmonary venous flow pattern recorded using transesophageal echocardiography. The S and D waves indicating flow into the left atrium are shown. There is a small atrial AR wave of retrograde flow out of the left atrium during atrial systole. On the right is an abnormal pulmonary venous flow pattern recorded in a patient with severe left ventricular hypertrophy. There is a large, prolonged AR wave with a peak velocity of more than 40 cm/sec. (Recordings courtesy of Dr. Abdel-Mohsen Nomeir of Bowman Gray School of Medicine of Wake Forest University.)

Assessment of Right Ventricular Performance

Although most attention in adult cardiology is appropriately focused on the performance of the left ventricle, the right ventricle may be an important contributor to cardiac dysfunction.[158] The concepts of preload, afterload, and contractility and most of the methods of evaluating left ventricular performance are also applicable to the right ventricle. The ejection of the thin-walled right ventricle is more sensitive to increases in afterload than is the left ventricle. Right ventricular dilatation in response to increased afterload is limited by the tethering of the right ventricle to the much thicker left ventricle and the limitations imposed by the pericardium. With increased afterload the thin-walled right ventricle dilates, causing functional tricuspid regurgitation.[159] Right ventricular performance can be importantly influenced by the presence and severity of such regurgitation.

Right ventricular volume and ejection fraction can be measured using echocardiography, radionuclear techniques, and angiography. In addition, right ventricular stroke volume and ejection fraction can be monitored on-line using the thermodilution technique[160–162] (p. 191). This is performed by injecting a bolus of cold saline solution into the right atrium, while the temperature in the pulmonary artery is recorded using a rapidly responding thermistor mounted on a catheter. This technique, which allows serial measurements, is convenient, reproducible, and reasonably accurate.

The right ventricular end-systolic pressure-volume relation can be determined with a manometer-tipped catheter in the right ventricle and either an impedance catheter or a radionuclide ventriculogram to provide simultaneous measurements of right ventricular volume while varying right ventricular load.[163,164] The right ventricular ESPVR behaves in a similar manner as the left ventricular ESPVR discussed above. The right ventricular ESPVR is linear in the physiological range and is shifted upward and leftward by the positive inotropic agent dobutamine.

INTEGRATED CARDIOVASCULAR PERFORMANCE

Cardiac Output (see p. 191)

The integrated pumping function of the cardiovascular system results ultimately in the cardiac output. The cardiac output can be measured using indicator dilution techniques, as described above. An alternate method to measure cardiac output is to use the Fick principle. Oxygen consumption is measured, or much less accurately assumed from the patient's height, weight, and age using a standard nomogram. The oxygen difference from the pulmonary artery to arterial circulation (A $-$ $\dot{V}_{O_2}$ difference) is measured. Then the cardiac output is calculated as:

$$\text{Cardiac Output} = \frac{O_2 \text{ Consumption}}{A - \dot{V}_{O_2} \text{ Difference}}$$

The cardiac output is usually corrected for body size and expressed as the cardiac index, i.e., the cardiac output per square meter of body surface area. The normal range for the cardiac index, in the basal (resting) state in the supine position is wide, between 2.5 and 4.2 liters/min/m^2. The wide normal range makes it possible for cardiac output to decline by almost 40 per cent and still remain within the normal limits. Thus, a cardiac index of less than 2.5 liters/min/m^2 usually represents a marked disturbance of cardiovascular performance and is almost always clinically apparent. Although the resting cardiac output (or index) is insensitive in detecting mild to moderate cardiac impairment, it provides a valuable measure of the integrated function of the cardiovascular system, especially in critically ill patients.

Arteriovenous Oxygen Difference

The most crucial function of the cardiovascular system is to supply the tissues with oxygen. This requires the integrated action of the heart, circulation, lungs, and the peripheral metabolism[165] (Fig. 14–26). As defined by the Fick principle, the oxygen delivered to the body is the product of the cardiac output and the difference in oxygen content of the arterial blood and the mixed venous blood (A $-$ $\dot{V}_{O_2}$ difference). Under normal circumstances at rest, adequate oxygen supply to the tissues is produced with a A $-$ $\dot{V}_{O_2}$ difference of 40 ± 10 ml O_2/liter. With nearly fully oxygenated arterial blood (>98 per cent saturation) and normal

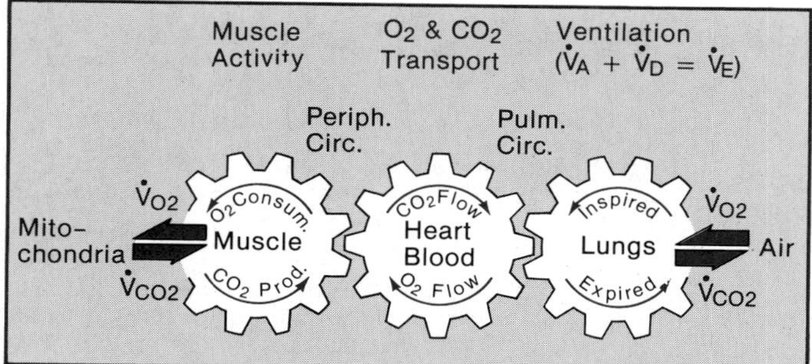

FIGURE 14–26. Interaction of physiological mechanisms coupling external to cellular respiration. Central role of circulation explains why cardiovascular diseases cause abnormalities in O_2 transport and O_2 uptake kinetics. O_2 consumption (O_2 consum.); CO_2 production (CO_2 prod.); alveolar ventilation ($\dot{V}_A$); physiological dead space ventilation ($\dot{V}_D$); expired ventilation ($\dot{V}_E$); O_2 uptake ($\dot{V}_{O_2}$); CO_2 output ($\dot{V}_{CO_2}$). (From Wasserman, K.: Measures of functional capacity in patients with heart failure. Circulation *81*(Suppl. 2):1, 1990. Reproduced by permission of the American Heart Association, Inc.)

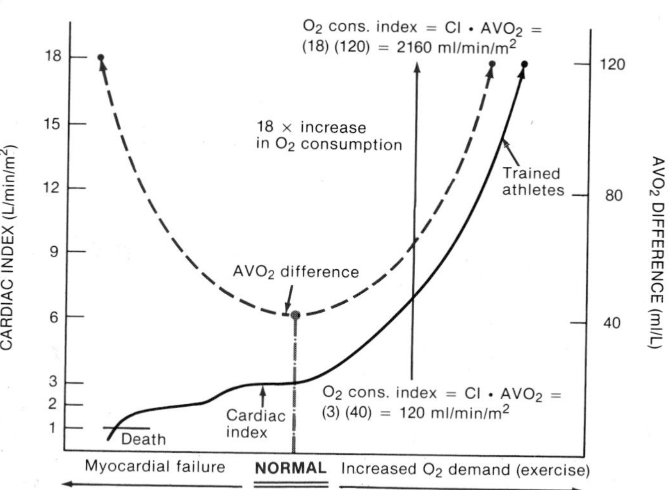

FIGURE 14–27. Relation between arteriovenous oxygen (AVO_2) difference *(broken line)* and cardiac index *(solid curve)* in normal subjects at rest *(center)* and during exercise *(right)*, and in the patient with progressively worsening myocardial failure *(left)*. (From Grossman, W.: Blood flow measurement: The cardiac output. *In* Grossman, W., and Baim, D. S.: Cardiac Catheterization, Angiography and Intervention. 4th ed. Philadelphia, Lea and Febiger, 1991, p. 106. Reproduced by permission.)

hemoglobin concentration and O_2-carrying capacity, the normal A $-$ $\dot{V}_{O_2}$ difference is achieved with a mixed venous O_2 saturation of >70 per cent. If the cardiac output is inadequate the tissues extract more O_2, and the A $-$ $\dot{V}_{O_2}$ difference increases. In this situation mixed venous O_2 saturation falls (Fig. 14–27). Thus, a normal mixed venous oxygen saturation (>70 per cent) indicates that the cardiac output is adequate to meet the body's demands.[166,167]

Reduced mixed venous O_2 saturation may result from an abnormality of cardiovascular function that is limiting the cardiac output, a deficiency in the O_2-carrying capacity of the blood, or pulmonary disease. When the ability to widen the A $-$ $\dot{V}_{O_2}$ difference and increase oxygen extraction is exhausted, anaerobic metabolism produces lactate, and venous lactate levels rise precipitously.[168]

It should be noted that the myocardium extracts oxygen nearly maximally from blood at rest. Thus, the coronary sinus oxygen saturation is low (<40 per cent), and the myocardium cannot use an increase in oxygen extraction as a compensatory mechanism for inadequate coronary flow.

During exercise the body's oxygen consumption increases dramatically. This increased need is met by a combination of an increase in cardiac output and widening of the A $-$ $\dot{V}_{O_2}$ difference.[169] For example, during very strenuous exercise, the oxygen consumption increases up to 18-fold. This is accomplished by a 6-fold increase in cardiac output (from 3 to 18 liters/min/m^2) and a 3-fold increase in the A $-$ $\dot{V}_{O_2}$ difference (from 40 to 120 ml/liter), with the mixed venous O_2 saturation decreasing from 75 to 25 per cent.

Cardiopulmonary Exercise Testing

(See also p. 153)

The integrated performance of the cardiovascular and pulmonary systems is evaluated by cardiopulmonary exercise testing.

A systematic approach to cardiopulmonary exercise testing requires the noninvasive assessment of total oxygen uptake ($\dot{V}_{O_2}$) and carbon dioxide production ($\dot{V}_{CO_2}$), while progressively increasing isotonic exercise is carried out on a treadmill or bicycle ergometer.[170–175] End-tidal O_2 and CO_2 concentrations and ventilation are measured continuously, allowing the monitoring of $\dot{V}_{O_2}$ and $\dot{V}_{CO_2}$ on a breath-by-breath basis. This permits determination of (1) the maximal oxygen uptake ($\dot{V}_{O_{2max}}$, or aerobic capacity),

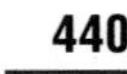

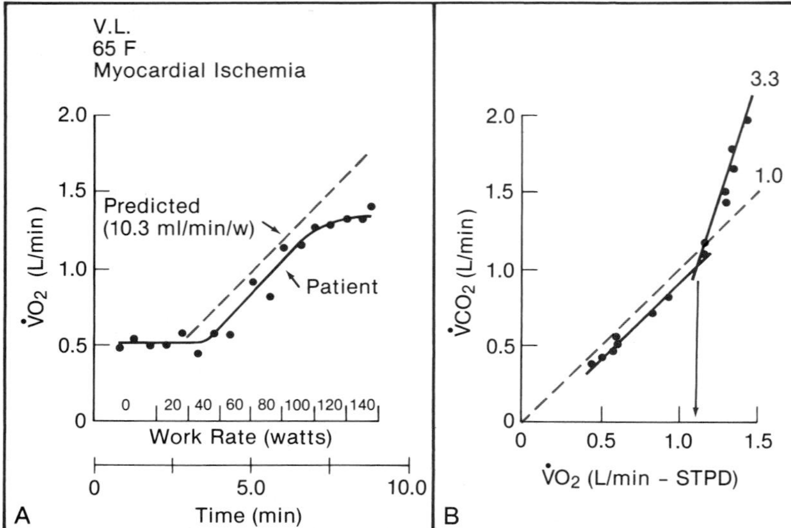

FIGURE 14–28. O_2 uptake ($\dot{V}_{O_2}$) plotted as the function of work rate *(panel A)* and CO_2 output ($\dot{V}_{CO_2}$) as function of $\dot{V}_{O_2}$ (V-slope plot) *(panel B)* of 64-year-old patient with shortness of breath at high altitude and ST-segment changes consistent with myocardial ischemia at 120 W cycle ergometer exercise, but without pain. Because of flattened $\dot{V}_{O_2}$ response *(panel A)* but continued steep rise in $\dot{V}_{O_2}$ above anaerobic threshold, the upper-component slope of $\dot{V}_{CO_2}$-$\dot{V}_{O_2}$ plot *(panel B)* is pathologically steep. Steep upper-component slope with a value of 3.3 suggests an exceptionally high rate of lactate release during exercise. Slope of 1 is drawn in *panel B* to provide visualization of steepening in the $\dot{V}_{CO_2}$-$\dot{V}_{O_2}$ plot reflecting the start of HCO_3 buffering of lactic acid. (From Wasserman, K., Beaver, W. L., and Whipp, B. J.: Gas exchange theory and the lactic acidosis (anaerobic) threshold. Circulation *81*(Suppl. 2):14, 1990. Copyright 1990 American Heart Association.)

defined as the value achieved when $\dot{V}_{O_2}$ remains stable despite an increase in the intensity of exercise (Figs. 14–28 and 5–1, p. 154), and (2) the anaerobic threshold. The latter is reached during the course of progressive exercise when the O_2 available to the tissues becomes inadequate. At this point, energy is generated inefficiently by anaerobic metabolism, a process producing lactate, which is buffered by bicarbonate, leading to increased production of CO_2. This can be recognized by a rise in $\dot{V}_{CO_2}$ that exceeds the rise in $\dot{V}_{O_2}$ producing a rise in the respiratory quotient (R), i.e., the ratio $\dot{V}_{CO_2}/\dot{V}_{O_2}$ (Fig. 14–28).

The anaerobic threshold indicates the maximum level of physical activity and O_2 uptake at which the cardiopulmonary system is able to provide sufficient O_2 to maintain aerobic metabolism in skeletal muscle. These two endpoints—the $\dot{V}_{O_2max}$ and the anaerobic threshold—can be determined objectively and are not affected by the bias of patient or examiner, which may limit the value of exercise tests. Although exercise capacity correlates with maximal $\dot{V}_{O_2}$, these correlations are not good enough to allow the former to serve as a substitute for the latter. The reproducibility of $\dot{V}_{O_2max}$ and the anaerobic threshold, when measured days or weeks apart in subjects whose condition has not changed, is excellent.[171,176] Normal values of $\dot{V}_{O_2max}$ and of the anaerobic threshold decline with age after 20 years and are higher in men than in women. Functional capacity has been conveniently categorized into five classes by Weber and his associates (A to E)[171]; impairment in group E is so severe that the patients cannot (or should not) exercise (Table 14–4).

The $\dot{V}_{O_2max}$ is a function of both the maximal cardiac output and the maximal extracton of O_2 by the tissues (maximal A − $\dot{V}$[O_2]). The latter does not vary systematically in patients of various classes and usually exceeds 70 per cent at $\dot{V}_{O_2max}$. Therefore, $\dot{V}_{O_2max}$ reflects the maximum cardiac output, which is a far more sensitive measurement than is the resting cardiac output in discriminating among patients in different degrees of cardiac disability.

Cardiopulmonary exercise testing is of clinical value in objectively assessing exercise tolerance and functional capacity, in evaluating the possible causes of exertional dyspnea and fatigue, in determining the severity of disability, in following its progress, and in assessing the response to therapy.[172,177] Impairment of pulmonary and/or musculoskeletal function can interfere with oxygen uptake during exertion. Therefore, in a patient with a reduced $\dot{V}_{O_2max}$ and clinical manifestations of lung disease, pulmonary function should be evaluated.[178]

When $\dot{V}_{O_2max}$ is reduced and arterial O_2 saturation declines during exercise, it is probably due to pulmonary dysfunction. Conversely, cardiac dysfunction can be recog-

TABLE 14–4 FUNCTIONAL IMPAIRMENT IN AEROBIC CAPACITY AND ANAEROBIC THRESHOLD AS MEASURED DURING INCREMENTAL EXERCISE TESTING

CLASS	DEGREE OF IMPAIRMENT	$\dot{V}O_2$ MAX (ml/min/kg)	ANAEROBIC THRESHOLD (ml/min/kg)
A	Mild to none	>20	>14
B	Mild to moderate	16 to 20	11 to 14
C	Moderate to severe	10 to 16	8 to 11
D	Severe	6 to 10	5 to 8
E	Very severe	<6	≤ 4

From Weber, K. T., Janicki, J. S., and McElroy, P. A.: Cardiopulmonary exercise (CPX) testing. *In* Weber, K. T., and Janicki, J. S. (eds.): Cardiopulmonary Exercise Testing. Philadelphia, W. B. Saunders Co., 1986, p. 153.

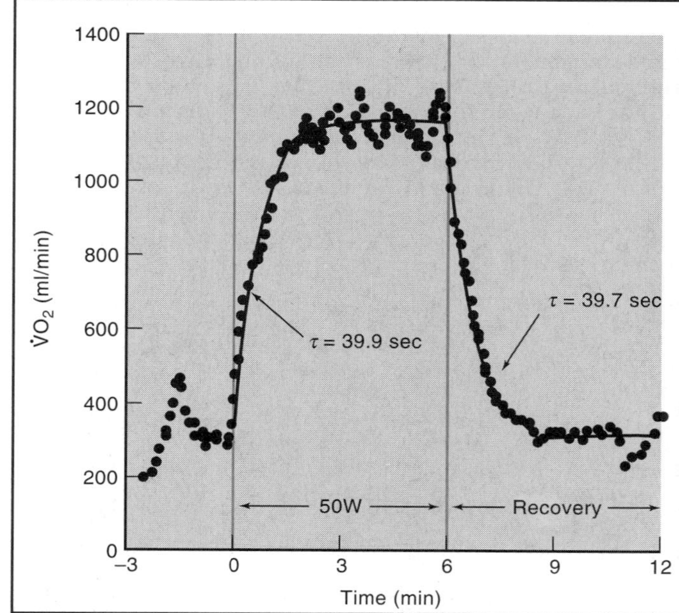

FIGURE 14–29. Plot of changes in oxygen uptake ($\dot{V}_{O_2}$) during 50 watts of constant work rate exercise and during recovery, along with the computer-derived line of the best fit to a single exponential model of the $\dot{V}_{O_2}$ response, for a representative normal subject. τ—time constant of upslope and downslope of $\dot{V}_{O_2}$. (From Koike, A., Yajima, T., Adachi, H., et al.: Evaluation of exercise capacity using submaximal exercise at a constant work rate in patients with cardiovascular disease. Circulation *91*:1719, 1995. Copyright 1995 American Heart Association.)

nized as the cause of reduced $\dot{V}_{O_{2max}}$ by measuring pulmonary capillary wedge pressure together with arterial pressure, cardiac output, and gas exchange at each stage of exercise. A triple-lumen balloon flotation thermodilution catheter can be used conveniently to make these measurements. As pump function deteriorates, wedge pressure rises and cardiac output declines at peak exercise.

A limitation of cardiopulmonary exercise testing is that many patients with heart disease, particularly ischemic heart disease, often do not attain a level of exercise in which $\dot{V}_{O_2}$ remains stable despite further increase in the intensity of exercise. The peak $\dot{V}_{O_2}$ they achieve is not the same as $\dot{V}_{O_2max}$, which by definition fails to rise despite a further increase in the intensity of exercise. Unlike $\dot{V}_{O_2max}$, peak $\dot{V}_{O_2}$ partially depends on the motivations of the patient and is subject to examiner bias.[179] On the other hand, the anaerobic threshold, which requires a lower level of activity than the $\dot{V}_{O_2max}$, can be more readily determined in patients with cardiac dysfunction and is quite reproducible.[176,180] Alterations in the anaerobic threshold reflect changes in the underlying condition.

The response of $\dot{V}_{O_2}$ to the onset and recovery from constant steady-state exercise is an alternate method of assessing exercise capacity (Fig. 14–29).[181] The time constant of the increase in $\dot{V}_{O_2}$ at the start of exercise is similar to the time constant of the fall in $\dot{V}_{O_2}$ after exercise (normal = 49 ± 10 sec). In patients with cardiovascular disease, this time constant is lengthened and inversely correlates with peak $\dot{V}_{O_2}$ and maximum work. The measurement of the time constant does not require the subject's maximum effort and may provide a useful measure of exercise capacity in patients with mild to moderate cardiovascular impairment.

REFERENCES

1. Braunwald, E.: On the difference between the heart's output and its contractile state (Editorial). Circulation *43*:171, 1971.
2. Ter Keurs, H. E., Buex, J. J., de Tombe, P. P., et al.: The effect of sarcomere length and Ca^{++} on force and velocity of shortening in cardiac muscle. Adv. Exp. Med. Biol. *226*:581, 1988.
3. de Tombe, P. P., and Little, W. C.: Inotropic effects of ejection are myocardial properties. Am. J. Physiol. *266*:H1202, 1994.
4. Suga, H., Kitabatake, A., and Sagawa, K.: End-systolic pressure determines stroke volume from fixed end-diastolic volume in the isolated canine left ventricle under a constant contractile state. Circ. Res. *44*:238, 1979.
5. Sagawa, K., Maughan, L., Suga, H., and Sunagawa, K.: Cardiac Contraction and the Pressure-Volume Relationship. New York, Oxford University Press, Inc. 1988.

MEASUREMENT OF KEY VARIABLES

6. Hipkins, S. F., Rutten, A. J., and Runciman, W. B.: Experimental analysis of catheter-manometer systems: In vitro and In vivo. Anesthesiology *71*:893, 1989.
7. Grossman, W.: Pressure measurement. *In* Grossman, W., and Baim, D. S. (eds.): Cardiac Catheterization, Angiography, and Intervention. Philadelphia, Lea and Febiger, 1991, p. 123.

7a. Courtois, M., Fattal, P. G., Kovacs, S. J., Jr., et al.: Anatomically and physiologically based reference level for measurement of intracardiac pressures. Circulation *92*:1994, 1995.

8. Sharir, T., Marmor, A., Ting, C. T., et al.: Validation of a method for noninvasive measurement of central arterial pressure. Hypertension *21*:74, 1993.
9. Bargiggia, G. S., Bertucci, C., Recusani, F., et al.: A new method for estimating left ventricular dP/dt by continuous wave Doppler echocardiography: Validation studies at cardiac catheterization. Circulation *80*:1287, 1989.
10. Nishimura, R. A., Schwartz, R. S., Tajik, A. J., and Holmes, D. R., Jr.: Noninvasive measurement of rate of left ventricular relaxation by Doppler echocardiography: Validation with simultaneous cardiac catheterization. Circulation *88*:146, 1993.
11. Yamamoto, K., Masuyama, T., Doi, Y., et al.: Noninvasive assessment of left ventricular relaxation using continuous-wave Doppler aortic regurgitant velocity curve: Its comparative value to the mitral regurgitation method. Circulation *91*:192, 1995.
12. Lange, R. A., Moore, D. M., Jr., Cigarroa, R. G., and Hillis, L. D.: Use of pulmonary capillary wedge pressure to assess severity of mitral stenosis: Is true left atrial pressure needed in this condition? J. Am. Coll. Cardiol. *13*:825, 1989.
13. Grossman, W.: Cardiac catheterization by direct exposure of artery and vein. *In* Grossman, W., and Baim, D. S. (eds.): Cardiac Catheterization, Angiography and Intervention. Philadelphia, Lea and Febiger, 1991, p. 47.
14. Schoenfeld, M. H., Palacios, I. F., Hutter, A. M., Jr., et al.: Underestimation of prosthetic mitral valve areas: Role of transseptal catheterization in avoiding unnecessary repeat mitral valve surgery. J. Am. Coll. Cardiol. *5*:1387, 1985.
15. Tobis, J., Nalcioglu, O., Seibert, A., et al.: Measurement of left ventricular ejection fraction by videodensitometric analysis of digital subtraction angiograms. Am. J. Cardiol. *52*:871, 1983.
16. Kronenberg, M. W., Price, R. R., Smith, C. W., et al.: Evaluation of left ventricular performance using digital subtraction angiography. Am. J. Cardiol. *51*:837, 1983.
17. Vine, D. L., Hegg, T. D., Dodge, H. T., et al.: Immediate effect of contrast medium injection of left ventricular volumes and ejection fraction. Circulation *56*:379, 1977.
18. Brogan, W. C., III, Hillis, L. D., and Lange, R. A.: Contrast agents for cardiac catheterization: Conceptions and misconceptions. Am. Heart J. *122*:1129, 1991.
19. Rackley, C. E., and Hood, W. P., Jr.: Quantitative angiographic evaluation and pathophysiological mechanisms in valvular heart disease. Prog. Cardiovasc. Dis. *15*:427, 1973.
20. Dodge, H. T., and Sheehan, F. H.: Quantitative contrast angiography for assessment of ventricular performance in heart disease. J. Am. Coll. Cardiol. *1*:73, 1983.
21. Baan, J., Van der Velde, E. T., Van Dijk, A. D., et al.: Ventricular volume measured from intracardiac dimensions with impedance catheter: Theoretical and experimental aspects. Cardiovascular System Dynamics: Models and Measurements. New York, Plenum Press, 1992, p. 569.
22. Burkhoff, D., Van der Velde, E., Kass, D., et al.: Accuracy of volume measurement by conductance catheter in isolated, ejecting canine hearts. Circulation *72*:440, 1984.
23. Kass, D. A., Yamazaki, T., Burkhoff, D., et al.: Determination of left ventricular end-systolic pressure-volume relationships by the conductance (volume) catheter technique. Circulation *73*:586, 1986.
24. Kass, D. A., Midei, M., Graves, W., et al.: Use of a conductance (volume) catheter and transient inferior vena caval occlusion for rapid determination of pressure-volume relationships in man. Cathet. Cardiovasc. Diagn. *15*:192, 1988.
25. Ferguson, J. J., Miller, M. J., Sahagian, P., et al.: Effects of respiration and vasodilation on venous volume in animals and man, as measured with an impedance catheter. Cathet. Cardiovasc. Diagn. *16*:25, 1989.
26. Boltwood, C., Jr., Appleyard, R., and Glantz, S.: Parallel conductance of LV depends on end-systolic volume. Circulation *80*:1360, 1989.
27. Applegate, R. J., Cheng, C. P., and Little, W. C.: Simultaneous conductance catheter and dimension assessment of left ventricle volume in the intact animal. Circulation *81*:638, 1990.
28. Glantz, S. A., Boltwood, C. M., Jr., Appleyard, R. F., et al.: Volume conductance catheter. Circulation *81*:703, 1990.
29. Steendijk, P., Van der Velde, E. T., and Baan, J.: Left ventricular stroke volume by single and dual excitation of conductance catheter in dogs. Am. J. Physiol. *264*:2198, 1993.
30. Herman, H. J., and Bartle, S. H.: Left ventricular volumes by angiocardiography: Comparison of methods and simplification of techniques. Cardiovasc. Res. *2*:404, 1968.
31. Rackley, C. E.: Quantitative evaluation of left ventricular function by radiographic techniques. Circulation *54*:862, 1976.
32. Wynne, J., Green, L. H., Mann, T., et al.: Estimation of left ventricular volumes in man from biplane cineangiograms filmed in oblique projections. Am. J. Cardiol. *41*:726, 1978.
33. Fifer, M. A., and Grossman, W.: Measurement of ventricular volumes, ejection fraction, mass and wall stress. *In* Grossman, E., and Baim, D. S. (eds.): Cardiac Catheterization, Angiography and Intervention. Philadelphia, Lea and Febiger, 1991, p. 300.
34. Dodge, H. T.: Hemodynamic aspects of cardiac failure. *In* Braunwald, E. (ed.): The Myocardium: Failure and Infarction. New York, HP Publishing Co., 1974, p. 70.
35. Schiller, N. B., Shah, P. M., Crawford, M., et al.: Recommendations for quantitation of the left ventricle by two-dimensional echocardiography. J. Am. Soc. Echocardiogr. *2*:358, 1989.
36. Collins, H. W., Kronenberg, M. W., and Byrd, B. F., III: Reproducibility of left ventricular mass measurements by two-dimensional and m-mode echocardiography. J. Am. Coll. Cardiol. *14*:672, 1989.
37. Reichek, N., Helak, J., Plappert, T., et al.: Validation of left ventricular mass estimates from clinical two-dimensional echocardiography: Initial results. Circulation *67*:348, 1983.
38. Bikkina, M., Levy, D., Evans, J. C., et al.: Left ventricular mass and risk of stroke in an elderly cohort: The Framingham Heart Study. JAMA *272*:33, 1994.
39. Krumholz, H. M., Larson, M., and Levy, D.: Prognosis of left ventricular geometric patterns in the Framingham Heart Study. J. Am. Coll. Cardiol. *25*:879, 1995.
40. Devereux, R. B.: Left ventricular geometry, pathophysiology and prognosis. J. Am. Coll. Cardiol. *25*:885, 1995.
41. Regen, D. M., Anversa, P., and Capasso, J. M.: Segmental calculation of left ventricular wall stresses. Am. J. Physiol. *264*:H1411, 1993.
42. Regen, D. M.: Calculation of left ventricular wall stress. Circ. Res. *67*:245, 1990.
43. Grossman, W., Jones, D., and McLaurin, L. P.: Wall stress and patterns of hypertrophy in the human left ventricle. J. Clin. Invest. *56*:56, 1974.
44. Peterson, K. L.: Instantaneous force-velocity-length relations of the left

ventricle: Methods, limitations and applications in humans. *In* Fishman, A. P. (ed.): Heart Failure. Washington, D.C., Hemisphere Publishing Co., 1978, p. 121.
45. Pomerantsev, E. V., Stertzer, S. H., and Shaw, R. E.: Quantitative left ventriculography: Methods of assessment of the regional contractility. J. Invas. Cardiol. *7:*11, 1995.
46. Dodge, H. T., Stewart, D. K., and Frimer, M.: Implications of shape, stress and wall dynamics in clinical heart disease. *In* Fishman, A. P. (ed.): Heart Failure. Washington, D. C., Hemisphere Publishing Co., 1978, p. 43.
47. Sheehan, F. H., Dodge, H. T., Mathey, D. G., et al.: IEEE Comput. Cardiol. 1982, p. 9.
48. Sheehan, F. H., Stewart, D. K., Dodge, H. T., et al.: Variability in the measurement of regional left ventricular wall motion from contrast angiograms. Circulation *68:*550, 1983.
49. Kass, D. A.: Measuring right ventricular volumes. Am. J. Physiol. *254:*H619, 1988.
50. Sandler, H., and Dodge, H. T.: Angiographic methods for determination of left ventricular geometry and volume. *In* Mirsky, I., Ghista, D. N., and Sandler, H. (eds.): Cardiac Mechanics: Physiological, Clinical and Mathematical Considerations. New York, John Wiley and Sons, 1974.
51. Hoit, B. D., Shao, Y., McMannis, K., et al.: Determination of left atrial volume using sonomicrometry: A cast validation study. Am. J. Physiol. *264:*H1011, 1993.

ASSESSMENT OF LEFT VENTRICULAR FUNCTION

52. Little, W. C., and Downes, T. R.: Clinical evaluation of left ventricular diastolic performance. Prog. Cardiovasc. Dis. *32:*273, 1990.
53. Applegate, R. J., and Little, W. C.: Systolic and diastolic left ventricular function. Prog. Cardiol. *4:*63, 1991.
54. Downes, T. R., Hackshaw, B. T., Kahl, F. R., et al.: Frequency of large "V" waves in the pulmonary artery wedge pressure in ventricular septal defect of acquired (during acute myocardial infarction) or congenital origin. Am. J. Cardiol. *60:*415, 1987.
55. Snyder, R. W., II, Glamann, D. B., Lange, R. A., et al.: Predictive value of prominent pulmonary arterial wedge V waves in assessing the presence and severity of mitral regurgitation. Am. J. Cardiol. *73:*568, 1994.
56. Glantz, S. A., and Parmley, W.: Factors which affect the diastolic pressure-volume curve. Circ. Res. *42:*171, 1978.
57. Glantz, S. A.: Computing indices of diastolic stiffness has been counterproductive. Fed. Proc. *39:*162, 1980.
58. Noordergraaf, A., and Melbin, J.: Ventricular afterload: A succinct yet comprehensive definition (Editorial). Am. Heart J. *95:*545, 1978.
59. Grossman, W.: Clinical measurement of vascular resistance and assessment of vasodilator drugs. *In* Grossman, W., and Baim, D. S. (eds.): Cardiac Catheterization, Angiography and Intervention. Philadelphia, Lea and Febiger, 1991, p. 143.
60. O'Rourke, M. F.: Steady and pulsatile energy losses in the systemic circulation under normal conditions and in simulated arterial disease. Cardiovasc. Res. *1:*313, 1967.
61. Nichols, W. W., Nicolini, F. A., and Pepine, C. J.: Determinants of isolated systolic hypertension in the elderly. J Hypertension *10:*S73, 1992.
62. Nichols, W. W., Conti, C. R., Walker, W. E., and Milnor, W. R.: Input impedance of the systemic circulation in man. Circ. Res. *40:*451, 1977.
63. Nichols, W. W., and O'Rourke, M. F.: McDonald's Blood Flow in Arteries. London, Arnold, 1990.
64. O'Rourke, M. F., and Brunner, H. R.: Introduction to arterial compliance and function. J. Hypertension *10:*S3, 1992.
65. Sunagawa, K., Maughan, W. L., and Sagawa, K.: Optimal arterial resistance for the maximal stroke work studied in isolated canine left ventricle. Circ. Res. *56:*586, 1985.
66. Little, W. C., and Cheng, C. P.: Left ventricular-arterial coupling in conscious dogs. Am. J. Physiol. *261:*H70, 1991.
67. Kelly, R. P., Ting, C. T., Yang, T. M., et al.: Effective arterial elastance as index of arterial vascular load in humans. Circulation *86:*513, 1991.
68. Carabello, B. A.: Clinical assessment of systolic dysfunction. ACC Curr. J. Rev. Jan/Feb:25, 1994.
69. Gleason, W. L., and Braunwald, E.: Studies on the first derivative of the ventricular pressure pulse in man. J. Clin. Invest. *41:*80, 1962.
70. Krayenbuehl, H. P., Rutishauser, W., Wirz, P., et al.: High-fidelity left ventricular pressure measurements for the assessment of cardiac contractility in man. Am. J. Cardiol. *31:*415, 1973.
71. Little, W. C.: The left ventricular dP/dt_{max}-end-diastolic volume relation in closed chest dogs. Circ. Res. *56:*808, 1985.
72. Burns, J. W., Covell, J. W., and Ross, J., Jr.: Mechanics of isotonic left ventricular contractions. Am. J. Physiol. *224:*725, 1973.
73. Fifer, M. A., Gunther, S., Grossman, W., et al.: Myocardial contractile function in aortic stenosis as determined from the rate of stress development during isovolumic stress. Am. J. Cardiol. *44:*1318, 1979.
74. Feldman, M. D., Alderman, J. D., Aroesty, J. M., et al.: Depression of systolic and diastolic myocardial reserve during atrial pacing tachycardia in patients with dilated cardiomyopathy. J. Clin. Invest. *82:*1661, 1988.
75. Mason, D. T., and Braunwald, E.: Studies on digitalis. IX: Effects of ouabain on the nonfailing human heart. J. Clin. Invest. *42:*1105, 1963.
76. Ross, J., Jr., and Sobel, B. E.: Regulation of cardiac contraction. Ann. Rev. Physiol. *34:*47, 1972.
77. Mason, D. T., Braunwald, E., Covell, J. W., et al.: Assessment of cardiac contractility: The relation between the rate of pressure rise and ventricular pressure during isovolumic systole. Circulation *44:*47, 1971.
78. Davidson, D. M., Covell, J. W., Malloch, C. I., and Rosse, J., Jr.: Factors influencing indices of left ventricular contractility in the conscious dog. Cardiovasc. Res. *8:*299, 1974.
79. Quinones, M. A., Gaasch, W. H., and Alexander, J. K.: Influence of acute changes in preload, afterload, contractile state and heart rate on ejection and isovolumic indices of myocardial contractility in man. Circulation *53:*293, 1976.
80. Kass, A., Maughan, W. L., Guo, A. M., et al.: Comparative influence of load versus inotropic states on indexes of ventricular contractility: Experimental and theoretical analysis based on pressure-volume relationships. Circulation *76:*1422, 1987.
81. Carabello, B. A., Mee, R., Collins, J. J., Jr., et al.: Contractile function in chronic gradually developing subcoronary aortic stenosis. Am. J. Physiol. *240:*H80, 1981.
82. Borow, K. M., Henderson, I. C., Neumann, A., et al.: Assessment of left ventricular contractility in patients receiving doxorubicin. Ann. Intern. Med. *99:*750, 1983.
83. Colan, S. D., Borow, K. M., and Neumann, A.: Left ventricular end-systolic wall stress-velocity of fiber shortening relation: A load independent index of myocardial contractility. J. Am. Coll. Cardiol. *4:*715, 1984.
84. Wisenbaugh, T., Booth, D., DeMaria, A., et al.: Relationship of contractile state to ejection performance in patients with chronic aortic valve disease. Circulation *73:*47, 1986.
85. Mirsky, I., Corin, W. J., Murakami, T., et al.: Correction for preload in assessment of myocardial contractility in aortic and mitral valve disease: Application of the concept of systolic myocardial stiffness. Circulation *78:*68, 1988.
86. Lang, R. M., Fellner, S. K., Neumann, A., et al.: Left ventricular contractility varies directly with blood ionized calcium. Ann. Intern. Med. *108:*524, 1988.
87. Borow, K. M., Neumann, A., Marcus, R. H., et al.: Effects of simultaneous alterations in preload and afterload on measurements of left ventricular contractility in patients with dilated cardiomyopathy: Comparisons of ejection phase, isovolumetric and end-systolic force-velocity indexes. J. Am. Coll. Cardiol. *20:*787, 1992.
88. Banerjee, A., Brook, M. M., Klautz, R. J. M., and Teitel, D. F.: Nonlinearity of the left ventricular end-systolic wall stress-velocity of fiber shortening relation in young pigs: A potential pitfall in its use as a single-beat index of contractility. J. Am. Coll. Cardiol. *23:*514, 1994.
89. Kass, D. A., and Maughan, W. L.: From "Emax" to pressure-volume relations: A broader view. Circulation *77:*1203, 1988.
90. Little, W. C., and Cheng, C. P.: Left ventricular systolic and diastolic performance. *In* Warltier, D. C. (ed.): Ventricular Function. Baltimore, Williams and Wilkins, 1995, p. 111.
91. Kass, D. A.: Clinical ventricular pathophysiology: A pressure-volume view. *In* Warltier, D.C. (ed.): Ventricular Function. Baltimore, Williams and Wilkins, 1995, p. 131.
92. Kass, D. A., Grayson, R., and Marino, P.: Pressure-volume analysis as a method for quantifying simultaneous drug (amrinone) effects on arterial load and contractile state in vivo. J. Am. Coll. Cardiol. *16:*726, 1990.
93. Starling, M. R.: Left ventricular-arterial coupling relations in the normal human heart. Am. Heart J. *125:*1659, 1993.
94. Starling, M. R., Kirsh, M. M., Montgomery, D. G., and Gross, M. D.: Impaired left ventricular contractile function in patients with long-term mitral regurgitation and normal ejection fraction. J. Am. Coll. Cardiol. *22:*239, 1993.
95. Little, W. C., Cheng, C. P., Peterson, T., and Vinten-Johansen, J.: Response of the left ventricular end-systolic pressure-volume relation in conscious dogs to a wide range of contractile states. Circulation *78:*736, 1988.
96. Kass, D. A., Beyar, R., Lankford, E., et al.: Influence of contractile state on curvilinearity of in situ end-systolic pressure-volume relations. Circulation *79:*167, 1989.
97. Little, W. C., and O'Rourke, R. A.: Effect of regional ischemia on the left ventricular end-systolic pressure-volume relationship in chronically instrumented dogs. J. Am. Coll. Cardiol. *5:*297, 1985.
98. Kass, D. A., Marino, P., Maughan, W. L., and Sagawa, K.: Determinants of end-systolic pressure-volume relations during acute regional ischemia in situ. Circulation *80:*1783, 1989.
99. Park, R. D., Little, W. C., and O'Rourke, R. A.: Effect of alteration of the left ventricular activation sequence on the left ventricular end-systolic pressure-volume relation in closed-chest dogs. Circ. Res. 57:706, 1986.
100. Little, W. C., Freeman, G. L., and O'Rourke, R. A.: Simultaneous determination of left ventricular end-systolic pressure-volume and pressure-dimension relationships in closed-chest dogs. Circulation *71:*1301, 1985.
101. Gorcsan, J., III, Romand, J. A., Mandarino, W. A., et al.: Assessment of left ventricular performance by on-line pressure-area relations using echocardiographic automated border detection. J. Am. Coll. Cardiol. 23:242, 1994.
102. Sodums, M. T., Badke, F. R., Starling, M. R., et al.: Evaluation of left ventricular contractile performance utilizing end-systolic pressure-volume relationships in conscious dogs. Circ. Res. *54:*731, 1984.
103. Freeman, G. L., Little, W. C., and O'Rourke, R. A.: Effect of vasoactive agents on the left ventricular end-systolic pressure-volume relation in closed-chest dogs. Circulation *74:*1107, 1986.
104. Brickner, M. E., and Starling, M. R.: Dissociation of end systole from end ejection in patients with long-term mitral regurgitation. Circulation *81:*1277, 1990.

105. Hsia, H. H., and Starling, M. R.: Is standardization of left ventricular chamber elastance necessary? Circulation *81:*1826, 1990.
106. Nakano, K., Sugawara, M., Ishihara, K., et al.: Myocardial stiffness derived from end-systolic wall stress and logarithm of reciprocal of wall thickness. Contractility index independent of ventricular size. Circulation *82:*1352, 1990.
107. Pirwitz, M. J., Lange, R. A., Willard, J. E., et al.: Use of the left ventricular peak systolic pressure/end-systolic volume ratio to predict symptomatic improvement with valve replacement in patients with aortic regurgitation and enlarged end-systolic volume. J. Am. Coll. Cardiol. *24:*1672, 1994.
108. Little, W. C., Cheng, C. P., Mumma, M., et al.: Comparison of measures of left ventricular contractile performance from pressure-volume loops in conscious dogs. Circulation *80:*1378, 1989.
109. Noda, T., Cheng, C. P., de Tombe, P. P., and Little, W. C.: Curvilinearity of the left ventricular end-systolic pressure-volume and dP/dt_{max}-end diastolic volume relations. Am. J. Physiol. *265:*H910, 1993.
110. Little, W. C., and Cheng, C. P.: Effect of exercise on left ventricular-arterial coupling assessed in the pressure-volume plane. Am. J. Physiol. *264:*H1629, 1993.
111. de Tombe, P. P., Jones, S., Burkhoff, D., et al.: Ventricular stroke work and efficiency both remain nearly optimal despite altered vascular loading. Am. J. Physiol. *264:*H1817, 1993.
112. Glower, D. D., Spratt, J. A., Snow, N. D., et al.: Linearity of the Frank-Starling relationship in the intact heart: The concept of preload recruitable stroke work. Circulation *71:*994, 1985.
113. Zile, M. R., Izzi, G., and Gaasch, W. H.: Left ventricular diastolic dysfunction limits use of maximum systolic elastance as an index of contractile function. Circulation *83:*674, 1991.
114. Kass, D. A., and Beyar, R.: Evaluation of contractile state by maximal ventricular power divided by the square of end-diastolic volume. Circulation *84:*1698, 1991.
115. Sharir, T., Feldman, M. D., Haber, H., et al.: Ventricular systolic assessment in patients with dilated cardiomyopathy by preload-adjusted maximal power. Validation and noninvasive application. Circulation *89:*2045, 1994.

LEFT VENTRICULAR PUMP FUNCTION

116. Starling, E. H.: Linacre Lecture on the Law of the Heart (1915). London, Longmans, 1918.
117. Sarnoff, S. J., and Mitchell, J. H.: Control of function of heart. *In* Hamilton, W. F., and Dow, P. (eds.): Handbook of Physiology. Washington, D. C., American Physiological Society, 1962, p. 489.
118. Little, W. C., and Applegate, R. J.: Congestive heart failure: Systolic and diastolic function. J. Cardiothor. Vasc. Anesth. *7*(Suppl. 2):2, 1993.
119. Grossman, W.: Diastolic dysfunction in congestive heart failure. N. Engl. J. Med. *325:*1557, 1991.
120. Litwin, S. E., and Grossman, W.: Diastolic dysfunction as a cause of heart failure. J. Am. Coll. Cardiol. *22:*49A, 1993.
121. Brutsaert, D., Sys, S. U., and Gillebert, T. C.: Diastolic failure: Pathophysiology and therapeutic implications. J. Am. Coll. Cardiol. *22:*318, 1993.
122. Gaasch, W. H.: Diagnosis and treatment of heart failure based on left ventricular systolic or diastolic dysfunction. JAMA *271:*1276, 1994.
123. Kitzman, D. W., Higginbotham, M. B., Cobb, F. R., et al.: Exercise intolerance in patients with heart failure and preserved left ventricular systolic function: Failure of the Frank-Starling mechanism. J. Am. Coll. Cardiol. *17:*1065, 1991.
124. Thomas, J. D., and Klein, A.: Doppler-echocardiographic evaluation of diastolic function. *In* Skorton, D. J. (eds.): Marcus Cardiac Imaging. Philadelphia, W. B. Saunders Co. 1996.
125. Bonow, R. O.: Radionuclide angiographic evaluation of left ventricular diastolic function. Circulation *84:*1208, 1991.
126. Myreng, Y., and Smiseth, O. A.: Assessment of left ventricular relaxation by Doppler echocardiography: Comparison of isovolumic relaxation time and transmitral flow velocities with time constant of isovolumic relaxation. Circulation *81:*260, 1990.
127. Weiss, J. L., Frederiksen, J. W., and Weisfeldt, M. L.: Hemodynamic determinants of the time-course of fall in canine left ventricular pressure. J. Clin. Invest. *58:*751, 1976.
128. Eichhorn, E. J., Willard, J. E., Alvarez, L., et al.: Are contraction and relaxation coupled in patients with and without congestive heart failure? Circulation *85:*2326, 1993.
129. Gilbert, J. C., and Glantz, S. A.: Determinants of left ventricular filling and of the diastolic pressure-volume relations. Circ. Res. *64:*827, 1989.
130. Gaasch, W. H., Carroll, J. D., Blaustein, A. S., and Bing, O. H. L.: Myocardial relaxation: Effects of preload on the time course of isovolumic relaxation. Circulation *73:*1037, 1986.
131. Freeman, G. L., Prabhu, S. D., Widman, L. E., and Colston, J. T.: An analysis of variability of left ventricular pressure decay. Am. J. Physiol. *264:*H262, 1993.
132. Grossman, W.: Evaluation of systolic and diastolic function of the myocardium. *In* Grossman, W., and Baim, D. S. (eds.): Cardiac Catheterization, Angiography and Intervention. Philadelphia, Lea and Febiger, 1991, p. 319.
133. Frais, M. A., Bergman, D. W., Kingma, I., et al.: The dependence of the time constant of left ventricular isovolumic relaxation (Tau) on pericardial pressure. Circulation. *81:*1071, 1990.
134. Yellin, E. L., Nikolic, S., and Frater, R. W. M.: Left ventricular filling dynamics and diastolic function. Prog. Cardiovasc. Dis. *32:*247, 1990.
135. Chen, C., Rodriguez, L., Guerrero, J. L., et al.: Noninvasive estimation of the instantaneous first derivative of left ventricular pressure using continuous-wave Doppler echocardiography. Circulation *83:*2101, 1991.
136. Mirsky, I.: Assessment of diastolic function: Suggested methods and future considerations. Circulation *69:*836, 1984.
137. Kennish, A., Yellin, E., and Frater, R. W.: Dynamic stiffness profiles in the left ventricle. J. Appl. Physiol. *39:*665, 1975.
138. Mirsky, I., and Pasipoularides, A.: Clinical assessment of diastolic function. Prog. Cardiovasc. Dis. *32:*291, 1990.
139. Keren, A., and Popp, R. L.: Assignment of patients into the classification of cardiomyopathies. Circulation *86:*1622, 1992.
140. Appleton, C. P.: Doppler assessment of left ventricular diastolic function: The refinements continue. J. Am. Coll. Cardiol. *21:*1697, 1993.
141. Pai, R. G., and Shah, P. M.: Echo-Doppler evaluation of left ventricular diastolic function. ACC Curr. J. Rev. 30, 1994.
142. Little, W. C., and Cheng, C. P.: Modulation of diastolic dysfunction in the intact heart. *In* Lorell, B. H., and Grossman, W. (eds.): Diastolic Relaxation of the Heart. Boston, Kluwer Academic Publishers, 1994, p. 167.
143. Cheng, C. P., Freeman, G. L., Santamore, W. P., et al.: Effect of loading conditions, contractile state, and heart rate on early diastolic left ventricular filling in conscious dogs. Circ. Res. *66:*814, 1990.
144. Little, W. C.: Enhanced load dependence of relaxation in heart failure: Clinical implications. Circulation *85:*2326, 1992.
145. Courtois, M., Mechem, C. J., Barzilai, B., et al.: Delineation of determinants of left ventricular early filling: Saline versus blood infusion. Circulation *90:*2041, 1994.
146. Little, R. C.: The mechanism of closure of the mitral valve: A continuing controversy. Circulation *59:*615, 1979.
147. Nishimura, R. A., Abel, M. D., Hatle, L. K., et al.: Significance of Doppler indices of diastolic filling of the left ventricle: Comparison with invasive hemodynamics in a canine model. Am. Heart J. *118:*1248, 1989.
148. Kono, T., Sabbah, H. N., Rosman, H., et al.: Left atrial contribution to ventricular filling during the course of evolving heart failure. Circulation *86:*1317, 1992.
149. Little, W. C., Kitzman, D., and Cheng, C. P.: Patterns of left ventricular filling indicating diastolic dysfunction: What is their importance? Choices Cardiol. *(in press).*
150. Appleton, C. P., and Hatle, L. K.: The natural history of left ventricular filling abnormalities: Assessment by two-dimensional and Doppler echocardiography. Echocardiography *9:*437, 1992.
151. Ohno, M., Cheng, C. P., and Little, W. C.: Mechanism of altered patterns of left ventricular filling during the development of congestive heart failure. Circulation *89:*2241, 1994.
152. Little, W. C., Ohno, M., Kitzman, D. W., et al.: Determination of left ventricular chamber stiffness from the time for deceleration of early left ventricular filling. Circulation *92:*1933, 1995.
153. Pinamonti, B., Di Lenardo, A., Sinagra, G., and Camerini, F.: Restrictive left ventricular filling pattern in dilated cardiomyopathy assessed by Doppler echocardiography; clinical, echocardiographic and hemodynamic correlations and prognostic implications. J. Am. Coll. Cardiol. *22:*808, 1993.
154. Oh, J. K., Hatle, L. K., Seward, J. B., et al.: Diagnostic role of Doppler echocardiography in constrictive pericarditis. J. Am. Coll. Cardiol. *23:*154, 1994.
155. Klein, A. L., Hatle, L. K., Taliercio, C. P., et al.: Prognostic significance of Doppler measures of diastolic function in cardiac amyloidosis. A Doppler echocardiography study. Circulation *83:*808, 1991.
156. Klein, A. L., and Tajik, A. J.: Doppler assessment of pulmonary venous flow in healthy subjects and in patients with heart disease. J. Am. Soc. Echocardiogr. *4:*379, 1991.
157. Basnight, M. A., Gonzalez, M. S., Kershenovich, S. C., and Appleton, C. P.: Pulmonary venous flow velocity: Relation to hemodynamics, mitral flow velocity and left atrial volume, and ejection fraction. J. Am. Soc. Echocardiol. *4:*547, 1991.
158. Dell'Italia, L. J.: The right ventricle: Anatomy, physiology, and clinical importance. Curr. Probl. Cardiol. *16:*653, 1991.
159. Morrison, D. A., Ovitt, T., Hammermeister, K. E., and Stoval, J. R.: Functional tricuspid regurgitation and right ventricular dysfunction in pulmonary hypertension. Am. J. Cardiol. *62:*108, 1988.
160. Voelker, W., Gruber, H. P., Ickrath, O., et al.: Determination of right ventricular ejection fraction by thermodilution technique—a comparison to biplane cineventriculography. Intensive Care Med. *14:*461, 1988.
161. Hurford, W. E., Zapol, W. M.: The right ventricle and critical illness: A review of anatomy, physiology, and clinical evaluation of its function. Intensive Care Med. *14:*448, 1988.
162. Spinale, F. G., Smith, A. C., Carabello, B. A., and Crawford, F. A.: Right ventricular function computed by thermodilution and ventriculography: A comparison of methods. J Thorac. Cardiovasc. Surg. *99:*141, 1990.
163. Brown, K. A., and Ditchey, R. V.: Human right ventricular end-systolic pressure-volume relation defined by maximal elastance. Circulation *78:*81, 1988.
164. Yamaguchi, S., Tsuiki, K., Miyawaki, H., et al.: Effect of left ventricular volume on right ventricular end-systolic pressure-volume relations: Resetting of regional preload in right ventricular free wall. Circ. Res. *65:*623, 1989.

165. Dell'Italia, L. J., Freeman, G. L., and Gaasch, W. H.: Cardiac function and functional capacity: Implications for the failing heart. Curr. Probl. Cardiol. *18*:705, 1993.
166. Sumimoto, S., Sugiura, T., Tarumi, N., and Taniguchi, H.: Mixed venous oxygen saturation as a guide to tissue oxygenation and prognosis in patients with acute myocardial infarction. Am. Heart J. *122*:27, 1991.
167. Inomata, S., Nishikawa, T., and Taguchi, M.: Continuous monitoring of mixed venous oxygen saturation for detecting alterations in cardiac output after discontinuation of cardiopulmonary bypass. Br. J. Anaesth. *72*:11, 1994.
168. Koike, A., Wasserman, K., Taniguchi, K., et al.: Critical capillary oxygen partial pressure and lactate threshold in patients with cardiovascular disease. J. Am. Coll. Cardiol. *23*:1644, 1994.
169. Grossman, W.: Blood flow measurement: The cardiac output. *In* Grossman, W., and Baim, D. S. (eds.): Cardiac Catheterization, Angiography and Intervention. Philadelphia, Lea and Febiger, 1990, p. 105.
170. Weber, K. T., and Janicki, J. S.: Lactate production during maximal and submaximal exercise in patients with chronic heart failure. J. Am. Coll. Cardiol. *6*:717, 1985.
171. Weber, K. T., Janicki, J. S., and McElroy, P. A.: Cardiopulmonary Exercise Testing. Philadelphia, W. B. Saunders Co., 1986.
172. Wasserman, K.: Measures of functional capacity in patients with heart failure. Circulation *81*(Suppl. 2):1, 1990.
173. Swedberg, K., and Gundersen, T.: The role of exercise testing in heart failure. J Cardiovasc. Pharmacol. *22*:S13, 1993.
174. Swedberg, K.: Exercise testing in heart failure: A critical review. Drugs *47*:14, 1994.
175. Weisman, I. M., and Zeballos, R. J.: An integrated approach to the interpretation of cardiopulmonary exercise testing. Clin. Chest Med. *15*:421, 1994.
176. Simonton, C. A., Higginbotham, M. B., and Cobb, F. R.: The ventilatory threshold: Quantitative analysis of reproducibility and relation to arterial lactate concentration in normal subjects and in patients with chronic congestive heart failure. Am. J. Cardiol. *62*:100, 1988.
177. Poole-Wilson, P. A.: Exercise as a means of assessing heart failure and its response to treatment. Cardiology *76*:347, 1989.
178. Franciosa, J. A., Baker, B. J., and Seth, L.: Pulmonary versus systemic hemodynamics in determining exercise capacity of patients with chronic left ventricular failure. Am. Heart J. *110*:807, 1985.
179. Jennings, G. L., and Esler, M. D.: Circulatory regulation at rest and exercise and the functional assessment of patients with congestive heart failure. Circulation *81*(Suppl. 2):5, 1990.
180. Sullivan, M. J., Cobb, F. R.: The anaerobic threshold in chronic heart failure: Relation to blood lactate, ventilatory basis, reproducibility, and response of exercise training. Circulation *81*(Suppl. 2):47, 1990.
181. Koike, A., Yajima, T., Adachi, H., et al.: Evaluation of exercise capacity using submaximal exercise at a constant work rate in patients with cardiovascular disease. Circulation *91*:1719, 1995.

Chapter 15

Clinical Aspects of Heart Failure: High-Output Heart Failure; Pulmonary Edema

EUGENE BRAUNWALD, WILSON S. COLUCCI, WILLIAM GROSSMAN

Heart failure is a principal complication of virtually all forms of heart disease. A panel of the National Heart, Lung and Blood Institute described this condition as follows: "Heart failure occurs when an abnormality of cardiac function causes the heart to fail to pump blood at a rate required by the metabolizing tissues or when the heart can do so only with an elevated filling pressure. The heart's inability to pump a sufficient amount of blood to meet the needs of the body tissues may be due to insufficient or defective cardiac filling and/or impaired contraction and emptying. Compensatory mechanisms increase blood volume and raise cardiac filling pressures, heart rate, and cardiac muscle mass to maintain the heart's pumping function and cause redistribution of blood flow. Eventually, however, despite these compensatory mechanisms, the ability of the heart to contract and relax declines progressively, and the heart failure worsens."[1]

An alternative definition, which focuses more on the clinical consequences of heart failure, has been offered by Packer as follows: "Congestive heart failure represents a complex clinical syndrome characterized by abnormalities of left ventricular function and neurohormonal regulation, which are accompanied by effort intolerance, fluid retention, and reduced longevity."[2] Included in these two definitions is a wide spectrum of clinicophysiological states, ranging from the rapid impairment of pumping function (occurring when, for example, a massive myocardial infarction, tachyarrhythmia, or bradyarrhythmia develops suddenly) to the gradual but progressive impairment of myocardial function, observed at first only during stress occurring in a patient whose heart sustains a pressure or volume overload for a prolonged period. Congestive heart failure is a relatively common disorder; it has been estimated that 2 million persons in the United States are being treated for heart failure and that there are 400,000 new cases each year.[3]

TABLE 15–1 FRAMINGHAM CRITERIA FOR CONGESTIVE HEART FAILURE

MAJOR CRITERIA
Paroxysmal nocturnal dyspnea or orthopnea
Neck-vein distention
Rales
Cardiomegaly
Acute pulmonary edema
S_3 gallop
Increased venous pressure >16 cm H_2O
Circulation time >25 sec
Hepatojugular reflux
MINOR CRITERIA
Ankle edema
Night cough
Dyspnea on exertion
Hepatomegaly
Pleural effusion
Vital capacity decrease 1/3 from maximum
Tachycardia (rate of >120/min)
MAJOR OR MINOR CRITERION
Weight loss >4.5 kg in 5 days in response to treatment

For establishing a definite diagnosis of congestive heart failure in this study, two major or one major and two minor criteria had to be present concurrently.

From McKee, P. A., Castelli, W. P., McNamara, P. M., and Kannel, W. B.: The natural history of congestive heart failure, the Framingham Study. N. Engl. J. Med. *285*:1441, 1971. Copyright Massachusetts Medical Society.

The clinical manifestations of heart failure vary enormously and depend on a variety of factors, including the age of the patient, the extent and rate at which cardiac performance becomes impaired, and the ventricle initially involved in the disease process.[4] A broad spectrum of severity of impairment of cardiac function is ordinarily included within the definition of heart failure, ranging from the mildest, which is manifest clinically only during stress, to the most advanced form, in which cardiac pump function is unable to sustain life without external support.

Useful criteria for the diagnosis of heart failure emerged from the Framingham study[5,6] (Table 15–1).

FORMS OF HEART FAILURE

Forward vs. Backward Heart Failure

The clinical manifestations of heart failure arise as a consequence of inadequate cardiac output and/or damming up of blood behind one or both ventricles. These two principal mechanisms are the basis of the so-called forward and backward pressure theories of heart failure. The *backward failure hypothesis,* first proposed in 1832 by James Hope, contends that when the ventricle fails to discharge its contents, blood accumulates and pressure rises in the atrium and the venous system emptying into it.[7] There is substantial physiological evidence in favor of this theory. As discussed on page 398, the inability of cardiac muscle to shorten against a load alters the relationship between ventricular end-systolic pressure and volume so that end-systolic (residual) volume rises. The following sequence then occurs that at first maintains cardiac output at a normal level: (1) ventricular end-diastolic volume and pressure increase; (2) the volume and pressure rise in the atrium behind the failing ventricle; (3) the atrium contracts more vigorously (a manifestation of Starling's law, operating on the atrium)[8]; (4) the pressure in the venous and capillary beds behind (upstream to) the failing ventricle rises; and (5) transudation of fluid from the capillary bed into the interstitial space (pulmonary or systemic) increases. Many of the symptoms characteristic of heart failure can be traced to this sequence of events and the resultant increase in fluid in the interstitial spaces of the lungs, liver, subcutaneous tissues, and serous cavities.

Cardiac output in the resting (basal) state is a relatively *insensitive* index of cardiac function (see p. 439). In many patients, the entire sequence of events outlined above may transpire while cardiac output *at rest* is still within normal limits. Indeed, the backward pressure theory of heart failure reflects one of the principal compensatory mechanisms in heart failure, i.e., the operation of Starling's law of the heart (see p. 378), in which distention of the ventricle helps to maintain cardiac output. The failing ventricle operates on an ascending, albeit depressed and flattened, function curve,[9] and the augmented ventricular end-diastolic volume and pressure characteristic of heart failure must be regarded as aiding in the maintenance of cardiac output. When this compensatory mechanism is interfered with (e.g., by means of dietary sodium restriction and treatment with diuretics), the patient may be less symptomatic owing to loss of extracellular fluid volume, with its accompanying reduction in congestion of the lungs, liver, and lower extremities. However, at the same time, cardiac output may decline,[10] and symptoms secondary to a reduction of cardiac output, such as fatigue, may actually intensify. Thus, although many of the clinical manifestations of heart failure are secondary to excessive retention of extracellular fluid, the elevation of ventricular preload associated with this excess fluid constitutes an important adaptive mechanism.

An important extension of the backward failure theory is the development of right ventricular failure as a consequence of left ventricular failure. According to this concept, the elevation of left ventricular diastolic, left atrial, and pulmonary venous pressures results in backward transmission of pressure and leads to pulmonary hypertension, which ultimately causes right ventricular failure. Often, pulmonary vasoconstriction plays a part in this form of pulmonary hypertension as well (see p. 780).

Eighty years after publication of Hope's work, Mackenzie proposed the *forward failure hypothesis,* which relates clinical manifestations of heart failure to inadequate delivery of blood into the arterial system.[11] According to this hypothesis, the principal clinical manifestations of heart failure are due to reduced cardiac output, which results in diminished perfusion of vital organs, including the brain, leading to mental confusion; skeletal muscles, leading to weakness; and kidneys, leading to sodium and water retention through a series of complex mechanisms[12] (Chap. 62). This retention of sodium and water, in turn, augments extracellular fluid volume and ultimately leads to symptoms of heart failure which are caused by congestion of organs and tissues.

Although these two seemingly opposing views concerning the pathogenesis of heart failure led to lively controversy during the first half of this century, it no longer seems fruitful to make a rigid distinction between backward and forward heart failure, since *both* mechanisms appear to operate in the majority of patients with *chronic* heart failure.[13] Exceptions may occur, however, and some patients, particularly those with *acute* decompensation, develop relatively pure forms of forward or backward failure.

For instance, a massive myocardial infarction may result in either (1) forward failure with a marked reduction of left ventricular output and cardiogenic shock (see p. 1238) and clinical manifestations secondary to impaired perfusion (e.g., hypotension, mental confusion, oliguria), or (2) backward failure with a transient inequality of output between the two ventricles, resulting in acute pulmonary edema. More commonly, patients with large myocardial infarctions develop a combination of forward and backward failure, with symptoms resulting from both inadequate cardiac output and pulmonary congestion. Early in the course of acute myocardial infarction, patients may succumb long before renal retention of salt and water can occur. However, if the patients survive the acute insult, expansion of the extracellular fluid volume and manifestations resulting therefrom usually occur.

RIGHT-SIDED VS. LEFT-SIDED HEART FAILURE

Implicit in the backward failure theory is the idea that fluid localizes behind the specific cardiac chamber that is *initially* affected. Thus, symptoms secondary to pulmonary congestion initially predominate in patients with left ventricular infarction, hypertension, and aortic and mitral valve disease; i.e., they manifest *left heart failure.* With time, however, fluid accumulation becomes generalized, and ankle edema, congestive hepatomegaly, ascites, and pleural effusion occur (i.e., the patients later exhibit *right heart failure* as well). Less commonly, prolonged right ventricular failure with massive accumulation of extracellular fluid may be associated with dyspnea, particularly when the patient is in the supine position and when large pleural effusions are present.

FLUID RETENTION IN HEART FAILURE. There is general agreement that fluid retention in heart failure is caused ultimately in part by reduction in glomerular filtration rate and in part by activation of the renin-angiotensin-aldosterone system. Reduced cardiac output is associated with a lowered glomerular filtration rate and an increased elaboration of renin, which, through the activation of angiotensin, results in the release of aldosterone (see p. 413). The combination of impaired hepatic function, owing to hepatic venous congestion, and reduced hepatic blood flow interferes with the metabolism of aldosterone,[12] further raising its plasma concentration and augmenting the retention of sodium and water.

As already noted, cardiac output (and glomerular filtration rate) may be normal in many patients with heart failure, particularly when they are at rest. However, during stress, such as physical exercise or fever, the cardiac output fails to rise normally, the glomerular filtration rate declines, and the renal mechanisms for salt and water retention described above come into play. In addition, ventricular filling pressure, and therefore pressures in the atrium and systemic veins behind (upstream to) the ventricle, may be normal at rest, only to rise abnormally during the stress. This, in turn, may cause transudation and symptoms of tissue congestion (pulmonary in the case of the left ventricle and systemic in the case of the right) during exercise. For this reason, simple rest may induce diuresis and relieve symptoms in many patients with mild heart failure.

ACUTE VS. CHRONIC HEART FAILURE

The clinical manifestations of heart failure depend importantly on the *rate* at which the syndrome develops and specifically on whether sufficient time has elapsed for compensatory mechanisms to become operative and for fluid to accumulate in the interstitial space (Table 15–2). For example, when a previously normal individual suddenly develops a serious anatomical or functional abnormality of the heart (such as massive myocardial infarction, heart block with a very slow ventricular rate [<35/min], a tachyarrhythmia with a very rapid rate [>180/min], rupture of a valve secondary to infective endocarditis, or

TABLE 15–2 COMPARISONS OF ACUTE VS CHRONIC HEART FAILURE

FEATURE	ACUTE HEART FAILURE	DECOMPENSATED CHRONIC HEART FAILURE	CHRONIC HEART FAILURE
Symptom severity	Marked	Marked	Mild to moderate
Pulmonary edema	Frequent	Frequent	Rare
Peripheral edema	Rare	Frequent	Frequent
Weight gain	None to mild	Frequent	Frequent
Whole-body fluid volume load	No change or mild increase	Markedly increased	Increased
Cardiomegaly	Uncommon	Usual	Common
Ventricular systolic function	Hypo-, normo-, or hypercontractile	Reduced	Reduced
Wall stress	Elevated	Markedly elevated	Elevated
Activation of sympathetic nervous system	Marked	Marked	Mild to marked
Activation of renin-angiotensin-aldosterone axis	Often increased	Marked	Mild to marked
Reparable, remedial causative lesion(s)	Common	Occasional	Occasional

Clinical and pathophysiological characteristics of the two major categories of unstable heart failure (acute heart failure and decompensated chronic heart failure) are compared with those of chronic heart failure.

From Leier, C. V.: Unstable heart failure. *In* Colucci, W. S. (ed.): Heart Failure: Cardiac Function and Dysfunction. *In* Braunwald, E. (Series ed.): Atlas of Heart Diseases, Vol. 4: Philadelphia, Current Medicine, 1995, pp. 9.1–9.15.

occlusion of a large segment of the pulmonary vascular bed by a pulmonary embolus), a marked, sudden reduction in cardiac output with symptoms due to inadequate organ perfusion and/or acute congestion of the venous bed behind the affected ventricle will occur. If the same anatomical abnormality develops gradually, or if the patient survives the acute insult, a number of adaptive mechanisms become operational, especially cardiac hypertrophy, and these allow the patient to adjust to and tolerate not only the anatomical abnormality but also a reduction in cardiac output with less difficulty.

Frequently, the important clinical manifestations of chronic heart failure secondary to tissue congestion may be suppressed by dietary sodium restriction and diuretics. Cardiac function may not have been improved, and such patients still are in "heart failure," albeit with fewer clinical manifestations thereof. Under these circumstances, an acute event such as an infection, an arrhythmia, or discontinuation of therapy may precipitate manifestations of acute heart failure.

LOW-OUTPUT VS. HIGH-OUTPUT HEART FAILURE

Low cardiac output at rest, or in milder cases only during exertion and other stresses, characterizes heart failure occurring in most forms of heart disease (i.e., congenital, valvular, rheumatic, hypertensive, coronary, and cardiomyopathic). A variety of high-output states, including thyrotoxicosis, arteriovenous fistulas, beriberi, Paget's disease of bone, anemia, and pregnancy (discussed later in this chapter), may lead to heart failure as well. Low-output heart failure is characterized by clinical evidence of impairment of the peripheral circulation, with systemic vasoconstriction and cold, pale, and sometimes cyanotic extremities; in advanced forms of low-output failure, as the stroke volume declines, the pulse pressure narrows.[14] In contrast, in high-output heart failure (see pp. 460 to 462), the extremities are usually warm and flushed, and the pulse pressure is widened or at least normal.

The ability of the heart to deliver the quantity of oxygen required by the metabolizing tissues is reflected in the arterial–mixed venous oxygen difference, which is abnormally widened (i.e., >5.0 ml/liter in the resting state) in patients with low-output heart failure. This difference may be normal or even reduced in high-output states, owing to elevation of the mixed venous oxygen saturation by the admixture of blood that has been shunted away from metabolizing tissues. However, regardless of the absolute level of the arterial–mixed venous oxygen, this difference still exceeds the level that existed *before* the development of heart failure, and cardiac output, regardless of its absolute level, is lower than it had been before the development of heart failure.

Systolic vs. Diastolic Heart Failure

(See also p. 403)

Implicit in the physiological definition of heart failure (inability to pump an adequate volume of blood and/or to do so only from an abnormally elevated filling pressure) is that heart failure can be caused by an abnormality in systolic function leading to a defect in the expulsion of blood (i.e., *systolic heart failure*), or by an abnormality in diastolic function leading to a defect in ventricular filling (i.e., *diastolic heart failure*) (Fig. 15–1). The former is the more familiar, classic heart failure in which an impaired inotropic state is responsible. Less familiar, but perhaps just as important, is diastolic heart failure, in which the ability of the ventricle(s) to accept blood is impaired.[15,16] This may be due to slowed or incomplete ventricular relaxation which may be transient, as occurs in acute ischemia, or sustained, as in concentric myocardial hypertrophy or re-

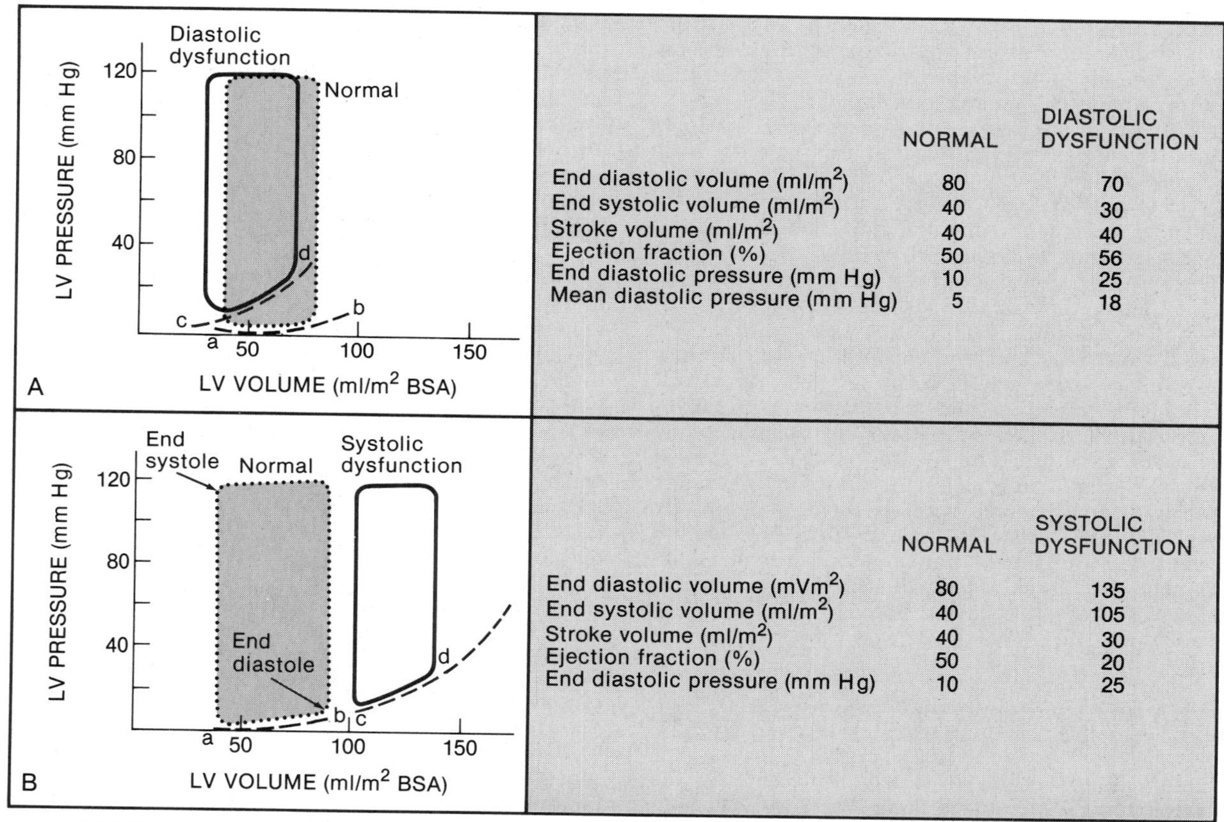

	NORMAL	DIASTOLIC DYSFUNCTION
End diastolic volume (ml/m^2)	80	70
End systolic volume (ml/m^2)	40	30
Stroke volume (ml/m^2)	40	40
Ejection fraction (%)	50	56
End diastolic pressure (mm Hg)	10	25
Mean diastolic pressure (mm Hg)	5	18

	NORMAL	SYSTOLIC DYSFUNCTION
End diastolic volume (mVm^2)	80	135
End systolic volume (ml/m^2)	40	105
Stroke volume (ml/m^2)	40	30
Ejection fraction (%)	50	20
End diastolic pressure (mm Hg)	10	25

FIGURE 15–1. *A,* Schematic of a pressure-volume loop from a normal subject (dotted line) and a patient with diastolic dysfunction (solid line). Dashed lines represent the diastolic pressure-volume relation. Isolated diastolic dysfunction is characterized by a shift in pressure-volume loop to the left. Contractile performance is normal (normal or increased ejection fraction, normal or slightly decreased stroke volume). However, LV pressures throughout diastole are increased; at a common diastolic volume = 70 ml/m². LV diastolic pressure is 25 mm Hg in the patient with diastolic failure compared with a diastolic pressure of 5 mm Hg in normal subject. Thus, diastolic dysfunction increases modulus of chamber stiffness. LV, left ventricular. *B,* Schematic of pressure-volume loop from a normal subject (dotted line) and a patient with systolic dysfunction (solid line). Dashed line represents diastolic pressure-volume relation. Systolic dysfunction is characterized by displacement of pressure-volume loop to the right. Despite compensatory dilation, stroke volume or ejection fraction remains low. LV diastolic pressures are increased as a result of large LV volume. LV, left ventricular. (From Zile, M. R.: Diastolic dysfunction: Detection, consequences, and treatment: 2. Diagnosis and treatment of diastolic dysfunction. Mod. Concepts Cardiovasc. Dis. *59:*1, 1990.)

TABLE 15–3 SYSTOLIC VS. DIASTOLIC DYSFUNCTION IN HEART FAILURE

A			B		
PARAMETERS	SYSTOLIC	DIASTOLIC	PARAMETERS	SYSTOLIC	DIASTOLIC
History			**Chest Roentgenogram**		
Coronary heart disease	++++	+	Cardiomegaly	+++	+
Hypertension	++	++++	Pulmonary congestion	+++	+++
Diabetes	+++	+	**Electrocardiograms**		
Valvular heart disease	++++	−	Low voltage	+++	−
Paroxysmal dyspnea	++	+++	Left ventricular hypertrophy	++	++++
Physical Examination			Q waves	++	+
Cardiomegaly	+++	+	**Echocardiograms**		
Soft heart sounds	++++	+	Low ejection fraction	++++	−
S_3 gallop	+++	+	Left ventricular dilation	++	−
S_4 gallop	+	+++	Left ventricular hypertrophy	++	++++
Hypertension	++	++++			
Mitral regurgitation	+++	+			
Rales	++	++			
Edema	+++	+			
Jugular venous distention	+++	+			

Certain aspects of the history and physical examination *(panel A)*, along with clinical measurements *(panel B)*, help to distinguish diastolic problems from those more often associated with systolic failure. Patients with hypertensive heart disease, for example, particularly severe left ventricular hypertrophy, often experience heart failure because of diastolic dysfunction. *Plus signs* indicate "suggestive" (the number reflects relative weight). *Minus signs* indicate "not very suggestive."

From Young, J. B.: Assessment of Heart Failure. *In* Colucci, W. S. (ed.): Heart Failure: Cardiac Function and Dysfunction. *In* Braunwald, E. (Series ed.): Atlas of Heart Diseases, Vol. 4: Philadelphia, Current Medicine, 1995, pp. 7.1–7.20.

strictive cardiomyopathy secondary to infiltrative conditions such as amyloidosis. The principal clinical manifestations of systolic failure result from an inadequate forward cardiac output, while the major consequences of diastolic failure relate to elevation of the ventricular filling pressure and the high venous pressure upstream to the ventricle, causing pulmonic and/or systemic congestion.

There are many examples of pure systolic or diastolic heart failure. Examples of the former are patients with acute massive pulmonary embolism or dilated cardiomyopathy, while examples of the latter are patients with hypertrophic cardiomyopathy or subendocardial fibrosis. However, in many patients, systolic and diastolic heart failure coexist. The most common form of heart failure, that caused by coronary atherosclerosis, is an example of combined systolic and diastolic failure. In this condition, systolic failure is caused by both the chronic loss of contracting myocardium secondary to myocardial necrosis resulting from previous infarction and the acute loss of myocardial contractility induced by a transient episode of ischemia. Diastolic failure is due to the ventricle's reduced compliance caused by replacement of normal, distensible myocardium with nondistensible fibrous scar tissue and by the acute reduction of diastolic distensibility of reversibly injured myocardium during a transient episode of ischemia. A number of clinical features and laboratory findings characterize these two forms of heart failure (Table 15–3).

CAUSES OF HEART FAILURE

From a clinical viewpoint, it is useful to classify the causes of heart failure into three broad categories: (1) *underlying causes,* comprising the structural abnormalities—congenital or acquired—that affect the peripheral and coronary vessels, pericardium, myocardium, or cardiac valves and lead to the increased hemodynamic burden or myocardial or coronary insufficiency responsible for heart failure; (2) *fundamental causes,* comprising the biochemical and physiological mechanisms through which either an increased hemodynamic burden or a reduction in oxygen delivery to the myocardium results in impairment of myocardial contraction (Chap. 13); and (3) *precipitating causes,* including the specific causes or incidents that precipitate heart failure in 50 to 90 per cent of episodes of clinical heart failure.

It is helpful for the clinician to identify both the underlying and the precipitating causes of heart failure. Appropriate management of the underlying heart disease (e.g., surgical correction of a congenital defect or an acquired valvular abnormality or pharmacological management of hypertension) may prevent the development or recurrence of heart failure. Similarly, treatment of a precipitating cause such as an infection with fever will often terminate an episode of heart failure and may be life-saving. More important, *prevention* of a precipitating cause can prevent heart failure.

Overt heart failure may, of course, also be precipitated if there is progression of the underlying heart disease. A previously stable, compensated patient may develop heart failure that is apparent clinically for the first time when the intrinsic process has advanced to a critical point, such as with progressive obliteration of the pulmonary vascular bed in a patient with cor pulmonale or further narrowing of a stenotic aortic valve. Alternatively, decompensation may occur as a result of failure or exhaustion of the compensatory mechanisms but without any change in the load on the heart in patients with persistent severe pressure or volume overload.

Precipitating Causes of Heart Failure

In one study of 101 patients admitted to an inner city municipal hospital with the diagnosis of heart failure, precipitating factors could be identified in 93 per cent[17] (Table 15–4).

INAPPROPRIATE REDUCTION OF THERAPY. Perhaps the most common cause of decompensation in a previously compensated patient with heart failure is inappropriate reduction in the intensity of treatment—be it dietary sodium restriction, reduced physical activity, a drug regimen, or, most commonly, a combination of these measures. Many patients with serious underlying heart disease, regardless of whether they previously experienced heart failure, may be relatively asymptomatic for as long as they carefully adhere to their treatment regimen. Dietary excesses of sodium, incurred frequently on vacations or holidays or during an illness of the spouse responsible for preparing the patient's meals, are frequent causes of sudden cardiac decompensation. Careful and repeated instruction of the patient is a

TABLE 15–4 PRECIPITATING FACTORS IN CHRONIC HEART FAILURE

PRECIPITANT	NO. OF PATIENTS
Lack of compliance	64
With diet	22
With drugs	6
With both (diet and drugs)	37
Uncontrolled hypertension	44
Cardiac arrhythmias	29
Atrial fibrillation	20
Atrial flutter	7
Multifocal atrial tachycardia	1
Ventricular tachycardia	1
Environmental factors	19
Inadequate therapy	17
Pulmonary infection	12
Emotional stress	7
Administration of inappropriate medications or fluid overload	4
Myocardial infarction	6
Endocrine disorders (thyrotoxicosis)	1

Adapted from Ghali, J. K., Kadakia, S., Cooper, R., and Ferlinz, J.: Precipitating factors leading to decompensation of heart failure: Traits among urban blacks. Arch. Intern. Med. *148*:2013, 1988.

simple yet effective measure to prevent this common clinical problem.

ARRHYTHMIAS (see also Chap. 22). Cardiac arrhythmias are far more common in patients with underlying structural heart disease than in normal subjects and commonly precipitate or intensify heart failure. The development of arrhythmias may precipitate heart failure through several mechanisms: (1) *Tachyarrhythmias,* most commonly atrial fibrillation (Table 15–4), reduce the time available for ventricular filling. When there is already an impairment of ventricular filling, as in mitral stenosis, or reduced ventricular compliance (diastolic failure; see below), tachycardia will raise atrial pressure and reduce cardiac output further. In addition, tachyarrhythmias increase myocardial oxygen demands and, in a patient with obstructive coronary artery disease, may induce or intensify myocardial ischemia, which, in turn, impairs both cardiac relaxation and systolic function, thereby raising left atrial and pulmonary capillary pressure further and causing symptoms secondary to pulmonary congestion. (2) *Marked bradycardia* in a patient with underlying heart disease usually depresses cardiac output, since stroke volume may already be maximal and cannot rise further to maintain cardiac output. (3) *Dissociation between atrial and ventricular contraction,* which occurs in many arrhythmias, results in loss of the atrial booster pump mechanism, which impairs ventricular filling, lowers cardiac output, and raises atrial pressure.[18] This loss is particularly deleterious in patients with impaired ventricular filling due to concentric cardiac hypertrophy (e.g., in systemic hypertension, aortic stenosis, and hypertrophic cardiomyopathy). (4) *Abnormal intraventricular conduction,* which occurs in many arrhythmias such as ventricular tachycardia, impairs myocardial performance because of loss of the normal synchronicity of ventricular contraction. In addition to precipitating heart failure, arrhythmias—sometimes fatal—may be *caused* by heart failure.

SYSTEMIC INFECTION. Although patients with congestive heart failure are particularly susceptible to pulmonary infections, presumably because of the diminished ability of congested lungs to expel respiratory secretions, *any* infection may precipitate cardiac failure. The mechanisms include increased total metabolism as a consequence of fever, discomfort, and cough, which increase the hemodynamic burden on the heart; the accompanying sinus tachycardia, secondary to fever and discomfort, plays an additional adverse role.

PULMONARY EMBOLISM (see also Chap. 46). Patients with congestive heart failure, particularly when confined to bed, are at high risk of developing pulmonary emboli. Such emboli may increase the hemodynamic burden on the right ventricle by elevating right ventricular systolic pressure further and may cause fever, tachypnea, and tachycardia, the deleterious effects of which have already been discussed.

PHYSICAL, ENVIRONMENTAL, AND EMOTIONAL EXCESSES. Intense, prolonged exertion or severe fatigue, such as may result from prolonged travel or emotional crises, and a severe climatic change, such as to a hot, humid environment, are relatively common precipitants of cardiac decompensation.

CARDIAC INFECTION AND INFLAMMATION. Myocarditis owing to a recurrence of acute rheumatic fever (Chap. 55) or to infective endocarditis (Chap. 33) or as a consequence of a variety of allergic inflammatory or infectious processes (including viral myocarditis) (Chap. 41) may impair myocardial function directly and exacerbate existing heart disease. The anemia, fever, and tachycardia that frequently accompany these processes are also deleterious. In patients with infective endocarditis, additional valvular damage also may precipitate cardiac decompensation.

DEVELOPMENT OF AN UNRELATED ILLNESS. Heart failure may be precipitated in patients with compensated heart disease when an unrelated illness develops. For example, the development of renal disease may impair further the ability of patients with heart failure to excrete sodium and thus may intensify the accumulation of fluid. Similarly, blood transfusion or the administration of sodium-containing fluid after a noncardiac operation may result in sudden heart failure in patients with underlying heart disease. Prostatic obstruction in the elderly male, parenchymal liver disease, and the administration of corticosteroids or estrogens with sodium-retaining properties also may precipitate heart failure in patients with underlying heart disease.

ADMINISTRATION OF CARDIAC DEPRESSANTS OR SALT-RETAINING DRUGS. A number of drugs depress myocardial function; among these are alcohol, beta-adrenoceptor blocking agents, many antiarrhythmic agents, verapamil, and antineoplastic drugs such as doxorubicin (Adriamycin) and cyclophosphamide (Chap. 42). Others, such as estrogens, androgens, glucocorticoids, and nonsteroidal antiinflammatory agents, may cause salt and water retention. Any of these drugs, when administered to a patient with heart disease, can precipitate or aggravate heart failure.

HIGH-OUTPUT STATES. Acute heart failure may be precipitated in patients with underlying heart disease, such as valvular heart disease, who develop one of the hyperkinetic circulatory states, such as pregnancy (see pp. 460 to 462).

DEVELOPMENT OF A SECOND FORM OF HEART DISEASE. Patients with one form of heart disease often remain compensated until they develop a second form. For example, a patient with chronic hypertension and left ventricular hypertrophy but without left ventricular failure may be asymptomatic until a myocardial infarction (which may be silent) develops and precipitates heart failure.

It is essential to search for these precipitating causes systematically in all patients with congestive heart failure, since lack of recognition or treatment or both may be responsible for otherwise refractory heart failure. In most instances, they can be treated effectively, after which appropriate measures should be instituted to avoid recurrence. When a precipitating cause of heart failure can be identified, it generally signifies a better prognosis than when a similar degree of heart failure is due simply to progression of the underlying cardiac disease.

Respiratory Distress

Breathlessness, a cardinal manifestation of left ventricular failure, may present with progressively increasing severity as (1) exertional dyspnea, (2) orthopnea, (3) paroxysmal nocturnal dyspnea, (4) dyspnea at rest, and (5) acute pulmonary edema.

EXERTIONAL DYSPNEA (see also p. 2). The principal difference between exertional dyspnea in normal subjects and in patients with heart failure is the degree of activity necessary to induce the symptom.[19] Indeed, as heart failure first develops, exertional dyspnea may simply appear to be an aggravation of the breathlessness that occurs in normal subjects during activity. An effort should be made to ascertain whether or not a *change* in the extent of exertion which causes dyspnea has actually occurred. As left ventricular failure advances, the intensity of exercise resulting in breathlessness declines progressively. However, there is no close correlation between subjective exercise capacity and objective measures of left ventricular performance at rest in patients with heart failure.[20] Exertional dyspnea may be absent in patients who are sedentary for a variety of reasons, such as habit, severe angina, intermittent claudication, or a noncardiovascular condition (e.g., crippling arthritis).

ORTHOPNEA. This symptom may be defined as dyspnea that develops in the recumbent position and is relieved by elevation of the head with pillows. Again, as in the case of exertional dyspnea, it is a *change* in the number of pillows required that is important. In the recumbent position there is reduced pooling of fluid in the lower extremities and abdomen; blood is displaced from the extrathoracic to the thoracic compartment. The failing left ventricle, operating on the flat portion of its depressed Starling curve (Fig. 14–18, p. 434), cannot accept and pump out the extra volume of blood delivered to it by the competent right ventricle without dilating, and pulmonary venous and capillary pressures rise further, causing interstitial pulmonary edema, reduced pulmonary compliance, increased airway resistance, and dyspnea. In contrast to paroxysmal nocturnal dyspnea (see below), orthopnea occurs rapidly, often within a minute or two of assuming recumbency, and develops when the patient is awake. It is a nonspecific symptom and may occur in any condition in which vital capacity is low; marked ascites, whatever its etiology, is an important cause of orthopnea.

The patient with orthopnea generally elevates his or her head and chest on several pillows to prevent nocturnal breathlessness and the development of paroxysmal nocturnal dyspnea (see below). In advanced left ventricular failure, orthopnea may be so severe that the patient cannot lie down and must spend the night in the sitting position. Often such patients are observed sitting at the side of the bed, slumped over a bedside table.

Cough may be caused by pulmonary congestion, occurs under the same circumstances as dyspnea (i.e., during exertion or recumbency), and is relieved by treatment of heart failure. Thus a nonproductive cough in patients with heart failure is often a "dyspnea equivalent," whereas a cough on recumbency may be considered an "orthopnea equivalent." Patients with severe chronic obstructive lung disease sometimes complain of orthopnea. *Trepopnea* is a rare form of orthopnea limited to one lateral decubitus position. It has been attributed to distortions of the great vessels in one position but not in the other.

PAROXYSMAL NOCTURNAL DYSPNEA. Attacks of paroxysmal dyspnea usually occur at night. The patient awakens, often quite suddenly, and with a feeling of severe anxiety and suffocation, sits bolt upright and gasps for breath. Bronchospasm, which may be caused by congestion of the bronchial mucosa and by interstitial pulmonary edema compressing the small bronchi, increases ventilatory difficulty and the work of breathing and is a common complicating factor of paroxysmal nocturnal dyspnea. The commonly associated wheezing is responsible for the alternate name of this condition, *cardiac asthma.* In contrast to orthopnea, which may be relieved immediately by sitting upright at the side of the bed with the legs dependent, attacks of paroxysmal nocturnal dyspnea may require 30 minutes or longer in this position for relief. Episodes of paroxysmal nocturnal dyspnea may be so frightening that the patient may be afraid to go back to sleep, even after the symptoms have abated.

The reason for the common occurrence of these episodes at night is not clear, but it seems likely that the combination of (1) the slow resorption of interstitial fluid from the dependent portion of the body and the resultant expansion of thoracic blood volume, (2) sudden elevation of thoracic blood volume and of the diaphragm which occurs immediately on assuming recumbency (as described above for orthopnea), (3) reduced adrenergic support of left ventricular function during sleep, and (4) normal nocturnal depression of the respiratory center all play major roles.

MECHANISMS OF DYSPNEA (Table 15–5)

Increased awareness of respiration or difficulty in breathing is commonly associated with pulmonary capillary hypertension caused by an elevation of left atrial or left ventricular filling pressure.[19] Patients with left ventricular failure typically exhibit a restrictive ventilatory defect, characterized by a reduction of vital capacity as a consequence of the replacement of the air in the lungs with blood or interstitial fluid or both. Consequently, the lungs become stiffer, air trapping occurs because of earlier than normal closure of dependent airways,[21] and the work of breathing is increased because higher intrapleural pressures are needed to distend the stiff lungs.[22] Tidal volume is reduced, and respiratory frequency rises in a compensatory fashion. Engorgement of blood vessels may reduce the caliber of the peripheral airways, increasing airway resistance. In addition, there are alterations in the distribution of ventilation and perfusion, resulting in widened alveolar-arterial differences for oxygen, hypoxemia, and an increased ratio of dead space to tidal volume. Thus, dyspnea (during exertion or at rest) and orthopnea are clinical expressions of pulmonary venous and capillary congestion. Paroxysmal nocturnal dyspnea reflects the presence of primarily *interstitial* edema, whereas pulmonary edema, in which there is transudation and expectoration of blood-tinged fluid (see p. 462), is often a manifestation of *alveolar* edema.

Whatever abnormalities in mechanics and gas exchange function of the lung that exist at rest are aggravated during exercise (and sometimes during recumbency) when pulmonary venous and capillary pressures rise further. Transudation of fluid from the intravascular to the extravascular space results in greater stiffening of the lungs, an augmentation in the work of breathing, and increased resistance to air flow.[23] There is an increased ventilatory drive, as a consequence of the stimulation of stretch receptors in the pulmonary vessels and interstitium, as well as a result of hypoxemia and metabolic acidosis. The increased work of breathing, combined with a low cardiac output and resulting impaired perfusion of the respiratory muscles, causes fatigue[21] and ultimately the sensation of dyspnea.

Dyspnea occurs whenever the work of respiration is excessive. Increased force generation is required for the respiratory muscles to move a given volume of air if the compliance of the lungs is reduced

TABLE 15–5 MECHANISMS OF DYSPNEA IN HEART FAILURE

1. DECREASED PULMONARY FUNCTION
Decreased compliance
Increased airway resistance
2. INCREASED VENTILATORY DRIVE
Hypoxemia- ↑PCW
V/Q mismatching- ↑PCW, ↓CO
↑CO_2 production- ↓CO-lactic acidosis
3. RESPIRATORY MUSCLE DYSFUNCTION
Decreased strength
Decreased endurance
Ischemia

Abbreviations: PCW, mean pulmonary capillary wedge pressure; V/Q, ventilation/perfusion; CO, cardiac output; CO_2, carbon dioxide production.

From Mancini, D. M.: Pulmonary factors limiting exercise capacity in patients with heart failure. Prog. Cardiovasc. Dis. *37*:347, 1995.

or the resistance to air flow is increased[22,23]; both of these changes occur in left heart failure. Dyspnea at rest also may occur in the late stages of heart failure when the combination of very low cardiac output, hypoxemia, and acidosis conspires to reduce the delivery of oxygen to the respiratory muscle.[24] Dyspnea may occur *without* pulmonary congestion in patients with right ventricular failure, a fixed low cardiac output, and/or a right-to-left shunt.

Differentiation Between Cardiac and Pulmonary Dyspnea

In most patients with dyspnea there is obvious clinical evidence of disease of either the heart *or* the lungs, but in some the differentiation between cardiac and pulmonary dyspnea may be difficult.[19] Like patients with heart failure, those with chronic obstructive lung disease also may waken at night with dyspnea, but this is usually associated with sputum production; the dyspnea is relieved after patients rid themselves of secretions by coughing rather than specifically by sitting up. When the dyspnea arises after a history of intensified cough and expectoration, it is usually primarily pulmonary in origin. *Acute cardiac asthma* (paroxysmal nocturnal dyspnea with prominent wheezing) usually occurs in patients who have obvious clinical evidence of heart disease and may be further differentiated from acute bronchial asthma by diaphoresis and bubblier airway sounds and the more common occurrence of cyanosis.

The difficulty in distinguishing between cardiac and pulmonary dyspnea may be compounded by the coexistence of diseases involving both organ systems. Thus, patients with a history of chronic bronchitis or asthma who develop left ventricular failure tend to develop particularly severe bronchoconstriction and wheezing in association with bouts of paroxysmal nocturnal dyspnea and pulmonary edema. Airway obstruction and dyspnea that respond to bronchodilators or smoking cessation favor a pulmonary origin of the dyspnea, while the response of these manifestations to diuretics supports heart failure as the cause of dyspnea.

PULMONARY FUNCTION TESTING. This testing should be carried out in patients in whom the etiology of dyspnea is unclear despite detailed clinical evaluation. The results may be helpful in determining whether dyspnea is produced by heart disease, lung disease, a combination of the two, or neither.

The major alterations in pulmonary function tests in congestive heart failure are reductions of vital capacity, total lung capacity, pulmonary diffusion capacity at rest and particularly during exercise, and pulmonary compliance; resistance to air flow is moderately increased; residual volume and functional residual volume are normal. Often there is hyperventilation at rest and during exercise, an increase in dead space, and some abnormalities of ventilation-perfusion relations with slight reductions in arterial P_{CO_2} and P_{O_2}. With pulmonary capillary hypertension, pulmonary compliance decreases and there is air trapping because of earlier than normal closure of dependent airways. The airway resistance rises,[25] as does the work of breathing.

Rarely, it may be difficult to differentiate among cardiac dyspnea, dyspnea based on *malingering,* and dyspnea caused by an *anxiety neurosis.* Careful observation for the appearance of effortless or irregular respiration during exercise testing often helps to identify the patient in whom dyspnea is related to the latter two noncardiac causes. Patients whose anxiety neurosis focuses on the heart may exhibit sighing respiration and difficulty in taking a deep breath as well as dyspnea at rest. Their breathing patterns are not rapid and shallow, as in cardiac dyspnea. Rarely a "therapeutic test" is helpful, and amelioration of dyspnea, accompanied by a weight loss exceeding 2 kg induced by administration of a diuretic, supports a cardiac origin for the dyspnea. Conversely, failure of these measures to achieve weight reduction in excess of 2 kg and to diminish dyspnea weighs heavily against a cardiac origin.

Reduced Exercise Capacity

MECHANISMS OF EXERCISE INCOMPETENCE. A nearly universal manifestation of heart failure is a reduction in exercise capacity. Although exercise capacity may be limited for a variety of reasons in patients with heart failure, the most common causes are the development of dyspnea due to pulmonary vascular congestion and the failure of the cardiovascular system to provide sufficient blood flow to exercising muscles. The latter reflects primarily an inadequate cardiac output response to exercise due to reductions in stroke volume and heart rate.[26,27] In addition to the impaired central hemodynamic response to exercise, a number of other factors may contribute to reduced exercise capacity in patients with heart failure, including an attenuated peripheral vascular response,[28–30] abnormal skeletal muscle metabolism,[31] deconditioning of skeletal and respiratory muscles,[32,33] and patient anxiety related to the development of exertional symptoms. The importance of these additional factors is emphasized by the observation that the improvement in exercise capacity that occurs with long-term pharmacological therapy (e.g., converting enzyme inhibitors) requires weeks to develop and is dissociated temporally from the acute improvement in hemodynamics that occurs with the initiation of therapy. There is evidence that the judicious use of cardiac rehabilitation can improve functional capacity in patients with heart failure,[34,35] possibly by improving peripheral muscle blood flow, promoting skeletal muscle conditioning, and improving psychological outlook (Chap. 40).

Exercise Testing

(See also Chap. 5 and p. 439)

MAXIMAL EXERCISE CAPACITY. Exercise stress testing may be an exceedingly useful adjunct in the *clinical assessment* of patients with suspected or known heart failure.[36,37] With use of a cycle ergometer or treadmill with a progressively increasing load, the maximum level of exercise which can be achieved can be determined; the latter correlates closely with the total oxygen uptake ($\dot{V}_{O_2}$). Close observation of the patient during an exercise test may disclose obvious difficulty in breathing at a low level of exercise (or the opposite). Thus this simple test may be considered to be an extension of the clinical examination.

A more formal assessment in which $\dot{V}_{O_2}$ is measured at each stage of exercise, or preferably in which $\dot{V}_{O_2}$ and $\dot{V}_{CO_2}$ are measured continuously, allows determination of maximum $\dot{V}_{O_2}$ and the anaerobic threshold (i.e., the point during the exercise test at which the respiratory quotient rises as a consequence of the production of excess lactate)[25] (Figs. 5–1, p. 154, and 5–2, p. 156, and Fig. 14–29, p. 440). When a progressive exercise test is carried out until (1) $\dot{V}_{O_2}$ fails to rise with further increases in activity or (2) the patient is limited by severe dyspnea and/or fatigue, a $\dot{V}_{O_2}$ less than 25 mg/kg/min represents a reduction of maximum $\dot{V}_{O_2}$. When this reduction is caused by a cardiac abnormality (rather than by pulmonary disease, anemia, peripheral vascular disease, skeletal muscle deformity, marked obesity, severe deconditioning, or malingering), it may be used to classify the severity of heart failure, to follow the progress of the patient, and to assess the efficacy of therapeutic maneuvers.[36–38]

SUBMAXIMAL EXERCISE CAPACITY. Because usual daily activities generally require much less than maximal exercise capacity,[39–41] the measurement of submaximal exercise capacity may provide information that is complementary to that provided by maximum exercise testing. In contrast to maximal exercise capacity, which reflects the adequacy of the central hemodynamic response, the ability to sustain a submaximal exercise effort may reflect abnormalities in the regulation of peripheral blood flow and at the level of the skeletal musculature. There is no consensus as to the optimal way of measuring submaximal exercise capacity. In the

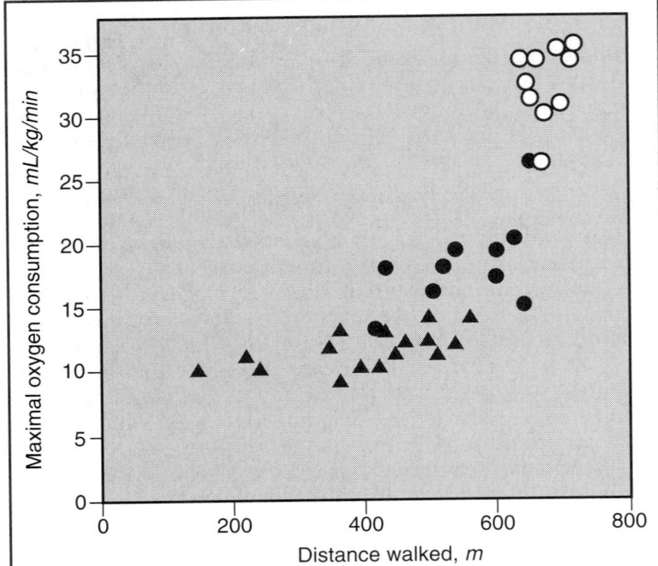

FIGURE 15–2. Relationship between the distance walked in 6 minutes and the peak $\dot{V}O_2$ in patients with mild (New York Heart Association functional Class II) symptoms of heart failure (triangles), moderate symptoms (NYHA Class III) (filled circles), and normal subjects (open circles) (×21). Because the 6-minute walk test involves only a submaximal exercise effort, it may be sensitive to changes in exercise function in the work range that is relevant to normal daily activities. (Adapted from Lipkin, D. P., et al.: Six minute walking test for assessing exercise capacity in chronic heart failure. BMJ *292*:653, 1986.)

exercise laboratory, submaximal exercise capacity can be assessed by measuring the duration of exercise at a constant workload that is generally chosen to be at or below the anaerobic threshold for the patient. A rough approximation of the submaximal exercise capacity can be obtained by measuring the distance walked in a fixed period of time. The "6-minute walk test," most common of the fixed-time tests, measures the distance walked on level ground in 6 minutes.[42–44] In this test, the patient is asked to walk in a level corridor as far as he or she can in 6 minutes. The patient can slow down or even stop, may be given a carefully controlled level of encouragement, and is told when 3 and 5 minutes have elapsed. The 6-minute walk test and other similar submaximal tests are being evaluated in clinical trials to determine if they are capable of detecting a therapeutic response. They appear to be predictive of maximal oxygen consumption (Fig. 15–2). Another form of submaximal exercise test measures the distance walked on a self-powered treadmill.[45]

Other Symptoms

FATIGUE AND WEAKNESS. These symptoms, often accompanied by a feeling of heaviness in the limbs, are generally related to poor perfusion of the skeletal muscles in patients with a lowered cardiac output. They may be associated with impaired vasodilation and altered metabolism in skeletal muscle.[24] Fatigue and weakness, of course, are notoriously nonspecific and may be caused by a variety of noncardiopulmonary diseases as well as by neurasthenia; they may be caused by sodium depletion, hypovolemia, or both, as a consequence of excessive treatment with diuretics and restriction of dietary sodium. Beta-adrenoreceptor blockers also may cause fatigue.

URINARY SYMPTOMS. *Nocturia* may occur relatively early in the course of heart failure. Urine formation is suppressed during the day when the patient is upright and active; this is due, at least in part, to a redistribution of blood flow away from the kidneys during activity.[46] When the patient rests in the recumbent position at night, the deficit in cardiac output in relation to oxygen demand is reduced, renal vasoconstriction diminishes, and urine formation increases. Nocturia may be troublesome in that it prevents the patient with heart failure from obtaining much-needed rest. The diurnal pattern of urine flow characteristic of heart failure contrasts sharply with that existing in renal failure, in which urine formation occurs at a reasonably constant rate, both day and night. *Oliguria* is a sign of late cardiac failure and is related to the suppression of urine formation as a consequence of severely reduced cardiac output.

CEREBRAL SYMPTOMS. Confusion, impairment of memory, anxiety, headache, insomnia, bad dreams or nightmares, and rarely, psychosis with disorientation, delirium, and even hallucinations may occur in elderly patients with advanced heart failure, particularly in those with accompanying cerebral arteriosclerosis.

SYMPTOMS OF PREDOMINANT RIGHT HEART FAILURE. Breathlessness is not as prominent in isolated right ventricular failure as it is in left heart failure because pulmonary congestion is usually absent. Indeed, when a patient with mitral stenosis or left ventricular failure develops right ventricular failure, the more severe forms of dyspnea (i.e., paroxysmal nocturnal dyspnea and episodic pulmonary edema) tend to diminish in frequency and intensity. This reduction results from an inability of the right ventricle to augment its output, which prevents the temporary imbalance between blood flow into and out of the pulmonary vascular bed. On the other hand, when cardiac output becomes markedly reduced in patients with terminal right heart failure, as may occur in isolated right ventricular infarction and in the late stages of primary pulmonary hypertension and of pulmonary thromboembolic disease, severe dyspnea (air hunger) may occur, presumably as a consequence of the reduced cardiac output, poor perfusion of respiratory muscles, hypoxemia, and metabolic acidosis. In addition, dyspnea may be a prominent symptom in some patients with right ventricular failure and anasarca, hydrothorax, and ascites as a consequence of lung compression; such patients may even have orthopnea.

Congestive hepatomegaly may produce discomfort, generally described as a dull ache or heaviness, in the right upper quadrant or epigastrium. This discomfort, which is caused by stretching of the hepatic capsule, may be severe when the liver enlarges rapidly, as in acute right heart failure. In contrast, chronic, slowly developing hepatic enlargement is generally painless. Other gastrointestinal symptoms, including anorexia, nausea, bloating, a sense of fullness after meals, and constipation, occur owing to congestion of the liver and gastrointestinal tract. In severe, preterminal heart failure, inadequate bowel perfusion can cause abdominal pain, distention, and bloody stools. Nausea, anorexia, and emesis also may be due to cardiac drugs, particularly digitalis (see p. 484).

Functional Classification

A classification of patients with heart disease based on the relation between symptoms and the amount of effort required to provoke them has been developed by the New York Heart Association.[47] Although there are obvious limitations to assigning numerical values to subjective findings, this classification is nonetheless useful in comparing groups of patients as well as the same patient at different times.

Class I—*No limitation:* Ordinary physical activity does not cause undue fatigue, dyspnea, or palpitation.

Class II—*Slight limitation of physical activity:* Such patients are comfortable at rest. Ordinary physical activity results in fatigue, palpitation, dyspnea, or angina.

Class III—*Marked limitation of physical activity:* Although patients are comfortable at rest, less than ordinary activity will lead to symptoms.

Class IV—*Inability to carry on any physical activity without discomfort:* Symptoms of congestive failure are present even at rest. With any physical activity, increased discomfort is experienced.

As discussed on page 13, the accuracy and reproducibility of this classification are limited. To overcome these limitations, Goldman et al. have developed a useful classification based on the estimated metabolic cost of various activities[48] (Table 1–7, p. 12).

QUALITY OF LIFE. A good "quality of life" implies the ability to live as one wants, free of physical, social, emotional, and economic limitations. Heart failure can have an enormous deleterious impact on the quality of life. Although a number of questionnaires are available to assess quality of life, the Minnesota Living with Heart Failure (MLHF) questionnaire was designed specifically for use in these patients[49–51] (Fig. 15–3). It consists of 21 brief questions, each of which is answered on a scale of 0 to 5. Eight questions have a strong relationship to the symptoms of dyspnea and fatigue and are referred to as *physical dimension measures.* Five other questions that are strongly related to emotional issues are referred to as *emotional dimension measures.* The test is self-administered and takes only 5 to 10 minutes to complete. For each question, the patient selects a number from 0 to 5. Zero indicates that heart failure had no effect, and 5 indicates a very large effect. Although such questionnaires have little role in routine clinical management of patients, they have provided valuable information in research settings by allowing the response to various therapies to be quantified.

Physical Findings

GENERAL APPEARANCE. Patients with mild or moderate heart failure appear to be in no distress after a few minutes of rest. However, they may be obviously dyspneic during and immediately after moderate activity. Patients with left ventricular failure may become uncomfortable if they lie flat without elevation of the head for more than a few minutes. Those with severe heart failure appear anxious and may exhibit signs of air hunger in this position. Patients with heart failure of recent onset appear acutely ill but are ordinarily well nourished, whereas those with chronic cardiac failure often appear malnourished and sometimes even cachectic. Chronic, marked elevation of systemic venous pressure may produce exophthalmos and severe tricuspid regurgitation and may lead to visible systolic pulsation of the eyes[52] and of the neck veins. Cyanosis, icterus, and a malar flush may be evident in patients with severe heart failure.

In mild or moderately severe heart failure, stroke volume is normal at rest; in severe heart failure, it is reduced, and this is reflected in a diminished pulse pressure and dusky discoloration of the skin. With very severe failure, particularly if cardiac output has declined acutely, systolic arterial pressure may be reduced. The pulse may be rapid, weak, and thready. The proportional pulse pressure (pulse pressure/systolic pressure) correlates reasonably well with cardiac output. In one study,[14] when it was less than 25 per cent, it usually reflected a cardiac index of less than 2.2 liters/min/m^2.

EVIDENCE OF INCREASED ADRENERGIC ACTIVITY. Increased activity of the adrenergic nervous system is an important accompaniment of heart failure. It is responsible for a number of physical signs, including peripheral vasoconstriction, which is manifested as pallor and coldness of the extremities and cyanosis of the digits. There may be diaphoresis with sinus tachycardia, loss of normal sinus rhythm, and obvious distention of the peripheral veins secondary to venoconstriction. Diastolic arterial pressure may be slightly elevated.

PULMONARY RALES. Moist rales result from the transudation into the alveoli of fluid, which then moves into the airways. Rales heard over the lung bases are characteristic of congestive heart failure of at least moderate severity. In acute pulmonary edema, coarse, bubbling rales and wheezes are heard over both lung fields and are accompanied by the expectoration of frothy, blood-tinged sputum (see p. 464). However, the absence of rales by no means excludes considerable elevation of pulmonary capillary pressure. With congestion of the bronchial mucosa, excessive bronchial secretions or bronchospasm or both may give rise to rhonchi and wheezes. Rales are usually heard at both lung bases, but if unilateral, they occur more commonly on the right side. When rales are audible *only* over the left lung in a patient with heart failure, they may signify the presence of pulmonary embolism to that lung.

SYSTEMIC VENOUS HYPERTENSION (see also p. 18). This can be detected more readily by inspection of the jugular veins, which provides a useful index of right atrial pressure.[53,54] The upper limit of normal of the jugular venous pressure is approximately 4 cm above the sternal angle when the patient is examined at a 45-degree angle. When tricuspid regurgitation is present, the *v* wave and *y* descent are most prominent; however, with impedance to right ventricular filling (tricuspid stenosis) or right ventricular emptying (pulmonary hypertension, pulmonic stenosis), the *a* wave is most prominent. The jugular venous pressure normally declines on exertion, but in patients with heart failure (and in those with constrictive pericarditis; see p. 1496) it rises, a finding known as *Kussmaul's sign.* Rarely, venous pressure may be so high that the peripheral veins on the dorsum of the hands or in the temporal region are dilated.

HEPATOJUGULAR REFLUX (see also p. 19). In patients with mild right heart failure, the jugular venous pressure may be normal at rest but rises to abnormal levels with compression of the right upper quadrant, a sign known as the *hepatojugular reflux.* To elicit this sign, the right upper quadrant should be compressed firmly, gradually, and continuously for 1 minute while the veins of the neck are observed. The patient should be advised to avoid straining, holding the breath, or carrying out a Valsalva maneuver. A positive test (i.e., expansion of the jugular veins during and immediately after compression) usually reflects the combination of a congested abdomen and inability of the right side of the heart to accept or reject the transiently increased venous return. Thus a positive abdominojugular reflux is helpful in differentiating hepatic enlargement caused by heart failure from that caused by other conditions.

CONGESTIVE HEPATOMEGALY. The liver often enlarges *before* overt edema develops, and it may remain so even after other symptoms of right-sided heart failure have disappeared. Inspection of the abdomen may reveal epigastric fullness and, on percussion, dullness in the right upper quadrant. If hepatomegaly has occurred rapidly and relatively recently, the liver is usually tender, owing to stretching of its capsule. In longstanding heart failure this tenderness disappears, even though the liver remains enlarged.

In patients with tricuspid regurgitation, the prominent right atrial *v* wave may be transmitted to the liver, which pulsates during systole. A prominent presystolic pulsation in the liver owing to an enlarged right atrial *a* wave can occur in tricuspid stenosis, constrictive pericarditis, restrictive cardiomyopathy involving the right ventricle, pulmonary hypertension, and pulmonic stenosis.

EDEMA. Although a cardinal manifestation of congestive heart failure, edema does not correlate well with the level of systemic venous pressure. In patients with chronic left ventricular failure and a low cardiac output, extracellular fluid volume may be sufficiently expanded to cause edema in the presence of only slight elevations of systemic venous pressure. A substantial gain of extracellular fluid volume, a minimum of 5 liters in adults, must usually take place

LIVING WITH HEART FAILURE QUESTIONNAIRE

These questions concern how your heart failure (heart condition) has prevented you from living as you wanted during the last month. The items listed below describe different ways some people are affected. If you are sure an item does not apply to you or is not related to your heart failure then circle 0 (No) and go on to the next item. If an item does apply to you, then circle the number rating how much it prevented you from living as you wanted. Remember to think about ONLY THE LAST MONTH.

DID YOUR HEART FAILURE PREVENT YOU FROM LIVING AS YOU WANTED DURING THE LAST MONTH BY:	NO	VERY LITTLE				VERY MUCH
1. causing swelling in your ankles, legs, etc?	0	1	2	3	4	5
2. making you sit or lie down to rest during the day?	0	1	2	3	4	5
3. making your walking about or climbing stairs difficult?	0	1	2	3	4	5
4. making your working around the house or yard difficult?	0	1	2	3	4	5
5. making your going places away from home difficult?	0	1	2	3	4	5
6. making your sleeping well at night difficult?	0	1	2	3	4	5
7. making your relating to or doing things with your friends or family difficult?	0	1	2	3	4	5
8. making your working to earn a living difficult?	0	1	2	3	4	5
9. making your recreational pastimes, sports or hobbies difficult?	0	1	2	3	4	5
10. making your sexual activities difficult?	0	1	2	3	4	5
11. making you eat less of the foods you like?	0	1	2	3	4	5
12. making you short of breath?	0	1	2	3	4	5
13. making you tired, fatigued, or low on energy?	0	1	2	3	4	5
14. making you stay in a hospital?	0	1	2	3	4	5
15. costing you money for medical care?	0	1	2	3	4	5
16. giving you side effects from medications?	0	1	2	3	4	5
17. making you feel you are a burden to your family or friends?	0	1	2	3	4	5
18. making you feel a loss of self-control in your life?	0	1	2	3	4	5
19. making you worry?	0	1	2	3	4	5
20. making it difficult for you to concentrate or remember things?	0	1	2	3	4	5
21. making you feel depressed?	0	1	2	3	4	5

FIGURE 15–3. The Minnesota Living with Heart Failure questionnaire. Improvement in quality of life is one of two primary goals of therapy (prolonged survival being the other). This measure of quality of life, which has been used in many investigations of treatments for heart failure, defines quality of life as living as one wants with minimal limitations secondary to heart failure and its treatment. Physical, social, emotional, and economic limitations are included. Patients self-administer the questions after listening to a standard set of instructions. The score is the sum of the responses for all 21 questions. Eight questions including dyspnea and fatigue are highly interrelated and their sum is called the *physical dimension.* Similarly, five interrelated questions comprise an *emotional dimension.* (Adapted from Rector, T. S., and Cohn, J. N.: Assessment of patient outcome with the Minnesota Living with Heart Failure questionnaire: Reliability and validity during a randomized, double-blind, placebo controlled trial of pimobendan. Am. Heart J. *124:*1017, 1992.)

before peripheral edema is manifested. Therefore, edema may develop over a number of days and may not be present initially in patients with acute heart failure and marked systemic venous hypertension.

Edema is usually symmetrical, pitting, and generally occurs first in the dependent portions of the body, where the systemic venous pressure rises to its highest levels. Accordingly, cardiac edema in ambulatory patients is usually first noted in the feet or ankles at the end of the day and generally resolves after a night's rest. In bedridden patients it is most commonly found over the sacrum. Facial edema seldom appears in adults with heart failure but may occur in infants and young children. Late in the course of heart failure, edema may become massive and generalized (anasarca). Longstanding edema results in pigmentation, reddening, and induration of the skin of the lower extremities, usually the dorsum of the feet and the pretibial areas.

HYDROTHORAX (PLEURAL EFFUSION). Because the pleural veins drain into both the systemic and the pulmonary venous beds, hydrothorax is observed most commonly in patients with hypertension involving both venous systems, but it also may occur when there is marked elevation of pressure in either venous bed. An increase in capillary permeability probably also plays a role in the pathogenesis of cardiac hydrothorax, since the protein content of the pleural fluid may be significantly greater (2 to 3 gm/dl) than that found in edema fluid (0.5 gm/dl). Hydrothorax is usually bilateral, but when unilateral it is usually confined to the right side of the chest. When hydrothorax develops, dyspnea usually intensifies, owing to a further reduction in vital capacity. Although the excess fluid in hydrothorax is usually resorbed as heart failure improves, sometimes interlobar effusions persist.

ASCITES. This finding occurs in patients with increased pressure in the hepatic veins and in the veins draining the peritoneum. Ascites usually reflects longstanding systemic venous hypertension. In patients with organic tricuspid valve disease and chronic constrictive pericarditis, ascites may be more prominent than subcutaneous edema. As in the case of hydrothorax, there is increased capillary permeability because the protein content is similar to that of hepatic lymph (i.e., four to six times that of edema fluid). Protein-losing enteropathy may occur in patients with visceral congestion,[55] and the resultant reduced plasma oncotic pressure may lower the threshold for the development of ascites.

Cardiac Findings

The presence of cardiac disease is usually readily evident on clinical examination of patients with congestive heart failure.

CARDIOMEGALY. This finding is nonspecific and occurs in the majority of patients with chronic heart failure. Notable exceptions are heart failure associated with chronic constrictive pericarditis, restrictive cardiomyopathy, and a variety of acute insults such as acute myocardial infarction, the sudden development of tachyarrhythmias or bradyarrhythmias, or rupture of a valve or chordae tendineae; in such circumstances heart failure may develop before the heart has had a chance to enlarge.

GALLOP SOUNDS. Protodiastolic sounds, generally emanating from the left ventricle (but occasionally from the right) and occurring 0.13 to 0.16 seconds after the second heart sound, are common findings in healthy children and young adults. Such physiological sounds are seldom audible in healthy persons after age 40 but occur in patients of all ages with heart failure and are referred to as *protodiastolic,* or *S_3, gallops.* In older adults they generally signify the presence of heart failure (see p. 35). In patients with mitral or tricuspid regurgitation or left-to-right shunts, rapid (torrential) flow into the ventricle in early diastole contributes to the generation of an S_3 (see p. 35), but under these conditions this sound is *not* to be interpreted as signifying the presence of heart failure. Thus, a protodiastolic gallop sound is an excellent sign of heart failure when other causes, such as a physiological S_3 occurring in a healthy child or young adult, constrictive pericarditis, mitral and tricuspid regurgitation, or a left-to-right shunt, can be excluded.

PULSUS ALTERNANS (see also p. 22). This sign is characterized by a regular rhythm with alternating strong and weak ventricular contractions. It should be distinguished from the alternation of strong and weak beats that occurs in pulsus bigeminus, in which the weak beat follows the strong beat by a shorter time interval than the strong beat follows the weak, whereas in pulsus alternans they are equally spaced or the weak beat is slightly closer to the succeeding than to the preceding beat. Severe pulsus alternans may be detected either by palpation of the peripheral pulses (the femoral more readily than the brachial, radial, or carotid) or by sphygmomanometry. As the cuff is slowly deflated, only alternate beats are audible for a variable number of millimeters of mercury below the systolic level, depending on the severity of the alternans, and then all beats are heard. Rarely, the weak beat is so small that the aortic valve is not opened, and this results in an apparent halving of the pulse rate, a condition referred to as *total alternans.* Pulsus alternans may be accompanied by alternation in the intensity of the heart sounds and of existing heart murmurs.

Pulsus alternans occurs most commonly in heart failure secondary to increased resistance to left ventricular ejection, as occurs in systemic hypertension and aortic stenosis, as well as in coronary atherosclerosis and dilated cardiomyopathy. It is usually associated with a ventricular protodiastolic gallop sound (S_3), signifies advanced myocardial disease, and often disappears with treatment of heart failure. In patients with heart failure, pulsus alternans often can be elicited by reduction in systemic venous return, as occurs with assumption of the erect posture or application of venous tourniquets, and it is reduced by an increase in venous return, as in recumbency or with exercise. Pulsus alternans tends to be present during tachycardia and is often initiated by a premature beat.

Pulsus alternans is attributed to an alternation in the stroke volume ejected by the left ventricle[56] and, ultimately, to a deletion in the number of contracting cells in every other cycle, presumably owing to incomplete recovery. Alternans is almost always concordant in the two sides of the circulation; i.e., the strong and weak beats occur simultaneously in the two ventricles. Rarely, pulsus alternans is accompanied by *electrical alternans;* however, the latter condition is usually not due to mechanical alternans but to alternating positions of the heart within the fluid-filled pericardial sac (Fig. 3–103, p. 93).

ACCENTUATION OF P_2 AND SYSTOLIC MURMURS. With the development of left ventricular failure, pulmonary artery pressure rises and P_2 becomes accentuated—often louder than A_2—and more widely transmitted. As left ventricular failure improves, P_2 becomes softer. *Systolic murmurs* are common in heart failure owing to the relative mitral or tricuspid regurgitation that may occur secondary to ventricular dilatation. Often these murmurs diminish or disappear when compensation is restored.

FEVER. A low-grade temperature (<38°C), which results from cutaneous vasoconstriction and therefore impairment of heat loss, may occur in severe heart failure; fever usually subsides when compensation is restored. Greater elevations of temperature usually signify the presence of an infection, pulmonary infarction, or infective endocarditis.

CARDIAC CACHEXIA. Longstanding, severe congestive heart failure, particularly of the right ventricle, may lead to anorexia, owing to hepatic and intestinal congestion and sometimes to digitalis intoxication. Occasionally, there is impaired intestinal absorption of fat[57] and rarely protein-losing enteropathy.[55] Patients with heart failure also may exhibit increased total metabolism secondary to (1) an augmentation of myocardial oxygen consumption, as occurs in patients with aortic stenosis and hypertension, (2) excessive work of breathing, (3) low-grade fever, and (4) elevated levels of circulating tumor necrosis factor.[58] This cytokine is produced by monocytes and causes cachexia and anorexia. The combination of reduced caloric intake and increased caloric expenditure, however produced, may lead to a reduction of tissue mass and, in severe cases, to cardiac cachexia.[59,60] In some patients the cachexia may be severe enough to suggest the presence of disseminated malignant disease. In others, the loss of lean body mass may be masked by the accumulation of edema. There is evidence that inflammatory cytokines, including tumor necrosis factor-alpha, may depress myocardial contractility,[61–63] modulate the growth and phenotype of various cells in the myocardium,[64] and contribute to cardiac cachexia.

CHEYNE-STOKES RESPIRATION. Also known as *periodic* or *cyclic respiration,* Cheyne-Stokes respiration is characterized by the combination of depression in the sensitivity of the respiratory center to carbon dioxide and left ventricular failure.[65,66] During the apneic phase, arterial PO_2 falls and PCO_2 rises; this combination excites the depressed respiratory center, resulting in hyperventilation and, subsequently, hypocapnia, followed by another period of apnea. The principal causes of depression of the respiratory center in patients with Cheyne-Stokes respiration are cerebral lesions such as cerebral arteriosclerosis, stroke, or head injury. These causes are often exaggerated by sleep, barbiturates, and narcotics, all of which further depress the sensitivity of the respiratory center. Left ventricular failure, which prolongs the circulation time from the lung to the brain, results in a sluggish response of the system and is responsible for the oscillations between apnea and hyperpnea and prevents return to a steady state of ventilation and blood gases. Usually patients are not aware of Cheyne-Stokes respiration. However, it can be readily observed in a sleeping patient, or a history can be elicited from the patient's bed partner. Cheyne-Stokes respiration may contribute to daytime sleepiness in such patients,[67] and occasionally the patient with heart failure awakens at night with dyspnea precipitated by Cheyne-Stokes respiration.[68] Ventilatory oscillations also may occur during exercise and appear to reflect oscillations in the circulation.[69]

LUNGS. In patients who have died of left ventricular failure, the lungs are enlarged, firm, and dark and may be filled with bloody fluid. With longstanding pulmonary congestion, they are brown with deposition of hemosiderin and usually do not seep edema fluid. On microscopic examination, the capillaries are engorged, and there is thickening of the alveolar septa as well as extravasation of large mononuclear cells containing red blood cells or hemosiderin granules or both.[70] Often the pulmonary vessels show medial hypertrophy and intimal hyperplasia.

LIVER. In acute right heart failure, the liver is enlarged, firm, and filled with fluid. On microscopic examination, the central hepatic veins and sinusoids are dilated.[71,72] With longstanding right heart failure, the liver returns to normal size, subsequently atrophies, and becomes "nutmeg" in appearance as a consequence of the dark red areas of central venous congestion and the lighter, fatty area in the periphery of the lobule. Cardiac cirrhosis is characterized by central lobular necrosis and atrophy as well as extensive fibrous retraction; sometimes there is sclerosis of the hepatic veins. Because cardiac cirrhosis is a function of the level of hepatic venous pressure and the duration of its elevation, it is not surprising that it occurs most commonly in patients with chronic constrictive pericarditis and organic tricuspid valve disease and in children after a Fontan procedure for tricuspid atresia (see p. 933),[73,74] who often have prolonged elevation of systemic venous pressure. In patients with left ventricular failure, central hepatic necrosis without evidence of passive congestion may be present.[75,76]

Liver biopsies in patients with acute heart failure exhibiting fulminant hepatic failure show replacement of hepatocytes by red blood cells. Presumably, the hypoxia caused by hypoperfusion produces hepatocyte necrosis[77,78]; erythrocytes may then enter the space of Disse between damaged endothelial cells. These changes resulting from acute heart failure may be transient if there is hemodynamic recovery.

OTHER VISCERA. Patients with chronic hepatic venous hypertension develop portal hypertension that results in congestive splenomegaly. On microscopic examination, the spleen shows dilatation of the sinusoids and fibrosis, and there is chronic passive congestion of the pancreas and of the veins and capillaries of the gastrointestinal tract. Rarely, intense mesenteric vasoconstriction without thrombotic or embolic occlusion of a mesenteric artery may lead to a hemorrhagic, nonbacterial enterocolitis, with hemorrhagic necrosis.

Chronic venous congestion also occurs in the kidney and brain, with dilation and engorgement of the capillaries. Small infarcts are frequently observed in the spleen and kidneys of patients with longstanding atrial fibrillation.

Laboratory Findings

Proteinuria and a high urine specific gravity are common findings in heart failure. Blood urea nitrogen and creatinine levels are often moderately elevated secondary to reductions in renal blood flow and glomerular filtration rate[12] (prerenal azotemia). The erythrocyte sedimentation rate is usually quite low, presumably secondary to impaired fibrinogen synthesis and resultant decreased fibrinogen concentrations.

SERUM ELECTROLYTES. Serum electrolyte values are generally normal in patients with mild or moderate heart failure before treatment. However, in severe heart failure, prolonged, rigid sodium restriction, coupled with intensive diuretic therapy as well as the inability to excrete water, may lead to dilutional hyponatremia, which occurs because of substantial expansion of extracellular fluid volume and a normal or increased level of total body sodium. It may be accompanied by, and presumably is caused in part by, elevated concentrations of circulating vasopressin.[79] Serum potassium levels are usually normal, although the prolonged administration of kaliuretic diuretics, such as the thiazides or loop diuretics, may result in hypokalemia (see p. 849). Hyperkalemia may occur in patients with severe heart failure[80] who show marked reductions in glomerular filtration rate and inadequate delivery of sodium to the distal tubular sodium-potassium exchange sites, particularly if such patients are also receiving potassium-retaining diuretics and/or converting enzyme.

LIVER FUNCTION TESTS. Congestive hepatomegaly and cardiac cirrhosis are often associated with impaired hepatic function, characterized by abnormal values of aspartate aminotransferase (AST), alanine aminotransferase (ALT), lactic dehydrogenase (LDH), and other liver enzymes.[81,82] Hyperbilirubinemia, secondary to an increase in both the directly and indirectly reacting bilirubins, is common, and in severe cases of acute (right or left) ventricular failure, frank jaundice may occur. *Acute* hepatic venous congestion can result in severe jaundice with a bilirubin level as high as 15 to 20 mg/dl, elevation of AST to more than 10 times the upper limit of normal, and elevation of the serum alkaline phosphatase level, as well as prolongation of the prothrombin time. Both the clinical and the laboratory pictures may resemble viral hepatitis, but the impairment of hepatic function is rapidly ameliorated by successful treatment of heart failure. In patients with longstanding cardiac cirrhosis, albumin synthesis may be impaired, with resultant hypoalbuminemia, intensifying the accumulation of fluid. Hepatic hypoglycemia, fulminant hepatic failure, and hepatic coma are uncommon, late, and sometimes terminal complications of cardiac cirrhosis. In general, disturbances of hepatic function are frequent when right atrial pressure rises above 10 mm Hg and cardiac index declines below 1.5/min/m^2.[82]

VENOUS PRESSURE. This can be conveniently measured with a spinal fluid manometer with the patient in the recumbent position and the arm abducted. The baseline for the measurement should be 5 cm below the sternal angle (i.e., the estimated position of the right atrium). The venous pressure is often elevated (i.e., >12 cm H_2O) at rest, but in mild or borderline cases it may be normal at rest but rises with hepatic compression or during exercise.

THE VALSALVA MANEUVER. Performance of this maneuver—forced expiration against a closed glottis—is helpful in the diagnosis of heart failure.[83,84] The test has been standardized as follows: The patient is asked to blow against an aneroid manometer and maintain a pressure of 40 mm Hg for 30 seconds. During the Valsalva maneuver, intrathoracic pressure rises, venous return to the heart diminishes, stroke volume falls, and venous pressure rises. Arterial pressure tracings normally show four distinct phases: (1) an initial rise in arterial pressure, which represents transmission to the periphery of the increased intrathoracic pressure; (2) with continuation of the strain and the accompanying reduction of venous return, reductions in systolic, diastolic, and pulse pressures accompanied by a reflex increase in heart rate; (3) on release of the strain, a sudden drop of arterial pressure equivalent to the fall in intrathoracic pressure; and (4) an overshoot of arterial pressure to above control levels, with a wide pulse pressure and bradycardia due to the combination of the inrush into the heart of blood that had been dammed up in the venous bed and reflex vasoconstriction and tachycardia secondary to the low perfusion pressure of the carotid and baroreceptors during phase 3.

In heart failure, phase 1 and 3 are normal; that is, there is normal transmission of the elevated intrathoracic pressure into the arterial tree during phase 1 and sudden loss of this with the release of the strain during phase 3. However, because the heart operates on the flat portion of its Starling curve (Fig. 13–2, p. 395), the impedance of venous return during phase 2 does not affect stroke volume. Therefore, the baroreceptor reflex is not activated, and there is no overshoot on release of the strain. This results in a "square-wave" appearance of the tracing. The abnormal blood pressure response is associated with "pseudonormalization" of the transmitral filling velocity pattern observed by Doppler echocardiography.

Although the Valsalva maneuver can be recorded most accurately through an indwelling needle, careful palpation of the pulse in normal individuals allows detection of phases 2 and 4 and their absence and slowing of the pulse in phase 4.[85] An automated device which monitors the arterial pulse in a finger has been used to detect an abnormal Valsalva response.[86]

The Chest Roentgenogram

(See also Chap. 7, pp. 228 to 229)

Two principal features of the chest roentgenogram are useful in the patient with congestive heart failure.

The *size and shape of the cardiac silhouette* provide important information concerning the precise nature of the underlying heart disease. Both the cardiothoracic ratio (Fig. 7–24, p. 220) and the heart volume determined on the plain film[87] are relatively specific but insensitive indicators of increased left ventricular end-diastolic volume.

In the presence of normal pulmonary capillary and venous pressure in the erect position, the lung bases are better perfused than the apices, and the vessels supplying the lower lobes are significantly larger than are those supplying the upper lobes.[88] With elevation of left atrial, pulmonary venous, and capillary pressures, interstitial and

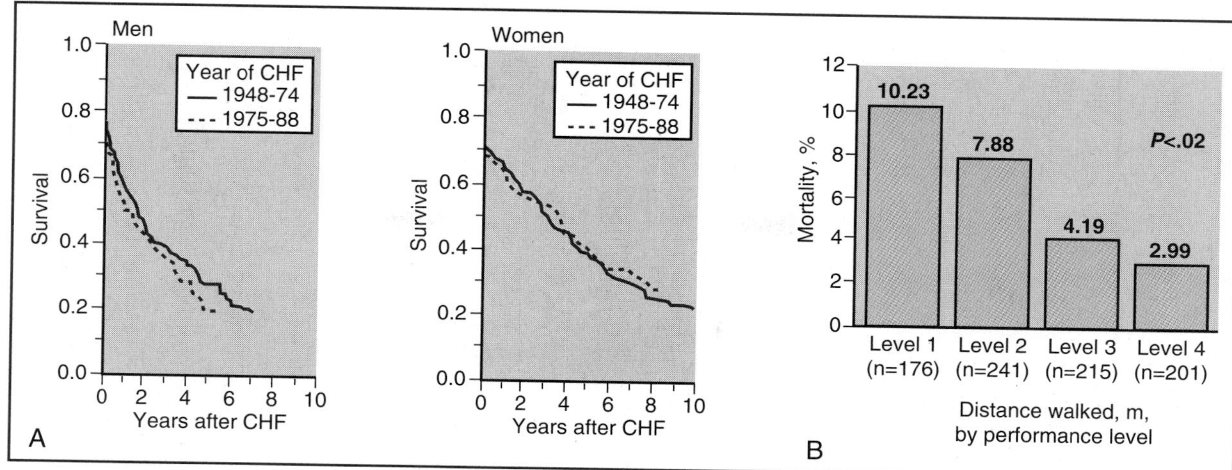

FIGURE 15–4. *A,* Graphs show age-adjusted survival rates after congestive heart failure (CHF) by calendar year of first diagnosis of CHF for men and women developing CHF during the calendar years 1948–1988. (From Ho, K. K. L., et al.: Survival after the onset of congestive heart failure in Framingham Heart Study subjects. Circulation *88:*107–115, 1993.) *B,* Mortality (%) as a function of performance level (base on distance walked). Mortality decreased as performance on the 6-minute walk test improved. (From Bittner, V., et al.: Prediction of mortality and morbidity with a 6-minute walk test in patients with left ventricular dysfunction. JAMA *270:*1702–1707, 1993. Copyright 1993 American Medical Association.)

perivascular edema develops and is most prominent at the lung bases because hydrostatic pressure is greater there. When pulmonary capillary pressure is slightly elevated, i.e., approximately 13 to 17 mm Hg,[89] the resultant compression of pulmonary vessels in the lower lobes causes equalization in size of the vessels at the apices and bases. With greater pressure elevation (approximately 18 to 23 mm Hg), actual pulmonary vascular redistribution occurs (i.e., further constriction of vessels leading to the lower lobes and dilatation of vessels leading to the upper lobes). When pulmonary capillary pressures exceed approximately 20 to 25 mm Hg, interstitial pulmonary edema occurs. This may be of several varieties: (1) *septal,* producing Kerley's lines (i.e., sharp, linear densities of interlobular interstitial edema) (p. 220); (2) *perivascular,* producing loss of sharpness of the central and peripheral vessels; and (3) *subpleural,* producing spindle-shaped accumulations of fluid between the lung and adjacent pleural surface. When pulmonary capillary pressure exceeds 25 mm Hg, alveolar edema, with a cloudlike appearance and concentration of the fluid around the hili in a "butterfly" pattern, and large pleural effusions may occur (Fig. 7–23, p. 219). With elevation of systemic venous pressure, the azygos vein and superior vena cava may enlarge.[90]

PROGNOSIS

SURVIVAL. Survival is reduced in patients with heart failure, which accounts for a substantial portion of all deaths from cardiovascular diseases. The Framingham Heart Study found that between the years of 1948 and 1988, patients with a diagnosis of heart failure had a median survival of 3.2 years for males and 5.4 years for females,[91] despite the fact that the patients with the poorest prognosis, i.e., those dying within 90 days of the diagnosis, were excluded from the analysis (Fig. 15–4*A*).

A large number of factors have been found to correlate with mortality in patients with congestive heart failure due to dilated cardiomyopathy (Table 15–6).[92] These fall into four major categories:

1. **Clinical.** In general, the presence of coronary artery disease as the etiology of heart failure, the presence of an audible S_3, low pulse and systolic arterial pressures, a high New York Heart Association Class, reduced exercise capacity, male gender (Figs. 15–4*B* and 15–5*A*), and the severity of symptoms (Fig. 15–6) have each been shown to be associated with a high mortality. When the NYHA Class is integrated with the maximal O_2 consumption determined during exercise, the mortality is 20 per cent per year in patients in Class III with a $\dot{V}O_{2\,max}$ of 10 to 15 ml/kg/min and rises to 60 per cent in patients in Class IV with a $\dot{V}O_{2\,max}$ of less than 10 ml/kg/min.[93–95] The distance walked in 6 minutes predicted both morbidity and mortality in the SOLVD trial[96] (Fig. 15–4*B*).

TABLE 15–6 FACTORS AFFECTING SURVIVAL IN PATIENTS WITH CONGESTIVE HEART FAILURE

1. CLINICAL
Coronary artery disease etiology
New York Heart Association Class
Exercise capacity
Heart rate at rest
Systolic arterial pressure
Pulse pressure
S_3
2. HEMODYNAMIC
LV ejection fraction
RV ejection fraction
LV stroke work index
LV filling pressure
Right atrial pressure
Maximal O_2 uptake
LV systolic pressure
Mean arterial pressure
Cardiac index
Systemic vascular resistance
3. BIOCHEMICAL
Plasma norepinephrine
Plasma renin
Plasma vasopressin
Plasma atrial natriuretic peptide
Serum sodium
Serum potassium
Total potassium stores
Serum magnesium
4. ELECTROPHYSIOLOGICAL
Frequent ventricular asystole
Complex ventricular arrhythmias
Ventricular tachycardia
Atrial fibrillation/flutter

Modified from Cohn, J. N., and Rector, T. S.: Prognosis of congestive heart failure and predictors of mortality. Am. J. Cardiol. *62:*25A, 1988.

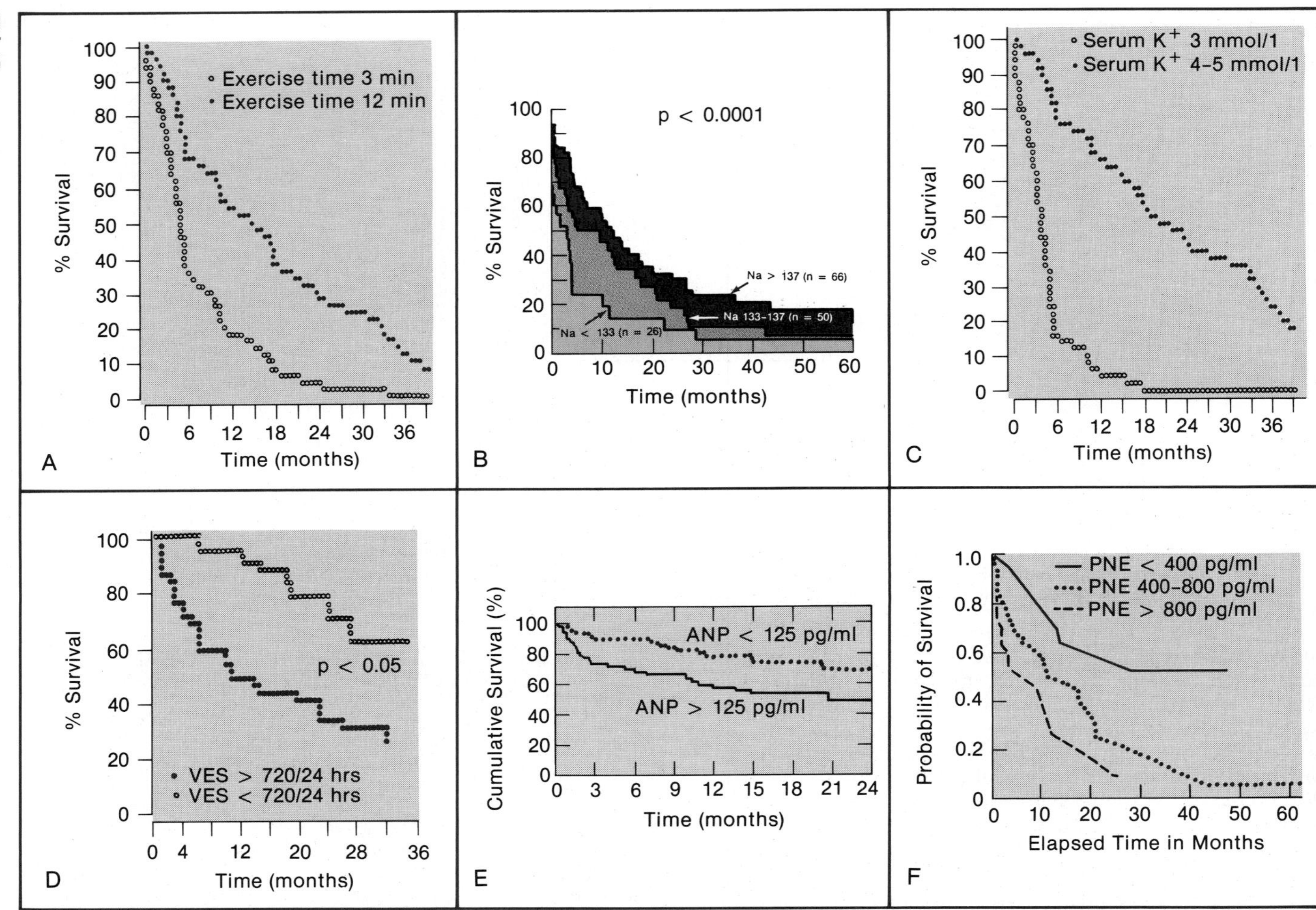

FIGURE 15–5. *A,* Estimated survival curve for patients with a short or a long exercise time in the modified Bruce protocol. Values were chosen arbitrarily. Patients had other important prognostic factors fixed at median values and were assumed to have coronary artery disease but not to be taking amiodarone. (From Cleland, J. G. F., Dargie, H. J., and Ford, I.: Mortality in heart failure: Clinical variables of prognostic value. Br. Heart J. *58*:572, 1987.) *B,* Kaplan-Meier analysis showing cumulative rates of survival in patients with severe chronic heart failure stratified into three groups based on pretreatment serum sodium concentration. Hyponatremic patients fared significantly worse than patients with a normal serum sodium concentration ($p < .0001$, Mantel-Cox). (From Packer, M., et al.: Role of neurohormonal mechanisms in determining survival in patients with severe chronic heart failure. Circulation *75* (Suppl. 4):80, 92, 1987, by permission of the American Heart Association, Inc.) *C,* Estimated survival curve for patients with a high or a low initial mean serum concentration of potassium. Values were chosen arbitrarily. Patients had other important prognostic factors fixed at median values and were assumed to have coronary artery disease but not to be taking amiodarone. (From Cleland, J. G. F., Dargie, H. J., and Ford, I.: Mortality in heart failure: Clinical variables of prognostic value. Br. Heart J. *58*:572, 1987.)

D, Relation between ventricular arrhythmia and survival in heart failure. VES = ventricular ectopic activity. (From Dargie, H. J., et al.: Relation of arrhythmias and electrolyte abnormalities to survival in patients with severe chronic heart failure. Circulation *75*:98, 1987, by permission of the American Heart Association, Inc.) *E,* Kaplan-Meier analysis of cumulative rates of survival in patients with heart failure stratified into two groups on the basis of median plasma concentration of atrial natriuretic peptide (ANP) (125 pg/ml). From Gottlieb, S. S., et al.: Prognostic importance of atrial natriuretic peptide in patients with chronic heart failure. Reprinted with permission from the American College of Cardiology. J. Am. Coll. Cardiol. *13*:1534, 1989.) *F,* Life-table analysis of survival, according to Tercile, based on level of plasma norepinephrine (PNE). Group 1 (<400 pg/ml) contained 27 patients, group 2 (400 to 800 pg/ml) 49 patients, and group 3 (>800 pg/ml) 30 patients. The probability of survival in each group was significantly different from the probabilities in the other two groups. (From Cohn, J. N., et al.: Plasma norepinephrine as a guide to prognosis in patients with chronic congestive heart failure. N. Engl. J. Med. *311*:822, 1984. Copyright Massachusetts Medical Society.)

2. **Hemodynamic.** Variables such as cardiac index, stroke work index, left ventricular cavity size, and both left and right ventricular ejection fraction[97–99] (Fig. 15–7) have been shown to correlate directly with survival in patients with heart failure, while systemic vascular resistance and heart rate correlate inversely. Combinations of hemodynamic abnormalities, such as depression of stroke work associated with elevation of filling pressure and systemic vascular resistance, are associated with a poor prognosis.[96]

3. **Biochemical.** The observation that there is activation of the neurohormonal axis in heart failure has prompted examination of the relations between a variety of biochemical measurements and clinical outcome. Strong inverse correlations have been reported between survival and plasma norepinephrine (Fig. 15–5*F*),[2,92,100–102] plasma renin,[92,102–104] vasopressin,[104] and atrial natriuretic peptide concentrations[105] (Fig. 15–5*E*). The concentrations of these substances reflect the severity of the underlying impair-

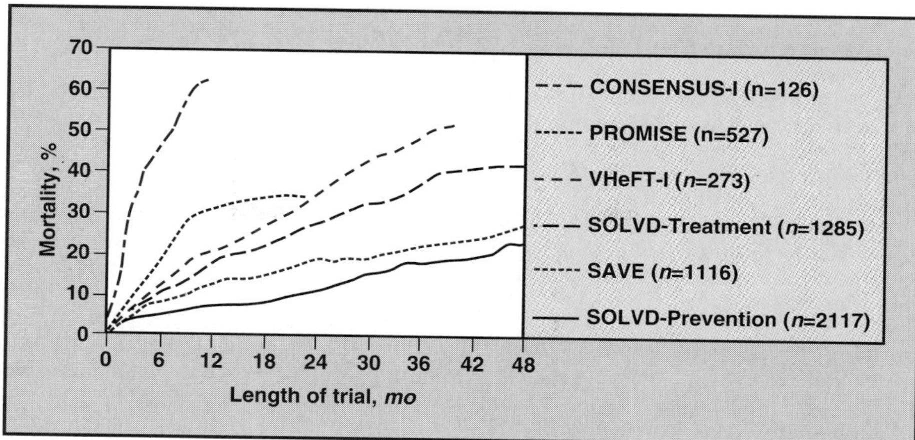

FIGURE 15–6. Based on data from several contemporary clinical trials which included placebo-treated groups, it can be estimated that the 1-year mortality is on the order of 50 to 60 per cent in patients with New York Heart Association (NYHA) functional Class IV symptoms, 15 to 30 per cent in patients with class II–III symptoms, and 5 to 10 per cent in asymptomatic patients with left ventricular dysfunction (×46–×51). Patients in CONSENSUS I were in NYHA Class IV treated with digitalis and diuretics; patients in SOLVD (prevention) and SAVE had reduced LV ejection fractions (< 35 and < 40 per cent, respectively) but no or mild limitation (NYHA Classes I and II). Patients in PROMISE, SOLD (treatment) and VHEFT I were in moderate failure (NYHA Classes II or III). (From Young, J. B.: Assessment of Heart Failure. *In* Colucci, W. S. (ed.): Heart Failure: Cardiac Function and Dysfunction. *In* Braunwald, E. (Series ed.): Atlas of Heart Disease. vol. 4. Philadelphia, Current Medicine, 1995, pp. 7.1–7.20.)

ment of circulatory function. In addition, some of these substances per se may exert adverse hemodynamic effects; norepinephrine, angiotensin II (the consequence of increasing renin concentration), and arginine vasopressin are potent vasoconstrictors, augmenting ventricular afterload and thereby reducing the shortening of myocardial fibers. Furthermore, they may be directly responsible for adverse bio-

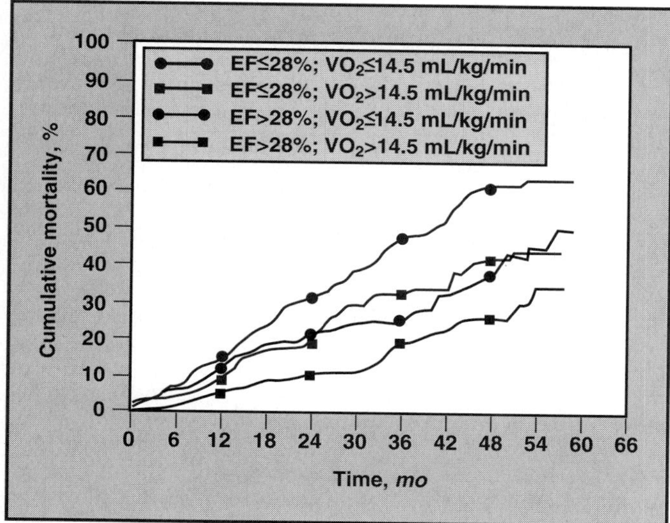

FIGURE 15–7. In a multivariate analysis of survival in the V-HEFT studies, the left ventricular ejection fraction (LVEF) and the peak oxygen consumption (peak $\dot{V}O_2$) were found to have independent prognostic value (×45). An LVEF < 0.28 and a peak $\dot{V}O_2$ < 14.5 ml/kg/min each predicted a poor survival, and the finding of both predicted a worse survival than if only one or the other were present. (From Rector, T. S., Cohn, J. N.: Prognosis, use of prognostic variables, and assessment of therapeutic responses. *In* Colucci, W. S. (ed.): Heart Failure: Cardiac Function and Dysfunction. *In* Braunwald, E. (Series ed.): Atlas of Heart Diseases, Vol. 4. Philadelphia, Current Medicine, 1995, pp. 8.1–8.10. Adapted from Cohn, J. N., et al.: Ejection fraction, peak exercise oxygen consumption, cardiothoracic ratio, ventricular arrhythmias, and plasma norepinephrine as determinants of prognosis in heart failure. Circulation *87*(Suppl. VI):5, 1993. Copyright 1993 American Heart Association.)

chemical effects on the myocardium. For example, the elevated norepinephrine concentration may be directly responsible for ventricular tachyarrhythmias,[100] as may the hypokalemia (Fig. 15–5*C*) and reduction of total body potassium stores resulting from the activation of the renin-angiotensin-aldosterone axis (and the administration of potassium-losing diuretics).[106] Hyponatremia also correlates well with high mortality[104] (Fig. 15–5*B*), but it is likely that this variable reflects activation of the renin-angiotensin-aldosterone axis; hyponatremic patients appear to be especially helped by angiotensin-converting enzyme inhibitors (see p. 494).

In most studies, the aforementioned variables have been assessed in a univariate manner, i.e., independently of one another, and there is still disagreement regarding whether each provides *independent* prognostic information. However, Cohn and Rector have shown that while ventricular function, as expressed in ejection fraction, appears to have the most profound effect on survival in patients with advanced heart failure, exercise tolerance (as reflected in peak O_2 consumption during a progressive exercise test) and activation of the sympathetic nervous system (as reflected in the plasma norepinephrine concentration) *each* provided important independent information.[92]

4. **Electrophysiological.** Death in patients with severe congestive heart failure occurs either by progressive pump failure or, in as many as one-half of all patients, suddenly and unexpectedly, presumably from an arrhythmia. When present, a variety of arrhythmias—especially frequent ventricular extrasystoles (Fig. 15–5*D*), ventricular tachyarrhythmias, left intraventricular conduction defects, as well as atrial flutter and fibrillation[92]—have been shown to be predictors of mortality. What is not yet clear is whether these arrhythmias are simply indicators of the severity of left ventricular dysfunction or whether they are responsible for and trigger fatal arrhythmias.[2] While there is some evidence that ventricular arrhythmias confer independent adverse prognostic effects,[100] routine treatment of patients with heart failure–associated arrhythmias with antiarrhythmic drugs has not yet been shown to exert a protective effect and reduce mortality. It has been speculated that repletion of potassium and magnesium stores will modify favorably the outcome in these patients.[2]

Although high-cardiac output states by themselves are seldom responsible for heart failure, their development in the presence of underlying heart disease often precipitates heart failure.[107] In these conditions, which are often characterized by arteriovenous shunting, the requirements of the peripheral tissues for oxygen can be satisfied only by an increase in cardiac output. While the normal heart is capable of augmenting its output on a long-term basis, this may not be true of the diseased heart.

Anemia

(See also p. 1786)

HISTORY. Chronic anemia in the absence of underlying heart disease produces surprisingly few symptoms, which may consist of easy fatigability, mild exertional dyspnea, and occasionally palpitations and cardiac awareness. Anemia, even when severe, rarely causes heart failure or angina pectoris, and when these are present, it is likely that the high cardiac output is superimposed on some specific cardiac abnormality, such as valvular or ischemic heart disease.

PHYSICAL EXAMINATION. The anemic patient generally has a pale, "pasty" appearance; in persons of color, the finding of paleness of the conjunctivae, mucous membranes, and palmar creases is helpful. Arterial pulses are bounding, "pistol shot" sounds can be heard over the femoral arteries (Duroziez's sign), and subungual capillary pulsations (Quincke's pulse) are present, as in patients with aortic regurgitation. A medium-pitched, midsystolic murmur along the left sternal border, generally Grade 1/6 to 3/6 in intensity (seldom accompanied by a thrill), is common. Heart sounds are accentuated, and the pulmonic component of the second heart sound may be particularly prominent in patients with sickle cell anemia and pulmonary hypertension; in such patients, a right ventricular lift can usually be palpated. A mid-diastolic flow murmur secondary to augmented blood flow across the mitral orifice, holosystolic murmurs resulting from tricuspid and mitral regurgitation secondary to ventricular dilatation, and rarely, diastolic murmurs resulting from aortic and pulmonic valve incompetence secondary to dilatation of these vessels may be heard. A protodiastolic gallop sound (S_3) frequently is audible at the cardiac apex. Jugular venous distention is uncommon, and although peripheral edema and hepatomegaly are occasionally present, they may be due not only to heart failure but also to accompanying abnormalities such as hypoproteinemia and nutritional deficiency.

Laboratory findings in patients with severe chronic anemia without underlying heart disease usually include mild to moderate cardiomegaly on the chest roentgenogram. The electrocardiogram usually does not show any specific changes but may show T-wave inversions in lateral precordial leads. The echocardiogram generally shows a modest and symmetrical increase in the size of all chambers, with large systolic excursions of the septal and posterior left ventricular walls. These findings are superimposed on those resulting from the underlying heart disease. Hematological and blood chemical findings reflect the specific type of anemia present.

MANAGEMENT OF HIGH-OUTPUT FAILURE DUE TO ANEMIA. Treatment of heart failure associated with severe anemia should be specific for the anemia (e.g., iron, folate, vitamin B_{12}, and so forth). When congestive heart failure is present, diuretics and cardiac glycosides are advisable, although some believe that the latter drugs are not helpful in this condition.

When both heart failure and anemia are severe, treatment must be carried out on an urgent basis and presents a difficult challenge. On the other hand, correction of the anemia is desirable to increase oxygen delivery to metabolizing tissues and thereby decrease the need for a sustained high cardiac output. On the other hand, a too-rapid expansion of the blood volume could intensify the manifestations of heart failure, and an increase in hematocrit will potentially depress cardiac output because of increased blood viscosity. The diagnostic steps for determining the etiology of the anemia should be taken immediately (e.g., blood drawn for serum iron, folate, and vitamin B_{12} measurements). The patient should be placed at bed rest and given supplementary oxygen. *Packed red blood cells* should then be transfused slowly (250 to 500 ml/24 hr), preceded or accompanied by vigorous diuretic therapy (e.g., furosemide, 40 mg intravenously immediately followed by 40 mg orally every 8 hours), and the patient should be observed closely for the development or exacerbation of dyspnea and pulmonary rales so that the transfusion can be discontinued immediately to avoid precipitating pulmonary edema. Vasodilator therapy is seldom helpful, since impedance to left ventricular emptying is already markedly reduced in most cases.

Systemic Arteriovenous Fistulas

Systemic arteriovenous fistulas may be congenital or acquired; the latter are either post-traumatic or iatrogenic. Increased cardiac output associated with such fistulas depends on the size of the communication and the magnitude of the resultant reduction in systemic vascular resistance.

The *physical findings* depend on the underlying disease and the location and size of the shunt. In general, a widened pulse pressure, brisk carotid and peripheral arterial pulsations, and mild tachycardia are present. *Branham's sign* (also called *Nicaladoni-Branham's sign*), which consists of slowing of the heart after manual compression of the fistula,[108,109] is present in the majority of cases; this maneuver also raises arterial and lowers venous pressure. It appears to result from the operation of a cardioaccelerator reflex with both afferent and efferent pathways in the vagus nerves.[110]

The skin overlying the fistula is warmer than normal, and a continuous "machinery" murmur and thrill are usually present over the lesion. Third and fourth heart sounds are commonly heard, as well as a precordial midsystolic murmur secondary to increased cardiac output. The electrocardiographic changes of left ventricular hypertrophy are often seen. Rarely, the fistula may become infected, leading to bacterial endarteritis.

ACQUIRED ARTERIOVENOUS FISTULAS. Acquired arteriovenous fistulas occur most frequently after such injuries as gunshot wounds and stab wounds and may involve any part of the body, most frequently the thigh.[111] Blood flow in the affected limb distal to the fistula diminishes after the creation of the fistula but then returns to normal and often increases with the passage of time. As a consequence, the affected limb is usually larger than its opposite member, and the overlying skin is warmer; cellulitis, venostasis, edema, and dermatitis with pigmentation frequently occur, in part as a consequence of chronically elevated venous pressure. Surgical repair or excision is generally advisable in fistulas that develop after gunshot wounds or trauma.

A rare form of acquired arteriovenous fistula results from spontaneous rupture of an aortic aneurysm into the inferior vena cava. This usually produces an enormous arteriovenous shunt and rapidly progressive left ventricular failure. On physical examination, a pulsating mass can be readily palpated superficially in the abdomen, and a continuous bruit is audible.

Massive fistulas may be associated with Wilms' tumors of the kidney, and these have been reported to cause high-output cardiac failure in children.[112]

High-output congestive heart failure resulting from the arteriovenous shunts surgically constructed for vascular access in patients undergoing long-term hemodialysis is not uncommon.[113,114] Cardiac outputs as high as 10 liters/min/m^2, which decrease substantially during temporary occlusion of the shunt, have been found in such patients. These values undoubtedly also reflect the chronic anemia present in many of these patients, but it is clear that it is the added hemodynamic burden imposed by the shunt that precipitates heart failure in patients who had previously tolerated chronic anemia without apparent impairment of cardiac function. It is usually possible to revise or band the fistula to reduce it to the appropriate size for dialysis without compromising cardiac function.[115]

CONGENITAL ARTERIOVENOUS FISTULAS. Congenital arteriovenous fistulas result from arrest of the normal embryonic development of the vascular system and are structurally similar to embryonic capillary networks. They range from barely noticeable strawberry birthmarks to enormous clusters of engorged vascular channels that may deform an entire extremity. Most frequently, the vessels of the lower extremities are involved.[116] When fistulas are large, patients generally complain of disfigurement as well as swelling and pain in the limb. On examination, erythema and cyanosis are usually apparent, as are venous varices, a continuous murmur, and thrill. Physical examination shows hemangiomatous changes associated with venous distention, deformity, and increased limb length. The fistulous connection may involve any vascular bed, including an internal mammary artery–pulmonary artery connection. *Left heart failure* occurs, particularly in patients with larger lesions that involve the pelvis as well as the extremities.[117,118] Angiography is useful in confirming the diagnosis and in determining the physical extent of the anomaly.

Surgical excision is the ideal treatment,[119] but in many instances the lesions are not sufficiently localized to permit this.[120] The results of ligation and excision have been unsatisfactory in the majority of cases, since the congenital arteriovenous communications are usually not confined to a single anatomical segment or to a circumscribed anatomical region. Complete cure of these lesions is possible in only a few instances. Embolization of Gelfoam pellets delivered through a catheter has been reported to obliterate multiple systemic arteriovenous fistulas and thereby diminish high-output heart failure.[119]

Hereditary Hemorrhagic Telangiectasia. Also known as *Osler-Weber-Rendu disease,* this condition may be associated with arteriovenous fistulas, particularly in the lungs and liver; the latter condition can produce a hyperkinetic circulation,[120–122] with heart failure as well as hepatomegaly with abdominal bruits. Because of the presence of oxygenated blood in the inferior vena cava and right atrium, this condition may be misdiagnosed as atrial septal defect.

The congenital arteriovenous communications resulting from *hemangioendothelioma of the liver* are commonly associated with marked increases in cardiac output, sometimes as high as 10 liters/min/m^2, and congestive heart failure.[123] These lesions, which are extremely difficult to treat surgically, may be quite large, increase in size with time, and lead to heart failure even in infancy. They are often associated with sizable cutaneous hemangiomas, which should alert the clinician to the possibility of their presence.

Hyperthyroidism

(See also p. 1891)

The principal findings on the physical examination of the cardiovascular system are tachycardia, a widened pulse pressure, brisk carotid and peripheral arterial pulsations, a hyperkinetic cardiac apex, and loud first heart sound. A midsystolic murmur along the left sternal border, secondary to increased flow is common; occasionally this murmur has an unusual scratchy component (the so-called Means-Lerman scratch) thought to be due to the rubbing together of normal pleural and pericardial surfaces as a consequence of hyperkinetic heart action. Rarely, systolic murmurs of mitral and tricuspid regurgitation, presumably secondary to papillary muscle dysfunction, may occur.

In patients with hyperthyroidism without heart disease, the *chest roentgenogram* is usually normal, although the *echocardiogram* may show increased left ventricular wall thickness and chamber dimensions and a normal or increased ejection fraction and velocity of shortening.[124] The *electrocardiogram* often shows widespread but nonspecific ST-segment elevation and upward coving, with terminal T-wave inversion in about one-fourth of patients and shortening of the Q-T interval.[125] Atrial fibrillation may occur and often is associated with an unusually rapid ventricular response (i.e., 170 to 220 beats/min). There is relative resistance to slowing of the ventricular rate with digitalis.[126] Spontaneous reversion to sinus rhythm is common when euthyroidism is restored.

THYROTOXIC HEART DISEASE

As in many other high-output states, the hyperkinetic state of hyperthyroidism does not usually lead to heart failure in the absence of underlying cardiac or coronary artery disease; the normal heart appears capable of tolerating the burden imposed by hyperthyroidism simply by means of dilatation and hypertrophy. A rare exception is the development of heart failure in patients with neonatal thyrotoxicosis without underlying heart disease.[127] However, when the elevated flow load of hyperthyroidism is superimposed on a reduced cardiovascular reserve (i.e., asymptomatic or only mildly symptomatic heart disease), congestive heart failure is likely to ensue. Similarly, in patients with obstructive coronary artery disease who are asymptomatic or who have only mild evidence of ischemia in the euthyroid state, the demand for increased coronary blood flow with hyperthyroidism frequently leads to an exacerbation of angina.

MANAGEMENT. Beta-adrenoceptor blockade may be both helpful and harmful in patients with thyrotoxic heart disease and heart failure. Although it may be beneficial by lowering the ventricular rate, particularly by prolonging the refractory period of the atrioventricular conduction system in patients with atrial fibrillation, it also may diminish myocardial contractility by blocking the adrenergic support of the heart. Therefore, it must be administered cautiously to the patient with thyrotoxic heart disease and heart failure and only after treatment with a digitalis glycoside, with the patient at rest and under careful observation. The initial dose should be small (e.g., propranolol, 0.5 mg intravenously or 10 mg orally), and the patient should be observed after the administration to be sure that heart failure is not intensified.

It is particularly important to recognize *apathetic hyperthyroidism,* a condition in the elderly in which the usual clinical manifestations of thyrotoxicosis, such as palpitations, tachycardia, and moist skin, are not present. In such patients, the first clinical signs of hyperthyroidism may be unexplained heart failure, an exacerbation of angina pectoris, or unexplained atrial fibrillation, usually but not always with a rapid ventricular rate.

Beriberi Heart Disease

PATHOGENESIS AND CLINICAL CONSIDERATIONS

(Table 15–7)

This condition is due to severe thiamine deficiency persisting for at least 3 months. Clinical beriberi is found most frequently in the Far East, although even in that part of the world it is far less prevalent now than in the past. It occurs predominantly in those individuals whose staple diet consists of polished rice, which is deficient in thiamine but high in carbohydrates. The presence of thiamine in the enriched flour used in white bread has virtually eradicated this disease in the United States and western Europe, where beriberi is found most commonly in diet faddists and alcoholics. Like polished rice, alcohol is low in vitamin B_1 but has a high carbohydrate content. In the West, alcoholics become thiamine deficient not only because of a low intake of the vitamin but also because they eat "junk" foods or drink large quantities of beer. The high carbohydrate content of these foods leads to a greater requirement for thiamine.

Patients in Asia present with edema ("wet beriberi"), general malaise, and fatigue. The elevation of cardiac output[128–132] is presumably secondary to the reduced systemic vascular resistance and augmented venous return.

TABLE 15–7 DIAGNOSTIC CRITERIA FOR BERIBERI HEART DISEASE

CLINICAL FEATURES
Dependent edema
Low peripheral vascular resistance: decreased minimum blood pressure and increased pulse pressure
Hyperkinetic circulatory state: midsystolic murmur and third heart sound
Enlarged heart
T-wave changes (inverted, diphasic, depressed) on electrocardiogram
Peripheral neuritis
Dietary deficiency for at least 3 months or chronic alcoholism
PRESENCE OF THIAMINE DEFICIENCY
Decrease in blood thiamine concentration
Decrease in erythrocyte transketolase activity
Increase in TPP effect
IMPROVEMENT AFTER ADEQUATE THIAMINE THERAPY

From Kawai, C., and Nakamura, Y.: The heart in nutritional deficiencies. *In* Abelmann, W. H. (ed.): Cardiomyopathies, Myocarditis, and Pericardial Disease. *In* Braunwald, E. (Series ed.): Atlas of Heart Diseases, Vol. 2: Philadelphia, Current Medicine, 1995, pp. 7.1–7.18.

PHYSICAL FINDINGS. In most cases in Western countries these are of the high-output state and usually of severe generalized malnutrition and vitamin deficiency. Evidence of peripheral neuropathy with sensory and motor deficits is common (so-called dry beriberi), as is the presence of nutritional cirrhosis characterized by paresthesias of the extremities, absence of decreased knee and ankle jerks, painful glossitis, the anemia of combined iron and folate deficiency, and hyperkeratinized skin lesions.

Beriberi heart disease[131–136] is characterized by evidence of biventricular failure, sinus rhythm, and marked edema (so-called wet beriberi). There is arteriolar vasodilatation, and the cutaneous vessels may be dilated, or in later cases with congestive heart failure, they may be constricted. Therefore, the absence of warm hands does not exclude the diagnosis of beriberi. A third heart sound and an apical systolic murmur are heard almost invariably, and there is a wide pulse pressure characteristic of the hyperkinetic state.

ELECTROCARDIOGRAM. This characteristically exhibits low voltage of the QRS complex, prolongation of the Q-T interval, and low voltage or inversion of T waves. The chest roentgenogram usually shows biventricular enlargement, pulmonary congestion, and pleural effusions. In alcoholics with beriberi heart disease, the left ventricular ejection fraction and peak left ventricular dP/dt are usually reduced.[131] The role played by alcoholic cardiomyopathy (see p. 1412) in this hemodynamic picture is not clear. The cardiac output falls, and the peripheral resistance rises acutely when thiamine is administered in the catheterization laboratory.[132]

Laboratory diagnosis can be made by demonstration of increased serum pyruvate and lactate levels in the presence of a low red blood cell transketolase level.[137] The thiamine concentration may be determined in biological fluids to confirm the diagnosis.[138–140]

At *postmortem examination,* the heart usually shows simple dilation without other changes. On microscopic examination, there is sometimes edema and hydropic degeneration of the muscle fibers. Nonspecific but abnormal histological and electron microscopic changes have been found in cardiac biopsy specimens.

Heart failure may develop explosively in beriberi, and some patients succumb to the illness within 48 hours of the onset of symptoms. *Shoshin beriberi,* seen most frequently in Asia and Africa,[133,134] is a fulminating form of the disease[141] characterized by hypotension, tachycardia, and lactic acidosis; if left untreated, the patients die of pulmonary edema. Thus, since the course of the disease may advance rapidly, treatment must be begun immediately once the diagnosis has been established. In the Western world, this fulminant form of the disease is uncommon.

TREATMENT. Akbarian and coworkers have reported careful hemodynamic studies which suggest that vasomotor depression or paralysis may be responsible for the depressed vascular resistance.[130] They studied four patients in whom ethanol excess was responsible for the thiamine deficiency. All had increased heart rate and cardiac output (averaging 6 liters/min/m^2) and reduced arterial–mixed venous oxygen difference and systemic vascular resistance. Right and left ventricular filling pressures and blood volume were also elevated.

Patients with beriberi heart disease fail to respond adequately to digitalis and diuretics alone. However, improvement after the administration of thiamine (up to 100 mg intravenously followed by 25 mg per day orally for 1 to 2 weeks) may be dramatic. Marked diuresis, decrease in heart rate and size, and clearing of pulmonary congestion may occur within 12 to 48 hours.[130,141,142] However, the acute reversal of the vasodilation induced by correction of the deficiency may cause the unprepared left ventricle to go into low-output failure. Therefore, patients should receive a glycoside and diuretic therapy along with thiamine.

Latent thiamine deficiency may occur in conditions such as alcoholic cardiomyopathy and in other forms of refractory congestive heart failure. The possibility of thiamine deficiency should be considered in many patients with heart failure of obscure origin, and patients with heart failure from other causes could develop superimposed beriberi heart disease unless adequate thiamine intake is maintained.

Paget's Disease

PATHOGENESIS. Paget's disease of bone is an asymmetrical process characterized by extremely rapid bone formation and resorption of the involved areas. Because of the increased vascularity of bone affected by Paget's disease, it has been assumed that this high flow occurred through the involved bone. However, it appears that the additional blood flow through an affected, resting limb passes through the *cutaneous tissue* overlying the involved bone, possibly secondary to local heat production resulting from the increased metabolic activity of affected bone.[143]

CLINICAL FINDINGS. These are a function of the extent of the disease and the specific bones involved. Involvement of at least 15 per cent of the skeleton by Paget's disease in an active stage, accompanied by a high alkaline phosphatase level, is necessary before a clinically significant augmentation of cardiac output is observed.

Such a high-output state may be well tolerated for years with the patient remaining asymptomatic. However, if a specific cardiac disorder (e.g., valvular disease, coronary stenosis) is present, the combination may cause rapid clinical deterioration.

The cardiovascular findings are not distinguishable from those in other conditions with high-output states. However, metastatic calcifications are characteristic. If they involve the heart, they may lead to sclerosis and calcification of the valve rings, with extension into the interventricular septum, and may produce abnormalities of atrioventricular or interventricular conduction.

Other Causes of High-Cardiac Output Failure

FIBROUS DYSPLASIA (ALBRIGHT SYNDROME). This condition, in which there is proliferation of fibrous tissue in bone, also may be associated with an elevated cardiac output, especially when multiple bones are involved.[144,145]

MULTIPLE MYELOMA. High-output heart failure also has been described in this condition.[146] The mechanism is not clear; it may be due to an associated anemia and/or hyperperfusion of the neoplastic tissue.

High-cardiac output failure also occurs in pregnancy (Chap. 59), renal disease, especially glomerulonephritis (Chap. 62), cor pulmonale (Chap. 43), polycythemia vera (Chap. 56), the carcinoid syndrome (Chap. 42), and obesity (Chap. 35).

PULMONARY EDEMA

Mechanism of Pulmonary Edema

ALVEOLAR-CAPILLARY MEMBRANE. Pulmonary edema develops when the movement of liquid from the blood to the interstitial space, and in some instances to the alveoli, exceeds the return of liquid to the blood and its drainage through the lymphatics.[147] The barrier between pulmonary capillaries and alveolar gas, the alveolar-capillary membrane, consists of three anatomical layers with distinct structural characteristics: (1) cytoplasmic projections of the capillary endothelial cells that join to form a continuous cytoplasmic tube; (2) the interstitial space, which varies in thickness and may contain connective tissue fibrils, fibroblasts, and macrophages between the capillary endothelium and the alveolar epithelium, terminal bronchioles, small arteries and veins, and lymphatic channels; and (3) the lining of the alveolar wall, which is continuous with the bronchial epithelium and is composed predominantly of large squamous cells (Type I) with thin cytoplasmic projections. There is normally a continuous exchange of liquid, colloid, and solutes between the vascular bed and interstitium.[148,149] A pathological state exists only when there is an increase in the net flux of liquid, colloid, and solutes from the vasculature into the interstitial space. Experimental studies have confirmed that the basic principles outlined in the classic Starling equation apply to the lung as well as to the systemic circulation.

$$\dot{Q}_{(iv\text{-}int)} = K_f[(P_{iv} - P_{int}) - \sigma_f(\Pi_{iv} - \Pi_{int})]$$

where

$\dot{Q}$ = net rate of transudation (flow of liquid from blood vessels to interstitial space)
P_{int} = interstitial hydrostatic pressures
P_{iv} = intravascular hydrostatic pressures
Π_{int} = interstitial colloid osmotic pressure
Π_{iv} = intravascular colloid osmotic pressure
σ_f = reflection coefficient for proteins
K_f = hydraulic conductance.

LYMPHATICS. These vessels serve to remove solutes, colloid, and liquid derived from the blood vessels. Because of a more negative pressure in the peribronchial and perivascular interstitial space and the increased compliance of this nonalveolar interstitium, liquid is more likely to increase here once the pumping capacity of the lymphatic channels is exceeded. As a consequence of the development of interstitial edema, small airways and blood vessels may become compressed.

The lymphatics play a key role in removing liquid from the interstitial space, and if the pumping capacity of the lymphatic channels is exceeded, edema will occur. It has been estimated that an average 70-kg person at rest has a Q_{lymph} of approximately 20 ml per hour,[150] and experimentally, lymph flow rates of up to 10 times control values have been reported. Thus it is possible that lymphatic pumping capacity can be as much as 200 ml per hour in an average-sized adult. With chronic elevations of left atrial pressure, the pulmonary lymphatic system hypertrophies and is able to transport greater quantities of capillary filtrate, thereby protecting the lungs from edema. Thus sudden marked increase in pulmonary capillary pressure can be rapidly fatal in a patient not preconditioned by growth of the lymphatic drainage system. The same hemodynamic abnormality may be well tolerated in the presence of well-developed lymphatics.

SEQUENCE OF FLUID ACCUMULATION DURING PULMONARY EDEMA. Whether initiated by an imbalance of Starling forces or by primary damage to the various components of the alveolar-capillary membranes, the sequence of liquid exchange and accumulation in the lungs is the same, and it can be represented as three stages. In *stage 1,* there is an increase in mass transfer of liquid and colloid from blood capillaries through the interstitium. Despite the increased filtration, there is no measurable increase in interstitial volume because there is an equal increase in lymphatic outflow. *Stage 2* occurs when the filtered load from the pulmonary capillaries is sufficiently large that the pumping capacity of the lymphatics is approached or exceeded, and liquid and colloid begin to accumulate in the more compliant interstitial compartment surrounding bronchioles, arterioles, and venules. In *stage 3,* further increments in filtered load exceed the volume limits of the loose interstitial spaces, causing distention of the less compliant interstitial space of the alveolar-capillary septum and resulting in alveolar flooding.

GRAVITY DEPENDENCE OF PULMONARY EDEMA. Since blood is more dense than gas-containing lung, the effects of gravity are much greater on the distribution of blood flow than on the distribution of tissue forces in the lung. From apex to base, the effective perfusion pressure of the pulmonary circulation (P_{pa}) increases by approximately 1.00 cm H_2O/cm vertical distance, whereas pleural pressures (P_{pl}) increase by only 0.25 cm H_2O/cm vertical distance.[151] Pulmonary capillaries (or alveolar vessels) are exposed to alveolar pressure (P_{alv}), which does not vary from apex to base. In contrast, pulmonary arteries, arterioles, veins, and venules (extraalveolar vessels) are exposed to pleural pressure, which does vary from apex to base. The consequences of these differences in forces on ventilation-perfusion relationships are described as three zones (Fig. 15–8). In *zone 1* (apex), pulmonary arterial pressure is less than alveolar pressure, and thus blood flow is strikingly diminished.[152] In *zone 2* (midlung), arterial pressure exceeds alveolar pressure, which in turn exceeds venous pressure. In *zone 3* (base), venous pressure exceeds alveolar pressure, resulting in distention of collapsible capillaries. Mean intravascular pressures are greatest in this zone; hence, with elevations of venous pressure or with disruption of alveolar-capillary membranes, edema formation is both more rapid and greatest here. It is only in this zone that the usual calculation of pulmonary vascular resistance is valid, and it is the only zone in which a valid pulmonary capillary wedge pressure measurement can be obtained.

In normal, erect humans, perfusion is greater in the basilar lung regions than in the apical ones. Deviation from this gravity-dependent pattern has been called *vascular redistribution,* a relative reduction in perfusion of the bases with a relative increase in apical perfusion. This phenomenon is most likely due to compression of the lumina of basilar vessels secondary to the greater and more rapid formation of edema at the lung bases and the tendency for extravascular liquid formed elsewhere to gravitate toward the bases. The situation with chronic elevations of left atrial pressure, as in mitral stenosis or chronic congestive heart failure, should be contrasted with that of acute pulmonary edema. Clinical experience with such chronic conditions suggests that redistribution of blood flow does occur, but with minimal or no evidence of interstitial edema and often in the absence of alveolar edema.

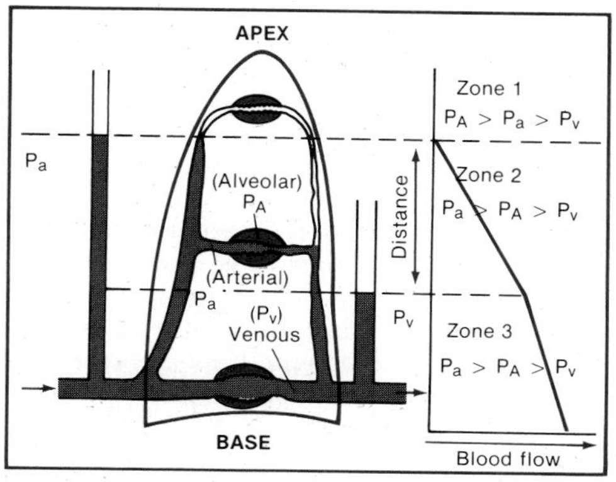

FIGURE 15–8. Schematic representation of the gravity-dependent, apex-to-base distribution of pulmonary blood flow in an upright lung. Pulmonary artery pressure (P_a) and pulmonary venous pressure (P_v) increase on a hydrostatic basis as the base is approached. Alveolar pressure (P_A) is constant with vertical distance. (The three zones are described at length in the text.)

Classification of Pulmonary Edema

The two most common forms of pulmonary edema are those initiated by an imbalance of Starling forces and those initiated by disruption of one or more components of the alveolar-capillary membrane (Table 15–8).[153–156] Less often, lymphatic insufficiency can be involved as a predisposing, if not initiating, factor in the genesis of edema. Although the initiating or primary mechanism may be clearly identifi-

TABLE 15–8 CLASSIFICATION OF PULMONARY EDEMA BASED ON INITIATING MECHANISM

I. IMBALANCE OF STARLING FORCES
A. Increased pulmonary capillary pressure
1. Increased pulmonary venous pressure without left ventricular failure (e.g., mitral stenosis)
2. Increased pulmonary venous pressure secondary to left ventricular failure
3. Increased pulmonary capillary pressure secondary to increased pulmonary arterial pressure (so-called overperfusion pulmonary edema)*
B. Decreased plasma oncotic pressure: Hypoalbuminemia secondary to renal, hepatic, protein-losing enteropathic, or dermatological disease or nutritional causes†
C. Increased negativity of interstitial pressure
1. Rapid removal of pneumothorax with large applied negative pressures (unilateral)
2. Large negative pleural pressures due to acute airway obstruction along with increased end-expiratory volumes (asthma)*
D. Increased interstitial oncotic pressure: No known clinical or experimental example
II. ALTERED ALVEOLAR-CAPILLARY MEMBRANE PERMEABILITY (ADULT RESPIRATORY DISTRESS SYNDROME)
A. Infectious pneumonia—bacterial, viral, parasitic
B. Inhaled toxins (e.g., phosgene, ozone, chlorine, Teflon fumes, nitrogen dioxide, smoke)
C. Circulating foreign substances (e.g., snake venom, bacterial endotoxins, alloxan,‡ alpha-naphthyl thiourea‡)
D. Aspiration of acidic gastric contents
E. Acute radiation pneumonitis
F. Endogenous vasoactive substances (e.g., histamine, kinins*)
G. Disseminated intravascular coagulation
H. Immunological—hypersensitivity pneumonitis, drugs (nitrofurantoin), leukoagglutinins
I. Shock lung in association with nonthoracic trauma
J. Acute hemorrhagic pancreatitis
III. LYMPHATIC INSUFFICIENCY
A. Post-lung transplant
B. Lymphangitic carcinomatosis
C. Fibrosing lymphangitis (e.g., silicosis)
IV. UNKNOWN OR INCOMPLETELY UNDERSTOOD
A. High-altitude pulmonary edema
B. Neurogenic pulmonary edema
C. Narcotic overdose
D. Pulmonary embolism
E. Eclampsia
F. Post-cardioversion
G. Post-anesthesia
H. Post-cardiopulmonary bypass

* Not certain to exist as a clinical entity. † Not certain that this, as a single factor, leads to clinical pulmonary edema. ‡ Predominantly an experimental technique.

able, multiple factors come into play during the development of edema, and irrespective of the initiating event, the stage of alveolar flooding is characterized to some degree by disruption of the alveolar-capillary membrane.

IMBALANCE OF STARLING FORCES

INCREASED PULMONARY CAPILLARY PRESSURE. Pulmonary edema will occur only when the pulmonary capillary pressure rises to values exceeding the plasma colloid osmotic pressure, which is approximately 28 mm Hg in the human. Since the normal pulmonary capillary pressure is about 8 mm Hg, there is a substantial margin of safety in the development of pulmonary edema.[150] Although pulmonary capillary wedge pressures must be abnormally high to increase the flow of interstitial liquid, at a time when edema is clearly present, these pressures may not correlate with the severity of pulmonary edema.[157] In fact, pulmonary capillary wedge pressures may have returned to normal at a time when there is still considerable pulmonary edema, since time is required for removal of both interstitial and alveolar edema. Other factors obscure the relationship between the severity of edema and measured pulmonary capillary pressures in addition to slower rates of removal after edema has collected. The rate of increase in lung liquid at any given elevation of capillary pressure is related to the functional capacity of lymphatics,[158] which may vary from patient to patient, and to variations in interstitial oncotic and hydrostatic pressures.

HYPOALBUMINEMIA. Pulmonary edema does not develop with hypoalbuminemia alone. However, hypoalbuminemia may alter the fluid conductivity of the interstitial gel so that liquid moves more easily between capillaries and lymphatics to add to the lymphatic safety factor.[159] Thus there must be, in addition to hypoalbuminemia, some elevations of pulmonary capillary pressure, but only small increases are necessary before pulmonary edema ensues. Indeed, in such patients, only moderate fluid overload can precipitate overt pulmonary edema in the absence of left ventricular failure.

INCREASED NEGATIVE INTERSTITIAL PRESSURE. When this is due to rapid removal of pleural air for relief of a pneumothorax, it may be associated with pulmonary edema. Usually, the pneumothorax has been present for several hours to days, allowing time for alterations in surfactant so that large negative pressures are necessary to open collapsed alveoli.[160] In this instance, the edema is unilateral and is most often only a radiographic finding with few clinical findings.

PRIMARY ALVEOLAR-CAPILLARY MEMBRANE DAMAGE

Many diverse medical and surgical conditions are associated with pulmonary edema that appears to be due not to primary alteration in Starling forces but rather to damage of the alveolar-capillary membrane (Table 15–8). These conditions include acute pulmonary infections and pulmonary effects of gram-negative septicemia and nonthoracic trauma as well as any condition associated with disseminated intravascular coagulation.[153,154,161–163] Despite the diversity of underlying causes, once diffuse alveolar-capillary injury has occurred, the pathophysiological and clinical sequence of events is quite similar in most patients. Because of the resemblance of the clinical picture to that seen with respiratory distress of the neonate, these conditions have been referred to as the *adult respiratory distress syndrome* (ARDS).

Direct evidence for increased capillary permeability has come mainly from experimental studies in which pulmonary edema has been produced by endotoxin infusion,[164] hemorrhagic shock,[165] infusion of oleic acid,[166,167] alloxan, thiourea, phorbol myristate acetate, complement fragments, cobra venom factor,[167–171] freebase cocaine smoking,[172] and inhalation of high concentrations of oxygen[173] or toxic gases, such as phosgene,[174] ozone,[175] and nitrogen dioxide.[176] It is probable, though not yet proved, that increased permeability of the alveolar-capillary membrane is an initiating event in most of the cases designated as ARDS.

Cardiogenic Pulmonary Edema

CLINICAL MANIFESTATIONS. During Stage 1, the distention and recruitment of small pulmonary vessels may actually improve gas exchange in the lung and augment slightly the diffusing capacity for carbon monoxide.[177] It is doubtful that any symptoms, except for exertional dyspnea, accompany these abnormalities, and physical findings in the lungs would be scarce except for mild inspiratory rales due to opening of closed airways. With progression to Stage 2, interstitial edema attributable to increased liquid in the loose interstitial space contiguous with the perivascular tissue of larger vessels may cause a loss of the normally sharp radiographic definition of pulmonary vascular markings, haziness and loss of demarcation of hilar shadows, and thickening of interlobular septa (Kerley B lines) (Fig. 7–35, p. 226). Competition for space between vessels, airways, and increased liquid within the loose interstitial space may compromise small airway lumina, particularly in the dependent portions of the lungs, and there may be reflex bronchoconstriction.[177] A mismatch exists between ventilation and perfusion that results in hypoxemia and more wasted ventilation. Indeed, in the setting of acute myocardial infarction, the degree of hypoxemia correlates with the degree of elevation of the pulmonary capillary wedge pressure.[178] Tachypnea is a frequent finding with interstitial edema and has been attributed to stimulation by the edema of interstitial J-type receptors or to stretch receptors in the interstitium rather than to hypoxemia, which is rarely of sufficient magnitude to stimulate breathing.[179] There are few changes in the standard spirometric indices.

With the onset of alveolar flooding, or Stage 3 edema, gas exchange is quite abnormal, with severe hypoxemia and often hypocapnia. Alveolar flooding can proceed to such a degree that many large airways are filled with blood-tinged foam that can be expectorated. Vital capacity and other lung volumes are markedly reduced. A right-to-left intrapulmonary shunt develops as a consequence of perfusion of the flooded alveoli. Although hypocapnia is the rule, hypercapnia with acute respiratory acidemia can occur in more severe cases. It is in such instances that morphine, with its well-known respiratory depressant effects, should be used with caution.

DIAGNOSIS. Acute cardiogenic pulmonary edema is the most dramatic symptom of left heart failure. Impaired left ventricular systolic and/or diastolic function, mitral stenosis, or whatever cause of elevated left atrial and pulmonary capillary pressures leading to cardiogenic pulmonary edema interferes with oxygen transfer in the lungs and, in turn, depresses arterial oxygen tension. Simultaneously, the sensation of suffocation and oppression in the chest intensifies the patient's fright, elevates heart rate and blood pressure, and further restricts ventricular filling. The increased discomfort and work of breathing place an additional load on the heart, and cardiac function becomes depressed further by the hypoxia. If this vicious circle is not interrupted, it may lead rapidly to death.

Acute cardiogenic pulmonary edema differs from orthopnea and paroxysmal nocturnal dyspnea in the more rapid and extreme development of pulmonary capillary hypertension. Acute pulmonary edema is a terrifying experience for the patient and often the bystander as well. Usually extreme breathlessness develops suddenly, and the patient becomes extremely anxious, coughs, and expectorates pink, frothy liquid, causing him or her to feel as if he or she is literally drowning. The patient sits bolt upright, or may stand, exhibits air hunger, and may thrash about. The respiratory rate is elevated, the alae nasi are dilated, and there is inspiratory retraction of the intercostal spaces and supraclavicular fossae that reflects the large negative intrapleural pressures required for inspiration. The patient often grasps the sides of the bed in order to allow use of the accessory muscles of respiration. Respiration is noisy, with loud inspiratory and expiratory gurgling sounds that are often easily audible across the room. Sweating is profuse, and the skin is usually cold, ashen, and cyanotic, reflecting low cardiac output and increased sympathetic drive.

On auscultation, the lungs are noisy, with rhonchi, wheezes, and moist and fine crepitant rales that appear at first over the lung bases but then extend upward to the apices as the condition worsens. Cardiac auscultation may be difficult because of the respiratory sounds, but a third heart sound and an accentuated pulmonic component of the second heart sound are frequently present.

The patient may suffer from intense precordial pain if the pulmonary edema is secondary to acute myocardial infarction. Unless cardiogenic shock is present, arterial pressure is usually elevated above the patient's normal level as a result of excitement and sympathetic vasoconstriction. Because of the presence of this systemic hypertension, it may be suspected (inappropriately) that the pulmonary edema is due to hypertensive heart disease. However, it should be noted that the latter condition is now quite rare, and if arterial pressure is elevated, examination of the fundi will usually indicate whether or not hypertensive heart disease is actually present.

DIFFERENTIATION FROM BRONCHIAL ASTHMA. It may be difficult to differentiate severe bronchial asthma from acute pulmonary edema, since both conditions may be associated with extreme dyspnea, pulsus paradoxus, demands for an upright posture, and diffuse wheezes that interfere with cardiac auscultation. In bronchial asthma, there is most often a history of previous similar episodes, and the patient is frequently aware of the diagnosis. During the acute attack, the asthmatic patient does not usually sweat profusely, and arterial hypoxemia, although present, is not usually of sufficient magnitude to produce cyanosis. In addition, the chest is hyperexpanded and hyperresonant, and use of accessory muscles is most prominent during respiration. The wheezes are more high-pitched and musical than in pulmonary edema, and other adventitious sounds such as rhonchi and rales are less prominent in asthma.

The patient with acute cardiogenic pulmonary edema most often perspires profusely and is frequently cyanotic owing to desaturation of arterial blood and decreased cutaneous blood flow. The chest is often dull to percussion, there is no hyperexpansion, accessory muscle use is less prominent than in asthma, and moist, bubbly rales and rhonchi are heard in addition to wheezes. As the patient recovers, the radiological appearance of pulmonary edema usually resolves more slowly than the elevated pulmonary capillary wedge pressure.

PULMONARY ARTERY WEDGE PRESSURE MEASUREMENTS. Measurement of pulmonary artery wedge pressure by means of a Swan-Ganz catheter may be critical to the differentiation between pulmonary edema secondary to an imbalance of Starling forces, i.e., cardiogenic pulmonary edema, and that secondary to alterations of the alveolar-capillary membrane. Specifically, a pulmonary capillary wedge or pulmonary artery diastolic pressure exceeding 25 mm Hg in a patient without previous pulmonary capillary pressure elevation (or exceeding 30 mm Hg in a patient with chronic pulmonary capillary pressure elevation) and with the clinical features of pulmonary edema strongly suggests that the edema is cardiogenic in origin.

Following effective treatment of the pulmonary edema, patients are often restored rapidly to the condition that existed before the attack, although they usually feel exhausted; between attacks of pulmonary edema, there may be few symptoms or signs of heart failure.

ADULT RESPIRATORY DISTRESS SYNDROME (ARDS)

There are many similarities between ARDS from diverse etiologies and the respiratory distress syndrome seen in infants, which is due only to immaturity of the surfactant system. Although surfactant deficiency cannot be assigned a primary role in the pathogenesis of ARDS, there are many data to support the idea that changes in the properties of surfactant are added to the initial impairment and serve to perpetuate pulmonary dysfunction. Impairment of surfactant has been shown to occur with cardiogenic pulmonary edema, exposure to various plasma constituents,[180] and high concentrations of oxygen[181] and in association with systemic hypotension.[182] Closely related to the pulmonary edema in the ARDS is that which is commonly associated with all forms of shock—the so-called *shock lung*.

POLYMORPHONUCLEAR LEUKOCYTES. Experimental and clinical data strongly imply a major role for interaction of polymorphonuclear leukocytes in the blood and circulating or cellular chemotactic macromolecules for the initiation, perpetuation, or amplification of lung injury leading to most forms of ARDS. Chemotaxins in the circulating blood (e.g., the fifth component of complement, C5a) or from alveolar macrophages can recruit polymorphonuclear leukocytes, cause them to adhere to the pulmonary capillary endothelium, and activate them to produce several toxic substances that alter alveolar-capillary membrane permeability or cause circulatory changes or both.

MONOCYTIC CELLS. Circulating monocytes and lymphocytes, tissue macrophages, and phagocytic cells along the vascular endothelium (reticuloendothelial cells) appear to play an important pathogenic and/or amplification role in ARDS. Upon being stimulated with several agents (e.g., endotoxin, these cells release cytokines, including interleukin-1 (IL-1), interleukin-6 (IL-6), and tumor necrosis factor (TNF), which may play a role in ARDS.

PLATELETS. Although it has not been possible to ascribe a major pathogenetic role to platelets, a secondary role seems probable. Nonetheless, heterologous platelet transfusions given to patients with ARDS and thrombocytopenia have no adverse effects on the extent or degree of lung injury.

LYMPHATIC DYSFUNCTION. It is not known whether alterations in lymphatic function, alone, ever account for pulmonary edema. However, lymphatic flow is impaired following endotoxin infusion in sheep.[183] Cessation of lymphatic pumping would be expected to result in a net gain of interstitial liquid, and this may leave a clinical counterpart of pulmonary edema following anesthesia or sedative drug overdose. More important, the paralytic effect following endotoxin infusion suggests that lymphatic dysfunction may play a significant role in lung injury.

COMBINATIONS OF MECHANISMS. In certain clinical settings, typified by gram-negative sepsis, several mechanisms combine to increase pulmonary edema. In addition to the mechanisms already discussed, endotoxin may release cytokines from reticuloendothelial cells and oxidant and arachidonic acid metabolites from polymorphonuclear leukocytes. These or other factors may depress cardiac function and thereby further contribute to edema formation.

Pulmonary Edema of Unknown Pathogenesis

HIGH-ALTITUDE PULMONARY EDEMA (HAPE). Victims of this disorder are usually persons mostly in their teens or early twenties who have quickly ascended to altitudes in excess of 2500 m and who then engage in strenuous physical exercise at that altitude before they have become acclimated.[184–188] Estimates place the incidence at 6.4 clinically apparent cases per 100 exposure to high altitude in persons less than 21 years of age and 0.4 cases per 100 exposures in those older than 21 years. The pathogenesis is shown in Figure 15–9. Gradual ascent, allowing time for acclimatization, and limiting physical exertion upon more rapid ascent are thought to be preventive. Usually within one day of ascent, affected patients complain of cough, dyspnea, and, in some cases, chest pain in association with tachycardia, bilateral rales, and cyanosis accompanied by radiographic evidence of discrete patches of pulmonary infiltrate.

Reversal of this syndrome is both rapid (less than 48 hours) and certain either by returning the patient to a lower altitude and/or by administering a high inspiratory concentration of oxygen. Sleeping below 2500 m, gradual acclimatization, and avoidance of heavy exertion for the first 2 or 3 days at high altitude appear to be preventive.

NEUROGENIC PULMONARY EDEMA. Central nervous system disorders ranging from head trauma to grand mal seizures can be associated with acute pulmonary edema (without detectable left ventricular disease.[189] The current idea is that sympathetic overactivity produces shifts of blood volume from the systemic to the pulmonary circulation, with secondary elevations of left atrial and pulmonary capillary pressures. Thus, an imbalance of Starling forces may be the basis for this form of pulmonary edema, although capillary pressure quickly returns to normal after the acute and transitory sympathetic discharge. It should be emphasized that although sympatholytics prevent neurogenic pulmonary edema, they appear to have no place in the treatment of this syndrome, since it appears that pulmonary capillary pressures have returned to near normal by the time the syndrome is diagnosed.

NARCOTIC OVERDOSE PULMONARY EDEMA. Acute pulmonary edema is a well-recognized sequela of heroin overdose.[190] Because of the illicit traffic in this drug, which is given by the intravenous route, the syndrome was initially thought to be due to injected impurities rather than to the heroin itself. However, since oral methadone and dextrapropoxyphene also can be associated with pulmonary edema,[191,192] the syndrome cannot be attributed entirely to injected impurities. The fact that edema fluid contains protein concentrations nearly identical to those found in

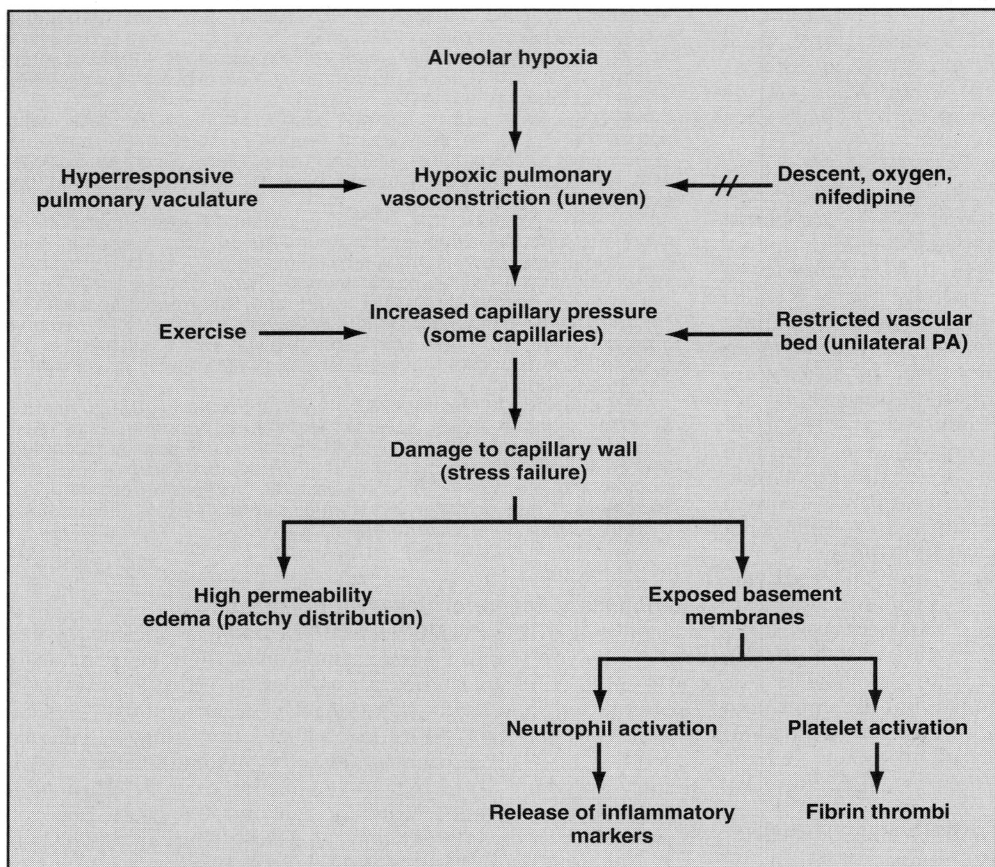

FIGURE 15–9. Diagram to show the sequence of events in the pathogenesis of HAPE. (From West, J. B., and Mathieu-Costello, O.: High-altitude pulmonary edema is caused by stress failure of pulmonary capillaries. Int. J. Sports Med. *13*:S54–S57, 1992.)

plasma,[193] and that pulmonary capillary wedge pressures, when measured, are normal,[194] argues for an alveolar-capillary membrane leak as the initiating cause. In animal experiments, histamine has been shown to be released in the lung after both heroin and morphine administration[195] and might play a role in this syndrome by increasing vascular permeability.

PULMONARY EMBOLISM (Chap. 46). Acute pulmonary edema in association with either a massive embolus or multiple smaller emboli has been well described and most often attributed to concomitant left ventricular dysfunction due to a combination of hypoxemia and encroachment of the interventricular septum on the left ventricular cavity. Although this sequence is quite likely to be applicable in the case of massive embolism, the mechanism of pulmonary edema in the case of microemboli has not been established. There are data to suggest, in the latter instance, that an increase in permeability of the alveolar-capillary membrane occurs.[162]

ECLAMPSIA (see p. 1852). Acute pulmonary edema frequently complicates eclampsia.[196] Multiple factors such as cerebral dysfunction with massive sympathetic discharge, left ventricular dysfunction secondary to acute systemic hypertension, hypervolemia, hypoalbuminemia (secondary to renal losses), and disseminated intravascular coagulation probably play a role in the pathogenesis.

POST-CARDIOVERSION. Although pulmonary edema has been documented to occur after cardioversion,[197] the mechanism is poorly understood. Ineffective left atrial function immediately following cardioversion has been suggested as a contributing factor, yet left ventricular dysfunction and neurogenic mechanisms are also possible.

POST-ANESTHESIA. In previously healthy subjects, pulmonary edema has been found in the early post-anesthesia period without a clear relationship to fluid overload or any subsequent evidence of left ventricular disease. The basis for this disorder is unknown, but it is tempting to invoke some role for temporary lymphatic dysfunction under anesthesia.

POST-CARDIOPULMONARY BYPASS. Although all patients who undergo cardiopulmonary bypass obviously have significant heart disease, the development of edema has been associated with normal left atrial pressures.[198,199] Alterations of surfactant due to prolonged collapse of the lung during the procedure, with subsequent need to apply high negative intrapleural pressures for reexpansion, and release of toxic substances have been suggested as mechanisms. Some data suggest that anaphylactic reactions to fresh frozen plasma may account for some episodes.[198] THe matter is far from settled, but the syndrome is fortunately rare.

Differential Diagnosis of Pulmonary Edema

The differentiation between the two principal forms of pulmonary edema, i.e., cardiogenic (hemodynamic) and noncardiogenic (caused by alterations in the pulmonary

TABLE 15–9 INITIAL DIFFERENTIATION OF CARDIOGENIC FROM NONCARDIOGENIC PULMONARY EDEMA

CARDIAC PULMONARY EDEMA	NONCARDIAC PULMONARY EDEMA
History	
Acute cardiac event	Acute cardiac event is uncommon in immediate history (but possible!)
	Underlying disease? (Table 15–1)
Clinical Examination	
Low-flow state = cool periphery	Usually high flow state = warm periphery
S_3 gallop/cardiomegaly	Bounding pulses
Jugular venous distention	No gallop
Crackles (wet)	No jugular venous distention
	Crackles (dry)
	Evidence of underlying disease (e.g., peritonitis)
Laboratory Tests	
ECG, ischemia/infarct?	ECG, usually normal
CXR, perihilar distribution	CXR, peripheral distribution
Cardiac enzymes may be ↑	Cardiac enzymes usually normal
PCWP $>$18 mm Hg	PCWP $<$18 mm Hg
Intrapulmonary shunting: small	Intrapulmonary shunting: large
Edema fluid/serum protein $<$0.5	Edema fluid/serum protein $>$0.7

From Sibbald, W. J., Cunningham, D. R., and Chin, D. N.: Noncardiac or cardiac pulmonary edema? A practical approach to clinical differentiation in critically ill patients. Chest *84*:460, 1983.

capillary membrane), usually can be made through assessment of the clinical context in which it occurs and through examination and consideration of the clinical data as shown in Table 15–9. Although this approach suggests an either/or situation, this may not be the case in reality. For example, sudden and large increases in intravascular pressure may disrupt the capillary and alveolar membranes leading to interstitial edema and alveolar loading with macromolecules that produce an edema liquid more compatible with noncardiogenic causes. Thus, a primary hemodynamic event can cause an alveolar-capillary membrane leak. Furthermore, high, normal, or only mild elevations in capillary hydrostatic pressures in the presence of alveolar capillary damage can cause an increase in the rate and extent of edema formation. Hence hemodynamic factors can and do play a role in increasing and perpetuating increased permeability.

REFERENCES

1. Report of the Task Force on Research in Heart Failure. National Heart, Lung and Blood Institute, 1994.
2. Packer, M.: Survival in patients with chronic heart failure and its potential modification by drug therapy. *In* Cohn, J. N. (ed.): Drug Treatment of Heart Failure, 2nd ed. Secaucus, N. J., ATC International, 1988, p. 273.
3. Kannel, W. B.: Epidemiologic aspects of heart failure. *In* Weber, K. T. (ed.): Heart Failure: Current Concepts and Management. Cardiology Clinics Series 7/1. Philadelphia, W. B. Saunders Co, 1989.
4. Braunwald, E., Mock, M. B., and Watson, J. (eds.): Congestive Heart Failure. Current Research and Clinical Applications. Orlando, Grune and Stratton, 1982.
5. McKee, P. A., Castell, W. P., McNamara, P. M., and Kannel, W. B.: The natural history of congestive heart failure, the Framingham Study. N. Engl. J. Med. *285*:1441, 1971.
6. Marantz, P. R., Tobin, J. N., Wassertheil-Smoller, S., et al.: The relationship between left ventricular systolic function and congestive heart failure diagnosed by clinical criteria. Circulation *77*:607, 1988.

FORMS AND CAUSES OF HEART FAILURE

7. Hope, J. A.: Treatise on the Diseases of the Heart and Great Vessels. London, Williams-Kidd, 1832.
8. Williams, J. F., Jr., Sonnenblick, E. H., and Braunwald, E.: Determinants of atrial contractile force in intact heart. Am. J. Physiol. *209*:1061, 1965.
9. Ross, J., Jr., and Braunwald, E.: Studies on Starling's law of the heart. IX. The effects of impeding venous return on performance of the normal and failing human left ventricle. Circulation *30*:719, 1964.
10. Stampfer, M., Epstein, S. E., Beiser, G. D., and Braunwald, E.: Hemodynamic effects of diuresis at rest and during intense upright exercise in patients with impaired cardiac function. Circulation 37:900, 1968.
11. Mackenzie, J.: Disease of the Heart, 3rd ed. London, Oxford University Press, 1913.
12. Moe, G. W., Legault, L., and Skorecki, K. L.: Control of extracellular fluid volume and pathophysiology of edema formation. *In* Brenner, B. M., and Rector, F. C., Jr. (eds.): The Kidney. 4th ed. Philadelphia, W. B. Saunders Company, 1991, pp. 623–676.
13. Braunwald, E.: The Pathogenesis of heart failure: Then and now. Medicine *70*:68, 1991.
14. Stevenson, L. W., and Perloff, J. K.: The limited reliability of physical signs for estimating hemodynamics in chronic heart failure. JAMA *261*:884, 1989.
15. Iriarte, M., Murga, N., Sagastagoitia, D., et al.: Congestive heart failure from left ventricular diastolic dysfunction in systemic hypertension. Am. J. Cardiol. *71*:308, 1993.
16. Gaasch, W. H.: Diagnosis and treatment of heart failure based on left ventricular systolic or diastolic dysfunction. JAMA *271*:1278, 1994.
17. Ghali, J. K., Kadakia, S., Cooper, R., and Ferlinz, J.: Precipitating factors leading to decompensation of heart failure: Traits among urban blacks. Arch. Intern. Med. *148*:2013, 1988.
18. Braunwald, E., and Frahm, C. J.: Studies on Starling's law of the heart: IV. Observations on the hemodynamic functions of the left atrium in man. Circulation *24*:633, 1961.

SYMPTOMS AND PROGNOSIS IN HEART FAILURE

19. Manning, H. L., and Schwartzstein, R. M.: Mechanisms of Disease: Pathophysiology of Dyspnea. N. Engl. J. Med. *333*:1547, 1995.
20. Geltman, E. M.: Mild heart failure: Diagnosis and treatment. Am. Heart J. *118*:1277, 1989.
21. Collins, J. V., Clark, T. J. H., and Brown, D. J.: Airway function in healthy subjects and in patients with left heart disease. Clin. Sci. Molec. Med. *49*:217, 1975.
22. Macklem, P. T.: Respiratory muscles: The vital pump. Chest *78*:753, 1980.
23. Fishman, A. P., and Ledlie, J. F.: Dyspnea. Bull. Eur. Physiopathol. Resp. *15*:789, 1979.
24. Poole-Wilson, P. A., and Buller, N. P.: Causes of symptoms in chronic congestive heart failure and implications for treatment. Am. J. Cardiol. *62*:31A, 1988.
25. Petermann, W., Barth, J., and Entzian, P.: Heart failure and airway obstruction. Int. J. Cardiol. *17*:207, 1987.
26. Weber, K., Kinasewitz G., Janicki, J., and Fishman, A.: Oxygen utilization and ventilation during exercise in patients with chronic cardiac failure. Circulation *65*:1213, 1982.
27. Colucci, W. S., Ribeiro, J. P., Rocco, M. B., et al.: Impaired chronotropic response to exercise in patients with congestive heart failure: Role of postsynaptic beta-adrenergic desensitization. Circulation *80*:314, 1989.
28. Kubo, S. H., Rector, T., Bank, A., and Heifetz, S.: Endothelium-dependent vasodilation is attenuated in patients with heart failure. Circulation *84*:1589, 1991.
29. Nakamura, M., Ishikawa, M., Funakoshi, T., et al.: Attenuated endothelium-dependent peripheral vasodilation and clinical characteristics in patients with chronic heart failure. Am. Heart J. *128*:1164, 1994.
30. Kraemer, M. D., Kubo, S. H., Rector, T. S., et al.: Pulmonary and peripheral vascular factors are important determinants of peak exercise oxygen uptake in patients with heart failure. J. Am. Coll. Cardiol. *21*:641, 1993.
31. Mancini, D. M., Walter, G., Reichek, N., et al.: Contribution of skeletal muscle atrophy to exercise intolerance and altered muscle metabolism in heart failure. Circulation *85*:1364, 1992.
32. Mancini, D. M., Wilson, J. R., Bolinger, L., et al.: In vivo magnetic resonance spectroscopy measurement of deoxymyoglobin during exercise in patients with heart failure: Demonstration of abnormal muscle metabolism despite adequate oxygenation. Circulation *90*:500, 1994.
33. Mancini, D. M., Henson, D., LaManca, J., and Levine, S.: Evidence of reduced respiratory muscle endurance in patients with heart failure. J. Am. Coll. Cardiol. *24*:972, 1994.
34. Sullivan, M., Higgenbotham, M., and Cobb, F.: Exercise training in patients with severe left ventricular dysfunction: Hemodynamic and metabolic benefits. Circulation *78*:506, 1988.
35. Coats, A. J., Adamopoulos, S., Raddaelli, A., et al.: Controlled trial of physical training in chronic heart failure. Exercise performance, hemodynamics, ventilation, and autonomic function. Circulation *85*:2119, 1992.
36. Weber, K. T., and Janicki, J. S.: Cardiopulmonary Exercise Testing. Philadelphia, W. B. Saunders Company, 1986.
37. Smith, R. F., Johnson, G., Ziesche, S., et al: Functional capacity in heart failure: Comparison of methods for assessment and their relation to other indexes of heart failure. The V-HeFT VA Cooperative Studies Group. Circulation *87*:VI88, 1993.
38. Wasserman, D.: Dyspnea on exertion: Is it the heart or the lungs? JAMA *248*:2042, 1982.
39. Oka, R. K., Stotts, N. A., Dae, M. W., et al.: Daily physical activity levels in congestive heart failure. Am. J. Cardiol. *71*:921, 1993.
40. Cross, A. M., Jr., and Higginbotham, M. B.: Oxygen deficit during exercise testing in heart failure. Relation to submaximal exercise tolerance. Chest *107*:904, 1995.
41. Francis, G. S., and Rector, T. S.: Maximal exercise tolerance as a therapeutic end point in heart failure—Are we relying on the right measure? (Editorial) Am. J. Cardiol. *73*:304, 1994.
42. Lipkin, D. P., Bayliss, J., and Poole-Wilson, P. A.: The ability of a submaximal exercise test to predict maximal exercise capacity in patients with heart failure. Eur. Heart J. *6*:829, 1985.
43. Guyatt, G. H., Sullivan, J. J., Thompson, P. J., et al.: The 6-minute walk: A new measure of exercise capacity in patients with chronic heart failure. Can. Med. Assoc. J. *132*:919, 1985.
44. Lipkin, P., Scriven, A. J., Crake, T., and Poole-Wilson, P. A.: Six-minute walking test for assessing exercise capacity in chronic heart failure. Br. Med. J. *292*:653, 1986.
45. Sparrow, J., Parameshwar, J., and Poole-Wilson, P. A.: Assessment of functional capacity in chronic heart failure: Time-limited exercise on a self-powered treadmill. Br. Heart J. *71*:391, 1994.
46. Higgins, C. B., Vatner, S. F., Franklin, D., and Braunwald, E.: Effects of experimentally produced heart failure on the peripheral vascular response to severe exercise in conscious dogs. Circ. Res. *31*:186, 1972.
47. Criteria Committee, New York Heart Association, Inc.: Diseases of the Heart and Blood Vessels. Nomenclature and Criteria for Diagnosis. 6th ed. Boston, Little, Brown and Co., 1964, p. 114.
48. Goldman, L., Hasimoto, B., Cook, E. F., and Loscalzo, A.: Comparative reproducibility and validity of symptoms for assessing cardiovascular functional class. Advantages of a new specific activity scale. Circulation *64*:1227, 1981.
49. Rector, T. S., Kubo, S. H., and Cohn, J. N.: Patients' self-assessment of their congestive heart failure: Content, reliability and validity of a new measure. The Minnesota Living with Heart Failure questionnaire. *In* Heart Failure, Vol. 3. 1987, p 198.
50. Rector, T. S., and Cohn, J. N.: Assessment of patient outcome with the Minnesota Living with Heart Failure questionnaire: Reliability and validity during a randomized, double-blind, placebo-controlled trial of pimobendan. Am. Heart J. *124*:1017, 1992.
51. Rector, T. S., Kubo, S. H., and Cohn, J. N.: Validity of the Minnesota Living with Heart Failure questionnaire as a measure of therapeutic response to enalapril or placebo. Am. J. Cardiol. *71*:1106, 1993.
52. Earnest, D. L., and Hurst, J. W.: Exophthalmos, stare and increase in

intraocular pressure and systolic propulsion of the eyeballs due to congestive heart failure. Am. J. Cardiol. *26*:351, 1970.
53. Chakko, S., Woska, D., Martinez, H., et al.: Clinical, radiographic, and hemodynamic correlations in chronic congestive heart failure: Conflicting results may lead to inappropriate care. Am. J. Med. *90*:353, 1991.
54. Butman, S. M., Ewy, G. A., Standen, J. R., et al.: Bedside cardiovascular examination in patients with severe chronic heart failure: Importance of rest or inducible jugular venous distension. J. Am. Coll. Cardiol. *22*:968, 1993.
55. Strober, W., Cohen, L. S., Waldmann, T. A., and Braunwald, E.: Tricuspid regurgitation: A newly recognized cause of protein-losing enteropathy, lymphocytopenia and immunologic deficiency. Am. J. Med. *44*:842, 1968.
56. Gleason, W. L., and Braunwald, E.: Studies on Starling's law of the heart: VI. Relationships between left ventricular end-diastolic volume and stroke volume in man with observations on the mechanism of pulsus alternans. Circulation *25*:841, 1962.
57. Berkowitz, D., Croll, M. N., and Likoff, W.: Malabsorption as a complication of congestive heart failure. Am. J. Cardiol. *11*:43, 1963.
58. Levine, B., Kalman, J., Mayer, L., et al.: Elevated circulating levels of tumor necrosis factor in severe chronic heart failure. N. Engl. J. Med. *323*:236, 1990.
59. Carr, J. G., Stevenson, L. W., Walden, J. A., and Heber, D.: Prevalence and hemodynamic correlates of malnutrition in severe congestive heart failure secondary to ischemic or idiopathic dilated cardiomyopathy. Am. J. Cardiol. *63*:709, 1989.
60. Pittman, J. G., and Cohen, P.: The pathogenesis of cardiac cachexia. N. Engl. J. Med. *27*:403, 1964.
61. Finkel, M. S., Oddis, C. V., Jacob, T. D., et al.: Negative inotropic effects of cytokines on the heart mediated by nitric oxide. Science *257*:387, 1992.
62. Yokoyama, T., Vaca, L., Rossen, R. D., et al.: Cellular basis for the negative inotropic effects of tumor necrosis factor-alpha in the adult mammalian heart. J. Clin. Invest. *92*:2303, 1993.
63. Mann, D. L., and Young, J. B.: Basic mechanisms in congestive heart failure: Recognizing the role of proinflammatory cytokines. Chest *105*:897, 1994.
64. Thaik, C. M., Calderone, A., Takahashi, N., and Colucci, W. S.: Interleukin-1 beta modulates the growth and phenotype of rat cardiac myocytes. J. Clin. Invest. *96*:1093, 1995.
65. Lange, R. L., and Hecht, H. H.: The mechanism of Cheyne-Stokes respiration. J. Clin. Invest. *41*:42, 1962.
66. Hanly, P., Zuberi, N., and Gray, R.: Pathogenesis of Cheyne-Stokes respiration in patients with congestive heart failure. Relationship to arterial Pco_2. Chest *104*:1079, 1993.
67. Hanly, P., and Zuberi-Khokhar, N.: Daytime sleepiness in patients with congestive heart failure and Cheyne-Stokes respiration. Chest *107*:952, 1995.
68. Rees, P. J., and Clark, T. J. H.: Paroxysmal nocturnal dyspnoea and periodic respiration. Lancet *2*:1315, 1979.
69. Ben-Dov, I., Sietsema, K. E., Casaburi, R., and Wasserman, K.: Evidence that circulatory oscillations accompany ventilatory oscillations during exercise in patients with heart failure. Am. Rev. Respir. Dis. *145*:776, 1992.
70. Friedman-Mor, Z., Chalon, J., Turndorf, H., and Orkin, L. R.: Cardiac index and incidence of heart failure cells. Arch. Pathol. Lab. Med. *102*:418, 1978.
71. Wolke, A. M., Brooks, K. M., and Schaffner, F.: The liver in congestive heart failure. Primary Cardiol. *8*:130, 1982.
72. Blasco, V. V.: Features of hepatic involvement in congestive heart failure. Cardiovasc. Rev. Rep. *4*:963, 1983.
73. Lemmer, J. H., Coran, A. G., Behrendt, D. M., et al.: Liver fibrosis (cardiac cirrhosis) five years after modified Fontan operation for tricuspid atresia. J. Thorac. Cardiovasc. Surg. *86*:757, 1983.
74. Matsuda, H., Covino, E., Hirose, H., et al.: Acute liver dysfunction after modified Fontan operation for complex cardiac lesions. J. Thorac. Cardiovasc. Surg. *96*:219, 1988.
75. Mace, S., Borkat, G., and Liebman, J.: Hepatic dysfunction and cardiovascular abnormalities: Occurrence in infants, children and young adults. Am. J. Dis. Child. *139*:60, 1985.
76. Kanel, G. C., Ucci, A. A., Kaplan, M. M., and Wolfe, H. J.: A distinctive perivenular hepatic lesion associated with heart failure. Am. J. Clin. Pathol. *73*:235, 1980.
77. Nouel, O., Henrion, J., Bernuau, J., et al.: Fulminant hepatic failure due to transient circulatory failure in patients with chronic heart disease. Dig. Dis. Sci. *25*:49, 1980.
78. Jenkins, J. G., Lynn, A. M., Wood, A. E., et al.: Acute hepatic failure following cardiac operation in children. J. Thorac. Cardiovasc. Surg. *84*:865, 1982.
79. Szatalowicz, V. L., Arnold, P. E., Chaimovitz, C., et al.: Radioimmunoassay of plasma arginine vasopressin in hyponatremic patients with congestive heart failure. N. Engl. J. Med. *305*:263, 1981.
80. Chakko, S. C., Frutchey, J., and Gheorghiade, M.: Life-threatening hyperkalemia in severe heart failure. Am. Heart J. *117*:1083, 1989.
81. Kaplan, M. M.: Liver dysfunction secondary to congestive heart failure. Practical Cardiol. *6*:39, 1980.
82. Kubo, S. H., Walter, B. A., John, D. H. A., et al.: Liver function abnormalities in chronic heart failure: Influence of systemic hemodynamics. Arch. Intern. Med. *147*:1227, 1987.
83. Gorlin, R., Knowles, J. H., and Storey, C. F.: The Valsalva maneuver as a test of cardiac function. Pathologic physiology and clinical significance. Am. J. Med. *22*:197, 1957.
84. Schmidt, D. E., and Shah, P. K.: Accurate detection of elevated left ventricular filling pressure by a simplified bedside application of the Valsalva maneuver. Am. J. Cardiol. *71*:462, 1993.
85. Elisberg, E. I.: Heart rate response to the Valsalva maneuver as a test of circulatory integrity. JAMA *186*:200, 1963.
86. McIntyre, K. M., Vita, J. A., Lambrew, C. T., et al.: A noninvasive method of predicting pulmonary-capillary wedge pressure. N. Engl. J. Med. *327*:1715, 1992.
87. Baron, M. G.: Radiological and angiographic examination of the heart. *In* Braunwald, E. (ed.): Heart Disease. 3rd ed. Philadelphia, W. B. Saunders Company, 1988, p. 148.
88. Chakko, S., Woska, D., Martinez, H., et al.: Clinical, radiographic, and hemodynamic correlations in chronic congestive heart failure: Conflicting results may lead to inappropriate care. Am. J. Med. *90*:353, 1991.
89. Evaluating the radiographic assessment of pulmonary venous hypertension in chronic heart disease. AJR *142*:877, 1984.
90. Daves, M. L.: Cardiac Roentgenology. Chicago, Year Book Medical Publishers, 1981, pp. 78–86.

PROGNOSIS

91. Ho, K. K., Anderson, K. M., Kannel, W. B., et al.: Survival after the onset of congestive heart failure in Framingham Heart Study subjects. Circulation *88*:107, 1993.
92. Cohn, J. N., and Rector, T. S.: Prognosis of congestive heart failure and predictors of mortality. Am. J. Cardiol. *62*:25A, 1988.
93. Sziachic, J., et al.: Correlates and prognostic implications of exercise capacity in chronic congestive heart failure. Am. J. Cardiol. *55*:1037, 1986.
94. Rahimtoola, S. H.: The pharmacologic treatment of chronic congestive heart failure. Circulation *80*:693, 1989.
95. Murali, S., and Thompson, M. E.: Pathophysiology and drug therapy in congestive heart failure. Cardiology *7*:41, 1990.
96. Gradman, A., Deedwania, P., Cody, R., et al.: Predictors of total mortality and sudden death in mild to moderate heart failure. J. Am. Coll. Cardiol. *14*:564, 1989.
97. Lee, T. H., Hamilton, M. A., Stevenson, L. W., et al.: Impact of left ventricular cavity size on survival in advanced heart failure. Am. J. Cardiol. *72*:672, 1993.
98. Di Salvo, T. G., Mathier, M., Semigran, M. J., and Dec, G. W.: Preserved right ventricular ejection fraction predicts exercise capacity and survival in advanced heart failure. J. Am. Coll. Cardiol. *25*:1143, 1995.
99. Parameshwar, J., Keegan, J., Sparrow, J., et al.: Predictors of prognosis in severe heart failure. Am. Heart J. *123*:421, 1992.
100. Cleland, J. G. F., and Dargie, H. J.: Arrhythmias, catecholamines and electrolyte. Am. J. Cardiol. *62*:55A, 1988.
101. Cleland, J. G. F., Dargie, H. J., and Ford, I.: Mortality in heart failure: Clinical variables of prognostic value. Br. Heart J. *58*:572, 1987.
102. Francis, G. S., Cohn, J. N., Johnson, G., et al.: Plasma norepinephrine, plasma renin activity, and congestive heart failure. Relations to survival and the effects of therapy in V-HeFT II. The V-HeFT VA Cooperative Studies Group. Circulation *87*:VI40, 1993.
103. Packer, M., Gottlieb, S. S., and Blum, M. A.: Immediate and long-term pathophysiologic mechanisms underlying the genesis of sudden cardiac death in patients with congestive heart failure. Am. J. Med. *82*(Suppl. 3a):4, 1987.
104. Packer, M., Lee, W. H., Kessler, P. D., et al.: Role of neurohormonal mechanisms in determining survival in patients with severe chronic heart failure. Circulation *75*:(Suppl. 4)80, 1987.
105. Gottlieb, S. S., Kukin, M. L., Ahern, D., and Packer, M.: Prognostic importance of atrial natriuretic peptide in patients with chronic heart failure. J. Am. Coll. Cardiol. *13*:1534, 1989.
106. Packer, M.: Potential role of potassium as a determinant of morbidity and mortality in patients with systemic hypertension and congestive heart failure. Am. J. Cardiol. *65*:45E, 1990.
107. Hyperdynamic States. *In* Fowler, N. O.: Diagnosis of Heart Disease. New York, Springer-Verlag, 1991, pp. 389–399.

HIGH OUTPUT HEART FAILURE

108. Nicoladoni, C.: Phlebarteriectasie der rechten oberen Extermitat. Arch. Klin. Chir. *18*:252, 1875.
109. Branham, H. H.: Aneurysmal varix of the femoral artery and vein following a gunshot wound. Int. J. Surg. *3*:250, 1890.
110. Gupta, P. D., and Singh, M.: Neural mechanism underlying tachycardia induced by non-hypotensive A-V shunt. Am. J. Physiol. *236*:H35, 1979.
111. Dorney, E. R.: Peripheral AV fistula of fifty-seven years' duration with refractory heart failure. Am. Heart J. *54*:778, 1957.
112. Sanyal, S. K., Saldivar, V., Coburn, T. P., et al.: Hyperdynamic heart failure due to A-V fistula associated with Wilms' tumor. Pediatrics *57*:564, 1976.
113. Ingram, C. W., Satler, L. F., and Rackley, C. E.: Progressive heart failure secondary to a high output state. Chest *92*:1117, 1987.
114. Fee, H. J., Levisman, J., Doud, R. B., and Golding, A. L.: High output congestive failure from femoral arteriovenous shunts for vascular access. Ann. Surg. *183*:321, 1976.
115. Anderson, C. B., Codd, J. R., Graff, R. A., et al.: Cardiac failure and upper extremity arteriovenous dialysis fistulas. Arch. Intern. Med. *136*:292, 1976.

116. Szilagyi, D. E., Smith, R. F., Elliott, J. P., and Hageman, J. H.: Congenital arteriovenous anomalies of the limbs. Arch. Surg. *111*:423, 1976.
117. Becker, D. G., Fish, C. R., and Juergen, S. J. L.: Arteriovenous fistulas of the female pelvis. Obstet. Gynecol. *31*:799, 1968.
118. Price, A. C., Coran, A. G., and Mattern, A. L.: Hemangioendothelioma of the pelvis: A cause of cardiac failure in the newborn. N. Engl. J. Med. *286*:647, 1972.
119. Coel, M. N., and Alksne, J. F.: Embolization to diminish high output failure secondary to systemic angiomatosis (Ullman's syndrome). Vasc. Surg. *12*:336, 1978.
120. Vaksmann, G., Rey, C., Marache, P., et al.: Severe congestive heart failure in newborns due to giant cutaneous hemangiomas. Am. J. Cardiol. *60*:392, 1987.
121. Gong, B., Baken, L. A., Julian, T. M., and Kubo, S. H.: High-output heart failure due to hepatic arteriovenous fistula during pregnancy: A case report. Obstet. Gynecol. *72*:440, 1988.
122. Baranda, M. M., Perez, M., DeAndres, J., et al.: High-output congestive heart failure as first manifestation of Osler-Weber-Rendu disease. J. Vasc. Dis. *35*:568, 1984.
123. Zavota, L., Bini, F., Carano, N., et al.: Hepatic hemangiomatosis with congestive cardiac failure and development into a cholestatic hepatopathy. Pediatr. Med. Chir. *6*:621, 1984.
124. Lewis, B. S., Ehrenfelk, E. N., Lewis, N., and Gotsman, M. S.: Echocardiographic left ventricular function in thyrotoxicosis. Am. Heart J. *97*:460, 1979.
125. Hoffman, I., and Lowrey, R. D.: The electrocardiogram in thyrotoxicosis. Am. J. Cardiol. *8*:893, 1960.
126. Braunwald, E., Mason, D. T., and Ross, J., Jr.: Studies of the cardiocirculatory actions of digitalis. Medicine *44*:233, 1965.
127. Shapiro, S., Steiner, M., and Dimich, I.: Congestive heart failure in neonatal thyrotoxicosis. A curable cause of heart failure in the newborn. Clin. Pediatr. *14*:1155, 1975.
128. Weiss, S., and Wilkinson, R. W.: The nature of the cardiovascular disturbances in nutritional deficiency states (beriberi). Ann. Intern. Med. *11*:104, 1937.
129. Burwell, C. S., and Dexter, L.: Beriberi heart disease. Trans. Assoc. Am. Physicians *60*:59, 1947.
130. Akbarian, M., Yankopoulos, N. A., and Abelmann, W. H.: Hemodynamic studies in beriberi heart disease. Am. J. Med. *41*:197, 1966.
131. Ayzenberg, O., Silber, M. H., and Bortz, D.: Beriberi heart disease. A case report describing the hemodynamic features. S. Afr. Med. J. *68*:263, 1985.
132. Akram, H., Maslowski, A. H., Smith, B. L., and Nichols, M. G.: The haemodynamic, histopathological and hormonal features of alcoholic beriberi. Q. J. Med. *50*:359, 1981.
133. Naidoo, D. P.: Beriberi heart disease in Durban. S. Afr. Med. J. *72*:241, 1987.
134. Naidoo, D. P., Rawat, R., Dyer, R. B., et al.: Cardiac beriberi: A report of four cases. S. Afr. Med. J. *72*:283, 1987.
135. Carson, P.: Alcoholic cardiac beriberi. Br. Med. J. *284*:1817, 1982.
136. Cardiovascular beriberi (editorial). Lancet *1*:1287, 1982.
137. Akbarian, M., and Dreyfus, P. M.: Blood trans-ketolase activity in beriberi heart disease. JAMA *203*:23, 1968.
138. Baker, H., quoted in Sauberlich, H. E.: Biochemical alterations in thiamine deficiency—their interpretation. Am. J. Clin. Nutr. *20*:543, 1967.
139. Brin, M.: Erythrocyte transketolase in early thiamine deficiency. Ann. N. Y. Acad. Sci. *98*:528, 1962.
140. Baker, H., and Frank, O.: Clinical Vitaminology: Methods and Interpretation. New York, Wiley Interscience, 1968.
141. Jeffrey, F. E., and Abelmann, W. H.: Recovery of proved Shoshin beriberi. Am. J. Med. *50*:123, 1971.
142. Whittemore, R., and Caddell, J. L.: Metabolic and nutritional diseases. *In* Moss, A. J., et al. (eds.): Heart Disease in Infants, Children and Adolescents. 2nd ed. Baltimore, Williams and Wilkins Co., 1977, pp. 590 and 591.
143. Heistad, D. D., Abboud, F. M., Schmid, P. G., et al.: Regulation of blood flow in Paget's disease of the bone. J. Clin. Invest. *55*:69, 1975.
144. Rutishauser, E., Veyrat, R., and Rouiller, C.: La vascularization de l'os pagé tique, étude anatomo-pathologique. Presse Méd. *62*:654, 1954.
145. Lequime, J., and Denolin, H.: Circulatory dynamics in osteitis deformans. Circulation *12*:215, 1955.
146. McBride, W., Jackman, J. D., Jr., Gammon, R. S., and Willerson, J. T.: High-output cardiac failure in patients with multiple myeloma. N. Engl. J. Med. *319*:1651, 1988.

PULMONARY EDEMA

147. Harris, P., and Heath, D.: Pulmonary edema. *In* The Human Pulmonary Circulation. 3rd ed. New York, Churchill Livingstone, 1986, pp. 373–383.
148. Guyton, A. C., Parker, J. C., Taylor, A. E., et al.: Forces governing water movement in the lung. *In* Fishman, A. P., and Renkin, E. M. (eds.): Pulmonary Edema. Bethesda, American Physiological Society, 1979, p. 70.
149. Guyton, A. C.: Textbook of Medical Physiology. 7th ed. Philadelphia, W. B. Saunders Company, 1986, p. 372.
150. Staub, N. C.: Pulmonary edema due to increased microvascular permeability to fluid and protein. Circ. Res. *43*:143, 1978.
151. Agostoni, E.: Mechanics of the pleural space. Physiol. Rev. *52*:57, 1972.
152. Dollery, C. T., Heimberg, P., and Hugh-Jones, P.: Relationships between blood flow and clearance rate of radioactive carbon dioxide and oxygen in normal and oedematous lungs. J. Physiol. (London) *162*:93, 1962.
153. Bernard, G. R., and Brigham, K. L.: Pulmonary edema. Pathophysiologic mechanisms and new approaches to therapy. Chest *89*:594, 1986.
154. Snapper, J. R., and Brigham, K. L.: Pulmonary edema. Hosp. Pract. *21*:87, 1986.
155. Sprung, C. L., Rackow, E. C., Fein, I. A., et al.: The spectrum of pulmonary edema: Differentiation of cardiogenic, intermediate, and noncardiogenic forms of pulmonary edema. Ann. Rev. Respir. Dis. *124*:718, 1981.
156. West, J. B., and Mathieu-Costello, O.: Pulmonary edema and hemorrhage: Recent advances. *In* Potchen, E. J., Grainger, R. G., and Greene, R. (eds.): *Pulmonary Radiology*. Philadelphia, W. B. Saunders Company, 1993, p. 125.
157. Minnear, F. L., Barie, P. S., and Malik, A. B.: Effects of large, transient increases in pulmonary vascular pressures on lung fluid balance. J. Appl. Physiol. *55*:983, 1983.
158. Cross, C. E., Shaver, J. A., Wilson, R. J., and Robin, E. D.: Mitral stenosis and pulmonary fibrosis: Special reference to pulmonary edema and lung lymphatic function. Arch. Intern. Med. *125*:248, 1970.
159. Kramer, G. C., Harms, B. A., Gunther, R. A., et al.: The effects of hypoproteinemia on blood-to-lymph fluid transport in sheep lung. Circ. Res. *49*:1173, 1981.
160. Mahfood, S., Hix, W. R., Aaron, B. L., et al.: Reexpansion pulmonary edema. Ann. Thorac. Surg. *45*:340, 1988.
161. Malik, A. B., and Staub, N. C. (eds.): Mechanisms of Lung Microvascular Injury. New York, New York Academy of Sciences, 1982.
162. Staub, N. C.: Pulmonary edema due to increased microvascular permeability. Ann. Rev. Med. *32*:291, 1981.
163. Carlson, R. W., Schaeffer, R. C., Jr., Puri, V. K., et al.: Hypovolemia and permeability pulmonary edema associated with anaphylaxis. Crit. Care Med. *9*:883, 1981.
164. Snell, J. D., Jr., and Ramsey, L. H.: Pulmonary edema as a result of endotoxemia. Am. J. Physiol. *217*:170, 1969.
165. Ratliff, N. B., Wilson, J. W., Horckel, D. B., and Martin, A. M., Jr.: The lung in hemorrhagic shock. II. Observations on alveolar and vascular ultrastructure. Am. J. Pathol. *58*:353, 1970.
166. Henning, R. J., Heyman, V., Alcover, I., and Romeo, S.: Cardiopulmonary effects of oleic acid-induced pulmonary edema and mechanical ventilation. Anesth. Analg. *65*:925, 1986.
167. Glauser, F. L., Fairman, R. P., Miller, J. E., and Falls, R. K.: Indomethacin blunts ethchloryne induced pulmonary hypertension but not pulmonary edema. J. Appl. Physiol. *53*:563, 1982.
168. Havill, A. M., Gee, M. H., Washburne, J. D., et al.: Alpha naphthyl thiourea produces dose dependent lung vascular injury in sheep. Am. J. Physiol. *243*:505, 1982.
169. Weinberg, P. F., Mathey, M. A., Webster, R. O., et al.: Biologically active products of complement in acute lung injury in patients with sepsis syndrome. Am. Rev. Resp. Dis. *130*:791, 1984.
170. Rinaldo, J. E., Dauber, G. H., Christman, J., and Rogers, R. M.: Neutrophil alveolitis endotoxemia. Am. Rev. Respir. Dis. *130*:1065, 1984.
171. Biermann, G. J., Dockey, B. F., and Thrall, R. S.: Polymorphonuclear leukocyte participation in acute oleic acid induced lung injury. Am. Rev. Respir. Dis. *128*:845, 1983.
172. Kline, J. N., and Hirasuna, J. D.: Pulmonary edema after freebase cocaine smoking—not due to an adulterant. Chest *97*:1009, 1990.
173. Kapanci, Y., Weibel, E. R., Kaplan, H. P., and Robinson, P. V. M.: Pathogenesis and reversibility of the pulmonary lesions of oxygen toxicity in monkey. II. Ultrastructural and morphometric studies. Lab. Invest. *20*:101, 1969.
174. Cameron, G. R., and Courtice, F. C.: The production and removal of oedema fluid in the lungs after exposure to carbonyl chloride (phosgene). J. Physiol. (London) *105*:175, 1946.
175. Bils, R. F.: Ultrastructural alterations of alveolar tissue of mice. III. Ozone. Arch. Environ. Health *20*:468, 1970.
176. Sherwin, R. P., and Richters, V.: Lung capillary permeability: nitrogen dioxide exposure and leakage of tritiated serum. Arch. Intern. Med. *128*:61, 1971.
177. Murray, J. F.: The lungs and heart failure. Hosp. Prac. *20*:55, 1985.
178. Fillmore, S. J., Giumaraes, A. C., Scheidt, S. S., and Killip, T.: Blood gas changes and pulmonary hemodynamics following acute myocardial infarction. Circulation *45*:583, 1972.
179. Szidon, J. P., Pietra, G. G., and Fishman, A. P.: The alveolar-capillary membrane and pulmonary edema. N. Engl. J. Med. *286*:1200, 1972.
180. Said, S. I., Avery, M. E., Davis, R. K., et al.: Pulmonary surface activity in induced pulmonary edema. J. Clin. Invest. *44*:458, 1965.
181. Miller, W. W., Waldhausen, J. A., and Rashkind, W. J.: Comparison of oxygen poisoning of the lung in cyanotic and acyanotic dogs. N. Engl. J. Med. *282*:943, 1970.
182. Henry, J. H.: The effect of shock on pulmonary alveolar surfactant: Its role in refractory respiratory insufficiency of the critically ill or severely injured patient. J. Trauma *8*:756, 1968.
183. Elias, R. M., and Johnston, M. G.: Modulation of lymphatic pumping by lymph borne factors after endotoxin administration in sheep. J. Appl. Physiol. *68*:199, 1990.
184. Schoene, R. B., Hackett, P. H., Henderson, W. R., et al.: High-altitude pulmonary edema. Characteristics of lung lavage fluid. JAMA *256*:63, 1986.

185. Naeije, R., Melot, C., and Lejeune, P.: Hypoxic pulmonary vasoconstriction and high altitude pulmonary edema. Am. Rev. Respir. Dis. *134*:332, 1986.
186. Sophocles, A. M., Jr.: High-altitude pulmonary edema in Vail, Colorado, 1975–1982. West. J. Med. *144*:569, 1986.
187. Lockhart, A., and Saiag, B.: Altitude and the human pulmonary circulation. Clin. Sci. *60*:599, 1981.
188. West, J. B., and Mathieu-Costello, O.: High altitude pulmonary edema is caused by stress failure of pulmonary capillaries. Int. J. Sports Med. *13*:S54, 1992.
189. Yabumoto, M., Kuriyama, T., Iwamoto, M., and Kinoshita, T.: Neurogenic pulmonary edema associated with ruptured intracranial aneurysm: Case report. Neurosurgery *19*:300, 1986.
190. Steinberg, A. D., and Karliner, J. S.: The clinical spectrum of heroin pulmonary edema. Arch. Intern. Med. *122*:122, 1968.
191. Fraser, D. W.: Methadone overdose: Illicit use of pharmaceutically prepared narcotics. JAMA *217*:1387, 1971.
192. Bogartz, L. J., and Miller, W. C.: Pulmonary edema associated with propoxyphene intoxication. JAMA *215*:259, 1971.
193. Katz, S., Aberman, A., Frand, U. I., et al.: Heroin pulmonary edema: Evidence for increased pulmonary capillary permeability. Am. Rev. Respir. Dis. *106*:472, 1972.
194. Gopinathan, K., Saroja, D., Spears, J. R., et al.: Hemodynamic studies in heroin induced acute pulmonary edema. Circulation *42*(Suppl. 3):44, 1970.
195. Brashear, R. E., Kelly, M. T., and White, A. C.: Elevated plasma histamine after heroin and morphine. J. Lab. Clin. Med. *83*:451, 1974.
196. Rovinsky, J. J., and Guttmacher, A. F.: Medical, Surgical, and Gynecologic Complications of Pregnancy. 2nd ed. Baltimore, Williams and Wilkins Co., 1965.
197. Goldbaum, T. S., Bacos, J. M., and Lindsay, J., Jr.: Pulmonary edema following conversion of tachyarrhythmia. Chest *89*:465, 1986.
198. Hashim, S. E., Kay, H. R., Hammond, G. L., et al.: Noncardiac pulmonary edema after cardiopulmonary bypass. Am. J. Surg. *147*:560, 1984.
199. Culliford, A. T., Thomas, S., and Spencer, F. C.: Fulminating noncardiogenic pulmonary edema: A newly recognized hazard during cardiac operations. J. Thorac. Cardiovasc. Surg. *80*:868, 1980.

ACKNOWLEDGEMENT

Dr. Roland H. Ingram and one of the authors of this chapter (E.B.) co-authored a chapter entitled "Pulmonary Edema: Cardiogenic and Non-cardiogenic" in the first four editions of this textbook. Portions of that chapter were updated, revised, and added to the present chapter. Dr. Ingram's important contributions to the present chapter are gratefully acknowledged.

Chapter 16
Drugs Used in the Treatment of Heart Failure

RALPH A. KELLY, THOMAS W. SMITH

VASODILATORS

The rationale for the use of vasodilators grew out of experience with parenteral sympatholytic agents and nitroprusside in patients with severe heart failure.[1] Studies of vasodilators demonstrated that they were well tolerated and effective in improving symptoms. The effectiveness of the isosorbide dinitrate–hydralazine combination[2] and of angiotensin-converting enzyme (ACE) inhibitors in reducing mortality in heart failure was demonstrated in several prospective randomized controlled trials in the 1980's (see Chap. 17, p. 495).[3] Table 16–1 lists those vasodilators commonly employed or under active investigation for the treatment of heart failure.

Vasodilators, as a class, reverse several of the characteristic physiological adaptations that accompany the development of heart failure (Fig. 16–1). These neurohumoral and physiological responses resemble, in some respects, those that accompany a fall in blood pressure due to hypovolemia. These include tachycardia and venous and arterial vasoconstriction, with shunting of blood toward the thorax and brain and away from the splanchnic, renal, and other peripheral vascular beds.[4] Although these responses provide a clear evolutionary advantage for survival with dehydration or following blood loss, they are maladaptive and deleterious in chronic heart failure.

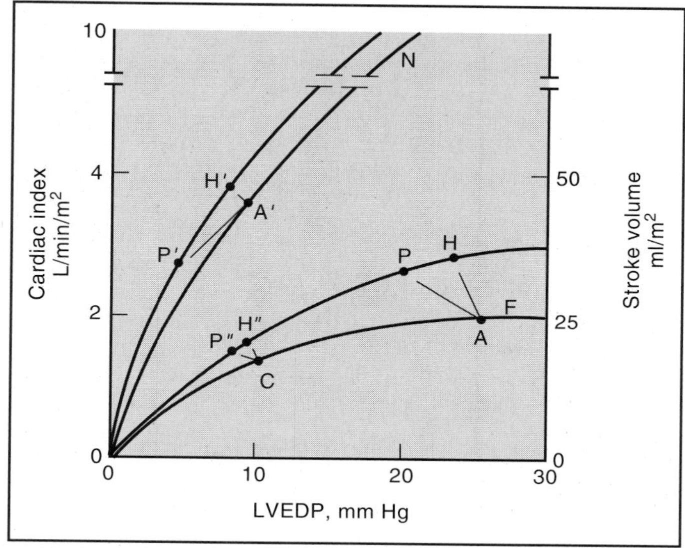

FIGURE 16–1. Effects of various vasodilators on the relationship between left ventricular end-diastolic pressure (LVEDP) and cardiac index or stroke volume in normal (N) and failing (F) hearts. "H" represents hydralazine or any other pure arterial vasodilator. It produces only a minimal increase in cardiac index in normal subjects (A′ → H′) or in patients with heart failure with a normal LVEDP (C → H″). In contrast, it elevates output in the patient with heart failure and elevated LVEDP (A → H). "C" represents a balanced vasodilator, such as sodium nitroprusside or captopril. It reduces filling pressure in all patients, elevates cardiac output in patients with heart failure and elevated LVEDP (A → C), lowers cardiac output in normal subjects (A′ → C′), and has little effect on cardiac output in heart failure patients with normal filling pressures (C → C″).

Renin-Angiotensin System Antagonists

RENIN-ANGIOTENSIN SYSTEMS. The importance of the renin-angiotensin system (RAS) in the pathophysiology of heart failure (see p. 413) has been underscored by the effectiveness of antagonists of this system in improving symptoms and in reducing mortality in this syndrome. Classically, this system has been viewed as a renin-angiotensin-aldosterone axis, the activity of which is determined by the rate of renin released into the systemic circulation from the juxtaglomerular apparatus in the glomerular afferent arterioles.[5] With the advent of highly specific and sensitive technologies for the detection and cellular localization of components of the renin-angiotensin system, such as autoradiography with radiolabeled ACE inhibitors, sensitive radioimmunoassay, in situ hybridization, quantitative polymerase chain reaction, and transgenic animal technology, it is now recognized that many "local" or "tissue" RAS exist throughout the vasculature and in parenchymal cells of most, if not all, organs.[5–9] Within the cellular components of blood vessels, for example, de novo synthesis and secretion of angiotensin II (Ang II) from aortic endothelial cells in vitro was described a decade ago by Kifor and Dzau,[10] and more recent evidence suggests that locally released Ang II acts within the vascular wall as a paracrine signalling peptide to promote the proliferation as well as the contraction of vascular smooth muscle cells.[5,11,12] Within the kidney, as well as within other organs classically associated with the renin-angiotensin-aldosterone axis, such as the adrenal cortex, all components of the classic systemic RAS (i.e., renin, angiotensinogen, and ACE) can be found, suggesting that the activity of Ang II within each of these tissues is largely, if not exclusively, determined by its local synthesis, activation, and release.

ANGIOTENSIN RECEPTORS. Two classes of Ang II receptors have been described to date, AT1 and AT2, both of which bind Ang II with roughly equal affinities and both of which are widely distributed in many tissues in a developmental and cell type–specific manner.[5,13–15] AT1 receptors are GTP-binding protein-linked integral membrane pro-

TABLE 16–1 VASODILATOR DRUGS USED IN THE TREATMENT OF HEART FAILURE

DRUG	MECHANISM	PRELOAD REDUCTION	AFTERLOAD REDUCTION	USUAL DOSE
RENIN-ANGIOTENSIN SYSTEM ANTAGONISTS				
Captopril	Inhibition of renal systemic and tissue generation of angiotensin II by	++	++	6.25–50 mg p.o. q8h
Enalapril	ACE; decreased metabolism of bradykinin	++	++	2.5–10 mg p.o. q12h
Enalaprilat				0.5–2.0 mg IV q12h
Quinapril		++	++	10–80 mg p.o. q.d.
Lisinopril		++	++	2.5–20 mg p.o. q12–24h
Ramipril		++	++	1.25–5 mg p.o. q.d.
Losartan	Blockade of angiotensin II (AT_1) receptors	++	++	25–50 mg q12h
NITROVASODILATORS				
				0.2–10 μg/kg/min IV
Nitroglycerin	Nitric oxide donors	+++	+	5–6 mg transdermal
Isosorbide Dinitrate		+++	+	10–60 mg q.i.d.
Nitroprusside		+++	+++	0.1–3 μg/kg/min IV
DIRECT VASODILATORS				
Hydralazine	Unclear	+	+++	10–100 p.o. q6h
Nicorandil*	Increased K^+ channel conductance	++	+++	Not determined
Minoxidil	and other mechanisms	+	+++	5–10 mg q.d.
Diazoxide		+	+++	1–3 mg/kg q4–24h
CALCIUM CHANNEL BLOCKING DRUGS				
Nifedipine	Inhibition of L-type voltage-sensitive	+	+++	10–30 mg p.o. t.i.d.
Amlodipine	Ca^{++} channels	+	+++	5–10 mg p.o. q.d.
Felodipine		+	+++	5–10 mg p.o. q.d.
PHOSPHODIESTERASE INHIBITORS				
Amrinone	Inhibition of type III cAMP phosphodiesterase(s) and other mechanisms	++	++	0.5 mg/kg, then 2–20 μg/kg/min IV
Milrinone		++	++	50 μg/kg, then 0.25–1 μg/kg/min IV
Vesnarinone*				Not determined
SYMPATHOMIMETICS				
Dobutamine	Myocardial and vascular beta-adrenergic agonist	+	++	2–20 μg/kg/min
Dopamine	Selective renal arterial vasodilation	–	– –	≤ 2 μg/kg/min
SYMPATHOLYTICS				
Prazosin (and other quinazoline derivatives)	$Alpha_1$-adrenergic receptor antagonist	+++	++	1–5 mg p.o. q12h
Phentolamine	Nonselective alpha-adrenergic blockade	++	++	0.5–1.0 mg/min I.V.
Labetalol	Beta-adrenergic and $alpha_1$-adrenergic blockade	+	++	100–400 mg b.i.d.
Carvedilol*		+	++	12.5–50 mg p.o. b.i.d.
Bucindolol*	Additional mechanisms	+	++	6.25–100 mg p.o. b.i.d.

* Investigational and not approved by the US Food and Drug Administration at the time of this writing.

Adapted from Kelly, R. A., and Smith, T. W.: The pharmacologic treatment of heart failure. *In* Hardman, J. G., Limbird, L. (eds.): Goodman & Gilman's Pharmacologic Basis of Therapeutics, 9th ed. New York, McGraw Hill Book Co., 1996. © 1996 the McGraw-Hill Companies, Inc.

teins with seven transmembrane-spanning domains that bind the diphenylimidazole derivative losartan.[13] The AT2 receptor is also a seven transmembrane-spanning domain receptor, although the cellular signalling pathways initiated by Ang II binding at this receptor are not clear at this time. Two groups have independently reported that the ratio of AT2 to AT1 receptors is 2:1 in normal human myocardium.[16,17] The number of Ang II receptors has been reported to be decreased by over 50 per cent in myocardial tissue obtained from patients with end-stage heart failure, with no change in the ratio of AT2 to AT1 receptors.[16] The present limited literature on the molecular pharmacology of angiotensin receptors in human heart failure is now likely to expand rapidly with the identification of specific receptor subtypes.

CARDIOVASCULAR ACTIONS OF ANGIOTENSINS

Despite the fact that the molecular components of the renin-angiotensin-aldosterone axis have been known for decades and that specific angiotensin and aldosterone antagonists have been available for over 20 years, the recognition that angiotensins appear to play a major role in vascular and cardiac cell biology and pharmacology has occurred only relatively recently. Several recent reviews and editorials have focused on possible direct or indirect effects of angiotensins on vascular and myocardial remodeling and improved myocardial energetics among other mechanisms.[18,19]

VASOCONSTRICTION. Angiotensins have direct vasoconstrictor activity in vascular smooth muscle. In addition, Ang II enhances the activity of the sympathetic nervous system by several mechanisms, including blockade of norepinephrine reuptake and facilitation of norepinephrine release. In normal subjects, a significant proportion of peripheral arterial vasoconstriction to an Ang II infusion is mediated by the local release of norepinephrine.[20,21] In addition, angiotensins have direct effects on coagulation and fibrinolytic pathways and on vascular smooth muscle proliferation.[22,23]

INOTROPY. A positive inotropic effect of Ang II, mediated by AT1 receptors, has been demonstrated in atrial and ventricular muscle strips in several species, including normal human myocardium, although it is not clear how relevant this is to human physiology.[17,24–26] Experiments in animal models of cardiac hypertrophy have suggested that an activated intracardiac RAS plays a role in mediating a decrease in ventricular compliance.[27–30]

CELLULAR PROLIFERATION. In vitro, Ang II is known to induce activation of signalling pathways that lead to cellular proliferation of fibroblasts isolated from cardiac muscle and that contribute to the increased fibrosis characteristic of some forms of cardiac hypertrophy and cardiomyopathy.[31–33] Ang II can induce hypertrophic growth of neonatal ventricular myocytes in vitro and may do so in vivo as well by potentiating the activity of the sympathetic nervous system and the release of norepinephrine, which is known to induce myocyte hypertrophy in vitro by acting through α_1-adrenergic receptors.[34–36] These two actions of Ang II, in addition to its arterial and venous vasoconstrictor properties, probably contribute importantly to the remodeling that occurs in surviving ventricular muscle following myocardial infarction, first documented by observations in rats with experimental myocardial infarction in the early 1980's with the ACE inhibitor captopril and since replicated in other species.[19,37,38]

RAS ANTAGONISTS. In addition to inhibition of intracardiac RAS, renin-angiotensin antagonists, by virtue of their vasodilating activity, also reduce intracavity pressures and diminish wall stress, thereby decreasing myocardial oxygen demand. They also inhibit Ang II stimulation of aldosterone release, which reduces intravascular volume and preload and may have direct actions on the extent of interstitial collagen deposition in the heart.[39] ACE inhibitors have also been shown to decrease sympathetic nervous system activity and improve parasympathetic nervous system tone, which could result in reduced electrophysiological instability in infarcted or cardiomyopathic muscle.[40]

RENAL ACTIONS OF ANGIOTENSIN II AND RAS ANTAGONISTS. In addition to the above diverse actions, RAS antagonists also exhibit beneficial pharmacological effects on sodium homeostasis in heart failure. This is due to the important role of angiotensin II in the regulation of intrarenal hemodynamics, glomerular filtration, and tubular resorption of solute and water in the kidney. Angiotensin II regulates glomerular efferent arteriolar tone, a major determinant of the filtration fraction—that is, the fraction of renal plasma flow that crosses the glomerular membrane and passes into the proximal tubule. Intrarenal Angiotensin II activity, in the absence of a marked decline in renal blood flow or perfusion pressure, increases filtration fraction, leading to increased solute resorption in the proximal tubule (Fig. 16–2). Angiotensin II also appears to have additional direct effects on renal tubular epithelial cell salt and water resorption. Angiotensin II induces the release of aldosterone from the adrenal cortex, increasing sodium resorption in the distal nephron (see p. 413). Finally, ACE inhibitors inhibit the intrarenal metabolism of bradykinin and increase intrarenal levels of this natriuretic autacoid.[6]

Although the unique intrarenal actions of renin-angiotensin system antagonists among vasodilators provide a pharmacological advantage for this class of drugs, there is an important caveat. Owing to their selective effects on efferent arteriolar tone, renin-angiotensin antagonists, unlike other vasodilators, limit the kidney's ability to autoregulate glomerular perfusion pressure and thereby maintain glomerular filtration. This may be particularly important in patients with a marginal cardiac output or blood pressure and can result in a decline in the glomerular filtration rate (GFR), resulting in an increase in serum creatinine levels. In the first *Co*operative *N*orth *S*candinavian *E*nalapril *Su*rvival *S*tudy (CONSENSUS I), in which the efficacy of enalapril was compared with placebo in patients with severe (NYHA class III and IV) heart failure, the serum creatinine increased by a factor of 2 or greater in 11 per cent of 123 patients compared with 3 per cent in the placebo group.[41] The maximal increase in serum creatinine correlated inversely with mean arterial pressure. Patients on higher daily doses of a Na,K,2Cl symport inhibitor (e.g., furosemide) were at a slightly higher risk for a significant elevation in serum creatinine.[42]

The factors associated with a decline in renal function in heart failure in patients receiving an ACE inhibitor are listed in Table 16–2. It should be noted that most patients in the CONSENSUS I trial tolerated enalapril well, and the serum creatinine in fact fell in 24 per cent of patients.[41] This has generally been the experience in most of the later trials involving ACE inhibitors, reviewed in Chapter 17, in which patients on average had less severe heart failure than those in the CONSENSUS I trial. In the arm of the SOLVD trial that examined symptomatic patients with heart failure, approximately 11 per cent of patients receiving enalapril had an increase in serum creatinine above 2 mg/dl compared with 8 per cent receiving placebo.[43] In the GISSI-3 trial, there was a small but significantly increased risk of renal dysfunction at 6 weeks in patients randomized to receive lisinopril who had normal renal function at the entry of study (0.6 per cent for lisinopril versus 0.3 per cent among controls).[44] A similar small, but statistically significant, increase in the incidence of moderate renal

TABLE 16–2 ACE INHIBITORS AND RENAL DYSFUNCTION IN HEART FAILURE

FACTORS FAVORING DETERIORATION IN RENAL FUNCTION
Na^+ depletion or poor renal perfusion
Large doses of diuretics
Increased urea/creatinine ratio
Mean arterial pressure < 80 mm Hg
Evidence of maximal neurohumoral activation
Presence of hyponatremia secondary to AVP activation
Interruption of counterregulatory mechanisms
Coadministration of prostaglandin inhibitors
Presence of adrenergic dysfunction (e.g., diabetes mellitus)
FACTORS FAVORING IMPROVEMENT IN RENAL FUNCTION
Maintenance of Na^+ balance
Reduction in diuretic dosage
Increase in sodium intake
Mean arterial pressure > 80 mm Hg
Minimal neurohumoral activation
Intact counterregulatory mechanisms

From Miller, J. A., Tobe, S. W., and Skorecki, K. L.: Control of extracellular fluid volume and the pathophysiology of edema. *In* Brenner, B. M., and Rector, F. C. (eds.): The Kidney, 5th ed. Philadelphia, W.B. Saunders Company, 1995.

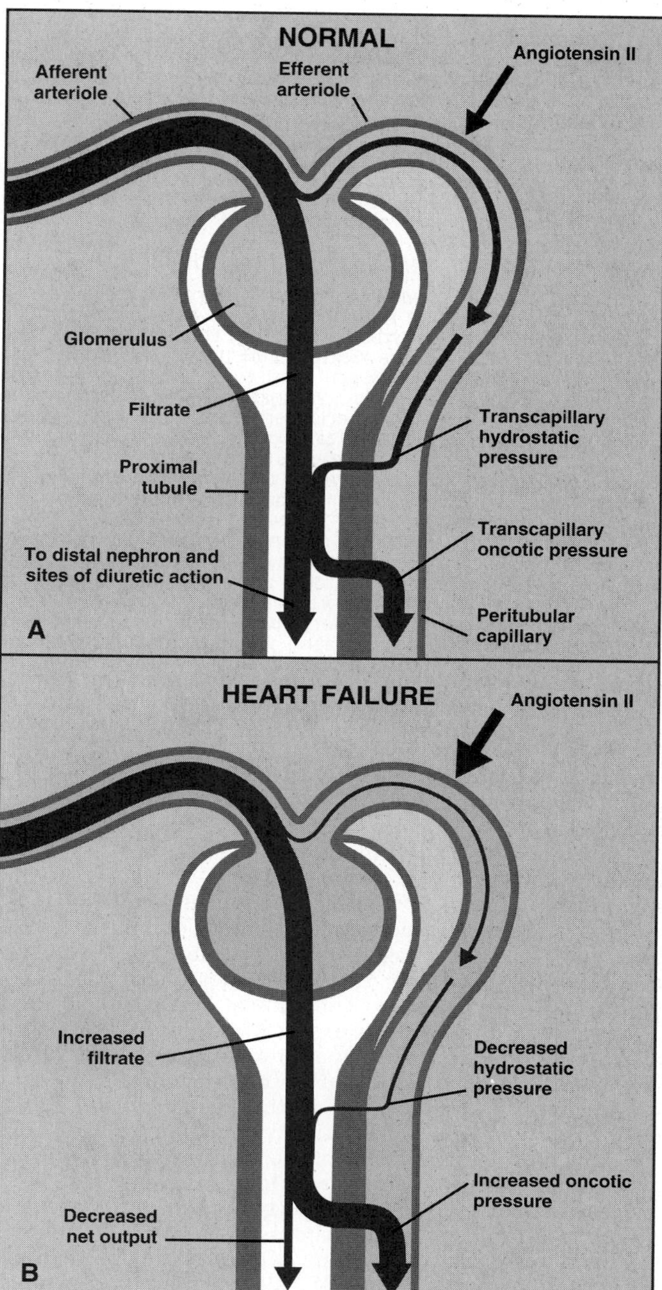

FIGURE 16–2. Renal function in the normal and heart failure states. Compared with normal glomerular function *(A)*, heart failure *(B)* is characterized by an increase in filtration fraction. This causes a fall in transcapillary hydrostatic pressure and increases oncotic pressure and thus promotes heightened solute and water reabsorption in the proximal tubule. This increase in filtration fraction is in large part mediated by increased constriction of the efferent arteriole by local intrarenal generation of angiotensin II. Renin angiotensin system antagonists can decrease the filtration fraction by causing relatively selective dilation of the efferent arteriole. (Adapted from Smith, T. W. and Kelly, R. A.: Therapeutic strategies for congestive heart failure in the 1990's. Hosp Pract 26:127, 1991. © 1991 The McGraw-Hill Companies, Inc.)

dysfunction was observed in the ISIS-4 trial with captopril (1.1 per cent for captopril versus 0.6 per cent with placebo).[45]

An increase in serum creatinine need not require discontinuation of an ACE inhibitor, particularly if the decline in urea or creatinine clearance does not lead to symptoms and urinary sodium excretion with or without diuretics does not decrease. More than a doubling of the serum creatinine should lead to a reduction in the ACE inhibitor dose or to a substitution with another class of vasodilator, provided that arterial perfusion pressure remains adequate. ACE inhibitors have been shown to improve or slow the decline in renal function in some patients with primary renal pathology.[46,47]

ANGIOTENSIN-CONVERTING ENZYME INHIBITORS

Ondetti has recently provided a personal history of the synthesis of the first orally bioavailable ACE inhibitor.[48] A synthetic nonapeptide analog, teprotide, was first studied in normal volunteers in the early 1970's, and its efficacy in the treatment of hypertension and heart failure was documented in several small trials. This agent was not orally bioavailable and remained investigational. Then, based on the observation that benzylsuccinic acid derivatives such as succinyl-L-proline were potent inhibitors of carboxyl peptidase A (ACE is a carboxyl peptidase), Ondetti and colleagues synthesized 3-mercaptopropanoyl-L-proline. This compound was 3000 times more potent as an ACE inhibitor than succinyl-L-proline, and its α-methyl analogue—given the generic name captopril—was well absorbed orally.

All orally active ACE inhibitors currently available fall into three general categories: (1) those with a sulfhydryl group that binds to the zinc moiety in ACE, including captopril and zofenapril*; (2) those in which the carboxyl group in the original succinyl-L-proline molecule was designed to bind the zinc moiety, and these include the majority of ACE inhibitors, including enalapril, lisinopril, ramipril, cilazapril, quinapril, and others; and (3) proline derivatives in which a phosphinic acid group is used to bind to the zinc moiety, of which fosinopril is the prototype. Several of these drugs are inactive esters or pro-drugs, such as zofenapril, enalapril, and fosinapril, and must be de-esterified to the active drug in vivo.

TISSUE ACTIONS OF ACE INHIBITORS. When tissue ACE levels are measured directly, significant differences have been noted in the extent of ACE inhibition in a given tissue or organ among ACE inhibitors, and specific tissues or organs exhibit different degrees of ACE inhibition to the same ACE inhibitor.[49–51] These differences in ACE activity and physiological responsiveness among members of the same class of RAS antagonists are probably due to the accessibility of active drug to cellular sites of Ang II generation within a given tissue. The clinical importance of these differences in the site and extent of accumulation of specific ACE inhibitors requires additional investigation. ACE inhibitors also effectively inhibit the systemic renin-angiotensin-aldosterone axis by preventing the conversion of angiotensin I to angiotensin II in the circulation.

CLINICAL USE. It is advisable to begin therapy for heart failure with an ACE inhibitor at low doses of a relatively short-acting drug (e.g., 6.25 mg captopril or 2.5 mg enalapril). An abrupt fall in blood pressure occasionally occurs following an initial dose of an ACE inhibitor, particularly in patients with depletion of this intravascular volume. This response is often unpredictable, and therefore caution is recommended when beginning these drugs in any patient who has significant left ventricular dysfunction or who has received large doses of diuretics.[52–54] Unacceptable hypotension can usually be reversed by intravascular volume expansion.

Few consistent and clinically important pharmacokinetic drug interactions exist between the ACE inhibitors and most other class of drugs that would be administered to patients with heart failure.[55] There is no consistent evidence for an important interaction between any ACE inhibitor and digoxin. Because most ACE inhibitors are cleared primarily by the kidney, a reduction in dose and/or increase in dosing interval may be necessary in patients with renal impairment. *Cough* is a relatively frequent side effect of ACE inhibitors that may develop after weeks or even months of therapy (see also p. 497). *Angioedema* is a rare but potentially life-threatening side effect of these drugs. ACE inhibitors are contraindicated in pregnancy because of drug-induced malformations of the kidney.

ANGIOTENSIN II RECEPTOR ANTAGONISTS. Although peptide Ang II antagonists such as saralasin (also a partial agonist) have been available for decades for experimental use, orally bioavailable angiotensin receptor antagonists have only recently become available.[13] The first of these to undergo dose-ranging and safety trials in humans with heart failure is the AT1-selective antagonist losartan. Despite its specificity for only one class of Ang II receptors (i.e., AT1) and the lack of bradykinin-potentiating activity that is characteristic of ACE inhibitors, losartan's spectrum of activity appears to be very similar to that of the ACE inhibitors,[56,57] although experience with patients in heart failure is limited to date. As with ACE inhibitors, there was no reflex tachycardia associated with the decline in blood pressure and no evidence of tolerance to the drug's hemodynamic effects over a 12-week period in one study.[57] In larger trials of losartan in the treatment of primary hypertension, there has been no increased frequency of cough associated with its use.

RENIN INHIBITORS. The pharmaceutical industry also has developed a number of agents that inhibit the enzymatic activity of renin, all of which are investigational at this time. The most promising of these are the transition state analogues of the peptide sequence at the renin cleavage site on angiotensinogen.[58,59] The data available to date do *not* suggest that either AT1 receptor antagonists or renin inhibitors have a spectrum of activity in heart failure that is importantly different from those of the ACE inhibitors. However, these agents may play an important role in the management of patients who cannot tolerate ACE inhibitors because of cough or angioedema.

Nitrovasodilators

The cellular mechanisms by which nitrovasodilators lead to the relaxation of vascular smooth muscle have become apparent only in the past decade despite the fact that these drugs are among the oldest vasodilators in clinical practice. It is now understood that these drugs mimic the activity of nitric oxide and its congeners. These are autocrine and paracrine signalling autacoids that are formed in endothelial and smooth muscle cells throughout the vasculature, as well as in many other cell types, including cardiac muscle cells.[60–63] Nitrogen oxides were originally identified as the bioactive factor(s) responsible for endothelium-dependent relaxation of blood vessels.[64] Their primary mechanism of action in vascular smooth muscle cells is probably based on their ability to bind to a heme moiety in soluble guanylate cyclase, resulting in an increase in intracellular cGMP. The pharmacological activity of each of the nitrovasodilators depends upon their biotransformation into nitrogen oxides within the blood and vascular tissues.[65]

Nitroprusside

Nitroprusside is an effective venous and arterial vasodilator and acts to reduce both ventricular preload and afterload. Owing to the fact that it is quickly metabolized to cyanide and nitric oxide, its onset of action is rapid and upward titration can usually be achieved expeditiously to achieve an optimal and predictable hemodynamic effect. For these reasons, nitroprusside is commonly used in intensive care settings for management of acutely decompensated heart failure when blood pressure is adequate to maintain cerebral, coronary, and renal perfusion. Ventricular filling pressures are rapidly reduced by an increase in venous compliance, resulting in a redistribution of blood volume from central (thoracic) to peripheral veins, particularly the splanchnic vasculature.[66]

Nitroprusside is among the most effective afterload-reducing agents due to its spectrum of vasodilating activity

---

* Not approved by the US Food and Drug Administration at the time of this writing.

on different vascular beds. It reduces systemic vascular resistance, increases aortic wall compliance, and, at optimal doses, improves ventricular-vascular coupling. Nitroprusside also decreases pulmonary vascular resistance, and improves other components of right ventricular afterload, including the amplitude and timing of reflected pressure waves during ejection.

Hydrocyanic acid and cyanide are byproducts of the biotransformation of nitroprusside. Cyanide toxicity is uncommon, however, because cyanide is rapidly metabolized by the liver to thiocyanate, which is cleared by the kidney. Thiocyanate and/or cyanide toxicity may occur in the presence of hepatic or renal failure, and following prolonged infusions of nitroprusside in patients with marginal cardiac output or passive congestion of the liver. Thiocyanate toxicity, which is more common in patients with renal insufficiency, should be suspected in any patient receiving this drug who has unexplained abdominal pain, mental status changes, or convulsions. Clinical manifestations of cyanide toxicity are more subtle in onset and are usually manifested by a decline in cardiac output accompanied by a metabolic acidosis due to accumulation of lactic acid.

Organic Nitrates and Molsidomine*

Owing to their relatively selective vasodilating effects on the epicardial coronary vasculature, the organic nitrates (nitroglycerin, isosorbide dinitrate, and isosorbide mononitrate) may improve systolic and diastolic ventricular function by improving coronary flow in patients with an ischemic cardiomyopathy, in addition to their activity in reducing ventricular filling pressures, wall stress, and oxygen consumption (see p. 497).[68] In acute myocardial infarction, however, the effect of the routine use of nitrovasodilators on mortality remains controversial (see p. 1211).[45,69]

The experience with newer nitrovasodilators, including isosorbide mononitrate and molsidomine in the treatment of heart failure, is limited compared with their use in the treatment of angina. Molsidomine given intravenously or orally is effective in reducing systemic vascular resistance, pulmonary capillary wedge pressure, and right atrial pressure.[70] Tolerance to the arteriolar and venular vasodilating effects of this drug does develop, although its extent and time course may differ from tolerance associated with organic nitrates. The spectrum of activity of 5-isosorbide mononitrate would not be expected to differ from that of isosorbide dinitrate in heart failure.

TOLERANCE TO NITROVASODILATORS IN HEART FAILURE. The rapid development of tolerance to the venous and arteriolar vasodilating effects of the nitrovasodilators has been known for over a century. The reader is referred to recent comprehensive reviews[71-73] and page 1304. Although nitrate tolerance is well documented, the mechanism(s) responsible is not clearly understood. It is likely that several mechanisms contribute to decreased responsiveness to nitrovasodilators with time, and that the importance of the relative contribution of each potential mechanism differs with the specific drug employed, the underlying disease (heart failure versus angina), and among specific vascular beds.[74-76]

Most of the data on the efficacy of intermittent or eccentric nitroglycerin dosing protocols have been obtained in patients with angina rather than chronic congestive failure symptoms.[77,78] Nevertheless, it seems prudent to recommend a daily nitrate-free interval in patients on chronic doses of isosorbide dinitrate, which can usually be achieved by providing the last dose of isosorbide dinitrate in the early evening.

Hydralazine

Although its cellular mechanism of action remains poorly understood, hydralazine is an effective antihypertensive drug (see p. 498), particularly when combined with other agents that blunt compensatory increases in sympathetic tone and salt and water retention. In heart failure, hydralazine reduces right and left ventricular afterload by reducing systemic as well as pulmonary artery input impedance and vascular resistance. Unless symptomatic hypotension occurs, this is usually accompanied only by minor reflex increases in sympathetic nervous system activity. These hemodynamic changes result in an augmentation of forward stroke volume and a reduction in ventricular systolic wall stress and in the regurgitant fraction in mitral insufficiency.

Hydralazine is effective in reducing renal vascular resistance and in increasing renal blood flow to a greater degree than most other vasodilators. Therefore, hydralazine may be the vasodilator of choice in heart failure patients with renal dysfunction who cannot tolerate an ACE inhibitor. Hydralazine has minimal effects on venous capacitance and therefore is most effective when combined with agents with venodilating activity (e.g., organic nitrates).

Side effects that may necessitate dose adjustment or withdrawal of hydralazine are common. The most common complaints—headache and dizziness—also may be due to nitrates that are usually administered concurrently with hydralazine. Often, with time, the symptoms diminish or respond to a reduction in dose.

Hydralazine metabolism is mediated primarily by hepatic acetylation, although many additional potential metabolic pathways have been described.[79] Therefore, patients with a "slow acetylater" phenotype have a prolonged elimination half-life of the drug. At the usual doses and dosing intervals of hydralazine, these patients are at greater risk of developing arthritis or other components of a lupus-like syndrome.

Calcium Channel Antagonists

Although all four classes of calcium channel antagonists now available (i.e., phenylalkylamine [e.g., verapamil], benzothiazepenes [e.g., diltiazem], diarylaminopropylamines [e.g., bepridil], and "first-generation" dihydropyridines [e.g., nifedipine, nimodipine, nitredipine]) are effective vasodilators (see also pp. 616 and 855), none has been shown to produce sustained improvement in symptoms in heart failure patients with predominant systolic ventricular dysfunction. Indeed, these drugs appear to worsen symptoms and may actually increase mortality in patients with systolic dysfunction. This includes patients with heart failure due to ischemic disease.[80] The reason for these adverse effects of calcium channel blockers in heart failure is unclear. It may be related to the known negative inotropic effects of these drugs, to reflex neurohumoral activation, or to a combination of these and other effects.

So-called second-generation calcium channel antagonists of the dihydropyridine class, particularly amlodopine and felodipine, appear to have fewer negative inotropic effects than earlier drugs, and are currently being evaluated in randomized prospective trials to determine their effects on both symptoms and mortality in heart failure patients already receiving standard medical management.[81,82]

K^+ CHANNEL ACTIVATORS

Despite the well-known role of outward K^+ currents in initiating repolarization and in the maintenance of membrane potential in most cell types, the molecular characterization of individual K^+ channel proteins has occurred only recently.[83] They comprise diverse families of integral plasma membrane proteins, the K^+ conductances of which are specific to each family and are regulated by a number of factors including changes in transmembrane voltage, intracellular Ca^{++} activity, and intracellular ATP levels, among other mechanisms.[83-85] The distribution of K^+ channel isoforms is tissue- and cell type–specific, permitting the possibility of relatively selective tissue pharmacological activity of drugs acting on a specific family of K^+ channels. In vascular smooth muscle, increased outward K^+ conductance causes cellular hyperpolarization and decreased Ca^{++} entry, resulting in vasorelaxation.[85] Diazoxide and minoxidil, classic direct-acting vasodilators, are now known to act at K^+ channels.

Nicorandil,* pinacidil,* and cromakalin* are representative of a new class of K^+ channel activators that exhibit a unique spectrum of activity among vasodilator drugs. Like minoxidil, nicorandil is primarily an arteriolar vasodilator, but it is also effective in dilating epicardial coronary arteries and in reducing preload in experimental animals and patients with heart failure.[86,87] Nicorandil, pinacidil, and cromakalin have been tested in humans, primarily for hypertension and angina, and are effective and relatively well tolerated with fewer adverse effects than older direct vasodilators of this class.

* Not approved by the US Food and Drug Administration at the time of this writing.

The experience to date with these agents in patients with heart failure has been less extensive. Unlike nitrovasodilators, tolerance has not been observed to the antianginal effect of nicorandil or the drug's ability to cause a sustained reduction in left ventricular filling pressures.[88] As with any novel class of vasodilators, the utility of nicorandil, and of other K^+ channel activators under development in the drug treatment of heart failure, must await the design and completion of large controlled efficacy and survival trials.

DIURETICS

The importance of diuretics in the treatment of the syndrome of congestive heart failure relates to the central role of the kidney as the target organ of many of the neurohumoral and hemodynamic changes that occur in response to a failing myocardium[89–92] (see also Chap. 62). Diuretics do not influence the natural history of the underlying heart disease responsible for the decline in cardiac output. However, they can improve symptoms of heart failure by acting directly on solute and water reabsorption by the kidney and may slow the progression of cardiac chamber dilation by reducing ventricular filling pressures (i.e., preload; Fig. 16–3).

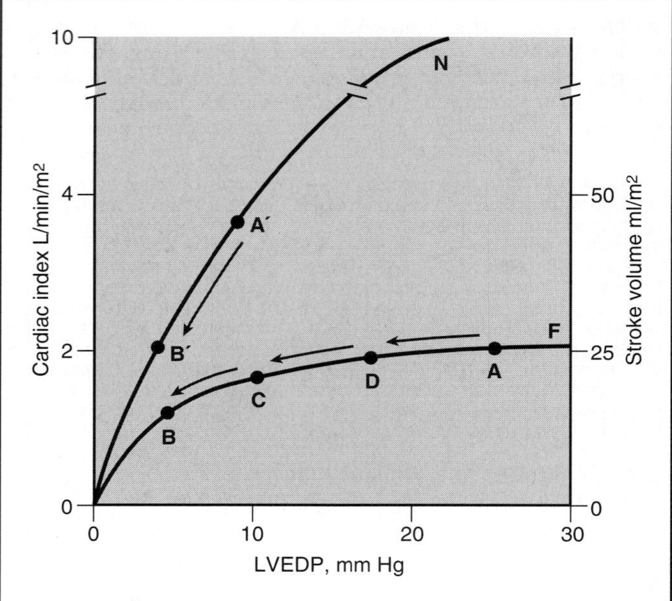

FIGURE 16–3. Effect of a venodilator (e.g., isosorbide dinitrate) or of diuretic therapy in a normal (N) subject (A′ → B′) and in a patient with heart failure (F) and markedly elevated left ventricular filling pressures (A → D), moderately elevated filling pressures (D → C), and normal filling pressures (C → B). In heart failure, a clinically significant decline in cardiac output usually does not occur until the LVEDP is below 10 mm Hg.

Renal Adaptations in Heart Failure

The increase in salt and water retention by the kidney in heart failure is due to characteristic alterations in intrarenal hemodynamics that occur in response to a decline in cardiac output, in addition to the activation of the sympathetic nervous system and of several hormonal as well as locally acting peptide and nonpeptide signalling pathways. A decrease in cardiac output, with or without an increase in intrapulmonary vascular pressures and decreased arterial oxygen saturation, results in an increase in peripheral and intrarenal vascular resistance, in the activation of intrarenal and other tissue renin-angiotensin systems, and in the release of arginine vasopressin (i.e., AVP, antidiuretic hormone). Increased adrenal cortical angiotensin II activity promotes aldosterone synthesis and release while increased intra-atrial and intraventricular pressures promote the release of atrial natriuretic peptide (ANP) and brain natriuretic peptide (BNP) from cardiac muscle.

INTRARENAL HEMODYNAMICS IN HEART FAILURE (See also Chap. 62). The changes in intrarenal hemodynamics that occur in early heart failure result in preservation of the GFR despite a decline in cardiac output and renal blood flow.[89,91] Although increases in sympathetic nervous system activity and local intrarenal release of angiotensin II act to increase resistance in both the afferent and efferent arterioles, this preservation of GFR is due in large part to a greater increase in efferent than in afferent arteriolar tone (Fig. 16–2). This results in an increase in the fraction of renal plasma flow that is filtered by the kidney (i.e., the filtration fraction). The increased filtration fraction also leads to an increase in hydrostatic pressure in the proximal tubule relative to the peritubular capillaries which, in addition to the increase in colloid osmotic pressure in this portion of the nephron, favors the reuptake of solute and water from the proximal tubule.[93]

In addition to their importance in mediating the increased renal salt and water resorption in heart failure, these characteristic alterations in glomerular hemodynamics are often importantly affected by several classes of drugs used in the treatment of heart failure. The kidney's ability to autoregulate and sustain GFR despite a falling cardiac output in worsening heart failure is compromised by any drug that lowers mean arterial pressure. Therefore, GFR may fall despite an increase in cardiac output following administration of some vasodilators. The importance of efferent arteriolar tone to the maintenance of GFR in heart failure also means that administration of renin-angiotensin system antagonists, including ACE inhibitors, could cause a decline in GFR in some patients despite an increase in cardiac output.

Mechanisms of Action

There are a number of classification schemes for diuretics based on their mechanism of action, their anatomical locus of action in the nephron, and the form of diuresis they elicit. Because the specific ion transport proteins that are the molecular targets for all the diuretics in common clinical use for the treatment of congestive heart failure recently have been identified and their amino acid sequence and intrarenal distribution characterized, a new classification of these drugs based on their molecular pharmacology has been advocated.[94] This classification scheme, rather than molecular structure (e.g., "thiazide" diuretic), site of action (e.g., "loop" diuretic), or efficacy and clinical outcome (e.g., "high-ceiling" diuretic and "potassium-sparing" diuretic) is employed in this chapter as well as the more traditional nomenclature. Diuretics currently available in the United States are listed in Table 16–3.

Diuretic Classes

OSMOTIC DIURETICS AND CARBONIC ANHYDRASE INHIBITORS. Mannitol, as an inert extracellular osmotic agent, increases the extracellular fluid volume; consequently, the drug is contraindicated in patients with decompensated congestive heart failure. Inducing a metabolic acidosis with a carbonic anhydrase inhibitor may be of use in edematous patients with hypochloremic metabolic alkalosis due to long-term use of loop diuretics, particularly if the acid-base status of these patients is complicated by hypercarbia.

INHIBITORS OF THE Na^+,K^+,2Cl SYMPORT (LOOP DIURETICS). These agents, traditionally classified as loop or high-ceiling diuretics, including furosemide, bumetanide, ethacrynic acid, and torsemide, have been known for over 10 years to reversibly inhibit a Na,K,2Cl symporter (cotransporter) when applied to the luminal membranes of epithe-

TABLE 16-3 DIURETICS: ACTION, DOSAGE, AND DRUG INTERACTIONS

DIURETIC	BRAND NAME	PRINCIPAL SITE AND MECHANISM OF ACTION	EFFECTS ON URINARY ELECTROLYTES	EFFECTS ON BLOOD ELECTROLYTES AND ACID-BASE BALANCE	EXTRARENAL EFFECTS	USUAL DOSAGE*	DRUG INTERACTIONS
OSMOTIC DIURETICS							
Mannitol	Osmitrol	Proximal tubule (primarily)	$\uparrow Na^+$ $\uparrow Cl^-$ $\uparrow H_2O$	$\uparrow$ Extracellular volume transiently	$\downarrow$ Intracranial pressure	50–200 gm/d	May enhance loop diuretic effectiveness by maintaining GFR
Glycerol	Glyrol				$\downarrow$ Intraocular pressure	1–1.5 gm/kg	
CARBONIC ANHYDRASE INHIBITORS							
Acetazolamide	Diamox	Proximal tubule	$\uparrow Na^+$ $\uparrow K^+$ $\uparrow HCO_3^-$	Metabolic acidosis	$\uparrow$ Ventilatory drive	250–500 mg/d	May be useful in alkalemia due to other diuretics
Dichlorphenamide	Doranide	Carbonic anhydrase inhibition			$\downarrow$ Intraocular pressure	10–20 mg/d	
Methazolamide	Neptazane					25–100 mg/d	
Na,K,2Cl SYMPORT INHIBITORS (LOOP DIURETICS)							
Furosemide	Lasix	Thick ascending limb of loop of Henle: Inhibition of Na/K/2Cl symport	$\uparrow Na^+$ $\uparrow Cl^-$	Hypochloremic alkalosis $\uparrow HCO_3$ $\downarrow K^+$, $\downarrow Na^+$ $\downarrow Cl^-$, $\downarrow Mg^{++}$ $\uparrow$ Uric acid	*Acute:* $\uparrow$ Venous capacitance	20–1000 mg/d	Tubular secretion delayed by competing organic acids (renal failure) and some drugs
Bumetanide	Bumex					0.5–20 mg/d	
Piretanide†	Arelix Diumax Tauliz				$\uparrow$ Systemic vascular resitance *Chronic:* $\downarrow$ Cardiac preload	6–20 mg/d	Effectiveness reduced by prostaglandin inhibitors
Ethacrynic acid	Edecrin				Ototoxicity	50–200 mg/d	Additive ototoxicity with aminoglycosides
Torsemide	Demadex					2.5–200 mg/d	Longer duration of action than furosemide
Na, Cl SYMPORT INHIBITORS (THIAZIDE AND THIAZIDE-LIKE DIURETICS)							
Chlorothiazide	Diuril	Distal tubule: Inhibit NaCl symport	$\uparrow Na^+$ $\uparrow Cl^-$ $\uparrow K^+$	$\downarrow Na^+$, particularly in elderly patients	$\uparrow$ Glucose $\uparrow$ LDL/triglycerides (may be dose related)	50–100 mg	Efficacy reduced by prostaglandin inhibitors Reduces renal clearance of lithium
Hydrochlorothiazide	Hydridiuril					25–50 mg/d	
Trichlormethiazide	Metahydrin					2–8 mg/d	
Chlorthalidone	Hygroton		$\uparrow Mg^{++}$ $\downarrow Ca^{++}$	$\downarrow Cl$, $\uparrow HCO_3^-$ (mild alkalosis) $\uparrow$ Uric acid $\uparrow Ca^{++}$ $\downarrow K^+$, $\downarrow Mg^{++}$		25–100 mg/d	Additive effect on NaCl and K^+ excretion with loop diuretics
Metolazone	Zaroxolyn					5–10 mg/d	
Hydroflumethiazide	Diucardin Saluron					25–200 mg/d	
Polythiazide	Renese					1–4 mg/d	
Quinethazone	Hydromox					50–100 mg/d	
Methyclothiazide	Enduron Aquatensen					2.5–10 mg/d	
Benzthiazide	Aquatag Exna					50–200 mg/d	
Bendroflumethiazide	Naturetin				Extrarenal effects less marked with indapamide	2.5–30 mg/d	
Indapamide	Lozol	Vasodilator				2.5–5 mg/d	
EPITHELIAL Na^+ CHANNEL INHIBITORS (POTASSIUM-SPARING DIURETICS)							
Triamterene	Dyrenium	Collecting duct Inhibit apical membrane Na^+ conductance	$\uparrow HCO_3^-$	$\downarrow$ GFR; metabolic acidosis $\uparrow Mg^{++}$		100–300 mg/d	Useful with K^+ wasting diuretics; may induce hyperkalemia with ACE inhibitors
Amiloride	Midamor					5–10 mg/d	
TYPE I MINERALOCORTICOID RECEPTOR ANTAGONIST (POTASSIUM-SPARING DIURETICS)							
Spironolactone	Aldactone	Collecting duct: Aldosterone antagonists	$\downarrow K^+$ $\uparrow Na^+$ $\uparrow Cl$	$\uparrow K^+$, particularly in patients	Gynecomastia	2 mg/d	Useful adjunct to therapy with K^+ wasting diuretics
Canrenone						24 mg/d	

* Dosages are p.o.
† Not yet licensed for use in the United States.

lial cells of the thick ascending limb of the loop of Henle.[95] Inhibition of this symporter results in marked increases in the fractional excretion of Na^+ and Cl^- and indirectly in the fractional excretion of Ca^{++} and Mg^{++}. By inhibiting the concentration of solute within the medullary interstitium, these drugs also reduce the driving force for water resorption in the collecting duct, regardless of the presence of AVP, resulting in the production of urine that is nearly isotonic with that of plasma at the height of the diuresis. The delivery of large amounts of Na^+ and fluid to the distal nephron increases both K^+ and H^+ secretion, a process that is accelerated by aldosterone.

The Na,K,2Cl symport inhibitors (loop diuretics) also exhibit several characteristic effects on intracardiac pressures and on systemic hemodynamics. An increase in venous capacitance and a lowering of pulmonary capillary wedge pressure within minutes of a bolus infusion of intravenous furosemide (0.5 to 1.0 mg/kg) have been well documented in patients with congestive symptoms following an acute myocardial infarction or with valvular heart disease.[96] All of the rapid hemodynamic actions of the loop diuretics are attenuated in patients with chronic congestive heart failure.

INHIBITORS OF THE Na^+,Cl^- SYMPORTER (THIAZIDE CLASS DIURETICS). Despite being the focus of intensive research by renal pharmacology and physiology laboratories for several decades, the site of action of thiazide diuretics within the distal convoluted tubule has only recently been identified as the Na^+,Cl^- symporter of the distal convoluted tubule.[97] This symporter (or related isoforms) is also present on cells within the vasculature and many cell types within other organs and tissues and may contribute to some of the other actions of these agents.

By blocking solute uptake in the distal convoluted tubule, Na^+/Cl^- symport inhibitors (thiazide class diuretics) prevent maximal dilution of the urine and decrease the kidney's ability to increase free water clearance. Thiazides increase Ca^{++} resorption in the distal nephron by several mechanisms, occasionally resulting in a small increase in the serum Ca^{++} concentration. In contrast, Mg^{++} resorption is diminished and hypomagnesemia may occur with prolonged use. Increased delivery of NaCl and fluid into the collecting duct directly enhances K^+ and H^+ secretion by this segment of the nephron and may lead to clinically important hypokalemia.

INHIBITORS OF EPITHELIAL Na^+ CHANNELS (POTASSIUM-SPARING DIURETICS). The apical (luminal) membranes of principal cells of the late distal convoluted tubule and the cortical collecting duct contain Na^+-selective channels that permit sodium entry from within the tubular lumen that is driven by the electrochemical gradient established by the Na,K-ATPase in the basolateral membranes of these cells.[98] Na^+ conductance by these channels is inhibited by amiloride and by triamterene, which subsequently diminish the electrochemical potential for K^+ secretion into the urine. Thus, these agents, along with mineralocorticoid inhibitors (below), are commonly referred to as "potassium-sparing" diuretics. Neither drug is effective in achieving a net negative Na^+ balance in heart failure when given alone.

INHIBITORS OF TYPE I MINERALOCORTICOID/GLUCOCORTICOID RECEPTORS (POTASSIUM-SPARING DIURETICS). Spironolactone and its active metabolites canrenone and potassium canrenoate bind to intracellular receptors that belong to a superfamily of cytosolic steroid receptor proteins. Upon ligand binding, these proteins translocate to the cell nucleus where they bind to specific DNA sequences and regulate the transcription and synthesis of a number of gene products, including apical membrane Na^+ channels, H,K-ATPase, and Na^+,K^+-ATPase, among others.[99,100] The spironolactone-bound type I receptor complex is inactive and diminishes K^+ and H^+ secretion by this portion of the nephron, particularly in patients with high plasma aldosterone levels, as in heart failure.[101] Hyperkalemia and, unusually, a metabolic acidosis, may result from the use of these drugs.

VASOPRESSIN ANTAGONISTS. Increased levels of circulating arginine vasopressin contribute to the increased systemic vascular resistance and positive solute and water balance in patients with advanced heart failure.[102] Classically, vasopressin receptors have been divided into V_1 and V_2 receptor subtypes, which exhibit different ligand-binding specificities. V_2 receptors are found largely in distal nephron segments within the kidney.[102] V_2-selective receptor antagonists inhibit recruitment of aquaporin-CD (aquaporin-2) water channels,[103,104] amiloride-sensitive Na^+ channels, and urea transporters into the apical membranes of collecting duct epithelial cells.

Orally bioavailable V_2-specific antagonists have been developed that induce in humans a marked increase in free water clearance and modest increases in Na^+, Cl^-, and urea clearance with no change in K^+ secretion.[105] Although the pharmacology of these drugs will undoubtedly prove to be complex in patients with heart failure, most of whom will be receiving other vasodilators and natriuretic drugs, these agents, all of which are currently investigational, are likely to be valuable adjuncts to the contemporary treatment of heart failure.

NATRIURETIC PEPTIDES. The contribution of the natriuretic peptides—ANP, BNP, and related proteins, including urodilatin and fragments of the proANP protein—in the physiological adaptations that accompany heart failure, and their potential role as drugs in the pharmacotherapy of this syndrome, have been the subject of intensive research over the past decade[106,107] (see also p. 414). Infusions of ANP have been shown to cause afferent arteriolar dilation and efferent arteriolar constriction, resulting in an increase in GFR.[106]

Even when infused at concentrations that do not affect GFR, ANP induces a natriuresis by inhibiting the resorptive capacity of the proximal tubular epithelium, largely by inhibiting the actions of locally acting antinatriuretic agents such as angiotensin II and by augmenting the activity of intrarenal dopamine. In the distal nephron, natriuretic peptides decrease Na^+ influx from the tubular lumen through amiloride-sensitive epithelial Na^+ channels. The result is a natriuresis with minimal effect on urinary potassium excretion.

Although these natriuretic peptides appear to have a favorable pharmacological profile in heart failure, their practical utility so far has been disappointing owing to their short biological half-life and the development of pharmacological tolerance, as well as undesirable hemodynamic effects, including symptomatic hypotension and bradycardia, and these agents remain investigational. There is little evidence for any clinically significant direct effect on ventricular function.[108] Receptor-mediated clearance pathways and metabolism by the zinc metallopeptidase neutral endopeptidase (NEP) comprise the two predominant mechanisms for natriuretic peptide inactivation and removal and are the target of new pharmaceutical strategies to lengthen the biological half-life of endogenous and exogenously infused natriuretic peptides.

Diuretic Resistance

Inhibitors of the Na,K,2Cl symport (loop diuretics) are the only diuretics that are effective as single agents in moderate and advanced heart failure due to the magnitude of their maximal ("ceiling") natriuretic effect and to the fact that the natriuretic effect of more distally acting drugs is limited by the increased resorption of solute and water in proximal nephron segments in heart failure (Fig. 16–4). The effectiveness of even the loop diuretics usually decreases with worsening heart failure, however. Although the absolute bioavailability of these drugs is not decreased in heart failure, their rate of absorption may be delayed, resulting in inadequate peak drug levels within the tubular lumen of the ascending loop of Henle to induce a maximal natriuresis.[109,110] Switching to an intravenous formulation obviates this problem (Table 16–4). Continuous intravenous infusions of loop diuretics may be particularly effective in some patients by providing continuously high intraluminal drug levels. Adding a second diuretic that acts at a site distal to the loop of Henle (e.g., Na,Cl symport inhibitors [thiazide class diuretics]) is also often effective, although rapid intravascular volume depletion and large K^+ losses can occur.

There is a shift of the sigmoid-shaped curve describing the relationship between the log of the diuretic concentration in the tubular lumen and its natriuretic effect in heart failure, as well as a lower maximal effect (Fig. 16–4).[109–111] This shift in the diuretic dose-response relationship has been termed "diuretic resistance" and is usually due to several contributing factors. Diuretic resistance should be distinguished from "diuretic adaptation" or the "braking" phenomenon that is observed even in normal subjects

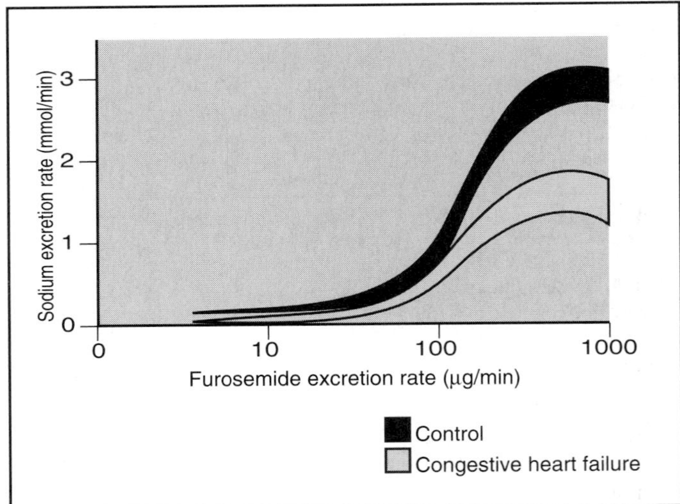

FIGURE 16–4. The relationship between urinary rate of excretion of furosemide and of sodium in normal subjects and in patients with congestive heart failure is shown. (Adapted from Knauf, H., and Matschler, E.: Functional state of the nephron and diuretic dose-response rationale for low dose combination therapy. Cardiology *84*(Suppl. 2):18, 1994.)

TABLE 16–4 MAXIMALLY EFFECTIVE ("CEILING") DOSES OF Na,K,2Cl SYMPORT INHIBITORS (LOOP DIURETICS)

	IV BOLUS DOSE (MG)		
	Furosemide	Bumetanide	Torsemide
Normal subjects	40	1	15–20
Congestive heart failure (normal GFR)	80–120	2–3	20–30
Renal insufficiency			
Moderate	80	3	60
Severe	200	10	200

GFR = glomerular filtration rate.

Adapted from Brater, D.C.: Diuretic resistance: Mechanisms and therapeutic strategies. Cardiology *84*(Suppl 2):57–67, 1994.

given multiple doses of a short-acting loop diuretic.[112] Diuretic-induced alterations in intrarenal hemodynamics, due to tubuloglomerular feedback and increased sympathetic-nerve activity, among other possible mechanisms, result in avid renal sodium retention by all nephron segments as intraluminal drug levels decline. This is now known to be due in part to hypertrophy of the tubular epithelium distal to the site of action of the loop diuretics, increasing the solute resorptive capacity of the kidney, as well as other adaptive mechanisms.[109,112,113]

The cause of apparent resistance to diuretics in patients who had achieved initially an acceptable natriuretic response and weight loss may be multifactorial. In the absence of an abrupt decline in cardiac or renal function, and if patient noncompliance with either the drug regimen or dietary salt restriction can be excluded, then the usual reason for diuretic resistance is the concurrent administration of other drugs. All nonsteroidal anti-inflammatory drugs (NSAIDs), including aspirin, can diminish diuretic efficacy. Most commonly, increasing doses of vasodilators, with or without a marked decline in intravascular volume due to concomitant diuretic therapy, is the cause of diuretic resistance.

It is often difficult to distinguish clinically between intravascular volume depletion following aggressive diuretic and vasodilator therapy and a decrease in cardiac output due to primary cardiac failure, although a more marked decline in urea clearance than in creatinine clearance suggests intravascular volume depletion. Pulmonary arterial and venous or left atrial pressure monitoring may be required to make this distinction. In addition, all vasodilators commonly employed as afterload-reducing agents in heart failure dilate a number of central and peripheral vascular beds, directing blood flow away from the kidney. Therefore, renal blood flow may be reduced despite a moderate increase in cardiac output, resulting in a decline in diuretic effectiveness.

Acid-Base and Electrolyte Disorders in Heart Failure: Complications of Diuretic Therapy

POTASSIUM HOMEOSTASIS. All of the diuretics discussed in this chapter, with the possible exception of V_2 vasopressin receptor antagonists, affect renal potassium handling.[112] In patients with congestive heart failure, both hypokalemia due to potassium-wasting diuretics and hyperkalemia due to potassium supplements administered with a potassium-sparing diuretic or a renin-angiotensin system antagonist may contribute to morbidity and mortality. Renal potassium losses due to diuretic use can be exacerbated by the hyperaldosteronism characteristic of patients with untreated heart failure and by the persistent chloride depletion and metabolic alkalosis that follows chronic use of loop diuretics. Long-term infusion of heparin, conversely, reduces aldosterone synthesis and may cause hyperkalemia, particularly in patients with insulin-dependent diabetes and in patients receiving potassium replacement and/or potassium-sparing drugs.

Despite the absence of conclusive data to determine whether routine administration of potassium supplements and/or potassium-sparing diuretics reduces serious morbidity or mortality in the treatment of patients with either primary hypertension or congestive heart failure, the standard of care, as represented by recent editorials and review articles on this topic, recommends that the serum K^+ be maintained between 3.5 and 5.0 mEq/liter.[114–116] This recommendation stems from the concern that alone among the major class of drugs used in the treatment of heart failure, the efficacy and safety of routine diuretic use has not been subjected to the rigors of prospective, randomized, and placebo-controlled clinical trials.[117,118] With the recognition that such trials would be practically impossible for all but asymptomatic patients with ventricular dysfunction, guidelines for potassium replacement and the other potential metabolic consequences of diuretic therapy must be established based on limited and potentially biased data.[119] Despite this limitation, the majority of the data that are available, much of it obtained from retrospective or subgroup analysis of clinical trials evaluating diuretic use in hypertension, is reassuring.[119–123] In addition to hypokalemia, it should also be emphasized that hyperkalemia also is a cause of morbidity in heart failure patients. Potassium supplements may not be necessary in patients receiving an ACE inhibitor with a diuretic. Automatic, "sliding-scale" prescriptions for potassium supplementation in hospitalized patients should not be used owing to the risk of severe hyperkalemia and cardiac arrhythmias.

HYPOMAGNESEMIA. Unlike urinary excretion of calcium, which is enhanced only by loop diuretics in volume-replete subjects, urinary magnesium wasting occurs with both thiazide and loop diuretics (although predominantly the latter), although not with potassium-sparing diuretics.[124,125] Magnesium deficiency is more commonly detected in patients with poor dietary magnesium intake (e.g., the elderly) and increased renal magnesium wasting due to diuretics as well as in patients with a history of a lengthy exposure to other drugs that exacerbate renal magnesium loss, including most commonly ethyl alcohol, but also cyclosporine, cisplatin, amphotericin B, and certain aminoglycoside antibiotics, including gentamicin and tobramycin.[124–126]

As emphasized by Leier et al.[114] and by Davies and Fraser,[127] despite a large and growing literature focusing on the importance of hypomagnesemia in diuretic use in heart failure, the absence of consistent use of a reliable test for magnesium deficiency and the reporting of data from poorly controlled, small, and statistically underpowered trials, have done little more than to further confuse this issue.

Unfortunately, the serum magnesium does not correlate well with other measures for determining magnesium homeostasis, as would be expected for this divalent cation that is largely bound to intracellular buffers or to bone (31 per cent and 67 per cent, respectively, of total body magnesium) with only approximately 1 per cent in the extracellular space. Although skeletal and cardiac muscle biopsies and/or measurements of free or total magnesium in circulating mononuclear cells are more reliable than serum magnesium levels, these measures are not readily available. The magnesium loading test is a reliable indicator of magnesium wasting in chronic malabsorption or renal magnesium losses due to intrinsic tubular defects. Nevertheless, the test requires careful patient compliance and has not been validated in the case of diuretic use. Newer techniques that measure either free or total magnesium in peripheral blood leukocytes are sufficiently sensitive and appear to be reliable indicators of total body magnesium depletion but are not yet widely available.

These issues notwithstanding, serial measurements of serum magnesium in a given patient reflect changes in total body magnesium homeostasis. For the clinician, a high index of suspicion (for example, a cachectic, elderly congestive heart failure patient receiving chronic loop diuretic therapy) coupled with a low normal serum magnesium level is sufficient to warrant beginning magnesium replacement therapy. If the total urinary magnesium excretion is less than 1 mEq/day (in the absence of diuretics), this also strongly increases the likelihood of significant magnesium depletion.

For the treatment of documented magnesium deficiency, which usually is found with concomitant potassium deficiency, enteric-coated $MgCl_2$ tablets, up to 32 mEq/day, may be safely given for a period of several months. Both epithelial Na^+ channel inhibitors and aldosterone receptor antagonists (potassium-sparing diuretics) reduce renal magnesium wasting caused by loop diuretics. By virtue of their antialdosterone activity, renin-angiotensin system antagonists also decrease diuretic-induced magnesium losses.

HYPONATREMIA. This is a common complication of diuretic therapy in patients with congestive heart failure. The origin of hyponatremia in these patients is multifactorial and includes diuretic-induced defects in renal diluting ability, inappropriately high vasopressin levels due to a reduced cardiac output, and elevated intracerebral angiotensin II levels, leading to excessive thirst. Hyponatremic patients tend to have a high plasma renin activity, elevated plasma norepinephrine and epinephrine levels, and reduced renal plasma flow compared with nonhyponatremic ($\geq$135 mEq/liter) patients. Mild hyponatremia (between 120 and 135 mEq/liter) generally responds to fluid restriction below urinary and insensible losses, usually less than 1500 ml/day, coupled with moderate (not severe) salt restriction. More severe hyponatremia ($<$120 mEq/liter) should be treated more rapidly but cautiously, with a combination of a loop diuretic and administration of 0.9 per cent NaCl (or, rarely, 3 per cent NaCl) administered intravenously. This may require concomitant monitoring of cardiac filling pressures. Administration of a loop diuretic transiently diminishes the kidney's ability to sustain a hypertonic medullary interstitium, thereby diminishing water reabsorption in the collecting duct. This results in a diuresis that is approximately isotonic with the patient's own plasma. Combined therapy with an ACE inhibitor and a loop diuretic may often result in improved control of hyponatremia in heart failure patients.

ACID-BASE DISTURBANCES. Because diuretics are commonly used in patients who may have multiple metabolic and respiratory acid-base problems, the contribution of diuretics to the clinical problem requires careful analysis. Of importance is the assessment of intravascular volume status; this may require invasive hemodynamic monitoring, particularly in edematous heart failure patients continuously treated with diuretics who display signs and symptoms of intravascular volume depletion and who have a hypochloremic metabolic alkalosis. Severe intravascular volume depletion with a marked hypochloremic alkalosis may require the administration of intravenous saline, with concurrent potassium and magnesium supplementation. Carbonic anhydrase inhibitors in relatively small doses (e.g., acetazolamide, 250 mg twice daily) may gradually reverse the metabolic alkalosis if a saline infusion is contraindicated, although potassium and magnesium repletion is still required.

ADVERSE EFFECTS OF DIURETIC THERAPY

CARBOHYDRATE INTOLERANCE. For many years, Na,Cl symport inhibitors (thiazide class diuretics) have been known to induce a mild form of carbohydrate intolerance, with the development of the typical clinical pattern of adult-onset diabetes in those individuals genetically predisposed to this disease. Ketoacidosis is rare in these patients, although nonketotic hyperosmolar coma may develop in volume-depleted type II diabetics receiving Na,Cl symport inhibitors. Although the development of clinically important diabetes may be unusual, it is now clear that some degree of insulin resistance can be documented in many patients receiving drugs of this diuretic class. Repletion of potassium losses has been shown to improve carbohydrate tolerance in more severely potassium-depleted patients.

HYPERLIPIDEMIA. Since the early 1980's, studies on the drug therapy of hypertension have documented an unfavorable effect of thiazide class diuretics on plasma lipid levels. Low-dose thiazide diuretic therapy had less impact on serum lipids than high doses as determined in a metaanalysis that examined the safety and efficacy of antihypertensive drugs, but the hyperlipidemic effect persisted, particularly in African-Americans and in men.[128] Nevertheless, advocates for the thiazide class diuretics, noting their proven efficacy and minimal side effect profile, particularly in older patients, and relative safety and low cost, question whether the modest changes in total cholesterol, triglyceride levels, and/or LDL-cholesterol of, at most, 1 to 5 per cent using low-dose diuretics, are of clinical importance.[118-122,129] Also, alpha$_1$-antagonists such as prazosin or terazosin (which have additive antihypertensive effects when prescribed with thiazide diuretics), as well as ACE inhibitors, appear to minimize or reverse the hyperlipidemic effects of the thiazides, whereas beta-adrenergic antagonists do not.

Diuretics and Renal Insufficiency

Many patients with congestive heart failure manifest some degree of renal insufficiency as a consequence of hypertensive glomerulosclerosis and/or atherosclerotic disease.[130] The pharmacokinetics of many drugs in common use in cardiovascular medicine are affected by a decline in renal function.[131] Renal dysfunction necessarily results in a decline in efficacy of diuretics. The loop diuretics remain the most effective class of diuretics in chronic renal failure, although their effectiveness is diminished by both pharmacokinetic and pharmacodynamic mechanisms. One useful approach to establishing an effective dose of a loop diuretic in congestive heart failure patients with chronic renal failure is to double the intravenous dose successively (i.e., from 40 mg furosemide, 1 mg bumetanide, or 20 mg torsemide intravenously) until a plateau is reached in NaCl excretion and urine volume (Table 16–4). Further increases in dose do not yield any greater immediate diuresis, although the duration of the natriuretic effect may be extended. The frequency of oral dosing can usually be diminished because of the prolonged elimination half-life of these drugs in chronic renal failure.

EXTRACORPOREAL ULTRAFILTRATION

In refractory heart failure, extracorporeal ultrafiltration has a place as a useful and relatively safe mechanism for removing fluid and electrolytes in a controlled fashion, whether or not there is underlying renal insufficiency.[132,133] Ultrafiltration also usually avoids the adverse hemodynamic effects of hemodialysis that can be difficult to manage in patients with heart failure and underlying ischemic heart disease. Ultrafiltration is far less effective in relieving symptoms attributable to uremia per se than is hemodialysis but is very effective in removing solutes and water.

Concurrent invasive hemodynamic monitoring is desirable, especially in unstable patients. Careful monitoring of plasma electrolytes and the hematocrit, which should not exceed 50 per cent, is required. Replacement electrolyte solutions are usually not necessary unless removal of intravascular volume has been excessive, or a specific electrolyte defect is being corrected (e.g., hyponatremia or hypokalemia). An improved response to diuretics has been reported following ultrafiltration, an effect that might be due to an improved cardiac output and reduced intracardiac filling pressures with a subsequent decline in the neurohumoral sodium-retaining signals to the kidney.

CARDIAC GLYCOSIDES

The chemical structure of this venerable class of drugs includes a steroid nucleus containing an unsaturated lactone at the C_{17} position and one or more glycosidic residues at C_3. Examples are found in a large number of plants and several toad species, typically serving as a venom or toxin that alters the future behavior of predators. William Withering's 1785 monograph contains the first comprehensive description of digitalis glycosides in the treatment of congestive heart failure.[134] This treatise describes the therapeutic efficacy and toxicities of the leaves of the common foxglove plant, *Digitalis purpurea.* Other digitalis glycosides are derived from the leaves of *Digitalis lanata* (digitoxin and digoxin), and from the seeds of *Strophanthus gratus* (ouabain). "Digitalis glycoside" and "cardiac glycoside" are often used interchangeably, although "cardiac glycoside" is the more inclusive term and "digitalis glycoside" should be reserved for compounds derived from *Digitalis* species. Digoxin is now the most commonly prescribed cardiac glycoside owing to its convenient pharmacokinetics, alternative routes of administration, and the widespread availability of serum drug level measurements. Both deslanoside, a rapidly acting agent available only for parenteral use, and digitoxin continue to be marketed in the United States.

Mechanisms of Action

INHIBITION OF MONOVALENT CATION ACTIVE TRANSPORT. All cardiac glycosides are potent and selective inhibitors of the active transport of Na^+ and K^+ across cell membranes. These drugs bind to specific high-affinity sites on the extracytoplasmic face of the alpha subunit of Na^+,K^+-ATPase, the enzymatic equivalent of the cellular "sodium pump."[135] The affinity of the alpha subunit for cardiac glycosides varies among species and among the three known mammalian alpha subunit isoforms, each of which is encoded by a separate gene.

The presence of the ouabain binding site on the alpha subunit of Na^+,K^+-ATPase has led to speculation that endogenous ouabain-like hormones or locally acting substances might exist that would serve as a regulatory ligand for the enzyme.[136] We have suggested the alternative possibility that the evolutionary persistence of the ouabain binding site could be due to a requirement for a specific amino acid sequence and conformation of the enzyme necessary for successful ion translocation, but which has also provided a target for evolutionary selection favoring certain plants and toads by serving as a means of poisoning animal predators.[137,138] There is evidence from site-directed mutagenesis studies that the affinity of Na^+,K^+-ATPase for cardiac glycosides is determined by the amino acid composition of the first transmembrane domain and the extracellular domain between the first and second (i.e., H_1 and H_2) transmembrane domains, and also the extracellular loop between the H_7 and H_8 transmembrane domains.[139]

Cardiac glycoside binding to and inhibition of the Na^+,K^+-ATPase sodium pump is reversible and entropically driven. Under physiological conditions these drugs bind preferentially to the enzyme following phosphorylation of a beta-aspartate on the cytoplasmic face of the alpha subunit, thus stabilizing this "E_2P" conformation.[135] Extracellular K^+ promotes dephosphorylation at this site as a step in this cation's active transport into the cytosol, accompanied by a decrease in the cardiac glycoside–binding affinity of the enzyme. This presumably explains why increased extracellular K^+ tends to reverse some manifestations of digitalis toxicity.

POSITIVE INOTROPIC EFFECT. For over 70 years cardiac glycosides have been known to increase the velocity and extent of shortening of cardiac muscle, resulting in a shift upward and to the left of the ventricular function (Frank-Starling) curve relating stroke work to filling volume or pressure. This occurs in normal as well as failing myocardium and in atrial as well as ventricular muscle. The effect appears to be sustained for periods of weeks or months without evidence of desensitization or tolerance.[140] This positive inotropic effect is due to an increase in the availability of cytosolic Ca^{++} during systole, thus increasing the velocity and extent of sarcomere shortening. This increase in intracellular Ca^{++} is a consequence of cardiac glycoside–induced inhibition of the sarcolemmal Na^+,K^+-ATPase.

Na^+ and Ca^{++} ions enter the cardiac muscle cell during each cycle of depolarization, contraction, and repolarization (Fig. 16–5 and Fig. 12–14, p. 370). Following activation of the fast Na^+ channel and the consequent depolarization, Ca^{++} enters the cell via the L-type Ca^{++} channel and triggers the release of additional Ca^{++} into the cytosol from the sarcoplasmic reticulum (SR). During repolarization and relaxation, Ca^{++} is again sequestered in the SR by a Ca^{++}-ATPase and is also extruded from the cell by the Na^+-Ca^{++} exchanger and by a sarcolemmal Ca^{++}-ATPase. Because the capacity of the Na^+-Ca^{++} exchanger to extrude Ca^{++} from the cell depends on the intracellular Na^+ activity, binding of a cardiac glycoside to the sarcolemmal Na^+,K^+-ATPase and inhibition of sodium pump activity reduces the rate of active Na^+ extrusion and cytosolic Na^+ content rises. This reduces the transmembrane Na^+ gradient driving the extrusion of intracellular Ca^{++} and more Ca^{++} is taken up by the SR and is available to activate contraction during the subsequent cell depolarization cycle. Evidence supporting this mechanism is available from studies using radionuclide tracers, cation-selective microelectrodes, and intracellular aequorin or ion-sensitive fluorescent dyes. Widespread acceptance of this mechanism of action awaited demonstration that small changes in intracellular Na^+ activity are accompanied by substantial increases in developed tension.[135,141]

ACTIONS ON VASCULAR SMOOTH MUSCLE. Alterations in peripheral arteriolar vascular smooth muscle Na^+-Ca^{++} exchange induced by cardiac glycosides have also been implicated as a mechanism by which these drugs could directly increase vascular tone and systemic vascular resistance, a rationale also promoted to link an endogenous circulating "digoxin-like" hormone to the pathogenesis of hypertension. Although this effect may occur transiently in normal humans following rapid increases in blood levels with bolus doses, no evidence exists that cardiac glycosides in the standard doses employed clinically affect blood pressure directly or "sensitize" the vasculature to endogenous or exogenous vasoconstrictors.[142] Indeed, as discussed below, digoxin administered chronically to patients with heart failure may decrease peripheral vascular resistance by decreasing centrally mediated sympathetic nervous system tone.

CARDIAC ENERGETICS. The immediate positive inotropic effect of cardiac glycosides, measured either in the intact heart in a conscious dog model or in isometrically contracting papillary muscle strips, is achieved with remarkable energy transfer efficiency and little oxygen wasting.[143,144] When compared with a beta-adrenergic agonist or a

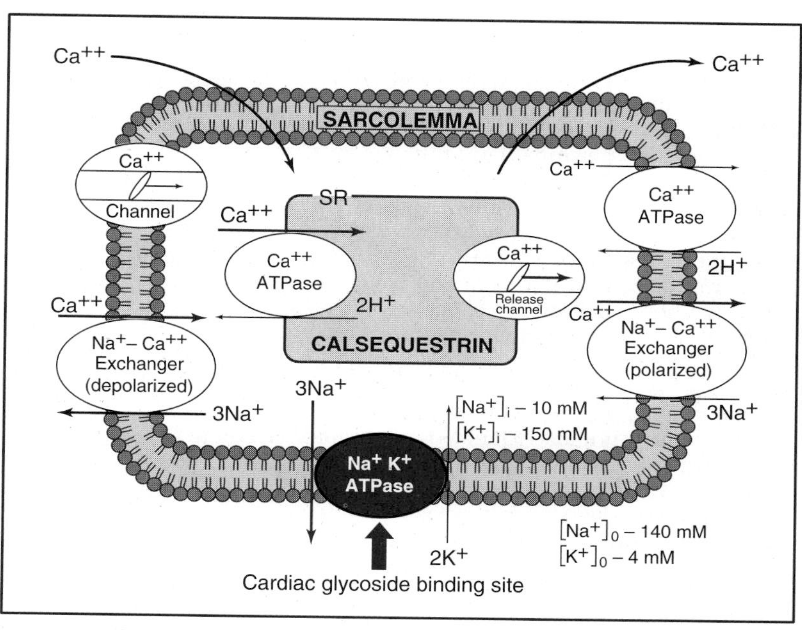

FIGURE 16–5. Selected components regulating cellular calcium homeostasis in cardiac myocytes. Structures on the left side of the diagram depict pathways of transmembrane calcium entry. From the upper left, the L-type calcium channel, a voltage-sensitive protein complex, carries the slow inward calcium current during phase 2 of the cardiac action potential and provides the pulse of intracellular calcium that triggers calcium-induced release of a larger amount of activator calcium from stores in the sarcoplasmic reticulum (SR). The arrow indicates the principal direction of ion movement when the channel is activated. Depolarization of the cell, activating this voltage-sensitive calcium channel, occurs by opening of the fast sodium channel (not shown).

In the center of the diagram is shown the SR with its ATP-driven calcium pump on the left and the calcium release channel on the right. On the right side of the diagram are shown the pathways for calcium extrusion across the sarcolemmal membrane, including the Ca-ATP-ase that pumps calcium from cardiac cells against a large electrochemical gradient and helps to maintain the low levels of free intracellular calcium that prevail during diastole. The Na^+-Ca^{2+} exchanger extrudes calcium from the cell in exchange for Na^+ entry under conditions of normal diastolic repolarization of the cell and constitutes the main route of Ca^{2+} extrusion. Arrows or concentrations shown in color denote pathways that increase or decrease in magnitude in the presence of cardiac glycosides.

cAMP phosphodiesterase inhibitor, ouabain caused no significant change for the same degree of tension development in the tension-time integral per unit initial heat, an index of the economy of isometric contraction in an isolated muscle preparation.[144]

With chronic administration of cardiac glycosides, it has been argued that the increase in cardiac output that accompanies the positive inotropic effect would eventually lead to reduced oxygen consumption as ventricular chamber size and pressures decline and wall stress diminishes. These new data indicate that, even in the short term, cardiac glycosides provide a moderate and metabolically efficient inotropic effect. This is an important consideration in patients with ischemic cardiomyopathies. Excessive increases in intracellular Ca^{++} are believed to contribute to cardiac glycoside toxicity when Ca^{++} overload results in spontaneous cycles of Ca^{++} release and reuptake. This may lead to Ca^{++}-induced activation of inward Ca^{++} current, resulting in transient late depolarizations (afterdepolarizations) that may be accompanied by after contractions and likely contribute to toxic electrophysiological effects.

OTHER INOTROPIC MECHANISMS. Other mechanisms that may contribute to the inotropic actions of cardiac glycosides include increased cytosolic Ca^{++} acting as a positive feedback signal to increase Ca^{++} entry through sarcolemmal L-type Ca^{++} channels. Cardiac glycosides have also been reported to increase Ca^{++}-triggered Ca^{++} release via cardiac (but not skeletal) muscle SR Ca^{++} release channels in isolated SR vesicles due to an increased probability of channel openings (not increased single channel conductance) when cardiac glycosides in nanomolar concentrations were present at the cytosolic face of oriented SR vesicle preparations inserted into planar lipid membranes.[145] Finally, experimental evidence indicates that cardiac glycosides may facilitate the release of norepinephrine from postganglionic receptor nerves through a Ca^{++}-dependent exocytotic process and inhibit norepinephrine reuptake, effects that could contribute to the drug's positive inotropic effect.[146]

REGULATION OF SYMPATHETIC NERVOUS SYSTEM ACTIVITY. Heart failure is often accompanied by an increase in sympathetic nervous system activity due, in part, to a reduction in the sensitivity of the arterial baroreflex response to blood pressure. This results in a decline in tonic baroreflex suppression of central nervous system–directed sympathetic activity. This loss of sensitivity of the normal baroreflex arc also appears to contribute to the sustained elevation in plasma norepinephrine, renin, and vasopressin levels characteristic of heart failure.

Mason et al.[147] observed that intravenous ouabain increased mean arterial pressure, forearm vascular resistance, and venous tone in normal human subjects, probably due to direct but transient effects on vascular smooth muscle (see above). In contrast, patients with heart failure responded with a decline in heart rate and other effects that were consistent with enhanced baroreflex responsiveness. Direct effects of cardiac glycosides on carotid baroreflex responsiveness to changes in carotid sinus pressure have been reported in isolated baroreceptor preparations from animals with experimentally induced heart failure.[148] Ferguson et al.[149] further demonstrated in patients with moderate to severe heart failure that infusion of deslanoside increased forearm blood flow and cardiac index and decreased heart rate, concomitant with a marked decrease in skeletal muscle sympathetic nerve activity measured as an indicator of centrally mediated sympathetic nervous system.

In an uncontrolled prospective study of 26 ambulatory patients with minimal to moderate (NYHA class I to III) heart failure, plasma norepinephrine levels declined significantly and analyses of heart rate variability before and after chronic therapy with digoxin revealed an increase in parasympathetic nervous system activity, consistent with decreased central sympathetic nervous system drive.[150]

Additional central and peripheral autonomic nervous system effects can be elicited by cardiac glycosides and include fatigue, malaise, abnormal dreams, anorexia, abdominal pain, and an enhanced respiratory drive to hypoxia. Psychiatric side effects of digitalis administration are uncommon with contemporary formulations and doses of these drugs.[151]

ELECTROPHYSIOLOGICAL ACTIONS (see also p. 500). Atrial and ventricular muscle and specialized cardiac pacemaker and conduction fibers differ in their responses and sensitivity to cardiac glycosides. These responses represent the sum of the direct effects on cardiac cells added to indirect, neurally mediated effects. At usual therapeutic serum concentrations (1.0 to 1.5 ng/ml), digoxin usually decreases automaticity and increases maximal diastolic resting membrane potential in atrial and atrioventricular (AV) nodal cells owing to augmented vagal tone and decreased sympathetic nervous system activity. This is accompanied by a prolongation of the effective refractory period and decreased AV nodal conduction velocity. At higher digoxin levels or in the presence of underlying disease, this may cause sinus bradycardia or arrest, prolongation of AV conduction, or heart block.

At toxic levels cardiac glycosides can increase sympathetic nervous system activity, potentially contributing to the generation of arrhythmias. Increased intracellular Ca^{++} loading and increased sympathetic tone both contribute to an increased rate of spontaneous (phase 4) diastolic depolarization and also to delayed afterdepolarizations (Fig. 16–5) that may reach threshold and generate propagated action potentials. The combination of increased automaticity and depressed conduction in the His-Purkinje network predisposes to arrhythmias, including ventricular tachycardia and fibrillation.

Pharmacokinetics and Dosing of Digoxin

The half-life for digoxin elimination of 36 to 48 hours in patients with normal or near-normal renal function permits once-a-day dosing. In the absence of loading doses, near steady-state blood levels are achieved in four to five half-lives, or about 1 week after initiation of maintenance therapy if normal renal function is present. Digoxin is largely excreted unchanged, with a clearance rate proportional to the GFR, resulting in the excretion of approximately one-third of body stores daily. In patients with heart failure and reduced cardiac reserve, increased cardiac output and renal blood flow in response to treatment with vasodilators or sympathomimetic agents may increase renal digoxin clearance, necessitating dosage adjustment. Digoxin is not removed effectively by peritoneal dialysis or hemodialysis because of its large (4 to 7 liter/kg) volume of distribution. The principal body reservoir is skeletal muscle and not adipose tissue. Accordingly, dosing should be based on estimated lean body mass. Neonates and infants tolerate and may require higher doses of digoxin for an equivalent therapeutic effect than older children or adults. Digoxin crosses the placenta and drug levels in maternal and umbilical vein blood are similar.

TABLE 16–5 FACTORS THAT ALTER PATIENT SENSITIVITY TO CARDIAC GLYCOSIDES

Serum electrolyte and acid-base disturbances
↑ Hypokalemia
↑ Hypomagnesemia
↑ Hypercalcemia
↑ Acidosis (typically respiratory)
↓ Hyperkalemia (may provoke AV block, however)
Thyroid status
↑ Hypothyroidism
↓ Hyperthyroidism
Underlying heart disease
↑ Ischemic cardiomyopathy
↑ Amyloid cardiomyopathy
Autonomic nervous system activity
↓ High sympathetic nervous system activity (but may exacerbate digoxin-induced arrhythmias)
↑ High parasympathetic (vagal) activity
Abnormal renal function
Decreases digoxin clearance
Decreases digoxin volume of distribution
Drug interactions (see Table 16–6)

Arrows indicate increased (↑) or decreased (↓) sensitivity to toxic effects of cardiac glycosides.

TABLE 16–6 DRUG INTERACTIONS WITH DIGOXIN

DRUG	MECHANISM	DIRECTION AND MAGNITUDE OF CHANGE IN BLOOD LEVEL	SUGGESTED CLINICAL MANAGEMENT
Cholestyramine, kaolin-pectin, neomycin, sulfasalazine	Decrease absorption	↓ 25%	Give 8 hr before digoxin, or use solution or gel form of digoxin
Antacids	Unclear	↓ 25%	Temporal dispersion of doses
Bran	Decreases absorption	↓ 25%	Temporal dispersion of doses
Propafenone, quinidine, verapamil, amiodarone	Decrease renal digoxin clearance, volume of distribution, or both	↑ 70–100%	Decrease digoxin by 50% and monitor serum digoxin levels as necessary
Thyroxine	Increases volume of distribution and renal clearance	Variable decreases in digoxin blood levels	Monitor serum digoxin levels
Erythromycin, omeprazole, tetracycline	Increase digoxin absorption	↑ 40–100%	Monitor serum digoxin levels
Albuterol	Increase volume of distribution	↓ 30%	Monitor serum digoxin levels
Captopril, diltiazem, nifedipine, nitrendipine	Variable moderate decrease in digoxin clearance and/or volume of distribution	Variable increase in blood levels	Monitor serum digoxin levels
Cyclosporine	May decrease renal function, and indirectly if renal function is impaired	Variable increase in blood levels	Monitor serum digoxin levels more frequently
Beta-blockers, verapamil, diltiazem, flecainide, disopyramide, bepridil	↓ SA or atrioventricular junctional conduction or automaticity		Monitor ECG for evidence of SA or AV block
Kaliuretic diuretics	Decreased serum and tissue K^+ increases automaticity and promotes inhibition of Na, K-ATPase by digoxin		Monitor ECG for arrhythmias consistent with digoxin toxicity
Sympathomimetic drugs	Increase automaticity		Monitor ECG for arrhythmia
Verapamil, diltiazem, beta-adrenergic blocking agents	Diminish cardiac contractile state		Discontinue or lower dose of Ca^{++} channel or beta-adrenergic antagonist

Current tablet preparations of digoxin average 70 to 80 per cent oral bioavailability, with elixir and encapsulated gel preparations approaching 90 to 100 per cent. Parenteral digoxin is available for intravenous use. Loading or maintenance doses can be given by intravenous injection, which should be carried out over at least 15 minutes to avoid vasoconstrictor responses to more rapid injection. Intramuscular digoxin is absorbed unpredictably, causes local pain, and is not recommended.

THERAPEUTIC DRUG MONITORING. Nomograms are available for estimating loading and maintenance doses of digoxin but are not widely used because of variability in individual patient responsiveness to cardiac glycosides and the ready availability in most clinical settings of serum digoxin concentration assays. Various clinical conditions and drug interactions that can alter digoxin's pharmacokinetics (Tables 16–5 and 16–6) are also reflected in the serum digoxin level. Reduced thyroid and renal function both decrease the volume of distribution of digoxin, necessitating downward adjustments in loading and maintenance doses. Hypochlorhydria (i.e., gastric pH >7), which is common in elderly patients and patients receiving histamine H_2 receptor antagonists or gastric H^+,K^+-ATPase inhibitors, reduces gastric metabolism of digoxin and the nonrenal clearance of the drug.[152] This may lead to higher steady-state blood levels in these patients with reduced renal function, particularly in the elderly.

Table 16–5 lists disease states and alterations in plasma and tissue electrolytes that can change patient susceptibility to toxicity at any given dose or serum level of the drug. Both hypokalemia and hypercalcemia can independently increase ventricular automaticity and lower the threshold for digoxin-induced cardiac arrhythmias. Hypomagnesemia may also contribute to arrhythmias with digoxin. Hyperkalemia may exacerbate digoxin-induced conduction disorders and cause high-grade AV nodal block.

Studies using noninvasive indices of ventricular function suggest a nonlinear relation between the serum digoxin concentration and the observed inotropic effect, with the majority of the increase in contractility occurring by the time steady-state levels around 1.8 nmol/liter (1.4 ng/ml) are reached (Fig. 16–6). The relation of serum digoxin level to therapeutic effect is less clear in the control of the ventricular rate among patients with atrial fibrillation. The effectiveness of cardiac glycosides given as single agents in controlling ventricular rate during exercise is limited at doses and serum levels in the usual therapeutic range.

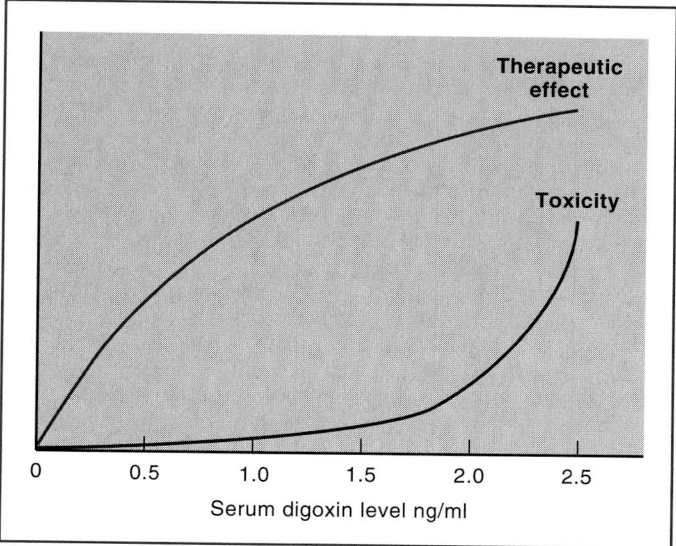

FIGURE 16–6. Schematic illustration of relationship between the therapeutic and toxic effects of digoxin and the serum digoxin level. Above a level of 1.8 nmol/L (1.5 ng/ml), there are minimal additional therapeutic effects and a substantial increase in the frequency of toxicity. (From Lewis, R. P.: Digitalis. *In* Leier, C. V. (ed.): Cardiotonic Drugs: A Clinical Survey. New York, Marcel Dekker, 1987, p. 85.)

Overt digitalis toxicity tends to emerge at two- to threefold higher serum concentrations than the target 1.8 nmol/liter, but it must always be remembered that a substantial overlap of serum levels exists among patients exhibiting symptoms and signs of toxicity and those with no clinical evidence of intoxication. If ready access to serum digoxin assays is available, a reasonable approach to the initiation of therapy is to begin at 0.125 to 0.375 mg/day, depending on lean body mass and estimated creatinine clearance, and to measure a serum digoxin level 1 week later with careful monitoring of clinical status in the interim. Patients with impaired renal function will not yet have reached steady state and need to be monitored closely until four to five clearance half-lives have elapsed (as long as 3 weeks). Oral or intravenous loading with digoxin, although generally safe, is rarely necessary as other safer and more effective drugs exist for short-term inotropic support or for initial treatment of supraventricular arrhythmias.

Blood samples for serum digoxin level measurement should be taken at least 6 to 8 hours following the last digoxin dose. Serum level monitoring is justified in patients with substantially altered drug clearance rates or volumes of distribution (e.g., very old, debilitated, or very obese patients). Adequacy of digoxin dosing and risk of toxicity in a given patient should never be based on a single isolated serum digoxin concentration measurement.[153]

DIGITOXIN, OUABAIN, AND DESLANOSIDE. Digitoxin is the principal native cardiac glycoside present in digitalis leaf. It is the least polar and most slowly excreted of all available cardiac glycosides. Oral bioavailability approaches 100 per cent and is less affected by malabsorption syndromes than is digoxin. Unlike digoxin, digitoxin is about 97 per cent bound to albumin in normal plasma and is extensively metabolized in the liver with minimal renal clearance of the native glycoside. Displacement of digitoxin from plasma protein by some drugs, including warfarin, can occur but rarely results in clinically important changes in serum levels at usual digitoxin doses. The elimination half-life is 4 to 6 days irrespective of renal function, resulting in a stable steady-state level of drug 3 to 4 weeks after initiation of a daily maintenance dose. Therapeutic serum or plasma concentrations are about 10-fold higher than those of digoxin owing to serum protein binding.

Ouabain undergoes predominantly renal clearance, although some gastrointestinal excretion does occur, with an elimination half-life of 18 to 24 hours in normal subjects. Deslanoside also is cleared primarily by the kidney. The plasma half-life is similar to that of digoxin, permitting once-daily maintenance dosing.

DIGITALIS TOXICITY. Although the incidence and severity of digitalis intoxication are decreasing,[154,155] vigilance for this important complication of therapy is essential. Disturbances of cardiac impulse formation, conduction, or both are the hallmarks of digitalis toxicity. Among the common electrocardiographic manifestations are ectopic beats of AV junctional or ventricular origin, first-degree atrioventricular block, an excessively slow ventricular rate response to atrial fibrillation, or an accelerated AV junctional pacemaker. These manifestations may require only a dosage adjustment and monitoring as clinically appropriate. Sinus bradycardia, sinoatrial arrest or exit block, and second- or third-degree atrioventricular conduction delay often respond to atropine, but temporary ventricular pacing is sometimes necessary and should be available. Potassium administration is often useful for atrial, AV junctional, or ventricular ectopic rhythms, even when the serum potassium is in the normal range, unless high-grade atrioventricular block is also present. Magnesium may be useful in patients with atrial fibrillation and an accessory pathway in whom digoxin administration has facilitated a rapid accessory pathway–mediated ventricular response. Lidocaine or phenytoin, which in conventional doses have minimal effects on atrioventricular conduction, are useful in the management of worsening ventricular arrhythmias that threaten hemodynamic compromise. Electrical cardioversion can precipitate severe rhythm disturbances in patients with overt digitalis toxicity, and should be used with particular caution.

ANTIDIGOXIN IMMUNOTHERAPY. Potentially life-threatening digoxin or digitoxin toxicity can be reversed by antidigoxin immunotherapy. Purified Fab fragments from digoxin-specific antisera are available at most poison control centers and larger hospitals in North American and Europe. The smaller (molecular weight 50,000) Fab fragments have a larger volume of distribution, more rapid onset of action, and more rapid clearance as well as reduced immunogenicity than does intact IgG.[156] Clinical experience in adults and children has established the effectiveness and safety of antidigoxin Fab in treating life-threatening digoxin toxicity, including cases of massive ingestion with suicidal intent.[157] Doses of Fab are calculated on the basis of a simple formula based on either the estimated dose of drug ingested or the total body digoxin burden and are administered intravenously in saline over 30 to 60 minutes. Recrudescent digoxin toxicity is unusual but can occur 24 to 48 hours after Fab administration in patients with normal renal function, or later in patients with renal impairment.[156–158] The efficacy and cost-effectiveness of less than complete neutralizing doses of digoxin-specific Fab fragments for suspected or moderate cases of digoxin toxicity need further assessment.

PHOSPHODIESTERASE INHIBITORS

Agents such as theophylline, 3-isobutyl-l-methyl xanthine (IBMX), and caffeine have long been recognized as nonspecific cGMP and cAMP phosphodiesterase (PDE) inhibitors. PDE use in heart failure, however, awaited the 1980's when a number of PDE isoenzyme subclass-specific inhibitors became available. The isoenzyme classification scheme initially devised by Beavo and Reifsnyder[159] now includes at least seven distinct but related gene families based on known cDNA sequences. Tissue and cell-specific PDE isoenzyme distribution, as well as subcellular localization and links to specific cGMP- and cAMP-dependent signalling pathways, are increasingly being recognized.[160,161] There are important differences in expression of specific classes of PDE inhibitors in the same tissue among species and in the same species during development.[162] Any specificity of selective inhibitors for most PDE isoenzymes exists only within a relatively narrow concentration range, with increasingly nonspecific inhibition at higher concentrations.

AMRINONE AND MILRINONE. Parenteral formulations of amrinone and milrinone are approved for short-term support of the circulation in advanced heart failure. Although both drugs have excellent oral bioavailability, longer-term prospective trials of oral formulations of these agents showed a high incidence of side effects, exhibited minimal long-term efficacy, and in the doses used caused increased mortality in heart failure patients.[163–165] Both agents are bipyridine derivatives and relatively selective inhibitors of the low K_m cGMP-inhibited, cAMP PDE (type III) group. Both cause vasodilation with a consequent fall in systemic vascular resistance, and they are powerful positive inotropic agents; they increase contractile force and velocity of relaxation of cardiac muscle.

Amrinone or milrinone is often used in combination with other oral or intravenous drugs for short-term treatment of patients with severe heart failure due to systolic right or left ventricular dysfunction. These drugs are commonly employed as adjuvant therapy with a sympathomimetic amine, usually dobutamine, for circulatory support following cardiopulmonary bypass, or as alternative therapy for hospitalized patients who have developed tolerance to dobutamine.[165–167] Although both dobutamine and the bipyridines increased intracellular cAMP and are positively inotropic, there are important differences. Only dobutamine, for example, consistently decreased both diastolic left ventricular filling pressures and volume, whereas a type III PDE inhibitor caused only a decrease in diastolic filling pressure.[168,169]

Both drugs are initiated by an intravenous loading dose followed by a continuous infusion. For amrinone this is typically a 0.5 to 0.75 mg/kg bolus infusion over 2 to 3 minutes and then 2 to 20 μg/kg/min. Milrinone is about 10-fold more potent, with a typical loading dose of 50 μg/kg over 10 minutes and an infusion rate from 0.25 to 1.0 μg/kg/min. Half-lives of amrinone and milrinone clearance are 4 to 5 hours and 2 to 3 hours, respectively, and are approximately doubled in patients with advanced heart failure. Clinically significant thrombocytopenia is reported in about 10 per cent of patients receiving amrinone but is rare with milrinone. Because of its greater selectively for PDE III isoenzymes, shorter half-life, and fewer side effects, milrinone is the agent of choice among currently available PDE inhibitors for short-term parenteral inotropic support in severe heart failure.

VESNARINONE.* This orally active positive inotropic agent with vasodilator activity appears to act via multiple mechanisms. In addition to relatively selective inhibition of an isoform of a type III cAMP PDE present in human myocardial and kidney tissue, vesnarinone also affects sarcolemmal membrane voltage-activated sodium and potassium channels. This could contribute to the drug's positive inotropic action as well as exerting electrophysiological effects. The net effect is a decrease in heart rate and prolongation of action potential duration, opposite to the results observed with other class III PDE inhibitors.

Vesnarinone has also been reported to decrease production by lymphocytes of some inflammatory cytokines and exhibits viricidal activity in experimental animals and in vitro models.[170] Neutropenia (absolute granulocyte count <1000 mm^3) is the most common important side effect of vesnarinone. The incidence in trials of vesnarinone in Europe and the United States has been approximately 3 per cent and several patients have died. The average daily dose of patients developing neutropenia was 60 mg/day and always occurred within the first 1 to 5 months of treatment.[171] Human recombinant granulocyte colony-stimulating factor (G-CSF) has been employed successfully in the treatment of severe neutropenia due to vesnarinone. Initially promising safety and efficacy data have been reported in heart failure patients for vesnarinone,[172] and trials are also underway for the related compound OPC-18790.*[173]

CALCIUM-SENSITIZING DRUGS

The classification of drugs as calcium-sensitizing agents refers to their ability to shift the relationship between the intracellular calcium concentration and the rate and extent of force development, producing increased force generation at any given intracellular calcium concentration. A calcium-sensitizing action of a drug can be detected and quantitated using several approaches; for example, force development in vitro over a range of Ca^{++} concentrations can be measured in skinned cardiac muscle fibers that have been made permeable to Ca^{++} using detergents. These drugs tend to be more energy efficient in generating increased force than agents that increase intracellular cAMP levels. This may prove advantageous in patients with heart failure due to an ischemic cardiomyopathy in whom cardiac ATP production is limited by O_2 delivery. However, these drugs may also adversely affect ventricular relaxation during diastole, an effect that depends on how Ca^{++}-sensitization is achieved and on which additional cardiovascular actions each drug may have.

PIMOBENDAN* AND SULMAZOLE.* Pimobendan and sulmazole have undergone extensive clinical testing in patients with heart failure.[174] Both inhibit type III cAMP PDEs and, like milrinone, are vasodilators. Unlike milrinone, these drugs also act as calcium sensitizers at clinically relevant concentrations. Pimobendan increased exercise tolerance and improved symptoms and quality of life in patients with heart failure in a series of relatively small prospective controlled trials.[175–177] However, these drugs, like milrinone, decreased survival in heart failure patients.

SIMENDAN* AND LEVOSIMENDAN.* Simendan is a type III PDE inhibitor that, like pimobendan, has also been shown to have Ca^{++}-sensitizing activity. This activity of racemic simendan was found to be due to its levo enantiomer, levosimendan, which is currently undergoing clinical testing. The cellular mechanisms by which levosimendan causes calcium sensitization are unknown, but recent data indicate that the drugs bind to a hydrophobic pocket on cardiac troponin C.[178]

* Not approved by the US Food and Drug Administration at the time of this writing.

In experimental animals, levosimendan decreased systemic vascular resistance and left ventricular end-diastolic pressure and increased myocardial contractility in a dose-dependent manner.[179,180] Importantly, the time constant of isovolumic relaxation and maximum segment lengthening velocity ($-dp/dt_{max}$) did not change significantly over a range of levosimendan concentrations.[180] This apparent lack of an effect on diastolic relaxation would not be predicted on the basis of the drug's Ca^{++}-sensitizing activity and may be due to its activity as a type III cAMP PDE inhibitor. Whether similar effects will be apparent in humans with heart failure is the subject of ongoing studies.

ADRENERGIC AND DOPAMINERGIC AGONISTS

A thorough grasp of the pharmacology of the peripheral adrenergic and dopaminergic signalling systems is essential to understanding the rationale for drug therapy of heart failure. Evidence for a generalized activation of the sympathetic nervous system in heart failure is reviewed on page 482. The reader is also referred to comprehensive reviews of the basic molecular pharmacology of G protein–linked receptors.[181–183]

A diminished cellular response to repeated or continuous administration of a drug or endogenous agonist is termed "desensitization" and represents a programmed response of the cell that typically involves several levels in the signal transduction sequence for that ligand. Desensitization for a given signalling pathway may be initiated by specific ligand-receptor signalling ("homologous desensitization") or by other endogenous agonists or drugs acting through different receptor pathways ("heterologous desensitization"). Desensitization of the beta-adrenergic signalling pathway has been the most extensively studied in heart failure[184–190] and is discussed on page 502.

DOBUTAMINE. This sympathomimetic amine is available for clinical use as a racemic mixture that stimulates both $beta_1$- and $beta_2$-adrenergic receptor subtypes and either binds but does not activate alpha-adrenergic receptors ([+] enantiomer) or stimulates $alpha_1$ and $alpha_2$ receptor subtypes ([−] enantiomer). Lower doses resulting in a clear positive inotropic effect in humans exert a predominant $beta_1$-adrenergic effect, while alpha-adrenergic agonist effects of the (−) enantiomer in the vasculature and myocardium appear to be blocked by the alpha receptor antagonist effect of the (+) enantiomer. Dobutamine does not stimulate dopaminergic receptors and unlike dopamine does not selectively alter renal blood flow (see below).

Racemic dobutamine also acts as a vasodilator to reduce aortic impedance and systemic vascular resistance, thus reducing afterload and improving ventricular-vascular coupling by reducing aortic impedance.[191–193] In contrast, dopamine may either have no effect or increase ventricular afterload by increasing systemic vascular resistance and by causing more rapid return of reflected aortic pressure waves, depending on the infusion rate of the drug. Therefore, dobutamine is preferable to dopamine for most patients with advanced heart failure who have not responded adequately to oral or intravenous vasodilators, digoxin, and diuretics.[193,194] Dobutamine infusions are initiated at 2 μg/kg/min and are titrated up according to a patient's hemodynamic response (usually not higher than 20 μg/kg/min; dosing is based on estimated lean body weight).

The importance of the vascular effects of dobutamine have been demonstrated by experiments in animals with an artificial (Jarvik 7) heart.[192] Even in the presence of a mechanical heart, dobutamine increased cardiac output by 10 to 15 per cent and decreased systemic vascular resistance. Interestingly, dobutamine also decreased venous capacitance and increased right atrial pressure, possibly owing to the $alpha_1$-adrenergic agonism of the (−) enantiomer. These experiments also demonstrated that the (+) enantiomer ("D-dobutamine") was responsible for the racemic drug's effects on aortic input impedance, wave reflectance, and systemic vascular resistance. These favorable actions on left ventricular afterload are also responsible for the reduction in functional mitral regurgitation often observed with dobutamine infusions in patients with large dilated ventricles and high left ventricular end-diastolic pressure.[195] Dobutamine also causes a decline in pulmonary vascular resistance that is present regardless of chronic background vasodilator therapy with organic nitrates, hydralazine, or captopril.

DOPAMINE. This endogenous catecholamine evokes vasodilatory responses by direct stimulation of dopaminergic D_1/D_5 postsynaptic as well as D_2 presynaptic receptors in the peripheral vasculature and on the luminal and basolateral membranes of renal tubular cells, particularly in the proximal tubule.[196] It causes relatively selective vasodilation of splanchnic and renal arterial beds at doses less than or equal to 2 μg/kg/min. This action may be useful in promoting renal blood flow and maintaining GFR in patients who become refractory to diuretics. At intermediate (2 to 10 μg/kg/min) infusion rates, dopamine enhances norepinephrine release from vascular sympathetic neurons, resulting in increased beta-adrenergic receptor activation in the heart. In patients with advanced heart failure, who often have depletion of intracardiac norepinephrine stores, dopamine may be a less effective positive inotropic drug than other direct-acting inotropes. At higher infusion rates (5 to 20 μg/kg/min) peripheral vasoconstriction occurs due to direct alpha-adrenergic receptor stimulation. Increases in systemic vascular resistance are common even at intermediate infusion rates. Tachycardia tends to be more pronounced than with dobutamine and may worsen systolic and diastolic function in patients with ischemic cardiomyopathies. Dose ranges noted above are based on estimated lean body weight rather than actual patient weight. Emergence of unexplained tachycardia or arrhythmias in a patient receiving "renal range" dopamine should raise the suspicion of an inappropriately high dopamine infusion rate.

DOPEXAMINE.* Dopexamine is a synthetic sympathomimetic agent designed as a dopamine analog for intravenous use that has a 60-fold higher affinity for $beta_2$ receptors than dopamine. Like dobutamine, dopexamine reduces pulmonary and systemic vascular resistance and has a positive inotropic effect at infusion rates of 0.25 μg/kg/min or higher.[197] Although dopexamine offers a hemodynamic profile that is intermediate between those of dobutamine and dopamine, no compelling evidence exists that this drug offers any important clinical advantages over the two older drugs.

ORAL DOPAMINE AGONISTS. Several orally bioavailable analogs of dopamine have been developed, including levodopa, fenoldopam,* and ibopamine.* Following absorption, ibopamine is converted into *N*-methyldopamine (epinine) and over 2 to 6 hours causes a gradual reduction in pulmonary and systemic vascular resistance.[198] Its use has been advocated in weaning patients off intravenous sympathomimetics while awaiting heart transplant.[199]

BETA-ADRENERGIC ANTAGONISTS

The development of intravenous and oral formulations of beta-adrenergic *agonists* for the support of the circulation in heart failure due to systolic ventricular dysfunction was based on the seemingly reasonable rationale that these drugs would improve contractile function and diastolic relaxation, much like endogenous catecholamines. However, results from clinical trials have indicated that beta-adrenergic agonists are not useful in the management of chronic heart failure and, except for temporary circulatory support in hospitalized patients, may actually be detrimental. In contrast, an increasing body of evidence indicates that beta-adrenergic *antagonists* improve symptoms, exercise tolerance, hemodynamics, and perhaps mortality in heart failure patients. Despite clinical and experimental animal data that these drugs have an initial negative inotropic effect and can worsen ventricular function, the introduction of beta-adrenergic antagonists in the treatment of heart failure has been based largely on empirical evidence from small observational studies.

* Not approved by the US Food and Drug Administration at the time of this writing.

PHARMACOLOGICAL CONSIDERATIONS (see also pp. 502 and 612). Beta-adrenergic antagonists are identified by their affinity for binding to beta-adrenergic receptors, which is sufficiently high to antagonize the binding of endogenous agonists (i.e., norepinephrine and epinephrine) at blood and tissue concentrations that do not cause other undesirable effects. Historically, these agents have been classified according to their relative selectivity for the $beta_1$- or $beta_2$-adrenergic receptors, their ability to bind other adrenergic receptors (usually alpha receptors), and their interactions with other molecular targets at clinically relevant doses (e.g., the K^+ channel antagonist activity of the [+]enantiomer of sotalol). In addition, many beta-adrenergic antagonists are characterized by their ability not only to prevent the binding of endogenous catecholamines but also to act as weak agonists (i.e., intrinsic sympathomimetic activity, or ISA), and also by chemical characteristics of the compound itself (e.g., lipophilicity) that determine the tissue distribution, oral bioavailability, and clearance mechanism(s) of each compound (Table 16–7).

This classification scheme recently has been made more complex with new evidence on the nature of drug binding to beta-adrenergic receptors. Although there has been evidence that cell-surface receptors linked to G protein signalling pathways might be capable of adapting an "active" conformation that initiates signal transduction even in the absence of agonist, conclusive proof has required the availability of experimental models in which the actions of endogenous catecholamines could be discounted or eliminated and which could exhibit an easily quantifiable biological signal. It is now known that the $beta_2$-adrenergic receptor appears to exist in equilibrium between two conformations, an inactive conformation (R) and an active conformation (R*). True agonists bind selectively to the R* conformation, stabilizing it and shifting the equilibrium toward the active signalling conformation, whereas "inverse agonists" favor the inactive conformation, shifting receptor equilibrium toward the conformation that does not initiate downstream signalling.[200,201] Neutral antagonists favor both conformations approximately equally, whereas partial agonists (i.e., beta-adrenergic antagonists with ISA) shift the binding equilibrium moderately toward the R* conformation.

Owing to their much higher affinities for the beta receptor than the endogenous catecholamines, all beta-adrenergic antagonists, regardless of whether they are "inverse agonists," neutral antagonists, or exhibit ISA, block the action of the endogenous catecholamines in vivo. Although the relevance of the distinction between neutral antagonists and drugs that exhibit inverse agonism for clinical cardiovascular pharmacology is not yet well defined, the acceptance of this model has broad implications for rational drug design beyond beta-adrenergic agonists and antagonists and is likely to be relevant to other G protein–coupled receptors.[201] Preliminary clinical data suggest that the distinction among agents with partial agonist, neutral antagonist, and inverse agonist properties also has clinical relevance.[202]

BETA BLOCKERS IN THE TREATMENT OF HEART FAILURE. In the 1970's, Waagstein and associates at the University of Göteberg in Sweden reported that the beta blockers alprenolol, metoprolol, and practolol improved symptoms and ventricular function over a period of several months in patients with mild to severe heart failure due to idiopathic dilated cardiomyopathy.[203] Although a number of smaller trials, many of which were not controlled, in the 1980's tended to support these observations, none was sufficiently large to provide definitive evidence regarding improvement in symptoms or exercise tolerance, or to have the statistical power to detect a change in mortality.[204–206]

Despite this accumulating evidence in support of the efficacy of long-term therapy with beta blockers in some patients with heart failure at the beginning of the 1990's, enthusiasm for this class of agents was clearly muted compared with that for ACE inhibitors and the promise of new classes of vasodilators and inotropic agents. This skepticism was reinforced by the early termination of the Xamoterol in Severe Heart Failure study, a beta-adrenergic antagonist with significant ISA properties, due to excess mortality in patients receiving active drug.[207,208] In addition, there has been no clear consensus as to why beta-adrenergic antagonists should be beneficial in heart failure. As reviewed by Bristow,[209] the characteristic downregulation of postsynaptic $beta_1$-adrenergic receptor in cardiac muscle

TABLE 16–7 PHARMACODYNAMIC PROPERTIES OF β-ADRENERGIC ANTAGONISTS

GENERIC NAME	PROPRIETARY NAME(S)	ADRENERGIC RECEPTOR SELECTIVITY	PARTIAL AGONISM (ISA)	INVERSE AGONISM‡	LIPID SOLUBILITY	VASODILATOR ACTIVITY	OTHER ACTIONS
Acebutol	Sectral	$+\beta_1$	+		+	+	
Atenolol	Tenormin	$+\beta_1$	0		0	0	
Betaxolol	Kerlone	$+\beta_1$	0		0		
Bevantolol*	—	$++\beta_1$	0		++	+	
Bisoprolol	Zebeta	$++\beta_1$	0		+	0	
Bucindolol*		$\beta_1\beta_2$	0		0	++	"Direct" vasodilator
Carteolol	Cartrol	$\beta_1\beta_2$	++		0	0	
Carvedilol	—	$(+)\beta_1, \alpha_1$	0	+	+	++	
Celiprolol*		$+\beta_1$	+		0	+	
Esmolol	Brevibloc	$+\beta_1$	0		0	+	
Labetalol	Trandate, Normodyne	$\beta_1, \beta_2\alpha_1$	0		++	++	
Metoprolol	Lopressor	$+\beta_1$	0	++	++	0	
Nadolol	Corgard	β_1, β_2	0		0	0	
Nebivelol*		$+\beta_1$	0		0	+	"Direct" vasodilator
Oxprenolol*	Trasicor	$\beta_1\beta_2$	++		+	0	
Penbutolol	Levatol	$\beta_1\beta_2$	++		+++	0	
Pindolol	Visken	$\beta_1\beta_2$	++		0		
Propranolol	Inderal	$\beta_1\beta_2$	0	++	+++	0	
Sotalol	Betapace	$\beta_1\beta_2$	0		0	0	Class III antiarrhythmic
Timolol	Blocadren	$\beta_1\beta_2$	0	+++	0	0	

ISA = Intrinsic sympathomimetic activity; + = mild effect; ++ = moderate effect; +++ = marked effect.
* Not approved by the US Food and Drug Administration at the time of this writing.
‡ Inverse agonism—the ability to bind and stabilize the inactive conformation of G protein–linked receptors—has not been well defined for beta-adrenergic antagonists to date in the context of human cardiovascular pharmacology. Adapted from Antman, E. M., and Kelly, R. A.: Pharmacological therapy of cardiac arrhythmias. *In* Antman, E. M., and Rutherford, J. D. (eds): Coronary Care Medicine: A Practical Approach. Norwell, MA, Kluwer Academic Press, 1996.

and moderate uncoupling of beta$_2$-adrenergic receptors could be viewed as an adaptive response of cardiac muscle that was designed to minimize the potential toxicity of high levels of catecholamines. However, this adaptation also compromises the ability of the heart to respond to appropriate increases in adrenergic tone, as with exercise.

The results of clinical trials in the 1990's (see p. 503), have tended to support the efficacy of these drugs in heart failure, although the mechanism(s) is not clear. It is not yet known, for example, whether long-term administration of beta-adrenergic antagonists increases beta receptor number in humans. Other mechanisms also may be operative that could increase the extent of activation of adenylate cyclase by endogenous beta-adrenergic agonists.[210] Thus, chronic beta-adrenergic antagonist administration could result in changes at a number of levels in the adrenergic signalling cascade that would favor improved cardiac function. There also is evidence that the favorable actions of these drugs in heart failure may be due to improved ventricular-arterial coupling, due in part to a decline in heart rate, but also a decrease in peak left ventricular end-systolic pressure and arterial elastance that reduces afterload.[211] Also, patients with idiopathic dilated cardiomyopathy receiving metoprolol had an increase in myocardial lactate extraction with exercise, suggesting either reduced ischemia and/or more efficient oxygen utilization.[212] Metoprolol also significantly decreased myocardial oxygen consumption and improved metabolic efficiency in patients undergoing acute atrial pacing studies both on the initiation of therapy and with long-term dosing (i.e., 3 months).[213] Beta-adrenergic antagonists may also reduce the incidence of sudden death due to primary ventricular arrhythmias, although this remains to be proven in heart failure. Detectable improvements in ventricular function usually are not apparent for a minimum of 1 to 3 months, and longer-term structural changes such as a decline in ventricular volume or mass may take 12 to 18 months (Fig. 16–7).[214]

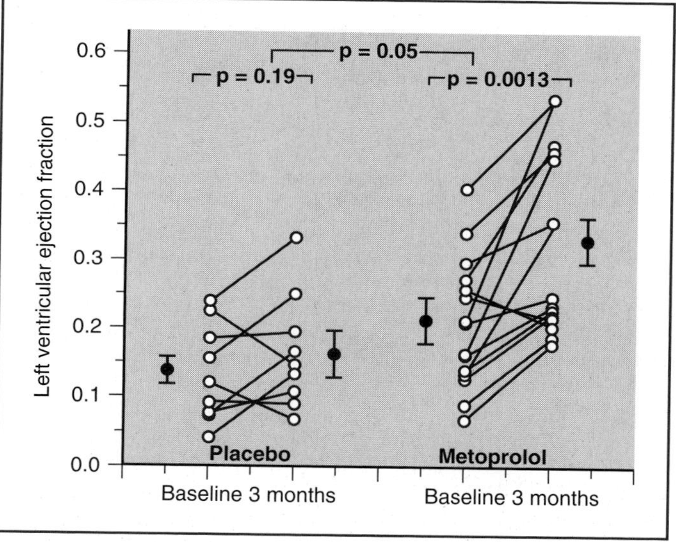

FIGURE 16–7. Changes in left ventricular ejection fraction between baseline and 3 months for placebo and metoprolol groups in patients with dilated cardiomyopathy. A significant increase in ejection fraction was seen only in the metoprolol group. Vertical bars are group mean value and standard error. (From Eichorn, E. J., Heesch, C. M. Barnett, J. H., et al.: Effect of metoprolol on myocardial function and energetics in patients with nonischemic dilated cardiomyopathy: A randomized, double-blind, placebo-controlled study. Reprinted with permission from the American College of Cardiology. J. Am. Coll. Cardiol. *24*:1310, 1994.)

Beta-adrenergic antagonists with vasodilator activity are also being evaluated for use in heart failure. *Labetalol,* a nonselective beta$_1$- and beta$_2$-antagonist that also blocks alpha$_1$ receptors and is already licensed in the United States for the treatment of hypertension, has been favorably evaluated in small trials of heart failure patients. *Carvedilol,** like labetolol, exhibits both alpha$_1$ and beta receptor antagonism with no partial agonist (ISA) activity, but modest beta$_1$ selectivity and an elimination half-life (2 to 8 hours) that permits once or twice daily dosing.[215,216] *Bucindolol** is a nonselective beta antagonist that is also a vasodilator, due to a mechanism other than alpha-adrenergic blockade in the vasculature.[217]

* Not approved by the US Food and Drug Administration at the time of this writing.

Carvedilol and bucindolol appear to be well tolerated in small trials of patients with both idiopathic and ischemic cardiomyopathies, and several preliminary reports support their efficacy in improving left ventricular ejection fraction, submaximal exercise tolerance, and symptoms. In a published report of 40 patients with idiopathic dilated cardiomyopathy randomized to receive either placebo or carvedilol (target dose, 25 mg twice a day) with background therapy of digoxin, diuretics, and an ACE inhibitor, carvedilol after 4 months improved symptoms, submaximal exercise capacity, and left ventricular ejection fraction (from 0.20 to 0.30) and decreased pulmonary artery wedge pressure.[218] Although pulmonary artery pressures and systemic vascular resistance both declined significantly after the first dose of carvedilol, resting pulmonary artery pressures and systemic vascular resistances declined little, if at all, upon readministration of the drug after several months of exposure. This suggests development of tolerance with time to the alpha$_1$ antagonist effects of this agent, an effect noted with chronic labetolol administration as well.

No clear consensus exists as yet on which of the pharmacological activities of beta-adrenergic antagonists listed in Table 16–7 are necessary or desirable in the treatment of heart failure. Nevertheless, the alpha$_1$ vasodilatory activity of carvedilol and the "direct" vasodilating action of bucindolol may make early upward dose titration of these drugs better tolerated than beta-adrenergic antagonists without vasodilator activity.

REFERENCES

VASODILATORS

1. Cohn, J. N., and Franciosa, J. A.: Vasodilator therapy of cardiac failure. N. Engl. J. Med. *297:*27, 1977.
2. Cohn, J. N., Archibald, D. G., Ziesche, S., et al.: Effect of vasodilator therapy on mortality in chronic congestive heart failure: Results of a Veterans Administration Cooperative Study. N. Engl. J. Med. *314:*1547, 1986.
3. CONSENSUS Trial Study Group: Effects of enalapril on mortality in severe congestive heart failure: Results of the Cooperative North Scandinavian Enalapril Survival Group (CONSENSUS). N. Engl. J. Med. *316:*1429, 1987.
4. Wang, S. Y., Manyari, D. E., Scott-Douglas, N., et al.: Splanchnic venous pressure-volume relation during experimental acute ischemic heart failure: Differential effects of hydralazine, enalaprilat, and nitroglycerin. Circulation *91:*1205, 1995.
5. Griendling, K. K., Murphy, T. J., and Alexander, R. W.: Molecular biology of the renin-angiotensin system. Circulation *87:*1816, 1993.
6. Linz, W., Wiemer, G., Gohlke, P., et al.: Contribution of kinins to the cardiovascular actions of angiotensin-converting enzyme inhibitors. Pharmacol. Rev. *47:*25, 1995.
7. Paul, M., Wagner, J., and Dzau, V. J.: Gene expression of the renin-angiotensin system in human tissues: Quantitative analysis by the polymerase chain reaction. J. Clin. Invest. *91:*2058, 1993.
8. Yang, G., Merrill, D. C., Thompson, M. W., et al.: Functional expression of the human angiotensinogen gene in transgenic mice. J. Biol. Chem. *269:*32497, 1994.
9. Dzau, V. J., and Re, R.: Tissue angiotensin system in cardiovascular medicine: A paradigm shift? Circulation *89:*493, 1994.
10. Kifor, I., and Dzau, V. J.: Endothelial renin-angiotensin pathways: Evidence for intracellular synthesis and secretion of angiotensins. Circ. Res. *60:*422, 1987.
11. Morishita, R., Gibbons, G. H., Ellison, K. E., et al.: Evidence for direct local effect of angiotensin in vascular hypertrophy: In vivo gene transfer of angiotensin converting enzyme. J. Clin. Invest. *94:*978, 1994.
12. Lee, M. A., Bohm, M., Paul, M., et al.: Tissue renin-angiotensin systems: Their role in cardiovascular disease. Circulation *87:*IV-7, 1993.
13. Smith, R. D., Chiu, A. T., Wong, P. C., et al.: Pharmacology of nonpeptide angiotensin II receptor antagonists. Annu. Rev. Pharmacol. Toxicol. *32:*135, 1992.
14. Timmermans, P., and Smith, R. D.: Angiotensin II receptor subtypes: Selective antagonists and functional correlates. Eur. Heart J. *15:*79, 1994.
15. Marrero, M. B., Schieffer, B., Paxton, W. G., et al.: Direct stimulation of Jak/STAT pathway by the angiotensin II AT$_1$ receptor. Nature *375:*247, 1995.
16. Regitz-Zagrosek, V., Friedel, N., Heymann, A., et al.: Regulation, chamber localization, and subtype distribution of angiotensin II receptors in human hearts. Circulation *91:*1461, 1995.
17. Holubarsch, C., Schmidt-Schweda, S., Knorr, A., et al.: Functional significance of angiotensin receptors in human myocardium: Significant differences between atrial and ventricular myocardium. Eur. Heart J. *15:*88, 1994.
18. Lonn, E. M., Yusuf, S., Jha, P., et al.: Emerging role of angiotensin-converting enzyme inhibitors in cardiac and vascular protection. Circulation *90:*2056, 1994.
19. Cohn, J. N.: Structural basis for heart failure: Ventricular remodeling and its pharmacological inhibition. Circulation *91:*2504, 1995.
20. Goldsmith, S. R., Hasking, G. J., and Miller, E.: Angiotensin II and sympathetic activity in patients with congestive heart failure. J. Am. Coll. Cardiol. *21:*1107, 1993.
21. Lyons, D., Webster, J., and Benjamin, N.: Angiotensin II: Adrenergic sympathetic constrictor action in humans. Circulation *91:*1457, 1995.
22. Vaughn, D. E., Lazos, S. A., and Tong, K.: Angiotensin II regulates the expression of plasminogen activator inhibitor-1 in cultured endothelial cells: A potential link between the renin-angiotensin system and thrombosis. J. Clin. Invest. *95:*995, 1995.
23. Feener, E. P., Northrup, J. M., Aiello, L. P., et al.: Angiotensin II induces plasminogen activator inhibitor-1 and -2 expression in vascular endothelial and smooth muscle cells. J. Clin. Invest. *95:*1353, 1995.
24. Ishihata, A., and Endo, M.: Pharmacological characteristics of the positive inotropic effect of angiotensin II in the rabbit ventricular myocardium. Br. J. Pharmacol. *108:*999, 1993.
25. Holubarsch, C., Hasenfuss, G., Schmidt-Schweda, S., et al.: Angiotensin I and II exert inotropic effects in atrial but not in ventricular human myocardium. Circulation *88:*1228, 1993.
26. Moravec, C. S., Schluchter, M. D., Paranaudi, L., et al.: Inotropic effects of angiotensin II and human cardiac muscle in vitro. Circulation *82:*1973, 1990.
27. Weinberg, E. O., Schoen, F. J., George, D., et al.: Angiotensin-converting enzyme inhibition prolongs survival and modifies the transition to heart failure in rats with pressure overload hypertrophy due to ascending aortic stenosis. Circulation *90:*1410, 1994.
28. Friedrich, S. P., Lorell, B. H., Rousseau, M. F., et al.: Intracardiac angiotensin-converting enzyme inhibition improves diastolic function in patients with left ventricular hypertrophy due to aortic stenosis. Circulation *90:*2761, 1994.
29. Hayashida, W., van Eyll, C., Rousseau, M. F., et al.: Regional remodeling and nonuniform changes in diastolic function in patients with left ventricular dysfunction: Modification by long-term enalapril treatment. J. Am. Coll. Cardiol. *22:*1403, 1993.
30. Pouleur, H., Rousseau, M. F., van Eyll, C., et al.: Effects of long-term enalapril therapy on left ventricular diastolic properties in patients with depressed ejection fraction. Circulation *88:*481, 1993.
31. Matsubara, H., Kanasaki, M., Murasawa, S., et al.: Differential gene expression and regulation of angiotensin II receptor subtypes in rat cardiac fibroblasts and cardiomyocytes in culture. J. Clin. Invest. *93:*1592, 1994.
32. Schorb, W., Peeler, T. C., Madigan, N. N., et al.: Angiotensin II–induced protein tyrosine phosphorylation in neonatal rat cardiac fibroblasts. J. Biol. Chem. *269:*19626, 1994.
33. Crabos, M., Roth, M., Hahn, A. W. A., et al.: Characterization of angiotensin II receptors in cultured adult rat cardiac fibroblasts: Coupling to signaling systems and gene expression. J. Clin. Invest. *93:*2372, 1994.
34. Waspe, L. E., Ordahl, C. P., and Simpson, P. C.: The cardiac β-myosin heavy chain isogene is induced selectively in α_1-adrenergic receptor-stimulated hypertrophy of cultured rat heart myocytes. J. Clin. Invest. *85:*1206, 1990.
35. Schunkert, H., Sadoshima, J.-I., Cornelius, T., et al.: Angiotensin II–induced growth responses in isolated adult rat hearts: Evidence for load-independent induction of cardiac protein synthesis by angiotensin II. Circ. Res. *76:*489, 1995.
36. LaMorte, V. J., Thorburn, J., Absher, D., et al.: G_q- and ras-dependent pathways mediate hypertrophy of neonatal rat ventricular myocytes following α_1-adrenergic stimulation. J. Biol. Chem. *269:*13490, 1994.
37. Pfeffer, J. M., Pfeffer, M. A., Mirsky, I., et al.: Regression of left ventricular hypertrophy and prevention of left ventricular dysfunction by captopril in the spontaneously hypertensive rat. Proc. Natl. Acad. Sci. U.S.A. *79:*3310, 1992.
38. Jufsurr, V. I., Khan, M. I., Jugdutt, S. J., et al.: Effect of enalapril on ventricular remodeling and function during healing after anterior myocardial infarction in the dog. Circulation *91:*802, 1995.
39. Weber, K. T., and Brilla, C. G.: Pathological hypertrophy and cardiac interstitium. Circulation *83:*1849, 1991.
40. Binkley, P. F., Haas, G. J., Starling, R. C., et al.: Sustained augmentation of parasympathetic tone with angiotensin converting enzyme inhibition in patients with congestive heart failure. J. Am. Coll. Cardiol. *21:*655, 1993.
41. Ljungman, S., Kjekshus, J., and Swedberg, K., for the CONSENSUS Group: Renal function in severe congestive heart failure during treatment with enalapril (the Cooperative North Scandinavian Enalapril Survival Study [CONSENSUS] Trial). Am. J. Cardiol. *70:*479, 1992.
42. Mandal, A. K., Markert, R. J., Saklayen, M. G., et al.: Diuretics potentiate angiotensin converting enzyme inhibitor–induced acute renal failure. Clin. Nephrol. *42:*170, 1994.
43. SOLVD Investigators: Effect of enalapril on survival in patients with reduced left ventricular ejection fractions and congestive heart failure. N. Engl. J. Med. *325:*293, 1991.
44. Gruppo Italiano per lo Studio della Sopravvivenza nell'Infarto Miocardico, GISSI-3 Investigators: Effects of lisinopril and transdermal glyceryl trinitrate singly and together on 6-week mortality and ventricular function after acute myocardial infarction. Lancet *343:*1115, 1994.
45. ISIS-4 (Fourth International Study of Infarct Survival) Collaborative Group: ISIS-4: A randomized factorial trial assessing early oral capto-

pril, oral mononitrate, and intravenous magnesium sulphate in 58,050 patients with suspected acute myocardial infarction. Lancet *345*:669, 1995.
46. Lewis, E. J., Hunsicker, I. G., Bain, R. P., et al.: The effect of angiotensin-converting-enzyme inhibition on diabetic nephropathy. N. Engl. J. Med. *329*:1456, 1993.
47. Keilani, T., Schlueter, M., and Batlle, D.: Selected aspects of ACE inhibitor therapy for patients with renal disease: Impact on proteinuria, lipids and potassium. J. Clin. Pharmacol. *35*:87, 1995.
48. Ondetti, M. A.: From peptides to peptidases: A chronicle of drug discovery. Annu. Rev. Pharmacol. Toxicol. *34*:1, 1994.
49. Zusman, R. M.: Fosinopril and cardiac performance. Rev. Contemp. Pharmacother. *4*:25, 1993.
50. Cushman, D. W., Wang, W. L., Fung, W. C., et al.: Differentiation of angiotensin converting enzyme inhibitors by their selective inhibition of ACE in physiologically important target organs. Am. J. Hypertens. *2*:294, 1989.
51. Zusman, R. M.: Angiotensin-converting enzyme inhibitors: More different than alike? Focus on cardiac performance. Am. J. Cardiol. *72*:25H, 1993.
52. Kostis, J. B., Shelton, B. J., Yusuf, S., et al.: Tolerability of enalapril initiation by patients with left ventricular dysfunction: Results of the medication challenge phase of the studies of left ventricular dysfunction. Am. Heart J. *128*:358, 1994.
53. Lang, R. M., DiBianco, R., Broderick, G. T., et al.: First-dose effects of enalapril 2.5 mg and captopril 6.25 mg in patients with heart failure: A double-blind, randomized, multicenter study. Am. Heart J. *128*:551, 1994.
54. Reid, J. L., MacFadyen, R. J., Squire, I. B., et al.: Blood pressure response to the first dose of angiotensin-converting enzyme inhibitors in congestive heart failure. Am. J. Cardiol. *71*:57E, 1993.
55. Shionoiri, H.: Pharmacokinetic drug interactions with ACE inhibitors. Clin. Pharamcokinet. *25*:20, 1993.
56. Sweet, C. S., and Rucinska, E. J.: Losartan in heart failure: Preclinical experiences and initial clinical outcomes. Eur. Heart J. *15*:139, 1994.
57. Crozier, I., Ikram, H., Awan, N., et al.: Losartan in heart failure: Hemodynamic effects and tolerability. Circulation *91*:691, 1995.
58. Wood, J. M., Cumin, F., and Maibaum, J.: Pharmacology of renin inhibitors and their application to the treatment of hypertension. Pharmacol. Ther. *61*:325, 1994.
59. Frishman, W. H., Fozailoff, A., Lin, C., et al.: Renin inhibition: A new approach to cardiovascular therapy. J. Clin. Pharmacol. *34*:873, 1994.
60. Stamler, J. S.: Redox signaling: Nitrosylation and related target interactions of nitric oxide. Cell *78*:931, 1994.
61. Nathan, C., and Xie, Q.-W.: Nitric oxide synthases: Roles, tolls, and controls. Cell *78*:915, 1994.
62. Balligand, J.-L., Kobzik, L., Han, X., et al.: Nitric oxide–dependent parasympathetic signalling in cardiac myocytes is due to activation of type III (constitutive endothelial) NO synthase. J. Biol. Chem. *270*:14582, 1995.
63. Hare, J. M., Loh, E., Creager, M. A., and Colucci, W. S.: Nitric oxide inhibits the positive inotropic response to β-adrenergic stimulation in humans with left ventricular dysfunction. Circulation *92*:2198, 1995.
64. Furchgott, R. F., and Zawadzki, J. V.: The obligatory role of endothelial cells in the relaxation of arterial smooth muscle by acetylcholine. Nature *288*:373, 1980.
65. Harrison, D. G., and Bates, J. N.: The nitrovasodilators: New ideas about old drugs. Circulation *87*:1461, 1993.
66. Risoe, C., Simonsen, S., Rootwelt, K., et al.: Nitroprusside and regional vascular capacitance in patients with severe congestive heart failure. Circulation *85*:997, 1992.
67. Heesch, C. M., Hatfield, B. A., Marcoux, L., et al.: Predictors of pressure and stroke volume response to afterload reduction with nitroprusside in patients with congestive heart failure secondary to idiopathic dilated cardiomyopathy. Am. J. Cardiol. *74*:951, 1994.
68. Fallen, E. L., Nahmias, C., Scheffel, A., et al.: Redistribution of myocardial blood flow with topical nitroglycerin in patients with coronary artery disease. Circulation *91*:1381, 1995.
69. European Study of Prevention of Infarct with Molsidomine (ESPRIM) Group: The ESPRIM trial: Short-term treatment of acute myocardial infarction with molsidomine. Lancet *344*:91, 1994.
70. Unger, P., Vachiery, J.-L., de Canniere, D., et al.: Comparison of the hemodynamic responses to molsidomine and isosorbide dinitrate in congestive heart failure. Am. Heart J. *128*:557, 1994.
71. Elkayam, U.: Tolerance to organic nitrates: Evidence, mechanisms, clinical relevance, and strategies for prevention. Ann. Intern. Med. *114*:667, 1991.
72. Mangione, N. J., and Glasser, S. P.: Phenomenon of nitrate tolerance. Am. Heart J. *128*:137, 1994.
73. Dupuis, J.: Nitrates in congestive heart failure. Cardiovasc. Drugs Ther. *8*:501, 1994.
74. Ignarro, L., Edwards, J., Gruetter, D. Y., et al.: Possible involvement of S-nitrosothiols in the activation of guanylate cyclase by nitrous compounds. FEBS Lett. *110*:275, 1980.
75. Mehra, A., Shotan, A., Ostrzega, E., et al.: Potentiation of isosorbide dinitrate effects with N-acetylcysteine in patients with chronic heart failure. Circulation *89*:2595, 1994.
76. Munzel, T., Sayegh, H., Freeman, B. A., et al.: Evidence for enhanced vascular superoxide anion production in nitrate tolerance. A novel mechanism underlying tolerance and cross-tolerance. J. Clin. Invest. *95*:187, 1995.
77. Parker, J. D., Parker, A. B., Farrell, B., et al.: Intermittent transdermal nitroglycerin therapy. Decreased anginal threshold during the nitrate-free interval. Circulation *91*:973, 1995.
78. Parker, J. O., Amies, M. H., Hawkinson, R. W., et al.: Intermittent transdermal nitroglycerin therapy in angina pectoris. Clinically effective without tolerance or rebound. Circulation *91*:1368, 1995.
79. Hofstra, A. H.: Metabolism of hydralazine: Relevance to drug-induced lupus. Drug Metab. Rev. *26*:485, 1994.
80. Elkayam, U., Shotan, A., Mehra, A., et al.: Calcium channel blockers in the heart. J. Am. Coll. Cardiol. *22*:139A, 1993.
81. Conti, C. R.: Use of calcium antagonists to treat heart failure. Clin. Cardiol. *17*:101, 1994.
82. Little, W. C., and Cheng, C.-P.: Vascular versus myocardial effects of calcium antagonists. Drugs *47*:41, 1994.
83. Kukuljan, M., Labarca, P., and Latorre, R.: Molecular determinants of ion conduction and inactivation in K^+ channels. Am. J. Physiol. *268*:C535, 1995.
84. Philipson, D. H., and Steiner, D. F.: Pas de deux or more: The sulfonylurea receptor and K^+ channels. Science *268*:372, 1995.
85. Nelson, M. T., and Quayle, J. M.: Physiological roles and properties of potassium channels in arterial smooth muscle. Am. J. Physiol. *268*:C799, 1995.
86. Kukovetz, W. R., Holzmann, S., and Poch, G.: Molecular mechanisms of the action of nicorandil. J. Cardiovasc. Pharmacol. *20*:S1, 1992.
87. Kato, K.: Hemodynamic and clinical effects of an intravenous potassium channel opener—a review. Eur. Heart J. *14*:40, 1993.
88. Tsutamoto, T., Kinoshita, M., Nakae, I., et al.: Absence of hemodynamic tolerance to nicorandil in patients with severe congestive heart failure. Am. Heart J. *127*:866, 1994.

DIURETICS

89. Awazu, M., and Ichikawa, I.: Alterations in renal function in experimental congestive heart failure. Semin. Nephrol. *14*:401, 1994.
90. Rouse, D., and Suki, W. N.: Effects of neural and humoral agents on the renal tubules in congestive heart failure. Sem. Nephrol. *14*:412, 1994.
91. Miller, J. A., Tobe, S. W., and Skorecki, K. L.: Control of extracellular fluid volume and the pathophysiology of edema. *In* Brenner, B. M., and Rector, F. C. (eds.): The Kidney. 5th ed. Philadelphia, W. B. Saunders Company, 1996.
92. Young, J. B., and Pratt, C. M.: Hemodynamic and hormonal alterations in patients with heart failure: Toward a contemporary definition of heart failure. Sem. Nephrol. *14*:427, 1994.
93. Maddox, D. A., and Brenner, B. M.: Glomerular ultrafiltration. *In* Brenner, B. M., and Rector, F. C. (eds.): The Kidney. 5th ed. Philadelphia, W. B. Saunders Company, 1996.
94. Jackson, E. K.: Diuretics and other agents employed in the mobilization of edema fluid. *In* Hardman, J. G., Limbird, L. (eds.): Goodman & Gilman's The Pharmacological Basis of Therapeutics, 9th ed. New York, McGraw-Hill Book Co., 1996.
95. Haas, M.: The Na-K-Cl cotransporters. Am. J. Physiol. *267*:C869, 1994.
96. Raftery, E. B.: Hemodynamic effects of diuretics in heart failure. Br. Heart J. *72*:44, 1994.
97. Gamba, G., Saltzberg, S. N., Lombardi, M., et al.: Primary structure and functional expression of a cDNA encoding the thiazide-sensitive, electroneutral sodium-chloride cotransporter. Proc. Natl. Acad. Sci. U.S.A. *90*:2749, 1993.
98. Palmer, L. G.: Epithelial Na channels and their kin. News Physiol. Sci. *10*:61, 1995.
99. Funder, J. W.: Mineralocorticoids, glucocorticoids, receptors and response elements. Science *259*:1132, 1993.
100. Funder, J. W.: Aldosterone action. Annu. Rev. Physiol. *55*:115, 1993.
101. Weber, K. T., and Villarreal, D.: Aldosterone and antialdosterone therapy in congestive heart failure. Am. J. Cardiol. *71*:3A, 1993.
102. Jackson, E. K.: Vasopressin and other agents affecting the renal conservation of water. *In* Hardman, J. G., Limbird, L. (eds.): Goodman & Gilman's The Pharmacological Basis of Therapeutics, 9th ed. New York, McGraw-Hill Book Co., 1996.
103. Nielsen, S., Chou, C.-L., Marples, D., et al.: Vasopressin increases water permeability of kidney collecting duct by inducing translocation of aquaporin-CD water channels to plasma membrane. Proc. Natl. Acad. Sci. U.S.A. *92*:1013, 1995.
104. Knoers, N. V. A., and van Os, C. H.: The clinical importance of the urinary excretion of aquaporin-2. N. Engl. J. Med. *332*:1575, 1995.
105. Ohnishi, A., Orita, Y., Takagi, N., et al.: Aquaretic effect of a potent, orally active, nonpeptide V_2 antagonist in men. J. Pharmacol. Exp. Therap. *272*:546, 1995.
106. Gunning, M. E., Ingelfinger, J. R., King, A. J., et al.: Vasoactive peptides and the kidney. *In* Brenner, B. M., and Rector, F. C. (eds.): The Kidney, 5th ed. Philadelphia, W. B. Saunders Company, 1996.
107. Deutsch, A., Frishman, W. H., Sukenik, D., et al.: Atrial natriuretic peptide and its potential role in pharmacotherapy. J. Clin. Pharmacol. *34*:1133, 1994.
108. Semigran, M. J., Aroney, C. N., Herrmann, H. C., et al.: Effects of atrial natriuretic peptide on myocardial contractile and diastolic function in patients with heart failure. J. Am. Coll. Cardiol. *20*:98, 1992.
109. Brater, D. C.: Diuretic resistance: Mechanisms and therapeutic strategies. Cardiology *84*:57, 1994.
110. Brater, D. C.: Pharmacokinetics of loop diuretics in congestive heart failure. Br. Heart J. *72*:S40, 1994.

111. Knauf, H., and Mutschler, E.: Functional state of the nephron and diuretic dose-response-rationale for low-dose combination therapy. Cardiology *84:*18, 1994.
112. Wilcox, C. S.: Diuretics. *In* Brenner, B. M., and Rector, F. C. (eds.): The Kidney, 5th ed. Philadelphia, W. B. Saunders Company, 1995.
113. Ellison, D. H.: The physiologic basis of diuretic synergism: Its role in treating diuretic resistance. Ann. Intern. Med. *114:*886, 1991.
114. Leier, C. V., Dei Cas, L., and Metra, M.: Clinical relevance and management of the major electrolyte abnormalities in congestive heart failure: Hyponatremia, hypokalemia, and hypomagnesemia. Am. Heart J. *128:*564, 1994.
115. Bigger, J. T., Jr.: Diuretic therapy, hypertension, and cardiac arrest. N. Engl. J. Med. *330:*1899, 1994.
116. Siscovick, D. S., Raghunathan, T. E., Psaty, B. M., et al.: Diuretic therapy for hypertension and the risk of primary cardiac arrest. N. Engl. J. Med. *330:*1852, 1994.
117. Siegel, D., Hulley, S. B., Black, D. M., et al.: Diuretics, serum and intracellular electrolyte levels, and ventricular arrhythmias in hypertensive men. JAMA *267:*1083, 1992.
118. Cody, R. J.: Clinical trials of diuretic therapy in heart failure: Research directions and clinical considerations. J. Am. Coll. Cardiol. *22:*165A, 1993.
119. Hampton, J. R.: Results of clinical trials with diuretics in heart failure. Br. Heart J. *72:*S68, 1994.
120. Ramsay, L. E., Yeo, W. W., and Jackson, P. R.: Metabolic effects of diuretics. Cardiology *84:*48, 1994.
121. Moser, M.: Effect of diuretics on morbidity and mortality in the treatment of hypertension. Cardiology *84:*27, 1994.
122. Silke, B.: Diuretic induced changes in symptoms and quality of life. Br. Heart J. *72:*S57, 1994.
123. Freis, E. D.: The efficacy and safety of diuretics in treating hypertension. Ann. Intern. Med. *122:*223, 1995.
124. Dorup, I.: Magnesium and potassium deficiency, its diagnosis, occurrence, and treatment in diuretic therapy and its consequences for growth, protein synthesis and growth factors. Acta Physiol. Scand. *150:*7, 1994.
125. Arsenian, M. A.: Magnesium and cardiovascular disease. Prog. Cardiovasc. Dis. *35:*271, 1993.
126. Al-Ghamdi, S. M. G., Cameron, E. C., and Sutton, R. A. L.: Magnesium deficiency: Pathophysiologic and clinical overview. Am. J. Kidney Dis. *24:*737, 1994.
127. Davies, D. L., and Fraser, R.: Do diuretics cause magnesium deficiency? Br. J. Clin. Pharmacol. *36:*1, 1993.
128. Materson, B. J., Reda, D. J., Cushman, W. C., et al.: Single-drug therapy for hypertension in men. A comparison of six antihypertensive agents with placebo. N. Engl. J. Med. *328:*914, 1993.
129. Kasiske, B. L., Ma, J. Z., Kalil, R. S. N., et al.: Effects of antihypertensive therapy on serum lipids. Ann. Intern. Med. *122:*133, 1995.
130. Lajoie, G., Laszik, Z., Nadasdy, T., et al.: The renal-cardiac connection: Renal parenchymal alterations in patients with heart disease. Sem. Nephrol. *14:*441, 1994.
131. Shuler, C., Golper, T. A., and Bennett, W. M.: Prescribing drugs in renal disease. *In* Brenner, B. M., and Rector, F. C. (eds.): The Kidney, 5th ed. Philadelphia, W. B. Saunders Company, 1996.
132. Kaplan, A. A.: Ultrafiltration in the treatment of congestive heart failure. Heart Failure *10:*192, 1994.
133. Agostoni, P., Marenzi, G., Lauri, G., et al.: Sustained improvement in functional capacity after removal of body fluid with isolated ultrafiltration in chronic cardiac insufficiency: Failure of furosemide to provide the same result. Am. J. Med. *96:*191, 1994.
134. Withering, W.: An account of the foxglove and some of its medical uses, with practical remarks on dropsy, and other diseases. *In* Willius, F. A., and Keys, T. E., (eds.): Classics of Cardiology. New York, Dover, *1:*231, 1941.
135. Eisner, D. A., and Smith, T. W.: The Na-K pump and its effectors in cardiac muscle. *In* Fozzard, H. A., Haber, E., Katz, A. M., et al.: (eds.): The Heart and Cardiovascular System. New York, Raven Press, 1992.
136. Blaustein, M. P.: Physiological effects of endogenous ouabain: Control of intracellular Ca^{2+} stores and cell responsiveness. Am. J. Physiol. *264:*C1367, 1993.
137. Kelly, R. A., and Smith, T. W.: The search for the endogenous digitalis: An alternative hypothesis. Am. J. Physiol. *256:*C937, 1989.
138. Kelly, R. A., and Smith, T. W.: Endogenous cardiac glycosides. Adv. Pharmacol. *25:*263, 1994.
139. Lingrel, J. B., Van Huysse, J., O'Brien, W., et al.: Structure-function studies of the Na,K-ATPase. Kidney Int. *45:*S32, 1994.
140. Schmidt, T. A., Allen, P. D., Colucci, W. S., et al.: No adaptation to digitalization as evaluated by digitalis receptor (Na,K-ATPase) quantification in explanted hearts from donors without heart disease and from digitalized recipients with end-stage heart failure. Am. J. Cardiol. *70:*110, 1992.
141. Harrison, S. M., McCall, E., and Boyett, M. R.: The relationship between contraction and intracellular sodium in rat and guinea-pig ventricular myocytes. J. Physiol. (London) *449:*517, 1992.
142. Pidgeon, G. B., Richards, A. M., Nicholls, M. G., et al.: Effect of ouabain on pressor responsiveness in normal man. Am. J. Physiol. *267:*E642, 1994.
143. Lucke, J. C., Elbeery, J. R., Koutlas, T. C., et al.: Effects of cardiac glycosides on myocardial function and energetics in conscious dogs. Am. J. Physiol. *267:*H2042, 1994.
144. Holubarsch, C., Hasenfuss, G., Just, H., et al.: Positive inotropism and myocardial energetics: Influence of β receptor agonist stimulation, phosphodiesterase inhibition, and ouabain. Cardiovasc. Res. *28:*994, 1994.
145. McGarry, S. J., and Williams, A. J.: Digoxin activates sarcoplasmic reticulum Ca^{2+} release channels: A possible role in cardiac inotropy. Br. J. Pharmacol. *108:*1043, 1993.
146. Kranzhofer, R., Haass, M., Kurz, T., et al.: Effect of digitalis glycosides on norepinephrine release in the heart. Dual mechanisms of action. Circ. Res. *68:*1628, 1991.
147. Mason, D. T., Braunwald, E., Karsh, R. B., et al.: Studies on digitalis. X. Effects of ouabain on forearm vascular resistance and venous tone in normal subjects and in patients in heart failure. J. Clin. Invest. *43:*532, 1964.
148. Wang, W., Chen, J.-S., and Zucker, I. H.: Carotid sinus baroreceptor sensitivity in experimental heart failure. Circulation *81:*1959, 1990.
149. Ferguson, D. W., Berg, W. J., Sanders, J. S., et al.: Sympathoinhibitory responses to digitalis glycosides in heart failure patients. Direct evidence from sympathetic neural recordings. Circulation *80:*65, 1989.
150. Krum, H., Bigger, J. T., Jr., Goldsmith, R. L., et al.: Effect of long-term digoxin therapy on autonomic function in patients with chronic heart failure. J. Am. Coll. Cardiol. *25:*289, 1995.
151. Patten, S. B., and Love, E. J.: Neuropsychiatric adverse drug reactions: Passive reports to Health and Welfare Canada's adverse drug reaction database (1965-Present). Intl. J. Psychiat. Med. *24:*45, 1994.
152. Hui, J., Geraets, D. R., Chandrasekaran, A., et al.: Digoxin disposition in elderly humans with hypochlorhydria. J. Clin. Pharmacol. *34:*734, 1994.
153. Kelly, R. A., and Smith, T. W.: Use and misuse of digitalis blood levels. Heart Dis. Stroke *1:*117, 1992.
154. Mahdyoon, H., Battilana, G., Rosman, H., et al.: The evolving pattern of digoxin intoxication: Observations at a large urban hospital from 1980 to 1988. Am. Heart J. *120:*1189, 1990.
155. Kelly, R. A., and Smith, T. W.: Recognition and management of digitalis toxicity. Am. J. Cardiol. *69:*108G, 1992.
156. Kelly, R. A., and Smith, T. W.: Antibody therapies for drug overdose. *In* Austen, K. F., Burakoff, S. J., Rosen, F. S., et al. (eds.): Therapeutic Immunology. Cambridge, Blackwell Scientific, 1996.
157. Bosse, G. M., and Pope, T. M.: Recurrent digoxin overdose and treatment with digoxin-specific Fab antibody fragments. J. Emerg. Med. *12:*179, 1994.
158. Clark, R. F., and Barton, E. D.: Pitfalls in the administration of digoxin-specific Fab fragments. J. Emerg. Med. *12:*233, 1994.
159. Beavo, J. A., and Reifsnyder, D. H.: Primary sequence of cyclic nucleotide phosphodiesterase isozymes and the design of selective inhibitors. Trends Pharmacol. Sci. *11:*150, 1990.
160. Nicholson, C. D., Challiss, R. A. J., and Shahid, M.: Differential modulation of tissue function and therapeutic potential of selective inhibitors of cyclic nucleotide phosphodiesterase isoenzymes. Trends Pharmacol. Sci. *12:*19, 1991.
161. Bode, D. C., Kanter, J. R., and Brunton, L. L.: Cellular distribution of phosphodiesterase isoforms in rat cardiac tissue. Circ. Res. *68:*1070, 1991.
162. Beavo, J. A.: cGMP inhibition of heart phosphodiesterase: Is it clinically relevant? J. Clin. Invest. *95:*444, 1995.
163. Packer, M., Carver, J. R., Rodeheffer, R. J., et al.: Effect of oral milrinone on mortality in severe chronic heart failure. N. Engl. J. Med. *325:*1468, 1991.
164. Packer, M.: The development of positive inotropic agents for chronic heart failure: How have we gone astray? J. Am. Coll. Cardiol. *22:*119A, 1993.
165. Nony, P., Boissel, J.-P., Lievre, M., et al.: Evaluation of the effect of phosphodiesterase inhibitors on mortality in chronic heart failure patients. Eur. J. Clin. Pharmacol. *46:*191, 1994.
166. Cheng, D. C. H., Asokumar, B., and Nakagawa, T.: Amrinone therapy for severe pulmonary hypertension and biventricular failure after complicated valvular heart surgery. Chest *104:*1618, 1993.
167. Wynands, J. E.: The role of amrinone in treating heart failure during and after coronary artery surgery supported by cardiopulmonary bypass. J. Cardiac Surg. *9:*453, 1994.
168. Installe, E., DeCoster, P., Gonzalez, M., et al.: Comparison between the positive inotropic effects of enoximone, a cardiac phosphodiesterase III inhibitor, and dobutamine in patients with moderate to severe congestive heart failure. Eur. Heart J. *12:*985, 1991.
169. Nagata, K., Iwase, M., Sobue, T., et al.: Differential effects of dobutamine and a phosphodiesterase inhibitor on early diastolic filling in patients with congestive heart failure. J. Am. Coll. Cardiol. *25:*295, 1995.
170. Matsui, S., Matsumori, A., Matoba, Y., et al.: Treatment of virus-induced myocardial injury with a novel immunomodulating agent, vesnarinone. Suppression of natural killer cell activity and tumor necrosis factor-α production. J. Clin. Invest. *94:*1212, 1994.
171. Bertolet, B. D., White, B. G., and Pepine, C. J.: Neutropenia occurring during treatment with vesnarinone (OPC-8212). Am. J. Cardiol. *74:*968, 1994.
172. Feldman, A. M., Bristow, M. R., Parmley, W. W., et al.: Effects of vesnarinone on morbidity and mortality in patients with heart failure. N. Engl. J. Med. *329:*149, 1993.
173. Hoit, B. D., Burwig, S., Eppert, D., et al.: Effects of a novel inotropic agent (OPC-18790) on systolic and diastolic function in patients with severe heart failure. Am. Heart J. *128:*1156, 1994.
174. Hagemeijer, F.: Calcium sensitization with pimobendan: Pharmacology,

hemodynamic improvement, and sudden death in patients with chronic congestive heart failure. Eur. Heart J. *14*:551, 1993.
175. Rector, T. S., and Cohn, J. N.: Assessment of patient outcome with the Minnesota Living with Heart Failure Questionnaire: Reliability and validity during a randomized, double-blind, placebo-controlled trial of pimobendan. Am. Heart J. *124*:1017, 1992.
176. Kubo, S. H., Gollub, S., Bourge, R., et al., for the Pimobendan Multicenter Research Group: Beneficial effects of pimobendan on exercise tolerance and quality of life in patients with heart failure. Results of a multicenter trial. Circulation *85*:942, 1992.
177. Remme, W. J., Krayenbuhl, H. P., Baumann, G., et al., for the Pimobendan-Enalapril Study Group: Long-term efficacy and safety of pimobendan in moderate heart failure. A double-blind parallel 6-month comparison with enalapril. Eur. Heart J. *15*:947, 1994.
178. Pollesello, P., Ovaska, M., Kaivola, J., et al.: Binding of a new Ca^{2+} sensitizer, levosimendan, to recombinant human cardiac troponin C. A molecular modelling, fluorescence probe, and protein nuclear magnetic resonance study. J. Biol. Chem. *269*:28584, 1994.
179. Rump, A. F. E., Acar, D., and Klaus, W.: A quantitative comparison of functional and anti-ischemic effects of the phosphodiesterase-inhibitors, amrinone, milrinone and levosimendan in rabbit isolated hearts. Br. J. Pharmacol. *112*:757, 1994.
180. Pagel, P. S., Harkin, C. P., Hettrick, D. A., et al.: Levosimendan (OR-1259), a myofilament calcium sensitizer, enhances myocardial contractility but does not alter isovolumic relaxation in conscious and anesthetized dogs. Anesthesiology *81*:974, 1994.

ADRENERGIC AGONISTS

181. Neer, E. J.: Heterotrimeric G proteins: Organizers of transmembrane signals. Cell *80*:249, 1995.
182. Clapham, D. E., and Neer, E. J.: New roles for G protein $\beta\gamma$ dimers in transmembrane signaling. Nature *365*:403, 1993.
183. Hoffman, B. R., and Lefkowitz, R. J.: Catecholamines, sympathomimetic drugs, and adrenergic receptor antagonists. *In* Hardman, J. G., Limbard, L. (eds.): Goodman & Gilman's The Pharmacological Basis of Therapeutics, 9th ed. New York, McGraw-Hill Book Co., 1996.
184. Muntz, K. H., Zhao, M., and Miller, J. C.: Downregulation of myocardial β-adrenergic receptors. Receptor subtype selectivity. Circ. Res. *74*:369, 1994.
185. Bristow, M. R., Minobe, W. A., Raynolds, M. V., et al.: Reduced β_1 receptor messenger RNA abundance in the failing human heart. J. Clin. Invest. *92*:2737, 1993.
186. Bristow, M. R.: Changes in myocardial and vascular receptors in heart failure. J. Am. Coll. Cardiol. *22*:61A, 1993.
187. Insel, P. A.: β-Adrenergic receptors in heart failure. J. Clin. Invest. *92*:2563, 1993.
188. Gurevich, V. V., Dion, S. B., Onorato, J. J., et al.: Arrestin interactions with G protein-coupled receptors. Direct binding studies of wild type and mutant arrestins with rhodopsin, $beta_2$-adrenergic, and m2 muscarinic cholinergic receptors. J. Biol. Chem. *270*:720, 1995.
189. Harding, S. E., Brown, L. A., Wynne, D. G., et al.: Mechanisms of β adrenoceptor desensitization in the failing human heart. Cardiovasc. Res. *28*:1451, 1994.
190. Hershberger, R. E.: Beta-adrenergic receptor agonists and antagonists in heart failure. *In* Hosenpud, J. D., and Greenberg, B. H. (eds.): Congestive Heart Failure. New York, Springer-Verlag, 1994, p. 454.
191. Binkley, P. F., VanFossen, D. V., Nunziata, E., et al.: Influence of positive inotropic therapy on pulsatile hydraulic load and ventricular-vascular coupling in congestive heart failure. J. Am. Coll. Cardiol. *15*:1127, 1990.
192. Binkley, P. F., Murray, K. D., Watson, K. M., et al.: Dobutamine increases cardiac output of total artificial heart. Implications for vascular contribution of inotropic agents to augmented ventricular function. Circulation *84*:1210, 1991.
193. Leier, C. V.: Current status of non-digitalis positive inotropic drugs. Am. J. Cardiol. *69*:120G, 1992.
194. Good, J., Frost, G., Oakley, C. M., et al.: The renal effects of dopamine and dobutamine in stable chronic heart failure. Postgrad. Med. J. *68*:S7, 1992.
195. Keren, G., Laniado, S., Sonnenblick, E. H., et al.: Dynamics of functional mitral regurgitation during dobutamine therapy in patients with severe congestive heart failure. A Doppler echocardiographic study. Am. Heart J. *118*:748, 1989.
196. Lokhandwala, M. F., and Amenta, F.: Anatomical distribution and function of dopamine receptors in the kidney. FASEB J. *5*:3023, 1991.
197. MacGregor, D. A., Butterworth, J. F., IV, Zaloga, G. P., et al.: Hemodynamic and renal effects of dopexamine and dobutamine in patients with reduced cardiac output following coronary artery bypass grafting. Chest *106*:835, 1994.
198. Leier, C. V., Hua Ren, J., Huss, P., et al.: The hemodynamic effects of ibopamine, a dopamine congener, in patients with congestive heart failure. Pharmacotherapy *6*:35, 1988.
199. Kleber, F. X., Sabin, G. V., Thyroff-Friesinger, U., et al.: Ibopamine as a valuable adjunct and substitute for dopamine in bridging therapy before heart transplantation. Cardiology *81*:121, 1992.

BETA-ADRENERGIC ANTAGONISTS

200. Bond, R. A., Leff, P., Johnson, T. D., et al.: Physiological effects of inverse agonists in transgenic mice with myocardial overexpression of the β_2-adrenoceptor. Nature *374*:272, 1995.
201. Black, J. W., and Shankley, N. P.: Inverse agonists exposed. Nature *374*:214, 1995.
202. Lowes, B. D., Chidiac, P., Olsen, S., et al.: Clinical relevance of inverse agonism and guanine nucleotide modulatable binding properties of β-adrenergic receptor blocking agents. Circulation *90*:I-543, 1994.
203. Waagstein, F., Hjalmarson, A., Varnauskas, E., et al.: Effect of chronic beta-adrenergic receptor blockade in congestive cardiomyopathy. Br. Heart J. *37*:1022, 1975.
204. Swedberg, K.: Initial experience with beta blockers in dilated cardiomyopathy. Am. J. Cardiol. *71*:30C, 1993.
205. Ikram, H., Fitzpatrick, D., and Crozier, I. G.: Therapeutic controversies with use of beta-adrenoceptor blockade in heart failure. Am. J. Cardiol. *71*:54C, 1993.
206. Doughty, R. N., MacMahon, S., and Sharpe, N.: Beta-blockers in heart failure: Promising or proved? J. Am. Coll. Cardiol. *23*:814, 1994.
207. The German and Austrian Xamoterol Study Group: Double-blind placebo-controlled comparison of digoxin and xamoterol in chronic heart failure. Lancet *1*:489, 1988.
208. The Xamoterol in Severe Heart Failure Study Group: Xamoterol in severe heart failure. Lancet *336*:1, 1990.
209. Bristow, M. R.: Pathophysiologic and pharmacologic rationales for clinical management of chronic heart failure with beta-blocking agents. Am. J. Cardiol. *21*:12C, 1993.
210. Ping, P., Gelzer-Bell, Roth, D. A., et al.: Reduced β-adrenergic activation decreases G-protein expression and β-adrenergic receptor kinase activity in porcine heart. J. Clin. Invest. *95*:1271, 1995.
211. Andersson, B., Hamm, C., Persson, S., et al.: Improved exercise hemodynamic status in dilated cardiomyopathy after beta-adrenergic blockade treatment. J. Am. Coll. Cardiol. *23*:1397, 1994.
212. Eichhorn, E. J., Heesch, C. M., Barnett, J. H., et al.: Effect of metoprolol on myocardial function and energetics in patients with nonischemic dilated cardiomyopathy: A randomized, double-blind, placebo-controlled study. J. Am. Coll. Cardiol. *24*:1310, 1994.
213. Heesch, C. M., Marcoux, L., Hatfield, B., et al.: Hemodynamic and energetic comparison of bucindolol and metoprolol for the treatment of congestive heart failure. Am. J. Cardiol. *75*:360, 1995.
214. Hall, S. A., Cigarroa, C. G., Marcoux, L., et al.: Time course of improvement in left ventricular function, mass and geometry in patients with congestive heart failure treated with beta-adrenergic blockade. J. Am. Coll. Cardiol. *25*:1154, 1995.
215. Fowler, M. B.: Beta-blockers in heart failure: Potential of carvedilol. J. Human Hypertens. *7*:S62, 1993.
216. Krum, H., Sackner-Bernstein, J. D., Goldsmith, R. L., et al.: Double-blind, placebo-controlled study of the long-term efficacy of carvedilol in patients with severe chronic heart failure. Circulation *92*:1499, 1995.
217. Bristow, M. R., O'Connell, J. B., Gilbert, E. M., et al., for the Bucindolol Investigators: Dose-response of chronic β-blocker treatment in heart failure from either idiopathic dilated or ischemic cardiomyopathy. Circulation *89*:1632, 1994.
218. Metra, M., Nardi, M., Giubbini, R., et al.: Effects of short- and long-term carvedilol administration on rest and exercise hemodynamic variables, exercise capacity and clinical conditions in patients with idiopathic dilated cardiomyopathy. J. Am. Coll. Cardiol. *24*:1678, 1994.

Chapter 17
Management of Heart Failure

THOMAS W. SMITH, RALPH A. KELLY, LYNNE WARNER STEVENSON, EUGENE BRAUNWALD

THERAPEUTIC STRATEGY FOR MANAGEMENT OF HEART FAILURE

The goals of therapy in patients with heart failure are to improve quality and length of life and to prevent progression of the syndrome. The relative importance of these goals and the design of therapy for each patient vary according to the clinical stage of heart failure (Fig. 17–1). Evidence for improvement in survival with medical therapy has now been shown for each stage from asymptomatic left ventricular dysfunction to severely symptomatic heart failure. Quality of life has been more difficult to assess, but objective measurement of functional capacity has shown improvement with therapy that is more dramatic as the severity of symptoms increases. The impact of therapy to reduce progression of disease, however, as measured by left-ventricular dimensions and ejection fraction, is most apparent before severe disease develops.

Table 17–1 classifies specific therapeutic targets in heart failure (HF) and the intensity with which they are pursued according to symptoms or functional class. The management of heart failure has three principal components: the removal or amelioration of the underlying cause, the removal of the precipitating cause, and the control of the heart failure state.

REMOVAL OF THE UNDERLYING CAUSE. All patients with heart failure should undergo evaluation for treatable causes of this condition. This includes the improvement of coronary blood flow through catheter-based intervention or coronary bypass surgery and repair of structural abnormalities such as congenital heart defects, valvular lesions, or left-ventricular aneurysms. When symptoms, such as dyspnea on exertion or orthopnea, are due to impairment of ventricular relaxation rather than diminished systolic contraction, specific measures may be indicated to reduce left ventricular hypertrophy or myocardial ischemia.

RECOGNITION AND REMOVAL OF PRECIPITATING CAUSES (see also p. 448). The recognition, prompt treatment, and, whenever possible, prevention of the specific entities that cause or exacerbate heart failure, such as infections, arrhythmias, and pulmonary emboli, are crucial to the successful management of heart failure. Excessive intake of alcohol, incessant tachycardia, or thyroid disease can serve as primary causes of heart failure and secondary causes of clinical deterioration in patients with heart failure due to other conditions such as chronic valvular or coronary artery disease.

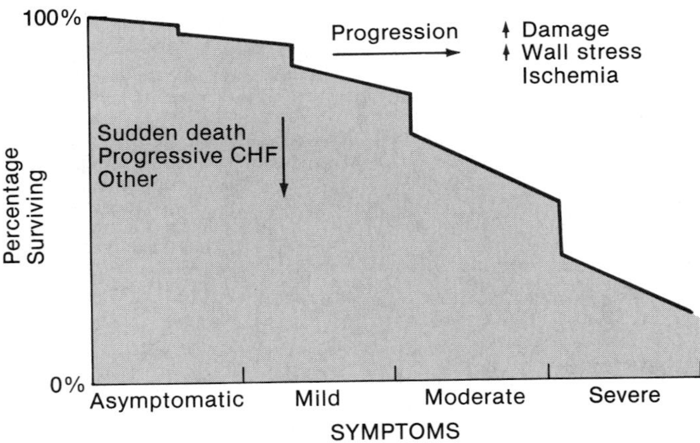

FIGURE 17–1. The natural history of congestive heart failure (CHF) is illustrated schematically. CHF usually progresses over time (either gradually or abruptly) from asymptomatic left ventricular dysfunction to severe CHF, as indicated on the horizontal axis. The mechanism of progression varies. The vertical axis indicates the proportion of patients surviving. Although mortality rates accelerate as CHF worsens, sudden death may occur at any stage (shown by the abrupt decreases in survival rate). Other deaths occur from progressive CHF and a variety of complications. (From Cheitlin, M. D. [ed.]: Dilemmas in Clinical Cardiology. Philadelphia, F.A. Davis, 1990, p. 256; with permission.)

General Approach to the Patient with Established Heart Failure

A condition as complex and variable as heart failure cannot be treated according to a simple formula; however, useful treatment guidelines have been developed[1] (i.e., pp. 1985 to 1989). Effective management depends not only on an appreciation of the nature of the underlying condition, but also on the tempo of progression; the presence of associated illnesses; the patient's age, occupation, personality, life style, family setting, and ability and motivation to cooperate with treatment; and, importantly, response to the therapeutic measures. The course of heart failure is rarely smoothly progressive; rather it is usually punctuated by a series of abrupt downward steps due to acute decompensation, generally as a consequence of one of the precipitating causes described on page 448 (see Fig. 17–1). When the precipitating cause has been removed and treatment has been intensified, the patient's previous condition may be restored. In other patients there are long periods—many months or even years—when the course is stable without any discernible deterioration.

After potentially reversible factors are addressed, the therapeutic regimen is designed according to the clinical stage (see Table 17–1), usually classified according to the New York Heart Association class (see p. 452). Most clinical studies addressing the efficacy of various interventions

TABLE 17–1 TARGETS OF THERAPY FOR HEART FAILURE

PATIENT DESCRIPTION Class		SYMPTOMS	MORTALITY Progressive Heart Failure	MORTALITY Unexpected	DISEASE PROGRESSION
I	Asymptomatic			++	+++
II	Mildly symptomatic *(with vigorous activity)*	(+)	(+)	++	++
III	Moderately to severely symptomatic *(with routine activity)*	++	++	+	+
IV	Decompensated *(bed and chair)*	+++	+++	+	(+)

+++ Very strong target for therapy.
++ Strong target.
+ Probable target.
(+) Possible target.

have described the heart failure in the populations under study as "asymptomatic" (NYHA Class I), "mild-to-moderate" (Classes II and III), or "severe (Class IV)." Once believed to be a hopeless condition, heart failure at every stage has now been shown to be influenced favorably by judicious intervention. Although much emphasis is still placed on the limited prognosis of patients with overt congestive heart failure, the current therapeutic armamentarium, carefully tailored to the individual patient, can yield good results even in severely symptomatic patients, as indicated by the ability of many patients to achieve functional capacity similar to that after transplantation. Two-year survival equivalent to that of cardiac transplantation can be achieved in many patients previously thought to have "end-stage heart failure" refractory to medical therapy.

The clinical features of heart failure reflect both the hemodynamic abnormalities and the disturbances of neurohormonal regulation that precede and may hasten the onset of symptoms. Therapy is initially directed at limitation of neurohormonal activation and broadened to address hemodynamic abnormalities as they become sufficiently severe to cause symptoms, first during activity and ultimately at rest.

Asymptomatic Patients with Ventricular Dysfunction

In asymptomatic patients (that is, patients with impaired cardiac function, NYHA Class I), therapy focuses on prevention of progression of disease (Fig. 17–2). Angiotensin-converting enzyme (ACE) inhibitors have been shown to diminish ventricular dilation in patients with symptomatic left-ventricular dysfunction who have suffered myocardial infarction, and they are useful in such patients because they delay the development of heart failure.[1a] Extended follow-up has shown that this therapy eventually translates into improved survival.[2–4] Recent trials have also demonstrated that ACE inhibitors reduce or delay the onset of congestive heart failure in asymptomatic patients with compromised ejection fractions from multiple causes.[5] Emphasis should also be placed on the reduction of factors that could hasten progression of disease such as hypertension, obesity, excessive use of alcohol, and, in the case of coronary artery disease, the risk factors for atherosclerosis. It is prudent to moderate salt intake in order to delay the onset of fluid retention that will lead to increased intracardiac filling pressures and eventually to congestive symptoms. The impact of digoxin is not well defined in these patients, who might derive benefit from the suppression of sympathetic tone caused by this drug but would be at some risk of developing arrhythmias.

Symptomatic Heart Failure

The cardinal symptoms of heart failure reflect the hemodynamic abnormalities of elevated filling pressures and reduced cardiac output that occur first with major exertion (Class II), then during routine activity (Class III), and ultimately at rest (Class IV). Less commonly, symptoms may relate to arrhythmias or embolic events associated with heart failure. As patients progress through cycles of compensation and decompensation, a consistent approach to clinical assessment, as described in detail in Chapter 15, provides the continuity necessary to optimize hemodynamic status and minimize symptoms.

Patients who describe symptoms of dyspnea and fatigue only with major exertion (NY Heart Association Class II) often demonstrate normal resting hemodynamics but reduced maximal oxygen uptake (see Ch. 5 and Fig. 14–26, p. 439), maximal cardiac output, and elevated intracardiac filling pressures during peak exercise. The distinction between this group and asymptomatic patients is frequently the result of differences in levels of activity and perception of fatigue. These patients should, in the absence of contraindications or side effects, receive ACE inhibitors to prevent progression of disease; therapy in this setting is designed primarily to reduce future risk rather than to improve clinical status. Although severe volume depletion should be avoided at the time that ACE inhibition is initiated, salt restriction is part of the regimen for these patients, consisting first of avoiding added salt then avoiding foods prepared with salt such as canned foods and processed foods. Levels of exertion that cause severe fatigue should be avoided, but patients should be encouraged to continue regular aerobic activity at a level that they can easily tolerate. Isometric exercise, associated with increases

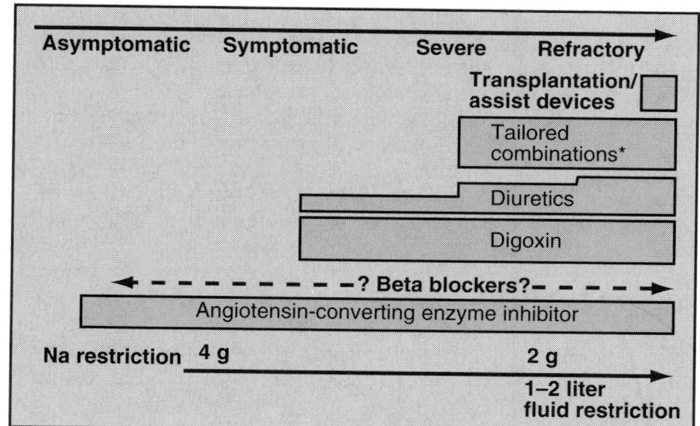

FIGURE 17–2. Escalation of therapy for left ventricular dysfunction in relation to the severity of symptoms and hemodynamic decompensation. Angiotensin-converting enzyme (ACE) inhibition has been demonstrated to improve prognosis for patients at all levels of heart failure. Digoxin decreases symptoms of heart failure once they have developed. It is not yet known which patients may benefit from beta-adrenergic blocking agents. Cardiac transplantation or implantable ventricular assist devices are considered only for a very small population with heart failure refractory to all other therapies.

*The term tailored combinations refers to the use of additional vasodilators (usually in combination with an ACE inhibitor) and, when necessary, short-term hemodynamic monitoring and use of intravenous nitroprusside, or dobutamine.

in peripheral resistance rather than the beneficial decreases during aerobic exercise, is generally proscribed.

SYMPTOMATIC TREATMENT. The general strategy in treating symptomatic heart failure is to use relatively simple means and then progressively stricter and more aggressive measures if clinical manifestations of heart failure persist or recur. An hour of supine rest in the afternoon frequently reduces overall fatigue. Depending on the level of symptoms and the physical demands of employment, some patients will need to restrict their hours or retire from work as symptoms become more severe. Initial symptoms can in many cases be treated with ACE inhibitors, which should be increased to target doses (Table 16–1, p. 472) or instituted if not previously prescribed. In addition to reducing progression of disease, ACE inhibitors help to address hemodynamic abnormalities through complex interactions involving inhibition of angiotensin II generation and aldosterone release, reducing sympathetic tone and thirst, and increasing bradykinin and prostaglandin levels.

Patients developing evidence of congestion despite adequate degrees of ACE inhibition and salt restriction should begin therapy with a *diuretic.* Although thiazide diuretics may restore fluid balance initially, many patients progress to need a loop diuretic. Patients with more advanced heart failure who are already on large doses of loop diuretics often respond to the addition of metolazone or a thiazide (see p. 477).

There is evidence of benefit from the use of *digoxin* in patients with symptomatic heart failure due to predominant systolic dysfunction, in whom ejection fraction and exercise capacity are improved, while rehospitalizations are decreased (see p. 501). Whether or not digoxin also improves survival in this population should be known after completion of the Digoxin Investigators Group (DIG) trial. A routine of regular exercise should continue.

Both the ACE inhibitors and the combination of hydralazine and isosorbide dinitrate have been shown to improve functional capacity and survival in mild-to-moderate heart failure.[4–7] Although ACE inhibitors offer additional survival benefits, the combination of hydralazine and isosorbide dinitrate represents a good alternative for the patient who cannot tolerate ACE inhibitors owing to cough, renal dysfunction, rash, angioneurotic edema, or other side effects. When symptoms and evidence of congestion persist during therapy with ACE inhibitors, the patient who is already receiving high doses of these agents (150 mg/day of captopril or 20 mg/day of enalapril) or the patient who develops symptomatic hypotension may benefit from individualized combinations of multiple vasodilator and diuretic agents as described below for refractory heart failure (see p. 507).

Careful adjustment of vasodilator, diuretic, and digoxin therapy can render the majority of patients with heart failure free from clinical evidence of congestion or hypoperfusion at rest. Relief of congestion usually improves not only the resting symptoms but also the symptoms of dyspnea and fatigue during minimal exertion. Patients with heart failure and severe fatigue *without* elevation of ventricular filling pressure often do not derive symptomatic benefit from additional modifications of a regimen that already includes standard doses of effective vasodilators and digoxin. Some patients with severe exertional dyspnea will derive benefit from the addition of oral nitrates (including a nitrate-free interval) to the baseline regimen or the use of prophylactic sublingual isosorbide dinitrate immediately before exertion.

When hypoperfusion becomes clinically evident (Table 17–2), outpatient therapy of symptomatic congestion is usually insufficient to achieve the patient's optimal condition. The cautious alterations in diuretic and vasodilator doses that are feasible in an outpatient setting usually have little effect or may precipitate hypotension and renal dysfunction. The presence of frequent angina or symptomatic ventricular arrhythmias should lower the threshold for hospital admission to adjust hemodynamic status (see Table 17–2). Hypotension, hyponatremia, and azotemia further identify patients who may be particularly difficult to stabilize without extensive redesign of the medical regimen. Unsuccessful attempts to address congestion and hypoperfusion simultaneously in the outpatient setting may lead to the erroneous conclusion that heart failure has become refractory to medical therapy. Similarly, repeated relapses after admissions for brief inotropic and diuretic infusions may indicate the need to redesign oral therapy during hemodynamic monitoring. Thus, these patients may be considered as refractory to outpatient management. Their treatment is discussed on page 507.

TABLE 17–2 CONDITIONS THAT MAY WARRANT HEMODYNAMIC MONITORING

Hypoperfusion suspected from:
Narrow pulse pressure
Cool extremities
Mental obtundation
Declining renal function with volume overload
Marked hyponatremia
Congestion in the presence of:
Angina or other evidence of active ischemia
Hemodynamically significant arrhythmias
Persistent systematic hypotension during ACEI therapy
Baseline renal impairment
Severe intrinsic pulmonary disease
Persistent congestion despite all of the following:
Salt and fluid restriction
High-dose loop diuretics
Metolazone or a thiazide
Evaluation for heart transplantation for advanced heart failure

VASODILATORS

A convenient framework in which to address the principles of vasodilator therapy include the concepts of preload and afterload reduction. Although this discussion focuses on heart failure due to predominant left-ventricular dysfunction, the general principles of vasodilator therapy are applicable to failure of either or both ventricles. There will be differences, however, in the specific drugs or other forms of therapy that can be used. For example, inhaled nitric oxide may effectively reduce pulmonary vascular resistance, whereas hydralazine reduces systemic vascular resistance. Nitroprusside decreases both pulmonary and systemic vascular resistance.

PRELOAD REDUCTION. Increases in heart rate as well as in diastolic intraventricular volume and pressure compensate for a decline in ventricular systolic performance. The relationship between ventricular filling pressures and cardiac stroke work is the familiar Frank-Starling curve (see p. 378) and is shown in Figure 17–3. In more advanced heart failure, there is often little augmentation of stroke volume with increasing filling pressures, and the transmission of increased pressure into the pulmonary and systemic venous beds produces edema and congestive symptoms.

These hemodynamic adaptations are often accompanied by worsening myocardial energy metabolism due to an increase in systolic and diastolic ventricular wall stress. They also result in a decrease in coronary blood flow, even in the absence of coronary artery disease, owing to the increase in heart rate, decline in mean arterial pressure, and increase in intracavitary and right atrial pressures. Therefore, agents that reduce ventricular filling pressures by selectively decreasing intravascular volume (e.g., diuretics) or by increasing venous capacitance (e.g., predominantly venous vasodilators such as nitrates) reduce pulmonary venous congestion with minimal effects on stroke volume and cardiac output.

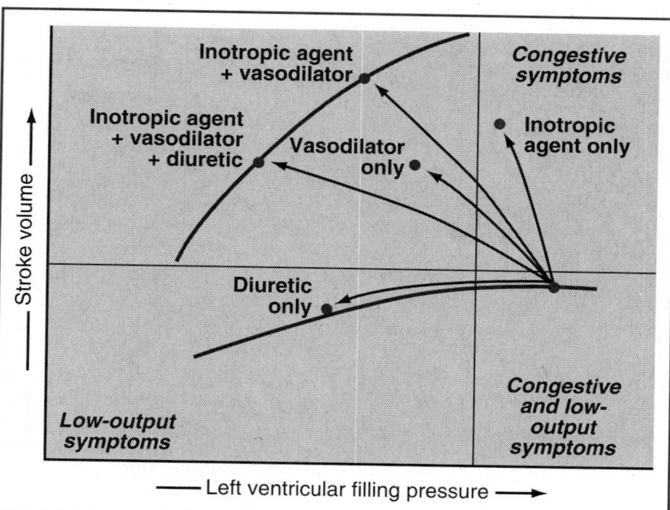

FIGURE 17–3. Frank-Starling ventricular function curves in heart failure due to systolic dysfunction. Predicted hemodynamic effects and consequent impact on symptoms of positive inotropic agents (e.g., digoxin), a balanced vasodilator (e.g., captopril), or a diuretic (e.g., furosemide) alone or in combination, in a patient with mild ventricular systolic dysfunction *(upper curve)* or severe ventricular systolic dysfunction *(lower curve)*. (Modified from: Smith, T. W., and Kelly, R. A.: Therapeutic strategies for CHF in the 1990's. Hosp. Pract. *26*:127, 1991. © 1991, The McGraw-Hill Companies, Inc.)

Preload reduction clearly improves symptoms due to systolic ventricular dysfunction and may also benefit patients with congestive symptoms due to impaired diastolic function (reduced compliance) (see p. 402). It should be kept in mind, however, that patients with diastolic dysfunction due to poorly compliant, hypertrophied ventricles may require elevated end-diastolic filling pressures to support an adequate forward stroke volume. In critical aortic stenosis, for example, a large decrease in preload may markedly reduce cardiac output, and therefore vasodilators and diuretics should be administered cautiously to these patients.

AFTERLOAD REDUCTION. Afterload, the sum of forces opposing ventricular emptying during systole, includes aortic and aortic outflow tract (including valvular) impedance and systemic vascular resistance. Afterload is also affected by the volume of blood in the ventricle at the initiation of systole and by ventricular-vascular coupling (i.e., the harmonics of reflected arterial pressure waves during systole). Hypertrophy of cardiac muscle is a physiological response to an increase in afterload and initially tends to preserve ventricular systolic function (Fig. 13–7, p. 399). A reduction in ventricular wall stress during systole, whether achieved by corrective surgery, intra-aortic balloon counterpulsation, or vasodilator drugs, results in improved systolic contractile function. The lowering of afterload improves forward stroke volume (Fig. 17–4) and reduces the regurgitant fraction due to functional mitral regurgitation, a common complicating factor in patients with enlarged left ventricles and severe heart failure secondary to systolic dysfunction.

Vasodilators are often classified as either predominantly "arteriolar" (afterload reducing) or predominantly "venous" (preload reducing), although many vasodilators exhibit activity in both vascular beds. The arteriolar vasodilator hydralazine, for example, may have little or no effect on venous capacitance despite causing a significant reduction in systemic vascular resistance. Nitroglycerin, a predominantly venous vasodilator, at lower doses may cause a pronounced increase in venous capacitance with little effect on the systemic arterial vasculature. The hemodynamic effects of vasodilators in current use are listed in Table 16–1, page 472. Nitroprusside is among the most effective afterload reducing agents because, in addition to reducing systemic vascular resistance, it increases aortic wall compliance and improves ventricular-vascular coupling. Direct intrarenal effects of several classes of these drugs, such as hydralazine and ACE inhibitors, may also prove effective in preserving renal blood flow and in promoting the effectiveness of diuretics.

Renin-Angiotensin System Antagonists

Survival Trials of ACE Inhibitors in Heart Failure

A number of well-designed prospective trials have demonstrated that ACE inhibitors improve survival in patients with overt heart failure due to systolic ventricular dysfunction regardless of the etiology or severity of symptoms. The COoperative Northern Scandinavian ENalapril SUrvival Study (CONSENSUS-1)[3] demonstrated a 40 per cent reduction in mortality at 6 months in patients with severe heart failure already treated with digoxin, diuretics, and other vasodilators, who were randomized to enalapril rather than placebo (Fig. 17–5). This finding, combined with those of smaller trials, convincingly demonstrates that ACE inhibitors improve survival of patients with severe heart failure (i.e., patients who were symptomatic at rest). Subsequent trials have examined the question of whether the much larger population of patients with left ventricular systolic dysfunction who have mild or moderate heart failure or who are asymptomatic also receive a survival benefit. The "treatment" arm of the Studies on Left Ventricular Dysfunction[4] (SOLVD) trial that randomized patients with symptomatic mild-to-moderate heart failure with left ventricular ejection fractions less than 35 per cent who received either enalapril or placebo reported a statistically significant 16 per cent reduction in overall mortality in the enalapril-treated group. Although the "prevention" arm of this trial that examined asymptomatic patients with a simi-

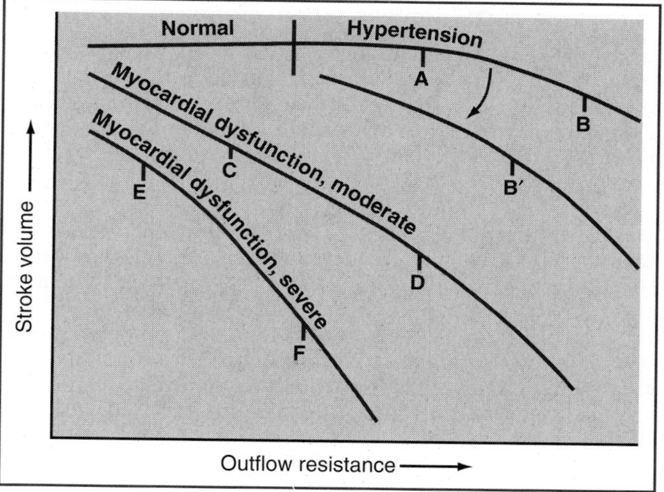

FIGURE 17–4. Relation of left ventricular stroke volume to systemic outflow resistance in normal and diseased hearts. A family of curves may be described, depending on the severity of the myocardial disease. If cardiac function is normal, a rise in resistance results in hypertension, as cardiac output remains fairly constant. Heart failure in a hypertensive patient could be shown by a move to either point B, a high resistance with normal function, or point B′, which represents a shift to a slightly depressed ventricular function curve. When myocardial dysfunction is more severe, as shown by the lower two curves, blood pressure is no longer directly determined by resistance, as stroke volume and resistance are inversely related. Consequently, arterial pressure may be similar at points E and F despite marked differences in cardiac output and resistance. It is also apparent that a reduction in outflow resistance will not affect significantly the stroke volume of the normal ventricle. However, it can produce a marked increase in the stroke volume on the failing ventricle (F → E). (From Cohn, J. N., and Franciosa, J. A.: Vasodilator therapy of cardiac failure. N. Engl. J. Med. *297*:27, 1977. Copyright 1977 Massachusetts Medical Society.)

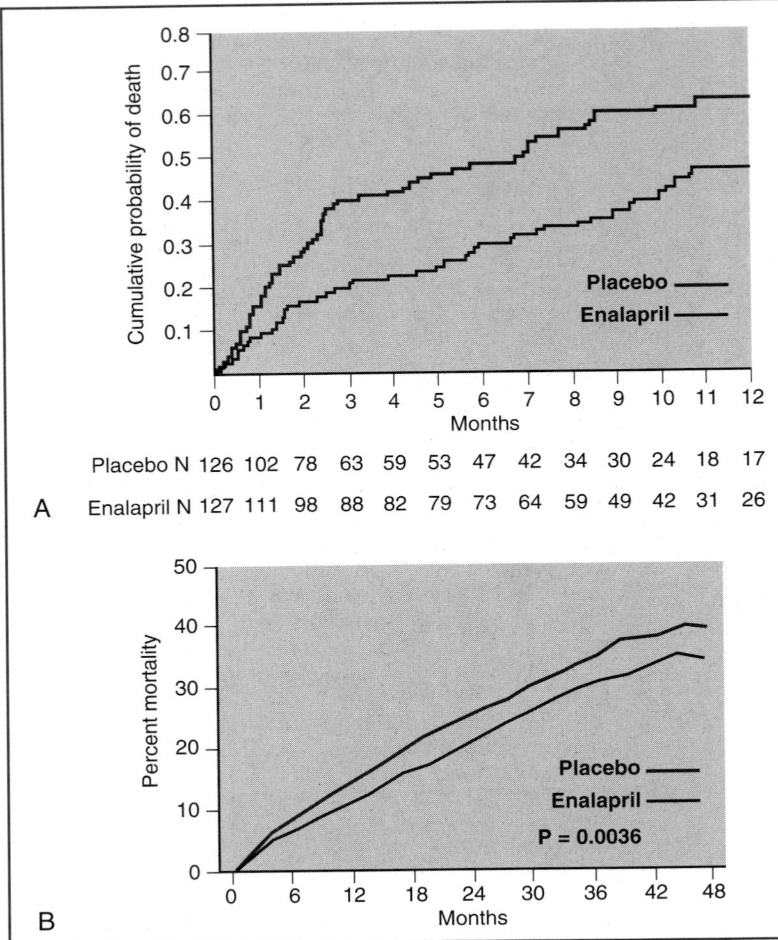

FIGURE 17–5. *A,* Cumulative probability of death in the placebo and enalapril groups in the CONSENSUS trial and *B,* in the SOLVD trial. (*A,* Reprinted from CONSENSUS Trial Study Group: Effects of enalapril on mortality in severe congestive heart failure: Results of the Cooperative North Scandinavian Enalapril Survival Study [CONSENSUS]. N. Engl. J. Med. *316:*1429, 1987, with permission. *B,* From SOLVD Investigators: Effect of enalapril on survival in patients with reduced left ventricular ejection fractions and congestive heart failure. N. Engl. J. Med. *325:*293, 1991. Copyright 1991 Massachusetts Medical Society.)

lar degree of left ventricular dysfunction failed to demonstrate a statistically significant reduction in mortality among enalapril-treated patients,[5] there was a significant (29 per cent) reduction in the combined endpoints of development of symptomatic heart failure and death due to any cause.

The second Veterans Administration Cooperative Vasodilator Heart Failure Trial[6] (V-HeFT-II) showed a small but clear survival benefit in patients with mild-to-moderate heart failure who had been randomized to receive enalapril rather than the combination of hydralazine and isosorbide dinitrate. A smaller randomized trial comparing captopril to hydralazine isosorbide dinitrate in patients with moderate-to-severe heart failure also demonstrated a significant survival advantage in patients receiving ACE inhibitors.[7]

The Survival And Ventricular Enlargement (SAVE) trial[8,9] studied patients with recent myocardial infarctions and ejection fractions of 40 per cent or less, but without overt heart failure, and showed a 20 per cent reduction in mortality and a 36 per cent reduction in the rate of progression to severe heart failure in the captopril-treated group after 48 months of follow-up. Both the SOLVD[10] and the SAVE trials[11] demonstrated that enalapril and captopril, respectively, markedly reduced or prevented the increases in left ventricular end-diastolic and end-systolic volumes and decline in ejection fraction observed in patients randomized to receive placebo. The Acute Infarction Ramipril Efficacy (AIRE) trial[12] had a study design similar to that of the SAVE trial, except that it randomized only patients who manifested clinical evidence of heart failure to either ramipril or placebo. There was a significant (27 per cent) reduction in mortality in the ACE inhibitor-treated group that was apparent within 30 days of treatment (unlike SAVE, in which the survival curves did not diverge until 1 year). The Trandelopril Cardiac Evaluation (TRACE) trial studied patients with severe left-ventricular dysfunction 3 to 7 days following myocardial infarction and reported a 20 per cent reduction in mortality.[13] Taken together, these trials indicate that ACE inhibitors prolong survival in a broad spectrum of patients with myocardial infarction and heart failure, ranging from those who are asymptomatic with ventricular dysfunction to those who have symptomatic heart failure but are normotensive and hemodynamically stable. The role of ACE inhibitors in the early treatment of patients with acute myocardial infarction is discussed in Chapter 37.

DOSES OF ACE INHIBITORS. There is no precisely defined relationship between dosage and long-term clinical effectiveness of these drugs.[2,14] The target dosages of an ACE inhibitor in several large prospective trials in which a positive effect was demonstrated on mortality as well as other endpoints were 50 mg of captopril three times daily,[8] 10 mg of enalapril twice daily,[6] 10 mg of lisinopril once daily,[15] 5 mg of ramipril twice daily,[12] or 30 mg of zofenopril twice daily.[16] Higher dosages are often used in the treatment of hypertension, but it is unclear whether increasing the dosage beyond that used in these trials will necessarily result in additional benefit.[14] Upward dosage titration may be prudent if a patient's blood pressure remains above a target level and may be of benefit in selected patients with significant functional mitral regurgitation. Despite the evidence for a class effect with these drugs, Pitt[14] has argued persuasively that it may be unwise to assume that all ACE inhibitors are equal or that dosages other than those shown to improve mortality in controlled clinical trials can be relied on to exert the demonstrated effects. Adding a second vasodilator (e.g., hydralazine, with or without nitrates) has been advocated by some investigators[17] in patients with advanced heart failure. However, this approach has not yet been evaluated in controlled clinical survival trials.

Yusuf et al.[18] and Lonn et al.,[19] in an overview of several clinical trials, have noted that ACE inhibitors appear to be reducing mortality by more than one mechanism. The most important reason for a reduction in mortality was a decrease in the rate of progression to worsening heart failure due in part to the direct hemodynamic effects of these drugs on ventricular remodeling and progressive dilation. However, both the SOLVD[4,5] and SAVE trials[8,9] also documented a reduction in acute myocardial infarction, an effect that could be due to improved myocardial energetics (due to decreased ventricular wall stress), prevention of myocardial hypertrophy, or a number of other mechanisms that are the subject of active investigation.

COST-BENEFIT RATIO. Paul et al.[20] have analyzed the cost-per-year of life extended of ACE inhibitors and combined hydralazine isosorbide dinitrate therapy for heart failure based on data from the SOLVD[4,5] and V-HeFT II[6] trials. Based on a decision analytic model, they estimated that enalapril added to standard heart failure therapy cost approximately $9700 per year of life extended (compared to $25,000 per year of life saved for the treatment of moderate hypertension), a cost that is well within the accepted range for many medical therapies. Although the combination of hydralazine and isosorbide dinitrate was more cost-effective than enalapril, the survival advantage with ACE inhibitors is significantly higher, and the cost differential will disappear as generic ACE inhibitors become available.

QUALITY OF LIFE. Despite the clear gains in survival, the impact of ACE inhibitors on quality of life measures, when compared to placebo or to other classes of vasodilators, has been less consistent. A marginal improvement in self-assessment of quality of life was observed in symptomatic patients randomized to receive enalapril in the SOLVD treatment trial.[21] However, there was no difference between symptomatic patients receiving enalapril and placebo in the SOLVD prevention trial or between patients with mild heart failure receiving either quinapril or placebo.[22] Quality of life measures were also not different in patients with more advanced heart failure randomized to receive either enalapril or the combination of hydralazine and isosorbide dinitrate in VeHeFT-II.[23] These data indicate that vasodilators probably have little impact on quality of life measures in patients with asymptomatic or mild heart failure (i.e., NYHA Class I or II), and that ACE inhibitors offer little or no advantage over other effective vasodilators in patients with more severe heart failure insofar as quality of life is concerned.

ACE Inhibitors and Valvular Regurgitation

The efficacy of ACE inhibitors in the treatment of chronic mitral or aortic regurgitation has been directly evaluated in a small number of studies (Chap. 32). Many patients with advanced heart failure secondary to ventricular systolic dysfunction have functional mitral regurgitation on the basis of dilation of the left ventricle and mitral valve ring. While treatment of mitral regurgitation with hydralazine or sodium nitroprusside is successful in short-term treatment, intravenous nitroprusside is impractical as chronic therapy, and hydralazine, when given alone, must be used at relatively high doses that often are associated with adverse effects. Intravenous enalapril has been shown to reduce the volume of regurgitant flow and to increase cardiac index significantly in patients with severe functional mitral regurgitation.[24] Captopril has been demonstrated to reduce functional mitral regurgitation in patients with heart failure and ischemic cardiomyopathy; significant improvements in stroke volume, systemic vascular resistance, left atrial size, and a daily activity status index were present in patients receiving 100 mg/day of captopril.[25] These findings, when combined with results of the SAVE study[8,11] and the SOLVD treatment trial[4,10] demonstrate that progressive left ventricular dilation, which is associated with functional mitral regurgitation, can often be reduced by ACE inhibitors and that these drugs are effective in the chronic management of this complication of left ventricular dysfunction.

Although less well documented, ACE inhibitors may also be of benefit in the medical management of left ventricular dysfunction secondary to aortic regurgitation. Enalapril (20 mg twice a day) was more effective than hydralazine in reducing left ventricular dimensions and left ventricular mass index in patients with mild-to-severe acute regurgitation.[26] Similar results were observed with quinapril (20 mg/day).[27]

FIRST-DOSE EFFECTS

It is advisable to begin therapy with an ACE inhibitor at low doses of a relatively short-acting drug (e.g., 6.25 mg of captopril or 2.5 mg of enalapril). An abrupt fall in blood pressure occasionally occurs following an initial dose of an ACE inhibitor, particularly in patients with depletion of intravascular volume. This response is often unpredictable; therefore, caution is recommended when beginning these drugs in any patient with significant left ventricular dysfunction, especially those who have received large doses of diuretics. Unacceptable hypotension can usually be reversed by intravascular volume expansion, although this is obviously not ideal in patients with heart failure.

The maximal hypotensive response to an initial oral dose of captopril occurs 1 to 2 hours after dosing, whereas the maximal response to oral enalapril occurs 4 to 6 hours after dosing. Among patients with left ventricular dysfunction without heart failure who, shortly after myocardial infarction, were given 12.5 mg of captopril in the SAVE trial, 5 per cent experienced dizziness, although the number of patients withdrawn from the trial owing to this symptom was not different from that of patients receiving placebo. Among patients in the SOLVD trials begun on 2.5 mg of enalapril, only 1.3 per cent experienced unacceptable side effects, most commonly symptoms of hypotension. In comparing the first-dose effects of enalapril (2.5 mg), captopril (6.25 mg), and quinapril (2.5 mg) in patients with mild-to-moderate heart failure, each drug dropped blood pressure to a comparable degree, although with a more rapid time course in the case of captopril.[28–31] Only approximately 4 per cent of patients experienced mild and transient side effects.

This favorable experience with oral captopril, enalapril, and quinapril may not be directly transferable to other ACE inhibitors owing to differences in the rate of activation of prodrugs and other pharmacokinetic considerations. For example, intravenous infusion of 1.5 mg of enalaprilat leads to a much more rapid decline in arterial pressure than does oral enalapril, causing a 15 to 20 per cent decline in mean arterial pressure within 60 minutes that typically persists for 4 to 6 hours.[32]

It is reasonable to initiate ACE inhibitor therapy in patients with chronic left ventricular dysfunction with those drugs for which extensive pharmacokinetic data exist in this patient population. (As of this writing, these include captopril, enalapril, lisinopril, and ramipril.) With careful observation of blood pressure, serum electrolytes, and serum creatinine levels, ACE inhibitor doses are customarily titrated upward over several days in hospitalized patients or a few weeks in ambulatory patients.

ACE INHIBITORS AND COUGH

Cough is an annoying side effect occurring in up to 5 per cent of patients on long-term therapy with ACE inhibitors.[33,34] The mechanism is unclear, but it is presumed to be due to inhibition of the metabolism of bradykinin and to substance P and inflammatory neuropeptides in the lung.[35] Patients with underlying structural lung disease or asthma are not at increased risk for this adverse effect. Cough often appears only after weeks or months of ACE inhibitor therapy, explaining why shorter prospective trials of these drugs reported a relatively low incidence of cough (i.e., 0.5 per cent in GISSI-3).[15] Approximately 3 per cent of patients in the SAVE study receiving active drug had to be withdrawn owing to cough compared with 1 per cent receiving placebo.[8] This symptom usually disappears within several days but may persist for up to 2 weeks after discontinuing the drug. Although switching to a different ACE inhibitor is rarely effective, some patients respond to a reduction in dosage.[34] Angiotensin receptor antagonists may be the best alternative for most patients with intractable cough. Inhaled sodium cromoglycate (40 mg/day in divided doses) has proved effective in reducing the frequency of cough in short-term trials.[36]

Nitrovasodilators

Nitrovasodilators have a well-established role in the management of heart failure (p. 474). Intravenous sodium nitroprusside (nitroprusside) is particularly useful in patients with advanced heart failure characterized by a reduced cardiac output and a high left ventricular filling pressure and systemic vascular resistance.[37,38] Although mean arterial pressure may be slightly reduced in these patients, most will respond to judicious administration of intravenous nitroprusside with a larger increase in stroke volume than patients with less severe ventricular dysfunction (see Fig. 17–4).[39] Forward stroke volume is often further enhanced by decreased "functional" mitral regurgitation as systemic vascular resistance and ventricular-filling pressures and volumes decrease; as a consequence, systemic arterial pressure can usually be sustained.[37] With continuous hemodynamic monitoring of right atrial, pulmonary capillary wedge, and systemic arterial pressures, sodium nitroprusside is often used as an initial strategy in the "tailored" medical management of advanced heart failure discussed on pages 508 to 509. The initial infusion rate is typically 0.3 μg/kg/min and is titrated upward depending on hemodynamic response. Cyanide and/or thiocyanate toxicities may be observed at infusion rates above 1.5 μg/kg/min.

As with most vasodilators, the most common adverse effect of nitroprusside is hypotension. The redistribution of blood flow from central organs to peripheral vascular beds may limit or prevent an increase in renal blood flow despite an increase in cardiac output. Nitroprusside-induced nonselective pulmonary arteriolar vasodilation may improve right ventricular function but also may worsen ventilation–perfusion mismatches in patients with advanced chronic obstructive pulmonary disease or large pleural effusions.[39] Coronary arteriolar dilation may reduce perfusion pressure to myocardium supplied by partially occluded vessels, creating a "coronary steal" in patients with heart failure and severe fixed obstructions in epicardial coronary arteries. This may account for an increase in the frequency of angina in response to nitroprusside in some patients with an ischemic cardiomyopathy despite a favorable hemodynamic response. An organic nitrate and hydralazine or an ACE inhibitor should then be substituted.

OTHER ORGANIC NITRATES. Despite its limited effects on systemic vascular resistance and the problem of pharmacological tolerance, isosorbide dinitrate has been shown to be more effective than placebo in improving capacity for exercise and in reducing symptoms when administered chronically to patients with heart failure. Isosorbide dinitrate has been shown to increase the clinical effectiveness of other vasodilators such as hydralazine, resulting in a sustained improvement in hemodynamics that exceeded that of either drug given alone. At a dose of 40 mg four times daily in combination with hydralazine, isosorbide dinitrate reduced overall mortality compared either to placebo or to the alpha$_1$-adrenergic receptor antagonist prazosin in the V-HeFT-I trial carried out in patients with mild-to-moderate heart failure concurrently treated with digoxin and diuretics.[40]

Hydralazine

As already mentioned, the combination of hydralazine (200 to 300 mg/day) and isosorbide dinitrate (120 to 160 mg/day) increased survival compared with placebo in V-HeFT I[40] but was less effective than enalapril in reducing mortality in heart failure patients in the V-HeFT II trial.[6] In another prospective trial comparing hydralazine with an ACE inhibitor, the Hydralazine versus ACE Inhibition with Captopril on Mortality in Advanced Heart Failure, or "Hy-C" study,[7] patients receiving captopril had a greater survival advantage than those receiving hydralazine (23 per cent cause mortality on captopril compared with 43 per cent on hydralazine at 8 months). However, hydralazine—with or without nitrates—may provide additional hemodynamic improvement for patients already being treated with conventional doses of an ACE inhibitor, digoxin, and diuretics,[17,41] although this has not yet been tested rigorously in clinical trials.

As with the ACE inhibitors, the most appropriate dosage of hydralazine has not been determined in heart failure. A target dosage of 300 mg daily was employed in the V-HeFT[14,40] trials and, in combination with isosorbide dinitrate, was documented to have a positive impact on survival. Although additional hemodynamic benefit may be demonstrable at higher dosages (the average dose of hydralazine in the Hy-C trial was 410 mg/day[7]), this has not been shown to translate into prolonged survival when compared to an ACE inhibitor.

DIURETICS

(See also pp. 849 to 851)

Unlike all other classes of drugs commonly employed in the treatment of heart failure, there have been no controlled prospective clinical trials designed to test the efficacy and safety of diuretics in the contemporary medical management of heart failure.[41a] Although recent evidence from studies of diuretic use in hypertension is reassuring regarding the safety of these drugs, these data cannot be directly applied to patients with heart failure.[42–45a] In our view, diuretics should not be used as first-line agents in the treatment of asymptomatic or mild heart failure (NYHA Class I and early Class II). Diuretics should be used periodically if signs or symptoms of heart failure persist or worsen on an optimal medical regimen of vasodilators and moderate salt restriction, with or without digoxin.

In patients with moderately severe heart failure (NYHA Class III), daily administration of loop diuretics will usually be necessary. Thiazide diuretics are usually ineffective as single agents in advanced heart failure. Potassium-sparing diuretics, particularly spironolactone or amiloride, or oral potassium (KCl) supplements, are often useful to prevent hypokalemia in patients on a daily loop diuretic regimen. However, their routine use is probably not necessary in patients receiving an ACE inhibitor and may be dangerous in patients with reduced renal function (i.e., a serum creatinine over 2 mg/dl).[46]

For patients with severe decompensated heart failure (NHYA Class IV), more aggressive use of loop diuretics alone or in combination with thiazide diuretics is warranted in the context of a tailored medical management approach to advanced heart failure. Sufficiently high doses of a loop diuretic need to be employed to exceed the threshold drug concentration within the renal tubular lumen needed to initiate and sustain a natriuresis. As in renal failure, this threshold response can be achieved by successive doubling of the intravenous dose until an adequate natriuretic response is achieved (Table 16–4, p. 479). For most patients with advanced heart failure, more than one "threshold" dose of a loop diuretic will be necessary each day to maintain a net negative sodium balance during the initial phase of a hospitalization. Adding a distally acting diuretic such as a thiazide is also effective but often is complicated by large urinary potassium losses. For a more detailed description of the metabolic complications of diuretic use in heart failure, see Chapter 16.

An alternative strategy in hospitalized patients is to administer the same daily parenteral dose of a loop diuretic by a continuous intravenous infusion.[47] This will lead to a sustained natriuresis due to the continual presence of high drug levels within the tubular lumen. This approach requires the use of a constant infusion pump but permits more precise control over the natriuretic effect. It also diminishes the potential for a too-rapid decline in intravascular volume and hypotension as well as the risk of ototoxicity in patients given large bolus intravenous doses of loop diuretics. A typical continuous furosemide infusion is initiated with a 20- to 40-mg intravenous loading dose as a bolus injection followed by a continuous infusion of 5 mg/hr, for a patient who had been receiving 200 mg of oral furosemide (or 100 mg intravenously) per day in divided doses.

USE OF DIURETICS IN THE ELDERLY. The age of patients with heart failure is increasing progressively. Elderly patients present special problems with diuretic use. In general, absorption of oral agents is delayed and renal clearance rates are lower in the elderly, thus slowing delivery of active drug to its renal tubular site of action. The decline in renal function that naturally occurs with aging diminishes the effectiveness of the thiazide diuretics earlier than the loop diuretics, since the thiazide diuretics are virtually ineffective at creatinine clearance rates below 30 to 40 ml/min. Epithelial Na^+ channel inhibitors (potassium-sparing diuretics), such as amiloride, also lose effectiveness as natriuretic agents in this range of creatinine clearance rate, although their potassium-sparing effects may be maintained. The elderly also have decreased baroreceptor responsiveness; reduced cerebral, renal, coronary, and splanchnic blood flow; and a tendency to electrolyte depletion.[48]

Elderly patients with congestive heart failure, with or without concomitant hypertension, often require multiple daily doses of a loop diuretic, often necessitating potassium and magnesium replacement.[48] Another important problem for which the elderly are probably at greater risk is hyponatremia. Although hyponatremia can occur with any diuretic, whether or not congestive heart failure is present, the longer-acting thiazide diuretics, alone or in combination with a potassium-sparing diuretic, appear to pose an unusually high risk. The decline in serum sodium is often exacerbated by poor dietary sodium and excessive free water intake and an inability to increase free water clearance (i.e., to dilute the urine appropriately), in part because of diuretic-induced hypovolemia. Hyponatremia may occur insidiously over weeks in the elderly and may be unassociated with any change in serum potassium levels. Mild confusion may go unnoticed in the elderly, but can rapidly degenerate into dementia, convulsions, and coma, even at serum sodium values near 130 mEq/liter, particularly if the fall in serum sodium has been rapid. Long-term administration of a loop diuretic may also lead to significant degrees of calcium depletion. Consequently, calcium supplements are recommended in elderly patients receiving these drugs. Magnesium losses, which occur with both thiazide and loop diuretics, may need to be replaced to increase serum ionized calcium and potassium levels (see Chap. 16).

DIGITALIS

Cardiac glycosides are of potential value in most patients with symptoms and signs of systolic heart failure secondary to ischemic, valvular, hypertensive, or congenital heart disease; dilated cardiomyopathies; and cor pulmonale. Improvement of depressed myocardial contractility by glycosides increases cardiac output, promotes diuresis, and reduces the filling pressure of the failing ventricle(s), with the consequent reduction of pulmonary vascular congestion and central venous pressure.

Digitalis is of no demonstrable benefit in isolated mitral stenosis with normal sinus rhythm unless right ventricular failure has supervened, or in patients with constrictive pericarditis except when there is invasion of the myocardium. There is no evidence that patients with left ventricular hypertrophy, normal left ventricular ejection fraction, and symptoms related to elevated filling pressures benefit from digitalis. Hypertrophic obstructive cardiomyopathy represents another condition in which digitalis is often of little value and may actually be deleterious because it can increase left ventricular outflow obstruction by augmenting the contractility of the hypertrophic outflow tract segment. In the later stages of hypertrophic cardiomyopathy, in which ventricular dilation and congestive problems occasionally predominate over obstructive hemodynamics, cardiac glycosides may be beneficial.

Evidence of Clinical Efficacy

It is widely accepted that cardiac glycosides are of benefit in the treatment of patients with heart failure accompanied by atrial fibrillation or atrial flutter and a rapid ventricular response. Since the turn of the century, however, there has been ongoing controversy surrounding the efficacy of cardiac glycosides in the treatment of patients with heart failure who are in sinus rhythm.[49] Several small observational trials in ambulatory patients with mild-to-moderate heart failure in sinus rhythm in the 1970's and early 1980's questioned the effectiveness of digoxin. However, during the past decade, the results of several randomized controlled trials support the use of digoxin when administered either alone or with vasodilators to patients with heart failure due to predominant systolic dysfunction. Although some of these trials were designed to test the safety and efficacy of a new therapeutic agent in the treatment of heart failure rather than to verify the effectiveness of digoxin, a prospective, randomized placebo group crossover design was typically included that permitted an independent assessment of the effectiveness of digoxin in each trial.[50,51]

The PROVED (Prospective Randomized Study of Ventricular Failure and Efficacy of Digoxin)[52] and RADIANCE (Randomized Assessment of Digoxin on Inhibition of ANgiotensin-Converting Enzyme)[53] trials are two prospective multicenter placebo-controlled trials that examined the effects of withdrawal of digoxin in patients with stable mild-to-moderate heart failure (i.e., New York Heart Association Classes II and III) and systolic ventricular dysfunction (left ventricular ejection fraction ≤ 0.35). All patients studied were in normal sinus rhythm. The target serum digoxin concentration in both studies during the baseline run-in phase was 0.7 to 2.0 ng/ml, with an average digoxin dose of 0.38 mg/day. Patients in the RADIANCE trial also received concurrent therapy with an ACE inhibitor. When patients were randomly assigned to either continue active digoxin therapy or to withdraw from active therapy and receive a matching placebo, 40 per cent of patients in the PROVED trial and 28 per cent of patients in the RADIANCE trial who received placebo noted a significant worsening of heart failure symptoms compared to 20 per cent and 6 per cent, respectively, in patients who continued to receive active drug (Fig. 17–6). This absolute risk reduction of 20 per cent in digoxin-treated patients constituted a substantial treatment effect.[54] Maximal treadmill exercise tolerance also declined significantly in patients withdrawn from digoxin in both trials, despite continuation of other medical therapies for heart failure, including ACE inhibitor therapy in RADIANCE.[53]

In the Dutch Ibopamine Multicenter Trial (DIMT), which was designed to test the efficacy of ibopamine (see p. 486) in ambulatory patients with heart failure with mild-to-moderate congestive heart failure compared to patients receiving digoxin or placebo, digoxin also significantly increased exercise time at 6 months, prevented clinical deterioration, and reduced plasma norepinephrine concentrations.[55]

These trials did not have the statistical power to detect an effect of digoxin therapy on the survival of patients with heart failure, an endpoint for which efficacy had already been established for the use of selected vasodilators in heart failure. The effect of digoxin on survival in both idiopathic dilated and ischemic cardiomyopathies was the pri-

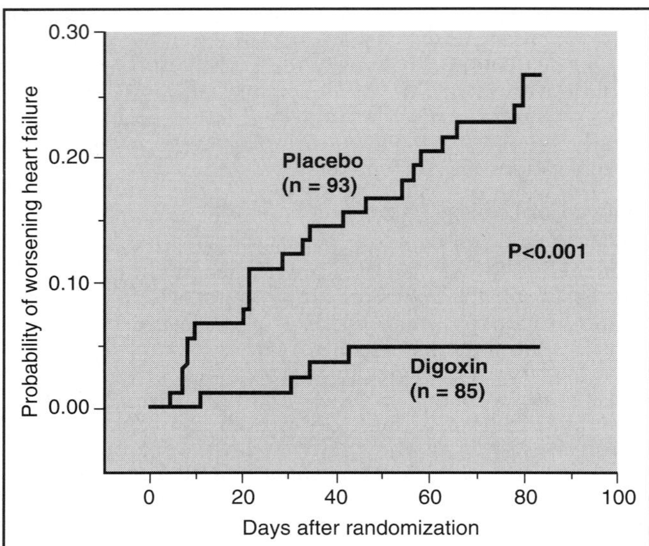

FIGURE 17–6. Kaplan-Meier analysis of the cumulative probability of worsening heart failure in patients continuing to receive digoxin and those switched to placebo. The patients in the placebo group had a higher risk of worsening heart failure throughout the 12-week study (relative risk, 5.9; 95 per cent confidence interval, 2.1 to 17.2; $P <$ 0.001). (From Packer, M., Gheorghiade, M., Young, J. B., et al.: Withdrawal of digoxin from patients with chronic heart failure treated with angiotensin-converting enzyme inhibitors. N. Engl. J. Med. *329*:1, 1993. Copyright Massachusetts Medical Society, with permission.)

mary endpoint for the multicenter National Insitutes of Health and Veterans Affairs Cooperative Studies Program-sponsored Digoxin Investigators' Group (DIG) trial, which enrolled 6800 patients with left ventricular ejection fractions of 45 per cent or lower, and who were receiving an ACE inhibitor (if tolerated) and diuretic. These patients and an additional group of 988 with a history of heart failure but with ejection fractions above 45 per cent were randomized to receive either digoxin or placebo.[56,57]

Follow-up at 3 to 5 years (mean 37 months) demonstrated no net impact on all-cause or cardiovascular mortality, with a lower incidence of mortality from progressive heart failure in the patients receiving digitalis being offset by an increased risk of presumed arrhythmia deaths. There was a substantial favorable effect of digoxin on the combined endpoint of death or hospitalization due to progressive heart failure. Treating 1000 patients with digoxin prevented 67 deaths or hospitalizations from worsening heart failure, while increasing risk of death or hospitalization from presumed arrhythmia for 15 patients.

Therapeutic Endpoints

The clinical use of cardiac glycosides is complicated by the absence of a readily measurable therapeutic endpoint except in atrial flutter or fibrillation, the lack of a reliable means to predict individual cardiac responses, and the difficulty in defining proximity to toxicity. The optimal dose of digitalis is not necessarily the largest dose that can be tolerated without the emergence of overt toxicity. The ratio of toxic to therapeutic effect for cardiac glycosides is small, and the availability of other measures of treating heart failure, particularly potent oral diuretics and vasodilators, usually obviates balancing therapy at the edge of toxicity. Electrocardiographic ST-segment and T-wave changes and slowing of sinus tachycardia are of little value in gauging the adequacy of digitalis dosage.

In patients with atrial flutter or fibrillation, control of the ventricular response provides a relatively straightforward endpoint, but digoxin alone does not provide adequate control of rate during exertion in many patients; ancillary use of a beta-adrenergic blocking agent, calcium channel blocker (verapamil or diltiazem), or amiodarone is often needed.

When congestive heart failure is the indication for use of digitalis, it is helpful to remember that positive inotropy is a graded response that is appreciable at dosages well short of "maximally tolerated doses." Available data suggest that further inotropic benefit may not occur clinically beyond serum digoxin levels in the range of 1.5 ng/ml. Improved autonomic balance with reduced sympathetic and enhanced vagal tone may occur at still lower serum levels, and it is our usual practice to target serum levels to the 1.0-ng/ml range. Oral maintenance doses predicted to produce a given serum digoxin concentration vary widely with renal function and lean body mass, as discussed on page 482. Carotid sinus massage can provide useful bedside clues to impending digitalis excess; for example, rhythm disorders such as second-degree atrioventricular block, accelerated atrioventricular junctional rhythm, and ventricular premature beats or bigeminy may emerge in response to carotid sinus stimulation before they occur spontaneously.[58]

Individual Sensitivity to Digitalis

A number of factors influencing individual sensitivity to cardiac glycosides are listed in Table 16–5, page 482.

Electrolyte and Acid-Base Disturbances

Disturbances of potassium homeostasis clearly influence the action of digitalis.[59] Myocardial concentrations of digoxin tend to decrease with increasing serum potassium concentration. Furthermore, hypokalemia has primary arrhythmogenic effects, both decreasing the effective refractory period of Purkinje cells and shortening the coupling interval for ventricular premature beats. Depression of atrioventricular nodal conduction can occur with both digitalis excess and either a very low or extremely high level of serum potassium.[60] Diuretics, catecholamines, insulin or carbohydrate loading, renal disease, and acid-base disturbances must all be considered as potential causes of clinically significant alterations in potassium homeostasis, which can in turn importantly affect the response to cardiac glycosides.

Administration of magnesium suppresses digitalis-induced arrhythmias, whereas hypomagnesemia appears to predispose to digitalis toxicity.[59,61] There is some evidence that the digitalis-induced potassium efflux from the myocardium is reduced by magnesium.[59] Magnesium depletion may become clinically important with the long-term administration of diuretic agents[61–63] and with gastrointestinal disease, diabetes mellitus, or poor nutritional states. Moreover, in patients with congestive heart failure, significant depletion of total body magnesium stores may occur owing to prolonged secondary aldosteronism.[61,64,65] Although the clinical importance of magnesium depletion in digitalis therapy remains unresolved, it deserves consideration in cases of suspected digitalis toxicity. Poor or no correlation was found between serum and tissue magnesium in patients with heart failure, leaving unsolved the problem of clinical assessment of magnesium stores.[64–68]

Type and Severity of Underlying Heart Disease

The effects of digitalis on the heart are modified by the type and severity of the underlying heart disease. This is dramatically demonstrated in otherwise healthy subjects who ingest massive doses of digitalis. Toxicity in such situations is frequently manifested by progressively impaired atrioventricular conduction or by sinoatrial exit block, rather than enhanced automaticity and ventricular ectopic activity as seen in patients with underlying heart disease.[69,70] In many patients with ischemic, myocardial, or valvular heart disease, the effects of digitalis are superimposed on an electrophysiologically unstable condition with preexisting abnormalities of impulse formation and conduction. The more severe and advanced the heart disease, the more likely the occurrence of focal ischemia, myocardial fibrosis, and ventricular dilation with stretching of the Purkinje fibers and resultant tendency toward increased automaticity. The observation that digitalis toxicity is particularly common in patients with amyloidosis involving the heart may be accounted for, at least in part, by digoxin binding by amyloid fibrils.[71]

CORONARY ARTERY DISEASE. Changes in myocardial oxygen consumption produced by digitalis are the net result of two opposing effects of the drug: a potential reduction in wall tension and an increase in contractility.[72] The increase in consumption of oxygen in response to digitalis in the normal heart results from increased velocity of contraction with little change in wall tension. In the failing heart, decreased consumption of oxygen typically occurs in response to cardiac glycosides and can be explained by a decrease in left ventricular end-diastolic pressure and volume and, consequently, on the basis of the Laplace relation, a decline in intramyocardial tension.

These considerations are of clinical importance when a decision must be made on whether to use digitalis in patients with coronary artery disease. Angina pectoris has been observed to improve after digitalization in patients with heart failure but occasionally to worsen in those who are well compensated. In patients with angina pectoris without heart failure, ouabain improved the depressed myocardial performance noted on exercise.[73] Despite these beneficial effects on left ventricular performance, there was no consistent alteration in exercise tolerance or the pressure-rate product at which angina occurred. Improved myocardial perfusion judged by means of thallium-201 scans was found in response to maintenance doses of digoxin in patients with coronary artery disease and left ventricular dysfunction.[74] The combination of a beta blocker and digoxin appears to be beneficial in patients with angina pectoris and abnormal ventricular function.[75] As a general rule, digoxin should be considered for use in patients with ischemic heart disease in the presence of atrial fibrillation or atrial flutter with a rapid ventricular response and in patients with symptomatic heart failure due to predominant systolic dysfunction who remain symptomatic on appropriate doses of an ACE inhibitor and diuretic.

ACUTE MYOCARDIAL INFARCTION (see also p. 1245). There is little to be gained from administration of digitalis to patients who have infarction uncomplicated by evidence of heart failure. There is limited clinical documentation of its value in cardiogenic shock, except in the management of supraventricular arrhythmias. Small increases in cardiac index and stroke work, as well as a reduction in left ventricular end-diastolic pressure, have been observed after digitalization of patients with left ventricular failure following myocardial infarction.[76] Although ouabain did not alter cardiac output in another series of patients with acute myocardial infarction,[77] it caused significant improvement in other indices of left ventricular performance such as end-diastolic pressure and stroke work. However, these hemodynamic changes have not been shown to be accompanied by improved survival.

Although the issue has been long debated, there appears to be no convincing evidence for an increased incidence of arrhythmias complicating digitalization in patients with acute infarction (when serum levels do not exceed the conventional therapeutic range).[78] The clearest indication for digitalis after acute myocardial infarction is in the treatment of atrial fibrillation with a rapid ventricular rate. Electrical cardioversion may be preferred in the treatment of other supraventricular tachyarrhythmias.[79]

Thus, current evidence indicates that digitalis has no well-defined role in the management of myocardial infarction without heart failure or supraventricular tachyarrhythmias. Insofar as the long-term management of patients with myocardial infarction is concerned, ACE inhibitor therapy is considered first-line therapy for left ventricular dysfunction and heart failure, followed by diuretics. Digitalis is indicated in the subgroup of patients with chronic congestive heart failure and a dilated left ventricle.

We recommend a three-part approach: (1) careful consideration whether any treatment of ventricular dysfunction is needed, (2) consideration of alternatives to digoxin therapy, and (3) restriction of digoxin use to the subgroup of patients with chronic congestive heart failure and systolic dysfunction who remain symptomatic on diuretics and an ACE inhibitor or other appropriate vasodilator regimen.

ADVANCED AGE. The diminished glomerular filtration rate in the elderly leads to a prolonged half-life and increased serum levels of digoxin and an increased probability of toxicity on a given dosage regimen. Advanced age is frequently associated with other factors that increase the likelihood of digitalis intoxication, including more severe heart disease; impairment of pulmonary, renal, and neurological function; and an increased number of concurrent medications.

RENAL FAILURE. The marked diminution of glomerular filtration rate with renal failure prolongs the half-life of digoxin and thus increases serum digoxin levels. Toxicity can be avoided by careful and frequent adjustments of dosage to correlate with the level of renal function present. Less predictably, dialysis can cause at least a transient decrease in serum potassium that increases the tendency toward digitalis-induced arrhythmias. Depending on the magnesium content of the dialysate and the use of magnesium-containing antacids, there may be significant aberrations of serum magnesium levels in patients undergoing dialysis. The minimum dose of digoxin that yields a serum digoxin level of about 1.0 ng/ml should be used in patients on dialysis, which is characterized by extreme fluctuations in fluid and electrolyte balance.

THYROID DISEASE. In hypothyroid patients the serum digoxin half-life is consistently prolonged, whereas in those with hyperthyroidism, serum digoxin levels tend to be decreased.[80] An increased distribution space for digoxin may exist in hyperthyroid patients. This is of interest in light of two experimental findings; the first is the demonstration of higher levels of Na^+, K^+-ATPase activity in the myocardium of hyperthyroid animals.[81] The second is increased tolerance to cardiac glycosides in heart cells grown in culture in the presence of high thyroid hormone concentrations, associated with an increased number of Na^+, K^+-ATPase sites and enhanced monovalent cation transport capacity.[82] Thus, the apparent resistance or sensitivity to digitalis in thyroid disease probably depends on changes in target organ responsiveness as well as on the pharmacokinetics of digoxin. Oral maintenance doses should be monitored with steady-state serum level measurements, and ventricular rate control in hyperthyroid patients with atrial fibrillation should be sought using approaches other than "pushing" digoxin to potentially toxic levels (e.g., additional use of beta blockers or verapamil).

PULMONARY DISEASE. Ventricular ectopic activity consistent with digitalis toxicity frequently occurs in patients with respiratory disease who are receiving digitalis.[83] However, respiratory failure and hypoxemia frequently provoke arrhythmias indistinguishable from those associated with an excess of digitalis. A total population of 931 patients admitted consecutively to a medical service and studied prospectively demonstrated an increased incidence of rhythm disturbance consistent with digitalis toxicity among the subset of patients with acute or chronic lung disease.[84] Excessive sensitivity to digitalis in patients with pulmonary disease generally correlates with overt cor pulmonale, hypercapnia, and hypoxemia. Thus, patients with a variety of pulmonary diseases may be sensitive to the arrhythmogenic effects of digitalis at relatively low serum concentrations.

DIGITALIS TOXICITY. Mechanisms, clinical manifestations, and treatment of digitalis toxicity are considered on page 484.

INTRAVENOUS SYMPATHOMIMETIC AGENTS

The pharmacology of these drugs is discussed on pages 485 to 486.

DOBUTAMINE. In patients with heart failure refractory to conventional oral medications, intravenous infusions of dobutamine up to several days in duration are usually well tolerated, although pharmacological tolerance generally limits long-term use. Dobutamine is typically initiated at 2 to 3 μg/kg/min without a loading dose and may be titrated according to symptoms and diuretic responsiveness or toward a hemodynamic target.[84a] Systemic arterial pressure may increase, remain constant, or decline depending on the extent of vasodilation and changes in cardiac output. Heart rate may fall after several hours if cardiac output is significantly increased and central sympathetic tone declines, although sinus tachycardia and supraventricular arrhythmias may also occur. Use of a flow-directed catheter to monitor pulmonary capillary wedge pressure as well as cardiac output allows more effective use of dobutamine alone or in conjunction with other vasodilators and diuretics.

The maximal effective dose of dobutamine depends on the individual patient. Teboul et al.[85] observed that in patients with severe heart failure, increasing the rate of infusion of dobutamine above 10 μg/kg/min resulted in no further increase in mixed venous oxygen saturation but was accompanied by a significant increase in myocardial oxygen consumption and could therefore be detrimental.

Outpatient therapy with dobutamine, administered continuously by a portable infusion pump through a central venous catheter, has been used successfully in patients with advanced heart failure and symptoms refractory to other drugs.[86–89] Although this approach has been useful in maintaining an acceptable functional status in some patients, it has not gained widespread clinical acceptance largely due to concern regarding its safety and the development of tolerance to a fixed-dose infusion rate. There have been no prospective controlled studies of this form of therapy for severe heart failure and no clear criteria have been established to identify those patients who, for reasons of safety, should be excluded from continuous dobutamine therapy.[86]

Intermittent use of dobutamine in a monitored setting may be appropriate for selected patients in order to minimize the development of tolerance. Periodic withdrawal of this synthetic sympathomimetic may prevent or diminish the onset of tolerance, although this strategy also has not been tested for efficacy or safety in patients with heart failure by prospective randomized clinical trials. Patients who become tolerant to dobutamine on continuous infusions may benefit from a Class III cAMP phosphodiesterase inhibitor (e.g., milrinone) for several days, after which dobutamine can be reinstituted.[90] Weaning patients from intravenous sympathomimetic agents is often difficult and may require aggressive use of vasodilators with continuous hemodynamic monitoring, as well as digoxin and diuretics (see p. 483).

DOPAMINE. The pharmacodynamic spectrum of activity of dobutamine is superior to that of dopamine for most patients with advanced heart failure, as discussed in Chapter 16. Therefore, dopamine is no longer a first-line agent for use in patients with decompensated congestive heart failure. There is also increasing debate regarding whether low-dose or "renal range" dopamine improves renal function and diuretic effectiveness in patients with heart failure and a depressed cardiac output.[91,92] There are no controlled trials that demonstrate the efficacy and safety of "renal range" dopamine infusions in patients with heart failure and declining renal function receiving vasodilators. Indeed, recent data from surgical intensive care patients do not support the contention that "renal range" dopamine is useful in preserving renal function or promoting a significant natriuresis in humans.[93–95]

Dopamine dosing must be based on an estimate of lean body weight and dosing based on actual body weight in heart failure patients may lead to toxic drug levels. As tachycardia and arrhythmias are frequent complications of dopamine administration in patients with heart failure, even if a correct dosing algorithm is used, this drug should only be used temporarily in hypotensive, decompensated patients with heart failure until other measures (e.g., an intra-aortic balloon pump) can be instituted.

OTHER PHARMACOLOGICAL AGENTS

Newer Inotropic Agents

PHOSPHODIESTERASE INHIBITORS. Development of *oral* formulations of phosphodiesterase (PDE) inhibitors for treatment of chronic heart failure has been deterred by the premature termination of the Prospective Randomized Milrinone Survival Evaluation (PROMISE) trial,[96] which showed a 53 per cent increase in mortality in patients with NYHA Class IV heart failure receiving milrinone. Unfavorable results were also evident in a smaller trial that compared oral milrinone to digoxin or placebo.[97] Sustained hemodynamic improvement was lacking in the milrinone group, and the incidence of adverse events, particularly cardiac arrhythmias, was greater.

Amrinone and milrinone are available for short-term circulatory support in patients with decompensated cardiac failure and following cardiac surgery. Milrinone, which is approximately tenfold more potent and has a shorter half life than amrinone, is also associated with a reduced risk of thrombocytopenia and therefore is the preferred drug in these patient groups. Milrinone, following a loading dose of 50 μg/kg and initiation of a maintenance infusion of between 0.25 to 1.0 μg/kg/min, acts both to reduce systemic vascular resistance and to increase cardiac contractility.[97a] As with all agents that mimic the activity of beta-adrenergic agonists, milrinone also accelerates the rate of relaxation of the heart (i.e., a positive lusitropic effect). Milrinone (or amrinone) may be used temporarily in decompensated hospitalized patients who have developed tolerance to dobutamine or, with dobutamine, as a bridge to transplantation or insertion of a ventricular assist device in end-stage heart failure.

VESNARINONE (see p. 485). Vesnarinone appeared to decrease mortality in one large placebo-controlled trial.[98] Patients on standard therapy for mild to moderately severe heart failure were randomized to placebo or vesnarinone at 60 mg or 120 mg/day. An increase in mortality in patients receiving the larger dose of active drug caused the early termination of that arm of the trial. The lower dose of 60 mg/day of vesnarinone, however, was associated with a greater than 50 per cent reduction in mortality at 12 weeks compared to placebo. Symptoms of heart failure and quality of life also improved in the 60-mg/day vesnarinone group, consistent with prior smaller trials.[98] Results of additional clinical trials in progress are awaited with interest.

Beta-Adrenergic Blocking Agents

The rationale for this approach is considered on pages 411 and 486. The Metoprolol in Dilated Cardiomyopathy (MDC) trial[99] compared metoprolol to placebo in patients with mild to moderate (Class II and III) heart failure due to an idiopathic dilated cardiomyopathy and an ejection fraction averaging 22 per cent who were already receiving optimal medical management, including an ACE inhibitor. Metoprolol therapy was initiated as a test dose of 5 mg. The target dose was 100 to 150 mg/day achieved over 7 weeks, and the mean dose of those on active drug was 108 mg at 3

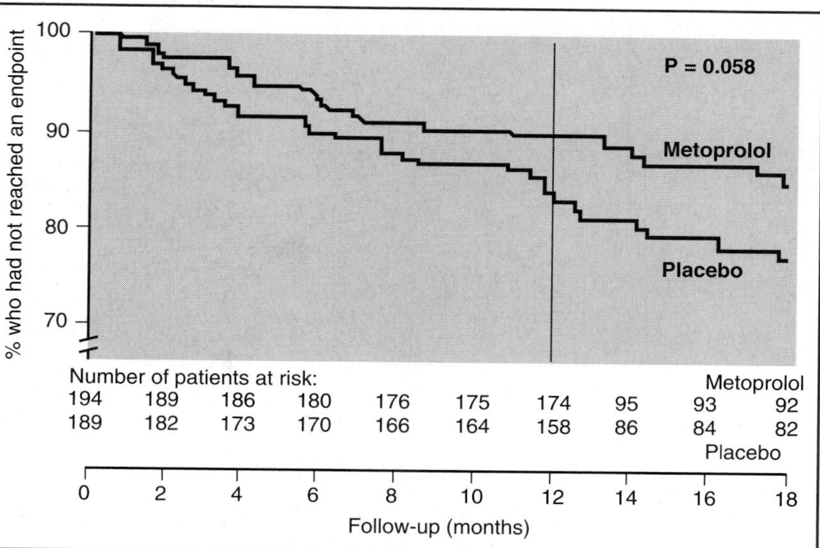

FIGURE 17–7. Percentage of patients who had not reached a primary endpoint (i.e., death or need for cardiac transplantation) in the metoprolol in dilated cardiomyopathy (MDC) trial. Although there was no difference in mortality between patients randomized to receive metoprolol or placebo, there was a significant reduction in the number of patients who required listing for cardiac transplantation (i.e., 19 in the placebo group versus two in the metoprolol group; $P < 0.001$). (From Waagstein, F., et al: Beneficial effects of metoprolol in idiopathic dilated cardiomyopathy. Lancet *342*:1441, 1993. © by The Lancet Ltd.)

months. Although there was no difference in mortality after 12 months of follow-up, the number of patients requiring hospitalization for worsening heart failure or listing for cardiac transplantation was significantly less in the metoprolol group (Fig. 17–7). Over 12 months, ejection fraction improved significantly more in patients receiving metoprolol (0.22 to 0.34) than patients receiving placebo (0.22 to 0.28).[99]

The Cardiac Insufficiency BIsoprolol Study (CIBIS)[100] examined the effects of this $beta_1$-selective antagonist in 641 patients with heart failure and NYHA Class III functional status, due to either an ischemic or a primary dilated cardiomyopathy. As in the MDC trial, mortality was not reduced, but functional status improved, and the incidence of clinical decompensation due to worsening heart failure declined. Eichhorn and Hjalmarson[101] have suggested that this trial was underpowered to detect a decrease in mortality. Interestingly, bisoprolol reduced mortality significantly in patients with idiopathic dilated cardiomyopathy, supporting the results of the MDC trial[99] but did not do so in patients with ischemic cardiomyopathy.

Fisher et al., on the other hand, have reported that both the functional status and the need for hospitalizations due to worsening heart failure were improved in patients with ischemic heart disease and an ejection fraction below 40 per cent who were randomized to receive metoprolol compared to placebo[102]; ejection fraction also improved significantly. Bucindolol, a nonselective beta-adrenergic antagonist with vasodilating activity, was superior to placebo in improving symptoms, NYHA functional class, and ejection fraction in patients with idiopathic cardiomyopathy over a 2-year follow-up period.[103,104] Maximal exercise tolerance declined on the highest dose of bucindolol, consistent with a decline in maximal heart rate achieved during active drug therapy from 150 beats/min on placebo to 110 beats/min.[105] However, there was a trend toward an improvement in submaximal exercise tolerance, which may be a more reliable indicator of functional status for patients receiving drug therapy for heart failure.[103,105] High-dose bucindolol (200 mg/day) significantly improved ejection fraction in patients with ischemic cardiomyopathy as well: results consistent with the report by Fisher et al. with metoprolol.[102] Preliminary reports of a large (1052 patients) multicenter, placebo-controlled trial of carvedilol, a nonselective beta-adrenergic antagonist with alpha-adrenergic antagonist (vasodilating) activity, has demonstrated a clear survival benefit as well as improved exercise tolerance for patients with mild as well as more severe (NYHA Class II-IV) symptoms of heart failure.[105a] Unlike previous trials of beta-antagonists in heart failure, a two-thirds reduction in mortality was identified in patients with ischemic as well as with idiopathic cardiomyopathies. While these data strongly support the use of beta-adrenergic agonists in most patients with heart failure, considerable care must be exercised both in the selection of patients and in the initiation of therapy, during which heart failure symptoms are often exacerbated. In another, smaller trial of carvedilol of heart failure, for example, 37 per cent of patients with advanced heart failure developed increasing dyspnea and fluid retention during initiation of low-dose therapy.[105b]

Thus, despite the lack of an understanding of underlying mechanisms, available evidence supports a potential role for beta-adrenergic antagonists in the treatment of patients with symptomatic heart failure. In all reported studies, which were conducted by investigators with substantial experience in the management of heart failure, the initial doses were low (e.g., 5-mg test doses for metoprolol, followed by 10 mg/day) and were slowly titrated upward over at least 4 to 6 weeks. Although this approach appears promising, as of this writing it is investigational, and beta blockers have not been approved by the U.S. Food and Drug Administration for the treatment of heart failure. A large-scale trial of bucindolol, the BEST trial, will further test this therapy on survival of patients with heart failure.

HEART FAILURE WITH PREDOMINANT DIASTOLIC VENTRICULAR DYSFUNCTION

The pathophysiology and assessment of diastolic dysfunction have been considered on pages 402, 434, and 447. The various abnormalities leading to diastolic dysfunction, shown in Figure 13–13, p. 402, stiffen the ventricles during diastole and/or diminish their rate of relaxation, elevating ventricular diastolic pressure and causing pulmonary and/or systemic venous congestion. The therapeutic approach to diastolic dysfunction has two major components.[106] The first involves attempts to reverse the heart's abnormal diastolic properties; the second is directed toward reducing filling pressure and thereby venous congestion (Table 17–3).

Examples of the first approach include pericardiectomy for constrictive pericarditis, the relief of ventricular systolic overload, and the subsequent regression of ventricular hypertrophy. Efforts to achieve such regression involve the aggressive control of hypertension and the relief of valvular, supravalvular, and subvalvular obstruction to ventricu-

TABLE 17–3 TREATMENT OF DIASTOLIC DYSFUNCTION

GOAL OF TREATMENT	METHOD OF TREATMENT
Produce hypertrophy progression:	Antihypertensive therapy Surgery (e.g., AVR for aortic stenosis)
Improve ventricular relaxation:	Systolic unloading Ischemia treatment Calcium channel blockers (?)
Prevent/treat ischemia:	Beta-adrenergic blockers Calcium channel blockers Nitrates Coronary bypass or angioplasty
Reduce venous pressure:	CBV decreased Diuretics Salt restriction Venodilation Nitrates ACE inhibitors Morphine Tourniquets
Decrease heart rate:	Digoxin in atrial fibrillation Beta-adrenergic blockers Verapamil, diltiazem
Maintain atrial contraction:	Cardioversion of atrial fibrillation Sequential AV pacing

AVR = aortic valve replacement; CBV = central blood volume.

Modified from Levine, H. J., and Gaasch, W. H.: Clinical recognition and treatment of diastolic dysfunction and heart failure. *In* Gaasch, W. H., and LeWinter, M. M. (eds.): Left Ventricular Diastolic Dysfunction and Heart Failure. Philadelphia, Lea and Febiger, 1994, p. 445.

lar outflow by operation[107] or balloon dilatation. There is some evidence that ACE inhibitors and aldosterone antagonists slow, arrest, or perhaps even reverse myocardial fibrosis in the presence of systolic overload,[108] and these agents might be useful in the management of diastolic dysfunction in such patients. The rapid relief of acute myocardial ischemia is often effective when diastolic dysfunction is secondary to this condition. Nitroglycerin, anti-ischemic agents (beta blockers and calcium antagonists), thrombolysis, mechanical revascularization, or a combination of these measures may be used, depending on the specific clinical circumstance. Calcium antagonists (see p. 1425), especially verapamil, have been shown to accelerate ventricular relaxation in patients with hypertrophic cardiomyopathy[109,110] and have been reported to be useful in the treatment of diastolic dysfunction characteristic of this condition (see p. 403).

Ventricular filling pressure and secondary venous congestion may be reduced by restriction of sodium intake and the administration of diuretics and venodilators. Even in the absence of myocardial ischemia, nitrates, by reducing preload, are useful in the management of diastolic ventricular dysfunction and in the treatment and prevention of consequent severe pulmonary congestion. Nitroglycerin may be administered intravenously or sublingually in emergency situations, and long-acting nitrates, such as isosorbide dinitrate, are often effective in the long term. In the long-term management of patients with diastolic dysfunction, however, excessive preload reduction should be avoided, because these patients often require higher-than-normal filling pressures to maintain an adequate stroke volume.

The maintenance of normal heart rate and rhythm is of critical importance in patients with predominant diastolic dysfunction. Tachycardia, whatever the underlying mechanism, must be controlled, thereby increasing the fraction of each cardiac cycle available for ventricular filling. Maintenance of sinus rhythm with synchronized atrioventricular sequential pacing may be critical in permitting atrial augmentation of ventricular filling, thereby raising ventricular filling pressure. Digoxin has no established place in the management of patients with predominant diastolic dysfunction and a well-preserved ventricular ejection fraction, and could, in principle, have an adverse effect in this group.

SUDDEN DEATH AND ARRHYTHMIAS

Sudden death accounts for 30 to 70 per cent of all deaths in patients with heart failure.[111] Sudden death increases in absolute frequency with the clinical severity of disease. Its relative importance, however, is substantial in patients with less advanced disease.[111] The incidence of sudden death ranges from 2 to 3 per cent yearly in patients with asymptomatic left-ventricular dysfunction[5,8] to 7 to 20 per cent yearly in patients with severe heart failure.[3,7] Death may occur unexpectedly in patients with heart failure for whom therapy has allowed the maintenance of good quality of life. The incidence of sudden death appears to be lower during therapy with ACE inhibitors.[6,7]

The multiple underlying causes of sudden death in this population have confounded attempts to predict or prevent it (Table 17–4). Sudden death can be caused not only by ventricular tachyarrhythmias, but also by bradyarrhythmias, which accounted for almost half of unexpected cardiac arrests in a series of ambulatory patients hospitalized during evaluation for cardiac transplantation.[112] Both tachyarrhythmias and bradyarrhythmias may occur without obvious underlying cause or result from another acute event such as myocardial infarction or pulmonary embolism.[112]

Substrate for Arrhythmias

The ventricular hypertrophy that commonly accompanies heart failure is associated with a variety of electrophysiological abnormalities that may enhance the potential for arrhythmias.[113–116] Prolonged duration of the action potential, slow impulse propagation, and heterogeneous recovery following depolarization facilitate reentry. Patchy interstitial fibrosis may decrease electrical coupling and slow impulse propagation between myocytes, establishing further the substrate for microreentrant ventricular arrhythmias.

Patients with heart failure consequent to previous myocardial infarctions have focal sites of fibrosis and adjacent

TABLE 17–4 CAUSES OF SUDDEN DEATH IN HEART FAILURE

UNDERLYING CAUSE	RHYTHM OBSERVED
Acute myocardial ischemia or infarction (coronary artery disease or embolus)	VT (usually polymorphic) or VF, bradycardia, EMD
Pulmonary embolism	Bradycardia, EMD
Embolic or hemorrhagic stroke	Bradycardia, polymorphic VT
Drugs prolonging QT interval	Polymorphic VT
Electrolyte depletion (potassium, magnesium)	Polymorphic VT
Hyperkalemia	Bradycardia Apparent VT*
Exaggerated vagal reflexes?	Sinus bradycardia Complete heart block
Primary arrhythmia	
Ventricular tachyarrhythmias	VT, VF
Conduction system disease	Sinus bradycardia Complete heart block

EMD = electromechanical dissociation; VF = ventricular fibrillation; VT = ventricular tachycardia.

* Rhythms during hyperkalemia are frequently diagnosed as ventricular tachycardia. These may also be "sinoventricular rhythms" in which the prolonged conduction causes absence of apparent atrial activity and marked widening of the QRS complex.

Adapted from Stevenson, W. G., Stevenson, L. W., Middlekauff, H. R., and Saxon, L. A.: Sudden death prevention in patients with advanced ventricular dysfunction. Circulation *88*:2953, 1993.

viable myocardium that may foster the occurrence of conduction block and macro-reentry arrhythmias, manifested usually as monomorphic ventricular tachycardia. Focal ischemia more commonly causes polymorphic ventricular tachycardia.

Ventricular hypertrophy and the accompanying abnormalities in intracellular calcium handling confer increased susceptibility to triggered activity from early afterdepolarizations, which in animal models have been strongly linked to polymorphic ventricular tachycardia (torsades de pointes).[114] Stretch of myocytes, as occurs in heart failure (Chap. 13), can also produce afterdepolarizations; animal models demonstrate increased susceptibility to ventricular fibrillation when intraventricular pressures are increased.[116]

Abnormalities of autonomic nervous system function in heart failure may also be arrhythmogenic. Increased beta-adrenergic stimulation augments intracellular calcium and increases delayed afterdepolarizations,[117] whereas alpha-adrenergic stimulation may promote early afterdepolarizations by prolonging action potential duration.[118] Sympathetic stimulation may cause heterogeneous changes in conduction and refractoriness, which predispose to reentrant ventricular arrhythmias. Reduced resting vagal tone also increases susceptibility to ventricular tachyarrhythmias. Abnormal autonomic balance may also predispose to sudden vasodepressor responses manifested as bradycardiac arrests. Depletion of potassium and magnesium during diuretic therapy has been associated with increased susceptibility to early afterdepolarizations and torsades de pointes.[119] Hypokalemia may specifically increase the risk of ventricular fibrillation during myocardial ischemia. Hyperkalemia causes slowing of conduction, which can lead to reentrant arrhythmias in addition to the more commonly recognized suppression of sinus and atrioventricular node function.

Approach to Ventricular Arrhythmias

EVALUATION OF CARDIAC ARREST SURVIVORS (see also Chap. 24). Among patients who have been resuscitated from ventricular fibrillation or ventricular tachycardia, those with left ventricular ejection fractions below 30 per cent have higher risk of recurrent sudden death than do patients with better ventricular function.[120,121] Once heart failure is severe, however, a history of prior cardiac arrest may not itself augur a worse outcome. One study of potential transplant candidates receiving selected antiarrhythmic therapy or an implantable defibrillator after previous resuscitation from cardiac arrest attributed to ventricular tachycardia or fibrillation showed a 17 per cent risk of sudden death during the next year, which was identical to the risk for potential candidates without such a history.[122]

The current diagnostic approach to cardiac arrest survivors with heart failure usually includes 24-hour electrocardiographic monitoring, exercise testing, and electrophysiological study to identify the responsible arrhythmia, which is often ventricular tachycardia but can be bradycardia due to conduction-system disease. Electrolyte abnormalities and active ischemia should also be sought as potential causes or contributing factors. Inducibility of ventricular tachycardia is more common in the patient with previous myocardial infarction than in the patient with nonischemic cardiomyopathy.[123] When ventricular tachycardia is inducible in patients with heart failure secondary to nonischemic cardiomyopathy, it may originate from bundle branch reentry in as many as a third of cases,[124] particularly if there is evidence of conduction system disease on the resting electrocardiogram. This type of ventricular tachycardia is particularly amenable to radiofrequency ablation techniques[125] (see Chap. 21).

Patients in whom ventricular tachycardia can be induced following cardiac arrest have a 15 to 50 per cent risk of recurrent cardiac arrest during the next 2 to 3 years during therapy with antiarrhythmic drugs. This risk includes both the risk of the underlying arrhythmia and the proarrhythmic risk of the drugs used to suppress arrhythmias. The choice of drug is often determined by efficacy of suppression of arrhythmia during serial electrophysiological testing. Amiodarone, however, may often be clinically effective despite continued inducibility of arrhythmias by programmed stimulation.[126] Cardiac arrest survivors with poor ventricular function in whom a cause cannot be found have a 30 per cent risk of recurrent arrest during the next 1 to 3 years.[120,127,128] Cardiac arrests attributed to factors such as hypoxia during pulmonary edema or torsades de pointes during antiarrhythmic drug therapy may identify patients at subsequent high risk despite the apparently transitory nature of the inciting cause. In one study of "secondary arrests" in advanced heart failure, the risk of sudden death was 39 per cent over the following year despite attempts to remove precipitating factors.[122]

PREVENTION OF RECURRENT VENTRICULAR TACHYARRHYTHMIAS. The risks of antiarrhythmic drug therapy are increased in patients with heart failure. With the exception of quinidine and amiodarone, most commonly used antiarrhythmic drugs depress contractility.[129] Heart failure was exacerbated by antiarrhythmic drug therapy in 3.8 per cent of patients enrolled in drug trials, most commonly in those with left ventricular ejection fractions below 25 per cent.[130] This observation is consistent with the finding that exacerbation of arrhythmias by drug therapy also occurs more commonly in patients with depressed ventricular function.[131] In the Cardiac Arrhythmia Suppression Trial (see p. 609), in patients with depressed ventricular function after myocardial infarction, the Type I agents flecainide, encainide, and moricizine suppressed ventricular ectopy but increased mortality.[132] Increased mortality has been suggested from other heart failure populations treated with Type I antiarrhythmic agents.[133] Thus, these drugs should be avoided when possible in patients with heart failure. Management objectives should include maintenance of potassium and magnesium balance and avoidance of noncardiac drugs such as phenothiazines or erythromycin that are known to cause Q-T prolongation.

Of currently available antiarrhythmic drugs, amiodarone appears to have the greatest potential to reduce sudden death in heart failure. Even in the presence of advanced heart failure, it is hemodynamically well tolerated and may actually improve ejection fraction.[134] Amiodarone has been reported to improve survival after myocardial infarction[135] and has been suggested to improve survival in the GESICA trial of severe heart failure[136,136a] (Fig. 17–8). The side effects of pulmonary and hepatic toxicity increase progressively over time (see p. 614) but are more easily accepted in a population with a 5-year survival of less than 50 per cent. In the absence of contraindications, amiodarone is generally the antiarrhythmic drug of choice for therapy of ventricular arrhythmias or atrial arrhythmias in patients with severe heart failure. In the absence of clinically significant arrhythmias, the role of amiodarone has not yet been clearly established.[136,137]

Unlike monomorphic ventricular tachycardia, polymorphic tachycardia usually cannot be reproduced with electrophysiological testing. It may result from ischemia or from factors that prolong the Q-T interval. A history of torsades de pointes in heart failure is associated with increased subsequent sudden death.[122] Although rarely incriminated as a primary cause of torsades de pointes, amiodarone may increase the risk of sudden death in patients with heart failure with a previous history of arrhythmias in the setting of Q-T prolongation.[138]

Implantable cardioverter debrillators offer a nonpharmacological approach for prevention of cardiac arrest due to ventricular arrhythmias[125] (see p. 621). The development of transvenous devices has markedly decreased the morbidity and mortality associated with implantation even in patients with severe heart failure, although induction and termina-

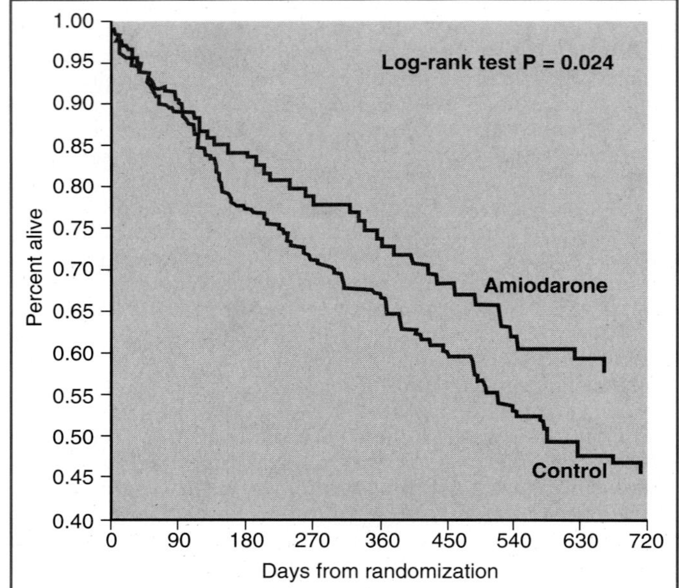

FIGURE 17–8. GESICA trial. Actuarial survival of patients with severe heart failure randomized to treatment with amiodarone (300 mg daily after loading dose of 600 mg daily for 14 days) or no treatment in addition to digitalis, diuretics, and, in most cases, ACE inhibitors. Reduction in mortality appeared to result equally from a decrease in sudden death and a decrease in death from progressive heart failure. (From Doval, H. C., Nul, D. R., Grancelli, H. O., et al.: Randomized trial of low-dose amiodarone in severe congestive heart failure. Lancet *344*:493, 1994.)

tion of ventricular tachyarrhythmias necessary to test the device may be poorly tolerated by patients with severe hemodynamic decompensation. Although effective in the majority of cases, these devices occasionally fail to defibrillate successfully, a problem that may be slightly more common in the population with heart failure. It should be emphasized that these devices do not prevent arrhythmias, and the discharges of the device may cause marked discomfort, the anticipation of which may severely limit activity in patients with frequent ventricular arrhythmias. Although these devices appear effective in reducing sudden death,[121] they have not yet been shown to reduce overall mortality in heart failure. Indeed, they may simply change the mode of death from arrhythmia to pump failure. At present, and pending the results of ongoing studies, there is no consensus regarding the relative efficacy of the use of amiodarone versus automatic implanted cardioverter defibrillators (AICDs) in patients with heart failure and symptomatic ventricular arrhythmias. Either would constitute a reasonable first choice, although most clinicians with extensive experience would proceed to placement of an AICD if events recur on amiodarone.

SYNCOPE. Loss of consciousness in a patient with depressed ventricular function warrants careful investigation (see p. 872). A history of such an episode, which occurs in up to 12 per cent of patients with heart failure, should not be casually attributed to fatigue or medications. In up to a third of cases, electrophysiological investigation may reveal ventricular tachycardia that requires specific therapy with drugs or devices. Implantation of a pacemaker may be indicated in patients found to have severe impairment of sinus or atrioventricular node function resulting from coronary artery disease or from cardiomyopathy of various causes. Syncope without obvious cause may represent an impaired ability to maintain adequate perfusion in response to stress, for which there is currently no specific therapy. In patients with advanced heart failure, a history of syncope was associated with a 45 per cent risk of sudden death at 1 year, whether or not a specific cause was identified.[139]

ASYMPTOMATIC VENTRICULAR ECTOPY AND NONSUSTAINED VENTRICULAR TACHYCARDIA. Ambulatory electrocardiographic monitoring reveals premature ventricular complexes in over 90 per cent of patients with heart failure, and nonsustained ventricular tachycardia (three or more consecutive beats) in up to 60 per cent.[125,140] In patients after myocardial infarction, frequent ventricular premature beats and nonsustained ventricular tachycardia are associated with more depressed left ventricular function, but the risk of sudden death with premature beats is increased independently of ejection fraction.[141] In contrast, patients with these asymptomatic arrhythmias in the presence of symptomatic heart failure due either to ischemic or nonischemic cardiomyopathy have a higher total mortality but not necessarily a higher risk of sudden death.[140] The ability to induce ventricular tachycardia in patients after myocardial infarction correlates with subsequent mortality.[142] In patients with heart failure, however, the ability to induce ventricular tachycardia with programmed ventricular stimulation did not predict subsequent sudden death.[123]

As with CAST, the postinfarction trial (see p. 600), suppression of asymptomatic ventricular arrhythmias with Type I antiarrhythmic agents not only fails to reduce mortality, but actually increases it.[132] Amiodarone, which is highly effective for suppression of ventricular ectopy and nonsustained ventricular tachycardia, does not worsen and may improve survival in heart failure patients.[136] The benefit shown from amiodarone, however, has been equal in groups with and without nonsustained ventricular tachycardia, and reduction was seen both in sudden death and heart failure endpoints.[136] There is currently no information that indicates a specific benefit from arrhythmia suppression in the absence of symptomatic ventricular arrhythmias.

ATRIAL FIBRILLATION. This arrhythmia, which occurs in approximately 20 per cent of patients with heart failure, has been associated with increased mortality in some[143] but not in all[144] studies of heart failure. Chronic atrial fibrillation in the presence of major left-ventricular dysfunction conferred a 16 per cent annual incidence of stroke, increasing to 20 per cent if the left atrial diameter was more than 2.5 cm/m^2.[133] This risk is decreased by anticoagulant therapy. In addition to the risk of emboli, atrial fibrillation decreases ventricular filling in heart failure, both through loss of the atrial booster pump and through reduction of filling time when the ventricular response is rapid. The regulation of the heart rate response to exercise is impaired in atrial fibrillation, and improved following successful cardioversion to sinus rhythm.[145] Digoxin is usually inadequate for the control of exercise heart rate response, which frequently increases to over 150 beats/min with minimal activity in patients with heart failure, even when the heart rate appears to be adequately controlled at rest. This degree of tachycardia may exacerbate ischemia and/or left ventricular dysfunction. Conversion to sinus rhythm has often been associated with improvement in symptoms and exercise capacity and at times in dramatic improvement in ejection fraction, which may deteriorate again with recurrence of atrial fibrillation.[146]

The risk of emboli, excessive ventricular rates, and possibly increased mortality mandate vigorous attempts to restore sinus rhythm in patients with heart failure, even when initial attempts have failed. Quinidine may maintain sinus rhythm in up to 50 per cent of patients.[133,147] However, concern has been raised based on data from meta-analyses and the Stroke Prevention in Atrial Fibrillation trial, indicating that quinidine may be associated with an up to threefold higher mortality.[133,147] Amiodarone has facilitated conversion to sinus rhythm in 80 per cent of patients with atrial fibrillation and heart failure, and sinus rhythm is maintained at a year in approximately 60 per cent of patients.[145] Amiodarone is generally preferred to quinidine both for efficacy and safety in patients with heart failure.

When sinus rhythm cannot be maintained, rate control is facilitated by amiodarone, usually combined with digoxin. Calcium antagonists may be deleterious, and the use of beta-blocking agents in this setting remains investigational. When pharmacological therapy is not tolerated or is inadequate to maintain adequate rate control, electrical ablation of the atrioventricular junction with placement of a rate-responsive ventricular pacemaker should be considered.[148]

REFRACTORY HEART FAILURE

Heart failure is usually considered to be refractory to medical therapy when severe symptoms persist despite therapy with ACE inhibitors and/or other vasodilators, as well as diuretics, and digoxin. Marked improvement can, however, frequently be achieved after further evaluation and intensification of therapy, which includes patient education as well as an individualized regimen of drugs, diet, and the judicious use of exercise.

The first step in dealing with a patient considered to be in refractory heart failure is to step back and take a fresh look to determine whether other conditions are responsible for the symptoms attributed to heart failure.

1. Could digitalis intoxication be present? Digitalis toxicity can occur despite a serum glycoside level in the usual therapeutic range and can cause fatigue, lethargy, and anorexia that may mimic refractory heart failure.
2. Are the symptoms due to electrolyte imbalance, such as hypokalemic alkalosis or hyponatremia, which may have developed as a consequence of excessive diuresis and restriction of sodium intake?
3. Could the patient with established heart disease be suffering from an unrelated illness such as occult neoplasm, viral hepatitis, or hepatic cirrhosis?
4. Has the patient been treated for predominant systolic dysfunction when the underlying pathophysiology is actually predominant diastolic dysfunction?

As in the initial evaluation of heart failure, heart failure that has become apparently refractory merits close evaluation for potentially reversible factors that could have precipitated or exacerbated circulatory decompensation. These include the following:

1. Could the patient be "cheating" on the restricted sodium diet or drinking excessive volumes of liquids?
2. Is the patient not complying with the medication schedule prescribed despite protestations to the contrary? A "pill count" is often helpful in determining compliance.
3. Is the patient receiving optimal doses of cardiac glycosides? Prescribed digoxin doses in the conventional range do not exclude the possibility of noncompliance or inadequate absorption. Benefit may derive from checking the serum digoxin concentration and adjusting the dose to maintain a steady-state serum level in the 1.0-ng/ml range without precipitating signs or symptoms of toxicity.
4. Could the patient be suffering from unrecognized pulmonary embolism (see Chap. 46)? This condition occurs frequently in heart failure, is often silent, and may be manifested only by slight tachycardia, anxiety, tachypnea, and intensification of heart failure. Dense areas on the chest roentgenogram may make it difficult or impossible to interpret lung scans, and a pulmonary angiogram may be required to establish the diagnosis. Although this procedure is not without risk, a positive result may lead to treatment with anticoagulants and/or interruption of the inferior vena cava that could prevent further emboli and prove to be life saving.
5. Could pulmonary infection be present? Pneumonitis, a frequent complication of left ventricular failure, may be difficult to recognize in patients with chronic congestive heart failure who often have increased interstitial markings on the chest roentgenogram and pulmonary rales on clinical examination. Is the suspicion of pulmonary infection high enough to warrant sputum culture and consideration of a course of antibiotics?
6. Could hyperthyroidism or infective endocarditis be present? Thyrotoxicosis (often apathetic in the elderly) and infective endocarditis may not have typical clinical manifestations in the presence of heart failure, but they can lead to refractory heart failure. Should thyroid function studies and/or multiple blood cultures be obtained?
7. Could alcohol, a potent myocardial depressant, be playing a role? In addition to producing cardiomyopathy (see p. 1412), alcohol can contribute to heart failure even when it is not the primary cause, but when its use is superimposed on some other form of heart disease.
8. Has the combination of ACE inhibition, other vasodilators, intensive diuretic therapy, and sodium restriction caused hypovolemia, low cardiac output, and hypotension?
9. Does the patient have inappropriate bradycardia due to sinus node dysfunction or atrioventricular block that could be corrected by means of a pacemaker? Could AV sequential pacing restore atrial augmentation of ventricular stroke volume?
10. Is the patient receiving any medications with salt-retaining effects, such as corticosteroids, estrogens, or nonsteroidal anti-inflammatory drugs, or drugs with undesired negative inotropic actions such as disopyramide or calcium antagonists?
11. Could therapy with vasodilators or other agents be responsible for an increased tendency to retention of salt and water that has not been adequately addressed by diuretic therapy?
12. Have the initial favorable hemodynamic effects of any drug in the regimen waned during long-term therapy (e.g., the development of nitrate tolerance)?
13. Can any aspect of therapy be intensified without producing adverse effects?

Management

If, after attention to these factors, patients are still in refractory heart failure, therapies that may initially have been considered to carry unacceptable risks for a stable patient may warrant reconsideration. For example, resection of a large ventricular aneurysm might have been deferred initially owing to high surgical risk in an otherwise stable patient, but reconsideration might be in order when the response to medical therapy wanes. Similar consideration may apply to patients with known multivessel coronary artery disease[149,150] or advanced valvular heart disease and poor left ventricular function. Other forms of surgically correctable heart failure that are not readily recognized on clinical examination include cardiac tumors (see Chap. 42), and constrictive pericarditis without calcification (see Chap. 43). Such conditions should be considered and excluded if possible. When other correctable factors have been addressed, a hemodynamic profile should be obtained and the potential for improvement with readjustment of loading conditions should be assessed.

Hemodynamic Goals

The dominant symptoms of severe heart failure usually reflect marked elevations in intracardiac filling pressures. Hospitalization for intravenous diuretics or brief infusions of inotropic agents facilitate fluid loss to achieve comfort at rest but often leave the patient just below the threshold for visceral congestion or pulmonary edema. Reversal of this cycle of decongestion and recongestion often requires more aggressive reduction of filling pressures. In severe heart failure, preload and afterload are interdependent.[151] Reduction of systemic vascular resistance (afterload) also reduces ventricular filling pressures (preload). Diuresis to reduce preload typically reduces the afterload faced by the ventricle. Therapy of severe persistent congestion requires careful adjustment of both vasodilator and diuretic therapy.

Reduction of intracardiac filling pressures has frequently been limited by concern that cardiac output will become further compromised. Cardiac output is closely related to filling pressures in the normal heart and in acute myocardial infarction.[152] In the chronically dilated ventricle, however, elevations in filling pressures can increase wall stress, compromise subendocardial perfusion, and worsen mitral regurgitation so that cardiac output actually decreases. Maximal stroke volumes are often achieved when the pulmonary capillary wedge pressures approach the normal range[153] (Fig. 17–9). In an average-sized adult, systemic vascular resistances of 1000 to 1200 dynes-sec-cm^{-5} are generally adequate for an optimal cardiac output while maintaining a systolic arterial pressure of at least 80 mm Hg. Most of the improvement in stroke volume with optimization of loading conditions in patients with severe heart failure results from a decrease in mitral regurgitant volume.[154] Similar considerations regarding tricuspid regurgitation apply to the right ventricle, in addition to which right ventricular contractility may actually improve acutely with the reduction of pulmonary vascular resistance. The level of right ventricular compensation determines the minimal levels of right atrial pressure, which may be below 5 mm Hg in some patients with left ventricular failure but in others cannot be reduced below 10 mm Hg owing to irreversible right ventricular dysfunction. Recognition of the importance of reducing filling pressures and secondary valvular regurgitation has led to the hemodynamic goals for refractory heart failure shown in Table 17–5.

Indications for Tailored Therapy with Hemodynamic Monitoring

In patients with severely symptomatic heart failure or with clinical evidence of hypoperfusion and/or congestion despite careful empiric adjustment of therapy (see Table 17–2), the insertion of a multilumen flotation catheter into the pulmonary artery often facilitates management. Right atrial and pulmonary artery pressures can be followed simultaneously, with intermittent brief inflation of a balloon-tipped distal end to obtain pulmonary capillary wedge pressures as an estimate of left ventricular filling pressures. Cardiac output is measured using temperature dilution between the right atrial port and pulmonary artery thermistor. This hemodynamic monitoring allows simultaneous optimization of filling pressures and systemic vascular resistance. This is often achieved first by the use of short-acting intravenous agents, such as nitroprusside or dobutamine, to reestablish a baseline of compensation upon which an oral regimen can then be imposed.[155–157] Nitroprusside is generally effective when the systemic vascular resistance is elevated. Dobutamine or dopamine may be required when the systemic vascular resistance is normal or low. Intravenous diuretics are administered concomitantly, guided in large part by the right atrial pressure and the presence of hepatomegaly or edema.

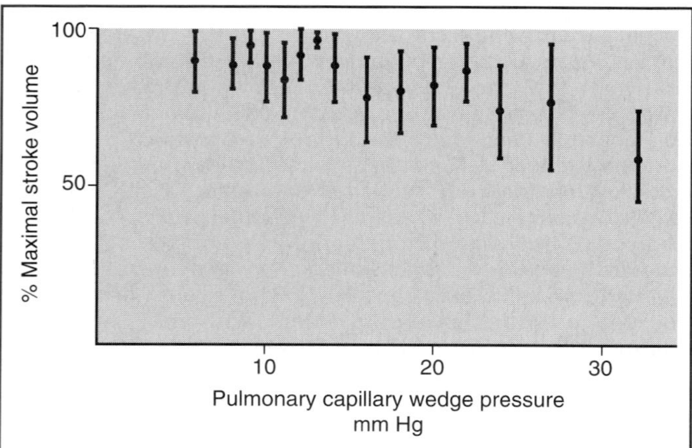

FIGURE 17–9. Maintenance of stroke volume with decreasing pulmonary capillary wedge pressures in 25 patients with advanced heart failure (average left-ventricular ejection fraction 18 per cent) presenting with clinical decompensation (initial average pulmonary capillary wedge pressure 31 ± 5 mm Hg, cardiac index 1.9 ± 4 liters/min/m^2). For each patient, the highest stroke volume measured was compared with that achieved with each pulmonary capillary wedge pressure achieved during therapy with intravenous nitroprusside and diuretics. (From Stevenson, L. W., and Tillisch, J. H.: Maintenance of cardiac output with normal filling pressures in dilated heart failure. Circulation *74*:1303, 1986; with permission.)

TABLE 17–5 PRINCIPLES OF HEART FAILURE MANAGEMENT BASED ON HEMODYNAMIC MONITORING

1. **Measurement of baseline hemodynamics**
2. **Intravenous nitroprusside and diuretics tailored to hemodynamic goals:**
   Pulmonary capillary wedge pressure ≤ 15 mm Hg
   Systemic vascular resistance ≤ 1000-1200 dynes-sec-cm^{-5}
   Right atrial pressure ≤ 7 mm Hg
   Systolic blood pressure ≥ 80 mm Hg
3. **Above hemodynamic goals achieved by 24 to 48 hours**
4. **Titration of high-dose oral vasodilators as nitroprusside weaned:**
   ACE inhibitor, isosorbide dinitrate
   Addition or substitution of hydralazine, if necessary
5. **Monitored ambulation and diuretic adjustment for 24 to 48 hours**
6. **Maintenance of digoxin levels at 1.0 to 1.5 ng/ml if no contraindication**
7. **Detailed patient education including salt and fluid restriction**
8. **Flexible outpatient diuretic regimen including occasional metolazone**
9. **Progressive walking or other exercise program**
10. **Vigilant follow-up**

ACE = angiotensin-converting enzyme.

The advantages of hemodynamic monitoring include the ability to alter both systemic vascular resistance and filling pressures simultaneously and safely. In the patient with a severely impaired left ventricle, refractory congestion often cannot be relieved by diuretics until the systemic vascular resistance is also effectively reduced. Intravenous nitroprusside is usually effective for improving hemodynamics in patients in whom the systemic vascular resistance is severely elevated and filling pressures are high, even in the presence of low systemic blood pressure.[156] Intravenous nitroprusside can be initiated at 20 μg/min (not per kilogram) titrating up to 200 to 300 μg/min as needed to reduce the systemic vascular resistance. Less commonly, the use of dobutamine may be required to improve cardiac output sufficiently to initiate vasodilation and diuresis.

Optimal hemodynamics are usually achieved within 48 hours of the aggressive institution of intravenous medications (see Table 17–5). Adjustment of oral vasodilators is performed under continuous hemodynamic monitoring, with oral diuretic doses estimated once the patient is considered to be euvolemic. Tailoring of therapy has allowed hospital discharge for almost 90 per cent of patients initially considered to be refractory to oral medical therapy. The sustained benefit of this approach has been demonstrated in terms of hemodynamic status, reduction of mitral regurgitation, freedom from congestive symptoms, improved exercise capacity, and reduced rehospitalizations.[155,158] Close outpatient supervision demonstrates clinical stability at one month in 60 to 70 per cent of patients undergoing tailored therapy for refractory heart failure, most of whom have been referred initially as potential candidates for transplantation.[159] As outlined in the

Bethesda guidelines for evaluation for cardiac transplantation: "Patients should not be considered to have *refractory* hemodynamic decompensation until therapy with intravenous followed by oral vasodilators and diuretic agents has been pursued using continuous hemodynamic monitoring to approach hemodynamic goals."[160]

Additional Considerations

The indications for anticoagulation in heart failure remain controversial (see p. 1988). In patients with Class II and III heart failure from the V-HeFT II trial,[6] the incidence of embolic events was 2.1/100 patient years, with 12 per cent of patients receiving anticoagulants. In ambulatory Class III and IV patients awaiting transplantation, the incidence was 3 per cent over an average follow-up of 301 days, with 37 per cent of patients receiving anticoagulation.[164] Anticoagulation is uniformly recommended in heart failure accompanied by atrial fibrillation or a history of embolic events, and considered in the presence of a mobile intracardiac thrombus. The risk/benefit ratio of anticoagulation for other patients with heart failure is unlikely to be defined in a randomized trial due to the low incidence of endpoints.

High-dose loop diuretics such as furosemide, bumetamide, and torsemide, with or without additional diuretics acting more distally (such as metolazone), may be used in patients with refractory heart failure. Ultrafiltration may be considered in patients with late-stage heart failure resistant to conventional treatment (see p. 480). Cheyne-Stokes respiration with severe sleep hypoxemia occurs relatively commonly in advanced heart failure. Supplemental oxygen therapy at night reduces Cheyne-Stokes respiration, correcting hypoxemia, and improves sleep by reducing arousals caused by the hyperpneic phase of the Cheyne-Stokes cycle.[161] Continuous positive airway pressure (CPAP) has been advocated as well in this setting.[162,163] In patients who do not have evidence of resting congestion but remain severely limited, a careful trial of exercise training may improve peak functional capacity by 20 per cent and lengthen submaximal exercise duration.[164]

Reestablishment of hemodynamic compensation with intravenous dobutamine and/or nitroprusside therapy often allows the reintroduction of ACE inhibitors that are not tolerated when angiotensin II is necessary to support arterial pressure in patients with a failing circulation. As oral vasodilators are substituted for intravenous agents after recompensation, the doses necessary to provide optimal loading conditions can be defined. Some patients, typically those with severe hyponatremia, develop symptomatic hypotension with very small (3 mg) doses of captopril, whereas others require doses as high as 100 mg every 6 hours. Patients who have not been stable on single vasodilators frequently demonstrate better hemodynamic responses to combination therapy, which may include nitrates and hydralazine in addition to or in place of ACE inhibitors.[7] Therapy can best be adjusted to meet the hemodynamic goals using agents with relatively rapid onset and short duration of action. Longer-acting inotrope vasodilators, such as milrinone or amrinone, may occasionally be necessary for prolonged intravenous support but patients are not easily weaned from these during titration of oral vasodilators. For similar reasons, captopril is the easiest drug to titrate acutely but can often be exchanged for longer-acting ACE inhibitors after patients have demonstrated stability at home.

SELECTION OF CANDIDATES FOR CARDIAC TRANSPLANTATION

(See also Chap. 18)

As the results of cardiac transplantation have improved to offer over 60 per cent survival after 6 years,[165] the pool of potential candidates has expanded to include patients with less immediate compromise and patients with conditions such as diabetes, who would once have been considered to have an absolute contraindication. At the same time, however, advances in medical therapy and revascularization procedures have challenged previous assumptions about when heart failure becomes "end-stage," allowing many patients once thought to need transplantation to maintain good quality of life without it, at least for a period of time. Current selection practice focuses on the identification of patients who truly have no option except transplantation and the selection of those patients who are most likely to derive major benefit in terms of both quality of life and survival.

INDICATIONS. Heart failure is the primary indication for cardiac transplantation. After potentially reversible factors, including myocardial ischemia, have been addressed, and the medical regimen has been optimized, the potential candidate for transplantation is evaluated in terms of an estimated 1-year mortality, which should generally exceed 25 to 50 per cent without transplantation.[166] The limitation of donor supply and of life span after transplantation require that indications for transplantation include a clearly improved early prognosis with transplantation.

Presentation with New York Heart Association Class IV symptoms is no longer sufficient indication for cardiac transplantation, as many patients respond favorably to redesign of their medical regimen during their evaluation for transplantation. Patients requiring continuing or repeated hospitalization to maintain hemodynamic compensation despite optimal medical management are considered to meet indications for transplantation without other functional assessment and are evaluated primarily for contraindications. The challenge is to identify from the population of ambulatory patients with heart failure those in greatest need of transplantation. Although survival of patients with severe heart failure on optimal management has improved, almost one-half of patients discharged after initial evaluation with Class IV symptoms will come to urgent transplantation or death within the next 2 years.[167] A left ventricular ejection fraction of 20 to 25 per cent was at one time also considered to be necessary and sufficient indication for transplantation. However, many patients with such values may exhibit a stable course when receiving optimal medical management.

Peak oxygen consumption ($\dot{V}_{O_2}$) in the ambulatory heart failure population (Fig. 5–21, p. 172) does provide a useful predictor of both mortality with heart failure and functional benefit from cardiac transplantation.[168] Measured through a mouthpiece and gas analyzer during bicycle or treadmill exercise, the peak $\dot{V}_{O_2}$ reflects cardiac reserve, integrative circulatory response, and the degree of peripheral muscle conditioning or deconditioning. Synthesis of several large experiences[166–168] yields a consensus that a peak $\dot{V}_{O_2}$ less than 10 to 12 ml/kg/min (the level required for walking and light household activity) confers a particularly poor prognosis, with 1-year mortality in the range of 50 per cent. Peak $\dot{V}_{O_2}$ exceeding 16 to 18 ml/kg/min (almost adequate for jogging) identifies a group of patients with a 2-year survival of over 80 per cent. This then leaves a middle group with a peak $\dot{V}_{O_2}$ of 12 to 16 ml/kg/min within which decisions regarding transplantation must be further refined by other factors, as well as by the patient's preference. For this intermediate group, the decision to proceed to transplantation must take into account the needs and resources of the individual patient. For example, although survival benefits from transplantation are predicted, many patients are not willing to accept the burdens of immunosuppression, biopsies, and intensive medical follow-up unless accompanied by a substantial improvement in the quality of life.

Quantification of functional capacity using peak $\dot{V}_{O_2}$ not only provides a valuable prognostic index but also allows

TABLE 17–6 SUMMARY OF GENERAL RECOMMENDATIONS: BETHESDA CONFERENCE ON CARDIAC TRANSPLANTATION

Functional status should not be assessed until patients have undergone aggressive therapy with combinations of vasodilators and diuretic agents. "Therapy should be adjusted until clinical congestion has been resolved or until further therapy has been repeatedly limited by severe hypotension (generally systolic blood pressure < 80 mm Hg) or marked azotemia. Patients should not be considered to have *refractory* hemodynamic decompensation until therapy with intravenous followed by oral vasodilators and diuretic agents has been pursued using continuous hemodynamic monitoring to approach hemodynamic goals."

SELECTION CRITERIA FOR BENEFITS FROM TRANSPLANTATION

I. Accepted Indications for Transplantation
1. Peak $\dot{V}_{O_2}$ < 10 ml/kg/min with achievement of anaerobic metabolism
2. Severe ischemia consistently limiting routine activity not amenable to bypass surgery or angioplasty
3. Recurrent symptomatic ventricular arrhythmias refractory to all accepted therapeutic modalities

II. Probable Indications for Cardiac Transplantation
1. Peak $\dot{V}_{O_2}$ < 14 mg/kg/min and major limitation of the patient's daily activities
2. Recurrent unstable ischemia not amenable to bypass or angioplasty
3. Instability of fluid balance/renal function not due to patient noncompliance with regimen of weight monitoring, flexible use of diuretic drugs and salt restriction

III. Inadequate Indications for Transplantation
1. Ejection fraction ≤ 20 per cent
2. History of functional Class III or IV symptoms of heart failure
3. Previous ventricular arrhythmias
4. Peak $\dot{V}_{O_2}$ > 15 m/kg/min without other indications

From Mudge, G. H., Goldstein, S., Addonizio, L. J., et al.: Cardiac transplantation: Recipient guidelines/prioritization. Reprinted with permission from the American College of Cardiology. J. Am. Coll. Cardiol. *22*:21, 1993.

comparison between pretransplant heart failure status and posttransplant status in recipients. Although the left ventricular ejection fraction is usually normal after transplantation, cardiac reserve is markedly limited. Many other factors, such as hypertension and the systemic effects of corticosteroids, also impair physical capacity. Most cardiac transplant recipients achieve a peak $\dot{V}_{O_2}$ in the range of 15 to 18 ml/kg/min, or 50 to 70 per cent of predicted, which is similar to that achieved by many patients with stable heart failure.[159] For comparison, the average healthy middle-aged man has a predicted maximal oxygen consumption of 25 to 35 ml/kg/min.

Considering both survival and functional benefits, very low peak $\dot{V}_{O_2}$ (≤10 ml/kg/min) is sufficient indication for transplantation in a patient on optimal therapy without contraindications (Table 17–6). Patients with higher peak oxygen consumption may still need transplantation for conditions such as recurrent severe myocardial ischemia not amenable to revascularization or refractory symptomatic ventricular arrhythmias. Although heart failure leading to cardiac transplantation is usually secondary to ischemic or idiopathic cardiomyopathy with a dilated left ventricle and depressed ejection fraction, these are neither necessary nor sufficient indications. Patients in New York Heart Association Class IV with restrictive cardiomyopathy, in which the left ventricle is minimally dilated and the ejection fraction is 30 to 40 per cent may be candidates for transplantation. Hypertrophic cardiomyopathy rarely requires transplantation when still in the hypercontractile stage during which drug therapy, pacemaker therapy, and other surgical options should be used. In the small percentage of patients in whom hypertrophic cardiomyopathy has become "burned out," congestive symptoms and exercise intolerance may become severe with only modest reductions in left ventricular ejection fraction.

CONTRAINDICATIONS (see Table 18–1, p. 516).

THE WAITING LIST FOR TRANSPLANTATION. The waiting list for cardiac transplantation continues to lengthen, as more than twice as many patients are listed monthly in the United States than actually receive donor hearts.[169] In 1984, there were 37 centers performing cardiac transplantation in the United States. The average waiting time was 6 weeks, and each center could identify the candidate in the greatest need when a donor heart became available. In 1994, there were 151 programs competing for donor hearts in the United States, which are distributed through the United Network of Organ Sharing (UNOS) according to priority and to time on the list.[170] In the United States, priority (Status I) is accorded first to hospitalized patients requiring

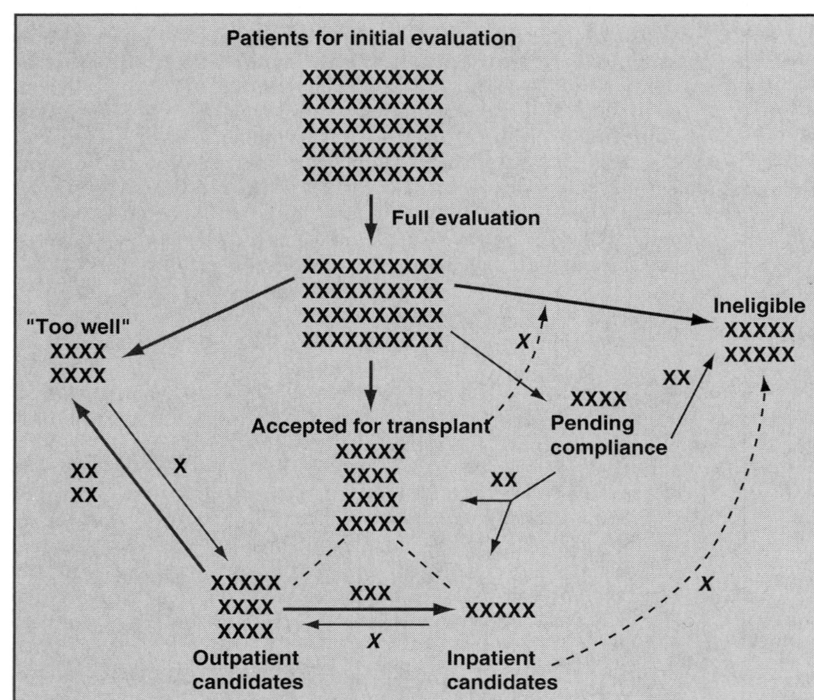

FIGURE 17–10. Diagram demonstrating dynamic nature of candidacy for transplantation. Patients may be "too well" at initial referral or as a result of improvement while on the waiting list. Accepted candidates may deteriorate from outpatient to critical status. One of the benefits of a combined heart failure transplant treatment and education program is the opportunity for ongoing assessment of compliance with a heart failure regimen that frequently allows eventual acceptance of patients previously considered ineligible due to noncompliance. Density of x's gives a semiquantitative estimate of patient flow.

TABLE 17–7 CRITERIA FOR CLINICAL STABILITY IN CANDIDATES AWAITING TRANSPLANTATION

Clinical Criteria
1. Stable fluid balance without orthopnea, elevated jugular venous pressure, or other evidence of congestion on the flexible diuretic regimen
2. Stable blood pressure with systolic pressure ≥ 80 mm Hg
3. Stable serum sodium concentration and renal function
4. Absence of symptomatic ventricular arrhythmias
5. Absence of frequent angina
6. Absence of severe drug side effects
7. Stable or improving activity level without dyspnea during self-care or 1 block exertion
Exercise Criteria (if initial peak $\dot{V}_{O_2}$ < 14 ml/kg/min)
1. Improvement in peak oxygen consumption of ≥ 2 ml/kg/min
2. Peak oxygen consumption ≥ 12 ml/kg/min

assist devices or intravenous inotropic therapy in intensive care units. All other patients are Status II, except in some regions in which variances exist allowing intermediate priority among hospitalized patients. Currently, over half of all transplanted hearts are distributed to hospitalized patients.

The average waiting time for patients at home is currently over 18 months and continues to lengthen. Sudden death occurs in 10 to 20 per cent of patients on the waiting list during this time.[111–112] A slightly higher proportion develop deterioration of cardiac function sufficient to require continued hospitalization until transplantation. Hospitalization may be indicated either to prevent imminent death or deterioration that would significantly increase perioperative mortality from transplantation. The approach to the hospitalized candidate with refractory heart failure includes hemodynamic monitoring to optimize supportive therapy as outlined above. Prolonged infusions of dobutamine, dopamine, or phosphodiesterase inhibitors may support patients in the hospital or occasionally at home, until transplantation. The need for more potent agents such as epinephrine should raise consideration of mechanical support devices as a bridge to transplantation (see pp. 517 and 538).

Clinical improvement may also occur while patients are on a waiting list. The highest risk of death is in the first 6 months after listing, after which some factors causing deterioration before referral may resolve and the benefits of optimized medical therapy may be realized. Ambulatory patients on the waiting list require periodic reevaluation, during which both clinical stability and functional capacity are assessed (Table 17–7). Up to 30 per cent of ambulatory transplant candidates may later meet criteria for stability and leave the active waiting list, with subsequent 2-year survival and exercise performance equivalent to that after cardiac transplantation.[171] Candidacy for transplantation is increasingly considered to be a dynamic state (Fig. 17–10).

Although cardiac transplantation was greeted in 1968 as a solution to the problem of end-stage heart failure,[172] the inevitable disparity between the donor supply and demand severely limits the application of this procedure. Implantable left ventricular devices (Chap. 19) provide not only bridges but eventually alternatives to transplantation and may thus lead to major revision of current criteria for selection and reevaluation of candidates for transplantation.

REFERENCES

THERAPEUTIC STRATEGY FOR MANAGEMENT OF HEART FAILURE

1. Williams, J. F., Jr., Bristow, M. R., Fowler, M. B., et al.: Guidelines for the evaluation and management of heart failure. Report of the American College of Cardiology/American Heart Association Task Force on Practical Guidelines (Committee on Evaluation and Management of Heart Failure). J. Am. Coll. Cardiol. *26*:1376, 1995.

1a. Cohn, J. N.: Structural basis for heart failure. Ventricular remodeling and its pharmacological inhibition. Circulation *91*:2504, 1995.

2. Pfeffer, M. A.: ACE inhibition in acute myocardial infarction. N. Engl. J. Med. *332*:118, 1995.

3. CONSENSUS Trial Study Group: Effects of enalapril on mortality in severe congestive heart failure. Results of the Cooperative North Scandinavian Enalapril Survival Group (CONSENSUS). N. Engl. J. Med. *316*:1429, 1987.

4. SOLVD Investigators: Effect of enalapril on survival in patients with reduced left ventricular ejection fractions and congestive heart failure. N. Engl. J. Med. *325*:293, 1991.

VASODILATORS

5. SOLVD Investigators: Effect of enalapril on mortality and the development of heart failure in asymptomatic patients with reduced left ventricular ejection fractions. N. Engl. J. Med. *327*:685, 1992.

6. Cohn, J. N., Johnson, G., Ziesche, S., et al.: A comparison of enalapril with hydralazine-isosorbide dinitrate in the treatment of chronic congestive heart failure. N. Engl. J. Med. *325*:303, 1991.

7. Fonarow, G. C., Chelimsky-Fallick, C., Stevenson, L. W., et al.: Effect of direct vasodilation with hydralazine versus angiotensin-converting enzyme inhibition with captopril on mortality in advanced heart failure: The Hy-C trial. J. Am. Coll. Cardiol. *19*:842, 1992.

8. Pfeffer, M. A., Braunwald, E., Moye, L. A., et al.: Effect of captopril on mortality and morbidity in patients with left ventricular dysfunction after myocardial infarction. N. Engl. J. Med. *327*:669, 1992.

9. Rutherford, J. D., Pfeffer, M. A., Moye, L. A., et al.: Effects of captopril on ischemic events after myocardial infarction. Results of the survival and ventricular enlargement trial. Circulation *90*:1731, 1994.

10. Konstam, M. A., Rousseau, M. F., Kronenberg, M. W., et al.: Effects of the angiotensin converting enzyme inhibitor enalapril on the long-term progression of left ventricular dysfunction in patients with heart failure. Circulation *86*:431, 1992.

11. St. John Sutton, M., Pfeffer, M. A., Plappert, T., et al.: Quantitative two-dimensional echocardiographic measurements are major predictors of adverse cardiovascular events after acute myocardial infarction. The protective effects of captopril. Circulation *89*:68, 1994.

12. Acute Infarction Ramipril Efficacy (AIRE) Study Investigators: Effect of ramipril on mortality and morbidity of survivors of acute myocardial infarction with clinical evidence of heart failure. Lancet *342*:821, 1993.

13. Kober, L., Torp-Pedersen, C., Carlsen, C., et al.: A clinical trial of the ACE inhibitor trandolapril in patients with left ventricular dysfunction after myocardial infarction. N. Engl. J. Med. *333*:1670, 1995.

14. Pitt, B.: Use of "xapril" in patients with chronic heart failure. A paradigm or epitaph for our times? Circulation *90*:1550, 1994.

15. Gruppo Italiano per lo Studio della Sopravvivenza nell'Infarto Miocardico. GISSI-3 Investigators: Effects of lisinopril and transdermal glyceryl trinitrate singly and together on 6-week mortality and ventricular function after acute myocardial infarction. Lancet *343*:1115, 1994.

16. Ambrosioni, E., Borghi, C., and Magnani, B., for the Survival of Myocardial Infarction Long-Term Evaluation (SMILE) Study Investigators: The effect of the angiotensin-converting-enzyme inhibitor zofenopril on mortality and morbidity after anterior myocardial infarction. N. Engl. J. Med. *332*:80, 1995.

17. Cohn, J. N.: Treatment of infarct related heart failure: Vasodilators other than ACE inhibitors. Cardiovasc. Drug Ther. *8*:119, 1994.

18. Yusuf, S., Garg, R., and McConachie, D.: Effect of angiotensin-converting enzyme inhibitors in left ventricular dysfunction: Results of the studies of left ventricular dysfunction in the context of other similar trials. J. Cardiovasc. Pharmacol. *22*:S28, 1993.

19. Lonn, E. M., Yusuf, S., Jha, P., et al.: Emerging role of angiotensin-converting enzyme inhibitors in cardiac and vascular protection. Circulation *90*:2056, 1994.

20. Paul, S. D., Kuntz, K. M., Eagle, K. A., et al.: Costs and effectiveness of enzyme inhibition in patients with heart failure. Arch. Intern. Med. *154*:1143, 1994.

21. Rogers, W. J., Johnstone, D. E., Yusuf, S., et al.: Quality of life among 5025 patients with left ventricular dysfunction randomized between placebo and enalapril: The studies of left ventricular dysfunction. J. Am. Coll. Cardiol. *23*:393, 1994.

22. Northridge, D. B., Rose, E., Raftery, E. D., et al.: A multicentre, double-blind, placebo-controlled trial of quinapril in mild, chronic heart failure. Eur. Heart J. *14*:403, 1993.

23. Rector, T. S., Johnson, G., Dunkman, W. B., for the V-HeFT VA Cooperative Studies Group: Evaluation by patients with heart failure of the effects of enalapril compared with hydralazine plus isosorbide dinitrate on quality of life. Circulation *87* (Suppl. VI):71, 1993.

24. Varriale, P., David, W., and Chryssos, B. E.: Hemodynamic response to intravenous enalaprilat in patients with severe congestive heart failure and mitral regurgitation. Clin. Cardiol. *16*:235, 1993.

25. Seneviratne, B., Moore, G. A., and West, P. D.: Effect of captopril on functional mitral regurgitation in dilated heart failure: A randomized double blind placebo controlled trial. Br. Heart J. *72*:63, 1994.

26. Lin, M., Chiang, H.-T., Lin, S.-L., et al.: Vasodilator therapy in chronic asymptomatic aortic regurgitation: Enalapril versus hydralazine therapy. J. Am. Coll. Cardiol. *24*:1046, 1994.

27. Schon, H. R.: Hemodynamic and morphologic changes after long-term angiotensin converting enzyme inhibition in patients with chronic valvular regurgitation. J. Hypertens. *12*:95, 1994.

28. Kostis, J. B., Shelton, B. J., Yusuf, S., et al.: Tolerability of enalapril initiation by patients with left ventricular dysfunction: Results of the

medication challenge phase of the studies of left ventricular dysfunction. Am. Heart J. *128:*358, 1994.

29. Lang, R. M., DiBianco, R., Broderick, G. T., et al.: First-dose effects of enalapril 2.5 mg and captopril 6.25 mg in patients with heart failure: A double-blind, randomized, multicenter study. Am. Heart J. *128:*551, 1994.
30. Squire, I. B., MacFadyen, R. J., Lees, K. R., et al.: Hemodynamic response and pharmacokinetics after the first dose of quinapril in patients with congestive heart failure. Br. J. Clin. Pharmacol. *38:*117, 1994.
31. Nussberger, J., Fleck, E., Bahrmann, H., et al.: Dose-related effects of ACE inhibition in man: Quinapril in patients with moderate congestive heart failure. Eur. Heart J. *15:*113, 1994.
32. Reid, J. L., MacFadyen, R. J., Squire, I. B., and Lees, K. R.: Blood pressure response to the first dose of angiotensin-converting enzyme inhibitors in congestive heart failure. Am. J. Cardiol. *71:*57, 1993.
33. Israili, Z. H., and Hall, W. D.: Cough and angioneurotic edema associated with angiotensin-converting enzyme inhibitor therapy. Ann. Intern. Med. *117:*234, 1992.
34. Ravid, D., Lishner, M., Lang, R., and Ravid, M.: Angiotensin-converting enzyme inhibitors and cough: A prospective evaluation in hypertension and in congestive heart failure. J. Clin. Pharmacol. *34:*1116, 1994.
35. Andersson, R. G. G., and Persson, K.: ACE inhibitors and their influence on inflammation, bronchial reactivity and cough. Eur. Heart J. *15:*52, 1994.
36. Hargreaves, M. R., and Benson, M. K.: Inhaled sodium cromoglycate in angiotensin-converting enzyme inhibitor cough. Lancet *345:*13, 1995.
37. Heesch, C. M., Hatfield, B. A., Marcoux, L., and Eichhorn, E. J.: Predictors of pressure and stroke volume response to afterload reduction with nitroprusside in patients with congestive heart failure secondary to idiopathic dilated cardiomyopathy. Am. J. Cardiol. *74:*951, 1994.
38. Risoe, C., Simonsen, S., Rootwelt, K., et al.: Nitroprusside and regional vascular capacitance in patients with severe congestive heart failure. Circulation *85:*997, 1992.
39. Haas, G. J., and Leier, C. V.: Vasodilators. *In* Hosenpud, J. D., and Greenberg, G. H. (eds.): Congestive Heart Failure. New York, Springer-Verlag, 1994, p. 400.
40. Cohn, J. N., Archibald, D. G., Ziesche, S., et al.: Effect of vasodilator therapy on mortality in chronic congestive heart failure. Results of a Veterans Administration Cooperative Study. N. Engl. J. Med. *314:*1547, 1986.
41. Massie, B. M., Packer, M., Hanlon, J. T., and Combs, D. T.: Hemodynamic responses to combined therapy with captopril and hydralazine in patients with severe heart failure. J. Am. Coll. Cardiol. *2:*338, 1983.

DIURETICS

41a. Cody, R. J.: Clinical trials of diuretic therapy in heart failure: Research directions and clinical considerations. J. Am. Coll. Cardiol. *22:*165A, 1993.
42. Bigger, J. T., Jr.: Diuretic therapy, hypertension, and cardiac arrest. N. Engl. J. Med. *330:*1899, 1994.
43. Siscovick, D. S., Raghunathan, T. E., Psaty, B. M., et al.: Diuretic therapy for hypertension and the risk of primary cardiac arrest. N. Engl. J. Med. *330:*1852, 1994.
44. Silke, B.: Diuretic induced changes in symptoms and quality of life. Br. Heart J. *72:*57, 1994.
45. Freis, E. D.: The efficacy and safety of diuretics in treating hypertension. Ann. Intern. Med. *122:*223, 1995.
45a. Jackson, E. K.: Diuretics. *In* Hardman, J. G., et al. (eds.): Goodman & Gilman's: The pharmacological basis of therapeutics. 9th ed. New York, McGraw-Hill, 1996, pp. 199–248.
46. Leier, C. V., Dei Cas, L., and Metra, M.: Clinical relevance and management of the major electrolyte abnormalities in congestive heart failure: Hyponatremia, hypokalemia, and hypomagnesemia. Am. Heart J. *128:*564, 1994.
47. Lahav, M., Regev, A., Ra'anani, P., and Theodor, E.: Intermittent administration of furosemide vs continuous infusion preceded by a loading dose for congestive heart failure. Chest *102:*725, 1992.
48. McMurray, J., and McDevitt, D. G.: Treatment of heart failure in the elderly. Br. Med. Bull. *46:*202, 1990.

DIGITALIS

49. Christian, H. A.: Digitalis effects in chronic cardiac cases with regular rhythm in contrast to auricular fibrillation. Med. Clin. North Am. *5:*117, 1922.
50. Kelly, R. A., and Smith, T. W.: Digoxin in heart failure: Implications of recent trials. J. Am. Coll. Cardiol. *22:*107, 1993.
51. Tauke, J., Goldstein, S., and Gheorghiade, M.: Digoxin for chronic heart failure: A review of the randomized controlled trials with special attention to the PROVED and RADIANCE trials. Prog. Cardiovasc. Dis. *37:*49, 1994.
52. Uretsky, B. F., Young, J. B., Shahidi, F. E., et al.: Randomized study assessing the effect of digoxin withdrawal in patients with mild to moderate chronic congestive heart failure: Results of the PROVED trial. J. Am. Coll. Cardiol. *22:*955, 1993.
53. Packer, M., Gheorghiade, M., Young, J. B., et al.: Withdrawal of digoxin from patients with chronic heart failure treated with angiotensin-converting enzyme inhibitors. N. Engl. J. Med. *329:*1, 1993.
54. Smith, T. W.: Digoxin in heart failure. N. Engl. J. Med. *329:*51, 1993.
55. van Veldhuisen, K. J., Man in 'T Veld, A. J., Dunselman, H. J., et al.: Double-blind placebo-controlled study of ibopamine and digoxin in patients with mild to moderate heart failure: Results of the Dutch Ibopamine Multicenter Trial (DIMT). J. Am. Coll. Cardiol. *22:*1564, 1993.
56. Yusuf, S., Garg, R., Held, P., et al.: Need for a large randomized trial to evaluate the effects of digitalis on morbidity and mortality in congestive heart failure. Am. J. Cardiol. *69:*64, 1992.
57. Digoxin Investigators' Group: The effect of digoxin on mortality and hospitalizations in patients with heart failure. Presentation at the 45th Annual Scientific Sessions, American College of Cardiology, Orlando, FL, March, 1996.
58. Lown, B., and Levine, S. A.: The carotid sinus: Clinical value of its stimulation. Circulation *23:*766, 1961.
59. Kelly, R. A.: Cardiac glycosides and congestive heart failure. Am. J. Cardiol. *65:*33, 1990.
60. Friedman, P. L.: Therapeutic and toxic electrophysiologic effects of cardiac glycosides. *In* Smith, T. W. (ed.): Digitalis Glycosides. Orlando, Grune & Stratton, 1985, p. 29.
61. Seelig, M.: Cardiovascular consequences of magnesium deficiency and loss: Pathogenesis, prevalence and manifestations: Magnesium and chloride loss in refractory potassium repletion. Am. J. Cardiol. *63:*4, 1989.
62. Cronin, R. E.: Magnesium disorders. *In* Kokko, J. P., and Tannen, R. L. (eds.): Fluids and Electrolytes. 2nd ed. Philadelphia, W. B. Saunders Company, 1990, p. 631.
63. Dorup, I., Skajaa, K., Clausen, T., and Kjeldsen, K.: Reduced concentrations of potassium, magnesium, and sodium-potassium pumps in human skeletal muscle during treatment with diuretics. Br. Med. J. *296:*455, 1988.
64. Gottlieb, S. S., Baruch, L., Kukin, M. L., et al.: Prognostic importance of the serum magnesium concentration in patients with congestive heart failure. J. Am. Coll. Cardiol. *16:*827, 1990.
65. Ralston, M. A., Murnane, M. R., Unverferth, D. V., and Leier, C. V.: Serum and tissue magnesium concentrations in patients with heart failure and serious ventricular arrhythmias. Ann. Intern. Med. *113:*841, 1990.
66. Gottlieb, S. S.: Importance of magnesium in congestive heart failure. Am. J. Cardiol. *63:*39, 1989.
67. Leier, C. V., Dei Cas, L., and Metra, M.: Clinical relevance and management of the major electrolyte abnormalities in congestive heart failure: Hyponatremia, hypokalemia, and hypomagnesemia. Am. Heart J. *128:*564, 1994.
68. Davies, D. L., and Fraser, R.: Do diuretics cause magnesium deficiency? Br. J. Clin. Pharmacol. *36:*1, 1993.
69. Smith, T. W., and Willerson, J. T.: Suicidal and accidental digoxin ingestion: Report of five cases with serum digoxin level correlations. Circulation *44:*29, 1971.
70. Smith, T. W., Butler, V. P., Jr., Haber, E., et al.: Treatment of life-threatening digitalis intoxication with digoxin-specific Fab fragments: Experience in 26 cases. N. Engl. J. Med. *307:*1357, 1982.
71. Rubinow, A., Skinner, M., and Cohen, A. S.: Digoxin sensitivity in amyloid cardiomyopathy. Circulation *63:*1285, 1981.
72. Braunwald, E.: 13th Bowditch Lecture. The determinants of myocardial oxygen consumption. The Physiologist *12:*65, 1969.
73. Glancy, D. L., Higgs, L. M., O'Brien, K. P., and Epstein, S. E.: Effects of ouabain on the left ventricular response to exercise in patients with angina pectoris. Circulation *43:*45, 1971.
74. Vogel, R., Kirch, D., LeFree, M., et al.: Effects of digitalis on resting and isometric exercise myocardial perfusion in patients with coronary artery disease and left ventricular dysfunction. Circulation *56:*355, 1977.
75. Crawford, M. H., LeWinter, M. M., O'Rourke, R. A., et al.: Combined propranolol and digoxin therapy in angina pectoris. Ann. Intern. Med. *83:*449, 1975.
76. Ratshin, R. A., Rackley, C. E., and Russell, R. O., Jr.: Hemodynamic evaluation of left ventricular function in shock complicating myocardial infarction. Circulation *45:*127, 1972.
77. Rahimtoola, S. H., Sinno, M. Z., Chuquimia, R., et al.: Effects of ouabain on impaired left ventricular function in acute myocardial infarction. N. Engl. J. Med. *287:*527, 1972.
78. Rahimtoola, S. H., and Gunnar, R. M.: Digitalis in acute myocardial infarction: Help or hazard? Ann. Intern. Med. *82:*234, 1975.
79. Selzer, A.: The use of digitalis in acute myocardial infarction. Prog. Cardiovasc. Dis. *10:*518, 1968.
80. Croxson, M. S., and Ibbertson, H. K.: Serum digoxin in patients with thyroid disease. Br. Med. J. *3:*566, 1975.
81. Curfman, G. D., Crowley, T. J., and Smith, T. W.: Thyroid-induced alterations in myocardial sodium- and potassium-activated adenosine triphosphatase, monovalent cation active transport, and cardiac glycoside binding. J. Clin. Invest. *59:*586, 1977.
82. Kim, D., and Smith, T. W.: Effects of thyroid hormone on sodium pump sites, sodium content, and contractile responses to cardiac glycosides in cultured chick ventricular cells. J. Clin. Invest. *74:*1481, 1984.
83. Green, L. H., and Smith, T. W.: The use of digitalis in patients with pulmonary disease. Ann. Intern. Med. *87:*459, 1977.
84. Beller, G. A., Smith, T. W., Abelmann, W. H., et al.: Digitalis intoxication: Prospective clinical study with serum level correlations. N. Engl. J. Med. *284:*989, 1971.
84a. Hoffman, B. B., and Lefkowitz, R. J.: Catecholamines, sympathomimetic drugs, and adrenergic receptor antagonists. *In* Hardman, J. G., et al.

(eds.): Goodman & Gilman's: The pharmacological basis of therapeutics. 9th ed. New York: McGraw-Hill, 1996, pp. 685–714.

INTRAVENOUS SYMPATHOMIMETIC AGENTS

85. Teboul, J.-L., Graini, L., Boujdaria, F., et al.: Cardiac index vs oxygen-derived parameters for rational use of dobutamine in patients with congestive heart failure. Chest *103:*81, 1993.
86. Sacher, H. L., Sacher, M. L., Landau, S. W., et al.: Outpatient dobutamine therapy: The rhyme and the riddle. J. Clin. Pharmacol. *32:*141, 1992.
87. Miller, L. W.: Outpatient dobutamine for refractory congestive heart failure: Advantages, techniques, and results. J. Heart Lung Transplant. *10:*482, 1991.
88. DeBroux, E., Lagace, G., Dumont, L., and Chartrand, C.: Efficacy of dobutamine in the failing transplanted heart. J. Heart Lung Transplant. *11:*1133, 1992.
89. Levy, D. K., Schwartz, J. M., Frishman, W. H., et al.: Ischemic hepatitis in a patient with congestive cardiomyopathy: An innovative approach to therapy using intravenous dobutamine. J. Clin. Pharmacol. *34:*270, 1994.
90. Thuillez, Ch., Richard, Ch., Teboul, J. L., et al.: Arterial hemodynamics and cardiac effects of enoximone, dobutamine, and their combination in severe heart failure. Am. Heart J. *125:*799, 1993.
91. Vendegna, T. R., and Anderson, R. J.: Are dopamine and/or dobutamine renoprotective in intensive care unit patients? Crit. Care Med. *22:*1893, 1994.
92. Thompson, B. T., and Cockrill, B. A.: Renal-dose dopamine: A siren song? Lancet *344:*7, 1994.
93. Duke, G. J., Briedis, J. H., and Weaver, R. A.: Renal support in critically ill patients: Low-dose dopamine or low-dose dobutamine? Crit. Care Med. *22:*1919, 1994.
94. Flancbaum, L., Choban, P. S., and Dasta, J. F.: Quantitative effects of low-dose dopamine on urine output in oliguric surgical intensive care unit patients. Crit. Care Med. *22:*61, 1994.
95. Baldwin, L., Henderson, A., and Hickman, P.: Effect of postoperative low-dose dopamine on renal function after elective major vascular surgery. Ann. Intern. Med. *120:*744, 1994.

NEWER INOTROPIC AGENTS

96. Packer, M.: The development of positive inotropic agents for chronic heart failure: How have we gone astray? J. Am. Coll. Cardiol. *22:*119, 1993.
97. DiBianco, R., Shabetai, R., Kostik, W., et al.: A comparison of oral milrinone, digoxin, and their combination in the treatment of patients with chronic heart failure. N. Engl. J. Med. *320:*677, 1989.
97a. Karlsberg, R. P., DeWood, M. A., DeMaria, A. N., et al.: Comparative efficacy of short-term intravenous infusions of milrinone and dobutamine in acute congestive heart failure following acute myocardial infarction. Clin. Cardiol. *19:*21, 1996.
98. Feldman, A. M., Bristow, M. R., Parmley, W. W., et al.: Effects of vesnarinone on morbidity and mortality in patients with heart failure. N. Engl. J. Med. *329:*149, 1993.

BETA-ADRENERGIC ANTAGONISTS

99. Waagstein, F., Bristow, M. R., Swedberg, K., et al.: Beneficial effects of metoprolol in idiopathic dilated cardiomyopathy. Lancet *342:*1441, 1993.
100. CIBIS Investigators and Committees: A randomized trial of β-blockade in heart failure. The Cardiac Insufficiency Bisoprolol Study (CIBIS). Circulation *90:*1765, 1994.
101. Eichhorn, E. J., and Hjalmarson, A.: β-Blocker treatment for chronic heart failure. The frog prince. Circulation *90:*2153, 1994.
102. Fisher, M. L., Gottlieb, S. S., Plotnick, G. D., et al.: Beneficial effects of metoprolol in heart failure associated with coronary artery disease: A randomized trial. J. Am. Coll. Cardiol. *23:*943, 1994.
103. Hjalmarson, A., and Waagstein, F.: The role of β-blockers in the treatment of cardiomyopathy and ischemic heart failure. Drugs *47:*31, 1994.
104. Woodley, S. L., Gilbert, E. M., and Anderson, J. L.: β-Blockade with bucindolol in heart failure due to ischemic vs idiopathic dilated cardiomyopathy. Circulation *84:*2426, 1991.
105. Bristow, M. R., O'Connell, J. B., Gilbert, E. M., et al., for the Bucindolol Investigators: Dose-response of chronic β-blocker treatment in heart failure from either idiopathic dilated or ischemic cardiomyopathy. Circulation *89:*1632, 1994.
105a. Packer, M., Bristow, M., and Cohn, J. N.: Effect of carvedilol on the survival of patients with chronic heart failure. Circulation *92*(Suppl. I):142, 1995.
105b. Krum, H., Sackner-Bernstein, J. D., Goldsmith, R. L., et al.: Double-blind placebo-controlled study of the long-term efficacy of carvedilol in patients with severe chronic heart failure. Circulation *92:*1499, 1995.

HEART FAILURE WITH PREDOMINANT DIASTOLIC VENTRICULAR DYSFUNCTION

106. Levine, H. J., and Gaasch, W. H.: Clinical recognition and treatment of diastolic dysfunction and heart failure. *In* Gaasch, W. H., and LeWinter, M. M. (eds.): Left Ventricular Diastolic Dysfunction and Heart Failure. Philadelphia: Lea and Febiger, 1994, p. 445.
107. Villari, B., Vasalli, G., Monrad, E. S., Chiariello, M., Turina, M., and Hess, O. M.: Normalization of diastolic dysfunction in aortic stenosis late after valve replacement. Circulation *91:*2353, 1995.
108. Brilla, C. G., Janicki, J. S., and Weber, K. T.: Cardioreparative effects of lisinopril in rats with genetic hypertension and left ventricular hypertrophy. Circulation *83:*1771, 1991.
109. Bonow, R. D., Frederick, T. M., Bacharach, S. L., et al.: Atrial systole and left ventricular filling in hypertrophic cardiomyopathy: Effect of verapamil. Am. J. Cardiol. *51:*1386, 1983.
110. Gilligan, D. M., Chan, W. L., Joshi, J., et al.: A double-blind, placebo-controlled crossover trial of nadolol and verapamil in mild and moderately symptomatic hypertrophic cardiomyopathy. J. Am. Coll. Cardiol. *21:*1672, 1993.

SUDDEN DEATH AND ARRHYTHMIAS

111. Stevenson, W. G., Stevenson, L. W., Middlekauff, H. R., and Saxon, L. A.: Sudden death prevention in patients with advanced ventricular dysfunction. Circulation *88:*2953, 1993.
112. Luu, M., Stevenson, W. G., Stevenson, L. W., et al.: Diverse mechanisms of unexpected cardiac arrest in advanced heart failure. Circulation *80:*1675, 1989.
113. Aronson, R. S.: Mechanisms of arrhythmias in ventricular hypertrophy. J. Cardiovasc. Electrophysiol. *14:*1735, 1991.
114. Charpentier, F., Baudet, S., and Le Marec, H.: Triggered activity as a possible mechanism for arrhythmias to ventricular hypertrophy. PACE Pacing Clin. Electrophysiol. *14:*1735, 1991.
115. Calkins, H., Maughan, L., Wiseman, H. F., et al.: Effect of acute volume load on refractoriness and arrhythmia development in isolated chronically infarcted canine hearts. Circulation *79:*687, 1989.
116. Franz, M. R., Cima, R., Wang, D., et al.: Electrophysiological effects of myocardial stretch and mechanical determinants of stretch-activated arrhythmias. Circulation *86:*968, 1992.
117. Lubbe, W. F., Podzuweit, T., and Opie, L. H.: Potential arrhythmogenic role of cyclic adenosine monophosphate (AMP) and systolic calcium overload: Implications for prophylactic effects of beta-blockers in myocardial infarction and proarrhythmic effects of phosphodiesterase inhibitors. J. Am. Coll. Cardiol. *19:*1622, 1992.
118. Ben-David, J., and Zipes, D. Alpha-adrenoceptor stimulation and blockade modulates cesium-induced early afterdepolarizations and ventricular tachyarrhythmias in dogs. Circulation *82:*225, 1990.
119. Gettes, L. S.: Electrolyte abnormalities underlying lethal ventricular arrhythmias. Circulation *85*(Suppl. 1):I-70, 1992.
120. Wilber, D., Garan, H., Finkelstein, D., et al.: Out-of-hospital cardiac arrest: Use of electrophysiologic testing in the prediction of long-term outcome. N. Engl. J. Med. *318:*19, 1988.
121. Kim, S. G., Fisher, J. D., Choue, C. W., et al.: Influence of left ventricular function on outcome of patients treated with implantable defibrillators. Circulation *85:*1304, 1992.
122. Stevenson, W. G., Middlekauff, H. M., Stevenson, L. W., et al.: Significance of aborted cardiac arrest and sustained ventricular tachycardia in patients referred for treatment therapy of advanced heart failure. Am. Heart J. *124:*123, 1992.
123. Stevenson, W. G., Stevenson, L. W., Weiss, J., and Tillisch, J. H.: Inducible ventricular arrhythmias and sudden death during vasodilator therapy of severe heart failure. Am. Heart J. *116:*1447, 1988.
124. Canceres, J., Jazayeri, M., McKinnie, J., et al.: Sustained bundle branch re-entry as a mechanism of clinical tachycardia. Circulation *79:*256, 1989.
125. Stevenson, W. G., Middlekauff, H. R., and Saxon, L. A.: Ventricular arrhythmias in heart failure. *In* Zipes D. P., and Jalife J., (eds.): Cardiac Electrophysiology: From Cell to Bedside. Philadelphia, W. B. Saunders Company, 1994, p. 848.
126. Horowitz, L. N., Greenspan, A. M., Spielman, S. R., et al.: Usefulness of electrophysiologic testing in evaluation of amiodarone therapy for sustained ventricular tachyarrhythmias associated with coronary heart disease. Am. J. Cardiol. *55:*367, 1985.
127. Weinberg, B. A., Miles, W. M., Klein, L. S., et al.: Five-year follow-up of 589 patients treated with amiodarone. Am. Heart J. *125:*109, 1993.
128. Sager, P. T., Choudhary, R., Leon, C., et al.: The long-term prognosis of patients with out-of-hospital cardiac arrest but no inducible ventricular tachycardia. Am. Heart J. *120:*1334, 1990.
129. Gottlieb, S. S., Kukin, M. L., Medina, N., et al.: Comparative hemodynamic effects of procainamides tocainide and encainide in severe chronic heart failure. Circulation *81:*860, 1990.
130. Ravid, S., Podrid, P. J., Lampert, S., et al.: Congestive heart failure induced by six of the newer antiarrhythmic drugs. J. Am. Coll. Cardiol. *14:*1326, 1989.
131. Stanton, M. S., Prystowsky, E. N., Fineberg, N. A., et al.: Arrhythmogenic effects of antiarrhythmic drugs: A study of 506 patients treated for ventricular tachycardia or fibrillation. J. Am. Coll. Cardiol. *14:*209, 1989.
132. The Cardiac Arrhythmia Suppression Trial (CAST) Investigators: CAST mortality and morbidity. Treatment versus placebo. N. Engl. J. Med. *324:*781, 1991.
133. Flaker, G. C., Blackshear, J. L., McBride, R., et al.: Predictors of thromboembolism in atrial fibrillation: Clinical features of patients at risk. The Stroke Prevention in Atrial Fibrillation Investigators. Ann. Intern. Med. *116:*2, 1992.

134. Hamer, A. W. F., Arkles, L. B., and Johns, J. A.: Beneficial effects of low dose amiodarone in patients with congestive heart failure: A placebo-controlled trial. J. Am. Coll. Cardiol. *14*:1768, 1989.
135. Pfisterer, M., Kiowski, W., Burckhardt, D., et al.: Beneficial effect of amiodarone on cardiac mortality in patients with asymptomatic complex ventricular arrhythmias after acute myocardial infarction and preserved, but not impaired left ventricular function. Am. J. Cardiol. *69*:1399, 1992.
136. Doval, H. C., Nul, D. R., Grancelli, H. O., et al.: Randomized trial of low-dose amiodarone in severe congestive heart failure. Lancet *344*:493, 1994.
136a. Hammill, S. C., and Packer, D. L.: Amiodarone in congestive heart failure unraveling the GESICA and CHF-STATE differences. Heart *75*:6, 1996.
137. Singh, S. N., Fletcher, R. D., Fisher, S. G., et al.: Amiodarone in patients with congestive heart failure and asymptomatic ventricular arrhythmia. N. Engl. J. Med. *333*:77, 1995.
138. Middlekauff, H. R., Stevenson, W. G., Saxon, L. A., and Stevenson, L. W.: Amiodarone and torsades de pointes in patients with advanced heart failure. Am. J. Cardiol. *76*:499, 1995.
139. Middlekauff, H. R., Stevenson, W. G., Stevenson, L. W., and Saxon, L. A.: Syncope in advanced heart failure: High sudden death regardless of etiology. J. Am. Coll. Cardiol. *21*:110, 1993.
140. Cohn, J. N., Johnson, G. R., Shabetai, R., et al.: Ejection fraction, peak exercise oxygen consumption, cardiothoracic ratio, ventricular arrhythmias, and plasma norepinephrine as determinants of prognosis in heart failure. Circulation *87*:5, 1993.
141. Hallstrom, A. P., Bigger, J. T., Doen, D., et al.: Prognostic significance of ventricular premature depolarizations measured 1 year after myocardial infarction in patients with early postinfarction asymptomatic ventricular arrhythmia. J. Am. Coll. Cardiol. *20*:259, 1992.
142. Bourke, J. P., Richards, D. A. B., Ross, D. L., et al.: Routine programmed electrical stimulation in survivors of acute myocardial infarction for prediction of spontaneous ventricular tachyarrhythmias during follow-up results, optimal stimulation protocol and cost-effective screening. J. Am. Coll. Cardiol. *18*:780, 1991.
143. Middlekauff, H. R., Stevenson, W. G., and Stevenson, L. W.: Prognostic significance of atrial fibrillation in advanced heart failure: A study of 390 patients. Circulation *84*:40, 1991.
144. Carson, P. E., Johnson, G. R., Dunkman, W. B., et al.: The influence of atrial fibrillation on prognosis in mild to moderate heart failure. Circulation *87*:VI-102, 1993.
145. Middlekauff, H. R., Wiener, I., and Stevenson, W. G.: Low-dose amiodarone for atrial fibrillation. Am. J. Cardiol. *72*:75, 1993.
146. Grogan, M., Smith, H. C., Gersh, B. J., and Wood, D. W.: Left ventricular dysfunction due to atrial fibrillation in patients initially believed to have idiopathic dilated cardiomyopathy. Am. J. Cardiol. *69*:1570, 1992.
147. Coplen, S. E., Antman, E. M., Berlin, J. A., et al.: Efficacy and safety of quinidine therapy for maintenance of sinus rhythm after cardioversion. Circulation *82*:1106, 1990.
148. Heinz, G., Siostrzonek, P., Kreiner, G., et al.: Improvement in left ventricular systolic function after successful radiofrequency His bundle ablation for drug refractory, chronic atrial fibrillation and recurrent atrial flutter. Am. J. Cardiol. *69*:489, 1992.

REFRACTORY HEART FAILURE

149. Elefteriades, J. A., Tolis, G., Levi, E., et al.: Coronary artery bypass grafting in severe left ventricular dysfunction: Excellent survival with improved ejection fraction and functional state. J. Am. Coll. Cardiol. *22*:1411, 1993.
150. Louie, H. W., Laks, H., Milgalter, E., et al.: Ischemic cardiomyopathy: Criteria for coronary revascularization and cardiac transplantation. Circulation *84*(Suppl. III):290, 1991.
151. Lang, R. M., Borow, K. M., Neumann, A., and Janzen, D.: Systemic vascular resistance: An unreliable index of left ventricular afterload. Circulation *74*:1114, 1989.
152. Forrester, J. S., Diamond, G., Chatterjee, K., and Swan, H. J. C.: Medical therapy of acute myocardial infarction by application of hemodynamic subsets. N. Engl. J. Med. *295*(24):1356, 1976.
153. Stevenson, L. W., and Tillisch, J. H.: Maintenance of cardiac output with normal filling pressures in dilated heart failure. Circulation *74*:1303, 1986.
154. Stevenson, L. W., Brunken, R. C., Belil, D., et al.: Afterload reduction with vasodilators and diuretics decreases mitral valve regurgitation during upright exercise in advanced heart failure. J. Am. Coll. Cardiol. *15*:174, 1990.
155. Stevenson, L. W.: Tailored therapy before transplantation for treatment of advanced heart failure: Effective use of vasodilators and diuretics. J. Heart Lung Transplant. *10*(3):468, 1991.
156. Guiha, N. H., Cohn, J. N., Mikulic, E., et al.: Treatment of refractory heart failure with infusion of nitroprusside. N. Engl. J. Med. *291*:587, 1974.
157. Pierpont, G. L., and Francis, G. S.: Medical management of terminal cardiomyopathy. Heart Transplant. *2*(1):18, 1982.
158. Fonarow, G. C., Stevenson, L. W., Walden, J. A., et al.: Impact of a comprehensive management program on the hospitalization rate for patients with advanced heart failure. J. Am. Coll. Cardiol. *25*:264, 1995.
159. Stevenson, L. W., Siestsema, K., Tillisch, J. H., et al.: Exercise capacity for survivors of cardiac transplantation or sustained medical therapy for stable heart failure. Circulation *81*:78, 1990.
160. Mudge, G. H., Goldstein, S., Addonizio, L. J., et al.: Cardiac transplantation: Recipient guidelines/prioritization. J. Am. Coll. Cardiol. *22*:21, 1993.
161. Hanly, P. J., Millnar, T. W., Steljes, D. G., et al.: The effect of oxygen on respiration and sleep in patients with congestive heart failure. Ann. Intern. Med. *111*:777, 1989.
162. Naughton, M. T., Liu, P. P., Benard, D. C., et al.: Treatment of congestive heart failure and Cheyne-Stokes respiration during sleep by CPAP. Am. J. Respir. Crit. Care Med. *152*:92, 1995.
163. Naughton, M. T., Rahman, A., Hara, K., et al.: Effect of CPAP on intrathoracic and left ventricular transmural pressures in patients with congestive heart failure. Circulation *91*:1725, 1995.
164. Sullivan, M. J., Higginbotham, M. B., and Cobb, F. R.: Exercise training in patients with chronic heart failure delays ventilatory anaerobic threshold and improves submaximal exercise performance. Circulation *79*:324, 1989.
164a. Natterson, P. D., Stevenson, W. G., Saxon, L. A., et al.: Risk of arterial embolization in 224 patients awaiting cardiac transplantation. Am. Heart J. *129*:564, 1995.
165. Hosenpud, J. D., Novick, R. J., Breen, T. J., and Daily, O. P.: The registry of the International Society for Heart and Lung Transplantation: Eleventh official report—1994. J. Heart Lung Transplant. *13*:561, 1994.
166. Kaye, M. P.: Registry of the International Society for Heart and Lung Transplantation: Tenth official report—1993. J. Heart Lung Transplant. *12*:541, 1993.
167. Stevenson, L. W., Couper, G., Natterson, B. J., et al.: Target heart failure population for new therapies. Circulation *92*:II-174, 1995.
168. Mancini, D. M., Eisen, H., Kussmaul, W., et al.: Value of peak exercise oxygen consumption for optimal timing of cardiac transplantation in ambulatory patients with heart failure. Circulation *83*:778, 1991.
169. Stevenson, L. W., Warner, S. L., Steimle, A. E., et al.: The impending crisis awaiting cardiac transplantation: Modeling a solution based on selection. Circulation *89*:450, 1994.
170. McManus, R. P., O'Hair, D. P., Beitzinger, J. M., et al.: Patients who die awaiting heart transplantation. J. Heart Lung Transplant. *12*:159, 1993.
171. Stevenson, L. W., Steimle, A. E., Fonarow, G., et al.: Improvement in exercise capacity of candidates awaiting heart transplantation. J. Am. Coll. Cardiol. *25*:163, 1995.
172. Moore, F. D. (Chairman): Fifth Bethesda Conference Report: Cardiac and other organ transplantation. Am. J. Cardiol. *22*:896, 1968.

Chapter 18
Heart and Heart-Lung Transplantation

MARK G. PERLROTH, BRUCE A. REITZ

Although cardiac transplantation in humans was first carried out in 1967, it is only since the early 1980's that it has been established as an accepted treatment for end-stage heart disease. The advances in immunosuppression and transplant management that have made this possible also have led to successful heart-lung and lung transplantation, which are continuing to evolve. The increasingly widespread application of thoracic organ transplantation has brought this therapy to many centers around the world and to an ever-increasing patient population.

The Registry of the International Society for Heart Transplantation in 1994 listed a cumulative total of more than 30,200 cardiac transplant procedures performed in 257 transplant centers.[1] The recent expansion of heart transplantation is emphasized by the fact that before 1980, fewer than 360 transplantations had been performed. The management philosophies and strategies discussed in this chapter are based in part on the experience of the Johns Hopkins Hospital and the Stanford University teams, and have been reviewed elsewhere.[2]

HISTORY

There are several mentions of heart transplantation in ancient Chinese mythology and biblical reference, but not until the pioneering work of Alexis Carrel at the beginning of the 20th century did surgeons have the ability to transplant organs such as the heart.[3] In a number of imaginative experiments, Carrel demonstrated that a heart could be transplanted and resume functioning in the new host. Not only did Carrel transplant hearts but he also suggested and performed the en bloc transplantation of heart and lungs,[4] both of these procedures being heterotopic transplants into the necks of recipient dogs.

With the advent of techniques for successful cardiac surgery in the 1950's, major attention was finally directed to the problem of transplantation of the heart in the chest in the normal, or orthotopic, position. The current most commonly used surgical technique for heart transplantation originated with the work of Lower and Shumway in 1959.[5] A number of important questions about transplants, including protocols for immunosuppression,[6] correlation of the surface electrocardiogram with allograft rejection,[7] and reversal of these changes with augmented immunosuppression, were subjects of early laboratory study. Despite this prior laboratory work, many were surprised when the first human heart transplant was performed by Christian Barnard in Capetown, South Africa in December 1967.[8] This transplant initiated a great amount of interest at other centers around the world, with 170 transplants by 65 surgical teams between December 1967 and March 1971. The one-year survival was only 15 per cent, and because of this, enthusiasm for heart transplantation rapidly waned by the end of 1971.

Only at Stanford University and the Medical College of Virginia did surgical teams continue with programs in heart transplantation. Working virtually alone through the decade of the 1970's, these investigators refined recipient selection criteria,[9] saw the development of the transvenous endomyocardial biopsy for diagnosing rejection,[10] developed rabbit antithymocyte globulin as an effective treatment of acute rejection,[11] and defined many of the late post-transplant complications and management principles.[12]

IMMUNOSUPPRESSIVE THERAPY. Widespread application of heart transplantation depended on the development of better immunosuppressive therapy (see pp. 522–523). This goal was reached with the discovery that cyclosporin A (cyclosporine), a novel cyclic undecapeptide of fungal origin, could selectively block the effect of interleukin-2 (IL-2) in stimulating T cells.[13–19]

Heart and lung transplantation has been extended to a large number of additional recipients, including neonates with hypoplastic left heart syndrome, the elderly (age 60 to 70), and patients with primary lung disease, such as emphysema and cystic fibrosis.

ORGANIZATION OF A TRANSPLANT PROGRAM

In 1994, there were 257 centers performing cardiac transplantation worldwide. Experience has shown that a successful program depends on both institutional commitment and participation of multiple professional groups within the institution that must work together in caring for the patient. Careful attention to detail in organizing a transplant program is crucial in obtaining and sustaining good outcomes in transplant patients.

The development of an effective cardiac transplant program requires careful organization and cooperation from both clinical and nonclinical personnel. Some but not all states require a certificate of need to initiate a new program of heart transplantation. The National Organ Transplantation Act of 1984 established certain minimum criteria for transplant programs to enroll in the nationwide computerized matching system.[20] To encourage excellent patient care and to discourage transplantation in centers with suboptimal results, the act established the United Network for Organ Sharing (UNOS), with membership limited to those centers that perform a minimum of 12 transplant procedures per year and that obtain a one-year survival rate of at least 70 per cent. In addition to these performance criteria, the center must have adequate operating room facilities and trained physicians and nursing personnel and be a participating member in a local organ procurement organization. The program must have established protocols and procedures for the selection of patients, the evaluation and distribution of donor organs, postoperative management, and long-term follow-up. Both surgeons and physicians involved in the care of the patient must meet certain criteria in terms of training and prior experience. The ability of an individual center to obtain funding from Medicare depends on similar criteria.[21]

RECIPIENT SELECTION

With improved outcomes in both quality of life and percentage of patients surviving, cardiac transplantation has become accepted therapy for many patients with end-stage heart disease. A fairly rigid selection process is required in order to obtain excellent results in individual patients. Although in recent years there has been a tendency to relax these criteria in an effort to extend the benefits of transplantation to a larger number of patients, this has heightened the problem of donor scarcity. The number of potential recipients rises exponentially with an extension of the upper age accepted, as shown in Figure 18–1. The diagnoses of patients undergoing heart transplantation are listed in Figure 18–2. The most frequent indications are

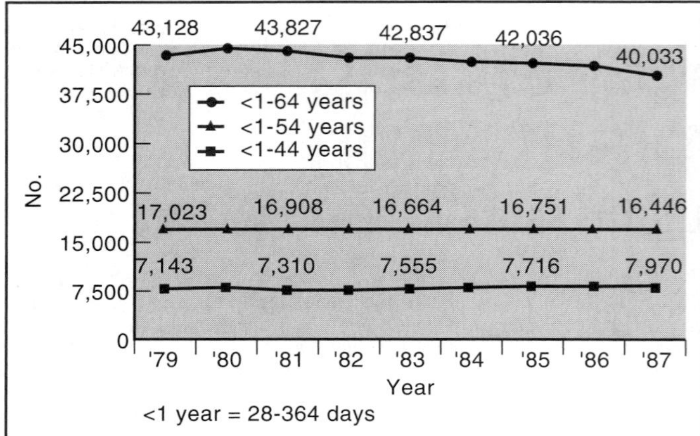

FIGURE 18–1. The need for heart transplantation in the United States, 1979 to 1987. (From O'Connell J. B., Gunnar, R. M., Evans, R. W., et al.: Task Force 1: Organization of Heart Transplantation in the U.S. J. Am. Coll. Cardiol. *22*(1):9, 1993. Reprinted with permission from the American College of Cardiology.)

equally divided between ischemic heart disease and cardiomyopathy. Contraindications (Table 18–1) vary somewhat by program. (See also pp. 509–511.)

An important aspect of evaluation is a comprehensive psychosocial evaluation by a clinical social worker or psychologist. The ability of the patient to follow a complex medical regimen is extremely important, as is the family support necessary to help the patient through multiple medical procedures and evaluations and to maintain the essential medical regimen after transplantation.

All conventional medical or surgical therapies should be used before consideration of transplantation. Evaluation might reasonably include endomyocardial biopsy to rule out other treatable causes of cardiomyopathy, especially for patients without ischemic heart disease. Occasionally, unsuspected sarcoidosis or myocarditis is detected that might respond favorably to an alternative therapy, and some patients with recurrent life-threatening arrhythmias may be best treated initially by placement of an automatic implantable cardiac defibrillator.

Although it may be easy to identify the most severely ill patients with a poor prognosis for six-month survival, there is a large group of patients with symptomatic cardiomyopathy and ominous objective findings (ejection fraction <20 per cent, stroke volume ≤40 ml, severe ventricular arrhythmias) for whom timing may be somewhat difficult. A further consideration may be the quality of life, which is a judgment of the patient and the physicians caring for the

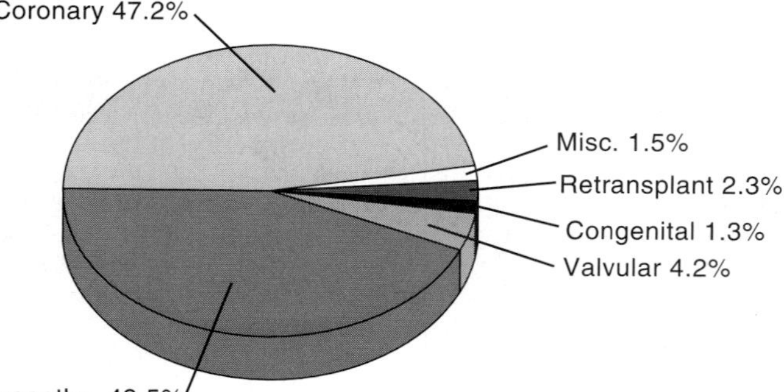

FIGURE 18–2. Adult heart transplantation indications. (From Hosenpud, J. D., Novick, R. J., Breen, T. J., and Daily, O. P.: The Registry of the International Society for Heart and Lung Transplantation: Eleventh Official Report—1994*. J. Heart Lung Transplant. *13*(4):561, 1994. Reprinted with permission from Mosby-Year Book, Inc.)

TABLE 18–1 CONTRAINDICATIONS TO HEART TRANSPLANTATION

Advanced age (>70 years)
Irreversible hepatic, renal, or pulmonary dysfunction
Severe peripheral vascular or cerebrovascular disease
Insulin-requiring diabetes mellitus with end-organ damage
Active infection
Recent cancer with uncertain status
Psychiatric illness, poor medical compliance
Systemic disease that would significantly limit survival or rehabilitation
Pulmonary hypertension with pulmonary vascular resistance >6 Wood units or 3 Wood units after treatment with vasodilators

patient. This comes into play in patients with intractable angina and coronary vessels that cannot be bypassed.

UPPER AGE LIMIT. One of the most controversial aspects of patient selection is the upper age limit for cardiac transplantation. The initial Stanford University criteria considered an upper age limit of 50 years. This was modified to include patients older than 55 and then up to age 60 during the era of improving results because of cyclosporine therapy in the early 1980's. Sufficient additional experience has now been reported in patients over age 55 to indicate that a strict chronological age criterion is not appropriate.[22–24] Older people can undergo transplantation with good expectation of survival and improvement in quality of life, although these patients should be optimal in every other respect. Some evidence has been reported suggesting that older patients may experience less rejection than younger patients.[25] The additional relative contraindication of diabetes or other systemic disease, such as chronic pulmonary disease, probably would eliminate most patients over 60 as potential candidates.

PULMONARY VASCULAR DISEASE. This is an important consideration. Orthotopic cardiac transplantation requires that the pulmonary vascular resistance be low, so that the normal right ventricle of the donor heart can adequately support the recipient's circulation after transplantation. A great deal of controversy has developed over the optimal measure of pulmonary vascular resistance. Most programs use the measurement of the traditional Wood unit, and limit the value to ≤6 units at rest or <3 with maximal vasodilation. Other centers use the pulmonary vascular resistance index (Wood units × body surface area) or transpulmonary pressure gradient (mean pulmonary artery pressure minus mean pulmonary capillary wedge pressure) ≤15 mm Hg.[26] Whatever measure of resistance is used, in those patients with values toward the upper limits, it is imperative to demonstrate in the catheterization laboratory that the resistance can be manipulated with either oxygen or vasodilators with or without inotropic agents.[27] If the pulmonary vascular resistance measurements remain elevated, strong consideration should be given to either heterotopic cardiac transplantation, which leaves the recipient's heart intact, or heart-lung transplantation. Because patients may remain on a waiting list for more than six months, repeat cardiac catheterization may be necessary semiannually to determine if the pulmonary vascular resistance has increased. Significantly elevated pulmonary vascular resistance and right heart failure remain problems after orthotopic cardiac transplantation and are major causes of early postoperative mortality.

CLINICAL CONSIDERATIONS. Ultimately, the selection of a candidate for heart transplantation results from a clinical assessment that a patient free of established contraindications (see Table 18–1) suffers severe cardiac disability refractory to expert management. The pathophysiology usually encompasses congestive heart failure but is occasionally dominated by recurrent lethal arrhythmias or intolerable ischemic symptoms. Reliance solely on a low (<20 per cent) ejection fraction has become less reliable since the introduction of aggressive vasodilator therapy. Some patients with extensive left ventricular dysfunction are remarkably symptom-free, and subgroups can experience one-year survivals of more than 60 per cent.[28] The success and acceptance of heart transplantation has encouraged enlistment of less severely ill candidates for this procedure to such an extent that expected survival has increased from almost none at 6 months to 50 per cent at 2 years.[29]

PEAK $\dot{V}O_2$. The measurement of peak oxygen consumption ($\dot{V}O_2$; ml/kg/min) (Figs. 5–1, p. 155, 5–2, p. 156, 14–29, p. 440) has been a useful supplementary criterion for the selection of recipients and the timing of transplantation.[30,31] Maximal exercise performance exceeding 14 ml/kg/min predicted a 1-year survival of greater than 90 per cent. The worst outlook was for those patients whose peak $\dot{V}O_2$ was <10 ml/kg/min, and they, if otherwise acceptable, should be recommended for cardiac transplantation. Those with intermediate values require additional evaluation based on disability, quality of life, and age.

COEXISTING DISEASES. Patients with involvement of other organs that precluded selection in the past, but that now respond to transplantation, may be considered candidates for *dual organ transplantation.* In addition to heart-lung, these include heart-kidney (notably for retransplantation of heart transplant recipients who have developed cyclosporine nephrotoxicity) and heart-liver (for homozygous familial hypercholesterolemia). Dual organ candidacy does not change a patient's status or position on the waiting list, but when patients become eligible for a heart or liver based on standard criteria, the second required organ may be allocated from the same donor.[32] The ethical dilemma of improving one life instead of two remains unresolved.

Patients with infective endocarditis (without metastatic infection) and patients with malignancy without evidence of recurrence (often with anthracycline cardiomyopathy) have successfully received heart transplants. Systemic amyloidosis, because of its frequent multiorgan involvement as well as documented recurrence in the allograft, remains an unlikely condition for transplantation at most centers.

Inevitably, all programs exercise some subjectivity in the selection process determined by the prior experience of the transplant team with the many clinical, physiological, and social variables involved. Although the evaluation of potential candidates for cardiac transplantation is difficult, these established criteria have led to certain predictable outcomes in terms of quality of life and actuarial survival. Deviations from these protocols usually produce less favorable results. As with any medical or surgical procedure, the final decision ultimately rests with the patient, in accordance with the concept of informed consent.

MANAGEMENT OF PATIENTS AWAITING TRANSPLANTATION

Because there are a number of patients awaiting transplantation at any point in time, their management is important. The UNOS patient waiting list for needed organs in August 1994 totaled 2892 patients awaiting heart transplantation and 214 United States patients awaiting heart-lung transplantation.[33] Because the current yearly number of procedures performed is about 2100, a number of awaiting recipients will not survive to receive a needed organ. Most centers experience between 20 and 30 per cent mortality of patients on the waiting list. United States heart-lung transplants, after peaking at 74 in 1988, have declined to approximately 50 to 60 per year, while lung transplants have steadily risen to an annual rate of more than 500.[34]

The management of end-stage congestive heart failure is described in Chapter 17. Although digitalis remains the only generally available oral inotropic agent, the use of intravenous low-dose dopamine or dobutamine has been a helpful tool for managing some of these patients.[35] Combined with brief hospitalizations for hemodynamic monitoring to optimize vasodilators, diuretics, and intravenous inotropes, patients will often sustain improvement lasting for weeks or even months. The use of anticoagulants as prophylaxis against systemic or pulmonary thromboembolism is practiced routinely at some centers.

MECHANICAL DEVICES FOR BRIDGING. Patients in whom conventional medical therapy fails may require intraaortic balloon counterpulsation or possibly a mechanical assist device for bridging to transplantation[36–38] (see Chap. 19). Growing experience has demonstrated that for short-term bridging, up to one week, the use of a centrifugal pump similar to types used during routine cardiac surgery can be effective. For longer-term mechanical support, ventricular assist devices have been successful. The use of the totally implantable heart has resulted in poor bridging to transplantation, with multiple complications owing to infections and/or thromboemboli.[39] Two long-term mechanical assist devices have been evaluated in multicenter studies, the Novacor and the ThermoCardiosystems, Inc. (TCI) HeartMate. Each was tested in approximately 100 patients for periods of up to a year or more. The Novacor required systemic anticoagulation, whereas the TCI did not. Thromboembolic complications were uncommon in both. Approximately 60 per cent of patients so treated went on to cardiac transplantation; of these, 85 to 89 per cent survived.[40]

Even before development of such sophisticated devices, the intraaortic balloon pump was and continues to be used successfully for this purpose. The first successful use of these mechanical devices occurred in 1984 for the left ventricular assist pump and in 1985 for a total artificial heart. Subsequently, more than 1000 patients have received one or the other device, and more than 500 have subsequently undergone cardiac transplantation. A recent review reported that 69 per cent of patients in whom the device was inserted as a bridge to transplantation ultimately underwent the transplant, with 95 per cent of these patients being discharged from the hospital. The one- and two-year survival estimates for patients requiring only univentricular mechanical support were equivalent to those of patients having isolated orthotopic cardiac transplantation alone. It is now accepted that ventricular assist devices are able to provide reasonable and safe circulatory support in patients dying of cardiac failure and have the potential to resuscitate and rehabilitate patients prior to undergoing cardiac transplantation.[41]

Once selected, patients are categorized on the basis of size, ABO blood group, time on the waiting list, and clinical status. The latter consists of two classes: In adults, status I comprises patients in an intensive care unit receiving parenteral inotropic drugs or mechanical support (i.e., ventilator, intraaortic balloon pump, or ventricular assist device). It does not automatically include patients with an intracardiac defibrillator or those who require continuous infusions of antiarrhythmic drugs. Status II comprises all other patients. Separate waiting lists are maintained for the two status classes.

Patients are "de-listed" if they improve or if they suffer complications (e.g., cerebral or pulmonary embolism) or superimposed illnesses (e.g., infections, gastrointestinal bleeding), which increase the risk of surgery and immunosuppression or which compromise rehabilitation or survival. They are reactivated when clinically appropriate.

EVALUATION AND MANAGEMENT OF THE HEART DONOR

The factor limiting the number of heart transplants performed is the availability of donor organs. Thus, it is imperative to obtain as high a percentage of potential donor organs as possible by increasing the donation rate and also to consider all donor organs that might possibly be suitable for transplantation. The cardiologist frequently is asked to take part in the donor evaluation process, so that the adequate function of the graft can be predicted before transplantation.

Brain death has been accepted as the legal definition of death throughout the United States.[42] The diagnosis should not involve physicians caring for the potential candidate, and it requires the absence of hypothermia (core temperature >32.5°C) or drugs capable of altering neurological or neuromuscular function.[43]

The specific neurological catastrophe that has resulted in brain death may include blunt traumatic injury to the head, intracranial hemorrhage, or penetrating traumatic injury. The characteristics of cardiac donors are listed in Table 18–2. Until fairly recently, heart and heart-lung transplant donor criteria were very selective. The upper age limit was usually 35 years of age, and there were a number of other

TABLE 18–2 CAUSES OF DEATH IN DONORS* FOR HEART TRANSPLANT PROCEDURES IN THE JOHNS HOPKINS SERIES (JULY 1983–JUNE 1990)

CAUSE OF DEATH	NO. DONORS
Head trauma	68
Gunshot wound	21
Cerebrovascular accident	23
Asphyxiation	5
Brain tumor	1
Liver failure	1
Heart-lung recipient	1

* Age, 24 years mean (0.7–47); sex, 92 males/28 females.

criteria.[44] With the need to increase the number of transplants, these criteria have been modified.[45,46] Most centers evaluate any potential donor up to as high as 55 years of age. Especially with the older or suboptimal donor, a careful cardiac history must be obtained from the next of kin and adequate cardiac function ensured, including potential evaluation with coronary arteriography for men older than 45 or women older than 55. The use of "on the operating table" coronary arteriography has been suggested because of the logistic requirements for performing coronary arteriography in a brain-dead patient.[47] Alternatively, simple inspection of the graft with palpation of the coronary arteries at the time of harvesting has been used by some groups to determine the presence of significant atherosclerosis. Sweeney and colleagues have reported on the use of hearts from donors who did not meet the standard criteria.[45] Recipients received grafts from older donors (> age 40) or from patients with a history of prolonged cardiac arrest or septicemia. Their results indicate that selective use of such donors is possible with reasonable outcomes. Hearts from older donors should, whenever possible, be reserved for older recipients because of inherent loss of function with age.

The evaluation of potential donors includes obtaining adequate background data, a physical examination, a 12-lead electrocardiogram, and an echocardiogram. Brain death and increased intracranial pressure often result in nonspecific ST- and T-wave changes. These also may be seen with hypothermia. The echocardiogram has assumed an even greater role in recent years in evaluating cardiac function. This evaluation should be done at a time when dosages of intravenous inotropic agents have been lowered to as low as is compatible with adequate blood pressure and cardiac output, and after adequate fluid resuscitation.

Current matching criteria of donors and recipients include only ABO compatibility and appropriate size match. A prospective specific cross-match between donor and recipient is performed only when recipients have been identified who have more than 5 per cent of reactivity when evaluated against a panel of random donors. When heart transplantation is performed across the ABO blood barrier, there is a significant risk of hyperacute rejection.[48]

With respect to size, fairly wide limits are acceptable, although donors who weigh less than 80 per cent of the recipient's weight should not be accepted for those patients who have higher levels of pulmonary vascular resistance. Similarly, hearts with ischemic times over two hours should be avoided in this situation.

Signs in patients with brain death usually are unstable and close attention is required to fluid balance, owing to diabetes insipidus. This necessitates monitoring of central venous pressure and adequate fluid resuscitation, administration of vasopressin, and replacement of fluid lost through urine output. If hypotension occurs despite adequate volume replacement, a vasopressor is infused. Dopamine is the standard inotropic agent used, but some donors will be better maintained on an alpha-adrenergic agent.

Donor evaluation currently also includes various serology results. These are for human immunodeficiency virus (HIV), hepatitis B antigen, cytomegalovirus (CMV), and toxoplasmosis. The finding of HIV antibody rules out a potential donor, and the presence of CMV antibody may disqualify a potential heart-lung donor for a CMV-negative recipient at some centers. UNOS guidelines suggest deferring organ donors who have received human pituitary-derived growth hormone.[49] Present consensus also excludes donors with carbon monoxide-hemoglobin levels above 20 per cent, arterial oxygen saturation less than 80 per cent, previous myocardial infarction, or severe coronary or structural heart disease. The presence of metastatic malignancy is also an exclusion at many centers, although those with primary brain tumors and skin cancers may be excepted. Relative contraindications include sepsis, prolonged (>6 hours) severe (<60 mm Hg) hypotension, noncritical coronary disease, hepatitis B surface antigen or hepatitis C antibodies (unless the organs are destined for recipients with the same serology), multiple resuscitations, severe left ventricular hypertrophy, or the need for inotropic support (dopamine >20 μg/kg/min) for 24 hours.[42]

Distant procurement of the heart and heart-lung for transplantation is now routine in almost all transplant centers.[50] The technique for heart preservation remains quite simple, with cold crystalloid or blood cardioplegia infusion combined with topical cold for extended preservation. Average ischemic times are between 3 and 4 hours, with excellent function in most cases. Data from the Registry of the International Society for Heart Transplantation show some relation between ischemic time and survival, although most experienced centers see no particular relation for up to 6 hours of ischemia.[51] Although laboratory work has shown satisfactory preservation using various techniques for up to 24 hours of ischemia, these have not been clinically applied.[52] The longest ex vivo preservation of the human heart has been 16 hours, but the heart was implanted heterotopically, so it did not supply all of the recipient's cardiac output immediately.[53]

Techniques for distant heart-lung procurement and preservation of isolated lung grafts include flush solutions in the pulmonary artery with potent pulmonary vasodilators,[54] the use of cold blood for flush,[55] placing the donor on cardiopulmonary bypass,[56] and the use of an autoperfusing heart-lung preparation for maintaining the organs at normothermia in a working state.[57] Again, distant procurement is limited to 6 hours or less, with most procurements having an ischemic period between 3 and 4 hours.

This length of allowable ischemic time has usually kept procurement between centers of not more than 1000 miles distance. The tendency to use donor organs within the local region also has limited times.

Allocation of organs begins with Status I patients in ever-widening zones. It is offered first to candidates in the local Organ Procurement Organization (OPO), then to patients within a 500-mile and then 1000-mile radius. If no recipient is found, the process is repeated for the Status II list.[58]

Regional organ procurement organizations (OPO) are available to assist doctors and hospitals with all medical and legal considerations involved in organ donation. Their telephone numbers (800 listings) have been listed by location.[58a]

OPERATIVE TECHNIQUE

The current technique for orthotopic heart transplantation was described in 1960 by Lower and Shumway.[5] The method involves retaining a large portion of the posterior wall of the right and left atrium in the recipient and implanting the donor heart with relatively long suture lines in the atria, together with direct end-to-end anastomoses of the aorta and the pulmonary artery. Modification of this technique with venous anastomoses at the level of the cavae and the pulmonary veins permits a more physiological atrial contribution to ventricular filling and causes less distortion of the mitral and tricuspid annuli, with less tendency to atrioventricular valve regurgitation; however, the long-term clinical advantage of this innovation remains

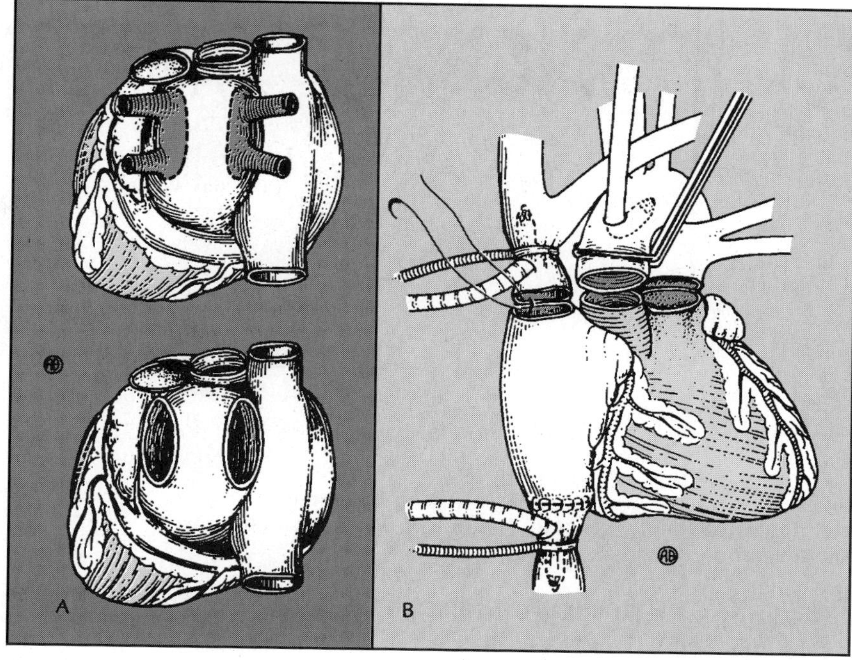

FIGURE 18–3. Total heart replacement by pulmonary venous anastomoses on right or left and caval anastomosis at the superior and inferior vena cava. Aorta and pulmonary artery attached as in the previous bi-atrial transplantation technique.

uncertain. No differences in patient survival can be demonstrated. The technique is illustrated in Figure 18–3.[59–61]

The operation is performed by way of a median sternotomy incision, with routine cannulation of the aorta and both venae cavae. Cardiopulmonary bypass is usually performed with moderate hypothermia of between 28° and 30°C. The implantation procedure usually requires from 45 to 60 minutes, and after careful attention to de-airing maneuvers and resuscitation of the heart, cardiopulmonary bypass is weaned. After placement of temporary pacing wires and chest drainage catheters, the incision is routinely closed.

RIGHT VENTRICULAR FAILURE. Because the pulmonary vascular resistance of the recipient may be elevated, acute right ventricular failure is a frequent cause of early morbidity and mortality. The normal donor right ventricle may be unable to meet the elevated resistance, and there is a high degree of both pulmonary and tricuspid valve insufficiency in the early post-transplant period.[62] This problem may be exacerbated by a relatively long ischemic time or by a donor heart somewhat smaller than that of the recipient. Isoproterenol is often routinely given for its chronotropic and inotropic effects, as well as for its beneficial lowering of pulmonary vascular resistance. Armitage and associates reported that elevated pulmonary vascular resistance could be successfully treated with an infusion of prostaglandin E_1.[63] Inhaled nitric oxide has also been utilized successfully.[64,65] Support of the transplanted heart with a right ventricular assist device helps overcome this early postoperative problem.[66]

Multiple types of congenital anomalies have been dealt with during cardiac transplantation. For example, absence of the right superior vena cava or persistent left superior vena cava can easily be accommodated.[67] Corrected transposition of the great vessels requires extra length of the donor aorta and pulmonary artery.[68]

HETEROTOPIC HEART TRANSPLANTATION. For certain rather limited indications, cardiac transplantation can be performed as a heterotopic graft. This procedure was first described by Demikhov[69] and in the early experimental work performed by McGough and colleagues.[70] It was introduced into clinical practice by Barnard in 1974, with the placement of a heterotopic heart in the right lower thorax, and the donor heart anastomosed in parallel with the retained recipient heart.[71] In cases in which the pulmonary vascular resistance remains severely elevated, the recipient's right heart can continue to function while the left heart is bypassed with the transplant.[71a] Other indications include a patient with a relatively small donor heart, a donor heart with a long ischemic time and anticipated poor early function, and a patient who has a reversible type of heart disease in which the graft may be removed when the native heart recovers. Heterotopic transplants account for about 2.5 per cent of the cardiac transplants currently performed. The operative technique includes left atrial-to-left atrial anastomosis, aorta-to-aorta anastomosis, superior vena cava-to-right atrium, and pulmonary artery-to-pulmonary artery connection.

Early Postoperative Recovery

Much of the early postoperative management is similar to that of other patients recovering from cardiac surgical procedures. Strict isolation precautions are no longer considered mandatory. The patient is weaned from the ventilator and from inotropic drugs, as tolerated. Early mobilization and use of physical therapy are begun as soon as tolerated.

The most important feature of early management is the institution of the immunosuppressive regimen, which will be continued throughout the patient's lifetime. Numerous protocols exist for maintenance immunosuppression, and they are continually changing. Most patients receive cyclosporine in combination with several other medications. Currently, the most common protocol involves triple-drug therapy of cyclosporine, azathioprine, and prednisone. They are usually given in higher doses in the early post-transplant period, with weaning to lower and less toxic levels for chronic administration. A typical protocol for immunosuppression is shown in Table 18–3. At the Stanford University Hospital, patients are given 500 mg of methylprednisolone intraoperatively. Postoperatively, patients receive cyclosporine at 6 to 8 mg/kg/day in divided doses, depending on serum levels and renal function, and intravenous methylprednisolone. After the third dose of methylprednisolone, oral prednisone is begun in doses of 1 mg/kg of body weight and is tapered to 0.4 mg/kg over 2 weeks. Azathioprine is given at about 2 mg/kg and is lowered if the white blood cell count falls below 4000/mm^3.

The demonstration of certain advantages has popularized prophylactic induction therapy,[72] although randomized trials have revealed no significant differences in total number of rejection episodes, infections, or serum creatinine levels.[73] The Utah transplant group showed that the monoclonal antibody directed against the CD3 (helper) lymphocyte (Orthoclone, OKT3) results in excellent early renal function and almost a complete absence of early acute rejection, allowing the patient to recover from the surgical procedure and begin rehabilitation. There is a low incidence of sensitization against the mouse monoclonal antibody, so early prophylactic administration does not preclude later use of OKT3 for treatment of acute rejection, if necessary.[74] Detection of circulating antibody of OKT3 at titers >1:1000 in previously treated patients predicts a poor response. An alternative anti–T-cell antibody preparation should then be selected.

Chronic maintenance immunosuppression usually consists of either cyclosporine, azathioprine, and prednisone or cyclosporine and azathioprine alone. Withdrawal or marked reduction of corticosteroids is of particular benefit in diabetics and in the presence of severe osteoporosis or aseptic necrosis of bone. In children, a corticosteroid-free

TABLE 18–3 IMMUNOSUPPRESSION FOR HEART TRANSPLANTATION PROTOCOLS

	POSTOPERATIVE	
DRUG	Early	Late
Cyclosporine	6–10 mg/kg/day PO* *or* 0.5–2 mg/kg/day IV	3–6 mg/kg/day PO†
or		
Tacrolimus (FK506)	0.15–0.30 mg/kg/day PO	0.15–0.30 mg/kg/day PO†
Methylprednisolone	500 mg IV after cardiopulmonary bypass 125 mg q8h × 3	
Prednisone	1 mg/kg/day PO tapered to 0.4 mg/kg	0.1–0.2 mg/kg/day PO
Azathioprine	2 mg/kg/day PO‡	1–2 mg/kg/day PO

* Omit if preoperative serum creatinine level is greater than 1.5 mg/dl and use IV.
† Or as modified by blood levels.
‡ Omit if white blood count < 4000/mm³.

regimen permits normal axial growth and prevents the development of the cushingoid features and acne which contribute to noncompliance in adolescents.[75]

Detection of Rejection

Detection and treatment of allograft rejection remain perhaps the most crucial aspects of transplant management. The most reliable and frequent technique to assess allograft rejection is the endomyocardial biopsy. Other less invasive techniques have relied on the detection of activated circulating lymphoblasts,[76] changes in the appearance of the heart by echocardiography[77] or in the voltage of the electrocardiogram,[78] and experimental techniques looking at the energy state of the myocardium by nuclear magnetic resonance (NMR) spectroscopy.[79]

NONINVASIVE TECHNIQUES

Imaging techniques rely on demonstration of myocardial depression as a result of injury from the rejection process. Myocyte necrosis is a relatively late manifestation of rejection, emphasizing the need for more sensitive and specific early signs.

In 1965, Lower and associates noted a consistent drop in the summed values of electrocardiographic voltage, coincident with rejection in 20 untreated dogs with heart transplants.[7] Later, electrocardiographic monitoring was used for patients treated with prednisone and azathioprine and found to be helpful. A decrease in the summed QRS voltage by 20 per cent was thought to be indicative of rejection.[80] However, a number of other conditions influence the QRS voltage, including myocardial and pulmonary edema, pulmonary infiltrates owing to a variety of causes, and pericardial effusion. Furthermore, cyclosporine-treated patients have less cardiac tissue edema, and thus the standard electrocardiogram is less sensitive. A directly implanted epicardial electrode with a telemetry monitoring system for following heart transplant patients' electrocardiograms has been successfully used by the Berlin transplant group, but it has not been widely adopted because of the need to implant electrodes and to maintain equipment for telemetry.[81,82]

ECHOCARDIOGRAPHY. This can aid in diagnosing rejection episodes. Dubroff and others have shown that there is an increase in left ventricular wall thickness during episodes of cardiac rejection.[77] Further studies have shown that this is a relatively insensitive technique. The appearance of rejection can be correlated with a decrease in the isovolumetric relaxation time[83]; however, the use of diastolic parameters is complicated by changes in heart rate between measurements, as well as by the unsynchronized hemodynamic contribution of the recipient atrial remnant. Thus, changes associated with rejection are an increase in posterior wall thickness, an increase in left ventricular mass, and a decrease in diastolic compliance. Unfortunately, most of these changes are indicative of advanced stages of rejection and therefore have limited usefulness. Echocardiograms are currently obtained as baseline studies early after transplantation and are correlated with those obtained during moderate or severe rejection to assess left ventricular performance during treatment and to ensure that left ventricular function is stable or improving. Patients' echocardiograms are recorded on their own individual tapes, which allows easy review and increases the sensitivity of Doppler echocardiographic studies for identifying subtle changes in ventricular performance.

RADIONUCLIDE TESTS. Among radionuclide tests, *technetium-99m pyrophosphate scintigraphy* (see p. 278) is a sensitive and specific indication of myocardial injury caused by ischemia. With increasingly severe cardiac rejection, there is a progressive increase in myocardial uptake in laboratory animals.[84] Other studies with thallium-201 or indium-111 have suggested some usefulness in experimental laboratory studies, but none of the nuclear scans are used clinically on a routine basis.[85]

Antimyosin antibodies (see p. 296), which are monoclonal Fab fragments directed against myosin, can be used to evaluate myosin exposure during the cell death associated with cardiac rejection.[86]

Nuclear magnetic resonance spectroscopy is a recent noninvasive technique for evaluating tissue biochemical characteristics. In rejecting dog and human hearts, there is a decline in phosphocreatine detected by NMR spectroscopy during the course of allograft rejection. The ratio of phosphocreatine to inorganic phosphorus declines, and these changes occur 24 to 48 hours before the appearance of myocyte necrosis on endomyocardial biopsies.[79] Although these techniques hold promise for a less invasive measure and would be particularly helpful in pediatric recipients, a low-cost, sensitive, and reliable technique has yet to be developed.

Other investigators have examined urinary byproducts of cellular degradation, such as urinary *thromboxane* B_2[87] and *putrescine*; however, these studies show minimal changes in cyclosporine-treated patients, and the techniques are not widely used.

Measurement of lymphocyte subsets has been a potentially attractive method for detecting rejection. In general, these techniques have not been sensitive or specific.[88] Recipients of heart and heart-lung transplants were followed for one year but demonstrated no reproducible correlation of CD4 to CD8 ratios with rejection episodes. These lymphocyte subsets were found to be affected more by viral infections than by rejection episodes.

Endomyocardial Biopsy

With the inadequacy of these noninvasive tests, the endomyocardial biopsy remains the standard method for the detection of rejection and its effective treatment with augmented immunosuppression. The technique was introduced for cardiac transplantation by Caves and associates in 1973.[89] The relatively diffuse interstitial infiltrate associated with rejection makes it possible for the focal biopsy to be a good reflection of events throughout the myocardium.[90] Although the endomyocardial biopsy is an invasive procedure, it seems relatively well-tolerated and can be performed in a sequential manner. Complications are usually mild, and include pneumothoraces, transient rhythm disturbances, and a rare instance of myocardial perforation or tricuspid regurgitation due to chordal interruption. Because it is a percutaneous and transvenous technique, there is no operative incision and only local anesthetic is required with minimal discomfort. The procedure is rapidly performed, usually through the right internal jugular vein, and can be repeated on many occasions through the same access site. It can also be placed from the left jugular vein or from the subclavian vein, and from the femoral veins, as shown in Figure 18–4. Fluoroscopy is usually used, although some operators prefer echocardiography for bioptome guidance.

To get an adequate sample for examination, four to six biopsy specimens are taken at each examination.[90] A typical post-transplant biopsy schedule is shown in Table 18–4. Patients who demonstrate allograft rejection are treated with an appropriate immunosuppressive regimen (see

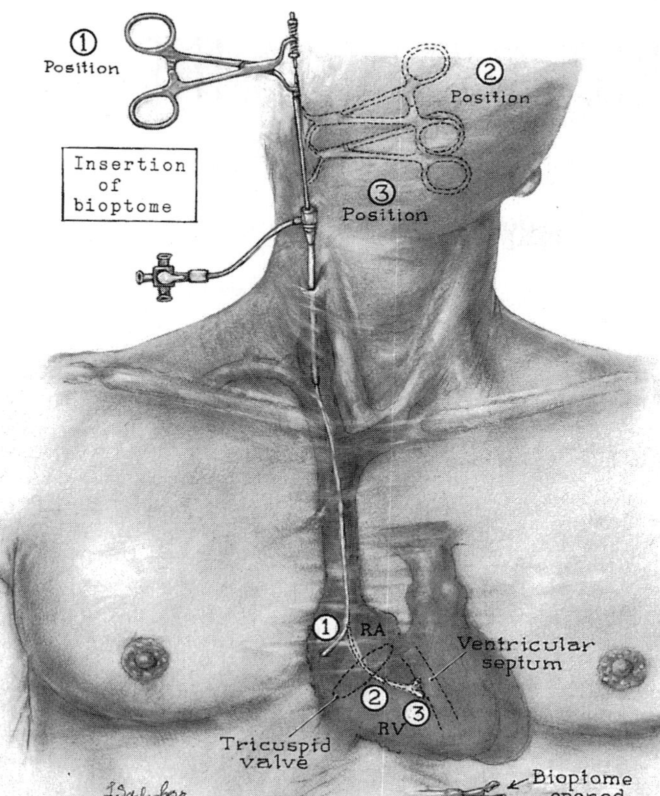

FIGURE 18–4. Positioning of the bioptome for endomyocardial biopsy. 1. Bioptome is inserted with the tip pointed toward the lateral wall of the right atrium. 2. At the level of the mid-right atrium, the bioptome is rotated anteriorly about 180° and is advanced through the tricuspid valve apparatus toward the right ventricle. 3. The bioptome is advanced to the interventricular septum with the jaws opened. (From Baughman, K. L.: History and current techniques of endomyocardial biopsy. *In* Baumgartner, W. A., Reitz, B. A., and Achuff, S. A. [eds.]: Heart and Heart-Lung Transplantation. Philadelphia, W.B. Saunders Company, 1990.)

below) and repeat endomyocardial biopsy is performed again after an interval of 10 to 14 days. The effect of treatment during this time is usually followed by echocardiographic and clinical assessment.

The variety and significance of the observed histological changes in cardiac allografts have now been reasonably well-defined. Multiple grading systems have been advocated by different transplant groups, but recently the International Society for Heart and Lung Transplantation has adopted uniform criteria.[91] The tissue fragments are embedded together in a single block, processed, and sectioned. Most biopsies are assessed using standard hematoxylin and eosin stains, but other special stains may be useful for additional information, such as the amount of collagen present or identification of specific subtypes of infiltrating lymphocytes.

The most important feature of most post-transplant biopsies is the detection of lymphocyte infiltration and the presence of myocyte necrosis. The continuum of histological findings from a normal biopsy to one showing severe acute rejection will include a variety of subtle findings, which are listed in Table 18–5. Figure 18–5 shows examples of acute rejection of varying grades.

A certain number of confusing histopathological changes can be seen in some biopsy specimens and be unrelated to rejection. For example, in specimens taken early after transplantation, there may be necrotic myocytes undergoing macrophagic removal because of ischemia at the time of the transplant procedure itself. Necrosis may also be secondary to infectious agents, such as CMV and toxoplasmosis. Oc-

TABLE 18–4 RECOMMENDED FREQUENCY OF ENDOMYOCARDIAL BIOPSY FOR ROUTINE MONITORING OF HEART TRANSPLANT REJECTION*

TIME AFTER TRANSPLANT	INTERVAL	NO. BIOPSIES
0–4 weeks	Every week	4
4–8 weeks	Every 2 weeks	2
8–16 weeks	Every month	2
6 months to indefinite	Every 3 months	

* Rebiopsy if indeterminate and 10 days after conclusion of rejection treatment.

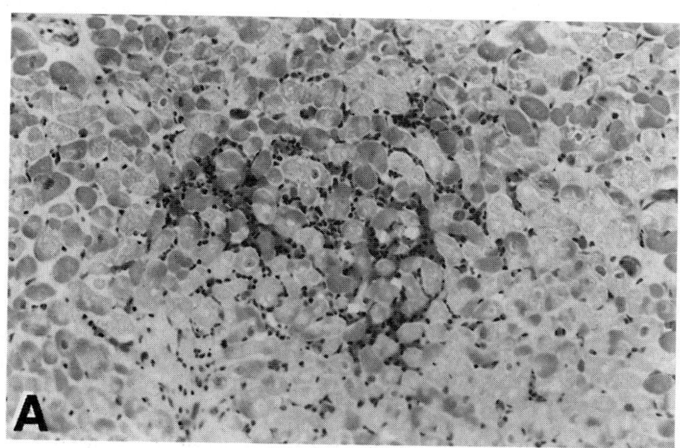

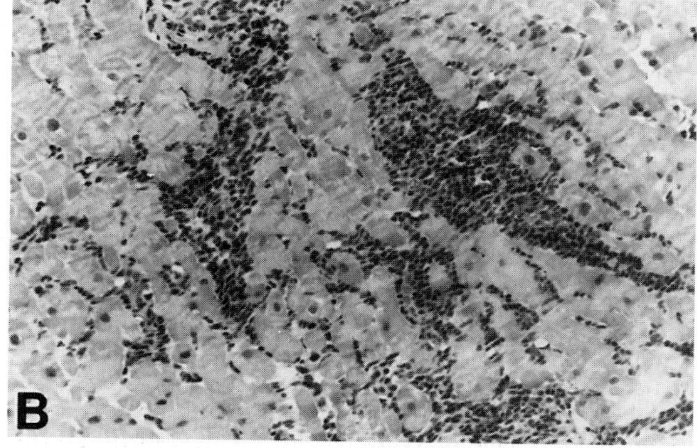

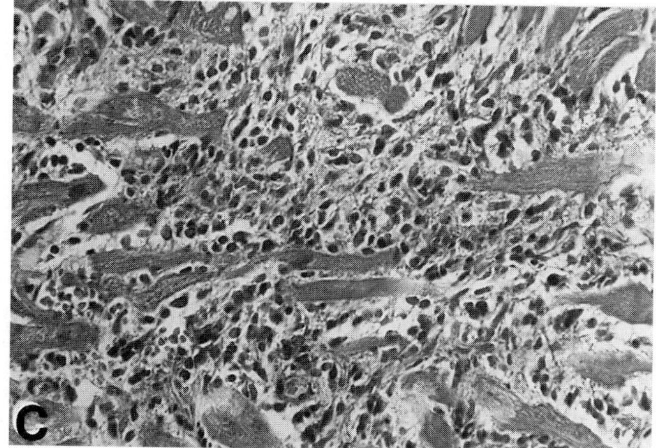

FIGURE 18–5. Composite photomicrograph showing different stages of acute cardiac rejection: *A,* Shows mild acute rejection, with a sparse interstitial lymphocytic infiltrate (Grade 1B, ISHLT) (Hematoxylin and eosin, original magnification × 200). *B,* Shows moderate acute rejection with islands of lymphocytes replacing myocardial tissue (Grade 3A, ISHLT) (Hematoxylin and eosin, original magnification × 200). *C,* Shows severe acute rejection with marked myocyte damage and a mixed inflammatory infiltrate (Grade 4, ISHLT) (Hematoxylin and eosin, original magnification × 300). (Courtesy of Margaret Billingham, M. D.)

TABLE 18–5 STANDARDIZED CARDIAC BIOPSY GRADING (ISHLT SCALE)

GRADE	FINDINGS
0	No rejection
1	1A = focal (perivascular or interstitial) infiltrate without necrosis
	1B = diffuse but sparse infiltrate without necrosis
2	One focus only with aggressive infiltration and/or focal myocyte damage
3	3A = multifocal aggressive infiltrates and/or myocyte damage
	3B = diffuse inflammatory process with necrosis
4	Diffuse aggressive polymorphous infiltrate, ± edema, ± hemorrhage, ± vasculitis, with necrosis

ISHLT = International Society for Heart and Lung Transplantation.
Modified from Miller, L.W., Schlant, R.C., Kobashigawa J., et al.: Task Force 5: Complications. J. Am. Coll. Cardiol. *22*(1):43, 1993. Reprinted with permission from the American College of Cardiology.

casional infections with these agents have been first diagnosed by the endomyocardial biopsy. Perhaps the most frequent abnormality is a biopsy taken from a previous biopsy site that may contain contraction bands and evidence of inflammation and collagen formation as a result of healing of the previous biopsy site. The findings associated with previous biopsy site histology are described in more detail elsewhere.[92]

In addition to classical cell-mediated rejection, occasional cases of hyperacute rejection due to preformed circulating antibodies from prior transfusion, pregnancy, or ABO incompatibility may occur within hours of surgery and require prompt retransplantation. In established allografts, vascular damage in the absence of lymphocytic infiltration has been accompanied by deposition of complement and IgG on endothelial cells that are swollen or disrupted.[93] The specificity of these findings remains somewhat controversial;[93a] however, when they are accompanied by clinical deterioration, treatment with an augmented immunosuppressive regimen and plasmapheresis has been used successfully.[94]

Treatment of Acute Rejection

Immunosuppression to prevent allograft rejection begins at the time of the transplant procedure and continues throughout the life of the recipient. Although a number of strategies are being developed to enhance the induction of immunosuppression and to maximize the potential for developing tolerance in the recipient, virtually every patient probably experiences some acute allograft rejection during the first post-transplant year. The balance between effective immunosuppression and excess immunosuppression with multiple opportunistic infections requires careful tailoring of the immunosuppressive therapy to the specific needs of the individual recipient. Although a number of new immunosuppressive agents will probably become available in the next few years, as of this writing acute rejection episodes are treated by a relatively small number of standard therapies.

The highest incidence of acute rejection occurs within the first 3 months after transplantation. Of patients receiving standard triple-drug therapy that includes cyclosporine, azathioprine, and prednisone, the authors found that 84 per cent have at least one episode of rejection during the first 3 months. After 3 months, the incidence of rejection diminishes significantly to about one episode per patient-year. Those patients with a relatively good match between donor and recipient, and who do not experience rejection within the first 3 months, usually have a lower incidence of late rejection. Recent combined data from 25 institutions covering 911 patients receiving their first heart transplant were more favorable, with 40 per cent of patients free of rejection at one year. There was a higher likelihood of rejection associated with younger recipients and female donors.[95]

The timing and severity of rejection episodes dictate the appropriate therapy. A representative algorithm for treatment is shown in Figure 18–6. Episodes that occur within the first 3 months or that are moderate to severe are best treated by pulse therapy with methylprednisolone. Methylprednisolone sodium succinate is administered intravenously at a dose of 1000 mg/day for 3 consecutive days. Rejection that occurs later than one month may be treated by augmenting oral steroid intake to 100 mg of prednisone per day for 3 consecutive days, tapered gradually back to a baseline over 2 weeks. Several studies have demonstrated that an equivalent oral dose of prednisone may be as effective as intravenous methylprednisolone in early acute rejection.[96] In children or small adults, the dosage of methylprednisolone and prednisone should be decreased proportionate to body size.

SEVERE REJECTION. Because of the side effects of increased corticosteroid therapy, the patient should be carefully monitored for infections, increased fluid retention, glucose intolerance, and psychological or mood changes. When prednisone treatment is ineffective or in particularly severe cases of rejection associated with hemodynamic changes, more aggressive therapy is given. The use of ATGAM (horse anti-thymocyte globulin), rabbit ATG, or OKT3 monoclonal antibody constitutes rescue therapy after unsuccessful use of prednisone or methylprednisolone. Unfortunately, the availability of commercial preparations of ATGAM is limited. Similarly, the availability of rabbit ATG preparations is erratic because such preparations are not commercially available and require special local arrange-

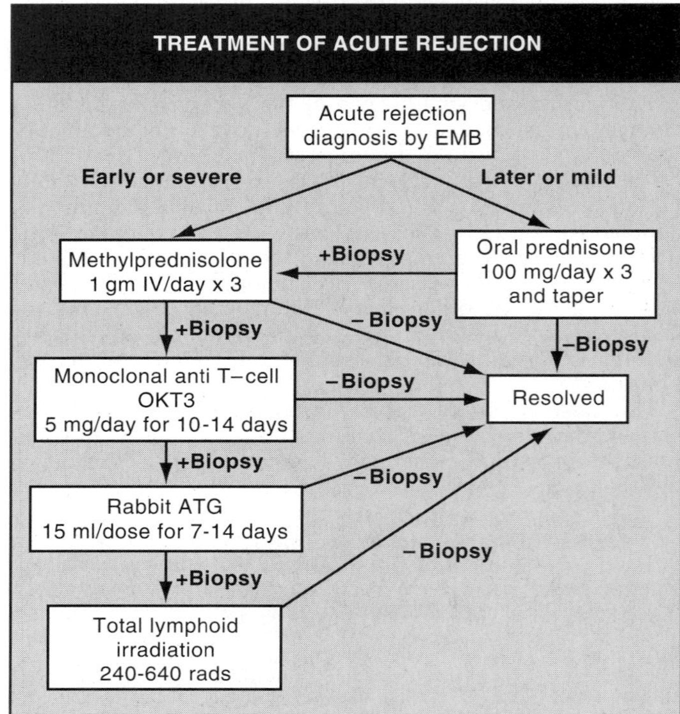

FIGURE 18–6. Algorithm for treating acute allograft rejection. EMB = endomyocardial biopsy; ATG = antithymocyte globulin.

ments for preparation. Consequently, OKT3 therapy is probably the most frequent type of rescue therapy being used, and is an effective treatment for most resistant rejection episodes.[97] Treatment with OKT3 is costly ($3,000 for a 10-day course). Because it stimulates the CD3 receptors to which it binds, it releases lymphokines, and initial doses may cause hypotension, fever, bronchospasm, diarrhea, or sterile meningitis. For these reasons, patients are transferred to acute care settings and pretreated with antihistamines, acetaminophen, and intravenous corticosteroids.

MILD REJECTION. Additional strategies for treatment of early or mild rejection have been advocated. Kobashigawa and associates treated patients with mild acute rejection with increases in oral cyclosporine, treating 40 episodes in 28 patients.[98] In their study of those patients with an actual increase in serum cyclosporine levels, 90 per cent had no progression of rejection or clearing of rejection, whereas 37 per cent of those who had no increase in levels progressed with more evidence of acute rejection requiring treatment. An alternative approach is simply to observe the patient in cases of grade IA or IB rejection and rebiopsy in 2 weeks, since almost two-thirds of patients with stable cyclosporine levels reverted to normal spontaneously. Olsen and coworkers from the University of Utah reported using methotrexate in the treatment of persistent low-grade rejection.[99] Methotrexate was given three times a week for an average of 8 weeks to 16 patients. All rejections were reversed, and the dose of prednisone could be reduced. Although there were no infections, azathioprine dosage had to be reduced in 10 patients because of leukopenia. Methotrexate has also been advocated for recurrent acute, as well as refractory, rejection in doses up to 15 mg/week.[100]

PERSISTENT OR RECURRENT REJECTION. For patients with persistent recurrent rejection episodes despite multiple courses of conventional therapy, Hunt and colleagues at Stanford[101] and Kirklin's group at Alabama[102] have supported the use of total lymphoid irradiation (TLI). It was administered according to standard protocols. Total doses varied from 240 to 1200 cGy (rads) over 5 to 10 weeks and were adjusted in response to leukopenia and thrombocytopenia. Measurement of absolute T-cell counts may also be helpful. Azathioprine should be discontinued or diminished during TLI. The frequency of rejection episodes eventually fell to 5 per cent of the pretreatment rate.

NEW IMMUNOSUPPRESSIVE AGENTS

TACROLIMUS (FK-506). The introduction of cyclosporine in the early 1980's was the stimulus for the tremendous growth in heart transplantation. Attention has subsequently focused on a variety of other agents, which also have selective effects and which may have a different side effect profile. The first of these new agents to be introduced into clinical practice is the macrolide antibiotic compound tacrolimus (FK-506), identified by the Fujisawa Company of Japan[103] and now approved by the Food and Drug Administration. This compound is produced by *Streptomyces tsukubaensis*. It appears to be about 100 times more effective per unit dose than cyclosporine. It too interacts with cyclophilin and binds calcineurin, preventing helper cell amplification by blocking IL-2 synthesis.[16]

Only 25 per cent of the oral dose is absorbed, and, like cyclosporine, it is metabolized by the hepatic P450 cytochrome system and then excreted in the bile. Drugs influencing the P450 system may alter clearance of tacrolimus. Adverse effects include nephrotoxicity, gastrointestinal disturbances, neurotoxicity, hyperglycemia, headache, and hypertension.[19,104] Preliminary experience in thoracic transplantation suggests that it has a definite role in both primary and rescue therapy.[105,106]

MYCOPHENOLATE MOFETIL. This immunosuppressant is now FDA-approved. It is a pro-drug, which is converted in vivo to mycophenolic acid, which interferes with the synthesis of guanosine. This purine is essential for the production of DNA, as well as cell surface glycoprotein adhesion molecules by both B and T cells. Nonimmune cells utilize the salvage pathway for guanosine synthesis and are therefore relatively insensitive to mycophenolate. Because its site of action differs from that of cyclosporine and tacrolimus, it may be synergistic with them in both acute and chronic rejection.[107] Side effects are primarily limited to gastrointestinal distress, but renal function seems unaffected.[108]

RAPAMYCIN. This investigative compound of fungal origin also binds to the FK-binding protein; however, its mode of action is not linked to calcineurin. Instead, it interferes with the action of growth factors on T cells. It selectively targets only those cells responsive to IL-2 and similar lymphokines and does not inhibit the replication of other rapidly dividing cells. Its mechanism complements that of cyclosporine and tacrolimus.[107] The availability of multiple agents for selective immunosuppression will almost certainly enhance the early and late acceptance of cardiac allografts, minimize toxicities, and increase the safety of cardiac transplantation.

Infection After Cardiac Transplantation

In most centers, infectious complications are the most common cause of death after transplantation. Despite the fact that more effective immunosuppressive therapy has reduced the incidence and severity of infections, they still remain a major problem.[109] The overall incidence of infections ranges from 41 to 71 per cent in various series, and multiple infections are frequent. In a multicenter analysis of 814 consecutive patients undergoing primary heart transplantation between 1990 and 1991, approximately half suffered acute infection at 6 months. This rose to almost two-thirds by one year.[110]

With the extensive experience now available from both kidney, liver, and heart transplant recipients, certain typical infection patterns can be described. Infections in the first postoperative month tend to involve bacterial pathogens encountered in surgical patients in general. Infections in the time from 1 to 4 months after surgery usually involve opportunistic pathogens, especially CMV. After this period, a mixture of both conventional and opportunistic infections is found.

In contradistinction to renal transplant recipients, cardiac recipients must receive somewhat higher levels of pharmacological immunosuppression, which cannot be significantly reduced at the time of infectious complications. This emphasizes the need for early diagnosis and aggressive therapy for any type of infection.

The role of immunization in preventing post-transplant infections is too often overlooked. If given before the institution of immunosuppressive regimens, immunization is more likely to be successful. Pretransplant inoculation with pneumococcal and hepatitis B vaccines, boosters for DPT, and, for young people not previously immunized, MMR and polio vaccines are recommended. Since these last two are live virus vaccines, they should be avoided by patients (and immediate family members) after transplantation when immunosuppression may enhance their virulence. The regular use of influenza vaccine every two years is controversial but has been advocated for HIV-infected patients, and may be useful in transplant patients as well.

EARLY INFECTION. Infections in the first month after transplantation are commonly bacterial and most frequently pulmonary. This is especially true for patients with lung transplants, in addition to heart. Typically, nosocomial organisms, such as *Legionella, Staphylococcus epidermidis, Pseudomonas aeruginosa, Proteus, Klebsiella,* and *Escherichia coli,* are encountered. The incidence of significant mediastinitis is between 0.4 and 4.5 per cent in heart transplant recipients. Treatment includes prolonged courses of antibiotics, debridement of devitalized bone, and the use of vascularized muscle flaps for subsequent wound closure. Other typical causes of early postoperative infection, such as urinary tract infections, bacteremias, and pneumonia, should be suspected. The clinical diagnosis of pneumonia is made on the basis of typical clinical features, including cough, fever, sputum production, and chest radiographs showing a new pulmonary infiltrate. An aggressive approach to early diagnosis is recommended. This may include bronchoscopy with washings and culture. The results of these cultures will determine specific antibiotic therapy, but early broad-spectrum coverage started immediately after obtaining appropriate cultures is recommended.

LATE INFECTION. Late post-transplant infections are more diverse. These are frequently of the opportunistic variety, including viruses (CMV, Herpes), *Pneumocystis carinii* (PCP), and fungi (e.g., *Candida* and *Aspergillus*), as well as more exotic varieties. Occasionally, *Nocardia* or *Toxoplasma gondii* are encountered. The variety of late post-transplant pneumonias may vary from center to center, depending on local prevalences and the use of prophylactic treatments. For example, in some series, *Pneumocystis carinii* is the most common late pulmonary infection, whereas in other series it is absent. The regular prophylactic administration of trimethoprim-sulfamethoxazole (TMP-SMZ) three times per week on a long-term basis is now routinely recommended by most transplant programs to prevent PCP and *Toxoplasma* infection (or if TMP-SMZ is not tolerated, monthly pentamidine aerosol inhalation for PCP prophylaxis).[111]

CYTOMEGALOVIRUS INFECTION. CMV infection is the most frequent and important viral infection in transplant recipients, with an incidence in cardiac recipients of between 73 and 100 per cent.[112,113] It is the single most frequent infecting organism, accounting for 26 per cent of all infections in a large cooperative study.[110] This can be minimized in CMV-negative patients by the use of CMV-negative blood products, but a CMV-positive donor will almost invariably transmit infection. It may be detected in some patients only by seroconversion or, if they are seropositive preoperatively, by a rise in IgG titers or the appearance of an IgM antibody. Some infections remain subclinical. When clinical disease is present, it may present as leukopenia, pneumonia, gastroenteritis, hepatitis, or retinitis in varying combinations. Of these, pneumonia is the most lethal (13 per cent mortality), while retinitis is the most refractory and requires indefinite maintenance therapy. Most cases are responsive to ganciclovir (DHPG) or foscarnet. The addition of hyperimmune globulin has further improved therapeutic outcome and decreased mortality, particularly from CMV pneumonia. Although seronegative recipients who accept allografts from CMV-positive donors are the most vulnerable, prior seropositivity does not offer protection from infection (15 per cent disease frequency) and late reactivation, reflecting the persistence of this member of the Herpesvirus family, may occur.

Unfortunately, diagnostic tests are not always positive. Viral cultures may be negative in the presence of infection, and serological responses may be diminished due to immunosuppression. The recent addition of polymerase chain reaction (PCR) technology for the detection of CMV viremia has added a more sensitive diagnostic method, but greater experience is needed before it becomes the standard.[114] Because of these limitations, CMV should always be suspected in the event of unexplained fevers, gastroenteritis, or culture-negative interstitial pneumonitis. Endoscopy with biopsy may establish the diagnosis promptly in these latter cases.[114a] Early prophylaxis with ganciclovir in the setting of positive CMV graft into a negative recipient includes the use of ganciclovir and hyperimmune globulin for 6 to 8 weeks post-transplant. Prophylaxis against CMV infection decreased the incidence of CMV disease in recipients who were seropositive pretransplant, but not in those who were seronegative.[115]

The importance of CMV infection cannot be overemphasized because of its relation to the development of late graft atherosclerosis. The availability of newer antiviral treatments may help to minimize the complications of this particular infection in the future.

FUNGAL INFECTIONS. Although less common than viral and bacterial infections, fungal infections are more serious, less responsive to therapy, and more likely to be lethal. (*Pneumocystis carinii,* originally thought to be a protozoan, has now been reclassified as fungus by ribosomal DNA analysis.[116]) *Candida* and *Aspergillus* are the most commonly encountered pathogens. Treatment with imidazoles is often effective for *Candida* and coccidioidomycosis, but their use may raise cyclosporine levels. Infections of vital organs usually require amphotericin B and flucytosine, which compromise renal function and potentiate leukopenia, respectively.

Toxoplasmosis is uncommon but responds to pyrimethamine.[117]

OTHER COMPLICATIONS OF IMMUNOSUPPRESSION

The cardiologist following cardiac transplant patients should be aware of the multiple complications of the immunosuppressive drugs. All of the commonly used drugs increase the risk of infection and are also associated with neoplasia.[118]

CYCLOSPORINE TOXICITY. Cyclosporine is associated with a number of complications. The most clinically significant effect of cyclosporine involves the kidneys. Almost all patient groups receiving cyclosporine have a fall in creatinine clearance, an increase in serum creatinine level, and hypertension.[119,120] Histopathological changes after chronic administration are found in the proximal convoluted tubule and in the distal tubules and consist of vacuolization of cells, epithelial swelling, hydropic degeneration, and necrosis. Increasing clinical and experimental evidence exists that cyclosporine produces a derangement in the prostaglandin system in the renal tubules. Indomethacin exacerbates renal dysfunction after cyclosporine administration.

Cyclosporine may act by increasing urinary thromboxane B_2 levels in a dose-dependent manner, with local vasoconstriction, platelet aggregation, and release of platelet-produced thromboxane. This may explain the development of hypertension, renal ischemia, and the dysfunction that is seen clinically, although azotemia and hypertension are occasionally independent of one another.[121] Acute elevation of cyclosporine to three to four times customary maintenance levels may cause acute oliguria and rapid decline in renal function. This is probably due to vasoconstriction and is promptly reversible with adjustment of dosage or removal of drugs hindering cyclosporine catabolism. Chronic interstitial fibrosis and nephron loss is common but is usually stable. It may be intermittently exacerbated by nephrotoxins used for therapy (e.g., amphotericin B, nonsteroidal anti-inflammatory drugs) or diagnosis (radiocontrast agents).

Early after transplant, many patients have oliguria. Thus, many transplant groups restrict the use of cyclosporine to continuous intravenous administration with careful control of circulating levels during the early post-transplant period, or omit cyclosporine altogether and use induction therapy with OKT3 until serum creatinine is normal and the patient has recovered from the effects of cardiopulmonary bypass.[120,122,123]

Hepatotoxicity, although uncommon, is usually acute and secondary to exceptionally high levels of cyclosporine. It is evidenced by an increase in bilirubin and by increases in serum liver enzymes. There are no characteristic cellular pathological alterations except for centrilobular fatty changes. The hepatotoxicity is dose-related and reverts to normal after the dose of cyclosporine is lowered or eliminated. In general, hepatotoxicity is uncommon after cardiac transplantation, and, so far, no long-term sequelae of cyclosporine on liver function have been reported.

Neurotoxic reactions are manifested by a fine tremor, paresthesias, and occasionally seizures. Most of these events are dose-related and reversible. Other unusual side effects include the development of hirsutism or hypertrichosis, observed in almost all patients who receive cyclosporine. These effects tend to regress as the dosage of cyclosporine is lowered. Similarly, gingival hyperplasia has been observed. A combination of cyclosporine and nifedipine has resulted in an increased rate of gingival hyperplasia (51 per cent) when compared with cyclosporine alone (8 per cent).[124] Because cyclosporine is metabolized almost exclusively by the liver, hepatic dysfunction can cause abrupt elevations of blood levels of cyclosporine, precipitating renal dysfunction. Many commonly used compounds can influence the hepatic P450 cytochrome system, which is responsible for cyclosporine catabolism. Drugs that raise cyclosporine levels include the antimicrobials erythromycin, doxycycline, imipenem, cilastatin, ticarcillin, norfloxacin, ketoconazole, and itraconazole; the calcium channel blockers diltiazem, verapamil, nifedipine, and nicardipine; hormone products such as danazol, androgens, estradiol, and oral contraceptives, as well as other commonly utilized medications such as cimetidine, ranitidine, warfarin, acetazolamide, metoclopramide, and amiodarone. (Diltiazem and ketoconazole have been used adjunctively to lower the consumption and cost of cyclosporine maintenance.[125])

Conversely, a drop in circulating cyclosporine levels, with the danger of causing rejection, may be precipitated by omeprazole, by the antibiotics rifampin and nafcillin, and by the anticonvulsants phenytoin, carbamazepine, valproic acid, primidone, and methsuximide.[126,127] The use of lovastatin to control hypercholesterolemia in patients on cyclosporine has rarely been associated with rhabdomyolysis.[128]

CORTICOSTEROID TOXICITY. Perhaps the most troublesome side effects of immunosuppressive therapy are associated with long-term administration of corticosteroids. In patients who require relatively high doses of steroids, these can be especially severe and include adrenal cortical atrophy, cushingoid appearance, cataracts, skin fragility, severe osteoporosis, peptic ulcers, aseptic necrosis of bone, weight gain, psychiatric effects, diabetes, elevated serum lipid levels, and heightened susceptibility to infection of all types. In children, axial growth may be impaired. Perhaps the major advance in transplantation will come when corticosteroid therapy can be completely eliminated, a strategy under investigation.[129]

AZATHIOPRINE TOXICITY. The major morbidity of long-term azathioprine administration is bone marrow suppression. Severe granulocytopenia has resulted from inadvertent coadministration of allopurinol for the treatment of CyA-induced hyperuricemia and gout and has been life-threatening. Azathioprine also causes hepatotoxicity in some patients, which may be so severe that the drug must be discontinued with substitution of an alkylating agent, such as cyclophosphamide.

NEOPLASMS IN IMMUNOSUPPRESSED CARDIAC TRANSPLANT RECIPIENTS

Cancer is an unfortunate consequence of chronic immunosuppression.[118] In general, transplant recipients have a threefold increase in the incidence of various cancers when compared with age-matched controls. Some specific cancers are more than 100 times more frequent in immunosuppressed patients than in the general population. For all tumors, the average time of appearance of the cancer after transplantation is 58 months, although some tumors may characteristically appear at other intervals. Cardiac transplant recipients have a somewhat higher incidence of cancer than do renal transplant patients, perhaps because of the higher levels of immunosuppression. The most common tumors among transplant patients are those of the skin and lips, non-Hodgkin's lymphomas, Kaposi's sarcomas, and uterine, cervical, vulval, and perineal neoplasms.[118] The frequency of common adenocarcinomas, such as those of breast, lung, prostate, and colon, does not exceed that of the general population.[130]

Perhaps the most important neoplasms are the lymphoproliferative tumors that occur early after transplantation, more frequently in younger recipients. Most of these tumors are thought to be the result of Epstein-Barr viral infection and consist of B-cell proliferation unchecked because of T-cell suppression or depletion.[131] The recurrent use of OKT3 has been identified as a risk factor in some programs,[132] but this has not been confirmed by others.[133] Approximately 15 per cent are of T-cell origin, and some of these also carry EBV markers.[130,134]

The tumors typically arise in extranodal sites, such as lung, gut, or central nervous system. Treatment has included diminishing immunosuppression, adding antiviral therapy with acyclovir or ganciclovir,[135] and irradiation or surgical removal for monofocal tumor. Closer surveillance by cardiac echocardiography and biopsy is essential during this period. If rejection occurs or if the tumor is refractory, additional therapy with alpha-interferon, chemotherapy, and monoclonal B cell antibodies have been employed with success.[136] Roughly one-third of patients will respond, and recurrence is uncommon.

Graft Atherosclerosis

The major long-term problem after cardiac transplantation, assuming greater importance as the number of survivors increases, is the development of significant coronary artery disease in the transplanted heart. Graft atherosclerosis was first observed by Thomson in 1969 in the first long-term survivor reported from South Africa.[137] Nineteen months after transplantation for ischemic cardiomyopathy, the patient died with extensive coronary artery disease. A variety of reports show an incidence of between 20 and 50 per cent at 5 years.[138–142]

With the advent of protocols using cyclosporine for immunosuppression, there has been no significant decline in the incidence of this disease.[143]

Graft atherosclerosis has been observed as an incidental finding at autopsy as early as 3 months after transplantation. Significant coronary disease may produce arrhythmias, myocardial infarction, sudden death, or impaired left ventricular function with congestive heart failure.[144] Angina pectoris is extremely rare because the cardiac allograft remains essentially denervated, although a patient has been reported who had angina pectoris in the presence of coronary artery disease.[145] The disease tends to be rather diffuse and concentric, and coronary angiograms must be closely inspected and compared with previous studies to appreciate the reduction in coronary diameter. The recent introduction of intravascular ultrasound to assess thickness and composition of the coronary arterial wall, as well as precise measurement of lumen diameter, has demonstrated the presence of disease which was not visible angiographically (Fig. 18–7*A*). Definite intimal thickening was present in one-quarter of patients at Stanford at 1 year and its prevalence increased to approximately 80 per cent at 5 years post-transplant. Calcification was uncommon (<10 per cent) up to 5 years, but approached 25 per cent at 6 to 10 years and 50 per cent at 11 to 15 years.[146]

Noninvasive stress imaging with thallium and sestaMIBI scans has been generally disappointing, probably because of the diffuse nature of the vascular lesion.

PATHOGENESIS. The cause of graft atherosclerosis remains controversial and is probably multifactorial.[147] Vascular endothelium is known to be immunologically active, and similar vascular changes are seen late after kidney and liver transplantation. The early stages of cardiac allograft rejection are characterized by lymphocytic perivascular infiltration, and vasculitis frequently is a prominent part of moderate to severe allograft rejection. Vascular changes with deposition of immunoglobulin, complement, and fibrin have been demonstrated both in patients and in animals. Platelet-derived growth factor producing activation and aggregation of platelets, as well as proliferation of mononuclear cells, has been demonstrated to occur during acute rejection. These data strongly support a complex immune mechanism for the development of graft atherosclerosis. Histological features of graft arteriopathy demonstrate extensive concentric intimal proliferation (Fig. 18–8) with hyperplasia of smooth muscle and lipid-laden macrophages.[148] Grossly, the vessels show diffuse disease extending symmetrically into distal branches with few collateral vessels. Proximal stenoses occur rarely.[149] Angiography may not be sensitive enough to show this disease (Fig. 18–7*B*).

RISK FACTORS. Several clinical studies have attempted to identify risk factors. In the most comprehensive report of patients treated with prednisone and azathioprine, significant clinical factors were donor age over 35, incompatibility at HLA-A1 and A2 loci, and serum triglyceride concentration greater than 280 mg/dl.[150] Lipoprotein(a) concentration in one study was more than three times higher in patients with angiographic coronary disease than in those with normal angiograms.[151] In other reports, which include experience with cyclosporine, the development of graft atherosclerosis was correlated with two or more rejection episodes, but not with lipid levels or donor age.[138]

Cytomegalovirus (CMV) Infection. Several reports emphasize the possible role of CMV infection in atherogenesis in general[152] and graft atherosclerosis in particular. In a review of 301 cardiac transplant recipients during the cyclosporine era, the Stanford group divided patients into two groups based on freedom from CMV infection.[153] Two hundred and ten patients were included in this group and 91 patients in the CMV infection group. The incidence of graft rejection was significantly higher in the CMV infection group and, using angiographic criteria or autopsy examination, graft atherosclerosis was also found to be significantly more severe. Intimal proliferation has been linked to the inactivation of p53 (a tumor suppressor) by CMV, permitting enhanced proliferation of smooth muscle cells.[154] Actuarial 5-year survival in the CMV infection–free group was 68.3 per cent, compared with only 32.2 per cent for the CMV infection group. Data from Johns Hopkins Hospital indicate that the presence of CMV infection and donor age were the two factors in a multifactorial analysis that correlated with the development of graft atherosclerosis.

In addition to measures to limit CMV, strategies have been directed toward limiting the amount of steroid administered. Hypercholesterolemia is a known risk factor for the development of coronary artery disease in general, and the use of prednisone[155] and cyclosporine[156] is correlated with elevated serum cholesterol levels in cardiac transplant recipients.

PREVENTION. Most centers use some preventive measures in the hope of reducing the incidence of graft atherosclerosis. These include modification of known risk factors,

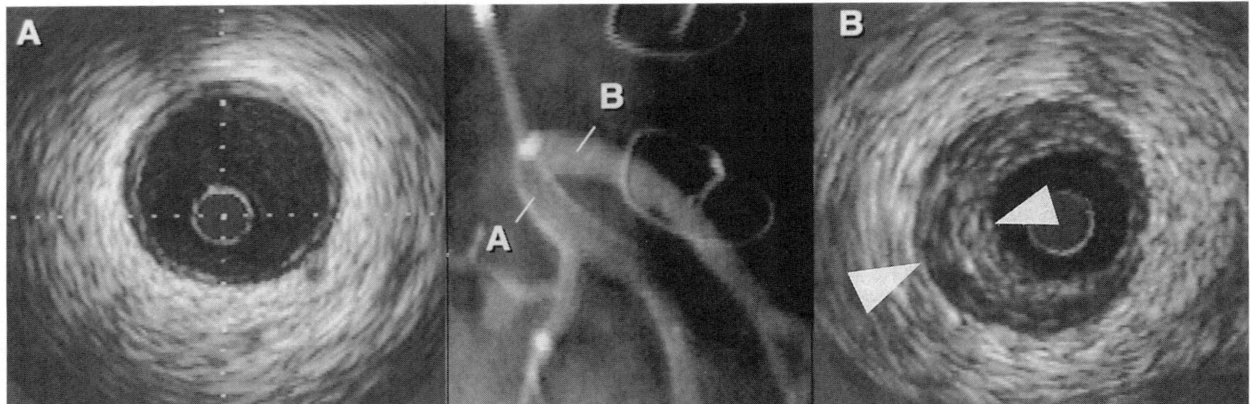

FIGURE 18–7. *A,* Intravascular ultrasound of the left anterior descending coronary artery in a transplant patient at the site shown at A in the middle panel depicting the coronary angiogram. *B,* Intravascular ultrasound in the proximal circumflex coronary artery at the point marked in the coronary angiogram in the central panel at B. Arrows show thickened intima. (Courtesy of Peter Fitzgerald, M.D.)

maintenance of ideal body weight through dietary restriction, reduced intake of cholesterol and saturated fats, the use of lipid-lowering agents such as pravastatin,[156a] cessation of smoking, regular exercise, and the use of an antiplatelet agent such as low-dose aspirin. The addition of diltiazem to the post-transplant regimen has retarded progression of allograft coronary disease, and its cyclosporine-sparing effect has also reduced costs.[157]

TREATMENT. The existence of more discrete proximal lesions has been treated by percutaneous transluminal coronary angioplasty in some cases, and even coronary artery bypass grafting has been reported.[158–161] However, retransplantation is the major alternative once diffuse graft atherosclerosis develops. The results of retransplantation are less good than for the primary procedure, with a reported patient survival rate of approximately 48 per cent at one year (n = 449) reported by the International Society for Heart and Lung Transplantation. Uncontrolled rejection and an interval of less than 6 months between operation and the need for pretransplant mechanical support were listed as risk factors.[162]

Late Follow-up

The late follow-up of cardiac transplant recipients requires a coordinated and systematic approach. The drug regimen for late follow-up is shown in Table 18–6. The two leading causes of early morbidity and mortality are rejection and infection. Later surveillance should focus also on graft atherosclerosis and cancer. The frequency and timing of transplant follow-up visits are determined by the general condition of the patient and the time after transplant. Endomyocardial biopsy remains a necessity and is performed every 3 to 4 months indefinitely. The authors currently recommend performing coronary arteriography on a yearly basis, although some programs alternate this with noninvasive studies of myocardial function or ischemia.

In addition to the objective laboratory data, a detailed interval history and physical examination are important to detect other complicating illnesses at an early stage. Patients may minimize new symptoms, and the physician

TABLE 18–6 DRUG REGIMEN FOR LONG-TERM RECIPIENT

Prednisone 0.1–0.2 mg/kg/day
Cyclosporine 3–6 mg/kg/day
Diltiazem 120–240 mg/kg/day
Sulfamethoxazole-trimethoprim b.i.d. 3 days/week
Azathioprine 1–2 mg/kg/day
Miscellaneous
Furosemide
Potassium supplements
Antacids
Aspirin
Additional antihypertensives p.r.n.

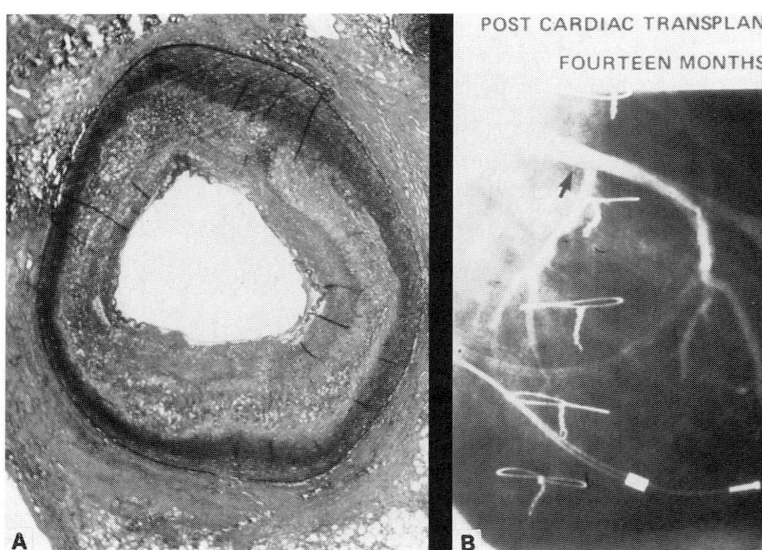

FIGURE 18–8. *A,* Histologic section of left main coronary artery showing concentric atheromatous plaque composed of a fibrous cap overlying a basal layer of extracellular and intracellular lipid. (Original magnification ×15.) *B,* Coronary arteriogram performed 4 days prior to death, 14 months after transplantation. (From Johnson, D. E., Alderman, E. L., Schroeder, J. S. et al.: Transplant coronary artery disease: Histopathologic correlations with angiographic morphology. J. Am. Coll. Cardiol. *17*:449, 1991. Reprinted with permission from the American College of Cardiology.)

must be constantly alert to the possibility of an occult, but potentially life-threatening, infectious complication. A detailed inquiry into all medications that the patient is taking should be performed to avoid errors of omission, dosage misunderstanding, or unexplained additions that might alter the metabolism or excretion of immunosuppressive drugs, potentially causing rejection (e.g., rifampin), nephropathy (e.g., erythromycin), or bone marrow suppression (e.g., allopurinol). A sampling of other late problems routinely encountered includes aseptic necrosis of bone, azotemia, cataracts, cholelithiasis, gout, heart failure, herpes zoster, impotence, obesity, rejection, vertebral compression fractures, and an assortment of skin lesions. A typical drug regimen for the long-term recipient is listed in Table 18–6.

Survival Expectations

Long-term survival and complete rehabilitation can be attained by most patients currently undergoing heart transplantation. Several studies have attempted to define the rehabilitation potential of surviving patients. In a reported series of 56 patients at Stanford, 51 (91 per cent) were classified as successfully rehabilitated; however, only 26 out of 51 patients (46 per cent of the total) returned to full-time work.[163] This may reflect planned early retirement, unwillingness to give up disability and insurance benefits, or the employer's resistance to hiring someone with a chronic disorder, rather than any physical limitation. In another study, 90 per cent of surviving patients were judged to be in a functional New York Heart Association Class I.[164] In a study by Lough and associates, a measure of life satisfaction demonstrated that 89 per cent of recipients rated their quality of life as good to excellent[165] and 86 per cent thought that they led "normal lives." [166]

Simple survival statistics, as reported by the International Society for Heart and Lung Transplantation, indicate a one-year actuarial survival of slightly greater than 80 per cent.[1,166] Individual programs may report survivals up to 90 to 95 per cent at one year. The current data from the International Society are shown in Figure 18–9. Survival was somewhat lower in patients below the age of 5 and above 65.[167] Other factors that may play a role in marginally decreasing survival are longer donor ischemic time, older donor age, and non-O blood type.[168] The probability of lethal rejection within 2 years was 5 per cent when three to six HLA mismatches were present.[169]

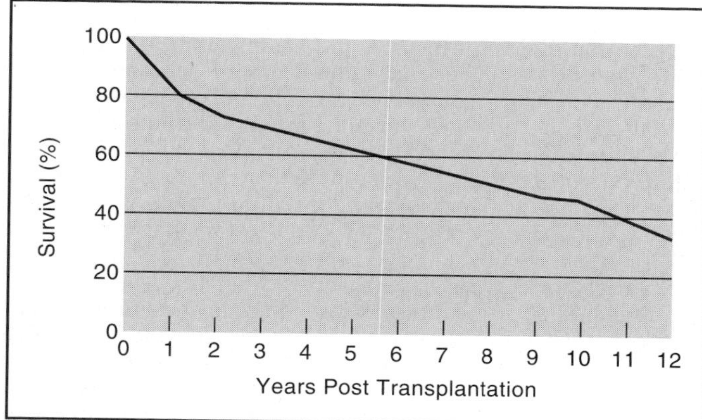

FIGURE 18–9. Heart transplantation actuarial survival for all patients reported to the Registry of the International Society for Heart Transplantation from 1975 to 1993. (From Hosenpud, J. D., Novick, R. J., Breen, T. J., and Daily, O. P.: The Registry of the International Society for Heart and Lung Transplantation: Eleventh Official Report —1994. J. Heart Lung Transplant. *13*(4):561, 1994. Reprinted with permission from Mosby-Year Book, Inc.)

Physiology of the Transplanted Heart

The transplanted heart remains largely,[170] but not entirely,[171] denervated throughout the life of the recipient. A variety of studies document the cardiac response to exercise or stress, which is less than normal but adequate for almost all activities (Fig. 18–10).[172–174] The heart rate accelerates slowly during the first stages of exercise, accompanied by an immediate increase in filling pressures as a result of augmented venous return from exercising muscles and decreased compliance. The latter may result from rejection, arteriopathy, arterial hypertension, small donor heart size, or cyclosporine. Atrial contribution to end-diastolic filling is compromised by the dissociation between host and donor atrial contractions. The mid-atrial anastomosis may partially deform the atrioventricular annuli, leading to mitral and tricuspid regurgitation. In the absence of hypertension or rejection, ventricular ejection fractions are normal to high.[175,176]

The effect of denervation is to isolate the heart from anatomically mediated reflexes while enhancing its sensitivity to circulating norepinephrine. The resting heart rate is generally higher due to absence of vagal tone. Respiratory sinus arrhythmia and carotid reflex bradycardia are absent. The more gradual increase of heart rate with exercise parallels the rise in circulating catecholamines, which also leads to an increase in the inotropic state of the myocardium. With augmented venous return and higher filling pressures, the stroke volume increases, contributing to the necessary increase in cardiac output during exercise.

Cardiac denervation results in an increase in beta-adrenergic receptor density.[177] In laboratory animals, denervation results in an increased responsiveness to noradrenaline and isoproterenol. This supersensitivity appears to be due both to upregulation of beta receptors and to a loss of norepinephrine uptake in postganglionic sympathetic neurones. In a study by Borow and associates, the heart

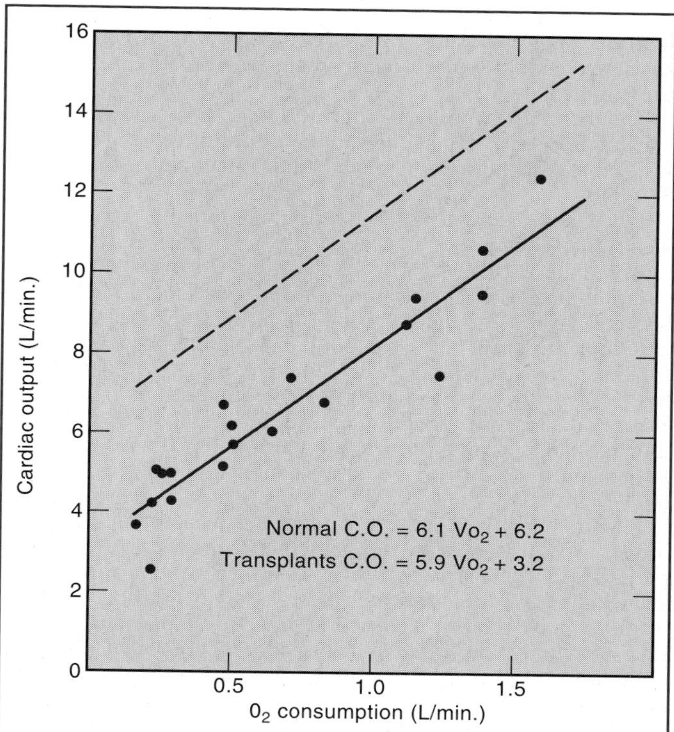

FIGURE 18–10. The relationship between cardiac output (C.O.) and oxygen consumption in seven patients one year after cardiac transplantation *(dots and solid line)*, and in 27 normal subjects age 14 to 41 *(dashed line)*. (From Hosenpud, J. D., Novick, R. J., Breen, T. J., and Daily, O. P.: The Registry of the International Society for Heart and Lung Transplantation: Eleventh Official Report—1994. J. Heart Lung Transplant. *13*(4):561, 1994. Reprinted with permission from Mosby-Year Book, Inc.)

rate response to dobutamine was compared with that of normal subjects pretreated with atropine and found to be greater in the transplanted group.[178] In other studies, infusions of isoproterenol produced a greater increase in heart rate than in normal controls.[179] This slight supersensitivity of the chronically denervated heart may be important in maintaining the necessary inotropic and chronotropic response to exercise and other stresses. All of the mechanisms underlying this supersensitivity have not been fully defined. Denervation of the allograft also blunts systemic responses to volume changes. Failure to reduce sympathetic tone during hypervolemia may contribute to hypertension and persistence of edema,[180] while blunted rate response to hypovolemia may predispose to orthostatic hypotension.

Arrhythmias are uncommon. Sinus node dysfunction occurs in 10 to 20 per cent of patients in the immediate perioperative period but is readily repaired in most cases with theophylline.[181] When this fails, permanent pacing may be necessary.

Pronounced sinus tachycardia (>120) at rest in an afebrile patient without obvious cause suggests physiological distress and warrants a search for hypovolemia, hypoglycemia, rejection, silent myocardial infarction, pulmonary emboli, adrenal insufficiency, tamponade, or abdominal catastrophe masked by corticosteroids.

Atrial arrhythmias—particularly atrial flutter—may signal rejection and are a sufficient indication for heart biopsy. Ventricular arrhythmias are uncommon except with ischemic disease or severe rejection. Ventricular fibrillation is often refractory to resuscitation.

With respect to the coronary circulation, it has been shown that coronary vasodilator reserve of the transplanted heart is normal in the absence of rejection, hypertrophy, or regional wall motion abnormalities. During periods of acute rejection, coronary flow reserve is impaired.

Cost Considerations

The cost of care has been divided into pretransplantation, evaluation and candidacy, transplantation, and posttransplantation by Evans.[182] Pretransplantation costs derive from the care needs of patients with end-stage heart disease and are multiplied by the steadily increasing time spent on waiting lists, which reached a median in 1993 of 208 days (22 per cent waited 6 to 12 months and 42 per cent waited more than a year).[183] Depending on the need for hospitalization, intensive care, or mechanical support, such costs easily exceed $100,000. These costs are considerably higher for Status 1 patients.[183a]

The cost of candidacy, including catheterization, myocardial biopsy, social service evaluation, special studies,[184] and professional fees totals between $10,000 to $20,000.

The median charge for a heart transplant in 1993 dollars was $123,000, with a median length of hospital stay of 23 days (range 1 to 554). The charge, when separated into its components, was distributed as follows: hospital charges $84,000, donor organ acquisition $17,000, surgeons' fees $13,000, and other professional fees $9000. The extremes for these figures varied by factors of 5 to 10.[182] Charges for the entire first year have been estimated at $209,000. Yearly follow-up thereafter, including angiography and regular biopsies (three to four/year), probably exceeds $15,000, with immunosuppressive drugs alone costing $4000 to $6000 annually.[185]

The increasing numbers of patients on waiting lists, the longer waiting periods, the growing proportion of Status 1 patients,[183a] the increased survival after surgery, and steady inflation guarantee continued increases in the total expenditure for each patient undergoing heart transplantation. Fortunately, there has been widespread acceptance of this burden, and, as early as 1985, the majority of private insurers[186] and, by 1990, 78 per cent of state Medicaid programs[187] covered heart transplantation. Medicare also pays for care at designated centers which meet Federal operational criteria.[21]

Reimbursement is usually less than 80 per cent of charges and long-term medication costs are not always recovered.[187] Insurance contracts that pay ongoing costs only when linked to claims of continued disability necessarily inhibit return to work.

Heart Transplantation in Children

Although the total number of heart transplant procedures has remained relatively constant since 1988, the number of children undergoing heart transplantation is increasing yearly. Approximately 320 patients under the age of 18 years received a heart transplant in 1993, with over 100 being younger than 1 year of age. The most common indication for heart transplantation in children has been cardiomyopathy, although congenital heart disease is rapidly increasing as an indication. The largest segment of children having transplant for congenital defects are those less than 1 year of age who frequently have hypoplastic left heart syndrome.

Various other indications have included severe Ebstein's anomaly, single ventricle, and tricuspid and pulmonary atresia with coronary artery sinusoids. Other patients with previous palliative operations may develop cardiomyopathy or late tricuspid valve insufficiency, which makes them inappropriate candidates for further palliative operations.[188]

The use of heart transplantation for this indication was pioneered by Bailey, who initially began with a xenograft procedure using a donor baboon.[189] Human heart donors subsequently have been utilized, although the availability of donors is limited.[190] The longest surviving pediatric heart transplant patient is just over 17 years. A one-year survival of about 85 per cent has been reported, with excellent early growth and development.[191] There is some evidence that rejection complications are less frequent in children in whom transplant occurs before one month of age. After that time, rejection is clearly common and appears to be no less than in adult patients.

A major drawback to transplantation in children is the need for invasive endomyocardial biopsy to monitor the function of the transplanted heart. Because of these difficulties, Bailey and coworkers have advocated using clinical signs together with echocardiography as a means of diagnosing rejection episodes. Rejection in neonatal patients may be associated with fever, fussiness, and difficulty feeding, together with thickening of the left ventricular free wall on echocardiogram and slight depression of function. There has not been a good study of concomitant endomyocardial biopsy and of clinical events such as these to prove the utility of this approach. The lack of careful monitoring and treatment of rejection may result in an increased incidence of graft coronary artery disease in these patients, but the frequency of this complication has yet to be determined in the neonatal transplants.

With continual improvements in immunosuppression, the consequence of long-term administration of these drugs may be lessened, and the need for retransplantation later in life may also be alleviated. These issues, together with limited donor resources, remain the major stumbling blocks to more widespread use of transplantation in infants and children.

Retransplantation

An important consideration in cardiac transplantation is the question of retransplantation. The major indications are (1) the development of graft coronary atherosclerosis, (2) treatment of severe acute early rejection, and (3) treatment of early acute right heart failure. All of these patient groups are less desirable potential recipients than are primary transplant candidates, either because of chronic immunosuppression or the circumstances surrounding early graft failure.

These patients should meet the same standard criteria as initial candidates. These include a lack of evidence of systemic infection, no other irreversible major organ system failure, and the potential for adequate rehabilitation. Recipients should be screened for the presence of pre-existing cytotoxic antibodies. If a sufficient percentage is determined against a panel of random donor cells, a specific cross-match will be required for the retransplantation procedure.

A variety of reports have demonstrated that the survival of retransplant procedures is less than for primary procedures. Survival has been reported from between 0 and 75 per cent, depending on the center, the number of patients treated, and the indication for retransplantation.[192,193] In the largest report, 63 patients underwent 66 retransplantations out of 792 total procedures at the Stanford University Medical Center. Seventeen patients were treated for early rejection and 37 patients for development of coronary artery disease. Causes of death were similar to those for other transplant recipients, and survival was 55 ± 8 per cent at one year. A major determinant of patient survival was a

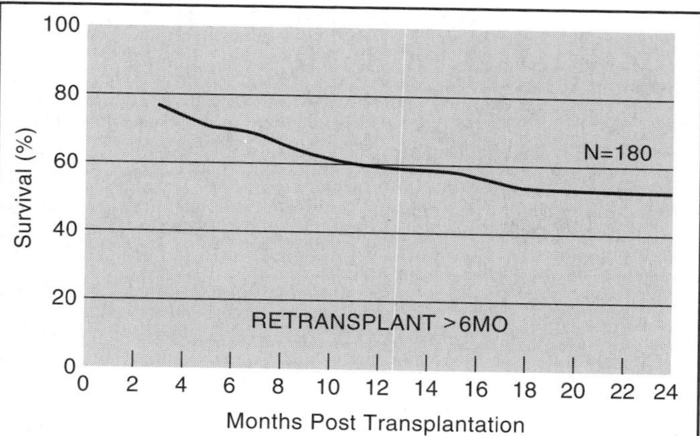

FIGURE 18–11. Actuarial survival for patients undergoing heart retransplantation reported to the Registry of the International Society for Heart Transplantation. (From Hosenpud, J. D., Novick, R. J., Breen, T. J., and Daily, O. P.: The Registry of the International Society for Heart and Lung Transplantation: Eleventh Official Report—1994. J. Heart Lung Transplant. *13*(4):561, 1994. Reprinted with permission from Mosby-Year Book, Inc.)

serum creatinine level of less than 2.0 mg/dl.[194] The actuarial survival of patients undergoing retransplant procedures reported to the Registry of the International Society for Heart and Lung Transplantation is shown in Figure 18–11. One-year survival in this group of 180 patients retransplanted after 6 months was 60 per cent. (Survival was 40 per cent for earlier retransplantation.)

HEART AND LUNG TRANSPLANTATION

Transplantation of the entire cardiopulmonary axis was accomplished experimentally even before orthotopic heart transplantation.[69,195] Despite early experimental attempts, it was a difficult clinical endeavor because of problems inherent with lung transplantation. The rather diffuse and nonspecific immunosuppression available before cyclosporine therapy led to major problems with pulmonary infections and delayed healing of the trachea or bronchus, such that no truly therapeutic and extended lung transplant had been reported.[196] The availability of cyclosporine-based protocols led to success in primate allografts in the laboratory[197] and then a clinical series initiated at Stanford University Medical Center. The first reported therapeutic success in heart-lung transplantation was reported in 1981.[18]

The indications for heart-lung transplantation initially were severe pulmonary vascular disease, either primary or secondary to congenital heart disease. Later, heart-lung transplantation was extended to patients with a variety of diffuse pulmonary diseases, such as emphysema, lymphangioleiomyomatosis, diffuse pulmonary atriovenous fistulas, and cystic fibrosis.[198,199] Long-term survival figures for heart-lung transplantation (Fig. 18–12) are not as favorable as for heart transplantation (Fig. 18–9).

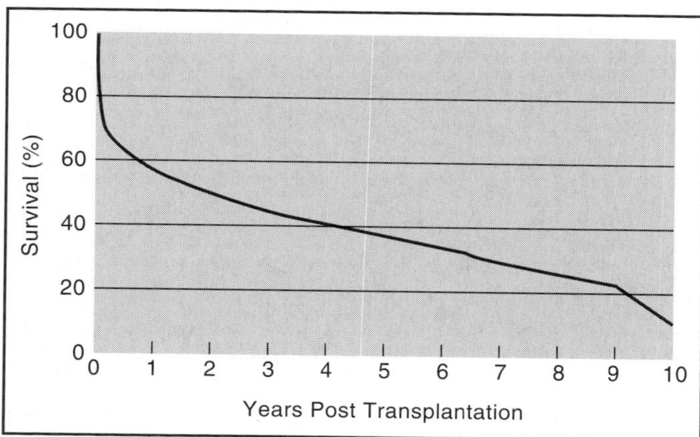

FIGURE 18–12. Survival of patients receiving heart-lung transplants, as reported to the Registry for the International Society for Heart Transplantation. (From Hosenpud, J. D., Novick, R. J., Breen, T. J., and Daily, O. P.: The Registry of the International Society for Heart and Lung Transplantation: Eleventh Official Report—1994. J. Heart Lung Transplant. *13*(4):561, 1994. Reprinted with permission from Mosby-Year Book, Inc.)

Single Lung Transplantation

Based on work with cyclosporine-based immunosuppressive protocols, single lung transplantation has been reported for interstitial pulmonary fibrosis[200] and double lung transplantation for emphysema and cystic fibrosis, among other indications.[201] Lung transplantation currently is undergoing a widespread renaissance with ever-increasing survival expectations. A number of centers are offering lung transplant procedures, and the availability of organ donors is also improving with an increasing awareness of the value and success of lung transplantation.

Current data show that the most frequent indication for single lung transplantation is interstitial pulmonary fibrosis, with the second indication being emphysema (Fig. 18–13). More diffuse pulmonary diseases are being treated by either bilateral single lung transplantation, en bloc double lung transplantation, or heart-lung transplantation in which the recipient's relatively normal heart is used as a donor for a second recipient (the "domino donor" procedure).[202,203]

INDICATIONS. Patient selection for lung transplantation follows the guidelines for heart transplants. Most patients over age 60 are excluded, as are patients who are ventilator-dependent or who have irreversible hepatic or renal disease, insulin-dependent diabetes, or a history of cancer or other systemic disease that might limit rehabilitation. Chronic pulmonary disease is somewhat difficult to gauge for potential timing of transplantation, but patients who are severely oxygen-dependent and demonstrate a course of clinical deterioration should be considered. A good indication of disability suggesting the need for transplant is a marked decrease in oxygen saturation with exercise.

THE DONOR LUNGS. Potential donors for lung transplant procedures must be infection-free, have good pulmonary gas exchange, lack a significant smoking history, and have a lung volume similar to or less than that of the intended recipient. Lung volumes can be judged by measurements on the chest film or by the lung volume determined by standard tables based on weight and height, comparing them with ideal similar measurements of lung volume for the intended recipient. In bilateral lung transplants, the volume of donor lungs should be the same or less than that of the intended recipient, although larger lungs in single lung transplantation can be placed on the left side, where the diaphragm has the potential to descend because of the absence of the liver under the left hemidiaphragm. Infection remains a major consideration, since this is the greatest source of morbidity and mortality. The presence of CMV in the donor

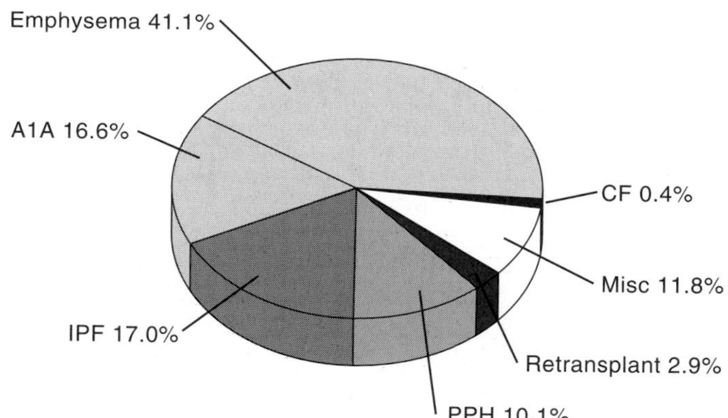

FIGURE 18–13. The indications for adult single lung transplantation. PPH = primary pulmonary hypertension, IPF = idiopathic pulmonary fibrosis, CF = cystic fibrosis, A1A = alpha$_1$-antitrypsin deficiency. (From Hosenpud, J. D., Novick, R. J., Breen, T. J., and Daily, O. P.: The Registry of the International Society for Heart and Lung Transplantation: Eleventh Official Report—1994. J. Heart Lung Transplant. *13*(4):561, 1994. Reprinted with permission from Mosby-Year Book, Inc.)

when transplanted into a CMV negative recipient has resulted in significant morbidity.[204–206] Other donor-transmitted pathogens are frequent, as well.

PREVENTION OF REJECTION. Immunosuppression protocols are similar to those for cardiac transplantation, with the exception that prednisone is often omitted for the first several weeks due to its effect on retardation of bronchial healing. Induction therapy with polyclonal ATG preparations or monoclonal OKT3 prophylaxis is advocated by some groups to allow for a rejection-free interval without the use of steroids. Ultimately, most patients are maintained on triple-drug therapy, which has been shown to correlate with better long-term survival and a reduced incidence of bronchiolitis obliterans.[207]

The diagnosis of rejection remains somewhat imprecise and is based in large degree on clinical grounds. The use of fiberoptic bronchoscopy with transbronchial parenchymal lung biopsy has been most successful in following recipients.[208] Transbronchial biopsy can usually differentiate infection from rejection. It is performed in a prospective surveillance manner, as well as for specific indications. When used for specific indications, it usually gives a higher percentage of positive results, which are about equally divided between the diagnosis of infection or rejection.[209,210] When cardiac biopsies and transbronchial biopsies are compared, pulmonary and cardiac rejection were present synchronously on six occasions and asynchronously on 16 occasions (nine pulmonary and seven cardiac). Thus, cardiac biopsy alone is insufficient to follow the heart-lung transplant patient.

Early acute pulmonary rejection usually is manifested by an interstitial infiltrate, a decrease in lung volume and in pulmonary compliance, a low-grade fever, cough, and a feeling of breathlessness. These changes can all be rapidly reversed by using intravenous methylprednisolone, usually 1 gram intravenously daily for 3 days. It is not uncommon for recipients to undergo two or three rejection episodes in the first month after transplantation. Later, more chronic episodes of rejection may present without a pulmonary infiltrate on x-ray film, and long-term follow-up requires careful attention to pulmonary function testing. Patients frequently use a home spirometer to check for expiratory indices, such as the forced expiratory volume at 1 second, which will show a decline as a consequence of chronic rejection. When suspected, these changes need to be followed up by transbronchial parenchymal biopsy or augmented immunosuppression to preserve pulmonary function as much as possible.

OTHER COMPLICATIONS. *Infection* is an important complication of lung transplantation. The absence of cough reflex in the denervated lung surely contributes to a frequency of pulmonary infection at least three times more frequently than that of heart transplant recipients, and is the major cause of death in long-term surviving patients.[211] The transplanted lung may have deficiencies in lymphatic drainage, especially early after transplant, and ciliary function may be depressed. Patients frequently develop chronic bronchitis and may lack bronchus-associated lymphatic tissue as a result of chronic rejection.[212]

The late development of *bronchiolitis obliterans* limits the results in long-term surviving patients.[209–213] The incidence was reported as high as 50 per cent from the initial Stanford series, and is 20 to 30 per cent in most recent reports. The causes are almost certainly immunological; there is a demonstrated higher incidence in patients with a poor human leukocyte antigen match and in patients treated with a two-drug protocol, as compared with a three-drug protocol. Bronchiolitis obliterans is partially reversed or arrested by an aggressive increase in immunosuppression. This complication has been reported to occur both after isolated single lung and double lung transplantation, as well as after heart-lung transplantation.[214]

The therapeutic potential of lung transplant procedures is readily apparent. Patients are able to exercise without oxygen, to have a much greater feeling of well-being, and to resume active lifestyles. Late pulmonary function is usually quite satisfactory. Most reports show a progressive improvement in pulmonary function over time, and gas exchange and ventilation are essentially normal at 1 and 2 years.[215] Continuing improvement in immunosuppressive protocols will certainly lead to an even more reliable and safer long-term result in such patients.[216]

REFERENCES

1. Hosenpud, J. D., Novick, R. J., and Breen, T. J., et al.: The Registry of the International Society for Heart and Lung Transplantation: Eleventh Official Report—1994. J. Heart Lung Transplant. *13*:561, 1994.
2. Baumgartner, W. A., Reitz, B. A., and Achuff, S. A.: Heart and Heart-Lung Transplantation. Philadelphia, W.B. Saunders Company, 1990.
3. Carrel, A., and Guthrie, C. C.: The transplantation of veins and organs. Am. J. Med. *10*:1101, 1905.
4. Carrel, A.: The surgery of blood vessels. Johns Hopkins Hosp. Bull. *18*:18, 1907.
5. Lower, R. R., and Shumway, N. E.: Studies on the orthotopic homotransplantation of the canine heart. Surg. Forum *11*:18, 1960.
6. Lower, R. R., Dong, E., and Shumway, N. E.: Long-term survival of cardiac homografts. Surgery *58*:110, 1965.
7. Lower, R. R., Dong, E., and Shumway, N. E.: Suppression of rejection crises in the cardiac homograft. Ann. Thorac. Surg. *1*:645, 1965.
8. Barnard, C. N.: A human cardiac transplant: An interim report of a successful operation performed at Groote Shuur Hospital, Capetown. S. Afr. Med. J. *41*:1271, 1967.
9. Griepp, R. B., Stinson, E. B., and Dong, E., et al.: Determinants of operative risk in human heart transplantation. Am. J. Surg. *122*:192, 1971.
10. Caves, P. K., Stinson, E. B., and Billingham, M. E., et al.: Percutaneous endomyocardial biopsy in human heart recipients. Ann. Thorac. Surg. *16*:325, 1973.
11. Bieber, C. P., Griepp, R. B., and Oyer, P. E., et al.: Use of rabbit antithymocyte globulin in cardiac transplantation: Relationship of serum clearance rates in clinical outcomes. Transplantation *22*:478, 1976.
12. Baumgartner, W. A., Reitz, B. A., and Oyer, P. E., et al.: Cardiac homotransplantation. Curr. Probl. Surg. *16*:24, 1979.
13. Kostakis, A. J., White, D. J. G., and Calne, R. Y.: Prolongation of the rat heart allograft survival by cyclosporine-A. IRCS Med. Sci. *5*:280, 1977.
14. Borel, J. F.: The history of cyclosporine-A and its significance. *In* White, D. J. G. (ed.): Cyclosporine-A: Proceedings of an International Conference on Cyclosporin-A. New York, Elsevier North Holland, Inc., 1982.
15. Calne, R. Y., Rolles, K., and White, D. J. G., et al.: Cyclosporin-A initially as the only immunosuppressant in 34 recipients of cadaveric organs: Thirty-two kidneys, two pancreases, two livers. Lancet *2*:1033, 1979.
16. Schreiber, S. L., and Crabtree, G. R.: The mechanism of action of cyclosporin A and FK506. Immunol. Today *13*:136, 1992.
17. Oyer, P. E., Stinson, E. B., and Jamieson, S. W., et al.: Cyclosporine in cardiac transplantation: A two and a half year follow-up. Transplant. Proc. *15*:2546, 1983.
18. Reitz, B. A., Wallwork, J. L., and Hunt, S. A., et al.: Heart-lung transplantation: Successful therapy for patients with pulmonary vascular disease. N. Engl. J. Med. *306*:557, 1982.
19. Abramowicz, M. (ed.): Medical Letter *36*:82, 1994.
20. Annas, G. J.: Regulating the introduction of heart and liver transplantation. Am. J. Public Health *75*:93, 1985.
21. Medicare Program: Criteria for Medicare coverage of heart transplants. Fed. Reg. *52*:10935, 1987.
22. Miller, L. W., Vitale-Noedel, N., Pennington, D. G., et al.: Heart transplantation in patients over age 55 years. J. Heart Transplant. *7*:254, 1988.
23. Olivari, M. T., Antolick, A., Kaye, M. P., et al.: Heart transplantation in elderly patients. J. Heart Transplant. *7*:258, 1988.
24. Loebe, M., Schueler, S., Warnecke, H., et al.: The effect of older age on the outcome of heart transplantation. J. Heart Transplant. *8*:107, 1989.
25. Renlund, D. G., Gilbert, E. M., O'Connell, J. B., et al.: Age-associated decline in cardiac allograft rejection. Am. J. Med. *83*:391, 1987.
26. Murali, S., Uretsky, B. F., Reddy, P. S., et al.: The use of transpulmonary pressure gradient in the selection of cardiac transplantation candidates. J. Am. Coll. Cardiol. *11*:45, 1988.
27. Deeb, G. M., Bolling, S. F., Guynn, T. P., et al.: Amrinone versus conventional therapy in pulmonary hypertensive patients awaiting cardiac transplantation. Ann. Thorac. Surg. *48*:665, 1989.
28. Stevenson, L. W., Tillisch, J. H., Hamilton, M., Luu, M., et al.: Importance of hemodynamic response to therapy in predicting survival with ejection fraction ≤20% secondary to ischemic or non-ischemic dilated cardiomyopathy. Am. J. Cardiol. *66*:1348, 1990.
29. Stevenson, L. W., Dracup, K. A., and Tilliach, J. H.: Efficacy of medical therapy tailored for severe congestive heart failure in patients transferred for urgent cardiac transplantation. Am. J. Cardiol. *58*:1046, 1988.
30. Mancini, D. M., Eisen, H., Kussmaul, W., et al.: Value of peak exercise oxygen consumption for optimal timing of cardiac transplantation in ambulatory patients with heart failure. Circulation *83*:778, 1991.
31. Kermani, M., Stevenson, L. W., Chelimsky-Fallick, C., et al.: Importance of serial exercise testing after evaluation for cardiac transplantation. J. Heart Lung Transplant. *11*:191, 1992.
32. UNOS 1994 Annual Report of the U.S. Scientific Registry of Transplant Recipients and the Organ Procurement and Transplantation Network. Transplant Data: 1988–1993. U.N.O.S., Richmond, Va, and the Division of Organ Transplantation, Bureau of Health Resources Development, Health Resources and Services Administration, and Services Administration, U.S. Department of Health and Human Services, Bethesda, Md., L-7.
33. UNOS Update. 11:30–31, June 1995.
34. UNOS Update. 11:50–53, March 1995.
35. Applefeld, M. M., Newman, K. A., Grove, W. R., et al.: Intermittent, continuous outpatient dobutamine infusion in the management of congestive heart failure. Am. J. Cardiol. *51*:455, 1983.
36. Miller, C. A., Pae, W. E., and Pierce, W. S.: Combined registry for the clinical use of mechanical ventricular assist pumps and the total artificial heart in conjunction with heart transplantation: 4th official report—1989. J. Heart Transplant. *9*:453, 1990.
37. Shumway, S. J., and Bolman, R. M., III: Cardiac transplantation and ventricular assist devices. Curr. Opin. Cardiol. *6*:269, 1991.
38. Farrar, D. J., Hill, J. D., Gray, L. A., et al.: Heterotopic prosthetic ventricles as a bridge to cardiac transplantation: A multi-center study in 29 patients. N. Engl. J. Med. *318*:33, 1988.
39. Griffith, B. P., Kormos, R. L., Hardesty, R. L., et al.: The artificial heart: Infection-related morbidity and its effect on transplantation. Ann. Thorac. Surg. *45*:409, 1988.
40. Costanzo-Nordin, M. R., Cooper, D. K. C., Jessup, M., et al.: 24th Bethesda Conference: Cardiac Transplantation, Report Task Force 6: Future Developments. J. Am. Coll. Cardiol. *22*:54, 1993.

41. Pae, W. E.: Ventricular assist devices and total artificial hearts: A combined registry experience. Ann. Thorac. Surg. *55:*295, 1993.
42. Baldwin, J. C., Anderson, J. L., Boucek, M. M., et al.: 24th Bethesda Conference: Cardiac Transplantation, Report Task Force 2: Donor Guidelines. J. Am. Coll. Cardiol. *22:*15, 1993.
43. Presidential Commission for the Study of Ethical Problems in Medicine and Biomedical and Behavioral Research. Guidelines for the determination of death. JAMA *246:*2184, 1981.
44. Griepp, R. B., Stinson, E. B., Clark, D. A., et al.: The cardiac donor. Surg. Gynecol. Obstet. *133:*792, 1971.
45. Sweeney, M. S., Lammermeier, D. E., Frazier, O. H., et al.: Extension of donor criteria in cardiac transplantation: Surgical risk vs. supply-side economics. Ann. Thorac. Surg. *50:*7, 1990.
46. Schueler, S., Warneke, H., Leob, E. M., et al.: Extended donor age in cardiac transplantation. Circulation *3:*133, 1989.
47. Robicsek, F., Masters, T. N., Thomley, A. M., et al.: Bench coronary cineangiography. J. Thorac. Cardiovasc. Surg. *103:*490, 1992.
48. Cooper, D. K. C., Human, P. A., Rose, A. G., et al.: Can cardiac allografts and xenografts be transplanted against the ABO blood group barrier? Transplant. Proc. *21:*549, 1989.
49. UNOS 1994 Annual Report of the U.S. Scientific Registry of Transplant Recipients and the Organ Procurement and Transplantation Network. Transplant Data: 1988–1993. U.N.O.S., Richmond, Va, and the Division of Organ Transplantation, Bureau of Health Resources Development, Health Resources and Services Administration, U.S. Department of Health and Human Services, Bethesda, Md., L-8.
50. Baumgartner, W. A.: Evaluation and management of the heart donor. *In* Baumgartner, W. A., Reitz, B. A., and Achuff, S. A. (eds.): Heart and Heart-Lung Transplantation. Philadelphia, W. B. Saunders Company, 1990, p. 86.
51. Kaye, M. P.: The Registry of the International Society for Heart Transplantation: Fourth Official Report—1987. J. Heart Transplant. *6:*63, 1987.
52. Yacoub, M., Mancad, P., and Ledingham, S.: Donor procurement and surgical techniques for cardiac transplantation. Semin. Thorac. Cardiovasc. Surg. *2:*153, 1990.
53. Wicomb, W. N., Cooper, D. K. C., Novitsky, D., et al.: Cardiac transplantation following storage of the donor heart by a portable hypothermic perfusion system. Ann. Thorac. Surg. *37:*243, 1984.
54. Baldwin, J. C., Frist, W. H., Starkey, T. D., et al.: Distant graft procurement for combined heart and lung transplantation using pulmonary artery flush and simple topical hypothermia for graft preservation. Ann. Thorac. Surg. *43:*670, 1987.
55. Wallwork, J., Jones, K., Cavarocchi, N., et al.: Distant procurement of organs for clinical heart-lung transplantation using a single flush technique. Transplantation *44:*654, 1987.
56. Hardesty, R. L., and Griffith, B. P.: Autoperfusion of the heart and lungs for preservation during distant procurement. J. Thorac. Cardiovasc. Surg. *93:*11, 1987.
57. Baumgartner, W. A., Williams, G. M., Fraser, C. D., et al.: Cardiopulmonary bypass with profound hypothermia: An optimal preservation method for multi-organ procurement. Transplantation *47:*123, 1989.
58. UNOS 1994 Annual Report of the U.S. Scientific Registry of Transplant Recipients and the Organ Procurement and Transplantation Network. Transplant Data: 1988–1993. U.N.O.S., Richmond, Va, and the Division of Organ Transplantation, Bureau of Health Resources Development, Health Resources and Services Administration, U.S. Department of Health and Human Services, Bethesda, Md., R-43.
58a. Abramowicz, M.: Medical Letter *37:*61, 1995.
59. Dreyfus, G., Jebaara, V., Mihaileanu, S., and Carpentier, A.: Total orthotopic heart transplantation: An alternative to the standard technique. Ann. Thorac. Surg. *52:*1181, 1991.
60. Kendall, S., Ciulli, F., Mullin, S. P., et al.: Total orthotopic heart transplantation: An alternative to the standard technique (Letter). Ann. Thorac. Surg. *54:*187, 1992.
61. Rees, A. P., Milani, R. V., Lavie, C. J., et al.: Valvular regurgitation and right-sided cardiac pressures in heart transplant recipients by complete Doppler and color flow evaluation. Chest *104:*82, 1993.
62. Bhatia, S. J. S., Kirshenbaum, J. M., Shemin, R. J., et al.: Time course of resolution of pulmonary hypertension and right ventricular remodeling after orthotopic cardiac transplantation. Circulation *76:*819, 1987.
63. Armitage, J. M., Hardesty, R. L., and Griffith, B. P.: Prostaglandin E_1: An effective treatment of right heart failure after orthotopic heart transplantation. J. Heart Transplant. *6:*348, 1987.
64. Girard, C., Durand, P. G., Vedrinne, C., et al.: Inhaled nitric oxide for right ventricular failure after heart transplantation. J. Cardiothorac. Vasc. Anesth. *7:*481, 1993.
65. Foubert, L., Latimer, R., Oduro, A., et al.: Use of inhaled nitrous oxide to reduce pulmonary hypertension after heart transplantation. J. Cardiothorac. Vasc. Anesth. *7:*640, 1993.
66. Fonger, J. D., Borkon, A. M., Baumgartner, W. A., et al.: Acute right ventricular failure following heart transplantation. Improvement with prostaglandin E_1 and right ventricular assist. J. Heart Transplant. *5:*317, 1986.
67. McGriffin, D. C., and Carp, R. B.: Cardiac transplantation in a patient with a persistent left superior vena cava and an absent right superior vena cava. J. Heart Transplant. *3:*115, 1984.
68. Reitz, B. A., Jamieson, S. W., Gaudiani, V. A., et al.: Method for cardiac transplantation in corrected transposition of the great arteries. J. Cardiovasc. Surg. (Torino) *23:*293, 1982.
69. Demikhov, V. P.: Experimental Transplantation of Vital Organs. New York, Consultants Bureau, 1962.
70. McGough, E. C., Brener, P. L., and Reemstma, K.: The parallel heart studies of intrathoracic auxiliary cardiac transplants. Surgery *60:*153, 1966.
71. Barnard, C. N., Losman, J. G.: Left ventricular bypass. S. Afr. Med. J. *49:*303, 1985.
71a. Cochrane, A. D., Adams, D. H., Radley-Smith, R., et al.: Heterotopic heart transplantation for elevated pulmonary vascular resistance in pediatric patients. J. Heart Lung Transplant. *14:*296, 1995.
72. Renlund, D. G., O'Connell, J. B., and Bristow, M. R.: Early rejection prophylaxis in heart transplantation: Is cytolytic therapy necessary? J. Heart Transplant. *8:*191, 1989.
73. Kobashigawa, J. A., Stevenson, L. W., Brownfield, E., et al.: Does short-course induction with OKT3 improve outcome after heart transplantation? A randomized trial. J. Heart Lung Transplant. *12:*205, 1993.
74. First, M. R., Schroeder, T. J., Hurtubise, P. E., et al.: Successful retreatment of allograft rejection with OKT3. J. Transplant. *47:*88, 1989.
75. Livi, U., Luciani, G. B., Boffa, G. M., et al.: Clinical results of steroid-induction immunosuppression after heart transplantation. Ann. Thorac. Surg. *55:*1160, 1993.
76. Reichenspurner, H., Ertel, W., Hammer, C., et al.: Immunologic monitoring of heart transplant patients under cyclosporine immunosuppression. Transplant. Proc. *16:*1251, 1984.
77. Dubroff, J. M., Clark, M. B., Wong, C. Y. H., et al.: Changes in left ventricular mass associated with the onset of acute rejection after cardiac transplantation. J. Heart Transplant. *3:*105, 1984.
78. Haberl, R., Weber, M., Reichenspurner, H., et al.: Frequency analysis of the surface electrocardiogram for recognition of acute rejection after orthotopic cardiac transplantation in man. Circulation *76:*101, 1987.
79. Fraser, C. D., Jr., Chacko, V. P., Jacobus, W. E., et al.: Evidence of 31p nuclear magnetic resonance studies of cardiac allografts that early rejection is characterized by reversible biochemical changes. Transplantation *48:*1068, 1989.
80. Griepp, R. B., Stinson, E. B., Dong, E., Jr., et al.: Acute rejection of the allografted human heart: Diagnosis and treatment. Ann. Thorac. Surg. *12:*1113, 1971.
81. Warnecke, H., Muller, J., Cohnert, T., et al.: Clinical heart transplantation without routine endomyocardial biopsy. J. Heart Lung Transplant. *11:*1093, 1992.
82. Muller, J., Warnecke, H., Spiegelsberger, S., et al.: Reliable noninvasive rejection diagnosis after heart transplantation in childhood. J. Heart Lung Transplant. *12:*189, 1993.
83. Valentine, H. A., Fowler, M. B., Hunt, S. A., et al.: Changes in Doppler echocardiographic indexes of left ventricular function as potential markers of acute cardiac rejection. Circulation *76*(Suppl. 5):V-86, 1987.
84. Golitsin, A., Pinedo, J. I., Cienfuegos, J. A., et al.: Thallium-201 uptake: A useful method for assessing heart transplantation. Transplant. Proc. *16:*1262, 1984.
85. McKillop, J. H., McDougall, I. R., Goris, M. L., et al.: Failure to diagnose cardiac transplant rejection with Tc-99m-pyp images. Clin. Nucl. Med. *6:*375, 1981.
86. Hesse, B., Mortensen, S. A., Folke, M., et al.: Ability of antimyosin scintigraphy monitoring to exclude acute rejection during the first year after heart transplantation. J. Heart Lung Transplant. *14:*23, 1995.
87. Foegh, M. L., Khirabadi, B. S., Shapiro, R., et al.: Monitoring of rat heart allograft rejection by urinary thromboxane. Transplant. Proc. *16:*1606, 1984.
88. O'Toole, C. M., Maher, P., Spiegelhalter, D., et al.: "Rejection or Infection" predictive value of T-cell subset ratio before and after heart transplantation. Heart Transplant. *4:*518, 1985.
89. Caves, P. K., Billingham, M. E., Schultz, W. P., et al.: Transvenous biopsy from canine orthotopic heart allografts. Am. Heart J. *85:*525, 1973.
90. Billingham, M. E.: The pathology of transplanted hearts. Semin. Thorac. Cardiovasc. Surg. *2:*233, 1990.
91. Billingham, M. E., Cary, N. R., Hammond, M. E., et al.: A working formulation for the standardization of nomenclature in the diagnosis of heart and lung rejection: Heart Rejection Study Group. J. Heart Transplant. *9:*587, 1990.
92. Hutchins, G. M.: The pathology of heart transplantation. *In* Baumgartner, W. A., Reitz, B. A., and Achuff, S. A. (eds.): Heart and Heart-Lung Transplantation. Philadelphia, W.B. Saunders Company, 1990, p. 183.
93. Normann, S. J., Salomon, D. R., Leelachaikul, P., et al.: Acute vascular rejection of the coronary arteries in human heart transplantation: Pathology and correlations with immunosuppression and cytomegalovirus infection. J. Heart Lung Transplant. *10:*674, 1991.
93a. Lones, M. A., Czer, L. S. C., Trento, A., et al.: Clinical-pathologic features of humoral rejection in cardiac allografts: A study in 81 consecutive patients. J. Heart Lung Transplant. *14:*151, 1995.
94. Czerska, B., Hobbs, R. E., James, K. B., et al.: Clinical manifestation of acute vascular rejection in cardiac transplant recipients. J. Heart Lung Transplant. *14:*S46, 1995.
95. Kobashigawa, J. A., Kirklin, J. K., Naftel, D. C., et al.: Pretransplantation risk factors for acute rejection after heart transplantation: A multi-institutional study. The Transplant Cardiologists Research Database Group. J. Heart Lung Transplant. *12:*355, 1993.
96. Michler, R. E., Smith, C. R., Drusin, R. E., et al.: Reversal of cardiac transplant rejection without massive immunosuppression. Circulation *74:*III-68, 1986.

97. Haverty, T. P., Sanders, M., and Sheahan, M.: OKT_3 treatment of cardiac allograft rejection. J. Heart Lung Transplant. *12*:591, 1993.
98. Kobashigawa, J., Stevenson, L. W., Moriguchi, J., et al.: Randomized study of high-dose oral cyclosporine therapy for mild acute cardiac rejection. J. Heart Transplant. *8*:53, 1989.
99. Olsen, S. L., O'Connell, J. B., Bristow, M. R., et al.: Methotrexate in the treatment of persistent cardiac allograft rejection. J. Heart Transplant. *8*(abstr):96, 1989.
100. Bourge, R. C., Kirklin, J. K., White-Williams, C., et al.: Methotrexate pulse therapy in the treatment of recurrent acute heart rejection. J. Heart Lung Transplant. *11*:1116, 1992.
101. Hunt, S., Strober, S., Hoppe, R., et al.: Use of total lymphoid irradiation for therapy of intractable cardiac allograft rejection. J. Heart Transplant. *8*(abstr):104, 1989.
102. Salter, M. M., Kirklin, J. K., Bourge, R. C., et al.: Total lymphoid irradiation in the treatment of early or recurrent heart rejection. J. Heart Lung Transplant. *11*:902, 1992.
103. Todo, S., Fung, J. J., Demetris, A. J., et al.: Early trials with FK506 as primary treatment in liver transplantation. Transplant. Proc. *22*:13, 1990.
104. Peters, D. H., Fitton, A., Plosker, G. L., et al.: Tacrolimus. A review of its pharmacology and therapeutic potential in hepatic and renal transplantation. Drugs *46*:746, 1993.
105. Armitage, J. M., Kormos, R. L., Fung, J., et al.: Preliminary experience with FK506 in thoracic transplantation. Transplantation *52*:164, 1991.
106. Griffith, B. P., Bando, K., Hardesty, R. L., et al.: A prospective randomized trial of FK506 versus cyclosporine after human pulmonary transplantation. Transplantation *57*:848, 1994.
107. Morris, R. E.: New small molecule immunosuppressants for transplantation: Review of essential concepts. J. Heart Lung Transplant. *12*:S275, 1993.
108. Kirklin, J. K., Bourge, R. C., Naftel, D. C., et al.: Treatment of recurrent heart rejection with mycophenolate mofetil (RS-61443): Initial clinical experience. J. Heart Lung Transplant. *13*:444, 1994.
109. Horn, J. E., and Bartlett, J. G.: Infectious complications following heart transplantation. *In* Baumgartner, W. A., Reitz, B. A., and Achuff, S. A. (eds.): Heart and Heart-Lung Transplantation. Philadelphia, W.B. Saunders Company, 1990, p. 220.
110. Miller, L. W., Naftel, D. C., Bourge, R. C., et al.: Infection after heart transplantation: A multi-international study. Cardiac Transplant Research Database Group. J. Heart Lung Transplant. *13*:381, 1994.
111. Fox, B. C., Sollinger, H. W., Belzer, F. O., et al.: Prospective randomized double-blind study of trimethoprim-sulfamethoxazole for prophylaxis of infection in renal transplantation: Clinical efficacy, absorption of trimethoprim-sulfamethoxazole, effects of microflora, and the cost-benefit of prophylaxis. Am. J. Med. *89*:225, 1990.
112. Dummer, J. S., Gardy, A., Poorsattar, A., et al.: Early infections in kidney, heart, and liver transplant recipients on cyclosporine. Transplantation *36*:259, 1983.
113. Onorato, I. M., Morens, D. M., Martone, W. J., et al.: Epidemiology of cytomegaloviral infections: Recommendations for prevention and control. Rev. Infect. Dis. *7*:479, 1985.
114. Wolf, D. G., and Spector, S. A.: Early diagnosis of CMV disease in transplant recipients by DNA amplification in plasma. Transplantation *56*:330, 1993.
114a. Macdonald, P. S., Keogh, A. M., Marshman, D., et al.: A double-blind placebo-controlled trial of low-dose ganciclovir to prevent cytomegalovirus disease after heart transplantation. J. Heart Lung Transplant. *14*:32, 1995.
115. Merigan, T. C., Renlund, D. G., Keay, S., et al.: A controlled trial of ganciclovir to prevent cytomegalovirus disease after heart transplantation. N. Engl. J. Med. *326*:1182, 1992.
116. Edman, J. C., Kovacs, J. A., Strand, M., et al.: Ribosomal RNA sequence shows *Pneumocystis carinii* to be a member of the fungi. Nature *334*:519, 1988.
117. Holliman, R. E., Johnson, J. D., Adams, S., et al.: Toxoplasmosis and heart transplantation. J. Heart Transplant. *10*:608, 1991.
118. Penn, I., and Brunson, M. E.: Cancers after cyclosporine therapy. Transplant. Proc. *20*:85, 1988.
119. Myers, B. D., Ross, J., Newton, L., et al.: Cyclosporine-associated chronic nephropathy. N. Engl. J. Med. *311*:699, 1984.
120. McGiffin, D. C., Kirklin, J. K., and Naftel, D. C.: Acute renal failure after heart transplantation and cyclosporine therapy. J. Heart Transplant. *4*:396, 1985.
121. Luke, R. G.: Mechanisms of cyclosporine-induced hypertension. Am. J. Hypertens. *4*:468, 1991.
122. Renlund, D. G., O'Connell, J. B., Gilbert, E. M., et al.: A prospective comparison of murine monoclonal CD-3 antibody-based and equine antithymocyte globulin-based rejection prophylaxis in cardiac transplantation: Decreased rejection and less corticosteroid use with OKT_3. Transplantation *47*:599, 1989.
123. Copeland, J. G., Emery, R. W., Levinson, M. M., et al.: Cyclosporine: An immunosuppressive panacea? J. Thorac. Cardiovasc. Surg. *91*:26, 1986.
124. Slavin, J., and Taylor, J.: Cyclosporine, nifedipine, and gingival hyperplasia. Lancet *2*:739, 1987.
125. Patton, P. R., Brunson, M. E., Pfaff, W. W., et al.: A preliminary report of diltiazem and ketoconazole: Their cyclosporine-sparing effect and impact on transplant outcome. Transplantation *57*:889, 1994.
126. Cockburn, I. T., and Krupp, P.: An appraisal of drug interactions with Sandimmune. Transplant. Proc. *21*:385, 1989.
127. Henricsson, S., Lindholm, A., and Aravoglou, M.: Cyclosporine metabolism in human liver microsomes and its inhibition by other drugs. Pharmacol. Toxicol. *66*:49, 1990.
128. East, C., Alivizato, P. A., Grundy, S. M., et al.: Rhabdomyolysis in patients receiving lovastatin after cardiac transplantation (letter). N. Engl. J. Med. *318*:47, 1988.
129. Olivari, M-T., Jessen, M. E., Baldwin, B. J., et al.: Triple-drug immunosuppression with steroid discontinuation by six months after heart transplantation. J. Heart Lung Transplant. *14*:127, 1995.
130. Penn, I.: Tumors after renal and cardiac transplantation. Hematol. Oncol. Clin. North Am. *7*:431, 1993.
131. Hanto, D. W., Frizzera, G., Gajl-Peczalska, K. J., et al.: Epstein-Barr virus, immunodeficiency, and B-cell lymphoproliferation. Transplantation *39*:461, 1985.
132. Swinnen, L. J., Costanzo-Nordin, M. R., Fisher, S. G., et al.: Increased incidence of lymphoproliferative disorder after immunosuppression with monoclonal antibody OKT_3 in cardiac transplant recipients. N. Engl. J. Med. *323*:1723, 1990.
133. Miller, L. W., Schlant, R. C., Kobashigawa, J., et al.: 24th Bethesda Conference: Cardiac Transplantation, Report Task Force 5: Complications. J. Am. Coll. Cardiol. *22*:41, 1993.
134. van Gorp, J., Dornewaard, H., Verdonck, L. F., et al.: Post-transplant T-cell lymphoma. Cancer *73*:3064, 1994.
135. Oettle, H., Wilborn, F., Schmidt, C. A., et al.: Treatment with ganciclovir and Ig for acute Epstein-Barr infection after allogenic bone marrow transplantation (letter). Blood *82*:2257, 1993.
136. Benkerrou, M. D., Durandy, A., and Fischer, A.: Therapy for transplant-related lymphoproliferative diseases. Hematol. Oncol. Clin. North Am. *7*:467, 1993.
137. Thomson, J. G.: Production of severe atheroma in a transplanted human heart. Lancet *2*:1088, 1969.
138. Billingham, M. E.: Cardiac transplant atherosclerosis. Transplant. Proc. *19* (Suppl. 5):19, 1987.
139. Hess, M. L., Hastillo, A., Thompson, J. A., et al.: Lipid mediators in organ transplantation: Does cyclosporine accelerate coronary atherosclerosis? Transplant. Proc. *19* (Suppl. 5):71, 1987.
140. Uretsky, B. F., Murali, S., Reedy, S., et al.: Development of coronary artery disease in cardiac transplant patients receiving immunosuppressive therapy with cyclosporine and prednisone. Circulation *76*:827, 1987.
141. Nitkin, R. S., and Schroeder, J. S.: Accelerated coronary artery disease risk in heart transplant patients. J. Am. Coll. Cardiol. *5* (Suppl. II):535, 1985.
142. Johnson, D. E., Alderman, E. L., Schroeder, J. S., et al.: Transplant coronary artery disease: Histopathologic correlations with angiographic morphology. J. Am. Coll. Cardiol. *17*:449, 1991.
143. Grattan, M. T., Moreno-Cabral, C. E., Starnes, V. A., et al.: Eight-year results of cyclosporine-treated patients with cardiac transplants. J. Thorac. Cardiovasc. Surg. *99*:500, 1990.
144. Gao, S. Z., Schroeder, J. S., Hunt, S. A., et al.: Myocardial infarction in cardiac transplant recipients: A clinicopathologic correlation. Am. J. Cardiol. *64*:1093, 1989.
145. Banner, N. R., and Yacoub, M. H.: Physiology of the orthotopic cardiac transplant recipient. Semin. Thorac. Cardiovasc. Surg. *2*:259, 1990.
146. Rickenbacher, P. R., Pinto, F. J., Chenzbraun, A., et al.: Incidence and severity of transplant coronary artery disease early and up to 15 years after transplantation, as detected by intravascular ultrasound. J. Am. Coll. Cardiol. *25*:171, 1995.
147. Gao, S., Hunt, S. A., and Schroeder, J. S.: Accelerated transplant coronary artery disease. Semin. Thorac. Cardiovasc. Surg. *2*:241, 1990.
148. Billingham, M. E.: Graft coronary disease: The lesions and the patients. Transplant. Proc. *21*:3665, 1989.
149. Gao, S.-Z., Alderman, E. A., Schroeder, J. S., et al.: Accelerated coronary vascular disease in the heart transplant patient: Coronary arteriographic findings. J. Am. Coll. Cardiol. *12*:334, 1988.
150. Bieber, C. P., Hunt, S. A., Schwinn, D. A., et al.: Complications in long-term survivors of cardiac transplantation. Transplant. Proc. *13*:207, 1981.
151. Barbir, M., Kushwaha, S., Hunt, B., et al.: Lipoprotein(a) and accelerated coronary artery disease in cardiac transplant patients. Lancet *340*:(8834)1500, 1992.
152. Melnick, J. L., Adam, E., and DeBakey, M. E.: Possible role of cytomegalovirus in atherogenesis. JAMA *263*:2204, 1990.
153. Grattan, M. T., Moreno-Cabral, C. E., Starnes, V. A., et al.: Cytomegalovirus infection is associated with cardiac allograft rejection and atherosclerosis. JAMA *261*:3561, 1989.
154. Speir, E., Modali, R., Huang, E. S., et al.: Potential role of human cytomegalovirus and P53 interaction in coronary restenosis. Science *265*:391, 1994.
155. Butman, S. M.: Hyperlipidemia after cardiac transplantation: Be aware and possibly wary of drug therapy for lowering of serum lipids. Am. Heart J. *121*:1585, 1991.
156. Superko, H. R., Haskell, W. L., and DiRicco, C. D.: Lipoprotein and hepatic lipase activity and high-density lipoprotein subclasses after cardiac transplantation. Am. J. Cardiol. *66*:1131, 1990.
156a. Kobashigawa, J. A., Katznelson, S., Laks, H., et al.: Effect of pravastatin on outcomes after cardiac transplantation. N. Engl. J. Med. *333*:621, 1995.
157. Schroeder, J. S., Gao, S.-Z., Alderman, E. A., et al.: A preliminary study of diltiazem in the prevention of coronary artery disease in heart transplant recipients. N. Engl. J. Med. *328*:164, 1993.
158. Vetrovec, G. W., Cowley, M. J., Newton, C. M., et al.: Applications of

percutaneous transluminal coronary angioplasty in cardiac transplantation: Preliminary results in 5 patients. Circulation *78*(Suppl. III):83, 1988.
159. Copeland, J. G., Butman, S. M., and Cethi, G.: Successful coronary artery bypass grafting for high-risk left main coronary artery atherosclerosis after cardiac transplantation. Ann. Thorac. Surg. *49*:106, 1990.
160. Halle, A. A., DiSciascio, G., Massin, E. K., et al.: Coronary angioplasty, atherectomy and bypass surgery in cardiac transplant recipients. J. Am. Coll. Cardiol. *26*:120, 1995.
161. Dunning, J. J., Kendall, S. W., Mullins, P. A., et al.: Coronary artery bypass grafting nine years after cardiac transplantation. Ann. Thorac. Surg. *54*:571, 1992.
162. Karawande, S. V., Ensley, R. D., Renlund, D. G., et al.: Cardiac retransplantation: A viable option? The Registry of the International Society for Heart and Lung Transplantation. Ann. Thorac. Surg. *54*:840, 1992.
163. Christopherson, L. K., Griepp, R. B., and Stinson, E. B.: Rehabilitation after heart transplantation. JAMA *236*:2082, 1976.
164. Hunt, S. A., Rider, A. K., Stinson, E. B., et al.: Does cardiac transplantation prolong life and improve its quality? Cardiovasc. Surg. *54*:56, 1975.
165. Lough, M. E., Lindsey, A. M., and Shinn, J. A., et al.: Life satisfaction following heart transplantation. J. Heart Transplant. *4*:446, 1985.
166. UNOS 1994 Annual Report of the U.S. Scientific Registry of Transplant Recipients and the Organ Procurement and Transplantation Network. Transplant Data: 1988–1993. U.N.O.S., Richmond, Va, and the Division of Organ Transplantation, Bureau of Health Resources Development, Health Resources and Services Administration, U.S. Department of Health and Human Services, Bethesda, Md., VII-9.
167. UNOS. Annual Report of the U.S. Scientific Registry for Organ Transplantation and the Organ Procurement and Transplantation Network. U.S. Department of Health and Human Services, 1990.
168. O'Connell, J. B., Gunnar, R. M., Evans, R. W., et al.: 24th Bethesda Conference: Cardiac Transplantation. Task Force 1. Organization of Heart Transplantation in the U.S. J. Am. Coll. Cardiol. *22*:8, 1993.
169. Jarcho, J., Naftel, D. C., Shroyer, T. W., et al.: Influence of HLA mismatch on rejection after heart transplantation: A multi-institutional study. J. Heart Lung Transplant. *13*:583, 1994.
170. Mason, J. W., and Harrison, D. C.: Electrophysiology and electropharmacology of the transplanted human heart. *In* Narula OS (ed.): Cardiac Arrhythmias: Electrophysiology, Diagnosis, Management. Baltimore, Williams and Wilkins, 1979, p. 66.
171. Burke, M. N., McGinn, A. L., Homans, D. C., et al.: Evidence for functional sympathetic reinnervation of left ventricle and coronary arteries after orthotopic cardiac transplantation in humans. Circulation *91*:72, 1995.
172. Banner, N. R., Lloyd, M. H., Hamilton, R. D., et al.: Cardiopulmonary response to dynamic exercise after heart and combined heart-lung transplantation. Br. Heart J. *61*:215, 1989.
173. Kavanagh, T., Yacoub, M. H., Mertens, D. J., et al.: Cardiorespiratory responses to exercise training after orthotopic cardiac transplantation. Circulation *77*:162, 1988.
174. von Scheidt, W., Neudert, J., Erdmann, E., et al.: Contractility of the transplanted, denervated human heart. Am. Heart J. *121*:1480, 1991.
175. Uretsky, B. F.: Physiology of the transplanted heart. Cardiovascular. Clin. *20*:23, 1990.
176. Verani, M. S., George, S. E., Leon, C. A., et al.: Systolic and diastolic ventricular performance at rest and during exercise in heart transplant recipients. J. Heart Transplant. *7*:145, 1988.
177. Naurie, K. G., Bristow, M. R., and Reitz, B. A.: Increased beta adrenergic receptor density in an experimental model of cardiac transplantation. J. Thorac. Cardiovasc. Surg. *86*:195, 1983.
178. Borow, K. M., Neumann, A. A., Arensman, F. W., et al.: Cardiac and peripheral vascular responses to adrenoceptor stimulation and blockage after cardiac transplantation. J. Am. Coll. Cardiol. *14*:1229, 1989.
179. Yusuf, S., Theodoropoulos, S., Mathias, C. J., et al.: Increased sensitivity of the denervated transplanted human heart to isoprenaline both before and after beta-adrenergic blockade. Circulation *75*:696, 1987.
180. Scherrer, U., Vissing, S. F., Morgan, B. J., et al.: Cyclosporine induced sympathetic activation and hypertension after heart transplantation. N. Engl. J. Med. *323*:693, 1990.
181. Redmond, J. M., Zehr, K. J., Gillinov, M. A., et al.: Use of theophylline for treatment of prolonged sinus node dysfunction in human orthotopic heart transplantation. J. Heart Lung Transplant. *12*(1 Pt 1):133, 1993.
182. Evans, R. W.: Measuring the costs of heart transplantation. Primary Cardiol. *20*:48, 1994.
183. UNOS 1994 Annual Report of the U.S. Scientific Registry of Transplant Recipients and the Organ Procurement and Transplantation Network. Transplant Data: 1988–1993. U.N.O.S., Richmond, Va, and the Division of Organ Transplantation, Bureau of Health Resources Development, Health Resources and Services Administration, U.S. Department of Health and Human Services, Bethesda, Md., F-29.
183a. Votapka, T. V., Swartz, M. T., Reedy, J. E., et al.: Heart transplantation charges: Status 1 versus Status 2 patients. J. Heart Lung Transplant. *14*:366, 1995.
184. Mudge, G. H., Goldstein, S., Addonizio, I. J., et al.: 24th Bethesda Conference: Cardiac Transplantation. Task Force 3: Recipient guidelines/prioritization. J. Am. Coll. Cardiol. *22*:21, 1993.
185. Evans, R. W.: Social, economic, and insurance issues in heart transplantation. *In* O'Connell, J. B., and Kaye, M. P., (eds.) Intrathoracic Transplantation 2000. Austin, Tx: RG Landes *1*:17, 1993.
186. Evans, R. W.: Cost-effectiveness of transplantation. Surg. Clin. North Am. *66*(3):603, 1986.
187. Evans, R. W.: Executive summary: The National Cooperative Transplantation Study: BHARC-100-91-020. Seattle, Battelle-Seattle Research Center, June 1991.
188. Cameron, D. E., and Gardner, T. J.: Heart transplantation in children. *In* Baumgartner, W. A., Reitz, B. A., and Achuff, S. A. (eds.): Heart and Heart-Lung Transplantation. Philadelphia, W.B. Saunders Company, 1990, p. 293.
189. Bailey, L. L., Nehlsen-Cannarella, S. L., Concepcion, W., et al.: Baboon to human cardiac xenotransplantation in a neonate. JAMA *254*:3321, 1985.
190. Boucek, M. M., Kanakriyeh, M. S., Mathis, C. M., et al.: Cardiac transplantation in infancy: Donors and recipients. J. Pediatr. *116*:171, 1990.
191. Bernstein, D., Baum, D., Hunt, S., Miller, J., Reitz, B., and Stinson, E. B.: Long-term (>5-year) survivors of pediatric heart transplantation. J. Heart Lung Transplant *(in press)*.
192. Watson, D. C., Reitz, B. A., Oyer, P. E., et al.: Sequential orthotopic heart transplantation in man. Transplantation *30*:401, 1980.
193. Novitsky, D., Cooper, D. K. C., Brink, J. G., et al.: Sequential second and third transplants in patients with heterotopic heart allografts. Clin. Transplant. *1*:57, 1987.
194. Smith, J. A., Ribakove, G. H., Hunt, S. A., Miller, J., Stinson, E. B., Oyer, P. E., Robbins, R. C., Shumway, N. E., and Reitz, B. A.: Cardiac retransplantation: The 25-year experience at a single institution. J. Heart Lung Transplant *(in press)*.
195. Neptune, W. B., Cookson, B. A., Bailey, C. P., et al.: Complete homologous heart transplantation. Arch. Surg. *66*:174, 1953.
196. Veith, F. J.: Lung transplantation. Surg. Clin. North Am. *58*:357, 1978.
197. Reitz, B. A., Burton, N. A., Jamieson, S. W., et al.: Heart and lung transplantation, autotransplantation, and allotransplantation in primates with extended survival. J. Thorac. Cardiovasc. Surg. *80*:360, 1980.
198. Wellens, F., Estenne, M., deFrancquen, P., et al.: Combined heart-lung transplantation for terminal pulmonary lymphangioleiomatosis. J. Thorac. Cardiovasc. Surg. *89*:872, 1985.
199. Jones, D. K., Higgenbottam, T. W., and Wallwork, J.: Long-term survival after heart-lung transplantation in cystic fibrosis. Chest *93*:644, 1988.
200. Toronto Lung Transplant Group: Experience with single lung transplantation for pulmonary fibrosis. JAMA *259*:2258, 1988.
201. Cooper, J. D., Patterson, G. A., Grosman, R., et al.: Double lung transplant for advanced chronic obstructive lung disease. Am. Rev. Respir. Dis. *139*:303, 1989.
202. Baumgartner, W. A., Traill, T. A., Cameron, D. E., et al.: Unique aspects of heart and lung transplantation exhibited in the "domino-donor" operation. JAMA *261*:3121, 1989.
203. Yacoub, M. H., Banner, N. R., Khaghani, A., et al.: Heart-lung transplantation for cystic fibrosis and subsequent domino heart transplantation. J. Heart Transplant. *9*:459, 1990.
204. Burke, C. M., Glanville, A. R., Macoviak, J. A., et al.: The spectrum of cytomegalovirus infection following human heart-lung transplantation. J. Heart Transplant. *5*:267, 1986.
205. Dummer, J. S., White, L. T., Monto, H. O., et al.: Morbidity of cytomegalovirus infection in recipients of heart or heart-lung transplant who received cyclosporine. J. Infect. Dis. *152*:1182, 1985.
206. Hutter, J. A., Scott, J. P., Wreghitt, T., et al.: The importance of cytomegalovirus in heart-lung transplantation. Chest *95*:627, 1989.
207. McCarthy, P. M., Starnes, V. A., Theodore, J., et al.: Improved survival after heart-lung transplantation. J. Thorac. Cardiovasc. Surg. *99*:54, 1990.
208. Higgenbottam, T., Stewart, S., Penketh, A., et al.: Transbronchial lung biopsy for the diagnosis of rejection in heart-lung transplant patients. Transplantation *46*:532, 1988.
209. Starnes, V. A., Theodore, J., Oyer, P. E., et al.: Pulmonary infiltrates after heart-lung transplantation: Evaluation by serial transbronchial biopsies. J. Thorac. Cardiovasc. Surg. *98*:945, 1989.
210. Starnes, V. A., Theodore, J., Oyer, P. E., et al.: Evaluation of heart-lung transplant recipients with prospective, serial, transbronchial biopsies in pulmonary function studies. J. Thorac. Cardiovasc. Surg. *98*:683, 1989.
211. Dummer, J. S., Montero, C. G., Griffith, B. P., et al.: Infections in heart-lung recipients. Transplantation *41*:725, 1986.
212. Ren, H., Hruban, R. H., Baumgartner, W. A., et al.: Hemorrhagic infarction of hilar lymph nodes associated with combined heart-lung transplantation. J. Thorac. Cardiovasc. Surg. *99*:861, 1990.
213. Allen, M. D., Burke, C. M., McGregor, C. G. A., et al.: Steroid-responsive bronchiolitis after human heart-lung transplantation. J. Thorac. Cardiovasc. Surg. *92*:449, 1986.
214. LoCicero, J., Robinson, P. G., Fisher, M.: Chronic rejection in single lung transplantation manifested by obliterative bronchiolitis. J. Thorac. Cardiovasc. Surg. *99*:1059, 1990.
215. Theodore, J., Morris, A. J., Burke, C. M., et al.: Cardiopulmonary function at maximum tolerable constant work rate exercise following human heart-lung transplantation. Chest *92*:433, 1987.
216. Davis, R. D., and Pasque, M. K.: Pulmonary transplantation. Ann. Surg. *221*(1):14, 1995.

Chapter 19
Assisted Circulation and the Mechanical Heart

WAYNE E. RICHENBACHER, WILLIAM S. PIERCE

Four hundred thousand new cases of congestive heart failure are diagnosed in the United States annually.[1] According to the Framingham Heart Study, the 5-year mortality rate for patients with congestive heart failure was 75 per cent in men and 62 per cent in women.[2] Standard medical and surgical therapies benefit only a small percentage of patients with ventricular dysfunction. Potential cardiac transplant recipients with hemodynamic instability may receive temporary mechanical circulatory support as a bridge to cardiac transplantation. Best estimates suggest that 17,000 to 66,000 patients in the United States may benefit from a permanent implantable blood pump each year.[3] Once they are perfected, not only will mechanical blood pumps be immediately accessible but they will ultimately provide a cost-effective alternative to cardiac transplantation or long-term medical treatment of patients in New York Heart Association (NYHA) functional Classes III and IV.[4]

Another population of patients who would benefit from mechanical circulatory support are individuals with reversible ventricular dysfunction. Two to 6 per cent of patients who undergo an open heart operation develop postcardiotomy cardiogenic shock.[5] Aggressive medical management, including intraaortic balloon (IAB) counterpulsation, allows 75 to 85 per cent of these patients to be weaned from cardiopulmonary bypass. Thus, approximately 1 per cent of patients who undergo an open heart procedure would benefit from interval support with a mechanical blood pump.

Patients with cardiovascular disease in whom hemodynamic deterioration is evident first receive conventional medical therapy. Conventional management is directed toward correction of any electrolyte or acid-base imbalance, hypoxemia, rhythm disturbance, or hypovolemic state. Cardiogenic shock, as defined in Table 19–1, is next treated with inotropic and, if systemic blood pressure permits, afterload-reducing agents. Patients who manifest ongoing hemodynamic instability, and who fulfill the selection criteria outlined in Table 19–2, may qualify for an advanced form of mechanical circulatory support.

Mechanical circulatory support devices can be roughly divided into three major groups. The IAB is a readily available, catheter-mounted intravascular device designed to improve the balance between myocardial oxygen supply and demand while increasing systemic perfusion to a modest degree. The ventricular assist device (VAD) is a blood pump that is designed to assist or replace the function of either the right or left ventricle. A right VAD will support the pulmonary circulation, while a left VAD provides systemic perfusion, in the absence of right or left ventricular ejection, respectively. Implantable VADs are positioned intracorporeally—in the anterior abdominal wall or within a body cavity other than the pericardium. Extracorporeal VADs may be located in a paracorporeal position, along the patient's anterior abdominal wall, or externally, at the patient's bedside. Two VADs have received Food and Drug Administration (FDA) approval for clinical use, although access to the majority of these devices is controlled by clinical trials as of this writing. The total artificial heart (TAH) is an orthotopically positioned cardiac replacement device. The pneumatic TAH is used infrequently, and only with FDA approval, as a mechanical bridge to cardiac transplantation. Completely implantable electric artificial hearts have been successfully implanted in experimental animals but are not expected to reach the clinical arena until the year 2000.

HISTORY

Extracorporeal counterpulsation was introduced by Clauss and coworkers in 1961.[6] The concept was modified by Moulopoulos and colleagues who described an intravascular counterpulsation balloon in 1962.[7] The first successful clinical application of balloon counterpulsation was reported by Kantrowitz et al. in 1968.[8] IAB insertion originally required a surgical procedure. In 1980, Bregman and Casarella described percutaneous IAB insertion utilizing a sheath and dilators.[9] The IAB is now a standard form of therapy for a variety of patients with cardiovascular disease. In 1993, nearly 100,000 IABs were inserted in the United States alone.[10]

The dawn of complete, clinical mechanical circulatory support occurred on May 6, 1953 when Gibbon successfully closed a secundum atrial septal defect in a patient supported with cardiopulmonary bypass.[11] The majority of patients with ventricular dysfunction, however, do not require pulmonary support with an in-line oxygenator. Roller-pump left ventricular assistance using atrial transseptal uptake and femoral arterial return was introduced by Dennis et al. in 1962.[12] Subsequently, DeBakey successfully employed left atrial to aortic bypass in patients who could not be weaned from cardiopulmonary bypass.[13] By the late 1970's, a variety of intracorporeal and extracorporeal mechanical blood pumps were being tested for both "support to weaning"[14] and "bridge to transplant"[15] indications. Patient selection and hemodynamic criteria were developed, and cannulation techniques, blood-biomaterial interactions, and control strategies evaluated. During the 1980's patient management was refined and clinical results improved. Advances in myocardial preservation resulted in fewer blood pumps being required for postcardiotomy cardiogenic shock. However, a disparity in the ratio of cardiac donors to recipients increased the need for long-term circulatory support in patients requiring a bridge to cardiac transplantation. Results in this patient population proved gratifying, with survival statistics approaching those achieved with conventional cardiac transplantation.[16] The early 1990's have seen research efforts focus on the development of implantable VADs suitable for permanent implantation in patients with end-stage cardiomyopathy.

While IAB and VAD development were in their infancy, investigators also initiated laboratory efforts to develop a cardiac replacement device. In 1958, Akutsu and Kolff described an experiment in which a pneumatic TAH was implanted in a dog.[17] By the mid 1960's, Kolff and Nosé had achieved 24-hour survival with sac-type hearts implanted in calves.[18] By the end of the decade, survival times approached 3 to 5 days.[19] Experimental animals with TAHs have now lived for up to 1 year. The TAH entered the clinical arena in 1969 when Cooley and associates introduced the concept of staged cardiac replacement.[20] DeVries and coworkers were the first to implant a TAH as a permanent cardiac replacement.[21]

TABLE 19–1 DEFINITION OF CARDIOGENIC SHOCK

Cardiac output index	<1.8 liters/min/m^2
Systolic blood pressure	<90 mm Hg
Left or right atrial pressure	>20 mm Hg
Urine output	<20 ml/hr
Systemic vascular resistance	>2100 dynes-sec/cm^5

INTRAAORTIC BALLOON COUNTERPULSATION

The design and function of the IAB have not changed substantially during the past three decades. The IAB is an intravascular catheter-mounted counterpulsation device with a balloon volume between 30 and 50 ml. A central lumen allows passage of the balloon catheter over a small-diameter guidewire and subsequent monitoring of central aortic blood pressure. The IAB is attached to a small bedside console and triggered to the patient's arterial pressure curve or electrocardiogram. The shuttle gas is helium, as its viscosity allows rapid balloon inflation and deflation, which facilitates counterpulsation in patients with tachyarrhythmias.

The IAB is positioned in the descending thoracic aorta and set to inflate at the dicrotic notch of the arterial pressure waveform when monitoring the aortic pressure (Fig. 19–1). The diastolic rise in aortic root pressure augments coronary blood flow and myocardial oxygen supply. The increase in systemic perfusion may be less than 0.5 liter/min. The IAB is deflated during the isovolumetric phase of left ventricular contraction. The reduction in the afterload component of cardiac work decreases peak left ventricular pressure and myocardial oxygen consumption. The net effect is a favorable shift in the myocardial oxygen supply/demand ratio, with a small increase in systemic perfusion.

Indications and Results of Clinical Use

Traditional indications for IAB counterpulsation include refractory cardiogenic shock following cardiac surgery or an acute myocardial infarction (see p. 1239). The latter indication includes patients suffering from primary pump failure in addition to those with mechanical complications, such as acute mitral regurgitation or a postinfarction ventricular septal defect.

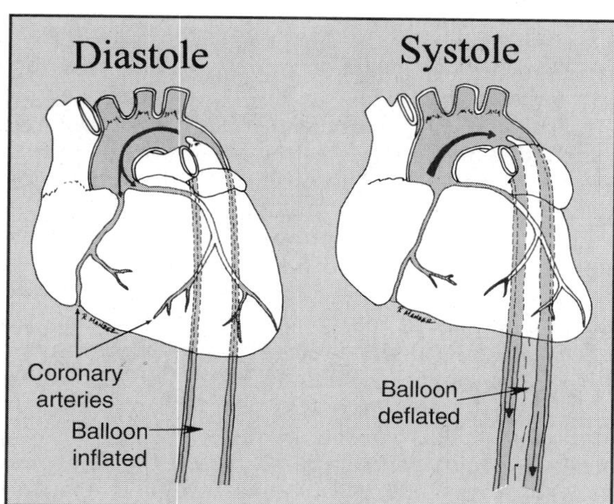

FIGURE 19–1. The intraaortic balloon is inserted via the common femoral artery and positioned in the descending thoracic aorta. The tip is located just distal to the left subclavian artery. The balloon is inflated during cardiac diastole, thereby increasing coronary artery perfusion. Left ventricular afterload is decreased as the balloon is deflated during cardiac systole. Proper balloon timing improves the ratio between myocardial oxygen supply and demand. (Courtesy of Arrow International, Inc. Redrawn by Richard Manzer.)

Seventy-five per cent of patients with an acute myocardial infarction who develop cardiogenic shock not amenable to conventional medical therapy will improve hemodynamically with IAB counterpulsation.[22] Outcome, however, is largely determined by the underlying coronary artery pathology. Patients with operable disease who undergo prompt revascularization achieve an early survival rate as high as 93 per cent.[23] Patients who develop a mechanical complication following an acute myocardial infarction are best managed with IAB counterpulsation, urgent cardiac catheterization, and immediate surgical repair. IAB counterpulsation will reduce the left-to-right shunt and maintain coronary perfusion in patients with a postinfarction *ventricular septal defect* (see p. 1243). Hospital mortality in patients managed with an IAB and urgent operation is 20 per cent to 27 per cent.[24] Patients with postinfarction *mitral regurgitation* secondary to papillary muscle dysfunction or rupture also benefit from IAB insertion (see p. 1243). IAB counterpulsation will increase coronary perfusion and reduce ischemic ventricular dysfunction, mitral regurgitation, and the pulmonary capillary wedge pressure. Outcome is related to the extent of cardiac dysfunction with surgical mortality approaching 55 per cent.[25]

Refractory *postcardiotomy cardiogenic shock* is related to preoperative left ventricular dysfunction, inadequate myocardial preservation, intraoperative myocardial infarction, prolonged cardiopulmonary bypass, and ischemic times, or technical difficulties with the conduct of the operation. With maximal medical support and IAB counterpulsation, survival rates average 52 to 66 per cent.[26]

An additional group of patients in cardiogenic shock who benefit from IAB counterpulsation are approved *cardiac transplant recipients* with hemodynamic decompensation before a donor heart becomes available (see p. 1239). The rationale for IAB counterpulsation in this clinical setting is to maintain systemic perfusion and preserve end-organ function until cardiac transplantation occurs. One-year actuarial survival in patients who require IAB counterpulsation prior to cardiac transplantation is 72 to 77 per cent.[27,28]

More recently the indications for IAB support have been expanded to include patients who do not fulfill hemodynamic selection criteria but who suffer from *unstable angina* or *malignant ventricular tachyarrhythmias.* Although nonrandomized trials suggest that IAB counterpulsation and subsequent myocardial revascularization may be of some benefit in patients with preinfarction angina,[29] aggressive preoperative medical management and judicious use of a cardiac anesthetic may eliminate the need for an IAB with equally good results. The role of IAB counterpulsation in patients with postinfarction angina is equally controversial.[30] In general, IAB support is reserved for patients with deteriorating hemodynamics or ongoing ischemia, as evidenced by rest pain or electrocardiographic changes in the region of the infarct, before myocardial revascularization.

TABLE 19–2 MECHANICAL CIRCULATORY SUPPORT SELECTION CRITERIA

Patient fulfills hemodynamic criteria (Table 19–1)
Maximal inotropic support and IAB counterpulsation
Exclude patient if:
Blood urea nitrogen > 100 mg/dl
Serum creatinine > 5.0 mg/dl
Chronic lung disease
Chronic liver disease
Metastatic cancer
Sepsis
Neurological deficit
Technically incomplete cardiac operative procedure (if postcardiotomy cardiogenic shock)
Age > 60 yr (if bridge to transplant)

IAB = Intraaortic balloon.

IAB counterpulsation may be beneficial in patients with *ventricular tachyarrhythmias*, particularly when these abnormalities are related to ischemia.[31] Ectopic impulses originate in the ischemic area surrounding an infarct zone, and the IAB may reduce the frequency of such arrhythmias by increasing myocardial perfusion and oxygenation in the ischemic zone. The role of perioperative IAB counterpulsation in hemodynamically stable patients with left main coronary artery disease or severe left ventricular dysfunction, and in high-risk patients undergoing a general surgical procedure, is less well defined.

Absolute contraindications to IAB counterpulsation include aortic insufficiency and aortic dissection. Contraindications to IAB insertion via the femoral arterial route include the presence of an abdominal aortic aneurysm or severe calcific aortoiliac or femoral arterial disease. The percutaneous insertion technique should not be employed in a patient who has a recent groin incision with violation of the subcutaneous tissue at the proposed puncture site.

INSERTION TECHNIQUE

The IAB is most commonly inserted in a percutaneous fashion via the common femoral artery.[32] Preinsertion evaluation of the patient's femoral arterial and pedal pulses facilitates rapid recognition of limb ischemia following balloon insertion. With the use of strict aseptic technique the femoral artery is accessed by means of the Seldinger approach. The femoral arterial puncture should occur below the inguinal ligament, to avoid a transperitoneal puncture, and above the profunda femoris artery, to reduce the potential for superficial femoral arterial cannulation.

The common femoral artery is dilated and the final dilator and sheath advanced over a J wire into the descending thoracic aorta. The final dilator is withdrawn and the IAB inserted into the introducer sheath. The radiopaque tip of the IAB is positioned just distal to the left subclavian artery. The balloon is unwound, purged, connected to the bedside console, and pulsed. Proper augmentation is best accomplished with the IAB synchronized 1:2 with the patient's arterial pressure trace. Once inflation and deflation times are determined, augmentation is set at 1:1. Postinsertion anticoagulation is usually accomplished with low molecular weight (10 per cent) dextran (20 ml/hr). Prophylactic heparin sodium administration is recommended in patients who have not had surgical intervention.

Alternatively the IAB may be inserted into the femoral artery using an open technique. The femoral artery is exposed and a 5-cm segment of an 8- to 10-mm diameter vascular graft anastomosed, at a 45-degree angle, to the common femoral artery. The IAB is passed through the vascular graft into the artery and positioned as already described. The IAB is fixed in position by tying umbilical tapes around the vascular graft.

When an abdominal aortic aneurysm or severe peripheral vascular disease precludes femoral arterial insertion, the IAB may be inserted directly into the ascending aorta or transverse arch.[33] Access is obtained through a median sternotomy, usually at the time of cardiotomy. The balloon is inserted through a vascular graft in a manner identical to that described in the open femoral arterial technique. The balloon is advanced across the transverse arch into the descending thoracic aorta. Alternatively, the IAB can simply be inserted through two, concentric pursestring sutures.

When greater patient mobility is desired, the IAB may be inserted into the subclavian or iliac artery.[34,35] These insertion sites are particularly applicable when long-term IAB support is anticipated, as in patients who require a mechanical bridge to cardiac transplantation. In the authors' opinion, however, hemodynamically unstable potential cardiac transplant recipients are best managed with a brief trial of IAB counterpulsation using the femoral arterial approach. If the patient's condition fails to improve within 48 to 72 hours, VAD implantation should be considered.

REMOVAL TECHNIQUE

As the patient's hemodynamic status improves, balloon augmentation is serially decreased. If the patient tolerates augmentation of every fourth to eighth heartbeat (1:4 to 1:8), the IAB can be safely withdrawn.[32] Balloon inflation is discontinued and the balloon aspirated to ensure deflation is complete. The balloon is withdrawn into the sheath. Manual pressure is applied to the femoral artery distal to the insertion site, and the balloon and insertion sheath withdrawn as a single unit. Blood is permitted to eject from the insertion site for one or two heart beats to clear any thrombotic debris from the vascular space. Pressure is then applied to the insertion site: manually for 30 minutes and with a sandbag for an additional 8 hours. One should make certain that the limb is adequately perfused during IAB removal. Withdrawal of an IAB inserted by the open technique requires surgical groin exploration, balloon and vascular graft removal, and femoral artery repair, usually with a vein patch. Open removal is also recommended when there has been high (proximal) percutaneous insertion, in morbidly obese patients, and in patients who develop limb ischemia following percutaneous insertion.

Balloons inserted into the ascending aorta can be removed under local anesthesia if the side arm graft is brought into the subcutaneous space.[36] The authors of this chapter, however, recommend repeat sternotomy with direct visualization of the insertion site.

COMPLICATIONS OF IAB USE

The complication rate from IAB counterpulsation varies from 6 to 46 per cent.[37] Major complications, including limb ischemia necessitating thrombectomy or amputation, aortic dissection, aortoiliac laceration or perforation, and deep wound infection requiring debridement, occur in 4 to 17 per cent of patients. Major complications lead to an additional operative procedure, prolonged hospitalization, long-term morbidity, or death. Minor complications, including bleeding at the insertion site, superficial wound infections, asymptomatic loss of peripheral pulse, or lymphocele, occur in 7 to 42 per cent of patients. Minor complications are usually self-limited or resolve following IAB removal.

The most common complications related to femoral IAB use are vascular.[37–39] Vascular complication rates vary from 6 to 24 per cent, and are usually related to the initial insertion procedure rather than the presence of the IAB within the vascular space. Risk factors for developing a major vascular complication following femoral IAB insertion include diabetes mellitus, systemic hypertension, female gender, and peripheral vascular disease. Interestingly, percutaneous IAB insertion has a major vascular complication rate similar to IAB insertion using an open surgical technique.[40,41] The risk of vascular complications associated with percutaneous insertion is related to the possibility of superficial, rather than common, femoral arterial cannulation and the potential for intimal disruption at the time of arterial cannulation.

LEG ISCHEMIA. This is the most common vascular complication of femoral IAB insertion, occurring in 5 to 19 per cent of patients.[37–39] When a patient develops leg ischemia following femoral IAB insertion, the IAB should be removed. Persistent ischemia following IAB removal requires emergent femoral arterial exploration, thrombectomy, and patch angioplasty. Balloon-dependent patients with limb ischemia benefit from moving the IAB to the contralateral leg or a femoral-femoral crossover graft.[42] Modified IABs, intended for sheathless insertion, may reduce the incidence of leg ischemia, particularly in patients with small femoral arteries.

Aortic dissection occurs in fewer than 5 per cent of patients[37]; however, the majority of patients who develop this complication do not survive. Aortic dissection occurs at the time of femoral IAB insertion and is managed by IAB removal. The incidence of aortic dissection may be reduced by using a guidewire and fluoroscopy and avoiding excessive force during IAB insertion.

The complication rate of transthoracic IAB counterpulsation is 0 to 13 per cent.[33,37] Complications associated with IAB insertion in the ascending aorta include side arm graft infection with mediastinitis, coronary artery or arch vessel embolization, and inability to close the sternum secondary to mechanical tamponade.

THE VENTRICULAR ASSIST DEVICE

Unlike the IAB that is designed to improve the ratio between myocardial oxygen supply and demand while supporting systemic perfusion to only a modest degree, the VAD is designed to effectively unload either the right or left ventricle while completely supporting the pulmonary or systemic circulation. The term *VAD* describes any of a variety of mechanical blood pumps employed singly to replace the function of either the right or left ventricle. Two blood pumps can be utilized for biventricular support. For right ventricular assistance, blood is withdrawn from the right atrium and returned to the main pulmonary artery. For left ventricular assistance, blood is withdrawn from either the left atrium or the apex of the left ventricle. The blood passes through the left VAD and is returned to the ascending aorta.

There is a wealth of information in the literature regarding the advantages and disadvantages of left atrial versus left ventricular inflow (with respect to the VAD) cannulation.[43,44] In general, left atrial inflow cannulation is technically easier to perform and may employ cannulas readily available to any open heart surgical team; however, it is thought to provide incomplete ventricular decompression. Left ventricular inflow cannulation requires a custom-designed cannula but provides very effective left ventricular decompression. The reduction in myocardial oxygen de-

TABLE 19–3 COMPARISON OF VENTRICULAR ASSIST PUMPS

VAD TYPE	ADVANTAGE	DISADVANTAGE
Roller	Readily available Simple to use Inexpensive	Flow limitation Blood trauma Tubing spallation Nonpulsatile Systemic anticoagulation Short-term use Constant supervision required
Centrifugal	Readily available Simple to use Relatively inexpensive Blood handling characteristics	Nonpulsatile Systemic anticoagulation Constant supervision required Not FDA approved as a VAD
Pulsatile	No blood trauma +/− anticoagulation Pulsatile flow Minimal supervision required Patient mobility	Expensive

VAD = Ventricular assist device; FDA = Food and Drug Administration.

mand is offset by the fact that left ventricular apical cannulation damages the myocardium, an important consideration in a patient with marginal ventricular function. A left ventricular apex cannula is, however, ideally suited to patients who receive mechanical circulatory support as a bridge to cardiac transplantation. In this patient population, ventricular recovery is not expected, and the apical cannula is removed in its entirety at the time of recipient cardiectomy.

REGULATORY AFFAIRS

To better understand the enormous amount of effort that has been expended developing mechanical blood pumps, and limitations imposed on clinicians who desire access to a VAD, it is important to become familiar with the process by which medical devices are evaluated and approved for clinical use.[45,46] In the United States the Medical Device Amendment of 1976 amended the Federal Food, Drug and Cosmetic Act to require the FDA to approve clinical investigation of new medical devices and to approve new medical devices before they could be sold for general use. To prove that a new medical device is both safe and effective, the device must be the subject of a carefully controlled clinical trial.

An investigator/manufacturer first conducts extensive in vitro device testing followed by in vivo animal experimentation. The data derived from the preclinical evaluation are submitted to the FDA along with results, if any, from foreign clinical trials. The investigator must also submit a formal clinical protocol and informed consent material that have been approved by the Institutional Review Board at the site of the proposed clinical trial. If the application for clinical investigation of the device is deemed satisfactory by the FDA, an Investigational Device Exemption (IDE) is granted to the investigator. It is expected that the clinical protocol will answer specific questions concerning the proposed indications and contraindications for use of the device.

Because of the inordinate expense of device research and development, and the cost incurred during the conduct of a clinical trial (under an approved IDE), most investigators have an industrial partner. Assuming that the clinical trial shows the device to be safe and effective for a well-defined set of indications, the next step is to seek approval from the FDA for commercial sale of the device. In general, the industrial partner will submit a Pre Market Approval (PMA) request to the FDA. The focus of the PMA application is to provide more extensive durability testing, an important consideration in devices intended for long-term clinical use.

Durability testing is most often accomplished by accelerated in vitro experimentation, frequently performed under conditions more severe than those experienced when the device is in actual clinical use. Approval of a PMA by the FDA allows the manufacturer to release the medical device for commercial sale.

Description of Devices

Mechanical blood pumps capable of replacing the function of a single ventricle can be divided into four categories. The advantages and disadvantages of each category of blood pump are summarized in Table 19–3. Representative members of each class of VAD are listed in Table 19–4. Specific design features and functional characteristics of each VAD are described below. Specific details regarding implantation and explanation technique are described in the section entitled Management Considerations.

ROLLER PUMP. The roller pump employs cannulas, tubing, and a roller head, all of which are readily available to any cardiac surgeon.[47,48] The inflow and outflow cannulas employed for roller pump ventricular assistance are the same as those employed for cardiopulmonary bypass in any open heart operation. The cannulas are connected to a length of $\frac{3}{8}$ inch ID medical grade silicone rubber tubing. The tubing is placed in the roller head and forward flow imparted to blood by the rotating, occlusive rollers. Cannula and tubing size frequently limit total blood flow, while the occlusive roller head is responsible for hemolysis and trauma to formed blood elements, in addition to tubing spallation and fatigue.[49,50] The system provides nonpulsatile flow, requires that the patient be fully anticoagulated, and is not pressure limited, which demands that the drive unit receive constant supervision. A fall in atrial pressure can lead to air embolism as air is drawn into the atrium around the atrial cannula. A sudden obstruction to VAD

TABLE 19–4 REPRESENTATIVE MEMBERS OF EACH VAD TYPE

VAD TYPE	NAME	MANUFACTURER
Roller	Roller	Many
Centrifugal	Bio-Pump Delphin Isoflow	Medtronic Bio-Medicus, Inc. Sarns, Inc./3M Aries Medical/St. Jude
Pulsatile (Pneumatic)	BVS 5000 Bi-ventricular Support System HeartMate 1000 IP LVAS Thoratec VAD System	Abiomed, Inc. ThermoCardiosystems, Inc. Thoratec Laboratories Corp.
Pulsatile (Electric)	Novacor N-100 HeartMate 1000 VE LVAS Penn State	Novacor Medical Division, Baxter Healthcare Corp. ThermoCardiosystems, Inc. Arrow International, Inc.

VAD = Ventricular assist device.

outflow can result in rapid system pressurization and tubing disruption. The roller pump is capable of providing right or left ventricular support, and two pumps can be employed for biventricular support. The limitations preclude use of this system beyond a few hours or days.

CENTRIFUGAL PUMPS. Centrifugal pumps are also simple to use and readily available to most cardiac surgeons (Fig. 19–2*A*).[51,52] Standard cardiopulmonary bypass atrial and arterial cannulas are connected to the centrifugal head by short lengths of medical grade polyvinylchloride tubing. Unlike the roller head, however, the centrifugal head imparts forward flow to blood by creating a vortex with a rapidly spinning series of cones or impeller blades that are located within the rigid pump housing (Fig. 19–2*B*). The nonocclusive pump head reportedly has better blood handling characteristics than a roller head, and the system is pressure limited, virtually eliminating the potential for air embolus or tubing disruption.[49,53] Centrifugal blood pumps provide nonpulsatile blood flow and require full systemic anticoagulation and constant driver supervision.[54] The pump can provide left or right heart support, or two pumps can be used for biventricular assistance.

Centrifugal pumps entered the clinical arena prior to the Medical Device Amendment of 1976. However, centrifugal blood pumps are considered a Class III medical device, subject to the constraints imposed by this amendment to the Federal Food, Drug and Cosmetic Act. Currently, centrifugal blood pumps are approved only for up to 6 hours of use, suitable for cardiopulmonary bypass, but not for short-term temporary ventricular assistance. Recently a coalition of centrifugal blood pump manufacturers formed the Health Industries Manufacturers Task Force to petition the FDA to reclassify centrifugal blood pumps as a Class II medical device, thereby removing the time constraints for ventricular support. This down-class petition is based upon the proven track record of centrifugal blood pumps in providing safe and effective ventricular assistance in non-FDA-approved clinical experience.

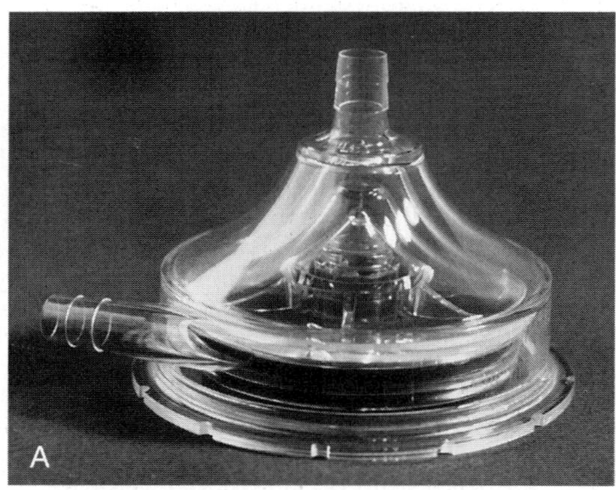

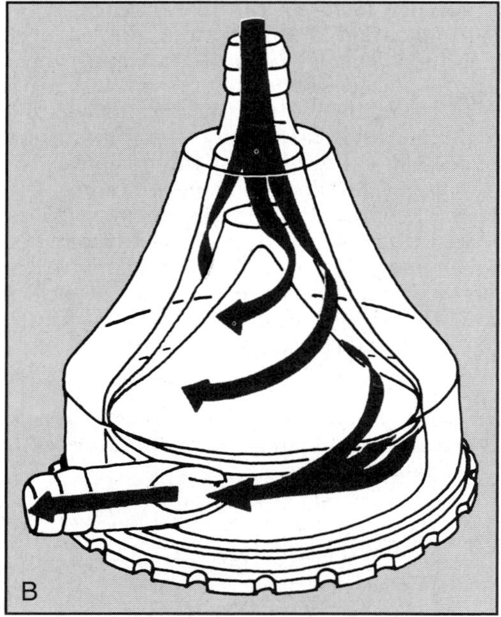

FIGURE 19–2. The Bio-Pump centrifugal pump. *A,* This extracorporeal blood pump can be used for either right or left ventricular assistance. Two pumps can be used for biventricular assistance. *B,* The Bio-Pump centrifugal blood pump imparts forward flow to blood by creating a vortex with a rapidly spinning series of cones. (Courtesy of Medtronic Bio-Medicus, Inc.)

Pneumatic Pulsatile Blood Pumps

Complex air-driven pulsatile VADs are considerably more expensive than either roller or centrifugal pumps and until recently were available only to centers participating in a clinical trial. These devices produce pulsatile flow with no trauma to formed blood elements. Furthermore, integral sophisticated control systems are largely self-regulating, and beyond the first few days following device insertion minimal supervision is required. As drive units become more refined and portable drivers are developed, patient mobility and life style have improved dramatically.

ABIOMED BVS 5000 BIVENTRICULAR SUPPORT SYSTEM. This system received PMA approval from the FDA in 1992 for treatment of patients with postcardiotomy cardiogenic shock (Fig. 19–3).[55–57] The BVS 5000 (Abiomed, Inc., Danvers, MA) is an external dual-chamber device that is capable of providing short-term univentricular or biventricular circulatory support. Each chamber contains a 100-ml polyurethane blood sac. Trileaflet polyurethane valves are located at the inlet and outlet side of the ventricular chamber. The atrial chamber fills passively throughout pump systole and diastole, while the ventricular chamber is intermittently pulsed with air from the drive console. Custom-designed cannulas provide right or left atrial inflow. The distal portion of the outlet cannula is a coated vascular prosthesis that is anastomosed to either the pulmonary artery or aorta. The cannulas traverse the skin subcostally. The drive unit functions asynchronously with respect to the patient's native cardiac rhythm. The control system maintains a constant 80-ml stroke volume by automatically adjusting the duration of pump systole and diastole in response to changes in preload and afterload.

THE HEARTMATE 1000 IP LVAS. This system received PMA approval from the FDA in 1994 for use as a mechanical bridge to cardiac transplantation (Fig. 19–4).[58–60] This implantable blood pump (ThermoCardiosystems, Inc., Woburn, MA) is connected to an external drive unit by a percutaneous air drive line. The titanium VAD housing contains a flexible segmented polyurethane diaphragm that is bonded to a rigid pusher plate. The unique, textured blood-containing surface promotes the formation of a stable neointima.[61] Patients do not require systemic anticoagulation and instead receive only antiplatelet agents. Intermittent air pulses from the external drive console actuate the pusher-plate diaphragm and eject blood from the VAD housing. The pump has a maximum stroke volume of 83 ml and a maximum pump output of 11 liters/min. Valved conduits containing 25-mm porcine valves are located at the inlet and outlet ports of the VAD housing. The VAD is designed only for left ventricular support, withdrawing blood from the left ventricular apex. Blood is returned to the ascending aorta. The device was originally designed to be implanted in the left upper quadrant of the patient's abdomen. However, in selected patients the device may be positioned preperitoneally, in the abdominal wall.[62] When the blood pump is placed in a preperitoneal position, the potential visceral complications associated

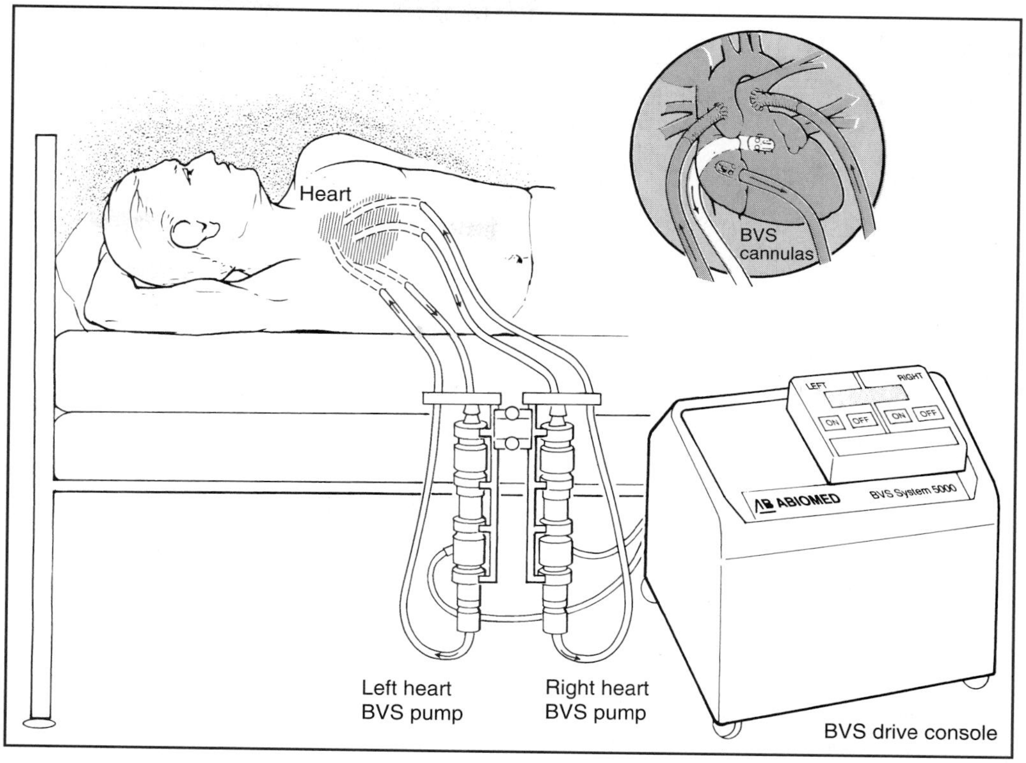

FIGURE 19–3. The Abiomed BVS 5000 Bi-ventricular Support System can support either right or left ventricular function. The system is simple in design and relatively inexpensive by pulsatile blood pump standards. The dual chamber, gravity-fed device restricts patient mobility more than implantable pulsatile blood pumps, but is ideally suited for use in postcardiotomy cardiogenic shock patients in whom the duration of support is less than 1 week. (From Shook, B.J.: The Abiomed BVS 5000 Bi-ventricular Support System. System description and clinical summary. Cardiac Surgery State of the Art Reviews *7*:309, 1993. Reproduced with permission.)

with peritoneal implantation are avoided. The drive console runs on standard alternating current, as well as internal rechargeable batteries. The batteries provide up to 40 minutes of support. The control system allows the VAD to function in a fixed rate or pump-on-full mode. The latter is a rate-responsive mode in which the VAD is automatically pulsed when the pump chamber is 90 per cent filled.

PIERCE-DONACHY SYSTEMS. The prototypical pneumatic, pulsatile VAD, and the device that has probably seen the largest US clinical experience, is the Thoratec Ventricular Assist Device (Thoratec Laboratories Corp., Berkeley, CA) based on the Pierce-Donachy design (Fig. 19–5).[63–65] In 1994 the Circulatory System Devices Advisory Panel to the FDA recommended approval of this paracorporeal blood pump as a bridge to cardiac transplantation; in 1995 the FDA granted full commercial approval. This versatile blood pump can be used for right, left, or biventricular assistance (Fig. 19–6). In the case of left ventricular assistance, custom-designed cannulas allow blood to be withdrawn from either the left atrium or the apex of the left ventricle. The blood pump consists of a machined polysulfone housing that contains a polyurethane blood sac and Sorin monostrut inlet and outlet valves (Sorin Biomedical, Inc., Irvine, CA). Patients are maintained on sodium warfarin. The blood pump has a stroke volume of 65 ml with a dynamic ejection fraction of approximately 0.75. Air pulses from the

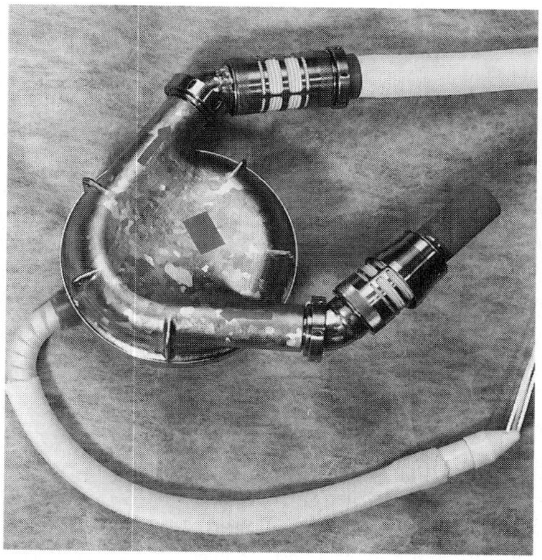

FIGURE 19–4. The implantable HeartMate 1000 IP LVAS blood pump has a percutaneous air drive line located at the bottom of this photograph. The short left ventricular apex inlet conduit, at right, and the outlet conduit at the top of this photograph, contain bioprosthetic valves that ensure a unidirectional flow of blood through the blood pump. The vascular graft on the outlet conduit is cut to length and sutured to the ascending aorta. (Courtesy of ThermoCardiosystems, Inc.)

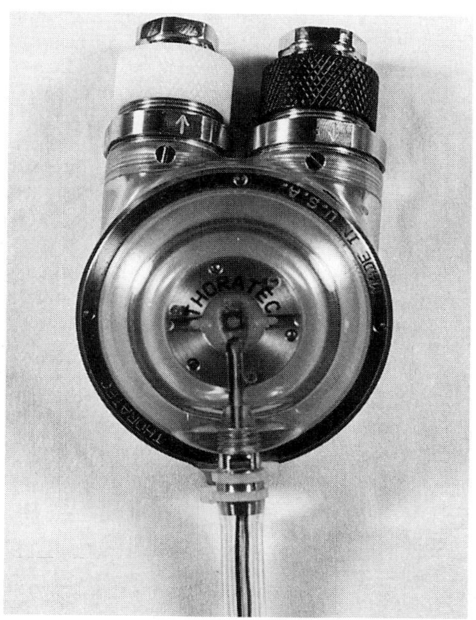

FIGURE 19–5. The paracorporeal Thoratec blood pump is positioned on the patient's anterior abdominal wall. The inlet and outlet cannulas (not shown) traverse the skin subcostally. The air drive line is located at the bottom of this photograph. The device can be used for either right or left heart support. Two devices can be used to provide biventricular assistance. (Courtesy of Thoratec Laboratories, Corp.)

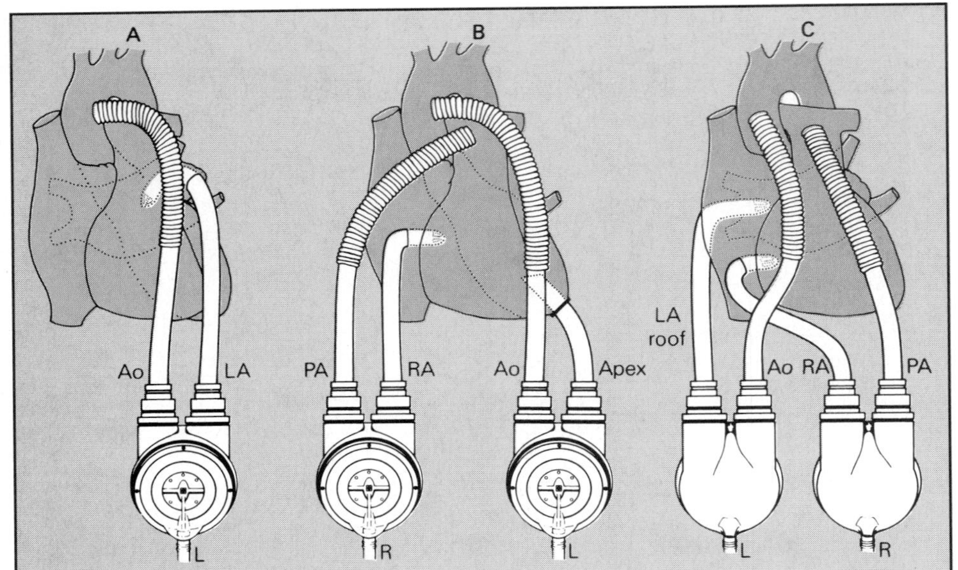

FIGURE 19–6. Cannulation configurations for the Thoratec ventricular assist device. *A*, Left atrial appendage to aortic left ventricular assistance. *B*, Left ventricular apex to aortic, and right atrium to main pulmonary artery biventricular assistance. *C*, Biventricular assistance where the left ventricular assist device inflow cannula is inserted into the left atrium via the right superior pulmonary vein. (*L* = left, *R* = right, *LA* = left atrium, *Ao* = aorta, *RA* = right atrium, *PA* = pulmonary artery. (From Farrar, D. J., Hill, J. O., Gray, L. A., Jr., et al.: Heterotopic prosthetic ventricles as a bridge to cardiac transplantation: A multicenter study in 29 patients. N. Engl. J. Med. *318*:333, 1988. Copyright Massachusetts Medical Society.)

drive unit intermittently compress the flexible blood sac ejecting blood from the VAD housing. The control system allows the device to function in one of three modes: a manual fixed-rate mode, a synchronized mode in which the R wave of the patient's electrocardiogram serves as an electronic trigger, and an asynchronous full-to-empty mode in which the VAD enters systole each time the blood sac fills. The last mode maximizes cardiac output by allowing the VAD pump rate to be determined by preload.

Electric Pulsatile Blood Pumps

The electric VAD will ultimately be completely implantable and capable of providing years of left ventricular support. These devices provide left-ventricular-apex to aortic flow and are not designed for right ventricular assistance. In addition to a mechanical blood pump, the electric VAD system will have an implantable controller and back-up battery. An external, portable battery pack will serve as the primary power source. The external battery pack will be carried in a shoulder bag and transfer energy to the implantable controller and blood pump using transcutaneous energy transmission.[66] Energy will be passed from an external primary coil located on the surface of the skin to a subcutaneous secondary coil by inductive coupling. There will be no break in the integument, eliminating the potential for an ascending drive line infection. The internal, rechargeable battery will allow brief periods of entirely tether-free VAD function. As these systems will be completely sealed, air displaced from the blood pump housing during diastole will move to an implanted reservoir known as a compliance chamber.[67] As the final technological barriers to the development of implantable electric VADs are overcome, these systems will be permanently implanted in patients with unreconstructable coronary artery disease or end stage cardiomyopathy not amenable to cardiac transplantation.

NOVACOR N-100 LEFT VENTRICULAR ASSIST SYSTEM. This system contains a polyurethane blood sac that is compressed by dual symmetrically opposed pusher plates.[68] In this system (Novacor Medical Division, Baxter Healthcare Corp., Oakland, CA), the pump is actuated by a spring-decoupled solenoid energy converter. The blood pump and energy converter are contained within a lightweight housing that is implanted in a preperitoneal position in the left upper quadrant of the patient's abdomen.[69] The inflow conduit and outflow conduit each contains a bioprosthetic pericardial valve. Patients require full anticoagulation with sodium warfarin.

The Novacor blood pump has a maximum stroke volume of 67 ml. The tethered configuration, the subject of an ongoing clinical trial that began in 1984, employs a percutaneous vented tube containing power and control wires.[68] The external console-based controller typically allows the device to function in a fill-rate trigger mode that provides synchronized counterpulsation to the native heart. Recently the clinical trial protocol was amended to allow testing of the wearable microprocessor-based controller.[70,71] The compact controller and rechargeable batteries are worn as a belt or carried in a "camera bag" and can support the blood pump for up to 7 hours.

HEARTMATE 1000 VE LVAS. This system (ThermoCardiosystems, Inc., Woburn, MA) utilizes a blood pump similar to that employed in the pneumatically powered ventricular assist system produced by the same manufacturer.[72,73] In the vented electric version, however, the

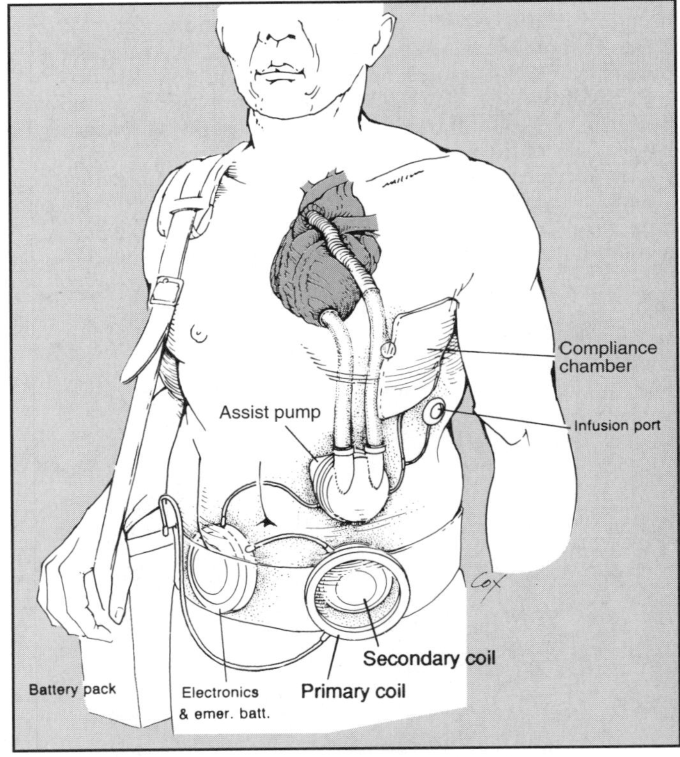

FIGURE 19–7. The completely implantable electric ventricular assist system being developed at Pennsylvania State University. The blood pump and energy converter are located preperitoneally in the patient's left upper quadrant. The implantable control system and rechargeable back-up battery are powered by an external battery pack. Energy passes from the superficial primary coil to the subcutaneous secondary coil using inductive coupling. Air displaced from the blood pump housing during diastole will enter the intrathoracic compliance chamber. Air that diffuses out of the compliance chamber over time is replenished using the subcutaneous infusion port.

TABLE 19–5 RESULTS OF CENTRIFUGAL BLOOD PUMP SUPPORT FOR POSTCARDIOTOMY CARDIOGENIC SHOCK

AUTHOR	DEVICE	NO. PATIENTS	WEANED (%)	SURVIVED (%)
Golding[78]	Bio-Pump	79	49 (62)	20 (25)
Lee[77]	Bio-Pump	28	N/A	9 (32)
Noon[79]*	Bio-Pump	89	42 (47)	19 (21)
Killen[76]	Bio-Pump	41	17 (41)	8 (20)
Curtis[52]	Delphin	60	23 (38)	12 (20)
Registry[5]	Centrifugal	559	254 (45)	143 (26)

* Includes 61 postcardiotomy patients.

diaphragm pusher-plate mechanism is pulsed by a low-speed high-torque motor. The percutaneous electrical leads connect the blood pump to the external controller and batteries. The rechargeable batteries are carried in a shoulder holster, or the device may be connected to a stationary control console. The clinical trial of the VE LVAS began in 1991, with selected patients managed in an outpatient setting.[73]

PENNSYLVANIA STATE UNIVERSITY SYSTEM. The completely implantable sealed system being developed at Pennsylvania State University contains a segmented polyurethane blood sac enclosed in a rigid polysulfone housing (Fig. 19–7).[74,75] Björk-Shiley inlet and outlet valves provide unidirectional blood flow. The blood sac is compressed by a pusher plate driven by a brushless direct current motor. Air displaced from the pump housing during VAD diastole is managed by a polyurethane compliance chamber.[67] Control electronics and a 30-minute battery pack are contained in an implantable cannister that receives power from a subcutaneous energy transmission coil. The external battery pack carried by the patient transfers energy to the implanted coil using transcutaneous energy transmission.[66] The device has a stroke volume of 62 ml and can pump up to 8.5 liters/min. The controller adjusts the VAD beat rate in response to physiologic conditions, ensuring that the blood pump functions in a full-to-empty mode.

The Penn State electric VAD has run continuously for more than one year on a mock circulatory system.[74] The system has provided circulatory support for more than one week in 26 Holstein calves. The average duration of support was 62 days; the longest nearly 8 months.

Indications and Results of Clinical Use

POSTCARDIOTOMY CARDIOGENIC SHOCK. The original indication for VAD support was postcardiotomy cardiogenic shock. One per cent of patients cannot be removed from cardiopulmonary bypass despite maximum medical therapy and IAB counterpulsation.[76,77] These patients are considered potential candidates for VAD insertion. The goal of mechanical circulatory support in this clinical setting is to alter the balance between myocardial oxygen supply and demand to create a milieu that favors myocardial recovery. At the same time, systemic perfusion is maintained. The endpoint in this situation is a return of ventricular function, with the expectation that following a few days of mechanical circulatory support the VAD(s) could be removed.

Reports describing the use of roller pumps to support patients with postcardiotomy ventricular dysfunction are dated and are mentioned primarily out of historical interest. In 1985, Litwak and associates reported the use of roller pump left-atrial-to-aortic-bypass in 27 patients who could not be weaned from cardiopulmonary bypass.[47] Eighteen patients (67 per cent) were separated from the device, and nine patients (33 per cent) were discharged from the hospital. Seven of the nine patients were alive and well at the time of the report, the longest survivor having been observed for more than a decade. Also in 1985, Rose and coworkers described left-atrial-to-aortic bypass in 46 patients with refractory postoperative cardiac failure.[48] Twenty-one patients (46 per cent) were weaned from the device. Five patients died within 90 days of device removal, with two additional deaths occurring 4 months and 4 years postoperatively. Of the 16 long-term survivors, who were observed for 6 to 54 months, 14 had excellent cardiac function, with 13 patients being in NYHA functional Class I or II. These excellent results, reported more than a decade ago, compare favorably with recent reports using more advanced forms of mechanical blood pumps.

The results achieved with centrifugal blood pump support for postcardiotomy cardiogenic shock are summarized in Table 19–5. The Combined Registry for the Clinical Use of Mechanical Ventricular Assist Devices and the Total Artificial Heart was developed in 1988 under the auspices of the International Society for Heart Transplantation and the American Society for Artificial Internal Organs.[5] Investigators from 70 centers worldwide voluntarily submit data to this registry. Although the registry gathers data from patients who receive support with either a centrifugal or pulsatile VAD, only patients who received centrifugal blood pump support are recorded in Table 19–5.

To summarize lessons learned from the use of centrifugal blood pumps in the management of postcardiotomy cardiogenic shock: Approximately 58 per cent of patients require left ventricular assistance alone, 15 per cent require right ventricular assistance alone, and 27 per cent require biventricular assistance.[52,76–79] The duration of support is brief, varying between 1.7 and 3.6 days.[52,76–78] In general, lower survival is associated with biventricular failure,[78] renal failure,[78] and age over 64 years.[76] Registry data show no significant difference in weaning from support or hospital discharge rates between the groups of patients supported with a pneumatic pulsatile device and those supported with a nonpulsatile centrifugal blood pump.[5] The Registry combines data from patients supported with centrifugal and pulsatile blood pumps, but supports the conclusion that advanced age (greater than 70 years) negatively affects patient survival.

Paracorporeal pulsatile VADs are ideally suited to provide circulatory support for patients with postcardiotomy cardiogenic shock, as they are designed to provide either left or right ventricular assistance, and they do not require left ventricular apex cannulation for left heart support. Results achieved with pulsatile blood pump support for postcardiotomy cardiogenic shock are summarized in Table 19–6 and are similar to those achieved with centrifugal blood pumps. Approximately 49 per cent of patients re-

TABLE 19–6 RESULTS OF PULSATILE VAD SUPPORT FOR POSTCARDIOTOMY CARDIOGENIC SHOCK

AUTHOR	DEVICE	NO. PATIENTS	WEANED (%)	SURVIVED (%)
Gray and Champsauer[55]	Abiomed BVS 5000	211	87 (41)	N/A
Guyton[56]	Abiomed BVS 5000	31	17 (55)	9 (29)
Pennington[80]	Thoratec	30	15 (50)	11 (37)
Farrar[81]	Thoratec	123	47 (38)	27 (22)
Registry[5]	Pneumatic	272	117 (43)	57 (21)

VAD = Ventricular assist device.

TABLE 19–7 RESULTS OF VAD SUPPORT AS A BRIDGE TO CARDIAC TRANSPLANTATION

AUTHOR	DEVICE	NO. PATIENTS	TRANSPLANTED (%)	SURVIVED (%)
McBride[83]	Centrifugal	77	56 (73)	36 (47)
Gray and Champsauer[55]	Abiomed BVS 5000	94	66 (70)	39 (41)
Hill[84]	Thoratec	300	187/287 (65)	159/287 (55)
Kormos[85]	Novacor N-100	43	30 (70)	28 (65)
Myers and Macris[60]*	Heartmate 1000 IP	39	21/33 (64)	19/33 (58)
Burton[59]	Heartmate 1000 IP	11	9 (82)	9 (82)

VAD = Ventricular assist device.
* Includes 7 VE LVAS patients.

quire left ventricular assistance alone, 7 per cent require right ventricular assistance alone, and 44 per cent require biventricular assistance.[55,56,80,81] The mean duration of support varied between 3.6 days and 4 days.[55,80] Survival was negatively influenced by presupport cardiac arrest events,[56] myocardial infarction, and renal failure.[80] Although an overall salvage rate of 25 per cent seems low, it must be understood that without mechanical circulatory support patients with refractory postcardiotomy cardiogenic shock would die. More importantly, 82 per cent of Registry patients who survived to hospital discharge were alive at 2 years (including both centrifugal and pulsatile blood pump patients)[5]; 86 per cent of those patients were in NYHA functional Class I or II.

ADJUNCT TO CARDIAC TRANSPLANTATION. With the introduction of cyclosporine-based immunosuppressive regimens and the resurgence of interest in cardiac transplantation in the early 1980's, a second patient population was identified who could potentially benefit from mechanical ventricular assistance. The number of patients with end-stage cardiomyopathy quickly exceeded the number of donor hearts available. The list of approved cardiac transplant candidates grew, and the time a patient spent waiting for a donor heart increased. In 1993, 3775 potential cardiac transplant recipients were listed with the United Network for Organ Sharing (UNOS).[82] During the same year, 730 potential cardiac transplant recipients died while on the UNOS waiting list.[82] Cardiac transplant recipients in whom there is hemodynamic decompensation before availability of a donor heart are potential candidates for VAD implantation. The role of mechanical circulatory support in this clinical setting would be to maintain systemic perfusion and end-organ function until a donor heart was available.[83] The recipient's heart and VAD would be removed at the time of cardiac transplantation.

Results of mechanical blood pump support as a bridge to cardiac transplantation are summarized in Table 19–7. Although the time a cardiac transplant candidate will wait for a suitable donor heart varies with status, blood type, and weight, the average waiting time is a number of months and can be as long as 1 to 2 years. The average duration of support for the series summarized in Table 19–7 varied between 23 and 98 days.[55,59,60,84,85] Pulsatile devices, and in particular implantable VADs, are designed to provide long-term support; 54 per cent of patients who receive support with a pulsatile device survive to hospital discharge following cardiac transplantation.[55,59,60,84,85] Some would question the wisdom of allocating hearts to this critically ill patient population, when the 1-year survival following conventional heart transplantation now exceeds 80 per cent.[86] Interestingly, 87 per cent of patients who receive VAD support, and are successfully transplanted, will survive to hospital discharge.[59,60,84,85] Thereafter, the clinical course of patients requiring interim circulatory support prior to cardiac transplantation parallels the course of patients who undergo conventional cardiac transplantation. All VAD patients are in NYHA functional Class IV at the time of implantation. Following transplantation the majority of patients return to NYHA functional Class I.[58] One- and two-year actuarial survival following transplantation averages 80 to 100 per cent.[60,84,85]

The benefits of an extended period of VAD support are well defined. Patients undergo vigorous nutritional and physical rehabilitation.[87] Exercise tolerance and end-organ dysfunction improve.[88–90] The vented electric version of the ThermoCardiosystems HeartMate has recently entered a clinical trial.[73] Although this device is still intended to serve as a bridge to cardiac transplantation, the protocol was amended to allow patients enrolled in this trial to be discharged from the hospital. The first four patients have been able to manage the system at home without assistance from medical or engineering personnel. Tether-free device function in an outpatient setting represents a dramatic improvement in quality of life[91,92] and health care economics.[3]

Mechanical circulatory support has been employed in two additional subpopulations of patients requiring cardiac transplantation—both following donor heart implantation. According to the Registry, 40 patients have been treated with circulatory support during a rejection episode complicated by hemodynamic compromise.[93] Only 23 patients (58 per cent) underwent a second cardiac transplant. Eight of the 23 patients (35 per cent) were discharged from the hospital. This represents an absolute salvage rate of 20 per cent. Sixty-eight other post-transplant patients suffered from presumed reversible cardiogenic shock unrelated to rejection.[93] VAD support in this patient population resulted in an absolute salvage rate of 19 per cent, statistically *equal* to the survival rate when ventricular assistance was employed in patients with postcardiotomy cardiogenic shock after other types of procedures.

ACUTE MYOCARDIAL INFARCTION. Patients in cardiogenic shock following acute myocardial infarction treated with mechanical circulatory support alone have a mortality rate of 80 per cent, the same as patients treated medically.[94] However, ventricular assistance may stabilize the patient's condition to allow cardiac catheterization and emergent revascularization. Mortality in certain subsets of patients may be reduced to 40 per cent.[94] Poor results with this patient population, however, leave the role for mechanical circulatory support in this clinical setting less well defined.

Complications Associated with VAD Use

Hemorrhage occurs in 27 to 87 per cent of patients who require mechanical ventricular assistance[5,76–78,83,95] and is related to hematologic abnormalities associated with prolonged cardiopulmonary bypass in postcardiotomy cardiogenic shock patients, and to platelet activation and disseminated intravascular coagulation secondary to blood-biomaterial interaction.[96] Stasis of blood within the blood pump and inadequate anticoagulation, however, may lead to thrombus deposition.[97] Thromboembolic complications occur in 9 to 44 per cent of patients,[5,76,78,83] although device-related thromboembolic events in patients supported with the HeartMate occur infrequently.[58,60,61,98] Multisystem organ failure is usually related to preimplantation end-organ hypoperfusion, but may be exacerbated by postimplantation low-flow states. Significant renal and hepatic dysfunction occur in 15 to 47 per cent of patients.[5,76,78,83,95] The degree to which pre-existing end-organ dysfunction is reversible is unknown. Following left VAD insertion, systemic hypoperfusion is most often related to right ventricular failure and inadequate left VAD filling.[99,100] Rapid recognition of profound right ventricular dysfunction and implantation of a right VAD may reduce the incidence of this lethal complication. Infection occurs in 7 to 25 per cent of patients and is attributable to prolonged hospitalization, indwelling lines and catheters, and percutaneous cannulas or drive lines.[5,76,77,83,95,101]

In a group of 965 patients supported with an external VAD for postcardiotomy cardiogenic shock, univariant analysis indicated that bleeding, renal and biventricular failure, systemic arterial desaturation secondary to an unrecognized patent foramen ovale, and inadequate cardiac output were associated with inability to wean a patient from mechanical circulatory support regardless of type of VAD employed.[93] From 27 to 45 per cent of patients who require a VAD as a bridge to cardiac transplantation develop a complication that precludes subsequent heart transplant.[102] Stepwise logistic regression analysis of data gathered from 544 patients who received mechanical circulatory support in conjunction with cardiac transplantation indicated, in decreasing order of importance, that bleeding, neurologic events, and biventricular and renal failure had a significant negative effect on future cardiac transplantation.[93]

Management Considerations

POSTCARDIOTOMY CARDIOGENIC SHOCK. Patients who have preexisting ventricular dysfunction and who are at risk for intractable heart failure following an open heart procedure have a femoral arterial line placed before initiation of cardiopulmonary bypass. The presence of a femoral arterial line facilitates subsequent IAB insertion. Selected patients also undergo a cursory pretransplant evaluation. Of 965 postcardiotomy cardiogenic shock patients reported to the Registry for Mechanical Circulatory Support, 43 patients (4.5 per cent) were activated as potential cardiac transplant recipients when they developed device dependency and had no contraindication to transplant.[5]

Upon completion of the cardiac operation, acid-base balance and electrolyte abnormalities are corrected. A functional cardiac rhythm is restored utilizing temporary cardiac pacing, if necessary. A patient is considered a candidate for VAD insertion when he or she fulfills the hemodynamic criteria outlined in Table 19–1, has no contraindication to VAD insertion as outlined in Table 19–2, and cannot be weaned from cardiopulmonary bypass despite moderate inotropic support[103] and IAB counterpulsation. It is imperative that operative decision-making be performed rapidly, and VAD insertion undertaken expeditiously, to avoid the complications associated with prolonged cardiopulmonary bypass time.[104]

Standard cardiopulmonary bypass cannulas are employed for roller or centrifugal VAD support.[105] Custom-designed cannulas are utilized with pulsatile VADs. For left ventricular assistance, left atrial cannulation is preferred, as myocardium is spared, and decannulation following a return of ventricular function can be performed without cardiopulmonary bypass (see Fig. 19–6). With a left VAD in place, cardiopulmonary bypass is discontinued. Simultaneous monitoring of left and right atrial pressures aids in the distinction among inflow cannula obstruction, hypovolemia, and right ventricular failure, should left VAD filling be less than satisfactory (Table 19–8). Right ventricular failure can be managed with judicious volume loading and intravenous isoproterenol hydrochloride or prostaglandin E_1. Intractable right heart failure mandates insertion of a right VAD. The goal is to achieve a cardiac index >2.2 liters/min/m^2. The IAB may be left in place to impart a degree of pulsatility to nonpulsatile roller or centrifugal left ventricular assistance. To avoid septic complications, however, the IAB is usually withdrawn in the immediate postoperative period.

Postoperatively, abnormal coagulation studies are aggressively corrected with protamine sulfate and blood product administration. When mediastinal tube drainage slows, anticoagulation is effected with continuous intravenous administration of heparin sodium. Sodium warfarin is not usually employed as the time course for ventricular recovery is measured in days. Various weaning protocols have been employed.[47,106] In general, ventricular support is periodically decreased to assess a patient's native ventricular function. This can be accomplished with Swan-Ganz catheter measurements of cardiac output, or observations of wall motion using transesophageal echocardiography,[107] or radionuclide imaging.[108] When ventricular recovery is complete, the patient is returned to the operating room for device explantation. Management is conventional thereafter.

BRIDGE TO CARDIAC TRANSPLANTATION. To be considered for mechanical circulatory support before cardiac transplantation, patients must not only fulfill VAD selection criteria but must also meet cardiac transplant selection and exclusion criteria (Chap. 18). When investigators were bound by clinical trial protocols, VAD implantation was often performed as a salvage procedure on an urgent or emergent basis. In the authors' opinion, prospective transplant recipients whose condition deteriorates to the point where they require an IAB should be considered for VAD insertion in the next 48 to 72 hours. VAD implantation can be accomplished on a semi-elective basis and the patient rehabilitated, rather than endure a prolonged debilitating intensive care unit admission.

Pulsatile devices are most frequently employed in this clinical setting. Implantation techniques are highly specialized, but well documented.[62,69,106] Cardiopulmonary bypass times are often brief, but postoperative bleeding can be troublesome. Consideration should be given to the use of aprotinin.[109] However, sensitization to aprotinin does occur; it may be prudent to use aminocaproic acid at the first operation, reserving aprotinin for VAD explantation and cardiac transplantation. Management of right ventricular failure in the presence of a pulsatile VAD can be problematic. Should a right VAD be necessary, device selection is limited. The versatile Thoratec device can be employed for either right- or left-sided support.[64] If an implantable device is employed on the left, right ventricular support can be provided only with a hybrid pump configuration utilizing a paracorporeal Thoratec VAD or nonpulsatile blood pump.

Postoperatively the patient should be rapidly extubated and all invasive monitoring lines removed as soon as medically allowed, to avoid nosocomial infection.[101] Fastidious cannula–drive line care will delay tract colonization.[110]

TABLE 19–8 HEMODYNAMIC STATUS DURING MECHANICAL LEFT VENTRICULAR ASSISTANCE

CVP (mm Hg)	LAP (mm Hg)	SYSTOLIC AoP (mm Hg)	CI (liters/min/m^2)	DIAGNOSIS
15–20	<15	>90	>2.0	Satisfactory pumping
<15	<15	<90	<2.0	Hypovolemia
15–20	>20	<90	<2.0	Inlet cannula obstruction
>20	<15	<90	<2.0	Right ventricular failure

CVP = Central venous pressure; LAP = left atrial pressure; AoP = aortic pressure; CI = cardiac output index.

Blood transfusions should be minimized and only leukodepleted blood administered. Interval panel reactive antibody determinations will detect the presence of preformed antibodies to human lymphocyte antigens and determine the need for a prospective crossmatch with the cardiac donor. Aggressive nutritional and physical rehabilitation will prepare the patient for the subsequent cardiac transplant.[87,92] It is probably wise to delay cardiac transplantation for 2 to 4 weeks following VAD insertion to allow time for end-organ recovery.[89,90] The VAD is explanted at the time of recipient cardiectomy.

TOTAL ARTIFICIAL HEART

The total artificial heart (TAH) is a biventricular device capable of supporting both the pulmonary and systemic circulations. It is implanted within the patient's pericardium (orthotopic position) in a manner very similar to donor heart implantation at the time of cardiac transplantation. The TAH must be compact and possess a control system capable of balancing the output of the two prosthetic ventricles, while varying cardiac output with physiologic need.

Pneumatic Total Artificial Heart

At least 11 different TAHs have been employed clinically worldwide (Fig. 19–8).[111] All possess similar design characteristics. Each prosthetic ventricle contains a flexible blood sac that is housed in a rigid case. Air pulses, generated by a bedside drive unit, are transmitted through small-diameter percutaneous drive lines and periodically compress the flexible blood sacs. Inlet and outlet valves ensure a unidirectional flow of blood through the prosthetic ventricle. Cardiac output and output balance between the ventricles are achieved with a sophisticated control system. A manual fixed-rate control system functions using the Starling mechanism. The prosthetic ventricles completely empty during systole, but heart rate and diastolic fill time are modified to limit diastolic filling. Any increase in preload results in more complete ventricular filling, a higher stroke volume, and increased cardiac output. An automatic control system employs two negative feedback servomechanisms.[112] The left ventricle pumps a full stroke with each beat, varying the rate to maintain systemic pressure within normal limits. The right ventricular beat rate varies to maintain a left atrial pressure of 5 to 12 mm Hg.

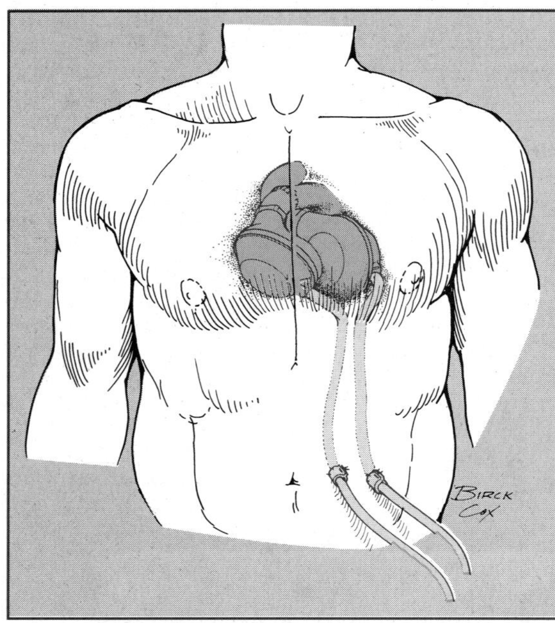

FIGURE 19–8. The pneumatic artificial heart is a biventricular device that is positioned within the patient's pericardium. Small-diameter percutaneous drive lines traverse the skin in the left subcostal region. (From Richenbacher, W. E., Pennock, J. L., Pae, W. E., and Pierce, W. S.: Artificial heart implantation for end-stage cardiac disease. J. Cardiovasc. Surg. *1*:3, 1986.)

TAH implantation is carried out using cardiopulmonary bypass, with bicaval venous and aortic cannulation.[113,114] The patient's heart is excised by transecting the great vessels just distal to the semilunar valves, and the atria along the atrioventricular groove. Prosthetic atrial cuffs are sutured to the atrial remnants. Vascular grafts are anastomosed to the aorta and pulmonary artery. The prosthetic ventricles are attached to the atrial cuffs and outlet grafts with snap-on quick connects or a threaded union nut. The ventricles are de-aired, pumping initiated, and cardiopulmonary bypass discontinued.

The pneumatic TAH has been employed extensively as a mechanical bridge to transplantation. Patient selection criteria are identical to those outlined in the VAD section. The sole exception is patient size. Patients must weigh at least 150 pounds and have an adequate anteroposterior thoracic dimension to avoid atrial compression and inflow obstruction at the time of sternal closure.[115] A recent Registry report includes 189 patients who received TAH support as a bridge to cardiac transplantation[93]: 135 patients (71.4 per cent) underwent transplantation and 67 patients (49.6 per cent) were discharged from the hospital. Transplantation rates were statistically equal regardless of whether the patient was supported with a right or left VAD, two VADs, or the TAH.[93] However, there was a highly statistically significant difference in outcome, with the best outcome obtained with univentricular support and least favorable outcome with the TAH. The only pneumatic TAH still employed as a bridge to transplantation under an investigational device exemption in the United States is the CardioWest (Jarvik) Artificial Heart (CardioWest, Tucson, AZ).[116] Between January 1990 and December 1994, the CardioWest TAH was implanted in 49 patients.[116] Follow-up was available in 46 patients, 17 (37 per cent) of whom were long-term survivors following cardiac transplantation.

Of historical interest, four patients received the Jarvik-7-100 TAH under an FDA-approved protocol, as a permanent form of circulatory replacement.[117] The longest-term survivor lived for 620 days, and all four patients succumbed to hematological, thromboembolic, and infectious complications. Currently, infectious complications secondary to percutaneous drive lines, and life style issues related to the requisite bulky external drive unit, preclude the use of pneumatic TAHs as a permanent form of circulatory support. Although the TAH can provide safe and effective hemodynamic support to a patient before transplant, the TAH is more expensive and technically more difficult to implant than a VAD. Furthermore, univentricular support will suffice in the majority of patients who require a mechanical bridge to cardiac transplantation. In the authors' opinion, transplant recipients in whom there is hemodynamic decompensation prior to cardiac transplantation are best served by VAD insertion. The TAH, if available, should be reserved for selected patients with a postinfarction ventricular septal defect, valvular heart disease, or intractable arrhythmias.

Electric Total Artificial Heart

When available for clinical use, the electric TAH will serve as a readily available cardiac replacement for patients with irreparable acute or chronic heart failure. The electric TAH is being designed for permanent use and, as such, will be completely implantable. Size constraints represent the most significant hurdle to device development. Two blood pumps are located within the pericardium, and un-

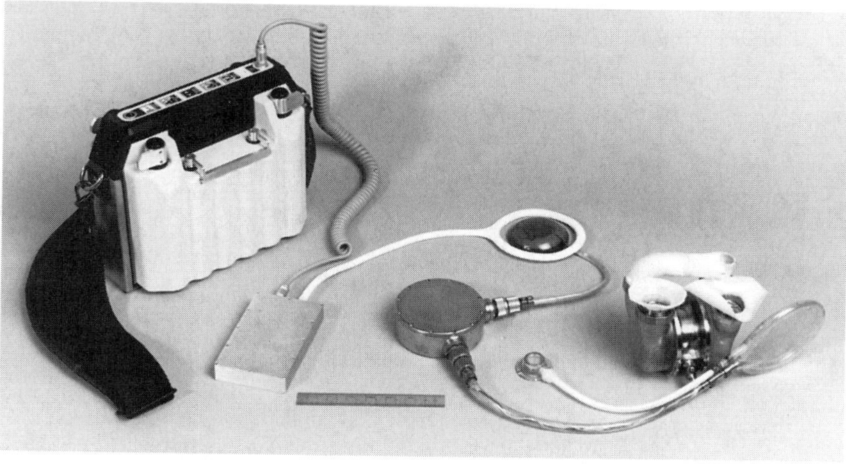

FIGURE 19–9. The electric motor-driven artificial heart being developed at Pennsylvania State University. Components from *left* to *right*: portable external electronics and battery pack with superficial primary transcutaneous energy transmission coil *(white ring)*, circular can containing control electronics and back-up battery connected to the subcutaneous secondary transcutaneous energy transmission coil (beneath the white primary coil), subcutaneous access port, artificial heart containing two prosthetic ventricles, and interposed energy converter, compliance chamber.

like the pneumatic TAH that employs a separate external drive unit for each ventricle, the electric TAH uses a single implantable energy converter to drive both ventricles, greatly increasing the complexity of device control. The electric TAH has a minimum energy requirement of 14 watts. Implantable batteries cannot provide the power required. Thus, currently available electric TAHs will rely on an external power source and transcutaneous energy transmission, with a small rechargeable implantable back-up battery capable of serving as a power source for 30 to 60 minutes. In the future, higher-energy density batteries may reduce or eliminate the need for a primary external power source altogether.[118,119]

Three research teams consisting of both a medical and industrial partner are currently developing an electric TAH under a contract program established by the National Heart, Lung, and Blood Institute in 1988.[120] The Abiomed/Texas Heart Institute TAH (Abiomed, Inc., Danvers, MA) is an electrohydraulically actuated device capable of providing cardiac output in excess of 10 liters/min.[121] An atrial flow balancing chamber is used to control the left-right blood flow balance.[122] Animal implantation has begun only recently, with survival exceeding 3 months.[123]

The Cleveland Clinic Foundation/Nimbus TAH (Nimbus, Inc., Rancho Cordova, CA) employs an electrohydraulic energy converter[124] and biolized blood contacting surface.[125] The device has been implanted in 12 calves for up to 120 days.[125] Two embolic events were attributed to fungal infections in the outlet grafts, while the gelatin-coated pump surfaces were clean despite nonuse of anticoagulants or antiplatelet agents postoperatively.

The Pennsylvania State University/Sarns (Sarns/3M Health Care, Ann Arbor, MI) TAH employs a dual pusher plate roller screw energy converter (Fig. 19–9).[126] Left-right output balance is achieved with an implanted control algorithm that adjusts the left-pump diastolic fill time and speed of systole, to just barely allow complete left pump filling while maximizing pump rate.[112] The device, in its current design, has been implanted in 14 calves with survival times exceeding 3 months.[126] The investigators are prepared to embark on long-term device durability testing using a mock circulatory loop.[127] At the current rate of development, the electric TAH is expected to enter a clinical trial within the next 5 to 10 years.

Acknowledgment

The authors gratefully acknowledge the assistance of Phyllis B. Jones in the preparation of this manuscript.

REFERENCES

1. Gillum, R. F.: Epidemiology of heart failure in the United States. Am. Heart J. *126*:1042, 1993.
2. Ho, K. K. L., Anderson, K. M., Kannel, W. B., et al.: Survival after the onset of congestive heart failure in Framingham Heart Study subjects. Circulation *88*:107, 1993.
3. Poirier, V.: The economic burden of artificial hearts. *In* Nosé, Y., Kjellstrand, C., and Ivanovich, P. (eds.): Progress in Artificial Organs—1985. Cleveland, ISAO Press, 1986, p. 96.
4. Frazier, O. H.: Ventricular assistance: A perspective on the future. Heart Failure *10*:259, 1995.
5. Pae, W. E., Jr., Miller, C. A., Matthews, Y., and Pierce, W. S.: Ventricular assist devices for postcardiotomy cardiogenic shock. J. Thorac. Cardiovasc. Surg. *104*:541, 1992.
6. Clauss, R. H., Birtwell, W. C., Albertal, G., et al.: Assisted circulation: I. The arterial counterpulsator. J. Thorac. Cardiovasc. Surg. *41*:447, 1961.
7. Moulopoulos, S. D., Topaz, S., and Kolff, W. J.: Diastolic balloon pumping (with carbon dioxide) in the aorta—A mechanical assistance to the failing circulation. Am. Heart J. *63*:669, 1992.
8. Kantrowitz, A., Tjonneland, S., Freed, P. S., et al.: Initial clinical experience with intraaortic balloon pumping in cardiogenic shock. JAMA *203*:135, 1968.
9. Bregman, D., and Casarella, W. J.: Percutaneous intraaortic balloon pumping: Initial clinical experience. Ann. Thorac. Surg. *29*:153, 1980.
10. U.S.A. Market for Diagnostic and Interventional Catheters and Allied Vascular Devices. D & MD Reports. Southborough, International Business Communications, Inc., 1994, Exhibit #6–16, pp. 6–48.
11. Gibbon, J. H., Jr.: Application of a mechanical heart and lung apparatus to cardiac surgery. Minn. Med. *37*:171, 1954.
12. Dennis, C., Carlens, E., Senning, A., et al.: Clinical use of a cannula for left heart bypass without thoracotomy: Experimental protection against fibrillation by left heart bypass. Ann. Surg. *156*:623, 1962.
13. DeBakey, M. E.: Left ventricular bypass pump for cardiac assistance. Clinical experience. Am. J. Cardiol. *27*:3, 1971.
14. Pierce, W. S., Parr, G. V. S., Myers, J. L., et al.: Ventricular-assist pumping in patients with cardiogenic shock after cardiac operations. N. Engl. J. Med. *305*:1606, 1981.
15. Normal, J. C., Cooley, D. A., Kahan, B. D., et al.: Total support of the circulation of a patient with post-cardiotomy stone-heart syndrome by a partial artificial heart (ALVAD) for 5 days followed by heart and kidney transplantation. Lancet *1*:1125, 1978.
16. Reedy, J. E., Pennington, D. G., Miller, L. W., et al.: Status I heart transplant patients: Conventional versus ventricular assist device support. J. Heart Lung Transplant. *11*:246, 1992.
17. Akutsu, T., and Kolff, W. J.: Permanent substitutes for valves and hearts. Trans. Am. Soc. Artif. Intern. Organs *4*:230, 1958.
18. Nosé Y., Topaz, S., SenGupta, A., et al.: Artificial hearts inside the pericardial sac in calves. Trans. Am. Soc. Artif. Intern. Organs. *11*:255, 1965.
19. Klain, M., Mrava, G. L., Tajima, K., et al.: Can we achieve over 100 hours' survival with a total mechanical heart? Trans. Am. Soc. Artif. Intern. Organ. *17*:437, 1971.
20. Cooley, D. A., Liotta, D., Hallman, G. L., et al.: Orthotopic cardiac prosthesis for two-staged cardiac replacement. Am. J. Cardiol. *24*:723, 1969.
21. Joyce, L. D., DeBries, W. C., Hastings, W. L., et al.: Response of the human body to the first permanent implant of the Jarvik-7 total artificial heart. Trans. Am. Soc. Artif. Intern. Organs *29*:81, 1983.

INTRAAORTIC BALLOON COUNTERPULSATION

22. Pae, W. E., Jr., and Pierce, W. S.: Intra-aortic balloon counterpulsation, ventricular assist pumping, and the artificial heart. *In* Baue, A. E., Geha, A. S., Hammond, G. L., et al. (eds.): Glenn's Thoracic and Cardiovascular Surgery. East Norwalk, Conn., Appleton and Lange, 1991, p. 1585.
23. Allen, B. S., Rosenkranz, E., Buckberg, G. D., et al.: Studies on prolonged acute regional ischemia: VI. Myocardial infarction with left ventricular power failure: A medical/surgical emergency requiring urgent revascularization with maximal protection of remote muscle. J. Thorac. Cardiovasc. Surg. *98*:691, 1989.

24. Komeda, M., Fremes, S. E., and David, T. E.: Surgical repair of postinfarction ventricular septal defect. Circulation *82:*IV-243, 1990.
25. Tepe, N. A., and Edmunds, L. H., Jr.: Operation for acute postinfarction mitral insufficiency and cardiogenic shock. J. Thorac. Cardiovasc. Surg. *89:*525, 1985.
26. Naunheim, K. S., Swartz, M. T., Pennington, D. G., et al.: Intraaortic balloon pumping in patients requiring cardiac operations. Risk analysis and long-term follow-up. J. Thorac. Cardiovasc. Surg. *104:*1654, 1992.
27. Peric, M., Frazier, O. H., Macris, M., and Radovancevic, B.: Intra-aortic balloon pump as a bridge to transplantation. J. Heart Transplant. *5:*380, 1986.
28. Birovljev, S., Radovancevic, B., Burnett, C. M., et al.: Heart transplantation after mechanical circulatory support: Four years' experience. J. Heart Lung Transplant. *11:*240, 1992.
29. Levine, F. H., Gold, H. K., Leinbach, R. C., et al.: Management of acute myocardial ischemia with intraaortic balloon pumping and coronary bypass surgery. Circulation *58:*(suppl. I):69, 1978.
30. Bardet, J., Rigaud, M., Kahn, J. C., et al.: Treatment of post-myocardial infarction angina by intra-aortic balloon pumping and emergency revascularization. J. Thorac. Cardiovasc. Surg. *74:*299, 1977.
31. Hanson, E. C., Levine, F. H., Kay, H. R., et al.: Control of postinfarction ventricular irritability with the intraaortic balloon pump. Circulation *62:*(Suppl. I):130, 1980.
32. Bregman, D., and Kaskel, P.: Advances in percutaneous intra-aortic balloon pumping. Crit. Care Clin. *2:*221, 1986.
33. McGeehin, W., Sheikh, F., Donahoo, J. S., et al.: Transthoracic intraaortic balloon pump support: Experience in 39 patients. Ann. Thorac. Surg. *44:*26, 1987.
34. Rubenstein, R. B., and Karhade, N.V.: Supraclavicular subclavian technique of intra-aortic balloon insertion. J. Vasc. Surg. *1:*577, 1984.
35. Buchanan, S. A., Langenburg, S. E., Mauney, M. C., et al.: Ambulatory intraaortic balloon counterpulsation. Ann. Thorac. Surg. *58:*1547, 1994.
36. Krause, A. H., Jr., Bigelow, J. C., and Page, U. S.: Transthoracic intraaortic balloon cannulation to avoid repeat sternotomy for removal. Ann. Thorac. Surg. *21:*562, 1976.
37. Richenbacher, W. E., and Pierce, W. S.: Management of complications of intraaortic balloon counterpulsation. *In* Waldhausen, J. A., and Orringer, M. B. (eds.): Complications in Cardiothoracic Surgery. St. Louis, Mosby-Year Book, Inc., 1991, p. 97.
38. Iverson, L. I. G., Herfindahl, G., Ecker, R. R., et al.: Vascular complications of intraaortic balloon counterpulsation. Am. J. Surg. *154:*99, 1987.
39. Gottlieb, S. O., Brinker, J. A., Borkon, A. M., et al.: Identification of patients at high risk for complications of intraoartic balloon counterpulsation: A multivariate risk factor analysis. Am. J. Cardiol. *53:*1135, 1984.
40. Shahian, D. M., Neptune, W. B., Ellis, F. H., Jr., and Maggs, P. R.: Intraaortic balloon pump morbidity: A comparative analysis of risk factors between percutaneous and surgical techniques. Ann. Thorac. Surg. *36:*644, 1983.
41. Gol, M. K., Bayazit, M., Emir, M., et al.: Vascular complications related to percutaneous insertion of intraaortic balloon pumps. Ann. Thorac. Surg. *58:*1476, 1994.
42. Friedell, M. L., Alpert, J., Parsonnet, V., et al.: Femorofemoral grafts for lower limb ischemia caused by intra-aortic balloon pump. J. Vasc. Surg. *5:*180, 1987.

THE VENTRICULAR ASSIST DEVICE

43. Lohmann, D. P., Swartz, M. T., Pennington, D. G., et al.: Left ventricular versus left atrial cannulation for the Thoratec ventricular assist device. Trans. Am. Soc. Artif. Intern. Organs *36:*M545, 1990.
44. Cohen, D. J., Kress, D. C., Swanson, D. K., et al.: Effect of cannulation site on the primary determinants of myocardial oxygen consumption during left heart bypass. J. Surg. Res. *47:*159, 1989.
45. Rahmoeller, G. A.: FDA requirements for clinical approval of left ventricular assist devices. *In* Attar, S. (ed.): New Developments in Cardiac Assist Devices. New York, Praeger Publishers, 1985, p. 36.
46. Kessler, D. A.: Hastings lecture, December 10, 1993, Rockville, Maryland, USA. Artif. Organs *18:*718, 1994.
47. Litwak, R. S., Koffsky, R. M., Jurado, R. A., et al.: A decade of experience with a left heart assist device in patients undergoing open intracardiac operation. World J. Surg. *9:*18, 1985.
48. Rose, D. M., Laschinger, J., Grossi, E., et al.: Experimental and clinical results with a simplified left heart assist device for treatment of profound left ventricular dysfunction. World J. Surg. *9:*11, 1985.
49. Oku, T., Harasaki, H., Smith, W., and Nosé, Y.: Hemolysis: A comparative study of four nonpulsatile pumps. Trans. Am. Soc. Artif. Intern. Organs *34:*500, 1988.
50. Noon, G. P., Kane, L. E., Feldman, L., et al.: Reduction of blood trauma in roller pumps for long-term perfusion. World J. Surg. *9:*65, 1985.
51. Magovern, G. J., Jr.: The Biopump and postoperative circulatory support. Ann. Thorac. Surg. *55:*245, 1993.
52. Curtis, J. J.: Centrifugal mechanical assist for postcardiotomy ventricular failure. Semin. Thorac. Cardiovasc. Surg. *6:*140, 1994.
53. Nishinaka, T., Nishida, H., Endo, M., and Koyanagi, H.: Less platelet damage in the curved vane centrifugal pump: A comparative study with the roller pump in open heart surgery. Artif. Organs *18:*687, 1994.
54. Morin, B. J., and Riley, J. B.: Thrombus formation in centrifugal pumps. J. Extra-Corporeal Technol. *24:*20, 1992.
55. Gray, L. A., Jr., and Champsaur, G. G.: The BVS 5000 biventricular assist device. The worldwide registry experience. ASAIO H *40:*M460, 1994.
56. Guyton, R. A., Schonberger, J. P. A. M., Everts, P. A. M., et al.: Postcardiotomy shock: Clinical evaluation of the BVS 5000 biventricular support system. Ann. Thorac. Surg. *56:*346, 1993.
57. Shook, B. J.: The Abiomed BVS 5000 biventricular support system. System description and clinical summary. Cardiac Surgery: State of the Art Reviews *7:*309, 1993.
58. Frazier, O. H., Rose, E. A., Macmanus, Q., et al.: Multicenter clinical evaluation of the HeartMate 1000 IP left ventricular assist device. Ann. Thorac. Surg. *53:*1080, 1992.
59. Burton, N. A., Lefrak, E. A., Macmanus, Q., et al.: A reliable bridge to cardiac transplantation: The TCI left ventricular assist device. Ann. Thorac. Surg. *55:*1425, 1993.
60. Myers, T. J., and Macris, M. P.: Clinical experience with the HeartMate left ventricular assist device. Heart Failure *10:*247, 1995.
61. Rose, E. A., Levin, H. R., Oz, M. C., et al.: Artificial circulatory support with textured interior surfaces. A counterintuitive approach to minimizing thromboembolism. Circulation *90:*II-87, 1994.
62. McCarthy, P. M., Wang, N., and Vargo, R.: Preperitoneal insertion of the HeartMate 1000 IP implantable left ventricular assist device. Ann. Thorac. Surg. *57:*634, 1994.
63. Farrar, D. J., Lawson, J. H., Litwak, P., and Cedarwall, G.: Thoratec VAD system as a bridge to heart transplantation. J. Heart Transplant. *9:*415, 1990.
64. Farrar, D. J., and Hill, J. D.: Univentricular and biventricular Thoratec VAD support as a bridge to transplantation. Ann. Thorac. Surg. *55:*276, 1993.
65. Holman, W. L., Bourge, R. C., McGiffin, D. C., and Kirklin, J. K.: Ventricular assist: Experience with a pulsatile heterotopic device. Semin. Thorac. Cardiovasc. Surg. 6:147, 1994.
66. Weiss, W. J., Rosenberg, G., Snyder, A. J., et al.: In vivo performance of a transcutaneous energy transmission system with the Penn State motor driven ventricular assist device. Trans. Am. Soc. Artif. Intern. Organs *35:*284, 1989.
67. Wisman, C. B., Rosenberg, G., Weiss, W. J., et al.: Development and successful application of an intrathoracic compliance chamber for the implantable electric motor-driven ventricular-assist pump. Surg. Forum *34:*253, 1983.
68. Starnes, V. A., Oyer, P. E., Portner, P. M., et al.: Isolated left ventricular assist as bridge to cardiac transplantation. J. Thorac. Cardiovasc. Surg. *96:*62, 1988.
69. Pennington, D. G., McBride, L. R., and Swartz, M. T.: Implantation technique for the Novacor left ventricular assist system. J. Thorac. Cardiovasc. Surg. *108:*604, 1994.
70. Loisance, D. Y., Deleuze, P. H., Mazzucotelli, J. P., et al.: Clinical implantation of the wearable Baxter Novacor ventricular assist system. Ann. Thorac. Surg. *58:*551, 1994.
71. Miller, P. J., Billich, T. J., LaForge, D. H., et al.: Initial clinical experience with a wearable controller for the Novacor left ventricular assist system. ASAIO J. 40:M465, 1994.
72. Frazier, O. H.: Chronic left ventricular support with a vented electric assist device. Ann. Thorac. Surg. *55:*273, 1993.
73. Myers, T. J., Dasse, K. A., Macris, M. P., et al.: Use of a left ventricular assist device in an outpatient setting. ASAIO J. 40:M471, 1994.
74. Pierce, W. S., Snyder, A. J., Rosenberg, G., et al.: A long-term ventricular assist system. J. Thorac. Cardiovasc. Surg. *105:*520, 1993.
75. Weiss, W. J., Rosenberg, G., Snyder, A., et al.: Results of in vivo testing of a completely implanted ventricular assist device. Proceedings, Cardiovascular Science and Technology Conference. Arlington, Association for the Advancement of Medical Instrumentation, 1993, p. 154.
76. Killen, D. A., Piehler, J. M., Borkon, A. M., and Reed, W. A.: Bio-Medicus ventricular assist device for salvage of cardiac surgical patients. Ann. Thorac. Surg. *52:*230, 1991.
77. Lee, W. A., Gillinov, A. M., Cameron, D. E., et al.: Centrifugal ventricular assist device for support of the failing heart after cardiac surgery. Crit. Care Med. *21:*1186, 1993.
78. Golding, L. A. R., Crouch, R. D., Stewart, R. W., et al.: Postcardiotomy centrifugal mechanical ventricular support. Ann. Thorac. Surg. *54:*1059, 1992.
79. Noon, G. P.: Bio-Medicus ventricular assistance. Ann. Thorac. Surg. *52:*180, 1991.
80. Pennington, D. G., McBride, L. W., Swartz, M. T., et al.: Use of the Pierce-Donachy ventricular assist device in patients with cardiogenic shock after cardiac operations. Ann. Thorac. Surg. *47:*130, 1989.
81. FDA panel recommends approval. Thoratec's Heartbeat *8.3:*6, 1994.
82. United Network for Organ Sharing: Personal communication. 1995.
83. McBride, L. R.: Bridging to cardiac transplantation with external ventricular assist devices. Semin. Thorac. Cardiovasc. Surg. *6:*169, 1994.
84. Hill, J. D., Farrar, D. J., and Thoratec VAD Principal Investigators: Multicenter clinical results with the Thoratec VAD system as a bridge to cardiac transplant. Proceedings, ASAIO Cardiovascular Science and Technology Conference. Boca Raton, The American Society for Artificial Internal Organs, 1994, p. 41.
85. Kormos, R. L., Pham, S. M., Hattler, B. G., and Griffith, B. P.: Evolution of bridge to cardiac transplantation from intermediate inpatient use to chronic outpatient care. Proceedings, ASAIO Cardiovascular Science and Technology Conference. Boca Raton, The American Society for Artificial Internal Organs, 1994, p. 41.
86. United Network for Organ Sharing. 1994 center specific report: Heart data. Overall survival rates. UNOS Update *11:*24, 1995.

87. Vega, J. D., Poindexter, S. M., Radovancevic, B., et al.: Nutritional assessment of patients with extended left ventricular assist device support. Trans. Am. Soc. Artif. Intern. Organs *36*:M555, 1990.
88. Levin, H. R., Chen, J. M., Oz, M. C., et al.: Potential of left ventricular assist devices as outpatient therapy while awaiting transplantation. Ann. Thorac. Surg. *58*:1515, 1994.
89. Farrar, D. J., and Hill, J. D.: Recovery of major organ function in patients awaiting heart transplantation with Thoratec ventricular assist devices. J. Heart Lung Transplant. *13*:1125, 1994.
90. Burnett, C. M., Duncan, J. M., Frazier, O. H., et al.: Improved multiorgan function after prolonged univentricular support. Ann. Thorac. Surg. *55*:65, 1993.
91. Dew, M. A., Kormos, R. L., Roth, L. H., et al.: Life quality in the era of bridging to cardiac transplantation. Bridge patients in an outpatient setting. ASAIO J. *39*:145, 1993.
92. Kormos, R. L., Murali, S., Dew, M. A., et al.: Chronic mechanical circulatory support: Rehabilitation, low morbidity, and superior survival. Ann. Thorac. Surg. *57*:51, 1994.
93. Pae, W. E., Jr.: Ventricular assist devices and total artificial hearts: A combined registry experience. Ann. Thorac. Surg. *55*:295, 1993.
94. Moritz, A., and Wolner, E.: Circulatory support with shock due to acute myocardial infarction. Ann. Thorac. Surg. *55*:238, 1993.
95. Oaks, T. E., Pae, W. E., Jr., Miller, C. A., and Pierce, W. S.: Combined registry for the clinical use of mechanical ventricular assist pumps and the total artificial heart in conjunction with heart transplantation. Fifth official report—1990. J. Heart Lung Transplant. *10*:621, 1991.
96. Bick, R. L.: Hemostasis defects associated with cardiac surgery, prosthetic devices, and other extracorporeal circuits. Semin. Thromb. Hemostas. *11*:249, 1985.
97. Copeland, J. G., III, Frazier, O. H., McBride, L. R., et al.: Panel II. Anticoagulation. Ann. Thorac. Surg. *55*:213, 1993.
98. McCarthy, P. M., James, K. B., Savage, R. M., et al.: Implantable left ventricular assist device. Approaching an alternative for end-stage heart failure. Circulation *90*(Suppl. II):83, 1994.
99. Fukuda, S., Takano, H., Taenaka, Y., et al.: Chronic effect of left ventricular assist pumping on right ventricular function. Trans. Am. Soc. Artif. Intern. Organs *34*:712, 1988.
100. Elbeery, J. R., Owen, C. H., Savitt, M. A., et al.: Effects of the left ventricular assist device on right ventricular function. J. Thorac. Cardiovasc. Surg. *99*:809, 1990.
101. Hill, J. D., Griffith, B. P., Meli, M., and Didisheim, P.: Panel III. Infections-prophylaxis and treatment. Ann. Thorac. Surg. *55*:217, 1993.
102. Richenbacher, W. E., and Pierce, W. S.: Management of complications of mechanical circulatory assistance. *In* Waldhausen, J. A., and Orringer, M. B. (eds.): Complications in Cardiothoracic Surgery. St. Louis, Mosby-Year Book, Inc., 1991, p. 103.
103. Emery, R. W., and Joyce, L. D.: Directions in cardiac assistance. J. Card. Surg. *6*:400, 1991.
104. Anstadt, M. P., Tedder, M., Hegde, S. S., et al.: Intraoperative timing may provide criteria for use of post-cardiotomy ventricular assist devices. ASAIO J. *38*:M147, 1992.
105. Magovern, G. J., Jr., Wampler, R. W., Joyce, L. D., and Wareing, T. H.: Nonpulsatile circulatory support: Techniques of insertion. Ann. Thorac. Surg. *55*:266, 1993.
106. Aufiero, T. X., and Pae, W. E., Jr.: Extracorporeal pneumatic ventricular assistance for postcardiotomy cardiogenic shock. Cardiac Surgery: State of the Art Reviews *7*:277, 1993.
107. Barzilai, B., Davila-Roman, V. G., Eaton, M. H., et al.: Transesophageal echocardiography predicts successful withdrawal of ventricular assist devices. J. Thorac. Cardiovasc. Surg. *104*:1410, 1992.
108. Sekela, M. E., Verani, M. S., and Noon, G. P.: Comparison of hemodynamics and ejection fraction during left heart bypass. Ann. Thorac. Surg. *51*:804, 1991.
109. Pae, W. E., Jr., Aufiero, T. X., Weldner, P. W., et al.: Aprotinin therapy for insertion of ventricular assist devices for staged heart transplantation. J. Heart Lung Transplant. *13*:811, 1994.
110. Hravnak, M., George, E., and Kormos, R. L.: Management of chronic left ventricular assist device percutaneous lead insertion sites. J. Heart Lung Transplant. *12*:856, 1993.

THE ARTIFICIAL HEART

111. Johnson, K. E., Prieto, M., Joyce, L. D., et al.: World experience with total artificial heart (TAH) implantation: A registry report. *In* Cardiovascular Science and Technology: Basic and Applied, II. Boston, Oxymoron Press, 1990, p. 32.
112. Snyder, A. J., Rosenberg, G., and Pierce, W. S.: Noninvasive control of cardiac output for alternately ejecting dual-pusherplate pumps. Artif. Organs *16*:189, 1992.
113. Richenbacher, W. E., Pennock J. L., Pae, W. E., Jr., and Pierce, W. S.: Artificial heart implantation for end-stage cardiac disease. J. Card. Surg. *1*:3, 1986.
114. DeVries, W. C.: Surgical technique for implantation of the Jarvik-7-100 total artificial heart. JAMA *259*:875, 1988.
115. Jarvik, R. K., DeVries, W. C., Semb, B. K. H., et al.: Surgical positioning of the Jarvik-7 artificial heart. J. Heart Transplant. *5*:184, 1986.
116. Arabia, F. A., Rosado, L. J., Sethi, G. K., et al.: CardioWest (Jarvik) artificial heart. Proceedings, ASAIO Cardiovascular Science and Technology Conference. Boca Raton, The American Society for Artificial Internal Organs, 1994, p. 42.
117. DeVries, W. C.: The permanent artificial heart. Four case reports. JAMA *259*:849, 1988.
118. Eisenberg, M.: High energy nickel-zinc batteries for LVAD applications. *In* Cardiovascular Science and Technology: Basic and Applied, II. Boston, Oxymoron Press, 1990, p. 273.
119. MacLean, G. K., Aiken, P. A., Adams, W. A., and Mussivand, T.: Comparison of rechargeable lithium and nickel/cadmium battery cells for implantable circulatory support devices. Artif. Organs *18*:331, 1994.
120. Sapirstein, J. S., Pae, W. E., Jr., Rosenberg, G., and Pierce, W. S.: The development of permanent circulatory support systems. Semin. Thorac. Cardiovasc. Surg. *6*:188, 1994.
121. Parnis, S. M., Yu, L. S., Ochs, B. D., et al.: Chronic in vivo evaluation of an electrohydraulic total artificial heart. ASAIO J. *40*:M489, 1994.
122. Kung, R. T. V., Yu, L. S., Ochs, B., et al.: An atrial hydraulic shunt in a total artificial heart. A balance mechanism for the bronchial shunt. ASAIO J. *39*:M213, 1993.
123. Kung, R. T. V., Yu, L. S., Ochs, B. D., et al.: Progress in the Abiomed total artificial heart. Proceedings, ASAIO Cardiovascular Science and Technology Conference. Boca Raton, The American Society for Artificial Internal Organs, 1994, p. 38.
124. Massiello, A., Kiraly, R., Butler, K., et al.: The Cleveland Clinic–Nimbus total artificial heart. Design and in vitro function. J. Thorac. Cardiovasc. Surg. *108*:412, 1994.
125. Harasaki, H., Fukamachi, K., Massiello, A., et al.: Progress in Cleveland Clinic–Nimbus total artificial heart development. ASAIO J. *40*:M494, 1994.
126. Snyder, A. J., Rosenberg, G., Weiss, W. J., et al. In vivo testing of a completely implanted total artificial heart system. ASAIO J. *39*:M177, 1993.
127. Weiss, W. J., Rosenberg, G., Snyder, A. J., et al.: Design improvements to the completely implantable Penn State total artificial heart. Proceedings, ASAIO Cardiovascular Science and Technology Conference. Boca Raton, The American Society for Artificial Organs, 1994, p. 38.

Chapter 20

Genesis of Cardiac Arrhythmias: Electrophysiological Considerations

DOUGLAS P. ZIPES

ANATOMY OF THE CARDIAC CONDUCTION SYSTEM

Sinus Node

In humans, the sinus node is a spindle-shaped structure composed of a fibrous tissue matrix with closely packed cells. It is 10 to 20 mm long, 2 to 3 mm wide, and thick, tending to narrow caudally toward the inferior vena cava. It lies less than 1 mm from the epicardial surface, laterally in the right atrial sulcus terminalis, at the junction of the superior vena cava and right atrium (Figs. 20–1 and 20–2). The artery supplying the sinus node branches from the right (55 to 60 per cent of the time) or the left circumflex (40 to 45 per cent) coronary artery, approaching the node from a clockwise or counterclockwise direction around the superior vena caval–right atrial junction.

CELLULAR STRUCTURE. Cell types in the sinus node include nodal cells, transitional cells, and atrial muscle cells. *Nodal cells,* also called "P cells," thought to be the source of normal impulse formation, are small (5 to 10 μm), ovoid, primitive-appearing cells with relatively few organelles, mitochondria, and myofibrils. They are grouped in elongated clusters located centrally in the sinus node. No transverse tubular system exists. Contact between nodal cells appears to occur via nexus connections.

TRANSITIONAL CELLS. Also known as "T cells," these are elongated cells intermediate in size and complexity between nodal cells and atrial muscle cells. T cells near nodal cells have simple intercellular connections, while more fully developed intercalated discs exist between T cells and atrial myocardium. Since nodal cells make contact only with each other or T cells, the latter may provide the only functional pathway for distribution of the sinus impulse formed in the nodal cells to the rest of the atrial myocardium.

ATRIAL MYOCARDIAL CELLS. These cells extend as peninsulas into the nodal boundaries, with overlapping zones of sinus and atrial cells most prominent on the nodal surface that abuts the crista terminalis.

GAP JUNCTIONS. Gap junctional channels (see p. 555) formed by connexin 45, 43, and 40, depending on the species and tissue type, electrically couple sinus node cells and probably account for their synchronized electrical activity.[1–3] Relative paucity and small size of gap junctions may account for slow conduction in the sinus node.[3] Few gap junctions may be required for frequency entrainment.[4] Although most gap junctions contain connexin 40, 43, and 45, the sinus and AV nodes are virtually devoid of connexin 43 but contain connexin 40 and connexin 45.[5–7] Abnormalities can cause arrhythmias.[8]

FUNCTION. Very probably no single cell in the sinus node serves as *the* pacemaker. Rather, sinus nodal cells function as electrically coupled oscillators, discharging synchronously because of mutual entrainment. Thus, faster-discharging cells are slowed by cells firing more slowly, while they themselves are sped so that a "democratically derived" discharge rate occurs.[9] In humans, sinus rhythm may result from impulse origin at widely separated sites, creating two or three individual wavefronts that merge to form a single widely disseminated wavefront.[10] Modulated parasystole can occur.[9]

INNERVATION. The sinus node is richly innervated with postganglionic adrenergic and cholinergic nerve terminals.[11–16] Discrete vagal efferent pathways innervate both the sinus and atrioventricular (AV) regions of the dog and nonhuman primate. The concentration of norepinephrine is two to four times higher in atrial than in ventricular tissue in canine and guinea pig hearts. Although the sinus nodal region contains amounts of norepinephrine equivalent to those in other parts of the right atrium, acetylcholine, acetylcholinesterase, and choline acetyltransferase (the enzyme necessary for the synthesis of acetylcholine) have all been found in greatest concentration in the sinus node, with the next highest concentration in the right and then the left atrium. The concentration of acetylcholine in the ventricles is only 20 to 50 per cent of that in the atria.

Vagal stimulation, by releasing acetylcholine, slows sinus nodal discharge rate and prolongs intranodal conduction time, at times to the point of sinus nodal exit block. Acetylcholine increases and norepinephrine decreases refractoriness in the center of the sinus node. Adrenergic stimulation speeds sinus discharge rate. The phase (timing) in the cardiac cycle at which vagal discharge occurs and the background sympathetic tone importantly influence vagal effects on sinus rate and conduction (see below). Negative chronotropic effects of acetylcholine are due to inhibition of the hyperpolarization-activated pacemaker current i_f,[17–21] probably mediated by a G protein (see p. 372). Acetylcholine also activates the muscarinic m_2 receptor in the pacemaker cell, which in turn activates a specific G protein (G_K) that activates the K channel [I_K(Ach)], which also modulates discharge rate.[22] The m_2 receptor also inhibits adenylate cyclase via G_i to antagonize adrenergic effects on the sinus node. After cessation of vagal stimulation, sinus nodal automatically may accelerate transiently (postvagal tachycardia).

Internodal and Intraatrial Conduction

Whether impulses travel from the sinus to the AV node over preferentially conducting pathways has been contested. Anatomical evidence has been interpreted to indicate the presence of three intraatrial pathways. The *anterior internodal pathway* begins at the anterior margin of the sinus node and curves anteriorly around the superior vena cava to enter the anterior interatrial band, called *Bachmann's bundle.* This band continues to the left atrium, with the anterior internodal pathway entering the superior margin of the AV node. *Bachmann's bundle* is a large muscle bundle that appears to conduct the cardiac impulse preferentially from right to left atrium. The *middle interno-*

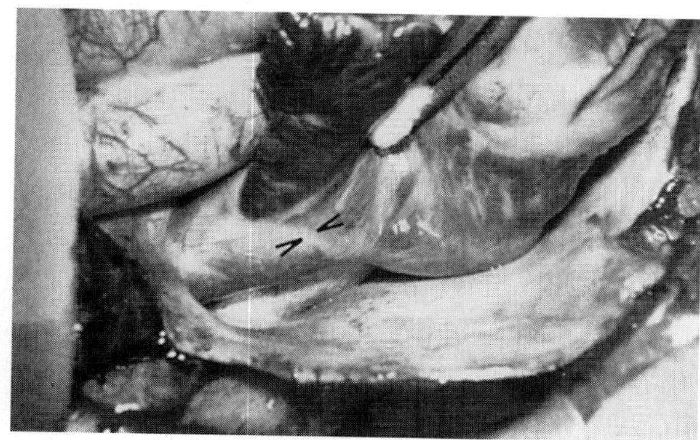

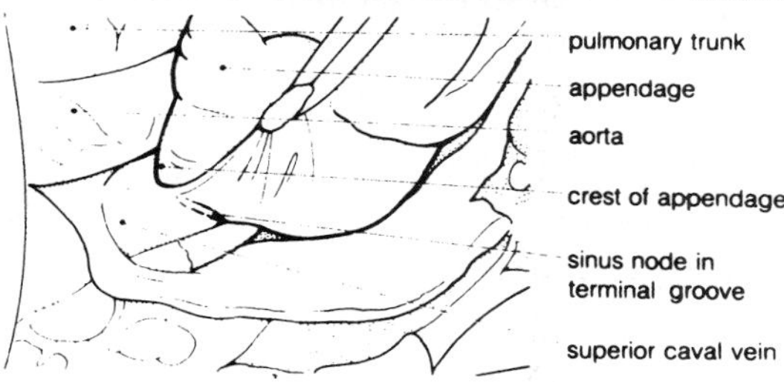

FIGURE 20–1. **The human sinus node. This photograph, taken in the operating room, shows the location of the normal cigar-shaped sinus node along the lateral border of the terminal groove at the superior vena cava–atrial junction (arrowheads). (From Anderson, R. H., Wilcox, B. R., and Becker, A. E.: Anatomy of the normal heart. *In* Hurst, J. W., Anderson, R. H., Becker, A. E., and Wilcox, B. R. [eds.]: Atlas of the Heart. New York, Gower Medical Publishing, 1988, p. 1.2.)**

dal tract begins at the superior and posterior margins of the sinus node and travels behind the superior vena cava to the crest of the interatrial septum, descending in the interatrial septum to the superior margin of the AV node. The *posterior internodal tract* starts at the posterior margin of the sinus node and travels posteriorly around the superior vena cava and along the crista terminalis to the eustachian ridge and then into the interatrial septum above the coronary sinus, joining the posterior portion of the AV node. Some fibers from all three tracts bypass the crest of the AV node and enter its more distal segment. These groups of internodal tissue are best referred to as *internodal atrial myocardium*, not tracts, because they do not appear to be histologically discrete specialized tracts, only plain atrial myocardium.

The basis for specialized tracts stems from finding cell types in the atrium that differ electrophysiologically and anatomically, but it is not clear that these different cells are responsible for more rapid conduction velocity. Also, differential sensitivity of atrial fibers to potassium, giving rise to an apparent sinoventricular rhythm[23] (i.e., impulse propagation from the sinus node to the ventricle without activating atrial myocardium), and activation changes following localized surgical lesions designed to interrupt discrete pathways provide further functional data to support the presence of specialized tracts. However, the *weight of evidence does not support the presence of specialized internodal tracts resembling the bundle branches, i.e., discrete histologically identifiable tracts of tissue.*

Preferential internodal conduction, i.e., more rapid conduction velocity between the nodes in some parts of the atrium compared with other parts, does exist and may be due to fiber orientation, size, geometry, or other factors rather than to specialized tracts located between the nodes. Importantly, the atrial anterosuperior and posteroinferior inputs or approaches to the AV node may be the anatomical substrates comprising the fast and anterograde slow pathways of AV nodal reentry, the upper end of the retrograde fast pathway being located at the apex of Koch's triangle, near the His bundle, and the upper end of the anterograde pathway being located near the coronary sinus os.[24–26]

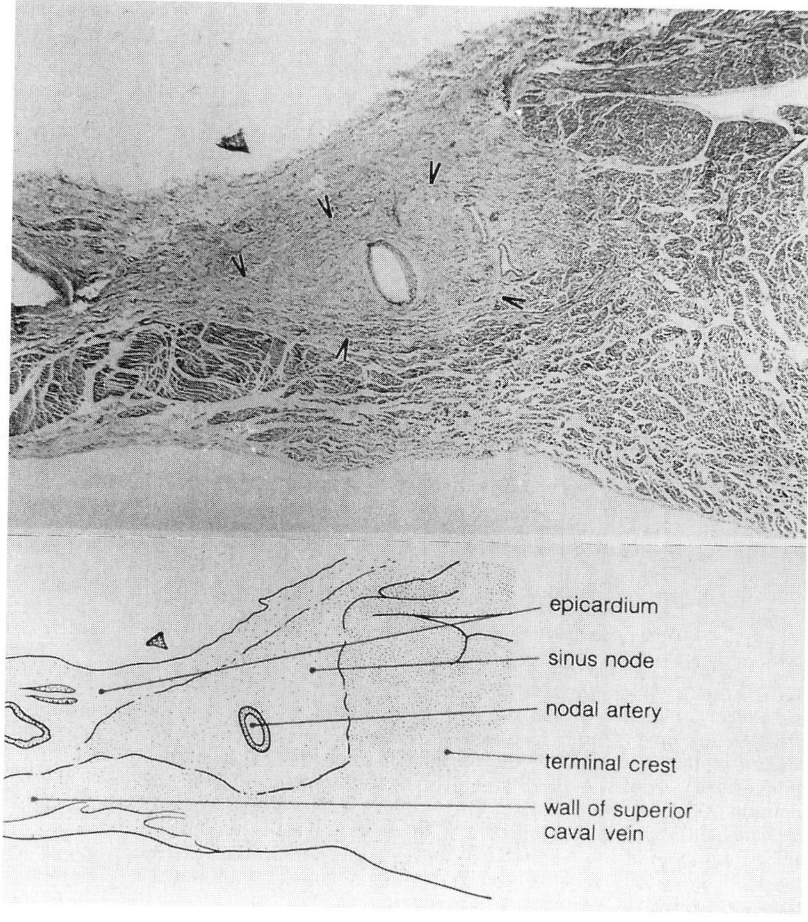

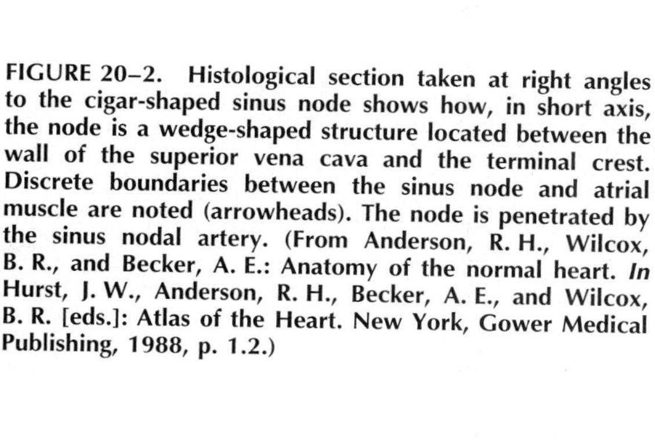

FIGURE 20–2. **Histological section taken at right angles to the cigar-shaped sinus node shows how, in short axis, the node is a wedge-shaped structure located between the wall of the superior vena cava and the terminal crest. Discrete boundaries between the sinus node and atrial muscle are noted (arrowheads). The node is penetrated by the sinus nodal artery. (From Anderson, R. H., Wilcox, B. R., and Becker, A. E.: Anatomy of the normal heart. *In* Hurst, J. W., Anderson, R. H., Becker, A. E., and Wilcox, B. R. [eds.]: Atlas of the Heart. New York, Gower Medical Publishing, 1988, p. 1.2.)**

The Atrioventricular Junctional Area and Intraventricular Conduction System

The normal AV junctional area (Figs. 20–3 and 20–4) can be divided into distinct regions: transitional cell zone, also called nodal approaches; compact portion, or the AV node itself; and the penetrating part of the AV bundle (His bundle), which continues as a nonbranching portion.

TRANSITIONAL CELL ZONE. In the rabbit AV node, the transitional cells or nodal approaches are located in posterior, superficial, and deep groups of cells. They differ histologically from atrial myocardium and connect the latter with the compact portion of the AV node. Some fibers may pass from the posterior internodal tract to the distal portion of the AV node or His bundle and provide the anatomical substrate for conduction to bypass AV nodal slowing. However, the importance of this structure is unclear (see p. 574).

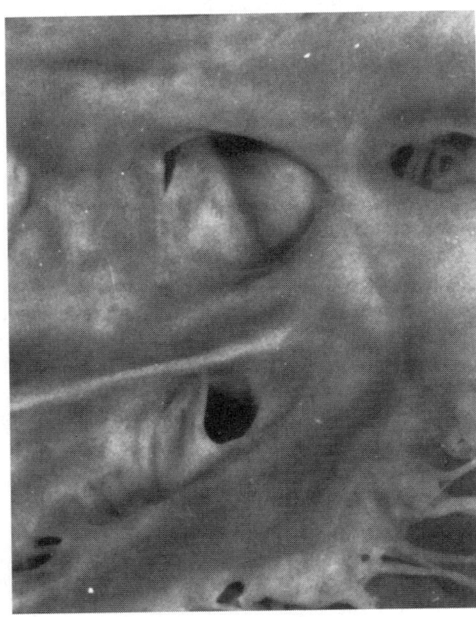

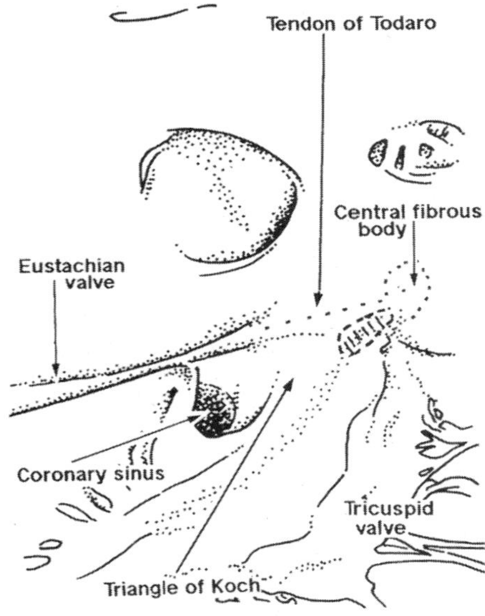

FIGURE 20–3. A photograph of a normal human heart showing the anatomical landmarks of the triangle of Koch. This triangle is delimited by the tendon of Todaro superiorly, which is the fibrous commissure of the flap guarding the openings of the inferior vena cava and coronary sinus, by the attachment of the septal leaflet of the tricuspid valve inferiorly and by the mouth of the coronary sinus at the base. The stippled area adjacent to the central fibrous body is the approximate site of the compact AV node. (From Janse, M. J., Anderson, R. H., McGuire, M. A., et al.: "AV nodal" reentry: I. "AV nodal" reentry revisited. J. Cardiovasc. Electrophysiol. *4*:561, 1993.)

THE AV NODE. The compact portion of the AV node is a superficial structure, lying just beneath the right atrial endocardium, anterior to the ostium of the coronary sinus, and directly above the insertion of the sepal leaflet of the tricuspid valve. It is at the apex of a triangle formed by the tricuspid annulus and the tendon of Todaro, which originates in the central fibrous body and passes posteriorly through the atrial septum to continue with the eustachian valve[24,25,27,28] (Figs. 20–3 and 20–4). The compact portion of the AV node is divided from and becomes the penetrating portion of the His bundle at the point where it enters the central fibrous body. In 85 to 90 per cent of human hearts, the arterial supply to the AV node is a branch from the right coronary artery that originates at the posterior intersection of the AV and interventricular grooves (crux). A branch of the circumflex coronary artery provides the AV nodal artery in the remaining hearts. Fibers in the lower part of the AV node may exhibit automatic impulse formation.

THE BUNDLE OF HIS, OR PENETRATING PORTION OF THE AV BUNDLE. This connects with the distal part of the compact AV node and perforates the central fibrous body, continuing through the annulus fibrosis, where it is called the nonbranching portion as it penetrates the membranous septum (Fig. 20–4). Proximal cells of the penetrating portion are heterogeneous, resembling those of the compact AV node, while distal cells are similar to cells in the proximal bundle branches. Connective tissue of the central fibrous body and membranous septum encloses the penetrating portion of the AV bundle, which may send out extensions into the central fibrous body.[24,25,27,28] However, large well-formed fasciculoventricular connections between the penetrating portion of the AV bundle and the ventricular septal crest are rarely found in adult hearts. Branches from the anterior and posterior descending coronary arteries supply the upper muscular interventricular septum with blood, making the conduction system at this site more impervious to ischemic damage unless the ischemia is extensive.

THE BUNDLE BRANCHES, OR BRANCHING PORTION OF THE AV BUNDLE. These structures begin at the superior margin of the muscular interventricular septum, immediately beneath the membranous septum, with the cells of the left bundle branch cascading downward as a continuous sheet onto the septum beneath the noncoronary aortic cusp (Fig. 20–5). The AV bundle then may give off other left bundle branches, sometimes constituting a true bifascicular system with an anterosuperior branch, in other hearts giving rise to a group of central fibers, and in still others appearing more as a network without a clear division into a fascicular system. The right bundle branch continues intramyocardially as an unbranched extension of the AV bundle down the right side of the interventricular septum to the apex of the right ventricle and base of the anterior papillary muscle. In some human hearts, the His bundle traverses the right interventricular crest, giving rise to a right-sided narrow stem origin of the left bundle branch. The anatomy of the left bundle branch system may be variable and may not conform to a constant bifascicular division. However, the concept of a trifascicular system remains useful to both the electrocardiographer and the clinician (Fig. 20–5).

TERMINAL PURKINJE FIBERS. These fibers connect with the ends of the bundle branches to form interweaving networks on the endocardial surface of both ventricles that transmit the cardiac impulse almost simultaneously to the entire right and left ventricular endocardium. Purkinje fibers tend to be less concentrated at the base of the ventricle and at the papillary muscle tips. They penetrate the myocardium for varying distances depending on the animal species; in humans, they apparently penetrate only the inner third of the endocardium, while in the pig they almost reach the epicardium. Such variations could influence changes produced by myocardial ischemia, for example, since Purkinje fibers appear more resistant to ischemia than are ordinary myocardial fibers.

CELLULAR COMPOSITION OF THE AV JUNCTIONAL AREA. Transitional cells in the rabbit are elongated, smaller than atrial cells, stain more palely, and are separated by numerous strands of connective tissue. They merge at the entrance of the compact portion of the AV node, where the cells are small and spherical, not separated by muscle or connective tissue, and have very few nexuses. They interweave in interconnecting whorls of fasciculi. The AV node is divided, based on electrophysiological characteristics, into AN, N, and NH regions[29] (Fig. 20–6).

In the rabbit, the AN region corresponds to the transitional cell groups of the posterior portion of the node, the NH region to the anterior portion of the bundle of lower nodal cells, and the N region to the small enclosed node where transitional cells merge with midnodal cells. *Dead-end pathways*—groups of cells that form an apparent electrophysiological cul-de-sac that does not contribute to overall conduction in the node—are also found at several sites. Cells in

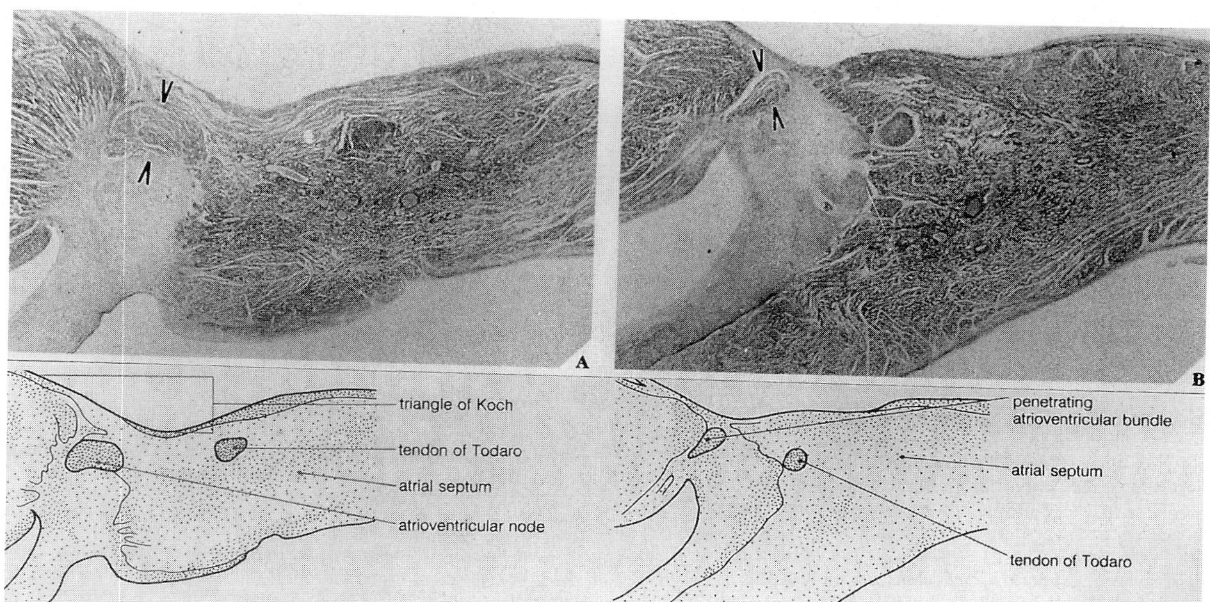

FIGURE 20–4. Sections through the atrioventricular junction show the position of the atrioventricular node (arrowhead) within the triangle of Koch *(A)* and the penetrating atrioventricular bundle of His (arrowheads) within the central fibrous body *(B)*. (From Anderson, R. H., Wilcox, B. R., and Becker, A. E.: Anatomy of the normal heart. *In* Hurst, J. W., Anderson, R. H., Becker, A. E., and Wilcox, B. R. [eds.]: Atlas of the Heart. New York, Gower Medical Publishing, 1988, p. 1.2.)

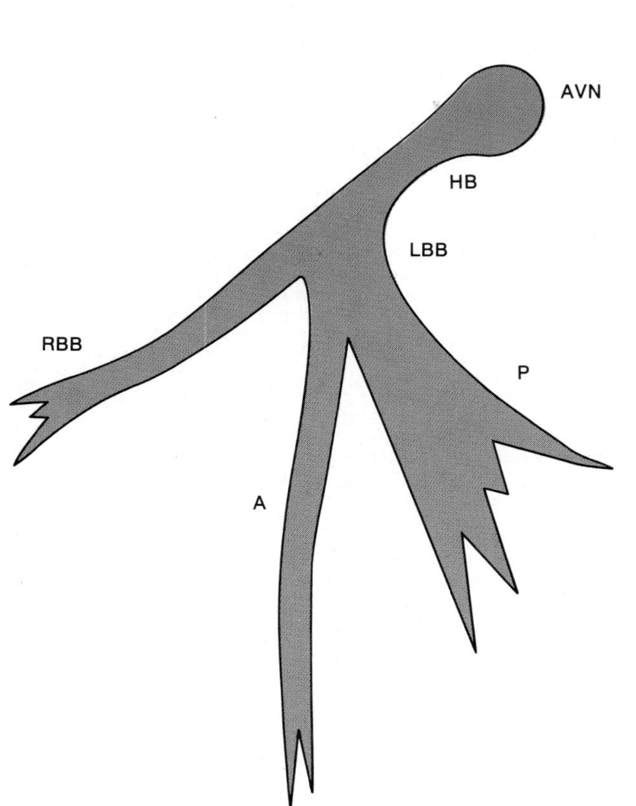

FIGURE 20–5. Schematic representation of the trifascicular bundle branch system. AVN, atrioventricular node; HB, His bundle; LBB, main left bundle branch; A, anterosuperior fascicle of the left bundle; P, posteroinferior fascicle of the left bundle branch; RBB, right bundle branch. (Modified from Rosenbaum, M. B., Elizari, M. V., and Lazzari, J. O.: The Hemiblocks. Oldsmar, FL, Tampa Tracings, 1970, cover illustration.)

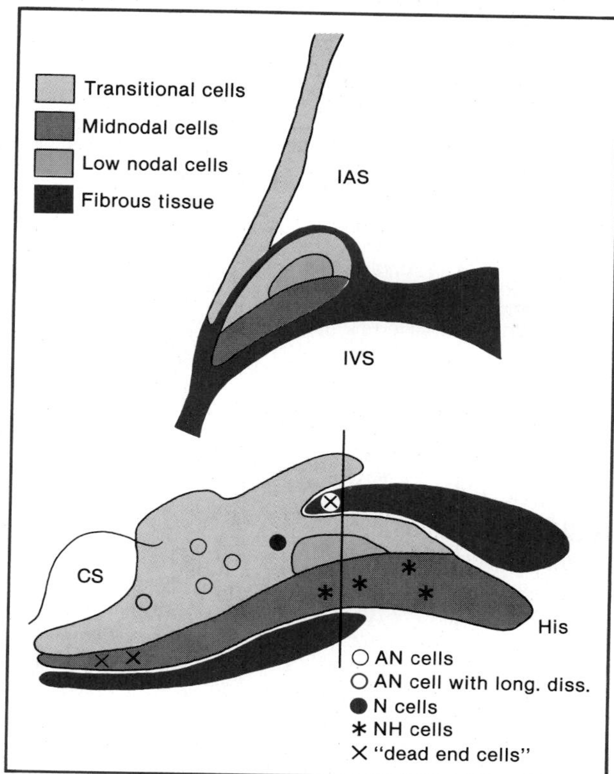

FIGURE 20–6. Diagram showing distribution of morphologically different cell types in AV node. *Upper panel,* Transverse section showing trilaminar appearance of the interior part of the node. The level of sectioning is indicated by the vertical dark line in the lower panel. *Lower panel,* Diagram of the AV node indicating the different sites identified histologically after recording typical action potentials. (From Janse, M. J., et al.: Electrophysiology and structure of the atrioventricular node of the isolated rabbit heart. *In* Wellens, J. H. H., et al. [eds.]: The Conduction System of the Heart. Philadelphia, Lea and Febiger, 1976, p. 296.)

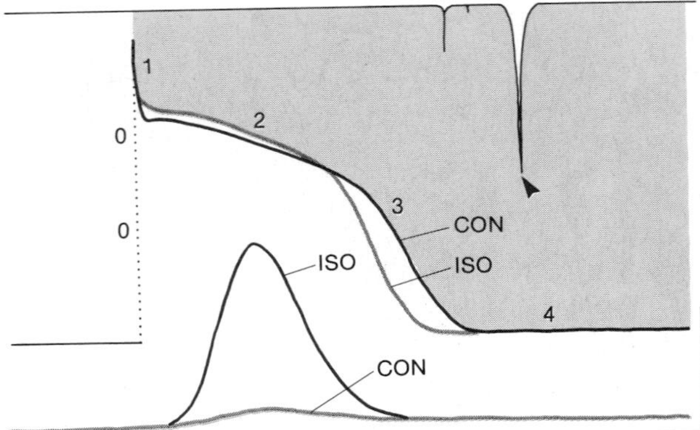

FIGURE 20–7. Recordings of canine Purkinje fiber action potential and developed tension before and during isoproterenol administration. Tracings from above downward show upstroke velocity of phase 0 (V_{max}, arrowhead), action potential configuration of Purkinje fiber, and developed tension in the Purkinje fiber bundle during control (CON) and after exposure to isoproterenol (ISO, 0.1 ml/10^{-5} M, added directly to the tissue bath). The five phases of the action potential are indicated by the large numerals. The short horizontal line to the left with a zero near the peak of the action potential indicates the zero voltage potential. Vertical calibration: 400 V/sec for $\dot{V}_{max}$/sec, 50 mV for action potential amplitude, and 400 mg for the developed tension, respectively. Horizontal calibration: 4 msec for the upper record and 100 msec for the middle and lower records. (V = volts; mV = millivolts; msec = milliseconds.) Isoproterenol increased plateau height of the action potential and developed tension and decreased action potential duration during the terminal phase of repolarization, without significantly affecting resting membrane potential or phase 0. (From Gilmour, R. F., Jr., and Zipes, D. P.: Basic electrophysiology of the slow inward current. *In* Antman, E., and Stone, P. [eds.]: Calcium Blocking Agents in the Treatment of Cardiovascular Disorders. Mt. Kisco, N.Y., Futura, 1983, pp. 1–37.)

the penetrating bundle remain similar to compact AV nodal cells. In the dog, P cells, similar to those found in the sinus node, and several types of transitional cells have been noted and related to the automaticity and conduction properties of the AV node.[24,25]

Purkinje cells are found in the His bundle and bundle branches, cover much of the endocardium of both ventricles, and align to form multicellular bundles in longitudinal strands separated by collagen. They are large, clear cells (10 to 30 μm in diameter, 20 to 50 μm long) with loosely arrayed mitochondria distributed between few linearly aligned myofibrils that have few myofilaments. Round nuclei occupy the center of the cell. Although conduction of the cardiac impulse appears to be their major function, free-running Purkinje fibers, sometimes called *false tendons,* which are composed of many Purkinje cells in a series, are capable of contraction (Fig. 20–7). Extensive lateral and end-to-end gap junctions, made up primarily of connexin 43, apparently transform the individual Purkinje cells into functioning like a cable.[3,6,7,30]

Innervation of AV Node and His Bundle

PATHWAYS OF INNERVATION. The AV node and His bundle region are innervated by a rich supply of cholinergic and adrenergic fibers with a density exceeding that found in the ventricular myocardium. Ganglia, nerve fibers, and nerve nets lie close to the AV node. Parasympathetic nerves to the AV node region enter the canine heart at the junction of the inferior vena cava and the inferior left atrium, adjacent to the coronary sinus entrance. Nerves in direct contact with AV nodal fibers have been noted, along with agranular and granular vesicular processes, presumably representing cholinergic and adrenergic processes. Acetylcholine release may be concentrated around the N region of the AV node.[13–15]

In general, autonomic neural input to the heart exhibits some degree of "sidedness," with the right sympathetic and vagal nerves affecting the sinus node more than the AV node and the left sympathetic and vagal nerves affecting the AV node more than the sinus node. The distribution of the neural input to the sinus and AV nodes is complex because of substantial overlapping innervation. Despite the overlap, specific branches of the vagal and sympathetic nerves can be shown to innervate certain regions preferentially, and sympathetic or vagal nerves to the sinus node can be interrupted discretely without affecting AV nodal innervation. Similarly, vagal or sympathetic neural input to the AV node can be interrupted without affecting sinus innervation. Supersensitivity to acetylcholine follows vagal denervation. Stimulation of the right stellate ganglion produces sinus tachycardia with less effect on AV nodal conduction, while stimulation of the left stellate ganglion generally produces a shift in the sinus pacemaker to an ectopic site and consistently shortens AV nodal conduction time and refractoriness but inconsistently speeds the sinus nodal discharge rate. Stimulation of the right cervical vagus nerve primarily slows the sinus nodal discharge rate, while stimulation of the left vagus primarily prolongs AV nodal conduction time and refractoriness when "sidedness" is present. While neither sympathetic nor vagal stimulation affects normal conduction in the His bundle, either can affect abnormal AV conduction.

Most efferent sympathetic impulses reach the canine ventricles over the ansae subclaviae, branches from the stellate ganglia. Sympathetic nerves then synapse primarily in the caudal cervical ganglia and form individual cardiac nerves that innervate relatively localized parts of the ventricles. On the right side, the major route to the heart is the recurrent cardiac nerve, and on the left, the ventrolateral cardiac nerve. In general, the right sympathetic chain shortens refractoriness primarily of the anterior portion of the ventricles, while the left affects primarily the posterior surface of the ventricles, although overlapping areas of distribution occur.

The intraventricular route of sympathetic nerves generally follows coronary arteries. Functional data suggest that afferent and efferent sympathetic nerves travel in the superficial layers of the epicardium and dive to innervate the endocardium, and anatomical observations support this conclusion. Vagal fibers travel intramurally or subendocardially, rising to the epicardium at the AV groove[13–15,31] (Fig. 20–8).

EFFECTS OF VAGAL STIMULATION. The vagus modulates cardiac sympathetic activity at prejunctional and postjunctional sites by regulating the amount of norepinephrine released and by inhibiting cyclic AMP-induced phosphorylation of cardiac proteins such as phospholamban.[22] The latter inhibition occurs at more than one level in the series of reactions comprising the adenylate cyclase, cyclic AMP–dependent, protein kinase system. Neuropeptides released from nerve fibers of both autonomic limbs also modulate autonomic responses. For example, neuropeptide Y released from sympathetic nerve terminals inhibits cardiac vagal effects.[11,12]

Tonic vagal stimulation produces a greater absolute reduction in sinus rate in the presence of tonic background sympathetic stimulation, a sympathetic-parasympathetic interaction termed *accentuated antagonism*. In contrast, changes in AV conduction during concomitant sympathetic and vagal stimulation are essentially the *algebraic sum* of the individual AV conduction responses to tonic vagal and sympathetic stimulation alone. Cardiac responses to brief vagal bursts begin after a short latency and dissipate quickly; in contrast, cardiac responses to sympathetic stimulation commence and dissipate slowly. The rapid onset and offset of responses to vagal stimulation allow for dynamic beat-to-beat vagal modulation of heart rate and AV conduction, whereas the slow temporal response to sympathetic stimulation precludes any beat-to-beat regulation by sympathetic activity. Periodic vagal bursting (as may occur each time a systolic pressure wave arrives at the baroreceptor regions in the aortic and carotid sinuses) induces phasic changes in sinus cycle length and can entrain the sinus node to discharge faster or slower at periods that are identical to those of the vagal burst. In a similar phasic manner, vagal bursts prolong AV nodal conduction time and are influenced by background levels of sympathetic tone. Because the peak vagal effects on sinus rate and AV nodal conduction occur at different times in the cardiac cycle, a brief vagal burst can slow the sinus rate without affecting AV nodal conduction or can prolong AV nodal conduction time and not slow the sinus rate.[9,11,12]

EFFECTS OF SYMPATHETIC STIMULATION. Stimulation of sympathetic ganglia shortens the refractory period equally in the epicardium and underlying endocardium of the left ventricular free wall, although dispersion of recovery properties occurs, i.e., different degrees of shortening of refractoriness occur when measured at different epicardial sites. Nonuniform distribution of norepinephrine may, in part, contribute to some of the nonuniform electrophysiological effects, since the ventricular content of norepinephrine is greater at the base than at the apex of the heart, with greater distribution to muscle than to Purkinje fibers. Afferent vagal activity appears to be greater in the posterior ventricular myocardium. This may account for the vagomimetic effects of inferior myocardial infarction.[13–15]

The vagi exert minimal but measurable effects on ven-

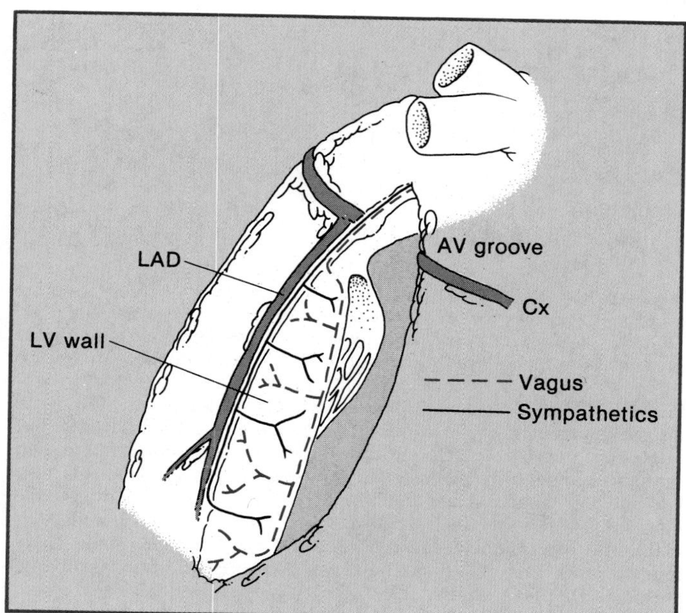

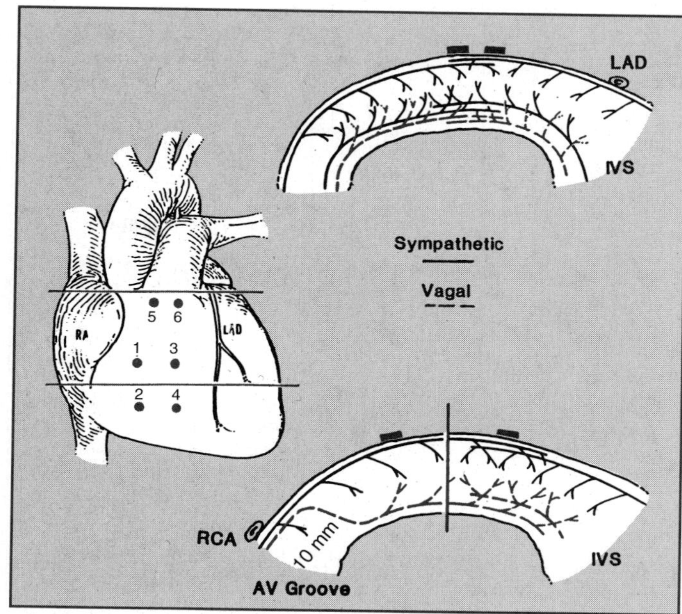

FIGURE 20–8. *Left panel,* Intraventricular route of sympathetic and vagal nerves to the left ventricle. *Right panel,* Schematic of the transverse views of the right ventricular wall showing functional pathways of efferent sympathetic and vagal nerves. *Top right,* Transverse view of the RV outflow tract at the upper horizontal line on the left. *Bottom right,* Transverse view of the anterolateral wall at the lower horizontal line on the left. Vertical solid line indicates center of RV anterolateral wall. Closed circles indicate positions of plunge electrodes labeled 1–6. IVS, interventricular septum; LAD, left anterior descending coronary artery; RCA, right coronary artery; RA, right atrium. (Reproduced with permission from Ito, M., and Zipes, D. P.: Efferent sympathetic and vagal innervation of the canine right ventricle. Circulation *90:*1459, 1994. Copyright 1994 American Heart Association.)

tricular tissue, decreasing the strength of myocardial contraction and prolonging refractoriness. Under some circumstances, acetylcholine can cause a positive inotropic effect. It is now clear that the vagus (acetylcholine) can exert direct effects on some types of ventricular fibers, as well as exert indirect effects by modulating sympathetic influences.[14,32]

ARRHYTHMIAS AND THE AUTONOMIC NERVOUS SYSTEM. Alterations in vagal and sympathetic innervation can influence the development of arrhythmias.[14,32] Damage to nerves extrinsic to the heart, such as the stellate ganglia, as well as to intrinsic cardiac nerves from diseases that may affect nerves primarily, e.g., viral infections, or secondarily, from diseases that cause cardiac damage, may produce cardioneuropathy. Such neural changes may create electrical instability via a variety of electrophysiological mechanisms. For example, myocardial infarction can interrupt afferent and efferent neural transmission and create areas of sympathetic supersensitivity that may be conducive to the development of arrhythmias.[13,14]

BASIC ELECTROPHYSIOLOGICAL PRINCIPLES

Cell Membrane (Sarcolemma)

(See also p. 369)

The cell membrane constitutes a bilayer boundary of phospholipid molecules[33] (Fig. 20–9). The tail end of the phospholipid molecules is nonpolar and hydrophobic, pointing toward the center of the membrane, while the head end is polar and hydrophilic, pointing toward the outer and inner layers of the membrane, in contact with the aqueous extracellular and intracellular environment. The sarcolemma, particularly the hydrophobic core, provides a high-resistance, insulated wrapping around the cell that exhibits selective permeability to ions—a property responsible for creating an electrical potential across the cell membrane. Ions are positively (cations) or negatively (anions) charged atoms such as Na^+, K^+, Ca^{++}, or Cl^- and other molecules whose movement inside the cell or across the cell membrane creates a flow of current that generates signals in excitable membranes.

At rest, the resistance to ion flow is greater across the cell membrane than in the cytoplasm of the cell interior. The cell membrane has openings called *channels* that span the cell membrane and serve as conduits through which ions move. The different protein or phospholipoprotein channels are selective, favoring passage of one ion over another. In contrast to the membrane lipids that act primarily as inert barriers, membrane proteins appear to be responsible for most of the known biological activities of membranes. Some kinds of channels open as a result of a neurotransmitter binding to their extracellular site and are called *receptor-operated channels.* Others open in response to a voltage change and are called *voltage-operated channels.* Gates, influenced by the electric field and by time, control ion movement through the channels and, when opened or closed, permit or prevent ion travel. Drugs can bind to sites within the channel and prevent ion passage. Sodium[34–37] and calcium[38–50] membrane channels cycle through three states during each action potential that include the closed or resting state, the open or activation state, and the closed or inactivation state (Fig. 20–10). Voltage-dependent ion channels are glycosylated proteins. Each subunit of these channels contains four covalently linked domains (except for potassium channels) designated I to IV (Fig. 20–9, *left*), and each domain contains six alpha-helical transmembrane segments designated S_1 to S_6 (Fig. 20–9, *right*). S_4 is thought to represent the m gate (see p. 558), and the cytoplasmic loop connecting the S_6 transmembrane segment of domain III to the S_1 segment of domain IV may be to the h gate.[35]

In addition to the channels, pumps and carriers (e.g., Na-K pump, which is blocked by digitalis [see p. 499], Ca^{++} pump, Na/Ca countertransport system, Na/H exchanger), receptors (e.g., α, β, muscarinic, and purinergic), and cytoplasmic regulators of second messengers (e.g., cyc-

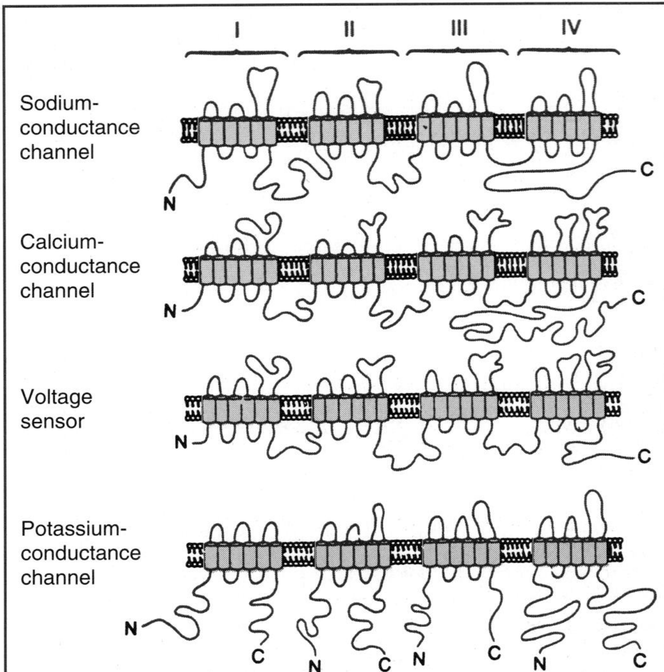

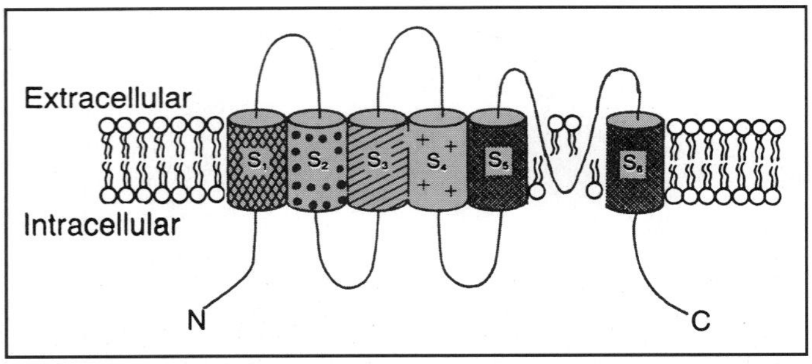

FIGURE 20–9. ***Left panel,*** **Four members of the family of ion-channel proteins. The major subunits of the calcium and sodium channels are tetramers made up of four covalently linked domains that are numbered I–IV. The voltage sensor that initiates contraction in the depolarized mammalian skeletal muscle resembles the calcium channel but is smaller, because it lacks the portion of the C-terminal amino acid sequence present in the calcium channel. Potassium channels also contain four domains, but unlike calcium and sodium channels, the domains are not covalently linked.** ***Right panel,*** **An ion channel domain. The ion channels shown on the left are tetramers made up of four domains, each of which contains six alpha-helical transmembrane segments. The S_4 segment, which is rich in positively charged amino acids, is believed to open the channel in response to membrane depolarization. The transmembrane segments S_5 and S_6, along with the intervening peptide chain, probably surround the pore through which ions cross the lipid barrier in the core of the membrane bilayer. (Modified from Katz, A. M.: Molecular biology in cardiology, a paradigmatic shift. J. Mol. Cell. Cardiol.** ***20:*****355, 1988.)**

lic AMP–phosphodiesterase) influence electrophysiological function.[51] Some protein complexes penetrate only the outer cell membrane and may serve as receptor sites for neurotransmitters and hormones, while others, such as the adenylate cyclase system, protrude through the inner cell membrane and may be involved in various enzymatic activities. Protein molecules protruding through the entire cell membrane, such as the Na-K pump, may help regulate ionic fluxes. The Na-K pump requires adenosine triphosphate (ATP) to extrude intracellular Na against its concentration and electrical gradients and to move K intracellularly, against its concentration gradient, resulting in high concentrations of K inside and of Na outside the cell (Table 20–1).

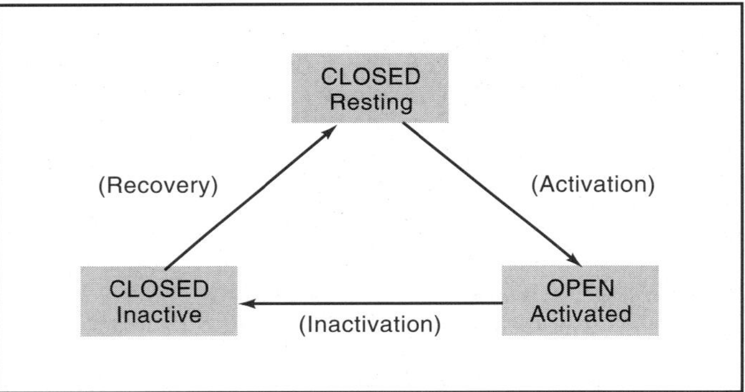

FIGURE 20–10. Three states through which ion channels cycle.

INTERCALATED DISCS

The cell membranes of some types of adjacent cells form close margins called *intercalated discs.* Three types of specialized junctions make up each intercalated disc. The macula adherens or desmosome and fascia adherens form the areas of strong adhesions between cells and may provide a linkage for the transfer of mechanical energy from one cell to the next. The *nexus,* also called *tight* or *gap junction,* is a region in the intercalated disc where cells are in functional contact with each other. Membranes at these junctions are separated by only about 10 to 20 Å and are connected by a series of hexagonally packed subunit bridges. Gap junctions provide low-resistance electrical coupling between adjacent cells by establishing aqueous pores that directly link the cytoplasms of these adjacent cells. The gap junctions allow movement of ions and perhaps of small molecules between cells, linking interiors of adjacent cells.

The gap junctions permit a multicellular structure such as the heart to function electrically like an orderly, synchronized, interconnected unit and are probably responsible in part for the fact that conduction in the myocardium is *anisotropic;* i.e., its anatomical and biophysical properties vary according to the direction in which they are measured. Usually, conduction velocity is two to three times faster longitudinally, i.e., in the direction of the long axis of the fiber, than it is

TABLE 20–1 INTRACELLULAR AND EXTRACELLULAR ION CONCENTRATIONS IN CARDIAC MUSCLE

ION	EXTRACELLULAR CONCENTRATION	INTRACELLULAR CONCENTRATION	RATIO OF EXTRACELLULAR TO INTRACELLULAR CONCENTRATION	E_i
Na	145 mM	15 mM	9.7	+60 mV
K	4 mM	150 mM	0.027	−94 mV
Cl	120 mM	5 mM	24	−83 mV
Ca	2 mM	10^{-7} M	2×10^4	+129 mV

E_i = equilibrium potential for a particular ion.

Although intracellular Ca content is about 2 mM, most of this is bound or sequestered in intracellular organelles (mitochondria and sarcoplasmic reticulum). For the same reason, the actual free Na concentration may be less. Intracellular Cl concentration depends on the average membrane potential, if Cl is passively distributed, and therefore on heart rate.

From Sperelakis, N.: Origin of the cardiac resting potential. *In* Berne, R. M., et al. (eds.): Handbook of Physiology, The Cardiovascular System, Bethesda, Md., American Physiological Society, 1979, p. 193.

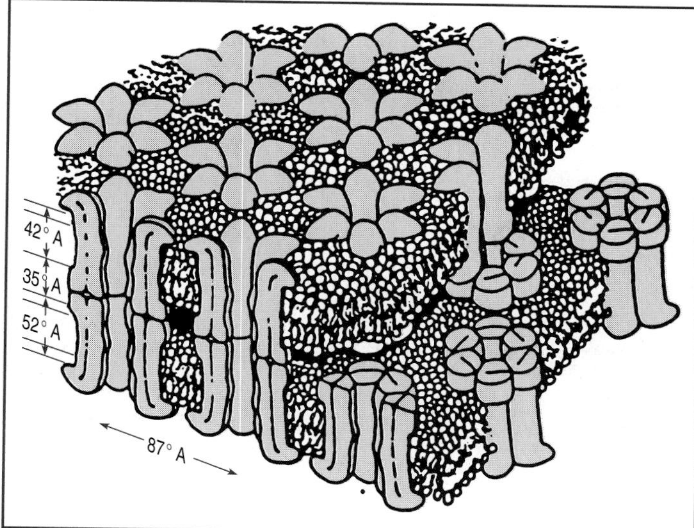

FIGURE 20–11. A model of the structure of a gap junction based on results of x-ray diffraction studies. Individual channels are composed of paired hexamers that travel in the membranes of adjacent cells and adjoin in the extracellular gap to form an aqueous pore that provides continuity of the cytoplasm of the two cells. (From Saffitz, J. E.: Cell-to-cell communication in the heart. Cardiol. Rev. *3*:86, 1995.)

transversely, i.e., in the direction perpendicular to this long axis. Resistivity is lower longitudinally than transversely. Interestingly, the safety factor for propagation is greater transversely than horizontally. Conduction delay or block occurs more commonly in the longitudinal direction than it does transversely. Because of anisotropy, propagation is discontinuous and can be a cause of reentry.

Gap junctions also may provide "biochemical coupling" that might permit cell-to-cell movement of ATP on other high-energy phosphates. Gap junctions also can change their electrical resistance. When intracellular calcium rises, as in myocardial infarction, the gap junction may close to help "seal off" the effects of injured from noninjured cells. Acidosis increases and alkalosis decreases gap junctional resistance. Increased gap junctional resistance tends to slow the rate of action potential propagation, a condition that could lead to conduction delay or block.[3,6–8,52–56]

Connexins are the proteins that form the intercellular channels of gap junctions. An individual channel (connexin) is created by two hemichannels, each located in the plasma membrane of adjacent cells, that are composed of six integral membrane protein subunits (connexins) that surround an aqueous pore, creating a transmembrane channel (Fig. 20–11). Connexin 43, a 43-kDa polypeptide, is the most abundant cardiac connexin, with connexin 40 and 45 found in smaller amounts. Gap junctions in the distal His bundle and proximal bundle branches have large amounts of connexin 40 and 43. Atrial gap junctions have large amounts of all three connexins, while ventricular gap junctions have large amounts of connexin 43 and 45 and much less connexin 40 (see p. 548).[3,6]

Phases of the Cardiac Action Potential

The cardiac transmembrane potential consists of five phases: phase 0—the upstroke or rapid depolarization; phase 1—early rapid repolarization; phase 2—plateau; phase 3—final rapid repolarization; and phase 4—resting membrane potential and diastolic depolarization (see Fig. 20–7). These phases are the result of passive ion fluxes moving down electrochemical gradients established by active ion pumps and exchange mechanisms. Each ion moves primarily through its own ion-specific channel. Impulses spread from one cell to the next without requiring neural input. The transplanted heart dramatically demonstrates this fact. The following discussion will explain the electrogenesis of each of these phases. For in-depth coverage, the reader is referred to other reference sources.[57,58]

Phase 4—The Resting Membrane Potential

Intracellular electrical activity can be recorded by inserting a glass microelectrode with a tip diameter less than 0.5 μm into a single cell. The electrode produces minimal damage, its entry point apparently being sealed by the cell. The transmembrane potential is recorded using this electrode in reference to an extracellular ground electrode placed in the tissue bath near the cell membrane and represents the potential difference between intracellular and extracellular voltages (Fig. 20–12, *left*). A variety of other techniques, including voltage and patch clamp procedures, can be used to study the passage of individual ionic species across specific channels in the cell membrane (Figs. 20–12, 20–13, and 20–14).

Intracellular potential during electrical quiescence in diastole is −50 to −95 mV, depending on the cell type (Table 20–2). This means that the inside of the cell is 50 to 95 mV negative relative to the outside of the cell owing to the distribution of ions such as K^+, Na^+, Cl^-, and Ca^{++} across the cell membrane.

K^+ is the major ion determining the resting potential.[59–65] During diastole, the cell membrane is quite permeable to K^+ and relatively impermeable to Na^+. Because of the Na-K pump, which pumps Na^+ out of the cell against its electrochemical gradient and simultaneously pumps K^+ into the cell against its chemical gradient, intracellular K^+ concentration remains high and intracellular Na^+ concentration remains low. This pump, fueled by an Na^+, K^+-ATPase enzyme that hydrolyzes ATP for energy, is bound to the membrane. It requires both Na^+ and K^+ to function and can transport three Na^+ ions outward for two K^+ ions inward. Therefore, the pump can be electrogenic, generating a net outward movement of positive charges. The rate of Na^+-K^+ pumping to maintain the same ionic gradients must increase as heart rate increases, since the cell gains a slight amount of Na^+ and loses a slight amount of K^+ with each depolarization. Cardiac glycosides block this pump.

THE NERNST EQUATION. Little Na^+, despite its concentration gradient, can diffuse into the cell, owing to the relative impermeability to Na^+ of the polarized cell membrane. However, K^+ can diffuse freely out of the cell down its concentration gradient and does so, removing with it a positive charge and leaving the inside of the cell more negative. Negative intracellular charges, presumably due to large polyvalent ions such as proteins, do not cross the membrane and help maintain intracellular negativity. K^+ continues to leave the cell until the forces driving it down its concentration gradient are balanced by the negative intracellular electrical charges that attract K^+ back into the cell. The transmembrane voltage at which the electrical

TABLE 20–2 PROPERTIES OF TRANSMEMBRANE POTENTIALS IN MAMMALIAN HEARTS

	SINUS NODAL CELL	ATRIAL MUSCLE CELL	AV NODAL CELL	PURKINJE FIBER	VENTRICULAR MUSCLE CELL
Resting potential (mV)	−50 to −60	−80 to −90	−60 to −70	−90 to −95	−80 to −90
Action potential					
Amplitude (mV)	60 to 70	110 to 120	70 to 80	120	110 to 120
Overshoot (mV)	0 to 10	30	5 to 15	30	30
Duration (msec)	100 to 300	100 to 300	100 to 300	300 to 500	200 to 300
Vmax (V/S)	1 to 10	100 to 200	5 to 15	500 to 700	100 to 200
Propagation velocity (M/sec)	<0.05	0.3 to 0.4	0.1	2 to 3	0.3 to 0.4
Fiber diameter (μm)	5 to 10	10 to 15	5 to 10	100	10 to 16

Modified from Sperelakis, N.: Origin of the cardiac resting potential. *In* Berne, R. M., Sperelakis, N., and Geiger, S. R. (eds.): Handbook of Physiology, The Cardiovascular System, Bethesda, Md., American Physiological Society, 1979, p. 190.

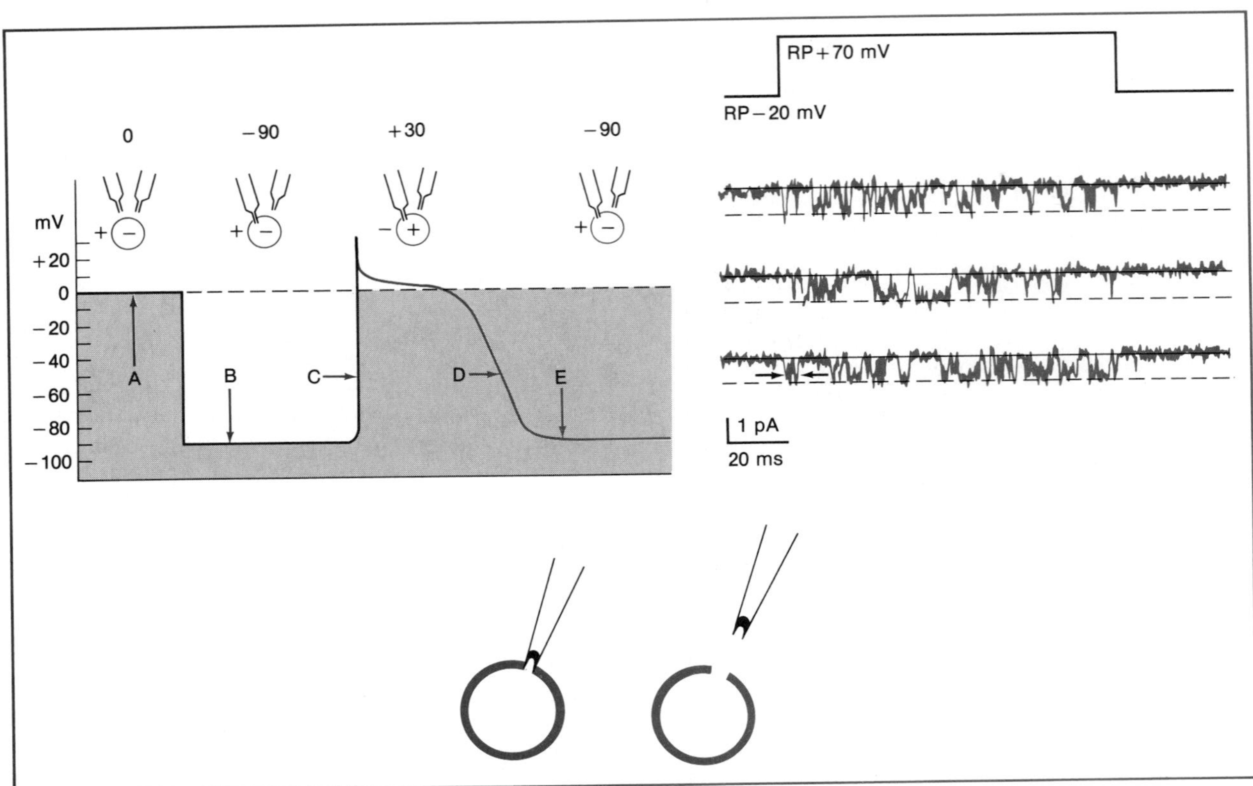

FIGURE 20–12. *Left,* A demonstration of action potentials recorded during impalement of a cardiac cell. The upper row of diagrams shows a cell (circle), two microelectrodes, and stages during impalement of the cell and its activation and recovery. *A,* Both microelectrodes are extracellular, and no difference in potential exists between them (0 potential). The environment inside the cell is negative and the outside is positive, since the cell is polarized. *B,* One microelectrode has pierced the cell membrane to record the intracellular resting membrane potential, which is − 90 mV with respect to the outside of the cell. *C,* The cell has depolarized and the upstroke of the action potential is recorded. At its peak voltage, the inside of the cell is about + 30 mV with respect to the outside of the cell. *D,* Phase of repolarization, returning the membrane to its former resting potential *(E)* (From Cranefield, P. F.: The Conduction of the Cardiac Impulse. Mt. Kisco, N.Y., Futura, 1975.)

Right, Calcium channel recording. A portion or patch of the sarcolemmal membrane from a single guinea pig ventricular muscle cell is sucked up into a micropipette to record the opening and closing of single calcium channels. The pipette is filled with 110 mM Ba^{++}. The Ba^{++} crosses the membrane through the calcium channel when it opens and generates a current, recorded as the large downward pulses that reach the interrupted line (first in the bottom tracing). The solid line indicates average baseline current while the interrupted line (about 1 pA) indicates average single channel current. The channel stays open for brief but varied durations and then closes (upward deflection back to solid line, second). Three sequentially obtained current records are shown. Resting membrane potential (RP) was near − 60 mV by addition of 10 mM [K]o. The RP was then reduced by 20 mV (RP − 20 mV) and virtually no Ca^{++} channel openings occurred. When RP was made 70 mV more positive (RP + 70 mV) Ca^{++} channel activity was generated. (Square wave-shaped tracing at very top indicates RP changes). Thus, this figure illustrates opening and closing of single calcium channels when the RP is reduced to the range at which the slow inward current functions. (From Tsien, R.: Excitable tissues: The heart. *In* Andreoli, T. E., et al. [eds.]: Physiology of Membrane Disorders. New York, Plenum Press, 1986, p. 478.)

Bottom insert shows micropipette technique used to study single channels in a portion of the membrane still attached to the cell *(left).* Membrane studied after being detached from the rest of the cell *(right).*

gradient is equal and opposite to the concentration gradient so that the algebraic sum of these two passive forces equals zero, is the K^+ electrochemical equilibrium potential E_K, and is described by the *Nernst equation:*

$$E_K = \frac{RT}{F} \ln \frac{[K^+]_o}{[K^+]_i} \quad (1)$$

where R is the gas constant, T is the absolute temperature, F is the Faraday number, ln is the logarithm to the base e, $[K^+]_o$ is the extracellular K^+ concentration, and $[K^+]_i$ is the intracellular K^+ concentration.[57,58]

Solving this equation predicts a transmembrane voltage of about −96 mV in cardiac muscle, which is very near the observed voltages. However, certain factors make the equation an approximation. Because the $[K^+]_o/[K^+]_i$ ratio primarily determines transmembrane voltage, the cell membrane is said to behave as a K^+ electrode during diastole and more closely follows the values predicted by the Nernst equation at $[K^+]_o$ greater than 10 mM. When $[K^+]_o$ is reduced, membrane permeability to K^+ also decreases, the small inward movement of Na^+, negligible at high $[K^+]_o$, becomes more important, and the actual resting membrane voltage becomes less than that predicted by the Nernst equation for a K^+ electrode. The difference between predicted and observed voltages increases as $[K^+]_o$ is reduced further.

The contribution of the minimal inward movement of Na^+ to the resting membrane potential can be incorporated into an equation called the *Goldman constant-field equation* and is a slight modification of the Nernst equation. If one assumes that the membrane is permeable to only Na^+ and K^+, the resting membrane potential (V_r) would be

$$V_r = \frac{RT}{F} \ln \frac{[K^+]_o + P_{Na}/P_K\,[Na]_o}{[K^+]_i + P_{Na}/P_K\,[Na]_i} \quad (2)$$

where P_{Na}/P_K is the ratio of the sodium to the potassium permeability coefficient of the cell membrane, $[Na]_o$ is the extracellular sodium concentration, and $[Na]_i$ is the intracellular sodium concentration. The equation can be modified further to include the minimal contributions of other ions.

Calcium contributes little to the resting membrane potential, although changes in Ca concentration can affect the permeability of the cell membrane to other ions. An increase in $[Ca]_i$ increases potassium conductance. Ca^{++} is handled by several mechanisms, including uptake by the sarcoplasmic reticulum. Also, there appears to be a passive transsarcolemmal Ca^{++}-Na^+ exchange reaction. This exchange depends in part on maintenance of the Na^+ concentration gradient by the Na^+-K^+ pump. Under normal conditions, one internal Ca^{++} ion is probably exchanged for three or more external Na^+ ions. Na^+-Ca^{++}

exchange generates a current across the cell membrane. Under some pathological conditions or drug actions when $[Na^+]_i$ is abnormally high, external Ca^{++} may be exchanged for internal Na^+. Cells that gain Na^+, in general, gain Ca^{++}—a reaction important to the genesis of some digitalis-induced arrhythmias. The role of Ca^{++} is further considered on page 366.

Phase 0—Upstroke or Rapid Depolarization

A stimulus delivered to excitable tissue evokes an action potential characterized by a sudden voltage change due to transient depolarization followed by repolarization. The action potential is conducted throughout the heart and is responsible for initiating each "heartbeat." Electrical changes of the action potential follow a relatively fixed time and voltage relationship that differs according to specific cell types (Figs. 20–13, 20–14, and 20–15). In nerve, the entire process takes several milliseconds, while action potentials in cardiac fibers last several hundred milliseconds. Normally, the action potential is independent of the size of the depolarizing stimulus, if the latter exceeds a certain threshold potential. Small subthreshold depolarizing stimuli depolarize the membrane in proportion to the strength of the stimulus. However, once the stimulus is sufficiently intense to reduce membrane potential to a threshold value in the range of − 70 to − 65 mV for normal Purkinje fibers, more intense stimuli do not produce larger action potential responses, and an "all-or-none" response results. In contrast, hyperpolarizing pulses, i.e., stimuli that render the membrane potential more negative, elicit a response proportional to the strength of the stimulus.

MECHANISM OF PHASE 0. The upstroke of the cardiac action potential in atrial and ventricular muscle and His-Purkinje fibers is due to a sudden increase in membrane conductance to Na^+. An externally applied stimulus or a spontaneously generated local membrane circuit current in advance of a propagating action potential depolarizes a sufficiently large area of membrane at a sufficiently rapid rate to open the Na^+ channels and depolarize the membrane further. When the membrane voltage reaches threshold, Na^+ rushes through ion-specific channels into the cell, down its electrochemical gradient—i.e., Na^+ is "drawn" into the cell by the low $[Na^+]_i$ and the negatively charged intracellular environment. The excited membrane no longer behaves like a K^+ electrode, i.e., exclusively permeable to K^+, but more closely approximates an Na^+ electrode, and the membrane moves toward the Na^+ equilibrium potential.

The rate at which depolarization occurs during phase 0, i.e., the maximum rate of change of voltage over time, is indicated by the expression dV/dt_{max} or $\dot{V}_{max}$ (Table 20–2), which is a reasonable ap-

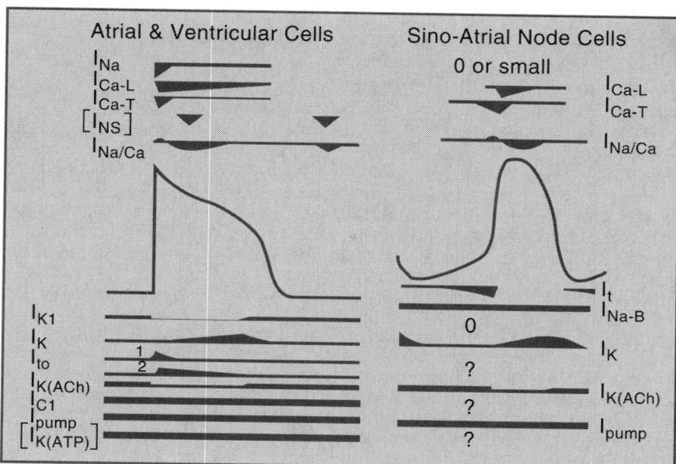

FIGURE 20–13. Currents and channels involved in generating the resting and action potential. The time course of a stylized action potential of atrial and ventricular cells is shown on the left and of sinoatrial node cells on the right. Above and below are the various channels and pumps that contribute the currents underlying the electrical events. See Table 20–3 for identification of the symbols and description of the channels or currents. Where possible, the approximate time courses of the currents associated with the channels or pumps are shown symbolically without effort to represent their magnitudes relative to each other. I_K incorporates at least two currents, $I_{K\text{-}R}$ and $I_{K\text{-}S}$. There appears to be an ultrarapid component as well, designated $I_{K\text{-}UR}$.

The heavy bars for I_{Cl}, I_{pump}, and $I_{K(ATP)}$ only indicate the presence of these channels or pump, without implying magnitude of currents, since that would vary with physiological and pathophysiological conditions. The channels identified by brackets (I_{NS} and $I_{K(ATP)}$) imply that they are active only under pathological conditions. For the sinoatrial node cells, I_{Na} and I_{K1} are small or absent. Question marks indicate that experimental evidence is not yet available to determine the presence of these channels in sinoatrial cell membranes. Although it is likely that other ionic current mechanisms exist, they are not shown here because their roles in electrogenesis are not sufficiently well defined. (From Members of the Sicilian Gambit: Antiarrhythmic Therapy: A Pathophysiologic Approach. Mt. Kisco, N.Y., Futura, 1994, p. 13.)

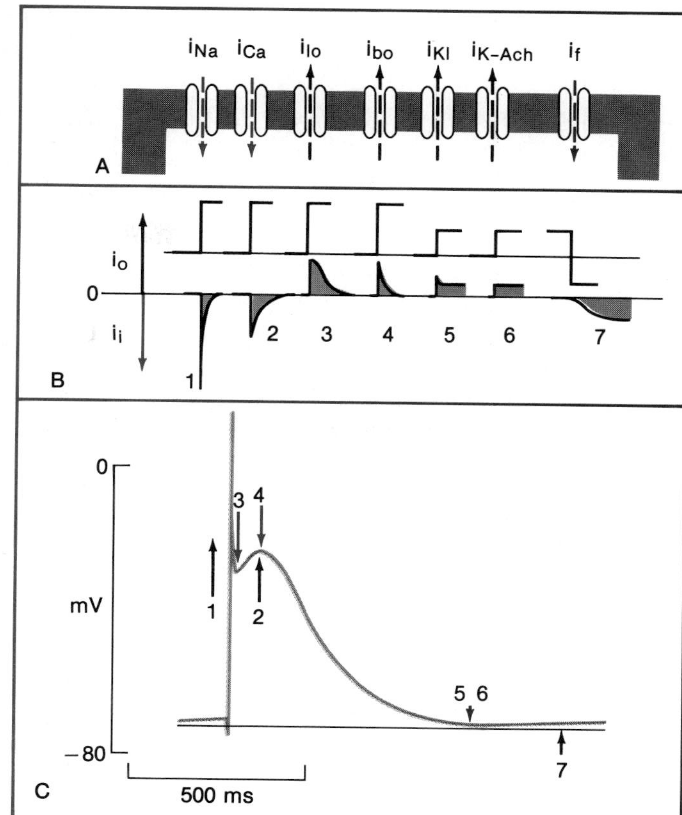

FIGURE 20–14. Schematic diagram of ionic channels *(A)* and corresponding transmembrane currents *(B)* presently known in human atrial myocardium and their influences on development of cellular action potential *(C)*. *A*, Currents crossing different channels under normal conditions are either inward (downward arrows) and therefore depolarize the membrane or outward (upward arrows) and therefore repolarize the membrane. i_{Na}, sodium current; i_{ca}, calcium current; i_{lo} and i_{bo}, long-lasting and brief transient potassium currents; i_{K1}, background potassium current; $i_{K\text{-}ACh}$, potassium current flowing through muscarinic cholinergic receptor channels; i_f, pacemaker current carried by both sodium and potassium ions. *B*, Time course of different transmembrane ionic currents (hatched areas) occurring when the membrane is submitted to rectangular (top traces) depolarizing pulses (1–6) or repolarizing pulses (7). Currents i_{Ki} and $i_{K\text{-}ACh}$ are shown here as outward currents, but because of the inward rectification, they are much smaller in the outward than in the inward direction. i_o, outward current; i_i, inward current. C, 1–7 correspond to the currents shown in *A* and *B*, and arrows indicate effect of each ionic current on the action potential; upward arrows, depolarizing effect; downward arrows, repolarizing or hyperpolarizing effects. (From Coraboeuf, E., and Escande, D.: Ionic currents in the human myocardium. NIPS *5*:28, 1990.)

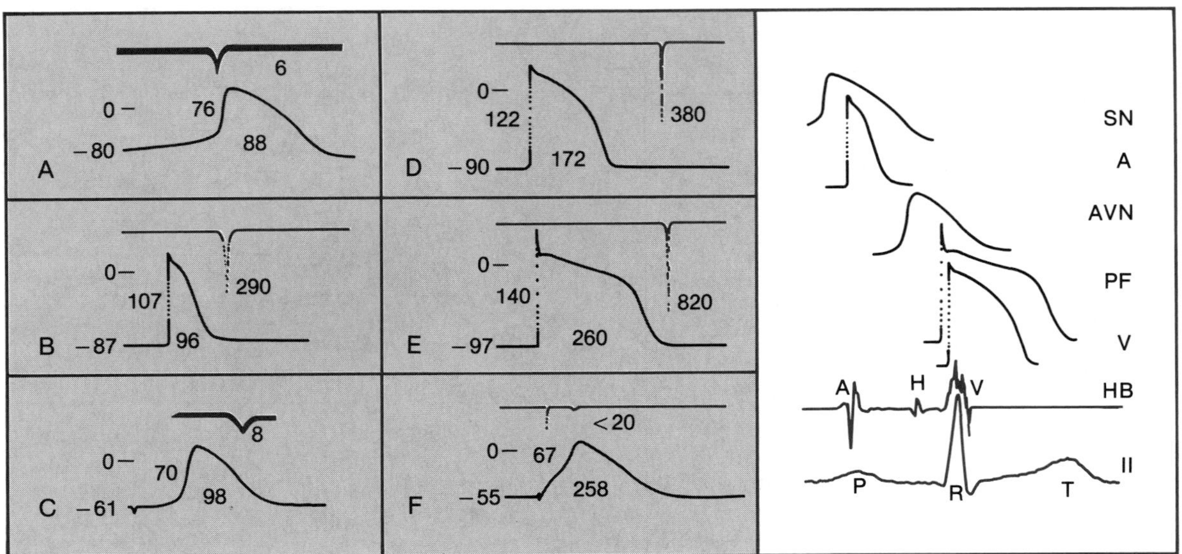

FIGURE 20–15. Action potentials recorded from different tissues in the heart *(left)*, remounted along with a His bundle recording and scalar ECG from a patient *(right)* to illustrate the timing during a single cardiac cycle. In panels *A* to *F*, the top tracing is dV/dt of phase 0 and the second tracing is the action potential. For each panel, the numbers (from left to right) indicate maximum diastolic potential (mV), action potential amplitude (mV), action potential duration at 90 per cent of repolarization (msec), and $\dot{V}_{max}$ of phase 0 (V/sec). Zero potential is indicated by the short horizontal line next to the zero on the upper left of each action potential. *A*, Rabbit sinoatrial node; *B*, canine atrial muscle; *C*, rabbit atrioventricular node; *D*, canine ventricular muscle; *E*, canine Purkinje fiber; *F*, diseased human ventricle. Note that the action potentials recorded in *A*, *C*, and *F* have reduced resting membrane potentials, amplitudes, and $\dot{V}_{max}$ compared with the other action potentials. In the *right panel*, SN = sinus nodal potential; A = atrial muscle potential; AVN = atrioventricular nodal potential; PF = Purkinje fiber potential; V = ventricular muscle potential; HB = His bundle recording; II = lead II. Horizontal calibration on the left: 50 msec for *A* and *C*, 100 msec for *B*, *D*, *E*, and *F*; 200 msec on the right. Vertical calibration on the left: 50 mV. Horizontal calibration on the right: 200 msec. (Modified from Gilmour, R. F., Jr., and Zipes, D. P.: Basic electrophysiology of the slow inward current. *In* Antman, E., and Stone, P. H. [eds.]: Calcium Blocking Agents in the Treatment of Cardiovascular Disorders. Mt. Kisco, N.Y., Futura, 1983, pp. 1–37.)

proximation of the rate and magnitude of Na^+ entry into the cell and a determinant of conduction velocity for the propagated action potential. The transient increase in sodium conductance lasts 1 to 2 msec. The action potential, or more properly the Na^+ current (I_{Na}), is said to be regenerative; that is, intracellular movement of a little Na^+ depolarizes the membrane more, which increases conductance to Na^+ more, which allows more Na^+ to enter, and so on. As this is occurring, however, $[Na^+]_i$ and positive intracellular charges increase and reduce the driving force for Na^+. When the equilibrium potential for Na^+ (E_{Na}) is reached, Na^+ no longer enters the cell, i.e., when the driving force acting on the ion to enter the cell balances the driving force acting on the ion to exit the cell, no current will flow. In addition, Na^+ conductance is time dependent so that when the membrane spends some time at voltages less negative than the resting potential, Na^+ conductance decreases. Therefore, an intervention that reduces membrane potential for a time—but not to threshold—partially inactivates Na^+ channels, and if threshold is now achieved, the magnitude and rate of Na^+ influx are reduced.

In cardiac Purkinje fibers and to a lesser extent in ventricular muscle, two different populations of Na^+ channels, or two different modes of operation of the same Na^+ channel, exist. One is responsible for the brief Na^+ current of phase 0, while the other, which is longer lasting, participates in the action potential plateau. Tetrodotoxin (TTX) and local anesthetics block both types of channels, diminishing the rate of rise of phase 0 and shortening action potential duration.[35] Further, there may be a background Na^+ current ($I_{Na\text{-}B}$) through a voltage-independent channel in sinus nodal cells that contributes to pacemaker behavior.[66]

At this point, several concepts need to be expanded. Ohm's law states that voltage equals current times resistance. The term *conductance* (g) is the inverse or reciprocal of resistance and is related to the ease with which ions can cross the cell membrane when driven by a potential difference across the membrane. As resistance of the membrane to passage of an ion increases, conductance decreases. Membrane permeability or conductance of the Na^+ channel during phase 0 is regulated hypothetically by two types of gates, the m gate and the h gate, which modulate Na ion passage through the channel (Fig. 20–16).

THE GATED SYSTEM—A HYPOTHETICAL MODEL. In this hypothetical model, three m (activation) gates and one h (inactivation) gate can be considered to be lined up in series in the membrane Na^+ channel (Fig. 20–16), with the m gate on the extracellular side and the h gate on the intracellular side of the membrane. When the membrane is in a resting polarized state, the m gates are almost completely closed, the h gate is open, and no Na^+ can cross the membrane. Although depolarization of the membrane opens the m gates and closes the h gate, the m gates open faster than the h gate closes, i.e., activation of the channel proceeds faster than inactivation can occur, and Na^+ flows through the Na^+ channel for about 1 msec while both gates are open simultaneously (Fig. 20–16, *left panel*, red arrow).

When the membrane repolarizes to fairly high negative values, i.e., membrane potential becomes more negative than about −60 mV, the gates shut rapidly, the h gate opens more slowly (reactivation or recovery from inactivation), and the membrane is once again capable of depolarization. Until that time, the cell is absolutely refractory; i.e., no stimulus, regardless of intensity, can activate the cell. If the membrane is activated a second time before reaching a large negative value, all the h gates have not yet reopened so that the maximum number of Na^+ channels that can open is reduced. The resulting action potential will have reduced $\dot{V}_{max}$, amplitude, duration, and conduction velocity. The state of the gates at any time depends on the membrane potential and the length of time the potential has been maintained.[35]

A sequence of positively charged amino acids has been identified as the activation (m) gate that opens the channel in response to depolarization, while an intracellular peptide loop is the inactivation (h) gate. When it dangles free, ions can move in or out of the channel. When the protein ball plugs the mouth of the pore, ion flow stops and inactivation results[37] (Fig. 20–17).

Using this model, the amount of current (I) generated by a specific ion (I_i) equals the membrane conductance for the ion (g_i) multiplied by the driving force for that ion. The driving force is the difference between the actual membrane voltage (V_m) and the equilibrium potential for that ion (E_i). Thus

$$I_i = g_i\,(V_m - E_i)$$

Conductance can be determined by rearranging the equation:

$$g_i = Ii\,(V_m - E_i)$$

The equations indicate that the current flow is voltage dependent; i.e., as the voltage of the membrane (V_m) changes relative to the equilibrium potential (E_i), the electrical driving force for an ion ($V_m - E_i$) changes and so does the current. The relationship between membrane voltage (V_m) at the time of depolarization and I_{Na}, measured in terms of $\dot{V}_{max}$ (maximum rate of rise of phase 0), is indicated by the so-called membrane responsiveness curve. When depolarization occurs at reduced membrane potentials, it results in decreased I_{Na} and $\dot{V}_{max}$.

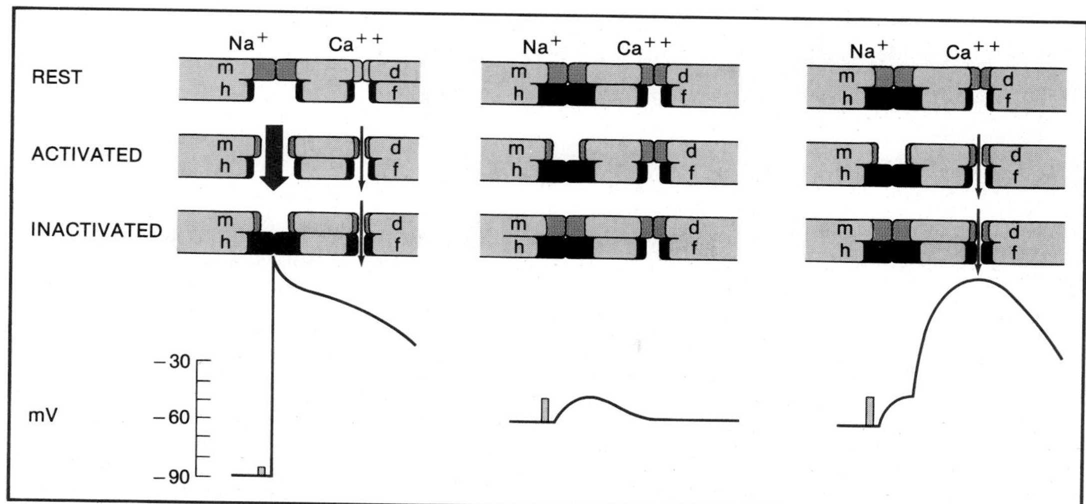

FIGURE 20–16. Schematic representation of membrane channels for rapid and slow inward currents at resting membrane potential *(top row)*, during the activated state *(middle row)*, and during the inactivated state *(bottom row)*. Vertically separated panels depict fibers with a normal resting potential of −90 mV *(left)*, with resting membrane potential reduced to less than −60 mV *(middle)*, and after stimulation of the cell with catecholamines *(right)*. The activation (m) and inactivation (h) gates of the fast channel and the activation (d) and inactivation (f) gates of the slow channel are depicted.

During the resting state *(left panel)*, the activation gates of both channels are closed while the inactivation gates are open. When the cell is stimulated, the m gates of the fast channel open, and for a brief period of time, the open m gates and h gates allow inward sodium current to flow, depolarize the cell, and produce its upstroke. The action potential is depicted below. The h gates then close the channel and inactivate sodium conductance. When the upstroke of the action potential exceeds the threshold for activation of the slow inward current, the d gates open, allowing ingress of the slow inward current that contributes to the plateau phase of the action potential. The f gates of the slow channel close more slowly than the h gates. Although the slow inward channel remains open longer than does the fast channel, less total current flows.

When the resting membrane potential is reduced below −60 mV by increasing $[K]_o$ from 4.0 to 14.0 mm *(middle panel)*, the cell depolarizes to −60 mV and the fast channel becomes inactivated because the h gates remain closed. Even though the m gate may open during activation, the amount of sodium current is too small to elicit an action potential. The inactivation gates of the slow channel (f gates) are only partially closed, and when the cell is excited after addition of catecholamine *(right panel)*, the d gates open and permit flow of a slow inward current that causes a slow-response action potential. This action potential resembles those in panels *A, C,* and *F* of Figure 20–15. (Reproduced by permission from Wit, A. L., and Bigger, J. T., Jr.: Possible electrophysiological mechanisms for lethal arrhythmias accompanying myocardial ischemia and infarction. Circulation *52* (Suppl. 3):96, 1975. Copyright 1975 American Heart Association.)

Membrane voltage also may regulate current flow by altering the status of the channel gates, thereby altering conductance. For the Na^+ channel,

$$gi_{Na} = \bar{g}_{Na}\, m^3h$$

where gi_{Na} is the conductance of the Na^+ channel at a given voltage, $\bar{g}_{Na}$ is the maximum possible conductance of the channel, m^3 represents the status of the activation gate (m = 1, the gate is open; m = 0, the gate is closed), and h represents the status of the inactivation gate (h = 1, gate open; h = 0, gate closed). Since the opening and closing of the gates are voltage and time dependent, the conductance of the channel (g) will be some fraction of the maximum possible conductance ($\bar{g}_{Na}$), depending on membrane voltage and the period during which the membrane has been at that voltage. $\dot{V}_{max}$ in Purkinje fibers approximates the Na^+ current. The state of the channel influences the effects of drugs (Fig. 20–18; see also Chap. 21).

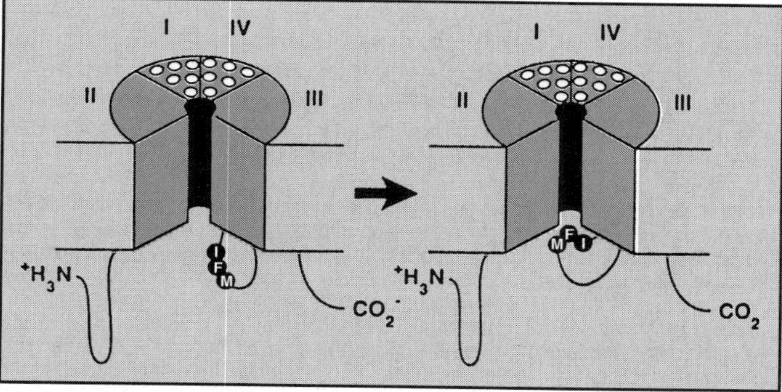

FIGURE 20–17. Mechanism of inactivation of sodium channels. The hinged-lid mechanism of sodium channel inactivation is illustrated. The intracellular loop connecting domains III and IV of the sodium channel is depicted as forming a hinged lid. The critical residue (Phe 1489 F) is shown as occluding the intracellular mouth of the pore. (From Catteral, W. A.: Molecular analysis of voltage gated sodium channels in the heart and other tissues. *In* Zipes, D. P., and Jalife, J. [eds.]: Cardiac Electrophysiology: From Cell to Bedside. 2nd ed. Philadelphia, W. B. Saunders Company, 1994, p. 1.)

UPSTROKE OF THE ACTION POTENTIAL. In normal atrial and ventricular muscle and in the fibers in the His-Purkinje system, action potentials have very rapid upstrokes with a large $\dot{V}_{max}$ and are called *fast responses.* Action potentials in the normal sinus and atrioventricular (AV) nodes have very slow upstrokes with a reduced $\dot{V}_{max}$ and are called *slow responses*[30] (Fig. 20–15 and Table 20–3). Upstrokes of "slow responses" are mediated by a slow inward, predominantly Ca^{++} current (I_{Ca}) rather than the fast inward I_{Na} (Table 20–4). These potentials received the name *slow response* because the time required for activation and inactivation of the slow inward current (I_{si}) is approximately an order of magnitude slower than that for the fast inward Na^+ current (I_{Na}). Recovery from inactivation also takes longer. Calcium entry and $[Ca^{++}]_i$ help promote inactivation. Thus the slow channel opens (activation gates d) and closes (inactivation gates f) more slowly than the fast channel, remains open for a longer time, and requires more time following a stimulus to be reactivated (see Fig. 20–16). In fact, recovery of excitability outlasts full restoration of maximum diastolic potential. This means that even though the membrane potential has returned to normal, the cell has not recovered excitability completely because the latter depends on elapse of a certain amount of time (i.e., is time

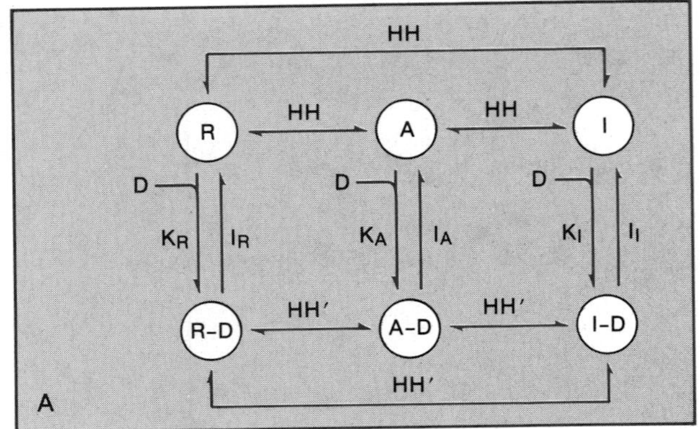

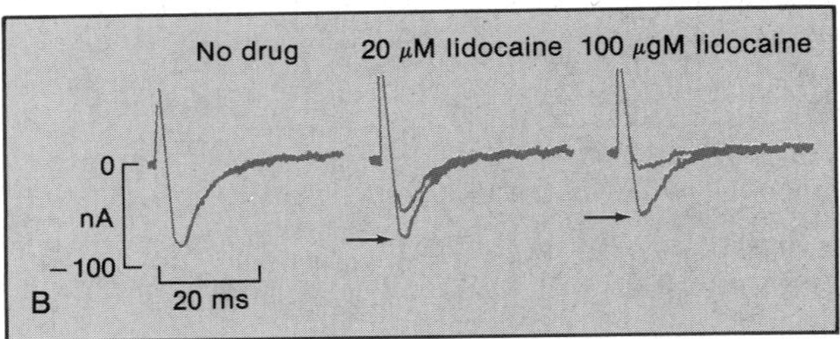

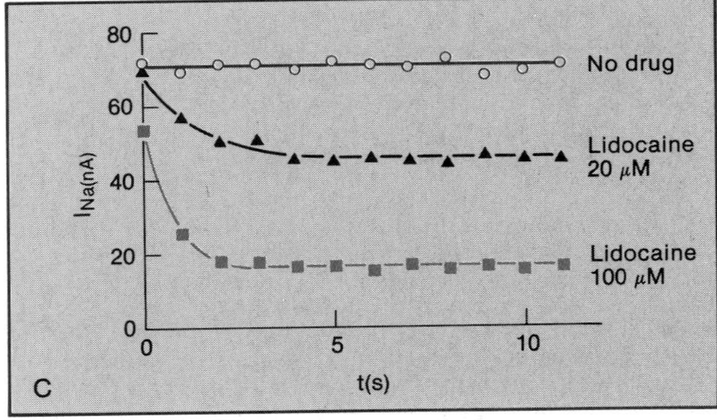

FIGURE 20–18. **Interaction between sodium channels and lidocaine.** ***A,*** **Schematic of the modulated receptor hypothesis is presented. Sodium channel gating is represented by transitions between a resting state (R), an open state (A), and an inactivated state (I). The rate constants for binding and unbinding of drug to the channel (k's, l's) depend on the gating state. The presence of bound drug alters the gating transitions from their normal kinetics (HH for Hodgkin-Huxley) to modified kinetics (HH′). Application of this hypothesis explains why some drugs affect cardiac electrophysiological properties according to different channel states, e.g., depolarized or repolarized conditions. (From Hondeghem, L. M., and Katzung, B. G.: Antiarrhythmic agents: The modulated receptor mechanism of action of sodium and calcium-blocking drugs. Annu. Rev. Pharmacol. Toxicol.** ***24:***387, **1984).**

B, **An example of use dependent block of I_{Na} by lidocaine is demonstrated. I_{Na} was measured (nA) during trains of 500 msec pulses when the cell was depolarized from a holding potential of −105 mV to −35 mV at 1 Hz following a period of rest. The traces show membrane currents associated with the 1st and 12th pulses superimposed, and the graph** ***(C)*** **plots measured I_{Na} amplitudes for each of the 12 pulses. Lidocaine exerted relatively little effect on the first inward current signal following the rest period (arrows,** ***B*****), but it substantially reduced peak I_{Na} following repetitive depolarizations. Lidocaine exerted a greater effect at the higher concentration. This figure illustrates that lidocaine blocks the sodium channel and reduces I_{Na} to a greater degree after repeated depolarizations of the cell compared with the first depolarization when the cell has been resting (use-dependence). (From Bean, B. P., Cohen, C. J., and Tsien, R. W.: Lidocaine block of cardiac sodium channels. J. Gen. Physiol.** ***81:***613, **1983.)**

dependent) and not just on recovery of a particular membrane potential (i.e., voltage dependence).

Calcium channels are much more selective for Ca^{++} than sodium channels are for Na^+. Selectivity results from the presence of binding sites for which the permeant ions must compete, and under physiological conditions, more than 90 per cent of the inward current through the calcium channel is carried by Ca^{++}. Other divalent cations such as barium and strontium also can carry I_{si}. The magnitude of I_{si} is determined by the probability of calcium channel opening (P), the current through an open channel (i), and the number of channels (N): $I_{si} = N \cdot P \cdot i$. There are estimated to be 1 to 10 functional Ca^{++} channels/μM^2 surface area. At 3 mM $[Ca^{++}]_o$ and a membrane potential of 0 mV, i approximates 0.05 pA.

The threshold for activation of I_{si}, i.e., the voltage the cell must reach to "turn on" the slow inward current, is about −30 to −40 mV. In fast-response type fibers, I_{si} is normally activated during phase 0 by the regenerative depolarization caused by the fast sodium current. Current flows through both fast and slow channels during the latter part of the action potential upstroke. However, I_{si} is much smaller than the peak Na^+ current and therefore contributes little to the action potential until the fast Na^+ current is inactivated, after completion of phase 0. Thus, I_{si} affects mainly the plateau of action potentials recorded in atrial and ventricular muscle and His-Purkinje fibers. When the fast Na^+ current inactivates rapidly, such as in frog ventricle, I_{si} may contribute noticeably to the peak of phase 0. In addition, I_{si} can be activated and may play a prominent role in partially depolarized cells in which the fast Na^+ channels have been inactivated, if conditions are appropriate for slow-channel activation.

At least two types of calcium currents exist: a slowly inactivating high-threshold dihydropyridine-sensitive current (slow or L current, $I_{Ca\text{-}L}$) and a fast inactivating low-threshold dihydropyridine-insensitive current (fast or T current, $I_{Ca\text{-}T}$). $I_{Ca\text{-}L}$ produces repolarization and propagation in sinus and AV nodal cells and contributes to the plateau, triggering calcium release from the sarcoplasmic reticulum in atrial, ventricular, and His-Purkinje cells. Calcium channel blockers block this channel, which is strongly modulated by neurotransmitters. $I_{Ca\text{-}T}$ is activated at thresholds intermediate between I_{Na} and $I_{Ca\text{-}L}$ and probably contributes inward current to the later stages of phase 4 depolarizations in the sinus node and His-Purkinje cells.[41,43–50]

Other significant differences exist between the fast and slow channels (Table 20–4). Drugs that elevate cyclic AMP levels such as beta-adrenoceptor agonists, phosphodiesterase inhibitors such as theophylline, and the lipid-soluble derivative of cyclic AMP, dibutyryl cyclic AMP, increase $I_{Ca\text{-}L}$. The beta-adrenoceptor agonist, binding to specific sarcolemmal receptors, facilitates the dissociation of two subunits of a regulatory protein (G protein, p. 372), one of which (G_s) activates adenylate cyclase and thus increases intracellular levels of cyclic AMP. The latter binds to a regulatory subunit of a cyclic AMP–dependent protein kinase that promotes phosphorylation of specific membrane proteins controlling the permeability of the slow channel. This putative conformational change in the channel increases the magnitude of the current or the conductance to the ion, presumably by increasing the amount of time the individual channels are open, without increasing the total number of calcium channels. The probability of channel opening increases.

The alpha subunit of the regulatory protein G_s can activate Ca channels directly. Acetylcholine reduces $I_{Ca\text{-}L}$ by decreasing adenylate cyclase activity. However, acetylcholine stimulates cGMP accumula-

TABLE 20–3 CARDIAC CURRENTS

INWARD CURRENTS	
I_{Na}	Fast inward current carried by Na^+ through a voltage-activated sodium channel.
$I_{Na\text{-}B}$	Proposed background Na^+ current through a voltage-independent channel in sinus nodal cells.
$I_{Ca\text{-}L}$	L-type (long-lasting) calcium current blocked by verapamil, diltiazem, and dihydropyridines, produces depolarization and propagation in SA and AV nodal cells, and contributes to the plateau of atrial, His-Purkinje, and ventricular cells; may induce early afterdepolarizations and calcium overload that could induce delayed afterdepolarizations.
$I_{Ca\text{-}T}$	T-type (transient) calcium current, may contribute inward current to the later stages of phase 4 depolarization in SA nodal and His-Purkinje cells.
I_f	Inward current carried by Na^+ and K^+ that is activated by polarization to negative membrane potentials in SA and AV nodal cells and His-Purkinje cells, generating phase 4 depolarization; increases the rate of impulse initiation in pacemaker cells.
I_{NS}	Inward current carried by Na^+ and, under some conditions, activated by Ca^{++} release from the sarcoplasmic reticulum during intracellular Ca^{++} overload, contributes to delayed afterdepolarizations; also can be the I_{T1}, the transient inward current.
OUTWARD CURRENTS	
I_{K1}	K^+ current responsible for maintaining resting potential near the K^+ equilibrium potential in atrial, AV nodal, His-Purkinje, and ventricular cells; also called the inward rectifier.
I_K	K^+ current carried through voltage-gated channels; also called delayed rectifier; major current causing repolarization; enhancement shortens repolarization while blockade lengthens it. This current is subdivided into a current with rapid activation and inactivation kinetics ($I_{K\text{-}R}$), a current with ultrarapid kinetics ($I_{K\text{-}UR}$), and a current with slow kinetics ($I_{K\text{-}S}$).
I_{to}	K^+ current turns on rapidly after depolarization and then inactivates; one type is voltage activated and modulated by neurotransmitters; the other type is activated by intracellular Ca^{++}.
$I_{K(ACh)}$	K^+ current whose channel is activated by the muscarinic (M_2) receptor via GTP regulatory (G) protein signal transduction; particularly important in SA and AV nodal cells and in atrial cells, where it can produce significant hyperpolarization, and in atrium, where it produces marked shortening of repolarization; appears identical to the channel opened by purinergic (adenosine) receptor and also designated $I_{K(Ado)}$.
$I_{K(ATP)}$	K^+ channel blocked by ATP and strongly activated during hypoxia and ischemia when intracellular ATP concentration falls; may contribute to shortening of action potential duration during ischemia.
I_{Cl}	Cl^- current increased by adrenergic stimulation, contributing to repolarization.
$I_{K(Ca)}$	K^+ current carried through a channel that is activated by intracellular Ca^{++}, accelerating repolarization in calcium-overloaded heart.
$I_{K(Na)}$	K^+ current activated by high cytosolic sodium concentrations and may promote repolarization in sodium overloaded heart.
I_{Arach}	Current activated by arachidonic acid and other fatty acids, especially in acid pH, for example, when these metabolites are liberated during ischemia.
PUMPS	
Na-K	Blocked by digitalis; generates small outward $I_{Na\text{-}K\ pump}$ current; when fully operative, $3Na^+$ leave and $2K^+$ enter the cell.
Ca	Found in sarcoplasmic reticulum; ATP-dependent.
CARRIERS	
Na/Ca	Countertransport system in sarcolemma and mitochondria; generates $I_{Na/Ca}$ by exchanging $1Ca^{++}$ for $3Na^+$; may contribute to generation of delayed afterdepolarizations during Ca^{++} overload.
Na/H	Exchanger blocked by amiloride.
Na/K/Cl	Cotransporter blocked by amiloride.
Cl/HCO_3	Exchanger.

tion. cGMP has negligible effects on the basal $I_{Ca\text{-}L}$ but decreases $I_{Ca\text{-}L}$ that has been elevated by beta-adrenoceptor agonists. This effect is mediated by cyclic AMP hydrolysis via a cGMP-stimulated cyclic nucleotide phosphodiesterase.[22]

DIFFERENCES BETWEEN CHANNELS. Fast and slow channels can be differentiated on the basis of their pharmacological sensitivity. Drugs that block the slow channel with a *fair* degree of specificity include verapamil, nifedipine, diltiazem, D-600 (a methoxy derivative of verapamil), and compounds such as manganese, lanthanum, nickel, and cobalt. Antiarrhythmic agents such as lidocaine, quinidine, procainamide, and disopyramide (see Chap. 21) affect the fast channel and not the slow channel. The puffer fish poison tetrodotoxin (TTX), which is too toxic to be used clinically, blocks the fast channel with considerable specificity (Table 20–4).

While fast-response action potentials are characteristic of atrial and ventricular muscle and His-Purkinje tissue, slow-response type action potentials are found in the normal sinus and AV nodes and many kinds of diseased tissue (Table 20–4). Normal action potentials recorded from the sinus node and the N region of the AV node have a reduced resting membrane potential, action potential amplitude, overshoot, upstroke, and conduction velocity compared with action potentials in muscle or Purkinje fibers (Fig. 20–15).

Slow-channel blockers, but not TTX, suppress sinus and AV nodal action potentials. The prolonged time for reactivation of the $I_{Ca\text{-}L}$ probably accounts for the fact that sinus and AV nodal cells remain refractory longer than the time it takes for full voltage repolarization to occur. Thus premature stimulation immediately after the membrane potential reaches full repolarization leads to action potentials with reduced amplitudes and upstroke velocities. Therefore, slow conduction and prolonged refractoriness are characteristic features of nodal cells. These cells also have a reduced "safety factor for conduction," which means that the stimulating efficacy of the propagating impulse is low and conduction block occurs easily. Membranes of nodal cells probably do have Na channels that are inactivated by the relatively depolarized range of potentials over which activity takes place. Hyperpolarization exposes a fast TTX-sensitive sodium current in nodal cells.

INWARD CURRENTS. Thus I_{Na} and I_{Ca} represent two important inward currents. Another important inward current is I_f, also called the *pacemaker current*.[17–21] This current is activated by hyperpolarization and is carried by Na^+ and K^+. It generates phase 4 diastolic depolarization in the sinus node. I_f activation is the major mechanism by which beta-adrenergic and cholinergic neurotransmitters regulate the cardiac rhythm under physiologic conditions (see p. 63). Catecholamines increase the probability of channel opening, with no change in single channel amplitude, and increase the discharge rate, with cholinergic action, in general, having an opposite effect.

A variety of manipulations, including those which block or inactivate I_{Na} (such as administration of TTX or depolarization of the cell membrane with K^+), combined with those that increase $I_{Ca\text{-}L}$ (such as administration of Ca^{++} or catecholamines), or those that decrease the outward potassium currents (such as barium), can transform a fast-channel–dependent fiber (e.g., a Purkinje fiber) to a slow-channel–dependent fiber. Whether these artificial in vitro alterations have clinical relevance is not known, but it is possible that myocardial ischemia or infarction, for example, can produce this transformation (Fig. 20–15*F*).

The electrophysiological changes accompanying *acute* myocardial ischemia may represent a depressed form of a fast response in the center of the ischemic zone and a slow response in the border area.[67] Probable slow-response activity has been shown in myocardium resected from patients undergoing surgery for recurrent ventricular tachyarrhythmias (Fig. 20–19). Whether and how slow responses play a role in the genesis of ventricular arrhythmias in these patients has not been established. I_{Na} is another inward current gated by $[Ca^{++}]$ that contributes to delayed afterdepolarizations (Table 20–3).

TABLE 20–4 CHARACTERISTICS OF FAST AND SLOW INWARD CURRENTS IN CARDIAC TISSUE

	FAST	SLOW
Primary charge carrier	NA	Ca (Na)
Activation threshold	− 70 to − 55 mV	− 55 to − 30 mV
Magnitude	1 to 30 μA	0.1 to 3.0 μA
Time constant of		
Activation	<1 msec	10 to 20 msec
Inactivation	<1 msec	50 to 500 msec
Inhibitors	Tetrodotoxin, local anesthetics, sustained depolarization at < − 40 mV	Verapamil, D-600, nifedipine, diltiazem, Mn, Co, Ni, La
Resting membrane potential	− 80 to − 95 mV	− 40 to − 70 mV
Conduction velocity	0.3 to 3.0 M/sec	0.01 to 0.10 M/sec
Rate of rise ($\dot{V}_{max}$) of action potential upstroke	200 to 1000 V/sec	1 to 10 V/sec
Action potential amplitude	100 to 130 mV	35 to 75 mV
Response to stimulus	All-or-none	Affected by characteristics of stimulus
Recovery of excitability	Prompt, ends with repolarization	Delayed, outlasts full repolarization
Safety factor for conduction	High	Low
Major current of action potential upstroke in the following:		
SA node	−	+
Atrial myocardium	+	−
AV node (N region)	−	+
His-Purkinje system	+	−
Ventricular myocardium	+	−
Neurotransmitter influence		
Beta-adrenergic	−	↑↑
Alpha-adrenergic	−	↑
Muscarinic cholinergic	−	↓ In atrium ↓ In ventricle

Phase 1—Early Rapid Repolarization

Following phase 0, the membrane repolarizes rapidly and transiently to near 0 mV, partly owing to inactivation of I_{Na} or activation of a transient outward current carried mostly by K ions. I_{to},[65] a K^+ current (Table 20–3), turns on rapidly after depolarization and then inactivates. One type of I_{to} is activated by $[Ca^{++}]_i$, and the other is voltage activated and modulated by neurotransmitter. I_{to} can modulate action potential duration and is nonuniformly distributed, being found in subepicardial but not subendocardial ventricular muscle cells. M cells are in a uniform subepicardial sheet and have repolarization characteristics similar to Purkinje fibers. They have sparse $I_{k\text{-}s}$ and may be important in the development of early afterdepolarizations and torsades de pointes[68–70] (see p. 566). They may be responsible for the U wave in the electrocardiogram (ECG). Cl^- moving intracellularly through a Cl channel also may affect the plateau. Beta-adrenoceptor stimulation via cyclic AMP–dependent protein kinase, activation of adenylate cyclase, and histamine activate the chloride current.[71] The increase in intra-

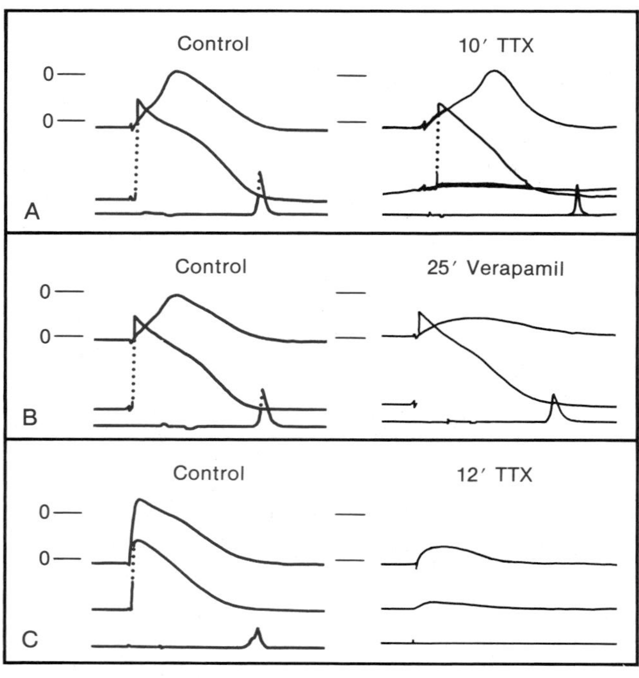

FIGURE 20–19. Effects of tetrodotoxin (TTX) and verapamil on action potentials in diseased human ventricle, removed from a patient at the time of endocardial resection for recurrent ventricular tachycardia. *A,* Action potentials and upstroke velocity recordings from an abnormal cell (upper action potential recording) and a relatively normal cell (lower action potential recording) before *(left)* and after *(right)* exposure to TTX for 10 minutes. $\dot{V}_{max}$ for the lower cell is shown in the bottom tracing. TTX produced activation delay and intermittent conduction block in the normal cell but had little effect on the action potential of the abnormal cell *(right panel).* Two consecutive cycles are superimposed in the right panel. *B,* After washout of TTX, the same two cells were exposed to verapamil for 25 minutes. Verapamil reduced both the action potential and the amplitude of the abnormal cell without affecting its resting membrane potential and slightly reduced both the action potential amplitude and V_{max} in the normal cell *(right panel). C,* Effects of TTX on a different specimen of myocardium from the same patient. Control recordings are shown on the left. In these cells, TTX markedly reduced action potential amplitude and $\dot{V}_{max}$ *(right panel),* while verapamil only slightly reduced action potential amplitude (not shown). (From Gilmour, R. F., Jr., et al.: Cellular electrophysiological abnormalities of diseased human ventricular myocardium. Am. J. Cardiol. *51:*137, 1983.)

cellular negative ions reduces the positive membrane voltage, and the membrane potential returns to near 0 mV, from which the plateau, or phase 2, arises. Sometimes a slight transient depolarization follows phase 1 repolarization. Phase 1 is well defined and separated from phase 2 in Purkinje fibers and some muscle fibers.

Phase 2—Plateau

During the plateau phase, which may last several hundred milliseconds, membrane conductance to all ions falls to rather low values. Potassium conductance (g_K) falls almost immediately upon depolarization, in spite of the large electrochemical gradient for K^+, owing to "inward-going rectification." *Rectification* simply means voltage dependence of membrane resistance. Inward-going rectification means that when the membrane depolarizes, it passes inward current more easily than it passes outward current, or in this instance, K^+ can enter the cell more easily than it can exit, and therefore, despite multiple important outward K^+ currents and a large electrochemical gradient, g_K is low and few K^+ ions leave the cell. Sodium conductance (g_{Na}) is low because of inactivation of sodium channels. Minor contributions to repolarization include a small inward Cl^- flux and electrogenic Na^+-K^+ exchange, pumping out 3 Na^+ in exchange for 2 K^+. The Na^+-K^+ exchange does not turn on and off with each single action potential but restores the ionic gradient over a cumulative time period. $I_{Ca\text{-}L}$, active during the plateau, supplies a small (compared with I_{Na}) inward current and balances these outward currents, and membrane voltage remains near zero for more than 100 msec. An inward Na^+ current, mentioned earlier, is blocked by tetrodotoxin, and also contributes to the plateau.

Phase 3—Final Rapid Repolarization

In this portion of the action potential, repolarization proceeds rapidly, owing at least in part to two currents: time-dependent inactivation of $I_{Ca\text{-}L}$, so that intracellular movement of positive charges decreases, and activation of an outward K^+ current (called the *delayed rectifier* or I_K, the major current-causing repolarization) (Table 20–3), so that extracellular movement of positive charges increases. The net membrane current becomes more outward, and the membrane potential shifts in a negative direction. As repolarization continues, g_K increases, and these repolarization changes self-perpetuate in a regenerative manner.

Phase 4—Diastolic Depolarization

(See also p. 557)

Under normal conditions, the membrane potential of atrial and ventricular muscle cells remains steady throughout diastole. I_{K1} is the current responsible for maintaining the resting potential near the K^+ equilibrium potential in atrial, AV nodal, His-Purkinje, and ventricular cells. I_{K1} is the inward rectifier, shutting off during depolarization. It is absent in sinus nodal cells. In other fibers found in certain parts of the atria, in the muscle of the mitral and tricuspid valves, in His-Purkinje fibers, and in the sinus node and distal portion of the AV node, the resting membrane potential does not remain constant in diastole but gradually depolarizes (Fig. 20–15*A*). If a propagating impulse does not depolarize the cell or group of cells, it may reach threshold by itself and produce a spontaneous action potential. The property possessed by spontaneously discharging cells is called *phase 4 diastolic depolarization;* when it leads to initiation of action potentials, automaticity results. The discharge rate of the sinus node normally exceeds the discharge rate of other potentially automatic pacemaker sites and thus maintains dominance of the cardiac rhythm. Discharge rate of the sinus node is more sensitive to the effects of norepinephrine and acetylcholine than is the discharge rate of ventricular muscle cells (Fig. 20–20). Normal or abnormal automaticity at other sites can discharge at rates faster than the sinus nodal discharge rate and can usurp control of the cardiac rhythm for one cycle or many.

Normal Automaticity

The ionic basis of automaticity is explained by a net gain in intracellular positive charges during diastole. Contributing to this change is a voltage-dependent channel activated by potentials negative to −50 to −60 mV, i.e., a hyperpolarization-activated inward pacemaker current. At this potential an inward current called I_f becomes activated and is carried by a channel relatively nonselective for monovalent cations. Hyperpolarization increases its rate of activation, and at −70 mV, the time constant ranges from 2 to 4 sec. I_f probably underlies the slow diastolic depolarization that occurs between −90 and −60 mV in Purkinje fibers. Although either K^+ or Na^+ can serve as ion transporters, I_f carries largely Na^+ at the more negative intracellular voltages. Extracellular K^+ ions activate I_f, but $[Na^+]_o$ does not influence its conductance.[17–21]

AUTOMATICITY IN SINUS NODAL CELLS. At the reduced membrane potentials of sinus nodal cells, I_f contributes only about 20 per cent of the pacemaker current, and automaticity is primarily dependent on I_K and $I_{Ca\text{-}L}$. However, sinus nodal cells exhibit significant I_f current if they are hyperpolarized in the range of −50 to −100 mV. Conversely, I_K in normally polarized Purkinje fibers adds little to the pacemaker current. The decay of I_K, together with the presence of an unidentified background inward current, and $I_{Ca\text{-}L}$ are the essential processes governing the rate of

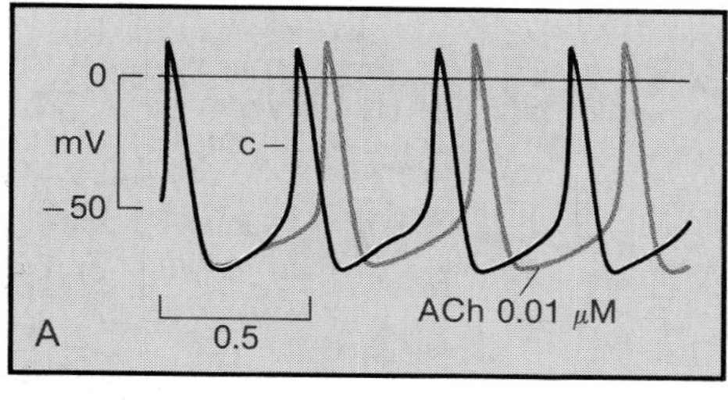

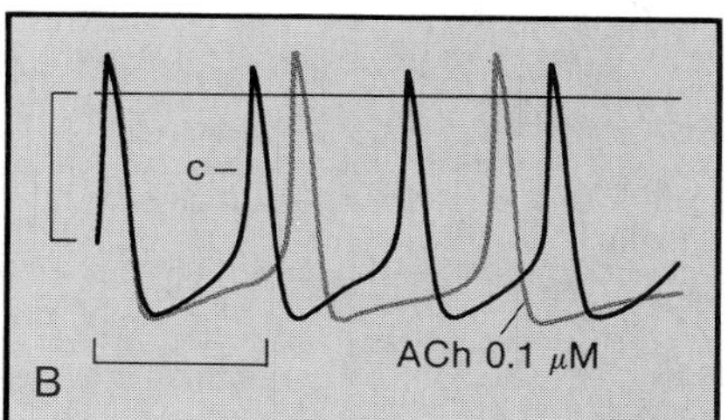

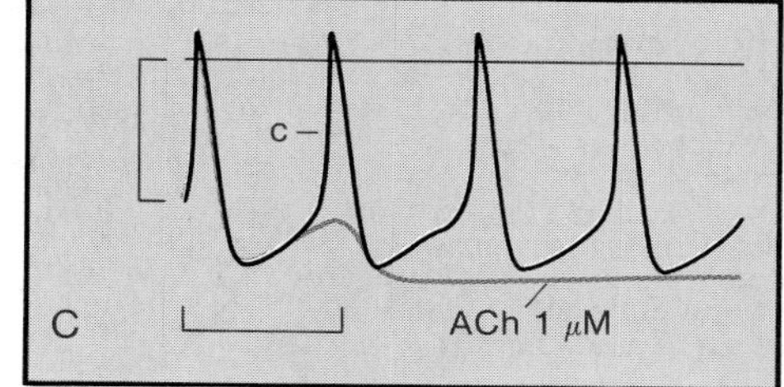

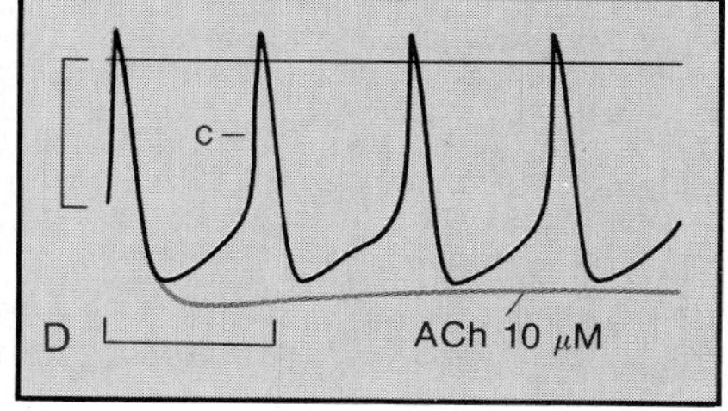

FIGURE 20–20. Effects of different doses of ACh on spontaneous activity in single SA node cell. *A–D,* Activity in the control Tyrode solution *(C)* is compared with that in the presence of 0.01, 0.1, 1.0, and 10 μM ACh, respectively. Each concentration of ACh was perfused for about 20 sec. Note that slowing occurred with 0.01 and 0.1 μM ACh and that the cell ceased to beat at higher concentrations, at which point hyperpolarization of the maximum diastolic depolarization also clearly appeared. (From DiFrancisco, D.: Current i_f and the neuronal modulation of heart rate. *In* Zipes, D. P., and Jalife, J. [eds.]: Cardiac Electrophysiology. From Cell to Bedside. Philadelphia, W. B. Saunders Company, 1990.)

pacemaker depolarization in sinus and AV nodal cells and in Purkinje fibers whose membrane potential has been depolarized to voltages largely positive to the activation range of I_f.[72]

Sinus nodal discharge rate maintains dominance over latent pacemaker sites because it depolarizes more rapidly and because of the mechanism called *overdrive suppression*, a phenomenon characterized by prolonged suppression of normal pacemakers in proportion to the duration and rate of stimulation by a more rapidly discharging pacemaker. The mechanism may relate to active Na extrusion during the more rapid rate that maintains diastolic depolarization of latent pacemakers at a level more negative than the threshold potential for automatic discharge.

The rate of sinus nodal discharge can be varied by several mechanisms in response to autonomic or other influences. The pacemaker locus can shift within or outside the sinus node to cells discharging faster or more slowly. If the pacemaker site remains the same, alterations in the slope of the diastolic depolarization, maximum diastolic potential, or threshold potential can speed or slow the discharge rate (Fig. 20–20). For example, if the slope of diastolic depolarization steepens, and if the resting membrane potential becomes less negative or the threshold potential more negative (within limits), discharge rate increases. Opposite changes slow the discharge rate.

Passive Membrane Electrical Properties

We have just discussed many of the features of active membrane properties. In addition, it is important to be aware of some features of the passive membrane properties, such as membrane resistance, capacitance, and cable properties.[35,57] The important difference between the active and passive states is that the active system responds out of proportion to the applied stimulus and thereby adds energy to the electrical system; the passive system responds proportionately to the size of the stimulus and does not add energy.

Although the cardiac cell membrane is resistant to current flow, it also has capacitative properties, which means it behaves like a battery and can store charges of opposite sign on its two sides: an excess of negative charges inside the membrane balanced by equivalent positive charges outside the membrane. These resistive and capacitative properties cause the membrane to take a certain amount of time to respond to an applied stimulus, rather than responding instantly, because the charges across the capacitative membrane must be altered first. A subthreshold rectangular-shaped current pulse applied to the membrane produces a slowly rising and decaying membrane-voltage change rather than a rectangular voltage change. A value called the *time constant of the membrane* reflects this property and is the time taken by the membrane voltage to reach 63 per cent of its final value after application of a steady current.

When aligned end to end, cardiac cells, particularly the His-Purkinje system, behave like a long cable in which current flows more easily inside the cell and to the adjacent cell across the gap junction than it does across the cell membrane to the outside. When current is injected at a point, most of it flows along the cell, but some leaks out. Because of this loss of current, the voltage change of a cell at a site distant from the point of applied current is less than the change in membrane voltage where the stimulus was given. A measure of this property of a cable is called the space or length constant λ; it is the distance along the cable from the point of stimulation that the voltage at steady state is 1/e (37 per cent) of its value at the point of introduction.

Restated, λ describes how far current flows before leaking passively across the surface membrane to a value about one-third its initial value. This distance is normally about 2 mm for Purkinje fibers, 0.5 mm for the sinus node, and 0.8 mm for ventricular muscle fibers. λ is about 10 times the length of an individual cell. As an example, if e is about 2.7 and a hyperpolarizing current pulse in a Purkinje fiber produces a membrane-voltage change of 15 mV at the site of current injection, the membrane potential change one space constant (2 mm) away would be $15/2.7 = 5.5$ mV.

Since the current loop in any circuit must be closed, current must flow back to its point of origin. Local circuit currents pass across gap junctions between cells and exit across the sarcolemmal membrane to close the loop and complete the circuit. Inward excitation currents in one area (carried by Na^+ in most regions) flow intracellularly along the length of the tissue (carried mostly by K^+), escape across the membrane, and flow extracellularly in a longitudinal direction. The outside local circuit current is the current recorded in an electrocardiogram. Through these local circuit currents the transmembrane potential of each cell influences the transmembrane potential of its neighbor because of the passive flow of current from one segment of the fiber to another across the low-resistance gap junctions.

If two cells having different resting membrane potentials are coupled to one another, the resting potentials of each cell will equalize; i.e., one cell will depolarize and the other will hyperpolarize. This "electrotonic" influence of neighboring cells on each other is determined chiefly by the length constant of the fiber and is due to the passive spread of current.

As discussed earlier, the speed of conduction depends on active membrane properties such as the magnitude of the Na^+ current, a measure of which is $\dot{V}_{max}$. Passive membrane properties also contribute to conduction velocity and include excitability threshold, which influences the capability of cells adjacent to the one that has been discharged to reach threshold; the intracellular resistance of the cell, which is determined by the free ions in the cytoplasm; the resistance of the gap junction, and the cross-sectional area of the cell. Direction of propagation is crucial due to the influence of anisotropy, as mentioned earlier.

Loss of Membrane Potential and Arrhythmia Development

Most acquired abnormalities of cardiac muscle or specialized fibers that result in arrhythmias produce a loss of membrane potential; i.e., maximum diastolic potential becomes less negative. This change should be viewed as a symptom of an underlying abnormality, analogous to fever or jaundice, rather than a diagnostic category in and of itself, because both the ionic changes resulting in cellular depolarization and the more fundamental biochemical or metabolic abnormalities responsible for the ionic alterations are probably multicausal. Cellular depolarization can result from elevated $[K^+]_o$ or decreased $[K^+]_i$, an increase in membrane permeability to Na^+ (P_{Na} increases), or a decrease in membrane permeability to K^+ (P_K decreases). Reference to Equation 2 (see p. 556) illustrates that these changes alone or in combination make V_r less negative.

Normal cells perfused by an abnormal milieu (e.g., hyperkalemia), abnormal cells perfused by a normal milieu (e.g., healed myocardial infarction), or abnormal cells perfused by an abnormal milieu (e.g., acute myocardial ischemia and infarction) may exist alone or in combination to reduce resting membrane voltage. Each of these changes can have one or more biochemical or metabolic causes. For example, acute myocardial ischemia results in decreased $[K^+]_i$[73–75] and increased $[K^+]_o$, norepinephrine release, and acidosis that may be related to an increase in intracellular Ca^{++} and Ca-induced membrane oscillations and accumulation of amphipathic lipid metabolites and oxygen-free radicals. All these changes can contribute to the development of abnormal electrophysiological environment and arrhythmias during ischemia and reperfusion. Knowledge of these changes may provide insight into therapy that actually reverses basic defects and restores membrane potential or other abnormalities to normal.

EFFECTS OF REDUCED RESTING POTENTIAL. The reduced resting membrane potential alters depolarization and repolarization phases of the cardiac action potential. For example, partial membrane depolarization prevents complete recovery from inactivation (h gate) of the rapid Na^+ channel. This reduces the number of available Na^+ channels for depolarization and decreases the magnitude of the rapid Na^+ current during phase 0. The subsequent reduction in $\dot{V}_{max}$ and action potential amplitude prolongs conduction time of the propagated impulse, at times to the point of block.

Action potentials with upstrokes dependent on the rapid Na^+ current flowing through partially inactivated Na^+ channels are called *depressed fast responses* (Fig. 20–19*C*). Their contours often resemble, and may be difficult to distinguish from, slow responses, in which upstrokes are due to $I_{Ca\text{-}L}$ (Fig. 20–15*F*). Membrane depolarization to levels of -60 to -70 mV may inactivate half the Na^+ channels, while depolarization to -50 mV or less may inactivate all the Na^+ channels. At membrane potentials positive to -50 mV, $I_{Ca\text{-}L}$ can be activated to generate phase 0 if conditions are appropriate. These action potential changes are

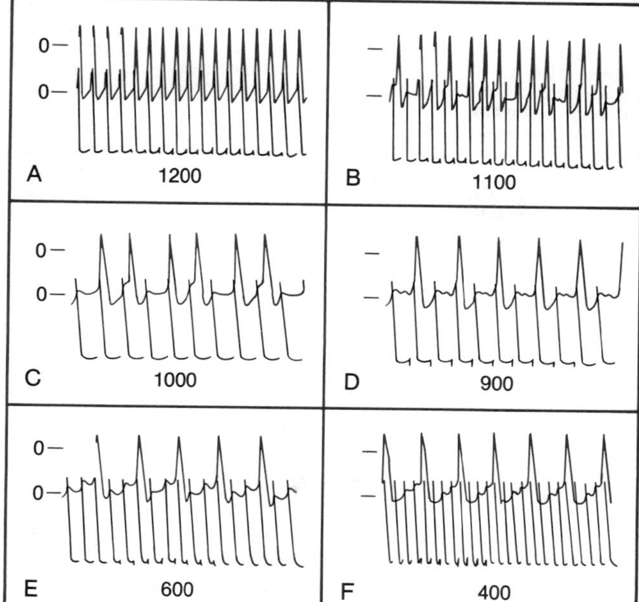

FIGURE 20–21. Rate-dependent conduction from the normal zone into the abnormal zone. When the pacing cycle length in the normal zone was shortened from 1200 to 400 msec *(panels A to F),* increasing degrees of entrance block into the abnormal area occurred, progressing from 1:1 conduction at a cycle length of 1200 msec, to 4:3 conduction at 1100 msec, 3:2 conduction at 1000 msec, 2:1 conduction at 900 msec, 3:1 conduction at 600 msec, and 4:1 conduction at 400 msec. Pacing the abnormal zone (not shown) resulted in block to the normal zone (unidirectional propagation). Vertical calibration: 50 mV. Horizontal calibration: 4 sec in *A* and *B* and 2 sec in *C* to *F.* (From Gilmour, R. F., Jr., et al.: Cellular electrophysiologic abnormalities of diseased human ventricular myocardium. Am. J. Cardiol. *51*:137, 1983.)

likely to be heterogeneous with unequal degrees if Na^+ inactivation that create areas with minimally reduced velocity, more severely depressed zones, and areas of complete block. These uneven changes are propitious for the development of arrhythmias (Fig. 20–21).

In these cells with reduced membrane potential, refractoriness may outlast voltage recovery of the action potential; i.e., the cell may still be refractory or partially refractory after the resting membrane potential returns to its most negative value. Further, if block of the cardiac impulse occurs in a fairly localized area without significant slowing of conduction proximal to the site of block, cells in this proximal zone exhibit short action potentials and refractory periods because unexcited cells distal to the block (still in a polarized state) electrotonically speed recovery in cells proximal to the site of block.

If conduction slows gradually proximal to the site of block, the duration of these action potentials and their refractory periods may be prolonged. Some cells may exhibit abnormal electrophysiological properties even though they have a relatively normal resting membrane potential.

TABLE 20–5 MECHANISMS OF ARRHYTHMOGENESIS

I. DISORDERS OF IMPULSE FORMATION
- A. Automaticity
  - 1. Normal automaticity
    - a. Experimental examples—Normal in vivo or in vitro sinus node, Purkinje fibers, others
    - b. Clinical examples—Sinus tachycardia or bradycardia inappropriate for the clinical situation, possibly ventricular parasystole
  - 2. Abnormal automaticity
    - a. Experimental example—Depolarization-induced automaticity in Purkinje fibers or ventricular muscle
    - b. Clinical example—Possibly accelerated ventricular rhythms after myocardial infarction
- B. Triggered Activity
  - 1. Early afterdepolarizations (EADs)
    - a. Experimental examples—EADs produced by barium, hypoxia, high concentrations of catecholamines, drugs such as sotalol, *N*-acetylprocainamide, cesium
    - b. Clinical examples—Possibly idiopathic and acquired long Q-T syndromes and associated ventricular arrhythmias
  - 2. Delayed afterdepolarizations (DADs)
    - a. Experimental example—DADs produced in Purkinje fibers by digitalis
    - b. Clinical example—Possibly some digitalis-induced arrhythmias

II. DISORDERS OF IMPULSE CONDUCTION
- A. Block
  - 1. Bidirectional or unidirectional without reentry
    - a. Experimental example—SA, AV, bundle branch, Purkinje-muscle, others
    - b. Clinical example—SA, AV, bundle branch, others
  - 2. Unidirectional block with reentry
    - a. Experimental examples—AV node, Purkinje-muscle junction, infarcted myocardium, others
    - b. Clinical examples—Reciprocating tachycardia in WPW syndrome, AV nodal reentry, VT due to bundle branch reentry, others
  - 3. Reflection
    - a. Experimental example—Purkinje fiber with area of inexcitability
    - b. Clinical example—Unknown

III. COMBINED DISORDERS
- A. Interactions between automatic foci
  - 1. Experimental examples—Depolarizing or hyperpolarizing subthreshold stimuli speed or slow automatic discharge rate
  - 2. Clinical examples—Modulated parasystole
- B. Interactions between automaticity and conduction
  - 1. Experimental examples—Deceleration-dependent block, overdrive suppression of conduction, entrance and exit block
  - 2. Clinical examples—Similar to experimental

MECHANISMS OF ARRHYTHMOGENESIS

(Table 20–5)

The mechanisms responsible for cardiac arrhythmias are generally divided into categories of disorders of impulse formation, disorders of impulse conduction, or combinations of both.[58,76–79] It is important to realize, however, that our present diagnostic tools do not permit unequivocal determination of the electrophysiological mechanisms responsible for most clinically occurring arrhythmias or their ionic bases. This is especially true for ventricular arrhythmias. It is very difficult to separate reentry from automaticity clinically. At best, one can postulate that a particular arrhythmia is "most consistent with" or "best explained by" one or the other electrophysiological mechanism. Some tachyarrhythmias can be started by one mechanism and perpetuated by another. For example, premature ventricular depolarization due to abnormal automaticity can precipitate an episode of ventricular tachycardia sustained by reentry. An episode of tachycardia due to one mechanism can precipitate another episode due to a different mechanism.[80]

Disorders of Impulse Formation

This category is defined as inappropriate discharge rate of the normal pacemaker, the sinus node (e.g., sinus rates too fast or too slow for the physiological needs of the patient), or discharge of an ectopic pacemaker that controls the atrial or ventricular rhythm. Pacemaker discharge from ectopic sites, often called *latent* or *subsidiary pacemakers,* can occur in fibers located in several parts of the atria, the coronary sinus, atrioventricular valves, portions of the AV junction, and the His-Purkinje system. Ordinarily kept from reaching the level of threshold potential because of overdrive suppression by the more rapidly firing sinus node or electrotonic depression from contiguous fibers, ectopic pacemaker activity at one of these latent sites can become manifest when sinus nodal discharge rate slows or block occurs at some level between the sinus node and the ectopic pacemaker site, permitting *escape* of the latent pacemaker at the latter's normal discharge rate. A clinical example would be sinus bradycardia to a rate of 45 beats/min that permits an AV junctional escape complex to occur at a rate of 50 beats/min.

Alternatively, the discharge rate of the latent pacemaker can speed up inappropriately and usurp control of the cardiac rhythm from the sinus node that has been discharging at a normal rate. A clinical example would be interruption of normal sinus rhythm by a premature ventricular complex or a burst of ventricular tachycardia. It is important to remember that such disorders of impulse formation can be due to a speeding or slowing of a *normal* pacemaker mechanism (e.g., phase 4 diastolic depolarization that is ionically normal for the sinus node or for an ectopic site such as a Purkinje fiber but occurs inappropriately fast or slow) or due to an ionically *abnormal* pacemaker mechanism.

The patient with persistent sinus tachycardia at rest or sinus bradycardia during exertion exhibits inappropriate sinus nodal discharge rates, but the ionic mechanisms responsible for sinus nodal discharge may still be normal, although the kinetics or magnitude of the currents may be altered. Conversely, when a patient experiences ventricular tachycardia during an acute myocardial infarction, ionic mechanisms ordinarily not involved in formation of spontaneous impulses for this fiber type may be operative to generate this tachycardia. For example, although pacemaker activity generally is not found in ordinary working myocardium, the effects of myocardial infarction perhaps can depolarize these cells to membrane potentials at which inactivation of I_K and activation of $I_{Ca\text{-}L}$ cause automatic discharge. Recent experimental evidence suggests that some areas of the ventricle during *acute* myocardial ischemia can enhance, while others suppress, automaticity and afterdepolarizations.[67] Areas of conduction block that may produce entrance block to the automatic focus can protect it from the effects of overdrive suppression and favor the development of automatic discharge. Because the maximum rate that can be achieved by adrenergic stimulation of normal automaticity is generally less than 200 beats/min, it is likely that episodes of faster tachycardia are not due to enhanced normal automaticity.

ABNORMAL AUTOMATICITY. Mechanisms responsible for *normal* automaticity were described earlier (see p. 563). *Abnormal* automaticity can arise from cells that have reduced maximum diastolic potentials, often at membrane potentials positive to −50 mV, when I_K and $I_{Ca\text{-}L}$ may be operative.

Automaticity at membrane potentials more negative than −70 mV may be due to I_f. When the membrane potential is between −50 and −70 mV, the cell may be quiescent. Electrotonic effects from surrounding normally polarized or more depolarized myocardium will influence the development of automaticity. Abnormal automaticity has been found in Purkinje fibers removed from dogs subjected to myocardial infarction, in rat myocardium damaged by epinephrine, in human atrial samples, and in ventricular myocardial specimens from patients undergoing aneurysmectomy and endocardial resection for recurrent ventricular tachyarrhythmias.

Abnormal automaticity can be produced in normal muscle or Purkinje fibers by appropriate interventions such as current passage that reduces diastolic potential. Automatic discharge rate speeds up with progressive depolarization, while hyperpolarizing pulses slow the spontaneous firing. Other interventions, such as barium administration, produce automaticity during which action potentials are similar to those produced by current passage. Both may be due to I_K and $I_{Ca\text{-}L}$. It is possible that partial depolarization and failure to reach normal maximal diastolic potential can induce automatic discharge in most if not all cardiac fibers. Although this type of spontaneous automatic activity has been found in human atrial and ventricular fibers, its relation to the genesis of clinical arrhythmias has not been established.

Rhythms due to automaticity may be slow atrial, junctional and ventricular escape rhythms, certain types of atrial tachycardias (such as those produced by digitalis), accelerated junctional (nonparoxysmal junctional tachycardia), and idioventricular rhythms and parasystole (see Chap. 22).

Triggered Activity

Automaticity is the property of a fiber to initiate an impulse *spontaneously,* without need for prior stimulation, so that electrical quiescence does not occur. *Triggered activity* is initiated by afterdepolarizations that are depolarizing oscillations in membrane voltage induced by one or more preceding action potentials. Thus triggered activity is pacemaker activity that results *consequent* to a preceding impulse or series of impulses, without which electrical quiescence occurs (Figs. 20–22 and 20–23). This is not an automatic self-generating mechanism, and the term *triggered automaticity* is therefore contradictory. These depolarizations can occur before (Fig. 20–22) or after (Fig. 20–23) full repolarization of the fiber and are best termed *early afterdepolarizations* (EADs)[81–94] when they arise from a reduced level of membrane potential during phases 2 (type 1) and 3 (type 2) of the cardiac action potential and *late* or *delayed afterdepolarizations* (DADs) when they occur after completion of repolarization (phase 4) generally at a more negative membrane potential than from which EADs arise[95] (Table 20–6). All afterdepolarizations may not reach threshold potential, but if they do, they can trigger another afterdepolarization and thus self-perpetuate.

Early Afterdepolarizations (EADS)

A variety of interventions, each of which results in an increase in intracellular positivity, can cause EADs.[81–85] EADs may be responsible for the lengthened repolarization time and ventricular tachyarrhythmias in several clinical situations, such as the acquired and congenital forms of the long Q-T syndrome.[86–94] Left ansae subclaviae stimulation (Fig. 20–24) increases the amplitude of cesium-induced EADs in dogs and the prevalence of ventricular tachyarrhythmias more than does right ansae subclaviae stimulation. This is possibly because of a greater quantitative effect that the left stellate ganglion exerts on the left ventricle compared with the right stellate ganglion.

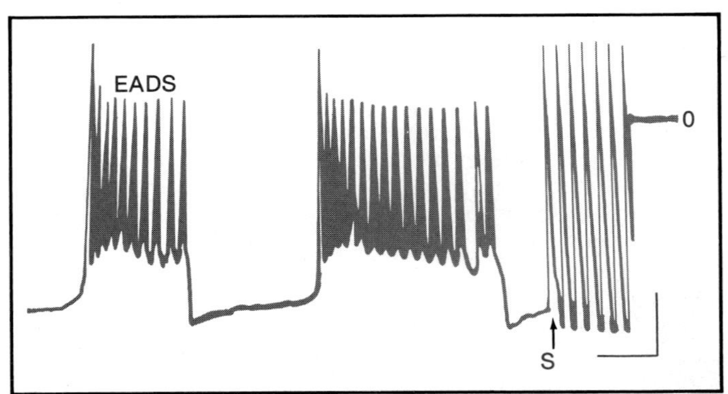

FIGURE 20–22. Early afterdepolarizations (EADs). Early afterdepolarizations occur spontaneously in an isolated canine cardiac Purkinje fiber when exposed to reduced extracellular potassium concentration. Note spontaneous phase four diastolic depolarization is present. In the initial two action potentials, a series of spontaneous depolarizations (EADs) result before the membrane returns to its maximum diastolic potential. Following the second series of EADs, pacing is begun (S) and normal action potentials follow. Horizontal calibration bar = 5 seconds, vertical bar = 25 mV. (From Kovacs, R. J., Bailey, J. C., and Zipes, D. P.: Mechanisms of cardiac arrhythmias. *In* Parmley, W. W., et al. [eds.]: Cardiology. Philadelphia, J. B. Lippincott, 1989.)

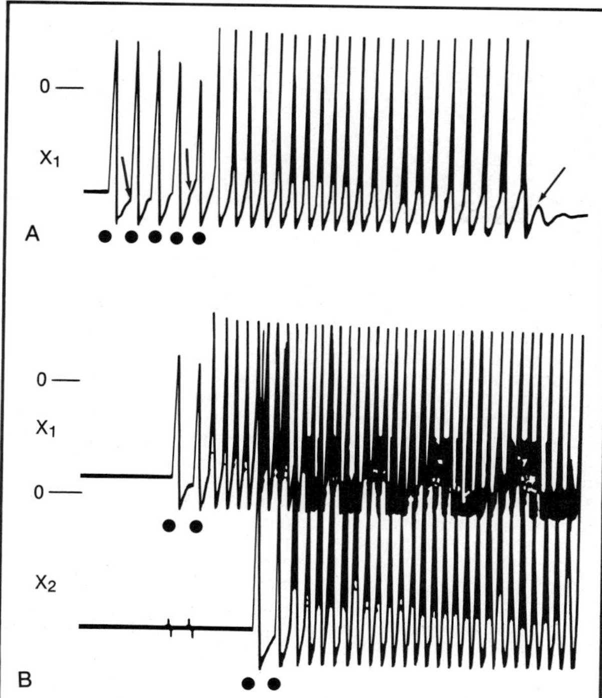

FIGURE 20–23. Triggered sustained rhythmic activity and delayed afterdepolarizations in diseased human ventricle. *A*, Spontaneous activity triggered by a series of driven action potentials (indicated by the dots) at a recording site X1. Note the gradual increase in size of the delayed afterdepolarizations (arrows) until the afterdepolarizations reaches threshold and maintains sustained rhythmic activity after cessation of pacing. The sustained rhythmic activity finally terminates when the last afterdepolarization fails to reach threshold (arrow). *B*, Initiation of triggered activity by intracellular current injection (indicated by dots beneath the respective action potential recordings) at sites X1 and X2, which lie along the same trabeculum. Although sites X1 and X2 were only about 4 mm apart, triggered sustained rhythmic activity from one site did not propagate to the other site, indicating complete dissociation between these two sites. For current pulses, cycle length = 2000 msec; pulse duration = 10 msec; pulse intensity = 200 na. Vertical calibration: 50 mV. Horizontal calibration: 10 sec. (From Gilmour, R. F., Jr., et al.: Cellular electrophysiological abnormalities of diseased human ventricular myocardium. Am. J. Cardiol. *51*:137, 1983.)

Patients with the idiopathic congenital long Q-T syndrome may have a myocardial defect in repolarization, e.g., involving an outward potassium current or an inward slow calcium current, rather than "sympathetic imbalance."[90,91,93,94] Sympathetic stimulation, primarily left, could periodically increase the EAD amplitude to provoke ventricular tachyarrhythmias (Fig. 20–24). Alpha-adrenoceptor stimulation also increases the amplitude of cesium-induced EADs and the prevalence of ventricular tachyarrhythmias, both of which are suppressed

TABLE 20–6 DETERMINANTS OF THE AMPLITUDE OF AFTERDEPOLARIZATIONS

INTERVENTION	EFFECT ON AMPLITUDE OF EADs	DADs
Long cycles (basic and premature)	↑	↓
Long action potential duration	↑	↑
Reduced membrane potential	↑	↓
Na channel blockers	No effect	↓
Ca channel blockers	↓	↓
Catecholamines	↑	↑

↑ Increase amplitude
↓ Decrease amplitude
EADs = Early afterdepolarizations
DADs = Delayed afterdepolarizations

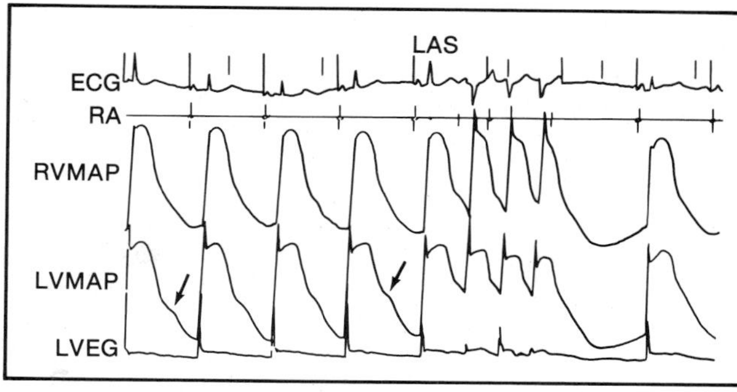

FIGURE 20–24. Following cesium administration during left ansae subclaviae stimulation (LAS), early afterdepolarizations increase in amplitude (arrows), culminating in a short run of nonsustained ventricular tachycardia. RVMAP, right ventricular monophasic action potential recording; LVMAP, left ventricular monophasic action potential recording; LVEG, left ventricular electrograms; time lines, one second. (Reproduced by permission from Ben-David, J., and Zipes, D. P.: Differential response to right and left stellate stimulation of early afterdepolarizations and ventricular tachycardia in the dog. Circulation *78*:1241, 1988. Copyright 1988 American Heart Association.)

by magnesium. Alpha-adrenoceptor blockade may be helpful in suppressing arrhythmias in some of these patients (see Chap. 22).

The ionic basis of EADs is unclear but may be via the L-type calcium channel.[81,82,85,95–98] EADs that arise at voltages close to the plateau (phase 2) appear to result from time- and voltage-dependent reactivation of L-type Ca^{++} channels. Lengthening action potential by a variety of ways allows development of this type of EAD. They may occur preferentially in Purkinje cells and M cells of ventricular myocardium.[83] EADs that arise at voltages negative to the action potential plateau appear to have separable time- and voltage-dependent properties, and the mechanism is uncertain. Short coupling intervals and rapid rates suppress EADs.

In patients with the acquired long Q-T syndrome and torsades de pointes due to drugs such as quinidine, N-acetyl procainamide, erythromycin,[99] and some class III antiarrhythmic agents, EADs also may be responsible. Such drugs easily elicit EADs experimentally and clinically, while magnesium suppresses them (Figs. 20–25 and 20–26). It is possible that multiple drugs can cause summating effects to provoke EADs and torsades de pointes in patients.[100] The potassium channel activators pinacidil and chromakalim can eliminate EADs.

Delayed Afterdepolarizations (DADs)

DADs and triggered activity have been demonstrated in Purkinje fibers, specialized atrial fibers and ventricular muscle fibers exposed to digitalis preparations, normal Purkinje fibers exposed to Na-free surperfusates from the endocardium of the intact heart, ventricular myocardial cells,[101] and endocardial preparations 1 day after a myocardial infarction. When fibers in the rabbit, canine, simian, and human mitral valves and in the canine tricuspid valve and coronary sinus are superfused with norepinephrine, they exhibit the capacity for sustained triggered rhythmic activity. It has been produced by palmitoyl carnitine in isolated ventricular myocytes.[102]

Triggered activity due to DADs also has been noted in diseased human atrial and ventricular fibers (Fig. 20–23) studied in vitro. Left stellate ganglion stimulation can elicit DADs in canine ventricles. In vivo, atrial and ventricular arrhythmias apparently due to triggered activity have been reported in the dog and possibly in humans. It is tempting to ascribe certain clinical arrhythmias to DADs, such as some arrhythmias precipitated by digitalis. The accelerated idioventricular rhythm one day after experimental canine myocardial infarction may be due to DADs, and some evidence suggests that certain ventricular tachycardias, such as that arising in the right ventricular outflow tract, may be due to DADs,[103] while other data suggest that EADs[104] are responsible.

IONIC BASIS OF DELAYED AFTERDEPOLARIZATIONS. DADs appear to be caused by a transient inward current (I_{TI}) that is small or absent under normal physiological conditions. When intracellular calcium overload occurs,[97,98,102] as during extensive sympathetic stimulation,[101] high $[Ca^{++}]_o$, or after large doses of digitalis, oscillatory release of Ca^{++} from the sarcoplasmic reticulum activates a nonselective cation channel (or an electrogenic Na^+-Ca^{++} exchange). This results in a transient inward current, carried primarily by Na^+, that generates the DAD. Drugs that block the diastolic Ca^{++} transient, by reducing Ca^{++} overload (e.g., Ca^{++} channel blockers, beta receptor blockers) or by inhibiting Ca^{++} release from the sarcoplasmic reticulum (caffeine, ryanodine), inhibit the DAD. Drugs that reduce the Na^+ current also reduce $[Na^+]_i$ (tetrodotoxin, lidocaine, phenytoin), relieve the Ca^{++} overload, and also can abolish DADs.

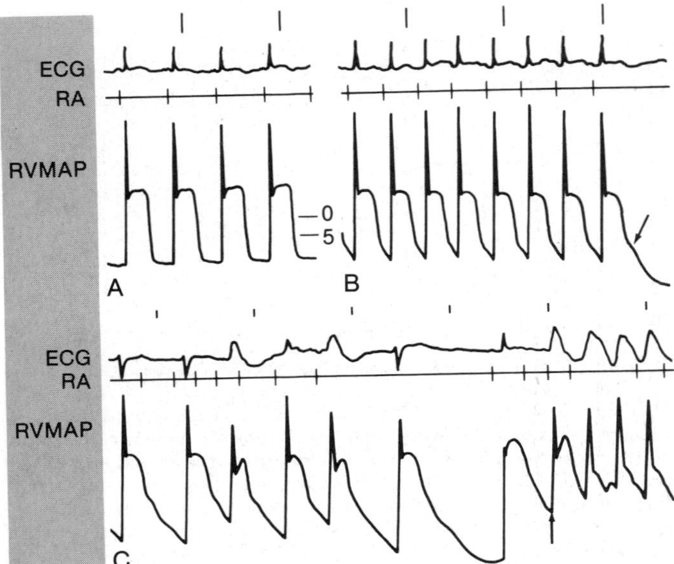

FIGURE 20–25. Induction of early afterdepolarizations in the dog by cesium chloride. Monophasic action potentials recorded from the right ventricle (RVMAP) initially show uniform contour with rapid upstroke, plateau, smooth continuous repolarization, and isoelectric interval for the resting potential (*panel A,* control). A prominent early afterdepolarization is apparent several seconds after cesium administration (*panel B,* arrow). *Panel C* shows development of premature ventricular complexes and long-short RR cycle grouping, culminating in the onset of ventricular tachycardia. A particularly prominent early afterdepolarization (arrow) follows a QRS complex that terminates the long cycle. Paper speed, 50 mm per second; time lines, one second intervals; ECG, electrocardiogram lead II; RA, right atrial electrogram; RVMAP, monophasic action potentials recorded from the apex of the right ventricle. Numbers in millivolts. (Reproduced by permission from Baillie, D. S., Inoue, H., Kaseda, S., et al.: Magnesium suppresses early depolarizations and ventricular tachyarrhythmias induced in dogs by cesium. Circulation *77*:1395, 1989. Copyright 1989 American Heart Association.)

DADs due to *digitalis toxicity* (see p. 484) behave differently from DADs due to catecholamines. Catecholamine-induced triggering often slows slightly after initiation, then regularizes, but slows still further prior to termination, without a progressive increase in maximum diastolic potential. A subthreshold DAD often follows termination of

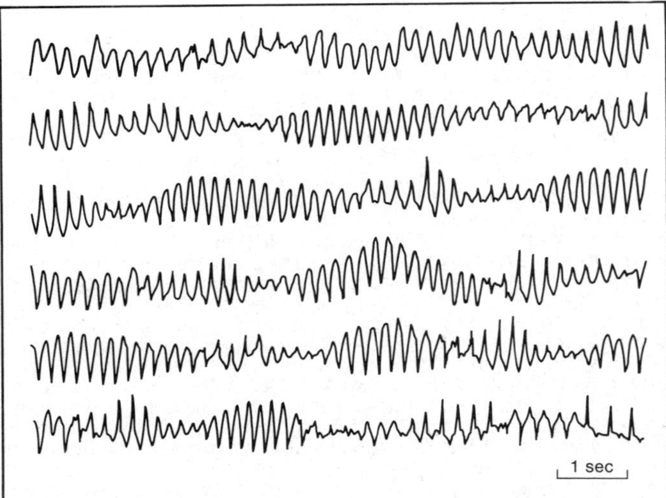

FIGURE 20–26. Torsades de pointes. Ventricular tachycardia initiated in Figure 20–25 continued, with varying morphology characteristic of torsades de points. Continuous recording of lead II. (Reproduced by permission from Zipes, D. P., and Ben-David, J.: Autonomic neural modulation of cardiac rhythm: 2. Mechanisms and examples. Mod. Concepts Cardiovasc. Dis. *57*:47, 1988. Copyright 1988 American Heart Association.)

TABLE 20–7 EFFECTS OF ELECTRICAL STIMULATION ON AUTOMATICITY AND TRIGGERED ACTIVITY

	NORMAL AUTOMATICITY	EADs	DADs
Suppressed by overdrive pacing	Yes	Not usually	Not usually
Terminated by premature stimulation	Not usually	Not usually	Usually

EADs = early afterdepolarizations; DADs = delayed afterdepolarizations

triggered activity. Spontaneous termination may be due, in part, to an increase in the rate of electrogenic sodium extrusion. Termination of digitalis-induced triggering is often characterized by speeding of the rate, decrease in action potential amplitude, and decrease in membrane potential, possibly due to $[Na^+]_i$ or $[Ca^{++}]_i$ accumulation.

Short coupling intervals or pacing at rates more rapid than the triggered activity rate (overdrive pacing) increases the amplitude and shortens the cycle length of the DAD following cessation of pacing (overdrive acceleration) rather than suppressing and delaying the escape rate of the afterdepolarization, as in normal automatic mechanisms (Table 20–7). Premature stimulation exerts a similar effect; the shorter the premature interval, the larger the amplitude and shorter the escape interval of the triggered event.

The clinical implication might be that tachyarrhythmias due to DAD-triggered activity may not be suppressed easily or, indeed, may be precipitated by rapid rates, either spontaneous (such as a sinus tachycardia) or pacing induced. Finally, because a single premature stimulus can both initiate and terminate triggered activity, differentiation from reentry (see below) becomes quite difficult. The response to overdrive pacing may help separate triggered arrhythmias from reentrant ones.

Parasystole

(See also p. 693)

Classically, parasystole has been likened to the function of a fixed-rate asynchronously discharging pacemaker: Its timing is not altered by the dominant rhythm, it produces depolarization when the myocardium is excitable, and the intervals between discharges are multiples of a basic interval.[105] Complete *entrance block,* constant or intermittent, insulates and protects the parasystolic focus from surrounding electrical events and accounts for such behavior. Occasionally, the focus may exhibit *exit block,* during which it may fail to depolarize excitable myocardium. In fact, the dominant cardiac rhythm may modulate parasystolic discharge to speed up or slow down its rate. Experimental simulations of parasystole demonstrate that the discharge rate of an isolated, "protected" focus can be modulated by electrotonic interactions with the dominant rhythm across an area of depressed excitability. Brief subthreshold depolarizations induced during the first half of the cardiac cycle of a spontaneously discharging pacemaker will delay the subsequent discharge, while similar depolarizations induced in the second half of the cardiac cycle will accelerate it (Fig. 20–27).

The ionic basis for these rate changes is not totally established, but it is probable that early depolarizing stimuli reactivate outward potassium currents and retard depolarization, while late stimuli contribute depolarizing current that enables the cell to reach threshold more quickly. Early hyperpolarizing subthreshold stimuli accelerate, while late hyperpolarizing stimuli retard discharge. Similar examples have been noted in human ventricular tissue, and interactions may be predicted according to the general rules of biological oscillators. Numerous clinical examples have been published to support these experimental observations.

DISORDERS OF IMPULSE CONDUCTION

Conduction delay and block[106] can result in bradyarrhythmias or tachyarrhythmias, the former when the propagating impulse blocks and is followed by asystole or a slow escape rhythm and the latter when the delay and block produce reentrant excitation (see below). Various factors,

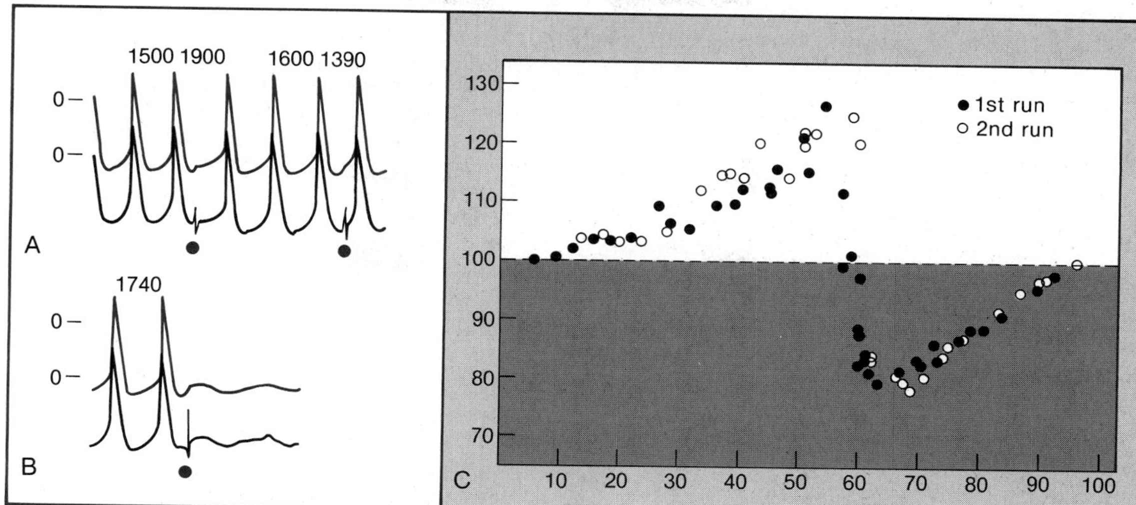

FIGURE 20–27. *Left,* Modulation of pacemaker activity by subthreshold current pulses in diseased human ventricle. *Panel A,* Two recording sites along the same trabeculum in a spontaneously active preparation. Current pulses (indicated by the dots) of 30 msec duration were injected through the lower microelectrode at various times. The interval between the spontaneous action potentials is given in milliseconds above each cycle. Injection of a subthreshold current pulse through the lower microelectrode relatively early in the spontaneous cycle (about 680 msec after initiation of the rapid portion of the preceding action potential upstroke) produced a subthreshold depolarization in the upper recording and delayed the next spontaneous discharge by 400 msec to 1900 msec. This response curve would fall in the first half of the curve indicated in panel *C.* The current pulse of the same intensity and duration delivered later in the spontaneous cycle (950 msec after the preceding upstroke) accelerated the next discharge by 210 msec to 1390 msec, relative to the previous two action potentials. The response to this current injection falls in the second half of the graph depicted in panel *C.*

Panel B, A stimulus at a precise interval in the cardiac cycle (called the singular point, in this example, 930 msec after the preceding action potential upstroke) abolishes pacemaker activity. (From Gilmour, R. F., Jr., et al.: Cellular electrophysiological abnormalities of diseased human ventricular myocardium. Am. J. Cardiol. *51:*137, 1983.) *Panel C,* Phase response curves from experimental data obtained in canine Purkinje fibers in a manner similar to the human experiment shown in panels *A* and *B.* Two different runs are shown. Ordinate: Percentage increase or decrease in the spontaneous cycle length of the "parasystolic focus" (control cycle length equals 100 per cent), Abscissa: Percentage of the "parasystolic focus" spontaneous cycle length during which stimulation was performed. The spontaneous cycle length was maximally prolonged (by 26 per cent) or shortened (by 20 per cent) by subthreshold depolarizations that entered the "parasystolic focus" after approximately 50 and 60 per cent of cycle had elapsed, respectively. Very similar curves can be plotted for patients with parasystole (for example, see Figures 9 and 10 from Zipes, D. P.: Plenary lecture. Cardiac electrophysiology: Promises and contributions. J. Am. Coll. Cardiol. *13:*1329, 1989). (Reproduced by permission from Jalife, J., and Moe, G. K.: Effect of electronic potentials on pacemaker activity of canine Purkinje fibers and relation to parasystole. Circ. Res. *39:*801, 1976. Copyright 1976 American Heart Association.)

involving both active and passive membrane properties, determine the conduction velocity of an impulse and whether or not conduction is successful. Among these factors are the stimulating efficacy of the propagating impulse, which is related to the amplitude and rate of rise of phase 0, the excitability of the tissue into which the impulse conducts, and the geometry of the tissue.

DECELERATION-DEPENDENT BLOCK. Diastolic depolarization has been suggested as a cause of conduction block at slow rates, so-called bradycardia or deceleration-dependent block (see p. 126). Yet excitability *increases* as the membrane depolarizes until about −70 mV, despite a reduction in action potential amplitude and $\dot{V}_{max}$. Evidently depolarization-induced inactivation of fast Na^+ channels is offset by other factors such as reduction in the difference between membrane potential and threshold potential. A more probable explanation of deceleration-dependent block is the reduction in action potential amplitude and excitability at long diastolic intervals. Rapid pacing also can produce overdrive suppression of conduction, with a similar mechanism related to the depression of action potential amplitude and excitability.

PHASE 3 OR TACHYCARDIA-DEPENDENT BLOCK. More commonly, impulses block at rapid rates or short cycle lengths, due to incomplete recovery of refractoriness, because of incomplete time- or voltage-dependent recovery of excitability (see p. 125). For example, this is the usual mechanism responsible for a nonconducted premature P wave or one that conducts with functional bundle branch block.

DECREMENTAL CONDUCTION. This term is used commonly in the clinical literature but often is misapplied to describe any Wenckebach-like conduction block, i.e., responses similar to block in the AV node during which progressive conduction delay precedes the nonconducted impulse. Correctly used, *decremental conduction* refers to the situation in which the properties of the fiber change along its length so that the action potential loses its efficacy as a stimulus to excite the fiber ahead of it. Thus the stimulating efficacy of the propagating action potential diminishes progressively, possibly as a result of its decreasing amplitude and $\dot{V}_{max}$.

Reentry

Electrical activity during each normal cardiac cycle begins in the sinus node and continues until the entire heart has been activated. Each cell becomes activated in turn, and the cardiac impulse dies out when all fibers have been discharged and are completely refractory. During this absolute refractory period, the cardiac impulse has "no place to go." It must be extinguished and restarted by the next sinus impulse. If, however, a group of fibers not activated during the initial wave of depolarization recovers excitability in time to be discharged before the impulse dies out, they may serve as a link to reexcite areas that were just discharged and have now recovered from the initial depolarization. Such a process is given various names, all meaning approximately the same thing: reentry, reentrant excitation, circus movement, reciprocal or echo beat, or reciprocating tachycardia.

ANATOMICAL REENTRY. The earliest studies on reentry were with models that had anatomically defined separate pathways in which it could be shown that there was (1) an area of unidirectional block, (2) recirculation of the impulse to its point of origin, and (3) elimination of the arrhythmia by cutting the pathway. In models with anatomically defined pathways, because the two (or more) pathways have different electrophysiological properties, e.g., a refractory period longer in one pathway than the other, the impulse (1) blocks in one pathway (site A in Fig. 20–28*A*) and (2) propagates slowly in the adjacent pathway (serpentine arrow, D to C, Fig. 20–28*A*). If conduction in this alternative route is sufficiently depressed, the slowly propagating impulse excites tissue beyond the blocked pathway (horizontal lined area in Fig. 20–28*A*) and returns in a reversed direction along the pathway initially blocked (B to A in Fig. 20–28*A*) to (3) reexcite tissue proximal to the site of block (A to D in Fig. 20–28*A*).

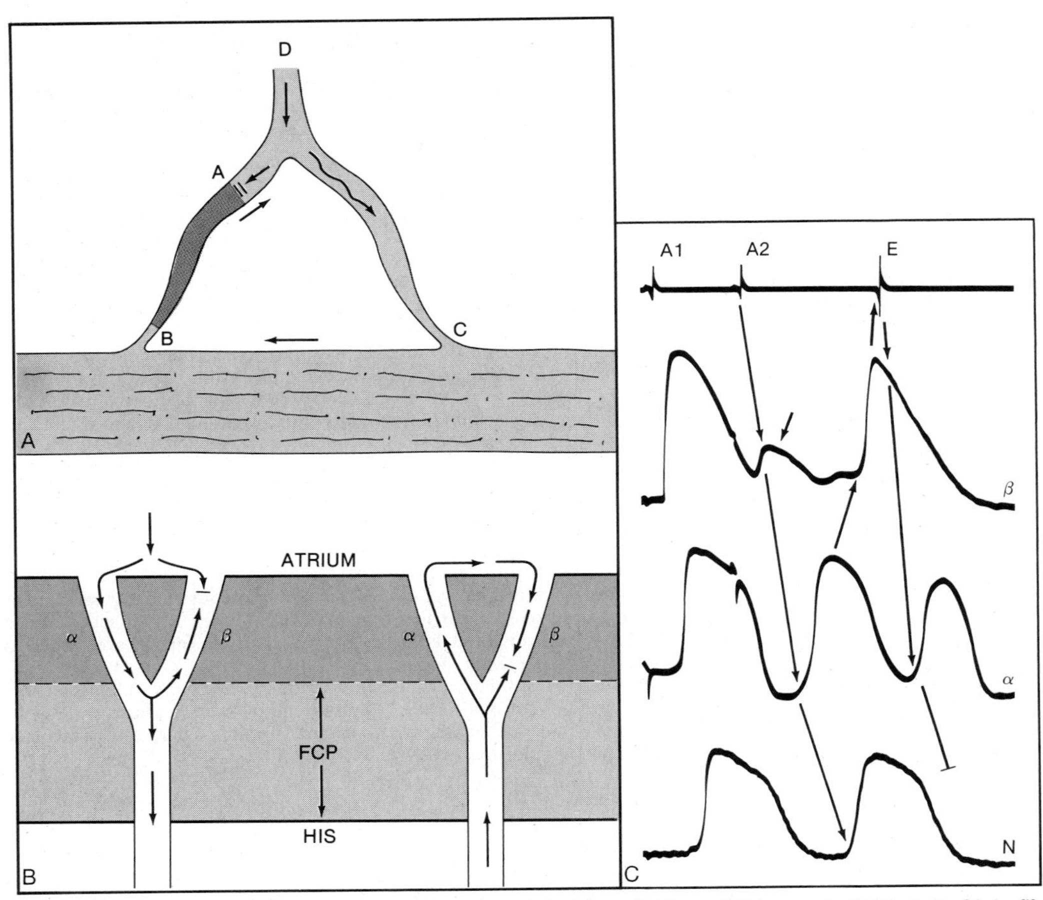

FIGURE 20–28. *Top left, A,* A diagram of reentry published by Schmitt and Erlanger in 1928. A Purkinje fiber (D) divides into two pathways (B and C), both of which join ventricular muscle. It is assumed that the original impulse travels down D, blocks in its anterograde direction at site A (arrow followed by double bar), but continues slowly down C (serpentine arrow) to excite ventricular muscle. The impulse then reenters the Purkinje twig at B and retrogradely excites A and D. If the impulse continues to propagate through D to the ventricular myocardium and elicits ventricular depolarization, a reentrant ventricular extrasystole results. Continued reentry of this type would produce ventricular tachycardia.

Bottom left, B, Atrial echoes. Schematic representation of intranodal dissociation responsible for an atrial echo *(left diagram).* A premature atrial response fails to penetrate the beta pathway, which exhibits unidirectional block, but propagates anterogradely through the alpha pathway. Once the final common pathway (FCP) is engaged, the impulse may return to the atrium via the now recovered beta pathway to produce an atrial echo. The neighboring *(right)* diagram illustrates the pattern of propagation during generation of a ventricular echo. A premature response in the His bundle traverses the final common pathway, encounters a refractory beta pathway (unidirectional block), reaches the atrium over the alpha pathway, and returns through a now recovered beta pathway to produce a ventricular echo.

Right, C, Actual recordings from the atrium (top tracing), cells impaled in the beta region (second tracing), alpha region (third tracing), and N portion of the AV node (bottom tracing) in an isolated rabbit preparation. The basic response to A_1 activated both alpha and beta pathways and the N cell (first tier of action potentials). The premature atrial response, A_2, caused only a local response in the beta cell (heavy arrow), was delayed in transmission to the alpha cell, and was further delayed in propagation to the N cell. Following the alpha response, a retrograde spontaneous response occurred in the beta cell and propagated to the atrium (E). This atrial response represents an atrial echo. The echo returned to stimulate the alpha cell but was not propagated to the N cell. It is important that while intranodal reentry has been shown to occur within the rabbit AV node, AV nodal reentry in humans probably occurs over extranodal pathways. (Reproduced by permission from Mendez, C., and Moe, G. K.: Demonstrations of a dual AV nodal conduction system in the isolated rabbit heart. Circ. Res. *19*:378, 1966. Copyright 1966 American Heart Association.)

For reentry of this type to occur, the time for conduction within the depressed but unblocked area and for excitation of the distal segments must exceed the refractory period of the initially blocked pathway (A in Fig. 20–28*A*) and the tissue proximal to the site of block (D in Fig. 20–28*A*). Stated another way, continuous reentry requires the anatomical length of the circuit traveled to equal or exceed the reentrant wavelength. The latter is equal to mean conduction velocity of the impulse multiplied by the longest refractory period of the elements in the circuit.

CONDITIONS FOR REENTRY. The length of the pathway is fixed and determined by the anatomy. Conditions that depress conduction velocity or abbreviate the refractory period will promote the development of reentry in this model, while prolonging refractoriness and speeding conduction velocity can hinder it. For example, if conduction velocity (0.30 m/sec) and refractoriness (350 m/sec) for ventricular muscle were normal, a pathway of 105 mm (0.30 m/sec × 0.35 sec) would be necessary for reentry to occur. However, under certain conditions, conduction velocity in ventricular muscle and Purkinje fibers can be very slow (0.03 m/sec), and if refractoriness is not greatly prolonged (600 msec), a pathway of only 18 mm (0.03 m/sec × 0.60 sec) may be necessary. Such reentry frequently exhibits an excitable gap, i.e., a time interval between the end of refractoriness from one cycle and beginning of depolarization in the next, when tissue in the circuit is excitable. This results because the wavelength of the reentrant circuit is less than the pathway length. Electrical stimulation during this time period can invade the reentrant circuit and reset its timing or terminate the tachycardia.

Rapid pacing can entrain the tachycardia, i.e., continuously reset it by entering the circuit and propagating around it in the same way as the reentrant impulse, increasing the tachycardia rate to the pacing rate without terminating the tachycardia. In reentrant circuits with an excitable gap, conduction velocity determines the revolution time of the impulse around the circuit and hence the rate of the tachycardia. Prolongation of refractoriness, unless it is great enough to eliminate the excitable gap and make the impulse propagate in relatively refractory tissue, will not influence the revolution time around the circuit or the rate of the tachycardia. Anatomical reentry occurs in patients with the Wolff-Parkinson-White syndrome, AV nodal reentry, in some atrial flutters, and in some ventricular tachycardias.

FUNCTIONAL REENTRY. Functional reentry lacks confining anatomical boundaries and can occur in contiguous fibers that exhibit functionally different electrophysiological properties. This depends on heterogeneous electrophysiological properties of cardiac muscle caused by local differences in the transmembrane action potentials. Dispersion of excitability and/or refractoriness, as well as anisotropic distributions of intercellular resistances, permits initiation and maintenance of reentry.[107–109]

Leading Circle Reentry. Leading circle reentry, important in atrial fibrillation, is reentrant excitation during which the reentrant circuit propagates around a functionally refractory core and follows a course along fibers that have a shorter refractory period, blocking in one direction in fibers with a longer refractory period (Fig. 20–29).

The pathway length of a functional circuit is determined by the smallest circuit in which the leading wavefront is just able to excite tissue ahead that is still relatively refractory. If these parameters change, the size of the circuit may change also, altering the rate of the tachycardia. Shorter wavelengths may predispose to fibrillation. No or a very short excitable gap exists, and the duration of the refractory period of the tissue in the circuit primarily determines the cycle length of the tachycardia because the stimulating efficacy of the head of the next impulse is just sufficient to excite the relatively refractory tissue in the wake of the preceding impulse. Propagating impulses originating outside the circuit cannot easily enter the circuit to reset, entrain, or terminate the reentry.[110]

Theoretically, drugs that prolong refractoriness and do not delay conduction would slow tachycardia due to the leading circle mechanism and not affect tachycardia with an excitable gap until the prolongation of refractoriness exceeded the duration of the excitable gap. Drugs that pri-

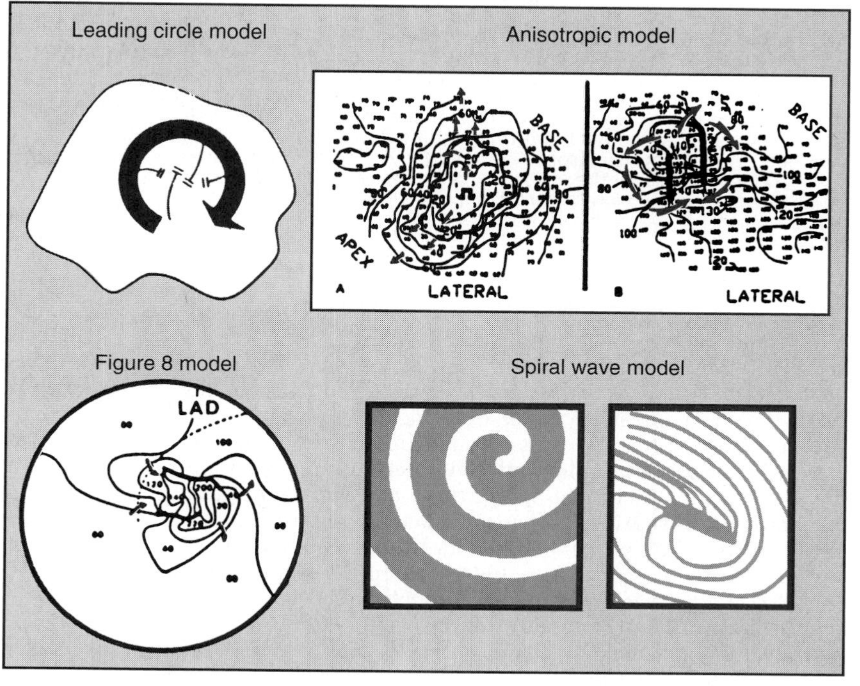

FIGURE 20–29. Functional models of reentry. *Leading circle model,* a diagrammatic representation of the leading circle model of reentry in isolated left atrium of the rabbit. The central area is activated by converging centripetal wavelets. (Reproduced with permission from Allessie, M. A., Bonke, F. I. M., and Schopman, F. J. G.: Circus movement in rabbit atrial muscle as a mechanism of tachycardia: III. The "leading circle" concept: A new model of circus movement in cardiac tissue without the involvement of an anatomical obstacle. Circ. Res. *41*:9, 1977. Copyright 1977 American Heart Association.)

Figure-of-8 model, activation map (in 20-msec isochrones) of a figure-of-8 circuit in the surviving epicardial layer of a dog 4 days after ligation of the left anterior descending coronary artery (LAD). The circuit consists of clockwise and counterclockwise wavefronts around two functional arcs of block that coalesce into a central common front that usually represents the slow zone of the circuit. (From El-Sherif, N.: The figure 8 model of reentrant excitation in the canine post-infarction heart. *In* Zipes, D. P., and Jalife, J. [eds.]: Cardiac Electrophysiology and Arrhythmias. New York, Grune and Stratton, 1985, p. 363.)

Anisotropic model, showing stimulation from the center of a multiple electrode array (at the pulse symbol, *A*) on the epicardial border zone of a 4-day-old canine infarct, producing an elliptical pattern of activation characteristic of conduction in an anisotropic medium. Arrows indicate the direction of the fast axes of conduction and the longitudinal orientation of the myocardial fibers. *B,* activation map of a reentrant circuit on the epicardial border obtained with the same electrode array during sustained ventricular tachycardia in the same heart. Arrows indicate the sequence of isochrones and thus the direction of movement of activation. (From Wit, A. L., and Janse, M. J.: The Ventricular Arrhythmias of Ischemia and Infarction: Electrophysiological Mechanisms. Mt. Kisco, N.Y., Futura, 1992.)

Spiral wave model, activation map of spiral wave activity in a thin slice of isolated ventricular muscle from a sheep heart *(right panel).* Isochrone lines were drawn from raw data by overlaying transparent paper on snapshots of video images during spiral wave activity (*left panel,* not from same experiment). Each line represents consecutive positions of the activation front recorded every 16.6 msec. (From Krinsky, V. I., et al.: Proc. R. Soc. Lond. [A] *437*:645, 1992.) (Entire figure modified from El-Sherif, N.: Reentrant mechanisms in ventricular arrhythmias. *In* Zipes, D. P., and Jalife, J. [eds.]: Cardiac Electrophysiology: From Cell to Bedside. Philadelphia, W. B. Saunders Company, 1994, p. 567.)

marily slow conduction would have major effects on tachycardia with an excitable gap and not on tachycardias due to the leading circle concept. Mixed circuits with both anatomical and functional pathways obfuscate these differences.

Random Reentry. Random reentry, also important in atrial fibrillation, occurs when the reentry propagates continuously and randomly, reexciting areas that were excited shortly before by another wavelet.

Anisotropic Reentry. Anisotropic reentry is due to the structural features responsible for variations in conduction velocity and time course of repolarization, such as concentration of gap junctions at the ends rather than on the side of cells, that can result in block and slowed conduction causing reentry[99] (Fig. 20–29). Even in normal cardiac tissue showing normal transmembrane potentials and uniform refractory periods, conduction can block in the direction parallel to the long axis of fiber orientation, propagate slowly in the direction transverse to the long axis of fiber orientation, and reenter the area of block. Spatial differences in refractoriness may not be necessary for reentry to occur. Such anisotropic reentry has been shown in atrial and ventricular muscle and may be responsible for ventricular tachycardia in epicardial muscle surviving myocardial infarction. An excitable gap may be present.[109]

Figure-of-Eight Reentry. This is reentry consisting of clockwise and counterclockwise wavefronts around two functional arcs of block that coalesce into a central common front commonly representing the slow zone of the circuit. Such reentry has been shown in both atrial and ventricular muscle[107] (Fig. 20–29).

Spiral Wave Reentry. Spiral waves of excitation have been demonstrated in cardiac muscle and represent a two-dimensional form of reentry; in three dimensions, spiral waves may be represented by scroll waves. Spiral waves may be stationary when the shape, size, and location of the arc remain unchanged throughout the episode; drifting, when the arc migrates away from its site of origin; or anchoring, when the drifting core becomes anchored to some small obstacle, such as a blood vessel. One can speculate that a stationary spiral wave could be responsible for a monomorphic tachycardia, a drifting spiral wave responsible for rhythm with changing contours such as torsades de pointes, and an anchoring spiral wave responsible for the transition from a polymorphic to a monomorphic tachycardia[110a–112] (Fig. 20–29).

REFLECTION. This can be considered a special subclass of reentry. As in reentry, an area of conduction delay is required, and the total time for the impulse to leave and return to its site of origin must exceed the refractory period of the proximal segment.

Reflection differs from reentry in that the impulse does not require a circuit but appears to travel along the *same* pathway in both directions. The impulse travels in one direction and meets an area of impaired conduction where active transmission pauses. Electrotonically, the impulse spans the zone of impairment, activates the distal segment, and returns electrotonically across the zone of impaired conduction to reexcite the proximal segment. A single reflection could cause a coupled premature complex, while continued reflection back and forth across an inexcitable zone could cause a tachycardia.

Tachycardias Due to Reentry

Reentry is probably the cause of many tachyarrhythmias, including various kinds of supraventricular and ventricular tachycardias, flutter, and fibrillation. However, in complex preparations, such as large pieces of tissue in vitro or the intact heart, it becomes much more difficult to prove unequivocally that reentry exists. In addition, many other factors, such as stretch, autonomic stimulation, and a host of modulating influences can act on these electrophysiological mechanisms, obscuring the cause of many arrhythmias. Initiation or termination of tachycardia by pacing stimuli, the demonstration of electrical activity bridging diastole, fixed coupling, and a variety of other clinically used techniques such as entrainment and resetting curves, while consistent with reentry, do not constitute absolute proof of its existence. The most compelling evidence probably is provided by entrainment.[113]

ATRIAL FLUTTER (see also p. 652). Reentry is the most likely cause of the usual form of atrial flutter, with the reentrant circuit confined to the right atrium, where it travels counterclockwise, in a caudocranial direction in the interatrial septum and in a craniocaudal direction in the right atrial free wall.[113–123] An area of slow conduction is present in the posterolateral to posteromedial inferior right atrium with a central area of block that can include an anatomical (inferior vena cava) and functional component. It is possible that several different reentrant circuits exist in patients with atrial flutter. However, this area of slow conduction is rather constant and represents the site of successful ablation of atrial flutter. It is also important in the conversion of atrial flutter to fibrillation.[117] Double potentials can be recorded from this area, with each one reflecting activation on either side of the block.[121] Ventricular activation can modulate the atrial flutter rate, probably through mechanotechnical coupling, and atrial volume changes.[123,124] Ablation results are consistent with a macroreentry circuit.[125–132]

ATRIAL AND VENTRICULAR FIBRILLATION (see also pp. 654 and 686). A critical mass of myocardium appears to be required to maintain fibrillation. Ventricular myocardium cut into small pieces ceases fibrillating when the pieces reach a critically small size. Partitioning the atrium into small segments presents atrial fibrillation, a concept that has led to a corrective surgical[133,134] and ablation[135,135a,b] procedure (see p. 621).

Ventricles of small animals stop fibrillating spontaneously, while this seldom occurs in the canine or human heart. In the canine ventricle, the left ventricular free wall and septum appear to be required as a critical mass to maintain fibrillation, since, if they are depolarized, the right ventricle stops fibrillating spontaneously. Fibrillation in the atrial appendage stops when it is clamped off from the rest of the atria in which fibrillation is induced by rapid atrial pacing and vagal stimulation. These observations support Moe's hypothesis that multiple wavelets of reentry, influenced by the mass of the tissue, refractory periods, and conduction velocity, maintain fibrillation.[110,136] These factors determine the number of wavelets present and the likelihood of continuation of fibrillation. One or more wavelets propagating in different directions characterize pacing-induced atrial fibrillation in humans.

Intraatrial reentry of the leading circle type appears responsible for multiple wavelets and has a short excitable gap.[110,136] Rapid pacing can regionally entrain portions of the atria but cannot terminate atrial fibrillation.[137,138] New-onset atrial fibrillation shortens atrial refractory period within 24 hours and can facilitate maintenance of atrial fibrillation. Atrial fibrillation begets atrial fibrillation and cellular adaptive changes result.[139,140,140a] Some patients may have rapidly discharging foci that maintain fibrillation.[141] Autonomic influences may be important in some patients.[142]

SINUS REENTRY (see also p. 649). The sinus node shares with the AV node electrophysiological features such as the potential for *dissociation of conduction;* i.e., an impulse can conduct in some nodal fibers but not in others, permitting reentry to occur.[143] The reentrant circuit may be located entirely within the sinus node or involve both the sinus node and atrium. Supraventricular tachycardias due to sinus node reentry generally may be less symptomatic than other supraventricular tachycardias because of slower rates. Ablation of the sinus node may be necessary in an occasional refractory tachycardia.[144]

ATRIAL REENTRY (see also p. 656). Reentry within the atrium, unrelated to the sinus node, may be a cause of supraventricular tachycardia in humans.[145–150] Atrial reentry appears to be less frequently encountered than other types of supraventricular tachycardia.[148] It has been shown to be due to reentry,[145,150] automaticity,[151] and afterdepolarizations causing triggered activity. There does not appear to be a relationship between the site of origin and mechanism. Adenosine has been used to probe for mechanism.[147] Distinguishing atrial tachycardia due to automaticity from atrial tachycardia sustained by reentry over quite small areas, i.e., microreentry of the leading circle type, is difficult. Multiple foci can be present.[152]

AV NODAL REENTRY (AVNR) (see also p. 661). Longitudinal dissociation of the AV node into two or more pathways has been demonstrated in animal studies.[153] For example, microelectrode studies on isolated rabbit AV nodal preparations reveal that cells in the upper portion of the AV node can be dissociated during propagation of premature stimuli so that one group of cells, called *alpha,* can discharge in response to a premature stimulus at a time when another group of cells, called *beta,* fails to discharge. The impulse can then propagate to the middle and lower portions of the AV node and turn around (without needing to activate the His bundle) to reexcite the beta group of cells and produce an atrial echo (Fig. 20–28*B*) or sustained tachycardia.

Dual AV nodal pathways also have been supported by finding that an impulse traveling from ventricle to atrium, if timed properly, can reach the atrium at the same time that another impulse is traveling from atrium to ventricle (Fig. 20–30). For this event to occur, the impulses traveling in opposite directions without colliding must be conducting in different AV nodal pathways. Another convincing fact is the finding of two ventricular responses to a single atrial depolarization or of two atrial responses to a single ventricular depolarization, due to simultaneous transmission over both the slow and fast AV nodal pathways.[154,155] Finally, the onset of AVNR is consistent with dual AV nodal pathways.[156–164]

Usually, a premature atrial response that can block anterogradely in one AV nodal pathway which conducts more rapidly (fast pathway, or beta pathway in Fig. 20–28*B*), but has a longer refractory period than a second pathway (slow pathway, or alpha pathway in Fig. 20–28*B*). The premature atrial response travels to the ventricle over the slow (alpha) pathway, prolonging the A-H interval, and back to the atrium over the fast (beta) pathway, with a short H-A interval, so-called slow-fast AVNR. Less commonly, the slow pathway has a long refractory period, and the premature atrial response can block anterogradely in the slow pathway and travel in the fast pathway, using the slow pathway retrogradely; this is called the *uncommon form* of AVNR, so-called fast-slow AVNR. Finally, some patients can have both anterograde and retrograde conduction over slowly conducting AV nodal fibers, so-called slow-slow AVNR.[164,165] Some patients may have more than two pathways. The nodal anatomic structure in patients with AVNR appears to be normal.[166,167]

LOCATION OF AV NODAL PATHWAYS. While the presence of dual AV nodal pathways in AVNR is indisputable,[23–25] the question is, Where are they located—intranodal and due to longitudinal dissociation or extranodal, involving separate atrial inputs into the AV node? The results from radiofrequency (RF) catheter ablation,[168–182] as well as surgery,[183–187] to treat patients with AVNR leaves little doubt that the fast and slow pathways have their origins well outside the limits of the compact portion of the AV node and, at the point they are interrupted, are composed of ordinary working atrial myocardium. While low[168] and high[26] amplitude potentials have been recorded in the posteroinferior right atrium, the evidence[187] suggests that these potentials may be due to local atrial activity and serve as markers of the posterior septal space rather than representing depolarizations of the slow pathway or its connections.

LH (low followed by high) frequency potentials are caused by asynchronous activation of muscle bundles above and below the coronary sinus orifice, while HL (high followed by low) frequency potentials are caused by asynchronous activation of atrial cells and a band of nodal-type cells that may represent the substrate of the slow pathway.[185,186] Thus, the slow and fast pathways are likely to be atrionodal approaches or connections rather than discreet intranodal pathways.

During the common form of AVNR, anterograde conduction occurs over a posteroinferior atrial approach, or "slow" pathway, whose upper end is located posteroinferiorly to the AV node, toward the coronary sinus orifice. RF lesions in this area eliminate AVNR by selectively affecting conduction over the slow pathway. The lower end of this pathway enters the compact portion of the AV node, where the impulse is able to "turn around" and retrogradely enter the "fast" or anterosuperior atrial approach, whose upper end inserts at the apex of Koch's triangle near the His bundle. This pathway also can be selectively ablated (Fig. 20–31).

During sinus rhythm, anterograde conduction probably occurs over the anterosuperior atrial approaches. A premature atrial impulse can block in this pathway, because of its longer refractory period, and now conduct anterogradely over the posteroinferior approaches, causing the "jump" in

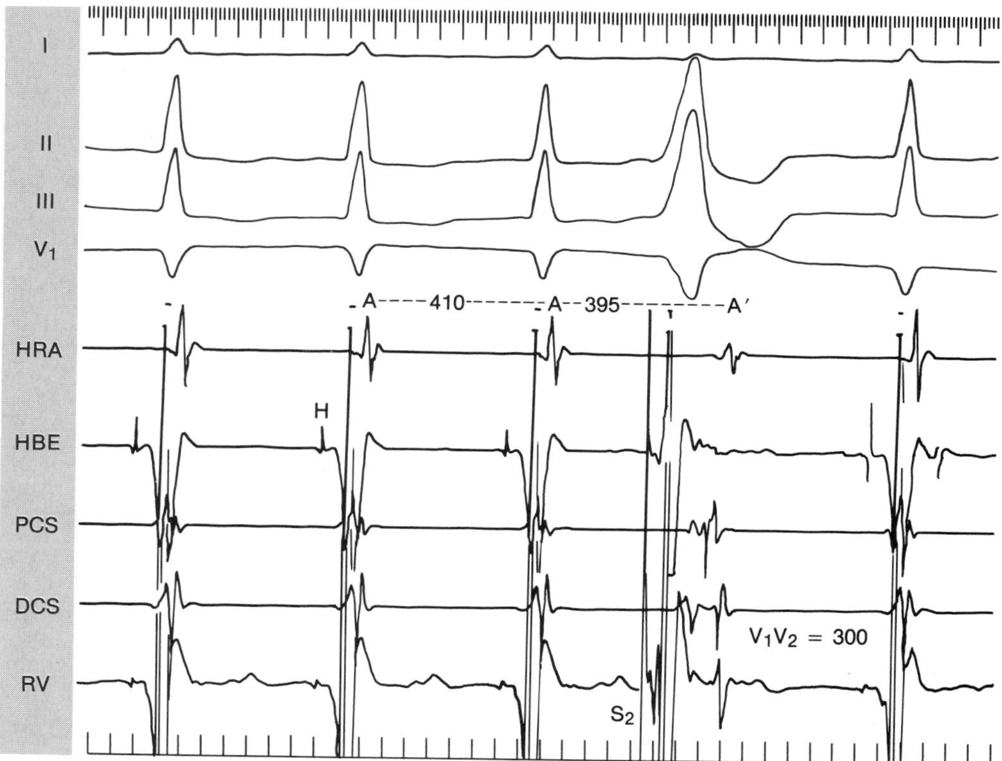

FIGURE 20–30. Atrial preexcitation during AV nodal reentry. AV nodal reentrant tachycardia is present with a cycle length of 410 msec. A premature ventricular complex (S2) from the right ventricular outflow tract with a coupling interval of 300 msec is introduced during the tachycardia before His is activated and penetrates the AV node retrogradely to shorten the AA interval to 395 msec. Shorter V1V2 intervals decreased the AA interval to 355 msec. Dual AV nodal pathways best explain how two impulses can travel in opposite directions in the AV node, i.e., the impulse from the tachycardia traveling anterogradely and the impulse from premature ventricular stimulation traveling retrogradely and not collide. Surface leads I, II, III, V1 are displayed along with high right atrial (HRA), His bundle (HBE), proximal coronary sinus (PCS), distal coronary sinus (DCS), and right ventricular (RV) electrograms. Numbers indicated in msec. Premature ventricular stimulus indicated by S2. His bundle activation indicated by H and atrial activation indicated by A. Large time 50 msec, small time 10 msec. (Reproduced with permission from Miles, W. M., Yee, R., Klein, G., et al.: The preexcitation index: An aid in determining the mechanism of supraventricular tachycardia and localizing accessory pathways. Circulation *74*:493, 1986. Copyright 1986 American Heart Association.)

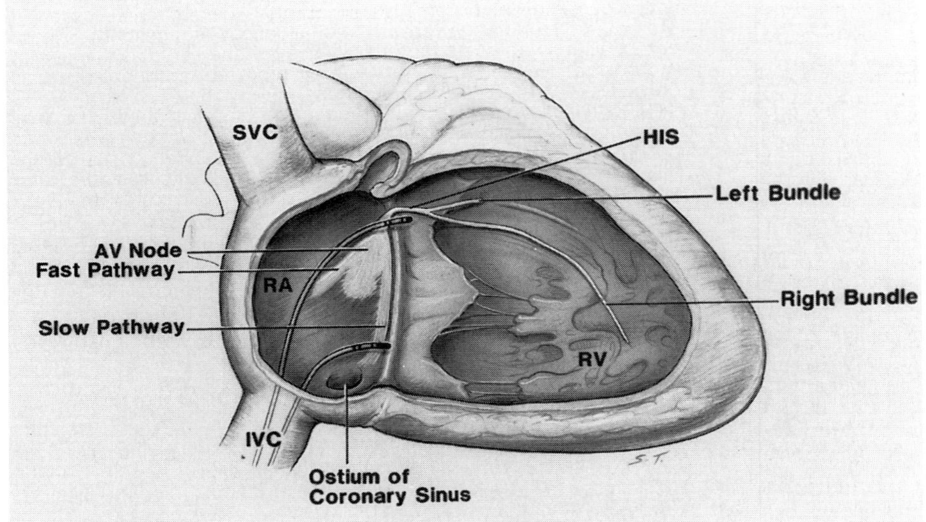

FIGURE 20–31. Schematic diagram of atrial approaches to the AV node that constitute the fast and slow pathways. AV node and pathways greatly enlarged for graphic purposes. Lower catheter lies posteroinferiorly over the slow pathway, while the upper catheter lies anterosuperiorly over the His bundle. SVC, superior vena cava; RA, right atrium; IVC, inferior vena cava; and RV, right ventricle.

the AH interval. At this point AVNR can occur. In the uncommon form of AVNR, anterograde conduction occurs over the fast pathway and retrograde conduction over the slow pathway, and in the slow-slow form, over two slow pathways.

In patients who have dual AV nodal physiology, both pathways exhibit electrophysiological responses in the anterograde direction characteristic of AV nodal fibers. However, the electrophysiological features of the pathway conducting retrogradely during the tachycardia differ from those of either anterogradely conducting pathways, in response not only to atrial or ventricular pacing but also to various drugs.[188] For example, drugs such as procainamide prolong conduction time in the retrogradely conducting, but not in either anterogradely conducting, pathway. Also, pacing at short cycle lengths prolongs anterograde, but not retrograde, AV nodal conduction time. Yet verapamil prolongs retrograde AV nodal conduction time, consistent with an effect on nodal fibers. The area of slow conduction in AVNR is located in the same region as the area of slow conduction in atrial flutter.[189]

While it is clear that activation of the ventricle is not necessary for AVNR (Fig. 20–32) and activation of the His bundle is also probably not required in some patients, the necessary role of atrial participation in the reentrant circuit is still debated.[156,157,163] The obligatory role of the atrium in the reentry is implicit in the diagram in Figure 20–28*B*. Figure 20–33 is an example of *apparent* dissociation of the atrium with uninterrupted continuation of the supraventricular tachycardia, leading to the conclusion that the atrium may *not* be a necessary part of the reentrant circuit in humans. However, data refuting the role of the atrium as a necessary link in the reentrant pathway must be obtained from studies in which both atria are carefully mapped for the presence of localized atrial activity, particularly near the upper AV node.

PREEXCITATION SYNDROME (see also p. 667). Atrioventricular reentry is the mechanism responsible for about 80 per

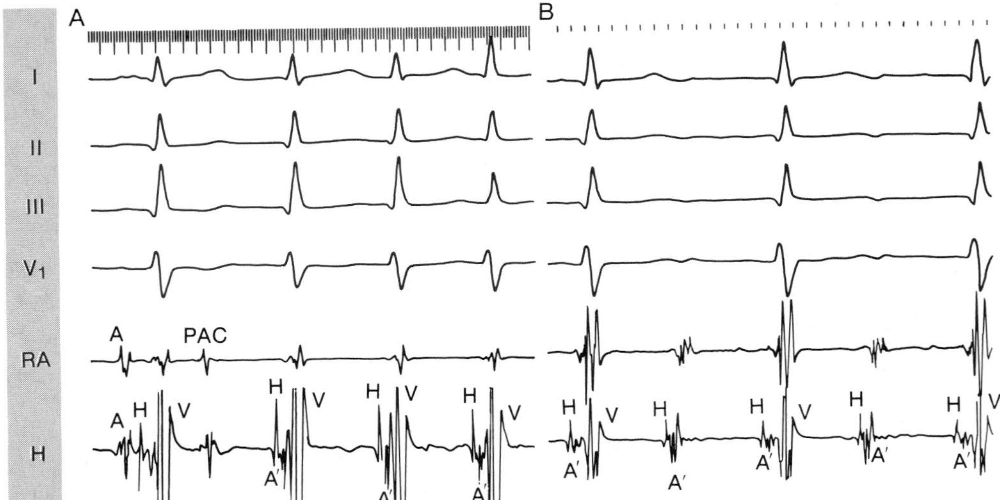

FIGURE 20–32. His-Purkinje block during AV nodal reentry. In panel *A*, a spontaneous premature atrial complex (PAC) is followed by PR (AH) prolongation and the initiation of AV nodal reentry. Retrograde atrial activation (A′) occurs simultaneously with the onset of the QRS complex. In panel *B*, 2:1 block distal to the His bundle recording site is present, with continuation of the AV nodal reentry, indicating that activation of the ventricle is not required for perpetuation of the tachycardia. Such an event could not occur during reciprocating tachycardia utilizing an accessory atrioventricular connection in the Wolff-Parkinson-White syndrome. Conventions as in Figure 20–30.

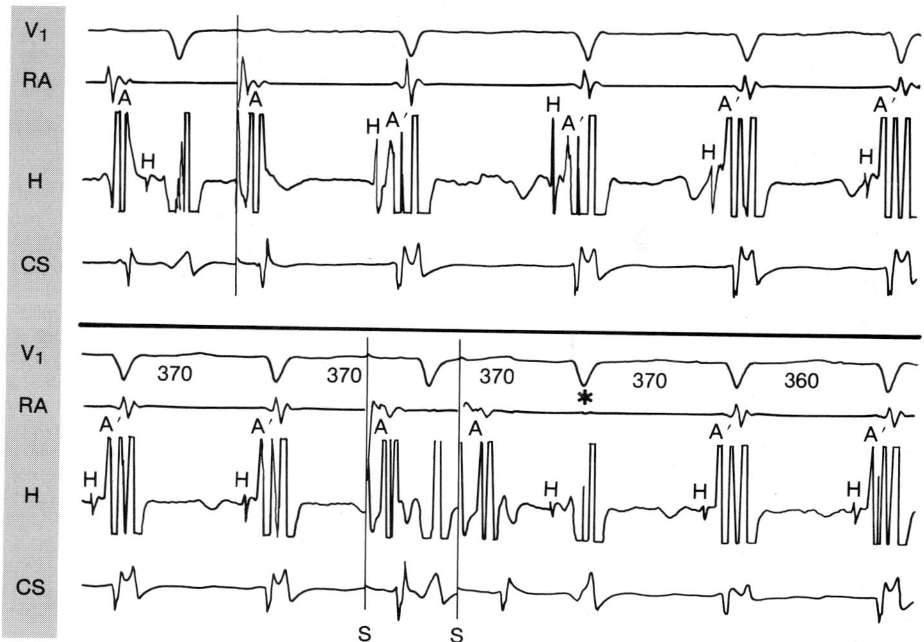

FIGURE 20–33. Dissociation of atria from ventricles without interrupting AV nodal reentrant supraventricular tachycardia. During sinus rhythm, a single premature atrial complex (S, *top panel*) was conducted with AV nodal delay (prolonged A-H interval) and initiated an AV nodal reentrant supraventricular tachycardia. Note that retrograde atrial activation (A′) occurred prior to onset of the QRS complex. Two premature atrial stimuli (S-S, *bottom panel*) captured the atria on both occasions without altering the regular cycle length of the AV nodal reentrant supraventricular tachycardia. Note that the QRS complex marked by an asterisk has no accompanying atrial complex, suggesting that atrial participation in the reentrant circuit was not required. V_1 = scalar lead; RA = right atrial electrogram; H = His bundle electgrogram; CS = coronary sinus electrogram.

cent of the tachycardias related to an accessory pathway.[190] In fact, the bundle described by Kent[191,192] was used to explain a reentrant mechanism for paroxysmal tachycardia even before the preexcitation syndrome was ever described in humans.

In most patients who have reciprocating tachycardias associated with the Wolff-Parkinson-White syndrome, the accessory pathway conducts more rapidly than does the normal AV node but takes a longer time to recover excitability; i.e., the anterograde refractory period of the accessory pathway exceeds that of the AV node at long cycles.[193,194] Consequently, a premature atrial complex that occurs sufficiently early blocks anterogradely in the accessory pathway and continues to the ventricle over the normal AV node and His bundle. After the ventricles have been excited, the impulse is able to enter the accessory pathway retrogradely and return to the atrium. A continuous conduction loop of this kind establishes the circuit for the tachycardia. The usual (orthodromic) activation wave during such a reciprocating tachycardia in a patient with an accessory pathway occurs in this manner: anterogradely over the normal AV node–His-Purkinje system and retrogradely over the accessory pathway, resulting in a normal QRS complex (Fig. 20–34).

Because the circuit requires both atria and ventricles, the term *supraventricular tachycardia* is not precisely correct, and the tachycardia is more accurately called *atrioventricular reciprocating tachycardia* (AVRT). The reentrant loop can be interrupted by ablation of the normal AV node–His bundle pathway *or* the accessory pathway.[195–204] Occasionally, the activation wave travels in a reverse (antidromic) direction to the ventricles over the accessory pathway and to the atria retrogradely up the AV node.[193,194] Two accessory pathways may form the circuit in some patients with antidromic AVRT. In some patients, the accessory pathway can be capable only of retrograde conduction ("concealed"), but the circuit and mechanism of AVRT remain the same. Less commonly, the accessory pathway can conduct only anterogradely. The pathway can be localized by analysis of the scalar ECG.[205–209,209a] Patients can have atrial fibrillation as well as AVRT.[210]

Unusual accessory pathways with AV nodal–like electrophysiological properties, nodofascicular or nodoventricular fibers, can constitute the circuit for reciprocating tachycardias in patients who have some form of the Wolff-Parkinson-White syndrome. Tachycardia in patients with nodoventricular fibers can be due to reentry using these fibers as the anterograde pathway and the His-Purkinje fibers and a portion of the AV node retrogradely.[194,195] In the Lown-Ganong-Levine syndrome (short P-R interval and normal QRS complex), conduction over a James fiber that connects atrium to the distal portion of the AV node and His bundle has been *proposed,* although little functional evidence to support the presence of this entity has been published, except in a rare patient with an unusual atrio–His connection (see p. 672).

VENTRICULAR TACHYCARDIA DUE TO REENTRY (see also p. 667). Reentry in the ventricle, both anatomical and functional, as a cause of sustained ventricular tachycardia has been supported by many animal[211–218] and clinical[219–222] studies (Fig. 20–29). Reentry in ventricular muscle, with or without contribution from specialized tissue, is responsible for many or most ventricular tachycardias in patients with ischemic heart disease. The area of microreentry appears to be quite small, and only uncommonly is a macroreentry found around the infarct scar. Surviving myocardial tissue (Fig. 20–35) separated by connective tissue provides serpentine routes of activation traversing infarcted areas that can establish reentry pathways. Bundle branch reentry can cause sustained ventricular tachycardia, particularly in patients with dilated cardiomyopathy.[221,223]

Both figure-of-eight[215] (Fig. 20–29) and single-circle[219] (Fig. 20–36) reentrant loops have been described, circulating around an area of functional block in a manner consistent with the leading circle hypothesis or conducting slowly across an apparent area of block created by anisotropy.[213]

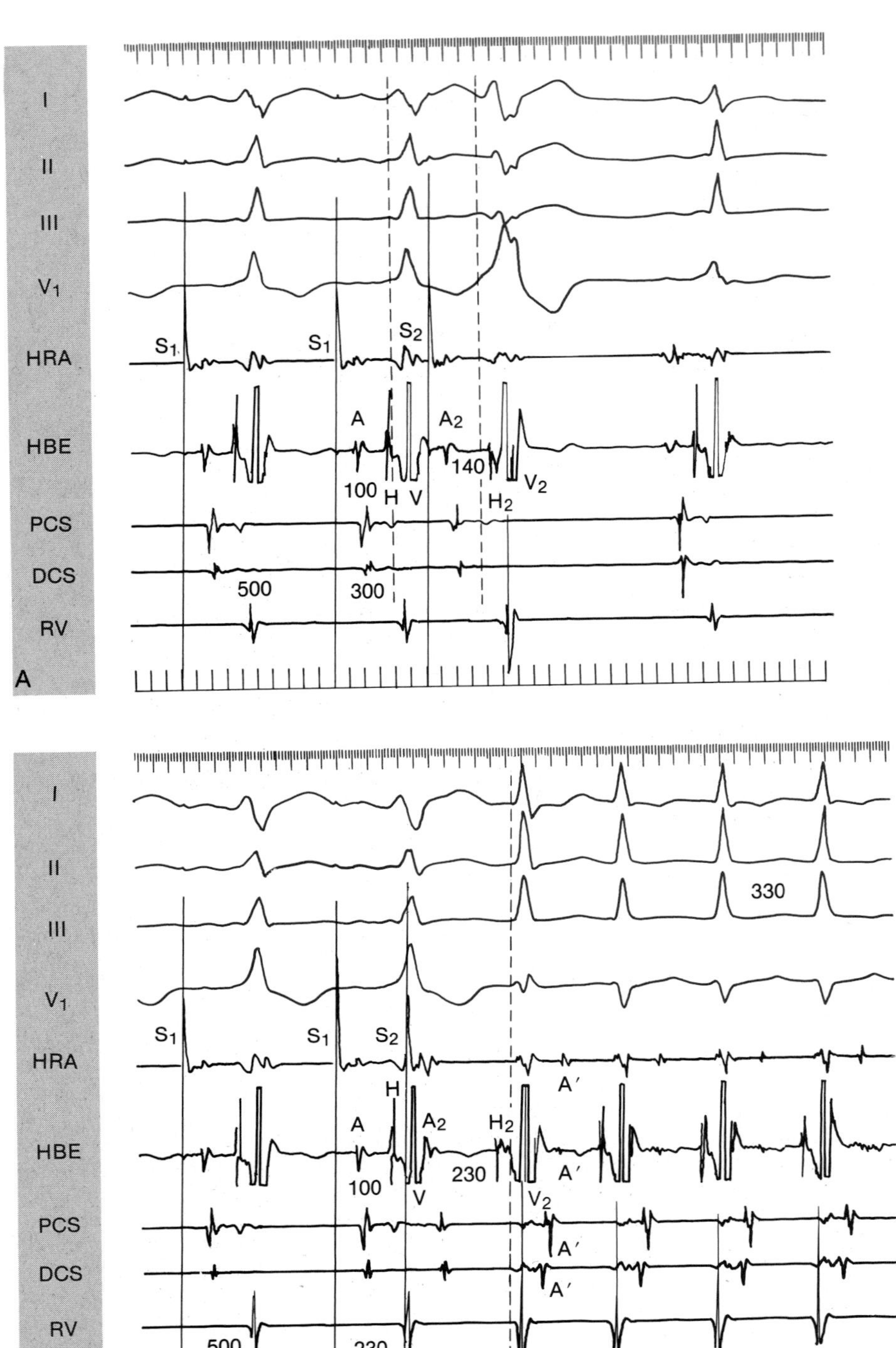

FIGURE 20–34. *A*, Wolff-Parkinson-White syndrome. Following high right atrial pacing at a cycle length of 500 msec (S_1-S_1), premature stimulation at a coupling interval of 300 msec (S_1-S_2) produces physiological delay in AV nodal conduction resulting in an increase in the AH interval from 100 to 140 msec but no delay in the AV interval. Consequently, activation of the His bundle occurs following activation of the QRS complex (second interrupted line) and the QRS complex becomes more anomalous in appearance due to increased ventricular activation over the accessory pathway. I, II, III, and V_1 and scalar leads. HRA, high right atrium; HBE, His bundle electrogram; PCS, proximal coronary sinus electrogram; DCS, distal coronary sinus electrogram; RV, right ventricular electrogram. Time lines 50 and 10 msec intervals. S_1, stimulus of the drive train; S_2, premature stimulus. A, H V, atrial His bundle, and ventricular activation during the drive train. A_2, H_2, V_2, atrial His bundle, and ventricular activation during the premature stimulus.

B, Induction of reciprocating atrioventricular tachycardia. Premature stimulation at a coupling interval of 230 msec prolongs the AH interval to 230 msec and results in anterograde block in the accessory pathway and normalization of the QRS complex (slight functional aberrancy in the nature of incomplete right bundle branch block occurs). Note that H2 precedes the onset of the QRS complex (interrupted line). Following V_2, the atria are excited retrogradely (A′) beginning in the distal coronary sinus, then followed by atrial activation in leads recording from the proximal coronary sinus, His bundle, and high right atrium. A supraventricular tachycardia is initiated at a cycle length of 330 msec. Conventions as in panel A. (From Zipes, D. P., Mahomed, Y., King, R. D., et al.: Wolff-Parkinson-White syndrome: Cryosurgical treatment. Indiana Med. *89*:432, 1986.)

When intramural myocardium survives, it may form part of the reentrant loop. Structural discontinuities that separate muscle bundles, owing to naturally occurring myocardial fiber orientation and anisotropic conduction as well as to collagen matrices formed from the fibrosis after a myocardial infarction, establish the basis for slowed conduction, fragmented electrograms, and continuous electrical activity that can lead to reentry. After the infarction, action potential recordings from surviving cells return to normal, suggesting that depressed activity in these cells does not account for the slowed conduction. However, ventricular myocardium resected from humans with recurrent ventricular tachycardia demonstrates abnormal action potentials, suggesting that causes of depressed conduction in humans may be multifactorial (Figs. 20–21 and 20–23). During acute ischemia, a variety of factors, including elevated $[K]_o$ and reduced pH, combine to create depressed action potentials in ischemic cells that retards conduction and can lead to reentry.[67,213,222]

Ventricular Tachycardias Due to Nonreentrant Mechanisms

In some instances of ventricular tachycardias related to coronary artery disease, but especially in patients without coronary artery disease, nonreentrant mechanisms are important causes of ventricular tachycardias. Experimentally, nonreentrant forms of ventricular tachycardia appear to cause 25 per cent of acute ischemic-induced ventricular tachycardias and 75 per cent of ventricular tachycardias due to reperfusion; rapidly firing nonreentrant foci are responsible for the transition to ventricular fibrillation.[224,224a] Nonreentrant mechanisms also can cause ventricular tachycardias clinically. However, in many patients, the mechanism of the ventricular tachycardia remains unknown.[225]

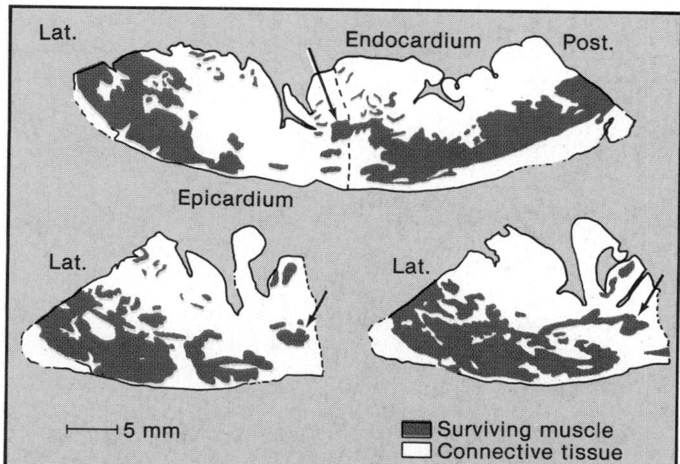

FIGURE 20–35. *Top panel* is a schematic drawing illustrating left ventricular myocardial sections of a human heart studied electrophysiologically and histologically after removal for cardiac transplant. Dark areas mark surviving cardiac tissue, while light areas point to fibrotic and fatty tissue. Note the irregularity of the surviving cardiac tissue interspersed with fibrotic tissue. Lower two panels are schematic drawings of sections from the lateral left ventricular wall 500 *(left)* and 1000 *(right)* μm, respectively, beneath the level of those shown in the top panel. Note that bulge of viable tissue at the left of the surviving posterior wall (arrow in the top panel) becomes isolated in the *lower left panel* (arrow). In the *lower right panel,* this isolated area merges with the bulk of surviving tissue in the lateral wall (arrow). (From deBakken, J. M. T., Coronel, R., Tisserons, S., et al.: Ventricular tachycardia in the infarcted Langendorff-perfused human heart: Role of the arrangement of surviving cardiac fibers. J. Am. Coll. Cardiol. *15:*1594, 1990. Reprinted with permission from the American College of Cardiology.)

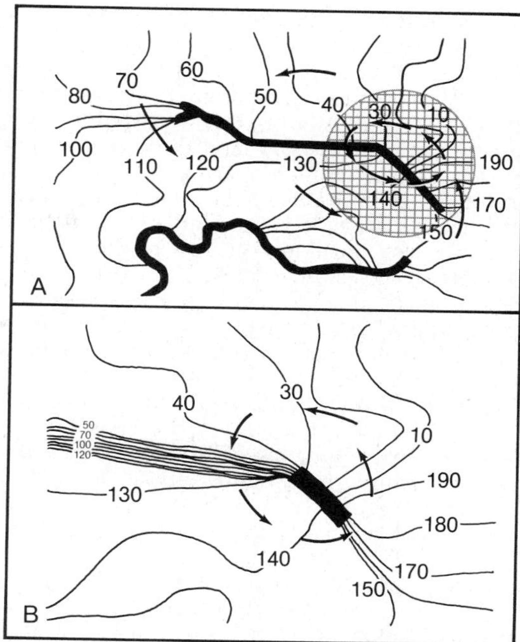

FIGURE 20–36. Model of anisotropic reentry in the epicardial border zone. *A,* The activation map of the single reentrant circuit is shown. The large arrows point out the general activation pattern; activation appears to occur around a long line of block. However, parallel isochrones adjacent to the line (isochrones 130 and 140) suggest that activation is also occurring across the line, resulting in the smaller circuit shown by the small arrows. *B,* This circuit is shown enlarged. Rapid activation occurs parallel to the long axis of the fiber orientation (isochrones 10–40 and at 130–150), whereas very slow activation (closely bunched isochrones 50–120) occurs transverse to fiber orientation in the circuit. The dark black rectangle is an area of either functional or anatomical block that forms the fulcrum of the circuit. (From Wit, A. L., and Dillon, S. M.: Anisotropic reentry. *In* Zipes, D. P., and Jalife, J. [eds.]: Cardiac Electrophysiology. From Cell to Bedside. Philadelphia, W. B. Saunders Company, 1990.)

TRIGGERED ACTIVITY. Early afterdepolarizations and triggered activity may be responsible for torsade de pointes.[226] A group of probably nonreentrant ventricular tachycardias occurring in the absence of structural heart disease can be initiated and terminated by programmed stimulation. They are catecholamine dependent and are terminated by Valsalva, adenosine, and verapamil. These ventricular tachycardias are generally but not exclusively located in the right ventricular outflow tract and may be due to triggered activity, possibly delayed afterdepolarizations that are cyclic AMP dependent.[96,103,227–229] Early afterdepolarizations have been recorded in this tachycardia as well.[104] Left ventricular fascicular tachycardias can be suppressed by verapamil but generally not adenosine,[229] and some may be due to triggered activity[230] and others due to reentry.[231] Adenosine can be a useful pharmacological probe to uncover arrhythmias dependent on adenylyl cyclase,[103] which is inhibited by the regulatory protein G_i[232]; adenosine can suppress some left ventricular tachycardias as well.[233] Early afterdepolarizations may not necessarily be the cause of reperfusion arrhythmias.[233a]

AUTOMATICITY. Automatic discharge can be responsible for some ventricular tachycardias[234,235] and does not appear to be suppressed by adenosine.[103] Unless invasive studies are undertaken, mechanisms of ventricular tachycardias can only be conjectured.[236–238]

APPROACH TO THE DIAGNOSIS OF CARDIAC ARRHYTHMIAS

It is important to remember that the physician evaluates a *patient* who has a rhythm disturbance and does not evaluate a rhythm disturbance in isolation.[239] Some arrhythmias are hazardous to the patient regardless of the clinical setting, while others are hazardous *because* of the clinical setting. Evaluation of the patient begins with a careful history[240] and physical examination and should usually progress from the simplest to the most complex test, from the least invasive and safest to the most invasive and risky, and from the least expensive out-of-hospital evaluations to those which require hospitalization and sophisticated, costly procedures. Occasionally, depending on the clinical circumstances, the physician may wish to proceed directly to a high-risk, expensive procedure, such as an electrophysiological study, prior to obtaining a 24-hour ECG recording.

Patients with cardiac rhythm disturbances may present with a variety of complaints, but commonly symptoms such as palpitations, syncope, presyncope, or congestive heart failure cause them to seek a physician's help. Their awareness of regular or irregular cardiac rhythm varies greatly. Some patients perceive slight variations in their heart rhythm with uncommon accuracy, while others are oblivious even to sustained episodes of ventricular tachycardia; still others complain of palpitations when they actually have regular sinus rhythm. The following tests can be used to evaluate patients who have cardiac arrhythmias.

Exercise Testing

(See also Chap. 5)

Exercise can induce various types of supraventricular and ventricular tachyarrhythmias and, uncommonly, bradyarrhythmias.[241–246] About one-third of normal subjects develop ventricular ectopy in response to exercise testing. Ectopy is more likely to occur at faster heart rates, usually in the form of occasional premature ventricular complexes (PVCs) of constant morphology, or even pairs of PVCs, and is often not reproducible from one stress test to the next.

Three to six beats of nonsustained ventricular tachycardia can occur in normal patients, especially the elderly, and its occurrence does not establish the existence of ischemic or other forms of heart disease or predict increased cardiovascular morbidity or mortality. Supraventricular premature complexes are often more common during exercise than at rest and increase in frequency with age; their occurrence does not suggest the presence of structural heart disease.

Approximately 50 per cent of patients who have coronary artery disease develop PVCs in response to exercise testing. Ventricular ectopy appears in these patients at lower heart rates (less than 130 beats/min) than in the normal population and often occurs in the early recovery period as well. In one study, exercise reproduced sustained ventricular tachycardia (VT) or ventricular fibrillation (VF) in only 11 per cent of patients with spontaneous VT or VF late after myocardial infarction,[243] but those who had it experienced a worse outcome. The relation of exercise to ventricular arrhythmia in patients with structurally normal hearts has no prognostic implications.[244] Stress testing with Holter monitoring has been used to assess antiarrhythmic drug efficacy.[247–249]

Patients who have symptoms consistent with an arrhythmia induced by exercise (e.g., syncope, sustained palpitation) should be considered for stress testing. Stress testing may be indicated to uncover more complex grades of ventricular arrhythmia, to provoke supraventricular arrhythmias, to determine the relationship of the arrhythmia to activity, to aid in choosing antiarrhythmic therapy and uncovering proarrhythmic responses, and possibly to provide some insight into the mechanism of the tachycardia. The test can be performed safely[245] and appears more sensitive than a standard 12-lead resting ECG to detect ventricular ectopy. However, prolonged ambulatory recording is more sensitive than exercise testing in detecting ventricular ectopy. Since either technique may uncover serious arrhythmias that the other technique misses, both examinations may be indicated for selected patients.

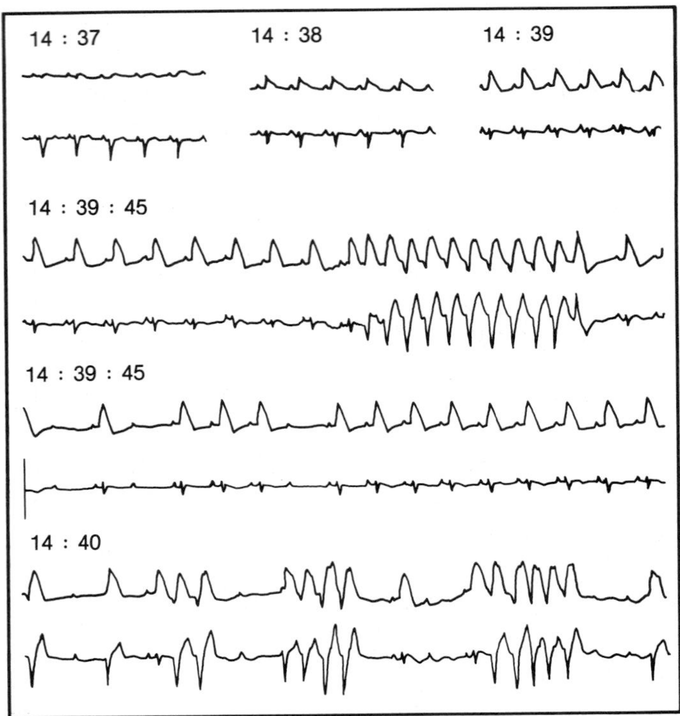

FIGURE 20–37. Long-term ECG recording in a patient with atypical angina. The top channel reflects an inferior lead while the bottom channel records an anterior lead. Note progressive ST-segment elevation in the inferior lead, eventually resembling a monophasic action potential. Bursts of nonsustained ventricular tachycardia result. Then, sinus slowing and Wenckebach AV block occur from a vasodepressor reflex response elicited by ischemia of the inferior myocardial wall, or possibly caused by ischemia of the sinus and AV nodes. In the bottom tracing, both AV block and ventricular arrhythmias are apparent. Numbers indicate time, e.g., 2:37 P.M. (Tracing of a patient of D. A. Chilson, M.D.)

Long-Term Electrocardiographic Recording

Prolonged ECG recording in patients engaged in normal daily activities is the most useful noninvasive method to document and quantitate frequency and complexity of arrhythmia, correlate arrhythmia with the patient's symptoms, and evaluate the effect of antiarrhythmic therapy on spontaneous arrhythmia. For example, recording normal sinus rhythm during the patient's typical symptomatic episode effectively excludes cardiac arrhythmia as a cause. In addition, some recorders can document alterations in QRS, ST, and T contours (Fig. 20–37).

Several modes of recordings are available[250]: (1) A recording can be continuous. If a tape recorder is used, every beat is recorded and is available for analysis. A real-time analysis device also can be used. (2) A recording can be patient activated. This is useful if the patient is able to perceive symptoms of the arrhythmia and activate the recorder. (3) A recording can be arrhythmia (event) activated. This is an effective mode, but it depends on the accuracy and reliability of the device's arrhythmia-detection algorithm. Many implantable pacemakers and defibrillators have the capability of long-term ECG (and device function) recording, and there is a recording device that can actually be implanted subcutaneously for long-term monitoring.

Transmitters that send an electrocardiographic signal transtelephonically to a receiver unit can be used to transmit on-line or stored electrocardiographic information. This device may be indicated when the rhythm disturbance is sufficiently infrequent and short lasting that continuous ECG recording is impractical. The arrhythmia must be of sufficient duration to permit real-time actual transmission or for storage and later transmission. It must not be associated with syncope or other symptoms that prevent the patient from transmitting or recording, or the patient must have another individual available to record the event. A disadvantage is that this approach relies on the patient's perception of a cardiac rhythm disturbance, and many patients may be unaware of significant or serious bradyarrhythmias and tachyarrhythmias. In addition, the technique requires access to a receiver 24 hours a day. Such an approach can be adapted for continuous monitoring. Home monitoring systems, presently not widely available, operate in a fashion similar to telemetry monitoring in a hospital, but transmit ECG data over telephone lines.

HOLTER MONITORING. Continuous ECG tape recorders represent the traditional Holter "monitor" and typically record on tape two ECG channels for 24 hours. Interpretative accuracy of long-term tape recordings varies with the system used, but most computers that scan the tapes are sufficiently accurate to meet clinical needs. All systems can potentially record more information than the physician needs or can assimilate.[251] So long as the system detects important episodes of ectopic activity, ventricular tachycardia, or asystolic intervals and semiquantitates these abnormalities, the physician probably receives all the clinical information that is needed. Approximately 25 to 50 per cent of patients experience a complaint during a 24-hour recording, caused by an arrhythmia in 2 to 15 per cent.

Significant rhythm disturbances are fairly uncommon in healthy young persons. However, sinus bradycardia with heart rates of 35 to 40 beats/min, sinus arrhythmia with pauses exceeding 3 sec, sinoatrial exit block, Wenckebach second-degree AV block (often during sleep), a wandering atrial pacemaker, junctional escape complexes, and premature atrial complexes (PACs) and PVCs are not necessarily abnormal. Frequent and complex atrial and ventricular rhythm disturbances are less commonly observed, however, and type II second-degree AV conduction disturbances are not recorded in normal patients. Elderly patients may have a greater prevalence of arrhythmias, some of which may be responsible for neurological symptoms. The long-term prognosis in asymptomatic healthy subjects with frequent and complex PVCs resembles that of the healthy U.S. population without an increased risk of death.

A majority of patients who have ischemic heart disease, particularly those after myocardial infarction, exhibit PVCs when monitored for periods of 6 to 24 hours[252,253] (p. 675). The frequency of PVCs progressively increases over the first several weeks, decreasing at about 6 months after infarction. Frequent and complex PVCs are an independent risk factor and are associated with a two- to fivefold increased risk of cardiac or sudden death in patients after myocardial infarction. Recent evidence from the Cardiac Arrhythmia Suppression Trial (CAST) raises the possibility that the ventricular ectopy may be a *marker* identifying the patient at risk rather than being *causally related* to sudden death, since PVC suppression with flecainide, encainide, or moricizine was associated with increased mortality compared with placebo. Thus the PVC may be an *innocent bystander,* unrelated to the tachyarrhythmia producing sudden death. Although the mechanism responsible for the drug-induced exacerbation of mortality is not clear, it may relate to an increase in ischemia-produced conduction delay due to sodium channel blocking drugs.

Holter recordings have been used to determine antiarrhythmic drug efficacy. In one study, Holter recordings led to predictions of antiarrhythmic drug efficacy more often than did electrophysiological testing in patients with sustained ventricular tachyarrhythmias, and there was no significant difference in the success of drug therapy as selected by the two methods.[247] The study also found sotalol to be the most efficacious of the seven antiarrhythmic drugs tested.[248] The beneficial results of noninvasive compared with invasive assessment of drug efficacy in this study have been challenged.[254,255]

Long-term ECG recording also has exposed potentially serious arrhythmias and complex ventricular ectopy in patients with left ventricular hypertrophy,[256] in those with mitral valve prolapse (see p. 1033), in those who have otherwise unexplained syncope (Chap. 22) or transient vague cerebrovascular symptoms, and in those with conduction disturbances, sinus node dysfunction, the bradycardia-tachycardia syndrome, the Wolff-Parkinson-White syndrome, Q-T dispersion,[257] pacemaker malfunction, and after thrombolytic therapy.[258,259] It has shown that asymptomatic atrial fibrillation occurs far more often than symptomatic atrial fibrillation in patients with that arrhythmia.[260]

HEART RATE VARIABILITY. Heart rate variability is used to evaluate vagal and sympathetic influences on the heart and to identify patients at risk for a cardiovascular event or death.[261–269] Frequency domain analysis resolves parasympathetic and sympathetic influences better than does time domain analysis, but both types of spectral analyses are useful. R-R variability predicts all-cause mortality as well as does left ventricular ejection fraction or nonsustained VT in patients after myocardial infarction[270–274] and can be added to other measures of risk to enhance prediction accuracy.[275–283] Perceived high- and low-frequency components of R-R interval variability suggest that both vagal and sympathetic activities, respectively, are at physiological levels. However, reduced R-R interval variability, the marker of increased risk,[284] merely indicates loss or reduction of the physiological periodic fluctuations, which can be due to many different influences, and cannot necessarily be interpreted to represent a particular shift in autonomic modulation.[284a]

T-WAVE ALTERNANS. Beat-to-beat alternation in the amplitude and/or morphology of the ECG measurement of repolarization, the ST segment and T wave, has been found in conditions favoring the development of ventricular tachyarrhythmias such as ischemia[285–289] and long Q-T interval syndrome,[32,290–292] and in patients with ventricular arrhythmias.[288,289] The electrophysiological basis of the alternation is not known and may vary with different disease states. T-wave alternans may represent a fundamental marker of an electrically unstable myocardium prone to developing VT or VF, and as such, ST-T wave analysis for alternans may be useful in the future as a method to stratify risk patients.

Invasive Electrophysiological Studies

An invasive electrophysiological procedure involves introducing multipolar catheter electrodes into the venous and/or arterial system, positioning the electrodes at various intracardiac sites to record electrical activity from portions of the atria or ventricles, from the region of the His bundle, bundle branches, accessory pathways, and other structures, and stimulating the atria, ventricles, or other sites electrically. Such studies are performed *diagnostically* to provide information on the type of rhythm disturbance and insight into its electrophysiological mechanism; *therapeutically* to terminate a tachycardia by electrical stimulation or electroshock, to evaluate effects of therapy by determining whether a particular intervention modifies or prevents electrical induction of a tachycardia or whether an electrical device properly senses and terminates an induced tachyarrhythmia, and to ablate myocardium involved in the tachycardia. Finally, these tests have been used *prognostically* to identify patients at risk for sudden cardiac death. The study may be helpful in patients who have AV block, intraventricular conduction disturbance, sinus node dysfunction, tachycardia, and unexplained syncope or palpitations.[293]

False-negative responses—not finding a particular electrical abnormality known to be present—as well as false-positive ones—induction of a nonclinical arrhythmia—may complicate interpretation of the results, as may lack of reproducibility. Altered autonomic tone in a supine patient undergoing study, hemodynamic or ischemic influences, changing anatomy (e.g., new infarction) after the study, day-to-day variability, and the fact that the test employs an artificial "trigger" (electrical stimulation) to induce the arrhythmia are several of many factors that may explain the disparity between test results and spontaneous clinical occurrences. Overall, these studies are quite safe when performed by skilled clinical electrophysiologists.

AV Block

(See also pp. 687–692)

In patients with AV block, the site of block usually dictates the clinical course of the patient and whether or not a pacemaker is needed.[106] Generally, the site of AV block can be determined from an analysis of the scalar ECG. When the site of block cannot be determined from such an analysis, and when knowing the site of block is imperative for patient management, an invasive electrophysiological study is indicated. Candidates include symptomatic patients in whom His-Purkinje block is suspected but not established and patients with AV block treated with a pacemaker who continue to be symptomatic, to search for a causal ventricular tachyarrhythmia. Possible candidates are those with second- or third-degree AV block in whom knowledge of the site of block or its mechanism may help direct therapy or assess prognosis, and patients suspected of having concealed His extrasystoles (Fig. 20–38). Patients with block in the His-Purkinje system more commonly become symptomatic because of periods of bradycardia or asystole and require pacemaker implantation than do patients who have AV nodal block.[294] Wenckebach (type I) AV block in older patients may have clinical implications similar to type II AV block.

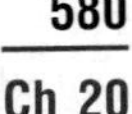

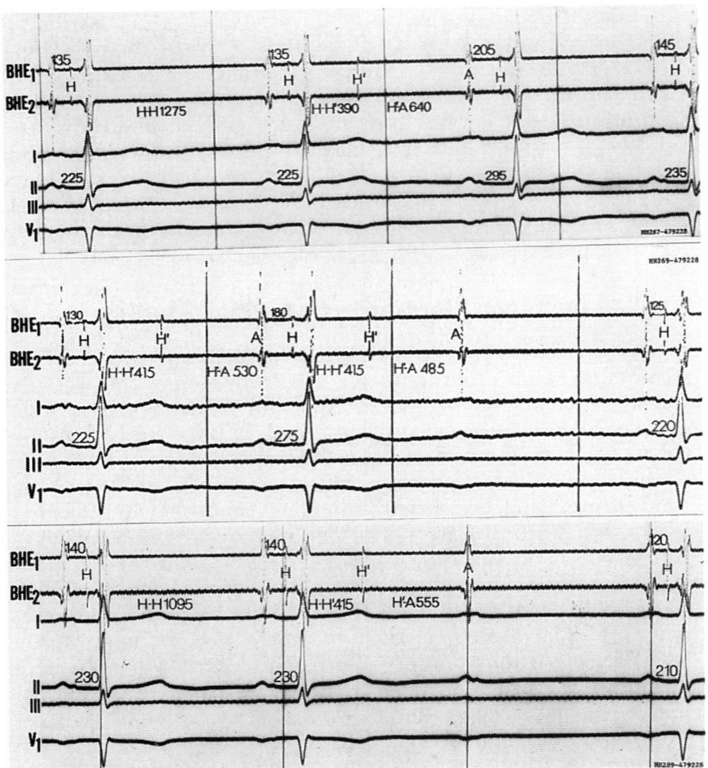

FIGURE 20–38. Concealed discharge from the bundle of His mimicking first-degree *(top)*, type I *(middle)*, and type II *(bottom)* second-degree AV block. Numbers are in milliseconds. Time lines are one second. (Magnification differs in the three panels.) Numbers in the bipolar His electrogram (BHE_1) indicate A-H intervals; the H-V interval is constant. Numbers in lead II indicate the P-R interval. H-H = interval between His responses in normal conducted cycles. H-H′ = interval between the last normal His discharge and the premature His discharge. H′ − A = interval between the premature His depolarization and the next normal sinus-initiated atrial discharge. H′ invaded the AV node and lengthened the A-H interval or produced AV nodal block of the next atrial depolarization. (From Bonner, A. J., and Zipes, D. P.: Lidocaine and His bundle extrasystoles. His bundle discharge conducted normally, conducted with functional right or left branch block, or blocked entirely (concealed). Arch. Intern Med. *136:*700, 1976. Copyright 1976 American Medical Association.)

Intraventricular Conduction Disturbance

For patients with an intraventricular conduction disturbance, an electrophysiological study provides information on the duration of the H-V interval, which can be prolonged with a normal P-R interval or normal with a prolonged P-R interval. A prolonged H-V interval (>55 msec) is associated with a greater likelihood of developing trifascicular block (but the rate of progression is slow, 2 to 3 per cent annually), having structural disease, and higher mortality. Finding very long H-V intervals (>80 to 90 msec) identifies patients at increased risk of developing AV block. The H-V interval has a high specificity (about 80 per cent) but low sensitivity (about 66 per cent) for predicting the development of complete AV block. During the study, atrial pacing is used to uncover abnormal His-Purkinje conduction.[295] A positive response is provocation of distal His block during 1:1 AV nodal conduction. Once again, sensitivity is low but specificity is high. Functional His-Purkinje block due to normal His-Purkinje refractoriness is not a positive response. Drug infusion, such as with procainamide or ajmaline, sometimes exposes abnormal His-Purkinje conduction. Ajmaline can cause arrhythmias and should be used cautiously.

An electrophysiological study is indicated in the patient with symptoms (syncope or presyncope) that appear to be related to a bradyarrhythmia or tachyarrhythmia when no other cause of symptoms is found. For many of these patients, ventricular *tachyarrhythmias* rather than AV block might be the cause of their symptoms.[296]

Sinus Nodal Dysfunction

The demonstration of slow sinus rates, sinus exit block, or sinus pauses temporally related to symptoms suggests a causal relationship and usually obviates further diagnostic studies.[297–301] Carotid sinus pressure that results in complete cardiac asystole or AV block with the patient's usual symptoms exposes the presence of a hypersensitive carotid sinus reflex (see p. 647). Carotid sinus massage must be done cautiously. Rarely, carotid sinus massage can precipitate a stroke. Neurohumoral agents, adenosine,[302] or stress testing can be employed to evaluate effects of autonomic tone on sinus node automaticity and sinoatrial conduction time. Electrophysiological studies should be considered in patients who have symptoms attributable to bradycardia or asystole, such as presyncope or syncope, and for whom noninvasive approaches have provided no explanation for the symptoms.[303]

SINUS NODE RECOVERY TIME (SNRT). This technique can be a useful test to evaluate sinus node function. The interval between the last paced high right atrial response and the first spontaneous (sinus) high right atrial response after termination of pacing is measured to determine the *sinus node recovery time* (SNRT). Because the spontaneous sinus rate influences the SNRT, the value is corrected by subtracting the spontaneous sinus node cycle length (prior to pacing) from the sinus recovery time (CSNRT) (Fig. 20–39). Normal CSNRT values are generally less than 525 msec. Prolonged CSNRT has been found in patients suspected of having sinus node dysfunction. Direct recordings of sinus node electrogram have documented that SNRT is influenced by prolongation of sinoatrial conduction time, as well as by changes in sinus nodal automaticity, especially in the first beat after cessation of pacing. After cessation of pacing, the first return sinus cycle can be normal and can be followed by secondary pauses (Fig. 20–39). Secondary pauses appear to be more common in patients whose sinus node dysfunction is caused by sinoatrial exit block. Sinoatrial exit block can cause some sinus pauses. It is important to evaluate AV nodal and His-Purkinje function in patients with sinus node dysfunction, since many also exhibit impaired AV conduction.

SINOATRIAL CONDUCTION TIME (SACT). This time can be estimated, based on the assumptions that (1) conduction times into and out of the sinus node are equal, (2) no depression of sinus node automaticity occurs, and (3) the pacemaker site does not shift following premature stimulation. These assumptions may be erroneous, particularly in patients with sinus nodal dysfunction; SACT can be measured directly with extracellular electrodes placed in the region of the sinus node and correlates well with the CSACT measured indirectly in patients with normal sinus node function. The sensitivity of the SACT and SNRT tests

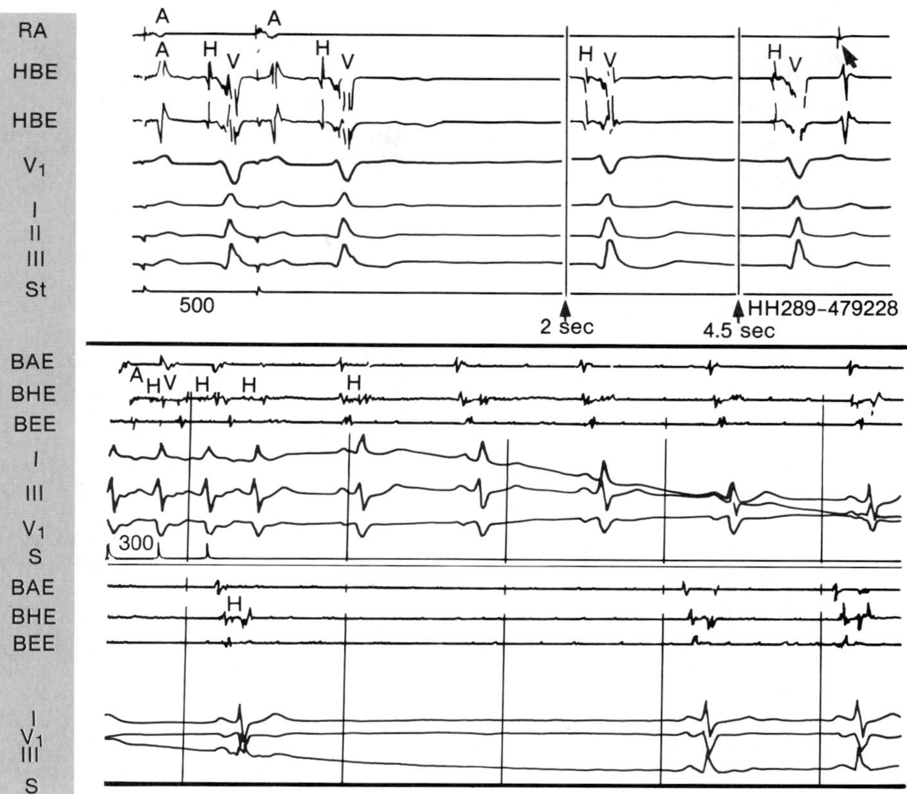

FIGURE 20–39. Abnormal response of sinus node to overdrive pacing. ***Top,*** **After 30 sec of right atrial pacing at a cycle length of 500 msec, sinus nodal discharge is suppressed for more than 8 sec. (Sections of 2 sec and 4.5 sec removed for mounting.)** ***Bottom,*** **Right atrial pacing at a cycle length of 300 msec was followed by initial P waves occurring at an appropriate rate. The rate then slowed progressively, with P-P prolongation reaching 3 seconds and reproducing the patient's symptoms. Continuous recording; time lines = 1 sec. RA and BAE = bipolar right atrial electrogram; HBE and BHE = bi-polar His electrogram; BEE = bipolar esophageal electrogram; I, II, III, and V = scalar leads; St and S = stimulus. (Modified from Zipes, D. P., and Noble, R. J.: Assessment of electrical abnormalities.** ***In*** **Hurst, J. W. [ed.]: The Heart. 5th ed. New York, McGraw-Hill Book Co., 1982, pp. 333–357.)**

is only about 50 per cent for each test alone and about 65 per cent when combined. The specificity, when combined, is about 88 per cent, with a low predictive value. Thus, if they are abnormal, the likelihood of the patient having sinus nodal dysfunction is great. However, if they are normal, that does not exclude the possibility of sinus node disease. Candidates for invasive electrophysiological study are symptomatic patients in whom sinus node dysfunction has not been established as a cause of the symptoms. Potential candidates are those requiring pacemakers to determine the pacing modality, patients with sinus node dysfunction to determine the mechanism and response to therapy, and patients in whom other causes of symptoms, e.g., tachyarrhythmias, are to be excluded.

Tachycardia

In patients with tachycardias, an electrophysiological study may be used to diagnose the arrhythmia, determine and deliver therapy, determine anatomical site(s) involved in the tachycardia, identify patients at high risk for developing serious arrhythmias, and gain insights into mechanisms responsible for the arrhythmia. The study can differentiate aberrant supraventricular conduction from ventricular tachyarrhythmias.[304] Since the electrocardiographic manifestations of ventricular tachycardia can be mimicked by aberrantly conducted supraventricular tachycardia, exceptions exist to the criteria that help to differentiate supraventricular tachyarrhythmias with abnormal QRS complexes from ventricular tachyarrhythmias.[237]

A *supraventricular tachycardia* is recognized electrophysiologically by the presence of an H-V interval equaling or exceeding that recorded during normal sinus rhythm (Fig. 20–40). In contrast, during *ventricular tachycardia,* the H-V interval is shorter than normal, or more commonly, the His deflection cannot be recorded clearly. Only two situations exist when a consistently short H-V interval occurs: during retrograde activation of the His bundle from activation originating in the ventricle, i.e., ventricular premature complex or tachycardia (see p. 677), or during conduction over an accessory pathway (preexcitation syndrome; see p. 667). Atrial pacing at rates exceeding the tachycardia rate can demonstrate ventricular origin of the wide QRS tachycardia by producing fusion and capture beats and normalization of the H-V interval (Fig. 20–41). The only ventricular tachycardia that exhibits an H-V interval resembling the normal sinus H-V interval is bundle branch reentry (see p. 686), but His activation will be in the retrograde direction.

INDICATIONS FOR TACHYCARDIA. An electrophysiological study should be considered (1) in patients who have symptomatic, recurrent, or drug-resistant supraventricular or ventricular tachyarrhythmias to help select optimal therapy; (2) in patients with tachyarrhythmias occurring too infrequently to permit adequate diagnostic or therapeutic assessment; (3) to differentiate supraventricular tachycardia and aberrant conduction from ventricular tachycardia; (4) whenever nonpharmacological therapy such as the use of electrical devices, catheter ablation, or surgery is contemplated; and (5) in patients surviving an episode of cardiac arrest occurring ≥ 48 hours after an acute myocardial infarction or without evidence of an acute Q-wave myocardial infarction. Electrophysiological studies are generally *not* indicated in patients with the long Q-T syndrome and torsades de pointes, although recent information about early afterdepolarizations (see p. 566) may make such studies useful in the future.

The process of initiation and termination of supraventricular or ventricular tachycardia with programmed electrical stimulation to test the potential efficacy of pharmacological, electrical, or surgical therapy represents an important application of electrophysiological studies in patients with tachycardia. Arrhythmia-free survival is higher among patients in whom a drug prevents electrical reinduction of a sustained monomorphic ventricular tachycardia that was induced during the predrug control state. Among patients in whom ventricular tachycardia remains inducible, characteristics of the induced arrhythmia predict features of future recurrences. When the tachycardia and its hemodynamic response are not altered, an adverse risk for recurrence and mortality is predicted. When the tachycardia cycle length prolongs more than 100 msec and stable hemodynamics result, mortality improves.

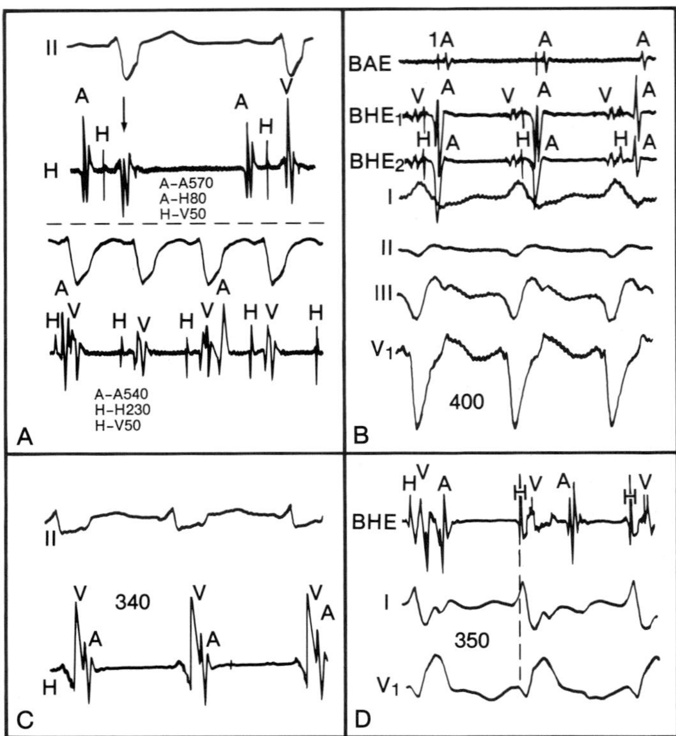

FIGURE 20–40. His bundle recording in four different patients with tachycardias. *A*, The top portion of the tracing shows His bundle recording during sinus rhythm. The H-V interval is 50 msec. The bottom portion shows His bundle recording during tachycardia. Since the QRS complex and H-V interval are the same as those recorded during sinus rhythm, this is a supraventricular tachycardia. Of note is the fact that the atria discharged at a rate that was different from (not a multiple of) the ventricular rate. Thus AV dissociation is present during this supraventricular tachycardia. *B*, His bundle activity occurred after the onset of the QRS complex, during ventricular tachycardia. (WPW had been excluded.) The R-P interval remained constant, and the atria were captured retrogradely from the ventricles. Thus AV dissociation is not present during this ventricular tachycardia. *C*, His bundle activity was not recorded despite careful exploration of the His bundle area with the catheter electrode tip. This most likely represents ventricular tachycardia with 1:1 retrograde atrial capture, but the diagnosis cannot be as clear as in panels *B* and *D*. In panel *D*, His bundle activity (interrupted line) preceded the onset of ventricular septal depolarization but followed the onset of the QRS complex. Thus this must be ventricular tachycardia. Retrograde (VA) Wenckebach conduction (not shown in its entirety) also was present. (From Zipes, D. P., et al.: Clinical electrophysiology and electrocardiography. *In* Willerson, J. T., and Sanders, C. A. [eds.]: Clinical Cardiology. New York, Grune and Stratton, 1977, pp. 235–248.)

Determination of drug efficacy based on results from long-term ECG recordings may be insufficient to predict a patient's therapeutic response when a low frequency of spontaneous ventricular arrhythmias are present. However, recently two studies have concluded that noninvasive assessment of drug efficacy testing beta blockers[305] and amiodarone[306] may be superior to the results of programmed electrical stimulation using conventional antiarrhythmic agents. Another controlled randomized study comparing invasive and noninvasive assessments of conventional drugs[248] found both techniques to be equivalent.[247] As of this writing both invasive and noninvasive methods should be considered appropriate approaches for guiding drug therapy.

Patients with Unexplained Syncope

(See p. 868)

The three common arrhythmic causes of syncope include sinus node dysfunction, tachyarrhythmias, and AV block. Of the three, tachyarrhythmias are most reliably initiated in the electrophysiology laboratory, followed by sinus node abnormalities and then His-Purkinje block.[307]

The cause of syncope goes undetected in up to 50 per cent of patients, depending in part on the extent of the evaluation. A careful, accurately performed history and physical examination begin the evaluation,[239] followed by noninvasive tests, including a 12-lead and 24-hour ECG recording, and can lead to a diagnosis in half or more of the patients.[307–311] The 1-year mortality is about 6 per cent in patients with unknown cause, 1 to 12 per cent in patients with noncardiovascular causes, but 19 to 30 per cent in patients with cardiovascular causes. The incidence of sudden death is also higher in patients with a cardiovascular cause of syncope. A small percentage (<5 per cent) of patients develop an arrhythmia coincident with syncope or presyncope during a 24-hour ECG recording, while a large percentage (15 per cent) have symptoms without an arrhythmia, excluding an arrhythmic cause. Prolonged ECG monitoring with patient-activated transtelephonic event recorders that have memory loops may increase the yield. Signal averaging (see p. 583) has a high sensitivity (about 75 per cent) and specificity (about 90 per cent) for predicting patients with syncope in whom ventricular tachycardia can be induced at electrophysiological study.[312] Tilt table testing[313–315,315a] and stress testing[316] can be useful in some patients, as can long-term ECG recordings.[317]

The electrophysiological study helps explain the cause of syncope or palpitations when it induces an arrhythmia that replicates the patient's symptoms. Syncopal patients with a nondiagnostic electrophysiological study have a low incidence of sudden death and 80 per cent remission rate. In those with recurrent syncope, the test is falsely negative in ≥20 per cent, due to failure to find AV block or sinus node dysfunction.

Syncopal patients considered for electrophysiological study are those whose spells remain undiagnosed despite general, neurological, and noninvasive cardiac evaluation, particularly if the patient has structural heart disease. The diagnostic yield is about 70 per cent in that group but only about 12 per cent in patients without structural heart disease. Prevention of syncope is economically important.[318] Mortality and incidence of sudden cardiac death are mainly determined by the presence of underlying heart disease.[319] Therapy of a putative cause found during electrophysiological testing prevents recurrence of syncope in about 80 per cent of patients. At times, empiric pacing is justified.

Palpitations

An electrophysiological study is indicated in patients with palpitations[240,320,321] who have had a pulse rate that medical personnel documented to be inappropriately rapid without electrocardiographic recording or in those suspected of having clinically significant palpitations without ECG documentation.

In patients with syncope or palpitation, the sensitivity of the electrophysiological test may be very low but may be increased at the expense of specificity. For example, more aggressive pacing techniques (e.g., using three or four premature stimuli), administration of drugs (e.g., isoproterenol), or left ventricular pacing can increase the success rate of ventricular tachycardia induction, but by precipitating nonclinical ventricular tachyarrhythmias such as nonsustained polymorphic or monomorphic ventricular tachycardia or ventricular fibrillation. Similarly, aggressive techniques during atrial pacing can induce nonspecific episodes of atrial flutter or atrial fibrillation. A diagnostic dilemma arises when the patient's clinical, symptom-producing arrhythmia is one of these nonspecific arrhythmias that can be produced in the normal patient who has no arrhythmia. Induction of *sustained* supraventricular (e.g., AV nodal reentry, AV reciprocating tachycardia) or monomorphic ventricular tachycardia in patients who are not subject

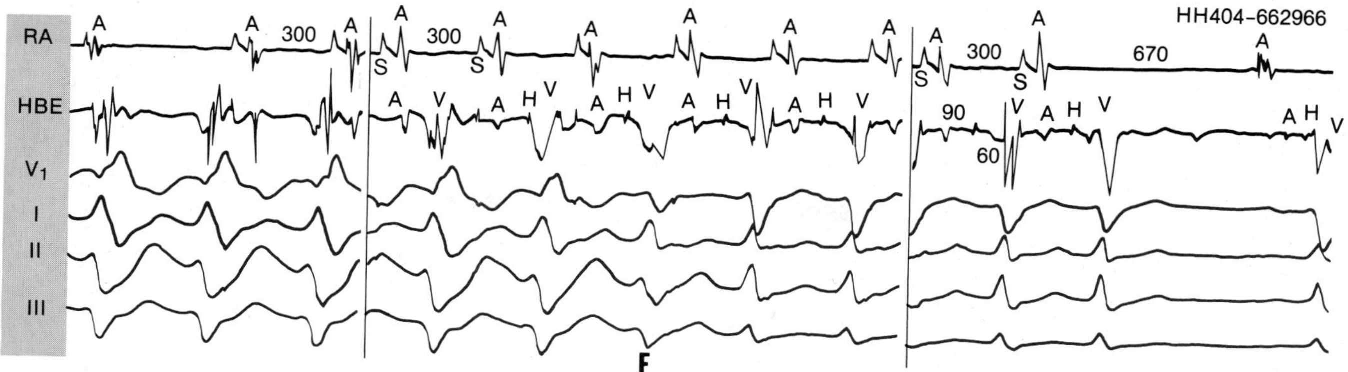

FIGURE 20–41. Termination of ventricular tachycardia by rapid atrial pacing. Ventricular tachycardia *(left panel)* with AV dissociation became captured by rapid atrial pacing (200 bpm) *(middle panel)* and was terminated after cessation of atrial pacing *(right panel)*. Note fusion beat (F) in the midportion of panel 2 and normalization of the H-V interval. (From Foster, P. R., and Zipes, D. P.: Pacing and cardiac arrhythmias. *In* Mandel, W. J. [ed.]: Cardiac Arrhythmias: Their Mechanisms, Diagnosis and Management. Philadelphia, J. B. Lippincott, 1980, pp. 605–624.)

to the spontaneous development of the tachycardia appears to be uncommon and provides important information that the induced tachyarrhythmia may be clinically significant and responsible for the patient's symptoms. Generally, other abnormalities such as prolonged sinus pauses following overdrive atrial pacing or His-Purkinje AV block are not induced in patients who do not or may not experience these abnormalities spontaneously. Induction of these arrhythmias has a high degree of specificity.

Complications of Electrophysiological Studies

The risks of undergoing only an electrophysiological study are small. Adding therapeutic maneuvers, e.g., ablation, to the procedure increases the incidence of complications. In a European survey[322] published in 1993 based on 4398 patients reported from 68 institutions, procedure-related complications ranged from 3.2 to 8 per cent. Five deaths occurred within the perioperative period of the ablation. In an NASPE survey[323] of 164 hospitals reporting in 1994 on over 10,000 patients who received RF ablation, complications ranged from 1 to 3 per cent, with procedure-related deaths about 0.2 per cent. The improvement in the complication rate probably reflects the learning curve for RF ablation.

OTHER DIAGNOSTIC ELECTROCARDIOGRAPHIC TECHNIQUES

ESOPHAGEAL ELECTROCARDIOGRAPHY. Esophageal electrocardiography is a useful noninvasive technique to diagnose arrhythmias.[324,325] The esophagus is adjacent to the posterior atria, and an electrode inserted into the esophagus can record atrial potentials. Bipolar recording is superior to unipolar recording. In addition, atrial and occasionally ventricular pacing can be performed via a catheter electrode inserted into the esophagus, and initiation and termination of tachycardias can be accomplished. Optimal electrode position for pacing correlates with patient height and is within about 1 cm of the site at which the maximum amplitude of the atrial electrogram is recorded. No serious immediate complications of transesophageal pacing have been reported. A capsule electrode that is easily swallowed has been used to record continuous atrial electrograms from the esophagus.

The esophageal atrial electrogram is useful to differentiate supraventricular tachycardia with aberrancy from ventricular tachycardia (see p. 677) and to define the mechanism of supraventricular tachycardias. For example, if atrial and ventricular depolarization occur simultaneously during a narrow QRS tachycardia, reentry utilizing an accessory AV pathway (Wolff-Parkinson-White) can be excluded, and AV nodal reentry is the most likely mechanism for the tachycardia (see p. 661).

BODY SURFACE MAPPING. Isopotential body surface maps are used to provide a complete picture of the effects of the currents from the heart on the body surface. The potential distributions are represented by contour lines of equal potential, and each distribution is displayed instant by instant throughout activation or recovery, or both.[327–329]

Body surface maps have been used clinically to localize and size areas of myocardial ischemia, localize ectopic foci or accessory pathways, differentiate aberrant supraventricular conduction from ventricular origin, recognize the patient prone to developing arrhythmias, and possibly understand the mechanisms involved.[330–337] Although these procedures are of interest, their clinical utility has not yet been established.

DIRECT CARDIAC MAPPING: RECORDING POTENTIALS DIRECTLY FROM THE HEART. Cardiac mapping is a method whereby potentials recorded directly from the heart are spatially depicted as a function of time in an integrated manner. The location of recording electrodes (epicardial, intramural, or endocardial) and the recording mode used (unipolar versus bipolar) as well as the method of display (isopotential versus isochrone maps) depend upon the problem under consideration. Special electrodes can record monophasic action potentials.[338]

Direct cardiac mapping via catheter electrodes or at the time of cardiac surgery can be used to identify and localize the site of rhythm disturbances in patients with supraventricular and ventricular tachyarrhythmias for electrical or surgical ablation, isolation, or resection, such as accessory pathways associated with the Wolff-Parkinson-White syndrome, the slow pathway in AV nodal reentry, and VT circuits, or to delineate the anatomical course of the His bundle to avoid injury during open-heart surgery. These approaches are discussed in greater detail in Chap. 21 under nonpharmacological approaches and in Chap. 22 under the individual arrhythmias.

SIGNAL-AVERAGING TECHNIQUES. Signal averaging is a method that improves signal-to-noise ratio when signals are recurrent and the noise is random.[339] In conjunction with appropriate filtering and other methods of noise reduction, signal averaging can detect cardiac signals of a few microvolts in amplitude, reducing noise amplitude, such as muscle potentials that are typically 5 to 25 μV, to less than 1 μV. With this method, electrical potentials generated by the sinus and AV nodes, His bundle, and bundle branches are detectable at the body surface.

Signal averaging has been applied clinically most often to detect late ventricular potentials of 1 to 25 μV, which

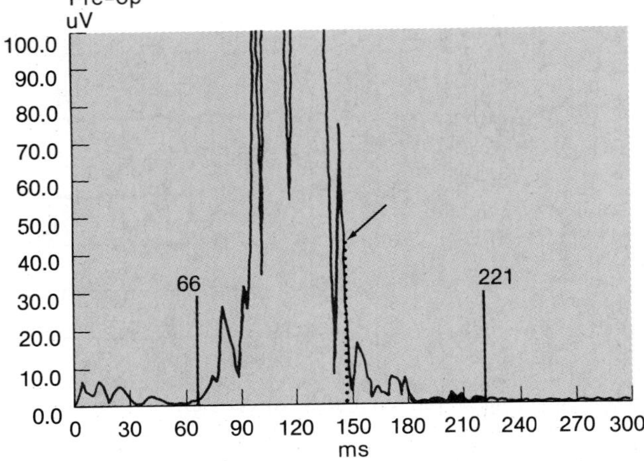

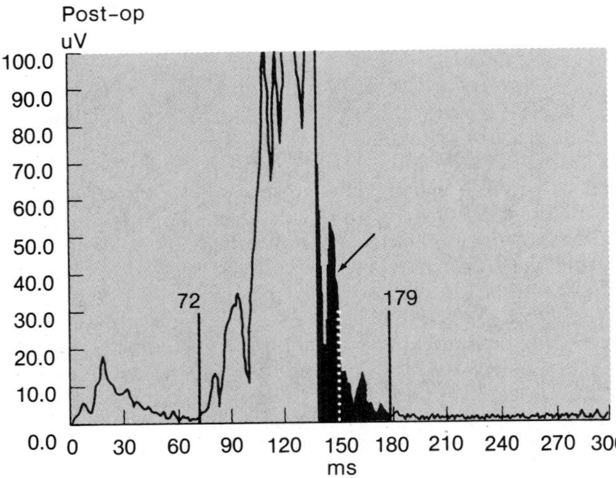

FIGURE 20–42. Signal-averaged ECG showing the presence of prolonged QRS duration due to late potentials (dark filled components in the terminal portion of the complex) present preoperatively but not postoperatively. RMS, root mean square (in mV); IN, integral of wave form delineated by the onset and offset markers; LAS, low amplitude signal. MN, mean value in the terminal QRS. Arrow indicates the 40 mV mark, after which the presence of low amplitude signals is determined. Scale = number of mV per notch.

are microvolt waveforms continuous with the QRS complex, probably corresponding to delayed and fragmented conduction in the ventricle[340–343] (Fig. 20–42). Criteria for late potentials are (1) filtered QRS complex duration >114 to 120 msec, (2) <20 μV of signal in the last 40 msec of the filtered QRS complex, and (3) the terminal filtered QRS complex remains below 40 μV for longer than 39 msec. These late potentials have been recorded in 70 to 90 per cent of patients with sustained and inducible ventricular tachycardia after myocardial infarction, in only 0 to 6 per cent of normal volunteers, and in 7 to 15 per cent of patients after myocardial infarction who do not have ventricular tachycardia. Late potentials can be detected as early as 3 hours after the onset of chest pain and increase in prevalence in the first week after infarction and may disappear in some patients after 1 year. If not present initially, late potentials usually do not appear later. Early use of thrombolytic agents may reduce the prevalence of late potentials after coronary occlusion.

Late potentials also have been recorded in patients with ventricular tachycardia not related to ischemia, such as dilated cardiomyopathies. Successful surgical resection of the ventricular tachycardia can eliminate late potentials but is not necessary to cause tachycardia suppression. Antiarrhythmic drug therapy, on the other hand, decreases the amplitude of the late potentials without abolishing them. Late potentials after myocardial infarction are an independent risk factor that identifies patients prone to develop ventricular tachycardia and can be combined with other data such as ejection fraction, spontaneous ventricular ectopy on a 24-hour ECG recording, or response to stress testing to recognize with high sensitivity and specificity patients at risk for ventricular tachycardia or sudden cardiac death. It also can be used to identify patients with nonsustained ventricular tachycardia or syncope who may develop sustained ventricular tachycardia at electrophysiological study.

The high-pass filtering used to record late potentials meeting the criteria just noted is called *time domain analysis* because the filter output corresponds in time with the input signal. Since late potentials are high-frequency signals, Fourier transform can be applied to extract high-frequency content from the signal-averaged ECG, called *frequency domain analysis*. Some but not all data suggest that frequency domain analysis provides useful information not available in the time domain analysis. The preferable alternative has not been determined.

UPRIGHT TILT TESTING (see also p. 870). The tilt test is used to identify patients who have a vasodepressor and/or a cardioinhibitory response as a cause of syncope.[344,345] Patients are positioned on a tilt table in the supine position and are tilted upright to a maximum of 60 to 80 degrees for 20 to 45 minutes, or longer if necessary. Isoproterenol,[346–348] a bolus or an infusion, may provoke syncope in patients asymptomatic after initial upright tilt testing or after just several minutes of tilt to shorten the time of the test necessary to produce a positive response. An initial intravenous isoproterenol dose of 2 μg can be increased in 2-μg steps until symptoms occur or a maximum of 8 μg is given. Isoproterenol induces a vasodepressor response in upright susceptible patients generally consisting of a decrease in heart rate and blood pressure along with near syncope or syncope. Intravenous edrophonium,[349] nitroglycerin,[344] and esmolol[350] withdrawal have been used. Atropine can block the early bradycardia but not the hypotension. Beta blockers[351,352] can inhibit the latter. Tilt test results are positive in two-thirds to three-quarters of patients susceptible to neurally mediated syncope, are repro-

TABLE 20–8 CLASSIFICATION OF HEART RATE AND HEMODYNAMIC RESPONSES TO HEAD-UP TILT TABLE TESTING

Type I: Mixed
Heart rate rises initially and then falls, but the ventricular rate does not fall to less than 40 beats/min or falls to 40 beats/min for less than 10 seconds with or without asystole for less than 3 seconds.

Blood pressure rises initially and then falls before heart rate falls.

Type IIA: Cardioinhibitory
Heart rate rises initially and then falls to a ventricular rate of less than 40 beats/min for greater than 10 seconds, or asystole occurs for greater than 3 seconds.

Blood pressure rises initially and then falls before heart rate falls.

Type IIB: Cardioinhibitory
Heart rate rises initially and then falls to a ventricular rate of less than 40 beats/min for more than 10 seconds, or asystole occurs for more than 3 seconds.

Blood pressure rises initially and only falls to hypotensive levels less than 80 mm Hg systolic at or after onset of rapid and severe heart rate fall.

Type III: Pure vasodepressor
Heart rate rises progressively and does not fall more than 10 per cent from peak at time of syncope.

Blood pressure falls to cause syncope.

ducible in about 80 per cent,[353–356] but have a 10 to 15 per cent false-positive response rate. Positive can be divided into mixed, cardioinhibitory, and vasodepressor categories[357] (Table 20–8). Therapy with beta blockers,[351,352] disopyramide,[358] and theophylline has been tried.

Mechanism. Vasodepressor reactions, which are thought to be caused by activation of unmyelinated left ventricular vagal C fibers, can be excited by a variety of substances, including increased left ventricular pressure. Stimulation of C fibers from vigorous left ventricular contraction on an empty cavity reduces efferent sympathetic tone while increasing efferent vagal tone, possibly producing vasodepression and paradoxic bradycardia. Isoproterenol increases left ventricular contractility while reducing left ventricular volume. A passive upright tilt exaggerates these responses because the tilt also reduces venous return and prevents isoproterenol from increasing cardiac output. Some patients may experience profound bradycardia while others may have a prominent vasodepressor component (Table 20–8).

BARORECEPTOR REFLEX SENSITIVITY TESTING. Acute blood pressure elevation triggers a baroreceptor reflex that augments vagal "tone" to the heart and slows the sinus rate. The increase in sinus cycle length per mm Hg increase is a measure of the sensitivity of the baroreceptor reflex (BRS) and identifies patients susceptible to developing VT and VF.[32] The mechanism of the redirection in BRS is not known. However, this test may be useful to identify patients at risk for developing a serious ventricular arrhythmia after myocardial infarction.

REFERENCES

ANATOMY OF THE CARDIAC CONDUCTION SYSTEM

1. Trabka-Janik, E., Coombs, W., Lemanski, L. F., et al.: Immunohistochemical focalization of gap junction protein channels in hamster sinoatrial node in correlation with electrophysiologic mapping of the pacemaker region. J. Cardiovasc. Electrophysiol. *5:*125, 1994.
2. Opthof, T.: Gap junctions in the sinoatrial node: Immunohistochemical focalization and correlation with activation pattern. J. Cardiovasc. Electrophysiol. *5:*138, 1994.
3. Saffitz, J. E.: Cell-to-cell communication in the heart. Cardiol. Rev. *3:*86, 1995.
4. Cai, D., Winslow, R. L., and Noble, D.: Effects of gap junction conductance on dynamics of the sinoatrial node cells: T-cell and large scale network models. IEEE Trans. Biomed. Eng. *41:*217, 1994.
5. Davis, L. M., Kanter, H. L., Beyer, E. C., et al.: Distinct gap junction protein phenotypes in cardiac tissues with disparate conduction properties. J. Am. Coll. Cardiol. *24:*1124, 1994.
6. Beyer, E. C., Veenstra, R. D., Kanter, H. L., et al.: Molecular structure and patterns of expression of cardiac gap junction proteins. *In* Zipes, D. P., and Jalife, J. (eds.): Cardiac Electrophysiology: From Cell to Bedside. 2nd ed. Philadelphia, W. B. Saunders Company, 1994, p. 31.
7. Pressler, M. L., Munster, P. N., and Haung, X.: Gap junction distribution in the heart: Functional relevance. *In* Zipes, D. P., and Jalife, J. (eds.): Cardiac Electrophysiology: From Cell to Bedside. 2nd ed. Philadelphia, W. B. Saunders Company, 1994, p. 144.
8. Severs, N. J.: Pathophysiology of gap junctions in heart disease. J. Cardiovasc. Electrophysiol. *5:*462, 1994.
9. Anumonwo, J. M. B., and Jalife, J.: Cellular and subcellular mechanisms of pacemaker activity initiation and synchronization in the heart. *In* Zipes, D. P., and Jalife, J. (eds.): Cardiac Electrophysiology: From Cell to Bedside. 2nd ed. Philadelphia, W. B. Saunders Company, 1994, p. 151.
10. Schuessler, R. B., Boineau, J. P., Bromberg, B. I., et al.: Normal and abnormal activation of the atrium. *In* Zipes, D. P., and Jalife, J. (eds.): Cardiac Electrophysiology: From Cell to Bedside. 2nd ed. Philadelphia, W. B. Saunders Company, 1994, p. 543.
11. Pappano, A. J.: Modulation of the heart beat by the vagus nerve. *In* Zipes, D. P., and Jalife, J. (eds.): Cardiac Electrophysiology: From Cell to Bedside. 2nd ed. Philadelphia, W. B. Saunders Company, 1994, p. 411.
12. Levy, M. N.: Time dependency of the autonomic interactions that regulate heart rate and rhythms. *In* Zipes, D. P., and Jalife, J. (eds.): Cardiac Electrophysiology: From Cell to Bedside. 2nd ed. Philadelphia, W. B. Saunders Company, 1994, p. 454.
13. Mitrani, R. D., and Zipes, D. P.: Clinical neurocardiology: Arrhythmias. *In* Ardell, J. L., and Armour, J. A. (eds.): Neurocardiology. Oxford, England, Oxford University Press, 1994, pp. 365–395.
14. Zipes, D. P.: Autonomic modulation of cardiac arrhythmias. *In* Zipes, D. P., and Jalife, J. (eds.): Cardiac Electrophysiology: From Cell to Bedside. 2nd ed. Philadelphia, W. B. Saunders Company, 1994, p. 441.
15. Elvan, A., and Zipes, D. P.: Functional anatomy of autonomic innervation of the atria. *In* Waldo, A., and Touboul, P. (eds.): Recent Advances in Atrial Flutter. Mt. Kisco, N. Y., Futura *(in press).*
16. Levy, M. N., and Schwartz, P. J. (eds.): Vagal Control of the Heart: Experimental Basis and Clinical Implications. Mt. Kisco, N. Y., Futura, 1994.
17. DiFrancesco, D.: A contribution of the hyperpolarization-activated current (I_f) to the generation of spontaneous activity in rabbit sinoatrial node myocytes. J. Physiol. *434:*23, 1991.
18. DiFrancesco, D., and Tortora, P.: Direct activation of cardiac pacemaker channels by intracellular cyclic AMP. Nature *351:*145, 1991.
19. DiFrancesco, D., and Zaza, A.: The cardiac pacemaker current I_f. J. Cardiovasc. Electrophysiol. *3:*334, 1992.
20. DiFrancesco, D.: Pacemaker mechanisms in cardiac tissue. Annu. Rev. Physiol. *55:*451, 1993.
21. DiFrancesco, D., Mangoni, M., and Maccaferri, G.: The pacemaker current in cardiac cells. *In* Zipes, D. P., and Jalife, J. (eds.): Cardiac Electrophysiology: From Cell to Bedside. 2nd ed. Philadelphia, W. B. Saunders Company, 1994, p. 96.
22. Kuarmby, L. M., and Hartzell, H. C.: Molecular biology of G proteins and their role in cardiac excitability. *In* Zipes, D. P., and Jalife, J. (eds.): Cardiac Electrophysiology: From Cell to Bedside. 2nd ed. Philadelphia, W. B. Saunders Company, 1994, p. 38.
23. Racker, D. K.: Transmission and reentrant activity in the sinoventricular conducting system and in the circumferential lamina of the tricuspid valve. J. Cardiovasc. Electrophysiol. *4:*513, 1993.
24. Janse, M. J., Anderson, R. H., McGuire, M. A., et al.: "AV nodal" reentry: 1. "AV nodal" reentry revisited. J. Cardiovasc. Electrophysiol. *4:*561, 1993.
25. McGuire, M. A., Janse, M. J., and Ross, D. L.: "AV nodal" reentry: 2. AV nodal, AV junctional or atrial nodal reentry? J. Cardiovasc. Electrophysiol. *4:*573, 1993.
26. Jackman, W. M., Beckman, K. J., McClelland, J. H., et al.: Treatment of supraventricular tachycardia due to atrioventricular nodal reentry by radiofrequency ablation of slow-pathway conduction. N. Engl. J. Med. *327:*313, 1992.

27. Ho, S. Y., McComb, J. M., Scott, C. D., et al.: Morphology of the cardiac conduction system in patients with electrophysiologically proven dual atrioventricular nodal pathways. J. Cardiovasc. Electrophysiol. *4*:504, 1993.
28. Ho, S. Y., Kilpatrick, L., Kanai, T., et al.: The architecture of the atrioventricular conduction axis in dogs compared to humans: Its significance to ablation of the atrioventricular nodal approaches. J. Cardiovasc. Electrophysiol. *6*:26, 1995.
29. Paes de Carvalho, A., and de Almeida, D. F.: Spread of activity through the atrioventricular node. Circ. Res. *8*:801, 1960.
30. Jongsma, H. J., and Rook, M. B.: Morphology and electrophysiology of cardiac gap junction channels. *In* Zipes, D. P., and Jalife, J. (eds.): Cardiac Electrophysiology: From Cell to Bedside. 2nd ed. Philadelphia, W. B. Saunders Company, 1994, p. 115.
31. Ito, M., and Zipes, D. P.: Efferent sympathetic and vagal innervation of the canine right ventricle. Circulation *90*:1459, 1994.
32. DeFerrari, G. M., Vanoli, E., and Schwartz, P. J.: Cardiac vagal activity, myocardial ischemia, and sudden death. *In* Zipes, D. P., and Jalife, J. (eds.): Cardiac Electrophysiology: From Cell to Bedside. 2nd ed. Philadelphia, W. B. Saunders Company, 1994, p. 422.
33. Spooner, P. M., and Brown, A. M.: Ion Channels in the Cardiovascular System. Mt. Kisco, N. Y., Futura, 1994.

BASIC ELECTROPHYSIOLOGICAL PRINCIPLES

34. Grant, A. O.: Evolving concepts of cardiac sodium channel function. J. Cardiovasc. Electrophysiol. *1*:53, 1990.
35. Katz, A. M.: Cardiac ion channels. N. Engl. J. Med. *328*:1244, 1993.
36. Hanck, D. A.: Biophysics of sodium channels. *In* Zipes, D. P., and Jalife, J. (eds.): Cardiac Electrophysiology: From Cell to Bedside. 2nd ed. Philadelphia, W. B. Saunders Company, 1994, p. 65.
37. Catterall, W. A.: Molecular analysis of voltage gated sodium channels in the heart and other tissues. *In* Zipes, D. P., and Jalife, J. (eds.): Cardiac Electrophysiology: From Cell to Bedside. 2nd ed. Philadelphia, W. B. Saunders Company, 1994, p. 1.
38. Marban, E., and O'Rourke, B.: Calcium channels: Structure, function and regulation. *In* Zipes, D. P., and Jalife, J. (eds.): Cardiac Electrophysiology: From Cell to Bedside. 2nd ed. Philadelphia, W. B. Saunders Company, 1994, p. 11.
39. Alvarez, J., and Vassort, G.: Cardiac T-type Ca current: Pharmacology and emphasis on its roles in cardiac tissues. J. Cardiovasc. Electrophysiol. *5*:376, 1994.
40. Borgatta, L., Watras, J., Katz, A. M., et al.: Regional differences in calcium-release channels from heart. Proc. Natl. Acad. Sci. U.S.A. *88*:2486, 1991.
41. January, C. T., Cunningham, P. M., and Zhou, Z.: Pharmacology of L- and T-type calcium channels in the heart. *In* Zipes, D. P., and Jalife, J. (eds.): Cardiac Electrophysiology: From Cell to Bedside. 2nd ed. Philadelphia, W. B. Saunders Company, 1994, p. 269.
42. Campbell, D. L., Rasmusson, R. L., Comer, M. B., et al.: The cardiac calcium-independent transient outward potassium current: Kinetics, molecular properties and role in ventricular repolarizations. *In* Zipes, D. P., and Jalife, J. (eds.): Cardiac Electrophysiology: From Cell to Bedside. 2nd ed. Philadelphia, W. B. Saunders Company, 1995, p. 83.
43. Rose, W. C., Balke, C. W., Wier, W. G., et al.: Macroscopic and unitary properties of physiological ion flux through L-type Ca channels in guinea-pig heart cells. J. Physiol. *456*:267, 1992.
44. Tang, S., Mikala, G., Bahinski, A., et al.: Molecular focalization of ion selectivity sites within the pore of a human cardiac L-type calcium channel. J. Biol. Chem. *286*:13026, 1993.
45. Clapham, D. E.: Control of intracellular calcium. *In* Zipes, D. P., and Jalife, J. (eds.): Cardiac Electrophysiology: From Cell to Bedside. 2nd ed. Philadelphia, W. B. Saunders Company, 1994, p. 127.
46. Hartzell, H. C., and Buchatelle-Gourdon, I.: Structure and neuromodulation of cardiac calcium channels. J. Cardiovasc. Electrophysiol. *3*:567, 1992.
47. Cohen, N. M., and Lederer, W. J.: Calcium current in single human cardiac myocytes. J. Cardiovasc. Electrophysiol. *4*:422, 1993.
48. Ming, Z., Nordin, C., and Aronson, R. S.: Role of L-type calcium channel window current in generating current-induced early afterdepolarizations. J. Cardiovasc. Electrophysiol. *5*:323, 1994.
49. Singh, B. N., Wellens, H. J. J., and Hiraoka, M. (eds.): Electropharmacological Control of Cardiac Arrhythmias. To Delay Conduction or Prolong Refractoriness? Edited by Mt. Kisco, N. Y., Futura, 1994.
50. Vassort, G., and Alvarez, J.: Cardiac T-type calcium current: Pharmacology and roles in cardiac tissues. J. Cardiovasc. Electrophysiol. *5*:376, 1994.
51. Members of the Sicilian Gambit: Antiarrhythmic Therapy: A Pathophysiologic Approach. Mt. Kisco, N. Y., Futura, 1994.
52. Pressler, M. L., and Rardon, D. P.: Molecular basis for arrhythmias: Role of two nonsarcolemmal ion channels. J. Cardiovasc. Electrophysiol. *1*:464, 1990.
53. Veenstra, R. D.: Physiological modulation of cardiac gap junction channels. J. Cardiovasc. Electrophysiol. *1*:168, 1990.
54. Brink, P. R.: Gap junction channels and cell-to-cell messengers in myocardium. J. Cardiovasc. Electrophysiol. *2*:360, 1991.
55. Shenasa, M., Borggrefe, M., and Breithardt, G. (eds.): Cardiac Mapping. Mt. Kisco, N. Y., Futura, 1993.
56. Delmar, M., Liu, S., and Morley, G. E.: Toward a moleculum model for the pH regulation of intercellular communication in the heart. *In* Zipes, D. P., and Jalife, J. (eds.): Cardiac Electrophysiology: From Cell to Bedside. 2nd ed. Philadelphia, W. B. Saunders Company, 1994, p. 135.
57. Fozzard, H. A., Haber, E., Jennings, R. B., Katz, A. M., and Morgan, H. E.: The Heart and Cardiovascular System. New York, Raven Press, 1991.
58. Zipes, D. P., and Jalife, J. (eds.): Cardiac Electrophysiology: From Cell to Bedside. 2nd ed. Philadelphia, W. B. Saunders Company, 1994.
59. Carmeliet, E.: Potassium channels in cardiac cells. Cardiovasc. Drugs Ther. *6*:305, 1992.
60. Tamkun, M. M., Bennett, T. B., and Snyder, S. D. J.: Cloning and expression of human cardiac potassium channels. *In* Zipes, D. P., and Jalife, J. (eds.): Cardiac Electrophysiology: From Cell to Bedside. 2nd ed. Philadelphia, W. B. Saunders Company, 1994, p. 21.
61. Lazdunski, M.: Potassium channels: Structure-function relationships, diversity and pharmacology. Cardiovasc. Drugs Ther. *6*:313, 1992.
62. Kass, R. S.: Delayed potassium channels in the heart: Cellular molecular and regulatory properties. *In* Zipes, D. P., and Jalife, J. (eds.): Cardiac Electrophysiology: From Cell to Bedside. 2nd ed. Philadelphia, W. B. Saunders Company, 1994, p. 74.
63. Joho, R. H.: Toward a molecular understanding of voltage-gaited potassium channels. J. Cardiovasc. Electrophysiol. *3*:589, 1992.
64. Delmar, M.: Role of potassium currents on cell excitability in cardiac ventricular myocytes. J. Cardiovasc. Electrophysiol. *3*:474, 1992.
65. Nabauer, M., Beuckelmann, D. J., and Erdmann, E.: Characteristics of transient outward current in human ventricular myocytes from patients with terminal heart failure. Circ. Res. *73*:386, 1993.
66. Hagiwara, N., Irisawa, H., Kasanuki, H., et al.: Background inward current sensitive to sodium ion in the sinoatrial node of rabbit heart. J. Physiol. (Lond.) *(in press)*.
67. Fleet, W. F., Johnson, T. A., Cascio, W. E., et al.: Marked activation delay caused by ischemia initiated after regional K^+ elevation in in situ pig hearts. Circulation *90*:3009, 1994.
68. Sicouri, S., Fish, J., and Antzelevitch, C.: Distribution of M cells in the canine ventricle. J. Cardiovasc. Electrophysiol. *5*:824, 1994.
69. Antzelevitch, C., Sicouri, S., Lukas, A., et al.: Regional differences in the electrophysiology of ventricular cells: Physiological and clinical implications. *In* Zipes, D. P., and Jalife, J. (eds.): Cardiac Electrophysiology: From Cell to Bedside. 2nd ed. Philadelphia, W. B. Saunders Company, 1994, p. 228.
70. Antzelevitch, C., and Sicouri, S.: Clinical relevance of cardiac arrhythmias generated by afterdepolarizations: The role of M cells in the generation of U waves, triggered activity and torsade de point. J. Am. Coll. Cardiol. *23*:259, 1994.
71. Harvey, R. D., and Hume, J. R.: Histamine activates the chloride current in cardiac ventricular myocytes. J. Cardiovasc. Electrophysiol. *1*:309, 1990.
72. Irisawa, H., and Hagiwara, N.: Ionic current in sinoatrial node cells. J. Cardiovasc. Electrophysiol. *2*:531, 1991.
73. Cohen, N. M., Lederer, W. J., and Nichols, C. G.: Activation of ATP-sensitive potassium channels underlies contractile failure in single human cardiac myocytes during complete metabolic inhibition. J. Cardiovasc. Electrophysiol. *3*:56, 1993.
74. Lederer, W. J., and Nichols, C. G.: Regulation and function of adenosine triphosphate-sensitive potassium channels in the cardiovascular system. *In* Zipes, D. P., and Jalife, J. (eds.): Cardiac Electrophysiology: From Cell to Bedside. 2nd ed. Philadelphia, W. B. Saunders Company, 1994, p. 103.
75. Ho, K., Nichols, C. G., Lederer, W. J., et al.: Cloning and expression of an inwardly rectifying ATP-regulated potassium channel. Nature *362*:31, 1993.

MECHANISMS OF ARRHYTHMOGENESIS

76. Wit, A. L., and Janse, M. J. (eds.): The Ventricular Arrhythmias of Ischemia and Infarction: Electrophysiological Mechanisms. Mt. Kisco, N. Y., Futura, 1993.
77. Akhtar, M., Myerburg, R. J., and Ruskin, J. N. (eds.): Sudden Cardiac Death: Prevalence, Mechanisms, and Approaches to Diagnosis and Management. Baltimore, Williams & Wilkins, 1994.
78. Josephson, M. E.: Clinical Cardiac Electrophysiology: Techniques and Interpretations. 2nd ed. Philadelphia, Lea and Febiger, 1993.
79. Podrid, P. J., and Kowey, P. R.: Cardiac Arrhythmia: Mechanisms, Diagnosis, and Management. Baltimore, Williams & Wilkins, 1995.
80. Zipes, D. P., Miles, W. M., and Klein, L. S.: Assessment of the patient with a cardiac arrhythmia. *In* Zipes, D. P., and Jalife, J. (eds.): Cardiac Electrophysiology: From Cell to Bedside. 2nd ed. Philadelphia, W. B. Saunders Company, 1994, p. 1009.
81. El-Sherif, N., and Craelius, W.: Early afterdepolarizations and arrhythmogenesis. J. Cardiovasc. Electrophysiol. *1*:145, 1990.
82. January, C. T., and Shorofsky, S.: Early afterdepolarizations: Newer insights into cellular mechanisms. J. Cardiovasc. Electrophysiol. *1*:161, 1990.
83. Sicouri, S., and Antzelevitch, C.: Drug-induced afterdepolarizations and triggered activity occur in a discreet subpopulation of ventricular muscle cells (M cells) in the canine heart: Quinidine and digitalis. J. Cardiovasc. Electrophysiol. *4*:48, 1993.
84. Boutjdir, M., Restivo, M., Wei, Y., et al.: Early afterdepolarization formation in cardiac myocytes: Analysis of phase plane patterns, action potential and membrane currents. J. Cardiovasc. Electrophysiol. *5*:609, 1994.

85. Rozanski, G. J., and Witt, R. C.: Alterations in repolarization of cardiac Purkinje fibers recovering from ischemic-like conditions: Genesis of early afterdepolarizations. J. Cardiovasc. Electrophysiol. *4*:134, 1993.
86. Jackman, W. M., Szabo, B., Friday, K. J., et al.: Ventricular tachyarrhythmias related to early afterdepolarization and triggered firing: Relationship to QT interval prolongation and potential therapeutic role for calcium channel blocking agents. J. Cardiovasc. Electrophysiol. *1*:170, 1990.
87. Zipes, D. P.: Monophasic action potentials in the diagnosis of triggered arrhythmia. Prog. Cardiovasc. Dis. *33*:385, 1991.
88. Zipes, D. P.: The long QT syndrome: A Rosetta stone for sympathetic related arrhythmias (Editorial). Circulation *84:* 1414, 1991.
89. Ben-David, J., and Zipes, D. P.: Torsades de pointes and proarrhythmia. Lancet *341*:1578, 1993.
90. Schwartz, P. J., Locati, E. H., Napolitano, C., et al.: The long QT syndrome. *In* Zipes, D. P., and Jalife, J. (eds.): Cardiac Electrophysiology: From Cell to Bedside. 2nd ed. Philadelphia, W. B. Saunders Company, 1994, p. 788.
91. Zhou, J., Zheng, L., Liu, W., et al.: Early afterdepolarizations in the familial long QTU syndrome. J. Cardiovasc. Electrophysiol. *3*:431, 1992.
92. Aaronson, R. S.: Mechanisms of arrhythmias in ventricular hypertrophy. J. Cardiovasc. Electrophysiol. *2*:249, 1991.
93. Krause, P. C., Rardon, D. P., Miles, W. M., et al.: Characteristics of $Ca2^+$-activated K^+ channels isolated from the left ventricle of a patient with idiopathic long QT syndrome. Am. Heart J. *126*:1134, 1993.
94. Shimizu, W., Ohe, T., Kurita, T., et al.: Epinephrine-induced ventricular premature complexes due to early afterdepolarizations and effects of verapamil and propanolol in a patient with congenital long QT syndrome. J. Cardiovasc. Electrophysiol. *5*:438, 1994.
95. Ming, Z., Aronson, R., and Nordin, C.: Mechanism of current-induced early afterdepolarizations in guinea pig ventricular myocytes. Am. J. Physiol. *267*:H1419, 1994.
96. Furukawa, T., Bassett, A. L., Furukawa, N., et al.: The ionic mechanism of reperfusion-induced early afterdepolarizations in feline left ventricular hypertrophy. J. Clin. Invest. *91*:1521, 1993.
97. Luo, Z. H., and Rudy, Y.: A dynamic model of the cardiac ventricular action potential: II. Afterdepolarizations, triggered activity and potentiations. Circ. Res. *74*:1097, 1994.
98. Luo, Z. H., and Rudy, Y.: A dynamic model of the cardiac ventricular action potential: I. Simulations of ionic currents and concentration changes. Circ. Res. *74*:1071, 1994.
99. Rubart, M., Pressler, M. L., Pride, H. P., and Zipes, D. P.: Electrophysiological mechanisms in a canine model of erythromycin-associated long QT syndrome. Circulation *88*:1832, 1993.
100. Zipes, D. P.: Unwitting exposure to risk (Editorial). Cardiol. Rev. *1*:1, 1993.
101. Marchi, S., Szabo, B., and Lazzara, R.: Adrenergic induction of delayed afterdepolarizations in ventricular myocardial cells: Beta induction and alpha modulation. J. Cardiovasc. Electrophysiol. *2*:476, 1991.
102. Wu, J., and Corr, P. B.: Palmitoyl carnitine modifies sodium currents and induces transient inward current in ventricular myocytes. Am. J. Physiol. *266*:H1034, 1994.
103. Lerman, B. B.: Response of nonreentrant catecholamine-mediated ventricular tachycardia to endogenous adenosine and acetylcholine: Evidence for myocardial receptor-mediated effects. Circulation *87*:382, 1993.
104. Nakagawa, H., Mukai, J., Nagata, K., et al.: Early afterdepolarizations in a patient with idiopathic monomorphic right ventricular tachycardia. PACE *16*:2067, 1993.
105. Castellanos, A., Saoubi, N., Moleiro, F., et al.: Parasystole. *In* Zipes, D. P., and Jalife, J. (eds.): Cardiac Electrophysiology: From Cell to Bedside. 2nd ed. Philadelphia, W. B. Saunders Company, 1994, p. 942.

DISORDERS OF IMPULSE CONDUCTION

106. Rardon, D. P., Miles, W. M., Mitrani, R. D., et al.: Atrioventricular block and dissociation. *In* Zipes, D. P., and Jalife, J. (eds.): Cardiac Electrophysiology: From Cell to Bedside. 2nd ed. Philadelphia, W. B. Saunders Company, 1994, p. 935.
107. El-Sherif, N.: Reentrant mechanisms in ventricular arrhythmias. *In* Zipes, D. P., and Jalife, J. (eds.): Cardiac Electrophysiology: From Cell to Bedside. 2nd ed. Philadelphia, W. B. Saunders Company, 1994, p. 567.
108. Janse, M. J., and Opthof, T.: Mechanisms of ischemia induced arrhythmias. *In* Zipes, D. P., and Jalife, J. (eds.): Cardiac Electrophysiology: From Cell to Bedside. 2nd ed. Philadelphia, W. B. Saunders Company, 1994, p. 489.
109. Wit, A. L., Dillon, S. M., and Coromilas, J.: Anisotropic reentry as a cause of ventricular tachyarrhythmias in myocardial infarction. *In* Zipes, D. P., and Jalife, J. (eds.): Cardiac Electrophysiology: From Cell to Bedside. 2nd ed. Philadelphia, W. B. Saunders Company, 1994, p. 511.
110. Allessie, M. A.: Reentrant mechanisms underlying atrial fibrillation. *In* Zipes, D. P., and Jalife, J. (eds.): Cardiac Electrophysiology: From Cell to Bedside. 2nd ed. Philadelphia, W. B. Saunders Company, 1994, p. 562.
110a. Winfree, A. T.: Theory of spirals. *In* Zipes, D. P., and Jalife, J. (eds.): Cardiac Electrophysiology: From Cell to Bedside. 2nd ed. Philadelphia, W. B. Saunders Company, 1994, p. 279.
111. Pertsov, A. M., and Jalife, J.: Three-dimensional vortex-like reentry. *In* Zipes, D. P., and Jalife, J. (eds.): Cardiac Electrophysiology: From Cell to Bedside. 2nd ed. Philadelphia, W. B. Saunders Company, 1994, p. 403.

112. Davidenko, J. M.: Spiral waves in the heart: Experimental demonstration of a theory. *In* Zipes, D. P., and Jalife, J. (eds.): Cardiac Electrophysiology: From Cell to Bedside. 2nd ed. Philadelphia, W. B. Saunders Company, 1994, p. 478.
113. Waldo, A. L.: Atrial flutter: Mechanisms, clinical features, and management. *In* Zipes, D. P., and Jalife, J. (eds.): Cardiac Electrophysiology: From Cell to Bedside. 2nd ed. Philadelphia, W. B. Saunders Company, 1994, p. 666.
114. Schoels, W., Offner, B., Brachmann, J., et al.: Circus movement atrial flutter in the canine sterile pericarditis model: Relation of characteristics of the surface electrocardiogram and conduction properties of the reentrant pathway. J. Am. Coll. Cardiol. *23*:799, 1994.
115. Ortiz, J., Nozaki, A., Shimizu, A., et al.: Mechanism of interruption of atrial flutter by moricizine: Electrophysiological and multiplexing studies in the canine sterile pericarditis model of atrial flutter. Circulation *89*:2860, 1994.
116. Cosio, F. G., Lopez, G. M., Arribas, F., et al.: Mechanisms of entrainment of human common flutter studied with multiple endocardial recordings. Circulation *89*:2117, 1994.
117. Lammers, W. J. E. P., Ravelli, F., Disertori, M., et al.: Variations in human atrial flutter cycle length induced by ventricular beats: Evidence of a reentrant circuit with a partially excitable gap. J. Cardiovasc. Electrophysiol. *2*:375, 1991.
118. Ravelli, F., Disertori, M., Cozzi, F., et al.: Ventricular beats induce variations in cycle length of rapid (type II) atrial flutter in humans: Evidence of leading circle reentry. Circulation *89*:2107, 1994.
119. Ortiz, J., Niwano, S., Abe, H., et al.: Mapping the conversion of atrial flutter to atrial fibrillation and atrial fibrillation to atrial flutter. Insights into mechanisms. Circ. Res. *74*:882, 1994.
120. Pinto, J. M., Graziano, J. N., and Boyden, T. A.: Endocardial mapping of reentry around an anatomical barrier in the canine right atrium: Observations during the action of the class IC agent, flecainide. J. Cardiovasc. Electrophysiol. *4*:672, 1993.
121. Shimizu, A., Nozaki, A., Rudy, Y., et al.: Characterization of double potentials in a functionally determined reentrant circuit: Multiplexing studies during interruption of atrial flutter in the canine pericarditis model. J. Am. Coll. Cardiol. *22*:2022, 1993.
122. Scholes, W., Kuebler, W., Yang, H., et al.: A unified functional/anatomic substrate for circus movement atrial flutter: Activation and refractory patterns in the canine right atrial enlargement model. J. Am. Coll. Cardiol. *21*:73, 1993.
123. Waxman, M. B., Yao, L., Cameron, D. A., et al.: Effects of posture, Valsalva maneuver and respiration on atrial flutter rate: An effect mediated through cardiac volume. J. Am. Coll. Cardiol. *17*:1545, 1991.
124. Waxman, M. B., Kirsh, J. A., Yao, L., et al.: Slowing of the atrial flutter rate during 1:1 atrioventricular conduction in humans and dogs: An effect mediated through atrial pressure and volume. J. Cardiovasc. Electrophysiol. *3*:544, 1992.
125. Lesh, M. D., VanHare, G. F., Epstein, L. M., et al.: Radiofrequency catheter ablation of atrial arrhythmias: Results and mechanisms. Circulation *89*:1074, 1994.
126. Epstein, L. M., Chiesa, N., Wong, M. N., et al.: Radiofrequency catheter ablation in the treatment of supraventricular tachycardia in the elderly. J. Am. Coll. Cardiol. *23*:1356, 1994.
127. Toboul, T., Saoudi, N., Atallah, G., et al.: Catheter ablation for atrial flutter: Current concepts and results. J. Cardiovasc. Electrophysiol. *3*:641, 1992.
128. Calkins, H., Leon, A. R., Deam, A. G., et al.: Catheter ablation of atrial flutter using radiofrequency energy. Am. J. Cardiol. *73*:353, 1994.
129. Isber, N., Restivo, M., Gough, W. B., et al.: Circus movement atrial flutter in the canine sterile pericarditis model: Cryothermal termination from the epicardial site of the slow zone of the reentrant circuit. Circulation *87*:1649, 1993.
130. Cosio, F. G., Lopez-Gil, M., Giocolea, A., et al.: Radiofrequency ablation of the inferior vena cava-tricuspid valve isthmus in common atrial flutter. Am. J. Cardiol. *71*:705, 1993.
131. Interian, A., Jr., Cox, M. M., Jimenez, R. A., et al.: A shared pathway in atrioventricular nodal reentrant tachycardia and atrial flutter: Implications for pathophysiology and therapy. Am. J. Cardiol. *71*:297, 1993.
132. Feld, G. K., Fleck, R. P., Chen, P. S., et al.: Radiofrequency catheter ablation for the treatment of human type I atrial flutter: Identification of a critical zone in the reentrant circuit by endocardial mapping techniques. Circulation *86*:1233, 1992.
133. Cox, J. L., Boineau, J. P., and Schuessler, R. D.: A review of surgery for atrial fibrillation. J. Cardiovasc. Electrophysiol. *2*:541, 1991.
134. Cox, J. L., Boineau, J. P., Schuessler, R. B., et al.: Five-year experience with the maze procedure for atrial fibrillation. Ann. Thorac. Surg. *56*:814, 1993.
135. Elvan, A., Pride, H. B., Eble, J. N., and Zipes, D. P.: Radiofrequency catheter ablation of the atria reduces the inducibility and duration of atrial fibrillation in dogs. Circulation *91*:2235, 1995.
135a. Haissaguerre, M., Gencel, L., Fischer, B., et al.: Successful catheter ablation of atrial fibrillation. J. Cardiovasc. Electrophysiol. *5*:1045, 1994.
135b. Swartz, J. F., Pellersels, G., Silvers, J., et al.: Catheter-based curative approach to atrial fibrillation in humans. Circulation *(in press).*

136. Konings, K. T., Kirchhof, C. J., Smeets, J. R., et al.: High-density mapping of electrically induced atrial fibrillation in humans. Circulation *89:*1665, 1994.
137. Kirchhof, C. J., Chorro, F., Scheffer, G. J., et al.: Regional entrainment of atrial fibrillation studied by high-resolution mapping in open-chest dogs. Circulation *88:*736, 1993.
138. Allessie, M. A., Kirchhof, C. J., Scheffer, G. J., et al.: Regional control of atrial fibrillation by rapid pacing in conscious dogs. Circulation *84:*1689, 1991.
139. Wijffels, M., Dorland, R., Kirchhof, C. J., et al.: What causes electrical remodeling of the atria due to atrial fibrillation? Circulation *90* (Suppl. 4):I-41 (Abs.), 1994.
140. Borgers, M., Ausma, J., Wijffels, M., et al.: Atrial fibrillation in the goat: A model for chronic hibernating myocardium. Circulation *90* (Suppl. 4):I-467 (Abs.), 1994.
140a. Wijffels, M. C. E. F., Kirchof, C. J. H. J., Dorland, R., et al.: Atrial fibrillation begets atrial fibrillation. Circulation *92:*1954, 1995.
141. Haissaguerre, M., Marcus, F. I., Fischer, B., et al.: Radiofrequency catheter ablation in unusual mechanisms of atrial fibrillation: Report of three cases. J. Cardiovasc. Electrophysiol. *9:*743, 1994.
142. Coumel, T.: Paroxysmal atrial fibrillation: A disorder of autonomic tone? Eur. Heart J. *15* (Suppl. A):9, 1994.
143. Naccarelli, G. V., Shih, H. T., and Jalal, S.: Sinus node reentry and atrial tachycardias. *In* Zipes, D. P., and Jalife, J. (eds.): Cardiac Electrophysiology: From Cell to Bedside. 2nd ed. Philadelphia, W. B. Saunders Company, 1994, p. 607.
144. Sperry, R. E., Ellenbogen, K. A., Wood, M. A., et al.: Radiofrequency catheter ablation of sinus node reentrant tachycardia. PACE *16:*2202, 1993.
145. Haines, D. E., and DiMarco, J. P.: Sustained intraatrial reentrant tachycardia: Clinical, electrocardiographic and electrophysiologic characteristics and long-term follow-up. J. Am. Coll. Cardiol. *15:*1345, 1990.
146. Chen, S. A., Chiang, C. E., Yang, C. J., et al.: Sustained atrial tachycardia in adult patients: Electrophysiological characteristics, pharmacological response, possible mechanisms, and effects of radiofrequency ablation. Circulation *90:*1262, 1994.
147. Engelstein, E. D., Lippman, N., Stein, K. M., et al.: Mechanism specific effects of adenosine on atrial tachycardia. Circulation *89:*2645, 1994.
148. Wellens, H. J. J.: Atrial tachycardia: How important is the mechanism? Circulation *90:*1576, 1994.
149. Chen, S. A., Chiang, C. E., Yang, C. J., et al.: Radiofrequency catheter ablation of sustained intra-atrial reentrant tachycardia in adult patients: Identification of electrophysiological characteristics and endocardial mapping techniques. Circulation *88:*578, 1993.
150. Kay, G. N., Chong, F., Epstein, A. E., et al.: Radiofrequency ablation for treatment of primary atrial tachycardias. J. Am. Coll. Cardiol. *21:*901, 1993.
151. DeBakker, J. M. T., Hauer, R. N. W., Bakker, P. F. A., et al.: Abnormal automaticity as mechanism of atrial tachycardia in the human heart—Electrophysiologic and histologic correlation: A case report. J. Cardiovasc. Electrophysiol. *5:*335, 1994.
152. Garsoń, A., Jr., Gillette, P. C., Moak, J. P., et al.: Supraventricular tachycardia due to multiple atrial ectopic foci: A relatively common problem. J. Cardiovasc. Electrophysiol. *1:*132, 1990.
153. Watanabe, Y., and Watanabe, M.: Impulse formulation and conduction of excitation in the atrioventricular node. J. Cardiovasc. Electrophysiol. *5:*517, 1994.
154. Kalbfleisch, S. J., Strickberger, S. A., Hummel, J. D., et al.: Double retrograde atrial response after radiofrequency ablation of typical AV nodal reentrant tachycardia. J. Cardiovasc. Electrophysiol. *4:*695, 1993.
155. Sakurada, H., Sakamoto, M., Hiyoshi, Y., et al.: Double ventricular responses to a single atrial depolarization in a patient with dual AV nodal pathways. PACE *15:*28, 1992.
156. Akhtar, M., Jazayeri, M. R., Sra, J., et al.: Atrioventricular nodal reentry: Clinical, electrophysiological and therapeutic considerations. Circulation *88:*282, 1993.
157. Josephson, M. E., and Miller, J. M.: Atrioventricular nodal reentry: Evidence supporting an intranodal location. PACE *16:*599, 1993.
158. Elizari, M. V., Sanchez, R. A., and Chiale, T. A.: Manifest fast and slow pathway conduction patterns and reentry in a patient with dual AV nodal physiology. J. Cardiovasc. Electrophysiol. *2:*98, 1991.
159. Ward, D. E., and Garratt, C. J.: The substrate for atrioventricular "nodal" reentrant tachycardia: Is there a "third pathway"? J. Cardiovasc. Electrophysiol. *4:*62, 1993.
160. Jazayeri, M. R., Sra, J. S., Deshpande, S. S., et al.: Electrophysiologic spectrum of atrioventricular nodal behavior in patients with atrioventricular nodal reentrant tachycardia undergoing selective fast or slow pathway ablation. J. Cardiovasc. Electrophysiol. *4:*99, 1993.
161. Perry, J. C., and Garson, A., Jr.: Complexities of junctional tachycardias. J. Cardiovasc. Electrophysiol. *4:*224, 1993.
162. Billette, J., and Nattel, S.: Dynamic behavior of the atrioventricular node: A functional model of interaction between recovery, facilitation, and fatigue. J. Cardiovasc. Electrophysiol. *5:*90, 1994.
163. Spach, M. S., and Josephson, M. E.: Initiating reentry: The role of nonuniform anisotropy in small circuits. J. Cardiovasc. Electrophysiol. *5:*182, 1994.
164. Jackman, W. M., Nakagawa, H., Heidbuchel, H., et al.: Three forms of atrioventricular nodal (junctional) reentrant tachycardia: Differential diagnosis, electrophysiological characteristics, and implications for anatomy of the reentrant circuit. *In* Zipes, D. P., and Jalife, J. (eds.): Cardiac Electrophysiology: From Cell to Bedside. 2nd ed. Philadelphia, W. B. Saunders Company, 1994, p. 620.
165. Silka, M. J., Kron, J., Park, J. K., et al.: Atypical forms of supraventricular tachycardia due to atrioventricular node reentry in children after radiofrequency modification of slow pathway conduction. J. Am. Coll. Cardiol. *23:*1363, 1994.
166. Yen, S., McComb, J. M., Scott, C. B., et al.: Morphology of the cardiac conduction system in patients with electrophysiologically proven dual atrioventricular nodal pathways. J. Cardiovasc. Electrophysiol. *4:*504, 1993.
167. McGuire, M. A., Yip, A. S., Robotin, M., et al.: Surgical procedure for the cure of atrioventricular junctional (AV node) reentrant tachycardia: Anatomic and electrophysiologic effects of dissection of the anterior atrionodal connections in a canine model. J. Am. Coll. Cardiol. *24:*784, 1994.
168. Haissaguerre, M., Gaita, F., Fischer, B., et al.: Elimination of atrioventricular nodal reentrant tachycardia using discreet slow potentials to guide applicaiton of radiofrequency energy. Circulation *85:*2162, 1992.
169. Langberg, J. J.: Radiofrequency catheter ablation of AV nodal reentry: The anterior approach. PACE *16:*615, 1993.
170. Lee, M. A., Morady, F., Kadish, A., et al.: Catheter modification of the atrioventricular junction with radiofrequency energy for control of atrioventricular nodal reentry tachycardia. Circulation *83:*827, 1991.
171. Gursoy, S., Schluter, M., and Kuck, K. H.: Radiofrequency current catheter ablation for control of supraventricular arrhythmias. J. Cardiovasc. Electrophysiol. *4:*194, 1993.
172. Kay, G. N., Epstein, A. E., Dailey, S. M., et al.: Role of radiofrequency ablation in the management of supraventricular arrhythmias: Experience in 760 consecutive patients. J. Cardiovasc. Electrophysiol. *4:*371, 1993.
173. Miles, W. M., Hubbard, J. E., Zipes, D. P., et al.: Elimination of AV nodal reentrant tachycardia with 2 : 1 VA block by posteroseptal ablation. J. Cardiovasc. Electrophysiol. *5:*510, 1994.
174. Strickberger, S. A., Daoud, E., Niebauer, M., et al.: Effects of partial and complete ablation of the slow pathway on fast pathway properties in patients with atrioventricular nodal reentrant tachycardia. J. Cardiovasc. Electrophysiol. *5:*645, 1994.
175. Baker, J. H., II, Plumb, V. J., Epstein, A. E., et al.: Predictors of recurrent atrioventricular nodal reentry after selective slow pathway ablation. Am. J. Cardiol. *73:*765, 1994.
176. Natale, A., Wathen, M., Wolfe, K., et al.: Comparative atrioventricular node properties after radiofrequency ablation and operative therapy of atrioventricular node reentry. PACE *16:*971, 1993.
177. Jazayeri, M. R., Hempe, S. L., Sra, J. S., et al.: Selective transcatheter ablation of the fast and slow pathways using radiofrequency energy in patients with atrioventricular nodal reentrant tachycardia. Circulation *85:*1318, 1992.
178. Natale, A., Kline, G., Yee, R., et al.: Shortening of fast pathway refractoriness after slow pathway ablation: Effects of autonomic blockade. Circulation *89:*1103, 1994.
179. Mitrani, R. D., Klein, L. S., Hackett, F. K., et al.: Radiofrequency ablation for atrioventricular node reentrant tachycardia: Comparison between fast (anterior) and slow (posterior) pathway ablation. J. Am. Coll. Cardiol. *21:*432, 1993.
180. Wu, D., Yeh, S. J., Wang, C. C., et al.: Nature of dual atrioventricular node pathways and the tachycardia circuit as defined by radiofrequency ablation technique. J. Am. Coll. Cardiol. *20:*884, 1992.
181. Langberg, J. J., Kim, Y. N., Goyal, R., et al.: Conversion of typical to atypical atrioventricular nodal reentrant tachycardia after radiofrequency catheter modification of the atrioventricular junction. Am. J. Cardiol. *69:*503, 1992.
182. Kalbfleisch, S. J., and Morady, F.: Catheter ablation of atrioventricular nodal reentrant tachycardia. *In* Zipes, D. P., and Jalife, J. (eds.): Cardiac Electrophysiology: From Cell to Bedside. 2nd ed. Philadelphia, W. B. Saunders Company, 1994, p. 1477.
183. Mahomed, Y., King, R. D., Zipes, D. P., et al.: Surgery for atrioventricular node reentry tachycardia: Results with surgical skeletonization of the atrioventricular node and discreet perinodal cryosurgery. J. Thorac. Cardiovasc. Surg. *104:*1035, 1992.
184. Mahomed, Y.: Surgery for atrioventricular nodal reentrant tachycardia. *In* Zipes, D. P., and Jalife, J. (eds.): Cardiac Electrophysiology: From Cell to Bedside. 2nd ed. Philadelphia, W. B. Saunders Company, 1994, p. 1577.
185. DeBakker, J. M., Coronel, R., McGuire, M. A., et al.: Slow potentials in the atrioventricular junctional area of patients operated on for atrioventricular node tachycardias and in isolated hearts. J. Am. Coll. Cardiol. *23:*709, 1994.
186. McGuire, M. A., DeBakker, J. M., Vermeulen, J. T., et al.: Origin and significance of double potentials near the atrioventricular node: Correlation of extracellular potentials, intracellular potentials and histology. Circulation *89:*2351, 1994.
187. McGuire, M. A., Bourke, J. P., Robotin, M. C., et al.: HIgh resolution mapping of Koch's triangle using 60 electrodes in humans with atrioventricular junctional (AV nodal) reentrant tachycardia. Circulation *88:*2315, 1993.
188. Philippon, F., Plumb, V. J., and Kay, G. N.: Differential effect of esmolol on the fast and slow AV nodal pathways in patients with AV nodal reentrant tachycardia. J. Cardiovasc. Electrophysiol. *5:*810, 1994.
189. Kalbfleisch, S. J., El-Atassi, R., Calkins, H., et al.: Associations between atrioventricular node reentrant tachycardia and inducible atrial flutter. J. Am. Coll. Cardiol. *22:*80, 1993.

190. Munger, T. M., Packer, D. L., Hammill, S. C., et al.: A population study of the natural history of Wolff-Parkinson-White syndrome in Olmsted County, Minnesota, 1953–1989. Circulation *87*:866, 1993.
191. Kent, A. F. S.: Researches on the structure and function of mammalian heart. J. Physiol. *14*:233, 1893.
192. Kent, A. F. S.: Observation on the auriculo-ventricular junction of the mammalian heart. Q. J. Exp. Physiol. *7*:193, 1913.
193. Packer, D. L., and Prystowsky, E. N.: Anatomical and physiological substrate for antidromic reciprocating tachycardia. *In* Zipes, D. P., and Jalife, J. (eds.): Cardiac Electrophysiology: From Cell to Bedside. 2nd ed. Philadelphia, W. B. Saunders Company, 1994, p. 655.
194. Miles, W. M., Klein, L. S., Rardon, D. P., et al.: Atrioventricular reentry and variants: Mechanisms, clinical features, and management. *In* Zipes, D. P., and Jalife, J. (eds.): Cardiac Electrophysiology: From Cell to Bedside. 2nd ed. Philadelphia, W. B. Saunders Company, 1994, p. 638.
195. Haissaguerre, M., Clementy, J., and Warin, J. F.: Catheter ablation of atrioventricular reentrant tachycardias. *In* Zipes, D. P., and Jalife, J. (eds.): Cardiac Electrophysiology: From Cell to Bedside. 2nd ed. Philadelphia, W. B. Saunders Company, 1994, p. 1487.
196. Guiraudon, G. M., Guiraudon, C. M., Klein, G. J., et al.: Operation for the Wolff-Parkinson-White syndrome in the catheter ablation era. Ann. Thorac. Surg. *57*:1084, 1994.
197. Ferguson, T. B., Jr., and Cox, J. L.: Surgery for atrial fibrillation. *In* Zipes, D. P., and Jalife, J. (eds.): Cardiac Electrophysiology: From Cell to Bedside. 2nd ed. Philadelphia, W. B. Saunders Company, 1994, p. 1563.
198. Guiraudon, G. M., Klein, G. J., Yee, R., et al.: Surgery for the Wolff-Parkinson-White syndrome. *In* Zipes, D. P., and Jalife, J. (eds.): Cardiac Electrophysiology: From Cell to Bedside. 2nd ed. Philadelphia, W. B. Saunders Company, 1994, p. 1553.
199. Jackman, W. M., Wang, W., Friday, K., et al.: Catheter ablation of accessory atrioventricular pathways (Wolff-Parkinson-White syndrome) by radiofrequency current. N. Engl. J. Med. *324*:1605, 1991.
200. Calkins, H., Souza, J., El-Atassi, R., et al.: Diagnosis and cure of the Wolff-Parkinson-White syndrome of paroxysmal supraventricular tachycardias during a simple electrophysiologic test. N. Engl. J. Med. *324*:1612, 1991.
201. Misaki, T., Watanabe, G., Iwa, T., et al.: Surgical treatment of Wolff-Parkinson-White syndrome in infants and children. Ann. Thorac. Surg. *58*:103, 1994.
202. Chen, S. A., Cheng, C. C., Chiang, C. E., et al.: Radiofrequency ablation in a patient with tachycardia incorporating triple free wall accessory pathways and atrioventricular nodal reentrant tachycardia. Am. Heart J. *127*:1656, 1994.
203. Chen, S. A., Chiang, C. E., Yang, C. J., et al.: Accessory pathway and atrioventricular node reentrant tachycardia in elderly patients: Clinical features, electrophysiologic characteristics and results of radiofrequency ablation. J. Am. Coll. Cardiol. *23*:702, 1994.
204. Yeh, S. J., Wang, C. C., Wen, M. S., et al.: Characteristics and radiofreqency ablation therapy of intermediate septal accessory pathway. Am. J. Cardiol. *73*:50, 1994.
205. Xie, B., Heald, S. C., Bashir, Y., et al.: Localization of accessory pathways from the 12-lead electrocardiogram using a new algorithm. Am. J. Cardiol. *74*:161, 1994.
206. Damle, R. S., Choe, W., Kanaan, N. M., et al.: Atrial and accessory pathway activation direction in patients with orthodromic supraventricular tachycardia: Insights from vector mapping. J. Am. Coll. Cardiol. *23*:684, 1994.
207. Rodriguez, L. M., Smeets, J. L., deChillou, C., et al.: The 12-lead electrocardiogram in mid-septal, anteroseptal, posteroseptal and right free wall accessory pathways. Am. J. Cardiol. *72*:1274, 1993.
208. Young, C., Lauer, M. R., Liem, L. B., et al.: A characteristic electrocardiographic pattern indicative of manifest left-sided posterior septal/paraseptal accessory atrioventricular connections. Am. J. Cardiol. *72*:471, 1993.
209. deChillou, C., Rodriguez, L. M., Schlapfer, J., et al.: Clinical characteristics and electrophysiologic properties of atrioventricular accessory pathways: Importance of the accessory pathway location. J. Am. Coll. Cardiol. *20*:666, 1992.
209a. Fitzpatrick, A.: The ECG in Wolff-Parkinson-White syndrome. PACE *18*:1469, 1995.
210. Clair, W. K., Wilkinson, W. E., McCarthy, E. A., et al.: Spontaneous occurrence of symptomatic paroxysmal atrial fibrillation and paroxysmal supraventricular tachycardia in untreated patients. Circulation *87*:1114, 1993.
211. Davidenko, J. M.: Spiral waves in the heart: Experimental demonstration of a theory. *In* Zipes, D. P., and Jalife, J. (eds.): Cardiac Electrophysiology: From Cell to Bedside. 2nd ed. Philadelphia, W. B. Saunders Company, 1994, p. 478.
212. Janse, M. J., and Opthof, T.: Mechanisms of ischemia-induced arrhythmias. *In* Zipes, D. P., and Jalife, J. (eds.): Cardiac Electrophysiology: From Cell to Bedside. 2nd ed. Philadelphia, W. B. Saunders Company, 1994, p. 489.
213. Wit, A. L., Dillon, S. M., and Coromilas, J.: Anisotropic reentry as a cause of ventricular tachyarrhythmias in myocardial infarction. *In* Zipes, D. P., and Jalife, J. (eds.): Cardiac Electrophysiology: From Cell to Bedside. 2nd ed. Philadelphia, W. B. Saunders Company, 1994, p. 511.
214. Witkowski, F. X., Penkoske, P. A., and Kavanagh, K. M.: Activation patterns during ventricular fibrillation. *In* Zipes, D. P., and Jalife, J. (eds.): Cardiac Electrophysiology: From Cell to Bedside. 2nd ed. Philadelphia, W. B. Saunders Company, 1994, p. 539.
215. El-Sherif, N.: Reentrant mechanisms in ventricular arrhythmias. *In* Zipes, D. P., and Jalife, J. (eds.): Cardiac Electrophysiology: From Cell to Bedside. 2nd ed. Philadelphia, W. B. Saunders Company, 1994, p. 567.
216. Watanabe, M., and Gilmour, R. F., Jr.: Dynamics of reentry in a ring-like Purkinje-muscle preparation. *In* Zipes, D. P., and Jalife, J. (eds.): Cardiac Electrophysiology: From Cell to Bedside. 2nd ed. Philadelphia, W. B. Saunders Company, 1994, p. 583.
217. Davidenko, J. M.: Spiral wave activity: A possible common mechanism for polymorphic and monomorphic ventricular tachycardias. J. Cardiovasc. Electrophysiol. *4*:730, 1993.
218. Dillon, S. M., Coromilas, J., Waldecker, B., et al.: Effects of overdrive stimulation on functional reentrant circuits causing ventricular tachycardia in the canine heart: Mechanisms for resumption or alteration of tachycardia. J. Cardiovasc. Electrophysiol. *4*:393, 1993.
219. Callans, D. J., and Josephson, M. E.: Ventricular tachycardias in the setting of coronary artery disease. *In* Zipes, D. P., and Jalife, J. (eds.): Cardiac Electrophysiology: From Cell to Bedside. 2nd ed. Philadelphia, W. B. Saunders Company, 1994, p. 732.
220. Marchlinski, F. E., Schwartzman, D., Gottlieb, C. D., et al.: Electrical events associated with arrhythmia initiation and stimulation techniques for arrhythmia prevention. *In* Zipes, D. P., and Jalife, J. (eds.): Cardiac Electrophysiology: From Cell to Bedside. 2nd ed. Philadelphia, W. B. Saunders Company, 1994, p. 863.
221. Blanck, Z., Sra, J., Dhala, A., et al.: Bundle branch reentry: Mechanisms, diagnosis, and treatment. *In* Zipes, D. P., and Jalife, J. (eds.): Cardiac Electrophysiology: From Cell to Bedside. 2nd ed. Philadelphia, W. B. Saunders Company, 1994, p. 878.
222. Gettes, L. S., Cascio, W. E., and Sanders, W. E.: Mechanisms of sudden cardiac death. *In* Zipes, D. P., and Jalife, J. (eds.): Cardiac Electrophysiology: From Cell to Bedside. 2nd ed. Philadelphia, W. B. Saunders Company, 1994, p. 527.
223. Blanck, Z., Dahla, A., Desphande, S., et al.: Bundle branch reentrant ventricular tachycardia: Cumulative experience in 48 patients. J. Cardiovasc. Electrophysiol. *4*:253, 1993.
224. Pogwizd, S. M., and Corr, P.: The contribution of nonreentrant mechanisms to malignant ventricular arrhythmias. Basic Res. Cardiol. *87* (Suppl. 2):115, 1992.
224a. Pogwizd, S. M.: Nonreentrant mechanisms underlying spontaneous ventricular arrhythmias in a model of nonischemic heart failure in rabbits. Circulation *92*:1034, 1995.
225. Belhassen, B., and Viskin, S.: Idiopathic ventricular tachycardia and fibrillation. J. Cardiovasc. Electrophysiol. *4*:356, 1993.
226. Ben-David, J., Zipes, D. P., Ayers, G. M., et al.: Canine left ventricular hypertrophy predisposes to ventricular tachycardia induction by phase II early afterdepolarizations after administration of BAY K 8644. J. Am. Coll. Cardiol. *20*:1576, 1992.
227. Wilber, D. J., Baerman, J., Olshansky, B., et al.: Adenosine-sensitive ventricular tachycardia: Clinical characteristics and response to catheter ablation. Circulation *87*:126, 1993.
228. Kobayashi, Y., Kikushima, S., Tanno, K., et al.: Sustained left ventricular tachycardia terminated by dipyridamole: Cyclic AMP-mediated triggered activity as a possible mechanism. PACE *17*:377, 1994.
229. Griffith, M. J., Garratt, C. J., Rowland, E., et al.: Effects of intravenous adenosine on verapamil-sensitive idiopathic ventricular tachycardia. Am. J. Cardiol. *73*:759, 1994.
230. Gonzalez, R. P., Scheinman, M. N., Lesh, M. D., et al.: Clinical and electrophysiologic spectrum of fascicular tachycardias. Am. Heart J. *128*:146, 1994.
231. Lauer, M. R., Liem, L. D., Young, C., et al.: Cellular and clinical electrophysiology of verapamil-sensitive ventricular tachycardias. J. Cardiovasc. Electrophysiol. *3*:500, 1992.
232. Priori, S. G., Napolitano, C., and Schwartz, P. J.: Cardiac receptor activation and arrhythmogenesis. Eur. Heart J. *14* (Suppl. E):20, 1993.
233. DeLacey, W. A., Nath, S., Haines, D. E., et al.: Adenosine and verapamil-sensitive ventricular tachycardia orginating from the left ventricle: Radiofrequency catheter ablation. PACE *15*:2240, 1992.
233a. Vera, Z., Pride, H. P., and Zipes, D. P.: Reperfusion arrhythmias: Role of early afterdepolarizations studied by monophasic action potential recordings in the intact canine heart during autonomically denervated and stimulated states. J. Cardiovasc. Electrophysiol. *6*:532, 1995.
234. Tai, Y. T., Lau, C. P., Fong, P. C., et al.: Incessant automatic ventricular tachycardia complicating acute coxsackie B myocarditis. Cardiology *80*:339, 1992.
235. James, T. N.: Congenital disorders of cardiac rhythm and conduction. J. Cardiovasc. Electrophysiol. *4*:702, 1993.
236. Leenhardt, A., Coumel, P., and Slama, R.: Torsades de pointes. J. Cardiovasc. Electrophysiol. *3*:281, 1992.
237. Miller, J. M.: The many manifestations of ventricular tachycardia. J. Cardiovasc. Electrophysiol. *3*:88, 1992.
238. Morady, F.: Further insight into mechanisms of ventricular tachycardia from the clinical electrophysiology laboratory. J. Cardiovasc. Electrophysiol. *2*:207, 1991.

APPROACH TO THE DIAGNOSIS OF CARDIAC ARRHYTHMIAS

239. Zipes, D. P., Miles, W. M., and Klein, L. S.: Assessment of the patient with a cardiac arrhythmia. *In* Zipes, D. P., and Jalife, J. (eds.): Cardiac

Electrophysiology: From Cell to Bedside. 2nd ed. Philadelphia, W. B. Saunders Company, 1994, p. 1009.
240. Barsky, A. J., Cleary, P. D., Barnett, M. C., et al.: The accuracy of symptom reporting by patients complaining of palpitations. Am. J. Med. *97:*214, 1994.
241. Sung, R. J., and Lauer, M. R.: Exercise-induced cardiac arrhythmias. *In* Zipes, D. P., and Jalife, J. (eds.): Cardiac Electrophysiology: From Cell to Bedside. 2nd ed. Philadelphia, W. B. Saunders Company, 1994, p. 1013.
242. Kobayashi, S., Yoshida, K., Nishimura, M., et al.: Paradoxical bradycardia during exercise and hypoxic exposure: The possible direct effect of hypoxia on sinoatrial node activity in humans. Chest *102:*1893, 1992.
243. O'Hara, G. E., Brugada, P., Rodriguez, L. M., et al.: Incidence, pathophysiology and prognosis of exercise-induced sustained ventricular tachycardia associated with healed myocardial infarction. Am. J. Cardiol. *70:*875, 1992.
244. Mont, L., Seixas, T., Brugada, P., et al.: Clinical and electrophysiologic characteristics of exercise-related idiopathic ventricular tachycardia. Am. J. Cardiol. *68:*897, 1991.
245. Yang, J. C., Wesley, R. C., Jr., and Froelicher, Z. F.: Ventricular tachycardia during routine treadmill testing: Risk and prognosis. Arch. Intern. Med. *151:*349, 1991.
246. Tuininga, Y. S., Orijns, H. J., Wiesfeld, A. C., et al.: Electrocardiographic patterns relative to initiating mechanisms of exercise-induced ventricular tachycardia. Am. Heart J. *126:*359, 1993.
247. Mason, J. W.: A comparison of electrophysiologic testing with Holter monitoring to predict antiarrhythmic-drug efficacy for ventricular tachyarrhythmias: Electrophysiologic study versus electrocardiographic monitoring. N. Engl. J. Med. *329:*445, 1993.
248. Mason, J. W.: A comparison of seven antiarrhythmic drugs in patients with ventricular arrhythmias: Electrophysiologic study versus electrocardiographic monitoring. N. Engl. J. Med. *329:*452, 1993.
249. Wever, E. F., Hauer, R. N., Oomen, A., et al.: Unfavorable outcome in patients with primary electrical disease who survived an episode of ventricular fibrillation. Circulation *88:*1021, 1993.
250. Kennedy, H. L.: Ambulatory (Holter) electrocardiography recordings. *In* Zipes, D. P., and Jalife, J. (eds.): Cardiac Electrophysiology: From Cell to Bedside. 2nd ed. Philadelphia, W. B. Saunders Company, 1994, p. 1024.
251. Kotar, S. L., and Gessler, J. E.: Full-disclosure monitoring: A concept that will change the way arrhythmias are detected and interpreted in the hospitalized patient. Heart Lung *22:*482, 1993.
252. Manolio, T. A., Furberg, C. D., Rautaharju, T. M., et al.: Cardiac arrhythmias on 24-h ambulatory electrocardiography in older women and men: The Cardiovascular Health Study. J. Am. Coll. Cardiol. *23:*916, 1994.
253. Marino, P., Nidasio, G., Golia, G., et al.: Frequency of predischarge ventricular arrhythmias in post myocardial infarction patients depends on residual left ventricular pump performance and is independent of the occurrence of acute reperfusion. The GISSI-2 investigators. J. Am. Coll. Cardiol. *23:*290, 1994.
254. Lazzara, R.: Results of Holter ECG guided therapy for ventricular arrhythmias: The ESVEM trial. PACE *17:*473, 1994.
255. Wyse, D. G., and Mitchell, B.: Selection of antiarrhythmic therapy: ESVEM in focus and in context. Cardiol. Rev. *2:*291, 1994.
256. Bikkina, M., Larson, M. G., and Levy, D.: Asymptomatic ventricular arrhythmias and mortality risk in subjects with left ventricular hypertrophy. J. Am. Coll. Cardiol. *22:*1111, 1993.
257. Statters, D. J., Malik, M., Ward, D. E., et al.: QT dispersion: Problems in methodology and clinical significance. J. Cardiovasc. Electrophysiol. *5:*672, 1994.
258. Berger, P. B., Ruocco, N. A., Ryan, T. J., et al.: Incidence and significance of ventricular tachycardia and fibrillation in the absence of hypotension or heart failure in acute myocardial infarction treated with recombinant tissue-type plasminogen activator: Results from the Thrombolysis in Myocardial Infarction (TIMI) phase II trial. J. Am. Coll. Cardiol. *22:*1773, 1993.
259. Maggioni, A. P., Zuanetti, G., Franzosi, M. G., et al.: Prevalence and prognostic significance of ventricular arrhythmias after acute myocardial infarction in the fibrinolytic era. Circulation *87:*312, 1993.
260. Page, R. L., Wilkinson, W. E., Clair, W. K., et al.: Asymptomatic arrhythmias in patients with symptomatic paroxysmal atrial fibrillation and paroxysmal supraventricular tachycardia. Circulation *89:*224, 1994.
261. Hohnloser, S. H., Klingenheben, T., vandeLoo, A., et al.: Reflex versus tonic vagal activity as a prognostic parameter in patients with sustained ventricular tachycardia or ventricular fibrillation. Circulation *89:*1068, 1994.
262. Fei, L., Anderson, M. H., Katritsis, D., et al.: Decreased heart rate variability in survivors of sudden cardiac death not associated with coronary artery disease. Br. Heart J. *71:*16, 1994.
263. Moise, N. S., Meyers-Wallen, V., Flohive, W. J., et al.: Inherited ventricular arrhythmias and sudden death in German Shepherd dogs. J. Am. Coll. Cardiol. *24:*233, 1994.
264. Vybiral, T., Glaeser, D. H., Goldberger, A. L., et al.: Conventional heart rate variability analysis of ambulatory electrocardiographic recordings fails to predict imminent ventricular fibrillation. J. Am. Coll. Cardiol. *22:*557, 1993.
265. Stein, K. M., Borer, J. S., Hochriter, C., et al.: Prognostic value and physiological correlates of heart rate variability in chronic severe mitral regurgitation. Circulation *88:*127, 1993.
266. Huikuri, H. V., Valkama, J. D., Airaksinen, K. E., et al.: Frequency domain measures of heart rate variability before the onset of nonsustained and sustained ventricular tachycardia in patients with coronary artery disease. Circulation *84:*1220, 1993.
267. Bigger, J. T.: Spectral analysis of R-R variability to evaluate autonomic physiology and pharmacology and to predict cardiovascular outcomes in humans. *In* Zipes, D. P., and Jalife, J. (eds.): Cardiac Electrophysiology: From Cell to Bedside. 2nd ed. Philadelphia, W. B. Saunders Company, 1994, p. 1151.
268. Coumel, P., Maison-Blanche, P., and Catuli, D.: Heart rate and heart rate variability in normal young adults. J. Cardiovasc. Electrophysiol. *5:*899, 1994.
269. Malliani, A., Lombardi, F., Pagani, M., et al.: Power spectral analysis of cardiovascular variability in patients at risk for sudden cardiac death. J. Cardiovasc. Electrophysiol. *5:*274, 1994.
270. Yarnold, P. R., Soltysik, R. C., and Martin, G. J.: Heart rate variability and susceptibility for sudden cardiac death: An example of multivariable optimal discriminate analysis. Stat. Med. *13:*1015, 1994.
271. Sandrone, G., Mortara, A., Torzillo, D., et al.: Effects of beta blockers (atenolol or metoprolol) on heart rate variability after acute myocardial infarction. Am. J. Cardiol. *74:*340, 1994.
272. Odemuyiwa, O., Poloniecki, J., Malik, M., et al.: Temporal influences on the prediction of post infarction mortality by heart rate variability: A comparison with the left ventricular ejection fraction. Br. Heart J. *71:*521, 1994.
273. Zabel, M., Klingenheben, T., and Hohnloser, S. H.: Changes in autonomic tone following thrombolytic therapy for acute myocardial infarction: Assessment by analysis of heart rate variability. J. Cardiovasc. Electrophysiol. *5:*211, 1994.
274. Niemela, M. J., Airaksinen, K. E., and Huikuri, H. V.: Effect of beta-blockade on heart rate variability in patients with coronary artery disease. J. Am. Coll. Cardiol. *23:*1370, 1994.
275. Adamson, P. B., Huang, M. H., Vanoli, et al.: Unexpected interaction between beta-adrenergic blockade and heart rate variability before and after myocardial infarction: A longitudinal study in dogs at high and low risk for sudden death. Circulation *90:*976, 1994.
276. Moser, M., Lehofer, M., Sedminek, A., et al.: Heart rate variability as a prognostic tool in cardiology: A contribution to the problem from a theoretical point of view. Circulation *90:*1078, 1994.
277. Huikuri, H. V., Niemela, M. J., Ojala, S., et al.: Circadian rhythms of frequency domain measures of heart rate variability in healthy subjects and patients with coronary artery disease: Effects of arousal and upright posture. Circulation *90:*121, 1994.
278. McClements, B. M., and Adgey, A. A.: Value of signal-averaged electrocardiography, radionuclide ventriculography, Holter monitoring and clinical variables for prediction of arrhythmic events in survivors of acute myocardial infarction in the thrombolytic era. J. Am. Coll. Cardiol. *21:*1419, 1993.
279. Mortara, A., LaRovere, M. T., Signorini, M. G., et al.: Can power spectral analysis of heart rate variability identify a high risk subgroup of congestive heart failure patients with excessive sympathetic activation? A pilot study before and after heart transplantation. Br. Heart J. *71:*422, 1994.
280. Goldberger, J. J., Ahmed, M. W., Parker, M. A., et al.: Dissociation of heart rate variability from parasympathetic tone. Am. J. Physiol. *266:*H2152, 1994.
281. Fei, L., Keeling, P. J., Gill, J. S., et al.: Heart rate variability and its relation to ventricular arrhythmias in congestive heart failure. Br. Heart J. *71:*322, 1994.
282. Griffin, M. P., Scollan, D. F., and Moorman, J. R.: The dynamic range of neonatal heart rate variability. J. Cardiovasc. Electrophysiol. *5:*112, 1994.
283. Bootsma, M., Swenne, C. A., vanBolhuis, H. H., et al.: Heart rate and heart rate variability as indexes of sympathovagal balance. Am. J. Physiol. *266:*H1565, 1994.
284. Tsuji, H., Venditti, F. J., Jr., Manders, E. S., et al.: Reduced heart rate variability and mortality risk in an elderly cohort: The Framingham Heart Study. Circulation *90:*878, 1994.
284a. Malik, M., and Camm, A. J.: Components of heart rate variability: What they really mean and what we really measure. Am. J. Cardiol. *72:*821, 1993.
285. Nearing, B. D., Huang, A. H., and Verrier, R. L.: Dynamic tracking of cardiac vulnerability by complex demodulation of the T wave. Science *252:*437, 1991.
286. Verrier, R. L., and Nearing, B. B.: Electrophysiologic basis for T wave alternans as an index of vulnerability to ventricular fibrillation. J. Cardiovasc. Electrophysiol. *5:*445, 1994.
287. Verrier, R. L., and Nearing, B. D.: T wave alternans as a harbinger of ischemia-induced sudden cardiac death. *In* Zipes, D. P., and Jalife, J. (eds.): Cardiac Electrophysiology: From Cell to Bedside. 2nd ed. Philadelphia, W. B. Saunders Company, 1994, p. 467.
288. Rosenbaum, D. S., He, B., and Cohen, R. J.: New approaches for evaluating cardiac electrical activity: Repolarization alternans and body surface Laplacian imaging. *In* Zipes, D. P., and Jalife, J. (eds.): Cardiac Electrophysiology: From Cell to Bedside. 2nd ed. Philadelphia, W. B. Saunders Company, 1994, p. 1187.
289. Rosenbaum, D. S., Jackson, L. E., Smith, J. M., et al.: Electrical alternans and vulnerability to ventricular arrhythmias. N. Engl. J. Med. *330:*235, 1994.
290. Zareba, W., Moss, A. J., leCessie, S., et al.: T wave alternans in idiopathic long QT syndrome. J. Am. Coll. Cardiol. *23:*1541, 1994.

291. Kanemoto, N., Goto, Y., Iwasaki, M., et al.: Torsades de pointes in patients with electrical alternans of T-U wave without change in QRS complex. Jpn. Circ. J. *56*:551, 1992.
292. Kothari, S. S., Patel, T., and Patel, T. K.: T-U wave alternans: A case report and review of the literature. Jpn. Heart J. *32*:843, 1991.
293. Zipes, D. P., DiMarco, J., Gillette, P., et al.: Guidelines to perform electrophysiologic studies. Circulation *92*:673, 1995.
294. Behar, S., Zissman, E., Zion, M., et al.: Prognostic significance of second-degree atrioventricular block in inferior wall acute myocardial infarction. SPRINT Study Group. Am. J. Coll. Cardiol. *72*:831, 1993.
295. Chiale, T. A., Sanchez, R. A., Franco, D. A., et al.: Overdrive prolongation of refractoriness and fatigue in the early stages of human bundle branch disease. J. Am. Coll. Cardiol. *23*:724, 1994.
296. Brugada, P., and Brugada, J.: Right bundle branch block, persistent ST segment elevation and sudden cardiac death: A distinct clinical and electrocardiographic syndrome. J. Am. Coll. Cardiol. *20*:1391, 1992.
297. Benditt, D. G., Sakaguchi, S., Goldstein, M. A., et al.: Sinus node dysfunction: Pathology, clinical features, evaluation, and treatment. *In* Zipes, D. P., and Jalife, J. (eds.): Cardiac Electrophysiology: From Cell to Bedside. 2nd ed. Philadelphia, W. B. Saunders Company, 1994, p. 1215.
298. deMarneffe, M., Gregoire, J. M., Waterschoot, P., et al.: The sinus node function: Normal and pathological. Eur. Heart J. *14*:649, 1993.
299. Lee, W. J., Wu, M. H., Young, M. L., et al.: Sinus node dysfunction in children. Acta Paediatr. Scand. *33*:159, 1992.
300. Asseman, P., Berzin, B., Desry, D., et al.: Postextrasystolic sinoatrial exit block in human sick sinus syndrome: Demonstration by direct recording of sinus node electrograms. Am. Heart J. *122*:1633, 1991.
301. Marcus, B., Gillette, P. C., and Garson, A., Jr.: Electrophysiologic evaluation of sinus node dysfunction in postoperative children and young adults utilizing combined autonomic blockade. Clin. Cardiol. *14*:33, 1991.
302. Resh, W., Feuer, J., and Wesley, R. C., Jr.: Intravenous adenosine: A noninvasive diagnostic test for sick sinus syndrome. PACE *15*:2068, 1992.
303. Wu, D. L., Yeh, S. J., Lin, F. C., et al.: Sinus automaticity and sinoatrial conduction in severe symptomatic sick sinus syndrome. J. Am. Coll. Cardiol. *19*:355, 1992.
304. Suyama, A. C., Sunagawa, K., Sugimachi, M., et al.: Differentiation between aberrant ventricular conduction and ventricular ectopy in atrial fibrillation using RR intervals scattergram. Circulation *88*:2307, 1993.
305. Steinbeck, G., Andersen, D., Bach, P., et al.: Comparison of electrophysiologically guided antiarrhythmic therapy with beta-blocker therapy in patients with symptomatic sustained ventricular tachyarrhythmias. N. Engl. J. Med. *327*:987, 1992.
306. CASCADE Investigators: Randomized antiarrhythmic drug therapy in survivors of cardiac arrest (the CASCADE Study). Am. J. Cardiol. *72*:280, 1993.
307. Brooks, R., and Ruskin, J.: Evaluation of the patient with unexplained syncope. *In* Zipes, D. P., and Jalife, J. (eds.): Cardiac Electrophysiology: From Cell to Bedside. 2nd ed. Philadelphia, W. B. Saunders Company, 1994, p. 1247.
308. Lerman-Sagie, T., Lerman, T., Mukamel, M., et al.: A prospective evaluation of pediatric patients with syncope. Clin. Pediatr. *33*:67, 1994.
309. Strieper, M. J., Auld, D. O., Hulse, J. E., et al.: Evaluation of recurrent pediatric syncope: Role of tilt table testing. Pediatrics *93*:660, 1994.
310. Kapoor, W. N.: Evaluation and management of the patient with syncope. J. A. M. A. *268*:2553, 1992.
311. Wilmshurst, T. T., Willicombe, P. R., and Webb-Peploe, M. M.: Effect of aortic valve replacement on syncope in patients with aortic stenosis. Br. Heart J. *70*:542, 1993.
312. Steinberg, J. S., Prystowsky, E., Freedman, R. A., et al.: Use of the signal-averaged electrocardiogram for predicting inducible ventricular tachycardia in patients with unexplained syncope: Relation to clinical variables in a multi-variate analysis. J. Am. Coll. Cardiol. *23*:99, 1994.
313. Sneddon, J. F., Counihan, P. J., Bashir, Y., et al.: Assessment of autonomic function in patients with neurally mediated syncope: Augmented cardiopulmonary baroreceptor responses to graded orthostatic stress. J. Am. Coll. Cardiol. *21*:1193, 1993.
314. Gilligan, D. M., Nihoyannopoulos, P., Chan, W. L., et al.: Investigation of a hemodynamic basis for syncope in hypertrophic cardiomyopathy: Use of head-up tilt test. Circulation *85*:2140, 1992.
315. Balaji, S., Oslizlok, P. C., Allen, M. C., et al.: Neurocardiogenic syncope in children with a normal heart. J. Am. Coll. Cardiol. *23*:779, 1994.
315a. Sutton, R., and Petersen, M. E. V.: The clinical spectrum of neurocardiogenic syncope. J. Cardiovasc. Electrophysiol. *6*:569, 1995.
316. Dilsizian, V., Bonow, R. O., Epstein, S. E., et al.: Myocardial ischemia detected by thallium scintigraphy is frequently related to cardiac arrest and syncope in young patients with hypertrophic cardiomyopathy. J. Am. Coll. Cardiol. *22*:796, 1993.
317. Aronow, W. S., Mercando, A. D., and Epstein, S.: Prevalence of arrhythmias detected by 24-hour ambulatory electrocardiography and value of antiarrhythmic therapy in elderly patients with unexplained syncope. Am. J. Cardiol. *70*:408, 1992.
318. Calkins, H., Byrne, M., and El-atassi, R.: The economic burden of unrecognized vasodepressor syncope. Am. J. Med. *95*:473, 1993.
319. Middlekauff, H. R., Stevenson, W. G., Stevenson, L. W., et al.: Syncope in advanced heart failure: High risk of sudden death regardless of origin of syncope. J. Am. Coll. Cardiol. *21*:110, 1993.
320. Brugada, P., Gursoy, S., Brugada, J., et al.: Investigation of palpitations. Lancet *341*:1254, 1993.
321. Biffi, A., Ammirati, F., Caselli, G., et al.: Usefulness of transesophageal pacing during exercise for evaluating palpitations in professional athletes. Am. J. Cardiol. *72*:922, 1993.
322. Hindricks, G., on behalf of the Multicenter European Radiofrequency Survey (MERFS) Investigators of the Working Group on Arrhythmias of the European Society of Cardiology: The Multicenter European Radiofrequency Survey (MERFS): Complications of radiofrequency catheter ablation of arrhythmias. Eur. Heart J. *14*:1644, 1993.
323. Scheinman, M. M.: Patterns of catheter ablation practice in the United States: Results of the 1992 NASPE Survey. PACE *17*:873, 1994.

OTHER DIAGNOSTIC ELECTROCARDIOGRAPHIC TECHNIQUES

324. Katz, A., Guetta, V., and Ovsyshcher, I. A.: Transesophageal electrocardiography using a temporary pacing balloon-tipped electrode in acute cardiac care. Ann. Emerg. Med. *20*:961, 1991.
325. Klein, L. S., Miles, W. M., Rardon, D. P., et al.: Transesophageal recording. *In* Zipes, D. P., and Jalife, J. (eds.): Cardiac Electrophysiology: From Cell to Bedside. 2nd ed. Philadelphia, W. B. Saunders Company, 1994, p. 1112.
327. Flowers, N. C., and Horan, L. G.: Body surface potential mapping. *In* Zipes, D. P., and Jalife, J. (eds.): Cardiac Electrophysiology: From Cell to Bedside. 2nd ed. Philadelphia, W. B. Saunders Company, 1994, p. 1049.
328. Franzone, P. C., Guerri, L., and Taccardi, B.: Spread of excitation in a myocardial volume: simulation studies in a model of anisotropic ventricular muscle activated by point stimulation. J. Cardiovasc. Electrophysiol. *4*:144, 1993.
329. Franzone, P. C., Guerri, L., and Taccardi, B.: Potential distributions generated by point stimulation in a myocardial volume: Simulation studies in a model of anisotropic ventricular muscle. J. Cardiovasc. Electrophysiol. *4*:438, 1993.
330. Green, L. S., Lux, R. L., Ershler, P. R., et al.: Resolution of pace mapping stimulus site separation using body surface potentials. Circulation *90*:462, 1994.
331. SippensGroenewegen, A., Spekhorst, H., vanHemel, N. M., et al.: Localization of the site of origin of post infarction ventricular tachycardia by endocardial pace mapping: Body surface mapping compared with a 12-lead electrocardiogram. Circulation *88*:2290, 1993.
332. DeAmbroggi, L., and Santambrogio, C.: Clinical use of body surface potential mapping in cardiac arrhythmias. Physiol. Res. *42*:137, 1993.
333. He, B., Kirby, D. A., Mullen, T. J., et al.: Body surface Laplacian mapping of cardiac excitation in intact pigs. PACE *16*:1017, 1993.
334. Dubuc, M., Nadeau, R., Tremblay, G., et al.: Pace mapping using body surface potential maps to guide catheter ablation of accessory pathways in patients with Wolff-Parkinson-White syndrome. Circulation *87*:135, 1993.
335. SippensGroenewegen, A., Spekhorst, H., vanHemel, N. M., et al.: Body surface mapping of ectopic left ventricular activation: QRS spectrum in patients with prior myocardial infarction. Circ. Res. *71*:1361, 1992.
336. Mitchell, L. B., Hubley-Koszey, C. L., Smith, E. R., et al.: Electrocardiographic body surface mapping in patients with ventricular tachycardia: Assessment of utility in the identification of effective pharmacologic therapy. Circulation *86*:383, 1992.
337. Liebeman, J., Zeno, J. A., Olshansky, B., et al.: Electrocardiographic body surface potential mapping in the Wolff-Parkinson-White syndrome: Noninvasive determination of the ventricular insertion sites of accessory atrioventricular connections. Circulation *83*:886, 1991.
338. Franz, M. R.: Bridging the gap between basic and clinical electrophysiology: What can be learned from monophasic action potential recordings? J. Cardiovasc. Electrophysiol. *5*:699, 1994.
339. Simson, M. B.: Signal-averaged electrocardiography. *In* Zipes, D. P., and Jalife, J. (eds.): Cardiac Electrophysiology: From Cell to Bedside. 2nd ed. Philadelphia, W. B. Saunders Company, 1994, p. 1038.
340. Shenasa, M., Fetsch, T., Martinez-Rubio, A., et al.: Signal averaging in patients with coronary artery disease: How helpful is it? J. Cardiovasc. Electrophysiol. *4*:609, 1993.
341. Berbari, E. J., Lander, P., Geselowitz, D. B., et al.: Identifying the end of ventricular activation: Body surface late potentials versus electrogram measurements in a canine infarction model. J. Cardiovasc. Electrophysiol. *5*:28, 1994.
342. Jordaens, L., Schoenfeld, P., Demeester, C., et al.: Late potentials and ejection fraction at hospital discharge: Prognostic value in thrombolyzed and non-thrombolyzed patients. A preliminary report. Acta Cardiol. *46*:531, 1991.
343. Kremers, M. S., Hsia, H., Wells, P., et al.: Diastolic potentials recorded by surface electrocardiographic signal averaging during sustained ventricular tachycardia: Possible origin from the reentrant circuit. PACE *14*:1000, 1991.
344. Benditt, D. G., Lurie, K. G., Adler, S. W., et al.: Rationale and methodology of head-up tilt table testing for evaluation of neurally mediated (cardioneurogenic) syncope. *In* Zipes, D. P., and Jalife, J. (eds.): Cardiac Electrophysiology: From Cell to Bedside. 2nd ed. Philadelphia, W. B. Saunders Company, 1994, p. 1115.
345. Kapoor, W. N., Smith, M. A., and Miller, N. L.: Upright tilt testing in evaluating syncope: A comprehensive literature review. Am. J. Med. *97*:78, 1994.
346. Tonnessen, G. E., Haft, J. I., Fulton, J., et al.: The value of tilt table testing with isoproterenol in determining therapy in adults with syn-

cope and presyncope of unexplained origin. Arch. Intern. Med. *154:*1613, 1994.
347. Sra, J. S., Murphy, V., Natale, A., et al.: Circulatory and catecholamine changes during head-up tilt testing in neurocardiogenic (vasovagal) syncope. Am. J. Cardiol. *73:*33, 1994.
348. Sheldon, R.: Evaluation of single-stage isoproterenol-tilt table test in patients with syncope. J. Am. Coll. Cardiol. *22:*114, 1993.
349. Lurie, K. G., Dutton, J., Mangat, R., et al.: Evaluation of edrophonium as a provocative agent for vasovagal syncope during head-up tilt-table testing. Am. J. Cardiol. *72:*1286, 1993.
350. Ovadia, M., and Thoele, D.: Tilt testing with esmolol withdrawal for the evaluation of syncope in the young. Circulation *89:*228, 1994.
351. Leor, J., Rotstein, Z., Vered, Z., et al.: Absence of tachycardia during tilt test predicts failure of beta-blocker therapy in patients with neurocardiogenic syncope. Am. Heart J. *127:*1539, 1994.
352. O'Marcaigh, A. S., MacLellan-Tobert, S. G., and Porter, C. J.: Tilt-table testing and oral metoprolol therapy in young patients with unexplained syncope. Pediatrics *93:*278, 1994.
353. Blanc, J. J., Mansourati, J., Maheu, B., et al.: Reproducibility of a positive passive upright tilt test at 7-day interval in patients with syncope. Am. J. Cardiol. *72:*469, 1993.
354. Brooks, R., Ruskin, J. N., Powell, A. C., et al.: Prospective evaluation of day-to-day reproducibility of upright tilt-table testing in unexplained syncope. Am. J. Cardiol. *71:*1289, 1993.
355. deBuitlier, M., Grogan, E. W., Jr., Picone, M. F., et al.: Immediate reproducibility of the tilt-table test in adults with unexplained syncope. Am. J. Cardiol. *71:*304, 1993.
356. Chen, X. C., Chen, M. Y., Remole, S., et al.: Reproducibility of head-up tilt-table testing for eliciting susceptibility to neurally mediated syncope in patients without structural heart disease. Am. J. Cardiol. *69:*755, 1992.
357. Sutton, R., and Petersen, M.E.V.: The clinical spectrum of neurocardiogenic syncope. J. Cardiovasc. Electrophysiol. *6:*569, 1995.
358. Morillo, C. A., Leitch, J. W., Yee, R., et al.: A placebo-controlled trial of intravenous and oral disopyramide for prevention of neurally mediated syncope induced by head-up tilt. J. Am. Coll. Cardiol. *22:*1843, 1993.

Chapter 21
Management of Cardiac Arrhythmias: Pharmacological, Electrical, and Surgical Techniques

DOUGLAS P. ZIPES

PHARMACOLOGICAL THERAPY

PRINCIPLES OF CLINICAL PHARMACOKINETICS

Pharmacological treatment of a patient with a cardiac arrhythmia has as its primary objective to reach an effective and well-tolerated plasma drug concentration as rapidly as possible and to maintain this concentration for as long as required without producing adverse effects. In many but not all situations and not with all drugs, plasma concentration after equilibration correlates with the pharmacodynamic as well as adverse effects of the drug. Therapeutic serum concentrations for the most important available antiarrhythmic agents are listed in Table 21–1 and are based on concentrations of drugs that exert therapeutic effects on often benign arrhythmias such as premature ventricular complexes (PVCs), without adverse effects in a majority of patients. However, the therapeutic concentration for any individual patient is the amount of drug required *for that patient* to suppress or terminate the specific cardiac arrhythmia requiring treatment without producing adverse effects.

For a specific patient, one must consider the response both of the patient and of the arrhythmia to the drug; the actual plasma concentration of the drug is often of secondary importance. Low drug concentrations can exert a therapeutic or toxic effect in some patients, while drug concentrations higher than the normal range may be needed and tolerated in another patient. In some patients, measured plasma concentrations can be useful to establish concentrations needed for prophylaxis, to judge the sensitivity or resistance of the arrhythmia to the drug, and to evaluate symptoms that suggest drug toxicity. Plasma concentrations also can be used to determine the effects of changing physiological states on drug concentrations, establish drug compliance or abuse, search for drug interactions that affect the pharmacokinetics, and establish the importance of physiologically active metabolites of the parent compound.[1,2] Active metabolites may be suspected when the clinical effect of the drug outlasts the therapeutic serum concentration of the parent compound or when results immediately following intravenous drug administration differ from those after oral administration of the drug.

Normally, because antiarrhythmic agents have a narrow toxic-therapeutic relationship, important complications of therapy can result from amounts of drug that only slightly exceed the amount necessary to produce beneficial effects; lesser concentrations are often subtherapeutic. It is obvious that careful dosing with these agents is essential to maintain adequate but nontoxic amounts of drug in the body, a task facilitated by understanding drug pharmacokinetics.[3–5] The latter consists of a quantitative assessment of drug dose-concentration factors, including drug absorption, distribution, metabolism, and excretion. Alterations in the rate of any of these processes can account for significant intra- and interpatient variations in plasma concentrations. In addition, changes in the functional status of any of the organs involved, e.g., the heart, liver, or kidneys, can significantly alter dose requirements in a given patient. The latter concerns a study of pharmacodynamics, or drug concentration-response issues.[2,6]

ABSORPTION

Drug absorption from the intestinal tract occurs for most drugs with a half-life of absorption in the range of 20 to 30 minutes. Completeness of absorption can vary between 50 and over 90 per cent, depending on the drug, with most absorption occurring in the small intestine. Different preparations of the same drug can undergo different rates of absorption in the same patient because the tablet preparations have different dissolution rates. Thus different brands of drug may not result in the same serum concentration. By altering the properties of the tablet, a slow-release form of a drug ordinarily rapidly absorbed and metabolized, such as procainamide, can be developed. Large amounts of some orally administered drugs, such as propranolol or verapamil, are transformed to inactive metabolites in the liver before they reach the systemic circulation—the so-called first-pass hepatic effect.[5] For such an agent, much more drug must be administered orally than intravenously to achieve the same physiological effect.

ABSORPTION ABNORMALITIES. Disease states and other factors can alter the rate and completeness of drug absorption. For example, heart failure can cause mucosal edema of the gut and impair the

TABLE 21–1 DOSAGE AND THERAPEUTIC SERUM CONCENTRATIONS FOR ANTIARRHYTHMIC AGENTS

	USUAL DOSE RANGES			
	Intravenous (mg)		Oral (mg)	
DRUG	*Loading*	*Maintenance*	*Loading*	*Maintenance*
Quinidine	6 to 10 mg/kg at 0.3 to 0.5 mg/kg/min	600 to 1000	300 to600 q6h	
Procainamide	6 to 13 mg/kg at 0.2 to 0.5 mg/kg/min	2 to 6 mg/min	500 to 1000	350 to 1000 q3–6h
Disopyramide	1 to 2 mg/kg over 15–45 min*	1 mg/kg/h		100 to 400 q6–8h
Lidocaine	1 to 3 mg/kg at 20 to 50 mg/min	1 to 4 mg/min	N/A	N/A
Mexiletine	500 mg*	0.5 to 1.0 gm/24 h	400 to 600	150 to 300 q6–8h
Tocainide	750 mg*		400 to 600	400 to 600 q8–12h
Phenytoin	100 mg q5min for ≤1000 mg		1000	100 to 400 q12–24h
Flecainide	2 mg/kg*	100 to 200 q12h		
Propafenone	1 to 2 mg/kg		600 to 900	150 to 300 q8–12h
Moricizine			300	100 to 400 q8h
Propranolol	0.25 to 0.5 mg, q5min for ≤0.15 to 0.20 mg/kg			10 to 200 q6–8h
Amiodarone	15mg/kg for 10 min, 1 mg/kg for 360 min, 0.5 mg/kg thereafter		800 to 1600 q.d. for 1 to 3 weeks	200 to 400 q.d.
Bretylium	5 to 10 mg/kg at 1 to 2 mg/kg/min	½ to 2 mg/min	N/A	4 mg/kg/day†
Verapamil	10 mg over 1 to 2 min	0.005 mg/kg/min		80 to 120 q6–8h
Adenosine	6–12 mg (rapidly)		N/A	N/A
Sotalol			N/A	80 mg q12h to start incrementing gradually to 320 mg/day as needed

* Investigational; IV.
† Investigational only.

absorption of orally administered drugs, as can decreased intestinal blood flow. Renal or hepatic hypoperfusion can reduce drug elimination and metabolism. Reduced volume of distribution and impaired clearance can increase elimination half-life, requiring a reduction in loading and maintenance doses (Table 21–2). Malabsorption syndromes, concomitant use of other drugs, or changes in gut motility or flora caused by diarrheal states, antibiotics, or the use of cathartics can alter absorption. Since most antiarrhythmic agents are basic compounds, they are ionized and poorly absorbed at normal gastric pH, and some drugs can decompose at gastric pH. Conditions that delay gastric emptying increase the absorption lag phase between ingestion of these drugs and their arrival in the small intestine, where most absorption takes place, and therefore can decrease absorption. In patients with severe hypotension, shock, or cardiac arrest, impaired tissue perfusion prevents reliable absorption of intramuscularly administered agents; these patients should receive all medications by the intravenous (IV) route.

TABLE 21–2 KNOWN INFLUENCE OF DISEASE STATES AND OTHER CONDITIONS ON ANTIARRHYTHMIC DRUG PHARMACOKINETICS

DISEASE OR CONDITION	EFFECTS
Congestive heart failure	Reduced clearance of: lidocaine, procainamide, flecainide Reduced volume of distribution of: lidocaine
Liver disease	Reduced clearance of: lidocaine, disopyramide, phenytoin, propranolol
Renal disease	Reduced clearance of: disopyramide, procainamide, bretylium, tocainide, flecainide Altered protein binding (with usually unchanged drug requirements) of: phenytoin
Post-myocardial infarction	Reduced clearance of: procainamide Altered protein binding of: lidocaine, quinidine
Prolonged administration	Reduced clearance of: lidocaine
Obesity	Increased volume of distribution of: lidocaine

From Roden, D.: New concepts in antiarrhythmic drug pharmacokinetics. Progr. Cardiol. *15*:19, 1987.

BIOAVAILABILITY

The rate of drug absorption, determined by the time required to achieve maximum plasma concentration, and the fraction of drug absorbed influence the drug's *bioavailability*, which is a measure of the amount of drug that reaches the systemic circulation intact. Bioavailability of a drug is influenced by factors such as pill dissolution, metabolism by gut mucosa, hepatic metabolism and binding, and absorption. It is a most important property of the drug. Absorption is thus only one component affecting bioavailability.

The fraction of an orally administered drug reaching the systemic circulation intact, or *systemic availability*, can be calculated (assuming equal clearances for IV and oral forms of drug) by comparing the areas under the plasma concentration curve achieved with oral and intravenous administrations using the following relationship. Systemic availability equals the area under the plasma concentration curve following oral administration divided by the area under the plasma concentration curve following IV administration times 100 (assuming equal IV and oral doses).

DRUG DISTRIBUTION

Most antiarrhythmic drugs in the therapeutic range are eliminated according to *first-order kinetics*, which means that the amount of drug eliminated per unit of time is directly proportional to the amount (or concentration) of drug in the body. More drug in the body results in more drug excreted by the kidneys or metabolized by the liver so that the *fraction* of drug eliminated per unit of time remains constant regardless of the amount of drug in the body. For example, one-half the drug may be eliminated in 6 hours whether the total amount of drug in the body is 4 gm or 10 gm, resulting in

TIME TO PEAK PLASMA CONCENTRATION (ORAL) (h)	EFFECTIVE SERUM OR PLASMA CONCENTRATION (μg/ml)	ELIMINATION HALF-LIFE (h)	BIOAVAILABILITY (%)	MAJOR ROUTE OF ELIMINATION
1.5 to 3.0	3 to 6	5 to 9	60 to 80	Liver
1	4 to 10	3 to 5	70 to 85	Kidneys
1 to 2	2 to 5	8 to 9	80 to 90	Kidneys
N/A	1 to 5	1 to 2	N/A	Liver
2 to 4	0.75 to 2	10 to 17	90	Liver
0.5 to 2	4 to 10	11	90	Liver
8 to 12	10 to 20	18 to 36	50 to 70	Liver
3 to 4	0.2 to 1.0	20	95	Liver
1 to 3	0.2 to 3.0	5 to 8	25 to 75	Liver
	0.1			
4	1 to 2.5	50 days	35 to 65	Liver
	0.5 to 1.5	8 to 14	25	Kidneys
2 to 4	0.04 to 0.90	3 to 6	20 to 50	Liver
1 to 2	0.10 to 0.15	3 to 8	10 to 35	Liver
2.5 to 4	2.5	12	90 to 100	Kidneys

Note: Results presented may vary according to doses, disease state, and IV or oral administration.

elimination of 2 gm in the first example and 5 gm in the second. As a consequence, the elimination half-life, or time required to eliminate half the body load (or to halve the plasma concentration) of such a drug, is constant and independent of the total-body load. The following discussion will assume first-order kinetics unless otherwise stated. (*Zero-order kinetics* indicates that the reaction occurs at a constant, usually maximal, rate and cannot increase further despite increased drug concentrations. Such nonlinear or saturable kinetics can occur at high concentrations of a drug that at usual concentrations exhibits first-order kinetics.[2])

The One-Compartment Model

Generally, two models, a *one-compartment open model* and a *two-compartment open model,* are used with relative accuracy to describe and predict serum concentrations at a given time for a variety of dose regimens. Even though these models are oversimplified representations of drug disposition, they provide guidelines for choosing loading doses and maintenance dose schedules for a given patient. In the one-compartment open model, drugs are considered to enter and to be eliminated from a single homogeneous unit that represents the entire body. Drugs entering the compartment are considered to be distributed immediately throughout the compartment, making the concentration of the drug equal to the amount of drug in the compartment divided by the volume of the compartment. The latter equals the amount of the drug in the compartment divided by the drug concentration.

In reality, a one-compartment open model is not entirely appropriate because a certain amount of time is needed to distribute the drug throughout the volume of the compartment. However, the one-compartment model predicts plasma concentration as a function of time and dose if distribution is significantly faster than the rate of administration or of excretion, which is the case for many antiarrhythmic drugs.

The Two-Compartment Model

If the rate of drug administration is rapid in relation to drug distribution (e.g., intravenous administration), a two-compartment open model more accurately predicts drug concentrations (Fig. 21–1). In this model the drug enters the system by the central compartment and can leave the system only by distribution into a peripheral compartment or elimination from the central compartment. The central compartment, in dynamic equilibrium with the more slowly equilibrating peripheral compartment, is assumed to consist of the blood volume and extracellular fluid of highly perfused tissues such as heart, lungs, kidneys, and liver, while the peripheral compartment, acting as a reservoir, consists of less well perfused tissue such as muscle, skin, and adipose tissue. The first-order rate constants $K_{1\rightarrow 2}$ and $K_{2\rightarrow 1}$ determine the rate of transfer of drug between the central and peripheral compartments or vice versa, with Ke representing the overall elimination rate constant. Ke relates the sum of all methods of irreversible drug elimination from the central compartment to the concentration of drug in that compartment (Fig. 21–1).

For antiarrhythmic drugs, the peripheral compartment is generally larger than the central compartment. The concepts of distribution

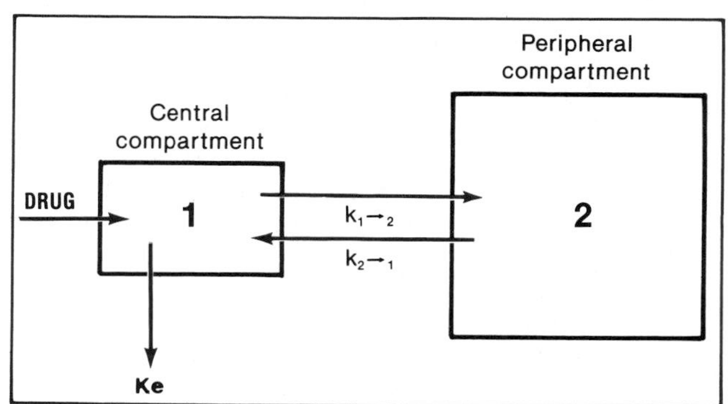

FIGURE 21–1. Two-compartment open model. A smaller central compartment into which drug is administered and from which it is eliminated (Ke) connects in dynamic equilibrium with a larger peripheral compartment.

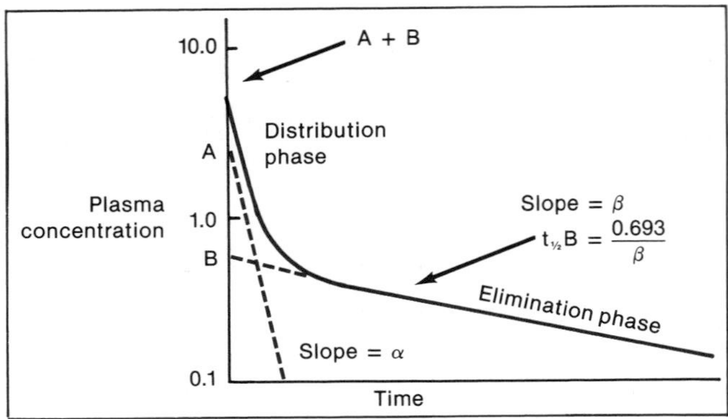

FIGURE 21–2. Schematic diagram of the semilogarithmic plot of drug plasma concentration as a function of time following rapid intravenous injection, according to the principles outlined for a two-compartment open model. (From Gibaldi, M., and Perrier, D.: Drugs and the pharmaceutical sciences. *In* Pharmacokinetics, Vol. 1. New York, Marcel Dekker, 1975.)

volumes and drug movement are more complex in the two-compartment open model than in the one-compartment open model. The two-compartment model may behave similarly to the one-compartment model when drugs are infused slowly or given orally and K_1 approximates K_2, but pronounced differences exist when injections are given rapidly.

DISTRIBUTION AND ELIMINATION PHASES. Following administration of drugs for which the kinetics are described by a two-compartment model, the curve of plasma drug concentration demonstrates two distinct phases: an early phase (alpha, or distribution, phase), characterized by rapidly falling plasma drug concentrations due to distribution between the central compartment and the peripheral compartment, and a second phase (beta, or elimination, phase) of slower decline in plasma drug concentration, representing primarily elimination of drugs from the central compartment (Fig. 21–2). *Alpha* is often referred to as the *rate constant for distribution* and *beta* as the *rate constant for elimination*. During the latter beta phase, when the drug is in distribution equilibrium, serum concentrations correlate with the pharmacological effects of the drug. The distribution of quinidine is shown in Figure 21–3.

VOLUME OF DISTRIBUTION. The extent of extravascular distribution of a drug is obtained by measuring the apparent *volume of distribution*, which is the hypothetical volume into which a dose of drug would have to be diluted to give the observed plasma concentration. It is determined by the dose administered divided by the plasma concentration at time 0. The latter equals the sum of A and B on the logarithmic plasma concentration axis obtained by extrapolating the alpha and beta phases back to 0 time (Fig. 21–2). It is also calculated by dividing the systemic clearance of the drug by beta, the rate constant of elimination. A large volume of distribution indicates a wide distribution and extensive tissue uptake of the drug and often exceeds by several times the actual amount of total-body water. The large volume of distribution for most antiarrhythmic agents indicates that they are present in higher concentrations in some tissues than in the plasma. The volume of distribution is dependent on the relative serum and tissue binding characteristics of the drug and can be constricted in some patients, such as those with renal failure, during which a change in serum protein or tissue binding can occur. Quinidine decreases the volume of distribution of digoxin, probably as a result of a decrease in tissue binding of digoxin.

DRUG METABOLISM AND EXCRETION. Approximately 97 per cent of the dose of any drug is removed from the body in a time equal to five half-lives. *Serum elimination half-life* is defined as the time interval for 50 per cent of the drug present in the body at the beginning of the interval to be eliminated. After one half-life, 50 per cent of the drug remains in the body (assuming no further drug is administered), after two half-lives 25 per cent remains, after three half-lives 12.5 per cent remains, and so forth. Half-life is determined from the relation-

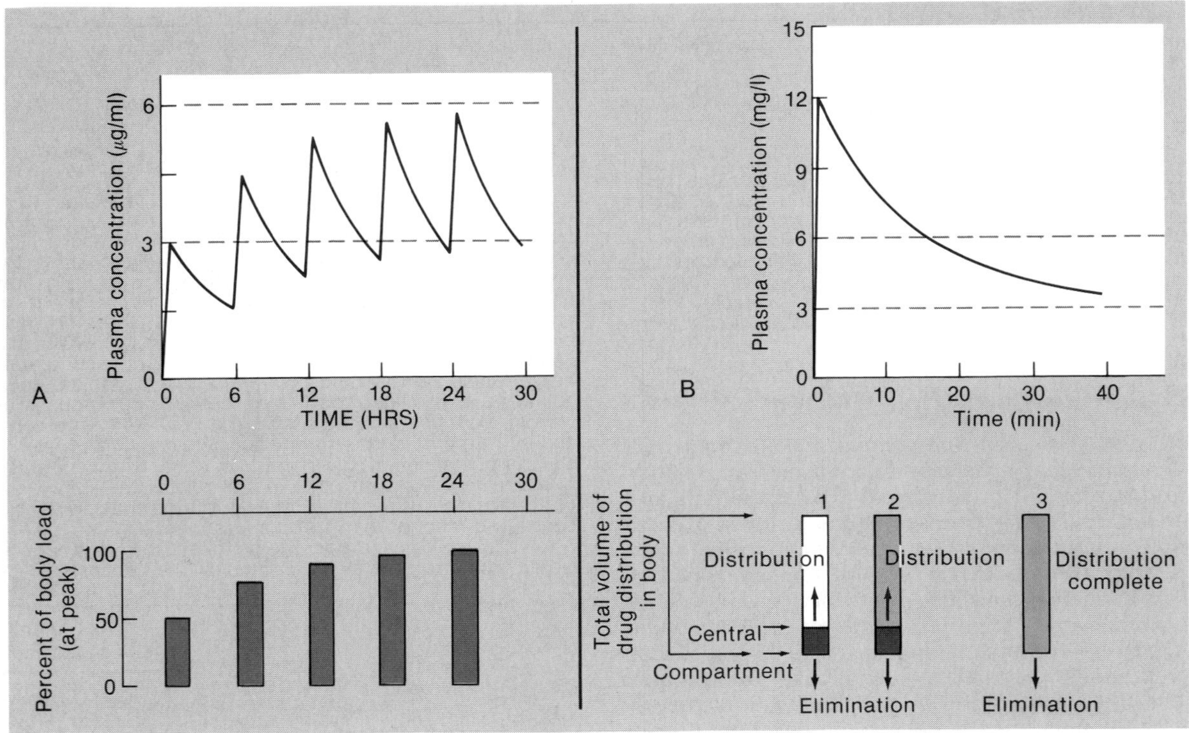

FIGURE 21–3. *A*, Changes in plasma concentration over time after beginning treatment with quinidine. *Top*, Quinidine plasma concentration over time, with the dashed line indicating the therapeutic range. *Bottom*, The hatched bars represent the body load immediately after each dose of quinidine, expressed as a percentage of the load after a dose when a steady state has been achieved. Quinidine is administered every 6 hours (the half-life in this case). Four half-lives, or 24 hours, are required to achieve a body load of quinidine that exceeds 90 per cent of the load at steady state. *B, Top*, Plasma concentrations produced by administering a full intravenous loading dose of quinidine as a bolus, with the therapeutic range shown by a dashed line. *Bottom*, The numbered vertical boxes indicate the volume of distribution of quinidine. Just after the drug is given, it is dissolved only in the small central compartment, as in box 1, and very high peak concentrations are achieved (in the toxic range). The drug then distributes throughout the rest of the body. Distribution has a half-life of about 8 minutes and is complete by 30 minutes (box 3). Quinidine concentration is now in the therapeutic range, and further decreases in plasma concentration are due solely to drug elimination. (From Nattel, S., and Zipes, D. P.: Clinical pharmacology of old and new antiarrhythmic drugs. Cardiovasc. Clin. *11*:221, 1980.)

ship t½ = 0.693/beta for a two-compartment model (Fig. 21–2). Since changes in drug distribution influence elimination half-life, the equation can be rewritten as t½ = 0.693 × volume of distribution/total-body clearance.

DRUG CLEARANCE. This is analogous to renal clearance and is the volume of blood totally cleared of drug per unit of time. It is the sum of the clearances for each process by which the drug is eliminated and can be calculated from the relationship: clearance = dose of the drug/area under the plasma concentration time curve (AUC). Expressed differently, clearance equals volume of distribution × beta, or volume of distribution × 0.693/half-life. A larger volume of distribution increases the elimination half-life at a given clearance. The larger volume of distribution of antiarrhythmic drugs accounts for the relatively long half-life despite their high clearance rates. Quinidine prolongs digitoxin's half-life by decreasing total-body clearance. Clearance of drugs with high extraction ratios strongly depends on blood flow to the organ from which they are eliminated, such as propranolol, verapamil, or lidocaine in the liver. For antiarrhythmic drugs that have a high renal extraction ratio, such as procainamide and quinidine, reduction of renal flow decreases their clearance.

ELIMINATION HALF-LIFE. Function of the organ system that eliminates a given drug from the body determines the elimination half-life. Primary routes of elimination are hepatic metabolism and renal clearance. The kidneys can remove unchanged drug or metabolites. For drugs rapidly metabolized in the liver, hepatic blood flow limits the rate of drug elimination. Disorders that reduce liver blood flow (e.g., low cardiac output, hepatic disease with portacaval shunting) markedly slow the elimination of such drugs. Drugs with a short half-life are convenient to use by intravenous infusion but not by chronic oral dosing, since the short half-life requires frequent oral doses to maintain a fairly constant plasma concentration. Generally, maintenance dosing involves giving a certain amount of the drug at a time interval that equals the elimination half-life. However, with drugs that have very long half-lives, such as 12 hours, this can result in excessive peak values shortly after administration and consequent side effects. Maintaining constant plasma concentrations is necessary because of the narrow toxic-therapeutic ratios exhibited by antiarrhythmic agents.

Some drugs have active metabolites with half-lives considerably longer than the parent compound, allowing dosing intervals to be more widely spaced than those predicted by the half-life of the parent drug. Procainamide (see p. 603) has an active metabolite, *N*-acetylprocainamide (NAPA), that is eliminated unchanged by the kidneys and can accumulate in high concentrations in patients with renal disease. The rate and extent of metabolism of the same drug can vary greatly from patient to patient owing to a variety of factors, including environment, genetics, age, disease states, and influence of other drugs given concomitantly. A genetically controlled acetyltransferase enzyme system influences the metabolism of some drugs making about half the American population "rapid" and half "slow acetylators." Rapid acetylators metabolize a greater proportion of a drug dose than do slow acetylators, who may require less drug to achieve any desired serum level or pharmacological effect. Also, rapid acetylators may be more prone to develop reactions from the metabolites of drugs or are less likely to develop side effects from the parent compound for a constant drug dose.

DRUG BINDING

Drugs exist in plasma both in the free form and bound to plasma proteins. Only free drug is capable of distributing into tissues and exerting a pharmacological action. Some drugs, e.g., verapamil, sotalol, and disopyramide, have optical isomers, with different potencies and effects. Virtually all assays for drug concentration in the blood measure *both* free and protein-bound drug. For antiarrhythmic drugs, the fraction of drug that is bound varies greatly among the different agents but is fairly constant for individual drugs over the clinically relevant range of plasma concentrations with the exception of phenytoin, lidocaine, propafenone, and disopyramide. With these drugs, binding sites become saturated at high concentrations, and therefore, a doubling of total drug concentration represents more than a doubling of unbound drug. Total plasma concentrations of a given drug generally correlate well with its clinical effects, and it has not been necessary to develop assays to measure free drug concentrations for antiarrhythmic agents. Some drugs, such as quinidine and lidocaine, bind to an α1-glycoprotein that increases in acute disease states such as myocardial infarction, which may decrease the concentration of free drug.

When a constant dose of a drug is administered repeatedly (orally or parenterally) at a constant dosing interval, accumulation occurs until drug concentration approaches a constant steady-state level, at which time the rate of drug administration equals the rate of drug elimination. The time it takes to reach steady state is a function of the half-life of the drug; 94 per cent of steady state is achieved after four half-lives and 99 per cent after seven half-lives. A drug with a long half-life takes longer to reach steady state than does one with a short half-life. The average steady-state concentration of a drug equals the fraction of the dose absorbed (F) × the maintenance dose ($dose_m$) divided by the total-body clearance (Cl_s) × the dosing interval (τ).

Average steady-state concentration

$$= \frac{F \times dose_m}{Cl_s \times \tau} = \frac{F \times dose_m t\frac{1}{2}}{0.693 \times V_{d\tau}}$$

If the drug is given intravenously,

$$\text{Steady-state concentration} = \frac{\text{infusion rate}}{Cl_s} = \frac{\text{infusion rate } t\frac{1}{2}}{0.693\ V_d}$$

Finally, it is important to stress that drug pharmacokinetics may differ in normal healthy volunteers compared with patients who have a variety of illnesses. Therefore, information derived from patients as well as normal subjects must be considered when one is planning dosing regimens.

GENERAL CONSIDERATIONS REGARDING ANTIARRHYTHMIC DRUGS

Most of the available antiarrhythmic drugs (Table 21–1) can be classified according to whether they exert blocking actions predominantly on sodium, potassium, or calcium channels and whether they block beta-adrenoceptors.[6,7] The commonly used Vaughan Williams classification is limited because it is based on the electrophysiological effects exerted by an arbitrary concentration of the drug, generally on normal cardiac tissue. Actually, the actions of these drugs are quite complex and depend on tissue type, species, the degree of acute or chronic damage, heart rate, membrane potential, the ionic composition of the extracellular milieu, and other factors (Table 21–2). Many drugs exhibit actions that belong in multiple categories or operate indirectly, such as by altering hemodynamics, myocardial metabolism, or autonomic neural transmission. Some drugs have active metabolites that exert different effects from the parent compound. Not all drugs in the same class have identical effects, e.g., bretylium, sotalol, and amiodarone are dramatically different, while some drugs in different classes have overlapping actions, e.g., class IA and IC drugs. In vitro studies on healthy fibers usually establish the properties of antiarrhythmic agents rather than their antiarrhythmic properties.

Despite these limitations, the Vaughan Williams classification[8] is widely known and provides a useful communication shorthand. It is listed here, but the reader is cautioned that drug actions are more complex than depicted by the classification. A more realistic view of antiarrhythmic agents is provided by the "Sicilian gambit."[9,10] This approach to drug classification is an attempt to identify the mechanisms of a particular arrhythmia, determine the vulnerable parameter of the arrhythmia most susceptible to modification, define the target most likely to affect the vulnerable parameter, and then select a drug that will modify the target. This concept provides a framework in which to consider antiarrhythmic drugs (Table 21–3 and 21–4).

DRUG CLASSIFICATION. According to the Vaughan Williams classification, *class I* drugs block the fast sodium channel. They, in turn, may be divided into three subgroups:

Class IA. Drugs that reduce $\dot{V}_{max}$ and prolong action potential duration: quinidine, procainamide, disopyramide; kinetics of onset and offset in blocking the Na^+ channel are of intermediate rapidity (<5 sec).

Class IB. Drugs that do not reduce $\dot{V}_{max}$ and that shorten action potential duration: mexiletine, phenytoin, and lidocaine; fast onset and offset kinetics (<500 msec).

TABLE 21–3 CLASSIFICATION OF DRUG ACTIONS ON ARRHYTHMIAS BASED ON MODIFICATION OF VULNERABLE PARAMETER

ARRHYTHMIA	MECHANISMS	VULNERABLE PARAMETER	DRUGS
	Automaticity		
	(a) Enhanced normal		
Inappropriate sinus tachycardia Some idiopathic ventricular tachycardias		Phase 4 depolarization (decrease)	β-adrenergic blocking agents Na^+-channel blocking agents
	(b) Abnormal		
Atrial tachycardia		Maximal diastolic potential (hyperpolarization) or Phase 4 depolarization (decrease)	M_2-agonist Ca^{++}- or Na^+-channel blocking agents M_2 agonists
Accelerated idioventricular rhythms		Phase 4 depolarization (decrease)	Ca^{++}- or Na^+-channel blocking agents
	Triggered activity		
	(a) EAD		
Torsades de pointes		Action potential duration (shorten) or EAD (suppress)	β-agonists; vagolytic agents (increase rate) Ca^{++}-channel blocking agents; Mg^{++}; β-adrenergic blockers
	(b) DAD		
Digitalis-induced arrhythmias		Calcium overload (unload) or DAD (suppress)	Ca^{++}-channel blocking agents Na^+-channel blocking agents
Certain autonomically mediated ventricular tachycardias		Calcium overload (unload) or DAD (suppress)	β-adrenergic blocking agents Ca^{++}-channel blocking agents, adenosine
	Reentry		
	(Na^+ channel-dependent)		
	(a) Long excitable gap		
Atrial flutter type I		Conduction and excitability (depress)	Na^+-channel blocking agents (except lidocaine, mexiletine, tocainide)
Circus movement tachycardia in WPW		Conduction and excitability (depress)	Na^+-channel blocking agents (except lidocaine, mexiletine, tocainide)
Sustained monomorphic ventricular tachycardia		Conduction and excitability (depress)	Na^+-channel blocking agents
	(b) Short excitable gap		
Atrial flutter type II		Refractory period (prolong)	K^+-channel blockers
Atrial fibrillation		Refractory period (prolong)	K^+-channel blockers
Circus movement tachycardia in WPW		Refractory period (prolong)	Amiodarone, sotalol
Polymorphic and sustained monomorphic ventricular tachycardia		Refractory period (prolong)	Quinidine, procainamide, disopyramide
Bundle branch reentry		Refractory period (prolong)	Quinidine, procainamide,
Ventricular fibrillation		Refractory period (prolong)	disopyramide, bretylium
	Reentry		
	(Ca^{++}-channel-dependent)		
AV nodal reentrant tachycardia		Conduction and excitability (depress)	Ca^+-channel blocking agents
Circus movement tachycardia in WPW		Conduction and excitability (depress)	Ca^+-channel blocking agents
Verapamil-sensitive ventricular tachycardia		Conduction and excitability (depress)	Ca^+-channel blocking agents

Reproduced with permission from Task Force of the Working Group on Arrhythmias of the European Society of Cardiology: The Sicilian gambit. A new approach to the classification of antiarrhythmic drugs based on their actions on arrhythmogenic mechanisms. Circulation *84*:1831, 1991. Copyright 1991, American Heart Association.

Class IC. Drugs that reduce $\dot{V}_{max}$, primarily slow conduction, and can prolong refractoriness minimally: flecainide, propafenone, and probably moricizine; slow onset and offset kinetics (10 to 20 sec).

Class II drugs block beta-adrenergic receptors and include propranolol, timolol, metoprolol, and others (Table 38–7, p. 1307).

Class III drugs block potassium channels and prolong repolarization. They include sotalol, amiodarone, bretylium, and *N*-acetylprocainamide.

Class IV drugs block the slow calcium channel and include verapamil, diltiazem, nifedipine, and others.

A recently proposed model suggests that antiarrhythmic drugs cross the cell membrane and interact with receptors in the membrane channels when the latter are in the rested, activated, or inactivated state (Table 20–1) and that each of these interactions is characterized by a different association and dissociation rate constant (Figs. 20–10, p. 554 and 20–16, p. 559). Such interactions are voltage- and time-dependent. Transitions among rested, activated, and inactivated states are governed by standard Hodgkin-Huxley–type equations. When the drug is bound (associated) to a receptor site at or very close to the ionic channel (the drug probably does not actually plug the channel), the latter cannot conduct, even in the activated state.

USE-DEPENDENCE. Some drugs exert greater inhibitory effects on the upstroke of the action potential at more rapid rates of stimulation and after longer periods of stimulation, a characteristic called *use-dependence.* Use-dependence

TABLE 21–4 ACTIONS OF ANTIARRHYTHMIC DRUGS

	CHANNELS						RECEPTORS				PUMPS	CLINICAL EFFECTS			ECG EFFECTS		
	NA																
DRUG	*Fast*	*Med*	*Slow*	Ca	K	I_f	α	β	M_2	P	Na-K ATPase	Left ventricular function	Sinus Rate	Extracardiac	P-R interval	QRS width	J-T interval
Lidocaine	○											→	→	◎			↓
Mexiletine	○											→	→	◎			↓
Tocainide	○											→	→	●			↓
Moricizine	● I											↓	→	○		↑	
Procainamide		● A			◎							↓	→	●	↑	↑	↑
Disopyramide		● A			◎				○			↓	→	◎	↑↓	↑	↑
Quinidine		● A			◎		○		○			→	↑	◎	↑↓	↑	↑
Propafenone		● A						◎				↓	↓	○	↑	↑	
Flecainide			● A		○							↓	→	○	↑	↑	
Encainide			● A									↓	→	○	↑	↑	
																	↑
Bepridil	○			●	◎							?	↓	○			↑
Verapamil	○			●			◎					↓	↓	○	↑		↑
Diltiazem				◎								↓	↓	○	↑		
Bretylium					●		◩	◩				→	↓	○			↑
Sotalol					●			●				↓	↓	○	↑		↑
Amiodarone	○			○	●		◎	◎				→	↓	●	↑		↑
Alinidine					◎	●						?	↓	●			
Nadolol								●				↓	↓	○	↑		
Propranolol	○							●				↓	↓	○	↑		
Atropine									●			→	→	◎	↓		
Adenosine										□		?	↓	○	↓		
Digoxin									□		●	↑	↓	●	↑		↓

Relative potency of block: ○ Low ◎ Moderate ● High
□ = Agonist ◩ = Agonist/Antagonist
A = Activated state blocker
I = Inactivated state blocker

From Schwartz, P. J., and Zaza, A.: Eur. Heart J. *13*:26, 1992.

means that depression of $\dot{V}_{max}$ is greater after the channel has been "used," i.e., after action potential depolarization rather than after a rest period. It is possible that this use-dependence results from preferential interaction of the antiarrhythmic drug with either the open or the inactive channel and little interaction with the resting channels of the unstimulated cell. Agents in class IB exhibit fast kinetics of onset and offset or use-dependent block of the fast channel; that is, they bind and dissociate quickly from the receptors. Class IC drugs have slow kinetics, and class IA drugs are intermediate. With increased time spent in diastole (slower rate), a greater proportion of receptors become drug-free, and the drug exerts less effect. Cells with reduced membrane potentials recover more slowly from drug actions than cells with more negative membrane potentials (Fig. 20–15, p. 558).

REVERSE DRUG DEPENDENCE. Some drugs exert greater effects at slow rates than at fast rates. This is particularly true for drugs that lengthen repolarization. The Q-T interval becomes prolonged more at slow than fast rates. This is opposite to what the ideal antiarrhythmic agent would do, since prolongation of refractoriness should be increased at fast rates so as to interrupt or prevent a tachycardia and should be maximal at slow rates to avoid precipitating torsades de pointes.[11]

MECHANISMS OF ARRHYTHMIA SUPPRESSION. Given the fact that enhanced automaticity, triggered activity, or reentry can cause cardiac arrhythmias (see Chap. 20), mechanisms by which antiarrhythmic agents suppress arrhythmias can be postulated.[9,10] Antiarrhythmic agents can slow the spontaneous discharge frequency of an automatic pacemaker by depressing the slope of diastolic depolarization, shifting the threshold voltage toward zero, or hyperpolarizing the resting membrane potential. Mechanisms by which different drugs suppress normal or abnormal automaticity may not be the same. In general, however, most antiarrhythmic agents in therapeutic doses depress the automatic firing rate of spontaneously discharging ectopic sites while minimally affecting the discharge rate of the normal sinus node. Slow-channel blockers like verapamil, beta blockers like propranolol, and some antiarrhythmic agents like amiodarone also depress spontaneous discharge of the normal sinus node, while drugs that exert vagolytic effects, such as disopyramide or quinidine, can increase the sinus discharge rate. Drugs can also suppress early or delayed afterdepolarizations (see pp. 566 and 567) and eliminate triggered arrhythmias due to these mechanisms.

As mentioned earlier (see p. 571), reentry depends critically on the timing interrelationships between refractoriness and conduction velocity, the presence of unidirectional block in one of the pathways, and other factors that influence refractoriness and conduction, such as excitability. An antiarrhythmic agent can stop reentry that is already present or prevent it from starting if the drug improves or depresses conduction. For example, *improved conduction* can (1) eliminate the unidirectional block so that reentry cannot begin or (2) facilitate conduction in the reentrant loop so that the returning wavefront reenters too quickly, encroaches on fibers still refractory, and becomes extinguished. A drug that *depresses conduction* can transform the unidirectional block to bidirectional block and thus terminate reentry or prevent it from occurring by creating an area of complete block in the reentrant pathway. Conversely, a drug that slows conduction without producing block or lengthening refractoriness significantly can promote reentry. Finally, most antiarrhythmic agents share the ability to prolong refractoriness relative to their effects on action potential duration; i.e., the ratio of effective refractory period to action potential duration exceeds 1.0. If a drug *prolongs refractoriness* of fibers in the reentrant pathway, the pathway may not recover excitability in time to be depolarized by the reentering impulse, and the reentrant propagation ceases. The different types of reentry (see pp. 571 and 572) influence the effects and effectiveness of a drug.

When one is discussing any of the properties of a drug, it is important that the situation and/or model from which conclusions are drawn be defined with care. Electrophysiological, hemodynamic, autonomic, pharmacokinetic, and adverse effects all may differ in normal subjects compared with patients, in normal tissue compared with abnormal tissue, in muscle compared with specialized fibers, and in different species.

STEREOSELECTIVITY. Drug interactions with a channel, receptor, or enzyme may depend on the three-dimensional geometry of the drug.[12] Many drugs have stereoisomers, molecules with the same atomic composition but different spatial arrangement, that can influence drug effects, metabolism, binding, clearance, and excretion. Most drugs are prescribed as 50/50 mixtures of their two forms (racemates), which may make 50 per cent of the dose ineffective for some drugs. Except for timolol, virtually all beta blockers are racemates. d-Propranolol exerts antiarrhythmic actions unrelated to beta-adrenoceptor blockade, while l-propranolol blocks the beta receptor. Both enantiomers (mirror images) of sotalol block the potassium channel to prolong action potential duration and suppress arrhythmias equally, but d-sotalol does not block the beta-adrenoceptor. Racemic propafenone exhibits beta-blocking actions due to the S-enantiomer. Other drugs with notable stereoselective differences include disopyramide with one form (S [+]) prolonging repolarization and having greater antiarrhythmic effects than R (−), which shortens repolarization. The latter form has less anticholinergic effects. The (−) enantiomer of verapamil exerts much more negative inotropic and dromotropic effects than does the (+) form and may have more potent antiarrhythmic actions. Stereoselectivity affects sodium channel blocking drugs less than it affects beta-adrenoceptor, potassium, and calcium blockers.

DRUG METABOLITES. Drug metabolites may add to or alter the effects of the parent compound by exerting similar actions, competing with the parent compound, or mediating drug toxicity. Quinidine has at least four active metabolites, but none with a potency exceeding the parent drug and none preliminarily implicated in causing torsades de pointes. About 50 per cent of procainamide is metabolized to NAPA. Only the parent drug blocks cardiac sodium channels and slows impulse propagation in the His-Purkinje system. NAPA prolongs repolarization and is a less effective antiarrhythmic drug but competes with procainamide for renal tubular secretory sites and can increase the parent's elimination half-life. Lidocaine's metabolite can compete with lidocaine for sodium channels and partially reverse block produced by lidocaine.

Genetically determined metabolic pathways account for many of the differences in patients' responses to some drugs. The genetically determined activity of hepatic *N*-acetyltransferase regulates the development of antinuclear antibodies and development of the lupus syndrome in response to procainamide. Slow acetylator phenotypes appear more prone to develop lupus than do rapid acetylators.[13–15] About 7 per cent of white and black subjects lack debrisoquin 4-hydroxylase. This enzyme is needed to metabolize debrisoquin (an antihypertensive drug) and propafenone, to hydroxylate several beta blockers, and to biotransform flecainide. The gene coding for this enzyme (termed $P450_{dbl}$) is on human chromosome 22. Lack of this enzyme reduces metabolism of the parent compound, leading to increased plasma concentrations of the parent drug and reduced concentrations of metabolites. Quinidine in low doses can inhibit this enzyme and thereby alter concentrations of the drugs and metabolites given in combination that are affected by the $P450_{dbl}$ enzyme, such as propafenone or flecainide. Understanding stereoselectivity and pharmacogenetics can provide major clues to understanding differences in drug efficacy and toxicity from one patient to the next. Cimetidine and ranitidine also affect drug metabolism, probably by inhibiting hepatic P450-metabolizing enzymes (Table 21–5).

SIDE EFFECTS. Antiarrhythmic drugs produce one group of side effects that relate to excessive dosage and plasma concentrations, resulting in both noncardiac (e.g., neurological defects) and cardiac (e.g., heart failure, some arrhythmias) toxicity, and another group of side effects unrelated to plasma concentrations, termed *idiopathic.* Examples of the latter include procainamide-induced lupus syndrome, amiodarone-induced pulmonary toxicity (although a recent publication relates maintenance dose to this side effect), and some arrhythmias such as quinidine-induced torsades de pointes.

PROARRHYTHMIA. Drug-induced or drug-aggravated cardiac arrhythmias (proarrhythmia) are a major clinical problem.[16–21] Electrophysiological mechanisms probably relate to prolongation of repolarization, the development of early afterdepolarizations to cause torsades de pointes,[22–31] and alterations in reentry pathways[32] to initiate or sustain ventricular tachyarrhythmias. Proarrhythmic events can occur in as many as 5 to 10 per cent of patients. Heart failure increases proarrhythmic risk. Patients with atrial fibrillation treated with antiarrhythmic agents had a 4.7 relative risk of cardiac death if they had a history of heart failure compared with patients not so treated who had a 3.7 relative risk of arrhythmic death. Patients without a history of congestive heart failure had no increased risk of cardiac mortality during antiarrhythmic drug treatment.[33] Reduced left ventricular function, treatment with digitalis and diuretics, and longer pretreatment Q-T interval characterize patients who develop drug-induced ventricular fibrillation. The more commonly known proarrhythmic events occur within several days of beginning drug therapy or changing dosage and are represented by such developments as incessant ventricular tachycardia, long Q-T syndrome, and torsades de pointes. However, in the Cardiac Arrhythmia Suppression Trial (CAST),[34–36] encainide and flecainide reduced spontaneous ventricular arrhythmias but were associated with a total mortality of 7.7 versus 3.0 per cent in the group receiving placebo. Deaths were equally distributed throughout the treatment period, raising the im-

TABLE 21–5 PHARMACOKINETIC INTERACTIONS OF ANTIARRHYTHMIC DRUGS

AGENTS	EFFECTS
Phenytoin Phenobarbital Rifampin	Increase clearance of: quinidine disopyramide mexiletine digitoxin
Cimetidine	Reduces clearance of: quinidine lidocaine procainamide flecainide moricizine
Amiodarone	Reduces clearance of: warfarin phenytoin quinidine procainamide digoxin
Digoxin	Clearance reduced by: quinidine verapamil amiodarone Volume of distribution reduced by: quinidine
Lidocaine	Clearance reduced by: propranolol cimetidine

From Roden, D.: New concepts in antiarrhythmic drug pharmacokinetics. Progr. Cardiol. *15*:19, 1987.

portant consideration that another kind of proarrhythmic response can occur some time after the beginning of drug therapy. Such late proarrhythmic effects may relate to drug-induced exacerbation of regional myocardial conduction delay due to ischemia and heterogeneous drug concentrations that may promote reentry. Moricizine also increased mortality, leading to termination of CAST II.[34–36]

CLASS IA ANTIARRHYTHMIC AGENTS

Quinidine

Quinidine and quinine are isometric alkaloids isolated from the cinchona bark.[37] Although quinidine shares the antimalarial, antipyretic, and vagolytic actions of quinine, the latter lacks the significant electrophysiological and antiarrhythmic effects of quinidine.

ELECTROPHYSIOLOGICAL ACTIONS (Tables 21–6 and 21–7). Quinidine exerts little effect on automaticity of the isolated or denervated normal sinus node but suppresses automaticity in normal Purkinje fibers, especially in ectopic pacemakers, by decreasing the slope of phase 4 diastolic depolarization and shifting threshold voltage toward zero. In patients with the sick sinus syndrome, quinidine can depress sinus nodal automaticity. It does not affect abnormal automaticity in depolarized Purkinje fibers. Quinidine produces early afterdepolarizations in experimental preparations and in humans, which may be responsible for torsades de pointes.[22–31] Because of its significant anticholinergic effect and reflex sympathetic stimulation resulting from alpha-adrenergic blockade that causes peripheral vasodilation, quinidine can increase sinus nodal discharge rate and can improve atrioventricular (AV) nodal conduction in the innervated heart in vivo. Direct myocardial effects can prolong AV nodal and His-Purkinje conduction times and refractoriness in the accessory pathway. Quinidine prolongs the duration of action potential of atrial and ventricular muscle and Purkinje fibers slightly (quinine shortens it) while also prolonging the effective refractory period without significantly changing resting membrane potential. Prolongation of repolarization is more prominent at slow heart rates (reverse use dependence)[38,39] owing to block of I_K.[40] Action potential amplitude, overshoot, and $\dot{V}_{max}$ of phase 0 are reduced, more so during ischemia, hypoxia, and in depolarized fibers, especially at fast rates. The open channel has a high affinity for quinidine, resulting in block of a fraction of sodium channels with each action potential upstroke.[41] The time for unblocking by IA drugs (about 4 sec) is slower than for IB drugs but faster than for IC drugs. For the duration of the plateau of the action potential (inactivated state) or in depolarized fibers, the rate of unblocking is slow, proceeding much faster in polarized fibers. Therefore, faster rates result in more block of sodium channels and less unblocking because of a lesser percentage of time spent in a polarized state (use-dependence). Isoproterenol can modulate the effects of quinidine on reentrant circuits in humans.[42]

HEMODYNAMIC EFFECTS. Quinidine decreases peripheral vascular resistance and can cause significant hypotension because of its alpha-adrenergic receptor blocking effects. Concomitant administration of vasodilators can exaggerate the potential for hypotension. In some patients, quinidine can increase cardiac output, possibly by reducing afterload and preload. No significant direct myocardial depressant action occurs unless large doses are given rapidly, intravenously. Most of the adverse effects of intravenous quinidine are probably the result of excessive vasodilation.

PHARMACOKINETICS (Table 21–1). Although orally administered quinidine sulfate and quinidine gluconate exhibit similar degrees of systemic availability, plasma quinidine concentrations peak at about 90 minutes after oral administration of quinidine sulfate and at 3 to 4 hours after oral administration of quinidine gluconate. Intramuscular quinidine produces a higher and an earlier peak plasma concentration but results in incomplete absorption and tissue necrosis. Quinidine may be given intravenously if it is infused slowly. Approximately 80 per cent of plasma quinidine is protein-bound, especially to α1-acid glycoprotein, which increases in heart failure. Both the liver and the kidneys remove quinidine, and dose adjustments may be made according to the creatinine clearance.[43,44] Metabolism is via the P450 cytochrome system. Approximately 20 per cent is excreted unchanged in the urine. Because congestive heart failure, hepatic disease, or poor renal function can reduce quinidine elimination and increase plasma concentration, dosage probably should be reduced and the drug given cautiously to patients with these disorders while serum quinidine concentration is monitored. Elimi-

TABLE 21–6 IN VIVO ELECTROPHYSIOLOGICAL CHARACTERISTICS OF ANTIARRHYTHMIC DRUGS

	ELECTROCARDIOGRAPHIC INTERVALS						ELECTROPHYSIOLOGICAL INTERVALS				
DRUG	Sinus Rate	P-R	QRS	Q-T	A-H	H-V	ERP AVN	ERP HPS	ERP A	ERP V	ERP AP
Quinidine	0 ↑	↓ 0 ↑	↑	↑	↓ 0 ↑	↑	0 ↑	↑	↑	↑	↑
Procainamide	0	0 ↑	↑	↑	0 ↑	↑	0 ↑	↑	↑	↑	↑
Disopyramide	0 ↑	↓ 0 ↑	↑	↑	↓ 0 ↑	↑	↑ 0	↑	↑	↑	↑
Lidocaine	0	0	0	0 ↓	0 ↓	0 ↑	0 ↓	0 ↑	0	0	0
Mexiletine	0	0	0	0 ↓	0 ↑	0 ↑	0 ↑	0 ↑	0	0	0
Tocainide	0	0	0	0 ↓	0	0	0	0	0	0	0
Phenytoin	0	0	0	0 ↓	0 ↓	0	0 ↓	↓	0	0	0
Moricizine	0 ↓	0 ↑	0 ↑	0	↑	↑	0	0	0 ↑	0 ↑	↑
Flecainide	0 ↓	↑	↑	0 ↑	↑	↑	↑	↑	↑	↑	↑
Propafenone	0 ↓	↑	↑	0 ↑	↑	↑	0 ↑	0 ↑	0 ↑	↑	↑
Amiodarone	↓	0 ↑	↑	↑	↑	↑	↑	↑	↑	↑	↑
Bretylium	↑ 0 ↓	0	0	0 ↑			0	↑	↑	↑	0
Propranolol	↓	0 ↑	0	0 ↓	0	0	↑	0	0	0	0 ↑
Verapamil	0 ↓	↑	0	0	↑	0	↑	0	0	0	0 ↑
Adenosine	↓ then ↑	↑	0	0	↑	0	↑	0	↓	0	0 ↓
Sotalol	↓	0 ↑	0	↑	↑	0	↑	↑	↑	↑	↑

Results presented may vary according to tissue type, experimental conditions, and drug concentration. ↑ = increase; ↓ = decrease; 0 = no change; 0 ↑ or 0 ↓ = slight inconsistent increase or decrease. A = atrium; AVN = AV node; HPS = His-Purkinje system; V = ventricle; AP = accessory pathway (WPW); ERP = effective refractory period—longest S_1–S_2 interval at which S_2 fails to produce a response.

TABLE 21–7 IN VITRO ELECTROPHYSIOLOGICAL CHARACTERISTICS OF ANTIARRHYTHMIC DRUGS

DRUG	APA	APD	dV/dt	MDP	ERP	CONDUCTION VELOCITY	PF PHASE 4	SINUS NODAL AUTOMATICITY
Quinidine	↓	↑	↓	0	↑	↓	↓	0
Procainamide	↓	↑	↓	0	↑	↓	↓	0
Disopyramide	↓	↑	↓	0	↑	↓	↓	↑ 0 ↓
Lidocaine	0 ↓	↓	0 ↓	0	↓	0 ↓	↓	0
Mexiletine	0	↓	0 ↓	0	↓	↓	↓	0
Tocainide	0	↓	0 ↓	0	↓	↓	0	↓
Phenytoin	0	↓	↑ 0 ↓	0	↓	0	↓	0
Moricizine	↓	↓	↓	0	↓	↓	0	0
Flecainide	↓	0 ↑	↓	0	↑	↓ ↓	↓	0
Propafenone	↓	0 ↑	↓	0	↑	↓ ↓	↓	↓
Propranolol	0 ↓	0 ↓	0 ↓	0	↓	0	↓ *	↓
Amiodarone	0	↑	0 ↓	0	↑	↓	↓	↓
Bretylium	0	↑	0	0	↑	0	0 ↓ *	0 ↓
Verapamil	0	↓	0	0	0	0	↓ *	↓
Adenosine	0	0	0	0	0	0	0	↓
Sotalol	0 ↓	↑	0 ↓	0	↑	0	0 ↓	↓

* With a background of sympathetic activity.

APA = action potential amplitude; APD = action potential duration; dV/dt = rate of rise of action potential; MDP = maximum diastolic potential; ERP = effective refractory period; PF = Purkinje fibers.

nation half-life is 5 to 8 hours after oral administration. Quinidine can increase plasma concentrations of flecainide by inhibiting the P450 enzyme system.[12]

DOSAGE AND ADMINISTRATION (Table 21–1). The usual oral dose of quinidine sulfate for an adult is 300 to 600 mg four times daily, which results in a steady-state level within about 24 hours. A loading dose of 600 to 1000 mg produces an earlier effective concentration. Similar doses of quinidine gluconate are used intramuscularly, while the intravenous dose of quinidine gluconate is about 10 mg/kg given at a rate of about 0.5 mg/kg/min as blood pressure and electrocardiographic (ECG) parameters are checked frequently. Oral doses of the gluconate are about 30 per cent greater than those of sulfate. Important interactions with other drugs occur (Table 21–2).

INDICATIONS. Quinidine is a versatile antiarrhythmic agent, useful for treating premature supraventricular and ventricular complexes and sustained tachyarrhythmias. It may prevent spontaneous recurrences or electrical induction of AV nodal reentrant tachycardia by prolonging atrial and ventricular refractoriness and depressing conduction in the retrograde fast pathway. In patients with the Wolff-Parkinson-White syndrome, quinidine prolongs the effective refractory period of the accessory pathway and, by so doing, can prevent reciprocating tachycardias and slow the ventricular response from conduction over the accessory pathway during atrial flutter or atrial fibrillation. Quinidine and other antiarrhythmic agents also can prevent recurrences of tachycardia by suppressing the "trigger," i.e., the premature atrial or ventricular complex that initiates a sustained tachycardia.

Quinidine successfully terminates atrial flutter or atrial fibrillation in about 10 to 20 per cent of patients, with higher success rates if the arrhythmia is of more recent onset and if the atria are not enlarged. Before quinidine is administered to these patients, the ventricular response should be slowed sufficiently with digitalis, propranolol, or verapamil, since quinidine-induced slowing of the atrial flutter rate—e.g., over the range of 300 to 200 beats/min—plus its vagolytic effect on AV nodal conduction may convert a 2:1 atrioventricular response (two atrial impulses for each QRS complex) to a 1:1 atrioventricular response, with an *increase* in the ventricular rate. Before elective cardioversion of patients with atrial fibrillation, quinidine probably should be given for 1 to 2 days, since this regimen restores sinus rhythm in some patients, thus obviating the need for direct-current cardioversion, and helps maintain sinus rhythm once it is achieved. A metaanalysis of six studies testing the effects of quinidine versus control in maintaining sinus rhythm in patients with atrial fibrillation showed that quinidine-treated patients remained in sinus rhythm longer than did the control group but had an increased total mortality over the same period. This important conclusion needs to be verified in a controlled, prospective study.

Quinidine has prevented sudden death in some patients resuscitated after out-of-hospital cardiac arrest and may be combined with other antiarrhythmic agents for increased efficacy in suppressing ventricular tachyarrhythmias. No published data from controlled, randomized studies indicate improved survival in quinidine-treated patients after myocardial infarction (Fig. 21–5). Cardiac arrest can occur despite quinidine therapy.[45,46] Because it crosses the placenta, quinidine can be used to treat arrhythmias in the fetus.

ADVERSE EFFECTS. The most common adverse effects of chronic oral quinidine therapy are gastrointestinal, including nausea, vomiting, diarrhea, abdominal pain, and anorexia. Gastrointestinal side effects may be milder with the gluconate form. Central nervous system toxicity includes tinnitus, hearing loss, visual disturbances, confusion, delirium, and psychosis. *Cinchonism* is the term usually applied to these side effects. Allergic reactions may be manifested as rash, fever, immune-mediated thrombocytopenia, hemolytic anemia, and rarely, anaphylaxis. Thrombocytopenia is due to the presence of antibodies to quinidine-platelet complexes, causing platelets to agglutinate and lyse. In patients receiving oral anticoagulants, quinidine may cause bleeding. Side effects may preclude long-term administration of quinidine in 30 to 40 per cent of patients.

Quinidine can slow cardiac conduction, sometimes to the point of block, manifested as prolongation of the QRS duration or sinoatrial (SA) or AV nodal conduction disturbances. Quinidine-induced cardiac toxicity can be treated with molar sodium lactate. Quinidine can prolong the Q-T interval and cause torsades de pointes in 1 to 3 per cent of patients.[19–30]

Quinidine may produce syncope in 0.5 to 2.0 per cent of patients, most often the result of a self-terminating episode of torsades de pointes (see pp. 684 and 767). Torsades de pointes may be due to the development of early afterdepolarizations, as noted above. Quinidine prolongs the Q-T interval in most patients, whether or not ventricular arrhythmias occur, but significant Q-T prolongation (Q-T interval of 500 to 600 msec) is often a characteristic of quinidine syncope. Many of these patients are also receiving digitalis or diuretics. Syncope is unrelated to plasma concentrations of quinidine or duration of therapy. Hypokalemia often is a prominent feature. Therapy for quinidine syncope requires immediate discontinuation of the drug and avoidance of

DRUG	MEMBRANE RESPONSIVENESS	ET	VFT	CONTRACTILITY	SLOW INWARD CURRENT	AUTONOMIC NERVOUS SYSTEM	LOCAL ANESTHETIC EFFECT
Quinidine	↓	↑	↑	0	0	Antivagal; alpha blocker	Yes
Procainamide	↓	↑	↑	0	0	Slight antivagal	Yes
Disopyramide	↓	↑	↑	↓	0	Central: antivagal, antisympathetic	Yes
Lidocaine	0 ↓	0 ↑	↑	0	0	0	Yes
Mexiletine	↓	↑	↑	↓	0	0	Yes
Tocainide	↓	↑	↑	0	0	0	Yes
Phenytoin	0 ↑	0			0	0	No
Moricizine	↓	↑	0		0	0	No
Flecainide	↓			↓	0	0	Yes
Propafenone	↓	↑	↑	↓	May inhibit	Antisympathetic	Yes
Propranolol	↓			↓	0 ↓	Antisympathetic	No
Amiodarone	0	0	↑	0 ↑	0	Antisympathetic	Yes
Bretylium	0 ↑	0	0 ↑	↓	0	Antisympathetic	Yes
Verapamil	0	0	0	↓	Inhibit	? Block alpha receptors; enhance vagal	Yes
Adenosine	0	0	0	0	May inhibit	Vagomimetic	No
Sotalol	0 ↓	0	0	↓	0 ↓	Antisympathetic	No

ET = excitability threshold; VFT = ventricular fibrillation threshold.

other drugs that have similar pharmacological effects, such as disopyramide, since cross-sensitivity exists in some patients. Magnesium given intravenously (2 gm over 1 to 2 min, followed by an infusion of 3 to 20 mg/min) is probably the initial drug treatment of choice. Atrial or ventricular pacing can be used to suppress the ventricular tachyarrhythmia and may act by suppressing afterdepolarizations. For some patients, drugs that do not prolong the Q-T interval, such as lidocaine or phenytoin, can be tried. When pacing is not available, isoproterenol can be given *with caution.*

Drugs that induce hepatic enzyme production, such as phenobarbital and phenytoin, can shorten the duration of quinidine's action by increasing its rate of elimination. Quinidine may elevate serum digoxin and digitoxin concentrations by decreasing total-body clearance of digitoxin and by decreasing the clearance, volume of distribution, and affinity of tissue receptors for digoxin (see p. 499).

Procainamide

ELECTROPHYSIOLOGICAL ACTIONS (Tables 21–6 and 21–7). The cardiac actions of procainamide on automaticity, conduction, excitability, and membrane responsiveness resemble those of quinidine. Procainamide predominantly blocks the inactivated state of I_{Na}. It also blocks I_K and $I_{K\,ATP}$.[47] Like quinidine, procainamide usually prolongs the effective refractory period (ERP) more than it prolongs the action potential duration (APD) and thus prevents early responses from occurring, arising from less negative resting potentials that might conduct slowly or block and cause an arrhythmia. Compared with disopyramide and quinidine, procainamide exerts the least anticholinergic effects but does produce more local anesthetic effects than quinidine. It does not affect normal sinus nodal automaticity. In vitro, procainamide decreases abnormal automaticity, with less effect on triggered activity or catecholamine-enhanced normal automaticity.

The electrophysiogical effects of NAPA,[48] procainamide's major metabolite, differ from those of the parent compound. NAPA (10 to 40 mg/liter) does not suppress the rate of phase 4 diastolic depolarization of Purkinje fibers and does not alter resting membrane potential, action potential amplitude, or $\dot{V}_{max}$ of phase 0 of the action potential of Purkinje fibers or ventricular muscle. However, NAPA, a K^+ channel blocker, exerts a class III action and prolongs the action potential duration of ventricular muscle and Purkinje fibers in a dose-dependent manner. Toxic doses produce early afterdepolarizations, triggered activity, and ventricular tachyarrhythmias, including torsades de pointes. Procainamide appears to exert greater electrophysiological effects than NAPA.

HEMODYNAMIC EFFECTS. Procainamide can depress myocardial contractility in high doses. It does not produce alpha blockade but can result in peripheral vasodilation, possibly via antisympathetic effects on brain or spinal cord that can impair cardiovascular reflexes.[49]

PHARMACOKINETICS (Table 21–1). Oral administration produces peak plasma concentration in about 1 hour. Absorption may be reduced in the first week after myocardial infarction. Approximately 80 per cent of oral procainamide is bioavailable, with 20 per cent bound to serum proteins. The overall elimination half-life for procainamide is 3 to 5 hours, with 50 to 60 per cent of the drug eliminated by the kidney and 10 to 30 per cent eliminated by hepatic metabolism. A prolonged-release form of procainamide given every 6 hours provides steady-state plasma levels of the drug equivalent to an equal total daily dose of short-acting procainamide given every 3 hours.

The drug is acetylated to NAPA, which is excreted almost exclusively by the kidneys. As renal function decreases and in patients with heart failure, procainamide levels—and particularly NAPA levels—increase and, because of the risk of serious cardiotoxicity, need to be carefully monitored in such situations. NAPA has an elimination half-life of 7 to 8 hours but exceeds 10 hours if high doses are used. Small amounts of procainamide are present in patients receiving NAPA because of deacetylation. Increased age, congestive heart failure, and reduced creatinine clearance lower the procainamide clearance and necessitate reduced dosage.

DOSAGE AND ADMINISTRATION (Table 21–1). Procainamide can be given by the oral, intravenous, or intramuscular route to achieve plasma concentrations that produce an antiarrhythmic effect in the range of 4 to 10 μg/ml. Occasionally, plasma concentrations exceeding 10 μg/ml have been required, but the probability of adverse effects generally precludes long-term administration at these higher plasma concentrations. Several intravenous regimens have been used to administer procainamide. Twenty-five to 50 mg can be given over a 1-minute period and then repeated every 5 minutes until the arrhythmia is controlled, hypotension results, or the QRS complex is prolonged more than 50 per cent. Doses of 10 to 15 mg/kg at 50 mg/min are commonly used during electrophysiological testing.[50,51] Using this method, plasma concentration falls rapidly during the first 15 minutes after the loading dose, with parallel effects on refractoriness and conduction. A constant-rate intravenous infusion of procainamide can be given at a dose of 2 to 6 mg/min. The upper limits regarding total IV dose are flexible and range between 1000 and 2000 mg depending on the patient's response.

Oral administration of procainamide requires a 3- to 4-hour dosing interval at a total daily dose of 2 to 6 gm, with a steady state reached within 1 day. When a loading dose is used, it should be twice the maintenance dose. Frequent dosing is required because of the short elimination half-life in normal subjects. For the prolonged-release form of procainamide, dosing is at 6-hour intervals. While a longer half-life may be seen in some cardiac patients, allowing longer intervals between drug administration, this needs to be documented for the individual patient. Procainamide is well absorbed after intramuscular injection, with virtually 100 per cent of the dose bioavailable.

INDICATIONS. Procainamide is used to treat both supraventricular and ventricular arrhythmias in a manner comparable with that of quinidine.[52] Although both drugs have similar electrophysiological actions, either drug can effectively suppress a supraventricular or ventricular arrhythmia that is resistant to the other drug.

Procainamide can be used to convert atrial fibrillation of recent onset to sinus rhythm.[53] As with quinidine, prior treatment with digitalis, propranolol, or verapamil is recommended to prevent acceleration of the ventricular response following procainamide therapy. In patients with paroxysmal supraventricular tachycardia, procainamide can inhibit the induction of sustained AV nodal reentrant tachycardia as a result of selective depression of retrograde AV nodal conduction in the fast pathway. Procainamide can block conduction in the accessory pathway of patients with the Wolff-Parkinson-White syndrome and is particularly useful in patients with atrial fibrillation and a rapid ventricular response due to conduction over the accessory pathway (see p. 655). Whether it can be used intravenously to identify those patients who have a short anterograde effective refractory period is not resolved. It can produce His-Purkinje block (see p. 750).

Procainamide is more effective than lidocaine in preventing the induction of ventricular tachycardia by programmed stimulation[54] and in acutely terminating sustained ventricular tachycardia. The electrophysiological response to procainamide given intravenously appears to predict the response to the drug given orally. Patients with ejection fractions ≥40 per cent whose ventricular tachycardia procainamide renders noninducible have a high likelihood of responding to the drug given orally. High doses, 500 to 1000 mg orally every 4 hours, resulting in a plasma concentration exceeding 10.0 μg/ml, may be necessary to suppress ventricular tachycardia in some patients. Most consistently, procainamide slows the rate of the induced ventricular tachycardia, a change correlated with the increase in QRS duration. Adding amiodarone to procainamide slows the ventricular tachycardia cycle length further but increases the noninducibility success rate only slightly. Procainamide appears to affect preferentially the reentrant circuit of the ventricular tachycardia compared with other areas of myocardium. The antiarrhythmic response to procainamide does not predict the response to NAPA.

ADVERSE EFFECTS. Multiple adverse noncardiac effects have been reported with procainamide administration and include skin rashes, myalgias, digital vasculitis, and Raynaud's phenomenon. Fever and agranulocytosis may be due to hypersensitivity reactions, and white blood cell and differential blood counts should be performed at regular intervals. Gastrointestinal side effects are less frequent than with quinidine, and adverse central nervous system side effects are less frequent than with lidocaine. Procainamide can cause giddiness, psychosis, hallucinations, and depression. Toxic concentrations of procainamide can diminish myocardial performance and promote hypotension. A variety of conduction disturbances or ventricular tachyarrhythmias[55] can occur similar to those produced by quinidine, including prolonged Q-T syndrome and polymorphous ventricular tachycardia. NAPA also can induce Q-T prolongation and torsades de pointes. In the absence of sinus node disease, procainamide does not adversely affect sinus node function. In patients with sinus dysfunction, procainamide tends to prolong corrected sinus node recovery time and can worsen symptoms in some patients who have the bradycardia-tachycardia syndrome. Procainamide does not increase the serum digoxin concentration.

Arthralgia, fever, pleuropericarditis, hepatomegaly, and hemorrhagic pericardial effusion with tamponade have been described in a systemic lupus erythematosus (SLE)–like syndrome. The syndrome can occur more frequently and earlier in patients who are "slow acetylators" of procainamide and is influenced by genetic factors.[13] The aromatic amino group on procainamide appears important for induction of SLE syndrome, since acetylating this amino group to form NAPA appears to block the SLE-inducing effect. Sixty to 70 per cent of patients who receive procainamide on a chronic basis develop antinuclear antibodies, with clinical symptoms in 20 to 30 per cent, but this is reversible when procainamide is stopped. When symptoms occur, SLE cell preparations are often positive. Positive serological tests are not necessarily a reason to discontinue drug therapy; however, the development of symptoms or a positive anti-DNA antibody is, except for patients whose life-threatening arrhythmia is controlled only by procainamide. Steroid administration in these patients may eliminate the symptoms. In contrast to naturally occurring SLE, the brain and kidney are spared, and there is no predilection for females.

Disopyramide

Disopyramide has been approved in the United States for oral but not intravenous administration to treat patients with ventricular arrhythmias.

ELECTROPHYSIOLOGICAL ACTIONS (Tables 21–6 and 21–7). Although structurally different from quinidine and procainamide, disopyramide produces similar electrophysiological effects in vitro. It causes use-dependent block of I_{Na} and non-use-dependent block of I_K.[40] Along with quinidine, low concentrations tend to prolong action potential duration and induce early afterdepolarizations (EADs) just as do higher concentrations.[31] Disopyramide also inhibits $I_{K\,ATP}$.[47] It decreases the slope of phase 4 diastolic depolarization in Purkinje fibers, produces a rate-dependent depression of $\dot{V}_{max}$ of phase 0, prolongs the effective refractory period more than it prolongs the action potential duration, lengthens conduction time in normal and depolarized Purkinje fibers, and does not affect calcium-dependent action potentials, except possibly at very high concentrations, or suppress late potentials in the signal-averaged ECG. Disopyramide, like procainamide, reduces the differences in action potential duration between normal and infarcted tissue by lengthening the action potential of normal cells more than it lengthens the action potential of cells from infarcted regions of the heart.

Stereochemical properties influence the effects of disopyramide. Racemic (clinically used) and (+)-disopyramide prolong canine Purkinje fiber action potential, while (−)-disopyramide shortens it. The (+) isomer exerts approximately three times more vagolytic effects than does the (−) isomer. Disopyramide, as a muscarinic blocker, can speed the sinus nodal discharge rate and shorten AV nodal conduction time and refractoriness when the nodes are restrained by cholinergic influences. Disopyramide also can slow the sinus nodal discharge rate by a direct action when given in high concentration and can significantly depress sinus nodal activity in patients with sinus node dysfunction. Disopyramide exerts greater anticholinergic effects than quinidine and does not appear to affect alpha- or beta-adrenoceptors.

Atrial and ventricular refractory periods increase, as do conduction time and refractoriness of the accessory pathway in patients with the Wolff-Parkinson-White syndrome. Disopyramide's effect on AV nodal conduction and refractoriness in vivo is not consistent. Disopyramide prolongs His-Purkinje conduction time, but infra-His block results infrequently. Disopyramide can be administered safely to patients who have first degree AV block and narrow QRS complexes.

HEMODYNAMIC EFFECTS. Disopyramide administered intravenously reduces systemic blood pressure and cardiac and stroke index and increases right atrial pressures and total peripheral resistance. Profound hemodynamic deterioration can occur, and patients who have abnormal ventricular function tolerate the negative inotropic effects of IV and oral disopyramide quite poorly. In these patients, the drug should be used with extreme caution or not at all.

PHARMACOKINETICS (Table 21–1). Disopyramide is 80 to 90 per cent absorbed, with a mean elimination half-life of 8 to 9 hours in healthy volunteers but almost 10 hours in patients with heart failure and sometimes longer in some patients with ventricular arrhythmias. Total-body clearance and volume of distribution decrease in patients, and mean serum concentration is higher than reported in normal subjects. Renal insufficiency prolongs the elimination time. Thus, in patients who have renal, hepatic, or cardiac insufficiency, loading and maintenance doses need to be reduced. Peak blood levels after oral administration result in 1 to 2 hours, and bioavailability exceeds 80 per cent. The fraction of disopyramide bound to serum protein varies inversely with the total plasma concentration of the drug but may be more stable (30 to 40 per cent) at clinically relevant concentrations of 3 μg/ml. It is bound to α1-acid glycoprotein and passes through the placenta. About half an oral dose is recovered unchanged in the urine, with about 30 per cent as the mono-*N*-dealkylated metabolite. The metabolites appear to exert less effect than the parent compound. Erythromycin inhibits its metabolism.[56]

DOSAGE AND ADMINISTRATION (Table 21–1). Doses are generally 100 to 200 mg orally every 6 hours with a range of 400 to 1200 mg/day. A controlled-release preparation can be given as 200 to 300 mg every 12 hours. The intravenous (investigational) dose is 1 to 2 mg/kg as an initial bolus given over 5 to 10 minutes, which may be followed by an infusion of 1 mg/kg/h.

INDICATIONS. Disopyramide appears comparable to quinidine and procainamide in reducing the frequency of premature ventricular complexes and effectively preventing recurrence of ventricular tachycardia in selected patients. Disopyramide has been combined with other drugs such as mexiletine to treat patients who do not respond or only partially respond to one drug.

Disopyramide terminates and prevents recurrent episodes of paroxysmal supraventricular tachycardia due to AV and AV nodal reentry. It prolongs the anterograde and retrograde refractory period of the accessory pathway in patients with the Wolff-Parkinson-White syndrome, helps prevent recurrence of atrial fibrillation after successful cardioversion as effectively as quinidine, and may terminate atrial flutter. In treating patients with atrial fibrillation, and particularly atrial flutter, the ventricular rate must be controlled prior to administering disopyramide, or the atrial rate may decrease sufficiently, aided by the vagolytic effects of disopyramide, to create 1:1 conduction during atrial flutter. Disopyramide may be useful in preventing inducible and spontaneous neurally mediated syncope.

ADVERSE EFFECTS. Three categories of adverse effects follow disopyramide administration. The most common relates to the drug's potent parasympatholytic properties and includes urinary hesitancy or retention, constipation, blurred vision, closed-angle glaucoma, and dry mouth. Symptoms may be minimized by concomitant administration of pyridostigmine. Second, disopyramide can produce ventricular tachyarrhythmias that are commonly associated with Q-T prolongation and torsades de pointes. Some patients can have "cross-sensitivity" to both quinidine and disopyramide and develop torsades de pointes while receiving either drug. When drug-induced torsades de pointes occurs, agents that prolong the Q-T interval should be used very cautiously or not at all. Finally, disopyramide can reduce contractility of the normal ventricle, but the depression of ventricular function is much more pronounced in patients with preexisting ventricular failure. Occasionally, cardiovascular collapse can result.

CLASS IB ANTIARRHYTHMIC AGENTS

Lidocaine

ELECTROPHYSIOLOGICAL ACTIONS (Tables 21–6 and 21–7). Lidocaine blocks I_{Na}, predominantly in the open or possibly inactivated state.[57] It has rapid onset and offset kinetics and does not affect normal sinus nodal automaticity but does depress both normal and abnormal forms of automaticity, as well as early and late afterdepolarizations in Purkinje fibers in vitro. Lidocaine exhibits only a modest depressant effect on $\dot{V}_{max}$ and has no effect on maximal diastolic potential of normal muscle and specialized tissue in concentrations of about 1.5 μg/ml. However, faster rates of stimulation, reduced pH,[58] increased extracellular K^+ concentration, and reduced membrane potential—all changes that can result from ischemia—increase the ability of lidocaine to block I_{Na}. Lidocaine reduces the magnitude of the transient inward current responsible for some forms of afterdepolarizations. Intracellular calcium activity may be reduced because of the sodium-calcium exchange mechanism. Lidocaine can convert areas of unidirectional block into bidirectional block during ischemia and prevent development of ventricular fibrillation by preventing fragmentation of organized large wavefronts into heterogeneous wavelets. Lidocaine may be arrhythmogenic if it depresses conduction but not to the point of bidirectional block, but this does not appear to be an important clinical problem.

Lidocaine, except in very high concentrations, does *not* affect slow-channel-dependent action potentials despite its moderate suppression of the slow inward current. In fact, its depressant effect on electrical potentials from ischemic myocardium supports the notion that these ischemic potentials are depressed fast responses rather than slow responses. Lidocaine significantly reduces the action potential duration and the effective refractory period of Purkinje fibers and ventricular muscle due to blocking of tetrodotoxin-sensitive sodium channels, and decreasing entry of sodium into the cell. It has little effect on atrial fibers and does not affect conduction in accessory pathways. In some in vitro preparations, lidocaine can improve conduction by hyperpolarizing tissues depolarized as a result of stretch or low external potassium concentration.

In vivo, lidocaine has a minimal effect on automaticity or conduction except in unusual circumstances. Patients with preexisting sinus nodal dysfunction, abnormal His-Purkinje conduction, or junctional or ventricular escape rhythms may develop depressed automaticity or conduction. Part of its effects may be to inhibit cardiac sympathetic nerve activity.

HEMODYNAMIC EFFECTS. Clinically significant adverse hemodynamic effects are rarely noted at usual drug concentrations unless left ventricular function is severely impaired.

PHARMACOKINETICS (Table 21–1). Lidocaine is used only parenterally because oral administration results in extensive first-pass hepatic metabolism and unpredictable, low plasma levels with excessive metabolites that can produce toxicity. Hepatic metabolism of lidocaine depends greatly on hepatic blood flow, so clearance of this drug almost equals (and can be approximated by) measurements of this flow. Severe hepatic disease or reduced hepatic blood flow, as in heart failure or shock, can markedly decrease the rate of lidocaine metabolism. Beta-adrenoceptor blockers can decrease hepatic blood flow and increase lidocaine serum concentration. Prolonged infusion can reduce lidocaine clearance. Its elimination half-life averages about 1 to 2 hours in normal subjects, more than 4 hours in patients after relatively uncomplicated myocardial infarction, more than 10 hours in patients after myocardial infarction complicated by cardiac failure, and even longer in the presence of cardiogenic shock. Maintenance doses should be reduced by one-third to one-half for patients with low cardiac output. Lidocaine is 50 to 80 per cent protein-bound and binds to α1-acid glycoprotein, which may increase in heart failure and myocardial infarction. Intravenous infusions should be discontinued as far in advance of electrophysiological studies as possible to avoid residual lidocaine effects. A two-compartment model accurately predicts serum concentrations.[59]

DOSAGE AND ADMINISTRATION (Table 21–1). Although lidocaine can be given intramuscularly, the intravenous route is most commonly used (Fig. 21–4). Intramuscular lidocaine is given in doses of 4 to 5 mg/kg (250 to 350 mg), resulting in effective serum levels at about 15 minutes and lasting for about 90 minutes. Intravenously, lidocaine is given as an initial bolus of 1 to 2 mg/kg of body weight at a rate of approximately 20 to 50 mg/min, with a second injection of one-half the initial dose 20 to 40 minutes later. Patients treated with an initial bolus followed by a maintenance infusion may experience transient subtherapeutic plasma concentrations at 30 to 120 minutes after initiation of therapy. A second bolus of about 0.5 mg/kg without increasing the maintenance infusion rate reestablishes therapeutic serum concentrations.

If recurrence of arrhythmia appears after a steady state has been achieved (e.g., 6 to 10 hours after starting therapy), a similar bolus should be given and the maintenance infusion rate increased. Increasing the maintenance infusion rate alone without an additional bolus results in a very slow increase in plasma lidocaine concentrations, reaching a new plateau in over 6 hours (four elimination half-lives), and is therefore not recommended. Another recommended intravenous dosing is 1.5 mg/kg initially and 0.8 mg/kg at 8-minute intervals for three doses. Doses are reduced by about 50 per cent for patients with heart failure.

If the initial bolus of lidocaine is ineffective, up to two more boluses of 1 mg/kg may be administered at 5-minute intervals. Patients who require more than one bolus to achieve a therapeutic effect have arrhythmias that respond only to higher lidocaine plasma concentrations, and a greater maintenance dose may be necessary to sustain these higher concentrations. Patients requiring only a single initial bolus of lidocaine should probably receive a maintenance infusion of 30 μg/kg/min, while those requiring two or three boluses may need infusions at 40 to 50 μg/kg/min.

Loading doses also may be administered by rapid infusion, and a constant-rate intravenous infusion may be used to maintain an effective concentration. Maintenance infusion rates in the range of 1 to 4 mg/min produce steady-state plasma levels of 1 to 5 μg/ml in patients with uncomplicated myocardial infarction, but these rates must be reduced during heart failure or shock because of concomitant reduced hepatic blood flow. A loading dose of approximately 75 mg followed by an initial infusion rate of 5.33 mg/min that declines exponentially to 2 mg/min with a half-life of 25 min also has been recommended.

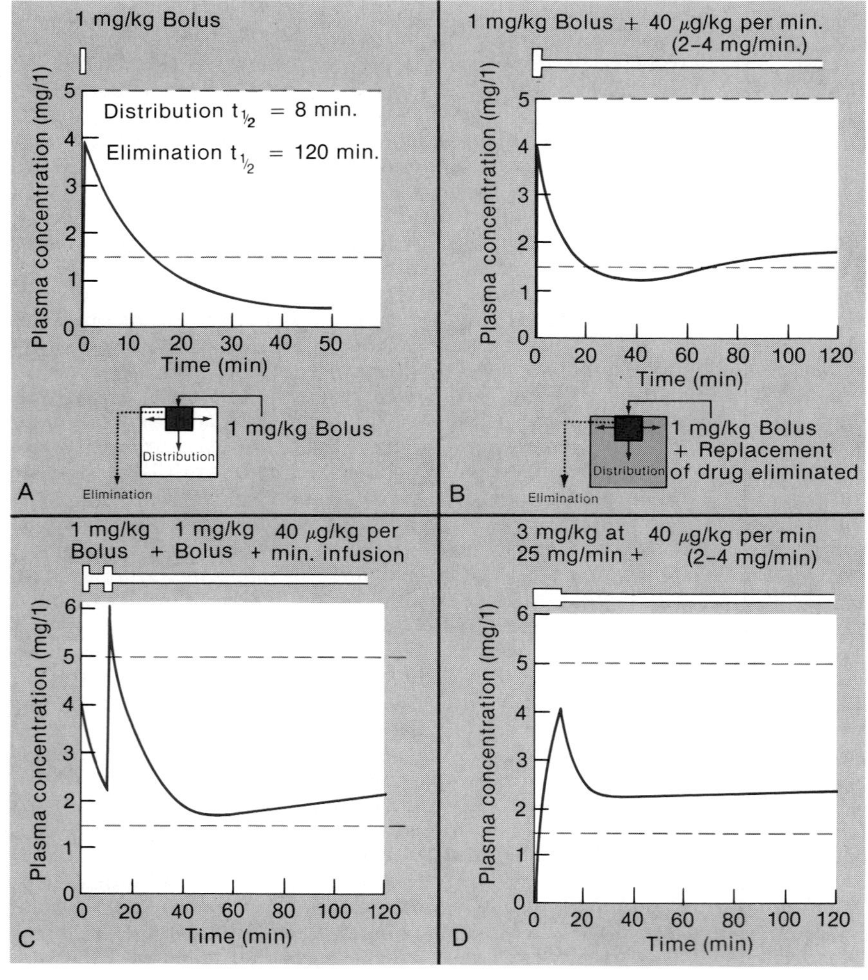

FIGURE 21–4. *A, Top,* Plasma concentrations after a bolus of lidocaine, with the therapeutic range indicated by a dashed line. *Bottom,* The disposition of the drug in the body, with the larger box indicating the total volume of distribution and the smaller box the central compartment. The bolus initially produces therapeutic lidocaine concentrations in the small central compartment. Rapid distribution of the drug to the rest of the body produces subtherapeutic concentrations within 15 minutes. *B,* Lidocaine is administered by an initial bolus as in *A,* with a maintenance infusion begun just after the bolus. The maintenance infusion replaces drug eliminated from the body, but drug is also lost from the central compartment by distribution, which is more rapid than elimination. As a result, plasma concentrations decrease transiently. In this instance, lidocaine concentration is subtherapeutic between 30 and 70 minutes after initiation of therapy. *C,* Subtherapeutic lidocaine concentrations after an initial bolus (as in *B*) can be prevented by giving a second lidocaine bolus 10 minutes after the first. A maintenance infusion should be started after the second bolus rather than after the first, as shown here. This will prevent excessive lidocaine concentrations after the second bolus. *D,* An alternative method to produce therapeutic lidocaine concentrations rapidly. This illustration indicates plasma concentrations after the administration of a loading dose of lidocaine given over 10 minutes. A maintenance infusion is begun after the loading dose has been given. (From Nattel, S., and Zipes, D. P.: Clinical pharmacology of old and new antiarrhythmic drugs. Cardiovasc. Clin. *11*:221, 1980.)

INDICATIONS. Lidocaine demonstrates efficacy against ventricular arrhythmias of diverse etiology, the ability to achieve effective plasma concentrations rapidly, and a fairly wide toxic-to-therapeutic ratio with a low incidence of hemodynamic complications and other side effects. However, its first-pass hepatic effect precludes oral use, and it is generally ineffective against supraventricular arrhythmias. In patients with the Wolff-Parkinson-White syndrome, for whom the effective refractory period of the accessory pathway is relatively short, lidocaine generally has no significant effect and may even accelerate the ventricular response during atrial fibrillation.

Lidocaine is used primarily for patients with acute myocardial infarction[60,61] or recurrent ventricular tachyarrhythmias. It has been effective in patients resuscitated from out-of-hospital ventricular fibrillation[62] and in patients after coronary revascularization.[63] Lidocaine prophylaxis in patients with acute myocardial infarction is controversial. However, most data suggest that the benefits of prophylactic lidocaine therapy in reducing the incidence of ventricular fibrillation in hospitalized patients who have had acute myocardial infarction have not been clearly established[60,61] (see p. 1248). Drug-induced side effects and a possible increase in the risk of developing asystole lead to the conclusion that prophylaxis is probably not indicated for all patients. Subcutaneous lidocaine can affect inducibility of ventricular arrhythmias by programed electrical stimulation.[64]

ADVERSE EFFECTS. The most commonly reported adverse effects of lidocaine are dose-related manifestations of central nervous system toxicity: dizziness, paresthesias, confusion, delirium, stupor, coma, and seizures.[65] Occasional sinus node depression and His-Purkinje block have been reported. In patients with atrial tachyarrhythmias, ventricular rate acceleration has been noted. Rarely, lidocaine can cause malignant hyperthermia.[66] Both lidocaine and procainamide can elevate defibrillation thresholds.[67]

Mexiletine

Mexiletine, a local anesthetic congener of lidocaine with anticonvulsant properties, is used for oral treatment of patients with symptomatic ventricular arrhythmias.

ELECTROPHYSIOLOGICAL ACTIONS (Table 21–6 and 21–7). Mexiletine is similar to lidocaine in many of its electrophysiological actions. In vitro, mexiletine shortens the duration of the action potential and refractory period of Purkinje fibers and to a lesser extent of ventricular muscle. It depresses $\dot{V}_{max}$ of phase 0 by blocking I_{Na}, especially at faster rates, and depresses automaticity of Purkinje fibers but not of the normal sinus node. Its onset and offset kinetics are rapid. Hypoxia or ischemia can increase its effects on $\dot{V}_{max}$.

Mexiletine can result in severe bradycardia and abnormal sinus nodal recovery time in patients with sinus node disease but not in patients with a normal sinus node. It does not affect AV nodal conduction and can depress His-Purkinje conduction, but not greatly, unless conduction was abnormal initially. Mexiletine does not appear to affect the refractory period of human atrial and ventricular muscle. The duration of the Q-T interval does not increase. Because of its rate-dependent effects, theoretically, mexiletine might be expected to suppress closely coupled rather than late coupled ventricular extrasystoles or faster tachycardias.

HEMODYNAMIC EFFECTS. Mexiletine exerts no major hemodynamic effects. It does not depress myocardial performance when given orally, although intravenous administration can produce hypotension.

PHARMACOKINETICS. Mexiletine has been reported to be rapidly and almost completely absorbed after oral ingestion by volunteers, with peak plasma concentrations attained in 2 to 4 hours. Elimination half-life in healthy subjects is approximately 10 hours and in patients after myocardial infarction, 17 hours. Therapeutic plasma levels of 1 to 2 μg/ml are maintained by oral doses of 200 to 300 mg every 6 to 8 hours. Absorption with less than 10 per cent first-pass hepatic effect occurs in the upper small intestine and is delayed and incomplete in patients who have myocardial infarction and in patients receiving narcotic analgesics, antacids, or atropine-like drugs that retard gastric emptying. Bioavailability of orally administered mexiletine is approximately 90 per cent, and about 70 per cent of the drug is protein-bound. The apparent volume of distribution is large, reflecting extensive tissue uptake. Normally, mexiletine is eliminated metabolically by the liver, with less than 10 per cent excreted unchanged in the urine. Doses probably should be reduced in patients with cirrhosis and those with left ventricular failure. Renal clearance of mexiletine decreases as urinary pH increases. Known metabolites exert no electrophysiological effects. Metabolism can be increased by phenytoin, phenobarbital, and rifampin and reduced by cimetidine. It is influenced by the genotype for the CYP206 gene.[3]

DOSAGE AND ADMINISTRATION. Recommended starting dose is 200 mg orally every 8 hours when rapid arrhythmia control is not essential. Doses may be increased or decreased by 50 to 100 mg every 2 to 3 days and are better tolerated when given with food. Total daily dose should not exceed 1200 mg. In some patients, administration every 12 hours can be effective. For rapid loading, 400 mg followed in 8 hours by a 200-mg dose is suggested.

INDICATIONS. Mexiletine is an effective antiarrhythmic agent for treating patients with both acute and chronic ventricular tachyarrhythmias but not with supraventricular tachycardias. Success rates vary from 6 to 60 per cent and can be increased in some patients if mexiletine is combined with other drugs such as procainamide, beta blockers, quinidine, disopyramide, or amiodarone. Most studies show no clear superiority of mexiletine over other class I agents. In the Electrophysiologic Study Versus Electrocardiographic Monitoring (ESVEM) investigation, sotalol was more effective than mexiletine.[68,69] It may be very useful in children with congenital heart disease and serious ventricular arrhythmias. In treating patients with a long Q-T interval, mexiletine probably would be safer than drugs such as quinidine that increase the Q-T interval further. It does not appear to alter the prognosis of patients with inducible ventricular tachyarrhythmias after myocardial infarction. It may be effectively combined with propafenone.[70,71] Mexiletine does not alter late potentials.[72]

ADVERSE EFFECTS. Thirty to 40 per cent of patients may require a change in dose or discontinuation of mexiletine therapy as a result of adverse effects, including tremor, dysarthria, dizziness, paresthesia, diplopia, nystagmus, mental confusion, anxiety, nausea, vomiting, and dyspepsia. Cardiovascular side effects are seen most often after intravenous dosing and include hypotension, bradycardia, and exacerbation of arrhythmia. Adverse effects of mexiletine appear to be dose-related, and toxic effects occur at plasma concentrations only slightly higher than therapeutic levels. Therefore, effective use of this antiarrhythmic drug requires careful titration of dose and monitoring of plasma concentration. Lidocaine should be avoided, or dose reduced, in patients also receiving lidocaine congeners like mexiletine.[73]

Tocainide

Tocainide is a primary amine analog of lidocaine that lacks two ethyl groups; this characteristic protects it from first-pass hepatic elimination and makes it effective orally.

ELECTROPHYSIOLOGICAL AND HEMODYNAMIC ACTIONS (Tables 21–6 and 21–7). Electrophysiological effects are virtually the same as those exerted by lidocaine and mexiletine. It has a small negative inotropic effect and increases peripheral vascular resistance slightly. Oral administration in patients after myocardial infarction does not appear to affect hemodynamic compensation adversely.

PHARMACOKINETICS. Bioavailability of tocainide is almost 100 per cent. The drug is rapidly and completely absorbed, yielding peak plasma concentrations 0.5 to 2 hours after oral ingestion. Approximately 40 per cent is excreted unchanged in the urine. Protein binding is 10 to 50 per cent, and there are no known active metabolites. Enantiomers may be more effective than the racemic mixture. Mean elimination half-life is 11 hours in normal volunteers, possibly longer in patients. There appears to be no pharmacokinetic interaction with other drugs, but caution must be used when combining drugs because of additive antiarrhythmic effects.

DOSAGE AND ADMINISTRATION. Oral regimens of 400 to 600 mg every 8 hours produce therapeutic plasma concentrations of 4 to 10 μg/ml. Dosing increases should not be made more often than every 3 or 4 days. Twice-daily doses can be tried in patients who respond to dosing three times a day. Doses should be reduced in patients with heart failure, or liver or renal disease.

INDICATIONS. Although tocainide effectively reduces the frequency of premature ventricular complexes, it has been less effective in preventing chronic recurrent ventricular tachycardia–ventricular fibrillation because of inefficacy and side effects. Tocainide and mexiletine may be acceptable choices for patients with ventricular arrhythmias in whom the Q-T interval is prolonged.

ADVERSE EFFECTS. Adverse effects are dose-related, similar to those produced by lidocaine, and include nausea, vomiting, anorexia, tremulousness, memory impairment, skin rash, sweating, paresthesia, diplopia, dizziness, anxiety, and tinnitus. Dosing with meals may reduce side effects, possibly by reducing peak serum concentrations of the drug. Occasionally, tocainide may produce pulmonary fibrosis or induce or aggravate ventricular arrhythmias. Hematological disorders including agranulocytosis, bone marrow depression, leukopenia, hypoplastic anemia, and thrombocytopenia have been reported with an estimated incidence of 0.18 per cent and may seriously limit the use of tocainide.[74]

Phenytoin (Diphenylhydantoin)

Phenytoin was employed originally to treat seizure disorders. Its value as an antiarrhythmic agent remains limited.

ELECTROPHYSIOLOGICAL ACTIONS (Tables 21–6 and 21–7). Therapeutic concentrations of phenytoin do not alter the discharge rate of rabbit sinus nodal tissue but may depress normal automaticity in cardiac Purkinje fibers in vitro or spontaneous ventricular rate in vivo. Phenytoin effectively abolishes abnormal automaticity caused by digitalis-induced delayed afterdepolarizations in cardiac Purkinje fibers and suppresses certain digitalis-induced arrhythmias in humans. Similar to lidocaine, phenytoin abbreviates Purkinje fiber action potential duration more than it shortens the effective refractory period, thus increasing the ratio of effective refractory period to action potential duration. Phenytoin can cause depolarized cells to repolarize by increasing potassium conductance and, in so doing, may increase the $\dot{V}_{max}$ of phase 0 in Purkinje fibers, particularly when these are depressed by digitalis.

The rate of rise of action potentials initiated early in the relative refractory period is increased, as is membrane responsiveness, possibly reducing the chance for impaired conduction and block. Phenytoin may slow conduction at high potassium concentrations but minimally affects sinus discharge rate and AV conduction in humans. As with other class IB agents, it has little effect on $\dot{V}_{max}$ in normally polarized fibers at slow rates and shows use dependence and rapid kinetics for onset and termination of effects.

Some of phenytoin's antiarrhythmic effects may be neurally mediated, since phenytoin may reduce the increase in impulse traffic in cardiac sympathetic nerves caused by ouabain toxicity and protect against some arrhythmias when it is injected into the central nervous system. The drug also may modulate vagal efferent activity centrally. It has no peripheral cholinergic or beta-adrenergic blocking actions.

Phenytoin exerts minimal *hemodynamic effects.*

PHARMACOKINETICS (Table 21–7). The pharmacokinetics of phenytoin are less than ideal. Absorption following oral administration is incomplete and varies with the brand of drug. Plasma concentrations peak 8 to 12 hours after an oral dose. Ninety per cent of the drug is protein-bound. Phenytoin has limited solubility at physiological pH, and intramuscular administration is associated with pain, muscle necrosis, sterile abscesses, and variable absorption. Therapeutic serum concentrations of phenytoin (10 to 20 μg/ml) are similar for treating both cardiac arrhythmias and epilepsy. Lower concentrations can suppress certain digitalis-induced arrhythmias or other arrhythmias when decreased plasma protein binding occurs (as in uremia), since a larger fraction of drug is free and pharmacologically active.

METABOLISM. Over 90 per cent of a dose is hydroxylated in the liver to presumably inactive compounds. Some families have a genetically determined inability to hydroxylate phenytoin, while others have a higher than usual capability for hydroxylation. Elimination half-time is about 24 hours and can be slowed in the presence of liver disease or when phenytoin is administered concomitantly with drugs such as phenylbutazone, dicumarol, isoniazid, chloramphenicol, and phenothiazines that compete with phenytoin for hepatic enzymes (Table 21–2). Because of the large number of medications that can increase or decrease phenytoin levels during chronic therapy, phenytoin plasma concentration should be determined frequently when changes are made in other medications. In some patients, maintenance dose regimens of phenytoin are difficult to predict because the enzyme system that metabolizes phenytoin becomes saturated at plasma concentrations within the therapeutic range. The half-life then increases with increasing phenytoin load. Above the saturation point, phenytoin elimination follows zero-order kinetics, so only a fixed amount of drug is eliminated per unit time. These concentration-dependent kinetics for elimination can cause unexpected toxicity, since disproportionately large changes in plasma concentration can follow dose increases.

DOSAGE AND ADMINISTRATION (Table 21–7). To achieve therapeutic plasma concentration rapidly, 100 mg of phenytoin should be administered intravenously every 5 minutes until the arrhythmia is controlled, about 1 gm has been given, or adverse side effects result. Generally, 700 to 1000 mg will control the arrhythmia. A large central vein should be used to avoid pain and development of phlebitis produced by the severely alkalotic (pH 11.0) vehicle in which phenytoin is dissolved. Orally, phenytoin is given as a loading dose of approximately 1000 mg the first day, 500 mg on the second and third days, and 400 mg daily thereafter. All maintenance doses can be given once or twice daily, depending on the brand, because of the long half-life of elimination.

INDICATIONS. Phenytoin has been used successfully to treat atrial and ventricular arrhythmias caused by digitalis toxicity but is much less effective in treating ventricular arrhythmias in patients with ischemic heart disease or with atrial arrhythmias not due to digitalis toxicity. The drug has been somewhat more successful in treating ventricular arrhythmias associated with general anesthesia and cardiac surgery. It can be tried in patients with the long Q-T syndrome.

ADVERSE EFFECTS. The most common manifestations of phenytoin toxicity are central nervous system effects of nystagmus, ataxia, drowsiness, stupor, and coma. Progression of such symptoms can be correlated with increases in plasma drug concentration. Neurological signs, such as nystagmus on lateral gaze, develop at plasma drug levels of about 20 μg/ml. Nausea, epigastric pain, and anorexia are also relatively common effects of phenytoin. Long-term administration can result in hyperglycemia, hypocalcemia, skin rashes, megaloblastic anemia, gingival hypertrophy, lymph node hyperplasia (a syndrome resembling malignant lymphoma), peripheral neuropathy, pneumonitis,[75] and drug-induced systemic lupus erythematosus. Birth defects also can result.[76,77]

CLASS IC ANTIARRHYTHMIC AGENTS

Flecainide

Flecainide is approved by the FDA for the treatment of patients with life-threatening ventricular arrhythmias.

ELECTROPHYSIOLOGICAL ACTIONS. Flecainide exhibits marked use-dependent depressant effects on the rapid sodium channel,[78] decreasing $\dot{V}_{max}$ with slow onset and offset kinetics. Drug dissociation from the sodium channel is very slow, with time constants of 10 to 30 sec (compared with 4 to 8 sec for quinidine and <1 second for lidocaine). Marked drug effects occur at physiological heart rates. Flecainide shortens the duration of Purkinje fiber action potential but prolongs it in ventricular muscle, actions that, depending on the circumstances, could enhance or reduce electrical heterogeneity and create or suppress arrhythmias. Flecainide profoundly slows conduction in all cardiac fibers and, in high concentrations, inhibits the slow channel. Conduction time in the atria, ventricles, AV node, and His-Purkinje system is prolonged. It can terminate experimental atrial reentry by causing conduction block in the reentry pathway[79–81] and eliminate atrial tachycardia by producing exit block from the focus.[82] Flecainide also can promote reentry.[83] Minimal increases in atrial or ventricular refractoriness or in the Q-T interval result. Anterograde and retrograde refractoriness in accessory pathways can increase significantly in a use-dependent fashion.[84] Normal sinus node function remains unchanged, but abnormal sinus node discharge may be depressed. Pacing thresholds are increased.

HEMODYNAMIC EFFECTS. Flecainide depresses cardiac performance, particularly in patients with compromised myocardial function. Left ventricular ejection fraction decreases after oral (single dose of 200 to 250 mg) or intravenous (1 mg) administration. Caution is warranted, particularly in patients with a history of heart failure. Flecainide should be used cautiously, if at all, in patients with severely compromised cardiac function.

PHARMACOKINETICS. Flecainide is at least 90 per cent absorbed with peak plasma concentrations in 3 to 4 hours. Elimination half-life in patients with ventricular arrhythmias is 20 hours, 85 per cent of the drug being excreted unchanged or as an inactive metabolite in urine. Two major metabolites exert fewer effects than the parent drug. Rate of elimination is slower in patients with renal disease and heart failure, and doses should be reduced in these situations. Therapeutic plasma concentrations range from 0.2 to 1.0 μg/ml. About 40 per cent of the drug is protein-bound. Increases in serum concentrations of digoxin (15 to 25 per cent) and propranolol (30 per cent) result during coadministration with flecainide. Propranolol, quinidine, and amiodarone may increase flecainide serum concentrations. Five to 7 days of dosing may be required to reach steady-state in some patients.

DOSAGE AND ADMINISTRATION. Starting dose is 100 mg every 12 hours, increased in increments of 50 mg twice daily, no sooner than every 3 to 4 days, until efficacy is achieved, an adverse effect is noted, or to a maximum of 400 mg/day. Cardiac rhythm and QRS duration should be monitored.

INDICATIONS. Flecainide is indicated for the treatment of life-threatening ventricular tachyarrhythmias.[85,86] Therapy should begin in the hospital while the ECG is being monitored because of the high incidence of proarrhythmic events (see below). Serum concentration should not exceed 1.0 μg/ml. Flecainide is particularly effective, more so than quinidine, in almost totally suppressing premature ventricular complexes and short runs of nonsustained ventricular tachycardia, although the importance of such a response on the subsequent outcome of the patient has not been established. As with other class I antiarrhythmic drugs, there are no data from controlled studies to indicate that the drug favorably affects survival or sudden cardiac death. Flecainide prevents electrical induction of ventricular tachyarrhythmias in a small percentage of patients (10 to 30 per cent) and eliminates recurrence of life-threatening ventricular tachyarrhythmias in about 40 per cent. However, it produces a use-dependent prolongation of ventricular tachycardia cycle length that improves hemodynamic tolerance.[86]

Flecainide may be very useful in a variety of supraventricular tachycardias,[87–90] such as atrial flutter[91] and atrial fibrillation,[87,92–94] in Wolff-Parkinson-White syndrome,[95] and for atrial tachycardia.[96] Flecainide may be more effective than procainamide in the acute termination of atrial fibrillation.[87] It is important to slow the ventricular rate before treating with flecainide to avoid 1:1 conduction.[97] Isoproterenol can reverse some of these effects. Flecainide has been used to treat fetal arrhythmias[98,99] and arrhythmias in children.[100] It may increase defibrillation thresholds.[101]

ADVERSE EFFECTS. Proarrhythmic effects are one of the most important adverse effects of flecainide. Its marked slowing of conduction precludes its use in patients with second degree AV block without a pacemaker and warrants cautious administration in patients with intraventricular conduction disorders. Aggravation of existing ventricular arrhythmias or onset of new ventricular arrhythmias can occur in 5 to 30 per cent of patients, the increased percentage in patients with preexisting sustained ventricular tachycardia, cardiac decompensation, and higher doses of the drug. Failure of the flecainide-related arrhythmia to respond to therapy, including electrical cardioversion-defibrillation, may result in a mortality as high as 10 per cent in patients who develop proarrhythmic events. Negative inotropic effects can cause or worsen heart failure. Patients with sinus node dysfunction may experience sinus arrest, and those with pacemakers may develop an increase in pacing threshold. In the Cardiac Arrhythmia Suppression Trial, patients treated with flecainide had 5.1 per cent mortality or nonfatal cardiac arrest compared with 2.3 per cent in the placebo group over 10 months.[34] Mortality was highest in those with non-Q-wave infarction, frequent premature ventricular complexes, and faster heart rates, raising the possibility of drug interaction with ischemia and electrical instability.[35,102,103] Exercise can amplify the conduction slowing in the ventricle produced by flecainide and in some cases can precipitate a proarrhythmic response. Therefore, exercise testing has been recommended to screen for proarrhythmia. Central nervous system complaints, including confusion and irritability, represent the most frequent noncardiac adverse effect.

Propafenone

Propafenone has been approved by the FDA for treatment of patients with life-threatening ventricular tachyarrhythmias.

ELECTROPHYSIOLOGICAL ACTIONS (Tables 21–6 and 21–7). Propafenone blocks the fast sodium current in a use-dependent manner, as well as at rest, in Purkinje fibers and to a lesser degree in ventricular muscle. Use-dependent effects contribute to its ability to terminate experimental atrial fibrillation.[104] The dissociation constant is slow, like that of flecainide. Effects are greater in ischemic than normal tissue and at reduced membrane potentials. Propafenone decreases excitability and suppresses spontaneous automaticity and triggered activity. It terminates experimental ventricular tachycardia by producing conduction block or by collision of the impulse with an echo wave.[105] Effects on action potential duration are variable in that guinea pig action potential duration is shortened, while rabbit action potential duration is prolonged. Although ventricular refractoriness increases, conduction slowing is the major effect. The active metabolites of propafenone exert important actions, reducing $\dot{V}_{max}$, action potential amplitude, and duration in canine Purkinje fibers. In contrast to propafenone and the *N*-depropylpropafenone metabolite, the 5-hydroxypropafenone metabolite suppressed ventricular tachycardia in the postinfarct canine model. Propafenone depresses sinus nodal automaticity. In patients, the A-H, H-V, P-R, and QRS intervals increase, as do refractory periods of the atria, ventricles, AV node, and accessory pathways. The corrected Q-T interval increases only as a function of increased QRS duration.

HEMODYNAMIC EFFECTS. Propafenone and 5-hydroxypropafenone exhibit negative inotropic properties at high concentrations in vitro, and large doses depress left ventricular function in vivo.[106] In patients with ejection fractions exceeding 40 per cent, the negative inotropic effects are well tolerated, but patients with preexisting left ventricular dysfunction and congestive heart failure may have symptomatic worsening of their hemodynamic status.

PHARMACOKINETICS. With more than 95 per cent of the drug absorbed, propafenone's maximum plasma concentration occurs in 2 to 3 hours. Systemic bioavailability is dose-dependent and ranges from 3 to 40 per cent due to variable presystemic clearance. Bioavailability increases as the dose increases, and plasma concentration is therefore nonlinear. A threefold increase in dosage (300 to 900 mg/day) results in a tenfold increase in plasma concentration, presumably due to saturation of hepatic metabolic mechanisms. Propafenone is 97 per cent bound to α1-acid glycoprotein with an elimination half-life of 5 to 8 hours. Maximum therapeutic effects occur at serum concentrations of 0.2 to 1.5 μg/ml. Marked interpatient variability of pharmacokinetics and pharmacodynamics may be due to genetically determined differences in metabolism. About 93 per cent of the population are extensive metabolizers and exhibit shorter elimination half-lives (5 to 6 hours), lower plasma concentrations of the parent compound, and higher concentrations of metabolites. Poor metabolizers, due to diminished capacity of the microsomal cytochrome P450 enzyme system in the liver (see earlier), exhibit an elimination half-life of 15 to 20 hours for the parent compound and virtually no 5-hydroxypropafenone.[3] Low-dose quinidine may inhibit the metabolism of propafenone, and stereoselectivity may be important with the (+)-enantiomer, providing nonspecific beta-adrenergic receptor blockade approximately 2.5 to 5 per cent the potency of propranolol. Poor metabolizers have a greater beta-adrenergic receptor blocking effect than extensive metabolizers. Since plasma propafenone concentrations may be 50 times or more propranolol levels, these beta-blocking properties may be relevant.[107] Propafenone also blocks the slow calcium channel to a degree about 100 times less than verapamil.

DOSAGE AND ADMINISTRATION. Most patients respond to oral doses of 150 to 300 mg every 8 hours, not exceeding 1200 mg/day. Doses are similar for both patients of both phenotypes. Concomitant food administration increases bioavailability, as does hepatic dysfunction. No good correlation between plasma propafenone concentration and arrhythmia suppression has been shown. Doses should not be increased more often than every 3 to 4 days. Propafenone increases plasma concentrations of warfarin, digoxin, and metoprolol.

INDICATIONS. Propafenone is indicated for the treatment of life-threatening ventricular tachyarrhythmias and effectively suppresses spontaneous premature ventricular complexes[108] and nonsustained and sustained ventricular tachycardia.[109] Spontaneous sinus rate during exercise is reduced. Although propafenone has not been approved by the FDA for treatment of patients with supraventricular tachycardias, the drug is effective in patients with atrial tachycardia,[109,110] AV nodal reentry, AV reentry,[111] and atrial flutter[112] or fibrillation.[108,113–116] It has been used effectively in the pediatric age group.[117–120] Propafenone increases the pacing threshold[121,122] but minimally affects the defibrillation threshold. Propafenoul is associated with a higher mortality in cardiac arrest survivors compared with an implantable defibrillator.[124] Sotalol was less effective than propafenone in the ESVEM trial.[68] Propafenone has been combined effectively with mexiletine.[70,71]

ADVERSE EFFECTS. Minor noncardiac effects occur in about 15 per cent of patients, with dizziness, disturbances in taste, and blurred vision the most common and gastrointestinal side effects next. Exacerbation of bronchospastic lung disease can occur. Cardiovascular side effects occur in 10 to 15 per cent of patients, including conduction abnormalities such as AV block, sinus node depression, and worsening of heart failure. Proarrhythmic responses, more often in patients with a history of sustained ventricular tachycardia and decreased ejection fractions, appear less commonly than with flecainide and may be in the range of 5 per cent. The applicability of data from the Cardiac Arrhythmic Suppression Trial about flecainide to propafenone is not clear, but limiting propafenone's application in a manner similar to other IC drugs seems prudent at present until more information is available. Its beta-blocking actions may make it different, however.[107]

Moricizine HCl (Ethmozine)

Moricizine HCl is a phenothiazine derivative used for treatment of patients with ventricular tachyarrhythmias. It was formerly discussed as a IB antiarrhythmic drug because it shortens Purkinje fiber action potential. However, the intensity of its effect on the Na^+ channel is more like that of a IA antiarrhythmic drug, while the time constants for onset and offset resemble those of class IC agents.

ELECTROPHYSIOLOGICAL ACTIONS. Moricizine decreases I_{Na} predominantly in the inactivated state, with a resultant decrease in $\dot{V}_{max}$ of phase 0, action potential amplitude, and action potential duration in canine cardiac Purkinje fibers (Tables 21–6 and 21–7). Maximum diastolic potential is not changed. Moricizine blocks $I_{Ca\text{-}L}$ and I_K and prolongs AV nodal and His-Purkinje conduction time and QRS duration. The J-T interval shortens slightly, while the Q-T_C prolongs <5 per cent due to QRS prolongation. Ventricular refractoriness prolongs slightly with no consistent atrial change. No alterations in sinus node automaticity result. In vitro, moricizine slows spontaneous automaticity in normal Purkinje fibers and suppresses abnormal automaticity arising from depolarized fibers and delayed afterdepolarizations. It terminates experimental flutter by causing block in the area of slow conduction.[126] Moricizine decreases R-R interval variability, which does not predict mortality.[127] Moricizine minimally raises the defibrillation threshold.[128]

HEMODYNAMIC EFFECTS. Moricizine exerts minimal effects on cardiac performance in patients with impaired left ventricular function. Exercise tolerance and ejection fraction do not change. A small but consistent increase in blood pressure and heart rate results. An occasional patient with significant left ventricular dysfunction may have worsening of heart failure.

PHARMACOKINETICS. Following oral ingestion, moricizine undergoes extensive first-pass metabolism resulting in absolute bioavailability of 35 to 40 per cent. Peak plasma concentrations are reached in 0.5 to 2 hours and later if the drug is taken after meals. Extent of absorption is not changed. Proportionality exists between dose and plasma concentrations in the therapeutic range. Protein binding is 95 per cent to α1-acid glycoprotein and albumin. Antiarrhythmic and electrophysiological actions do not relate to plasma concentrations or to any identified metabolite, of which there are more than 20. At least two metabolites are pharmacologically active but are in small concentrations. Moricizine induces its own metabolism,[129] and plasma concentrations decrease with multiple dosing. Plasma elimination half-life is 1.5 to 3.5 hours, with slightly more than half the drug excreted in the feces and slightly less than half excreted in the urine.

DOSAGE AND ADMINISTRATION. The usual adult dose is 600 to 900 mg/day, given every 8 hours in three equally divided doses. Increments of 150 mg/day at 3-day intervals can be tried. Some patients may be treated every 12 hours. Dose reductions in patients with hepatic or neural disease, AV conduction disturbances, or sick sinus syndrome without a pacemaker and with significant congestive heart failure should be observed.

INDICATIONS. Moricizine exerts an efficacy that is about comparable with those of quinidine and disopyramide.[130] It is less effective in preventing ventricular tachycardia initiation at electrophysiological study and may have proarrhythmic effects. It caused an increase in mortality compared with placebo during initial treatment of patients who had symptomatic or minimally symptomatic ventricular arrhythmias after myocardial infarction[35,134] (see p. 677). Risk was greater in patients taking diuretics.[36]

ADVERSE EFFECTS. Usually the drug is well tolerated. Noncardiac adverse effects primarily involve the nervous system and include tremor, mood changes, headache, vertigo, nystagmus, and dizziness. Gastrointestinal side effects include nausea, vomiting, and diarrhea. Worsening of congestive heart failure is uncommon but can happen. Proarrhythmic effects have been reported in about 3 to 15 per cent of patients[135,136] and appear to be more common in patients with severe ventricular arrhythmias. Advancing age increases the susceptibility to adverse effects.[137]

CLASS II ANTIARRHYTHMIC AGENTS

Beta-Adrenoceptor Blocking Agents

Although many beta-adrenoceptor blockings drugs have been approved for use in the United States (see Table 21–8), acebutolol (PVCs), esmolol (SVT), metoprolol (post-myocardial infarction), atenolol (post-myocardial infarction), propranolol (post-myocardial infarction, SVT, ventricular tachycardia [VT]), and timolol (post-myocardial infarction) have been approved to treat arrhythmias or to prevent sudden death after myocardial infarction.[138] While it is generally considered that no beta blocker offers distinct advantages over the others and that, when titrated to

TABLE 21–8 PHARMACODYNAMIC PROPERTIES OF BETA-ADRENOCEPTOR BLOCKING DRUGS

DRUG	β_2-BLOCKADE POTENCY RATIO (PROPRANOLOL = 1.0)	RELATIVE β_2-SELECTIVITY	INTRINSIC SYMPATHOMIMETIC ACTIVITY	CLASS I ACTIVITY
Acebutolol	0.3	+	+	+
Atenolol	1.0	++	0	0
Bevantolol	0.3	++	0	0
Bisoprolol	10.3	++	0	0
Bucindolol*		0	+	0
Carteolol	10.0	0	+	0
Carvedilol†	10.0	0	0	++
Celiprolol‡	9.4	+	+	0
Dilevalol§	1.0	0	+	0
Esmolol	0.02	++	0	0
Labetalol*	0.3	0	+	0
Metoprolol	1.0	++	0	0
Nadolol	1.0	0	0	0
Oxprenolol	0.5–1.0	0	+	+
Penbutolol	1.0	0	+	0
Pindolol	6.0	0	++	+
Propranolol	1.0	0	0	++
Sotalol¶	0.3	0	0	0
Timolol	6.0	0	0	0

* Bucinodolol and labetalol have additional α_1-adrenergic blocking activity and direct vasodilatory actions (β_2-agonism).
† Carvedilol has additional α_1-adrenergic blocking activity without peripheral β_2-agonism.
‡ Celiprolol may have additional peripheral α_2-adrenergic blocking activity at high doses.
§ Dilevalol is an isomer of labetalol adrenergic with peripheral β_2-agonism but no α_1-blocking activity.
¶ Sotalol has an additional type of antiarrhythmic activity.
Adapted from Duran, A., and Myerburg, R. J.: *In* Singh, B. N., et al. (eds.): Cardiovascular Pharmacology and Therapeutics. New York, Churchill Livingstone, 1994, pp. 665–674.

the proper dose, all can be used effectively to treat cardiac arrhythmias, hypertension, or other disorders, differences in pharmacokinetic or pharmacodynamic properties that confer safety, reduce adverse effects, or affect dosing intervals or drug interactions influence the choice of agent. Also, some beta blockers such as sotalol exert unique actions.

Beta receptors can be separated into those that affect predominantly the heart ($beta_1$) or the bronchi and those that affect predominantly blood vessels ($beta_2$). In low doses, selective beta blockers can block $beta_1$ receptors more than they block $beta_2$ receptors and might be preferable for treating patients with pulmonary or peripheral vascular diseases. In high doses, the selective $beta_1$ blockers also block $beta_2$ receptors.

Some beta blockers exert intrinsic sympathomimetic activity; i.e., they slightly activate the beta receptor. These drugs appear to be as efficacious as beta blockers without intrinsic sympathomimetic actions and may cause less slowing of heart rate at rest and less prolongation of AV nodal conduction time. They have been shown to induce less depression of left ventricular function than beta blockers without intrinsic sympathomimetic activity. Only nonselective beta blockers without intrinsic sympathomimetic activity have been demonstrated to reduce mortality in patients after myocardial infarction[138a] (Fig. 21–5).

The following discussion will concentrate on the use of propranolol as a prototypical antiarrhythmic agent.

ELECTROPHYSIOLOGICAL ACTIONS. Beta blockers exert an electrophysiological action by competitively inhibiting catecholamine binding at beta-adrenoceptor sites, an effect almost entirely due to the (−) levorotatory stereoisomer, or by their quinidine-like or direct membrane-stabilizing action (Tables 21–6 and 21–7). The latter is a local anesthetic effect that depresses I_{Na} and membrane responsiveness in cardiac Purkinje fibers, occurs at concentrations generally 10 times that necessary to produce beta blockade, and most likely plays an insignificant antiarrhythmic role. Thus major effects of beta blockers will take place in cells most actively stimulated by adrenergic actions. At beta-blocking concentrations, propranolol slows spontaneous automaticity in the sinus node or in Purkinje fibers that are being stimulated by adrenergic tone, producing block of I_f. Beta blockers also block $I_{Ca\text{-}L}$ stimulated by beta-agonists. In the absence of adrenergic stimulation, only high concentrations of propranolol slow normal automaticity in Purkinje fibers, probably by a direct membrane action.

Concentrations that cause beta-receptor blockade but no local anesthetic effects do not alter the normal resting membrane potential, maximum diastolic potential amplitude, $\dot{V}_{max}$, repolarization, or refractoriness of atrial, Purkinje, or ventricular muscle cells when these tissues are not being superfused with catecholamines. However, in the presence of isoproterenol, a pure beta-receptor stimulator, beta blockers reverse isoproterenol's accelerating effects on repolarization; in the presence of norepinephrine, beta blockade permits unopposed alpha-adrenoceptor stimulation to prolong action potential duration in Purkinje fibers.

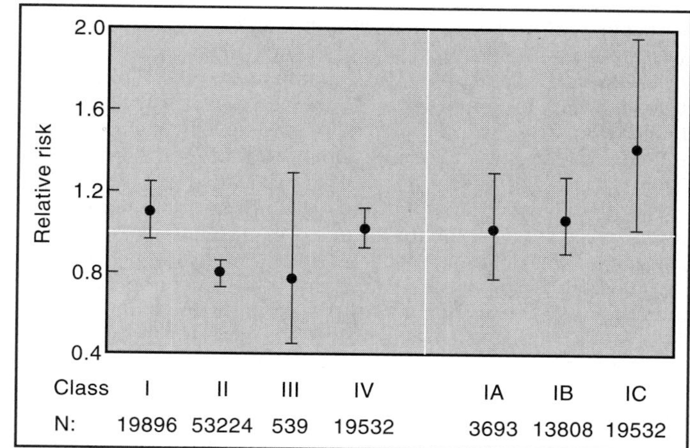

FIGURE 21–5. Meta-analytical data from randomized clinical trials of antiarrhythmic drugs in survivors of acute myocardial infarction. The relative risk is compared with placebo therapy (mean and 95 per cent confidence interval) for death during therapy with various electrophysiological classes of compounds. Class IA agents, particularly IC, increase mortality, while beta blockers and class III agents (essentially amiodarone) decrease mortality. (Data from Teo, K. K., and Yusuf, S. *In* Singh, B. N., et al. [eds.]: Cardiovascular Pharmacology and Therapeutics. New York, Churchill-Livingstone, 1994, pp. 631–643.)

Propranolol (2×10^{-6} M) reduces the amplitude of digitalis-induced delayed afterdepolarizations and suppresses triggered activity in Purkinje fibers.

Propranolol upregulates beta adrenoceptors in part by externalizing receptors from a light vesicle fraction to the sarcolemma. Beta blockers do not blunt heart rate variability in dogs after myocardial infarction.[139]

Concentrations exceeding 3 μg/ml are required to depress $\dot{V}_{max}$ action potential amplitude, membrane responsiveness, and conduction in normal atrial, ventricular, and Purkinje fibers without altering resting membrane potential. These effects probably result from depression of I_{Na}. Propranolol shortens the action potential duration of Purkinje fibers and, to a lesser extent, of atrial and ventricular muscle fibers. Long-term administration of propranolol may lengthen action potential duration. Similar to the effects of lidocaine, acceleration of repolarization of Purkinje fibers is most marked in areas of the ventricular conduction system in which the action potential duration is greatest. The reduction in refractory period is not as great as the reduction in action potential duration (effective refractory period duration/action potential duration >1.0). At least one beta blocker, sotalol, markedly increases the time course of repolarization in Purkinje fibers and ventricular muscles (see p. 615). Smaller doses of propranolol are required to prevent sympathetically induced shortening of ventricular refractoriness than are required to prevent sympathetically induced sinus acceleration.

Propranolol slows the sinus discharge rate in humans by 10 to 20 per cent, while severe bradycardia occasionally results if the heart is particularly dependent on sympathetic tone or if sinus node dysfunction is present. The slowing is probably due to beta blockade because D-propranolol does not significantly slow the sinus discharge rate in doses comparable to the racemic mixture. The P-R interval lengthens, as do AV nodal conduction time and effective and functional refractory periods (if the heart rate is maintained constant), but refractoriness and conduction in the normal His-Purkinje system remain unchanged even after high doses of propranolol. Therefore, therapeutic doses of propranolol in humans do not exert a direct depressant or "quinidine-like" action but influence cardiac electrophysiology via a beta-blocking action. Beta blockers do not affect conduction in normal ventricular muscle, as evidenced by their lack of effect on the QRS complex, and they insignificantly prolong the right ventricular effective refractory period and uncorrected Q-T interval.

Because administration of beta blockers that do not have direct membrane action prevents many arrhythmias resulting from activation of the autonomic nervous system, it is thought that the beta-blocking action is responsible for their antiarrhythmic effects.[140–144] However, the possible importance of direct membrane effect of some of these drugs cannot be discounted totally because beta blockers with direct membrane actions can affect transmembrane potentials of diseased cardiac fibers at much lower concentrations than are needed to affect normal fibers directly. However, indirect actions on arrhythmogenic effects of ischemia are probably quite important. Beta blockers reduce myocardial injury during experimental cardiopulmonary resuscitation.[145]

HEMODYNAMIC EFFECTS. Beta blockers exert negative inotropic effects and can precipitate or worsen heart failure. By blocking beta receptors, these drugs may cause peripheral vasoconstriction and exacerbate coronary artery spasm in some patients.

PHARMACOKINETICS (Table 21–1). Although various types of beta blockers exert similar pharmacological effects, their pharmacokinetics differ substantially. Propranolol is almost 100 per cent absorbed, but the effects of first-pass hepatic metabolism reduce bioavailability to about 30 per cent and produce significant interpatient variability of plasma concentration for a given dose. Reduction in hepatic blood flow, as in patients with heart failure, decreases the hepatic extraction of propranolol, and in these patients propranolol may further decrease its own elimination rate by reducing cardiac output and hepatic blood flow. Beta blockers eliminated by the kidney tend to have longer half-lives and exhibit less interpatient variability of drug concentration than do those beta blockers metabolized by the liver.

DOSAGE AND ADMINISTRATION (Table 21–7). The appropriate dose of propranolol is best determined by a measure of the patient's physiological response, such as changes in resting heart rate or in the prevention of exercise-induced tachycardia, since wide individual differences exist between the observed physiological effect and plasma concentration. For example, intravenous dosing is best achieved by titrating the dose to a clinical effect, beginning with doses of 0.25 to 0.50 mg, increasing to 1.0 mg if necessary, and administering doses every 5 minutes until either a desired effect or toxicity is produced or a total of 0.15 to 0.20 mg/kg has been given. In many instances, the short-acting effects of esmolol are preferred. Orally, propranolol is given in four divided doses, usually ranging from 40 to 160 mg a day to more than 1 gm a day. A once-daily long-acting propranolol preparation is available. Generally, if one agent in adequate doses proves to be ineffective, other beta blockers will be ineffective also.

INDICATIONS. Arrhythmias associated with thyrotoxicosis, pheochromocytoma, and anesthesia with cyclopropane or halothane, or arrhythmias largely due to excessive cardiac adrenergic stimulation, such as those initiated by exercise or emotion, often respond to propranolol therapy. Beta-blocking drugs usually do not convert chronic atrial flutter or atrial fibrillation to normal sinus rhythm but may do so if the arrhythmia is of recent onset. The rate of the atrial flutter/fibrillation is not changed, but the ventricular response decreases because beta blockade prolongs AV nodal conduction time and refractoriness. Esmolol combined with digoxin has been useful.[146] In the absence of heart failure, beta blockers can be more effective than digoxin to control the rate.[147] For reentrant supraventricular tachycardias using the AV node as one of the reentrant pathways, such as AV nodal reentrant tachycardia[148,149] and orthodromic reciprocating tachycardias in Wolff-Parkinson-White syndrome or inappropriate sinus tachycardia,[150,151] or for sinus reentrant tachycardia, propranolol may slow or terminate the tachycardia and be used prophylactically to prevent a recurrence. Combining propranolol with digitalis, quinidine, or a variety of other agents may be effective when propranolol as a single agent fails. *Metoprolol* and *esmolol* may be useful in patients with multifocal atrial tachycardia.[152]

Propranolol may be effective for digitalis-induced arrhythmias such as atrial tachycardia, nonparoxysmal AV junctional tachycardia, premature ventricular complexes, or ventricular tachycardia. If a significant degree of AV block is present during a digitalis-induced arrhythmia, lidocaine or phenytoin may be preferable to propranolol. Propranolol also may be useful to treat ventricular arrhythmias associated with the prolonged Q-T interval syndrome[153–155] and with mitral valve prolapse. For patients with ischemic heart disease, propranolol generally does not prevent episodes of chronic recurrent monomorphic ventricular tachycardia that occur in the absence of acute ischemia but may be effective in some patients, usually at a beta-blocking concentration. It is well accepted that propranolol, timolol, and metoprolol reduce the incidence of overall death and sudden cardiac death after myocardial infarction[156–158] (Fig. 21–5). The mechanism of this reduction in mortality is not entirely clear and may relate to reduction in the extent of ischemic drainage, autonomic effects, a direct antiarrhythmic effect, or combinations of these factors. Beta blockers may have been protective against proarrhythmic responses in CAST[159] and may be more effective in some patients than electrophysiologically guided antiarrhythmic drug therapy[160] for ventricular tachyarrhythmias. Labetalol has been used for ventricular arrhythmias in eclampsia.[161]

Labetalol is an $alpha_1$- and beta-blocking drug. *Esmolol* is an ultra-short-acting (elimination half-life 9 min) cardioselective beta-adrenoceptor blocker useful for the rapid control of the ventricular rate in patients with atrial flutter/fibrillation.[162] Its withdrawal has been used in tilt-table testing.[163]

ADVERSE EFFECTS. Adverse cardiovascular effects from propranolol include unacceptable hypotension, bradycardia, and congestive heart failure. The bradycardia may be due to sinus bradycardia or AV block. Sudden withdrawal of propranolol in patients with angina pectoris can precipitate or worsen angina and cardiac arrhythmias and cause an acute myocardial infarction, possibly owing to heightened sensitivity to beta-agonists caused by previous beta blockade (upregulation). Heightened sensitivity may begin several days after cessation of propranolol therapy and may last 5 or 6 days. Other adverse effects of propranolol include worsening of asthma or chronic obstructive pulmonary disease, intermittent claudication, Raynaud's phenomenon, mental depression, increased risk of hypoglycemia among insulin-dependent diabetic patients, easy fatigability, disturbingly vivid dreams or insomnia, and impaired sexual function.

CLASS III ANTIARRHYTHMIC AGENTS

Amiodarone

Amiodarone is a benzofuran derivative approved by the FDA for the treatment of patients with life-threatening ventricular tachyarrhythmias when other drugs are ineffective or are not tolerated.

ELECTROPHYSIOLOGICAL ACTIONS (Tables 21–6 and 21–7). When chronically given orally, amiodarone prolongs action potential duration and refractoriness of all cardiac fibers without affecting resting membrane potential. When acute effects are evaluated, amiodarone and its metabolite, desethylamiodarone, prolong the action potential duration of ventricular muscle but shorten the action potential duration of Purkinje fibers. Injected into the sinus and AV nodal arteries, amiodarone reduces sinus and junctional discharge rates and prolongs AV nodal conduction time. It decreases the slope of diastolic depolarization of the sinus node and markedly depresses $\dot{V}_{max}$ in guinea pig papillary muscle in a rate- or use-dependent manner. Such depression of $\dot{V}_{max}$ is caused by blocking of inactivated sodium channels, an effect that is accentuated by depolarized and reduced by hyperpolarized membrane potentials. Amiodarone also inhibits depolarization-induced automaticity. Amiodarone depresses conduction at fast rates more than at slow rates (use or frequency dependence),[164–166] not only by depressing $\dot{V}_{max}$ but also by increasing resistance to passive current flow. It does not prolong repolarization more at slow than fast rates (does not exert reverse use or frequency dependence) but does exert time-dependent effects on refractoriness, which may in part explain the low incidence of torsades de pointes and high efficacy.[164,165]

Desethylamiodarone has relatively greater effects on fast-channel tissue and probably contributes importantly to antiarrhythmic efficacy. The delay to build up adequate concentrations of this metabolite may explain in part the delay in amiodarone's antiarrhythmic action.

In vivo, amiodarone noncompetitively antagonizes alpha and beta receptors and blocks conversion of thyroxine (T_4) to triiodothyronine (T_3), which may account for some of its electrophysiological effects. Amiodarone exhibits slow-channel blocking effects, and chronic oral therapy slows the spontaneous sinus nodal discharge rate in anesthetized dogs even after pretreatment with propranolol and atropine. With oral administration it prolongs the Q-T interval, at times changing the contour of the T wave and producing U waves, and slows the sinus rate by 20 to 30 per cent.

Effective refractory periods of all cardiac tissues are prolonged. His-Purkinje conduction time increases and QRS duration lengthens, especially at fast rates. Amiodarone given intravenously modestly prolongs the refractory period of atrial and ventricular muscle. P-R interval and AV nodal conduction time lengthen. The duration of the QRS complex lengthens at increased rates but less than after oral amiodarone. Thus, far less increase in prolongation of conduction time (except for the AV node), duration of repolarization, and refractoriness occurs after intravenous administration compared with the oral route. Considering these actions, it is clear that amiodarone has class I (blocks I_{Na}), class II (antiadrenergic), and class IV (blocks $I_{Ca\text{-}L}$) actions, in addition to class III effects (blocks I_K). Amiodarone's actions approximate those of a theoretically ideal drug that exhibits use-dependence of Na^+ channels with fast diastolic recovery from block and use-dependent prolongation of action potential duration. It does not increase[167] and may decrease[168] Q-T dispersion. Catecholamines can partially reverse some of the effects of amiodarone.[164,169]

HEMODYNAMIC EFFECTS. Amiodarone is a peripheral and coronary vasodilator. When administered intravenously in doses of 2.5 to 10 mg/kg, amiodarone decreases heart rate, systemic vascular resistance, left ventricular contractile force, and left ventricular dP/dt. Left ventricular output may increase. Oral doses of amiodarone sufficient to control cardiac arrhythmias do not depress left ventricular ejection fraction, even in patients with reduced ejection fractions measured by radionuclide ventriculography. However, because antiadrenergic actions of amiodarone may block I_{si} to some degree, and because it does exert some negative inotropic action, it should be given cautiously, particularly intravenously, to patients with marginal cardiac compensation.

PHARMACOKINETICS. Amiodarone is slowly, variably, and incompletely absorbed, with systemic bioavailability of 35 to 65 per cent. Plasma concentrations peak 3 to 7 hours after a single oral dose. There is minimal first-pass effect, indicating little hepatic extraction. Elimination is by hepatic excretion into bile with some enterohepatic recirculation. Extensive hepatic metabolism occurs with desethylamiodarone as a major metabolite. The plasma concentration ratio of parent to metabolite is 3:2. Both extensively accumulate in liver, lung, fat, "blue" skin, and other tissues. Myocardium develops a concentration 10 to 50 times that found in the plasma. Plasma clearance of amiodarone is low, and renal excretion negligible. Doses need not be reduced in patients with renal disease. Amiodarone and desethylamiodarone are not dialyzable. Volume of distribution is large but variable, averaging 60 liters/kg. Amiodarone is highly protein-bound (96 per cent), crosses the placenta (10 to 50 per cent), and is found in breast milk.

The onset of action after intravenous administration generally is within several hours. Following oral administration, the onset of action may require 2 to 3 days, often 1 to 3 weeks, and, on occasion, even longer. Loading doses reduce this time interval. Plasma concentrations relate well to oral doses during chronic treatment, averaging about 0.5 μg/ml for each 100 mg/day at doses between 100 and 600 mg/day. Elimination half-life is multiphasic with an initial 50 per cent reduction in plasma concentration 3 to 10 days after cessation of drug ingestion (probably representing elimination from well-perfused tissues) followed by a terminal half-life of 26 to 107 days (mean 53 days), with most patients in the 40- to 55-day range. To achieve steady state without a loading dose takes about 265 days. Interpatient variability of these pharmacokinetic parameters mandates close monitoring of the patient. Therapeutic serum concentrations range from 1 to 2.5 μg/ml. Greater suppression of arrhythmias may occur up to 3.5 μg/ml, but the risk of side effects increases.

DOSAGE AND ADMINISTRATION. An optimal dosing schedule for all patients has not been achieved.[170–173] One recommended approach is to treat with 800 to 1600 mg daily for 1 to 3 weeks,[174] reduced to 800 mg daily for the next 2 to 4 weeks, then 600 mg daily for 4 to 8 weeks, and finally, after 2 to 3 months of treatment, a maintenance dose of 400 mg or less per day. Maintenance drug can be given once or twice daily and should be titrated to the *lowest effective dose* to minimize the occurrence of side effects.[175] Doses as low as 100 mg/day can be effective in some patients.[176] Regimens must be individualized for a given patient and clinical situation. Amiodarone may be administered intravenously[177] to achieve more rapid loading and effect in emergencies at initial doses of 15 mg/min for 10 minutes, followed by 1 mg/min for 6 hours, and then 0.5 mg/min for the remaining 18 hours and for the next several days, as necessary. Supplemental infusions of 150 mg over 10 minutes can be used for breakthrough VT or ventricular fibrillation (VF). IV infusions have been continued safely for 2 to 3 weeks. Patients with depressed ejection fractions should receive intravenous amiodarone with great caution because of hypotension. High-dose oral loading (800 to 2000 mg two or three times a day to maintain trough serum concentrations of 2 to 3 μg/ml) may suppress ventricular arrhythmias in 1 to 2 days.

INDICATIONS. Amiodarone has been used to suppress a wide spectrum of supraventricular and ventricular tachyarrhythmias in utero,[178,179] in adults,[175] and in children,[180,181] including AV nodal and AV entry, junctional tachycardia,[182] atrial flutter and fibrillation,[183–188] ventricular tachycardia and ventricular fibrillation associated with coronary artery disease,[189–192] and hypertrophic cardiomyopathy. Success rates vary widely depending on patient population,[193] arrhythmia, underlying heart disease, length of follow-up, definition and determination of success, and other factors. In general, however, amidarone's efficacy equals or exceeds that of all other antiarrhythmic agents and may be in the range of 60 to 80 per cent for most supraventricular tachyarrhythmias (including those associated with the Wolff-Parkinson-White syndrome) and 40 to 60 per cent for ventricular tachyarrhythmias. Amiodarone may be useful in improving survival in patients with hypertrophic cardiomyopathy, asymptomatic ventricular arrhythmias after myocardial infarction, and ventricular tachyarrhythmia after resuscitation.

Patients who have an internal cardioverter-defibrillator receive fewer shocks if they are treated with amiodarone compared with conventional drugs.[194] Amiodarone may facilitate defibrillation experimentally[195] but increases the electrical defibrillation threshold.[196,197] Because of its long half-life and the difficulty involved in starting another antiarrhythmic drug (while not knowing if amiodarone's effects are still present), as well as its side effects profile, amiodarone is generally among the last antiarrhythmic agents tried.

A number of prospective, randomized, controlled trials with amiodarone have been performed recently.[191,198] They have demonstrated the superiority of amiodarone over placebo[199–201] and metoprolol[202] on mortality in patients after myocardial infarction, documented an effect not different from placebo in patients with congestive heart failure in one study,[203] showed a benefit in another,[204] and found a greater improvement in mortality in patients resuscitated from ventricular fibrillation compared with conventional drugs.[205,206] Several studies are in progress, including the European Myocardial Infarction Amiodarone Trial (EMIAT)[207] that compares amiodarone with placebo in patients with reduced left ventricular function after myocardial infarction, the Canadian Amiodarone Myocardial Infarction Arrhythmia Trial (CAMIAT),[208] similar to EMIAT in patients with ventricular ectopy, and trials comparing amiodarone with implantable defibrillators.[137,209,210]

Some controversy exists regarding the ability to predict effectiveness of amiodarone in patients with ventricular tachyarrhythmias. Clinical assessment, suppression of spontaneous ventricular arrhythmias as documented by 24-hour ECG recordings, and response to electrophysiological testing have served as endpoints to judge therapy. In the patient with a history of sustained ventricular tachycardia or fibrillation and minimal spontaneous ventricular arrhythmias in between symptomatic episodes, an invasive electrophysiological study is indicated to judge drug efficacy. The answer to when, after amiodarone therapy is started, such a study should be done is still not entirely resolved but probably should be 1 week or longer. In the 10 to 40 per cent of patients whose electrically induced clinical ventricular tachyarrhythmias become no longer inducible while they are receiving amiodarone, the chances for a spontaneous recurrence of the arrhythmias are low while the patients are taking amiodarone, probably less than 5 to 10 per cent at 1 year. For those patients whose ventricular tachyarrhythmias are still inducible, the recurrence rate is 40 to 50 per cent at 1 year. However, in this latter group, greater difficulty in inducing the arrhythmias may predict a less likely possibility of a recurrence.

Patients' hemodynamic responses to the induced arrhythmia also may predict how they tolerate a spontaneous recurrence. Amiodarone slows the ventricular tachycardia,[211,212] but it is important to remember that the supine patient in the electrophysiology laboratory may tolerate the same tachycardia better than when in an erect position. The arrhythmia's response to sotalol may predict its response to amiodarone.[213] An ejection fraction ≥ 0.4 may predict a good response to amiodarone in patients with ventricular tachycardia or ventricular fibrillation.[214]

Because of the serious nature of the arrhythmias being treated, the unusual pharmacokinetics of the drug, and its adverse effects (see below), amiodarone therapy should be started with the patient hospitalized and monitored for several days to a week. Combining other antiarrhythmic agents with amiodarone may improve efficacy in some patients.[215,216]

ADVERSE EFFECTS. Adverse effects are reported by about 75 per cent of patients treated with amiodarone for 5 years but compel stopping the drug in 18 to 37 per cent. The most frequent side effects requiring drug discontinuation involve pulmonary and gastrointestinal complaints.[175] Most adverse effects are reversible with dose reduction or cessation of treatment. Adverse effects become more frequent when therapy is continued long term. Of the noncardiac adverse reactions, pulmonary toxicity is the most serious; in one study it occurred between 6 days and 60 months of treatment in 33 of 573 patients, with 3 deaths. The mechanism is unclear but may relate to a hypersensitivity reaction and/or widespread phospholipidosis. Dyspnea, nonproductive cough, and fever are common symptoms, with rales, hypoxia, a positive gallium scan, reduced diffusion capacity,[217] and radiographic evidence of pulmonary infiltrates noted. Amiodarone must be discontinued if such pulmonary inflammatory changes occur. Steroids can be tried, but no controlled studies have been done to support their use. A 10 per cent mortality in patients with pulmonary inflammatory changes results, often in patients with unrecognized pulmonary involvement that is allowed to progress. Chest roentgenograms at 3-month intervals for the first year and then twice a year for several years have been recommended. At maintenance doses less than 300 mg daily, pulmonary toxicity is uncommon. Advanced age, high drug maintenance dose, and reduced predrug diffusion capacity (DL_{co}) are risk factors for developing pulmonary toxicity. An unchanged DL_{co} volume may be a negative predictor of pulmonary toxicity.

Although asymptomatic elevations of liver enzymes are found in most patients, the drug is not stopped unless values exceed two or three times normal in a patient with initially abnormal values. Cirrhosis occurs uncommonly but may be fatal. Neurological dysfunction, photosensitivity (perhaps minimized by sunscreens), bluish skin discoloration, corneal microdeposits (in almost 100 per cent of adults receiving the drug more than 6 months), gastroenterological disturbances, and hyperthyroidism[218,219] (1 to 2 per cent) or hypothyroidism (2 to 4 per cent) can occur. Amiodarone appears to inhibit the peripheral conversion of T_4 to T_3 so that chemical changes result, characterized by a slight increase in T_4, reverse T_3 and thyroid-stimulating hormone (TSH), and a slight decrease in T_3. Reverse T_3 concentration has been used as an index of drug efficacy. During hypothyroidism, TSH increases greatly while T_3 increases in hyperthyroidism.

Cardiac side effects include symptomatic bradycardias in about 2 per cent, aggravation of ventricular tachyarrhythmias (with occasional development of torsades de pointes) in 1 to 2 per cent,[220] possibly higher in women,[221] and worsening of congestive heart failure in 2 per cent. Possibly due to interactions with anesthetics, complications after open-heart surgery have been noted by some,[222] but not all,[223] investigators, including pulmonary dysfunction, hypotension, hepatic dysfunction, and low cardiac output.

Important interactions with other drugs occur, and when given concomitantly with amiodarone, the dose of warfarin, digoxin, and other antiarrhythmic drugs should be reduced by one-third to one-half and the patient watched closely. Drugs with synergistic actions, such as beta blockers or calcium channel blockers, must be given cautiously.

Bretylium Tosylate

Bretylium is a quaternary ammonium compound that is approved by the FDA for parenteral use only in patients with life-threatening ventricular tachyarrhythmias.

ELECTROPHYSIOLOGICAL ACTIONS (Tables 21–6 and 21–7). Bretylium is selectively concentrated in sympathetic ganglia and their postganglionic adrenergic nerve terminals. After initially *causing* norepinephrine release, bretylium *prevents* norepinephrine release by depressing sympathetic nerve terminal excitability without depressing pre- or postganglionic sympathetic nerve conduction, impairing conduction across sympathetic ganglia, depleting the adrenergic neuron of norepinephrine, or decreasing the responsiveness of adrenergic receptors. It produces a state resembling chemical sympathectomy. During chronic bretylium treatment, the beta-adrenergic responses to circulating catecholamines are increased. The initial release of catecholamines results in several transient electrophysiological responses such as an increase in the discharge rates of the isolated perfused sinus node and of in vitro Purkinje fibers, often making quiescent fibers automatic.

Bretylium initially increases conduction velocity and excitability and decreases refractoriness in the rabbit atrium, and partially depolarized fibers may hyperpolarize. Pretreatment with reserpine or propranolol prevents these early changes. Initial catecholamine release can aggravate some arrhythmias, such as those caused by digitalis excess or myocardial infarction. Prolonged drug administration lengthens the duration of the action potential and refractoriness of atrial and ventricular muscle and Purkinje fibers, possibly by blocking one or more repolarizing potassium currents. The ratio of effective refractory period to action potential duration does not change, nor do membrane responsiveness and conduction velocity. Bretylium exerts little effect on diastolic excitability but increases ventricular fibrillation thresholds in some studies[224,225] but not others.[226] It is not clear whether the chemical sympathectomy-like state alone or together with other actions exerts the antifibrillatory effect. Reduced disparity between action potential duration and refractory period in regions of normal and infarcted myocardium may account for some of its antifibrillatory effects. Bretylium has no effect on vagal reflexes and does not alter the responsiveness of cholinergic receptors in the heart.

HEMODYNAMIC EFFECTS. Bretylium does not depress myocardial contractility. After an initial increase in blood pressure, the drug can cause significant hypotension by blocking the efferent limb of the baroceptor reflex. Hypotension results most commonly when patients are sitting or standing but also can occur in the supine position in seriously ill patients. Bretylium reduces the extent of the vasoconstriction and tachycardia reflexes during standing. Orthostatic hypotension can persist for several days after the drug has been discontinued.

PHARMACOKINETICS (Table 21–1). Bretylium is effective orally as well as parenterally, but it is absorbed poorly and erratically from the gastrointestinal tract. Bioavailability may be less than 50 per cent, and elimination is almost exclusively by renal excretion without significant metabolism or active metabolites being recognized. Elimination half-life is 5 to 10 hours but with fairly wide variability. Doses should be reduced in patients with renal insufficiency. In survivors of ventricular tachycardia or ventricular fibrillation, bretylium had an elimination half-life of 13.5 hours following single intravenous dosing, which was similar to previous results in normal subjects. Renal clearance accounted for virtually all elimination. Onset of action after intravenous administration occurs within several minutes, but full antiarrhythmic effects may not be seen for 30 minutes to 2 hours.

DOSAGE AND ADMINISTRATION (Table 21–1). Bretylium can be given intravenously in doses of 5 to 10 mg/kg of body weight diluted in 50 to 100 ml of 5 per cent dextrose in water and administered over 10 to 20 minutes or more quickly in a life-threatening state. This dose can be repeated in 1 to 2 hours if the arrhythmia persists. The total daily dose probably should not exceed 30 mg/kg. A similar initial dose, but undiluted, can be given intramuscularly. The maintenance intravenous dose is 0.5 to 2.0 mg/min. Intramuscular injection during cardiopulmonary resuscitation from cardiac arrest and in shock states should be avoided because of unreliable absorption during reduced tissue perfusion. In this situation, bretylium should be given intravenously.

INDICATIONS. Bretylium is used in patients who are in an intensive care setting and who have life-threatening recurrent ventricular tachyarrhythmias that have not responded to other antiarrhythmic drugs. Bretylium has been effective in treating some patients with drug-resistant tachyarrhythmias and in treating victims of out-of-hospital ventricular fibrillation.

ADVERSE EFFECTS. Hypotension, most prominently orthostatic but also supine, appears to be the most significant side effect and can be prevented with tricyclic drugs such as protriptyline. Transient hypertension, increased sinus rate, and worsening of arrhythmias, often those due to digitalis excess or ischemia, may follow initial drug administration and may be due to initial release of catecholamines. Bretylium should be used cautiously or not at all in patients who have a relatively fixed cardiac output, such as those with severe aortic stenosis. Vasodilators or diuretics can enhance these hypotensive effects. Nausea and vomiting can occur following parenteral administration. Parotid pain primarily during meals commonly occurs after 2 to 4 months of oral therapy and is associated with increased salivation without parotid swelling or inflammation.

Sotalol

Sotalol is a nonspecific beta-adrenoceptor blocker without intrinsic sympathomimetic activity that prolongs repolarization. It was approved in 1992 by the FDA to treat patients with life-threatening ventricular tachyarrhythmias.[191,227]

ELECTROPHYSIOLOGICAL ACTIONS. Both d- and l-isomers

have similar effects on prolonging repolarization, while the l-isomer is responsible for virtually all the beta-blocking activity. Sotalol does not block alpha adrenoceptors and does not block the sodium channel (no membrane-stabilizing effects) but does prolong atrial and ventricular repolarization times[228] by reducing I_K thus prolonging the plateau of the action potential. Action potential prolongation is greater at slower rates (reverse use dependence). Resting membrane potential, action potential amplitude, and $\dot{V}_{max}$ are not significantly altered. Sotalol prolongs atrial and ventricular refractoriness, A-H and Q-T intervals, and sinus cycle length. It narrows the excitable gap in reentrant ventricular tachycardia.[229]

HEMODYNAMICS. Sotalol exerts a negative inotropic effect only through its beta-blocking action. It can increase the strength of contraction by prolonging repolarization, which will occur maximally at slow heart rates. In patients with reduced cardiac function, sotalol can cause a decrease in cardiac index, an increase in filling pressure, and overt heart failure. Therefore, it must be used cautiously in patients with marginal cardiac compensation but appears to be well tolerated in patients with normal cardiac function.[230–232]

PHARMACOKINETICS. Sotalol is completely absorbed and not metabolized, making it 90 to 100 per cent bioavailable. It is not bound to plasma proteins, is excreted unchanged primarily by the kidneys, and has an elimination half-life of 10 to 15 hours. The plasma concentrations occur 2.5 to 4.0 hours after oral ingestion, with steady state attained after five or six doses. Effective antiarrhythmic plasma concentration is in the range of 2.5 μg/ml. There is very little intersubject variability in plasma levels. Over the dose range of 160 to 640 mg, sotalol displays dose proportionality with plasma concentration. The dose must be reduced in patients with renal disease. The beta-blocking effect is half maximal at 80 mg/day and maximal at ≥320 mg/day. Significant beta-blocking action occurs at 160 mg/day.

DOSAGE. The typical oral dose is 80 to 160 mg every 12 hours, allowing 2 to 3 days between dose adjustments to attain steady state and monitor the ECG for arrhythmias and Q-T prolongation. Doses exceeding 320 mg/day can be used in patients when the potential benefits outweigh the risk of proarrhythmia.

INDICATIONS. Approved only to treat patients with ventricular tachyarrhythmias,[233–235] sotalol is also useful to prevent recurrence of a wide variety of supraventricular tachycardias, including atrial flutter and fibrillation,[236,237] atrial tachycardia, AV nodal reentry, and AV reentry. It also shows the ventricular response to atrial tachyarrhythmias.[238] It appears to be more effective than conventional antiarrhythmic drugs and comparable with amiodarone in treating patients with ventricular tachyarrhythmias.[68] Sotalol has been shown to be superior to lidocaine for acute termination of sustained ventricular tachycardia[239] and is useful in patients with arrhythmogenic right ventricular dysplasia.[240] It can prolong the duration of late potentials.[241] Sotalol may be effective in pediatric patients.[242] It may reduce the defibrillation threshold.[196]

ADVERSE EFFECTS. Proarrhythmia is the most serious adverse effect. Overall, new or worsened ventricular tachyarrhythmias occur in about 4 per cent, and this response is due to torsades de pointes in about 2.5 per cent. The incidence of torsades de pointes increases to 4 per cent in patients with a history of sustained ventricular tachycardia and is dose related, reportedly only 1.6 per cent at 320 mg/day but 4.4 per cent at 480 mg/day.[243] Other adverse effects commonly seen with other beta blockers also apply to sotalol. Sotalol should be used with caution or not at all in combination with other drugs that prolong the Q-T interval. However, such combinations have been used successfully.[244]

CLASS IV ANTIARRHYTHMIC AGENTS

The Calcium Channel Antagonists: Verapamil and Diltiazem

Verapamil, a synthetic papaverine derivative, is the prototype of a class of drugs that block the slow calcium channel and reduce I_{Ca-L} in cardiac muscle. *Diltiazem* has electrophysiological actions similar to those of verapamil.[138] *Nifedipine* (see p. 1308) exhibits minimal electrophysiological effects at clinically used doses and will not be discussed here.

ELECTROPHYSIOLOGICAL ACTIONS (Tables 21–6 and 21–7). By blocking the slow inward current in all cardiac fibers, verapamil reduces the plateau height of the action potential, slightly shortens muscle action potential, and slightly prolongs total Purkinje fiber action potential. It does not appreciably affect the action potential amplitude, $\dot{V}_{max}$ of phase 0, or resting membrane voltage in cells that have fast-response characteristics due to I_{Na} (atrial and ventricular muscle, the His-Purkinje system). Verapamil suppresses slow responses elicited by a variety of experimental methods as well as triggered sustained rhythmic activity and early and late afterdepolarizations (see pp. 566 to 567). Verapamil and other slow-channel blockers suppress electrical activity in the normal sinus and AV nodes in concentrations that do not suppress action potentials of fast-channel-dependent cells. Verapamil depresses the slope of diastolic depolarization in sinus nodal cells, $\dot{V}_{max}$ of phase 0, maximum diastolic potential, and action potential amplitude in the sinus and AV nodal cells and prolongs conduction time and the effective and functional refractory periods of the AV node. The AV nodal blocking effects of verapamil and diltiazem[245] are more apparent at faster rates of stimulation (use-dependence) and in depolarized fibers (voltage-dependence). Verapamil slows the activation and delays recovery from inactivation of the slow channel. Unbinding of the drug from its receptor occurs more rapidly in tissue that is hyperpolarized.

Verapamil does exert some local anesthetic activity because the dextrorotatory stereoisomer of the clinically used racemic mixture exerts slight blocking effects on I_{Na}. The levorotatory stereoisomer blocks the slow inward current carried by calcium, as well as other ions, traveling through the slow channel. Verapamil does not modify calcium uptake, binding, or exchange by cardiac microsomes, nor does it affect calcium-activated ATPase. Verapamil does not block beta receptors and may block alpha receptors and potentiate vagal effects on the AV node. Verapamil also may cause other effects that indirectly alter cardiac electrophysiology, such as decreasing platelet adhesiveness or reducing the extent of myocardial ischemia.

In vivo, both in experimental animals and in humans, verapamil prolongs conduction time through the AV node (the A-H interval) without affecting the P-A, H-V, or QRS interval and lengthens the anterograde and retrograde functional and effective refractory periods of the AV node. Spontaneous sinus rate may decrease slightly, an event only partially reversed by atropine. More commonly, the sinus rate does not change significantly in vivo because verapamil causes peripheral vasodilation, transient hypotension, and reflex sympathetic stimulation that mitigates any direct slowing effect verapamil may exert on the sinus node. If verapamil is given to a patient who is also receiving a beta blocker, the sinus nodal discharge rate may slow because reflex sympathetic stimulation is blocked. Verapamil does not exert a direct effect on atrial or ventricular refractoriness or on anterograde or retrograde properties of accessory pathways. However, reflex sympathetic stimulation may increase the ventricular response over the accessory pathway during atrial fibrillation in patients with the Wolff-Parkinson-White syndrome.

HEMODYNAMIC EFFECTS. Since verapamil interferes with excitation-contraction coupling, it inhibits vascular smooth muscle contraction and causes marked vasodilation in coronary and other peripheral vascular beds. Propranolol does not block the vasodilation produced by verapamil. Reflex sympathetic effects may reduce in vivo the marked negative inotropic action of verapamil on isolated cardiac muscle, but direct myocardial depressant effects of verapamil may predominate when the drug is given in high doses. In patients with well-preserved left ventricular function, combined therapy with propranolol and verapamil appears to be well tolerated, but beta blockade can accentuate the hemodynamic depressant effects produced by oral verapamil. Patients who have reduced left ventricular function may not tolerate the combined blockade of beta receptors and of slow channels, and the combined use of verapamil and propranolol in these patients must be undertaken cautiously or not at all. Verapamil decreases myocardial oxygen demand while decreasing coronary vascular resistance and reduces the extent of ischemic damage in experimental preparations. Such changes may be antiarrhythmic. Diltiazem also reduces ventricular arrhythmias during coronary occlusion in the dog, possibly by preventing calcium overload. In a hamster model of hereditary cardiomyopathy, verapamil prevents progression of the disease and the secondary heart failure.

Peak alterations in hemodynamic variables occur 3 to 5 minutes after completion of the verapamil injection, the major effects being dissipated within 10 minutes. Mean arterial pressure decreases and left ventricular end-diastolic pressure increases; systemic resistance decreases and left ventricular dP/dt max decreases. Heart rate, cardiac index, left ventricular minute work, and mean pulmonary artery pressure do not change significantly. Thus afterload reduction produced by verapamil significantly minimizes its negative inotropic action so that cardiac index may not be reduced. In addition, when verapamil slows the ventricular rate in a patient with a tachycardia, cardiac slowing also may improve hemodynamics. Nevertheless, caution should be exercised when giving verapamil to patients with severe myocardial depression or those receiving beta blockers or disopyramide because hemodynamic deterioration may progress in some patients.

PHARMACOKINETICS (Table 21–1). Following single oral doses of verapamil, measurable prolongation of AV nodal conduction time occurs in 30 minutes and lasts 4 to 6 hours. After intravenous administration, AV nodal conduction delay occurs within 1 to 2 minutes, and A-H interval prolongation is still detectable after 6 hours. Effective plasma concentrations necessary to terminate supraventricular tachycardia are in the range of 125 ng/ml following doses of 0.075 to 0.150 mg/kg. After oral administration, absorption is almost complete, but an overall bioavailability of 20 to 35 per cent suggests substantial first-pass metabolism in the liver, particularly of the l-isomer. The elimination half-life of verapamil is 3 to 7 hours, with up to 70 per cent of the drug excreted by the kidneys. Norverapamil is a major metabolite that may contribute to verapamil's electrophysiological actions. Serum protein binding is approximately 90 per cent. With diltiazem, percentage of heart rate reduction in atrial fibrillation relates to plasma concentration.[246]

DOSAGE AND ADMINISTRATION (Table 21–1). The most commonly used intravenous dose is 10 mg infused over 1 to 2 minutes while cardiac rhythm and blood pressure are monitored. A second injection of equal dose may be given 30 minutes later. The initial effect achieved with the first bolus injection, such as slowing of the ventricular response during atrial fibrillation, may be maintained by a continuous infusion of the drug at a rate of 0.005 mg/kg/min. The oral dose is 240 to 480 mg/day in divided doses. Diltiazem is given intravenously at a dose of 0.25 mg/kg as a bolus over 2 minutes, with a second dose in 15 minutes if necessary. Orally, doses must be adjusted to the patient's needs with a 120- to 360-mg range. Various long-acting preparations exist for verapamil and diltiazem.

INDICATIONS. After simple vagal maneuvers have been tried and adenosine given, intravenous verapamil or diltiazem[247] is the next treatment of choice for terminating sustained sinus nodal reentry, AV nodal reentry, or orthodromic AV reciprocating tachycardia associated with the Wolff-Parkinson-White syndrome. Verapamil is as effective as adenosine for termination of these arrhythmias.[248] Verapamil should definitely be tried prior to attempting termination by digitalis administration, pacing, electrical direct-current cardioversion, or acute blood pressure elevation with vasopressors. Verapamil and diltiazem terminate 60 to more than 90 per cent of episodes of paroxysmal supraventricular tachycardias within several minutes. Verapamil may be of use in some fetal supraventricular tachycardias as well. Although intravenous verapamil has been given along with intravenous propranolol, this combination should be used only with great caution.

Verapamil and diltiazem decrease the ventricular response over the AV node during atrial fibrillation or atrial flutter, possibly converting a small number of episodes to sinus rhythm, particularly if the atrial flutter or fibrillation is of recent onset.[126] Some patients who exhibit atrial flutter may develop atrial fibrillation following verapamil administration. Quinidine, flecainide, and esmolol appear to be more effective than verapamil in establishing and maintaining sinus rhythm in patients with atrial fibrillation. As noted earlier, in patients with atrial fibrillation associated with the Wolff-Parkinson-White syndrome, intravenous verapamil may *accelerate* the ventricular response, and therefore, the intravenous route is contraindicated in this situation. Verapamil can terminate some atrial tachycardias. Even though verapamil terminates a left septal ventricular tachycardia,[249] hemodynamic collapse can occur if intravenous verapamil is given to patients with the more common forms of ventricular tachycardia. *A general rule to avoid complications, however, is to not give intravenous verapamil to any patient with wide-QRS tachycardia unless one is absolutely certain of the nature of the tachycardia and its response to verapamil.*

Orally, verapamil or diltiazem may prevent the recurrence of AV nodal reentrant and orthodromic AV reciprocating tachycardias[247,248,250] associated with the Wolff-Parkinson-White syndrome as well as help maintain a decreased ventricular response during atrial flutter or atrial fibrillation in patients without an accessory pathway.[251–253] In this regard, the effectiveness of verapamil appears to be enhanced when given concomitantly with quinidine, and diltiazem when given with digoxin.[254] Verapamil generally has not been effective in treating patients who have recurrent ventricular tachyarrhythmias, although it may suppress some forms of ventricular tachycardia such as a left septal ventricular tachycardia,[249,254a,255–258] as noted above. It may be useful in about two-thirds of patients with idiopathic ventricular tachycardia that has a left bundle branch block morphology,[254a] in patients with hypertrophic cardiomyopathy who have experienced cardiac arrest,[259] in patients with a short-coupled variant of torsades de pointes,[260] in patients with right ventricular dysplasia,[240] and in patients with ventricular arrhythmias due to coronary artery spasm.[261] While data from animal models suggest that verapamil may be useful in reducing or preventing ventricular arrhythmias due to acute myocardial ischemia, calcium antagonists have not been shown to reduce mortality or prevent sudden cardiac death in patients after acute myocardial infarction, except for diltiazem in patients with non-Q-wave infarctions. Verapamil abolishes the wall motion abnormality found in patients with the long Q-T syndrome.[262]

ADVERSE EFFECTS. Verapamil must be used cautiously in patients with significant hemodynamic impairment or in those receiving beta blockers, as previously noted. Hypotension, bradycardia, AV block, and asystole are more likely to occur when the drug is given to patients who are already receiving beta-blocking agents. Hemodynamic collapse has been noted in infants, and verapamil should be used cautiously in patients less than 1 year old. Verapamil also should be used with caution in patients with sinus node abnormalities, since marked depression of sinus nodal function or asystole can result in some of these patients. Isoproterenol, calcium, glucagon infusion, dopamine, or atropine (which may be only partially effective) or temporary pacing may be necessary to counteract some of the adverse effects of verapamil. Isoproterenol may be more effective for treating bradyarrhythmias and calcium for treating hemodynamic dysfunction secondary to verapamil. AV nodal depression is common in overdoses.[263] Contraindications to the use of verapamil and diltiazem include the presence of advanced heart failure, second or third degree AV block without a pacemaker in place, atrial fibrillation and anterograde conduction over an accessory pathway, significant sinus node dysfunction, most ventricular tachycardias, cardiogenic shock, and other hypotensive states. While the drugs probably should not be used in patients with manifest heart failure, if the latter is due to one of the supraventricular tachyarrhythmias noted earlier, verapamil or diltiazem may restore sinus rhythm or significantly decrease the ventricular rate, leading to hemodynamic improvement. Finally, it is important to note that verapamil can decrease the excretion of digoxin by about 30 per cent. Hepatotoxicity may occur on occasion.

OTHER ANTIARRHYTHMIC AGENTS

Adenosine

Adenosine is an endogenous nucleoside present throughout the body and has been approved by the FDA to treat patients with supraventricular tachycardias.[264]

ELECTROPHYSIOLOGICAL ACTIONS (Tables 21–6 and 21–7). Adenosine interacts with A_1 receptors present on the extracellular surface of cardiac cells, activating K^+ channels ($I_{K\ Ach}$, $I_{K\ Ado}$) in a fashion similar to that produced by acetylcholine. The increase in K^+ conductance shortens atrial action potential duration, hyperpolarizes the membrane potential, and decreases atrial contractility. Similar changes occur in the sinus and AV nodes. In contrast to these direct effects mediated through guanine nucleotide regulatory proteins G_i and G_o, adenosine antagonizes catecholamine-stimulated adenylate cyclase to decrease cyclic AMP accumulation and to decrease $I_{Ca\text{-}L}$ and the pacemaker current i_f in sinus nodal cells. $\dot{V}_{max}$ is reduced. Shifts in pacemaker site within the sinus node and sinus exit block may occur. Reflex-mediated sinus tachycardia can follow adenosine administration. In the N region of the AV node, conduction is depressed, along with decreases in action potential amplitude, duration, and $\dot{V}_{max}$. Adenosine slows the sinus rate in humans, which is followed by a reflex increase in sinus discharge. Transient prolongation of the A-H interval results, often with transient first, second, or third degree AV nodal block. Delay in AV nodal conduction is rate-dependent.[265] His-Purkinje conduction is generally not directly affected. Adenosine does not affect conduction in normal accessory pathways. Conduction may be blocked in accessory pathways that have long conduction times or decremental conduction properties. Patients with heart transplants exhibit a supersensitive response to adenosine.[266] Adenosine may mediate the phenomenon of preconditioning ischemia.[264]

PHARMACOKINETICS. Adenosine is removed from the extracellular space by washout, enzymatically by degradation to inosine, by phosphorylation to AMP, or by reuptake into cells via a nucleoside transport system. The vascular endothelium and the formed blood elements contain these elimination systems that result in very rapid clearance of adenosine from the circulation. Elimination half-life is 1 to 6 seconds. Most of adenosine's effects are produced during its first passage through the circulation. Important drug interactions occur. Methyl xanthines are competitive antagonists, and therapeutic concentrations of theophylline totally block the exogeneous adenosine effect. Dipyridamole is a nucleoside transport blocker that blocks reuptake of adenosine, delaying its clearance from the circulation or interstitial space and potentiating its effect. Smaller adenosine doses should be used in patients receiving dipyridamole.

DOSAGE AND ADMINISTRATION. To terminate tachycardia, a bolus of adenosine is injected intravenously rapidly into a central vein (if possible) at doses of 6 to 12 mg. When given into a central vein, and in patients after heart transplantation, or in patients receiving dipyridamole, the initial dose should be reduced to 3 mg.[267] Transient sinus slowing or AV nodal block results.

INDICATIONS. Adenosine has become the drug of first choice to terminate acutely a supraventricular tachycardia such as AV junctional tachycardias[268] or AV nodal or AV reentry.[269–273] It is useful in pediatric patients[274,275] and to judge the effectiveness of ablation of accessory pathways.[276] Adenosine can produce AV block or terminate atrial tachycardias[277,278] and sinus node reentry. It results in transient AV block during atrial flutter or fibrillation. Adenosine terminates a group of ventricular tachycardias whose maintenance depends on adrenergic drive, most often located in the right ventricular outflow tract, but found at other sites as well.[256,279–281] Adenosine has less potential than verapamil for lowering the blood pressure should tachycardia persist after injection.

Doses as low as 2.5 mg terminate some tachycardias; doses of 12 mg or less terminate 92 per cent of supraventricular tachycardias, usually within 30 seconds. Successful termination rates with adenosine are comparable with those achieved with verapamil. Because of its effectiveness and extremely short duration of action, adenosine is preferable to verapamil in most instances, particularly in patients who previously have received intravenous beta-adrenoceptor blockers, in those having poorly compensated heart failure or severe hypotension, and in neonates. Verapamil might be chosen first in patients receiving drugs, such as theophylline, known to interfere with adenosine's actions or metabolism, in patients with active bronchoconstriction, and in those with inadequate venous access. Adenosine produces transient AV nodal block in patients with atrial flutter, atrial fibrillation, and some types of atrial tachycardia, facilitating the diagnosis by exposing the atrial rhythm.

Adenosine may be useful to help differentiate wide-QRS tachycardias,[281] since it terminates many supraventricular tachycardias with aberrancy or reveals the underlying atrial mechanism, and it does not block conduction over the accessory pathway or terminate most ventricular tachycardias. Adenosine does terminate some ventricular tachycardias, and therefore tachycardia termination is not completely diagnostic for a supraventricular tachycardia.[282] This agent may predispose to the development of atrial fibrillation and possibly can increase the ventricular response in patients with atrial fibrillation conducting over an accessory pathway. Adenosine also may be useful in differentiating conduction over the AV node versus an accessory pathway during ablative procedures designed to interrupt the accessory pathway. Endogenously released adenosine may be important in ischemia and hypoxia-induced AV nodal block and in postdefibrillation bradyarrhythmias.

ADVERSE EFFECTS. Transient side effects occur in almost 40 per cent of patients with supraventricular tachycardia given adenosine and are most commonly flushing, dyspnea, and chest pressure. These symptoms are fleeting, generally less than 1 minute, and are well tolerated. Premature ventricular complexes, transient sinus bradycardia, sinus arrest, and AV block are common when a supraventricular tachycardia abruptly terminates. Induction of atrial fibrillation can be problematic in patients with the Wolff-Parkinson-White syndrome or rapid AV conduction.[283,284]

ELECTRICAL THERAPY OF CARDIAC ARRHYTHMIAS

DIRECT-CURRENT CARDIOVERSION

Electrical cardioversion offers obvious advantages over drug therapy in terminating tachycardia. Under conditions optimal for close supervision and monitoring, a precisely regulated "dose" of electricity can restore sinus rhythm immediately and safely. The distinction between supraventricular and ventricular tachyarrhythmias—crucial to the proper medical management of arrhythmias—becomes less significant, and the time-consuming titration of drugs with potential side effects is abolished.[285]

MECHANISMS. Electrical cardioversion appears to terminate most effectively those tachycardias presumed to be due to reentry, such as atrial flutter and atrial fibrillation, AV nodal reentry, reciprocating tachycardias associated with Wolff-Parkinson-White syndrome, most forms of ventricular tachycardia, ventricular flutter, and ventricular fibrillation. The electrical shock, by depolarizing all excitable myocardium, and possibly by prolonging refractoriness, interrupts reentrant circuits, discharges foci, and establishes electrical homogeneity that terminates reentry. The mechanism by which a shock successfully terminates ventricular fibrillation has not been completely explained. If the precipitating factors are no longer present, interrupting the tachyarrhythmia for only the brief time produced by the shock may prevent its return for long duration even though the anatomical and electrophysiological substrates required for the tachycardia are still present.

Tachycardias thought to be due to disorders of impulse formation (automaticity) include parasystole, some forms of atrial tachycardia, nonparoxysmal AV junctional tachycardia, and accelerated idioventricular rhythms. An attempt to cardiovert these tachycardias electrically is not indicated in most instances. It has not been established whether the shock can terminate tachycardias due to enhanced automaticity or triggered activity.

TECHNIQUE. Prior to elective cardioversion, a careful physical examination, including palpation of all pulses, should be performed, A 12-lead electrocardiogram is obtained before and after cardioversion, as well as a rhythm strip during the electroshock. The patient, who should be informed completely about what to expect, is in a fasting state and "metabolically balanced," i.e., blood gases, pH, and electrolytes should be normal with no evidence of drug toxicity. Withholding digitalis for several days before elective cardioversion in patients without clinical evidence of digitalis toxicity is not necessary. Maintenance antiarrhythmic drug administration 1 to 2 days before electrical cardioversion of patients with atrial fibrillation may revert some patients to sinus rhythm, may help prevent recurrence of atrial fibrillation once sinus rhythm is restored, and may help determine patient tolerance to the drug.

Self-adhesive pads applied in the standard apex-anterior or apex-posterior paddle positions have transthoracic impedances similar to paddles and are very useful in elective cardioversions or other situations in which there is time for their application, such as at the start of an electrophysiological study.[286] Paddles 12 to 13 cm in diameter can be used to deliver maximum current to the heart, but the benefits of these paddles as compared with those of 8 to 9 cm diameter have not been clearly established. Larger paddles may distribute the intracardiac current over a wider area and may reduce shock-induced myocardial necrosis.

A synchronized shock, i.e., one delivered during the QRS complex, is used for all cardioversions except for very rapid ventricular tachyarrhythmias, such as ventricular flutter or fibrillation. Recent data suggest that for internal cardioversion, shocks delivered late in the QRS complex during ventricular tachycardia are more effective and have a lower risk of acceleration than those delivered near QRS onset.[287] Because myocardial damage increases directly with increases in applied energy, the minimum effective energy should be used. Therefore, shocks are "titrated" when the clinical situation permits. Except for atrial fibrillation, shocks in the range of 25 to 50 joules successfully terminate most supraventricular tachycardias and should be tried initially. If unsuccessful, a second shock of higher energy can be delivered. The starting level to terminate atrial fibrillation should probably be 50 to 100 joules. Intracardiac defibrillation can be tried if external cardioversion fails.[288–290] For patients with stable ventricular tachycardia, starting levels in the range of 25 to 50 joules can be employed. If there is some urgency to terminate the tachyarrhythmia, one can begin with higher energies. To terminate ventricular fibrillation, 200 to 400 joules generally are used, although much lower energies (<100 joules) terminate ventricular fibrillation when the shock is delivered at the *very onset* of the arrhythmia, using adhesive pads in the electrophysiology laboratory, for example. Research in new waveforms will likely improve defibrillation capabilities.[291–294]

During elective cardioversion, a short-acting barbiturate such as methohexital or an amnesic such as diazepam or midazolam can be used. A physician skilled in airway management should be in attendance, an intravenous route should be established, and all equipment necessary for emergency resuscitation should be immediately accessible. Before cardioversion, 100 per cent oxygen may be administered for 5 to 15 minutes and is continued throughout the procedure. Manual ventilation of the patient may be necessary to avoid hypoxia during periods of deepest sleep.

INDICATIONS. As a rule, any tachycardia that produces hypotension, congestive heart failure, or angina and does not respond promptly to medical management should be terminated electrically. Very rapid ventricular rates in patients with atrial fibrillation and the Wolff-Parkinson-White syndrome are often best treated by electrical cardioversion. In almost all instances, the patient's hemodynamic status improves after cardioversion. An occasional patient may develop hypotension, reduced cardiac output, or congestive heart failure following the shock. This may be related to complications of the cardioversion, such as embolic events, myocardial depression resulting from the anesthetic agent or the shock itself,[295,296] hypoxia, lack of restoration of left atrial contraction despite return of electrical atrial systole,[297] or post-shock arrhythmias. Direct-current countershock of digitalis-induced tachyarrhythmias is contraindicated.

Favorable candidates for electrical cardioversion of atrial fibrillation include those patients who (1) have symptomatic atrial fibrillation of less than 12 months' duration and derive significant hemodynamic benefits from sinus rhythm, (2) have embolic episodes, (3) continue to have atrial fibrillation after the precipitating cause has been removed (e.g., following treatment of thyrotoxicosis), and (4) have a rapid ventricular rate that is difficult to slow.

Unfavorable candidates include patients with (1) digitalis toxicity, (2) no symptoms and a well-controlled ventricular rate without therapy, (3) sinus node dysfunction and various unstable supraventricular tachyarrhythmias or bradyarrhythmias (often the bradycardia-tachycardia syndrome) who finally develop and maintain atrial fibrillation (which in essence represents a "cure" of the sick sinus syndrome), (4) little or no benefit from normal sinus rhythm who promptly revert to atrial fibrillation after cardioversion despite drug therapy, (5) a large left atrium and longstanding atrial fibrillation, (6) infrequent episodes of atrial fibrillation that revert spontaneously to sinus rhythm, (7) no mechanical atrial systole after the return of electrical atrial systole, (8) atrial fibrillation and advanced heart block, (9) cardiac surgery planned in the near future, and (10) antiarrhythmic drug intolerance. Atrial fibrillation is likely to recur after cardioversion in patients who have significant chronic obstructive lung disease, congestive heart failure, mitral valve disease (particularly mitral regurgitation), atrial fibrillation longer than 1 year, and an enlarged left atrium.

In patients with atrial flutter, slowing the ventricular rate by administering digitalis or terminating the flutter with an antiarrhythmic agent may be difficult, so electrical cardioversion is often the initial treatment of choice. For the patient with other types of supraventricular tachycardia, electrical cardioversion may be employed when (1) vagal maneuvers or simple medical management (e.g., intravenous adenosine and verapamil) has failed to terminate the tachycardia and (2) the clinical setting indicates that fairly prompt restoration of sinus rhythm is desirable because of hemodynamic decompensation or electrophysiological consequences of the tachycardia. Similarly, in patients with ventricular tachycardia, the hemodynamic and electrophysiological consequences of the arrhythmias determine the need and urgency for direct-current cardioversion (see p. 680). Electrical countershock is the *initial* treatment of choice for ventricular flutter or ventricular fibrillation.[285,298,299] Speed is essential.

If, after the first shock, reversion to sinus rhythm does not occur, a higher energy level should be tried. When transient ventricular arrhythmias result after an unsuccessful shock, a bolus of lidocaine can be given prior to delivering a shock at the next energy level. If sinus rhythm returns only transiently and is promptly supplanted by the tachycardia, a repeat shock can be tried, depending on the tachyarrhythmia being treated and its consequences. Administration of an antiarrhythmic agent intravenously may be useful prior to delivering the next cardioversion shock. After cardioversion, the patient should be monitored at least until full consciousness has been restored and preferably for several hours thereafter.

RESULTS. Cardioversion restores sinus rhythm in 70 to 95 per cent of patients depending on the type of tachyarrhythmia. However, sinus rhythm remains after 12 months in less than one-third to one-half the patients with chronic atrial fibrillation. Thus, maintenance of sinus rhythm, once established, is the difficult problem, not the immediate termination of the tachycardia, and depends on the particular arrhythmia, the presence of underlying heart disease, and the response to antiarrhythmic drug therapy. Atrial size decreases following termination of atrial fibrillation and restoration of sinus rhythm,[300,301] and functional capacity improves.[302–304]

COMPLICATIONS. Arrhythmias induced by the cardioversion generally are caused by inadequate synchronization, with the shock occurring during the ST segment or T wave. Occasionally, a properly synchronized shock can produce ventricular fibrillation (Fig. 21–6). Post-shock arrhythmias usually are transient and do not require therapy. Embolic episodes are reported to occur in 1 to 3 per cent of the patients converted from atrial fibrillation to sinus rhythm. Prior anticoagulation for 2 to 3 weeks should be considered for patients who have no contraindication to such therapy and have atrial fibrillation present for longer than 2 to 3 days. This is particularly true for those who are at high risk for emboli, such as those with mitral stenosis and atrial fibrillation of recent onset, a history of recent or recurrent emboli, a prosthetic mitral valve, enlarged heart (including left atrial enlargement), or congestive heart failure. Anticoagulation with warfarin for several weeks afterward is recommended. Importantly, exclusion of left atrial thrombus by transesophageal echocardiography does not preclude embolism after cardioversion of atrial fibrillation.[305–308] Atrial thrombi may be present in patients with nonfibrillation atrial tachyarrhythmias and congenital heart disease.[309]

Although direct-current shock has been demonstrated in animals to cause cardiac injury, studies in humans indicate that elevations of myocardial enzymes after cardioversion are not common. ST-segment elevation can occur with elective direct-current cardioversion, although cardiac enzymes and myocardial scintigraphy may be unremarkable. A decrease in serum K^+ and Mg^{++} can occur after cardioversion of ventricular tachycardia.[310]

Cardioversion of ventricular tachycardia also can be achieved by a chest thump. Its mechanism of termination probably relates to a mechanically induced premature atrial or ventricular complex that interrupts a tachycardia. The thump cannot be timed very well and is probably only effective when delivered during a nonrefractory part of the cardiac cycle. Care must therefore be taken, because the thump can alter a ventricular tachycardia and possibly induce ventricular flutter or fibrillation if it occurs during the vulnerable period of the T wave.

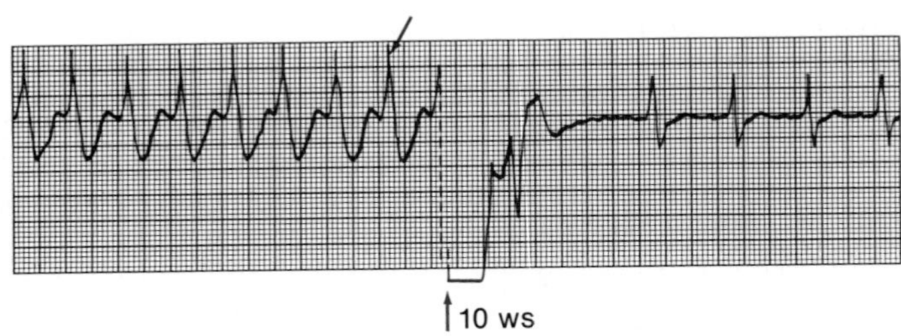

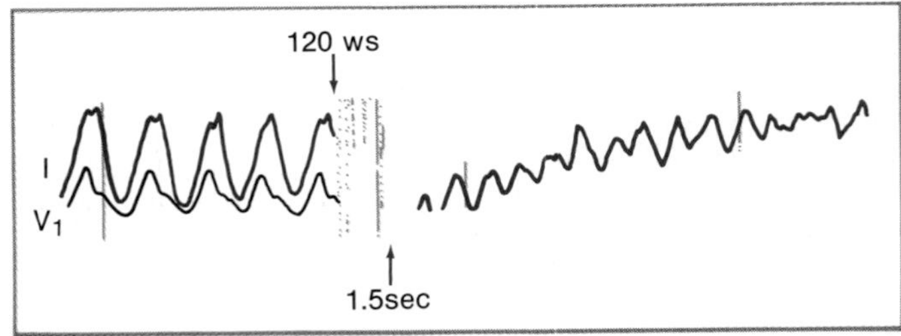

FIGURE 21–6. *Top,* A synchronized shock (note synchronization marks in the apex of the QRS complex [↓]) during ventricular tachycardia is followed by a single repetitive ventricular response and then normal sinus rhythm. *Bottom,* A shock synchronized to the terminal portion of the QRS complex in a patient with atrial fibrillation and conduction to the ventricle over an accessory pathway (WPW syndrome) results in ventricular fibrillation that was promptly terminated by a 400 joule shock. Recording was lost for 1.5 sec (↑) owing to baseline drift after the shock.

IMPLANTABLE ELECTRICAL DEVICES FOR TREATMENT OF CARDIAC ARRHYTHMIAS

Implantable devices that monitor the cardiac rhythm and can deliver competing pacing stimuli and low- and high-energy shocks have been used effectively in selected patients and are discussed fully in Chapter 23.

ABLATION THERAPY OF CARDIAC ARRHYTHMIAS

Ablation Therapy

The purpose of catheter ablation is to destroy myocardial tissue by delivering electrical energy over electrodes on a catheter placed next to an area of the endocardium integrally related to the onset and/or maintenance of the arrhythmia. Lasers, cryothermy, and microwave energy sources have been used, but not commonly. RF catheter ablation (Fig. 21–7) has largely replaced the DC shock. RF energy is delivered from an external generator and destroys tissue by controlled heat production (Fig. 21–8).

Radiofrequency Catheter Ablation of Accessory Pathways

LOCATION OF PATHWAYS. The safety, efficacy, and cost-effectiveness of RF catheter ablation of an accessory atrioventricular pathway[311–314] have made ablation the treatment of choice in most adult and many pediatric patients who have AV reentrant tachycardia[315] or atrial flutter/fibrillation associated with a rapid ventricular response over the accessory pathway.[316–319] However, the fact that the lesion size, when RF energy is delivered to an immature heart, can increase as the heart grows makes the long-term outlook for ablation less certain in the very young.[320–324] RF energy has replaced DC shock as the optimal energy source.[325–327]

An electrophysiological study is performed initially, to determine that the accessory pathway is part of the tachycardia circuit and to locate the optimal site for ablation. Pathways can be located in the right or left free wall or septum of the heart (Fig. 21–9). Septal accessory pathways are classified as anteroseptal, midseptal, and posteroseptal.[328–331] Parahissian pathways can be distinguished from anteroseptal pathways.[329] Midseptal locations are true septal pathways, while those classified as anteroseptal generally have no septal connection but are located anteriorly along the central fibrous body or the right fibrous trigone at the right anterior free wall. Pathways classified as posteroseptal are located posterior to the central fibrous body within the pyramidal space. Anteroseptal pathways are found near the His bundle, and accessory pathway activation potential as well as a His bundle potential can be recorded simultaneously from a catheter placed at the His bundle region. Midseptal pathways are classified as right midseptal if an accessory pathway potential is recorded through a catheter located in an area bounded anteriorly by the tip electrode of the His bundle catheter and posteriorly by the coronary sinus ostium. For left midseptal pathways, the accessory pathway potential recording catheter is

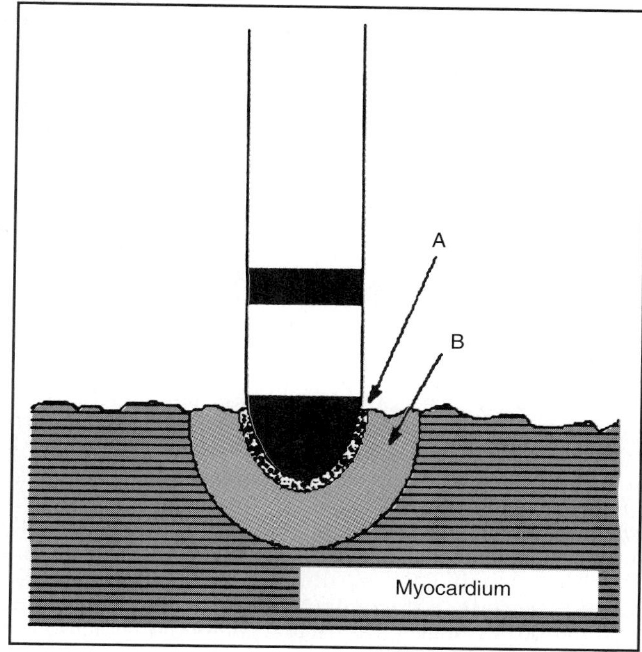

FIGURE 21–8. Mechanism of heating during radiofrequency catheter ablation. Because current density drops off rapidly as a function of distance from the electrode surface, only a small shell of myocardium adjacent to the distal electrode *(A)* is heated directly. The major portion of the lesion *(B)* is produced by conduction of heat away from the electrode-tissue interface into surrounding tissue. (From Langberg, J. J., and Leon, A.: Energy sources for catheter ablation. *In* Zipes, D. P., and Jalife, J. [eds.]: Cardiac Electrophysiology: From Cell to Bedside. 2nd ed. Philadelphia, W. B. Saunders Company, 1994, pp. 1434–1441.)

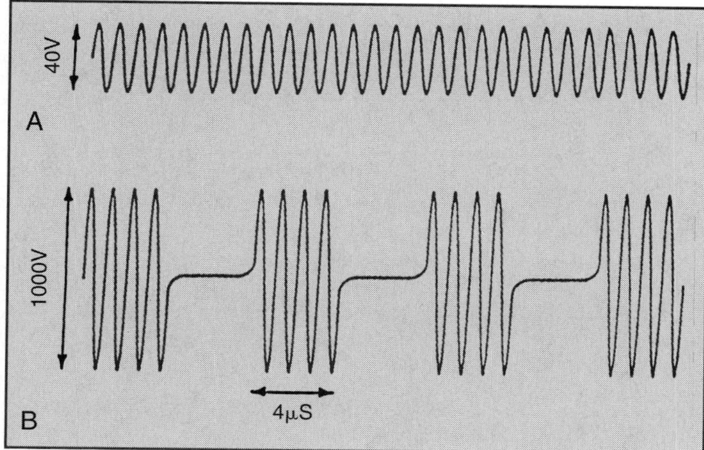

FIGURE 21–7. Comparison of output waveforms used for radiofrequency catheter ablation *(A)* and electrosurgical cutting *(B)*. Resistive heating during ablation is produced by a relatively low voltage (40 to 70 V) delivered in a continuous unmodulated fashion. The brief, high-voltage pulses used during electrosurgery promote arcing and coagulum formation. (From Kalbfleisch, S. J., and Langberg, J. J.: Catheter ablation with radiofrequency energy: biophysical aspects and clinical applications. J. Cardiovasc. Electrophysiol. *3:*173, 1992.)

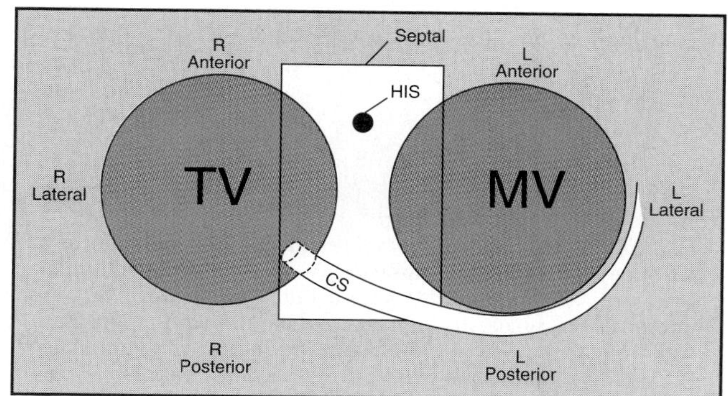

FIGURE 21–9. Schematic of free wall accessory pathway locations around the mitral and tricuspid annuli as visualized in the left anterior oblique projection. TV = tricuspid valve; MV = mitral valve; CS = coronary sinus; and His = His bundle. (From Miles, W. M., Zipes, D. P., and Klein, L. S.: Ablation of free wall accessory pathways. *In* Zipes, D. P. [ed.]: Catheter Ablation of Arrhythmias. Armonk, N.Y., Futura Publishing Company, 1994, pp. 211–230.)

placed at the left side of the septum within a similar region. Right posteroseptal pathways insert along the tricuspid ring in the immediate vicinity of the coronary sinus ostium, while left posteroseptal pathways are close to the terminal portion of the coronary sinus and may be located at a subepicardial site around the proximal coronary sinus, within a middle cardiac vein, or subendocardially along the ventricular aspect of the mitral annulus. Pathways at all locations and in all age groups can be ablated successfully.[332,333] Multiple pathways are present in about 5 per cent of patients.[334,335] Epicardial locations may be more easily approached from within the coronary sinus.[336] Conduction block after ablation usually occurs between the local atrial electrogram and the accessory pathway potential.[337]

ABLATION SITE. The optimal ablation site can be found by direct recordings of the accessory pathway (Fig. 21–10). The ventricular insertion site can be determined by finding the site of the earliest onset of the ventricular electrogram in relation to the onset of the delta wave, while the atrial insertion site can be found by locating the region of the shortest ventriculoatrial interval. Other helpful guidelines are unfiltered unipolar recordings that register a QS wave and the shortest AV conduction time during maximal preexcitation. A major ventricular potential synchronous with the onset of the delta wave can be a target site in left-sided preexcitation, while earlier ventricular excitation in relation to the delta wave is to be found for right-sided preexcitation. Reproducible mechanical inhibition of accessory pathway conduction[338] and subthreshold stimulation[339] also have been used to determine the optimal site. Accidental catheter trauma should be avoided, however.[340] Intracardiac echocardiography can be helpful at times.[341,342]

Accessory pathways often cross the left atrioventricular groove obliquely, with the atrial insertion site located closer to the ostium of the coronary sinus.[343] Therefore, a retrograde accessory pathway potential is recorded proximally close to the atrial potential at the atrial insertion site of the accessory pathway and recorded distally close to the ventricular potential at the ventricular insertion site. Consequently, the earliest site of retrograde atrial activation and the earliest site of anterograde ventricular activation are not directly across the AV groove from each other. Thus, if ablation of the accessory pathway is from the atrial aspect of the mitral annulus, the site of earliest atrial activation is the optimal site for ablation, while if the ventricular aspect of the mitral annulus is the ablation target, the site of earliest ventricular activation would be the optimal position. Identification of the earliest site of atrial activation is usually performed during orthodromic atrioventricular reentrant tachycardia (AVRT).

. Successful ablation sites should exhibit stable fluoroscopic and electrical characteristics. During orthodromic AVRT, the interval between the onset of ventricular activation in any lead and local atrial activation is usually 70 to 90 msec at the successful ablation site. When thermistor-tipped ablation catheters are used, a stable rise in catheter tip temperature is a helpful adjunct to insure catheter stability and adequate catheter-tissue contact. In such an instance, the tip temperature generally exceeds 50°C.[344] The retrograde transaortic and transseptal approaches have been used with equal success to ablate accessory pathways located on the left side of the heart.[345,346] Routine electrophysiological study performed weeks after the ablation procedure is generally not indicated but should be considered in patients who have recurrent delta wave or symptoms of tachycardia.[347,348]

Patients with atriofascicular accessory pathways have connections consisting of a proximal portion responsible for conduction delay and decremental conduction properties and a long distal segment located along the endocardial surface of the right ventricular free wall that has electrophysiological properties similar to the right bundle branch. The distal end of the right atriofascicular accessory pathway can insert into the apical region of the right ventricular free wall close to the distal right bundle branch or can actually fuse with the latter.[349] Right atriofascicular accessory pathways actually may represent a duplication of the AV conduction system and can be localized for ablation by recording potentials from the rapidly conducting distal component extending from the tricuspid annulus to the apical region of the right ventricular free wall.[350] Ablation attempts should be performed more proximally to avoid inadvertently ablating the distal right bundle branch, which could actually be proarrhythmic and create incessant tachycardia by lengthening the reentrant circuit.[351–353]

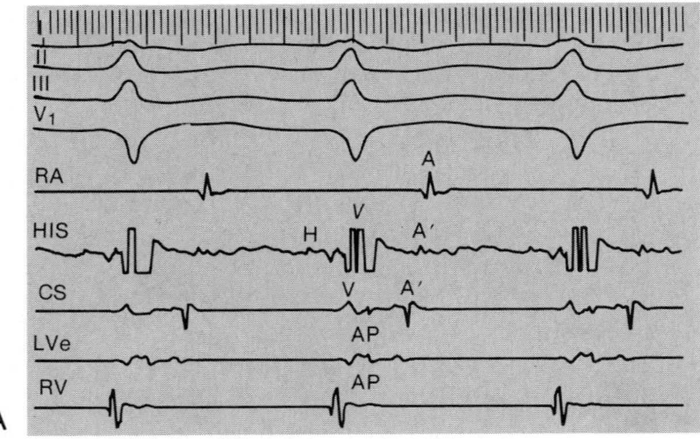

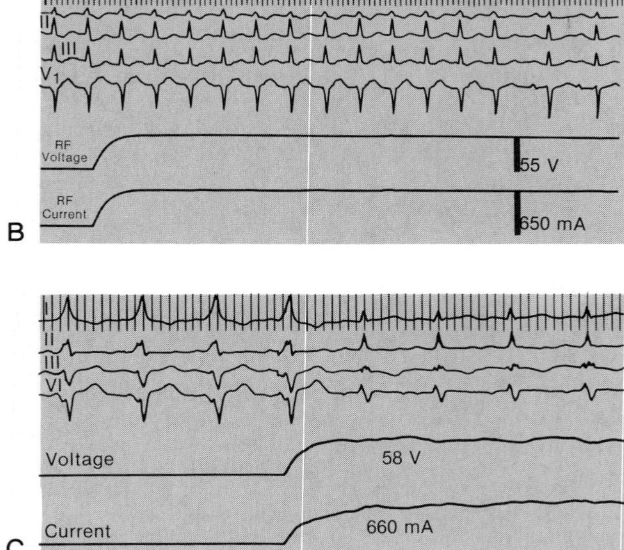

FIGURE 21–10. ***A*** **and** ***B*****, Radiofrequency (RF) ablation of a left free-wall accessory pathway.** ***A*****, Depicts atrioventricular reentrant tachycardia with anterograde conduction over the normal pathway and retrograde conduction over the left free-wall accessory pathway. The electrodes in the coronary sinus (CS) record activation over the accessory pathway (AP), which is apposed by the catheter positioned in the left ventricular endocardium (LV_e).** ***B*****, RF energy is delivered during the tachycardia and produces termination after 3.8 seconds. The delta wave has disappeared and tachycardia can no longer be initiated (not shown). Conventions as in Figure 21–11.** ***C*****, Radiofrequency catheter ablation of a right free-wall accessory pathway. Elimination of accessory pathway conduction almost immediately after delivery of radiofrequency energy indicates that the catheter is positioned virtually on the accessory pathway and best insures a successful ablation. Leads I, II, III, V scalar recordings. (From Zipes, D. P., et al.: Nonpharmacologic therapy: Can it replace antiarrhythmic drug therapy? J. Cardiovasc. Electrophysiol.** ***2*****:S255, 1991.)**

INDICATIONS. Ablation of accessory pathways is indicated in patients with symptomatic AV reentrant tachycardia that is drug resistant or when the patient is drug intolerant or does not desire long-term drug therapy. It is also indicated in patients with atrial fibrillation (or other atrial tachyarrhythmias) and a rapid ventricular response via accessory pathway when the tachycardia is drug resistant or when the patient is drug intolerant or does not desire long-term drug therapy. Other candidates might include patients with AVRT or atrial fibrillation with rapid ventricular rates identified during electrophysiological study of another arrhythmia; asymptomatic patients with ventricular preexcitation whose livelihood, profession, and important activities, insurability, mental well-being, or the public safety would be affected by spontaneous tachyarrhythmias or by the presence of the electrocardiographic abnormality; patients with atrial fibrillation and a controlled ventricular response via the accessory pathway; and patients with a family history of sudden cardiac death.[354]

RESULTS. From the results of a NASPE survey,[355] successful ablation of left free wall accessory pathways was obtained in 2312 of 2527 (91 per cent) patients; for septal accessory pathways, 1115 of 1279 (87 per cent); and for right free wall accessory pathways, 585 of 715 (82 per cent). Significant complications were reported in 94 of 4521 patients (2.1 per cent) and there were 13 procedure-related deaths in 4521 patients studies (0.2 per cent). In Europe, the complication rate was 4.4 per cent, with 3 deaths in 2222 patients.[356]

Radiofrequency Catheter Modification of the AV Node for AV Nodal Reentrant Tachycardias (AVNRT)

FAST-PATHWAY ABLATION. Ablation can be performed to eliminate conduction in the fast pathway or the slow pathway.[357–368] Ablation of the latter is preferred because the complication of heart block is minimized, patients with slow-slow reentry can be effectively treated and residual 1° AV block is avoided. Nevertheless, for fast-pathway ablation, the electrode tip is positioned along the AV node–His bundle axis in the anterosuperior portion of the tricuspid annulus. The catheter is gradually withdrawn until the atrial electrogram amplitude equals or exceeds that of the ventricular electrogram and the His bundle recording is either absent or extremely small (<0.05 mV). During energy delivery, the ECG is monitored for PR prolongation and/or the occurrence of AV block. If accelerated junctional rhythm is noted during delivery of RF energy, the atrium can be paced at a faster rate to ensure integrity of AV conduction. The initial RF pulse is delivered at 15 to 20 watts for 10 to 15 seconds and gradually increased. Endpoints are P-R prolongation, elimination of retrograde fast-pathway conduction, and noninducibility of AVNRT. An alternative approach is to apply RF current at the site of earliest retrograde atrial activation during tachycardia. RF current should be discontinued if the P-R interval prolongs by more than 50 per cent or if AV block results.[357,358]

The major electrophysiological effects of fast-pathway ablation are elimination or marked attenuation of ventriculoatrial conduction, an increase in the A-H interval, and elimination of dual AV nodal physiology (Fig. 21–11). Titrating the energy may reduce the risk of complete AV block, which is the most important complication associated with ablation of the fast pathway. If it is going to occur, complete AV block usually occurs during the ablation procedure, but some episodes have occurred 24 hours or more after the procedure, possibly as a result of the extension of the RF lesion over time. Tachycardia recurrence rate after successful fast-pathway ablation is approximately 10 to 15 per cent.[357,358]

SLOW-PATHWAY ABLATION. The slow pathway can be located by mapping along the posteromedial tricuspid annulus close to the coronary sinus os. Electrogram recordings

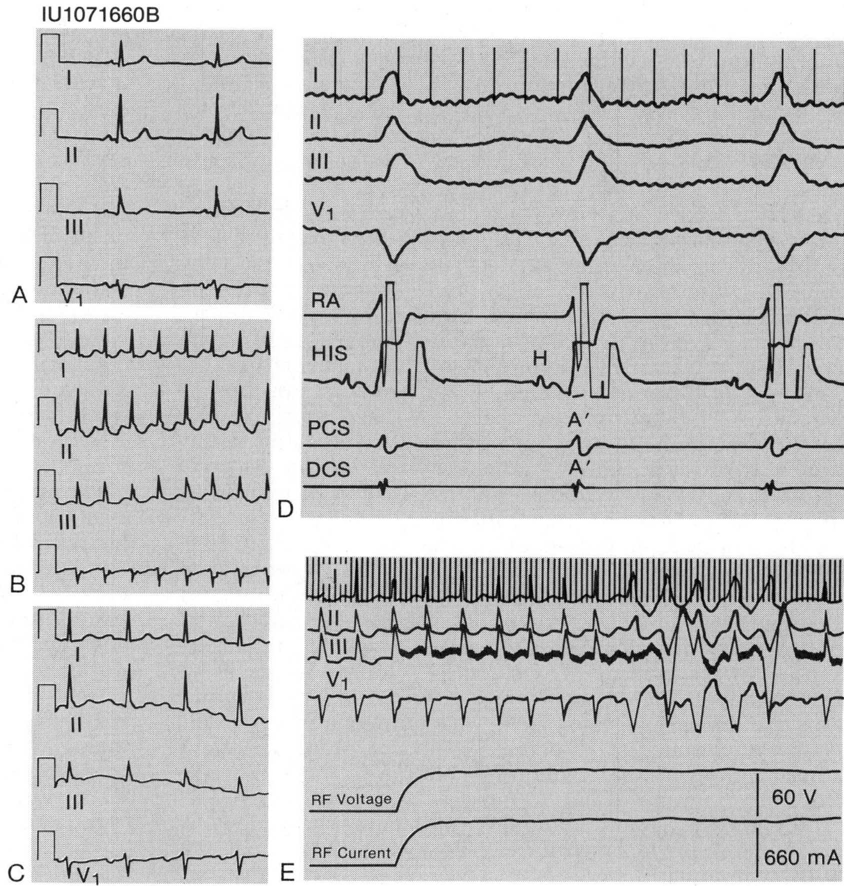

FIGURE 21–11. Radiofrequency (RF) AV nodal modification for AV nodal reentrant tachycardia. Panel *A*, Normal sinus rhythm. Panel *B*, AV nodal reentrant tachycardia. Panel *C*, Normal sinus rhythm following AV nodal ablation. Note prolonged P-R interval. Panel *D*, AV nodal reentrant tachycardia with intracavitary recordings. Note virtually simultaneous activation of atria and ventricles, consistent with AV nodal reentrant tachycardia. Panel *E*, Radiofrequency ablation with catheter placed in the anterior region of the AV node producing selective ablation of the anterogradely conducting fast pathway. Leads I, II, III, and V_1, scalar recordings. RA, right atrial electrogram; His, His bundle electrogram; PCS, electrogram recorded from the proximal electrodes of the coronary sinus catheter; DCS, electrogram recorded from the distal electrode of the coronary sinus catheter. Large time lines 50 msec; small time lines 10 msec. Vertical bars, calibration for RF voltage and current. Square wave for ECG = 1 mV, 200 msec.

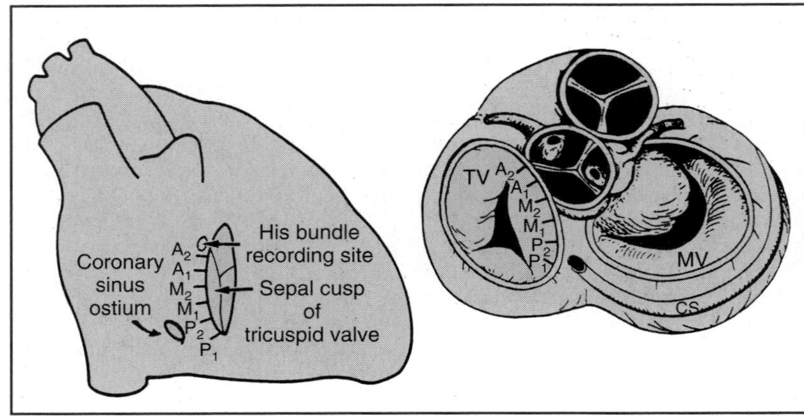

FIGURE 21–12. Radiographic and anatomical correlation during selective modification of the AV node. Schematic representations of right anterior oblique *(left)* and left anterior oblique *(right)* views. The most posterior location (P_1) is initially targeted for selective slow pathway ablation. Depending on the response, the catheter can be advanced progressively to a more anterior location (from P_1 to P_2 and then to M_1 and M_2). TV = tricuspid valve; MV = mitral valve; CS = coronary sinus. (Reproduced with permission from Akhtar, M., Jazayeri, M. R., Sra, J. S., et al.: Atrioventricular nodal reentry: Clinical, electrophysiologic and therapeutic considerations. Circulation *88*:282, 1993. Copyright 1993 American Heart Association.)

are obtained with an atrial-to-ventricular electrogram ratio of less than 0.5 and either a multicomponent atrial electrogram or a recording of possible slow-pathway potential.[362,362a] In the anatomical approach,[357,363] target sites are selected fluoroscopically by dividing the level of the coronary sinus os and the His bundle electrogram recording position into six anatomical regions (Fig. 21–12). Serial RF lesions are created in each region starting at the most posterior site and progressing to the more anterior locus. Finally, the slow pathway can be localized during ventricular pacing. The success rate with the anatomical or electrogram mapping approach is equivalent, and most often, combinations of both are used, yielding success rates approaching 100 per cent with less than 1 per cent chance of complete heart block.

Slow-pathway ablation results in an increase in the anterograde AV block cycle length and AV nodal effective refractory period without a change in the A-H interval or retrograde conduction properties of the AV node (see Chap. 22). Approximately 40 per cent of patients may have evidence of residual slow-pathway function after successful elimination of sustained AVNRT, usually manifested as persistent dual AV nodal physiology and single AV nodal echos during atrial extrastimulation. The endpoint for slow-pathway ablation is the elimination of sustained AVNRT both with and without an infusion of isoproterenol.[359,365,367]

AVNRT recurs in about 5 per cent of patients after slow-pathway ablation. In some patients, the effective refractory period of the fast pathway decreases after slow-pathway ablation, possibly due to electrotonic interaction between the two pathways.[369,370] Atypical forms of reentry can result following ablation,[371] as can apparent parasympathetic denervation, resulting in inappropriate sinus tachycardia.[372]

At present, the fast-pathway approach is appropriate when the slow-pathway approach has been found unsuccessful and perhaps in some patients in whom the induction of AVNRT is not reproducible, because fast-pathway ablation provides a reliable endpoint of P-R prolongation, in contrast to slow-pathway ablation, for which the only reliable endpoint is elimination of tachycardia. Ablation of the slow pathway is a safe and effective means for treating atypical AVNRT. In patients with AVNRT undergoing slow-pathway ablation, junctional ectopy during application of RF energy is a sensitive but nonspecific marker of successful ablation,[373–375] occurring in longer bursts at effective target sites than at ineffective sites. VA conduction should be expected during the junctional ectopy, and poor VA conduction or actual block is a predictor of AV block in patients undergoing RF ablation of the slow pathway.

INDICATIONS. Radiofrequency catheter ablation for AV nodal reentrant tachycardia can be considered in patients with symptomatic sustained AVNRT that is drug resistant or when the patient is drug intolerant or does not desire long-term drug treatment. The procedure also can be considered in patients with sustained AVNRT identified during electrophysiological study or catheter ablation of another arrhythmia or when finding dual AV nodal pathway physiology and atrial echos but without AVNRT during electrophysiological study in a patient suspected to have AVNRT clinically.[354]

RESULTS. Results of the NASPE survey indicate that 3052 patients had slow-pathway ablation with a 96 per cent reported success rate, while 255 had fast-pathway ablation that was successful in 229 (90 per cent). Significant complications occurred in 0.96 per cent, but no procedure-related deaths were reported.[355] In Europe, the complication rate was 8.0 per cent, mostly due to AV block following fast-pathway ablation, and there were no deaths in 815 patients.[356]

Radiofrequency Catheter Ablation of Atrial Tachycardia, Sinus Node Reentry/Inappropriate Sinus Tachycardia, and Atrial Flutter

Atrial arrhythmias amenable to catheter ablation include atrial tachycardias that are automatic or reentrant,[376–379] sinus node reentry,[380] incessant/inappropriate sinus tachycardia, junctional tachycardias,[381] and typical and atypical atrial flutter.[382–384] Activation mapping is used to determine the site of the atrial tachycardia by recording the earliest onset of local activation. Ten to 15 per cent of patients may have multiple atrial foci. Sites tend to cluster near the pulmonary veins in the left atrium and the mouths of the atrial appendages and along the crista terminalis on the right. Reentrant atrial tachycardia appears to occur more commonly in the setting of structural heart disease, specifically following prior atrial surgery. The region of slow conduction is not in a constant anatomical location but varies from patient to patient depending on the operation performed. Therefore, careful review of operative reports and electrophysiological mapping is essential. The atriotomy scar often plays an important role in the genesis of the tachycardia. When the sinus node area is to be ablated, it can be identified anatomically as well as electrophysiologically, and ablation lesions are usually placed between the superior vena cava and crista terminalis.

Understanding the reentrant pathway for typical atrial flutter (negative sawtooth waves in leads II, III, and aV_f at a rate of about 300/min) has been essential to developing an ablation approach. Reentry in the right atrium, with the left atrium passively activated, constitutes the mechanism of typical atrial flutter with a caudocranial activation along the right atrial septum and a craniocaudal activation of the right atrial free wall. A zone of slow conduction in the low right atrium, typically bounded by the tricuspid annulus, the inferior vena cava, and the coronary sinus, exists in the

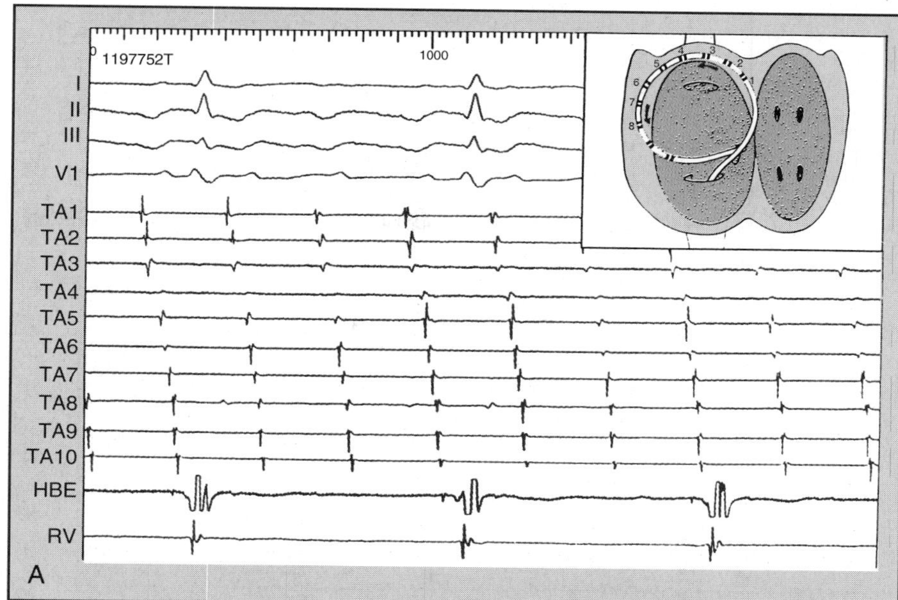

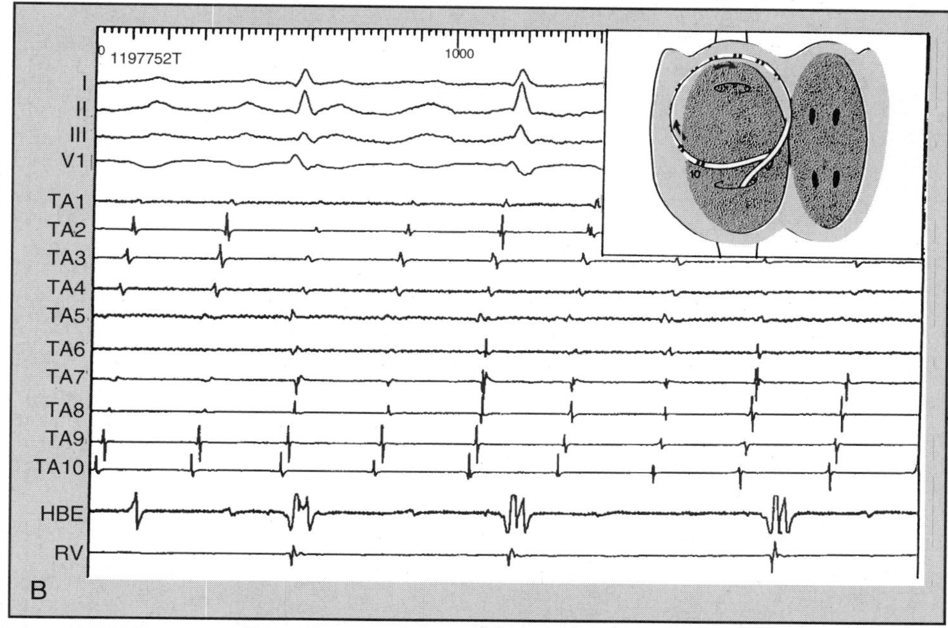

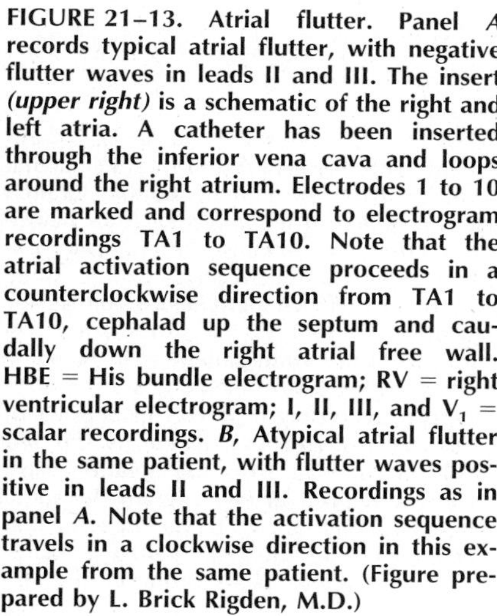
FIGURE 21–13. Atrial flutter. Panel *A* records typical atrial flutter, with negative flutter waves in leads II and III. The insert *(upper right)* is a schematic of the right and left atria. A catheter has been inserted through the inferior vena cava and loops around the right atrium. Electrodes 1 to 10 are marked and correspond to electrogram recordings TA1 to TA10. Note that the atrial activation sequence proceeds in a counterclockwise direction from TA1 to TA10, cephalad up the septum and caudally down the right atrial free wall. HBE = His bundle electrogram; RV = right ventricular electrogram; I, II, III, and V_1 = scalar recordings. *B,* Atypical atrial flutter in the same patient, with flutter waves positive in leads II and III. Recordings as in panel *A.* Note that the activation sequence travels in a clockwise direction in this example from the same patient. (Figure prepared by L. Brick Rigden, M.D.)

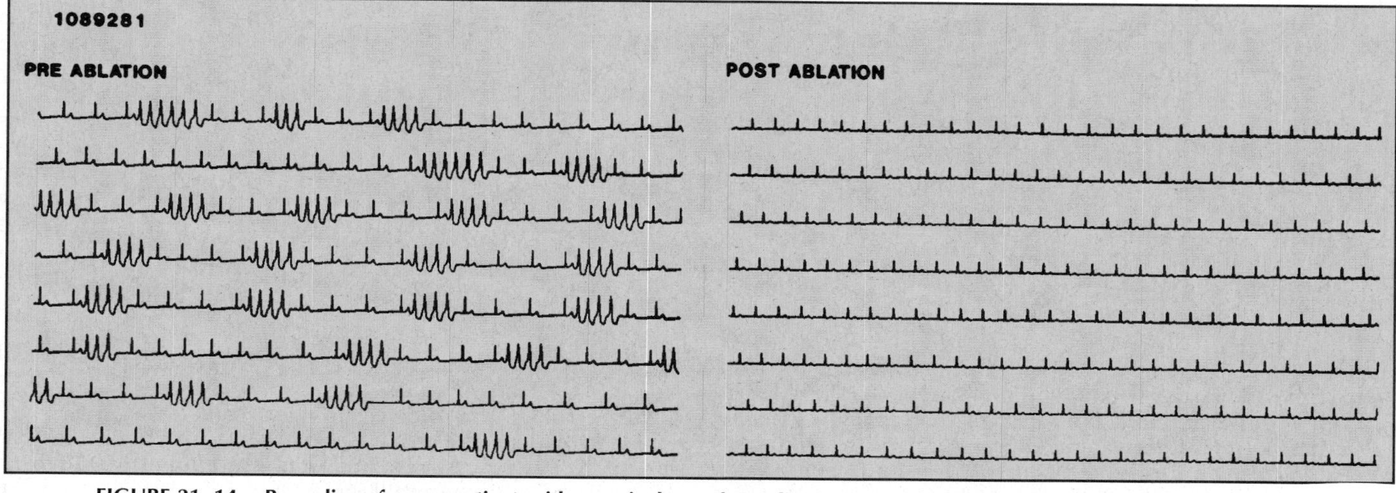

FIGURE 21–14. Recordings from a patient with ventricular tachycardia arising from the right ventricular outflow tract. Before the ablation procedure, frequent runs of symptomatic nonsustained ventricular tachycardia were recorded (*top half*). After ablation, all spontaneous episodes of ventricular tachycardia were eliminated *(bottom half).* (From Klein, L. S., Miles, W. M., and Zipes, D. P.: Ablation of idiopathic ventricular tachycardia and bundle branch reentry. *In* Zipes, D. P. [ed.]: Catheter Ablation of Arrhythmias. Armonk, N.Y., Futura Publishing Company, 1994, pp. 259–276.)

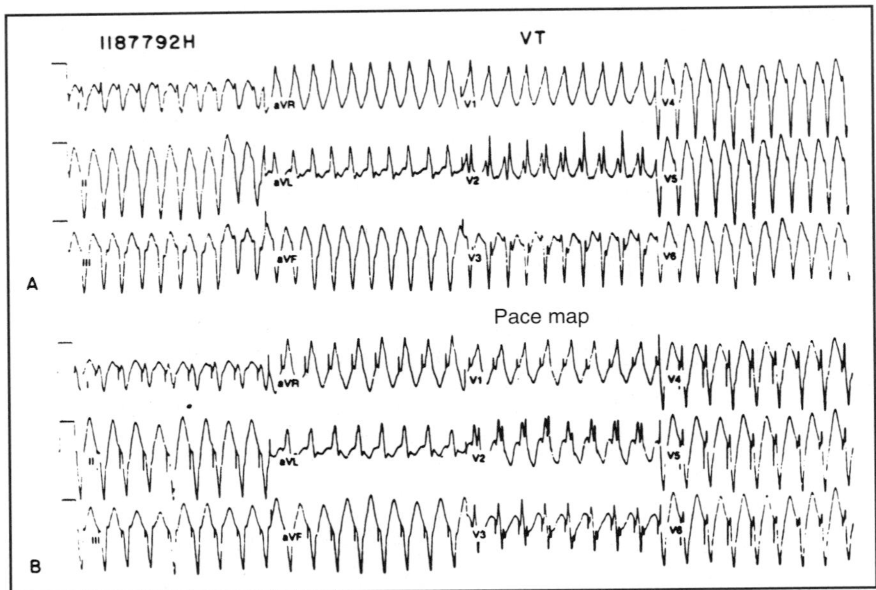

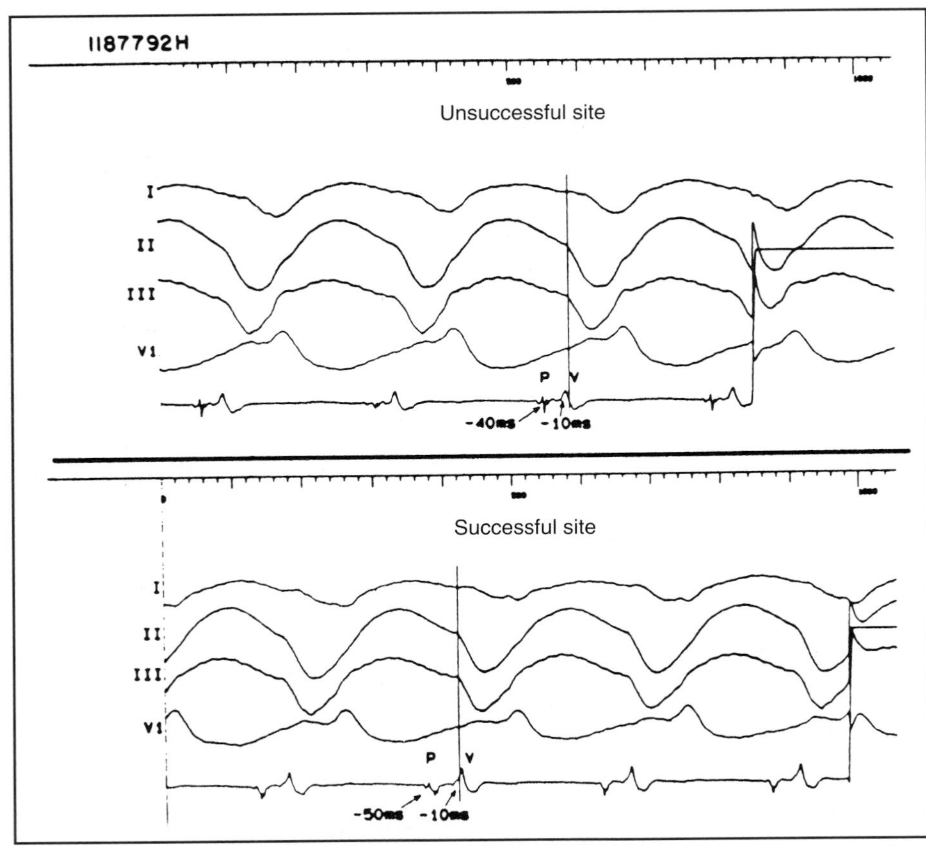

FIGURE 21–15. *Top panel,* Scalar ECG from a patient with verapamil-sensitive VT having the morphology of a right bundle branch block with extreme left axis deviation before (A) and during (B) pacing. *Bottom,* Left ventricular pacing at electrophysiological study exactly replicated the spontaneous ventricular tachycardia. *Bottom panel,* Intracardiac recordings from the same patient as in panel *A.* Four surface leads are shown along with an intracardiac recording from the distal poles of an ablation catheter positioned in the left ventricle. Recordings from the ablation catheter show a ventricular electrogram (V) and a Purkinje potential (P). Ablation, delivered at the vertical line at the right, failed to eliminate the ventricular tachycardia in the top panel but did so in the bottom panel. Note that the timing of the ventricular electrogram to the onset of the QRS complex during VT (vertical line) is the same at both successful and unsuccessful ablation sites, but the Purkinje potential is recorded earlier from the site at which VT was ultimately eliminated.

region of the slow pathway.[385–387] Placing an ablation lesion across the zone of slow conduction abolishes the atrial flutter. This can be accomplished near the entrance of the slow zone in the low posterolateral right atrium, at the midpoint of the slow zone in the posterior right atrium, or near the exit at the posteromedial right atrium. Lesions can be guided anatomically or electrophysiologically. Atypical atrial flutter may be more difficult to ablate and has a clockwise rotation, cephalad up the right atrial free wall and caudad down the septum, with upright flutter waves in the inferior leads (Fig. 21–13).

INDICATIONS. Candidates for RF catheter ablation include patients with atrial tachycardia, sinus node reentry, inappropriate sinus tachycardia, or atrial flutter that is drug resistant, those who are drug intolerant, or those who do not desire long-term drug therapy.[354]

RESULTS. From the U.S. NASPE survey, 371 patients underwent ablation for atrial tachycardia and atrial flutter

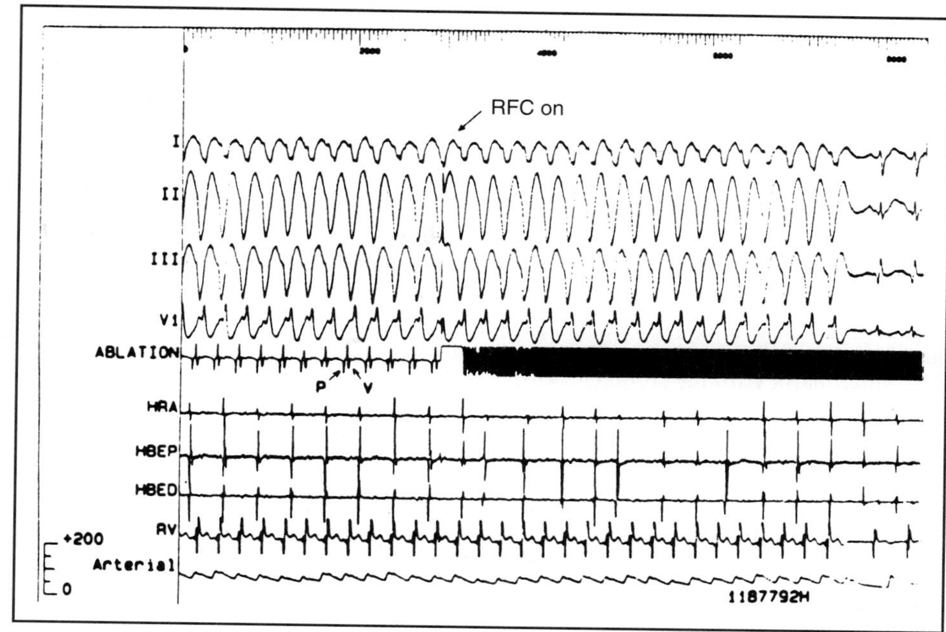

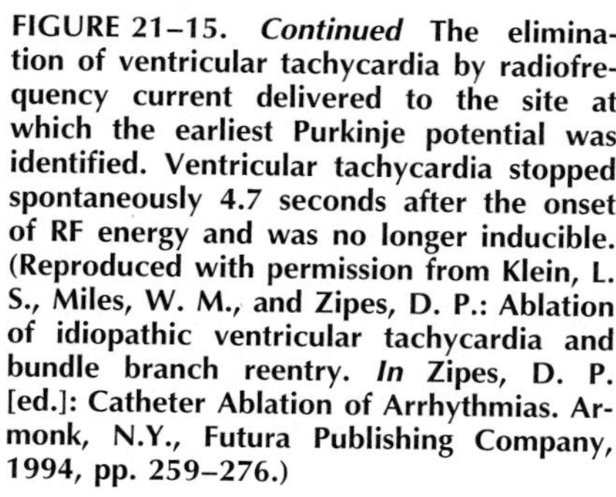
FIGURE 21–15. ***Continued*** **The elimination of ventricular tachycardia by radiofrequency current delivered to the site at which the earliest Purkinje potential was identified. Ventricular tachycardia stopped spontaneously 4.7 seconds after the onset of RF energy and was no longer inducible. (Reproduced with permission from Klein, L. S., Miles, W. M., and Zipes, D. P.: Ablation of idiopathic ventricular tachycardia and bundle branch reentry.** ***In*** **Zipes, D. P. [ed.]: Catheter Ablation of Arrhythmias. Armonk, N.Y., Futura Publishing Company, 1994, pp. 259–276.)**

with a success rate of 75 per cent and three significant complications (0.8 per cent) with no deaths.[355] The complication rate was 5 per cent in the European survey, and there were no deaths in 141 patients.[356]

Radiofrequency Catheter Ablation of Atrial Fibrillation

Although surgical procedures involving incision and isolation of atrial myocardium have been devised to eliminate atrial fibrillation, and their feasibility demonstrated catheter techniques for eliminating atrial fibrillation are in the relatively early stage of development, but preliminary success has been reported.[388–392]

Ablation and Modification of Atrioventricular Conduction for Atrial Tachyarrhythmias

To achieve RF catheter ablation of AV conduction, a catheter is placed across the tricuspid valve and positioned to record the largest His bundle electrogram associated with the largest atrial electrogram. RF energy is applied until complete AV block is achieved and is continued for an additional 30 seconds. If no change in AV conduction is observed after 60 seconds of RF ablation, the catheter is repositioned and the attempt is repeated. Patients who fail conventional RF ablation attempts from the right ventricle can undergo an attempt from the left ventricle with a catheter positioned along the posterior interventricular septum to record a large sharp His bundle electrogram. Energy is applied between the catheter electrode and the skin patch or between catheters in the left and right ventricles. Success rates approach 100 per cent in most studies today, with recurrence of AV conduction in less than 5 per cent.[393] Improved left ventricular function can result.[394]

More recently, the AV junction has been modified to slow the ventricular rate without producing complete AV block by ablating in the region of the slow pathway, as described under AV nodal modification for AV nodal reentry. Success rates for slowing the ventricular response vary but this procedure can be tried prior to producing complete AV block.[395–397]

INDICATIONS. Ablation and modification of atrioventricular conduction can be considered in (1) patients with symptomatic atrial tachyarrhythmias who have inadequately controlled ventricular rates unless primary ablation of the atrial tachyarrhythmia is possible, (2) similar patients when drugs are not tolerated or the patient does not wish to take them, even though the ventricular rate can be controlled, (3) patients with symptomatic nonparoxysmal junctional tachycardia that is drug resistant or by whom drugs are not tolerated or are not desired, (4) patients resus citated from sudden cardiac death due to atrial flutter or atrial fibrillation with a rapid ventricular response in the absence of an accessory pathway, and (5) patients with a dual-chamber pacemaker and a pacemaker-mediated tachycardia that cannot be treated effectively by drugs or by reprograming the pacemaker.[354]

RESULTS. Results from the U.S. survey indicated that the procedure was successful in producing complete AV block in 95 per cent of 1600 patients, with significant complications occurring in 21 (1.3 per cent) and 2 procedure-related deaths (0.1 per cent).[355] In Europe, the complication rate was 3.2 per cent, and there was 1 death in 900 patients.[356]

Radiofrequency Catheter Ablation of Ventricular Tachycardia

In general, the success rate for ablation of ventricular tachycardias is lower than for AV nodal or AV reentry.[398–410] This may be related to the fact that this procedure is often a last-ditch effort in patients with drug-resistant ventricular tachycardias but also relates to very difficult mapping and ablation requirements in the thick-walled ventricles. Further, the ventricular tachycardia must be reproducibly inducible, monomorphic, sustained, and hemodynamically stable so that the patient can tolerate the ventricular tachycardia during the procedure. Also, the origin of the ventricular tachycardia must be fairly circumscribed and endocardially situated. Very rapid ventricular tachycardias, polymorphic ventricular tachycardias, and infrequent nonsustained episodes are not amenable to this form of therapy at this time.[398,399]

Radiofrequency catheter ablation of ventricular tachycardia must be divided into idiopathic ventricular tachycardia that occurs in patients with essentially normal hearts,[399,402–404,406,408,410] ventricular tachycardia that occurs in a variety of disease settings but without coronary artery disease, and ventricular tachycardia in patients with coronary artery disease.[398,400,405,407,409] In the first group, the ventricular tachycardias occur most commonly in the right ventricular outflow tract (Fig. 21–14) and less often in the inflow tract. Left ventricular tachycardias are characteristically septal in origin (Fig. 21–15). Abnormal patterns of sympathetic innervation may be present.[411] Ventricular tachycardias in abnormal hearts without coronary artery disease can be due to bundle branch reentry, a characteristic of dilated cardiomyopathies. In these patients, ablation of the right bundle branch eliminates the tachycardia.[412] Ventricular tachycardia can occur in right ventricular dysplasia, hypertrophic cardiomyopathy, and a host of other noncoronary disease problems (see p. 679).

Activation mapping[401,407] and pace mapping are effective in patients with idiopathic ventricular tachycardias to locate the site of origin of the ventricular tachycardia. Purkinje potentials (Fig. 21–15) can be recorded in some patients with left ventricular tachycardias.[399,406] Pace mapping involves stimulation of various ventricular sites to initiate a QRS contour that duplicates the QRS contour of the spontaneous ventricular tachycardia, thus establishing the apparent site of origin of the arrhythmia. This technique is limited by several methodological problems but may be useful when the tachycardia cannot be initiated and when a 12-lead ECG has been obtained during the spontaneous ventricular tachycardia. Localization of the site of origin of ventricular tachycardia in patients with coronary artery disease is more difficult than in patients with structurally normal hearts because of the altered anatomy and electrophysiology. Pace mapping is not as helpful as it is for idiopathic ventricular tachycardia. Further, reentry circuits can sometimes be large and resistant to the relatively small lesions produced by RF catheter ablation. Finding the area of slow conduction used as part of the reentrant circuit is helpful, since ablation at this site has a good chance of eliminating the tachycardia.

In patients without structural heart disease, only a single ventricular tachycardia is usually present, and catheter ablation of that ventricular tachycardia is curative. In patients with extensive structural heart disease, especially those with prior myocardial infarction, multiple ventricular tachycardias are often present. Catheter ablation of a single ventricular tachycardia in such patients may only be palliative and may not eliminate the need for further antiarrhythmic therapy.

INDICATIONS. Patients considered for RF catheter ablation of ventricular tachycardia are those with symptomatic sustained monomorphic ventricular tachycardia when the tachycardia is drug resistant, when the patient is drug intolerant, or when the patient does not desire long-term drug therapy; patients with bundle branch reentrant ventricular tachycardia; and patients with sustained monomorphic ventricular tachycardia and an implantable cardioverter-defibrillator who are receiving multiple shocks not manageable by reprograming or concomitant drug therapy. Occasionally, nonsustained ventricular tachycardia or even severely symptomatic premature ventricular complexes can be eliminated by RF catheter ablation.[354]

RESULTS. In the U.S. NASPE survey, 429 patients underwent ablation with an overall success rate of 71 per cent. In 224 patients with structurally normal hearts, the success rate was 85 per cent. The success rate was 54 per cent in 115 patients with ventricular tachycardia due to ischemic heart disease and 61 per cent in 90 patients with idiopathic cardiomyopathy. There were 13 significant complications (3.0 per cent) and, interestingly, considering the nature of the disease, no procedure-related deaths.[355] The complication rate was 7.5 per cent in the European survey, and there was 1 death in 320 patients.[356]

Chemical Ablation

Chemical ablation with alcohol or phenol of an area of myocardium involved in a tachycardia has been used to create AV block in patients not responding to catheter ablation and to eliminate atrial and ventricular tachycardias.[413,414] Excessive myocardial necrosis is the major complication, and alcohol ablation should be considered only when other ablative approaches fail or cannot be done.

SURGICAL THERAPY OF TACHYARRHYTHMIAS

The objectives of a surgical approach to treating a tachycardia are to excise, isolate, or interrupt tissue in the heart critical for the initiation, maintenance, or propagation of the tachycardia while preserving or even improving myocardial function. In addition to a direct surgical approach to the arrhythmia, indirect approaches such as aneurysmectomy, coronary artery bypass grafting, and relief of valvular regurgitation or stenosis can be useful in selected patients by improving cardiac hemodynamics and myocardial blood flow. Cardiac sympathectomy alters adrenergic influences on the heart and has been effective in some patients, particularly those who have recurrent ventricular tachycardia with the long Q-T syndrome.

Supraventricular Tachycardias

Surgical procedures[415–420] exist for patients (adults and children) with atrial tachycardias,[420] atrial flutter, AV nodal reentry,[416] and AV reentry,[417,421,422] (Fig. 21–16). Radiofrequency (RF) catheter ablation adequately treats the majority of these patients except for those with atrial fibrillation. Therefore, RF catheter ablation has replaced direct surgical intervention except for the occasional patient in whom RF catheter ablation fails or who is having concomitant cardiovascular surgery. In some instances, a prior attempt at RF catheter ablation complicates surgery by obliterating the normal tissue planes that exist in the AV groove of the heart or by rendering tissues too friable. Occasionally, pa-

FIGURE 21–16. Schematic diagram showing the two approaches for surgical interruption of the accessory pathway. The left panel depicts the left atrioventricular groove and its vascular contents, the coronary sinus (C.S.) and circumflex coronary artery (C.A.). Multiple accessory pathways (AP) course through the fat pad. The middle panel shows the epicardial dissection approach while the right panel exhibits the endocardial dissection. Both approaches clear out the fat pad and interrupt any accessory pathways. (From Zipes, D.P.: Cardiac electrophysiology: promises and contributions. Reprinted by permission of the American College of Cardiology. J. Am. Coll. Cardiol. *13*:1329, 1989.)

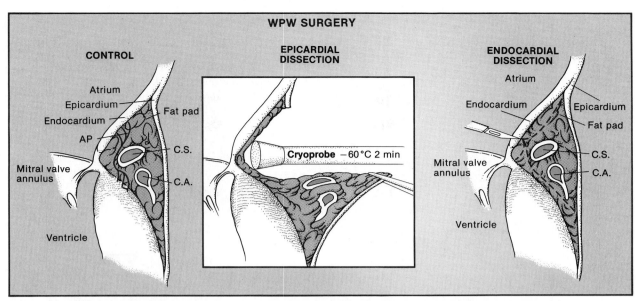

tients with atrial tachycardias have multiple foci that require surgical intervention.[420]

The Maze procedure,[418,423] developed to treat patients with atrial fibrillation (see p. 656), eliminates the arrhythmia by reducing atrial tissue mass to a size at any instant in time too small to perpetuate the reentrant circuits responsible for atrial fibrillation. It forces atrial activation to proceed along a surgically determined pathway, thus maintaining sinus rhythm with AV nodal conduction. The Maze procedure permits organized electrical depolarization of the atria, restores atrial transport function, and in so doing decreases the risk of thromboembolism. Maintenance of sinus rhythm more than 3 months after the procedure approaches 100 per cent, although 30 to 40 per cent of patients require pacemakers because of chronotropic incompetence of the sinus node. The advent of minimally invasive endoscopic and endovascular techniques may make it possible to perform an equivalent of the Maze procedure without thoracotomy in the future.

Ventricular Tachycardia

In contrast to patients with supraventricular arrhythmias, candidates for surgical therapy of ventricular arrhythmias often have severe left ventricular dysfunction, generally caused by coronary artery disease. The etiology of the underlying heart disease influences the type of surgery performed. Candidates are patients with drug-resistant, symptomatic recurrent ventricular tachyarrhythmias who, ideally, have a localized abnormality, scar, or aneurysm with good left ventricular function. Poorer surgical results are obtained in patients with a history of congestive heart failure and left ventricular dysfunction.

Ischemic Heart Disease

In almost all patients who have ventricular tachycardia associated with ischemic heart disease, the arrhythmia, regardless of its configuration on the surface ECG, arises in the left ventricle or on the left ventricular side of the interventricular septum. The contour of the ventricular tachycardia can change from a right bundle branch block to a left bundle branch block pattern without a change in the 1earliest activation site, suggesting that the left ventricular site of origin remains the same, often near the septum, but its exit pathway is altered.

Indirect surgical approaches, including cardiac thoracic sympathectomy, coronary artery bypass grafting (CABG), and ventricular aneurysm or infarct resection with or without CABG, have been successful in about 60 per cent of reported cases. Coronary artery bypass grafting as a primary therapeutic approach generally has been limited to patients who experience ventricular tachycardia during ischemia

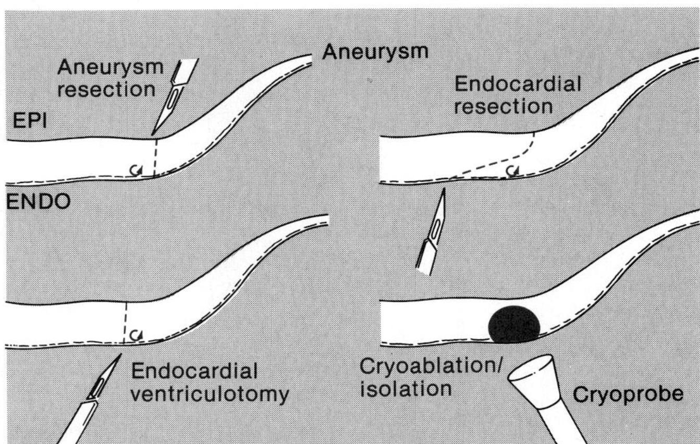

FIGURE 21–17. Schematic diagram showing the surgical approaches to ventricular tachycardia surgery in a patient with a left ventricular aneurysm. In the top left, the aneurysm is resected but the area of ventricular tachycardia origin remains (small circle with arrow) and tachycardia can recur. Bottom left panel demonstrates the technique for endocardial encircling ventriculotomy, no longer used. A nontransmural incision is made, which isolates the area of arrhythmia development. Top right panel demonstrates the method for endocardial resection. The aneurysm and a strip of endocardium containing the tachycardia focus are removed. Bottom right panel demonstrates cryoablation of the ventricular tachycardia focus. (From Zipes, D. P.: Cardiac electrophysiology: promises and contributions. Reprinted by permission of the American College of Cardiology. J. Am. Coll. Cardiol. *13*:1329, 1989.)

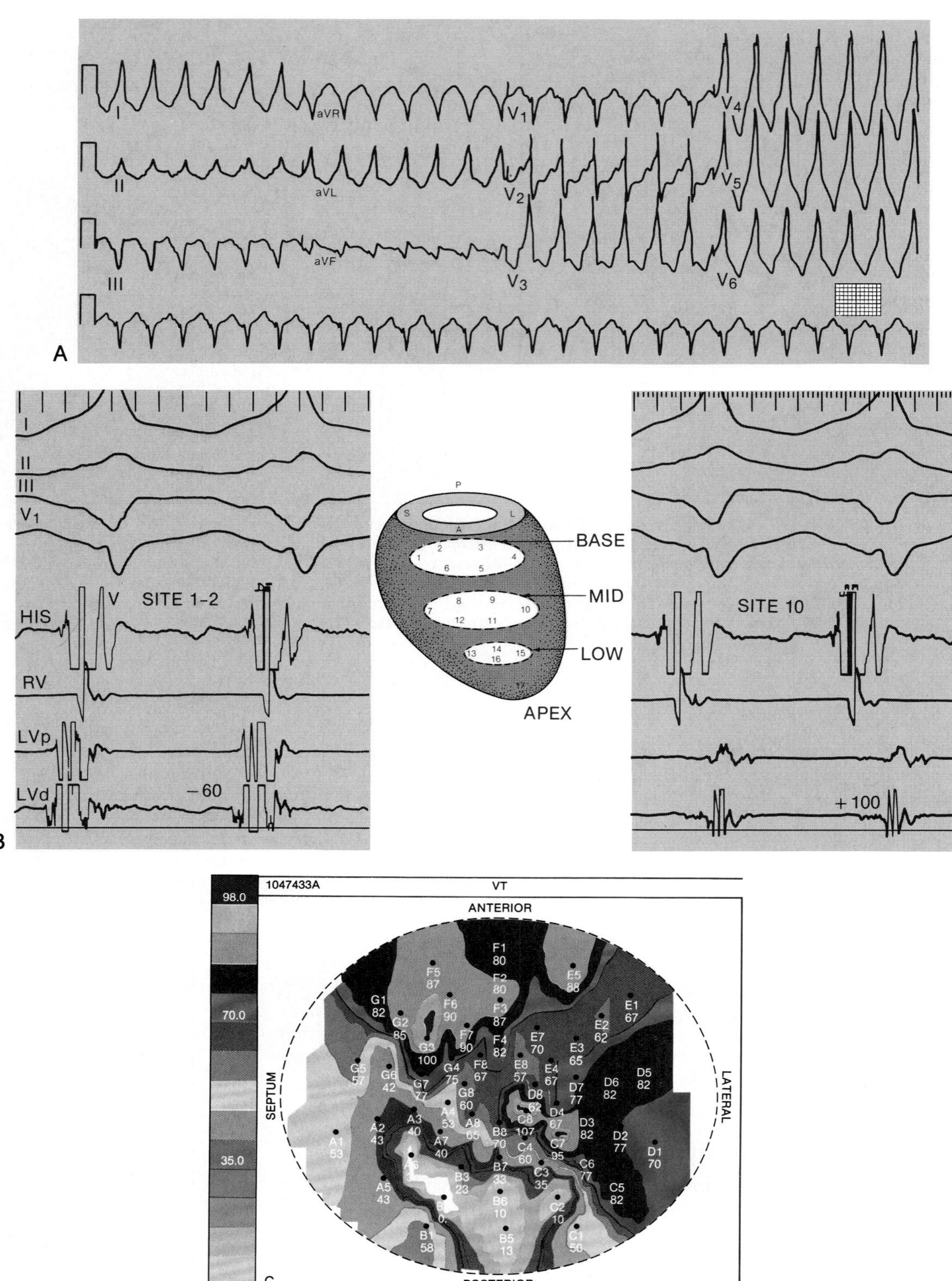

FIGURE 21–18. Mapping of a ventricular tachycardia. *A,* The 12-lead ECG demonstrates a ventricular tachycardia with a normal axis and left bundle branch block contour. *B,* A left ventricular catheter placed in the posteroseptal region of the left ventricle (positions 1, 2 in the schematic insert) records electrical activity from the distal electrodes of the left ventricular catheter (LVd) 60 msec in advance of the onset of the QRS complex. This illustrates that the tip of the catheter is close to the "origin" of the ventricular tachycardia. Electrical activity in the proximal left ventricular electrodes (LVp) and in the right ventricular recording (RV) is quite late (left panel). In the right panel, electrical activity recorded at site 10 in the midlateral left ventricle occurs well after the onset of the QRS complex, indicating that it is far from the origin of the tachycardia. *C,* At the time of surgery, a balloon studded with electrodes was inflated in the left ventricle and recorded an isopotential map that confirmed the origin of the ventricular tachycardia at a posteroseptal position in the left ventricle. (Schematic in *B* reproduced with permission from Dusman, R. E., et al.: Electrophysiological directed endocardial resection and cryoablation in the treatment of ventricular tachyarrhythmias. Indiana Med. *81:*242, 1988.)

but can be useful in patients with coronary disease resuscitated from sudden death who have no inducible arrhythmias at electrophysiological study. Patients with sustained monomorphic ventricular tachycardia or only polymorphic ventricular tachycardia or ventricular fibrillation uncommonly have their arrhythmia affected by coronary bypass surgery, although the latter can reduce the frequency of the arrhythmic episodes in some patients and prevent new ischemic events.

SURGICAL TECHNIQUES. Generally two types of direct surgical procedures are used: resection and ablation (Fig. 21–17). The *encircling endocardial ventriculotomy* (EEV) involving a transmural ventriculotomy to isolate areas of endocardial fibrosis that are recognized visually is no longer employed. The rationale for *endocardial resection* is based on animal and clinical data indicating that arrhythmias after myocardial infarction arise mostly in the subendocardial borders between normal and infarcted tissue. Endocardial resection involves peeling off a layer of endocardium, often in the rim of an aneurysm, that has been demonstrated by means of mapping procedures to be the site of earliest activation recorded during the ventricular tachycardia (Fig. 21–18). Some ventricular tachycardias can arise from the epicardium. Tachycardias arising from the base of the papillary muscles are cryoablated. Cryoablation also can be used to isolate areas of the ventricle that cannot be resected and is often combined with resection. *Laser approaches* are experimental but appear promising.

RESULTS. For ventricular tachyarrhythmias, operative mortality ranges from 6 to 23 per cent, with success rates defined as absence of recurrence of spontaneous ventricular arrhythmias ranging from 59 to 98 per cent. In experienced centers, operative mortality may be as low as 5 per cent in stable patients undergoing elective procedures, with 85 to 95 per cent of survivors free of inducible or spontaneous ventricular tachyarrhythmias. Recurrence rates range from 2 to 38 per cent. Postoperative survival is strongly influenced by the degree of left ventricular dysfunction. Patients with less favorable anatomy who are poor surgical candidates and who fail drug treatment are generally considered for an implantable cardioverter-defibrillator. By no longer having to operate on these patients, surgeons have improved the overall operative mortality.[419,424]

Operative mortality for nonthoracotomy implantable cardioverter-defibrillator (ICD) implantation is less than 1 per cent, with an annual sudden cardiac death mortality rate of less than 1 per cent.[425] Nevertheless, the latter patients are obligated to a lifetime of ICD therapy, which, naturally, does not prevent the arrhythmia but only terminates it after its onset. Some experts recommend surgery for patients with ventricular tachycardia who have discrete aneurysms that are amenable to intraoperative mapping and resection because such patients have a very high probability for cure of their arrhythmia.[426]

Electrophysiological Studies

PREOPERATIVE ELECTROPHYSIOLOGICAL STUDY. This involves induction of the ventricular tachycardia and electrophysiological mapping to pinpoint the area to be resected. A resolution of 4 to 8 cm^2 of ventricular endocardium is probably achieved, although more accurate anatomical localization of the mapping electrode tip in the ventricle may be possible. Tachycardias that are too rapid, short in duration, or polymorphic cannot be mapped accurately unless multiple catheters or a multielectrode array is used. Administering a drug such as procainamide may slow the ventricular tachycardia and transform a nonsustained pleomorphic ventricular tachycardia into a sustained ventricular tachycardia of uniform contour that can be mapped.

INTRAOPERATIVE VENTRICULAR MAPPING. Electrophysiological mapping is also performed at the time of surgery, with the operator using a handheld probe or an electrode array coupled with on-line computer techniques that instantaneously provide an activation map cycle by cycle. The sequence of activation during ventricular tachycardia can be plotted and the area of earliest activation determined (Fig. 21–18).

During ventricular tachycardia, the origin of the arrhythmia is generally ascribed to electrical activity recorded 25 to 50 msec in advance of the QRS complex. However, that is an arbitrary value, and it is quite clear that such activity can be late following the preceding cycle or early in advance of the next cycle. In addition, when such activity is recorded well after termination of the QRS complex, it becomes important to determine whether the deflections represent depolarization or repolarization. Potentials recorded prior to the onset of the surface QRS complex suggest that the origin of the tachycardia is nearby. When the earliest recordable electrical activity occurs after the onset of the QRS complex, the site of origin may be in the interventricular septum.

It is important to emphasize that the area of earliest recorded electrical activity during ventricular tachycardia may not actually represent the site of origin of the tachycardia, since the latter may originate several centimeters away, e.g., in a small scarred area, and be conducted very slowly until it reaches more normally excitable tissue where it exits the endocardium and generates a recordable extracellular complex. However, this area of early activation is probably closely related to the origin of the tachycardia which, based on present state of knowledge and results from surgery, warrants surgical intervention at that site. Finding an area of "continuous electrical activity" does not necessarily mean that reentry is present or that this is the origin of the tachycardia, since similar activity can be produced by automatically discharging foci, by recording slowly propagating, overlapping, or fragmented wavefronts from several areas, or by recording repolarization activity. However, it is likely that the origin of the tachycardia is close to the area of continuous electrical activity. In some patients, intramural mapping using a plunge needle electrode can be useful, particularly if the origin of the tachycardia is not located in the subendocardium.

Acknowledgments

Some of the illustrations were taken from studies performed by William M. Miles and Lawrence S. Klein.

REFERENCES

CLINICAL PHARMACOKINETICS

1. Follath, F.: The utility of serum drug level monitoring during therapy with class III antiarrhythmic agents. J. Cardiovasc. Pharmacol. *20* (Suppl. II):S41, 1992.
2. Roden, D. M., and Murray, K. T.: Pharmacokinetics, pharmacodynamics, and pharmacogenetics. *In* Zipes, D. P., and Jalife, J. (eds.): Cardiac Electrophysiology: From Cell to Bedside. 2nd ed. Philadelphia, W. B. Saunders Company, 1994, pp. 1287–1296.
3. Buchert, E., and Woosley, R. L.: Clinical implications of variable antiarrhythmic drug metabolism. Pharmacogenetics *2*:2, 1992.
4. Roden, D. M.: Are pharmacokinetics helpful for the clinician? J. Cardiovasc. Electrophysiol. *2*:S178, 1991.
5. Lalka, D., Griffith, R. K., and Cronenberger, C. L.: The hepatic first-pass metabolism of problematic drugs. J. Clin. Pharmacol. *33*:657, 1993.
6. Stanton, M. S.: Class I antiarrhythmic drugs: Quinidine, procainamide, disopyramide, lidocaine, mexiletine, tocainide, phenytoin, moricizine, flecainide, propafenone. *In* Zipes, D. P., and Jalife, J. (eds.): Cardiac Electrophysiology: From Cell to Bedside. 2nd ed. Philadelphia, W. B. Saunders Company, 1994, pp. 1296–1317.
7. Nattel, S.: Antiarrhythmic drug classifications: A critical appraisal of their history, present status and clinical relevance. Drugs *41*:672, 1991.
8. Vaughan Williams, E. M.: The relevance of cellular to clinical electrophysiology in classifying antiarrhythmic actions. J. Cardiovasc. Pharmacol. *20* (Suppl. 2):S1, 1992.
9. Rosen, M. R., Strauss, H. C., and Janse, M. J.: The classification of antiarrhythmic drugs. *In* Zipes, D. P., and Jalife, J. (eds.): Cardiac Electrophysiology: From Cell to Bedside. 2nd ed. Philadelphia, W. B. Saunders Company, 1994, pp. 1277–1286.
10. Members of the Sicilian Gambit: Antiarrhythmic Therapy: A Pathophysiologic Approach. Armonk, N.Y., Futura Publishing Company, 1994.
11. Sadanaga, T., Ogawa, S., Okada, Y., et al.: Clinical evaluation of the use-dependent QRS prolongation and the reverse use-dependent QT prolongation of class I and class III antiarrhythmic agents and their value in predicting efficacy. Am. Heart J. *126*:114, 1993.
12. Birgersdotter, U. M., Wong, W., Turgeon, J., et al.: Stereoselective genetically determined interaction between chronic flecainide and quinidine in patients with arrhythmias. Br. J. Clin. Pharmacol. *33*:275, 1992.
13. Adams, L. E., Baldkrishnan, K., Roberts, S. M., et al.: Genetic, immunologic and biotransformation studies of patients on procainamide. Lupus *2*:89, 1993.
14. Danielly, J., DeJong, R., Radke-Mitchell, L. C., et al.: Procainamide-associated blood dyscrasias. Am. J. Cardiol. *74*:1179, 1994.
15. Skaer, T. L.: Medication-induced systemic lupus erythematosus. Clin. Ther. *14*:496, 1992.
16. Falk, R. H.: Proarrhythmia in patients treated for atrial fibrillation or flutter. Ann. Intern. Med. *117*:141, 1992.
17. Kidwell, G. A.: Drug-induced ventricular proarrhythmia. Cardiovasc. Clin. *22*:317, 1992.
18. Patterson, E., Szabo, B., Scherlag, B. J., et al.: Arrhythmogenic effects of antiarrhythmic drugs. *In* Zipes, D. P., and Jalife, J. (eds.): Cardiac Elec-

trophysiology: From Cell to Bedside. 2nd ed. Philadelphia, W. B. Saunders Company, 1994, pp. 496–511.
19. Benditt, D. G., Bailin, S., Remole, S., et al.: Proarrhythmia: Recognition of patients at risk. J. Cardiovasc. Electrophysiol. *2*:S221, 1991.
20. Bhein, S., Muller, A., Gerwin, R., et al.: Comparative study on the proarrhythmic effects of some antiarrhythmic agents. Circulation *87*:617, 1993.
21. Morganroth, J.: Early and late proarrhythmia from antiarrhythmic drug therapy. Cardiovasc. Drugs Ther. *6*:11, 1992.
22. Ben-David, J., and Zipes, D. P.: Torsades de pointes and proarrhythmia. Lancet *341*(8860):1578, 1993.
23. Roden, D. M.: Torsade de pointes. Clin. Cardiol. *16*:683, 1993.
24. Lazzara, R.: Antiarrhythmic drugs and torsade de pointes. Eur. Heart J. *14* (Suppl. H):88, 1993.
25. Roden, D. M.: Early after-depolarizations and torsade de pointes: Implications for the control of cardiac arrhythmias by prolonging repolarization. Eur. Heart J. *14* (Suppl. H):56, 1993.
26. Banai, S., and Tzivoni, D.: Drug therapy for torsade de pointes. J. Cardiovasc. Electrophysiol. *4*:206, 1993.
27. Weissenburger, J., Davy, J. M., and Chezalviel, F.: Experimental models of torsades de pointes. Fund. Clin. Pharmacol. *7*:29, 1993.
28. Lazzara, R.: Mechanistic and clinical aspects of acquired long QT syndromes. Ann. N.Y. Acad. Sci. *644*:48, 1992.
29. Sicouri, S., and Antzelevitch, C.: Drug-induced afterdepolarizations and triggered activity occur in a discreet subpopulation of ventricular muscle cells (M cells) in the canine heart: Quinidine and digitalis. J. Cardiovasc. Electrophysiol. *4*:48, 1993.
30. Faber, T. S., Zehender, M., Van de Loo, A., et al.: Torsade de pointes complicating drug treatment of low-malignant forms of arrhythmia: Four case reports. Clin. Cardiol. *17*:197, 1994.
31. Wyse, K. R., Ye, V., and Campbell, T. J.: Action potential prolongation exhibits simple dose-dependence for sotalol, but reverse dose-dependence for quinidine and disopyramide: Implications for proarrhythmia due to triggered activity. J. Cardiovasc. Pharmacol. *21*:316, 1993.
32. Fast, V. G., and Pertsov, A. M.: Shift and termination of functional reentry in isolated ventricular preparations with quinidine-induced inhomogeneity in refractory period. J. Cardiovasc. Electrophysiol. *3*:255, 1992.
33. Flaker, G. C., Blackshear, J. L., McBride, R., et al.: Antiarrhythmic drug therapy and cardiac mortality in atrial fibrillation. The Stroke Prevention in Atrial Fibrillation Investigators. J. Am. Coll. Cardiol. *20*:527, 1992.
34. Epstein, A. E., Halstrom, A. P., Rogers, W. J., et al.: Mortality following ventricular arrhythmia suppression by encainide, flecainide and moricizine after myocardial infarction: The original design concept of the Cardiac Arrhythmia Suppression Trial (CAST). JAMA *270*:2451, 1993.
35. Cardiac Arrhythmia Suppression Trial II Investigators: Effect of the antiarrhythmic agent moricizine on survival after myocardial infarction. N. Engl. J. Med. *327*:227, 1992.
36. Anderson, J. L., Platia, E. V., Hallstrom A., et al.: Interaction of baseline characteristics with the hazard of encainide, flecainide and moricizine therapy in patients with myocardial infarction. A possible explanation for increased mortality in the Cardiac Arrhythmia Suppression Trial (CAST). Circulation *90*:2843, 1994.

CLASS IA AGENTS

37. Levy, S., and Azoulay, S.: Stories about the origin of quinquina and quinidine. J. Cardiovasc. Electrophysiol. *5*:635, 1994.
38. Cappato, R., Alboni, P., Codeca, L., et al.: Direct and autonomically mediated effects of oral quinidine on RR/QT relation after an abrupt increase in heart rate. J. Am. Coll. Cardiol. *22*:99, 1993.
39. Hondeghem, L. M.: Ideal antiarrhythmic agents: Chemical defibrillators. J. Cardiovasc. Electrophysiol. *2*:S169, 1991.
40. Carmeliet, E.: Use-dependent block of the delayed K^+ current in rabbit ventricular myocytes. Cardiovasc. Drugs Ther. *7* (Suppl. 3):599, 1993.
41. Grant, A. O., and Wendt, D. J.: Blockade of ion channels by antiarrhythmic drugs. J. Cardiovasc. Electrophysiol. *2*:S153, 1991.
42. Markel, M. L., Miles, W. M., Luck, J. C., et al.: Differential effects of isoproterenol on sustained ventricular tachycardia before and during procainamide and quinidine antiarrhythmic drug therapy. Circulation *87*:783, 1993.
43. Allen, N. M.: Relationship between serum quinidine concentration and quinidine dosage. Pharmacol. Ther. *12*:189, 1992.
44. Packer, M.: Hemodynamic consequences of antiarrhythmic drug therapy in patients with chronic heart failure. J. Cardiovasc. Electrophysiol. *2*:S240, 1991.
45. Hook, B. G., Rosenthal, M. E., Marchlinski, F. E., et al.: Results of electrophysiological testing and long-term follow-up in patients sustaining cardiac arrest only while receiving type IA antiarrhythmic agents. PACE *15*:324, 1992.
46. Sager, P. T., Pearlmutter, R. A., Rosenfeld, L. E., et al.: Antiarrhythmic drug exacerbation of ventricular tachycardia inducibility during electrophysiologic study. Am. Heart J. *123*:926, 1992.
47. Wu, B., Sato, T., Kiyosue, T., et al.: Blockade of two, four-dinotrophenol induced ATP sensitive potassium currents in guinea pig ventricular myocytes by class I antiarrhythmic drugs. Cardiovasc. Res. *26*:1095, 1992.
48. Kar, P. M., Kellner, K., Ing, T. S., et al.: Combined high-efficiency hemodialysis and charcoal hemoperfusion in severe *N*-acetylprocainamide intoxication. Am. J. Kidney Dis. *20*:403, 1992.
49. Dibner-Dunlap, M. E., Cohen, M. D., Yuih, S. N., et al.: Procainamide inhibits sympathetic nerve activity in rabbits. J. Lab. Clin. Med. *119*:211, 1992.
50. Grimm, W., Cho, J.-G., and Marchlinski, F. E.: Effects of incremental doses of procainamide in patients with sustained uniform ventricular tachycardia. J. Cardiovasc. Electrophysiol. *5*:313, 1994.
51. Brautigam, R. T., Porter, S., and Kutalek, S. P.: The effects of programmed ventricular stimulation on plasma procainamide levels: An experimental model. J. Clin. Pharmacol. *34*:184, 1994.
52. Ellenbogen, K. A., Wood, M. A., and Stambler, B. S.: Procainamide: A perspective on its value and danger. Heart Dis. Stroke *2*:473, 1993.
53. Edvardsson, N.: Comparison of class I and class III action in atrial fibrillation. Eur. Heart J. *14* (Suppl. H):62, 1993.
54. Kudenchuk, P. J., Halperin, B., Kron, J., et al.: Serial electropharmacologic studies in patients with ischemic heart disease and sustained ventricular tachyarrhythmias: When is drug testing sufficient. Am. J. Cardiol. *72*:1400, 1993.
55. Steinberg, J. S., Sahar, B. I., Rosenbaum, M., et al.: Proarrhythmic effects of procainamide and tocainide in a canine infarction model. J. Cardiovasc. Pharmacol. *19*:52, 1992.
56. Echizen, H., Kawasaki, H., Chiba, K., et al.: A potent inhibitory effect of erythromycin and other macrolide antibiotics on the mono-*N*-dealkylation metabolism of disopyramide with human liver microsomes. J. Pharmacol. Exp. Ther. *264*:1425, 1993.

CLASS IB AGENTS

57. Chahine, M., Chen, L. Q, Barchi, R. L., et al.: Lidocaine block of human heart sodium channels expressed in *Zenopus* oocytes. J. Mol. Cell Cardiol. *24*:1231, 1992.
58. Ye, V. Z., Wyse, K. R., and Campbell, T. J.: Lidocaine shows greater selective depression of depolarized and acidotic myocardium than propafenone: Possible implications for proarrhythmia. J. Cardiovasc. Pharmacol. *21*:47, 1993.
59. Destache, C. J., Hilleman, D. E., Mohiuddin, S. J., et al.: Predictive performance of Bayesian and nonlinear least-squares regression programs for lidocaine. Ther. Drug Monit. *14*:286, 1992.
60. Nattel, S., and Arenal, A.: Antiarrhythmic prophylaxis after acute myocardial infarction: Is lidocaine still useful? Drugs *45*:9, 1993.
61. Jaffe, A. S.: Prophylatic lidocaine for suspected acute myocardial infarction? Heart Dis. Stroke *1*:179, 1992.
62. Jaffe, A. S.: The use of antiarrhythmics in advanced cardiac life support. Ann. Emerg. Med. *22*:307, 1993.
63. Johnson, R. G., Goldberger, A. L., Thurer, R. L., et al.: Lidocaine prophylaxis in coronary revascularization patients: A randomized, prospective trial. Ann. Thorac. Surg. *55*:1180, 1993.
64. Buckles, D. S., Ick, B., and Gillette, P. C.: Subcutaneous lidocaine affects inducibility in programmed electrophysiology testing in children: A follow-up study. Am. Heart J. *124*:1241, 1992.
65. McCaughey, W.: Adverse effects of local anesthetics. Drug Saf. *7*:178, 1992.
66. Tatsukawa, H., Okuda, J., Kondoh, M., et al.: Malignant hyperthermia caused by intravenous lidocaine for ventricular arrhythmia. Ann. Intern. Med. *31*:1069, 1992.
67. Echt, D. S., Gremillion, S. T., Lee, J. T., et al.: Effects of procainamide and lidocaine on defibrillation energy requirements in patients receiving implantable cardioverter defibrillator devices. J. Cardiovasc. Electrophysiol. *5*:752, 1994.
68. Mason, J. W.: A comparison of seven antiarrhythmic drugs in patients with ventricular tachyarrhythmias: Electrophysiologic Study Versus Electrocardiographic Monitoring investigators. N. Engl. J. Med. *329*:452, 1993.
69. Lazzara, R.: Results of Holter ECG guided therapy for ventricular arrhythmias: The ESVEM trial. PACE *17*:473, 1994.
70. Takanaka, C., Nonokawa, M., Machii, T., et al.: Mexiletine and propafenone: A comparative study of monotherapy, low and full dose combination therapy. PACE *15*:2130, 1992.
71. Yeung-Lai-Wah, J. A., Murdock, C. J., Boone, J., et al.: Propafenone-mexiletine combination for the treatment of sustained ventricular tachycardia. J. Am. Coll. Cardiol. *20*:547, 1992.
72. Lombardi, F., Finocciaro, M. L., DallaVecchia, L., et al.: Effects of mexiletine, propafenone and flecainide on signal-averaged electrocardiogram. Eur. Heart J. *13*:517, 1992.
73. Geraets, D. R., Scott, S. D., and Ballew, K. A.: Toxicity potential of oral lidocaine in a patient receiving mexiletine. Ann. Pharmacol. Ther. *26*:1380, 1992.
74. Gelfand, M. S., Yunus, F., and White, F. L.: Bone marrow granulomas, fever, pancytopenia, and lupus-like syndrome due to tocainide. South. Med. J. *87*:839, 1994.
75. Kahn, A. S., Dadparvar, S., Brown, S. J., et al.: The role of gallium-67-citrate in the detection of phenytoin-induced pneumonitis. J. Nucl. Med. *35*:471, 1994.
76. Danielson, M. K., Danielson, B. R., Marchner, H., et al.: Histopathological and hemodynamic studies supporting hypoxia and vascular disruption as explanation to phenytoin teratogenicity. Teratology *46*:485, 1992.
77. Lindhout, D., and Omtzigt, J. G.: Pregnancy and the risk of teratogenicity. Epilepsia 33 (Suppl. 4):S41, 1992.

78. Wang, Z., Fremini, B., and Nattel, S.: Mechanism of flecainide's rate-dependent actions on action potential duration in canine atrial tissue. J. Pharmacol. Exp. Ther. *267*:575, 1993.
79. Yamashita, T., Inoue, H., Nozaki, A., et al.: Role of anisotropy in determining the selective action of antiarrhythmics in atrial fluttter in the dog. Cardiovasc. Res. *26*:244, 1992.
80. Crijns, H. J., deLangen, C. D., Grandjean, J. G., et al.: Sustained atrial flutter around the tricuspid valve in pigs: Differentiation of procainamide (class IA) from flecainide (class IC) and their rate-dependent effects. J. Cardiovasc. Pharmacol. *21*:462, 1993.
81. Pinto, J. M., Graziano, J. N., and Boyden, P. A.: Endocardial mapping of reentry around an anatomical barrier in the canine right atrium: Observations during the action of the class IC agent, flecainide. J. Cardiovasc. Electrophysiol. *4*:672, 1993.
82. Windle, J. R., Witt, R. C., and Rozanski, G. J.: Effects of flecainide on ectopic atrial automaticity and conduction. Circulation *88*:1878, 1993.
83. Krishnan, S. C., and Antzelevitch, C.: Flecainide-induced arrhythmia in canine ventricular epicardium. Phase II reentry? Circulation *87*:562, 1993.
84. Goldberger, J., Helmy, I., Katzung, B., et al.: Use-dependent properties of flecainide acetate in accessory atrioventricular pathways. Am. J. Cardiol. *73*:43, 1994.
85. Gill, J. S., Mehta, D., Ward, D. E., et al.: Efficacy of flecainide, sotalol and verapamil in the treatment of right ventricular tachycardia in patients without overt cardiac abnormality. Br. Heart J. *68*:392, 1992.
86. Kidwell, G. A., Greenspon, A. J., Greenberg, R. M., et al.: Use-dependent prolongation of ventricular tachycardia cycle length by type I antiarrhythmic drugs in humans. Circulation *87*:118, 1993.
87. Madrid, A. H., Moro, C., Marin-Huerta, E., et al.: Comparison of flecainide and procainamide in conversion of atrial fibrillation. Eur. Heart J. *14*:1127, 1993.
88. Hohnloser, S. H., and Zabel, M.: Short- and long-term efficacy and safety of flecainide acetate for supraventricular arrhythmias. Am. J. Cardiol. *70*:3A, 1992.
89. A symposium: Use of flecainide for the treatment of supraventricular arrhythmias. Am. J. Cardiol. *70*:1A, 1992.
90. Anderson, J. L., Platt, M. L., Guarnier, I. T., et al.: Flecainide acetate for paroxysmal supraventricular tachyarrhythmias: The flecainide supraventricular tachycardia study group. Am. J. Cardiol. *74*:578, 1994.
91. Balaji, S., Johnson, T. B., Sade, R. M., et al.: Management of atrial flutter after the Fontan procedure. J. Am. Coll. Cardiol. *23*:1209, 1994.
92. Lau, C. P., Leung, W. H., and Wong, C. K.: A randomized double-blind crossover study comparing the efficacy and tolerability of flecainide and quinidine in the control of patients with symptomatic paroxysmal atrial fibrillation. Am. Heart J. *124*:645, 1992.
93. Grey, E., and Silverman, D. I.: Efficacy of type IC antiarrhythmic agents for treatment of resistant atrial fibrillation. PACE *16*:2235, 1993.
94. LeClercq, J. F., Chouty, F., Denjoy, I., et al.: Flecainide in quinidine-resistant atrial fibrillation. Am. J. Cardiol. *70*:62A, 1992.
95. Auricchio, A.: Reversible protective effect of propafenone or flecainide during atrial fibrillation in patients with an accessory atrioventricular connection. Am. Heart J. *124*:932, 1992.
96. vonBernuth, G., Engelhardt, W., Kramer, H. H., et al.: Atrial automatic tachycardia in infancy and childhood. Eur. Heart J. *13*:1410, 1992.
97. Ahsan, A., Aldridge, R., and Bowes, R.: 1:1 Atrioventricular conduction in atrial flutter with digoxin and flecainide. Int. J. Cardiol. *39*:88, 1993.
98. vanEngelen, A. D., Weijtens, O., Brenner, J. I., et al.: Management outcome and follow-up of fetal tachycardia. J. Am. Coll. Cardiol. *24*:1371, 1994.
99. Ito, S., Magee, L., and Smallhorn, J.: Drug therapy for fetal arrhythmias. Clin. Perinatol. *21*:543, 1994.
100. Perry, J. C., and Garson, A., Jr.: Flecainide acetate for treatment of tachyarrhythmias in children: Review of world literature on efficacy, safety and dosing. Am. Heart J. *124*:1614, 1992.
101. Manz, M., Jung, W., and Luderitz, B.: Interactions between drugs and devices: Experimental and clinical studies. Am. Heart J. *127*:978, 1994.
102. Stramba-Badiale, M., Lazzarotti, M., Facchini, M., et al.: Malignant arrhythmias and acute myocardial ischemia: Interaction between flecainide and the autonomic nervous system. Am. Heart J. *128*:973, 1994.
103. Sadanaga, T., and Ogawa, S.: Ischemia enhances use-dependent sodium channel blockade by pilsicainide, a class IC antiarrhythmic agent. J. Am. Coll. Cardiol. *23*:1378, 1994.
104. Wang, J., Bourne, G. W., Wang, Z., et al.: Comparative mechanisms of antiarrhythmic drug action in experimental atrial fibrillation: Importance of use-dependent effects on refractoriness. Circulation *88*:1030, 1993.
105. Brugada, J., Boersma, L., Abdollah, H., et al.: Echo-wave termination of ventricular tachycardia: A common mechanism of termination of reentrant arrhythmias by various pharmacological interventions. Circulation *85*:1879, 1992.
106. Santinelli, V., Arnese, M., Oppo, I., et al.: Effects of flecainide and propafenone on systolic performance in subjects with normal cardiac function. Chest *103*:1068, 1993.
107. Lombardi, F., Torzillo, D., Sandrone, G., et al.: Beta-blocking effect of propafenone based on spectral analysis of heart rate variability. Am. J. Cardiol. *70*:1028, 1992.
108. Zehender, M., Hohnloser, S., Geibel, A., et al.: Short-term and long-term treatment with propafenone: Determinance of arrhythmia suppression, persistence of efficacy, arrhythmogenesis, and side effects in patients with symptoms. Br. Heart J. *67*:491, 1992.
109. Bryson, H. M., Palmer, K. J., Langtry, H. D., et al.: Propafenone: A reappraisal of its pharmacology, pharmacokinetics and therapeutic use in cardiac arrhythmias. Drugs *45*:85, 1993.
110. Paul, T., Reimer, A., Janousek, J., et al.: Efficacy and safety of propafenone in congenital junctional ectopic tachycardia. J. Am. Coll. Cardiol. *20*:911, 1992.
111. Furlanello, F., Guarnerio, M., Inama, G., et al.: Long-term follow-up of patients with inducible supraventricular tachycardia treated with flecainide or propafenone: Therapy guided by transesophageal electropharmacologic testing. Am. J. Cardiol. *70*:19A, 1992.
112. Balaji, S., Johnson, T. B., Sade, R. M., et al.: Management of atrial flutter after Fontan procedure. J. Am. Coll. Cardiol. *23*:1209, 1994.
113. Kingma, J. H., and Suttorp, M. J.: Acute pharmacologic conversion of atrial fibrillation and flutter: The role of flecainide, propafenone and verapamil. Am. J. Cardiol. *70*:56A, 1992.
114. Capucci, A., Boriani, G., Boto, G. L., et al.: Conversion of recent-onset atrial fibrillation by a single or loading dose of propafenone or flecainide. Am. J. Cardiol. *74*:503, 1994.
115. Reimold, S. C., Cantillon, C. O., Friedman, P. L., et al.: Propafenone versus sotalol for suppression of recurrent symptomatic atrial fibrillation. Am. J. Cardiol. *71*:558, 1993.
116. Gentili, C., Giordano, F., Alois, A., et al.: Efficacy of intravenous propafenone in acute atrial fibrillation complicating open-heart surgery. Am. Heart J. *123*:1225, 1992.
117. Paul, T., and Janousek, J.: New antiarrhythmic drugs in pediatric use: Propafenone. Pediatr. Cardiol. *15*:190, 1994.
118. Heusch, A., Kramer, H. H., Krogmann, O. N., et al.: Clinical experience with propafenone for cardiac arrhythmias in the young. Eur. Heart J. *15*:1050, 1994.
119. Janousek, J., Paul, T., Reimer, A., et al.: Usefulness of propafenone for supraventricular arrhythmias in infants and children. Am. J. Cardiol. *72*:294, 1993.
120. Vignati, G., Mauri, L., and Figini, A.: The use of propafenone in the treatment of tachyarrhythmias in children. Eur. Heart J. *14*:546, 1993.
121. Cornacchia, D., Fabbri, M., Maresta, A., et al.: Effect of steroid eluting versus conventional electrodes on propafenone induced rise in chronic ventricular pacing threshold. PACE *16*:2279, 1993.
122. Bianconi, L., Boccadamo, R., Toscano, S., et al.: Effects of oral propafenone therapy on chronic myocardial pacing threshold. PACE *15*:148, 1992.
123. Natale, A., Montenero, A. S., Bombardieri, G., et al.: Effects of acute and prolonged administration of propafenone on internal defibrillation in the pig. Am. Heart J. *124*:104, 1992.
124. Siebels, J., and Kuck, K. H.: Implantable cardioverter defibrillator compared with antiarrhythmic drug treatment in cardiac arrest survivors (The Cardiac Arrest Study, Hamburg). Am. Heart J. *127*:1139, 1994.
125. Yamane, T., Sunami, A., Sawanobori, T., et al.: Use-dependent block of Ca^{2+} current by moricizine in guinea-pig ventricular myocytes: A possible ionic mechanism of action potential shortening. Br. J. Pharmacol. *108*:812, 1993.
126. Ortiz, J., Nozaki, A., Shimizu, A., et al.: Mechanism of interruption of atrial flutter by moricizine: Electrophysiological and multiplexing studies in the canine sterile pericarditis model of atrial flutter. Circulation *89*:2860, 1994.
127. Bigger, J. T., Jr., Rolnitzky, L. M., Steinman, R. C., et al.: Predicting mortality after myocardial infarction from the response of RR variability to antiarrhythmic drug therapy. J. Am. Coll. Cardiol. *23*:733, 1994.
128. Ujhelyi, M. R., O'Rangers, E. A., Kluger, J., et al.: Defibrillation energy requirements during moricizine and moricizine-lidocaine therapy. J. Cardiovasc. Pharmacol. *20*:932, 1992.
129. Benedek, I. H., Davidson, A. F., and Pieniaszek, H. J., Jr.: Enzyme induction by moricizine: Time course and extent in healthy subjects. J. Clin. Pharmacol. *34*:167, 1994.
130. Clyne, C. A., Estes, N. A., III, and Wang, P. J.: Moricizine. N. Engl. J. Med. *327*:255, 1992.
131. Damle, R., Levine, J., Matos, J., et al.: Efficacy and risks of moricizine in inducible sustained ventricular tachycardia. Ann. Intern. Med. *116*:375, 1992.
132. Powell, A. C., Gold, M. R., Brooks, R., et al.: Electrophysiologic response to moricizine in patients with sustained venricular arrhythmias. Ann. Intern. Med. *116*:382, 1992.
133. Bhandari, A. K., Lerman, R., Erlich, S., et al.: Electrophysiological evaluation of moricizine in patients with sustained ventricular tachyarrhythmias: Low efficacy and high incidence of proarrhythmia. PACE *16*:1853, 1993.
134. Greene, H. L., Roden, D. M., Katz, R. J., et al.: The Cardiac Arrhythmia Suppression Trial: First CAST then CAST-II. J. Am. Coll. Cardiol. *19*:894, 1992.
135. Nazari, J., Bauman, J., Pham, T., et al.: Exercise induced fatal sinusoidal ventricular tachycardia secondary to moricizine. PACE *15*:1421, 1992.
136. Tschaidse, O., Graboys, T. B., Lown, B., et al.: The prevalence of proarrhythmic events during moricizine therapy. Am. Heart J. *124*:912, 1992.
137. Akiyama, T., Pawitan, Y., Campbell, W. B., et al.: Effects of advancing age on the efficacy and side effects of antiarrhythmic drugs in post-myocardial infarction patients with ventricular arrhythmias: The CAST Investigators. J. Am. Geriatr. Soc. *40*:666, 1992.

138. Singh, B. N.: Beta-blockers and calcium channel blockers as antiarrhythmic drugs. *In* Zipes, D. P., and Jalife, J. (eds.): Cardiac Electrophysiology: From Cell to Bedside. 2nd ed. Philadelphia, W. B., Saunders Company, 1994, pp. 1317–1330.
138a. Kendall, M. J., Lynch, K. P., and Hjalmarson, A.: β-Blockers and sudden cardiac death. Ann. Intern. Med. *123:*358, 1995.
139. Adamson, P. B., Huang, M. H., Vanolie, E., et al.: Unexpected interaction between beta-adrenergic blockade and heart rate variability before and after myocardial infarction: A longitudinal study in dogs at high and low risk for sudden death. Circulation *90:*976, 1994.
140. Patel, J., Lee, W., Fusilli, L., et al.: Anti-arrhythmic efficacy of beta-adrenergic blockade during acute ischemia in the myocardium with scar. Am. J. Med. Sci. *307:*259, 1994.
141. Lubbe, W. F., Todzuweit, T., and Opie, L. H.: Potential arrhythmogenic role of cyclic adenosine monophosphate (AMP) and cytosolic calcium overload: Implications for prophylactic effects of beta-blockers in myocardial infarction and proarrhythmic effects of phosphodiesterase inhibitors. J. Am. Coll. Cardiol. *19:*1622, 1992.
142. Krishnan, S., and Levy, M. N.: Effects of coronary artery occlusion and reperfusion on the idioventricular rate in anesthetized dogs. J. Am. Coll. Cardiol. *23:*1484, 1994.
143. Aronow, W. S., Ahn, C., Mercando, A. D., et al.: Decrease in mortality by propranolol in patients with heart disease and complex ventricular arrhythmias is more an anti-ischemic than an antiarrhythmic effect. Am. J. Cardiol. *74:*613, 1994.
144. Hopson, J. R., and Martins, J. B.: Hemodynamic and reflex sympathetic control of transmural activation and rate of ventricular tachycardia in ischemic and hypertrophic ventricular myocardium of the dog. Circulation *86:*618, 1992.
145. Ditchey, R. V., Rubio-Perez, A., and Slinker, B. K.: Beta-adrenergic blockade reduces myocardial injury during experimental cardiopulmonary resuscitation. J. Am. Coll. Cardiol. *24:*804, 1994.
146. Shettigar, U. R., Toole, J. G., and Appunn, D. O.: Combined use of esmolol and digoxin in the acute treatment of atrial fibrillation or flutter. Am. Heart J. *126:* 368, 1993.
147. Sarter, D. H., and Marchlinski, F. E.: Redefining the role of digoxin in the treatment of atrial fibrillation. Am. J. Cardiol. *69:*71G, 1992.
148. Natale, A., Klein, G., Yee, R., et al.: Shortening of fast pathway refractoriness after slow pathway ablation: Effects of autonomic blockade. Circulation *89:*1003, 1994.
149. Elvas, L., Gursoy, S., Brugada, J., et al.: Atrioventricular nodal reentrant tachycardia: A review. Can. J. Cardiol. *10:*342, 1994.
150. Skeberis, V., Simonis, F., Tsakonas, K., et al.: Inappropriate sinus tachycardia following radiofrequency ablation of AV nodal tachycardia: Incidence and clinical significance. PACE *17:*924, 1994.
151. Morillo, C. A., Klein, G. J., Thakur, R. K., et al.: Mechanism of "inappropriate" sinus tachycardia: Role of sympathovagal balance. Circulation *90:*873, 1994.
152. Hill, G. A., and Owens, S. D.: Esmolol in the treatment of multifocal atrial tachycardia. Chest *101:*1726, 1992.
153. Garson, A., Jr., Dick, M., II, Fournier, A., et al.: The long QT syndrome in children. An international study of 287 patients. Circulation *87:*1866, 1993.
154. Malfatto, G., Beria, G., Sala, S., et al.: Quantitative analysis of T wave abnormalities and their prognostic implications in the idiopathic long QT syndrome. J. Am. Coll. Cardiol. *23:*296, 1994.
155. Moss, A. J., and Robinson, J.: Clinical features of the idiopathic long QT syndrome. Circulation *85* (Suppl. 1):1140, 1992.
156. Hjalmarson, Å.: Empiric therapy with beta-blockers. PACE *17:*460, 1994.
157. Sweeney, M. O., Moss, A. J., and Eberly, S.: Instantaneous cardiac death in the posthospital period after acute myocardial infarction. Am. J. Cardiol. *70:*1375, 1992.
158. Pitt, B.: The role of beta-adrenergic blocking agents in preventing sudden cardiac death. Circulation *85* (Suppl. 1):1107, 1992.
159. Kennedy, H. L., Brooks, A. H., Bergstrand, R., et al.: Beta-blocker therapy in the Cardiac Arrhythmia Suppression Trial: CAST Investigators. Am. J. Cardiol. *74:*674, 1994.
160. Steinbeck, G., Andresen, D., Bach, P., et al.: A comparison of electrophysiologically guided antiarrhythmic drug therapy with beta-blocker therapy in patients with symptomatic sustained ventricular tachyarrhythmias. N. Engl. J. Med. *327:*987, 1992.
161. Bhorat, I. E., Naidoo, D. P., Rout, C. C., et al.: Malignant ventricular arrhythmias in eclampsia: A comparison of labetalol with dihydralazine. Am. J. Obstet. Gynecol. *168:*1292, 1993.
162. Ko, W. J., and Chu, S. H.: A new dosing regimen for esmolol to treat supraventricular tachyarrhythmia in Chinese patients. J. Am. Coll. Cardiol. *23:*302, 1994.
163. Ovadia, M., and Thoele, D.: Esmolol tilt testing with esmolol withdrawal for the evaluation of syncope in the young. Circulation *89:*228, 1994.

CLASS III AGENTS

164. Sager, P. T., Follmer, C., Uppal, P., et al.: The effects of beta-adrenergic stimulation on the frequency-dependent electrophysiologic actions of amiodarone and sematilide in humans. Circulation *90:*1811, 1994.
165. Sager, P. T., Uppal, P., Follmer, C., et al.: Frequency-dependent electrophysiologic effects of amiodarone in humans. Circulation *88:*1063, 1993.
166. Chiamvimonvat, N., Mitchell, L. B., Gillis, A. M., et al.: Use-dependent electrophysiologic effects of amiodarone in coronary artery disease and inducible ventricular tachycardia. Am. J. Cardiol. *70:*598, 1992.
167. Hii, J. T., Wyse, B. G., Gillis, A. M., et al.: Precordial QT interval dispersion as a marker of torsade de pointes: Disparate effects of class IA antiarrhythmic drugs and amiodarone. Circulation *86:*1376, 1992.
168. Cui, G., Sen, L., Sager, P., et al.: Effects of amiodarone, sematilide, and sotalol on QT dispersion. Am. J. Cardiol. *74:*896, 1994.
169. Calkins, H., Sousa, J., el-Atassi, R., et al.: Reversal of antiarrhythmic drug effects by epinephrine: Quinidine versus amiodarone. J. Am. Coll. Cardiol. *19:*347, 1992.
170. Kalbfleisch, S. J., Williamson, B., Man, K. C., et al.: Prospective, randomized comparison of conventional and high dose loading regimens of amiodarone in the treatment of ventricular tachycardia. J. Am. Coll. Cardiol. *22:*1723, 1993.
171. Summitt, J., Morady, F., and Kadish, A.: A comparison of standard and high-dose regimens for the initiation of amiodarone therapy. Am. Heart J. *124:*366, 1992.
172. Kim, S. G., Mannino, M. M., Chou, R., et al.: Rapid suppression of spontaneous ventricular arrhythmias during oral amiodarone loading. Ann. Intern. Med. *117:*197, 1992.
173. Evans, S. J., Myers, M., Zaher, C., et al.: High dose oral amiodarone loading: Electrophysiologic effects and clinical tolerance. J. Am. Coll. Cardiol. *19:*169, 1992.
174. Russo, A. M., Beauregard, L. M., and Waxman, H. L.: Oral amiodarone loading for the rapid treatment of frequent refractory sustained ventricular arrhythmias associated with coronary artery disease. Am. J. Cardiol. *72:*1395, 1993.
175. Weinberg, B. A., Miles, W. M., Klein, L. S., et al.: Five-year follow-up of 589 patients treated with amiodarone. Am. Heart J. *125:*109, 1993.
176. Mahmarian, J. J., Smart, F. W., Moye, L. A., et al.: Exploring the minimal dose of amiodarone with antiarrhythmic and hemodynamic activity. Am. J. Cardiol. *74:*681, 1994.
177. Perry, J. C., Knilans, T. K., Marlow, D., et al.: Inravenous amiodarone for life-threatening tachyarrhythmias in children and young adults. J. Am. Coll. Cardiol. *22:*95, 1993.
178. Flack, N. J., Zosmer, N., Bennet, P. R., et al.: Amiodarone given by three routes to terminate fetal atrial flutter associated with severe hydrops. Obstet. Gynecol. *82:*714, 1993.
179. Azancot-Benisty, A., Jacqz-Aigrain, E., Guirgis, N. M., et al.: Clinical and pharmacologic study of fetal supraventricular tachyarrhythmias. J. Pediatr. *121:*608, 1992.
180. Shuler, C. O., Case, C. L., and Gillette, P. C.: Efficacy and safety of amiodarone in infants. Am. Heart J. *125:*430, 1993.
181. Figa, F. H., Gow, R. M., Hamilton, R. M., et al.: Clinical efficacy and safety of intravenous amiodarone in infants and children. Am. J. Cardiol. *74:*573, 1994.
182. Raja, P., Hawker, R. E., Chaikitpinyo, A., et al.: Amiodarone management of junctional ectopic tachycardia after cardiac surgery in children. Br. Heart J. *72:*261, 1994.
183. Disch, D. L., Greenberg, M. L., and Holzberger, P. T.: Managing chronic atrial fibrillation: A Markov decision analysis comparing warfarin, quinidine and low-dose amiodarone. Ann. Intern. Med. *120:*449, 1994.
184. Skoularigis, J., Rothlisberger, C., Skudicky, D., et al.: Effectiveness of amiodarone and electrical cardioversion for chronic rheumatic atrial fibrillation after mitral valve surgery. Am. J. Cardiol. *72:*423, 1992.
185. Estes, N. A., III: Evolving strategies for the management of atrial fibrillation: The role of amiodarone. JAMA *267:*3332, 1992.
186. Gosselink, A. T., Crijns, H. J., VanGelder, I. C., et al.: Low-dose amiodarone for maintenance of sinus rhythm after cardioversion of atrial fibrillation or flutter. JAMA *267:*3289, 1992.
187. Zehender, M., Hohnloser, S., Muller, B., et al.: Effects of amiodarone versus quinidine and verapamil in patients with chronic atrial fibrillation: Results of a comparative study and 2-year follow-up. J. Am. Coll. Cardiol. *19:*1054, 1992.
188. Middlekauff, H. R., Wiener, I., and Stevenson, W. G.: Low-dose amiodarone for atrial fibrillation. Am. J. Cardiol. *72:*75F, 1993.
189. Butler, J., Harriss, D. R., Sinclair, M., et al.: Amiodarone prophylaxis for tachycardias after coronary artery surgery: A randomized double-blind placebo control trial. Br. Heart J. *70:*56, 1993.
190. Roden, D. M.: Current status of class III antiarrhythmic drug therapy. Am. J. Cardiol. *72:*44B, 1993.
191. Nora, M., and Zipes, D. P.: Empiric use of amiodarone and sotalol. Am. J. Cardiol. *72:*62F, 1993.
192. Singh, B. N.: Controlling cardiac arrhythmias by lengthening repolarization: Historical overview. Am. J. Cardiol. *72:*18F, 1993.
193. Stevenson, W. G., Stevenson, L. W., Middlekauff, H. R., et al.: Sudden death prevention in patients with advanced ventricular dysfunction. Circulation *88:*2953, 1993.
194. Dolack, G. L.: Clinical predictors of implantable cardioverter-defibrillator shocks (results of the CASCADE trial). Cardiac Arrest in Seattle, Conventional versus Amiodarone Drug Evaluation. Am. J. Cardiol. *73:*237, 1994.
195. Anastasiou-Nana, M. I., Nanas, J. N., Nanas, S. N., et al.: Effects of amiodarone on refractory ventricular fibrillation in acute myocardial infarction: Experimental study. J. Am. Coll. Cardiol. *23:*253, 1994.
196. Dorian, P., and Newman, D.: Effect of sotalol on ventricular fibrillation and defibrillation in humans. Am. J. Cardiol. *72:*72A, 1993.

197. Jung, W., Manz, M., Pizzulli, L., et al.: Effects of chronic amiodarone therapy on defibrillation threshold. Am. J. Cardiol. *70:*1023, 1992.
198. Nademanee, K., Singh, B. N., Stevenson, W. G., et al.: Amiodarone in post-MI patients. Circulation *88:*264, 1993
199. Ceremuzynski, L.: Secondary prevention after myocardial infarction with class III antiarrhythmic drugs. Am. J. Cardiol. *72:*82F, 1993.
200. Pfisterer, M. E., Kiowski, W., Brunner, H., et al.: Long-term benefit of one-year amiodarone treatment for persistent complex ventricular arrhythmias after myocardial infarction. Circulation *87:*309, 1993.
201. Zarenbski, D. G., Nolan, P. E., Jr., Slack, M. K., et al.: Empiric long-term amiodarone prophylaxis following a myocardial infarction. A meta-analysis. Arch. Intern. Med. *153:*2661, 1993.
202. Navarro-Lopez, F., Cosin, J., Marrugat, J., et al.: Comparison of the effects of amiodarone versus metoprolol on the frequency of ventricular arrhythmias and on mortality after acute myocardial infarction: Spanish study on sudden death. Am. J. Cardiol. *72:*1243, 1993.
203. Singh, S. N., Fletcher, R. D., Fisher, S., et al.: Amiodarone in patients with congestive heart failure and symptomatic arrhythmia. N. Engl. J. Med. *333:*77, 1995.
204. Doval, H. C., Nul, D. R., Grancelli, H. O., et al.: Randomized trial of low-dose amiodarone in severe congestive heart failure: Grupo de Estudio de la Sobrevida en la Insuficiencia Cardiaca en Argentina (GESICA). Lancet *344:*493, 1994.
205. Greene, H. L.: The CASCADE Study: Randomized antiarrhythmic drug therapy in survivors of cardiac arrest in Seattle. CASCADE Investigators. Am. J. Cardiol. *72:*70F, 1993.
206. The CASCADE Investigators: Randomized antiarrhythmic drug therapy in survivors of cardiac arrest (The CASCADE Study). Am. J. Cardiol. *72:*280, 1993.
207. Camm, A. J., Julian, D., Janse, G., et al.: The European Myocardial Infarct Amiodarone Trial (EMIAT). EMIAT Investigators. Am. J. Cardiol. *72:*95F, 1993.
208. Cairns, J. A., Connolly, S. J., Roberts, R., et al.: Canadian Amiodarone Myocardial Infarction Arrhythmia Trial (CAMIAT): Rationale and protocol. CAMIAT Investigators. Am. J. Cardiol. *72:*87F, 1993.
209. Connolly, S. J., Gent, M., Roberts, R. S., et al.: Canadian Implantable Defibrillator Study (CIDS): Study design and organization. CIDS Co-investigators. Am. J. Cardiol. *72:*103F, 1993.
210. AVID Investigators: Antiarrhythmics Versus Implantable Defibrillators (AVID): Rationale, design and methods. Am. J. Cardiol. *75:*470, 1995.
211. Man, K. C., Williamson, B. D., Niebauer, M., et al.: Electrophysiologic effects of sotalol and amiodarone in patients with sustained monomorphic ventricular tachycardia. Am. J. Cardiol. *74:*1119, 1994.
212. Pastor, A., Almendral, J. M., Arenal, A., et al.: Comparison of electrophysiologic effects of quinidine and amiodarone in sustained ventricular tachyarrhythmias associated with coronary artery disease. Am. J. Cardiol. *72:*1389, 1993.
213. Martinez-Rubio, A., Shenasa, M., Chen, X., et al.: Response to sotalol predicts the response to amiodarone during serial drug testing in patients with sustained ventricular tachycardia and coronary artery disease. Am. J. Cardiol. *73:*357, 1994.
214. Olson, P. J., Woelfel, A., Simpson, R. J., Jr., et al.: Stratification of sudden death risk in patients receiving long-term amiodarone treatment for sustained ventricular tachycardia or ventricular fibrillation. Am. J. Cardiol. *71:*823, 1993.
215. Kerin, N. Z., Ansari-Leesar, M., Faitel, K., et al.: The effectiveness and safety of the simultaneous administration of quinidine and amiodarone in the conversion of chronic atrial fibrillation. Am. Heart J. *125:*1017, 1993.
216. Bashir, Y., Paul, V. E., Griffith, M. J., et al.: A prospective study of the efficacy and safety of adjuvant metoprolol and xamoterol in combination with amiodarone for resistant ventricular tachycardia associated with impaired left ventricular function. Am. Heart J. *124:*1233, 1992.
217. Ulrik, C. S., Backer, V., Aldershvile, J., et al.: Serial pulmonary function tests in patients treated with low-dose amiodarone. Am. Heart J. *123:*1550, 1992.
218. Davies, P. H., Franklyn, J. A., and Sheppard, M. C.: Treatment of amiodarone induced thyrotoxicosis with carbimazole alone and continuation of amiodarone. B.M.J. *305:*224, 1992.
219. Trip, M. D., Duren, D. R., and Wiersinga, W. M.: Two cases of amiodarone-induced thyrotoxicosis successfully treated with a short course of antithyroid drugs while amiodarone was continued. Br. Heart J. *72:*266, 1994.
220. Hohnloser, S. H., Klingenheben, T., and Singh, B. N.: Amiodarone-associated proarrhythmic effects: A review with special reference to torsade de pointes tachycardia. Ann. Intern. Med. *121:*529, 1994.
221. Makkar, R. R., Fromm, B. S., Steinman, R. T., et al.: Female gender as a risk factor for torsades de pointes associated with cardiovascular drugs. JAMA *270:*2590, 1993.
222. Mickleborough, L. L., Maruyiama, H., Mohamed, S., et al.: Are patients receiving amiodarone at increased risk for cardiac operations? Ann. Thorac. Surg. *58:*622, 1994.
223. Chelimsky-Fallick, C., Middlekauff, H. R., Stevenson, W. G., et al.: Amiodarone therapy does not compromise subsequent heart transplantation. J. Am. Coll. Cardiol. *20:*1556, 1992.
224. Quesada, A., Sanchis, J., Charro, F. J., et al.: Changes in canine ventricular fibrillation threshold induced by verapamil, flecainide and bretylium. Eur. Heart J. *14:*712, 1993.
225. Usui, M., Inoue, H., Saihara, S., et al.: Antifibrillatory effects of class III antiarrhythmic drugs: Comparative study with flecainide. J. Cardiovasc. Pharmacol. *21:*376, 1993.
226. Jones, D. L., Kim, Y. H., Natale, A., et al.: Bretylium decreases and verapamil increases defibrillation threshold in pigs. PACE *17:*1380, 1994.
227. Hohnloser, S. H., and Woosley, R. L.: Sotalol. N. Engl. J. Med. *331:*31, 1994.
228. Singh, B. N.: Electrophysiologic basis for the antiarrhythmic actions of sotalol and comparison with other agents. Am. J. Cardiol. *72:*8A, 1993.
229. Reiter, M. J., Zetelaki, Z., Kirchhof, C. J., et al.: Interaction of acute ventricular dilation and d-sotalol during sustained reentrant ventricular tachycardia around a fixed obstacle. Circulation *89:*423, 1994.
230. Alboni, P., Razzolini, R., Scarfo, S., et al.: Hemodynamic effects of oral sotalol during both sinus rhythm and atrial fibrillation. J. Am. Coll. Cardiol. *22:*1373, 1993.
231. Winters, S. L., Kukin, M. K., Tee, E., et al.: Effects of oral sotalol on systemic hemodynamics and programmed electrical stimulation in patients with ventricular arrhythmias and structural heart disease. Am. J. Cardiol. *72:*38A, 1993.
232. Hohnloser, S. H., Zabel, M., Krause, T., et al.: Short- and long-term antiarrhythmic and hemodynamic effects of d,l-sotalol in patients with symptomatic ventricular arrhythmias. Am. Heart J. *123:*1220, 1992.
233. Kehoe, R. F., MacNeil, D. J., Zheutlin, T. A., et al.: Safety and efficacy of oral sotalol for sustained ventricular tachyarrhythmias refractory to other antiarrhythmic agents. Am. J. Cardiol. *72:*56A, 1993.
234. Young, G. D., Kerr, C. R., Mohama, R., et al.: Efficacy of sotalol guided by programmed electrical stimulation for sustained ventricular arrhythmias secondary to coronary artery disease. Am. J. Cardiol. *73:*677, 1994.
235. Sotalol in life-threatening ventricular arrhythmias: An unique class III antiarrhythmic. Symposium proceedings. Am. J. Cardiol. *72:*1A, 1993.
236. Wang, J., Bourne, G. W., Wang, Z., et al.: Comparative mechanisms of antiarrhythmic drug action in experimental atrial fibrillation. Importance of use-dependent effects on refractoriness. Circulation *88:*1030, 1993.
237. Wang, J., Feng, J., and Nattel, S.: Class III antiarrhythmic drug action in experimental atrial fibrillation: Differences in reverse use dependence and effectiveness between d-sotalol and the new antiarrhythmic drug ambasilide. Circulation *90:*2032, 1994.
238. Brodsky, M., Saini, R., Bellinger, R., et al.: Comparative effects of the combination of digoxin and dl-sotalol therapy versus digoxin monotherapy for control of ventricular response in chronic atrial fibrillation. Am. Heart J. *127:*572, 1994.
239. Ho, D. S., Zecchin, R. P., Richards, D. A., et al.: Double-blind trial of lignocaine versus sotalol for acute termination of spontaneous sustained ventricular tachycardia. Lancet *344:*18, 1994.
240. Wichter, T., Borggrefe, M., Haverkamp, W., et al.: Efficacy of antiarrhythmic drugs in patients with arrhythmogenic right ventricular disease: Results in patients with inducible and noninducible ventricular tachycardia. Circulation *86:*29, 1992.
241. Freedman, R. A., Karagounis, L. A., and Steinberg, J. S.: Effects of sotalol on the signal-averaged electrocardiogram in patients with sustained ventricular tachycardia: Relation to suppression of inducibility and changes in tachycardia cycle length. J. Am. Coll. Cardiol. *20:*1213, 1992.
242. Maragnes, P., Tipple, M., and Fournier, A.: Effectiveness of oral sotalol for treatment of pediatric arrhythmias. Am. J. Cardiol. *69:*751, 1992.
243. MacNeil, D. J., Davies, R. O., and Beitchman, D.: Clinical safety profile of sotalol in the treatment of arrhythmias. Am. J. Cardiol. *72:*44A, 1993.
244. Dorian, P., Newman, D., Berman, N., et al.: Sotalol and type IA drugs in combination prevent recurrence of sustained ventricular tachycardia. J. Am. Cardiol. *22:*106, 1993.

CLASS IV AGENTS

245. Talajic, M., Lemery, R., Roy, D., et al.: Rate-dependent effects of diltiazem on human atrioventricular nodal properties. Circulation *86:*870, 1992.
246. Dias, V. C., Weir, S. J., and Ellenbogen, K. A.: Pharmacokinetics and pharmacodynamics of intravenous diltiazem in patients with atrial fibrillation or atrial flutter. Circulation *86:*1421, 1992.
247. Dougherty, A. H., Jackman, W. M., Naccarelli, G. V., et al.: Acute conversion of paroxysmal supraventricular tachycardia with intravenous diltiazem. IV Diltiazem Study Group. Am. J. Cardiol. *70:*587, 1992.
248. Hood, M. A., and Smith, W. M.: Adenosine versus verapamil in the treatment of supraventricular tachycardia: A randomized double-crossover trial. Am. Heart J. *123:*1543, 1992.
249. Ohe, T., Aihara, N., Kamakura, S., et al.: Long-term outcome of verapamil-sensitive sustained left ventricular tachycardia in patients without structural heart disease. J. Am. Cardiol. *25:*54, 1995.
250. Lai, W. T., Voon, W. C., Yen, H. W., et al.: Comparison of the electrophysiologic effects of oral sustained-release and intravenous verapamil in patients with paroxysmal supraventricular tachycardia. Am. J. Cardiol. *71:*405, 1993.
251. Ellenbogen, K. A.: Role of calcium antagonists for heart rate control in atrial fibrillation. Am. J. Cardiol. *69:*36B, 1992.
252. Ellenbogen, K. A., Dias, V. C., and Cardello, F. P.: Safety and efficacy of intravenous diltiazem in atrial fibrillation or atrial flutter. Am. J. Cardiol. *75:*45, 1995.
253. Goldenberg, I. F., Lewis, W. R., Dias, V. C., et al.: Intravenous diltiazem for the treatment of patients with atrial fibrillation or flutter and moderate to severe congestive heart failure. Am. J. Cardiol. *74:*884, 1994.
254. Koh, K. K., Kwan, K. S., Park, H. B., et al.: Efficacy and safety of digoxin alone and in combination with low-dose diltiazem or betaxolol

to control ventricular rate in chronic atrial fibrillation. Am. J. Cardiol. *75*:88, 1995.

254a. Gill, J. S., Blaszyk, K., Ward, D. E., et al.: Verapamil for the suppression of idiopathic ventricular tachycardia of left bundle branch block-like morphology. Am. Heart J. *126*:1126, 1993.

255. Griffith, M. J., Garrett, C. J., Rowland, E., et al.: Effects of intravenous adenosine on verapamil-sensitive idiopathic ventricular tachycardia. Am. J. Cardiol. *73*:759, 1994.

256. Wen, M. S., Yeh, S. J., Wang C. C., et al.: Radiofrequency ablation therapy in idiopathic left ventricular tachycardia with no obvious structural heart disease. Circulation *89*:1690, 1994.

257. Nakagawa, H., Beckman, K. J., McClelland, J. H., et al.: Radiofrequency catheter ablation of idiopathic left ventricular tachycardia guided by a Purkinje potential. Circulation *88*:2607, 1993.

258. Bhadha, K., Marchlinski, F. E., and Iskandrian, A. S.: Ventricular tachycardia in patients without structural heart disease. Am. Heart J. *126*:1194, 1993.

259. Dilsizian, V., Bonow, R. O., Epstein, S. E., et al.: Myocardial ischemia detected by thallium scintigraphy is frequently related to cardiac arrest and syncope in young patients with hypertrophic cardiomyopathy. J. Am. Coll. Cardiol. *22*:796, 1993.

260. Leenhardt, A., Glaser, E., Burguera, M., et al.: Short-coupled variant of torsade de pointes: A new electrocardiographic entity in the spectrum of idiopathic ventricular tachyarrhythmias. Circulation *89*:206, 1994.

261. Myerburg, R. J., Kessler, K. M., Mallon, S. M., et al.: Life-threatening ventricular arrhythmias in patients with silent myocardial ischemia due to coronary artery spasm. N. Engl. J. Med. *326*:1451, 1992.

262. DeFerrari, G. M., Mador, F., Beria, G., et al.: Effect of calcium channel block on the wall motion abnormality of the idiopathic long QT syndrome. Circulation *89*:2126, 1994.

263. Ramoska, E. A., Spiller, H. A., Winter, M., et al.: A 1-year evaluation of calcium channel blocker overdoses: Toxicity and treatment. Ann. Emerg. Med. *22*:196, 1993.

OTHER ANTIARRHYTHMIC AGENTS

264. DiMarco, J. P.: Adenosine. *In* Zipes, D. P., and Jalife, J. (eds.): Cardiac Electrophysiology: From Cell to Bedside. 2nd ed. Philadelphia, W. B. Saunders Company, 1994, pp. 1336–1344.

265. Nayebpour, M., Billette, J., Amellal, F., et al.: Effects of adenosine on rate-dependent atrioventricular nodal function: Potential roles in tachycardia termination and physiological regulation. Circulation *88*:2632, 1993.

266. O'Nuanin, S., Jennison, S., Bashir, Y., et al.: Effects of adenosine on atrial repolarization in the transplanted human heart. Am. J. Cardiol. *71*:248, 1993.

267. McIntosh-Yellin, N. L., Drew, B. J., and Scheinman, M. M.: Safety and efficacy of central intravenous bolus administration of adenosine for termination of supraventricular tachycardia. J. Am. Coll. Cardiol. *22*:741, 1993.

268. Scheinman, M. M., Gonzalez, R. P., Cooper, M. W., et al.: Clinical and electrophysiologic features and role of catheter ablation techniques in adult patients with automatic atrioventricular junctional tachycardia. Am. J. Cardiol. *74*:565, 1994

269. Akhtar, M., Jazayeri, M. R., Sra, J., et al.: Atrioventricular nodal reentry: Clinical, electrophysiological and therapeutic considerations. Circulation *88*:282, 1993.

270. Lauer, M. R., Young, C., Liem, L. B., et al.: Efficacy of adenosine in terminating catecholamine-dependent supraventricular tachycardia. Am. J. Cardiol. *73*:38, 1994.

271. Klein, L. S., Hackett, F. K., Zipes D. P., et al.: Radiofrequency catheter ablation of Mahaim fibers at the tricuspid annulus. Circulation *87*:738, 1993.

272. Li, H. G., Morillo, C. A., Zardini, M., et al.: Effect of adenosine or adenosine triphosphate on antidromic tachycardia. J. Am. Coll. Cardiol. *24*:728, 1994.

273. Garratt, C. J., O'Nunain, S., Griffith, M. J., et al.: Effects of intravenous adenosine in patients with preexcited junctional tachycardias: Therapeutic efficacy and incidence of proarrhythmic events. Am. J. Cardiol. *74*:401, 1994.

274. Ralston, M. A., Knilans, T. K., Hannon, D. W., et al.: Use of adenosine for diagnosis and treatment of tachyarrhythmias in pediatric patients. J. Pediatr. *124*:139, 1994.

275. Reyes, G., Stanton, R., and Galvis, A. G.: Adenosine in the treatment of paroxysmal supraventricular tachycardia in children. Ann. Emerg. Med. *21*:1499, 1992.

276. Keim, S., Curtis, A. B., Belardinelli, L., et al.: Adenosine-induced atrioventricular block: A rapid and reliable method to assess surgical and radiofrequency catheter ablation of accessory atrioventricular pathways. J. Am. Coll. Cardiol. *19*:1005, 1992.

277. Chen, S. A., Chiang, C. E., Yang, C. J., et al.: Sustained atrial tachycardia in adult patients: Electrophysiological characteristics, pharmacological response, possible mechanisms, and effective radiofrequency ablation. Circulation *90*:1262, 1994.

278. Engelstein, E. D., Lippman, N., Stein, K. M., et al.: Mechanism-specific effects of adenosine on atrial tachycardia. Circulation *89*:2645, 1994.

279. Griffith, M. J., Garratt, C. J., Rowland, E., et al.: Effects of intravenous adenosine on verapamil-sensitive idiopathic ventricular tachycardia. Am. J. Cardiol. *73*:759, 1994.

280. Lerman, B. B.: Response of nonreentrant catecholamine-mediated ventricular tachycardia to endogenous adenosine and acetylcholine. Evidence for myocardial receptor-mediated effects. Circulation *87*:382, 1993.

281. Wilber, D. J., Baerman, J., Olshansky, B., et al.: Adenosine-sensitive ventricular tachycardia. Clinical characteristics and response to catheter ablation. Circulation *87*:126, 1993.

282. Crosson, J. E., Etheridge, S. P., Milstein, S., et al.: Therapeutic and diagnostic utility of adenosine during tachycardia evaluation in children. Am. J. Cardiol. *74*:155, 1994.

283. Cowell, R. T., Paul, V. E., and Ilsley, C. D.: Hemodynamic deterioration after treatment with adenosine. Br. Heart J. *71*:569, 1994.

284. Exner, D. V., Muzigka, T., and Gillis, A. M.: Proarrhythmia in patients with the Wolff-Parkinson-White syndrome after standard doses of intravenous adenosine. Ann. Intern. Med. *122*:351, 1995.

ELECTRICAL THERAPY OF CARDIAC ARRHYTHMIAS

285. Kerber, R. E.: External direct current cardioversion-defibrillation. *In* Zipes, D. P., and Jalife, T. (eds.): Cardiac Electrophysiology: From Cell to Bedside. 2nd ed. Philadelphia, W. B. Saunders Company, 1994, pp. 1360–1365.

286. Ewy, G. A.: The optimal technique for electrical cardioversion of atrial fibrillation. Clin. Cardiol. *17*:79, 1994.

287. Li, H. G., Yee, R., Mehra, R., et al.: Effect of shock timing on efficacy and safety of internal cardioversion for ventricular tachycardia. J. Am. Coll. Cardiol. *24*:703, 1994.

288. Alt, E., Schmitt, C., Ammer, R., et al.: Initial experience with intracardiac atrial defibrillation in patients with chronic atrial fibrillation. PACE *17*:1067, 1994.

289. Wharton, J. M., and Johnson, F. E.: Catheter based atrial defibrillation. PACE *17*:1058, 1994.

290. Levy, S., and Richard, P.: Is there any indication for an intracardiac defibrillator for the treatment of atrial fibrillation? J. Cardiovasc. Electrophysiol. *5*:982, 1994.

291. Kerber, R. E., Spencer, K. T., Kallok, M. J., et al.: Overlapping sequential pulses: A new waveform for transthoracic defibrillation. Circulation *89*:2369, 1994.

292. Hillsley, R. E., Wharton, J. M., Cates, A. W., et al.: Why do some patients have high defibrillation thresholds at defibrillator implantation? Answers from basic research. PACE *17*:222, 1994.

293. Blanchard, S. M., and Ideker, R. E.: Mechanisms of electrical defibrillation: Impact of new experimental defibrillator waveforms. Am. Heart J. *127*:970, 1994.

294. Hoch, D. H., Batsford, W. P., Greenberg, S. M., et al.: Double sequential external shocks for refractory ventricular fibrillation. J. Am. Coll. Cardiol. *23*:1141, 1994.

295. Grimm, R. A., Stewart, W. J., Maloney, J. D., et al.: Impact of electrical cardioversion for atrial fibrillation on left atrial appendage function and spontaneous echo contrast: Characterization by simultaneous transesophageal echocardiograhy. J. Am. Coll. Cardiol. *22*:1359, 1993.

296. Ito, M., Pride, H. P., and Zipes, D. P.: Defibrillating shocks delivered to the heart heterogeneously impair efferent sympathetic responsiveness. Circulation *88*:2661, 1993.

297. Manning, W. J., Silverman, D. I., Katz, S. E., et al.: Impaired left atrial mechanical function after cardioversion: Relation to duration of atrial fibrillation. J. Am. Coll. Cardiol. *23*:1535, 1994.

298. Schneider, T., Mauer, D., Diehl, P., et al.: Early defibrillation by emergency physicians or emergency medical technicians? A controlled, prospective multi-center study. Resuscitation *27*:297, 1994.

299. Ekstrom, L., Herlitz, J., Wennerblom, D., et al.: Survival after cardiac arrest outside hospital over a 12-year period in Gothenburg. Resuscitation *27*:181, 1994.

300. Welikovitch, L., Lafreniere, G., Burggraf, G. W., et al.: Change in atrial volume following restoration of sinus rhythm in patients with atrial fibrillation: A prospective echocardiographic study. Can. J. Cardiol. *10*:993, 1994.

301. Gosselink, A. T., Crijns, H. J., Hamer, H. P., et al.: Changes in left and right atrial size after cardioversion of atrial fibrillation: Role of mitral valve disease. J. Am. Coll. Cardiol. *22*:1666, 1993.

302. Shite, J., Yokota, Y., and Yokoyama, M.: Heterogeneity and time course of improvement in cardiac function after cardioversion in chronic atrial fibrillation: Assessment of serial echocardiographic indices. Br. Heart J. *70*:154, 1993.

303. VanGelder, I. C., Orijns, H. J., Blanksma, P. K., et al.: Time course of hemodynamic changes and improvement of exercise tolerance after cardioversion of chronic atrial fibrillation unassociated with cardiac valve disease. Am. J. Cardiol. *72*:560, 1993.

304. Gosselink, A. T., Orijns, H. J., VandenBerg, M. P., et al.: Functional capacity before and after cardioversion of atrial fibrillation: A controlled study. Br. Heart J. *72*:161, 1994.

305. Missault, L., Jordaens, L., Gheeraert, P., et al.: Embolic stroke after an anticoagulated cardioversion despite prior exclusion of atrial thrombi by transesophageal echocardiography. Eur. Heart J. *15*:1279, 1994.

306. Black, I. W., Fatkin, D., Sagar, K. B., et al.: Exclusion of atrial thrombus by transesophageal echocardiography does not preclude embolism after cardioversion of atrial fibrillation: A multicenter study. Circulation *89*:2509, 1994.

307. Fatkin, D., Kurchar, D. L., Thorburn, C. W., et al.: Transesophageal echocardiography before and during direct current cardioversion of atrial fibrillation: Evidence of atrial stunning as a mechanism of thromboembolic complications. J. Am. Coll. Cardiol. *23*:307, 1994.

308. Grimm, R. A., Stewart, W. J., Black, I. W., et al.: Should all patients undergo transesophageal echocardiography before electrical cardioversion of atrial fibrillation? J. Am. Coll. Cardiol. *23*:533, 1994.
309. Feltes, T. F., and Friedman, R. A.: Transesophageal echocardiographic detection of atrial thrombi in patients with nonfibrillation atrial tachyarrhythmias and congenital heart disease. J. Am. Coll. Cardiol. *24*:1365, 1994.
310. Salerno, D. M., Katz, A., Dunbar, D. N., et al.: Serum electrolytes and catecholamines after cardioversion from ventricular tachycardia and atrial fibrillation. PACE *16*:1862, 1993.

ABLATION THERAPY

311. Catheter ablation for cardiac arrhythmias: Clinical applications, personnel and facilities. American College of Cardiology Cardiovascular Technology Assessment Committee. J. Am. Coll. Cardiol. *24*:828, 1994.
312. Manolis, A. S., Wang, P. J., and Estes, N. A., III: Radiofrequency catheter ablation for cardiac tachyarrhythmias. Ann. Intern. Med. *121*:452–461, 1994.
313. Zipes, D. P. (ed.): Catheter Ablation of Arrhythmias. Armonk, N.Y., Futura Publishing Company, 1994.
313a. Jackman, W. M., Wang, X., Friday, K. J., et al.: Catheter ablation of accessory atrioventricular pathways (Wolff-Parkinson-White syndrome) by radiofrequency current. N. Engl. J. Med. *324*:1605, 1991.
313b. Calkins, H., Sousa, J., el-Atassi, R., et al.: Diagnosis and cure of the Wolff-Parkinson-White syndrome or paroxysmal supraventricular tachycardias during a single electrophysiologic test. N. Engl. J. Med. *324*:1612, 1991.
314. Haissaguerre, M., Gaita, F., Marcus, F. I., et al.: Radiofrequency catheter ablation of accessory pathways: A contemporary review. J. Cardiovasc. Elecrophysiol. *5*:532, 1994.
315. Haissaguerre, M., Clementy, J., and Warin, J. F.: Catheter ablation of atrioventricular reentrant tachycardias. *In* Zipes, D. P., and Jalife, J. (eds.): Cardiac Electrophysiology: From Cell to Bedside. 2nd ed. Philadelphia, W. B. Saunders Company, 1994, pp. 1487–1499.
316. Miles, W. M., Zipes, D. P., and Klein, L. S.: Ablation of free wall accessory pathways. *In* Zipes, D. P. (ed.): Catheter Ablation of Arrhythmias. Armonk, N.Y., Futura Publishing Company, 1994, pp. 211–230.
317. Kuck, K., Schleuter, M., Cappato, R., et al.: Ablation of septal accessory pathways. *In* Zipes, D. P. (ed.): Catheter Ablation of Arrhythmias. Armonk, N.Y., Futura Publishing Company, 1994, pp. 231–257.
318. Ganz, L. I., and Friedman, P. L.: Supraventricular tachycardia. N. Engl. J. Med. *332*:162, 1995.
319. Thakur, R. K., Klein, G. K., and Yee, R.: Radiofrequency catheter ablation in patients with Wolff-Parkinson-White syndrome. Can. Med. Assoc. J. *151*:771, 1994.
320. Park, J. K., Halperin, B. D., McAnulty, J. H., et al.: Comparison of radiofrequency catheter ablation procedures in children, adolescents and adults and the impact of accessory pathway location. Am. J. Cardiol. *74*:786, 1994.
321. Sreeram, N., Smeets, J. L., Pulles-Heintzberger, C. F., et al.: Radiofrequency catheter ablation of accessory atrioventricular pathways in children and young adults. Br. Heart J. *70*:160, 1993.
322. Saul, J. P., Hulse, J. E., Papagiannis, J., et al.: Late enlargement of radiofrequency lesions in infant lambs: Implications for ablation procedures in small children. Circulation *90*:492, 1994.
323. Kugler, J. D., Danford, D. A., Deal, B. J., et al.: Radiofrequency catheter ablation for tachyarrhythmias in children and adolescents: The Pediatric Electrophysiology Society. N. Engl. J. Med. *330*: 1481, 1994.
324. vanHare, G. F., Witherell, C. L., and Lesh, M. D.: Follow-up of radiofrequency catheter ablation in children: Results in 100 consecutive patients. J. Am. Coll. Cardiol. *23*:1651, 1994.
325. Nath, S., Whayne, J. G., Kaul, S., et al.: Effects of radiofrequency catheter ablation on regional myocardial blood flow: Possible mechanism for late electrophysiological outcome. Circulation *89*:2667, 1994.
326. Nath, S., Redick, J. A., Whayne, J. G., et al.: Ultrastructural observations in the myocardium beyond the reach of an acute coagulation necrosis following radiofrequency catheter ablation. J. Cardiovasc. Electrophysiol. *5*:838, 1994.
327. Nath, S., DiMarco, J. P., and Haines, D. E.: Basic aspects of radiofrequency catheter ablation. J. Cardiovasc. Electrophysiol. *5*:863, 1994.
328. Xie, B., Heald, S. C., Bashir, Y., et al.: Radiofrequency catheter ablation of septal accessory atrioventricular pathways. Br. Heart J. *72*:281, 1994.
329. Haissaguerre, M., Marcus, F., Poquet, F., et al.: Electrocardiographic characteristics and catheter ablation of parahissian accessory pathways. Circulation *90*:1124, 1994.
330. Scheinman, M. M., Wang, Y. S., vanHare, G. F., et al.: Electrocardiographic and electrophysiologic characteristics of anterior, midseptal and right anterior free wall accessory pathways. J. Am. Coll. Cardiol. *20*:1220, 1992.
331. Dhala, A. A., Deshpande, S. S., Bremner, S., et al.: Transcatheter ablation of posteroseptal accessory pathways using a venous approach and radiofrequency energy. Circulation *90*:1799, 1994.
332. Epstein, L. M., Chiesa, N., Wong, M. N., et al.: Radiofrequency catheter ablation in the treatment of supraventricular tachycardia in the elderly. J. Am. Coll. Cardiol. *23*:1356, 1994.
333. Chen, S. A., Chiang, C. E., Yang, C. J., et al.: Accessory pathway and atrioventricular node reentrant tachycardia in elderly patients: Clinical features, electrophysiologic characteristics and results of radiofrequency ablation. J. Am. Coll. Cardiol. *23*:702, 1994.
334. Cappato, R., Schluter, M., Mont, L., et al.: Anatomic, electrical, and mechanical factors affecting bipolar endocardial electrograms: Impact on catheter ablation of manifest left free-wall accessory pathways. Circulation *90*:884, 1994.
335. Shih, H. T., Miles, W. M., Klein, L. S., et al.: Multiple accessory pathways in the permanent form of junctional reciprocating tachycardia. Am. J. Cardiol. *73*:361, 1994.
336. Langberg, J. J., Man, K. C., Varperian, V. R., et al.: Recognition and catheter ablation of subepicardial accessory pathways. J. Am. Coll. Cardiol. *22*:1100, 1993.
337. Calkins, H., Mann, C., Kalbfleisch, S., et al.: Site of accessory pathway block after radiofrequency catheter ablation in patients with the Wolff-Parkinson-White syndrome. J. Cardiovasc. Electrophysiol. *5*:20, 1994.
338. Cappato, R., Schluter, M., Weiss, C., et al.: Catheter-induced mechanical conduction block of right-sided accessory fibers with Mahaim-type preexcitation to guide radiofrequency ablation. Circulation *90*:282, 1994.
339. Willems, S., Hendricks, G., Shenasa, M., et al.: Termination of orthodromic tachycardia using direct current sub-threshold stimulation in patients with concealed accessory pathways. Eur. Heart J. *14*(Abs.):294, 1993.
340. Chiang, C. E., Chen, S. A., Wu, T. J., et al.: Incidence, significance, and pharmacological responses of catheter-induced mechanical trauma in patients receiving radiofrequency ablation for supraventricular tachycardias. Circulation *90*:1847, 1994.
341. Chu, E., Kalman, J. M., Kwasman, M. A., et al.: Intracardiac echocardiography during radiofrequency catheter ablation of cardiac arrhythmias in humans. J. Am. Coll. Cardiol. *24*:1351, 1994.
342. Chu, E., Fitzpatrick, A. P., Chin, M. C., et al.: Radiofrequency catheter ablation guided by intracardiac echocardiography. Circulation *89*:1301, 1994.
343. Damle, R. S., Choe, W., Kanaan, N. M., et al.: Atrial and accessory pathway activation direction in patients with orthodromic supraventricular tachycardia: Insights from vector mapping. J. Am. Coll. Cardiol. *23*:684, 1994.
344. Calkins, H., Prystowsky, E., Carlson, M., et al.: Temperature monitoring during radiofrequency catheter ablation procedures using a closed loop control. Atakar Multicenter Investigators Group. Circulation *90*:1279, 1994
345. Lesh, M. D., vanHare, G. F., Scheinman, M. M., et al.: Comparison of the retrograde and transseptal methods for ablation of left freewall accessory pathways. J. Am. Coll. Cardiol. *22*:542, 1993.
346. Deshpande, S. S., Bremner, S., Sra, J. S., et al.: Ablation of left free-wall accessory pathways using radiofrequency energy at the atrial insertion site: Transseptal versus transaortic approach. J. Cardiovasc. Electrophysiol. *5*:219, 1994.
347. Wagshal, A. B., Pires, L. A., and Young, P. G.: Usefulness of follow-up electrophysiologic study and event monitoring after successful radiofrequency catheter ablation of supraventricular tachycardia. Am. J. Cardiol. *75*:50, 1995.
348. Chen, S. A., Chiang, C. E., Yang, C. J., et al.: Usefulness of serial follow-up electrophysiologic studies in predicting late outcome of radiofrequency ablation for accessory pathways and atrioventricular nodal reentrant tachycardia. Am. Heart J. *126*:619, 1993.
349. Jackman, W. M., McClelland, J. H., Nakagawa, H., et al.: Ablation of right atriofascicular (Mahaim) accessory pathways. *In* Zipes, D. P. (ed.): Catheter Ablation of Arrhythmias. Armonk, N.Y., Futura Publishing Company, 1994, pp. 187–210.
350. McClelland, J. H., Wang, X., Beckman, K. J., et al.: Radiofrequency catheter ablation of right atrial fascicular (Mahaim) accessory pathways guided by accessory pathway activation potentials. Circulation *89*:2655, 1994.
351. Klein, L. S., Hackett, F. K., Zipes, D. P., and Miles, W. M.: Radiofrequency catheter ablation of "Mahaim fibers" at the tricuspid annulus. Circulation *87*:738, 1993.
352. Li, H. G., Klein, G. K., Thakur, R. K., et al.: Radiofrequency ablation of decremental accessory pathways mimicking nodal ventricular conduction. Am. J. Cardiol. *74*:829, 1994.
353. Grogin, H. R., Lee, R. J., Kwasman, M., et al.: Radiofrequency catheter ablation of atriofascicular and nodoventricular Mahaim tracts. Circulation *90*:272, 1994.
354. Zipes, D. P., DiMarco, J. P., Gillette, P. C., et al.: ACC/AHA guidelines for clinical intracardiac electrophysiologic procedures. Circulation *92*:673, 1995; J. Am. Coll. Cardiol. *26*:555, 1995; J. Cardiovasc. Electrophysiol. *6*:652, 1995.
355. Scheinman, M. M.: Patterns of catheter ablation practice in the United States: Results of the 1992 NASPE survey. PACE *17*:873, 1994.
356. Hindricks, G., on behalf of the Multicentre European Radiofrequency Survey (MERFS) Investigators of the Working Group on Arrhythmias of the European Society of Cardiology: The Multicentre European Radiofrequency Survey (MERFS): Complications of radiofequency catheter ablation of arrhythmias. Eur. Heart J. *14*:1644, 1993.
357. Deshpande, S., Jazayeri, M., Dahla, A., et al.: Selective transcatheter modification of the atrioventricular node. *In* Zipes, D. P. (ed.): Catheter Ablation of Arrhythmias. Armonk, N.Y., Futura Publishing Company, 1994, pp. 151–186.
357a. Jackman, W., Beckman, K. J., McClelland, J. H., et al.: Treatment of supraventricular tachycardia due to atrioventricular nodal reentry by radiofrequency catheter ablation of the slow-pathway conduction. N. Engl. J. Med. *327*:313, 1992.

358. Kalbfleisch, S. J., and Morady, F.: Catheter ablation of atrioventricular nodal reentrant tachycardia. *In* Zipes, D. P., and Jalife, J. (eds.): Cardiac Electrophysiology: From Cell to Bedside. 2nd ed. Philadelphia, W. B. Saunders Company, 1994, pp. 1477–1487.
359. Manolis, A. S., Wang, P. J., and Estes, N. A. M., III: Radiofrequency ablation of slow pathway in patients with atrioventricular nodal reentrant tachycardia: Do arrhythmia recurrences correlate with persistent slow pathway conduction or site of successful ablation? Circulation *90:*2815, 1994.
360. Dhala, A., Bremner, S., Deshpande, S., et al.: Efficacy and safety of atrioventricular nodal modification for atrioventricular nodal reentrant tachycardia in the pediatric population. Am. Heart J. *128:*903, 1994.
361. Sra, J. S., Jazayeri, M. R., Blanck, Z., et al.: Slow pathway ablation in patients with atrioventricular node reentrant tachycardia and a prolonged PR interval. J. Am. Coll. Cardiol. *24:*1064, 1994.
362. DeBakker, J. N., Coronel, R., McGuire, M. A., et al.: Slow potentials in the atrioventricular junctional area of patients operated on for atrioventricular node tachycardias and in isolated porcine hearts. J. Am. Coll. Cardiol. *23:*709, 1994.
362a. McGuire, M. A., deBakker, J. M., Vermeulen, J. T., et al.: Origin and significance of double potentials near the atrioventricular node. Correlation of extracellular potentials, intracellular potentials and histology. Circulation *89:*2351, 1994.
363. Kalbfleisch, S. J., Strickberger, S. A., Williamson, B., et al.: Randomized comparison of anatomic and electrogram mapping approaches to ablation of the slow pathway of atrioventricular node reentrant tachycardia. J. Am. Coll. Cardiol. *23:*716, 1994.
364. Li, H. G., Klein, G. J., Stites, H. W., et al.: Elimination of slow pathway conduction: An accurate indicator of clinical success after radiofrequency atrioventricular node modification. J. Am. Coll. Cardiol. *22:*1849, 1993.
365. Lindsay, B. D., Chung, M. K., Gamache, M. C., et al.: Therapeutic endpoints for the treatment of atrioventricular node reentrant tachycardia by catheter-guided radiofrequency current. J. Am. Coll. Cardiol. *22:*733, 1993.
366. Langberg, J. J., Leon, A., Borganelli, M., et al.: A randomized, prospective comparison of anterior and posterior approaches to radiofrequency catheter ablation of atrioventricular nodal reentry tachycardia. Circulation *87:*1551, 1993.
367. Mitrani, R. D., Klein, L. S., Hackett, F. K., et al.: Radiofrequency ablation for atrioventricular node reentrant tachycardia: Comparison between fast (anterior) and slow (posterior) pathway ablation. J. Am. Coll. Cardiol. *21:*432, 1993.
368. Miles, W. M., Hubbard, J. E., Zipes, D. P., et al.: Elimination of AV nodal reentrant tachycardia with 2:1 VA block by posteroseptal ablation. J. Cardiovasc. Electrophysiol. *5:*510, 1994.
369. Strickberger, S. A., Daoud, E., Niebauer, M., et al.: Effects of partial and complete ablation of the slow pathway on fast pathway properties in patients with atrioventricular nodal reentrant tachycardia. J. Cardiovasc. Electrophysiol. *5:*645, 1994.
370. Natale, A., Klein, G., and Yee, R.: Shortening of fast pathway refractoriness after slow pathway ablation: Effects of autonomic blockade. Circulation *89:*1103, 1994.
371. Silka, M. J., Kron, J., Park, J. K., et al.: Atypical forms of supraventricular tachycardia due to atrioventricular node reentry in children after radiofrequency modification of slow pathway conduction. J. Am. Coll. Cardiol. *23:*1363, 1994.
372. Kocovic, D. Z., Harada, T., Shea, J. B., et al.: Alterations of heart rate and of heart rate variability after radiofrequency catheter ablation of supraventricular tachycardia. Circulation *88:*1671, 1993.
373. Alison, J. F., Yeung-Lai-Wah, J. A., Schulzer, M., et al.: Characterization of junctional rhythm after atrioventricular node ablation. Circulation *91:*84, 1995.
374. Gentzer, J. H., Goyal, R., Williamson, B. D., et al.: Analysis of junctional ectopy during radiofrequency ablation of the slow pathway in patients with atrioventricular nodal reentrant tachycardia. Circulation *90:*2820, 1994.
375. Thakur, R. K., Klein, G. J., Yee, R., et al.: Junctional tachycardia: A useful marker during radiofrequency ablation for atrioventricular node reentrant tachycardia. J. Am. Coll. Cardiol. *22:*1706, 1993.
376. Chen, S. A., Chiang, C. E., Yang, C. J., et al.: Sustained atrial tachycardia in adult patients: Electrophysiological characteristics, pharmacological response, possible mechanisms, and effects of radiofrequency ablation. Circulation *90:*1262, 1994.
377. Lesh, M. D., vanHare, G. F., Epstein, L. M., et al.: Radiofrequency catheter ablation of atrial arrhythmias: Results and mechanisms. Circulation *89:*1074, 1994.
378. Tracy, C. M., Swartz, J. F., Fletcher, R. D., et al.: Radiofrequency catheter ablation of ectopic atrial tachycardia using paced activation sequence mapping. J. Am. Coll. Cardiol. *21:*910, 1993.
379. Kay, G. N., Chong, F., Epstein, A. E., et al.: Radiofrequency ablation for treatment of primary atrial tachycardias. J. Am. Coll. Cardiol. *21:*901, 1993.
380. Sanders, W. E., Jr., Sorrentino, R. A., Greenfield, R. A., et al.: Catheter ablation of sinoatrial node reentrant tachycardia. J. Am. Coll. Cardiol. *23:*926, 1994.
381. Scheinman, M. M., Gonzalez, R. P., Cooper, M. W., et al.: Clinical and electrophysiologic features and role of catheter ablation techniques in adult patients with automatic atrioventricular junctional tachycardia. Am. J. Cardiol. *74:*565, 1994.
382. Kirkorian, G., Mancada, E., Chevalier, P., et al.: Radiofrequency ablation of atrial flutter: Efficacy of an anatomically guided approach. Circulation *90:*2804, 1994.
383. Calkins, H., Leon, A. R., Dean, A. G., et al.: Catheter ablation of atrial flutter using radiofrequency energy. Am. J. Cardiol. *73:*353, 1994.
384. Cosio, F. G., Lopez, G. M., Goicholea, A., et al.: Radiofrequency ablation of the inferior vena cava-tricuspid valve isthmus in common atrial flutter. Am. J. Cardiol. *71:*705, 1993.
385. Kalbfleisch, S. J., el-Atassi, R., Calkins, H., et al.: Association between atrioventricular node reentrant tachycardia and inducible atrial flutter. J. Am. Coll. Cardiol. *22:*80 1993.
386. Interian, A., Jr., Cox, M. M., Jimenez, R. A., et al.: A shared pathway in atrioventricular nodal reentrant tachycardia and atrial flutter: Implications for pathophysiology and therapy. Am. J. Cardiol. *71:*297, 1993.
387. Olshansky, B., Okumura, K., Hess, P. G., et al.: Demonstration of an area of slow conduction in human atrial flutter. J. Am. Coll. Cardiol. *16:*1639, 1990.
388. Haissaguerre, M., Marcus, F. I., Fischer, B., et al.: Radiofrequency catheter ablation in unusual mechanisms of atrial fibrillation: Report of three cases. J. Cardiovasc. Electrophysiol. *5:*743, 1994.
389. Haissaguerre, M., Gencel, L., Fischer, B., et al.: Successful catheter ablation of atrial fibrillation. J. Cardiovasc. Electrophysiol. *5:*1045, 1994.
390. Swartz, J. F., Pellersels, G., Silvers, J., et al.: Catheter-based curative approach to atrial fibrillation in humans. Circulation *90* (Suppl. 1): I335, 1994.
391. Elvan, A., Pride, H. P., Eble, J. N., et al.: Radiofrequency catheter ablation of the atria reduces the inducibility and duration of atrial fibrillation in dogs. Circulation *91:*2235, 1995.
392. Morillo, C. A., Klein, G. J., Jones, D. L., et al.: Chronic rapid atrial pacing: Structural, functional and electrophysiological characteristics of a new model of sustained atrial fibrillation. Circulation *91:*1588, 1995.
393. Olgin, J., and Scheinman, M.: Catheter ablation of the atrioventricular node for treatment of supraventricular tachyarrhythmias. *In* Zipes, D. P., and Jalife, J. (eds.): Cardiac Electrophysiology: From Cell to Bedside. 2nd ed. Philadelphia, W. B. Saunders Company, 1994, pp. 1453–1460.
394. Rodriguez, L. M., Smeets, J. L., Xie, B., et al.: Improvement in left ventricular function by ablation of atrioventricular nodal conduction in selected patients with lone atrial fibrillation. Am. J. Cardiol. *72:*1137, 1993.
395. Feld, G. K., Fleck, R. P., Fujimura, O., et al.: Control of rapid ventricular response by radiofrequency catheter modification of the atrioventricular node in patients with medically refractory atrial fibrillation. Circulation *90:*2299, 1994.
396. DellaBella, P., Carbucicchio, C., Tondo, C., et al.: Modulation of atrioventricular conduction by ablation of the slow atrioventricular node pathway in patients with drug-refractory atrial fibrillation or flutter. J. Am. Coll. Cardiol. *25:*39, 1995.
397. Williamson, B. D., Man, K. C., Daoud, E., et al.: Radiofrequency catheter modification of atrioventricular conduction to control the ventricular rate during atrial fibrillation. N. Engl. J. Med. *331:*910, 1994.
398. Borggrefe, M., Chen, X., Hindricks, G., et al.: Catheter ablation of ventricular tachycardia in patients with coronary heart disease. *In* Zipes, D. P., and Jalife, J. (eds.): Cardiac Electrophysiology: From Cell to Bedside. 2nd ed. Philadelphia, W. B. Saunders Company, 1994, pp. 1502–1517.
399. Klein L. S., Miles, W. M., Mitrani, R. D., et al.: Ablation of ventricular tachycardia in patients with structurally normal hearts. *In* Zipes, D. P., and Jalife, J. (eds.): Cardiac Electrophysiology: From Cell to Bedside. 2nd ed. Philadelphia, W. B. Saunders Company, 1994, pp. 1518–1523.
400. Gonska, B. D., Cao, K., Schauman, N. A., et al.: Catheter ablation of ventricular tachycardia in 136 patients with coronary artery disease: Results and longterm follow-up. J. Am. Coll. Cardiol. *24:*1506, 1994.
401. Davis, L. M., Cooper, M. W., Johnson, D. C., et al.: Simultaneous 60-electrode mapping of ventricular tachycardia using percutaneous catheters. J. Am. Coll. Cardiol. *24:*709, 1994.
402. Gill, J. S., deBelder, M., and Ward, D. E.: Right ventricular outflow tract ventricular tachycardia associated with an aneurysmal malformation: Use of transesophageal echocardiography during low-energy direct-current ablation. Am. Heart J. *128:*620, 1994.
403. Coggins, D. L., Lee, R. J., Sweeney, J., et al.: Radiofrequency catheter ablation as a cure for idiopathic tachycardia of both left and right ventricular origin. J. Am. Coll. Cardiol. *23:*1333, 1994.
404. Wen, M. S., Yeh, S. J., Wang, C. C., et al.: Radiofrequency ablation therapy in idiopathic left ventricular tachycardia with no obvious structural heart disease. Circulation *89:*1690, 1994.
405. Kim, Y. H., Sosa-Suarez, G., Trouton, T. G., et al.: Treatment of ventricular tachycardia by transcatheter radiofrequency ablation in patients with ischemic heart disease. Circulation *89:*1094, 1994.
406. Nakagawa, H., Beckman, K. J., McClelland, J. H., et al.: Radiofrequency catheter ablation of idiopathic left ventricular tachycardia guided by a Purkinje potential. Circulation *88:*2607, 1993.
407. Stevenson, W. G., Kahn, H., Sager, P., et al.: Identification of reentry circuit sites during catheter mapping and radiofrequency ablation of ventricular tachycardia late after myocardial infarction. Circulation *88:*1647, 1993.
408. Calkins, H., Kalbfleisch, S. J., el-Atassi, R., et al.: Relation between efficacy of radiofrequency catheter ablation and site of origin of idiopathic ventricular tachycardia. Am. J. Cardiol. *71:*827, 1993.
409. Morady, F., Harvey, M., and Kalbfleisch, S. J.: Radiofrequency catheter

ablation of ventricular tachycardia in patients with coronary artery disease. Circulation *87*:363, 1993.

410. Kottkamp, H, Chen, X., Hindricks, G., et al.: Radiofrequency catheter ablation of idiopathic left ventricular tachycardia: Further evidence for microreentry as the underlying mechanism. J. Cardiovasc. Electrophysiol. *5*:268, 1994.
411. Mitrani, R. D., Klein, L. S., Miles, W. M., et al.: Regional cardiac sympathetic denervation in patients with ventricular tachycardia in the absence of coronary artery disease. J. Am. Coll. Cardiol. *22*:1344, 1993.
412. Blanck, Z., Dhala, A., Deshpande, S., et al.: Bundle branch reentrant ventricular tachycardia: Cumulative experience in 48 patients. J. Cardiovasc. Electrophysiol. *4*:253, 1993.
413. Haines, D. E., Verow, A. F., Sinusas, A. J., et al.: Intracoronary ethanol ablation in swine: Characterization of myocardial injury in target and remote vascular beds. J. Cardiovasc. Electrophysiol. *5*:41, 1994.
414. Haines, D. E.: Chemical ablative therapy for arrhythmias. *In* Zipes, D. P., and Jalife, J. (eds.): Cardiac Electrophysiology: From Cell to Bedside. 2nd ed. Philadelphia, W. B. Saunders Company, 1994, pp. 1537–1546.

SURGICAL THERAPY

415. Crawford, F. A., Jr., and Gillette, P. C.: Surgical treatment of cardiac dysrhythmias in infants and children. Ann. Thorac. Surg. *58*:1262, 1994.
416. Mahomed, Y.: Surgery for atrioventricular nodal reentrant tachycardia. *In* Zipes, D. P., and Jalife, J. (eds.): Cardiac Electrophysiology: From Cell to Bedside. 2nd ed. Philadelphia, W. B. Saunders Company, 1994, pp. 1577–1583.
417. Guiraudon, G. M., Klein, G. J., Yee, R., et al.: Surgery for the Wolff-Parkinson-White syndrome. *In* Zipes, D. P., and Jalife, J. (eds.): Cardiac Electrophysiology: From Cell to Bedside. 2nd ed. Philadelphia, W. B. Saunders Company, 1994, pp. 1553–1563.
418. Ferguson, T. B., Jr., and Cox, J. L.: Surgery for atrial fibrillation. *In* Zipes, D. P., and Jalife, J. (eds.): Cardiac Electrophysiology: From Cell to Bedside. 2nd ed. Philadelphia, W. B. Saunders Company, 1994, pp. 1563–1576.
419. Lawrie, G. M., and Pacifico, A.: Surgery for ventricular tachycardia. *In* Zipes, D. P., and Jalife, J. (eds.): Cardiac Electrophysiology: From Cell to Bedside. 2nd ed. Philadelphia, W. B. Saunders Company, 1994, pp. 1547–1552.
420. Ferguson, T. B., Jr.: The future of arrhythmia surgery. J. Cardiovasc. Electrophysiol. *5*:621, 1994.
421. Misaki, T., Watanabe, G., Iwa, T., et al.: Surgical treatment of Wolff-Parkinson-White syndrome in infants and children. Ann. Thorac. Surg. *58*:103, 1994.
422. Guiraudon, G. M., Guiraudon, C. M., Klein, G. J., et al.: Operation for the Wolff-Parkinson-White syndrome in the catheter ablation era. Ann. Thorac. Surg. *57*:1084, 1994.
423. Cox, J. L., Boineau, J. P., Schuessler, R. B., et al.: Five-year experience with the Maze procedure for atrial fibrillation. Ann. Thorac. Surg. *56*:814, 1993.
424. DiMarco, J. P.: Management of sudden cardiac death survivors. Role of surgical and catheter ablation. Circulation *85* (Suppl. I):I125, 1992.
425. Zipes, D. P., Roberts, D., for the PCD Investigators: Results of the World Wide Study of the Implantable Pacemaker, Cardioverter, Defibrillator: A comparison of epicardial and endocardial lead systems. Circulation *92*:59, 1995.
426. Ferguson, T. B., Jr., Smith, J. M., Cox, J. L., et al.: Direct operation versus ICD therapy for ischemic ventricular tachycardia. Ann. Thorac. Surg. *58*:1291, 1994.

Chapter 22
Specific Arrhythmias: Diagnosis and Treatment

DOUGLAS P. ZIPES

DIAGNOSTIC AND THERAPEUTIC CONSIDERATIONS

History

The initial evaluation of the patient suspected of having a cardiac arrhythmia begins with a careful history, specifically questioning the patient regarding the presence of palpitations, syncope, spells of lightheadedness, chest pain, or symptoms of congestive heart failure. Palpitations,[1] an awareness of the heartbeat (see p. 9), may result from irregularities in cardiac rate or rhythm or a change in contractility of the heart. Some patients are able to reproduce this sensation by tapping their hand on their chest, knee, or a table top in a fashion similar to the perceived palpitation or recognize a cadence tapped out by a physician. Such a maneuver can help establish the rate and rhythm of the arrhythmia, narrowing it to a particular rate range, a regular or irregular arrhythmia, or one in which a regular rhythm is interrupted by premature beats. The latter often are perceived only upon the contraction that ends the pause that follows the premature beat. The patient may feel as if the heart has stopped for a moment. A rapid, irregular tapping can suggest the ventricular response to atrial fibrillation, while a rapid, regular tapping can suggest an atrioventricular (AV) nodal reentrant supraventricular tachycardia, for example, particularly in a young person, or ventricular tachycardia in an older person. Information regarding the nature of onset and termination of the rhythm disturbance is particularly important. Knowing the rate of the arrhythmia is crucial, and a brief demonstration by the physician of how to determine heart rate can yield important dividends. The patient, and sometimes a close relative, should be instructed in how to count the pulse.

Answers by the patient to key questions can provide clues to the type of rhythm disturbance, particularly if the physician has some additional information, such as physical findings and a 12-lead electrocardiogram. For example, a young adult with presyncope, normal physical findings, and electrocardiographic changes indicating Wolff-Parkinson-White (WPW) syndrome (see p. 667) should be asked whether the palpitations are regular or irregular, how fast they are, and how they start and stop. If the tachycardia is regular, with a rate of approximately 200 beats per minute, and of sudden onset and termination, it is likely that the patient is experiencing an AV reciprocating tachycardia (see p. 669); on the other hand, if the rhythm is irregular, the patient may have atrial fibrillation, a potentially more serious arrhythmia in the presence of WPW syndrome. In an older patient with presyncope, especially with a history of myocardial infarction, the physician should suspect ventricular tachycardia (see p. 675) if the ventricular rate is rapid and AV heart block (see p. 684) or sinus nodal disease (see p. 648) if the rate is slow. The ventricular rhythm can be regular or irregular. Premature atrial or ventricular beats, perceived as dropped or skipped beats by the patient, are probably the most common cause of palpitations.

The physician should inquire about circumstances that can trigger the arrhythmia, such as emotionally upsetting events, ingestion of caffeine-containing beverages, cigarette smoking, exercise, excessive alcohol intake, or gastrointestinal problems (Fig. 22–1). A careful diet and drug history can be useful, for example, in revealing that the patient develops palpitations only after using a nasal decongestant that contains a sympathomimetic vasoconstrictor or that the patient has been exposed to "street" drugs such as cocaine. States conducive to the genesis of arrhythmias should be considered, such as thyrotoxicosis, pericarditis, mitral valve prolapse, hypokalemia secondary to diuretics, and so forth. Family history can be helpful. A variety of familial disorders can result in arrhythmias, including myotonic dystrophy, Duchenne muscular dystrophy (see p. 1865), and dilated cardiomyopathy (see p. 1407). Congenital conduction system disorders can result in sudden death.

Physical Examination

In addition to recording cardiac rate and rhythm, a number of physical findings can be helpful. For example, findings accompanying AV dissociation (see p. 692) include variable peak systolic blood pressure as the atria alter their contribution to ventricular filling, variable intensity of the first heart sound as the P-R interval changes despite a regular ventricular rhythm, intermittent cannon *a* waves in the jugular venous pulse as atrial contraction occurs against closed AV valves, and apparent "intermittent" gallop sounds when atrial systole occurs at various times of the cardiac cycle. The *venous pulse* provides a window through which to judge atrial and ventricular rates and relative timing relationships. It is of interest that Wenckebach first noted the two types of second degree AV block that bear his name (see p. 689) by recording the jugular phlebogram before the electrocardiogram was available.

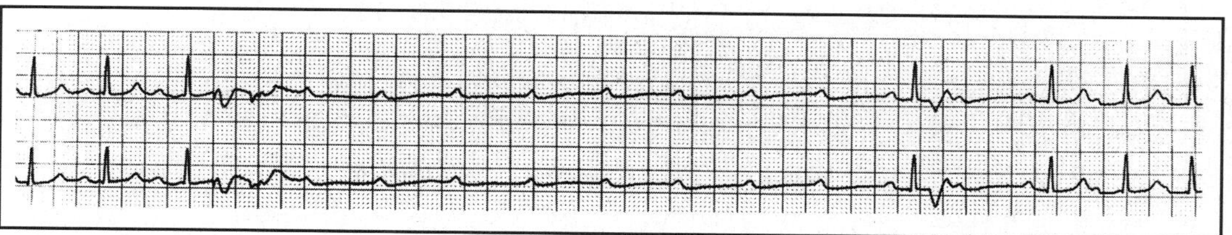

FIGURE 22–1. Transient AV block. This monitor lead recording demonstrates transient AV block during a period of nausea and vomiting, most probably due to excessive vagal stimulation.

Examining the *second heart sound* can be helpful (p. 32). A paradoxically split second heart sound can occur during a QRS complex with a left bundle branch block contour that results from ventricular tachycardia or supraventricular tachycardia with aberration. A widely split second heart sound that does not become single during expiration can accompany right bundle branch block. Unfortunately, similar physical findings occur with different cardiac arrhythmias. For example, progressive diminution of the intensity of the first heart sound results as the P-R interval lengthens, which can occur during AV dissociation when the atrial rate exceeds the ventricular rate or during Wenckebach second degree AV block. Similarly, constant cannon *a* waves can occur with 1:1 atrioventricular relationships during ventricular or supraventricular tachycardia. Since AV dissociation can occur (uncommonly) during a supraventricular tachycardia and VA association can occur during a ventricular tachycardia, the clues provided by physical findings can be only suggestive.

CAROTID SINUS MASSAGE. The response to carotid sinus massage or the Valsalva maneuver provides important diagnostic information by increasing vagal tone and primarily slowing the rate of sinus nodal discharge and prolonging AV nodal conduction time and refractoriness. Sinus tachycardia slows gradually during carotid massage and then returns to the previous rate when massage is discontinued; AV nodal reentry and AV reciprocating tachycardias that involve the AV node in one of its pathways can slow slightly, terminate abruptly, or not change; and ventricular response to atrial flutter, atrial fibrillation, and some atrial tachycardias usually decreases (Table 22–1). Rarely, carotid sinus massage terminates a ventricular tachycardia.

To perform carotid massage, the patient is placed in a supine position, with the neck hyperextended and the head turned away from the side being tested, the sternocleidomastoid muscles relaxed or gently pushed out of the way, and the carotid impulse felt at the angle of the jaw. The carotid bifurcation is touched gently initially with the palmar portion of the fingertips to detect hypersensitive responses. Then, if no change in cardiac rhythm occurs, pressure is applied more firmly for approximately 5 seconds, first on one side and then on the other (*never* on both sides simultaneously) with a gentle rotating massaging motion. External pressure stimulates baroreceptors in the carotid sinus to trigger a reflex increase in vagal activity and sympathetic withdrawal. Responses can occur with right-sided massage and not left, or vice versa, so each side should be tested separately. Generally, the maximal response occurs with the first massage if repeated attempts are performed at short intervals. Some risk is associated with carotid sinus massage, particularly in older patients, and cerebral emboli can occur.[2] Before massage, the carotid artery should be auscultated so that massage is not performed in patients who have carotid bruits indicative of carotid arterial disease.

Electrocardiography

The ECG remains the most important and definitive single noninvasive diagnostic test. Initially, a 12-lead electrocardiogram is recorded, and a long recording employing the lead that shows distinct P waves is obtained for proper analysis. If P waves are not clearly visible, atrial activity can be recorded by placing the right and left arm leads in various chest positions to discern P waves (so-called Lewis leads) using esophageal electrodes or intracavitary right atrial leads. An echocardiogram showing atrial contraction can be helpful.

Each arrhythmia must be approached in a systematic manner to answer the following questions: Are P waves present? What are the atrial and ventricular rates? Are they identical? Are the P-P and R-R intervals regular or irregular? If irregular, is it a consistent, repeating irregularity? Is there a P wave related to each ventricular complex? Does the P wave precede or follow the QRS complex? Is the resultant P-R or R-P interval constant? Is the R-P interval long and the P-R interval short, or vice versa? Are all P waves and QRS complexes identical and normal in contour? To determine the significance of changes in P-wave or QRS contour, or amplitude, one must know the lead being recorded. Are P, P-R, QRS, and Q-T durations normal? Considering the clinical setting, what is the significance of the arrhythmia? Should it be treated and, if so, how? For supraventricular tachycardias with a normal QRS complex, a branching decision tree may be useful.

THE LADDER DIAGRAM. This is employed to depict depolarization and conduction schematically. Straight or slightly slanting lines drawn on a tiered framework beneath an ECG trace represent electrical events occurring in the various cardiac structures (Fig. 22–2*A* and *B*). Since the ECG and therefore the ladder diagram represent electrical activity against a time base, conduction is indicated by the lines of the ladder diagram sloping in a left-to-right direction. A less steep line depicts slower conduction. A short bar drawn perpendicular to a sloping line represents blocked conduction (Fig. 22–2*C*). Activity originating in an ectopic site such as the ventricle is indicated in another tier drawn beneath the ventricular tier. In general, atrial, AV junctional, or ventricular activity is diagrammed to begin in that particular tier. It is important to remember that sinus nodal discharge and conduction and, under certain circumstances, AV junctional discharge and conduction can only be assumed; their activity is not recorded on scalar ECG.

ELECTROPHYSIOLOGICAL STUDY. When this study is indicated, it is performed by introducing multipolar catheter electrodes into the vascular system and positioning them in various parts of the heart. The catheters are used to record local electrical activity and to stimulate the heart. Multiple leads are recorded simultaneously, usually at a paper speed of 50 to 100 mm/sec. (Standard ECGs generally are recorded at a paper speed of 25 mm/sec.) Because of the rapid recording speed, intervals or complexes of normal duration may appear prolonged. An electrode positioned across the septal leaflet of the tricuspid valve records His bundle activity as well as low right atrial activity and high ventricular septal depolarization. Occasionally, a right bundle branch deflection also can be recorded. Three basic measurements are made using the ECG and the His bundle catheter recording: the P-A, A-H, and H-V intervals (Fig. 22–2*D*). The *P-A interval* is the time between the onset of the P wave in the surface tracing (which generally slightly precedes the onset of the high right atrial recording) and the low right atrial deflection, recorded in the His lead.

TABLE 22–1 ARRHYTHMIA CHARACTERISTICS*

TYPE OF ARRHYTHMIA	P WAVES			QRS COMPLEXES		
	Rate (bpm)	Rhythm	Contour	Rate	Rhythm	Contour
Sinus rhythm	60 to 100	Regular**	Normal	60 to 100	Regular	Normal
Sinus bradycardia	<60	Regular	Normal	<60	Regular	Normal
Sinus tachycardia	100 to 180	Regular	May be peaked	100 to 180	Regular	Normal
AV nodal reentry	150 to 250	Very regular except at onset and termination	Retrograde; difficult to see; lost in QRS complex	150 to 250	Very regular except at onset and termination	Normal
Atrial flutter	250 to 350	Regular	Sawtooth	75 to 175	Generally regular in absence of drugs or disease	Normal
Atrial fibrillation	400 to 600	Grossly irregular	Baseline undulation, no P waves	100 to 160	Grossly irregular	Normal
Atrial tachycardia with block	150 to 250	Regular; may be irregular	Abnormal	75 to 200	Generally regular in absence of drugs or disease	Normal
AV junctional rhythm	40 to 100‡	Regular	Normal	40 to 60	Fairly regular	Normal
Reciprocating tachycardias using an accessory (WPW) pathway	150 to 250	Very regular except at onset and termination	Retrograde; difficult to see; follow the QRS complex	150 to 250	Very regular except at onset and termination	Normal
Nonparoxysmal AV junctional tachycardia	60 to 100‡	Regular	Normal	70 to 130	Fairly regular	Normal
Ventricular tachycardia	60 to 100‡	Regular	Normal	110 to 250	Fairly regular; may be irregular	Abnormal, >0.12 second
Accelerated idioventricular rhythm	60 to 100‡	Regular	Normal	50 to 110	Fairly regular; may be irregular	Abnormal, >0.12 second
Ventricular flutter	60 to 100‡	Regular	Normal; difficult to see	150 to 300	Regular	Sine wave
Ventricular fibrillation	60 to 100‡	Regular	Normal; difficult to see	400 to 600	Grossly irregular	Baseline undulations; no QRS complexes
First degree AV block	60 to 100¶	Regular	Normal	60 to 100	Regular	Normal
Type I second degree AV block	60 to 100¶	Regular	Normal	30 to 100	Irregular‖	Normal
Type II second degree AV block	60 to 100¶	Regular	Normal	30 to 100	Irregular‖	Abnormal, >0.12 second
Complete AV block	60 to 100‡	Regular	Normal	<40	Fairly regular	Abnormal, >0.12 second
Right bundle branch block	60 to 100	Regular	Normal	60 to 100	Regular	Abnormal, >0.12 second
Left bundle branch block	60 to 100	Regular	Normal	60 to 100	Regular	Abnormal, >0.12 second

* In an effort to summarize these arrhythmias in a tabular form, generalizations have to be made. For example, response to carotid sinus massage may be slightly different from what is listed. Acute therapy to terminate a tachycardia may be different from chronic therapy to prevent a recurrence. Some of the exceptions are indicated in the footnotes; the reader is referred to the text for a complete discussion.

** P waves initiated by sinus node discharge may not be precisely regular because of sinus arrhythmia.

† Often, carotid sinus massage fails to slow a sinus tachycardia.

‡ Any independent atrial arrhythmia may exist or the atria may be captured retrogradely.

§ Constant if atria are captured retrogradely.

¶ Atrial rhythm and rate may vary, depending on whether sinus bradycardia or tachycardia, etc., is the atrial mechanism.

‖ Regular or constant if block is unchanging.

Modified from Zipes, D. P.: Arrhythmias. *In* Andreoli, K., et al. (eds): Comprehensive Cardiac Care. 6th ed. St. Louis, C. V. Mosby, 1987.

This interval reflects intraatrial conduction and has not proved to be of much clinical value.

The A-H Interval. This is timed from the onset of the first rapid deflection recorded in the atrial electrogram (A) in the His bundle lead to the beginning of the His (H) deflection. Since the low right atrium and His bundle anatomically delineate the boundaries of the AV node, the A-H interval closely approximates AV nodal conduction time. The A-H interval is affected by various interventions: atropine and isoproterenol shorten the A-H interval, while vagal maneuvers, digitalis, propranolol, verapamil, adenosine, and rapid or premature atrial pacing lengthen it. Normal range for the A-H interval is 55 to 130 msec, depending on heart rate, autonomic tone, and other factors.

The H-V Interval. This is the time from the beginning of the H deflection to the earliest onset of ventricular depolarization recorded in *any* lead. This interval represents conduction from the His bundle through the bundle

TABLE 22–1 ARRHYTHMIA CHARACTERISTICS* *(Continued)*

VENTRICULAR RESPONSE TO CAROTID SINUS MASSAGE	P WAVES / PHYSICAL EXAMINATION		QRS COMPLEXES	
	Intensity of S_1	Splitting of S_2	*a* Waves	Treatment
Gradual slowing and return to former rate	Constant	Normal	Normal	None
Gradual slowing and return to former rate	Constant	Normal	Normal	None, unless symptomatic; atropine
Gradual slowing† and return to former rate	Constant	Normal	Normal	None, unless symptomatic; treat underlying disease
Abrupt slowing caused by termination of tachycardia, or no effect	Constant	Normal	Constant cannon *a* waves	Vagal stimulation, adenosine, verapamil, digitalis, propranolol, DC shock, pacing
Abrupt slowing and return to former rate; flutter remains	Constant; variable if AV block changing	Normal	Flutter waves	DC shock, digitalis, quinidine, propranolol, verapamil, adenosine
Slowing; gross irregularity remains	Variable	Normal	No *a* waves	Digitalis, quinidine, DC shock, verapamil, adenosine
Abrupt slowing and return to normal rate; tachycardia remains	Constant; variable if AV block changing	Normal	More *a* waves than *c-v* waves	Stop digitalis if toxic; digitalis if not toxic; possibly verapamil
None; may be slight slowing	Variable§	Normal	Intermittent cannon waves§	None, unless symptomatic; atropine
Abrupt slowing caused by termination of tachycardia, or no effect	Constant but decreased	Normal	Constant cannon waves	(See AV nodal reentry above)
None, may be slight slowing	Variable§	Normal	Intermittent cannon waves§	None, unless symptomatic; stop digitalis if toxic
None	Variable§	Abnormal	Intermittent cannon waves§	Lidocaine, procainamide, DC shock, quinidine, amiodarone
None	Variable§	Abnormal	Intermittent cannon waves§	None, unless symptomatic; lidocaine, atropine
None	Soft or absent	Soft or absent	Cannon waves	DC shock
None	None	None	Cannon waves	DC shock
Gradual slowing caused by sinus slowing	Constant, diminished	Normal	Normal	None
Slowing caused by sinus slowing and an increase in AV block	Cyclic decrease then increase after pause	Normal	Normal; increasing *a-c* interval; *a* waves without *c* waves	None, unless symptomatic; atropine
Gradual slowing caused by sinus slowing	Constant	Abnormal	Normal; constant *a-c* interval; *a* waves without *c* waves	Pacemaker
None	Variable§	Abnormal	Intermittent cannon waves§	Pacemaker
Gradual slowing and return to former rate	Constant	Wide	Normal	None
Gradual slowing and return to former rate	Constant	Paradoxical	Normal	None

branch–Purkinje system to the point of ventricular muscle activation and is usually constant—between 30 and 55 msec—regardless of heart rate or autonomic tone. Other intervals are discussed under the individual tachycardias.

CONSEQUENCES OF ARRHYTHMIAS. The ventricular rate and duration of an arrhythmia, its site of origin, and the cardiovascular status of the patient primarily determine the electrophysiological and hemodynamic consequences of a particular rhythm disturbance. Electrophysiological consequences, often influenced by the presence of underlying heart disease such as acute myocardial infarction, include the development of serious arrhythmias as a result of rapid or slow rates, initiation of sustained arrhythmias by premature systoles, or the progression of rhythms such as ventricular tachycardia to ventricular fibrillation. Extremes of heart rate or loss of the atrial contribution to ventricular filling can alter circulatory dynamics. Rapid rates greatly shorten the diastolic filling time, and particularly in diseased hearts, the increased heart rate can fail to compensate for the reduced stroke output; as a consequence, arterial pressure, cardiac output, and coronary blood flow decline. Arrhythmias that prevent sequential AV contraction mitigate the hemodynamic benefits of the atrial booster pump, whereas atrial fibrillation causes complete loss of atrial contraction and can reduce cardiac output. Chronic tachycardias can cause cardiac dilation and heart failure from a tachycardia-induced cardiomyopathy.

Management

The therapeutic approach to a patient with a cardiac arrhythmia begins with an accurate electrocardiographic *interpretation* of the arrhythmia and continues with determination of the *cause* of the arrhythmia (if possible), the

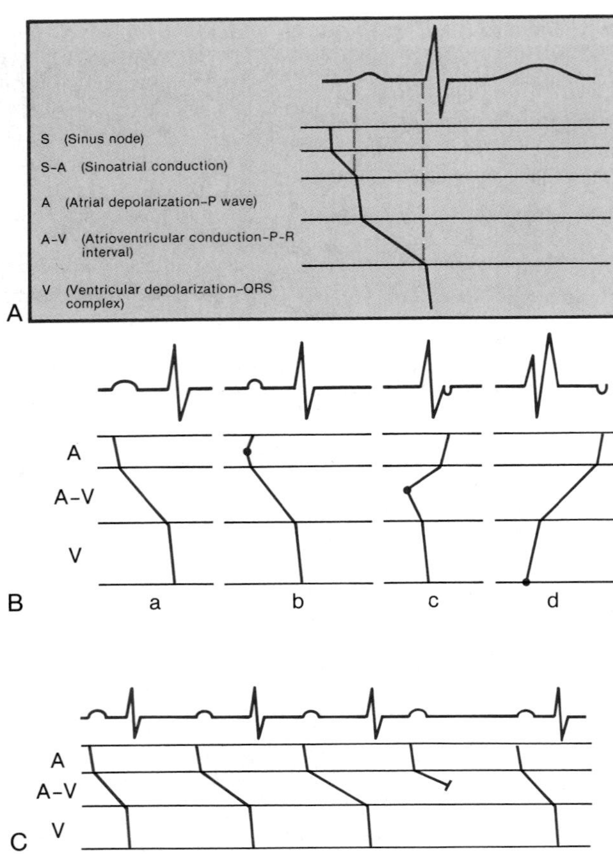

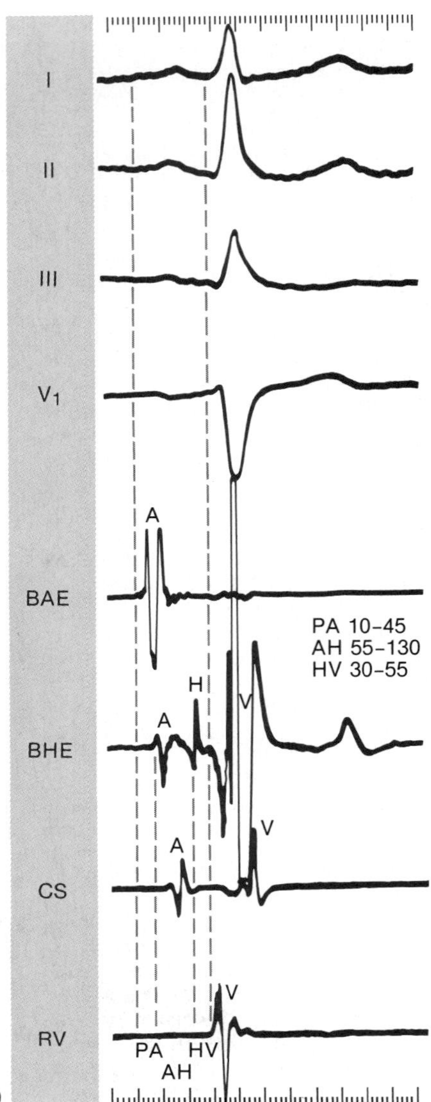

FIGURE 22–2. *A*, Ladder diagram. Straight or slightly sloping lines beginning with the P wave and QRS complex indicate atrial and ventricular depolarization. The instants at which the sinus node discharges and the duration of sinoatrial conduction cannot be measured in the surface ECG and are therefore assumed. The sloping line connecting A and V, delimited by the interrupted lines, represents AV conduction.

B, Normal and ectopic beats. a = Normal sinus rhythm; b = ectopic atrial beat; c = AV junctional beat; d = ventricular ectopic beats. All are drawn with appropriate ladder diagrams beneath (T waves omitted). Retrograde atrial conduction is inscribed for the latter two beats. As with the sinus node, the exact discharge time of the AV junctional focus and conduction time from that point to the ventricles and atria are assumed.

C, Second degree Wenckebach type I AV block. The P-R interval lengthens progressively until finally the fourth P wave fails to reach the ventricles. As the P-R interval is prolonged, note decreasing slope of the line representing AV conduction and the small line perpendicular to the fourth sloping line indicating that the P wave is blocked. (*A* to *C* reproduced with permission from Zipes, D. P., and Fisch, C.: ECG Analysis: 1. Introduction. Premature ventricular complexes. Arch. Intern. Med. *128:*140, 1971. Copyright American Medical Association.)

D, A single cardiac cycle showing the intervals measured during an electrophysiological study. In this and in similar subsequent figures, BAE indicates bipolar atrial electrogram recording high right atrial activity; BHE indicates the bipolar His electrogram recording low right atrial activity (A), His bundle activity (H), and ventricular septal activity (V); CS indicates bipolar electrogram recording of left atrial activity in coronary sinus lead; RV indicates right ventricular electrogram recording right ventricular activity; I = lead I; II = lead II; III = lead III; V_1 = lead V_1; PA = interval representing intraatrial conduction time; AH = interval representing AV nodal conduction time; HV = interval representing His-Purkinje conduction time. All values are in milliseconds. Normal values for P-A, A-H, and H-V intervals are given at the upper right. Paper speed = 100 mm/sec unless otherwise stated. Interrupted lines demarcate the various intervals. Note the normal sequence of atrial activation recorded with this technique: high right atrial activity (BAE) precedes low right atrial activity recorded in the BHE lead, which precedes left atrial activity recorded in the CS lead. Large time lines = 50 msec. Small time lines = 10 msec.

nature of the underlying *heart disease* (if any), and the *consequences* of the arrhythmias in the individual patient. Thus one does not treat arrhythmias as isolated events without having knowledge of the entire clinical situation. *Patients* who have arrhythmias, rather than the arrhythmias themselves, are treated.

When a patient develops a tachyarrhythmia, slowing the ventricular rate is the initial and often most important therapeutic maneuver. Therapy can differ radically for the same arrhythmia in two different patients because the consequences of tachycardia in individual patients differ. For example, a supraventricular tachycardia at a rate of 200 beats/min can produce few or no symptoms in a healthy young adult and therefore requires little or no therapy because it is usually self-limited. The same arrhythmia can precipitate pulmonary edema in a patient with mitral stenosis, syncope in a patient with aortic stenosis, shock in a patient with acute myocardial infarction, or hemiparesis in a patient with cerebrovascular disease. In these situations, the tachycardia requires prompt electrical conversion.

The *cause* of the arrhythmia can influence therapy greatly. Electrolyte imbalance (potassium, magnesium, calcium), acidosis or alkalosis, hypoxemia, and many drugs can produce rhythm disturbances, and their identification and treatment can abolish or prevent these arrhythmias. Because heart failure can cause arrhythmias, treatment of this condition with digitalis, diuretics, or vasodilators can suppress some of the arrhythmias that accompany cardiac decompensation. Similarly, arrhythmias secondary to hypotension may respond to leg elevation or vasopressor therapy. Mild sedation or reassurance can be successful in treating some arrhythmias related to emotional stress. Precipitating or contributing disease states such as myocarditis, infection, hypokalemia, anemia, and thyroid disorders should be sought and treated when possible. Since therapy always involves some risk, one must be sure—particularly as the therapeutic regimen escalates—that the risks of *not* treating the arrhythmia continue to outweigh the risks of therapy with potentially hazardous antiarrhythmic measures.

INDIVIDUAL CARDIAC ARRHYTHMIAS

SINUS NODAL DISTURBANCES

NORMAL SINUS RHYTHM

Normal sinus rhythm is arbitrarily limited to impulse formation beginning in the sinus node at frequencies between 60 and 100 beats/min. A range of 50 to 90 beats/min has been suggested recently.[3] Infants and children generally have faster heart rates than do adults, both at rest and during exercise. The P wave is upright in leads I, II, and aV_f and negative in lead aV_r, with a vector in the frontal plane between 0 and +90 degrees. In the horizontal plane, the P vector is directed anteriorly and slightly leftward and therefore can be negative in leads V_1 and V_2 but positive in V_3 to V_6. The P-R interval exceeds 120 msec and can vary slightly with rate. If the pacemaker site shifts, a change in the morphology of the P wave can occur. The rate of sinus rhythm varies significantly and depends on many factors, including age, sex, and physical activity.

The sinus nodal discharge rate responds readily to autonomic stimuli and depends on the effect of the two opposing autonomic influences. Steady vagal stimulation decreases the spontaneous sinus nodal discharge rate and predominates over steady sympathetic stimulation, which increases the spontaneous sinus nodal discharge rate. Single or brief bursts of vagal stimulation can speed, slow, or entrain sinus nodal discharge. A given vagal stimulus produces a greater absolute reduction in heart rate when the basal heart rate has been increased by sympathetic stimulation, a phenomenon known as *accentuated antagonism.*

SINUS TACHYCARDIA

ELECTROCARDIOGRAPHIC RECOGNITION (Fig. 22–3*A*). *Tachycardia* in the adult is defined as a rate exceeding 100 beats/min. During sinus tachycardia, the sinus node exhibits a discharge frequency between 100 and 180 beats/min, but it may be higher with extreme exertion. The maximum heart rate achieved during strenuous physical activity decreases with age from near 200 beats/min to less than 140 beats/min. Sinus tachycardia generally has a gradual onset and termination. The P-P interval can vary slightly from cycle to cycle. P waves have a normal contour but can develop a larger amplitude and become peaked. They appear before each QRS complex with a stable P-R interval unless concomitant AV block ensues.

Accelerated phase 4 diastolic depolarization of sinus nodal cells generally is responsible for sinus tachycardia. Rate changes can result from a shift in pacemaker cells to a different locus within the sinus node. Carotid sinus massage and Valsalva or other vagal maneuvers gradually slow a sinus tachycardia, which then accelerates to its previous rate upon cessation of enhanced vagal tone. More rapid sinus rates can fail to slow in response to a vagal maneuver.

CLINICAL FEATURES. Sinus tachycardia is common in infancy and early childhood and is the normal reaction to a variety of physiological or pathophysiological stresses such as fever, hypotension, thyrotoxicosis, anemia, anxiety, exertion, hypovolemia, pulmonary emboli, myocardial ischemia, congestive heart failure, or shock. It can occur during REM sleep[4] and can be an adverse prognostic sign after heart transplantation.[5] Drugs, such as atropine, catecholamines,[6] thyroid medications,[7] alcohol, nicotine, or caffeine, or inflammation can produce sinus tachycardia. Persistent sinus tachycardia can be a manifestation of heart failure.

In patients with mitral stenosis or severe ischemic heart disease, sinus tachycardia can result in a reduced cardiac output or angina or can precipitate another arrhythmia, in part related to the abbreviated ventricular filling time and compromised coronary blood flow. Sinus tachycardia can be a cause of inappropriate defibrillator discharge.[8] *Chronic inappropriate sinus tachycardia* has been described in otherwise healthy persons, possibly owing to increased automaticity of the sinus node or an automatic atrial focus located near the sinus node.[9] The abnormality can result from a defect in either sympathetic or vagal nerve control of sinoatrial automaticity, or there can be an abnormality of the intrinsic heart rate.[10] It has been noted following radiofrequency catheter ablation of AV nodal tachycardia.[11–13]

MANAGEMENT. This should focus on the *cause* of the sinus tachycardia. Elimination of tobacco, alcohol, coffee, tea, or other stimulants, such as the sympathomimetic agents in nose drops, may be helpful. Drugs such as propranolol or verapamil or fluid replacement in a hypovolemic patient or fever reduction in a febrile patient can be used to help slow the sinus nodal discharge rate. Treatment of inappropriate sinus tachycardia requires beta blockers, calcium channel blockers, or digitalis, alone or in combination. In severe cases, sinus node radiofrequency[14] or surgical[15] ablation may be indicated. Occlusion of the sinus node artery has been attempted as treatment.[16]

SINUS BRADYCARDIA

ELECTROCARDIOGRAPHIC RECOGNITION (Fig. 22–3*B*). Sinus bradycardia exists in the adult when the sinus node discharges at a rate less than 60 beats/min. P waves have a normal contour and occur before each QRS complex with a constant P-R interval exceeding 120 msec

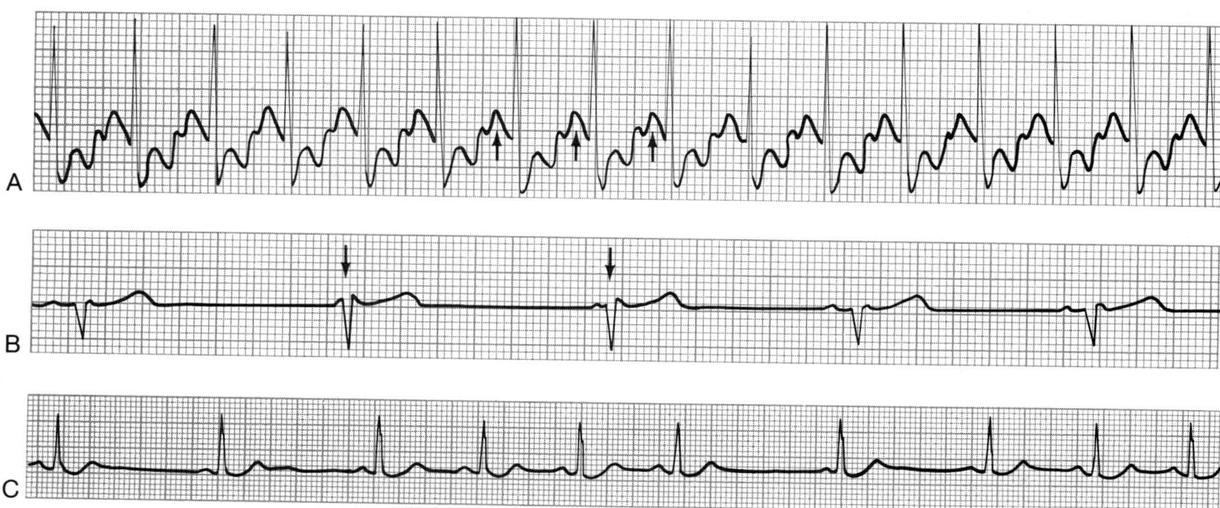

FIGURE 22–3. *A,* Sinus tachycardia (150 beats/min) in a patient during acute myocardial ischemia; note ST-segment depression. P waves are indicated by arrows. *B,* Sinus bradycardia at a rate of 40 to 48 beats/min. The second and third QRS complexes (arrows) represent junctional escape beats. Note P waves at onset of QRS complex. *C,* Nonrespiratory sinus arrhythmia occurring as a consequence of digitalis toxicity. Monitor leads.

unless concomitant AV block is present. Sinus arrhythmia often coexists.

CLINICAL FEATURES. Sinus bradycardia can result from excessive vagal or decreased sympathetic tone as well as from anatomical changes in the sinus node (see Sick Sinus Syndrome, p. 648). Sinus bradycardia frequently occurs in healthy young adults, particularly well-trained athletes (who also can have tachyarrhythmias), and decreases in prevalence with advancing age. It may be present in patients with anorexia nervosa[17] and following cardiac transplantation.[18] During sleep, the normal heart rate can fall to 35 to 40 beats/min, especially in adolescents and young adults, with marked sinus arrhythmia sometimes producing pauses of 2 seconds or longer. Eye surgery, coronary arteriography, meningitis, intracranial tumors, increased intracranial pressure, cervical and mediastinal tumors, and certain disease states such as severe hypoxia, Chagas' disease,[19] myxedema, hypothermia, fibrodegenerative changes, convalescence from some infections, gram-negative sepsis, and mental depression can produce sinus bradycardia. Obstructive jaundice is considered to cause sinus bradycardia, but the evidence is not clear. Sinus bradycardia also occurs during vomiting or vasovagal syncope (see p. 863) and can be produced by carotid sinus stimulation or by administration of parasympathomimetic drugs, lithium, amiodarone, beta-adrenoceptor blocking drugs, clonidine, propafenone, or calcium-antagonists. Conjunctival instillation of beta blockers for glaucoma can produce sinus or AV nodal abnormalities.

In most instances, sinus bradycardia is a benign arrhythmia and actually can be beneficial by producing a longer period of diastole and increasing ventricular filling time. It can be associated with syncope due to an abnormal reflex.[20] Sinus bradycardia occurs in 10 to 15 per cent of patients with acute myocardial infarction and may be even more prevalent when patients are seen in the early hours of infarction. Unless accompanied by hemodynamic decompensation or arrhythmias, sinus bradycardia generally is associated with a more favorable outcome following myocardial infarction than is the presence of sinus tachycardia. It usually is transient and occurs more commonly during inferior than anterior myocardial infarction; it has been noted during reperfusion with thrombolytic agents. Bradycardia following resuscitation from cardiac arrest is associated with a poor prognosis.

MANAGEMENT. Treatment of sinus bradycardia per se is usually not necessary. For example, if the patient with an acute myocardial infarction is asymptomatic, it is probably best not to speed up the sinus rate. If cardiac output is inadequate or if arrhythmias are associated with the slow rate, atropine (0.5 mg IV as an initial dose, repeated if necessary) is usually effective. Lower doses of atropine, particularly when given subcutaneously or intramuscularly, can exert an initial parasympathomimetic effect, possibly via a central action. Ephedrine, hydralazine, or theophylline can be useful in managing some patients with symptomatic sinus bradycardia. These drugs should be given with caution so as not to "overshoot" and produce too rapid a rate. In some patients who experience congestive heart failure or symptoms of low cardiac output as a result of chronic sinus bradycardia, electrical pacing may be needed. Atrial pacing is usually preferable to ventricular pacing in order to preserve sequential atrioventricular contraction and is preferable to drug therapy for long-term management of sinus bradycardia. As a general rule, no available drugs increase the heart rate reliably and safely over long periods without important side effects.

SINUS ARRHYTHMIA

Sinus arrhythmia (Fig. 22–3*C*) is characterized by a phasic variation in sinus cycle length during which the maximum sinus cycle length minus minimum sinus cycle length exceeds 120 msec or the maximum sinus cycle length minus minimum sinus cycle length divided by the minimum sinus cycle length exceeds 10 per cent. It is the most frequent form of arrhythmia and is considered to be a normal event. P-wave morphology usually does not vary, and the P-R interval exceeds 120 msec and remains unchanged, since the focus of discharge remains relatively fixed within the sinus node. Occasionally, the pacemaker focus can wander within the sinus node, or its exit to the atrium may change, producing P waves of slightly different contour (but not retrograde) and a slightly changing P-R interval that exceeds 120 msec.

Sinus arrhythmia commonly occurs in the young, especially with slower heart rates or following enhanced vagal tone, such as after the administration of digitalis or morphine, and decreases with age or with autonomic dysfunction, such as diabetic neuropathy. Sinus arrhythmia appears in two basic forms. In the *respiratory* form, the P-P interval cyclically shortens during inspiration, primarily as a result of reflex inhibition of vagal tone, and slows during expiration; breath-holding eliminates the cycle-length variation. Efferent vagal effects alone have been suggested as responsible for respiratory sinus arrhythmias. *Nonrespiratory* sinus arrhythmia is characterized by a phasic variation in P-P interval unrelated to the respiratory cycle and may be the result of digitalis intoxication. Loss of sinus rhythm variability is a risk factor for sudden cardiac death (see p. 750). Loss of sinus arrhythmia can occur in patients with acute intracranial lesions.[21]

Symptoms produced by sinus arrhythmia are uncommon, but on occasion, if the pauses between beats are excessively long, palpitations or dizziness may result. Marked sinus arrhythmia can produce a sinus pause sufficiently long to produce syncope if not accompanied by an escape rhythm.

Treatment is usually unnecessary. Increasing the heart rate by exercise or drugs generally abolishes sinus arrhythmia. Symptomatic individuals may experience relief from palpitations with sedatives, tranquilizers, atropine, ephedrine, or isoproterenol administration, as in the treatment of sinus bradycardia.

VENTRICULOPHASIC SINUS ARRHYTHMIA. This arrhythmia occurs when the ventricular rate is slow. The most common example occurs during complete AV block, when P-P cycles that contain a QRS complex are shorter than P-P cycles without a QRS complex. Similar lengthening can be present in the P-P cycle that follows a premature ventricular complex with a compensatory pause. Alterations in the P-P interval are probably due to the influence of the autonomic nervous system responding to changes in ventricular stroke volume.

Sinus Pause or Sinus Arrest

Sinus pause or sinus arrest (Fig. 22–4) is recognized by a pause in the sinus rhythm. The P-P interval delimiting the pause does not equal a multiple of the basic P-P interval. Differentiation of sinus arrest, which is thought to be due to a slowing or cessation of spontaneous sinus nodal automaticity and therefore a disorder of impulse formation, from sinoatrial exit block (see below) in patients with sinus arrhythmia can be quite difficult without direct recordings of sinus node discharge.[22,23]

Failure of sinus nodal discharge results in absence of atrial depolarization and in periods of ventricular asystole if escape beats initiated by latent pacemakers do not occur (Fig. 22–4). Involvement of the sinus node by acute myocardial infarction,[24] degenerative fibrotic changes, effects of digitalis toxicity, stroke, or excessive vagal tone all can produce sinus arrest. Transient sinus arrest may have no clinical significance by itself if latent pacemakers promptly escape to prevent ventricular asystole or the genesis of other arrhythmias precipitated by the slow rates. Sinus arrest and AV block have been demonstrated in as many as 30 per cent of patients with sleep apnea.[25]

Treatment is as outlined above for sinus bradycardia. In patients who have a chronic form of sinus node disease characterized by marked sinus bradycardia or sinus arrest, permanent pacing is often necessary.

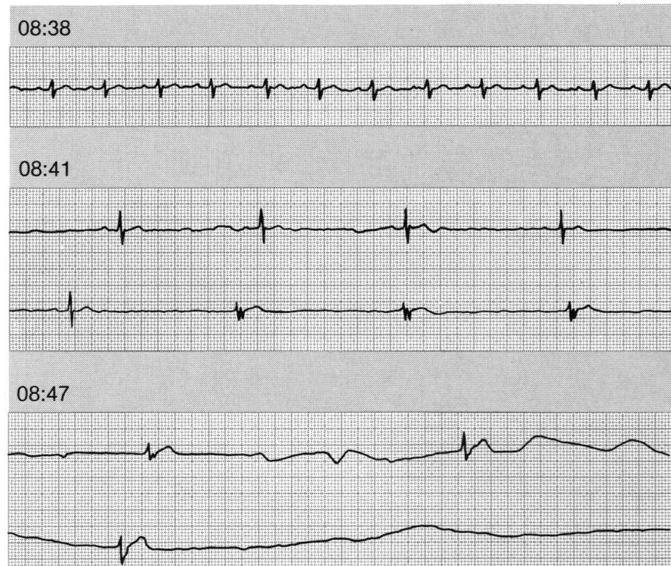

FIGURE 22–4. Sinus arrest. The patient had a long-term ECG recorder connected when he died suddenly due to cardiac standstill. The rhythms demonstrate progressive sinus bradycardia and sinus arrest at 08:41. The rhythm then becomes a ventricular escape rhythm which progressively slows and finally ceases at 08:47. Monitor lead. Double ECG strips are continuous recordings.

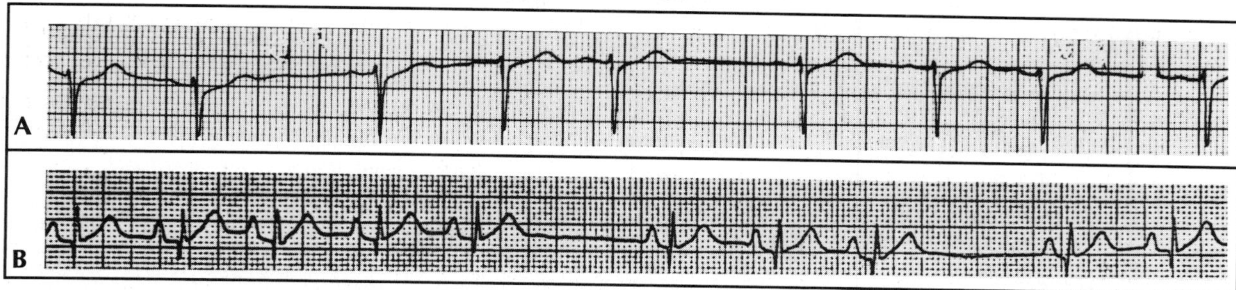

FIGURE 22–5. Sinus nodal exit block. *A*, Type I SA nodal exit block has the following features: the P-P interval shortens from the first to the second cycle in each grouping, followed by a pause. The duration of the pause is less than twice the shortest cycle length, and the cycle after the pause exceeds the cycle before the pause. The P-R interval is normal and constant. Lead V_1. *B*, The P-P interval varies slightly because of sinus arrhythmia. Two pauses in sinus nodal activity occur, equalling twice the basic P-P interval and are consistent with type II 2:1 SA nodal exit block. The P-R interval is normal and constant. Lead III.

Sinoatrial (SA) Exit Block

This arrhythmia is recognized electrocardiographically by a pause due to the absence of the normally expected P wave[23,26] (Fig. 22–5). The duration of the pause is a multiple of the basic P-P interval. SA exit block is due to a conduction disturbance during which an impulse formed within the sinus node fails to depolarize the atria or does so with delay[27] (Fig. 22–6). An interval without P waves that equals approximately two, three, or four times the normal P-P cycle characterizes type II second degree SA exit block. During type I (Wenckebach) second degree SA exit block, the P-P interval progressively shortens prior to the pause, and the duration of the pause is less than two P-P cycles. (See p. 689 and Fig. 22–52, p. 689, for further discussion of Wenckebach intervals.) First degree SA exit block cannot be recognized electrocardiographically because SA nodal discharge is not recorded. Third degree SA exit block can present as complete absence of P waves and is difficult to diagnose with certainty without sinus node electrograms.

Excessive vagal stimulation, acute myocarditis, infarction, or fibrosis involving the atrium as well as drugs such as quinidine, procainamide, or digitalis can produce SA exit block. SA exit block is usually transient. It may be of no clinical importance except to prompt a search for the underlying cause. Occasionally, syncope can result if the SA block is prolonged and unaccompanied by an escape rhythm. SA exit block can occur in well-trained athletes[28] and can be a factor in sick sinus syndrome.[27]

Therapy for patients who have symptomatic SA exit block is as outlined for sinus bradycardia.

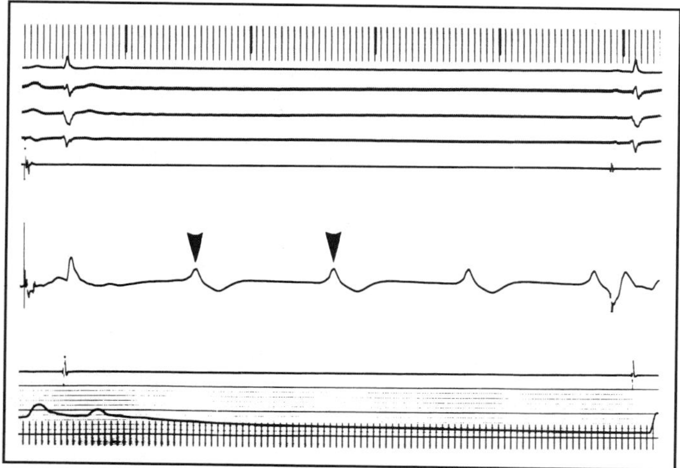

FIGURE 22–6. Sinus node exit block. Following a period of atrial pacing (only the last paced cycle is shown), the patient developed sinus node exit block. The tracing demonstrates sinus node potentials (arrowheads), recorded with a catheter electrode, not conducting to the atrium until the last complex. Recordings are leads I, II, III, and V_1, right atrial recording, sinus node recording, and right ventricular apical recording. The bottom tracing is femoral artery blood pressure.

Wandering Pacemaker

This variant of sinus arrhythmia involves the passive transfer of the dominant pacemaker focus from the sinus node to latent pacemakers that have the next highest degree of automaticity located in other atrial sites or in AV junctional tissue. Thus only one pacemaker at a time controls the rhythm, in sharp contrast to AV dissociation (see p. 692). As with other forms of sinus arrhythmia, the change occurs in a gradual fashion over the duration of several beats. The ECG (Fig. 22–7) displays a cyclical increase in R-R interval, a P-R interval that gradually shortens and can become less than 120 msec, and a change in the P-wave contour, which becomes negative in lead I or II (depending on the site of discharge) or is lost within the QRS complex. Generally, these changes occur in reverse as the pacemaker shifts back to the sinus node. Rarely, the rate may remain unchanged during these P-wave transitions.

Wandering pacemaker is a normal phenomenon that often occurs in the very young and particularly in athletes, presumably because of augmented vagal tone. Persistence of an AV junctional rhythm for long periods of time, however, may indicate underlying heart disease. *Treatment* is usually not indicated but, if necessary, is the same as that for sinus bradycardia (see above).

Hypersensitive Carotid Sinus Syndrome

(See also p. 865)

ELECTROCARDIOGRAPHIC RECOGNITION (Fig. 22–8). This condition is characterized most frequently by ventricular asystole due to cessation of atrial activity from sinus arrest or SA exit block. AV block is observed less frequently, probably in part because the absence of atrial activity due to sinus arrest precludes the manifestations of AV block. However, if an atrial pacemaker maintained an atrial rhythm during the episodes, a higher prevalence of AV block probably would be noted. In symptomatic patients, AV junctional or ventricular escapes generally do not occur or are present at very slow rates, suggesting that heightened vagal tone and sympathetic withdrawal can suppress subsidiary pacemakers located in the ventricles as well as supraventricular structures.

CLINICAL FEATURES. Two types of hypersensitive carotid sinus responses are noted. *Cardioinhibitory* carotid sinus hypersensitivity is generally defined as ventricular asystole exceeding 3 seconds during carotid sinus stimulation, although normal limits have not been carefully established. In fact, asystole exceeding 3 seconds during carotid

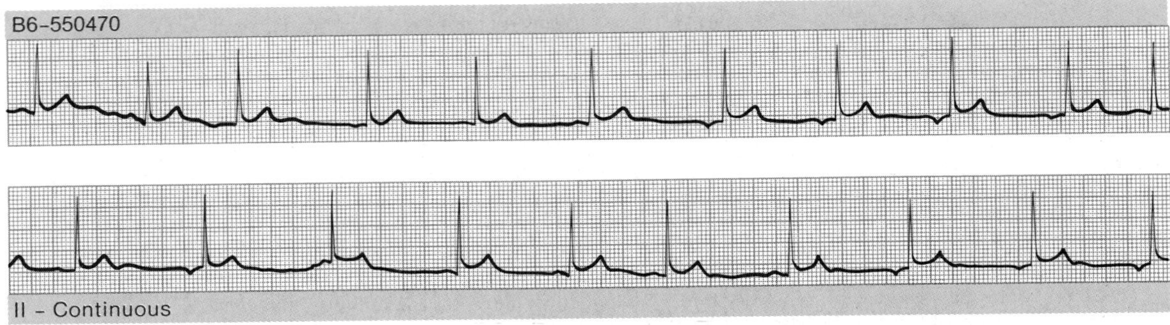

FIGURE 22–7. Wandering atrial pacemaker. As the heart rate slows, the P waves become inverted and then gradually revert toward normal when the heart rate speeds up again. The P-R interval shortens to 0.14 sec with the inverted P wave and is 0.16 sec with the upright P wave. This phasic variation in cycle length with varying P-wave contour suggests a shift in pacemaker site and is characteristic of wandering atrial pacemaker.

sinus massage is not common but can occur in asymptomatic subjects (Fig. 22–8). *Vasodepressor* carotid sinus hypersensitivity is generally defined as a decrease in systolic blood pressure of 50 mm Hg or more without associated cardiac slowing or a decrease in systolic blood pressure exceeding 30 mm Hg when the patient's symptoms are reproduced.

Even if a hyperactive carotid sinus reflex is elicited in patients, particularly in older patients who complain of syncope or presyncope, the hyperactive reflex elicited with carotid sinus massage may not necessarily be responsible for these symptoms. Direct pressure or extension on the carotid sinus from head turning, neck tension, and tight collars also can be a source of syncope by reducing blood flow through the cerebral arteries.

Hypersensitive carotid sinus reflex is most commonly associated with coronary artery disease. The mechanism responsible for hypersensitive carotid sinus reflex is not known, but possibilities include a high level of resting vagal tone, hyperresponsiveness to acetylcholine, excessive release of acetylcholine, baroreflex hypersensitivity, inadequate cholinesterase activity to metabolize the acetylcholine released, and concomitant sympathetic abnormality. Carotid sinus receptors, autonomic centers of the brain stem, and the afferent limb of the reflex have all been incriminated.

MANAGEMENT. Atropine abolishes cardioinhibitory carotid sinus hypersensitivity. However, the majority of symptomatic patients require pacemaker implantation. It must be stressed that because AV block can occur during the periods of hypersensitive carotid reflex, some form of *ventricular* pacing, with or without atrial pacing, is generally required. Atropine and pacing do not prevent the decrease in systemic blood pressure in the vasodepressor form of carotid sinus hypersensitivity,[29] which may result from inhibition of sympathetic vasoconstrictor nerves and possibly activation of cholinergic sympathetic vasodilator fibers. Combinations of vasodepressor and cardioinhibitory types can occur, and vasodepression can account for continued syncope after pacemaker implantation in some patients. Patients who have a hyperactive carotid sinus reflex that does not cause symptoms require no treatment. Drugs such as digitalis, alpha-methyldopa, clonidine, and propranolol can enhance the response to carotid sinus massage and be responsible for symptoms in some patients. Severe vasodepressor or mixed vasodepressor and cardioinhibitory responses may require treatment with either radiation therapy or surgical denervation of the carotid sinus. Elastic support hose and sodium-retaining drugs may be helpful in patients with vasodepressor responses.

Sick Sinus Syndrome

This term is applied to a syndrome encompassing a number of sinus nodal abnormalities[23] that include (1) persistent spontaneous sinus bradycardia not caused by drugs and inappropriate for the physiological circumstance, (2) sinus arrest or exit block,[26,27,30] (3) combinations of SA and AV conduction disturbances, or (4) alternation of paroxysms of rapid regular or irregular atrial tachyarrhythmias and periods of slow atrial and ventricular rates (bradycardia-tachycardia syndrome, Fig. 22–9). More than one of these conditions can be recorded in the same patient on different occasions, and often their mechanisms can be shown to be causally interrelated and combined with an abnormal state of AV conduction or automaticity.

More than one pathophysiological mechanism can produce the clinical manifestations of sick sinus syndrome. The spontaneous clinical arrhythmia and the response to electrophysiological testing (see Chap. 20) depend on the underlying mechanism of sinus nodal dysfunction. Patients who have sinus node disease can be categorized as having intrinsic sinus node disease unrelated to autonomic abnormalities or combinations of intrinsic and autonomic abnormalities. Symptomatic patients with sinus pauses and/or

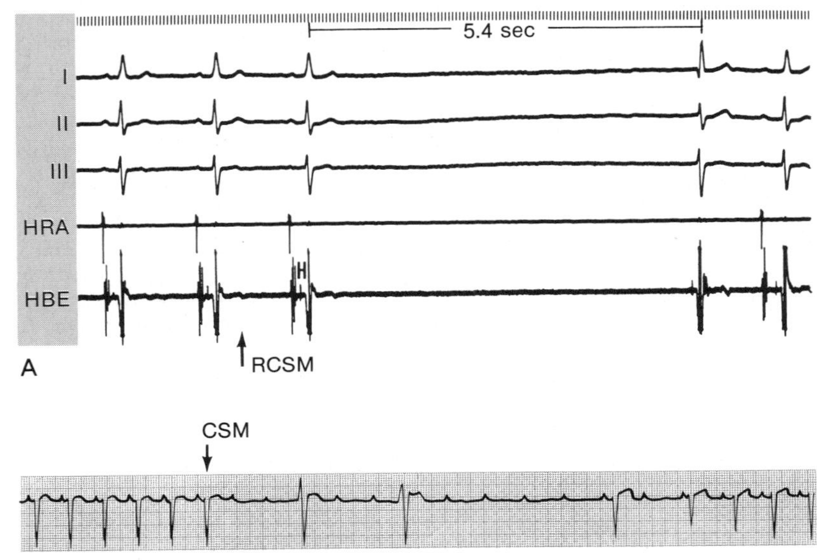

FIGURE 22–8. *A,* Right carotid sinus massage (arrow, RCSM) results in sinus arrest and a ventricular escape beat (probably fascicular) 5.4 sec later. Sinus discharge then resumes. *B,* (Monitor lead) carotid sinus massage (see arrow, CSM) results in slight sinus slowing but, more importantly, advanced AV block. Obviously, an atrial pacemaker without ventricular pacing would be inappropriate for this patient.

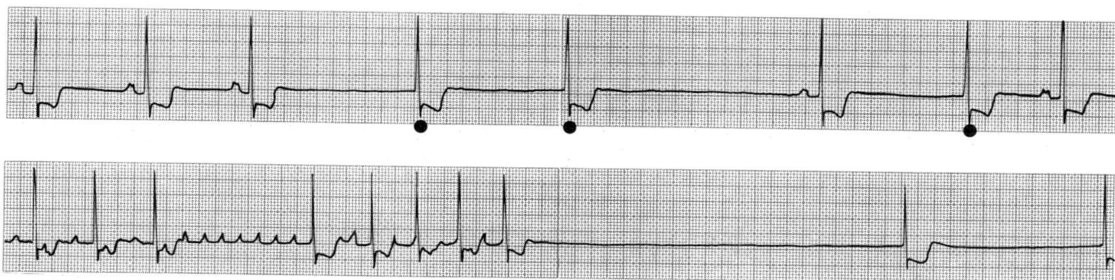

FIGURE 22–9. Sick sinus syndrome with bradycardia-tachycardia. Intermittent sinus arrest is apparent with junctional escape beats at irregular intervals (filled circles, *top*). In the bottom panel of this continuous monitor lead recording, a short episode of atrial flutter is followed by almost 5 sec of asystole before a junctional escape rhythm resumes. The patient became presyncopal at this point.

SA exit block frequently show abnormal responses on electrophysiological testing and can have a relatively high incidence of atrial fibrillation[31] and/or embolic episodes.[32] In children, sinus node dysfunction most commonly occurs in those with congenital or acquired heart disease, particularly following corrective cardiac surgery.[33–35] A familial disorder has been suggested. However, sick sinus syndrome can occur in the absence of other cardiac abnormalities. The course of the disease is frequently intermittent and unpredictable, influenced by the severity of the underlying heart disease. Excessive physical training can heighten vagal tone and produce syncope related to sinus bradycardia or AV conduction abnormalities in otherwise normal individuals.

The anatomical basis of sick sinus syndrome can involve total or subtotal destruction of the sinus node, areas of nodal-atrial discontinuity, inflammatory or degenerative changes of the nerves and ganglia surrounding the node, and pathological changes in the atrial wall. Fibrosis and fatty infiltration occur, and the sclerodegenerative processes generally involve the sinus node and the AV node or the bundle of His and its branches or distal subdivisions.[36] Occlusion of the sinus node artery may be important.[37]

MANAGEMENT. For patients with sick sinus syndrome, treatment depends on the basic rhythm problem but generally involves permanent pacemaker implantation when symptoms are manifested[38] (see Chap. 23). DDD pacing may be preferable.[39] Theophylline has been used.[40] Pacing for the bradycardia combined with drug therapy to treat the tachycardia is required in those with the bradycardia-tachycardia syndrome. In these patients, drug therapy without pacing can aggravate the bradycardia. Digitalis and other drugs that can affect sinus discharge should be used cautiously in patients with sick sinus syndrome without a pacemaker. Beta blockers with intrinsic sympathetic activity may help prevent bradycardia.[41] Prolonged sinoatrial conduction time or sinus nodal recovery time at electrophysiological study in the absence of symptoms is not an indication for prophylactic pacing, since therapy is directed toward control of symptoms. Adenosine has been suggested as a noninvasive test of sinus node function.[42,43]

SINUS NODAL REENTRY TACHYCARDIA

The rate of sinus nodal reentrant tachycardia varies from 80 to 200 beats/min but is generally slower than the other forms of supraventricular tachycardia, with an average rate of 130 to 140 beats/min[44] (Fig. 22–10) (see also p. 581). Electrocardiographically, P waves are identical or very similar to the sinus P-wave morphologically; the P-R interval is related to the tachycardia rate, but generally the R-P interval is long, with a shorter P-R interval (Fig. 22–11*D*). AV block can occur without affecting the tachycardia, and vagal maneuvers can slow and then abruptly terminate the tachycardia. Electrophysiologically, the tachycardia can be initiated and terminated by premature atrial and, uncommonly, premature ventricular stimulation (Fig. 22–10). Initiation of sinus nodal reentry does not depend on a critical degree of intraatrial or AV nodal conduction delay, and the atrial activation sequence is the same as during sinus rhythm. AV nodal Wenckebach block during the tachycardia is common. The development of bundle branch block does not affect the cycle length or P-R interval during tachycardia. Prolongation of AV nodal conduction time or development of AV nodal block can occur prior to termination of the tachycardia but does not affect the sinus nodal reentry.

Sinus nodal reentry may account for 5 to 10 per cent of cases of supraventricular tachycardia. It occurs in all age groups, without sex predilection. Patients may be slightly older and have a higher incidence of heart disease than patients with supraventricular tachycardia due to other mechanisms. Many may not seek medical attention because the relatively slow rate of the tachycardia does not result in serious symptoms. On the other hand, sinus nodal reentry may be responsible for apparent "anxiety-related sinus tachycardia" in some patients. Drugs such as propranolol, verapamil, and digitalis may be effective in terminating and preventing recurrences of sinus node reentrant tachycardia. Surgery or radiofrequency catheter ablation[45] to destroy all or part of the sinus node is occasionally necessary.

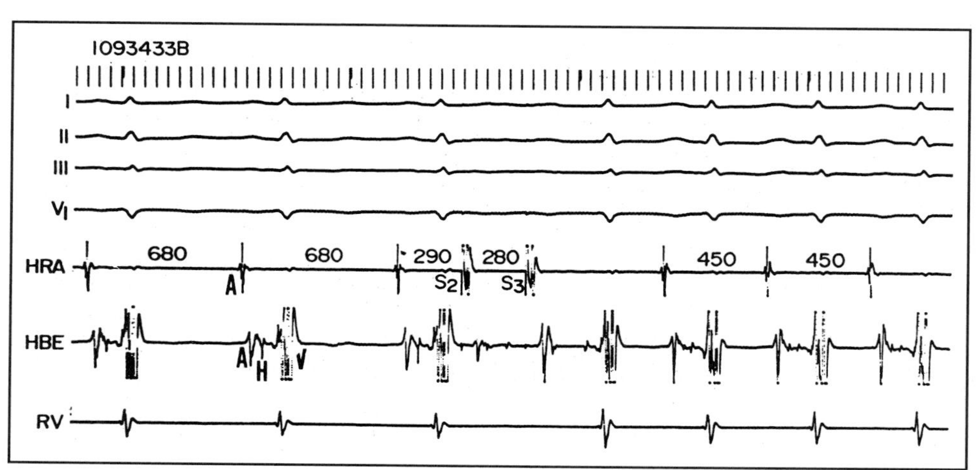

FIGURE 22–10. Sinus node reentry. Following three spontaneous sinus-initiated beats, premature stimulation of the high right atrium (S_2, S_3) initiates a sustained tachycardia at a cycle length of 450 msec that has the identical high-low atrial activation sequence characteristic of sinus node discharge. This is sinus node reentry. Leads I, II, III, and V_1 are scalar leads; HRA, high right atrial electrogram; HBE, His bundle electrogram; RV, right ventricular electrogram. Numbers in milliseconds. A, atrial electrogram; H, His electrogram; V, ventricular electrogram.

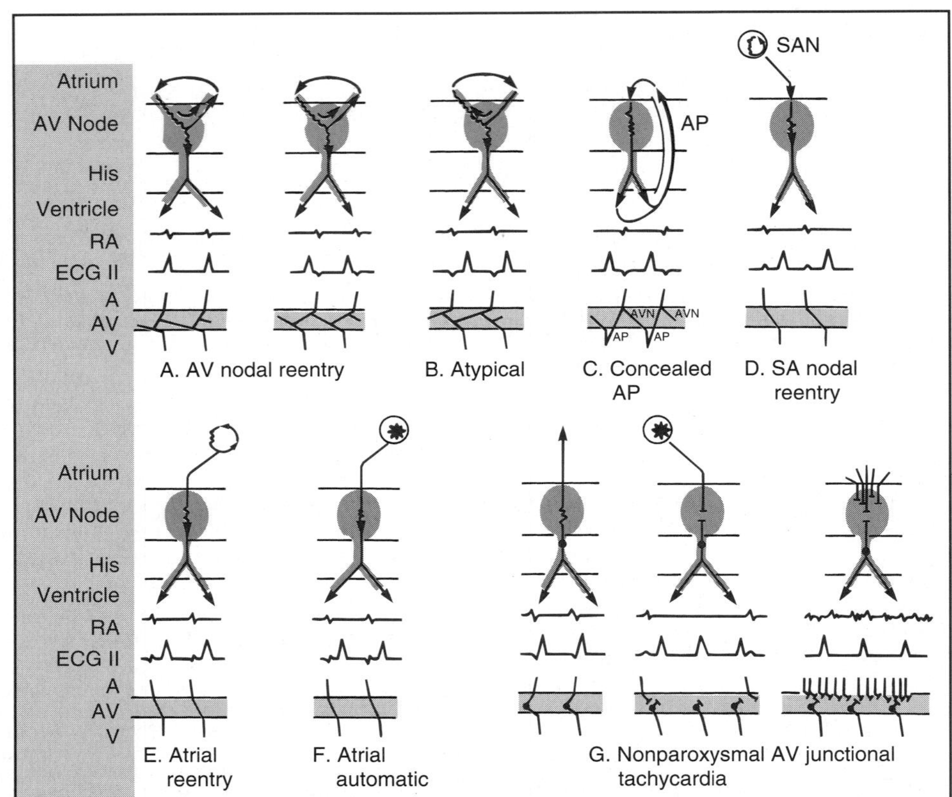

FIGURE 22–11. Diagrammatic representation of various tachycardias. In the top portion of each example, a schematic of the presumed anatomical pathways is drawn; in the bottom half, the ECG presentation and the explanatory ladder diagram are depicted. *A,* AV nodal reentry. In the left example, reentrant excitation is drawn with retrograde atrial activity occurring simultaneously with ventricular activity owing to anterograde conduction over the slow AV nodal pathway (SP) and retrograde conduction over the fast AV nodal pathway (FP). In the right example, atrial activity occurs slightly later than ventricular activity, owing to retrograde conduction delay. *B,* Atypical AV nodal reentry due to anterograde conduction over a fast AV nodal pathway and retrograde conduction over a slow AV nodal pathway. *C,* Concealed accessory pathway. Reciprocating tachycardia is due to anterograde conduction over the AV node and retrograde conduction over the accessory pathway. Retrograde P waves occur after the QRS complex. *D,* Sinus nodal reentry. The tachycardia is due to reentry within the sinus node, which then conducts to the rest of the heart. *E,* Atrial reentry. Tachycardia is due to reentry within the atrium, which then conducts to the rest of the heart. *F,* Automatic atrial tachycardia. Tachycardia is due to automatic discharge in the atrium, which then conducts to the rest of the heart; it is difficult to distinguish from atrial reentry. *G,* Nonparoxysmal AV junctional tachycardia. Various presentations of this tachycardia are depicted with retrograde atrial capture, AV dissociation with the sinus node in control of the atria, and AV dissociation with atrial fibrillation.

DISTURBANCES OF ATRIAL RHYTHM

Premature Atrial Complexes

Premature complexes are among the most common causes of an irregular pulse. They can originate from any area in the heart—most frequently from the ventricles, less often from the atria and from the AV junctional area, and rarely from the sinus node. Although premature complexes arise commonly in normal hearts, they are more often associated with structural heart disease and increase in frequency with age.

ELECTROCARDIOGRAPHIC RECOGNITION (Fig. 22–12). The diagnosis of premature atrial complexes is indicated on the ECG by a premature P wave with a P-R interval exceeding 120 msec (except in WPW syndrome, in which the P-R interval is usually less than 120 msec). Although the contour of the premature P wave can resemble that of the normal sinus P wave, it generally differs. While variations in the basic sinus rate at times can make the diagnosis of prematurity difficult, differences in the contour of the P waves are usually apparent and indicate a different focus of origin. When a premature atrial complex occurs early in diastole, conduction may not be completely normal. The AV junction may still be refractory from the preceding beat and prevent propagation of the impulse (blocked or nonconducted premature atrial complex, Fig. 22–12*A*) or cause conduction to be slowed (premature atrial complex with a prolonged P-R interval). As a general rule, the R-P interval is inversely related to the P-R interval; thus a short R-P interval produced by an early premature atrial complex occurring close to the preceding QRS complex is followed by a long P-R interval. When premature atrial complexes occur early in the cardiac cycle, the premature P waves can be difficult to discern because they are superimposed on T waves. Careful examination of tracings from several leads may be necessary before the premature atrial complex is recognized as a slight deformity of the T wave. Often such premature atrial complexes block before reaching the ventricle and can be misinterpreted as a sinus pause or sinus exit block (Fig. 22–12*A*).

The length of the pause following any premature complex or series of premature complexes is determined by the interaction of several factors. If the premature atrial complex occurs when the sinus node and perinodal tissue are not refractory, the impulse can conduct into the sinus node, discharge it prematurely, and cause the next sinus cycle to begin from that time. The interval between the

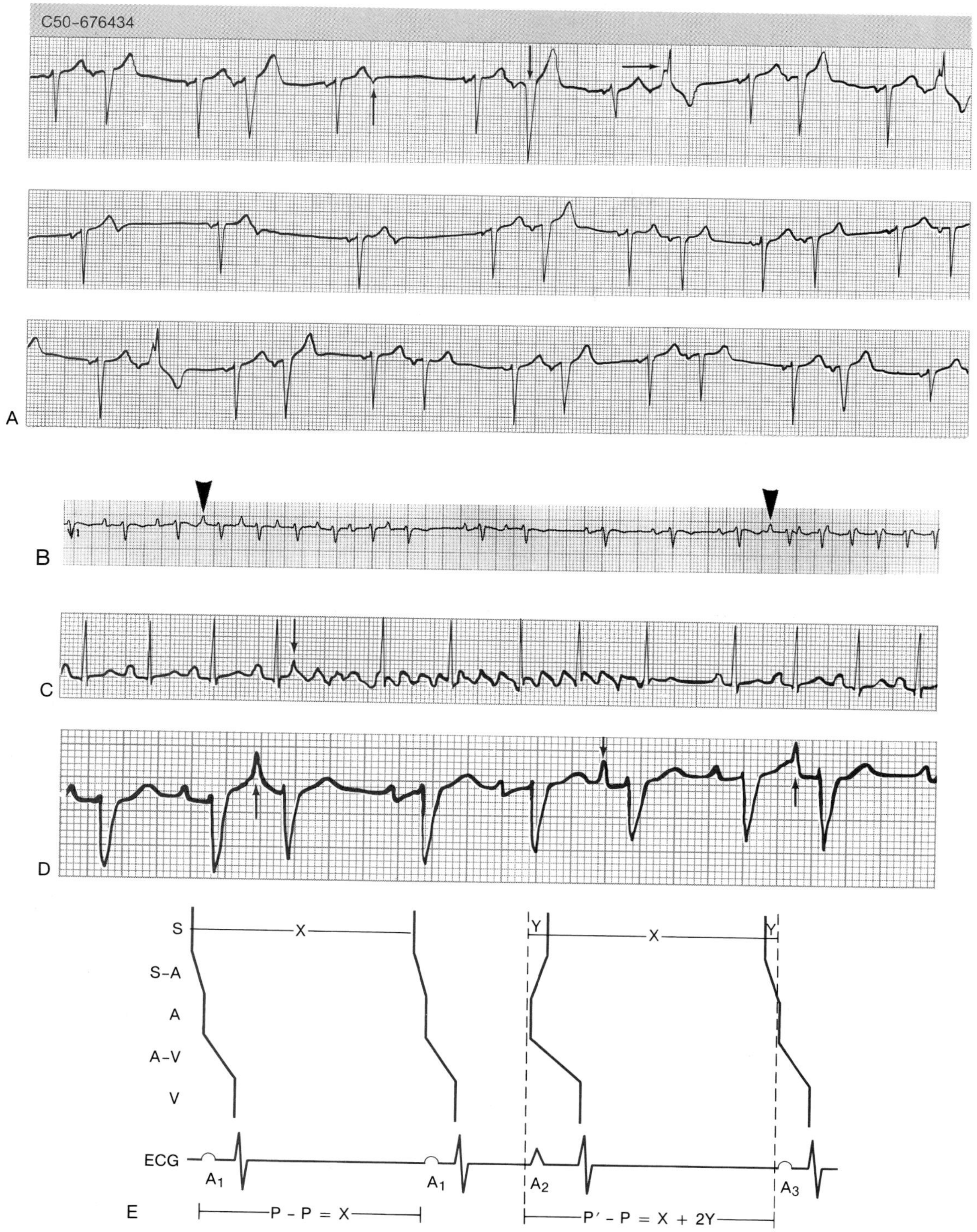

FIGURE 22–12. *A*, Premature atrial complexes that block entirely or conduct with functional right or functional left bundle branch block. Depending on preceding cycle length and coupling interval of the premature atrial complex, the latter blocks entirely in the AV node (↑) or conducts with functional left bundle branch block (↓) or functional right bundle branch block (→).

B, Premature atrial complex on the left (arrowhead) initiates AV nodal reentry that is due to reentry anterogradely and retrogradely over two slow AV nodal pathways, producing a retrograde P wave midway in the cardiac cycle. On the right, a premature atrial complex initiates AV nodal reentry due to anterograde conduction over the slow pathway and retrograde conduction over the fast pathway (Fig. 22–11*A*), producing a retrograde P wave in the terminal portion of the QRS complex, simulating an R prime.

C and *D*, A premature atrial complex (↓) initiating a short run of atrial flutter (*C*) and a premature atrial complex (↑) depressing the return of the next sinus nodal discharge (*D*). A slightly later premature atrial complex (↓) in *D* does not depress sinus nodal automaticity. Panels *B–D*, Monitor leads.

E, Diagrammatic example of effects of a premature atrial complex. Sinus interval (A_1-A_1) equals X. Third P wave represents premature atrial complex (A_2) that reaches and discharges SA node, causing the next sinus cycle to begin at that time. Therefore, the P′-P (A_2-A_3) equals X + 2Y msec, assuming no depression of SA nodal automaticity. (Modified from Zipes, D. P., and Fisch, C.: Premature atrial contraction. Arch. Intern. Med. *128*:453, 1971.)

two normal P waves flanking a premature atrial complex that has reset the timing of the basic sinus rhythm is less than twice the normal P-P interval, and the pause after the premature atrial complex is said to be "noncompensatory." Referring to Figure 22–12*E*, reset (noncompensatory pause) occurs when A_1-A_2 interval + A_2-A_3 interval is less than two times the A_1-A_1 interval, and A_2-A_3 interval is greater than A_1-A_1 interval. The interval between the premature atrial complex (A_2) and the following sinus-initiated P wave (A_3) exceeds one sinus cycle but is less than "fully compensatory" (see below), because the A_2-A_3 interval is lengthened by the time it takes the ectopic atrial impulse to conduct to the sinus node and depolarize it and then for the sinus impulse to return to the atrium. These factors lengthen the return cycle, i.e., the interval between the premature atrial complex (A_2) and the following sinus-initiated P wave (A_3) (Fig. 22–12*E*). Premature discharge of the sinus node by an early premature atrial complex can temporarily depress sinus nodal automatic activity, causing the sinus node to beat more slowly initially (Fig. 22–12*D*). Often when this happens the interval between the A_3 and the next sinus-initiated P wave exceeds the A_1-A_1 interval.

Less commonly, the premature atrial complex encounters a refractory sinus node or perinodal tissue, in which case the timing of the basic sinus rhythm is not altered, since the sinus node is not reset by the premature atrial complex, and the interval between the two normal, sinus-initiated P waves flanking the premature atrial complex is twice the normal P-P interval. The interval following this premature atrial discharge is said to be a "full compensatory pause," i.e., of sufficient duration so that the P-P interval bounding the premature atrial complex is twice the normal P-P interval. However, sinus arrhythmia can lengthen or shorten this pause. Rarely, an *interpolated premature atrial* complex may occur. In this case, the pause after the premature atrial complex is very short, and the interval bounded by the normal sinus-initiated P waves on each side of the premature atrial complex is only slightly longer than or equals one normal P-P cycle length. The interpolated premature atrial complex fails to affect the sinus nodal pacemaker, and the sinus impulse following the premature atrial complex is conducted to the ventricles, often with a slightly lengthened P-R interval. An interpolated premature complex of any type represents the only type of premature systole that does not actually replace the normally conducted beat. Premature atrial complexes can originate in the sinus node and are identified by premature P waves that have a contour identical to the normal sinus P wave. The cycle after the premature sinus complex equals or is slightly shorter than the basic sinus cycle. Premature sinus complexes are not commonly recognized.

On occasion, when the AV node has had sufficient time to repolarize and conduct without delay, the supraventricular QRS complex initiated by the premature atrial complex can be aberrant in configuration because the His-Purkinje system or ventricular muscle has *not* completely repolarized and conducts with functional delay or block (Fig. 22–12*A*). It is important to remember that the refractory period of cardiac fibers is related directly to cycle length. (In the adult, the AV nodal effective refractory period is prolonged at shorter cycle lengths.) A slow heart rate (long cycle length) produces a longer His-Purkinje refractory period than does a faster heart rate. As a consequence, a premature atrial complex that follows a long R-R interval (long refractory period) can result in functional bundle branch block (aberrant ventricular conduction). Since the right bundle branch at long cycles has a longer refractory period than the left bundle branch, aberration with a right bundle branch block pattern at slow rates occurs more commonly than aberration with a left bundle branch block pattern. At shorter cycles, the refractory period of the left bundle branch exceeds that of the right bundle branch, and a left bundle branch block pattern may be more likely to occur.

CLINICAL FEATURES. Premature atrial complexes can occur in a variety of situations, e.g., during infection, inflammation, or myocardial ischemia, or they can be provoked by a variety of medications, by tension states, or by tobacco, alcohol, or caffeine. Premature atrial complexes can precipitate or presage the occurrence of sustained supraventricular (Fig. 24–12*B* and *C*) and rarely ventricular tachyarrhythmias.

MANAGEMENT. Premature atrial complexes generally do not require therapy.[46] In symptomatic patients or when the premature atrial complexes precipitate tachycardias, treatment with digitalis, a beta blocker, or a calcium antagonist can be tried.

Atrial Flutter

(See also p. 572)

ELECTROCARDIOGRAPHIC RECOGNITION. The atrial rate during typical (sometimes called *type I*) atrial flutter is usually 250 to 350 beats/min, although class IA and IC antiarrhythmic drugs and amiodarone can reduce the rate to the range of 200 beats/min. If this occurs, the ventricles can respond in a 1:1 fashion to the slower atrial rate. Ordinarily, the atrial rate is about 300 beats/min, and in untreated patients the ventricular rate is half the atrial rate, i.e., 150 beats/min (Fig. 22–13*A*). A significantly slower ventricular rate (in the absence of drugs) suggests abnormal AV conduction. In children, in patients with the preexcitation syndrome (see p. 667), occasionally in patients with hyperthyroidism, and in those whose AV nodes conduct rapidly, atrial flutter can conduct to the ventricle in a 1:1 fashion, producing a ventricular rate of 300 beats/min. The rate in atypical (sometimes called *type II*) flutter, is 350 to 450 beats/min. Reentry is probably responsible for most atrial flutters.[47]

In typical atrial flutter, the ECG reveals identically recurring regular sawtooth flutter waves (Figs. 22–12*C* and 22–13*B*) and evidence of continual electrical activity (lack of an isoelectric interval between flutter waves), often best visualized in leads II, III, aV_f, or V_1 (Fig. 22–14). The flutter waves for (type I) typical atrial flutter are inverted (negative) in these leads because of a counterclockwise reentrant pathway, and sometimes they are upright (positive) when the reentrant loop is clockwise (see Chap. 20). If the AV conduction ratio remains constant, the ventricular rhythm will be regular; if the ratio of conducted beats varies (usually the result of a Wenckebach AV block), the ventricular rhythm will be irregular. Alternation between 2:1 and 4:1 AV conduction often occurs and may be due to two levels of block—2:1 high in the AV node and 3:2 lower down. The irregular ventricular response is frequently due to Wenckebach periodicity. Recurrent alternation of short and long ventricular intervals can be due to concealed conduction (see p. 693). Various degrees of penetration into the AV junction by the flutter impulses also can influence AV conduction. The ratio of flutter waves to conducted ventricular complexes most often is an even number (e.g., 2:1, 4:1, and so on). Impure flutter (flutter-fibrillation, or "flitter"), occurring at a rate faster than pure flutter, shows variability in the contour and spacing of the flutter waves and in some instances can represent dissimilar atrial rhythms, i.e., fibrillation in one atrium and a slower, more regular rhythm resembling atrial flutter in the opposite atrium. Prolonged atrial conduction time has been found to be a predisposing factor for the development of atrial flutter.

CLINICAL FEATURES. Atrial flutter is less common than atrial fibrillation. Paroxysmal atrial flutter can occur in patients without structural heart disease, while chronic (persistent) atrial flutter is usually associated with underlying heart disease such as rheumatic or ischemic heart disease or cardiomyopathy. It can occur as a result of atrial dilation from septal defects, pulmonary emboli, mitral or tricuspid valve stenosis or regurgitation, or chronic ventricular failure. Toxic and metabolic conditions that affect the heart, such as thyrotoxicosis, alcoholism, and pericarditis, can cause atrial flutter. Occasionally, it can be congenital or follow surgery for congenital heart disease,[48] or even occur in utero.[49,50] Atrial flutter tends to be unstable, reverting to sinus rhythm or degenerating into atrial fibrillation. Less commonly, the atria can continue to flutter for months or years. In atrial flutter, the atria contract, which may, in part, account for fewer systemic emboli than in atrial fibrillation. In children, continued episodes of atrial flutter are associated with an increased possibility of sudden death.

Atrial flutter usually responds to carotid sinus massage with a decrease in ventricular rate in stepwise multiples, returning in a reverse manner to the former ventricular rate at the termination of carotid massage (Fig. 22–13*A*). Very rarely, sinus rhythm follows carotid sinus massage. Exercise, by enhancing sympathetic or lessening parasympathetic tone, can reduce the AV conduction delay and produce a doubling of the ventricular rate.

Physical examination may reveal rapid flutter waves in

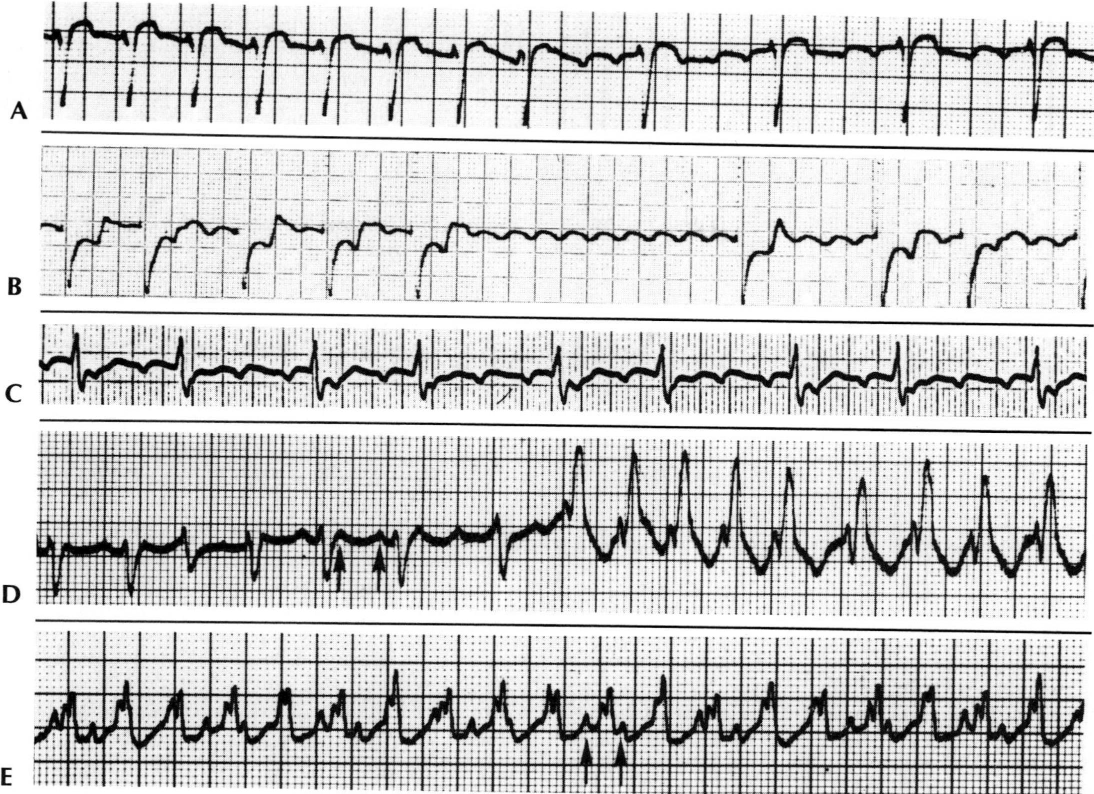

FIGURE 22–13. Various manifestations of atrial flutter. *A,* Atrial flutter at a rate of 300 beats/min conducts to ventricles with 2:1 block. In the midportion of the tracing, carotid sinus massage converts the block to 4:1 and the ventricular rate slows to 75 beats/min. *B,* Carotid sinus massage produces a transient period of AV block clearly revealing the flutter waves. *C,* Quinidine has slowed the atrial flutter rate to approximately 188 beats/min. The block is variable. *D,* Wide QRS complexes with an RSR′ configuration in V_1 begin after a short cycle that follows a long cycle in the midportion of the ECG strip. This represents functional right bundle branch block. Arrows indicate flutter waves. *E,* The QRS complexes are 0.12 sec in duration and have a regular interval at a rate of 200 beats/min. Atrial activity is also regular at a rate of 300 beats/min and independent from the ventricular activity (arrows). Thus atrial flutter is present with a probable ventricular tachycardia, an example of complete AV dissociation. Monitor leads in *A, B, C,* and *E.*

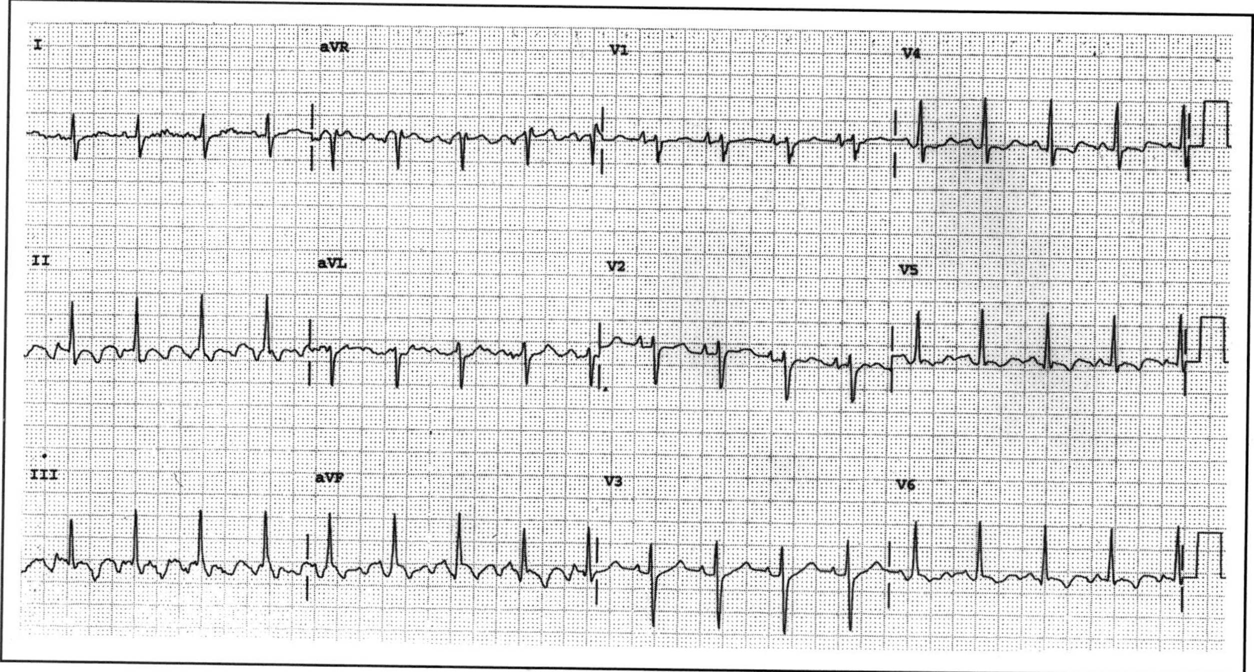

FIGURE 22–14. Simultaneous atrial flutter and sinus rhythm. In this patient with a heart transplant, the recipient atrium exhibits atrial flutter, best seen in leads II, III and aV_f, while the donor atrium exhibits sinus rhythm (best seen in the chest leads). (Tracing courtesy of Sharon Hunt.)

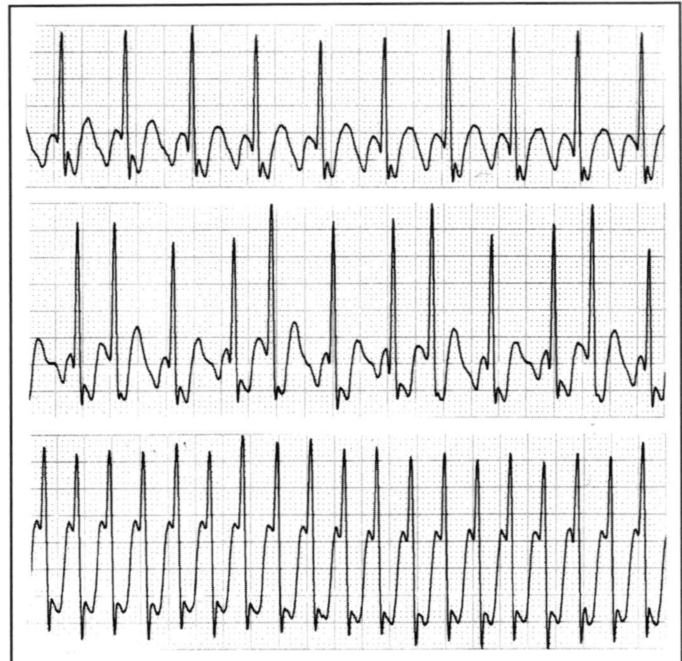

FIGURE 22–15. Atrial flutter with 1:1 conduction caused by flecainide. In the top panel, atrial flutter occurs with 2:1 conduction. In the middle panel, 2:1 conduction alternates with 3:2 conduction. In the bottom panel, flecainide has been started and the atrial flutter rate slows, resulting in 1:1 conduction.

the jugular venous pulse. If the relationship of flutter waves to conducted QRS complexes remains constant, the first heart sound will have a constant intensity. Occasionally, sounds caused by atrial contraction can be auscultated.

MANAGEMENT. Synchronous direct-current (DC) cardioversion (see p. 619) is commonly the initial treatment of choice for atrial flutter, since cardioversion promptly and effectively restores sinus rhythm, often requiring relatively low energies (< 50 joules). If the electrical shock results in atrial fibrillation, a second shock at a higher energy level is used to restore sinus rhythm or, depending on the clinical circumstances, the atrial fibrillation can be left untreated. The latter can revert to atrial flutter or sinus rhythm. If the patient cannot be electrically cardioverted or if electrical cardioversion is contraindicated—for example, after large amounts of digitalis are administered—*rapid atrial pacing* with a catheter in the esophagus[51] or the right atrium can terminate type I (but not type II) atrial flutter effectively in most patients, producing sinus rhythm or atrial fibrillation with a slowing of the ventricular rate and concomitant clinical improvement.[52–54]

Verapamil (see p. 616), given as an initial bolus of 5 to 10 mg IV, followed by a constant infusion at a rate of 5 μg/kg/min, or *diltiazem,* 0.25 mg/kg, to slow the ventricular response, can be tried. Calcium antagonists can restore sinus rhythm in patients with atrial flutter of recent onset but less commonly terminate chronic atrial flutter. *Adenosine* produces transient AV block and can be used to reveal flutter waves if the diagnosis of the arrhythmias is in doubt. It generally will not terminate the atrial flutter and can provoke atrial fibrillation.[55] Esmolol, a beta-adrenergic blocker with a 9-min elimination half-life, can be used in doses of 200 μg/kg/min to slow the ventricular rate.[56]

If the flutter cannot be electrically cardioverted, terminated by pacing, or slowed by the preceding drugs, a *short-acting digitalis preparation* (such as digoxin or deslanoside) can be tried alone or with a calcium antagonist or beta blocker. The dose of digitalis necessary to slow the ventricular response varies and at times can result in toxic levels because it is often difficult to slow the ventricular rate during atrial flutter. Frequently, atrial fibrillation develops after digitalis administration and can revert to normal sinus rhythm upon withdrawal of digitalis; occasionally, normal sinus rhythm may occur without intervening atrial fibrillation. Intravenous amiodarone has been shown to slow the ventricular rate as effectively as digoxin.[57]

If the atrial flutter persists, class IA or IC drugs (see Chap. 20) can be tried to restore sinus rhythm and to prevent a recurrence of atrial flutter.[58] Amiodarone, also, especially in low doses of 200 mg/day, can prevent recurrences. Side effects of these drugs, especially proarrhythmic responses, must be carefully considered and are dealt with at length in Chapter 21. Sometimes treatment of the underlying disorder, such as thyrotoxicosis, is necessary to effect conversion to sinus rhythm. In certain instances, atrial flutter can continue, and if the ventricular rate can be controlled with drugs, conversion to sinus rhythm may not be indicated. Class I and III drugs should be discontinued if flutter remains.

It is important to reemphasize that class I or III drugs should *not* be used unless the ventricular rate during atrial flutter has been *slowed* with digitalis or a calcium antagonist or beta-blocking drug.[59] Because of the vagolytic action of quinidine, procainamide, and disopyramide (see Chap. 21), but primarily because of the ability of class I drugs to slow the flutter rate, AV conduction can be *facilitated* sufficiently to result in a 1:1 ventricular response to the atrial flutter (Fig. 22–15).

Prevention of recurrent atrial flutter is often difficult to achieve but should be approached as outlined for the prevention of paroxysmal supraventricular tachycardia due to AV nodal reentry (see p. 661). If recurrences cannot be prevented, therapy is directed toward controlling the ventricular rate when the flutter does recur, with digitalis alone or combined with beta blockers or calcium antagonists. The risks of emboli in type I atrial flutter appear to be low, presumably because the atria contract, and therefore anticoagulation is usually not necessary.[60] However, carefully controlled studies are lacking. Radiofrequency catheter ablation (see p. 624) can eliminate typical atrial flutter with a success rate of about 75 to 90 per cent.[61–70]

Atrial Fibrillation

(See also p. 627)

ELECTROCARDIOGRAPHIC RECOGNITION (Fig. 22–16). This arrhythmia is characterized by wavelets propagating in different directions,[71] causing disorganized atrial deploarizations without effective atrial contraction.[72–74] Electrical activity of the atrium can be detected electrocardiographically as small irregular baseline undulations of variable amplitude and morphology, called f waves, at a rate of 350 to 600 beats/min. At times, small, fine, rapid f waves can occur and are detectable only by right atrial leads or by

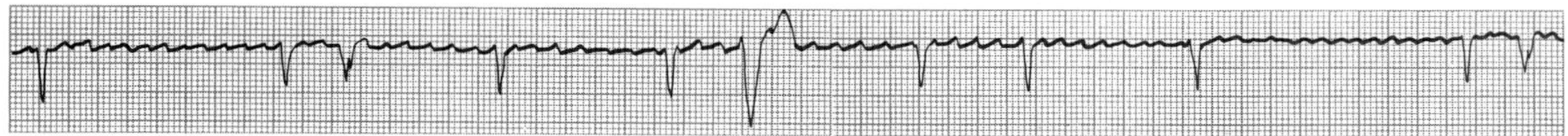

FIGURE 22–16. Atrial fibrillation with ventricular extrasystoles following the longer pauses (monitor lead). Fibrillatory waves are quite obvious. When the ventricular cycle lengths prolong, ventricular extrasystoles result. This phenomenon has been called the "rule of bigeminy."

intracavitary or esophageal electrodes. The ventricular response is grossly irregular ("irregularly irregular") and, in the untreated patient with normal AV conduction, is usually between 100 and 160 beats/min. In patients with the WPW syndrome (see p. 667), the ventricular rate during atrial fibrillation at times can exceed 300 beats/min and lead to ventricular fibrillation. Atrial fibrillation should be suspected when the ECG shows supraventricular complexes at an irregular rhythm and no obvious P waves. The recognizable f waves probably do not represent total atrial activity but depict only the larger vectors generated by the multiple wavelets of depolarization that occur at any given moment.

Each recorded f wave is not conducted through the AV junction, so a rapid ventricular response comparable with the atrial rate does not occur. Many atrial impulses are canceled, owing to a collision of wavefronts, or are blocked in the AV junction without reaching the ventricles (i.e., concealed conduction [see p. 693]), which accounts for the irregular ventricular rhythm. The refractory period and conductivity of the AV node are determinants of the ventricular rate. When the ventricular rate is very rapid or very slow, it may appear to be more regular. Even though the conversion of atrial fibrillation to atrial flutter is accompanied by slowing of the atrial rate, an increase in the ventricular response can result, since more atrial impulses are transmitted to the ventricle because of less concealed conduction. Also, it is easier to slow the ventricular rate during atrial fibrillation than during atrial flutter with drugs such as digitalis, calcium antagonists, and beta blockers, because the increased concealed conduction makes it easier to produce AV block.

It has been suggested that transmission of impulses across the AV node during atrial fibrillation occurs electrotonically and that the distal portion of the AV node behaves as a pacemaker, producing the ventricular rhythm during atrial fibrillation.[74a] This postulate has not been proven.[75]

CLINICAL FEATURES. Atrial fibrillation is a common arrhythmia, found in 1 per cent of persons older than 60 years to more than 5 per cent in patients over 69 years old.[76] The overall chance of atrial fibrillation developing over 2 decades in patients more than 30 years old, according to Framingham data, is 2 per cent. Estimates are that 1 to 1.5 million Americans have atrial fibrillation, occurring more commonly in men than in women.[77] In one study[78] of men and women 65 years or older, atrial fibrillation had a prevalence of 9.1 per cent in those with clinical cardiovascular disease, 4.6 per cent in those with subclinical cardiovascular disease, and 1.6 per cent in those without cardiovascular disease. A history of congestive heart failure, valvular heart disease and stroke, left atrial enlargement, abnormal mitral or aortic valve function, treated systemic hypertension, and advanced age was independently associated with the prevalence of atrial fibrillation. Four important aspects of atrial fibrillation are etiology, control of the ventricular rate, prevention of recurrences, and prevention of thromboembolic episodes. Occult or manifest thyrotoxicosis should be considered in patients with recent-onset atrial fibrillation.[79,80] Atrial fibrillation can be intermittent or chronic and may be influenced by autonomic activity.[81] Atrial fibrillation, whether it is persistent or intermittent, is a predictor of stroke. Symptoms as a result of atrial fibrillation are determined by multiple factors, including the underlying cardiac status, the rapid ventricular rate, and loss of atrial contraction.

Physical findings include a slight variation in the intensity of the first heart sound, absence of *a* waves in the jugular venous pulse, and an irregularly irregular ventricular rhythm. Often, with fast ventricular rates, a significant pulse deficit appears, during which the auscultated or palpated apical rate is faster than the rate palpated at the wrist (pulse deficit) because each contraction is not sufficiently strong to open the aortic valve or to transmit an arterial pressure wave through the peripheral artery. If the ventricular rhythm becomes regular in patients with atrial fibrillation, conversion to sinus rhythm, atrial tachycardia, atrial flutter with a constant ratio of conducted beats, or development of junctional or ventricular tachycardia should be suspected.

EMBOLIZATION AND ANTICOAGULATION (see also Ch. 48). In addition to hemodynamic alterations, the risk of systemic emboli, probably arising in the left atrial cavity or appendage due to circulatory stasis, is an important consideration. Nonvalvular atrial fibrillation is the most common cardiac disease associated with cerebral embolism. In fact, almost half of cardiogenic emboli in the United States occur in patients with nonvalvular atrial fibrillation. The risk of stroke in patients with nonvalvular atrial fibrillation is 5 to 7 times greater than in controls without atrial fibrillation. Overall, 20 to 25 per cent of ischemic strokes are due to cardiogenic emboli.

Many studies have evaluated the risk of stroke in patients with nonvalvular atrial fibrillation and the benefits of anticoagulation and antiplatelet therapy.[82–91] Certain patients with atrial fibrillation appear at higher risk of emboli.[92] For example, patients with mitral stenosis and atrial fibrillation have a 4 to 6 per cent incidence of embolism per year. Risk factors that predict stroke in patients with nonvalvular atrial fibrillation include a history of previous stroke or transient ischemic attack (relative risk 22.5), diabetes (relative risk 1.7), history of hypertension (relative risk 1.6), and increasing age (relative risk 1.4 for each decade). Patients with any of these risk factors have an annual stroke risk of at least 4 per cent if untreated. Patients whose only stroke risk factor is congestive heart failure or coronary artery disease have stroke rates approximately three times higher than do patients without any risk factors.[93] Left ventricular dysfunction and a left atrial size greater than 2.5 cm/m^2 on echocardiographic examination are associated with thromboembolism. Patients younger than age 60 who have a normal echocardiogram and no risk factors have an extremely low risk for stroke (1 per cent per year).[94]

Patients younger than age 65 with no risk factors have an annual rate of stroke of 1 per cent. Therefore, the risk of stroke in patients with *lone atrial fibrillation,* i.e., idiopathic atrial fibrillation in the absence of any structural heart disease or any of the above risk factors, is quite low.

The annual rate of stroke for the unanticoagulated control group in five large anticoagulation trials[95] was 4.5 per cent and was reduced to 1.4 per cent (68 per cent risk reduction) for the warfarin-treated group (60 per cent risk reduction in men; 84 per cent risk reduction in women). Aspirin, 325 mg per day, produced a risk reduction of 44 per cent. The annual rate of major hemorrhage was 1 per cent for the control group, 1 per cent for the aspirin group, and 1.3 per cent for the warfarin group. There was no difference in stroke risk when patients with paroxysmal (intermittent) atrial fibrillation were compared with those with constant (chronic) atrial fibrillation. Anticoagulation therapy was approximately 50 per cent more effective than aspirin therapy for prevention of ischemic stroke in atrial fibrillation patients. Risk factors for anticoagulant-associated intracranial hemorrhage included excessive anticoagulation and poorly controlled hypertension. Elderly individuals were at increased risk for anticoagulant-associated brain hemorrhage, especially if overanticoagulated.[95]

From these and other data, it appears that individuals less than 60 years of age without any clinical risk factors (lone atrial fibrillation) do not require antithrombotic therapy for stroke prevention because of their low risk. The stroke rate is also low (about 2 per cent per year) in patients with lone atrial fibrillation between the ages of 60 and 75 years. These patients appear to be adequately protected from stroke with aspirin therapy. In very elderly (over 75 years of age) patients with atrial fibrillation, anticoagulation should be used with caution and carefully monitored because of the potential increased risk of intracranial hemorrhage. Despite this, elderly patients with atrial fibrillation are still likely to benefit from anticoagulation because they are at particularly high stroke risk.[96] Food[97] and drugs such as antibiotics and antiarrhythmics (e.g., amiodarone) can influence the effects of warfarin (see p. 615).

The following recommendations for antithrombotic therapy can be made[93,96]: Any patient with atrial fibrillation who has risk factors for stroke (prior stroke or transient ischemic attack, significant valvular heart disease, hypertension, diabetes, age greater than 75 years, left atrial enlargement, coronary artery disease, or congestive heart failure) should be treated with warfarin anticoagulation to achieve an INR of 2.0 to 3.0 for stroke prevention if the individual is a good candidate for oral anticoagulation. Patients with contraindications to anticoagulation and unreliable individuals should be considered for aspirin treatment. Patients with atrial fibrillation who do not have any of the preceding risk factors have a low stroke risk (2 per cent per year or less) and can be protected from stroke with aspirin. In patients over the age of 75 years, anticoagulation should be used with caution and monitored carefully to keep the INR less than 3.0 because of the risk of intracranial hemorrhage.[98–103]

The risk of embolism following cardioversion to sinus rhythm in patients with atrial fibrillation varies from 0 to 7 per cent, depending on the underlying risk factors. Patients at high risk are those with prior embolism, a mechanical valve prosthesis, or mitral stenosis. Low-risk patients are those younger than age 60 without underlying heart disease. The high-risk group should receive chronic anticoagulation (see below), whether or not they will undergo cardioversion, while anticoagulation may not be necessary in the low-risk group. Patients not in the low-risk group with atrial fibrillation longer in duration than 2 days should receive warfarin to achieve an INR of 2.0 to 3.0 for 3 weeks before elective cardioversion and for 3 to 4 weeks after reversion to sinus rhythm.[104] Anticoagulation with heparin has been recommended for emergency cardioversion. Risk stratification with transesophageal echocardiography may be useful,[105] but the absence of a left atrial thrombus on echocardiography is not necessarily assurance that the patient will not have an embolus at or after cardioversion.[106,107]

It is important to emphasize that these suggestions must be individualized for a given patient. For example, patients at risk of trauma by virtue of occupation, participation in sports, and episodes of dizziness or syncope are at increased risk of bleeding if given anticoagulants and probably should not receive warfarin. Patients should be warned about taking any new drugs, e.g., nonsteroidal antiinflammatory agents, if they are receiving warfarin.

For patients with intermittent atrial fibrillation, guidelines are unclear. A reasonable approach would be to treat them according to the recommendations noted above, particularly if recurrences are frequent.

MANAGEMENT. The atria are often abnormal in patients with atrial fibrillation, showing increased conduction time or enlargement. Maintenance of sinus rhythm after cardioversion is influenced by the duration of atrial fibrillation and, in some adults, atrial dilatation. Animal studies[73,108–110a] indicate that atrial fibrillation begets atrial fibrillation; the longer the patient has atrial fibrillation, the greater is the likelihood that it will remain.

The patient with atrial fibrillation discovered for the first time should be evaluated for a precipitating cause, such as thyrotoxicosis, mitral stenosis, pulmonary emboli, or pericarditis. The patient's clinical status determines initial therapy, the objectives being to slow the ventricular rate and to restore atrial systole. If the sudden onset of atrial fibrillation with a rapid ventricular rate results in acute cardiovascular decompensation, electrical cardioversion is the initial treatment of choice. High-energy shock over a right atrial catheter can be successful when transthoracic shocks fail. Atrial contraction may not return immediately after restoration of electrical systole, and clinical improvement may be delayed.[111,112] DC cardioversion establishes normal sinus rhythm in over 90 per cent of patients, but sinus rhythm remains for 12 months in only 30 to 50 per cent. Patients with atrial fibrillation of less than 12 months' duration have a greater chance of maintaining sinus rhythm after cardioversion. In the absence of decompensation, the patient can be treated with drugs such as digitalis, beta blockers, or calcium antagonists to maintain a resting apical rate of 60 to 80 beats/min that does not exceed 100 beats/min after slight exercise.[113] The combined use of digitalis and a beta blocker[56] or calcium antagonist can be helpful in slowing the ventricular rate. Digitalis may be more effective if associated left ventricular dysfunction is present; without this, a beta blocker may be preferable to control the ventricular rate.[114] Clonidine has been used to slow the rate.[115]

Classes IA, IC,[116] and III (amiodarone, sotalol[117]) agents can be used to terminate acute-onset atrial fibrillation and prevent recurrences of atrial fibrillation.[58] No one drug, with the possible exception of amiodarone,[99] appears clearly superior, and selection is often based on side effect profile and risk of proarrhythmia.[118–120] These drugs increase the likelihood of maintaining sinus rhythm from about 30 to 50 per cent to 50 to 70 per cent of patients per year after cardioversion. However, whether it is preferable to allow atrial fibrillation to continue with just rate control has not been established.[121] Before electrical cardioversion, an antiarrhythmic agent is often administered for a few days to help prevent relapse of atrial fibrillation, as well as to convert some patients to sinus rhythm.[122] Rapid atrial pacing will not terminate atrial fibrillation.[108,123] In some patients with frequent recurrence and rapid ventricular rates not controlled by drugs, AV node modification[124] or interruption by radiofrequency catheter ablation and implantation of a rate-adaptive VVI (VVIR) pacemaker can be acceptable therapy[125,126] (see Chap. 23). Whenever possible, atrial or dual-chamber pacing is preferable, since the incidence of atrial fibrillation and stroke is reduced compared with VVI pacing. Application of the maze procedure,[127] the atrial compartment operation,[128] and new ablation approaches have been used to eliminate atrial fibrillation[129–132] (see p. 628). An atrial defibrillator also has received interest recently (see Chap. 23).[133–135] Atrial or dual-chamber pacing may reduce recurrence of atrial fibrillation in some patients who have intermittent episodes.[136]

Many elderly patients tolerate atrial fibrillation well without therapy because the ventricular rate is slow as a result of concomitant AV nodal disease. These patients often have associated sick sinus syndrome, and the development of atrial fibrillation represents a cure of sorts. Such patients may demonstrate serious supraventricular and ventricular arrhythmias or asystole after cardioversion, so the likelihood of establishing and maintaining sinus rhythm should be weighed against the risks of cardioversion or other forms of therapy.

Atrial Tachycardias

ELECTROCARDIOGRAPHIC RECOGNITION (Fig. 22–17). Atrial tachycardia has an atrial rate of generally 150 to 200 beats/min with a P-wave contour different from that of the sinus P wave. P waves are usually in the second half of the tachycardia cycle (long R-P/short P-R tachycardia).[44] When the tachycardia is due to digitalis excess, the atrial rate can increase gradually as the digitalis is continued (a similar

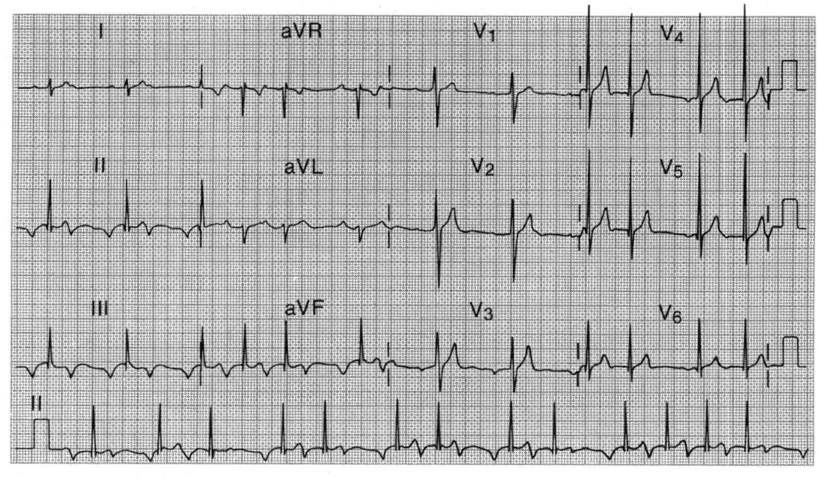

FIGURE 22–17. Atrial tachycardia. This 12-lead ECG and rhythm strip (*bottom*) demonstrate an atrial tachycardia at a cycle length of approximately 520 msec. Conduction varies between 3:2 and 2:1. Note the negative P waves in leads 2, 3, and aVF and, when consecutive P waves conduct, that the R-P interval exceeds the P-R interval. Note also that the tachycardia persists despite the development of AV block, an important finding that excludes the participation of an atrioventricular accessory pathway and sharply differentiates this tachycardia from the one shown in Figure 22–34, p. 673.

response can occur in nonparoxysmal AV junctional tachycardia); this increase may be associated with gradual prolongation of the P-R interval. If the atrial rate is not excessive and AV conduction is not significantly depressed by the digitalis, each P wave may conduct to the ventricles. As the atrial rate increases and AV conduction becomes impaired, Wenckebach (Mobitz type I) second degree AV block (see p. 689) can ensue. This is sometimes called *atrial tachycardia with block.* Frequently, other manifestations of digitalis excess, such as premature ventricular complexes, are present. In nearly half the cases of atrial tachycardia with block, the atrial rate is irregular. Characteristic isoelectric intervals between P waves, in contrast to atrial flutter, are usually present in all leads. However, at rapid atrial rates, the distinction between atrial tachycardia with block and atrial flutter can be difficult. Analysis of P-wave configuration during tachycardia indicates that a positive or biphasic P wave in aVL predicts a right atrial focus, whereas a positive P wave in V_1 predicts a left atrial focus.

CLINICAL FEATURES. Atrial tachycardia occurs most commonly in patients with significant structural heart disease, such as coronary artery disease, with or without myocardial infarction, cor pulmonale, or digitalis intoxication. Potassium depletion can precipitate the arrhythmia in patients taking digitalis. The signs, symptoms, and prognosis are usually related to underlying cardiovascular status.

Physical findings include a variable rhythm and intensity of the first heart sound, owing to the varying AV block and P-R interval. An excessive number of *a* waves may be seen in the jugular venous pulse. Carotid sinus massage increases the degree of AV block by slowing the ventricular rate in a stepwise fashion without terminating the tachycardia, as in atrial flutter. It should be performed cautiously in patients who have digitalis toxicity because serious ventricular arrhythmias can result.

MANAGEMENT. Atrial tachycardia with block in a patient not receiving digitalis is treated in a manner similar to other atrial tachyarrhythmias. Depending on the clinical situation, digitalis, a beta blocker, or a calcium channel blocker can be administered to slow the ventricular rate, and then if atrial tachycardia remains, class IA, IC, or III drugs can be added. Ablation procedures can be tried, including surgical isolation and radiofrequency catheter ablation[62,137,138] (see p. 621). Tachycardias can recur at a different site following a successful ablation attempt. If atrial tachycardia appears in a patient receiving digitalis, the drug initially should be assumed to be responsible for the arrthythmia. Therapy includes cessation of digitalis and administration of potassium chloride orally or intravenously if serum [K^+] is not abnormally elevated or a drug such as lidocaine, propranolol, and phenytoin while cardiac rhythm is monitored. Often, the ventricular response is not excessively fast, and simply withholding digitalis is all that is necessary.

Mechanisms: Automatic Atrial Tachycardia

Three types of atrial tachycardias have been distinguished experimentally: automatic, triggered, and reentrant atrial tachycardia. The characteristics of automatic and reentrant tachycardias will be discussed separately. Entrainment, resetting curve patterns in response to overdrive pacing,[139] and recording monophasic action potentials can be used to help distinguish one mechanism from the other.[140,141] Adenosine has been used to distinguish mechanisms.[142] However, there are no clear clinical distinctions between tachycardias of different mechanisms.

ELECTROCARDIOGRAPHIC FEATURES (Fig. 22–11*F*). Automatic atrial tachycardia is characterized electrocardiographically by a supraventricular tachycardia that generally accelerates after its initiation, with heart rates less than 200 beats/min. The P-wave contour differs from the sinus P wave, the P-R interval is influenced directly by the tachycardia rate, and AV block can exist without affecting the tachycardia; i.e., it continues uninterrupted. Vagal maneuvers generally do not terminate the tachycardia, even though they can produce AV nodal block. Thus pharmacological or physiological maneuvers that selectively result in AV block do not affect the automatic focus nor does the development of bundle branch block alter the P-R or R-P interval unless it is associated with prolongation of the H-V interval.

Initiation of tachycardia with premature atrial stimulation is generally not possible but is independent of intra-atrial or AV nodal conduction delay when it occurs. The atrial activation sequence usually differs from a sinus-initiated P wave, and the A-H interval is related to the tachycardia rate. The first P wave of the tachycardia is the same as the subsequent P waves of the tachycardia in contrast to most forms of reentrant supraventricular tachycardias, in which the initial and subsequent P waves differ.[143] Usually the tachycardia cannot be terminated by pacing, although it can exhibit overdrive suppression. The introduction of premature atrial complexes during tachycardia merely resets the timing of the tachycardia. It is very difficult to differentiate this mechanism from microreentry, using the leading-circle concept (see p. 571).

CLINICAL FEATURES. Many supraventricular tachycardias associated with AV block are probably due to automatic atrial tachycardia,[143] including atrial tachycardia due to digitalis intoxication (Fig. 22–17). Automatic atrial tachycardia occurs in all age groups and is seen in settings of myocardial infarction, chronic lung disease (especially with acute infection), acute alcohol ingestion, and a variety of

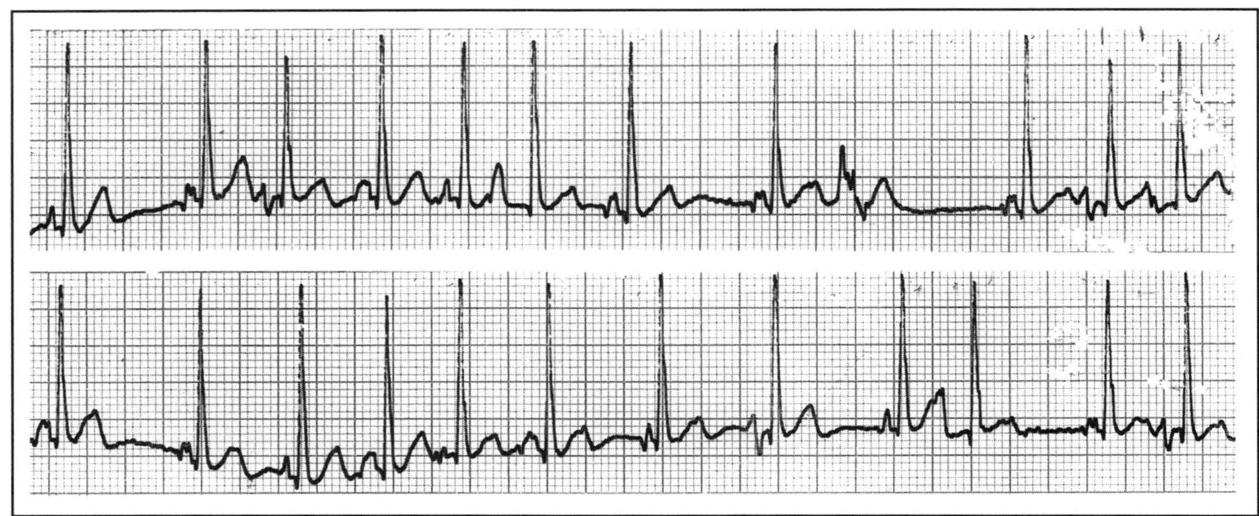

FIGURE 22–18. Chaotic (multifocal) atrial tachycardia. Premature atrial complexes occur at varying cycle lengths and with differing contours.

metabolic derangements. Abnormal histology can be present.[143] Differentiation from other tachycardias such as sinus nodal reentry (if the P waves of the automatic atrial tachycardia resemble the sinus-initiated P waves), atrial reentry (particularly if caused by microreentry), and some other mechanisms can be difficult.

Management is as discussed under atrial tachycardia due to digitalis.

Mechansims: Atrial Tachycardia Due to Reentry

ELECTROCARDIOGRAPHIC RECOGNITION (Fig. 22–11*E*). This arrhythmia presents electrocardiographically with a P wave that has a contour different from the sinus P wave, a P-R interval influenced directly by the tachycardia rate, and the ability to develop AV block without interrupting the tachycardia. Reentry can exist around a surgical scar, anatomical defect, or atriotomy incision.[62] Electrophysiologically, initiation of the tachycardia occurs with premature stimulation during the atrial relative refractory period, resulting in a critical degree of intraatrial conduction delay, an atrial activation sequence different from that which occurs during sinus rhythm, and an AV nodal conduction time related to the tachycardia rate. Vagal maneuvers generally do not terminate the tachycardia and can produce AV block.

CLINICAL FEATURES. The relative infrequency of published reports suggests that atrial reentry is not a commonly recognized cause of supraventricular tachycardia. The tachycardia can be started and stopped by an atrial extrastimulus. Spontaneous termination can be either sudden, with progressive slowing, or with alternating long-short cycle lengths.

Chaotic Atrial Tachycardia

Chaotic (sometimes called *multifocal*) atrial tachycardia is characterized by atrial rates between 100 and 130 beats/min, with marked variation in P-wave morphology and totally irregular P-P intervals (Figs. 22–18). Generally, at least three P-wave contours are noted, with most P waves conducted to the ventricles. This tachycardia occurs commonly in older patients with chronic obstructive pulmonary disease and congestive heart failure and may eventually develop into atrial fibrillation. Digitalis appears to be an unusual cause, while theophylline administration has been implicated. Chaotic atrial tachycardia can occur in childhood.

MANAGEMENT. This is primarily directed toward the underlying disease. Antiarrhythmic agents are often ineffective in slowing either the rate of the atrial tachycardia or the ventricular response. Beta-adrenoreceptor blockers should be avoided in patients with bronchospastic pulmonary disease but can be effective if tolerated. Verapamil and amiodarone have been useful. Potassium and magnesium replacement may suppress the tachycardia.

AV Junctional Rhythm Disturbances

AV Junctional Escape Beats

MECHANISM. Automatic fibers that are prevented from initiating depolarization by a pacemaker such as the sinus node, which possesses a more rapid rate of firing, are called *latent pacemakers.* Such latent pacemakers are found in some parts of the atrium, in the AV node–His bundle area, in the right and left bundle branches, and in the Purkinje system. Under usual conditions, automatic fibers are *not* found in atrial or ventricular myocardium. It is possible that the N region of the AV node is automatic, at least in some species, but is kept suppressed by neighboring atrial tissue. A latent pacemaker can become the dominant pacemaker by default or usurpation, i.e., by passive or active mechanisms. A decrease in the number of impulses arriving at a latent pacemaker site, the result of slowing of the sinus node or interruption of the propagation of the normal impulse anywhere along its course, allows the latent pacemaker to escape and initiate depolarization passively, by default. An increase in the discharge rate of a latent pacemaker can capture pacemaker control actively, by usurpation. As will be seen, the implication of the two different mechanisms of ectopic impulse formation is important therapeutically.

ELECTROCARDIOGRAPHIC RECOGNITION. An AV junctional escape beat occurs when the rate of impulse formation of the primary pacemaker, generally the sinus node, becomes less than that of the AV junctional region or when impulses from the primary pacemaker do not penetrate to the region of the escape focus and allow the AV junctional focus to reach threshold and discharge. The interval from the last normally conducted beat to the AV junctional escape beat is a measure of the initial discharge rate of the AV junctional focus and generally corresponds to a rate of 35 to 60 beats/min (Fig. 22–3*B*). Although an AV junctional escape rhythm is usually fairly regular, intervals between subsequent escape beats after the initial escape beat can gradually shorten as the rate of discharge of the escape focus increases, the so-called *rhythm of development* or *warm-up phenomenon.*

The electrocardiogram displays pauses longer than the normal P-P interval, interrupted by a QRS complex of supraventricular configuration with absent, retrograde, fusion, or sinus P waves that do not conduct to the ventricle. If P waves precede the QRS, they have a P-R interval generally less than 0.12 sec. The exact site of impulse formation (i.e., AN, N, or NH regions; low atrium; or His bundle) is not known and may differ from patient to patient and be influenced by the cause of the arrhythmia.

Treatment, if any, lies in increasing the discharge rate of the higher pacemakers and improving AV conduction and can require pacing. Frequently, no treatment is necessary.

Premature AV Junctional Complexes

Premature AV junctional complexes are characterized by an impulse that arises prematurely in the AV junction (the exact site—i.e., AN, N, or NH regions; low atrium; or His bundle—is not known and may vary from patient to patient) and that attempts conduction in

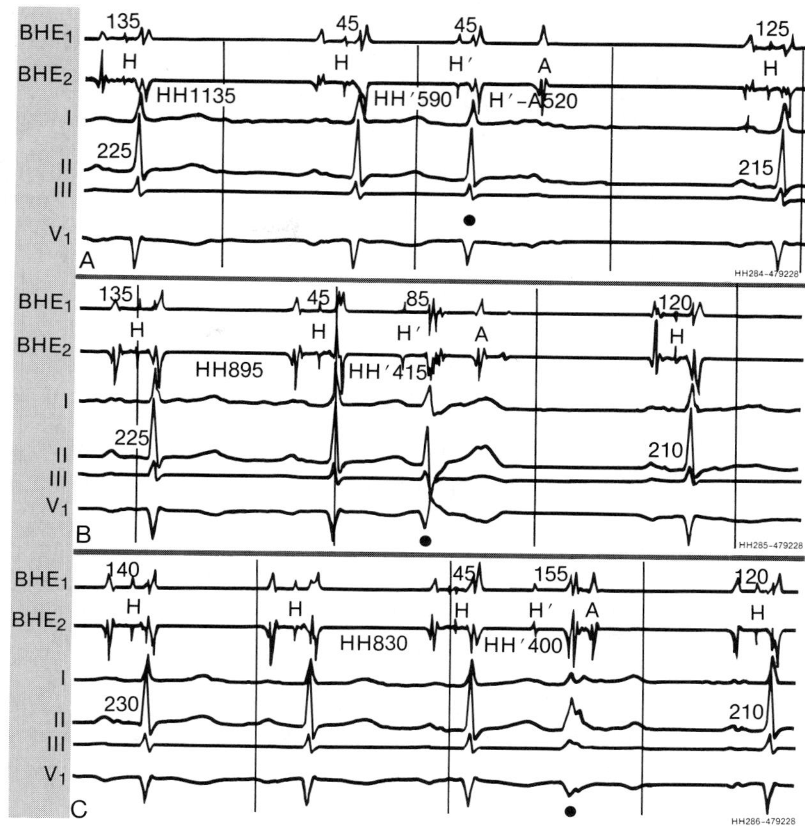

FIGURE 22–19. Premature AV junctional complexes arising in or near the bundle of His (H′) conduct normally *(A)* or with *(B)* functional right or *(C)* functional left bundle branch block. The filled circles indicate the premature junctional complex. Anterograde conduction of the premature junctional (H′) discharges depends on the coupling interval between the last normal His discharge (H) and H-H′ interval and the spontaneous cycle length (H-H) that preceded H′. When H′ follows a shorter preceding cycle length and occurs at longer coupling intervals, a normal QRS complex results. As the preceding H-H cycle lengthens or as the H-H′ interval shortens, a zone of functional right bundle branch block occurs, followed by a zone of functional left bundle branch block. Not shown are premature His discharges that fail to conduct entirely. Numbers in milliseconds. Time lines = 1 sec in each panel. (Magnification is not the same in all three panels.) (From Bonner, A. J., and Zipes, D. P.: Lidocaine and His bundle extrasystoles. His bundle discharge conducted normally, conducted with functional right or left bundle branch block, or blocked entirely [concealed]. Arch. Intern. Med. *136*:700, 1976. Copyright American Medical Association.)

anterograde and retrograde directions. If unimpeded in its course, the impulse discharges the atrium to produce a premature retrograde P wave and a premature QRS complex with a supraventricular contour. The retrograde P wave can occur before, during, or after the QRS complex. Alterations in conduction time can influence the P-R or R-P relationships without a change in the site of origin of the impulse. Premature AV junctional complexes that conduct aberrantly are difficult to distinguish from premature ventricular complexes using the scalar ECG (Fig. 22–19).

Treatment of premature AV junctional complexes is generally not necessary. However, since they may arise distal to the AV node, they can occur early in the cardiac cycle and can initiate a ventricular tachyarrhythmia in some instances. Under these circumstances therapy is approached as for premature ventricular complexes (see p. 675).

AV Junctional Rhythm

If the AV junctional escape beats continue for a period of time, the rhythm is called an *AV junctional rhythm* (Fig. 22–20). Since the inherent rate of the AV junctional tissue is 35 to 60 beats/min, the AV junctional tissue can assume the role of the dominant pacemaker at this rate only by passive default of the sinus pacemaker. The ECG displays a normally conducted QRS complex, which can conduct retrogradely to the atrium or can occur independently of atrial discharge, producing AV dissociation (see p. 692).

An AV junctional escape rhythm can be a normal phenomenon in response to the effects of vagal tone, or it can occur during pathological sinus bradycardia or heart block. The escape beat or rhythm serves as a safety mechanism to prevent the occurrence of ventricular asystole. *Physical findings* vary depending on the P-QRS relationship. Large *a* waves in the jugular venous pulse and a loud, soft, or changing intensity of the first heart sound may be present if atrial contraction occurs when the tricuspid valve is shut.

Therapy is discussed under AV junctional escape beats (see above).

Nonparoxysmal AV Junctional Tachycardia

ELECTROCARDIOGRAPHIC RECOGNITION (Figs. 22–21 and 22–22). To usurp dominant pacemaker status, the AV junctional tissue must exhibit enhanced discharge rate such

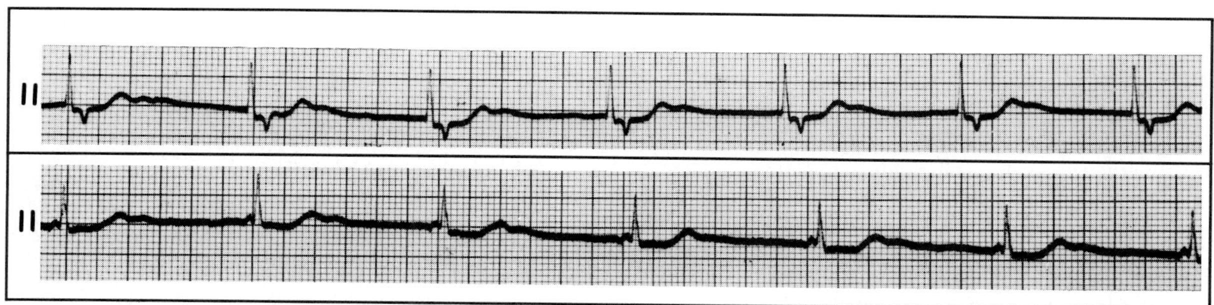

FIGURE 22–20. AV junctional rhythm. *Top,* AV junctional discharge occurs fairly regularly at a rate of approximately 50 beats/min. Retrograde atrial activity follows each junctional discharge. *Bottom,* Recording made on a different day in the same patient; the AV junctional rate is slightly more variable, and retrograde P waves precede the onset of the QRS complex. The positive terminal portion of the P wave gives the appearance of AV dissociation, which was not present.

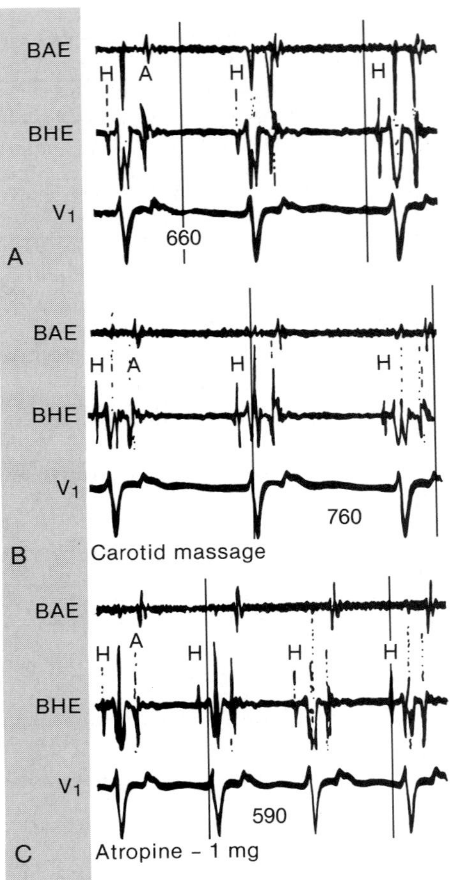

FIGURE 22–21. Nonparoxysmal AV junctional tachycardia. *A*, Control; *B*, response to carotid sinus massage; *C*, response to atropine, 1 mg intravenously. Note that His bundle depolarization is the earliest recordable electrical activity in each cycle. The atria are depolarized retrogradely (low right atrial activity recorded in BHE precedes high right atrial activity recorded in BAE). Note also that carotid sinus massage slows the junctional discharge rate while atropine speeds it up. From these tracings alone one could not distinguish the rhythm from some other types of supraventricular tachycardias. However, onset and termination of this tachycardia were typical of nonparoxysmal AV junctional tachycardia.

as during nonparoxysmal AV junctional tachycardia. The tachycardia is usually of gradual onset and termination, hence the modifier *nonparoxysmal*. On occasion, nonparoxysmal AV junctional tachycardia can become manifest abruptly because of slowing of the dominant pacemaker that may then allow sudden capture and control of the rhythm by the AV junctional focus.

Nonparoxysmal AV junctional tachycardia is recognized by a QRS of supraventricular configuration at a fairly regular rate of 70 to 130 beats/min but can be faster. Accepted terminology assigns the label of tachycardia to rates exceeding 100 beats/min. The term *nonparoxysmal AV junctional tachycardia,* although not entirely correct when the rate is 70 to 100 beats/min, has generally been accepted, since rates exceeding 60 beats/min represent in effect a tachycardia for the AV junctional tissue. Enhanced vagal tone can slow while vagolytic agents can speed up the discharge rate. Although retrograde activation of the atria can occur, the atria commonly are controlled by an independent sinus, atrial, or on occasion a second AV junctional focus resulting in AV dissociation (Fig. 22–11*G*). The electrocardiographic diagnosis can be complicated by the presence of entrance and exit blocks at the AV junctional tissue level and incomplete forms of AV dissociation.

The cause of this arrhythmia probably is *accelerated automatic discharge* in or near the His bundle. It is possible that nonparoxysmal AV junctional tachycardia originates in atrial fibers without recognition of the latter's role from analysis of the scalar ECG or on intracardiac electrograms, unless a careful search is made. Wenckebach periods can occur (Fig. 3–50, color plate 2), but the presence of exit block has not yet been demonstrated by His bundle recording in humans, and the block can be in the AV node with the origin of the nonparoxysmal AV junctional tachycardia proximal to the site of the His bundle recording.

CLINICAL FEATURES. Nonparoxysmal AV junctional tachycardia occurs most commonly in patients with underlying heart disease, such as inferior infarction or myocarditis (often the result of acute rheumatic fever), or after open-heart surgery.[144–146] An important cause is excessive digitalis, which also can produce the ECG manifestations of varying degrees of exit block (usually Wenckebach type) from the accelerated AV junctional focus. Junctional tachycardia occurs commonly during radiofrequency catheter ab-

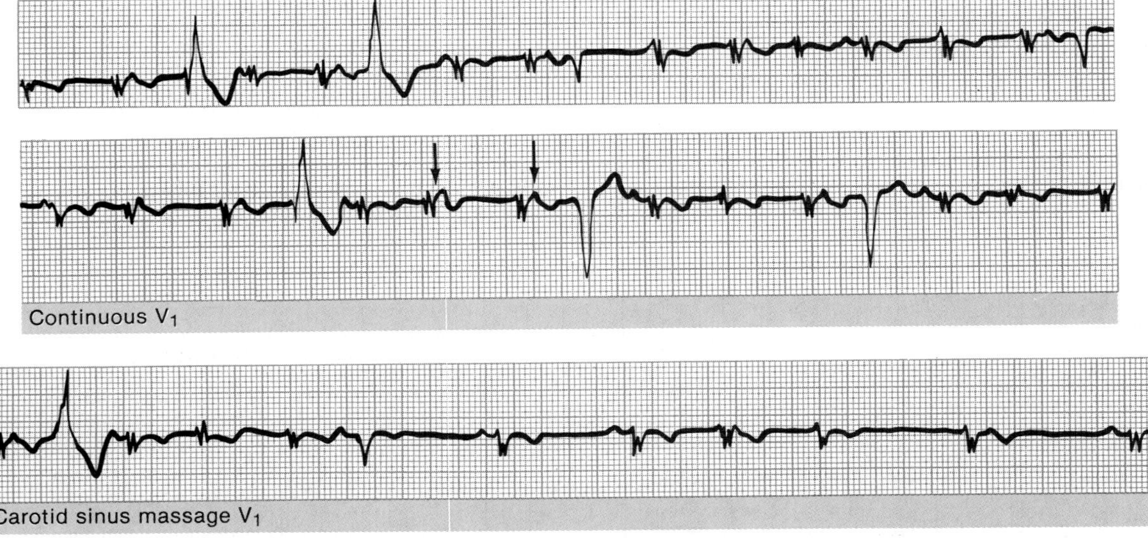

FIGURE 22–22. Nonparoxysmal AV junctional tachycardia in a healthy young adult. This tachycardia occurs at a fairly regular interval ("W-shaped" complexes) and is interrupted intermittently with sinus captures that produce functional right and left bundle branch block. Two P waves are indicated by arrows. The junctional discharge rate is approximately 120 beats/min (cycle length = 500 msec) and the rhythm irregular, sometimes shortened by sinus captures or delayed by concealed conduction that resets and displaces the junctional focus. In the bottom panel, carotid sinus massage slows the junctional as well as the sinus discharge rate.

lation of the slow pathway[147] (see p. 623). Nonparoxysmal AV junctional tachycardia can occur in otherwise healthy individuals without symptoms (Fig. 22–22) or can be a serious and difficult-to-control tachycardia, occasionally chronic, rapid, and long-lasting. It can occur congenitally in infants or children, with a relatively high mortality.[148,149]

The clinical features vary depending on the rate of the arrhythmia and the underlying etiology and severity of heart disease. As in most arrhythmias, the physical signs are determined by the relationship of the P wave to the QRS complex and the rate of atrial and ventricular discharge. The first heart sound can therefore be constant or varying, and cannon *a* waves may or may not occur in the jugular venous pulse.

The ventricular rhythm can be regular or irregular, often in a constant fashion. It is especially important to recognize slowing and regularization of the ventricular rhythm in a patient with atrial fibrillation as being caused by nonparoxysmal AV junctional tachycardia and as a possible early sign of *digitalis intoxication* (see p. 484). Initially, during atrial fibrillation, the regular ventricular rhythm can result from an AV junctional escape rhythm because the depressed AV conduction caused by digitalis blocks the passage of impulses from the fibrillating atria (Fig. 22–11*G*). As digitalis administration is continued, the ventricular rate can then speed because of increased discharge of the AV junctional pacemaker but can still be regular. Further digitalis administration can produce a rate that is slow and irregular because of varying degrees of AV junctional exit block. The rhythm can be misdiagnosed as resumption of conduction from the fibrillating atria. The rate then can increase further because of development of a ventricular tachycardia.

MANAGEMENT. Therapy is directed toward the underlying etiological factor and functional support of the cardiovascular system. If the rhythm is regular, the cardiovascular status is not compromised, and if the patient is not taking digitalis, digitalis administration could be considered. Electrical cardioversion can be tried if necessary and if digitalis toxicity is excluded; theoretically, however, if the nonparoxysmal AV junctional tachycardia is due to enhanced automaticity, cardioversion may be ineffective. If the patient tolerates the arrhythmia well, careful monitoring and attention to the underlying heart disease are usually all that are required in the adult. The arrhythmia usually will abate spontaneously. If digitalis toxicity is the cause, the drug must be stopped, and potassium, lidocaine, phenytoin, or propranolol administered. Drug therapy includes agents from classes IA, IC, and III.[144,148–150] Catheter ablation of the junctional site can be effective.[151–154]

Tachycardias Involving the AV Junction

Much confusion exists regarding the nomenclature of tachycardias characterized by a supraventricular QRS complex, a regular R-R interval, and no evidence of ventricular preexcitation. Because it is now apparent that a variety of electrophysiological mechanisms can account for these tachycardias (Fig. 22–11), the nonspecific term *paroxysmal supraventricular tachycardia* (PSVT) has been proposed to encompass the entire group. This term may be inappropriate because tachycardias in patients with accessory pathways (see below) are no more supraventricular than they are ventricular in origin, since they may require participation of both the atria and the ventricles in the reentrant pathway, and they exhibit a QRS complex of normal contour and duration only because anterograde conduction occurs over the normal AV node–His bundle pathways (Fig. 22–11*C*). If conduction over the reentrant pathway reverses direction and travels in an "antidromic" direction—i.e., to the ventricles over the accessory pathway and to the atria over the AV node–His bundle—the QRS complex exhibits a prolonged duration, although the tachycardia is basically the same. The term *reciprocating tachycardia* has been offered as a substitute for paroxysmal supraventricular tachycardia, but use of such a term presumes the mechanism of the tachycardia to be reentrant (which is probably the case for many supraventricular tachycardias). Reciprocating tachycardia is probably the mechanism of many ventricular tachycardias as well. Thus no universally acceptable nomenclature exists for these tachycardias. In this chapter, descriptive titles, although cumbersome, will be used for the sake of clarity. In addition, the mechanism of reentry will be assumed operative when the weight of evidence supports its presence even though unequivocal proof is lacking.

Atrioventricular (AV) Nodal Reentrant Tachycardia

ELECTROCARDIOGRAPHIC RECOGNITION. Reentrant tachycardia in the AV node is characterized by a tachycardia with a QRS complex of supraventricular origin, with sudden onset and termination generally at rates between 150 and 250 beats/min (commonly 180 to 200 beats/min in adults) and with a regular rhythm. Uncommonly, the rate may be as low as 110 beats/min and occasionally, especially in children, may exceed 250. Unless functional aberrant ventricular conduction or a previous conduction defect exists, the QRS complex is normal in contour and duration. P waves are generally buried in the QRS complex. AV nodal reentry recorded at the onset begins abruptly, usually following a premature atrial complex that conducts with a prolonged P-R interval (see Figs. 22–11*A* and 22–12*B* and Figs. 20–28 through 20–33), pp. 570 through 575. The abrupt termination, usually with a retrograde P wave, is sometimes followed by a brief period of asystole or bradycardia. The R-R interval can shorten over the course of the first few beats at the onset or lengthen during the last few beats preceding termination of the tachycardia. Variation in cycle length is usually caused by variation in anterograde AV nodal conduction time. Cycle-length and/or QRS alternans can occur, usually when the rate is very fast. Carotid sinus massage can slow the tachycardia slightly prior to its termination or, if termination does not occur, can produce only slight slowing of the tachycardia.

ELECTROPHYSIOLOGICAL FEATURES

An atrial complex that conducts with a critical prolongation of AV nodal conduction time generally precipitates AV nodal reentry (see Figs. 22–23, 22–24, and 22–25). Premature ventricular stimulation also can induce AV nodal reentry in about one-third of patients. Data from radiofrequency catheter ablation results[157,158] and mapping[159–162] support the presence of separate atrial inputs into the AV node, the fast and slow pathways,[155,156] to explain this tachycardia (see Chap. 20). In Figure 20–31 (p. 574), and Figure 22–11*A* and *B* (p. 650), the atria are shown as a necessary link between the fast and slow pathways. In most examples, the retrograde P wave occurs at the onset of the QRS complex, clearly excluding the possibility of an accessory pathway. If an accessory pathway in the ventricle were part of the tachycardia circuit, the ventricles would have to be activated anterogradely before the accessory pathway could be activated retrogradely and depolarize the atria, placing the retrograde P wave no earlier than during the ST segment (see Preexcitation Syndrome, p. 667).

In approximately 30 per cent of instances, atrial activation begins at the end of, or just after, the QRS complex, giving rise to a discrete P wave on the surface ECG (often appearing as a nubbin of an R′ in V_1) (Fig. 22–11*A*), while in the majority of patients P waves are not seen, since they are buried within the inscription of the QRS complex. In the most common variety of AV nodal reentrant tachycardia, the V-A interval (i.e., interval between onset of QRS and onset of atrial activity) is less than 50 per cent of the R-R interval, and the ratio of A-V to V-A interval exceeds 1.0. Most of these patients during tachycardia have a V-A minimum value of ≤ 61 msec measured to the earliest recorded atrial activity and of ≤ 95 msec measured to atrial activity recorded in the high right atrial electrogram. These V-A intervals are longer in patients with tachycardia related to accessory pathways as well as in atypical forms of AV nodal reentry (Fig. 22–11*B*).

SLOW AND FAST PATHWAYS. In the majority of patients, anterograde conduction occurs to the ventricle over the slow (alpha) pathway and retrograde conduction over the fast (beta) pathway (see Fig. 20–28*B* and Fig. 22–11*A* and *B*). To initiate tachycardia, an

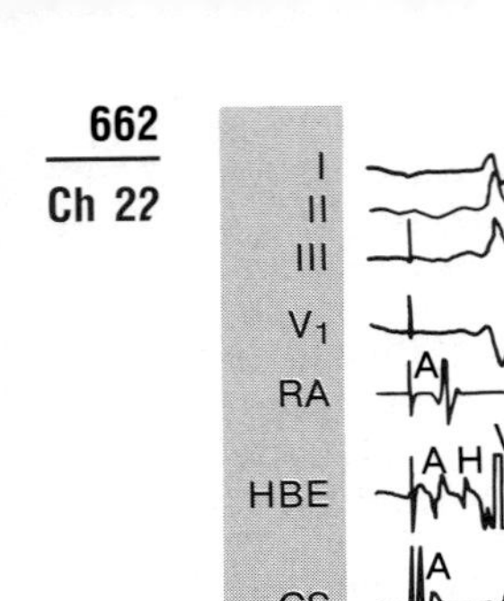

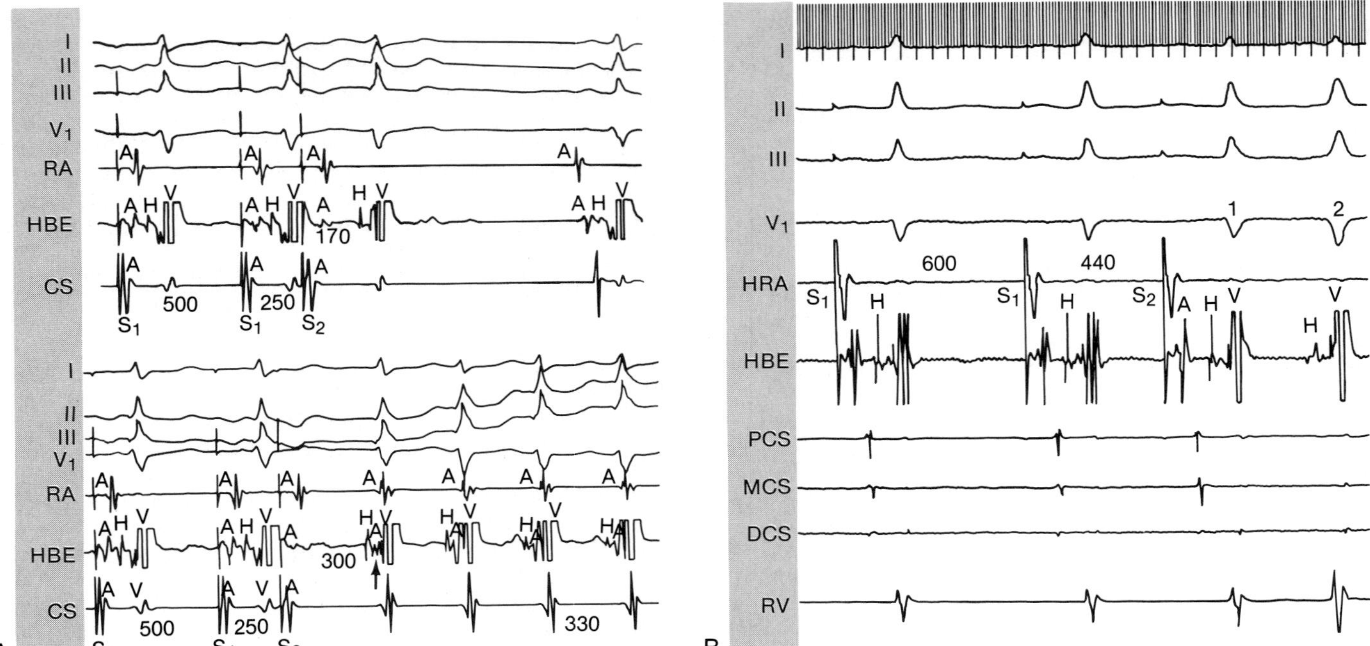

FIGURE 22–23. *A*, Initiation of AV nodal reentrant tachycardia in a patient with dual atrioventricular nodal pathways. Upper and lower panels show the last two paced beats of a train of stimuli delivered to the coronary sinus at a pacing cycle length of 500 msec. The results of premature atrial stimulation at an S_1-S_2 interval of 250 msec on two occasions are shown. In the upper panel, S_2 was conducted to the ventricle with an A-H interval of 170 msec and then was followed by a sinus beat. In the lower panel, S_2 was conducted with an A-H interval of 300 msec and initiated AV nodal reentry. Note that the retrograde atrial activity occurs (arrow) prior to the onset of ventricular septal depolarization and is superimposed on the QRS complex. Retrograde atrial activity begins first in the low right atrium (HBE lead) and then progresses to the high right atrium (RA) and coronary sinus (CS) recordings.

B, Two QRS complexes in response to a single atrial premature complex. Following a basic train of S_1 stimuli at 600 msec, an S_2 at 440 msec is introduced. The first QRS complex in response to S_2 occurs following a short (95 msec) A-H interval due to anterograde conduction over the fast AV nodal pathway. The first QRS complex is labeled number 1 (in lead V_1). The second QRS complex in response to the S_2 stimulus (labeled number 2) follows a long A-H interval (430 msec) due to anterograde conduction over the slow AV nodal pathway.

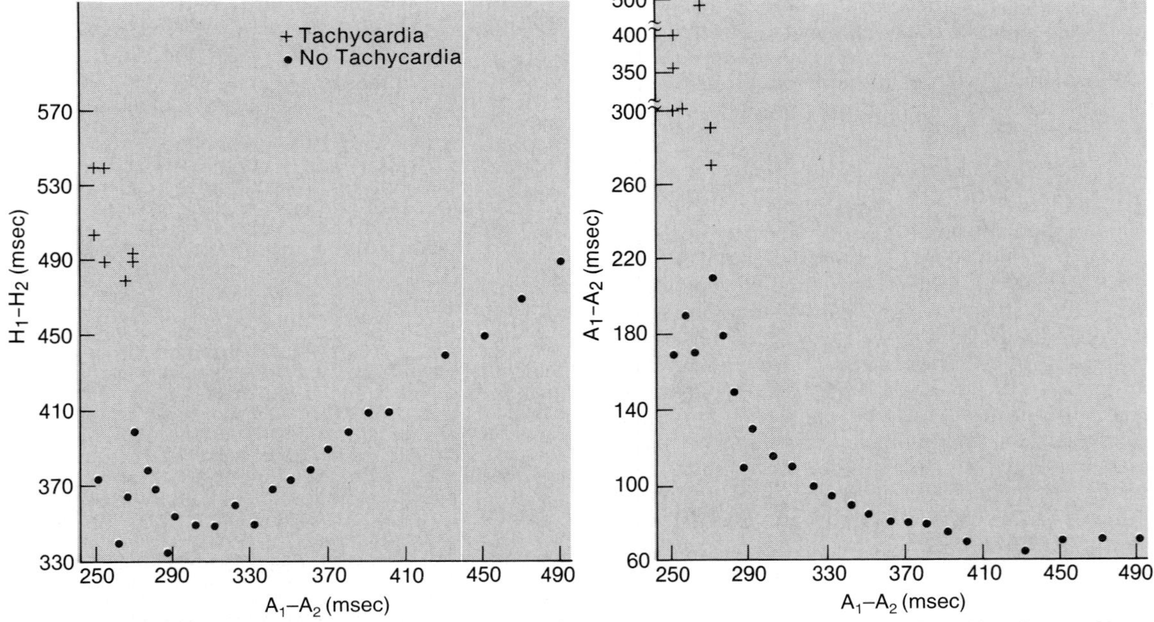

FIGURE 22–24. H_1-H_2 intervals *(left)* and A_2-H_2 intervals *(right)* at various A_1-A_2 intervals. Discontinuous AV nodal curve. At a critical A_1-A_2 interval the H_1-H_2 interval and the A_1-H_2 intervals increase markedly. At the break in the curves, AV nodal reentrant tachycardia is initiated.

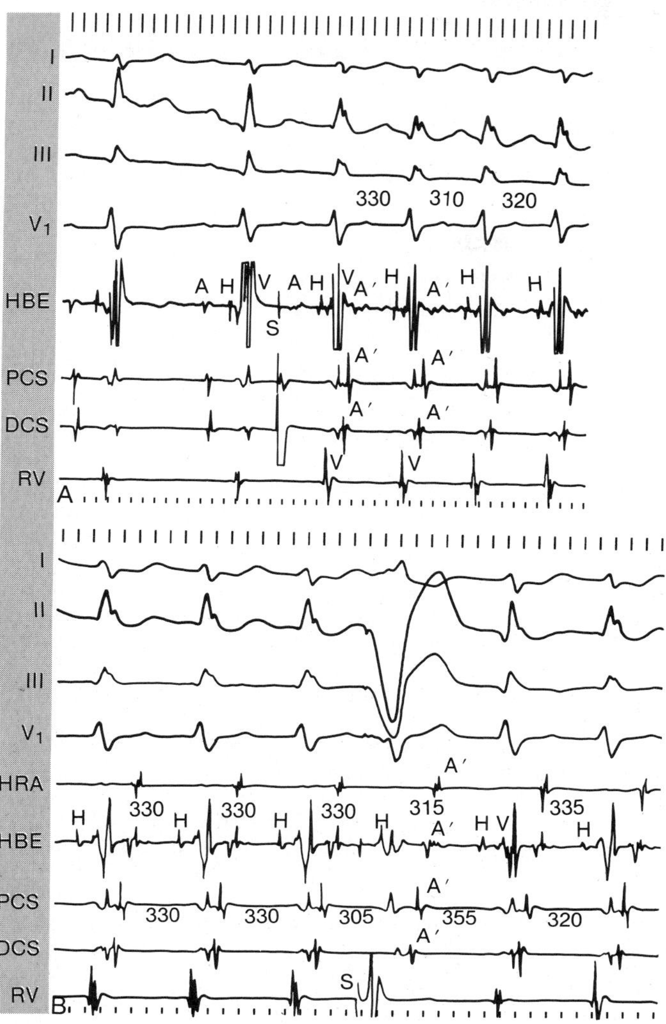

FIGURE 22–25. Atrial preexcitation during atrioventricular reciprocating tachycardia (AVRT) in a patient with a concealed accessory pathway. No evidence of an accessory pathway conduction is present in the two sinus-initiated beats shown in panel *A*. A premature stimulus in the coronary sinus (S) precipitates a supraventricular tachycardia at a cycle length of approximately 330 msec. The retrograde atrial activation sequence begins first in the distal coronary sinus (A′, DCS), followed by activation recorded in the proximal coronary sinus (PCS), low right atrium (HBE), and then high right atrium (not shown). The QRS complex is normal and identical to the sinus-initiated QRS complex. (The terminal portion is slightly deformed by the superimposition of the retrograde atrial recording.) Note that the R-P interval is short and the P-R interval is long. The shortest V-A interval exceeds 65 msec, consistent with conduction over a retrogradely conducting atrioventricular pathway.

In panel *B*, premature ventricular stimulation at a time when the His bundle is still refractory from anterograde activation during tachycardia shortens the A-A interval from 330 to 305 msec without a change in the retrograde atrial activation sequence. (Note that no change occurs in the H-H interval when the right ventricular stimulus, S, is delivered. H-H intervals are in msec in HBE lead.) Thus the ventricular stimulus, despite His bundle refractoriness, still reaches the atrium and produces an identical retrograde atrial activation sequence. The only way this can be explained is via conduction over a retrogradely conducting accessory pathway. Therefore, the patient has a concealed accessory pathway with the Wolff-Parkinson-White syndrome.

atrial complex blocks in the fast pathway anterogradely, travels to the ventricle over the slow pathway, and returns to the atrium over the previously blocked fast pathway. The proximal and distal final pathways for this circus movement appear to be located within the AV node so that, as currently conceived, the circus movement occurs over the two atrial approaches and the AV node (Fig. 22–11*A* and *B*). The reentrant loop for typical AV nodal reentry is anterograde slow AV nodal pathway → final distal common pathway (probably distal AV node) → retrograde fast AV nodal pathway → atrial myocardium. In atypical AV node reentry, the reentry occurs in an opposite direction.[163] In some patients, the His bundle may be incorporated in the reentrant circuit. Less commonly, the reentry pathway can be over two slow pathways, so-called slow-slow AV node reentry (Fig. 22–12*B*). Some data are consistent with intranodal activity.[164]

The cycle length of the tachycardia generally depends on how well the slow pathway conducts, because the fast pathway usually exhibits excellent capability for retrograde conduction and has the shorter refractory period in the retrograde direction. Therefore, conduction time in the anterograde slow pathway is a major determinant of the cycle length of the tachycardia.

THE DUAL PATHWAY CONCEPT. The evidence supporting the dual pathway concept derives from several observations, the most compelling of which is that radiofrequency catheter ablation of *either* the slow pathway or the fast pathway eliminates AV nodal reentry without eliminating AV nodal conduction. Other observations provide supporting proof. For example, in these patients, a plot of the A_1-A_2 versus the A_2-H_2 or A_1-A_2 versus the H_1-H_2 intervals shows a discontinuous curve (Fig. 22–24). The explanation is that at a crucial A_1-A_2 interval the impulse suddenly blocks in the fast pathway and conducts with delay over the slow pathway, with sudden prolongation of the A_2-H_2 (or H_1-H_2) interval. Generally, the A-H interval increases at least 50 msec with only a 10- to 20-msec decrease in the coupling interval of the premature atrial complex. Less commonly, dual pathways may be manifested by different P-R or A-H intervals during sinus rhythm or at identical paced rates or by a sudden jump in the A-H interval during atrial pacing at a constant cycle length. Two QRS complexes in response to one P wave provide additional evidence[165] (Fig. 22–23*B*).

Some patients with AV nodal reentry may not have discontinuous refractory period curves, and some patients who do not have AV nodal reentry can exhibit discontinuous refractory curves. In the latter patients, dual AV nodal pathways can be a benign finding. Many of these patients also exhibit discontinuous curves retrogradely. Similar mechanisms of tachycardia can occur in children. Triple AV nodal pathways can be demonstrated in occasional patients. Virtually irrefutable proof of dual AV nodal pathways is the simultaneous propagation in opposite directions of two AV nodal wavefronts without collision (Fig. 20–30, p. 573) or the production of two QRS complexes from one P wave (Fig. 22–23*B*) or two P waves from one QRS complex.[166]

In fewer than 5 to 10 per cent of patients with AV nodal reentry, anterograde conduction proceeds over the fast pathway and retrograde conduction over the slow pathway (termed the *unusual form* of AV nodal reentry or atypical AV node reentry), producing a long V-A interval and a relatively short A-V interval[156–163] (generally A-V/V-A < 0.75; Fig. 22–11*B*). Finally, it is possible to have tachycardias that use either the anterograde slow or fast pathways and conduct retrogradely over an accessory pathway (see below).

The ventricles are not needed to maintain AV nodal reentry in humans, and spontaneous AV block has been noted on occasion, particularly at the onset of the arrhythmia. Such block can take place in the AV node distal to the reentry circuit, between the AV node and bundle of His, within the bundle of His, or distal to it[167] (see Fig. 20–32, p. 574). Rarely, the block can be located between the reentry circuit in the AV node and the atrium. Most commonly, when block appears, it is below the bundle of His. Termination of the tachycardia generally results from block in the anterogradely conducting slow pathway ("weak link") so that a retrograde atrial response is not followed by a His or ventricular response.

RETROGRADE ATRIAL ACTIVATION. The sequence of retrograde atrial activation is normal during AV nodal reentrant supraventricular tachycardia. This means that the earliest site of atrial activation during retrograde conduction over the fast pathway is recorded in the His bundle electrogram followed by electrograms recorded from the os of the coronary sinus and then spreading to depolarize the rest of the right and left atria. During retrograde conduction over the slow pathway in the atypical type of AV nodal reentry, atrial activation recorded in the proximal coronary sinus precedes atrial activation recorded in the low right atrium, suggesting that the slow and fast pathways can enter the atria at slightly different positions. Mapping at the time of surgery confirms this conclusion. Functional bundle branch block during AV nodal reentrant tachycardia does not modify the tachycardia significantly.

CLINICAL FEATURES. AV nodal reentry commonly occurs in patients who have no structural heart disease. Symptoms frequently accompany the tachycardia and range from feelings of palpitations,[168] nervousness, and anxiety to angina, heart failure, syncope, or shock depending on the duration and rate of the tachycardia and the presence of structural heart disease. Tachycardia can cause syncope because of the rapid ventricular rate, reduced cardiac output, and cerebral circulation or because of asystole when the tachycardia terminates, owing to tachycardia-induced depression of sinus node automaticity. The prognosis for patients without heart disease is usually good.

Hemodynamic consequences of supraventricular tachyarrhythmias in patients with normal ventricular function are due primarily to a marked decrease in left ventricular end-diastolic and stroke volumes with an increase in ejection rate and cardiac output without a significant change in ejection fraction as heart rate is increased and the atrial contribution to ventricular filling is lost. Heart disease or tachycardia can reduce the ejection fraction. Initial hypotension during tachycardia can evoke a sympathetic response that increases blood pressure and in turn causes a rise in vagal tone that can terminate the tachycardia.

MANAGEMENT

THE ACUTE ATTACK (Table 22–2). This depends on the underlying heart disease, how well the tachycardia is tolerated, and the natural history of previous attacks in the individual patient. For some patients, rest, reassurance, and sedation may be all that are required to abort an attack. Vagal maneuvers, including carotid sinus massage, Valsalva and Mueller maneuvers, gagging, and occasionally exposure of the face to ice water serve as the first line of therapy. These maneuvers may slightly slow the tachycardia rate, which then may speed up to the original rate following cessation of the attempt, or may terminate it. Vagal maneuvers should be tried *again* after each pharmacological approach. Digitalis, calcium antagonists, beta-adrenoceptor blockers, and adenosine normally depress conduction in the anterogradely conducting slow AV nodal pathway, while class IA and IC drugs depress conduction in the retrogradely conducting fast pathway.

Adenosine (see p. 619), 6 to 12 mg given rapidly IV, is the initial drug of choice.[169] *Verapamil* (see p. 616), 5 to 10 mg IV, or diltiazem, 0.25 to 0.35 mg/kg IV, terminates AV nodal reentry successfully in about 2 minutes in about 90 per cent of instances and is given when simple vagal manuevers and adenosine fail.

Cholinergic drugs, such as *edrophonium chloride* (Tensilon), a short-acting cholinesterase inhibitor, can terminate AV nodal reentry when administered initially at a trial dose of 3 to 5 mg IV. If unsuccessful, a dose of 10 mg IV may be given. Edrophonium is infrequently needed. Similarly, *intravenous digitalis* administration is usually not necessary to terminate AV nodal reentry. If digitalis is used, digoxin can be given, 0.5 to 1.0 mg IV over 10 to 15 min, followed by 0.25 mg every 2 to 4 hours, with a total dose less than 1.5 mg within any 24-hour period. *Oral digitalis* administration to terminate an acute attack is generally not indicated. Vagal maneuvers that were ineffective previously can terminate the tachycardia following digitalis administration and therefore should be repeated.

If a beta-adrenoceptor antagonist is selected, esmolol (50 to 200 μg/kg/min) would seem preferable because of its shorter duration of action. *Propranolol* can be tried. Recommended IV dosing is best achieved by titrating the dose to the clinical effect, begun with doses of 0.25 to 0.5 mg, increasing to 1.0 mg if necessary, and administering doses every 5 minutes until either a desired effect or toxicity is produced or a total of 0.15 to 0.2 mg/kg is given. Beta-adrenoceptor blockers must be used cautiously, if at all, in patients with heart failure, chronic lung disease, or a history of asthma because its beta-adrenoceptor blocking action depresses myocardial contractility and can produce bronchospasm. Digitalis, calcium antagonists, beta blockers, and adenosine normally depress conduction in the anterogradely conducting slow pathway, whereas class 1A and 1C drugs depress conduction in the retrogradely conducting fast pathway.

TABLE 22–2 DRUGS THAT SLOW CONDUCTION IN, AND PROLONG REFRACTORINESS OF, ACCESSORY PATHWAY AND AV NODE

AFFECTED TISSUE	DRUGS
Accessory pathway	Class IA
AV node	Class II Class IV Adenosine Digitalis
Both	Class IC Class III (amiodarone)

DC CARDIOVERSION. Before digitalis or a beta blocker is administered, it is advisable to reassess the clinical status of the patient and consider whether DC cardioversion may be advisable. DC shock administered to patients who have received excessive amounts of digitalis can be dangerous and can result in serious postshock ventricular arrhythmias (see p. 621). Particularly if signs or symptoms of cardiac decompensation occur, DC electrical shock should be considered early. DC shock, synchronized to the QRS complex to avoid precipitating ventricular fibrillation, successfully terminates AV nodal reentry with energies in the range of 10 to 50 joules; higher energies can be required in some instances (see p. 623).

In the event that digitalis has been given in large doses and DC shock is contraindicated, competitive *atrial* or *ventricular pacing* can restore sinus rhythm. In some instances, esophageal pacing can be useful (see p. 705).

Class IA, IC, and III drugs are usually not required to terminate AV nodal reentry. Unless contraindicated, DC cardioversion generally should be employed before using these agents, which are more often administered to prevent recurrences.

Pressor drugs can terminate AV nodal reentry by inducting reflex vagal stimulation mediated by baroreceptors in the carotid sinus and aorta when the systolic blood pressure is acutely elevated to levels of about 180 mm Hg. One of the following drugs, diluted in 5 to 10 ml of 5 per cent dextrose and water, can be given over 1 to 3 minutes: phenylephrine (Neo-Synephrine), 0.5 to 1.0 mg; methoxamine (Vasoxyl), 3 to 5 mg; or metaraminol (Aramine), 0.5 to 2.0 mg. Pressor drugs should be used cautiously or not at all in the elderly and in patients who have structural heart disease, significant hypertension, hyperthyroidism, or acute myocardial infarction. This potentially dangerous and almost always uncomfortable mode of therapy is rarely needed unless the patient is also hypotensive.

PREVENTION OF RECURRENCES. Initially, one must decide whether the frequency and severity of the attacks warrant long-term therapy. If the attacks of paroxsymal tachycardia are infrequent, well tolerated, short lasting, and either terminate spontaneously or are easily terminated by the patient, no prophylactic therapy may be necessary. If the attacks are sufficiently frequent and/or long lasting to necessitate therapy, the patient can be treated with drugs empirically or on the basis of serial electrophysiological testing. If empirical testing is desirable, digitalis, a long-acting calcium antagonist, or long-acting beta-adrenoceptor blocker is a reasonable initial choice. The clinical situation and potential contraindications, e.g., beta blockers in an asthmatic, usually dictate the selection. If digitalis is used, rapid oral digitalization can be accomplished in 24 to 36 hours with digoxin at an initial dose of 1.0 to 1.5 mg, followed by 0.25 to 0.5 mg every 6 hours for a total dose of 2.0 to 3.0 mg. A less rapid oral regimen digitalizes in 2 to 3 days with an initial dose of 0.75 to 1.0 mg, followed by 0.25 to 0.50 mg every 12 hours for a total dose of 2.0 to 3.0 mg. Alternatively, digoxin administered as a maintenance dose of 0.125 to 0.500 mg achieves digitalization in about 1 week.

Sustained-release verapamil in the range of 240 mg per day, long-acting diltiazem 60 to 120 mg twice daily, or long-acting propranolol in doses of 80 to 120 mg per day can be tried. If these drugs are ineffective taken singly, combinations can be tested.

Because it is preferable to *cure* the patient of the tachycardia rather than to use potentially toxic drugs to suppress it or to implant an antitachycardia device that only terminates the tachycardia after its onset (Chap. 23), radiofrequency catheter ablation should be considered early in the management of patients with symptomatic recurrent episodes of AV node reentry. For patients who do not wish to take drugs, are drug intolerant, or in whom drugs are ineffective, radiofrequency catheter ablation is the treatment of choice.[170,171] It should be considered before long-term therapy with class IA, IC, or III antiarrhythmic drugs. Ablation has replaced surgery[162,172,173] in virtually all instances.[70,174–183]

Reentry Over a Retrogradely Conducting (Concealed) Accessory Pathway

ELECTROCARDIOGRAPHIC RECOGNITION (Fig. 22–25). The presence of an accessory pathway that conducts unidirectionally from the ventricle to the atrium but not in the reverse direction is not apparent by analysis of the scalar ECG during sinus rhythm because the ventricle is not preexcited.[184,185] Therefore, the ECG manifestations of the Wolff-Parkinson-White (WPW) syndrome are absent, and the accessory pathway is said to be "concealed." Since the mechanism responsible for most tachycardias in patients who have the WPW syndrome is macroreentry caused by anterograde conduction over the AV node–His bundle pathway and retrograde conduction over an accessory pathway, the latter, even if it only conducts retrogradely, can still participate in the reentrant circuit to cause an *AV reciprocating* tachycardia. Electrocardiographically, a tachycardia due to this mechanism can be *suspected* when the QRS complex is normal and the retrograde P wave occurs *after* completion of the QRS complex, in the ST segment, or early in the T wave (Fig. 22–11*C*).

MECHANISMS. The cause of unidirectional propagation is not clear and can relate to multiple factors. During sinus rhythm, the atrial impulse probably enters the accessory pathway but blocks near the ventricular insertion site with both right- and left-sided concealed accessory pathways. During functional block in patients with anterograde conduction over accessory pathways, block occurs near the ventricular insertion site most commonly with left-sided pathways but more often near the atrial insertion site with right-sided accessory pathways.

The P wave follows the QRS complex during tachycardia because the ventricle must be activated before the propagating impulse can enter the accessory pathway and excite the atria retrogradely. Therefore, the retrograde P wave must occur after ventricular excitation, in contrast to AV nodal reentry, in which the atria usually are excited during ventricular activation (Fig. 22–11*A*). Also, the contour of the retrograde P wave can differ from the usual retrograde P wave, since the atria may be activated eccentrically, i.e., in a manner other than the normal retrograde activation sequence, which starts at the low right atrial septum as in AV nodal reentry. This occurs because the concealed accessory pathway in most instances is left-sided, i.e., inserts into the left atrium, making the left atrium the first site of retrograde atrial activation and causing the retrograde P wave to be negative in lead I (Fig. 22–25).

Finally, since the tachycardia circuit involves the ventricles, if functional bundle branch block occurs in the same ventricle in which the accessory pathway is located, the V-A interval and cycle length of the tachycardia can become longer (see Fig. 22–30*B*). This important change ensues because the bundle branch block lengthens the reentrant circuit (see Preexcitation Syndrome). For example, the normal activation sequence for a reciprocating tachycardia circuit with a left-sided accessory pathway without functional bundle branch block progresses from atrium → AV node–His bundle → right and left ventricles → accessory pathway → atrium. However, during functional left bundle branch block, for example, the tachycardia circuit travels from atrium → AV node–His bundle → right ventricle → septum → left ventricle → accessory pathway → atrium. This increase in the V-A interval provides definitive proof that the ventricle and accessory pathway are part of the reentry circuit. The additional time required for the impulse to travel across the septum from the right to the left ventricle before reaching the accessory pathway and atrium lengthens the V-A interval, which lengthens the cycle length of the tachycardia by an equal amount, assuming no other changes in conduction times occur within the circuit. Thus lengthening of the tachycardia cycle length by more than 35 msec during ipsilateral functional bundle branch block is diagnostic of a free wall accessory pathway if the lengthening can be shown to be due to V-A prolongation only and not to prolongation of the H-V interval (which can develop with the appearance of bundle branch block). In an occasional patient, the increase in cycle length due to prolongation of VA conduction can be nullified by a simultaneous decrease in the P-R (A-H) interval.

The presence of ipsilateral bundle branch block can facilitate reentry and cause an incessant AV reentrant tachycardia.[186] Functional bundle branch block in the ventricle contralateral to the accessory pathway does not lengthen the tachycardia cycle if the H-V interval does not lengthen.

Septal Accessory Pathway. An exception to these observations occurs in the patient with a concealed septal accessory pathway (see Preexcitation Syndrome, p. 667). First, retrograde atrial activation is normal because it occurs retrogradely up the septum. Second, the V-A interval and the cycle length of the tachycardia increase 25 msec or less with the development of ipsilateral functional bundle branch block.

Functional bundle branch block, particularly functional left bundle branch block, during tachycardia occurs more commonly in patients who have an accessory pathway than in those with AV nodal reentry, possibly because in the latter, slow pathway anterograde conduction allows for longer recovery time of the His-Purkinje system, while in tachycardias associated with accessory pathways, anterograde conduction over the AV node may be more rapid. Functional left bundle branch block can occur more commonly during rapid tachycardias, perhaps because the refractory period of the right bundle branch appears to be shorter than that of the left bundle branch at short cycle lengths. Premature right ventricular stimulation that starts an AV reciprocating tachycardia is more likely to induce functional left bundle branch block than is premature atrial stimulation.

Vagal maneuvers, by acting predominantly on the AV node, produce a response on AV reentry similar to AV nodal reentry, and the tachycardia can transiently slow and sometimes terminate. Generally, termination occurs in the anterograde direction so that the last retrograde P wave fails to conduct to the ventricle.

ELECTROPHYSIOLOGICAL FEATURES. Electrophysiological criteria supporting the diagnosis of tachycardia involving reentry over a concealed accessory pathway include the fact that initiation of tachycardia depends on a critical degree of atrioventricular delay (necessary to allow time for the accessory pathway to recover excitability so that it can conduct retrogradely), but the delay can be in the AV node or His-Purkinje system; i.e., a critical degree of A-H delay is not necessary. Occasionally, a tachycardia can start with little or no measurable lengthening of AV nodal or His-Purkinje conduction time. The AV nodal refractory period curve is smooth, in contrast to the discontinuous curve found in many patients with AV nodal reentry. Dual AV nodal pathways occasionally can be noted as a concomitant but unrelated finding.

DIAGNOSIS OF ACCESSORY PATHWAYS. This can be accomplished by demonstrating that during ventricular pacing, premature ventricular stimulation activates the atria before retrograde depolarization of the His bundle, indicating that the impulse reached the atria before it depolarized the His bundle and must have traveled a different pathway to do so. Also, if the ventricles can be stimulated prematurely during tachycardia at a time when the His bundle is refractory, and the impulse still conducts to the atrium, this indicates that retrograde propagation traveled to the atrium over a pathway other than the bundle of His (Fig. 22–25*B*). If the premature ventricular complex depolarizes the atria without lengthening of the V-A interval and with the same retrograde atrial activation sequence, one assumes that the stimulation site (i.e., ventricle) is within the reentrant circuit without intervening His-Purkinje or AV nodal tissue that might increase the V-A interval and therefore the A-A interval. In addition, if a premature ventricular complex delivered at a time when the His bundle is refractory terminates the tachycardia without activating the atria retrogradely, it most likely invaded, and blocked in, an accessory pathway.

The V-A interval (a measurement of conduction over the accessory pathway) generally is constant over a wide range of ventricular paced rates and coupling intervals of premature ventricular complexes as well as during the tachycardia in the absence of aberration. Similar short V-A intervals can be observed in some patients during AV nodal reentry, but if the VA conduction time or R-P interval is the same during tachycardia *and* ventricular pacing at comparable rates, an accessory pathway is almost certainly present. The V-A interval is usually less than 50 per cent of the R-R interval. The tachycardia can be easily initiated following premature ventricular stimulation that conducts retrogradely in the accessory pathway but blocks in the AV node or His bundle. Atria and ventricles are required components of the macroreentrant circuit, and therefore continuation of the tachycardia in the presence of AV or VA block excludes an accessory atrioventricular pathway as part of the reentrant circuit.

CLINICAL FEATURES. The presence of concealed accessory pathways is estimated to account for about 30 per cent of patients with apparent supraventricular tachycardia referred for electrophysiological evaluation. The great majority of these accessory pathways are located between the left ventricle and left atrium and in the posteroseptal area, less

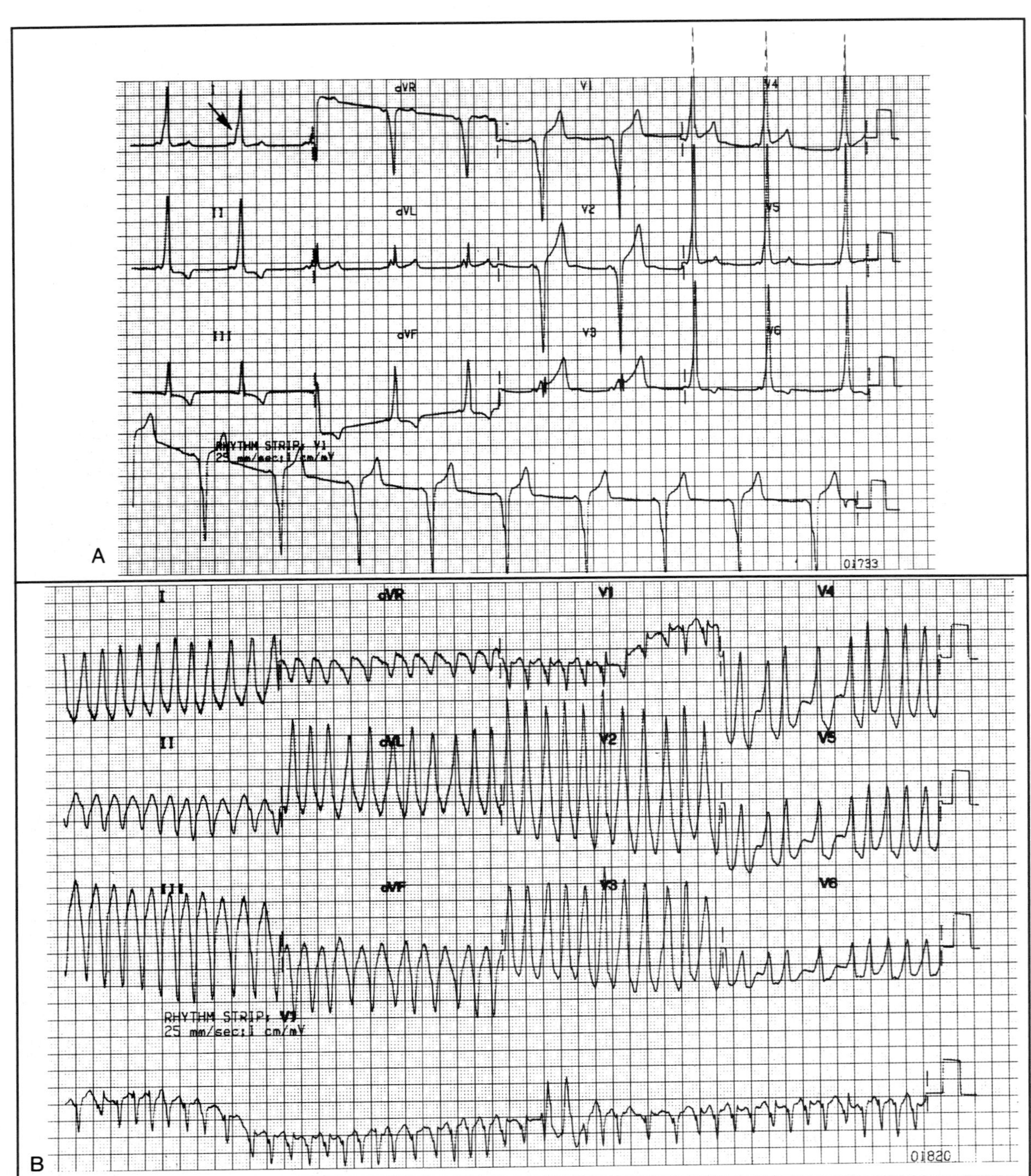

FIGURE 22–26. *A*, Right anteroseptal accessory pathway. The 12-lead ECG characteristically exhibits a normal to inferior axis. The delta wave is negative in V_1 and V_2, upright in leads I, II, aV_l, and aV_f, isoelectric in lead III, and negative in aV_r. Location verified at surgery. Arrow indicates delta wave (lead I).

B, Right posteroseptal accessory pathway. Negative delta waves in leads II, III, and AVF, upright in I and AVL, localize this pathway to the posteroseptal region. The negative delta wave in V_1 with sharp transition to an upright delta wave in V_2 pinpoint it to the right posteroseptal area. Atrial fibrillation is present. Location verified at surgery.

commonly between the right ventricle and right atrium. It is important to be aware of a concealed accessory pathway as a possible cause for apparently "routine" supraventricular tachycardia, since the therapeutic response at times may not follow the usual guidelines. The tachycardia rates tend to be somewhat faster than those occurring in AV nodal reentry (≥200 beats/min), but a great deal of overlap exists between the two groups.

Paroxysmal supraventricular tachycardia can be followed by polyuria after termination due to atrial dilatation and release of atrionatriuretic factor. Syncope can occur because the rapid ventricular rate fails to provide adequate cerebral circulation or because the tachyarrhythmia depresses the sinus pacemaker, causing a period of asystole when the tachyarrhythmia terminates. Physical examination reveals an unvarying, regular ventricular rhythm with constant intensity of the first heart sound. The jugular venous pressure can be elevated, but the waveform generally remains constant.

MANAGEMENT. The therapeutic approach to terminate

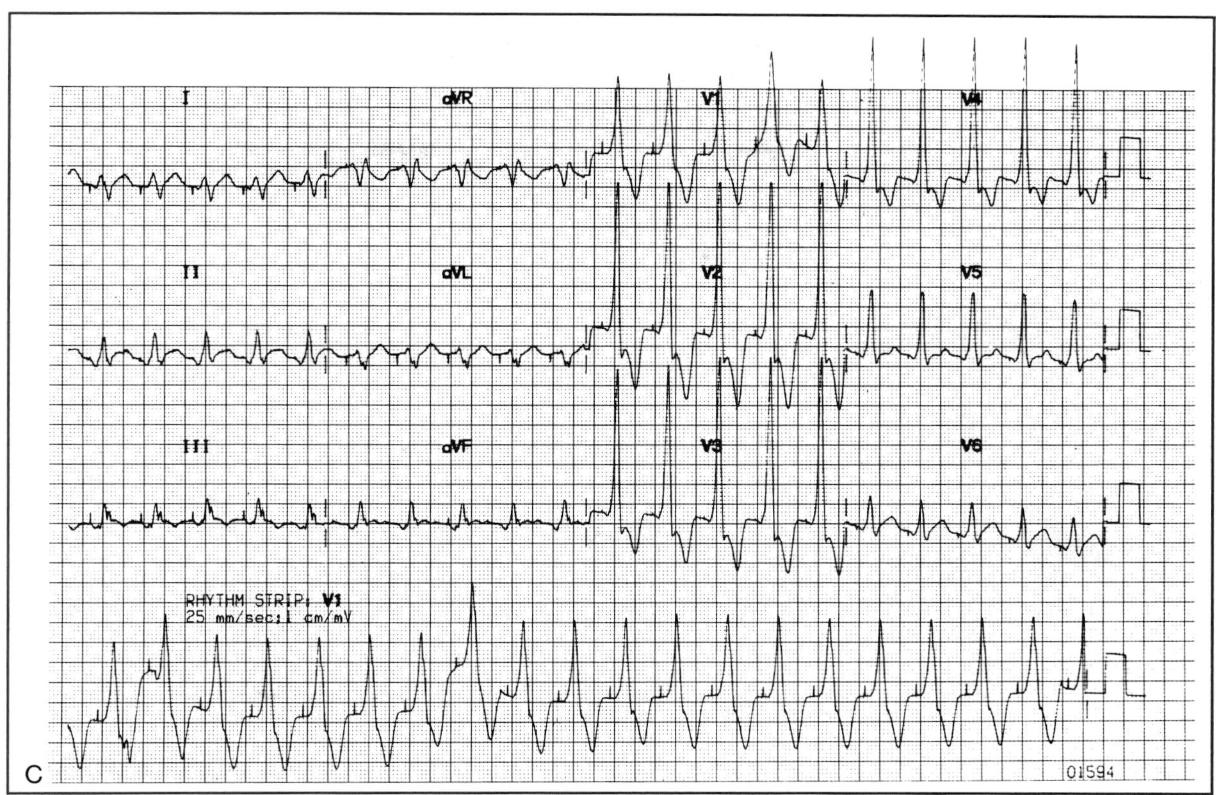

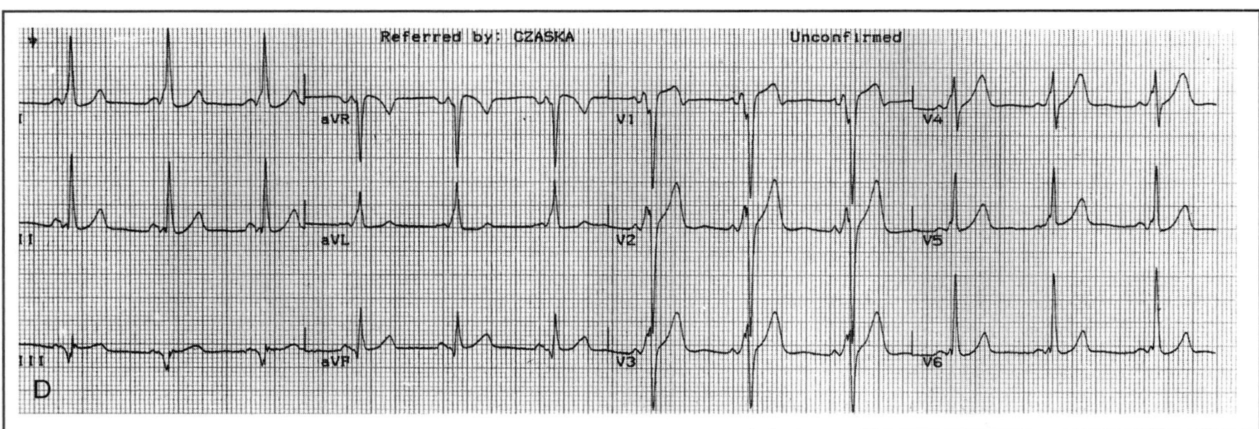

FIGURE 22–26 ***Continued C,*** **Left lateral accessory pathway. Positive delta wave in the anterior precordial leads and in leads II, III, and AVF, positive or isoelectric in lead I and AVL, and isoelectric or negative in V_5 and V_6 are typical of a left lateral accessory pathway. Rapid coronary sinus pacing (450 msec cycle length) was used to enhance preexcitation (negative P wave I, II, III, aVf, V_{3-6}). Location verified at surgery.**

D, **Right free wall accessory pathway. Predominantly negative delta wave in V_1 and axis more leftward than in panel *A* indicate the presence of a right free wall accessory pathway.**

Illustration continued on following page

this form of tachycardia acutely is as outlined for AV nodal reentry (see p. 664). It is necessary to achieve block of a single impulse from atrium to ventricle or ventricle to atrium. Generally, the most successful method is to produce transient AV nodal block; therefore, vagal maneuvers, IV adenosine, verapamil or diltiazem, digitalis, and beta blockers are acceptable choices. Radiofrequency catheter ablation and conventional antiarrhythmic agents that prolong activation time or refractory period in the accessory pathway need to be considered for chronic prophylactic therapy, similar to that discussed for reciprocating tachycardias associated with the preexcitation syndrome. Radiofrequency catheter ablation is curative, has low risk, and should be considered early for symptomatic patients[70,184,185,187–189] (see p. 621). The presence of atrial fibrillation in patients with a *concealed accessory pathway* should not be a greater therapeutic challenge than in patients who do not have such a pathway, because anterograde AV conduction occurs only over the AV node and not over an accessory pathway. Intravenous verapamil and digitalis are not contraindicated. However, it must be remembered that under some circumstances, such as catecholamine stimulation, anterograde conduction in the apparently concealed accessory pathway can occur.

Preexcitation Syndrome

ELECTROCARDIOGRAPHIC RECOGNITION (Fig. 22–26). Preexcitation or the Wolff-Parkinson-White electrocardiographic abnormality occurs when the atrial impulse activates the

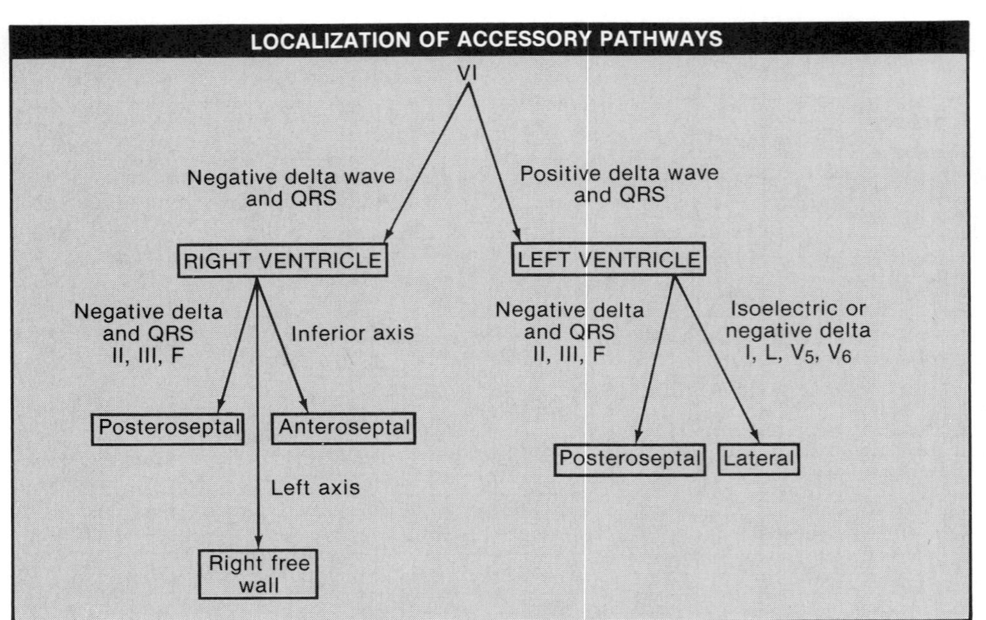

FIGURE 22–26 *Continued E,* Logic diagram to determine location of accessory pathways. Begin with analysis of V_1 to determine whether the delta wave and the QRS complex are negative or positive. That establishes the ventricle in which the accessory pathway is located. Next, determine whether the delta wave and QRS complex are negative in leads II, III and AVF. If so, then the accessory pathway is located in a posteroseptal position. If the accessory pathway is located in the right ventricle, an inferior axis indicates an anteroseptal location while left axis indicates a right free wall location. If the accessory pathway is located in the left ventricle, an isoelectric or negative delta wave and QRS complex in leads I, aVl, V_5, and V_6 indicate a left lateral (free wall) location.

whole or some part of the ventricle, or the ventricular impulse activates the whole or some part of the atrium, earlier than would be expected if the impulse traveled by way of the normal specialized conduction system only.[184,185] This is caused by muscular connections composed of working myocardial fibers that exist outside the specialized conducting tissue and connect the atrium and ventricle, bypassing AV nodal conduction delay. They are named *accessory atrioventricular pathways* or connections, commonly called *Kent bundles,* and are responsible for the most common variety of preexcitation (incidentally noted in other species such as monkeys, dogs, and cats). The term *syndrome* is attached to this disorder when tachyarrhythmias due to the accessory pathway occur. Three basic features typify the ECG abnormalities of patients with the usual form of WPW conduction caused by an AV connection: (1) P-R interval less than 120 msec during sinus rhythm, (2) QRS complex duration exceeding 120 msec with a slurred, slowly rising onset of the QRS in some leads (delta wave) and usually a normal terminal QRS portion, and (3) secondary ST-T wave changes that are generally directed opposite to the major delta and QRS vectors. Analysis of the scalar ECG can be used to localize the accessory pathway[190,191] (Fig. 22–26*D*). Body surface mapping can be useful.[192]

In the *Wolff-Parkinson-White* (WPW) *syndrome,* the most common tachycardia is characterized by a normal QRS, a regular rhythm, ventricular rates of 150 to 250 beats/min

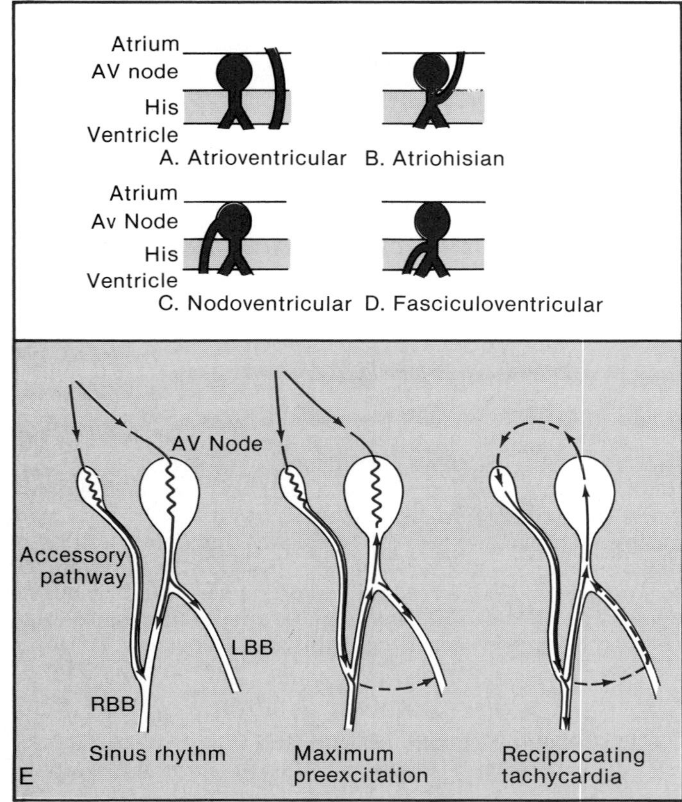

FIGURE 22–27. Schematic representation of accessory pathways. Panel A demonstrates the "usual" atrioventricular accessory pathway giving rise to most clinical presentations of tachycardia associated with Wolff-Parkinson-White syndrome. Panel B illustrates the very uncommon atriohisian accessory pathway. If the LGL syndrome exists, it would have this type of anatomy which has been demonstrated on occasion histopathologically. Panel C, nodoventricular pathways, original concept, in which anterograde conduction travels down the accessory pathway with retrograde conduction in the bundle branch–His bundle–AV node (see below). Panel D demonstrates the fasciculoventricular connections, not thought to play an important role in the genesis of tachycardias. Panel E illustrates the current concept of nodoventricular accessory pathway in which the accessory pathway is an atrioventricular communication with AV nodal–like properties. Sinus rhythm results in a fusion QRS complex, as in the usual form of WPW shown in panel A. Maximum preexcitation results in ventricular activation over the accessory pathway and the His bundle is activated retrogradely. During reciprocating tachycardia, anterograde conduction occurs over the accessory pathway with retrograde conduction over the normal pathway. (Panel E reproduced with permission from Benditt, D. G., and Milstein, S.: Nodoventricular accessory connection: A misnomer or a structural/functional spectrum. J. Cardiovasc. Electrophys. *1:*231, 1990.)

(generally faster than AV nodal reentry), and sudden onset and termination, behaving in most respects like the tachycardia described for conduction utilizing a concealed pathway (see p. 665). The major difference between the two is the capacity for anterograde conduction over the accessory pathway during atrial flutter or atrial fibrillation (see below).

Variants

A variety of other anatomical substrates exist that provide the basis for different ECG manifestations of several variations of the preexcitation syndrome[184] (Fig. 22–27). Fibers from atrium to His bundle bypassing the physiological delay of the AV node are called *atriohisian tracts* (Fig. 22–27*B*) and are associated with a short P-R interval and a normal QRS complex. Although demonstrated anatomically (see below), the electrophysiological significance of these tracts in the genesis of tachycardias with a short P-R interval and a normal QRS complex (Lown-Ganong-Levine, or LGL, syndrome) remains to be established. Indeed, evidence does *not* support the presence of a specific LGL syndrome comprising a short P-R interval, normal QRS complex, and tachycardias related to an atriohisian bypass tract.

Two varieties of Mahaim fibers include those passing from the AV node to the ventricle, called *nodoventricular fibers* (or nodofascicular if the insertion is into the right bundle branch rather than ventricular muscle (Fig. 22–27*C*), and those arising in the His bundle or bundle branches and inserting in the ventricular myocardium, called *fasciculoventricular fibers* (Fig. 22–27*D*). For nodoventricular connections, the P-R interval may be normal or short, and the QRS complex is a fusion beat. Nodoventricular connections can be involved in tachycardias, but fasciculoventricular pathways generally are not.

In patients who have an atriohisian tract, theoretically, the QRS complex would remain normal and the short A-H interval fixed or show very little increase during atrial pacing at more rapid rates. The author has found this response to be uncommon. Rapid atrial pacing in patients who have nodoventricular or nodofascicular connections shortens the H-V interval and widens the QRS complex, producing a left bundle branch block contour, but in contrast to the situation in patients who have an atrioventricular connection (Fig. 22–28), the A-V interval also lengthens. In patients who have fasciculoventricular connections, the H-V interval remains short and the QRS complex unchanged and anomalous during rapid atrial pacing.

ATRIOFASCICULAR ACCESSORY PATHWAYS. These fibers almost always represent a duplication of the AV node and the distal conducting system and are located in the right ventricular free wall. The apical end lies close to the lateral tricuspid annulus and conducts slowly, with AV node–like properties. After a long course, the distal portion of these fibers, which conducts rapidly, inserts into the distal right bundle branch or the apical region of the right ventricle.[184,193] No preexcitation is generally apparent during sinus rhythm but can be exposed by premature right atrial stimulation. The absence of retrograde conduction in these pathways produces only an antidromic AV reentry tachycardia ("preexcited" tachycardia) characterized by anterograde conduction over the accessory pathway and retrograde conduction over the right bundle branch–His bundle–AV node, making the atrium a necessary part of the circuit. The preexcited tachycardia has a left bundle branch block pattern, long A-V interval (due to the long conduction time over the accessory pathway), and short V-A interval. Right bundle branch block can be proarrhythmic by increasing the length of the tachycardia circuit (V-A interval prolongs due to delay in retrograde activation of the His bundle), and the tachycardia can become incessant.[184,193]

ELECTROPHYSIOLOGICAL FEATURES OF PREEXCITATION (Figs. 22–27 to 22–36; see also p. 665). If the Kent bundle accessory pathway is capable of anterograde conduction, two parallel routes of AV conduction are possible, one subject to physiological delay over the AV node and the other passing directly without delay from atrium to ventricle. This produces the typical QRS complex that is a fusion beat, due to depolarization of the ventricle in part by the wavefront traveling over the accessory pathway and in part by the wavefront traveling over the normal AV node–His bundle route. The delta wave represents ventricular activation from input over the accessory pathway. The extent of contribution to ventricular deplorization by the wavefront over each route depends on their relative activation times. If AV nodal conduction delay occurs, for example, because of a rapid atrial pacing rate or premature atrial complex, more of the ventricle becomes activated over the accessory pathway, and the QRS complex becomes more anomalous in contour. Total activation of the ventricle over the accessory pathway can occur if the AV nodal conduction delay is sufficiently long. In contrast, if the accessory pathway is relatively far from the sinus node, for example, a left lateral accessory pathway, or if AV nodal conduction time is relatively short, more of the ventricle may be activated by conduction over the normal pathway (Fig. 22–28). The normal fusion beat during sinus rhythm has a short H-V interval, or His bundle activation actually begins after the onset of ventricular depolarization, because part of the atrial impulse bypasses the AV node and activates the ventricle early, at a time when the atrial impulse traveling the nor-

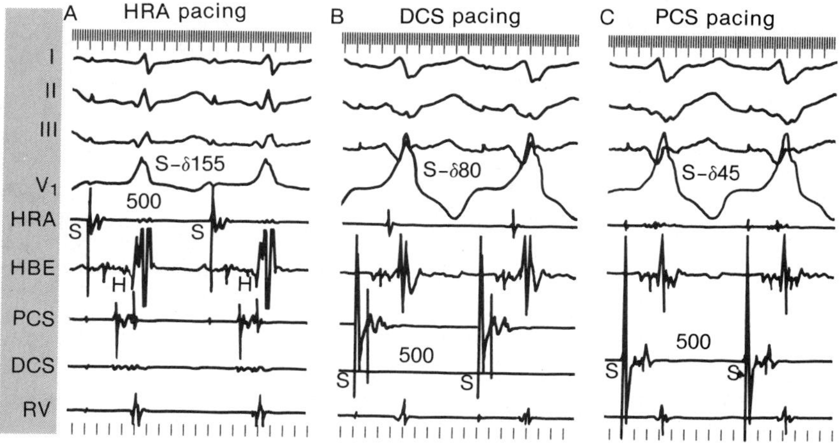

FIGURE 22–28. **Atrial pacing at different atrial sites illustrating different conduction over the accessory pathway. In panel A, high right atrial pacing at a cycle length of 500 msec produces anomalous activation of the ventricle (note upright QRS complex in V_1) and a stimulus-delta interval of 155 msec. This indicates that the time from the onset of the stimulus to the beginning of the QRS complex is relatively long because the stimulus is delivered at a fairly large distance from the accessory pathway. Note that the His bundle activation (H) occurs at about the onset of the QRS complex. In panel B atrial pacing occurs through the distal coronary sinus electrode (DCS). At the same pacing cycle length, DCS pacing results in more anomalous ventricular activation and a shorter stimulus-delta interval (80 msec). His bundle activation is now buried within the inscription of the ventricular electrogram in the HBE lead. Panel C, Pacing from the proximal coronary sinus electrode (PCS) results in the shortest stimulus-delta interval (45 msec) indicating that the pacing stimulus is being delivered very close to the atrial insertion of the accessory pathway, which is located in the left posteroseptal region of the atrioventricular groove.**

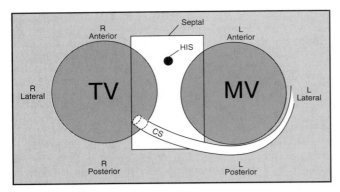

FIGURE 22–29. Schematic representation of the tricuspid (TV) and mitral (MV) valves, and the position of the coronary sinus (CS). This figure indicates the quadrants in which accessory pathways can be located. (Reproduced with permission from Miles, W. M., Zipes, D. P., and Klein, L. S.: Ablation of free wall accessory pathways. *In* Zipes, D. P. [eds.]: Catheter Ablation of Arrhythmias. Armonk, N.Y., Futura, 1994, p. 212.)

mal route just reaches the His bundle. This finding of a short or negative H-V interval occurs *only* during conduction over an accessory pathway or from retrograde His activation during a complex originating in the ventricle, such as a ventricular tachycardia.

Pacing the atrium at rapid rates, at premature intervals, or from a site close to the atrial insertion of the Kent bundle accentuates the anomalous activation of the ventricles and shortens the H-V interval even more (His activation may become buried in the ventricular electrogram, as in Fig. 22–28*B*). The position of the accessory pathway can be determined by a careful analysis of the spatial direction of the delta wave in the 12-lead ECG in maximally preexcited beats[190,191] (Figs. 22–26 and 22–29). T-wave abnormalities can occur after disappearance of preexcitation with orientation of the T wave according to the site of preexcitation (T-wave memory). A variety of electrical (Fig. 22–30), radionuclide, and echocardiographic techniques can be used to localize the insertion site of the accessory pathway (Chap. 21). The location of the pathway may be associated with specific electrophysiological responses.[194]

KENT BUNDLE CONDUCTION. Even though the Kent bundle conducts more rapidly than does the AV node (conduction velocity is faster in the accessory pathway), the Kent bundle usually has a longer refractory period during long cycle lengths (e.g., sinus rhythm)—i.e., it takes longer for the accessory pathway to recover excitability than it does for the AV node. Consequently, a premature atrial complex can occur sufficiently early to block anterogradely in the accessory pathway and conduct to the ventricle only over the normal AV node–His bundle (Figs. 22–31*A,B* and 20–34). The resultant H-V interval and the QRS complex become normal. Such an event can initiate the most common type of reciprocating tachycardia, which is characterized by anterograde conduction over the normal pathway and retrograde conduction over the accessory pathway *(orthodromic AV reciprocating tachycardia)* (Figs. 22–31 and 20–34). The accessory pathway, blocking in an anterograde direction, recovers excitability in time to be activated following the QRS complex, in a retrograde direction, completing the reentrant loop.

Much less commonly, patients can have tachycardias called *antidromic* tachycardias during which anterograde conduction occurs over the accessory pathway and retrograde conduction over the AV node. The resultant QRS complex is abnormal owing to total ventricular activation over the accessory pathway (Figs. 22–31*C* and 22–32). In both tachycardias, the accessory pathway is an obligatory part of the reentrant circuit. In patients with bidirectional conduction over the accessory pathway, different fibers may be used anterogradely and retrogradely.

Five to ten per cent of patients have multiple accessory pathways often suggested by various ECG clues, and on occasion, tachycardia can be due to a reentrant loop conducting anterogradely over one accessory pathway and retrogradely over the other. Interestingly, 15 to 20 per cent of patients may exhibit AV nodal echoes or AV nodal reentry after interruption of the accessory pathway.

PERMANENT FORM OF AV JUNCTIONAL RECIPROCATING TACHYCARDIA (PJRT). An incessant form of supraventricular tachycardia has been recognized that generally occurs with a long R-P interval that exceeds the P-R interval (Figs. 22–33 and 22–34). Usually, a posteroseptal accessory pathway (most often right ventricular but other locations as well[194a]) that conducts very slowly, possibly due to a long and tortuous route, appears responsible. Tachycardia is maintained by anterograde AV nodal conduction and retrograde conduction over the accessory pathway (Fig. 22–31*D*). While anterograde conduction over this pathway has been demonstrated, the long anterograde conduction time over the accessory pathway ordinarily prevents ECG manifestations of accessory pathway conduction during sinus rhythm. Therefore, during sinus rhythm, the QRS is prolonged from conduction over this accessory pathway only when conduction times

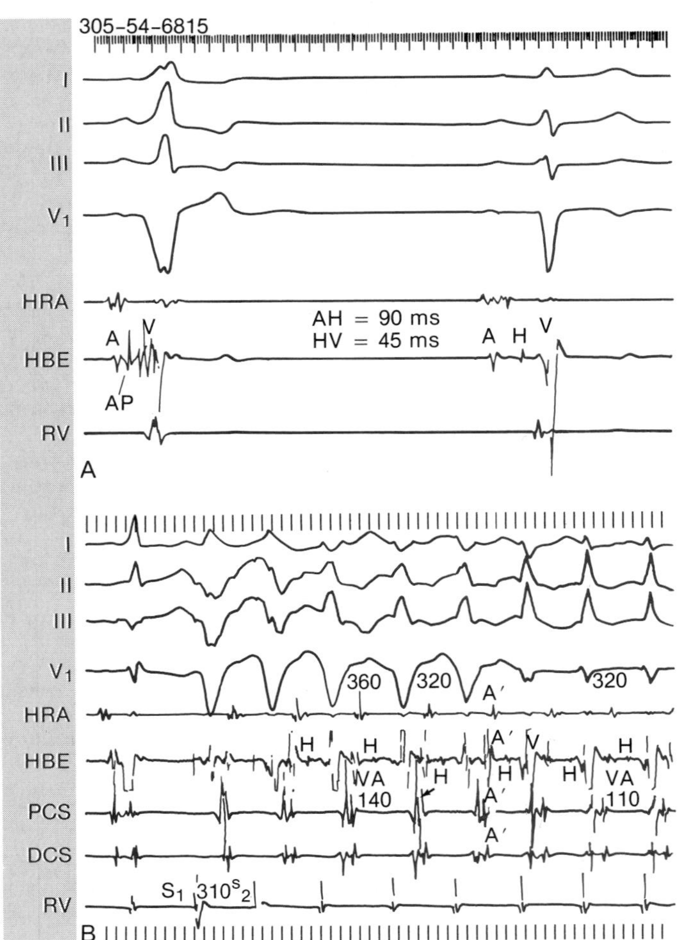

FIGURE 22–30. *A*, Recording of depolarization of an accessory pathway (AP) with a catheter electrode. The first QRS complex illustrates conduction over the accessory pathway (AP). In the scalar ECG a short P-R interval and delta wave (best seen in leads I and V_1) are apparent. His bundle activation is buried within the ventricular complex. In the following complex, conduction has blocked over the accessory pathway and a normal QRS complex results. His bundle activation clearly precedes the onset of ventricular depolarization by 45 msec. The A-H interval for this complex is 90 msec. (From Prystowsky, E. N., Browne, K. F., and Zipes, D. P.: Intracardiac recording by catheter electrode of accessory pathway depolarization. Reprinted with permission from the American College of Cardiology. J. Am. Coll. Cardiol. *1*:468, 1983.)

B, Influence of functional ipsilateral bundle branch block on the V-A interval during an atrioventricular reciprocating tachycardia (AVRT). Partial preexcitation can be noted in the sinus-initiated complex (first complex). Two premature ventricular stimuli (S_1, S_2) initiate a sustained supraventricular tachycardia that persists with a left bundle branch block for several complexes, finally reverting to normal. The retrograde atrial activation sequence is recorded first in the proximal coronary sinus lead (arrow, PCS), then in the distal coronary sinus lead (DCS) and low right atrium (HBE) and then high right atrium (HRA). During the functional bundle branch block, the V-A interval in the PCS lead is 140 msec, shortening to 110 msec when the QRS complex reverts to normal. Such behavior is characteristic of a left-sided accessory pathway with prolongation of the reentrant pathway by the functional left bundle branch block.

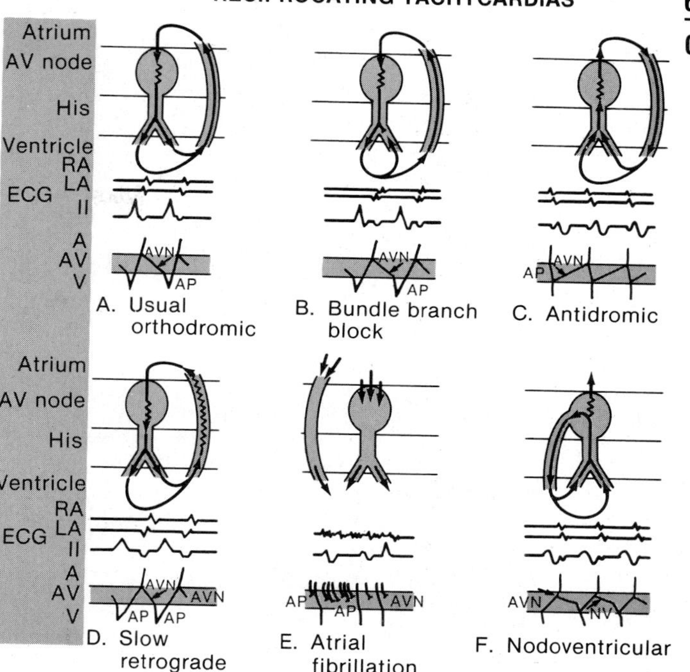

FIGURE 22–31. Schematic diagram of tachycardias associated with accessory pathways. Format as in Figure 22–11. *A*, Orthodromic tachycardia with anterograde conduction over the AV node–His bundle route and retrograde conduction over the accessory pathway (left-sided for this example as depicted by LA activation preceding RA activation). *B*, Orthodromic tachycardia and ipsilateral functional bundle branch block. *C*, Antidromic tachycardia with anterograde conduction over the accessory pathway and retrograde conduction over the AV node–His bundle. *D*, Orthodromic tachycardia with a slowly conducting accessory pathway. *E*, Atrial fibrillation with the accessory pathway as a bystander. *F*, Anterograde conduction over a portion of the AV node and a nodoventricular pathway and retrograde conduction over the AV node.

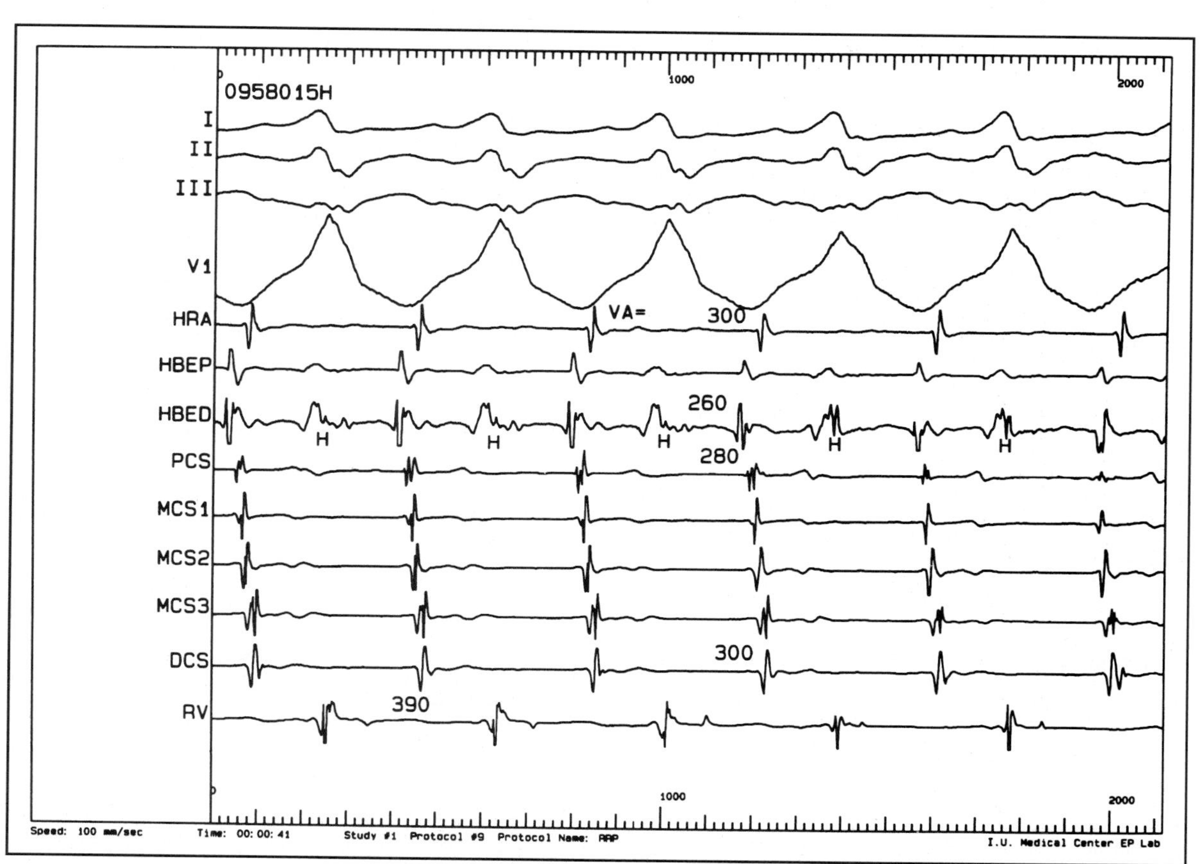

FIGURE 22–32. Antidromic atrioventricular reciprocating tachycardia. Tachycardia in this example is due to anterograde conduction over the accessory pathway (note the abnormal QRS complex of a left posterior accessory pathway) and a normal retrograde atrial activation sequence (beginning first in the HBED lead) due to retrograde conduction over the atrioventricular node. Tachycardia cycle length is 390 msec, with a VA interval of 300 msec measured in the high right atrial lead, 260 msec in the distal His lead and 280 msec in the proximal coronary sinus lead. I, II, III, and V_1 are scalar leads; HRA, high right atrial electrogram; HBEP and HBED leads are His bundle electrogram proximal and distal, respectively; PCS, proximal coronary sinus; MCS1-3, midcoronary sinus leads; DCS, distal coronary sinus lead; RV, right ventricular electrogram.

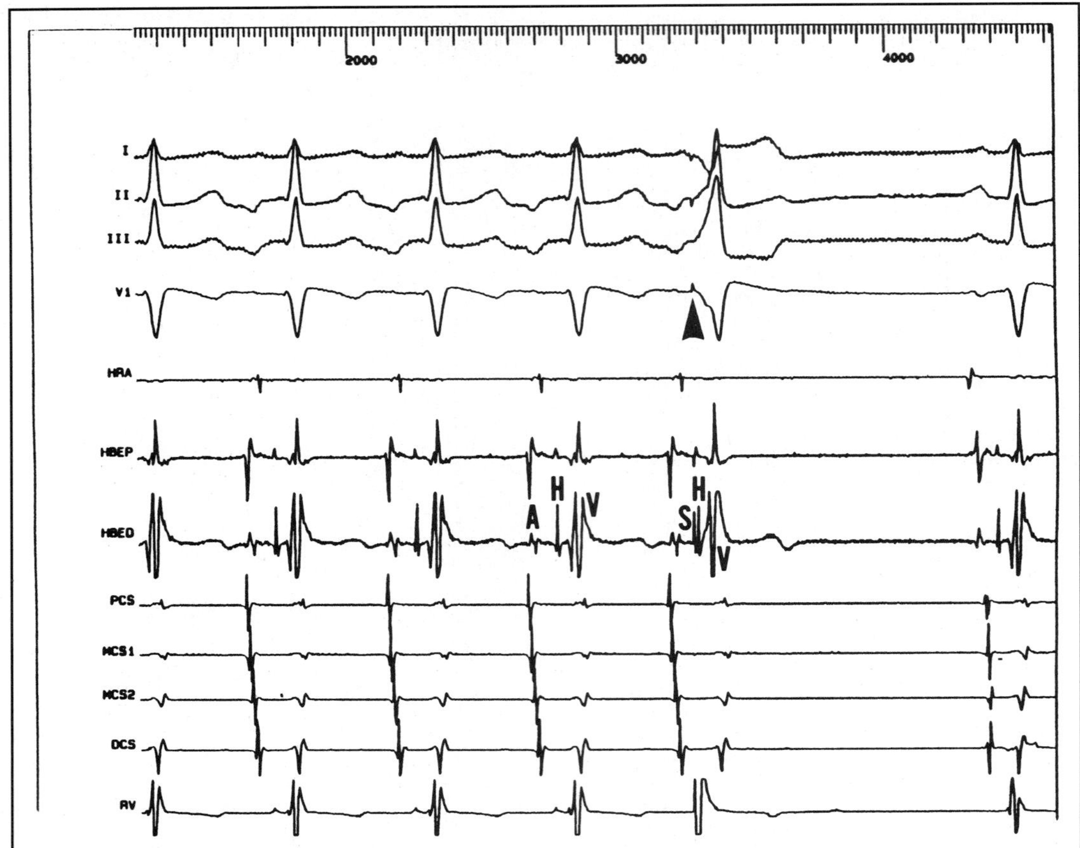

FIGURE 22–33. Termination of the permanent form of AV junctional reciprocating tachycardia (PJRT). In the left portion of this example, PJRT is present. The atrial activation sequence is indistinguishable from atypical AV nodal reentry and atrial tachycardia originating in the low right atrium. The response to premature stimulation(s) identifies the tachycardia as PJRT. Premature ventricular stimulation (arrowhead) occurs at a time when the His bundle is refractory from depolarization during the tachycardia (second labeled H). Therefore, premature ventricular stimulation cannot enter the AV node. Further, premature ventricular stimulation does not reach the atrium. Yet premature ventricular stimulation terminates the tachycardia. This can only be explained by the premature ventricular complex invading and blocking in a retrogradely conducting accessory pathway. I, II, III, and V_1 are scalar ECG leads; HRA, high right atrial electrogram; HBEP, HBED, His bundle electrogram proximal and distal, respectively; PCS, proximal coronary sinus electrogram; MCS1, MCS2, midcoronary sinus electrograms; DCS, distal coronary sinus electrograms; RV, right ventricular electrogram.

through the AV node–His bundle exceed those in the accessory pathway.[184,185]

RECOGNITION OF ACCESSORY PATHWAYS. When retrograde atrial activation during tachycardia occurs over an accessory pathway that connects the left atrium to the left ventricle, the earliest retrograde activity is recorded from a left atrial electrode usually positioned in the coronary sinus (Fig. 22–25). When retrograde atrial activation during tachycardia occurs over an accessory pathway that connects the right ventricle to the right atrium, the earliest retrograde atrial activity generally is recorded from a lateral right atrial electrode. Participation of a septal accessory pathway creates earliest retrograde atrial activation in the low right atrium situated near the septum, anterior or posterior, depending on the insertion site. These mapping techniques with catheter electrodes and at the time of surgery (see p. 583) provide accurate assessments of the position of the accessory pathway, which can be anywhere in the AV groove except in the intervalvular trigone between the mitral valve and the aortic valve annuli. Recording electrical activity directly from the accessory pathway obviously provides precise localization (Fig. 22–30*A*).

It may be difficult to distinguish AV nodal reentry from participation of a septal accessory connection using the retrograde sequence of atrial activation because activation sequences during both tachycardias are similar. Other approaches to demonstrate retrograde atrial activation over the accessory pathway must be tried and can be accomplished by inducing premature ventricular complexes during tachycardia to determine whether retrograde atrial excitation can occur from the ventricle at a time when the His bundle is refractory (Fig. 22–25*B*). Since ventriculoatrial conduction cannot occur over the normal conduction system because the His bundle is refractory, an accessory pathway must be present for the atria to become excited and is most likely participating in the tachycardia circuit. No patient with a reciprocating tachycardia due to an accessory AV pathway has a V-A interval of less than 70 msec measured from the onset of ventricular depolarization to the onset of the earliest atrial activity recorded on an esophageal lead or of less than 95 msec when measured to the high right atrium. In contrast, in the majority of patients with reentry in the AV node, intervals from the onset of ventricular activity to the earliest onset of atrial activity recorded in the esophageal lead are less than 70 msec.

OTHER FORMS OF TACHYCARDIA IN PATIENTS WITH WPW SYNDROME

Patients can have other types of tachycardia during which the accessory pathway is a "bystander," i.e., uninvolved in the mechanism responsible for the tachycardia, such as AV nodal reentry or an atrial tachycardia that conducts to the ventricle over the accessory pathway. In patients with atrial flutter or atrial fibrillation, the accessory pathway is not a requisite part of the mechanism responsible for tachycardia, and the flutter or fibrillation occurs in the atrium unrelated to the accessory pathway (Fig. 22–31*E*). Propagation to the ventricle during atrial flutter or atrial fibrillation therefore can occur over the normal AV node–His bundle or accessory pathway. Patients with WPW syndrome who have atrial fibrillation almost always have inducible reciprocating tachycardias as well, which can develop into the atrial fibrillation (Fig. 22–35). In fact, interruption of the accessory pathway and elimination of AV reciprocating tachycardia usually prevent recurrence of the atrial fibrillation. Atrial fibrillation presents a potentially serious risk because of the possibility for very rapid conduction over the accessory pathway. At more rapid rates, the refractory period of the accessory pathway can shorten significantly and permit an extremely rapid ventricular response during atrial flutter or atrial fibrillation (Figs. 22–26*B* and 22–30) that can lead to ventricular fibrillation. The rapid ventricular response can exceed the ability of the ventricle to follow in an organized manner, resulting in fragmented, disorganized ventricular activation and hypotension, and can lead to ventricular fibrillation (Fig. 22–36). Alternatively, supraventricular discharge bypassing AV nodal delay can activate the ventricle during the vulnerable period of the antecedent T wave and precipitate ventricular fibrillation. Patients who have had ventricular fibrilla-

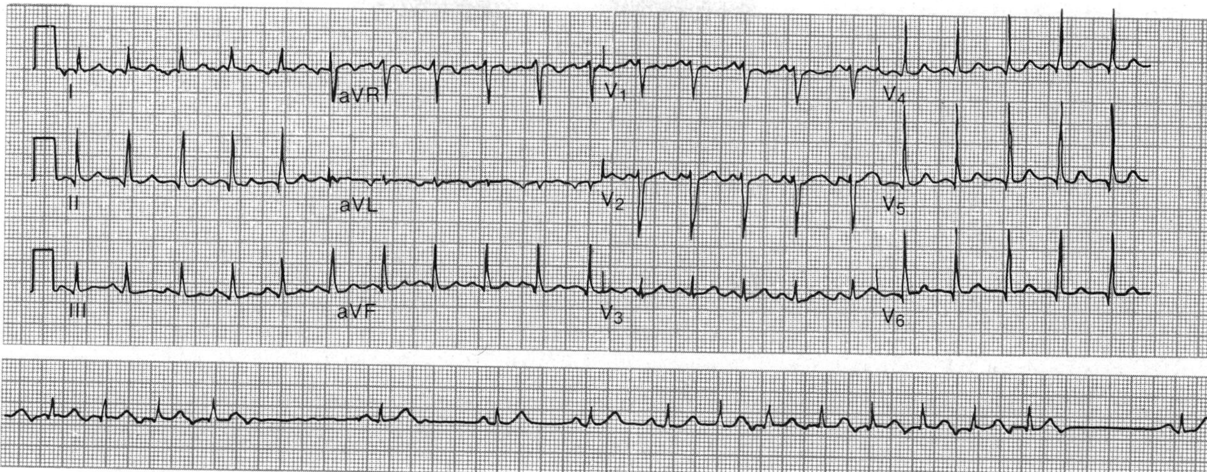

FIGURE 22–34. Permanent form of junctional reciprocating tachycardia (PJRT) in a patient with a left-sided accessory pathway. The 12-lead ECG demonstrates a long R-P interval–short PR interval tachycardia, which, in contrast to the usual form of PJRT, exhibits negative P waves in leads I and aVL. The rhythm strips below (lead I) indicate that whenever a nonconducted P wave occurs, the tachycardia always terminates, only to begin again after several sinus beats. This is in marked contrast to Figure 22–13, in which the tachycardia continues despite nonconducted P waves.

tion have ventricular cycle lengths during atrial fibrillation in the range of 200 msec or less.

Patients with preexcitation syndrome can have other causes of tachycardia such as AV nodal reentry, sometimes with dual AV nodal curves, sinus nodal reentry, or even ventricular tachycardia unrelated to the accessory pathway. Some accessory pathways can conduct anterogradely only, and others retrogradely only. If the pathway conducts only anterogradely, it cannot participate in the usual form of reciprocating tachycardia (Fig. 22–31*A*). It can, however, participate in antidromic tachycardia (Fig. 22–31*C*) as well as conduct to the ventricle during atrial flutter or atrial fibrillation (Fig. 22–31*E*). Some data suggest that the accessory pathway demonstrates automatic activity, which could conceivably be responsible for some instances of tachycardia.

"WIDE QRS TACHYCARDIAS." In patients with the preexcitation syndrome, so-called wide QRS tachycardias can be due to multiple mechanisms, including sinus or atrial tachycardias, AV nodal reentry, atrial flutter or fibrillation with anterograde conduction over the accessory pathway; orthodromic reciprocating tachycardia with functional or preexisting bundle branch block; antidromic reciprocating tachycardia; reciprocating tachycardia with anterograde conduction over one accessory pathway and retrograde conduction over a second one; tachycardias using Mahaim fibers; or ventricular tachycardia.[195]

CLINICAL FEATURES. The reported incidence of preexcitation syndrome depends on large measure on the population studied, varying from 0.1 to 3.0 per thousand in apparently healthy subjects, with an average of about 1.5 per thousand. The incidence of the electrocardiographic pattern of WPW conduction in 22,500 healthy aviation personnel was 0.25 per cent with a prevalence of documented tachyarrhythmias of 1.8 per cent. Left free wall accessory pathways are most common, followed in frequency by posteroseptal, right free wall, and anteroseptal locations. WPW syndrome is found in all age groups, from fetal and neonatal periods to the elderly, and in identical twins. The prevalence is higher in males and decreases with age, apparently due to loss of preexcitation. The majority of adults with preexcitation syndrome have normal hearts, although a variety of acquired and congenital cardiac defects have been reported, including Ebstein's anomaly,[196] mitral valve prolapse,[197] and cardiomyopathies. Patients with Ebstein's anomaly (see p. 934) often have multiple accessory pathways, right-sided either in the posterior septum or posterolateral wall, with preexcitation localized to the atrialized ventricle. They often have reciprocating tachycardia with a long V-A interval and a right bundle branch block morphology.

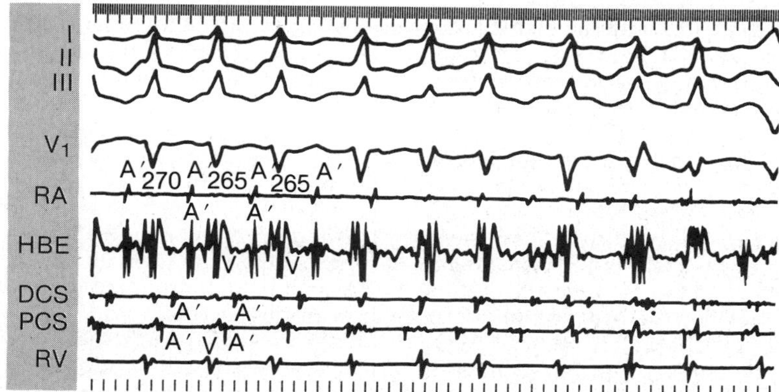

FIGURE 22–35. AV reciprocating tachycardia disorganizing into atrial fibrillation. During sustained atrioventricular reciprocating tachycardia at a cycle length of approximately 265 msec, retrograde atrial activation sequence began first in the right paraseptal region (not shown in this example; location proven at surgery) and was then recorded in the proximal coronary sinus electrogram, followed by atrial activity in the distal coronary sinus, in the low right atrium recorded in the His bundle lead and then in the high right atrium. Spontaneously, the atrial activation sequence becomes irregular (after the last A′) and atrial fibrillation begins. Note that the last QRS complex reflects conduction over the accessory pathway. Such a transformation occurred repeatedly in this patient and was associated with a quickening of the ventricular rate. Atrial fibrillation did not recur following surgical interruption of the accessory pathway.

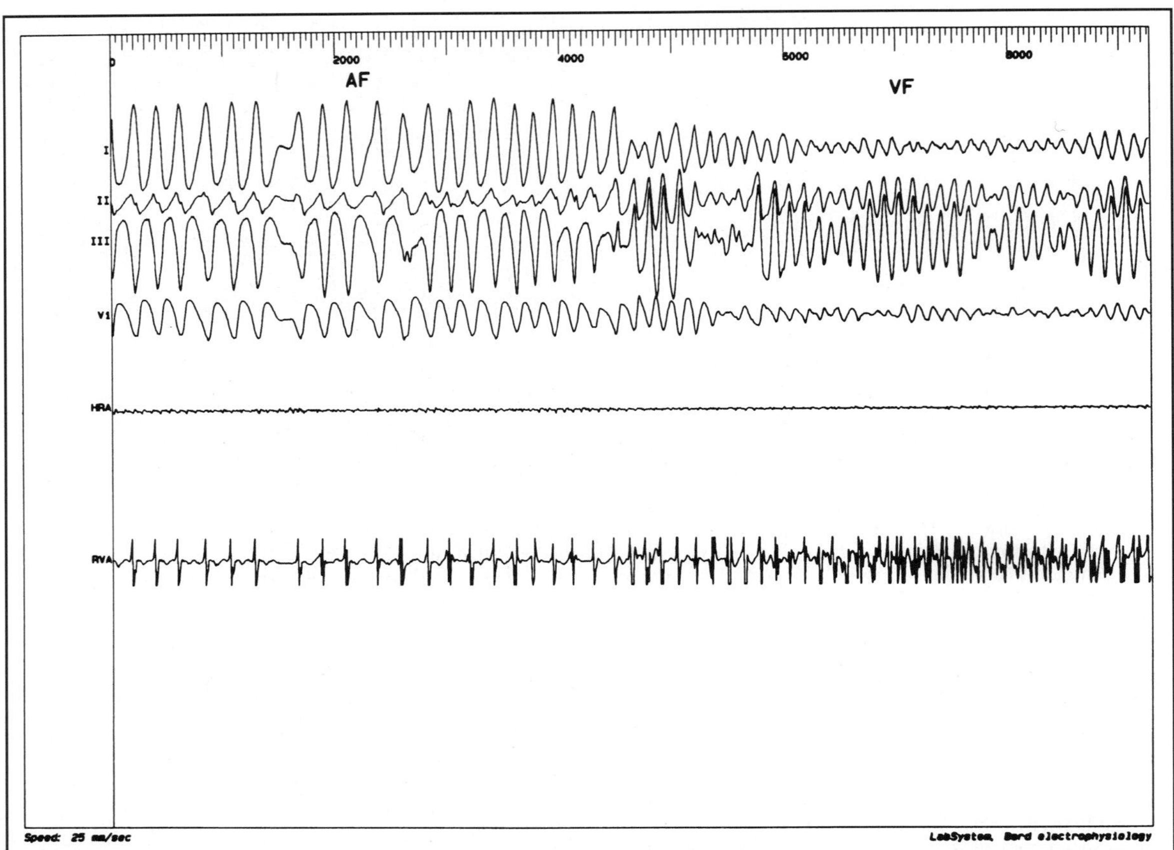

FIGURE 22–36. Atrial fibrillation becoming ventricular fibrillation. In the left portion of this panel, the ECG demonstrates atrial fibrillation with conduction over an accessory pathway producing a rapid ventricular response, at times in excess of 350 beats/min. In the midportion of the tracing, ventricular fibrillation develops. I, II, III, and V_1 are scalar ECG leads; HRA, high right atrial electrogram; RVA, right ventricular apex electrogram; AF, atrial fibrillation; VF, ventricular fibrillation.

The frequency of paroxysmal tachycardia apparently increases with age, from 10 per 100 patients with WPW syndrome in a 20- to 39-year age group to 36 per 100 in patients more than 60 years old. Approximately 80 per cent of patients with tachycardia have a reciprocating tachycardia, 15 to 30 per cent have atrial fibrillation, and 5 per cent atrial flutter. Ventricular tachycardia occurs uncommonly. The anomalous complexes can mask or mimic myocardial infarction (see p. 135), bundle branch block, or ventricular hypertrophy, and the presence of the preexcitation syndrome can call attention to an associated cardiac defect. The prognosis is excellent in patients without tachycardia or an associated cardiac anomaly. For most patients with recurrent tachycardia the prognosis is good, but sudden death occurs rarely,[198] with an estimated frequency of <0.1 per cent.[199]

It is very likely that an accessory pathway is congenital, although its manifestations can be detected in later years and appear to be "acquired." Relatives of patients with preexcitation, particularly those with multiple pathways, have an increased prevalence of preexcitation, suggesting a hereditary mode of acquisition. Some children and adults can lose their tendency to develop tachyarrhythmias as they grow older, possibly owing to fibrotic or other changes at the site of the accessory pathway insertion. Pathways can lose their ability to conduct anterogradely. Tachycardia beginning in infancy can disappear but frequently recurs. Tachycardia still present after age 5 years persists in 75 per cent of patients, regardless of accessory pathway location. Intermittent preexcitation during sinus rhythm and abrupt loss of conduction over the accessory pathway after intravenous ajmaline or procainamide and with exercise suggest that the refractory period of the accessory pathway is long and that the patient is not at risk of developing a rapid ventricular rate should atrial flutter or fibrillation develop. These approaches are relatively specific, but not very sensitive, with a low positive predictive accuracy. Exceptions to these safeguards can occur.

TREATMENT. Patients with ventricular preexcitation who have only the electrocardiographic abnormality, without tachyarrhythmias, do not require electrophysiological evaluation or therapy. However, for the patient with frequent episodes of symptomatic tachyarrhythmias, therapy should be initiated.

Three therapeutic options exist: electrical (see p. 619) or surgical (see p. 628) ablation and pharmacological therapy. Drugs are chosen to prolong conduction time and/or refractoriness in the AV node, the accessory pathway, or both to prevent rapid rates from occurring. If successful, this would prevent maintenance of an AV reciprocating tachycardia or a rapid ventricular response to atrial flutter or atrial fibrillation. Some drugs might suppress premature complexes that precipitate the arrhythmias.

Adenosine, verapamil, propranolol, and digitalis all prolong conduction time and refractoriness in the AV node. Verapamil and propranolol do not directly affect conduction in the accessory pathway, while digitalis has had variable effects. Because digitalis has been reported to shorten refractoriness in the accessory pathway and speed the ventricular response in some patients with atrial fibrillation, it is advisable *not* to use digitalis as a single drug in patients with the WPW syndrome who have or may develop atrial flutter or atrial fibrillation. Since many patients can develop atrial fibrillation *during* the reciprocating tachycardia (Fig. 22–35), this caveat probably applies to *all* patients who have tachycardia and WPW syndrome. Rather, drugs that prolong the refractory period in the accessory pathway such as class IA and IC drugs (Chap. 21) should be used.

Class IC[200,201] drugs, amiodarone[202], and sotalol can affect both the AV node and the accessory pathway. Lidocaine does not prolong refractoriness of the accessory pathway in patients whose effective refractory period is ≤300 msec. Verapamil and IV lidocaine can *increase* the ventricular rate during atrial fibrillation in patients with the WPW syndrome. Intravenous verapamil can precipitate *ventricular fibrillation* when given to a patient with the WPW syndrome who has a rapid ventricular rate during atrial fibrillation. This does not appear to happen with *oral* verapamil. Catecholamines can expose WPW syndromes, shorten the refractory period of the accessory pathway, and reverse the effects of some antiarrhythmic drugs.[203]

Termination of an Acute Episode. Termination of the acute episode of reciprocating tachycardia, suspected electrocardiographically from a normal QRS complex, regular R-R intervals, a rate of about 200 beats/min, and a retrograde P wave in the ST segment, should be approached as for AV nodal reentry. After vagal maneuvers, adenosine followed by intravenous verapamil or diltiazem is the initial treatment of choice. It is important to note that atrial fibrillation can occur after drug administration, particularly adenosine, with a rapid ventricular response. An external cardioverter-defibrillator should be immediately available if necessary. For atrial flutter or fibrillation, the latter suspected from an anomalous QRS complex and grossly irregular R-R intervals (Figs. 22–26*B* and 22–35), drugs that prolong refractoriness in the accessory pathway, often coupled with drugs that prolong AV nodal refractoriness (e.g., procainamide and propranolol), must be used. In many patients, particularly those with a very rapid ventricular response and any signs of hemodynamic impairment, electrical cardioversion is the *initial* treatment of choice.

Prevention. For long-term therapy to prevent a recurrence, it is not always possible to predict which drugs may be most effective for an individual patient. Some drugs actually can increase the frequency of episodes of reciprocating tachycardia by prolonging the duration of anterograde and not retrograde refractory periods of the accessory pathway, thereby making it easier for a premature atrial complex to block anterogradely in the accessory pathway and initiate tachycardia. Oral administration of two drugs, such as quinidine and propranolol or procainamide and verapamil, to decrease conduction capabilities in both limbs of the reentrant circuit can be beneficial. Class IC drugs, amiodarone, or sotalol, which prolong refractoriness in both the accessory pathway and the AV node, can be effective.[204,205] Depending on the clinical situation, empirical drug trials or serial electrophysiological drug testing can be employed to determine optimal drug therapy for patients with reciprocating tachycardia. For patients who have atrial fibrillation with a rapid ventricular response, induction of atrial fibrillation while the patient is receiving therapy is essential to be certain that the ventricular rate is controlled. Patients who have accessory pathways with very short refractory periods may be poor candidates for drug therapy, since the refractory periods may be prolonged insignificantly in response to the standard agents.

Electrical or Surgical Ablation (see Chap. 21). Radiofrequency catheter ablation of the accessory pathway is advisable for patients with frequent symptomatic arrhythmias that are not fully controlled by drugs, in patients who are drug intolerant, or in those who do not wish to take drugs. This option should be considered early in the course of therapy of the symptomatic patient because of its high success rate and low frequency of complications and potential cost-effectiveness.[63,65,70,206–208] Rarely, surgical interruption of the accessory pathway may be necessary[209,210] (see p. 631).

Summary of Supraventricular Tachycardias

Electrocardiographic clues are often present that permit differentiation among the various supraventricular tachycardias. P waves during tachycardia identical to sinus P waves and occurring with a long R-P interval and a short P-R interval are most likely due to sinus nodal reentry. Retrograde (inverted in II, III, and aV_f) P waves generally represent reentry involving the AV junction, either AV nodal reentry or reciprocating tachycardia using a paraseptal accessory pathway. Tachycardia without manifest P waves is probably due to AV nodal reentry (P waves buried in QRS), while a tachycardia with an R-P interval exceeding 60 to 70 msec may be due to an accessory pathway. AV dissociation or AV block during tachycardia excludes the presence of a functioning AV accessory pathway and makes AV nodal reentry less likely. Multiple tachycardias can occur at different times in the same patient. QRS alternans, thought to be a feature of AV reciprocating tachycardia, is more likely a rapid rate–related phenomenon, independent of the tachycardia mechanism. RP-PR relationships (Table 22–3) help differentiate supraventricular tachycardias.

TABLE 22–3 SUPRAVENTRICULAR TACHYCARDIAS

SHORT R-P/LONG P-R	LONG R-P/SHORT P-R
AV node reentry	Atrial tachycardia
AV reentry	Sinus node reentry Atypical AV node reentry AVRT with a slowly conducting accessory pathway (e.g., PJRT)

VENTRICULAR RHYTHM DISTURBANCES

Premature Ventricular Complexes

ELECTROCARDIOGRAPHIC RECOGNITION. A premature ventricular complex is characterized by the premature occurrence of a QRS complex that is bizarre in shape and has a duration usually exceeding the dominant QRS complex, generally greater than 120 msec. The T wave is commonly large and opposite in direction to the major deflection of the QRS. The QRS complex is not preceded by a premature P wave but can be preceded by a nonconducted sinus P wave occurring at its expected time. The diagnosis of a premature ventricular complex can never be made with unequivocal certainty from the scalar electrocardiogram, since a supraventricular beat or rhythm can mimic the manifestations of ventricular arrhythmia (Figs. 22–19 and 22–37). Retrograde transmission to the atria from the premature ventricular complex occurs fairly frequently but is often obscured by the distorted QRS complex and T wave. If the retrograde impulse discharges and resects the sinus node prematurely, it produces a pause that is not fully compensatory. More commonly, the sinus node and atria are not discharged prematurely by the retrograde impulse, since interference of impulses frequently occurs at the AV junction (see p. 692), establishing a collision between the anterograde impulse conducted from the sinus node and the retrograde impulse conducted from the premature ventricular complex. Therefore, a fully compensatory pause usually follows a premature ventricular complex: the R-R interval produced by the two sinus-initiated QRS complexes on either side of the premature complex equals twice the normally conducted R-R interval. The premature ventricular complex may not produce any pause and may therefore be interpolated (Fig. 22–37*E*), or it may produce a postponed compensatory pause when an interpolated premature complex causes P-R prolongation of the first postextrasystolic beat to such a degree that the P wave of the second postextrasystolic beat occurs at a very short R-P interval and is therefore blocked.[211]

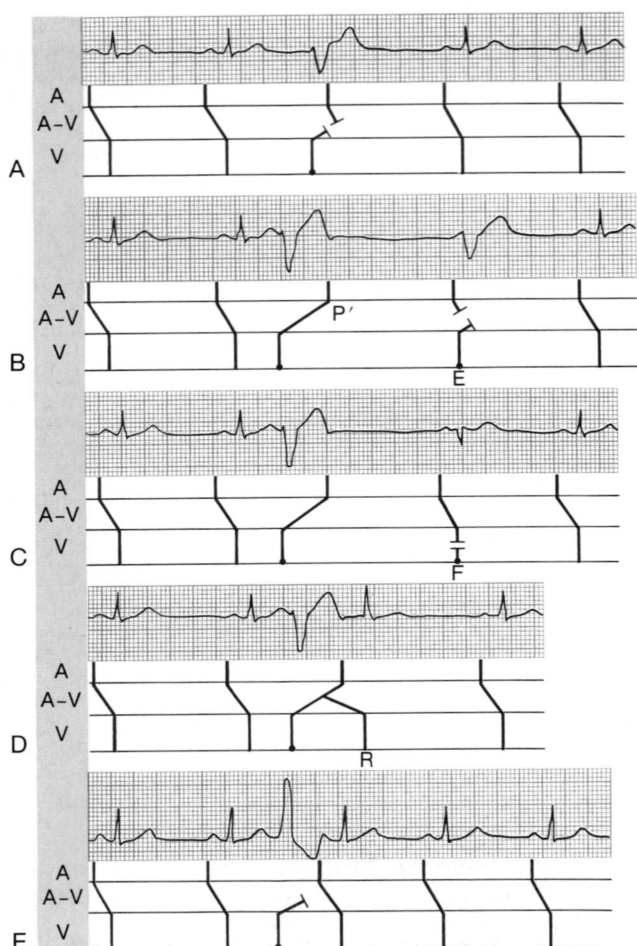

FIGURE 22–37. Premature ventricular complexes. *A* to *D* were recorded in the same patient. *A,* A late premature ventricular complex results in a compensatory pause. *B,* A slower sinus rate and a slightly earlier premature complex results in retrograde atrial excitation (P′). The sinus node is reset, producing a noncompensatory pause. Before the sinus-initiated P wave that follows the retrograde P wave can conduct to the ventricle, a ventricular escape (E) occurs. *C,* Events are similar to those in *B* except that a ventricular fusion beat (F) results following the premature ventricular complex owing to a slightly faster sinus rate. *D,* The impulse propagating retrogradely to the atrium reverses its direction after a delay and returns to reexcite the ventricles (R) to produce a ventricular echo. *E,* An interpolated premature ventricular complex is followed by a slightly prolonged P-R interval of the sinus-initiated beat. Lead II.

Interference within the ventricle can result in *ventricular fusion beats* (see p. 712) due to the simultaneous activation of the ventricle by two foci, one of them from the supraventricular impulse and the other from the premature ventricular complex. On occasion, a fusion beat can be narrower than the dominant sinus beat. This occurs when a right bundle branch block pattern of a premature ventricular complex arising in the left ventricle fuses with the sinus-initiated complex conducting through the AV junction or when the ventricle with a left bundle branch block pattern is paced artificially, producing a narrow ventricular fusion beat between the paced and the sinus-conducted beats. Narrow premature ventricular complexes also have been explained as originating at a point equidistant from each ventricle in the ventricular septum and by arising high in the fascicular system. Whether a compensatory or noncompensatory pause, retrograde atrial excitation, or an interpolated complex, fusion complex, or echo beat occurs (Fig. 22–37), it is merely a function of how the AV junction conducts and the timing of the events taking place.

The term *bigeminy* refers to pairs of complexes and indicates a normal and premature complex; *trigeminy* indicates a premature complex following two normal beats; a premature complex following three normal beats is called *quadrigeminy;* and so on. Two successive premature ventricular complexes are termed a *pair* or a *couplet,* while three successive premature ventricular complexes are called a *triplet.* Arbitrarily, three or more successive premature ventricular complexes are termed *ventricular tachycardia.* Premature ventricular complexes can have different contours and often are called *multifocal* (Fig. 22–38). More properly they should be called "multiform," "polymorphic," or "pleomorphic," since it is not known whether multiple foci are discharging or whether conduction of the impulse originating from one site is merely changing.

Premature ventricular complexes can exhibit fixed or variable coupling; i.e., the interval between the normal QRS complex and the premature ventricular complex can be relatively stable or variable. Fixed coupling can be due to reentry, triggered activity (see p. 566), or other mechanisms. Variable coupling can be due to parasystole[212] (see p. 693), to changing conduction in a reentrant circuit, or to changing discharge rates of triggered activity. Usually, it is difficult to determine the precise mechanism responsible for the premature ventricular complex based on either constant or variable coupling intervals. Focal mechanism can be important, without macroreentry.[213]

CLINICAL FEATURES. The prevalence of premature complexes increases with age and is associated with male sex and reduced serum potassium concentration.[214] They are more frequent in the morning in patients after myocardial infarction, but this circadian variation is absent in patients with severe left ventricular dysfunction.[215] Symptoms of palpitations or discomfort in the neck or chest can result because of the greater-than-normal contractile force of the postextrasystolic beat or the feeling that the heart has stopped during the long pause after the premature complex. Long runs of frequent premature ventricular complexes in patients with heart disease can produce angina or hypotension. Frequent interpolated premature ventricular complexes actually represent a doubling of the heart rate and can compromise the patient's hemodynamic status. Activity that increases the heart rate can decrease the patient's awareness of the premature systole or reduce their number. Exercise can increase the number of premature complexes in some patients. Premature systoles can be quite uncomfortable in patients who have aortic regurgitation because of the large stroke volume. Sleep is usually associated with a decrease in the frequency of ventricular arrhythmias, but some patients can experience an increase.

Premature ventricular complexes occur in association with a variety of stimuli and can be produced by direct mechanical, electrical, and chemical stimulation of the myocardium. Often they are noted in patients with left ventricular false tendons, during infection, in ischemic or inflamed myocardium, and during hypoxia, anesthesia, or surgery. They can be provoked by a variety of medications, by electrolyte imbalance, by tension states, by myocardial stretch,[216,217] and by excessive use of tobacco, caffeine, or

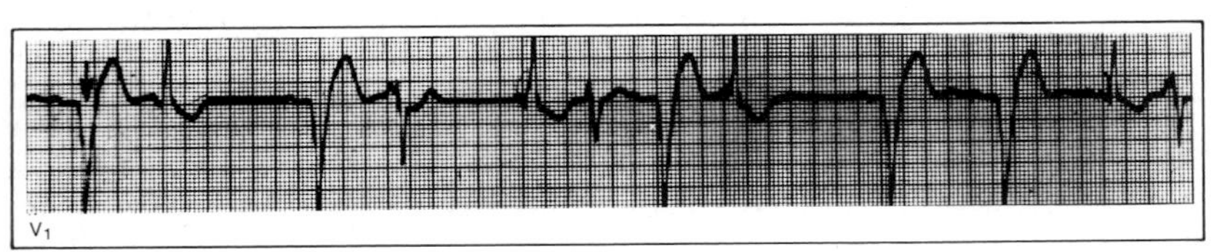

FIGURE 22–38. Multiform premature ventricular complexes. The normally conducted QRS complexes exhibit a left bundle branch block contour (arrow) and are followed by premature ventricular complexes with three different morphologies.

alcohol. Both central and peripheral autonomic stimulation have profound effects on heart rate, which can produce or suppress premature complexes. Almost 20 per cent of patients recovering from acute myocardial infarction treated by fibrinolytic drugs have more than 10 premature ventricular complexes per hour.[218] Increased premature ventricular complexes during anitarrhythmic drug titration in the CAST study predicted patients at increased risk of arrhythmic death despite antiarrhythmic drug treatment.[219]

Physical examination reveals the presence of a premature beat followed by a pause that is longer than normal. A fully compensatory pause can be distinguished from one that is not fully compensatory, since the former does not change the timing of the basic rhythm. The premature beat is often accompanied by a decrease in intensity of the heart sounds, often with auscultation of just the first heart sound, which can be sharp and snapping, and a decreased or absent peripheral (e.g., radial) pulse. The relationship of atrial to ventricular systole determines the presence of normal *a* waves or giant *a* waves in the jugular venous pulse, and the length of the P-R interval determines the intensity of the first heart sound. The second heart sound can be abnormally split, depending on the origin of the ventricular complex.

The importance of premature ventricular complexes varies depending on the clinical setting. In the absence of underlying heart disease, the presence of premature ventricular complexes usually has no impact on longevity or limitation of activity; antiarrhythmic drugs are not indicated.[220,221] The patient should be reassured if he or she is symptomatic (see Chap. 20, Exercise Testing and Long-Term ECG Recording). In men without apparent coronary disease, the incidental detection of ventricular arrthymias is associated with a twofold increase in risk for all-cause mortality and myocardial infarction or death due to coronary disease.[222] However, it has not been demonstrated that premature ventricular systoles or complex ventricular arrhythmias play a *precipitating* role in the genesis of sudden death in these patients, and the arrhythmias may simply be a marker of heart disease. Results from electrophysiologic testing suggest that patients with premature ventricular complexes who do not have ventricular tachycardia induced at electrophysiological study have a low incidence of subsequent sudden death. Antiarrhythmic therapy given to suppress the premature ventricular systoles or complex ventricular arrhythmias has not been shown to reduce the incidence of sudden death in such apparently healthy men.

In patients suffering from acute myocardial infarction, premature ventricular complexes considered to presage the onset of ventricular fibrillation, such as those occurring close to the preceding T wave, more than five or six per minute, bigeminal or multiform complexes, or those occurring in salvoes of two, three, or more, do not occur in about half the patients who develop ventricular fibrillation, and about half of those patients who have these premature ventricular complexes do not develop ventricular fibrillation. Thus these premature ventricular complexes are not particularly helpful prognostically. The presence of one[223] to more than ten ventricular extrasystoles per hour[224] can identify patients at increased risk of developing ventricular tachycardia or sudden cardiac death after myocardial infarction.[225]

MANAGEMENT. Both fast and slow heart rates can provoke the development of premature ventricular complexes. Premature ventricular complexes accompanying slow ventricular rates can be abolished by increasing the basic rate with atropine or isoproterenol or by pacing, whereas slowing the heart rate in some patients with sinus tachycardia can eradicate premature ventricular complexes. In the hospitalized patient, intravenous lidocaine (see p. 605) is generally the initial treatment of choice to suppress premature ventricular complexes. If maximum dosages of lidocaine are unsuccessful, then procainamide given intravenously can be tried. Quinidine can be given intravenously slowly and cautiously. Propranolol can be tried if the other drugs have been unsuccessful. Intravenous magnesium can be useful.[226] For long-term oral maintenance, a variety of class I,[205] II,[227] and III[202,228] drugs can be useful, to prevent ventricular tachycardia. Class IC drugs seem particularly successful in suppressing premature ventricular complexes, but flecainide and moricizine have been shown to increase mortality in patients treated after myocardial infarction.[229] Amiodarone[202,230–234] can be quite effective. Athletes with structural heart disease and ventricular extrasystoles who are in high-risk groups can participate in low-intensity sports only.[46] In patients with isolated systolic hypertension, chlorthalidone in doses that are effective in decreasing stroke and cardiovascular event rates do not increase the frequency of ventricular extrasystole.[235] Thrombolysis therapy does not influence the frequency of ventricular extrasystoles,[236] which are related to residual left ventricular pump performance after myocardial infarction.[237] Low levels of serum potassium and magnesium are associated with higher prevalence rates of ventricular arrhythmias.[238] Metroprolol and diltiazem but not enalapril or hydrochlorothiazide reduce premature ventricular complexes in patients with hypertension.[239]

Ventricular Tachycardia

ELECTROCARDIOGRAPHIC RECOGNITION. Ventricular tachycardia arises distal to the bifurcation of the His bundle, in the specialized conduction system, in ventricular muscle, or in combinations of both tissue types.[240] The mechanisms include disorders of impulse formation and conduction considered earlier (Chap. 20). Autonomic modulation can be important. The electrocardiographic diagnosis of ventricular tachycardia is suggested by the occurrence of a series of three or more consecutive, bizarrely shaped premature ventricular complexes whose duration exceeds 120 msec, with the ST-T vector pointing opposite to the major QRS deflection. The R-R interval can be exceedingly regular or can vary. Patients can have ventricular tachycardias with multiple morphologies originating at the same or closely adjacent sites, probably with different exit paths. Others have multiple sites of origin. Atrial activity can be independent of ventricular activity (AV dissociation, p. 692), or the atria can be depolarized by the ventricles retrogradely (VA association). Depending on the particular type of ventricular tachycardia, the rates range from 70 to 250 beats/min, and the onset can be paroxysmal (sudden) or nonparoxysmal. QRS contours during the ventricular tachycardia can be unchanging (uniform, monomorphic), can vary randomly (multiform, polymorphic, or pleomorphic), can vary in a more or less repetitive manner (torsades de pointes), can vary in alternate complexes (bidirectional ventricular tachycardia), or can vary in a stable but changing contour (i.e., right bundle branch contour changing to left bundle branch contour). Ventricular tachycardia can be sustained, defined arbitrarily as lasting longer than 30 sec or requiring termination because of hemodynamic collapse, or nonsustained, when it stops spontaneously in less than 30 sec. Most commonly, very premature stimulation is required to initiate ventricular tachycardia electrically, while late coupled ventricular complexes usually initiate its spontaneous onset[240] (Fig. 22–39).

Making the electrocardiographic distinction between supraventricular tachycardia with aberration and ventricular tachycardia can be difficult at times, since features of both arrhythmias overlap, and under certain circumstances a supraventricular tachycardia can mimic the criteria established for ventricular tachycardia.[241–243] Ventricular complexes with a bizarre or prolonged configuration indicate only that conduction through the ventricle is abnormal, and such complexes can occur in supraventricular rhythms due to preexisting bundle branch block, aberrant conduc-

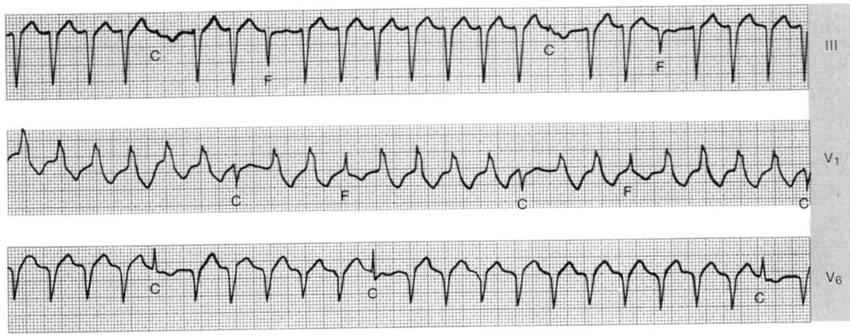

FIGURE 22–39. Fusion and capture beats during a ventricular tachycardia. The QRS complex is prolonged, and the R-R interval is regular except for occasional capture beats (C) that have a normal contour and are slightly premature. Complexes intermediate in contour represent fusion beats (F). Thus, even though atrial activity is not clearly apparent, AV dissociation is present during a ventricular tachycardia and produces intermittent capture and fusion beats.

tion during incomplete recovery of repolarization, conduction over accessory pathways, and several other conditions. These complexes do not necessarily indicate the origin of impulse formation or the reason for the abnormal conduction. Conversely, ectopic beats originating in the ventricle uncommonly can have a fairly normal duration and shape. However, it is important to emphasize that ventricular tachycardia is the most common cause of a wide QRS complex tachycardia. A past history of myocardial infarction makes the diagnosis even more likely.

During the course of a tachycardia characterized by widespread, bizarre QRS complexes, the presence of fusion beats and capture beats provides maximum support for the diagnosis of ventricular tachycardia (Table 22–4). *Fusion beats* indicate activation of the ventricle from two different foci, implying that one of the foci had a ventricular origin. *Capture* of the ventricle by the supraventricular rhythm with a normal configuration of the captured QRS complex at an interval shorter than the tachycardia in question indicates that the impulse has a supraventricular origin (Fig. 22–39). Atrioventricular dissociation (see p. 692) has long been considered a hallmark of ventricular tachycardia. However, retrograde VA conduction to the atria from ventricular beats occur in at least 25 per cent of patients, and therefore, ventricular tachycardia may not exhibit AV dissociation. Atrioventricular dissociation can occur uncommonly during supraventricular tachycardias. Even if a P wave appears to be related to each QRS complex, it is at times difficult to determine whether the P wave is conducted anterogradely to the next QRS complex (i.e., supraventricular tachycardia with aberrancy and a long P-R interval) or retrogradely from the preceding QRS complex (i.e., a ventricular tachycardia). As a general rule, however, AV dissociation during a wide QRS tachycardia is strong presumptive evidence that the tachycardia is of ventricular origin.

DIFFERENTIATION BETWEEN VENTRICULAR AND SUPRAVENTRICULAR TACHYCARDIA. Some electrocardiographic features characterizing supraventricular arrhythmia with aberrancy are (1) consistent onset of the tachycardia with a premature P wave, (2) a very short R-P interval ($\leq$0.1 sec) often requiring an esophageal recording to visualize the P waves, (3) a QRS configuration the same as that which occurs from known supraventricular conduction at similar rates, (4) P-wave and QRS rate and rhythm linked to suggest that ventricular activation depends on atrial discharge (e.g., AV Wenckebach block), and (5) slowing or termination of the tachycardia by vagal maneuvers.

TABLE 22–4 MAJOR FEATURES IN THE DIFFERENTIAL DIAGNOSIS OF WIDE QRS BEATS VERSUS TACHYCARDIA

SUPPORTS SVT	SUPPORTS VT
Slowing or termination by ↑ vagal tone	Fusion beats
Onset with premature P wave	Capture beats
RP interval $\leq$ 100 msec	AV dissociation
P and QRS rate and rhythm linked to suggest ventricular activation depends on atrial discharge, e.g., 2:1 AV block	P and QRS rate and rhythm linked to suggest atrial activation depends on ventricular discharge, e.g., 2:1 VA block
RSR′ V_1	
Long-short cycle sequence	"Compensatory" pause
	Left axis deviation; QRS duration > 140 msec
	Specific QRS contours (see text)

SVT = supraventricular tachycardia; VT = ventricular tachycardia.

Analysis of specific QRS contours also can be helpful in diagnosing ventricular tachycardia and localizing its site of origin. For example, QRS contours suggesting a ventricular tachycardia include the left-axis deviation in the frontal plane and a QRS duration exceeding 140 msec with a QRS of normal duration during sinus rhythm. During ventricular tachycardia with a right bundle branch block appearance, (1) the QRS complex is monophasic or biphasic in V_1 with an initial deflection different from sinus-initiated QRS complex, (2) the amplitude of the R wave in V_1 exceeds the R′, and (3) small R and large S wave or a QS pattern in V_6 may be present. With a ventricular tachycardia having a left bundle branch block contour, (1) the axis can be rightward with negative deflections deeper in V_1 than in V_6, (2) a broad prolonged (>40 msec) R wave in V_1, and (3) a small Q–large R-wave or QS pattern in V_6 can exist. A QRS complex that is similar in V_1 through V_6, either all negative or all positive, favors a ventricular origin as does the presence of 2:1 ventriculoatrial block. (An upright QRS complex in V_1 through V_6 also can occur due to conduction over a left-sided accessory pathway.) Supraventricular beats with aberration often have a triphasic pattern in V_1, an initial vector of the abnormal complex similar to that of the normally conducted beats, and a wide QRS complex that terminates a short cycle length that follows a long cycle (long-short cycle sequence). During atrial fibrillation, fixed coupling, short coupling intervals, a long pause after the abnormal beat, and runs of bigeminy rather than a consecutive series of abnormal complexes all favor ventricular origin of the premature complex rather than supraventricular origin with aberration. A grossly irregular, wide QRS tachycardia with ventricular rates exceeding 200 beats/min should raise the question of atrial fibrillation with conduction over an accessory pathway (Figs. 22–6*B* and 22–30). In the presence of preexisting bundle branch block, a wide QRS tachycardia with a contour different from that which occurred during sinus rhythm is most likely a ventricular tachycardia. Exceptions exist to all the aforementioned criteria, especially in patients who have preexisting conduction disturbances or preexcitation syndrome; when in doubt, one must rely on sound clinical judgment, considering the ECG as only one of several helpful ancillary tests.

Termination of a tachycardia by triggering vagal reflexes is considered diagnostic of supraventricular tachycardias. However, ventricular tachycardia rarely can be stopped in a similar manner.

ELECTROPHYSIOLOGICAL FEATURES. Electrophysiologically, ventricular tachycardia can be distinguished by a short or negative H-V interval (i.e., H begins after the onset of ventricular depolarization) because of retrograde activa-

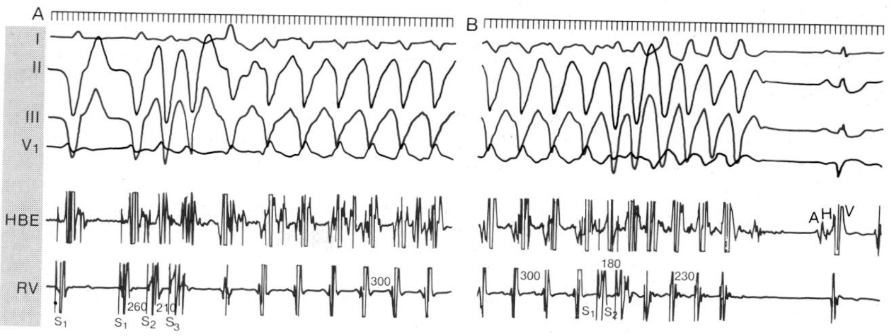

FIGURE 22–40. Initiation and termination of ventricular tachycardia using programed ventricular stimulation. The last two ventricular-paced beats at a cycle length of 600 msec are shown in panel A. A premature stimulus (S_2) at an S_1-S_2 interval of 260 msec and another premature stimulus (S_3) at a cycle length of 210 msec initiate a sustained monomorphic ventricular tachycardia at a cycle length of 300 msec. Two premature ventricular stimuli (S_1-S_2) in panel B create an unstable ventricular tachycardia which persists for several beats at a shorter cycle length (230 msec) and then terminates, followed by sinus rhythm.

tion from the ventricles (see Fig. 20–40, p. 582). His bundle deflections usually are not apparent during ventricular tachycardia because they are obscured by simultaneous ventricular septal depolarization or because of inadequate catheter position. The latter must be determined during supraventricular rhythm before the onset or after the termination of ventricular tachycardia (Fig. 22–40). His bundle deflections dissociated from ventricular activation are diagnostic, with rare exception. Ventricular tachycardia can produce QRS complexes of narrow duration and of short H-V interval, most likely when the site of origin is close to the His bundle in the fascicles.

Successful electrical induction of ventricular tachycardia by premature stimulation of the ventricle (Fig. 22–40) depends on the characteristics of the ventricular tachycardia and the anatomical substrate. Patients with sustained, hemodynamically stable ventricular tachycardia and ventricular tachycardia due to chronic coronary artery disease have monomorphic ventricular tachycardia induced (>90 per cent) more frequently than patients who present with nonsustained ventricular tachycardia, ventricular tachycardia due to noncoronary-related causes or acute ischemia, and cardiac arrest (40 to 75 per cent).[244] In general, it is more difficult to induce ventricular tachycardia with late premature ventricular stimuli compared with early premature stimuli, during sinus rhythm compared with ventricular pacing, and with one premature stimulus compared with two or three.[245] The specificity of ventricular tachycardia induction using more than two premature ventricular stimuli begins to decrease (while the sensitivity increases), and nonsustained polymorphic ventricular tachycardia or ventricular fibrillation can be induced in patients who have no history of ventricular tachycardia. Of patients who present with stable ventricular tachycardia who have inducible sustained monomorphic ventricular tachycardia, the latter is induced in about 25 per cent with single extra stimuli, 50 per cent with double extrastimuli, and 25 per cent with triple extrastimuli.[246] A recent study suggests that using a single basic cycle length of 400 msec and up to four extrastimuli can be an adequate induction technique.[247] Occasionally, ventricular tachycardia can be initiated only from the left ventricle or from specific sites in the right ventricle. Multiple premature stimuli reduce the need for left ventricular stimulation. Drugs such as isoproterenol, various antiarrhythmic agents, and alcohol can facilitate the induction of ventricular tachycardia. Coughing during ventricular tachycardia that causes hypotension can help to maintain blood pressure.

Termination by pacing depends significantly on the rate of the ventricular tachycardia and the site of pacing.[248] Slower ventricular tachycardias are terminated more easily and with fewer stimuli than are more rapid ones. An increasing number of stimuli are required to terminate more rapid ventricular tachycardias, which increases the risks of pacing-induced acceleration of the ventricular tachycardia. Subthreshold stimulation and transthoracic stimulation can terminate ventricular tachycardia. Atrial pacing, at times, also can induce and terminate ventricular tachycardia (see Fig. 20–41, p. 583).

CLINICAL FEATURES. Symptoms occurring during ventricular tachycardia depend on the ventricular rate, duration of tachycardia, the presence and extent of the underlying heart disease and peripheral vascular disease. Ventricular tachycardia can be in the form of short, asymptomatic, nonsustained episodes,[249] sustained, hemodynamically stable events, generally occurring at slower rates or in otherwise normal hearts, or unstable runs, often degenerating into ventricular fibrillation. Some patients who have nonsustained ventricular tachycardias initially, later develop sustained episodes or ventricular fibrillation.[246] The location of impulse formation and therefore the way in which the depolarization wave spreads across the myocardium also can be important. Physical findings depend in part on the P-to-QRS relationship. If atrial activity is dissociated from the ventricular contractions, the findings of AV dissociation (see p. 692) are present. If the atria are captured retrogradely, regularly occurring cannon *a* waves appear when atrial and ventricular contractions occur simultaneously and the signs of AV dissociation are absent.

More than half the patients treated for symptomatic recurrent ventricular tachycardia have ischemic heart disease. The next biggest group has cardiomyopathy (both congestive[250–252] and hypertrophic[253–255]) with lesser percentages divided among those with primary electrical disease,[256] mitral valve prolapse,[257] valvular heart disease, congenital heart disease,[258] and miscellaneous causes. Left ventricular hypertrophy can lead to ventricular arrhythmias.[259,260] Coronary artery spasm can cause transient myocardial ischemia with severe ventricular arrhythmias (during ischemia as well as during the apparent reperfusion period) in some patients.[244] Complex ventricular arrhythmias can occur *after* coronary artery bypass grafting. In patients resuscitated from sudden cardiac death (Chap. 24), the majority (75 per cent) have severe coronary artery disease, and ventricular tachyarrhythmias can be induced by premature ventricular stimulation in approximately 75 per cent. When ventricular tachycardia occurs in the ambulatory patient, it is uncommonly induced by R-on-T premature ventricular complexes (see Ventricular Fibrillation, p. 686). Patients who have sustained ventricular tachycardia are more likely to have reduced ejection fraction, slowed ventricular conduction and electrogram abnormalities, left ventricular aneurysm, abnormal signal-averaged ECGs, and previous myocardial infarction than are patients who have ventricular fibrillation, indicating different electrophysiological and anatomical substances. When sustained ventricular tachycardia can be induced electrically, patients who present with cardiac arrest have faster rates than do patients who present with ventricular tachycardia. Cycle length of induced ventricular tachycardia correlates with whether the patient presents with cardiac arrest or sustained ventricular tachycardia.[246] Young patients also can suffer cardiac arrest from ventricular tachycardia or ventricular fibrillation, and persistent electrical inducibility of arrhythmias in these patients connotes a poor prognosis. In patients with coronary artery disease, sustained ventricular tachycardia displays a circadian variation, with peak frequency in the morning.[261]

Many approaches have been used to assess prognosis in patients with ventricular arrhythmias. Reduced baroreceptor sensitivity and heart period variability apparently due to reduced vagal activity may indicate an increased risk of ventricular tachycardia or sudden cardiac death.[262,263] The presence of nonsustained ventricular tachycardia after myocardial infarction often presages sudden cardiac death. Findings of reduced left ventricular function, spontaneous ventricular arrhythmias, late potentials on signal-averaged ECG,[264] Q-T interval dispersion,[265,266] and inducible sustained ventricular tachyarrhythmias at electrophysiological study all carry increased risk, further exaggerated when two or more of these features are present in the same patient. Also, clinical presentation of cardiac arrest during the first spontaneous episode of ventricular arrhythmia identifies patients at increased risk. Ventricular fibrillation is more likely to occur earlier than sustained ventricular tachycardia in patients after myocardial infarction. Electrophysiological testing can be used to stratify patients according to risk and to help guide therapy in cardiac arrest survivors and patients with sustained or nonsustained ventricular tachycardia, unexplained syncope after myocardial infarction, and cardiomyopathy.

MANAGEMENT. The most important decision involves whether or not to treat. Because reduction in sudden death with antiarrhythmic drug therapy (excluding beta blockers and perhaps amiodarone[202,267]) has not been demonstrated in controlled studies, therapy of asymptomatic patients should, in general, be discouraged. Treatment is reserved for prevention or reduction of symptoms produced by sustained and at times nonsustained ventricular tachyarrhythmias; it can be divided into approaches used to terminate sustained ventricular tachycardia and to prevent recurrences.

Termination of Sustained Ventricular Tachycardia. Ventricular tachycardia that does not cause hemodynamic decompression can be treated medically to achieve acute termination by administering intravenous lidocaine or procainamide, followed by an infusion of the successful drug. Lidocaine is often ineffective[232]; sotalol[268,269] and procainamide appear to be superior. Although quinidine can be used intravenously, great caution is needed because of hypotension. Amiodarone is effective intravenously.[270–274a]

If the arrhythmia does not respond to medical therapy, electrical DC cardioversion can be employed. Ventricular tachycardia that precipitates hypotension, shock, angina, or congestive heart failure or symptoms of cerebral hypoperfusion should be treated *promptly* with DC cardioversion (see p. 619). Very low energies can terminate ventricular tachycardia, beginning with a synchronized shock of 10 to 50 joules. Digitalis-induced ventricular tachycardia is best treated pharmacologically. After conversion of the arrhythmia to a normal rhythm, it is essential to institute measures to prevent a recurrence.

Striking the patient's chest, sometimes called "thumpversion" (see p. 762), can terminate ventricular tachycardia by mechanically inducing a premature ventricular complex that presumably interrupts the reentrant pathway necessary to support it. Chest stimulation at the time of the vulnerable period during the arrhythmia can accelerate the ventricular tachycardia or possibly provoke ventricular fibrillation.

In patients with recurrent ventricular tachycardia, competitive ventricular pacing via a pacing catheter inserted into the right ventricle or transcutaneously can be used. This procedure incurs the risk of accelerating the ventricular tachycardia to ventricular flutter or ventricular fibrillation. Synchronized cardioversion via a catheter electrode in the ventricle can be performed. Intermittent ventricular tachycardia, interrupted by several supraventricular beats, is generally best treated pharmacologically.

A search for reversible conditions contributing to the initiation and maintenance of ventricular tachycardia should be made and the conditions corrected if possible. For example, ventricular tachycardia related to ischemia, hypotension, or hypokalemia at times can be terminated by antianginal treatment, vasopressors, or potassium, respectively. Correction of heart failure can reduce the frequency of ventricular arrhythmias.[252] Slow ventricular rates that are caused by sinus bradycardia or AV block can permit the occurrence of premature ventricular complexes and ventricular tachyarrhythmias that can be corrected by administering atropine, by temporary isoproterenol administration, or by transvenous pacing. Supraventricular tachycardia can initiate ventricular tachyarrhythmias and should be prevented if possible.

Prevention of Recurrences. This is generally more difficult than is terminating the acute episode, and there is no "right" drug to choose. Often, because of similar levels of efficacy, drugs are selected on the basis of potential side effects, e.g., avoiding procainamide for long-term therapy because of the development of drug-induced lupus, avoiding flecainide and disopyramide in patients with reduced left ventricular function, not giving disopyramide to patients with prostate enlargement, and withholding flecainide and moricizine from patients after myocardial infarction. Positive attributes of drugs are helpful. For example, class IB drugs might be chosen early for a patient whose Q-T interval is prolonged. Moricizine, sotalol,[269,275,276] and propafenone are well tolerated by patients and have minimal side effects, allowing for an early choice. One group of patients may have a unique form of ventricular tachycardia that may be precipitated by physical activity and is mediated or triggered by catecholamines and cyclic AMP and is suppressed by adenosine, vagal maneuvers, beta-adrenoceptor blockade, and verapamil[277,278] (see p. 616). Verapamil can be effective in some other types of ventricular tachycardia. Verapamil-sensitive ventricular tachycardias often have a right bundle branch block morphology with left-axis deviation, often arise in the left ventricular septum in patients without structure heart disease, and are precipitated when critical heart rates are achieved (see p. 683). Usually, however, verapamil is not effective in the vast majority of patients with ventricular tachycardia. Although amiodarone is very effective, side effects can limit its use.[202,267] While propranolol reduces sudden death after myocardial infarction, it does not do so to a greater degree in patients with complex ventricular arrhythmias. This suggests that it may be effective via an anti-ischemic mechanism.

When single drugs fail, combinations of drugs with different mechanisms of action can be successful, allowing use of low doses of both agents rather than high or toxic doses of one drug. Most of the combinations represent empirical trials, but I generally attempt to combine drugs to which the patient has exhibited a partial therapeutic response. Evaluating the effectiveness of drug therapy is often difficult. Whether serial drug testing by electrophysiological methods is preferable to the use of endpoints obtained by electrocardiographic methods is unsettled, and both invasive and noninvasive techniques should be considered appropriate for guiding drug selection.[70] One recent study suggests that a noninvasive assessment is less expensive.[239]

Different thresholds for arrhythmic suppression can exist. For example, the serum concentration of procainamide necessary to suppress spontaneous ventricular tachycardia can be lower than the concentration necessary to achieve a significant suppression of premature ventricular complexes.

Ventricular or *atrial pacing,* combined with antiarrhythmic agents if necessary, can be tried, but generally, unless the ventricular tachycardia is initiated by significant bradycardia, such as ventricular rates less than 40 due to complete AV block, attempts at "overdrive" pacing are ineffective over the long term.

Implantable devices that pace, cardiovert, and defibrillate,[280–284] surgery,[285–293] and ablation[294–299] techniques are used frequently in patients for whom drugs are ineffective or not tolerated due to side effects (see Chaps. 21 and 23). Revascularization procedures can be beneficial in selected patients.

Specific Types of Ventricular Tachycardia

A number of fairly specific types of ventricular tachycardia have been identified, related either to a constellation of distinctive electrocardiographic and electrophysiological features or to a specific set of clinical events. While our understanding of electrophysiological mechanisms responsible for clinically occurring ventricular tachycardias is still naive, being able to identify different kinds of ventricular tachycardias is the first step toward understanding their mechanisms.

ARRHYTHMOGENIC RIGHT VENTRICULAR DYSPLASIA. These patients present with ventricular tachycardia that generally has a left bundle branch block contour, often with right-axis deviation, with T waves inverted over the right precordial leads[300] (Fig. 22–41*A*). The ventricular tachycardia may be due to reentry.[301] Supraventricular arrhythmias also

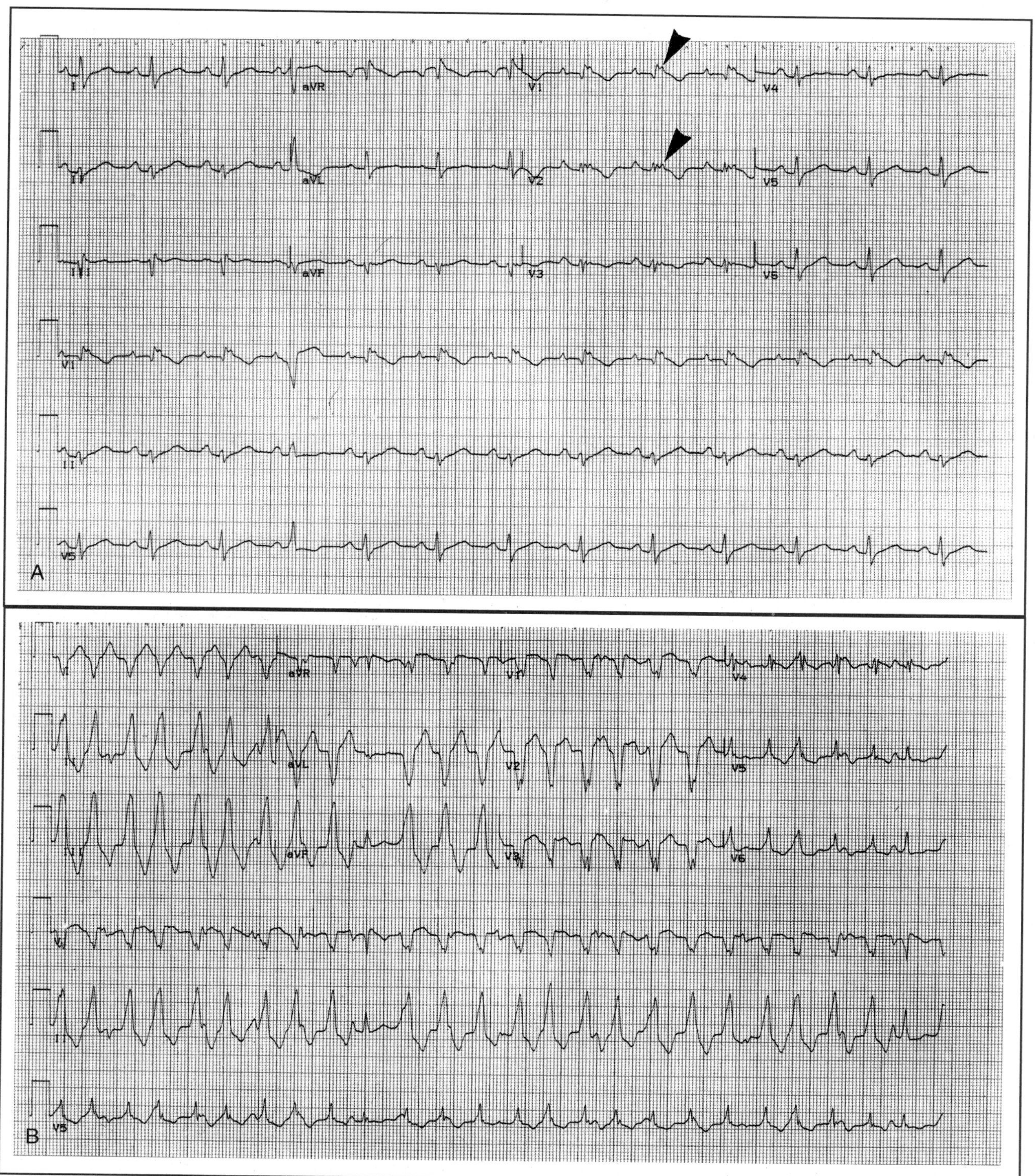

FIGURE 22–41. *A,* Normal sinus rhythm in a patient with arrhythmogenic right ventricular dysplasia. The arrowheads point to late right ventricular activation called an *epsilon wave. B,* Ventricular tachycardia in the same patient with right ventricular dysplasia.

can occur, and exercise can induce the ventricular tachycardia in some patients.

Arrhythmogenic right ventricular dysplasia is due to a type of cardiomyopathy,[302] possibly familial in some patients,[303] with hypokinetic areas involving the wall of the right ventricle. In the familial form, the genetic abnormality has been mapped to an unknown gene[303a] on chromosome 14. It can be an important cause of ventricular arrhythmias in children and young adults with an apparently normal heart, as well as in older patients. Initial presentation can be subtle.[304] Right heart failure or asymptomatic right ventricular enlargement can be present with normal pulmonary vasculature. Males predominate, and all patients usually show an abnormal right ventricle by echocardiography,[305] computed tomography,[306] right ventricular angiography, or magnetic resonance imaging.[307,308] Sympathetic innervation appears to be abnormal.[309] ECG during sinus rhythm exhibits complete or incomplete right bundle branch block.[310] Signal-averaged ECG is abnormal.[311,312] Although the conventional pharmacological approaches to therapy may be appropriate, surgical manipulations have been successful in some of these patients,[289,290,313] as has been implantable defibrillator therapy.[314] Radiofrequency catheter ablation can be tried.

TETRALOGY OF FALLOT (see also pp. 929 and 968). Chronic serious ventricular arrhythmias can occur in patients some years after repair of *tetralogy of Fallot*.[258] Sustained ventricular tachycardia after repair can be caused by reentry at the site of previous operation in the right ventricular outflow tract and can be cured by resection[292] or catheter ablation[315,316] of this area. The signal-averaged ECG can be abnormal.[317] Decreased cardiac output can occur during ventricular tachycardia and residual right ventricular outflow obstruction, leading to ventricular fibrillation.[318]

CARDIOMYOPATHIES (see also Ch. 41)

Dilated Cardiomyopathy (see also p. 1407). Both dilated and hypertrophic cardiomyopathies can be associated with ventricular tachycardias and an increased risk of sudden cardiac death. The use of the signal-averaged ECG in identifying patients with dilated cardiomyopathy at risk for sudden death is controversial, with positive[319] and negative[320,321] results. Induction of ventricular tachycardia by programed stimulation[322] does not appear to identify high-risk patients,[250,323] while Q-T dispersion may.[265] Because it is difficult to predict patients at risk of sudden death or those who might respond favorably to an antiarrhythmic drug, implantable cardioverter-defibrillators have been advocated for the patient with life-threatening ventricular arrhythmias and dilated cardiomyopathy.[324,325] Bundle branch reentry may be the basis of some ventricular tachycardias in this population and can be treated by ablating the right bundle branch.[326–328] Asymptomatic ventricular arrhythmias are common.[329]

Hypertrophic Cardiomyopathy (see also p. 1414). The risk of sudden death in patients with hypertrophic cardiomyopathy is increased by the presence of syncope, family history of sudden death in first-degree relatives, or the presence of nonsustained ventricular tachycardia on 24-hour ECG recordings.[255,330] Asymptomatic or mildly symptomatic patients with brief and infrequent episodes of nonsustained ventricular tachycardia have a low mortality.[331] Results of electrophysiological testing can help identify patients at increased risk of ventricular arrhythmias and sudden death.[332,333] Triggering events such as supraventricular tachycardia and atrial fibrillation[334] and ischemia[335] may be important. Amiodarone has been useful in some patients with mildly symptomatic, nonsustained ventricular tachycardia[330,336] but not in patients with nonarrhythmic problems.[337] Q-T dispersion is increased in those with ventricular arrhythmias and sudden death.[338] DDD pacing has been useful to reduce the outflow gradient, and its role in affecting ventricular arrhythmia is being evaluated.

MITRAL VALVE PROLAPSE (see also p. 1029). Patients with mitral valve prolapse[257] frequently have ventricular arrhythmias, although a causal relationship is not clearly established between the arrhythmia and the mitral valve prolapse. The prognosis for most patients appears good, although sudden death can occur.[339]

IDIOPATHIC VENTRICULAR TACHYARRHYTHMIAS. *Idiopathic ventricular fibrillation* may occur in about 1 per cent of cases of out-of-hospital ventricular fibrillation, affecting mostly men and those in middle

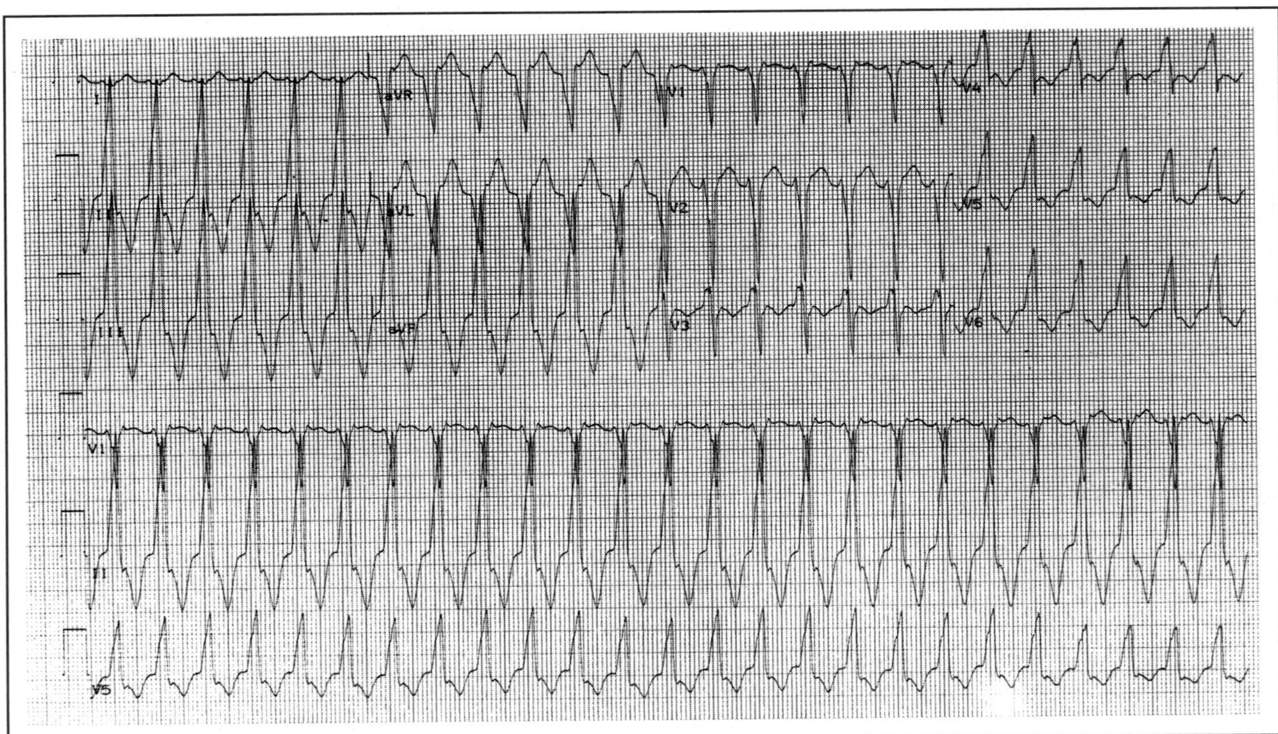

FIGURE 22–42. Ventricular tachycardia originating from the right ventricular outflow tract. This tachycardia is characterized by a left bundle branch block contour in V_1 and an inferior axis.

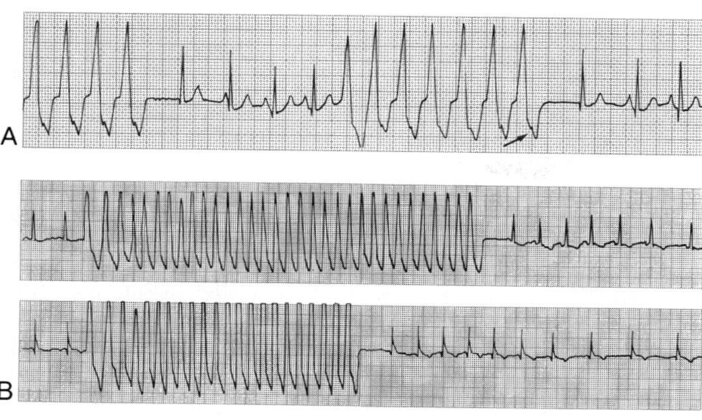

FIGURE 22–43. Panel *A*, Repetitive monomorphic ventricular tachycardia. Short episodes of a monomorphic ventricular tachycardia at a rate of 160 beats/min repeatedly interrupt the normal sinus rhythm. Retrograde atrial capture probably occurs (arrow points to the deflection in the ST segment) and the retrograde P wave of the last complex of the repetitive monomorphic ventricular tachycardia conducts over the normal pathway to produce a normal contour QRS complex. In panel B, short runs of a very rapid (260 beats/min) ventricular tachycardia of uniform contour occur. They probably provoke a compensatory sympathetic response because each is followed by a brief period of sinus tachycardia. The sinus pacemaker appears unstable as changes in P-wave morphology result.

age.[340] Cardiovascular evaluation is normal except for the arrhythmia. Monomorphic ventricular tachycardia is rarely induced at electrophysiological study. The natural history is incompletely known, but recurrences are not uncommon.[341,342] Antiarrhythmic drugs and implantable defibrillators[343] are useful therapeutic choices. Some patients may have right bundle branch block and ST-segment elevation.[344,345] It is important in this entity, as well as in patients with idiopathic ventricular tachycardias (see below), to remember that the arrhythmia at times may be an early manifestation of a developing cardiomyopathy, at least in some of the patients.

Idiopathic ventricular tachycardias with monomorphic contours can be divided into at least three types. Two types, paroxysmal ventricular tachycardia and repetitive monomorphic ventricular tachycardia,[346] appear to originate from the region of the right ventricular outflow tract (Figs. 22–42 and 22–43). Right ventricular outflow tract ventricular tachycardias have a characteristic ECG appearance of left bundle branch block contour in V_1 and an inferior axis in the frontal plane. Vagal maneuvers, including adenosine,[347] terminate the ventricular tachycardia, while exercise, stress, isoproterenol infusion, and rapid or premature stimulation can initiate or perpetuate the tachycardia. Beta blockers and verapamil[348] can suppress this tachycardia as well. The responsible mechanism may be cyclic adenosine monophosphate–triggered activity due to early[349] or delayed[350] afterdepolarizations. The paroxysmal form is exercise or stress induced, while the repetitive monomorphic type occurs at rest with sinus beats interposed between runs of nonsustained ventricular tachycardia that may be precipitated by transient increases in sympathetic activity unrelated to exertion.[350] The prognosis for most patients is quite good. Radiofrequency catheter ablation effectively eliminates this focal tachycardia in symptomatic patients.[351] In others, antiarrhythmic drugs can be effective.[352] An anatomic abnormality in the outflow tract of the right ventricle has been recognized in some patients.[353,354] In a small number of patients, the tachycardia seems to arise in the inflow tract or apex of the right ventricle.[351]

A *left septal ventricular tachycardia* has been described as arising in the left posterior septum, often preceded by a fascicular potential,[355] and is sometimes called a *fascicular tachycardia* (Fig. 22–44). Entrainment has been demonstrated, suggesting reentry as a cause of some of the tachycardias.[356] Verapamil[277,278] or dilitiazem[357] suppresses this tachycardia, while adenosine does so only rarely.[358–360] The response to verapamil suggests that the slow inward current may be important, possibly in a reentrant circuit or via delayed afterdepolarizations. Several mechanisms may be operative, and the group may not be homogeneous.[361] Oral verapamil is not as effective as intravenous verapamil. Once initiated, the tachycardia is paroxysmal and sustained. It can be started by rapid atrial or ventricular pacing and sometimes by exercise or isoproterenol. Generally, the prognosis is good.[277,278] Radiofrequency catheter ablation is effective in symptomatic patients.[297,351,355] Late potentials have been reported in one-third of patients.[362]

Sudden unexplained nocturnal death syndrome (SUNDS) occurs in apparently healthy young Southeast Asians, sometimes associated with nightmares. Thiamine deficiency has been suggested.[362a]

Accelerated Idioventricular Rhythm

ELECTROCARDIOGRAPHIC RECOGNITION. The ventricular rate, commonly between 60 and 110 beats/min, usually

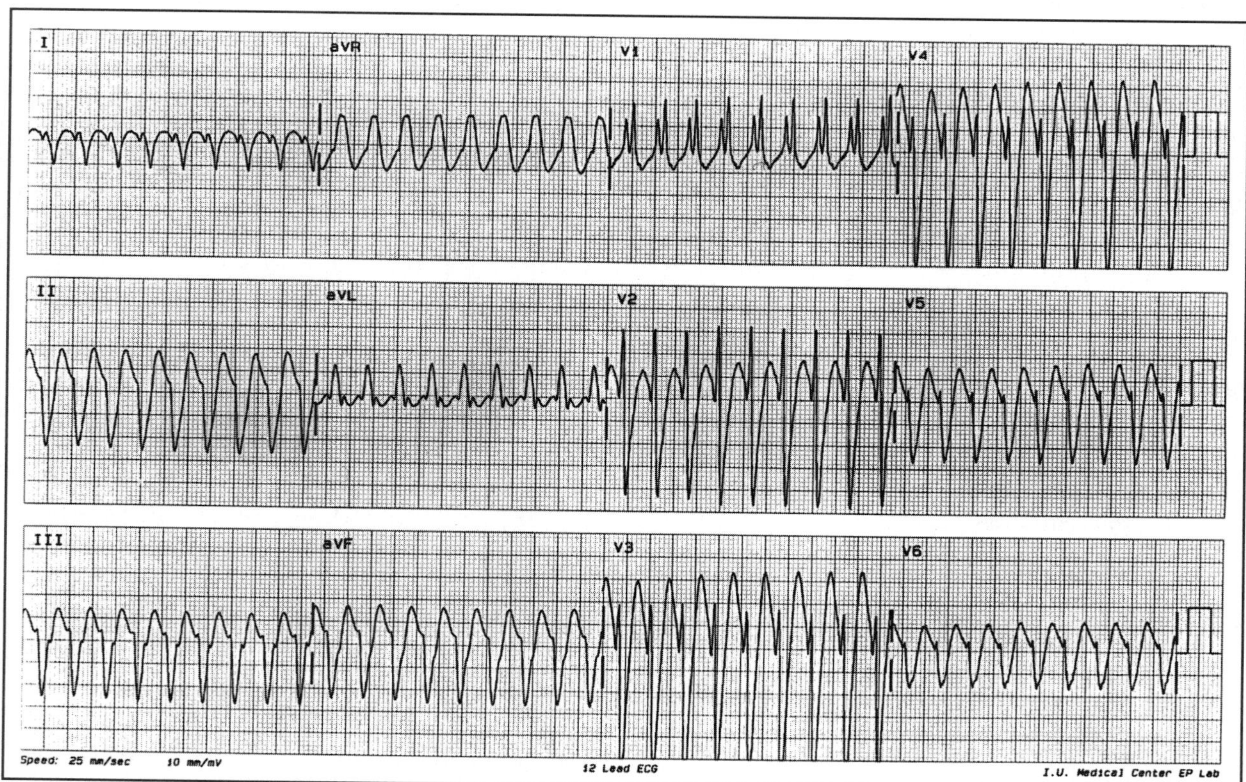

FIGURE 22–44. Left septal ventricular tachycardia. This tachycardia is characterized by a right bundle branch block contour. In this instance, the axis was rightward. The site of the ventricular tachycardia was established to be in the left posterior septum by electrophysiological mapping and ablation.

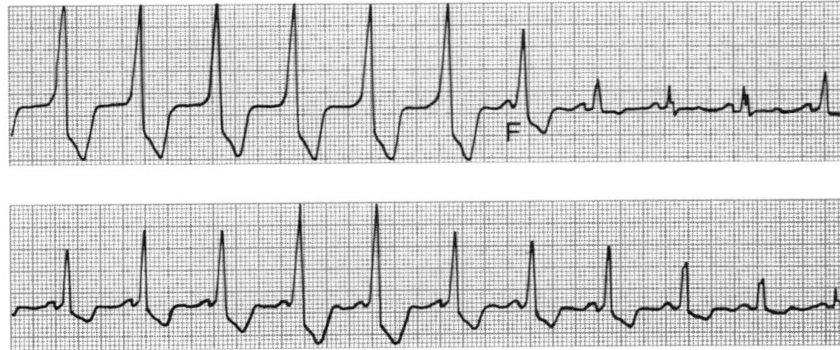

FIGURE 22–45. Accelerated idioventricular rhythm. In this continuous monitor-lead recording, an accelerated idioventricular rhythm competes with the sinus rhythm. Wide QRS complexes at a rate of 90 beats/min fuse (F) with the sinus rhythm, which takes control briefly, generating the narrow QRS complexes, and then yields once again to the accelerated idioventricular rhythm as the P waves move "in and out" of the QRS complex. This example of isorhythmic AV dissociation may be due to hemodynamic modulation of the sinus rate via the autonomic nervous system.

hovers within 10 beats of the sinus rate so that control of the cardiac rhythm is passed back and forth between these two competing pacemaker sites.[363] Consequently, fusion beats often occur at the onset and termination of the arrhythmia as the pacemakers vie for control of ventricular depolarization (Fig. 22–45). Because of the slow rate, capture beats are common. The onset of this arrhythmia is generally gradual (nonparoxysmal) and occurs when the rate of the ventricular tachycardia exceeds the sinus rate because of sinus slowing or SA or AV block. The ectopic mechanism also can begin after a premature ventricular complex, or the ectopic ventricular focus can simply accelerate sufficiently to overtake the sinus rhythm. The slow rate and nonparoxysmal onset avoid the problems initiated by excitation during the vulnerable period, and consequently, precipitation of more rapid ventricular arrhythmias is rarely seen. Termination of the rhythm generally occurs gradually as the dominant sinus rhythm accelerates or as the ectopic ventricular rhythm decelerates. The ventricular rhythm can be regular or irregular and occasionally can show sudden doubling, suggesting the presence of exit block. Many characteristics incriminate enhanced automaticity as the responsible mechanism.

The arrhythmia occurs as a rule in patients who have heart disease, e.g., those with acute myocardial infarction or with digitalis toxicity. It is transient and intermittent, with episodes lasting a few seconds to a minute, and does not appear to affect seriously the patient's clinical course or the prognosis. It commonly occurs at the moment of reperfusion of a previously occluded coronary artery,[364] and it can be found during resuscitation.[365]

MANAGEMENT. Suppressive therapy rarely is necessary because the ventricular rate is generally less than 100 beats/min. The following conditions exist during which therapy may be considered: (1) when AV dissociation results in loss of sequential AV contraction and with it the hemodynamic benefits of atrial contribution to ventricular filling, (2) when accelerated idioventricular rhythm occurs together with a more rapid ventricular tachycardia, (3) when accelerated idioventricular rhythm begins with a premature ventricular complex that has a short coupling interval, which causes discharge in the vulnerable period of the preceding T wave, (4) when the ventricular rate is too rapid and produces symptoms, and (5) if ventricular fibrillation develops as a result of the accelerated idioventricular rhythm. This last event appears to be fairly rare. Therapy, when indicated, should be as already noted for ventricular tachycardia. Often simply increasing the sinus rate with atropine or atrial pacing suppresses the accelerated idioventricular rhythm.

Torsades de Pointes

ELECTROCARDIOGRAPHIC RECOGNITION. The term *torsades de pointes* refers to a ventricular tachycardia characterized by QRS complexes of changing amplitude that appear to twist around the isoelectric line and occur at rates of 200 to 250/min[366–368] (Fig. 22–46*A*). Originally described in the setting of bradycardia due to complete heart block,[369] the term *torsades de pointes* is usually used to connote a *syndrome,* not simply an ECG description of the QRS complex of the tachycardia, characterized by prolonged ventricular repolarization with Q-T intervals usually exceeding 500 msec. The U wave also can become prominent, but its role in this syndrome and in the long Q-T syndrome is not clear. Long-short R-R cycle sequences commonly precede the onset of torsades de pointes due to acquired causes.[370] Relatively late premature ventricular complexes can discharge during the termination of the long T wave, precipitating successive bursts of ventricular tachycardia during which the peaks of the QRS complexes appear successively on one side and then on the other or the isoelectric baseline, giving the typical twisting appearance with continuous and progressive changes in QRS contour and amplitude.[371] Recently, a tachycardia resembling torsades de pointes has been described in which the Q-T interval is normal, and premature ventricular complexes with short coupling intervals initiate the tachycardia.[372] Torsades de

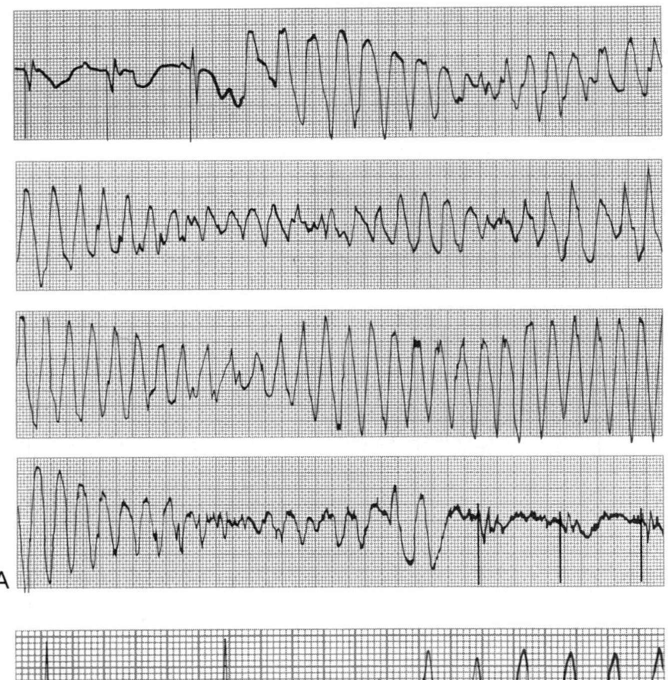

FIGURE 22–46. Torsades de pointes. *A,* Continuous-recording monitor lead. A demand ventricular pacemaker (VVI) had been implanted because of type II second degree AV block. After treatment with amiodarone for recurrent ventricular tachycardia, the Q-T interval became prolonged (about 640 msec during paced beats), and the patient developed episodes of torsades de pointes. In this recording, the tachycardia spontaneously terminates and a paced ventricular rhythm is restored. Motion artifact is noted at the end of the recording as the patient lost consciousness. *B,* Tracing from a young boy with a congenital long Q-T syndrome. The Q-TU interval in the sinus beats is at least 600 msec. Note TU wave alternans in the first and second complexes. A late premature complex occurring in the downslope of the TU wave initiates an episode of ventricular tachycardia.

pointes can terminate with progressive prolongation of cycle lengths and larger and more distinctly formed QRS complexes, ending with a return to the basal rhythm, a period of ventricular standstill, a new attack of torsades de pointes, or ventricular fibrillation.

Ventricular tachycardia that is similar morphologically to torsades de pointes and occurs in patients *without* Q-T prolongation, whether spontaneous or electrically induced, generally should be classified as polymorphic ventricular tachycardia, not as torsades de pointes. The distinction has important therapeutic implications (see below).

ELECTROPHYSIOLOGICAL FEATURES. Electrophysiological mechanisms responsible for torsades de pointes are not completely understood.[373,374] Most data suggest that early afterdepolarizations (see Fig. 20–22, p. 566) are responsible for both the long Q-T and the torsades de pointes or at least its initiation.[375–377] Perpetuation may be due to triggered activity, reentry due to dispersion of repolarization[378] produced by the early afterdepolarizations, or abnormal automaticity. Two out-of-phase discharging foci have been shown experimentally to produce a tachycardia similar to torsades de pointes, as have drifting rotors[379] (see p. 1378).

CLINICAL FEATURES. While many predisposing factors have been cited, the most common causes are congenital, severe bradycardia, potassium depletion, and use of class IA and some IC drugs. Clinical features depend on whether the torsades de pointes is due to the acquired or congenital (idiopathic) long Q-T syndrome (see below). Symptoms from the tachycardia depend on its rate and duration, as with other ventricular tachycardias, and range from palpitations to syncope and death. Females, perhaps because of a longer Q-T interval, are at greater risk for developing torsades de pointes than are males.[380]

MANAGEMENT. The approach to ventricular tachycardia with a polymorphic pattern depends on whether or not it occurs in the setting of a prolonged Q-T interval. For this practical reason and because the mechanism of the tachycardia can differ depending on whether or not a long Q-T interval is present, it is important to restrict the definition of torsades de pointes to the typical polymorphic ventricular tachycardia in the setting of a long Q-T and/or U wave in the basal complexes. In all patients with torsades de pointes, administration of class IA, possibly some class IC, and class III antiarrhythmic agents (amiodarone and sotalol) can increase the abnormal Q-T interval and worsen the arrhythmia. Intravenous magnesium is the initial treatment of choice for torsades de pointes due to an acquired cause,[281,282] followed by temporary ventricular or atrial pacing. Isoproterenol, given cautiously because it can exacerbate the arrhythmia, can be used until pacing is instituted. Lidocaine, mexiletine, or phenytoin can be tried. Potassium channel openers may be useful.[383–385] The cause of the long Q-T should be determined and corrected if possible. When the Q-T interval is normal, polymorphic ventricular tachycardia *resembling* torsades de pointes is diagnosed, and standard antiarrhythmic drugs can be given. In borderline cases, the clinical context may help determine whether treatment should be initiated with antiarrhythmic drugs. Torsades de pointes due to the congenital long Q-T interval syndrome is treated with beta blockade, surgical sympathetic interruption, pacing, and implantable defibrillators (see below). ECGs taken on close relatives can help secure the diagnosis of long Q-T syndrome in borderline cases.

Long Q-T Syndrome

ELECTROCARDIOGRAPHIC RECOGNITION (Fig. 22–46*B*). The upper limit for the duration of the normal Q-T interval *corrected* for heart rate (Q-Tc) is often given as 0.44 sec. However, the normal corrected Q-T interval actually may be longer, 0.46 for men and 0.47 for women, with a normal range ±15 per cent of the mean value.[386] The nature of the U-wave abnormality and its relationship to the long Q-T syndrome are not clear. M cells may be responsible for the U wave (see p. 562).[387] The probable risk of developing life-threatening ventricular arrhythmias in patients with the idiopathic long Q-T syndrome is exponentially related to the length of the Q-Tc interval.[386] T-wave "humps" in the ECG suggest the presence of the long Q-T syndrome[388] and may be caused by early afterdepolarizations.[389] A point score system has been suggested to aid in the diagnosis.[390] Two-to-one AV block (because of the long repolarization time) and T-wave alternans can occur.[391,392]

CLINICAL FEATURES. The long Q-T syndrome can be divided into idiopathic (congenital) and acquired forms.[368] The idiopathic form is a familial disorder (see p. 951) that can be associated with sensorineural deafness (Jervell and Lange-Nielsen syndrome, autosomal recessive) or normal hearing (Romano-Ward syndrome, autosomal dominant). A nonfamilial form with normal hearing has been called the sporadic form.

The hypothesis that the idiopathic long Q-T syndrome results from a preponderance of left sympathetic tone has been replaced by genetic information linking the disorder in different families to sites in chromosomes 3p21–24, 4, 7q35–36, and 11p15.5,[393–399] and recently establishing two genes, HERG on chromosome 7, a putative potassium gene,[400] and SCN5A on chromosome 3,[401] the cardiac sodium gene, as potential causes.[401a] Clear evidence for genetic heterogeneity exists (see p. 750) and can be responsible for different shaped T waves. Chromosome 3 abnormality is associated with the longest Q-Tc durations and delay in onset of the T wave, while chromosome 7 abnormality results in T waves of low amplitude.[401b,401c] Thus it is likely that an intrinsic cardiac repolarization abnormality gives rise to early afterdepolarizations that prolong the Q-T interval and produce torsades de pointes. The acquired form has a long Q-T interval caused by various drugs such as quinidine, procainamide, *N*-acetylprocainamide, sotalol,[402] amiodarone, disopyramide,[403] phenothiazines, or tricyclic antidepressants; nonsedating antihistamines such as astemizole and terfenedine,[404–406] whose actions can be exacerbated by drugs affecting their metabolism such as ketoconazoles; drugs such as erythromycin,[407–409] pentamidine,[410,411] and some antimalarials; electrolyte abnormalities such as hypokalemia and hypomagnesemia; the results of a liquid protein diet and starvation; central nervous system lesions; significant bradyarrhythmias; cardiac ganglionitis; mitral valve prolapse; and probucol.[412]

Patients with congenital long Q-T syndrome can present with syncope, at times misdiagnosed as epilepsy,[413,414,414a] due to ventricular tachycardias that are often caused by torsades de pointes. Sudden death can occur in this group of patients, and it occurs in 9 per cent of pediatric patients without preceding symptoms.[414,415] It is obvious that in some the ventricular arrhythmia becomes sustained and probably results in ventricular fibrillation. Patients with idiopathic long Q-T syndrome who are at increased risk for sudden death include those with family members who died suddenly at an early age and those who have experienced syncope. They commonly develop ventricular tachyarrhythmias during periods of adrenergic stimulation such as fright or exertion. Syndactyly has been described recently in some patients with the idiopathic form.[416] Stress testing can prolong the Q-T interval and produce T-wave alternans, the latter indicative of electrical instability.[417] Electrocardiograms should be obtained for all family members when the propositus presents with symptoms. Patients should undergo prolonged ECG recording,[418,419] with various stresses designed to evoke ventricular arrhythmias, such as auditory stimuli, psychological stress, cold pressor stimulation, and exercise. The Valsalva maneuver can lengthen the Q-T interval and cause T-wave alternans and ventricular tachycardia in patients who have prolonged Q-T syndromes. Catecholamines[420,421,421a] can be infused in some patients, but this challenge must be performed cautiously, with resuscitative equipment along with alpha and beta antagonists close at hand. Stellate ganglion stimulation and blockade have been useful to provoke or abolish arrhythmias. Premature ventricular stimulation electrically generally does not induce arrhythmias in this syndrome. Patients with the acquired form commonly develop torsades de pointes during periods of bradycardia or after a long pause in the R-R interval, while those with the idiopathic form can have a sinus tachycardia preceding the ventricular arrhythmia. Competitive sports are generally contraindicated for patients with the congenital long Q-T syndrome.[46] An interesting contractile abnormality has been described in patients with the idiopathic long Q-T syndrome that is abolished by verapamil.[422] Cardiac sympathetic innervation appears to be normal,[423] although this is not completely resolved.[424]

Recently, a dog colony with sudden death and ventricular tachyarrhythmias, apparently due to early afterdepolarizations with a normal Q-T interval, has been described.[425,425a] In humans with normal Q-T intervals, ventricular tachyarrhythmias resembling torsades de pointes also have been noted.[426]

MANAGEMENT. For patients who have the idiopathic long Q-T syndrome but do not have syncope, complex ventricular arrhythmias, or a family history of sudden cardiac death, no therapy is recommended. In asymptomatic patients with complex ventricular arrhythmias or a family history of early sudden cardiac death, beta-adrenoceptor blockers at maximally tolerated doses are recommended. In patients with syncope, beta blockers at maximally tolerated doses, perhaps combined with a class IB antiarrhythmic drug, are suggested. For patients who continue to have syncope despite maximum drug therapy, left-sided cervicothoracic sympathetic ganglionectomy that interrupts the stellate ganglion and the first three or four thoracic ganglia may be helpful, and permanent pacing[427] also has been used. Implantation of a cardioverter-defibrillator seems advisable in patients who have syncope despite sympathetic interruption[368,428] (Chap. 23). For patients with the acquired form and torsades de pointes, IV magnesium and atrial or ventricular pacing are initial choices. Class IB antiarrhythmic drugs or isoproterenol (cautiously) to increase heart rate can be tried. Avoidance of precipitating drugs is mandatory. Potassium channel activating drugs such as pinacidil and cromakalim may be useful[383–385] in both forms of long Q-T syndrome. Interventions that reduce Q-T dispersion may be beneficial.[427]

BIDIRECTIONAL VENTRICULAR TACHYCARDIA

This is an uncommon type of ventricular tachycardia characterized by QRS complexes with a right bundle branch block pattern, alternating polarity in the frontal plane from −60 to −90 degrees to +120 to +130 degrees, and a regular rhythm. The ventricular rate is between 140 and 200 beats/min. Although the mechanism and site of origin of this tachycardia have remained somewhat controversial, most evidence supports a ventricular origin.

Bidirectional ventricular tachycardia is usually but not exclusively a manifestation of digitalis excess, typically in older patients and in those with severe myocardial disease. When the tachycardia is due to digitalis, the extent of toxicity is often advanced, with a poor prognosis.

Drugs useful to treat digitalis toxicity such as lidocaine, potassium, phenytoin, and propranolol should be considered if excessive digitalis administration is suspected. Otherwise, the usual therapeutic approach to ventricular tachycardia (see p. 680) is recommended.

BUNDLE BRANCH REENTRANT VENTRICULAR TACHYCARDIA

Ventricular tachycardia due to bundle branch reentry is characterized by a QRS morphology determined by the circuit established over the bundle branches or fascicles. Retrograde conduction over the left bundle branch system and anterograde conduction over the right bundle branch create a QRS complex with a left bundle branch block contour and constitute the most common form. The frontal plane axis may be about +30 degrees. Conduction in the opposite direction produces a right bundle branch block contour. Reentry also can occur over the anterior and posterior fascicles. Electrophysiologically, bundle branch reentrant complexes are started after a critical S_2-H_2 or S_3-H_3 delay. The H-V interval of the bundle branch reentrant complex equals or exceeds the H-V interval of the spontaneous normally conducted QRS complex.

Bundle branch reentry is a form of monomorphic sustained ventricular tachycardia usually seen in patients with structural heart disease, such as dilated cardiomyopathy. During follow-up, congestive heart failure is the most common cause of death in this population.[430,431] Myocardial ventricular tachycardias also can be present. Uncommonly, bundle branch reentry can occur in the absence of myocardial disease.[430,431]

The therapeutic approach is as for other types of ventricular tachycardia, except that creation of bundle branch block interrupts the reentry circuit and can eliminate the tachycardia.[294]

Ventricular Flutter and Fibrillation

(See also Chap. 24)

ELECTROCARDIOGRAPHIC RECOGNITION. These arrhythmias represent severe derangements of the heartbeat that usually terminate fatally within 3 to 5 minutes unless corrective measures are undertaken promptly. Ventricular flutter presents as a sine wave in appearance: regular large oscillations occurring at a rate of 150 to 300/min (usually about 200) (Fig. 22–47*A*). The distinction between rapid ventricular tachycardia and ventricular flutter can be difficult and is usually of academic interest only. Hemodynamic collapse is present with both. Ventricular fibrillation is recognized by the presence of irregular undulations of varying contour and amplitude (Fig. 22–47*B*). Distinct QRS complexes, ST segments, and T waves are absent. Fine-amplitude fibrillatory waves (<0.2 mV) are present with prolonged ventricular fibrillation. These five waves identify patients with worse survival rates, and are sometimes confused with asystole.[432]

MECHANISMS. Ventricular fibrillation occurs in a variety of clinical situations, most commonly associated with coronary artery disease and as a terminal event. Intracellular calcium accumulation,[433] action

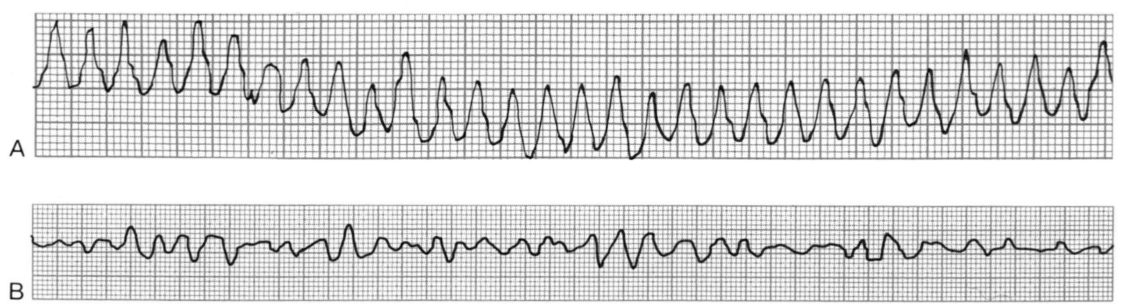

FIGURE 22–47. Ventricular flutter and ventricular fibrillation. *A*, The sine wave appearance of the complexes occurring at a rate of 300 beats/min is characteristic of ventricular flutter. *B*, The irregular undulating baseline typifies ventricular fibrillation.

of free radicals, metabolic alterations, and autonomic modulation are some important influences on development of ventricular fibrillation during ischemia. Thrombolytic agents reduce the incidence of ventricular arrhythmias[433a] and of inducible ventricular tachycardia after myocardial infarction. Cardiovascular events, including sudden cardiac death due to ventricular fibrillation, but not asystole,[434] occur most frequently in the morning and may be related to increased platelet aggregability. Aspirin reduces this mortality. Ventricular fibrillation can occur during antiarrhythmic drug administration, hypoxia, ischemia, atrial fibrillation and very rapid ventricular rates in the preexcitation syndrome (see p. 667) after electrical shock administered during cardioversion (see p. 619) or accidentally by improperly grounded equipment, and during competitive ventricular pacing to terminate ventricular tachycardia.

CLINICAL FEATURES. Ventricular flutter or ventricular fibrillation results in faintness, followed by loss of consciousness, seizures, apnea, and eventually, if the rhythm continues untreated, death. The blood pressure is unobtainable, and heart sounds are usually absent. The atria can continue to beat at an independent rhythm for a time or in response to impulses from the fibrillating ventricles. Eventually, electrical activity of the heart ceases.

In patients resuscitated from out-of-hospital cardiac arrest, 75 per cent have ventricular fibrillation. Bradycardia and asystole can occur in 15 to 25 per cent of these patients and is associated with a worse prognosis than is ventricular fibrillation. Ventricular tachycardia commonly precedes the onset of ventricular fibrillation, although frequently no consistent premonitory patterns emerge. Heart rate variability may be decreased.[435,436]

While 75 per cent of resuscitated patients exhibit significant coronary artery disease, only 20 to 30 per cent develop acute transmural myocardial infarction. In one study,[437] 73 per cent had recent thrombosis. Those who do *not* develop a myocardial infarction have an increased recurrence rate for sudden cardiac death or nonfatal ventricular fibrillation. Patients who have ventricular fibrillation and acute myocardial infarction have a recurrence rate at 1 year of 2 per cent. In the past 20 years, there appears to have been an overall decrease in the incidence of sudden cardiac death, parallel to the decrease in death from coronary heart disease. In some studies, patients at risk for sudden cardiac death have ischemia, reduced left ventricular function, 10 or more premature ventricular complexes per hour, spontaneous and induced ventricular tachycardia, hypertension and left ventricular hypertrophy, obesity, and elevated cholesterol levels; smoking, male sex, increased age, and excess alcohol consumption also predispose to sudden cardiac death.

Predictors of death for resuscitated patients include reduced ejection fraction,[438,439] abnormal wall motion, history of congestive heart failure, history of myocardial infarction but no acute event, and the presence of ventricular arrhythmias. Patients discharged after an anterior myocardial infarction complicated by ventricular fibrillation appear to represent a subgroup at high risk of sudden death. Ventricular fibrillation can occur in infants, young people, athletes, persons without known structural heart disease,[440,441] and in unexplained syndromes. Survival chances for the elderly are reasonable if ventricular tachycardia/fibrillation is the presenting rhythm. Severe bradycardia or asystole bodes a reduced survival rate for most patients. Transcutaneous pacing does not seem to be helpful.[442] Persons in lower socioeconomic strata are at greater risk for cardiac mortality and are less likely to survive an episode of out-of-hospital cardiac arrest.[443]

MANAGEMENT (see also pp. 619 and 731). *Immediate* nonsynchronized DC electrical shock using 200 to 400 joules is mandatory treatment for ventricular fibrillation and for ventricular flutter that has caused loss of consciousness. Cardiopulmonary resuscitation is employed only until defibrillation equipment is readied. *Time should not be wasted with cardiopulmonary resuscitation maneuvers if electrical defibrillation can be done promptly.* Defibrillation requires fewer joules if done early. If the circulation is markedly inadequate despite return to sinus rhythm, closed-chest massage with artificial ventilation as needed should be instituted. The use of anesthesia during electrical shock obviously is dictated by the patient's condition and is generally not required. After conversion of the arrhythmia to a normal rhythm, it is essential to monitor the rhythm continuously and to institute measures to prevent a recurrence.

Metabolic acidosis quickly follows cardiovascular collapse. If the arrhythmia is terminated within 30 to 60 seconds, significant acidosis does not occur. The use of sodium bicarbonate to reverse the acidosis may be necessary, but its efficacy is presently being reevaluated (see p. 766). Intravenous calcium generally is recommended only for situations characterized by hypocalcemia, hyperkalemia, calcium-antagonist overdose, and possibly electromechanical dissociation.

In this short period of time, artificial ventilation by means of a tightly fitting rubber face mask and an Ambu bag is quite satisfactory and eliminates the delay attending intubation by inexperienced personnel. If such a mask and bag are not available, mouth-to-mouth or mouth-to-nose resuscitation is indicated. It is important to reemphasize that there should be *no delay in instituting electrical shock*. If the patient is not monitored and it cannot be established whether asystole or ventricular fibrillation caused the cardiovascular collapse, the electrical shock should be administered *without* wasting precious seconds attempting to obtain an electrocardiogram. The DC shock may cause the asystolic heart to begin discharging and also terminate ventricular fibrillation, if the latter is present. Lidocaine administration may be associated with asystole.

A search for conditions contributing to the initiation of ventricular flutter or fibrillation should be made and the conditions corrected, if possible. Initial medical approaches to prevent a recurrence of ventricular fibrillation include intravenous administration of lidocaine, bretylium, procainamide, or amiodarone. Ventricular fibrillation rarely terminates spontaneously, and death results unless countermeasures are instituted immediately. Subsequent therapy is necessary to prevent a recurrence. Antiischemic approaches are useful in selected patients.[444] Catheter ablation techniques are useful in only well-tolerated monomorphic ventricular arrhythmias.[445]

HEART BLOCK

Heart block is a disturbance of impulse conduction that can be permanent or transient owing to anatomical or functional impairment. It must be distinguished from *interference,* a normal phenomenon that is a disturbance of impulse conduction caused by physiological refractoriness due to inexcitability from a preceding impulse. Either interference or block can occur at any site where impulses are conducted, but they are recognized most commonly between the sinus node and atrium (SA block), between the atria and ventricles (AV block), within the atria (intraatrial block), or within the ventricles (intraventricular block). During AV block, the block can occur in the AV node, His bundle, or bundle branches. In some instances of bundle branch block the impulse may only be delayed and not completely blocked in the bundle branch, yet the resulting QRS complex may be indistinguishable from a QRS complex generated by complete bundle branch block.

The conduction disturbance is classified by severity in three categories. During *first degree heart block,* conduction time is prolonged but all impulses are conducted. *Second degree heart block* occurs in two forms: Mobitz type I (Wenckebach) and type II. Type I heart block is characterized by a progressive lengthening of the conduction time until an impulse is not conducted. Type II heart block denotes occasional or repetitive sudden block of conduction of an impulse without prior measurable lengthening of conduction time. When no impulses are conducted, *complete* or *third degree block* is present. The degree of block may depend in part on the direction of impulse propagation. For unknown reasons, normal retrograde conduction can occur in the presence of advanced anterograde AV block. The reverse also can occur. Some electrocardiographers use the term *advanced heart block* to indicate blockage of two or more consecutive impulses.[445a]

Certain features of type I second degree block deserve special emphasis because when actual conduction times are not apparent in the electrocardiogram, e.g., during SA, junctional, or ventricular exit block (Fig. 22–48), type I conduction disturbance can be difficult to recognize. During typical type I block, the increment in conduction time is greatest in the second beat of the Wenckebach group, and the absolute *increase* in conduction time *decreases* progressively over subsequent beats. These two features serve to establish the characteristics of classic Wenckebach group beating: (1) the interval between successive beats progressively decreases, although the conduction time increases (but by a decreasing function), (2) the duration of the pause produced by the nonconducted impulse is less than twice the interval preceding the blocked impulse (which is usually the shortest interval), and (3) the cycle following the nonconducted beat (beginning the Wenckebach group) is longer than the cycle preceding the blocked impulse. Although much emphasis has been placed on this characteristic grouping of cycles, primarily to be able to diagnose Wenckebach exit block, this typical grouping occurs in fewer than 50 per cent of patients who have type I Wenckebach AV nodal block.

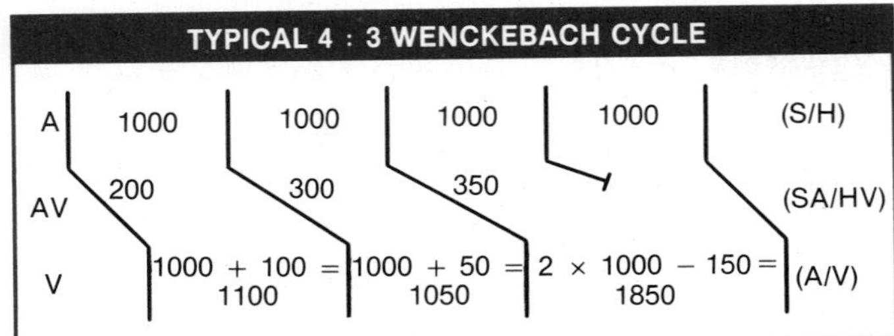

FIGURE 22–48. Typical 4:3 Wenckebach cycle. P waves ("A" tier) occur at a cycle length of 1000 msec. The P-R interval ("A-V" tier) is 200 msec for the first beat and generates a ventricular response ("V" tier). The P-R interval increases by 100 msec in the next complex, resulting in an R-R interval of 1100 msec (1000 + 100). The increment in the P-R interval is only 50 msec for the third cycle, and the P-R interval becomes 350 msec. The R-R interval shortens to 1050 msec (1000 + 50). The next P wave blocks, creating an R-R interval that is less than twice the P-P interval by an amount equal to the increments in the P-R interval. Thus, the Wenckebach features explained in the text can be found in this diagram. If the increment in the P-R interval of the last conducted complex *increased* rather than decreased (e.g., 150 msec rather than 50 msec) then the last R-R interval before the block would increase (1150 msec) rather than decrease and thus become an example of atypical Wenckebach (Fig. 22–43).

If this were a Wenckebach exit block from the sinus node to the atrium, the sinus node cycle length (S) would be 1000 msec, and the S-A interval would increase from 200 to 300 to 350 msec, culminating in block. These events would be inapparent in the scalar ECG. However, the P-P interval in the ECG would shorten from 1100 to 1050 msec and finally there would be a pause of 1850 msec (A) (Fig. 22–4). If this were a junctional rhythm arising from the His bundle and conducting to the ventricle, the junctional rhythm cycle length would be 1000 msec (H), and the H-V interval would progressively lengthen from 200 to 300 to 350 msec, while the R-R interval would decrease from 1100 to 1050 msec and then increase to 1850 msec (V). The only clue to the Wenckebach exit block would be the cycle length changes in the ventricular rhythm.

Differences in these cycle-length patterns can result from changes in pacemaker rate (e.g., sinus arrhythmia), in neurogenic control of conduction, and in the increment of conduction delay. For example, if the P-R increment in the last cycle *increases*, the R-R cycle of the last conducted beat can lengthen rather than shorten. In addition, since the last conducted beat is often at a critical state of conduction, it can become blocked, producing a 5:3 or 3:1 conduction ratio instead of a 5:4 or 3:2 ratio. During a 3:2 Wenckebach structure, the duration of the cycle following the nonconducted beat will be the same as the duration of the cycle preceding the nonconducted beat.

Atrioventricular (AV) Block

AV block exists when the atrial impulse is conducted with delay or is not conducted at all to the ventricle at a time when the AV junction is not physiologically refractory.

FIRST DEGREE AV BLOCK. During first degree AV block, every atrial impulse conducts to the ventricles, producing a regular ventricular rate, but the P-R interval exceeds 0.20 sec in the adult. P-R intervals as long as 1.0 sec have been noted and at times can exceed the P-P interval, a phenomenon known as "skipped" P waves. Clinically important P-R interval prolongation can result from conduction delay in the AV node (A-H interval), in the His-Purkinje system (H-V interval), or at both sites. Equally delayed conduction over both bundle branches uncommonly can produce P-R prolongation without significant QRS complex aberration. Occasionally, intraatrial conduction delay can result in P-R prolongation. If the QRS complex in the scalar ECG is normal in contour and duration, the AV delay almost always resides in the AV node, rarely within the His bundle itself.

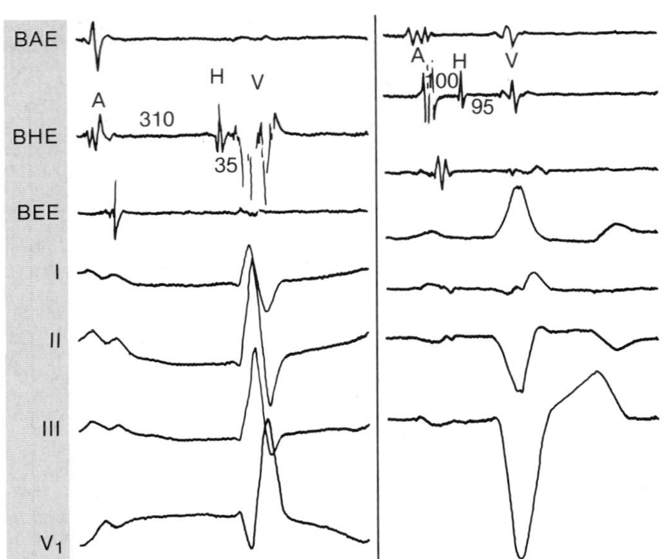

FIGURE 22–49. First degree AV block. One complex during sinus rhythm is shown. The P-R interval in the left panel measured 370 msec (P-A = 25 msec; A-H = 310 msec; H-V = 35 msec) during a right bundle branch block. Conduction delay in the AV node causes the first degree AV block. In the panel on the right, the P-R interval is 230 msec (P-A = 35 msec; A-H = 100 msec; H-V = 95 msec) during a left bundle branch block. The conduction delay in the His-Purkinje system causes the first degree AV block.

If the QRS complex shows a bundle branch block pattern, conduction delay may be within the AV node and/or His-Purkinje system (Fig. 22–49). In this latter instance, His bundle electrocardiography is necessary to localize the site of conduction delay. Acceleration of the atrial rate or enhancement of vagal tone by carotid massage can cause first degree AV nodal block to progress to type I second degree AV block. Conversely, type I second degree AV nodal block can revert to first degree block with deceleration of the sinus rate.

SECOND DEGREE AV BLOCK (Figs. 22–48, 22–50, and 22–51). The block of some atrial impulses conducted to the ventricle at a time when physiological interference is not involved constitutes second degree AV block. The nonconducted P wave can be intermittent or frequent, at regular or irregular intervals, and can be preceded by fixed or lengthening P-R intervals. A distinguishing feature is that conducted P waves relate to the QRS complex with recurring P-R intervals; i.e., the association of P with QRS is not random. Wenckebach and Hay, by analyzing the *a-c* and *v* waves in the jugular venous pulse, described two types of second degree AV block. After the introduction of the electrocardiograph, Mobitz classified them as type I and type II. Electrocardiographically, typical type I second degree AV block is characterized by progressive P-R prolongation culminating in a nonconducted P wave (Figs. 22–50 and 22–51), while in type II second degree AV block, the P-R interval remains constant prior to the blocked P wave (Fig.

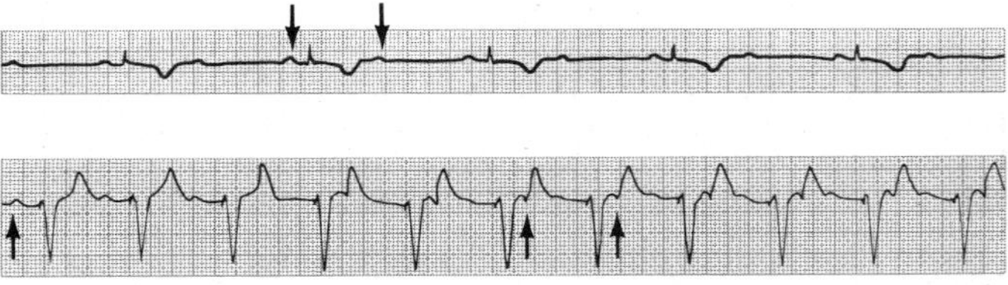

FIGURE 22–50. Unidirectional block. *Top,* During spontaneous sinus rhythm at a rate of 68 beats/min, 2:1 anterograde AV conduction occurs. In the bottom ECG, during ventricular pacing at a rate of 70 beats/min, 1:1 retrograde conduction is seen. P waves are indicated by arrows.

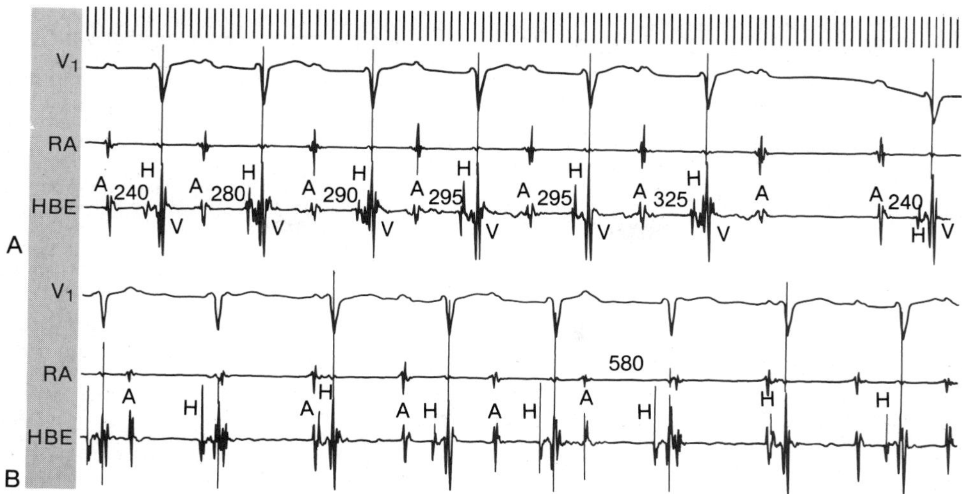

FIGURE 22–51. Type I (Wenckebach) atrioventricular nodal block (panel A). During spontaneous sinus rhythm, progressive P-R prolongation occurs, culminating in a nonconducted P wave. From the His bundle recording (HBE), it is apparent that the conduction delay and subsequent block occurs within the AV node. Since the increment in conduction delay does not consistently decrease, the R-R intervals do not reflect the classic Wenckebach structure diagrammed in Figure 22–42. Panel B was recorded 5 min following 0.6 mg IV atropine. Atropine has had its predominant effect on sinus and junctional automaticity at this time, with little improvement in AV conduction. Consequently, more P waves are blocked and AV dissociation, due to a combination of AV block and enhanced junctional discharge rate, is present. At 8 min (not shown), when atropine finally improved AV conduction, 1:1 atrioventricular conduction occurred.

22–52*A*). In both instances the AV block is intermittent and generally repetitive and can block several P waves in a row. Often, the eponyms *Mobitz type I* and *Mobitz type II* are applied to the two types of block, while the term *Wenckebach block* refers to type I block only. Wenckebach block in the His-Purkinje system in a patient with a bundle branch block can resemble AV nodal Wenckebach block very closely (Fig. 22–52*B*).

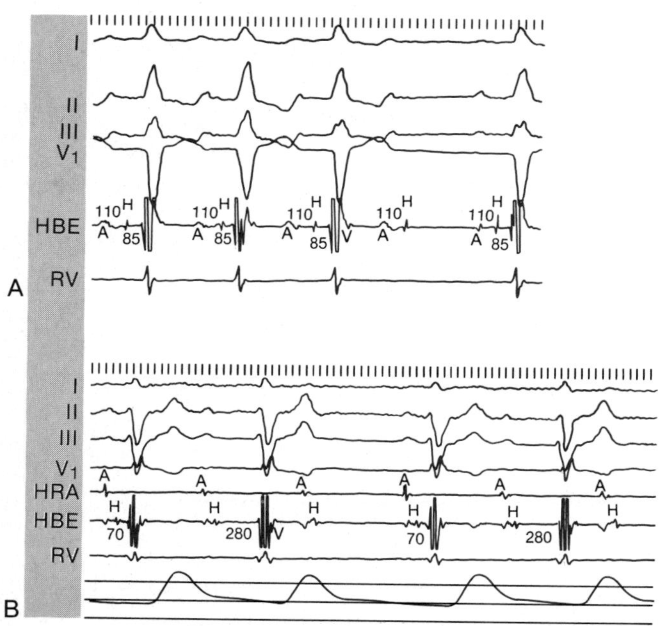

FIGURE 22–52. Type II AV block. *A,* Sudden development of His-Purkinje block is apparent. The A-H and H-V intervals remain constant, as does the P-R interval. Left bundle branch block is present. *B,* Wenckebach AV block in the His-Purkinje system. The QRS complex exhibits a right bundle branch block morphology. However, note that the second QRS complex in the 3:2 conduction exhibits a slightly different contour from the first QRS complex, particularly in V_1. This is the clue that the Wenckebach AV block might be in the His-Purkinje system. The HV interval increases from 70 msec to 280 msec, and then block distal to His results.

Although it has been suggested that type I and type II AV block are different manifestations of the same electrophysiological mechanism, differing only quantitatively in the size of the increments, clinically separating second degree AV block into type I and type II serves a useful function, and in most instances, the differentiation can be made easily and reliably from the surface ECG. Type II AV block often antedates the development of Adams-Stokes syncope and complete AV block, while type I AV block with a normal QRS complex is generally more benign and does not progress to more advanced forms of AV conduction disturbance. In older people, type I AV block with or without bundle branch block has been associated with a clinical picture similar to that in type II AV block.

In the patient with an acute myocardial infarction, type I AV block usually accompanies inferior infarction (perhaps more often if a right ventricular infarction also occurs), is transient, and does not require temporary pacing, whereas type II AV block occurs in the setting of an acute anterior myocardial infarction, can require temporary or permanent pacing, and is associated with a high rate of mortality, generally due to pump failure.[446] A high degree of AV block can occur in patients with acute inferior myocardial infarction and is associated with more myocardial damage and a higher mortality rate compared with those without AV block.

While type I conduction disturbance is ubiquitous and can occur in any cardiac tissue in vivo, as well as in vitro, the site of block for the usual forms of second degree AV block can be judged from the surface ECG with sufficient reliability to permit clinical decisions without requiring invasive electrophysiological studies in most instances. Type I AV block with a normal QRS complex almost always takes place at the level of the AV node, proximal to the His bundle. An exception is the uncommon patient with type I intrahisian block. Type II AV block, particularly in association with a bundle branch block, is localized to the His-Purkinje system. Type I AV block in a patient with a bundle branch block can be due to block in the AV node or in the His-Purkinje system. Type II AV block in a patient with a normal QRS complex can be due to intrahisian AV block, but the block is likely to be type I AV nodal block, which exhibits small increments in AV conduction time.

The preceding generalizations encompass the vast majority of patients who present with second degree AV block. However, certain caveats must be heeded to avoid misdiagnosis because of subtle ECG changes or exceptions:

1. The 2:1 AV block can be a form of type I or type II AV block (Fig. 22–53). If the QRS complex is normal, the block is more likely to be type I, located in the AV node, and one should search for a transition of the 2:1 block to 3:2 block, during which the P-R interval lengthens in the second cardiac cycle. If a bundle branch block is present, the block can be located either in the AV node or in the His-Purkinje system.
2. AV block can occur simultaneously at two or more levels and can cause difficulty in distinguishing between types I and II.[447]
3. If the atrial rate varies, it can alter conduction times and cause type I AV block to stimulate type II or change type II AV block into type I.[448] For example, if the shortest atrial cycle length that just achieved 1:1 AV nodal conduction at a constant P-R interval is decreased by as little as 10 or 20 msec, the P wave of the shortened cycle can block at the level of the AV node without an apparent increase in the antecedent P-R interval. Apparent type II AV block in the His-Purkinje system can be converted to type I in the His-Purkinje system in some patients by increasing the atrial rate.
4. Concealed premature His depolarizations can create electrocardiographic patterns that simulate type I or type II AV block (see Fig. 20–38, p. 580).
5. Abrupt, transient alterations in autonomic tone can cause sudden block of one or more P waves without altering the P-R interval of the conducted P wave before or after block. Thus apparent type II AV block would be produced at the AV node. Clinically, a burst of vagal tone usually lengthens the P-P interval as well as producing AV block.
6. The response of the AV block to autonomic changes either spontaneous or induced to distinguish type I from type II AV block, can be misleading. Although vagal stimulation generally increases and vagolytic agents decrease the extent of type I AV block, such conclusions are based on the assumption that the intervention acts primarily on the AV node and fail to consider rate changes. For example, atropine can minimally improve conduction in the AV node and markedly increase the sinus rate, resulting in an *increase* in AV nodal-conduction time and the degree of AV block as a result of the faster atrial rate (Fig. 22–51*B*). Conversely, if an increase in vagal tone minimally prolongs AV conduction time but greatly slows the heart rate, the net effect on type I AV block may be to improve conduction. In general, however, carotid sinus massage improves and atropine worsens AV conduction in patients with His-Purkinje block, while the opposite results are to be expected in patients who have AV nodal block. These two interventions can help differentiate the site of block without invasive study, although damaged His-Purkinje tissue may be influenced by changes in autonomic tone.
7. During type I AV block with high ratios of conducted beats, the increment in P-R interval can be quite small, suggesting type II AV block if only the last few P-R intervals before the blocked P wave are measured. By comparing the P-R interval of the first beat in the long Wenckebach cycle with that of the beats immediately preceding the blocked P wave, the increment in AV conduction becomes readily apparent.
8. The classic AV Wenckebach structure depends on a stable atrial rate and a maximal increment in AV conduction time for the second P-R interval of the Wenckebach cycle, with a progressive decrease in subsequent beats. Unstable or unusual alterations in the increment of AV conduction time or in the atrial rate, often seen with long Wenckebach cycles, result in atypical forms of type I AV block in which the last R-R interval can lengthen because the P-R increment *increases;* these are common.
9. Finally, it is important to remember that the P-R interval in the scalar ECG is made up of conduction through the atrium, the AV node, and the His-Purkinje system. An increment in HV conduction, for example, can be masked in the scalar ECG by a reduction in the A-H interval, and the resulting P-R interval will not reflect the entire increment in His-Purkinje conduction time. Very long P-R intervals (>200 msec) are more likely to result from AV nodal conduction delay (and block), with or without concomitant His-Purkinje conduction delay, although an H-V interval of 350 msec is quite possible.

First degree and type I second degree AV block can occur in normal healthy children, and Wenckebach AV block can be a normal phenomenon in well-trained athletes, probably related to an increase in resting vagal tone. Occasionally, progressive worsening of the Wenckebach AV conduction disorder can result so that the athlete becomes symptomatic and has to decondition. In patients who have chronic second degree AV nodal block (proximal to the His bundle)

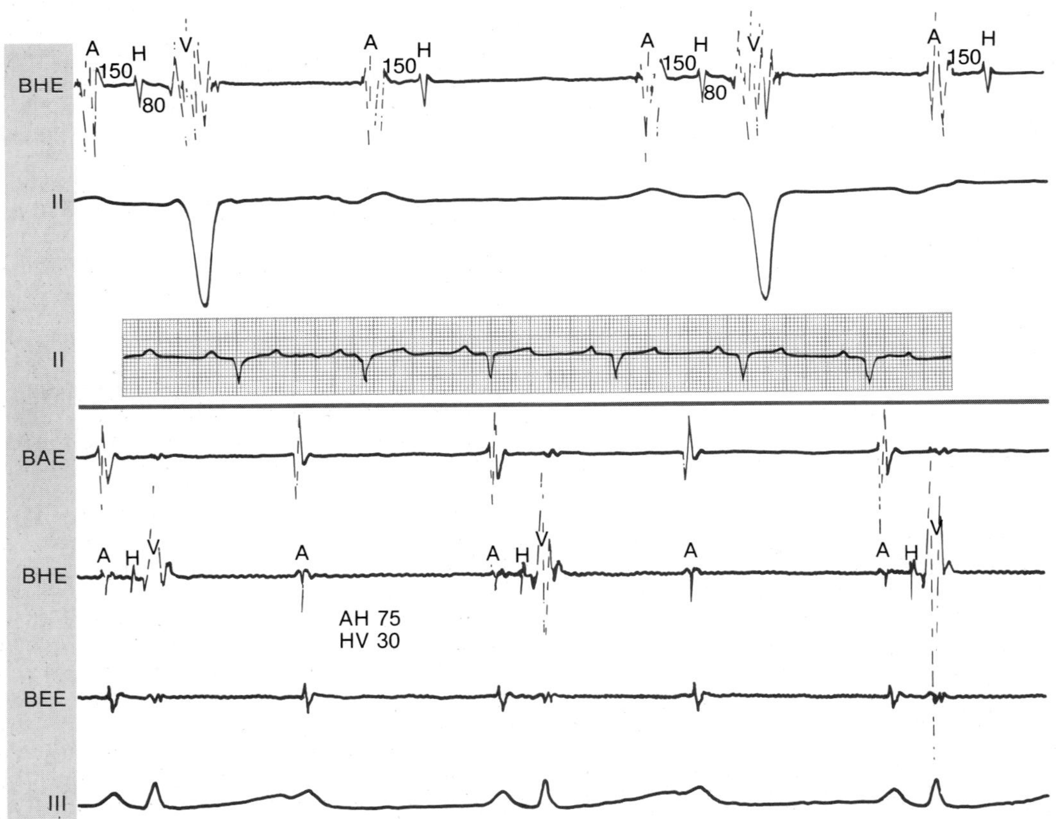

FIGURE 22–53. **2:1 AV block proximal and distal to the His bundle deflection in two different patients.** ***Top,*** **2:1 AV block seen in the scalar ECG occurs distal to the His bundle recording site in a patient with right bundle branch block and anterior hemiblock. The A-H interval (150 msec) and H-V interval (80 msec) are both prolonged.** ***Bottom,*** **2:1 AV block occurs proximal to the bundle of His in a patient with a normal QRS complex. The A-H interval (75 msec) and the H-V interval (30 msec) remain constant and normal.**

without structural heart disease, the course is relatively benign (except in older age groups), while in those who have structural heart disease the prognosis is poor and related to underlying heart disease. *Advanced AV block* indicates block of two or more consecutive P waves.

Complete AV Block

ELECTROCARDIOGRAPHIC RECOGNITION. Complete AV block occurs when no atrial activity conducts to the ventricles, and therefore, the atria and ventricles are controlled by independent pacemakers. Thus, complete AV block is one type of complete AV dissociation (see p. 692). The atrial pacemaker can be sinus or ectopic (tachycardia, flutter, or fibrillation) or can result from an AV junctional focus occurring above the block with retrograde atrial conduction. The ventricular focus is usually located just below the region of block, which can be above or below the His bundle bifurcation. Sites of ventricular pacemaker activity that are in, or closer to, the His bundle appear to be more stable and can produce a faster escape rate than those located more distally in the ventricular conduction system. The ventricular rate in acquired complete heart block is less than 40 beats/min but can be faster in congenital complete AV block. The ventricular rhythm, usually regular, can vary owing to premature ventricular complexes, a shift in the pacemaker site, an irregularly discharging pacemaker focus, or autonomic influences.

CLINICAL FEATURES. Complete AV block can result from block at the level of the AV node (usually congenital) (Fig. 22–54), within the bundle of His, or distal to it in the Purkinje system (usually acquired) (Fig. 22–55). Block proximal to the His bundle generally exhibits normal QRS complexes and rates of 40 to 60 beats/min because the escape focus that controls the ventricle arises in or near the His bundle. In complete AV nodal block, the P wave is not followed by a His deflection, but each ventricular complex is preceded by a His deflection (Fig. 22–54). His bundle electrocardiography can be useful to differentiate AV nodal from intrahisian block, since the latter may carry a more serious prognosis than the former. Intrahisian block is recognized infrequently without invasive studies. In patients with AV nodal block, atropine usually speeds both the atrial and the ventricular rates. Exercise can reduce the extent of AV nodal block. Acquired complete AV block occurs most commonly distal to the bundle of His owing to trifascicular conduction disturbance. Each P wave is followed by a His deflection, and the ventricular escape complexes are not preceded by a His deflection (Fig. 22–55). The QRS complex is abnormal, and the ventricular rate is usually less than 40 beats/min.

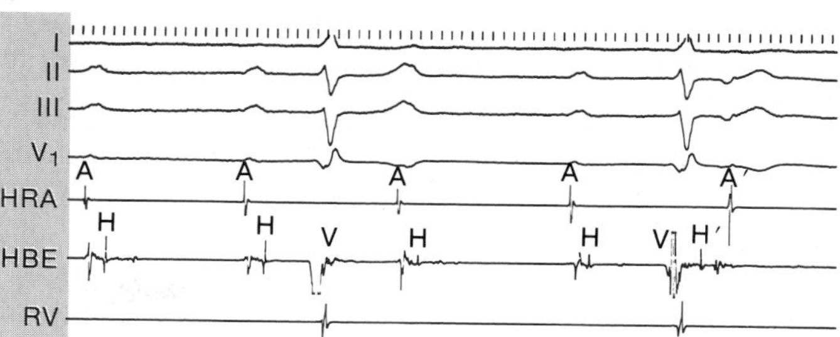

FIGURE 22–55. **Complete anterograde AV block with retrograde VA conduction. All the sinus P waves block distal to His, consistent with acquired complete AV block. The ventricles escape at a cycle length of approximately 1800 msec (33 beats/min) and are not preceded by His bundle activation. The ventricular escape rhythm produces a QRS contour with left axis deviation and right bundle branch block, possibly due to impulse origin in the posterior fascicle of the left bundle branch. Of interest is the fact that the second ventricular escape beat conducts retrogradely through His (H′) and to the atrium (note the low-high atrial activation sequence and the negative P wave in leads II and III). The first ventricular complex does not conduct retrogradely, probably because the His bundle is still refractory from the immediately atrial impulse.**

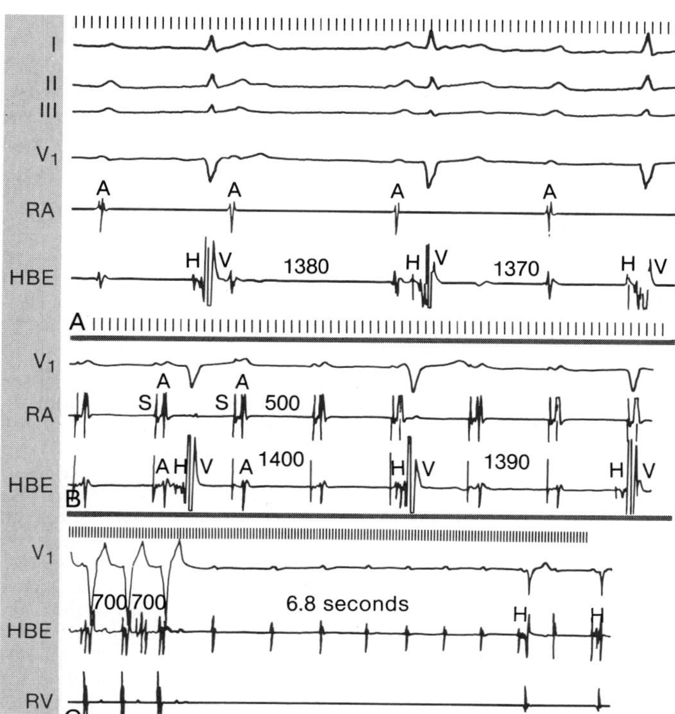

FIGURE 22–54. **Congenital third degree AV block. In panel *A*, complete AV nodal block is apparent. No P wave is followed by a His bundle potential, while each ventricular depolarization is preceded by a His bundle potential. In panel *B*, atrial pacing (cycle length 500 msec) fails to alter cycle length of the functional rhythm. Still, no P wave is followed by a His bundle potential. In panel *C*, after 30 sec of ventricular pacing (cycle length 700 msec), suppression of the junctional focus results for almost 7 sec (overdrive suppression of automaticity; see Chapter 20).**

Unusual forms such as paroxysmal AV block or AV block following a period of rapid ventricular rate can occur. Paroxysmal AV block in some instances can be due to hyperresponsiveness of the AV node to vagotonic reflexes. Surgery, electrolyte disturbances, myoendocarditis,[449] tumors, Chagas' disease, rheumatoid nodules, calcific aortic stenosis, myxedema, polymyositis, infiltrative processes (such as amyloid, sarcoid, or scleroderma), and an almost endless assortment of common and unusual conditions can produce AV block. In the adult, drug toxicity, coronary disease, and degenerative processes appear to be the most common causes of AV heart block. The degenerative process produces partial or complete anatomical or electrical disruption within the AV nodal region, the AV bundle, or both bundle branches. Rapid rates can sometimes be followed by block, an event known as *overdrive suppression* of conduction. This form of block may be important as a cause of paroxysmal AV block after cessation of a tachycardia.

AV Block in Children. In children, the most common cause of AV block is congenital (Chap. 29). Under such circumstances, the AV block can be an isolated finding or associated with other lesions. Connective tissue disease (see p. 1667) and the presence of anti–Rh_0 negative antibodies in maternal sera of patients with congenital complete AV block raise the possibility that placentally transmitted antibodies play a role in some instances.[450–452] Anatomical disruption between the atrial musculature and peripheral parts of the conduction system and nodoventricular discontinuity are two common histological findings. Children are most often asymptomatic; however, some develop symptoms that require pacemaker implantation. Mortality from congenital AV block is highest in the neonatal period, is much lower during childhood and adolescence, and increases slowly later in life. Adams-Stokes attacks can occur in patients with congenital heart block at any age. It is difficult to predict the prognosis in the individual patient. A persistent heart rate at rest of 50 beats/min or less correlates with the incidence of syncope, and extreme bradycardia can contribute to the frequency of Adams-Stokes attacks in children with congenital complete AV block. The site of block may not distinguish symptomatic children who have congenital or surgically induced complete heart block from those without symptoms. Prolonged recovery times of escape foci following rapid pacing (Fig. 22–54*C*) (see discussion of sinus node recovery time, p. 648) slow heart rates on 24-hour ECG recordings, and the occurrence of paroxysmal tachycardias may be predisposing factors to the development of symptoms.

CLINICAL FEATURES. Many of the signs of AV block are evidenced at the bedside. First degree AV block can be recognized by a long *a-c* wave interval in the jugular venous pulse and by diminished intensity of the first heart sound as the P-R interval lengthens. In type I second degree AV block, the heart rate may increase imperceptibly with gradually diminishing intensity of the first heart sound, widening of the *a-c* interval, terminated by a pause, and an *a* wave not followed by a *v* wave. Intermittent ventricular pauses and *a* waves in the neck not followed by *v* waves characterize type II AV block. The first heart sound maintains a constant intensity. In complete AV block, the findings are the same as those in AV dissociation (see below).

Significant clinical manifestations of first and second degree AV block usually consist of palpitations or subjective feelings of the heart "missing a beat." Persistent 2:1 AV block can produce symptoms of chronic bradycardia. Complete AV block can be accompanied by signs and symptoms of reduced cardiac output, syncope or presyncope, angina, or palpitations due to ventricular tachyarrhythmias. It can occur in twins.[453]

MANAGEMENT. As discussed in Chapter 23, drugs cannot be relied on to increase the heart rate for more than several hours to several days in patients with symptomatic heart block without producing significant side effects. Therefore, temporary or permanent pacemaker insertion is indicated in patients with symptomatic bradyarrhythmias.[454] Long-term pacing can alter cardiac function.[455] For short-term therapy when the block is likely to be evanescent but still requires treatment or until adequate pacing therapy can be established, vagolytic agents such as atropine are useful for patients who have AV nodal disturbances, while catecholamines such as isoproterenol can be used transiently to treat patients who have heart block at any site (see treatment for Sinus Bradycardia, above). Isoproterenol should be used with extreme caution or not at all in patients who have acute myocardial infarction. The use of transcutaneous pacing is preferable.

Atrioventricular (AV) Dissociation

CLASSIFICATION. As the term indicates, dissociated or independent beating of atria and ventricles defines AV dissociation. AV dissociation is never a *primary* disturbance of rhythm but is a "symptom" of an underlying rhythm disturbance produced by one of three causes or a combination of causes (Fig. 22–56) that prevent the normal transmission of impulses from atrium to ventricle, as follows:

1. Slowing of the dominant pacemaker of the heart (usually the sinus node), which allows escape of a subsidiary or latent pacemaker. AV dissociation by *default* of the primary pacemaker to a subsidiary one in this manner is often a normal phenomenon. It may occur during sinus arrhythmia or sinus bradycardia, permitting an independent AV junction rhythm to arise (Fig. 22–3*B*).
2. Acceleration of a latent pacemaker that *usurps* control of the ventricles. Abnormally enhanced discharge rate of a usually slower subsidiary pacemaker is pathological and commonly occurs during nonparoxysmal AV junctional tachycardia or ventricular tachycardia without retrograde atrial capture (see Figs. 22–22 and 22–39).
3. Block, generally at the AV junction, that prevents impulses formed at a normal rate in a dominant pacemaker from reaching the ventricles and allows the ventricles to beat under the control of a subsidiary pacemaker. Junctional or ventricular escape rhythm during AV block, without retrograde atrial capture, is a common example in which block gives rise to AV dissociation. It is important to remember that complete AV block is *not* synonymous with complete AV dissociation; patients who have complete AV block have complete AV dissociation, but patients who

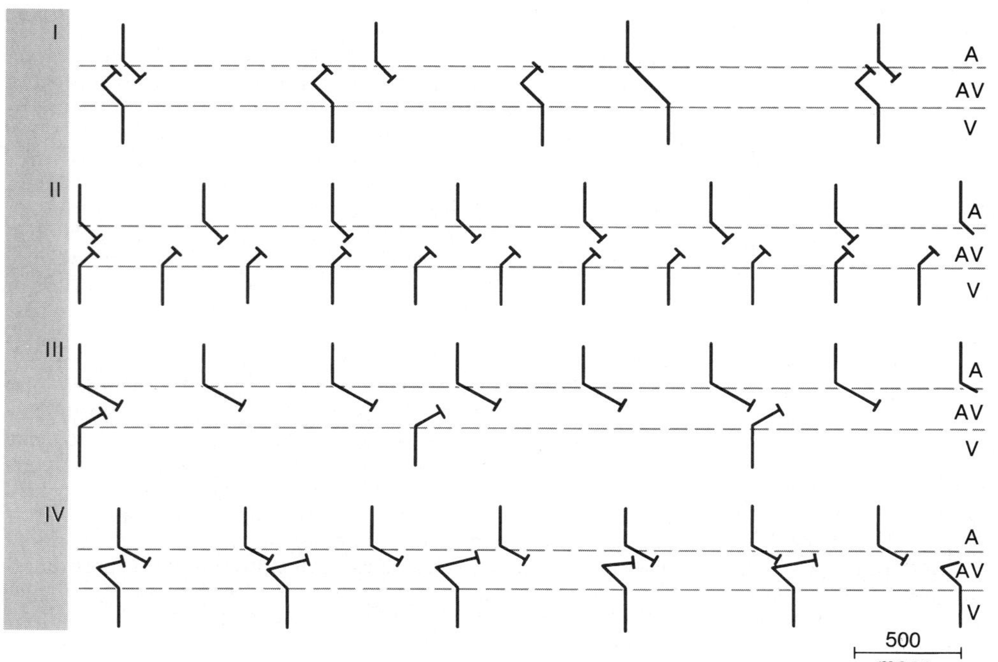

FIGURE 22–56. Diagrammatic illustration of the causes of AV dissociation. A sinus bradycardia that allows the escape of an AV junctional rhythm which does not capture the atria retrogradely illustrates cause I (top panel). Intermittent sinus captures occur (third P wave) to produce incomplete AV dissociation (see Fig. 22–3*B*). For cause II, a ventricular tachycardia without retrograde atrial capture produces complete AV dissociation (see Figs. 22–22 and 22–39). As the third cause, complete AV block with a ventricular escape rhythm is diagrammed (see Figs. 22–54 and 22–55). The combination of causes II and III is shown in panel IV, representing a nonparoxysmal AV junctional tachycardia and some degree of AV block.

have complete AV dissociation may or may not have complete AV block (see Figs. 22–54 and 22–55).

4. A combination of causes. For example, when digitalis excess results in the production of nonparoxysmal AV junctional tachycardia associated with SA or AV block.

MECHANISMS. With this classification in mind, it is important to emphasize that the term *AV dissociation* is *not* a diagnosis and is analogous to the term *jaundice* or *fever.* One must state that "AV dissociation is present *due to . . .*" and then give the cause. The accelerated rate of a slower, normally subsidiary pacemaker or the slower rate of a faster, normally dominant pacemaker that prevents conduction due to physiological collision and mutual extinction of opposing wavefronts (interference) or the manifestations of AV block are the basic disturbances producing AV dissociation. The atria in all these cases beat independently from the ventricles, under control of the sinus node or ectopic atrial or AV junctional pacemakers, and can exhibit any type of supraventricular rhythms. If a single pacemaker establishes control of both atria and ventricles for one beat (capture) or a series of beats (sinus rhythm, AV junctional rhythm with retrograde atrial capture, ventricular tachycardia with retrograde atrial capture, and so forth), AV dissociation is abolished for that period. Conversely, as stated above, whenever the atria and ventricles fail to respond to a single impulse for one beat (premature ventricular complex without retrograde capture of the atrium) or a series of beats (ventricular tachycardia without retrograde atrial capture), AV dissociation exists for that period. The interruption of AV dissociation by one or a series of beats under the control of one pacemaker, either anterogradely or retrogradely, indicates that the AV dissociation is incomplete. Complete or incomplete dissociation also can occur in association with all forms of AV block. Commonly, when AV dissociation occurs as a result of AV block, the atrial rate exceeds the ventricular rate. For example, a subsidiary pacemaker with a rate of 40 beats/min can escape in the presence of a 2:1 AV block when the atrial rate is 78. If the AV block is bidirectional, AV dissociation results.

ELECTROCARDIOGRAPHIC AND CLINICAL FEATURES. The electrocardiogram demonstrates the independence of P waves and QRS complexes. The P-wave morphology depends on the rhythm controlling the atria (sinus, atrial tachycardia, junctional, flutter, or fibrillation). During complete AV dissociation, both the QRS complex and the P waves appear regularly spaced without a fixed temporal relationship to each other. When the dissociation is incomplete, a QRS complex of supraventricular contour occurs early and is preceded by a P wave at a P-R interval exceeding 0.12 sec and within a conductable range. This indicates ventricular capture by the supraventricular focus. Similarly, a premature P wave with a retrograde morphology and a conductable R-P interval may indicate retrograde atrial capture by the subsidiary focus.

The physical findings include a variable intensity of the first heart sound as the P-R interval changes, atrial sounds, and *a* waves in the jugular venous pulse lacking a consistent relationship to ventricular contraction. Intermittent large (cannon) *a* waves may be seen in the jugular venous pulse when atrial and ventricular contractions occur simultaneously. The second heart sound can split normally or paradoxically, depending on the manner of ventricular activation. A premature beat representing a ventricular capture can interrupt a regular heart rhythm. When the ventricular rate exceeds the atrial rate, a cyclic increase in intensity of the first heart sound is produced as the P-R interval shortens, climaxed by a very loud sound (bruit de canon). This intense sound is followed by a sudden reduction in intensity of the first heart sound and the appearance of giant *a* waves as the P-R interval shortens and P waves "march through" the cardiac cycle.

MANAGEMENT. This is directed toward the underlying heart disease and precipitating cause. The individual components *producing the AV dissociation*—not the AV dissociation per se—determine the specific type of antiarrhythmic approaches. Therapy ranges from pacemaker insertion in a patient who has AV dissociation due to complete AV block to antiarrhythmic drug administration in a patient who has AV dissociation due to a ventricular tachycardia.

OTHER ELECTROPHYSIOLOGICAL ABNORMALITIES LEADING TO CARDIAC ARRHYTHMIAS

SUPERNORMAL CONDUCTION AND EXCITATION

SUPERNORMAL CONDUCTION. This is the term applied to situations characterized by conduction that is better than expected but generally not as good as normal.[456–459] The phenomenon almost always occurs when conduction is depressed but can be present in normal cardiac tissues as well. It generally occurs when conduction takes place during the relative refractory period of the preceding complex (Fig. 22–57). The electrophysiological basis can relate, in some examples, to supernormal excitability (see below) but probably to other mechanisms as well. Supernormal conduction commonly has been invoked to explain AV (most probably His-Purkinje rather than AV nodal) conduction that is more rapid than expected or AV conduction that results when AV block is expected.

SUPERNORMAL EXCITATION. This phenomenon results when a stimulus, normally subthreshold, occurs during the supernormal period of recovery of the preceding complex and produces a propagated response. Stimuli occurring earlier or later fail to produce a propagated response. Demonstrated in vitro in Purkinje fibers but not ventricular muscle, supernormal excitation occurs during phase 3 of the cardiac action potential when the membrane potential, closer to threshold at the end of repolarization, requires less current to produce a propagated response. A similar phenomenon occurs during phase 4 diastolic depolarization or during afterdepolarizations that reduce the membrane potential closer to threshold. The phenomenon is most easily recognized when a nonsensing pacemaker, failing because of battery exhaustion and reduced output, produces a propagated response only when discharge falls during a specific time period in a cardiac cycle (Fig. 22–58). Similar phenomena probably occur spontaneously with "weak" automatic foci, but the recognition of these events clinically is difficult and often speculative.

CONCEALED CONDUCTION

Concealed conduction describes the phenomenon during which impulses penetrate an area of the conduction tissue, the AV node commonly but other areas as well, without emerging.[460] Since the transmission of the impulse is concealed, i.e., electrically silent in the standard electrocardiogram, concealed conduction becomes manifested only by its *effects* on the conduction and/or formation of subsequent impulses.[461] The most common example follows a premature ventricular complex. Partial retrograde penetration of the AV node by the premature ventricular complex is *deduced* because the following sinus-initiated P wave blocks to produce a compensatory pause (Fig. 22–59) or conducts with a longer P-R interval if the premature ventricular complex is interpolated. The slower ventricular response when the atrial rate increases from atrial flutter to atrial fibrillation is due to a greater number of atrial impulses blocking (conducting into, without emerging) in the AV node and is a manifestation of concealed conduction.[462] Concealed conduction occurs in WPW syndrome and can be manifested by unidirectional block anterogradely or retrogradely in an accessory pathway[463] (see p. 665). Concealed junctional extrasystoles (Fig. 20–38, p. 580) can create electrocardiographic manifestations of apparent AV block. Strict confirmation of concealed conduction should be the demonstration of conduction, such as in the form of conducted junctional extrasystoles (Fig. 22–19, p. 659).

PARASYSTOLE (Fig. 22–60)

This refers to a cardiac arrhythmia characterized electrocardiographically by (1) varying coupling interval between the ectopic (parasystolic) complex and the dominant (generally, sinus-initiated) complex, (2) a common minimal time interval between interectopic intervals, with the longer interectopic intervals being multiples of this minimal interval, (3) fusion complexes, and (4) the presence of the parasystolic impulse whenever the cardiac chamber is excitable. Parasystole with exit block is suspected when the parasystolic discharge focus fails to appear even though cardiac tissue is excitable. The analogy commonly invoked to represent parasystole is the behavior of a fixed-rate nonsensing (VOO) pacemaker (Chap. 23). Parasystole can occur in the sinus and AV nodes, atrium and ventricle, and AV junction. The parasystolic mechanism presumably results from the regular discharge of an automatic focus that is independent of, and protected from, discharge by the dominant cardiac rhythm. A

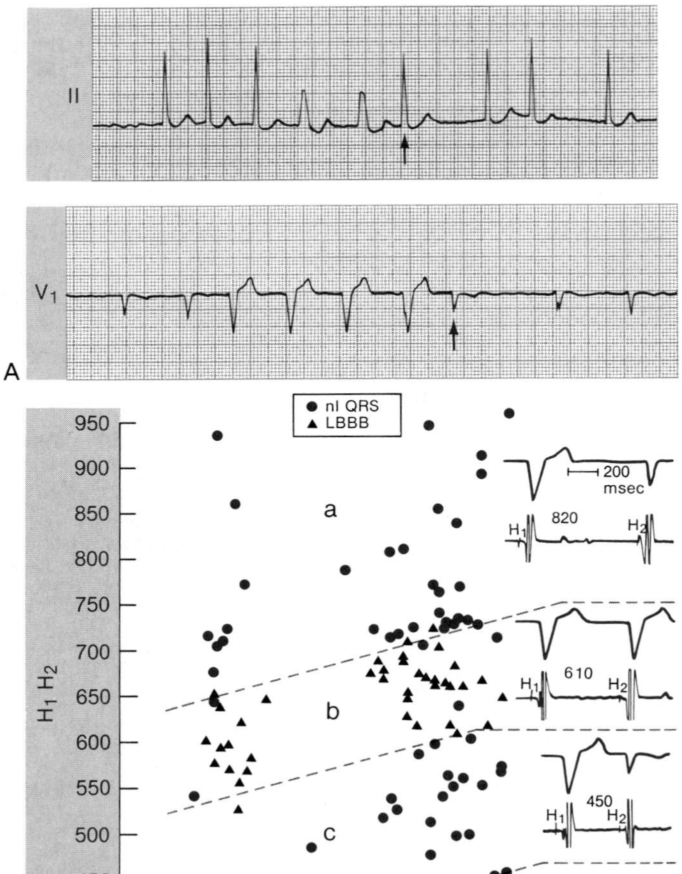

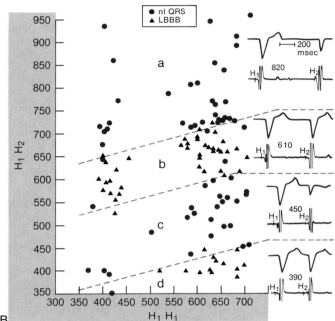

FIGURE 22–57. Supernormal conduction. Panel *A* illustrates atrial fibrillation with long-short R-R cycle sequences giving rise to QRS complexes conducted with a functional left bundle branch block. In each example, however, a shorter R-R cycle length is terminated by a normal QRS complex (arrow), an example of supernormal conduction.

Panel *B* shows a graph of the intervals and illustrative recordings during an electrophysiological study of the patient whose ECG is shown in panel *A*. The H-V interval of the complexes conducted with a left bundle branch block morphology is 45 msec, while the H-V interval of those conducted with a normal morphology is 35 msec. The graph indicates the premature interval (H_1-H_2, ordinate) plotted against the preceding cycle length (H_1-H_1, abscissa). All H_1-H_1 intervals were taken from complexes with a left bundle branch block morphology. Normal complexes are represented by filled circles and left bundle branch block contours by filled triangles. Four zones of conduction are identified, and illustrated by the four examples to the right. The longest H_1-H_2 intervals are followed by a normal intraventricular conduction (zone A), while at shorter intervals, left bundle branch block occurs (zone B). When the H_1-H_2 interval shortens further, normal intraventricular conduction returns and the H-V intervals shorten to 35 msec (zone C, supernormal conduction). At the shortest H_1-H_2 interval, left bundle branch block again appears (zone D). (From Miles, W. M., Prystowsky, E. N., Heger, J. J., and Zipes, D. P.: Evaluation of the patient with wide QRS tachycardia. Med. Clin. North Am. *68:*1015, 1984.)

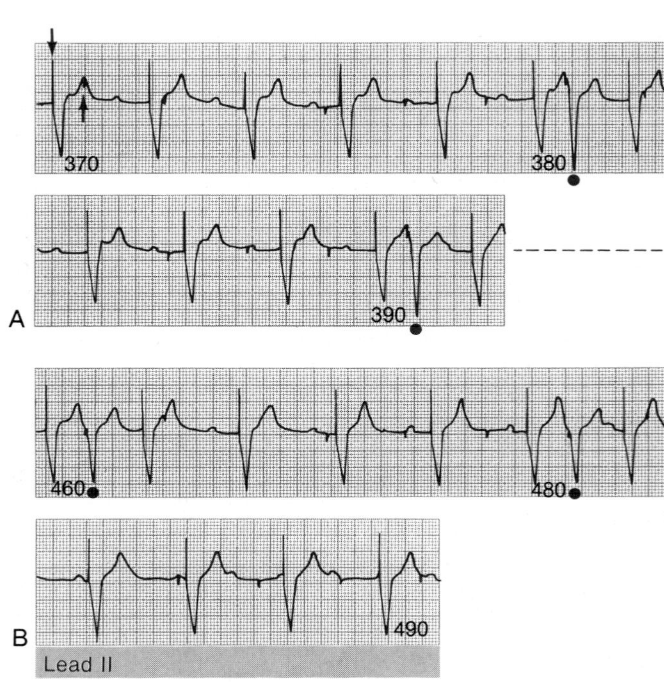

FIGURE 22–58. Supernormal excitation. Panels *A* and *B* represent noncontiguous portions of a continuous ECG recording with a middle segment removed (dotted line). The patient presented with a bipolar pacemaker that had exceeded end-of-life and was no longer consistently producing ventricular depolarization (small negative deflections indicated by the upright arrow). A temporary pacemaker was implanted and set at a fixed rate (asynchronous, V00). These large deflections are indicated by the inverted arrow. The numbers in msec indicate the interval between the onset of the QRS complex and the following subthreshold pacemaker stimulus. At intervals of 370 msec (beginning, panel *A*) and 490 msec (end, panel *B*), the subthreshold stimulus fails to produce a propagated ventricular response. However, at intervals between 380 and 480 msec, ventricular depolarizations result (filled circles). Thus the period of supernormal excitation is 100 msec duration, from 380 to 480 msec after the onset of the QRS complex.

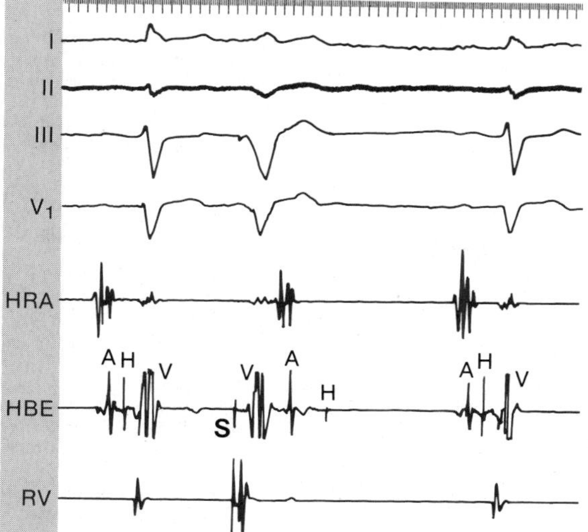

FIGURE 22–59. Concealed conduction. Following the first normally conducted sinus-initiated complex, a premature ventricular complex is stimulated (S). The next spontaneous sinus-initiated P wave blocks to produce a fully compensatory pause. The third sinus-initiated P wave conducts normally. From the His bundle recording it is obvious that the nonconducted sinus beat blocks distal to the His bundle recording site. Note that the A-H interval of the nonconducted sinus P wave beat is prolonged, suggesting that the premature ventricular complex retrogradely activated His and invaded the AV node, making it partially refractory to the next sinus beat. Since retrograde conduction into the AV node is not recorded, and can only be surmised on the basis of the increase in the following A-H interval, it is an example of concealed conduction. Further, since retrograde His and AV node activation by the premature ventricular complex would not be apparent in the scalar ECG but is responsible for the compensatory pause, the blocked P wave is an example of concealed conduction.

number of mechanisms have been postulated to explain the apparent protection enjoyed by the parasystolic rhythm.[464]

These "classic" definitions of parasystole now need to be modified because it has been well established that the dominant sinus beats can modulate the discharge rate of the parasystolic rhythm despite entrance block. Thus wide variations in the modulated parasystolic cycle may occur. The "true" or unmodulated parasystolic cycle length can be determined by finding two consecutive parasystolic complexes without intervening beats. Phase response curves can be generated. Fixed coupling between the dominant and parasystolic rhythms can occur due to a variety of mechanisms, including entrainment. It is possible that modulated parasystole in the presence of supernormal excitability can trigger ventricular fibrillation.

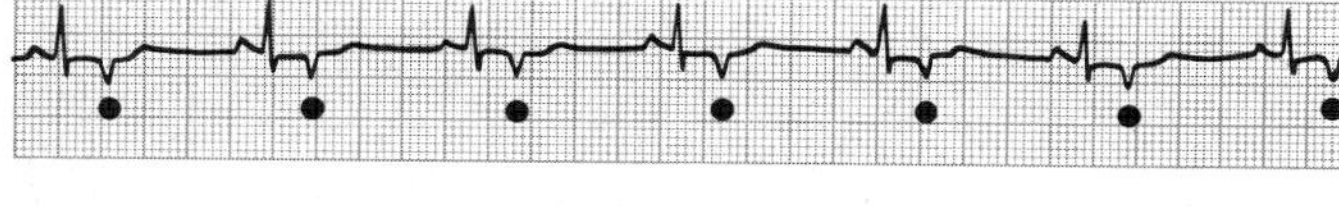

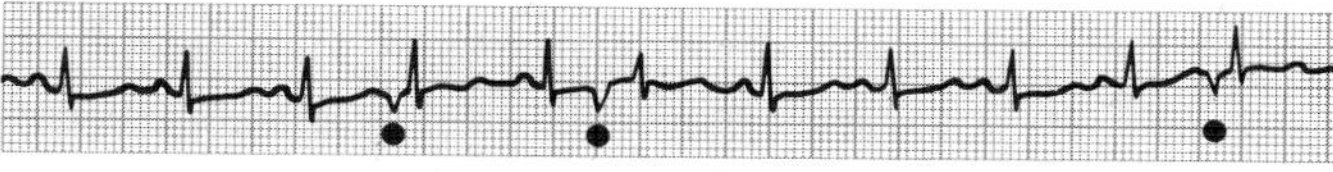

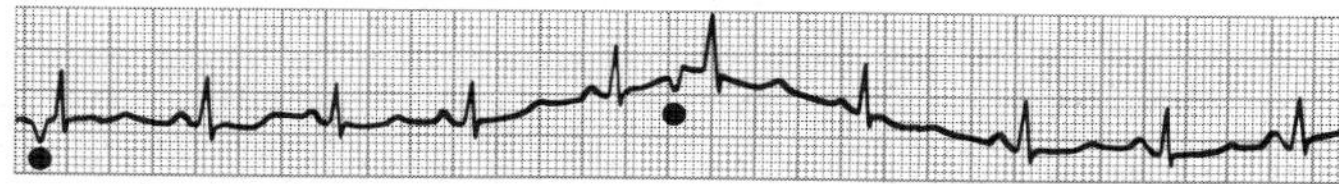

FIGURE 22–60. Atrial parasystole. *Top panel,* The atrial parasystolic impulses (filled circles under the negative P waves) are present at a fixed coupling interval to the dominant sinus rhythm. The reason for the fixed coupling is as follows: Each time the parasystolic impulse depolarizes the atrium, it also discharges the sinus node. Diastolic depolarization in the sinus node begins at that point (reset) and results in the following sinus P wave (positive P wave). Thus the constant parasystolic discharge rate (interectopic interval approximately 960 msec), resetting of the sinus node, and constant phase 4 diastolic depolarization in the sinus node combine to result in fixed coupling. *Middle and bottom panels,* The sinus discharge rate is slightly faster. It is no longer discharged by the parasystolic impulse which is still occurring at approximately 960 msec (slightly longer interval in the bottom tracing). Variable coupling, the usual presentation of parasystole, results. Lead II.

Acknowledgments

The author thanks William M. Miles, M.D., and Lawrence S. Klein, M.D., for critical comments and Joan Zipes and Robin Reid for secretarial assistance.

REFERENCES

1. Barsky, A. J., Cleary, P. D., Barnett, M. C., et al.: The accuracy of symptom reporting by patients complaining of palpitations. Am. J. Med. *97*:214, 1994.
2. Munro, N. C., McIntosh, S., Lawson, J., et al.: Incidence of complications after carotid sinus massage in older patients with syncope. J. Am. Geriatr. Soc. *42*:1248, 1994.

SINUS NODAL DISTURBANCES

3. Spodick, D. H.: Normal sinus heart rate: Sinus tachycardia and sinus bradycardia redefined. Am. Heart J. *124*:1119, 1992.
4. Dickerson, L. W., Huang, A. H., Thurnher, M. M., et al.: Relationship between coronary hemodynamic changes and the phasic events of rapid eye movement sleep. Sleep *16*:1550, 1993.
5. Scott, C. D., McComb, J. M., and Dark, J. H.: Heart rate and late mortality in cardiac transplant recipients. Eur. Heart J. *14*:530, 1993.
6. Tsai, J., Chern, T. L., Hu, S. C., et al.: The clinical implication of theophylline intoxication in the emergency department. Hum. Exp. Toxicol. *13*:651, 1994.
7. Sills, I. N.: Hyperthyroidism. Pediatr. Rev. *15*:417, 1994.
8. Johnson, N. J., and Marchlinski, F. E.: Arrhythmias induced by device antitachycardia therapy due to diagnostic nonspecificity. J. Am. Coll. Cardiol. *18*:1418, 1991.
9. Gelb, B. D., and Garson, A., Jr.: Noninvasive discrimination of right atrial ectopic tachycardia from sinus tachycardia in dilated cardiomyopathy. Am. Heart J. *120*:886, 1990.
10. Morillo, C. A., Klein, G. J., Thakur, R. K., et al.: Mechanism of "inappropriate" sinus tachycardia: Role of sympathovagal balance. Circulation *90*:873, 1994.
11. Skeberis, V., Simonis, F., Tsakonas, K., et al.: Inappropriate sinus tachycardia following radiofrequency ablation of AV nodal tachycardia: Incidence and clinical significance. PACE *17*:924, 1994.
12. Kocovic, D. Z., Harada, T., Shea, J. B., et al.: Alterations of heart rate and of heart rate variability after radiofrequency catheter ablation of supraventricular tachycardia: Delineation of parasympathetic pathways in the human heart. Circulation *88*:1671, 1993.
13. Ehlert, F. A., Goldberger, J. J., Brooks, R., et al.: Persistent inappropriate sinus tachycardia after radiofrequency current catheter modification of the atrioventricular node. Am. J. Cardiol. *69*:1092, 1992.
14. Waspe, L. E., Chien, W. W., Merillat, J. C., et al.: Sinus node modification using radiofrequency current in a patient with persistent inappropriate sinus tachycardia. PACE *17*:1569, 1994.
15. Hendry, P. J., Packer, D. L., Anstadt, M. P., et al.: Surgical treatment of automatic atrial tachycardias. Ann. Thorac. Surg. *42*:253, 1990.
16. DePaola, A. A. G., Horowitz, L. N., Vattimo, A. C., et al.: Sinus node artery occlusion for treatment of chronic nonparoxysmal sinus tachycardia. Am. J. Cardiol. *70*:128, 1992.
17. Kollai, M., Bonyhay, I., Jokkel, G., et al.: Cardiac vagal hyperactivity in adolescent anorexia nervosa. Eur. Heart J. *15*:1113, 1994.
18. Scott, C. D., Dark, J. H., and McComb, J. M.: Sinus node function after cardiac transplantation. J. Am. Coll. Cardiol. *24*:1334, 1994.
19. Caeiro, T., and Iosa, D.: Chronic Chagas' disease: Possible mechanism of sinus bradycardia. Can. J. Cardiol. *10*:765, 1994.
20. Alboni, T., Menozzi, C., Brignole, M., et al.: An abnormal neuroreflex plays a role in causing syncope in sinus bradycardia. J. Am. Coll. Cardiol. *22*:1130, 1993.
21. Frank, J. I., Ropper, A. H., and Zuniga, G.: Acute intracranial lesions and respiratory sinus arrhythmia. Arch. Neurol. *49*:1200, 1992.
22. Sneddon, J. F., and Camm, A. J.: Sinus node disease: Current concepts in diagnosis and therapy. Drugs. *44*:728, 1992.
23. Benditt, D. G., Sakaguchi, S., Goldstein, M. A., et al.: Sinus node dysfunction: Pathophysiology, clinical features, evaluation and treatment. *In* Zipes, D. P., and Jalife, J. (eds.): Cardiac Electrophysiology: From Cell to Bedside. 2nd ed. Philadelphia, W. B. Saunders Company, 1994, p. 1215.
24. Kyrickidis, M., Barbetseas, J., Antonopoulos, A., et al.: Early atrial arrhythmias in acute myocardial infarction: Role of the sinus node artery. Chest *101*:944, 1992.
25. Becker, H., Brandenburg, U., Peter, J. H., et al.: Reversal of sinus arrest and atrioventricular conduction block in patients with sleep apnea during nasal continuous positive airway pressure. Am. J. Respir. Crit. Care Med. *151*:215, 1995.
26. Fisch, C.: Electrocardiographic manifestations of exit block. *In* Zipes, D.P., and Jalife, J. (eds.): Cardiac Electrophysiology: From Cell to Bedside. 2nd ed. Philadelphia, W. B. Saunders Company, 1994, p. 955.

27. Wu, D. L., Yeh, S. J., Lin, F. C., et al.: Sinus automaticity and sinoatrial conduction in severe symptomatic sick sinus syndrome. J. Am. Coll. Cardiol. *19*:355, 1992.
28. Bjornstad, H., Storstein, L., Meen, H. D., et al.: Ambulatory electrocardiographic findings in top athletes, athletic students and controlled subjects. Cardiology *84*:42, 1994.
29. Benditt, D. G., Petersen, M., Lurie, K. G., et al.: Cardiac pacing for prevention of recurrent vasovagal syncope. Ann. Intern. Med. *122*:204, 1995.
30. Asseman, P., Berzin, B., Desry, D., et al.: Postextrasystolic sinoatrial exit block in human sick sinus syndrome: Demonstration by direct recording of sinus node electrograms. Am. Heart J. *122*:1633, 1991.
31. Centurion, O. A., Fukatani, M., Konoe, A., et al.: Different distribution of abnormal endocardial electrograms within the right atrium in patients with sick sinus syndrome. Br. Heart J. *68*:596, 1992.
32. Sgarbossa, E. B., Pinski, S. L., Maloney, J. D., et al.: Chronic atrial fibrillation and stroke in paced patients with sick sinus syndrome: Relevance of clinical characteristics and pacing modalities. Circulation *88*:1045, 1993.
33. Marcus, B., Gillette, P. C., and Garson, A., Jr.: Electrophysiologic evaluation of sinus node dysfunction in postoperative children and young adults utilizing combined autonomic blockade. Clin. Cardiol. *14*:33, 1991.
34. Matthys, D., and Verhaaren, H.: Exercise-induced bradycardia after Mustard repair for complete transposition. Int. J. Cardiol. *36*:126, 1992.
35. Lee, W. J., Wu, M. H., Young, M. L., et al.: Sinus node dysfunction in children. Acta Paediatr. Sin. *33*:159, 1992.
36. Bharati, S., and Lev, M.: The pathologic changes in the conduction system beyond the age of 90. Am. Heart J. *124*:486, 1992.
37. Alboni, P., Baggioni, G. F., Scarfo, S., et al.: Role of sinus node artery disease in sick sinus syndrome in inferior wall acute myocardial infarction. Am. J. Cardiol. *67*:1180, 1991.
38. Haywood, G. A., Katritsis, D., Ward, J., et al.: Atrial adaptive rate pacing in sick sinus syndrome: Effects on exercise capacity and arrhythmias. Br. Heart J. *69*:174, 1993.
39. Hesselson, A. B., Parsonnet, V., Bernstein, A. D., et al.: Deleterious effects of long-term single-chamber ventricular pacing in patients with sick sinus syndrome: The hidden benefits of dual-chamber pacing. J. Am. Coll. Cardiol. *19*:1542, 1992.
40. Saito, D., Matsubara, K., Yamanari, H., et al.: Effects of oral theophylline on sick sinus syndrome. J. Am. Coll. Cardiol. *21*:1199, 1993.
41. Strickberger, S. A., Fish, R. D., Lamas, G. A., et al.: Comparison of the effects of propanolol versus pindolol on sinus rate and pacing frequency in sick sinus syndrome. Am. J. Cardiol. *71*:53, 1993.
42. Resh, W., Feuer, J., and Wesley, R. C., Jr.: Intravenous adenosine: A noninvasive diagnostic test for sick sinus syndrome. PACE *15*:2068, 1992.
43. Saito, D., Yamanari, H., Matsubara, K., et al.: Intravenous injection of adenosine triphosphate for assessing sinus node dysfunction in patients with sick sinus syndrome. Arzneimittelforschung *43*:1313, 1993.
44. Naccarelli, G. V., Shih, H., and Jalal, S.: Sinus node reentry and atrial tachycardias. *In* Zipes, D. P., and Jalife, J. (eds.): Cardiac Electrophysiology: From Cell to Bedside. 2nd ed. Philadelphia, W. B. Saunders Company, 1994, p. 607.
44a. Tang, C. W., Scheinman, M. M., Van Hare, G. F., et al.: Use of P wave configuration during atrial tachycardia to predict site of origin. J. Am. Coll. Cardiol. *26*:1315, 1995.
45. Sperry, R. E., Ellenbogen, K. A., Wood, M. A., et al.: Radiofrequency catheter ablation of sinus node reentrant tachycardia. PACE *16*:2202, 1993.

DISTURBANCES OF ATRIAL RHYTHM

46. Zipes, D. P., and Garson, A., Jr.: Twenty-sixth Bethesda Conference: Recommendation for determining eligibility for competition in athletes with cardiovascular abnormalities. Task force 6: Arrhythmias. J. Am. Coll. Cardiol. *24*:892, 1994.
47. Waldo, A. L.: Atrial flutter: Mechanisms, clinical features and management. *In* Zipes, D. P., and Jalife, J. (eds.): Cardiac Electrophysiology: From Cell to Bedside. 2nd ed. Philadelphia, W. B. Saunders Company, 1994, p. 666.
48. Balaji, S., Johnson, T. B., Sade, R. M., et al.: Management of atrial flutter after the Fontan procedure. J. Am. Coll. Cardiol. *23*:1209, 1994.
49. Flack, N. J., Zosmer, N., Bennett, P. R., et al.: Amiodarone given by three routes to terminate fetal atrial flutter associated with severe hydrops. Obstet. Gynecol. *82* (4 Pt. 2, Suppl.):714, 1993.
50. Chang, J. S., Chen, V. C., Tsai, C. H., et al.: Successful conversion of fetal atrial flutter with digoxin: Report of one case. Acta Paediatr. Sin. *35*:229, 1994.
51. Tucker, K. J., and Wilson, C.: A comparison of transesophageal atrial pacing and direct current cardioversion for the termination of atrial flutter: A prospective randomized clinical trial. Br. Heart J. *69*:530, 1993.
52. Yoshitake, N., Tanoiri, T., Nomoto, J., et al.: Patterns of interruption of atrial flutter induced by rapid atrial pacing. Jpn. Circ. J. *58*:181, 1990.
53. Baeriswyl, G., Zimmerman, M., and Adamec, R.: Efficacy of rapid atrial pacing for conversion of atrial flutter in medically treated patients. Clin. Cardiol. *17*:246, 1994.
54. Cosio, F. G., Lopez-Gill, M., Arribas, F., et al.: Mechanisms of entrainment of human common flutter studied with multiple endocardial recordings. Circulation *89*:2117, 1994.
55. Botteron, G. W., and Smith, J. M.: Spatial and temporal inhomogeneity of adenosine's effect on atrial refractoriness in humans: Using atrial fibrillation to probe atrial refractoriness. J. Cardiovasc. Electrophysiol. *5*:477, 1994.
56. Shettigar, U. R., Toole, J. G., and Appunn, A. O.: Combined use of esmolol and digoxin in the acute treatment of atrial fibrillation or flutter. Am. Heart J. *126*:368, 1993.
57. Cochrane, A. D., Siddins, M., Rosenfeldt, F. L., et al.: A comparison of amiodarone and digoxin for treatment of supraventricular arrhythmias after cardiac surgery. Eur. J. Cardiothorac. Surg. *8*:194, 1994.
58. Crijns, H. J., VanGelder, I. C., and Lie, K. I.: Benefits and risks of antiarrhythmic drug therapy after DC electrical cardioversion of atrial fibrillation or flutter. Eur. Heart J. *15* (Suppl. A):17, 1994.
59. Till, J. A., Baxendall, M., and Benetar, A.: Acceleration of the ventricular response to atrial flutter by amiodarone in an infant with Wolff-Parkinson-White syndrome. Br. Heart J. *70*:84, 1993.
60. Santiago, D., Warshofsky, M., LiMandri, G., et al.: Left atrial appendage function and thrombus formation in atrial fibrillation-flutter: A transesophageal echocardiographic study. J. Am. Coll. Cardiol. *24*:159, 1994.
61. American College of Cardiology Cardiovascular Technology Assessment Committee: Catheter ablation for cardiac arrhythmias: Clinical applications, personnel and facilities. J. Am. Coll. Cardiol. *24*:828, 1994.
62. Lesh, M. D., and VanHare, G. F.: Status of ablation in patients with atrial tachycardia and atrial flutter. PACE *17*:1026, 1994.
63. Scheinman, M. M.: Patterns of catheter ablation practice in the United States: Results of the 1992 NASPE survey. North American Society of Pacing and Electrophysiology. PACE *17*:873, 1994.
64. Epstein, L. M., Chiesa, N., Wong, M. N., et al.: Radiofrequency catheter ablation in the treatment of supraventricular tachycardia in the elderly. J. Am. Coll. Cardiol. *23*:1356, 1994.
65. Hindricks, G.: The Multicenter European Radiofrequency Survey (MERFS): Complications of radiofrequency catheter ablation of arrhythmias. The Multicenter European Radiofrequency Survey (MERFS) Investigators of the Working Group on Arrhythmias of the European Society of Cardiology. Eur. Heart J. *14*:1644, 1993.
66. Lesh, M. D., VanHare, G. F., Epstein, L. M., et al.: Radiofrequency catheter ablation of atrial arrhythmias: Results and mechanisms. Circulation *89*:1074, 1994.
67. Calkins, H., Leon, A. R., Deam, A. G., et al.: Catheter ablation of atrial flutter using radiofrequency energy. Am. J. Cardiol. *73*:353, 1994.
68. Kay, G. N., Epstein, A. E., Dailey, S. M., et al.: Role of radiofrequency ablation in the management of supraventricular arrhythmias: Experience in 760 consecutive patients. J. Cardiovasc. Electrophysiol. *4*:371, 1993.
69. Olshansky, B., Wilber, D. J., and Hariman, R. J.: Atrial flutter: Update on the mechanism and treatment. PACE *15*:2308, 1992.
70. Zipes, D. P., DiMarco, J. P., Gillette, P. C., et al.: AHA/ACC guidelines for clinical intracardiac electrophysiologic procedures. Circulation *92*:673, 1995.
71. Konings, K. T., Kirchhof, C. J., Smeets, J. R., et al.: High-density mapping of electrically induced atrial fibrillation in humans. Circulation *89*:1665, 1994.
72. Ruffy, R.: Atrial fibrillation. *In* Zipes, D. P., and Jalife, J. (eds.): Cardiac Electrophysiology: From Cell to Bedside. 2nd ed. Philadelphia, W. B. Saunders Company, 1994, p. 682.
73. Allessie, M. A.: Reentrant mechanisms underlying atrial fibrillation. *In* Zipes, D. P., and Jalife, J. (eds.): Cardiac Electrophysiology: From Cell to Bedside. 2nd ed. Philadelphia, W. B. Saunders Company, 1994, p. 562.
74. Falk, R. H., and Podrid, P. J. (eds.): Atrial Fibrillation: Mechanisms and Management. New York, Raven Press, 1992.
74a. Meijler, F. L., Wittkampf, F. H., Brennen, K. R., et al.: Electrocardiogram of the humpback whale (Megaptera novaengliae), with specific reference to atrioventricular transmission and ventricular excitation. J. Am. Coll. Cardiol. *20*:475, 1992.
75. Watanabe, Y., and Watanabe, M.: Impulse formation and conduction of excitation in the atrioventricular node. J. Cardiovasc. Electrophysiol. *5*:517, 1994.
76. The National Heart Lung and Blood Institute Working Group on Atrial Fibrillation: Atrial fibrillation: Current understandings and research imperatives. J. Am. Coll. Cardiol. *22*:1830, 1993.
77. Domanski, M. J.: The epidemiology of atrial fibrillation. Coronary Artery Dis. *6*:95, 1995.
78. Furberg, C. D., Psaty, B. M., Manolio, T. A., et al.: Prevalence of atrial fibrillation in elderly subjects (The Cardiovascular Health Study). Am. J. Cardiol. *74*:236, 1994.
79. Sawin, C. T., Geller, A., Wolf, P. A., et al.: Low serum thyrotropin concentrations as a risk factor for atrial fibrillation in older persons. N. Engl. J. Med. *331*:1249, 1994.
80. Woeber, K. A.: Thyrotoxicosis and the heart. N. Engl. J. Med. *327*:94, 1992.
81. Coumel, P.: Paroxysmal atrial fibrillation: A disorder of autonomic tone. Eur. Heart J. *15* (Suppl. A):9, 1994.
82. Warfarin versus aspirin for prevention of thromboembolism in atrial fibrillation: Stroke Prevention in Atrial Fibrillation II. Lancet *343*:687, 1994.

83. EAFT (European Atrial Fibrillation Trial) Study Group: Secondary prevention in non-rheumatic atrial fibrillation after transient ischemic attack or minor stroke. Lancet *342*:1255, 1993.
84. Ezekowitz, M. D., Bridgers, S. L., James, K. E., et al.: Warfarin in the prevention of stroke associated with nonrheumatic atrial fibrillation. N. Engl. J. Med. *327*:1406, 1992.
85. Connolly, S. J., Laupacis, A., Gent, M., et al.: Canadian Atrial Fibrillation Anti-Coagulation (CAFA) Study. J. Am. Coll. Cardiol. *18*:349, 1991.
86. The Boston Area Anticoagulation Trial for Atrial Fibrillation Investigators: The effect of low-dose warfarin on the risk of stroke in patients with nonrheumatic atrial fibrillation. N. Engl. J. Med *323*:1505, 1990.
87. Stroke Prevention in Atrial Fibrillation Study Group Investigators: Preliminary report of the Stroke Prevention in Atrial Fibrillation Study. N. Engl. J. Med *322*:863, 1990.
88. Petersen, P., Boisen, G., Godtfredsen, J., et al.: Placebo-controlled, randomized trial of warfarin and aspirin for prevention of thromboembolic complications in chronic atrial fibrillation. The Copenhagen AFASAK Study. Lancet *1*:175, 1989.
89. Stroke Prevention in Atrial Fibrillation Investigators: Stroke Prevention in Atrial Fibrillation Study: Final results. Circulation *84*:527, 1991.
90. The Stroke Prevention in Atrial Fibrillation Investigators: Predictors of thromboembolism in atrial fibrillation: I. Clinical features of patients at risk. Ann. Intern. Med. *116*:1, 1992.
91. The Stroke Prevention in Atrial Fibrillation Investigators: Predictors of thromboembolism in atrial fibrillation: II. Echocardiographic features of patients at risk. Ann. Intern. Med. *116*:6, 1992.
92. Chimowitz, M. I., DeGeorgia, M. A., Poole, R. M., et al.: Left atrial spontaneous echo contrast is highly associated with previous stroke in patients with atrial fibrillation or mitral stenosis. Stroke *25*:1295, 1994.
93. Albers, G. W.: Atrial fibrillation and stroke: Three new studies, three remaining questions. Arch. Intern. Med. *154*:1443, 1994.
94. Matchar, D. B., McCrory, D. C., Barnett, H. J., et al.: Medical treatment for stroke prevention. Ann. Intern. Med. *121*:41, 1994.
95. Risk factors for stroke and efficacy of antithrombotic therapy in atrial fibrillation: Analysis of pooled data from five randomized controlled trials. Atrial Fibrillation Investigators: Atrial Fibrillation, Aspirin, Anticoagulation Study; Boston Area Anticoagulation Trial for Atrial Fibrillation Study; Canadian Atrial Fibrillation Anticoagulation Study; Stroke Prevention in Atrial Fibrillation Study; Veterans Affairs Stroke Prevention in Nonrheumatic Atrial Fibrillation Study. Arch. Intern. Med. *154*:1449, 1994.
96. Albers, G. W., and Hirsh, J.: Anticoagulation/platelet inhibition for atrial fibrillation. Coronary Artery Dis. *6*:129, 1995.
97. Wells, T. S., Holbrook, A. M., Crowther, N. R., et al.: Interactions of warfarin with drugs and food. Ann. Intern. Med. *121*:676, 1994.
98. Guidelines for medical treatment for stroke prevention. Ann. Intern. Med. *121*:54, 1994.
99. Disch, D. L., Greenberg, M. L., Holzberger, P. T., et al.: Managing chronic atrial fibrillation: A Markov decision analysis comparing warfarin, quinidine and low-dose amiodarone. Ann. Intern. Med. *120*:449, 1994.
100. Fuster, V., Dyken, M. L., Vokonas, P. S., et al.: Aspirin as a therapeutic agent in cardiovascular disease. Circulation *87*:659, 1993.
101. Patrono, C.: Aspirin as an antiplatelet drug. N. Engl. J. Med. *330*:1287, 1994.
102. Pritchett, E. L. C.: Management of atrial fibrillation. N. Engl. J. Med. *326*:1264, 1992.
103. Hirsh, J.: Oral anticoagulant drugs. N. Engl. J. Med. *324*:1865, 1991.
104. Laupacis, A., Albers, G. W., Dunn, M., et al.: Antithrombotic therapy in atrial fibrillation. Chest *102*:426S, 1992.
105. Leung, D. Y., Black, I. W., Cranney, G. B., et al.: Prognostic implications of left atrial spontaneous echo contrast in nonvalvular atrial fibrillation. J. Am. Coll. Cardiol. *24*:755, 1994.
106. Black, I. W., Fatkin, D., Sagar, K. B., et al.: Exclusion of atrial thrombus by transesophageal echocardiography does not preclude embolism after cardioversion of atrial fibrillation: A multicenter study. Circulation *89*:2509, 1994.
107. Manning, W. J., Silverman, D. I., and Gordon, S. P. F.: Cardioversion from atrial fibrillation without prolonged anticoagulation with use of transesophageal echocardiography to exclude the presence of atrial thrombi. N. Engl. J. Med. *328*:750, 1993.
108. Allessie, M. A., Wijffels, M. C., and Kirchhof, C. J.: Experimental models of arrhythmias: Toys or truth? Eur. Heart J. *15* (Suppl. A):2, 1994.
109. Janse, M. J.: Electrophysiology of atrial fibrillation. Coronary Artery Dis. *6*:101, 1995.
110. Morillo, C. A., Klein, G. J., Jones, D. L., et al.: Chronic rapid atrial pacing: Structural, functional, and electrophysiological characteristics of a new model of sustained atrial fibrillation. Circulation *91*:1588, 1995.
110a. Wijffels, M. C. E. F., Kirchhef, C. J. H. J., Dorland, R., et al.: Atrial fibrillation begets atrial fibrillation: A study in awake chronically instrumented goats. Circulation *92*:1954, 1995.
111. Shite, J., Yokota, Y., and Yokoyama, M.: Heterogeneity and time course of improvement in cardiac function after cardioversion of chronic atrial fibrillation: Assessment of serial echocardiographic indices. Br. Heart J. *70*:154, 1993.
112. Manning, W. J., Silverman, D. I., and Katz, S. E.: Impaired left atrial mechanical function after cardioversion: Relation to the duration of atrial fibrillation. J. Am. Coll. Cardiol. *23*:1535, 1994.
113. Lundstrom, T., Moor, E., and Ryden, L.: Differential effects of xamoterol and verapamil on ventricular rate regulation in patients with chronic atrial fibrillation. Am. Heart J. *124*:917, 1992.
114. Sarter, B. H., and Marchlinski, F. E.: Redefining the role of digoxin in the treatment of atrial fibrillation. Am. J. Cardiol. *69*:71G, 1992.
115. Roth, A., Kaluski, E., Felner, S., et al.: Clonidine for patients with rapid atrial fibrillation. Ann. Intern. Med. *116*:388, 1992.
116. Weiner, P., Ganam, R., Ganem, R., et al.: Clinical course of recent-onset atrial fibrillation treated with oral propafenone. Chest *105*:1013, 1994.
117. Ruffy, R.: Sotalol. J. Cardiovasc. Electrophysiol. *4*:81, 1993.
118. Falk, R. H.: Proarrhythmia in patients treated for atrial fibrillation or flutter. Ann. Intern. Med. *117*:141, 1992.
119. Hohnloser, S. H., Klingenhaben, T., and Singh, B. N.: Amiodarone-associated proarrhythmic effects: A review with special reference to torsades de pointes tachycardia. Ann. Intern. Med. *121*:529, 1994.
120. Roden, D. M.: Risks and benefits of antiarrhythmic therapy. N. Engl. J. Med. *331*:785, 1994.
121. Sopher, M., and Camm, A. J.: Therapy for atrial fibrillation: Control of the ventricular response and prevention of recurrence. Coronary Artery Dis. *6*:105, 1995.
122. Fujiki, A., Yoshida, S., Tani, M., et al.: Efficacy of class IA antiarrhythmic drugs in converting atrial fibrillation unassociated with organic heart disease and their relation to atrial electrophysiologic characteristics. Am. J. Cardiol. *74*:282, 1994.
123. Kirchhof, C., Charro, F., Scheffer, G. J., et al.: Regional entrainment of atrial fibrillation studied by high-resolution mapping in open-chest dogs. Circulation *88*:736, 1993.
124. Williamson, B. D., Man, K. C., Daoud, E., et al.: Radiofrequency catheter modification of atrioventricular conduction to control the ventricular rate during atrial fibrillation. N. Engl. J. Med. *331*:910, 1994.
125. Brignole, M., Gianfranchi, L., Menozzi, C., et al.: Influence of atrioventricular junction radiofrequency ablation in patients with chronic atrial fibrillation and flutter on quality of life and cardiac performance. Am. J. Cardiol. *74*:242, 1964.
126. Harvey, M. N., and Morady, F.: Radiofrequency catheter ablation for atrial fibrillation. Coronary Artery Dis. *6*:114, 1995.
127. Ferguson, T. B., Jr.: Surgery for atrial fibrillation. Coronary Artery Dis. *6*:120, 1995.
128. Shyu, K. G., Cheng, J. J., Chen, J. J., et al.: Recovery of atrial function after atrial compartment operation for chronic atrial fibrillation in mitral valve disease. J. Am. Coll. Cardiol. *24*:392, 1994.
129. Haissaguerre, M., Marcus, F. I., Fischer, B., et al.: Radiofrequency catheter ablation in unusual mechanisms of atrial fibrillation: Report of three cases. J. Cardiovasc. Electrophysiol. *5*:743, 1994.
130. Haissaguerre, M., Gencel, L., Fischer, B., et al.: Successful catheter ablation of atrial fibrillation. J. Cardiovasc. Electrophysiol. *5*:1045, 1994.
131. Swartz, J. F., Pollersels, G., Silvers, J., et al.: A catheter-based curative approach to atrial fibrillation in humans. Circulation *90* (Suppl. I): (Abs.):1335, 1994.
132. Elvan, A., Pride, H. P., Eble, J. N., et al.: Radiofrequency catheter ablation of the atria reduces the inducibility and duration of atrial fibrillation in dogs. Circulation *91*:2235, 1995.
133. Keane, B., Boyd, E., Anderson, D., et al.: Comparison of biphasic and monophasic waveforms in epicardial atrial defibrillation. J. Am. Coll. Cardiol. *24*:171, 1994.
134. Benditt, B. G., Dunbar, B., Fetter, J., et al.: Low-energy transvenous cardioversion defibrillation of atrial tachyarrhythmias in the canine: An assessment of electrode configurations and monophasic pulse sequencing. Am. Heart J. *127*:994, 1994.
135. Ayers, G. M., Alferness, C. A., Ilina, M., et al.: Ventricular proarrhythmic effects of ventricular cycle length and shock strength in a sheep model of transvenous atrial defibrillation. Circulation *89*:413, 1994.
136. Pollak, A., and Falk, R. H.: Pacemaker therapy in patients with atrial fibrillation. Am. Heart J. *125*:824, 1993.
137. Kay, G. N., Chong, F., Epstein, A. E., et al.: Radiofrequency ablation for treatment of primary atrial tachycardias. J. Am. Coll. Cardiol. *21*:901, 1993.
138. Chen, S. A., Chiang, C. E., Yang, C. J., et al.: Radiofrequency catheter ablation of intraatrial reentrant tachycardia in adult patients: Identification of electrophysiological characteristics and endocardial mapping techniques. Circulation *88*:578, 1993.
139. Kadish, A. H., and Morady, F.: The response of paroxysmal supraventricular tachycardia to overdrive atrial and ventricular pacing: Can it help determine the tachycardia mechanism? J. Cardiovasc. Electrophysiol. *4*:239, 1993.
140. Case, C. L., and Gillette, P. C.: Automatic atrial and junctional tachycardias in the pediatric patient: Strategies for diagnosis and management. PACE *16*:1323, 1993.
141. Chen, S. A., Chiang, C. E., Yang, C. J., et al.: Sustained atrial tachycardia in adult patients: Electrophysiological characteristics, pharmacological response, possible mechanisms and effects of radiofrequency ablation. Circulation *90*:1262, 1994.
142. Engelstein, E. D., Littman, N., Stein, K. M., et al.: Mechanism-specific effects of adenosine on atrial tachycardia. Circulation *89*:2645, 1994.
143. DeBakker, J. M. T., Hauer, R. N. W., Bakker, P. F. A., et al.: Abnormal automaticity as mechanism of atrial tachycardia in the human heart—Electrophysiologic and histologic correlation: A case report. J. Cardiovasc. Electrophysiol. *5*:335, 1994.

144. Raja, T., Hawker, R. E., Chaikitpinyo, A., et al.: Amiodarone management of junctional ectopic tachycardia after cardiac surgery in children. Br. Heart J. *72*:261, 1994.
145. Till, J. A., Ho, S. Y., and Rowland, E.: Histopathological findings in three children with His bundle tachycardia occurring subsequent to cardiac surgery. Eur. Heart J. *13*:709, 1992.
146. Braunstein, P. W., Jr., Sade, R. M., and Gillette, P. C.: Life-threatening postoperative junctional ectopic tachycardia. Ann. Thorac. Surg. *53*:726, 1992.
147. Gentzer, J. H., Goyal, R., Williamson, B. D., et al.: Analysis of junctional ectopy during radiofrequency ablation of the slow pathway in patients with atrioventricular nodal reentrant tachycardia. Circulation *90*:2820, 1994.
148. Heusch, A., Kramer, H. H., Krogmann, O. N., et al.: Clinical experience with propafenone for cardiac arrhythmias in the young. Eur. Heart J. *15*:1050, 1994.
149. Case, C. L., and Gillette, P. C.: Automatic atrial and junctional tachycardias in the pediatric patient: Strategies for diagnosis and management. PACE *16*:1323, 1993.
150. Paul, T., Reimer, A., Janousek, J., et al.: Efficacy and safety of propafenone in congenital junctional ectopic tachycardia. J. Am. Coll. Cardiol. *20*:911, 1992.
151. Scheinman, M. M., Gonzalez, R. P., Cooper, M. W., et al.: Clinical and electrophysiologic features and role of catheter ablation techniques in adult patients with automatic atrioventricular junctional tachycardia. Am. J. Cardiol. *74*:565, 1994.
152. Gonzalez, R. V., and Scheinman, M. M.: Paroxysmal junctional and fascicular tachycardia in adults: Clinical presentation course and therapy. *In* Zipes, D. P., and Jalife, J. (eds.): Cardiac Electrophysiology: From Cell to Bedside. 2nd ed. Philadelphia, W. B. Saunders Company, 1994, p. 691.
153. Kuck, K. H., and Schluter, M.: Junctional tachycardia and the role of catheter ablation. Lancet *341*:1386, 1993.
154. Ehlert, F. A., Goldberger, J. J., Deal, B. J., et al.: Successful radiofrequency energy ablation of automatic junctional tachycardia preserving normal atrioventricular nodal conduction. PACE *16*:54, 1993.
155. Akhtar, M., Jazayeri, M. R., Sra, J., et al.: Atrioventricular nodal reentry. Clinical, electrophysiological, and therapeutic considerations. Circulation *88*:282, 1993.
156. Jackman, W. M., Nakagawa, H., and Heidbuchel, H.: Three forms of atrioventricular nodal (junctional) reentrant tachycardia: Differential diagnosis, electrophysiological characteristics, and implications for anatomy of the reentrant circuit. *In* Zipes, D. P., and Jalife, J. (eds.): Cardiac Electrophysiology: From Cell to Bedside. 2nd ed. Philadelphia, W. B. Saunders Company, 1994, p. 620.
157. Gamache, M. C., Bharati, S., Lev, M., et al.: Histopathological study following catheter guided radiofrequency current ablation of the slow pathway in a patient with atrioventricular nodal reentrant tachycardia. PACE *17*:247, 1994.
158. Langberg, J. J.: Radiofrequency catheter ablation of AV nodal reentry: The anterior approach. PACE *16*:615, 1993.
159. DeBakker, J. M., Coronel, R., McGuire, M. A., et al.: Slow potentials in the atrioventricular junctional area of patients operated on for atrioventricular node tachycardias and in isolated porcine hearts. J. Am. Coll. Cardiol. *23*:709, 1994.
160. Janse, M. J., Anderson, R. H., McGuire, M. A., et al.: AV nodal reentry: I. AV nodal reentry revisited. J. Cardiovasc. Electrophysiol. *4*:561, 1993.
161. McGuire, M. A., Janse, M. J., and Ross, D. L.: AV nodal reentry: II. AV nodal, AV junctional or atrial nodal reentry? J. Cardiovasc. Electrophysiol. *4*:573, 1993.
162. McGuire, M. A., Yit, A. S., Robotin, M., et al.: Surgical procedure for the cure of atrioventricular junctional (AV node) reentrant tachycardia: Anatomic and electrophysiologic effects of dissection of the anterior atrial nodal connections in a canine model. J. Am. Coll. Cardiol. *24*:784, 1994.
163. Silka, M. J., Kron, J., Park, J. K., et al.: Atypical forms of supraventricular tachycardia due to atrioventricular node reentry in children after radiofrequency modification of slow pathway conduction. J. Am. Coll. Cardiol. *23*:1363, 1994.
164. Josephson, M. E., and Miller, J. M.: Atrioventricular nodal reentry: Evidence supporting an intranodal location. PACE *16*:599, 1993.
165. Suzuki, F., Tanaka, K., Ishihara, N., et al.: Double ventricular responses during extrastimulation of atrioventricular nodal reentrant tachycardia. Eur. Heart J. *15*:285, 1994.
166. Kalbfleisch, S. J., Strickberger, S. A., Hummel, J. D., et al.: Double retrograde atrial response after radiofrequency ablation of typical AV nodal reentrant tachycardia. J. Cardiovasc. Electrophysiol. *4*:695, 1993.
167. Abe, H., Ohkita, T., Fujita, M., et al.: Atrioventricular (AV) nodal reentry associated with 2:1 infra-His conduction block during tachycardia in a patient with AV nodal triple pathways. Jpn. Heart J. *35*:241, 1994.
168. Gursoy, S., Steurer, G., Brugada, J., et al.: Brief report: The hemodynamic mechanism of pounding in the neck in atrioventricular nodal reentrant tachycardia. N. Engl. J. Med. *327*:772, 1992.
169. Nayebpour, M., Billette, J., Amellal, F., et al.: Effects of adenosine on rate-dependent atrioventricular nodal function: Potential roles in tachycardia termination and physiological regulation. Circulation *88*:2632, 1993.
170. Jackman, W. M., Beckman, K. J., McClelland, J. H., et al.: Treatment of supraventricular tachycardia due to atrioventricular nodal reentry by radiofrequency catheter ablation of the slow-pathway conduction. N. Engl. J. Med. *327*:313, 1992.
171. Lee, M. A., Morady, F., Kadish, A., et al.: Catheter modification of the atrioventricular junction with radiofrequency energy for control of atrioventricular nodal reentrant tachycardia. Circulation *83*:827, 1991.
172. Mahomed, Y., King, R. D., Zipes, D. P., et al.: Surgery for atrioventricular node reentry tachycardia: Results with surgical skeletonization of the atrioventricular node and discrete perinodal cryosurgery. J. Thorac. Cardiovasc. Surg. *104*:1035, 1992.
173. McGuire, M. A., Bourke, J. P., Robotin, M. C., et al.: High resolution mapping of Koch's triangle using 60 electrodes in humans with atrioventricular junctional (AV nodal) reentrant tachycardia. Circulation *88*:2315, 1993.
174. Mitrani, R. D., Klein, L. S., Hackett, F. K., et al.: Radiofrequency ablation for atrioventricular node reentrant tachycardia: Comparison between fast (anterior) and slow (posterior) pathway ablation. J. Am. Coll. Cardiol. *21*:432, 1993.
175. Miles, W. M., Hubbard, J. E., Zipes, D. P., et al.: Elimination of AV nodal reentrant tachycardia with 2:1 VA block by posteroseptal ablation. J. Cardiovasc. Electrophysiol. *5*:510, 1994.
176. Kalbfleisch, S. J., and Morady, F.: Catheter ablation of atrioventricular nodal reentrant tachycardia. *In* Zipes, D. P., and Jalife, J. (eds.): Cardiac Electrophysiology: From Cell to Bedside. 2nd ed. Philadelphia, W. B. Saunders Company, 1994, p. 1477.
177. Baker, J. H., II, Plumb, V. J., Epstein, A. E., et al.: Predictors of recurrent atrioventricular nodal reentry after selective slow pathway ablation. Am. J. Cardiol. *73*:765, 1994.
178. Kay, G. N., Epstein, A. E., Dailey, S. M., et al.: Role of radiofrequency ablation in the management of supraventricular arrhythmias: Experience in 760 consecutive patients. J. Cardiovasc. Electrophysiol. *4*:371, 1993.
179. Jazayeri, M. R., Sra, J. S., Deshpande, S. S., et al.: Electrophysiologic spectrum of atrioventricular nodal behavior in patients with atrioventricular nodal reentrant tachycardia undergoing selective fast or slow pathway ablation. J. Cardiovasc. Electrophysiol. *4*:99, 1993.
180. Gursoy, S., Schluter, M., and Kuck, K. H.: Radiofrequency current catheter ablation for control of supraventricular arrhythmias. J. Cardiovasc. Electrophysiol. *4*:194, 1993.
181. Li, H. G., Klein, G. J., Stites, H. W., et al.: Elimination of slow pathway conduction: An accurate indicator of clinical success after radiofrequency atrioventricular node modification. J. Am. Coll. Cardiol. *22*:1849, 1993.
182. Lindsay, D. D., Chung, M. K., Gamache, M. C., et al.: Therapeutic endpoints for the treatment of atrioventricular node reentrant tachycardia by catheter-guided radiofrequency current. J. Am. Coll. Cardiol. *22*:733, 1993.
183. Wu, D., Yeh, S. J., Wang, C. C., et al.: A simple technique for selective radiofrequency ablation of the slow pathway in atrioventricular node reentrant tachycardia. J. Am. Coll. Cardiol. *21*:1612, 1993.
184. Miles, W. M., Klein, L. S., Rardon, D. P., et al.: Atrioventricular reentry and variants: Mechanisms, clinical features, and management. *In* Zipes, D.P., and Jalife, J. (eds.): Cardiac Electrophysiology: From Cell to Bedside. 2nd ed. Philadelphia, W. B. Saunders Company, 1994, p. 638.
185. Yee, R., Klein, G. J., and Guiraudon, G. M.: The Wolff-Parkinson-White syndrome. *In* Zipes, D. P., and Jalife, J. (eds.): Cardiac Electrophysiology: From Cell to Bedside. 2nd ed. Philadelphia, W. B. Saunders Company, 1994, p. 1199.
186. Stanke, A., Storti, C., DePonti, R., et al.: Spontaneous incessant AV reentrant tachycardia related to left bundle branch block and concealed left-sided accessory AV pathway. J. Cardiovasc. Electrophysiol. *5*:777, 1994.
187. Calkins, H., Langberg, J., Sousa, J., et al.: Radiofrequency catheter ablation of accessory atrioventricular connections in 250 patients. Abbreviated therapeutic approach to Wolff-Parkinson-White syndrome. Circulation *85*:1337, 1992.
188. Kuck, K. H., Schluter, M., and Gursoy, S.: Preservation of atrioventricular nodal conduction during radiofrequency current catheter ablation of midseptal accessory pathways. Circulation *86*:1743, 1992.
189. Bashir, Y., Heald, S. C., O'Nunain, S., et al.: Radiofrequency current delivery by way of a bipolar tricuspid annulus-mitral annulus electrode configuration for ablation of posteroseptal accessory pathways. J. Am. Coll. Cardiol. *22*:550, 1993.
190. Xie, B., Heald, S. C., Bashir, Y., et al.: Localization of accessory pathways from the 12-lead electrocardiogram using a new algorithm. Am. J. Cardiol. *74*:161, 1994.
191. Rodriguez, L. M., Smeets, J. L., deChillou, C., et al.: The 12-lead electrocardiogram in midseptal, anteroseptal, posteroseptal and right free wall accessory pathways. Am. J. Cardiol. *72*:1274, 1993.
192. Dubuc, M., Nadeau, R., Tremblay, G., et al.: Pace mapping using body surface potential maps to guide catheter ablation of accessory pathways in patients with Wolff-Parkinson-White syndrome. Circulation *87*:135, 1993.
193. Jackman, W. M., McClelland, J. H., Nakagawa, H., et al.: Ablation of right atriofascicular (Mahaim) accessory pathways. *In* Zipes, D. P. (ed.): Catheter Ablation of Arrhythmias. Armonk, N.Y., Futura, 1994, p. 187.

194. deChillou, C., Rodriguez, L. M., Schlapfer, J., et al.: Clinical characteristics and electrophysiologic properties of atrioventricular accessory pathways: Importance of the accessory pathway location. J. Am. Coll. Cardiol. *20*:666, 1992.
194a. Shih, H. T., Miles, W. M., Klein, L. S., et al.: Multiple accessory pathways in the permanent forms of junctional reciprocating tachycardia. Am. J. Cardiol. *73*:361, 1994.
195. Wienecke, M., Case, C., Buckles, D., et al.: Inducible ventricular tachyarrhythmia in children with Wolff-Parkinson-White syndrome. Am. J. Cardiol. *73*:396, 1994.
196. Pressley, J. C., Wharton, J. M., Tang, A. S., et al.: Effect of Ebstein's anomaly on short- and long-term outcome of surgically treated patients with Wolff-Parkinson-White syndrome. Circulation *86*:1147, 1992.
197. Rechavia, E., Mager, A., Birnbaum, Y., et al.: Mitral valve prolapse, sick sinus and Wolff-Parkinson-White syndromes: Interrelationships with respect to sudden cardiac death. Isr. J. Med. Sci. *29*:654, 1993.
198. Munger, T. M., Packer, D. L., Hammill, S. C., et al.: A population study of the natural history of Wolff-Parkinson-White syndrome in Olmstead County, Minnesota, 1953–1989. Circulation *87*:866, 1993.
199. Zardini, M., Yee, R., Thakur, R. K., et al.: Risk of sudden arrhythmic death in the Wolff-Parkinson-White syndrome: Current perspectives. PACE *17*:966, 1994.
200. Camm, A. J., Katritsis, D., and Nunain, S. O.: Effects of flecainide on atrial electrophysiology in the Wolff-Parkinson-White syndrome. Am. J. Cardiol. *70*:33A, 1992.
201. Crozier, I.: Flecainide in the Wolff-Parkinson-White syndrome. Am. J. Cardiol. *70*:26A, 1992.
202. Podrid, P. J.: Amiodarone. Ann. Intern. Med. *122*:689, 1995.
203. Manolis, A. S., Katsaros, C., and Kokkinos, D. V.: Electrophysiological and electropharmacological studies in preexcitation syndromes: Results with propafenone therapy and isoproterenol infusion testing. Eur. Heart J. *13*:1489, 1992.
204. Auricchio, A.: Reversible protective effect of propafenone or flecainide during atrial fibrillation in patients with an accessory atrioventricular connection. Am. Heart J. *124*:932, 1992.
205. Stanton, M. S.: Class I antiarrhythmic drugs: Quinidine, procainamide, disopyramide, lidocaine, mexiletine, tocainide, phenytoin, moricizine, flecainide, propafenone. *In* Zipes, D. P., and Jalife, J. (eds.): Cardiac Electrophysiology: From Cell to Bedside. 2nd ed. Philadelphia, W. B. Saunders Company, 1994, p. 1296.
206. Haissaguerre, M., Clementy, J., and Warin, J. F.: Catheter ablation of atrioventricular reentrant tachycardias. *In* Zipes, D. P., and Jalife, J. (eds.): Cardiac Electrophysiology: From Cell to Bedside. 2nd ed. Philadelphia, W. B. Saunders Company, 1994, p. 1487.
207. Hogenhuis, W., Stevens, S. K., Wang, P., et al.: Cost-effectiveness of radiofrequency ablation compared with other strategies in Wolff-Parkinson-White syndrome. Circulation *88*:11437, 1993.
208. Kalbfleisch, S. J., el-Atassi, R., Calkins, H., et al.: Safety, feasibility and cost of outpatient radiofrequency catheter ablation of accessory atrioventricular connections. J. Am. Coll. Cardiol. *21*:567, 1993.
209. Guiraudon, G. M., Klein, G. J., Yee, R., et al.: Surgery for the Wolff-Parkinson-White syndrome. *In* Zipes, D. P., and Jalife, J. (eds.): Cardiac Electrophysiology: From Cell to Bedside. 2nd ed. Philadelphia, W. B. Saunders Company, 1994, p. 1553.
210. Guiraudon, G. M., Guiraudon, C. M., Klein, G. J., et al.: Operation for the Wolff-Parkinson-White syndrome in the catheter ablation era. Ann. Thorac. Surg. *57*:1084, 1994.

VENTRICULAR RHYTHM DISTURBANCES

211. Wang, K., and Hodges, M.: The premature ventricular complex as a diagnostic aid. Ann. Intern. Med. *117*:766, 1992.
212. Murakawa, Y., Inoue, H., Koide, T., et al.: Reappraisal of the coupling interval of ventricular extrasystoles as an index of ectopic mechanisms. Br. Heart J. *68*:589, 1992.
213. Pogwizd, S. M.: Focal mechanisms underlying ventricular tachycardia during prolonged ischemic cardiomyopathy. Circulation *90*:1441, 1994.
214. Kostis, J. B., Allen, R., Berkson, D. M., et al.: Correlates of ventricular ectopic activity in isolated systolic hypertension. SHEP Cooperative Research Group. Am. Heart J. *127*:112, 1994.
215. Gillis, A. M., Peters, R. W., Mitchell, L. B., et al.: Effects of left ventricular dysfunction on the circadian variation of ventricular premature complexes in healed myocardial infarction. Am. J. Cardiol. *69*:1009, 1992.
216. Franz, M. R., Cima, R., Wang, D., et al.: Electrophysiological effects of myocardial stretch and mechanical determinants of stretch-activated arrhythmias. Circulation *86*:968, 1992.
217. Wang, Z., Taylor, L. K., Denney, W. D., et al.: Initiation of ventricular extrasystoles by myocardial stretch in chronically dilated and failing canine left ventricle. Circulation *90*:2022, 1994.
218. Maggioni, A. P., Zuanetti, G., Franzosi, M. G., et al.: Prevalence and prognostic significance of ventricular arrhythmias after acute myocardial infarction in the fibrinolytic area. GISSI-2 results. Circulation *87*:312, 1993.
219. Wyse, D. G., Morganroth, J., Ledingham, R., et al.: New insights into the definition and meaning of proarrhythmia during initiation of antiarrhythmic drug therapy from the Cardiac Arrhythmia Suppression Trial and its private study. The CAST Investigators. J. Am. Coll. Cardiol. *23*:1130, 1994.
220. Fleg, J. L., and Kennedy, H. L.: Long-term prognostic significance of ambulatory electrocardiographic findings in apparently healthy subjects greater than or equal to 60 years of age. Am. J. Cardiol. *70*:748, 1992.
221. Kennedy, H. L.: Ambulatory (Holter) electrocardiography recordings. *In* Zipes, D. P., and Jalife, J. (eds.): Cardiac Electrophysiology: From Cell to Bedside. 2nd ed. Philadelphia, W. B. Saunders Company, 1994, p. 1024.
222. Bikkina, M., Larson, M. G., and Levy, D.: Prognostic implications of asymptomatic ventricular arrhythmias: The Framingham Heart Study. Ann. Intern. Med. *117*:990, 1992.
223. Wilson, A. C., and Kostis, J. B.: The prognostic significance of very low frequency ventricular ectopic activity in survivors of acute myocardial infarction. The BHAT Study Group. Chest *102*:732, 1992.
224. Odemuyiwa, O., Farrell, T. G., Malik, M., et al.: Influence of age on the relation between heart rate variability, left ventricular ejection fraction, frequency of ventricular extrasystoles, and sudden death after myocardial infarction. Br. Heart J. *67*:387, 1992.
225. Hallstrom, A. P., Bigger, J. T., Jr., Roden, D., et al.: Prognostic significance of ventricular premature depolarizations measured one year after myocardial infarction in patients with early post infarction asymptomatic ventricular arrhythmia. J. Am. Coll. Cardiol. *20*:259, 1992.
226. Sueta, C. A., Clarke, S. W., Dunlop, S. H., et al.: Effect of acute magnesium administration on the frequency of ventricular arrhythmia in patients with heart failure. Circulation *89*:660, 1994.
227. Singh, B. N.: Beta-blockers and calcium channel blockers as anti-arrhythmic drugs. *In* Zipes, D. P., and Jalife, J. (eds.): Cardiac Electrophysiology: From Cell to Bedside. 2nd ed. Philadelphia, W. B. Saunders Company, 1994, p. 1317.
228. Hondeghem, L. M.: Class III agents: Amiodarone, bretylium and sotalol. *In* Zipes, D. P., and Jalife, J. (eds.): Cardiac Electrophysiology: From Cell to Bedside. 2nd ed. Philadelphia, W. B. Saunders Company, 1994, p. 1330.
229. The Cardiac Arrhythmia Suppression Trial II Investigators: Effect of the antiarrhythmic agent moricizine on survival after myocardial infarction. N. Engl. J. Med. *327*:227, 1992.
230. Navarro-Lopez, F., Kosin, J., Marrugat, J., et al.: Comparison of the effects of amiodarone versus metoprolol on the frequency of ventricular arrhythmias and on mortality after acute myocardial infarction. SSSD Investigators. Spanish Study on Sudden Death. Am. J. Cardiol. *72*:1243, 1993.
231. Zarembski, D. G., Nolan, P. E., Jr., Slack, M. K., et al.: Empiric long-term amiodarone prophylaxis following myocardial infarction: A metaanalysis. Arch. Intern. Med. *153*:2661, 1993.
232. Nasir, N., Jr., Taylor, A., Doyle, T. K., et al.: Evaluation of intravenous lidocaine for the termination of sustained monomorphic ventricular tachycardia in patients with coronary artery disease with or without healed myocardial infarction. Am. J. Cardiol. *74*:1183, 1994.
233. Nasir, N., Jr., Doyle, T. K., Wheeler, S. H., et al.: Usefulness of Holter monitoring in predicting efficacy of amiodarone therapy for sustained ventricular tachycardia associated with coronary artery disease. Am. J. Cardiol. *73*:554, 1994.
234. Man, K. C., Williamson, B. D., Niebauer, M., et al.: Electrophysiologic effects of sotalol and amiodarone in patients with sustained monomorphic ventricular tachycardia. Am. J. Cardiol. *74*:1119, 1994.
235. Kostis, J. B., Lacy, C. R., Hall, W. D., et al.: The effect of chlorthalidone on ventricular ectopic activity in patients with isolated systolic hypertension. The SHEP Study Group. Am. J. Cardiol. *74*:464, 1994.
236. Dorian, P., Langer, A., Morgan, C., et al.: Importance of ST-segment depression as a determinant of ventricular premature complex frequency after thrombolysis for acute myocardial infarction. Tissue Plasminogen Activator: Toronto (TPAT) Study Group. Am. J. Cardiol. *74*:419, 1994.
237. Marino, P., Nidasio, G., Golia, G., et al.: Frequency of predischarge ventricular arrhythmias in post myocardial infarction patients depends on residual left ventricular pump performance and is independent of the occurrence of acute reperfusion. The GISSI-2 Investigators. J. Am. Coll. Cardiol. *23*:290, 1994.
238. Tsuji, H., Venditti, F. J., Jr., Evans, J. C., et al.: The associations of levels of serum potassium and magnesium with ventricular premature complexes. The Framingham Heart Study. Am. J. Cardiol. *74*:232, 1994.
239. Papademetriou, V., Narayan, P., and Kokkinos, P.: Effects of diltiazem, metoprolol, enalapril, and hydrochlorothiazide on frequency of ventricular premature complexes. Am. J. Cardiol. *73*:242, 1994.
240. Shenasa, M., Borggrefe, M., Haverkamp, W., et al.: Ventricular tachycardia. Lancet *341*(8859):512, 1993.
241. Griffith, M. J., Garratt, C. J., Mounsey, P., et al.: Ventricular tachycardia as default diagnosis in broad complex tachycardia. Lancet *343*(8894):386, 1994.
242. Miller, J. M.: Recognition of ventricular tachycardia. *In* Zipes, D. P., and Jalife, J. (eds.): Cardiac Electrophysiology: From Cell to Bedside. 2nd ed. Philadelphia, W. B. Saunders Company, 1994, p. 990.
243. Jazayeri, M. R., and Akhtar, M.: Wide QRS complex tachycardia: Electrophysiological mechanisms and electrocardiographic features. *In* Zipes, D. P., and Jalife, J. (eds.): Cardiac Electrophysiology: From Cell to Bedside. Philadelphia, W. B. Saunders Company, 1994, p. 977.
244. Myerburg, R. J., Kessler, K. M., Kimura, S., et al.: Life-threatening ventricular arrhythmias: The link between epidemiology and pathophysiology. *In* Zipes, D. P., and Jalife, J. (eds.): Cardiac Electrophysiology: From Cell to Bedside. 2nd ed. Philadelphia, W. B. Saunders Company, 1994, p. 723.

245. Hummel, J. D., Strickberger, S. A., Daoud, E., et al.: Results and efficiency of programmed ventricular stimulation with four extrastimuli compared with one, two and three extrastimuli. Circulation *90*:2827, 1994.
246. Cossú, S. F., and Buxton, A. E.: The clinical spectrum of ventricular tachyarrhythmias in patients with coronary artery disease: Relationship between clinical and electrophysiologic characteristics in patients with nonsustained ventricular tachycardia and cardiac arrest. Cardiol. Rev. *3*:240, 1995.
247. Ho, D. S., Cooper, M. J., Richards, D. A., et al.: Comparison of number of extrastimuli versus change in basic cycle length for induction of ventricular tachycardia by programmed ventricular stimulation. J. Am. Coll. Cardiol. *22*:1711, 1993.
248. Callans, D. J., and Josephson, M. E.: Ventricular tachycardias in the setting of coronary artery disease. *In* Zipes, D. P., and Jalife, J. (eds.): Cardiac Electrophysiology: From Cell to Bedside. 2nd ed. Philadelphia, W. B. Saunders Company, 1994, p. 732.
249. Mitra, R. L., and Buxton, A. E.: The clinical significance of nonsustained ventricular tachycardia. J. Cardiovasc. Electrophysiol. *4*:490, 1993.
250. Turitto, G., Ahuja, R. K., Caref, E. B., et al.: Risk stratification for arrhythmic events in patients with nonischemic dilated cardiomyopathy and nonsustained ventricular tachycardia: Role of programmed ventricular stimulation and the signal-averaged electrocardiogram. J. Am. Coll. Cardiol. *24*:1523, 1994.
251. Roelke, M., and Ruskin, J. N.: Dilated cardiomyopathy: Ventricular arrhythmias and sudden death. *In* Zipes, D. P., and Jalife, J. (eds.): Cardiac Electrophysiology: From Cell to Bedside. 2nd ed. Philadelphia, W. B. Saunders Company, 1994, p. 744.
252. Stevenson, W. G., Middlekauff, H. R., and Saxon, L. A.: Ventricular arrhythmias in heart failure. *In* Zipes, D. P., and Jalife, J. (eds.): Cardiac Electrophysiology: From Cell to Bedside. 2nd ed. Philadelphia, W. B. Saunders Company, 1994, p. 848.
253. Spirito, P., Rapezzi, C., Autore, C., et al.: Prognosis of asymptomatic patients with hypertrophic cardiomyopathy and nonsustained ventricular tachycardia. Circulation *90*:2743, 1994.
254. Dilsizian, V., Bonow, R. O., Epstein, S. E., et al.: Myocardial ischemia detected by thallium scintigraphy is frequently related to cardiac arrest and syncope in young patients with hypertrophic cardiomyopathy. J. Am. Coll. Cardiol. *22*:796, 1993.
255. Fananapazir, L., McAreavy, D., and Epstein, N. D.: Hypertrophic cardiomyopathy. *In* Zipes, D. P., and Jalife, J. (eds.): Cardiac Electrophysiology: From Cell to Bedside. 2nd ed. Philadelphia, W. B. Saunders Company, 1994, p. 769.
256. Wellens, H. J. J., Rodriguez, L. M., and Smeets, J. L.: Ventricular tachycardia in structurally normal hearts. *In* Zipes, D. P., and Jalife, J. (eds.): Cardiac Electrophysiology: From Cell to Bedside. 2nd ed. Philadelphia, W. B. Saunders Company, 1994, p. 780.
257. Hauer, R. N. W., and Wilde, A. A. W.: Mitral valve prolapse. *In* Zipes, D. P., and Jalife, J. (eds.): Cardiac Electrophysiology: From Cell to Bedside. 2nd ed. Philadelphia, W. B. Saunders Company, 1994, p. 833.
258. Perry, J. C., and Garson, A., Jr.: Arrhythmias following surgery for congenital heart disease. *In* Zipes, D. P., and Jalife, J. (eds.): Cardiac Electrophysiology: From Cell to Bedside. 2nd ed. Philadelphia, W. B. Saunders Company, 1994, p. 838.
259. Rials, S. J., Wu, Y., Ford, N., et al.: Effect of left ventricular hypertrophy in its regression on ventricular electrophysiology and vulnerability to inducible arrhythmia in the feline heart. Circulation *91*:426, 1995.
260. Ben-David, J., Zipes, D. P., Ayers, G. M., et al.: Canine left ventricular hypertrophy predisposes to ventricular tachycardia induction by phase-II early afterdepolarizations after administration of BAY K 8644. J. Am. Coll. Cardiol. *20*:1576, 1992.
261. Lampert, R., Rosenfeld, L., Batsford, W., et al.: Circadian variation of sustained ventricular tachycardia in patients with coronary artery disease and implantable cardioverter-defibrillators. Circulation *90*:241, 1994.
262. Fei, L., Satters, D. J., Hnatkova, K., et al.: Change of autonomic influence on the heart immediately before the onset of spontaneous idiopathic ventricular tachycardia. J. Am. Coll. Cardiol. *24*:1515, 1994.
263. Hohnloser, S. H., Klingenheben, T., vandeLoo, A., et al.: Reflex versus tonic vagal activity as a prognostic parameter in patients with sustained ventricular tachycardia or ventricular fibrillation. Circulation *89*:1068, 1994.
264. Elami, A., Merin, G., Flugelman, M. Y., et al.: Usefulness of late potentials on the immediate postoperative signal-averaged electrocardiogram in predicting ventricular tachyarrhythmias early after isolated coronary artery bypass grafting. Am. J. Cardiol. *74*:33, 1994.
265. Pye, M., Quinn, A. C., and Cobbe, S. M.: QT interval dispersion: A non-invasive marker of susceptibility to arrhythmia in patients with sustained ventricular arrhythmias? Br. Heart J. *71*:511, 1994.
266. Hingham, P. D., Furniss, S. S., and Campbell, R. W.: QT dispersion and components of the AT interval in ischemia and infarction. Br. Heart J. *73*:32, 1995.
267. Nora, M., and Zipes, D. P.: Empiric use of amiodarone and sotalol. Am. J. Cardiol. *72*:62F, 1993.
268. Ho, D. S., Zecchin, R. P., Richards, D. A., et al.: Double-blind trial of lignocaine versus sotalol for acute termination of spontaneous sustained ventricular tachycardia. Lancet *344*(8914):18, 1994.
269. Sotalol in life-threatening ventricular arrhythmias: A unique class III antiarrhythmic. Symposium proceedings. Am. J. Cardiol. *72*:1A, 1993.
270. Perry, J. C., Knilans, T. K., Marlow, D., et al.: Intravenous amiodarone for life-threatening tachyarrhythmias in children and young adults. J. Am. Coll. Cardiol. *22*:95, 1993.
271. Wolfe, C. L., Nibley, C., Bhandari, A., et al.: Polymorphous ventricular tachycardia associated with acute myocardial infarction. Circulation *84*:1543, 1991.
272. Nalos, P. C., Ismail, Y., Pappas, J. M., et al.: Intravenous amiodarone for short-term treatment of refractory ventricular tachycardia or fibrillation. Am. Heart J. *122*:1629, 1991.
273. Kowey, P. R., Mirinchak, R. A., Rials, S. J., et al.: Electrophysiologic testing in patients who respond acutely to intravenous amiodarone for incessant ventricular tachyarrhythmias. Am. Heart J. *125*:1628, 1993.
274. Figa, F. H., Gow, R. M., Hamilton, R. M., et al.: Clinical efficacy and safety of intravenous amiodarone in infants and children. Am. J. Cardiol. *74*:573, 1994.
274a. Scheinman, M. M.: Parenteral antiarrhythmic drug therapy in ventricular tachycardia / ventricular fibrillation: Evolving role of class III agents—focus on amiodarone. J. Cardiovasc. Electrophysiol. *6*(Part 2):914, 1995.
275. Hohnloser, S. H., and Woosley, R. L.: Sotalol. N. Engl. J. Med. *331*:31, 1994.
276. Young, G. D., Kerr, C. R., Mohama, R., et al.: Efficacy of sotalol guided by programmed electrical stimulation for sustained ventricular arrhythmias secondary to coronary artery disease. Am. J. Cardiol. *73*:677, 1994.
277. Ohe, T., Aihara, N., Kamakura, S., et al.: Long-term outcome of verapamil-sensitive sustained left ventricular tachycardia in patients without structural heart disease. J. Am. Coll. Cardiol. *25*:54, 1995.
278. Sung, R. J., Lauer, M. R., and Lai, W. T.: Verapamil-responsive ventricular tachycardia: Adenosine sensitivity and role of catecholamines. *In* Zipes, D. P., and Jalife, J. (eds.): Cardiac Electrophysiology: From Cell to Bedside. 2nd ed. Philadelphia, W. B. Saunders Company, 1994, p. 907.
279. Omoigui, N. A., Marcus, F. I., Mason, J. W., et al.: Cost of initial therapy in the Electrophysiological Study Versus ECG Monitoring Trial (ESVEM). Circulation *91*:1070, 1995.
280. Kudenchuk, P. J., Bardy, G. H., Dolack, G. L., et al.: Efficacy of a single-lead unipolar transvenous defibrillator compared with a system employing an additional coronary sinus electrode: A prospective, randomized study. Circulation *89*:2641, 1994.
281. Choue, C. W., Kim, S. G., Fischer, J. D., et al.: Comparison of defibrillator therapy and other therapeutic modalities for sustained ventricular tachycardia or ventricular fibrillation associated with coronary artery disease. Am. J. Cardiol. *73*:1075, 1994.
282. Strickberger, S. A., Hummel, J. D., Daoud, E., et al.: Implantation by electrophysiologists of 100 consecutive cardioverter defibrillators with nonthoracotomy lead systems. Circulation *90*:868, 1994.
283. Sweeney, M. O., and Ruskin, J. N.: Mortality benefits and the implantable cardioverter-defibrillator. Circulation *89*:1851, 1994.
284. Zipes, D. P., Roberts, D., for the PCD Investigators: Results of the world wide study of the implantable pacemaker, cardioverter defibrillator: A comparison of epicardial and endocardial lead systems. Circulation *92*:59, 1995.
285. Ferguson, T. D., Jr., Smith, J. M., Cox, J. L., et al.: Direct operation versus ICD therapy for ischemic ventricular tachycardia. Ann. Thorac. Surg. *58*:1291, 1994.
286. Crawford, F. A., Jr., and Gillette, P. C.: Surgical treatment of cardiac dysrhythmias in infants and children. Ann. Thorac. Surg. *58*:1262, 1994.
287. Guiraudon, G. M., Thakur, R. K., Klein, G. J., et al.: Encircling endocardial cryoablation for ventricular tachycardia after myocardial infarction: Experience with 33 patients. Am. Heart J. *128*:982, 1994.
288. Morris, J. J., Rastogi, A., Stanton, M. S., et al.: Operation for ventricular tachyarrhythmias: Refining current treatment strategies. Ann. Thorac. Surg. *58*:1490, 1994.
289. Misaki, T., Watanabe, G., Iwa, T., et al.: Surgical treatment of arrhythmogenic right ventricular dysplasia: Long-term outcome. Ann. Thorac. Surg. *58*:1380, 1994.
290. Misaki, T., Watanabe, G., Iwa, T., et al.: Surgical treatment of arrhythmogenic right ventricular dysplasia: Long-term outcome. Ann. Thorac. Surg. *58*:1380, 1994.
291. Rokkas, C. K., Nitta, T., Schuessler, R. B., et al.: Human ventricular tachycardia: Precise intraoperative localization with potential distribution mapping. Ann. Thorac. Surg. *57*:1628, 1994.
292. Misaki, T., Tsubota, M., Watanabe, G., et al.: Surgical treatment of ventricular tachycardia after surgical repair of tetralogy of Fallot: Relation between intraoperative mapping and histological findings. Circulation *90*:264, 1994.
293. Lee, R., Mitchell, J. B., Garan, H., et al.: Operation for recurrent ventricular tachycardia: Predictors of short- and long-term efficacy. J. Thorac. Cardiovasc. Surg. *107*:732, 1994.
294. Klein, L. S., and Miles, W. M.: Ablative therapy for ventricular arrhythmias. Prog. Cardiovasc. Dis. *37*:225, 1995.
295. Gonska, D. D., Cao, K., Schaumann, A., et al.: Catheter ablation of ventricular tachycardia in 136 patients with coronary artery disease: Results and long-term follow-up. J. Am. Coll. Cardiol. *24*:1506, 1994.
296. Blanck, Z., Dhala, A., Deshpande, S., et al.: Catheter ablation of ventricular tachycardia. Am. Heart J. *127*:1126, 1994.

297. Wen, M. S., Yeh, S. J., Wang, C. C., et al.: Radiofrequency ablation therapy in idiopathic left ventricular tachycardia with no obvious structural heart disease. Circulation *89*:1690, 1994.
298. Borggrefe, M., Chen, X., Hindricks, W., et al.: Catheter ablation of ventricular tachycardia in patients with coronary heart disease. *In* Zipes, D. P., and Jalife, J. (eds.): Cardiac Electrophysiology: From Cell to Bedside. Philadelphia, W. B. Saunders Company, 1994, p. 1502.
299. Klein, L. S., Miles, W. M., Mitrani, R. D., et al.: Ablation of ventricular tachycardia in patients with structurally normal hearts. *In* Zipes, D. P., and Jalife, J. (eds.): Cardiac Electrophysiology: From Cell to Bedside. Philadelphia, W. B. Saunders Company, 1994, p. 1518.
300. Fontaine, G., Fontaliran, F., Lascault, G., et al.: Arrhythmogenic right ventricular dysplasia. *In* Zipes, D. P., and Jalife, J. (eds.): Cardiac Electrophysiology: From Cell to Bedside. Philadelphia, W. B. Saunders Company, 1994, p. 754.
301. Yamabe, H., Okumura, K., Tsuchiya, T., et al.: Demonstration of entrainment and presence of slow conduction during ventricular tachycardia in arrhythmogenic right ventricular dysplasia. PACE *17*:172, 1994.
302. Lee, A. H., Morgan, J. M., and Gallagher, P. J.: Arrhythmogenic right ventricular cardiomyopathy. J. Pathol. *171*:157, 1993.
303. Solenthaler, M., Ritter, M., Candinas, R., et al.: Arrhythmogenic right ventricular dysplasia in identical twins. Am. J. Cardiol. *74*:303, 1994.
303a. Rampazzo, A., Nava, A., Danieli, G. A., et al.: The gene for arrhythmogenic right ventricular cardiomyopathy maps to chromosome 14g23-q24. Hum. Mol. Genet. *3*:959, 1994.
304. Mehta, D., Davies, M. J., Ward, D. E., et al.: Ventricular tachycardias of right ventricular origin: Markers of subclinical right ventricular disease. Am. Heart J. *127*:360, 1994.
305. Rolov, M. V., Brodsky, M. A., Allen, B. J., et al.: Spectrum of right heart involvement in patients with ventricular tachycardia unrelated to coronary artery disease or left ventricular dysfunction. Am. Heart J. *126*:1348, 1993.
306. Hamada, S., Tamamiya, M., Ohe, T., et al.: Arrhythmogenic right ventricular dysplasia: Evaluation with electron-beam CT. Radiology *187*:723, 1993.
307. Auffermann, W., Wichter, T., Breithardt, G., et al.: Arrhythmogenic right ventricular disease: MR imaging versus angiography. A.J.R. *161*:549, 1993.
308. Blake, L. M., Scheinman, M. M., and Higgins, C. B.: MR features of arrhythmogenic right ventricular dysplasia. A.J.R. *162*:809, 1994.
309. Wichter, T., Hendricks, G., Lerch, H., et al.: Regional myocardial sympathetic dysinnervation in arrhythmogenic right ventricular cardiomyopathy. An analysis using ^{123}I-meta-iodobenzylguanidine scintigraphy. Circulation *89*:667, 1994.
310. Metzger, J. T., deChillou, C., Cherieax, E., et al.: Value of the 12-lead electrocardiogram in arrhythmogenic right ventricular dysplasia, and absence of correlation with echocardiographic findings. Am. J. Cardiol. *72*:964, 1993.
311. Kinoshita, O., Kamakura, S., Ohe, T., et al.: Frequency analysis of signal-averaged electrocardiogram in patients with right ventricular tachycardia. J. Am. Coll. Cardiol. *20*:1230, 1992.
312. Kinoshita, O., Fontaine, G., Rosas, F., et al.: Optimal high-pass filter settings of the signal-averaged electrocardiogram in patients with arrhythmogenic right ventricular dysplasia. Am. J. Cardiol. *74*:1074, 1994.
313. McLay, J. S., Norris, A., Campbell, R. W., et al.: Arrhythmogenic right ventricular dysplasia: An uncommon cause of ventricular tachycardia in young and old? Br. Heart J. *69*:158, 1993.
314. Breithardt, G., Wichter, T., Haverkamp, W., et al.: Implantable cardioverter defibrillator therapy in patients with arrhythmogenic right ventricular cardiomyopathy, long QT syndrome or no structural heart disease. Am. Heart J. *127*:1151, 1994.
315. Burton, M. E., and Leon, A. R.: Radiofrequency catheter ablation of right ventricular outflow tract tachycardia late after complete repair of tetralogy of Fallot using the pace mapping technique. PACE *16*:2319, 1993.
316. Biblo, L. A., and Carlson, M. D.: Transcatheter radiofrequency ablation of ventricular tachycardia following surgical correction of tetralogy of Fallot. PACE *17*:1556, 1994.
317. Matsuoka, S., Akita, H., Hayabuchi, Y., et al.: Abnormal signal averaged ECG after surgical repair of tetralogy of Fallot: A combined analysis in the time and frequency domain. Jpn. Circ. J. *57*:841, 1993.
318. Dreyer, W. J., Paridon, S. M., Fisher, D. J., et al.: Rapid ventricular pacing in dogs with right ventricular outflow tract obstruction: Insights into a mechanism of sudden death in postoperative tetralogy of Fallot. J. Am. Coll. Cardiol. *21*:1731, 1993.
319. Mancini, D. M., Wong, K. L., and Simson, M. B.: Prognostic value of an abnormal signal-averaged electrocardiogram in patients with nonischemic congestive cardiomyopathy. Circulation *87*:1083, 1993.
320. Keeling, P. J., Kulakowski, T., Yi, G., et al.: Usefulness of signal-averaged electrocardiogram in idiopathic dilated cardiomyopathy for identifying patients with ventricular arrhythmias. Am. J. Cardiol. *72*:78, 1993.
321. Turitto, G., Ahuja, R. K., Bekheit, S., et al.: Incidence and prediction of induced ventricular tachyarrhythmias in idiopathic dilated cardiomyopathy. Am. J. Cardiol. *73*:770, 1994.
322. Marchlinski, F. E., Schwartzman, D., Gottlieb, C. D., et al.: Electrical events associated with arrhythmia initiation and stimulation techniques for arrhythmia prevention. *In* Zipes, D. P., and Jalife, J. (eds.): Cardiac Electrophysiology: From Cell to Bedside. Philadelphia, W. B. Saunders Company, 1994, p. 863.
323. Chen, X., Shenasa, M., Borggrefe, M., et al.: Role of programmed ventricular stimulation in patients with idiopathic dilated cardiomyopathy and documented sustained ventricular tachyarrhythmias: Inducibility and prognostic value in 102 patients. Eur. Heart J. *15*:76, 1994.
324. Borggrefe, M., Chen, X., Martinez-Rubio, A., et al.: The role of implantable cardioverter defibrillators in dilated cardiomyopathy. Am. Heart J. *127*:1145, 1994.
325. Lessmeier, T. J., Lehmann, M. H., Steinman, R. T., et al.: Outcome with implantable cardioverter-defibrillator therapy for survivors of ventricular fibrillation secondary to idiopathic dilated cardiomyopathy or coronary artery disease without myocardial infarction. Am. J. Cardiol. *72*:911, 1993.
326. Blanck, Z., Deshpande, S., Mohammad, R., et al.: Catheter ablation of the left bundle branch for the treatment of sustained bundle branch reentrant ventricular tachycardia. J. Cardiovasc. Electrophysiol. *6*:40, 1995.
327. Blanck, Z., Sra, J., Dhala, A., et al.: Bundle branch reentry: Mechanisms, diagnosis and treatment. *In* Zipes, D. P., and Jalife, J. (eds.): Cardiac Electrophysiology: From Cell to Bedside. Philadelphia, W. B. Saunders Company, 1994, p. 878.
328. Callans, D. J., Schwartzman, D., Gottlieb, C. B., et al.: Insights into the electrophysiology of ventricular tachycardia gained by the catheter ablation experience: Learning while burning. J. Cardiovasc. Electrophysiol. *5*:877, 1994.
329. Larsen, L., Markham, J., and Haffajee, C. I.: Sudden death in idiopathic dilated cardiomyopathy: Role of ventricular arrhythmias. PACE *16*:1051, 1993.
330. McKenna, W. J., Sadoul, N., Slade, A. K., et al.: The prognostic significance of nonsustained ventricular tachycardia in hypertrophic cardiomyopathy. Circulation *90*:3115, 1994.
331. Spirito, P., Rapezzi, C., Autore, C., et al.: Prognosis of asymptomatic patients with hypertrophic cardiomyopathy and nonsustained ventricular tachycardia. Circulation *90*:2743, 1994.
332. Fananapazir, L., Chang, A. C., Epstein, S. E., et al.: Prognostic determinants in hypertrophic cardiomyopathy: Prospective evaluation of a therapeutic strategy based on clinical, Holter, hemodynamic, and electrophysiological findings. Circulation *86*:730, 1992.
333. Saumarez, R. C., Camm, A. J., Panagos, A., et al.: Ventricular fibrillation in hypertrophic cardiomyopathy is associated with increased fractionation of paced right ventricular electrograms. Circulation *86*:467, 1992.
334. Shakespeare, C. F., Keeling, P. J., Slade, A. K., et al.: Arrhythmias and hypertrophic cardiomyopathy. Arch. Mal. Coeur Vaiss *87*:31, 1992.
335. Dilsizian, V., Bonow, R. O., Epstein, S. E., et al.: Myocardial ischemia detected by thallium scintigraphy is frequently related to cardiac arrest and syncope in young patients with hypertrophic cardiomyopathy. J. Am. Coll. Cardiol. *22*:796, 1993.
336. Stewart, J. T., and McKenna, W. J.: Management of arrhythmias in hypertrophic cardiomyopathy. Cardiovasc. Drugs. Ther. *8*:95, 1994.
337. Almendral, J. M., Ormaetxe, J., and Martinez-Alday, J. D.: Treatment of ventricular arrhythmias in patients with hypertrophic cardiomyopathy. Eur. Heart J. *14* (Suppl. J):71, 1993.
338. Buja, G., Miroelli, M., Turrini, P., et al.: Comparison of QT dispersion in hypertrophic cardiomyopathy between patients with and without ventricular arrhythmias and sudden death. Am. J. Cardiol. *72*:973, 1993.
339. Vohra, J., Sathe, S., Warren, R., et al.: Malignant ventricular arrhythmias in patients with mitral valve prolapse and mild mitral regurgitation. PACE *16*:387, 1993.
340. Belhassen, B., and Viskin, S.: Idiopathic ventricular tachycardia and fibrillation. J. Cardiovasc. Electrophysiol. *4*:356, 1993.
341. Tung, R. T., Shen, W. K., Hammill, S. C., et al.: Idiopathic ventricular fibrillation in out-of-hospital cardiac arrest survivors. PACE *17*:1405, 1994.
342. Almendral, J., Ormaetxe, J., and Delcan, J. L.: Idiopathic ventricular tachycardia and fibrillation: Incidence, prognosis and therapy. PACE *15*:627, 1992.
343. Masrani, K., Cowley, C., Bekheit, S., et al.: Recurrent syncope for over a decade due to idiopathic ventricular fibrillation. Chest *106*:1601, 1994.
344. Sumiyoshi, M., Nakata, Y., Hisaoka, T., et al.: A case of idiopathic ventricular fibrillation with incomplete right bundle branch block and persistent ST segment elevation. Jpn. Heart J. *34*:661, 1993.
345. Brugada, P., and Brugada, J.: Right bundle branch block, persistent ST segment elevation and sudden cardiac death: A distinct clinical and electrocardiographic syndrome. J. Am. Coll. Cardiol. *20*:1391, 1992.
346. Katritsis, D. G., Jaswinder, S. G., and Camm, A. J.: Repetitive monomorphic ventricular tachycardia. *In* Zipes, D. P., and Jalife, J. (eds.): Cardiac Electrophysiology: From Cell to Bedside. 2nd ed. Philadelphia, W. B. Saunders Company, 1994, p. 900.
347. Lerman, B. B.: Response of nonreentrant catecholamine-mediated ventricular tachycardia to endogenous adenosine and acetylcholine: Evidence of myocardial receptor-mediated effects. Circulation *87*:382, 1993.
348. Gill, J. S., Mehta, D., Ward, D. E., et al.: Efficacy of flecainide, sotalol, and verapamil in the treatment of right ventricular tachycardia in patients without overt cardiac abnormality. Br. Heart J. *68*:392, 1992.

349. Nakagawa, H., Mukai, J., Nagata, K., et al.: Early afterdepolarizations in a patient with idiopathic monomorphic right ventricular tachycardia. PACE *16:*2067, 1993.
350. Lerman, B. B., Stein, K., Engelstein, E. D., et al.: Mechanism of repetitive monomorphic ventricular tachycardia. Circulation *92:*421, 1995.
351. Klein, L. S., Miles, W. M., Mitrani, R. D., et al.: Catheter ablation of ventricular tachycardia. *In* Smith, T. W., Antman, E. M., Bittl, J. A., Colucci, W. S., Gotto, A. M., Loscalzo, J., Williams, G. H., and Zipes, D. P. (eds.): Cardiovascular Therapeutics. Philadelphia, W. B. Saunders Company, 1996.
352. Gill, J. S., Blaszyk, K., Ward, D. E., et al.: Verapamil for the suppression of idiopathic ventricular tachycardia of left bundle branch block-like morphology. Am. Heart J. *126:*1126, 1993.
353. Carlson, M. D., White, R. D., Trohman, R. G., et al.: Right ventricular outflow tract ventricular tachycardia: Detection of previously unrecognized anatomic abnormalities using cine magnetic resonance imaging. J. Am. Coll. Cardiol. *24:*720, 1994.
354. Gill, J. S., DeBelder, M., and Ward, D. E.: Right ventricular outflow tract ventricular tachycardia associated with an aneurysmal malformation: Use of transesophageal echocardiography during low-energy direct-current ablation. Am. Heart J. *128:*620, 1994.
355. Nakagawa, H., Beckman, K. J., McClelland, J. H., et al.: Radiofrequency catheter ablation of idiopathic left ventricular tachycardia guided by a Purkinje potential. Circulation *88:*2607, 1993.
356. Kottkamp, H., Chen, X., Hindricks, G., et al.: Radiofrequency catheter ablation of idiopathic left ventricular tachycardia: Further evidence for microreentry as the underlying mechanism. J. Cardiovasc. Electrophysiol. *5:*268, 1994.
357. Gill, J. S., Ward, D. E., and Camm, A. J.: Comparison of verapamil and diltiazem in the suppression of idiopathic ventricular tachycardia. PACE *15:*2122, 1992.
358. DeLacey, W. A., Nath, S., Haines, D. E., et al.: Adenosine and verapamil-sensitive ventricular tachycardia originating from the left ventricle: Radiofrequency catheter ablation. PACE *15:*2240, 1992.
359. Kobayashi, Y., Kikushima, S., Tanno, K., et al.: Sustained left ventricular tachycardia terminated by dipyridamole: Cyclic AMP-mediated triggered activity as a possible mechanism. PACE *17:*377, 1994.
360. Griffith, M. J., Garratt, C. J., and Rowland, E.: Effects of intravenous adenosine on verapamil-sensitive idiopathic ventricular tachycardia. Am. J. Cardiol. *73:*759, 1994.
361. Gonzalez, R. P., Scheinman, M. M., Lesh, M. D., et al.: Clinical and electrophysiologic spectrum of fascicular tachycardias. Am. Heart J. *128:*147, 1994.
362. Gaita, F., Giustetto, C., Leclercq, J. F., et al.: Idiopathic verapamil-responsive left ventricular tachycardia: Clinical characteristics and long-term follow-up of 33 patients. Eur. Heart J. *15:*1252, 1994.
362a. Munger, R. G., and Booton, E. A.: Thiamine and sudden death in sleep of South-East Asian refugees. Lancet *335:*1154, 1990.
363. Grimm, W., and Marchlinski, F. E.: Accelerated idioventricular rhythm, bidirectional ventricular tachycardia. *In* Zipes, D. P., and Jalife, J. (eds.): Cardiac Electrophysiology: From Cell to Bedside. 2nd ed. Philadelphia, W. B. Saunders Company, 1994, p. 920.
364. Zipes, D. P.: Unwitting exposure to risk (Editorial). Cardiol. Rev. *1:*1, 1993.
365. Pepe, P. E., Levine, R. L., Fromm, R. E., Jr., et al.: Cardiac arrest presenting with rhythms other than ventricular fibrillation: Contribution of resuscitative efforts toward total survivorship. Crit. Care Med. *21:*1838, 1993.
366. Roden, D. M.: Torsade de pointes. Clin. Cardiol. *16:*683, 1993.
367. Ben-David, J., and Zipes, D. P.: Torsades de pointes and proarrhythmia. Lancet *341:*1578, 1993.
368. Schwartz, P. J., Locati, E. H., Napolitano, C., et al.: The long QT syndrome. *In* Zipes, D. P., and Jalife, J. (eds.): Cardiac Electrophysiology: From Cell to Bedside. Philadelphia, W. B. Saunders Company, 1994, p. 788.
369. Fontaine, G.: A new look at torsades de pointes. Ann. N.Y. Acad. Sci. *644:*157, 1992.
370. Kurita, T., Ohe, T., Marui, N., et al.: Bradycardia-induced abnormal QT prolongation in patients with complete atrioventricular block with torsades de pointes. Am. J. Cardiol. *69:*628, 1992.
371. Haverkamp, W., Shenasa, M., Borggrefe, M., et al.: Torsades de pointes. *In* Zipes, D. P., and Jalife, J. (eds.): Cardiac Electrophysiology: From Cell to Bedside. 2nd ed. Philadelphia, W. B. Saunders Company, 1994, p. 885.
372. Leenhardt, A., Glaser, E., Burguera, M., et al.: Short-coupled variant of torsade de pointes: A new electrocardiographic entity in the spectrum of idiopathic ventricular tachyarrhythmias. Circulation *89:*206, 1994.
373. Napolitano, C., Priori, S. G., and Schwartz, P. J.: Torsade de pointes: Mechanisms and management. Drugs *47:*51, 1994.
374. Tan, H. L., Hou, C. J. Y., Lauer, M. R., et al.: Electrophysiologic mechanisms of the long QT interval syndromes and torsade de pointes. Ann. Intern. Med. *122:*701, 1995.
375. Miwa, S., Inoue, T., and Yokoyama, M.: Monophasic action potentials in patients with torsades de pointes. Jpn. Circ. J. *58:*248, 1994.
376. Roden, D. M.: Early after-depolarizations and torsade de pointes: Implications for the control of cardiac arrhythmias by prolonging repolarization. Eur. Heart J. *14* (Suppl. H):56, 1993.
377. Weissenburger, J., Davy, J. M., and Chezalviel, F.: Experimental models of torsades de pointes. Fund. Clin. Pharmacol. *7:*29, 1993.
378. Hii, J. T., Wyse, D. G., Gillis, A. M., et al.: Precordial QT interval dispersion as a marker of torsade de pointes: Disparate effects of class IA antiarrhythmic drugs and amiodarone. Circulation *86:*1376, 1992.
379. Pertsov, A. M., and Jalife, J.: Three-dimensional vortex-like reentry. *In* Zipes, D. P., and Jalife, J. (eds.): Cardiac Electrophysiology: From Cell to Bedside. 2nd ed. Philadelphia, W. B. Saunders Company, 1994, p. 403.
380. Makkar, R. R., Fromm, B. S., Steinman, R. T., et al.: Female gender as a risk factor for torsades de pointes associated with cardiovascular drugs. J.A.M.A. *270:*2590, 1993.
381. Perticone, F., Ceravolo, R., DeNovara, G., et al.: New data on the antiarrhythmic value of magnesium treatment: Magnesium and ventricular arrhythmias. Magnet. Reson. *5:*265, 1992.
382. Banai, S., and Tzivoni, D.: Drug therapy for torsade de pointes. J. Cardiovasc. Electrophysiol. *4:*206, 1993.
383. Carlsson, L., Abrahamsson, C., and Drews, L.: Antiarrhythmic effects of potassium channel openers in rhythm abnormalities related to delayed repolarization. Circulation *85:*1491, 1992.
384. Vos, M. A., Gorgels, A. P., Lipcsei, G. C., et al.: Mechanism-specific antiarrhythmic effects of the potassium channel activator levcromakalim against repolarization-dependent tachycardias. J. Cardiovasc. Electrophysiol. *5:*731, 1994.
385. Sato, T., Yoshiki, H., Yamamoto, M., et al.: Early afterdepolarization abolished by potassium channel opener in a patient with idiopathic long QT syndrome. J. Cardiovasc. Electrophysiol. *6:*279, 1995.
386. Moss, A. J.: Measurement of the QT interval and the risk associated with QTc interval prolongation: A review. Am. J. Cardiol. *72:*23B, 1993.
387. Antzelevitch, C., and Sicouri, S.: Clinical relevance of cardiac arrhythmias generated by afterdepolarizations: Role of M cells in the generation of U waves, triggered activity and torsade de pointes. J. Am. Coll. Cardiol. *23:*259, 1994.
388. Lehmann, M. H., Suzuki, F., Fromm, B. S., et al.: T wave humps as a potential electrocardiographic marker of the long QT syndrome. J. Am. Coll. Cardiol. *24:*746, 1994.
389. Krause, P. C., Rardon, D. P., Miles, W. M., et al.: Characteristics of Ca^{2+}-activated K^+ channels isolated from the left ventricle of the patient with idiopathic long QT syndrome. Am. Heart J. *126:*1134, 1993.
390. Schwartz, P. J., Moss, A. J., Vincent, G. M., et al.: Diagnostic criteria for the long QT syndrome: An update. Circulation *88:*782, 1993.
391. Habbab, M. A., and El-Sherif, N.: TU alternans, long QTU and torsade de pointes: Clinical and experimental observations. PACE *15:*916, 1992.
392. Rosenbaum, M. B., and Acunzo, R. S.: Pseudo 2:1 atrioventricular block and T wave alternans in the long QT syndromes. J. Am. Coll. Cardiol. *18:*1363, 1991.
393. Keating, M.: Genetics of the long QT syndrome. J. Cardiovasc. Electrophysiol. *5:*146, 1994.
394. Vincent, G. M.: Hypothesis for the molecular physiology of the Romano-Ward long QT syndrome. J. Am. Coll. Cardiol. *20:*500, 1992.
395. Tanaka, T., Nakahara, K., Kato, N., et al.: Genetic linkage analyses of Romano-Ward syndrome (RWS) in 13 Japanese families. Hum. Genet. *94:*380, 1994.
396. Weitkamp, L. R., Moss, A. J., Lewis, R. A., et al.: Analysis of HLA and disease susceptibility: Chromosome 6 genes and sex influence on long-QT phenotype. Am. J. Hum. Genet. *55:*1230, 1994.
397. Towbin, J. A., Li, H., Taggart, R. T., et al.: Evidence of genetic heterogeneity in Romano-Ward long QT syndrome: Analysis of 23 families. Circulation *90:*2635, 1994.
398. Desmyttere, S., Bonduelle, M., DeWolf, D., et al.: A case of term mors in utero in chromosome 11p linked long QT syndrome family. Genet. Couns. *5:*289, 1994.
399. Jiang, C., Atkinson, D., Towbin, J. A., et al.: Two long QT syndrome loci map to chromosomes 3 and 7 with evidence for further heterogeneity. Nat. Genet. *8:*141, 1994.
400. Curran, M. E., Splawski, I., Timothy, K. W., et al.: A molecular basis for cardiac arrhythmia: HERG mutations cause long QT syndrome. Cell *80:*795, 1995.
401. Wang, Q., Shen, J., Splawski, I., et al.: SCN5A mutations associated with an inherited cardiac arrhythmia, long QT syndrome. Cell *80:*805, 1995.
401a. Roden, D. M., George, A. L., Jr., and Bennett, P. B.: Recent advances in understanding the molecular mechanism of the long QT syndrome. J. Cardiovasc. Electrophysiol. *6:*1023, 1995.
401b. Grace, A. A., and Chien, K. R.: Congenital long QT syndromes. Toward molecular dissection of arrhythmia substrates. Circulation *92:*2786, 1995.
401c. Moss, A. J., Zareba, W., Benhorin, J., et al.: ECG T-wave patterns in genetically distinct forms of the hereditary long QT syndrome. Circulation *92:*2929, 1995.
402. Vos, M. A., Verduyn, S. C., Gorgels, A. P., et al.: Reproducible induction of early afterdepolarizations and torsade de pointes arrhythmias by d-sotalol and pacing in dogs with chronic atrioventricular block. Circulation *91:*864, 1995.
403. Lazzara, R.: Antiarrhythmic drugs and torsade de pointes. Eur. Heart J. 14 (Suppl. H):88, 1993.
404. Woosley, R. L., Chen, Y., Freiman, J. P., et al.: Mechanism of the cardiotoxic actions of terfenadine. JAMA *269:*1532, 1993.
405. Smith, J.: Cardiovascular toxicity of antihistamines. Otolaryngol. Head Neck Surg. *111:*348, 1994.
406. Herings, R. M., Stricker, B. H., Leufkens, H. G., et al.: Public health problems and the rapid estimation of the size of the population at risk:

Torsades de pointes and the use of terfenadine and astemizole in The Netherlands. Pharm. World Sci. *15*:212, 1993.
407. Brandriss, M. W., Richardson, W. S., and Barold, S. S.: Erythromycin-induced QT prolongation and polymorphic ventricular tachycardia (torsades de pointes): Case report and review. Clin. Infect. Dis. *18*:995, 1994.
408. Rubart, M., Pressler, M. L., Pride, H. P., et al.: Electrophysiological mechanisms in a canine model of erythromycin-associated long QT syndrome. Circulation *88*:1832, 1993.
409. Gitler, B., Berger, L. S., and Buffa, S. D.: Torsades de pointes induced by erythromycin. Chest *105*:368, 1994.
410. Mani, S., Kocheril, A. G., and Andriole, V. T.: Case report: Pentamidine and polymorphic ventricular tachycardia revisited. Am. J. Med. Sci. *305*:236, 1993.
411. Eisenhauer, M. D., Eliasson, A. H., Taylor, A. J., et al.: Incidence of cardiac arrhythmias during intravenous pentamidine therapy in HIV-infected patients. Chest *105*:389, 1994.
412. Tamura, M., Ueki, Y., Ohtsuka, E., et al.: Probucol-induced QT prolongation and syncope. Jpn. Circ. J. *58*:374, 1994.
413. Singh, B., al Shahwan, S. A., Habbab, M. A., et al.: Idiopathic long QT syndrome: Asking the right question. Lancet *341*:741, 1993.
414. Villain, E., Levy, M., Kachaner, J., et al.: Prolonged QT interval in neonates: Benign, transient, or prolonged risk of sudden death. Am. Heart J. *124*:194, 1992.
414a. Pacia, S. V., Devinsky, O., Luciano, D. J., et al.: The prolonged QT syndrome presenting as epilepsy: A report of two cases and literature review. Neurology *44*:1408, 1994.
415. Garson, A., Jr., Dick, M., II, Fournier, A., et al.: The long QT syndrome in children: An international study of 287 patients. Circulation *87*:1866, 1993.
416. Marks, M. L., Whisler, S. L., Clericuzio, C., et al.: A new form of long QT syndrome associated with syndactyly. J. Am. Coll. Cardiol. *25*:59, 1995.
417. Zareba, W., Moss, A. J., leCessie, S., et al.: T wave alternans in idiopathic long QT syndrome. J. Am. Coll. Cardiol. *23*:1541, 1994.
418. Buckingham, T. A., Bhutto, Z. R., Telfer, E. A., et al.: Differences in corrected QT intervals at minimal and maximal heart rate may identify patients at risk for torsades de pointes during treatment with antiarrhythmic drugs. J. Cardiovasc. Electrophysiol. *5*:408, 1994.
419. Eggeling, T., Osterhues, H. H., Hoeher, M., et al.: Value of Holter monitoring in patients with the long QT syndrome. Cardiology *81*:107, 1992.
420. Ohe, T., Kurita, T., Shimizu, W., et al.: Introduction of TU abnormalities in patients with torsades de pointes. Ann. N.Y. Acad. Sci. *644*:178, 1992.
421. Shimizu, W., Ohe, T., Kurita, T., et al.: Epinephrine-induced ventricular premature complexes due to early afterdepolarizations and effects of verapamil and propanolol in a patient with the congenital long QT syndrome. J. Cardiovasc. Electrophysiol. *5*:438, 1994.
421a. Shimizu, W., Ohe, T., Kurita, T., et al.: Effects of verapamil and propranolol on early afterdepolarizations and ventricular arrhythmias induced by epinephrine in congenital long QT syndrome. J. Am. Coll. Cardiol. *26*:1299, 1995.
422. DeFerrari, G. M., Nador, F., Beria, G., et al.: Effect of calcium channel block on the wall motion abnormality of the idiopathic long QT syndrome. Circulation *89*:2126, 1994.
423. Calkins, H., Lehmann, M. H., Allman, K., et al.: Scintigraphic pattern of regional cardiac sympathetic innervation in patients with familial long QT syndrome using positron emission tomography. Circulation *87*:1616, 1993.
424. Muller, K. D., Jakob, H., Neuzner, J., et al.: ^{123}I-metaiodobenzylguanidine scintigraphy in the detection of irregular regional sympathetic innervation in long QT syndrome. Eur. Heart J. *14*:316, 1993.
425. Moise, N. S., Meyers-Wallen, V., Flahive, W. J., et al.: Inherited ventricular arrhythmias and sudden death in German Shepherd dogs. J. Am. Coll. Cardiol. *24*:233, 1994.
425a. Moise, M. D., Moon, P. F., Flahive, W. J., et al.: Phenylprine-induced ventricular arrhythmias in dogs with inherited sudden death. J. Cardiovasc. Electrophysiol. (*In press*).
426. Leenhardt, A., Lucet, V., Denjoy, I., et al.: Catecholaminergic polymorphic ventricular tachycardia in children: A seven-year follow-up of 21 patients. Circulation *91*:1512, 1995.
427. Eldar, M., Griffin, J. C., VanHare, G. F., et al.: Combined use of beta-adrenergic blocking agents and long-term cardiac pacing for patients with the long QT syndrome. J. Am. Coll. Cardiol. *20*:830, 1992.
428. Moss, A. J., and Robinson, J.: Clinical features of the idiopathic long QT syndrome. Circulation *85* (Suppl. 1):1140, 1992.
429. Malfatto, G., Beria, G., Sala, S., et al.: Quantitative analysis of T wave abnormalities and their prognostic implications in the idiopathic long QT syndrome. J. Am. Coll. Cardiol. *23*:296, 1994.
430. Blanck, Z., Dhala, A., Deshpande, S., et al.: Bundle branch reentrant ventricular tachycardia: Cumulative experience in 48 patients. J. Cardiovasc. Electrophysiol. *4*:253, 1993.
431. Blanck, Z., Jazayeri, M., Dhala, A., et al.: Bundle branch reentry: A mechanism of ventricular tachycardia in the absence of myocardial or valvular dysfunction. J. Am. Coll. Cardiol. *22*:1718, 1993.
432. Epstein, A. E., and Ideker, R. E.: Ventricular fibrillation. *In* Zipes, D. P., and Jalife, J. (eds.): Cardiac Electrophysiology: From Cell to Bedside. 2nd ed. Philadelphia, W. B. Saunders Company, 1994, p. 927.
433. Lubbe, W. F., Podzweit, T., and Opie, L. H.: Potential arrhythmogenic role of cyclic adenosine monophosphate (AMP) and cytosolic calcium overload: Implications for prophylactic effects of beta-blockers in myocardial infarction and proarrhythmic effects of phosphodiesterase inhibitors. J. Am. Coll. Cardiol. *19*:1622, 1992.
433a. Tobe, T. J., deLangen, C. D., Crijns, H. J., et al.: Effects of streptokinase during acute myocardial infarction on the signal-averaged electrocardiogram and on the frequency of late arrhythmias. Am. J. Cardiol. *72*:647, 1993.
434. Arntz, H. R., Willich, S. N., Oeff, M., et al.: Circadian variation of sudden cardiac death reflects age-related variability in ventricular fibrillation. Circulation *88*:2284, 1993.
435. Fei, L., Anderson, M. H., Katritsis, D., et al.: Decreased heart rate variability in survivors of sudden cardiac death not associated with coronary artery disease. Br. Heart J. *71*:16, 1994.
436. Dougherty, C. M., and Burr, R. L.: Comparison of heart rate variability in survivors and nonsurvivors of sudden cardiac arrest. Am. J. Cardiol. *70*:441, 1992.
437. Davies, M. J.: Anatomic features in victims of sudden coronary death: Coronary artery pathology. Circulation *85* (Suppl. 1):119, 1992.
438. Rodriguez, L. M., Smeets, J., O'Hara, G. E., et al.: Incidence and timing of recurrences of sudden death and ventricular tachycardia during antiarrhythmic drug treatment after myocardial infarction. Am. J. Cardiol. *69*:1403, 1992.
439. Kim, S. G., Fisher, J. D., Choue, C. W., et al.: Influence of left ventricular function on outcome of patients treated with implantable defibrillators. Circulation *85*:1304, 1992.
440. Wever, E. F., Hauer, R. N., Oomen, A., et al.: Unfavorable outcome in patients with primary electrical disease who survived an episode of ventricular fibrillation. Circulation *88*:1021, 1993.
441. Meissner, M. D., Lehmann, M. H., Steinman, R. T., et al.: Ventricular fibrillation in patients without significant structural heart disease: A multicenter experience with implantable cardioverter-defibrillator therapy. J. Am. Coll. Cardiol. *21*:1406, 1993.
442. Cummins, R. O., Graves, J. R., Larsen, M. P., et al.: Out-of-hospital transcutaneous pacing by emergency medical technicians in patients with asystolic cardiac arrest. N. Engl. J. Med. *328*:1377, 1993.
443. Hallstrom, A., Boutin, P., and Cobb, L.: Socioeconomic status and prediction of ventricular fibrillation survival. Am. J. Public Health *83*:245, 1993.
444. Every, N. R., Fahrenbruch, C. E., Hallstrom, A. P., et al.: Influence of coronary bypass surgery on subsequent outcome of patients resuscitated from out of hospital cardiac arrest. J. Am. Coll. Cardiol. *19*:1435, 1992.
445. Kim, Y. H., Sosa-Suarez, G., Trouton, T. G., et al.: Treatment of ventricular tachycardia by transcatheter radiofrequency ablation in patients with ischemic heart disease. Circulation *89*:1094, 1994.

HEART BLOCK

445a. Rardon, D. P., Miles, W. M., Mitrani, R. D., et al.: Atrioventricular block and dissociation. *In* Zipes, D. P., and Jalife, J. (eds.): Cardiac Electrophysiology: From Cell to Bedside. 2nd ed. Philadelphia, W. B. Saunders Company, 1994, p. 935.
446. Behar, S., Zissman, E., Zion, M., et al.: Prognostic significance of second-degree atrioventricular block in inferior wall acute myocardial infarction. SPRINT Study Group. Am. J. Cardiol. *72*:831, 1993.
447. Castellanos, A., Cox, M. M., Fernandez, P. R., et al.: Mechanisms and dynamics of episodes of progression of 2:1 atrioventricular block in patients with documented 2-level conduction disturbances. Am. J. Cardiol. *70*:193, 1992.
448. Gonzalez, M. D., Scherlag, B. J., Mabo, P., et al.: Functional dissociation of cellular activation as a mechanism of Mobitz type II atrioventricular block. Circulation *87*:1389, 1993.
449. Terasaki, F., James, T. N., and Nakayama, Y.: Ultrastructural alterations of the conduction system in mice exhibiting sinus arrest or heart block during coxsackievirus B3 acute myocarditis. Am. Heart J. *123*:439, 1992.
450. Alexander, E., Buyon, J. P., and Provost, T. T.: Anti-Ro/SS-A antibodies in the pathophysiology of congenital heart block in neonatal lupus syndrome, an experimental model: In vitro electrophysiologic and immunocytochemical studies. Arthritis Rheum *35*:176, 1992.
451. Frohn-Mulder, I. M., Meilof, J. F., Szatmari, A., et al.: Clinical significance of maternal anti-Ro/SS-A antibodies in children with isolated heart block. J. Am. Coll. Cardiol. *23*:1677, 1994.
452. Julkunen, H., Kurki, T., Kaaja, R., et al.: Isolated congenital heart block: Long-term outcome of mothers and characterization of the immune response to SS-A/Ro and to SS-B/La. Arthritis Rheum *36*:1588, 1993.
453. Antretter, H., Dapunt, O. E., Robl, W., et al.: Third-degree atrioventricular block in adult identical twins. Lancet *343*:1576, 1994.
454. Shen, W. K., Hammill, S. C., Hayes, D. L., et al.: Long-term survival after pacemaker implantation for heart block in patients greater than or equal to 65 years. Am. J. Cardiol. *74*:560, 1994.
455. Lee, M. A., Dae, M. W., Langberg, J. J., et al.: Effects of long-term right ventricular apical pacing on left ventricular perfusion, innervation, function and histology. J. Am. Coll. Cardiol. *24*:225, 1994.

OTHER ELECTROPHYSIOLOGICAL ABNORMALITIES LEADING TO CARDIAC ARRHYTHMIAS

456. Oreto, G., Smeets, J. L., and Rodriguez, L. M.: Supernormal conduction in the left bundle branch. J. Cardiovasc. Electrophysiol. *5*:345, 1994.

457. Centurion, O. A., Isomoto, S., Shimizu, A., et al.: Supernormal atrial conduction and its relation to atrial vulnerability and atrial fibrillation in patients with sick sinus syndrome and paroxysmal atrial fibrillation. Am. Heart J. *128:*88, 1994.
458. Moore, E. N., Spear, J. F., and Fisch, C.: Supernormal conduction and excitability. J. Cardiovasc. Electrophysiol. *4:*320, 1993.
459. Chen, P. S., Wolf, P. L., Cha, Y. M., et al.: Effects of subendocardial ablation on anodal supernormal excitation and ventricular vulnerability in open-chest dogs. Circulation *87:*216, 1993.
460. Liu, Y., Zeng, W., Delmar, M., et al.: Ionic mechanisms of electrotonic inhibition and concealed conduction in rabbit atrioventricular nodal myocytes. Circulation *88:*1634, 1993.
461. Fisch, C.: Electrocardiographic manifestations of exit block, concealed conduction and "supernormal" conduction. *In* Zipes, D. P., and Jalife, J. (eds.): Cardiac Electrophysiology: From Cell to Bedside. 2nd ed. Philadelphia, W. B. Saunders Company, 1994, p. 955.
462. Fujiki, A., Mizumaki, K., and Tani, M.: Effects of diltiazem on concealed atrioventricular nodal conduction in relation to ventricular response during atrial fibrillation in anesthetized dogs. Am. Heart J. *125:*1284, 1993.
463. Martinez-Alday, J. D., Almendral, J., Arenal, A., et al.: Identification of concealed posteroseptal Kent pathways by comparison of ventriculoatrial intervals from apical and posterobasal right ventricular sites. Circulation *89:*1060, 1994.
464. Castellanos, A., Saoudi, N., Moleiro, F., et al.: Parasystole. *In* Zipes, D. P., and Jalife, J. (eds.): Cardiac Electrophysiology: From Cell to Bedside. 2nd ed. Philadelphia, W. B. Saunders Company, 1994, p. 942.

Chapter 23
Cardiac Pacemakers and Antiarrhythmic Devices

S. SERGE BAROLD, DOUGLAS P. ZIPES

Since the first pacemaker implantation in 1958, cardiac pacing has continued to grow so that presently more than 500,000 patients in the United States have pacemakers. Almost 400,000 pacemakers are implanted worldwide each year. In addition to pacemakers that treat bradyarrhythmias with the aim of restoring normal or near-normal hemodynamics at rest and exercise, electrical therapy of ventricular tachyarrhythmias with devices capable of pacing, cardioversion, and defibrillation has become very important.[1]

A pacemaker is a device that delivers battery-supplied electric stimuli over leads with electrodes in contact with the heart. Virtually all leads are inserted transvenously. There are two types of leads: (1) unipolar, with only one electrode in the heart (cathode) and the other on the pacemaker casing, and (2) bipolar, with two electrodes in the heart (the tip is usually the cathode). All leads serve as two-way conductors for delivery of electrical impulses to the heart and the detection of spontaneous electrical activity. Electronic circuitry regulates the timing and characteristics of the stimuli. The power source is a lithium-iodine battery that has a high-energy density (energy content/volume), low interval losses caused by self-discharge, and a long shelf life; it can be hermetically sealed to prevent ingress of body fluids. Importantly, the lithium-iodine battery has predictable characteristics that permit early warning of battery depletion. As the voltage drops near end of life, the pacing rate on magnet application declines as an indicator of the elective replacement time. For single-chamber pulse generators the expected life is 7 to 12 years and for dual-chamber pulse generators it is 5 to 10 years, depending on function and appropriate programming to conserve battery life.

PACEMAKER MODALITIES AND FUNCTION

Pacemakers are categorized with a basic three-letter identification code according to the site of the pacing electrodes and the mode of pacing[1a]: V = ventricle, A = atrium, D = dual (A and V), I = inhibited, T = triggered, and O = none. The first position denotes the chamber paced, and the second position indicates the chamber sensed. The third position indicates the response to sensing, if any, with I indicating an inhibited response (pacemaker discharge suppressed by a sensed signal), T indicating a triggered response (pacemaker discharge triggered by a sensed signal), and D indicating both inhibited and triggered functions. I and T responses reset the timing circuit controlling the pacemaker lower rate interval. Occasionally, the letter S is used for the first or second position to indicate that a single-chamber device is suitable for either atrial or ventricular pacing, depending on how the parameters are programmed. For most pacemakers, the first three positions contain all the information of practical importance. Fourth and fifth positions are available to describe additional functions; however, the letters are infrequently stated in practice except for R, which indicates a rate-adaptive pulse generator driven by a nonatrial sensor (Table 23–1).

Cardiac pacing can be performed to treat patients who have bradyarrhythmias and tachyarrhythmias. Temporary pacing is used when an arrhythmia is transient, and permanent pacing is used when an arrhythmia is likely to be recurrent or permanent.

TEMPORARY PACING

Temporary cardiac pacing can be accomplished transvenously, via the esophagus, transcutaneously, epicardially, and via a coronary artery. *Transvenous* pacing is usually done through percutaneous puncture of the internal jugular, subclavian, or femoral vein using balloon-tipped and semifloating catheters without fluoroscopy or stiffer catheters with fluoroscopy.[2,3] The (intracardiac) electrogram from the distal electrode identifies the location of the lead.[4] For atrial pacing, a preformed J-catheter is positioned in the right atrial appendage. Atrioventricular (AV) sequential pacing usually requires two leads. Single-lead atrial synchronous ventricular inhibited (VDD) pacing is feasible, but atrial pacing from floating electrodes requires further development.[5] VDD pacing also can be achieved with atrial sensing via an esophageal electrode.[6] An electrode in the *esophagus* uniformly achieves atrial pacing with a 10-msec stimulus. Pacing is relatively noninvasive, safe, and simple and can be useful to treat sinus bradycardia or arrest, to initiate and terminate some supraventricular tachycardias, and to provide overdrive suppression of ventricular tachyarrhythmias.[7–9] Current technology cannot provide reliable esophageal ventricular pacing.

Transcutaneous ventricular pacing is used during emergency treatment of asystole or severe bradycardia; it involves large-surface-area, high-impedance electrodes placed on the anterior and posterior chest walls, stimuli of long duration (20 to 40 msec), and high current (50 to 100 mA).[10–12] Barring terminal asystole from severe metabolic derangement, failure to pace is almost always due to incorrect electrode placement. Identification of ventricular capture requires a filtered electrocardiogram (ECG). Some patients cannot tolerate transcutaneous pacing because of severe pain from skeletal muscle stimulation despite analgesics. Transcutaneous pacing produces a hemodynamic response similar to that of transvenous ventricular pacing,

TABLE 23–1 THE NASPE/BPEG GENERIC (NBG) PACEMAKER CODE

POSITION:	I	II	III	IV	V
Category:	Chamber(s) Paced	Chamber(s) Sensed	Response to Sensing	Programmability, Rate Modulation	Antitachyarrhythmia Function(s)
Letters:	0 = none A = atrium V = ventricle D = dual (A + V)	0 = none A = atrium V = ventricle D = dual (A + V)	0 = none T = triggered I = inhibited D = dual (T + I)	0 = none P = simple programmable M = multiprogrammable C = communicating R = rate modulation	0 = none P = pacing (antitachyarrhythmia) S = shock D = dual (P + S)
Manufacturers' designation only:	S = single (A or V)	S = single (A or V)			

Note: Positions I through III are used exclusively for antibradyarrhythmia function. NASPE = North American Society of Pacing and Electrophysiology; BPEG = British Pacing and Electrophysiology Group.

Modified from Bernstein, A.D., Camm, A.J., Fletcher, R.D., et al.: The NASPE/BPEG generic pacemaker code for antibradyarrhythmia and adaptive-rate pacing and antitachyarrhythmia devices. PACE *10*:794, 1987.

and demand pacing can be accomplished by sensing the surface QRS complex. Pacing can initiate and terminate many reentrant supraventricular and ventricular tachyarrhythmias.[13,14] Transcutaneous pacing may be useful when endocardial pacing is contraindicated and avoids some of the possible complications associated with temporary endocardial pacing such as infection, phlebitis, venous thrombosis, and perforation of the right ventricle. *Epicardial* pacing using ventricular and/or atrial pacing wires implanted at surgery is done in postoperative cardiac surgical patients, while pacing via a *coronary artery* (or the left ventricle) can be accomplished during percutaneous transluminal coronary angioplasty.[15,16]

INDICATIONS. Temporary pacing is indicated prophylactically in patients with a high risk of developing high-degree AV block, severe sinus node dysfunction, or asystole in acute myocardial infarction, after cardiac surgery, at times after cardioversion, during cardiac catheterization, and occasionally before implantation or replacement of a permanent pacemaker. Asymptomatic patients with bifascicular block who only undergo surgery with general anesthesia do not need prophylactic pacing. Pacing is also indicated when temporary bradycardia causes symptomatic, hemodynamic, or electrophysiological consequences as in acute myocardial infarction (discussed later), hyperkalemia, drug-induced bradycardia or toxicity (e.g., digitalis), bradycardia-dependent ventricular tachycardia, before implantation of a permanent pacemaker in a patient with unstable rhythm, and at times in myocarditis such as Lyme disease. Finally, rapid (burst) temporary pacing can be used to terminate tachycardias such as atrial flutter, AV nodal and AV reentry, and sustained monomorphic ventricular tachycardia (see p. 683). Atrial fibrillation, ventricular fibrillation, and very rapid ventricular tachycardias cannot be treated by pacing techniques. Cardioversion by transvenous leads designed for low energy delivery can terminate ventricular tachycardia, atrial flutter, and atrial fibrillation.[17] Pacing at relatively fast rates can prevent some ventricular tachycardias that are bradycardia-dependent or associated with Q-T prolongation and torsades de pointes. Less frequent uses include atrial pacing at a rate faster than a supraventricular tachycardia to increase the degree of AV block, synchronized atrial pacing to restore AV synchrony during incessant ventricular tachycardia, and coupled ventricular pacing with an early stimulus timed to provide an electrical but not a mechanical response to slow the effective rate.

TEMPORARY PACING IN ACUTE MYOCARDIAL INFARCTION (see also p. 1252). The role of temporary pacing in AV block during acute myocardial infarction is still controversial because the risk/benefit ratio is unclear. Death is generally not related directly to the conduction disturbance, and the prognosis depends more on the size of the myocardial infarction than on the degree of AV block. AV block in *inferior infarction* is almost always localized in the AV node and is relatively benign. Inferior infarction does not cause narrow QRS type II second degree AV block.[18,19] Most hemodynamically stable patients with second degree AV block can be treated without pacing but require monitoring. Pacing is rarely necessary in hemodynamically stable patients with complete AV block and a ventricular rate around 40 to 45 per minute in the absence of ventricular arrhythmia. Temporary ventricular pacing is indicated in second or third degree AV block only in the presence of an excessively slow ventricular rate, ventricular arrhythmia, hypotension, signs of hypoperfusion, or congestive heart failure. Dual-chamber pacing may sometimes be required to improve hemodynamics, especially when there is right ventricular infarction.[20] *Right ventricular infarction* causes an acute increase in diastolic stiffness so that the right ventricle becomes far more dependent on preload and acts more or less as a passive conduit for the atrial pump. Right ventricular infarction can be associated with hypotension or shock, partly or entirely due to AV block and loss of AV synchrony. Ventricular pacing may not improve the hemodynamic state, but AV sequential pacing with restoration of AV synchrony can cause a dramatic increase in the blood pressure, cardiac output, and stroke volume.

The development of second or third degree AV block associated with bundle branch block during *anterior infarction* necessitates temporary pacing, but the mortality rate is nonetheless quite high because these conduction disturbances generally occur in patients with very large infarcts. Dual-chamber pacing should be used in pacemaker-dependent patients.[20] Prophylactic pacing traditionally has been recommended in the presence of new right bundle branch block with left-axis deviation (left anterior hemiblock), right bundle branch block with right-axis deviation (left posterior hemiblock), left bundle branch block with first degree AV block, and alternating right and left bundle branch block because these patients are at higher risk of suddenly developing high-degree AV block with catastrophic consequences. Vagally induced AV block with a narrow QRS complex (such as during vomiting) does not require pacing.

The role of pacing for *right bundle branch block* with a normal axis or *left bundle branch block* with a normal P-R interval is more controversial. Preexisting right or left bundle branch block is usually not an indication for temporary pacing. During prophylactic pacing in anterior infarction, the pacemaker can be turned off in some patients until needed to avoid ventricular fibrillation that may result from delivery of a stimulus in the vulnerable period if the pacemaker is not inhibited appropriately by spontaneous ventricular activity. Furthermore, continuous ventricular pacing can mask the development of transient second or third degree AV block, considered by many to be an indication for permanent pacing.

The advent of reliable external transcutaneous pacing has diminished the need in many patients for prophylactic temporary right ventricular pacing in acute myocardial infarction, an important consideration in patients treated with thrombolytic therapy and anticoagulants. Patients with anterior myocardial infarction and bifascicular block can be managed simply by application of large pacing electrodes on the chest and keeping an external pulse generator close by for transcutaneous pacing.

PERMANENT PACING

Indications for permanent pacing were published by a Joint Committee in the American College of Cardiology (ACC) and the American Heart Association (AHA) in 1984 and 1991.[21] The ACC/AHA document recognizes the fact that indications for permanent pacing in an individual patient may not always be clear-cut; however, they have been grouped according to the following classifications: Class I, conditions for which there is general agreement that permanent pacemakers should be implanted; Class II, conditions for which permanent pacemakers are used frequently but opinion diverges on whether they are necessary; and Class III, conditions for which there is general agreement that pacemakers are unnecessary. The ACC/AHA guidelines also indicate that in those patients being considered for pacemakers, decision making may be influenced by a number of additional factors. Despite their shortcomings,[22,23] the 1991 ACC/AHA guidelines provide a useful framework on which Table 23–2 is based (see also p. 1963).

AV Block

Type II second degree AV block is defined as the occurrence of a single nonconducted P wave associated with constant PR intervals before and after the blocked impulse, provided that the sinus rate or the P-P interval is constant and there are at least two consecutive conducted P waves (i.e., 3:2 AV block) to determine the behavior of the P-R interval.[22,24] The definitions of type I and type II second degree AV block are purely descriptive and do not refer to the site of block. However, type II AV block invariably occurs below the AV node, while type I AV block in the setting of a normal QRS complex generally occurs in the AV node. Although 2:1 AV block can occur in either the AV node or the His-Purkinje system, it cannot be classified into type I or type II. Advanced second degree AV block refers to 2:1, 3:1, or 4:1 AV block, and the like.

Although the meaning of bifascicular block is obvious, that of trifascicular block is not as simple.[22] In this respect, the ACC/AHA guidelines use the term *trifascicular block* rather loosely. The combination of bifascicular block (right bundle branch block + left anterior hemiblock, right bundle branch block + left posterior hemiblock or left bundle branch block) and first degree AV block on the surface electrocardiogram must not be designated as trifascicular block because the site of AV block can be either in the AV node or in the His-Purkinje system. Electrocardiographic documentation of trifascicular block during 1:1 AV conduction is rare and occurs usually in the presence of alternating right bundle branch block and left bundle branch block or fixed right bundle branch block with alternating left anterior hemiblock and left posterior hemiblock. In Table 23–2, left bundle branch block is bifascicular block, while right bundle branch block is described as bundle branch block rather than unifascicular block to avoid confusion with left anterior or left posterior hemiblock.

Before pacemaker implantation, reversible causes of AV block such as Lyme disease, athletic heart,[25] hypervagotonia, ischemia, and drug, metabolic, or electrolyte imbalance must be excluded. There is general (although not unanimous) agreement that permanent pacing is indicated in asymptomatic patients with acquired complete AV block. It is also indicated in asymptomatic patients with alternating right and left bundle branch block and those with well-documented second degree AV block in the His-Purkinje system, often associated with bundle branch block, because symptoms usually develop in a relatively short time. His bundle recordings are often required to demonstrate the site of block (AV node or His-Purkinje system) in patients with bundle branch block and type I or advanced second degree AV block. Some symptomatic patients with marked first degree AV block may benefit from dual-chamber pacing with a more physiological AV interval.[26,27]

ACUTE MYOCARDIAL INFARCTION (see also p. 1252). Permanent pacing is rarely, if ever, indicated in AV block due to inferior infarction because it is almost always transient, occasionally lasting as long as 2 to 3 weeks. Pacing is not required in anterior infarction complicated by permanent bundle branch or bifascicular block but can be considered (although this is still controversial) to prevent sudden death from asystole in those patients who develop transient trifascicular block (second or third degree AV block) even though 1:1 AV conduction returns.

CONGENITAL AV BLOCK (see also p. 966). Permanent pacing in asymptomatic patients with congenital AV block is recommended if there is (1) a mean daytime junctional rate slower than 50/min, (2) no or little change in the junctional rate with physical activity, (3) long periods of asystole during sleep secondary to junctional exit block, (4) cardiomegaly, (5) depressed left ventricular function detected echocardiographically, and (6) electrocardiographic evidence of atrial enlargement. Pacing can be considered if the patient has a prolonged QRS complex (≥ 0.12 sec), frequent multiformed or repetitive ventricular ectopy, or Q-Tc > 0.45 sec.[28–30]

BUNDLE BRANCH BLOCK. Eighty per cent of patients with asymptomatic bundle branch block have associated heart disease, with coronary artery disease found in almost half. Half the deaths are sudden and are usually not due to bradycardia but rather to myocardial infarction or ventricular tachycardia. H-V interval prolongation is found in 40 to 50 per cent of patients with bundle branch block and bifascicular block. However, a prolonged H-V interval that is shorter than 100 msec generally is not predictive of future events such as syncope and death. Although the development of AV block is more frequent in patients with H-V interval prolongation (1 to 2 per cent per year), the low incidence militates against investigation or treatment of the asymptomatic patient.[30]

INDUCIBLE AV BLOCK. His-Purkinje block induced by atrial pacing, though an insensitive sign of conduction system disease, may constitute an indication for permanent pacing provided that functional infranodal block is excluded.[30] Exercise-induced AV block is an indication for pacing because it is almost always infranodal and most asymptomatic patients eventually develop serious problems.[30] Rarely, exercise-induced AV block is secondary to myocardial ischemia and does not require pacing unless ischemia cannot be alleviated.[31] The use of drugs such as ajmaline and procainamide that depress His-Purkinje conduction to provoke His-Purkinje block in susceptible patients is still controversial.[32,33]

BUNDLE BRANCH BLOCK AND SYNCOPE. In patients with bundle branch block and syncope, it is important to perform a complete electrophysiological study because sustained monomorphic ventricular tachycardia is the cause of symptoms in 20 to 30 per cent of patients.[30] An abnormal electrophysiological study including the induction of ventricular tachycardia is associated with a greater incidence of total and sudden death during follow-up, while a normal or nondiagnostic study correlates with a higher rate of symptomatic remission and a better prognosis with a low risk of dying from an arrhythmia. Obviously, a negative

TABLE 23–2 INDICATIONS FOR PERMANENT PACING

1. Acquired AV Block in Adults

Class 1
- A. Permanent or intermittent complete AV block at any anatomic level in the absence of reversible causes, regardless of symptoms.*†
- B. Permanent or intermittent second degree AV block regardless of the type or the site of block, with symptomatic bradycardia.†
- C. Permanent or intermittent asymptomatic type II second degree AV block.†‡
- D. Asymptomatic type I or advanced second degree AV block at intra-His or infra-His levels.†‡
- E. Exercise-induced second or complete AV block regardless of symptoms but without reversible ischemia.†
- F. Atrial fibrillation, atrial flutter, or rare cases of supraventricular tachycardia with AV block and bradycardia associated with congestive heart failure or periods of asystole ≥3.0 sec or escape rate <40 beats/min or alternating tachycardia and bradycardia difficult to control pharmacologically. The bradycardia must be unrelated to drugs known to impair AV conduction.

Class II
Symptomatic first degree AV block improved by temporary dual-chamber pacing.

Class III
- A. Asymptomatic first degree AV block.
- B. Asymptomatic type I second degree AV block at the supra-His (AV node) level.

2. After Acute Myocardial Infarction

Class I
Persistent or transient second degree or complete AV block in the His-Purkinje system.

Class II
Persistent advanced or complete AV block at the AV node (longer than 16 days).

Class III
- A. Transient AV conduction disturbances without intraventricular conduction defects.
- B. Transient AV block in the presence of isolated left anterior hemiblock.
- C. Acquired left anterior hemiblock, bundle branch block, or bifascicular block with or without first degree AV block, but in the absence of second degree or complete AV block.

3. Chronic Intraventricular Block

Class I
- A. Bundle branch block or bifascicular block with second or complete AV block associated with symptomatic bradycardia.
- B. Bundle branch block or bifascicular block with intermittent type II second degree AV block without symptoms (see section 1).
- C. Bundle branch block or bifascicular block with infranodal block without symptoms: type I, advanced second degree, or complete AV block (see section 1).
- D. Trifascicular block during 1:1 AV conduction regardless of symptoms such as (1) alternating left bundle branch block and right bundle branch block, (2) fixed right bundle branch block with alternating left anterior hemiblock and left posterior hemiblock.
- E. Exercise-induced second or complete AV block regardless of symptoms, but without demonstrable ischemia as a cause of AV block.

Class II
- A. Bundle branch block or bifascicular block with syncope that is not proved to be due to complete AV block but other possible causes of syncope are not identified.
- B. Markedly prolonged HV (≥100 msec).
- C. Pacing-induced infra-His block.

Class III
- A. Hemiblock, bundle branch block, or bifascicular block without second degree or complete AV block or symptoms.
- B. Hemiblock, bundle branch block, or bifascicular block with first degree AV block without symptoms.

study does not exclude transient bradycardia as a cause of syncope or the possibility of sudden death, although the risk is quite low, and recurrence of syncope does not correlate with a higher mortality or sudden death. An H-V interval ≥ 100 msec identifies patients with a higher risk of AV block who require pacing.[32] Pacing can be considered in patients who have an H-V between 70 and 100 msec and no identifiable cause for syncope.[33]

Sick Sinus Syndrome

About half of all pacemakers are used to treat sick sinus syndrome (see p. 648). A pacemaker should be implanted only when a causal relationship has been demonstrated between bradycardia and symptoms, which may be difficult to accomplish in elderly patients with vague symptoms. If in doubt about the need for pacing, it is usually safe to wait because arrhythmias associated with sick sinus syndrome rarely result in sudden cardiac death. In the bradycardia-tachycardia syndrome (Chap. 22), drugs alone may worsen the bradycardia; symptomatic patients are usually best managed by a combination of pacemaker and antiarrhythmic drugs.[34] When bradycardia is secondary to necessary drug therapy, e.g., beta blocker or amiodarone, a pacemaker can be used to treat the consequences of the drug. Permanent pacing should not be considered when there is transient bradycardia due to an increase in vagal tone or drug therapy that can be discontinued or reduced. In the sick sinus syndrome, pacing improves the quality of life and facilitates treatment of supraventricular tachycardias exhibited by over a third of the patients. Most patients have structural heart disease, and single-chamber ventricular pacing (as opposed to atrial-based pacing, discussed later) is no longer recommended.

The role of prophylactic pacing in asymptomatic patients with ECG evidence of sick sinus syndrome has not been established. Asymptomatic patients should be followed closely, and drugs that depress sinus node function should be avoided. Two-second pauses are usually harmless. During sleep, the sinus rate normally may fall to 30/min and exhibit pauses of 3 sec. While it is often stated that sinus pauses are abnormal if they exceed 3 sec without intervening escape beats, the validity of such a conclusion has not been established; neither has the validity of permanent pacing in these asymptomatic patients.

Hypersensitive Carotid Sinus Syndrome and Neurally Mediated (Vasovagal) Syncope

HYPERSENSITIVE CAROTID SINUS SYNDROME. In the carotid sinus syndrome (see p. 865), patients with a predominant cardioinhibitory reflex response (slowing of sinus rate and/or prolongation of AV conduction with AV block) benefit from permanent pacing. The AAI mode is contraindicated, and the VVI mode generally is poorly tolerated. Most patients require dual-chamber pacing with the DDI or DDD mode, preferably with hysteresis (discussed later). In pre-

TABLE 23–2 INDICATIONS FOR PERMANENT PACING—*Continued*

4. Sick Sinus Syndrome

Class I

Sinus node dysfunction with documented symptomatic bradycardia. (In some patients this will occur as a consequence of long-term essential drug therapy of a type and dose for which there are no acceptable alternatives.)

Class II

Sinus node dysfunction, occurring spontaneously or as a result of necessary drug therapy, with heart rate <40 beats/min when a clear association between significant symptoms consistent with bradycardia and the actual presence of bradycardia has not been documented.

Class III

A. Sinus node dysfunction in asymptomatic patients, including those in whom substantial sinus bradycardia (heart rate <40 beats/min) is a consequence of long-term drug treatment.
B. Sinus node dysfunction in patients in whom symptoms suggestive of bradycardia are clearly documented *not* to be associated with a slow heart rate.

5. Hypersensitive Carotid Sinus and Malignant Vasovagal Syndromes

Class I

Recurrent syncope associated with clear, spontaneous events provoked by carotid sinus stimulation; minimal carotid sinus pressure induces asystole of >3 sec duration in the absence of any medication that depresses the sinus node or AV conduction.

Class II

A. Recurrent syncope without clear, provocative events and with a hypersensitive cardioinhibitory response.
B. Syncope with associated bradycardia reproduced by a head-up tilt with or without isoproterenol or other forms of provocative maneuvers and in which a temporary pacemaker and a second provocative test can establish the likely benefits of a permanent pacemaker. Pacing should be considered only in patients refractory to drug therapy.

Class III

A. A hyperactive cardioinhibitory response to carotid sinus stimulation in the absence of symptoms.
B. Vague symptoms such as dizziness or lightheadedness, or both, with a hyperactive cardioinhibitory response to carotid sinus stimulation.
C. Recurrent syncope, lightheadedness or dizziness in the absence of a cardioinhibitory response.

* Asymptomatic complete AV block, permanent or intermittent, at any anatomic site is a Class II indication in the 1991 ACC/AHA guidelines when the ventricular rate ≥40 beats/min in asymptomatic patients and a Class I indication when the ventricular rate <40 beats/min or there is asystole ≥3 sec in asymptomatic patients. The 1991 ACC/AHA guidelines classify permanent or intermittent complete AV block at any level as a Class I indication when associated with (1) symptomatic bradycardia, (2) congestive heart failure, (3) conditions requiring therapy with drugs that suppress automacity.

† A number of conditions are listed in the 1991 ACC/AHA guidelines in both the section on acquired AV block and the sections on bifascicular and trifascicular block (chronic intraventricular block). The same format was adopted in this table to facilitate comparison with the ACC/AHA guidelines.

‡ Class II indication in the 1991 ACC/AHA guidelines.

Adapted from Dreifus, L. S., et al.: ACC/AHA guidelines for implantation of cardiac pacemakers and antiarrhythmia devices. Reprinted with permission from American College of Cardiology. J. Am. Coll. Cardiol. *18*:1, 1991.

dominant vasodepressor syncope, dual-chamber pacing may not abolish symptoms.[35–37]

NEURALLY MEDIATED SYNCOPE. *Neurally mediated syncope* refers to vasovagal syncope often reproducible by tilt-table testing. Pacing should not be first-line therapy because many patients respond to drug therapy with beta blockers or other agents. In drug-refractory patients who show a significant bradycardia component during syncope, dual-chamber pacing with hysteresis may prolong the time from onset of symptoms to loss of consciousness or may prevent syncope altogether. Pacing may permit a more gradual blood pressure decline during the attacks that would be perceived by the patient, who can then take appropriate protective measures (such as lying down, stopping car driving, and the like).[37–39] Thus pacing can be beneficial by retarding symptoms. The AAI, VVI, or VDD modes are contraindicated.[37–40]

Pacing Without Conduction System Disease

Dual-chamber pacing with a short A-V interval has emerged as effective therapy for many patients with obstructive hypertrophic cardiomyopathy and a resting or provocable left ventricular outflow tract gradient ≥ 30 mm Hg[41,42] (see p. 1426). Pacing produces apical preexcitation, and a favorable response is closely tied to optimization of the A-V interval to ensure pacing-induced ventricular depolarization at all times. Preliminary results of dual-chamber pacing with a short A-V interval in a small number of patients with end-stage idiopathic dilated cardiomyopathy are promising.[43] Such therapy presently remains investigational. The benefit of dual-chamber pacing with a short A-V interval in patients with congestive heart failure due to left ventricular systolic dysfunction (regardless of etiology) has not yet been determined. Permanent pacing combined with beta-blocker therapy appears highly effective in patients with the long Q-T syndrome (see p. 685) who do not respond to beta-blocker therapy alone and/or cardiac sympathectomy. Pacing at a rate designed to normalize the Q-T interval provides adjunctive therapy because complete protection requires the implantation of an automatic defibrillator.[44] Finally, rapid atrial pacing in conjunction with drug therapy may benefit patients with drug-refractory orthostatic hypotension.[45,46]

METHODS OF PACEMAKER IMPLANTATION

Virtually all pacemakers are implanted transvenously under local anesthesia using either the cephalic vein exposed by cutdown or blind percutaneous puncture of the subclavian vein.[47–49] The pacemaker pocket is fashioned over the pectoralis major muscle. The cephalic vein is often of sufficient size to accept one or two pacing leads. If not, passage of a flexible guidewire followed by a standard subclavian vein introducer provides simple and direct access to the subclavian vein. Although blind percutaneous subclavian vein puncture is potentially more dangerous than insertion through the cephalic vein, in skilled hands it is remarkably safe. It reduces the time required for implantation, facilitates implanting two leads, reduces the need for surgical expertise (especially with peel-away sheaths), and has made the implantation of most sophisticated pacemakers a relatively simple surgical procedure.[50] Many of the complications (some lethal) of blind subclavian puncture, which include pneumothorax, subclavian arterial puncture with hemothorax, air embolism, hemopneumomediastinum, subcutaneous emphysema, nerve injury, and thoracic duct injury, are preventable. Leads inserted via medial subclavian puncture are susceptible to compression damage in the tight costoclavicular angle (subclavian crush).[49,51,52]

With contemporary transvenous leads, complications are related more to the skill and experience of the implanter and implantation technique than to lead design because all leads now possess good performance characteristics. Epicardial leads are used only if there is no venous access, in

TABLE 23–3 TECHNICAL ASPECTS OF PACEMAKER IMPLANTATION

1. Pacing threshold (also during cough and deep respiration) in terms of voltage and pulse width with matching external pacemaker. The voltage threshold at a single pulse width of 0.5 to 0.6 msec is usually sufficient.
2. Lead impedance at 5-V output and 0.5- to 0.6-msec pulse width.
3. Recording of atrial and ventricular electrograms: unipolar, bipolar (if applicable), morphology, amplitude and current of injury (ST-segment elevation associated with good contact) during normal and deep inspiration. The signal amplitude also can be measured with a PSA.
4. Determination of slew rate (dV/dt) if signal is small.
5. High-voltage pacing (10 V) to detect left diaphragmatic stimulation from ventricular electrode and right phrenic nerve–diaphragmatic stimulation from atrial electrode.
6. Blood pressure measurement during ventricular pacing to determine susceptibility to pacemaker syndrome.
7. Atrial and ventricular pacing to determine antegrade AV and retrograde VA conduction.
8. Interrogation and reprogramming of the pulse generator before implantation.
9. ECG recordings with and without magnet application to demonstrate atrial and/or ventricular pacing and normal atrial and/or ventricular sensing.
10. Chest x-ray immediately after implantation to exclude pneumothorax when applicable.

certain pediatric patients, or in patients undergoing open-heart surgery. Alternatively, endocardial leads can be introduced via a transatrial approach with a limited thoracotomy.[48,53] The operative techniques and intraoperative measurements necessary for safe and long-term pacing (Table 23–3) are straightforward compared with the technical knowledge required to understand the electrophysiology of pacing and follow-up of patients so as to make the best use of the important programmable functions.

Capture Thresholds, Sensing, and Leads

DETERMINATION OF THE PACING THRESHOLD

This is crucial to optimize pacemaker longevity and is determined at the time of implantation using an external testing device (pacing system analyzer, or PSA) with circuitry similar to that of the implantable pulse generator. Most implantable pulse generators are constant voltage sources; the leading edge of the voltage pulse remains constant regardless of the impedance (resistance). The threshold should be determined in volts at a given pulse width of 0.5 to 0.6 msec. To measure the threshold, the PSA is set at 5 V and pulse width 0.5 msec (usually the nominal parameters of an implantable device). The pacing rate is increased until consistent pacing capture is achieved. The voltage is then slowly reduced until loss of capture occurs outside the myocardial refractory period. The lowest voltage at a given pulse width capable of causing consistent capture outside the myocardial refractory period defines the stimulation threshold (Fig. 23–1). Ventricular capture near the pacing threshold may occur only when stimuli fall in the supernormal phase (Fig. 23–1).

The current delivered to the myocardium is determined by the impedance (resistance) according to Ohm's law. Normal lead impedance, ranging between 250 and 1000 ohms, typically is 500 to 700 ohms at the nominal output of 5 V. The relationship of threshold voltage and pulse width is not linear and establishes the strength-duration curve; the shorter the pulse width, the higher is the voltage threshold.

THE STRENGTH-DURATION CURVE (Fig. 23–2). This is steep, with a short pulse width, and becomes essentially flat at a pulse width exceeding 2 msec (rheobase). The acute ventricular pacing threshold should be ≤ 0.8 V at 0.5 msec, and the acute atrial pacing threshold should be ≤ 1.5 V at 0.5 msec. Lower values are often obtained. A high initial threshold value requires lead repositioning. The lowest threshold possible at implantation should be sought because ultimately it may determine the threshold at maturity and hence the voltage required for long-term pacing.

After implantation, the output of the pulse generator is usually left at 5 V and 0.5 msec or at a longer pulse width for the first 8 weeks. At 8 weeks, when the chronic threshold has been attained in most cases, the output voltage and pulse width should be programmed to reduce current drain from the battery and yet maintain an adequate margin of safety. A low output voltage and/or short pulse width enhances battery longevity. The safety margin for capture is the amount by which the pulse generator voltage output exceeds the chronic threshold value at a given pulse duration and should be 1.75; i.e., the output voltage should be at least 1.75 times the chronic threshold voltage at the same pulse width.[50] In practice, a voltage safety margin of 2 is often used, so the output voltage is set at twice the chronic threshold voltage at the same pulse width. An output voltage exceeding 5 V should not be used routinely because of reduced pulse generator efficiency and longevity.

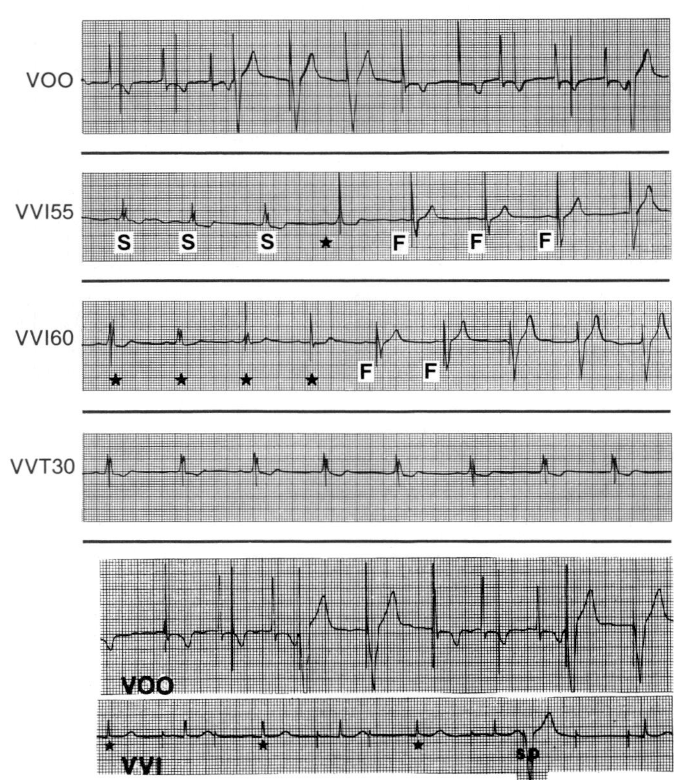

FIGURE 23–1. VOO, VVI, and VVT pacing. *Top strip:* VOO pacing. The pacemaker competes with the spontaneous rhythm and stimuli capture the ventricle only beyond the myocardial refractory period.

Second strip: VVI pacemaker, rate = 55/min. The first three beats are sensed (S) and the 4th beat (star) is a ventricular pseudofusion beat. The 5th, 6th, and 7th complexes are ventricular fusion beats (F).

Third strip: VVI pacemaker, rate = 60/min. The first three beats (stars) are ventricular pseudofusion beats. The 4th beat (star) appears to be a ventricular pseudofusion beat because the initial QRS vector occurs just before the stimulus. The T wave of the 4th beat is identical to that of the previous beat, suggesting that depolarization was also identical, providing further proof for pseudofusion. The 5th and 6th complexes are ventricular fusion beats (F) while the last three beats are pure ventricular-paced beats.

Fourth strip: Same patient as in third strip. The pacemaker was programmed to the VVT mode, rate = 30/min. The pacemaker emits or triggers a ventricular stimulus immediately upon sensing each QRS complex. Thus, the stimulus marks the precise time of sensing the VVT mode. This may be correlated with the ventricular pseudofusion beats in the third strip where the first pseudofusion beat is deformed by a ventricular stimulus just before the R wave returns to baseline, i.e., just before sensing would have occurred as determined from the VVT mode in the 4th strip.

Bottom strip: VVI pacemaker with ineffectual stimuli but normal sensing. The high pacing threshold was close to the output of the pulse generator. The 3rd to the last stimulus captures the ventricle in the supernormal phase (SP) when the excitability threshold attains its lowest value. Spontaneous QRS complexes falling within the pacemaker refractory period (for sensing—350 ms after the stimulus) are not sensed; those beyond the pacemaker refractory period are sensed and recycle the pacemaker.

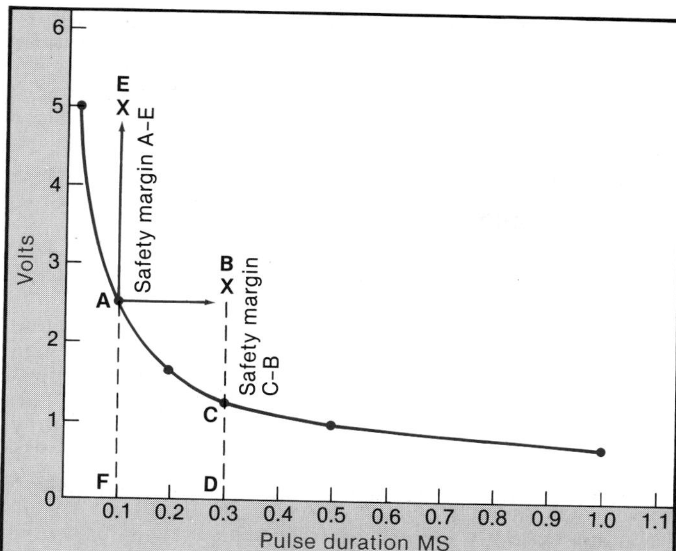

FIGURE 23–2. Strength-duration curve relating voltage and pulse width at the chronic pacing threshold. Values above the curve pace the heart while values below the curve fail to capture. The threshold for pacing at A is 2.5 V at a pulse width of 0.1 ms. Consequently, starting from the threshold at A, the output voltage of the pulse generator could be doubled to 5 V while the pulse width is kept constant at 0.1 ms, i.e, going to E. This would provide a voltage safety margin of EF/AF = 2. Alternatively, the output voltage could be left at 2.5 V and the pulse width increased to 0.3 ms to B. This would yield a voltage safety margin of BD/CD or slightly more than 2. The second option consumes less battery current and is to be preferred.

ADJUSTMENT OF PULSE WIDTH. If the pulse width is varied without a programmable voltage output, it should be adjusted to 3 times the value at threshold provided that the pulse width at threshold is ≤ 0.2 msec. Because of the configuration of the strength-duration curve, with a pulse width at threshold ≥ 0.3 msec, tripling the pulse width (keeping the voltage constant) may or may not provide a voltage safety margin of 2 and probably should not be used in pacemaker-dependent patients.

The relatively flat characteristic of the voltage strength-duration curve from 0.5 to 1.5 msec means that an increase in the pulse width alone in this range will not provide a sufficient margin of safety in terms of volts. Therefore, when the voltage at threshold requires a pulse width ≥ 0.4 to 0.5 msec, an adequate safety margin cannot be obtained by programming pulse width alone. With a threshold of 2.5 V/0.1 msec, the pulse generator could be programmed to 2.5 V/0.3 msec or 5 V/0.1 msec to provide a voltage safety factor of at least 2. However, pulse widths < 0.2 msec situated on the steep portion of the voltage strength-duration curve are not recommended because shifts of the curve in response to the vagaries of daily living become more pronounced, while fluctuations of pulse width (electronic jitter) cannot always be discounted at short pulse widths. In terms of battery current drain, multiplying the voltage output by 2 (keeping the pulse width constant) is equivalent to multiplying the pulse width by 4 (keeping the voltage constant). Consequently, if the pacemaker circuit is more efficient at 2.5 V than at 5 V, with a threshold of 2.5 V/0.2 msec, an output of 2.5 V/0.6 msec is preferable to 5.0 V/0.2 msec. With a voltage threshold of 2.5 V/0.3 msec, an output of 5.0 V/0.3 msec is usually recommended. With a relatively high chronic threshold exceeding 3 to 3.5 V at a pulse width of 0.5 msec at the time of pacemaker replacement or during follow-up, the output voltage should exceed 5 V. In this situation, use of a new lead or (less preferably) a pulse generator programmable to a high voltage (10 V) should be considered.

LEAD IMPEDANCE. In addition to testing thresholds, the integrity of new and old leads can be evaluated by determining the voltage threshold and lead impedance either directly or noninvasively by telemetry. Lead impedance normally remains constant or falls slightly over time. Lead fracture (with apposed ends) elevates both the voltage threshold and the lead impedance (> 1000 ohms), while with an insulation defect the voltage threshold may be low or normal and the lead impedance will be low (< 250 ohms). A high voltage threshold due to lead displacement or an excessive tissue reaction around the electrode (exit block) is associated with a normal lead impedance.

CHANGES IN THE PACING THRESHOLD. With conventional leads, this variable rises shortly after implantation because edema and inflammation separate the tip from the myocardium. Most of the threshold increase appears to result from the formation of nonexcitable fibrous tissue around the electrode, increasing the effective size of the "virtual" electrode at the interface with the myocardium.[54,55] The threshold usually reaches its maximum value 10 to 20 days after implantation and stabilizes to about 2 to 4 times the acute value at 1 to 2 months. Small electrodes have lower initial thresholds and a greater proportional rise during the initial reaction, but the chronic threshold is lower than that of larger electrodes.

Threshold evolution sometimes takes longer than expected, and on rare occasions, the threshold continues to rise gradually with ultimate failure to capture. If there is no lead displacement, such failure to capture is often called *exit block;* this is a relatively rare complication. Exercise, sympathomimetic drugs, and glucocorticoids decrease the threshold, while food, sleep, insulin, ischemia, hypothyroidism, hyperkalemia, mineralocorticoids, and certain antiarrhythmic agents increase the threshold. Type 1C (see p. 608) antiarrhythmic drugs (especially flecainide),[56–58] toxic levels of Type 1A antiarrhythmic agents, and hyperkalemia may cause exit block.[59] Amiodarone has no important effect on the threshold.[59] Isoproterenol infusion or systemic steroids can be used to treat a high threshold temporarily until the underlying condition is corrected.

SENSING. A pacemaker senses the potential difference between the two electrodes used for pacing. In a bipolar system, the bipolar electrogram should be recorded to determine adequate electrode position for sensing. In a unipolar system, the unipolar electrogram is recorded from the tip electrode and closely reflects the cardiac signal because the anodal contribution from the pacemaker plate is generally negligible. The amplitude and slew rate (dV/dt) of the electrogram must exceed the sensitivity of the pulse generator to ensure reliable sensing.[55,60,61]

SIGNAL AMPLITUDE. The ventricular signal is often 6 to 15 mV, a range that exceeds the sensitivity threshold of a pulse generator. The ventricular electrogram should measure at least 5 to 6 mV and the atrial electrogram at least 1.5 to 2 mV. A signal with a gradual slope (lower slew rate) is more difficult to sense than is a sharp upstroke signal. Determination of the slew rate may be useful when the signal is low or borderline (3 to 5 mV for ventricular signals) but is not necessary if the amplitude of the signal is large. A low electrographic signal may require repositioning of the lead. Rarely, unipolar and bipolar ventricular electrograms are too small for sensing at nominal sensitivity because of chronic ischemia or cardiomyopathy. In this situation, a bipolar pulse generator programmable to a high sensitivity should be used.

Following initial lead placement, the ventricular electrogram from the tip electrode shows an initial current of injury (ST-segment elevation) that reflects good endocardial contact and disappears after a few days.[61] Over the long term, the amplitude of the QRS signal from conventional leads diminished slightly, but the slew rate can diminish further (about 40 per cent).[60,61] These changes normally are of no clinical importance for ventricular sensing but can be important in the case of smaller atrial signals, although studies with contemporary leads have documented the stability of the atrial signal chronically.[62]

LEAD DESIGN

New lead technology and design have improved bipolar leads sufficiently to eliminate the previous advantages of unipolar leads over bipolar leads. Generally, bipolar leads are preferred because of greater signal-to-noise ratio, less sensitivity to extraneous interference (especially skeletal myopotentials), less frequent crosstalk (atrial stimulus sensed by ventricular lead in a dual-chamber system), and avoidance of muscle stimulation occasionally seen at the anodal site of unipolar pulse generators.[60,63,64] Improvement in the design of lead fixation mechanisms has reduced the incidence of dislodgment to 0.5 to 1.5 per cent or less with ventricular leads and about 1 to 5 per cent with atrial leads. Adhering leads utilize either passive fixation with tines or fins to enhance entanglement in trabeculae or active fixation with myocardial penetration by grasping screws or small jaws. Tined and screw-in leads are the most popular and exhibit equally good performance. Active fixation leads are particularly useful in right ventricular dilatation, in tricuspid insufficiency, and when pacing of the right ventricular outflow tract is needed. Screw-in leads exhibit a decrease in the pacing threshold and an increase in signal amplitude in the first 30 minutes after implantation because of partial resolution of the initial local injury.

Contemporary electrodes have a small surface area that reduces stimulation thresholds because of a higher current density. Porous electrodes with a small surface area yield a low pacing threshold and yet provide a greater surface area for improved sensing. Steroid-eluting leads have a reservoir within the electrode tip that elutes a trace of dexamethasone directly at the electrode-tissue interface and reduces the local tissue reaction and the thickness of the fibrous capsule surrounding the tip electrode.[54,64–68] Steroid-eluting leads are associated with very low pacing thresholds and lack of initial peaking and excellent sensing with less chronic degradation of the endocardial signal,[55] and they have virtually eliminated so-called exit block with ineffectual pacemaker stimuli. Such leads permit low output pacing and conservation of battery life.[67]

Single-Chamber Pacemakers

AOO AND VOO MODES. In the AOO and VOO modes, the pacemaker stimuli are generated at a fixed rate (asynchronously) with no relationship to the spontaneous rhythm. Stimuli capture the atrium or ventricle only when they fall outside the refractory period following spontaneous beats (Fig. 23–1). Ventricular fibrillation induced by a pacemaker stimulus falling in the ventricular vulnerable period is extremely rare unless myocardial ischemia or severe electrolyte abnormalities are present. AOO or VOO pacing is used only temporarily during pacemaker testing with application of the magnet or for competitive pacing to terminate some tachycardias.

VVI MODE. A VVI (ventricular demand) pacemaker prevents the ventricular rate from decreasing below a predetermined programmed level (Fig. 23–1). If the spontaneous rate decreases below the set rate, the pacemaker paces at a cycle length appropriate to maintain the preset rate. A faster spontaneous rate inhibits pacemaker discharge. The timing cycle (or internal clock) of a VVI pulse generator begins with either a sensed or a paced ventricular event. The initial portion of the cycle consists of a refractory period (usually 200 to 350 msec) during which the pulse generator is insensitive to any signals so as to avoid sensing its own stimulus, the paced or spontaneous QRS complex, T waves, and the decaying residual voltage at the electrode-myocardial interface. Beyond the pacemaker refractory period, a sensed spontaneous QRS complex inhibits the pacemaker, and its timing clock returns to the baseline; a new pacing style is initiated, and the output circuit remains inhibited for a period equal to the programmed pacemaker interval. If no spontaneous QRS complex is sensed, the timing cycle ends with the delivery of a ventricular stimulus, and a new cycle is started. The sensing function conserves battery capacity and prevents competition between the pacemaker and the intrinsic rhythm. VVI (or VVIR, p. 723) pacing is still the most common mode of pacing worldwide. A VVI pacemaker is simple, inexpensive, and reliable and has a small size and long life. However, its inability to maintain AV synchrony and provide an increased rate on exercise constitutes an important disadvantage.

AAI MODE. This (atrial demand) mode is similar to the VVI mode except that the pacemaker senses atrial electrical activity and paces the atrium (Fig. 23–3). AAI units must have a greater sensitivity than VVI units because the atrial electrogram is considerably smaller than the ventricular electrogram and the refractory period should be longer (400 msec) to avoid sensing the "far-field" ventricular electrogram via the atrial lead. AAI pacing is used for patients with sick sinus syndrome and intact AV conduction.

VVT MODE. In the VVT mode, upon sensing a spontaneous QRS complex, the pacemaker immediately discharges (rather than inhibits) its stimulus during the absolute refractory period of the ventricular myocardium (Fig. 23–1). If no QRS complex is sensed, the pacemaker delivers its impulse at the end of the interval corresponding to the programmed (lower) rate. The maximum pacing rate that can be generated by continual sensing is either factory-set or programmable. The triggered mode can be used to activate discharge of an implanted pacemaker by the application of chest wall stimuli (generating signals for sensing) from an external pacemaker. In this way, appropriately timed stimuli to the chest wall can be used to initiate or terminate some tachycardias by triggering corresponding stimuli from the implanted pacemaker.

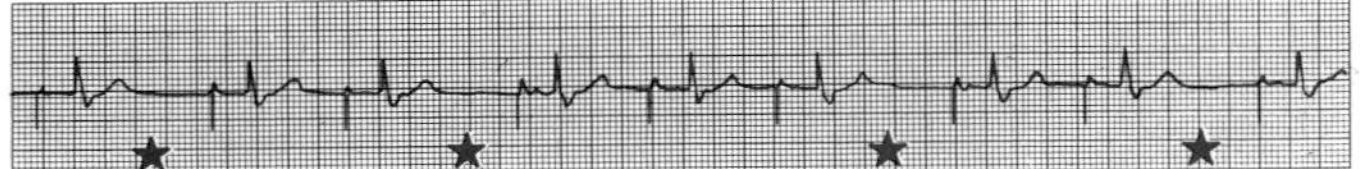

FIGURE 23–3. AAI pacemaker, rate = 70/min (automatic interval = 857 msec) and refractory period = 250 msec. There is intermittent prolongation of the interstimulus interval (stars) because the atrial lead senses the farfield QRS complex just beyond the 250 msec pacemaker refractory period. When the refractory period was programmed to 400 msec, the irregularity disappeared, with restoration of regular atrial pacing at a rate of 70/min.

Intervals and Rates

Three pacemaker intervals are important. The *automatic interval* is the period between two consecutive stimuli during continuous pacing. The *escape interval* is measured from the onset of the sensed surface QRS complex (in a ventricular pacemaker) to the following stimulus and exceeds the automatic interval by a few milliseconds to almost the duration of the entire QRS complex, depending on when during the surface QRS complex the intracardiac electrogram is sensed by the pacemaker. A special magnet held over a pulse generator closes a magnetic reed switch that eliminates the sensing function with conversion to the AOO/VOO mode. The *magnet interval* varies according to the manufacturer and is generally shorter than the automatic interval so as to override the spontaneous rhythm. The magnetic interval is often used to assess battery status and lengthens with impending battery depletion.

Some pacemakers have a hysteresis interval; i.e., the escape interval is significantly longer than the automatic interval. Its purpose is to maintain sinus rhythm (and AV synchrony) by preventing the onset of pacing for as long as possible at a rate lower than the automatic rate of the pacemaker. However, hysteresis appears to have no advantage over a simple decrease in the pacing rate, and its advantages are more theoretical than real during single-chamber pacing.

Electrocardiogram During Pacing

Evaluation of the pacemaker stimulus recorded on digital ECG machines is meaningless because the recording circuitry distorts stimuli with striking changes in amplitude and polarity. The vector of the pacemaker stimulus in the frontal plane when recorded with an analog ECG machine correlates with lead position, and amplitude changes are meaningful. A change from small bipolar stimuli to large-amplitude spikes suggests an insulation defect, while spike attenuation of a unipolar stimulus in several ECG leads during held respiration suggests an increase in lead impedance due to a fracture or loose connection

FUSION AND PSEUDOFUSION BEATS. During ventricular pacing, ventricular fusion beats occur when the ventricles are activated simultaneously by a spontaneous depolarization and a paced impulse. A ventricular fusion beat is often narrower than a pure paced beat and can exhibit various morphologies depending on the relative contribution of the two foci to ventricular depolarization (Fig. 23–1). Pseudofusion beats consist of the superimposition of an ineffectual pacemaker spike on the spontaneous QRS complex originating from a single focus and represent a normal manifestation of VVI pacing. A large portion of the surface QRS complex may be inscribed before its intracardiac counterpart (electrogram) generates the necessary voltage (about 3 to 4 mV) capable of inhibiting a VVI pacemaker (Fig. 23–4). Therefore, a normally functioning VVI pacemaker can deliver its impulse within a spontaneous surface QRS complex (mimicking undersensing) before the pulse generator has the opportunity to sense the somewhat late intracardiac electrogram in the right ventricle.[69]

In a pseudofusion beat, the pacemaker stimulus occurs too late to cause true fusion because it falls within the absolute refractory period of the myocardium initiated by the spontaneous depolarization. In the presence of normal sensing, striking examples of pseudofusion beats with

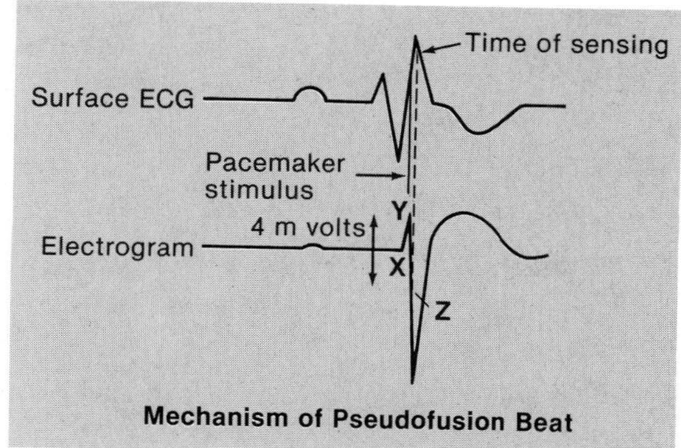

FIGURE 23–4. Mechanism of pseudofusion beat. The surface ECG and the ventricular electrogram are recorded simultaneously. The electrogram generates the necessary intracardiac voltage to inhibit the pacemaker (yz assumed at 4 mV) at a point corresponding with the descending limb of the surface QRS complex in its second half (dotted line). Consequently, it is possible for a pacemaker stimulus to occur at the apex of the R deflection just before the dotted line (which depicts the time of sensing) because the ventricular electrogram has not yet generated the required voltage to reach the sensitivity of the pulse generator and inhibit it. (From Barold, S. S., Falkoff, M. D., Ong, L. S., and Heinle, R. A.: Electrocardiographic analysis of normal and abnormal pacemaker function. Cardiovasc. Clin. *14*:97, 1983.)

pacemaker stimuli occurring late within the QRS complex can be seen in right bundle branch block, left ventricular extrasystoles, and any condition causing delayed intraventricular conduction. True sensing failure must be excluded whenever pseudofusion beats are observed. Pacemaker spikes falling clearly after termination of the surface QRS complex indicate sensing failure. Atrial fusion and pseudofusion beats also can occur with atrial pacing but are more difficult to recognize in view of the smaller size of the P wave in the ECG.

PATTERNS OF VENTRICULAR ACTIVATION

RIGHT VENTRICULAR PACING. Right ventricular (RV) pacing produces a left bundle branch block (LBBB) pattern of depolarization. During RV pacing, paced beats usually exhibit a typical LBBB pattern in leads 1 and aV_l, but leads V_5 and V_6 sometimes show deep S waves because the main electrical forces may be moving away from the horizontal level where V_5 and V_6 are recorded. The mean electrical axis of the paced QRS complex in the frontal plane is oriented superiorly (more often in the left than in the right upper quadrant) because the sequence of activation travels from apex to base, away from the inferior leads. As the pacing electrode moves toward the RV outflow tract, activation travels simultaneously to the base superiorly and the apex inferiorly, and the mean axis of the paced QRS complex in the frontal plane may point to the left lower quadrant. RV outflow tract stimulation immediately below the pulmonary valve causes right-axis deviation of the paced QRS complex in the frontal plane because most of the activation travels from base to apex, but the pattern in the left precordial lead always remains that of LBBB. Paced beats from the RV outflow tract not uncommonly exhibit qR, QR, or Qr configuration leads 1 and aV_l, but the inferior leads show a dominant R wave. In this situation, the precordial leads do not exhibit Qr, qR, or QR complexes.

LEFT VENTRICULAR PACING. Epicardial or endocardial stimulation of the left ventricle produces late activation of the RV and therefore a right bundle branch block (RBBB) pattern.[70,71] Pacing from the distal coronary sinus produces the same pattern.

MYOCARDIAL INFARCTION. Because the QRS complex during RV pacing resembles that of spontaneous LBBB (except for the initial forces), the diagnosis of myocardial infarction often can be made during RV pacing by applying the criteria used in complete LBBB.[72] Ventricular fusion beats must be absent. Large unipolar stimuli can mask Q waves. An extensive anteroseptal myocardial infarction can cause a q wave in leads 1, aV_l, V_5 and V_6, producing a qR pattern following the stimulus (not to be confused with a normal QS pattern). Although the sensitivity of the qR change is low, its specificity approaches 100 per cent because it is never seen in leads V_5 and V_6 during uncomplicated pacing. A QR or Qr complex in leads II, III, and aV_f is also diagnostic of an inferior myocardial infarction. Also, an anterior myocardial infarction can be associated with late notching of the ascending limb of the QRS complex in the left precordial leads, indicating an extensive infarction.

During RV apical pacing, the inferior leads and the anterior leads (V_1 to V_3) often record secondary ST-segment elevation. ST-segment depression can occur as a normal finding in leads 1, aV_l, V_5, and V_6. Relatively stable ST–T-wave changes resembling primary abnormalities occasionally can be seen during uncomplicated RV pacing. Dis-

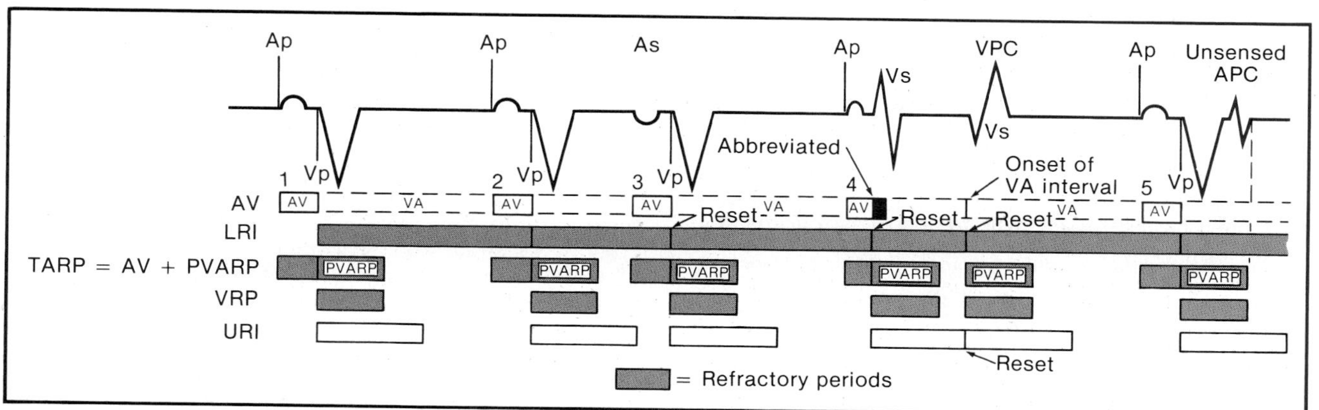

FIGURE 23–5. Diagram showing the function and timing intervals of a simple DDD pacemaker (with ventricular-based lower rate timing) consisting of only four fundamental intervals: lower rate interval = LRI; ventricular refractory period = VRP; atrioventricular delay = AV; postventricular atrial refractory period = PVARP. These provide two derived intervals: atrial escape interval (AEI or pacemaker VA interval) = LRI − AV, and total atrial refractory period (TARP) = AV + PVARP. Ap = atrial paced event; Vp = ventricular paced event; As = atrial sensed event; Vs = ventricular sensed event. Reset refers to the termination and reinitiation of a timing interval before it has timed out to its completion according to its programmed duration. Premature termination of the programmed AV delay by a ventricular sensed event (Vs) is indicated by its abbreviation. The upper rate interval (URI) is equal to the TARP. An atrial sensed event, As (third beat), initiates an A-V interval, terminating with a ventricular paced beat (Vp); As also aborts the AEI initiated by the second Vp. The third Vp resets the LRI and starts the PVARP, VRP, URI, AEI, and LRI. The fourth beat consists of an atrial paced beat (Ap) that terminates the AEI initiated by the third ventricular paced beat (Vp). The atrial paced beat (Ap) is followed by a sensed conducted QRS (Vs) that occurs before the expected release of Vp. Vs inhibits the release of Vp and the AV interval is abbreviated.

The QRS of the fourth beat sensed (Vs) initiates the AEI, LRI, PVARP, VRP, and URI. The fifth beat is a ventricular extrasystole (VPC) that initiates an AEI, PVARP, and VRP; it resets the LRI and URI. The last beat is followed by an atrial extrasystole (APC) unsensed by the atrial channel because it falls within the PVARP. Such a simple DDD pacemaker equipped with six timing cycles functions quite well provided that crosstalk (sensing of atrial stimulus by ventricular channel) does not occur.

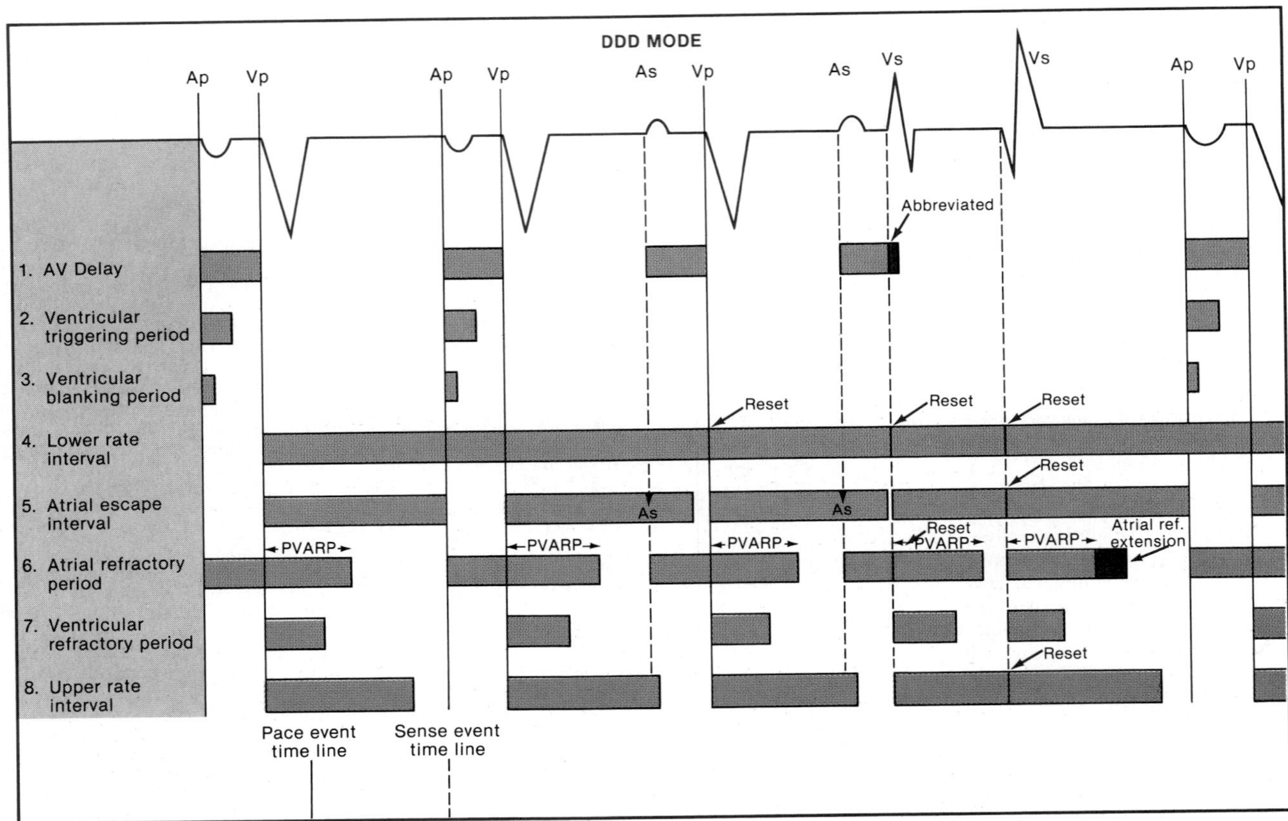

FIGURE 23–6. DDD mode. Diagrammatic representation of timing cycles. Ventricular triggering period = ventricular safety pacing. The second Vs (ventricular sensed event) is a ventricular extrasystole. The fourth A-V interval initiated by As (atrial sensed event) is abbreviated because the conducted QRS (Vs) occurs before the A-V interval has timed out. The postventricular atrial refractory (ref) period (PVARP) generated by the ventricular extrasystole is automatically extended by the atrial refractory period extension. (This design is based on the concept that most episodes of endless-loop tachycardia are initiated by a ventricular extrasystole with retrograde ventriculoatrial conduction.) The arrow pointing down within the atrial escape (pacemaker VA) interval indicates that an atrial sensed event (As) has taken place; the atrial escape interval actually terminates at this point, but the atrial escape interval is depicted in its entirety (as if As had not occurred) for the sake of clarity. The signal As inhibits release of the atrial stimulus otherwise expected at the completion of the atrial escape interval. Ap = atrial paced beat; Vp = ventricular paced beat; As = atrial sensed event; Vs = ventricular sensed event. The abbreviations and format used in this illustration are the same for Figs. 23–9 to 23–11 and 23–13. (From Barold, S. S., et al.: All dual-chamber pacemakers function in the DDD mode. Am. Heart J. *115:*1353, 1988.)

cordant T waves are of no diagnostic value. Sequential electrocardiograms are often needed to determine the significance of the ST–T-wave abnormalities.

ST–T-wave abnormalities occur more commonly in acute myocardial infarction than the qR pattern or QRS notching noted earlier. Pronounced primary ST-segment elevation with convex configuration clinches the diagnosis of myocardial infarction. When less obvious, the diagnosis becomes fairly certain only when the polarity of the T wave is opposite to that of the ST-segment elevation. ST-segment depression concordant with the QRS complex occasionally can occur in V_3 to V_6 during uncomplicated RV pacing and rarely in leads V_1 and V_2. Consequently, obvious ST-segment depression in leads V_1 and V_2 should be considered abnormal and indicative of anterior or inferior myocardial infarction (or ischemia). Inhibition of the pacemaker by chest wall stimulation or by reduction of the rate or output may allow the emergence of the spontaneous rhythm and reveal diagnostic Q waves. Continuous ventricular pacing per se can induce striking ST–T-wave abnormalities in the underlying spontaneous beats.[73]

Dual-Chamber Pacemakers

Types, Rates, and Intervals

TIMING INTERVALS. In the various types of dual-chamber pacemakers, the timing intervals are best understood by focusing first on the DDD mode. A DDD pulse generator paces and senses in both the atrium and the ventricle. Simple dual-chamber pacing modes are then derived by the removal of "building blocks" from the DDD mode and equalization of the various timing intervals.[69] These simpler pacing modes are important because a DDD pacemaker may have to be downgraded for treatment of certain complications.

As in a standard VVI pacemaker, the ventricular channel of a DDD device requires two basic timing cycles: the lower rate interval and the ventricular refractory period. A simple DDD system consists of the VVI mode with an added atrial channel (Fig. 23–5). This arrangement necessitates two new intervals, an atrioventricular (A-V) interval (the electronic analog of the P-R interval) and an upper rate interval (equal to the pacemaker total atrial refractory period, discussed later), to control the response of the ventricular channel to sensed atrial activity and maintain 1:1 AV synchrony between the lower and upper rates (Fig. 23–5). The atrial escape interval is obtained by subtracting the programmed AV delay from the lower rate interval. The atrial escape interval starts with a ventricular paced or sensed event and terminates with the release of an atrial stimulus.

Most dual-chamber pulse generators are designed with ventricular-based (V-V) lower rate timing controlled by ventricular events and a constant atrial escape interval, as in all examples discussed in this chapter.[74] An atrial sensed event triggers a ventricular stimulus after the completion of the AV interval (provided that no ventricular sensed event occurs during the A-V interval) and inhibits release of the atrial stimulus expected at completion of the atrial escape interval. A ventricular sensed event beyond the A-V interval inhibits both the atrial and ventricular

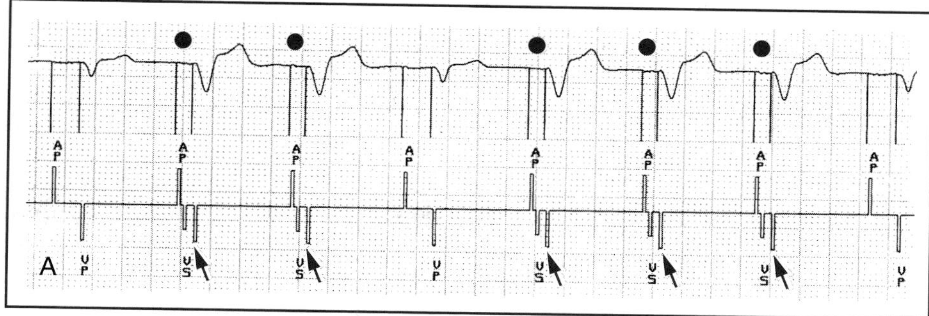

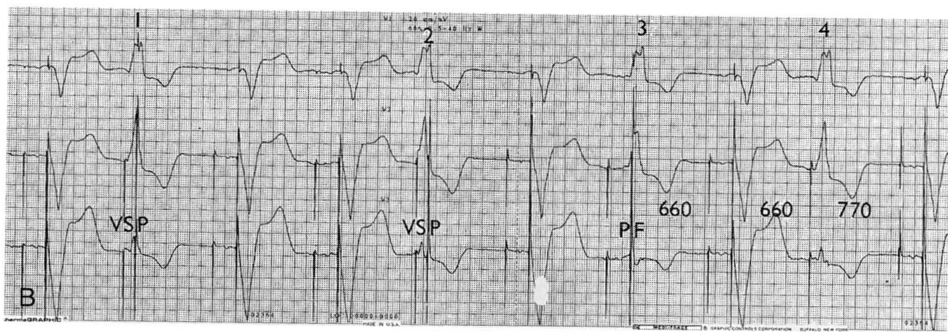

FIGURE 23–7. Ventricular safety pacing during DDD pacing (ECG leads V_1, V_2, and V_3). *A*, In the absence of crosstalk, the first, fourth, and last A-V intervals are equal to the programmed value of 200 msec. Intermittent crosstalk (solid black circles) leads to activation of the ventricular safety pacing mechanism so that the A-V interval of the second, third, fifth, sixth, and seventh beats (solid black circles) is abbreviated to 110 msec. The marker channel below the ECG confirms the presence of crosstalk with ventricular sensing (Vs) of the atrial stimulus (Ap) within the ventricular safety pacing period but beyond the short ventricular blanking period initiated by Vp. The arrows point to Vp triggered at the end of the ventricular safety pacing period (110 msec after the release of Ap). In a DDD pulse generator with ventricular-based lower rate timing, activation of the ventricular safety pacing mechanism due to continual crosstalk leads to an increase in the pacing rate (although the atrial escape interval remains constant).

B, Activation of the ventricular safety pacing (VSP) mechanism of a DDD pulse generator by sensed ventricular extrasystoles. The ECG was recorded at double speed and double standardization. Lower-rate interval = 857 msec, A-V = 200 msec. The first and second ventricular extrasystoles (1 and 2) are sensed by the ventricular channel of the DDD pacemaker. The onset of these two ventricular extrasystoles is deformed by an atrial stimulus; the atrial stimulus occurs because the ventricular electrogram has not yet generated sufficient voltage for sensing by the ventricular channel to inhibit the atrial and ventricular channels. The mechanism is identical to that of ventricular pseudofusion beats (Fig. 23–4). This particular pseudofusion beat is created by events occurring in different chambers (atrial stimulus and spontaneous ventricular depolarization). The ventricular channel senses the ventricular electrogram of the first and second ventricular extrasystoles within the ventricular safety pacing period but beyond the short ventricular blanking period initiated by the atrial stimulus. The pacemaker therefore triggers a ventricular stimulus at the completion of the ventricular safety pacing period, producing an abbreviated A-V interval of 110 msec: the ventricular stimulus therefore falls at the end of the QRS complex (1 and 2). This ECG represents normal function of a DDD pacemaker with a ventricular safety pacing mechanism. The third ventricular extrasystole (3) is deformed by a ventricular stimulus delivered after the onset of the QRS deflection on the surface ECG, thereby producing a pseudofusion beat. The fourth ventricular extrasystole (4) is also sensed by the ventricular channel. Note that the preceding atrial stimulus occurs at the termination of the atrial escape interval (about 660 msec) and almost simultaneously with the onset of the QRS complex. The interval from Ap preceding the fourth ventricular extrasystole to the last Ap measures 770 to 780 msec. This interval indicates that the pacemaker senses the fourth ventricular extrasystole (4) just beyond the ventricular safety pacing period of 110 msec initiated by the preceding Ap.

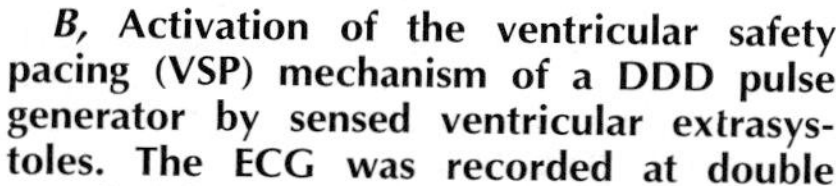

channels and initiates new lower rate and atrial escape intervals. An atrial paced or sensed event initiates the atrial refractory period because the atrial channel must remain refractory during the A-V interval to prevent initiation of a new A-V interval when one is already in progress.[69,75] The A-V interval must terminate with a paced or sensed ventricular event that continues the atrial refractory period. The second part, called the *postventricular atrial refractory period* (PVARP), must be programmed appropriately to prevent sensing of retrograde P waves due to ventriculoatrial (VA) conduction. The total atrial refractory period is equal to the sum of the AV delay and the PVARP.

In a simple DDD pulse generator, the upper rate interval is equal to the total atrial refractory period. The A-V interval, PVARP, and upper rate interval are interrelated according to the formula: upper rate (ppm) = 60/total atrial refractory period (sec). Consequently, a pacemaker with an upper rate of 120/min can sense atrial signals only 500 msec or longer apart.

LOWER RATE TIMING. Some pacemakers exhibit atrial-based lower rate timing in response to certain combinations of atrial and ventricular activity that make up the P-R or A-V interval. With atrial-based timing, the lower rate interval starts with an atrial sensed or paced event and terminates with a subsequent atrial paced event so that the atrial escape interval must vary to maintain constancy of the lower rate interval.[74]

CROSSTALK. Also known as *self-inhibition*, this refers to the inappropriate detection of the atrial stimulus by the ventricular channel.[69] Crosstalk depends on the amplitude of the atrial stimulus and the sensitivity of the ventricular channel and is less frequent with bipolar leads. Crosstalk often can be eliminated by reduction of the atrial output and/or ventricular sensitivity. The prevention of crosstalk also requires a ventricular blanking (refractory) period (10 to 60 msec) that starts coincidentally with the atrial stimulus[69] (Fig. 23–6). In some DDD pacemakers, the first part of the A-V interval (beyond the blanking period) initiated by an atrial stimulus contains an additional backup system known as *ventricular safety pacing* (VSP) (Fig. 23–6).

During the VSP interval (or its initial portion), any signal (atrial stimulus, QRS, and the like) sensed by the ventricular channel triggers a ventricular stimulus at the completion of the VSP period (usually lasting 100 to 120 msec from the atrial stimulus). Activation of the VSP mechanism produces characteristic abbreviation of the paced A-V interval (Fig. 23–7). Crosstalk without a VSP mechanism produces unexpected prolongation of the interval from the atrial stimulus to the succeeding spontaneous QRS complex (if any) to a value longer than the programmed A-V interval (Fig. 23–8). In patients without underlying spontaneous rhythm, crosstalk without a VSP mechanism can cause asystole (Fig. 23–8); however, with appropriate programming of the ventricular blanking period and the VSP mechanism, crosstalk is rarely a clinical problem.

UPPER RATE RESPONSE OF DDD PULSE GENERATORS. The programmed upper rate of a DDD pulse generator depends on the patient's activity level, age, left ventricular function, and the presence of coronary artery disease, atrial tachyarrhythmias, and retrograde VA conduction. The maximal rate of a DDD pacemaker can be defined by either the duration of the total atrial refractory period (causing fixed-ratio pacemaker AV block such as 2:1, 3:1, and so on) or a separate upper rate timing circuit causing Wenckebach-like AV block (6:5, 5:4, and so on).[69,75]

FIXED-RATIO AV BLOCK. This provides the simplest way of controlling the upper rate by programming the total atrial refractory period. The number of unsensed P waves depends on the atrial rate and where the P waves occur in the pacemaker cycle (Fig. 23–9). The A-V interval always remains constant. This response is often called 2:1 AV block. Actually, the paced ventricular rate will be exactly half the atrial rate or equal to the lower rate of the pacemaker, whichever is higher. An upper rate using fixed-ratio AV block only may be inappropriate in some patients, especially young and physically active individuals, because the sudden reduction of the ventricular rate with 2:1 AV block on exercise may be poorly tolerated.

WENCKEBACH UPPER RATE RESPONSE. This mode avoids sudden reduction of the paced ventricular rate and maintains some degree of AV synchrony. A Wenckebach response can occur only if the upper rate interval is programmed to a value longer than the total atrial refractory period (Fig. 23–10). Prolongation of the A-V interval (atrial

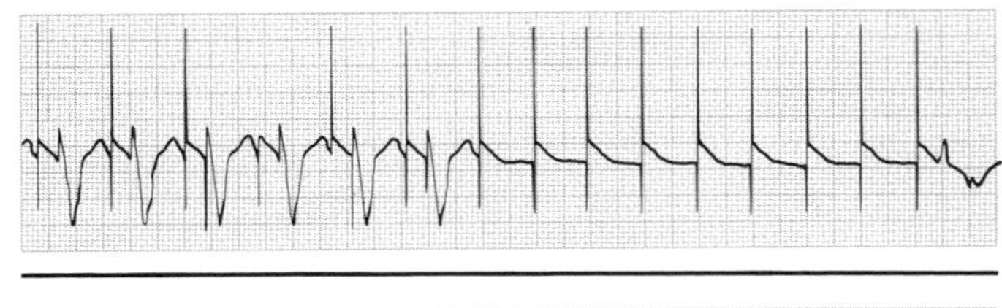

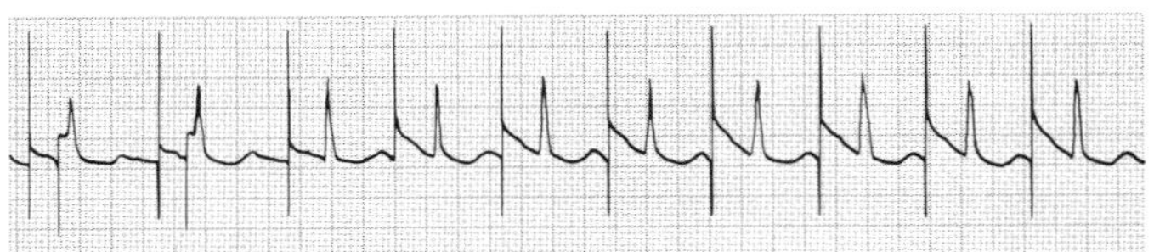

FIGURE 23–8. Crosstalk during DDD pacing without a ventricular safety pacing mechanism. *Top strip,* The lower rate was increased to test for crosstalk. Lower rate interval = 580 msec, AV = 170 msec. The interval between atrial stimuli on the right is shorter than the lower rate interval. Crosstalk causes an increase in the atrial pacing rate faster than the freerunning (lower) AV sequential rate on the left. Continual crosstalk causes prolonged ventricular asystole. *Bottom strip,* Crosstalk with AV conduction. Lower rate interval = 857 msec, AV interval = 200 msec. Crosstalk occurs with the third atrial stimulus and prolongs the interval between the atrial stimulus and the succeeding conducted QRS complex to a value longer than the programmed AV interval. The rate of atrial pacing increases because the sensed atrial stimulus by the ventricular channel initiates a new atrial escape interval just beyond termination of the ventricular blanking period. Consequently, the interval between two consecutive atrial stimuli becomes equal to the atrial escape interval of 657 msec (857–200) plus the duration of the ventricular blanking period (50 msec), providing a total of about 700 msec.

sensed, ventricular paced) occurs only when the upper rate interval > P-P interval > total atrial refractory period. With a progressive increase in atrial rate, when the P-P interval is less than or equal to the total atrial refractory period, the Wenckebach response switches to 2:1 fixed-ratio AV block.[69,75]

OTHER DUAL-CHAMBER PACING MODES

DVI MODE. The DVI mode can be considered as the DDD mode with the PVARP extending through the entire atrial escape interval.[69] No atrial sensing occurs because the total atrial refractory period extends through the entire lower rate interval. Asynchronous atrial pacing can precipitate atrial fibrillation. Three types of DVI function are possible: uncommitted, partially committed, and committed. In the uncommitted DVI mode the ventricular channel can sense through the entire duration of the A-V interval, while in the partially committed DVI mode the ventricular channel can sense only beyond an initial ventricular blanking period. In contrast, a committed DVI pacemaker possesses a ventricular blanking period encompassing the entire A-V interval, making crosstalk impossible. In the committed DVI mode, AV sequential pacing occurs in an all-or-none manner; i.e., two sequential stimuli always occur together, while sensing spontaneous ventricular activity inhibits the release of both stimuli.

VDD MODE. The VDD mode functions like the DDD mode except

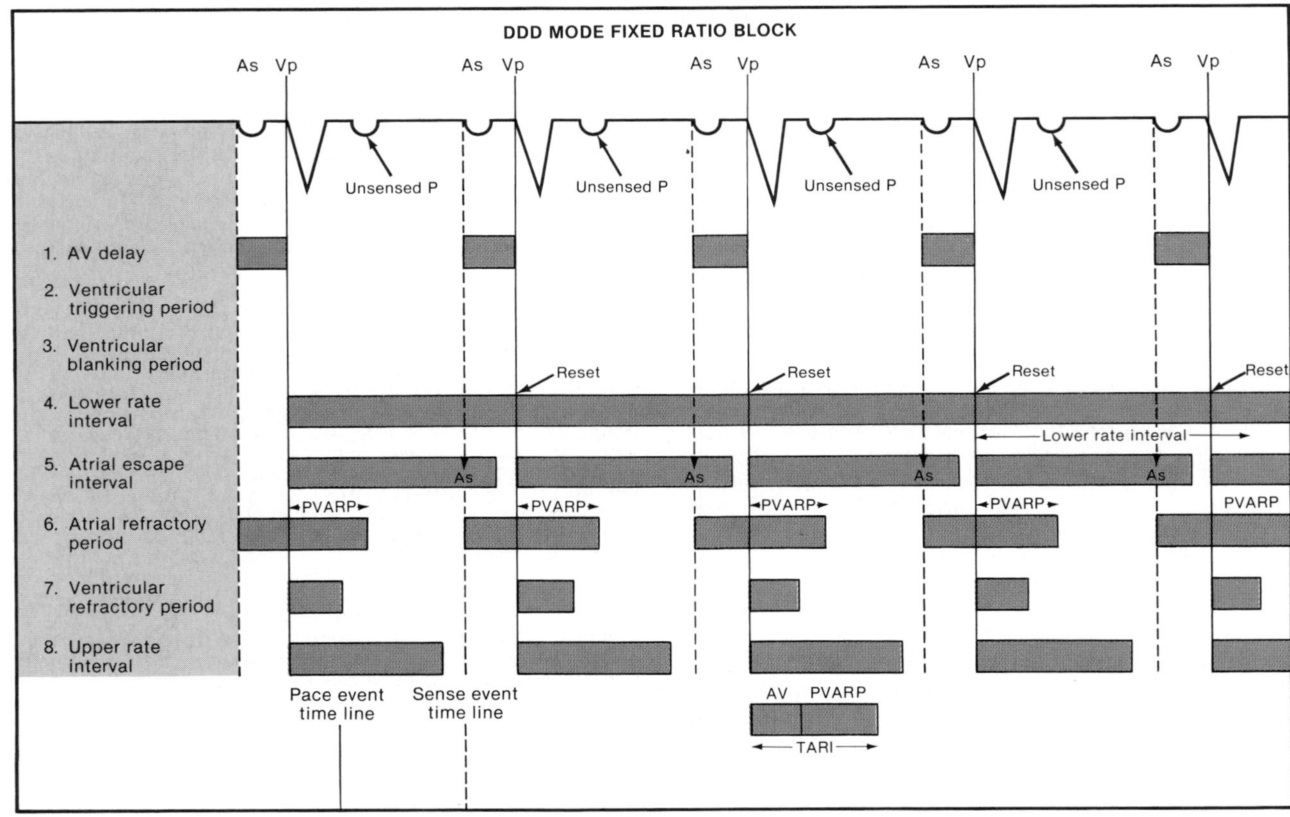

FIGURE 23–9. Upper rate response of DDD pacemaker with fixed-ratio AV block. The upper rate interval is longer than the total atrial refractory period (AV + postventricular atrial refractory period, or PVARP), and the P-P interval (As-As) is shorter than the total atrial refractory period (TARP). The arrow pointing down within the atrial escape (pacemaker VA) interval indicates that an atrial sensed event (As) has taken place; the atrial escape interval actually terminates at this point but the atrial escape interval is depicted in its entirety (as if As had not occurred) for the sake of clarity. Every second P wave falls within the PVARP and is unsensed. The AV interval remains constant. An upper rate response with fixed ratio pacemaker AV block occurs in two types of DDD pacemakers. (1) A device without a separately progammable upper rate interval in which the TARP is equal to the upper rate interval. (2) A device with a separately programmable upper rate interval (i.e., upper rate interval > TARP) only when the P-P interval < TARP as shown in this figure. In such a device, an upper rate response with pacemaker Wenckebach AV block can only occur when the P-P interval > TARP as shown in Figure 25–10. (From Barold, S. S.: Management of patients with dual chamber pulse generators: Central role of pacemaker atrial refractory period. Learning Center Highlights, Heart House, American College of Cardiology 5:[4], 8, 1990, with permission.) (See Fig. 23–6 for abbreviations.)

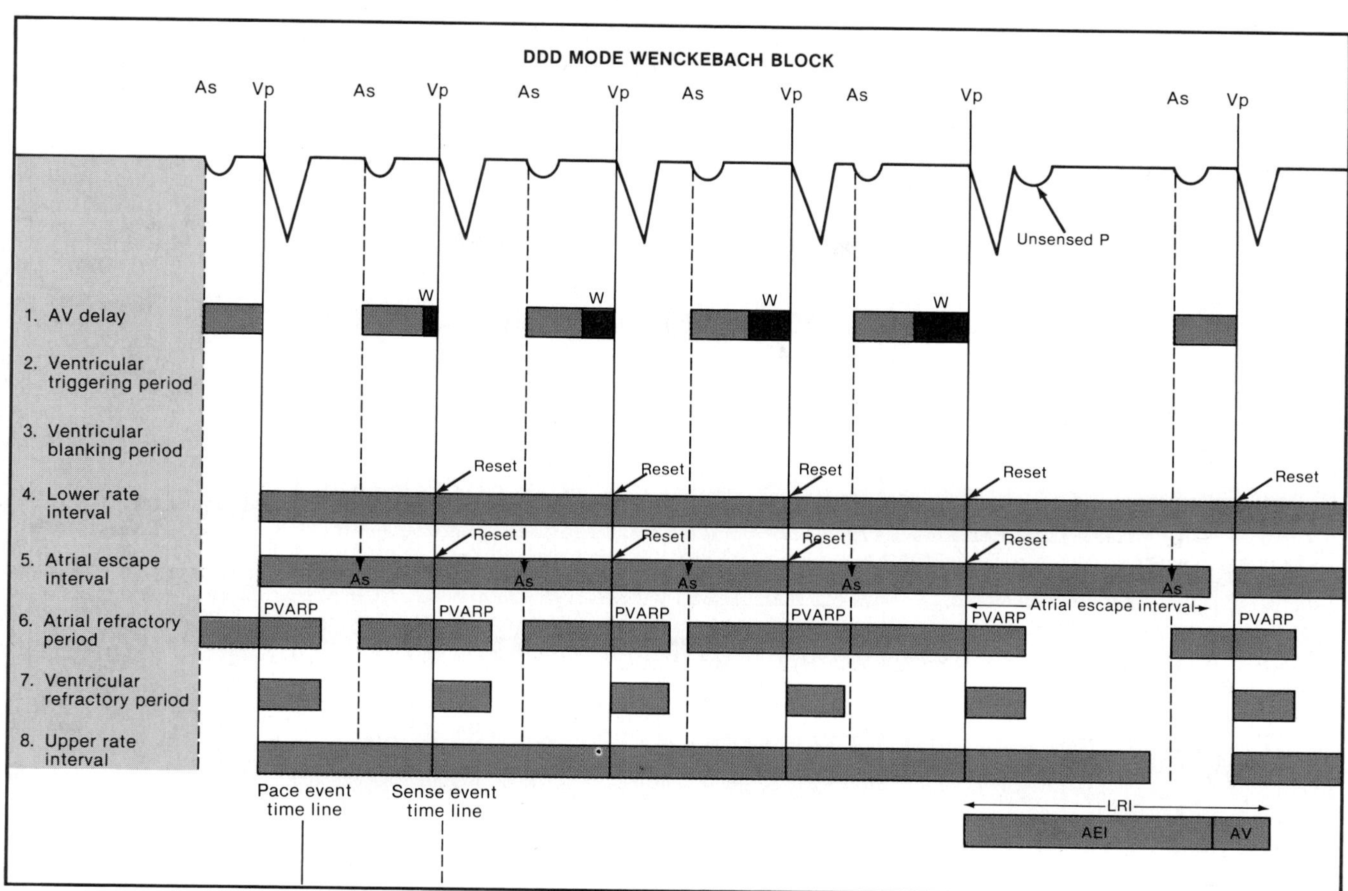

FIGURE 23–10. DDD mode. Upper rate response with pacemaker Wenckebach AV block. The upper rate interval is *longer* than the programmed total atrial refractory period, a mandatory prerequisite for a Wenckebach upper rate response. The P-P interval (As-As) is *longer* than the programmed total atrial refractory period. The As-Vp (atrial sensed–ventricular paced) interval lengthens by a varying period to conform to the upper rate interval. During the Wenckebach sequence, the pacemaker synchronizes a ventricular paced beat (Vp) to an atrial sensed event (As). Because the pacemaker cannot violate its programmed (ventricular) upper rate interval, the ventricular paced beat (Vp) can be released only at the completion of the upper rate interval. The AV delay (As-Vp) becomes progressively longer (than the programmed value) as the ventricular channel waits to deliver its ventricular stimulus (Vp) until the upper rate interval has timed out. The maximum prolongation of the AV delay (As-Vp) represents the difference between the upper rate interval and the total atrial refractory period. The As-Vp (atrial sensed–ventricular paced) interval lengthens during the pacemaker Wenckebach sequence as long as the As-As interval (P-P) remains longer than the total atrial refractory period. The sixth P wave falls within the postventricular atrial refractory period (PVARP) and is unsensed and thus not followed by a ventricular stimulus (Vp). A pause occurs and the Wenckebach cycle restarts. In the first four pacing cycles, the intervals between pacemaker stimuli (Vp-Vp) are constant and equal to the upper rate interval. When the P-P interval becomes shorter than the programmed total atrial refractory period, Wenckebach pacemaker AV block cannot occur and fixed ratio pacemaker AV block, e.g., 2:1, will supervene as in Figure 23–9. The arrow pointing down within the atrial escape interval (AEI) indicates that an atrial sensed event (As) has taken place; the atrial escape interval actually terminates at this point, but for the sake of clarity the atrial escape interval is depicted as if As had not occurred. LRI = lower rate interval. AEI = Atrial escape interval. (From Barold, S. S., et al.: All dual chamber pacemakers function in the DDD mode. Am. Heart J. *115*:1353, 1988.)

that the generated atrial stimulus is diverted internally rather than emitted.[69] Therefore, no atrial pacing occurs. The absence of the atrial stimulus eliminates the need for crosstalk intervals (Fig. 23–11). The omitted atrial stimulus nevertheless begins an "implied" A-V interval that must be refractory in its entirety so that in most contemporary designs a P wave occurring within the "implied" A-V interval is not sensed. Without sensed atrial activity, the VDD mode paces effectively in the VVI mode at the lower rate of the pacemaker.

DDI MODE. The DDI mode generally has been described as an improved DVI mode or a hybrid of the DVI and DDD modes. Sensing and pacing occur in both atrium and ventricle. The DDI mode is best considered as a DDD mode with identical upper and lower rate intervals (provided that the lower rate is controlled by ventricular events, i.e., V-V timing)[69] (Fig. 23–12). Atrial sensing occurs beyond the PVARP. An atrial sensed event initiates an A-V interval that terminates (as in the DDD mode) only at the completion of the upper rate interval (identical to the lower rate interval). Although atrial sensing occurs, the pacemaker cannot increase the ventricular pacing rate in response to a faster atrial rate, so ventricular pacing always occurs at the programmed lower rate. In other words, there is no atrial tracking. For this reason, the DDI mode is useful in patients with the sick sinus syndrome and paroxysmal atrial tachyarrhythmias. The DDI mode provides atrial pacing and AV synchrony (in the absence of atrial tachyarrhythmias) with the potential of preventing atrial tachyarrhythmias by overdrive suppression.

During atrial tachyarrhythmia with continual atrial sensing, the DDI pacemaker simply paces the ventricle at its constant rate and becomes functionally identical to the VVI mode (Fig. 23–12). In patients with AV block and a sinus rate faster than the programmed pacing rate, the DDI mode produces an unfavorable hemodynamic situation identical to the VVI mode with AV dissociation (with occasional delivery of an atrial stimulus when the preceding P wave occurs in the PVARP).[76,77] The DDI mode has become less useful than in the past because a number of DDD or DDDR devices now respond to supraventricular tachyarrhythmias by automatic mode conversion to a slower, nonatrial tracking mode (VVI, VVIR, DDI, DDIR). Upon cessation of the arrhythmia, these devices revert to the DDD or DDDR mode with AV synchrony over a relatively broad range of atrial rates.[78,79]

RETROGRADE VA CONDUCTION AND ENDLESS-LOOP TACHYCARDIA. Endless-loop tachycardia (sometimes incorrectly called *pacemaker-mediated tachycardia*) is a well-known complication of dual-chamber pacing (VDD, DDD, or

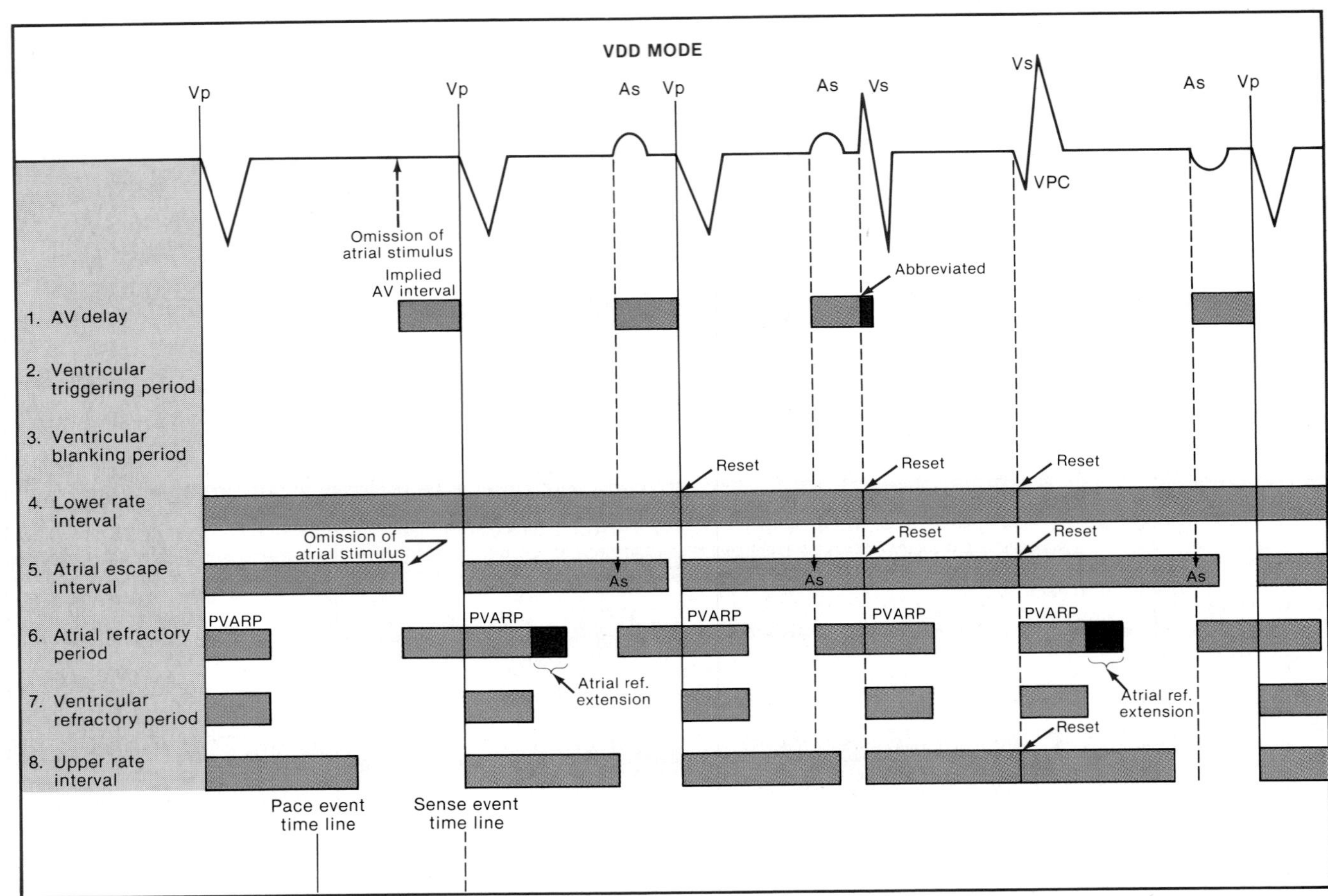

FIGURE 23–11. VDD mode. In the DDD mode, an atrial stimulus is released at the completion of the atrial escape interval whenever an atrial sensed event (As) or ventricular sensed event does not occur within the atrial escape interval. This atrial stimulus is omitted in the VDD mode. Nevertheless, the pulse generator initiates an implied AV interval with the same characteristics as in the DDD mode. In the first ventricular cycle (Vp-Vp) because the ventricular paced beat (Vp) terminating the implied AV interval is not preceded by an atrial paced beat or atrial sensed event (As), the post-ventricular atrial refractory period (PVARP) is automatically extended as occurs after a sensed ventricular extrasystole (depicted as VPC) (Fig. 23–6). Ventricular blanking and ventricular triggering (ventricular safety pacing) periods are not needed because there are no atrial stimuli in the VDD mode. In the absence of atrial sensed events (As), the pulse generator effectively paces in the VVI mode at the programmed lower rate interval (first cycle). The atrial escape interval terminates at the onset of the implied AV interval.

To promote AV synchrony for as long as possible, atrial sensing can occur in the implied AV interval of some contemporary dual chamber pacemakers functioning in the VDD mode. In such a situation, As (in the implied AV interval) initiates an entirely new AV interval so that the pacemaker releases Vp beyond the lower rate interval. The maximal extension of the lower rate interval by this response is equal to the programmed As-Vp interval. The arrow pointing down within the atrial escape interval indicates that an atrial sensed event (As) has taken place; the atrial escape interval actually terminates at this point, but for the sake of clarity it is depicted as if As had not occurred. (From Barold, S. S., et al.: All dual chamber pacemakers function in the DDD mode. Am. Heart J. *115*:1353, 1988.)

DDDR) and starts with sensing of a retrograde P wave usually linked to a ventricular extrasystole[69] (Fig. 23–13). Endless-loop tachycardia can be sustained or unsustained and often occurs at the programmed upper rate of the pacemaker. When the sum of the retrograde VA conduction time and the programmed A-V interval exceeds the upper rate interval, the tachycardia is slower than the programmed upper rate. Intact retrograde VA conduction occurs in approximately two-thirds or more of patients with sinus node dysfunction and in 15 to 35 per cent of patients with AV block. Thus 35 to 50 percent of all patients receiving dual-chamber pacemakers may be susceptible to endless-loop tachycardia. Absent retrograde VA conduction at the time of implantation or even later provides no guarantee of protection because a few patients may exhibit VA conduction subsequently, particularly during states of sympathetic stimulation. Rarely, VA conduction occurs only with exercise. Any condition capable of separating the sinus P wave from the QRS complex, coupled with retrograde VA conduction, can initiate endless-loop tachycardia.[69,80] These include a ventricular extrasystole, loss of atrial capture, myopotential sensing by the atrial channel of unipolar devices, undersensing of sinus P waves (with preserved sensing of retrograde P waves), an excessively long A-V interval, and application and removal of the magnet.

Endless-loop tachycardia can be induced when the atrial output is programmed below the pacing threshold, PVARP is at its minimum value, and there is a lower rate above the spontaneous rate (Fig. 23–14). When atrial capture persists at the lowest output, endless-loop tachycardia can be induced by chest wall stimulation (delivered by a temporary pacemaker) provided that the external signals are sensed selectively by the atrial channel. Conversion to the asynchronous mode with the magnet over the pacemaker terminates endless-loop tachycardia with rare exceptions.

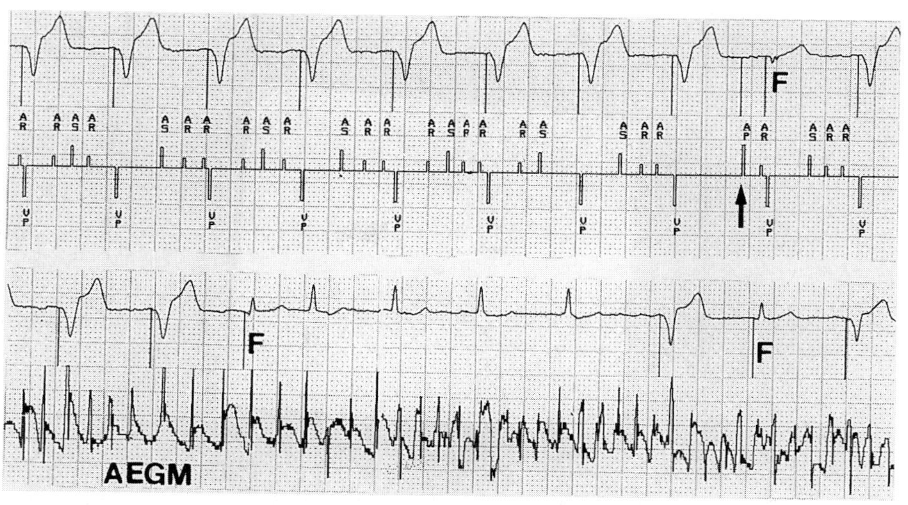

FIGURE 23–12. DDI pacing during atrial fibrillation. The DDI mode is equivalent to the DDD mode with identical lower rate interval and upper rate interval (provided there is ventricular-based lower rate timing). *Top,* ECG recorded simultaneously with event markers. *Bottom,* ECG recorded simultaneously with the telemetered atrial electrogram (AEGM). F = fusion beat; As = atrial sensed event; AR = atrial event detected in the postventricular atrial refractory period; Vp = ventricular paced event. Lower rate interval = 750 msec, A-V interval = 200 msec, postventricular atrial refractory period = 250 msec. Sensed events in the atrial refractory period (AR) do not initiate any timing cycles. Although the pacemaker senses atrial events (As), it does not track atrial activity so that ventricular pacing can occur only at the programmed lower rate of 80 beats/min. The As-Vp intervals are always longer than the programmed Ap-Vp interval, a characteristic feature of the DDI mode. There is intermittent sensing of the f waves. The arrow points to a cycle where the pacemaker does not sense f waves and therefore releases Ap at the completion of the atrial escape interval. Except for this cycle, the ECG cannot be distinguished from VVI pacing.

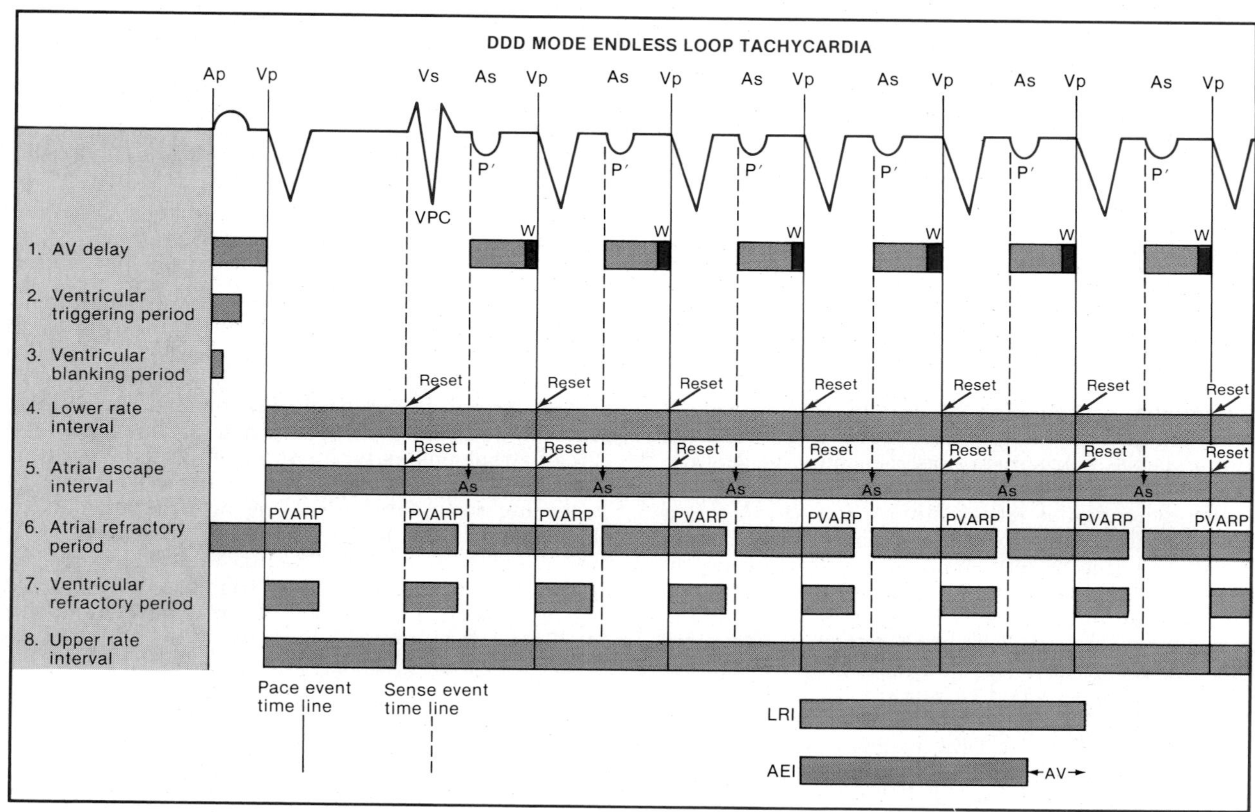

FIGURE 23–13. DDD mode. Endless loop (reentrant) tachycardia initiated by a ventricular extrasystole (VPC, second beat) with retrograde ventriculoatrial (VA) conduction (P′ or As). The atrial channel senses the retrograde P wave (P′) and a ventricular pacemaker stimulus (Vp) is issued after extension of the As-Vp (atrial sensed–ventricular paced) interval to conform to the supremacy of the upper rate interval (as in Fig. 23–10). The ventricular paced beat (Vp) generates another retrograde P wave, again sensed by the pulse generator outside its postventricular atrial refractory period (PVARP) and the process perpetuates itself. The pulse generator itself provides the anterograde limb of the macroreentrant process because it functions as an artificial AV junction. Retrograde VA conduction (P′) following a ventricular paced beat (Vp) provides the retrograde limb of the reentrant process. The cycle length of the endless loop tachycardia is equal to the upper rate interval. However, the cycle length of an endless loop tachycardia may occasionally be longer than the upper rate interval if retrograde VA conduction is prolonged. In this situation when the AV interval is *not* extended, the retrograde VA conduction time (as seen by the pacemaker) may be calculated by subtracting the AV interval from the cycle length of the tachycardia. Disruption of either the anterograde limb (by eliminating atrial sensing) or the retrograde limb (by eliminating retrograde VA conduction) terminates endless loop tachycardia. The arrow pointing down within the atrial escape interval indicates that an atrial sensed event (As) has taken place. Although the atrial escape interval actually terminates at this point, for the sake of clarity it is depicted as if As had not occurred. LRI = lower rate interval; AEI = atrial escape interval. (From Barold, S. S., et al.: All dual chamber pacemakers function in the DDD mode. Am. Heart J. *115:*1353, 1988.)

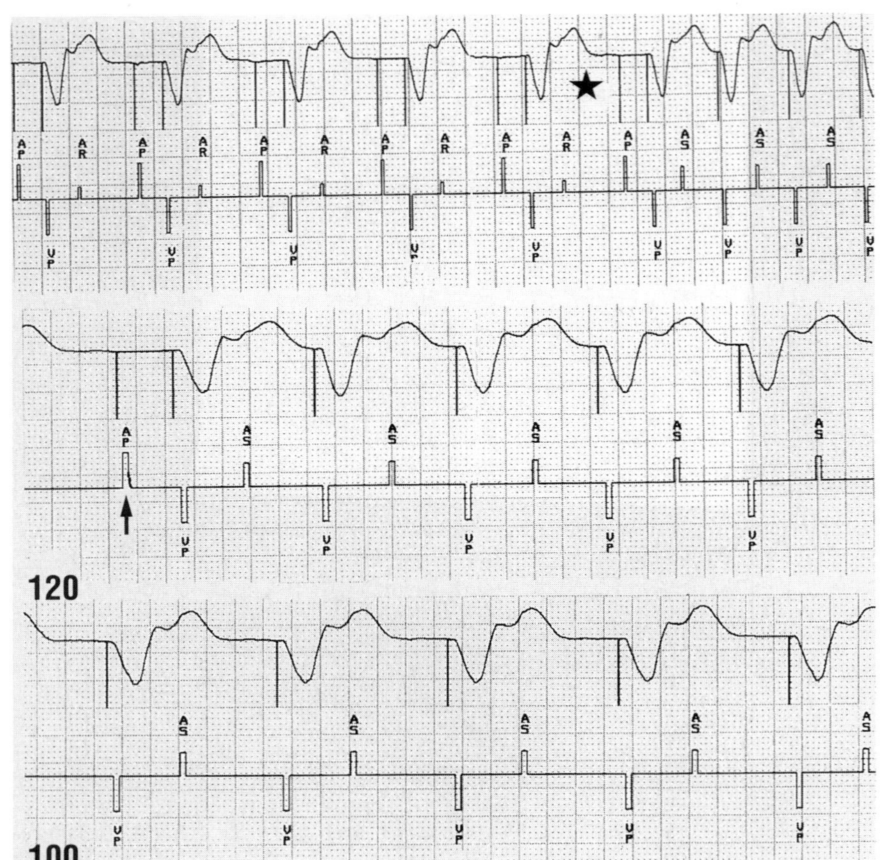

FIGURE 23–14. *Top,* DDD pacing with endless loop tachycardia. Lower rate interval = 857 msec, A-V = 200 msec after atrial pacing and 150 msec after atrial sensing, postventricular atrial refractory period (PVARP) = 300 msec; upper rate interval = 500 msec (120 beats/min). *Top,* Subthreshold atrial stimulation (Ap). Ventricular pacing causes retrograde VA conduction. On the left, the retrograde P waves fall within the PVARP and are unsensed. The PVARP was shortened to 200 msec at the star. The pacemaker then senses the retrograde P waves and initiates endless-loop tachycardia (recorded at a speed of 25 mm/sec).

Bottom, This panel (recorded at a speed of 50 mm/sec) also shows the initiation of endless-loop tachycardia by subthreshold atrial stimulation. The markers indicate that the retrograde VA time measures approximately 240 msec. The As-Vp interval is prolonged to conform to the upper rate interval, i.e., Vp-Vp interval = upper rate interval = 500 msec (120 beats/min). In the bottom panel (also recorded at 50 mm/sec), the upper rate interval was programmed to 600 msec (100 beats/min). The retrograde VA conduction time during endless-loop tachycardia remains constant at 240 msec, but the As-Vp interval lengthens further to conform to the upper rate interval, i.e., Vp-Vp interval = 600 msec. Endless-loop tachycardia was no longer induced by subthreshold atrial stimulation when the PVARP was again programmed to 300 msec, as in the top panel on the left.

To prevent endless-loop tachycardia, the PVARP should be programmed to 50 msec beyond the duration of retrograde VA conduction determined noninvasively by pacemaker programming. Other measures include a shorter A-V interval, differential discrimination of a larger anterograde P wave from smaller retrograde atrial depolarization, and activation of a special mechanism upon sensing a ventricular event (outside AV delay) that is interpreted as a ventricular extrasystole: synchronous atrial stimulation (to preempt retrograde atrial depolarization) or automatic PVARP extension for one cycle (Fig. 23–8). Some pacemakers possess an automatic tachycardia-terminating algorithm (e.g., omission of a ventricular stimulus, temporary PVARP prolongation, or shortening of a single A-V interval) activated when ventricular pacing occurs at designated rates (usually the programmed upper rate) for a certain duration.

TACHYCARDIA DURING DDD PACING. Various types of tachycardia can occur during DDD pacing.[80] The diagnosis is usually simple and facilitated by telemetry of event markers or electrograms (discussed later). Tachycardias other than endless-loop tachycardia return upon removal of the magnet. The magnet, by producing a slower rate in the DOO or VOO mode, permits identification of P or f waves. Programming to slow VVI pacing allows analysis of atrial activity. Atrial flutter or fibrillation can cause regular or irregular atrial and ventricular pacing due to intermittent lack of atrial sensing with consequent release of atrial stimuli. This response, coupled with periods of rapid ventricular pacing secondary to sensing rapid atrial activity, produces a chaotic pattern virtually diagnostic of atrial fibrillation or flutter (Fig 23–15). Tachycardia triggered by myopotentials sensed by the atrial channel of a unipolar device is easily reproducible with isometric exercise (Fig. 23–16).

Multiprogrammability

A programmable pulse generator is capable of noninvasive adjustment of its function so that an appropriate pacemaker "prescription" can be "written" by the physician. The available technology, which is reliable and cost-effective, is mandatory in modern pacemaker prac-

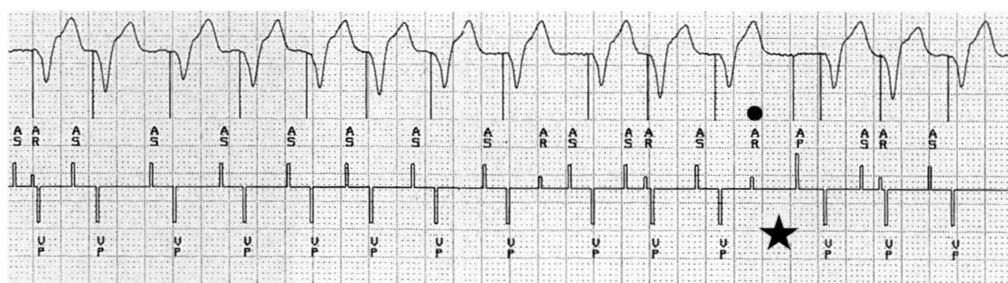

FIGURE 23–15. DDD pacing with atrial fibrillation causing rapid and irregular ventricular pacing. Lower rate interval = 750 msec, upper rate interval = 440 msec, As-Vp interval = 160 msec, Ap-Vp interval = 200 msec, PVARP = 250 msec. The constantly changing pattern of ventricular pacing is due to intermittent sensing of f waves. When the pacemaker fails to sense f waves beyond the PVARP, it delivers an atrial stimulus (Ap) at the completion of the atrial escape interval (star). This chaotic pattern is virtually diagnostic of atrial fibrillation or flutter during DDD pacing. AR = atrial sensing during the atrial refractory period. AR cannot initiate any timing cycles.

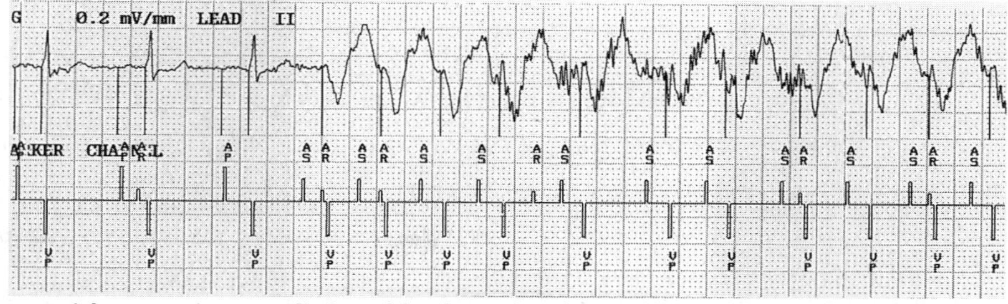

FIGURE 23–16. Unipolar DDD pacing with myopotential triggering induced by arm exercise. The atrial channel senses myopotentials, whereupon ventricular stimulation is delivered at an irregular and rapid rate, sometimes at the programmed upper rate of 140 beats/min (upper rate interval = approximately 430 msec). Lower rate interval = 857 msec, As-Vp interval = 150 msec, Ap-Vp interval = 150 msec, postventricular atrial refractory period = 250 msec. AR represents atrial sensing during the postventricular atrial refractory period. AR cannot initiate any timing intervals. Myopotential oversensing was eliminated by decreasing the sensitivity of the atrial channel without compromising P-wave sensing.

tice because it reduces the need for secondary interventions and increases device longevity by optimizing output. A program change should always be confirmed by telemetry to reduce the likelihood of error and should be entered in the patient's chart. Programmability after pacemaker implantation is often underutilized. It offers the opportunity to create an optimal pacing system for a specific clinical situation. Like chronic pharmacological therapy requiring dosage adjustment according to changing circumstances, pacemaker parameters appropriate at the time of implantation may cease to be adequate in the future and may need modification. Programmability has simplified troubleshooting many pacemaker problems and often obviates operative revision to treat many pacemaker complications (Table 23–4).

SINGLE-CHAMBER PACEMAKERS. The three most important parameters for single-chamber pacing are rate, output (voltage and pulse width), and sensitivity. The ability to program other parameters such as refractory period, mode, polarity, and hysteresis is also desirable in certain clinical circumstances.

Programming an increase in output may be necessary when the acute or chronic pacing threshold rises disproportionately. When the pacing threshold has stabilized several weeks after implantation, decreasing output is important to conserve battery life and increase longevity of the pulse generator. For most patients, the nominal output delivered by the pacemaker is excessive and wasteful. Reducing voltage rather than pulse width often minimizes or eliminates undesirable diaphragmatic pacing or muscle stimulation at the anodal site of normally functioning and positioned unipolar pacemakers (in the absence of insulation leak). Programming the output to subthreshold levels (or very low rate) permits study of the underlying rhythm.

The pacemaker should be programmed to be twice as sensitive as the value of the sensing threshold. This corresponds to a numerical setting at least half the threshold value. For example, if the sensitivity threshold, i.e., the lowest setting associated with regular sensing during deep inspiration, is 8 mV, the sensitivity value should be programmed to 4 mV. Oversensing the T wave and/or residual voltage at the electrode-myocardial interface (afterpotential) is easily remedied by decreasing the sensitivity (increasing the numerical value) and/or prolonging the refractory period. Oversensing myopotentials by a unipolar pacemaker requires reduction of sensitivity; however, if this is associated with undersensing the QRS, programming to the triggered (VVT, AAT) mode may be required.

DUAL-CHAMBER PACEMAKERS. The programming of DDD pacemakers requires special considerations. Most of the parameters in Table 23–4 must be programmed individually in each chamber. The PVARP must be programmed to prevent sensing retrograde P waves and the possibility of endless-loop tachycardia. Programming the ventricular blanking period may be desirable to prevent crosstalk. The upper rate (interval) must be programmed according to the patient's age, activity, retrograde VA conduction, nature of heart disease, and propensity to supraventricular tachycardia. Programming the sensor response of rate-adaptive pacemakers requires special care. The A-V interval should be programmed to obtain a maximum hemodynamic advantage.[81] Some pulse generators possess algorithms that shorten the A-V interval during exercise as the normal heart does. Electrical events on the right side of the heart must be translated into optimal timing of atrial and ventricular mechanical activity on the left side of the heart.[82–84]

It may be reasonable to start with an A-V interval of 100 to 150 msec after atrial sensing and to prolong the A-V interval after atrial

TABLE 23–4 MULTIPROGRAMMABILITY IN SINGLE-CHAMBER PACEMAKERS*

PARAMETER	VARIABILITY	PURPOSE
Rate	Increase	To optimize output, to overdrive or terminate tachyarrhythmias, to adapt pediatric needs, to test AV conduction with AAI pacemakers, to confirm atrial capture during AAI pacing by observing concomitant change in ventricular rate
	Decrease	To assess underlying rhythm and dependency status, to adjust rate below angina threshold, to allow emergence of normal sinus rhythm and preservation of atrial transport, to test sensing function
Output	Increase	To adapt to pacing threshold
	Decrease	To test threshold for pacing, to conserve battery longevity according to threshold for pacing, to reduce extracardiac stimulation (pectoral muscle, diaphragm), to assess underlying rhythm and dependency status
Sensitivity	Increase (reduction of numerical value)	To sense low electrographic signals (P and QRS)
	Decrease (increase of numerical value)	To test sensing threshold, to avoid T-wave or afterpotential sensing, to avoid sensing extracardiac signals, e.g., myopotentials
Refractory period	Increase	To minimize farfield QRS sensing (AAI pacing), to minimize T-wave sensing (VVI pacing), to minimize afterpotential sensing
	Decrease	To maximize QRS sensing (VVI pacing), to detect early premature ventricular complexes
Hysteresis		To delay onset of ventricular pacing to preserve atrial transport function
Polarity	Conversion to unipolar mode	To amplify the signal for sensing in the presence of a low bipolar electrogram, to compensate temporarily for lead fracture in the other electrode
	Conversion to bipolar mode	To decrease electromagnetic or myopotential interference, to evaluate oversensing, to eliminate extracardiac anodal stimulation
Mode	VVT/AAT	To perform noninvasive electrophysiologic study and to terminate reentrant tachycardias (chest wall stimulation with external pacemaker), to prevent inhibition of unipolar pacemaker by extracardiac interference, to evaluate oversensing by "marking" sensed signals
	VOO/AOO	To prevent inhibition of pacemaker by interference (usually as a temporary measure) when triggered mode is not available or is undesirable

* Also applicable to dual-chamber pacemakers when each channel is considered individually.

pacing by 50 msec to produce basically the same effective A-V interval as that initiated by atrial sensing.[85] Abnormal depolarization from ventricular pacing results in an altered contraction pattern that can decrease LV function.[81,86,87] Consequently, one should try initially to program an A-V interval that allows spontaneous AV conduction and native ventricular activation (associated with increased battery longevity).[88] However, an excessively long A-V interval can be counterproductive. The optimal A-V interval can vary considerably from patient to patient and depends on many factors, including LV compliance, LV filling pressure, atrial size and contractility, mitral valve function, heart rate, and variability of the interatrial conduction time.[83,88,89] The optimal A-V interval can change with time due to progressive delay in interatrial conduction or changes in LV function.[90] Two-dimensional and Doppler echocardiography can be useful to optimize the A-V interval at rest and on exercise.

Programming a dual-chamber pacemaker to different modes may be necessary to respond to changing circumstances or complications. Chronic atrial fibrillation is the most important cause of change in the pacing mode to VVI(R) pacing. About 85 to 90 per cent of DDD and DDDR pulse generators should remain in the original programmed mode at 5 years because of improved atrial sensitivity, better leads, and increasing experience.[81,91–93] In the absence of automatic mode conversion or fallback (to a slower rate), the DDI or DDIR mode is useful in patients with atrial chronotropic incompetence and paroxysmal supraventricular tachyarrhythmias.[76] The VDD mode may be useful in patients with relatively normal atrial response to activity when atrial pacing is not functioning appropriately owing to a high pacing threshold or atrial lead displacement. If the VDD mode is not available, the DDD mode can be used with the atrial output turned off or programmed to the lowest value for subthreshold stimulation.

HEMODYNAMICS OF CARDIAC PACING

In a normal subject, increase in cardiac output with exercise is provided by a rate increase (300 per cent) with only a modest contribution from the increased stroke volume (50 per cent). Advancing age changes the relative contributions; however, increase in heart rate at age 70 still provides approximately two-thirds of the total increase in cardiac output with maximum exercise. Although patients with fixed-frequency pacing (VVI) may tolerate loss of AV synchrony, their effort tolerance is limited because in them cardiac output increase relies solely on an increase in stroke volume. This limitation is worse in patients with severe LV dysfunction because their stroke volume is fixed, making an increase in cardiac output dependent solely on rate augmentation.[94]

In the normal heart, AV synchrony at rest contributes about 20 to 30 per cent of the cardiac output. In some patients with congestive heart failure, atrial systole may contribute little to the resting cardiac output because of a substantial increase in LV filling pressure. However, such patients should not be denied AV sequential pacing; medical therapy can improve their ventricular performance, reduce LV filling pressure, and restore their responsiveness to the benefits of atrial systole. AV synchrony is quite important in patients with LV diastolic dysfunction (and normal systolic function), contributing 30 to 40 per cent to end-diastolic volume and cardiac output at rest. Loss of AV synchrony in such patients leads to marked reduction in cardiac output and produces serious hemodynamic changes, including pulmonary venous congestion. Consequently, AV sequential pacing should be used in all patients with LV diastolic dysfunction (aortic stenosis, hypertrophic cardiomyopathy, and LV hypertrophy secondary to hypertension).

Most studies showing the negligible contribution of AV synchrony during relatively high levels of exercise were conducted predominantly in patients with AV block, normal LV function, and devices with a fixed A-V interval.[81,83,95–97] It seems that AV synchrony is important at lesser levels of exercise, particularly in patients with borderline heart failure, LV dysfunction, or decreased LV compliance. The P-R interval normally shortens on exercise (4 to 5 msec/10 beats/min). Pacemakers designed with a rate-adaptive automatic shortening of the A-V interval on exercise are associated with better exercise performance, especially if exercise is begun with the optimal A-V interval determined at rest.[98–101]

Many studies have shown that during exercise an increase in the pacing rate provided by VVIR, VDD, DDD, or DDDR modes increases the cardiac output and duration of exercise more than does fixed-frequency VVI pacing.[81,89,94] In addition to superior hemodynamic effects, an increase in maximum oxygen consumption, reduced AV oxygen difference, and an increase in subjective well-being result.[81,89] The hemodynamic advantage is retained on an ongoing basis, because studies have shown no difference between acute and long-term results. Furthermore, rate-adaptive pacemakers actually may lead to improved LV function over time.[81,94]

Pacemaker Syndrome

Pacemaker syndrome is a clinical constellation of signs and symptoms produced by adverse hemodynamic and electrophysiological responses to pacing because of inadequate timing of atrial and ventricular contractions.[81,102–106] During VVI pacing, the pacemaker syndrome most commonly occurs in patients with normal or near-normal LV function and retrograde VA conduction. Early reports suggested that during VVI pacing, only 15 per cent of patients with preserved VA conduction develop symptoms suggestive of the pacemaker syndrome, with about half exhibiting its full-blown form. Its true incidence now seems higher because about two-thirds of patients with dual-chamber pulse generators prefer the dual-chamber mode to the VVI mode.[77,107–112] Thus the obvious cases during VVI pacing represent the tip of a much larger "iceberg" of cardiac dysfunction, often with subtle, unrecognized manifestations. Indeed, "asymptomatic" patients often feel better when their VVI pacemaker is upgraded to a DDD system, suggesting the existence of a "subclinical" pacemaker syndrome.[77]

The prominent symptoms of the pacemaker syndrome are due mostly to reduction in cardiac output, hypotension (more pronounced in the upright position), and higher ventricular filling pressures,[104,105] but many patients have subtle manifestations. Symptoms include orthostatic hypotension (especially in the first few seconds of ventricular pacing taking over from normal sinus rhythm), syncope or near syncope (due to reduction in cerebral flow), fatigue, exercise intolerance, lightheadedness, malaise, weakness, lethargy, dyspnea, induction of congestive heart failure, cough, patient awareness of beat-to-beat variations of cardiac response (from spontaneous to paced beats), neck pulsations or pressure sensation or fullness in the chest, neck, or head, headache, chest pain, impaired exercise capacity, and disturbed mentation. Many nonspecific symptoms similar to those of the pacemaker syndrome are common in the elderly and complicate the diagnosis. Physical examination may show cannon waves in the jugular venous pulse and palpable liver pulsations.

MECHANISM. Loss of AV synchrony can decrease cardiac output by 20 to 30 per cent at rest, but hemodynamic compromise in the pacemaker syndrome is more complex because retrograde VA conduction causes a "negative atrial kick" with more profound hemodynamic disadvantage than simple loss of AV synchrony. Atrial contraction against closed mitral and tricuspid AV valves causes systemic and pulmonary venous regurgitation and congestion (cannon *a* waves), sometimes leading to the development of congestive heart failure in previously compensated patients. In addition to the marked reduction in cardiac output, retrograde VA conduction leads to atrial distension and activation of stretch receptors that produce a reflex vasodepressor effect mediated by the autonomic nervous system.[104,105] Thus, in the face of hypotension due to low cardiac output, compensatory mechanisms that ordinarily increase the peripheral resistance become attenuated. In some cases involving profound hypotension there can even be a net reduction in peripheral resistance, and for this reason, concomitant treatment of congestive heart failure with vasodilators can precipitate the pacemaker syndrome during VVI pacing.

The relatively small group of patients who have pacemaker syndrome without VA conduction often exhibit venous cannon *a* waves that probably initiate the same hemodynamic disturbance as retrograde VA conduction. Patients intolerant of VVI or VVIR pacing demonstrate increased variability of anterograde Doppler-determined left atrial flow during VVI compared with DDD pacing.[113] The precise role of atrial natriuretic peptide in the genesis of the pacemaker syndrome is unclear. The high atrial natriuretic peptide level may be a marker of the pacemaker syndrome rather than contributing to its pathophysiology.[114,115]

Implantation of a VVIR pacemaker (see below) does not protect the patient from retrograde VA conduction and the pacemaker syndrome. It can develop on exercise when sinus rhythm gives way to ventricular pacing in patients with atrial chronotropic incompetence. On exercise, VA conduction can persist, or if absent at rest, it can occasionally appear with exercise under the influence of catecholamines. Atrial-based pacemakers (single-lead atrial and dual-chamber) also can produce the pacemaker syndrome at rest and/or exercise whenever inappropriate programming and/or selection of the pacing mode result in "inadequate timing of atrial and ventricular contractions."[103] If left atrial activation is delayed, the programmed A-V interval may not provide adequate time for effective left atrial systole before LV systole, and in extreme cases, left atrial systole may actually begin after the onset of LV systole.[85,88,116] Simultaneous atrial pacing from the right atrial appendage and coronary sinus can restore optimal timing of left atrial and left ventricular systole in patients with severe interatrial conduction delay.[117,118] In patients with complete AV block, the pacemaker syndrome can occur in the DDI mode secondary to AV dissociation whenever the sinus rate exceeds the programmed lower rate.

MANAGEMENT. The pacemaker syndrome due to VVI (VVIR) pacing is an iatrogenic condition[106] and can be eliminated by restoring AV synchrony either with atrial pacing alone (if AV conduction is normal) or dual-chamber pacing with an appropriate AV delay. Occasionally, restoration of AV synchrony during VVI pacing can be achieved by reducing the pacing rate (or using hysteresis) to minimize competition with sinus rhythm. At the time of pacemaker implantation, the lack of a drop in blood pressure with VVI pacing does not eliminate the potential for pacemaker syndrome.

Rate-Adaptive Pacemakers

Atrial chronotropic incompetence is the inability to increase the heart rate to appropriate levels that satisfy body needs. Guidelines such as the inability to achieve a heart rate exceeding 70 per cent of the maximum heart rate predicted for a given level of metabolic demand and the inability to reach a heart rate of 100/min on exercise provide practical definitions of atrial chronotropic incompetence. Testing can be by treadmill or long-term ambulatory ECG recordings during walking or ordinary activities. About 40 per cent of patients with sick sinus syndrome exhibit varying degrees of atrial chronotropic incompetence.[119] It is also found in some patients with AV block. The rate of a pacemaker can be designed to respond to the activity of a biological parameter that varies in parallel with the need for greater cardiac output. Such a rate-responsive system is called *rate-modulated, rate-adaptive,* or *sensor-driven* and is designated by the letter R in the fourth position of the pacemaker code, e.g., VVIR is a rate-adaptive ventricular demand pacemaker and DDDR is a rate-adaptive DDD device (Fig. 23–17). The magnitude and rate of change of the sensor-driven response are programmable. The ideal sensor should be stable, reliable long-term, and easy to implant, program, and troubleshoot. It also should respond in direct proportion to metabolic demand, use a standard lead, consume little battery current, be autoprogrammable, respond quickly, and decelerate gradually at the end of exercise. No existing single sensor satisfies all of these criteria.

Types of Rate-Adaptive Pacemakers

Of the many sensors in clinical use or investigation[120–122] (Table 23–5), currently approved devices in the United States respond to activity, minute ventilation, or temperature.

ACTIVITY-SENSING PACEMAKERS. This is the most commonly used system. It employs a piezoelectric sensor bonded to the inner surface of the pacemaker to detect

TABLE 23–5 CATEGORIES OF SENSORS FOR RATE-ADAPTIVE PACING

FUNCTIONAL-ORGANIC SOURCE	SIGNAL	SENSOR/METHOD OF DETECTION
1. Activity	Vibration generated by body movement	Piezoelectric
	Horizontal motion	Piezoelectric or silicone integrated accelerometer-accelerometric
	Vertical motion	Encapsulated mercury droplet gravimetric acceleration
2. Respiration	Respiratory rate	Transthoracic impedance
	Minute ventilation	Transthoracic impedance
3. Evoked (paced) parameters	Paced ventricular repolarization (Q-T interval)	Electrogram
	Paced ventricular depolarization integral*	Calculates area under the paced ventricular deflection electrogram
4. Hemodynamic parameters	Right ventricular pressure (dP/dt)	Piezoelectric crystal on ventricular lead tip
	Preejection interval	Intracardiac impedance and electrogram—onset of ventricular signal to beginning of ejection (preejection interval)
	Right ventricular volume	Intracardiac impedance—peak to peak voltage amplitude (relative stroke volume)
	Rate of change in right ventricular volume (dV/dt)	Intracardiac impedance (relative contractility)
5. Central venous blood	Temperature	Thermistor, electrical
	H^+ ion concentration	pH, electrical
	O_2 saturation	Reflectance of blood

* Withdrawn as a single-sensor system but incorporated with minute ventilation in a dual-sensor system.
Adapted from Benedek, Z. M., Gross, J., Furman, S: Rate-modulated pacemakers. The Newspaper of Cardiology, April 1993, with permission.

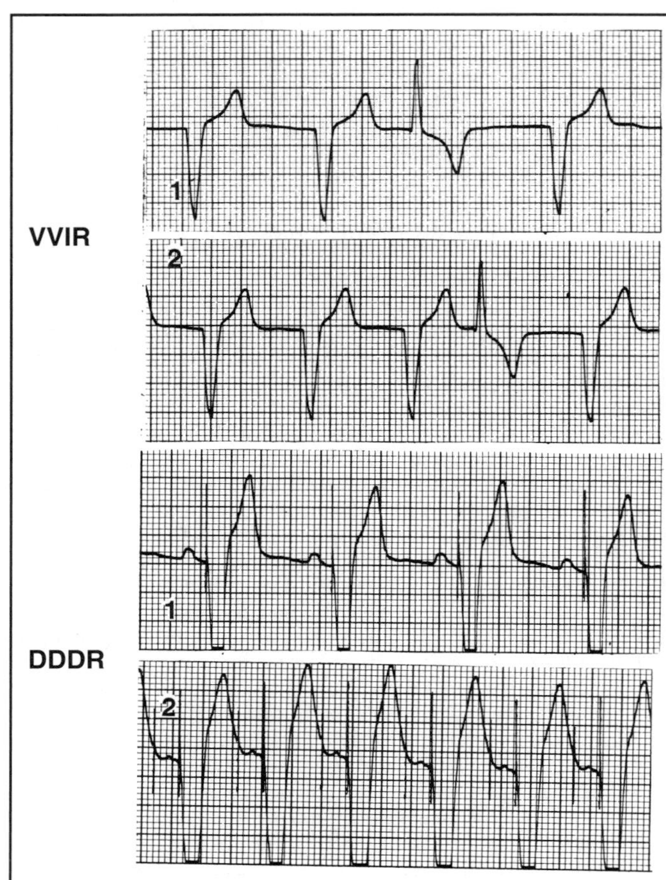

FIGURE 23–17. Response of rate-adaptive VVIR and DDDR pacemakers to exercise. *Top,* VVIR. The tiny bipolar stimuli cannot be discerned. *Panel 1* shows pacing at the programmed lower rate interval (LRI) = 857 mscec (corresponding to a rate of 70/min). The third beat is a ventricular extrasystole sensed by the pacemaker. The escape interval is essentially equal to the automatic interval. *Panel 2* shows the response on exercise when the ventricular rate increases to about 88/min (sensor-driven interval = 680 msec) so that a sensed ventricular extrasystole now resets the pacemaker with an escape interval of about 680 ms. *Bottom panels,* DDDR. *Panel 1* shows DDD pacing with sensing of P waves (LRI = 1000 msec). In *panel 2* during exercise the AV sequential (Ap-Vp) pacing rate increases to 107/min (cycle length 560 msec). (Reproduced with permission from Barold, S. S., et al.: Pacing in the nineties: Technologic, hemodynamic and electrophysiologic considerations in the selection of the optimal mode of pacing. *In* Rackley, C. E. [ed.]: Challenges in Cardiology 1, Mt. Kisco, N.Y., Futura, 1992, p. 39.)

mechanical forces or vibrations (body movements but not myopotentials) that are transformed to electrical energy to control the pacing rate. The pacing rate is increased in proportion to the detected vibration. The sensor is nonmetabolic and therefore nonphysiological. It does not respond to an increase in metabolic demand such as with emotional stimuli that are unrelated to exercise. Nevertheless, it works well in practice. The system is simple, reliable, stable, easy to program, uses a standard lead, and exhibits a fast response to brief periods of exercise. The sensor is unaffected by drugs or disease. Its main advantage is the precise recognition of onset and end of exercise, an important characteristic in older patients who do not exercise much and do so primarily in short bursts of physical work such as walking or climbing stairs. Other sensor-driven systems that exhibit a delayed response at the onset of exercise and reach a maximum rate after the end of the exercise are less desirable for the elderly. Several disadvantages exist. Pacing rate plateaus after the initial increase despite continued exercise. The pacing rate depends on the type of activity and does not correlate with the level of exercise or the amount of work, particularly at high levels of exercise. Rate change does not occur during mental exercise, emotional stress, or isometric exercise. Physical pressure on the pacemaker such as lying on it can cause an inappropriate rate increase during sleep. Pacing rate may be slower when stairs are climbed compared with when they are descended. External vibrations such as occur when riding in a vehicle in rough terrain or in a train or a helicopter can increase the pacing rate. Generally, these aberrations are innocuous. To overcome the limitations of vibration-sensitive pacemakers, some manufacturers have replaced the activity sensor with an accelerometer (itself containing a piezoelectric crystal) integrated within the circuitry rather than on the inner surface of the device. Accelerometer-based pacemakers respond to changes (velocity) in motion (not deflections of the casing) and exhibit less susceptibility to environmental noise and more specificity than conventional activity sensors.[123–126]

OTHER TYPES OF SENSORS

RESPIRATORY-DEPENDENT PACEMAKER. The original system that measured only respiratory rate[127] has been supplanted by devices calculating minute ventilation volume (tidal volume × respiratory rate) derived from the transthoracic impedance. The system injects a small current between the pacemaker casing and the proximal electrode of a standard bipolar lead and determines impedance between the tip electrode and the pacemaker casing. The pacemaker ignores the impedance change related to stroke volume by appropriate filtering. The transthoracic impedance increases with inspiration and decreases with expiration, and its amplitude varies according to the tidal volume. The calculated minute ventilation volume (and the generated pacing rate) correlates closely with metabolic demand or workload. The system is highly physiological, reliable, and works well clinically.[128–130] Programming generally requires a treadmill stress test. Drawbacks include a delayed reaction to the onset and bursts of exercise (recently improved with new algorithms[131]), inappropriately fast rates after the end of exercise, additional battery current for sensor function that may reduce the life of the pulse generator, and excessive pacing rates in patients with tachypnea from congestive heart failure or other causes, as well as a response to swinging of the arms, shoulder movements, or coughing. Electrocautery can increase the sensor-driven rate to its upper limit.

TEMPERATURE-SENSING PACEMAKER. This pacemaker's operation is based on an increase in metabolic rate with activity that produces heat transported in the blood. A small thermistor totally incorporated into a special pacing lead can detect the rate of change of blood temperature (not the absolute value) in the right ventricle. A slow rise in central venous temperature as a result of fever, emotion, or high external temperature is generally disregarded by the pacemaker. A special algorithm compensates for the decrease in blood temperature at the onset of exercise as the cooler blood returns from the extremities. Temperature accurately reflects oxygen consumption in the middle and late stages of exercise. Thus, while central venous temperature correlates well with metabolic demand at high workloads, the rate response is insufficient at low workloads such as brief everyday activities because of the relatively slow and minimal increase in central venous temperature.[132] In some patients with congestive heart failure, a very gradual (slow) and prolonged temperature dip (due to sluggish flow of blood from extremities) early during exercise may cause a paradoxical drop in the pacing rate. Also, the heat-dissipation mechanism at the end of exercise is often impaired in patients with heart failure. The drawbacks of this system have made it far less popular than activity, minute ventilation, and Q-T sensors.

Q-T INTERVAL–SENSING PACEMAKER. This unipolar ventricular system operates on the principle that the Q-T interval shortens with physical exercise due to the release of catecholamines.[121,133–135] Mental stress also increases the pacing rate.[136] The Q-T system provides a stable, rugged sensor using a standard pacemaker lead. Its disadvantages include a relatively slow response, nonsustained rate changes, and some difficulty in ensuring reliable T-wave sensing, especially with chronic leads. Type 1A and 3 antiarrhythmic drugs and beta blockers may interfere with pacemaker response, while myocardial ischemia or infarction may cause an inappropriate increase in the pacing rate.

SENSOR COMBINATIONS. New generation devices utilize two nonatrial sensors to overcome the drawbacks (false-positive or false-negative response) of each sensor used alone. Data from the sensors are crosschecked to avoid an unphysiological response.[137–140] Activity sensors react quickly and, while nonspecific, are more suitable to determine the onset of exercise. An activity sensor can therefore be combined with another, more physiological but slower-reacting sensor. Such combinations include (1) activity and Q-T interval, (2) activity and minute ventilation volume, and (3) activity and temperature. The Q-T sensor is best suited for detection of increased catecholamine effect during emotional circumstances, but an increase in rate in this situation may constitute a disadvantage in some patients with heart disease. Experience with dual-sensor devices is limited, and their clinical superiority over single-sensor devices with refined algorithms and optimally programmed parameters has not yet been established. Some dual-sensor devices may not require more complex programming because they can adapt their rate response automatically by a process of "learning" according to memorized patterns of patient activity.[41]

PROGRAMMING RATE-ADAPTIVE PACEMAKERS. The rate-adaptive pulse generator should be programmed so that a casual 2- to 3-min walk increases the rate 10 to 25/min to about 90/min and a fast walk or stair climbing increases the rate 20 to 45/min to about 100 to 120/min.[142,143] Stress testing and Holter recordings can be useful to set appropriate functions, and telemetered paced-derived histograms can help assess rate response. Pacemaker function in elderly patients should be evaluated at low exercise loads to correspond with their activities of daily living and not with maximum exercise, which obviously represents an artificial situation. Overprogramming causes unpleasant palpitations with minimal effort. Very rapid rate increases and decreases generally should be avoided. Care should be taken that fast rates do not precipitate angina in patients with coronary artery disease, worsening of congestive heart failure, and hypotension in patients with cardiomyopathy or atrial or ventricular tachyarrhythmias.[144] In patients with bradycardia-tachycardia syndrome, the sensor-controlled upper rate of a DDDR device can be programmed to a faster value than the atrial controlled upper rate to prevent rapid paced ventricular rates from tracking of a supraventricular tachyarrhythmia.

EVOLVING SENSOR APPLICATIONS. These include (1) detection of unphysiological atrial rates (crosschecking) to activate a protective mechanism preventing rapid ventricular pacing as in automatic mode conversion, (2) automatic capture detection, e.g., presence or absence of a Q-T interval,[145,146] and (3) optimization of timing intervals such as AV delay or refractory periods to adjust the pacemaker to changing physiological circumstances.[140,147]

Selection of Pacing Mode

ATRIAL-BASED PACING. Atrial-based pacing is gaining popularity because atrial pacing and sensing are reliable on a long-term basis and atrial lead dislodgment is relatively rare. It can provide normal or near-normal hemodynamics at rest and on exercise with enhancement of quality of life and avoidance of pacemaker syndrome. Atrial and AV pacing are preferable to single-chamber ventricular pacing because they reduce the incidence of chronic (and perhaps paroxysmal) atrial fibrillation, particularly in patients with the bradycardia-tachycardia syndrome.[81,148–152] If supraventricular tachyarrhythmia recurs after pacemaker implantation, increasing the atrial pacing rate to 80/min may help. If not, antiarrhythmic drug therapy is indicated because poor arrhythmia control predisposes to systemic embolism. Atrial arrhythmias seem to respond better to antiarrhythmic agents in patients with atrial or dual-chamber pacemakers than in those with single-lead ventricular devices. Long-term anticoagulation should be strongly considered in patients with refractory paroxysmal atrial fibrillation (see p. 655). Atrial and AV pacing also decrease the risk of embolization and stroke, the incidence of congestive heart failure, and overall mortality,[81,148,151,153–158] especially in sick sinus patients older than 70 years.[148,151,154] Single-chamber ventricular pacing should therefore be avoided in most patients, especially those with sick sinus syndrome.

VVIR VERSUS DDD PACING. In patients with atrial chronotropic incompetence, maintenance of AV synchrony at rest in the DDD mode contributes more to quality of life than improved exercise tolerance in the VVIR mode.[159,160] Most patients spend their lives predominantly at rest, punctuated by relatively short periods of mild exercise during the course of the day when a moderate rate response would be clearly beneficial. In patients with complete AV block (normal atrial chronotropic function) and without significant LV dysfunction, VDD, DDD, and VVIR pacing provide almost the same degree of enhanced exercise performance.[95,161,162] Yet a substantial number of patients remain intolerant of VVIR pacing *at rest*.

VVIR VERSUS DDDR PACING. In patients with atrial chronotropic incompetence, the VVIR and DDDR modes are clearly superior to the DDD mode in terms of exercise performance because the sensor increases the pacing rate according to activity.[163,164] Many studies[98,112,165–169] (but not all[170,171]) of patients with atrial chronotropic incompetence and DDDR pulse generators have shown superior performance on exercise, improved sense of well-being, and patient preference of the DDDR mode compared with the VVIR mode. In some cases, patients describe a subjective improvement in their sense of well-being or quality of life and elimination of bothersome nonspecific symptoms when DDDR mode is used instead of the VVIR mode, even though the patients have no demonstrable objective improvement in functional exercise capacity.[112]

AAI AND AAIR PACING. In the United States, perhaps 1 per cent or less of patients requiring pacing receive a single-chamber atrial pacemaker. AAI and AAIR pacemakers are underutilized despite the wealth of information showing their superiority over VVI pacing in sick sinus patients without AV block.[62,149,150,172,173] The concern that patients with AAI (AAIR) pacemakers may develop AV block is largely unfounded. Second or third degree AV block has an annual incidence of about 1 per cent in carefully selected patients with AAI (AAIR) pacemakers, and its occurrence is rarely catastrophic and often related to drug therapy. Guidelines for selecting AAI or AAIR pacing include 1:1 AV conduction with atrial pacing to rates 120 to 140/min (despite its poor predictive value for the development of AV block), P-R interval ≤ 0.24 sec at rest, and absence of bundle branch block.[172–174] With careful patient selection, AAI or AAIR pacing could be used safely in probably 40 per cent of patients with sick sinus syndrome, and of these, about 40 per cent may require rate-adaptive devices (AAIR) because of atrial chronotropic incompetence.[94,119]

Individual Patient Considerations

When deciding the type of pacemaker to be used, the physician needs to determine whether the atrium can be paced and/or sensed, whether latent or overt AV block exists, and whether atrial chronotropic incompetence is present[175] (Fig. 23–18). The majority of patients with atria that can be paced and/or sensed should be considered for single-chamber atrial or dual-chamber pacing (AAI, AAIR, VDD, DDD, or DDDR) because VVI or VVIR pacing causes greater morbidity and mortality. Single-lead ventricular pacing should be reserved primarily for patients with chronic atrial fibrillation and AV block. A VVI pacemaker programmed to a low rate may be justified in the occasional patient with infrequent episodes of bradycardia. Replacement of a depleted VVI pacemaker with another VVI or VVIR unit is reasonable in many asymptomatic patients.

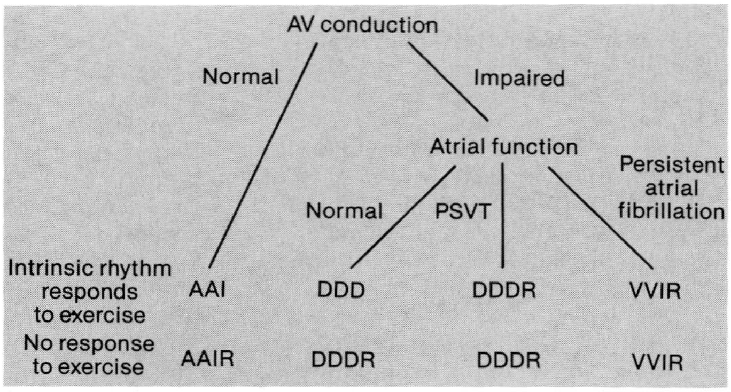

FIGURE 23–18. Algorithm for determining the optimal pacemaker mode for an individual patient. PSVT = paroxysmal supraventricular arrhythmias of all types including atrial fibrillation. A DDDR should be considered in patients with the bradycardia-tachycardia syndrome with intrinsic or drug-induced AV conduction delay to provide greater flexibility because (1) drug therapy of supraventricular tachyarrhythmias may further depress the atrial chronotropic response on exercise and (2) troublesome paroxysmal atrial tachyarrhythmias may necessitate programming to the DDIR mode or using a device with a fallback or automatic mode conversion mechanism to control the paced ventricular rate during supraventricular tachyarrhythmia. (From Griffin, J. C.: The optimal pacing mode for the individual patient: The role of DDDR. *In* Barold, S. S., and Mugica, J. [eds.]: New Perspectives in Cardiac Pacing 2, Mt. Kisco, N.Y., Futura, 1991, p. 325.)

Single-lead ventricular pacing is appropriate in patients who are incapacitated and inactive as well as those with a short life expectancy. VVIR does not improve survival when compared with the VVI mode.

It is important to assess what is best for the patient's level of activity, whether there is underlying coronary artery disease or LV dysfunction, what is affordable, what is the simplest system that will optimize hemodynamics, what is the natural history of the condition for which pacing is being used, and what is the impact of present and future drug therapy. Advanced age is not an indication for a simpler (and cheaper) VVI or VVIR system.[111,176,177] Active elderly patients benefit greatly from restoration of AV synchrony because the atrial contribution to cardiac output normally increases with advanced age. Dual-chamber pacemakers in the elderly appear cost-effective on a long-term basis by avoiding or reducing the complications associated with single-lead ventricular pacing.

Patients with angina pectoris generally tolerate DDD, DDDR, or VVIR modes better than the VVI mode, provided the upper rate is not excessively high. The increased MVO_2 related to rate increase on exercise is counterbalanced by the increase in MVO_2 during fixed-frequency VVI pacing, probably secondary to enhanced contractility (from increased sympathetic activity) and wall tension, which increase stroke volume.[178] The DDI or DDD mode with search hysteresis is preferred for carotid sinus hypersensitivity or neurally mediated syncope. For example, pacing might occur at a relatively fast rate of 100 beats/min when the spontaneous rate drops below a certain value such as 50 beats/min. After a given period of pacing, the pacemaker "searches" for the return of normal rhythm (>50 beats/min) by intermittent prolongation of one or more pacing intervals.[69] Pacing ceases if the spontaneous R-R interval is <1200 msec. This feature avoids continuation of pacing at 100 beats/min until it is inhibited by a spontaneous rhythm >100 beats/min, as with conventional hysteresis function. Patients with paroxysmal supraventricular tachyarrhythmias require a DDD or DDDR system with automatic mode conversion or fallback to slower paced ventricular rates to avoid tracking of unphysiological atrial rates. A single-lead VDD pacing system may provide a relatively simple and less expensive VDD/VVIR pacemaker for patients with AV block and normal atrial chronotropic function.[179–182]

Cost considerations aside, either a sensor-driven single-chamber or a sensor-driven dual-chamber pacemaker with extensive programmability of pacing modes would meet the needs of all patients given the high incidence of atrial chronotropic incompetence in the elderly and its progression or development over time.

COMPLICATIONS OF PACEMAKERS

Complications of venous entry, complications of lead placement and pocket formation, and electrical complications or pacemaker malfunction constitute three major groups of complications associated with permanent pacemaker implantation.

Complications of Lead Placement and Pocket Formation

Lead displacement can produce loss of pacing and/or sensing. Whereas myocardial perforation is rare with contemporary leads, it is more common with stiff temporary leads. Perforation may produce no symptoms or may cause intermittent or complete failure to pace and/or diaphragmatic pacing. A friction rub may be audible. If the lead has migrated to the left ventricle, paced beats can have a right bundle branch block contour in lead V_1. Echocardiography can be diagnostic. Although cardiac tamponade is rare, if it does occur, it is usually at the time of lead insertion and rarely after the first 24 hours; at this time, the lead may be withdrawn and safely repositioned under careful observation.

The incidence of symptomatic venous thrombosis is quite low despite the fact that contrast venography is abnormal in 30 to 45 per cent of patients, with total subclavian vein obstruction in 8 to 20 per cent. Subclavian venous obstruction probably occurs gradually, so the development of collaterals makes symptomatic obstruction rare. Should symptoms occur, treatment with anticoagulants is required for several weeks. Superior vena caval obstruction is a rare complication and has been treated successfully with thrombolytic agents, while superior vena caval stenosis has been treated successfully with balloon angioplasty alone or with stents.[183–186] Symptomatic pacemaker-related right atrial thrombus also can be treated with a thrombolytic agent.[187]

Contraction of the left diaphragm in synchrony with a paced stimulus can occur with or without lead perforation and is generally eliminated or minimized by programming the pacemaker output to a lower value. Contraction of the right diaphragm is due to phrenic nerve stimulation from a malpositioned right atrial electrode. Invariably, left intercostal muscle stimulation is due to lead perforation of the right ventricle. An insulation break causing a current leak either from the extravascular portion of the lead or the pulse generator can be associated with pectoral muscle twitching at or near the site of implantation. Some normally functioning unipolar pulse generators can cause pectoral muscle stimulation by the indifferent (anodal) plate without an insulation leak, particularly if the pacemaker has flipped over in a large pocket.

Twiddler's syndrome usually occurs when there is a relatively large pacemaker pocket and the patient repeatedly rotates the implanted pulse generator under the skin. The lead may retract from the heart to produce pacemaker failure. A pulse generator can erode through the skin or migrate, usually because of suboptimal implantation technique. Early infections are rare. *Staphylococcus aureus* is the most common offending organism in early infections, and *S. epidermidis* is most common in late infections. Transesophageal echocardiography may confirm vegetations related to a pacemaker lead.[188,189] The eradication of infection often requires removal of the entire pacing system, now feasible without thoracotomy with intravascular techniques that should be performed by an experienced operator because of the risk of bleeding, cardiac tamponade, and death.[190]

Pacemaker Malfunction

LOSS OF CAPTURE. The causes of loss of capture by visible pacemaker stimuli and pacemaker failure with no stimuli are listed in Table 23–6. Many of the abnormalities with visible stimuli are due to changes in the electrode-tissue interface that can be overcome by reprogramming or correcting any reversible metabolic or drug-related abnormalities[191] (Fig. 23–1). In some cases of chronic progressive increases in pacing threshold, lead replacement can be required. Absence of stimuli is often due to interruption of electric circuit with no current flow related to a broken electrode with intact insulation or less commonly due to pulse generator failure (battery component). Wire breakage is not always evident radiologically, while an insulation defect is not visible. A tight ligature on polyurethane leads can compress the insulation and spread the coil of wire without interfering with function, giving the appearance of a fracture (pseudofracture) radiologically.[192] A particular design feature without malfunction of one type of bifurcated bipolar lead resembles a pseudofracture.[192] Compression or distortion of the conductor coil identifies a point of stress on the lead.

ABNORMAL PACING RATE. A change in the pacing rate or erratic pacing can occur due to normal function (Table 23–7). Abnormal causes due to pacemaker malfunction are often found by exclusion. A constantly changing spike-to-spike interval during pacing often is caused by oversensing and/or a problem with the electrode rather than component failure. "Runaway pacemakers" with very rapid, life-threatening rates of stimulation are now rare but can still occur. At extremely rapid rates, stimulation is either ineffectual or can occur intermittently, producing bursts of tachycardia. This situation requires immediate disconnection and removal of the pacemaker.

TABLE 23–6 CAUSES OF LOSS OF CAPTURE BY VISIBLE PACEMAKER STIMULI AND LOSS OF PACING STIMULI

Loss of Capture
1. *Normal situation:* Stimuli in myocardial refractory period
2. *Electrode-tissue interface:* Early displacement or unstable position of pacing leads (most common cause); perforation (sometimes inapparent); malposition into coronary sinus or middle cardiac vein; elevated threshold (acute or chronic); inapparent displacement (exit block); subcutaneous emphysema (with loss of anodal contact of unipolar pacemakers), Twiddler's syndrome; myocardial infarction, elevation of pacing threshold after defibrillation or cardioversion; electrolyte abnormalities, e.g., hyperkalemia; drug toxicity, e.g., type 1A antiarrhythmic agents or drug effect, e.g., 1C antiarrhythmic agents (flecainide and propafenone)
3. *Electrode:* Fracture, short circuit, and insulation break
4. *Pulse generator:* Normally functioning pulse generator with inappropriate programming of output parameters, spontaneous pacemaker failure due to battery exhaustion or component failure, component failure from iatrogenic causes such as defibrillation, therapeutic radiation, and electrocautery
Loss of Pacing Stimuli
1. *Normal situation:* Total inhibition of pulse generator when the intrinsic rate is faster than the preset pacemaker rate.
2. *Hysteresis with normal function:* Escape interval > automatic interval
3. *Pseudomalfunction:* Overlooking tiny bipolar pacemaker stimuli in the ECG
4. *Lead:* Fracture, loose connection, or set screw problems
5. *Pulse generator:* Total battery depletion, component failure, sticky magnetic reed switch (application of magnet produces no effect). Subcutaneous emphysema (unipolar systems)
6. *Extreme electromagnetic interference*
7. *Oversensing* (signals originating from outside or inside the pulse generator)

TABLE 23–7 CAUSES OF CHANGES IN PACING RATE

Normal Function
1. Low programmed rate
2. Application of the magnet
3. Inaccurate speed of ECG machine drive
4. Apparent malfunction in special function pulse generators, e.g., triggered mode (AAT, VVT)
5. Reversion to interference rate (in response to electromagnetic or other signals) with either a faster or a slower rate than the spontaneous freerunning or magnet rate (according to manufacturer)
Abnormal Function
1. Battery failure (slowing of rate)
2. Runaway pacemaker: Spontaneous or due to therapeutic radiation or electrocautery
3. Component failure, e.g., erratic delivery of pacemaker stimuli; spontaneous or due to therapeutic radiation, electrocautery, or defibrillation
4. Permanent or temporary change in mode after therapeutic radiation, electrocautery, or defibrillation. If functionally reset from electromagnetic interference, the device can be reprogrammed to its original mode.
5. Phantom reprogramming (done without documentation), misprogramming
6. Oversensing

UNDERSENSING. Low-amplitude electrograms and/or signals with a low slew rate (inappropriate frequency content) represent the most common cause of undersensing. An inadequate signal can be due to poor lead position at the time of implantation, lead displacement, or lead maturation with attenuation of a previously small but adequate electrogram. Lead dislodgment, low-amplitude signal from premature ventricular complexes, and myocardial infarction are common causes, often correctable by programming a higher sensitivity. Undersensing also can occur with component failure of a pulse generator, an abnormal (jammed) magnetic reed switch (that fails to restore sensing upon magnet removal), or inappropriate programming of sensitivity or refractory period. A DDD pacemaker will not sense an adequate ventricular signal falling within the blanking period designed to prevent crosstalk. Asynchronous pacing (noise mode) also can occur at a preset rate as a protective response to continually sensed interference. Insulation or wire fracture defects also can attenuate the effective electrogram detected by a pulse generator. Hyperkalemia, toxic effects of antiarrhythmic drugs (especially antiarrhythmic drugs in classes 1A and 1C) and cardioversion and defibrillation also can lead to transient undersensing. Oversensing of an extraneous signal that initiates a new refractory period can lead to undersensing if the electrogram falls within the refractory period initiated by the sensed extraneous event. Occasionally, oversensing can present only with undersensing when the relatively fast spontaneous rhythm precludes pacemaker pauses.

OVERSENSING. This is by far the most common cause of pacemaker pauses, i.e., failure of delivery of a ventricular pacemaker stimulus at the anticipated time according to the programmed automatic (escape) interval; its occurrence is confirmed by magnet-induced conversion to the asynchronous mode. Unwanted signals causing oversensing arise from several sources.[193] For example, atrial depolarization can be sensed during VVI pacing when the ventricular lead becomes displaced toward the RV inflow tract.

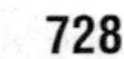

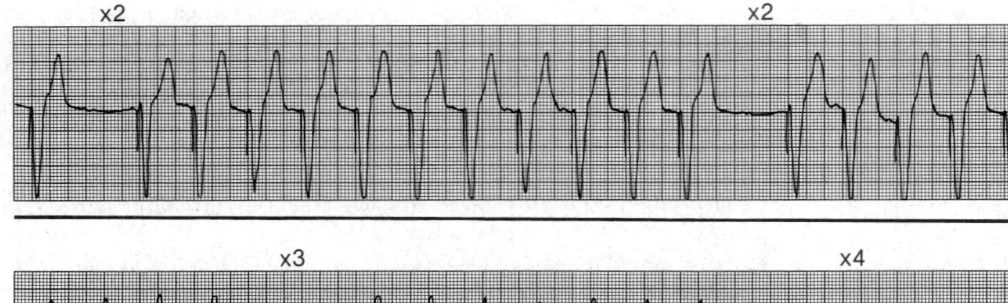

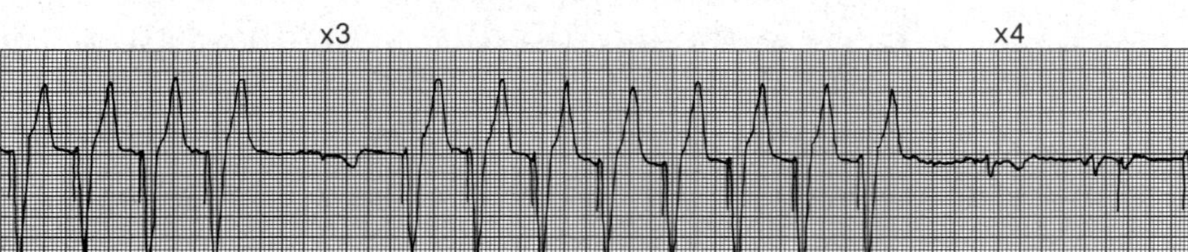

FIGURE 23–19. Electrocardiographic diagnosis of intermittent lead fracture or loose connection during VVI pacing. During spontaneous pacing an ECG (not shown) revealed intermittent pacemaker pauses of varying duration. The ECG shows asynchronous pacing at 100/min upon application of the magnet over the pulse generator. Wriggling the pulse generator in its pocket produces pauses that are exact multiples of the magnet interval (×2, ×3, and ×4) a response diagnostic of an intermittent electrode problem because it reflects the correct timing of a normally functioning pulse generator delivering its impulse into a transiently disrupted circuit with high impedance. (From Barold, S. S. et al.: Differential diagnosis of pacemaker pauses. *In* Barold S. S. [ed.]: Modern Cardiac Pacing. Mt. Kisco, NY, Futura Publishing Co., 1985, p. 592.)

Prevention of asystole requires magnet application or programming to the VOO or VVT mode. T-wave sensing often represents detection of the voltage at the electrode-myocardial interface generated by a pacemaker stimulus (discussed later) and the natural T wave and can be corrected by programming a lesser sensitivity and/or a longer pacemaker refractory period.

The pacing system itself can generate signals that are sensed and inhibit delivery of the pacemaker stimulus. For example, the electrode-tissue interface can act as a capacitor that generates voltage (polarization voltage or afterpotential) that is subsequently dissipated over a relatively long period. The decay of the "afterpotential" constitutes a time-changing voltage that can be sensed when the pacemaker refractory period terminates. Also, abrupt changes in resistance within a pacing system can produce corresponding voltage changes that generate signals often invisible on the surface ECG. Such "make-break," or false, signals can occur from loose connections, wire fractures with intermittent contact, short circuits, insulation defects, or the interaction of two pacemaker catheters lying side by side and touching each other within the heart.

Intermittent electrode problems, especially oversensing due to an intermittent fracture, constitute the "great imitator" in cardiac pacing and often cause a chaotic pattern of pacing. Indeed, erratic behavior with pauses of varying lengths suggests a defective lead system rather than pacemaker component malfunction. False signals tend to occur at random, producing inhibition of stimuli for relatively long and constantly changing periods. Magnet application eliminates only pauses caused by oversensing. The demonstration of pacemaker pauses that are exact multiples of the *magnet* interval during asynchronous pacing is virtually diagnostic of an intermittent wire fracture (or electrode problem) (Fig. 23–19). Sometimes this irregularity can be demonstrated only by wriggling the pacemaker in its pocket.

Oversensing skeletal muscle potentials (myopotential interference) remains the most common cause of pacemaker pauses and occurs almost invariably with unipolar pulse generators[194–196] (Fig. 23–20). Although myopotential interference can be demonstrated in as many as 50 per cent of patients with unipolar pulse generators, only 10 per cent report symptoms and require pacemaker reprogramming.[194] Oversensing of diaphragmatic potentials on deep inspiration is uncommon and associated with short pauses. The incidence of myopotential interference has remained unchanged over the last 25 years because absolute discrimination between the cardiac electrogram and myopotentials is difficult. The problem will disappear as bipolar systems eventually replace unipolar ones. In the meantime, myopotential oversensing can be corrected by reducing the input sensitivity, converting to the triggered VVT (AAT) or VOO (AOO) mode, programming from unipolar to bipolar sensing, and rarely, pacemaker replacement. In the DDD mode, myopotential oversensing by the atrial channel can result in rapid paced ventricular rates.

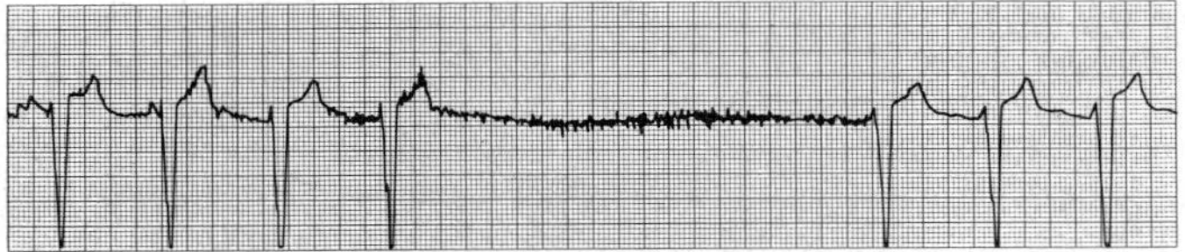

FIGURE 23–20. Prolonged inhibition of unipolar VVI pacemaker (rate = 70 ppm) from myopotential oversensing.

INTERFERENCE

Transthoracic cardioversion or defibrillation delivers a large amount of energy to the heart. Circuitry designed to protect the pulse generator shunts energy to the lead. Contemporary pulse generators, especially unipolar systems, are more susceptible than in the past to disturbance from this type of electric discharge.[197,198] The shock can damage circuitry, with partial or complete destruction of the pulse generator, which can result in a runaway state, induction of end-of-life behavior, and reversible or irreversible alteration of the microprocessor program. It also can cause an acute, temporary (usual), or chronic increase in the pacing threshold, probably due to myocardial burns; undersensing abnormalities, usually temporary but sometimes lasting as long as 10 days; reprogramming to another mode, even with different parameters; and reset to the VOO or VVI mode (with change of polarity from bipolar to unipolar in some designs) in response to high-level interference. A reset pacemaker returns to normal when reprogrammed.

Similar problems can occur from discharge of an implanted cardioverter-defibrillator.[199] Patients with an implanted cardioverter-defibrillator (ICD) should receive a dedicated bipolar pacing system that can be reset only to the bipolar VVI or VOO mode because large unipolar stimuli can interfere with sensing of ventricular fibrillation by an ICD. While thermal electrical burns at the electrode-myocardial interface can theoretically precipitate ventricular fibrillation, this has not yet been clearly documented in humans with external shocks. Paddles or patches for cardioversion must be placed well away from the pacemaker along a line perpendicular to the axis of the ventricular lead inside the heart, as with anterior and posterior paddles.

ELECTROCAUTERY. This is the most common form of interference in the hospital environment.[198] Apart from the expected response during its application (temporary inhibition, reversion to asynchronous interference mode, or reset to the VVI or VOO mode as a normal response to high-intensity interference), electrical and thermal burns at the electrode-myocardial interface can cause ventricular fibrillation or chronic elevation of pacing thresholds. Damage to a pulse generator can result with permanent loss of output, runaway behavior, random failure, and reprogramming. Application of the magnet over the pulse generator or programming to an asynchronous mode may prevent oversensing but does not protect the pacemaker from irreversible malfunction. During electrocautery, patients must be managed according to a careful protocol, with pacemaker testing before and after the procedure. Radiofrequency catheter ablation of arrhythmias potentially can cause similar disturbances of pacemaker behavior and can produce upper-rate pacing in a minute ventilation–driven DDDR pacemaker.[198]

RADIATION THERAPY. This can damage pacemaker electronics and cause unpredictable transient or permanent malfunction including unaway behavior. The effect is cumulative and similar whether the dose is given at one time or spread over several treatments. Given a sufficiently high cumulative absorbed dose, all pulse generators will fail catastrophically.[199–202] Appropriate shielding of the pulse generator during radiation therapy is mandatory. Barring reset and other responses related to sensing electromagnetic interference, malfunction requires pacemaker replacement because long-term reliability becomes questionable.

MAGNETIC RESONANCE IMAGING (MRI). This can cause rapid pacing, inhibition, resetting of DDD pulse generators, and transient reed switch malfunction with asynchronous pacing. MRI is generally contraindicated in patients with pacemakers.[199,203,204] Serious malfunction with no output or rapid pacing may occur because pulsed energy from MRI can enter the lead by capacitive coupling and cause rapid ventricular pacing. Permanent component damage has not been reported. When an MRI is considered absolutely essential, it is reasonable to program the pacemaker to its lowest voltage and pulse width or to the OOO mode, provided the patient has an adequate underlying rhythm.[191]

Pacemaker Follow-up

Despite the reliability of modern pacemakers, a follow-up program is mandatory because complications are not uncommon and pacemaker failure is ultimately inevitable. Good follow-up should provide improved pacemaker longevity by appropriate programming and should identify impending pacemaker failure in most instances. The frequency and type of follow-up depend on the projected battery life, type, mode, and programming of pulse generators, the stability of pacing and sensing, the need for programming changes, the underlying rhythm (pacemaker dependency), travel logistics, and the use of alternative methods of follow-up such as the telephone.[205]

Transtelephonic pacemaker monitoring is the simplest method of pacemaker follow-up, and its main function is to detect changes in pacemaker rate as an indirect reflection of battery depletion.[205,206] Transtelephonic monitoring should complement and not replace comprehensive follow-up and is generally used to document satisfactory pacing function between visits. Transtelephonic monitoring usually is performed every 2 to 3 months until the first indication of battery depletion, when it may be performed once a month. The ECG is recorded with and without magnet placement. Free-running and magnet intervals and pulse width are measured. In dual-chamber pacemakers, rate and pulse widths are measured along with the A-V interval. Complex ECGs from DDD pulse generators transmitted by phone are often uninterpretable. As a rule, transtelephonic follow-up does not allow programming or transmission of telemetered data.

When the patient is discharged after pacemaker implantation, the pulse generator is programmed to optimize function during the expected physiological changes in the early phase. The patient should be seen about 2 weeks after implantation, when the operative site is also inspected. The pacing system is evaluated 2 months after implantation, when pacing and sensing thresholds have stabilized, and in virtually all patients, definitive programming can be performed for long-term function. Follow-up in the clinic should be done every 6 to 12 months for single-chamber and every 3 to 6 months for dual-chamber pacemakers. The complexity of contemporary pacemakers requires meticulous record keeping (Table 23–8). Periodic transtelephonic pacemaker monitoring should supplement these visits. More frequent follow-up can become necessary when impending battery depletion is detected.

Pacemaker follow-up requires equipment such as a multichannel ECG machine, magnet, digital counter for interval measurement, programmers, temporary pacemaker and chest electrodes for chest wall stimulation, Doppler echocardiography, long-term ECG recorders, closed-loop event recorders, and equipment for cardiopulmonary resuscitation. First, a 12-lead ECG is obtained with and without application of the magnet. Various intervals (lower rate, pulse width, and so on) are measured with an electronic counter. If telemetry is available, the pulse generator is interrogated to document initial pacemaker parameters. The following aspects of pacemaker function are then evaluated systematically.

Battery voltage can be evaluated directly by telemetry or indirectly. When it reaches a critical level, the elective replacement indicator (ERI) is activated, and the pacing rate in the free-running and/or magnet mode slows. This change can be gradual or stepwise (sudden). The ERI of some DDD pulse generators consists of reversion to a simpler VVI or VOO mode to reduce current drain from the battery. Approximately 6 months exist between activation of the ERI and the dangerous end-of-life state. Ventricular pacing is documented from the control ECG and the ECG after application of the magnet. Ventricular pacing threshold is best determined in the VVI mode (or DDD with short A-V interval to ensure ventricular capture) by programming voltage and/or pulse width until capture is lost. Ventricular sensing is also best confirmed in the VVI mode by reducing the pacing rate to allow the spontaneous rhythm to emerge. The ventricular sensing threshold can be determined by decreasing the ventricular sensitivity gradually until sensing failure occurs.

In patients with dual-chamber pacemakers, provided there is an underlying ventricular rhythm, using the AAI or AOO mode at various rates confirms atrial capture (Fig. 23–21). If a paced P wave is not visible with double stan-

TABLE 23–8 DATA REQUIRED IN PACEMAKER CHART

Pacemaker data: Date(s) of implant(s), model and serial number of pacemaker lead(s), model and serial number of pulse generator

Data from implant: Indication, pacing threshold(s), sensing threshold(s), intracardiac electrograms, lead impedance(s), presence of retrograde ventriculoatrial (VA) conduction, presence of diaphragmatic or accessory muscle stimulation at 5- and 10-V output, chest x-ray soon after implantation

Technical specifications: Pacemaker behavior in the magnet mode, record of elective replacement indicator, magnet and/or freerunning rate, mode change, telemetered battery data (impedance and voltage)

Data from pacemaker clinic: Programmed parameters from time of implant and most recent changes, 12-lead ECG and long rhythm strips showing pacing and inhibition of pacing (if possible) to determine underlying rhythm (by programming very low output, OOO mode, low rate or with chest wall stimulation). Degree of pacemaker dependency. 12-lead ECG on application of the magnet. Rhythm strip of magnet mode for at least 1 min. Electronic rate intervals and pulse widths freerunning and upon application of the magnet before programming. Interrogation and printout of telemetry, e.g., memory or programmed and real-time data.

Systematic evaluation of pacing system: Atrial and/or ventricular pacing and sensing thresholds documented by rhythm strip. Retrograde ventriculoatrial conduction and propensity to endless loop tachycardia in dual chamber systems. Crosstalk in dual chamber systems. Myopotential interference (record best way of reproducing abnormality). Printouts showing pacemaker function when a parameter is programmed. Evaluation of atrial chronotropic response. Evaluation of sensor function with exercise protocols. Histograms or other data to demonstrate heart rate response in the rate-adaptive mode. Efficacy of rate-adaptive parameters. Response to onset and cessation of exercise. Doppler echocardiography to optimize AV interval (rest and exercise). Final telemetry printout at end of pacemaker evaluation and date. Check that any changes in parameters are intentional by comparing the final parameters with those obtained at the time of initial pacemaker interrogation.* Any discrepancy must be justified in the record.

Ancillary data: Symptoms and potential problems, e.g., accessory muscle stimulation. ECG with event marker recorders, telemetered electrogram and diagnostic diagrams. Holter recordings. Transtelephonic data. Special functions such as automatic PVARP extension, tachycardia terminating algorithms, automatic mode conversion, etc. Intolerance of VOO pacing on application of magnet.

* In one system an arrow points to a parameter when its final programmed value differs from the value at the initial interrogation.

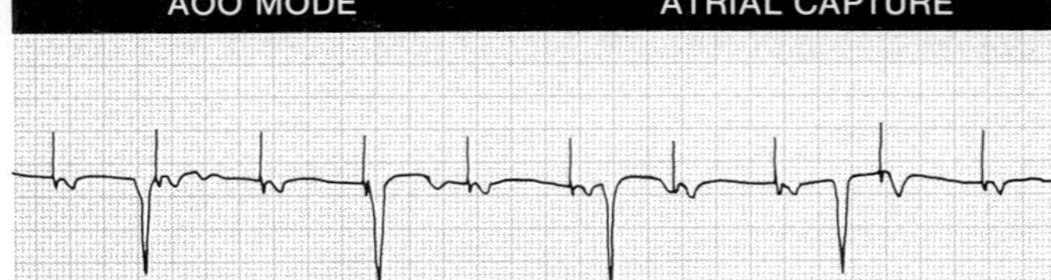

FIGURE 23–21. Determination of atrial capture in a patient with a DDD pulse generator and complete AV block. The pulse generator was first reprogrammed to the VVI mode and the rate was gradually decreased to 30/min, whereupon a ventricular escape rhythm at a rate of 45/min emerged. The pulse generator was then programmed to the AOO mode at a rapid rate. The atrial stimuli dissociated from the QRS complex demonstrate successful atrial capture. This maneuver is contraindicated in pacemaker-dependent patients.

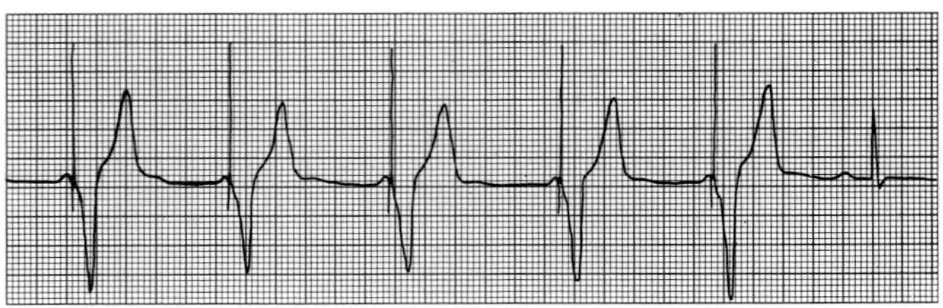

FIGURE 23–22. Semiquantitative assessment of atrial signal amplitude by programming the sensitivity of a DDD pulse generator. To demonstrate atrial sensing, the pulse generator was programmed to a lower rate of 50 ppm and AV = 50 msec. With an atrial sensitivity of 1.2 mV, all the P waves were sensed (not shown). At an atrial sensitivity of 1.6 mV, the tracing shows intermittent failure of atrial sensing (last P wave, i.e., if it had been sensed the ventricular stimulus would have occurred near the apex of the P wave). In this case, the lowest sensitivity (corresponding to the highest numerical value) causing consistent P wave sensing was 1.2 mV. Consequently, the atrial sensitivity should be programmed to 0.6 mV.

dardization of the ECG and/or lengthening of the A-V interval, echocardiography or esophageal electrocardiography can be used to document atrial systole. Alternatively, evaluation of atrial capture can be determined by competitive atrial pacing in the DVI mode at a slow rate. Evaluating atrial sensing is extremely important because atrial undersensing is one of the most common problems in DDD pacing. To evaluate atrial sensing, the pacemaker lower rate should be reduced below that of spontaneous atrial activity and the AV delay shortened to 50 to 100 msec to guarantee that any sensed P wave will trigger a ventricular stimulus. Atrial sensing can be assessed by decreasing the atrial sensitivity from the lowest numerical value (or most sensitive) to the highest numerical value (or least sensitive) until P wave tracking is lost (Fig. 23–22). The final programmed value should be double the atrial sensing threshold (half the numerical value). Telemetry, when available, provides proof of atrial sensing and its exact timing by transmitted event markers (Fig. 23–23). Random rather than sustained loss of atrial sensing is not uncommon in Holter recordings but rarely is of any clinical significance. Changes in body position, respiration, congestive heart failure, and exercise may alter the amplitude of the P-wave signal and affect atrial sensing.

Myopotential interference in unipolar pulse generators should be evaluated routinely with isometric exercise and 24-hour Holter recordings. In DDD pacing, myopotential interference can inhibit the ventricular channel (Fig. 23–20), can increase the ventricular pacing rate when the atrial channel senses myopotentials (Fig. 23–16), can cause the pacemaker to revert to the asynchronous interference mode at a predetermined rate, and can activate the ventricular safety pacing mechanism.

Evaluating retrograde VA conduction is important in patients prone to development of endless-loop tachycardia. Susceptibility to crosstalk should be determined as previously discussed.

Telemetry is an indispensable feature of contemporary pulse generators and provides information on all programmed values as well as real-time or measured data on how the pacemaker is operating at the time of interrogation. These data include information on the output circuit, battery parameters, sensor activity for rate-adaptive pacemakers, event markers, and transmission of electrograms. Telemetered battery voltage and impedance correlate with battery depletion. Pacing impedance reflects lead integrity. Telemetry also provides diagnostic data about the interaction between the pulse generator and the patient over an extended period of time. Cumulative totals of sensed and paced events are useful in programming the pacemaker.

Advanced telemetry systems can memorize the occurrence and duration of certain arrhythmias and document

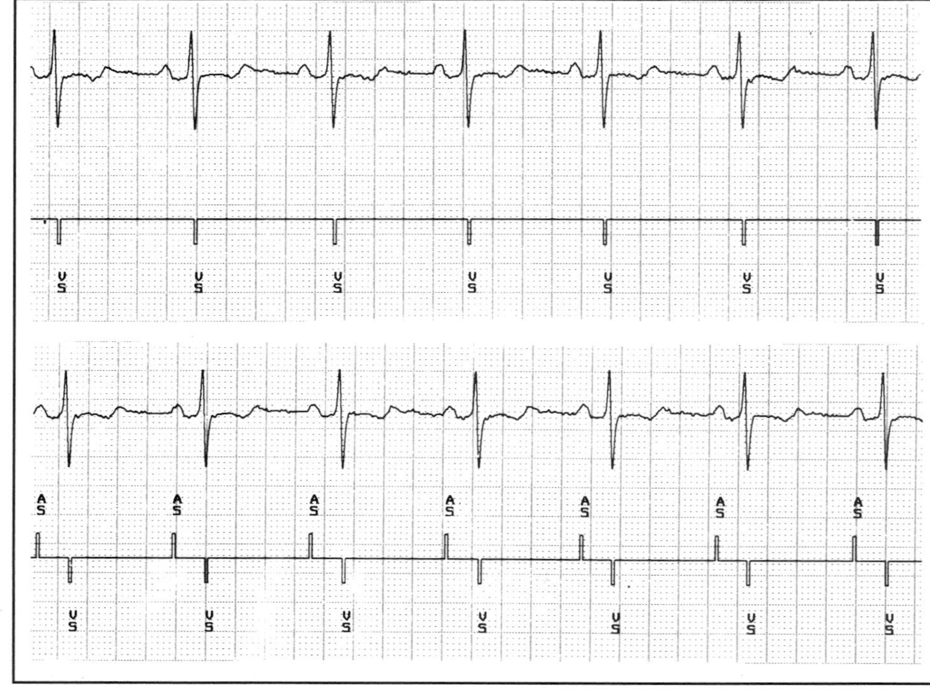

FIGURE 23–23. ECGs with annotated marker channel during DDD pacing. As = atrial sensed event; Vs = ventricular sensed event. Lower rate interval = 1200 msec, A-V delay = 200 msec after atrial sensing and atrial pacing, atrial escape interval = 1000 msec. *Top,* The marker channel shows appropriate inhibition of ventricular stimulation by sensed ventricular depolarizations (Vs). There is loss of atrial sensing because there are no markers consistent with atrial sensing. *Bottom,* The atrial sensitivity was increased and atrial sensing was restored. In the top panel the atrial stimulus is inhibited because the Vs-Vs interval is shorter than the atrial escape interval; i.e., Vs resets the atrial escape interval and the lower rate interval continually.

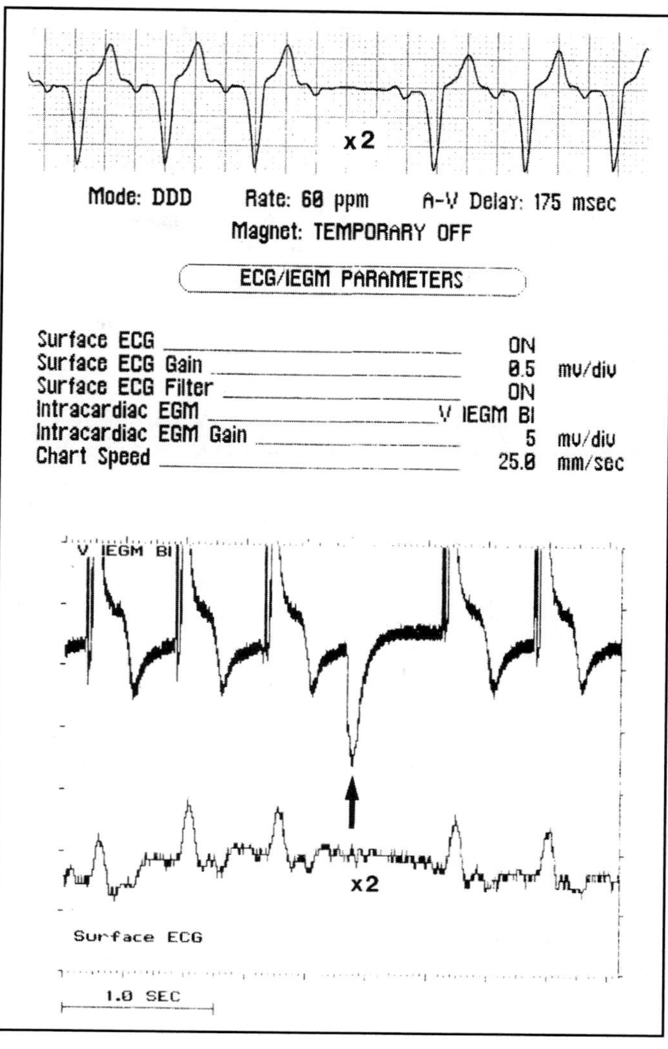

FIGURE 23–24. *Top,* DDD pacing with intermittent inhibition of the ventricular channel by false signals caused by defective lead insulation. The tiny bipolar stimuli are not discernible. A-V delay = 175 msec. The pacemaker senses the P wave and triggers an appropriate ventricular stimulus. Oversensing of a false signal from an intermittent insulation defect causes a pause (x2) exactly double the duration of the undisturbed Vp-Vp interval during 1:1 atrial tracking.

Bottom, Simultaneous recording of telemetered bipolar ventricular electrogram (V IEGM BI) and surface ECG. The ventricular electrogram registers a false signal (arrow) generated by the insulation defect. The signal measures approximately 10 mV. and is invisible on the surface ECG. The ventricular channel senses the false signal and inhibits the release of Vp. The prolonged Vp-Vp interval is an exact multiple of the atrial-driven Vp-Vp interval because timing of the P wave or sinus rhythm remains undisturbed. In contrast, during continual AV sequential (Ap-Vp) pacing (without magnet application), oversensing of a false signal produces pauses that are not multiples of the Vp-Vp interval because the timing of Ap (terminating the atrial escape interval) depends on the timing of the false signal that initiates the atrial escape interval. (Compare with Fig. 23–19.)

the time and duration of changes in pacemaker function such as automatic mode conversion in response to supraventricular tachyarrhythmias. Event markers depicting pacing and sensing are recorded simultaneously with the ECG and permit real-time evaluation of the pacing system and facilitate troubleshooting (Figs. 23–7A, 23–12, 23–14 to 23–16, and 23–23). Although the actual sensed signal cannot be identified, event markers indicate how the pacemaker interprets a specific paced or sensed event and provide precise representation of timing intervals. While the telemetered endocardial electrogram is generally less useful than event markers, it may demonstrate the nature of a malfunction caused by lead displacement or fracture, undersensing due to a poor signal, or oversensing, especially when the nature of the signal cannot be determined from the ECG (Figs. 23–12 and 23–24). The telemetered atrial electrogram or atrial event markers can easily document the existence of retrograde VA conduction and its precise duration (Fig. 23–14). In the future, replay of stored electrograms will improve the diagnosis of arrhythmias and pacemaker malfunction.

Finally, long-term ECG recordings help to investigate pacemaker function and the significance of syncope, dizziness, and palpitations.[207] Syncope in pacemaker patients is often due to causes other than pacemaker malfunction.[207,208]

ELECTRICAL DEVICES TO TREAT TACHYCARDIAS

Electric devices can be used to treat tachycardias by preventing the tachycardia onset or terminating the tachycardia after it has developed. Techniques to prevent tachycardia onset are applicable to a very small number of patients and include pacing at normal or increased rates to suppress bradycardia-dependent tachyarrhythmias such as torsades de pointes associated with a long Q-T syndrome (see p. 685). In the absence of bradycardia, an increase in pacing rate rarely successfully suppresses refractory ventricular tachyarrhythmias chronically. Dual-chamber pacing with a short A-V interval can prevent some AV nodal or AV reciprocating tachycardias, and rapid continuous atrial pacing can be used to produce a fast atrial tachycardia with a high degree of AV block to override a slower atrial tachycardia associated with a faster ventricular rate, but ablative cures are preferable.

SUPRAVENTRICULAR TACHYCARDIA. Rapid pacing and/or premature stimulation can be used to terminate AV nodal and AV reciprocating tachycardias, atrial flutter, and some atrial tachycardias. Automatic tachycardia-terminating pacemakers are no longer popular for most patients with supraventricular tachycardias because ablation procedures can be curative (see p. 621). Only when drug therapy is ineffective or not tolerated and the patient has undergone an unsuccessful curative procedure or refuses to have it should an antitachycardia pacemaker be considered. Considering the fact that catheter ablative therapy and surgery successfully eliminate AV nodal and AV reentry in over 95 per cent of patients with a mortality close to zero, success rates of antitachycardia pacing are not impressive.

IMPLANTABLE CARDIOVERTER-DEFIBRILLATORS (ICDs)

Table 23–9 outlines the indications for ICD implantation. These guidelines are more liberal than those drawn up in 1991 by two separate task forces before the general availability of third-generation transvenous ICDs.[21,209] The efficacy of antitachycardia pacing for ventricular tachycardia (VT) termination by an easily implantable transvenous device with backup defibrillation has encouraged the use of ICDs often as first-line therapy for hemodynamically tolerated VT with or without antiarrhythmic agents. ICDs are powered by lithium silver vanadium pentoxide cells and have decreased in weight and volume from 250 to 280 gm (150 cm^3) to 132 gm (83 cm^3), and future devices will soon be 60 cm^3.

While longevity varies depending on the use of the ICD in an individual patient, it is in the range of 4 to 5 years with the ability to deliver about 300 shocks. ICDs utilize a hierarchical approach to the treatment of VT with multiprogrammable tiered therapy (antitachycardia pacing, low-energy cardioversion, defibrillation, and backup VVI pacing) together with advanced diagnostic and telemetry function and the capability of testing therapy through noninvasive programmed stimulation by the induction of VT and ventricular fibrillation (VF)[210–212] (Fig. 23–25). The maximum output is usually delivered for defibrillation when synchronization of the shock is not necessary. Therapy can be programmed to escalate from pacing to low-energy synchronized cardioversion to high-energy defibrillation, depending on the arrhythmia and the patient's response. Energy of the shocks is programmable, generally 0.1 to 35 or 40 J. The number of consecutive cycles before tachycardia recognition is programmable, and therefore the time to respond with therapy, is variable. Charging to about 30 J takes 5 to 15 seconds (depending on circumstances). The number of times the device retries therapy is programmable. For VF, if the first shock fails, the device will recharge and deliver up to three to six additional shocks according to the manufacturer. In early "committed" ICDs, delivery of therapy occurred despite spontaneous termination of arrhythmia during capacitor charging. Such a response can cause unnecessary shocks that may occasionally induce VT or VF (device proarrhythmia). To prevent shocks for nonsustained arrhythmias, newer devices are "uncommitted." A "second look" confirms that the arrhythmia is still present during capacitor charging and immediately before the shock is to be delivered. A shock is therefore aborted if an arrhythmia terminates spontaneously.

ARRHYTHMIA SENSING. ICDs contain complex sensing circuitry that permits reliable sensing of small signals during VF without oversensing in normal sinus rhythm.[213,214] ICDs are biased for high detection sensitivity (rather than specificity). Most commonly, rate only (for a programmable duration) is used for VT and VF detection. Rate sensing alone is quite sensitive but not specific because therapy can be delivered for supraventricular tachycardia when the rate exceeds the programmed upper rate cutoff (Fig. 23–26). Some ICDs possess a rate or interval *stability* criterion that defines how widely the R-R interval can vary and still be sensed as VT or VF. This feature improves device diagnosis of atrial fibrillation and can prevent unnecessary shocks.[215] A less helpful feature is the *sudden onset* criterion to differentiate the sudden onset of a high-rate VT from the more gradual increase in ventricular rate with sinus tachycardia. These and other measures to improve specificity must be used with care because they reduce the sensitivity of the detection algorithm.[216] Spurious shocks due to supraventricular tachyarrhythmias remain an important problem. Future ICDs will incorporate improved

TABLE 23–9 INDICATIONS FOR ICDs

ICD Implantation Generally Indicated
1. Patients with hypotensive ventricular tachycardia (VT) or ventricular fibrillation (VF) not associated with acute ischemia/infarction, severe electrolyte imbalance, or drug toxicity in whom EP-guided therapy or ambulatory monitoring cannot be used to accurately predict efficacy of therapy (e.g., in patients in whom VT/VF is noninducible during EP testing, patients with nonischemic cardiomyopathy) and in patients who remain at high risk despite guided antiarrhythmic drug therapy (e.g., patients with severe left ventricular dysfunction).
2. VF or hypotensive VT with contraindications to drug or surgical therapy (including drug intolerance and noncompliance).
3. Persistently inducible clinically relevant VT or VF during EP testing despite drug therapy, corrective surgery, or catheter ablation.
4. Recurrent episodes of spontaneous VT or VF despite EP- or Holter-guided antiarrhythmic drug therapy.
5. Unexplained syncope in a patient with hypotensive VT inducible during EPS with characteristics 1, 2, or 3 above.
6. Highly symptomatic long Q-T interval syndromes despite medical therapy (with or without permanent pacemaker implantation).
ICD Implantation an Option but No Medical Consensus
1. Hypotensive VT or VF in a patient in whom serial drug testing is possible but ICD implantation is preferred over drug/ablative therapy.
2. Inducible nonclinical VT following drug, ablative, or surgical therapy in high-risk patients.
3. VT/VF apparently controlled by drug, surgical, or ablative therapy in a patient in whom the longterm efficacy of such treatment is unknown (e.g., hypertrophic cardiomyopathy).
ICD Implantation Generally Not Indicated
1. Frequent recurrent (e.g., daily) or incessant VT or VF.
2. VT or VF attributable to acute ischemia/infarction, severe electrolyte imbalance, drug toxicity or other reversible causes.
3. Recurrent syncope of undetermined etiology without inducible VT/VF during EP testing.
4. VF secondary to atrial fibrillation in the Wolff-Parkinson-White syndrome.
5. Hemodynamically significant VT/VF in a patient with limited life expectancy (<6 months). This may include patients with Class IV heart failure who are not heart transplant candidates.
6. Surgical, medical, or psychiatric contraindications.

Reproduced with permission from Roelke, M., O'Nunain, S., Ruskin, J. N.: Implantable cardioverter-defibrillator: A clinician's guide to patient and device selection, The Newspaper of Cardiology, Sept/Oct 1994.

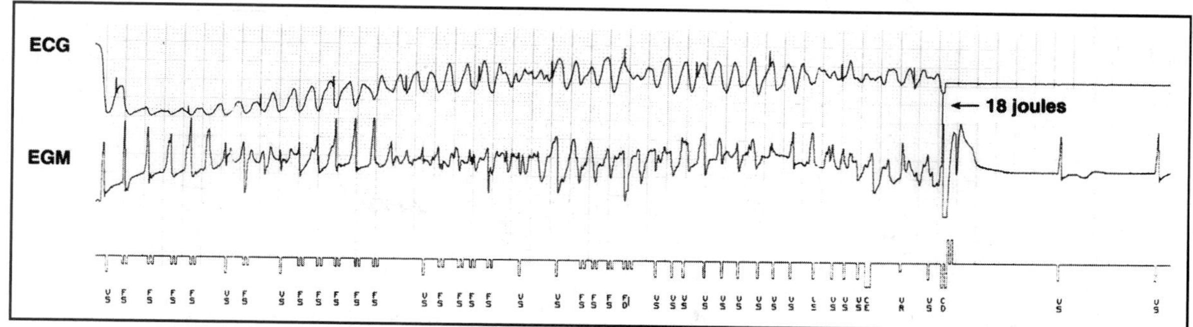

FIGURE 23–25. Termination of ventricular fibrillation by ICD. Scalar ECG and intracavitary electrogram record ventricular fibrillation. Marker channel senses fibrillation (FS) for most, but not all, impulses. Only 75 per cent of the intervals need to be counted for device diagnosis of ventricular fibrillation. Defibrillation (CD) is accomplished with an 18-J shock.

electrogram recognition and an atrial lead for better diagnosis of arrhythmias (also for atrial pacing and/or atrial defibrillation), and biosensors will provide on-line hemodynamic monitoring to better detect life-threatening arrhythmias.[217–219]

ICD Implantation

THORACOTOMY IMPLANTATION. ICDs were originally implanted by thoracotomy, now an outmoded approach. Two to three defibrillating patches were applied inside or outside the pericardium. Additional pacemaker electrodes were applied epicardially and less often transvenously. All leads were then tunneled subcutaneously to the device implanted in an abdominal pocket in the left upper quadrant.

NONTHORACOTOMY IMPLANTATION. Most ICDs are now implanted transvenously, and small devices can now be placed pectorally.[220] Transvenous systems generally utilize two relatively long intravascular spring or coil electrodes (with or without subcutaneous patches) for defibrillation. Earlier systems with a monophasic waveform were successful in 70 to 80 per cent of patients.[215,221–225] Contemporary devices with a biphasic waveform (reversal of shock polarity) are associated with a lower energy requirement for defibrillation and allow successful transvenous ICD implantation in virtually all patients[220,225–232] (including epicardial systems[233]). It is not known why a biphasic waveform is superior to a monophasic one for transvenous and epicardial defibrillation. There are presently three transvenous systems according to lead configuration: (1) single right ventricular (RV) lead (two spring electrodes, one in the RV and one in the superior vena cava, and a third tip electrode that participates in the pacing/sensing functions)[234]; (2) an RV lead (one spring electrode in the RV and distal electrodes that participate in the pacing/sensing functions) and a second lead (spring electrode) placed in the superior vena cava, right atrium, right atrial appendage, coronary sinus, or left inominate vein[215,221,235]; and (3) an RV lead as in (2), with an electrically "active" pacemaker titanium shell that obviates the need for a second spring electrode.[236,237] Subcutaneous patches can be used to provide a variety of configurations to lower the defibrillation threshold. Most monophasic systems require a tripolar lead arrangement with a subcutaneous patch (bidirectional shock).[215,221,238] The introduction of biphasic shock devices has greatly reduced the number of VF inductions during implantation and the need for subcutaneous patches, required in only 5 to 15 per cent of cases.[217,220,228,230,231,239,239a]

Careful testing at the time of implantation must establish adequate electrograms (voltage and slew rate) for sensing during sinus rhythm, VT, and VF, as well as appropriate pacing thresholds. The optimal pulse duration of the shock is calculated from the defibrillation impedance derived by delivering a low-energy test shock during the patient's normal rhythm. The lowest energy that consistently defibrillates (LED) is determined by inducing VF and delivering a test shock (usually starting with 15 to 20 J 10 to 15 sec after VF induction).[240,241] The LED should be at least 10 J less than the maximum output of the device.[223] As a rule, LED testing requires three consecutive successful shocks delivered at least 5 min apart. Even if the ICD is being used to treat VT alone, it must be shown to defibrillate as well. In contrast to the LED, the actual defibrillation threshold (DFT) is a more complex parameter that characterizes the probability of successful defibrillation (in the form of a dose-response sigmoid curve).[240,241] Precise DFT testing requires too many shocks to be practical clinically. Although it is strictly incorrect, the terms LED and DFT are often used interchangeably.

Antiarrhythmic drugs can alter the LED and DFT. Chronic amiodarone administration raises the DFT.[36,37] Class 1B agents (lidocaine and rarely mexiletine)[243,244] and class 1C agents (flecainide and moricizine)[245] also can increase the DFT. Animal data for propafenone are conflicting.[246,247] Propanolol (but not timolol) and verapamil increase DFT,[248–250] while class 1A agents have little effect. Sotalol decreases DFT.[244,251] Continuing efficacy of the ICD should be reevaluated whenever antiarrhythmic therapy is altered.

Antitachycardia Pacing and Low-Energy Synchronized Cardioversion

Rapid pacing often can terminate VT with a cycle length >250 msec.[252] Antitachycardia pacing (ATP) is best used in patients with hemodynamically stable VT with a cycle length equal to or more than 300 msec. ICDs can deliver a large number of ATP algorithms. A common method, adaptive burst pacing, starts with a cycle length shorter than that of the VT by a given percentage, usually 80 to 90 per cent. Pacing bursts can be fixed (constant cycle length) or autodecremental (ramp pacing), where each successive cycle in the burst is decremented[253,254] (Fig. 23–26). Both methods are commonly used and equally effective.[215,254–257] Other variations include a scanning function that introduces each burst with increasing prematurity and a program that adds a stimulus to each successive burst. All these therapies, number of stimuli in a burst, and the number of ATP attempts are programmable. The success of ATP increases in parallel with increase in VT cycle length.[256,257] ATP is successful in 60 to 90 per cent of carefully selected cases,[215,254,256–260] but the risk of acceleration or inducing VF ranges from 3 to 35 per cent and is inversely related to VT cycle length.[230,253,254,256–258,261]

The success and complications of low-energy synchronized cardioversion are similar to those of

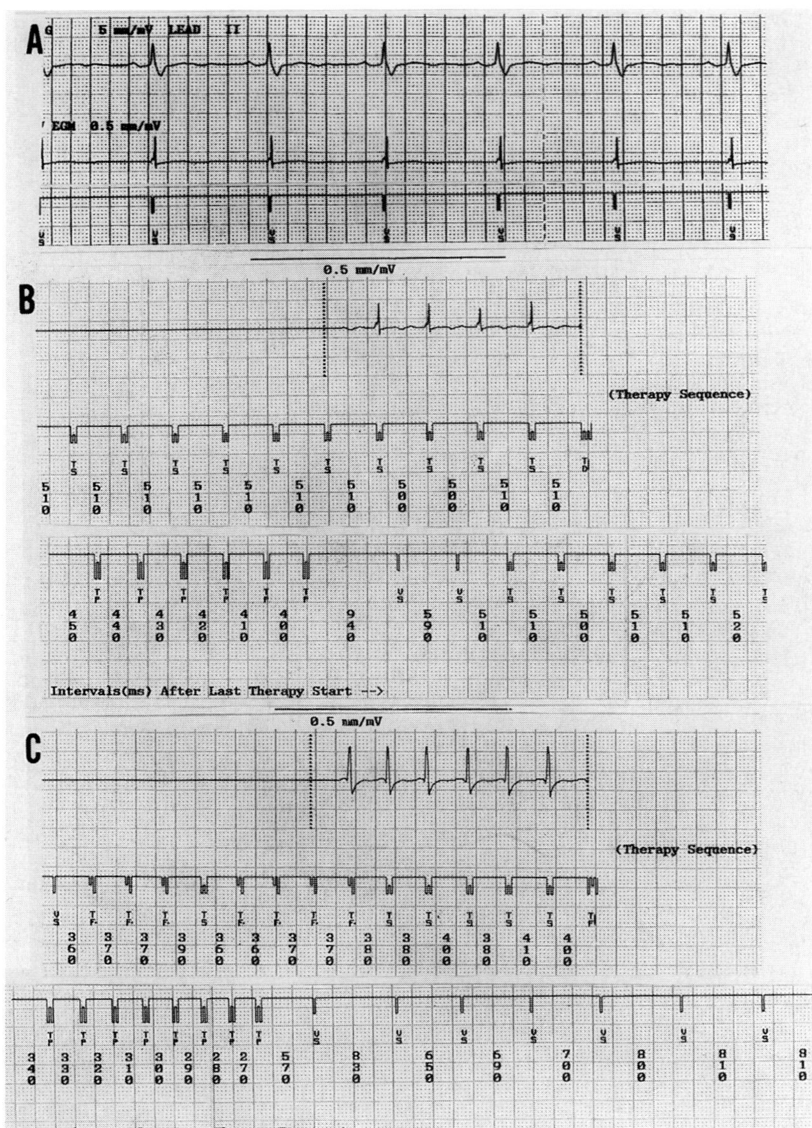

FIGURE 23–26. Electrogram recordings from a Medtronic Jewel ICD. Two different tachycardia zones were programmed for detection and therapy. In the top panel, (*A*) lead II is recorded simultaneously with the ventricular electrogram and an event channel that registers ventricular sensing (VS). In the middle panel (*B*), the contour of the ventricular electrogram is unchanged, indicating a supraventricular rhythm, but the rate is about 120/min. (Msec are given vertically beneath each cycle). This supraventricular tachycardia (probably a sinus tachycardia) falls in the tachycardia sensing zone, as indicated by the tachycardia sensing (TS) markings. When a sufficient number of cycles meet the criteria for tachycardia detection (TD), therapy in the form of rapid pacing at decreasing cycle lengths (450 to 400 msec) is delivered. Sinus tachycardia resumes after a pause of 940 msec. In the bottom panel, (*C*) the device detects a ventricular tachycardia (note electrogram change) that hovers between fast (TF) and slow (TS) ventricular tachycardia zones. Antitachycardia pacing at decreasing cycle lengths (340 to 270 msec) terminates the ventricular tachycardia, with restoration of a slower rhythm, probably sinus.

ATP.[218,253,256,257,260,262,263] Low-energy synchronized cardioversion sometimes works better than ATP. However, shocks of 0.5 to 3.0 J are generally painful and poorly tolerated, so low-energy synchronized cardioversion is often used as secondary therapy.[218] ATP saves the patient the discomfort of shock delivery and can lead to a significant reduction in the number of shocks. Both ATP and low-energy synchronized cardioversion must be carefully individualized. An ICD automatically switches to more aggressive therapy (including defibrillation) whenever it identifies failure of programmed therapy with ATP or low-energy synchronized cardioversion or when VT acceleration or VF occurs as a result of therapy.

COMPLICATIONS. The mortality of ICD implantation by thoracotomy is about 3 to 5 per cent and is less than 1 per cent when implanted transvenously.[264] The morbidity of the transvenous procedure is considerably less than that associated with thoracotomy. The complications of transvenous ICDs include those of venous access and pocket formation (as with pacemakers), infection, and lead problems such as perforation, displacement, fracture, or insulation breakdown, as well as migration or fracture, crinkling, and erosion of subcutaneous patches.[221,264–268] Other complications include high DFT, component or battery failure, inappropriate shocks for unsustained VT or sinus tachycardia or supraventricular tachyarrhythmias (that may precipitate VT or VF), undersensing, oversensing (T wave, signals from lead fracture or loose connection with or without myopotential oversensing, counting of non-ICD pacemaker stimuli), and the induction of atrial fibrillation by a shock.[222,269–272] Psychological complications are important and include the fear of painful shocks, anxiety, and depression that may respond to psychological counseling and rarely may lead to explantation.[273,274]

Follow-up

Acceptable ICD function, including its ability to defibrillate, is tested before the patient is discharged. After implantation, about half the patients require antiarrhythmic drug therapy to control sustained or nonsustained VT to avoid repeated device therapy. However, when an implanted ICD is in place, the number of drugs and dosages can be reduced to avoid side effects, with the knowledge that the ICD will adequately treat an occasional "breakthrough" tachycardia. Patients should be seen every 2 to 3 months, depending on individual responses. In older ICDs, the capacitors of the device needed periodic reformation (charged and discharged) for proper continuing function. Newer devices provide for automatic capacitor reformation at programmable intervals.

Periodic chest x-rays should be done in the first 6 months to detect transvenous lead and patch displacement. The DFT of transvenous systems can rise in the first 2 months, so DFT testing should be repeated at 2 months, especially in patients with a relatively high DFT at the time of implantation.[275,276] At the time of each visit, the device is investigated to determine the number and type of events, type of therapy delivered, and the patient's response. Event registers, stored intervals, and/or electrograms (from the sensing electrodes) allow retrospective validation of events that activate the ICD. The pacing and sensing functions are evaluated in the usual manner, together with determination of pacing lead impedance and recording of the ventricular electrogram. Unfortunately, at the time of follow-up, the high-voltage shock impedance (of the defibrillating leads) cannot be measured without delivery of a shock. The elective replacement time of the device is indicated by increase in battery voltage and an increase in the charge time. The majority of patients receive shocks during long-term follow-up.[277] The likelihood of appropriate shocks increases with decreasing left ventricular ejection fraction, inducible sustained VT before treatment, inducible sustained VT while on drug therapy, and the induction of VT by only one or two stimuli. Multiple ICD discharges, especially by devices with limited memory, usually require hospitalization for further investigation.

STORED ELECTROGRAMS. Replay of stored electrograms (and simultaneous display of event markers) provides data similar to Holter monitoring or an ECG loop recorder in that it allows review of device diagnosis of arrhythmias, triggering mechanism of arrhythmias, and response to therapy.[54,278–280] Significant changes in electrogram morphology allow differentiation of VT from supraventricular tachycardia in 93 per cent of cases[278] (Figs. 23–26 and 23–27). Electrogram analysis is also useful in troubleshooting and for management decisions to prevent the delivery of unnecessary shocks, e.g., spurious shocks from lead fracture (Fig. 23–28), and double counting of QRS and T wave. The incidence of shocks for non-life-threatening rhythms is about 20 to 30 per cent, often due to atrial fibrillation.[260] Device reprogramming or antiarrhythmic drug therapy (beta blockers for sinus tachycardia and digitalis for atrial fibrillation) based on analysis of stored electrograms has led to a dramatic reduction of ICD response to non-VT rhythms.[279] Stored electrograms also can document abnormalities leading to aborted shocks in uncommitted ICDs. Stored electrograms have indicated that preceding symptoms are not always a reliable indicator of the arrhythmia that triggered ICD therapy. Some patients with rapid VT or even VF can receive appropriate therapy before the development of significant symptoms such as syncope.[281] Severe symptoms preceding a shock suggest VT or VF as the underlying rhythm.

Impact on Survival

It is generally accepted that the ICD reduces the incidence of sudden death to ≤1 to 2 per cent annually in high-risk patients.[264,282] The impact of ICD therapy on overall cardiovascular survival is uncertain because no controlled randomized trials comparing the ICD with other forms of therapy have been reported. Total mortality of ICD patients is high because of poor LV function, myocardial infarction, and congestive heart failure.[283–285] A number of large trials are underway to determine the effectiveness of drug therapy versus ICD and whether prophylactic ICD implantation might benefit patients with a high risk of sudden death.[286–296]

Future Directions

With the "active" system, the DFT is 24 J or less in 98 per cent of patients.[236] The system promises to be nearly as simple to implant as a VVI pacemaker, with profound implications for safety (low number of VF inductions), cost, reliability, and use. Pectoral implantation should increase lead longevity by avoiding the stress imposed on tunneled leads to the abdomen. This and elimination of subcutaneous patches and the use of a single incision will reduce complications, infection, and surgical implantation time to <1 hour. Local anesthesia with sedation will largely re-

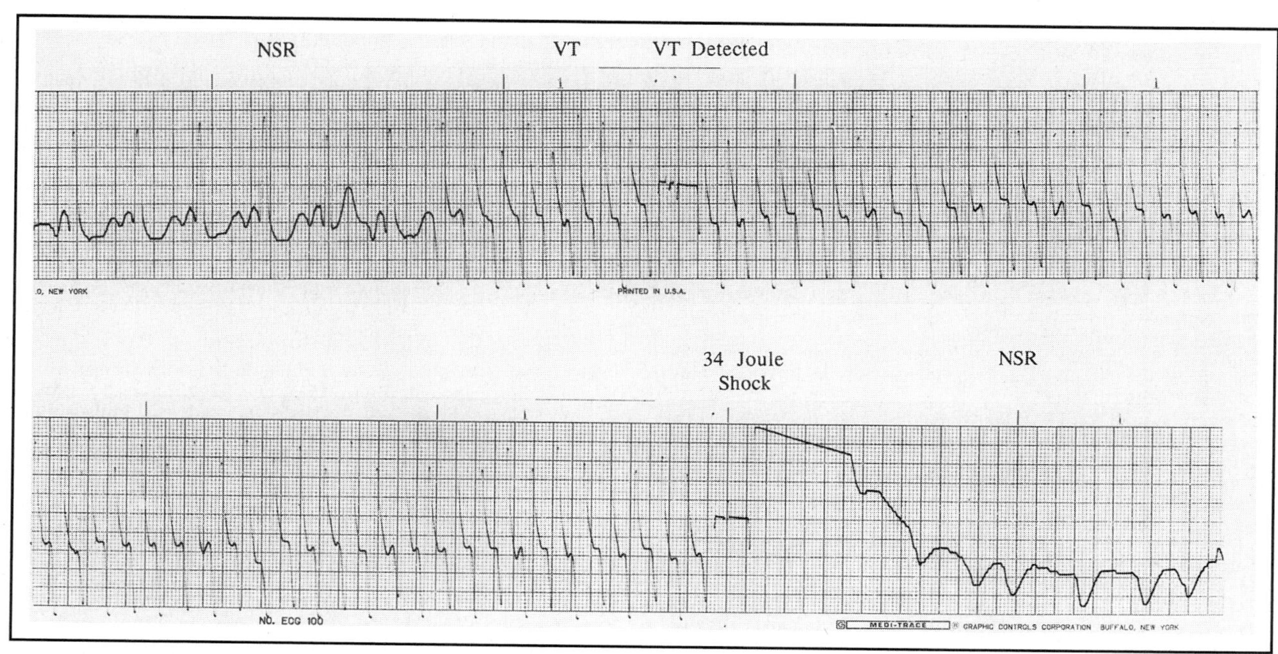

FIGURE 23–27. Intracavitary electrogram recordings from an AICD P2 Endotak demonstrating the transition from sinus rhythm (NSR, note negative P wave preceding each ventricular depolarization) to ventricular tachycardia (VT, note change in electrogram and loss of preceding P wave), prompting, in the lower tracing, a 34-J shock with restoration of sinus rhythm. This device uses an integrated bipolar sensing system from the distal tip electrode to the large right ventricular shocking coil, and is able to record P waves.

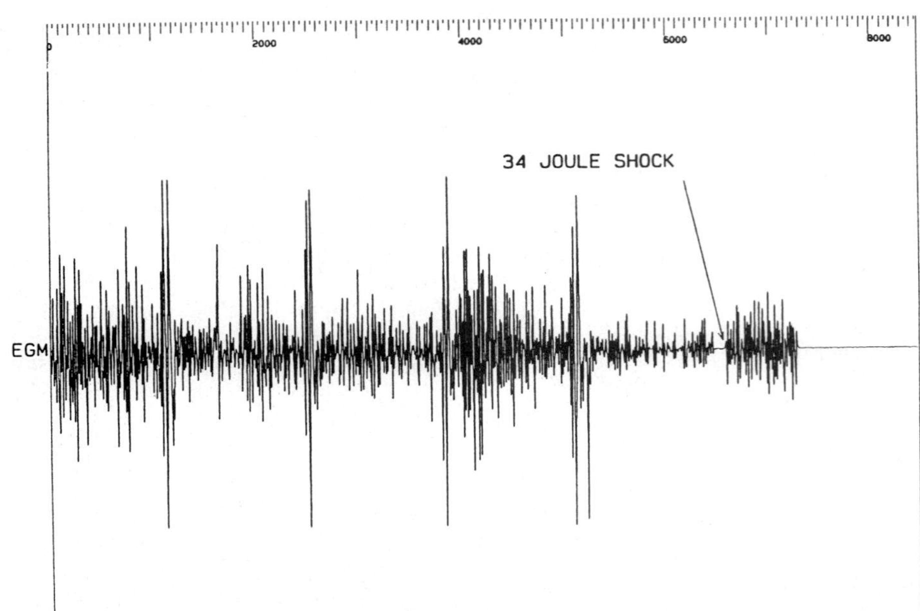

FIGURE 23–28. Electrogram recordings from a Cadence ICD demonstrating recording artifacts due to a lead insulation break. The ICD erroneously sensed these artifacts as ventricular depolarizations and delivered a 34-J shock.

place general anesthesia. These advances will further broaden the indications for ICDs. Future ICDs will be smaller (60 to 70 cm^3), especially if more efficient waveforms and better leads permit a maximum output of 20 to 25 J. Leads of different design will be smaller, while new subcutaneous patch arrays will ensure transvenous implantation in 100 per cent of cases. The devices will incorporate dual-chamber pacing (now required in 5 to 15 per cent of patients[210]), improved sensing and diagnostic algorithms, and more memory with extended electrogram storage. Transtelephonic monitoring and programming will be available. Overall costs will drop because of brief hospitalizations, fewer complications, and the use of less sophisticated "shock-only devices" with backup VVI pacing in selected patients.

REFERENCES

PACEMAKER MODALITIES AND FUNCTION

1. Kusumoto, F. M., and Goldschlager, N.: Medical progress: Cardiac pacing. N. Engl. J. Med. *334*:89, 1996.
1a. Bernstein, A. D., Camm, A. J., Fletcher, R. D., et al.: The NASPE/BPEG generic pacemaker code for antibradyarrhythmia and adaptive-rate pacing and antitachyarrhythmia devices. PACE *10*:794, 1987.
2. Bartecchi, C. E.: Temporary pacing catheter electrodes. *In* Bartecchi, C. E., and Mann, D. E. (eds.): Temporary Cardiac Pacing. Chicago, Precept Press, 1990, p. 268.
3. Fitzpatrick, A., and Sutton, R.: A guide to temporary pacing. Br. Med. J. *304*:365, 1992.
4. Goldberger, J., Kruse, J., Ehlert, F. A., and Kadish, A.: Temporary transvenous pacemaker placement: What criteria constitute an adequate pacing site? Am. Heart J. *126*:488, 1993.
5. Bongiorni, M. G., and Bedendi, N.: Atrial stimulation by means of floating electrodes: A multicenter experience, The Multicenter Study Group. PACE *15*:1977, 1992.
6. Vrouchos, G. T., and Vardas, P. E.: Sensing through the esophagus for temporary atrial synchronous ventricular VDD pacing. PACE *14*:511, 1991.
7. Santini, M., Ansalone, G., Cacciatore, G., and Turitto, G.: Transesophageal pacing. PACE *13*:298, 1990.
8. Guarnerio, M., Furlanello, F., Vergara, G., et al.: Electropharmacological testing by transesophageal atrial pacing in inducible supraventricular tachyarrhythmias: A good approach for selection of long-term antiarrhythmic therapy. Eur. Heart J. *13*:763, 1992.
9. Biffi, A., Ammirati, F., Caselli, G., et al.: Usefulness of transesophageal pacing during exercise for evaluating palpitations in top-level athletes. Am. J. Cardiol. *72*:922, 1993.
10. Zoll, P. M.: Noninvasive cardiac stimulation revisited. PACE *13*:2014, 1990.
11. Luck, J. C., and Markel, M. L.: Clinical applications of external pacing: A renaissance? PACE *14*:1299, 1991.
12. Trigano, J. A., Birkui, P. J., and Mugica, J.: Noninvasive transcutaneous cardiac pacing: Modern instrumentation and new perspectives. PACE *15*:1937, 1992.
13. Grubb, B. P., Markel, M. L., Artman, S. E., et al.: Observations on induction and termination of paroxysmal supraventricular tachycardia by external pacing. PACE *15*:1944, 1992.
14. Grubb, B. P., Temesy-Armos, P., Hahn, H., and Elliott, L.: The use of external, noninvasive pacing for the termination of ventricular tachycardia in the emergency department setting. Ann. Emerg. Med. *21*:174, 1992.
15. de la Serna, F., Meier, B., Pande, A. K., et al.: Coronary and left ventricular pacing as standby in invasive cardiology. Cathet. Cardiovasc. Diagn. *25*:285, 1992.
16. Laird, J. R., Hull, R., Stajduhar, K. C., et al.: Transcoronary cardiac pacing during myocardial ischemia. Cathet. Cardiovasc. Diagn. *30*:162, 1993.
17. Lévy, S., Lauribe, P., Dolla, E., et al.: A randomized comparison of external and internal cardioversion of chronic atrial fibrillation. Circulation *86*:1415, 1992.
18. Barold, S. S.: Narrow QRS Mobitz type II second-degree AV block in acute myocardial infarction: True or false? Am. J. Cardiol. *67*:1291, 1991.
19. Behar, S., Zissman, E., Zion, M., et al.: Prognostic significance of second-degree block in inferior wall acute myocardial infarction. Am. J. Cardiol. *72*:831, 1993.
20. Murphy, P., Morton, P., Murtagh, J. G., et al.: Hemodynamic effects of different temporary pacing modes for the management of bradycardias complicating acute myocardial infarction. PACE *15*:381, 1992.
21. Dreifus, L. S., Fisch, C., Griffin, J. C., et al.: Guidelines for implantation of cardiac pacemakers and antiarrhythmia devices: A report of the American College of Cardiology/American Heart Association Task Force on Assessment of Diagnostic and Therapeutic Procedures (Committee on Pacemaker Implantation). J. Am. Coll. Cardiol. *18*:1, 1991.
22. Barold, S. S.: ACC/AHA guidelines for implantation of cardiac pacemakers: How accurate are the definitions of atrioventricular and intraventricular conduction blocks? PACE *16*:1221, 1993.
23. Barold, S. S.: Indications for permanent pacemakers: Comments on the 1991 ACC/AHA and BPEG guidelines. *In* Santini, M., Pistolese, M., and Alliegro, A. (eds.): Progress in Clinical Pacing 1992. Mt. Kisco, N.Y., Futura, 1993, p. 439.
24. Rardon, D. P., Miles, W. M., Mitrani, R. D., et al.: Atrioventricular block and dissociation. *In* Zipes, D. P., and Jalife, J. (eds.): Cardiac Electrophysiology: From Cell to Bedside. 2nd ed. Philadelphia, W. B. Saunders Company, 1995, p. 935.
25. Cooper, J. P., Fraser, A. G., and Penny, W. J.: Reversibility and benign recurrence of complete heart block in athletes. Int. J. Cardiol. *35*:118, 1992.
26. Kim, Y. H., O'Nunain, S., Trouton, T., et al.: Pseudo-pacemaker syndrome following inadvertent fast pathway ablation for atrioventricular nodal reentrant tachycardia. J. Cardiovasc. Electrophysiol. *4*:178, 1993.
27. Mabo, P., DePlace, C., Gras, D., et al.: Isolated first degree AV block: An indication for permanent DDD pacing. PACE *16*(Abs.):1123, 1993.
28. Odemuyiwa, O., and Camm, A. J.: Prophylactic pacing for prevention of sudden death in congenital complete heart block? PACE *15*:1526, 1992.
29. Solti, F., Szatmary, L., Vecsey, T., et al.: Congenital complete heart block associated with QT prolongation. Eur. Heart J. *13*:1080, 1992.
30. Barold, S. S., Falkoff, M. D., Ong, L. S., et al.: Atrioventricular block: New insights. *In* Barold, S. S., and Mugica, J. (eds.): New Perspectives in Cardiac Pacing 2. Mt. Kisco, N.Y., Futura, 1991, p. 23.

31. Coplan, N. L., Morales, M. C., Romanello, P., et al.: Exercise-induced atrioventricular block: Influence of myocardial ischemia. Chest *100:*1728, 1991.
32. Gaggioli, G., Bottoni, N., Brignole, M., et al.: Progression to 2d and 3d grade atrioventricular block in patients after electrostimulation for bundle-branch block and syncope: A long-term study. G. Ital. Cardiol. *24:*409, 1994.
33. Bergfeldt, L., Edvardsson, N., Rosenqvist, M., et al.: Atrioventricular block progression in patients with bifascicular block assessed by repeated electrocardiography and a bradycardia-detecting pacemaker. Am. J. Cardiol. *74:*1129, 1994.
34. Sneddon, J. F., and Camm, A. J.: Sinus node disease: Current concepts in diagnosis and therapy. Drugs *44:*728, 1992.
35. Katritsis, D., Ward, D. E., and Camm, A. J.: Can we treat carotid sinus syndrome? PACE *14:*1367, 1991.
36. Benditt, D. G., Remole, S., Asso, A., et al.: Cardiac pacing for carotid sinus syndrome and vasovagal syncope. *In* Barold, S. S., and Mugica, J. (eds.): New Perspectives in Cardiac Pacing 3. Mt. Kisco, N.Y., Futura, 1993, p. 15.
37. Maloney, J. D., Jaeger, F. J., Rizo-Patron, C., and Zhu, D. W.: The role of pacing for the management of neurally mediated syncope: Carotid sinus syndrome and vasovagal syncope. Am. Heart J. *127:*1030, 1994.
38. Petersen, M. E., Chamberlain-Webber, R., Fitzpatrick, A. P., et al.: Permanent pacing for cardioinhibitory malignant vasovagal syndrome. Br. Heart J. *71:*274, 1994.
39. Benditt, D. G., Petersen, M., Lurie, K. G., et al.: Cardiac pacing for prevention of recurrent vasovagal syncope. Ann. Intern. Med. *122:*204, 1995.
40. Petersen, M. E., Price, D., Williams, T., et al.: Short AV interval VDD pacing does not prevent tilt induced vasovagal syncope in patients with cardioinhibitory vasovagal syndrome. PACE *17:*882, 1994.
41. Fananapazir, L., Epstein, N. D., Curiel, R. V., et al.: Long-term results of dual-chamber (DDD) pacing in obstructive hypertrophic cardiomyopathy: Evidence for progressive symptomatic and hemodynamic improvement and reduction of left ventricular hypertrophy. Circulation *90:*2731, 1994.
42. Jeanrenaud, X., Goy, J. J., and Kappenberger, L.: Effects of dual-chamber pacing in hypertrophic obstructive cardiomyopathy. Lancet *339:*1318, 1992.
43. Hochleitner, M., Hörtnagl, H., Hörtnagl, H., et al.: Long-term efficacy of physiologic dual chamber pacing in the treatment of end-stage idiopathic dilated cardiomyopathy. Am. J. Cardiol. *70:*1320, 1992.
44. Eldar, M., Griffin, J. C., VanHare, G. F., et al.: Combined use of beta-adrenergic blocking agents and long-term cardiac pacing for patients with the long QT syndrome. J. Am. Coll. Cardiol. *20:*830, 1992.
45. Weisman, P., Chin, M. T., and Moss, A. J.: Cardiac tachypacing for severe refractory orthostatic hypotension. Ann. Intern. Med. *16:*650, 1992.
46. Grubb, B. P., Wolfe, D. A., Samoil, D., et al.: Adaptive rate pacing controlled by right ventricular preejection interval for severe refractory orthostatic hypotension. PACE *16:*801, 1993.

METHODS OF PACEMAKER IMPLANTATION

47. Byrd, C. L.: Clinical experience with the extrathoracic introducer insertion technique. PACE *16:*1781, 1993.
48. Belott, P. H., and Reynolds, D. W.: Permanent pacemaker implantation. *In* Ellenbogen, K. A., Kay, G. N., and Wilkoff, B. L. (eds.): Clinical Cardiac Pacing. Philadelphia, W. B. Saunders Company, 1995, p. 447.
49. Magney, J. E., Staplin, D. H., Flynn, D. M., and Hunter, D. W.: A new approach to percutaneous subclavian venipuncture to avoid lead fracture or central venous catheter occlusion. PACE *16:*2133, 1993.
50. Hayes, D. L., Naccarelli, G. V., Furman, S., and Parsonnet, V.: Report of the NASPE policy conference training requirements for permanent pacemaker implantation and follow-up, North American Society of Pacing and Electrophysiology. PACE *17:*6, 1994.
51. Fyke, F. E., III.: Infraclavicular lead failure: Tarnish on a golden route. PACE *16:*445, 1993.
52. Jacobs, D. M., Fink, A. S., Miller, R. P., et al.: Anatomical and morphological evaluation of pacemaker lead compression. PACE *16:*434, 1993.
53. Hoyer, M. H., Beerman, L. B., Ettedgui, J. A., et al.: Transatrial lead placement for endocardial pacing in children. Ann. Thorac. Surg. *58:*97, 1994.
54. Stokes, K. B., and Kay, G. N.: Artificial electric cardiac stimulation. *In* Ellenbogen, K. A., Kay, G. N., and Wilkoff, B. L. (eds.): Clinical Cardiac Pacing. Philadelphia, W. B. Saunders Company, 1995, p. 3.
55. Kay, G. N.: Basic aspects of cardiac pacing. *In* Ellenbogen, K. A. (ed.): Cardiac Pacing. Boston, Blackwell Scientific, 1992, p. 32.
56. Soriano, J., Almendral, J., Arenal, A., et al.: Rate-dependent failure of ventricular capture in patients treated with oral propafenone. Eur. Heart J. *13:*269, 1992.
57. Bianconi, L., Boccadamo, R., Toscano, S., et al.: Effects of oral propafenone therapy on chronic myocardial pacing threshold. PACE *15:*148, 1992.
58. Cornacchia, D., Fabbri, M., Maresta, A., et al.: Effect of steroid eluting versus conventional electrodes on propafenone induced rise in chronic ventricular pacing threshold. PACE *16:*2279, 1993.
59. Barold, S. S., McVenes, R., and Stokes, K.: Effect of drugs on pacing threshold in man and in canines: Old and new facts. *In* Barold, S. S., and Mugica, J. (eds.): New Perspectives in Cardiac Pacing 3. Mt. Kisco, N.Y., Futura, 1993, p. 57.
60. Kay, G. N., and Ellenbogen, K. A.: Sensing. *In* Ellenbogen, K. A., Kay, G. N., and Wilkoff, B. L. (eds.): Clinical Cardiac Pacing. Philadelphia, W. B. Saunders Company, 1995, p. 38.
61. Furman, S.: Sensing and timing the cardiac electrogram. *In* Furman, S., Hayes, D. L., and Holmes, D. R., Jr. (eds.): A Practice of Cardiac Pacing. 3rd ed. Mt. Kisco, N.Y., Futura, 1993, p. 89.
62. Santini, M., Ansalone, G., Cacciatore, G., and Turitto, G.: Status of single chamber atrial pacing. *In* Barold, S. S., and Mugica, J. (eds.): New Perspectives in Cardiac Pacing 2. Mt. Kisco, N.Y., Futura, 1991, p. 273.
63. Hayes, D. L.: Pacemaker polarity configuration: What is best for the patient? PACE *15:*1099, 1992.
64. Mond, H. G., and Helland, J. R.: Engineering and clinical aspects of clinical leads. *In* Ellenbogen, K. A., Kay, G. N., and Wilkoff, B. L. (eds.): Clinical Cardiac Pacing. Philadelphia, W. B. Saunders Company, 1995, p. 69.
65. Mond, H., and Stokes, K.: The electrode-tissue interface: The revolutionary role of steroid elution. PACE *15:*95, 1992.
66. Rhoden, W. E., Llewellyn, M. J., Schofield, S. W., and Bennett, D. H.: Acute and chronic performance of a steroid eluting electrode for ventricular pacing. Int. J. Cardiol. *37:*209, 1992.
67. Stamato, N. J., O'Toole, M. F., Fetter, J. G., and Enger, E. L.: The safety and efficacy of chronic ventricular pacing at 1.6 volts using a steroid eluting lead. PACE *15:*248, 1992.
68. Gillis, A. M., Rothschild, J. M., Hillier, K., et al.: A randomized comparison of a bipolar steroid-eluting electrode and a bipolar microporous platinum electrode: Implications for long-term programming. PACE *16:*964, 1993.

TYPES OF PACEMAKERS

69. Barold, S. S.: Timing cycles and operational characteristics of pacemakers. *In* Ellenbogen, K. A., Kay, G. N., and Wilkoff, B. L. (eds.): Clinical Cardiac Pacing. Philadelphia, W. B. Saunders Company, 1995, p. 567.
70. Ghani, M., Thakur, R. K., Boughner, D., et al.: Malposition of transvenous pacing lead in the left ventricle. PACE *16:*1800, 1993.
71. Shmuely, H., Erdman, S., Strasberg, B., and Rosenfeld, J. B.: Seven years of left ventricular pacing due to malposition of pacing electrode. PACE *15:*369, 1992.
72. Barold, S. S., Falkoff, M. D., Ong, L. S., and Heinle, R. A.: Electrocardiographic diagnosis of myocardial infarction during ventricular pacing. Cardiol. Clin. *5:*403, 1987.
73. Fu, L., Imai, K., Okabe, A., et al.: A possible mechanism for pacemaker-induced T-wave changes. Eur. Heart J. *13:*1173, 1992.
74. Barold, S. S.: Ventricular- versus atrial-based lower rate timing in dual chamber pacemakers: Does it really matter? PACE *18:*83, 1995.
75. Furman, S.: Comprehension of pacemaker cycles. *In* Furman, S., Hayes, D. L., and Holmes, D. R., Jr. (eds.): A Practice of Cardiac Pacing. 3rd ed. Mt. Kisco, N.Y., Futura, 1993, p. 135.
76. Irwin, M., Harris, L., Cameron, D., et al.: DDI pacing: Indications, expectations, and follow-up. PACE *17:*274, 1994.
77. Sulke, N., Drisas, A., Bostock, J., et al.: "Subclinical" pacemaker syndrome: A randomized study of symptom free patients with ventricular demand (VVI) pacemakers upgraded to dual chamber devices. Br. Heart J. *67:*57, 1992.
78. Barold, S. S., and Mond, H. G.: Fallback responses of dual chamber (DDD and DDDR) pacemakers: A proposed classification. PACE *17:*1160, 1994.
79. Mond, H. G., and Barold, S. S.: Dual chamber rate adaptive pacing in patients with paroxysmal supraventricular tachyarrhythmias: Protective measures for rate control. PACE *16:*2168, 1993.
80. Barold, S. S., Falkoff, M. D., Ong, L. S., and Heinle, R. A.: Electrocardiography of contemporary DDD pacemakers: Basic concepts, upper rate response, retrograde ventriculoatrial conduction and differential diagnosis of pacemaker tachycardias. *In* Saksena, S., and Goldschlager, N. (eds.): Electrical Therapy for Cardiac Arrhythmias: Pacing, Antitachycardia Devices, Catheter Ablation. Philadelphia, W. B. Saunders Company, 1990, p. 225.
81. Barold, S. S.: The fourth decade of cardiac pacing: Hemodynamic, electrophysiological and clinical considerations in the selection of the optimal pacemaker. *In* Zipes, D. P., and Jalife, J. (eds.): Cardiac Electrophysiology: From Cell to Bedside. 2nd ed. Philadelphia, W. B. Saunders Company, 1995, p. 1366.
82. Chirife, R., Ortega, D. F., and Salazar, A. I.: Nonphysiological left heart AV intervals as a result of DDD and AAI "physiological" pacing. PACE *14:*1752, 1991.
83. Frielingsdorf, J., Gerber, A. E., and Hess, O. M.: Importance of maintained atrioventricular synchrony in patients with pacemakers. Eur. Heart J. *15:*1431, 1994.
84. Chirife, R.: Proposal of a method for automatic optimization of left heart atrioventricular interval applicable to DDD pacemakers. PACE *18:*49, 1995.
85. Camous, J. P., Raybaud, F., Dolisi, C., et al.: Interatrial conduction in patients undergoing AV stimulation: Effects of increasing right atrial stimulation rate. PACE *16:*2082, 1993.
86. Prinzen, F. W., Delhaas, T., Arts, T., and Reneman, R. S.: Asymmetrical changes in ventricular wall mass by asynchronous electrical activation of the heart. Adv. Exp. Med. Biol. *346:*257, 1993.

87. Lee, M. A., Dae, M. W., Langberg, J. J., et al.: Effects of long-term right ventricular apical pacing on left ventricular perfusion, innervation, function and histology. J. Am. Coll. Cardiol. *24*:225, 1994.
88. Daubert, C., Ritter, P., Mabo, P., et al.: AV delay optimization in DDD and DDDR pacing. *In* Barold, S. S., and Mugica, J. (eds.): New Perspectives in Cardiac Pacing 3. Mt. Kisco, N.Y., Futura, 1993, p. 259.
89. Buckingham, T. A., Janosik, D. L., and Pearson, A. C.: Pacemaker hemodynamics: Clinical implications. Prog. Cardiovasc. Dis. *34*:347, 1992.
90. Pierantozzi, A., Bocconcelli, P., and Sgarbi, E.: DDD pacemaker syndrome and atrial conduction time. PACE *17*:374, 1994.
91. Benditt, D. G., Wilbert, L., Hansen, R., et al.: Late follow-up of dual-chamber rate-adaptive pacing. Am. J. Cardiol. *71*:714, 1993.
92. Detollenaere, M., vanWassenhove, E., and Jordaens, L.: Atrial arrhythmias in dual chamber pacing and their influence on long-term mortality. PACE *15*:1846, 1992.
93. Ray, S. G., Connelly, D. T., Hughes, M., et al.: Stability of the DDD pacing mode in patients 80 years of age and older. PACE *17*:1218, 1994.

HEMODYNAMICS OF CARDIAC PACING

94. Maloney, J. D., Helguera, M. E., and Woscoboinik, J. R.: Physiology of rate-responsive pacing. Cardiol. Clin. *10*:619, 1992.
95. Oldroyd, K. G., Rae, A., Carter, R., et al.: Double blind crossover comparison of the effects of dual chamber pacing (DDD) and ventricular rate adaptive (VVIR) pacing on neuroendocrine variables, exercise performance and symptoms in complete heart block. Br. Heart J. *65*:188, 1991.
96. Griffin, J. C.: VVIR or DDDR: Does it matter? Clin. Cardiol. *14*:257, 1991.
97. Janosik, D. L., and Labovitz, A. J.: Basic physiology of cardiac pacing. *In* Ellenbogen, K. A., Kay, G. N., and Wilkoff, B. L. (eds.): Clinical Cardiac Pacing. Philadelphia, W. B. Saunders Company, 1995, p. 367.
98. Sulke, A. N., Chambers, J. B., and Sowton, E.: The effect of atrio-ventricular delay programming in patients with DDDR pacemakers. Eur. Heart J. *13*:464, 1992.
99. Mabo, P., Ritter, P., Varin, C., et al.: Intérêt d'un algorithme d'adaptation automatique du délai auriculo-ventriculaire à la fréquence atriale instantanée en stimulation cardiaque DDD. Arch. Mal. Coeur *85*:1001, 1992.
100. Ritter, P. H., Vai, F., Bonnet, J. L., et al.: Rate adaptive atrio-ventricular delay improves cardio-pulmonary performance in patients implanted with a dual chamber pacemaker for complete heart block. Eur. J. Cardiac Pacing Electrophysiol. *1*:31, 1991.
101. Potratz, J., Stierle, U., Djonlagic, H., et al.: The hemodynamic effect of a rate responsive AV delay in dual chamber pacing. PACE *16*(Abs.):920, 1993.
102. Schüller, N., and Brandt, J.: The pacemaker syndrome: Old and new causes. Clin. Cardiol. *14*:336, 1991.
103. Barold, S. S.: Pacemaker syndrome during atrial-based pacing. *In* Aubert, A. E., Ector, H., and Stroobandt, R. (eds.): Cardiac Pacing and Electrophysiology: A Bridge to the 21st Century. Dordrecht, Holland, Kluwer Academic Publishers, 1994, p. 251.
104. Ellenbogen, K. A., and Stambler, B. D.: Pacemaker syndrome. *In* Ellenbogen, K. A., Kay, G. N., and Wilkoff, B. L. (eds.): Clinical Cardiac Pacing. Philadelphia, W. B. Saunders Company, 1995, p. 419.
105. Ellenbogen, K. A., Wood, M. A., and Stambler, B.: Pacemaker syndrome: Clinical, hemodynamic and neurohumoral features. *In* Barold, S. S., and Mugica, J. (eds.): New Perspectives in Cardiac Pacing 3. Mt. Kisco, N.Y., Futura, 1993, p. 85.
106. Travill, C. M., and Sutton, R.: Pacemaker syndrome: An iatrogenic condition. Br. Heart J. *68*:163, 1992.
107. Heldman, D., Mulvihill, D., Nguyen, H., et al.: True incidence of pacemaker syndrome. PACE *13*:1742, 1990.
108. Rediker, D. E., Eagle, K. A., Homma, S., et al.: Clinical and hemodynamic comparison of VVI versus DDD pacing in patients with DDD pacemakers. Am. J. Cardiol. *63*:323, 1988.
109. Linde-Edelstam, C., Nordlander, R., Pehrsson, K., and Rydén, L.: A double-blind study of submaximal exercise tolerance and variation in paced rate in atrial synchronous compared to activity sensor modulated ventricular pacing. PACE *15*:905, 1992.
110. Linde, C.: Is atrioventricular synchronous pacing the superior treatment in patients with high degree atrioventricular block? Eur. J. Cardiac Pacing Electrophysiol. *3*:42, 1993.
111. Channon, K. M., Hargreaves, M. R., Cripps, T. R., et al.: DDD vs. VVI pacing in patients aged over 75 years with complete heart block: A double-blind crossover comparison. Q. J. Med. *87*:245, 1994.
112. Sulke, N., Chambers, J., Dritsas, A., and Sowton, E.: A randomized double-blind crossover comparison of four rate-responsive pacing modes. J. Am. Coll. Cardiol. *17*:696, 1991.
113. Sulke, N., Chambers, J., and Sowton, E.: Variability of left atrial bloodflow predicts intolerance of ventricular demand pacing and may cause pacemaker syndrome. PACE *17*:1149, 1994.
114. Theodorakis, G. N., Kremastinos, D. T., Markianos, M., et al.: Total sympathetic activity and natriuretic factor levels in VVI and DDD pacing with different atrioventricular delays during daily activity and exercise. Eur. Heart J. *13*:1477, 1992.
115. Clemo, H. F., Baumgarten, C. M., Stambler, B. S., et al.: Atrial natriuretic factor: Implications for cardiac pacing and electrophysiology. PACE *17*:70, 1994.
116. Grant, S. C. D., and Bennett, D. H.: Atrial latency in a dual chambered pacing system causing inappropriate sequence of cardiac chamber activation. PACE *15*:116, 1992.
117. Daubert, C., Mabo, P., and Leclercq, C.: Physiologic pacing systems in patients with sick sinus syndrome. *In* Benditt, D. G. (ed.): Rate-Adaptive Pacing. Cambridge, MA, Blackwell Scientific Publications, 1993, p. 151.
118. Daubert, C., Mabo, P., Berder, V., et al.: Atrial tachyarrhythmias associated with high degree interatrial conduction block: Prevention by permanent atrial resynchronisation. Eur. J. Pacing Electrophysiol. *3*:35, 1994.
119. Brandt, J., and Schüller, H.: Consideration for the selection of rate-adaptive single lead atrial (AAIR) pacing. *In* Barold, S. S., and Mugica, J. (eds.): New Perspectives in Cardiac Pacing 3. Mt. Kisco, N.Y., Futura, 1993, p. 349.
120. Katritsis, D., and Camm, A. J.: Adaptive-rate pacemakers: Comparison of sensors and clinical experience. Cardiol. Clin. *10*:671, 1992.
121. Lau, C. P.: The range of sensors and algorithms used in rate adaptive cardiac pacing. PACE *15*:1177, 1992.
122. Katritsis, D., Shakespeare, C. F., and Camm, A. J.: New and combined sensors for adaptive rate pacing. Clin. Cardiol. *16*:240, 1993.
123. Lau, C. P., Tai, Y. T., Fong, P. C., et al.: Clinical experience with an activity sensing DDDR pacemaker using an accelerometer sensor. PACE *15*:334, 1992.
124. Bacharach, D. W., Hilden, T. S., Millerhagen, J. O., et al.: Activity-based pacing: Comparison of a device using an accelerometer versus a piezoelectric crystal. PACE *15*:188, 1992.
125. Charles, R. G., Heemels, J. P., and Westrum, B. L.: Accelerometer-based adaptive-rate pacing: A multicenter study, European EXCEL Study Group. PACE *16*:418, 1993.
126. Alt, E., and Matula, M.: Comparison of two activity-controlled rate-adaptive pacing principles: Acceleration versus vibration. Cardiol. Clin. *10*:635, 1992.
127. Santomauro, M., Fazio, S., Ferraro, S., et al.: Follow-up of a respiratory rate modulated pacemaker. PACE *15*:17, 1992.
128. Nappholz, T., Maloney, J. D., and Kay, G. N.: Rate-adaptive pacing based on impedance derived minute ventilation. *In* Ellenbogen, K. A., Kay, G. N., and Wilkoff, B. L. (eds.): Clinical Cardiac Pacing. Philadelphia, W. B. Saunders Company, 1995, p. 219.
129. Li, H., Neubauer, S. A., and Hayes, D. L.: Follow-up of a minute ventilation rate adaptive pacemaker. PACE *15*:1826, 1992.
130. Abrahamsen, A. M., Barvik, S., Aarsland, T., and Dickstein, K.: Rate responsive cardiac pacing using a minute ventilation sensor. PACE *16*:1650, 1993.
131. Slade, A. K. B., Pee, S., Jones, S., et al.: New algorithms to increase initial rate response in a minute ventilation volume rate adaptive pacemaker. PACE *17*:1960, 1994.
132. Sellers, T. D., Fearnot, N. E., and Smith, H. J.: Temperature controlled rate-adaptive pacing. *In* Ellenbogen, K. A., Kay, G. N., and Wilkoff, B. L. (eds.): Clinical Cardiac Pacing. Philadelphia, W. B. Saunders Company, 1995, p. 201.
133. Bellamy, C. M., Roberts, D. H., Hughes, S., and Charles, R. G.: Comparative evaluation of rate modulation in new generation evoked QT and activity sensing pacemaker. PACE *15*:993, 1992.
134. Connelly, D. T., and Rickards, A. F.: The evoked QT interval. *In* Ellenbogen, K. A., Kay, G. N., and Wilkoff, B. L. (eds.): Clinical Cardiac Pacing. Philadelphia, W. B. Saunders Company, 1995, p. 250.
135. Connelly, D. T., and Rickards, A. F.: Rate-responsive pacing using electrographic parameters as sensors. Cardiol. Clin. *10*:659, 1992.
136. Frais, M. A., Dowie, A., McEwen, B., et al.: Response of the QT-sensing, rate-adaptive ventricular pacemaker to mental stress. Am. Heart J. *126*:1219, 1993.
137. Cowell, R., Morris-Thurgood, J., Paul, V., et al.: Are we being driven to two sensors? Clinical benefits of sensor cross-checking. PACE *16*:1441, 1993.
138. Connelly, D. T.: Initial experience with a new single chamber, dual sensor rate responsive pacemaker, the Topaz Study Group. PACE *16*:1833, 1993.
139. Provenier, F., vanAcker, R., Backers, J., et al.: Clinical observations with a dual sensor rate adaptive single chamber pacemaker. PACE *15*:1821, 1992.
140. Benditt, D. G., Mianulli, M., Lurie, K., et al.: Multiple-sensor systems for physiologic cardiac pacing. Ann. Intern. Med. *121*:960, 1994.
141. VanKrieken, F. M., Perrins, J. P., and Sigmund, M.: Clinical results of automatic slope adaptation in a dual sensor VVIR pacemaker. PACE *15*:1815, 1992.
142. Provenier, F., and Jordaens, L.: Evaluation of six minute walking test in patients with single chamber rate responsive pacemakers. Br. Heart J. *72*:192, 1994.
143. Hayes, D. L., VonFeldt, L., and Higano, S. T.: Standardized informal exercise testing for programming rate adaptive pacemakers. PACE *14*:1772, 1991.
144. Lefroy, D. C., Crake, T., and Davies, D. W.: Ventricular tachycardia: An unusual pacemaker-mediated tachycardia. Br. Heart J. *71*:481, 1994.
145. Alt, E., Kriegler, C., Fotuhi, P., et al.: Feasibility of using intracardiac impedance measurements for capture detection. PACE *15*:1873, 1992.
146. Bolz, A., Hubmann, M., Hardt, R., et al.: Low polarization pacing lead for detecting the ventricular-evoked response. Med. Prog. Technol. *19*:192, 1993.

147. Chirife, R., Ortega, D. F., and Salazar, A. I.: Feasibility of measuring relative right ventricular volumes and ejection fraction with implantable rhythm control devices. PACE *16*:1673, 1993.
148. Santini, M., Alexidou, G., Ansalone, G., et al.: Relation of prognosis in sick sinus syndrome to age, conduction defect, and modes of permanent cardiac pacing. Am. J. Cardiol. *65*:729, 1990.
149. Andersen, H. R., Thuesen, L., Bagger, J. P., et al.: Prospective randomized trial of atrial versus ventricular pacing in sick-sinus syndrome. Lancet *344*:1523, 1994.
150. Barold, S. S., and Santini, M.: Natural history of sick sinus syndrome after pacemaker implantation. *In* Barold, S. S., and Mugica, J. (eds.): New Perspectives in Cardiac Pacing 3. Mt. Kisco, N.Y., Futura, 1993, p. 169.
151. Hesselson, A. B., Parsonnet, V., Bernstein, A. D., and Bonavita, G. J.: Deleterious effect of long-term single-chamber ventricular pacing in patients with sick sinus syndrome: The hidden benefits of dual chamber pacing. J. Am. Coll. Cardiol. *19*:1542, 1992.
152. Sgarbossa, E. B., Pinski, S. L., Maloney, J. D., et al.: Chronic atrial fibrillation and stroke in paced patients with sick sinus syndrome: Relevance of clinical characteristics and pacing modalities. Circulation *88*:1045, 1993.
153. Linde-Edelstam, C., Gullberg, B., Nordlander, R., et al.: Longevity in patients with high degree atrioventricular block paced in the atrial synchronous or the fixed-rate ventricular-inhibited mode. PACE *15*:304, 1992.
154. Shen, W. K., Neubauer, S. A., Espinosa, R. E., et al.: Should age be a consideration in mode selection in permanent pacing? A survival analysis. J. Am. Coll. Cardiol. (Abs. Suppl.):13A, 1995.
155. Rosenqvist, M., Brandt, J., and Schüller, H.: Long-term pacing in sinus node disease: Effects of stimulation mode on cardiovascular morbidity and mortality. Am. Heart J. *116*:16, 1988.
156. Witte, J., v. Knorre, G. H., Volkman, H. J., et al.: Survival rate in sinus syndrome patients: AAI/DDD versus VVI pacing. *In* Santini, M., Pistolese, M., and Alliegro, A. (eds.): Progress in Clinical Pacing 1992. Mt. Kisco, N.Y., Futura, 1993, p. 175.
157. Sethi, K. K., Mohan, J. C., and Khalilullah, M.: Pacing in sick sinus syndrome. PACE *16*(Abs.):1543, 1993.
158. Lamas, G. A., Pashos, C. L., Normand, S. L. T., and McNeil, B. J.: Factors affecting 2-year survival in Medicare pacemaker patients. PACE *16*(Abs.):919, 1993.
159. Lukl, J., Doupal, V., and Heinc, P.: Quality-of-life during DDD and dual sensor VVIR pacing. PACE *17*:1844, 1994.
160. Lau, C. P., Tai, Y. T., Lee, P. W. E., et al.: Quality-of-life in DDDR pacing: Atrioventricular synchrony or rate adaptation? PACE *17*:1838, 1994.
161. Menozzi, C., Brignole, M., Moracchini, P. V., et al.: Inpatient comparison between chronic VVIR and VDD pacing in patients affected by high degree AV block without heart failure. PACE *13*:1816, 1990.
162. Lascault, G., Frank, R., Iwa, T., et al.: Comparison of DDD and "VVIR like" pacing during moderate exercise: Echo-Doppler study. Eur. Heart J. *13*:914, 1992.
163. Jutzy, R. V., Isaeff, D. M., Bansal, R. C., et al.: Comparison of VVIR, DDD, and DDDR pacing. J. Electrophysiol. *3*:194, 1989.
164. Batey, R., Sweesy, M. W., Scala, G., and Forney, R. C.: Comparison of low rate dual chamber pacing to activity responsive rate variable ventricular pacing. PACE *13*:646, 1990.
165. Landzberg, J. S., Franklin, J. O., Mahawar, S. K., et al.: Benefits of physiologic atrioventricular synchronization for pacing with an exercise rate response. Am. J. Cardiol. *66*:193, 1990.
166. Jutzy, R. V., Florio, J., Isaeff, D. M., et al.: Comparative evaluation of rate modulated dual chamber and VVIR pacing. PACE *13*:1838, 1990.
167. Alagona, P., Jr., Batey, R., Sweesy, M., et al.: Improved exercise tolerance with dual chamber versus single chamber rate adaptive pacing. PACE *13*:532, 1990.
168. Higano, S. T., and Hayes, D. L.: Hemodynamic importance of atrioventricular synchrony during low levels of exercise. PACE *13*(Abs.):509, 1990.
169. Adornato, E., Bacca, F., Polimeni, R. M., and DeSeta, F.: Ventricular single chamber RR pacing in comparison to dual chamber RR pacing: Preliminary results of an Italian multicenter trial. PACE *16*(Abs.):1147, 1993.
170. Lemke, B., Dryander, S. V., Jager, D., et al.: Aerobic capacity in rate modulated pacing. PACE *15*:1914, 1992.
171. Windle, J., Plath, R., Eisenger, G., and Easley, A., Jr.: Effect of pacing mode in patients with left ventricular dysfunction. PACE *14*(Abs.):684, 1991.
172. Brandt, J., Anderson, H., Fåhraeus, T., and Schüller, H.: Natural history of sinus node disease treated with atrial pacing in 213 patients: Implications for selection of stimulation mode. J. Am. Coll. Cardiol. *20*:633, 1992.
173. Brandt, J., and Schüller, H.: Pacing for sinus node disease: A therapeutic rationale. Clin. Cardiol. *17*:495, 1994.
174. Katritsis, D., and Camm, A. J.: AAI pacing mode: When is it indicated and how can it be achieved? Clin. Cardiol. *16*:339, 1993.
175. Clarke, M., Sutton, R., Ward, D., et al.: Recommendations for pacemaker prescription for symptomatic bradycardia: Report of a working party of the British Pacing and Electrophysiology Group. Br. Heart J. *66*:185, 1991.
176. Payne, G. E., and Skehan, J. D.: Issues in cardiac pacing: Can agism be justified? Br. Heart J. *72*:102, 1994.
177. Bush, D. E., and Finucane, T. E.: Permanent cardiac pacemakers in the elderly. J. Am. Geriatr. Soc. *42*:326, 1994.
178. Barold, S. S.: Cardiac pacing in special and complex situations: Indications and modes of stimulation. Cardiol. Clin. *10*:573, 1992.
179. Sutton, R.: The second coming of VDD. Eur. J. Cardiac Pacing Electrophysiol. *1*:225, 1992.
180. Antonioli, G. E., Ansani, L., Barbieri, D., et al.: Italian multicenter study on a single lead VDD pacing system using a narrow atrial dipole spacing. PACE *15*:1890, 1992.
181. Lau, C. P., Tai, Y. T., Li, J. P., et al.: Initial clinical experience with a single pass VDDR pacing system. PACE *15*:1894, 1992.
182. Varriale, P., and Chryssos, B. E.: Atrial sensing performance of the single-lead VDD pacemaker during exercise. J. Am. Coll. Cardiol. *22*:1854, 1993.

COMPLICATIONS OF PACEMAKERS

183. Lindsay, H. S., Chennells, P. M., and Perrins, E. J.: Successful treatment by balloon venoplasty and stent insertion of obstruction of the superior vena cava by an endocardial pacemaker lead. Br. Heart J. *71*:363, 1994.
184. Sunder, S. K., Ekong, E. A., Sivalingam, K., and Kumar, A.: Superior vena cava thrombosis due to pacing electrodes: Successful treatment with combined thrombolysis and angioplasty. Am. Heart J. *123*:790, 1992.
185. Mazzetti, H., Dussaut, A., Tentori, C., et al.: Superior vena cava occlusion and/or syndrome related to pacemaker leads. Am. Heart J. *125*:831, 1993.
186. Spittell, P. C., and Hayes, D. L.: Venous complications after insertion of a transvenous pacemaker. Mayo Clinic Proc. *67*:258, 1992.
187. Cooper, C. J., Dweik, R., and Gabbay, S.: Treatment of pacemaker-associated right atrial thrombus with 2-hour rTPA infusion. Am. Heart J. *126*:228, 1993.
188. Vilacosta, I., Zamorano, J., Camino, A., et al.: Infected transvenous permanent pacemakers: Role of transesophageal echocardiography. Am. Heart J. *125*:904, 1993.
189. Vilacosta, I., Sarria, C., San Roman, J. A., et al.: Usefulness of transesophageal echocardiography for diagnosis of infected transvenous permanent pacemakers. Circulation *89*:2684, 1994.
190. Smith, H. J., Fearnot, N. E., Byrd, C. L., et al.: Five-years experience with intravascular lead extraction. PACE *17*:2016, 1994.
191. Hayes, D. L., and Vliestra, R. E.: Pacemaker malfunction. Ann. Intern. Med. *119*:828, 1993.
192. Castle, L. W., and Cook, S.: Pacemaker radiography. *In* Ellenbogen, K. A., Kay, G. N., and Wilkoff, B. L. (eds.): Clinical Cardiac Pacing. Philadelphia, W. B. Saunders Company, 1995, p. 538.
193. Barold, S. S.: Oversensing by single-chamber pacemakers: Mechanisms, diagnosis, and treatment. Cardiol. Clin. *3*:565, 1985.
194. Barold, S. S., Falkoff, M. D., Ong, L. S., and Heinle, R. A.: Interference in cardiac pacemakers: Endogenous sources. *In* El Sherif, N., and Samet, P. (eds.): Cardiac Pacing and Electrophysiology. 3rd ed. Philadelphia, W. B. Saunders Company, 1991, p. 634.
195. Gross, J. N., Platt, S., Ritacco, R., et al.: The clinical relevance of electromyopotential oversensing in current unipolar devices. PACE *15*:2023, 1992.
196. Jain, P., Kaul, U., and Wasir, H. S.: Myopotential inhibition of unipolar demand pacemakers: Utility of provocative manoeuvres in assessment and management. Int. J. Cardiol. *34*:33, 1992.
197. Altamura, G., Bianconi, L., LoBiano, F., et al.: Transthoracic DC shock may represent a serious hazard in pacemaker dependent patients. PACE *18*:194, 1995.
198. van Gelder, B. M., Bracke, F. A., and el Gamal, M. I.: Upper rate pacing after radiofrequency catheter ablation in a minute ventilation rate adaptive DDD pacemaker. PACE *17*:1437, 1994.
199. Barold, S. S., Falkoff, M. D., Ong, L. S., and Heinle, R. A.: Interference in cardiac pacemakers: Exogenous sources. *In* El Sherif, N., and Samet, P. (eds.): Cardiac Pacing and Electrophysiology. 3rd ed. Philadelphia, W. B. Saunders Company, 1991, p. 608.
200. Epstein, A. E., and Wilkoff, B. L.: Pacemaker-defibrillator interactions. *In* Ellenbogen, K. A., Kay, G. N., and Wilkoff, B. L. (eds.): Clinical Cardiac Pacing. Philadelphia, W. B. Saunders Company, 1995, p. 757.
201. Souliman, S. K., and Christie, J.: Pacemaker failure induced by radiotherapy. PACE *17*:270, 1994.
202. Raitt, M. H., Stelzer, K. J., Laramore, G. E., et al.: Runaway pacemaker during high-energy neutron radiation therapy. Chest *106*:955, 1994.
203. Lauck, G., vonSmekal, A., Jung, W., et al.: Influence of nuclear magnetic resonance imaging on software-controlled cardiac pacemakers. PACE *16*(Abs.):1140, 1993.
204. Tobisch, R. J., Irnich, W., and Batz, L.: Electromagnetic compatibility of pacemakers and nuclear magnetic resonance imaging. PACE *16*(Abs.):1140, 1993.
205. Bernstein, A. D., Irwin, M. E., Parsonnet, V., et al.: NASPE Policy Conference Report: Antibradycardia pacemaker follow-up: Effectiveness, needs and resources. PACE *17*:1714, 1994.
206. Sweesy, W., Erickson, S. L., Crago, J. A., et al.: Analysis of the effectiveness of in-office and transtelephonic follow-up in terms of pacemaker system complications. PACE *17*:2001, 1994.
207. Barold, S. S.: Evaluation of pacemaker function by Holter recordings. *In* Moss, A., and Stern, S. (eds.): Non-invasive electrocardiology. London, W. B. Saunders Company, 1996, p. 107.

208. Sgarbossa, E. B., Pinski, S. L., Jaeger, F. J., et al.: Incidence and predictors of syncope in paced patients with sick sinus syndrome. PACE *15*:2055, 1992.

ELECTRICAL DEVICES TO TREAT TACHYCARDIAS

209. Lehman, M. H., and Saksena, S.: Implantable cardioverter defibrillators in cardiovascular practice: Report of the Policy Conference of the North American Society of Pacing and Electrophysiology, NASPE Policy Conference Committee. PACE *14*:969, 1991.
210. Mitrani, R. D., Klein, L. S., Rardon, D. P., et al.: Current trends in the implantable cardioverter defibrillator. *In* Zipes, D. P., and Jalife, J. (eds.): Cardiac Electrophysiology: From Cell to Bedside. Philadelphia, W. B. Saunders Company, 1995, p. 1393.
211. Naccarelli, G. V.: Implantable cardioverter/defibrillator. *In* Willerson, J. T., and Cohn, J. N. (eds.): Cardiovascular Medicine. New York, Churchill-Livingstone, 1995, p. 1441.
212. Cannom, D. S.: Internal cardioverter-defibrillator: Newer technology and newer devices. *In* Podrid, P. J., and Kowey, P. R. (eds.): Cardiac Arrhythmia: Mechanisms, Diagnosis, and Treatment. Baltimore, Williams & Wilkins, 1995, p. 708.
213. Olson, W. H.: Tachyarrhythmia sensing and detection. *In* Singer, I. (ed.): Implantable Cardioverter-Defibrillator. Armonk, N.Y., Futura, 1994, p. 71.
214. Estes, N. A. M., III: Overview of the implantable cardioverter-defibrillator. *In* Estes, N. A. M., III, Manolis, A. S., and Wang, P. J. (eds.): Implantable Cardioverter-Defibrillator: A Comprehensive Textbook. New York, Marcel Dekker, 1994, p. 635.
215. Saksena, S., for the PCD Investigator Group: Clinical outcome of patients with malignant ventricular tachyarrhythmias and a multiprogrammable implantable cardioverter-defibrillator implanted with or without thoracotomy: An international multicenter study. J. Am. Coll. Cardiol. *23*:1521, 1994.
216. Swerdlow, C. D., Ahern, T., Chen, P. S., et al.: Underdetection of ventricular tachycardia by algorithms to enhance specificity in a tiered-therapy cardioverter-defibrillator. J. Am. Coll. Cardiol. *24*:416, 1994.
217. Luceri, R. M., Zilo, P., and the United States and Canadian Enguard Investigators: Initial clinical experience with a dual lead endocardial defibrillation system with atrial pace/sense capability. PACE *18*:163, 1995.
218. Saksena, S., Krol, R. B., and Kaushik, R. R.: Innovations in pulse generators and lead systems: Balancing complexity with clinical benefit and long-term results. Am. Heart J. *127*:1010, 1994.
219. Duffin, E. G., and Barold, S. S.: Implantable cardioverter-defibrillators: An overview and future directions. *In* Singer, I. (ed.): Implantable Cardioverter Defibrillator. Armonk, N.Y., Futura Publishing Co., 1994, p. 751.
220. Stanton, M. S., Hayes, D. L., Munger, T. M., et al.: Consistent subcutaneous prepectoral implantation of a new implantable cardioverter defibrillator. Mayo Clin. Proc. *69*:309, 1994.
221. Bardy, G. H., Hofer, B., Johnson, G., et al.: Implantable transvenous cardioverter-defibrillators. Circulation *87*:1152, 1993.
222. Brachmann, J., Sterns, L. D., Hilbel, T., et al.: Acute efficacy and chronic follow-up of patients with non-thoracotomy third generation implantable defibrillators. PACE *17*:499, 1994.
223. Brooks, R., Garan, H., Torchiana, D., et al.: Three-year outcome of a nonthoracotomy approach to cardioverter-defibrillator implantation in 198 consecutive patients. Am. J. Cardiol. *74*:1011, 1994.
224. Camunas, J., Mehta, D., Ip, J., et al.: Total pectoral implantation: A new technique for implantation of transvenous defibrillator lead systems and implantable cardioverter defibrillator. PACE *16*:380, 1993.
225. Natale, A., Sra, J., Axtell, K., et al.: Preliminary experience with a hybrid nonthoracotomy defibrillating system that includes a biphasic device: Comparison with a standard monophasic device using the same lead system. J. Am. Coll. Cardiol. *24*:406, 1994.
226. Neuzner, J., Pitschner, H. F., Huth, C., and Schlepper, M.: Effect of biphasic waveform pulse on endocardial defibrillation efficacy in humans. PACE *17*:207, 1994.
227. Marks, M. L., Johnson, G., Hofer, B. O., and Bardy, G. H.: Biphasic waveform defibrillation using a three-electrode transvenous lead system in humans. J. Cardiovasc. Electrophysiol. *5*:103, 1994.
228. Heuzner, J., for the European Ventak P_2 Investigator Group: Clinical experience with a new cardioverter defibrillator capable of biphasic waveform pulse and enhanced data storage: Results of a prospective multicenter study, European Ventak P_2 Investigator Group. PACE *17*:1243, 1994.
229. Wyse, D. G., Kavanagh, K. M., Gillis, A. M., et al.: Comparison of biphasic and monophasic shocks for defibrillation using a nonthoracotomy system. Am. J. Cardiol. *71*:197, 1993.
230. Trappe, H. J., Fieguth, H. G., Pfitzner, P., et al.: Epicardial and nonthoracotomy defibrillation lead systems combined with a cardioverter defibrillator. PACE *18*:127, 1995.
231. Manolis, A. S., Rastegar, H., Wang, P. J., and Estes, N. A., 3rd: Fully transvenous cardioverter defibrillators: Rare need for subcutaneous patch with two newer-generation systems. Am. Heart J. *128*:808, 1994.
232. Saksena, S., An, H., Mehra, R., et al.: Prospective comparison of biphasic and monophasic shocks for implantable cardioverter defibrillators using endocardial leads. Am. J. Cardiol. *70*:304, 1992.
233. Thakur, R. K., Souza, J. J., Troup, P. J., et al.: A direct comparison of epicardial and nonthoracotomy defibrillation using monophasic and biphasic shocks. PACE *18*:70, 1995.
234. Manolis, A. S.: Implantable cardioverter-defibrillators lead systems. *In* Estes, N. A. M., III, Manolis, A. S., and Wang, P. J. (eds.): Implantable Cardioverter-Defibrillator: A Comprehensive Textbook. New York, Marcel Dekker, 1994, p. 607.
235. Accorti, P. R., Jr.: Lead technology. *In* Singer, I. (ed.): Implantable Cardioverter-Defibrillator. Armonk, N.Y., Futura, 1994, p. 179.
236. Bardy, G. H., Dolack, G. L., Kudenchuk, P. J., et al.: Prospective, randomized comparison in humans of a unipolar defibrillation system with that using an additional superior vena cava electrode. Circulation *89*:1090, 1994.
237. Raitt, M. H., and Bardy, G. H.: Advances in implantable cardioverter defibrillator therapy. Curr. Opin. Cardiol. *9*:23, 1994.
238. Saksena, S., DeGroot, P., Krol, R. B., et al.: Low-energy endocardial defibrillation using an axillary or a pectoral thoracic electrode location. Circulation *88*:2655, 1993.
239. Neuzner, J., Pitschner, H. F., and Steinmetz, F.: 100% successful implantation of nonthoracotomy lead systems with biphasic cardioverter/defibrillator: European multicenter results in 832 patients. PACE *17*(Abs.):760, 1994.
239a. Villacastin, J., Almendral, J., Arenal, A., et al.: Incidence and clinical significance of multiple consecutive, appropriate, high-energy discharges in patients with implanted cardioverter-defibrillators. Circulation *93*:753, 1996.
240. Jones, D. L.: The defibrillation threshold: A reliable method for rapid determination of defibrillation efficacy. *In* Estes, N. A. M., III, Manolis, A. S., and Wang, P. J. (eds.): Implantable Cardioverter-Defibrillator: A Comprehensive Textbook. New York, Marcel Dekker, 1994, p. 29.
241. Austin, E., and Singer, I.: Operative techniques for implantation and testing of implantable cardioverter-defibrillators. *In* Singer, I. (ed.): Implantable Cardioverter-Defibrillator. Armonk, N.Y., Futura, 1994, p. 327.
242. Jung, W., Manz, M., Pizzulli, L., et al.: Effects of chronic amiodarone therapy on defibrillation threshold. Am. J. Cardiol. *70*:1023, 1992.
243. Jung, W., Manz, M., Pfeiffer, D., et al.: Effects of antiarrhythmic drugs on epicardial defibrillation energy requirements and the rate of defibrillator discharge. PACE *16*:198, 1992.
244. Manz, M., Jung, W., and Lüderitz, B.: Interactions between drugs and devices: Experimental and clinical studies. Am. Heart J. *127*:978, 1994.
245. Avitall, B., Hare, J., Zander, G., et al.: Cardioversion, defibrillation, and overdrive pacing of ventricular arrhythmias: The effect of Moricizine in dogs with sustained monomorphic ventricular tachycardia. PACE *16*:2092, 1993.
246. Peters, W., Gang, E. S., Solrngen, S., et al.: Acute effects of intravenous propafenone on the internal ventricular defibrillation energy requirements in the anesthetized dog. J. Am. Coll. Cardiol. *17*(Abs.):129A, 1991.
247. Natale, A., Montenero, A. S., Bombardieri, G., et al.: Effects of acute and prolonged administration of propafenone on internal defibrillation in the pig. Am. Heart J. *124*:104, 1992.
248. Schrader, R., Brooks, M., and Echt, D. S.: Effects of verapamil and Bay K 8644 on defibrillation energy requirements in dogs. J. Cardiovasc. Pharmacol. *19*:839, 1992.
249. Jones, D. L., Klein, G. J., Guiraudon, G. M., et al.: Effects of lidocaine and verapamil on defibrillation in humans. J. Electrocardiol. *24*:299, 1991.
250. Barold, S. S.: Effect of drugs on defibrillation threshold. *In* Antonioli, G. E., Aubert, A. E., and Ector, H. (eds.): Pacemaker Leads 1991. Amsterdam, Elsevier, 1991, p. 59.
251. Dorian, P., and Newman, D.: Effect of sotalol on ventricular fibrillation and defibrillation in humans. Am. J. Cardiol. *72*:72A, 1993.
252. Akhtar, M., Jazayeri, M., Sra, J., et al.: Role of implantable cardioverter-defibrillator in the management of patients with ventricular tachycardia and ventricular fibrillation. *In* Akhtar, M., Myerburg, R. J., and Ruskin, J. N. (eds.): Sudden Cardiac Death: Prevalence, Mechanisms, and Approaches to Diagnosis and Management. Baltimore, Williams and Wilkins, 1994, p. 588.
253. Bardy, G. H., Poole, J. E., Kudenchuk, P. J., et al.: A prospective, randomized repeat-crossover comparison of antitachycardia pacing with low-energy cardioversion. Circulation *87*:1889, 1993.
254. Kantoch, M. J., Green, M. S., and Tang, A. S.: Randomized cross-over evaluation of two adaptive pacing algorithms for the termination of ventricular tachycardia. PACE *16*:1664, 1993.
255. Calkins, H., el-Atassi, R., Kalbfleisch, S., et al.: Comparison of fixed burst versus decremental burst pacing for termination of ventricular tachycardia. PACE *16*:26, 1993.
256. Estes, N. A., 3rd, Naugh, C. J., Wang, P. J., and Manolis, A. S.: Antitachycardia pacing and low-energy cardioversion for ventricular tachycardia termination: A clinical perspective. Am. Heart J. *127*:1038, 1994.
257. Hammill, S. C., Packer, D. L., Stanton, M. S., Fetter, J., and the Multicenter PCD Investigator Group: Termination and acceleration of ventricular tachycardia with autodecremental pacing, burst pacing and cardioversion in patients with an implantable cardioverter defibrillator. PACE *18*:3, 1995.
258. Heisel, A., Neuzner, J., Himmrich, E., et al.: Safety of antitachycardia pacing in patients with implantable cardioverter defibrillators and severely depressed left ventricular function. PACE *18*:137, 1995.
259. Rabinovich, R., Muratore, C., Iglesias, R., et al.: Results of delivered

therapy for VT or VF in patients with third-generation implantable cardioverter defibrillators. PACE *18:*133, 1995.
260. Rankin, A. C., Zaim, S., Powell, A., et al.: Efficacy of a tiered therapy defibrillator system used to treat recurrent ventricular arrhythmias refractory to drugs. Br. Heart J. *70:*61, 1993.
261. Callans, D. J., and Josephson, M. E.: Future developments in implantable cardioverter defibrillators: The optimal device. Progr. Cardiovasc. Dis. *36:*227, 1993.
262. Nathan, A. W.: The role of cardioversion therapy in patients with implanted cardioverter defibrillators. Am. Heart J. *127:*1046, 1994.
263. Lauer, M. R., Young, C., Liem, L. B., et al.: Ventricular fibrillation induced by low-energy shock from programmable implantable cardioverter-defibrillators in patients with coronary artery disease. Am. J. Cardiol. *73:*559, 1994.
264. Zipes, D. P., Roberts, D., for the PCD Investigators: Results of the worldwide study of the implantable cardioverter-defibrillator: A comparison of epicardial and endocardial lead systems. Circulation *92:*59, 1995.
265. Timmis, G. C.: The development of implantable cardioversion defibrillation systems: The clinical chronicle of defibrillation leads. Am. Heart J. *127:*1003, 1994.
266. Fahy, G. J., Kleman, J. M., Wilkoff, B. L., et al.: Low incidence of lead related complications associated with nonthoracotomy implantable cardioverter defibrillator systems. PACE *18:*172, 1995.
267. Pfeiffer, D., Jung, W., Fehske, W., et al.: Complications of pacemaker-defibrillator devices: Diagnosis and management. Am. Heart J. *127:*1073, 1994.
268. Spratt, K. A., Blumenberg, E. A., Wood, C. A., et al.: Infections of implantable cardioverter defibrillators: Approach to management. Clin. Infect. Dis. *17:*679, 1993.
269. Kelly, P. A., Mann, D. E., Damle, R. S., and Reiter, M. J.: Oversensing during ventricular pacing in patients with a third-generation implantable cardioverter-defibrillator. J. Am. Coll. Cardiol. *23:*1531, 1994.
270. Sandler, M. J., and Kutalek, S. P.: Inappropriate discharge by an implantable cardioverter defibrillator: Recognition of myopotential sensing using telemetered intracardiac electrograms. PACE *17:*665, 1994.
271. Manz, M., Jung, W., Hogl, B., et al.: Atrial fibrillation following defibrillator discharge: Comparison of two lead systems. Eur. Heart J. *13*(Suppl.):152A, 1992.
272. Jung, W., Mletzko, R., Hugl, B., et al.: Incidence of atrial tachyarrhythmias following shock delivery of implantable cardioverter/defibrillators. Circulation *84*/4(Abs.):II-612, 1991.
273. Fricchione, G. L., Vlay, L. C., and Vlay, S. C.: Cardiac psychiatry and the management of malignant ventricular arrhythmias with the internal cardioverter-defibrillator. Am. Heart J. *128:*1050, 1994.
274. Quill, T. E., Barold, S. S., and Sussman, B. L.: Discontinuing an implantable cardioverter defibrillator as a life sustaining treatment. Am. J. Cardiol. *74:*205, 1994.
275. Venditti, F. J., Jr., Martin, D. T., Vassolas, G., and Bowen, S.: Rise in chronic defibrillation thresholds in nonthoracotomy implantable defibrillator. Circulation *89:*216, 1994.
276. Hsia, H. H., Mitra, R. L., Flores, B. T., and Marchlinski, F. E.: Early postoperative increase in defibrillation threshold with nonthoracotomy system in humans. PACE *17:*1166, 1994.
277. Tchou, P. J., Keim, S. G., Mehdirad, A. A., and Rist, K. E.: ICDs: Clinical outcome in the first decade. *In* Naccarelli, G. V., and Veltri, E. P. (eds.): Implantable Cardioverter-Defibrillators. Boston, Blackwell Scientific, 1993, p. 216.
278. Marchlinski, F. E., Gottlieb, C. D., Sarter, B., et al.: ICD data storage: Value in arrhythmia management. PACE *16:*527, 1993.
279. Hook, B. G., Callans, D. F., Kleiman, R. B., et al.: Implantable cardioverter-defibrillator therapy in the absence of significant symptoms: Rhythm diagnosis and management aided by stored electrogram analysis. Circulation *87:*1897, 1993.
280. Roelke, M., Garan, H., McGovern, B. A., and Ruskin, J. N.: Analysis of the initiation of spontaneous monomorphic ventricular tachycardia by stored intracardiac electrograms. J. Am. Coll. Cardiol. *23:*117, 1994.
281. Grimm, W., Flores, B. F., and Marchlinski, F. E.: Symptoms and electrocardiographically documented rhythm preceding spontaneous shocks in patients with implantable cardioverter-defibrillator. Am. J. Cardiol. *71:*1415, 1993.
282. Klein, L. S., Miles, W. M., and Zipes, D. P.: Antitachycardia devices: Realities and promises. J. Am. Coll. Cardiol. *18:*1349, 1991.
283. Powell, A. C., Fuchs, T., Finkelstein, D. M., et al.: Influence of implantable cardioverter-defibrillators on the long-term prognosis of survivors of out-of-hospital cardiac arrest. Circulation *88:*1083, 1993.
284. Grimm, W., Flores, B. T., and Marchlinski, F. E.: Shock occurrence and survival in 241 patients with implantable cardioverter-defibrillator therapy. Circulation *87:*1880, 1993.
285. Sweeney, M. O., and Ruskin, J. N.: Mortality benefits and the implantable cardioverter-defibrillator. Circulation *89:*1851, 1994.
286. Zipes, D. P.: Implantable cardioverter-defibrillator: Lifesaver or a device looking for a disease? Circulation *89:*2934, 1994.
287. Zipes, D. P.: The implantable cardioverter defibrillator revolution continues. Mayo Clin. Proc. *69:*395, 1994.
288. Kim, S. G., Fisher, J. D., and Furman, S.: Hypothetical death rates of patients with implantable defibrillators remain very hypothetical. Am. J. Cardiol. *72:*1453, 1993.
289. Kim, S. G.: Implantable defibrillator therapy: Does it really prolong life? How can we prove it? Am. J. Cardiol. *71:*1213, 1993.
290. Dorian, P., Connolly, S., and Yusuf, S.: The impact of left ventricular dysfunction on outcomes with the implantable defibrillator. Am. Heart J. *127:*1159, 1994.
291. Bigger, J. T., Jr.: Prediction and prevention of sudden cardiac death. *In* Estes, N. A. M., III, Manolis, A. S., and Wang, P. J. (eds.): Implantable Cardioverter Defibrillator: A Comprehensive Textbook. New York, Marcel Dekker, 1994, p. 557.
292. Kim, S. G.: Impact of implantable cardioverter-defibrillator therapy on patient survival. Cardiol. Rev. *2:*113, 1994.
293. O'Nunain, S., and Ruskin, J.: Cardiac arrest. Lancet *341:*1641, 1993.
294. Moss, A. J.: Influence of the implantable cardioverter-defibrillator on survival: Retrospective studies and prospective trials. Progr. Cardiovasc. Dis. *36:*85, 1993.
295. Kolettis, T. M., and Saksena, S.: Prophylactic implantable cardioverter defibrillator therapy in high-risk patients with coronary artery disease. Am. Heart J. *127:*1164, 1994.
296. Zipes, D. P.: Are implantable cardioverter defibrillators better than conventional antiarrhythmic drugs for survivors of cardiac arrest? Circulation *91:*2115, 1995.

Chapter 24

Cardiac Arrest and Sudden Cardiac Death

ROBERT J. MYERBURG, AGUSTIN CASTELLANOS

DEFINITION

Sudden cardiac death (SCD) is natural death due to cardiac causes, heralded by abrupt loss of consciousness within 1 hour of the onset of acute symptoms. Preexisting heart disease may or may not have been known to be present, but the time and mode of death are unexpected. This definition incorporates the key elements of "natural," "rapid," and "unexpected." It consolidates previous definitions which have conflicted,[1–20a] largely because the most useful operational definition of SCD differs for the clinician, the cardiovascular epidemiologist, the pathologist, and the scientist attempting to define pathophysiological mechanisms.

Four elements must be considered in the construction of a definition of SCD to satisfy medical, scientific, legal, and social considerations: (1) prodromes, (2) onset, (3) cardiac arrest, and (4) biological death (Fig. 24–1). Because the proximate cause of SCD is a disturbance of cardiovascular function, which is incompatible with maintaining consciousness because of abrupt loss of cerebral blood flow, any definition must recognize the brief time interval between the onset of the mechanism directly responsible for cardiac arrest and the consequent loss of consciousness (Fig. 24–1*C*). The 1-hour definition, however, refers to the duration of the "terminal event" (Fig. 24–1*B*), which defines the interval between the onset of symptoms signalling the pathophysiological disturbance leading to cardiac arrest and the onset of the cardiac arrest itself (Fig. 24–1*B* and *C*).

Premonitory signs and symptoms, which may occur during the days or weeks before a cardiac arrest,[17] tend to be nonspecific for the impending event.[8] *Prodromes* (Fig. 24–1*A*), which may be more specific for an imminent cardiac arrest, are relatively abrupt changes that begin during an arbitrarily defined period of up to 24 hours before the cardiac arrest.[4,21] The fourth element, *biological death* (Fig. 24–1*D*), is an immediate consequence of the clinical cardiac arrest in the past, occurring within minutes. However, since the development of community-based intervention systems, and long-term life support systems, patients may

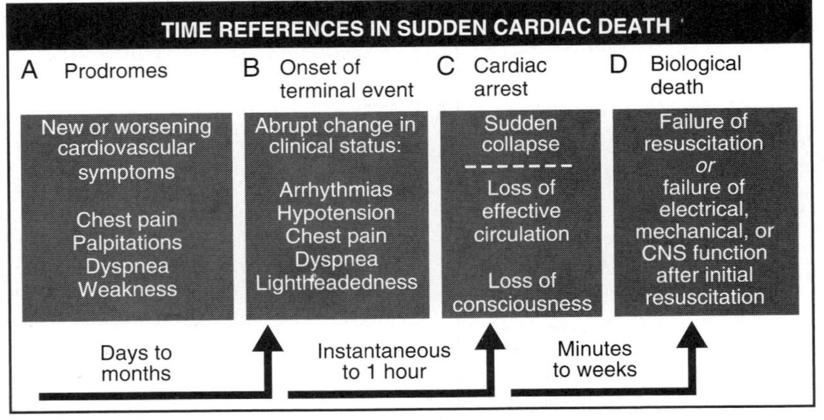

FIGURE 24–1. Sudden cardiac death is viewed from four temporal perspectives: *(A)* prodromes, *(B)* onset of the terminal event, *(C)* cardiac arrest, and *(D)* progression to biological death. Individual variability of the components influence clinical expression: some victims experience no prodromes, with onset leading almost instantaneously to cardiac arrest; others may have an onset which lasts up to 1 hour before clinical arrest; some patients may live weeks after the cardiac arrest before progression to biological death if there has been irreversible brain damage and life-support systems are used. These modifying factors influence interpretation of the 1-hour definition. From the perspective of the clinician, the two most relevant factors are the onset of the terminal event *(B)* and the clinical cardiac arrest itself *(C)*. In contrast, legal and social considerations focus on the time of biological death *(D)*.

TABLE 24–1 DEFINITION OF TERMS RELATED TO SUDDEN CARDIAC DEATH

TERM	DEFINITION	QUALIFIERS OR EXCEPTIONS
Death	Irreversible cessation of all biological functions	None
Cardiac arrest	Abrupt cessation of cardiac pump function which may be reversible by a prompt intervention but will lead to death in its absence	Rare spontaneous reversions; likelihood of successful intervention relates to mechanism of arrest and clinical setting
Cardiovascular collapse	A (sudden) loss of effective blood flow due to cardiac and/or peripheral vascular factors which may revert spontaneously (e.g., vasodepressor syncope) or only with interventions (e.g., cardiac arrest)	Nonspecific term which includes cardiac arrest and its consequences and also events which characteristically revert spontaneously

now remain biologically alive for a long period of time after the onset of a pathophysiological process which has caused irreversible damage and will ultimately lead to death.[18–20,22] In this circumstance, the causative pathophysiological and clinical event is the cardiac arrest itself, rather than the factors responsible for the delayed biological death. However, in legal, forensic, and certain social circumstances, biological death must continue to be used as the absolute definition of death. Finally, the forensic pathologist studying *unwitnessed deaths* may use the definition of sudden death for a person known to be alive and functioning normally 24 hours before,[4] and this remains appropriate within its obvious limits because unwitnessed death cannot be ignored in their studies.[23] Thus the generally accepted clinical-pathophysiological definition of up to 1 hour between onset of the terminal event and biological death requires qualifications for specific circumstances.

The development of community-based intervention systems also has led to inconsistencies in the use of terms considered absolute. *Death* is defined biologically, legally, and literally as an absolute and irreversible event. Thus SCD may be aborted, or a patient may survive cardiac arrest or cardiovascular collapse; however, survival after (sudden) death is a contradiction in terms. Table 24–1 provides definitions for events and terms related to the concept of SCD—death, cardiac arrest, and cardiovascular collapse.

EPIDEMIOLOGY AND CAUSES OF SUDDEN DEATH

EPIDEMIOLOGY

The worldwide incidence of SCD is difficult to estimate because it varies largely as a function of coronary heart disease prevalence in different countries.[24] Estimates for the United States range from 300,000 to nearly 400,000 SCDs annually,[25] the variation based in part on the definition of sudden death used in individual studies.[5,16] The most widely used estimate is 300,000 SCDs annually,[26] a figure which represents 50 per cent or more of all cardiovascular deaths in the United States.[24–28]

The influence of the temporal definition of SCD on epidemiological data[4] is demonstrated by a retrospective death certificate study in a large metropolitan area in the United States reported by Kuller et al.[4] When the temporal definition was restricted to death less than 2 hours after the onset of symptoms, 12 per cent of all natural deaths were sudden, and 88 per cent of the sudden natural deaths were due to cardiac causes. This estimate is similar to observations in a large prospective cohort study—the Framingham study—in which 13 per cent of all deaths observed during a 26-year period were "sudden," defined as death within 1 hour of the onset of symptoms.[29,30] In contrast to deaths occurring less than 2 hours after the onset of symptoms, the application of the 24-hour definition of sudden death to the data from Kuller et al.[4] increased the fraction of all natural deaths falling into the "sudden" category to 32 per cent but reduced the proportion of all sudden natural deaths which were cardiac deaths to 75 per cent.

Prospective studies demonstrate that about 50 per cent of all coronary heart disease deaths are sudden and unexpected, occurring shortly (instantaneous to 1 hour) after the onset of symptoms. In the prospective combined Albany-Framingham study of 4120 males, sudden deaths within 1 hour of an observed collapse were analyzed for a population of men dying between 45 and 74 years of age.[9] During a 16-year follow-up, there were 234 total coronary deaths/1000 population observed, of which 109 (47 per cent) were sudden and unexpected. Because coronary heart disease dominates sudden and total cardiac deaths in the United States, the fraction of total cardiac deaths which are sudden is similar to the fraction of coronary heart disease deaths which are sudden, although there does appear to be a geographical variation in the fraction of coronary deaths which are sudden.[31] This 50 per cent fraction may not apply to other nations or to subcultures which have a lower prevalence of coronary heart disease. It also is of interest that the recent decline in coronary heart disease mortality in the United States[32] has not changed the fraction of coronary deaths that are sudden and unexpected,[33] even though there may be a decline in out-of-hospital deaths compared with emergency department deaths.[27]

POPULATION POOLS AND TIME-DEPENDENCE OF RISK

Two factors are of primary importance for identifying populations at risk and when considering strategies for primary prevention of SCD: (1) the size of denominators of population subgroups (Fig. 24–2*A*), and (2) time-dependence of risk (Fig. 24–2*B*).

POPULATION SUBGROUPS AND SCD. The more than 300,000 adult SCDs which occur annually in the United States can be viewed in terms of incidence in an unselected adult population. Because of the large denominator which this population pool represents, the overall incidence is 1 to 2/1000 population (0.1–0.2 per cent) per year. This large population base includes both those victims whose SCDs occur as a first cardiac event and those whose SCDs may be predicted with greater accuracy because they are included in higher-risk subgroups. Any intervention designed for the *general* population must, therefore, be applied to the 99/1000 who will not have an event to reach and possibly influence the 1/1000 who will. The cost and risk-to-benefit uncertainties limit the nature of such broad-based interventions and demand a higher resolution of risk identification. Figure 24–2*A* highlights this problem by expressing the incidence (per cent/year) of SCD among various subgroups and comparing the incidence figures to the total number of events which occur annually in each subgroup. By moving from the total adult population to a subgroup with high risk because of the presence of selected coronary risk factors, there may be a 10-fold or greater increase in the incidence of events annually, with the mag-

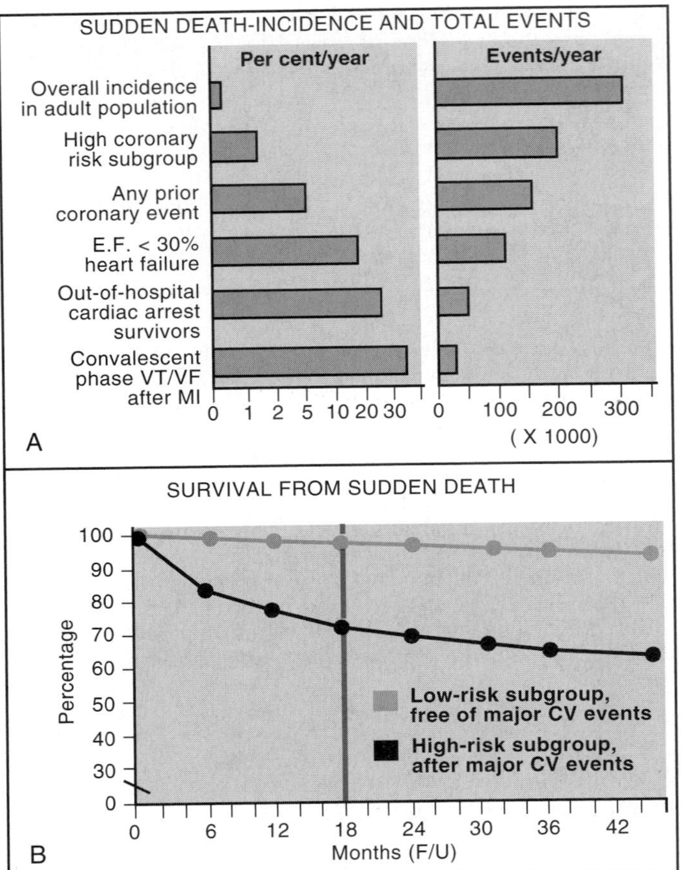

FIGURE 24–2. Impact of population pools and time-from-events on the clinical epidemiology of sudden cardiac death. The top panel *(A)* compares incidence and total numbers of sudden cardiac deaths in different subgroups; the lower panel *(B)* demonstrates time-dependence of risk for sudden death after major cardiovascular events.

In the top panel (*A*), estimates of incidence figures (per cent/year) and the total number of events/year are shown for the overall adult population in the United States, and for increasingly higher-risk subgroups. The overall adult population has an estimated sudden death incidence of 0.1 to 0.2 per cent/year, accounting for a total number of events of more than 300,000/year. With the identification of increasingly powerful risk factors, the incidence *increases* progressively, but it is accomplished by a progressive *decrease* in the total number of patients identified. The inverse relation between incidence and total number of events occurs because of the progressively smaller denominator pool in the highest subgroup categories.

Successful interventions among larger population subgroups will require identification of specific markers to increase the ability to identify specific patients who will be at particularly high risk for a future event (*Note:* The horizontal axis for the incidence figures is not linear, and should be interpreted accordingly.)

In the lower panel *(B),* idealized curves of survival from sudden death are shown for a population of patients with known cardiovascular disease but at low risk because of freedom from major cardiovascular (CV) events *(top curve),* and for populations of patients who have survived a major cardiovascular event *(bottom curve).* Attrition over time is accelerated in both absolute and relative terms for the initial 6 to 18 months after the major cardiovascular event. After the initial attrition, the slopes of the curves for the high-risk and low-risk populations parallel each other, highlighting both the early attrition and the attenuation of risk after 18 to 24 months.

These relations have been observed in diverse high-risk subgroups (cardiac arrest survivors, post-myocardial infarction patients with high-risk markers, recent onset of heart failure), and highlight the changing risk pattern as a function of time and the importance of the time dimension for recognition and intervention in strategies designed to alter outcome. (Modified from Myerburg, R. J., et al.: Sudden cardiac death: Structure, function and time-dependence of risk. Circulation *85*(Suppl. I):I-2, 1992. Copyright 1992 American Heart Association.)

nitude of increase dependent on the number of risk factors operating in the subgroup. The size of the denominator pool, however, remains very large, and implementation of interventions remains problematic, even at this heightened level of risk. Higher resolution is desirable and can be achieved by identification of more specific subgroups. The corresponding absolute number of deaths becomes progressively smaller as the subgroups become more focused (Fig. 24–2*A*), limiting the potential benefit of interventions to the much smaller subgroups.

TIME-DEPENDENCE OF RISK. Risk of SCD is not linear as a function of time after a change in cardiovascular status.[26,34,35] Survival curves after major cardiovascular events, which identify populations at high risk for both sudden and total cardiac death, usually demonstrate that the most rapid rate of attrition occurs during the first 6 to 18 months (Fig. 24–2*B*). Thus there is a time-dependence of risk which focuses the opportunity for effective intervention to the early period after a conditioning event. Curves that have these characteristics have been generated from among survivors of out-of-hospital cardiac arrest, new onset of heart failure, and unstable angina, and from high-risk subgroups of patients having recent myocardial infarction. *The addition of time as a dimension for measuring risk may increase the resolution within subgroups.*

AGE, HEREDITY, GENDER, AND RACE

AGE. There are two ages of peak incidence of sudden death: between birth and 6 months of age (the sudden infant death syndrome) and between 45 and 75 years of age.[3] In the adult population the *incidence* of sudden death owing to coronary heart disease increases as a function of advancing age,[33,36–38] in parallel with the age-related increase in incidence of total coronary heart disease deaths.[32] However, the *proportion* of deaths caused by coronary heart disease that are sudden and unexpected decreases with advancing age.[19,33,36–38] Kuller et al.[39] reported that 76 per cent of coronary heart disease deaths in the 20-to-39-year age group were sudden and unexpected, and the Framingham data demonstrated that 62 per cent of all coronary heart disease deaths were sudden in the 45-to-54 year age group in men. The proportion fell progressively to 58 per cent in the 55-to-64-year age group and to 42 per cent in the 65-to-74-year age group.[36,37] Age also influences the proportion of cardiovascular causes among all causes of natural sudden death in that the proportion of coronary deaths and of all cardiac causes of death which are sudden is highest in the younger age groups, whereas the fraction of total sudden natural deaths which are due to any cardiovascular cause is higher in the older age groups.[40] In their study of sudden death in children and young adults, Neuspiel and Kuller[40] reported that only 19 per cent of sudden natural deaths in children between 1 and 13 years of age were cardiac deaths; the proportion increased to 30 per cent in the 14-to-21-year age group. All of these studies of age factors used a 24-hour definition of sudden death.

HEREDITY. To the extent that SCD is an expression of underlying coronary heart disease, hereditary factors that contribute to coronary heart disease risk operate nonspecifically for the SCD syndrome.[41]

Among the less common causes of SCD, hereditary patterns have been reported for some specific syndromes. Such patterns are described for some forms of congenital and hereditary Q-T interval prolongation (see p. 951),[42] hypertrophic obstructive cardiomyopathy,[43] and familial SCD in children and young adults.[44] Although stable congenital conducting system abnormalities have a good prognosis,[45] progressive familial conducting system disease, which appears to have a hereditary pattern, carried an increased risk of SCD.[46] Familial sudden death associated with cardiac ganglionitis has been reported,[47] but an inheritance pattern has not been demonstrated in the reports to date. Linkage analyses in families with long Q-T interval syndromes have provided a major advance in the understanding of a genetic basis for one cause of sudden death (see p. 1667). Abnormalities on three different chromosomes (loci on chromosomes 11, 7, and 3) each associate with congenital long Q-T syndrome. Two of the three (on chromosomes 7 and 3) encode a membrane channel abnormality that can prolong repolarization.[48–50] This observation may provide a screening tool for individuals at risk, as well as the potential for specific therapeutic strategies.

GENDER. The SCD syndrome has a huge preponderance in males compared with females because of the protection females enjoy from coronary atherosclerosis before advanced years.[29,30,37] During the first 14 years of follow-up in the Framingham study, 59 of 66 (89 per cent) sudden unexpected coronary deaths (<1 hour) occurred in men.[8] The Framingham study at 20 years of follow-up demonstrated a 3.8-fold excess incidence of sudden coronary death in men compared with women.[37] This male/female ratio is similar to data recorded in three prospective studies of prehospital cardiac arrest in which the percentages of males observed were 75 per cent (mean age 63 years),[18] 85 per cent (mean age 60 years),[19] and 89 per cent (mean age 58 years),[51] respectively. In the study by Kuller et al.,[4] 75 per cent of all SCDs (using the 24-hour definition) in a 40-to-64-year-old population were in men. When the data in another study by Kuller et al. were analyzed for survival of less than 2 hours, the proportion of men increased to 80 per cent.[52] In the Framingham study[37] the excess risk in men peaked at 6.75:1 in the 55-to-64-year age group and then fell to 2.17:1 in the 65-to-74-year age group. Even though the overall risk is much lower in women, the classic coronary risk factors are expressed in them.[29,30,53,54] Cigarette smoking, diabetes, use of oral contraceptives,[55] and reduced vital capacity[30] are particularly strong factors.

RACE. A number of studies comparing racial differences and relative risk of SCD in whites and blacks with coronary heart disease in the United States have yielded conflicting and inconclusive data.[4,56,57] However, a recent large study from an urban area demonstrated excess risk of cardiac arrest and SCD in blacks compared with whites.[57] An excess was observed across all age groups, but the magnitude of excess risk among adults decreased with increasing age.

Data on the prevalence of coronary heart disease in Japanese men living in the United States have demonstrated that the low rates reported in those living in Japan tend to increase toward, but do not reach, levels observed in white men in the United States.[58] Thus, an interplay between race and environmental factors may be operative.

BIOLOGICAL RISK FACTORS AND SUDDEN DEATH

The known coronary risk factors cannot be used to distinguish the patients at risk for SCD from those at risk for other manifestations of coronary heart disease.[9] Using a multivariate analysis of selected risk factors (i.e., age, systolic blood pressure, heart rate, electrocardiographic abnormalities, vital capacity, relative weight, cigarette consumption, and serum cholesterol) from the population in the Framingham data, Kannel and Schatzkin[33] determined that 53 per cent of the SCDs in men and 42 per cent of those in women occurred among the 10 per cent of the population in the highest risk decile (Fig. 24–3). The comparison of risk factors in the victims of SCD with those in people who developed any manifestations of coronary artery disease did not provide useful patterns, by either univariate or multivariate analysis, to distinguish victims of SCD from the overall pool.[9] In addition, data from 19,946 patients in the Coronary Artery Surgery Study identified no angiographic or hemodynamic patterns that discriminated sudden from nonsudden cardiac deaths.[38]

Hypertension is a clearly established risk factor for coronary heart disease and also emerges as a highly significant risk factor for incidence of SCD.[9] However, there is no influence of increasing systolic blood pressure levels on the ratio of sudden deaths to total coronary heart disease

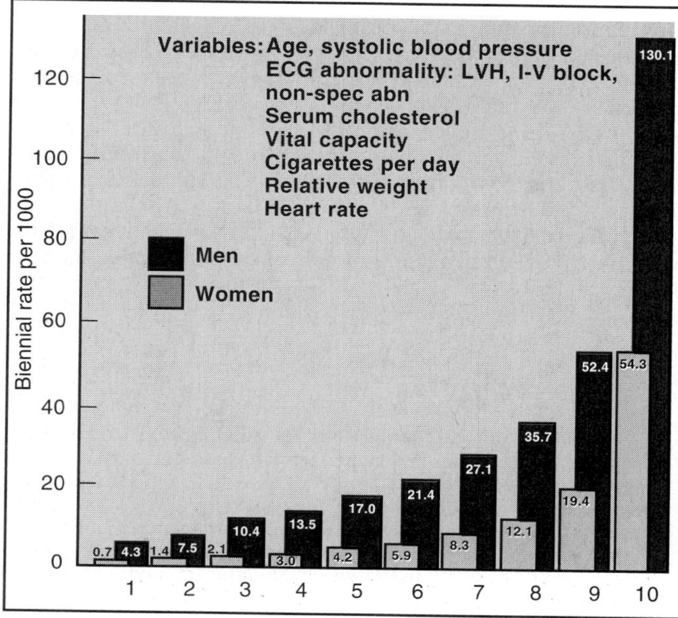

FIGURE 24–3. Risk of sudden death by decile of multivariant risk: 26-year follow-up, the Framingham Study. ECG = electrocardiographic; I-V = intraventricular; LVH = left ventricular hypertrophy; non-spec abn = nonspecific abnormality. (From Kannel, W. B., and Shatzkin, A.: Sudden death: Lessons from subsets in population studies. Reprinted by permission of the American College of Cardiology. J. Am. Coll. Cardiol. *5*[Suppl. 6]:141B, 1985.)

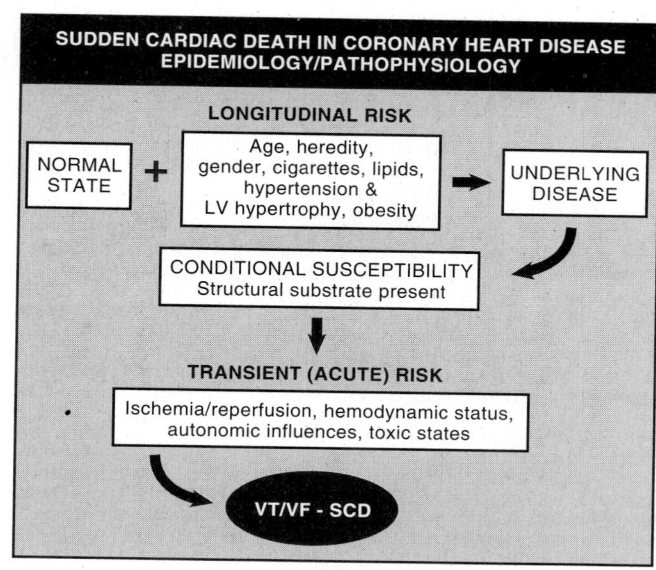

FIGURE 24–4. Epidemiology of SCD: conventional (conditioning) risk factors versus transient (triggering) risk factors. Conventional risk factors predict risk of the disease underlying SCD; transient risk factors predict risk of the pathophysiological event that initiates the fatal event. (Modified from Myerburg, R. J., Kessler, K. M., Kimura, S., et al.: Life-threatening ventricular arrhythmias: The link between epidemiology and pathophysiology. *In* Zipes, D. P., and Jalife, J. [eds.]: Cardiac Electrophysiology, 2nd ed. Philadelphia, W. B. Saunders Company, 1995.)

deaths.[36] No relationship has been observed between cholesterol concentration and the proportion of coronary deaths that were sudden.[37] Neither the electrocardiographic pattern of left ventricular hypertrophy nor nonspecific ST-T wave abnormalities influence the proportion of total coronary deaths that are sudden and unexpected[36]; *only intraventricular conduction abnormalities are suggestive of a disproportionate number of SCDs.*[37] A low vital capacity also suggests a disproportionate risk for sudden versus total coronary deaths.[37] This is of interest because such a relation was particularly striking in the analysis of data on women in the Framingham study who had died suddenly.[29,30] A high hematocrit also was predictive in women.[31]

The conventional risk factors used in most studies of SCD are the risk factors for coronary artery disease. The rationale is based upon two facts: (1) Coronary disease is the structural basis for 80 per cent of SCDs in the United States, and (2) the coronary risk factors are easy to identify because they tend to be present continuously over time (Fig. 24–4). However, risk factors specific for fatal arrhythmias are dynamic pathophysiological events and occur transiently.[59] Transient pathophysiological events are being modeled epidemiologically,[60] in an attempt to express and use them as clinical risk factors[61] for both profiling and intervention.[62]

LIFE STYLE AND PSYCHOSOCIAL FACTORS

LIFE STYLE. There is a strong association between *cigarette smoking* and all manifestations of coronary heart disease. The Framingham study demonstrates that cigarette smokers have a two- to threefold increase in sudden death risk in each decade of life at entry between 30 and 59 years, and that this is one of the few risk factors in which the proportion of coronary heart disease deaths that are sudden increases in association with the risk factor.[37] In addition, in a study of 310 survivors of out-of-hospital cardiac arrest, Hallstrom et al.[63] observed a 27 per cent incidence of recurrent cardiac arrest at 3 years in those who continued to smoke after their index event, compared with 19 per cent in those who stopped ($P < .04$). Obesity is a second factor which appears to influence the proportion of coronary deaths that occur suddenly.[30,37] With increasing relative weight, the percentage of coronary heart disease deaths that were sudden in the Framingham study increased linearly from a low of 39 per cent to a high of 70 per cent. Total coronary heart disease deaths increased with increasing relative weight as well.

Epidemiological observations suggest a relationship between *low levels of physical activity* and increased coronary heart disease death risk.[64] The Framingham study, however, showed an *insignificant* relationship between low levels of physical activity and incidence of sudden death but a high proportion of sudden to total cardiac deaths at higher levels of physical activity.[37] An association between acute physical exertion (especially in physically inactive individuals) and the onset of myocardial infarction has been suggested,[62] but it is not yet known if this also applies to SCD.

PSYCHOSOCIAL FACTORS. These appear to influence the risk for SCDs. Rahe and coworkers[65] recorded recent life changes in the realms of health, work, home and family, and personal and social factors, relating the magnitude of such changes to myocardial infarction and SCD. There was an association between significant elevations of life-change scores during the 6 months before a coronary event, and the association was particularly striking in victims of SCD. In a study of sudden death in women,[66] those who died suddenly were less often married, had fewer children, and had greater educational discrepancies with their spouses than did age-related controls living in the same neighborhood as the sudden death victims. A history of psychiatric treatment, cigarette smoking, and greater quantities of alcohol consumption than the controls also characterized the sudden death group.[66] Ruberman and coworkers reported on the influences of psychosocial factors on sudden and total death after myocardial infarction in 2320 male survivors of myocardial infarction.[67] Controlling for other major prognostic factors, including frequency of premature ventricular contractions, a greater than fourfold increase in risk of sudden and total deaths was predicted by *social isolation* and a *high level of life stress.* These psychosocial factors were inversely related to levels of education. In an earlier study, a more than threefold increase of sudden death risk during follow-up after myocardial infarction had been reported in men who had complex ventricular ectopy and low levels of education compared with better-educated men with the same arrhythmias.[68] Interestingly, there was no relation between educational level and recurrent myocardial infarction.

In a survey of life style, it was found that people with lower educational levels smoked more cigarettes, drank more alcohol, exercised less, and were more overweight.[69] The studies by Friedman and Rosenman[70] on the time-oriented, aggressive *type A personality* characteristics have suggested an increased incidence of all manifestations of coronary heart disease in such patients, including the incidence of sudden cardiac death. The validity of the discrimination of a high-risk subgroup based on type A personality characteristics has recently been challenged.[71]

FUNCTIONAL CLASSIFICATION AND SUDDEN DEATH. The Framingham study demonstrated a striking relation between functional classification and death during a 2-year follow-up period. However, the proportion of deaths that were sudden did not vary with functional classification, ranging from 50 to 57 per cent in all groups, ranging from those free of clinical heart disease to those in functional Class IV.[37]

Sudden Death and Previous Coronary Heart Disease

Although SCD is the first clinical manifestation of coronary heart disease in 20 to 25 per cent or more of all coronary heart disease patients,[9,16,23,26] a previous myocardial infarction can be identified in as many as 75 per cent of patients who die suddenly. The high incidence of both clinical and unrecognized prior myocardial infarction in victims of SCD has led to a search for predictors of SCD in survivors of myocardial infarction, as well as in patients with other clinical manifestations of coronary heart disease.

LEFT VENTRICULAR EJECTION FRACTION IN CHRONIC ISCHEMIC HEART DISEASE. A marked depression of the left ventricular ejection fraction is the most powerful predictor of SCD in patients with chronic ischemic heart disease, as well as those whose SCD results from other causes (see below). Increased risk, independent of other risk factors, is measurable at ejection fractions greater than 40 per cent, but the greatest rate of change of risk is between 30 and 40 per cent.[72] An ejection fraction equal to or less than 30 per cent is the single most powerful predictor for SCD, but it has a low specificity. Low ejection fraction data parallel risk data based on arrhythmias, but ejection fraction remains an independent predictor.[72]

VENTRICULAR ECTOPY IN CHRONIC ISCHEMIC HEART DISEASE. Most forms of ventricular ectopic activity (premature ventricular contractions, PVCs) in the absence of heart disease[73] are prognostically benign. When present in people over the age of 30, however, PVCs select a subgroup with a higher probability of coronary artery disease and of SCD.[74] In addition, the occurrence of PVCs in survivors of myocardial infarction,[75] particularly if frequent and of complex forms such as multiform or repetitive PVCs,[72,76] predicts an increased risk of SCD on long-term follow-up. Most of these studies have identified both *frequency* and *forms* of ventricular ectopic activity as indicators of risk, but uniformity for such classifications is lacking.[77] Although most studies cite a frequency cutoff of 10 PVCs/hour as a threshold level for increased risk, some have identified frequency cutoffs in the range of 1 to 9 PVCs/hour, 10 PVCs/1000 sinus beats, and more than 20 PVCs/hour. Forms suggestive of high risk include multiform PVCs, bigeminy, short coupling intervals (R-on-T phenomenon), and salvos of three or more ectopic beats.[77] Several investigators have emphasized that the most powerful predictors among the various forms of PVCs are salvos of three or more complexes.[72,76,78]

Many of the reported studies have been based on a single ambulatory monitor sample recorded 1 week to several months after the onset of acute myocardial infarction, and the duration of the samples has ranged from 1 hour to 48 hours. Ruberman et al.[78] reported that repeated short-term (1-hour) ambulatory recordings at 6-month intervals beginning 1 month after myocardial infarction reestablished the increased risk imparted by complex forms of PVCs for the ensuing 3½-year interval, as long as complex forms remained on the interval recordings.

All early drug intervention studies were limited by design features which made interpretation of therapeutic efficacy (mortality reduction) impossible.[79] The results of the Cardiac Arrhythmia Suppression Trial (CAST) (see p. 1265), designed to test the hypothesis that PVC suppression by antiarrhythmic drugs alters risk of SCD after myocardial

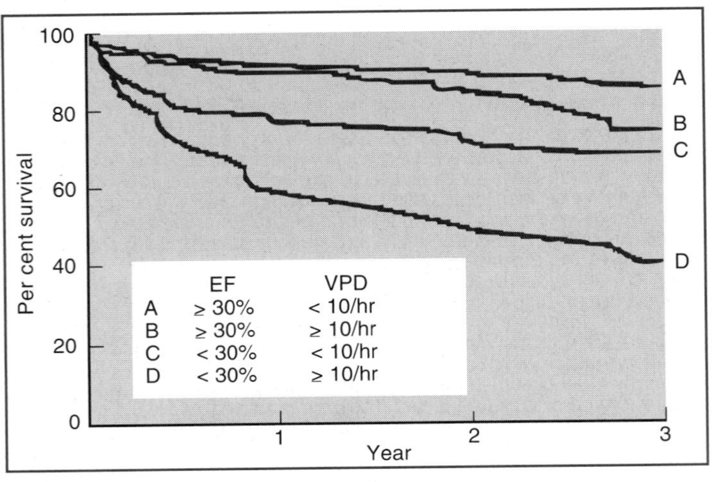

FIGURE 24–5. Survival during 3 years of follow-up after acute myocardial infarction as a function of left ventricular dysfunction (ejection fraction, EF) and ventricular arrhythmias (VPDs/hour as measured by Holter monitoring). The survival curves were calculated as Kaplan-Meier estimates. With higher PVC frequencies and lower ejection fractions, the mortality rates increase. The number of patients in groups A, B, C, and D were 536, 136, 80, and 37, respectively. (From Bigger, J. T.: Relation between left ventricular dysfunction and ventricular arrhythmias after myocardial infarction. Am. J. Cardiol. *57*:8B, 1986.)

infarction, were surprising for two reasons.[80] First, the death rate in the randomized placebo group was lower than expected, and second, the rate among patients in the encainide and flecainide arms exceeded control rates by more than three times. Thus, for these two Class IC drugs, treatment had an adverse effect for a population dominated by frequent single PVCs, and with a mean ejection fraction of about 40 per cent. Subgroup analysis demonstrated increased risk in the placebo group for patients with nonsustained ventricular tachycardia and with ejection fraction of 30 per cent or less, but excess risk in the treated group was still observed. The role of antiarrhythmic drugs for patients with the latter characteristics (ejection fraction less than 30 per cent and nonsustained ventricular tachycardia) requires prospective study, but CAST has shown that antiarrhythmics can have an adverse effect in lower-risk groups. In the continuation of CAST (CAST II), comparing moricizine with placebo and altering enrollment to favor patients with more advanced disease, no adverse effect (other than short-term proarrhythmic risk at initiation of therapy) was observed, but no long-term benefit emerged either.[81] Whether the conclusions from CAST and CAST II extend beyond the drugs studied or to other diseases remains to be learned.[82]

Left ventricular dysfunction is a major co-factor for the risk implied by chronic PVCs after myocardial infarction,[72] and complex forms of both PVCs and left ventricular dysfunction are independent predictors which exert lethal expressions most powerfully in different time periods after myocardial infarction. The risk of death indicated by post-myocardial infarction PVCs is therefore enhanced by the presence of left ventricular dysfunction (Fig. 24–5); the latter appears to exert its influence most strongly in the first 6 months after infarction.[72] Finally, there are data suggesting that the risk associated with post-infarction complex PVCs is higher in patients who have non-Q-wave infarctions than in those with transmural infarctions.[83]

Causes of Sudden Cardiac Death

Coronary heart disease and its consequences account for at least 80 per cent of SCDs in Western cultures. It also is the most common cause in many areas of the world in which the prevalence of coronary heart disease is lower. Despite the established relation between coronary heart disease and SCD,[18–20,34] a complete understanding of SCD requires recognition of other causes which, although less common and often quite rare (Table 24–2), may be recognizable before death, have therapeutic implications, and provide broad insight into the sudden death problem.

CORONARY ARTERY ABNORMALITIES. Although structural abnormalities of coronary arteries other than coronary atherosclerosis are infrequent causes of SCD, the relative risk of SCD may be quite high for specific abnormalities. Nonatherosclerotic coronary artery abnormalities include congenital lesions, coronary artery embolism, coronary arteritis, and mechanical abnormalities of the coronary arteries. Among the congenital lesions, *anomalous origin of a left coronary artery from the pulmonary artery* (see p. 909) is relatively common[84] and has a high death rate in childhood if not surgically treated.[85] The early risk for SCD is not excessively high,[84] but patients who survive to adulthood without surgical intervention are at risk.[85] Other forms of coronary AV fistulas are much less frequent and have a low incidence of SCD. *Anomalous origin of a left coronary artery from the right or noncoronary aortic sinus of Valsalva* (see p. 260) appears to have increased risk of SCD,[86–88] particularly when the anomalous artery passes between the aortic and the pulmonary artery roots. *Anomalous origin of the right coronary artery from the left sinus of Valsalva* also has been reported in association with SCD[86–88] but may not have the same risk as origin of the left coronary from the right sinus of Valsalva. Congenitally hypoplastic, stenotic, or atretic left coronary arteries are uncommon abnormalities which have a high risk of myocardial infarction but not of SCD.[84]

Embolism to the coronary arteries occurs most commonly in aortic valve endocarditis and from thrombotic material on diseased or prosthetic aortic or mitral valves.[89] Emboli also may originate from left ventricular mural thrombi or as a consequence of surgery or cardiac catheterization. Symptoms and signs of myocardial ischemia or infarction are the most common manifestations. In each of these categories SCD is a risk resulting from the electrophysiological consequences of the embolic ischemic event. Although embolism of platelet aggregates is a pathophysiological mechanism which has not clearly been demonstrated to be associated with SCD in clinical settings, some observations have focused attention on the feasibility of such a mechanism.

The *mucocutaneous lymph node syndrome* (Kawasaki's disease)[91] (see p. 994) carries a risk of SCD in association with coronary arteritis. Polyarteritis nodosa and related vasculitis syndromes (see p. 1783) can cause SCD presumably because of coronary arteritis,[92] as can coronary ostial stenosis in syphilitic aortitis[45] (see p. 1441). The latter has become a very rare manifestation of syphilis.[93]

Several types of mechanical obstruction to coronary arteries must be listed among causes of SCD. Coronary dissection, with or without dissection of the aorta, occurs in the Marfan syndrome[94] (see p. 1669) and has also been reported in the peripartum period of pregnancy.[95] Among the rare mechanical causes of SCD is prolapse of myxomatous polyps from the aortic valve into coronary ostia[96] as well as dissection or rupture of a sinus of Valsalva aneurysm, with involvement of the coronary ostia and proximal coronary arteries.[97] Finally, deep myocardial bridges over coronary arteries (see p. 258) have been reported in association with SCD occurring during strenuous exercise,[98] possibly due to dynamic mechanical obstruction.

Coronary artery spasm (see p. 1340) may cause serious arrhythmias and SCD[99–101] with or without concomitant coronary atherosclerotic lesions.[100] Painless myocardial ischemia, associated with either spasm or fixed lesions, may be a cause of heretofore unexplained sudden death.[101–103] Different patterns of silent ischemia (e.g., totally asymptomatic, post-myocardial infarction, and mixed silent/anginal pattern) may have different prognostic implications.[104]

VENTRICULAR HYPERTROPHY. Left ventricular hypertrophy is an independent risk factor for SCD,[6] accompanies many causes of SCD,[105] and may be a physiological contributor to mechanisms of potentially lethal arrhythmias.[105,106] The underlying states resulting in hypertrophy include hypertensive heart disease with or without atherosclerosis, valvular heart disease, obstructive and nonobstructive hypertrophic cardiomyopathy, primary pulmonary hypertension with right ventricular hypertrophy, and advanced right ventricular overload secondary to congenital heart disease. Each of these conditions is associated with risk of SCD, and it has been suggested that patients with severely hypertrophic ventricles are particularly susceptible to arrhythmic death.[105]

HYPERTROPHIC OBSTRUCTIVE CARDIOMYOPATHY (see p. 1414). Risk of SCD in hypertrophic obstructive cardiomyopathy was identified in the early clinical and hemodynamic studies of this entity.[107] Two subsequent large series have yielded similar data on the magnitude of this risk. Goodwin[108] observed 48 deaths, of which 36 (67 per cent) were sudden, among a cohort of 254 patients followed for a mean of 6 years, while Shah et al.[109] reported that 26 of 49 deaths (55 per cent) among 190 patients were sudden. Cardiac arrest survivors in this etiological group may have better long-term outcome than do survivors with other etiologies. In one report only 11/33 (33 per cent) had recurrent cardiac arrest or death during a mean follow-up of 7 years.[110]

Specific clinical markers have not been especially predictive of SCD in individual patients, although young age at onset,[108,111] strong family history,[43,108] and worsening symptoms[108] appear to indicate higher risk. In one study, however, 54 per cent of the sudden deaths occurred in patients without any functional limitations.[111] The mechanism of SCD in patients with hypertrophic obstructive cardiomyopathy was initially thought to involve outflow tract obstruction, possibly as a consequence of catecholamine stimulation, but more recent data have focused on lethal arrhythmias as the common mechanism of sudden death in this disease.[105,111–116] These studies have demonstrated a high prevalence of PVCs and nonsustained ventricular tachycardia on ambulatory monitoring,[112,114] or the inducibility of potentially lethal arrhythmias during programed electrical stimulation.[115,116] However, stable and asymptomatic nonsustained ventricular tachycardia has limited predictive power for SCD in these patients. Rapid and/or polymorphic symptomatic nonsustained tachycardias have better predictive power.

The question of whether the pathogenesis of the arrhythmias represents an interaction between electrophysiological and hemodynamic abnormalities or is a consequence of electrophysiological

TABLE 24–2 CAUSES AND CONTRIBUTING FACTORS IN SUDDEN CARDIAC DEATH

I. CORONARY ARTERY ABNORMALITIES
  A. Coronary atherosclerosis
    1. Chronic ischemic heart disease with transient supply/demand imbalance—thrombosis, spasm, physical stress
    2. Acute myocardial infarction
    3. Chronic atherosclerosis with change in myocardial substrate
  B. Congenital abnormalities of coronary arteries
    1. Anomalous origin from pulmonary artery
    2. Other coronary AV fistula
    3. Origin of left coronary artery from right sinus of Valsalva
    4. Origin of right coronary artery from left sinus of Valsalva
    5. Hypoplastic or aplastic coronary arteries
    6. Coronary-intracardiac shunt
  C. Coronary artery embolism
    1. Aortic or mitral endocarditis
    2. Prosthetic aortic or mitral valves
    3. Abnormal native valves or LV mural thrombus
    4. Platelet embolism
  D. Coronary arteritis
    1. Polyarteritis nodosa, progressive systemic sclerosis, giant cell arteritis
    2. Mucocutaneous lymph node syndrome (Kawasaki's disease)
    3. Syphilitic coronary ostial stenosis
  E. Miscellaneous mechanical obstruction of coronary arteries
    1. Coronary artery dissection in Marfan syndrome
    2. Coronary artery dissection in pregnancy
    3. Prolapse of aortic valve myxomatous polyps into coronary ostia
    4. Dissection or rupture of sinus of Valsalva
  F. Functional obstruction of coronary arteries
    1. Coronary artery spasm with or without atherosclerosis
    2. Myocardial bridges
II. HYPERTROPHY OF VENTRICULAR MYOCARDIUM
  A. Left ventricular hypertrophy associated with coronary heart disease
  B. Hypertensive heart disease without significant coronary atherosclerosis
  C. Hypertrophic myocardium secondary to valvular heart disease
  D. Hypertrophic cardiomyopathy
    1. Obstructive
    2. Nonobstructive
  E. Primary or secondary pulmonary hypertension
    1. Advanced chronic right ventricular overload
    2. Pulmonary hypertension in pregnancy (highest risk peripartum)
III. MYOCARDIAL DISEASES AND HEART FAILURE
  A. Chronic congestive heart failure
    1. Ischemic cardiomyopathy
    2. Idiopathic congestive cardiomyopathy
    3. Alcoholic cardiomyopathy
    4. Hypertensive cardiomyopathy
    5. Post-myocarditis cardiomyopathy
    6. Postpartum cardiomyopathy
  B. Acute cardiac failure
    1. Massive acute myocardial infarction
    2. Acute myocarditis
    3. Acute alcoholic cardiac dysfunction
    4. Ball-valve embolism in aortic stenosis or prosthesis
    5. Mechanical disruptions of cardiac structures
      (a) Rupture of ventricular free wall
      (b) Disruption of mitral apparatus
        (1) Papillary muscle
        (2) Chordae tendineae
        (3) Leaflet
      (c) Rupture of interventricular septum
    6. Acute pulmonary edema in noncompliant ventricles
IV. INFLAMMATORY, INFILTRATIVE, NEOPLASTIC, AND DEGENERATIVE PROCESSES
  A. Acute viral myocarditis with or without ventricular dysfunction
  B. Myocarditis associated with the vasculitides
  C. Sarcoidosis
  D. Progressive systemic sclerosis
  E. Amyloidosis
  F. Hemochromatosis
  G. Idiopathic giant cell myocarditis
  H. Chagas' disease
  I. Cardiac ganglionitis
  J. Arrhythmogenic right ventricular dysplasia; right ventricular cardiomyopathy
  K. Neuromuscular diseases (e.g., muscular dystrophy, Friedreich's ataxia, myotonic dystrophy)
  L. Intramural tumors
    1. Primary
    2. Metastatic

derangement of hypertrophied muscle[105,106] is unanswered. The observation that patients with nonobstructive hypertrophic cardiomyopathy have high-risk arrhythmias and are at increased risk for SCD[112] suggests that an electrophysiological mechanism secondary to the hypertrophied muscle itself plays some role. Stafford and colleagues[117] reported exercise-related cardiac arrest in nonobstructive hypertrophic cardiomyopathy. Ventricular fibrillation (VF) was reproduced during electrophysiological testing after induction of atrial fibrillation with a rapid ventricular response. In athletes under 35 years of age, hypertrophic cardiomyopathy is the most common cause of SCD, in contrast to athletes over the age of 35, among whom ischemic heart disease is the most common cause.[87,88,118–120]

SUDDEN DEATH IN DILATED CARDIOMYOPATHY AND HEART FAILURE. The advent of therapeutic interventions which provide better long-term control of congestive heart failure has begun to improve long-term survival of such patients (see p. 493). However, the proportion of heart failure patients with stable hemodynamics who die suddenly appears to be increasing.[121] In reports to date, as many as 47 per cent of deaths in heart failure patients are categorized as SCDs, and the risk of SCD increases with deteriorating left ventricular function.[122] The mechanism (VT/VF versus bradyarrhythmias/asystole) appears to relate to cause—i.e., ischemic versus nonischemic.[122] Among patients with cardiomyopathy who have good functional capacity (Class I and II), total mortality risk is considerably better than for those with poor functional capacity (Class III and IV). However, the proportional risk of death being sudden and unexpected is higher in the better functional class group[123] (Fig. 24–6). In contrast, unexplained syncope has been observed to be a powerful predictor of SCD in patients who are functional Class II or IV due to any etiology.[124] The actuarial 1-year probability of SCD was 45 per cent in this study.

The interaction between post-myocardial infarction ventricular arrhythmia and depressed ejection fraction in determining risk for SCD has been described.[72] The majority of studies addressing the relation between chronic congestive heart failure and SCD focused on patients with ischemic, idiopathic, and alcoholic congestive cardiomyopathy.[121,123,125–127] A chronic myopathic syndrome after myocarditis has been cited as an infrequent but well-documented cause of SCD.[128] Peripartum cardiomyopathy (see p. 1851) also may cause SCD.

Acute Heart Failure. All causes of acute cardiac failure, in the absence of prompt interventions, may result in SCD caused by either the circulatory failure itself or secondary arrhythmias. The electrophysiological mechanisms involved have been proposed to be related to acute stretching of myocardial fibers and/or the His-Purkinje system, with its experimentally demonstrated arrhythmogenic effect,[129] but the roles of neurohumoral mechanisms and acute electrolyte shifts have not been fully evaluated.[121] Among the causes of acute cardiac failure which are associated with SCD are massive acute myocardial infarction, acute myocarditis, acute alcoholic cardiac dysfunction, and a number of mechanical causes of heart failure such as massive pulmonary embolism, mechanical disruption of intracardiac

TABLE 24–2 CAUSES AND CONTRIBUTING FACTORS IN SUDDEN CARDIAC DEATH—*Continued*

M. Obstructive intracavitary tumors
   1. Neoplastic
   2. Thrombotic

V. DISEASES OF THE CARDIAC VALVES
   A. Valvular aortic stenosis/insufficiency
   B. Mitral valve disruption
   C. Mitral valve prolapse
   D. Endocarditis
   E. Prosthetic valve dysfunction

VI. CONGENITAL HEART DISEASE
   A. Congenital aortic or pulmonic valve stenosis
   B. Right-to-left shunts with Eisenmenger's physiology
      1. Advanced disease
      2. During labor and delivery
   C. After surgical repair of congenital lesions, e.g., tetralogy of Fallot

VII. ELECTROPHYSIOLOGICAL ABNORMALITIES
   A. Abnormalities of the conducting system
      1. Fibrosis of the His-Purkinje system
         (a) Primary degeneration (Lenegre's disease)
         (b) Secondary to fibrosis and calcification of the "cardiac skeleton" (Lev's disease)
         (c) Post-viral conducting system fibrosis
         (d) Hereditary conducting system disease
      2. Anomalous pathways of conduction
   B. Prolonged Q-T interval syndrome
      1. Congenital
         (a) With deafness
         (b) Without deafness
      2. Acquired
         (a) Drug effect
            (1) Cardiac, antiarrhythmic
            (2) Noncardiac
         (b) Electrolyte abnormality
         (c) Toxic substances
         (d) Hypothermia
         (e) Central nervous system injury
   C. Ventricular fibrillation of unknown or uncertain cause
      1. Absence of identifiable structural or functional causes
         (a) "Idiopathic" ventricular fibrillation
         (b) Short-coupled torsades de pointes, polymorphic VT
         (c) Nonspecific (?) fibrofatty infiltration in previously healthy victim
      2. Sleep-death in Southeast Asians
         (a) Bangungut
         (b) Pokkuri
         (c) Nonlaitai

VIII. ELECTRICAL INSTABILITY RELATED TO NEUROHUMORAL AND CENTRAL NERVOUS SYSTEM INFLUENCES
   A. Catecholamine-dependent lethal arrhythmias
   B. Central nervous system–related
      1. Psychic stress, emotional extremes
      2. Auditory-related
      3. "Voodoo" death in primitive cultures
      4. Diseases of the cardiac nerves
      5. Congenital Q-T interval prolongation

IX. SUDDEN INFANT DEATH SYNDROME AND SUDDEN DEATH IN CHILDREN
   A. Sudden infant death syndrome
      1. Immature respiratory control functions
      2. Susceptibility to lethal arrhythmias
      3. Congenital heart disease
      4. Myocarditis
   B. Sudden death in children
      1. Eisenmenger syndrome, aortic stenosis, hypertrophic cardiomyopathy, pulmonary atresia
      2. After corrective surgery for congenital heart disease
      3. Myocarditis
      4. No identified structural or functional cause

X. MISCELLANEOUS
   A. Sudden death during extreme physical activity
   B. Mechanical interference with venous return
      1. Acute cardiac tamponade
      2. Massive pulmonary embolism
      3. Acute intracardiac thrombosis
   C. Dissecting aneurysm of the aorta
   D. Toxic/metabolic disturbances
      1. Electrolyte disturbances
      2. Metabolic disturbances
      3. Proarrhythmic effects of antiarrhythmic drugs
      4. Proarrhythmic effects of noncardiac drugs
   E. Mimics of sudden cardiac death
      1. "Cafe coronary"
      2. Acute alcoholic states ("holiday heart")
      3. Acute asthmatic attacks
      4. Air or amniotic fluid embolism

structures secondary to infarction or infection, and ball-valve embolism in aortic or mitral stenosis (Table 24–2).

INFLAMMATORY, INFILTRATIVE, NEOPLASTIC, AND DEGENERATIVE DISEASES OF THE HEART. Almost all diseases in this category have been associated with SCD, with or without concomitant cardiac failure. Acute viral myocarditis with left ventricular dysfunction (see p. 1437) is commonly associated with cardiac arrhythmias, including potentially lethal arrhythmias. It is now recognized that serious ventricular arrhythmias or SCD can occur in myocarditis in the absence of clinical evidence of left ventricular dysfunction.[45,128,130] In a report of 19 SCDs among 1,606,167 previously screened US Air Force recruits, 8 of the 19 (42 per cent) had evidence of myocarditis (5 nonrheumatic, 3 rheumatic) at postmortem examination, and 15 (79 per cent) suffered their cardiac arrests during strenuous exertion.[131] Viral carditis also may cause damage isolated to the specialized conducting system and result in a propensity to arrhythmias; the rare association of this process with SCD has been reported.[132] The risk of potentially lethal arrhythmias is not limited to the acute phase of the disease.[128]

Myocardial involvement in collagen-vascular disorders, tumors, chronic granulomatous diseases, infiltrative disorders, and protozoan infestations varies widely, but in all instances SCD may be the initial or terminal manifestation of the disease process. Among the granulomatous diseases, *sarcoidosis* (see p. 1431) stands out because of the frequency of SCD associated with it. Roberts et al.[133] reported that SCD was the terminal event in 67 per cent of sarcoid heart disease deaths; the occurrence of SCD has been related to the extent of cardiac involvement.[134] In a report on the pathological findings in nine patients who died of *progressive systemic sclerosis*, (see p. 1781), eight who died suddenly had evidence of transient ischemia and reperfusion histologically, suggesting that this might represent Raynaud-like involvement of coronary vessels.[135] *Amyloidosis* of the heart (see p. 1421) may also cause sudden death. An incidence of 30 per cent has been reported[139]; diffuse involvement of ventricular muscle or of the specialized conducting system may be associated with SCD.

Arrhythmogenic Right Ventricular Dysplasia (see p. 681). This condition is associated with a high incidence of ventricular arrhythmias, particularly recurrent ventricular tachycardia.[136] Although symptomatic ventricular tachycardia has been well recognized in the syndrome for many years, the risk of SCD was unclear[136] and thought to be relatively low. However, isolated right ventricular *cardiomyopathy* has histopathological features similar to right ventricular dysplasia and may be a variant, or advanced form, of the same process. Right ventricular cardiomyopathy carries a high risk of SCD,[137,138] suggesting that selection may have influenced the perception in the past that risk of SCD was low in right ventricular displasia.

VALVULAR HEART DISEASE (see Chap. 32). Before the advent of surgery for valvular heart disease, *aortic stenosis* was one of the more common noncoronary causes of SCD. Campbell reported in 1968 that 44 of 70 (73 per cent) deaths in patients with aortic stenosis were sudden.[141] The advent of safe and effective procedures for aortic valve replacement has reduced the incidence of this cause of sudden death,[142] but patients with prosthetic or heterograft aortic valve replacements remain at some risk for SCD caused by arrhythmias, prosthetic valve dysfunction, or coexistent coronary heart disease.[143] SCD has been reported to be the second most common mode of death after valve replacement surgery, accounting for 62 of 298 deaths (21 per cent).[144] The incidence peaked 3 weeks after operation and then plateaued after 8 months. Nonetheless, the risk is appreciably lower than in those patients who had not had the advantage of valvular surgery in prior years. In another report analyzing outcome in patients receiving prosthetic

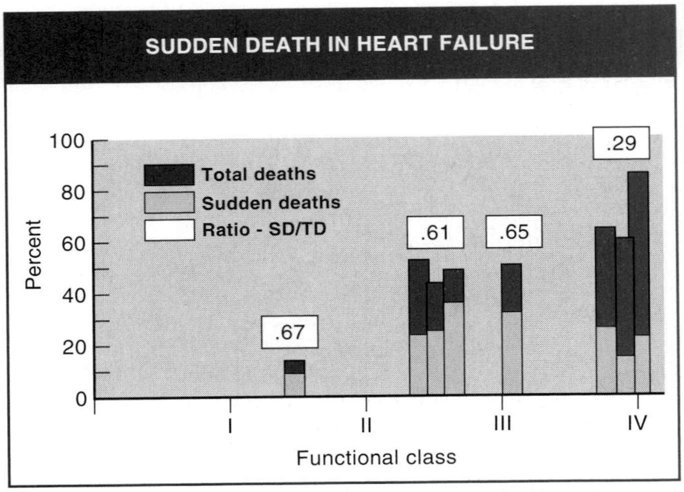

FIGURE 24–6. Risk of sudden cardiac death related to functional classification in heart failure. The relative probability of death being sudden is higher in the patients with better functional capacity who are at lower total mortality risk. (Modified from Kjekshus, J.: Arrhythmia and mortality in congestive heart failure. Am. J. Cardiol. *65*:42-I, 1990.)

valves for isolated severe aortic stenosis, SCD occurred at a rate of only 0.3 per cent/year and was responsible for only 18 per cent of late deaths.[145] A high incidence of ventricular arrhythmia has been observed during follow-up of patients with valve replacement,[145,146] especially in those who had aortic stenosis, multiple valve surgery, or cardiomegaly.[146] Sudden death during follow-up was associated with ventricular arrhythmias and thromboembolism. Hemodynamic variables were less predictive. Stenotic lesions of other valves imply much lower risk of SCD. Regurgitant lesions, particularly chronic aortic regurgitation and acute mitral regurgitation, may cause SCD, but the risk is also lower than with aortic stenosis.

Mitral valve prolapse (see p. 1029) is prevalent and associated with a high incidence of cardiac arrhythmias; however, the incidence of SCD is quite low.[147] This uncommon complication appears to correlate with nonspecific ST-T wave changes in the inferior leads on the ECG.[148] In data reviewed from 17 reported instances of SCD in mitral valve prolapse patients, these nonspecific ST-T wave changes were present in 6 of 8 who had had prior electrocardiograms.[149] An association with redundancy of mitral leaflets on echocardiogram also has been suggested.[150] Reported associations between Q-T interval prolongation or preexcitation and SCD in mitral prolapse syndrome are less consistent.[147]

Endocarditis of the aortic and mitral valves (see Chap. 33) may be associated with rapid death resulting from acute disruption of the valvular apparatus, coronary embolism, or abscesses of valvular rings or the septum; however, such deaths are rarely true sudden deaths as conventionally defined.

CONGENITAL HEART DISEASE. The congenital lesions most commonly associated with SCD are aortic stenosis (see p. 1035)[130,151,152] and communications between the left and right sides of the heart with the Eisenmenger physiology (see p. 799).[153] In the latter the risk of SCD is a function of pulmonary vascular disease severity; also, there is an extraordinarily high risk of maternal mortality during labor and delivery in the pregnant patient with Eisenmenger syndrome (see p. 975).[154] Potentially lethal arrhythmias and SCD have been described as late complications after surgical repair of complex congenital lesions, particularly tetralogy of Fallot (see p. 929), transposition of the great arteries, and atrioventricular canal.[155,156] These patients should be followed closely and treated aggressively when cardiac arrhythmias are identified, although the late risk of SCD may not be as high as previously thought.[157]

ELECTROPHYSIOLOGICAL ABNORMALITIES. Acquired disease of the AV node and His-Purkinje system and the presence of accessory pathways of conduction are two groups of structural abnormalities of specialized conduction which may be associated with SCD. Epidemiological studies have suggested that intraventricular conduction disturbances in coronary heart disease are one of the few factors that may increase the proportion of SCD in coronary heart disease.[37] A specific clinical example is the risk of VF during the first 30 days after myocardial infarction in patients with anterior infarctions and bundle branch block. Lie et al.[158] reported that 47 per cent of patients who had late hospital VF had had anteroseptal infarcts with bundle branch block, and that these 14 were from a total pool of only 40 patients with the combination of bundle branch block and anterior myocardial infarction. Thus there was a 35 per cent incidence of VF in this subgroup, which represented only 4.1 per cent of a total of 966 myocardial infarctions. This risk persists for 6 weeks after the infarction and then abates.[159] AV block or intraventricular conduction abnormalities were found in 9 of 10 patients who had recurrent VF during hospitalization after resuscitation from prehospital cardiac arrest.[20]

Primary fibrosis (Lenegre's disease)[160] or secondary mechanical injury (Lev's disease)[161] of the His-Purkinje system is commonly associated with intraventricular conduction abnormalities and symptomatic AV block, and less commonly with SCD. The identification of people at risk and the efficacy of pacemakers for preventing SCD, rather than only ameliorating symptoms, have been the subjects of debate.[162,163] However, current prevailing thought is that survival may depend more on the nature and extent of the underlying disease than on the conduction disturbance itself.[164]

Patients with congenital AV block (see p. 966) or nonprogressive congenital intraventricular block usually have a low risk of SCD.[165] Progressive congenital intraventricular blocks predict a high risk,[165] as does the coexistence of structural congenital defects. A hereditary form has been reported in association with a familial propensity to SCD.[46,165]

The anomalous pathways of conduction, bundles of Kent in the Wolff-Parkinson-White syndrome, and Mahaim fibers, are commonly associated with nonlethal arrhythmias. However, when the anomalous pathways of conduction have short refractory periods, the occurrence of atrial fibrillation may allow the induction of VF during very rapid conduction across the bypass tract.[166] The incidence of SCD in patients with short refractory period bypass tracts is not yet known. Patients who have multiple pathways appear to be at higher risk of SCD,[166] as do patients with a familial pattern of anomalous pathways and premature SCD.[167]

Q-T Prolongation (see also pp. 685 and 1667). The prolonged Q-T interval syndrome is a functional abnormality, perhaps associated with neurogenic influences, that may cause lethal arrhythmias.[168] In the hereditary *congenital form* two varieties have been reported: those with autosomal recessive inheritance and associated deafness, the Jervell and Lange-Nielsen syndrome,[169] and those without deafness, the Romano-Ward syndrome.[42] Some patients have prolonged Q-T intervals throughout life without any manifest arrhythmias, whereas others are highly susceptible to symptomatic and potentially fatal ventricular arrhythmias, particularly the torsades de pointes form of ventricular tachycardia.[170] Patients at higher risk are characterized by deafness, female gender, syncope, and documented torsades depointes or prior ventricular fibrillation, and they require aggressive medical or surgical interventions.[171,172] Moreover, making an effort to identify relatives at risk is an important preventive measure, given the familial pattern of the entity. A recent major advance has been the identification of three specific genetic markers by linkage analyses[48–50] (see p. 1667).

The *acquired form* of prolonged Q-T interval may be due to drug idiosyncrasies (particularly antiarrhythmics and psychotropic drugs), electrolyte abnormalities, hypothermia, toxic substances, and central nervous system injury.[172] It also has been reported both in intensive weight reduction programs that involve the use of liquid protein diets[173] and in anorexia nervosa.[174] Lithium carbonate may prolong the Q-T interval and has been reported to be associated with an increased incidence of SCD in cancer patients with preexisting heart disease.[175] Drug interactions recently have been recognized as a mechanism of prolongation of the Q-T interval and torsades de pointes. For example, terfenadine (Seldane), which can prolong the Q-T interval, is normally converted by a hepatic P450 enzyme to a metabolite that retains antihistamine activity, but not Q-T prolonging effects. It may be arrhythmogenic when the hepatic enzyme is blocked by another substance, such as ketoconazole.[176] Acquired prolonged Q-T intervals usually carry a risk of serious arrhythmias and SCD, but the risk is abolished when the inciting factor is removed. In acquired prolonged Q-T syndrome, as in the congenital form, the torsades de pointes form of ventricular tachycardia is commonly the specific arrhythmia that triggers or degenerates into lethal VF.

ELECTRICAL INSTABILITY RESULTING FROM NEUROHUMORAL AND CENTRAL NERVOUS SYSTEM INFLUENCES. Catecholamine-dependent lethal arrhythmias in the absence of Q-T interval prolongation, with control by beta-adrenoceptor blocking agents, have been described.[177] Several central nervous system–related interactions with cardiac electrical stability have been suggested (see p. 1878). The hereditary forms of prolonged Q-T interval syndrome, discussed above, appear to have a relation to sympathetic nervous system imbalance.[168,178] Lown and coworkers identified psychic stress as a mediating factor for advanced cardiac arrhythmias and perhaps SCD.[179] Epidemiological data also suggest an association between behavioral abnormalities and the risk of SCD, particularly in women[67,68]; emotional extremes have been suggested as a triggering mechanism for SCD.[3,180] Associations between auditory stimulation[130] and auditory auras[181] and SCD have been reported.[130] The auditory abnormalities in some forms of congenital Q-T prolongation have already been cited.[169]

A variant of torsades de pointes, characterized by short coupling intervals between a normal impulse and the initiating impulse, has been described (Fig. 24–7). It appears to have familial trends and to be related to alterations in autonomic nervous system activity. The 12-lead ECG demonstrates normal Q-T intervals; but ventricular fibrillation and sudden death are common.

The syndrome of "voodoo death" in developing countries has been studied extensively.[183,184] There appears to be an association between isolation from the tribe, a sense of hopelessness, severe bradyarrhythmias, and sudden death. With cultural changes in many of these areas, the syndrome has become less amenable to observation and study; however, there do remain pockets of cultural isolation in which the syndrome no doubt still exists.

SUDDEN INFANT DEATH SYNDROME AND SCD IN CHILDREN

The sudden infant death syndrome (SIDS) occurs between birth and 6 months of age, more commonly in males, and has an incidence of 0.1 to 0.3 per cent of live births.[185] Because of its abrupt nature, a cardiac mechanism has been suspected for many years,[186] but a variety of causes, with central respiratory dysfunction playing a major role, are considered likely.[187] Many cases of the sudden infant death syndrome are believed to represent a form of "sleep apnea" which, if prolonged, may lead to hypoxia, cyanosis, and cardiac arrhythmias. Experience with "near-misses" and the results of respiratory monitoring, in conjunction with the propensity of the syndrome to occur in premature infants, all suggest impaired central nervous system respiratory control reflexes, possibly owing to immaturity.[185,187–189] There has recently been interest, however, in the possibility of obstructive apnea as another mechanism.[187] Identification of individual infants at risk is difficult, but the risk does not persist beyond the first 6 months of life.

Despite the current focus on the respiratory mechanisms involved in the syndrome, their role has not yet been explicitly established. Furthermore, the question of whether or not an identifiable subset of infants who have apneic spells are particularly prone to genesis of cardiac arrhythmias remains conjectural.[188–190] A primary cardiac cause is still considered the basis of this syndrome in some victims.[186,190] Marino and Kane[191] observed either accessory pathways (two cases)

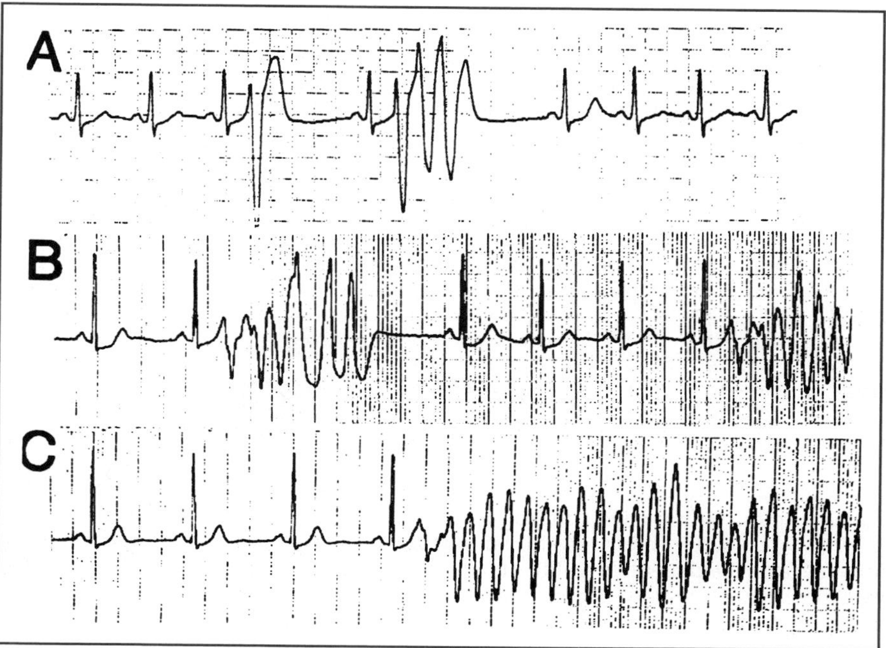

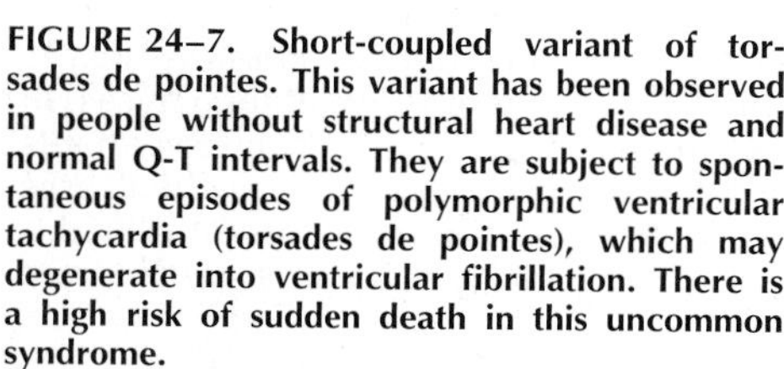
FIGURE 24–7. Short-coupled variant of torsades de pointes. This variant has been observed in people without structural heart disease and normal Q-T intervals. They are subject to spontaneous episodes of polymorphic ventricular tachycardia (torsades de pointes), which may degenerate into ventricular fibrillation. There is a high risk of sudden death in this uncommon syndrome.

or dispersed or immature AV nodal or bundle branch cells in the annulus fibrosus (four cases) among a group of seven sudden infant death syndrome victims studied by detailed histopathology.

Sudden death in children beyond the age group at risk for SIDS often is associated with identifiable heart disease,[129,192] although one study identified cardiac causes in only 25 per cent of sudden natural death victims between the ages of 1 and 21 years.[40] About 25 per cent of SCDs in children occur in those who have undergone previous surgery for congenital cardiac disease. Of the remaining 75 per cent, more than one-half occur in children who have one of four lesions: congenital aortic stenosis, Eisenmenger syndrome, pulmonary stenosis or atresia, or obstructive hypertrophic cardiomyopathy.[192] Neuspiel and Kuller[40] observed 14 cases of myocarditis among 51 SCDs in children (27 per cent).

OTHER CAUSES OF SUDDEN DEATH

SCD in athletes during or after extreme physical activity is infrequent but receives a great deal of attention when it does occur. The special position of prominent athletes in society has created unusual, conflicting, and sometimes inconsistent attitudes in response to SCD risk in these individuals.[193] The majority of such individuals have a previously unrecognized cardiac abnormality, with hypertrophic cardiomyopathy with or without obstruction, valvular aortic stenosis, and occult coronary artery disease as the most common causes identified after death.[88,118–120,194,195] A surprisingly large fraction of people who died suddenly during exertion had unsuspected myocarditis, according to a report of a large cohort of US Air Force recruits.[131] A small group of such victims, however, have neither previously determined functional abnormality nor structural abnormalities at postmortem examination.[20,87,88,128,129]

There are rare instances of idiopathic VF causing SCD in the absence of any identifiable structural or functional abnormality of the heart.[196] Although long-term survival after a potentially fatal event appears to be good, some degree of risk appears to remain.[197] Limited data suggest that risk persists primarily in patients with subtle cardiac abnormalities, in contrast to patients who are truly normal.[198] In addition, these events tend to occur in young, otherwise healthy people. A specific variation of this syndrome has been observed in southeast Asians. Many years ago syndromes referred to as *Bangungut* in young Filipino males,[199] *Pokkuri* in young Japanese males,[200] and *Nonlaitai* in young Laotian males[201] were reported. In each there was a tendency for sudden death to occur during sleep, and at one time a toxic cause was suspected.[199,200] Documented cases have now been reported in Laotians who came to the United States after the Vietnam war. The mechanism was identified to be ventricular fibrillation in some of these cases; in at least one instance electrophysiological study demonstrated inducible ventricular arrhythmia by programmed electrical stimulation.[202] Pathological examinations have revealed a high incidence of mild to significant cardiomegaly (14 of 18) and a variety of structural abnormalities of specialized conducting tissue.[203] The fact that these cases continue to occur in a new cultural setting suggests that there may be a hereditary predisposition.

There also are a number of noncardiac conditions which *mimic* SCD. These include the so-called *cafe coronary*,[204,205] in which food, usually an unchewed piece of meat, lodges in the oropharynx and causes an abrupt obstruction at the glottis. The classic description of a cafe coronary is sudden cyanosis and collapse in a restaurant, during a meal accompanied by lively conversation. The *holiday heart syndrome* is characterized by cardiac arrhythmias, most commonly atrial, and other cardiac abnormalities associated with acute alcoholic states.[206] It has not been determined whether potentially lethal arrhythmias occurring in such settings account for reported sudden deaths associated with acute alcoholic states.[3] *Massive pulmonary embolism* (Chap. 46) may cause acute cardiovascular collapse and sudden death; sudden death in severe acute asthmatic attacks, without prolonged deterioration of the patient's condition, is well recognized.[207] Air or amniotic fluid embolism at the time of labor and delivery may cause sudden death on rare occasions, with the clinical picture mimicking sudden cardiac death.[208] Peripartum air embolism caused by an unusual sexual practice has been reported as a cause of such sudden deaths.[209]

Proarrhythmic effects of antiarrhythmic drugs have received particular attention,[210] but psychotropic drugs, arrhythmogenic effects of toxic substances, and electrolyte disturbances—particularly hypokalemia, hypocalcemia, and hypomagnesemia—also have been implicated.[172] Classic proarrhythmia is an event which tends to appear within days after the initiation of antiarrhythmic therapy.[211] The pattern of SCD over time among patients treated with two of the drugs used in the Cardiac Arrhythmia Suppression Trial suggests a different pattern of proarrhythmic risk, likely caused by a different mechanism.[59,82] This form of risk appears to be a continuous function extending over 1 or more years of exposure.

Finally, a number of abnormalities that do not directly involve the heart may cause SCD or mimic it. These include aortic dissection (see p. 1564), acute cardiac tamponade (see p. 1503), and rapid exsanguination (see p. 1539).

PATHOLOGY AND PATHOPHYSIOLOGY

Pathological observations in SCD victims reflect the epidemiological and clinical preponderance of coronary heart disease as the major structural predisposing factor.[212] Liberthson and coworkers[213] reported that 81 per cent of 220 autopsied victims of SCD had significant coronary heart disease, defined as more than one coronary vessel with greater than 75 per cent stenosis as the primary pathological feature. At least one vessel with more than 75 per cent stenosis was found in 94 per cent of victims, acute coronary occlusion in 58 per cent, healed myocardial infarction in 44 per cent, and acute myocardial infarction in 27 per cent. These observations are consistent with many other studies of the frequency of coronary disease in sudden death victims. All of the other causes of SCD (Table 24–2) collectively account for no more than 10 to 20 per cent of cases, but they have provided a large base of enlightening pathological data.[45,128]

THE PATHOLOGY OF SUDDEN DEATH CAUSED BY CORONARY HEART DISEASE

THE CORONARY ARTERIES. Extensive atherosclerosis is the most common pathological finding in the coronary arteries of victims of SCD (Table 24–3). In postmortem examinations of 169 hearts, sites of 75 per cent or more stenosis were present in three or four major vessels in 61 per cent of the hearts studied; two vessels with at least 75 per cent stenosis were found in 15 per cent; and 24 per cent of the hearts had either single-vessel disease or no vessels having lesions producing 75 per cent stenosis.[214] A distinctly higher proportion of hearts having three or four vessels with 75 per cent stenotic lesions was observed in white men (70 per cent) compared with white women (34 per cent). In contrast, 58 per cent of the hearts of both black men and black women had three or four vessels with 75 per cent or more stenoses. Consistent with clinical findings in survivors of out-of-hospital cardiac arrest,[20] there was no special predilection of disease distribution for any coronary artery, and there was no quantitative difference between proximal and distal distribution of disease.

Kuller et al.[52] pointed out that 90 per cent or greater narrowing of at least one coronary artery was found in 77 per cent of autopsied victims of sudden *coronary* death, compared with 8 per cent of victims of other causes of sudden death. Davies[45] reported that 61 per cent of patients dying suddenly because of coronary heart disease had three vessels with 75 per cent or more stenosis at any one point; an additional 18 (23 per cent) had two vessels with 75 per

TABLE 24–3 PATHOLOGICAL FINDINGS IN SUDDEN DEATH DUE TO CORONARY HEART DISEASE

THE CORONARY ARTERIES	VENTRICULAR MYOCARDIUM
A. Chronic atherosclerosis	A. Healed myocardial infarction
B. Acute lesions	B. Left ventricular hypertrophy
1. Plaque fissuring	C. Ventricular aneurysm
2. Platelet aggregates	D. Acute myocardial infarction
3. Organizing thrombus	
4. Coronary artery spasm	

cent or more stenosis. Among 100 age- and sex-matched controls who died of trauma or cerebral tumors, only 27 per cent had two- or three-vessel disease, and 52 per cent had no vessels with lesions of 75 per cent or more. In the same study the majority of sudden deaths caused by coronary heart disease were associated with at least one point of more than 85 per cent stenosis, and Davies suggested that this parameter provided the best discrimination between hearts of SCD victims and controls.

Several studies have demonstrated no specific pattern of distribution of coronary artery lesions which preselect for SCD. In a quantitative analysis comparing coronary artery narrowing at postmortem examination in SCD victims and controls, 36 per cent of the 5-mm segments of the coronary arteries from the SCD group had 76 to 100 per cent cross-sectional area reductions compared with 3 per cent in the controls.[215] An additional 34 per cent of the sections from the SCD group had 51 to 75 per cent reductions in cross-sectional areas. Only 7 per cent of the sections from the SCD patients had 0 to 25 per cent reductions in cross-sectional areas. The *distribution* of the lesions causing greater than 75 per cent narrowing was similar in the three major coronary arteries, but quantitative differences between proximal and distal halves of the vessels were inconsistent.[215] Similar conclusions resulted from pathological observations of out-of-hospital cardiac arrest victims who were not successfully resuscitated.[213] These studies indicate that extensive coronary artery disease is the pathological hallmark of SCDs caused by coronary heart disease and that no specific anatomical pattern of distribution of the disease preselects SCD victims.

The role of acute (active) *coronary artery* lesions, such as plaque fissuring, platelet aggregation, and thrombosis, in the onset of cardiac arrest leading to SCD, is becoming clarified.[216,217] In one study of 100 consecutive sudden coronary death victims, 44 per cent had major (more than 50 per cent luminal occlusion) recent coronary thrombi, 30 per cent had minor occlusive thrombi, and 21 per cent had plaque fissuring.[216] Only 5 per cent had no acute coronary artery changes; 65 per cent of the thrombi occurred at sites of preexisting high-grade stenoses, and an additional 19 per cent were found at sites of more than 50 per cent stenosis. In a subsequent study by the same investigators, 50/168 victims (30 per cent) had occlusive intraluminal coronary thrombi, and 73 (44 per cent) had mural intraluminal thrombi.[217] Single-vessel disease, acute infarction at postmortem examination, and prodromal symptoms were associated with the presence of thrombi.

An overview of the major studies on the incidence of acute thrombotic occlusions, in which the definition of sudden death ranges from 15 minutes to 24 hours, reveals wide variation in the reported frequency of recent coronary thrombosis in sudden death. It ranges from 15 to 64 per cent, but the majority of studies which used 6 hours or less as the definition of "sudden" had frequencies of less than 40 per cent.[212,213,216–219] Factors which confound the analysis of such data include relations between platelet aggregates and thrombus formation and the spontaneous lysis of clots.

Baba et al.[219] reported the presence of *organizing* thrombus in about 31 per cent of 121 sudden coronary heart disease deaths. They were commonly associated with sites of more than 75 per cent chronic obstruction and with concomitant acute lesions at the same sites, leading to the speculation that clinical events 5 to 7 days before death might create a substrate for fatal acute coronal events. *Coronary artery spasm,* an established cause of acute ischemia, also may cause SCD and is recognizable in rare instances at postmortem examination.[220]

THE MYOCARDIUM. Myocardial pathology in SCD caused by coronary heart disease reflects the extensive atherosclerosis which usually is present. Studies in victims of out-of-hospital SCD and from epidemiological sources both indicate that healed myocardial infarction is a common finding in sudden coronary death victims, with most investigators reporting frequencies ranging from 40 to more than 70 per cent.[8,196,221,222] For example, Newman and coworkers[221,222] reported that 72 per cent of men in a 25-to-44-year age group who died suddenly (24 or fewer hours) with no previous clinical history of coronary heart disease had scars of large (63 per cent) or small (less than 1 cm cross-sectional area, 9 per cent) areas of healed myocardial necrosis. The incidence of acute myocardial infarction is considerably less, with cytopathological evidence of recent myocardial infarction averaging about 20 per cent. This estimate corresponds well with studies in out-of-hospital cardiac arrest survivors, who have an incidence of new myocardial infarction in the range of 20 to 30 per cent.

VENTRICULAR HYPERTROPHY. Myocardial hypertrophy may coexist and interact with acute or chronic ischemia but appears to confer an independent mortality risk.[223] There is not a close correlation between increased heart weight and severity of coronary heart disease in SCD victims[214]; heart weights are higher in SCD victims than in those with non–sudden death despite similar prevalence of history of hypertension before death.[8] Hypertrophy-associated mortality risk is also independent of left ventricular function and extent of coronary artery disease.[223] Anderson[105] suggests that left ventricular hypertrophy itself may be a predisposing factor to SCD. Experimental data also suggest increased susceptibility to potentially lethal ventricular arrhythmias in left ventricular hypertrophy with ischemia and reperfusion.[224] A study of massively enlarged hearts (i.e., weighing more than 1000 gm), however, did not indicate an excess incidence of SCD,[225] but the underlying pathology in that study was dominated by lesions that produce volume overload.

SPECIALIZED CONDUCTING SYSTEM IN SCD

Pathological data on the specialized conducting system of victims of SCD are relatively sparse. Lie[226] studied the specialized conducting system of 49 of 120 SCD patients with no previous history of coronary heart disease who died within 6 hours of onset of symptoms. Thirty-nine patients had acute myocardial infarction and 10 did not. Two patients with acute anteroseptal infarctions had hemorrhage and/or infarction involving the AV node and peripheral bundle branches. Luminal narrowing of the artery to the AV node was present in 50 per cent, but there were no thromboses of vessels to the specialized conducting system. Evidence of ischemic injury was present with an equal frequency in SCD[226] and myocardial infarction patients.[227]

Fibrosis of the specialized conducting system is a common but nonspecific endpoint of multiple causes. Although this process is associated with AV block or intraventricular conduction abnormalities, its role in SCD is uncertain. Lev's and Lenegre's diseases, ischemic injury caused by small-vessel disease, and numerous infiltrative or inflammatory processes all may result in such changes. In addition, active inflammatory processes such as myocarditis and infiltrative processes such as amyloidosis, scleroderma, hemochromatosis, and morbid obesity all may damage or destroy the AV node and/or bundle of His and result in AV block.[228]

Focal diseases such as sarcoidosis, Whipple's disease, and rheumatoid arthritis also may involve the conducting system. These various categories of conducting system disease have been considered as possible pathological substrates for SCD which may be overlooked because of the difficulty in doing careful postmortem examinations of the conducting system routinely.[228] Focal involvement of conducting tissue by tumors (especially mesothelioma of the AV node but also lymphoma, carcinoma, rhabdomyoma, and fibroma) also has been reported,[228] and rare cases of SCD have been associated with these lesions. It has been suggested that abnormal postnatal morphogenesis of the specialized conducting system may be a significant factor in some SCDs in infants and children.[228]

CARDIAC NERVES AND SCD

Diseases of cardiac nerves have been postulated to have a role in SCD.[229,230] Neural involvement may be the result of random damage to neural elements within the myocardium (i.e., "secondary" cardioneuropathy), or may be "primary," as in a selective cardiac viral neuropathy.[230] Secondary involvement may be a consequence of ischemic neural injury in coronary heart disease and has been postulated to result in autonomic destabilization, enhancing the propensity to arrhythmias. Some experimental data support this hypothesis, and a clinical technique for imaging cardiac neural fibers suggests a changing pattern over time after myocardial infarction.[231-234] Involvement of neural plexuses, with or without conducting system involvement, has been observed at necropsy in 54 per cent of patients who died within 24 hours of onset of myocardial infarction.[229] Specific causes for primary cardioneuropathies are less obvious. Viral, neurotoxic, and hereditary causes (e.g., progressive muscular dystrophy and Friedreich's ataxia) have been emphasized.

Disordered extrinsic neural involvement of the heart usually is considered to be functional, such as in prolonged Q-T interval syndrome. However, a primary role for neural dysfunction in hereditary long Q-T syndrome is open to question now that genetic abnormalities that alter specific membrane ion channels involved in repolarization processes have been demonstrated in a number of families (see p. 1667).[48-50] Nonetheless, stellate ganglion inflammation has been observed in some tissues removed surgically for symptomatic Q-T prolongation in hereditary Q-T syndrome[235] or after myocardial infarction.[236] The possible significance of such extrinsic cardiac neural involvement is not yet clear.[236]

MECHANISMS AND PATHOPHYSIOLOGY

The occurrence of potentially lethal tachyarrhythmias, or of severe bradyarrhythmia or asystole, is the end of a cascade of pathophysiological abnormalities which result from complex interactions between coronary vascular events, myocardial injury, variations in autonomic tone, and/or the metabolic and electrolyte state of the myocardium. There is no uniform hypothesis regarding mechanisms by which these elements interact to lead to the final pathway of lethal arrhythmias. However, Figure 24–8 shows a model of the pathophysiology of SCD, in which the central event is the initiation of a potentially fatal arrhythmia. The possibility of this event is increased by a variety of *structural abnormalities* and modulated by *functional variations*.[237]

Pathophysiological Mechanisms of Lethal Tachyarrhythmias

CORONARY ARTERY STRUCTURE AND FUNCTION. In that large majority of SCDs associated with coronary atherosclerosis, the distribution of chronic arterial narrowing has been well defined by pathological studies.[45,212,213] However, the specific mechanisms by which these lesions lead to potentially lethal disturbances of electrical stability are poorly understood. Steady-state reductions in regional myocardial blood flow, in the absence of superimposed acute lesions, may create a setting in which alterations in the metabolic or electrolyte state of the myocardium or neural fluctuations result in loss of electrical stability.[121] Increased myocardial oxygen demand with a fixed supply may be the mechanism of exercise-induced arrhythmias and sudden death during intense physical activity in athletes or others whose heart disease had not previously become clinically manifested.[87,88,118-120,131,194,195,238] Vasoactive events leading to acute reduction in regional myocardial blood flow in the presence of a normal or previously compromised circulation constitute a common cause of transient ischemia, angina pectoris, arrhythmias, and perhaps SCD.[101-104] Coronary artery spasm or modulation of coronary collateral flow exposes the myocardium to the double hazard of transient ischemia and reperfusion (Fig. 24–9).[101,224,239] The mechanism of production of spasm is unclear, although sites of endothelial disease appear to predispose.[240] A role of the autonomic nervous system, particularly mechanisms related to alpha-adrenoceptor activity, has been suggested[241]; vagal activity also may be involved in the production of spasm,[242] possibly due to failure of acetylcholine to trigger release of nitrous oxide in areas of endothelial disease. However, neurogenic influences do not appear to be a sine qua non for the production of spasm. Vessel susceptibility and humoral factors, particularly those related to platelet activation and aggregation,[243] also appear to be important mechanisms.

Transition of stable atherosclerotic plaques to an "active" state because of endothelial damage, with plaque fissuring leading to platelet activation and aggregation followed by thrombosis, appears to contribute to mechanisms of SCD. In addition to initiating the thrombus, platelet activation produces a series of biochemical alterations which may enhance or retard susceptibility to VF by means of vasomotor modulation. Hammon and Oates studied the effects of thromboxane synthetase inhibitors[244] and demonstrated protection against the induction of experimental VF, presumably by blocking conversion of prostaglandin H_2 (PGH_2) to thromboxane A_2, which theoretically shunts accumulated PGH_2 to metabolic pathways that favor conversion to prostacyclin. Inhibition of cyclo-oxygenase by concurrent indomethacin administration gave further support to the hypothesis that PGH_2 shunting to other prostaglandin pathways might protect against VF by prostacyclin production. The possibility that inhibition of prostacyclin production might enhance the risk of VF[244] is supported by the finding from the Aspirin–Myocardial Infarction Study that the incidence of recurrent myocardial infarction was reduced by aspirin, but the relative and perhaps absolute numbers of SCD tended to increase.[245]

A number of pieces of indirect evidence support the possibility that more than the mechanical consequences to flow is involved in platelet-activated thrombosis of coro-

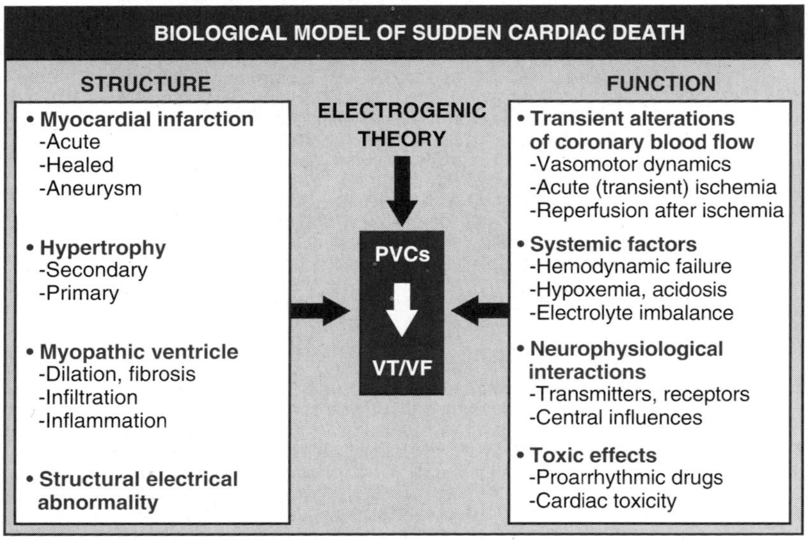

FIGURE 24–8. Biological model of sudden cardiac death. Structural cardiac abnormalities are commonly defined as the causative basis for SCD. However, functional alterations of the abnormal anatomic substrate usually are required to alter stability of the myocardium, permitting a potentially fatal arrhythmia to be initiated. In this conceptual model, short- or long-term structural abnormalities interact with functional modulations to influence the probability that premature ventricular contractions (PVCs) initiate ventricular tachycardia or fibrillation (VT/VF). (From Myerburg, R. J., et al.: A biological approach to sudden cardiac death: Structure, function, and cause. Am. J. Cardiol. *63:*1512, 1989.)

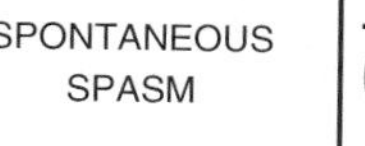

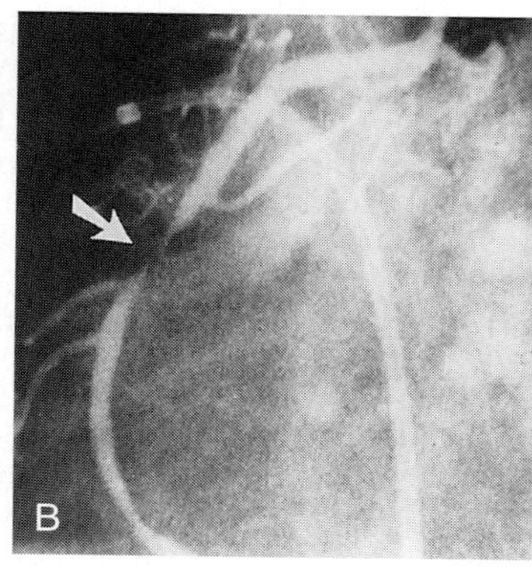

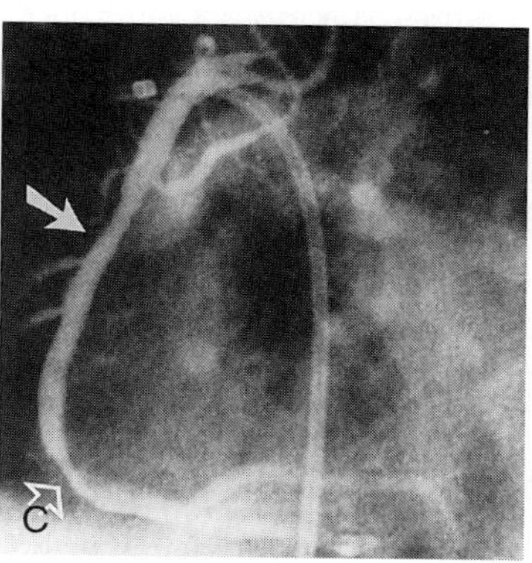

FIGURE 24–9. Life-threatening ventricular arrhythmias associated with acute myocardial ischemia due to coronary artery spasm and with reperfusion. *A,* Continuous lead II electrocardiographic monitor recording during ischemia [time 0 to 55 sec] due to spasm of the right coronary artery *(B).* There is an abrupt transition [time 56 sec to 72 sec] from repetitive ventricular ectopy to a rapid polymorphic, prefibrillatory tachyarrhythmia [time 80 sec to 130 sec] associated with nitroglycerin-induced reversal of the spasm *(C).*

nary arteries in SCD. Davies and Thomas[216] pointed out that 95 of 100 subjects who died suddenly (fewer than 6 hours after the onset of symptoms) had acute coronary thrombi, plaque fissuring, or both. This incidence was considerably higher than in many previous reports, but it is noteworthy that only 44 per cent of the patients had the largest thrombus occluding 51 per cent or more of the cross-sectional area of the involved vessel, and only 18 per cent of the patients had more than 75 per cent occlusion. This raises questions whether mechanical obstruction to flow was dominant, or whether the high incidence of nonoccluding thrombi simply reflected the state of activation of the platelets. The discrepancy between the relatively high incidence of acute thrombi in postmortem studies and the low incidence of evolution of new myocardial infarction among survivors of out-of-hospital VF[18–20,246] highlights this question. Spontaneous thrombolysis, a dominant role of spasm induced by platelet products, or a combination may explain this discrepancy.

ACUTE ISCHEMIA AND INITIATION OF LETHAL ARRHYTHMIAS. The onset of acute ischemia produces immediate electrical, mechanical, and biochemical dysfunction of cardiac muscle (Fig. 24–8). The specialized conducting tissue is more resistant to acute ischemia than is working myocardium, and therefore the electrophysiological consequences are less intense and delayed in onset in this tissue.[247] Experimental studies also have provided data on the long-term consequences of left ventricular hypertrophy and healed experimental myocardial infarction. Tissue exposed to chronic stress produced by long-term left ventricular pressure overload[248] and tissue which has healed after ischemic injury[249,250] both show lasting cellular electrophysiological abnormalities, including regional changes in transmembrane action potentials and refractory periods. Moreover, acute ischemic injury or acute myocardial infarction in the presence of healed myocardial infarction is more arrhythmogenic than is the same extent of acute ischemia in previously normal tissue.[250,251] In addition to the direct effect of ischemia on normal or previously abnormal tissue, it is possible that reperfusion after transient ischemia may cause lethal arrhythmias.[101,252,253] Reperfusion of ischemic areas may occur by three mechanisms: (1) spontaneous thrombolysis, (2) collateral flow from other coronary vascular beds to the ischemic bed, and (3) reversal of vasospasm. Some mechanisms of reperfusion-induced arrhythmogenesis appear to be related to the duration of ischemia prior to reperfusion.[253,254] Experimentally, there is a window of vulnerability beginning 5 to 10 minutes after the onset of ischemia and lasting up to 20 to 30 minutes.

ELECTROPHYSIOLOGICAL EFFECTS OF ACUTE ISCHEMIA. Within the first minutes after experimental coronary ligation there is a propensity to ventricular arrhythmias which abates after 30 minutes and reappears after several hours.[255] The initial 30 minutes of arrhythmias is divided into two periods, the first of which lasts for about 10 minutes and is presumably directly related to the initial ischemic injury. The second period (20 to 30 minutes) may be related either to reperfusion of ischemic areas or to the evolution of differing injury patterns in the epicardial and endocardial muscle. Multiple mechanisms of reperfusion arrhythmias have been observed experimentally.[224,256,257]

At the level of the myocyte, the immediate consequences of ischemia, which include loss of integrity of cell membranes with efflux of K^+, influx of Ca^{++}, acidosis, reduction of transmembrane resting potentials, and enhanced automaticity in some tissues, are followed by a separate series of changes during reperfusion. Those of particular current interest are the possible continued influx of Ca^{++} which may produce electrical instability,[253,258] responses to alpha- and/or beta-adrenoceptor stimulation,[233,234,259–261] and neurophysiologically induced afterdepolarization as triggering responses for Ca^{++}-dependent arrhythmias.[258,260] Other possible mechanisms studied experimentally include formation of superoxide radicals in reperfusion arrhythmias[262,263] and differential responses of endocardial and epicardial muscle activation times and refractory periods during ischemia or reperfusion.[256,264]

The importance of the myocardial response to the onset of ischemia has been emphasized, on the basis of the demonstration of dramatic cellular electrophysiological changes during the early period after coronary occlusion.[255,256,265] However, the state of the myocardium at the time of onset of ischemia is a critical additional factor. Tissue healed after previous injury appears to be more susceptible to the electrical destabilizing effects of acute ischemia, as is chronically hypertrophied muscle. Of more direct clinical relevance is the suggestion that K^+ depletion by diuretics and clinical hypokalemia may make ventricular myocardium more susceptible to potentially lethal arrhythmias.[266,267]

The association of metabolic and electrolyte abnormalities, as well as neurophysiological and neurohumoral changes,[268–271] with SCD emphasizes the importance of changes in the myocardial substrate in the propensity to lethal arrhythmias. Most direct among myocardial metabolic changes in response to ischemia are acute increase in interstitial K^+ levels to values exceeding 15 mM, a fall in tissue pH to below 6.0, changes in adrenoceptor activity, and alterations in autonomic nerve traffic,[129] all of which tend to create and maintain electrical instability, especially if regional in distribution. Other metabolic changes such as cyclic adenosine monophosphate elevation, accumulation of free fatty acids and their metabolites, formation of lysophosphoglycerides, and impaired myocardial glycolysis also have been suggested as myocardial destabilizing influences.[272]

Local myocardial and systemic influences integrate to establish operational mechanisms. Associations between systemic patterns of autonomic fluctuation are expressed as patterns of heart rate variability,[273,274] identifying subsets of patients at higher risk for SCD.

TRANSITION FROM MYOCARDIAL INSTABILITY TO LETHAL ARRHYTHMIAS. *The combination of a triggering event and a susceptible myocardium is evolving as a fundamental electrophysiological concept for the mechanism of initiation of potentially lethal arrhythmias* (Figs. 24–4 and 24–8). The endpoint of their interaction is disorganization of patterns of myocardial activation, usually by premature impulses (i.e., the "trigger"), into multiple uncoordinated reentrant pathways (i.e., ventricular fibrillation). Clinical,[77,275] experimental,[249,276] and pharmacological[276] data all suggest that triggering events and the myocardial instability permitting the evolution of lethal arrhythmias may be dissociated from one another. In the absence of myocardial vulnerability, many triggering events, such as frequent and complex PVCs, may be innocuous.[237]

The onset of ischemia is accompanied by abrupt reduction in transmembrane resting potential and amplitude and in duration of the action potential in the affected area,[265] with little change in remote areas. When ischemic cells depolarize to resting potentials less than −60 mV, they may become inexcitable and of little electrophysiological importance. As they are depolarizing to that range, however, or repolarizing as a consequence of reperfusion, the membranes pass through ranges of reduced excitability, upstroke velocity, and time courses of repolarization. These characteristics result in slow conduction and electrophysiological instability. These events that occur regionally in ischemic myocardium, adjacent to nonischemic tissue, create a setting for the key elements of reentry—slow conduction and unidirectional block—which makes them vulnerable to reentrant arrhythmias. When premature impulses are generated in this environment, they may further alter the dispersion of recovery between ischemic tissue, chronically abnormal tissue, and normal cells,[250] ultimately leading to complete disorganization and VF. VF is probably not a consequence only of reentry.[129] Rapid-enhanced automaticity caused by ischemic injury to the specialized conducting tissue, or slow-channel–triggered activity in partially depolarized tissue, may result in rapid bursts of automatic activity which also could lead to failure of coordinated conduction and VF.

The dispersion of refractory periods produced by acute ischemia, which provides the substrate for reentrant tachycardias and VF, may be further enhanced by a healed ischemic injury. The time course of repolarization is lengthened after healing of ischemic injury[249,250] and shortened by acute ischemia.[250,253,265] The coexistence of the two appears to make the ventricle more susceptible to sustained arrhythmias in some experimental models.[250]

Bradyarrhythmias and Asystolic Arrest

The basic electrophysiological mechanism in this form of arrest is failure of normal subordinate automatic activity to assume pacemaking function of the heart in the absence of normal function of the sinus node and/or AV junction. Bradyarrhythmic and asystolic arrests are more common in severely diseased hearts and probably represent diffuse involvement of subendocardial Purkinje fibers. Systemic influences which increase extracellular K^+ concentration, such as anoxia, acidosis, shock, renal failure, trauma, and hypothermia, may result in partial depolarization of normal or already diseased pacemaker cells in the His-Purkinje system, with a decrease in the slope of spontaneous phase 4 depolarization and ultimate loss of automaticity.[277] These processes usually produce global dysfunction of automatic cell activity, in contrast to the regional dysfunction more common in acute ischemia. Functionally depressed automatic cells (e.g., owing to increased extracellular K^+ concentration) are more susceptible to overdrive suppression. Under these conditions, brief bursts of tachycardia may be followed by prolonged asystolic periods, with further depression of automaticity by the consequent acidosis and increased local K^+ concentration, or by changes in adrenergic tone. The ultimate consequence may be degeneration into VF or persistent asystole.

Pulseless Electrical Activity

Pulseless electrical activity, formerly called electromechanical dissociation (EMD), is separated into *primary* and *secondary* forms. The common denominator in both is continued electrical rhythmicity of the heart in the absence of effective mechanical function. The secondary form includes those causes which result from an abrupt cessation of cardiac venous return, such as massive pulmonary embolism, acute malfunction of prosthetic valves, exsanguination, and cardiac tamponade from hemopericardium. The primary form is the more familiar; in it none of these obvious mechanical factors are present, but ventricular muscle fails to produce an effective contraction despite continued electrical activity (i.e., *failure of electromechanical coupling*).[278] It usually occurs as an end-stage event in advanced heart disease, but it may occur in patients with acute ischemic events or, more commonly, after electrical resuscitation from a prolonged cardiac arrest. Although not thoroughly understood, it appears that diffuse disease, metabolic abnormalities, or global ischemia provides the pathophysiological substrate. The proximate mechanism for failure of electromechanical coupling may be abnormal intracellular Ca^{++} metabolism, intracellular acidosis, or perhaps adenosine triphosphate depletion.

CLINICAL CHARACTERISTICS OF THE PATIENT WITH CARDIAC ARREST

Before the development of coronary care units, the in-hospital mortality owing to acute myocardial infarction was in the range of 25 to 30 per cent.[279] The current in-hospital mortality rate (see Chap. 37) is lower in large part because of prevention of in-hospital sudden deaths, now that acute potentially lethal arrhythmias in this setting are preventable or reversible.[280] However, the prior relationship between acute myocardial infarction and SCD in the hospitalized patient ingrained the concept of the association between the two, which was then extrapolated to the victims of out-of-hospital cardiac arrest. The advent of community-based emergency rescue systems generated cohorts of survivors of out-of-hospital cardiac arrest, and it soon became apparent that the majority of these cardiac arrests were, in fact, *not* associated with the evolution of a new transmural myocardial infarction.

Studies from Seattle[19] and from Miami[246] demonstrated that only a minority of survivors of out-of-hospital VF had clinical evidence indicating that a new transmural myocardial infarction was associated with the cardiac arrest. In the Seattle study, only one of five survivors had new transmural infarctions.[19] These studies led to the conclusion that in the majority of such patients, transient pathophysiological events were responsible for cardiac arrest. That this conclusion is reasonable and has clinical relevance is supported by the fact that the recurrence rate in survivors of out-of-hospital cardiac arrest is low in the subgroup of patients who had documentation of a new transmural myocardial infarction. It was found to be 30 per cent at 1 year and 45 per cent at 2 years in those survivors who did not have a new transmural myocardial infarction.[18,19] Recurrence rates decreased subsequently,[51] possibly owing in part to long-term interventions. However, it is not known whether this results from a change in the natural history, changes in preventive strategies for underlying disease, or long-term interventions for controlling arrhythmic risk.[26]

Clinical cardiac arrest and SCD are best described in the framework of the same four phases of the event used to establish definitions (Fig. 24–1): prodromes, onset of the terminal event, the cardiac arrest, and progression to biological death or survival.

Prodromal Symptoms

Patients risk for SCD may have prodromes such as chest pain, dyspnea, weakness or fatigue, palpitations, and a number of nonspecific complaints. Several epidemiological and clinical studies demonstrated that such symptoms may presage coronary events, particularly myocardial infarction and SCD,[8,52,281] and result in contact with the medical system weeks to months before SCD.

In a prospective study in Edinburgh, Scotland, however, only 12 per cent of victims of SCD had consulted a physician because of new or worsening angina pectoris during periods of up to 6 months before death.[282] In contrast, 33 per cent of myocardial infarction patients had consulted their physicians for this complaint. Nonetheless, 46 per cent of victims of SCD had seen a physician within 4 weeks before death, but three-fourths of them had sought medical help for complaints which appeared to be unrelated to the heart. Liberthson et al.,[18] in a study of patients successfully resuscitated after out-of-hospital cardiac arrest, noted that 28 per cent reported retrospectively that they had had new or changing angina pectoris or dyspnea in the 4 weeks before arrest, and that 31 per cent had seen a physician during this time but only 12 per cent because of these symptoms.

Patients who have chest pain as a prodrome to SCD appear to have a higher probability of intraluminal coronary thrombosis at postmortem examination.[217] Attempts to identify early prodromal symptoms which are more specific for the patient at risk for SCD have not yet been successful. Fatigue has been a particularly common symptom in the days or weeks before SCD in a number of studies,[281] but this symptom is nonspecific. The symptoms that occur within the last hours or minutes before cardiac arrest are more specific for heart disease and may include symptoms of arrhythmias, ischemia, or heart failure.[21,283] Liberthson et al.[213] reported specific cardiac symptoms at a mean interval of about 3.8 hours before collapse in 24 per cent of victims of SCD. However, most studies have reported such symptoms even less commonly, particularly when victims whose deaths were instantaneous are included.[8]

Onset of the Terminal Event

The period of 1 hour or less between acute changes in cardiovascular status and the cardiac arrest itself, which has been defined as the "onset of the terminal event," is a subject about which there is limited information. Reports from ambulatory monitor recordings fortuitously obtained at the time of unexpected cardiac arrest indicate dynamic change in cardiac electrical activity during the minutes or hours before the onset of cardiac arrest.[284–286] These reports suggest that increasing heart rate and advancing grades of ventricular ectopy are common antecedents of VF. Although these recordings suggest transient electrophysiological destabilization of the myocardium, the extent to which these objective observations are paralleled by clinical symptoms is less well documented. SCDs caused by either arrhythmias or acute circulatory failure mechanisms involve a high incidence of acute myocardial disorders at the onset of the terminal event; such disorders are more likely to be ischemic when the death is due to arrhythmias and to be associated with low-output states or myocardial anoxia when the deaths are due to circulatory failure.[21,287]

Abrupt, unexpected loss of effective circulation may be caused by cardiac arrhythmias or mechanical disturbances, but the majority of such events that terminate in SCD are arrhythmic in origin. Hinkle and Thaler[287] classified cardiac deaths among 142 subjects who died during a follow-up of 5 to 10 years. Class I was labeled arrhythmic death and Class II was death caused by circulatory failure. The distinction between the two classes was based on whether circulatory failure preceded (Class II) or followed (Class I) the disappearance of the pulse. Among deaths which occurred less than 1 hour after the onset of the terminal illness, 93 per cent were due to arrhythmias; in addition, 90 per cent of deaths caused by heart disease were initiated by arrhythmic events rather than circulatory failure. Table 24–4 demonstrates that deaths caused by circulatory failure occurred predominantly in patients who could be identified as having terminal illnesses (95 per cent were comatose), were associated more fre-

TABLE 24–4 DIFFERENCES IN CLINICAL STATUS IMMEDIATELY BEFORE DEATH IN PATIENTS DYING OF ARRHYTHMIA AND CIRCULATORY FAILURE

CLINICAL STATUS IMMEDIATELY BEFORE DEATH	ARRHYTHMIC DEATHS (N = 82) (CLASS I)	CIRCULATORY FAILURE DEATHS (N = 59) (CLASS II)
Comatose	0/82 (0%)	56/59 (95%)
Standing or actively moving	39/82 (48%)	0/59 (0%)
Terminal arrhythmia		
• Ventricular fibrillation	15/18 (83%)	3/9 (33%)
• Asystole	3/18 (17%)	6/9 (67%)
Duration of terminal illness		
• <1 hour	53/82 (65%)	4/59 (7%)
• >24 hours	17/82 (21%)	48/59 (81%)
Nature of terminal illness		
• Acute cardiac events	80/82 (98%)	8/59 (14%)
• Noncardiac events	1/82 (1%)	51/59 (86%)

Data from Hinkle, L. E. and Thaler, H. T.: Clinical classification of cardiac deaths. Circulation *65*:457, 1982.

quently with bradyarrhythmias than with VF as the terminal arrhythmias, and were dominated by noncardiac events as the terminal illness. In contrast, 98 per cent of the arrhythmic deaths were associated primarily with cardiac disorders.

Clinical Features of Cardiac Arrest

The cardiac arrest itself is characterized by abrupt loss of consciousness owing to lack of adequate cerebral blood flow. It is an event which uniformly leads to death in the absence of an active intervention, although spontaneous reversions occur rarely. The most common cardiac mechanism is VF, followed by bradyarrhythmias or asystole, and sustained VT.[20] Other, less frequent mechanisms include electromechanical dissociation, rupture of the ventricle,[288] cardiac tamponade, acute mechanical obstruction to flow, and acute disruption of a major blood vessel.[3,45,128]

The potential for successful resuscitation is a function of the setting in which cardiac arrest occurs, the mechanism of the arrest, and the underlying clinical status of the victim.[289] Closely related to the potential for successful resuscitation is the decision of whether or not to attempt to resuscitate.[290]

At present there are fewer low-risk patients with otherwise uncomplicated myocardial infarctions weighting in-hospital cardiac arrest statistics than previously.[288] Bedell and coworkers[291] reported that only 14 per cent of in-hospital CPR patients were discharged from the hospital alive, and that 20 per cent of these died within the ensuing 6 months. Although 41 per cent of the patients had suffered an acute myocardial infarction, 73 per cent had a history of congestive heart failure, and 20 per cent had had prior cardiac arrests. The mean age of 70 years (10 years older than the populations in several major prehospital cardiac arrest studies[18,19,51]) may have influenced the outcome statistics, but the patient population at risk for in-hospital cardiac arrest was heavily influenced by patients with high-risk complicated myocardial infarction or patients with other high-risk markers. Noncardiac clinical diagnoses were dominated by renal failure, pneumonia, sepsis, diabetes, and a history of cancer. The strong male preponderance consistently reported in out-of-hospital cardiac arrest studies is not present in in-hospital patients, but the better prognosis of ventricular tachycardia (VT) or VF mechanisms, compared with bradyarrhythmic or asystolic mechanisms, persists (27 per cent survival versus 8 per cent survival). However, the proportion of arrests which are due to in-hospital VT or VF is considerably less (33 per cent), with the combination of respiratory arrest, asystole, and electromechanical dissociation dominating the statistics (61 per cent).

The important risk factors for death after CPR are listed in Table 24–5. The facts that the fraction of out-of-hospital cardiac arrest survivors who are discharged from the hospital alive may now equal or exceed the fraction of in-hospital cardiac arrest victims who are discharged alive,[292] and that the postdischarge mortality rate for in-hospital cardiac arrest survivors is higher than that for out-of-hospital cardiac arrest survivors,[51,291,293] are telling clinical statistics. Not only do they emphasize the success of preventive measures for cardiac arrest in low-risk in-hospital patients, causing those statistics to be dominated by higher-risk patients, but they also emphasize the improvement in prehospital and in-hospital care of out-of-hospital cardiac arrest victims.[294]

TABLE 24–5 PREDICTORS OF MORTALITY AFTER IN-HOSPITAL CARDIOPULMONARY RESUSCITATION

BEFORE ARREST
Hypotension (systolic BP < 100 mm Hg)
Pneumonia
Renal failure (BUN > 50 mg/dl)
Cancer
Homebound life style
DURING ARREST
Arrest duration > 15 minutes
Intubation
Hypotension (systolic BP < 100 mm Hg)
Pneumonia
Homebound life style
AFTER RESUSCITATION
Coma
Need for pressors
Arrest duration > 15 minutes

Modified from Bedell, S. E., et al.: Survival after cardiopulmonary resuscitation in the hospital. N. Engl. J. Med. *309*:569, 1983. Copyright Massachusetts Medical Society.

Cardiac arrest associated with coronary heart disease in the hospitalized elderly patient has a similar outcome. Gulati et al.[295] reported that 14 of 52 (27 per cent) elderly patients (mean age 76 years) were successfully resuscitated, although only 9 (17 per cent) remained alive after 1 week. Similar outcome was observed in another report comparing patients younger and older than 70 years.[296] Coronary heart disease was the cause in 48 patients (92 per cent); 5 of 22 patients (23 per cent) with VF arrests survived and only 1 of 19 (5 per cent) with asystole survived.[295] Among those 70 years of age or older, survival to discharge from hospital after out-of-hospital cardiac arrest was lower (29 per cent) than among younger patients (47 per cent).[297] However, long-term neurological status, survival, and length of hospitalization were similar among older and younger patients.

Progression to Biological Death

The time course for progression from cardiac arrest to biological death relates to the mechanism of the cardiac arrest, the nature of the underlying disease process, and the delay between onset and resuscitative efforts. Unattended VF characteristically leads to the onset of irreversible brain damage within 4 to 6 minutes, and biological death follows within a matter of minutes. In large series, however, it has been demonstrated that a limited number of victims may remain biologically alive for longer periods and may be resuscitated after delays in excess of 8 minutes before beginning basic life support and in excess of 16 minutes before advanced life support.[298] Despite these exceptions, it is clear that the probability for a favorable outcome deteriorates rapidly as a function of time after unattended cardiac arrest. Younger patients with less severe cardiac disease and the absence of coexistent multisystem disease appear to have a higher probability of a favorable outcome after such delays. Irreversible injury of the central nervous system usually occurs before biological death, and the interval may extend to a period of weeks in those patients who are resuscitated during the temporal gap between brain damage and biological death (see Definition, p. 742). In-hospital cardiac arrest caused by VF is less likely to have a protracted course between the arrest and biological death, with patients either surviving after a prompt intervention or succumbing rapidly because of inability to stabilize cardiac rhythm or hemodynamics.[291]

Those patients whose cardiac arrest is due to sustained VT with cardiac output inadequate to maintain consciousness may remain in VT for considerably longer periods, with flow which is marginally sufficient to maintain viability. This allows a longer interval between the onset of cardiac arrest and the end of the period, which will allow successful resuscitation. The lives of such patients usually end in VF or an asystolic arrest if the VT is not actively or spontaneously reverted. Once the transition from VT to VF or to a bradyarrhythmia occurs, the subsequent course to biological death is similar to that in patients in whom VF or bradyarrhythmias are the initiating event.

The progression in patients with asystole or bradyarrhythmias as the initiating event is more rapid. Such patients, whether in an in-hospital[291] or out-of-hospital[20,299] environment, have a very poor prognosis because of advanced heart disease or coexistent multisystem disease. They tend to respond poorly to interventions, even if the heart is successfully paced.[300] Although a small subgroup of patients with bradyarrhythmias associated with electrolyte or pharmacological abnormalities may respond well to interventions, the majority progress rapidly to biological death.[299] The infrequent cardiac arrests caused by mechanical factors such as tamponade, structural disruption, and impedance to flow by major thromboembolic obstructions to right or left ventricular outflow are reversible only in those instances in which the mechanism is recognized and an intervention is feasible. The vast majority of these events lead to rapid biological death, although prompt relief of tamponade may save some lives.

Hospital Course of Survivors of Cardiac Arrest

The hospital course of survivors of cardiac arrest is characterized by an initial period of instability, followed by clinical features which are determined by the electrical and hemodynamic status of the patient, and the consequence of central nervous system injury occurring during the cardiac arrest.[20,22] The conditions of patients who are resuscitated immediately from *primary* VF associated with acute myocardial infarction usually stabilize promptly, and they require no special management after the early phase of the infarction (Chap. 37). The management after *secondary cardiac arrest in myocardial infarction* is dominated by the hemodynamic status of the patient. Among survivors of *out-of-hospital cardiac arrest,* the initial 24 to 48 hours of hospitalization are characterized by a tendency to ventricular arrhythmias, which usually respond well to antiarrhythmic therapy.[20,246,283] The overall rate of recurrent cardiac arrest is low, about 10 to 20 per cent, but the mortality rate in patients who have recurrent cardiac arrests is about 50 per cent.[18–20] Only 5 to 10 per cent of in-hospital deaths after prehospital resuscitation are due to recurrent cardiac arrhythmias.[20,22] Patients who have recurrent cardiac arrest have a high incidence of either new or preexisting AV or intraventricular conduction abnormalities.[20]

The most common causes of death in hospitalized survivors of out-of-hospital cardiac arrest are noncardiac events related to central nervous system injury suffered during the cardiac arrest itself. These include anoxic encephalopathy and sepsis related to prolonged intubation and hemodynamic monitoring lines.[20,22] Fifty-nine per cent of deaths during index hospitalization after prehospital resuscitation have been reported to be due to such causes.[20] It has been reported that 39 per cent of 457 consecutive patients in coma never awakened after admission to the hospital and died after a median survival of 3.5 days.[301] Two-thirds of the 61 per cent who awakened had no gross deficits, and an additional 21 per cent had persisting cognitive deficits only. Of the patients who did awaken, 25 per cent had done so by admission, 71 per cent by the first hospital day, and 92 per cent by the third day. A small number of patients awakened after prolonged hospitalization. Of the 206 hospital deaths (45 per cent of the 457 patients), 80 per cent had not awakened before death.

Cardiac causes of delayed death during hospitalization after out-of-hospital cardiac arrest are most commonly related to hemodynamic deterioration, which accounts for about one-third of deaths in-hospital.[20,22] Among all deaths, those that occurred within the first 48 hours of hospitalization usually were due to hemodynamic deterioration or arrhythmias, regardless of the neurological status; later deaths were related to neurological complications. Admission characteristics most predictive of subsequent awakening included motor response, pupillary light response, spontaneous eye movement, and blood sugar below 300 mg/dl.[302]

Clinical Profile of Survivors of Out-of-Hospital Cardiac Arrest

The clinical features of survivors of out-of-hospital cardiac arrest are heavily influenced by the type and extent of the underlying disease associated with the event. Causation is dominated by coronary heart disease, which accounts for approximately 80 per cent of out-of-hospital cardiac arrest in the United States[246] and is commonly extensive. The cardiomyopathies collectively account for another 10 to 15 per cent, with all other structural heart diseases, plus functional and toxic/environmental causes, accounting for the remainder (Table 24–2, p. 748).

Complex PVCs have been reported in the majority of survivors of prehospital cardiac arrest who had serial ambulatory monitor recordings.[246,303,304] These arrhythmias are difficult to suppress[303] and show trends to higher grades of ventricular ectopy in victims of recurrent cardiac arrest compared with long-term survivors.[51,304] Complex forms were strongly associated with a history of congestive heart failure or previous myocardial infarction. The strongest predictors of subsequent mortality were use of digitalis, elevated BUN, cerebrovascular accident, previous myocardial infarction, and age; however, the presence of complex PVCs or frequent ectopy (≥25 PVCs/hour) added strongly to risk.

LEFT VENTRICULAR FUNCTION. This is abnormal in the majority of survivors of out-of-hospital cardiac arrest, often severely so, but there is a wide variation, ranging from severe dysfunction to normal or near-normal measurements, with as many as 50 per cent ranging from normal to moderate dysfunction (Fig. 24–10).[51] The author found that the ejection fraction of those who died during follow-up was lower than that of the long-term survivors (38 versus 45 per cent, respectively).[20,51] From data reported in a number of large series, the mean ejection fraction has been in the range of 32 to 35 per cent. Patients who died of recurrent cardiac arrest had higher ejection fractions than those who died non-sudden cardiac deaths (43 versus 25 per cent). Ritchie et al.[305] reported on studies of left ventricular function by radionuclide techniques in 154 survivors of out-of-hospital VF, 91 of whom had both rest and exercise studies. The mean ejection fraction at rest was 40 per cent, with 20 per cent having values greater than 50 per cent. Only 3 of 91 patients (3 per cent) studied had a normal increase (>5 per cent) in ejection fraction during exertion; 18 per cent had normal resting wall motion. The ejection fraction at rest was the best predictor of death during follow-up.[305] Fifty per cent of survivors studied by cardiac catheterization and angiography had ejection fractions below 50 per cent, and 30 per cent had left ventricular end-diastolic pressures greater than 15 mm Hg[306]; in this study, ejection fraction and severity of wall motion abnormality correlated with risk of recurrent cardiac arrest.

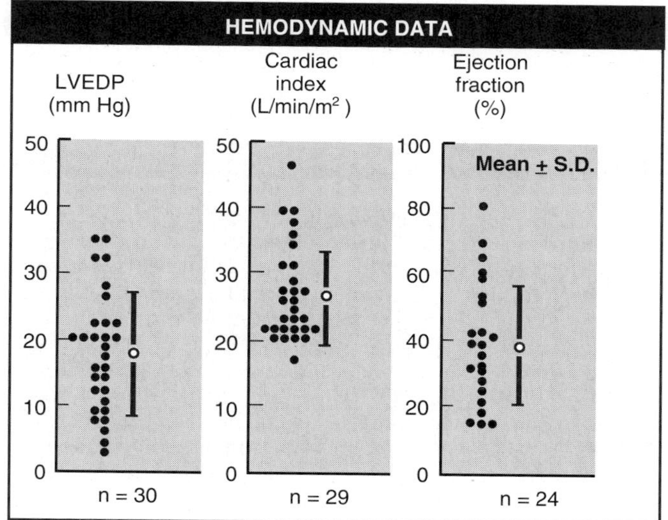

FIGURE 24–10. Hemodynamic data from prehospital cardiac arrest victims studied during initial post-arrest hospitalization, and the relation between ejection fraction (EF) at initial study and long-term outcome. These data indicate a broad range of cardiac function and a statistically insignificant difference between EF at entry in long-term survivors and in recurrent cardiac arrest victims. (From Myerburg, R. J., et al.: Clinical, electrophysiologic, and hemodynamic profile of patients resuscitated from prehospital cardiac arrest. Am. J. Med. *68*:568, 1980.)

CORONARY ANGIOGRAPHY. Studies in survivors of out-of-hospital cardiac arrest have shown that as a group, this population tends to have extensive disease but no specific pattern of abnormalities. Moderate to severe stenosis of the left main coronary artery was present in only 8 per cent of the patients in one series,[306] and only 9 per cent in another,[20] frequencies not different from those in the overall population of coronary heart disease patients. Significant lesions in two or more vessels were present in 74 per cent of the patients who had any coronary lesions in one study,[20] and 94 per cent of the patients in another had 70 per cent or greater degrees of stenosis in one or more arteries.[306] Among patients who had recurrent cardiac arrests, the incidence of triple-vessel disease was higher than among those who did not.

EXERCISE TESTING. This is commonly used to evaluate the need for and response to antiischemic therapy in survivors of out-of-hospital cardiac arrest. The incidence of positive tests related to ischemia is relatively low, although termination of testing because of fatigue is common.[246,303,307] Mortality during follow-up was greater in patients who had angina or failure of a normal rise in systolic blood pressure occurring during exercise.[307]

ELECTROCARDIOGRAPHIC OBSERVATIONS. In survivors of out-of-hospital cardiac arrest these have proved of value only for discriminating risk of recurrence among those whose cardiac arrest was associated with new transmural myocardial infarction. Patients who develop documented new Q waves, in association with a clinical picture suggesting that an acute ischemic event began prior to the cardiac arrest itself, are at much lower risk for recurrence.[18,246,308] A higher incidence of repolarization abnormalities (ST-segment depression, flat T waves, prolonged Q-T_c) occurs in out-of-hospital cardiac arrest survivors than in post-myocardial infarction patients, and these might be markers for increased risk.[309]

Lower serum K^+ levels were observed in survivors of cardiac arrest than in patients with acute myocardial infarction or stable coronary heart disease.[310] The investigators concluded that this was a consequence of resuscitation interventions, rather than a preexisting state owing to chronic diuretic use. Low ionized Ca^{++} levels, with normal total calcium levels, also were observed during resuscitation from out-of-hospital cardiac arrest.[311] Higher resting lactate levels have been reported in out-of-hospital cardiac arrest survivors than in normal subjects.[312] Lactate levels correlated inversely with ejection fractions and directly with PVC frequency and complexity.

Studies from the early 1970's in both Miami[18] and Seattle[19] indicated that the risk of recurrent cardiac arrest in the first year after surviving an initial event was about 30 per cent and at 2 years was 45 per cent. Total mortality at 2 years was about 60 per cent in both studies. In both of these studies, less than half of the patients followed were being treated with long-term antiarrhythmic therapy; beta-adrenoceptor blocker therapy was in its infancy, and Ca^{++}-entry blockers were not yet available. Thus these figures appear to be as close to valid natural history figures as possible. However, they can serve only as historical control figures for current observations, and thus are of limited value, because the risk of recurrent cardiac arrest likely is lower now than it was in the early 1970's.[313] Moreover, the risk of recurrent cardiac arrest/SCD appears to be lower for survivors with hypertrophic cardiomyopathy—about 33 per cent during a mean follow-up period of 7 years.[110] In a recent report of cardiac arrest survivors with and without successful medical and/or surgical antiarrhythmic endpoints, the 1-year recurrent cardiac arrest rate was 14.5 per cent and the 2-year cumulative rate was 21.1 per cent, with a clustering of events within the first 6 to 12 months (i.e., time-dependent risk) (Fig. 24–11).[314]

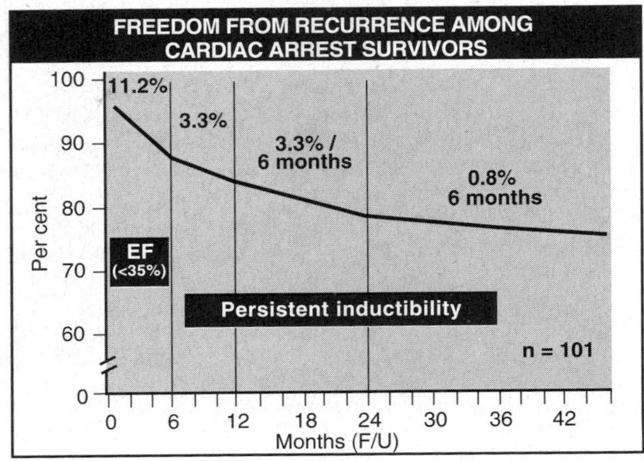

FIGURE 24–11. Time-dependence of recurrences among survivors of cardiac arrest. Actuarial analysis of occurrences among a population of 101 cardiac arrest survivors with coronary artery disease is demonstrated. The risk was highest in the first 6 months (11.2 per cent) and then fell to 3.3 per cent/6 months for the next three 6-month blocks. After 24 months the rate fell to 0.8 per cent/6 months. A low ejection fraction (EF) was the most powerful predictor of death during the first 6 months; subsequently, persistent inducibility during programmed stimulation, despite drug therapy or surgery, was the most powerful predictor. (Modified from Furukawa, T., et al.: Time-dependent risk of and predictors for cardiac arrest recurrence in survivors of out-of-hospital cardiac arrest with chronic coronary artery disease. Circulation *80*:599, 1989. The figure is reproduced from Myerburg, R. J., et al.: Sudden cardiac death: Structure, function and time-dependence of risk. Circulation *85*(Suppl. I):I-2, 1992. Copyright 1992 American Heart Association.)

MANAGEMENT OF CARDIAC ARREST

COMMUNITY-BASED INTERVENTIONS

Systems for intervention in out-of-hospital cardiac arrest have their roots in the development of the coronary care unit (CCU) approach to the management of potentially lethal arrhythmias.[315] Previously, cardiac arrest in the setting of acute coronary events was almost uniformly fatal, wherever it occurred. With the confluence of the key elements of the CCU in the late 1950's and early 1960's (i.e., continuous monitoring, CPR, effective acute drug therapy, and electrical management of tachycardias, bradycardias, and VF), there was a dramatic reduction in the immediate in-hospital mortality from potentially lethal arrhythmias occurring in the course of acute coronary events.[316] The next step toward the development of community-based intervention for cardiac arrest was the concept of the mobile coronary care unit,[317] which was based on the rationale of providing a CCU environment during the high-risk prehospital phase of acute myocardial infarction. Only a small extension in concept in the late 1960's led to the development of community-based intervention systems designed to respond routinely to out-of-hospital cardiac arrests.

The systems as developed in the United States are largely integrated into fire departments as emergency rescue systems. They employ paramedical personnel or emergency medical technicians trained in CPR and the use of telemetered monitoring equipment, defibrillators, and specific intravenous drug therapy. Although the initial out-of-hospital intervention experience in Miami and Seattle[18,19] reported in the early 1970's yielded only 14 and 10 per cent survivals to discharge, respectively, later data indicate that such systems are becoming increasingly effective in saving lives (Fig. 24–12).[292,308] By the mid-1970's, both had increased survival rates to about 25 per cent,[20,292] and by the early 1980's to 30 per cent or more.[292] Survival rates in these centers appear to have decreased since then, presumably because of the extension of rescue systems into less densely populated regions.[318]

Conversely, recent reports from very densely populated areas (i.e., Chicago and New York City) have provided disturbing outcomes data. The Chicago study reported that only 9 per cent of out-of-hospital cardiac arrest victims survived to be hospitalized and that only 2 per cent were discharged alive.[57] Moreover, outcomes in blacks were far worse than in whites (0.8 per cent versus 2.6 per cent). The fact that a large majority had bradyarrhythmias, asystole, or

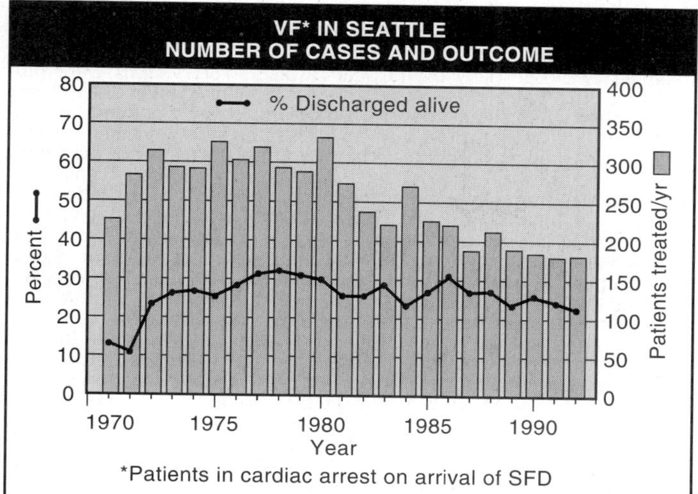

FIGURE 24–12. Annual number of emergency rescue responses to out-of-hospital cardiac arrest *(vertical bars)* and the percent of patients discharged alive *(solid line)*, from 1970 through 1992 in Seattle, Washington. Patients were in cardiac arrest when initially examined by emergency rescue personnel. (Courtesy of Leonard A. Cobb, M.D., Seattle, Washington.)

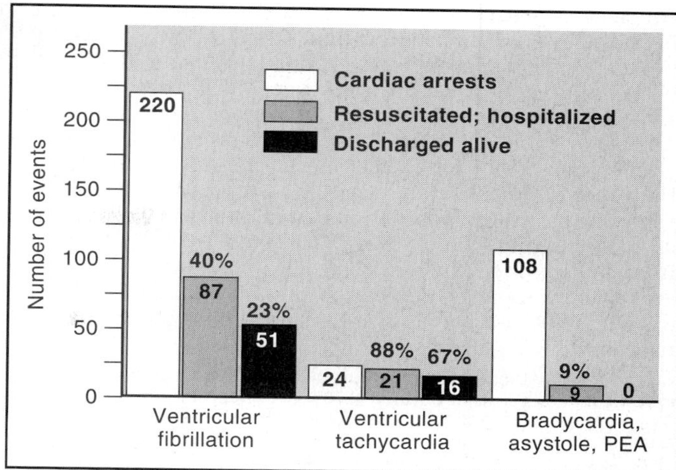

FIGURE 24–13. Survival after out-of-hospital cardiac arrest as function of the intial electrophysiological mechanism recorded by emergency rescue personnel. The mechanisms among 352 out-of-hospital cardiac arrest victims are separated into three categories: ventricular fibrillation (n = 220; 62 per cent), ventricular tachycardia (n = 24; 7 per cent), and bradycardia/asystole/pulseless electrical activity (PEA) (n = 108; 31 per cent). The white bars illustrate the total number of events in each category. The light-colored bars illustrate the number and per cent of patients who were initially resuscitated in the field and reached the hospital alive in each category, and the dark bars illustrate the percentage of total events in which patients were discharged from the hospital alive for each category. The data are derived from the Miami, Florida experience.[20]

pulseless electrical activity on initial emergency medical services contact suggests prolonged times between collapse and emergency medical services arrival and/or absent or ineffective bystander interventions. The New York City report indicated a survival-to-hospital-discharge rate of only 1.4 per cent.[319] Among those who had bystander CPR, the rate increased to 2.9 per cent, and bystander CPR plus VF as the initial rhythm yielded a further increase to 5.3 per cent. Finally, for those whose arrests occurred after emergency medical services arrival, the success rate increased further to 8.5 per cent. This trend, together with the fact that (as in Chicago) nontachyarrhythmic events constituted a majority, suggests that delays and breaks in the "chain of survival"[294] exert a major negative impact on emergency medical services results in densely populated areas.

IMPORTANCE OF ELECTRICAL MECHANISMS. The electrical mechanism of out-of-hospital cardiac arrest, as defined by the initial rhythm recorded by emergency rescue personnel, has a powerful impact on success of initial resuscitation and outcome, the latter measured in terms of patients discharged from the hospital alive. The subgroup of patients who are in sustained VT at the time of first contact, although the smallest group statistically, has the best outcome (Fig. 24–13). Eighty-eight per cent of patients in cardiac arrest due to VT were successfully resuscitated and admitted to the hospital alive, and 67 per cent were ultimately discharged alive.[20] However, this relatively low-risk group represents only 7 to 10 per cent of all cardiac arrests in studies reported to date. Because of the inherent time lag between collapse and initial recordings, it is possible that many more cardiac arrests begin as rapid sustained VT and degenerate into VF before arrival of emergency rescue personnel.

Patients who are in a bradyarrhythmia or asystole at initial contact have the worst prognosis; only 9 per cent of such patients in the Miami study were admitted to the hospital alive and none was discharged.[20] In a later experience there was some improvement in outcome, although the improvement was strictly limited to those patients in whom the initial bradyarrhythmia recorded was an idioventricular rhythm which responded promptly to chronotropic agents in the field.[299] Bradyarrhythmias also have adverse prognostic implications after defibrillation from VF in the field. Patients who were defibrillated to an initial heart rate less than 60 beats/min, regardless of the specific bradyarrhythmic mechanism, had a poor prognosis, with 95 per cent of such patients dying either before hospitalization or in the hospital (Fig. 24–14).[18] In contrast, an initial heart rate in excess of 100 beats/min yielded a 43 per cent rate of discharge from hospital, with only 17 per cent of such patients dying before hospitalization, and 40 per cent during hospitalization. Heart rates between 60 and 100 beats/min after defibrillation yield intermediate results.

The outcome in the largest group of patients, those in whom VF is the initial rhythm recorded, is intermediate

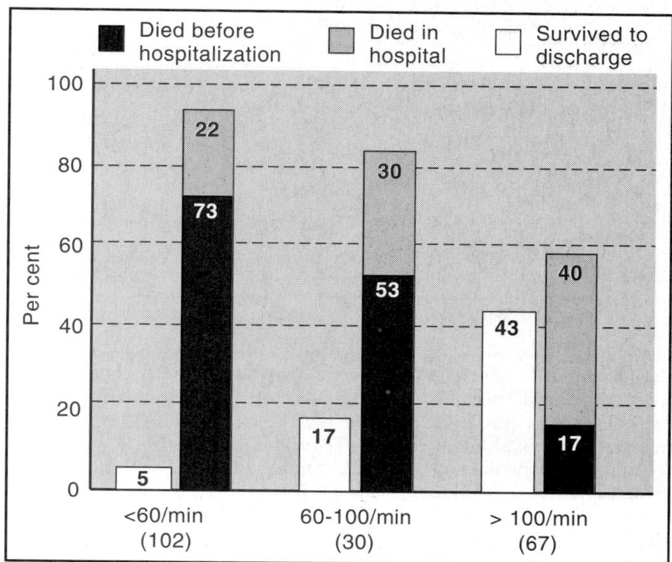

FIGURE 24–14. Prognostic implication of initial heart rate after prehospital defibrillation. Prehospital and in-hospital deaths and long-range survival (i.e., discharged survivors) are compared with the initial postdefibrillation heart rate: <60 beats/min, 60 to 100 beats/min, or >100 beats/min. Numbers in parentheses represent the number of patients in each group. (Modified from Liberthson, R. R., et al.: Prehospital ventricular fibrillation: Prognosis and follow-up course. Reprinted by permission of N. Engl. J. Med. *291*:317, 1974. Copyright Massachusetts Medical Society.)

between sustained VT and bradyarrhythmia and asystole. Figure 24–13 demonstrates that 40 per cent of such patients were successfully resuscitated and admitted to the hospital alive, and 23 per cent were ultimately discharged alive.[20] More recent data indicate improvement in outcome. The proportion of each of the electrophysiological mechanisms responsible for cardiac arrest varied among the earlier reports, with VF ranging from 65 to greater than 90 per cent of the study populations, and bradyarrhythmia and asystole ranging from 10 to 30 per cent.[20,283,292,308] However, in recent reports from very densely populated metropolitan areas, the ratios of tachyarrhythmic to bradyarrhythmic/pulseless activity events were reversed, and outcomes were far worse.[57,319]

The factors which have contributed to improved outcome since the first observations in the early 1970's are incompletely understood. Both improved prehospital care and improvements in in-hospital technology and practices may contribute, as described in the "chain of survival" concept.[294] Of these two general factors, the influence of prehospital care has been studied in more detail. Eisenberg and coworkers[320] compared initial resuscitation and ultimate discharge alive in two subgroups of patients, those who had standard CPR continuously from the arrival of emergency rescue personnel through transport to an emergency department where defibrillation took place, and another group in whom paramedics or emergency rescue personnel trained to defibrillate were allowed to do so at the scene of the cardiac arrest. The standard CPR technique resulted in only 23 per cent of patients arriving at the hospital alive and 7 per cent discharged alive, in contrast to the immediate defibrillation group in which 53 per cent arrived at the hospital alive and 26 per cent were discharged alive. Subsequent data continue to support the concept that early defibrillation is a key element in improving survival rates (Fig. 24–15).[292,298] Immediate defibrillation by ambulance technicians is especially important in rural communities, where it yields a 19 per cent survival, compared with only 3 per cent from standard CPR.[318]

A second element in prehospital care which appears to contribute to outcome is the role of bystander CPR by laypeople awaiting the arrival of emergency rescue personnel. It has been reported that

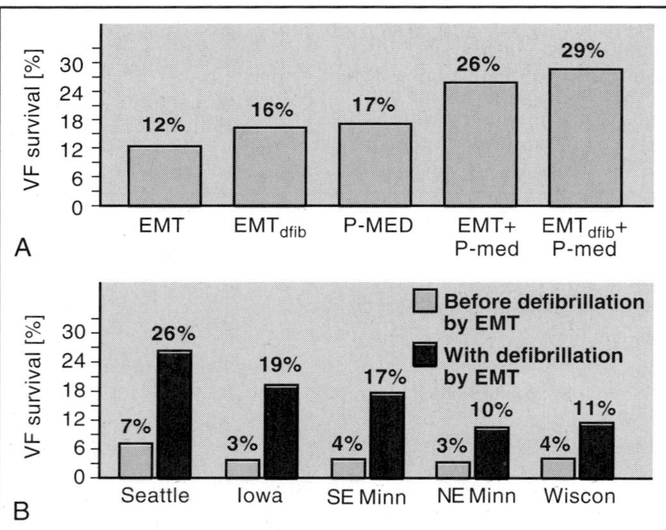

FIGURE 24–15. Impact of emergency rescue system design and immediate defibrillation on out-of-hospital cardiac arrest survival. *A,* Per cent survival to hospital discharge with rescue activities by standard emergency medical technician (EMT) trained in CPR, EMTs allowed to defibrillate immediately (EMT_{dfib}), initial response by paramedics (P-MED), two-tiered system with EMT and P-MED, and two-tiered system with EMT allowed to defibrillate if they are the first responders plus P-MED. Training of first-responders (EMT_{dfib}) and a two-tiered system have the best outcome. *B,* Comparison of outcomes observed in five geographic areas with EMT providing only CPR (dark color) versus EMT trained to defibrillate as first-responders (light color). In each group, there was a marked improvement in outcome when EMT personnel were trained and permitted to defibrillate. (Modified from Ornato, J. P., and Om, A.: Community experience in treating out-of-hospital cardiac arrest. *In* Akhtar, M., Myerburg, R. J., and Ruskin, J. N. [eds.]: Sudden Cardiac Death: Prevalence, Mechanisms and Approach to Diagnosis and Management. Baltimore, Williams & Wilkins, 1994, p. 450, with permission of the publisher.)

although there was no significant difference in the percentage of patients successfully resuscitated and admitted to the hospital alive with (67 per cent) or without (61 per cent) bystander intervention, almost twice as many prehospital cardiac arrest victims were ultimately discharged alive when they had had bystander CPR (43 per cent) than when such support was not provided (22 per cent).[22] Central nervous system protection, expressed as early regaining of consciousness, appears to be the major protective element of bystander CPR.[22] The rationale for bystander intervention is further highlighted by the relation between time to defibrillation and survival, when analyzed as a function of time to initiation of basic CPR. It has been reported that more than 40 per cent of victims whose defibrillation and other advanced life support activities were instituted more than 8 minutes after collapse survived if basic CPR had been initiated less than 2 minutes after onset of the arrest. A delay of more than 5 minutes to basic CPR was associated with no survivors.[292]

The time from onset of cardiac arrest to advanced life support influences outcome statistics. Mayer[321] reported improved short-term (to hospital admission) and long-term (to hospital discharge) survival rates for prehospital VF victims with short paramedic response times compared with those with long response times. Improvement in both early neurological status and survival occurs in the patient defibrillated by first responders, even if they are minimally trained emergency technicians allowed to carry out defibrillation as part of basic life support, compared with outcomes associated with awaiting more highly trained paramedics.[322] Thus the time to defibrillation plays a central role in determining outcome in cardiac arrest caused by VF. The development and deployment of automatic external defibrillators (see p. 1252) in the community holds promise for progress in the future.[323] This technology is a natural extension of lay bystander CPR.

MANAGEMENT OF THE INDIVIDUAL PATIENT

Management of the cardiac arrest victim is divided into five elements: (1) initial assessment, (2) basic life support, (3) advanced life support and definitive resuscitative efforts, (4) post–cardiac arrest care, and (5) long-term management. The first of these can be applied by a broad population base, which includes physicians and nurses as well as paramedical personnel, emergency rescue technicians, and laypeople educated in bystander intervention. The requirements for specialized knowledge and skills become progressively more focused as the patient moves through post–cardiac arrest management and into long-term follow-up care.

Initial Assessment and Basic Life Support

This activity includes both diagnostic maneuvers and elementary interventions. The first action of the person(s) in attendance when an individual collapses unexpectedly must be *confirmation that collapse is due to (or suspected to be due to) a cardiac arrest.* A few seconds of observation for response to voice, respiratory movements, and skin color, and simultaneous palpation of major arteries for the presence or absence of a pulse, yield sufficient information to determine whether a life-threatening incident is in progress. Once suspected or confirmed, contact with an available emergency medical rescue system (911) should be an immediate priority.[324]

The absence of carotid or femoral pulse, particularly if confirmed by the absence of an audible heartbeat, is the primary diagnostic criterion and can be performed accurately by trained laypeople. Skin color may be pale or intensely cyanotic. Absence of respiratory efforts, or the presence of only agonal respiratory efforts, in conjunction with an absent pulse, is diagnostic of cardiac arrest; however, respiratory efforts may persist for a minute or more after the onset of the arrest. In contrast, absence of respiratory efforts or severe stridor with persistence of a pulse suggests a primary respiratory arrest which will lead to a cardiac arrest in a short time. In the latter circumstance, initial efforts should include exploration of the oropharynx in search of a foreign body and the Heimlich maneuver, particularly if this occurs in a setting in which aspiration is likely (e.g., restaurant death or "cafe coronary").[204,205]

THUMPVERSION. Once the diagnosis of a pulseless collapse (presumed cardiac arrest) is established, a blow to the chest (precordial thump, "thumpversion"[325]) may be attempted by a properly trained rescuer. It has been recommended to be reserved as an advanced life support activity.[289] Caldwell and coworkers supported its use on the basis of a prospective study in 5000 patients.[325] In their study precordial thumps successfully reverted VF in 5 events, VT in 11, asystole in 2, and undefined cardiovascular collapse in 2 others in whom the electrical mechanism was unknown. In no instance was conversion of VT to VF observed. Because the latter is the only major concern of the precordial thump technique, and electrical activity can be initiated by mechanical stimulation in the asystolic heart,[326] the technique is considered optional for responding to a *pulseless* cardiac arrest in the absence of monitoring when a defibrillator is not immediately available. It should not be used unmonitored for the patient with a rapid tachycardia without complete loss of consciousness. For attempted thumpversion in cardiac arrest, one or two blows should be delivered firmly to the junction of the middle and lower thirds of the sternum from a height of 8 to 10 inches, but the effort should be abandoned if the patient does not immediately develop a spontaneous pulse and begin breathing. Another mechanical method, which requires that the patient is still conscious, is "cough-induced cardiac compression"[327] or "cough-version."[325] In the former a conscious act of forceful coughing by the patient in VF may support forward flow by cyclic increases in intrathoracic pressure[327]; the same act during sustained VT may cause conversion.[325,328]

THE ABCs OF CPR. The goal of this activity is to maintain viability of the central nervous system, heart, and other vital organs until definitive intervention can be achieved. The activities included within basic life support encompass both the initial responses outlined above and their natural flow into establishing ventilation and perfusion.[289] This range of activities can be carried out not only by professional and paraprofessional personnel, but also by trained emergency technicians and laypeople. Time is the key issue, and there should be no delay between the diagnosis and preparatory efforts in the initial response and the institution of basic life support.

AIRWAY. Clearing the airway is a critical step in preparing for successful resuscitation. This includes tilting the head backward and lifting the chin, in addition to seeking foreign bodies—including dentures—and removing them. The Heimlich maneuver should be performed if there is reason to suspect a foreign body lodged in the oropharynx. This entails wrapping the arms around the victim from the back and delivering a sharp thrust to the upper abdomen with a closed fist.[329] If it is not possible for the person in attendance to carry out the maneuver because of insufficient physical strength, mechanical dislodgment of the foreign body can sometimes be achieved by abdominal thrusts with the unconscious patient in a supine position. The Heimlich maneuver is not entirely benign: Ruptured abdominal viscera in the victim have been reported,[330] as has an instance in which the rescuer disrupted his own aortic root and died.[331]

If there is strong suspicion that respiratory arrest precipitated cardiac arrest, particularly in the presence of a mechanical airway obstruction, a second precordial thump should be delivered after the airway is cleared.

BREATHING. With the head properly placed and the oropharynx clear, mouth-to-mouth respiration can be initiated if no specific rescue equipment is available. To a large extent, the procedure used for establishing ventilation depends on the site at which the cardiac arrest occurs. A variety of devices are available, including plastic oropharyngeal airways, esophageal obturators, the masked AMBU bag, and endotracheal tubes. Intubation is the preferred procedure, but time should not be sacrificed even in the in-hospital setting while awaiting an endotracheal tube or a person trained to insert it quickly and properly. Thus, in the in-hospital setting, temporary support with AMBU bag ventilation is the usual method until endotracheal intubation can be carried out, and in the out-of-hospital setting mouth-to-mouth resuscitation is used while awaiting emergency rescue personnel. The effect of the acquired immunodeficiency syndrome and hepatitis B transmission on attitudes toward mouth-to-mouth resuscitation by bystanders and even professional personnel in hospitals is an area of concern,[289] but currently available data assessing risk of infection suggest that it is minimal.[332,333] The impact of this concern on attitudes toward, and outcomes of, resuscitative efforts has not been assessed.

Conventional CPR ventilatory techniques require that the lungs be inflated 10 to 12 times/minute whether one or two rescuers are present.[289] For one-rescuer resuscitation, a pause for ventilation (two breaths) is taken after every 15 chest compressions; for two rescuers, one breath is administered after every fifth compression. Techniques of CPR based on the hypothesis that increased intrathoracic pressure is the prime mover of blood, rather than cardiac compression itself,[334,335] have been evaluated; the cyclic ventilatory techniques are altered in these procedures (see below). However, clinical applicability is still not clarified.

CIRCULATION (Fig. 24–16). This element of basic life support is intended to maintain blood flow (i.e., circulation)

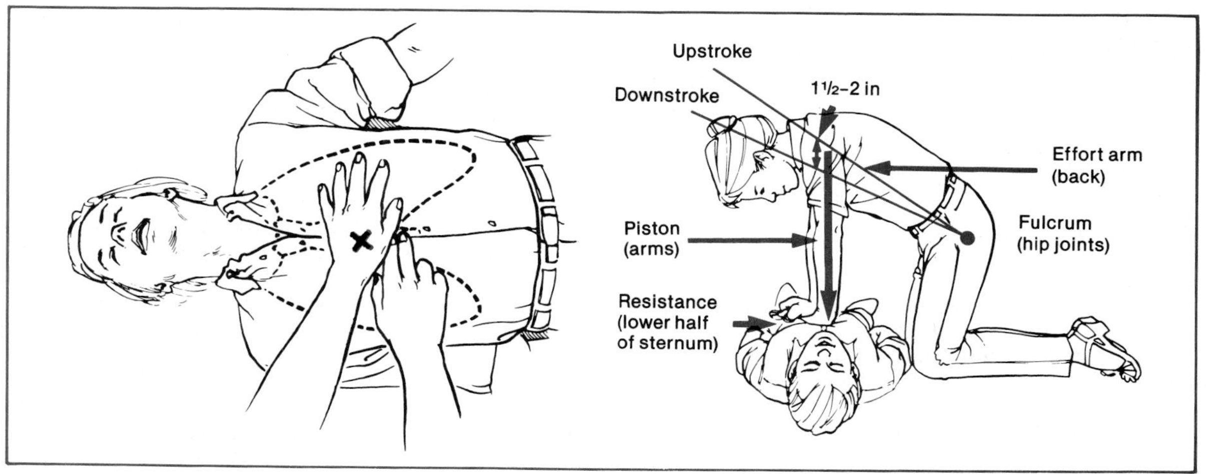

FIGURE 24–16. External chest compression. *Left,* Locating the correct hand position on the lower half of the sternum. *Right,* Proper position of the rescuer, with shoulders directly over the victim's sternum and elbows locked. (From Standards and guidelines for cardiopulmonary resuscitation [CPR] and emergency cardiac care [ECC]. JAMA *255*:2906, 1986. Copyright 1986, the American Medical Association.)

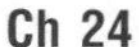

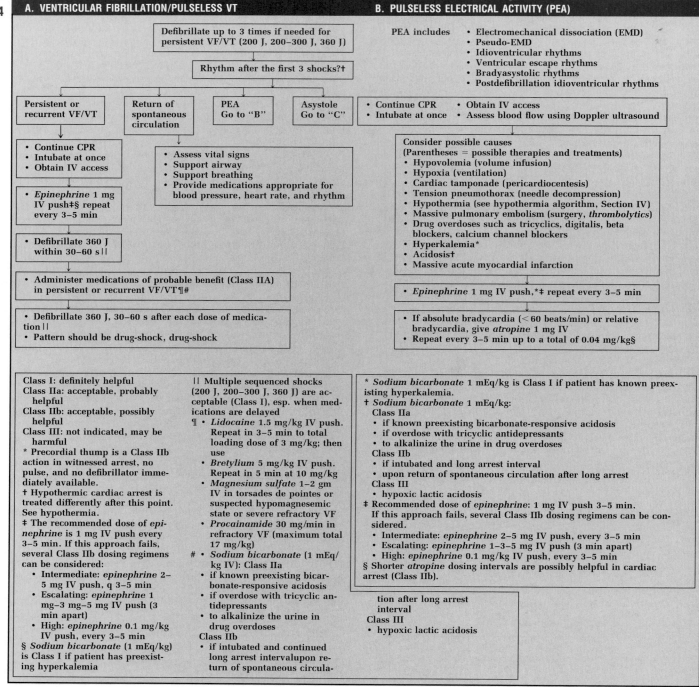

A. VENTRICULAR FIBRILLATION/PULSELESS VT

Defibrillate up to 3 times if needed for persistent VF/VT (200 J, 200–300 J, 360 J)

↓

Rhythm after the first 3 shocks?†

↓

- Persistent or recurrent VF/VT
  ↓
  - Continue CPR
  - Intubate at once
  - Obtain IV access

  ↓
  - *Epinephrine* 1 mg IV push‡§ repeat every 3–5 min

  ↓
  - Defibrillate 360 J within 30–60 s||

  ↓
  - Administer medications of probable benefit (Class IIA) in persistent or recurrent VF/VT¶#

  ↓
  - Defibrillate 360 J, 30–60 s after each dose of medication||
  - Pattern should be drug-shock, drug-shock
- Return of spontaneous circulation
  ↓
  - Assess vital signs
  - Support airway
  - Support breathing
  - Provide medications appropriate for blood pressure, heart rate, and rhythm
- PEA Go to "B"
- Asystole Go to "C"

B. PULSELESS ELECTRICAL ACTIVITY (PEA)

PEA includes
- Electromechanical dissociation (EMD)
- Pseudo-EMD
- Idioventricular rhythms
- Ventricular escape rhythms
- Bradyasystolic rhythms
- Postdefibrillation idioventricular rhythms

- Continue CPR
- Intubate at once
- Obtain IV access
- Assess blood flow using Doppler ultrasound

↓

Consider possible causes
(Parentheses = possible therapies and treatments)
- Hypovolemia (volume infusion)
- Hypoxia (ventilation)
- Cardiac tamponade (pericardiocentesis)
- Tension pneumothorax (needle decompression)
- Hypothermia (see hypothermia algorithm, Section IV)
- Massive pulmonary embolism (surgery, *thrombolytics*)
- Drug overdoses such as tricyclics, digitalis, beta blockers, calcium channel blockers
- Hyperkalemia*
- Acidosis†
- Massive acute myocardial infarction

↓

- *Epinephrine* 1 mg IV push,*‡ repeat every 3–5 min

↓

- If absolute bradycardia (<60 beats/min) or relative bradycardia, give *atropine* 1 mg IV
- Repeat every 3–5 min up to a total of 0.04 mg/kg§

Class I: definitely helpful
Class IIa: acceptable, probably helpful
Class IIb: acceptable, possibly helpful
Class III: not indicated, may be harmful

* Precordial thump is a Class IIb action in witnessed arrest, no pulse, and no defibrillator immediately available.

† Hypothermic cardiac arrest is treated differently after this point. See hypothermia.

‡ The recommended dose of *epinephrine* is 1 mg IV push every 3–5 min. If this approach fails, several Class IIb dosing regimens can be considered:
- Intermediate: *epinephrine* 2–5 mg IV push, q 3–5 min
- Escalating: *epinephrine* 1 mg–3 mg–5 mg IV push (3 min apart)
- High: *epinephrine* 0.1 mg/kg IV push, every 3–5 min

§ *Sodium bicarbonate* (1 mEq/kg) is Class I if patient has preexisting hyperkalemia

|| Multiple sequenced shocks (200 J, 200–300 J, 360 J) are acceptable (Class I), esp. when medications are delayed

¶
- *Lidocaine* 1.5 mg/kg IV push. Repeat in 3–5 min to total loading dose of 3 mg/kg; then use
- *Bretylium* 5 mg/kg IV push. Repeat in 5 min at 10 mg/kg
- *Magnesium sulfate* 1–2 gm IV in torsades de pointes or suspected hypomagnesemic state or severe refractory VF
- *Procainamide* 30 mg/min in refractory VF (maximum total 17 mg/kg)

\#
- *Sodium bicarbonate* (1 mEq/kg IV): Class IIa
- if known preexisting bicarbonate-responsive acidosis
- if overdose with tricyclic antidepressants
- to alkalinize the urine in drug overdoses

Class IIb
- if intubated and continued long arrest intervalupon return of spontaneous circulation after long arrest interval

Class III
- hypoxic lactic acidosis

* *Sodium bicarbonate* 1 mEq/kg is Class I if patient has known preexisting hyperkalemia.

† *Sodium bicarbonate* 1 mEq/kg:
Class IIa
- if known preexisting bicarbonate-responsive acidosis
- if overdose with tricyclic antidepressants
- to alkalinize the urine in drug overdoses

Class IIb
- if intubated and long arrest interval
- upon return of spontaneous circulation after long arrest

Class III
- hypoxic lactic acidosis

‡ Recommended dose of *epinephrine*: 1 mg IV push 3–5 min. If this approach fails, several Class IIb dosing regimens can be considered.
- Intermediate: *epinephrine* 2–5 mg IV push, every 3–5 min
- Escalating: *epinephrine* 1–3–5 mg IV push (3 min apart)
- High: *epinephrine* 0.1 mg/kg IV push, every 3–5 min

§ Shorter *atropine* dosing intervals are possibly helpful in cardiac arrest (Class IIb).

Modified from Guidelines for cardiopulmonary resuscitation and emergency cardiac care. JAMA *268*:2171, 1992.

until definitive steps can be taken. The rationale as originally developed was based on the hypothesis that chest compression allows the heart to maintain an externally driven pump function by sequential emptying and filling of its chambers, with competent valves favoring the forward direction of flow. In fact, the application of this technique has proved successful when used as recommended.[289] The palm of one hand is placed over the lower sternum and the heel of the other rests on the dorsum of the lower hand. The sternum is then depressed with the resuscitator's arms straight at the elbows to provide a less tiring and more forceful fulcrum at the junction of the shoulders and back (Fig. 24–16). Using this technique, sufficient force is applied to depress the sternum about 3 to 5 cm, with abrupt relaxation, and the cycle is carried out at a rate of about 80 to 100 compressions/min.[289] Despite the fact that this conventional technique produces measurable carotid artery flow and a record of successful resuscitations, the absence of a pressure gradient across the heart in the presence of an extrathoracic arterial-venous pressure gradient has led to a concept that it is not cardiac compression per se, but rather a pumping action produced by pressure changes in the entire thoracic cavity that optimizes systemic blood flow during resuscitation.[334–337] Experimental work in which the chest is compressed during ventilations rather than between them (simultaneous compression-ventilation, SCV) demonstrates better extrathoracic arterial flow.[334,337,338] However, increased carotid artery flow does not necessarily

TABLE 24–6 ADVANCED LIFE SUPPORT FOR CARDIAC ARREST VICTIMS—*Continued*

C. ASYSTOLE/SEVERE BRADYCARDIA

- Continue CPR
- Intubate at once
- Obtain IV access
- Confirm asystole in more than one lead

↓

Consider possible causes
- Hypoxia
- Hyperkalemia
- Hypokalemia
- Preexisting acidosis
- Drug overdose
- Hypothermia

↓

Consider immediate transcutaneous pacing (TCP)*

↓

- *Epinephrine* 1 mg IV push,†‡ repeat every 3–5 min

↓

- *Atropine* 1 mg IV, repeat every 3–5 min up to a total of 0.04 mg/kg§ ||

↓

Consider
- Termination of efforts¶

* TCP is a Class IIb intervention. Lack of success may be due to delays in pacing. To be effective TCP must be performed early, simultaneously with drugs. Evidence does not support routine use of TCP for asystole.

† The recommended dose of *epinephrine* is 1 mg IV push every 3–5 min. If this approach fails, several Class IIb dosing regimens can be considered:
- Intermediate: *epinephrine* 2–5 mg IV push, every 3–5 min
- Escalating: *epinephrine* 1 mg–3 mg–5 mg IV push (3 min apart)
- High: *epinephrine* 0.1 mg/kg IV push, every 3–5 min

‡ *Sodium bicarbonate* 1 mEq/kg is Class I if patient has known preexisting hyperkalemia.

§ Shorter *atropine* dosing intervals are Class IIb in asystolic arrest.

|| *Sodium bicarbonate* 1 mEq/kg:

Class IIa
- if known preexisting bicarbonate-responsive acidosis
- if overdose with tricyclic antidepressants
- to alkalinize the urine in drug overdoses

Class IIb
- if intubated and continued long arrest interval
- upon return of spontaneous circulation after long arrest interval

Class III
- hypoxic lactic acidosis

¶ If patient remains in asystole or other agonal rhythms after successful intubation and initial medications and no reversible causes are identified, consider termination of resuscitative efforts by a physician. Consider interval since arrest.

equate with improved cerebral perfusion,[335,339,340] and the reduction in coronary blood flow caused by elevated intrathoracic pressures by certain techniques[335,341] may be too high a price for the improved peripheral flow. In addition, a high thoracoabdominal gradient has been demonstrated during experimental SCV,[342] which could divert flow from the brain in the absence of concomitant abdominal binding. The comparative hemodynamics of models of conventional cardiac compression and techniques based on chest (thoracic) compression suggest that blood movement is based on both mechanisms in experimental[343] and clinical[344] studies. Based upon these observations, new mechanically assisted techniques for improving circulation during CPR are being evaluated.[344–346] More clinical studies are needed before establishing their general clinical applications.

Advanced Life Support and Definitive Resuscitation

This next step in the sequence of resuscitative efforts is designed to achieve definitive support and stabilization of the patient.[289] The implementation of advanced life support does not indicate abrupt cessation of basic life support activities, but rather a transition from one level of activity to the next. In the past, advanced life support required judgments and technical skills which removed it from the realm of activity of lay bystanders and even emergency medical technicians, limiting these activities to specifically trained paramedical personnel, nurses, and physicians. With further education of emergency technicians, most community-based CPR programs now permit them to carry out advanced life support activities.[289,298,320] In addition, the development and testing of equipment—the automatic external defibrillator—which has the ability to sense and analyze air flow, sense cardiac electrical activity, and provide definitive electrical intervention[323,347] may provide a role for less highly trained rescue personnel (i.e., police, ambulance drivers) and perhaps even trained lay bystanders in advanced life support.

The general goals of advanced life support are to optimize ventilation, revert the cardiac rhythm to one which is hemodynamically effective, and maintain and support the restored circulation. Thus, during advanced life support, the patient (1) is intubated and well oxygenated, (2) is defibrillated, cardioverted, or paced, and (3) has an intravenous line established to deliver necessary medications. After intubation, the goal of ventilation is to reverse hypoxemia and not merely achieve a high alveolar pO_2. Thus oxygen rather than room air should be used to ventilate the patient; if possible, the arterial pO_2 should be monitored. Respirator support in hospital and AMBU bag by means of an endotracheal tube or face mask in the out-of-hospital setting usually are used.

DEFIBRILLATION-CARDIOVERSION (Table 24–6*A*). Rapid conversion to an effective cardiac electrical mechanism is a key step for successful resuscitation.[292,308] Delay should be minimal, even when conditions for CPR are optimal. When VF or a rapid VT is recognized on a monitor or by telemetry, defibrillation should be carried out immediately with a shock of 200 joules. Up to 90 per cent of VF victims weighing up to 90 kg can be successfully resuscitated with a 200-joule shock,[348] and a 300- or 360-joule shock may be used if this is not successful.[289] Failure of the initial shocks to successfully cardiovert to an effective rhythm is a poor prognostic sign.[289] After failure of three shocks up to a maximum of 360 joules of energy, CPR should be continued while the patient is intubated and intravenous access achieved. Epinephrine, 1 mg IV, is administered and followed by repeated defibrillation attempts at 360 joules. Epinephrine may be repeated at 3- to 5-minute intervals with defibrillator shocks in between. Simultaneously, the rescuer should focus on ventilation to correct the biochemistry of the blood, efforts which render the heart more likely to reestablish a stable rhythm (i.e., improved oxygenation, reversal of acidosis, and improvement of the underlying electrophysiological condition). Although adequate oxygenation of the blood is crucial in the immediate management of the metabolic acidosis of cardiac arrest, additional correction may be achieved if necessary by intravenous administration of sodium bicarbonate. This is recommended for circumstances of known or suspected preexisting bicarbonate-responsive causes of acidosis, certain drug overdoses, and prolonged resuscitation runs.[289] The more general role for bicarbonate during cardiac arrest has been questioned[349–351]; but in any circumstance, much less sodium bicarbonate than was previously recommended is adequate for treatment of acidosis in this setting.[352] Excessive quantities can be deleterious.[351,352] Although some investigators have questioned the use of sodium bicarbonate at all because risks of alkalosis, hypernatremia, and hyperosmolality may outweigh its benefits,[353] the circumstances cited may benefit from administration of 1 mEq/kg of sodium bicarbonate while CPR is being carried out. Up to 50 per cent of this dose may be repeated every 10 to 15 minutes during the course of CPR.[354] When possible, arterial pH, pO_2, and pCO_2 should be monitored during the resuscitation.

PHARMACOTHERAPY. For the patient who remains in VT or VF despite direct current (DC) cardioversion after epinephrine, electrical stability of the heart may be achieved by intravenous administration of antiarrhythmic agents during continued resuscitation. As a matter of routine, lidocaine is tried first as an IV bolus, at a dose of 1.0 to 1.5 mg/kg (p. 605), with the dose repeated in 3 to 5 minutes in those in whom resuscitation remains unsuccessful or unstable electrical activity persists. If a total loading dose of 3.0 mg/kg has failed to support successful defibrillation, bretylium tosylate,[355] 5 mg/kg IV, should be given next. It can be repeated 5 minutes later in a dose of 10 mg/kg. Continued failure is an indication for other intravenous antiarrhythmic drugs, such as *procainamide hydrochloride* (see p. 1248)[356] or IV amiodarone (see p. 1248).[357] Procainamide is administered as a 30 mg/min intravenous infusion, to a maximum of 17 mg/kg. Intravenous amiodarone (see p. 1248), given as a 150- to 500-mg bolus and a 10 mg/kg/day infusion, may also be effective for refractory VT and VF.[357] In patients in whom acute hyperkalemia is the triggering event for resistant VF, or who are hypocalcemic or toxic from Ca^{++}-entry blocking drugs, 10 per cent calcium gluconate, 5 to 20 ml infused at a rate of 2 to 4 ml/min, may be helpful.[289] Calcium should *not* be used routinely during resuscitation,[358] even though ionized Ca^{++} levels may be low during resuscitation from cardiac arrest.[311] Some resistant forms of polymorphic VT or torsades de pointes, rapid monomorphic VT or ventricular flutter (rate $\geq$260/min), or resistant VF may respond to intravenous beta-blocker therapy (propranolol, 1 mg IV boluses to a total dose of up to 15 to 20 mg; metoprolol, 5 mg IV, up to 20 mg) or intravenous $MgSO_4$, 1 to 2 gm IV given over 1 to 2 minutes.

BRADYARRHYTHMIC AND ASYSTOLIC ARREST; PULSELESS ELECTRICAL ACTIVITY (Table 24–6*B* and *C*). The approach to the patient with bradyarrhythmic or asystolic arrest, or pulseless electrical activity, differs from the approach to patients with tachyarrhythmic events (VT/VF). Once this form of cardiac arrest is recognized, efforts should focus first on gaining control of the cardiorespiratory status (i.e., continue CPR, intubate, and establish IV access), then reconfirming the rhythm (in two leads if possible), and finally on taking actions which are likely to favor the emergence of a stable spontaneous rhythm, or attempts should be made to pace the heart. Possible reversible causes, particularly for bradyarrhythmia and asystole, should be considered and excluded (or treated) promptly. These include hypovolemia, hypoxia, cardiac tamponade, tension pneumothorax, preexisting acidosis, drug overdose, hypothermia, and hyperkalemia. Epinephrine (1.0 mg IV every 3 to 5 minutes) and atropine, 1.0 to 2.0 mg intravenously, are commonly used in an attempt to elicit spontaneous electrical activity or increase the rate of a bradycardia. These have had only limited success, as have intravenous isoproterenol infusions in doses up to 15 to 20 μg/min. In the absence of an intravenous line, epinephrine (1 mg [i.e., 10 ml of a 1:10,000 solution]) may be given by the intracardiac route, but there is danger of coronary or myocardial laceration. Sodium bicarbonate, 1 mEq/kg, may be tried for known or strongly suspected preexisting hyperkalemia or bicarbonate-responsive acidosis.

Pacing of the bradyarrhythmic or asystolic heart has been limited in the past by the unavailability of personnel capable of carrying out such procedures at the scene of cardiac arrests. With the development of more effective external pacing systems in recent years,[359] the role of pacing and its influence on outcome must now be reevaluated. Unfortunately all data to date suggest that the *asystolic* patient continues to have a very poor prognosis, despite new techniques.[291,299,360]

A recently published update on standards for CPR and emergency cardiac care[289] included a series of teaching algorithms to be used as guides to appropriate care. Table 24–6 provides the algorithms for VF and pulseless VT, asystole (or cardiac standstill), and pulseless electrical activity. These general guides are not to be interpreted as inclusive of all possible approaches or contingencies. The special circumstance of CPR in pregnant women requires additional attention to effects of drugs on the gravid uterus and the fetus, mechanical and physiological influences of pregnancy on efficacy of CPR, and risk of complications such as ruptured uterus and lacerated liver.[361]

STABILIZATION. As soon as electrical resuscitation from VT, VF, bradycardia, asystole, or pulseless electrical activity is achieved, the focus of attention shifts to maintaining a stable electrical and hemodynamic status. For electrical stability, a continuous infusion of an effective drug, based on observation during the cardiac arrest run, is commonly used. This may be lidocaine, 1 to 4 mg/min depending on size and clinical factors, or procainamide, 2 to 4 mg/min. Occasionally, a continuous infusion of propranolol or esmolol is used. Catecholamines are used in cardiac arrest not only in an attempt to achieve better electrical stability (e.g., conversion from fine to coarse VF, or increasing the rate of spontaneous contraction during bradyarrhythmias), but also for their inotropic and peripheral vascular effects. Epinephrine is the first choice among the catecholamines for use in cardiac arrest because it increases myocardial contractility, elevates perfusion pressure, may convert electromechanical dissociation to electromechanical coupling, and improves chances for defibrillation. Because of its adverse effects on renal and mesenteric flow, norepinephrine is a less desirable agent despite its inotropic effects. When the chronotropic effect of epinephrine is undesirable, dopamine or dobutamine is preferable to norepinephrine for inotropic effect. Isoproterenol may be used for the treatment of primary or postdefibrillation bradycardia when heart rate control is the primary goal of therapy intended to improve cardiac output. Calcium chloride, 2 to 4 mg/kg, is sometimes used in patients with pulseless electrical activity which persists after administration of catecholamines. The efficacy of this intervention is uncertain. Stimulation of alpha-adrenoceptors may be important during definitive resuscitative efforts.[362,363] For instance, the alpha-adrenoceptor stimulating effects of epinephrine and higher dosages of dopamine, producing elevation of aortic diastolic pressures by peripheral vasoconstriction[363] with increased cerebral[362] and myocardial flow,[362] have recently been reemphasized.[335,362] The importance of stimulating alpha-adrenoceptors in defibrillation in experimental VF also has been suggested.[363]

Post–Cardiac Arrest Care

For successfully resuscitated cardiac arrest victims, whether the event occurred in or out of hospital, post–cardiac arrest care includes admission to an intensive care unit and continuous monitoring for a minimum of 48 to 72 hours. Some elements of post-arrest management are common to all resuscitated patients, but prognosis and certain details of management are specific for the clinical setting in which the cardiac arrest occurred. The major management categories include (1) primary cardiac arrest in acute myocardial infarction, (2) secondary cardiac arrest in acute myocardial infarction, (3) cardiac arrest associated with noncardiac disorders, and (4) survival of out-of-hospital cardiac arrest.

PRIMARY CARDIAC ARREST IN ACUTE MYOCARDIAL INFARCTION (see also p. 1208). VF in the absence of preexisting hemodynamic complications (i.e., primary VF) currently is less common in hospitalized patients than the 15 to 20 per cent incidence which existed before availability of cardiac care units (CCUs). Early aggressive antiarrhythmic treatment is probably responsible,[364] and those events which do occur are almost always successfully reverted by prompt interventions in properly equipped emergency departments or CCUs.[365] After resuscitation, patients are often maintained on a lidocaine infusion at 2 to 4 mg/min. Antiarrhythmic support is usually discontinued after 24 hours if arrhythmias do not recur (see p. 1245). The occurrence of VF in the early phase of myocardial infarction is not an indication for long-term antiarrhythmic therapy.[366] Rapid VT producing the clinical picture of cardiac arrest in acute myocardial infarction is treated similarly; its intermediate and long-term implications are the same as those of VF. Cardiac arrest caused by bradyarrhythmias or asystole in acute inferior wall myocardial infarction, in the absence of primary hemodynamic consequences, is uncommon and may respond to either atropine or pacing. The prognosis is good, with no special long-term care required in most instances. Rarely, symptomatic bradyarrhythmias that require permanent pacemakers persist in survivors. In contrast to inferior myocardial infarction, bradyarrhythmic cardiac arrest associated with large anterior wall infarctions (and atrioventricular or intraventricular block) has a very poor prognosis (see p. 1250).

SECONDARY CARDIAC ARREST IN ACUTE MYOCARDIAL INFARCTION (see also p. 1233). This is defined as cardiac arrest occurring in association with, or as a result of, hemodynamic or mechanical dysfunction. The immediate mortality among patients in this setting ranges from 59 to 89 per cent, depending on severity of the hemodynamic abnormalities and size of the myocardial infarction.[367] Resuscitative efforts commonly fail in such patients, and when they are successful, the post–cardiac arrest management often is difficult. When secondary cardiac arrest occurs by the mechanisms of VT or VF, lidocaine in standard dosages is used, although the dose may have to be reduced in the presence of severe heart failure.[368] Other antiarrhythmics may have to be used in addition to or instead of lidocaine if complex arrhythmias persist or cardiac arrest recurs. The success of interventions and prevention of recurrent cardiac arrest relate closely to the outcome of managing the hemodynamic status. The incidence of cardiac arrest caused by bradyarrhythmias or asystole, or by electromechanical dissociation, is higher in the secondary form of cardiac arrest in acute myocardial infarction.[369] Such patients usually have large myocardial infarctions and major hemodynamic abnormalities and may be acidotic and hypoxemic. Even with aggressive therapy the prognosis after a bradyarrhythmic or asystolic arrest in such patients is very poor, and patients are resuscitated only rarely from electromechanical dissociation. All patients in circulatory failure at the onset of arrest are in a high-risk category, with only a 2 per cent survival rate among hypotensive patients in one study.[291]

CARDIAC ARREST AMONG IN-HOSPITAL PATIENTS WITH NONCARDIAC ABNORMALITIES. These patients fall into two major categories: (1) those with life-limiting diseases such as malignancies, sepsis, organ failure, end-stage pulmonary disease, and advanced central nervous system disease; and (2) those with acute toxic or proarrhythmic states which are potentially reversible. In the former category, the ratio of tachyarrhythmic to bradyarrhythmic cardiac arrest is low,[291] and the prognosis for surviving cardiac arrest is poor. Although the data may be somewhat skewed by the practice of assigning "do not resuscitate" orders to patients with end-stage disease, available data for attempted resuscitations show a poor outcome. Bedell et al.[291] reported that only 7 per cent of cancer patients, 3 per cent of renal failure patients, and no patients with sepsis or acute central nervous system disease were successfully resuscitated and discharged from the hospital alive. For the few successfully resuscitated patients in these categories, postarrest management is dictated by the underlying precipitating factors, such as transient hypoxia, electrolyte imbalances, and acidosis. Additional supportive cardiac care is directed to stabilizing hemodynamic, respiratory, and cardiac electrical states.

Most antiarrhythmic drugs (see Chap. 21),[170,172,210,211] a number of drugs used for noncardiac purposes,[172,175,176] and electrolyte disturbances may precipitate potentially lethal arrhythmias and cardiac arrest. Quinidine[370] and the other Class IA antiarrhythmic drugs, and the Class III drugs, are proarrhythmic by the generation of torsades de pointes, the Class IA drugs generally producing a dose-independent idiosyncratic response and the Class III, a dose-dependent adverse effect. The Class IC drugs rarely, if ever, cause torsades de pointes[371] but cause excess SCD risk in patients with recent myocardial infarction,[80] possibly by interacting with ischemia[372,373] or other transient risk factors.[374] Among other categories of drugs,[172,375] the phenothiazines, tricyclic antidepressants, lithium,[175] terfenadine,[176] pentamidine,[376] cocaine,[377] and cardiovascular drugs which are not antiarrhythmics—such as phenylamine and lidoflazine—are recognized causes. Beyond these, a broad array of pharmacological and pathophysiological/metabolic causes have been reported.[375] Hypokalemia, hypomagnesemia, and perhaps hypocalcemia are the electrolyte disturbances most closely associated with cardiac arrest. Acidosis and hypoxia may potentiate the vulnerability associated with electrolyte disturbances. Proarrhythmic effects may be foreshadowed by prolongation of the Q-T interval, although this electrocardiographic change is often not present.[173]

The torsades de pointes form of VT is a common manifestation of proarrhythmic effects of Class IA drugs. This arrhythmia usually is unstable and self-limiting and may terminate spontaneously, degenerate to VF, or evolve into a sustained VT. Cardiac arrest caused by this mechanism is managed by pacing, isoproterenol, and removal of the offending agent. Class IC drugs may cause a rapid, sinusoidal VT pattern, especially among patients with poor left ventricular function. This VT has a tendency to recur repetitively after cardioversion until the drug has begun to clear; this proarrhythmic form has been controlled by propranolol in some patients.[378]

When the patient's condition can be stabilized until the offending factor is removed (e.g., proarrhythmic drugs) or corrected (e.g., electrolyte imbalances, hypothermia), the prognosis is excellent. The recognition of torsades de pointes (see p. 684) and the identification of its risk by prolongation of the Q-T interval in association with the offending agent are helpful in managing these patients. No long-term prophylaxis is required in most patients. In contrast, beta-adrenoceptor blocking drugs or stellate ganglionectomy is required for long-term management of patients with the congenital form of Q-T interval prolongation who have been resuscitated after life-threatening arrhythmias.

POST–CARDIAC ARREST CARE IN SURVIVORS OF OUT-OF-HOSPITAL CARDIAC ARREST. The initial management of survivors of out-of-hospital cardiac arrest centers on stabilizing the cardiac electrical status, supporting hemodynamics, and providing supportive care for reversal of organ damage which has occurred as a consequence of the cardiac arrest. Frequent complex ventricular arrhythmias are common during the first 48 to 72 hours after resuscitation[20]; however, they often are manageable by conventional treatment. The risk of recurrent cardiac arrest is relatively low, and arrhythmias account for only 10 per cent of in-hospital deaths after successful prehospital resuscitation.[20,320] However, the mortality rate among those who do have recurrent cardiac arrest during the index hospitalization is 50 per cent. Antiarrhythmic therapy is used in an attempt to prevent recurrent cardiac arrest in patients who demonstrate residual electrophysiological instability and recurrent arrhythmia during the first 48 hours of post-arrest hospitalization. Lidocaine is the drug of choice for initial management, followed by intravenous procainamide or bretylium if initial drug therapy fails. Patients who have either preexisting or new atrioventricular or intraventricular conduction disturbances are at particularly high risk for recurrent cardiac arrest.[20] The routine use of temporary pacemakers has been evaluated in such patients but was not found to be useful for preventing early recurrent cardiac arrest. Invasive techniques for hemodynamic monitoring are used in unstable patients but not routinely for those who are stable on admission.

Respiratory support by conventional methods is used as necessary. During the convalescent period, attention to central nervous system status, including physical rehabilitation, is of primary importance to an optimal outcome. Bass[379] has recently summarized the neurological sequelae to cardiac arrest, including a review of various interventions. Preliminary data which suggested a beneficial effect of barbiturate loading for reversal of ischemic brain injury during and after cardiac arrest[380] have not been supported by a multicenter study of thiopental loading in comatose post-arrest patients[381] Management of other organ system injury (e.g., renal, hepatic), as well as early recognition and treatment of infectious complications, also contributes to ultimate survival.

LONG-TERM MANAGEMENT OF SURVIVORS OF OUT-OF-HOSPITAL CARDIAC ARREST. When the survivor of an out-of-hospital cardiac arrest has awakened and achieved electrical and hemodynamic stability, usually between 1 and 7 days after the event, decisions must be made regarding the nature and extent of the work-up required to establish a long-term management strategy. The goals of the work-up are to identify the specific etiological and triggering cause of the cardiac arrest[374] (if not already evident), clarify the functional status of the patient's cardiovascular system, and establish long-term therapeutic strategies. The extent of the work-up is largely dictated by the degree of central nervous system recovery and the factors already known to have contributed to the cardiac arrest. For instance, patients who have limited return of central nervous system function usually do not undergo extensive work-ups, and patients whose cardiac arrests were triggered by an acute transmural myocardial infarction have work-ups similar to those for other patients with acute myocardial infarction.

Survivors of out-of-hospital cardiac arrest not associated with acute myocardial infarction who have good return of neurological function undergo extensive diagnostic work-ups and carefully designed long-term therapy. The work-up normally includes cardiac catheterization with coronary angiography, an evaluation of functional significance of coronary lesions by stress-imaging techniques, determination of functional and hemodynamic status, and estimation of baseline susceptibility to life-threatening arrhythmias and of the expected response to long-term therapy.

GENERAL CARE. The general management of survivors of cardiac arrest is determined by the specific cause and the pathophysiology of the underlying process. For patients with ischemic heart disease (who constitute approximately 80 per cent of this population), control of episodes of myocardial ischemia, optimization of therapy for left ventricular dysfunction, and attention to general medical status are all addressed. Ischemic risk may be managed pharmacologically, surgically, or by catheter intervention techniques, depending on the anatomy and physiology of the disease process. Although there are limited data suggesting that coronary bypass surgery may improve the recurrence rate and total mortality rates after survival from out-of-hospital cardiac arrest,[382-384] no properly controlled prospective studies have validated this impression for either bypass surgery or angioplasty. Therefore, indications for surgery are limited to two groups of patients: (1) those who have a generally accepted indication for surgery[246] (including a documented ischemic mechanism for the cardiac arrest), and (2) those who meet specific criteria for surgery directed to arrhythmia control.[385]

Medical antiischemic therapy includes nitrates, beta-adrenoceptor blocking agents, and Ca^{2+}-entry blockers. Beta-adrenoceptors may have an antianginal effect and also influence the role of sympathetic nervous system activity on the genesis of potentially lethal arrhythmias. Although no placebo-controlled data are available to define a benefit of beta-blockers or other medical antiischemic therapy for long-term survival after out-of-hospital cardiac arrest, Morady and colleagues[99] suggested that medical or surgical antiischemic therapy, rather than antiarrhythmic therapy, should be the primary approach to long-term management of the subgroup of prehospital cardiac arrest survivors in whom transient myocardial ischemia was the inciting factor. Moreover, in an uncontrolled observation comparing cardiac arrest survivors who had ever been on beta-blockers after the index event with those who had not received the drug, a significant improvement in long-term outcome was observed among those who had received beta-blockers.[386]

In a report from the Coronary Artery Surgery Study (CASS), Holmes et al.[387] compared sudden death rates in medically and surgically treated patients in the CASS registry. This study did not directly address the issue of surgery in survivors of out-of-hospital cardiac arrest, but there was a significant difference at 5 years, with a 98 per cent sudden death–free survival in the surgical group versus 94 per cent in the medical group ($P < .0001$). The differences were minimal in the groups with one- or two-vessel disease and no history of heart failure, but expanded to 91 and 69 per cent, respectively, in patients with three-vessel disease and a history of heart failure. The question of how to apply these data to indications for surgery for cardiac arrest survivors remains unanswered at this time. The problem is further confounded by the fact that assignment of the 13,476 analyzable patients to medical versus surgical groups was not randomized (i.e., it was based instead on clinical judgment). Further evaluation of the specific role of coronary surgery *after* out-of-hospital cardiac arrest is needed.

The long-term management of the consequences of left ventricular dysfunction by conventional means such as digitalis preparations and chronic diuretic use has been evaluated in several studies. Data from the Multiple Risk Factor Intervention Trial (MRFIT) suggested a higher mortality rate in the special intervention group,[388] presumably related to diuretic use and K^+ depletion, and other data regarding the relation between K^+ depletion and arrhythmias have focused attention on routine use of such drugs. Although the facts currently are far from conclusive,[266] use of diuretics should be accompanied by careful monitoring of electrolytes. Similar concerns have been raised in respect to digitalis use in high-risk patients after acute myocardial infarction.[389-392] The use of digoxin in survivors of prehospital cardiac arrest should be tailored to specific indications for left ventricular dysfunction.

PREVENTION OF RECURRENT CARDIAC ARREST

In a survivor of out-of-hospital cardiac arrest, the risk of recurrent cardiac arrest not associated with acute transmural myocardial infarction was 30 per cent at 1 year and 45 per cent at 2 years in the early 1970's.[18,19] Although it is not known whether this natural history risk is the same currently, it is generally believed that the risk of recurrence remains substantial (Fig. 24–17). Long-term therapeutic strategies intended to prevent recurrences of potentially lethal arrhythmias have been based on several medical approaches, on antiarrhythmic surgery, and on the use of implantable devices. Antiarrhythmic surgery evolved in parallel with programmed stimulation approaches to management, and most recently antitachycardiac and antifibrillatory devices have been developed for use in subgroups of these patients. A problem which impinges on all long-term strategies is the lack of a reliable current natural history denominator against which to compare the results of any intervention (Fig. 24–17).

LONG-TERM ANTIARRHYTHMIC THERAPY. The antiarrhythmic approach to long-term management of survivors of out-of-hospital cardiac arrest was based initially on two assumptions: (1) that the high frequency of chronic PVCs identified in cardiac arrest survivors constitutes a triggering mechanism for potentially lethal arrhythmias, and (2) that electrophysiological instability of the myocardium predisposing to potentially lethal arrhythmias can be modified by antiarrhythmic drugs.[275,303] Therapeutic strategies derived from these assumptions included endpoints identified by the ability to suppress induction of VT/VF by programmed electrical stimulation,[393,394] suppression of ambient arrhythmias on ambulatory monitors,[395,396] and by empiric therapy using amiodarone,[397,398] beta blockers,[386,399] or membrane-active antiarrhythmic drugs.[275,303,386]

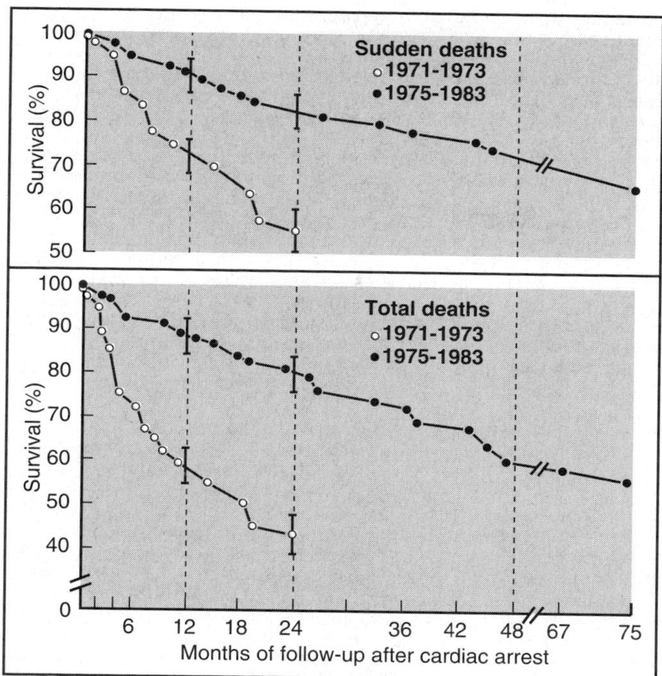

FIGURE 24–17. Sudden deaths and total deaths in survivors of prehospital cardiac arrest during an 8-year follow-up period *(closed circles)*, compared with 1970–1973 historical experience during the initial Miami studies *(open circles)*. The more recent experience indicates a 67 per cent reduction in recurrent cardiac arrest rate in the first year of follow-up. Whether this was due to aggressive antiarrhythmic therapy or other factors in the patient populations or their management cannot be determined from comparison to historical controls. However, the 10 per cent 1-year mortality rate is similar to outcome with other forms of antiarrhythmic intervention in recent years. (From Myerburg, R. J., and Kessler, K. M.: Management of patients who survive cardiac arrest. Mod. Concepts Cardiovasc. Dis. *55*:61, 1986.)

One major limitation hovers over the interpretation of all antiarrhythmic drug studies in patients who have survived out-of-hospital cardiac arrest—namely, the lack of randomized, concurrent placebo-controlled studies. This limitation derives from the ethical consideration of withholding active therapy from patients known to be at high risk for recurrent cardiac arrest, when a drug could reasonably be expected to provide a benefit. The results of CAST,[80,81] and of other antiarrhythmic drug observations in out-of-hospital cardiac arrest survivors,[386] give reason to question this limitation, but no concurrent placebo-controlled data are currently forthcoming using any of the methods listed above. Accordingly, studies have been designed in which outcomes after suppression of inducibility by programmed electrical stimulation or suppression of "high-risk" ventricular ectopic activity on ambulatory monitoring, are compared with outcomes after failure of suppression. In another type of study design, one antiarrhythmic therapeutic strategy serves as a positive control for another (e.g., empiric amiodarone versus electrophysiologically guided antiarrhythmic therapy). Each of these approaches remains limited by the inability to identify a mortality benefit in a positively controlled study design.[26,400] Relative efficacy may be identified, but not an absolute mortality benefit.

PROGRAMMED ELECTRICAL STIMULATION. The use of programmed electrical stimulation (see p. 720) to identify benefit on the basis of suppression of inducibility by an antiarrhythmic drug gained early popularity for evaluating long-term therapy among survivors of out-of-hospital cardiac arrest.[393,394,401–406] It evolved as the preferred method of management, despite problems relative to sensitivity and specificity of the various pacing protocols[407] and concerns about the extent to which the myocardial status at the time of the programmed electrical stimulation study reflected that present at the time of the clinical cardiac arrest. Imponderables such as the extent to which electrode catheter–stimulated extrasystoles mimic spontaneous PVCs, and the ischemic, autonomic, and biochemical status of the heart at the time of the study, may influence the data.[408] Nonetheless, among a series of six reports,[393,394,401–404] induction of sustained VT or VF at baseline study ranged from 31 to 79 per cent, and successful suppression of inducibility has ranged from 18 to 78 per cent. The mortality rate during follow-up on those patients in whom inducibility was suppressed by antiarrhythmic therapy ranged from 0 to 22 per cent (mean = 9 per cent), compared with the range of 22 to 78 per cent (mean = 43 per cent) in those patients in whom VT or VF was still inducible on any antiarrhythmic therapy.

The evaluation of these data is significantly influenced by definitions of inducibility and noninducibility, and also by the clinical features of the patient population in each of the studies, which varied considerably. In most reports VF or sustained VT could not be induced in 25 to 30 per cent of the patients. It is probable that differences are determined in part by the numbers of patients who have anatomically discrete versus ischemic substrates among various populations studied.[313] Careful attention to protocol details, anatomy of the disease processes, and definitions of inducibility may help to clarify these discrepancies in the future. For the present, however, 50 to 70 per cent of *unselected* survivors of cardiac arrest caused by VF or sustained VT can be anticipated to be inducible into sustained arrhythmias. For the subgroup with discrete ventricular aneurysms, more than 90 per cent may be inducible.[246,401] The clinical significance of induced VF, as opposed to a sustained VT or VF which evolves from an induced VT, is often difficult to interpret. Induced VF is commonly considered nonspecific when the induction protocol is aggressive and the patient has not had a clinical cardiac arrest. However, most accept it as a valid positive study in survivors of out-of-hospital cardiac arrest, especially when the protocol is less aggressive (e.g., double extrastimuli or triple extrastimuli in which coupling intervals are not excessively short) and the induction is reproducible.

Most investigators agree that inducibility into a *sustained* clinical arrhythmia provides an indication of risk and that its prevention is an endpoint for therapy, but the implications of induced *nonsustained* forms are more controversial. While it has been suggested that induction of nonsustained rhythms may indicate risk, it often is nonspecific if an aggressive protocol is used.[407] The use of the suppression of nonsustained arrhythmias as an endpoint of therapy is not considered valid. The significance of *noninducibility* at baseline electrophysiological stimulation testing in relation to risk and long-term management also is a controversial issue. Opinions have ranged from the conclusion that patients showing noninducibility are not electrophysiologically unstable and require no long-term antiarrhythmic therapy[99,393,404,414] to the other extreme that such patients remain at risk but do not provide an objective endpoint of therapy by this method, and therefore must be treated by other techniques.[51,246,303,395] Some patients in this category have had cardiac arrest clearly resulting from transient ischemia and require only antiischemic therapy.[99] In the 6 reports, 24-month mortality in patients who had noninducibility ranged from 3 to 38 per cent, higher than in patients in whom inducibility could be suppressed by antiarrhythmic therapy (average 9 per cent) but lower than in those in whom inducibility could not be suppressed (average 43 per cent). In one study, left ventricular ejection fraction discriminated high risk from low risk in noninducible patients; in another, reversible causes of the index event predicted noninducibility.[406,415] A recent report[416] demonstrated that patients in whom ventricular arrhythmias could not be induced were at risk for recurrent cardiac arrest, although the risk is lower than would be anticipated for patients in whom arrhythmias could be induced. There was a 12 per cent event rate at 24 months in the patient population reported. When patients with structural heart disease and low ejection fractions cannot be induced into VT or VF after cardiac arrest, it is generally agreed that high risk of recurrence persists.

AMBULATORY ELECTROCARDIOGRAPHIC MONITORING. The development of detailed methods of analysis of ambulatory monitor recordings[395] led some investigators to study suppressibility of ambient arrhythmias as a specific and individualized means of evaluating drug therapy. Graboys et al.[395] reported outcome in a group of 123 patients with advanced ambient ventricular arrhythmias who had survived one or more cardiac arrests. Suppression of specific forms of complex ventricular ectopy (then defined as three or more consecutive beats and early-cycle PVCs) identified on either ambulatory monitoring or exercise testing was accompanied by a significantly lower mortality rate compared with those in whom such suppression was not achieved. The mortality rate was more than 80 per cent at 3 years in patients whose complex forms could not be suppressed compared with a nearly 90 per cent survival among the patients in whom complex PVCs were suppressed. A subsequent report confirmed the original observation.[396]

Other investigators provided data suggesting the possibility that ambient arrhythmia suppression might be equivalent to suppression of inducible arrhythmias by programmed electrical stimulation in predicting outcome.[409–411] Moreover, analysis of the CAST data base also suggested an association between the ease of suppression of ambient ventricular arrhythmias and survival,[412] supporting the notion of a meaningful relationship between *suppressibility* of ambient arrhythmias and survival. Data from the Electrophysiologic Study versus Electrocardiographic Monitoring (ESVEM) trial[410] did demonstrate a benefit favoring outcome prediction by programmed stimulation compared with ambulatory monitoring techniques in coronary artery disease patients, most evident in the interval of the first 2 years of follow-up. For nonischemic diseases, the opposite was true. In another randomized trial comparing invasive and noninvasive techniques among patients who had symptomatic tachyarrhythmias, the invasive technique was superior in prevention of recurrences.[413] However, the qualifying arrhythmias were not restricted to cardiac arrests, and therefore the applicability to cardiac arrest survivors remains uncertain.

While a high fraction of patients will have successful suppression of the therapeutic targets using ambulatory monitor techniques compared to programmed electrical stimulation, more patients will have programmed electrical stimulation–inducible arrhythmias than ambient ectopy targets,[409–411] and programmed electrical stimulation still maintains preference as the method of choice for evaluating antiarrhythmic therapy. The question of whether *suppressibility* rather than *suppression* is the meaningful marker remains uncertain[412] for both techniques.

Finally, empiric antiarrhythmic therapy predominantly using amiodarone has been supported as having a relative benefit in several studies.[397,398] Whether it has an absolute mortality benefit can only be determined by placebo-controlled data, which are not available.

SURGICAL INTERVENTION

Direct antiarrhythmic surgical techniques (see p. 619) which were originally conceived for control of recurrent sustained VT, such as map-guided endocardial resection[417] and encircling endocardial ventriculotomy,[418] have largely yielded to the technology of intraoperative map-guided cryoablation techniques.[419] This approach is limited primarily to those patients who have inducible, hemodynamically stable sustained monomorphic VT during electrophysiological testing and are unresponsive to drug therapy and have suitable ventricular and coronary artery anatomy. While the outcome using this technique has been much better than that of previous techniques,[419] it has very little applicability to survivors of out-of-hospital cardiac arrest because the type of arrhythmia favoring this surgical approach is infrequently observed among cardiac arrest survivors. The less specific antiarrhythmic surgical techniques used previously demonstrate less efficacy and higher mortality.

In contrast, coronary revascularization procedures have a clearly defined role for cardiac arrest survivors in whom an ischemic mechanism was responsible for the event and suitable surgical anatomy is present.[99,420]

Platia et al.[421] evaluated the concomitant use of ventricular endocardial resection with implantable defibrillators for patients with refractory ventricular arrhythmias. During a mean 25-month follow-up, 4 of 25 patients (16 per cent) had recurrent tachycardia which was successfully reverted by the device, but 1 patient died because the device malfunctioned. The practice of implanting cardioverter-defibrillator patches at the time of antiarrhythmic or antiischemic surgery in anticipation of a possible need at a later time based on results of postsurgical electrophysiological studies has now largely been abandoned because of the success of transvenous defibrillator lead systems.

IMPLANTABLE DEVICES (see Chap. 23)

The development of a reliable implantable cardioverter-defibrillator added a new dimension to the management of patients at high risk of cardiac arrest.[422] In their initial report,[423] Mirowski and coworkers evaluated the results in 52 patients who had survived an arrhythmic cardiac arrest plus at least one recurrence not associated with acute myocardial infarction. Other forms of preventive management had failed in all these patients, and the group had a mean of 3.9 cardiac arrests per patient. The analysis is complicated by the fact that concomitant cardiovascular surgical procedures were carried out in 15 patients, and about the same number had previous surgery, plus pacemaker implantation in 9. Although 12 of these 52 very high-risk patients died during a 14-month mean follow-up period, producing a 23 per cent 1-year total mortality rate, the 1-year sudden death rate was 8.5 per cent. Devices were triggered 62 times in 17 patients. Assuming death would have followed in these patients without the device, the total 1-year mortality rate would have been 48 per cent.

Subsequently, Echt and colleagues[424] reported their experience in 70 patients. Because 35 of their patients (50 per cent) had had no previous cardiac arrests (14 patients with uncontrollable recurrent ventricular tachycardia) or only 1 previous arrest (21 patients), this population may have been less "unstable" than Mirowski's group.[423] There was a mean of 1.9 ± 1.7 cardiac arrests/patient, 3.1 ± 2.3 arrhythmic episodes/patient, and 4.0 ± 2.1 drug failures/patient. During an average follow-up period of 8.9 months (range, 1 to 33 months), 37 patients (53 per cent) received one or more shocks. The 12-month total death rate was 10 per cent, the sudden death rate was less than 2 per cent, and the complication rate was acceptably low. Subsequent reports have confirmed that implantable cardioverter-defibrillators can achieve sudden death rates consistently less than 5 per cent at 1 year, and total death rates in the 10 to 20 per cent range, among populations who have high mortality risks, as predicted by mortality surrogates such as historical controls or time to first appropriate shock.[425–430]

The interpretation of the benefit of implantable defibrillator devices for automated intervention during onset of cardiac arrest, and for a mortality benefit, remain uncertain and debated.[400,431] While the studies cited above document the ability of implantable devices to successfully revert potentially fatal arrhythmias, the absence of placebo-controlled trials limits the ability to identify a true mortality benefit because of confounding factors such as competing risks for sudden and nonsudden death,[26] the degree to which appropriate shocks represent the interruption of an event that would have been fatal,[400] and the lack of ability of a positive control to determine mortality benefit of either or both interventions.[79] Despite these limitations, implantable defibrillator therapy has continued to increase its relative position among other forms of therapy for survivors of out-of-hospital cardiac arrest because of the issues of efficacy and safety of antiarrhythmic therapy cited earlier, and the limited applicability of antiarrhythmic surgical therapy. Issues that leave major questions unanswered and could affect the defibrillator approach for survivors of out-of-hospital cardiac arrest include relative benefit of amiodarone versus defibrillators, the role of beta blockers as antiadrenergic therapy, and the role of antiischemic surgical and medical therapy as definitive approaches.

A much larger issue, and one that has not yet been defined, is the use of implantable defibrillators among patients who are at high risk for cardiac arrest, but who have not yet had an event. A number of trials are under way to attempt to determine whether preventive defibrillator therapy is an effective means of preventing the first cardiac arrest. Many of the trials are studying cost efficacy in addition to medical efficacy. One of the more important strategies being tested is a comparison of defibrillator therapy versus empiric amiodarone therapy.

MANAGEMENT ALGORITHM

The options for diagnostic evaluation and long-term management of cardiac arrest survivors are complex, with specific problems unique both to patient subgroups and to the various therapeutic strategies. A two-tiered algorithm has been developed as a guide to management.[432] Management stage I (Fig. 24–18) addresses diagnostic evaluation and general management, and stage II (Fig. 24–19) is oriented to strategies specifically for control of potentially lethal arrhythmias. Endpoints of management are reached in stage I for those patients in whom cardiac arrest was precipitated by acute myocardial infarction, those who have some form of noncoronary heart disease or cardiac arrest clearly related to transient ischemia, and those who have cardiac arrest caused by proarrhythmic factors, such as adverse drug effect or electrolyte imbalances. Patients with life-limiting concurrent morbid states and those who have major post-arrest residual damage of the central nervous system also reach their management endpoints in stage I, without progressing to Stage II, except for the possible use of empiric therapy such as amiodarone.

Among the remainder, who constitute the majority of survivors and most commonly have chronic ischemic heart disease, electrophysiological stimulation studies should be performed (Fig. 24–19). In that subgroup of patients among whom sustained VT with or without degeneration to VF is inducible, a primary endpoint of therapy is prevention of inducibility by an appropriate antiarrhythmic agent or drug combination. The former practice of testing multiple antiarrhythmic drugs and drug combinations has largely been abandoned. Most Class I antiarrhythmic drugs have been effective in no more than 20 per cent of patients who have programmed electrical stimulation–inducible ventricular arrhythmias and up to 40 to 50 per cent of ambient arrhythmias evaluated by ambulatory monitoring. A possible exception is sotalol, which showed greater efficacy in one study.[411] The combination of limited short-term endpoint efficacy, uncertain long-term benefit (especially among patients with advanced heart disease[414]), and safety issues[80,81] has led to a trend away from the use of these drugs. Evaluation of beta-blocker therapy by programmed electrical stimulation in selected cardiac arrest survivors has been suggested.[433] The Class III drugs, including amiodarone, sotalol, and newly developing agents, are being evaluated.

Among those patients in whom the programmed electrical stimulation approach is not feasible because of noninducibility of sustained VT or VF, another objective approach should be used (Fig. 24–19). Some patients who have salvos or nonsustained VT on ambulatory monitoring may be treated with antiarrhythmic drugs in an attempt to suppress repetitive forms[395,409–411] or treated with amiodarone empirically.[397,398] If this is successful, it may be used as the endpoint of therapy.[409] Those patients who have neither inducibility by electrophysiological stimulation nor complex forms on ambulatory monitoring in conjunction with low (<35 per cent) ejection fractions should receive implantable cardioverter-defibrillator devices[414,421,423,424] in lieu of empiric therapy.

Antiarrhythmic surgical intervention is preferred only in patients who have inducible and intraoperatively mappable VT that appears related to the cardiac arrest event and cannot be managed by antiarrhythmic drugs. The results of surgery in such patients have been encouraging.[385,419]

An implantable device is therapy of choice for an increasing number of cardiac arrest survivors.[434] Candidates include cardiac arrest survivors who fail endpoints for antiarrhythmic drug therapy, survivors who are not inducible into VT/VF and do not have a defined ischemic mechanism or do have an ejection fraction less than 35 per cent, and all patients who fall into either of the two previous

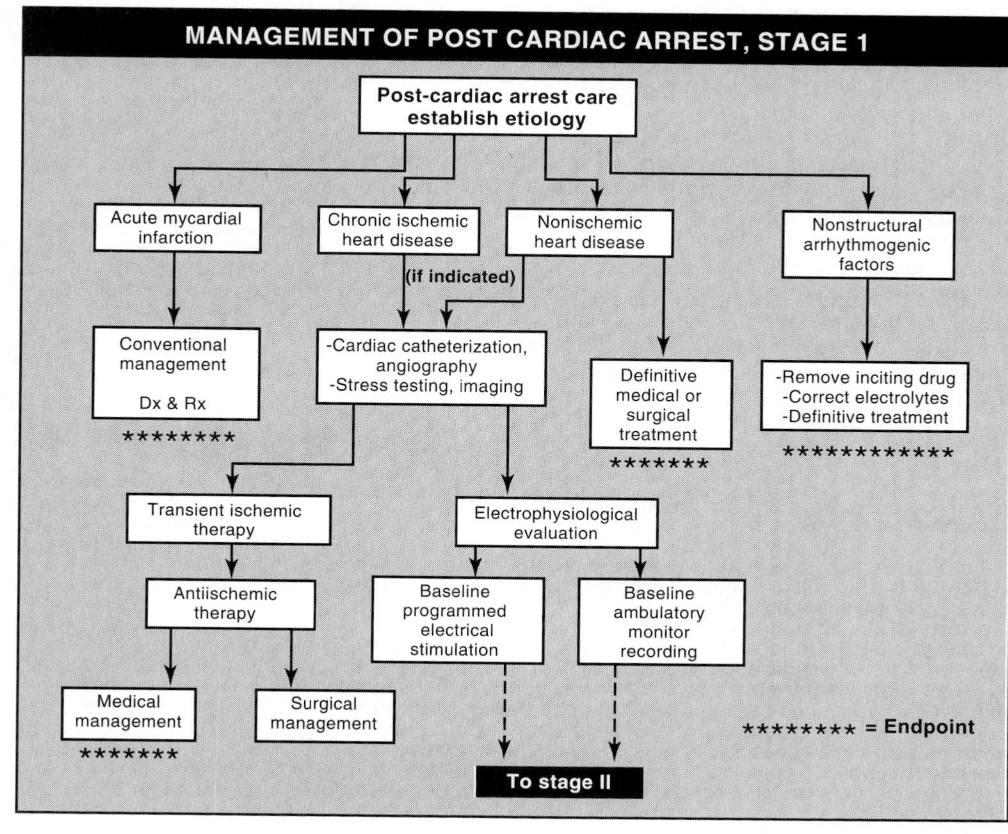

FIGURE 24–18. Management algorithm—stage I. Flow diagram for initial management and diagnostic activities in survivors of prehospital cardiac arrest. Patients whose arrests were associated with new acute transmural myocardial infarction or nonstructural arrhythmogenic factors are managed by conventional techniques. All patients with chronic ischemic heart disease, and many with nonischemic heart disease, enter a pathway which leads to advanced electrophysiological study and management. (From Myerburg, R. J., and Kessler, K. M.: Management of patients who survive cardiac arrest. Mod. Concepts Cardiovasc. Dis. *55*:61, 1986.)

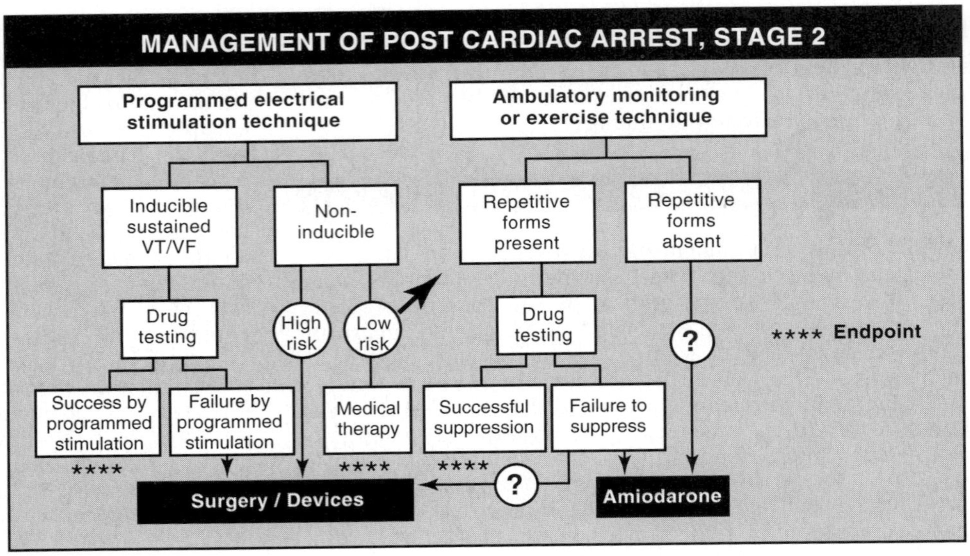

FIGURE 24–19. Management algorithm—stage II. Advanced electrophysiological evaluation of survivors of out-of-hospital cardiac arrest. Patients enter the programmed electrical stimulation (or ambulatory monitor) pathway and are initially evaluated by drug testing using this technique. If the heart is inducible into sustainted VT or VF (with some limitations of interpretation for the latter), and drug testing results in successful prevention of inducibility, an acceptable endpoint of therapy has been achieved (****). If the arrhythmia remains inducible (failure by programmed stimulation), antiarrhythmic surgery or an implantable device is considered. If the heart is noninducible into an arrhythmia at baseline and the patient is at low risk for recurrence because of either (1) an identifiable and controllable ischemic mechanism, (2) reversible metabolic mechanisms, or (3) no more than moderate depression of ejection fraction, the patient may be managed by appropriate medical therapy. Ambulatory monitoring techniques are applicable if repetitive forms are present.

When programmed stimulation is not available or not applicable to an individual patient, the ambulatory monitoring or exercise techniques may be used. For drug testing, repetitive forms must be identified as the target arrhythmia and successful suppression by conventional drug therapy is considered an acceptable endpoint, perhaps equivalent to electrophysiological testing under some conditions.[409–411] Failure to suppress repetitive forms in high-risk patients should lead to considerations for implantable devices and possibly some forms of surgical intervention. Among others in this category, amiodarone is an acceptable therapeutic approach. If repetitive forms are absent and the patient is at high risk (e.g., very low EF), amiodarone or implantable devices are the therapies of choice. (From Myerburg, R. J., and Kessler, K. M.: Management of patients who survive cardiac arrest. Med. Concepts Cardiovasc. Dis. *55*:61, 1986.)

categories and are not candidates for antiarrhythmic surgery. Moreover, despite the fact that there may be a statistical benefit for successful programmed electrical stimulation–guided antiarrhythmic therapy in cardiac arrest survivors with ejection fractions less than 30%,[406] the mortality rate in such patients remains substantial,[406,414] and such patients *may* have a better outcome with implantable-device therapy. However, it must be reiterated that mortality benefit for implantable defibrillators in this circumstance has not been proven.

When used according to defined indications, the recent statistics for each of the approaches outlined above are intriguing. Each method has now been recognized to yield a 1-year survival rate of 90 per cent or better, compared with the 70 per cent survival cited earlier. Whether this means that each of the methods is equally effective or whether some other uncontrolled factor is influencing outcome has not been defined and requires further evaluation. However, high risk is attendant on indiscriminate changes in pharmacological therapy which has been determined appropriate by any of the endpoints used. Swerdlow et al.[401] and Myerburg et al.,[51] using different therapeutic approaches, both have reported that arbitrary cessation, or changes in therapy without retesting for the endpoint used to establish the initial therapy, is accompanied by a high risk of recurrent cardiac arrest.

SUDDEN DEATH AND PUBLIC SAFETY

The unexpectedness of SCD has raised questions concerning secondary risk to the public created by people in the throes of a cardiac arrest. There are no controlled data available to guide public policy regarding people at high risk for potentially lethal arrhythmias and for abrupt incapacitation. Myerburg and Davis[435] reported observations on 1348 sudden deaths caused by coronary heart disease in people 65 years of age or less during a 7-year period in Dade County, Florida. One hundred one (7.5 per cent) of these deaths occurred in people who were engaged in activities at the time of death which were potentially hazardous to the public (e.g., 56 driving private automobiles or taxis, 15 driving trucks, 10 working at altitude, 2 piloting aircraft) and 122 (9.1 per cent) of the victims had occupations which could create potential hazards to others if an abrupt loss of consciousness had occurred while at work (e.g., 57 taxi and truck drivers, 8 aircraft pilots, 9 bus drivers, 9 policemen and firemen). There were no catastrophic events as a result of these cardiac arrests, only minor property damage in 19 and minor injuries in 5.

Levy et al.[436] reported a case of a bus driver with a strong history of coronary heart disease who caused the deaths of himself and several others, but they did not conclusively demonstrate that unexpected cardiac arrest was the proximate cause of the accident. Furthermore, Waller[437] studied an elderly population and demonstrated that cardiac disease alone was not responsible for a significant increase in accident risk: *senility*, or *senility plus cardiovascular disease, was much more important*. Several other studies also have led to the conclusion that risk to the public is small.[438] In specific reference to private automobile drivers, most of the data show that sudden death at the wheel usually involves enough of a prodrome to allow the driver to get to the roadside before losing consciousness.[435,438–440] A recent analysis of recurrent VT/VF events among cardiac arrest survivors suggested limitation of driving privileges for the first 8 months after the index event,[35] based on the clustering of recurrent event rates early after the index event.[34,35] Therefore, although there are likely to be isolated instances in which cardiac arrest causes public hazards in the future, the risk appears to be small, and because it is difficult to identify specific individuals at risk, sweeping restrictions to avoid such risks appear unwarranted. The exceptions are people with multisystem disease, particularly senility, and individual circumstances that require specific consideration, such as high-risk patients who have special responsibilities—school bus drivers, aircraft pilots, trainmen, and truck drivers.

REFERENCES

DEFINITION

1. Weiss, S.: Instantaneous "physiologic" death. N. Engl. J. Med. *223*:793, 1940.
2. Spain, D. M., Bradess, V. A., and Mohr, C.: Coronary atherosclerosis as a cause of unexpected and unexplained death: An autopsy study from 1949–1959. JAMA *174*:384, 1960.
3. Burch, G. E., and DePasquale, N. P.: Sudden, unexpected, natural death. Am. J. Med. Sci. *249*:86, 1965.
4. Kuller, L., Lilienfeld, A., and Fisher, R.: An epidemiological study of sudden and unexpected deaths in adults. Medicine *46*:341, 1967.
5. Paul, O., and Schatz, M.: On sudden death. Circulation *43*:7, 1971.
6. Gordon, T., and Kannel, W. B.: Premature mortality from coronary heart disease. The Framingham Study. JAMA *215*:1617, 1971.
7. Biorck, C., and Wikland, B.: Sudden death—what are we talking about? Circulation *45*:256, 1972.
8. Friedman, M., Manwaring, J. H., Rosenman, R. H., et al.: Instantaneous and sudden deaths: Clinical and pathological differentiation in coronary artery disease. JAMA *225*:1319, 1973.
9. Kannel, W. B., Doyle, J. T., McNamara, P. M., et al.: Precursors of sudden coronary death: Factors related to the incidence of sudden death. Circulation *51*:606, 1975.

10. Helmers, C., Lundman, T., Maasing, R., and Wester, P. O.: Mortality pattern among initial survivors of acute myocardial infarction using a life-table technique. Acta Med. Scand. *200*:469, 1976.
11. Mitchell, J. R. A., and Schwartz, C. J.: Arterial Disease. Oxford, Blackwell, 1965.
12. Ruberman, W., Weinblatt, E., Goldberg, J. D., et al.: Ventricular premature beats and mortality after myocardial infarction. N. Engl. J. Med. *297*:750, 1977.
13. Myerburg, R. J.: Sudden death. J. Cont. Ed. Cardiol. *14*:15, 1978.
14. Lovegrove, T., and Thompson, P.: The role of acute myocardial infarction in sudden cardiac death—a statistician's nightmare. Am. Heart J. *96*:711, 1978.
15. Thomas, A. C., Davies, M. J., and Popple, A. W.: A pathologist's view of sudden cardiac death. *In* Kulbertus, H. E., and Wellens, H. J. J. (eds.): Sudden Death. The Hague, Netherlands, Martinus Nijhoff, 1980, pp. 34–48.
16. Goldstein, S.: The necessity of a uniform definition of sudden coronary death: Witnessed death within 1 hour of the onset of acute symptoms. Am. Heart J. *103*:156, 1982.
17. Kuller, L. H.: Prodromata of sudden death and myocardial infarction. Adv. Cardiol. *25*:61, 1978.
18. Liberthson, R. R., Nagel, E. L., Hirschman, J. C., and Nussenfeld, S. R.: Prehospital ventricular fibrillation: Prognosis and follow-up course. N. Engl. J. Med. *291*:317, 1974.
19. Baum, R. S., Alvarez, H., and Cobb, L. A.: Survival after resuscitation from out-of-hospital ventricular fibrillation. Circulation *50*:1231, 1974.
20. Myerburg, R. J., Conde, C. A., Sung, R. J., et al.: Clinical, electrophysiologic, and hemodynamic profile of patients resuscitated from prehospital cardiac arrest. Am. J. Med. *68*:568, 1980.
20a. Sequiera, R. F., and Myerburg, R. J.: Sudden cardiac death. *In* Fuster, V., Ross, R., and Topol, E. J. (eds.): Atherosclerosis and coronary artery disease. Philadelphia, Lippincott-Raven Publishers, 1996, pp. 1031–1050.
21. Hinkle, L. E.: The immediate antecedents of sudden death. Acta Med. Scand. *210*:207, 1981.
22. Thompson, R. G., Hallstrom, A. P., and Cobb, L. A.: Bystander-initiated cardiopulmonary resuscitation in the management of ventricular fibrillation. Ann. Intern. Med. *90*:737, 1979.
23. Kuller, L. H.: Sudden death: Definition and epidemiologic considerations. Prog. Cardiovasc. Dis. *23*:1, 1980.

EPIDEMIOLOGY AND CAUSES OF SUDDEN DEATH

24. Epstein, F. H., and Pisa, Z.: International comparisons in ischemic heart disease mortality. Proc. Conf. Decline in Coronary Heart Disease Mortality. DHEW, NIH Publication No. 79–1610, Washington, D.C., U.S. Government Printing Office, 1979, pp. 58–88.
25. Report of the Working Group on Arteriosclerosis of the National Heart, Lung, and Blood Institute (Volume 2): Patient Oriented Research—Fundamental and Applied, Sudden cardiac death. DHEW, NIH Publication No. 82–2035, Washington, D.C., U.S. Government Printing Office, 1981, pp. 114–122.
26. Myerburg, R. J., Kessler, K. M., and Castellanos, A.: Sudden cardiac death: Epidemiology, transient risk, and intervention assessment. Ann. Intern. Med. *119*:1187, 1993.
27. Gillum, R. F.: Sudden coronary death in the United States; 1980–1985. Circulation *79*:756, 1989.
28. Epstein, S. E., Quyyumi, A. A., and Bonow, R. O.: Sudden cardiac death without warning: Possible mechanisms and implications for screening asymptomatic populations. N. Engl. J. Med. *321*:321, 1989.
29. Schatzkin, A., Cupples, L. A., Heeren, T., et al.: The epidemiology of sudden unexpected death: Risk factors for men and women in the Framingham Heart Study. Am. Heart J. *107*:1300, 1984.
30. Schatzkin, A., Cupples, L. A., Heeren, T., et al.: Sudden death in the Framingham Heart Study: Differences in incidence and risk factors by sex and coronary disease status. Am. J. Epidemiol. *120*:888, 1984.
31. Gillum, R. F.: Geographic variations in sudden coronary death. Am. Heart J. *119*:380, 1990.
32. Rosenberg, H. M., and Klebbs, A. J.: Trends in cardiovascular mortality with a focus on ischemic heart disease: United States, 1950–1976. Proc. Conf. Decline in Coronary Heart Disease Mortality. DHEW, NIH Publication No. 79–1610, Washington, D.C., U.S. Government Printing Office, 1979, pp. 11–41.
33. Kannel, W. B., and Schatzkin, A.: Sudden death: Lessons from subsets in population studies. J. Am. Coll. Cardiol. *5*(Suppl. 6):141B, 1985.
34. Myerburg, R. J., Kessler, K. M., Castellanos, A.: Sudden cardiac death: Structure, function, and time-dependence of risk. Circulation *85*(Suppl. I):I-2, 1992.
35. Larsen, G. C., Stupey, M. R., Walance, C. G., et al.: Recurrent cardiac events in survivors of ventricular fibrillation or tachycardia: Implications for driving restrictions. JAMA *271*:1335, 1994.
36. Doyle, J. T., Kannel, W. B., McNamara, P. M., et al.: Factors related to suddenness of death from coronary disease: Combined Albany-Framingham studies. Am. J. Cardiol. *37*:1073, 1976.
37. Kannel, W. B., and Thomas, H. E.: Sudden coronary death: The Framingham study. Ann. N.Y. Acad. Sci. *382*:3, 1982.
38. Holmes, D. R., Davis, K., Gersh, B. J., et al.: Rich factor profiles of patients with sudden cardiac death and death from other cardiac causes: A report from the Coronary Artery Surgery Study (CASS). J. Am. Coll. Cardiol. *13*:524, 1989.
39. Kuller, L., Lilienfeld, A., and Fischer, R.: Sudden and unexpected deaths in young adults: An epidemiologic study. JAMA *198*:158, 1966.
40. Neuspiel, D. R., and Kuller, L. H.: Sudden and unexpected natural death in childhood and adolescence. JAMA *254*:1321, 1985.
41. Neufeld, H. N., and Goldbourt, V.: Coronary heart disease: Genetic aspects. Circulation *67*:943, 1983.
42. Garza, L. A., Vick, R. L., Nora, J. J., and McNamara, D. G.: Heritable Q-T prolongation without deafness. Circulation *41*:39, 1970.
43. Clark, C. E., Henry, W. L., and Epstein, S. E.: Familial prevalence and genetic transmission of idiopathic hypertrophic subaortic stenosis. N. Engl. J. Med. *289*:709, 1973.
44. Green, J. R., Krovetz, M. J., Shanklin, D. R., et al.: Sudden unexpected death in three generations. Arch. Intern. Med. *124*:359, 1969.
45. Davies, M. J.: Pathological view of sudden cardiac death. Br. Heart J. *45*:88, 1981.
46. Brookfield, L., Bharati, S., Denes, P., et al.: Familial sudden death: Report of a case and review of the literature. Chest *94*:989, 1988.
47. James, T. N., and MacLean, W. A. H.: Paroxysmal ventricular arrhythmias and familial sudden death associated with neural lesions in the heart. Chest *78*:24, 1980.
48. Keating, M. T., Atkinson, D., Dunn, C., et al.: Linkage of a cardiac arrhythmia, the long QT syndrome, and the Harvey *ras*-1 gene. Science *252*:704, 1991.
49. Curran, M. E., Splawski, I., Timothy, K. W., et al.: A molecular basis for cardiac arrhythmia; HERG mutations cause long QT syndrome. Cell *80*:795, 1995.
50. Wang, O., Shen, J., Splawski, I., et al.: SCN5A mutations associated with an inherited cardiac arrhythmia, long QT syndrome. Cell *80*:805, 1995.
51. Myerburg, R. J., Kessler, K. M., Estes, D., et al.: Long-term survival after prehospital cardiac arrest: Analysis of outcome during an 8-year study. Circulation *70*:538, 1984.
52. Kuller, L., Cooper, M., and Perper, J.: Epidemiology of sudden death. Arch. Intern. Med. *129*:714, 1972.
53. Krueger, D. E., Ellenberg, S. S., Bloom, S., et al.: Risk factors for fatal heart attack in young women. Am. J. Epidemiol. *113*:357, 1981.
54. Wenger, N. K.: Coronary disease in women. Annu. Rev. Med. *36*:285, 1985.
55. Jick, H., Dinan, B., Herman, R., and Rothman, K. J.: Myocardial infarction and other vascular diseases in young women: Role of estrogens and other factors. JAMA *240*:2548, 1978.
56. Hagstrom, R. M., Federspiel, C. F., and Ho, Y. C.: Incidence of myocardial infarction and sudden death from coronary heart disease in Nashville, Tennessee. Circulation *44*:884, 1971.
57. Becker, L. B., Han, B. H., Mayer, P. M., et al.: Racial differences in the incidence of cardiac arrest and subsequent survival. N. Engl. J. Med. *329*:600, 1993.
58. Marmot, M. E., Syme, S. L., Kagan, A., et al.: Epidemiologic studies of coronary heart disease and stroke in Japanese men living in Japan, Hawaii, and California: Prevalence of coronary and hypertensive heart disease and associated risk factors. Am. J. Epidemiol. *102*:514, 1975.
59. Myerburg, R. J., Kessler, K. M., Kimura, S., et al.: Life-threatening ventricular arrhythmias: The link between epidemiology and pathophysiology. *In* Zipes, D. P., and Jalife, J. (eds.): Cardiac Electrophysiology. 2nd ed. Philadelphia, W. B. Saunders Company, 1995, p. 723.
60. Maclure, M.: The case-crossover design: A method for studying transient effects on the risk of acute events. Am. J. Epidemiol. *33*:144, 1991.
61. Muller, J. E., Tofler, G. H., and Stone, P. H.: Circadian variation and triggers of onset of acute cardiovascular disease. Circulation *79*:733, 1989.
62. Mittleman, M. A., Maclure, M., Tofler, G. H., et al.: Triggering of acute myocardial infarction by heavy physical exertion: Protection against triggering by regular exertion. N. Engl. J. Med. *329*:1677, 1993.
63. Hallstrom, A. P., Cobb, L. A., and Ray, R.: Smoking as a risk factor for recurrence of sudden cardiac arrest. N. Engl. J. Med. *314*:271, 1986.
64. Paffenbarger, R. S., Hale, W. E., Brand, R. J., and Hyde, R. T.: Work energy level, personal characteristics, and fatal heart attack: A birth-cohort effect. Am. J. Epidemiol. *105*:200, 1977.
65. Rahe, R. H., Romo, M., Bennett, L., and Siltman, P.: Recent life changes, myocardial infarction, and abrupt coronary death. Arch. Intern. Med. *133*:221, 1974.
66. Talbott, E., Kuller, L. H., Petre, K., and Perper, J.: Biologic and psychosocial risk factors of sudden death from coronary disease in white women. Am. J. Cardiol. *39*:858, 1977.
67. Ruberman, W., Weinblatt, E., Goldberg, J. D., and Chaudhary, B. S.: Psychosocial influences on mortality after myocardial infarction. N. Engl. J. Med. *311*:552, 1984.
68. Weinblatt, E., Ruberman, W., Goldberg, J. D., et al.: Relation of education to sudden death after myocardial infarction. N. Engl. J. Med. *299*:60, 1978.
69. Lambert, C. A., Netherton, D. R., Finison, L. J., et al.: Risk factors and life style: A statewide health-interview survey. N. Engl. J. Med. *306*:1048, 1982.
70. Friedman, M., and Rosenman, R. H.: Association of specific overt behavior pattern with blood and cardiovascular findings. JAMA *169*:1286, 1959.
71. Shekelle, R. B., Gale, M., and Norosis, M.: Type A score (Jenkins Activity Survey) and risk of recurrent coronary heart disease in the aspirin-myocardial study. Am. J. Cardiol. *56*:221, 1985.

72. Bigger, J. T., Fleiss, J. L., Kleiger, R., et al.: The relationships among ventricular arrhythmias, left ventricular dysfunction, and mortality in the 2 years after myocardial infarction. Circulation *69:*250, 1984.
73. Kennedy, H. L., Whitlock, J. A., Sprague, M. K., et al.: Long-term follow-up of asymptomatic healthy subjects with frequent and complex ventricular ectopy. N. Engl. J. Med. *312:*193, 1985.
74. Chiang, B. N., Perlman, L., Ostrander, L. D., and Epstein, F.: Relation of premature systole to coronary heart disease and sudden death in the Tecumseh epidemiologic study. Ann. Intern. Med. *70:*1159, 1969.
75. PrattA, C. M., Theroux, P., Slymen, D., et al.: Spontaneous variability of ventricular arrhythmias in patients at increased risk for sudden death after acute myocardial infarction: Consecutive ambulatory electrocardiographic recordings of 88 patients. Am. J. Cardiol. *59:*278, 1987.
76. Ruberman, W., Weinblatt, E., Goldberg, J. D., et al.: Ventricular premature complexes and sudden death after myocardial infarction. Circulation *64:*297, 1981.
77. Myerburg, R. J., Kessler, K. M., Luceri, R. M., et al.: Classification of ventricular arrhythmias based on parallel hierarchies of frequency and form. Am. J. Cardiol. *54:*1355, 1984.
78. Ruberman, W., Weinblatt, E., Frank, C. W., et al.: Repeated 1-hour electrocardiographic monitoring of survivors of myocardial infarction at 6-month intervals: Arrhythmia detection and relation to prognosis. Am. J. Cardiol. *47:*1197, 1981.
79. Myerburg, R. J., Kessler, K. M., Chakko, S., et al.: Future evaluation of antiarrhythmic therapy. Am. Heart J. *127:*1111, 1994.
80. Echt, D. S., Liebson, P. R., Mitchell, L. B., et al.: Mortality and morbidity in patients receiving encainide, flecainide, or placebo: The Cardiac Arrhythmia Suppression Trial. N. Engl. J. Med. *324:*781, 1991.
81. The Cardiac Arrhythmia Suppression Trial II Investigators: Effect of the antiarrhythmic agent moricizine on survival after myocardial infarction. N. Engl. J. Med. *327:*227, 1992.
82. Akhtar, M., Breithardt, G., Camm, A. J., et al.: CAST and beyond: Implications of the Cardiac Arrhythmia Suppression Trial. Circulation *81:*1123, 1990.
83. Maisel, A. S., Scott, N., Gilpin, E., et al.: Complex ventricular arrhythmias in patients with Q wave versus non-Q wave myocardial infarction. Circulation *72:*963, 1985.
84. Levin, D. C., Fellows, K. E., and Abrams, H. L.: Hemodynamically significant primary anomalies of the coronary arteries: Angiographic aspects. Circulation *58:*25, 1978.
85. Harthorne, J. W., Scannell, J. G., and Dinsmore, R. E.: Anomalous origin of the left coronary artery: Remedial cause of sudden death in adults. N. Engl. J. Med. *275:*660, 1966.
86. Roberts, W. C., Siegel, R. J., and Zipes, D. P.: Origin of the right coronary artery from the left sinus of Valsalva and its functional consequences: Analysis of 10 necropsy patients. Am. J. Cardiol. *49:*863, 1982.
87. Maron, B. J., Epstein, S. E., and Roberts, W. C.: Causes of sudden death in competitive athletes. J. Am. Coll. Cardiol. *7:*204, 1986.
88. Waller, B. F.: Exercise-related sudden death in young (age $\leq$ 30 years) and old (age > 30 years) conditioned subjects. *In* Wenger, N. K. (ed.): Exercise and the Heart, Philadelphia, F. A. Davis Co., 1985, pp. 9–73.
89. Roberts, W. C.: Coronary embolism: A review of causes, consequences, and diagnostic considerations. Cardiovasc. Med. *3:*699, 1978.
90. El Maraghi, N., and Genton, E.: The relevance of platelet and fibrin thromboembolism of the coronary microcirculation, with special reference to sudden cardiac death. Circulation *62:*936, 1980.
91. Kegel, S. M., Dorsey, T. J., Rowen, M., and Taylor, W. F.: Cardiac death in mucocutaneous lymph node syndrome. Am. J. Cardiol. *40:*282, 1977.
92. Thiene, G., Valente, M., and Rossi, L.: Involvement of the cardiac conduction system in panarteritis nodosa. Am. Heart J. *95:*716, 1978.
93. Heggveit, H. A.: Syphilitic aortitis—a clinicopathological autopsy of 100 cases. Circulation *29:*346, 1964.
94. Roberts, W. C., and Honig, H. S.: The spectrum of cardiovascular disease in the Marfan syndrome. Am. Heart J. *104:*115, 1982.
95. Shaver, P. J., Carrig, T. F., and Baker, W. P.: Postpartum coronary artery dissection. Br. Heart J. *40:*83, 1978.
96. Harris, L. S., and Adelson, L.: Fatal coronary embolism from a myxomatous polyp of the aortic valve. An unusual cause of sudden death. Am. J. Clin. Pathol. *43:*61, 1965.
97. Roberts, W. C.: Pathology of arterial aneurysms. *In* Bergan, J. J., and Yao, S. T. (eds.): Aneurysms, Diagnosis and Treatment. New York, Grune and Stratton, 1982, pp. 17–43.
98. Morales, A. R., Romanelli, R., and Boucek, R. J.: The mural left anterior descending coronary artery, strenuous exercise, and sudden death. Circulation *62:*230, 1980.
99. Morady, F., DiCarlo, L., Winston, S., et al.: Clinical features and prognosis of patients with out-of-hospital cardiac arrest and a normal electrophysiologic study. J. Am. Coll. Cardiol. *4:*39, 1984.
100. Nakamura, M., Takeshita, A., and Nose, Y.: Clinical characteristics associated with myocardial infarction, arrhythmias, and sudden death in patients with vasospastic angina. Circulation *75:*1110, 1987.
101. Myerburg, R. J., Kessler, K. M., Mallon, S. M., et al.: Life-threatening ventricular arrhythmias in patients with silent myocardial ischemia due to coronary artery spasm. N. Engl. J. Med. *326:*1451, 1992.
102. Sharma, B., Francis, G., Hodges, M., and Asinger, R.: Demonstration of exercise-induced ischemia without angina in patients who recover from out-of-hospital ventricular fibrillation. Am. J. Cardiol. *47*(Abs.):445, 1981.
103. Maseri, A., Severi, S., and Marzullo, P.: Role of coronary arterial spasm in sudden coronary ischemic death. Ann. N.Y. Acad. Sci. *382:*204, 1982.
104. Sheps, D. S., and Heiss, G.: Sudden death and silent myocardial ischemia. Am. Heart J. *117:*177, 1989.
105. Anderson, K. P.: Sudden death, hypertension, and hypertrophy. J. Cardiovasc. Pharmacol. *6*(Suppl. 3):S498, 1984.
106. Messerli, F. H., Ventura, H. O., Elizardi, D. J., et al.: Hypertension and sudden death: Increased ventricular ectopic activity in left ventricular hypertrophy. Am. J. Med. *77:*18, 1984.
107. Braunwald, E., Morrow, A. G., Cornell, W. P., et al.: Idiopathic hypertrophic subaortic stenosis: Clinical, hemodynamic, and angiographic manifestations. Am. J. Med. *29:*924, 1960.
108. Goodwin, J. F.: The frontiers of cardiomyopathy. Br. Heart J. *48:*1, 1982.
109. Shah, P. M., Adelman, A. G., Wigle, E. D., et al.: The natural (and unnatural) history of hypertrophic obstructive cardiomyopathy. Circ. Res. *35*(Suppl. 2):179, 1974.
110. Cecchi, F., Maron, B. J., and Epstein, S. E.: Long-term outcome of patients with hypertrophic cardiomyopathy successfully resuscitated after cardiac arrest. J. Am. Coll. Cardiol. *13:*1283, 1989.
111. Maron, B. J., Roberts, W. C., and Epstein, S. E.: Sudden death in hypertrophic cardiomyopathy: A profile of 78 patients. Circulation *65:*1388, 1982.
112. Savage, D. D., Seides, S. F., Maron, B. J., et al.: Prevalence of arrhythmias during 24-hour electrocardiographic monitoring and exercise testing in patients with obstructive and non-obstructive hypertrophic cardiomyopathy. Circulation *59:*866, 1979.
113. Goodwin, J. F., and Krikler, D. M.: Arrhythmia as a cause of sudden death in hypertrophic cardiomyopathy. Lancet *2:*937, 1976.
114. Maron, B. J., Savage, D. D., Wolfson, J. K., and Epstein, S. E.: Prognostic significance of 24 hour ambulatory electrocardiographic monitoring in patients with hypertrophic cardiomyopathy: A prospective study. Am. J. Cardiol. *48:*252, 1981.
115. Fananapazir, L., and Epstein, S. E.: Hemodynamic and electrophysiologic evaluation of patients with hypertrophic cardiomyopathy surviving cardiac arrest. Am. J. Cardiol. *67:*280, 1991.
116. Kowey, P. R., Eisenberg, R., and Engel, T. R.: Sustained arrhythmias in hypertrophic obstructive cardiomyopathy. N. Engl. J. Med. *310:*156, 1984.
117. Stafford, W. J., Trohman, R. G., Bilsker, M., et al.: Cardiac arrest in an adolescent with atrial fibrillation and hypertrophic cardiomyopathy. J. Am. Coll. Cardiol. *7:*701, 1986.
118. Maron, B. J., Epstein, S. E., and Roberts, W. C.: Hypertrophic cardiomyopathy: A common cause of sudden death in the young competitive athlete. Eur. Heart J. *4*(Suppl. F):135, 1983.
119. Waller, B. F.: Sudden death in midlife. Cardiovasc. Med. *10:*55, 1985.
120. Northcote, R. J., Flannigan, C., and Ballantyne, D.: Sudden death and vigorous exercise: A study of 60 deaths associated with squash. Br. Heart J. *55:*198, 1986.
121. Packer, M.: Sudden unexpected death in patients with congestive heart failure: A second frontier. Circulation *72:*681, 1985.
122. Stevenson, W. E., Stevenson, L. W., Middlekauff, H. R., et al.: Sudden death prevention in patients with advanced ventricular dysfunction. Circulation *88:*2953, 1993.
123. Kjekshus, J.: Arrhythmia and mortality in congestive heart failure. Am. J. Cardiol. *65:*42-I, 1990.
124. Middlekauff, H. R., Stevenson, W. G., Stevenson, L. W., et al.: Syncope in advanced heart failure: High sudden death risk regardless of syncope etiology. J. Am. Coll. Cardiol. *21:*110, 1993.
125. Huang, S. K., Messer, J. V., and Denes, P.: Significance of ventricular tachycardia in idiopathic dilated cardiomyopathy: Observations in 35 patients. Am. J. Cardiol. *51:*507, 1983.
126. Meinertz, T., Hoffmann, T., Kasper, W., et al.: Significance of ventricular arrhythmias in idiopathic dilated cardiomyopathy. Am. J. Cardiol. *53:*902, 1984.
127. Poll, D. S., Marchinski, F. E., Buxton, A. E., et al.: Sustained ventricular tachycardia in patients with idiopathic dilated cardiomyopathy: Electrophysiologic testing and lack of response to antiarrhythmic drug therapy. Circulation *70:*451, 1984.
128. Warren, J. V.: Unusual sudden death. Cardiol. Ser. *8*(4):5, 1984.
129. Surawicz, B.: Ventricular fibrillation. J. Am. Coll. Cardiol. *51*(Suppl. B):43, 1985.
130. Topaz, O., and Edwards, J. E.: Pathologic features of sudden death in children, adolescents, and young adults. Chest *87:*476, 1985.
131. Phillips, M., Rabinowitz, M., Higgins, J. R., et al.: Sudden cardiac death in air force recruits. JAMA *256:*2696, 1986.
132. Robboy, S. J.: Atrioventricular node inflammation: Mechanisms of sudden death in protracted meningococcemia. N. Engl. J. Med. *286:*1091, 1972.
133. Roberts, W. C., McAllister, H. A., and Farrans, V. J.: Sarcoidosis of the heart: A clinicopathologic study of 35 necropsy patients (group I) and review of 78 previously described necropsy patients (group II). Am. J. Med. *63:*86, 1977.
134. Silverman, K. J., Hutchins, G. M., and Bulkley, B. H.: Cardiac sarcoid: A clinicopathologic study of 84 unselected patients with systemic sarcoidosis. Circulation *58:*1204, 1978.
135. Bulkley, B. H., Klacsman, P. G., and Hutchins, G. M.: Angina pectoris, myocardial infarction and sudden cardiac death with normal coronary arteries: A clinicopathological study of nine patients with progressive systemic sclerosis. Am. Heart J. *95:*563, 1978.
136. Marcus, F. L., Fontaine, G. H., Guiraudon, G., et al.: Right ventricular dysplasia: A report of 24 adult cases. Circulation *65:*384, 1982.

137. Ibsen, H. H. W., Baandrup, U., and Simonsen, E. E.: Familial right ventricular dilated cardiomyopathy. Br. Heart J. *54:*156, 1985.
138. Thiene, G., Nava, A., Corrado, D., et al.: Right ventricular cardiomyopathy and sudden death in young people. N. Engl. J. Med. *318:*129, 1988.
139. Wright, J. R., and Calkins, E.: Clinical-pathologic differentiation of common amyloid syndromes. Medicine *60:*429, 1981.
140. Ridolfi, R. L., Bulkley, B. H., and Hutchins, G. M.: The conduction system in cardiac amyloidosis: Clinical and pathologic features of 23 patients. Am. J. Med. *62:*677, 1977.
141. Campbell, M.: Calcific aortic stenosis and congenital bicuspid aortic valves. Br. Heart J. *30:*606, 1968.
142. Smith, N., McAnulty, J. G., and Rahimtoola, S. H.: Severe aortic stenosis with impaired left ventricular function and clinical heart failure: Results of valve replacement. Circulation *58:*255, 1978.
143. Rahimtoola, S. H.: Valvular heart disease: A perspective. J. Am. Coll. Cardiol. *1:*199, 1983.
144. Blackstone, E. H., and Kirklin, J. W.: Death and other time-related events after valve replacement. Circulation *72:*753, 1985.
145. Gohlke-Barwolf, C., Peters, K., Petersen, J., et al.: Influence of aortic valve replacement on sudden death in patients with pure aortic stenosis. Eur. Heart J. *9*(Suppl. E):139, 1988.
146. Konishi, Y., Matsuda, K., Nishiwaki, N., et al.: Ventricular arrhythmias late after aortic and/or mitral valve replacement. Jpn. Cir. J. *49:*576, 1985.
147. Chesler, E., King, R. A., and Edwards, J. E.: The myxomatous mitral valve and sudden death. Circulation *67:*632, 1983.
148. Campbell, R. W. F., Godman, M. G., Fiddler, G. I., et al.: Ventricular arrhythmias in the syndrome of balloon deformity of mitral valve: Definition of possible high-risk group. Br. Heart J. *38:*1053, 1976.
149. Pocock, W. A., Bosman, C. K., Chesler, E., et al.: Sudden death in primary mitral valve prolapse. Am. Heart J. *107:*378, 1984.
150. Nishimura, R. A., McGoon, M. D., Shub, C., et al.: Echocardiographically documented mitral valve prolapse: Long-term follow-up of 237 patients. N. Engl. J. Med. *313:*1305, 1985.
151. Glew, R. H., Varghese, P. J., Krovetz, L. J., et al.: Sudden death in congenital aortic stenosis: A review of 8 cases with an evaluation of premonitory clinical features. Am. Heart J. *78:*615, 1969.
152. Hoffman, J. I. E.: The natural history of congential isolated pulmonic and aortic stenosis. Annu. Rev. Med. *20:*15, 1969.
153. Young, D., and Marks, H.: Fate of the patient with the Eisenmenger syndrome. Am. J. Cardiol. *28:*658, 1971.
154. Jones, A. M., and Howitt, G.: Eisenmenger syndrome in pregnancy. Br. Med. J. *1:*1627, 1965.
155. Garson, A., Nihill, M. R., McNamara, D. G., and Cooley, D. A.: Status of the adult and adolescent after repair of tetralogy of Fallot. Circulation *59:*1232, 1979.
156. Gillette, P. C., Kugler, J. D., Garson, A., et al.: The mechanism of cardiac dysrhythmia after Mustard operation for transposition of the great arteries. Am. J. Cardiol. *45:*1225, 1980.
157. Murphy, J. G., Gersh, B. J., Mair, D. D., et al.: Long-term outcome in patients undergoing surgical repair of tetralogy of Fallot. N. Engl. J. Med. *329:*593, 1993.
158. Lie, K. I., Leim, K. L., Schuilenberg, R. M., et al.: Early identification of patients developing late in-hospital ventricular fibrillation after discharge from the coronary care unit. Am. J. Cardiol. *41:*674, 1978.
159. Hauer, R. N. W., Lie, K. I., Liem, K. L., and Durrer, D.: Long-term prognosis in patients with bundle branch block complicating acute anteroseptal infarction. Am. J. Cardiol. *49:*1581, 1982.
160. Lenegre, J.: The pathology of complete atrioventricular block. Prog. Cardiovasc. Dis. *6:*317, 1964.
161. Lev, M.: Anatomic basis for atrioventricular block. Am. J. Med. *37:*742, 1964.
162. Denes, P., Dhingra, R. C., Wu, D., et al.: Sudden death in patients with chronic bifascicular block. Arch. Intern. Med. *137:*1005, 1977.
163. McAnulty, J. H., Rahimtoola, S. H., Murphy, E. S., et al.: A prospective study of sudden death in "high risk" bundle branch block. N. Engl. J. Med. *299:*209, 1978.
164. McAnulty, J. H., Rahimtoola, S. H., Murphy, E., et al.: Natural history of "high-risk" bundle-branch block: Final report of a prospective study. N. Engl. J. Med. *307:*137, 1982.
165. Stephan, E.: Hereditary bundle branch system defect. Survey of a family with four affected generations. Am. Heart J. *95:*89, 1978.
166. Kline, G. J., Bashore, T. M., Sellers, T. D., et al.: Ventricular fibrillation in the Wolff-Parkinson-White syndrome. N. Engl. J. Med. *301:*1080, 1979.
167. Vidaillet, H. J., Pressley, J. C., Henke, E., et al.: Familial occurrence of accessory atrioventricular pathways (preexicitation syndrome). N. Engl. J. Med. *317:*65, 1987.
168. Schwartz, P. J., Periti, M., and Malliani, A.: The long Q-T syndrome. Am. Heart J. *89:*378, 1975.
169. Fraser, G. R., Froggatt, P., and James, T. N.: Congenital deafness associated with electrocardiographic abnormalities, fainting attacks and sudden death. Q. J. Med. *33:*362, 1964.
170. Smith, W. M., and Gallagher, J. J.: Les torsades de pointes. Ann. Intern. Med. *93:*578, 1980.
171. Moss, A. J., Schwartz, P. J., Crampton, R. S., et al.: The long-QT syndrome: A prospective international study. Circulation *71:*17, 1985.
172. Bhandari, A. K., and Scheinman, M.: The long QT syndrome. Mod. Concepts Cardiovasc. Dis. *54:*45, 1985.
173. Isner, J. M., Sours, H. E., Paris, A. L., et al.: Sudden, unexpected death in avid dieters using the liquid-protein-modified-fast diet: Observations in 17 patients and the role of the prolonged QT interval. Circulation *60:*1401, 1979.
174. Isner, J. M., Roberts, W. C., Heymsfield, S. B., and Yager, J.: Anorexia nervosa and sudden death. Ann. Intern. Med. *102:*49, 1985.
175. Lyman, G. H., Williams, C. C., Dinwoodie, W. R., and Schocken, D. D.: Sudden death in cancer patients receiving lithium. J. Clin. Oncol. *2:*1270, 1984.
176. Woosley, R. L., Chen, Y., Freiman, J. P., and Gillis, R. A.: Mechanism of cardiotoxic actions of terfenadine. JAMA *269:*1532, 1993.
177. Coumel, P., Rosengarten, M. D., Leclercq, J. F., and Attuel, P.: Role of sympathetic nervous system in nonischemic ventricular arrhythmias. Br. Heart J. *47:*137, 1982.
178. Schwartz, P. J.: The idiopathic long Q-T syndrome. Ann. Intern. Med. *99:*561, 1982.
179. Lown, B., DeSilva, R. A., and Lenson, R.: Role of psychologic stress and autonomic nervous system changes in provocation of ventricular premature complexes. Am. J. Cardiol. *41:*979, 1977.
180. Engel, G. L.: Psychologic stress, vasodepressor vasovagal syncope, and sudden death. Ann. Intern. Med. *89:*403, 1978.
181. Sheps, D. S., Conde, C. A., Mayorga-Cortes, A., et al.: Primary ventricular fibrillation: Some unusual features. Chest *72:*235, 1977.
182. Leenhardt, A., Glaser, E., Burguera, M., et al.: Short-coupled variant of *torsade de pointes:* A new electrocardiographic entity in the spectrum of idiopathic ventricular tachyarrhythmias. Circulation *89:*206, 1994.
183. Burrell, R. J. W.: The possible bearing of curse death and other factors in Bantu culture in the etiology of myocardial infarction. *In* James, T. N., and Keyes, J. W. (eds.): The Etiology of Myocardial Infarction. Boston, Little, Brown, 1963.
184. Cannon, W. B.: "Voodoo" death. Psychosom. Med., *19:*182, 1957.
185. Baba, N., Quattrochi, J. J., Reiner, C. B., et al.: Possible role of the brain stem in sudden infant death syndrome. JAMA *249:*2789, 1983.
186. Valdes-Dapena, M. A.: Sudden infant death syndrome: A review of the medical literature. Pediatrics *66:*597, 1980.
187. Valdes-Dapena, M. A.: Are some sudden crib deaths sudden cardiac deaths? J. Am. Coll. Cardiol. *5*(Suppl. B):113B, 1985.
188. Brooks, J. G.: Apnea of infancy and sudden infant death syndrome. Am. J. Dis. Child. *136:*1012, 1982.
189. Hodgman, J. E., Hoppenbrouwers, T., Geidel, S., et al.: Respiratory behavior in near-miss sudden infant death syndrome. Pediatrics *69:*785, 1982.
190. Southall, D. P., Richard, J. M., de Swiet, M., et al.: Identification of infants destined to die unexpectedly during infancy: Evaluation of predictive importance of prolonged apnea and disorders of cardiac rhythm or conduction. Br. Med. J. *286:*1092, 1983.
191. Marino, T. A., and Kane, B. M.: Cardiac atrioventricular junctional tissues in hearts from infants who died suddenly. J. Am. Coll. Cardiol. *5:*1178, 1985.
192. Lambert, E. C., Menon, V. A., Wagner, H. R., and Viad, P.: Sudden unexpected death from cardiovascular disease in children. Am. J. Cardiol. *34:*89, 1974.
193. Maron, B. J.: Sudden death in young athletes—lessions from the Hank Gathers affair. N. Engl. J. Med. *329:*55, 1993.
194. Roberts, W. C., and Maron, B. J.: Sudden death while playing professional football. Am. Heart J. *102:*1061, 1981.
195. Waller, B. F., Csere, R. S., Baker, W. P., and Roberts, W. C.: Running to death. Chest *79:*346, 1981.
196. Reichenbach, D. D., Moss, N. S., and Meyer, E.: Pathology of the heart in sudden cardiac death. Am. J. Cardiol. *39:*865, 1977.
197. Meissner, M. D., Lehmann, M. H., and Steinman, R. T.: Ventricular fibrillation in patients without significant structural heart disease: A multicenter experience with implantable cardioverter-defibrillator therapy. J. Am. Coll. Cardiol. *21:*1406, 1993.
198. Deal, B. J., Miller, S. W., Scagliotti, D., et al.: Ventricular tachycardia in a young population without overt heart disease. Circulation *73:*1111, 1986.
199. Aponte, C.: The enigma of "bangungut." Ann. Intern. Med. *52:*1259, 1960.
200. Sugai, M.: A pathologic study on sudden and unexpected death, especially on the cardiac death autopsied by medical examiners in Tokyo, Acute Pathol. Jpn. *9:*723, 1959.
201. Baron, R. C., Thacker, S. B., Gorelkin, L., et al.: Sudden death among Southeast Asian refugees: An unexplained nocturnal phenomenon. JAMA *250:*2947, 1983.
202. Otto, C. M., Tauxe, R. V., Cobb, L. A., et al.: Ventricular fibrillation causes sudden death in Southeast Asian immigrants. Ann. Intern. Med. *101:*45, 1984.
203. Kirschner, R. H., Eckner, F. A. A., and Baron, R. C.: The cardiac pathology of sudden, unexplained nocturnal death in Southeast Asian refugees. JAMA *256:*2700, 1986.
204. Haugen, R. K.: The cafe coronary: Sudden deaths in restaurants. JAMA *186:*142, 1963.
205. Eller, W. C., and Haugen, R. K.: Food asphyxiation—restaurant rescue. N. Engl. J. Med. *289:*81, 1973.
206. Ettinger, P. O., Wu, C. F., De La Cruz, C., et al.: Arrhythmias and the "holiday heart": Alcohol-associated cardiac rhythm disorders. Am. Heart J. *95:*555, 1978.
207. Benatar, S. R.: Fatal asthma. N. Engl. J. Med. *314:*243, 1986.
208. Morgan, M.: Amniotic fluid embolism. Anaesthesia *34:*20, 1979.
209. Aronson, M. E., and Nelson, P. K.: Fatal air embolism in pregnancy resulting from an unusual sexual act. Obstet. Gynecol. *30:*127, 1967.

210. Ruskin, J. N., McGovern, B., Garan, H., et al.: Antiarrhythmic drugs: A possible cause of out-of-hospital cardiac arrest. N. Engl. J. Med. *309*:1302, 1983.
211. Minardo, J. D., Heger, J. J., Miles, W. M., et al.: Clinical characteristics of patients with ventricular fibrillation during antiarrhythmia drug therapy. N. Engl. M. Med. *319*:257, 1988.

PATHOLOGY AND PATHOPHYSIOLOGY OF SUDDEN DEATH

212. Baroldi, G., Falzi, G., and Mariani, F.: Sudden coronary death: A postmortem study in 208 selected cases compared to 97 "control" subjects. Am. Heart J. *98*:20, 1979.
213. Liberthson, R. R., Nagel, E. L., Hirschman, J. C., et al.: Pathophysiologic observations in prehospital ventricular fibrillation and sudden cardiac death. Circulation *49*:790, 1974.
214. Perper, J. A., Kuller, L. H., Cooper, M.: Arteriosclerosis of coronary arteries in sudden, unexpected deaths. Circulation *52*(Suppl. 3):27, 1975.
215. Warnes, C. A., and Roberts, W. C.: Sudden coronary death: Relation of amount and distribution of coronary narrowing at necropsy to previous symptoms of myocardial ischemia, left ventricular scarring, and heart weight. Am. J. Cardiol. *54*:65, 1984.
216. Davies, M. J., and Thomas, A.: Thrombosis and acute coronary artery lesions in sudden cardiac ischemic death. N. Engl. J. Med. *310*:1137, 1984.
217. Davies, M. J., Bland, J. M., Hangartner, J. R. W., et al.: Factors influencing the presence or absence of acute coronary artery thrombi in sudden ischaemic death. Eur. Heart J. *10*:203, 1989.
218. Baroldi, G., Falzi, A., Mariani, F., and Baroldi, L. A.: Morphology, frequency, and significance of intramural arterial lesions in sudden coronary death. G. Ital. Cardiol. *10*:644, 1980.
219. Baba, N., Bashe, W. J., Jr., Keller, M. D., et al.: Pathology of atherosclerotic heart disease in sudden death. I. Organizing thrombus and acute coronary vessel lesions. Circulation *52*(Suppl. 3):53, 1975.
220. Roberts, W. C., Currey, R. C., Isner, J. M., et al.: Sudden death in Prinzmetal's angina with coronary spasm documented by angiography. Analysis of three necropsy patients. Am. J. Cardiol. *50*:203, 1982.
221. Newman, W. P., Strong, J. P., Johnson, W. D., et al.: Community pathology of atherosclerosis and coronary heart disease in New Orleans: Morphologic findings in young black and white men. Lab. Invest. *44*:496, 1981.
222. Newman, W. P., Tracy, R. E., Strong, J. P., et al.: Pathology of sudden cardiac death. Ann. N.Y. Acad. Sci. *382*:39, 1982.
223. Cooper, R. S., Simmons, B. E., Castaner, A., et al.: Left ventricular hypertrophy is associated with worse survival independent of ventricular function and number of coronary arteries severely narrowed. Am. J. Cardiol. *65*:441, 1990.
224. Furukawa, T., Bassett, A. L., Furukawa, N., et al.: The ionic mechanism of reperfusion-induced early afterdepolarizations in the feline left ventricular hypertrophy. J. Clin. Invest. *91*:1521, 1993.
225. Roberts, W. C., and Podolak, N. J.: The king of hearts: Analysis of 23 patients with hearts weighing 1,000 grams or more. Am. J. Cardiol. *55*:485, 1985.
226. Lie, J. T.: Histopathology of the conduction system in sudden death from coronary heart disease. Circulation *51*:446, 1975.
227. Lie, J. T., and Hunt, D.: The cardiac conduction system in acute myocardial infarction. Aust. N.Z. J. Med. *4*:331, 1974.
228. James, T. N.: Neural variations and pathologic changes in structure of the cardiac conduction system and their functional significance. J. Am. Coll. Cardiol. *5*(Suppl.):71B, 1985.
229. Rossi, L.: Pathologic changes in the cardiac conduction and nervous system in sudden coronary death. Ann. N.Y. Acad. Sci. *382*:50, 1982.
230. James, T. N.: Primary and secondary cardioneuropathies and their functional significance. J. Am. Coll. Cardiol. *2*:983, 1983.
231. Tuli, M., Minardo, J., Mock, B. H., et al.: SPECT with high purity I-123-MIBG after transmural myocardial infarction (TMI), demonstrating sympathetic denervation following reinnervation in a dog model. J. Nucl. Med. *28*:669, 1987.
232. Stanton, M. S., Tuli, M. M., Radtke, N. L., et al.: Regional sympathetic denervation after myocardial infarction in humans detected noninvasively using ^{123}I-metaiodobenzlguanidine (MIBG). J. Am. Coll. Cardiol. *14*:1519, 1989.
233. Barber, M. J., Mueller, T. M., Henry, D. P., et al.: Transmural myocardial infarction in the dog produces sympathectomy in non-infarcted myocardium. Circulation *67*:787, 1982.
234. Gaide, M. S., Myerburg, R. J., Kozlovskis, P. L., and Bassett, A. L.: Elevated sympathetic response of epicardium proximal to healed myocardial infarction. Am. J. Physiol. *14*:646, 1983.
235. Diederick, K., Djoniagic, H., Schreiner, W. B., and Bos, I.: Hereditares QT syndrom: ein weiterer Fall mit Grenzstrang Ganglionitis. Herz-Kreis *3*:149, 1982.
236. Rossi, L.: Cardioneuropathy and extracardiac neural disease. J. Am. Coll. Cardiol. *5*(Suppl.):66B, 1985.
237. Myerburg, R. J., Kessler, K. M., Bassett, A. L., and Castellanos, A.: A biological approach to sudden cardiac death: Structure, function, and cause. Am. J. Cardiol. *63*:1512, 1989.
238. Cobb, L. A., and Weaver, W. D.: Exercise: A risk for sudden death in patients with coronary heart disease. J. Am. Coll. Cardiol. *7*:215, 1986.
239. Schamroth, L.: Mechanism of lethal arrhythmias in sudden death. Possible role of vasospasm and release. Pract. Cardiol. *7*:105, 1981.
240. MacAlpin R. N.: Relation of coronary arterial spasm to sites of organic stenosis. Am. J. Cardiol. *46*:143, 1980.
241. Robertson, D., Robertson, R. M., Nies, A. S., et al.: Variant angina pectoris: Investigation of indexes of sympathetic nervous system function. Am. J. Cardiol. *43*:1080, 1979.
242. Endo, M., Hirosawa, K., Kaneko, N., et al.: Prinzmetal's variant angina. Coronary arteriogram and left ventriculogram during angina attack induced by methacholine, N. Engl. J. Med. *294*:252, 1976.
243. Buda, A. J., Fowles, R. E., Schroeder, J. S., et al.: Coronary artery spasm in the denervated transplanted human heart. A clue to underlying mechanisms. Am. J. Med. *70*:1144, 1981.
244. Hammon, J. W., and Oates, J. A.: Interaction of platelets with the vessel wall in the pathophysiology of sudden cardiac death. Circulation *73*:224, 1986.
245. Aspirin-Myocardial Infarction Study Research Group: A randomized controlled trial of aspirin in persons recovered from myocardial infarction. JAMA *243*:661, 1980.
246. Myerburg, R. J., Kessler, K. M., Zaman, L., et al.: Survivors of prehospital cardiac arrest. JAMA *247*:1485, 1982.
247. Cox, J. L., Daniel, T. M., and Boineau, J. P.: The electrophysiologic time-course of acute myocardial ischemia and the effects of early coronary artery reperfusion. Circulation *48*:971, 1973.
248. Cameron, J. S., Myerburg, R. J., Wong, S. S., et al.: Electrophysiologic consequences of chronic experimentally induced left ventricular pressure overload. J. Am. Coll. Cardiol. *2*:481, 1983.
249. Myerburg, R. J., Bassett, A. L., Epstein, K., et al.: Electrophysiologic effects of procainamide in acute and healed experimental ischemic injury of cat myocardium. Circ. Res. *50*:386, 1982.
250. Myerburg, R. J., Epstein, K., Gaide, M. S., et al.: Electrophysiologic consequences of experimental acute ischemia superimposed upon healed myocardial infarction in cats. Am. J. Cardiol. *49*:323, 1982.
251. Furukawa, T., Moroe, K., Mayrovitz, H. N., et al.: Arrhythmogenic effects of graded coronary blood flow reductions superimposed on prior myocardial infarction in dogs. Circulation *84*:368, 1991.
252. Kaplinsky, E., Ogawa, S., Michelson, E. L., and Dreifus, L. S.: Instantaneous and delayed arrhythmias after reperfusion of acutely ischemic myocardium: Evidence for multiple mechanisms. Circulation *63*:333, 1981.
253. Kimura, S., Bassett, A. L., Saoudi, N. C., et al.: Cellular electrophysiological changes and "arrhythmias" during experimental ischemia and reperfusion in isolated cat ventricular myocardium. J. Am. Coll. Cardiol. *7*:833, 1986.
254. Manning, A. S., and Hearse, D. J.: Reperfusion-induced arrhythmias: Mechanisms and prevention. J. Mol. Cell Cardiol. *16*:497, 1984.
255. Harris, A. S.: Delayed development of ventricular ectopic rhythms following experimental coronary occlusion. Circulation *1*:1318, 1950.
256. Kimura, S., Bassett, A. L., Kohya, T., et al.: Simultaneous recording of action potentials from endocardium and epicardium during ischemia in the isolated cat ventricle: Relation of temporal electrophysiological heterogeneities to arrhythmias. Circulation *74*:401, 1986.
257. Coronel, R., Wilms-Schopman, F. J. G., Opthof, T., et al.: Reperfusion arrhythmias in isolated perfused pig hearts: Inhomogeneities in extracellular potassium, ST and QT potentials, and transmembrane action potentials. Circ. Res. *71*:1131, 1992.
258. Sharma, A. D., Saffitz, J. E., Lee, B. L., et al.: Alpha adrenergic-mediated accumulation of calcium in reperfused myocardium. J. Clin. Invest. *72*:802, 1982.
259. Corr, P. B., Shayman, J. A., Kramer, J. B., and Kipnis, R. J.: Increased alpha-adrenergic receptors in ischemic cat myocardium. J. Clin. Invest. *67*:1232, 1981.
260. Sheridan, D. J., Penkoske, P. A., Sobel, B. E., and Corr, P. B.: Alpha-adrenergic contributions to dysrhythmia during myocardial ischemia and reperfusion in cats. J. Clin. Invest. *65*:161, 1980.
261. Schwartz, P. J., and Stone, H. L.: Left stellectomy in the prevention of ventricular fibrillation caused by acute myocardial ischemia in conscious dogs with anterior myocardial infarction. Circulation *62*:1256, 1980.
262. Gaudel, Y., and Duvelleroy, M.: Role of oxygen radicals in cardiac injury due to reoxygenation. J. Mol. Cell Cardiol. *16*:459, 1984.
263. Manning, A. S., Coltart, D. J., and Hearse, D. J.: Ischemia and reperfusion-induced arrhythmias in the rat: Effects of xanthine oxidase inhibition with allopurinol. Circ. Res. *55*:545, 1984.
264. Chilson, D. A., Peigh, P., Mahomed, Y., and Zipes, D. P.: Encircling endocardial ventriculotomy interrupts vagal-induced prolongation of endocardial and epicardial refractoriness in the dog. J. Am. Coll. Cardiol. *5*:290, 1985.
265. Janse, M. J., and Downer, E.: The effect of acute ischaemia on transmembrane potentials in the intact heart. Relation to re-entry mechanisms. *In* Kulbertus, H. E. (ed.): Re-entrant Arrhythmias. Lancaster, PA, MTP Press, 1977, pp. 195–209.
266. Kuller, L. H., Hulley, S. B., Cohen, J. D., and Neaton, J.: Unexpected effects of treating hypertension in men with electrocardiographic abnormalities: A critical analysis. Circulation *73*:114, 1986.
267. Struthers, A. D., Whitesmith, R., and Reid, J. L.: Prior thiazide diuretic treatment increases adrenaline-induced hypokalaemia. Lancet *1*:1358, 1983.
268. Skinner, J. E.: Regulation of cardiac vulnerability by the cerebral defense system. J. Am. Coll. Cardiol. *5*(Suppl. B):88, 1985.
269. Schwartz, P. J., Billman, G. E., and Stone, H. L.: Autonomic mechanisms in ventricular fibrillation induced by myocardial ischemia dur-

ing exercise in dogs with healed myocardial infarction. Circulation *69:*790, 1984.

270. Verrier, R. L., and Hagestad, E. L.: Role of the autonomic neuron system in sudden death. *In* Josephson, M. E. (ed.): Sudden Cardiac Death. Philadelphia, F. A. Davis Co., 1985, pp. 41–63.
271. Schwartz, P. J., and Stone, H. L.: The role of autonomic nervous system in sudden coronary death. Ann. N.Y. Acad. Sci. *382:*162, 1982.
272. Opie, L. H.: Products of myocardial ischemia and electrical instability of the heart. J. Am. Coll. Cardiol. *5*(Suppl. B):162, 1985.
273. Huikuri, H. V., Linnaluoto, M. K., Seppanen, T., et al.: Circadian rhythm of heart rate variability in survivors of cardiac arrest. Am. J. Cardiol. *70:*610, 1992.
274. Huikuri, H. V., Valkama, J. O., Airakainen, K. E., et al.: Frequency domain measures of heart rate variability before the onset of nonsustained and sustained ventricular tachycardia in patients with coronary artery disease. Circulation *87:*1220, 1993.
275. Myerburg, R. J., Kessler, K. M., Kiem, I., et al.: The relationship between plasma levels of procainamide, suppression of premature ventricular contractions, and prevention of recurrent ventricular tachycardia. Circulation *64:*280, 1981.
276. Task Force of the Working Group on Arrhythmias of the European Society of Cardiology: The Sicilian Gambit: A new approach to the classification of antiarrhythmic drugs based on their action on arrhythmogenic mechanisms. Circulation *84:*1831, 1991.
277. Vassalle, M.: On the mechanisms underlying cardiac standstill: Factors determining success or failure of escape pacemakers in the heart. J. Am. Coll. Cardiol. *5*(Suppl. B):35, 1985.
278. Fozzard, H. A.: Electromechanical dissociation and its possible role in sudden cardiac death. J. Am. Coll. Cardiol. *5*(Suppl. B):31, 1985.

CLINICAL CHARACTERISTICS OF THE PATIENT WITH CARDIAC ARREST

279. Pell, S., and D'Alonzo, C. A.: Immediate mortality and five-year survival of employed men with a first myocardial infarction. N. Engl. J. Med. *270:*915, 1964.
280. Kimball, J. J., and Killip, T.: Aggressive treatment of arrhythmias in acute myocardial infarction: Procedures and results. Prog. Cardiovasc. Dis. *10:*483, 1968.
281. Feinlieb, M., Simon, A. B., Gillum, J. R., and Margolis, J. R.: Prodromal symptoms and signs of sudden death. Circulation *52*(Suppl. 3):155, 1975.
282. Fulton, M., Lutz, W., Donald, K. W., et al.: Natural history of unstable angina. Lancet *1:*860, 1972.
283. Goldstein, S., Landis, J. R., Leighton, R., et al.: Characteristics of the resuscitated out-of-hospital cardiac arrest victim with coronary heart disease. Circulation *64:*977, 1981.
284. Nikolic, G., Bishop, R. L., and Singh, J. B.: Sudden death recorded during Holter monitoring. Circulation *66:*218, 1982.
285. Pratt, C. M., Francis, M. J., Luck, J. C., et al.: Analysis of ambulatory electrocardiograms in 15 patients during spontaneous ventricular fibrillation with special reference to preceding arrhythmic events. J. Am. Coll. Cardiol. *2:*789, 1983.
286. Bayes de Luna, A., Coumel, P., and Leclercq, J. F.: Ambulatory sudden death: Mechanisms of production of fatal arrhythmia on the basis of data from 157 cases. Am. Heart J. *117:*151, 1989.
287. Hinkle, L. E., and Thaler, H. T.: Clinical classification of cardiac deaths. Circulation *65:*457, 1982.
288. Bates, R. J., Beutler, S., Resnekov, L., and Anagnostopoulos, C. E.: Cardiac rupture: Challenge in diagnosis and management. Am. J. Cardiol. *40:*429, 1977.
289. Emergency Cardiac Care Committee and Subcommittees, American Heart Association: Guidelines for cardiopulmonary resuscitation and emergency cardiac care. JAMA *268:*2172, 1992.
290. Lo, B., and Steinbrook, R. L.: Deciding whether to resuscitate. Arch. Intern. Med. *143:*1561, 1983.
291. Bedell, S. E., Delbanco, T. L., Cook, E. F., and Epstein, F. H.: Survival after cardiopulmonary resuscitation in the hospital. N. Engl. J. Med. *309:*569, 1983.
292. Cobb, L. A., Weaver, W. D., and Fahrenbrush, C. E.: Community-based interventions for sudden cardiac death: Impact, limitations, and charges. Circulation *85*(Suppl. I):I-98, 1992.
293. Goldstein, S., Landis, J. R., Leighton, R., et al.: Predictive survival models for resuscitated victims of out-of-hospital cardiac arrest with coronary heart disease. Circulation *71:*873, 1985.
294. Cummins, R. O., Ornato, J. P., Thies, W. H., and Pepe, P. E.: Improving survival from sudden cardiac arrest: The "chain of survival" concept: A statement for heart professionals from the Advanced Cardiac Life Support Subcommittee and the Emergency Cardiac Care Committee, American Heart Association. Circulation *83:*1832, 1991.
295. Gulati, R. S., Bhan, G. L., and Horan, M. A.: Cardiopulmonary resuscitation of old people. Lancet *2:*267, 1983.
296. Taffet, G. E., Teasdale, T. A., and Luchi, R. J.: In-hospital cardiopulmonary resuscitation. JAMA *260:*2069, 1988.
297. Tresch, D. D., Thakur, R. K., Hoffmann, R. G., et al.: Should the elderly be resuscitated following out-of-hospital cardiac arrest? Am. J. Med. *86:*145, 1989.
298. Eisenberg, M. S., Bergner, L., and Hallstrom, A. P.: Cardiac resuscitation in the community: Importance of rapid provision and implications of program planning. JAMA *241:*1905, 1979.
299. Myerburg, R. J., Estes, D., Zaman, L., et al.: Outcome of resuscitation from bradyarrhythmic or asystolic prehospital cardiac arrest. J. Am. Coll. Cardiol. *4:*1118, 1984.
300. Jaggarao, N. S. V., Heber, M., Grainger, R., et al.: Use of an automated external defibrillator-pacemaker by ambulance staff. Lancet *2:*73, 1982.
301. Longstreth, W. T., Inui, T. S., Cobb, L. A., and Copass, M. K.: Neurologic recovery after out-of-hospital cardiac arrest. Ann. Intern. Med. *98:*588, 1983.
302. Longstreth, W. T., Diehr, P., and Inui, T. S.: Prediction of awakening after out-of-hospital cardiac arrest. N. Engl. J. Med. *308:*1378, 1983.
303. Myerburg, R. J., Conde, C. A., Sheps, D. S., et al.: Antiarrhythmic drug therapy in survivors of prehospital cardiac arrest: Comparison of effects on chronic ventricular arrhythmias and on recurrent cardiac arrest. Circulation *59:*855, 1979.
304. Weaver, W. D., Cobb, L. A., and Hallstrom, A. P.: Ambulatory arrhythmia in resuscitated victims of cardiac arrest. Circulation *66:*212, 1982.
305. Ritchie, J. L., Hallstrom, A. P., Troubaugh, G. B., et al.: Out-of-hospital sudden coronary death: Rest and exercise radionuclide left ventricular function in survivors. Am. J. Cardiol. *55:*645, 1985.
306. Weaver, W. D., Lorch, G. S., Alvarez, H. A., and Cobb, L. A.: Angiographic findings and prognostic indicators in patients resuscitated from sudden cardiac death. Circulation *54:*895, 1976.
307. Weaver, W. D., Cobb, L. A., and Hallstrom, A. P.: Characteristics of survivors of exertion- and nonexertion-related cardiac arrest: Value of subsequent exercise testing. Am. J. Cardiol. *50:*671, 1982.
308. Cobb, L. A., Werner, J. A., and Troubaugh, G. B.: Sudden cardiac death: I. A decade's experience with out-of-hospital resuscitation; and II. Outcome of resuscitation, management, and future directions. Mod. Concepts Cardiovasc. Dis. *49:*31, 1980.
309. Haynes, R. E., Hallstrom, A. P., and Cobb, L. A.: Repolarization abnormalities in survivors of out-of-hospital ventricular fibrillation. Circulation *57:*654, 1978.
310. Thompson, R. G., and Cobb, L. A.: Hypokalemia after resuscitation from out-of-hospital cardiac arrest. JAMA *248:*2860, 1982.
311. Urban, P., Scheidegger, D., Buchmann, B., and Barth, D.: Cardiac arrest and blood ionized calcium levels. Ann. Intern. Med. *109:*110, 1988.
312. Sheps, D. S., Conde, C., Cameron, B., et al.: Resting peripheral blood lactate elevation in survivors of prehospital cardiac arrest: Correlation with hemodynamic, electrophysiologic, and oxyhemoglobin dissociation indexes. Am. J. Cardiol. *44:*1276, 1979.
313. Myerburg, R. J., Kessler, K. M., Zaman, L., et al.: Factors leading to decreasing mortality among patients resuscitated from out-of-hospital cardiac arrest. *In* Brugada, P., and Wellens, H. J. J. (eds.): Cardiac Arrhythmias: Where to Go from Here? Mt. Kisko, N.Y., Futura, 1987, pp. 505–525.

MANAGEMENT OF CARDIAC ARREST

314. Furukawa, T., Rozanski, J. J., Nogami, J., et al.: Time-dependent risk of and predictors for cardiac arrest recurrence in survivors of out-of-hospital cardiac arrest with chronic coronary artery disease. Circulation *80:*599, 1989.
315. Goldman, L.: Coronary care units: A perspective on their epidemiologic impact. Int. J. Cardiol. *2:*284, 1982.
316. Killip, T., and Kimball, J. T.: Treatment of myocardial infarction in a coronary care unit: A two-year experience with 250 patients. Am. J. Cardiol. *20:*457, 1967.
317. Pantridge, J. F., and Adgey, A. A. J.: Pre-hospital coronary care. The mobile coronary care unit. Am. J. Cardiol. *24:*666, 1969.
318. Stults, K. R., Brown, D. D., Schug, V. L., and Bean, J. A.: Prehospital defibrillation performed by emergency medical technicians in rural communities. N. Engl. J. Med. *310:*219, 1984.
319. Lombardi, G., Gallagher, J., and Gennis, P.: Outcome of out-of-hospital cardiac arrest in New York City: The Pre-Hospital Arrest Survival Evaluation (PHASE) Study. JAMA *271:*678, 1994.
320. Eisenberg, M. S., Copass, M. K., Hallstrom, A. P., et al.: Treatment of out-of-hospital cardiac arrests with rapid defibrillation by emergency medical technicians. N. Engl. J. Med. *302:*1379, 1980.
321. Mayer, J. D.: Paramedic response time and survival from cardiac arrest. Soc. Sci. Med. *13D:*267, 1979.
322. Weaver, W. D., Copass, M. K., Bufi, D., et al.: Improved neurologic recovery and survival after early defibrillation. Circulation *69:*943, 1984.
323. Weaver, W. D., Hill, D., Fahrenbruch, C. E., et al.: Use of the automatic external defibrillator in the management of out-of-hospital cardiac arrest. N. Engl. J. Med. *318:*661, 1988.
324. Stults, K. R.: Phone first. J. Emerg. Med. Serv. *12:*28, 1987.
325. Caldwell, G., Miller, G., Quinn, E., et al.: Simple mechanical methods for cardioversion: Defense of the precordial thump and cough version. Br. Med. J. *291:*627, 1985.
326. Lown, B., and Taylor, J.: "Thumpversion" (editorial). N. Engl. J. Med. *283:*1223, 1970.
327. Criley, J. M., Blaufuss, A. N., and Kissel, J. L.: Cough-induced cardiac compression: Self-administered form of cardiopulmonary resuscitation. JAMA *263:*1246, 1976.
328. Wei, J. Y., Greene, H. L., and Weisfeldt, M. L.: Cough-facilitated conversion of ventricular tachycardia. Am. J. Cardiol. *45:*174, 1980.
329. Heimlich, H. J.: A life-saving maneuver to prevent food-choking. JAMA *234:*398, 1975.

330. Visintine, R. E., and Baick, C. H.: Ruptured stomach after Heimlich maneuver. JAMA *234:*415, 1975.
331. Feldman, T., Mallon, S. M., Bolooki, H., et al.: Fatal acute aortic regurgitation in a person performing the Heimlich maneuver (letter). N. Engl. J. Med. *315:*1613, 1986.
332. Centers for Disease Control: Guidelines for prevention and transmission of human immunodeficiency virus and hepatitis B virus to health-care and public-safety workers. M.M.W.R. *38*(Suppl. 6):1, 1989.
333. Sande, M. A.: Transmission of AIDS: The case against casual contagion. N. Engl. J. Med. *314:*380, 1986.
334. Weisfeldt, M. L., and Chandra, N.: Physiology of cardiopulmonary resuscitation. Annu. Rev. Med. *32:*435, 1981.
335. Ewy, G. A.: Current status of cardiopulmonary resuscitation. Mod. Concepts Cardiac Dis. *53:*43, 1984.
336. Weisfeldt, M. L., Chandra, N., and Tsitlik, J. E.: Increased intrathoracic pressure—not direct heart compression—causes the rise in intrathoracic vascular pressures during CPR in dogs and pigs. Crit. Care Med. *9:*377, 1981.
337. Rudikoff, M. T., Maughan, W. L., Effrom, M., et al.: Mechanisms of blood flow during cardiopulmonary resuscitation. Circulation *61:*345, 1980.
338. Chandra, N., Rudikoff, M., and Weisfeldt, M. L.: Simultaneous chest compression and ventilation at high airway pressure during cardiopulmonary resuscitation. Lancet *1:*175, 1980.
339. Ditchey, R. V., and Lindenfeld, J.: Potential adverse effects of volume loading on perfusion of vital organs during closed-chest resuscitation. Circulation *69:*181, 1984.
340. Michael, J. R., Guerci, D., Koehler, R. C., et al.: Mechanisms by which epinephrine augments cerebral and myocardial perfusion during cardiopulmonary resuscitation in dogs. Circulation *69:*822, 1984.
341. Sanders, A. B., Ewy, G. A., Alferness, A., et al.: Failure of one method of simultaneous chest compression, ventilation, and abdominal binding during CPR. Crit. Care Med. *120:*509, 1982.
342. Ducas, J., Roussos, C. H., Karsaidis, C., and Magder, S.: Thoraco-abdominal mechanisms during resuscitation maneuvers. Chest *84:*446, 1983.
343. Guerci, A. D., Halperin, H. R., Beyar, R., et al.: Aortic diameter and pressure-flow sequence identify mechanism of blood flow during external chest compression in dogs. J. Am. Coll. Cardiol. *14:*790, 1989.
344. Paradis, N. A., Martin, G. B., Goetting, M. B., et al.: Simultaneous aortic, jugular, and right atrial pressures during cardiopulmonary resuscitation in humans: Insights into mechanisms. Circulation *80:*361, 1989.
345. Sack, J. B., Kesselbrenner, M. B., and Bregman, D.: Survival from in-hospital cardiac arrest with interposed abdominal counterpulsation during cardiopulmonary resuscitation. JAMA *267:*379, 1992.
346. Cohen, T. J., Turaker, K. G., Lurie, K. G., et al.: Active compression-decompression: A new method of cardiopulmonary resuscitation. JAMA *267:*2916, 1992.
347. Cummins, R. O., Eisenberg, M., Bergner, L., and Murray, J. A.: Sensitivity, accuracy, and safety of an automatic external defibrillator. Lancet *2:*318, 1984.
348. Gascho, J. A., Crampton, R. S., Cherwek, M. L., et al.: Determinants of ventricular defibrillation in adults. Circulation *60:*231, 1979.
349. Federiuk, C. S., Sanders, A. B., Kern, K. B., et al.: The effect of bicarbonate on resuscitation from cardiac arrest. Ann. Emerg. Med. *20:*1173, 1991.
350. Aufderheide, T. P., Martin, D. R., Olson, D. W., et al.: Prehospital bicarbonate use in cardiac arrest: A 3-year experience. Am. J. Emerg. Med. *10:*4, 1992.
351. Kette, F., Weil, M. H., and Gazmuri, R. J.: Buffer solutions may compromise cardiac resuscitation by reducing coronary perfusion pressure. JAMA *266:*2121, 1991.
352. Sodium bicarbonate in cardiac arrest (editorial). Lancet *1:*946, 1976.
353. Weil, M. H., Trevino, R. P., and Rackow, E. C.: Sodium bicarbonate during CPR: Does it help or hinder? Chest *88:*487, 1985.
354. White, R. D.: Cardiovascular pharmacology: Part I. *In* McIntyre, K. M., and Lewis, A. J. (eds.): Textbook of Advanced Life Support. Dallas, American Heart Association, Inc., 1983, pp. 99–114.
355. Haynes, R. E., Chinn, T. L., Copass, M. K., and Cobb, L. A.: Comparison of bretylium tosylate and lidocaine in the resuscitation of patients from out-of-hospital ventricular fibrillation: A randomized clinical trial. Am. J. Cardiol. *487:*353, 1981.
356. Giardina, E. G., Heissenbuttel, R. H., and Bigger, J. T.: Intermittent intravenous procainamide to treat ventricular arrhythmias. Correlation of plasma concentration with effect on arrhythmia, electrocardiogram, and blood pressure. Ann. Intern. Med. *78:*183, 1973.
357. Williams, M. L., Woelfel, A., Cascio, W. E., et al.: Intravenous amiodarone during prolonged resuscitation from cardiac arrest. Ann. Intern. Med. *110:*839, 1989.
358. Hughes, W. G., and Ruedy, J. R.: Should calcium be used in cardiac arrest? Am. J. Med. *81:*285, 1986.
359. Zoll, P. M., Zoll, R. H., Clinton, J. E., et al.: External non-invasive temporary cardiac pacing: Clinical trials. Circulation *71:*937, 1985.
360. Knowlton, A. A., and Falk, R. H.: External cardiac pacing during in hospital cardiac arrest. Am. J. Cardiol. *51:*1295, 1986.
361. Lee, R. V., Rogers, B. D., White, L. M., and Harvey, R. C.: Cardiopulmonary resuscitation of pregnant women. Am. J. Med. *81:*311, 1986.
362. Holmes, H. R., Babbs, C. F., Voorhees, W. D., et al.: Influence of adrenergic drugs upon vital organ perfusion during CPR. Crit. Care Med. *8:*137, 1980.
363. Yakaitis, R. W., Otto, C. W., and Blitt, C. D.: Relative importance of alpha and beta-adrenergic receptors during resuscitation. Crit. Care Med. *7:*293, 1979.
364. Wyman, M. G., and Hammersmith, L.: Comprehensive treatment plan for the prevention of primary ventricular fibrillation in acute myocardial infarction. Am. J. Cardiol. *33:*661, 1974.
365. Conley, M. J., McNeer, J. F., Lee, K. L., et al.: Cardiac arrest complicating acute myocardial infarction: Predictability and prognosis. Am. J. Cardiol. *39:*7, 1977.
366. Vismara, L. A., Amsterdam, B. A., and Mason, D. T.: Relation of ventricular arrhythmias in the late-hospital phase of acute myocardial infarction to sudden death after hospital discharge. Am. J. Med. *59:*6, 1975.
367. Robinson, J. S., Sloman, G., Mathew, T. H., and Goble, A. J.: Survival after resuscitation from cardiac arrest in acute myocardial infarction. Am. Heart J. *69:*740, 1965.
368. Thompson, P. D., Melmon, K. L., Richardson, J. A., et al.: Lidocaine pharmocokinetics in advanced heart failure, liver disease, and renal failure in humans. Ann. Intern. Med. *78:*499, 1973.
369. Norris, R. M., and Mercer, C. J.: Significance of idioventricular rhythms in acute myocardial infarction. Prog. Cardiovasc. Dis. *16:*455, 1974.
370. Selzer, A., and Wray, H. W.: Quinidine syncope: Paroxysmal ventricular fibrillation occurring during treatment of chronic atrial arrhythmias. Circulation *30:*17, 1964.
371. The Cardiac Arrhythmia Pilot Study (CAPS) Investigators: Effects of encainide, flecainide, imipramine, and moricizine on ventricular arrhythmias during the year after myocardial infarction: The CAPS. Am. J. Cardiol. *61:*501, 1988.
372. Nattel, S., Pedersen, D. H., and Zipes, D. P.: Alterations in regional myocardial distribution and arrhythmogenic effects of aprindine produced by coronary artery occlusion in the dog. Cardiovasc. Res. *15:*80, 1981.
373. Starmer, C. F., Lastra, A. A., Nesterenko, V. V., and Grant, A. O.: Proarrhythmic response to sodium channel blockade: Theoretical model and numerical experiments. Circulation *84:*1364, 1991.
374. Myerburg, R. J., Kessler, K. M., Kimura, S., Castellanos, A.: Sudden cardiac death: Future approaches based on identification and control of transient risk factors. J. Cardiovasc. Electrophysiol. *3:*626, 1992.
375. Haverkamp, W., Shenasa, M., Borggrefe, M., and Breithardt, G.: Torsade de pointes. *In* Zipes, D. P., and Jalife, J. (ed.): Cardiac Electrophysiology: From Cell to Bedside. 2nd ed. Philadelphia, W.B. Saunders Company, 1995, p. 885.
376. Wharton, J. M., Demopulus, P. A., and Goldschlager, N.: Torsade de pointes during administration of pentamidine isethionate. Am. J. Med. *83:*571, 1987.
377. Kimura, S., Bassett, A. L., Xi, H., and Myerburg, R. J.: Early afterdepolarizations and triggered activity produced by cocaine: A possible mechanism of cocaine arrhythmogenesis. Circulation *85:*2227, 1992.
378. Myerburg, R. J., Kessler, K. M., Cox, M. M., et al.: Reversal of proarrhythmic effects of flecainide acetate and encainide hydrochloride by propranolol. Circulation *80:*1571, 1989.
379. Bass, E.: Cardiopulmonary arrest: Pathophysiology and neurologic complications. Ann. Intern. Med. *103:*920, 1985.
380. Breivik, H., Safar, P., Sands, P., et al.: Clinical feasibility trials of barbiturate therapy after cardiac arrest. Crit. Care Med. *6:*228, 1978.
381. Brain Resuscitation Clinical Trial I Study Group: Randomized clinical study of thiopental loading in comatose survivors of cardiac arrest. N. Engl. J. Med. *314:*397, 1986.
382. Cobb, L. A., Hallstrom, A. P., Zia, M., et al.: Influence of coronary revascularization on recurrent sudden cardiac death syndrome. J. Am. Coll. Cardiol. *1*(Abs.):688, 1983.
383. Kron, I. L., Lerman, B. B., Haines, D. E., et al.: Coronary bypass grafting in patients with ventricular fibrillation. Ann. Thorac. Surg. *48:*85, 1989.
384. O'Rourke, R. A.: Role of myocardial revascularization in sudden cardiac death. Circulation *85*(Suppl. I):I-112, 1992.
385. Harken, A. H., Wetstein, L., and Josephson, M. E.: Mechanisms and surgical management of ventricular tachyarrhythmias. *In* Josephson, M. E. (ed.): Sudden Cardiac Death. Philadelphia, F. A. Davis Co., 1985, pp. 287–300.
386. Hallstrom, A. P., Cobb, L. A., Yu, B. H., et al.: An antiarrhythmic drug experience in 941 patients resuscitated from an initial cardiac arrest between 1970 and 1985. Am. J. Cardiol. *68:*1025, 1991.
387. Holmes, D. R., Davis, K. B., Mock, B. B., et al.: The effect of medical and surgical treatment on subsequent sudden cardiac death in patients with coronary artery disease: A report from the Coronary Artery Surgery Study. Circulation *73:*1254, 1986.
388. Multiple Risk Factor Intervention Trial Research Group: Baseline rest electrocardiographic abnormalities, antihypertensive treatment, and mortality in the Multiple Risk Factor Intervention Trial. Am. J. Cardiol. *55:*1, 1985.
389. Bigger, J. T., Fleiss, J. L., Rolnitzky, L. M., et al.: Effect of digitalis treatment on survival after acute myocardial infarction. Am. J. Cardiol. *55:*623, 1985.
390. Ryan, T. J., Bailey, K. R., McCabe, C. H., et al.: The effects of digitalis on survival in high risk patients with coronary artery disease. The Coronary Artery Surgery Study (CASS). Circulation *67:*735, 1983.
391. Madsen, E. G., Gilpin, E., Henning, H., et al.: Prognostic importance of digitalis after acute myocardial infarction. J. Am. Coll. Cardiol. *3:*681, 1984.
392. Muller, J. E., Turi, Z. G., Stone, P. H., et al.: Digoxin therapy and mortality after myocardial infarction: Experience in the MILIS study. N. Engl. J. Med. *314:*265, 1986.

393. Ruskin, J. N., DiMarco, J. P., and Garan, H.: Out-of-hospital cardiac arrest: Electrophysiologic observations and selection of long-term antiarrhythmic therapy. N. Engl. J. Med. *303*:607, 1980.
394. Josephson, M. E., Horowitz, L. N., Spielman, S. C., and Greenspan, A. M.: Electrophysiologic and hemodynamic studies in patients resuscitated from cardiac arrest. Am. J. Cardiol. *46*:948, 1980.
395. Graboys, T. B., Lown, B., Podrid, P. J., and DeSilva, R.: Long-term survival of patients with malignant ventricular arrhythmias treated with antiarrhythmic drugs. Am. J. Cardiol. *50*:437, 1982.
396. Lampert, S., Lown, B., Graboys, T. B., et al.: Determinants of survival in patients with malignant ventricular arrhythmia associated with coronary artery disease. Am. J. Cardiol. *61*:791, 1988.
397. Herre, J., Sauve, M. J., Malone, P., et al.: Long-term results of amiodarone therapy in patients with recurrent sustained ventricular tachycardia or ventricular fibrillation. J. Am. Coll. Cardiol. *13*:442, 1989.
398. The CASCADE Investigators: Randomized antiarrhythmic drug therapy in survivors of cardiac arrest (The CASCADE Study). Am. J. Cardiol. *72*:280, 1993.
399. Steinbeck, G., Andresen, S., Bach, P., et al.: A comparison of electrophysiologically guided antiarrhythmic drug therapy with beta-blocker therapy in patients with symptomatic sustained ventricular tachyarrhythmias. N. Engl. J. Med. *327*:987, 1992.
400. Connolly, S. J., and Yusuf, S.: Evaluation of the implantable cardioverter defibrillator in survivors of cardiac arrest: The need for randomized trials. Am. J. Cardiol. *69*:959, 1992.
401. Swerdlow, C. R., Winkle, R. A., and Mason, J. W.: Determinants of survival in patients with ventricular tachycardia. N. Engl. J. Med. *308*:1436, 1983.
402. Roy, D., Waxman, H. L., Kienzle, M. G., et al.: Clinical characteristics and long-term follow-up in 119 survivors of cardiac arrest: Relation to inducibility at electrophysiologic testing. Am. J. Cardiol. *52*:969, 1983.
403. Benditt, D. G., Benson, D. W., Jr., Klein, G. J., et al.: Prevention of recurrent sudden cardiac arrest: Role of provocative electropharmacologic testing. J. Am. Coll. Cardiol. *2*:418, 1983.
404. Morady, F., Scheinman, M. M., Hess, D. S., et al.: Electrophysiologic testing in the management of survivors of out-of-hospital cardiac arrest. Am. J. Cardiol. *51*:85, 1983.
405. Skale, B. T., Miles, W. M., Heger, J. J., et al.: Survivors of cardiac arrest: Prevention of recurrence by drug therapy as predicted by electrophysiologic testing or electrocardiographic monitoring. Am. J. Cardiol. *57*:113, 1986.
406. Wilbur, D. J., Garan, H., Finkelstein, D., et al.: Out-of-hospital cardiac arrest: Use of electrophysiological testing in the prediction of long-term outcome. N. Engl. J. Med. *318*:19, 1988.
407. Wellens, H. J. J., Brugada, P., and Stevenson, W. G.: Programmed electrical stimulation of the heart in patients with life-threatening ventricular arrhythmias: What is the significance of induced arrhythmias and what is the correct stimulation protocol? Circulation *72*:1, 1985.
408. Myerburg, R. J., and Zaman, L.: Indications for intracardiac electrophysiologic studies in survivors of prehospital cardiac arrest. Circulation *75*:151, 1987.
409. Kim, S. O., Seiden, S. W., Felder, S. D., et al.: Is programmed stimulation of value in predicting the long-term success of antiarrhythmic therapy for ventricular tachycardia? N. Engl. J. Med. *315*:356, 1986.
410. Mason, J. W., for The Electrophysiologic Study versus Electrocardiographic Monitoring Investigators: A comparison of electrophysiologic testing with Holter monitoring to predict antiarrhythmic-drug efficacy for ventricular tachyarrhythmias. N. Engl. J. Med. *329*:445, 1993.
411. The ESVEM Investigators: Determinants of predicted efficacy of antiarrhythmic drugs in The Electrophysiologic Study versus Electrocardiographic Monitoring Trial. Circulation *87*:323, 1993.
412. Goldstein, S., Brooks, M. M., Ledingham, R., et al.: The association between ease of suppression of ventricular arrhythmias and survival. Circulation *91*:79, 1995.
413. Mitchell, L. B., Duff, H. J., Manyeri, D. E., and Wyse, D. G.: Randomized clinical trial of invasive and non-invasive approaches to drug therapy of ventricular tachycardia. N. Engl. J. Med. *317*:1681, 1987.
414. Akhtar, M., Guran, H., Lehmann, M. H., and Troup, P. J.: Sudden cardiac death: Management of high-risk patients. Ann. Intern. Med. *114*:499, 1991.
415. Zheutlin, T. A., Steinman, R. T., Mattioni, T. A., and Kehoe, R. F.: Long-term arrhythmic outcome in survivors of ventricular fibrillation with absence of inducible ventricular tachycardia. Am. J. Cardiol. *62*:1213, 1988.
416. Crandall, B. G., Morris, C. D., Cutler, J. E., et al.: Implantable cardioverter-defibrillator therapy in survivors of out-of-hospital sudden cardiac death without inducible arrhythmias. J. Am. Coll. Cardiol. *21*:1186, 1993.
417. Josephson, M. E., Harken, A. H., and Horowitz, L. N.: Endocardial excision: A new surgical technique for the treatment of recurrent ventricular tachycardia. Circulation *60*:1430, 1979.
418. Guiradon, G., Gontaine, G., Frank, R., et al.: Encircling endocardial ventriculotomy: A new surgical treatment for life-threatening ventricular tachycardias resistant to medical treatment following myocardial infarction. Ann. Thorac. Surg. *26*:438, 1978.
419. Bolooki, H., Horowitz, M. D., Interian, A., et al.: Long-term surgical syndrome associated with cardiac dysfunction after myocardial infarction. Ann. Surg. *216*:333, 1992.
420. Kelly, P., Ruskin, J. N., Vlahakes, G. J., et al.: Surgical coronary revascularization in survivors of prehospital cardiac arrest. J. Am. Coll. Cardiol. *15*:267, 1990.
421. Platia, E. V., Griffith, L. S. C., Watkins, L., et al.: Treatment of malignant ventricular arrhythmias with endocardial resection and implantation of the automatic cardioverter-defibrillator. N. Engl. J. Med. *314*:213, 1986.
422. Mirowski, M., Reid, P. R., Mower, M. M., et al.: Termination of malignant ventricular arrhythmias with an implanted automatic defibrillator in human beings. N. Engl. J. Med. *303*:322, 1980.
423. Mirowski, M., Reid, P. R., Winkle, R. A., et al.: Mortality in patients with implanted automatic defibrillators. Ann. Intern. Med. *98*:585, 1983.
424. Echt, D. S., Armstrong, K., Schmidt, P., et al.: Clinical experience, complications, and survival in 70 patients with the automatic implantable cardioverter/defibrillator. Circulation *71*:289, 1985.
425. Kelly, P. A., Cannom, D. S., Garan, H., et al.: The automatic implantable defibrillator (AICD): Efficacy, complications and survival in patients with malignant ventricular arrhythmias. J. Am. Coll. Cardiol. *11*:1278, 1988.
426. Tchou, P. J., Kadri, N., Anderson, J., et al.: Automatic implantable cardioverter-defibrillators and survival of patients with left ventricular dysfunction and malignant ventricular arrhythmias. Ann. Intern. Med. *109*:529, 1988.
427. Fogoros, R. N., Elson, J. J., and Bonnet, C. A.: Actuarial incidence and pattern of occurrence of shocks following implantation of the automatic implantable cardioverter-defibrillator. PACE *12*:1465, 1989.
428. Myerburg, R. J., Luceri, R. M., Thurer, R., et al.: Time to first shock and clinical outcome in patients receiving automatic implantable cardioverter-defibrillators. J. Am. Coll. Cardiol. *14*:508, 1989.
429. Newman, D., Sauve, M. J., Herre, J., et al.: Survival after implantation of the cardioverter defibrillator. Am. J. Cardiol. *69*:899, 1992.
430. Siebels, J., Kuck, K.-H., and the CASH Investigators: Implantable cardioverter defibrillator compared with antiarrhythmic drug treatment in cardiac arrest survivors (the Cardiac Arrest Study, Hamburg). Am. Heart. J. *127*:1139, 1994.
431. Kim, S. G., Fisher, J. D., Furman, S., et al.: Benefits of implantable defibrillators are overestimated by sudden death rates and better represented by the total arrhythmic death rate. J. Am. Coll. Cardiol. *17*:1587, 1991.
432. Myerburg, R. J., and Kessler, K. M.: Management of patients who survive cardiac arrest. Mod. Concepts Cardiovasc. Dis. *55*:61, 1986.
433. Huikuri, H. V., Cox, M., Interian, A., et al.: Efficacy of intravenous propranolol for significance of inducibility of ventricular tachyarrhythmias with different electrophysiological characteristics in coronary artery disease. Am. J. Cardiol. *64*:1305, 1989.
434. Lehmann, M. H., and Saksena, S., for the NASPE Policy Conference Committee: Implantable cardioverter defibrillators in cardiovascular practice: Report of the Policy Conference of the North American Society of Pacing and Electrophysiology. PACE *14*:969, 1991.
435. Myerburg, R. J., and Davis, J. H.: The medical ecology of public safety. I. Sudden death due to coronary heart disease. Am. Heart J. *68*:586, 1964.
436. Levy, R. I., De La Chapelle, C. E., and Richards, D. W.: Heart disease in drivers of public motor vehicles as a cause of highway accidents. JAMA *184*:143, 1963.
437. Waller, J. A.: Cardiovascular disease, aging, and traffic accidents. J. Chron. Dis. *20*:615, 1967.
438. Kerwin, A. J.: Sudden death while driving. Can. Med. Assoc. J. *131*:312, 1984.
439. Öström, M., and Eriksson, A.: Natural death while driving. J. Forensic Sci. *32*:988, 1987.
440. Christian, M. S.: Incidence and implications of natural deaths of road users. B.M.J. *297*:1021, 1988.

Chapter 25
Pulmonary Hypertension

STUART RICH, EUGENE BRAUNWALD, WILLIAM GROSSMAN

NORMAL PULMONARY CIRCULATION

During the passage of red blood cells through the lungs, hemoglobin is normally oxygenated to nearly full capacity and the blood is cleansed of much particulate matter and bacteria. The lungs, in addition to functioning as a blood oxygenator and filter, play a dominant role in achieving acid-base balance by excreting carbon dioxide, thereby helping to maintain an optimal blood pH.[1] Normally, the pulmonary vascular bed offers remarkably little resistance to flow. Pulmonary hypertension results from reductions in the caliber of the pulmonary vessels and/or increases in pulmonary blood flow.

PULMONARY BLOOD FLOW, PRESSURE, AND RESISTANCE

PULMONARY CIRCULATION IN THE NORMAL ADULT. *Pulmonary blood flow* refers to the volume of blood per unit of time that passes from the pulmonary artery through the capillary bed and into the pulmonary veins. However, it must be remembered that the lungs have a dual circulation and receive both systemic venous blood (the "pulmonary blood flow") through the pulmonary artery and arterial blood through the bronchial circulation. The bronchial arteries ramify normally into a capillary network drained by bronchial veins, some of which empty into the pulmonary veins, whereas the remainder empty into the systemic venous bed. Therefore, the bronchial circulation constitutes a physiological "right-to-left" shunt. The function of the bronchial circulation is to provide nutrition to the airways. Normally, blood flow through this system is quite low, amounting to approximately 1 per cent of cardiac output[2]; the resulting desaturation of left atrial blood is usually trivial. However, in some forms of pulmonary disease, e.g., severe bronchiectasis, and in the presence of many congenital cardiovascular malformations that cause cyanosis, the blood flow through the bronchial circulation can increase significantly, account for nearly 30 per cent of the left ventricular output,[3] and produce a significant right-to-left shunt. In pulmonary disease, significant right-to-left shunting through the bronchial circulation may also result in arterial desaturation. In cyanotic congenital heart disease, bronchial blood is not fully oxygenated; it may participate in gas exchange and improve systemic oxygenation.

The normal pulmonary artery pressure in a person living at sea level has a peak systolic value of 18 to 25 mm Hg, an end-diastolic value of 6 to 10 mm Hg, and a mean value ranging from 12 to 16 mm Hg (Chap. 6).* Definite pulmonary hypertension is present when pulmonary artery systolic and mean pressures exceed 30 and 20 mm Hg, respectively. The normal mean pulmonary venous pressure is 6 to 10 mm Hg; therefore, the normal arteriovenous pressure difference, which moves the entire cardiac output across the pulmonary vascular bed, ranges from 2 to 10 mm Hg. This small pressure gradient is all the more remarkable when one considers that to move the same amount of blood per minute through the systemic vascular bed a pressure differential of approximately 90 mm Hg (systemic arterial mean pressure minus right atrial mean pressure) is required.

Thus, the normal pulmonary vascular bed offers less than one-tenth the *resistance* to flow offered by the systemic bed. *Vascular resistance* is generally quantified, by analogy to Ohm's law, as the ratio of pressure drop (ΔP in mm Hg) to mean flow (Q in liters/min). The ratio is commonly multiplied by 79.9 (or 80 for simplification) to express the results in dynes-seconds-centimeters^{-5}. This conversion to metric units may be avoided, i.e., resistance may be expressed in units of mm Hg/liter/min, which are sometimes referred to as hybrid units, PRU (peripheral resistance units), or Wood units (after the English cardiologist Paul Wood). The calculated pulmonary vascular resistance in normal adults[4] is 67 ± 23 (S.D.) dynes-sec-cm^{-5}, or 1 Wood unit.

Vascular resistance reflects a composite of variables that includes, but is not limited to, the cross-sectional area of small muscular arteries and arterioles. Other determinants are blood viscosity, the total mass of lung tissue (i.e., resistance is higher in infants and children than in adults), proximal vascular obstruction (e.g., pulmonary coarctation, pulmonary embolism, peripheral pulmonic stenosis), and extramural compression of vessels (perivascular edema).

Because the pulmonary vascular bed contains considerable elastic tissue, the cross-sectional area of the bed varies directly with transmural pressure and flow. Therefore, pulmonary vascular resistance decreases passively with increases in flow. This fall in resistance results in part from the increase in the radius of distensible vessels secondary to increased flow. From a consideration of the Poiseuille relationship—in which $R = \Delta P/Q = 8\eta l/\pi r^4$, where R = resistance, ΔP = pressure drop, Q = flow, η = viscosity of fluid, and l and r = length and radius of the vessel, respectively—it is apparent that resistance can be effectively influenced by even small changes in the radius of the vessel. Recruitment of additional vascular channels also contributes to the fall in resistance that characterizes increased flow through the pulmonary circuit. This phenomenon is particularly prominent in the upright position, where vessels in the upper parts of the lungs are in a partially collapsed state owing to low hydrostatic pressure.

The reduction in resistance in a distensible vascular bed that occurs with increased flow has been offered as the explanation for the ab-

* All pressures discussed here are in reference to atmospheric pressure at the level of the heart. True transmural pressures are more physiologically meaningful, especially when pulmonary parenchymal disease is present, but these are rarely measured.

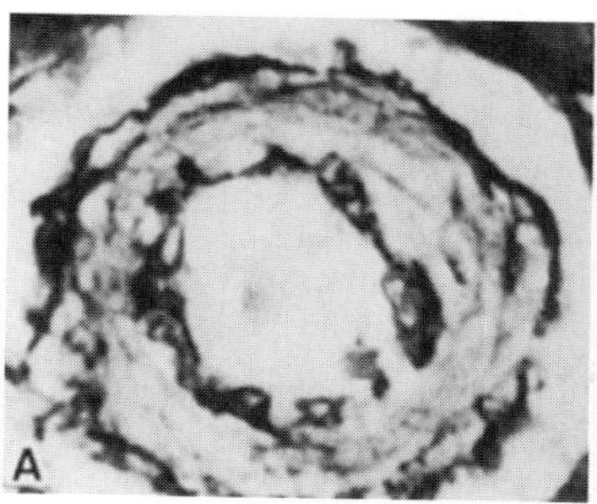

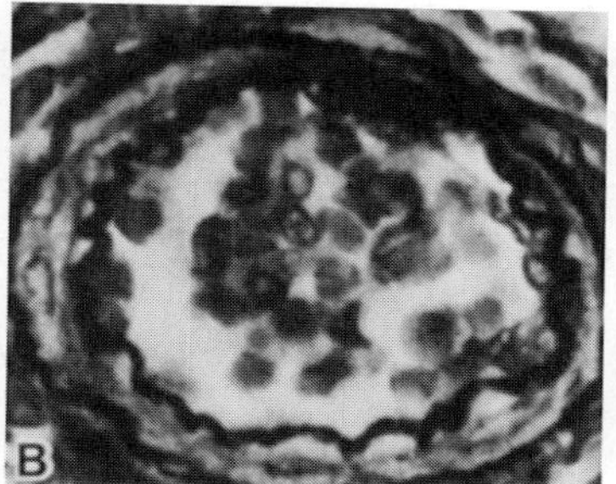

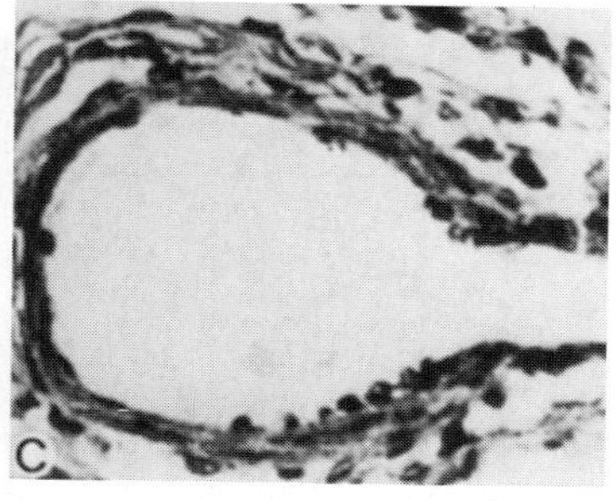

FIGURE 25–1. Changes in pulmonary arteries after birth. Comparison of relative medial thicknesses at birth *(A)*, at age 2 months *(B)*, and at age 7 months *(C)*. Elastic-van Gieson stain; magnification × 360; reduced 17 per cent. (From Petersen, R. C., and Edwards, W. D.: Pulmonary vascular disease in 57 necropsy cases of total anomalous pulmonary venous connections. Histopathology *7*:47, 1983, with permission of Blackwell Scientific Publications.)

sence of pulmonary hypertension in many patients with large left-to-right intracardiac shunts, particularly atrial septal defects. However, it must be pointed out that the increased distensibility of pulmonary vessels in such situations has developed over years and that this principle is not necessarily applicable to acute increase in pulmonary blood flow.[5] In this regard, the results of studies with unilateral occlusion of a pulmonary artery using a balloon catheter are relevant.[6] Acute increases in flow in the supine position were associated with increases in ΔP, so that vascular resistance of the lung (the slope of the line relating ΔP to flow) remained unchanged. In the upright position, however, blood vessels in the upper part of the lung usually are in a partially or fully collapsed state and with an increase in flow, these vessels may expand, thereby reducing vascular resistance.[5]

FETAL AND NEONATAL CIRCULATIONS (see also p. 1607). In the fetus, oxygenated blood enters the heart from the inferior vena cava and streams across the foramen ovale to the left atrium, left ventricle, ascending aorta, and cranial vessels. Desaturated blood returns from the superior vena cava and passes through the tricuspid valve into the right ventricle and pulmonary artery. Because the resistance of the pulmonary vascular bed in the collapsed fetal lung is extremely high, only 10 to 30 per cent of the total right ventricular output passes through the lungs, the remainder being shunted across the ductus arteriosus to the descending aorta and then back to the placenta. At birth, there is an abrupt change in the pulmonary circulation. With the first breath, expansion of the lungs and the abrupt rise in the Po_2 of blood lead to a release of pulmonary arteriolar vasoconstriction and a stretching and dilatation of muscular pulmonary arteries and arterioles, with a marked drop in vascular resistance.[7] This facilitates a large increase in pulmonary blood flow and raises left atrial volume and pressure. The latter closes the flap valve of the foramen ovale, so that interatrial right-to-left shunting ordinarily ceases within the first hour of life. Normally, the ductus arteriosus closes over the next 10 hours as a result of contraction of the thick smooth muscle bundles within its wall in response to a rising arterial oxygen tension and a change in the prostaglandin milieu.[8] Following the initial dramatic fall in pulmonary vascular resistance at birth, there is a continuous decline over the first few months of life associated with thinning of the media of muscular pulmonary arteries and arterioles until the normal adult pattern is achieved[29] (Fig. 25–1).

AGING AND THE PULMONARY CIRCULATION. Pulmonary artery pressure and pulmonary vascular resistance increase with advanced age, similar to increases that occur in systemic vascular resistance.[10–12] Reduced compliance of the pulmonary vascular bed secondary to intimal fibrosis or increased wall thickness in the muscular pulmonary arteries is a possible cause.[13] It is also possible that some of the changes in the pulmonary arteries relate to reduced compliance of left ventricular filling, which is passively reflected back on the pulmonary vascular bed.[14] The prevalence of mild pulmonary hypertension (mean pulmonary artery pressure $\geq$ 20 mm Hg) may be as high as 13 per cent in ages up to 45 years, and 28 per cent in ages up to 75 years.[15]

RESPONSE TO ANOXIA, DRUGS, AND NEURAL AND ENVIRONMENTAL FACTORS

HYPOXIA. It is well established that acute *hypoxia* elicits pulmonary vasoconstriction,[16,17] and there is general agreement that this response is part of a self-regulatory mechanism for adjusting capillary perfusion to alveolar ventilation. There appears to be an age dependency and a considerable species variability in the magnitude of this vasoconstrictor response, which is quite intense in cattle, intermediate in humans and the pig, and comparatively mild in dogs and sheep; hypoxic vasoconstriction is more profound in the infant or young mammal than in the adult. Variability exists within a given species as well, and there is strong evidence for a genetic determination of individual reactivity to hypoxia in animals.[18]

The mechanism of the acute pulmonary vasoconstriction that occurs in response to hypoxia is uncertain (Fig. 25–2). There is some evidence that hypoxia-induced local release of histamine may play an important role, with pulmonary vasoconstriction secondary to stimulation of pulmonary vascular H_1-receptors (cf. discussion of histamine below). There has been considerable speculation about the role of vascular endothelium as a mediator of hypoxia-induced pulmonary vasoconstriction.[19] This is based on recent findings concerning the role of vascular endothelium in the regulation of vascular smooth muscle contraction and relaxation.[20–22] Balanced release of endothelial-derived relaxing factor (EDRF)[20] and of the vasoconstrictor peptide endothelin[22] by endothelial cells plays a critical role in regulation of tone in systemic vascular resistance vessels and may be of considerable importance in the pulmonary circulation as well.

Considerable evidence suggests a role for increased Ca^{++} entry into vascular smooth muscle mediating hypoxic pulmonary vasoconstriction.[24] The concentration of Ca^{++} in the vicinity of the contractile machinery represents a balance between the inflow and outflow across the cell membrane and intracellular release and uptake. Within the cell Ca^{++} can be mobilized from the sarcoplasmic reticulum, mitochondrial membrane, or inner aspect of the cell membrane.[25] Although most of the evidence favors an influx of Ca^{++} from extracellular fluid, the relative contribution of differential mobilization from intracellular stores is unsettled. The mechanism responsible for intracellular mobilization of Ca^{++} is also unclear.[26,27]

Changes in alveolar oxygenation affect the oxygenation of blood in small pulmonary arteries and arterioles by direct gaseous diffusion from the alveoli, respiratory bronchioles, and alveolar ducts in the pulmonary arterioles, even though the latter are "upstream" in relation to the alveoli. This fact, taken together with evidence for a reduction in pulmonary arterial blood volume during hypoxia,[28] supports the view that the small pulmonary arteries and arterioles are the main sites of vasoconstriction and increased resistance during hypoxia.[28,29] Although alveolar oxygen tension is a major physiological determinant of pulmonary arteriolar tone, a reduction in the oxygen tension in the mixed venous blood flowing through the small pulmonary arteries and arterioles may also lead to pulmonary arterial vasoconstriction.[30] *Acidemia* appears to potentiate the effects of hypoxemia, whereas alkalosis may be protective.[31]

NEURAL REGULATION. The media and adventitia of the large elastic pulmonary arteries and of the large pulmonary veins are supplied by nerve fibers that may influence the distensibility of these capacitance vessels.[2,10] Although *neural regulation* of pulmonary vascular resistance can be

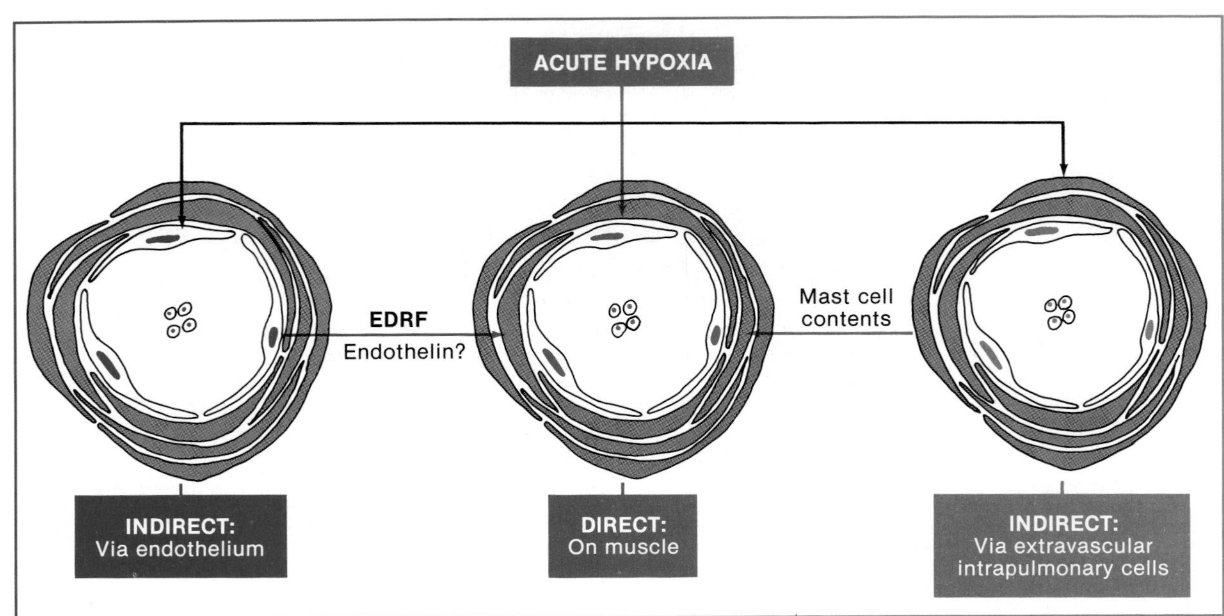

FIGURE 25–2. Possible mechanisms whereby acute hypoxia leads to pulmonary vasoconstriction. A small pulmonary artery can be affected in one of three ways: indirectly via the endothelium *(left),* indirectly via extravascular cells in the lung *(right),* or directly via an effect of hypoxia on vascular smooth muscle cells *(middle).* (From Fishman, A. P.: The enigma of hypoxic pulmonary vasoconstriction. *In* Fishman, A. P. [ed.]: The Pulmonary Circulation: Normal and Abnormal. Philadelphia, University of Pennsylvania Press, 1990, pp. 109–129.)

demonstrated[32] and may be particularly important in fetal life, its importance in the normal human adult is uncertain. *Chemical and hormonal regulation* of pulmonary vascular resistance is a complex and as yet incompletely understood subject, with roles having been reported for catecholamines, acetylcholine, prostaglandins, histamine, bradykinin, serotonin, and angiotensin.[2,19,33–45] The exact site of action of these agents within the pulmonary vascular tree (i.e., arterioles, venules, capillaries, and so on) is uncertain at present.

DRUGS. Controversy exists concerning the effects of *alpha-adrenergic agonists* on the pulmonary vascular bed. Some studies have shown that norepinephrine causes increases in pulmonary arterial and wedge pressures with no change in pulmonary blood flow or pulmonary vascular resistance.[41] Evidence exists for alpha-adrenergic–mediated constriction of small pulmonary arteries and veins induced by the stimulation of sympathetic nerves.[42]

Both the alpha-adrenergic blocking agent phentolamine and tolazoline (Priscoline), which also exhibits alpha-adrenergic blocking action, can lower pulmonary vascular resistance. *Beta-adrenergic stimulation* with isoproterenol has been shown repeatedly to cause pulmonary *vasodilatation.* In contrast, beta-adrenergic blockade does not produce any change in pulmonary vascular resistance, suggesting that there is no tonic activation of beta receptors for maintenance of the normal low pulmonary vascular resistance. *Acetylcholine* is also a potent relaxant of pulmonary arteries and arterioles[33] and transiently lowers pulmonary vascular resistance in patients with elevated pulmonary vascular resistance with a major reversible component. Whether this effect of acetylcholine is mediated by release

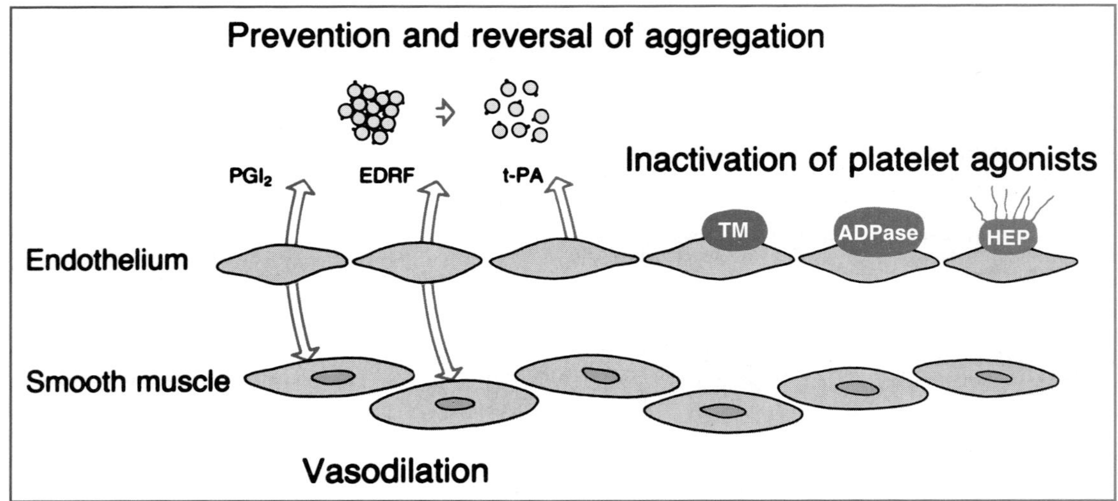

FIGURE 25–3. The vasoactive and anti-aggregatory properties of the normal vascular endothelium are illustrated. Endothelial cells both retain and release into the blood many substances that are anti-aggregatory and fibrinolytic. These include prostacyclin (PGI_2), endothelium-derived relaxing factor (EDRF), and tissue plasminogen activator (t-PA). Some endothelium-derived substances also diffuse from the endothelium to the vascular smooth muscle to produce vasodilation. (From Ware, J. A., and Heistadt, D. D.: Platelet-endothelium interactions. N. Engl. J. Med. *328*:628, 1993. Copyright Massachusetts Medical Society.)

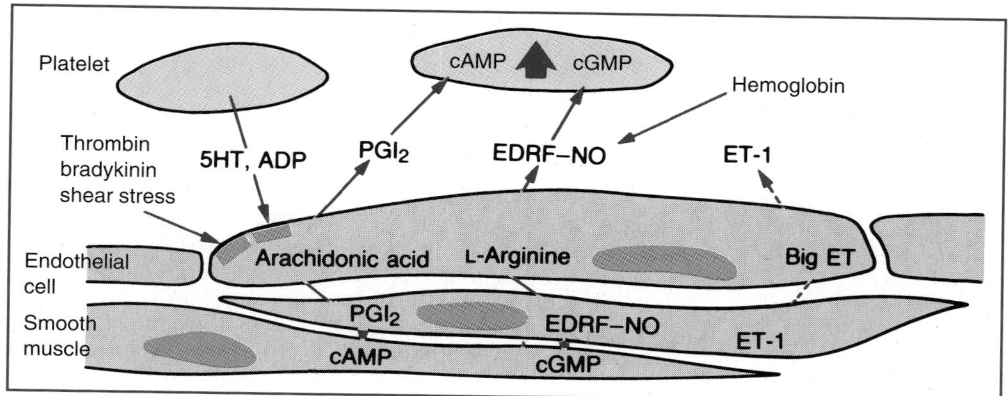

FIGURE 25–4. Generation of PGI_2, EDRF–nitric oxide (NO), and endothelin-1 (ET-1) in endothelial cells. Stimulation of receptors on the cells by serotonin or ADP released from platelets or by thrombin, bradykinin, or shear stress leads to the release of vasoactive mediators. Prostacyclin relaxes vascular smooth muscle and inhibits aggregation of platelets by increasing levels of cyclic AMP (cAMP). EDRF-NO relaxes vascular smooth muscle and inhibits platelet aggregation and adhesion, increasing levels of cyclic GMP (cGMP). The simultaneous increase in cAMP and cGMP inhibits platelet aggregation. (From Vane, J. R., Anggard, E. E., and Botting, R. M.: Regulatory functions of the vascular endothelium. N. Engl. J. Med. *323*:27, 1990. Copyright Massachusetts Medical Society.)

of EDRF from pulmonary vascular endothelium has not been determined.

Lung tissue is particularly active in the synthesis, metabolism, and release of a number of the *prostaglandins,* some of which may play a role in the regulation of pulmonary vascular resistance. Prostaglandins I_2 and E are active pulmonary vasodilators, whereas $F_2\alpha$ and A_2 are pulmonary vasoconstrictors.[34] Prostacyclin (PGI_2) is a powerful vasodilator that also inhibits platelet aggregation through activation of adenylate cyclase. Its metabolic half-life in the bloodstream is less than one circulation time with its metabolite 6-keto-prostaglandin $F_1\alpha$ having little biological activity.[35] A variety of drugs with diverse mechanisms of action are reported to encourage prostacyclin production and include calcium channel blockers, angiotensin-converting enzyme inhibitors, diuretics, and nitrates.[36] Physiologically, prostacyclin is a local hormone rather than a circulating one. The release of prostacyclin by endothelial cells causes relaxation of the underlying vascular smooth vessel and prevents platelet aggregation within the bloodstream. Because the biological actions of prostacyclin are the opposite from those of thromboxane, the balance between these two peptides appears to control the local environment within the vascular bed (Fig. 25–3).

The biological action of nitric oxide (EDRF), is quite similar to that of prostacyclin in that it relaxes vascular smooth muscle and potentially inhibits the aggregation and adhesions of platelets by raising platelet levels of cyclic GMP.[37,37a] The observation that activation of the same receptors or a change in membrane confirmation induced by shear stress leads to the release of both nitric oxide and prostacyclin suggests that these substances act in concert as a common mechanism that defends the vascular endothelium[38,38a] (Fig. 25–4).

Histamine, a vasodilator in the systemic circulation, is primarily a vasoconstrictor in the pulmonary vascular bed. Because large doses of histamine receptor blockers or histamine depletors attenuate the hypoxia-induced pulmonary vasoconstrictor response, it has been suggested that histamine may actually be the chemical mediator of hypoxia-induced vasoconstriction in animals.[39,40] This suggestion is supported by the observation that the periarterial mast cells in the rat and guinea pig lung lose their granules and apparently release histamine during hypoxia.[29] However, other experimental findings are contradictory,[16] and as a consequence, the role of histamine in the regulation of the pulmonary circulation in humans remains unclear. *Serotonin* is a potent pulmonary vasoconstrictor in experimental animals but apparently has little or no effect in humans. *Angiotensin II,* generated in the lung by means of enzymatic conversion of angiotensin I, is thought to be a potent pulmonary vasoconstrictor.[29] However, its role in the normal regulation of pulmonary vascular resistance in humans is unknown.

HIGH ALTITUDE. Life at high altitudes is associated with pulmonary hypertension of variable severity, reflecting the range of reactivities of different persons to the pulmonary vasoconstrictive effect of hypoxia.[44] As discussed earlier, pulmonary arterial pressure normally declines rapidly following birth at sea level. However, the fall in pulmonary artery pressure of infants born at high altitude may be slower in onset and of lesser magnitude. Mean pulmonary arterial pressure in normal adults living 10,000 feet above sea level is approximately 25 mm Hg[45] and increases to over 50 mm Hg with exercise.

PRIMARY PULMONARY HYPERTENSION

Primary pulmonary hypertension (PPH) is the diagnosis given to patients with pulmonary hypertension of unexplained etiology, making it essentially a diagnosis of exclusion.[46] However, PPH has well-characterized clinical features that allow a diagnosis to be made with reasonable precision if an orderly evaluation of the heart and lungs is made in affected patients.[47] The actual incidence of PPH appears to be approximately two cases per million population, thus qualifying it as an orphan disease.[48]

ETIOLOGY

Although the precise cause of PPH is, by definition, unknown, recent developments in our understanding of vascular biology point to an abnormality in the pulmonary vascular endothelium. The normal pulmonary vascular endothelial cell maintains the vascular smooth muscle in a state of relaxation.[36] The findings of increased pulmonary

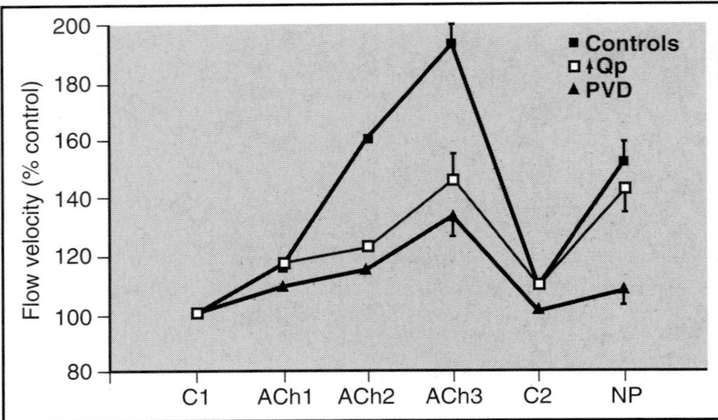

FIGURE 25–5. Relative effects of endothelium-dependent and independent vasodilators on injured pulmonary vessels. The vasodilator response to increasing doses of acetylcholine (ACh 1, 2, 3) and nitroprusside (NP) are shown in children with normal pulmonary vasculature, children with increased pulmonary blood flow but normal vasculature (↑ Qp), and children with pulmonary vascular disease (PVD). The response to acetylcholine, an endothelium-dependent vasodilator, is reduced in patients with increased pulmonary blood flow and pulmonary vascular disease, whereas the response to nitroprusside, an endothelium-independent vasodilator, is lost only in patients with pulmonary vascular disease. (Reproduced with permission from Celermajor, D. S., Cullen, S., and Deanfield, J. E.: Impairment of endothelium-dependent pulmonary artery relaxation in children with congenital heart disease and abnormal pulmonary hemodynamics. Circulation *87*:440, 1993. Copyright 1993 American Heart Association.)

vascular reactivity and vasoconstriction in patients with PPH suggest that a marked vasoconstrictive tendency underlies the development of PPH in predisposed individuals,[49] possibly as a result of loss of endothelial cell integrity[36] (Fig. 25–5) The autonomic nervous system has been considered a contributory factor in the development of PPH through stimulation of the pulmonary vascular bed by either neuronally released or circulating catecholamines. In some patients with PPH the response to vasodilators such as tolazoline, acetylcholine, or isoproterenol is a reduction in pulmonary artery pressure and pulmonary vascular resistance,[50–52] which supports the notion that the autonomic nervous system is at least in part maintaining a role in the constant elevation of the pulmonary vascular resistance.

As in the systemic circulation (see p. 1164), vascular endothelial cells promote relaxation or contraction of adjacent smooth muscle cells via elaboration of endothelium-derived relaxing factor (EDRF) and endothelin, respectively[20,21] (Fig. 36–4, p. 1164). The secretion of EDRF by vascular endothelium, which serves to dampen or counter many direct vasoconstrictor influences, is lost with endothelial dysfunction that may result from a variety of causes (e.g., shear stress). Studies of vasodilators in pulmonary-hypertension demonstrate that responsiveness to endothelium-dependent vasodilating agents is impaired before response to endothelium-dependent vasodilators[53,54] (Fig. 25–5). This may reflect the underlying severity of vascular damage. Conversely, endothelin, a potent vasoconstrictor peptide, may also play an important role in the regulation of pulmonary vascular tone.[55] Its secretion may be enhanced in the presence of vasoconstriction or in the setting of platelet aggregation. Because it has a long half-life, subtle disturbances in production or release could lead to sustained vasoconstriction.[22] Recently, endothelin ETA receptor antagonists have been reported to reduce pulmonary artery pressure in experimental animals.[56] Given that the major resistance vessels in the pulmonary vascular bed are at the arteriolar level, diffuse arteriolar vasoconstriction could easily cause chronically sustained elevations in pulmonary vascular resistance, resulting in pulmonary hypertension. In postmortem examinations in PPH, the pulmonary vasculature is typified by severe medial hypertrophy,[57] consistent with the appearance of chronic sustained pulmonary vasoconstriction.

A striking feature of the pulmonary vasculature in patients with PPH is intimal proliferation, and in some vessels it causes virtually complete vascular occlusion[57,58] (Fig. 25–6). Several growth factors have been implicated in the development of this type of vascular pathology, which includes basic fibroblast growth factor from the endothelium[59] and platelet derived growth factor[60] and transform-

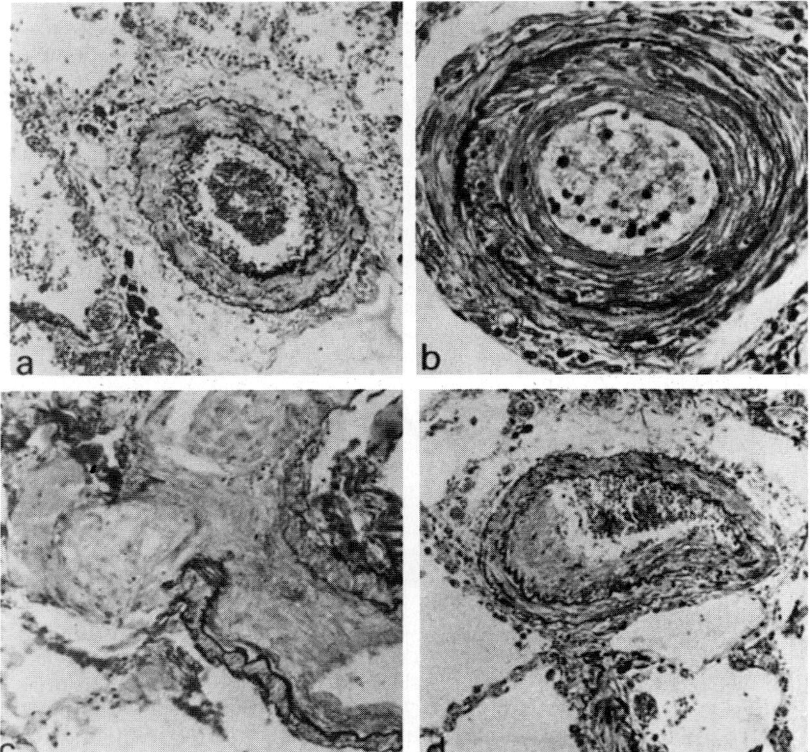

FIGURE 25–6. Photomicrographs of pulmonary arterial histologic lesions seen in clinically unexplained pulmonary hypertension. All slides were stained with Verhoeff-van Gieson stain. *A*, Medial hypertrophy (×100). *B*, Concentric laminal intimal fibrosis—seen most often in association with plexiform lesion (×200). *C*, Plexiform lesion demonstrating obstruction in the arterial lumen, aneurysmal dilatation, and proliferation of anastomosing vascular channels (×200). *D*, Eccentric intimal fibrosis—often seen in association with organized microthrombi but also present in many patients with plexiform lesions (×100). (Reproduced with permission from Palevsky, H. I., Schloo, B. L., Pietria, G. G., et al.: Primary pulmonary hypertension. Vascular structure, morphometry and responsiveness to vasodilator agents. Circulation *80*:1207, 1989. Copyright 1989 American Heart Association.)

ing growth factor-β[61] from platelets. Enhanced growth factor release, activation, and intracellular signaling may lead to smooth muscle cell proliferation and migration as well as extracellular matrix synthesis. Even advanced lesions show evidence of in situ activity of ongoing synthesis of connective tissue proteins such as elastin, collagen, and fibronectin.[62,63]

An equally important etiologic feature of PPH is the widespread development of thrombosis in situ of the small pulmonary arteries with resultant vascular obstruction.[57,58,64,65] Although it was once believed that recurrent, systemic venous microembolism could be an underlying mechanism in PPH,[46] this theory has been essentially rejected for lack of both animal and human data to support it as a clinical entity. Animal studies suggest that more than 22 million thromboemboli to the pulmonary arterioles would be required to raise the mean pulmonary artery pressure 5 mm Hg, yet no source of these emboli has ever been found in patients dying of PPH.[64] Various defects in coagulation, including abnormal platelet function and defective fibrinolysis, have been demonstrated in patients with PPH.[64,66–70] Increased production of biologically active von Willebrand factor in patients with PPH could predispose to platelet fibrin microthrombi,[71] and exposure of subendothelial cell surface structures due to injury may provide the substrate for ongoing vascular thrombosis in this condition.[72] Alterations of the normal physiological function of endothelial cells has been shown to create a local procoagulant environment[36] (Fig. 25–3).

Endothelial denudation results in platelet adherence to exposed tissue collagen, with release of platelet derived smooth muscle mitogens which also have vasoconstrictor properties. This process in turn leads to an inflammatory response and thrombosis, thereby narrowing the lumen of the pulmonary vessels. In a person who is susceptible—whether on a genetic or an acquired basis—intense vasoconstriction may lead to fibrinoid necrosis of the arteriolar wall and the development of plexiform lesions. Ultimately, the vessels are reduced in number, and the residua of these destroyed vessels can be seen histologically as "ghost vessels." Destruction of large numbers of pulmonary arterioles reduces the cross-sectional area of the pulmonary vascular bed, thus producing a permanent increase in pulmonary vascular resistance and fixed pulmonary hypertension. The latter, in turn, damages other blood vessels and initiates a vicious circle, with progressively rising pulmonary arterial pressure (Fig. 25–7).

An important emerging concept for the development of PPH is that patients with an underlying genetic predisposition develop the disease following exposure to specific stimuli, which serve as triggers. Predisposition to the development of pulmonary hypertension has been noted by the marked heterogeneity in responses of the pulmonary vasculature in a variety of disease states. Examples include the considerable variability among individuals to vasoconstrictive stimuli such as hypoxia or acidosis, which can produce marked pulmonary hypertension in one person and be essentially without effect in another.[44] The pulmonary arterial pressure response to hypoxia is particularly great in individuals with blood group A.[16] This variability in the responsiveness of the pulmonary vascular bed undoubtedly accounts for the fact that only a minority of individuals develop pulmonary edema on exposure to high altitude (see p. 462). Also, the severity of pulmonary hypertension and the level of pulmonary vascular resistance vary considerably among individuals with congenital heart

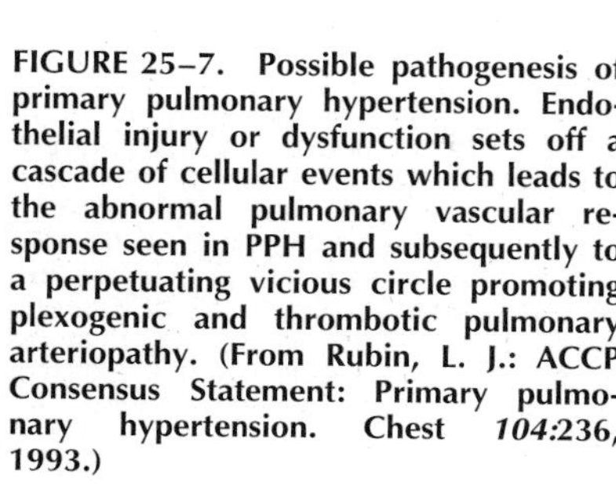
FIGURE 25–7. Possible pathogenesis of primary pulmonary hypertension. Endothelial injury or dysfunction sets off a cascade of cellular events which leads to the abnormal pulmonary vascular response seen in PPH and subsequently to a perpetuating vicious circle promoting plexogenic and thrombotic pulmonary arteriopathy. (From Rubin, L. J.: ACCP Consensus Statement: Primary pulmonary hypertension. Chest *104*:236, 1993.)

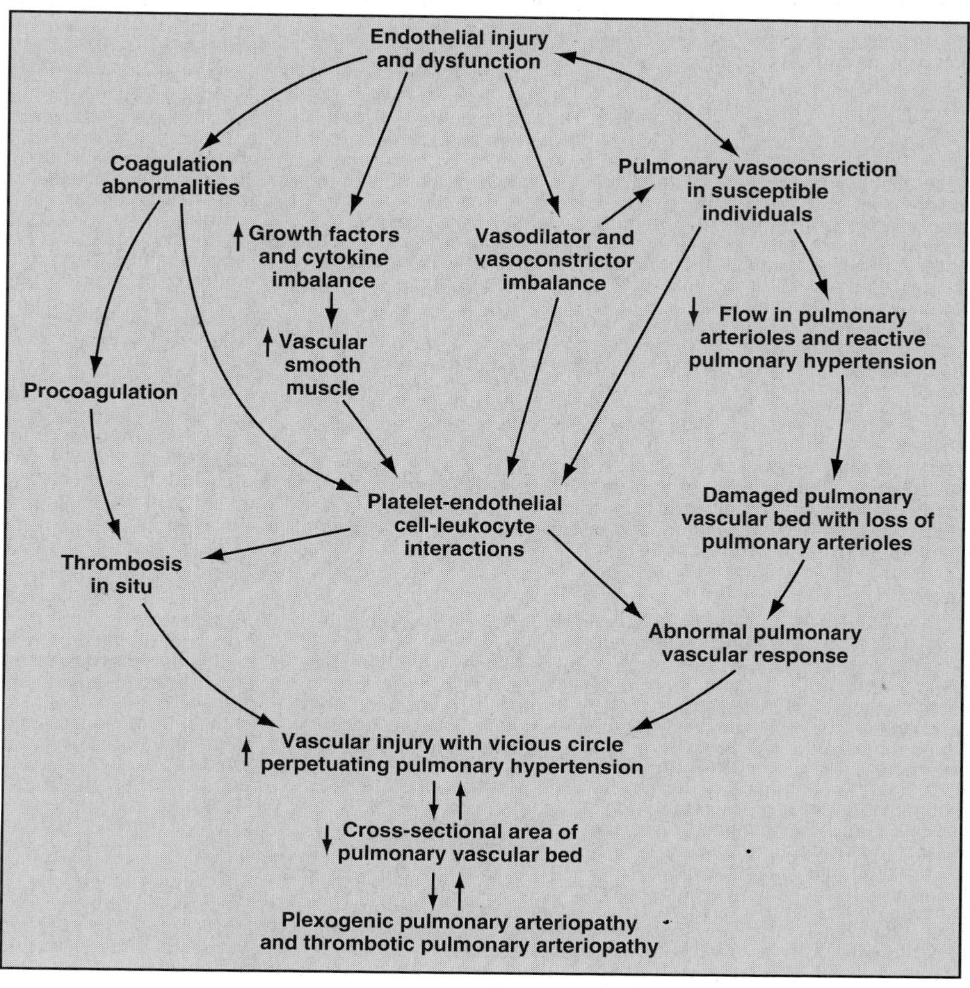

disease and comparably sized ventricular septal defects. Presumably there is a genetic basis for these differences in pulmonary vascular reactivity, just as there appears to be a genetic basis for the increased reactivity of the systemic vascular bed in essential systemic hypertension.

Specific Risk Factors in the Development of Pulmonary Hypertension

Although pulmonary hypertension can be the clear result of a disease process affecting the pulmonary parenchyma or vessels directly, a number of conditions have been identified that appear to be associated with the development of primary or unexplained pulmonary hypertension in which a clearly defined cause-and-effect relationship are lacking. Whereas risk factors for the development of PPH were once thought to be uncommon, a recent study suggests that it may be the rule rather than the exception.[48] Obesity,[48] portal hypertension,[73–82] anorexigens,[83–87] human immunodeficiency virus,[88–92] systemic hypertension,[93–96] and chronically increased pulmonary blood flow[97,98] have all been implicated as risk factors in the development of pulmonary hypertension. The translation into PPH may depend upon other clinical features such as the patient's age or gender at the time of disease expression. However, PPH should no longer be considered a constellation of distinct subtypes, but rather the expression of an entire spectrum of vascular responses to endothelial injury resulting in vasoconstriction and in situ thrombosis, with associated varying degrees of intimal proliferation.[64]

PORTAL HYPERTENSION

Pulmonary abnormalities have been commonly associated with the development of hepatic cirrhosis and portal hypertension. These include hypoxemia and intrapulmonary shunting,[73] portal-pulmonary shunting, impaired hypoxic pulmonary vasoconstriction,[73] and pulmonary hypertension.[74,78–82] Studies show that the liver plays an important role in regulating pulmonary vascular tone. Although the relative risk associated with the development of pulmonary hypertension in patients with portal hypertension is unknown, a large postmortem study from the Johns Hopkins Hospital showed that the prevalence of unexplained or pulmonary hypertension in patients with cirrhosis was 5.6 times higher than that of PPH alone.[74] There was early speculation that the mechanism related to recurrent thromboemboli originating from the portal vein which gain access to the pulmonary circulation via portal-systemic venous shunts, whereas others hypothesized that the development of pulmonary hypertension may be a result of the inability of cirrhotic livers to detoxify vasoactive substances normally absorbed from the gastrointestinal track and activated by the hepatic circulation.[83]

Elevated levels of tumor necrosis factor-α (TNF-α) have recently been reported in rats made portal-hypertensive by partial ligation of the portal vein.[75] TNF-α is a cytokine which, in addition to contributing to a hyperdynamic state, has been implicated in causing structural and metabolic damage to vascular endothelial cells.[76,77] Increased levels of platelet activating factor have also been reported in cirrhosis.

Patients who develop PPH in association with cirrhosis appear to be similar to patients without cirrhosis with the sole exception that they tend to have higher cardiac outputs and consequently lower calculated systemic and pulmonary vascular resistances, which are characteristic of the cirrhotic state.[78]

ANOREXIGENS

A marked increase in the incidence of PPH among the populations of Austria, Germany, and Switzerland in 1967, associated with the use of aminorex, suggested that in predisposed individuals aminorex could lead to the development of severe pulmonary vascular disease.[83] Aminorex has similarities to both adrenalin and ephedrine in its chemical structure and is a potent anorexigen. The influence of aminorex became apparent because of a marked increase in the number of patients with PPH admitted to hospitals between 1967 and 1973. The female to male incidence was 4.5:1 but may reflect the fact that aminorex was more often used by women than by men. The clinical features of pulmonary hypertension in affected patients were identical to those attributed to PPH. The mechanism by which aminorex may induce pulmonary hypertension has never been resolved, but the fact that it occurred in less than 1 per cent of patients exposed to the drug points to some underlying predisposition. Of note, however, is that the association occurred not only with aminorex but with other amphetamine-like agents as well.

More recently, PPH has been associated with the use of the appetite suppressants fenfluramine and dexfenfluramine.[84–87] A large series from France has shown an increased likelihood of developing pulmonary hypertension when exposed to these drugs, particularly for periods of greater than 3 months. Although they are known to decrease serotonin uptake, the mechanism by which they produce pulmonary hypertension remains unknown. As with aminorex, only a small percentage of the people exposed developed pulmonary hypertension. Whether or not the pulmonary hypertension is reversible upon discontinuation of usage remains unknown at this time.

HIV INFECTION

Over the past 5 years there have been reports of patients with HIV infection developing unexplained or primary pulmonary hypertension.[88–92] A series of 20 patients from France were recently reported,[91] but the majority of the them had a history of intravenous heroin abuse, raising the possibility of more than one risk factor contributing to the pulmonary hypertension. The patients with HIV tended to be younger, with less severe symptoms and lower values of pulmonary vascular resistance. However, in most other clinical parameters they were quite similar to patients with PPH. The mechanism by which HIV infection causes pulmonary hypertension is unclear, but it does not appear to be simply a phenomenon of immunodeficiency. Attempts to localize the HIV infection to the pulmonary vascular endothelium with electron microscopy, immunohistochemistry, DNA in situ hybridization, and polymerase chain reaction techniques have been unsuccessful.[92] The nonspecific finding of tubuloreticular intracytoplasmic inclusions on electron microscopy suggests that the HIV virus may be related to PPH via some mediator such as interferon-α and β that is released from the HIV infection.[92]

SYSTEMIC HYPERTENSION

Systemic hypertension is two to three times more common in patients with PPH than in an age-matched population.[48] The underlying mechanisms related to the development of essential hypertension are quite diverse, but the possibility exists that in some patients the mechanism that increases systemic vascular resistance similarly affects the pulmonary vascular bed.[93,94] It has been suggested that neurohumoral factors may play a role[95] or that the pulmonary vasculature is hypercontractile and overreacts to sympathetic stimulation.[96] Given that essential hypertension is extremely common in the general population, other confounding factors likely contribute to the development of pulmonary hypertension in affected individuals.

INCREASED PULMONARY BLOOD FLOW

For many years the observation has been made that patients with atrial septal defect can develop PPH as an adult.[97] However, the incidence of this is extremely low, raising the possibility that they are two completely unrelated events. It is possible that chronically increased pulmonary blood flow may have effects on the pulmonary endothelium through some type of mechanical means that would cause perturbations in the integrity of the vascular wall and lead to the development of pulmonary vascular disease. Recently increased pulmonary blood flow from hyperthyroidism and beriberi have been reported to be associated with the development of unexplained pulmonary hypertension, suggesting that high pulmonary blood flow,[98] rather than mere coincidence, is the basis for the development of pulmonary hypertension in patients with pre-tricuspid shunts such as atrial septal defect or anomalous pulmonary venous drainage.

FAMILIAL PPH

A familial incidence of PPH in a minority of patients (approximately 6 per cent) has been documented.[46] The transmission in families is unpredictable, and incomplete penetrance, in which the gene is transmitted to affected progeny by individuals who manifest no evidence of disease, is a major confounding feature.[99–102] The vertical transmission in some families strongly suggests the action of a single dominant gene. Recently, genetic anticipation, by which there is worsening of the disease in subsequent generations manifest by an earlier age of onset, has been described.[103] Genetic anticipation has been described in several unrelated neurologic diseases, in which the molecular basis has been attributed to trinucleotide repeat expansion. It is hoped that newer methodology designed to detect single copies of large trinucleotide repeats may lead to the discovery of a gene responsible for familial PPH.

The clinical features of familial PPH are identical to those in patients with the sporadic form with the exception that it typically has an earlier diagnosis from the onset of symptoms, likely due to an increased awareness by the patient or family.[104] Survival also appears similar between the sporadic and familial forms, as an analysis of 36 familial PPH patients found few differences from 41 patients with the sporadic disease. Pathologically all of the characteristics of patients with PPH have been described, including plexogenic arteriopathy, thrombotic arteriopathy, pulmonary veno-occlusive disease, and even pulmonary capillary hemangiomatosis.

The prevalence of antinuclear antibodies in patients with PPH is considerably higher than in the population at large.[105] Some investigators have suggested that PPH may be a forme fruste of an underlying collagen vascular disease. Recently an association between PPH and the major histocompatibility complex has been described in children.[106] Specifically, increased frequencies of HLA-DR3, DRw52, and DQw2 as well as decreased DR5 have been reported. The familial clustering of these HLA antigens in four families with PPH raises the possibility of a susceptibility factor for PPH located near the major histocompatibility locus on chromosome 6p21.3.

PATHOLOGICAL FINDINGS

In 1973 the World Health Organization (WHO) characterized PPH as three distinct subsets: plexogenic arteriopathy, recurrent thromboembolism, and pulmonary veno-occlusive disease.[46] Since that time, however, several large pathology series of patients with PPH have allowed better characterization and understanding of the pathological changes that occur in these patients[57,107,108] (Table 25–1). A classification developed by Heath and Edwards for pulmonary vascular disease from congenital heart disease has been adapted to patients with PPH because of the striking similarities in many of these patients.[109] However, the Heath and Edwards classification implies a natural progression of pulmonary vascular changes not typical of the patients with PPH.

Pathological changes of PPH can be limited to the pulmonary arteriolar circulation or involve the capillaries, venules, and veins (Fig. 25–6). The most common vascular changes can be best characterized as a *hypertensive pulmonary arteriopathy,* which is present in 85 per cent of cases.[57] These changes involve medial hypertrophy of the arteries and arterioles, often in conjunction with other vascular changes. Isolated medial hypertrophy is uncommon, and when it exists it has been assumed to represent an early stage in the disease. The presence of a plexogenic pulmonary arteriopathy is the most common type of hypertensive arteriopathy seen in patients with PPH.[107] It is characterized by medial hypertrophy along with intimal proliferation and other complex lesions. The intimal proliferation may be concentric laminar intimal fibrosis, eccentric intimal fibrosis, or concentric nonlaminar intimal fibrosis. The frequency of these findings differs from case to case and within regions in the same lung of the same patient. In addition, plexiform and dilatation lesions, as well as a necrotizing arteritis, may be seen throughout the lungs. These lesions, however, are not pathognomonic for PPH but representative of a chronic, severe pulmonary hypertensive state.

The other major classification of vascular changes in PPH is a *thrombotic pulmonary arteriopathy.*[57] The typical features include medial hypertrophy of the arteries and arterioles with both eccentric and concentric nonlaminar intimal fibrosis. The presence of colander lesions, representing recanalized thrombi, is also typical. These lesions are believed to arise as a result of a primary in situ thrombosis of the small vascular arteries and not from recurrent pulmonary embolism.

On rare occasion a diffuse pulmonary arteritis with secondary thrombosis has been reported in patients with PPH, predominantly in children.[108,109] Although the association has not been reported in patients with underlying collagen vascular diseases, it may reflect the vascular response to a specific but not clearly identified risk factor.

PULMONARY VENO-OCCLUSIVE DISEASE

Pulmonary veno-occlusive disease is a rare form of PPH, observed in approximately 5 per cent of cases.[57,58] The histopathological diagnosis is based on the presence of obstructive eccentric fibrous intimal pads within the pulmonary veins and venules. There is often arterialization of the pulmonary veins with associated alveolar capillary congestion. Other changes of chronic pulmonary hypertension such as medial hypertrophy and muscularization of the arterioles with eccentric intimal fibrosis may also be present.[110] The pulmonary venous obstruction explains the increased pulmonary capillary wedge pressure described in patients in the late stages of the disease, and the increase in basilar bronchovascular markings described on the chest radiograph. These clinical findings, along with a perfusion lung showing diffuse, patchy nonsegmental abnormalities, is highly suggestive of the diagnosis on a clinical basis.[111]

PULMONARY CAPILLARY HEMANGIOMATOSIS

This extremely rare condition is characterized by proliferation of the thin-walled microvessels that infiltrate the peribronchial and perivascular interstitium and lung parenchyma.[112–114] On occasion it may be confused with pulmonary veno-occlusive disease. The lesions are often patchy and the proliferating vessels may form small nodules within the alveolar interstitial space. These thin-walled vessels

TABLE 25–1 HISTOPATHOLOGIC CLASSIFICATION OF PRIMARY PULMONARY VASCULAR DISEASE

PRESENT CLASSIFICATION	PREVIOUS CLASSIFICATION	CHARACTERISTIC HISTOPATHOLOGIC FEATURES*
Primary Pulmonary Arteriopathy with		
Plexiform lesions with or without thrombotic lesions	Plexogenic pulmonary arteriopathy	Plexiform lesions; medial hypertrophy, eccentric or concentric-laminar intimal proliferation and fibrosis, fibrinoid degeneration, arteritis, dilatation lesions, and thrombotic lesions
Thrombotic lesions	Thromboembolic pulmonary arteriopathy	Thrombi (fresh, organizing, or organized, and recanalized-collander lesions); varying degrees of medial hypertrophy; no plexiform lesions
Isolated medial hypertrophy	Plexogenic pulmonary arteriopathy	Medial hypertrophy; increase of medial muscle, muscular arteries, muscularization of nonmuscularized intra-acinar arteries; no appreciable intimal or luminal obstructive lesions
Intimal fibrosis and medial hypertrophy	Plexogenic pulmonary arteriopathy	Eccentric or concentric-laminar proliferation and fibrosis; varying degrees of medial hypertrophy; no thrombotic or plexiform lesions
Isolated arteritis	Plexogenic pulmonary arteriopathy	Active or healed arteritis limited to pulmonary arteries; varying degrees of medial hypertrophy, intimal fibrosis, and thrombotic lesions; no plexiform lesions
Pulmonary veno-occlusive disease	Pulmonary veno-occlusive disease	Intimal fibrosis and recanalized thrombi (collander lesions); pulmonary veins and venules; arterialized veins, capillary congestion, alveolar edema and siderophages, dilated lymphatics, pleural and septal edema and arterial medial hypertrophy, intimal fibrosis, and thrombotic lesions
Pulmonary capillary hemangiomatosis	—	Infiltrating thin-walled blood vessels widespread throughout pulmonary parenchyma, pleura, bronchi, and walls of pulmonary veins and arteries

* Medial hypertrophy may be accompanied by muscularization of arterioles.

From Pietra, G. G., Edwards, W. D., Kay, J. M., et al.: Histopathology of primary pulmonary hypertension: A qualitative and quantitative study of pulmonary blood vessels from 58 patients in the National Heart, Lung, and Blood Institute Primary Pulmonary Hypertension Registry. Circulation *80:*1198, 1989. Copyright 1989 by American Heart Association.

are prone to bleeding and may be manifest clinically as overt hemoptysis in affected patients. The perfusion lung scan in these patients may show "hot spots" reflective of the local areas within the lung that have increased vascularity. These are typically seen at the lung periphery and can be confirmed by pulmonary angiography. The natural history of this form of PPH is not yet defined.

CLINICAL FEATURES

NATURAL HISTORY AND SYMPTOMATOLOGY. The most extensive study on the natural history of PPH was reported from the NIH Registry on Primary Pulmonary Hypertension from 1981 to 1987.[46] The study included the long-term follow-up of 194 patients in whom PPH was diagnosed by established clinical and hemodynamic criteria. Sixty-three per cent of the patients were female, with the mean age of 36 ± 15 years (range 1 to 81 years) at the time of diagnosis. The mean interval from the onset of symptoms to diagnosis was 2 years, and the most common presenting symptoms were dyspnea (60 per cent), fatigue (19 per cent), syncope or near syncope (13 per cent), and Raynaud's phenomenon (10 per cent). There was no ethnic differentiation, with 12.3 per cent being black and 2.3 per cent being Hispanic.

Syncope is a characteristic symptom of PPH, assumed to be due to a fixed cardiac output. A recent study on the systolic function and interactions of the left and right ventricles in patients with PPH revealed an increased right ventricular end-diastolic volume and reduced right ventricular ejection fraction, with a greater stroke volume than the left ventricle.[115] The mechanism for maintaining cardiac output with exercise was primarily through increased heart rate, as the stroke volume actually decreased. Right ventricular ejection fraction decreased with exercise, suggesting exercise-induced right ventricular failure. This is expected because pulmonary artery pressure increases with exercise in PPH. Left ventricular ejection fraction is maintained, however, but left ventricular end-diastolic volume decreases and left ventricular end-systolic volume becomes extremely small, suggesting that the left ventricle is shortening to its maximal extent. The fact that left ventricular end-diastolic and systolic volumes decreased, whereas right ventricular end-systolic and diastolic volumes remained unchanged, supports the concept that underfilling, and not external compression, accounts for the small left ventricular chamber size observed in PPH. Syncope occurs because of exercise-induced right ventricular failure whereby heart rate becomes the only mechanism by which to increase cardiac output, which has limited effectiveness.

On *physical examination* an increased pulmonic component of the second heart sound was the most common finding (93 per cent), with tricuspid regurgitation noted in 40 per cent and peripheral edema in 32 per cent. In 90 per cent of patients the chest radiograph revealed enlargement of the main pulmonary arteries, and the electrocardiogram revealed right ventricular hypertrophy in 87 per cent. The clinical profiles of these patients were remarkably similar to those in a previously reported retrospective study of 120 patients from the Mayo Clinic.[65] In the Mayo Clinic series, 75 per cent of the patients were women with a mean age of 34 years (range 3 to 64 years) and a mean interval from onset of symptoms to diagnosis of 1.9 years.

The NIH Registry also revealed that restrictive changes in pulmonary function testing and reduced diffusing capacity for carbon monoxide were very common, with the forced vital capacity approximately 80 per cent of predicted and the diffusing capacity 70 per cent of predicted. These changes, however, do not relate with any measure of severity of the pulmonary hypertension. An additional, virtually universal finding was mild to moderate hypoxemia (mean Po_2 72 ± 16 mm Hg), which is attributed to the effect of a low mixed venous oxygen from low cardiac output amplified by underlying ventilation-perfusion inequality.

The hemodynamic findings also suggested that the severity of the disease could be related to a rising right atrial pressure and falling cardiac index, both of which reflect underlying right ventricular dysfunction. The fact that the mean pulmonary artery pressure was similar in patients whose duration of symptoms was less than 1 year and those who were symptomatic for more than 3 years suggests that the pulmonary artery pressure rises to fairly high levels early in the course of the disease.

Univariate analysis from the Registry pointed to the mean right atrial pressure, mean pulmonary artery pressure, and cardiac index as well as the diffusing capacity from carbon monoxide as significantly related to mortality.[116] In addition, the New York Heart Association classification also has been shown to relate very strongly to survival (Fig. 25–8). Based on estimates obtained from the proportional hazards model, a regression equation was developed that describes the relation between these three hemodynamic variables and subsequent mortality.

$$P(t) = [(t)]A(x,y,z)$$
$$H(t) = [0.88 - 0.14t + 0.01t^2]$$
$$A(x,y,z) = e^{(0.007325x) + (0.0526y) - (0.3275z)}$$

Where p(t) = per cent survival at t years, t = number of years, x = mean pulmonary artery pressure, y = mean right atrial pressure, and z = cardiac index. This equation has since been validated in two subsequent studies,[117,118] suggesting that baseline hemodynamic characteristics are very predictive of outcome.

The most common cause of death in patients with PPH in the NIH Registry was progressive right heart failure (47 per cent). Sudden cardiac death (both witnessed and unwitnessed) occurred in 26 per cent. Of interest is that sudden cardiac death was limited to patients who were New York Heart Association Class IV, suggesting that it is a manifestation of end-stage disease rather than a phenomenon that occurs early or unpredictably in the clinical course of the disease. The remainder of the patients died of some other medical complication such as pneumonia or

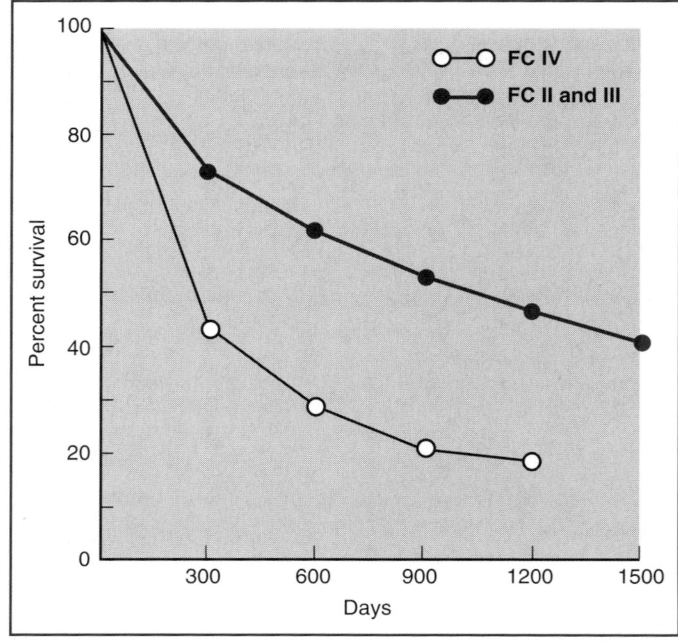

FIGURE 25–8. Five-year survival of patients enrolled in the NIH Registry on PPH based on New York Heart Association functional class. Survival of patients who were FC II and III was slightly greater than 3 years, whereas the mean survival of patients who were FC IV was approximately 6 months. (Adapted from D'Alonzo, G. E., Barst, R. G., Levy, P. S., et al.: Survival in patients with primary pulmonary hypertension: Results of a national prospective registry. Ann. Intern. Med. *115*:343, 1991.)

bleeding, suggesting that patients with PPH do not tolerate coexistent medical conditions well. In the Registry experience there were no deaths or sustained morbidity related to the diagnostic evaluation done at baseline assessment. It should be pointed out, however, that these were university centers with an established experience in the management of patients with PPH.

MECHANISMS FOR RIGHT VENTRICULAR FAILURE. It is presumed that right ventricular dysfunction in patients with chronic pulmonary hypertension is a result of chronic pressure overload and associated volume overload with the development of tricuspid regurgitation. However, animal studies suggest that right ventricular ischemia may also be a feature and potentially a very common one.[118–121] The mechanism of right ventricular failure in pulmonary hypertension is complex. The chronic pressure overload that induces right ventricular hypertrophy and reduced contractility has been shown to cause a reduction in coronary blood flow to the right ventricular myocardium, which can produce right ventricular ischemia, both acutely and chronically. This appears to be a result of a reduction in right ventricular coronary artery driving pressure. In an interesting animal study by Vlahakes et al.,[122] acute right ventricular failure due to right ventricular hypertension was overcome by increasing central aortic pressure, which resulted in increasing right ventricular coronary driving pressure. Murray and Vatner[123] reported that a moderate increase in aortic pressure was accompanied by a large increase in right ventricular myocardial perfusion only when the autonomic nervous system was blocked with an alpha blocker. As the symptom of angina associated with PPH is characteristic of myocardial ischemia, it likely represents ongoing ischemia due to this phenomenon.

The clinical course of patients with PPH can be highly variable. However, with the onset of overt right ventricular failure manifested by worsening symptoms and systemic venous congestion, patient survival is generally limited to approximately 6 months. Understanding the clinical course of patients with PPH is important especially when considering major interventional therapy such as organ transplantation.

PHYSICAL EXAMINATION. Findings are consistent with pulmonary hypertension and right ventricular pressure overload: a large *a* wave in the jugular venous pulse; a low-volume carotid arterial pulse with a normal upstroke; a left parasternal (right ventricular) heave; a systolic pulsation produced by a dilated, tense pulmonary artery in the second left interspace; an ejection click and flow murmur in the same area; a closely split second heart sound with a loud pulmonic component; and a fourth heart sound of right ventricular origin. Late in the course, signs of right ventricular failure (hepatomegaly, peripheral edema, and ascites) may be present. Patients with severe pulmonary hypertension may also have prominent *v* waves in the jugular venous pulse, owing to tricuspid regurgitation; a third heart sound of right ventricular origin; a high-pitched early diastolic murmur of pulmonic regurgitation; and a holosystolic murmur of tricuspid regurgitation. Cyanosis is a late finding in PPH and may be worsened by a patent foramen ovale with right-to-left shunting. Other causes for cyanosis include a markedly reduced cardiac output with systemic vasoconstriction and ventilation-perfusion mismatches in the lung. Uncommonly, the left laryngeal nerve becomes paralyzed as a consequence of compression by a dilated pulmonary artery (Ortner's syndrome).[124]

LABORATORY FINDINGS

HEMATOLOGICAL AND CHEMICAL STUDIES. Results of these studies are usually normal in patients with PPH. If there is chronic arterial oxygen desaturation, polycythemia may be present. A number of investigators have reported hypercoagulable states, abnormal platelet function, defects in fibrinolysis, and other abnormalities of coagulation in patients with PPH.[66,69] Abnormal liver function tests can indicate right ventricular failure with resultant systemic venous hypertension.

ELECTROCARDIOGRAPHY. The electrocardiogram in PPH usually exhibits right atrial and right ventricular enlargement. A direct correlation between the amplitude of the R in V_1, the R/S ratio in V_1, and the level of pulmonary arterial pressure has been reported.[125]

ROENTGENOGRAPHY. Radiographic examination of the chest in patients with PPH shows enlargement of the main pulmonary artery and its major branches, with marked tapering of peripheral arteries.[126,127] The right ventricle and atrium may also be enlarged. Fluoroscopic examination may disclose exaggerated pulsations of secondary pulmonary arterial branches, reflecting an elevation in pulmonary arterial pulse pressure. However, in contrast to the plethoric peripheral lung fields in patients with left-to-right shunts, oligemia is noted in these lung regions in patients with PPH. It has been suggested that survival in PPH correlates inversely with the size of the main pulmonary artery[127]—a reasonable suggestion because the latter correlates with the height of the pulmonary arterial pressure. The diameter of the pulmonary artery may be determined from computed tomographic (CT) scans and used to estimate pulmonary artery pressures.[128]

PULMONARY FUNCTION TESTS. Pulmonary function tests typically show mild restriction with a reduced diffusion capacity for carbon monoxide (DL_{CO}) and hypoxemia with hypocapnea. Some patients have increased residual volumes and reduced maximum voluntary ventilation.

ECHOCARDIOGRAPHY. This usually demonstrates enlargement of the right atrium and ventricle, normal or small left

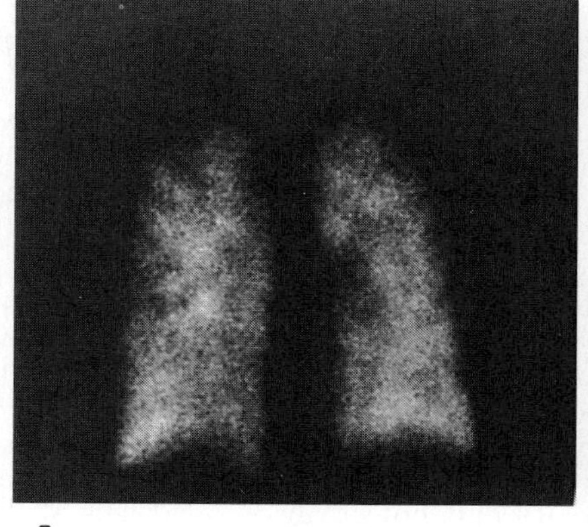
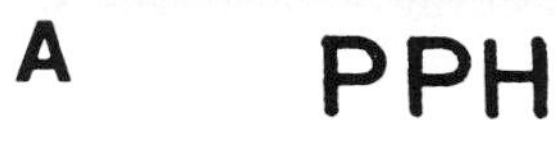

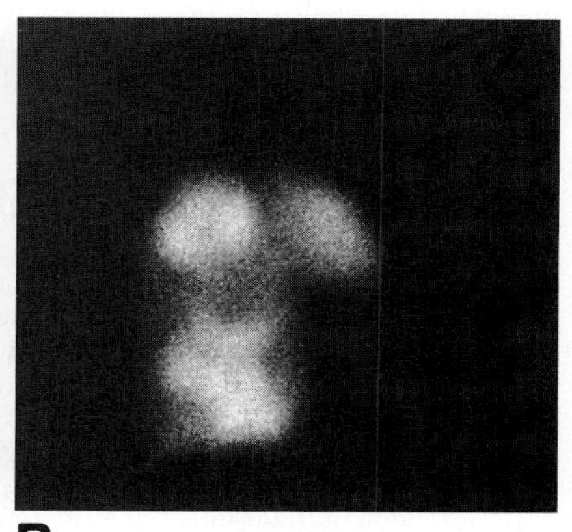

FIGURE 25–9. Perfusion lung scans in patients with pulmonary hypertension. *A*, Patient with primary pulmonary hypertension (PPH). *B*, Patient with pulmonary thromboembolism causing pulmonary hypertension (PTE). Both perfusion scans are abnormal. The scan on the patient with PPH shows a mottled distribution in a nonsegmental, nonanatomic manner. The scan on the patient with PTE reveals lobar, segmental, and subsegmental defects highly suggestive of an anatomic obstruction to pulmonary blood flow.

ventricular dimensions, and a thickened interventricular septum. The septal/posterior left ventricular wall ratio may be abnormally increased, as in hypertrophic obstructive cardiomyopathy, but the other echocardiographic signs characteristic of that condition are not present. Systolic prolapse of the mitral valve is frequently present, as is abnormal septal motion of the ventricular septum, due to chronic right ventricular pressure overload and reduced left ventricular filling.[129,130] Doppler echocardiographic evidence of right ventricular systolic hypertension may be obtained by measuring the velocity of the tricuspid regurgitant jet and using the Bernoulli formula (see p. 69). Doppler techniques have demonstrated left ventricular diastolic dysfunction with marked dependence on atrial contraction for ventricular filling.[130]

LUNG SCINTIGRAPHY. A perfusion lung scan is an essential component in making the correct diagnosis of PPH. It may reveal a relatively normal perfusion pattern or diffuse, patchy perfusion abnormalities.[131] The severity of the perfusion abnormality in lung scans does not parallel the hemodynamics, as serial lung scans performed in patients with PPH over time do not show progressive changes consistent with the patients' worsening clinical state.[131] A perfusion lung scan should help distinguish patients with PPH from those who have pulmonary hypertension secondary to chronic pulmonary thromboembolism[132] (Fig. 25–9). The risk associated with lung scans in PPH has been grossly overstated. The early literature reported three patients with pulmonary hypertension who died following lung scans, but it is not clear that the deaths were caused by the procedure. In the NIH Registry on PPH not one morbid clinical event was associated with the performance of lung scan in any of the patients with pulmonary hypertension.[46]

PULMONARY ANGIOGRAPHY. Pulmonary angiography is essential to establish the correct diagnosis in a patient with presumed PPH in whom the perfusion lung scan suggests segmental or lobar defects. Typically pulmonary angiography demonstrates large central pulmonary arteries with marked peripheral tapering. Postmortem arteriograms demonstrate the absence of "background haze" secondary to the loss of small, nonmuscular pulmonary arterioles[67] (Fig. 25–10). Although pulmonary angiography carries an increased risk in patients with PPH, it can be performed safely if adequate precautions are taken.[65] The NIH Registry contains no deaths or serious morbidity associated with pulmonary angiography.

Maintenance of adequate oxygenation by the administration of supplemental oxygen and the avoidance of vasovagal reactions (and rapid treatment of those that occur with intravenous atropine) should reduce the associated risk in this patient group. The placement of an arterial line for continuous arterial pressure monitoring is advised, and nonionic contrast agents appear to be better tolerated. Injections are preferably limited to the individual lungs or specific lobes to reduce the contrast load. Pulmonary wedge angiography, using a segmental angiographic technique with hand injection of small amounts of angiographic contrast through the terminal lumen of a balloon-flotation catheter while the balloon is inflated, is not a substitute for pulmonary angiography.

CARDIAC CATHETERIZATION. The diagnosis of PPH cannot be confirmed without cardiac catheterization (Table 25–2). Besides allowing the exclusion of other causes, it also establishes the severity of disease and allows the assessment of prognosis. By definition, patients with PPH should have a low or normal pulmonary capillary wedge pressure. Although it has often been stated that one may be unable to obtain an accurate wedge pressure in these patients, this is rarely the case in experienced hands.[133] However, when an increased wedge pressure is obtained, it must be correlated with left ventricular end-diastolic pressure and not attributed to a "falsely elevated" reading. It has been shown that left ventricular diastolic compliance becomes significantly

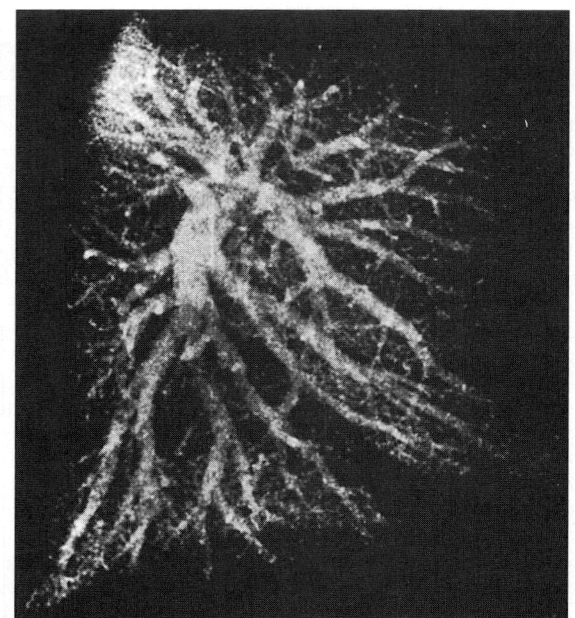

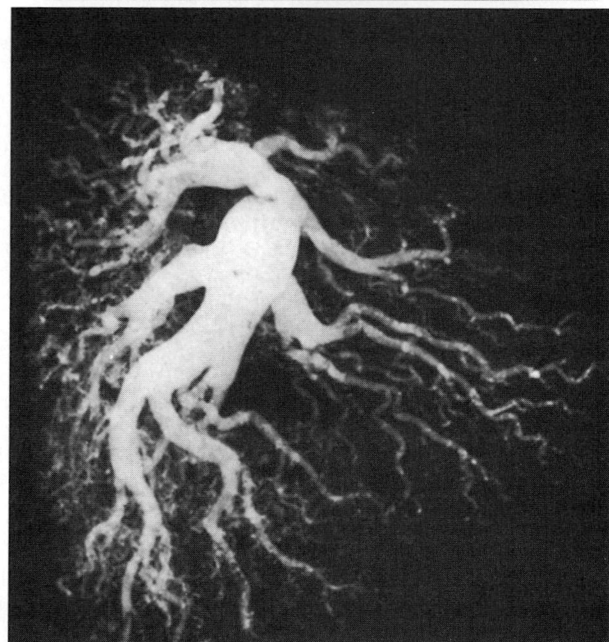

FIGURE 25–10. *A*, Postmortem pulmonary arteriogram of a normal lung in a 22-year-old man. The caliber of the pulmonary arteries tapers down gradually, and there is a rather dense background filling of vessels. *B*, Postmortem pulmonary arteriogram from an 18-year-old man with unexplained plexogenic pulmonary arteriopathy (primary pulmonary hypertension). The main branches are dilated. (From Wagenvoort, C. A., and Wagenvoort, N.: Pathology of Pulmonary Hypertension. New York, copyright 1977, reprinted by permission of John Wiley and Sons, Inc.)

impaired in PPH and parallels the severity of the disease; thus, pulmonary capillary wedge pressures tend to rise slightly in the late stages of PPH, although they rarely exceed 16 mm Hg.[134] The measurements of all right-sided pressures are properly made at expiration to avoid incorporating negative intrathoracic pressures.

It can be extremely difficult to pass a catheter into the pulmonary artery in patients with pulmonary hypertension owing to the tricuspid regurgitation, dilated right atrium and ventricle, and low cardiac output. The flow-directed thermodilution balloon catheters which are properly used also lack stiffness and can be difficult to place. A specific flow-directed thermodilution balloon catheter has been developed for patients with pulmonary hypertension (Ameri-

TABLE 25–2 APPLICATIONS OF CATHETERIZATION IN ESTABLISHING ETIOLOGIC DIAGNOSIS OF PULMONARY HYPERTENSION

CONDITION	TEST APPLIED	FINDING
Congenital heart disease	Step-up in O_2 saturation in right heart Step-down in O_2 saturation in left heart Cardiac angiography	Left-to-right shunt and location of shunt Right-to-left shunt and location of shunt Anatomic definition
Peripheral pulmonary artery stenoses	Intrapulmonary arterial pressure Pulmonary angiogram	Intrapulmonary arterial pressure gradients Pulmonary arterial branch stenoses
Major pulmonary arterial occlusion by clot, or tumor*	Continuous pressure recording from distal pulmonary artery to main pulmonary artery Selective or main pulmonary angiography	Focal pressure gradient in a lobar or larger pulmonary artery, intravascular filling defect or narrowing
Mitral stenosis Cor triatriatum Supravalvular mitral ring	Simultaneous wedge and left ventricular pressure recording	An elevated wedge pressure and mean mitral valve diastolic pressure gradient >3 mm Hg at rest, both of which increase with exercise
Mitral regurgitation	Simultaneous wedge and left ventricular pressure recording Left ventriculogram	Large systolic pressure wave in wedge tracing. Regurgitation of contrast from left ventricular angiogram into the left atrium.
Left ventricular diastolic dysfunction	Left ventricular pressure	Left ventricular end-diastolic pressure >15 mm Hg LVEDP response to intravenous fluid challenge; normalization of LVEDP with marked reduction in pulmonary artery pressure with intravenous nitroprusside.

* Ventilation and perfusion lung scans precede catheterization.
LVEDP = left ventricular end-diastolic pressure
Modified from Reeves, J. T., and Groves, B. M.: Approach to the patient with pulmonary hypertension. *In* Weir, E. K., and Reeves, J. T.: Pulmonary Hypertension. Mt. Kisco, NY, Futura Publishing Co., 1984, p. 20.

can Edwards Laboratories, Irvine, California) which has an extra port for the placement of a 0.32-inch guidewire to provide better stiffness to the catheter.[135] The risk associated with cardiac catheterization in patients with PPH is extremely low in experienced hands, but deaths have been reported.[65]

DIAGNOSIS

(Table 25–3)

It is essential that diagnostic efforts be pursued vigorously in patients with severe pulmonary hypertension in order to ensure that no patient with secondary pulmonary hypertension is erroneously classified as having PPH. Secondary pulmonary hypertension is often treatable in that the cause can be attacked directly. Patients with PPH may tolerate diagnostic procedures poorly. These individuals can experience sudden cardiovascular collapse and even death during or shortly after the induction of general anesthesia for surgical procedures, during cardiac catheterization and angiography.

The *differential diagnosis* of PPH includes a number of well-defined causes of secondary pulmonary hypertension. Exclusion of mitral stenosis, congenital cardiac defects (including cor triatriatum), pulmonary thromboembolism, and pulmonary venous obstruction by means of catheterization and angiography is imperative. "Silent" mitral stenosis, i.e., without the characteristic diastolic murmur, can be excluded by means of echocardiographic visualization of the motion of the mitral valve and the absence of a transvalvular pressure gradient (Chap. 32). *Congenital cardiac defects* with Eisenmenger syndrome can usually be ruled out if significant left-to-right or right-to-left shunts are absent, although occasional patients with equal pulmonary and systemic vascular resistances may have no detectable shunt at rest. Transesophageal echocardiography can reliably detect congenital cardiac defects and distinguish an atrial septal defect from a patent foramen ovale.[136] *Cor triatriatum* (see p. 923) is recognized by appropriate hemodynamic studies and angiographic visualization of the left atrial membrane. This entity presents a characteristic left atrial echocardiogram with normal mitral valve motion. Cardiac catheterization reveals a hemodynamic pattern similar in some ways to mitral stenosis, i.e., a diastolic pressure gradient between the left ventricle and the pulmonary capillary bed. *Pulmonary embolism* (Chap. 46) can be excluded by pulmonary angiography,[137] and *sickle cell disease with in situ pulmonary vascular thrombosis* (Chap. 57) can be evaluated by hemoglobin electrophoresis. The presence of severe *pulmonary parenchymal disease* can be recognized by the characteristic physical findings, chest roentgenogram, pulmonary function tests, and high-resolution chest computed tomography. *Collagen vascular disease* is suggested by the involvement of other organ systems or the presence of abnormal immunological phenomena, such as antinuclear antibodies and LE cells (Chap. 56).

TREATMENT

LIFE STYLE CHANGES. The diagnosis of PPH does not necessarily imply total disability for the patient. However, physical activity can be associated with elevated pulmonary artery pressures, as marked hemodynamic changes have been documented to occur early in the onset of increased physical activity.[138] For that reason, graded exercise activities, such as bike riding or swimming, in which patients can gradually increase their workload and easily limit the extent of their work, are thought to be safer than isometric activities. Isometric activities such as lifting weights or stair climbing can be associated with syncopal events and should be limited or avoided.

The subject of pregnancy should also be discussed with women of childbearing age. The physiological changes that occur in pregnancy can potentially activate the disease and result in the death of the mother and/or the child.[139] Besides the increased circulating blood volume and oxygen consumption that will increase right ventricular work, circulating procoagulant factors and the risk of pulmonary embolism from deep vein thrombosis and amniotic fluid are serious concerns. Syncope and cardiac arrest have also been reported to occur during active labor and delivery, and a syndrome of postpartum circulatory collapse has also been described.[140] For these reasons surgical sterilization should be given strong consideration by women with PPH or their husbands.

TABLE 25–3 DIAGNOSTIC STUDIES USEFUL FOR ELUCIDATING CAUSES OF PULMONARY HYPERTENSION

POTENTIAL CAUSE OF PULMONARY HYPERTENSION	POSSIBLE DIAGNOSTIC STUDIES
Pulmonary thromboembolic disease	Ventilation/perfusion scans and/or pulmonary angiography
Pulmonary venous thrombosis or obstruction	Chest x-ray, angiography, computed tomography, magnetic resonance imaging
Congenital intra-cardiac shunts causing increased pulmonary blood flow	Transesophageal echocardiography
Increased left atrial pressure; secondary to mitral or aortic valve disease, left ventricular dysfunction, or systemic hypertension	Pulmonary artery wedge pressure or left atrial pressure (via patent foramen ovale) (>15 mm Hg)
Pulmonary airways disease (e.g., chronic bronchitis and emphysema)	Respiratory function tests (FVC/FEV_1)
Hypoxic pulmonary hypertension associated with (i) impaired ventilation; either central (CNS) or peripheral (chest wall problems or upper airway obstruction); (ii) residence at high altitude	Sleep apnea studies and respiratory tests
Interstitial lung disease, pneumoconioses and fibrosis (e.g., silicosis, rheumatoid disease, and sarcoidosis)	Chest x-ray, spirometry and carbon monoxide diffusion, high-resolution chest computed tomography
Collagen disease (e.g., SLE, polyarteritis nodosa, scleroderma)	Serology, immunogenetic studies, skin, muscle, or other tissue biopsy, esophageal motility studies
Parasitic disease (schistosomiasis or filariasis)	Rectal biopsy, complement fixation, skin tests, blood smears
Cirrhosis or portal hypertension	Liver function tests
Peripheral pulmonary artery stenosis (including Takayasu's disease and fibrosing mediastinitis)	Selective pulmonary angiography, or pressure gradient at catheterization
Sickle cell disease	Erythrocyte morphology, hemoglobin electrophoresis
Choriocarcinoma and hydatidiform mole	Serum or urinary beta subunit of chorionic gonadotrophin
Intravenous injection of pulverized pills	Lung biopsy

Modified from Weir, E. K.: Diagnosis and management of primary pulmonary hypertension. *In* Weir, E. K., and Reeves, J. T.: Pulmonary Hypertension. Mt. Kisco, NY, Futura Publishing Co., 1984, p. 141.

DIGOXIN. The value of digoxin in patients with PPH has never been studied specifically. Animal studies performed on the utility of digoxin in right ventricular systolic overload show that prior administration helped prevent the reduction in contractility of the right ventricle.[141] More recently, digoxin has been shown to have sympatholytic properties and to restore baroreceptor tone toward normal in patients with congestive heart failure (see p. 499). Given that patients with advanced PPH have low cardiac outputs with resting tachycardia and systemic venous congestion, it makes intuitive sense to believe that digoxin may be as helpful in these patients as it is in patients with left ventricular failure.

DIURETIC THERAPY. Diuretics appear to be of marked benefit in symptom relief in patients with PPH. Their traditional role has been limited to patients manifesting right ventricular failure and systemic venous congestion. However, patients with advanced PPH can have increased left ventricular filling pressures that contribute to the symptoms of dyspnea and orthopnea which can be relieved with diuretics.[142] Diuretics may also serve to reduce right ventricular wall stress in patients with concomitant tricuspid regurgitation and volume overload. The fear that diuretics will induce systemic hypotension is unfounded, as the main factor limiting the cardiac output is pulmonary vascular resistance and not pulmonary blood volume. Patients with severe venous congestion may require high doses of loop diuretics or the use of combined diuretics. In these instances electrolytes need to be carefully watched for hyponatremia and hypokalemia.

SUPPLEMENTAL OXYGEN THERAPY. Hypoxic pulmonary vasoconstriction can contribute to pulmonary vascular disease in patients with alveolar hypoxia from parenchymal lung disease.[143,144] Supplemental low-flow oxygen alleviates arterial hypoxemia and attenuates the pulmonary hypertension in these disorders[143]; in contrast, most patients with PPH do not exhibit resting hypoxemia and derive little benefit from supplemental oxygen therapy.[145] Patients who experience arterial oxygen desaturation with activity, however, may benefit from ambulatory supplemental oxygen as they develop increased oxygen extraction in the face of a fixed oxygen delivery. Patients with severe right-sided heart failure and resting hypoxemia resulting from a markedly increased oxygen extraction at rest should be treated with continuous oxygen therapy to maintain their arterial oxygen saturation above 90 per cent. Patients with hypoxemia due to a right-to-left shunt via a patent foramen ovale do not improve their level of oxygenation to an appreciable degree with supplemental oxygen.

VASODILATOR TREATMENT

Because of early reports showing a reduction in pulmonary artery pressure following the acute administration of vasodilators,[50–52] it has been presumed that vasodilators are the mainstay of treatment in patients with PPH. This, however, is not supported by the published literature over the past two decades. Vasodilators appear to be effective in a subset of patients with PPH, but many complexities regarding vasodilator administration make their use in these patients very difficult.

The first principle in utilizing vasodilators in patients with PPH is to establish accurate baseline hemodynamics. Because substantial hemodynamic variability has been reported to exist in the pulmonary vascular bed which will produce changes in cardiac output and pulmonary artery pressure from moment to moment, serial baseline recordings are required in order to evaluate the magnitude of change in hemodynamics that may be attributed to variability rather than to drug effect.[146] The practice of attributing "peak" effect of the drug to an administered agent introduces bias into the assessment. Thus, by choosing the highest level of pulmonary artery pressure as the baseline and the subsequent lowest one as drug effect, one may be misled to attribute a favorable influence from a medication when, in fact, no effect, or even an adverse one, is occurring.

It must also be emphasized that the hemodynamic assessment of the entire circulatory system is essential when determining the influence of drugs in these patients. Small changes in pulmonary artery pressure are likely due to variability and are not related to direct drug influence. Changes in pulmonary vascular resistance cannot be directly measured but are computed by the change in pulmonary pressure and cardiac output simultaneously. Because thermodilution cardiac output, the method that is most commonly used in these patients, can have large errors in reproducibility, particular care should be taken in the methodology of thermodilution used in these patients. In addition, when an underlying right-to-left shunt exists or there is concern about severe tricuspid regurgitation, the Fick determination of cardiac output is preferred.

Changes in pulmonary capillary wedge pressure can have important influences on the determination of pulmonary vascular resistance. A

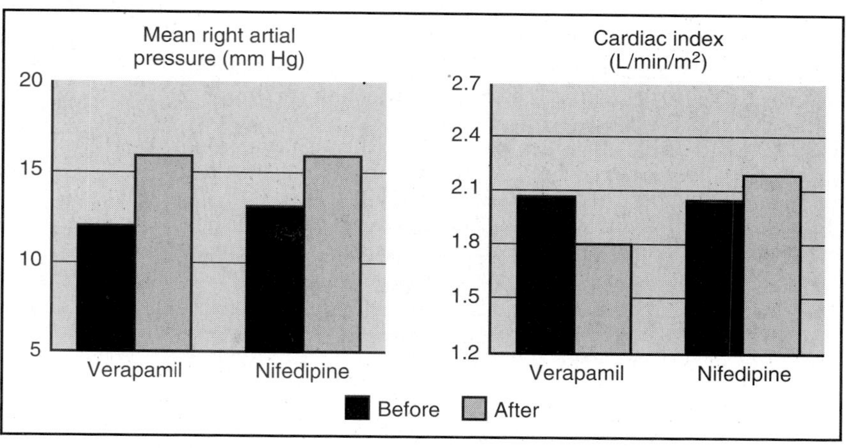

FIGURE 25–11. Adverse effects of calcium blockers in pulmonary hypertension. The hemodynamic effects of verapamil and nifedipine in patients with pulmonary hypertension are shown. An increase in right atrial pressure in association with no significant change in cardiac index as produced by nifedipine suggests that right ventricular dysfunction is occurring. The increased right atrial pressure associated with a fall in cardiac index, as produced by verapamil, suggests that negative inotropic effects are producing overt right ventricular failure. (Adapted from Packer, M., Medina, N., and Yushak, M.: Adverse hemodynamic and clinical effects of calcium channel blockade in pulmonary hypertension secondary to obliterative pulmonary vascular disease. Reprinted with permission from the American College of Cardiology. J. Am. Coll. Cardiol. *4*:890, 1994.)

rising capillary wedge pressure due to an increased cardiac output may be the first sign of impending left ventricular failure and an adverse effect of a drug, whereas the calculated pulmonary vascular resistance may become lower and suggest a beneficial effect. The right atrial pressure also reflects the filling characteristics of the right ventricle. Right atrial pressure increase in the face of a rising cardiac output suggests right ventricular diastolic dysfunction[147] (Fig. 25–11). Resting heart rate is a physiological parameter of marked importance in patients with congestive heart failure, and treatments that cause an increased heart rate are likely to yield deleterious long-term results. Finally, systemic arterial oxygen content should be evaluated in patients with PPH. Effective vasodilator drugs can result in vasodilatation of blood vessels supplying poorly ventilated areas of the lung and worsen hypoxemia.[148] This is particularly noticeable in patients with underlying chronic lung disease. For all of these reasons it has been advocated that vasodilators be initiated only in the hospital setting with central catheter placement for direct hemodynamic recordings and never initiated in the outpatient setting.[149]

ACUTE TESTING WITH INTRAVENOUS VASODILATORS

Intravenous vasodilators may be of value in the short-term assessment of pulmonary vasodilator reserve in patients with PPH. Historically, tolazoline received attention as an agent to acutely test the responsiveness of the pulmonary vascular bed in patients with pulmonary hypertension from several causes.[150,151] However, it is poorly tolerated acutely owing to its side effects and has largely been replaced by other agents. Acetylcholine was one of the first medications used to evaluate patients with PPH.[152,153] It is rapidly inactivated by the lung, which explains why the intravenous administration seems to produce selective pulmonary vasodilator effects. Although it has been reported to produce substantial acute reductions in pulmonary artery pressure in some patients, chronic therapy with this drug is not feasible. Isoproterenol is a potent beta-adrenergic agent that affects both the systemic and pulmonary vascular beds and increases cardiac output by chronotropic and inotropic mechanisms. It is considered a pulmonary vasodilator because it results in a lowering of the calculated pulmonary vascular resistance.[154] However, it rarely results in a substantial lowering of the pulmonary artery pressure in patients with pulmonary hypertension because of its more direct effect in increasing cardiac output.[155] Phentolamine is a potent alpha-adrenergic blocker that has been shown to cause pulmonary vasodilatation in animals and humans.[156,157] Its widespread use is limited by the profound systemic hypotension that occurs upon administration, and it is generally not used in the evaluation of PPH.[158] Sodium nitroprusside is a potent vasodilator that acts on arterial and venous beds. Its short half-life is also an advantage because the effects rapidly dissipate when infusion of the drug is stopped. Like phentolamine, its use as a test of vasodilator reserve is limited by the marked lowering in systemic blood pressure that occurs.

ADENOSINE. This substance is an intermediate product in the metabolism of adenosine triphosphate that has potent vasodilator properties through its action on specific vascular receptors.[159] In addition to pulmonary vasodilatation, it can also produce systemic and coronary vasodilatation.[160,161] It is believed to stimulate the endothelial cell and vascular smooth muscle receptors of the A2 type, which induce vascular smooth muscle relaxation by increasing cyclic AMP.[162] In patients with PPH, adenosine has been shown to be an extremely potent vasodilator and predictive of the subsequent effects of intravenous prostacyclin and oral calcium channel blockers[163,164] (Fig. 25–12). Adenosine has an extremely short half-life (less than 5 seconds), which provides a safety net by its rapid dissolution should any adverse side effects occur. It is administered intravenously in doses of 50 ng/kg/min and titrated upward every 2 minutes until the patient develops uncomfortable symptoms (such as chest tightness or dyspnea). It should be noted that adenosine is given as an infusion, and not as an intravenous bolus as is used to treat supraventricular tachyarrhythmias.

PROSTACYCLIN. This substance (epoprostenol sodium, or PGI_2) is a metabolite of arachidonic acid that is synthesized and released from vascular endothelium and smooth muscle.[35] The vasodilatory effects are thought to be mediated by activation of specific membrane PGI_2 receptors that are also coupled to the adenylate cyclase system.[35,165] Other effects include the inhibition of platelet activation and aggregation as well as leukocyte adhesion to the endothelium.[166] Prostacyclin has been used as an acute test of vasodilator reserve in patients with PPH.[167] Like adenosine, its short half-life allows the drug to be discontinued if any acute adverse effects result. Also similar to adenosine, it is administered incrementally, at 2 ng/kg/min and increased every 15 to 30 minutes until systemic effects such as headache, flushing, or nausea occur which limit the acute dose titration. Favorable acute effects from prostacyclin appears to be predictive of a favorable response to oral calcium channel blockers[168] and determination of this effect.

NITRIC OXIDE (NO). This substance, whose activity is identical to that of EDRF, is produced from L-arginine by NO synthase.[38a,169] NO diffuses to the vascular smooth muscle and mediates vasodilatation by stimulating soluble guanylate cyclase to produce cyclic GMP. Because it binds very rapidly to hemoglobin with a high affinity and is thereby inactivated, inhalation of NO gas results in selective pulmonary vascular effects without influencing the systemic circulation.[38a,169] The inhalation of NO by patients with PPH has been shown to produce a reduction in pulmonary vascular resistance acutely, similar to that achieved with intravenous adenosine.[170] NO has also been shown to be effective in patients with pulmonary hypertension secondary to congenital heart disease and the adult respiratory distress syndrome.[171] Although as yet untested, NO should produce vasodilatory effects similar to those of adenosine and prostacyclin in the initial assessment of pulmonary vasodilator reserve in these patients.

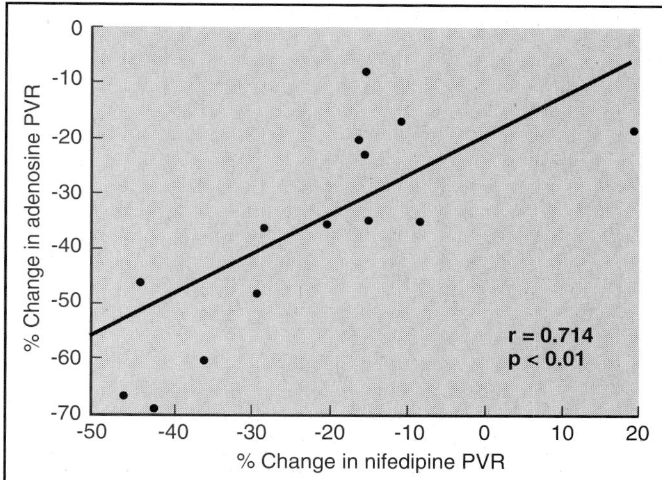

FIGURE 25–12. Testing of pulmonary vasodilator reserve with an infusion of intravenous adenosine. The per cent reduction in pulmonary vascular resistance (PVR) from intravenous adenosine challenge and the subsequent effect of nifedipine in patients with primary pulmonary hypertension are shown. The relative vasodilatory effect on PVR was greater for adenosine than for nifedipine. However, failure to respond to adenosine predicted failure to respond to nifedipine. (From Schrader, B., Inbar, S., Kaufmann, E., et al.: Comparison of the effects of adenosine and nifedipine in pulmonary hypertension. Reprinted with permission from the American College of Cardiology. J. Am. Coll. Cardiol. *19*:1060, 1992.)

CALCIUM CHANNEL BLOCKERS. Of the vasodilators tested in patients with PPH, the calcium channel blockers appear to have the widest usage. Early reports utilizing conventional doses failed to demonstrate a chronic sustained benefit.[172–175] Moreover, the calcium channel blockers have properties that could worsen the underlying pulmonary hypertension, including negative inotropic effects on right ventricular function (Fig. 25–11) and reflex sympathetic stimulation, which may increase resting heart rate.[147,176] Recently it has been reported that patients with PPH who are challenged with very high doses of calcium blockers may manifest a dramatic reduction in pulmonary artery pressure and pulmonary vascular resistance which, upon serial catheterization, has been maintained for over 5 years[117,177] (Fig. 25–13*A*). Importantly, the patient's quality of life is restored with improved functional class, and survival (94 per cent at 5 years) is improved compared with nonresponders and historical control subjects (36 per cent) (Fig. 25–13*B*).

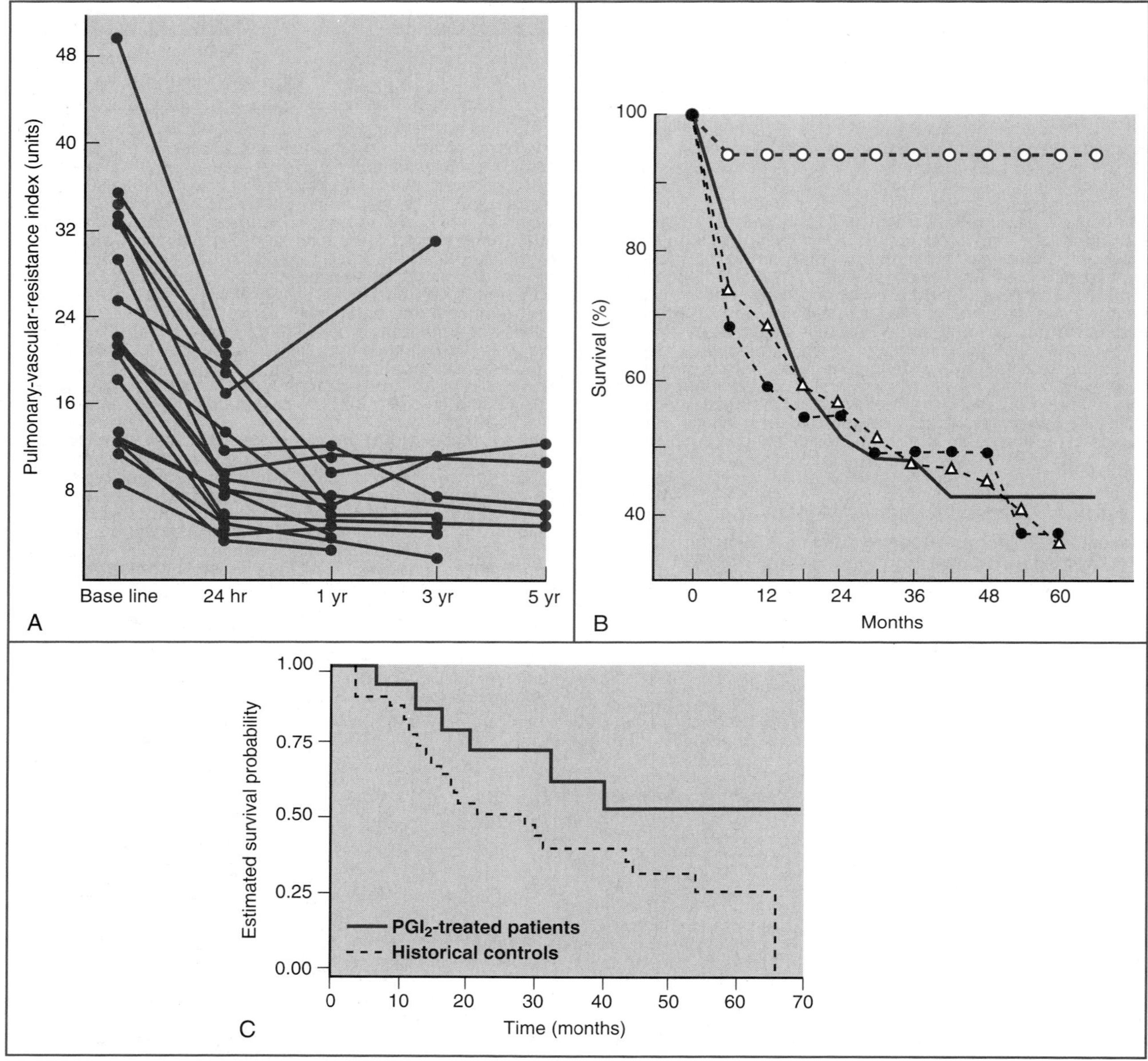

FIGURE 25–13. *A,* Hemodynamic effects of high doses of calcium channel blockers on patients with primary pulmonary hypertension followed over 5 years. The acute reduction in pulmonary vascular resistance that was achieved after 24 hours was maintained over 5 years, as documented by serial catheterizations. The patient who appeared not to have the sustained reduction in pulmonary vascular resistance was studied only after 3 years and was found not to be taking the high dose of calcium channel blockers as prescribed. *B,* The effect of high doses of calcium channel blockers on survival over 5 years in patients with primary pulmonary hypertension. Patients who responded to the high-dose regimen *(open circles)* had a 95 per cent 5-year survival compared with the nonresponders *(solid line),* who had a 36 per cent 5-year survival. This was similar to patients studied in the National Institutes of Health Registry on PPH *(triangles),* as well as patients from the University of Illinois only *(solid circles). C,* The effect of intravenous prostacyclin on survival in patients with primary pulmonary hypertension. The survival of patients given a chronic infusion of prostacyclin and followed out to 5.5 years is compared to functional class III and IV patients from the NIH Registry (historical controls). (*A* and *B* from Rich, S., Kaufmann, E., and Levy, P. S.: The effects of high doses of calcium channel blockers on survival of primary pulmonary hypertension. N. Engl. J. Med. *327:*76, 1992. *C,* from Barst, R. J., Rubin, L. J., McGoon, M. D., et al.: Survival of primary pulmonary hypertension with longterm continuous intravenous prostacyclin. Ann. Intern. Med. *121:*409, 1994.)

This experience suggests that some patients with PPH have the ability to have their pulmonary hypertension reversed and their quality of life and survival enhanced. It is unknown if the response to calcium channel blockers identifies two subsets of patients with PPH, or different stages of PPH, or a combination of both. However, it is essential to point out that patients who do not exhibit a dramatic hemodynamic response to calcium channel blockers do not appear to benefit from their long-term administration. Unfortunately, it is becoming common practice for physicians to prescribe calcium channel blockers at conventional doses to all patients with pulmonary hypertension, often without hemodynamic guidance. This unfortunate practice may result in a quicker deterioration of these patients and should be strongly discouraged.

CHRONIC PROSTACYCLIN INFUSION THERAPY. Continuous infusion prostacyclin therapy has now been shown in prospective randomized trials to improve quality of life and symptoms related to PPH, exercise tolerance, hemodynamics, and survival.[178–180,180a] The initial enthusiasm for prostacyclin was based on the demonstration of pulmonary vasodilator effects when administered to experimental animals with acute pulmonary vasoconstriction, and subsequently to patients with primary pulmonary hypertension.[181–185] More recently, however, a prospective treatment trial was undertaken in which patients were randomized to receive chronic intravenous prostacyclin therapy independent of any acute response to the drug, with substantial benefits noted as well[180] (Fig. 25–13*C*). The long-term effects of prostacyclin in PPH may be related to its ability to restore the integrity of the pulmonary vascular endothelium and to produce antithrombotic effects, as well as to its vasodilator properties.

Prostacyclin is generally administered through a central venous catheter that is surgically implanted and delivered by an ambulatory infusion system. The delivery system is complex and requires patients to learn the techniques of sterile drug preparation, operation of the pump, and care of the intravenous catheter. Most of the serious complications that have occurred with prostacyclin therapy have been attributable to the delivery system and include catheter-related infections and thrombosis and temporary interruption of the infusion due to pump malfunction. Anecdotal reports of rebound pulmonary hypertension occurring in patients in whom the infusion was interrupted suggest that great care must be taken to ensure that the infusion is never stopped.

Side effects related to the prostacyclin therapy include flushing, headache, nausea, diarrhea, and a unique type of jaw discomfort that occurs with eating. In most patients these symptoms are minimal and well tolerated. Tachyphylaxis to the drug also develops, requiring a constant periodic dose increase to maintain its efficacy. To date chronic prostacyclin has been given in patients with PPH for over 5 years with continued favorable effectiveness. In some patients (Class IV) who are critically ill, it serves as a bridge to lung transplantation, stabilizing the patient to a more favorable preoperative state. Patients who are less critically ill may do so well on prostacyclin that they may delay the need to consider transplantation, perhaps indefinitely. Currently prostacyclin has been used only in Class III and IV patients, and it is not known how effective it may be in patients with less advanced disease.

ANTICOAGULANTS. Oral anticoagulant therapy is widely recommended for patients with PPH, although its clinical efficacy as a therapy is difficult to prove. A retrospective review of patients with PPH followed over a 15-year period at the Mayo Clinic suggested that patients who received warfarin had improved survival over those who did not.[65] Recently, the influence of warfarin therapy was investigated in patients with PPH who failed to respond to high doses of calcium channel blockers.[117] A significant improvement in survival was observed in those patients who received anticoagulation, with a 1-year survival of 91 per cent and 3-year survival of 47 per cent, compared with 1 and 3 years of 62 per cent and 31 per cent, respectively, in patients who were not anticoagulated. The current recommendation is to use warfarin in relatively low doses, as has been recommended for prophylaxis of venous thromboembolism, controlling the INR to 1.5 to 2.5 times control.[47] Heparin, given its inhibitory effects on smooth muscle cell proliferation, might be a more suitable anticoagulant in PPH, although its use is more difficult. Adjusting to a partial thromboplastin time of 1.3 to 1.5 times control would make it a viable alternative treatment in patients considered to have a greater risk of hemorrhagic events (such as prior episodes of hemoptysis), or patients who for some reason cannot safely take warfarin.

ATRIAL SEPTOSTOMY

It has been presumed that intracardiac shunting, allowing blood flow from right to left, provides some type of protection to the right ventricle in the presence of pulmonary hypertension. It has also been noted that sudden cardiac death may be a more common occurrence in patients with PPH than in patients with Eisenmenger's physiology.[186]

Since 1983 there have been several reports of atrial septostomies performed in patients with PPH.[187–190] It has been suggested that it provides palliation to select patients, manifested primarily by improvement in the symptoms of syncope and right-sided heart failure, and possibly improving survival until more definitive therapy can be instituted. However, because it does not affect the underlying pulmonary vascular disease, it should be considered an adjunct palliative therapy only. Because it creates hypoxemia, only patients with fairly normal resting systemic arterial oxygen saturations can be considered candidates. At the present time this technique should be considered investigational. It is not an appropriate measure in the setting of acute right ventricular failure and impending cardiogenic shock.

HEART-LUNG AND LUNG TRANSPLANTATION

(See also p. 529)

Heart-lung transplantation has been performed successfully in patients with PPH for more than a decade.[191–194] Because these patients have pulmonary vascular disease and severe right ventricular dysfunction, it was originally believed that heart-lung transplant was the only transplantation option. The widespread application of heart-lung transplant, however, has been limited by the number of centers with expertise to perform the procedure, the scarcity of suitable donor organs, and the very long waiting times required for patients with end-stage right-heart failure. More recently, bilateral or double lung transplantation and single lung transplantation have been performed successfully in patients with PPH.[195,196] Hemodynamic studies have shown an immediate reduction in pulmonary artery pressure and

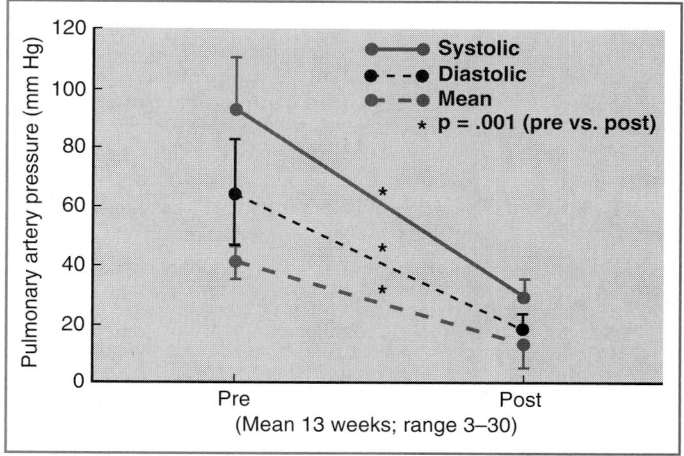

FIGURE 25–14. The hemodynamic effects of single lung transplantation in patients with pulmonary hypertension. The reduction in mean pulmonary artery pressure after a mean of 13 weeks following single lung transplantation in patients with pulmonary hypertension is shown. A significant reduction, approaching normal values, was achieved in almost all patients. (Reproduced with permission from Pasque, M. Q., Trulock, E. P., Kaiser, L. R., and Cooper, J. D.: Single lung transplantation for pulmonary hypertension. Circulation *84*:2275, 1991. Copyright 1991 American Heart Association.)

pulmonary vascular resistance associated with improvement in right ventricular function[196] (Fig. 25–14).

The advantage of bilateral lung transplantation is that pulmonary blood flow is relatively evenly distributed between both lungs postoperatively and thus there is greater reserve for the patient should the patient sustain rejection or infection. The advantage of single lung transplantation is that it is a simpler operation, and there would be more potential suitable donors and shorter waiting times. However, studies have shown that more than 90 per cent of the pulmonary blood flow postoperatively goes to the transplanted lung, thus leaving the potential for marked ventilation-perfusion mismatch and little reserve should the transplanted lung sustain perioperative problems.[197]

The concern regarding restoration of right ventricular function has lessened by the finding that, as in patients undergoing pulmonary thromboendarterectomy for pulmonary hypertension, marked regression of right ventricular hypertrophy occurs in the postoperative recovery period following lung transplantation, with a dramatic improvement in right ventricular performance.[196] The major long-term problem in patients who survive the operation is the high incidence of bronchiolitis obliterans in the transplanted lungs, acute organ rejection, and opportunistic infection. In most series 4-year survival remains below 60 per cent for lung transplantation, with patients being transplanted for pulmonary hypertension having the worst long-term outcome. This reason, as well as the expense of the operation and the early mortality rate, render lung transplantation a treatment of last resort for PPH. Many advocate that patients with PPH not undergo lung transplantation until they manifest clinical right ventricular failure. Early data suggest that prostacyclin may prove to be the ideal bridge to keep these patients alive and stable until organs become available.

SECONDARY PULMONARY HYPERTENSION

Several secondary causes of pulmonary hypertension have been well established, although the mechanisms for the pulmonary hypertension often remain in doubt (Table 25–4). In many instances, increased resistance to pulmonary blood flow downstream leads to what has been referred to as "passive" pulmonary hypertension, because in many cases there is elevation of the pulmonary artery pressure but no significant elevation in pulmonary vascular resistance. Reactive pulmonary hypertension often coexists in these states, elevating the pulmonary artery pressure and pulmonary vascular resistance to levels higher than can be accounted for purely by increased downstream resistance to blood flow. In some instances, relieving the downstream obstruction results in normalization of pulmonary artery pressure and pulmonary vascular resistance, whereas in other instances it may not. This has been believed to be related to the chronicity of the reactive pulmonary hypertension leading to irreversible vascular changes, although this hypothesis has never been proven. When reactive pulmonary hypertension occurs, it often results in right ventricular failure, which can predominate in the patient's clinical symptomology and lead to a marked deterioration in functional class and death.

INCREASED RESISTANCE TO PULMONARY VENOUS DRAINAGE

PATHOPHYSIOLOGY. Increased resistance to pulmonary venous drainage is a mechanism common to several conditions of diverse causes in which pulmonary arterial hypertension occurs. Altered resistance to pulmonary venous drainage may be the result of diseases affecting the left ventricle or pericardium, mitral or aortic valvular disease, or rare entities such as cor triatriatum, left atrial myxoma, or pulmonary veno-occlusive disease (see below).

The magnitude of pulmonary hypertension depends, in part, on the performance of the right ventricle. In response to an acute stress, such as pulmonary embolism, the normal right ventricle of an adult living at sea level can develop systolic pulmonary pressures of 45 to 50 mm Hg, above which right ventricular failure supervenes. Systolic pressures of 80 to 100 mm Hg can be generated only by a hypertrophied right ventricle that is normally perfused. If right ventricular infarction or ischemia has occurred,[198–200] or if the right and left ventricles are both affected by a myopathic process, right ventricular failure occurs at lower pulmonary vascular pressures, and significant pulmonary hypertension may not develop despite an increase in pulmonary vascular resistance.

In the presence of a healthy, nonischemic right ventricle, an increase in left atrial pressure from subnormal levels up to 7 mm Hg results in a fall in both pulmonary vascular resistance and the pressure gradient across the lungs. These reductions may reflect distention of a population of compliant small vessels or recruitment of additional vascular channels or both. With further increases in left atrial pressure, pulmonary arterial pressure rises along with pulmonary venous pressure; i.e., at a constant pulmonary blood flow, the pressure gradient between the pulmonary artery and veins and the pulmonary vascular resistance remains constant. Finally, when pulmonary venous pressure approaches or exceeds 25 mm Hg on a chronic basis, a disproportionate elevation of pulmonary artery pressure occurs; i.e., the pressure gradient between the pulmonary artery

TABLE 25–4 CLASSIFICATION OF PULMONARY HYPERTENSION BASED ON ESTABLISHED CAUSES

LEFT VENTRICULAR DIASTOLIC FAILURE
- Hypertension
- Aortic stenosis
- Coronary artery disease
- Constrictive pericarditis
- Cardiomyopathy
  - Hypertrophic
  - Restrictive
  - Dilated

LEFT ATRIAL HYPERTENSION
- Mitral stenosis
- Mitral regurgitation
- Cor triatriatum
- Left atrial myxoma or thrombus

LUNG DISEASE
- Parenchymal
  - Chronic obstructive pulmonary disease
  - Restrictive lung disease
  - Interstitial lung disease
- Disorders of ventilation
  - Obesity-hypoventilation syndromes
  - Neuromuscular disorders
  - Chest wall deformities
- Congenital anomalies
- Induced hypoxia

PULMONARY VASCULAR OBSTRUCTION
- Chronic thromboembolic pulmonary hypertension
- Mediastinal fibrosis
- Peripheral artery stenosis
- Foreign body embolization
- Tumor embolization

PULMONARY VASCULAR DISEASE
- Collagen vascular disease
- Congenital heart disease with post-tricuspid left-to-right shunting
- Increased pulmonary blood flow
  - Atrial septal defect
  - Anomalous pulmonary venous drainage
  - High-output cardiac failure
    - Beriberi
    - Arteriovenous fistula
- Persistent fetal circulation of the newborn
- Primary pulmonary hypertension

OTHER RARE VASCULAR DISEASES
- Takayasu's arteritis
- Sarcoidosis
- Hemoglobinopathies
- Alveolar proteinosis

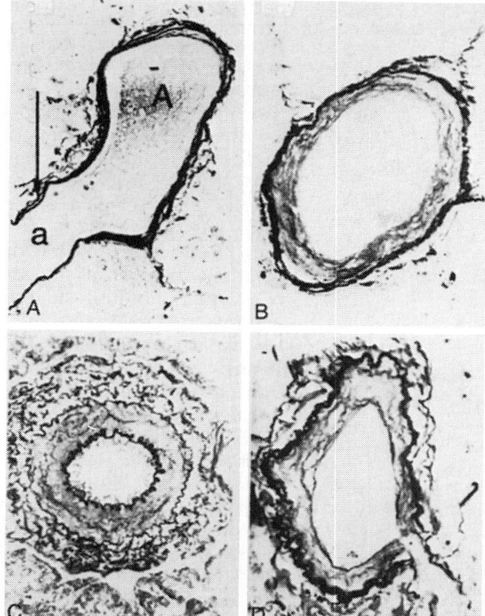

FIGURE 25–15. *A,* Oblique section through a muscular pulmonary artery, *A,* showing the characteristic thin media bounded by inner and outer elastic laminae. An arteriolar branch, a, arises from the parent vessel and passes downward and to the left. Its wall consists of a single elastic lamina except near its origin from its parent artery where the remains of a thin media bounded by two elastic laminae can still be seen *(arrow)* (Elastic–van Gieson × 284). *B,* Transverse section of a normal pulmonary venule. The wall consists of a single elastic lamina. There is considerable intimal fibrosis due to age change. (Elastic–van Gieson × 375). Muscular pulmonary artery *(C)* and venule *(D)* in a young woman with severe mitral stenosis. Note the marked hypertrophy in the artery and the crenated internal elastic lamina, suggesting constriction. The venule shows severe intimal fibrosis. (Modified from Harris, P., and Heath, D.: The Human Pulmonary Circulation. 3rd ed. New York, Churchill Livingstone, 1986, pp. 338 and 341.)

and veins rises while pulmonary blood flow remains constant or falls, indicating an elevation in pulmonary vascular resistance that is due, in part, to pulmonary vasoconstriction. The latter occurs to a variable extent in response to passive elevations of pulmonary venous pressure and probably reflects the reactivity of the pulmonary vasculature, which may be variable between and within species.

There is considerable variability in pulmonary arterial vasoconstriction in response to pulmonary venous hypertension. Marked reactive pulmonary hypertension, with pulmonary artery systolic pressures in excess of 80 mm Hg, occurs in somewhat less than one-third of patients with pulmonary venous pressures elevated chronically in excess of 25 mm Hg. The fact that less than one-third of patients with severe mitral stenosis develop severe reactive pulmonary hypertension also argues in favor of a spectrum of pulmonary vascular reactivity to chronic increases in pulmonary venous pressure.

The mechanism involved in elevating pulmonary vascular resistance is unclear. There may be a neural component; also, an elevation of pulmonary venous pressure may narrow or close airways, which may diminish ventilation and lead to hypoxia and, in turn, elevate pulmonary artery pressure. Finally, interstitial pulmonary edema secondary to pulmonary venous hypertension may encroach on the vascular lumen and contribute to the pulmonary arterial hypertension.

PATHOLOGY. Structural changes in the pulmonary vascular bed develop in association with chronic pulmonary venous hypertension, irrespective of its etiology. At the ultrastructural level, these changes include swelling of the pulmonary capillary endothelial cells, thickening of their basal lamina, and wide separation of groups of connective tissue fibrils, indicative of interstitial edema. With persistence of the edema, there is proliferation of reticular and elastic fibrils, so that the alveolar capillaries become embedded in dense connective tissue.[5] The permeability of interendothelial junctions depends on pulmonary capillary pressure, with leakage of large molecules (40,000 to 60,000 daltons) occurring at capillary pressures in excess of approximately 30 mm Hg.[201,202]

Light microscopic examination of the lungs of patients with pulmonary venous hypertension shows distention of pulmonary capillaries, thickening and rupture of the basement membranes of endothelial cells, and transudation of erythrocytes through these ruptured membranes into the alveolar spaces, which contain fragments of disintegrating erythrocytes. Pulmonary hemosiderosis is commonly observed and may progress to extensive fibrosis. In the late stages of pulmonary venous hypertension, areas of hemorrhage may be scattered throughout the lungs, edema fluid and coagulum may collect in the alveolar spaces, and there may be widespread organization and fibrosis of pulmonary alveoli. Occasionally, particularly in patients with chronic pulmonary venous hypertension due to mitral valve disease, ossification of alveolar spaces occurs.[203,204] Pulmonary lymphatics may become markedly distended, giving the appearance of lymphangiectasis, particularly when the pulmonary venous pressure chronically exceeds 30 mm Hg. Structural alterations in the small pulmonary arteries, arterioles, and venules include medial hypertrophy and intimal fibrosis and, rarely, necrotizing arteritis (Fig. 25–15). However, vasodilatation and plexiform lesions are not seen. The latter characterize the "irreversible" forms of pulmonary arterial hypertension, and their absence in that form of pulmonary hypertension associated with chronic pulmonary venous pressure elevation correlates with the reversibility of the pulmonary hypertension.

PULMONARY HYPERTENSION SECONDARY TO ELEVATION OF LEFT VENTRICULAR DIASTOLIC PRESSURE

LEFT VENTRICULAR DIASTOLIC FAILURE. This may result from hypertension; aortic stenosis; ischemic heart disease; hypertrophic, restrictive, and congestive cardiomyopathies; and constrictive pericarditis. Because chronic increases in mean left ventricular filling pressure exceeding 25 mm Hg are uncommon, the resulting pulmonary arterial hypertension is only moderate unless reactive pulmonary hypertension also occurs. In the absence of the latter, a normal pulmonary artery mean pressure of 15 mm Hg may rise to approximately 30 mm Hg as a result of left ventricular diastolic dysfunction. Because cardiac output is usually reduced in such patients, the mean pulmonary artery pressure would be considerably less than 30 mm Hg if pulmonary vascular resistance remains unchanged. However, many patients with left ventricular diastolic dysfunction exhibit increased pulmonary vascular resistance and moderately severe pulmonary hypertension.

PULMONARY HYPERTENSION SECONDARY TO LEFT ATRIAL HYPERTENSION

Mitral Valve Disease (see also Chap. 32)

MITRAL STENOSIS. This valvular lesion represents an important cause of pulmonary hypertension. Although the pulmonary hypertension associated with mitral stenosis is initially a result of an increase in resistance to pulmonary venous drainage and backward transmission of the elevated left atrial pressure, many patients subsequently exhibit marked pulmonary vasoconstriction and anatomical changes in vessels, so that the pulmonary hypertension is "reactive" as well as "passive." The elevation of pulmonary vascular resistance and the associated pulmonary hypertension may come to dominate the clinical picture in mitral stenosis (Fig. 25–16).[206,207] Thus, patients with mitral stenosis often develop what might be considered to be a more proximal obstruction at the level of the pulmonary arterioles and small muscular arteries, with resultant pulmonary hypertension equal to or exceeding systemic arterial pressure during exertion and sometimes even at rest. The clinical picture in such patients is characterized by right ventricular failure with distended neck veins, hepatomegaly, and ascites. These patients exhibit marked fatigue, occasionally a more serious complaint than dyspnea. The murmur of mitral stenosis may be soft or even inaudible, and the opening snap of the stenotic mitral valve may be indistinguishable from a loud pulmonic component of S_2, owing to narrowing of the S_2-opening snap interval. Pulmonary congestion and edema may not be prominent clinically. Cardiac output is usually markedly reduced. This constellation of findings may obscure the underlying diagnosis of mitral stenosis and suggest instead either PPH or pulmonary hypertension secondary to some other disorder.

Diagnostic Studies. The echocardiogram shows left atrial enlargement and thickened mitral valve leaflets whose mobility is markedly reduced (see p. 1012). At cardiac catheterization, the pulmonary arterial hypertension is associated with substantial elevations of the pulmonary wedge pressure, and there is generally a sizable (>10 mm

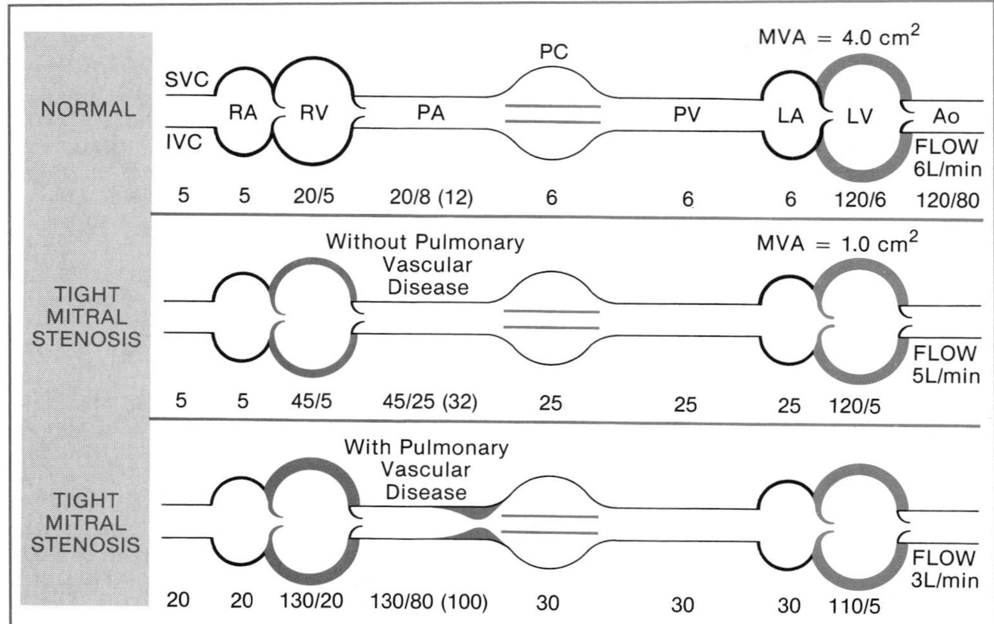

FIGURE 25–16. Schematic diagram of cardiopulmonary circulation in patients with tight mitral stenosis with and without pulmonary vascular disease. Pressures (in mm Hg) are listed for the superior and inferior venae cavae (SVC and IVC), right atrium (RA), right ventricle (RV), pulmonary arteries (PA), capillaries (PC), veins (PV), left atrium (LA), left ventricle (LV), and aorta (Ao) for the normal circulation *(upper panel)* and for the two types of mitral stenosis *(middle and lower panels).* Note that with pulmonary vascular disease (the "second stenosis") severe pulmonary hypertension occurs, and right ventricular failure develops. (Modified from Dexter, L.: Physiologic changes in mitral stenosis. N. Engl. J. Med. 254:829, 1956. Schlant, R. C.: Altered cardiovascular function of rheumatic heart disease and other acquired valvular disease. *In* Hurst, J. L., and Logue, R. B. (eds.): The Heart. 4th ed. New York, McGraw-Hill Book Co., 1978, p. 971.)

Hg) pressure gradient between pulmonary capillary wedge and left ventricular diastolic pressures. These findings are of key importance in distinguishing mitral stenosis from primary pulmonary hypertension, a condition in which left atrial size and the wedge pressure are normal and in which there is no diastolic pressure gradient between the wedge and left ventricular pressures.

Protection Against Pulmonary Edema. At least three mechanisms that tend to protect against pulmonary edema formation are operative in patients with mitral stenosis and chronic elevations of pulmonary venous pressure in excess of 25 mm Hg (Chap. 15). First, lymphatic drainage of the pulmonary interstitium increases abruptly when pulmonary venous pressure is increased to 25 mm Hg.[208,209] Acute increases in pulmonary lymph flow of up to eight times the resting level occur when pulmonary venous pressure is raised to 30 mm Hg for a 10-minute interval, and the increased lymphatic flow persists at high levels for 30 to 60 minutes after pulmonary venous pressure has returned to normal.[208] In models of *chronic* pulmonary venous pressure elevation, increases in pulmonary lymph flow of up to 28 times normal have been observed.[209]

Diminished permeability of the capillary alveolar barrier is a second protective mechanism that might be operative in patients with *chronic* pulmonary venous hypertension in excess of 25 mm Hg. There is morphological evidence of thickening of the layer between the capillary lumen and the alveolar space.[210–213] A third mechanism operating in patients with chronic increased resistance to pulmonary venous drainage is the reactive constriction of small muscular pulmonary arteries and arterioles (Fig. 25–15). This constriction, which results in considerable elevation of pulmonary artery pressure, is usually associated with a significant decline in right ventricular output (and therefore pulmonary blood flow). The lower pulmonary blood flow tends to diminish the formation of pulmonary edema because it results in substantially lower left atrial and pulmonary venous pressures at any given size of the mitral valve orifice[214] or for any given impairment of left ventricular function.

Effects of Surgery. After corrective surgery on the mitral valve or mitral balloon valvuloplasty (see p. 1014), both pulmonary vascular resistance and pulmonary hypertension decline,[215,216] the major extent of which is noted within the first postoperative week. The extent of reversal of pulmonary vascular obstruction has varied depending on the adequacy of the procedure in producing an increase in mitral orifice area and whether the patient develops mitral valve restenosis.[217]

MITRAL REGURGITATION. Although pulmonary hypertension is widely recognized as developing in patients with left atrial hypertension due to mitral stenosis, it can also occur in patients with pure mitral regurgitation.[218] In one series, nearly half of a cohort of 41 patients with severe mitral regurgitation had pulmonary artery systolic pressures in excess of 50 mm Hg. In this subgroup of patients, pulmonary vascular resistance was three times normal and cardiac output was substantially depressed, compared with that in patients in whom severe mitral regurgitation was associated with only minimal pulmonary artery pressure elevation.[218] Presumably, the pulmonary hypertension in these patients is reversible, just as it is in mitral stenosis, although data on this point have not been reported.

COR TRIATRIATUM (see also p. 923). This is a malformation in which partitioning of the left atrium creates two left atrial subchambers. The posterior subchamber receives the pulmonary venous inflow, which then drains through an opening in the partition into the anterior subchamber and then through the mitral orifice into the left ventricle. When the opening in the partition separating the two left atrial subchambers is small, severe pulmonary venous and pulmonary arterial hypertension result.[219]

INCREASED RESISTANCE TO FLOW THROUGH THE PULMONARY VASCULAR BED

Pulmonary Parenchymal Disease

Pulmonary hypertension is a common sequela to chronic bronchitis and emphysema (Chap. 47).[220] It had long been believed that the elevated pulmonary artery pressures in patients with emphysema resulted from destruction of the pulmonary vascular bed. Current views minimize this pathogenic pathway, because no direct correlation exists between the severity of the emphysema and the degree of right ventricular hypertrophy.[220,221]

PATHOPHYSIOLOGY. Hypoxia-induced vasoconstriction (see p. 781) probably plays a major role in producing pulmonary hypertension in patients with chronic bronchitis and emphysema.[222–224] There is also evidence for a pulmonary vasoconstrictive action by hydrogen ions, particularly in the presence of hypoxia. In this regard, in patients with chronic obstructive lung disease pulmonary artery pressure correlates inversely with arterial oxygen saturation and directly with arterial P_{CO_2},[225–228] providing indirect evidence for a role for hypoxia and hypercapnia in the production of pulmonary hypertension. When patients with chronic bronchitis and emphysema inspire high concentrations of oxygen acutely, there is only a modest decrease in pulmonary artery pressure and vascular resistance,[226,229–231] both of which remain considerably elevated. This suggests that muscular hypertrophy of pulmonary arterioles may in itself be of importance in maintaining the hypoxic pulmonary hypertension.

TRIALS WITH OXYGEN THERAPY. The results of two large trials designed to assess the role of long-term oxygen therapy in cor pulmonale due to chronic bronchitis and emphysema have been disappointing insofar as pulmonary vascular dynamics are concerned (see p. 1617).[232,233] Long-term domiciliary oxygen therapy in one study was associated with no change in mean pulmonary artery pressure after 500 days of oxygen treatment, compared with a 3-mm Hg increase in the control group.[232] In another study, nocturnal oxygen administration was associated with a 7 per cent increase in pulmonary vascular resistance after 6 months, compared with an 11 per cent decrease in patients receiving continuous oxygen.[233]

Blood volume and red cell mass, in particular, increase during acute respiratory failure and may contribute to the development of elevated pulmonary arterial pressures. By increasing blood viscosity, increases in hematocrit to within the range commonly seen in chronic bronchitis and emphysema (i.e., 50 to 55 per cent) result in 30 to 50 per cent increases in the transpulmonary arteriovenous pressure gradient at constant blood flow.

SPECIFIC DISORDERS

Progressive interstitial pulmonary fibrosis may be associated with pulmonary hypertension. The latter may occur in patients with *progressive systemic sclerosis* (see p. 1781), in whom the fibrotic process leads to major reduction in the cross-sectional area of the pulmonary vascular bed due to obliteration of alveolar capillaries and narrowing and obliteration of many small arteries and arterioles.[2,5] Moreover, a marked elevation of pulmonary artery pressure ($\geq$100 mm Hg systolic) and resistance ($\geq$2000 dynes-sec-cm^{-5}) in patients with a variant of scleroderma, the *CREST syndrome* (*c*alcinosis, *R*aynaud's phenomenon, *e*sophageal dysmotility, *s*clerodactyly, and *t*elangiectasia), has been reported[235] (see p. 1781). In patients with the CREST form of *scleroderma,* marked right ventricular dysfunction may be present with right ventricular ejection fractions less than 30 per cent, presumably reflecting systolic overload of the right ventricle due to severe pulmonary vascular disease,[154,236] in the absence of interstitial lung disease.

Fibrous obliteration of the pulmonary vascular bed and pulmonary hypertension have also been described in patients with various forms of pulmonary vasculitis (Table 25–5). These include isolated Raynaud's phenomenon,[237,238] dermatomyositis,[239] rheumatoid arthritis,[240] and systemic lupus erythematosus.[241,242] In the latter a *lupus anticoagulant* may be present in the IgG or IgM fractions of the serum; this may cause a paradoxical hypercoagulable state, intrapulmonary microthrombi, and pulmonary hypertension.[242] Pulmonary hypertension is an uncommon accompaniment of the Hamman-Rich syndrome,[243] desquamative interstitial pneumonia, idiopathic pulmonary hemosiderosis,[244] and sarcoidosis.[245] It is not clear whether significant pulmonary hypertension may result from pulmonary fibrosis due to radiation therapy.

Diffuse lymphatic spread of carcinoma may also cause pulmonary hypertension and right heart failure.[246] In many cases tumor microemboli and the attendant thrombotic and fibrotic reaction lead to vascular obstruction. Obstruction of the major pulmonary arteries by tumor (usually sarcoma) may be a cause of right ventricular and main pulmonary artery hypertension.[247] Congenital pulmonary aplasia or hypoplasia, the latter often observed in Down syndrome,[248] may be responsible for an elevation of pulmonary vascular resistance and pulmonary hypertension.

TABLE 25–5 PULMONARY VASCULITIDES

VASCULITIDES IN WHICH LUNG IS THE MAJOR ORGAN INVOLVED
Wegener's granulomatosis
Lymphomatoid granulomatosis
Lymphocytic angiitis and granulomatosis
Churg-Strauss syndrome
Overlap vasculitis
Necrotizing sarcoid granulomatosis
VASCULITIDES IN WHICH LUNG MAY BE INVOLVED
Henoch-Schönlein syndrome
Disseminated leukocytoclastic vasculitis
Cryoglobulinemia
Disseminated giant cell arteritis
Behçet's disease
Takayasu's disease
Polyarteritis nodosa
DISEASES IN WHICH PULMONARY VASCULITIS MAY BE PART OF THE SPECTRUM OF PATHOLOGY
Collagen-vascular disorders
Rheumatoid arthritis
Systemic lupus erythematosus
Progressive systemic sclerosis
Eosinophilic pneumonias
Sarcoidosis
Immunoblastic lymphadenopathy
Organic dust diseseases (hypersensitivity pneumonitides)
Bronchocentric granulomatosis
Ulcerative colitis
Ankylosing spondylitis
Hughes-Stovin syndrome

From Fulmer, J. D., and Kaltreider, H. B.: The pulmonary vasculitides. Chest *82*:615, 1982.

Eisenmenger Syndrome

(See also pp. 750 and 967)

Decreased cross-sectional area of the pulmonary arteriolar bed with irreversible pulmonary hypertension characterizes the so-called Eisenmenger syndrome. This term was used by Wood[249] to refer to patients with congenital cardiac lesions and severe pulmonary hypertension in whom reversal of a left-to-right shunt has occurred. Left-to-right shunts are due usually to congenital cardiovascular malformations[250–254] (e.g., atrial and ventricular septal defects, patent ductus arteriosus).

PATHOPHYSIOLOGY (see p. 967). Pulmonary hypertension in congenital heart disease may occur simply because of increased pulmonary blood flow. When chronic, the increased pulmonary flow is often associated with a passive reduction in pulmonary resistance and little elevation of pulmonary vascular pressures. In a normal adult with a pulmonary blood flow (PBF) of 5 liters/min, a pulmonary vascular resistance (PVR) of 60 dynes-sec-cm^{-5}, and a mean left atrial pressure (LA) of 6 mm Hg, the pulmonary artery mean pressure (PA) may be calculated from the expression

$$PVR = \frac{(PA - LA)80}{PBF} = \frac{(PA - 6)80}{5} = 60 \text{ dynes-sec-cm}^{-5}$$

$$PA = \frac{60 \times 5}{80} + 6 = 10 \text{ mm Hg}$$

If PBF is doubled, a reduction in PVR to 30 dynes-sec-cm^{-5} maintains PA mean pressure at a normal level of 10 mm Hg. However, if PBF is increased four- to sixfold, the reserve capacity of the pulmonary vascular bed is exceeded, and pulmonary artery pressure rises. Thus, if the PVR is 30 dynes-sec-cm^{-5}, a PBF of 30 liters/min is associated with a mean PA pressure that is only minimally elevated at 17 mm Hg, although the high right ventricular stroke volumes associated with the augmentation in pulmonary blood flow result in considerably higher values (40 to 45 mm Hg) for pulmonary artery and right ventricular systolic pressures. If no underlying arteriolar vascular disease exists, abolition of the shunt by corrective operation restores pulmonary blood flow and PA pressure to normal.

If a congenital cardiovascular defect causes pulmonary hypertension from the time of birth, the small, muscular arteries of the fetal lung may undergo delayed or only partial involution, resulting in persistently high levels of pulmonary vascular resistance (see p. 781). This is true especially in those lesions in which a left-to-right shunt enters the right ventricle or pulmonary artery directly (i.e., a post-tricuspid valve shunt, such as ventricular septal defect or patent ductus arteriosus); these patients experience a higher incidence of severe and irreversible pulmonary vascular damage than those in whom the shunt is proximal to the tricuspid valve (pre-tricuspid shunts, as in atrial septal defect and partial anomalous pulmonary venous drainage). In the latter category, pulmonary hypertension may result from a large pre-tricuspid left-to-right shunt, which enhances the risk of pulmonary vascular damage.

PATHOLOGY. The extent of reversibility of pulmonary vascular obstructive disease in the presence of congenital heart disease varies. From an anatomical point of view, reversible conditions are those in which the decreased pulmonary arteriolar cross-sectional area is the result of medial hypertrophy and vasoconstriction; irreversibility is associated with the presence of necrotizing arteritis and plexiform lesions in these small vessels.[250–253] The classification by Heath and Edwards[109] of six grades of structural change is widely employed to assess the potential reversibility of pulmonary vascular disease and is summarized as follows: *Grade I* is characterized by hypertrophy of the media of small muscular pulmonary arteries and arterioles.

In *Grade II,* intimal cellular proliferation is added to the medial hypertrophy. *Grade IIII* is characterized by advanced medial thickening with hypertrophy and hyperplasia, together with progressive intimal proliferation and concentric fibrosis that results in obliteration of many arterioles and small arteries. In *Grade IV,* dilatation and so-called "plexiform lesions" of the muscular pulmonary arteries and arterioles are observed (Fig. 25–17). The latter consist of a plexiform network of capillary-like channels within a dilated segment of a muscular pulmonary artery. The channels are separated by proliferating endothelial cells, which often contain thrombi; indeed, the network of capillary channels may constitute recanalization of a thrombus. *Grade V* changes include complex plexiform, angiomatous, and cavernous lesions and hyalinization of intimal fibrosis. Finally, *Grade VI* is characterized by the presence of necrotizing arteritis.

The Heath and Edwards classification implies that the morphological alterations are sequential, with Grade I being the earliest stage and Grade VI being the "end stage" of pulmonary vascular obliterative disease. That such an orderly progression may not in fact occur is suggested by the findings of Wagenvoort, which indicate that plexiform lesions develop gradually in areas affected by necrotizing arteritis. They have suggested that fibrinoid necrosis of a small segment of a pulmonary arterial branch leads to medial destruction and subsequent aneurysmal dilatation of the vessel as well as the formation of a fibrin clot in the lumen, often with admixture of platelets.[250] Organization of the fibrin clot by strands of intimal cells leads to formation of the plexus; the small capillary-like channels within the plexus (Fig. 25–17) provide continuity to the distal portion of the artery, which undergoes poststenotic dilatation. With time, the inflammatory component of the process subsides, fibrin disappears, and the strands of intimal cells become fibrotic. Wagenvoort's view is supported by animal experiments in which end-to-end systemic-pulmonary anastomoses resulted in arteritis and fibrinoid necrosis before the appearance of plexiform lesions.[255,256] Thus, although Heath-Edwards Grades I, II, and III may represent chronological progression, evidence exists that Grade VI (necrotizing arteritis) changes appear next, followed by Grades IV and V as end-stage alterations.

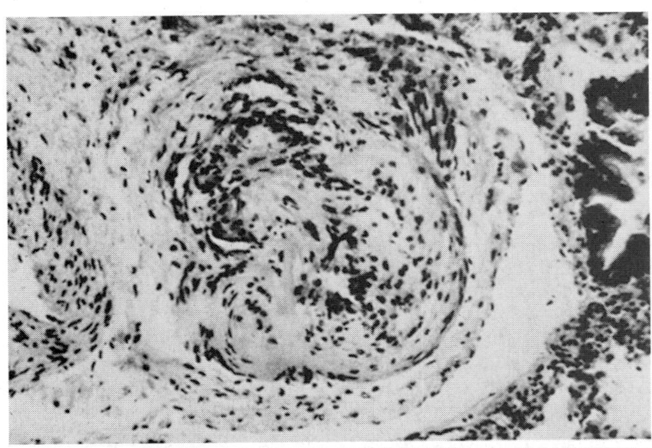

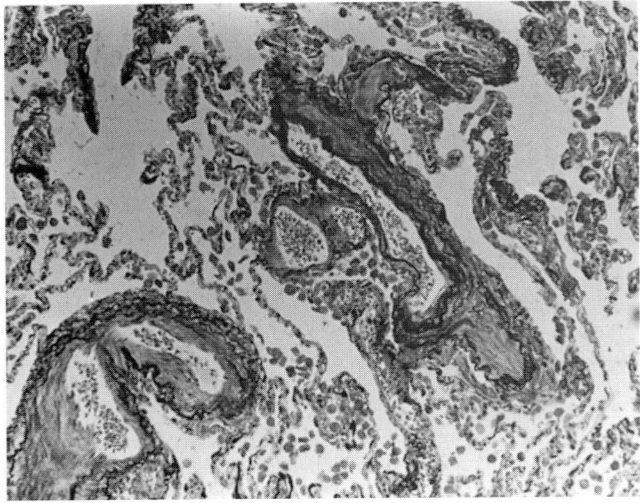

FIGURE 25–17. *Top,* Histological section from the lung of a 3-year-old boy with a common atrioventricular canal and severe pulmonary hypertension. A muscular pulmonary artery with an early plexiform lesion is seen as well as fibrinoid necrosis of the media and active proliferation of intimal cells. (From Wagenvoort, C. A., and Wagenvoort, N.: Pathology of Pulmonary Hypertension. 2nd ed. New York, John Wiley and Sons, 1977.) *Bottom,* Photomicrograph of a lung biopsy specimen from a 35-year-old man with a patent ductus arteriosus and systemic pulmonary hypertension. A predominance of advanced changes is seen, including plexiform and dilatation lesions.

CLINICAL CONSIDERATIONS. As already mentioned, *Eisenmenger syndrome* is the term used by Wood to refer to patients with congenital central communications with severe pulmonary hypertension, in whom reversal of a left-to-right shunt has occurred across the pulmonary-systemic communication.[249] The patients described originally by Eisenmenger had ventricular septal defects, and the term *Eisenmenger complex* is applied to patients with severe pulmonary hypertension and right-to-left shunt through such a defect. The broader term *Eisenmenger syndrome* is applied to any anomalous circulatory communication that leads to obliterative pulmonary vascular disease, including pre- and post-tricuspid shunts. Health-Edwards Grades IV to VI changes are usual in these patients; occasionally, lesser anatomical changes predominate and may be reversible after successful corrective operation.

When the pulmonary vascular resistance has increased so that it equals or exceeds systemic resistance, and the anatomical changes of the pulmonary vessels are predominantly those of Grades IV to VI, surgical closure of the anomalous circulatory communication will be associated with a prohibitive immediate risk and if the patient survives will usually fail to relieve pulmonary hypertension. Operation may, in fact, hasten death in most survivors who had either balanced shunts or predominant right-to-left shunts because closure of the right-to-left communication merely increases the load on an already overburdened right ventricle. Structural changes in the pulmonary vascular bed are evident in pulmonary arteriograms, which reveal dilated central pulmonary arteries and narrowing of the peripheral branches. These changes can be evaluated by means of quantitative analysis of the pulmonary wedge angiogram.[257] This technique has been employed successfully by Rabinovitch, Reid, and coworkers, who have demonstrated progressively more abrupt tapering of the pulmonary arteries in patients with increasingly abnormal hemodynamics and increasingly severe structural changes in lung biopsy tissue.[257]

OTHER CONDITIONS ASSOCIATED WITH DECREASED CROSS-SECTIONAL AREA OF THE PULMONARY VASCULAR BED

PERSISTENT FETAL CIRCULATION IN THE NEWBORN (see also p. 883). This condition has been reported as a cause of severe pulmonary hypertension.[260–262] Affected infants exhibit cyanosis, tachypnea, acidemia, normal pulmonary parenchymal markings on chest radiography, and anatomically normal hearts. Cyanosis is the result of right-to-left shunting across the foramen ovale and through a patent ductus arteriosus.[260] The condition may be due to persistence of extremely muscular small pulmonary arteries, a diminution in the absolute number of these resistance vessels, or a combination of the two.[262]

INCREASED RESISTANCE TO FLOW THROUGH LARGE PULMONARY ARTERIES

PULMONARY THROMBOEMBOLISM (Chap. 46). Pulmonary thromboembolism, as a single event or as repeated events, rarely leads to the development of chronic pulmonary hypertension.[263] However, in a subset of patients (believed to be less than 0.1 per cent of all patients suffering from pulmonary embolism), the outcome is unusual.[264] Rather than having inherent fibrinolytic resolution of the thromboembolism with restoration of vascular patency, the thromboemboli in these patients fail to resolve adequately (see p. 1598). They undergo organization and incomplete recanalization and become incorporated into the vascular wall. Commonly they are at the subsegmental and segmental and lobar vessels, although it is believed that the chronic thromboembolism tends to propagate retrogradely, leading to slowly progressive vascular obstruction.[263] It appears that the vast majority of these patients have suffered one major thromboembolic event rather than multiple recurrences.

The slowly progressive nature of the course of the disease allows right ventricular hypertrophy to ensue and compensate for the increased pulmonary vascular resistance. However, owing to either progressive thrombosis or vascular changes in the "uninvolved" vascular bed,[264,265] the pulmonary hypertension becomes progressive and the patients manifest the clinical symptoms of dyspnea, fatigue, hypoxemia, and right heart failure. It is particularly critical that these patients be identified and distinguished from patients with primary pulmonary hypertension or other causes, as a large proportion of patients are amenable to surgical thromboendarterectomy with an extraordinarily good outcome[264] (Fig. 46–16, p. 1599). The perfusion lung scan should adequately select out patients with this entity and is another reason why lung perfusion scanning is recommended for all patients who present with pulmonary hypertension (Fig.25–9).

Because the lung scan typically underestimates the severity of the central pulmonary arterial obstruction, any patient who presents with one or more mismatched segmental or larger defects should be considered to have this entity and should undergo pulmonary angiography.[262,263] Pulmonary angiography can be performed safely in these patients if particular attention is given to the hemodynamic state, and immediate treatment with atropine for any vagally induced response to contrast injection is considered.[263]

Patients suitable to undergo pulmonary thromboendarterectomy must have thrombi that are accessible to surgical removal and demonstrate a significant increase in pulmonary vascular resistance.[264] Although the published operative mortality is fairly high, survivors have immediate hemodynamic improvement with a good long-term prognosis. Right ventricular dysfunction of any magnitude is not a contraindication to surgery, as right ventricular function has been noted to improve once the obstruction of pulmonary blood flow is removed.

PERIPHERAL PULMONIC STENOSIS. This is a congenital lesion that occurs particularly in association with supravalvular aortic stenosis or as a sequela of the rubella syndrome (see p. 924). Hypertension in the proximal pulmonary arteries depends on the extent, location, and severity of the stenotic lesions.[266,267]

TAKAYASU'S (GIANT CELL) ARTERITIS (see also p. 1572). This frequently involves the pulmonary vessels; the pathological changes resemble those seen in systemic arteries. In the vast majority of these patients, the aorta and major arch vessels are involved as well. This condition can also be distinguished from PPH by the fact that the occlusive changes occur in the large and intermediate vessels rather than in the more distal vessels characteristic of PPH.[258,259]

HYPOVENTILATION

As discussed earlier (see p. 781), conditions associated with hypoxia may cause pulmonary hypertension, particularly if there is associated acidemia.[31] A number of disorders that affect the upper airways, neuromuscular control, or pulmonary parenchyma lead to hypoventilation and (in the setting of a reactive pulmonary vascular bed) pulmonary hypertension.

THE OBESITY-HYPOVENTILATION SYNDROME[270,271] (see also p. 1614). Also called the Pickwickian syndrome, this condition may lead to substantial pulmonary hypertension (mean pulmonary artery pressure $\geq$ 50 mm Hg), which correlates with the presence of hypoxemia and acidosis (Fig. 47–5, p. 1608). *Pharyngeal-tracheal obstruction* occurs in the presence of hypertrophied tonsils and adenoids[272,273] and may cause reversible pulmonary hypertension.

NEUROMUSCULAR DISORDERS. These include myasthenia gravis, poliomyelitis, and damage to the central respiratory center.[274] They may cause hypoventilation of sufficient severity to result in pulmonary hypertension (see p. 1877). *Disorders of the chest wall* (kyphoscoliosis, pectus excavatum) may also cause hypoventilation and pulmonary hypertension (see p. 1865).

The pulmonary hypertension in all of these conditions subsides with restoration of normal respiration and correction of the hypoxia. It should also be recognized that hypoxia may intensify pulmonary hypertension of other causes. For example, severe pulmonary hypertension occurring in children with a left-to-right shunt who reside at high altitude is often due to the combination of high pulmonary blood flow and superimposed hypoxic pulmonary vasoconstriction; pulmonary pressures may fall rapidly toward normal when residence is established at sea level.

OTHER CAUSES OF PULMONARY HYPERTENSION

HIGH-ALTITUDE PULMONARY EDEMA (see also p. 465). This entity is associated with reversible pulmonary hypertension. It is observed particularly in individuals acclimatized to high altitudes who, after a stay of some days or weeks at sea level, return to high altitude.[275] The finding of high-altitude pulmonary edema in four persons without a right pulmonary artery has been reported,[276] giving support to speculation concerning the combined role of hypoxia and hyperfusion in patients with this condition.[277]

HIGH-OUTPUT CARDIAC FAILURE. A chronic high-output cardiac state can lead to elevation in left ventricular end-diastolic filling pressure.[278] This, along with the chronically increased pulmonary blood flow, may lead to reactive pulmonary hypertension in some individuals.[97] Because these states are uncommon, pulmonary hypertension presenting in this way is rare. Two cases of high-output failure associated with pulmonary hypertension due to hyperthyroidism and cardiac beriberi have been reported.[98] In each instance the pulmonary hypertension subsided when the underlying high-output state was treated. We have recently seen a patient with a chronic arteriovenous fistula resulting in high-output cardiac failure with a similar profile of increased left ventricular end-diastolic pressure and severe reactive pulmonary hypertension. In this individual surgically correcting the arteriovenous fistula improved the high cardiac output state and pulmonary hypertension as well.

OTHER CONDITIONS. Severe pulmonary hypertension is an occasional but unusual finding in patients with *isolated partial anomalous pulmonary venous drainage.*[279] Speculation exists that the cause may be the increase in pulmonary blood flow associated perhaps with a reflex pulmonary arterial vasoconstriction secondary to distention of the right atrium.

The cause of the pulmonary hypertension that occasionally develops following surgical correction of *tetralogy of Fallot* is unclear. In these patients, pulmonary vascular thrombotic lesions are common and, if extensive, may predispose to pulmonary hypertension when operation—either complete correction or creation of a left-to-right shunt—causes a sudden increase in pulmonary blood flow.[280]

Sickle cell anemia may be complicated by in situ pulmonary thrombosis and infarction (see p. 1787), although this does not usually lead to pulmonary hypertension. There are two case reports of cor pulmonale associated with hemoglobin SC disease,[281,282] but the prevalence of pulmonary hypertension in patients with this condition is unknown.

Intravenous drug abuse may lead to diffuse pulmonary vascular occlusion and pulmonary hypertension. Moderately severe pulmonary hypertension developed in association with *alveolar proteinosis* has been reported.[284] Hypoxemia appears to be the mediating factor.

REFERENCES

NORMAL PULMONARY CIRCULATION

1. Comroe, J. H., Jr.: The main functions of the pulmonary circulation. Circulation *33:*146, 1966.
2. Wagenvoort, C. A., and Wagenvoort, N.: Pathology of Pulmonary Hypertension. 2nd ed. New York, John Wiley and Sons, 1977.
3. Fritts, H. W., Harris, P., Chidsey, C. A., et al.: Estimation of flow rate through bronchial–pulmonary vascular anastomoses with use of T-1824 dye. Circulation *23:*390, 1961.
4. Barratt-Boyes, B. G., and Wood, E. H.: Cardiac output and related measurements and pressure values in the right heart and associated vessels, together with an analysis of the hemodynamic response to the inhalation of high oxygen mixtures in healthy subjects. J. Lab. Clin. Med. *51:*72, 1958.
5. Harris, P., and Heath, D.: The Human Pulmonary Circulation. 3rd ed. New York, Churchill Livingstone, 1986, 702 pp.
6. Harris, P., Segel, N., and Bishop, J. M.: The relation between pressure and flow in the pulmonary circulation in normal subjects and in patients with chronic bronchitis and mitral stenosis. Cardiovasc. Res. *1:*73, 1968.
7. Rudolph, A. M.: The changes in the circulation after birth. Their importance in congenital heart disease. Circulation *41:*343, 1970.
8. Friedman, W. F., Molony, D. A., and Kirkpatrick, S. E.: Prostaglandins: Physiological and clinical correlations. Adv. Pediatr. *25:*151, 1978.
9. Naeye, R. L.: Arterial changes during the perinatal period. Arch. Pathol. *71:*121, 1961.
10. Davidson, W. R., Jr., and Fee, E. C.: Influence of aging on pulmonary hemodynamics in a population free of coronary artery disease. Am. J. Cardiol. *65:*1454, 1990.
11. Ghali, J. K., Liao, Y., Cooper, R. S., and Cao, G.: Changes in pulmonary hemodynamics with aging in a predominantly hypertensive population. Am. J. Cardiol. *70:*367, 1992.
12. Cacciapuoti, F., D'Avino, M., Lama, D., et al.: Hemodynamic change in pulmonary circulation induced by effort in the elderly. Am. J. Cardiol. *7:*1481, 1993.
13. Heath, D.: Structural changes in the pulmonary vasculature associated with aging. *In* Carder, L., and Moyer, J. H. (eds.): Aging of the Lung. New York, Grune & Stratton, 1964, pp. 70–76.
14. Spirito, P., and Maron, B. J.: Influence of aging on Doppler echocardiographic indices of left ventricular diastolic function. Br. Heart J. *59:*672, 1988.
15. Rich, S., Chomka, E., Hasara, L., et al.: The prevalence of pulmonary hypertension in the United States. Chest *96:*236, 1989.
16. Fishman, A. P.: Hypoxia on the pulmonary circulation: How and where it acts. Circ. Res. *38:*221, 1976.
17. Haneda, T., Nakajima, T., Shirato, K., et al.: Effects of oxygen breathing on pulmonary vascular input impedance in patients with pulmonary hypertension. Chest *83:*520, 1983.

18. Weir, E. K., Tucker, A., Reeves, J. T., and Will, D. H.: Pulmonary hypertension in cattle at high altitude. Cardiovasc. Res. *8:*745, 1975.
19. Fishman, A. P.: The enigma of hypoxic pulmonary vasoconstriction. *In* Fishman, A. P. (ed.): The Pulmonary Circulation: Normal and Abnormal. Philadelphia, University of Pennsylvania Press, 1990, pp. 109–129.
20. Griffith, T. M., Edwards, D. H., Davies, R. L., et al.: EDRF coordinates the behaviour of vascular resistance vessels. Nature *329:*442, 1987.
21. Hickey, K. A., Rubanyi, G., Paul, R. J., and Highsmith, R. F.: Characterization of a coronary vasoconstrictor produced by cultured endothelial cells. Am. J. Physiol. *248:*C550, 1985.
22. Stewart, D. J., Levy, R. D., Cernacek, P., and Langleben, D.: Increased plasma endothelin-1 in pulmonary hypertension: Marker or mediator of disease? Ann. Intern. Med. *114:*464, 1991.
23. Kotlikoff, M. I., and Fishman, A. P.: Endothelin: Mediator of hypoxic vasoconstriction? *In* Fishman, A. P. (ed.): The Pulmonary Circulation: Normal and Abnormal. Phildelphia, University of Pennsylvania Press, 1990, pp. 85–89.
24. McMurtry, I. F.: Bay K 8644, a Ca^{++} channel facilitator, potentiates hypoxic vasoconstriction in isolated rat lungs. Fed. Proc. *44:*2389, 1985.
25. McMurtry, I. F.: Humeral control. *In* Bergofsky, E. (ed.): Abnormal Pulmonary Circulation. New York, Churchill Livingstone, 1986, pp. 83–126.
26. Rabinovitch, M., Gamble, W., Nadas, A. S., et al.: Rat pulmonary circulation after chronic hypoxia: Hemodynamic and structural features. Am. J. Physiol. *236:*H818, 1979.
27. Rabinovitch, M., Gamble W. J., Miettinen, O. S., and Reid, L.: Age and sex influence on pulmonary hypertension of chronic hypoxia and on recovery. Am. J. Physiol. *240:*H62, 1981.
28. Glazier, J. B., and Murray, J. F.: Sites of pulmonary vasomotor reactivity in the dog during alveolar hypoxia and serotonin and histamine infusion. J. Clin. Invest. *50:*2550, 1971.
29. Bergofsky, E. H.: Mechanisms underlying vasomotor regulation of regional pulmonary blood flow in normal and disease states. Am. J. Med. *57:*378, 1974.
30. Hauge, A.: Hypoxia and pulmonary vascular resistance: The relative effects of pulmonary arterial and alveolar pO_2. Acta Physiol. Scand. *76:*121, 1969.
31. Enson, Y., Giuntini, C., Lewis, M. L., et al.: The influence of hydrogen ion concentration and hypoxia on the pulmonary circulation. J. Clin. Invest. *43:*1146, 1964.
32. Kadowitz, P. J., Joiner, P. D., and Hyman, A. L.: Effect of sympathetic nerve stimulation on pulmonary vascular resistance in the intact spontaneously breathing dog. Proc. Soc. Exp. Biol. Med. *147:*68, 1974.
33. Fritts, H. W., Harris, P., Clauss, R. H., et al.: The effect of acetylcholine on the human pulmonary circulation under normal and hypoxic conditions. J. Clin. Invest. *37:*99, 1958.
34. Kadowitz, P. J., and Hyman, A. L.: Differential effects of prostaglandins A_1 and A_2 on pulmonary vascular resistance in the dog. Proc. Soc. Exp. Biol. Med. *149:*282, 1975.
35. Moncada, S.: Prostacyclin, from discovery to clinical application. J. Pharmacol. *16*(Suppl):71, 1985.
36. Vane, J. R., Anggard, E. E., and Botting, R. M.: Regulatory functions of the vascular endothelium. N. Engl. J. Med. *323:*27, 1990.
37. Radomski, M. W., Palmer, R. M., and Moncada, S.: The anti-aggregating properties of vascular endothelium: Interactions between prostacyclin and nitric oxide. Br. J. Pharmacol. *92:*639, 1987.
37a. Cooper, C. J., Landzberg, M. J., Anderson, T. J., et al.: Role of nitric oxide in the local regulation of pulmonary vascular resistance in humans. Circulation *93:*266, 1996.
38. DeNucci, G., Gryglewski, R. J., Warner, T. D., and Vane, J. R.: Receptor-mediated release of endothelium-derived relaxing factor and prostacyclin from bovine aortic endothelial cells is coupled. Proc. Natl. Acad. Sci. U.S.A. *85:*2334, 1988.
38a. Mehta, S., Stewart, D. J., Langleben, D., and Levy, R. D.: Short-term pulmonary vasodilation with L-arginine in pulmonary hypertension. Circulation *92:*1539, 1995.
39. Kay, J. M., Waymire, J. C., and Grover, R. F.: Lung mast cell hyperplasia and pulmonary histamine forming capacity in hypoxic rats. Am. J. Physiol. *226:*178, 1974.
40. Haas, F., and Bergofsky, E. H.: Role of the mast cell in the pulmonary pressor response to hypoxia. J. Clin. Invest. *51:*3154, 1972.
41. Goldring, R. M., Turino, G. M., Cohen, G., et al.: The catecholamines in the pulmonary arterial pressor response to acute hypoxia. J. Clin. Invest. *41:*1211, 1962.
42. Long, W. A., and Brown, D. L.: Central neural regulation of the pulmonary circulation. *In* Fishman, A. P. (ed.): The Pulmonary Circulation: Normal and Abnormal. University of Pennsylvania Press, Philadelphia, 1990, pp. 131–149.
43. Tucker, A., Hoffman, E. A., and Weir, E. K.: Histamine receptor antagonism does not inhibit hypoxic pulmonary vasoconstriction in dogs. Chest *71*(Suppl):261, 1977.
44. Moret, P., Covarrubias, E., Coudert, J., and Duchosall, F.: Cardiocirculatory adaptation to chronic hypoxia. Acta Cardiol. (Brux.) *27:*596, 1972.
45. Vogel, J. H. K., Weaver, W. F., Rose, R. L., et al.: Pulmonary hypertension on exertion in normal men living at 10,150 feet (Leadville, Colorado). Med. Thorac. *19:*461, 1962.
46. Hatano, S., and Strasser, T. (eds.): Primary Pulmonary Hypertension. Geneva, World Health Organization, 1975, pp. 7–45.
47. Rubin, L. J.: ACCP concensus statement. Primary pulmonary hypertension. Chest *104:*236, 1993.
48. Abenhaim, L., Moride, Y., Rich, S., et al.: The International Primary Pulmonary Hypertension Study. Chest *105*(2):37S, 1994.
49. Wood, P.: Pulmonary hypertension with special reference to the vasoconstrictive factor. Br. Heart J. *20:*557, 1958.
50. Daoud, F. S., Reeves, J. T., and Kelly, D. B.: Isoproterenol as a potential pulmonary vasodilator in primary pulmonary hypertension. Am. J. Cardiol. *42:*817, 1978.
51. Shepherd, J. T., Edwards, J. E., Burchell, H. B., et al.: Clinical, physiological and pathological considerations in patients with idiopathic pulmonary hypertension. Br. Heart J. *19:*70, 1957.
52. Marshall, R. J., Helmholz, H. F., and Shepherd, J. T.: Effect of acetylcholine on pulmonary vascular resistance in a patient with idiopathic pulmonary hypertension. Circulation *20:*391, 1959.
53. Uren, N. G., Ludman, P. E., Crake, T., and Oakley, C. M.: Response of the pulmonary circulation to acetylcholine, calcitonin, gene-related peptide, substance P, and oral nicardipine in patients with primary pulmonary hypertension. J. Am. Coll. Cardiol. *19:*835, 1992.
54. Celermajer, D. S., Cullen, S., and Deanfield, J. E.: Impairment of endothelium-dependent pulmonary artery relaxation in children with congenital heart disease and abnormal pulmonary hemodynamics. Circulation *87:*440, 1993.
55. Luscher, T. F.: Endothelin: Systemic arterial and pulmonary effects of a new peptide with potent biologic properties. Am. Rev. Respir. Dis. *146:*S56, 1992.
56. Okada, M., Yamashita, C., Okada, M., and Okada, K.: Endothelin receptor antagonists in a beagle model of pulmonary hypertension: Contribution of possible potential therapy. J. Am. Coll. Cardiol. *25:*1213, 1995.
57. Pietra, G. G., Edwards, W. D., Kay, J. M., et al.: Histopathology of primary pulmonary hypertension. A qualitative and quantitative study of pulmonary blood vessels from 58 patients in the National Heart, Lung, and Blood Institute, Primary Pulmonary Hypertension Registry. Circulation *80:*1198, 1989.
58. Edwards, W. D., and Edwards, J. E.: Clinical primary pulmonary hypertension—three pathological types. Circulation *56:*884, 1977.
59. Lindner, V., et al.: Role of basic fibroblast growth factor in vascular lesion formation. Circ. Res. *63:*106, 1991.
60. Pierce, G. F., et al.: Platelet-derived growth factor β and transforming growth factors induce in vivo and in vitro tissue repair structures by unique mechanisms. J. Cell Biol. *109:*429, 1989.
61. Botney, M. D., et al.: Vascular remodeling in primary pulmonary hypertension. Potential role for transforming growth factor β. Am. J. Pathol. *144:*286, 1994.
62. Bodreau, N., and Rabinovich, M.: Developmentally regulated changes in extracellular matrix in endothelial and smooth muscle cells in the ductus arteriosus may be related to intimal proliferation. Lab. Invest. *64:*187, 1991.
63. Botney, M. D., et al.: Active collagen synthesis by pulmonary arteries in human primary pulmonary hypertension. Am. J. Pathol. *143:*121, 1993.
64. Rich, S., and Brundage, B. H.: Pulmonary hypertension: A cellular basis for understanding the pathophysiology and treatment. J. Am. Coll. Cardiol. *14:*545, 1989.
65. Fuster, V., Steele, P. M., Edwards, W. D., et al.: Primary pulmonary hypertension: Natural history and the importance of thrombosis. Circulation *70:*580, 1984.
66. Inglesby, T. V., Singer, J. W., and Gordon, D. S.: Abnormal fibrinolysis in familial pulmonary hypertension. Am. J. Med. *55:*5, 1973.
67. Anderson, E. G., Simon, G., and Reid, L.: Primary and thromboembolic pulmonary hypertension: A quantitative pathological study. J. Pathol. *110:*273, 1973.
68. Stuard, I. D., Heusinkveld, R. S., and Moss, A. J.: Microangiopathic hemolytic anemia and thrombocytopenia in primary pulmonary hypertension. N. Engl. J. Med. *287:*869, 1972.
69. Franz, R. C., Ziady, F., Coetzee, W. J. C., and Hugo, N.: A possible causal relationship between defective fibrinolysis and pulmonary hypertension. S. Afr. Med. J. *55:*170, 1979.
70. Tubbs, R. R., Levin, R. D., Shirey, E. K., and Hoffman, G. C.: Fibrinolysis in familial pulmonary hypertension. Am. J. Clin. Pathol. *71:*384, 1979.
71. Geggel, R. L., Carvalho, A. C., Hoyer, L. N., et al.: Von Willebrand factor abnormalities in primary pulmonary hypertension. Am. Rev. Respir. Dis. *135:*294, 1987.
72. Ware, J. A., and Helstad, D. D.: Platelet-endothelium interactions. N. Engl. J. Med. *328:*628, 1993.
73. Hopkins, W. E., Waggoner, A. D., and Barzilai, B.: Frequency and significance of intrapulmonary right-to-left shunting in end-stage hepatic disease. Am. J. Cardiol. *70:*516, 1992.
74. McDonnell, P. J., Toye, P. A., and Hutchins, G. M.: Primary pulmonary hypertension and cirrhosis: Are they related? Am. Rev. Respir. Dis. *127:*437, 1983.
75. Lopez-Talavera, J. C., Merrill, W. M., and Groszmann, R. J.: Tumor necrosis factor α: A major contributor to the hyperdynamic circulation in prehepatic portal-hypertensive rats. Gastroenterology *108:*761, 1995.
76. Stephens, K. E., Ishizaka, A., Larryk, J. W., and Raffin, T. A.: Tumor

necrosis factor causes increased pulmonary permeability and edema. Comparison to septic lung injury. Am. Rev. Respir. Dis. *137*:1364, 1988.
77. Goto, M., Takei, Y., Kuwano, S., et al.: Tumor necrosis factor and endotoxin in the pathogenesis of liver and pulmonary injuries after orthotopic liver transplantation in the rat. Hepatology *16*:487, 1992.
78. Groves, B. M., Brundage, B. H., Elliott, C. G., et al.: Pulmonary hypertension associated with hepatic cirrhosis. *In* Fishman, A. P. (ed.): The Pulmonary Circulation: Normal and Abnormal. Philadelphia, University of Pennsylvania Press, 1990, pp. 359–369.
79. Naeye, R. L.: "Primary" pulmonary hypertension with coexisting portal hypertension. A retrospective study of six cases. Circulation *22*:376, 1960.
80. Segel, N., Kay, J. M., Bayley, T. J., and Paton, A.: Pulmonary hypertension with hepatic cirrhosis. Br. Heart J. *30*:575, 1968.
81. Senior, R. M., Britton, R. C., Turino, G. M., et al.: Pulmonary hypertension associated with cirrhosis of the liver and with portacaval shunts. Circulation *37*:88, 1968.
82. Robalino, B. D., and Moodie, D. S.: Association between primary pulmonary hypertension and portal hypertension: Analysis of its pathophysiology and clinical, laboratory and hemodynamic manifestations. J. Am. Coll. Cardiol. *17*:492, 1991.
83. Gurtner, H. P.: Pulmonary hypertension, "plexogenic pulmonary arteriopathy" and the appetite depressant drug aminorex: Post or propter? Bull. Eur. Physiopathol. Resp. *15*:897, 1979.
84. Douglas, J. G., Monro, J. F., Kitchin, A. H., et al.: Pulmonary hypertension and fenfluramine. Br. Med. J. *283*:881, 1981.
85. McMurray, J., Bloomfield, P., and Miller, H. C.: Irreversible pulmonary hypertension after therapy with fenfluramine. Br. Med. J. *292*:239, 1986.
86. Brenot, F., Herve, P., Pettipretz, P., et al.: Primary pulmonary hypertension and fenfluramine use. Br. Heart J. *70*:537, 1993.
87. Roche, N., Labrune, S., Braune, J. M., and Huchon, G. J.: Pulmonary hypertension and dexfenfluramine. Lancet *339*:437, 1992.
88. Polos, P. G., Wolfe, D., Harley, R. A., et al.: Pulmonary hypertension and human immunodeficiency virus infection. Chest *101*:474, 1992.
89. Jacques, C., Richmond, G., Tierney, L., et al.: Primary pulmonary hypertension and human immunodeficiency virus infection in a non-hemophiliac man. Hum. Pathol. *23*:191, 1992.
90. Maliakkal, R., Freedman, S. A., and Sridhar, S.: Progressive pulmonary thromboembolism in association with HIV disease. N.Y. State J. Med. *92*:403, 1992.
91. Petitpretz, P., Brenot, F., Azarian, R., et al.: Pulmonary hypertension in patients with human immunodeficiency virus infection. Circulation *89*:2772, 1994.
92. Mette, S. A., Palevsky, H. I., Pietra, G. G., et al.: Primary pulmonary hypertension in association with human immunodeficiency virus infection. Am. Rev. Respir. Dis. *145*:1196, 1992.
93. Alpert, M. A., Bauer, J. H., Parker, B. M., et al.: Pulmonary hypertension in systemic hypertension. South Med. J. *78*:784, 1995.
94. Guazzi, M. D., Polese, A., Bartonelli, A., et al.: Evidence of a shared mechanism of vasoconstriction in pulmonary and systemic circulation in hypertension: A possible role of intracellular calcium. Circulation *66*:881, 1982.
95. Guazzi, M. D., DeCasare, N., Fiorentini, C., et al.: Pulmonary vascular supersensitivity to catecholamines in systemic high blood pressure. J. Am. Coll. Cardiol. *8*:1137, 1986.
96. Moruzzi, P., Sganzerla, P., and Guazzi, M. D.: Pulmonary vasoconstriction overreactivity in borderline systemic hypertension. Cardiovasc. Res. *23*:666, 1989.
97. Yamaki, S., Horiuchi, T., Miura, M., et al.: Pulmonary vascular disease in secundum atrial septal defect with pulmonary hypertension. Chest *89*:694, 1986.
98. Okura, H., and Takatsu, Y.: High-output heart failure as a cause of pulmonary hypertension. Intern. Med. *33*:363, 1994.
99. Robertson, B., Rosenhamer, G., and Lindberg, J.: Idiopathic pulmonary hypertension in two siblings. Acta Med. Scand. *186*:569, 1969.
100. Melmon, K. L., and Braunwald, E.: Familial pulmonary hypertension. N. Engl. J. Med. *269*:770, 1963.
101. Rogge, J. D., Mishkin, M. E., and Genovese, P. D.: The familial occurrence of primary pulmonary hypertension. Ann. Intern. Med. *65*:672, 1966.
102. Kingdon, H. S., Cohen, L. S., Roberts, W. C., and Braunwald, E.: Familial occurrence of primary pulmonary hypertension. Arch. Intern. Med. *118*:422, 1966.
103. Lloyd, J. E., Butler, M. G., Foroud, T. M., et al.: Fewer males at birth and genetic anticipation are features of familial primary pulmonary hypertension. Am. Rev. Respir. Dis. *147*:A928, 1993.
104. Lloyd, J. E., Primm, R. K., and Newman, J. H.: Transmission of familial primary pulmonary hypertension. Am. Rev. Respir. Dis. *129*:194, 1984.
105. Rich, S., Kieras, K., Hart, K., et al.: Antinuclear antibodies in primary pulmonary hypertension. J. Am. Coll. Cardiol. *8*:1307, 1986.
106. Barst, R. J., Flaster, E. R., Menom, A., et al.: Evidence for the association of unexplained pulmonary hypertension in children with the major histocompatibility complex. Circulation *85*:249, 1992.
107. Wagenvoort, C. A., and Wagenvoort, N.: Primary pulmonary hypertension: A pathologic study of the lung vessels in 156 clinically diagnosed cases. Circulation *42*:1163, 1970.
108. Bjornsson, J., and Edwards, W. D.: Primary pulmonary hypertension: A histopathologic study of 80 cases. Mayo Clin. Proc. *60*:16, 1969.
109. Clausen, K. P., and Geer, J. C.: Hypertensive pulmonary arteritis. Am. J. Dis. Child. *118*:718, 1969.
110. Wagenvoort, C. A.: Pulmonary veno-occlusive disease: Entity or syndrome. Chest *69*:82, 1976.
111. Rich, S.: Primary pulmonary hypertension. Prog. Cardiovasc. Dis. *31*:205, 1988.
112. Wagenvoort, C. A.: Capillary hemangiomatosis of the lung. Histopathology *2*:401, 1978.
113. Magee, F., Wright, J. L., Kay, M. J., et al.: Pulmonary capillary hemangiomatosis. Am. Rev. Resp. Dis. *132*:922, 1985.
114. Whittaker, J. S., Pickering, C. A. C., Heath, D., et al.: Pulmonary capillary hemangiomatosis. Diag. Histopathol. *6*:77, 1983.
115. Nootens, M., Wolfkiel, C. J., Chomka, E. V., and Rich, S.: Understanding right and left ventricular systolic function and interactions at rest and with exercise in primary pulmonary hypertension. Am. J. Cardiol. *75*:379, 1995.
116. D'Alonzo, G. E., Barst, R. J., Ayres, S. M., et al.: Survival in patients with primary pulmonary hypertension: Results from a national prospective registry. Ann. Intern. Med. *115*:343, 1991.
117. Rich, S., Kaufmann, E., and Levy, P. S.: The effect of high doses of calcium-channel blockers on survival in primary pulmonary hypertension. N. Engl. J. Med. *327*:76, 1992.
118. Sandoval, J., Bauerle, O., Palomar, A., et al.: Survival in primary pulmonary hypertension. Validation of a prognostic equation. Circulation *89*:1733, 1994.
119. Brooks, H., Kirk, E. S., Vokanas, P. S., et al.: Performance of the right ventricle under stress: Relation to right coronary flow. J. Clin. Invest. *50*:2176, 1971.
120. Murray, P. A., and Vatner, S. F.: Reduction of maximal coronary vasodilator capacity in conscious dogs with severe right ventricular hypertrophy. Circ. Res. *48*:27, 1981.
121. Doty, D. B., Wright, C. B., Hirratzka, L. F., et al.: Coronary reserve in volume-induced right ventricular hypertrophy from septal defect. Am. J. Cardiol. *54*:1059, 1984.
122. Vlhakes, G. J., Turley, K., and Hoffman, J. I. E.: The pathophysiology of failure in acute right ventricular hypertension: Hemodynamic and biochemical correlations. Circulation *63*:87, 1981.
123. Murray, P. A., and Vatner, S. F.: Carotid sinus baroreceptor control of right coronary circulation in normal, hypertrophied, and failing right ventricles of conscious dogs. Circ. Res. *49*:1339, 1981.
124. Wilmhurst, P. T., Webb-Peploe, M. M., and Corker, R. J.: Left recurrent laryngeal nerve palsy associated with primary pulmonary hypertension and recurrent pulmonary embolism. Br. Heart J. *49*:141, 1983.
124a. Chobanian, A. V., and Dzau, V. J.: Renin antiotensin system and atherosclerotic vascular disease. *In* Fuster, V., Ross, R., and Topol, E. J. (eds.): Atherosclerosis and coronary artery disease. Philadelphia, Lippincott-Raven Publishers, 1996, pp.237–242.
125. Kanemoto, N.: Electrocardiographic and hemodynamic correlations in primary pulmonary hypertension. Angiology *39*:781, 1988.
126. Kanemoto, N., Furuya, H., Etoh, T., Sasamoto, H., and Matsuyama, S.: Chest roentgenograms in primary pulmonary hypertension. Chest *76*:45, 1979.
127. Anderson, G., Reid, L., and Simon, G.: The radiographic appearances in primary and in thromboembolic pulmonary hypertension. Clin. Radiol. *24*:113, 1973.
128. Kuriyama, K., Gamsu, G., Stern, R. G., et al.: CT-determined pulmony artery diameters in predicting pulmonary hypertension. Invest. Radiol. *19*:16, 1984.
129. Goodman, D. J., Harrison, D. C., and Popp, R. L.: Echocardiographic features of primary pulmonary hypertension. Am. J. Cardiol. *33*:438, 1974.
130. Louie, E. K., Rich, S., and Brundage, B. H.: Doppler echocardiographic assessment of impaired left ventricular filling with right ventricular pressure overload due to primary pulmonary hypertension. J. Am. Coll. Cardiol. *8*:1298, 1986.
131. Rich, S., Pietra, G. G., Kieras, K., et al.: Primary pulmonary hypertension: Radiographic and scintigraphic patterns of histologic subtypes. Ann. Intern. Med. *105*:499, 1986.
132. Fishman, A. J., Moser, K. M., and Fedullo, P. F.: Perfusion lung scans vs pulmonary angiography in the evaluation of suspected primary pulmonary hypertension. Chest *84*:679, 1983.
133. Levin, R. I., and Glassman, E.: Left atrial-pulmonary artery wedge pressure relation: Effect of elevated pulmonary vascular resistance. Am. J. Cardiol. *55*:856, 1985.
134. Rozkovic, A., Montanes, D., and Oakley, C. M.: Factors that influence the outcome of primary pulmonary hypertension. Br. Heart J. *55*:449, 1986.
135. Groves, B. M., Ditchey, R. V., Reeves, J. T., et al.: Multicenter trial of a new guide wire thermodilution catheter. J. Am. Coll. Cardiol. *3*:599, 1984.
136. Nootens, M. T., Berarducci, L. A., Kaufmann, E., et al.: The prevalence and significance of a patent foramen ovale in pulmonary hypertension. Chest *104*:1673, 1993.
137. Benotti, J. R., and Grossman, W.: Pulmonary angiography. *In* Grossman, W., and Baim, D. S. (eds.): Cardiac Catheterization, Angiography and Intervention. 4th ed. Philadelphia, Lea and Febiger, 1991.
138. Janiki, J. S., Weber, K. T., Likoff, M. J., et al.: The pressure-flow response of the pulmonary circulation in patients with heart failure and pulmonary vascular disease. Circulation *72*:1270, 1985.

139. McCaffrey, R. M., and Dunn, L. J.: Primary pulmonary hypertension in pregnancy. Obstet. Gynecol. Surg. *19*:567, 1964.
140. Nelson, D. M., Main, E., Crafford, W., et al.: Peripartum heart failure due to primary pulmonary hypertension. Obstet. Gynecol. *62*:58S, 1983.
141. Spann, J. F., Buccino, R. A., Sonnenblick, E. H., et al.: Contractile state of cardiac muscle obtained from cats with experimentally produced ventricular hypertrophy. Circ. Res. *21*:431, 1967.
142. Fishman, A. P.: Chronic cor pulmonale. Am. Rev. Respir. Dis. *114*:775, 1976.
143. Abraham, A. S., Cole, R. B., and Bishop, J. B.: Reversal of pulmonary hypertension by prolonged oxygen administration to patients with chronic bronchitis. Circ. Res. *23*:147, 1968.
144. Swan, H. J. C., Burchell, H. B., and Wood, E. H.: Effect of oxygen on pulmonary vascular resistance in patients with pulmonary hypertension associated with atrial septal defect. Circulation *20*:66, 1959.
145. Morgan, J. M., Griffiths, M., du Bois, R. M., and Evans, T. W.: Hypoxic pulmonary vasoconstriction in systemic sclerosis and primary pulmonary hypertension. Chest *99*:551, 1991.
146. Rich, S., D'Alonzo, G. E., Dantzker, D. R., et al.: Magnitude and implications of spontaneous hemodynamic variability in primary pulmonary hypertension. Am. J. Cardiol. *55*:159, 1985.
147. Packer, M., Medine, N., and Yushak, M.: Adverse hemodynamic and clinical effects of calcium channel blockade in pulmonary hypertension secondary to obliterative pulmonary vascular disease. J. Am. Coll. Cardiol. *4*:890, 1984.
148. Melot, C., Hallemans, R., Naeije, R., et al.: Deleterious effect of nifedipine on pulmonary gas exchange in chronic obstructive pulmonary disease. Am. Rev. Respir. Dis. *130*:612, 1984.
149. Rich, S., and Kaufmann, L: High dose titration of calcium channel blocking agents for primary pulmonary hypertension: Guidelines for short-term drug testing. J. Am. Coll. Cardiol. *18*:1323, 1991.
150. Grover, R. F., Reeves, J. T., and Blount, S. F., Jr.: Tolazoline hydrochloride (Priscoline): An effective pulmonary vasodilator. Am. Heart J. *61*:5, 1961.
151. Rudolph, A. M., Paul, M. H., Sommer, L. S., et al.: Effects of tolazoline hydrochloride (Priscoline) on circulatory dynamics in patients with pulmonary hypertension. Am. Heart J. *56*:424, 1958.
152. Samet, P., Bernstein, W. H., and Widrich, J.: Intracardiac infusion of acetylcholine in primary pulmonary hypertension. Am. Heart J. *60*:433, 1960.
153. Charms, B. L.: Primary pulmonary hypertension: Effect of unilateral pulmonary artery occlusion and infusion of acetylcholine. Am. J. Cardiol. *99*:94, 1961.
154. Shettigar, U. R., Hultgren, H. N., Specter, M., et al.: Primary pulmonary hypertension: Favorable effect of isoproterenol. N. Engl. J. Med. *295*:1414, 1976.
154a. Morgan, J. M., Griffiths, M., du Bois, R. M., and Evans, T. W.: Hypoxic pulmonary vasoconstriction in systemic sclerosis and primary pulmonary hypertension. Chest *99*:551, 1991.
154b. Heath, D., and Edwards, J. E.: The pathology of hypertensive pulmonary vascular disease. A description of six grades of structural changes in the pulmonary arteries with special references to congenital cardiac septal defects. Circulation *18*:533, 1958.
155. Person, B., and Proctor, R. G.: Primary pulmonary hypertension: Responses to indomethacin, terbutaline and isoproterenol. Chest *76*:601, 1979.
156. Bergofsky, E. H.: Mechanisms underlying vasomotor regulation of regional pulmonary blood flow in normal and disease states. Am. J. Med. *57*:378, 1974.
157. Fishman, A. P.: Autonomic vasomotor tone in the pulmonary circulation. J. Anesthesiol. *45*:1, 1976.
158. Ruskin, J. N., and Hutter, A. M.: Primary pulmonary hypertension treated with oral phentolamine. Ann. Intern. Med. *90*:772, 1979.
159. Beladinelli, L., Linden, J., and Berne, M. R.: The cardiac effects of adenosine. Prog. Cardiovasc. Dis. *32*:73, 1989.
160. Watt, A. H., Penny, W. J., Singh, H., et al.: Adenosine causes transient dilatation of coronary arteries in man. Br. J. Clin. Pharmacol. *24*:665, 1987.
161. Bush, A., Busst, C. M., Clarke, B., and Barnes, P. J.: Effect of infused adenosine on cardiac output and systemic resistance in normal subjects. Br. J. Clin. Pharmacol. *27*:165, 1989.
162. McCormack, D. G., Clarke, B., and Barnes, P. J.: Characterization of adenosine receptors in human pulmonary arteries. Am. J. Physiol. *256*:H41, 1989.
163. Schrader, B., Inbar, S., Kaufmann, L., et al.: Comparison of the effects of adenosine and nifedipine in pulmonary hypertension. J. Am. Coll. Cardiol. *19*:1060, 1992.
164. Nootens, M., Schrader, B., Kaufmann, E., et al.: Comparative acute effects of adenosine and prostacyclin in primary pulmonary hypertension. Chest *107*:54, 1995.
165. Muller, B.: Pharmacology of thromboxane A_2, prostacyclin and other ecosanoids in the cardiovascular system. Therapie *46*:217, 1991.
166. Dusting, G. J., and MacDonald, P. S.: Prostacyclin and vascular function: Implications for hypertension and atherosclerosis. Pharmacol. Ther. *48*:323, 1990.
167. Rubin, L. J., Groves, B. M., Reeves, J. T., et al.: Prostacyclin-induced pulmonary vasodilation in primary pulmonary hypertension. Circulation *66*:334, 1982.
168. Barst, R. J.: Pharmacologically induced pulmonary vasodilatation in children and young adults with primary hypertension. Chest *89*:497, 1986.
169. Frostell, C., Fratacci, M. D., Wain, J. C., et al.: Inhaled nitric oxide: A selective pulmonary vasodilator reversing hypoxic pulmonary vasoconstriction. Circulation *83*:2038, 1991.
170. Pepke-Zaba, J., Higgenbottam, W., Tuan Ding-Xuan, A., et al.: Inhaled nitric oxide as a cause of selective pulmonary vasodilation in pulmonary hypertension. Lancet *338*:1173, 1991.
171. Roberts, J. D., Lang, P., Bigatello, L. M., et al.: Inhaled nitric oxide in congenital heart disease. Circulation *87*:447, 1993.
172. Rubin, L. J., Nicod, P., Hillis, L. D., and Firth, B. G.: Treatment of primary pulmonary hypertension with nifedipine. A hemodynamic and scintigraphic evaluation. Ann. Intern. Med. *99*:433, 1983.
173. Fisher, J., Borer, J. S., Moses, J. W., et al.: Hemodynamic effects of nifedipine versus hydralazine in primary pulmonary hypertension. Am. J. Cardiol. *54*:646, 1984.
174. Melot, C., Naejie, R., Mols, P., et al.: Effects of nifedipine on ventilation/perfusion matching in primary pulmonary hypertension. Chest *83*:203, 1983.
175. Olivari, M. T., Cohn, J. N., Carlyle, P., and Levine, T. B.: Beneficial hemodynamic and exercise response to nifedipine in primary pulmonary hypertension. J. Am. Coll. Cardiol. *1*:735, 1983.
176. Packer, M., Medina, N., Yushak, M., and Wiener, I.: Detrimental effects of verapamil in patients with primary hypertension. Br. Heart J. *52*:106, 1984.
177. Rich, S., and Brundage, B. H.: High-dose calcium channel-blocking therapy for primary pulmonary hypertension: Evidence of long-term reduction in pulmonary arterial pressure and regression of right ventricular hypertrophy. Circulation *76*:135, 1987.
178. Jones, D. K., Whigenbottam, T. W., and Wallwork, J.: Treatment of primary pulmonary hypertension with intravenous epoprostenol (prostacyclin). Br. Heart J. *57*:270, 1987.
179. Rubin, L. J., Mendoza, J., Hood, M., et al.: Treatment of primary pulmonary hypertension with continuous intravenous prostacyclin (epoprostenol). Ann. Intern. Med. *112*:485, 1990.
180. Barst, R. J., Rubin, L. J., McGoon, M. D., et al.: Survival in primary pulmonary hypertension with long-term continuous intravenous prostacyclin. Ann. Intern. Med. *121*:409, 1994.
180a. Raffy, O., Azarian, R., Brenot, F., et al.: Clinical significance of the pulmonary vasodilator response during short-term infusion of prostacyclin in primary pulmonary hypertension. Circulation *93*:484, 1996.
181. Guadagni, D. N., Ikram, H., and Maslowski, A. H.: Haemodynamic effects of prostacyclin (PGI_2) in pulmonary hypertension. Br. Heart J. *45*:385, 1981.
182. Rubin, L. J., Groves, B. M., Reeves, J. T., et al.: Prostacyclin-induced acute pulmonary vasodilation in primary pulmonary hypertension. Circulation *66*:334, 1982.
183. Groves, B. M., Rubin, L. J., Frosolono, M. F., et al.: A comparison of the acute hemodynamic effects of prostacyclin and hydralazine in primary pulmonary hypertension. Am. Heart J. *110*:1200, 1985.
184. Rozkovec, A., Stradling, J. R., Shepherd, G., et al.: Prediction of favourable responses to long term vasodilator treatment of pulmonary hypertension by short-term administration of epoprostenol (prostacyclin) or nifedipine. Br. Heart J. *59*:696, 1988.
185. Lock, J. E., Olley, P. M., Coceani, P. M., et al.: Use of prostacyclin in persistent fetal circulation. Lancet *1*:1343, 1979.
186. Young, D., and Mark, H.: Fate of the patient with Eisenmenger's syndrome. Am. J. Cardiol. *65*:655, 1971.
187. Rich, S., and Lam, W.: Atrial septostomy as palliative therapy for refractory primary pulmonary hypertension. Am. J. Cardiol. *51*:1560, 1983.
188. Nihill, M. R., O'Laughlin, M. P., and Mullins, C. E.: Effects of atrial septostomy in patients with terminal cor pulmonale due to pulmonary vascular disease. Cathet. Cardiovasc. Diagn. *24*:166, 1991.
189. Hausknecht, M. J., Sims, R. E., Nihill, M. R., and Cashion, W. R.: Successful palliation of primary pulmonary hypertension by atrial septostomy. Am. J. Cardiol. *65*:1045, 1990.
190. Kirstein, D., Levy, P. S., Hsui, D. T., et al.: Blade balloon atrial septostomy in patients with severe primary pulmonary hypertension. Circulation *91*:2028, 1995.
191. Jamieson, S. W., Stinson, E. B., Oyer, P. E., et al.: Heart and lung transplantation for pulmonary hypertension. Am. J. Surg. *147*:740, 1984.
192. Dawkins, K. D., Jamieson, S. W., Hunt, S. A., et al.: Long-term results, hemodynamics, and complications after combined heart and lung transplantation. Circulation *71*:919, 1985.
193. Dawkins, K. D., Haverich, A., Derby, G. C., et al.: Long-term hemodynamics following combined heart and lung transplantation in primates. J. Thorac. Cardiovasc. Surg. *89*:55, 1985.
194. Reitz, B. A., Wallwork, J. L., Hunt, S. A., et al.: Heart-lung transplantation: Successful therapy for patients with pulmonary vascular disease. N. Engl. J. Med. *306*:557, 1982.
195. Kaiser, L. R., and Cooper, J. D.: The current status of lung transplantation. Adv. Surg. *25*:259, 1992.
196. Pasque, M. K., Trulock, E. P., Kaiser, L. R., and Cooper, J. D.: Single-lung transplantation for pulmonary hypertension: Three-month hemodynamic follow-up. Circulation *84*:2275, 1991.
197. Levine, S. M., Jenkinson, S. G., Bryan, C. L., et al.: Ventilation-perfusion inequalities during graft rejection in patients undergoing single lung transplantation for primary pulmonary hypertension. Chest *101*:401, 1992.

198. Brooks, H. L., Kirk, E. S., Vokonas, P. S., et al.: Performance of the right ventricle under stress. J. Clin. Invest. *50:*2176, 1971.
199. Berman, J. L., Green, L. G., and Grossman, W.: Right ventricular diastolic pressure in coronary artery disease. Am. J. Cardiol. *44:*1263, 1979.
200. Lorell, B. H., Leinbach, R. C., Pohost, G. M., et al.: Right ventricular infarction. Am. J. Cardiol. *43:*463, 1979.
201. Kay, J. M., and Edwards, F. R.: Ultrastructure of the alveolar-capillary wall in mitral stenosis. J. Pathol. *111:*239, 1973.
202. Szidon, J. P., Pietra, G. G., and Fishman, A. P.: The alveolar-capillary membrane and pulmonary edema. N. Engl. J. Med. *286:*1200, 1972.
203. Hicks, J. D.: Acute arterial necrosis in the lungs. J. Pathol. Bacteriol. *65:*333, 1953.
204. Whitaker, W., Black, A., and Warrack, A. J. N.: Pulmonary ossification in patients with mitral stenosis. J. Fac. Radiol. (Lond.) *7:*29, 1955.
205. Jordan, S. C., Hicken, P., Watson, D. A., et al.: Pathology of the lungs in mitral stenosis in relation to respiratory function and pulmonary haemodynamics. Br. Heart J. *28:*101, 1966.
206. Grossman, W.: Profiles in valvular heart disease. *In* Grossman, W., and Baim, D. S. (eds.): Cardiac Catheterization, Angiography and Intervention. 4th ed. Philadelphia, Lea and Febiger, 1991.
207. Dexter, L.: Physiologic changes in mitral stenosis. N. Engl. J. Med. *254:*829, 1956.
208. Robin, E. R., and Meyer, E. C.: Cardiopulmonary effects of pulmonary venous hypertension with special reference to pulmonary lymphatic flow. Circ. Res. *8:*324, 1960.
209. Uhley, H. N., Leeds, S. E., Sampson, J. J., and Friedman, M.: Role of pulmonary lymphatics in chronic pulmonary edema. Circ. Res. *11:*966, 1962.
210. Parker, F., and Weiss, S.: The nature and significance of the structural changes in the lungs in mitral stenosis. Am. J. Pathol. *12:*573, 1936.
211. Coalson, J. J., Jacques, W. E., Campbell, G. S., and Thompson, W. M.: Ultrastructure of the alveolar capillary membrane in congenital and acquired heart disease. Arch. Pathol. *83:*377, 1967.
212. Kay, J. M., and Edwards, F. R.: Ultrastructure of the alveolar capillary wall in mitral stenosis. J. Pathol. *111:*239, 1973.
213. Heath, D., and Edwards, J. E.: Histological changes in the lung in diseases associated with pulmonary venous hypertension. Br. J. Dis. Chest *53:*8, 1959.
214. Carabello, B. A., and Grossman, W.: Calculation of stenotic valve orifice area. *In* Grossman, W., and Gaim, D. S. (eds.): Cardiac Catheterization, Angiography, and Intervention. 4th ed. Philadelphia, Lea and Febiger, 1991.
215. Braunwald, E., Braunwald, N. S., Ross, J., Jr., and Morrow, A. G.: Effects of mitral valve replacement on pulmonary vascular dynamics of patients with pulmonary hypertension. N. Engl. J. Med. *273:*509, 1965.
216. Dalen, J. E., Matloff, J. M., Evans, G. L., et al.: Early reduction of pulmonary vascular resistance after mitral valve replacement. N. Engl. J. Med. *277:*387, 1967.
217. Levine, M. J., Weinstein, J. S., Diver, D. J., et al.: Progressive improvement in pulmonary vascular resistance following percutaneous mitral valvuloplasty. Circulation *79:*1061, 1989.
218. Alexopoulos, D., Lazzam, C., Borrica, S., et al.: Isolated chronic mitral regurgitation with preserved systolic left ventricular function and severe pulmonary hypertension. J. Am. Coll. Cardiol. *14:*319, 1989.
219. Magidson, A.: Cor triatriatum. Severe pulmonary arterial hypertension and pulmonary venous hypertension in a child. Am. J. Cardiol. *9:*603, 1962.
220. Cromie, J. B.: Correlation of anatomic pulmonary emphysema and right ventricular hypertrophy. Am. Rev. Respir. Dis. *84:*657, 1961.
221. Hicken, P., Heath, D., and Brewer, D.: The relation between the weight of the right ventricle and the percentage of abnormal air space in the lung in emphysema. J. Pathol. Bacteriol. *92:*519, 1966.
221a. Burrow, B., Kettel, L. J., Niden, A. H., et al.: Patterns of cardiovascular dysfunction in chronic obstructive lung disease. N. Engl. J. Med. *286:*912, 1972.
222. Harvey, R. M., Ferrer, M. I., Richards, D. W., and Cournand, A.: Influence of chronic pulmonary disease on the heart and circulation. Am. J. Med. *10:*719, 1951.
223. Abraham, A. S., Cole, R. B., Green, I. D., et al.: Factors contributing to the reversible pulmonary hypertension in patients with acute respiratory failure studied by serial observation during recovery. Circ. Res. *24:*51, 1969.
224. Abraham, A. S., Cole, R. B., and Bishop, J.: Effects of prolonged oxygen administration on the pulmonary hypertension of patients with chronic bronchitis. Circ. Res. *23:*147, 1968.
225. Segel, N., and Bishop, J. M.: The circulation in patients with chronic bronchitis and emphysema at rest and during exercise with special reference to the influence of changes in blood viscosity and blood volumes on the pulmonary circulation. J. Clin. Invest. *45:*1555, 1966.
226. Horsfield, K., Segel, N., and Bishop, J. M.: The pulmonary circulation in chronic bronchitis at rest and during exercise breathing air and 80% oxygen. Clin. Sci. *34:*473, 1968.
227. Harvey, R. M., Ferrer, M. I., Richards, D. W., Jr., and Cournand, A.: Influence of chronic pulmonary disease on the heart and circulation. Am. J. Med. *10:*719, 1951.
228. Yu, P. N., Lovejoy, F. W., Joos, H. A., et al.: Studies of pulmonary hypertension. I. Pulmonary circulatory dynamics in patients with pulmonary emphysema at rest. J. Clin. Invest. *32:*130, 1953.
229. Kitchin, A. H., Lowther, C. P., and Matthews, M. B.: The effect of exercise and of breathing oxygen-enriched air on the pulmonary circulation in emphysema. Clin. Sci. *21:*93, 1961.
230. Wilson, R. H., Hoseth, W., and Dempsey, M. E.: The effects of breathing 99.6% oxygen on pulmonary vascular resistance and cardiac output in patients with pulmonary emphysema and chronic hypoxia. Ann. Intern. Med. *42:*629, 1955.
231. Aber, G. M., Harris, A. M., and Bishop, J. M.: The effect of acute changes in inspired oxygen concentration of cardiac, respiratory and renal function in patients with chronic obstructive airways disease. Clin. Sci. *26:*133, 1964.
232. Stuart-Harris, C., Bishop, J. M., Clark, T. J. H., et al.: Long-term domiciliary oxygen therapy in chronic hypoxic cor pulmonale complicating chronic bronchitis and emphysema. Lancet *1:*681, 1981.
233. Nocturnal Oxygen Therapy Trial Group: Continuous or nocturnal oxygen therapy in hypoxic chronic obstructive airways disease? Ann. Intern. Med. *93:*391, 1980.
234. Foreman, S., Weill, H., Duke, R., et al.: Bullous disease of the lung: Physiologic improvement after surgery. Ann. Intern. Med. *69:*757, 1968.
235. Salerni, R., Rodnan, G. P., Leon, D. F., and Shaver, J. A.: Pulmonary hypertension in the CREST syndrome variant of progressive systemic sclerosis (scleroderma). Ann. Intern. Med. *86:*394, 1977.
236. Follansbee, W. P., Curtiss, E. I., Medsger, T. A., et al.: Myocardial function and perfusion in the CREST syndrome variant of progressive systemic sclerosis. Am. J. Med. *77:*489, 1984.
237. Seldin, D. W., Ziff, M., and DeGraff, A. V., Jr.: Raynaud's phenomenon associated with pulmonary hypertension. Tex. State J. Med. *58:*654, 1962.
238. Winters, W. L., Jr., Joseph, R. R., and Lerner, N.: "Primary" pulmonary hypertension and Raynaud's phenomenon. Arch. Intern. Med. *114:*821, 1964.
239. Caldwell, I. W., and Aitchison, J. D.: Pulmonary hypertension in dermatomyositis. Br. Heart J. *18:*273, 1956.
240. Walker, W. C., and Wright, V.: Pulmonary lesions and rheumatoid arthritis. Medicine *47:*501, 1968.
241. Santini, D., Fox, D., Kloner, R. A., et al.: Pulmonary hypertension in systemic lupus erythematosus: Hemodynamics and effects of vasodilator therapy. Clin. Cardiol. *3:*406, 1980.
242. Asherson, R. A., Mackworth-Young, C. G., Boey, M. L., et al.: Pulmonary hypertension in systemic lupus erythematosus. Br. Med. J. *287:*1024, 1983.
243. Muschenheim, C.: Some observations on the Hamman-Rich disease. Am. J. Med. Sci. *241:*279, 1961.
244. Soergel, K. H., and Sommers, S. C.: Idiopathic pulmonary hemosiderosis and related syndromes. Am. J. Med. *32:*499, 1962.
245. Manglo, A., Fisher, J., Libby, D. M., and Saddekni, S.: Sarcoidosis, pulmonary hypertension, and acquired peripheral pulmonary artery stenosis. Cathet. Cardiovasc. Diagn. *11:*69, 1985.
246. Kane, R. D., Hawkins, H. K., Miller, J. A., and Noce, P. S.: Microscopic pulmonary tumor emboli associated with dyspnea. Cancer *36:*1473, 1975.
247. Jacques, J. E., and Barclay, R.: The solid sarcomatous pulmonary artery. Br. J. Dis. Chest *11:*123, 1974.
248. Cooney, T. P., and Thurlbeck, W. M.: Pulmonary hypoplasia in Down's syndrome. N. Engl. J. Med. *307:*1170, 1982.
249. Wood, P.: The Eisenmenger syndrome, or pulmonary hypertension with reversed central shunt. Br. Med. J. *2:*755, 1958.
250. Yamaki, S., and Wagenvoort, C. A.: Comparison of primary plexogenic arteriopathy in adults and children. A morphometric study in 40 patients. Br. Heart J. *54:*428, 1985.
251. Haworth, S. G.: Pulmonary vascular disease in different types of congential heart disease. Implications for interpretation of lung biopsy findings in early childhood. Br. Heart J. *52:*557, 1984.
252. Rabinovitch, M., Keane, J. F., Norwood, W. I., et al.: Vascular structure in lung tissue obtained at biopsy correlated with pulmonary hemodynamic findings after repair of congenital heart defects. Circulation *69:*655, 1984.
253. Davies, N. J. H., Shinebourne, E. A., Scallan, M. J., et al.: Pulmonary vascular resistance in children with congenital heart disease. Thorax *39:*895, 1984.
254. Takahashi, T., and Wagenvoort, C. A.: Density of muscularized arteries in the lung. Arch. Pathol. Lab. Med. *107:*23, 1983.
255. Harley, R. A., Friedman, P. J., Saldana, M., et al.: Sequential development of lesions in experimental extreme pulmonary hypertension. Am. J. Pathol. *52:*52A, 1968.
256. Saldana, M. E., Harley, R. A., Liebow, A. A., and Carrington, C. B.: Extreme experimental pulmonary hypertension in relation to polycythemia. Am. J. Pathol. *52:*935, 1968.
257. Rabinovitch, M., Keane, J. F., Fellows, K. E., et al.: Quantitative analysis of the pulmonary wedge angiogram in congenital heart defects. Circulation *63:*152, 1981.
258. Kawai, C., Ishikawa, K., Kato, M., et al.: Pulmonary pulseless disease: Pulmonary involvement in so-called Takayasu's disease. Chest *73:*651, 1978.
259. Lande, A., and Bard, R.: Takayasu's arteritis: An unrecognized cause of pulmonary hypertension. Angiography *27:*114, 1976.
260. Levin, D. E., Heymann, M. A., Kitterman, J. A., et al.: Persistent pulmonary hypertension of the newborn infant. J. Pediatr. *89:*626, 1976.

261. Finn, M. C., Williams, L. C., and King, T. D.: Persistent fetal circulation in the newborn. J. La. State Med. Soc. *129*:169, 1977.
262. Haworth, S. G., and Reid, L.: Persistent fetal circulation: Newly recognized structural features. J. Pediatr. *88*:614, 1976.
263. Rich, S., Levitsky, S., and Brundage, B. H.: Pulmonary hypertension from chronic pulmonary thromboembolism. Ann. Intern. Med. *108*:425, 1988.
264. Moser, K. M., Daily, P. O., Peterson, K., et al.: Thromboembolic pulmonary hypertension. Ann. Intern. Med. *107*:560, 1987.
265. Shure, D., Gregoratos, G., and Moser, K. M.: Fiberoptic angioscopy: Role in diagnosis of chronic pulmonary arterial obstruction. Ann. Intern. Med. *103*:844, 1985.
266. Delaney, T. B., and Nadas, A. S.: Peripheral pulmonic stenosis. Am. J. Cardiol. *13*:451, 1964.
267. McCue, C. M., Robertson, L. W., Lester, R. G., and Mauck, H. P.: Pulmonary artery coarctations. J. Pediatr. *67*:222, 1965.
268. Pool, P. E., Vogel, J. H. K., and Blount, S. G., Jr.: Congenital unilateral absence of a pulmonary artery. Am. J. Cardiol. *10*:706, 1962.
269. Cohn, L. H., Sanders, J. H., Jr., and Collins, J. J., Jr.: Surgical treatment of congenital unilateral pulmonary arterial stenosis with contralateral pulmonary hypertension. Am. J. Cardiol. *38*:257, 1976.
270. Burwell, C. S., Robin, E. D., Whaley, R. D., and Bickelmann, A. G.: Extreme obesity associated with alveolar hypoventilation. Am. J. Med. *21*:811, 1956.
271. James, T. N., Frame, B., and Coates, E. D.: De subitaneis mortibus. III. Pickwickian syndrome. Circulation *48*:1311, 1973.
272. Noonan, A. J.: Reversible cor pulmonale due to hypertrophied tonsils and adenoids: Studies in two cases. Circulation *32*(Suppl. II):164, 1965.
273. Menashe, V. D., Farrchi, C., and Miller, M.: Hypoventilation and cor pulmonale due to chronic upper airway obstruction. J. Pediatr. *57*:198, 1965.
274. Naeye, R. L.: Alveolar hypoventilation and cor pulmonale secondary to damage to the respiratory center. Am. J. Cardiol. *8*:416, 1961.
275. Hultgren, H. N., Lopez, C. E., Lundberg, E., and Miller, H.: Physiologic studies of pulmonary edema at high altitude. Circulation *29*:393, 1964.
276. Hackett, P. H., Creagh, C. E., Grover, R. F., et al.: High altitude pulmonary edema in persons without the right pulmonary artery. N. Engl. J. Med. *302*:1070, 1980.
277. Staub, N. C.: Pulmonary edema—Hypoxia and overperfusion. N. Engl. J. Med. *302*:1085, 1980.
278. Ingram, C., Satler, L. F., and Rackley, C. E.: Progressive heart failure secondary to a high output state. Chest *92*:1117, 1987.
279. Saaluke, M. G., Shapiro, S. R., Perry, L. W., and Scott, L. P.: Isolated partial anomalous pulmonary venous drainage associated with pulmonary vascular obstructive disease. Am. J. Cardiol. *39*:439, 1977.
280. Heath, D., DuShane, J. W., Wood, E. H., and Edwards, J. E.: The etiology of pulmonary thrombosis in cyanotic congenital heart disease with pulmonary stenosis. Thorax *13*:213, 1958.
281. Durant, J. R., and Cortes, F. M.: Occlusive pulmonary vascular disease associated with hemoglobin SC disease. Am. Heart J. *71*:100, 1966.
282. Rowley, P. T., and Enlander, D.: Hemoglobin SC disease presenting as acute cor pulmonale. Am. Rev. Respir. Dis. *98*:494, 1968.
283. Houck, R. J., Bailey, G. L., Doaroca, P. J., et al.: Pentazocine abuse: Report of a case with pulmonary arterial cellulose granulomas and pulmonary hypertension. Chest *77*:2, 1980.
284. Oliva, P. B., and Vogel, J. H. K.: Reactive pulmonary hypertension in alveolar proteinosis. Chest *58*:167, 1970.
285. Rose, A. G., Halper, J., and Factor, S. M.: Primary arteriopathy in Takayasu's disease. Arch. Pathol. Lab. Med. *108*:644, 1984.

Chapter 26
Systemic Hypertension: Mechanisms and Diagnosis

NORMAN M. KAPLAN

DEFINITIONS, PREVALENCE, AND CONSEQUENCES OF HYPERTENSION

Hypertension, despite its widely recognized high prevalence and associated danger, remains inadequately treated in the majority of patients. In the representative sample of the U.S. population examined in the 1988–1991 National Health and Nutrition Examination Survey (NHANES III), only 21 per cent of hypertensives had their blood pressure well controlled, as defined by a reading below 140/90 mm Hg[1] (Fig. 26–1). Although most hypertension had been identified previously, only about half of hypertensives were currently being treated. Even in a group of hypertensive health care workers with an insurance plan that covered all costs, only 12 per cent of those surveyed in 1992 had their blood pressure adequately managed.[2]

Despite these disturbing figures, the management of hypertension is now the leading indication for both visits to physicians and the use of prescription drugs in the United States. According to the National Ambulatory Care Survey, over 85 million office visits related to hypertension were made in 1991.[3] Clearly, more attention is being directed toward hypertension, but its adequate control remains elusive. This reflects, in large part, the asymptomatic nature of the disease for the first 15 to 20 years, even as it progressively damages the cardiovascular system.[4] Asymptomatic patients often are unwilling to alter life style or take medication to forestall some far-off, poorly perceived danger, particularly when they are made uncomfortable in the process.

In view of these built-in barriers to effective control of the individual patient, the population-wide application of preventive measures becomes inherently more attractive. Although the specific mechanisms for most hypertension remain unknown, it is highly likely that the process could be slowed, if not prevented, by the prevention of obesity, moderate reduction in sodium intake, higher levels of physical activity, and avoidance of excessive alcohol consumption.[5] Since most people will eventually develop hypertension during their lifetime, the need for more widespread adoption of potentially effective and totally safe preventive measures is obvious. In the meantime, better management of those already afflicted must be practiced, starting with careful documentation of the diagnosis.

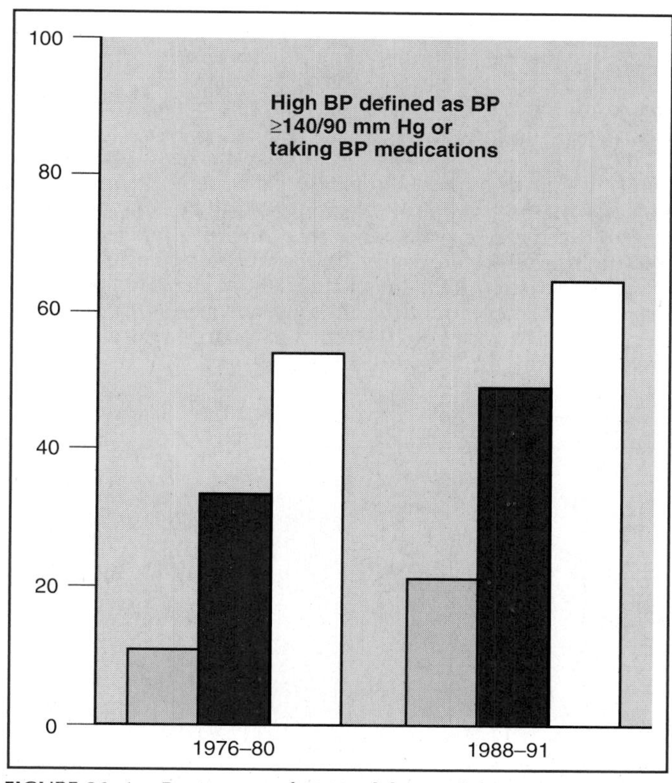

FIGURE 26–1. Percentage of U.S. adults aged 18 to 74 years surveyed in 1976–1980 and 1988–1991 with hypertension controlled *(left-hand bars)*, treated *(middle)*, and diagnosed *(right)*. Hypertension was defined as use of antihypertensive drug therapy or raised systolic (≥ 140) or diastolic (≥ 90) blood pressure on a single occasion. (Adapted from Joint National Committee on Detection, Evaluation, and Treatment of High Blood Pressure: The fifth report of the Joint National Committee on Detection, Evaluation, and Treatment of High Blood Pressure [JNC V]. Arch. Intern. Med. *153:*154, 1993. Copyright 1993 American Medical Association.)

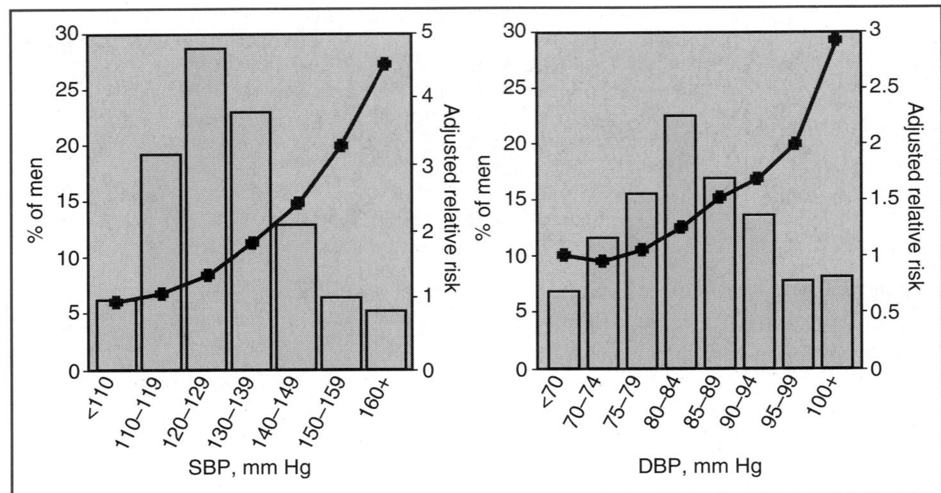

FIGURE 26–2. *Left,* Percentage distribution of systolic blood pressure (SBP) for men screened for the Multiple Risk Factor Intervention Trial who were aged 35 to 57 years and had no history of myocardial infarction (n = 347978) *(shaded bars)* and corresponding 12-year rates of cardiovascular mortality by SBP level adjusted for age, race, total serum cholesterol level, cigarettes smoked per day, reported use of medication for diabetes mellitus, and imputed household income (using census tract of residence). *Right,* Same as at left but for diastolic blood pressure (DBP) (n = 356222). (From National High Blood Pressure Education Program Working Group: National High Blood Pressure Education Program Working Group report on primary prevention of hypertension. Arch. Intern. Med. *153:*186, 1993. Copyright 1993 American Medical Association.)

DEFINITION OF HYPERTENSION

Blood pressure is distributed in a typical bell-shaped curve within the overall population (Fig. 26–2). As seen in the 12-year experience of the 350,000 men screened for the Multiple Risk Factor Intervention Trial (MRFIT) study, the long-term risks for cardiovascular mortality associated with various levels of pressure rise progressively over the entire range of blood pressure, with no threshold that clearly identifies potential danger. Therefore, the definition of hypertension is somewhat arbitrary, usually taken as that level of pressure associated with a doubling of long-term risk.[4] Perhaps the best operational definition is "the level at which the benefits (minus the risks and costs) of action exceed the risks and costs (minus the benefits) of inaction."[6]

The issue as to what blood pressure level should be taken to signify hypertension is further complicated by its typically marked variability. Such variability is seldom recognized by the relatively few office readings taken by most practitioners[7] but can easily be identified by automatically recorded measurements taken throughout the day and night (Fig. 26–3). This variability often can be attributed to physical activity or emotional stress but is frequently without obvious cause.

In a few patients, markedly elevated levels clearly indicate serious disease requiring immediate treatment. However, in most cases, initial readings are not high enough to indicate immediate danger, and the diagnosis of hypertension should be substantiated by repeated readings. The reason for such caution is obvious: The diagnosis of hypertension imposes psychological[8] and socioeconomic burdens on an individual and usually implies the need for a commitment to lifelong therapy.

Both transient and persistent elevations of pressure are common when it is taken in the physician's office or hospital.[7] To obviate "white coat" hypertension, more widespread use of out-of-the-office readings, either with semiautomatic inexpensive devices or automatic ambulatory recorders, is encouraged both to establish the diagnosis and to monitor the patient's response to therapy.[9] A large body of data provides normal ranges for both home self-recorded[10] and automatic ambulatory measurements.[11] Both average about 10/5 mm Hg lower than the average of multiple office readings. A closer correlation between the presence of various types of target organ damage, specifically left ventricular hypertrophy,[12] proteinuria, and retinopathy,[13] has been noted with ambulatory levels than with office levels. However, in the absence of adequate long-term follow-up evidence of the risks associated with either home or ambulatory monitoring, office readings should

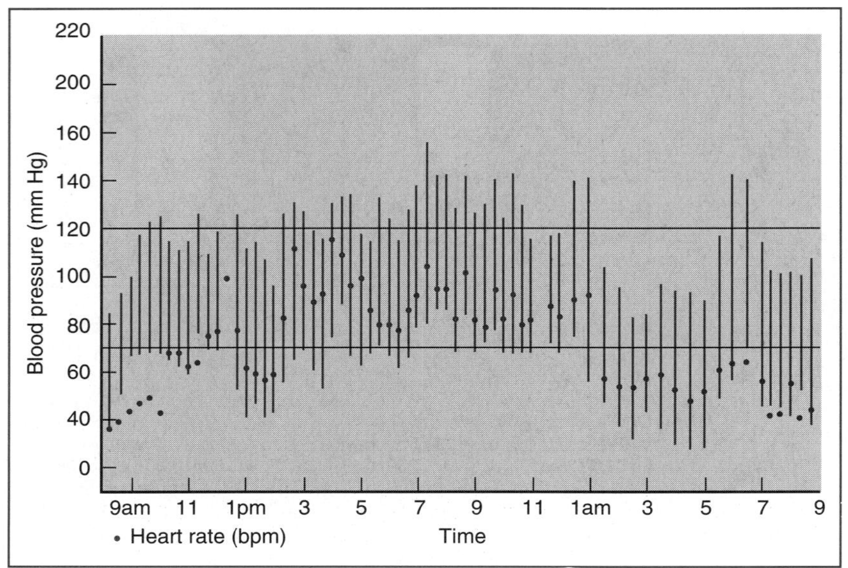

FIGURE 26–3. Computer printout of blood pressures obtained by ambulatory blood pressure monitoring over 24 hours beginning at 9 A.M. in a 50-year-old man with hypertension receiving no therapy. The patient slept from midnight until 6 A.M. *Solid circles,* Heart rate. (From Zachariah, P. K., Sheps, S. G., and Smith, R. L.: Defining the roles of home and ambulatory monitoring. Diagnosis *10:*39, 1988.)

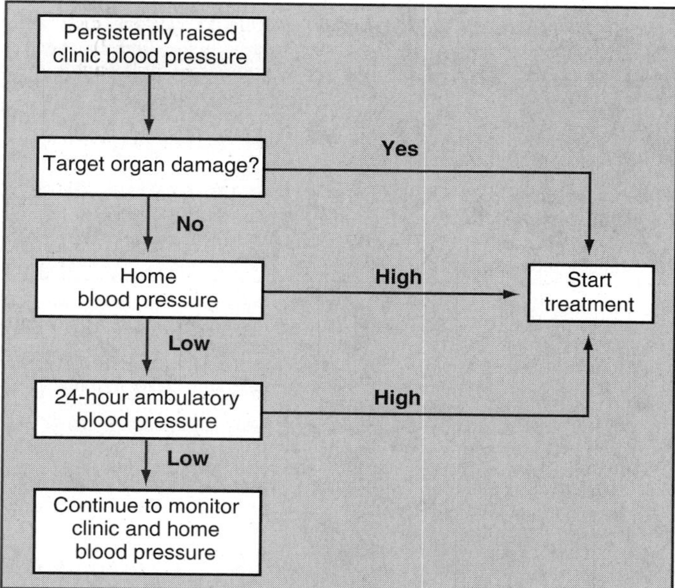

FIGURE 26–4. Schema for evaluation of hypertensive patients by use of clinic, home, and ambulatory monitoring of blood pressure. (From Pickering, T. G.: Blood pressure measurement and detection of hypertension. Lancet *344*:31, 1994.)

continue to be the basis for the diagnosis and management of hypertension.

Whenever possible, office readings should be supplemented by out-of-the-office measurements, particularly when there is an apparent discrepancy between the level of blood pressure and the degree of target organ damage, wherein white coat hypertension should be suspected. Pickering has provided a scheme for the use of home and ambulatory monitoring in such a circumstance[7] (Fig. 26–4). In as many as half of patients with office readings that remain elevated despite the use of three or more drugs, hypertension in as many as half is found to be well controlled by out-of-the-office readings.[14] Purely white coat hypertension, that is, persistently elevated office readings but persistently normal out-of-the-office readings, is found in 20 to 30 per cent of patients.[7] Most are found to be free of the target organ damage[15] and metabolic abnormalities (dyslipidemia, hyperinsulinemia)[16] that are often found in patients with sustained hypertension, so close observation and life style modifications but not antihypertensive drug therapy seem appropriate management for such patients.

In addition to their role in the recognition of white coat hypertension, out-of-the-office readings are essential for the recognition of persistently elevated pressures soon after awakening, when the largest proportion of sudden deaths, myocardial infarctions, and strokes occur.[17] Increased awareness of the role of the abrupt and marked rise of pressure after awakening in the etiology of these early morning cardiovascular catastrophes has prompted therapeutic strategies to ensure control of hypertension at that time, including late evening dosing with currently available medications[18] and the development of tablets that are delayed in releasing active drug so that they can be taken at bedtime but not become active until the hours before awakening.[19]

In view of the usual nocturnal fall in pressure (Fig. 26–3), the addition of the maximal antihypertensive effect of medication taken before bedtime could incite myocardial and cerebral ischemia during sleep. Therefore, the best way to blunt the early morning surge in pressure is to use formulations that provide full 24-hour coverage and to take them as early in the morning as possible.

Although a nocturnal fall in pressure is usual, various groups of hypertensives who have a more serious degree of target organ damage or subsequent major cardiovascular events[20] have been noted to have little or no nocturnal fall. These include patients with left ventricular hypertrophy,[21] diabetes,[22] or renal damage[23] and blacks.[24] The recognition of abnormal nocturnal patterns of blood pressure, presumably adding an additional stress to the cardiovascular system, is a potential indication for more widespread use of automatic recordings.

Another source of potentially useful prognostic information is the blood pressure response to exercise, usually ascertained in treadmill testing. An exaggerated response in normotensive adults, defined as a systolic pressure above 210 mm Hg in men or 190 mm Hg in women, has been found to be followed 5 years later by a 1.7 times increased incidence of hypertension over that seen in those with a normal response.[25] Over a 16-year follow-up, those middle-aged men with resting systolic pressures of 140 mm Hg or higher who increased their pressure to 200 mm Hg or higher within the first 6 minutes of a bicycle exercise test at a workload of 600 kpm/min had a cardiovascular death rate of 16.1 per cent compared with a rate of 6.0 per cent in those with a lesser pressure response.[26]

DOCUMENTATION OF HYPERTENSION. For most patients who are in no immediate danger from markedly elevated pressure, i.e., below approximately 170/110 mm Hg, the following guidelines are offered:

1. Multiple readings should be obtained using appropriate techniques (pp. 20 to 21, Table 26–1). If possible, the readings should be taken under varying conditions and at various times for at least 4 to 6 weeks with a semiautomatic home device. If there is a need to establish the diagnosis more rapidly, a set of readings obtained by an automatic monitor over a single 24-hour period will be adequate.
2. Although the logical approach would be to calculate the average values from multiple readings when deciding whether or not hypertension is present, even a single high measurement should not be disregarded. In large populations, a single set of casual measurements has been found to predict a greater likelihood of subsequent cardiovascular disease.[27] However, such elevated measurements do not necessarily predict either fixed hypertension or increased risk for each individual. For example, in one study, only 10.8 per cent of 719 men aged 18 to 30 with initial systolic values of 140 to 170 began to exhibit systolic pressures persistently above 140 over the next 12 to 15 years.[28] Nonetheless, persistently elevated pressures were found 2.3 times more often among those with initially high readings, obviously placing them at higher risk.
3. Systolic elevations pose a risk that is equal to or greater than that posed by diastolic elevations.[27] Isolated systolic hypertension, as is commonly seen among the elderly, presents a risk both for stroke and myocardial infarction.[29]
4. The elderly often have sclerotic brachial arteries that may not become occluded until very high pressures are exerted by the balloon; therefore, cuff diastolic levels may be considerably higher than those measured intraarterially. In patients with high cuff readings but little or no hypertensive retinopathy, cardiac hypertrophy, or other evidence of longstanding hypertension, "pseudohypertension" should be suspected and ruled out before treatment is begun.[30]
5. Elderly persons with elevated systolic pressure should be monitored carefully for significant falls in pressure either with sudden upright posture or after meals.[31] These changes probably reflect a progressive loss of baroreceptor responsiveness with age. This condition makes the elderly particularly susceptible to marked orthostatic hypotension after even small decreases in vascular volume.

For the individual patient, hypertension can be definitively diagnosed when most readings are at a level known to be associated with a significantly higher cardiovascular risk without treatment. The recommendations of the Fifth Joint National Committee are shown in Table 26–2.[32] Note that systolic levels of 130 to 139 mm Hg and diastolic levels of 85 to 89 mm Hg are classified as *high normal blood pressure,* a recommendation stemming from a prospective 8.6-year observation of over 7000 white American men aged 40 to 59. A 52 per cent increase in *relative risk* for coronary disease was noted among those in the middle quintile, whose diastolic pressures were between 80 and 87 mm Hg, compared with patients with diastolic pressures below 80 mm Hg.[33] Therefore, persons with relatively high systolic or diastolic pressures should be advised that they may be at increased risk and counseled to follow better health habits in the hope of slowing the progression toward definite hypertension.

The criteria shown in Table 26–2 are based on at least three sets of measurements taken over at least a 3-month interval. Even more readings may be needed to establish a patient's usual level.

Even though they are diagnosed as hypertensive, not all persons with usual levels above 140/90 mm Hg need be treated with drugs, although all should be advised to use the various life style modifications described in Chapter 27. The threshold level recommended by various expert committees for institution of drug therapy varies between diastolic levels of 90 to 100 mm Hg and systolic levels between

TABLE 26–1 GUIDELINES IN MEASURING BLOOD PRESSURE

I. CONDITIONS FOR THE PATIENT

A. Posture
1. For patients who are over age 65, diabetic, or receiving antihypertensive therapy, check for postural changes by taking readings immediately and 2 minutes after patient stands.
2. Sitting pressures usually are adequate for routine follow-up. Patient should sit quietly with back supported for 5 minutes and arm supported at level of heart.

B. Circumstances
1. No caffeine for preceding hour.
2. No smoking for preceding 15 minutes.
3. No exogenous adrenergic stimulants, e.g., phenylephrine in nasal decongestants or eye drops for pupillary dilation.
4. A quiet, warm setting.
5. Home readings taken under varying circumstances and 24-hour ambulatory recordings may be preferable and more accurate in predicting subsequent cardiovascular disease.

II. EQUIPMENT

A. Cuff size: The bladder should encircle and cover two-thirds of the length of the arm; if not, place the bladder over the brachial artery; if bladder is too small, spuriously high readings may result.
B. Manometer: Aneroid gauges should be calibrated every 6 months against a mercury manometer.
C. For infants, use ultrasound equipment, e.g., the Doppler method.

III. TECHNIQUE

A. Number of readings
1. On each occasion, take at least two readings, separated by as much time as is practical. If readings vary by more than 5 mm Hg, take additional readings until two are close.
2. For diagnosis, obtain at least 3 sets of readings at least a week apart.
3. Initially, take pressure in both arms; if pressure differs, use arm with higher pressure.
4. If arm pressure is elevated, take pressure in one leg, particularly in patients below age 30.

B. Performance
1. Inflate the bladder quickly to a pressure 20 mm Hg above the systolic, as recognized by disappearance of the radial pulse.
2. Deflate the bladder 3 mm Hg every second.
3. Record the Korotkoff phase V (disappearance) except in little children, in whom use of phase IV (muffling) may be preferable.
4. If Korotkoff sounds are weak, have the patient raise the arm, and open and close the hand 5 to 10 times, after which the bladder should be inflated quickly.

C. Recordings
1. Note the pressure, patient position, the arm, cuff size (e.g., 140/90, seated, right arm, large adult cuff).

140 and 170 mm Hg.[34] As will be noted on p. 813, the most rational approach is to incorporate age, gender, and the presence of other major cardiovascular risk factors in the decision process along with the level of blood pressure. The threshold for therapy is important, since over 60 per cent of all hypertensives have diastolic blood pressures between 90 and 100 mm Hg (Fig. 26–2).

BORDERLINE HYPERTENSION. In view of the usual variability in blood pressure levels, the term *labile* is inappropriate for describing diastolic pressures that only occasionally exceed 90 mm Hg. Instead, the term *borderline* should be used. In 30 to 40 per cent of patients whose initial diastolic measurement exceeds 90 mm Hg, repeat readings taken soon after will be well below this value.[35] Such patients should be advised that their blood pressure level is *borderline elevated* and should be checked at least annually while they follow general health measures. Tracking of patients with borderline hypertension has not been conducted for a sufficiently long period to provide firm data regarding the likelihood that persistent hypertension will develop.

TABLE 26–2 CLASSIFICATION OF BLOOD PRESSURE FOR ADULTS AGED 18 YEARS AND OLDER*

CATEGORY	SYSTOLIC	DIASTOLIC
Normal†	<130	<85
High normal	130–139	85–89
Hypertension‡		
Stage 1 (mild)	140–159	90–99
Stage 2 (moderate)	160–179	100–109
Stage 3 (severe)	180–209	110–119
Stage 4 (very severe)	>210	>120

From Joint National Committee: The fifth report of the Joint National Committee on Detection, Evaluation, and Treatment of High Blood Pressure (JNC V). Arch. Intern. Med. *153:*154, 1993.

* These definitions apply to adults who are not taking antihypertensive drugs and who are not acutely ill. When systolic and diastolic blood pressures fall into different categories, the higher category should be selected to classify the individual's blood pressure status. Isolated systolic hypertension is defined as a systolic blood pressure of 140 mm Hg or more and a diastolic blood pressure of less than 90 mm Hg and staged appropriately.

† Optimal blood pressure with respect to cardiovascular risk is less than 120 mm Hg systolic and less than 80 mm Hg diastolic. However, unusually low readings should be evaluated for clinical significance.

‡ Based on the average of two or more readings taken at each of two or more visits after an initial screening.

HYPERTENSION IN CHILDREN AND ADOLESCENTS (see also p. 822). Upper limits of normal in children of various ages were proposed in the Fifth Joint National Committee report[32] (Table 26–3). Premature labeling of children whose readings are above these limits as hypertensive should be avoided, since long-time tracking is only now being carried out.[36] Appropriate management for asymptomatic children with sustained elevations in blood pressure has not been established. Although many maintain similarly high readings over 3- to 4-year periods, most become normotensive. Such patients should be followed carefully, with particular emphasis placed on regular exercise and weight reduction for those who are overweight in the hope of preventing progression of the disease. If life style modifications are not successful, antihypertensive agents probably should be prescribed for those with sustained hypertension.

TABLE 26–3 CLASSIFICATION OF HYPERTENSION IN THE YOUNG*

AGE GROUP	≥95TH PERCENTILE	≥99TH PERCENTILE
Infants (≤2 y)		
SBP	≥112	≥118
DBP	≥74	≥82
Children, y		
3–5		
SBP	≥116	≥124
DBP	≥76	≥84
6–9		
SBP	≥122	≥130
DBP	≥78	≥86
10–12		
SBP	≥126	≥134
DBP	≥82	≥90
13–15		
SBP	≥136	≥144
DBP	≥86	≥92
Adolescents (16–18 y)		
SBP	≥142	≥150
DBP	≥92	≥98

From 1993 Joint National Committee: The 1993 report of the Joint National Committee on Detection, Evaluation, and Treatment of High Blood Pressure. Arch. Intern. Med. *153:*154, 1993. Copyright 1993, American Medical Association.

* SBP indicates systolic blood pressure; DBP, diastolic blood pressure. Classification based on report of Second Task Force on Blood Pressure Control in Children—1987. All values expressed as millimeters of mercury.

PREVALENCE OF HYPERTENSION

As noted previously, the criteria used for the diagnosis greatly affect the number of people considered hypertensive: The prevalence almost doubles when the level of 140/90 instead of 160/95 mm Hg is used. Most surveys prior to 1980 using single measurements assigned a level of 160/95 mm Hg as the minimum blood pressure denoting hypertension for adults. The levels used to define hypertension shown in Table 26–2 are lower; however, if the diagnosis is based on multiple measurements taken under reasonably controlled circumstances, as it should be, these lower levels seem appropriate. With the lower numbers, hypertension is common, and its frequency increases with the age of the population[5] (Fig. 26–5). The apparent decreases from the 1976–1980 survey may reflect more careful measurements or a true decrease in prevalence by adoption of preventive measures. The incidence of hypertension among blacks is greater at every age beyond adolescence, and they have a higher proportion of more severe disease[37] with a higher mortality rate than whites at every level of income.[38]

SECONDARY HYPERTENSION. Among the large number of people with hypertension, it is helpful to know whether some secondary process—perhaps curable by operation or more easily controlled by a specific drug—may be present (Table 26–4) so that the clinician can determine whether more definitive diagnostic testing is in order.[38a] Most surveys to determine the relative proportion of various secondary diseases are biased as a result of the selection process, with only the increasingly suspect population "funneled" to an investigator interested in a particular disease. Thus estimates as high as 20 per cent for certain secondary forms of hypertension have been reported; however, these do not reflect the incidence in the population at large. Estimates more likely to be indicative of the situation in usual clinical practice are shown in Table 26–5.[39–41] The closest approximation of usual medical practice is the survey by Rudnick et al. with middle-class white patients seen in a family practice in Hamilton, Canada, from 1965 to 1974.[39] In this as in the other surveys, many of the patients underwent intravenous pyelography in addition to providing a history and undergoing a physical examination and routine urine and blood tests. Although a few patients with secondary diseases may have been missed, the similarity of data strongly supports the view that in more than 90 per cent of all hypertensive persons there will be no recognizable cause; i.e., they have essential hypertension.

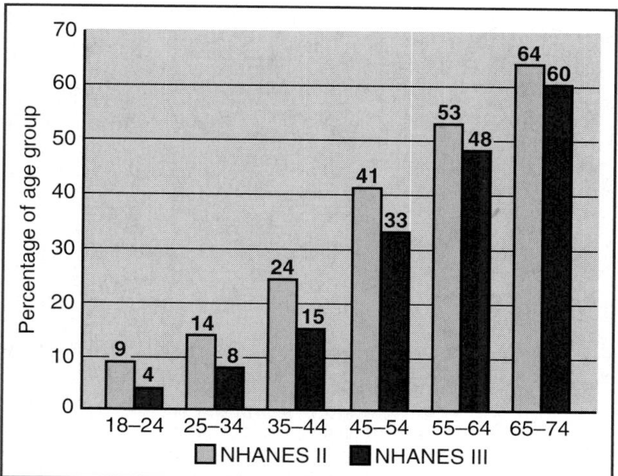

FIGURE 26–5. Incidence of hypertension in U.S. adults according to data from the National Health and Nutrition Examination Surveys conducted during 1976–1980 (NHANES II) and 1988–1991 (NHANES III). Hypertension is defined as mean blood pressure of 140/90 mm Hg or higher based on three readings taken on a single occasion or the use of antihypertensive mediations. (From Centers for Disease Control and Prevention, National Center for Health Statistics [Composed from National High Blood Pressure Education Program Working Group]): Report on primary prevention of hypertension. Arch. Intern. Med. *153*:186, 1993.)

TABLE 26–4 TYPES OF HYPERTENSION

I. SYSTOLIC AND DIASTOLIC HYPERTENSION

- A. Primary, essential, or idiopathic
- B. Secondary
  - 1. Renal
    - a. Renal parenchymal disease
      - (1) Acute glomerulonephritis
      - (2) Chronic nephritis
      - (3) Polycystic disease
      - (4) Diabetic nephropathy
      - (5) Hydronephrosis
    - b. Renovascular
      - (1) Renal artery stenosis
      - (2) Intrarenal vasculitis
    - c. Renin-producing tumors
    - d. Renoprival
    - e. Primary sodium retention (Liddle's syndrome, Gordon's syndrome)
  - 2. Endocrine
    - a. Acromegaly
    - b. Hypothyroidism
    - c. Hyperthyroidism
    - d. Hypercalcemia (hyperparathyroidism)
    - e. Adrenal
      - (1) Cortical
        - (a) Cushing's syndrome
        - (b) Primary aldosteronism
        - (c) Congenital adrenal hyperplasia
        - (d) Apparent mineralocorticoid excess (licorice)
      - (2) Medullary: Pheochromocytoma
    - f. Extraadrenal chromaffin tumors
    - g. Carcinoid
    - h. Exogenous hormones
      - (1) Estrogen
      - (2) Glucocorticoids
      - (3) Mineralocorticoids
      - (4) Sympathomimetics
      - (5) Tyramine-containing foods and monoamine oxidase inhibitors
  - 3. Coarctation of the aorta
  - 4. Pregnancy-induced hypertension
  - 5. Neurological disorders
    - a. Increased intracranial pressure
      - (1) Brain tumor
      - (2) Encephalitis
      - (3) Respiratory acidosis
    - b. Sleep apnea
    - c. Quadriplegia
    - d. Acute porphyria
    - e. Familial dysautonomia
    - f. Lead poisoning
    - g. Guillain-Barré syndrome
  - 6. Acute stress, including surgery
    - a. Psychogenic hyperventilation
    - b. Hypoglycemia
    - c. Burns
    - d. Pancreatitis
    - e. Alcohol withdrawal
    - f. Sickle cell crisis
    - g. Postresuscitation
    - h. Postoperative
  - 7. Increased intravascular volume
  - 8. Alcohol and drug use

II. SYSTOLIC HYPERTENSION

- A. Increased cardiac output
  - 1. Aortic valvular insufficiency
  - 2. A-V fistula, patent ductus
  - 3. Thyrotoxicosis
  - 4. Paget's disease of bone
  - 5. Beriberi
  - 6. Hyperkinetic circulation
- B. Rigidity of aorta

TABLE 26–5 FREQUENCY OF VARIOUS DIAGNOSES IN HYPERTENSIVE SUBJECTS

DIAGNOSIS	RUDNICK et al.[39]	SINCLAIR et al.[40]	ANDERSON et al.[41]*
Essential hypertension	94%	92.1%	89.5%
Chronic renal disease	5%	5.6%	1.8%
Renovascular disease	0.2%	0.7%	3.3%
Coarctation of aorta	0.2%		
Primary aldosteronism		0.3%	1.5%
Cushing's syndrome	0.2%	0.1%	0.6%
Pheochromocytoma		0.1%	0.3%
Oral contraceptive–induced	0.2%	1.0%	
No. of patients	665	3783	4429

Data from Rudnick, K. V., et al.: Hypertension in family practice. Can. Med. Assoc. J. *117*,492, 1977; Sinclair, A. M., et al.: Secondary hypertension in a blood pressure clinic. Arch. Intern. Med. *147*:1289, 1987; Anderson, G. H., Jr., et al.: The effect of age on prevalence of secondary forms of hypertension in 4429 consecutively referred patients. J. Hypertens. *12*:609, 1994.

* The patients screened by Anderson et al. were referred for evaluation of secondary causes; those screened by Rudnick and Sinclair were all those seen in a primary setting.

THE CHANGING NATURE OF CHILDHOOD HYPERTENSION (see also p. 822). Even among children, secondary hypertension is less common than indicated by previous surveys of hospital-based populations. As more apparently normal children are being screened and more are found to be hypertensive, the clinical presentation of childhood hypertension is changing from that of a rare and serious disease, usually related to renal damage, to a more common and usually asymptomatic process, in most cases without recognizable cause.[36] Some prepubertal hypertensive children do not have recognizable secondary diseases, whereas most identified after puberty have primary hypertension.

SCREENING FOR SECONDARY HYPERTENSION

Because of the relatively low frequency of the various secondary diseases, the clinician should be selective in carrying out various screening and diagnostic tests. The presence of features *inappropriate* for usual uncomplicated primary hypertension indicates the need for additional tests (Table 26–6). However, for the 9 out of 10 hypertensive patients without these features, a hematocrit, urine analysis, automated blood biochemical profile (including plasma glucose, potassium, creatinine, and total and high-density lipoprotein cholesterol), and an electrocardiogram are all that is required. Although some would include other tests, an inordinate number of screening tests for relatively rare diseases will increase the likelihood of a false-positive result. For example, according to Bayes' theorem (see p. 162), using a prevalence rate of 2 per cent for renovascular hypertension, which is probably higher than seen in the overall hypertensive population, the predictive value of an intravenous pyelogram (IVP) or isotopic renogram suggestive of this diagnosis is only 10 per cent, and an abnormal IVP or renogram is more likely to be a false-positive result than true-positive indicating a specific diagnosis.[42]

TABLE 26–6 FEATURES OF "INAPPROPRIATE" HYPERTENSION

1. Onset before age 20 or after age 50
2. Level of blood pressure >180/110 mm Hg
3. Organ damage
   a. Funduscopic findings of Grade 2 or higher
   b. Serum creatinine >1.5 mg/100 ml
   c. Cardiomegaly (on x-ray) or left ventricular hypertrophy (on electrocardiogram)
4. Features indicative of secondary causes
   a. Unprovoked hypokalemia
   b. Abdominal bruit
   c. Variable pressures with tachycardia, sweating, tremor
   d. Family history of renal disease
5. Poor response to therapy that is usually effective

NATURAL HISTORY OF UNTREATED HYPERTENSION

A meta-analysis of nine major prospective observational studies involving 420,000 individuals free of known coronary or cerebral vascular disease at baseline who were followed for 6 to 25 years (mean of 10 years) shows a "direct, continuous and apparently independent association" of diastolic blood pressure (DBP) with both stroke and coronary heart disease (CHD)[43] (Fig. 26–6). The data indicate that prolonged increases in usual DBP of 5 and 10 mm Hg were associated with at least 34 and 56 per cent increases in stroke risk and with at least 21 and 37 per cent increases in CHD risk, respectively.

SYMPTOMS AND SIGNS. Because uncomplicated hypertension is almost always asymptomatic, a person may be unaware of the consequent progressive cardiovascular damage for as long as 10 to 20 years. Only if blood pressure is measured frequently and people are made aware that hypertension may be harmful even if asymptomatic will the majority of people with unrecognized or inadequately

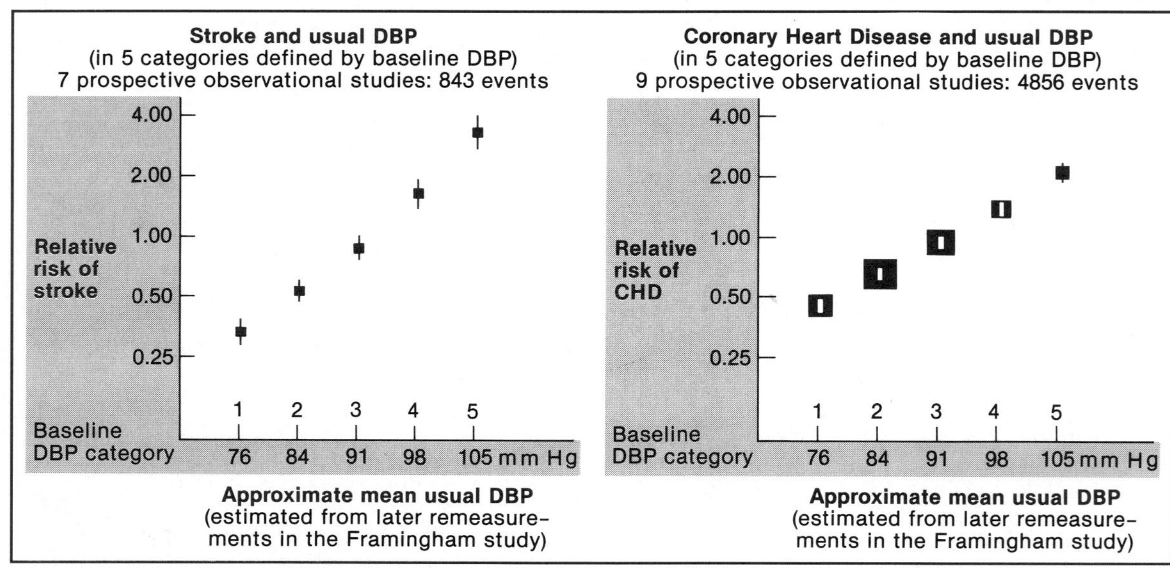

FIGURE 26–6. The relative risks of stroke and of coronary heart disease, estimated from the combined results of the prospective observational studies, for each of five categories of diastolic blood pressure. (Estimates of the usual DBP in each baseline DBP category are taken from mean DBP values 4 years post-baseline in the Framingham study.) The solid squares represent disease risks in each category relative to risk in the whole study population; the sizes of the squares are proportional to the number of events in each DBP category, and 95 per cent confidence intervals for the estimates of relative risk are denoted by vertical lines. (From MacMahon, S., Peto, R., Cutler, J., et al.: Blood pressure and coronary heart disease: Part I, prolonged differences in blood pressure: Prospective observational studies corrected for the regression dilution bias. Lancet *335*:765, 1990. © by the Lancet Ltd.)

treated hypertension be managed effectively. Symptoms often attributed to hypertension—headache, tinnitus, dizziness, and fainting—may be observed just as commonly in the normotensive population.[44] Moreover, many symptoms attributed to the elevated blood pressure are psychogenic in origin,[8] often reflecting hyperventilation induced by anxiety over the diagnosis of a lifelong, insidious disease which threatens well-being and survival. Even headache, long considered a frequent symptom of hypertension, is poorly related to the level of blood pressure,[45] as noted in 10 to 20 per cent of those with DBP levels from below 90 to above 120 mm Hg.

COURSE OF UNTREATED HYPERTENSION. As noted in Figure 26–6, even minimal hypertension is accompanied by significant increases in coronary disease and stroke. However, these figures may be misleading, since they seem to imply that most hypertensives, including those with minimally elevated pressures, will experience adverse consequences of hypertension, and rather quickly. The issue is well identified in the data from the Pooling Project,[33] which includes multiple prospective follow-up studies including the Framingham cohort. As noted previously, these data indicate that those white men with diastolic pressures of 80 to 87 mm Hg had a 52 per cent greater *relative* risk of having a major coronary event over an 8.6-year period than did those with diastolic pressures below 80. However, this large increased *relative* risk translates to an *absolute* excess risk of only 3.5 men per 100 over the 8.6-year interval. Obviously, the majority of those with even higher diastolic pressures did not suffer a major coronary event.

Nonetheless, because there are so many persons with hypertension, the fact that even a minority of them will suffer a premature cardiovascular event in the course of their disease makes hypertension a major societal problem. In fact, when the death rates for various levels of diastolic blood pressure are multiplied by the proportion of people in the population who have these various levels, the majority of excess deaths attributable to hypertension are found to occur among those with minimally elevated pressures[5] (Fig. 26–2).

As the public and the medical profession have become aware of the overall societal consequences of even mild hypertension, enthusiasm for its early recognition and aggressive treatment has continued to mount. A closer look at the issue of deciding on the need for therapy is provided in Chapter 27. However, further consideration of the natural course of hypertension, as it applies to the individual patient, is needed in order to answer a basic question: Are the blood pressure and the consequent risk high enough to justify medical intervention? Unless the risk is high enough to mandate some form of intervention, there seems to be no need to identify and label the person as hypertensive, since psychological and socioeconomic burdens accompany this label; unless risks clearly outweigh these burdens, caution is obviously advised. A cogent view of this issue has been offered by Rose[46]:

> In reality the care of the symptomless hypertensive person is preventive medicine, not therapeutics. If a preventive measure exposes many people to a small risk, the harm it does may readily . . . outweigh the benefits, since these are received by relatively few. . . . We may thus be unable to identify that small level of harm to individuals from long-term intervention that would be sufficient to make that line of prevention unprofitable or even harmful. Consequently we cannot accept long-term mass preventive medication.

We are thus left with a dilemma: For hypertensive individuals as a group, even those with the least elevated pressures, risk is increased; for the individual hypertensive, the risk may not justify the labeling or treatment of the condition.

Guidelines are available to help practitioners resolve this dilemma in dealing with the individual patient. These guidelines are based on the overall assessment of cardiovascular risk and the biological aggressiveness of the hypertension. They are intended to apply only to those with stage 1 (formerly referred to as mild) hypertension, that is, diastolic pressure between 90 and 99 mm Hg; those with diastolic levels persistently at or above 100 mm Hg have been shown to be at high enough risk from the hypertension per se to justify immediate intervention. Recall, however, that most hypertensives are in the range between 90 and 99 mm Hg (Fig. 26–2).

OVERALL CARDIOVASCULAR RISK. The Framingham Study and other epidemiological surveys have clearly defined certain risk factors for premature cardiovascular disease in addition to hypertension (see Chap. 35). For varying levels of blood pressure, the Framingham data (available in the *Coronary and Stroke Risk Handbooks* published by the American Heart Association) show the increasing likelihood of a vascular event over the next 10 years for both men and women at various ages as more and more risk factors are added[29] (Fig. 26–2). For example, a 55-year-old man with a systolic blood pressure of 160 mm Hg who is otherwise at low risk would have a 13.7 per cent chance of a vascular event in the next 10 years (Fig. 26–7). A man of the same age with the same pressure but with all the additional risk factors (elevated serum total cholesterol, low HDL-cholesterol, cigarette smoking, glucose intolerance, and left ventricular hypertrophy on the electrocardiogram) has a 59.5 per cent chance. Obviously, the higher the overall risk, the more intensive the interventions should be.

An interesting—and disturbing—connection between untreated hypertension and *hypercholesterolemia* has been noted in multiple populations.[47] This connection may be mediated through insulin resistance and hyperinsulinemia, anticipated in those with upper body obesity[48] but also found in nonobese hypertensives[49] (see p. 820). Clearly, through this association, hypertensives are often burdened with an even greater risk than that imposed by their blood pressure alone.

Complications of Hypertension

The higher the level of blood pressure, the more likely that various cardiovascular diseases will develop prematurely through acceleration of atherosclerosis, the pathological hallmark of uncontrolled hypertension. If untreated, about 50 per cent of hypertensive patients die of coronary heart disease or congestive failure, about 33 per cent of stroke, and 10 to 15 per cent of renal failure. Those with

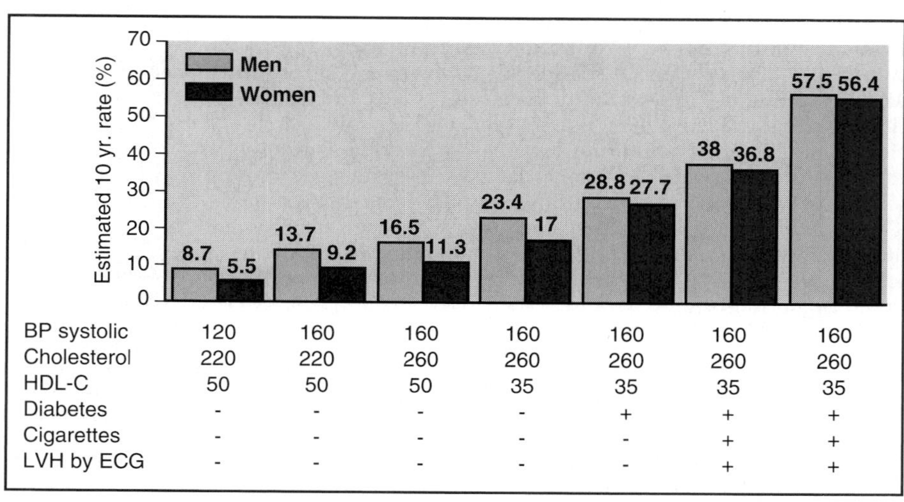

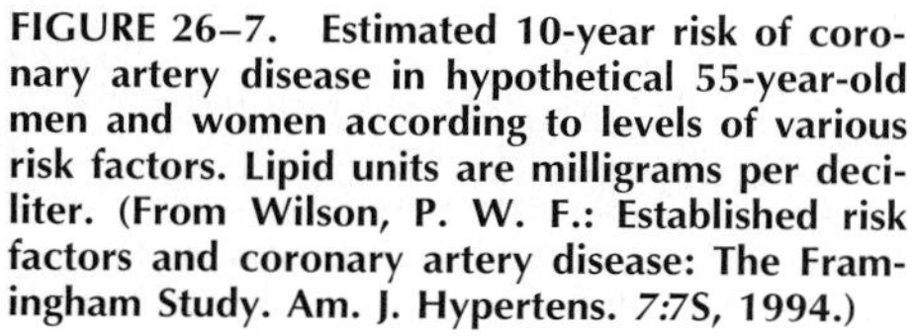
FIGURE 26–7. Estimated 10-year risk of coronary artery disease in hypothetical 55-year-old men and women according to levels of various risk factors. Lipid units are milligrams per deciliter. (From Wilson, P. W. F.: Established risk factors and coronary artery disease: The Framingham Study. Am. J. Hypertens. *7*:7S, 1994.)

TABLE 26–7 VASCULAR COMPLICATIONS OF HYPERTENSION

HYPERTENSIVE	ATHEROSCLEROTIC
Accelerated-malignant phase	Coronary heart disease
Hemorrhagic stroke	Sudden death
Congestive heart failure	Other arrhythmias
Nephrosclerosis	Atherothrombotic stroke
Aortic dissection	Peripheral vascular disease

Adapted from Smith, W. M.: Treatment of mild hypertension. Results of a ten-year intervention trial. Circ. Res. *25* (Suppl. I):98, 1977. Copyright 1977 by the American Heart Association.

rapidly accelerating hypertension die more frequently of renal failure, as do those who are diabetic, once proteinuria or other evidence of nephropathy develops. It is easy to underestimate the role of hypertension in producing the underlying vascular damage that leads to these cardiovascular catastrophes. Death is usually attributed to stroke or myocardial infarction instead of to the hypertension that was largely responsible. Moreover, hypertension may not persist after a myocardial infarction or stroke.

In general, the vascular complications of hypertension can be considered as either "hypertensive" or "atherosclerotic" (Table 26–7). The former are more directly caused by the increased blood pressure per se and can be prevented by lowering this level; the latter have more multiple causations (Chap. 35). Although hypertension may represent the most significant of the known risk factors of atherosclerosis in quantitative terms, lowering blood pressure may not by itself halt the atherosclerotic process.

The path from hypertension to vascular disease likely involves three interrelated processes: *pulsatile flow, endothelial cell dysfunction,* and *smooth muscle cell hypertrophy.* Higher systolic pressures are probably more responsible for these changes than are lower diastolic levels, providing an explanation for the closer approximation of cardiovascular risk to systolic pressure.

These three interrelated processes are probably responsible for the arteriolar and arterial sclerosis that is the usual consequence of longstanding hypertension leading to the target organ damage to be described as the features included in overall assessment of hypertension risks. Beyond the damage to eyes, heart, brain, and kidney, the large vessels such as the aorta may be directly affected, leading to aneurysms and dissection.

Target Organ Damage

The biological aggressiveness of a given level of hypertension varies among individuals. This inherent propensity to induce vascular damage can be ascertained best by examination of the eyes, heart, and kidney.

FUNDUSCOPIC EXAMINATION. As described by Keith et al. in 1939, vascular changes in the fundus reflect both hypertensive retinopathy and arteriosclerotic retinopathy (Fig. 2–1, p. 16).[50] The two processes induce first narrowing of the arteriolar lumen (Grade 1) and then sclerosis of the adventitia and/or thickening of the arteriolar wall, visible as arteriovenous nicking (Grade 2). Progressive hypertension induces rupture of small vessels, seen as hemorrhages and exudates (Grade 3) and eventually papilledema (Grade 4). The Grade 3 and 4 changes are clearly indicative of an accelerated-malignant form of hypertension, whereas the lesser changes have been correlated with other evidence of target organ damage.[51]

CARDIAC INVOLVEMENT. Hypertension places increased tension on the left ventricular myocardium, causing it to stiffen and hypertrophy, and accelerates the development of atherosclerosis within the coronary vessels.[51a] The combination of increased demand and lessened supply increases the likelihood of myocardial ischemia, leading to higher incidences of myocardial infarction, sudden death, arrhythmias, and congestive failure in hypertensives (Figs. 26–2 and 26–6).

Abnormalities of Left Ventricular Function. Even before left ventricular hypertrophy (LVH) develops, changes in both systolic and diastolic function may be seen. Those with minimally increased left ventricular muscle mass may have supernormal contractility reflecting an increased inotropic state with a high percentage of fractional shortening and increased wall stress.[52] The earliest functional cardiac changes in hypertension are in left ventricular diastolic function with prolongation and incoordination of isovolumic relaxation, reduced rate of rapid filling, and an increase in the relative amplitude of the *a* wave, probably caused by increased passive stiffness.[53]

With increasing hemodynamic load, either systolic or diastolic dysfunction may evolve, progressing to different forms of congestive heart failure[54] (Fig. 26–8) (see also p. 394). The syndrome of severe concentric hypertrophy with a small ventricular cavity leading to dyspnea and pulmonary congestion has been most frequently reported in black hypertensive women.[55] In addition, impaired coronary flow reserve and thallium perfusion defects may be observed in hypertensives without obstructive coronary disease.[56]

Left Ventricular Hypertrophy (LVH). Hypertrophy as a response to the increased afterload of an elevated systemic vascular resistance can be viewed as necessary and protective up to a certain point. Beyond that point, a variety of dysfunctions accompany LVH.

In the past, LVH was recognized by electrocardiography (Fig. 4–11, p. 116), based on increased voltage of QRS complexes, intrinsicoid deflection over lead V_5 or V_6 greater than 0.06 sec, and ST-segment depression greater than 0.5 mm (see p. 139). Increasingly, echocardiography is being used (see p. 66) because it is much more sensitive in recognizing early cardiac involvement. By echocardiography, left ventricular mass is shown to progressively increase with increases in blood pressure[57,58] (Fig. 26–9). LVH may be noted by echocardiography even before blood pressures become overtly abnormal in young offspring of hypertensive parents,[59] and larger left ventricular mass by echocardiography may identify subjects at risk of developing hypertension.[60] Left ventricular mass is greater in those whose pressure does not fall during sleep, reflecting a more persistent pressure load.[61]

The pathogenesis of LVH involves a number of variables other than the pressure load. One of these is hemodynamic volume load; Devereux et al.[62] found a closer correlation between left ventricular (LV) stroke volume and LV mass with diastolic than with systolic blood pressure. Other determinants are obesity,[63] levels of sympathetic nervous system and renin-angiotensin activity, and whole blood viscosity, presumably by way of its influence on peripheral resistance.[62] The

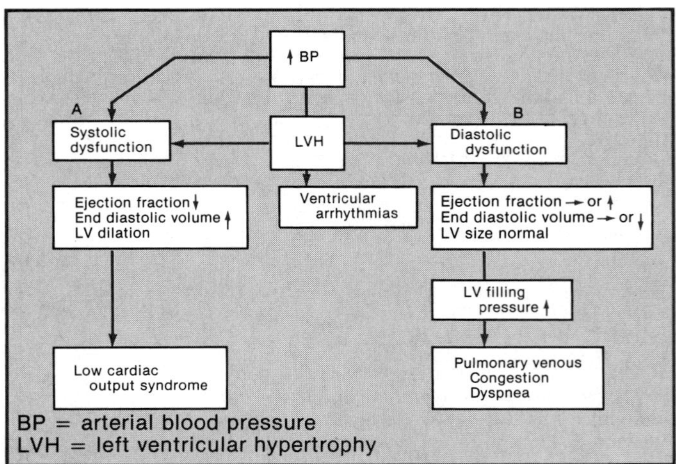

FIGURE 26–8. Consequences of systolic and diastolic dysfunction related to hypertension. *A,* Systolic dysfunction and congestive heart failure may occur late in the evolution of hypertensive heart disease, because of impaired ventricular contraction. *B,* Diastolic dysfunction is the most common manifestation of the effect of hypertension on cardiac function and also can lead to congestive heart failure due to increased filling pressures. LV = left ventricular. (From Shepherd, R. F. J., Zachariah, P. K., Shub, C.: Hypertension and left ventricular diastolic function. Mayo Clin. Proc. *64*:1521, 1989.)

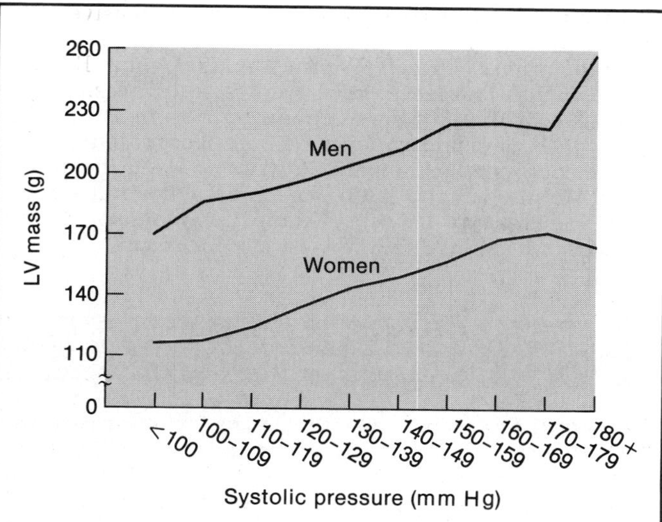

FIGURE 26–9. Mean left ventricular mass by sex and by systolic pressure, including participants taking antihypertensive medications, aged 17 to 90 years. These data were obtained by M-mode echocardiograms taken on 2226 men and 2746 women in the Framingham Study, cohort examination 16 and offspring cycle 2, 1979 to 1983. (From Savage, D. D., Levy, D., Danneberg, A. L., et al.: Association of echocardiographic left ventricular mass with body size, blood pressure and physical activity [the Framingham Study]. Am. J. Cardiol. *65:*371, 1990.)

correlation is much closer between LVH and pressures taken during the stresses of work by ambulatory monitoring than between LVH and casual pressures.[63] Blacks have more extensive LVH and more impairment of LV diastolic function than do whites with equal levels of blood pressure.[64]

The basic signals that initiate and maintain myocardial hypertrophy probably include a number of growth factors whose effects may be transmitted via the alpha$_1$-adrenergic receptor to activate intracellular transducing proteins and ribonucleic acid (RNA) transcription factors.[65] The renin-angiotensin-aldosterone mechanism may be involved in both functional[66] and structural[67] changes in the myocardium.

Different patterns of hypertrophy may evolve, often starting with asymmetrical LV remodeling due to isolated septal thickening, noted in 22 per cent of untreated hypertensives with normal LV mass.[68] The pattern of LVH may have important prognostic implications. In a 10-year follow-up of 253 hypertensives, all-cause mortality was higher and cardiovascular events were most frequent in those with *concentric* LVH.[69] The degree of increased muscle mass is a strong and independent risk factor for cardiac mortality over and above the extent of coronary artery disease.[70] In addition, the risk of ventricular arrhythmias is increased at least twofold in the presence of LVH.[71]

Since the presence of LVH may connote a number of deleterious effects of hypertension on cardiac function, a great deal of effort has been expended in showing that treatment of hypertension will cause LVH to regress. Treatment with all antihypertensive drugs except those which further activate sympathetic nervous system activity, e.g., diuretics and direct vasodilators such as hydralazine when used alone, has been shown to cause LVH regression.[72] With regression, left ventricular function usually improves.[73]

Features of Coronary Artery Disease. As detailed elsewhere (see p. 1168), hypertension is a major risk factor for myocardial ischemia and infarction.[27,29] Moreover, in the Framingham cohort, the prevalence of silent myocardial infarction was significantly increased in hypertensive subjects.[74] They are also more susceptible to silent ischemia[75] and sudden death.[74] Beyond these multiple additional risks associated with hypertension, a higher incidence of coronary events has been recognized when elevated diastolic blood pressures are reduced with either diuretic or beta-blocker–based therapies to levels below 85 to 90 mm Hg.[76] This J-shaped curve in the incidence of coronary disease probably reflects a reduction in perfusion pressure through coronary vessels either narrowed or having impaired vasodilatory reserve in the presence of a hypertrophied myocardium.

RENAL FUNCTION. Renal dysfunction, too subtle to be recognized, may be responsible for the development of most cases of essential hypertension. As discussed on p. 817, increased renal retention of salt and water may be a mechanism initiating primary hypertension, but the retention is so small that it escapes detection. With detailed study, both structural damage and functional derangements reflecting intraglomerular hypertension often reflected by microalbuminuria[77] can be found in almost all hypertensive persons. Microalbuminuria has been correlated with both high blood pressure and evidence of endothelial cell dysfunction.[78] In patients with longstanding hypertension, a loss of concentrating ability may be manifested by nocturia, creatinine clearance falls, and the development of more significant proteinuria. As hypertension-induced nephrosclerosis proceeds, the plasma creatinine level begins to rise, and eventually renal insufficiency with uremia may develop, making hypertension a leading cause for end-stage renal disease, particularly in blacks.[79]

CEREBRAL INVOLVEMENT. Hypertension, particularly systolic, is a major risk factor for initial and recurrent stroke and for transient ischemic attacks caused by extracranial atherosclerosis.[80] Usually with, but sometimes without, hypertension, increasing LV mass on echocardiography was associated with progressively higher risk for stroke in an elderly cohort.[81] The blood pressure usually rises further during the acute phases of a stroke, and caution is advised in lowering the blood pressure during this crucial period.[82]

PLASMA RENIN ACTIVITY AS A PROGNOSTIC GUIDE. In 1972, Bruner et al. published data showing that a group of hypertensives with low levels of plasma renin activity (PRA) had a benign course, with no heart attacks or strokes uncovered on retrospective analysis.[83] Subsequently, many investigators have examined the relationship between renin levels and cardiovascular complications and found that, with few exceptions,[84] patients with low PRA do *not* have a more benign course than do those with normal PRA.

On the basis of the aforementioned assessments of overall cardiovascular risk and severity of hypertension, it should be possible to determine the approximate risk status and prognosis for individual patients. This can most easily be accomplished with the Framingham data, as described on page 813.

SHORT-TERM COURSE OF LOW-RISK HYPERTENSION. Data on the 4-year experiences of over 1600 "low-risk" hypertensives who served as controls in the Australian Therapeutic Trial document the validity of this assessment.[85] To enter this placebo versus drug trial, the patients had to be free of all identifiable cardiovascular disease, with the second set of diastolic pressures between 95 and 109 mm Hg. Thus they could be considered "low-risk" hypertensives. Over the next 4 years, in the majority of these patients, who were given placebo tablets but neither nondrug nor drug therapy, blood pressures *dropped progressively,* from an average of 157/102 to 144/91 mm Hg. Diastolic pressure was below 95 mm Hg in 47.5 per cent at the end of the trial. The fall in blood pressure was not related to any recognizable change in the patients' status; similar decreases occurred independent of changes in or stability of body weight. Of great interest was the lack of excess morbidity or mortality among those whose diastolic pressures remained below 100 mm Hg.

These results support strongly the view that certain patients can be characterized as being at relatively low risk and can therefore safely do without drug therapy long enough for the clinician to monitor both their blood pressure levels over time and the effectiveness of nondrug measures, if indicated. The large number of patients whose pressures fell and the high average degree of fall may seem surprising, but none of these patients started with any identifiable cardiovascular disease or complications due to hypertension. Moreover, placebo may be more effective than no therapy.

Similar results were observed in the even larger Medical Research Council (MRC) trial in England, in which over 18,000 patients with pretreatment diastolic pressures between 95 and 109 mm Hg were randomly assigned to antihypertensive drugs or placebo.[86] At the end of 5 years, these pressures had dropped to below 90 mm Hg in 43 per cent of the men and 50 per cent of the women on placebo.

THE POTENTIAL FOR PROGRESSION. Although these data reflect the benign nature of "low-risk" hypertension over the short term, it should be noted that the diastolic blood pressure rose above 110 mm Hg in 12 per cent of the nondrug-treated patients in both the Australian and English trials. Therefore, continued monitoring of the blood pressure levels is obviously needed for all patients with even the mildest "low-risk" hypertension.

A SYNTHESIS OF RISK. In the MRC trial, older age, male sex, hypercholesterolemia, and cigarette smoking, along with an increased level of systolic blood pressure at entry, were related significantly to the subsequent development of cardiovascular complications.[86] Although the ability to discriminate between those who did and did not suffer a coronary or cerebrovascular event in this 5-year trial was not precise, the degree of risk from hypertension can be categorized with reasonable accuracy, taking into account (1) the level of blood pressure, (2) the biological nature of the hypertension, based on the degree of target organ damage, and (3) the coexistence of other risks. Although risk is increased for the hypertensive population as a whole, problems are more likely in those with higher levels of pressure (diastolic above 100 mm Hg), considerable target organ damage (retinopathy, cardiomegaly, renal damage), and other risk factors (hypercholesterolemia, cigarette smoking, diabetes). For them, immediate and effective reduction of pressure appears to be indicated. But for the majority, who are at relatively low risk, the more reasonable approach would be to continue to monitor the blood pressure while encouraging healthful habits, such as weight control, moderate sodium restriction, isotonic exercise, and relaxation, in hopes of slowing progression of the disease (Chap. 27).

A group of physicians from New Zealand has formalized this approach into a nomogram based on the concept that "decisions to treat raised blood pressure should be based primarily on the estimated absolute risk of cardiovascular disease rather than on blood pressure alone."[87] They separate patients by levels of blood pressure, gender, and age and take various risk factors and evidences of target organ damage into account. After consideration of the available data both on the ability of therapy to reduce cardiovascular risk and on the financial and other costs of therapy, they propose active drug therapy for those patients whose overall risk status of a major cardiovascular event in 10 years (based on the Framingham data) is more than about 20 per cent. They believe that at that level of absolute risk, "150 people would require treatment to reduce the annual number of cardiovascular events by about one."

Although one could argue that their limit for active therapy is too high, excluding some patients who would benefit from therapy, I believe that their concept is absolutely correct and should be followed in making the crucial decision for the institution of therapy, as will be detailed in the next chapter.

It is obvious that since there is no certain way to predict the course of the blood pressure, even hypertensives who are not treated should be followed, and recognition of their hypertension should motivate them to follow good health habits. In this way, no harm should be done, and the potential benefit may be considerable if progression of the disease can be slowed by life style modifications.

MECHANISMS OF PRIMARY (ESSENTIAL) HYPERTENSION

No single or specific cause is known for most hypertension, referred to as *primary* in preference to *essential.* Since persistent hypertension can develop only in response to an increase in cardiac output or a rise in peripheral resistance, defects may be present in one or more of the multiple factors that affect these two forces (Fig. 26–10). The interplay of various derangements in factors affecting cardiac output and peripheral resistance may precipitate the disease, and these may differ in both type and degree in different patients.

Hemodynamic Patterns

Before describing specific abnormalities in the various factors shown in Figure 26–10 to affect the basic equation BP = CO × PR, the hemodynamic patterns that have been measured in patients with hypertension will be considered. One cautionary factor should be kept in mind: The development of the disease is slow and gradual. By the time blood pressure becomes elevated, the initiating factors may no longer be apparent, because they may have been "normalized" by multiple compensatory interactions. Nonetheless, when a group of untreated young hypertensive patients was studied initially, cardiac output was normal or slightly increased and peripheral resistance was normal.[88] Over the next 20 years, cardiac output fell progressively, while peripheral resistance rose. In a much larger study involving over 2600 subjects in Framingham followed for 4 years by echocardiography, an increased cardiac index and

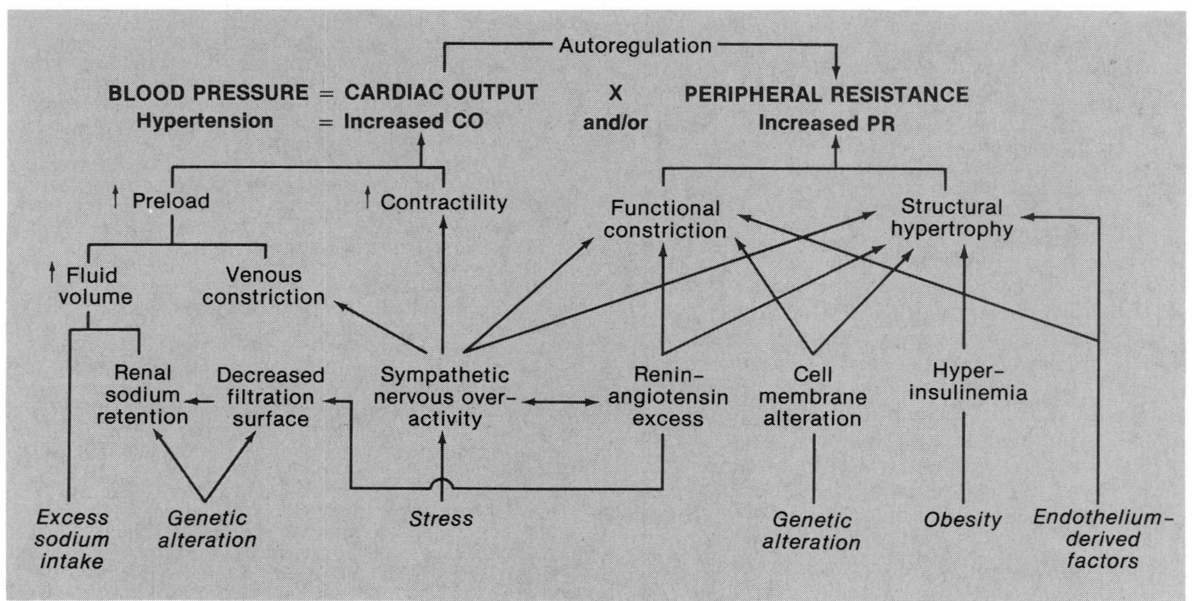

FIGURE 26–10. Some of the factors involved in the control of blood pressure that affect the basic equation: Blood pressure = cardiac output (CO) × peripheral resistance (PR). Cellular hyperplasia may be seen along with hypertrophy. (From Kaplan, N. M.: Clinical Hypertension. 6th ed. Baltimore, © by Williams and Wilkins, 1994, p. 57.)

end-systolic wall stress were related to the development of hypertension, but these hemodynamic measures were no longer significant predictors when adjustments for age and baseline blood pressure were made.[89]

Regardless of how hypertension begins, the eventual primacy of increased resistance can be shown even in models of hypertension that feature an initial increase in fluid volume and cardiac output.[90]

Genetic Predisposition

As discussed on p. 1677 and shown in Figure 26–10, genetic alterations may initiate the cascade to permanent hypertension. Clearly, heredity plays a role, although only one linkage has been described, involving regions within or close to the angiotensinogen gene.[91,91a] In studies of twins and family members in which the degree of familial aggregation of blood pressure levels is compared with the closeness of genetic sharing, the genetic contributions have been estimated to range from 30 to 60 per cent.[92] Unquestionably, environment plays some role, and Harrap[92] offers as a working model an interaction between genes and environment "in which the average population pressure is determined by environment, but blood pressure rank within the distribution is decided largely by genes."

If genetic markers of a predisposition to develop hypertension are found, specific environmental manipulations could then be directed toward those susceptible subjects. For now, children and siblings of hypertensives should be more carefully screened. They should be vigorously advised to avoid environmental factors known to aggravate hypertension and increase cardiovascular risk (e.g., smoking, inactivity, and excess sodium).

The Fetal Environment

Environmental factors may come into play very early. Low birth weight as a consequence of fetal undernutrition is followed by an increased incidence of high blood pressure later in life.[93] Increased postnatal feeding of low-birth-weight infants does not alter their blood pressure levels at 8 years of age,[94] suggesting that permanent imprinting has already occurred. Brenner and Chertow[95] hypothesize that a decreased number of nephrons could very well serve as this permanent, irreparable defect that eventuates in hypertension (Fig. 26–11). In their words: "This hypothesis draws on observations suggesting (1) a direct relationship between birth weight and nephron number, (2) an inverse relationship between birth weight and childhood, adolescent, and adult blood pressures, and (3) an inverse relationship between nephron number and blood pressure, irrespective of whether nephron number is reduced congenitally or in postnatal life (as from partial renal ablation or acquired renal disease)."

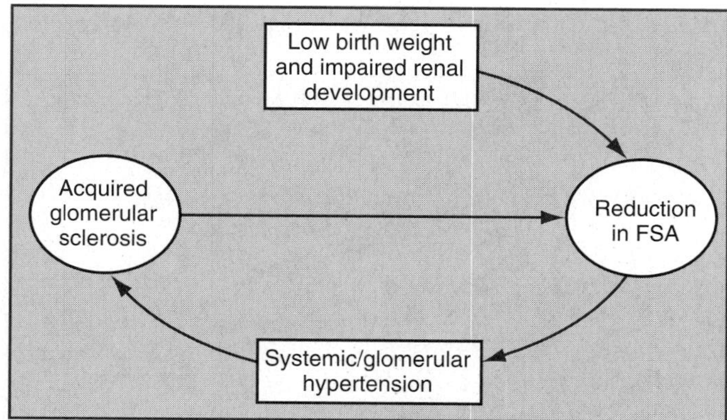

FIGURE 26–11. Hypothesis. The risks of developing essential hypertension and progressive renal injury in adult life are increased as a result of congenital oligonephropathy, an inborn deficit of filtration surface area (FSA) due to impaired renal development. Low birth weight, due to intrauterine growth retardation or prematurity, contributes to this oligonephropathy. Systemic and glomerular hypertension in later life results in progressive glomerular sclerosis, further reducing FSA and thereby perpetuating a vicious cycle, leading, in the extreme, to end-stage renal failure. (From Brenner, B. M., and Chertow, G. M.: Congenital oligonephropathy: An inborn cause of adult hypertension and progressive renal injury? Curr. Opin. Nephrol. Hypertens. *2*:691, 1993.)

This hypothesis fits nicely with Brenner's explanation for the inexorable progression of renal damage once it begins and the concept that hypertension may begin by renal sodium retention induced by the decreased filtration surface area.[96]

Renal Retention of Excess Sodium

A considerable amount of circumstantial evidence supports a role for sodium in the genesis of hypertension (Table 26–8). To induce hypertension, some of that excess sodium must be retained by the kidneys. Such retention could arise in a number of ways, including

- A decrease in filtration surface by a congenital or acquired deficiency in nephron number or function.[96]
- A resetting of the normal pressure-natriuresis relationship, wherein a rise in pressure invokes an immediate increase in renal sodium excretion, shrinking fluid volume and returning the pressure to normal. Guyton[97] has long argued for a resetting of this relationship as a fundamental defect that must be present to explain the persistence of an elevated pressure.
- Nephron heterogeneity, as hypothesized by Sealey et al.,[98] as the presence of "a subpopulation of nephrons that is ischemic either from afferent arteriolar vasoconstriction or from an intrinsic narrowing of the lumen. Renin secretion from this subgroup of nephrons is tonically elevated. This increased renin secretion then interferes with the compensatory capacity of intermingled normal nephrons to adaptively excrete sodium and, consequently, perturbs overall blood pressure homeostasis."
- An acquired inhibitor of the sodium pump that "affects sodium transport across cell membranes. In the kidney, it adjusts urinary sodium excretion so that sodium balance is near that of normal subjects on the same intake of sodium, thus making it difficult to demonstrate an increase in extracellular fluid volume. In the arteriole, it causes a rise in intracellular sodium concentration, which in turn raises the intracellular calcium concentration and thus increases vascular reactivity."[99] A great deal of work has gone into identification of a circulating sodium pump inhibitor. Some believe it to be ouabain,[100,101] but others do not.[102]

TABLE 26–8 EVIDENCE FOR A ROLE OF SODIUM IN PRIMARY (ESSENTIAL) HYPERTENSION

1. In multiple populations, the rise in blood pressure with age is directly correlated with increasing levels of sodium intake.
2. Multiple, scattered groups who consume little sodium (less than 50 mmol/day) have little or no hypertension. When they consume more sodium, hypertension appears.
3. Animals given sodium loads, if genetically predisposed, develop hypertension.
4. Some people, when given large sodium loads over short periods, develop an increase in vascular resistance and blood pressure.
5. An increased concentration of sodium is present in the vascular tissue and blood cells of most hypertensives.
6. Sodium restriction, to a level of 60 to 90 mmol per day, will lower blood pressure in most people. The antihypertensive action of diuretics requires an initial natriuresis.

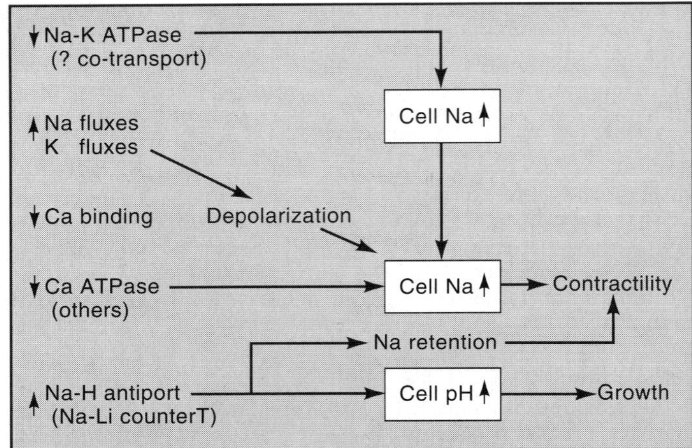

FIGURE 26–12. Hypotheses linking abnormal ionic fluxes to increased peripheral resistance through increases in cell sodium, calcium, or pH. *CounterT* = countertransport. (From Swales, J. D.: Functional disturbance of the cell membrane in hypertension. J. Hypertens. *8* [Suppl. 7]:S203, 1990.)

- A deficient responsiveness of the atrial natriuretic hormone.[103] Although the atrial and brain natriuretic peptides likely play an important role in maintenance of sodium balance and blood pressure regulation,[104] the evidence for their involvement in the genesis of hypertension is weak at best.

There are, then, more than enough possible ways to incite renal retention of even a very small bit of the excess sodium typically ingested that could eventually expand body fluid volume. Variations in sensitivity to sodium also have been noted and may explain why only some people respond to excess sodium and others do not.[105]

Defects in Cell Transport or Binding

A host of defects in various cell membrane functions has been shown mostly in red blood cells. Most involve increased movement of sodium into the cell, thereby increasing intracellular calcium, which, in turn, would increase vascular tone and contractility[106] (Fig. 26–12). John Swales questions their pathogenetic role, concluding that "the best unifying hypothesis is that all the reported abnormalities are markers for a disturbance of physicochemical properties of the cell membrane lipids of hypertensive patients."[107]

Vascular Hypertrophy

Both excess sodium intake and renal sodium retention would presumably work primarily on increasing fluid volume and cardiac output. A number of other factors may work primarily on the second part of the equation, BP = CO × PR (Fig. 26–10). Most of these can cause both functional contraction and structural remodeling and hypertrophy.

Multiple vasoactive substances act as growth factors for vascular hypertrophy.[108] As seen in Figure 26–13, these pressor-growth promoters may result in both vascular contraction and hypertrophy simultaneously, but the perpetuation of hypertension involves hypertrophy. The various hormonal mediators shown at the top of Figure 26–13 may serve as the initiator of what eventuates as increased peripheral resistance. From the study of certain "pure" forms of hormonally induced hypertension, Lever and Harrap[109] have postulated that "most forms of secondary hypertension have two pressor mechanisms: a primary cause, e.g., renal clip, and a second process, which is slow to develop, capable of maintaining hypertension after removal of the primary cause, and probably self-perpetuating in nature. We suggest that essential hypertension also has two mechanisms, both based upon cardiovascular hypertrophy: (1) a growth-promoting process in children (equivalent to the

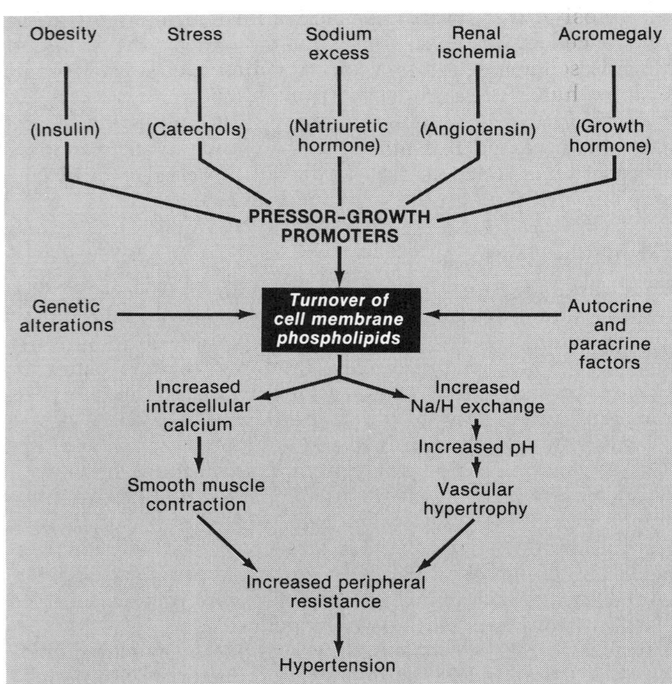

FIGURE 26–13. Scheme for the induction of hypertension by numerous pressor hormones that act as vascular growth promoters. (From Kaplan, N. M.: Clinical Hypertension. 6th ed. Baltimore, © by Williams and Wilkins, 1994, p. 84.)

primary cause in secondary hypertension) and (2) a self-perpetuating mechanism in adults."

These investigators have built on the original proposal of Folkow[110] of a "positive feedback interaction" wherein even mild functional pressor influences, if repeatedly exerted, may lead to structural hypertrophy, which, in turn, reinforces and perpetuates the elevated pressure (Fig. 26–14). Lever and Harrap[109] have added two hypotheses to Folkow's first: a reinforcement of the hypertrophic response to stimuli that initially raise the pressure, e.g., defects in the vascular cell membrane, and the action of various trophic mechanisms that may cause vascular hypertrophy directly, as the "slow pressor mechanism." Whereas the immediate pressor effect is mediated by increased free intracellular calcium, the slowly developing vascular hypertrophy is postulated to involve phosphati-

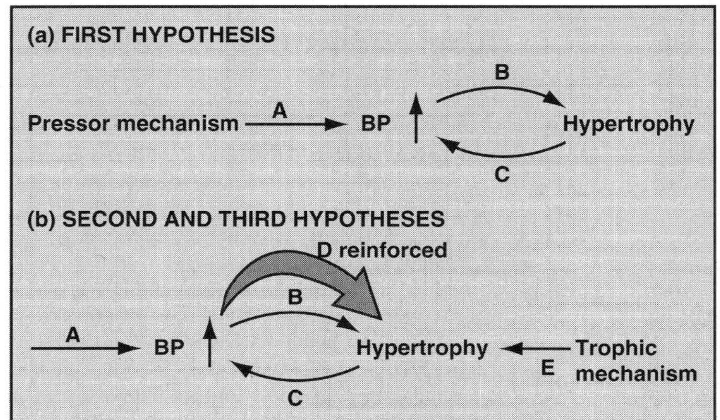

FIGURE 26–14. Hypotheses for the initiation and maintenance of hypertension: A, Folkow's first proposal that a minor overactivity of a pressor mechanism (A) raises blood pressure slightly, initiating positive feedback (BCB) and a progressive rise of blood pressure. B, As in A with two additional signals: D, an abnormal or "reinforced" hypertrophic response to pressure, and E, increase of a humoral agent causing hypertrophy directly. (From Lever, A. F., and Harrap, S. B.: Essential hypertension: A disorder of growth with origins in childhood? J. Hypertens. *10*:101, 1992.)

dyl-inositol metabolism and activation of tyrosine kinase[111] in the cell membrane.

This scheme to explain an immediate pressor action and a slow hypertrophic effect is thought to be common to the action of pressor-growth promoters. When present in high concentrations over long periods, as with angiotensin II in renal artery stenosis, each of these pressor-growth promoters causes hypertension. Moreover, when the source of the excess pressor-growth promoter is removed, hypertension may recede slowly, presumably reflecting the time needed to reverse vascular hypertrophy.

No marked excess of any known pressor hormone is identifiable in the majority of hypertensive patients. Nonetheless, a lesser excess of one or more may have been responsible for intiation of a process sustained by the positive feedback postulated by Folkow[110] and the trophic effects emphasized by Lever and Harrap.[109] This sequence encompasses a variety of specific initiating mechanisms that accentuate and maintain the hypertension by a nonspecific feedback-trophic mechanism (Fig. 26–14). If this double process is fundamental to the pathogenesis of primary hypertension, the difficulty in recognizing the initiating causal factor is easily explained. As formulated by Lever[112]:

> The primary cause of hypertension will be most apparent in the early stages; in the later stages, the cause will be concealed by an increasing contribution from hypertrophy. . . . A particular form of hypertension may wrongly be judged to have "no known cause" because each mechanism considered is insufficiently abnormal by itself to have produced the hypertension. The cause of essential hypertension may have been considered already but rejected for this reason.

A large number of circulating hormones and locally acting substances may be involved. Support exists for each of those shown as potential instigators in Figure 26–10. They will be considered in the order shown without attempting to prioritize their role.

Sympathetic Nervous Hyperactivity

Young hypertensives tend to have increased levels of circulating catecholamines,[113] augmented sympathetic nerve traffic in muscles,[114] faster heart rate,[115] and heightened vascular reactivity to norepinephrine.[116] These could raise blood pressure in a number of ways—either alone or in concert with stimulation of renin release by catecholamines—by causing arteriolar and venous constriction, by increasing cardiac output, or by altering the normal renal pressure-volume relationship. In addition to cardiac stimulation by sympathetic activity, vagal inhibitory responses to baroreceptors and other stimuli also may be important. In humans with denervated transplanted hearts, both pulse and blood pressure fail to display the usual nocturnal fall, and hypertension is frequent.[117] The transient increase in epinephrine during stress reactions may invoke a more prolonged pressor response by facilitating the release of norepinephrine from sympathetic neurons.[118]

Repetitive stress or an accentuated, exaggerated response to stress is the logical means by which sympathetic activation would arise. Young hypertensives tend to be hyperresponsive,[119] and at least among middle-aged men in Framingham, the development of hypertension over 18 to 20 years was associated with heightened anxiety and anger intensity and suppressed expression of anger at baseline.[120] Moreover, in the 29-year-old normotensives in the Tecumseh Blood Pressure Study, increased sympathetic activity was closely correlated with higher hematocrit levels (presumably reflecting a decrease in plasma volume from vasoconstriction), and higher hematocrits have been found repeatedly to be associated with higher blood pressures.[115]

The Tecumseh subjects with higher plasma catecholamines also tended to have higher plasma renin activity (PRA) levels. Other investigators have noted that hypertensives with high PRA had more anxiety, suppressed anger, and susceptibility to emotional distress.[121] Obviously, the sympathetic and renin mechanisms may be connected in various ways.

Sympathetic nervous activity could be activated from the brain without the mediation of stress or emotional distress. Hypertension has been induced in animals by various neurogenic defects. An intriguing association has been reported between essential hypertension and compression of the ventrolateral medulla by loops of the posterior inferior cerebellar artery or an ectatic vertebral artery seen by magnetic resonance tomography.[122]

Whatever the specific role of sympathetic activity in the pathogenesis of hypertension, it appears to be involved in the increased cardiovascular morbidity and mortality that affect hypertensive patients during the early morning hours. Increased alpha-sympathetic activity occurs in the early morning, associated with the preawakening increase in REM sleep[123] and the assumption of upright posture after overnight recumbency.[124] As a consequence of the increased sympathetic activity, blood pressure rises abruptly and markedly. This rise must be at least partly responsible for the increase in cardiovascular catastrophes in the early morning hours.[17]

The Renin-Angiotensin System

Both as a direct pressor and as a growth promoter, the renin-angiotensin mechanism also may be involved in the pathogenesis of hypertension.[124a] All functions of renin are mediated through the synthesis of angiotensin II. This system is the primary stimulus for the secretion of aldosterone and hence mediates the mineralocorticoid responses to varying sodium intakes and volume loads. When sodium intake is reduced or effective plasma volume shrinks, the increase in renin–angiotensin II stimulates aldosterone secretion, and this, in turn, is responsible for a portion of the enhanced renal retention of sodium and water (Fig. 26–15).

According to the feedback shown in Figure 26–15, any rise in blood pressure inhibits release of renin from the renal juxtaglomerular (JG) cells. Therefore, primary (essential) hypertension would be expected to be accompanied by low, suppressed levels of PRA. When large populations of hypertensives are surveyed, only about 30 per cent have low PRA, whereas 50 per cent have normal levels and the remaining 20 per cent high levels.[125]

NORMAL AND HIGH RENIN HYPERTENSION

A number of explanations have been offered for these "inappropriately normal" or high levels, beyond the proportion expected in a normal gaussian distribution curve. One of the more attractive is the concept of "nephron heterogeneity" described by Sealey et al.,[98] which assumes a mixture of normal and ischemic nephrons caused by afferent arteriolar narrowing. Excess renin from the ischemic nephrons could raise the total blood renin level to varying degrees and cause some persons to have normal or high renin hypertension.

This hypothesis is similar to that proposed by Goldblatt, who believed that "the primary cause of essential hypertension in man is intrarenal obliterative vascular disease, from any cause, usually arterial and arteriolar sclerosis, or any other condition which brings about the same disturbance of intrarenal hemodynamics."[126] When Goldblatt placed the clamp on the main renal arteries in canine studies, he was trying to explain the pathogenesis of primary (essential) hypertension rather than what he ended up explaining: the pathogenesis of renovascular hypertension.[126a] Nonetheless, his experimental concept is the basis for the more modern model of Sealey et al. The elevated renin from the ischemic population of nephrons, although diluted in the systemic circulation, provides the "normal" renin levels that are usual in patients with primary hypertension who would otherwise be expected to shut down renin secretion and in whom levels would be low. These diluted levels are still high enough to impair sodium excretion in the nonischemic hyperfiltering nephrons

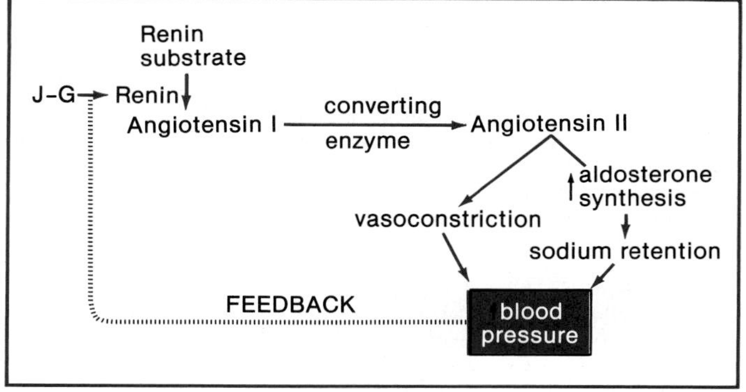

FIGURE 26–15. Overall scheme of the renin-angiotensin mechanism.

but are too low to support efferent tone in the ischemic nephrons, thereby reducing sodium excretion in them as well.

Sealey and associates' concept of nephron heterogeneity differs from Brenner and associates' concept of nephron scarcity previously noted. Nevertheless, Sealey et al. agree that "a reduction in nephron number related to either age or ischemia could amplify the impaired sodium excretion and promote hypertension."[98]

The renin-angiotensin system is active in multiple organs, either from in situ synthesis of various components or by transport from renal JG cells through the circulation. The presence of the complete system in endothelial cells, the brain, the heart, and the adrenal cortex[127] broadens the potential roles of this mechanism far beyond its previously accepted boundaries. Angiotensin may have a direct role in vascular hypertrophy: When local expression of vascular angiotensin-converting enzyme (ACE) was increased by in vivo gene transfer, local hypertrophy of the vessel way occurred, independent of systemic factors or hemodynamic effects.[128]

Hyperinsulinemia/Insulin Resistance

An association between hypertension and hyperinsulinemia has been recognized for many years, particularly with accompanying obesity,[49] but also in nonobese hypertensives.[129] The association does not apply to some ethnic groups such as Pima Indians but has been found in blacks and Asians as well as whites.[130]

All obese people are hyperinsulinemic secondary to insulin resistance and even more so if the obesity is predominantly visceral, i.e., abdominal or upper body, wherein decreased hepatic uptake of insulin contributes to the hyperinsulinemia.[131] The hyperinsulinemia of hypertension also arises as a consequence of resistance to the effects of insulin on peripheral glucose utilization.[132] The cause for the insulin resistance is unknown. It could reflect a simple inability of insulin to reach the skeletal muscle cells, wherein its major peripheral actions on glucose metabolism occur. This, in turn, may result from a defect in the usual vasodilatory effect of insulin, mediated through increased synthesis of nitric oxide,[133] which normally counters the multiple pressor effects of insulin[134] (Fig. 26–16). These pressor effects, in addition to activation of sympathetic activity, include a trophic action on vascular hypertrophy and increased renal sodium reabsorption.

The failure of vasodilation to antagonize the multiple pressor effects of insulin presumably eventuates in a rise in blood pressure that may be either a primary cause of hypertension or, at least, a secondary potentiator. In addition, the underlying insulin resistance is often associated with a full syndrome, including dyslipidemia and diabetes along with hypertension, which combine to be a major risk factor for premature coronary disease.[132]

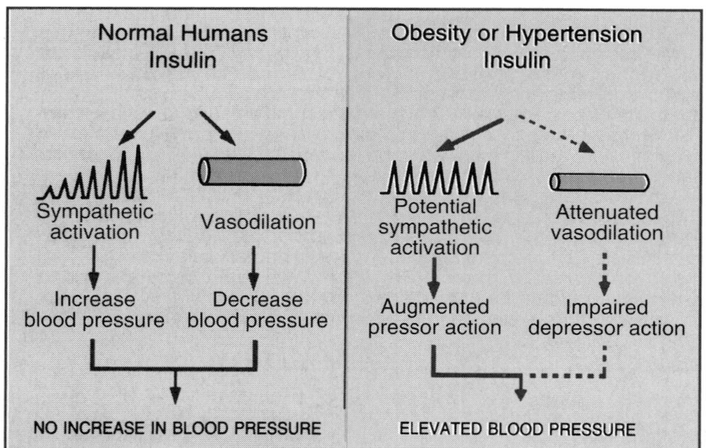

FIGURE 26–16. *Left panel,* Insulin's actions in normal humans. Although insulin causes a marked increase in sympathetic neural outflow which would be expected to increase blood pressure, it also causes vasodilation which would decrease blood pressure. The net effect of these two opposing influences is no change or a slight decrease in blood pressure. There may be an imbalance between the sympathetic and vascular actions of insulin in conditions such as obesity or hypertension. *Right panel,* Insulin may cause potentiated sympathetic activation or attenuated vasodilation. An imbalance between these pressor and depressor actions of insulin may result in elevated blood pressure. (From Anderson, E. A., and Mark, A. L.: Cardiovascular and sympathetic actions of insulin: The insulin hypothesis of hypertension revisited. Cardiovasc. Risk Factors *3:*159, 1993.)

Endothelial Cell Dysfunction

The impairment of normal vasodilation seen in the insulin resistance syndrome has been shown to involve a failure to synthesize the normal endothelium-derived relaxing factor nitric oxide (NO).[133] This is one of the rapidly increasing evidences for an active role for the endothelial cells, now known to be the source of multiple relaxing and constricting substances, most having a local, paracrine influence on the underlying smooth muscle cells[135] (Fig. 26–17).

NITRIC OXIDE (see also p. 1164). Hypertensive patients have been shown by some[136] but not all[137] to have a reduced vasodilatory response to various stimuli of NO release. In addition, hypertensives display a less pronounced decrease in forearm blood flow when an inhibitor of NO synthesis is infused, indicating a decreased basal release of NO by the endothelial cells of hypertensive endothelial cells. The forearm responsiveness has been restored by normalization of blood pressure by antihypertensive drugs with different modes of action.[138]

The previously noted frequent association of dyslipidemia with hypertension may be based on an inhibition of endothelium-dependent vasodilation by oxidized lipoproteins.[139]

ENDOTHELIN. A number of endothelium-derived constricting factors are shown in the middle portion of Figure 26–17. Of these, endothelin-1 appears to be of particular importance because it causes pronounced and prolonged vasoconstriction[140] and because inhibitors of its synthesis or binding cause significant vasodilation.[141] Its role in human hypertension, however, remains uncertain.

OTHER POSSIBLE MECHANISMS

The preceding description of the possible roles of the various mechanisms portrayed in Figure 26–10 does not exhaust the list of putative contributors to the pathogenesis of primary hypertension.

Other pressor hormones are known, including vasopressin,[142] but their possible role in human hypertension remains unknown. Similarly, a number of vasodepressor hormones are known, but their function, too, remains uncertain. These include kallikrein[143] and medullipin, a renomedullary lipid.[144]

Contributions from excesses of various minerals, particularly lead,[145] and changing ratios among dietary sodium, potassium, calcium, and magnesium also have been postulated.[146] Support for these and other postulated mechanisms is meager, and the overall schemes involving intracellular sodium and calcium and the pressor-growth promotor mechanisms for vascular hypertrophy seem more than adequate to explain the pathogenesis of primary hypertension. However, a number of associations between hypertension and other conditions have been noted and may offer additional insights into the potential causes and possible prevention of the disease.

ASSOCIATION OF HYPERTENSION WITH OTHER CONDITIONS

OBESITY. Even though obese hypertensives may have lower rates of coronary mortality than lean hypertensives,[147] hypertension is more common among obese individuals and probably adds to their increased risk of developing ischemic heart disease. In the Framingham offspring study, adiposity, as measured by subscapular skinfold thickness, was the major controllable contributor to hypertension.[148] This finding corroborates the crucial importance of the *distribution* of body fat, since blood pressure as well as blood lipids, glucose levels, and insulin levels tends to

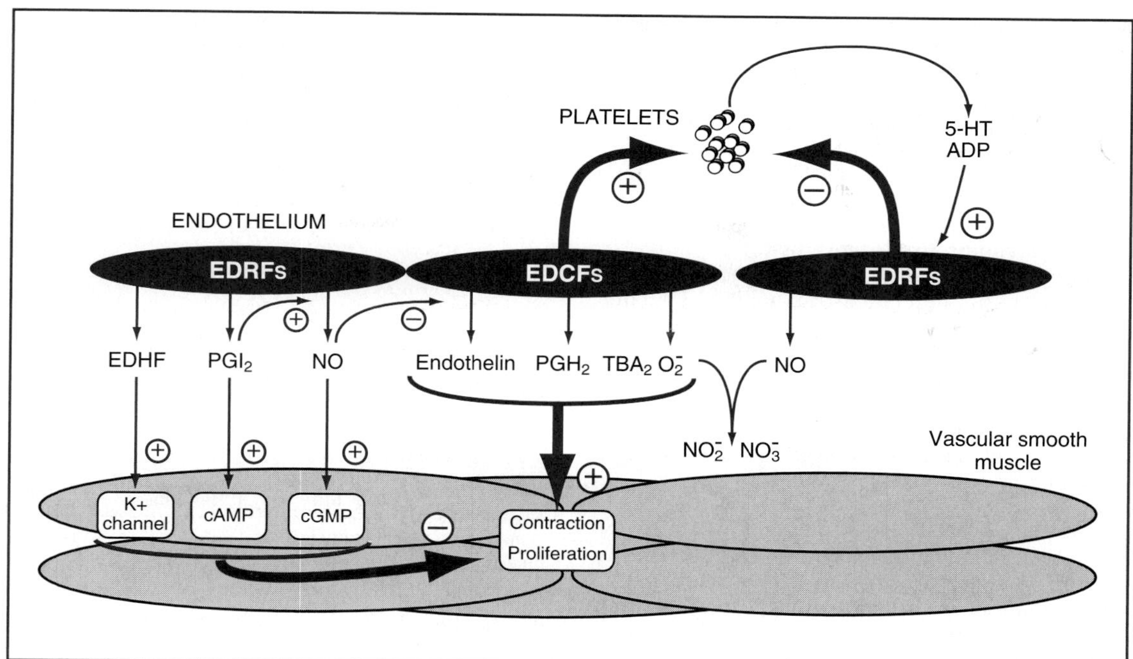

FIGURE 26–17. Schematic diagram of proposed interactions between endothelial mediators. ***PGI₂,*** **prostacyclin;** ***NO,*** **nitric oxide;** ***EDHF,*** **endothelium-derived hyperpolarizing factor;** ***PGH₂,*** **prostaglandin H₂;** ***TBA₂,*** **thromboxane A₂;** ***O₂⁻,*** **superoxide anion;** ***5-HT,*** **serotonin;** ***ADP,*** **adenosine diphosphate;** ***EDRFs,*** **endothelium-derived relaxing factors;** ***EDCFs,*** **endothelium-derived contracting factors. (From Flavahan, N. A.: Atherosclerosis or lipoprotein-induced endothelial dysfunction: Potential mechanism underlying reduction in EDRF/nitric oxide activity. Circulation** ***85:*****1927, 1992.)**

be highest in those with visceral or upper body obesity.[131] As noted previously, these may all be interconnected via insulin resistance and hyperinsulinemia. Children seem particularly vulnerable to the hypertensive effects of weight gain.[36] Therefore, avoidance of childhood obesity with the hope of avoiding subsequent hypertension seems important. The evidence that weight reduction will lower established hypertension is discussed on p. 844.

SLEEP APNEA. One of the contributors to the hypertension in obese people is sleep apnea. Snoring and sleep apnea are clearly associated with hypertension, and this, in turn, may be induced by increased sympathetic activity in response to hypoxemia during apnea.[149]

PHYSICAL INACTIVITY. Physical fitness may help prevent hypertension, and persons who are already hypertensive may lower their blood pressure by means of regular isotonic exercise. The relationship may involve insulin resistance, because increased resistance was coupled with low physical fitness in normotensive men with a family history of hypertension.[150] Regular exercise may prevent hypertension and thereby protect against the development of cardiovascular disease.[151] Among 16,936 Harvard male alumni followed for 16 to 50 years, those who did not engage in vigorous sports play were at 35 per cent greater risk for developing hypertension, whether or not they had higher blood pressures while at Harvard, a family history of hypertension, or obesity—factors that also increased the risk of hypertension.[152]

ALCOHOL INTAKE. Alcohol in small amounts (less than two usual portions a day) provides protection from coronary mortality[153] and atherosclerosis[154] but in larger amounts (more than two portions a day) increases blood pressure[155] and overall mortality.[153] The reduction in coronary disease in persons who ingest small amounts of alcohol may reflect an improvement in the lipid profile,[156] a reduction in factors that encourage thrombosis,[157] and an improvement in insulin sensitivity.[158]

The pressor effect of larger amounts of alcohol primarily reflects an increase in cardiac output and heart rate, possibly a consequence of increased sympathetic nerve activity.[159] Alcohol also alters cell membranes, allowing more calcium to enter, perhaps by inhibition of sodium transport.[160]

SMOKING (see also p. 844). Cigarette smoking raises blood pressure, probably through the nicotine-induced release of norepinephrine from adrenergic nerve endings. In addition, smoking causes an acute and marked reduction in radial artery compliance, independent of the increase in blood pressure.[161] When smokers quit, a trivial rise in blood pressure may occur, probably reflecting a gain in weight.[162]

HEMATOLOGIC FINDINGS. Polycythemia vera is frequently associated with hypertension (see p. 1792). More common is a "pseudo-" or "stress" polycythemia with a high hematocrit[115] and increased blood viscosity[163] but contracted plasma volume as well as normal red cell mass and serum erythropoietin levels. High white blood cell counts are predictive of the development of hypertension.[164]

HYPERURICEMIA. Hyperuricemia is present in 25 to 50 per cent of individuals with untreated primary hypertension, about five times the frequency found in normotensive persons. Hyperuricemia likely reflects decreased renal blood flow, presumably a reflection of nephrosclerosis.[165] In addition to these conditions which are often associated with hypertension, distinctive features of hypertension may be important in various special groups of people.

HYPERTENSION IN SPECIAL GROUPS

Blacks

Although, on average, blood pressure in blacks is not higher than that in whites during adolescence,[36] adult blacks have hypertension more frequently, producing higher rates of morbidity and mortality. These higher rates may reflect a lesser tendency for the pressure to fall during sleep[24] and greater degrees of left ventricular hypertrophy,[64] but the lower socioeconomic status and lesser access to adequate health care of blacks as a group are likely more important. In particular, blacks suffer more renal damage, even with effective blood pressure control, leading to a significantly greater prevalence of end-stage disease.[166] When given a high-sodium diet, blacks but not whites tend to have increases in glomerular filtration rates, providing a possible mechanism for increased glomerular sclerosis.[167] Hypertension in blacks has been characterized as having a relatively greater component of fluid volume excess, including a higher prevalence of low plasma renin activity and a greater responsiveness to diuretic therapy.[168]

Perhaps blacks evolved the physiological machinery that would offer protection in their ancestral habitat, i.e., hot, arid climates in which avid sodium conservation was necessary for survival because the diet was relatively low in sodium.[169] When they migrate to areas where sodium intake is excessive, they are then more susceptible to "sodium overload." In addition, blacks also may be more susceptible to hypertension because as a group they tend to ingest less potassium.[170]

Women

In general, women suffer less cardiovascular morbidity and mortality than men for any degree of hypertension.[171] Moreover, before menopause, hypertension is less common in women than in men. Perhaps the lower frequency and severity of hypertension reflect the lower blood volume afforded women by menses. Eventually, however, more women than men suffer a hypertension-related cardiovascular complication because there are more elderly women than elderly men and hypertension is both more common and dangerous in the elderly.[172]

Children and Adolescents

(See also Chap. 31)

As in adults, care is needed in establishing the presence of persistently elevated blood pressures in children using the upper limits of normal shown in Table 26–3. Recall that these are the averages of the first blood pressure value obtained; since the pressure usually falls on repeated measurements, levels below those shown in Table 26–3 may be abnormally high for a given child. In addition, the recent inclusion of height along with age and weight to the nomograms for children and adolescents likely improves their diagnostic accuracy.[173] Uncertainty remains as to the meaning of readings above the 95th percentile in an asymptomatic child, since the tracking of blood pressure as children grow older does not tend to be persistent; the positive predictive value of a blood pressure above the 95th percentile in a 10-year-old boy being at a hypertensive level at age 20 is only 0.44.[174] Moreover, the sensitivity of this high blood pressure in a 10-year-old to detect hypertension 10 years later is only 0.17.

Nonetheless, most authorities[36,175,176] agree that those with "significant" hypertension (levels above the 95th percentile) should be given a limited work-up for target organ damage and secondary causes (perhaps including an echocardiogram and likely including a renal isotopic scan); if these are negative, they should be carefully monitored and given nonpharmacological therapy. Those with "severe" hypertension (levels above the 99th percentile) should be more rapidly and completely evaluated and given appropriate pharmacological therapy.

EPIDEMIOLOGY. The older the child, the more likely the hypertension is of unknown cause, i.e., primary or essential. In prepubertal children, chronic hypertension is more likely caused by congenital or acquired renal parenchymal or vascular disease[176] (Table 26–9).

In adolescents, primary hypertension is the most likely diagnosis. Factors that increase the likelihood for early onset of hypertension include a positive family history of hypertension, obesity, poor physical fitness, and an increase in thickness of the interventricular septum during systole on echocardiography.[177,178] Among black children, a greater blood pressure reactivity to stress also may be predictive.[179]

TABLE 26–9 MOST COMMON CAUSES OF CHRONIC HYPERTENSION IN CHILDHOOD

- NEWBORN
  - Renal artery stenosis or thrombosis
  - Congenital renal structural abnormalities
  - Coarctation of the aorta
  - Bronchopulmonary dysplasia
- INFANCY TO 6 YEARS
  - Renal structural and inflammatory diseases
  - Coarctation of the aorta
  - Renal artery stenosis
  - Wilms' tumor
- 6–10 YEARS
  - Renal structural and inflammatory diseases
  - Renal artery stenosis
  - Essential (primary) hypertension
  - Renal parenchymal diseases
- ADOLESCENCE
  - Primary hypertension
  - Renal parenchymal diseases

From Loggie, J. M. H.: Hypertension in children. Heart Dis Stroke May/June:147, 1994.

MANAGEMENT. Once persistently elevated blood pressures are identified and an appropriate work-up has been performed, weight reduction if the patient is overweight and moderate restriction of dietary sodium should be encouraged. In particular, regular dynamic exercise should be encouraged with few restrictions except for those with severe hypertension.[180] Those deemed to be in need of drug therapy are usually treated in the way adults are managed, as described in the next chapter. Unfortunately, there are very few controlled trials of various therapies in children, so most have adopted newer drugs, i.e., ACE inhibitors and calcium channel blockers, as appropriate therapies.[181] The pharmacological management of life-threatening hypertension follows the guidelines given later in this chapter with appropriate reductions in doses.[36,182]

Elderly

As more people live longer, more hypertension, particularly systolic, will be seen. By the usual criteria of the average of three blood pressure measurements on one occasion at or above 140 mm Hg systolic and/or 90 mm Hg diastolic or the taking of antihypertensive medication, 54 per cent of men and women aged 65 to 74 have hypertension; among blacks, the prevalence is 72 per cent.[183] In elderly patients with significant hypertension of recent onset, chronic renal disease or atherosclerotic renovascular disease is more likely to be found.

The risks of both pure systolic and combined systolic and diastolic hypertension at every level are greater in the elderly than in younger patients, reflecting the adverse effects of age-related atherosclerosis and concomitant conditions. It comes as no surprise that the elderly achieved even greater reductions in coronary disease and heart failure by effective therapy than the younger hypertensives in multiple clinical trials.[183,184]

The elderly may display two features that reflect age-related cardiovascular changes. The first is pseudohypertension from markedly sclerotic arteries that do not collapse under the cuff, presenting much higher cuff pressures than are present within the vessels. If arteries feel rigid but there are few retinal or cardiac findings to go along with marked hypertension, direct intraarterial measurements may be needed before therapy is begun to avoid inordinate lowering of blood pressures that are not, in fact, elevated. The second feature, seen in about 20 per cent of the elderly, is postural and postprandial hypotension, usually reflecting a progressive loss of baroreceptor responsiveness with age.[31,184] A standing blood pressure should always be taken in patients over age 65, particularly if seated or supine hypertension is noted; if postural hypotension is present, maneuvers to overcome the precipitous falls in pressure should be utilized before the seated and supine hypertension is cautiously treated. More about the special therapeutic challenges often found in the elderly is provided in the next chapter.

Diabetes Mellitus

(See also p. 1900)

Hypertension and diabetes coexist more commonly than predicted by chance. They feed on each other to markedly accelerate cardiovascular damages that are, in turn, responsible for the premature disabilities and higher rates of mortality that afflict diabetics. Among some 1500 diabetics followed by Danish investigators, 51 per cent of the insulin-dependent diabetics and 80 per cent of the non-insulin-dependent diabetics had blood pressures above 140/90 mm Hg.[185] In more than half these hypertensive diabetics, isolated systolic hypertension was noted.

Not only is hypertension more common in diabetics, but it also tends to be more persistent, with less of the usual nocturnal fall in pressure.[22] The absence of a nocturnal fall in pressure may reflect autonomic neuropathy or incipient diabetic nephropathy.[186]

The presence of hypertension increases all the microvascular and macrovascular complications seen in diabetes. Even at the initial presentation of diabetes, the presence of hypertension is associated with about a doubling of the prevalence of microalbuminuria, left ventricular hypertrophy, and electrocardiographic signs of myocardial ischemia.[187] As these newly diagnosed diabetics were followed for about 5 years, those with hypertension suffered almost a twofold greater incidence of cardiovascular morbidity and mortality than did the nonhypertensive diabetics.

When hypertensive, patients with diabetes mellitus may confront some interesting problems. With progressive renal insufficiency, they may have few functional juxtaglomerular cells, and as a result, the syndrome of hyporeninemic hypoaldosteronism may appear, usually manifested by hyperkalemia. If hypoglycemia develops because of too much insulin or other drugs, severe hypertension may occur as a result of stimulated sympathetic nervous activity.

Diabetics are also susceptible to special problems associated with antihypertensive therapy. High doses of both diuretics and beta blockers may worsen diabetic control, probably by inducing further insulin resistance. Those who are prone to hypoglycemia may have difficulties with beta-blocking agents, since these drugs blunt their protective catecholamine response, and severe hypoglycemia may develop with sweating as the only warning. Diabetic neuropathy may add to the postural hypotension and impotence that frequently complicate antihypertensive therapy. Diabetic nephropathy will impair sodium excretion and diminish the effectiveness of diuretics. On the other hand, successful control of hyperglycemia and reduction of blood pressure will protect such patients from the otherwise inexorable progress of diabetic nephropathy. Angiotensin-converting enzyme inhibitors may be especially effective in reducing the high intraglomerular pressures that are probably responsible for the progressive glomerulosclerosis of diabetes.[188]

SECONDARY FORMS OF HYPERTENSION

(See Tables 26–4 and 26–5, pp. 811 and 812)

Oral Contraceptive and Postmenopausal Estrogen Use

The use of estrogen-containing oral contraceptive pills is probably the most common cause of secondary hypertension in young women. Most women who take them experience a slight rise in blood pressure, and about 5 per cent develop hypertension (i.e., blood pressure above 140/90 mm Hg) within 5 years of oral contraceptive use. This is more than twice the incidence seen among women of the same age who do not use these agents.[172] Although the hypertension is usually mild, it may persist after the oral contraceptive is discontinued, it may be severe, and it is almost certainly a factor in the increased cardiovascular mortality seen among young women who take these agents.[189] Despite these facts, these drugs have provided effective and safe birth control for millions of women, and the need for oral contraceptives remains.

The dangers of oral contraceptives should be kept in proper perspective. While it is true that use of these drugs is associated with increased morbidity and mortality, the absolute numbers are quite small, and overall mortality from cardiovascular disease has been declining progressively among women in the United States at a rate equal to that noted among American men. Moreover, the risks appear to have been lessened by more careful selection of users and lower doses of hormones.[190] Most adverse effects occur in women who smoke and have other cardiovascular risk factors and who take formulations with more than 50 μg of estrogen. Thus, the currently used low-estrogen and progesterone forms seem quite safe for the purposes of temporary birth control.

INCIDENCE. The best data on the incidence of oral contraceptive–induced hypertension came from a large study of the Royal College of General Practitioners. The incidence of hypertension was 2.6 times greater among 23,000 pill users compared with 23,000 nonusers, resulting in a 5 per cent incidence over 5 years of oral contraceptive use.[191] In addition, this incidence increased with long duration of pill use, being only slightly higher than that among controls during the first year but rising to almost three times higher by the fifth year. In a much smaller but more carefully performed prospective study of 186 Scottish women, systolic pressure rose in 164 (by more than 25 mm Hg in 8) and diastolic pressure rose in 150 (by more than 20 mm Hg in 2) during the first 2 years of oral contraceptive use.[192] After 3 years, the mean rise in 83 of these women was 9.2 mm Hg. The current use of smaller amounts of estrogen (20 to 35 μg) than the 50 μg taken by most of these women may induce less hypertension.

CLINICAL FEATURES. The likelihood of developing hypertension among women using oral contraceptives is much greater among those who are over age 35 or obese or who drink large quantities of alcohol.[193] The presence of hypertension during a prior pregnancy increases this likelihood but not enough to preclude pill use in such women who require contraception. In most women the hypertension is mild; however, in some it may accelerate rapidly and cause severe renal damage.[194] When the pill is discontinued, blood pressure falls to normal within 3 to 6 months in about half the patients. Whether the pill caused permanent hypertension in the other half or just uncovered primary hypertension at an earlier time is not clear.

MECHANISMS OF HYPERTENSION. Oral contraceptive use probably causes hypertension by renin-aldosterone–mediated volume expansion. Estrogens and the synthetic progestogens used in oral contraceptive pills both cause sodium retention.[195] In keeping with the probable role of hyperinsulinemia in other hypertensive states (see p. 820), this may be involved in oral contraceptive–induced hypertension as well because plasma insulin levels are increased after start of oral contraceptive use, reflecting peripheral insulin resistance.[196]

MANAGEMENT. The use of estrogen-containing oral contraceptives should be restricted in women over age 35, particularly if they also smoke or are hypertensive or obese. Women given the pill should be properly monitored as follows: (1) the supply should be limited initially to 3 months and thereafter to 6 months; (2) they should be required to return for a blood pressure check before an additional supply is provided; and (3) if blood pressure has risen, an alternative contraceptive should be offered. If the pill remains the only acceptable contraceptive, the elevated blood pressure can be reduced with appropriate therapy. In view of the probable role of aldosterone, use of a diuretic-spironolactone combination seems appropriate. In those who stop taking oral contraceptives, evaluation for secondary hypertensive diseases should be postponed for at least 3 months to allow the changes in the renin-angiotensin-aldosterone system to remit. If the hypertension does not recede, additional work-up and therapy may be needed.

POSTMENOPAUSAL ESTROGEN USE. Millions of women use estrogen for its potential benefits after menopause. It does not appear to induce hypertension, even though it does induce various changes in the renin-angiotensin-aldosterone system seen with oral contraceptive use.[197] Moreover, the majority of case-control studies have shown a significantly *lower* mortality rate from coronary artery disease among postmenopausal estrogen users than nonusers.[198] Such cardioprotection likely reflects improvement in endothelium-dependent, flow-mediated vasodilation, either from a direct effect on endothelial function or through changes in blood lipids.[199]

Renal Parenchymal Disease

In the overall population, renal parenchymal disease is the most common cause of secondary hypertension, responsible for 2 to 5 per cent of cases (Table 26–5). As chronic glomerulonephritis becomes less common, hypertensive nephrosclerosis and diabetic nephropathy have become the most common causes of end-stage renal disease (ESRD).[200] The higher prevalence of hypertension among U.S. blacks is probably responsible for their significantly higher rate of ESRD, with hypertension as the underlying cause in as many as one-half of these patients.[201]

Not only does hypertension cause renal failure and renal failure cause hypertension, but also more subtle renal dysfunction may be involved in patients with primary hypertension. As discussed earlier (see p. 817), the kidneys may initiate the hemodynamic cascade eventuating in primary hypertension. As that disease progresses, some renal dysfunction is demonstrable in most patients; progressive renal damage is the end result and is the cause of death in perhaps 10 per cent of hypertensives. Since early treatment of hypertension will likely protect against nephrosclerosis, there is hope that improved control of hypertension will slow the progression and reduce the frequency of ESRD.

In hypertension with renal parenchymal disease the sequence of progressively worsening renal damage is (1) acute renal diseases that are often reversible, (2) unilateral and bilateral diseases without renal insufficiency, (3) chronic renal disease with renal insufficiency, and (4) hypertension in the anephric state and after renal transplantation.

ACUTE RENAL DISEASES. Hypertension may appear with any sudden, severe insult to the kidneys that either markedly impairs the excretion of salt and water, which leads to volume expansion, or reduces renal blood flow, which sets off the renin-angiotension-aldosterone mechanism. Bilateral ureteral obstruction is an example of the former; sudden bilateral renal artery occlusion, as by emboli, is an example of the latter. Relief of either may dramatically reverse severe hypertension. This has been particularly striking in men with high-pressure chronic retention of urine, who may manifest both renal failure and severe hypertension, both of which may be relieved by relief of the obstruction.[202] Some of the collagen diseases also may produce rapidly progressive renal damage. The more common acute processes are glomerulonephritis and oliguric renal failure.

ACUTE GLOMERULONEPHRITIS. Although the classic syndrome of type-specific poststreptococcal nephritis has become much less common, glomerular lesions of various types may be associated with hypertension. Moreover, although the epidemic poststreptococcal disease is usually self-limited, the disease in some patients follows a progressive, smoldering course that may lead to renal insufficiency.[203] Typically, hypertension accompanies the fluid retention of acute renal injury and is best relieved by sodium and fluid restriction and potent diuretics. Dialysis and parenteral antihypertensive drugs may be needed if encephalopathy supervenes. In milder cases, the hypertension recedes as the edema is relieved.

ACUTE OLIGURIC RENAL FAILURE. Acute renal failure may occur after hypotension, particularly in patients in whom renin levels are already high, such as those with cirrhosis and ascites or at the end of pregnancy. The release of even more renin by decreased blood pressure and effective circulating blood volume may flood the renal vasculature and cause such intense renal vasoconstriction that renal function shuts down. Hypertension in this setting is usually not an important problem and can be controlled by preventing volume overload. High doses of furosemide may be helpful, but dialysis is often needed. When acute renal failure occurs in the setting of accelerated or malignant hypertension, aggressive therapy (including dialysis) may be followed by sustained recovery of renal function.[203] The use of nonsteroidal antiinflammatory agents (NSAIDs) may cause acute renal failure usually in the setting of chronic renal damage.[204]

VASCULITIS. Rapidly progressive renal deterioration with severe hypertension occurs not infrequently during the course of scleroderma and other forms of vasculitis (p. 799). Therapy with antihypertensives, particularly angiotensin-converting enzyme inhibitors, may reverse the process.[205]

EXTRACORPOREAL SHOCK WAVE LITHOTRIPSY. As this procedure has been utilized increasingly to treat nephrolithiasis, at least transient rises in blood pressure have been observed in from 20 to 30 per cent of patients,[206] but persistent hypertension is unusual.[207]

RENAL DISEASE WITHOUT RENAL INSUFFICIENCY

Although an entire kidney may be removed without obvious effect and no rise in blood pressure,[208] hypertension may be associated with unilateral and bilateral renal parenchymal diseases in the absence of significant renal insufficiency. Although such hypertension may reflect other unrecognized processes, most likely it is caused by activation of the renin-angiotensin-aldosterone mechanism. However, in some patients whose hypertension has been relieved by correction of a renal defect, the levels of renin have not been high.

UNILATERAL PARENCHYMAL RENAL DISEASE. A number of unilateral kidney diseases may be associated with hypertension, and in some of these the affected kidney may appear shrunken. Nonetheless, most small kidneys do not cause hypertension, and when they are indiscriminately removed from patients with hypertension, the condition is relieved in only about 25 per cent.[209] Of that 25 per cent, most have arterial occlusive disease, either as the primary cause of the renal atrophy or secondary to irregular scarring of the parenchyma.[210]

POLYCYSTIC KIDNEY DISEASE. Although patients with adult polycystic kidney disease usually progress to renal insufficiency, some retain reasonably normal glomerular filtration rates (GFR) and display no azotemia. Hypertension, although more common in those with renal failure, is present in perhaps half of those with a normal GFR and probably reflects variable degrees of both renin excess and fluid retention.[211]

CHRONIC PYELONEPHRITIS. The relationship between pyelonephritis and hypertension is multifaceted: Pyelonephritis, either unilateral or bilateral, may cause hypertension; hypertensive individuals may be more susceptible to renal infection. In pyelonephritic patients with hypertension but fairly normal renal function, renin levels are high,[212] probably from interstitial scarring with obstruction of intrarenal vessels.

CHRONIC RENAL DISEASES WITH RENAL INSUFFICIENCY. As dialysis and transplantation prolong the lives of more patients with renal insufficiency, their hypertension must be dealt with over much longer periods. Hypertension in most patients with renal insufficiency is predominantly caused by volume overload resulting from the inability of the reduced functioning renal mass to handle the usual sodium and water intake. With proper attention to sodium and water intake and, if needed, adequate dialysis, control of blood pressure may not be particularly difficult. Unfortunately, some patients are much more fragile, alternating between low and high pressures, and some are much more resistant, presumably because of a greater contribution of high renin levels to the hypertension. Moreover, their pressures may not fall much during sleep, posing an additional burden on the heart and vasculature.[23] Nonetheless, with judicious use of available therapy, hypertension should not be a major problem for most patients with renal insufficiency.

In view of increasing evidence that glomerular capillary hypertension is responsible for the progressive loss of renal function once renal damage begins (Fig. 26–11), aggressive reduction of intraglomerular hypertension in order to prevent further renal loss is being actively pursued. Angiotensin-converting enzyme (ACE) inhibitors may be particularly effective in this regard.[188]

Three aspects of hypertension with end-stage renal disease (ESRD) should be recognized: (1) hypertension contributes to the cardiovascular diseases that are the cause of death in about half of patients with ESRD;[213] (2) renal damage may progress despite apparent control of hypertension, particularly among blacks;[201] and (3) a significant proportion of ESRD may reflect bilateral renovascular disease that may be made worse by antihypertensive drug therapy but markedly improved by revascularization.[214]

Diabetic Nephropathy (see also p. 1900). Hypertension often accompanies diabetic nephropathy, reflecting inability to handle volume loads because of loss of nephrons as a result of progressive intercapillary glomerulosclerosis. As shown in Figure 26–18, intrarenal hypertension accelerates the progress of the glomerulosclerosis, and antihypertensive therapy has been shown to slow the progression of renal failure.[188] Although more effective relief of glomerular capillary hypertension may be possible with ACE inhibitors, long-term protection has been obtained with traditional antihypertensive drugs, not including ACE inhibitors.[215] As common as it is, hypertension may not be as severe or as likely to progress to an accelerated-malignant phase in diabetics with nephropathy for two reasons: first, these patients often have a diminished intravascular volume because of the hypoalbuminemia of the nephrotic syndrome; second, they have low renin levels, presumably owing to hyalinization of juxtaglomerular cells, which may present as hyporeninemic hypoaldosteronism.

Analgesic Nephropathy. In addition to acute renal insufficiency that may accompany the inhibition of renal prostaglandins by nonsteroidal antiinflammatory agents,[204] permanent interstitial renal damage may supervene after prolonged exposure to analgesics, particularly phenacetin and, to a lesser degree, acetaminophen.[216] Until late in their course, these patients have a greater propensity for salt wasting and therefore may have less severe hypertension.

HYPERTENSION DURING CHRONIC DIALYSIS AND AFTER RENAL TRANSPLANTATION. In patients with end-stage renal disease, blood pressure depends mainly upon body fluid volume. Hypertension may be accentuated by the accumulation of endogenous inhibitors of nitric oxide synthase, withdrawing the vasodilation provided by nitric oxide.[217] With neither the vasoconstrictor effects of renal renin nor the vasodepressor actions of various renal hormones, blood pressure may be particularly labile and sensitive to changes in adrenergic activity. Among patients receiving maintenance hemodialysis every 48 hours, elevated blood pressures tend to fall progressively after dialysis is completed, remain depressed during the remainder of the first 24 hours, and rise again during the second day.[218] Thus antihypertension therapy may be needed only on the days between dialyses.

Whereas successful renal transplantation may cure primary hypertension,[219] various problems may result, with about half the recipients becoming hypertensive within 1 year.[220] These problems include stenosis of the renal artery at the site of anastomosis, rejection reactions, high doses of adrenal steroids and cyclosporine, and excess renin derived from the retained diseased kidneys. ACE inhibitor therapy may obviate the need to remove the native diseased kidneys in order to relieve hypertension caused by their persistent secretion of renin.[221] The source of the donor kidney also may play a role in the subsequent development of hypertension in the recipient: More hypertension has been observed when donors had a family history of hypertension or when the donors had died of subarachnoid hemorrhage and had probably been hypertensive.[222]

Renovascular Hypertension

Renovascular hypertension is the most common secondary form of hypertension and is not easily recognizable. Although no more than 1 per cent of all adults with hypertension have renovascular hypertension (Table 26–5), the prevalence is much higher in those with sudden onset of severe hypertension and other suggestive features[223] (Table 26–10). Mann and Pickering classify patients into low, moderate, and high "clinical index of suspicion" as a guide to the selection of additional work-up for renovascular hypertension. Those with characteristics listed under moderate are considered to have a 5 to 15 per cent likelihood of the diagnosis and therefore are in need of a noninvasive screening test. Those with characteristics listed under high

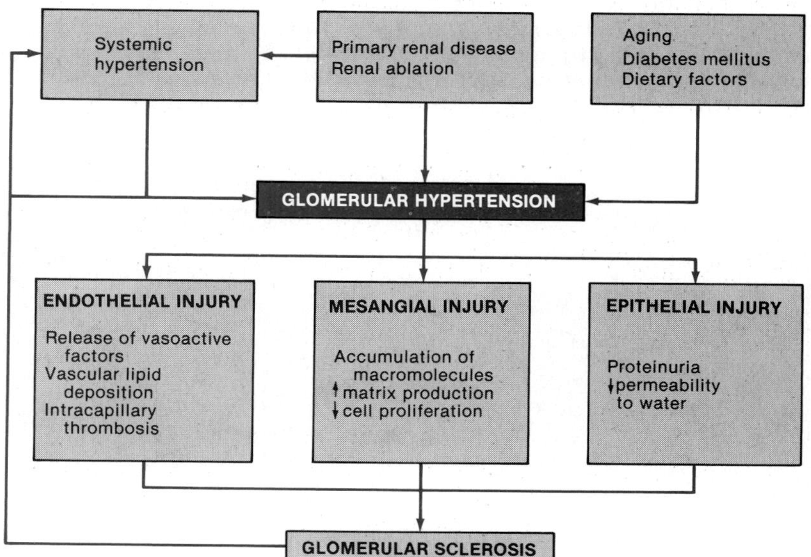

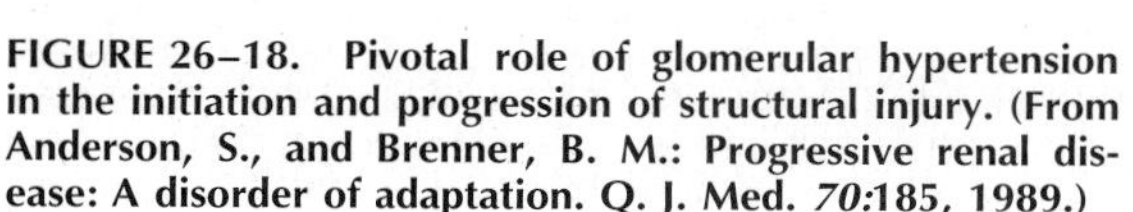
FIGURE 26–18. Pivotal role of glomerular hypertension in the initiation and progression of structural injury. (From Anderson, S., and Brenner, B. M.: Progressive renal disease: A disorder of adaptation. Q. J. Med. *70*:185, 1989.)

TABLE 26–10 TESTING FOR RENOVASCULAR HYPERTENSION: CLINICAL INDEX OF SUSPICION AS A GUIDE TO SELECTING PATIENTS FOR WORK-UP

LOW (SHOULD NOT BE TESTED): Borderline, mild, or moderate hypertension, in the absence of clinical clues
MODERATE (NONINVASIVE TESTS RECOMMENDED):
Severe hypertension (diastolic blood pressure greater than 120 mm Hg)
Hypertension refractory to standard therapy
Abrupt onset of sustained, moderate to severe hypertension at age < 20 or age > 50
Hypertension with a suggestive abdominal bruit (long, high-pitched, and localized to the region of the renal artery)
Moderate hypertension (diastolic blood pressure exceeding 105 mm Hg) in a smoker, in a patient with evidence of occlusive vascular disease (cerebrovascular, coronary, peripheral vascular), or in a patient with unexplained but stable elevation of serum creatinine
Normalization of blood pressure by an angiotensin-converting enzyme inhibitor in a patient with moderate or severe hypertension (particularly a smoker or a patient with recent onset of hypertension)
HIGH (MAY CONSIDER PROCEEDING DIRECTLY TO ARTERIOGRAPHY):
Severe hypertension (diastolic blood pressure greater than 120 mm Hg with either progressive renal insufficiency or refractoriness to aggressive treatment, particularly in a patient who has been a smoker or has other evidence of occlusive arterial disease)
Accelerated or malignant hypertension (grade III or IV retinopathy)
Hypertension with recent elevation of serum creatinine, either unexplained or reversibly induced by an angiotensin-converting enzyme inhibitor
Moderate to severe hypertension with incidentally detected asymmetry of renal size

From Mann, S. J., Pickering, T. G.: Detection of renovascular hypertension. State of the art: 1992. Ann. Intern. Med. *117*:845, 1992.

are considered to have a greater than 25 per cent likelihood of the diagnosis so that renal arteriography should be the initial test.

In multiple series, renovascular disease has been found less commonly in black hypertensives than in whites.[224,225] In the large series described by Novick et al.,[225] the blacks had more severe hypertension and extensive atherosclerosis in other vascular beds.

CLASSIFICATION. In adults, the two major types of renovascular disease tend to appear at different times and affect the sexes differently (Table 26–11). Atherosclerotic disease affecting mainly the proximal third of the main renal artery is seen mostly in older men. Fibroplastic disease involving mainly the distal two-thirds and branches of the renal arteries appears most commonly in younger women. Overall, about two-thirds of cases are caused by atherosclerotic disease and one-third by fibroplastic disease. While the nonatherosclerotic stenoses involve all layers of the renal artery, the most common is medial fibroplasia.

There are a number of other intrinsic and extrinsic causes of renovascular hypertension, including emboli within the renal artery or compression of this vessel by nearby tumors. Most renovascular hypertension develops from partial obstruction of one main renal artery, but only a branch need be involved; segmental disease was found in 11 per cent of cases in one large series.[226] On the other hand, if apparent complete occlusion of the renal artery is slow in developing, enough collateral flow will become available to preserve the viability of the kidney. In this way, the seemingly nonfunctioning kidney may be responsible for continued renin secretion and hypertension. If recognized, such totally occluded vessels can sometimes be repaired, with return of renal function and relief of hypertension.[227]

Renovascular stenosis is often bilateral, although usually one side is clearly predominant. In the Cooperative Study on Renovascular Hypertension, 25 per cent of the subjects had bilateral atherosclerotic or fibroplastic disease.[228] The possibility of bilateral disease should be suspected in those with renal insufficiency, particularly if rapidly progressive oliguric renal failure develops without evidence of obstructive uropathy and even more so if it develops after start of ACE inhibitor therapy.[228]

MECHANISMS. Since Goldblatt produced renovascular hypertension in the dog in 1934, the pathophysiology of this disease has been studied extensively. Confusion has arisen because of the use of one-kidney models, which are more appropriate to the study of renal parenchymal hypertension. The sequence of changes in the two-kidney (one-clip) model and in patients with renovascular hypertension almost certainly starts with the release of increased amounts of renin when sufficient ischemia is induced to diminish pulse pressure against the juxtaglomerular cells in the renal afferent arterioles. A reduction of renal perfusion pressure by 50 per cent leads to an immediate and persistent increase in renin secretion from the ischemic kidney, with suppression of secretion from the contralateral one. With time, renin levels fall (but not to the low levels expected based on the elevated blood pressure), accompanied by an expanded body fluid volume and increased cardiac output.[229]

DIAGNOSIS. The presence of the clinical features listed under moderate in Table 26–10 indicates the need for a screening test for renovascular hypertension in perhaps 5 to 10 per cent of all hypertensives. A positive screening test, or very strong clinical features, calls for more definitive confirmatory tests.

Some patients have renovascular hypertension but none of the clinical features listed in Table 26–10, clinically resembling patients with mild primary hypertension. Nonetheless, these features should be used to exclude the major-

TABLE 26–11 FEATURES OF THE TWO MAJOR FORMS OF RENAL ARTERY DISEASE

CAUSE	INCIDENCE (%)	AGE (yr)	LOCATION OF LESION IN RENAL ARTERY	NATURAL HISTORY
Atherosclerosis	65	>50	Proximal 2 cm; branch disease rare	Progression in 50 per cent, often to total occlusion
Fibromuscular dysplasias				
Intimal	1–2	Birth–25	Mid-main renal artery and/or branches	Progression in most cases; dissection and/or thrombosis common
Medial	30	25–50	Distal main renal artery and/or branches	Progression in 33 per cent; dissection and/or thrombosis rare
Periarterial	1–2	15–30	Middle to distal main renal artery or branches	Progression in most cases; dissection and/or thrombosis common

From Kaplan, N. M.: Clinical Hypertension. 6th ed. Baltimore, Williams and Wilkins, 1994, p. 326.

ity of hypertensives from additional work-up and to identify the 10 per cent or so who should undergo a work-up.

Functional Diagnostic Tests. Isotopic renography and plasma renin measurements after an oral captopril challenge are currently the best initial tests in patients with those suggestive clinical features listed under moderate in Table 26–10, to be followed by renal arteriography and then renal vein renin assays.[230,231] The latter procedure may not be needed if isotopic renography after captopril indicates significant renal ischemia in the kidney with renal artery disease by arteriography. In some centers with facilities dedicated to the performance of renal artery duplex sonography, that procedure is being utilized for initial screening.[230] In the future, magnetic resonance arteriography may be utilized.

The captopril challenge test depends on the abrupt inhibition of circulating angiotensin II by the ACE inhibitor removing the major support for perfusion through a stenotic renal artery to a kidney. The acutely ischemic kidney immediately releases more renin and undergoes a marked decrease in glomerular filtration and renal blood flow. Therefore, both plasma renin levels and the isotopic flow through the kidneys 1 hour after a single 50-mg dose of the ACE inhibitor should be measured. To measure the plasma renin response, the patient should be on normal sodium dietary intake and off diuretics and ACE inhibitors; if possible, other antihypertensive medications should be withdrawn for at least a week, although the test was originally found to be almost equally valid among those examined while on therapy.[232] After the patient sits for 30 minutes, venous blood is obtained for basal PRA, and 50 mg of captopril is given orally. At 60 minutes, another blood sample for stimulated PRA is obtained. The original criteria for a positive test for renovascular hypertension were (1) a stimulated PRA of 12 ng/ml/hr or more, (2) an absolute increase in PRA of 10 ng/ml/hr or more, and (3) a 150 per cent or greater increase in PRA or, if baseline PRA is below 3 ng/ml/hr, a 400 per cent increase. The authors have subsequently reported a high prevalence of false-positive responses in patients with high baseline renin levels.[233] Others report sensitivity ranging from 0.73 to 1.0 and specificity ranging from 0.73 to 0.95.[231]

The performance of isotopic renography 1 hour after the oral captopril dose provides additional diagnostic information that appears to be more accurate than the renin response.[234] The renogram may use labeled hippurate, a measure of renal blood flow, or diethylenetriaminepentaacetic acid (DTPA) or mercaptoacetyltriglycine (MAG3), measures of glomerular filtration rate. If the postcaptopril test shows a significant difference between the two kidneys, the procedure should be repeated without captopril to document the ischemic origin of the differences in blood flow or GFR. With captopril renography, renal vein renin measurements are needed less often to localize the affected side when renovascular disease is bilateral.

MANAGEMENT

Medical. The availability of ACE inhibitors (see p. 494) may be considered a two-edged sword; one edge provides better control of renovascular hypertension than may be possible with other antihypertensive medications, while the other edge exposes the already ischemic kidney to a further loss of blood flow by removing the high levels of angiotensin II that were supporting its circulation.[231] Calcium entry blockers and other antihypertensive drugs may be almost as effective as ACE inhibitors and considerably safer.[235]

Angioplasty. Angioplasty has been shown to improve 60 to 70 per cent of patients, more with fibromuscular disease than with atherosclerosis, as is also the case for surgery.[236] It is being performed more and more frequently as the initial procedure, particularly in patients who are poor candidates for major surgery, even in the presence of severe stenoses.[237]

Surgery. Surgical repair has been shown to relieve renovascular hypertension in an increasing number of patients, including the elderly[238] and those with renal insufficiency.[239] Most agree that surgery is indicated in patients whose hypertension is not well controlled or whose renal function deteriorates on medical therapy and in those with only a transient response to angioplasty or when lesions are not amenable to that procedure.

RENIN-SECRETING TUMORS

Made up of juxtaglomerular cells or hemangiopericytomas, these tumors have been found mostly in young patients with severe hypertension, very high renin levels in both peripheral blood and the kidney harboring the tumor, and secondary aldosteronism manifested by hypokalemia.[240] The tumor usually can be recognized by selective renal angiography, usually performed for suspected renovascular hypertension, although a few are extrarenal.[241] More commonly, children with Wilms' tumors (nephroblastoma) may have hypertension and high plasma renin and prorenin levels that revert to normal after nephrectomy.[242]

Adrenal Causes of Hypertension

(See Chap. 61)

Adrenal causes of hypertension include primary excesses of aldosterone, cortisol, and catecholamines; more rarely, excess deoxycorticosterone (DOC) is present along with congenital adrenal hyperplasia. Together these cause less than 1 per cent of all hypertensive diseases. Each can usually be recognized with relative ease, and patients suspected of having these disorders can be screened by means of readily available tests. More of a problem than the diagnosis of these adrenal disorders is the need to exclude their presence because of the increasing identification of incidental adrenal masses when abdominal computed tomography (CT) is done to diagnose intraabdominal pathology. Unsuspected adrenal tumors have been found in from 1 to 2 per cent of abdominal CT scans obtained for reasons unrelated to the adrenal gland. Most of these "incidentalomas" appear to be nonfunctional on the basis of normal basal adrenal hormone levels. However, when more detailed studies are done, a significant number show incomplete suppression of cortisol by dexamethasone, i.e., subclinical Cushing's disease which does not appear to progress to overt hypercortisolism, and a few have unsuspected catecholamine hypersecretion.[243] Nonfunctioning adenomas have significantly less lipid content than do functioning adenomas by chemical-shift magnetic resonance imaging,[244] so this procedure may have clinical usefulness. The threat of malignancy probably can be best excluded by adrenal scintigraphy with the radioiodinated derivative of cholesterol, NP-59.[245] Benign lesions almost always take up the isotope, while malignant ones almost always do not. Osella et al.[243] found lower plasma dehydroepiandrosterone sulfate (DHEA-S) levels in most with nonfunctioning benign adenomas and high levels in those with adrenal malignancies. Most tumors larger than 4 cm are resected, since a significant number of them are malignant.

Primary Aldosteronism

(See also p. 1895)

This disease is relatively rare in unselected populations (Table 26–5), although it has been recognized in considerably more patients screened by a plasma aldosterone/renin activity ratio.[246]

PATHOPHYSIOLOGY. Primary aldosterone excess usually arises from solitary benign adenomas. As diagnostic tests have improved and become more readily available, larger numbers of patients with minimal features have been recognized.[246] Many of these patients have been found to have bilateral adrenal hyperplasia, the number averaging about one-third of all cases of aldosteronism.

MINERALOCORTICAL HYPERTENSION. The pathogenesis of the familial glucocorticoid-suppressible aldosteronism has now been elucidated, and it is not as rare as once thought.[247] The syndrome is caused by a mutation in the genes involved in the coding for the aldosterone synthase enzyme normally found only in the outer zona glomerulosa and the 11-beta-hydroxylase enzyme in the zona fasciculata.[248] The chimeric gene induces an enzyme that catalyzes the synthesis of 18-hydroxylated cortisol in the zona fasciculata. Since this zone is under the control of ACTH, the glucocorticoid suppressibility of the syndrome is explained.

Another unusual form of mineralocorticoid hypertension also has been explained by the recognition of deficiency of the enzyme 11-beta-hydroxysteroid dehydrogenase (11-β-OHSD) in the renal tubule, where it normally converts cortisol (which has the ability to act on the mineralocorticoid receptor) to cortisone (which does not). The persistence of high levels of cortisol induces all the features of mineralocorticoid excess. The 11-β-OHSD enzyme may be congenitally absent (the syndrome of apparent mineralocorticoid excess)[249] or inhibited by the glycyrrhetenic acid contained in licorice.[250] More subtle deficiencies of 11-β-OHSD have been recognized in some patients with chronic renal disease[251] and low-renin essential hypertension.[252]

Whatever the source, excess mineralocorticoid usually causes hypertension and hypokalemia, defined as a plasma potassium level below 3.2 mEq/liter. Very rarely, mineralocorticoid excess has been recognized in normotensive persons.[246] Not so rarely, hypokalemia may be absent or only intermittent, but in most patients with adenomas, persistent hypokalemia is observed.[253]

The hypertension begins as a volume overload but soon converts, as do apparently all forms of hypertension, to increased peripheral resistance. Hypertension may be severe, with a mean pressure in one group of 136 patients of 205/123 mm Hg and 4 of the patients showing histological evidence of malignant hypertension on renal biopsy.[254] Furthermore, 23 per cent of these patients had a serious vascular complication such as stroke or myocardial infarction. In association with the increased pressure and expanded blood volume, renin secretion is suppressed. Although this finding has been almost invariable with hyperaldosteronism, the overwhelming majority of hypertensive patients with suppressed renin do not have mineralocorticoid excess.

DIAGNOSIS. Serious consideration should be given to the diagnosis of primary aldosteronism when hypertension and hypokalemia coexist. If normokalemic patients with the disease are thereby missed, little will be lost as long as the patients are protected by appropriate treatment of the hypertension. Since this is likely to include a diuretic, significant hypokalemia will likely soon become manifested, making the diagnosis obvious. If hypokalemia is present, excessive urinary potassium excretion (above 30 mmol/day) is strongly suggestive of mineralocorticoid excess.

A high plasma aldosterone/renin ratio in plasma is a useful screening test that can be performed immediately upon recognition of hypokalemia in a hypertensive patient, without special conditions or preparation.[246] Not only should plasma renin levels be low, but plasma aldosterone levels should be elevated, giving a ratio of well above 30.[255] Although this ratio is being used increasingly to screen for primary aldosteronism, it has not always been found to be abnormal in patients with the syndrome.[256] Therefore, the finding of increased urinary aldosterone levels or the failure to suppress plasma aldosterone levels by volume expansion also may be useful.

ESTABLISHING THE PATHOLOGY. Once the diagnosis of primary aldosteronism is made, the type of adrenal pathology should be determined, and only those patients with a tumor should be subjected to operation and those with bilateral hyperplasia kept on medical therapy. The best initial study is an adrenal CT or MRI scan (Fig. 26–19). However, the ability of these scans to identify hitherto hidden degrees of adrenal pathology may engender confusion; the usual modularity seen in the remainder of a gland that harbors a solitary adrenal adenoma may give the appearance of bilateral hyperplasia, and some larger hyperplastic modules may look like adenomas.[257] Therefore, unless the scan is unequivocal, additional tests to discriminate between adenoma and hyperplasia should be done (Fig. 26–19).

Various maneuvers are available.[253] Basal levels of serum 18-hydroxycorticosterone (18-OHB) and changes in plasma aldosterone levels after 2 hours of upright posture from 8 A.M. to 10 A.M. usually distinguish patients with adenomas (who usually have basal 18-OHB levels above 65 ng/dl and falls in upright plasma aldosterone) from those with bilateral hyperplasia (who usually have basal 18-OHB levels below 50 ng/dl and postural rises in plasma aldosterone presumably invoked by their supersensitivity to posture-mediated rises in renin-angiotensin). In addition, most adenomas but few hyperplastic glands secrete increased amounts of 18-hydroxylated cortisol, suggesting that they harbor similar mutant genes as found in the glucocorticoid-suppressible syndrome. If there is still uncertainty, bilateral adrenal vein catheterization with analysis of venous aldosterone and cortisol levels should be performed.

THERAPY. Once the diagnosis of primary aldosteronism is made and the type of adrenal disorder has been established, the choice of therapy is fairly easy: Patients with a solitary adenoma should have the tumor resected, now

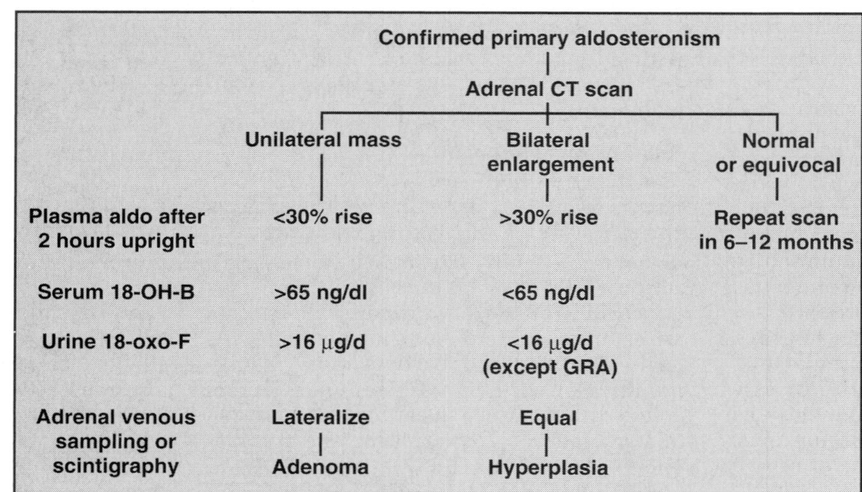

FIGURE 26–19. A flow diagram for the progressive work-up of confirmed primary aldosteronism, with additional steps for when initial studies are aberrant. Rare, angiotensin II–responsive adenomas may demonstrate features of hyperplasia but lateralize by venous sampling or scintigraphy. On the other hand, primary adrenal hyperplasia may demonstrate features of an adenoma except for equally high steroid levels by venous sampling. *18-OH-B,* 18-hydroxycorticosterone; *18-oxo-F,* 18-hydrocortisol; *GRA,* glucocorticoid-remediable aldosteronism. (From Kaplan, N. M.: Primary aldosteronism. *In* Kaplan, N. M. [ed.]: Clinical Hypertension. 6th ed. Baltimore, Williams and Wilkins, 1994, p. 404.)

more and more frequently done by laparoscopic surgery.[258] Those with bilateral hyperplasia should be treated with spironolactone (see p. 1897) and if necessary a thiazide diuretic or other antihypertensive drugs.[259] Fortunately, the doses of spironolactone required for chronic therapy are usually low enough to avoid bothersome side effects. When an adenoma is resected, about half of patients will become normotensive, while the others, though improved, remain hypertensive, either from preexisting primary hypertension or from renal damage due to prolonged secondary hypertension.[253]

CUSHING'S SYNDROME (see also p. 1896)

Hypertension occurs in about 80 per cent of patients with Cushing's syndrome. If left untreated, it can cause marked left ventricular hypertrophy and congestive heart failure.[260] As with hypertension of other endocrine causes, the longer it is present, the less likely it is to disappear when the underlying cause is relieved.

MECHANISM OF HYPERTENSION. Blood pressure may increase for a number of reasons. The secretion of mineralocorticoids also may be increased along with cortisol. The excess cortisol may overwhelm the renal 11-β-OHSD enzyme's ability to convert it to the inactive cortisone so that it activates renal mineralocorticoid receptors to retain sodium and expand fluid volume.[261] Cortisol stimulates the synthesis of renin substrate and the expression of angiotensin II receptors, which may be responsible for enhanced pressor effects.[262]

DIAGNOSIS. The syndrome should be suspected in patients with truncal obesity, thin skin, muscle weakness, and osteoporosis. If clinical features are suggestive, the diagnosis can be either ruled out or virtually ensured by the measurement of free cortisol in a 24-hour urine or the simple overnight *dexamethasone suppression test.*[263] In normal subjects, the level of plasma cortisol in a sample drawn at 8 A.M. after a bedtime dose of 1 mg of dexamethasone should be below 7 μg/100 mg. If the level is higher, additional work-up is in order to establish both the diagnosis of cortisol excess and the pathological type. Measurement of urine free cortisol levels is almost as good a screening test: Most patients who do not have Cushing's syndrome excrete less than 100 μg/24 hours.

When an abnormal screening test is found, some would immediately perform pituitary and adrenal CT or MRI scans to elucidate the type of pathology. However, most authorities continue to recommend longer dexamethasone suppression tests using 0.5 mg every 6 hours and then 2.0 mg every 6 hours, each for 2 days, measuring urinary free cortisol excretion and plasma cortisol levels on the second day of each dose. Patients with Cushing's syndrome fail to suppress urine free cortisol to below 25 μg/day on the 0.5-mg dose; if Cushing's syndrome is caused by excess pituitary ACTH drive with bilateral adrenal hyperplasia, urinary free cortisol will be suppressed to below 40 per cent of the control value on the 2.0-mg dose. Plasma ACTH assays provide an additional means of differentiating pituitary and ectopic ACTH excess from adrenal tumors with ACTH suppression.[264] The response to corticotropin-releasing hormone (CRH) and inferior petrosal sinus sampling may help identify the pituitary cause for the syndrome.[265]

THERAPY. In about two-thirds of patients with Cushing's syndrome, the process begins with overproduction of ACTH by the pituitary, which leads to bilateral adrenal hyperplasia. Although pituitary hyperfunction may reflect a hypothalamic disorder, the majority of patients have discrete pituitary adenomas that usually can be resected by selective transsphenoidal microsurgery.[266]

If an adrenal tumor is present, it should be removed surgically. With earlier diagnosis and more selective surgical therapy, it is hoped that more patients with Cushing's syndrome will be cured without the need for lifelong glucocorticoid replacement therapy and with permanent relief of their hypertension. Temporarily, and rarely permanently, therapy may require one of a number of medical approaches.[267]

CONGENITAL ADRENAL HYPERPLASIA (see also p. 1678). Two other enzymatic defects may induce hypertension by interfering with cortisol biosynthesis. The low levels of cortisol lead to increased ACTH, which increases the accumulation of precursors proximal to the enzymatic block, specifically deoxycorticosterone (DOC), which induces mineralocorticoid hypertension. The more common of these is *11-hydroxylase deficiency,* which leads to virilization (from excessive androgens) and hypertension with hypokalemia (from excessive DOC).[268] A partial deficiency has been recognized in 15 patients with what appeared to be ordinary primary hypertension.[269] The other is *17-hydroxylase deficiency,* which also causes hypertension from excess DOC but, in addition, causes failure of secondary sexual development because sex hormones are also deficient.[270] Affected children are hypertensive, but the defect in sex hormone synthesis may not become obvious until after puberty. Thereafter, affected males display ambiguity of sexual development and fail to mature.

PHEOCHROMOCYTOMA (see also p. 1897)

The wild fluctuations in blood pressure and dramatic symptoms of pheochromocytoma usually alert both the patient and the physician to the possibility of this diagnosis. However, such fluctuations may be missed or, as occurs in half the patients, the hypertension may be persistent. The symptoms may be incorrectly ascribed to psychoneurosis by practitioners not sensitized to "spells," which usually represent menopausal hot flushes or anxiety-induced hyperventilation. Unfortunately, if the diagnosis is missed, severe complications may arise from exceedingly high blood pressure and damage to the heart by catecholamines (see p. 1447). Stroke and hypertensive crises with encephalopathy and retinal hemorrhages may occur, probably because blood pressure levels soar in vessels unprepared by a chronic hypertensive condition. Fortunately, a simple and inexpensive test will detect the disease with virtual certainty, so that diagnostic indecision should be minimized.

PATHOPHYSIOLOGY. The cells of the sympathetic nervous system arise from the primitive neural crest as primitive stem cells, called *sympathogonia.* These cells differentiate into ganglion cells, neuroblasts, and chromaffin cells. Tumors develop from each of these cell types; ganglioneuromas and neuroblastomas usually occur in children, whereas tumors arising from chromaffin cells, i.e., pheochromocytomas, occur at all ages anywhere along the sympathetic chain and rarely in aberrant sites.[271] About 15 per cent of pheochromocytomas are extraadrenal; nonsecreting ones are called *paragangliomas* or *chemodectomas.*

Of the 85 per cent of pheochromocytomas that arise in the adrenal medulla, 10 per cent are bilateral and another 10 per cent are malignant. Multiple adrenal tumors are particularly common in patients with simple familial pheochromocytoma and multiple endocrine neoplasia (MEN) Type 2A in association with medullary carcinoma of the thyroid (Sipple's syndrome) or with mucosal ganglioneuromas in addition (Type 2B). The MEN2 syndromes are inherited as autosomal dominants with mutations at the same locus on chromosome 10.[272] Diffuse medullary hyperplasia may precede the development of tumors, and the tumors may, in fact, reflect extreme degrees of nodular hyperplasia.[273] Adrenal pheochromocytomas have been found to produce a number of other hormones in addition to catecholamines, which in turn are co-secreted with the soluble protein chromogranin A.[274]

Secretion from nonfamilial pheochromocytomas varies considerably, with small tumors tending to secrete larger proportions of active catecholamines. If the predominant secretion is epinephrine, which is formed primarily in the adrenal medulla, the symptoms reflect its effects—mainly systolic hypertension due to increased cardiac output, tachycardia, sweating, flushing, and apprehension. If norepinephrine is predominantly secreted, as from some of the adrenal tumors and from almost all the extraadrenal tumors, the symptoms include both systolic and diastolic hypertension from peripheral vasoconstriction but less tachycardia, palpitations, and anxiety. The hemodynamic features of 24 untreated patients with surgically proven pheochromocytomas were quite similar to those found in 24 untreated patients of similar sex, age, weight, and blood pressure with primary hypertension, with increased total peripheral resistance as the primary in both groups.[274]

The episodic hypertension often seen in patients with a pheochromocytoma may arise from catecholamines released from the tumor, stored in the sympathetic nerves, and released when the sympathetic nerves are activated by various stresses rather than directly from the tumor.[275]

DIAGNOSIS. Many more hypertensive patients have variable blood pressures and "spells" than the 0.1 per cent or so who harbor a pheochromocytoma. Spells with paroxysmal hypertension may occur with a number of stresses, and a large number of conditions may involve transient catecholamine release. A pheochromocytoma should be suspected in patients with hypertension that is either paroxysmal or persistent and accompanied by the symptoms and signs listed in Table 26–12. In addition, children and patients with rapidly accelerating hypertension should be screened. Those whose tumors secrete predominantly epinephrine are prone to postural hypotension from a contracted blood volume and blunted sympathetic reflex tone. Suspicion should be heightened if activities such as bending over, exercise, palpation of the abdomen, smoking, or dipping snuff cause repetitive spells that begin abruptly, advance rapidly, and subside within minutes.

High levels of catecholamines may induce myocarditis (Chap. 41), which may progress to cardiomyopathy and left ventricular failure.[276] Electrocardiographic changes of ischemia also may be seen.[277] Beta blockers given to such patients may raise the pressure and induce coronary spasm through blockade of beta-mediated vasodilation.[278]

LABORATORY CONFIRMATION. The easiest and best procedure is either a 24-hour or spot urine assay for total metanephrine. This catecholamine metabolite is least affected by various interfering sub-

TABLE 26–12 FEATURES SUGGESTIVE OF PHEOCHROMOCYTOMA

HYPERTENSION: PERSISTENT OR PAROXYSMAL
Markedly variable blood pressures (± orthostatic hypotension)
Sudden paroxysms (± subsequent hypertension) in relation to:
Stress: anesthesia, angiography, parturition
Pharmacological provocation: histamine, nicotine, caffeine, beta blockers, glucocorticoids, tricyclic antidepressants
Manipulation of tumors: abdominal palpation, urination
Rare patients persistently normotensive
Unusual settings
Childhood, pregnancy, familial
Multiple endocrine adenomas: medullary carcinoma of thyroid (MEN2), mucosal neuromas (MEN2B)
Neurocutaneous lesions: Neurofibromatosis

ASSOCIATED SYMPTOMS:
Sudden spells with headache, sweating, palpitations, nervousness, nausea, and vomiting
Pain in chest or abdomen

ASSOCIATED SIGNS:
Sweating, tachycardia, arrhythmia, pallor, weight loss

stances including antihypertensive drugs, with the exception of labetalol, which may cause markedly elevated levels of all catecholamines.[279] In addition to the effects of labetalol, urinary metanephrine excretion will be increased if patients are taking sympathomimetic or dopaminergic drugs or are under acute, severe stress such as an acute myocardial infarction or severe congestive heart failure. Interference with the measurement of metanephrine may occur for the next few days after use of radiograph contrast media containing methylglucamine, leading to a falsely low value. Therefore, the urine should be collected before coronary angiography or other such procedures are done.

If urine assays are equivocal, measurement of a plasma norepinephrine level 3 hours after a single 0.3-mg oral dose of the adrenergic inhibitor clonidine has been shown to separate the nonpheochromocytoma patients, whose levels are suppressed, from those with disease whose levels are not suppressed.[274]

LOCALIZATION OF THE TUMOR. Once the diagnosis has been made, medical therapy should be started and the tumor localized by CT or MRI scans, which usually demonstrate these typically large tumors with ease. Radioisotopes that localize in chromaffin tissue are available and are of additional help in the few patients in whom localization is not possible by CT or MRI.[274]

THERAPY. Once diagnosed and localized, pheochromocytomas should be resected. Great care should be taken in preparing patients for operation and managing them through the procedure.[274] The most important part of their preoperative management is alpha-adrenergic receptor blockade sufficient to overcome vasoconstriction and allow the reduced blood volume to reexpand. If the tumor is unresectable, chronic medical therapy with the alpha blocker phenoxybenzamine (Dibenzyline) or the inhibitor of catechol synthesis, α-methyl-tyrosine (Demser), can be used.

Other Causes of Hypertension

A host of other causes of hypertension are known (Table 26–4). One that is likely becoming more common is ingestion of various drugs—prescribed (e.g., cyclosporine[280] and erythropoietin[281]), over the counter (e.g., phenylpropanolamine[282]), and illicit (e.g., cocaine).

COARCTATION OF THE AORTA (see pp. 911 and 965). Congenital narrowing of the aorta may occur at any level of the thoracic or abdominal aorta. It is usually found just beyond the origin of the left subclavian artery or distal to the insertion of the ligamentum arteriosum. The coarctation may be localized or more diffuse. Other cardiac anomalies usually accompany the latter, giving rise to considerable mortality during the first year of life, although operative treatment of both the coarctation and associated anomalies may reduce this mortality rate. With less severe postductal lesions, damage is more insidious, and symptoms may not appear until the teenage years or later.

Hypertension in the arms and weak or absent femoral pulses are the classic features of coarctation. The pathogenesis of the hypertension may be more complicated than simple mechanical obstruction; a generalized vasoconstrictor mechanism is likely to be involved, which may be either renin-angiotensin or sympathetic nervous activity.[283] The lesion may be detected by two-dimensional echocardiography (Fig. 29–28, p. 912), and aortography proves the diagnosis. To diminish the development of congestive heart failure, endocarditis, and stroke, the obstruction should be corrected in early childhood either by surgery[284] or by angioplasty.[285] Immediately after either, the blood pressure may transiently rise even further, and mesenteric arteritis may develop. These changes may reflect very high levels of renin-angiotensin and catecholamines and can be prevented by the prophylactic use of beta blockers.[286]

HORMONAL DISTURBANCES

Hypertension is seen in as many as half of patients with a variety of hormonal disturbances, including acromegaly,[287] hypothyroidism,[41] and hyperparathyroidism.[288] The diagnosis of the latter two conditions has been made easier by readily available blood tests, and affected hypertensives may be relieved of their high blood pressure by correction of the hormonal disturbance. This happens more frequently with hypothyroidism than with hyperparathyroidism.[289]

Hypertension After Heart Surgery

(See also p. 1723)

Transient hypertension may develop postoperatively for various reasons: pain, physical and emotional excitement, hypoxia, hypercapnia, and excessive volume loads.[290] More severe hypertension has been noted to follow a number of cardiovascular surgical procedures:

1. *Coronary bypass surgery.* The incidence, exceeding 33 per cent, is far higher than after other major cardiac or noncardiac surgery.[291] The problem appears more commonly on the background of preexisting hypertension, greater than 50 per cent obstruction of the left main coronary artery, or the preoperative use of beta blockers. The hemodynamic pattern of increased peripheral resistance can be explained by the markedly elevated plasma catecholamine levels measured in such patients in the presence of normal renin-angiotensin levels.[292] In those patients who had previously received beta-blocker therapy, the postoperative hypertension also may reflect a rebound phenomenon. Therefore, continuation of beta-blocker therapy through the perioperative period is likely to reduce the frequency of the problem. If it occurs, parenteral therapy is often required, and intravenous nicardipine has been found to be very effective.[293]

2. *Aortic valve replacement.* Transient hypertension may give way to more permanent hypertension. In one series, 53 per cent of 116 patients were hypertensive 5 years after surgery, and hypertension was a major determinant of late failure of the homograft valve.[294]

3. *Closure of an atrial septal defect.*[295]

4. *Cardiac transplantation.* With current immunosuppression using cyclosporine and high doses of adrenal steroids, hypertension is almost invariable and can be resistant to intensive therapy.[296] Fortunately, with effective antihypertensive therapy, left ventricular hypertrophy may be prevented.[297]

HYPERTENSION DURING PREGNANCY

(See also p. 1852)

In as many as 10 per cent of first pregnancies in previously normotensive women, hypertension appears during the last trimester or immediately after delivery, in the syndrome called *preeclampsia, pregnancy-induced hypertension,* or *gestational hypertension.*[298] This disorder should be distinguished from chronic hypertension, although both may progress into eclampsia, defined as the occurrence of convulsions. Gestational hypertension is of unknown cause but occurs more frequently in primigravid women or in subsequent pregnancies with a different father,[299] suggesting an immunological mechanism. Additional predisposing factors include increased age, black race, multiple gestations, concomitant heart or renal disease, and chronic hypertension.[300]

The diagnosis is usually based on a rise in pressure of 30/15 mm Hg or more to a level above 140/90.[301] Though some measure the Korotkoff fourth sound (muffling), the fifth sound (disappearance) is closer to the true diastolic and should be used.[301]

CLINICAL FEATURES. The features shown in Table 26–13 should help distinguish gestational hypertension from chronic, primary hypertension. The distinction should be made because management and prognosis are different: Gestational hypertension is self-limited and rarely recurs in subsequent pregnancies, whereas chronic hypertension progresses and usually complicates subsequent pregnancies. The separation may be difficult because of a lack of knowledge of prepregnancy blood pressure and because of the usual tendency for high pressure to fall considerably during the middle trimester so that hypertension present before pregnancy may not be recognized.

In gestational hypertension, the blood pressure usually rises only late in pregnancy. Among 84 patients with the onset of hypertension before 37 weeks' gestation, 55 had renal disease documented by kidney biopsy 6 months post partum when morphological changes due solely to gestational hypertension should have subsided.[302] Gestational hypertension was the diagnosis in only 10 per cent of primiparous women with onset of hypertension before 37 weeks, whereas it was the diagnosis in three-fourths of primigravid women with onset of hypertension after 37 weeks.

The hemodynamic features of gestational hypertension are a further rise in cardiac output than that usually seen in normal pregnancy accompanied by profound vasoconstriction that reduces the intravascular capacity even more than blood volume.[298] The mother may be particularly vulnerable to encephalopathy because of her previously normal blood pressure. As is described in more detail on p. 832, cerebral blood flow is normally maintained constant over a fairly narrow range of mean arterial pressure, roughly between 60 to 100 mm Hg in normotensive individuals. In a previously normotensive young woman, an acute rise in blood pressure to 150/100 mm Hg may exceed the upper limit of autoregulation, resulting in a "breakthrough" of cerebral blood flow (acute dilation) that leads to cerebral edema, convulsions, and all the clinical manifestations of eclampsia.

TABLE 26–13 DIFFERENCES BETWEEN PREECLAMPSIA AND CHRONIC HYPERTENSION

	PREECLAMPSIA	CHRONIC HYPERTENSION
Age	Young (<20)	Older (>30)
Parity	Primigravida	Multigravida
Onset	After 20 weeks of pregnancy	Before 20 weeks of pregnancy
Weight gain and edema	Sudden	Gradual
Systolic blood pressure	<160	>160
Funduscopic findings	Spasm, edema	Arteriovenous nicking, exudates
Proteinuria	Present	Absent
Plasma uric acid	Increased	Normal
Blood pressure after delivery	Normal	Elevated

Beyond the common associations with proteinuria and edema, no other tests have been found to accurately predict the development of preeclampsia.[303]

PATHOGENESIS. The common factor that predisposes to development of gestational hypertension is *reduced uteroplacental perfusion.* Increasing evidence supports a failure of normal invasion of the uterus by trophoblasts as the mechanism.[304] As explained by D. A. Clark[305]:

> The key lesion in preeclampsia is failure of extravillous cytotrophoblast cells to invade the maternal uterine spiral arteries to a sufficient depth during the first and second trimester. Consequently, the arterial wall does not distend enough to allow sufficient blood flow to the placenta in late pregnancy. The placenta is thereby subjected to ischaemia, and compensatory mechanisms are activated which lead to increased vascular volume and blood pressure. Some of these mechanisms may involve release of prostacyclins, since administration of aspirin can reduce the incidence of preeclampsia. Endothelins, which are potent vasoconstrictors, may also be implicated in the systemic effects, and vascular spasm (leading to encephalopathy and seizures) may result from endothelial damage by shed trophoblast membrane vesicles in the bloodstream.

The defect in trophoblastic invasion may be prevented by suppression of maternal immune responses that produce antibodies against trophoblast antigens.[306] Support for this hypothesis comes from the observation that the incidence of preeclampsia is reduced by repeated exposure to semen,[299] presumably allowing the mother to develop immunological tolerance to the fetal antigenic load. The lesser degree of immunological reaction within the maternal decidua would thereby allow more extensive trophoblastic invasion.[306]

The failure of trophoblastic invasion may, as noted by Clark,[305] lead to a number of secondary phenomena that are responsible for the rise in blood pressure, renal damage, and edema. A decreased synthesis of nitric oxide may be involved,[307] along with increased levels of vasoconstricting prostaglandins.

PREVENTION. Along with more prolonged exposure to semen, as suggested by the data from Robillard et al.,[299] small doses of aspirin[308] and calcium supplements[309] have been found to reduce the incidence of preeclampsia in high-risk women.

Treatment

GESTATIONAL HYPERTENSION. Women with gestational hypertension and their fetuses can be protected from excessive morbidity and mortality by maneuvers that lower the blood pressure without impairing uteroplacental perfusion. These maneuvers include modified bed rest, a nutritious diet with normal amounts of sodium, and antihypertensive agents when diastolic blood pressure above 100 mm Hg indicates impairment of renal function and predisposition to overt eclampsia.

However, as noted by Redman and Roberts,[310] "The cure is achieved by delivery, which removes the diseased tissue—the placenta. In short, the need is to deliver before it is too late. To achieve this apparently simple end, the clinician must detect the symptomless prodromal condition by screening all pregnant women, admit to hospital those with advanced preeclampsia so as to keep track of an unpredictable situation, and time preemptive delivery to maximize the safety of mother and baby."

Caution is advised in the use of drugs for mild gestational hypertension, traditionally limited to methyldopa. In one of the few controlled studies comparing modified bed rest versus antihypertensive drug therapy, half of 200 primigravid women with relatively mild hypertension at 26 to 35 weeks' gestation were given labetalol and the other half were monitored while in the hospital.[311] Those given labetalol had a significant fall in blood pressure, whereas the controls did not, but those in both groups had some worsening of renal function. However, the number of small-for-gestational age infants was higher in the labetalol group (19 versus 9 per cent). Thus, drug treatment of maternal blood pressure did not improve perinatal outcome and was associated with fetal growth retardation. Most authorities recommend antihypertensive drugs if diastolic pressures remain above 100 mm Hg.[312] The only drugs that are contraindicated are ACE inhibitors because of their propensity to induce neonatal renal failure and hypotension.[313]

If the syndrome advances and eclampsia threatens before the 32nd week of gestation, expectant management (bed rest, oral antihypertensives, and intensive fetal monitoring) provides better eventual outcomes than more aggressive therapy (glucocorticoids for 48 hours followed by delivery either by induction or cesarean).[314] If parenteral antihypertensives are needed, hydralazine works well.[315]

CHRONIC HYPERTENSION. If pregnancy begins while a woman is on antihypertensive drug therapy, the medications, including diuretics, are usually continued, on the basis of the belief that the mother should be protected and that the fetus will not suffer from any sudden hemodynamic shifts such as occur when therapy is first begun. Among women with chronic hypertension who were not undergoing treatment, therapy with either hydralazine or methyldopa significantly reduced the incidence of gestational hypertension when compared with that in a placebo-treated group.[316] However, despite modern treatment, the incidence of perinatal mortality and fetal growth retardation remains higher in patients with chronic hypertension.[317]

MANAGEMENT OF ECLAMPSIA. With appropriate care of gestational hypertension, eclampsia hardly ever supervenes; when it does, however, maternal and fetal mortality remain very high.[318] Excellent results have been reported with the use of magnesium sulfate to prevent convulsions.[319] Patients with severe eclampsia who have persistent oliguria after a fluid challenge should undergo hemodynamic monitoring, since management may require additional volume or a reduction in preload or afterload.[320]

CONSEQUENCES OF PREGNANCY-RELATED HYPERTENSION. The long-term prognosis of women with gestational hypertension is excellent. When 200 women with the most severe form, eclampsia, were followed for up to 44 years, the distribution of blood pressure was identical to that in the general population.[321] Chesley concludes that "eclampsia neither is a sign of latent essential hypertension nor causes hypertension." The long-term mortality rate in black women having eclampsia and of white women having eclampsia as multiparas is increased, probably because they had underlying but previously unrecognized chronic hypertension or renal disease.

After delivery, women may develop transient or persistent hypertension. In many, early primary hypertension may have been masked by the hemodynamic changes of pregnancy. Some women develop postpartum heart failure that may be an idiopathic cardiomyopathy but is usually related to hypertension, preexisting heart disease, or complications of pregnancy.[322]

HYPERTENSIVE CRISES

DEFINITIONS. A number of clinical circumstances may require rapid reduction of the blood pressure (Table 26–14). These may be separated into *emergencies,* which require immediate reduction of blood pressure (within 1 hour), and *urgencies,* which can be treated more slowly. A persistent diastolic pressure exceeding 130 mm Hg is often associated with acute vascular damage; some patients may suffer vascular damage from lower levels of pressure, while others manage to withstand even higher levels without apparent harm. As discussed below, the rapidity of the rise may be more important than the absolute level in producing acute vascular damage. Therefore, in practice, all patients with diastolic blood pressures above 130 mm Hg should be treated, some more rapidly with parenteral drugs, others more slowly with oral agents, as described on p. 858.

TABLE 26–14 CIRCUMSTANCES REQUIRING RAPID TREATMENT OF HYPERTENSION

ACCELERATED-MALIGNANT HYPERTENSION WITH PAPILLEDEMA
CEREBROVASCULAR
Hypertensive encephalopathy
Atherothrombotic brain infarction with severe hypertension
Intracerebral hemorrhage
Subarachnoid hemorrhage
CARDIAC
Acute aortic dissection
Acute left ventricular failure
Acute or impending myocardial infarction
After coronary bypass surgery
RENAL
Acute glomerulonephritis
Renal crises from collagen-vascular diseases
Severe hypertension after kidney transplantation
EXCESSIVE CIRCULATING CATECHOLAMINES
Pheochromocytoma crisis
Food or drug interactions with monoamine-oxidase inhibitors
Sympathomimetic drug use (cocaine)
Rebound hypertension after sudden cessation of antihypertensive drugs
ECLAMPSIA
SURGICAL
Severe hypertension in patients requiring immediate surgery
Postoperative hypertension
Postoperative bleeding from vascular suture lines
SEVERE BODY BURNS
SEVERE EPISTAXIS

From Kaplan, N. M.: Management of hypertensive emergencies. Lancet *344:*1335, 1994. © by the Lancet Ltd.

When the rise in pressure causes acute damage to retinal vessels, the term *accelerated-malignant hypertension* is used. The separation has been based on the presence of retinal hemorrhages or exudates (accelerated) and papilledema (malignant). The clinical features and survival rates of those with or without papilledema are so similar that there is no reason to separate the two.[323]

Hypertensive encephalopathy is characterized by headache, irritability, alterations in consciousness, and other manifestations of central nervous dysfunction with sudden and marked elevations in blood pressure. Symptoms can be reversed by a reduction in the pressure.

INCIDENCE. In fewer than 1 per cent of patients with primary hypertension, the disease progresses to an accelerated-malignant phase. Although the incidence likely is falling as a consequence of more widespread treatment of hypertension, no difference was found in the numbers of patients seen in Birmingham, England, from 1970 to 1993.[324]

Any hypertensive disease can initiate a crisis. Some, including pheochromocytoma and renovascular hypertension, do so at a higher rate than does primary hypertension. However, since hypertension is of unknown cause in over 90 per cent of all patients, most hypertensive crises appear in the setting of preexisting primary hypertension.[324]

PATHOPHYSIOLOGY. Whenever blood pressure rises and remains above a critical level, various processes set off a series of local and systemic effects that cause further rises in pressure and vascular damage that eventuate in accelerated-malignant hypertension (Fig. 26–20).

Studies in animals and humans by Strandgaard and Paulson have elucidated the mechanism of hypertensive encephalopathy.[325] First, they directly measured the caliber of pial arterioles over the cerebral cortex in cats whose blood pressure was varied over a wide range of infusion by vasodilators or angiotensin II. As the pressure fell, the arterioles

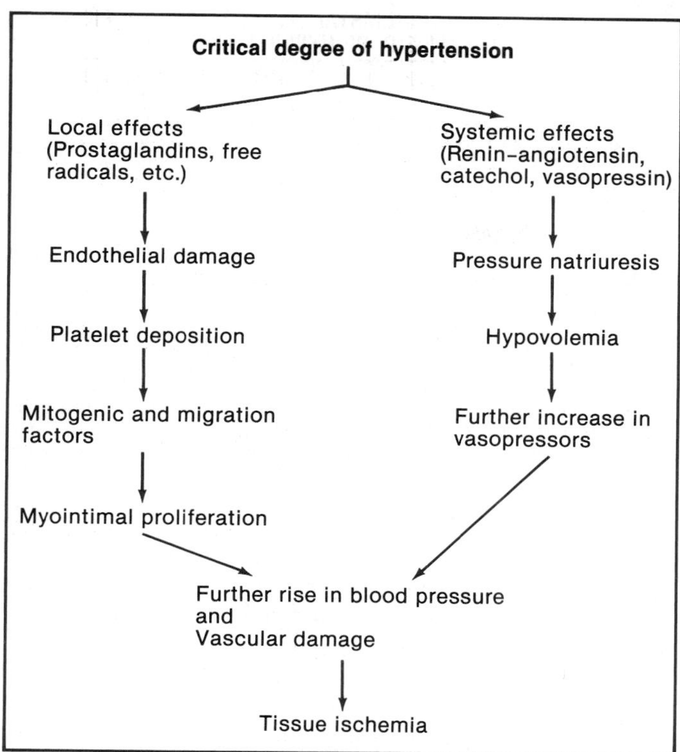

FIGURE 26–20. A scheme for the initiation and progression of malignant hypertension. (From Kaplan, N. M.: Clinical Hypertension. 6th ed. Baltimore, © by Williams and Wilkins, 1994, p. 283.)

became dilated; as the pressure rose, they become constricted. Thus a constant cerebral blood flow was maintained by means of autoregulation, which is dependent on the cerebral sympathetic nerves. However, when mean arterial pressure rose above 180 mm Hg, the tightly constricted vessels could no longer withstand the pressure and suddenly dilated. This began in an irregular manner, first in areas with less muscle tone and then diffusely, producing generalized vasodilatation. This "breakthrough" of cerebral blood flow hyperperfuses the brain under high pressure, causing leakage of fluid into the perivascular tissue and resulting in cerebral edema and the syndrome of hypertensive encephalopathy.

In human subjects, cerebral blood flow was measured repetitively by an isotopic technique while blood pressure was lowered or raised with vasodilators or vasoconstrictors in a manner similar to that employed in the animal studies.[325] Curves depicting cerebral blood flow as a function of arterial pressure demonstrated autoregulation with a constancy of flow over mean pressures in normotensive persons from about 60 to 120 mm Hg and in hypertensive patients from about 110 to 180 mm Hg (Fig. 26–21). This "shift to the right" in hypertensive patients is the result of structural thickening of the arterioles as an adaptation to the chronically elevated pressures. When pressures were raised beyond the upper limit of autoregulation, the same "breakthrough" with hyperperfusion occurred as was seen in the animal studies. In previously normotensive persons whose vessels have not been altered by prior exposure to high pressure, breakthrough occurred at a mean arterial pressure of about 120 mm Hg; in hypertensive patients, the breakthrough occurred at about 180 mm Hg.

These studies confirm clinical observations. In previously normotensive persons, severe encephalopathy occurs with relatively little hypertension. In children with acute glomerulonephritis and in women with eclampsia, convulsions may occur owing to hypertensive encephalopathy with blood pressures as low as 150/100 mm Hg. Obviously, chronically hypertensive patients withstand such pressures

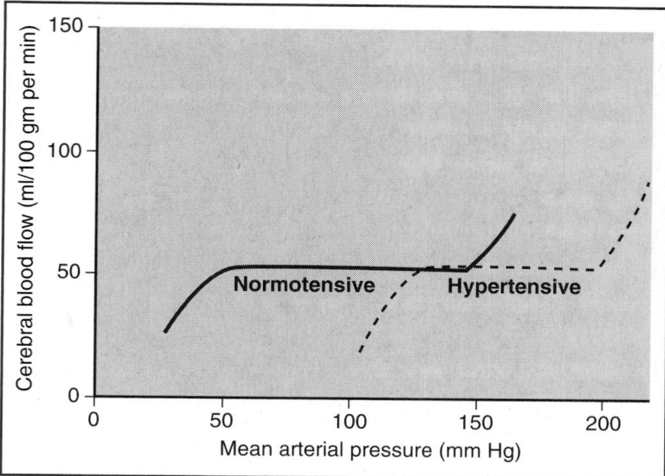

FIGURE 26–21. Idealized curves of cerebral blood flow at varying levels of systemic blood pressure in normotensive and hypertensive subjects. Rightward shift is shown in autoregulation with chronic hypertension. (Adapted from Strandgaard, S., Olesen, J., Skinhøj, and Lassen, N. A.: Autoregulation of brain circulation in severe arterial hypertension. Br. Med. J. *1*:507, 1973.)

without difficulty; however, when pressures increase significantly, they too may develop encephalopathy.

MANIFESTATIONS AND COURSE. The symptoms and signs of hypertensive crises are usually dramatic (Table 26–15). However, some patients may be relatively asymptomatic, despite markedly elevated pressures and extensive organ damage. Young black men are particularly prone to hypertensive crisis with severe renal insufficiency but little obvious prior distress. When the blood pressure is so high as to induce encephalopathy or accelerated-malignant hypertension, the following clinical features are frequently present:

1. Renal insufficiency with protein and red cells in the urine and azotemia; acute oliguric renal failure also may develop.
2. Elevated levels of plasma renin from the diffuse intrarenal ischemia, resulting in secondary aldosteronism, often manifested by hypokalemia. Although not causal, the secondarily elevated renin and aldosterone levels most likely exacerbate the hypertensive process.
3. Microangiopathic hemolytic anemia with red cell fragmentation and intravascular coagulation.
4. Cardiac size and function may *not* be abnormal in those who suddenly develop malignant hypertension.[326]

If left untreated, patients die quickly from brain damage or more gradually from renal damage. Before effective therapy was available, fewer than 25 per cent of patients with malignant hypertension survived 1 year and only 1 per cent survived 5 years.[327] With therapy including renal dialysis, over 90 per cent survive 1 year and about 80 per cent survive 5 years. Death in patients with severe hypertension is usually from stroke or renal failure if it occurs in the

TABLE 26–15 CLINICAL CHARACTERISTICS OF HYPERTENSIVE CRISIS

Blood pressure: Usually >140 mm Hg diastolic
Funduscopic findings: Hemorrhages, exudates, papilledema
Neurological status: Headache, confusion, somnolence, stupor, visual loss, focal deficits, seizures, coma
Cardiac findings: Prominent apical impulse, cardiac enlargement, congestive failure
Renal: Oliguria, azotemia
Gastrointestinal: Nausea, vomiting

From Kaplan, N. M.: Clinical Hypertension. 6th ed. Baltimore, © by Williams and Wilkins, 1994, p. 283.

TABLE 26–16 CONDITIONS TO BE DIFFERENTIATED FROM A HYPERTENSIVE CRISIS

Acute left ventricular failure
Uremia from any cause, particularly with volume overload
Cerebrovascular accident
Subarachnoid hemorrhage
Brain tumor
Head injury
Epilepsy (postictal)
Collagen diseases, particularly lupus, with cerebral vasculitis
Encephalitis
Overdose and withdrawal from narcotics, amphetamines, etc.
Hypercalcemia
Acute anxiety with hyperventilation syndrome

first few years after onset. If therapy keeps patients alive for longer than 5 years, death will usually be due to coronary artery disease, in which factors other than the high pressure per se are probably also involved.[323]

DIFFERENTIAL DIAGNOSIS. The presence of hypertensive encephalopathy or accelerated-malignant hypertension demands immediate, aggressive therapy to lower blood pressure effectively, often before the specific cause is known. However, certain serious diseases as well as psychogenic problems, i.e., acute anxiety with hyperventilation or panic attacks,[328] can mimic a hypertensive crisis (Table 26–16), and management of these conditions obviously requires different diagnostic and therapeutic approaches. In particular, blood pressure should not be lowered too abruptly in a patient with a stroke.[82,329] Specific therapy of hypertensive crises is described in the next chapter (p. 858).

REFERENCES

1. Whelton, P. K.: Epidemiology of hypertension. Lancet *344:*101, 1994.
2. Stockwell, D. H., Madhavan, S., Cohen, H., et al.: The determinants of hypertension awareness, treatment, and control in an insured population. Am. J. Public Health *84:*1768, 1994.
3. Schappert, S. M.: National ambulatory medical survey: 1991 summary. NCHS Advance Data, no. 230, Vital and Health Statistics of the National Center for Health Statistics, Hyattsville, MD, U.S. Department of Health and Human Services Publication (PHS) 93-1250. March 29, 1993.
4. Kaplan, N. M.: Clinical Hypertension. 6th ed. Baltimore, Williams and Wilkins, 1994.
5. National High Blood Pressure Education Program Working Group: National High Blood Pressure Education Program Working Group Report on Primary Prevention of Hypertension. Arch. Intern. Med. *153:*186, 1993.
6. Rose, G.: Epidemiology. *In* Marshall, A. J., and Barritt, D. W. (eds.): The Hypertensive Patient. Kent, England, Pitman Medical, 1980, p. 1.
7. Pickering, T. G.: Blood pressure measurement and detection of hypertension. Lancet *344:*31, 1994.
8. Alderman, M. H., and Lamport, B.: Labelling of hypertensives: A review of the data. J. Clin. Epidemiol. *43:*195, 1990.
9. Sheps, S. G., and Canzanello, V. J.: Current role of automated ambulatory blood pressure and self-measured blood pressure determinations in clinical practice. Mayo Clin. Proc. *69:*1000, 1994.
10. de Gaudemaris, R., Chau, N. P., and Mallion, J.-M.: Home blood pressure: Variability, comparison with office readings and proposal for reference values. J. Hypertens. *12:*831, 1994.
11. Staessen, J. A., O'Brien, E. T., Amery, A. K., et al.: Ambulatory blood pressure in normotensive and hypertensive subjects: Results from an international database. J. Hypertens. *12* (Suppl. 7):S1, 1994.
12. Clement, D. L., De Buyzere, M., and Duprez, D.: Prognostic value of ambulatory blood pressure monitoring. J. Hypertens. *12:*857, 1994.
13. Tseng, Y.-Z., Tseng, C.-D., Lo, H.-M., et al.: Characteristic abnormal findings of ambulatory blood pressure indicative of hypertensive target organ complications. Eur. Heart J. *15:*1037, 1994.
14. Mejia, A. D., Egan, B. M., Schork, N. J., and Zweifler, A. J.: Artifacts in measurement of blood pressure and lack of target organ involvement in the assessment of patients with treatment-resistant hypertension. Ann. Intern. Med. *112:*270, 1990.
15. Høegholm, A., Bank, L. E., Kristensen, K. S., et al.: Microalbuminuria in 411 untreated individuals with established hypertension, white coat hypertension, and normotension. Hypertension *24:*101, 1994.
16. Marchesi, E., Perani, G., Falaschi, F., et al.: Metabolic risk factors in white coat hypertensives. J. Hum. Hypertens. *8:*475, 1994.
17. Muller, J. E., Abela, G. S., Nesto, R. W., and Tofler, G. H.: Triggers, acute risk factors and vulnerable plaques: The lexicon of a new frontier. J. Am. Coll. Cardiol. *23:*809, 1994.
18. Pickering, T. G., Levenstein, M., and Walmsley, P.: Nighttime dosing of doxazosin has peak effect on morning ambulatory blood pressure: Results of the HALT study. Am. J. Hypertens. *7:*844, 1994.
19. Anders, R. J., White, W. B., Grimm, R. H., et al.: Pharmacodynamic profile of delayed release verapamil gastrointestinal therapeutic system (GITS) following nocturnal dosing. J. Hypertens. *12* (Suppl. 3):S25, 1994.
20. Verdecchia, P., Porcellati, C., Schillaci, G., et al.: Ambulatory blood pressure: An independent predictor of prognosis in essential hypertension. Hypertension *34:*793, 1994.
21. Palatini, P., Penzo, M., Racioppa, A., et al.: Clinical relevance of nighttime blood pressure and of daytime blood pressure variability. Arch. Intern. Med. *152:*1855, 1992.
22. Lurbe, A., Redón, J., Pascual, J. M., et al.: Altered blood pressure during sleep in normotensive subjects with type I diabetes. Hypertension *21:*227, 1993.
23. Rosansky, S. J., Johnson, K. L., Hutchinson, C., and Erdel, S.: Blood pressure changes during daytime sleep and comparison of daytime and nighttime sleep-related blood pressure changes in patients with chronic renal failure. J. Am. Soc. Nephrol. *4:*1172, 1993.
24. Gretler, D. D., Fumo, M. T., Nelson, K. S., and Murphy, M. B.: Ethnic differences in circadian hemodynamic profile. Am. J. Hypertens. *7:*7, 1994.
25. Manolio, T. A., Burke, G. L., Savage, P. J., et al.: Exercise blood pressure response and 5-year risk of elevated blood pressure in a cohort of young adults: The CARDIA Study. Am. J. Hypertens. *7:*234, 1994.
26. Mundal, R., Kjeldsen, S. E., Sandvik, L., et al.: Exercise blood pressure predicts cardiovascular mortality in middle-aged men. Hypertension *24:*56, 1994.
27. Neaton, J. D., and Wentworth, D.: Serum cholesterol, blood pressure, cigarette smoking, and death from coronary heart disease. Arch. Intern. Med. *152:*56, 1992.
28. Froom, P., Bar-David, M., Ribak, J., et al.: Predictive value of systolic blood pressure in young men for elevated systolic blood pressure 12 to 15 years later. Circulation *68:*467, 1983.
29. Wilson, P. W. F.: Established risk factors and coronary artery disease: The Framingham Study. Am. J. Hypertens. *7:*7S, 1994.
30. Zweifler, A. J., and Shahab, S. T.: Pseudohypertension: A new assessment. J. Hypertens. *11:*1, 1993.
31. Schutzman, J., Jaeger, F., Maloney, J., and Fouad-Tarazi, F.: Head-up tilt and hemodynamic changes during orthostatic hypotension in patients with supine hypertension. J. Am. Coll. Cardiol. *24:*454, 1994.
32. Joint National Committee on Detection, Evaluation, and Treatment of HIgh Blood Pressure: The fifth report of the Joint National Committee on Detection, Evaluation, and Treatment of High Blood Pressure (JNC V). Arch. Intern. Med. *153:*154, 1993.
33. The Pooling Project Research Group: Relationship of blood pressure, serum cholesterol, smoking habit, relative weight and ECG abnormalities to incidence of major coronary events: Final report of the pooling project. J. Chron. Dis. *31:*201, 1978.
34. Swales, J. D.: Guidelines on guidelines. J. Hypertens. *11:*899, 1993.
35. Hypertension Detection and Follow-up Program Cooperative Group: Blood pressure studies in 14 communities: A two-stage screen for hypertension. JAMA *237:*2385, 1977.
36. Lieberman, E.: Hypertension in childhood and adolescence. *In* Kaplan, N. M. (ed.): Clinical Hypertension. 6th ed. Baltimore, Williams and Wilkins, 1994, p. 437.
37. Cooper, R. S., and Liao, Y.: Is hypertension among blacks more severe or simply more common? Circulation *85*(Abs.):12, 1992.
38. Sorlie, P., Rogot, E., Anderson, R., et al.: Black-white mortality differences by family income. Lancet *340:*346, 1992.
38a. Frohlich, E. D.: Hypertension: Clinical classifications. *In* Fuster, V., Ross, R., and Topol, E. J. (eds.): Atherosclerosis and Coronary Artery Disease. Philadelphia, Lippincott-Raven Publishers, 1996, pp. 243–258.
39. Rudnick, J. V., Sackett, D. L., Hirst, S., and Holmes, C.: Hypertension in family practice. Can. Med. Assoc. J. *3:*492, 1977.
40. Sinclair, A. M., Isles, C. G., Brown, I., et al.: Secondary hypertension in a blood pressure clinic. Arch. Intern. Med. *147:*1289, 1987.
41. Anderson, G. H., Jr., Blakeman, N., and Streeten, D. H. P.: The effect of age on prevalence of secondary forms of hypertension in 4429 consecutively referred patients. J. Hypertens. *12:*609, 1994.
42. Coughlin, S. S., Trock, B., Criqui, M. H., et al.: The logistic modeling of sensitivity, specificity, and predictive value of a diagnostic test. J. Clin. Epidemiol. *45:*1, 1992.
43. MacMahon, S., Peto, R., Cutler, J., et al.: Blood pressure, stroke, and coronary heart disease: I. Prolonged differences in blood pressure: Prospective observational studies corrected for the regression dilution bias. Lancet *335:*765, 1990.
44. Weiss, N. S.: Relation of high blood pressure to headache, epistaxis, and selected other symptoms. N. Engl. J. Med. *287:*631, 1972.
45. Cooper, W. D., Glover, D. R., Hormbrey, J. M., and Kimber, G. R.: Head-

ache and blood pressure: Evidence of a close relationship. J. Hum. Hypertens. *3*:41, 1989.
46. Rose, G.: Strategy of prevention: Lessons from cardiovascular disease. Br. Med. J. *282*:1847, 1981.
47. Lemne, C., Hamsten, A., Karpe, F., et al.: Dyslipoproteinemic changes in borderline hypertension. Hypertension *24*:605, 1994.
48. Kaplan, N. M.: The deadly quartet: Upper-body obesity, glucose intolerance, hypertriglyceridemia, and hypertension. Arch. Intern. Med. *149*:1514, 1989.
49. Maheux, P., Jeppesen, J., Sheu, W. H.-H., et al.: Additive effects of obesity, hypertension, and type 2 diabetes on insulin resistance. Hypertension *24*:695, 1994.
50. Keith, N. M., Wagener, H. P., and Barker, N. W.: Some different types of essential hypertension: Their course and prognosis. Am. J. Med. Sci. *197*:332, 1939.
51. Dahlöf, B., Stenkula, S., and Hansson, L.: Hypertensive retinal vascular changes: Relationship to LV hypertrophy and arteriolar changes before and after treatment. Blood Press. *1*:35, 1992.
51a. Phillips, R. A., and Diamond, J. A.: Hypertensive Heart Disease. *In* Fuster, V., Ross, R., and Topol, E. J. (eds.): Atherosclerosis and Coronary Artery Disease. Philadelphia, Lippincott-Raven Publishers, 1996, pp. 275–302.
52. de Simone, G., Devereux, R. B., Roman, M. J., et al.: Assessment of left ventricular function by the midwall fractional shortening/end-systolic stress relation in human hypertension. J. Am. Coll. Cardiol. *23*:1444, 1994.
53. Ren, J.-F., Pancholy, S. B., Iskandrian, A. S., et al.: Doppler echocardiographic evaluation of the spectrum of left ventricular diastolic dysfunction in essential hypertension. Am. Heart J. *127*:906, 1994.
54. Shepherd, R. F. J., Zachariah, P. K., and Shub, C.: Hypertension and left ventricular diastolic function. Mayo Clin. Proc. *64*:1521, 1989.
55. Karam, R., Lever, H. M., and Healy, B. P.: Hypertensive hypertrophic cardiomyopathy or hypertrophic cardiomyopathy with hypertension? A study of 78 patients. J. Am. Coll. Cardiol. *13*:580, 1989.
56. Houghton, J. L., Frank, M. J., Carr, A. A., et al.: Relations among impaired coronary flow reserve, left ventricular hypertrophy and thallium perfusion defects in hypertensive patients without obstructive coronary artery disease. J. Am. Coll. Cardiol. *15*:43, 1990.
57. Savage, D. D., Levy, D., Dannenberg, A. L., et al.: Association of echocardiographic left ventricular mass with body size, blood pressure and physical activity (the Framingham Study). Am. J. Cardiol. *65*:371, 1990.
58. Devereux, R. B., Roman, M. J., Ganau, A., et al.: Cardiac and arterial hypertrophy and atherosclerosis in hypertension. Hypertension *23* (part 1):802, 1994.
59. Nielsen, J. R., Oxhøj, H., and Fabricius, J.: Left ventricular structural changes in young men at increased risk of developing essential hypertension: Assessment by echocardiography. Am. J. Hypertens. *2*:885, 1989.
60. Post, W. S., Larson, M. G., and Levy, D.: Impact of left ventricular structure on the incidence of hypertension. Circulation *90*:179, 1994.
61. Verdecchia, P., Schillaci, G., Guerrieri, M., et al.: Circadian blood pressure changes and left ventricular hypertrophy in essential hypertension. Circulation *81*:528, 1990.
62. Devereux, R. B., Koren, M. J., de Simone, G., et al.: LV mass as a measure of preclinical hypertensive disease. Am. J. Hypertens. *5*:175S, 1992.
63. Gottdiener, J. S., Reda, D. J., Materson, B. J., et al.: Importance of obesity, race and age to the cardiac structural and functional effects of hypertension. J. Am. Coll. Cardiol. *24*:1492, 1994.
64. Mayet, J., Shahi, M., Foale, R. A., et al.: Racial differences in cardiac structure and function in essential hypertension. Br. Med. J. *308*:1011, 1994.
65. Frohlich, E. D., Apstein, C., Chobanian, A. V., et al.: The heart in hypertension. N. Engl. J. Med. *327*:998, 1992.
66. Clarkson, P. B. M., Wheeldon, N. M., MacLeod, C., et al.: Effects of angiotensin II and aldosterone on diastolic function in vivo in normal man. Clin. Sci. *87*:397, 1994.
67. Weber, K. T., Sun, Y., and Guarda, E.: Structural remodeling in hypertensive heart disease and the role of hormones. Hypertension *23* (Part 2):869, 1994.
68. Verdecchia, P., Porcellati, C., Zampi, I., et al.: Asymmetric left ventricular remodeling due to isolated septal thickening in patients with systemic hypertension and normal left ventricular masses. Am. J. Cardiol. *73*:247, 1994.
69. Koren, M. J., Devereux, R. B., Casale, P. N., et al.: Relation of left ventricular mass and geometry to morbidity and mortality in uncomplicated essential hypertension. Ann. Intern. Med. *114*:345, 1991.
70. Ghali, J. K., Liao, Y., Simmons, B., et al.: The prognostic role of LV hypertrophy in patients with or without coronary artery disease. Ann. Intern. Med. *117*:831, 1992.
71. Schmieder, R. E., and Messerli, F. H.: Determinants of ventricular ectopy in hypertensive cardiac hypertrophy. Am. Heart J. *123*:89, 1992.
72. Dahlöf, B., Pennert, K., and Hansson, L.: Reversal of left ventricular hypertensive patients: A metaanalysis of 109 treatment studies. Am. J. Hypertens. *5*:95, 1992.
73. Habib, G. B., Mann, D. L., and Zoghbi, W. A.: Normalization of cardiac structure and function after regression of cardiac hypertrophy. Am. Heart J. *128*:333, 1994.
74. Kannel, W. B.: Contribution of the Framingham Study to preventive cardiology. J. Am. Coll. Cardiol. *15*:206, 1990.
75. Hedblad, B., and Janzon, L.: Hypertension and ST segment depression during ambulatory electrocardiographic recording: Results from the prospective population study "men born in 1914" in Malm, Sweden. Hypertension *20*:32, 1992.
76. Lindblad, U., Råstam, L., and Rydén, L.: The J-curve phenomenon: Inverse relation between achieved diastolic blood pressure and risk of acute myocardial infarction. *In* Kendall, M. J., Kaplan, N. M., and Horton, R. C. (eds.): Difficult Hypertension, Practical Management and Decision Making. London, Martin Dunitz, 1995, pp. 79–96.
77. Harvey, J. M., Howie, A. J., Lee, S. J., et al.: Renal biopsy findings in hypertensive patients with proteinuria. Lancet *340*:1435, 1992.
78. Pedrinelli, R., Giampietro, O., Carmassi, F., et al.: Microalbuminuria and endothelial dysfunction in essential hypertension. Lancet *344*:14, 1994.
79. Perneger, T. V., Klag, M. J., Feldman, H. I., and Whelton, P. K.: Projections of hypertension-related renal disease in middle-aged residents of the United States. JAMA *269*:1272, 1993.
80. Alter, M., Friday, G., Lai, S. M., et al.: Hypertension and risk of stroke recurrence. Stroke *25*:1605, 1994.
81. Bikkina, M., Levy, D., Evans, J. C., et al.: Left ventricular mass and risk of stroke in an elderly cohort. JAMA *272*:33, 1994.
82. O'Connell, J. E., and Gray, C. S.: Treating hypertension after stroke. Br. Med. J. *308*:1523, 1994.
83. Bruner, H. R., Laragh, J. H., Baer, L., et al.: Essential hypertension: Renin and aldosterone, heart attack and stroke. N. Engl. J. Med. *286*:441, 1972.
84. Alderman, M. H., Madhavan, S., Ooi, W. L., et al.: Association of the renin-sodium profile with the risk of myocardial infarction in patients with hypertension. N. Engl. J. Med. *324*:1098, 1991.
85. Management Committee: Untreated mild hypertension. Lancet *1*:185, 1982.
86. Medical Research Council Working Party: MRC trial of treatment of mild hypertension: Principal results. Br. Med. J. *291*:97, 1985.
87. Jackson, R., Barham, P., Bills, J., et al.: Management of raised blood pressure in New Zealand: A discussion document. Br. Med. J. *307*:107, 1993.

MECHANISMS OF ESSENTIAL HYPERTENSION

88. Lund-Johansen, P.: Central haemodynamics in essential hypertension at rest and during exercise: A 20-year follow-up study. J. Hypertens. *7* (Suppl. 6):S52, 1989.
89. Post, W. S., Larson, M. G., and Levy, D.: Hemodynamic predictors of incident hypertension. Hypertension *24*:585, 1994.
90. Julius, S., Mejia, A. D., Schork, N. J., and Krause, L. C.: Neurogenic hyperkinetic borderline hypertension (BHT) in Tecumseh, Michigan. Circulation *81*:16, 1990.
91. Jeunemaitre, X., Soubrier, F., Kotelevtsev, Y. V., et al.: Molecular basis of human hypertension: Role of angiotensinogen. Cell *71*:169, 1992.
91a. Hunt, S. C., Hopkins, P. N., and Williams, R. R.: Hypertension: Genetics and mechanisms. *In* Fuster, V., Ross, R., and Topol, E. J. (eds.): Atherosclerosis and Coronary Artery Disease. Philadelphia, Lippincott-Raven Publishers, 1996, pp. 209–236.
92. Harrap, S. B.: Hypertension: genes versus environment. Lancet *344*:169, 1994.
93. Law, C. M., de Sweit, M., Osmond, C., et al.: Initiation of hypertension in utero and its amplification throughout life. Br. Med. J. *306*:24, 1993.
94. Lucas, A., and Morley, R.: Does early nutrition in infants born before term programme later blood pressure? Br. Med. J. *309*:304, 1994.
95. Brenner, B. M., and Chertow, G. M.: Congenital oligonephropathy: An inborn cause of adult hypertension and progressive renal injury? Curr. Opin. Nephrol. Hypertens. *2*:691, 1993.
96. Brenner, B. M., and Anderson, S.: The interrelationships among filtration surface area, blood pressure, and chronic renal disease. J. Cardiovasc. Pharmacol. *19* (Suppl. 6):S1, 1992.
97. Guyton, A. C.: Kidneys and fluids in pressure regulation: Small volume but large pressure changes. Hypertension *19* (Suppl. I):I-2, 1992.
98. Sealey, J. E., Blumenfeld, J. D., Bell, G. M., et al.: On the renal basis for essential hypertension: Nephron heterogeneity with discordant renin secretion and sodium excretion causing a hypertensive vasoconstriction-volume relationship. J. Hypertens. *6*:763, 1988.
99. de Wardener, H. E., and MacGregor, G. A.: Dahl's hypothesis that a saluretic substance may be responsible for a sustained rise in arterial pressure: Its possible role in essential hypertension. Kidney Int. *18*:1, 1980.
100. Woolfson, R. G., Poston, L., and de Wardener, H. E.: Digoxin-like inhibitors of active sodium transport and blood pressure: The current status. Kidney Int. *46*:297, 1994.
101. Hamlyn, J. M., Laredo, J., Lu, Z., et al.: Do putative endogenous digitalis-like factors have a physiological role? Hypertension *24*:641, 1994.
102. Lewis, L. K., Yandle, T. G., Lewis, J. G., et al.: Ouabain is not detectable in human plasma. Hypertension *24*:549, 1994.
103. Richards, A. M.: The natriuretic peptides and hypertension. J. Intern. Med. *235*:543, 1994.
104. Buckley, M. G., Markandu, N. D., Sagnella, G. A., and MacGregor, G. A.: Brain and atrial natriuretic peptides: A dual peptide system of potential importance in sodium balance and blood pressure regulation in patients with essential hypertension. J. Hypertens. *12*:809, 1994.

105. Kimura, G., and Brenner, B. M.: A method for distinguishing salt-sensitive from non–salt-sensitive forms of human and experimental hypertension. Curr. Opin. Nephrol. Hypertens. *2:*341, 1993.
106. Resnick, L. M., Gupta, R. K., DiFabio, B., et al.: Intracellular ionic consequences of dietary salt loading in essential hypertension. J. Clin. Invest. *94:*1269, 1994.
107. Swales, J. D.: Membrane transport of ions in hypertension. Cardiovasc. Drug Ther. *4:*367, 1990.
108. Dzau, V. J., Gibbons, G. H., Cooke, J. P., and Omoigui, N.: Vascular biology and medicine in the 1990s: Scope, concepts, potentials, and perspectives. Circulation *87:*705, 1993.
109. Lever, A. F., and Harrap, S. B.: Essential hypertension: A disorder of growth with origins in childhood? J. Hypertens. *10:*101, 1992.
110. Folkow, B.: "Structural factor" in primary and secondary hypertension. Hypertension *16:*89, 1990.
111. Davis, M. G., Ali, S., Leikauf, G. D., and Dorn, G. W., II: Tyrosine kinase inhibition prevents deformation-stimulated vascular smooth muscle growth. Hypertension *24:*706, 1994.
112. Lever, A. F.: Slow pressor mechanisms in hypertension: A role for hypertrophy of resistance vessels? J. Hypertens. *4:*515, 1986.
113. Müller, R., Steffen, H. M., Weller, P., and Krone, W.: Plasma catecholamines and adrenoceptors in young hypertensive patients. J. Hum. Hypertens. *8:*351, 1994.
114. Floras, J. S., and Hara, K.: Sympathoneural and haemodynamic characteristics of young subjects with mild essential hypertension. J. Hypertens. *11:*647, 1993.
115. Smith, S., Julius, S., Jamerson, K., et al.: Hematocrit levels and physiologic factors in relationship to cardiovascular risk in Tecumseh, Michigan. J. Hypertens. *12:*455, 1994.
116. Ziegler, M. G., Mill, P., and Dimsdale, J. E.: Hypertensives' pressor response to norepinephrine: Analysis by infusion rate and plasma levels. Am. J. Hypertens. *4:*586, 1991.
117. Reeves, R. A., Shapiro, A. P., Thompson, M. E., and Johnsen, A.-M.: Loss of nocturnal decline in blood pressure after cardiac transplantation. Circulation *73:*401, 1986.
118. Vincent, H. H., Boomsma, F., Man in'T Veld, A. J., and Schalekamp, M. A. D. H.: Stress levels of adrenaline amplify the blood pressure response to sympathetic stimulation. J. Hypertens. *4:*255, 1986.
119. al'Absi, M., Lovallo, W. R., McKey, B. S., and Pincomb, G. A.: Borderline hypertensives produce exaggerated adrenocortical responses to mental stress. Psychosom. Med. *56:*245, 1994.
120. Markovitz, J. H., Matthews, K. A., Kannel, W. B., et al.: Psychological predictors of hypertension in the Framingham Study: Is there tension in hypertension? JAMA *270:*2439, 1993.
121. Perini, C., Smith, D. H. G., Neutel, J. M., et al.: A repressive coping style protecting from emotional distress in low-renin essential hypertensives. J. Hypertens. *12:*601, 1994.
122. Naraghi, R., Geiger, H., Crnac, J., et al.: Posterior fossa neurovascular anomalies in essential hypertension. Lancet *344:*1466, 1994.
123. Somers, V. K., Dyken, M. E., Mark, A. L., and Abboud, F. M.: Sympathetic-nerve activity during sleep in normal subjects. N. Engl. J. Med. *328:*303, 1993.
124. Cohen, M. C., and Muller, J. E.: Onset of acute myocardial infarction: Circadian variation and triggers. Cardiovasc. Res. *26:*831, 1992.
125. Brunner, H. R., Sealey, J. E., and Laragh, J. H.: Renin subgroups in essential hypertension. Circ. Res. *32/33* (Suppl. I):I-99, 1973.
126. Goldblatt, H.: Reflections. Urol. Clin. North Am. *2:*219, 1975.
126a. Jackson, E. K., and Garrison, J. C.: Renin and angiotensin. *In* Hardman, J. G., et al. (eds.): Goodman and Gilman's The pharmacological basis of therapeutics. 9th ed. New York, McGraw-Hill, 1996, pp. 733–758.
127. Johnston, C. J.: Renin-angiotensin system: A dual tissue and hormonal system for cardiovascular control. J. Hypertens. *10* (Suppl. 7):S13, 1992.
128. Morishita, R., Gibbons, G. H., Ellison, K. E., et al.: Evidence for direct local effect of angiotensin in vascular hypertrophy. J. Clin. Invest. *94:*978, 1994.
129. Nilsson, P. M., Lind, L., Andersson, P.-E., et al.: On the use of ambulatory blood pressure recordings and insulin sensitivity measurements in support of the insulin-hypertension hypothesis. J. Hypertens. *12:*965, 1994.
130. Wing, J. R., Van Der Merwe, M. T., Joffe, B. I., et al.: Insulin-mediated glucose disposal in black South Africans with essential hypertension. Q. J. Med. *87:*431, 1994.
131. Lemieux, S., Després, J. P., Moorjani, S., et al.: Are gender differences in cardiovascular disease risk factors explained by the level of visceral adipose tissue? Diabetologia *37:*757, 1994.
132. Reaven, G. M., and Laws, A.: Insulin resistance, compensatory hyperinsulinaemia, and coronary heart disease. Diabetologia *37:*948, 1994.
133. Steinberg, H. O., Brechtel, G., Johnson, A., et al.: Insulin-mediated skeletal muscle vasodilation is nitric oxide dependent. J. Clin. Invest. *94:*1172, 1994.
134. Anderson, E. A., and Mark, A. L.: Cardiovascular and sympathetic actions of insulin: The insulin hypothesis of hypertension revisited. Cardiovasc. Risk Factors *3:*159, 1993.
135. Flavahan, N. A.: Atherosclerosis or lipoprotein-induced endothelial dysfunction: Potential mechanisms underlying reduction in EDRF/nitric oxide activity. Circulation *85:*1927, 1992.
136. Panza, J. A., Casino, P. R., Kilcoyne, C. M., and Quyyumi, A. A.: Role of endothelium-derived nitric oxide in the abnormal endothelium-dependent vascular relaxation of patients with essential hypertension. Circulation *87:*1468, 1993.
137. Cockroft, J. R., Chowienczyk, P. J., Benjamin, N., and Ritter, J. M.: Preserved endothelium-dependent vasodilatation in patients with essential hypertension. N. Engl. J. Med. *330:*1036, 1994.
138. Lyons, D., Webster, J., and Benjamin, N.: The effect of antihypertensive therapy on responsiveness to local intra-arterial N^{G}-monomethyl-L-arginine in patients with essential hypertension. J. Hypertens. *12:*1047, 1994.
139. Galle, J., Öchslen, M., Schollmeyer, P., and Wanner, C.: Oxidized lipoproteins inhibit endothelium-dependent vasodilation. Hypertension *23:*556, 1994.
140. Kiowski, W., Linder, L., and Erne, P.: Vascular effects of endothelin-1 in humans and influence of calcium channel blockade. J. Hypertens. *12* (Suppl. 1):S21, 1994.
141. Haynes, W. G., and Webb, D. J.: Contribution of endogenous generation of endothelin-1 to basal vascular tone. Lancet *344:*852, 1994.
142. Henneberry, H. P., Slater, J. D. H., Eisen, V., and Führ, S.: Arginine vasopressin response to hypertonicity in hypertension studied by arginine vasopressin assay in unextracted plasma. J. Hypertens. *10:*221, 1992.
143. Fitzgibbon, W. R., Ploth, D. W., and Margolius, H. S.: Kinins and vasoactive peptides. Curr. Opin. Nephrol. Hypertens. *2:*283, 1993.
144. Muirhead, E. E., Brooks, B., and Byers, L. W.: Biologic differences between vasodilator prostaglandins and medullipin I. Am. J. Med. Sci. *303:*86, 1992.
145. Maheswaran, R., and Beevers, D. G.: Lead and blood pressure. J. Hypertens. *7* (Suppl. 6):S381, 1989.
146. Witteman, J. C. M., Willett, W. C., Stampfer, M. J., et al.: A prospective study of nutritional factors and hypertension among U.S. women. Circulation *80:*1320, 1989.
147. Carman, W. J., Barrett-Connor, E., Sowers, M., and Khaw, K.: Higher risk of cardiovascular mortality among lean hypertensive individuals in Tecumseh, Michigan. Circulation *89:*703, 1994.
148. Sonne-Holm, S., Sørensen, T. I. A., Jensen, G., and Schnohr, P.: Independent effects of weight change and attained body weight on prevalence of arterial hypertension in obese and non-obese men. Br. Med. J. *299:*767, 1989.
149. Hla, K. M., Young, T. B., Bidwell, T., et al.: Sleep apnea and hypertension. Ann. Intern. Med. *120:*382, 1994.
150. Endre, T., Mattiasson, I., Hulthén, U. L., et al.: Insulin resistance is coupled to low physical fitness in normotensive men with a family history of hypertension. J. Hypertens. *12:*81, 1994.
151. Blair, S. N., Kohl, H. W., III, Paffenbarger, R. S., Jr., et al.: Physical fitness and all-cause mortality: A prospective study of healthy men and women. JAMA *262:*2395, 1989.
152. Paffenbarger, R. S., Jr.: Contributions of epidemiology to exercise science and cardiovascular health. Med. Sci. Sports Exerc. *20:*426, 1988.
153. Grøbæk, M., Deis, A., Sørensen, T. I. A., et al.: Influence of sex, age, body mass index, and smoking on alcohol intake and mortality. Br. Med. J. *308:*302, 1994.
154. Kiechl, S., Willeit, J., Egger, G., et al.: Alcohol consumption and carotid atherosclerosis: Evidence of dose-dependent atherogenic and antiatherogenic effects. Stroke *25:*1593, 1994.
155. Marmot, M. G., Elliott, P., Shipley, M. J., et al.: Alcohol and blood pressure: The INTERSALT study. Br. Med. J. *308:*1263, 1994.
156. Gaziano, J. M., Buring, J. E., Breslow, J. L., et al.: Moderate alcohol intake, increased levels of high-density lipoprotein and its subfractions, and decreased risk of myocardial infarction. N. Engl. J. Med. *329:*1829, 1993.
157. Ridker, P. M., Vaughan, D. E., Stampfer, M. J., et al.: Association of moderate alcohol consumption and plasma concentration of endogenous tissue-type plasminogen activator. JAMA *272:*929, 1994.
158. Facchini, F., Chen, Y.-D. I., and Reaven, G. M.: Light-to-moderate alcohol intake is associated with enhanced insulin sensitivity. Diabetes Care *17:*115, 1994.
159. Grassi, G. M., Somers, V. K., Renk, W. S., et al.: Effects of oral alcohol intake on blood pressure and sympathetic nerve activity in normotensive humans: A preliminary report. J. Hypertens. *7* (Suppl. 6):S20, 1989.
160. Kojima, S., Kawano, Y., Abe, H., et al.: Acute effects of alcohol ingestion on blood pressure and erythrocyte sodium concentration. J. Hypertens. *11:*185, 1993.
161. Giannattasio, C., Mangoni, A. A., Stella, M. L., et al.: Acute effects of smoking on radial artery compliance in humans. J. Hypertens. *12:*691, 1994.
162. Terres, W., Becker, P., and Rosenberg, A.: Changes in cardiovascular risk profile during the cessation of smoking. Am. J. Med. *97:*242, 1994.
163. Smith, W. C. S., Lowe, G. D. O., Lee, A. J., and Tunstall-Pedoe, H.: Rheological determinants of blood pressure in a Scottish adult population. J. Hypertens. *10:*467, 1992.
164. Friedman, G. D., Selby, J. V., and Quesenberry, C. P., Jr.: The leukocyte count: A predictor of hypertension. J. Clin. Epidemiol. *43:*907, 1990.
165. Messerli, F. H., Frohlich, E. D., Dreslinski, G. R., et al.: Serum uric acid in essential hypertension: An indicator of renal vascular involvement. Ann. Intern. Med. *93:*817, 1980.

HYPERTENSION IN SPECIAL GROUPS

166. Walker, W. G., Neaton, J. D., Cutler, J. A., et al.: Renal function change in hypertensive members of the Multiple Risk Factor Intervention Trial. JAMA *268:*3085, 1992.

167. Parmer, R. J., Stone, R. A., and Cervenka, J. H.: Renal hemodynamics in essential hypertension: Racial differences in response to changes in dietary sodium. Hypertension *24:*752, 1994.
168. Luft, F. C., Miller, J. Z., Grim, C. E., et al.: Salt sensitivity and resistance of blood pressure. Hypertension *17* (Suppl. 1):102, 1991.
169. Wilson, T. W., and Grim, C. E.: Biohistory of slavery and blood pressure differences in blacks today. Hypertension *17* (Suppl. 1):122, 1991.
170. Barlow, R. J., Connel, M. A., and Milne, F. J.: A study of 48-hour faecal and urinary electrolyte excretion in normotensive black and white South African males. J. Hypertens. *401:*197, 1986.
171. Isles, C. G., Hole, D. J., Hawthorn, V. M., and Lever, A. F.: Relation between coronary risk and coronary mortality in women of the Renfrew and Paisley survey: Comparison of men. Lancet *339:*702, 1992.
172. Kaplan, N. M.: The treatment of hypertension in women. Arch. Intern. Med. *155:*563, 1995.
173. Rosner, B., Prineas, R. J., Loggie, J. M. H., and Daniels, S. R.: Blood pressure nomograms for children and adolescents, by height, sex, and age, in the United States. J. Pediatr. *123:*871, 1993.
174. Gillman, M. W., Cook, N. R., Rosner, B., et al.: Identifying children at high risk for the development of essential hypertension. J. Pediatr. *122:*837, 1993.
175. Morgenstern, B. Z.: Hypertension in pediatric patients: Current issues. Mayo Clin. Proc. *69:*1089, 1994.
176. Loggie, J. M. H.: Hypertension in children. Heart Dis. Stroke May/June:147, 1994.
177. Lauer, R. M., Burns, T. L., Clarke, W. R., and Mahoney, L. T.: Childhood predictors of future blood pressure. Hypertension *18* (Suppl. I):I-74, 1991.
178. Hansen, H. S., Nielsen, J. R., Nyldebrandt, N., and Froberg, K.: Blood pressure and cardiac structure in children with a parental history of hypertension: The Odense Schoolchild Study. J. Hypertens. *10:*677, 1992.
179. Murphy, J. K., Alpert, B. S., and Walker, S. S.: Ethnicity, pressor reactivity, and children's blood pressure. Hypertension *20:*327, 1992.
180. Kaplan, N. M., Deveraux, R. B., and Miller, H. S., Jr.: Task Force 4: Systemic hypertension. J. Am. Coll. Cardiol. *24:*885, 1994.
181. Gruskin, A. B., Dabbagh, S., Fleischmann, L. E., and Atiyeh, B. A.: Application since 1980 of antihypertensive agents to treat pediatric disease. J. Hum. Hypertens. *8:*381, 1994.
182. Deal, J. E.: Treatment of children with hypertension. *In* Kendall, M., Kaplan, N. M., and Horton, R. (eds.): Difficult Hypertension, Practical Management and Decision Making. London, Martin Dunitz, 1995, pp. 7–20.
183. National High Blood Pressure Education Program Working Group: National High Blood Pressure Education Program Working Group report on hypertension in the elderly. Hypertension *23:*275, 1994.
184. Kaplan, N. M.: The promises and perils of treating the elderly hypertensive. Am. J. Med. Sci. *305:*183, 1993.
185. Tarnow, L., Rossing, P., Gall, M.-A., et al.: Prevalence of arterial hypertension in diabetic patients before and after the JNC-V. Diabetes Care *17:*1247, 1994.
186. Berrut, G., Hallab, M., Bouhanick, B., et al.: Value of ambulatory blood pressure monitoring in type I (insulin-dependent) diabetic patients with incipient diabetic nephropathy. Am. J. Hypertens. *7:*222, 1994.
187. The Hypertension in Diabetes Study Group: Hypertension in diabetes study (HDS): I. Prevalence of hypertension in newly presenting type 2 diabetic patients and the association with risk factors for cardiovascular and diabetic complications. J. Hypertens. *11:*309, 1993.
188. Lewis, E. J., Hunsicker, L. G., Bain, R. P., and Rohde, R. D.: The effect of angiotensin-converting enzyme inhibition on diabetic nephropathy. N. Engl. J. Med. *329:*1456, 1993.

SECONDARY HYPERTENSION

189. Hannaford, P. C., Croft, P. R., and Kay, C. R.: Oral contraception and stroke. Evidence from the Royal College of General Practitioners' Oral Contraception Study. Stroke *25:*935, 1994.
190. Rosenberg, L., Palmer, J. R., and Shapiro, S.: Use of lower dose oral contraceptives and risk of myocardial infarction. Circulation *83*(Abs.):8, 1991.
191. Royal College of General Practitioners: Hypertension. *In* Oral Contraceptives and Health. From the Oral Contraceptive Study of the Royal College of General Practice. New York, Pitman Publishing, 1974, p. 37.
192. Weir, R. J.: Effect on blood pressure of changing from high to low dose steroid preparation in women with oral contraceptive induced hypertension. Scott. Med. J. *27:*212, 1982.
193. Wallace, R. B., Barrett-Connor, E., Criqui, M., et al.: Alteration in blood pressures associated with combined alcohol and oral contraceptive use: The Lipid Research Clinics Prevalence Study. J. Chron. Dis. *35:*251, 1982.
194. Lim, K. G., Isles, C. G., Hodsman, G. P., et al.: Malignant hypertension in women of childbearing age and its relation to the contraceptive pill. Br. Med. J. *294:*1057, 1987.
195. McAreavey, D., Cumming, A. M. M., Boddy, K., et al.: The renin-angiotensin system and total body sodium and potassium in hypertensive women taking estrogen-progestogen oral contraceptives. Clin. Endocrinol. *18:*111, 1983.
196. Gosland, I. F., Walton, C., Felton, C., et al.: Insulin resistance, secretion, and metabolism in users of oral contraceptives. J. Clin. Endocrinol. Metab. *74:*64, 1992.
197. Nabulsi, A. A., Folsom, A. R., White, A., et al.: Association of hormone-replacement therapy with various cardiovascular risk factors in postmenopausal women. N. Engl. J. Med. *328:*1069, 1993.
198. Rosenberg, L., Palmer, J. R., and Shapiro, S.: A case-control study of myocardial infarction in relation to use of estrogen supplements. Am. J. Epidemiol. *137:*54, 1993.
199. Lieberman, E. H., Gerhard, M. D., Uehata, A., et al.: Estrogen improves endothelium-dependent, flow-mediated vasodilation in postmenopausal women. Ann. Intern. Med. *121:*936, 1994.
200. Perneger, T. V., Brancati, F. L., Whelton, P. K., and Klag, M. J.: End-stage renal disease attributable to diabetes mellitus. Ann. Intern. Med. *121:*912, 1994.
201. Smith, S. R., Svetkey, K. P., and Dennis, V. W.: Racial differences in the incidence and progression of renal diseases. Kidney Int. *40:*815, 1991.
202. Ghose, R. R., and Harindra, V.: Unrecognized high pressure chronic retention of urine presenting with systemic arterial hypertension. Br. Med. J. *298:*1626, 1989.
203. Bakir, A. A., Bazilinski, N., and Dunea, G.: Transient and sustained recovery from renal shutdown in accelerated hypertension. Am. J. Med. *80:*173, 1986.
204. Shankel, S. W., Johnson, D. C., Clark, P. S., et al.: Acute renal failure and glomerulopathy caused by nonsteroidal anti-inflammatory drugs. Arch. Intern. Med. *152:*986, 1992.
205. Coruzzi, P., and Novarini, A.: Which antihypertensive treatment in renal vasculitis? Nephron *62:*372, 1992.
206. Hammond, J. J., Raffaele, J., Liddel, N., et al.: A prospective study to evaluate the effects of extracorporeal shock wave lithotripsy (ESWL) on blood pressure (BP), renal function (RF) and glomerular filtration (GFR). J. Am. Coll. Cardiol. *21*(Abs.):257, 1993.
207. Smith, L. H., Drach, G., Hall, P., et al.: National High Blood Pressure Education Program (NHBPEP) review paper on complications of shock wave lithotripsy for urinary calculi. Am. J. Med. *91:*635, 1991.
208. Najarian, J. S., Chavers, B. M., McHugh, L. E., and Matas, A. J.: 20 years or more of follow-up on living kidney donors. Lancet *340:*807, 1992.
209. Smith, H. W.: Unilateral nephrectomy in hypertensive disease. J. Urol. *76:*685, 1956.
210. Lüscher, T. F., Wanner, C., Hauri, D., et al.: Curable renal parenchymatous hypertension: Current diagnosis and management. Cardiology *72* (Suppl. 1):33, 1985.
211. Torres, V. E., Donovan, K. A., Scicli, G., et al.: Synthesis of renin by tubulocystic epithelium in autosomal-dominant polycystic kidney disease. Kidney Int. *42:*364, 1992.
212. Siamopoulos, K., Sellars, L., Mishra, S. C., et al.: Experience in the management of hypertension with unilateral chronic pyelonephritis: Results of nephrectomy in selected patients. Q. J. Med. *207:*34, 1983.
213. Rostand, S. G., Brunzell, J. D., Cannon, R. O., III, and Victor, R. G.: Cardiovascular complications in renal failure. J. Am. Soc. Nephrol. *2:*1053, 1991.
214. Breyer, J. A., and Jacobson, H. R.: Ischemic nephropathy. Curr. Opin. Nephrol. Hypertens. *2:*216, 1993.
215. Parving, H.-H., Smidt, U. M., Mathiesen, E. R., et al.: Effective antihypertensive treatment postpones renal insufficiency in diabetic nephropathy. Am. J. Kidney Dis. *22:*188, 1993.
216. Dubach, U. C., Rosner, B., and Stürmer, T.: An epidemiologic study of abuse of analgesic drugs: Effects of phenacetin and salicylate on mortality and cardiovascular morbidity (1968 to 1987). N. Engl. J. Med. *324:*155, 1991.
217. Brenner, B. M., and Yu, A. S. L.: Uremic syndrome revisited: A pathogenetic role for retained endogenous inhibitors of nitric oxide synthesis. Curr. Opin. Nephrol. Hypertens. *1:*3, 1992.
218. Henrich, W. L.: Hemodynamic instability during hemodialysis. Kidney Int. *30:*605, 1986.
219. Curtis, J. J., Luke, R. G., Dustan, H. P., et al.: Remission of essential hypertension after renal transplantation. N. Engl. J. Med. *309:*1009, 1983.
220. Raman, G. V.: Posttransplant hypertension. J. Hum. Hypertens. *5:*1, 1991.
221. Bresticker, M., Nelson, J., Wolf, J., and Anderson, B.: Plasma renin activity in renal transplant patients with hypertension. Am. J. Hypertens. *4:*623, 1991.
222. Strandgaard, S., and Hansen, U.: Hypertension in renal allograft recipients may be conveyed by cadaveric kidneys from donors with subarachnoid hemorrhage. Br. Med. J. *292:*1041, 1986.
223. Mann, S. J., and Pickering, T. G.: Detection of renovascular hypertension: State of the art: 1992. Ann. Intern. Med. *227:*845, 1992.
224. Svetkey, L. P., Kadir, S., Dunnick, N. R., et al.: Similar prevalence of renovascular hypertension in selected blacks and whites. Hypertension *17:*678, 1991.
225. Novick, A. C., Zaki, S., Goldfarb, D., and Hodge, E. E.: Epidemiologic and clinical comparison of renal artery stenosis in black patients and white patients. J. Vasc. Surg. *20:*1, 1994.
226. Bookstein, J. J.: Segmental renal artery stenosis in renovascular hypertension. Radiology *90:*1073, 1968.
227. Geyskes, G. G., Klinge, O. J., Kooiker, C. J., et al.: Renovascular hypertension: The small kidney updated. Q. J. Med. *66:*203, 1988.
228. Rimmer, J. M., and Gennari, F. J.: Atherosclerotic renovascular disease and progressive renal failure. Ann. Intern. Med. *228:*712, 1993.
229. Pickering, T. G.: Renovascular hypertension: Etiology and pathophysiology. Semin. Nucl. Med. *19:*79, 1989.
230. Canzanello, V. J., and Textor, S. C.: Noninvasive diagnosis of renovascular disease. Mayo Clin. Proc. *69:*1172, 1994.

231. Derkx, F. H. M., and Schalekamp, M. A. D. H.: Renal artery stenosis and hypertension. Lancet *344*:237, 1994.
232. Muller, F. B., Sealey, J. E., Case, D. B., et al.: The captopril test for identifying renovascular disease in hypertensive patients. Am. J. Med. *80*:6433, 1986.
233. Gerber, L. M., Mann, S. J., Müller, F. B., et al.: Response to the captopril test is dependent on baseline renin profile. J. Hypertens. *12*:173, 1994.
234. Elliott, W. J., Martin, W. B., and Murphy, M. B.: Comparison of two noninvasive screening tests for renovascular hypertension. Arch. Intern. Med. *153*:755, 1993.
235. Mimran, A.: Renal effects of antihypertensive agents in parenchymal renal disease and renovascular hypertension. J. Cardiovasc. Pharmacol. *19* (Suppl. 6):45, 1992.
236. Losinno, F., Zuccalà, A., Busato, F., and Zucchelli, P.: Renal artery angioplasty for renovascular hypertension and preservation of renal function: Long-term angiographic and clinical follow-up. A.J.R. *162*:853, 1994.
237. Tykarski, A., Edward, R., Dominiczak, A. F., and Reid, J. L.: Percutaneous transluminal renal angioplasty in the management of hypertension and renal failure in patients with renal artery stenosis. J. Hum. Hypertens. *7*:491, 1993.
238. Bedoya, L., Ziegelbaum, M., Vidt, D. G., et al.: Baseline renal function and surgical revascularization in atherosclerotic renal arterial disease in the elderly. Cleveland Clin. J. Med. *56*:415, 1989.
239. Libertino, J. A., Bosco, P. J., Ying, C. Y., et al.: Renal revascularization to preserve and restore renal function. J. Urol. *147*:1485, 1992.
240. McVicar, M., Carman, C., Chandra, M., et al.: Hypertension secondary to renin-secreting juxtaglomerular cell tumor: Case report and review of 38 cases. Pediatr. Nephrol. *7*:404, 1993.
241. Geddy, P. M., and Main, J.: Renin-secreting retroperitoneal leiomyosarcoma: An unusual cause of hypertension. J. Hum. Hypertens. *4*:57, 1990.
242. Leckie, B. J., Birnie, G., and Carachi, R.: Renin in Wilms' tumor: Prorenin as an indicator. J. Clin. Endocrinol. Metab. *79*:1742, 1994.
243. Osella, G., Terzolo, M., Borretta, G., et al.: Endocrine evaluation of incidentally discovered adrenal masses (incidentalomas). J. Clin. Endocrinol. Metab. *79*:1532, 1994.
244. Tsushima, Y.: Different lipid contents between aldosterone-producing and nonhyperfunctioning adrenocortical adenomas: In vivo measurement using chemical-shift magnetic resonance imaging. J. Clin. Endocrinol. Metab. *79*:1759, 1994.
245. Gross, M. D., Shapiro, B., Gouffard, J. A., et al.: Distinguishing benign from malignant euadrenal masses. Ann. Intern. Med. *109*:613, 1988.
246. Gordon, R. D.: Mineralocorticoid hypertension. Lancet *344*:240, 1994.
247. Rich, G. M., Ulick, S., Cook, S., et al.: Glucocorticoid-remediable aldosteronism in a large kindred: Clinical spectrum and diagnosis using a characteristic biochemical phenotype. Ann. Intern. Med. *116*:813, 1992.
248. Lifton, R. P., Dluhy, R. G., Powers, M., et al.: A chimaeric 11β-hydroxylase/aldosterone synthase gene causes glucocorticoid-remediable aldosteronism and human hypertension. Nature *355*:262, 1992.
249. Stewart, P. M., Corrie, J. E. T., Shackleton, C. H. L., and Edwards, C. R. W.: Syndrome of apparent mineralocorticoid excess: A defect in the cortisol-cortisone shuttle. J. Clin. Invest. *82*:340, 1988.
250. Stewart, P. M., Wallace, A. M., Valentino, R., et al.: Mineralocorticoid activity of liquorice: 11-Beta-hydroxysteroid dehydrogenase deficiency comes of age. Lancet *2*:821, 1987.
251. Vierhapper, H., Derfler, K., Nowotny, P., et al.: Impaired conversion of cortisol to cortisone in chronic renal insufficiency: A cause of hypertension or an epiphenomenon? Acta Endocrinol. *125*:160, 1991.
252. Walker, B. R., Stewart, P. M., Shackleton, C. H. L., et al.: Deficient inactivation of cortisol by 11β-hydroxysteroid dehydrogenase in essential hypertension. Clin. Endocrinol. *39*:221, 1993.
253. Blumenfeld, J. D., Sealey, J. E., Schlussel, Y., et al.: Diagnosis and treatment of primary hyperaldosteronism. Ann. Intern. Med. *121*:877, 1994.
254. Ferriss, J. B., Beevers, D. G., Brown, J. J., et al.: Clinical, biochemical and pathological features of low renin ("primary") hyperaldosteronism. Am. Heart J. *95*:375, 1978.
255. Weinberger, M. H., and Fineberg, N. S.: The diagnosis of primary aldosteronism and separation of two major subtypes. Arch. Intern. Med. *153*:2125, 1993.
256. Bravo, E. L., and Canale, M. P.: Clinical utility of some screening tests in the evaluation of suspected primary aldosteronism. Hypertension *24*(Abs.):58, 1994.
257. Radin, D. R., Manoogian, C., and Nadler, J. L.: Diagnosis of primary hyperaldosteronism: Importance of correlating CT findings with endocrinologic studies. A.J.R. *158*:553, 1992.
258. Guazzoni, G., Montorsi, F., Bergamaschi, F., et al.: Effectiveness and safety of laparoscopic adrenalectomy. J. Urol. *152*:1375, 1994.
259. Young, W. F., Jr.: Primary aldosteronism. *In* Rakel, R. E. (ed.): Conn's Current Therapy. Philadelphia, W. B. Saunders Company, 1993, p. 610.
260. Sugihara, N., Shimizu, M., Kita, Y., et al.: Cardiac characteristics and postoperative courses in Cushing's syndrome. Am. J. Cardiol. *69*:1475, 1992.
261. Ulick, S., Tedde, R., and Wang, J. Z.: Defective ring A reduction of cortisol as the major metabolic error in the syndrome of apparent mineralocorticoid excess. J. Clin. Endocrinol. Metab. *74*:593, 1992.
262. Sato, A., Suzuki, H., Murakami, M., et al.: Glucocorticoid increases angiotensin II type 1 receptor and its gene expression. Hypertension *23*:25, 1994.
263. Montwill, J., Igoe, D., and McKenna, T. J.: The overnight dexamethasone test is the procedure of choice in screening for Cushing's syndrome. Steroids *59*:296, 1994.
264. Orth, D. N.: Differential diagnosis of Cushing's syndrome. N. Engl. J. Med. *325*:957, 1991.
265. Trainer, P. J., and Grossman, A.: The diagnosis and differential diagnosis of Cushing's syndrome. Clin. Endocrinol. *34*:317, 1991.
266. Klibanski, A., and Zervas, N. T.: Diagnosis and management of hormone-secreting pituitary adenomas. N. Engl. J. Med. *324*:822, 1991.
267. Trainer, P. J., and Besser, M.: Cushing's syndrome: Therapy directed at the adrenal glands. Endocrinol. Metab. Clin. North Am. *23*:571, 1994.
268. Helmberg, A., Ausserer, B., and Kofler, R.: Frame shift by insertion of 2 basepairs in codon 394 of CYP11B1 causes congenital adrenal hyperplasia due to steroid 11β-hydroxylase deficiency. J. Clin. Endocrinol. Metab. *75*:1278, 1992.
269. de Simone, G., Tommaselli, A. P., Rossi, R., et al.: Partial deficiency of adrenal 11-hydroxylase: A possible cause of primary hypertension. Hypertension *7*:204, 1985.
270. Cottrell, D. A., Bello, F. A., and Falko, J. M.: Case report: 17-Alpha-hydroxylase deficiency masquerading as primary hyperaldosteronism. Am. J. Med. Sci. *300*:380, 1990.
271. Whalen, R. K., Althausen, A. F., and Daniels, G. H.: Extra-adrenal pheochromocytoma. J. Urol. *147*:1, 1992.
272. Nanes, M. S., and Catherwood, B. D.: The genetics of multiple endocrine neoplasia syndromes. Annu. Rev. Med. *43*:253, 1992.
273. Gagel, R. F., Tashjian, A. H., Jr., Cummings, T., et al.: The clinical outcome of prospective screening for multiple endocrine neoplasia type 2a: An 18-year experience. N. Engl. J. Med. *318*:478, 1988.
274. Bravo, E. L.: Evolving concepts in the pathophysiology, diagnosis, and treatment of pheochromocytoma. Endocrinol. Rev. *15*:356, 1994.
275. Atuk, N. O., Hanks, J. B., Weltman, J., et al.: Circulating dihydroxyphenylglycol and norpinephrine concentrations during sympathetic nervous system activation in patients with pheochromocytoma. J. Clin. Endocrinol. Metab. *79*:1609, 1994.
276. Scott, I., Parkes, R., and Cameron, D. P.: Phaeochromocytoma and cardiomyopathy. Med. J. Aust. *148*:94, 1988.
277. Haas, G. J., Tzagournis, M., and Boudoulas, H.: Pheochromocytoma: Catecholamine-mediated electrocardiographic changes mimicking ischemia. Am. Heart J. *116*:1363, 1988.
278. Goldbaum, T. S., Henochowicz, S., Mustafa, M., et al.: Pheochromocytoma presenting with Prinzmetal's angina. Am. J. Med. *81*:921, 1986.
279. Feldman, J. M.: Falsely elevated urinary excretion of catecholamines and metanephrines in patients receiving labetalol therapy. J. Clin. Pharmacol. *27*:288, 1987.
280. Textor, S. C., Canzanello, V. J., Taler, S. J., et al.: Cyclosporine-induced hypertension after transplantation. Mayo Clin. Proc. *69*:1182, 1994.
281. Fahal, I. H., Yaqoob, M., and Ahmad, R.: Phlebotomy for erythropoietin-induced malignant hypertension. Nephron *61*:214, 1992.
282. Lake, C. R., Gallant, S., Masson, E., and Miller, P.: Adverse drug effects attributed to phenylpropanolamine: A review of 142 case reports. Am. J. Med. *89*:195, 1990.
283. Ross, R. D., Clapp, S. K., Gunther, S., et al.: Augmented norepinephrine and renin output in response to maximal exercise in hypertensive coarctation patients. Am. Heart J. *123*:1293, 1992.
284. Stewart, A. B., Ahmed, R., Travill, C. M., and Newman, C. G. H.: Coarctation of the aorta—life and health 20–44 years after surgical repair. Br. Heart J. *69*:65–70, 1993.
285. Shaddy, R. E., Boucek, M. M., Sturtevant, J. E., et al.: Comparison of angioplasty and surgery for unoperated coarctation of the aorta. Circulation *87*:793, 1993.
286. Gidding, S. S., Rocchini, A. P., Beekman, R., et al.: Therapeutic effect of propranolol on paradoxical hypertension after repair of coarctation of the aorta. N. Engl. J. Med. *312*:1224, 1985.
287. Ritchie, C. M., Sheridan, B., Fraser, R., et al.: Studies on the pathogenesis of hypertension in Cushing's disease and acromegaly. Q. J. Med. *76*:855, 1990.
288. Lind, I., Hvarfner, A., Palmer, M., et al.: Hypertension in primary hyperparathyroidism in relation to histopathology. Eur. J. Surg. *157*:457, 1991.
289. Jespersen, B., Brock, A., Charles, P., et al.: Unchanged noradrenaline reactivity and blood pressure after corrective surgery in primary hyperparathyroidism. Scand. J. Clin. Lab. Invest. *53*:470, 1993.
290. Heuser, D., Guggenberger, H., and Fretschner, R.: Acute blood pressure increase during the perioperative period. Am. J. Cardiol. *63*:26C, 1989.
291. Colvin, J. R., and Kenny, G. N. C.: Automatic control of arterial pressure after cardiac surgery. Anaesthesia *44*:37, 1989.
292. Weinstein, G. S., Zabetakis, P. M., Clavel, A., et al.: The renin-angiotensin system is not responsible for hypertension following coronary artery bypass grafting. Ann. Thorac. Surg. *43*:74, 1987.
293. Kaplan, J. A.: Clinical considerations for the use of intravenous nicardipine in the treatment of postoperative hypertension. Am. Heart J. *119*:443, 1990.
294. Estafanous, F. G., Tarazi, R. C., Buckley, S., and Taylor, P. C.: Arterial hypertension in immediate postoperative period after valve replacement. Br. Heart J. *40*:718, 1978.
295. Cockburn, J. S., Benjamin, I. S., Thomson, R. M., and Bain, W. H.: Early systemic hypertension after surgical closure of atrial septal defect. J. Cardiovasc. Surg. *16*:1, 1975.
296. Brozena, S. C., Johnson, M. R., Ventura, J. O., and Naftel, D. C.: Effectiveness of diltiazem or lisinopril for treatment of hypertension in car-

diac transplant patients: A prospective, randomized multi-center trial. Circulation *88* (Part 2):480, 1993.
297. Leenen, F. H. H., Holliwell, D. L., and Cardella, C. J.: Blood pressure and left ventricular anatomy and function after heart transplantation. Am. Heart J. *122:*1087, 1991.
298. Roberts, J. M., and Redman, C. W. G.: Pre-eclampsia: More than pregnancy-induced hypertension. Lancet *341:*1447, 1993.
299. Robillard, P.-Y., Hulsey, T.C., Périanin, J., et al.: Association of pregnancy-induced hypertension with duration of sexual cohabitation before conception. Lancet *344:*973, 1994.
300. Eskenazi, B., Fenster, L., and Sidney, S.: A multivariate analysis of risk factors for preeclampsia. JAMA *266:*231, 1991.
301. Brown, M. A., Reiter, L., Smith, B., et al.: Measuring blood pressure in pregnant women: A comparison of direct and indirect methods. Am. J. Obstet, Gynecol. *171:*661, 1994.
302. Ihle, B. U., Long, P., and Oats, J.: Early onset pre-eclampsia: Recognition of underlying renal disease. Br. Med. J. *294:*79, 1987.
303. Dekker, G. A., and Sibai, B. M.: Early detection of preeclampsia. Am. J. Obstet. Gynecol. *165:*160, 1991.
304. Zhou, Y., Damsky, C. H., Chiu, K., et al.: Preeclampsia is associated with abnormal expression of adhesion molecules by invasive cytotrophoblasts. J. Clin. Invest. *91:*950, 1993.
305. Clark, D. A.: Does immunological intercourse prevent pre-eclampsia? Lancet *344:*969, 1994.
306. Chen, G., Wilson, R., Cumming, G., et al.: Immunological changes in pregnancy-induced hypertension. Eur. J. Obstet, Gynecol. *53:*21, 1994.
307. Seligman, S. P., Buyon, J. P., Clancy, R. M., et al.: The role of nitric oxide in the pathogenesis of preeclampsia. Am. J. Obstet. Gynecol. *171:*944, 1994.
308. Sibai, B. M., Caritis, S. N., Thom, E., et al.: Prevention of preeclampsia with low-dose aspirin in healthy, nulliparous pregnant women. N. Engl. J. Med. *329:*1213, 1993.
309. Carroli, G., Duley, L., Belizán, J. M., and Villar, J.: Calcium supplementation during pregnancy: A systematic review of randomised controlled trials. Br. J. Obstet. Gynaecol. *202:*753, 1994.
310. Redman, C. W. G., and Roberts, J. M.: Management of pre-eclampsia. Lancet *341:*1451, 1993.
311. Sibai, B. M., Gonzalez, A. R., Mabie, W. C., and Moretti, M.: A comparison of labetalol plus hospitalization versus hospitalization alone in the management of preeclampsia remote from term. Obstet. Gynecol. *70:*323, 1987.
312. National High Blood Pressure Education Program Working Group: Report on high blood pressure in pregnancy. Am. J. Obstet. Gynecol. *163:*1689, 1990.
313. Rosa, F. W., Bosco, L. A., Graham, C. F., et al.: Neonatal anuria with maternal angiotensin-converting enzyme inhibition. Obstet. Gynecol. *74:*371, 1989.
314. Sibai, B. M., Mercer, B. M., Schiff, E., and Friedman, S. A.: Aggressive versus expectant management of severe preeclampsia at 28 to 32 weeks' gestation: A randomized controlled trial. Am. J. Obstet. Gynecol. *171:*818, 1994.
315. Paterson-Brown, S., Robson, S. C., Redfern, N., et al.: Hydralazine boluses for the treatment of severe hypertension in pre-eclampsia. Br. J. Obstet. Gynaecol. *101:*409, 1994.
316. Welt, S. I., Dorminy, J. H., Jelovsek, F. R., et al.: The effect of prophylactic management and therapeutics on hypertension disease in pregnancy: Preliminary studies. Obstet. Gynecol. *57:*557, 1981.
317. Rey, E., and Couturier, A.: The prognosis of pregnancy in women with chronic hypertension. Am. J. Obstet. Gynecol. *171:*410, 1994.
318. Moodley, J.: Treatment of eclampsia. Br. J. Obstet. Gynaecol. *97:*99, 1990.
319. Pritchard, J. A., Cunningham, F. G., and Pritchard, S. A.: The Parkland Memorial Hospital protocol for treatment of eclampsia: Evaluation of 245 cases. Am. J. Obstet. Gynecol. *148:*951, 1984.
320. Clark, S. L., Greenspoon, J. S., Aldahl, D., and Phelan, J. P.: Severe preeclampsia with persistent oliguria: Management of hemodynamic subsets. Am. J. Obstet. Gynecol. *154:*490, 1986.
321. Chesley, L. C.: Hypertension in pregnancy: Definitions, familial factor, and remote prognosis. Kidney Int. *18:*234, 1980.
322. Marin-Neto, J. A., Maciel, B. C., Urbanetz, L. L. T., et al.: High output failure in patients with peripartum cardiomyopathy: A comparative study with dilated cardiomyopathy. Am. Heart J. *121:*134, 1991.

HYPERTENSIVE CRISES

323. Webster, J., Petrie, J. C., Jeffers, T. A., and Lovell, H. G.: Accelerated hypertension: Patterns of mortality and clinical factors affecting outcome in treated patients. Q. J. Med. *86:*485, 1993.
324. Lip, G. Y. H., Beevers, M., and Beevers, G.: The failure of malignant hypertension to decline: A survey of 24 years' experience in a multiracial population in England. J. Hypertens. *12:*1297, 1994.
325. Strandgaard, S., and Paulson, O. B.: Cerebral blood flow and its pathophysiology in hypertension. Am. J. Hypertens. *2:*486, 1989.
326. Shapiro, L. M., and Beevers, D. G.: Malignant hypertension: Cardiac structure and function at presentation and during therapy. Br. Heart J. *49:*477, 1983.
327. Kaplan, N. M.: Management of hypertensive emergencies. Lancet *344:*1335, 1994.
328. White, W. B., and Baker, L. H.: Episodic hypertension secondary to panic disorder. Arch. Intern. Med. *146:*1129, 1986.
329. Carlberg, B.: Blood pressure in acute stroke: Causes and consequences. Hypertens. Res. *17* (Suppl. I):S77, 1994.

Chapter 27
Systemic Hypertension: Therapy

NORMAN M. KAPLAN

As noted at the beginning of Chapter 26, the number of patients being treated for hypertension has expanded markedly over the last 25 years so that it is now the leading reason for office visits to physicians. Nonetheless, a recent survey of well-informed hypertensive patients whose costs were completely covered by insurance found that only 12 per cent had their disease under good control.[1] This apparent paradox of expanded coverage but continued poor control is not the consequence of either the ineffectiveness of available therapy or an unwillingness of physicians to provide it. In controlled trials, most patients with the most prevalent form of hypertension, previously called "mild" but now referred to as grade 1, i.e., diastolic blood pressure (DBP) between 90 and 100 mm Hg, achieve excellent control with one of multiple drugs.[2] Relatively few patients are truly resistant to therapy.[3] Moreover, physicians in the United States begin treatment of virtually all patients with blood pressure levels above 140/90 mm Hg.

The problem derives from the inherent nature of hypertension: induced by common but unhealthy life styles, asymptomatic and persistent, with overt consequences delayed by 10 to 30 years so that the costs of therapy, both in money and in adverse effects, seem to outweigh benefits to be derived from adherence to the regimen. Furthermore, behind the inherent nature of the disease that often interferes with patient adherence to their physician's requests, there lurks yet another disquieting feature to the therapy of most hypertension: it may not benefit the majority of patients who adhere faithfully to their treatment. Among "mild" hypertensives, only about one in 500 are saved from a serious adverse effect per year of therapy.[4] Moreover, in some population settings, those who take antihypertensive therapy have higher rates of coronary mortality than those who do not, particularly if they start with relatively mild hypertension.[5] Presumably, the minimum protection they could receive from lower blood pressure is negated by the adverse effects of therapy. Those with higher initial risk have more to gain even if these putative adverse effects persist. Such potential harm from misdirected therapy underscores the need for caution, as called for by Geoffrey Rose[6] and formalized by Jackson et al.,[7] in the use of medication as a preventive measure. Their advice, detailed in the next section, needs to be kept in mind as we consider the general principles and specific details of the treatment of hypertension.

Yet another element, the issue of cost-effectiveness, has been introduced into the debate about the value of treating all patients with any degree of hypertension.[8] As the escalating costs of health care consume a greater share of society's resources, two opposing forces have risen: one, the need for less expensive illness care and the other, the relatively large cost of prevention when indiscriminately applied to low-risk subjects. Therefore, it is likely that the calls for more selective and targeted antihypertensive therapy[7] will be more widely listened to in the future.

We will examine the evidence for benefits of therapy and then apply this evidence to the criteria for the initiation of therapy to individual patients.

BENEFITS OF THERAPY

The treatment of hypertension is aimed not at the simple reduction of blood pressure but at the prevention of the cardiovascular complications that are known to accompany the high pressure.[8a] Over the past 25 years, multiple randomized controlled trials have tested the ability of a limited number of antihypertensive drugs—primarily diuretics and adrenergic inhibitors—to prevent strokes and heart attacks.

A series of meta-analyses from 1986 on have portrayed the effects of therapy in a progressively enlarging number of completed trials.[9–11] They have shown a uniform and persistent reduction in morbidity and mortality from stroke averaging 40 per cent, a reduction that fits exactly to what was predicted from epidemiological evidence if the attributable risk had been completely reversed.[12] On the other hand, the impact on coronary heart disease reported in 1986 on the basis of data from nine trials was not significant, averaging only 8 per cent.[9] By 1990, with analysis of five more sets of data, the reduction was 14 per cent, still below the 20 to 25 per cent predicted if the risk attributed to blood pressure had been completely reversed.[12] By 1993, however, data from three recently reported trials in elderly patients[13–15,15a] brought the overall impact on coronary events to a 16 per cent reduction, with confidence limits of 8 to 23 per cent, which overlap the excess 20 to 25 per cent risk predicted from epidemiological evidence (Figure 27–1).

Some have assumed that these data now prove that treatment of hypertension completely reverses the risk of both stroke and coronary disease, providing "the maximum attainable reduction over a short interval."[16] Caution is advised in assuming that the diuretic and adrenergic blocking drugs used in all of the trials now completed have, in fact, provided all of the protection against coronary disease that could be obtained. Recall that the evidence for the impact on stroke is uniform and equal to that expected, but the evidence on coronary disease is spotty and less impressive. Moreover, only one of the trials involving patients under age 60 showed a significant reduction in coronary events. This trial, the Hypertension Detection and Follow-up Program (HDFP), has been faulted both for its design, by which the control group received less medical care beyond antihypertensive therapy, and for its loose criteria for the diagnosis of coronary events.[4] The large number of coro-

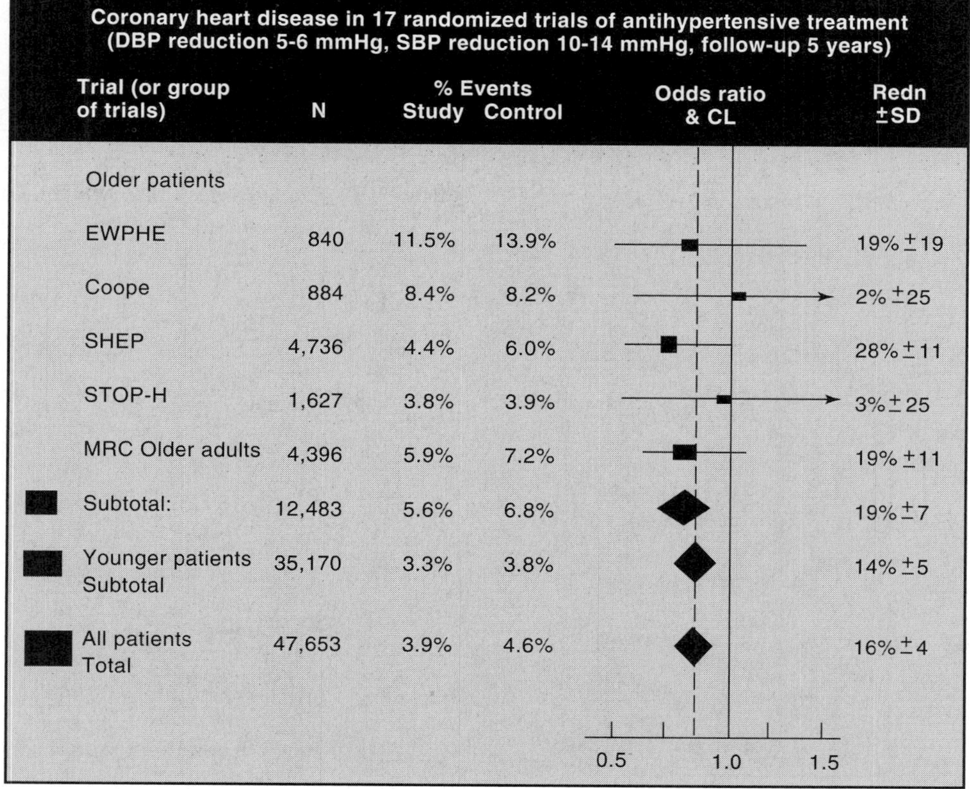

FIGURE 27–1. Effects of blood pressure reduction on coronary heart disease incidence in 12 randomized controlled trials of young patients (most under age 60) and 5 trials in older patients (all over age 60). Box size is proportional to number of events recorded. Horizontal lines denote 99 per cent confidence intervals of odds ratios from individual trial results and diamonds denote 95 per cent confidence intervals for odds ratios for combined trial results. (From MacMahon, S., and Rodgers, A.: The effects of blood pressure reduction in older patients: An overview of five randomized controlled trials in elderly hypertensives. Clin. Exper. Hypertens. *15:* 967, 1993.)

nary events in HDFP provided 31 per cent of the total included in the 1993 meta-analysis, suggesting that "there may have been a systematic bias as a result of flawed design."[4]

Swales concludes, "Despite such misgivings, the consistent trend in all the major trials for a reduction in coronary events, and the impressive significant impact in some trials, particularly in the elderly, allow us to conclude that treatment reduces the frequency of ischaemic heart disease. Nevertheless, the extent of that impact is uncertain and is likely to remain so for some years, and the observed effect may well be heterogeneous, depending on patient groups studied (particularly in relation to age) and classes of drugs used. Meta-analyses that pool disparate studies cannot help us to make such fine distinctions, but where findings are reasonably consistent, as for stroke, they provide robust overall conclusions."[4]

Just as the risks of untreated hypertension rise progressively with every increment in pressure (Fig. 27–2), so do the benefits of treatment increase progressively the higher the level.

BENEFITS FOR SEVERE HYPERTENSION. The evidence for protection from overall and cause-specific mortality by therapy of patients with more severe hypertension (DBP above 110 mm Hg, Table 26–2) is incontrovertible.[17] Whereas most patients with accelerated or malignant hypertension died within a year if left untreated, survival rates of well beyond 50 per cent after 10 years have been reported since effective therapy has been provided.[18] For those with nonmalignant but severe hypertension, the evidence is almost as impressive.[10]

BENEFITS FOR MODERATE HYPERTENSION. Those patients with initial DBP between 100 and 110 mm Hg (grade 2 or moderate) enrolled in the multiple clinical trials have generally been found to benefit from therapy.[10] Nonetheless, there is a need to ensure that their pressure is *persistently* elevated: Even among the patients enrolled in the Australian trial whose DBP was between 105 and 109 after two sets of readings 4 weeks apart, 11 per cent of those given only placebo pills had DBP persistently below 90 mm Hg for the next 4 years.[19] Their blood pressure fell mostly during the first 4 months. Therefore, unless there is an obvious need for the more immediate institution of drug therapy, such as progressive target organ damage or blood pressures so high as to threaten immediate danger, all patients should be given the opportunity to achieve a spontaneous reduction of their initially high pressures over a 4- to 6-month interval. During that time they should have their pressures carefully monitored, since if it goes up—as it did in 10 to 15 per cent of the placebo-treated patients in the multiple trials shown in Figure 27–1—immediate institution of drug therapy may be indicated.

As noted in the preceding chapter, the monitoring logically can be done at home and, for some, with ambulatory 24-hour monitoring, which may provide, in a condensed manner, better prognostic evidence than multiple blood pressure measurements taken in the office. While the blood pressure is being monitored, the use of appropriate nondrug therapies may help lower the pressure even more, without risk and with relatively little inconvenience. Such nondrug therapies may not only lower the blood pressure but also reduce overall cardiovascular risk by amelioration of such conditions as hyperlipidemia, glucose intolerance, and alcohol abuse.

BENEFITS FOR MILD HYPERTENSION. The majority of people with elevated blood pressure, defined as above 140/90 mm Hg, have "mild" hypertension (grade 1) with DBP between 90 and 100 mm Hg (see Chap. 26, Fig. 26–2). As shown in Figure 26–2, even though the risk rises progressively, the sheer number of patients with minimally elevated pressure causes them to make a major contribution to the overall population risk from hypertension. Therefore, the call for population-wide preventive measures makes sense and should be heeded.[20]

However, when individual patients are involved, the issues are not so simple and the answer not so obvious. The rate of cardiovascular complications falls progressively with lower levels of pressure, whether they are naturally lower or lowered by therapy. However, the fall in risk observed in the clinical trials is not a straight-line, linear one, shown as line A in Figure 27–2. Rather, in some studies it follows a curvilinear pattern, with a sharp downward trend at higher levels and a much lower rate of decrease in risk at lower levels, shown as line B in Figure 27–2. As we shall note subsequently, the data from most trials follow a J curve, with an upward trend below some crucial level, shown as line C in Figure 27–2. Disregarding the presence of this J curve for now, it is obvious that less benefit is provided when diastolic pressures are lowered below 100 mm Hg and much less when lowered below 95 mm Hg than when lowered from higher levels (Fig. 27–3). These data are from a trial comparing two forms of therapy[21] and are not included in the meta-analyses of placebo-controlled trials, although the data in them are similar. Thus, in the MRC trial,[22] to prevent one stroke, therapy had to be given for 1 year to 333 patients with entry blood pressure in the 105 to 109 range, but to 666 patients with blood pressure of 100 to 104 and to 2000 patients with blood pressure of 95 to 99 mm Hg.

Thus, lowering, the threshold of treatment from a DBP of 100 down to 95 means that an additional 1334 patients will be treated for 1 year without apparent benefit. The number will be far greater if the threshold is lowered to a DBP of 90. Not only will more patients be treated without apparent benefit, but a far greater number of patients will be treated if a lower threshold is used. In the large population screened for the HDFP, 25.3 per cent had a DBP of 90 or higher,

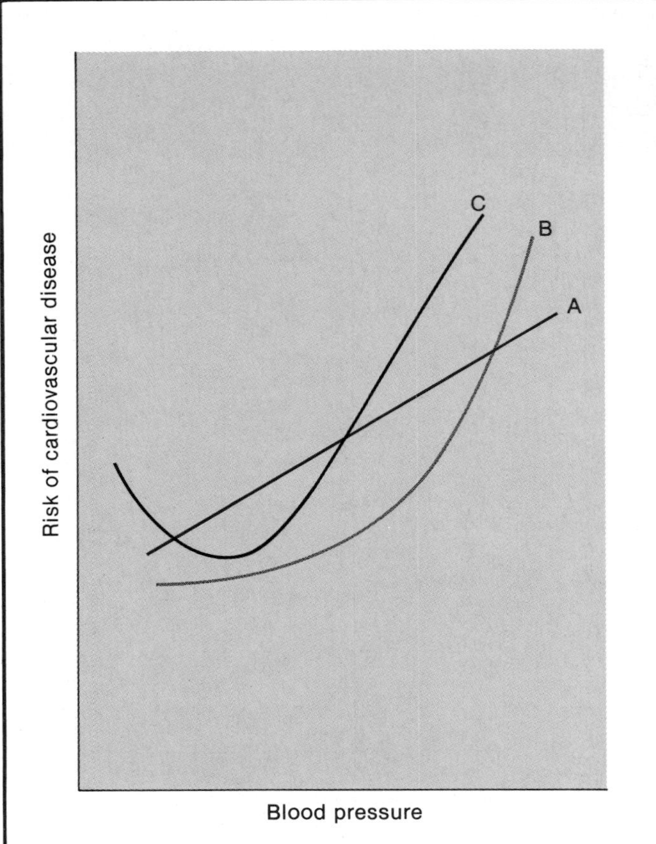

FIGURE 27–2. Three models representing hypothetical relationships between levels of blood pressure and risk of cardiovascular disease. (From Epstein, F. H.: Proceedings of the XVth International Congress of Therapeutics, September 5–9, 1979. Brussels, Excerpta Medica, 1980.)

but 40 per cent of these readings were between 90 and 94 and two-thirds were below 100 mm Hg.

RESULTS OF CLINICAL TRIALS

Whereas the evidence for overall protection of patients with DBP between 95 and 100 is reasonably strong, the evidence for those between 90 and 95 is weak at best and nonexistent in most trials that have included such patients.[23] Part of this failure may reflect the finding that many of the patients in these trials were not, in fact, hypertensive: None of the trials required more than a 2-month run-in period before randomization to active or placebo therapy, and it has been shown that readings in as many as one-third to one-half of patients with DBP above 95 mm Hg will be persistently below 90 mm Hg after 4 to 6 months without therapy.[19]

In addition, as noted, the risks are relatively small at such low levels of elevated blood pressure, and the trials, despite their size and duration, may not have been adequate to show protection with so little preexisting risk. Moreover, the trials mainly involved low-risk, otherwise healthy patients, unlike many seen in clinical practice. In the HDFP trial, those patients with initial DBP between 90 and 95 mm Hg whose pressures were lowered more aggressively (the stepped-care group) had fewer cardiovascular events than did those whose pressures were lowered less.[24] However, the more intensively treated (Special Intervention) half of the patients in the Multiple Risk Factor Intervention Trial (MRFIT) whose initial DBP was between 90 and 94 mm Hg had a *higher* total and coronary death rate than did those given less therapy (Usual Care),[25] so that the evidence from the two large nonplacebo-controlled trials done in the U.S. remains contradictory.

THRESHOLD FOR THERAPY

There is legitimate cause for the disagreement as to the level at which to institute drug therapy, some expert groups such as the U.S. Joint National Committee[26] believing that drug therapy should be given to most with DBP above 90 mm Hg, and others such as the British[27] and Canadian[28] expert committees believing that it should be given only to those with DBP above 100 mm Hg in the absence of coexisting risk factors or target organ damage. The disagreement is not only of academic interest. As many as 40 million persons in the United States alone are in that 90 to 100 mm Hg range, and so obviously the issue has great clinical and economic relevance.

A compromise position was adopted by a conference sponsored by the World Health Organization and the International Society of Hypertension.[29] In substance, it states that after 3 to 6 months of observation, 95 mm Hg DBP should be used as the level for institution of active drug therapy. Patients with DBP between 90 and 95 who are at high overall risk of developing coronary artery disease should be "considered" for treatment.

The recommendations of all these expert committees call for therapy at lower levels of blood pressure when other major risk factors or target organ damage is present. Although it is not possible to predict with certainty which patients will develop complications, the larger the number of other cardiovascular risk factors present, the larger the number of complications observed and the greater the potential for protection by the amelioration of these other risks as well.[30] Because of their relatively lower degree of risk at every level of pressure, women are relatively less in need of therapy than are men.[31]

A Rational Approach

A group of experts from New Zealand have taken into account all of these considerations—level of blood pressure, age, gender, other risk factors, and target organ damage (Table 27–1)—and have constructed a rational approach based on their assessment of the evidence of benefit that has been shown.[7]

Their recommendation is that "people with an estimated absolute risk of cardiovascular disease of about 20 per cent or more in 10 years and a sustained blood pressure greater than 150 mm Hg systolic or 90 mm Hg diastolic (phase 5) should be considered for treatment to lower blood pressure

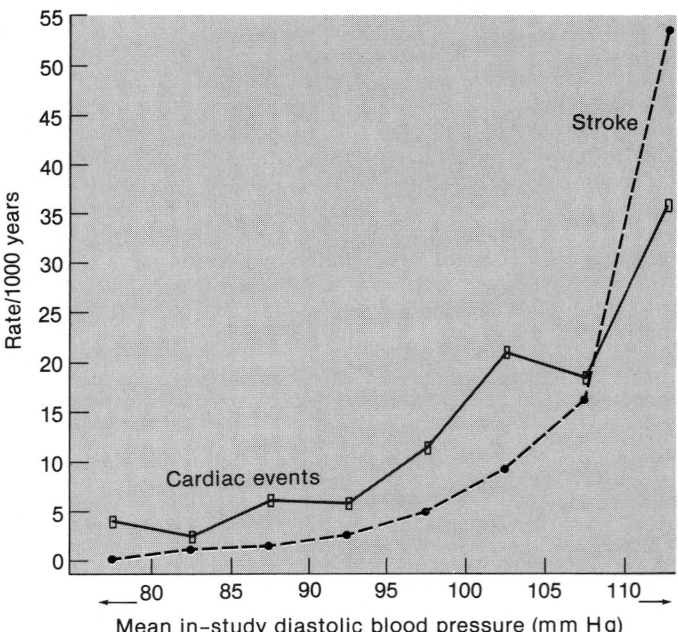

FIGURE 27–3. Absolute rate of cardiac events and stroke related to diastolic blood pressure during antihypertensive treatment. The extremes of the diastolic pressure scale include all values at or below 80 and above 110 mm Hg. Square = cardiac events; Circle = stroke. (From IPPPSH Collaborative Group: Cardiovascular risk and risk factors in a randomized trial of treatment based on the beta-blocker oxprenolol: The International Prospective Primary Prevention Study in Hypertension [IPPPSH]. J. Hypertens. *3*:388, 1985.)

TABLE 27–1 FEATURES CONSIDERED IN THE DECISION TO TREAT

OTHER RISK FACTORS
Cigarette smoking
Total cholesterol/HDL cholesterol ratio >6
Diabetes
Obesity (body mass index >30)
Family history of premature cardiovascular disease (in parent or sibling before age 55)
SYMPTOMATIC CARDIOVASCULAR DISEASE
Angina or silent ischemia
Myocardial infarction
Coronary angioplasty or bypass surgery
Heart failure
Left ventricular hypertrophy demonstrated by ECG or echocardiography
Transient ischemic attacks
Stroke
Peripheral vascular disease
Familial hyperlipidemia
Other target organ damage such as renal disease

From Jackson, R., et al.: Management of raised blood pressure in New Zealand: A discussion document. Br. Med. J. *307*:107, 1993.

(see Figure 27–4 to estimate risk). Lowering the blood pressure of these patients by an average of 5 to 6 mm Hg diastolic (and 10 mm Hg systolic) would reduce their risk of cardiovascular disease by about one-third. In those with an absolute risk of 20 per cent in 10 years, the risk would be reduced to about 13 per cent in 10 years, meaning that one event would be prevented for every 150 patients treated each year. Any adverse effects of treatment are unlikely to outweigh the benefits of treatment at this level of risk, and treatment is likely to be relatively cost-effective. The absolute benefits and cost-effectiveness of treatment would be greater if larger reductions of blood pressure could be achieved.

Notice from Figure 27–4 that the threshold for therapy decreases progressively with degree of hypertension, age, and numbers of other risk factors. Therapy is advised in all patients with sustained average blood pressures above 170/100 regardless of degree of absolute risk. They also recommend that patients under age 40 with levels above 150/90 be referred to a specialist for work-up of secondary causes. These recommendations, as rational as they are, may be too conservative for many practitioners who have accepted the need for "more aggressive" therapy at much lower levels of blood pressure and overall risk. Perhaps the absolute level of risk should be placed at 10 per cent or 15 per cent, but that would obviously expose many more patients to the potential adverse effects and financial costs of therapy without the expectation of benefit. Regardless of whether this really quite simple and rational approach gains widespread acceptance, there is little reason for patients or physicians to be concerned about "watchful waiting." Recall the experience of the placebo-treated half of the patients in the Australian trial[32]: Over 4 years, the average DBP fell below 95 in 47.5 per cent of patients with baseline DBP of 95 to 109, and increased morbidity and mortality were seen only in those whose average DBP remained above 100.

If drug therapy is not given, close surveillance of all patients must be provided, because from 10 to 17 per cent of the placebo-treated patients in various trials had progression of their blood pressure to a level above that considered an indication for active treatment. Moreover, all patients should be strongly advised to use the appropriate life style modifications described on p. 844.

Systolic Pressure in the Elderly

The New Zealand recommendations rationally recommend that therapy be given to the elderly at lower levels of pressure because they "generally have a higher absolute risk of cardiovascular disease and therefore derive greater benefit from treatment."[7] They recognize that little evidence about the value of therapy is available for people aged 80 or over. Since survival seems to be better at higher pressures in those over 80,[33] caution is obviously needed for the older elderly. As seen in Figure 27–1, the elderly achieved even greater protection from coronary disease in the three recently published trials. Furthermore, protection from congestive heart failure was even more impressive, therapy reducing the incidence by over 50 per cent.[13,14]

The New Zealand data include systolic levels in the decision to treat. This is based on the epidemiological evidence reviewed in Chapter 26 that systolic levels are more predictive of long-term prognosis than are diastolic levels and the evidence from the Systolic Hypertension in the Elderly Program (SHEP) trial,[13] wherein excellent protection was shown in a large group of elderly patients with isolated systolic hypertension, the average pretreatment blood pressure being 170/77. A consensus has been reached that systolic blood pressure over 160 mm Hg should be treated, at least to age 80. However, as seen in Figure 27–4, some older women with no other risk factors likely do not need therapy until systolic levels are above 170 mm Hg.

USE OF SURROGATE INDICATIONS. All of the preceding coverage of the benefits of therapy and the threshold for treatment has involved "hard" endpoints: morbidity and mortality. Some argue that softer endpoints should also be taken into account, using as surrogates one or another evidence of cardiovascular damage that may be easier to assess and quicker to appear. These include regression of left ventricular hypertrophy or carotid artery stenosis and reduction of proteinuria. Most, however, hold to the need for the hard endpoints.

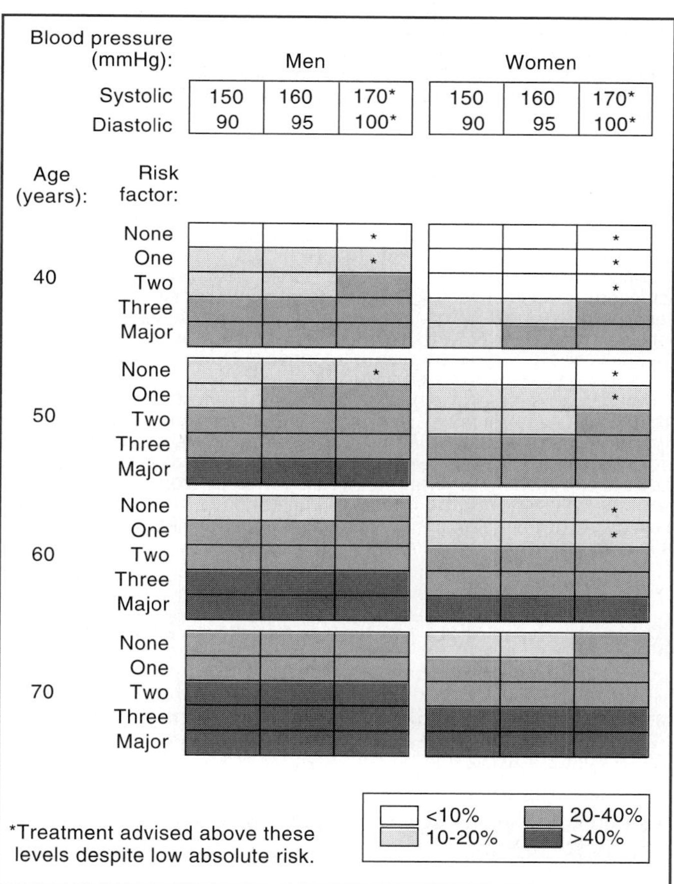

FIGURE 27–4. Absolute risk (percentage) of having a cardiovascular event in 10 years according to age, blood pressure, and other risk factors shown in Table 27–1. (From Jackson, R., et al.: Management of raised blood pressure in New Zealand: A discussion document. Br. Med. J. *307*:107, 1993.)

GOAL OF THERAPY

Once having decided to treat, the clinician must consider the goal of therapy. In the past, most physicians assumed that the effects of reduction of blood pressure on cardiovascular risk would fit a straight line downward (line A in Fig. 27–2),[34] justifying the opinion "the lower, the better." However, as noted, data from large trials indicated a more gradual decline in risk when pressures were reduced to moderate levels (line B in Fig. 27–2), around 95 mm Hg in the IPPPSH trial (Fig. 27–3).[21] Subsequently, Cruickshank[35] called attention to a J curve (line C in Fig. 27–2), reflecting a progressive fall in risk as pressure is lowered, but only to a certain level; below that level, the risk for coronary ischemic events goes back up.

Additional evidence for the J curve has been added to the six retrospective studies analyzed by Cruickshank, including two prospective studies of sizeable numbers of patients.[36,37] Recall, too, the data from HDFP and MRFIT showing higher coronary mortality rates among mild hypertensives with baseline ECG abnormalities if they were given more intensive therapy.[38,39] The apparent propensity to induce myocardial ischemia when pressures are lowered below a certain crucial threshold may not apply to other vital organs. Therefore, maximal protection against stroke or renal damage may require greater falls in pressure than the coronary circulation can safely handle.

The presence of a J curve has been stoutly defended[40] and almost as aggressively denied.[41] Some deny that it occurs except as an "irregularity" of small sets of data in a particularly vulnerable group of patients.[12] On the other hand, the denial of a J-curve on the basis of the absence of a lower threshold of risk in long-term observations on normotensive and mildly hypertensive people free of coronary artery disease and given no antihypertensive therapy[12] should be given no credence as evidence against the presence of such a threshold in more significantly hypertensive patients, often with preexisting coronary artery disease, who are given antihypertensive therapy and whose pressures are thereby "artificially" lowered. This is particularly important in the elderly, who may experience an increase in coronary events with even small decrements in blood pressure, whether induced by antihypertensive therapy or not.[42] The Hypertension Optimal Treatment (HOT) Trial should provide more conclusive evidence about the J curve in patients who were randomized to different target blood pressures.[43] For now, the prudent course is to accept the considerable evidence that a J curve does exist and hope to avoid it by careful, gradual reduction in pressure with agents that do not simultaneously incite other risks.

Once good control of blood pressure in a patient has been achieved, it may be possible to reduce or withdraw drug therapy. Perhaps one-fourth of patients with initially mild hypertension who achieve good control with therapy will remain normotensive for at least 1 year after their therapy is stopped.[44] However, such patients need to remain under observation.

There is no simple or single answer to the questions of whom to treat with drugs for mild hypertension and how much the pressure should be reduced. Each patient must be considered separately, taking various factors into account. The foregoing discussion should indicate the wisdom of withholding drug therapy from many of these patients, at least until the effects of time and life style modifications have been given a chance, thereby avoiding too fast and too great falls in pressure.

LIFE STYLE MODIFICATIONS

Interest in the use of various nondrug therapies, better called life style modifications, for the treatment of hypertension has risen markedly in the past few years. Yet many practitioners either do not use them or use them in a casual, perfunctory manner. This hesitant attitude can be attributed both to the sparseness of firm evidence indicating that these therapies succeed and to the difficulty many have faced in convincing patients to adhere to them. This situation is likely to change: Evidence for the effectiveness of these approaches in lowering blood pressure is growing,[2,45,46] techniques for improving adherence are being popularized, and patients seem increasingly willing to adopt changes in life style. These changes come at a propitious time, when many more people are being identified as hypertensive and are considered in need of lowering of blood pressure. Although most have turned first to drugs, the evidence presented in the previous section suggests that these can be safely withheld from many hypertensives to allow life style modifications a chance to be effective. The need for strong and immediately effective therapy was clear when the majority of patients had fairly severe hypertension; however, as a larger number of patients with mild hypertension have entered the picture, a more gradual approach to their management seems more appropriate. In addition, increasing awareness of the need to address other risk factors, such as dyslipidemia and glucose intolerance, along with hypertension has given additional emphasis to the value of life style modifications that can impact favorably on them as well.

Just as the increased awareness of the problem of patients' frequent poor adherence to drug therapy has led to attempts to improve the situation, similar attention toward adherence to life style modifications is likely to improve their effectiveness. These measures should be introduced gradually and gently. Too many and too drastic changes in life style may discourage patients from accepting them. Eventually, however, all hypertensive patients should benefit from moderate restriction of dietary salt, reduction of excess body weight, regular exercise, and moderation of alcohol intake.[26] As will be noted, when used together these can postpone the onset of hypertension and reduce the severity of existing disease. We will first examine the effect of each modification used alone. The data shown in Figure 27–5 are from the largest and best-controlled study comparing the effects of most of the individual modifications on blood pressure, not in hypertensives but in subjects with high-normal levels, DBP 80 to 89 mm Hg.[45] Altogether, 2182 men and women, aged 30 to 54, were randomly assigned to one of three life style changes (weight reduction, sodium restriction, or stress management) for 18 months or to one of four nutritional supplements (calcium, magnesium, potassium, or fish oil) for 6 months with placebo controls for each group. The results demonstrate a significant effect of weight loss, averaging 3.9 kg, and sodium restriction, averaging 44 mmol/day, but no effect of the other modalities. Obviously, different effects could be seen in various hypertensive patients.

AVOIDANCE OF TOBACCO. Until recently, the major pressor effect of tobacco was missed because patients have not been allowed to smoke in places where blood pressures are recorded. With automatic monitoring, the effect is easy to demonstrate[47] (Fig. 27–6). Patients who smoke or dip snuff should be strongly and repeatedly told to stop. Failing that, they should be advised to monitor their blood pressure while they smoke because such pressures are at least partially responsible for increased risks for cardiovascular disease and should be the target of antihypertensive therapy.

WEIGHT REDUCTION. In most published studies, weight loss has been shown to reduce blood pressure. In a review of adequately controlled intervention studies, a 1.0-kilogram decrease in body weight was accompanied by an average reduction of 1.6/1.3 mm Hg in blood pressure.[48] There may be a threshold, around 4 kg, to observe an effect,[49] but significant falls in pressure have been noted with only modest weight loss.[50] Use of a very low calorie supplement may achieve faster weight loss and marked falls in blood pressure.[51] Moreover, weight loss may reduce the sensitivity of blood pressure to sodium.[52] Although the rate of recidivism among obese people is high, an attempt at weight reduction in all obese hypertensive patients should be made, using whatever level of caloric restriction the patient is able to maintain.

DIETARY SODIUM RESTRICTION. On page 817 evidence was presented incriminating the typically high sodium content of the diet of people living in developed, industri-

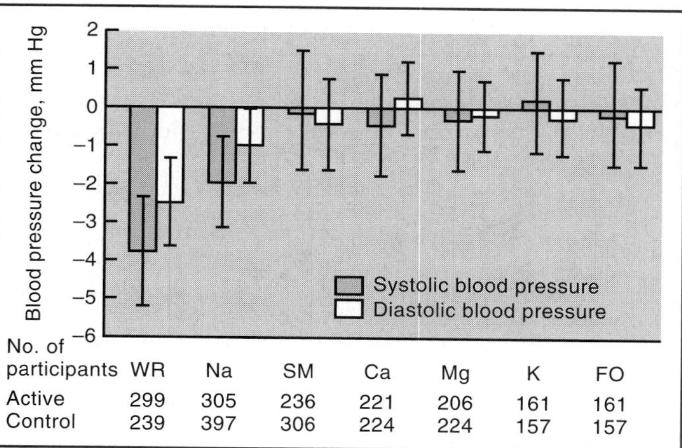

FIGURE 27–5. Net mean changes in systolic and diastolic blood pressure (baseline minus follow-up), with 95 per cent confidence intervals. WR = weight reduction; Na = sodium reduction; SM = stress management; Ca = calcium supplementation; Mg = magnesium supplementation; K = potassium supplementation; FO = fish oil supplementation. (From The Trials of Hypertension Prevention Collaborative Research Group: The effects of nonpharmacologic interventions on blood pressure of persons with high normal levels. Results of the Trials of Hypertension Prevention, Phase I. JAMA *267*:1213, 1992. Copyright 1992 American Medical Association.)

alized societies as a cause of hypertension. Once hypertension is present, modest salt restriction may help lower the blood pressure. In a review by Cutler et al. of 20 well-controlled intervention studies in which daily intake (based on urinary sodium excretion) was reduced by as little as 16 to as much as 171 mmol/day, blood pressure reductions (beyond those seen in controls) averaged 4.9/2.6 mm Hg.[53] There is probably a dose-response relation—the more sodium reduction, the greater the blood pressure fall. In a small but well-controlled study, the fall in blood pressure was shown to be 8/5 mm Hg on a daily sodium intake of 100 mmol and 16/9 mm Hg on a 50 mmol per day intake.[54]

However, rigid degrees of sodium restriction are not only difficult for patients to achieve but may also be counterproductive.[55] The marked stimulation of renin-aldosterone that accompanies rigid sodium restriction may prevent the blood pressure from falling and increase the amount of potassium wastage if diuretics are concomitantly used. Not all hypertensives will respond to a moderate degree of sodium restriction to a level of 70 to 100 mmol sodium, or approximately 2 gm per day. Blacks and elderly patients may be more responsive to sodium restriction, perhaps because of their usually lower renin responsiveness.[56]

Even if the blood pressure does not fall with moderate degrees of sodium restriction, the patient may still benefit: Improved beta-adrenergic responsiveness,[57] increased antihypertensive effectiveness of other drugs,[58] less diuretic-induced potassium wastage,[55] and reduction in left ventricular hypertrophy[59] have all been reported among patients on moderate sodium restriction. Although there is no certainty that moderate sodium restriction will help, there is little evidence that it will hurt.[55] For example, neither the intake of other vital nutrients[60] nor exercise tolerance in a hot environment[61] is reduced by a lower sodium intake.

Therefore, I consider it to be useful for all persons, as a preventive measure in those who are normotensive, and, more certainly, as partial therapy in those who are hypertensive. Population-wide reductions may be possible[62] with a considerable potential thereby to reduce cardiovascular mortality.[63] Although some believe that a "wholesale recommendation to add sodium restriction to antihypertensive therapy is not warranted,"[64] I believe that the potential benefits far outweigh the costs.

The easiest way to accomplish moderate sodium restriction is to substitute natural foods for processed foods, since natural foods are low in sodium and high in potassium, whereas most processed foods have had sodium added and potassium removed. Additional guidelines include the following:

1. Add no sodium chloride to food during cooking or at the table.
2. If a salty taste is desired, use a half sodium and half potassium chloride preparation (such as Lite Salt) or a pure potassium chloride substitute.
3. Avoid or minimize the use of "fast" foods, many of which have high sodium content.
4. Recognize the sodium content of some antacids and proprietary medications. (For example, Alka-Seltzer contains more than 500 mg of sodium; Rolaids are virtually sodium free.)

POTASSIUM SUPPLEMENTATION. Some of the advantages of a lower sodium intake may relate to its tendency to increase body potassium content, both by a coincidental increase in dietary potassium intake and by a decrease in potassium wastage if diuretics are being used. Potassium deficiency exerts multiple effects that may increase blood pressure,[65] and potassium infusions increase the vasodilating effect of acetylcholine, apparently through the nitric oxide pathway.[66] Potassium supplements have been shown to reduce the blood pressure an average of 8.2/4.5 mm Hg in 19 trials published up to 1990.[67] Nonetheless, potassium supplements are too costly and potentially hazardous for routine use in normokalemic hypertensives. Patients should be protected from potassium depletion and encouraged to increase dietary potassium intake, which may be enough to lower blood pressure.[68]

MAGNESIUM SUPPLEMENTATION. In controlled trials little effect on blood pressure is seen with magnesium supplements.[69] However, those who are magnesium depleted may not be able to replete concomitant potassium deficiency.[70]

CALCIUM SUPPLEMENTATION. As noted on page 818, an increase in free calcium concentration in vascular smooth muscle cells may be a final step in the pathogenesis of primary hypertension. Nonetheless, some hypertensive patients have a lower calcium intake and higher urinary calcium excretion than do normotensives.[71] In 22 mostly short-term studies, about one-third of hypertensives given 1 to 2 gm of supplemental calcium per day exhibited a fall in blood pressure.[72] Elderly hypertensives appeared to be even less responsive.[73] Because some given calcium supplements have a rise in blood pressure, the best course is to ensure that calcium intake is not inadvertently reduced by reduction of milk and cheese consumption in an attempt to reduce saturated fat and sodium intake when supplemental calcium is not taken.

OTHER DIETARY CHANGES. Some lowering of the blood pressure has been noted in studies of a lacto-ovo-vegetarian diet,[74] high fiber intake,[75] and high doses of omega-3 fatty acids from fish oil.[76] No additional effect of 6-gm daily supplements of fish oil was found in those who regularly ate fish three or more times a week.[77] Decreases in total dietary fat do not seem to alter blood pressure.[78] In the attempt to reduce calories and overall coronary risk, substitution of carbohydrate for fat may aggravate further the hyperinsulinemia often present in primary hypertension and therefore may be counterproductive.[79] Consumption of dried garlic powder lowered diastolic pressure in four of seven trials compared with placebo.[80]

When consumed by noncoffee drinkers, caffeine equivalent to the amount in two to three cups of coffee raises the blood pressure, probably by activation of the sympathetic nervous system.[81] However, chronic caffeine ingestion is *not* associated with significant rises in blood pressure because of tolerance to the hemodynamic effects.

MODERATION OF ALCOHOL. Moderate alcohol consumption, less than 1 oz of ethanol per day, does not increase the prevalence of hypertension. Heavier drinking clearly exerts a pressor effect that makes *alcohol abuse the most common cause of reversible hypertension.*[64] One to two portions of alcohol-containing beverages a day, containing 0.5 to 1.0 oz of ethanol, need not be prohibited, particu-

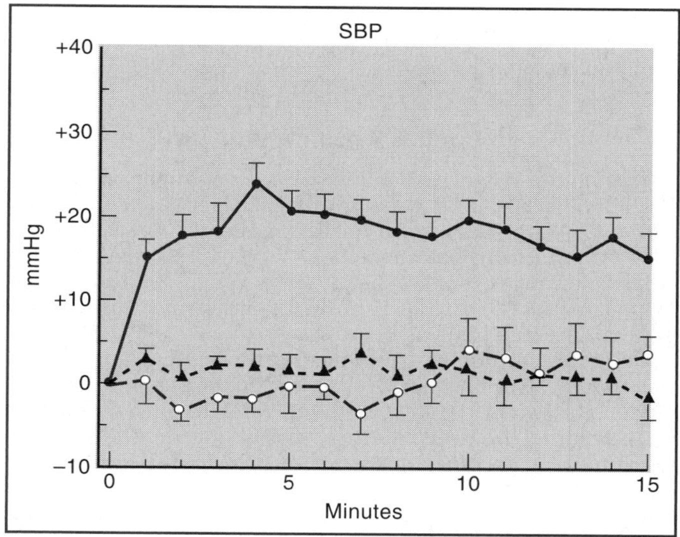

FIGURE 27–6. Changes in systolic blood pressure (SBP) over 15 minutes after smoking the first cigarette of the day within the first 5 minutes *(solid circles),* during no activity *(open circles),* and during sham-smoking *(triangles)* in normotensive smokers. (From Groppelli, A., et al.: Blood pressure and heart rate response to repeated smoking before and after beta blockade and selective α_1 inhibition. J. Hypertens. *10*:495, 1992.)

larly because fewer coronary events and lower mortality have been noted in those who consume that amount.[82]

PHYSICAL EXERCISE. Although the systolic pressure rises considerably during dynamic (aerobic) exercise, vascular compliance increases[83] and resting blood pressure usually falls[84] in hypertensives after regular exercise programs. Unfit patients are at increased risk for coronary ischemia if they engage in heavy exercise,[85] and so a gradual buildup is advisable. Although pure static exercise acutely raises both systolic and diastolic pressures, repetitive circuit weight training also lowers blood pressure.[86]

RELAXATION TECHNIQUES. A review of 26 reports of various forms of relaxation—transcendental meditation, yoga, biofeedback, psychotherapy—reports that they were no more effective in lowering blood pressure than were sham controls.[87]

COMBINED THERAPIES

When multiple life style modifications are combined, additional antihypertensive effects may be seen. The best study is the placebo arm of the Treatment of Mild Hypertension Study (TOMHS),[2] in which 234 mild hypertensives followed a 48-month regimen of moderate sodium restriction, weight loss, regular exercise, and moderation of alcohol. Despite relatively small changes in weight (average loss of 6.6 lbs), sodium intake (reduction of 10 per cent), exercise level, and alcohol consumption, these patients had an 8.6/8.6 mm Hg fall in blood pressure at the end of the 4-year program. Moreover, they experienced improvements in lipid profile and reduction in left ventricular mass.

THE POTENTIAL OF LIFE STYLE MODIFICATIONS

Part of the antihypertensive effect reported in this and other trials of life style modification may be attributable to the nonspecific fall in blood pressure so often seen when repeated readings are taken. Such decreases may reflect a statistical regression toward the mean, a placebo effect, or a relief of anxiety and stress with time. The same phenomenon is probably also responsible for much of the initial response to drug therapy, so that success may be attributed to both drugs and nondrugs when it is deserved by neither.

Nonetheless, increasingly long and strong evidence from controlled studies attests to the efficacy of multifaceted nondrug programs to reduce the blood pressure. Whether such success can be achieved by individual practitioners is uncertain. However, because help is available, including various educational materials for patients, professional assistants such as dietitians and psychologists, and groups organized for weight reduction, exercise, and relaxation therapies, the effort seems both increasingly easy and likely to be successful in lowering blood pressure.

TABLE 27–2 GENERAL GUIDELINES TO IMPROVE PATIENT ADHERENCE TO ANTIHYPERTENSIVE THERAPY

1. Be aware of the problem of nonadherence and be alert to signs of patient nonadherence.
2. Establish the goal of therapy: to reduce blood pressure to normotensive levels with minimal or no side effects.
3. Educate the patient about the disease and its treatment.
   a. Involve the patient in decision-making.
   b. Encourage family support.
4. Maintain contact with the patient.
   a. Encourage visits and calls to allied health personnel.
   b. Allow the pharmacist to monitor therapy.
   c. Give feedback to the patient via home BP readings.
   d. Make contact with patients who do not return.
5. Keep care inexpensive and simple.
   a. Do the least work-up needed to rule out secondary causes.
   b. Obtain follow-up laboratory data only yearly unless indicated more often.
   c. Use home blood pressure readings.
   d. Use nondrug, no-cost therapies.
   e. Use the fewest daily doses of drugs needed.
   f. If appropriate, use combination tablets.
   g. Tailor medication to daily routines.
6. Prescribe according to pharmacological principles.
   a. Add one drug at a time.
   b. Start with small doses, aiming for 5 to 10 mm Hg reductions at each step.
   c. Prevent volume overload with adequate diuretic and sodium restriction.
   d. Take medication immediately upon awakening or after 4 A.M. if patient awakens to void.
   e. Ensure 24-hour effectiveness by home or ambulatory monitoring.
   f. Continue to add effective and tolerated drugs, stepwise, in sufficient doses to achieve the goal of therapy.
   g. Be willing to stop unsuccessful therapy and try a different approach.
   h. Adjust therapy to ameliorate side effects that do not spontaneously disappear.

From Kaplan, N. M.: Clinical Hypertension. 6th ed. Baltimore, © Williams & Wilkins, 1994, p. 197.

ANTIHYPERTENSIVE DRUG THERAPY

If the life style modifications just described are not followed or prove to be ineffective, or if the level of hypertension at the onset is so high that immediate drug therapy is deemed necessary, the general guidelines listed in Table 27–2 should be helpful in improving patient adherence to lifelong treatment.

General Guidelines

The points listed in Table 27–2 are all aimed at providing effective, 24-hour control of hypertension in a manner that encourages adherence to the regimen. The approach is based on known pharmacological principles and proven ways to improve adherence. It is designed for the 90 per cent of patients with fairly mild hypertension, in whom a gradual approach is feasible.

Once the selection of the most appropriate agent for initial therapy has been made (by a process that will be discussed further in the next section), a relatively low dose of a single drug should be started, aiming for a reduction of 5 to 10 mm Hg in blood pressure at each step. Many physicians, by nature and training, desire to control a patient's hypertension rapidly and completely. Regardless of which drugs are used, this approach often leads to easy fatigability, weakness, and postural dizziness, which many patients find intolerable, particularly when they felt well before therapy was begun. Although hypokalemia and other electrolyte abnormalities may be responsible for some of these symptoms, a more likely explanation has been provided by the studies of Strandgaard and Haunsø.[88] As shown in Figure 27–7, they demonstrated the constancy of cerebral blood flow by autoregulation over a range of mean arterial pressures from about 60 to 120 mm Hg in normal subjects and from 110 to 180 mm Hg in patients with hypertension. This shift to the right protects the hypertensive patient from a surge of blood flow, which could cause cerebral edema. However, the shift also predisposes the hypertensive patient to cerebral ischemia when blood pressure is lowered.

The lower limit of autoregulation necessary to preserve a constant cerebral blood flow in hypertensive patients is a mean of about 110 mm Hg. Thus acutely lowering the pressure from 160/110 (mean = 127) to 140/85 (mean = 102) may induce cerebral hypoperfusion, although hypotension in the accepted sense has not been produced. This provides an explanation for what many patients experience at the start of antihypertensive therapy, i.e., manifestations of cerebral hypoperfusion, even though blood pressure levels do not seem inordinately low.

Thus, there should be a gradual approach to antihypertensive therapy in order to avoid symptoms related to overly aggressive blood pressure reduction. Fortunately, as shown in the middle of Figure 27–7, if therapy is continued for a period of time, the curve of cerebral autoregulation shifts back toward normal, allowing patients to tolerate greater reductions in blood pressure without experiencing symptoms.

STARTING DOSAGES. The need to start with a fairly small dosage also reflects a greater responsiveness of some patients to doses of medication that may be appropriate for the majority. All drugs exert increasing effect with increasing dosages, portrayed by a log-linear dose-response curve[89] (Fig. 27–8). However, different patients re-

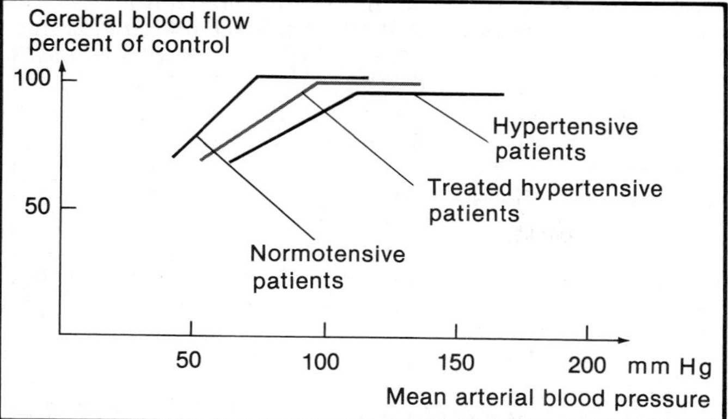

FIGURE 27–7. Mean cerebral blood flow autoregulation curves from normotensive, severely hypertensive, and effectively treated hypertensive patients are shown. (Modified from Strandgaard [Circulation *53*:720, 1976.] From Strandgaaard, S., Haunsø, S.: Why does antihypertensive treatment prevent stroke but not myocardial infarction? Lancet *2*:658, 1987. © by the Lancet Ltd.)

quire different absolute amounts of drug for their own dose response.

As a hypothetical example, for the majority of patients, 50 mg of the beta blocker atenolol would provide a moderate response, shown as point A on the Therapeutic Effect curve, whereas a dose of 25 mg would provide only a minimal response. At the dose A, providing the significant albeit partial response, the side effects would be minimal, as shown by point A′ on the curve of Toxic Effect. If a starting dose of 100 mg were used, the therapeutic effect would be near maximal (point B) but the side effects would be much greater as well (point B′). Therefore, a lower starting dose is preferable for most patients.

However, the response to a given dose is not the same for all patients but rather assumes a bell-shaped curve; some patients are very sensitive to that dose and some very resistant, the majority having a moderate response. Therefore, a significant minority of patients—the very sensitive ones—would obtain a near-maximal response to the 25-mg dose and would better be started on 12.5 mg in order to achieve a moderate therapeutic effect (point A) with minimal side effects (point A′). Without knowing how individual patients will respond, the safest and easiest approach is to start at a dose that probably is not enough for most patients.

The situation was well described by Herxheimer.[90] "For a new drug to penetrate the market quickly, it should be rapidly effective in a high proportion of patients and simple to use. To achieve this, the dosage of the first prescription is therefore commonly set at about the ED_{90} level, i.e., the dose which the early clinical (phase 2) studies have shown to be effective in 90 per cent of the target population, provided that the unwanted effects at this dose are considered acceptable. In 25 per cent of patients a smaller—perhaps much smaller—dose (the ED_{25}) will be effective. The patients in this quartile are the most sensitive to the drug and are liable to receive far more than they need if they are given the ED_{90}. They are also likely to be more sensitive to the dose-related side effects of the drug."

As I have written,[91] Herxheimer goes on to recommend a logical solution: starting doses should be less than the usual maximal effective dose. For this to be effective, however, physicians must be willing to start most patients with a dose of medication that will not be fully effective. As he states, "The disadvantage from the marketing standpoint is that for the majority of patients the dose must be titrated. That is time-consuming for doctors and patients and more difficult to explain to them. A drug requiring dose titration cannot be presented as the 'quick fix', the instant good news that marketing departments love."[90] The quick fix is inappropriate for most hypertensive patients. To allow for autoregulation of blood flow to maintain perfusion to vital organs when perfusion pressure is lowered, the fall in pressure should be relatively small and gradual.[88] More precipitous falls in pressure as frequently seen with larger starting doses may induce considerable hypoperfusion that results in symptoms that are at least bothersome (fatigue, impotence) and that may be potentially hazardous (postural hypotension, coronary ischemia). It is far better to start low and go slow.[91]

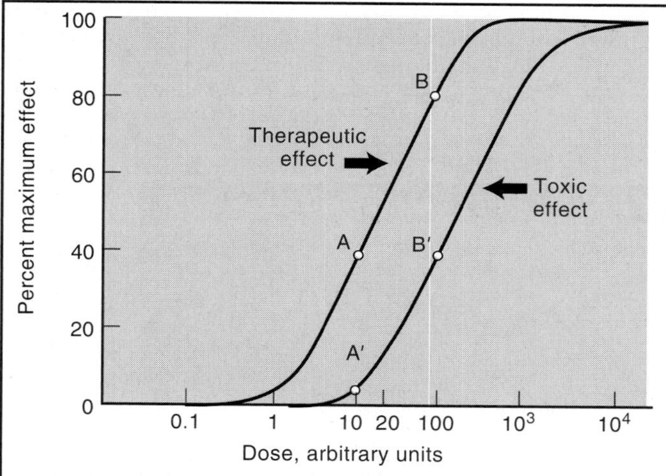

FIGURE 27–8. Theoretical therapeutic and toxic logarithmic-linear dose-response curves. The horizontal axis is a logarithmic scale with arbitrary dose units. The vertical axis is a linear scale showing percentage of maximum possible response. See text for discussion. (From Fagan, T. C.: Remembering the lessons of basic pharmacology. Arch. Intern. Med. *154*:1430, 1994. Copyright 1994 American Medical Association.)

DRUG COMBINATIONS. Combinations of smaller doses of two drugs from different classes have been marketed to take advantage of the differences in the dose-response curves for therapeutic and toxic (side) effects shown in Figure 27–8.[91a] By combining two drugs, each at a dose near point A, a greater antihypertensive effect will be provided (up to point B), but because the side effects are not additive for different classes of drugs, they remain at point A′. A combination of low doses of a beta blocker (bisoprolol) and a diuretic (hydrochlorothiazide) has been approved for initial therapy for hypertension, after it was shown to provide antihypertensive efficacy far beyond that of each component but with no more side effects than seen with each separately.[92] More and more low-dose combinations are likely to become available.

COMPLETE COVERAGE WITH ONCE DAILY DOSING. A number of choices within each of the six major classes of antihypertensive drugs now available provide full 24-hour efficacy. Therefore, single daily dosing should be feasible for virtually all patients, thereby improving adherence to therapy.[93] Moreover, the use of longer-acting agents avoids the potential of inducing too great a peak effect in order to provide an adequate effect at the end of the dosing interval (the trough). As seen in Figure 27–9, when the angiotensin-converting enzyme (ACE) inhibitor enalapril was given in a once-daily dose large enough to achieve a trough effect, the peak effect was greater than desired.[94] When the same total dosage of the drug was given in two doses, a much smoother effect with excellent peak and trough effects was obtained.

Rather than adding to the patient's burden (and expense) of taking two doses a day, the better way to accomplish the desired sustained effect is to use inherently longer-acting drugs (or sustained-release formulations of shorter-acting ones). As noted, such choices are available within each class.[95] However, because patients differ not only as to degree of response but also as to the duration of effect, the prudent course is to document the patient's response at the end of the dosing interval by home or ambulatory monitoring. With this approach the abrupt surge in blood pressure that occurs on awakening will be blunted, and, it is hoped, patients can be better protected from the increased incidence of cardiovascular catastrophes at this crucial time.

If medications are taken at bedtime in order to ensure coverage in the early morning, ischemia to vital organs might be induced by the combination of the maximal effect of the drug within the first 3 to 6 hours after intake and the usual nocturnal fall in pressure. Therefore, the safest course is to take medications with 24-hour duration of action as early in the morning as possible, as early as 4 or 5 A.M. if the patient awakens to urinate.

THE INITIAL CHOICE. The initial choice of antihypertensive therapy is perhaps the most important decision made in the treatment process. That drug is likely to be effective in about half the patients and, if no significant overt side

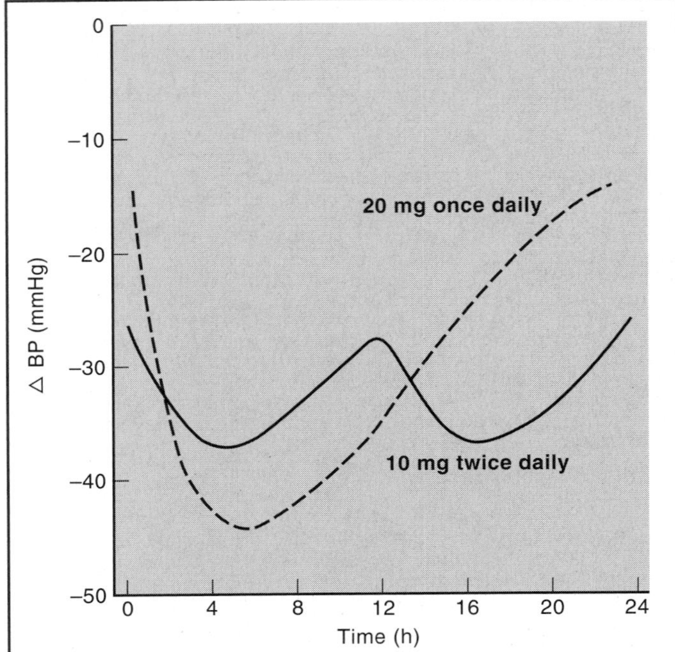

FIGURE 27–9. Comparison of blood pressure (BP) response profiles (placebo-controlled) in a representative patient following 20 mg enalapril once a day and 10 mg twice a day. (From Elliott, H.L.: Trough: Peak ratio and twenty-four-hour blood pressure control. J. Hypertens. *12*[Suppl. 5]:S29, 1994.)

effects occur, may be taken for many years. If the choice is ineffective or bothersome, the patient's confidence may be shaken, postponing or preventing adequate control. A number of guidelines by expert committees have been recently published. About half of them, including the U.S. Joint National Committee (JNC),[26] recommend diuretics or beta blockers for initial therapy.[96] The rationale is simple, as stated in the JNC-5 report: "Because diuretics and beta blockers are the only classes of drugs that have been used in long-term controlled clinical trials and have been shown to reduce morbidity and mortality, they are recommended as first-choice agents." The preference given to diuretics and beta blockers has been roundly criticized as a backward step, going against the rapidly rising use of newer agents.[97,98] However, the critics have failed to read the remainder of the JNC-5 statement: ". . . unless they are contraindicated or unacceptable, or unless there are special indications for other agents."[26]

There are multiple considerations listed in JNC-5 that may be taken into account when choosing initial therapy. These include demography, the presence of concomitant conditions, quality of life, physiological measurements, and cost. The importance of demography is nicely portrayed in the results of a large Veterans Administration cooperative trial in which younger and older and black and white hypertensive men were randomly assigned to a drug representing each of the six major classes or a placebo.[99] When the percentage of responders to each drug was determined for each demographic group, the same drug (the ACE inhibitor captopril) was found to be the most effective drug for the younger whites but the least effective drug for the older blacks.

INDIVIDUALIZED THERAPY. Perhaps the most crucial factor in the selection process is the presence of one or more concomitant conditions, some that could be worsened by the drug chosen, others that could be improved. Table 27–3 is my formulation of the relative appropriateness of members of the five major classes, not including centrally acting alpha-agonists, which are not included in the JNC-5 choices for initial therapy. Most of these preferences or contraindications are obvious; others will be defended later in this chapter. Regardless of the correctness of this formulation, the concept is absolutely valid: The choice of therapy should be individualized.

SUBSTITUTION. Even after a careful attempt to select the most appropriate drug for an individual patient, the choice may be either ineffectual in perhaps a third or unacceptable because of side effects in another 10 to 20 per cent of all patients. Although the overall effectiveness of all approved drugs is about equal in the general population,[2] individual patients show considerable variability in their response to different drugs.[100] Therefore, the physician must be willing to discontinue the initial choice and try a drug from another category. A more structured trial and error approach has been described in which each patient is put through multiple double-blind, randomized crossover trials against placebos to determine the best drug.[101] However, this approach probably is too much trouble for most physicians and patients. Other approaches have been recommended, including one based on the renin profile[102] and another on multiple hemodynamic features.[103] The general principles shown in Tables 27–2 and 27–3 should serve well to ensure that each patient receives a drug likely to provide good control and few side effects.

For patients with more severe hypertension, in whom the first choice can be expected to be only partially effective, the stepped-care approach is logical. A diuretic will enhance the effectiveness of most other drugs used, preventing the "pseudotolerance" that develops because of the fluid retention that frequently follows the use of some adrenergic blocking drugs and vasodilators. Increasingly, an

TABLE 27–3 INDIVIDUALIZED CHOICES OF THERAPY

COEXISTING CONDITION	DIURETIC	BETA BLOCKER	ALPHA BLOCKER	CALCIUM BLOCKER	ACEI
Older age (> 65)	++	+/−	+	+	+
Black race	++	+/−	+	+	+/−
Angina	+/−	++	+	++	+
Post-myocardial infarction	+	++	+	+/−*	++
Congestive failure	++	+/−	+	−	++
Cerebrovascular disease	+	+	+/−	++	+
Renal insufficiency	++	+/−	+	++	++
Diabetes	+/−	−	++	+	++
Dyslipidemia	−	−	++	+	+
Asthma or COPD	+	−	+	+	+
Benign prostatic hypertrophy			++		

++ = preferred; + = suitable; +/− = usually not preferred; − = usually contraindicated; * = dihydropyridines may be contraindicated; ACEI = angiotensin-converting enzyme inhibitors.

ACE inhibitor or calcium antagonist is being chosen as the second or third drug when triple therapy is needed.

THE GOAL OF THERAPY. As discussed earlier in the chapter, caution is advised in lowering diastolic pressure below 85 mm Hg, the apparent nadir of the J curve, particularly in patients prone to coronary disease. On the other hand, lower levels may prove to be maximally effective in other groups such as diabetics with nephropathy.

THE PLACE OF GUIDELINES. As noted, a number of guidelines on the treatment of hypertension by expert committees have recently been published (see p. 1991). Although considerable differences exist between them and a number of valid objections have been raised to the entire process of establishing such guidelines,[96] these structured recommendations are finding increased use in the rapidly expanding world of managed care.[104] Like them or not they have a place, and I believe they should be used, not as rigid legal documents but as gentle persuasions coming from the best-thinking of independent, informed experts who wish to ease the way for the harried practitioner.

DIURETICS

(See also pp. 498 to 499)

Diuretics useful in the treatment of hypertension may be divided into four major groups by their primary site of action within the tubule, starting in the proximal portion and moving to the collecting duct: (1) agents acting on the proximal tubule, such as carbonic anhydrase inhibitors, which have limited antihypertensive efficacy; (2) loop diuretics; (3) thiazides and related sulfonamide compounds; and (4) potassium-sparing agents (Fig. 16–3, p. 476). A thiazide is the usual choice, often in combination with a potassium-sparing agent. Loop diuretics should be reserved for those patients with renal insufficiency or resistant hypertension.

MECHANISM OF ACTION. All diuretics initally lower the blood pressure by increasing urinary sodium excretion and by reducing plasma volume, extracellular fluid volume, and cardiac output.[91a] Within 6 to 8 weeks the lowered plasma, extracellular fluid volume, and cardiac output return toward normal. At this point and beyond, the lower blood pressure is related to a fall in peripheral resistance, thereby improving the underlying hemodynamic defect of hypertension. The mechanism responsible for the lowered peripheral resistance is unknown, but there is a need for an initial diuresis, because diuretics fail to lower the blood pressure when the excreted sodium is returned or when given to chronic dialysis patients with nonfunctioning kidneys. With the shrinkage in blood volume and lower blood pressure, increased secretion of renin and aldosterone retards the continued sodium diuresis. Both renin-induced vasoconstriction and aldosterone-induced sodium retention prevent continued diminution of body fluids and progressive fall in blood pressure while diuretic therapy is continued.

CLINICAL EFFECTS. With continuous diuretic therapy, blood pressure usually falls about 10 mm Hg, although the degree depends on various factors, including the initial height of the pressure, the quantity of sodium ingested, the adequacy of renal function, and the intensity of the counterregulatory renin-aldosterone response. The antihypertensive effect of the diuretic persists indefinitely, although it may be overwhelmed by dietary sodium intake above 8 gm per day.

If other antihypertensive drugs are used, a diuretic may also be needed. Without a concomitant diuretic, antihypertensive drugs that do not block the renin-aldosterone mechanism may cause sodium retention. This mechanism probably reflects the success of the drugs in lowering the blood pressure and may involve the abnormal renal pressure–natriuresis relationship that is presumably present in primary hypertension. Just as it takes more pressure to excrete a given load of sodium in the hypertensive individual, so does a lowering of pressure toward normal incite sodium retention.

The crucial need for adequate diuretic therapy to keep intravascular volume diminished has been repeatedly documented.[105] Therefore, diuretics are likely to continue to be widely used in antihypertensive therapy. Drugs that inhibit the renin-aldosterone mechanism, such as ACE inhibitors, or drugs that induce some natriuresis themselves, such as calcium antagonists, may continue to work without the need for concomitant diuretics. However, a diuretic will enhance the effectiveness of all other types of drugs, including calcium antagonists.[106]

DOSAGE AND CHOICE OF AGENT. Most patients with mild to moderate hypertension and serum creatinine concentrations below 2.0 mg/dl will respond to the lower doses of the various diuretics listed in Table 27–4. An amount equivalent to 12.5 mg of hydrochlorothiazide is usually adequate; larger doses will have some additional antihypertensive effect but at the price of additional potassium wastage and insulin resistance.[107] For uncomplicated hypertension, a moderately long-acting thiazide is a logical choice, and a single morning dose of hydrochlorothiazide will provide a 24-hour antihypertensive effect. The nonthiazide agent indapamide has special properties that make it an attractive choice; it seldom disturbs lipid or glucose levels.[108] With renal failure, manifested by a serum creatinine level above 2.0 mg/dl or creatinine clearance below 25 ml/min, thiazides are usually not effective, and multiple doses of furosemide, one or two doses of torsemide,[109] or a single dose of metolazone will be needed.

SIDE EFFECTS. A number of biochemical changes often accompany successful diuresis, including a decrease in plasma potassium and increases in glucose, insulin, and cholesterol (Fig. 27–10).

Hypokalemia. Serum potassium falls an average of 0.67 mmol/liter after institution of continuous, daily diuretic

TABLE 27–4 DIURETICS AND POTASSIUM-SPARING AGENTS

AGENT	DAILY DOSAGE (mg)	DURATION OF ACTION (hr)
THIAZIDES		
Bendroflumethiazide (Naturetin)	2.5–5.0	More than 18
Benzthiazide (Aquatag, Exna)	12.5–50	12–18
Chlorothiazide (Diuril)	125–500	6–12
Cyclothiazide (Anhydron)	0.5–2	18–24
Hydrochlorothiazide (Esidrix, HydroDIURIL, Oretic)	6.25–50	12–18
Hydroflumethiazide (Saluron)	12.5–50	18–24
Methyclothiazide (Enduron)	2.5–5.0	More than 24
Polythiazide (Renese)	1–4	24–48
Trichlormethiazide (Metahydrin, Naqua)	1–4	More than 24
RELATED SULFONAMIDE COMPOUNDS		
Chlorthalidone (Hygroton)	12.5–50	24–72
Indapamide (Lozol)	2.5	24
Metolazone (Zaroxolyn, Diulo)	0.5–10	24
Quinethazone (Hydromox)	25–100	18–24
LOOP DIURETICS		
Bumetanide (Bumex)	0.5–5	4–6
Ethacrynic acid (Edecrin)	25–100	12
Furosemide (Lasix)	40–480	4–6
Torsemide (Demadex)	5–40	12
POTASSIUM-SPARING AGENTS		
Amiloride (Midamor)	5–10	24
Spironolactone (Aldactone)	25–100	8–12
Triamterene (Dyrenium)	50–100	12

From Kaplan, N. M.: Clinical Hypertension. 6th ed. Baltimore, © by Williams and Wilkins, 1994, p. 200.

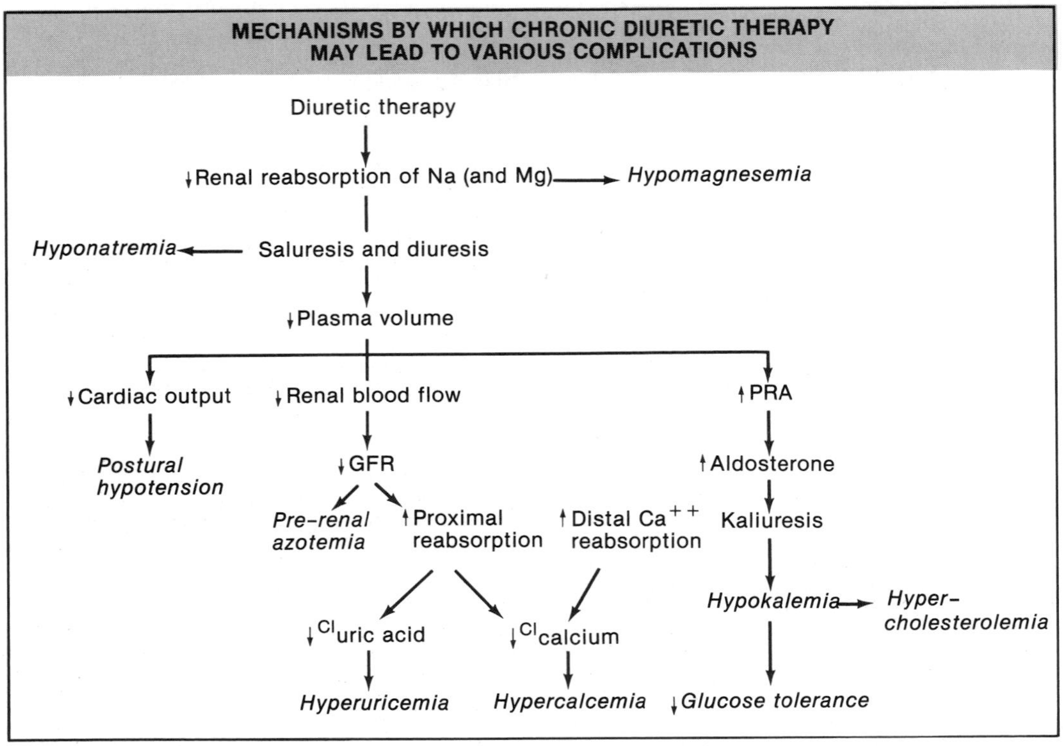

MECHANISMS BY WHICH CHRONIC DIURETIC THERAPY MAY LEAD TO VARIOUS COMPLICATIONS

Diuretic therapy

↓Renal reabsorption of Na (and Mg) → *Hypomagnesemia*

Hyponatremia ← Salluresis and diuresis

↓Plasma volume

↓Cardiac output → *Postural hypotension*

↓Renal blood flow → ↓GFR → *Pre-renal azotemia*; ↑Proximal reabsorption

↑PRA → ↑Aldosterone → Kaliuresis → *Hypokalemia* → *Hyper-cholesterolemia*

↑Distal Ca^{++} reabsorption

↓^{Cl}uric acid → *Hyperuricemia*

↓^{Cl}calcium → *Hypercalcemia*

Hypokalemia → ↓*Glucose tolerance*

FIGURE 27–10. The mechanisms by which chronic diuretic therapy may lead to various complications. The mechanism for hypercholesterolemia remains in question, although it is shown as arising via hypokalemia. Cl = clearance; PRA = plasma renin activity; GFR = Glomerular filtration rate. (From Kaplan, N. M.: Clinical Hypertension. 6th ed. Baltimore, © by Williams & Wilkins, 1994, p. 203.)

therapy for hypertension.[110] Among 158 hypertensives given diuretics for 2 years, plasma potassium levels fell to between 3.0 and 3.3 mmol/liter in 29 per cent and to between 2.6 and 2.9 mmol/liter in 7 per cent.[111] This fall in serum concentration may not reflect a significant decrease in total body potassium nor may it progress after the initial decline. Nevertheless, it may precipitate potentially hazardous ventricular ectopic activity and increase the risk of primary cardiac arrest,[112] even in patients not known to be susceptible because of concomitant digitalis therapy or myocardial irritability. The arrhythmogenic effect of diuretic-induced hypokalemia may become manifested only at times of stress, when catecholamines may lower the plasma potassium level another 0.5 to 1.0 mmol/liter or when beta-adrenergic agonists are used as bronchodilators.[113]

Most patients are unaware of mild diuretic-induced hypokalemia, although it may contribute to leg cramps, polyuria, and muscle weakness, but subtle interference with antihypertensive therapy may accompany even mild hypokalemia, and correction of hypokalemia may result in a fall in blood pressure.[114] In addition to increasing the propensity to ventricular ectopic activity, hypokalemia may be responsible for the worsening of insulin resistance, the loss of carbohydrate tolerance, and the rise in plasma lipids seen with diuretic use.[115]

Prevention of hypokalemia is preferable to correction of potassium deficiency. The following maneuvers should help prevent diuretic-induced hypokalemia:

- Use the smallest dose of diuretic needed.
- Use a moderately long-acting (12- to 18-hour) diuretic, such as hydrocholorothiazide, because longer-acting drugs (e.g., chlorthalidone) may increase potassium loss.
- Restrict sodium intake to less than 100 mmol per day (i.e., 2 gm sodium).
- Increase dietary potassium intake.
- Restrict concomitant use of laxatives.
- Use a combination of a thiazide with a potassium-sparing agent except in patients with renal insufficiency or in association with an ACE inhibitor.
- The concomitant use of a beta blocker or an ACE inhibitor will diminish potassium loss by blunting the diuretic-induced rise in renin-aldosterone.

If hypokalemia is to be treated, these principles should be followed, along with some form of supplemental potassium. Potassium chloride is preferred for correction of the associated alkalosis. If tolerated, granular potassium chloride can be given as a salt substitute; thereby, extra potassium will be provided while sodium intake is reduced. Caution is necessary when supplemental potassium chloride is given to older patients with borderline renal function in whom hyperkalemia may be induced.

HYPOMAGNESEMIA. In some patients concomitant diuretic-induced magnesium deficiency will prevent the restoration of intracellular deficits of potassium[116] so that hypomagnesemia should be corrected. Magnesium deficiency may also be responsible for some of the arrhythmias ascribed to hypokalemia.[117]

HYPERURICEMIA. The serum uric acid level is elevated in as many as one-third of untreated hypertensive patients. With chronic diuretic therapy, hyperuricemia appears in another third of patients, probably as a consequence of increased proximal tubular reabsorption accompanying volume contraction. Diuretic-induced hyperuricemia precipitates acute gout, most frequently in those who are obese and consume large amounts of alcohol.[118] Since asymptomatic hyperuricemia does not cause urate deposition, most investigators agree that it need not be treated. If therapy is used, a uricosuric drug such as probenecid should be given. Although allopurinol is often used, it is more likely to cause side effects and is a less rational choice, since the problem is a failure to excrete uric acid and not its overproduction.

HYPERLIPIDEMIA. Serum cholesterol levels often rise after diuretic therapy.[119] Although the rise in lipids can be prevented by a diet low in saturated fat, the propensity toward worsening of the lipid profile may inhibit the potential for diuretic therapy to reduce the incidence of coronary disease while it lowers blood pressure.

HYPERGLYCEMIA AND INSULIN RESISTANCE. Diuretics may impair glucose tolerance and precipitate diabetes mellitus,[115] probably because they increase insulin resistance and hyperinsulinemia.[120] The manner by which diuretics increase insulin resistance is uncertain, but in view of the multiple potential pressor actions of hyperinsulinemia (see p. 820), this could be a significant problem.

HYPERCALCEMIA. A slight rise in serum calcium, less than 0.5 mg/dl, is frequently seen with thiazide diuretic therapy, at least in part because increased calcium reabsorption accompanies the increased sodium reabsorption in the proximal tubule induced by contraction of extracellular fluid volume.[121] The rise is of little concern except in patients with previously unrecognized hyperparathyroidism, who may experience a much more marked rise. On the other hand, the diuretic-induced positive calcium balance is associated with a reduction in the incidence of osteoporosis in the elderly.[122]

IMPOTENCE. A high incidence of impotence (22.6 per cent) was found among men taking 10 mg of bendroflumethiazide per day, compared with a rate of 10.1 per cent among those on placebo and 13.2 per cent among those on propranolol in the large MRC trial.[123]

LOOP DIURETICS. Loop diuretics are usually needed in the treatment of hypertensive patients with renal failure defined here as a serum creatinine exceeding approximately 2.0 mg/dl. Furosemide has been most widely used, although either torsemide[109] or metolazone may be as effective, and each requires only a single daily dose. Many physicians use furosemide in the management of uncomplicated hypertension, but this drug provides less antihypertensive action when given once or twice a day than do longer-acting diuretics, which maintain a slight volume contraction.

POTASSIUM-SPARING AGENTS. These drugs are normally used in combination with a thiazide diuretic. Of the three currently available, one (spironolactone) is an aldosterone antagonist, while the other two (triamterene and amiloride) are direct inhibitors of potassium secretion. In combination with a thiazide diuretic, they will diminish the amount of potassium wasting. Although they are more expensive than thiazides alone, they may decrease the total cost of therapy by reducing the need to monitor and treat potassium depletion.

An Overview of Diuretics in Hypertension

Diuretics have been effective for the treatment of millions of hypertensive patients during the past 30 years. They reduce DBP and maintain it below 90 mm Hg in about half of all hypertensive patients, providing the same degree of effectiveness as most other antihypertensive drugs.[2] In two groups that constitute a rather large portion of the hypertensive population, the elderly[124] and blacks,[99] diuretics may be particularly effective. One-half of a diuretic tablet per day is usually all that is needed, minimizing cost and maximizing adherence to therapy. Even lower doses, i.e., 6.25 mg of hydrochlorothiazide, may be adequate when combined with other drugs.[92]

The side effects of high-dose diuretic therapy are usually not overtly bothersome, but the hypokalemia, hypercholesterolemia, hyperinsulinemia, and worsening of glucose tolerance that often accompany prolonged diuretic therapy gave rise to concerns about their long-term benignity. However, lower doses are usually just as potent as higher doses in lowering the blood pressure and less likely to induce metabolic mischief.[107] Therefore, the advocacy of low-dose diuretic therapy in the 1993 JNC-5 report[26] and by most expert committees[96] and reviewers[4] is appropriate.

ADRENERGIC INHIBITORS

A number of drugs that inhibit the adrenergic nervous system are available, including some that act centrally on vasomotor center activity, peripherally on neuronal catecholamine discharge, or by blocking alpha- and/or beta-adrenergic receptors (Table 27–5); some act at multiple sites. Figure 27–11, a schematic view of the ending of an adrenergic nerve and the effector cell with its receptors, depicts how some of these drugs act. When the nerve is stimulated, norepinephrine, which is synthesized intraneuronally and stored in granules, is released into the synaptic cleft. It binds to postsynaptic alpha- and beta-adrenergic receptors and thereby initiates various intracellular processes. In vascular smooth muscle, alpha stimulation causes constriction and beta stimulation causes relaxation. In the central vasomotor centers, sympathetic outflow is inhibited by alpha stimulation; the effect of central beta stimulation is unknown.

An important aspect of sympathetic activity involves the feedback of norepinephrine to alpha- and beta-adrenergic receptors located on the neuronal surface, i.e., presynaptic receptors. Presynaptic alpha-adrenergic receptor activation inhibits release, whereas presynaptic beta activation stimulates further norepinephrine release. The presynaptic receptors probably play a role in the action of some of the drugs to be discussed.

Elucidation and quantitation of the various actions of these drugs remain incomplete. The listing in Table 27–5 is based on the predominant site of action according to currently available data. The action of beta-adrenergic receptor blockers involves a peripheral effect, but they almost certainly also act on central vasomotor mechanisms.

TABLE 27–5 ADRENERGIC INHIBITORS USED IN TREATMENT OF HYPERTENSION

1. PERIPHERAL NEURONAL INHIBITORS
   a. Reserpine
   b. Guanethidine (Ismelin)
   c. Guanadrel (Hylorel)
   d. Bethanidine (Tenathan)
2. CENTRAL ADRENERGIC INHIBITORS
   a. Methyldopa (Aldomet)
   b. Clonidine (Catapres)
   c. Guanabenz (Wytensin)
   d. Guanfacine (Tenex)
3. α-RECEPTOR BLOCKERS
   a. α_1- and α_2-receptor
      (1) Phenoxybenzamine (Dibenzyline)
      (2) Phentolamine (Regitine)
   b. α_1-receptor
      (1) Doxazosin (Cardura)
      (2) Prazosin (Minipress)
      (3) Terazosin (Hytrin)
4. β-RECEPTOR BLOCKERS
   a. Acebutolol (Sectral)
   b. Atenolol (Tenormin)
   c. Betaxolol (Kerlone)
   d. Bisoprolol (Zebeta)
   e. Carteolol (Cartrol)
   f. Metoprolol (Lopressor, Toprol)
   g. Nadolol (Corgard)
   h. Penbutolol (Levatol)
   i. Pindolol (Visken)
   j. Propranolol (Inderal)
   k. Timolol (Blocadren)
5. α- AND β-RECEPTOR BLOCKER
   Labetalol (Normodyne, Trandate)

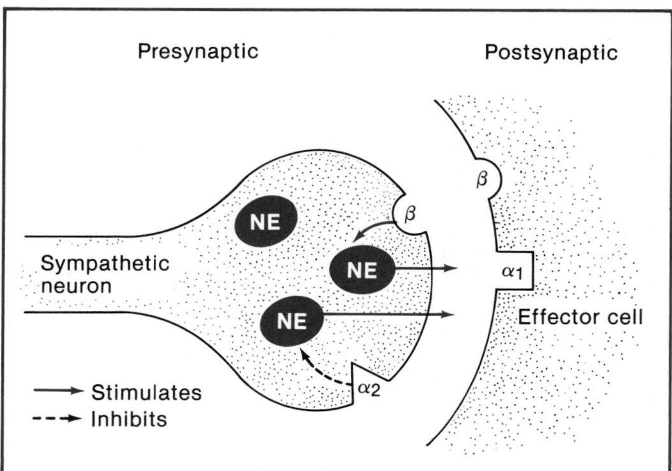

FIGURE 27–11. Simplified schematic view of the adrenergic nerve ending showing that norepinephrine (NE) is released from its storage granules when the nerve is stimulated and enters the synaptic cleft to bind to alpha$_1$ and beta receptors on the effector cell (postsynaptic). In addition, a short feedback loop exists, in which NE binds to alpha$_2$ and beta receptors on the neuron (presynaptic), to inhibit or to stimulate further release, respectively.

Reserpine, guanethidine, and related compounds act differently to inhibit the release of norepinephrine from peripheral adrenergic neurons.

RESERPINE. Reserpine, the most active and widely used of the derivatives of the rauwolfia alkaloids, depletes the postganglionic adrenergic neurons of norepinephrine by inhibiting its uptake into storage vesicles, exposing it to degradation by cytoplasmic monoamine oxidase. The peripheral effect is predominant, although the drug enters the brain and depletes central catecholamine stores as well. This probably accounts for the sedation and depression seen with reserpine use. The drug has certain advantages. Only one dose a day is needed; in combination with a diuretic, the antihypertensive effect is significant, greater than that noted with propranolol in one comparative study[125]; little postural hypotension is noted; and many patients experience no side effects. The drug has a relatively flat dose-response curve, so that a dose of only 0.05 mg per day will give almost as much antihypertensive effect as 0.125 or 0.25 mg per day but fewer side effects.[126] However, the psychological depression that occurs in perhaps 2 per cent of patients may be severe but difficult to recognize and treat. Although it remains popular in some places, the use of reserpine has declined progressively because it has no commercial sponsor.[127]

GUANETHIDINE. This agent and a series of related guanidine compounds, including guanadrel, bethanidine, and debrisoquine, act by inhibiting the release of norepinephrine from the adrenergic neurons, perhaps by a local anesthetic-like effect on the neuronal membrane. In order to act, the drug must be transported actively into the nerve through an amine pump. Various drugs, in particular tricyclic antidepressants, amphetamines, and ephedrine, competitively block the uptake of guanethidine into the nerves and thereby antagonize its effects.

Their low lipid solubility prevents guidance compounds from entering the brain, so that sedation, depression, and other side effects involving the central nervous system are not seen. Initially, the predominant hemodynamic effect is to decrease cardiac output; after continued use, peripheral resistance declines. Blood pressure is reduced further when the patient is upright, owing to gravitational pooling of blood in the legs, since compensatory sympathetic nervous system–mediated vasoconstriction is blocked. This results in the most common side effect, postural hypotension. Patients should be advised to arise slowly, sleep with the head of the bed elevated, and wear elastic hose to minimize this potential problem. Unlike reserpine, guanethidine has a steep dose-response curve, so that it can be successfully used in treating hypertension of any degree in daily doses of 10 to 300 mg. Like reserpine, it has a long biological half-life and may be given once daily. As other drugs have become available, guanethidine and related compounds have been relegated mainly to the treatment of severe hypertension unresponsive to all other agents.

Drugs That Act on Receptors

Predominantly Central Alpha Agonists

Until the mid-1980's, methyldopa was the most widely used of the adrenergic receptor blockers, but its use has fallen off as beta blockers and other drugs have become more popular. In addition, three other drugs—clonidine, guanabenz, and guanfacine, which act similarly to methyldopa but have fewer serious side effects—have become available.

METHYLDOPA. The primary site of action of methyldopa is within the central nervous system, where alpha-methylnorepinephrine, derived from methyldopa, is released from adrenergic neurons and stimulates central alpha-adrenergic receptors, reducing the sympathetic outflow from the central nervous system.[128] The blood pressure mainly falls as a result of a decrease in peripheral resistance with little effect on cardiac output. However, methyldopa, in concert with other antihypertensive agents that decrease sympathetic activity, may reduce the degree of left ventricular hypertrophy as noted by echocardiography.[129] Renal blood flow is well maintained, and significant postural hypotension is unusual. Therefore, the drug has been widely used in hypertensive patients with renal failure or cerebrovascular disease.

Methyldopa need be given no more than twice daily, in doses ranging from 250 to 3000 mg per day.

Side effects include some that are common to centrally acting drugs that reduce sympathetic outflow: sedation, dry mouth, impotence, and galactorrhea. However, methyldopa causes some unique side effects that are probably of an autoimmune nature, since a positive antinuclear antibody test is seen in about 10 per cent of patients who take the drug, and red cell autoantibodies occur in about 20 per cent. Clinically apparent hemolytic anemia is rare, probably because methyldopa also impairs reticuloendothelial function so that antibody-sensitized cells are not removed from the circulation and hemolyzed.[130] Inflammatory disorders in various organs have been reported, most commonly involving the liver (with diffuse parenchymal injury similar to viral hepatitis).[131]

CLONIDINE. Although of different structure, clonidine shares many features with methyldopa. It probably acts at the same central sites, has similar antihypertensive efficacy, and causes many of the same bothersome but less serious side effects (e.g., sedation, dry mouth). It does not, however, induce the autoimmune and inflammatory side effects.

As an alpha-adrenergic receptor agonist, the drug also acts on presynaptic alpha receptors and inhibits norepinephrine release (Fig. 27–11), and plasma catecholamine levels fall.[132] The drug has a fairly short biological half-life, so that when it is discontinued, the inhibition of norepinephrine release disappears within about 12 to 18 hours, and plasma catecholamine levels rise. This is probably responsible for the rapid rebound of the blood pressure to pretreatment levels and the occasional appearance of withdrawal symptoms, including tachycardia, restlessness, and sweating. Rarely, the blood pressure increases beyond the pretreatment level. If the rebound requires treatment, clonidine may be reintroduced or alpha-adrenergic receptor antagonists given. Similar "overshoots" have been reported less commonly after the discontinuation of a variety of other antihypertensives.[133]

Clonidine is available in a *transdermal* preparation, which may provide smoother blood pressure control for as long as 7 days with fewer side effects. However, bothersome skin rashes preclude its use in perhaps one-fourth of patients.[134]

GUANABENZ. This drug differs in structure but shares many characteristics with both methyldopa and clonidine, acting primarily as a central alpha agonist. It may differ, however, in not causing fluid retention,[135] so that it may turn out to be effective without the need for a concomitant diuretic. Moreover, unlike diuretics, guanabenz has been found to reduce serum cholesterol.[136]

GUANFACINE. This drug is also similar to clonidine but is longer acting, which enables once-a-day dosing and minimizes rebound hypertension.[137]

Alpha-Adrenergic Receptor Antagonists

Before 1977 the only alpha blockers used to treat hypertension were phenoxybenzamine (Dibenzyline) and phentolamine (Regitine). These drugs are effective in acutely lowering blood pressure, but their effects are offset by an accompanying increase in cardiac output, and side effects are frequent and bothersome. Their limited efficacy may reflect their blockade of presynaptic alpha-adrenergic receptors, which interferes with the feedback inhibition of norepinephrine release (Fig. 27–11). Increased catecholamine release would then blunt the action of postsynaptic alpha-adrenergic receptor blockade. Their use has largely been limited to the treatment of patients with pheochromocytomas.

PRAZOSIN. This was the first of a group of selective antagonists of the postsynaptic $alpha_1$ receptors. By blocking alpha-mediated vasoconstriction, prazosin induces a fall in peripheral resistance with both venous and arteriolar dilation. Because the presynaptic alpha-adrenergic receptor is left unblocked, the feedback loop for the inhibition of norepinephrine release is intact, an action that is also certainly responsible for the greater antihypertensive effect of the drug and the absence of concomitant tachycardia, tolerance, and renin release. The inhibition of norepinephrine release may also account for the propensity toward greater first-dose falls in blood pressure.

OTHER ALPHA BLOCKERS. Two other alpha blockers, terazosin[138] and doxazosin,[139] are available. Beyond longer duration of action and less propensity for first-dose hypotension, they appear to differ little from prazosin.

Selective alpha blockers are as effective as other first-line antihypertensives.[2] When given to patients whose condition is poorly controlled on standard triple therapy (diuretic, beta blocker, and vasodilator), they may reduce blood pressure even more than anticipated.[140] They can be safely and effectively used in patients with renal failure. The favorable hemodynamic changes—a fall in peripheral resistance with maintenance of cardiac output—make them an attractive choice for patients who wish to remain physically active. In addition, blood lipids are not adversely altered and may actually improve with alpha blockers, unlike the adverse effects observed with diuretics and beta blockers.[141] Moreover, improved insulin sensitivity with lesser rises in plasma glucose and insulin levels after a glucose load has been observed with alpha blockers.[142] Alpha blockers decrease the smooth muscle tone of the bladder neck and prostate, relieving the obstructive symptoms of prostatism.[143] They are then an excellent choice for older men with benign prostatic hypertrophy.

Side effects, beyond first-dose postural hypotension, include the nonspecific effects of lower blood pressure, such as dizziness, weakness, fatigue, and headaches. Most patients, however, find the drugs easy to take, with little sedation, dry mouth, or impotence.

Beta-Adrenergic Receptor Antagonists

(See also p. 610)

In the 1980's, beta-adrenergic receptor blockers became the most popular form of antihypertensive therapy after diuretics, reflecting their relative effectiveness and freedom from many bothersome side effects. For the majority of patients, beta blockers are usually easy to take, because somnolence, dry mouth, and impotence are seldom encountered. Because beta blockers have been found to reduce mortality if taken either before or after acute myocardial infarction,[144] i.e., secondary prevention, it was assumed that they might offer special protection against initial coronary events, i.e., primary prevention. However, in four large clinical trials, a beta blocker provided no more protection than did a diuretic.[15,123,145,146] In the continuation of the HAPPHY trial, the group who remained on metoprolol experienced a lower eventual coronary mortality and morbidity rate than did the one who continued on a diuretic.[147,148]

THE VARIETY OF BETA BLOCKERS. Beta blockers now available in the United States are listed in Table 27–5, and others are available in other countries. A number of agents with additional vasodilatory effects will probably soon be approved for use in the United States, and they may be free of many of the unfavorable hemodynamic and adverse effects of currently available agents.[149] Pharmacologically, those now available differ considerably from one another with respect to degree of absorption, protein binding, and bioavailability. However, the three most important differences affecting their clinical use are cardioselectivity, intrinsic sympathomimetic activity, and lipid solubility. Despite these differences, they all seem to be about equally as effective as antihypertensives.

Cardioselectivity. As seen in Figure 27–12, beta blockers can be classified by their degree of cardioselectivity relative to their blocking effect on the $beta_1$-adrenergic receptors in the heart compared with that on the $beta_2$ receptors in the bronchi, peripheral blood vessels, and elsewhere. Such cardioselectivity can be easily shown using small doses in acute studies; with the rather high doses used to treat hypertension, much of this selectivity is lost.

Intrinsic Sympathomimetic Activity (ISA). Some of these drugs have ISA, interacting with beta receptors to cause a measurable agonist response but at the same time blocking the greater agonist effects of endogenous catecholamines. As a result, while in usual doses they lower the blood pressure about the same degree as do other beta blockers, they cause a smaller decline in heart rate, cardiac output, and renin levels. As noted under Side Effects, ISA may blunt the adverse effects on lipid metabolism seen with non-ISA beta blockers.[150]

Lipid Solubility. Atenolol and nadolol are among the least lipid-soluble of the beta blockers. This could translate into two clinically important advantages. First, because they escape hepatic inactivation and are excreted virtually unchanged through the kidneys (Fig. 27–13), they remain as active drugs in the plasma much longer, allowing once-a-day dosage. Second, because they do not enter the brain as readily, they may cause fewer central nervous system side effects.[151]

Mechanism of Action. Despite these and other differences, the various beta blockers now available are approximately equipotent as antihypertensive agents. How they lower the blood pressure remains uncertain, although a number of possible mechanisms are likely to be involved. In those without ISA, cardiac output falls 15 to 20 per cent and renin release is reduced about 60 per cent. Central nervous system beta-adrenergic receptor blockade may reduce sympathetic discharge, but similar antihypertensive effects are seen with those drugs that are more lipid-soluble, and therefore in high concentration within the central nervous system, and those that are less lipid-soluble.

At the same time that beta blockers lower blood pressure through various means, their blockade of peripheral beta-adrenergic receptors inhibits vasodilation, leaving alpha receptors open to catecholamine-mediated vasoconstriction. However, over time, vascular resistance tends to return to normal, which presumably preserves the antihypertensive effect of a reduced cardiac output.[152]

Clinical Effects. Even in small doses, beta blockers begin to lower the blood pressure within a few hours, although their maximal effect may not be noted for some weeks. Even though progressively higher doses have usually been given, careful study has shown a near-maximal effect from smaller doses. For example, in a double-blind crossover study involving 24 patients, 40 mg of propranolol twice a day provided the same antihypertensive effects as 80, 160, or 240 mg twice a day.[153] The degree of blood pressure reduction is at least comparable to that noted with other antihypertensive drugs. Because beta blockers, along with diuretics, are the only class of antihypertensive drugs tested in large clinical trials and thereby shown to reduce mortality, they have been given preference in JNC-5 and elsewhere.[4] They may be particularly well suited for younger and middle-aged hypertensives, especially non-blacks, and in patients with myocardial ischemia and high levels of stress.[154] However, since the hemodynamic responses to stress are reduced, they may interfere with athletic performance.[155]

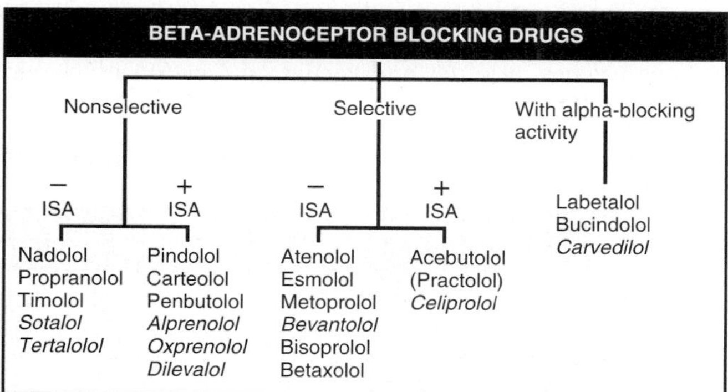

FIGURE 27–12. Classification of beta-adrenergic receptor blockers based on cardioselectivity and intrinsic sympathomimetic activity (ISA). Those not approved for use in the United States are in italics. (From Kaplan, N. M.: Clinical Hypertension. 6th ed. Baltimore, © by Williams & Wilkins, 1994, p. 221.)

SPECIAL USES FOR BETA BLOCKERS

COEXISTING ISCHEMIC HEART DISEASE. Even without evidence that beta blockers protect patients from initial coronary events, the antiarrhythmic and antianginal effects of these drugs make them especially valuable in hypertensive patients with coexisting coronary disease.

PATIENTS NEEDING ANTIHYPERTENSIVE VASODILATOR THERAPY. If a diuretic and an adrenergic receptor blocker are inadequate to control blood pressure, the addition of a vasodilator is a logical third step. When used alone, direct vasodilators induce reflex sympathetic stimulation of the heart. The simultaneous use of beta blockers prevents this undesirable increase in cardiac output, which not only

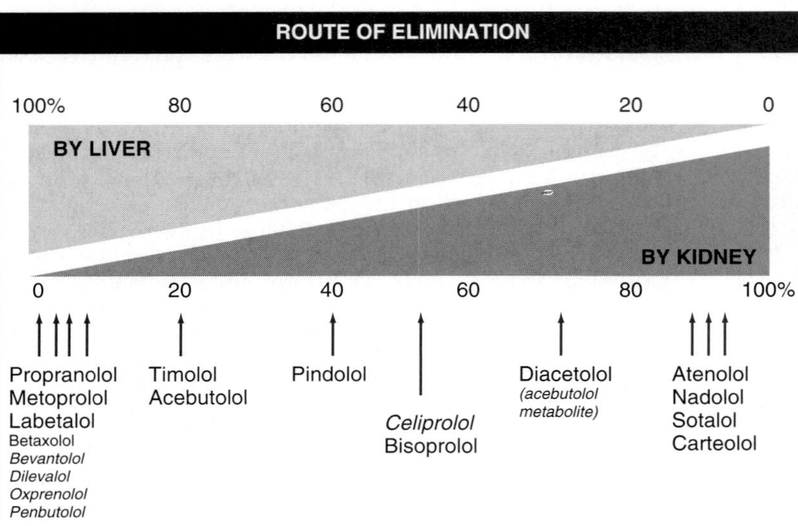

FIGURE 27–13. The relative degree of clearance by hepatic uptake and metabolism (liver) and renal excretion (kidney) of 10 beta-adrenoceptor blocking agents. The differences largely reflect differences in lipid solubility, which progressively diminishes from left to right. (Modified from Meier, J.: Beta-adrenoceptor-blocking agents: Pharmacokinetic differences and their clinical implications illustrated on pindolol. Cardiology *64*[Suppl. 1]:1, 1979.)

bothers the patient but also dampens the antihypertensive effect of the vasodilator.

PATIENTS WITH HYPERKINETIC HYPERTENSION. Some hypertensive patients have increased cardiac output that may persist for many years. Beta blockers are particularly effective in such patients, but a reduction in exercise capacity may necessitate restriction of their use in young athletes.

PATIENTS WITH MARKED ANXIETY. The somatic manifestations of anxiety—tremor, sweating, and tachycardia—can be helped, without the undesirable effects of methods commonly used to control anxiety, such as alcohol and tranquilizers.

PERIOPERATIVE STRESS. The ultra-short-acting cardioselective agent esmolol has been successfully used to prevent postintubation tachycardia and hypertension.[156]

SIDE EFFECTS. Most of the side effects of beta blockers relate to their major pharmacological action, the blockade of beta-adrenergic receptors. Certain concomitant problems may worsen when beta-adrenergic receptors are blocked. These include peripheral vascular disease, bronchospasm, and congestive heart failure. However, cautious use of beta blockers in patients with systolic dysfunction may prove to be valuable.[157]

Diabetics may have additional problems with beta blockers, more so with nonselective ones. The responses to hypoglycemia, both the symptoms and the counterregulatory hormonal changes that raise blood sugar levels, are partially dependent on sympathetic nervous activity. Diabetics who are susceptible to hypoglycemia may not be aware of the usual warning signals and may not rebound as quickly. The majority of noninsulin-dependent diabetics can take these drugs without difficulty, although their diabetes may be exacerbated, probably from beta blocker interference with insulin sensitivity.[142]

The most common side effect is fatigue, which is probably a consequence of decreased cardiac output and also of the decrease in cerebral blood flow that may accompany successful lowering of the blood pressure by any drug (Fig. 27–7). More direct effects on the central nervous system—insomnia, nightmares, and hallucinations—occur in some patients.[158] An association with depression appears to be accounted for by various confounding variables.[159]

When a beta blocker is discontinued, angina pectoris and myocardial infarction may occur.[160] Since patients with hypertension are more susceptible to coronary disease, they should be weaned gradually and given appropriate coronary vasodilator therapy. Perturbations of lipoprotein metabolism accompany the use of beta blockers.[141] Nonselective agents cause greater rises in triglycerides and falls in cardioprotective high-density lipoprotein-cholesterol levels, whereas ISA agents cause less or no effect and some agents such as celiprolol may raise HDL-cholesterol levels.[161] Patients with renal failure may take beta blockers without additional hazard, although modest falls in renal blood flow and glomerular filtration rate have been measured, presumably from renal vasoconstriction.

Caution is advised in the use of beta blockers in patients suspected of harboring a pheochromocytoma (see p. 828), because unopposed alpha-adrenergic agonist action may precipitate a serious hypertensive crisis if this disease is present. The use of beta blockers during pregnancy has been clouded by scattered case reports of various fetal problems. Moreover, prospective studies have found that the use of beta blockers during pregnancy may lead to fetal growth retardation.[162]

AN OVERVIEW OF BETA BLOCKERS IN HYPERTENSION. Beta blockers are likely to continue to be popular in the treatment of hypertension. If a beta blocker is chosen, those agents that have ISA and are more cardioselective and lipid-insoluble offer the likelihood of fewer perturbations of lipid and carbohydrate metabolism and greater patient adherence to therapy; only one dose a day is needed and side effects probably are minimized.

Alpha- and Beta-Adrenergic Receptor Antagonists

The combination of an alpha and a beta blocker in a single molecule is available in the form of labetalol, which combines both alpha- and beta-blocking actions in a ratio between 1:3 and 1:7. The fall in pressure mainly results from a decrease in peripheral resistance, with little or no fall in cardiac output.[163] The most bothersome side effects are related to postural hypotension; the most serious side effect is hepatotoxicity.[164] Intravenous labetalol is used to treat hypertensive emergencies.

VASODILATORS

Until recently, direct-acting arteriolar vasodilators were used mainly as third drugs, when combinations of a diuretic and adrenergic blocker failed to control blood pressure. However, with the availability of vasodilators of different types that can be easily tolerated when used as first or second drugs, a wider and earlier application of vasodilators in therapy of hypertension has begun (Table 27–6).

TABLE 27–6 VASODILATOR DRUGS USED TO TREAT HYPERTENSION

DRUG	RELATIVE ACTION ON ARTERIES (A) OR VEINS (V)
Direct	
Hydralazine	A > > V
Minoxidil	A > > V
Nitroprusside	A = V
Diazoxide	A > V
Nitroglycerin	V > A
Calcium entry blockers	A > > V
Converting enzyme inhibitors	A > V
Alpha blockers	A = V

Direct Vasodilators

Hydralazine is the most widely used agent of this type. Minoxidil is more potent but is usually reserved for patients with severe, refractory hypertension associated with renal failure.[91a] Diazoxide and nitroprusside are given intravenously for hypertensive crises and are discussed on page 858.

HYDRALAZINE. Since the early 1970's, hydralazine, in combination with a diuretic and a beta blocker, has been used increasingly to treat severe hypertension. The drug acts directly to relax the smooth muscle in precapillary resistance vessels with little or no effect on postcapillary venous capacitance vessels. As a result, blood pressure falls by a reduction in peripheral resistance, but in the process a number of compensatory processes, which are activated by the arterial baroreceptor arc, blunt the decrease in pressure and cause side effects.[165] When a diuretic is used to overcome the tendency for fluid retention and an adrenergic inhibitor is used to prevent the reflex increase in sympathetic activity and rise in renin, the vasodilator is more effective and causes few, if any, side effects. Without the protection conferred by concomitant use of an adrenergic blocker, numerous side effects (tachycardia, flushing, headache, and precipitation of angina) may be seen.

The drug need be given only twice a day. Its daily dosage should be kept below 400 mg to prevent the lupus-like syndrome that appears in 10 to 20 per cent of patients who receive more. This reaction, although uncomfortable to the patient, is almost always reversible. In fact, the reaction is uncommon with daily doses of 200 mg or less and is more common in slow acetylators of the drug.

MINOXIDIL. This drug vasodilates by opening potassium channels in vascular smooth muscle. Its hemodynamic effects are similar to those of hydralazine, but minoxidil is even more effective and may be used once a day. It is particularly useful in managing patients with severe hypertension and renal failure.[166] Even more than with hydralazine, diuretics and adrenergic receptor blockers must be used with minoxidil to prevent the reflex increase in cardiac output and fluid retention. Pericardial effusions have appeared in about 3 per cent of those given minoxidil, in some without renal or cardiac failure.[167] The drug also causes hair to grow profusely, and the facial hirsutism precludes use of the drug in most women.

Calcium Antagonists

(See also p. 475)

These drugs have become the most popular class of agents used in the treatment of hypertension. They differ in both their sites and modes of action (Table 27–7), with major pharmacological differences between the various dihydropyridines.[168] Dihydropyridines have the greatest peripheral vasodilatory action with little effect on cardiac automaticity, conduction, or contractility. However, comparative trials have shown that verapamil and diltiazem, which do affect these properties, are also effective antihypertensives, and they may cause fewer side effects related to vasodilation, such as flushing and ankle edema. Calcium antagonists are effective in hypertensive patients of all ages and races.[99]

Calcium antagonists may cause at least an initial natriuresis, probably by producing renal vasodilation,[169] which may obviate the need for concurrent diuretic therapy. In fact, unlike all other antihypertensive agents, they may have their effectiveness reduced rather than enhanced by concomitant dietary sodium restriction,[170] whereas most careful studies show an enhancement of their effect by concomitant diuretic therapy.[106] Their renal vasodilatory effect allows glomerular filtration rate and renal blood flow to be well maintained as they reduce systemic blood pressure.[171] Because they act primarily to dilate afferent arterioles, these agents could accelerate a decline in renal function by increasing flow within the glomeruli. Although they do not decrease proteinuria as well as ACE inhibitors,[172] they seem to preserve renal function as well[171] and, in some studies, better than the latter drugs.[173] They have been used successfully for treatment of hypertension associated with diabetes without altering glucose tolerance or lipid levels.[174]

TABLE 27–7 PHARMACOLOGICAL EFFECTS OF CALCIUM ANTAGONISTS*

	DILTIAZEM	VERAPAMIL	DIHYDROPYRIDINES
Heart rate	↓	↓	↑–
Myocardial contractility	↓	↓↓	↓–
Nodal conduction	↓	↓↓	–
Peripheral vasodilation	↑	↑	↑↑

* The ↓ indicates decrease; ↑, increase; and –, no change.

A potentially serious adverse effect from the use of calcium antagonists to treat hypertension was described in a case-control study wherein more hypertensives who had a myocardial infarction were taking short-acting calcium antagonists than were hypertensives who had not had an infarct.[174a] The most likely explanation for the finding is exclusion bias, which is an inherent problem with case-control studies wherein the cases are at greater risk for the complication than the controls; i.e., higher-risk patients are excluded from the control group but not from the case group. Specifically, short-acting calcium antagonists, which were not approved for the treatment of hypertension and which were more expensive and more difficult to use because they require three doses a day compared with the other approved antihypertensive agents, were probably given to patients considered at higher risk for coronary events. Similar case-control studies claiming that the use of reserpine was associated with a threefold increase in breast cancer were subsequently shown to be erroneous because of exclusion bias.[174b] No data incriminating the long-acting calcium antagonists approved for the treatment of hypertension have been presented.

Along with freedom from most of the side effects seen with other classes, calcium antagonists may be unique in not having their antihypertensive efficacy blunted by nonsteroidal antiinflammatory agents.[175]

Liquid nifedipine has been used effectively to reduce high levels of blood pressure quickly. Doses of 5 to 10 mg provide almost uniform reduction of blood pressure by 25 per cent within 30 minutes.[176] Intravenous nicardipine is available for hypertensive emergencies.[177]

Renin-Angiotensin Inhibitors

(See also p. 473)

Activity of the renin-angiotensin system may be inhibited in four ways (Fig. 27-14), three of which can be applied clinically.[177a] The first, use of adrenergic receptor blockers to inhibit the release of renin, was discussed earlier (p. 851). The second, direct inhibition of renin activity by specific renin inhibitors, is being actively investigated.[178] The third, inhibition of the enzyme that converts the inactive decapeptide angiotensin I to the active octapeptide angiotensin II (AII), is being widely utilized with orally effective ACE inhibitors. The fourth approach to inhibiting the renin-angiotensin system, blockade of angiotensin's actions by a

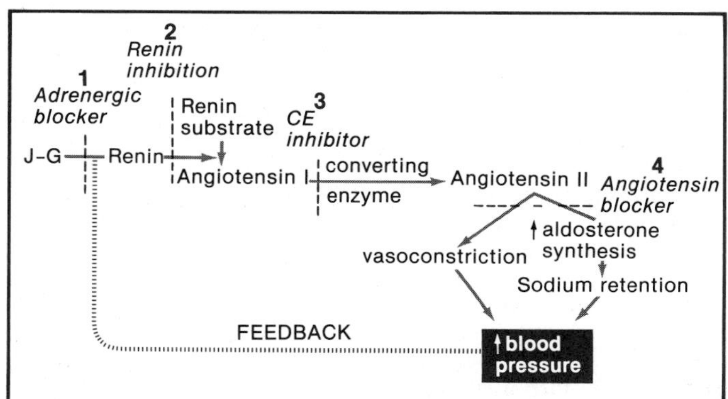

FIGURE 27–14. The four sites of action of inhibitors of the renin-angiotensin system. J-G = juxtaglomerular apparatus. (From Kaplan, N. M.: Clinical Hypertension. 6th ed. Baltimore, © by Williams & Wilkins, 1994, p. 241.)

competitive blocker, is now feasible, and orally effective AII receptor blockers are now approved for clinical use.[179] The AII receptor blockers may offer additional benefits, but their immediate advantage is the absence of cough and angioedema that often accompany ACE inhibitors. Because they are so widely used, the remainder of this section will examine ACE inhibitors.

MECHANISM OF ACTION. The first of these ACE inhibitors, captopril, was synthesized as a specific inhibitor of the converting enzyme that breaks the peptidyldipeptide bond in angiotensin I, preventing the enzyme from attaching to and splitting the angiotensin I structure. Because angiotensin II cannot be formed and angiotensin I is inactive, the ACE inhibitor paralyzes the renin-angiotensin system, thereby removing the effects of endogenous angiotensin II as both a vasoconstrictor and a stimulant to aldosterone synthesis. Subsequently, a number of other ACE inhibitors, differing primarily by the presence of a carboxyl or phosphoryl group rather than a sulfhydryl group, act in a similar manner but with a slower onset and a longer duration of action.

Interestingly, the plasma angiotensin II levels actually return to previous readings with chronic use of ACE inhibitors while the blood pressure remains lowered[180]; this suggests that the antihypertensive effect may involve other mechanisms. Since the same enzyme that converts angiotensin I to angiotensin II is also responsible for inactivation of the vasodepressor hormone bradykinin, by inhibiting the breakdown of bradykinin, ACE inhibitors increase the concentration of a vasodepressor hormone while they decrease the concentration of a vasoconstrictor hormone.[181] The increased plasma kinin levels may contribute to the improvement in insulin sensitivity observed with ACE inhibitors,[182] but they are also responsible for the most common and bothersome side effect of their use, a dry, hacking cough.[183] ACE inhibitors may also vasodilate by increasing levels of vasodilatory prostaglandins and decreasing levels of vasoconstricting endothelins.[184] Their effects may also involve inhibition of the renin-angiotensin system within the heart and other tissues.

Regardless of the manner in which they work, ACE inhibitors lower blood pressure mainly by reducing peripheral resistance with little, if any, effect on heart rate, cardiac output, or body fluid volumes. After a year of treatment with an ACE inhibitor, the structure and function of subcutaneous resistance vessels were improved whereas no changes were observed with a beta blocker.[185] The lack of a rise in heart rate despite a significant fall in blood pressure has been explained by a blunting of the adrenergic nervous system.[186]

CLINICAL USE. In patients with uncomplicated primary hypertension, ACE inhibitors provide antihypertensive effects that are equal to those seen with other classes, but they are less effective in blacks,[99] perhaps because blacks tend to have lower renin levels. They are equally effective in elderly and younger hypertensive patients.

The initial dose of ACE inhibitor may precipitate a rather dramatic but transient fall in blood pressure,[187] but the full effect may not be seen for 7 to 10 days. The initial dosage may be as little as 12.5 mg of captopril twice a day or 5 mg once a day of most of the other members of this class. The response to an ACE inhibitor is usually well maintained, perhaps because its suppression of aldosterone mitigates the tendency toward volume expansion that often antagonizes the effects of other antihypertensives.

These drugs have been a mixed blessing for patients with renovascular hypertension. On the one hand, the response of plasma renin to a single dose of captopril may provide a simple diagnostic test for the disease (see p. 827). More importantly, they usually control the blood pressure effectively.[188] On the other hand, the removal of the high levels of angiotensin II that they produce may deprive the stenotic kidney of the hormonal drive to its blood flow, thereby causing a marked fall of renal perfusion so that patients with solitary kidneys or bilateral disease may develop acute and sometimes persistent renal failure.[189]

Patients with intraglomerular hypertension, specifically those with diabetic nephropathy or reduced renal functional mass, may benefit especially from the reduction in efferent arteriolar resistance that follows reduction in angiotensin II. The clinical evidence for modulation of the progressive loss of renal function in diabetic nephropathy is now unequivocal.[190] Whether this effect is quantitatively better with ACE inhibitors than that provided by other drugs is less certain as is the ability of ACE inhibitors to also slow the progress of other forms of renal disease.[191] Because of their ability to improve insulin sensitivity, ACE inhibitors are particularly attractive for diabetics, with or without nephropathy,[192] and for hypertensives with visceral obesity.[193]

SIDE EFFECTS. Most patients who take an ACE inhibitor experience no side effects nor the biochemical changes often seen with other drugs that may be of even more concern even though they are not so obvious; neither rises in lipids, glucose, or uric acid nor falls in potassium levels are seen, and insulin sensitivity may improve.

To be sure, ACE inhibitors may cause both specific and nonspecific adverse effects. Among the specific ones are rash, loss of taste, glomerulopathy manifested by proteinuria, and leukopenia. In addition, these drugs may cause a hypersensitivity reaction with angioneurotic edema[194] or a cough, although often persistent, is infrequently associated with pulmonary dysfunction.[194a] The cough, seen in over 10 per cent of women and about half as many men,[195] may not disappear for 3 weeks after the ACE inhibitor is discontinued.[196] The recently approved angiotensin II receptor blockers do not induce the cough, which presumably arises from the increased levels of kinins that occur when the ACE enzyme is inhibited.

There is at least a potential problem for those patients taking an ACE inhibitor who coincidentally develop volume depletion, as from gastroenteritis, since they may be unable to marshal the compensatory homeostatic responses that involve increased angiotensin II and aldosterone. Lastly, patients on potassium supplements or sparing agents may not be able to excrete potassium loads and therefore may develop hyperkalemia.

AN OVERVIEW OF ACE INHIBITOR THERAPY. These drugs are widely used for all degrees and forms of hypertension. Their use is likely to increase further because of their particular ability to decrease intrarenal hypertension, to unload the hemodynamic burden of congestive heart failure, and to protect against ventricular dysfunction after myocardial infarction. Angiotensin II receptor blockers may offer all of the advantages of ACE inhibitors and fewer side effects.

Other Vasodilators

A variety of other forms of antihypertensive therapy are under investigation. These include endothelin receptor antagonists,[197] agents that serve as exogenous atrial natriuretic factor[198] or prolong its endogenous effectiveness,[199] and a host of renin inhibitors and angiotensin antagonists.[200,200a]

SPECIAL CONSIDERATIONS IN THERAPY

RESISTANT HYPERTENSION. There are multiple causes for resistance to therapy, usually defined as the failure of diastolic blood pressure to fall below 90 mm Hg despite the use of three or more drugs,[105] although some believe the definition should extend to the use of only two drugs in maximal doses.[201] Often patients do not respond well because they do not take their medications. On the other hand, what appears to be a poor response based on office readings of blood pressure may turn out to be an adequate response when home readings are obtained.[202] However, a number of factors may be responsible for a poor response even if the appropriate medication is taken regularly (Table 27–8). Most common is volume overload owing either to inadequate diuretic or excessive dietary sodium intake. Larger doses or more potent diuretics often bring resistant hypertension under control. On the other hand, blood pressure of a few patients is resistant to therapy because of overly vigorous diuresis, which contracts vascular volume and activates both renin and catecholamines.

Resistance is particularly common in patients with visceral obesity and associated insulin resistance.[203] A frequently overlooked cause is the interference with virtually all antihypertensive drugs (with the possible exception of calcium antagonists) by NSAIDs.[204]

Resistance can usually be overcome by adequate doses of a diuretic, a calcium antagonist, and an ACE inhibitor.

ANESTHESIA IN HYPERTENSIVE PATIENTS. In the absence of significant cardiac dysfunction, hypertension does not add to the cardiovascular risks of surgery.[205] However, if possible, hypertension should be well controlled by means of medications before anesthesia and surgery to reduce the risk of myocardial ischemia.[206] Therefore, patients taking antihypertensive medications should continue these drugs, as long as the anesthesiologist is aware of their use and takes reasonable precautions to prevent wide swings in pressure. The very short-acting beta blocker esmolol has been successful in preventing surges in blood pressure during intubation.[156] Patients receiving calcium antagonists may occasionally manifest adverse effects when inhalation agents such as halothane, enflurane, and isoflurane are used, either because the cardiovascular effects of these agents are similar to those of calcium antagonists or because these agents may increase the plasma levels of the calcium antagonists.[207]

Hypertension is often observed during and immediately after coronary bypass surgery (see p. 830); various intravenous agents have been successfully used to lower the pressure. Nitroprusside has been the usual choice during the postoperative period, but toxicity, often in the form of loss of consciousness and cyanide or thiocyanate toxicity, may develop in those who are critically ill and given the drug for prolonged periods.[208] Esmolol, labetalol, or nicardipine may be a better choice.[209]

HYPERTENSIVE CHILDREN (see also p. 822). Almost nothing is known about the effects of various antihypertensive medications given to children over long periods. In the absence of adequate data, an approach similar to that advocated for adults is advised.[210] The dosages of drugs are shown in Table 31–5, p. 998. Emphasis should be placed on weight reduction in hypertensive children who are obese, in the hope of attempting to control hypertension without the need for drug therapy.

HYPERTENSION DURING PREGNANCY. This topic is discussed in Chapter 59.

HYPERTENSION IN THE ELDERLY. As noted on page 822, a few elderly persons may have high blood pressure as measured by the sphygmomanometer but may have less or no hypertension when direct intraarterial readings are made. Presumably their pseudohypertension is related to the failure of the sphygmomanometer cuff to collapse the rigid artery beneath the cuff. The cuff systolic pressure may more frequently underestimate the intraarterial level, whereas the cuff diastolic level tends to be higher than the direct measurement.[211] If both systolic and diastolic pressures are elevated, elderly patients should be treated in a manner similar to that for younger persons; they seem to respond as well[11] but may have a number of problems with the medications[212] (Table 27–9). In view of the reduced effectiveness of the baroceptor reflex and the failure of peripheral resistance to rise appropriately with standing,[213] drugs with a propensity to cause postural hypotension

TABLE 27–8 CAUSES FOR INADEQUATE RESPONSIVENESS TO THERAPY

PSEUDORESISTANCE	
"White coat" or office elevations	
Pseudohypertension in elderly	
NONADHERENCE TO THERAPY	
Side effects of medication	
Cost of medication	
Lack of consistent and continuous primary care	
Inconvenient and chaotic dosing schedules	
Instructions not understood	
Inadequate patient education	
Organic brain syndrome (e.g., memory deficit)	
DRUG-RELATED CAUSES	
Doses too low	
Inappropriate combinations (e.g., two centrally acting adrenergic inhibitors)	
Rapid inactivation (e.g., hydralazine)	
Drug interactions	
Nonsteroidal antiinflammatory drugs	Oral contraceptives
	Adrenal steroids
Sympathomimetics	Licorice (chewing tobacco)
Nasal decongestants	
Appetite suppressants	Cyclosporine
Cocaine	Erythropoietin
Caffeine	Cholestyramine
Antidepressants (MAO inhibitors, tricyclics)	
Excessive volume contraction with stimulation of renin-aldosterone	
Hypokalemia (usually diuretic-induced)	
Rebound after clonidine withdrawal	
ASSOCIATED CONDITIONS	
Smoking	
Increasing obesity	
Sleep apnea	
Insulin resistance/hyperinsulinemia	
Ethanol intake more than 1 ounce a day (>3 portions)	
Anxiety-induced hyperventilation or panic attacks	
Chronic pain	
Intense vasoconstriction (Raynaud's, arteritis)	
SECONDARY HYPERTENSION	
Renal insufficiency	
Renovascular hypertension	
Pheochromocytoma	
Primary aldosteronism	
VOLUME OVERLOAD	
Excess sodium intake	
Progressive renal damage (nephrosclerosis)	
Fluid retention from reduction of blood pressure	
Inadequate diuretic therapy	

Modified from Joint National Committee. Fifth report of the Joint National Committee on detection, evaluation, and treatment of high blood pressure (JNC V). Arch. Intern. Med. *153*:154, 1993. Copyright 1993 American Medical Association.

TABLE 27–9 FACTORS THAT MIGHT CONTRIBUTE TO INCREASED RISK OF PHARMACOLOGICAL TREATMENT OF HYPERTENSION IN THE ELDERLY

FACTORS	POTENTIAL COMPLICATIONS
Diminished baroreceptor activity	Orthostatic hypotension
Decreased intravascular volume	Orthostatic hypotension, dehydration
Sensitivity to hypokalemia	Arrhythmia, muscular weakness
Decreased renal and hepatic function	Drug accumulation
Polypharmacy	Drug interaction
CNS changes	Depression, confusion

should be avoided, and all drugs should be given in slowly increasing doses to prevent extensive lowering of the pressure.

Including the data shown in Figure 27–1, the results of all 13 randomized trials lasting at least 1 year involving over 16,000 elderly hypertensives demonstrate that treating healthy old patients is highly efficacious.[214] By design, the patients enrolled in these trials were healthier than most elderly hypertensives so that caution is advised in extrapolating these excellent results to the patients usually seen in clinical practice.

Isolated systolic hypertension is common in the elderly and presents a serious risk, particularly for strokes. The results of the SHEP indicated that these risks could be significantly reduced by small doses of diuretic and, if needed, a beta blocker.[13] Calcium antagonists also work well in the elderly.[215] The average level of systolic pressure reached by the SHEP participants, 145 mm Hg, seems a reasonable goal for most elderly patients.

HYPERTENSION WITH CONGESTIVE HEART FAILURE. Cardiac output may fall so markedly in hypertensive patients who are in heart failure with systolic dysfunction that their blood pressure is reduced, obscuring the degree of hypertension; often, however, the diastolic pressure is raised by intense vasoconstriction while the systolic pressure falls as a result of the reduced stroke volume. Lowering the blood pressure may, by itself, relieve the heart failure. Chronic unloading has been most efficiently accomplished with ACE inhibitors[216] (see p. 856). Caution is needed for those elderly hypertensives with diastolic dysfunction related to marked left ventricular hypertrophy, because unloaders may worsen their status, whereas beta blockers or calcium antagonists may be beneficial.

As noted in Chapter 26, left ventricular hypertrophy (LVH) is frequently found by echocardiography, even in patients with mild hypertension. All antihypertensive drugs except direct vasodilators have been shown to regress LVH, and regression may continue for as long as 5 years of treatment.[217]

HYPERTENSION WITH ISCHEMIC HEART DISEASE. The coexistence of ischemic heart disease makes antihypertensive therapy even more essential, since relief of the hypertension may ameliorate the coronary disease. Beta blockers and calcium antagonists are particularly useful if angina or arrhythmias are present. Caution is needed to avoid decreased coronary perfusion that is likely to be responsible for the J curve seen in multiple trials[35–37] (see p. 841).

The often markedly high levels of blood pressure during the early phase of an acute myocardial infarction may reflect sympathetic nervous hyperreactivity to pain. Cautious use of antihypertensive drugs that do not decrease cardiac output may be useful in the immediate postinfarction period, whereas beta blockers and ACE inhibitors have been shown to provide long-term benefit.

THERAPY FOR HYPERTENSIVE CRISES

When diastolic blood pressure exceeds 140 mm Hg, rapidly progressive damage to the arterial vasculature is demonstrable experimentally, and a surge of cerebral blood flow may rapidly lead to encephalopathy (p. 832). If such high pressures persist or if there are any signs of encephalopathy, the pressures should be lowered using parenteral agents in those patients considered to be in immediate danger or with oral agents in those who are alert and in no other acute distress.

A number of drugs for this purpose currently are available (Table 27–10). If diastolic pressure exceeds 140 mm Hg and the patient has any complications, such as an aortic dissection, a constant infusion of nitroprusside is most effective and will almost always lower the pressure to the desired level. Constant monitoring with an intraarterial line is mandatory because a slightly excessive dose may lower the pressure abruptly to levels that will induce shock. The potency and rapidity of action of nitroprusside have made it the treatment of choice for life-threatening hypertension. However, nitroprusside acts as a venous and arteriolar dilator, so that venous return and cardiac output are lowered[218] and intracranial pressures may increase.[219] Therefore, other parenteral agents are being more widely used. These include labetalol[163] and the calcium antagonist nicardipine.[177]

With any of these agents, intravenous furosemide is often needed to lower the blood pressure further and prevent retention of salt and water. Diuretics should not be given if volume depletion is initially present.

For patients in less immediate danger, oral therapy may be used. Almost every drug has been used and most will, with repeated doses, reduce high pressures. The current

TABLE 27–10 PARENTERAL DRUGS FOR TREATMENT OF HYPERTENSIVE EMERGENCY (IN ORDER OF RAPIDITY OF ACTION)

DRUG	DOSAGE	ONSET OF ACTION	ADVERSE EFFECTS
VASODILATORS			
Nitroprusside (Nipride, Nitropress)	0.25–10 μg/kg/min as I.V. infusion	Instantaneous	Nausea, vomiting, muscle twitching, sweating, thiocyanate intoxication
Nitroglycerin	5–100 μg/min as I.V. infusion	2–5 min	Tachycardia, flushing, headache, vomiting, methemoglobinemia
Diazoxide (Hyperstat)	50–100 mg/I.V. bolus, repeated or 15–30 mg/min by I.V. infusion	2–4 min	Nausea, hypotension, flushing, tachycardia, chest pain
Nicardipine (Cardene)	2–10 mg/hr I.V.	5–10 min	Tachycardia, headache, flushing, local phlebitis
Hydralazine (Apresoline)	10–20 mg I.V. 10–50 mg I.M.	10–20 min 20–30 min	Tachycardia, flushing, headache, vomiting, aggravation of angina
Enalapril (Vasotec IV)	1.25–5 mg q 6 hr	15 min	Precipitous fall in BP in high renin states; response variable
ADRENERGIC INHIBITORS			
Phentolamine (Regitine)	5–15 mg I.V.	1–2 min	Tachycardia, flushing
Trimethaphan (Arfonad)	0.5–5 mg/min as I.V. infusion	1–5 min	Paresis of bowel and bladder, orthostatic hypotension, blurred vision, dry mouth
Esmolol (Brevibloc)	500 μg/kg/min for 4 min, then 150–300 μg/kg/min I.V.	1–2 min	Hypotension
Labetalol (Normodyne, Trandate)	20–80 mg I.V. bolus every 10 min 2 mg/min I.V. infusion	5–10 min	Vomiting, scalp tingling, burning in throat, postural hypotension, dizziness, nausea

preference of many is nifedipine, 10 mg by mouth or sublingually, repeated in 30 minutes if needed.[176] The sublingual route provides a slower route and probably, therefore, a safer one. The pressure almost always falls about 25 per cent within the first 30 minutes. Rarely, and not unexpectedly, a few patients may suffer tissue ischemia with such rapid and marked falls in pressure. A safer course for many patients, particularly if their current high pressures are simply a reflection of stopping previously effective oral medication, is simply to restart that medication and monitor their response closely. If their nonadherence to therapy was caused by side effects, appropriate changes should be made.

With some exceptions,[220] most centers are seeing fewer patients in hypertensive crisis, presumably because more patients are diagnosed and treated before the disease enters this malignant course. The continued successful treatment of many more hypertensive persons will prevent the more frequent long-range cardiovascular complications of hypertension.

REFERENCES

BENEFITS OF THERAPY

1. Stockwell, D. H., Madhavan, S., Cohen, H., et al.: The determinants of hypertension awareness, treatment, and control in an insured population. Am. J. Public Health *84:*1768, 1994.
2. Neaton, J. D., Grimm R. H., Jr., Prineas, R. J., et al.: Treatment of mild hypertension study. JAMA *270:*713, 1993.
3. Kaplan, N. M.: Treatment of hypertension: Drug therapy. *In* Kaplan, N. M. (ed.): Clinical Hypertension. 6th ed. Baltimore, Williams and Wilkins, 1994, p. 191.
4. Swales, J. D.: Pharmacological treatment of hypertension. Lancet *344:* 380, 1994.
5. Thürmer, H. H., Lund-Larsen, P. G., and Tverdal, A.: Is blood pressure treatment as effective in a population setting as in controlled trials? Results from a prospective study. J. Hypertens. *12:*481, 1994.
6. Rose, G.: The Strategy of Preventive Medicine. Oxford, Oxford University Press, 1992.
7. Jackson, R., Barham, P., Bills, J., et al.: Management of raised blood pressure in New Zealand: A discussion document. Br. Med. J. *307:*107, 1993.
8. Johannesson, M.: Economic evaluation of hypertension treatment—methods and empirical results. *In* Swales, J. D. (ed.): Textbook of Hypertension. Oxford, Blackwell Scientific Publications, 1994, p. 1292.
8a. Kaplan, N. M.: Management of hypertension. *In* Fuster, V., Ross, R., and Topol, E. J. (eds.): Atherosclerosis and Coronary Artery Disease. Philadelphia, Lippincott-Raven Publishers, 1996, pp. 259–274.
9. MacMahon, S. W., Cutler, J. A., Furberg, C. D., and Payne, G. H.: The effects of drug treatment for hypertension on morbidity and mortality from cardiovascular disease: A review of randomized controlled trials. Prog. Cardiovasc. Dis. *29:*99, 1986.
10. Collins, R., Peto, R., MacMahon, S., et al.: Blood pressure, stroke, and coronary heart disease. Part II: Short-term reductions in blood pressure: Overview of randomized drug trials in their epidemiological context. Lancet *335:*827, 1990.
11. MacMahon, S., and Rodgers, A.: The effects of blood pressure reduction in older patients: An overview of five randomized controlled trials in elderly hypertensives. Clin. Exper. Hypertens. *15:*967, 1993.
12. MacMahon, S., Peto, R., Cutler, J., et al.: Blood pressure, stroke and coronary heart disease: Part I. Prolonged differences in blood pressure: Prospective observational studies corrected for the regression dilution bias. Lancet *335:*765, 1990.
13. SHEP Cooperative Research Group: Prevention of stroke by antihypertensive drug treatment in older persons with isolated systolic hypertension. JAMA *265:*3255, 1991.
14. Dahlöf, B., Lindholm, L. H., and Hansson, L.: Morbidity and mortality in the Swedish Trial in Old Patients with Hypertension (STOP-Hypertension). Lancet *338:*1281, 1991.
15. Medical Research Council Working Party: Medical Research Council trial of treatment of hypertension in older adults: Principal results. Br. Med. J. *304:*405, 1992.
15a. Chobanian, A. V.: Have long-term benefits of antihypertensive therapy been underestimated? Provocative findings from the Framingham Heart Study. Circulation *93:*638, 1996.
16. Hebert, P. R., Moser, M., Mayer, J., et al.: Recent evidence on drug therapy of mild to moderate hypertension and decreased risk of coronary heart disease. Arch. Intern. Med. *153:*578, 1993.
17. Kaplan, N. M.: Management of hypertensive emergencies. Lancet *344:* 1335, 1994.
18. Bing, R. F., Heagerty, A. M., Russell, G. I., et al.: Prognosis in malignant hypertension. J. Hypertens. *4*(Suppl. 6):S42, 1986.
19. Management of Committee of the Australian Therapeutic Trial in Mild Hypertension: Untreated mild hypertension. Lancet *1:*185, 1982.
20. National High Blood Pressure Education Program Working Group: National High Blood Pressure Education Program Working Group Report on primary prevention of hypertension. Arch. Intern. Med. *153:*186, 1993.
21. IPPPSH Collaborative Group: Cardiovascular risk and risk factors in a randomized trial of treatment based on the beta-blocker oxprenolol: The International Prospective Primary Prevention Study in Hypertension (IPPPSH). J. Hypertens. *3:*379, 1985.
22. Medical Research Council Working Party: MRC trial of treatment of mild hypertension: principal results. Br. Med. J. *291:*97, 1985.
23. Kaplan, N. M. (ed.): Treatment of Hypertension: Rationale and Goals. Baltimore, Williams and Wilkins, 1994, p. 145.
24. Hypertension Detection and Follow-Up Program Cooperative Group: The effect of treatment on mortality in "mild" hypertension. N. Engl. J. Med. *307:*976, 1982.
25. Multiple Risk Factor Intervention Trial Research Group: Multiple risk factor intervention trial. Risk factor changes and mortality results. JAMA *248:*1465, 1982.

THRESHOLD FOR THERAPY

26. Joint National Committee on Detection, Evaluation, and Treatment of High Blood Pressure: The fifth report of the Joint National Committee on Detection, Evaluation and Treatment of High Blood Pressure (JNC V). Arch. Intern. Med. *153:*154, 1993.
27. Sever, P., Beevers, G., Bulpitt, C., et al.: Management guidelines in essential hypertension: Report of the second working party of the British Hypertension Society. Br. Med. J. *306:*983, 1993.
28. Haynes, R. B., Lacourcière, Y., Rabkin, S. W., et al.: Report of the Canadian Hypertension Society Consensus Conference: 2. Diagnosis of hypertension in adults, Can. Med. Assoc. J. *149:*409, 1993.
29. The Guidelines Subcommittee of the WHO/ISH Mild Hypertension Liaison Committee: 1993 Guidelines for the management of mild hypertension. Hypertension *22:*392, 1993.
30. Samuelsson, O.: Experiences from hypertension trials. Impact of other risk factors. Drugs *36*(Suppl. 3):9, 1988.
31. Kaplan, N. M.: The treatment of hypertension in women. Arch. Intern. Med. *155:*563, 1995.
32. Management Committee: The Australian therapeutic trial in mild hypertension. Lancet *1:*1261, 1980.
33. Bulpitt, C. J., and Fletcher, A. E.: Aging, blood pressure and mortality. J. Hypertens. *10*(Suppl. 7):45, 1992.
34. Epstein, F. H.: Proceedings of the XVth International Congress of Therapeutics, Sept. 5–9, 1979. Brussels, Excerpta Medica, 1980.
35. Cruickshank, J. M.: Coronary flow reserve and the J curve relation between diastolic blood pressure and myocardial infarction. Br. Med. J. *297:*1227, 1988.
36. Lindblad, U., Råstam, L., Rydén, L., et al.: Control of blood pressure and risk of first acute myocardial infarction: Skaraborg hypertension project. Br. Med. J. *308:*681, 1994.
37. Madhavan, S., Ooi, W. L., Cohen, H., and Alderman, M. H.: Relation of pulse pressure and blood pressure reduction to the incidence of myocardial infarction. Hypertension *23:*395, 1994.
38. Kuller, L. H., Hulley, S. B., Cohen, J. D., and Neaton, J.: Unexpected effects of treating hypertension in men with electrocardiographic abnormalities. A critical analysis. Circulation *73:*114, 1986.
39. Cooper, S. P., Hardy, R. J., Labarthe, D. R., et al.: The relation between degree of blood pressure reduction and mortality among hypertensives in the hypertension detection and follow-up program. Am. J. Epidemiol. *127:*387, 1988.
40. Cruickshank, J. M.: J curve in antihypertensive therapy: Does it exist? A personal point of view. Cardiovasc. Drug Ther. *8:*757, 1994.
41. Amery, A., Berglund, G., Cruickshank, J. M., et al.: How much should blood pressure be lowered? The problem of the J-shaped curve. J. Hypertens. *7*(Suppl. 6):S338, 1989.
42. Tervahauta, M., Pekkanen, J., Enlund, H., and Nissinen, A.: Change in blood pressure and 5-year risk of coronary heart disease among elderly men: The Finnish cohorts of the Seven Countries Study. J. Hypertens. *12:*1183, 1994.
43. The HOT Study Group: The Hypertension Optimal Treatment (HOT) Study: a prospective study of the optimal therapeutic goal and of the value of a low dose aspirin in anti-hypertensive treatment. Blood Press *2:*62, 1993.
44. Schmieder, R. E., Rockstroh, J. K., and Messerli, F. H.: Antihypertensive therapy. To stop or not to stop? JAMA *256:*1566, 1991.

LIFE STYLE MODIFICATIONS

45. The Trials of Hypertension Prevention Collaborative Research Group: The effects of nonpharmacologic interventions on blood pressure of persons with high normal levels. Results of the Trials of Hypertension Prevention, Phase I. JAMA *267:*1213, 1992.
46. Geleijnse, J. M., Witteman, J. C. M., Bak, A. A. A., et al.: Reduction in blood pressure with a low sodium, high potassium, high magnesium salt in older subjects with mild to moderate hypertension. Br. Med. J. *309:*436, 1994.
47. Groppelli, A., Giorgi, D. M. A., Omboni, S., et al.: Persistent blood pressure increase induced by heavy smoking. J. Hypertens. *10:*495, 1992.
48. Staessen, J., Fagard, R., Lijnen, P., and Amery, A.: Body weight, sodium intake and blood pressure. J. Hypertens. *7*(Suppl. 1):S19, 1989.

49. Smoller, S. W., Blaufox, M. D., Oberman, A., et al.: TAIM Study: Adequate weight loss as effective as drug therapy for mild hypertension. Circulation *81*:4, 1990.
50. Schotte, D. E., and Stunkard, A. J.: The effects of weight reduction on blood pressure in 301 obese patients. Arch. Intern. Med. *150*:1701, 1990.
51. Wadden, T. A., Foster, G. D., Letizia, K. A., and Stunkard, A. J.: A multicenter evaluation of a proprietary weight reduction program for the treatment of marked obesity. Arch. Intern. Med. *152*:961, 1992.
52. Rocchini, A. P., Key, J., Bondie, D., et al.: The effect of weight loss on the sensitivity of blood pressure to sodium in obese adolescents. N. Engl. J. Med. *321*:580, 1989.
53. Cutler, J. A., Follmann, D., Elliott, P., and Suh, I.: An overview of randomized trials of sodium reduction and blood pressure. Hypertension *17*(Suppl. I):I-27, 1991.
54. MacGregor, G. A., Markandu, N. D., Sagnella, G. A., et al.: Double-blind study of three sodium intakes and long-term effects of sodium restriction in essential hypertension. Lancet *2*:1244, 1989.
55. Alderman, M. H., Madhaven, S., Cohen, H., et al.: Low urinary sodium is associated with greater risk of myocardial infarction among treated hypertensive men. Hypertension *25*:1144, 1995.
56. Weinberger, M. H., and Fineberg, N. S.: Sodium and volume sensitivity of blood pressure. Age and pressure change over time. Hypertension *18*:67, 1991.
57. Feldman, R. D.: A low-sodium diet corrects the defect in β-adrenergic response in older subjects. Circulation *85*:612, 1992.
58. Singer, D. R. J., Markandu, N. D., Sugden, A. L., et al.: Sodium restriction in hypertensive patients treated with a converting enzyme inhibitor and a thiazide. Hypertension *17*:798, 1991.
59. Jula, A., Karanko, H., and Rönnemaa, T.: Effects of long-term sodium restriction on left ventricular hypertrophy in mild to moderate essential hypertension. (Abstract) J. Hypertens. *10*(Suppl. 4):104, 1992.
60. Nowson, C. A., and Morgan, T. O.: Change in blood pressure in relation to change in nutrients effected by manipulation of dietary sodium and potassium. Clin. Exp. Pharmacol. Physiol. *15*:225, 1988.
61. Hargreaves, M., Morgan, T. O., Snow, R., and Guerin, M.: Exercise tolerance in the heat on low and normal salt intakes. Clin. Sci. *76*:553, 1989.
62. Kumanyika, S. K., Hebert, P. R., Cutler, J. A., et al.: Feasibility and efficacy of sodium reduction in the Trials of Hypertension Prevention, Phase I. Hypertension *22*:502, 1993.
63. Joossens, J. V., and Kesteloot, H.: Trends in systolic blood pressure, 24-hour sodium excretion, and stroke mortality in the elderly in Belgium. Am. J. Med. *90*(Suppl. 3A):5, 1991.
64. Alderman, M. H.: Non-pharmacological treatment of hypertension. Lancet *344*:307, 1994.
65. Krishna, G. G., and Kapoor, S. C.: Potassium depletion exacerbates essential hypertension. Ann. Intern. Med. *115*:77, 1991.
66. Taddei, S., Mattei, P., Virdis, A., et al.: Effect of potassium on vasodilation to acetylcholine in essential hypertension. Hypertension *23*:485, 1994.
67. Cappuccio, F. P., and MacGregor, G. A.: Does potassium supplementation lower blood pressure? A meta-analysis of published trials. J. Hypertens. *9*:465, 1991.
68. Siani, A., Strazzullo, P., Giacco, A., et al.: Increasing the dietary potassium intake reduces the need for antihypertensive medication. Ann. Intern. Med. *115*:753, 1991.
69. Wirell, M. P., Wester, P. O., and Stegmayr, B. G.: Nutritional dose of magnesium in hypertensive patients on beta blockers lowers systolic blood pressure: A double-blind, cross-over study. J. Intern. Med. *236*:189, 1994.
70. Whang, R., Whang, D. D., and Ryan, M. P.: Refractory potassium repletion. A consequence of magnesium deficiency. Arch. Intern. Med. *152*:40, 1992.
71. Lind, L., Lithell, H., Gustafsson, I. B., et al.: Calcium metabolism and sodium sensitivity in hypertensive subjects. J. Hum. Hypertens. *7*:53, 1993.
72. Grobbee, D. E., and Waal-Manning, H. J.: The role of calcium supplementation in the treatment of hypertension. Current evidence. Drugs *39*:7, 1990.
73. Morris, C. D., and McCarron, D. A.: Effect of calcium supplementation in an older population with mildly increased blood pressure. Am. J. Hypertens. *5*:230, 1992.
74. Sciarrone, S. E. G., Strahan, M. T., Beilin, L. J., et al.: Ambulatory blood pressure and heart rate responses to vegetarian meals. J. Hypertens. *11*:277, 1993.
75. Eliasson, K., Ryttig, K. R., Hylander, B., and Rössner, S.: A dietary fibre supplement in the treatment of mild hypertension. A randomized, double-blind, placebo-controlled trial. J. Hypertens. *10*:195, 1992.
76. Morris, M. C., Sacks, F., and Rosner, B.: Does fish oil lower blood pressure? A meta-analysis of controlled trials. Circulation *88*:523, 1993.
77. Bønaa, K. H., Bjerve, K. S., Straume, B., et al.: Effect of eicosapentaenoic and docosahexaenoic acids on blood pressure in hypertension. A population-based intervention trial from the Tromsø study. N. Engl. J. Med. *322*:795, 1990.
78. Sacks, F. M.: Dietary fats and blood pressure: A critical review of the evidence. Nutr. Rev. *47*:291, 1989.
79. Parillo, M., Coulston, A., Hollenbeck, C., and Reaven, G.: Effect of a low fat diet on carbohydrate metabolism in patients with hypertension. Hypertension *11*:244, 1988.
80. Silagy, C. A., and Neil, H. A. W.: A meta-analysis of the effect of garlic on blood pressure. J. Hypertens. *12*:463, 1994.
81. Sung, B. H., Whitsett, T. L., Lovallo, W. R., et al.: Prolonged increase in blood pressure by a single oral dose of caffeine in mildly hypertensive men. Am. J. Hypertens. *7*:755, 1994.
82. Grønbæk, M., Deis, A., Sørensen, T. I. A., et al.: Influence of sex, age, body mass index, and smoking on alcohol intake and mortality. Br. Med. J. *308*:302, 1994.
83. Cameron, J. D., and Dart, A. M.: Exercise training increases total systemic arterial compliance in humans. Am. J. Physiol. *266*:H693, 1994.
84. Dubbert, P. M., Martin, M. E., Cushman, W. C., et al.: Endurance exercise in mild hypertension: Effects on blood pressure and associated metabolic and quality of life variables. J. Hum. Hypertens. *8*:265, 1994.
85. Shaper, A. G., Wannamethee, G., and Walker, M.: Physical activity, hypertension and risk of heart attack in men without evidence of ischaemic heart disease. J. Hum. Hypertens. *8*:3, 1994.
86. Steward K. J.: Weight training in coronary artery disease and hypertension. Prog. Cardiovasc. Dis. *35*:159, 1992.
87. Eisenberg, D. M., Delbanco, T. L., Berkey, C. S., et al.: Cognitive behavioral techniques for hypertension: Are they effective? Am. J. Hypertens. *4*:416, 1993.

ANTIHYPERTENSIVE DRUG THERAPY

88. Strandgaard, S., and Haunsø, S.: Why does antihypertensive treatment prevent stroke but not myocardial infarction? Lancet *2*:658, 1987.
89. Fagan, T. C.: Remembering the lessons of basic pharmacology. Arch. Intern. Med. *154*:1430, 1994.
90. Herxheimer, A.: How much drug in the tablet? Lancet *337*:346, 1991.
91. Kaplan, N. M.: The appropriate goals of antihypertensive therapy: Neither too much nor too little. Ann. Intern. Med. *116*:686, 1992.
91a. Oates, J. A.: Antihypertensive agents and the drug therapy of hypertension. *In* Hardman, J. G., et al. (eds.): Goodman and Gilman's The Pharmacological Basis of Therapeutics. 9th ed. New York, McGraw-Hill, 1996, pp. 781–808.
92. Frishman, W. H., Bryzinski, B. S., Coulson, L. R., et al.: A multifactorial trial design to assess combination therapy in hypertension. Arch. Intern. Med. *154*:1461, 1994.
93. Eisen, S. A., Miller, D. K., Woodward, R. S., et al.: The effect of prescribed daily dose frequency on patient medication compliance. Arch. Intern. Med. *150*:1881, 1990.
94. Elliott, H. L.: Trough: Peak ratio and 24-hour blood pressure control. J. Hypertens. *12*(Suppl. 5):S29, 1994.
95. Anderson, A., Morgan, O., and Morgan, T.: Effectiveness of blood pressure control with once daily administration of enalapril and perindopril. Am. J. Hypertens. *7*:371, 1994.
96. Swales, J. D.: Guidelines on guidelines. J. Hypertens. *11*:899, 1993.
97. Weber, M. A., and Laragh, J. H.: Hypertension: Steps forward and steps backward. Arch. Intern. Med. *153*:149, 1993.
98. Tobian, L., Brunner, H. R., Cohn, J. N., et al.: Modern strategies to prevent coronary sequelae and stroke in hypertensive patients differ from the JNC V consensus guidelines. J. Hypertens. *7*:859, 1994.
99. Materson, B. J., Reda, D. J., and Cushman, W. C.: Department of Veterans Affairs Single-Drug Therapy of Hypertension Study. Revised figures and new data. Am. J. Hypertens. *8*:189, 1995.
100. Attwood, S., Bird, R., Burch, K., et al.: Within-patient correlation between the antihypertensive effects of atenolol, lisinopril and nifedipine. J. Hypertens. *12*:1053, 1994.
101. Guyatt, G. H., Keller, J. L., Jaeschke, R., et al.: The n-of-1 randomized controlled trial: Clinical usefulness. Our three-year experience. Ann. Intern. Med. *112*:293, 1990.
102. Laragh, J. H.: Perspectives in choosing therapy for hypertension. *In* Kaplan, N. M., Brenner, B. M., and Laragh, J. H. (eds.): New Therapeutic Strategies in Hypertension. New York, Raven Press, 1989, p. 141.
103. Bravo, E. L.: Rational drug therapy based on understanding the pathophysiology of hypertension. Cleveland Clin. J. Med. *56*:362, 1989.
104. Woolf, S. H.: Practice guidelines: A new reality in medicine. III. Impact on patient care. Arch. Intern. Med. *153*:2646, 1993.

Diuretics

105. Kaplan, N. M.: Difficult to treat hypertension. Am. J. Med. Sci. *309*:339, 1995.
106. Burris, J. F., Weir, M. R., Oparil, S., et al.: An assessment of diltiazem and hydrochlorothiazide in hypertension. Application of factorial trial design to a multicenter clinical trial of combination therapy. JAMA *263*:1507, 1990.
107. Harper, R., Ennis, C. N., Sheridan, B., et al.: Effects of low dose versus conventional dose thiazide diuretic on insulin action in essential hypertension. Br. Med. J. 309:226, 1994.
108. Hall, W. D., Weber, M. A., Ferdinand, K., et al.: Lower dose diuretic therapy in the treatment of patients with mild to moderate hypertension. J. Hum. Hypertens. *8*:571, 1994.
109. Baumgart, P.: Torsemide in comparison with thiazides in the treatment of hypertension. Cardiovasc. Drug Ther. *7*:63, 1993.
110. Morgan, D. G., and Davidson, C.: Hypokalemia and diuretics: An analysis of publications. Br. Med. J. *280*:905, 1980.
111. Sandor, F. F., Pickens, P. T., and Crallan, J.: Variations of plasma potassium concentrations during long-term treatment of hypertension with diuretics without potassium supplements. Br. Med. J. *284*:711, 1982.

112. Siscovick, D. S., Raghunathan, T. E., Psaty, B. M., et al.: Diuretic therapy for hypertension and the risk of primary cardiac arrest. N. Engl. J. Med. *330*:1852, 1994.
113. Lipworth, B. J., McDevitt, D. G., and Struthers, A. D.: Electrocardiographic changes induced by inhaled salbutamol after treatment with bendrofluazide: Effects of replacement therapy with potassium, magnesium and triamterene. Clin. Sci. *78*:225, 1990.
114. Kaplan, N. M., Carnegie, A., Raskin, P., et al.: Potassium supplementation in hypertensive patients with diuretic-induced hypokalemia. N. Engl. J. Med. *312*:746, 1985.
115. Samuelsson, O., Hedner, T., Berglund, G., et al.: Diabetes mellitus in treated hypertension: Incidence, predictive factors and the impact of non-selective beta-blockers and thiazide diuretics during 15 years treatment of middle-aged hypertensive men in the Primary Prevention Trial Göteborg, Sweden. J. Hum. Hypertens. *8*:257, 1994.
116. Dørup, I., Skajaa, K., and Thybo, N. K.: Oral magnesium supplementation restores the concentrations of magnesium, potassium and sodium-potassium pumps in skeletal muscle of patients receiving diuretic treatment. J. Intern. Med. *233*:117, 1993.
117. Horner, S. M.: Efficacy of intravenous magnesium in acute myocardial infarction in reducing arrhythmias and mortality. Meta-analysis of magnesium in acute myocardial infarction. Circulation *86*:774, 1992.
118. Waller, P. C., and Ramsay, L. E.: Predicting acute gout in diuretic-treated hypertensive patients. J. Hum. Hypertens. *3*:457, 1989.
119. Kasiske, B. L., Ma, J. Z., Kalil, R. S. N., and Louis, T. A.: Effects of antihypertensive therapy on serum lipids. Ann. Intern. Med. *122*:133, 1995.
120. Pollare, T., Lithell, H., and Berne, C.: A comparison of the effects of hydrochlorothiazide and captopril on glucose and lipid metabolism in patients with hypertension. N. Engl. J. Med. *321*:868, 1989.
121. Gesek, F. A., and Friedman, P. A.: Mechanism of calcium transport stimulated by chlorothiazide in mouse distal convoluted tubule cells. J. Clin. Invest. *90*:429, 1992.
122. Morton, D. J., Barrett-Connor, E. L., and Edelstein, S. L.: Thiazides and bone mineral density in elderly men and women. Am. J. Epidemiol. *139*:1107, 1994.
123. Medical Research Council Working Party on Mild to Moderate Hypertension: Adverse reactions to bendrofluazide and propranolol for the treatment of mild hypertension. Lancet *2*:539, 1981.
124. Beard, K., Bulpitt, C., Mascie-Taylor, H., et al.: Management of elderly patients with sustained hypertension. Br. Med. J. *304*:412, 1992.

Adrenergic Inhibitors

125. Veterans Administration Cooperative Study Group on Antihypertensive Agents: Propranolol in the treatment of essential hypertension. JAMA *237*:2303, 1977.
126. Participating Veterans Administration Medical Centers: Low dose vs. standard dose of reserpine. JAMA *248*:2471, 1982.
127. Lederle, F. A., Applegate, W. B., and Grimm, R. H., Jr.: Reserpine and the medical marketplace. Arch. Intern. Med. *153*:705, 1993.
128. Struthers, A. D., Brown, M. J., Adams, E. F., and Dollery, C. T.: The plasma noradrenaline and growth hormone response to α-methyldopa and clonidine in hypertensive subjects. Br. J. Clin. Pharmacol. *19*:311, 1985.
129. Fouad, F. M., Nakashima, Y., Tarazi, R. C., and Salcedo, E. E.: Reversal of left ventricular hypertrophy in hypertensive patients treated with methyldopa. Am. J. Cardiol. *49*:795, 1982.
130. Kelton, J. G.: Impaired reticuloendothelial function in patients treated with methyldopa. Am. J. Cardiol. *49*:795, 1982.
131. Kaplowitz, N., Aw, T. Y., Simon, F. R., and Stolz, A.: Drug-induced hepatotoxicity. Ann. Intern. Med. *104*:826, 1986.
132. van Zwieten, P. A.: Different types of centrally acting antihypertensive drugs. Eur. Heart J. *13*:18, 1992.
133. Houston, M. C.: Abrupt cessation of treatment in hypertension: Consideration of clinical features, mechanisms, prevention and management of the discontinuation syndrome. Am. Heart J. *102*:415, 1981.
134. Schmidt, G. R., Schuna, A. A., and Goodfriend, T. L.: Transdermal clonidine compared with hydrochlorothiazide as monotherapy in elderly hypertensive males. J. Clin. Pharmacol. *29*:133, 1989.
135. Gehr, M., MacCarthy, E. P., and Goldberg, M.: Guanabenz: A centrally acting, natriuretic antihypertensive drug. Kidney Int. *29*:1203, 1986.
136. Kaplan, N. M., and Grundy, S.: Comparison of the effects of guanabenz and hydrochlorothiazide on plasma lipids. Clin. Pharmacol. Ther. *44*: 297, 1988.
137. Lewin, A., Alderman, M. H., and Mathur, P.: Antihypertensive efficacy of guanfacine and prazosin in patients with mild to moderate essential hypertension. J. Clin. Pharmacol. *30*:1081, 1990.
138. Lenz, M. L., Pool, J. L., Laddu, A. R., et al.: Combined terazosin and verapamil therapy in essential hypertension: Hemodynamic and pharmacokinetic interactions. Am. J. Hypertens. *8*:133, 1995.
139. Pickering, T. G., Levenstein, M., and Walmsley, P.: Nighttime dosing of doxazosin has peak effect on morning ambulatory blood pressure. Results of the HALT study. Am. J. Hypertens. *7*:844, 1994.
140. Heagerty, A. M., Russell, G. I., Bing, R. F., et al.: The addition of prazosin to standard triple therapy in the treatment of severe hypertension. Br. J. Clin. Pharmacol. *13*:539, 1982.
141. Rabkin, S. W., Huff, M. W., Newman, C., et al.: Lipids and lipoproteins during antihypertensive drug therapy. Comparison of doxazosin and atenolol in a randomized, double-blind trial: The Alpha Beta Canada study. Hypertension *24*:241, 1994.
142. Andersson, P.-E., Johansson, J., Berne, C., and Lithell, H.: Effects of selective $alpha_1$ and $beta_1$-adrenoreceptor blockade on lipoprotein and carbohydrate metabolism in hypertensive subjects, with special emphasis on insulin sensitivity. J. Hum. Hypertens. *8*:219, 1994.
143. Monda, J. M., and Oesterling, J. E.: Medical treatment of benign prostatic hyperplasia: 5α-reductase inhibitors and α-adrenergic antagonists. Mayo Clin. Proc. *68*:670, 1993.
144. Viscoli, C. M., Horwitz, R. I., and Singer, B. H.: Beta-blockers after myocardial infarction: influence of first-year clinical course on long-term effectiveness. Ann. Intern. Med. *118*:99, 1993.
145. IPPPSH Collaborative Group: Cardiovascular risk and risk factors in a randomized trial of treatment based on the beta-blocker oxprenolol: The International Prospective Primary Prevention Study in Hypertension (IPPPSH). J. Hypertens. *3*:379, 1985.
146. Wilhelmsen, L., Berglund, G., Elmfeldt, D., et al.: Beta-blockers versus diuretics in hypertensive men: Main results from the HAPPHY Trial. J. Hypertens. *5*:561, 1987.
147. Wikstrand, J., Warnold, I., Olsson, G., et al.: Primary prevention with metoprolol in patients with hypertension. Mortality results from the MAPHY study. JAMA *259*:1976, 1988.
148. Wikstrand, J., Warnold, I., Tuomilehto, J., et al.: Metoprolol versus thiazide diuretics in hypertension. Hypertension *17*:579, 1991.
149. Fitzgerald, J. D.: The applied pharmacology of beta-adrenoceptor antagonists (beta blockers) in relation to clinical outcomes. Cardiovasc. Drug Ther. *5*:561, 1991.
150. Lithell, H., Pollare, T., and Vessby, B.: Metabolic effects of pindolol and propranolol in a double-blind cross-over study in hypertensive patients. Blood Pressure *1*:92, 1992.
151. Yudofsky, S. C.: β-blockers and depression. The clinician's dilemma. JAMA *267*:1295, 1991.
152. Man in't Veld, A. J., Van Den Meiracker, A. H., and Schalekamp, M. A.: Do beta-blockers really increase peripheral vascular resistance? Review of the literature and new observations under basal conditions. Am. J. Hypertens. *1*:91, 1988.
153. Serlin, M. M., Orme, M. L' E., Baber, N. A., et al.: Propranolol in the control of blood pressure: A dose-response study. Clin. Pharmacol. Ther. *27*:586, 1980.
154. Cruickshank, J. M.: The case for beta-blockers as first-line antihypertensive therapy. J. Hypertens. *10*:S21, 1992.
155. Gullestad, L., Birkeland, K., Nordby, G., et al.: Effects of selective β_2-adrenoceptor blockade on serum potassium and exercise performance in normal men. Br. J. Clin. Pharmacol. *32*:201, 1991.
156. Oxorn, D., Knox, J. W. D., and Hill, J.: Bolus doses of esmolol for the prevention of perioperative hypertension and tachycardia. Can. J. Anaesth. *37*:206, 1990.
157. Eichhorn, E. J., and Hjalmarson, A.: β-Blocker treatment for chronic heart failure. The frog prince. Circulation *90*:2153, 1994.
158. Dahlöf, C., and Dimenäs, E.: Side effects of β-blocker treatments as related to the central nervous system. Am. J. Med. Sci. *299*:236, 1990.
159. Bright, R. A., and Everitt, D. E.: β-blockers and depression. Evidence against an association. JAMA *267*:1783, 1992.
160. Psaty, B. M., Koepsell, T. D., Wagner, E. H., et al.: The relative risk of incident coronary heart disease associated with recently stopping the use of β-blockers. JAMA *263*:1653, 1990.
161. Dujovne, C. A., Ferraro, L., Goldstein, R. J., et al.: Comparative effects of atenolol versus celiprolol on serum lipids and blood pressure in hyperlipidemic and hypertensive subjects. Am. J. Cardiol. *72*:1131, 1993.
162. Butters, L., Kennedy, S., and Rubin, P. C.: Atenolol in essential hypertension during pregnancy. Br. Med. J. *301*:587, 1990.
163. Goa, K. L., Benfield, P., and Sorkin, E. M.: Labetalol. A reappraisal of its pharmacology, pharmacokinetics and therapeutic use in hypertension and ischaemic heart disease. Drugs *37*:583, 1989.
164. Clark, J. A., Zimmerman, H. J., and Tanner, L. A.: Labetalol hepatotoxicity. Ann. Intern. Med. *113*:210, 1990.

Vasodilators

165. Shepherd, A. M. M., and Irving, N. A.: Differential hemodynamic and sympathoadrenal effects of sodium nitroprusside and hydralazine in hypertensive subjects. J. Cardiovasc. Pharmacol. *8*:527, 1986.
166. Halstenson, C. E., Opsahl, J.A., Wright, E., et al.: Disposition of minoxidil in patients with various degrees of renal function. J. Clin. Pharmacol. *29*:798, 1989.
167. Houston, M. C., McChesney, J. A., and Chatterjee, K.: Pericardial effusion associated with minoxidil therapy. Arch. Intern. Med. *131*:69, 1981.
168. Kelly, J. G., and O'Malley, K.: Clinical pharmacokinetics of calcium antagonists. Clin. Pharmacokinet. *22*:416, 1992.
169. Cappuccio, F. P., Antonios, T. F. T., Markandu, N. D., et al.: Acute natriuretic effect of nifedipine on different sodium intakes in essential hypertension: Evidence for distal tubular effect? J. Hum. Hypertens. *8*:627, 1994.
170. Luft, F. C., Fineberg, N. S., and Weinberger, M. H.: Long-term effect of nifedipine and hydrochlorothiazide on blood pressure and sodium homeostasis at varying levels of salt intake in mildly hypertensive patients. Am. J. Hypertens. *4*:752, 1991.
171. ter Wee, P. M., De Micheli, A. G., and Epstein, M.: Effects of calcium antagonists on renal hemodynamics and progression of nondiabetic chronic renal disease. Arch. Intern. Med. *154*:1185, 1994.
172. Ranieri, G., Andriani, A., Lamontanara, G., and De Cesaris, R.: Effects

of lisinopril and amlodipine on microalbuminuria and renal function in patients with hypertension. Clin. Pharmacol. Ther. *56*:323, 1994.

173. Siewert-Delle, A., Ljungman, S., Hartford, M., and Wikstrand, J.: Effects of intensified blood-pressure reduction on renal function and albumin excretion in primary hypertension. Addition of felodipine or ramipril to long-term treatment with β-blockade. Am. J. Hypertens. *8*:113, 1995.
174. Zanetti-Elshater, F., Pingitore, R., Beretta-Piccoli, C., et al.: Calcium antagonists for treatment of diabetes-associated hypertension. Am. J. Hypertens. *7*:36, 1994.
174a. Psaty, B. M., Heckbert, S. R., Koepsell, T. D., et al.: The risk of myocardial infarction associated with antihypertensive drug therapies. JAMA *274*:620, 1995.
174b. Horwitz, R. I., Feinstein, A. R.: Exclusion bias and the false relationship of reserpine use and breast cancer. Arch. Intern. Med. *145*:1873, 1995.
175. Klassen, D. K., Jane, L. H., Young, D. Y., and Peterson, C. A.: Assessment of blood pressure during naproxen therapy in hypertensive patients treated with nicardipine. Am. J. Hypertens. *8*:146, 1995.
176. Jaker, M., Atkin, S., Soto, M., et al.: Oral nifedipine vs oral clonidine in the treatment of urgent hypertension. Arch. Intern. Med. *149*:260, 1989.
177. Neutel, J. M., Smith, D. H. G., Cook, W. E., et al.: A comparison of intravenous nicardipine and sodium nitroprusside in the immediate treatment of severe hypertension. Am. J. Hypertens. *7*:623, 1994.
177a. Jackson, E. K., and Garrison, J. C.: Renin and angiotensin. *In* Hardman, J. G., et al. (eds.): Goodman and Gilman's The Pharmacological Basis of Therapeutics. 9th ed. New York; McGraw-Hill, 1996, pp. 733–758.
178. Kobrin, I., Viskoper, R. J., Laszt, A., et al.: Effects of an orally active renin inhibitor, RO 42-5892, in patients with essential hypertension. Am. J. Hypertens. *6*:349, 1993.
179. Grossman, E., Peleg, E., Carroll, J., et al.: Hemodynamic and humoral effects of the angiotensin II antagonist losartan in essential hypertension. Am. J. Hypertens. *7*:1041, 1994.
180. van den Meiracker, A. H., Man in't Veld, A. J., Admiraal, P. J. J., et al.: Partial escape of angiotensin converting enzyme (ACE) inhibition during prolonged ACE inhibitor treatment: Does it exist and does it affect the antihypertensive response? J. Hypertens. *10*:803, 1992.
181. Pellacani, A., Brunner, H. R., and Nussberger, J.: Plasma kinins increase after angiotensin-converting enzyme inhibition in human subjects. Clin. Sci. *87*:567, 1994.
182. Tomiyama, H., Kushiro, T., Abeta, H., et al.: Kinins contribute to the improvement of insulin sensitivity during treatment with angiotensin converting enzyme inhibitor. Hypertension *23*:450, 1994.
183. Fletcher, A. E., Palmer, A. J., and Bulpitt, C. J.: Cough with angiotensin converting enzyme inhibitors: how much of a problem? J. Hypertens. *12*(Suppl. 2):S43, 1994.
184. Ferri, C., Laurenti, O., Bellini, C., et al.: Circulating endothelin-1 levels in lean noninsulin-dependent diabetic patients: Influence of ACE-inhibition. Am. J. Hypertens. *8*:40, 1995.
185. Schiffrin, E. L., Deng, L. Y., and Larochelle, P.: Effects of a β-blocker or a converting enzyme inhibitor on resistance arteries in essential hypertension. Hypertension *23*:83, 1994.
186. Giannattasio, C., Cattaneo, B. M., Omboni, S., et al.: Sympathomoderating influence of benazepril in essential hypertension. J. Hypertens. *10*:373, 1992.
187. Postma, C. T., Dennesen, P. J. W., de Boo, T., and Thien, T.: First dose hypotension after captopril; Can it be predicted? A study of 240 patients. J. Hum. Hypertens. *6*:205, 1992.
188. Kaplan, N. M.: Renal vascular hypertension. *In* Kaplan, N. M. (ed.): Clinical Hypertension. 6th ed. Baltimore, Williams & Wilkins, 1994, p. 319.
189. Devoy, M. A. B., Tomson, C. R. V., Edmunds, M. E., et al.: Deterioration in renal function associated with angiotensin converting enzyme inhibitor therapy is not always reversible. J. Intern. Med. *232*:493, 1992.
190. Lewis, E. J., Hunsicker, L. G., Bain, R. P., and Rohde, R. D.: The effect of angiotensin-converting-enzyme inhibition on diabetic nephropathy. N. Engl. J. Med. *329*:1456, 1993.
191. Buzio, C., Regolisti, G., Perazzoli, F., et al.: Renal effects of nifedipine and captopril in patients with essential hypertension and reduced renal reserve. Hypertension *24*:763, 1994.
192. Hypertension in Diabetes Study Group: Hypertension in Diabetes Study III. Prospective study of therapy of hypertension in type 2 diabetic patients: Efficacy of ACE inhibition and β-blockade. Diabetic Med. *11*:773, 1994.
193. Raccah, D., Pettenuzzo-Mollo, M., Provendier, O., et al.: Comparison of the effects of captopril and nicardipine on insulin sensitivity and thrombotic profile in patients with hypertension and android obesity. Am. J. Hypertens. *7*:731, 1994.
194. Chu, T. J., and Chow, N.: Adverse effects of ACE inhibitors. Ann. Intern. Med. *118*:313, 1993.
194a. Wood, R.: Bronchospasm and cough as adverse reactions to the ACE inhibitors captopril, enalapril and lisinopril. Br. J. Clin. Pharmacol. *39*:265, 1995.
195. Os, I., Bratland, B., Dahlöf, B., et al.: Female preponderance for lisinopril-induced cough in hypertension. Am. J. Hypertens. *7*:1012, 1994.
196. Lip, G. Y. H., Zarifis, J., Beevers, M., and Beevers, D. G.: Duration of cough following cessation of ACE inhibitor therapy. Am. J. Hypertens. *8*:98, 1995.
197. Warner, T. D., Battistini, B., Doherty, A. M., and Corder, R.: Endothelin receptor antagonists: Actions and rationale for their development. Biochem. Pharmacol. *48*:625, 1994.
198. Vesely, D. L., Douglass, M. D., Dietz, J. R., et al.: Three peptides from the atrial natriuretic factor prohormone amino terminus lower blood pressure and produce diuresis, natriuresis, and/or kaliuresis in humans. Circulation *90*:1129, 1994.
199. Ogihara, T., Rakugi, H., Masuo, K., et al.: Antihypertensive effects of the neutral endopeptidase inhibitor SCH 42495 in essential hypertension. Am. J. Hypertens. *7*:943, 1994.
200. Cody, R. J.: The clinical potential of renin inhibitors and angiotensin antagonists. Drugs *47*:586, 1994.
200a. Awan, N. A., and Mason, D. T.: Direct selective blockade of the vascular angiotensin II receptors in therapy for hypertension and severe congestive heart failure. Am. Heart J. *131*:177, 1996.

SPECIAL CONSIDERATIONS IN THERAPY

201. Setaro, J. F., and Black, H. R.: Refractory hypertension. N. Engl. J. Med. *8*:543, 1992.
202. Mejia, A. D., Egan, B. M., Schork, N. J., and Zwiefler, A. J.: Artefacts in measurement of blood pressure and lack of target organ involvement in the assessment of patients with treatment-resistant hypertension. Ann. Intern. Med. *117*:270, 1990.
203. Isaksson, H., Cederholm, T., Jansson, E., et al.: Therapy-resistant hypertension associated with central obesity, insulin resistance, and large muscle fibre area. Blood Pressure *2*:46, 1993.
204. Johnson, A. G., Nguyen, T. V., and Day, R. O.: Do nonsteroidal anti-inflammatory drugs affect blood pressure? Ann. Intern. Med. *121*:289, 1994.
205. Estafanous, F. G.: Hypertension in the surgical patient: Management of blood pressure and anesthesia. Cleveland Clin. J. Med. *56*:385, 1989.
206. Wolfsthal, S. D.: Is blood pressure control necessary before surgery? Med. Clin. North Am. *77*:349, 1993.
207. Haworth, R. A., Goknur, A. B., and Berkoff, H. A.: Inhibition of Na-Ca exchange by general anesthetics. Circ. Res. *65*:1021, 1989.
208. Patel, C. G., Laboy, V., Venus, B., et al.: Use of sodium nitroprusside in post-coronary bypass surgery. A plea for conservatism. Chest *80*:663, 1986.
209. Halpern, N. A., Goldberg, M., Neely, C., et al.: Postoperative hypertension: A multicenter, prospective, randomized comparison between intravenous nicardipine and sodium nitroprusside. Crit. Care Med. *20*:1637, 1992.
210. Lieberman, E.: Hypertension in childhood and adolescence. *In* Kaplan, N. M. (ed.): Clinical Hypertension. 6th ed. Baltimore, Williams and Wilkins, 1994, p. 437.
211. Lewis, R. R., Evans, P. J., McNabb, W. R., and Padayachee, T. S.: Comparison of indirect and direct blood pressure measurements with Osler's manoeuvre in elderly hypertensive patients. J. Hum. Hypertens. *8*:879, 1994.
212. Kaplan, N. M.: The promises and perils of treating the elderly hypertensive. Am. J. Med. Sci. *305*:183, 1993.
213. Lye, M., Vargas, E., Faragher, E. B., et al.: Haemodynamic and neurohumoral responses in elderly patients with postural hypotension. Eur. J. Clin. Invest. *20*:90, 1990.
214. Mulrow, C. D., Cornell, J. A., Herrera, C. R., et al.: Hypertension in the elderly. Implications and generalizability of randomized trials. JAMA *272*:1932, 1994.
215. Stein, G. H., Hamilton, B. P., Hamilton, J. H., et al.: One year experience of elderly hypertensive patients with isradipine therapy. J. Hum. Hypertens. *8*:911, 1994.
216. Groden, D. L.: Vasodilator therapy for congestive heart failure. Arch. Intern. Med. *153*:445, 1993.
217. Franz, I.-W., Ketelhut, R., Behr, U., and Tönnesmann, U.: Time course of reduction in left ventricular mass during long-term antihypertensive therapy. J. Hum. Hypertens. *8*:191, 1994.
218. Brush, J. E., Jr., Udelson, J. E., Bacharach, S. L., et al.: Comparative effects of verapamil and nitroprusside on left ventricular function in patients with hypertension. J. Am. Coll. Cardiol. *14*:515, 1989.
219. Cottrell, J. E., Patel, K., Turndorf, H., and Ransohoff, J.: Intracranial pressure changes induced by sodium nitroprusside in patients with intracranial mass lesions. J. Neurosurg. *48*:329, 1978.
220. Lip, G. Y. H., Beevers, M., and Beevers, G.: The failure of malignant hypertension to decline: A survey of 24 years' experience in a multiracial population in England. J. Hypertens. *12*:1297, 1994.

Chapter 28
Syncope and Hypotension

WISHWA N. KAPOOR

Syncope is defined as a sudden temporary loss of consciousness associated with a loss of postural tone with spontaneous recovery not requiring electrical or chemical cardioversion. Syncope is a common symptom accounting for 1 to 6 per cent of hospital admissions and up to 3 per cent of emergency department visits. Loss of consciousness is also common in healthy young adults (12 to 48 per cent), although most do not seek medical attention. Syncope is a frequent symptom in the elderly; a 6 per cent incidence and 23 per cent previous lifetime episodes were reported in one long-term care institution.

CLINICAL AND PATHOPHYSIOLOGICAL CLASSIFICATION

Although syncope has a large differential diagnosis, the causes can be classified into four major categories (Table 28–1).

Reflex-Mediated Vasomotor Instability Syndromes

Neurally mediated, neurocardiogenic, reflex, and neuroregulatory syncope are broad terms, used synonymously, referring to syncope resulting from reflex mechanisms associated with inappropriate vasodilatation and/or bradycardia.[1] These terms incorporate more specific syndromes such as vasovagal, vasodepressor, situational, or carotid sinus syncope. Currently, various neurally mediated syndromes are believed to have common pathophysiological elements as well as differences in triggering factors, afferent and efferent neural arcs, and central nervous system (CNS) processing that ultimately result in hypotension and loss of consciousness[1] (Fig. 28–1). For all of these syndromes, there are facilitating factors, such as emotional state, volume status, and posture, predisposing to syncope.

TABLE 28–1 ETIOLOGIES OF SYNCOPE

REFLEX-MEDIATED VASOMOTOR INSTABILITY	DECREASED CARDIAC OUTPUT
Vasovagal	**Obstruction to Flow**
Situational	Obstruction to LV outflow
Micturition	Aortic stenosis, HCM
Cough	Mitral stenosis, myxoma
Swallowing	Obstruction to RV outflow
Defecation	Pulmonic stenosis
Carotid sinus syncope	PE, pulmonary hypertension
Neuralgias	Myxoma
High altitude	**Other Heart Disease**
Psychiatric disorders	Pump failure
Others (exercise, selected drugs)	MI, CAD, coronary spasm
	Tamponade, aortic dissection
ORTHOSTATIC HYPOTENSION	**Arrhythmias**
NEUROLOGICAL DISEASES	Bradyarrhythmias
Migraines	Sinus node disease
TIAs	Second and third degree atrioventricular block
Seizures	Pacemaker malfunction
	Drug-induced bradyarrhythmias
	Tachyarrhythmias
	Ventricular tachycardia
	Torsades de pointes (e.g., associated with congenital long Q-T syndromes or acquired Q-T prolongation)
	Supraventricular tachycardia

LV = left ventricle; HCM = hypertrophic cardiomyopathy; MI = myocardial infarction; TIA = transient ischemic attack; CAD = coronary artery disease.

Receptors that respond to pain, mechanical stimuli, and temperature appear to serve as the origins of the afferent signals triggering the various neurally mediated syncopal syndromes.[1–3] For example, in carotid sinus hypersensitivity, carotid artery baroreceptors and in vasovagal syncope, left ventricular baroreceptors (mechanoreceptors) serve as triggers. Similar receptors in the aortic arch, carotid arteries, atrial and ventricular myocardium, respiratory tree, bladder, and gastrointestinal tract may trigger various other neurally mediated syndromes.[1] The afferent pathway consists of neural fibers (e.g., vagal C fibers in vasovagal syncope) that transmit signals to the CNS sites (in the medulla, particularly the nucleus tractus solitarius). The efferent outflow results in vasodilation and bradycardia. Ventricular mechanoreceptors are sensitized by catecholamines and arginine vasopressin, high levels of which are often found before vasovagal syncope. Provocation of syncope with upright tilt testing after heart transplantation has raised questions about this mechanism, because evidence for reinnervation is not found in some patients.[4–6] Central inhibition of sympathetic excitatory neurons has been considered to be an alternative mechanism with vasopressin release and opiate receptor activation playing possible roles.[7,8] Additionally, the role of serotonin[2,9] and endogenous nitric oxide as mediators of central inhibitory activity has been postulated.[2] More complete understanding of the mechanism of neurally mediated syncope has to await further studies. Current understanding of the clinical and pathophysiological mechanism of specific entities is described below.

VASOVAGAL SYNCOPE. Vasodepressor or vasovagal syncope is characterized by a sudden fall in blood pressure with or without bradycardia in association with autonomic and humoral activity such as pallor, nausea, sweating, mydriasis, bradycardia, hyperventilation, and antidiuresis. Vasodepressor syncope often occurs in young people and generally in response to fear or injury. Predisposing factors include fatigue, prolonged standing, venipuncture, blood donation, heat, dental surgery, and eye surgery. Vasovagal syncope may also occur without any identifiable predisposing factors and may be provoked by standing still in an upright posture in susceptible individuals.

Vasovagal syncope has three phases. During the first phase, blood pressure and heart rate increase largely owing to a baroreceptor-mediated rise in sympathetic tone. This is followed by abrupt hypotension and bradycardia (occasionally asystole of 10 to 20 sec or greater) with premonitory symptoms culminating in syncope. The third phase consists of rapid recovery upon recumbency.

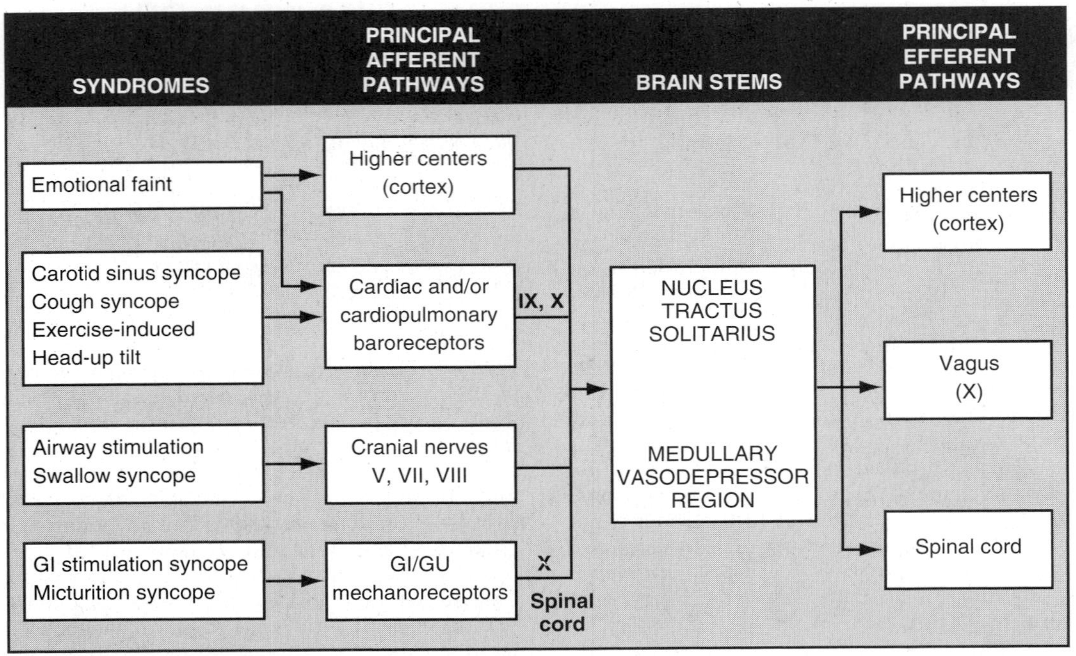

FIGURE 28–1. The mechanisms for various reflex-mediated vasomotor syndromes showing similarities and differences in the mechanisms of these entities IX and X refer to the ninth and tenth cranial nerves. (Adapted from Benditt, D.G., et al.: Tilt table testing for evaluation of neurally mediated (cardioneurogenic) syncope: Rationale and proposed protocols. PACE *14*:1528, 1991.)

Generally, vasovagal syncope occurs in an upright posture. During upright standing, there is decreased venous return, stroke volume, and arterial pressure leading to compensatory responses mediated by arterial and cardiopulmonary baroreceptors. Normally, afferent neural input from baroreceptors is relayed to the medullary centers; this results in increased sympathetic and decreased parasympathetic activity. However, occasionally abrupt decrease in venous return (e.g., with hemorrhage) may result in a relatively "empty ventricle" that contracts vigorously, leading to excessive stimulation of ventricular mechanoreceptors and paradoxical vasodilatation and bradycardia.[2,3] Increased circulating epinephrine level and higher CNS centers may augment this response.

SITUATIONAL SYNCOPE. Syncope in association with various daily activities (e.g., micturition, defecation, cough, and swallowing) is termed *situational syncope.*

Micturition syncope was originally described in healthy young men who, after rising from bed in the early morning hours, experienced sudden loss of consciousness during or immediately after urination. Predisposing factors having a facilatatory role include reduced food intake, recent upper respiratory tract infection, fatigue, and ingestion of alcohol. Older patients (mean age 60 years) with multiple acute and chronic medical problems may experience micturition syncope[10] often associated with orthostatic hypotension. Isolated case reports have associated micturition syncope and presyncope with bladder neck obstruction, psychomotor epilepsy, complete AV block, and pheochromocytoma of the bladder.

The mechanism of micturition syncope is probably similar to that of vasovagal syncope except for the site or nature of the trigger factors. Mechanoreceptors in the bladder have been implicated in micturition syncope. A combination of physiological changes during sleep and urination may predispose to micturition syncope. These changes include sudden decompression of the bladder, a decline of blood pressure and heart rate mediated by decreased peripheral resistance during sleep, possible Valsalva maneuver during micturition, and orthostatic hypotension (in the elderly).

In *defecation syncope,* vagal afferents transmit neural impulses from gut wall tension receptors. These signals are then presumably transmitted to the CNS, resulting in hypotension and bradycardia. A variety of gastrointestinal tract conditions (Meckel's diverticulum, ruptured appendix) and cardiovascular diseases (ventricular arrhythmias), as well as orthostatic hypotension and transient ischemic attacks, have been reported to contribute to syncope.[11] Cases of association with pulmonary embolism and foreign body (toothpick) in the rectum have been reported. Syncope in association with rectal and pelvic examination and during sigmoidoscopy probably has a similar mechanism.

Syncope in association with *swallowing* probably results from afferent neural impulses in the upper gastrointestinal tract served by the glossopharyngeal or vagus nerves with transmission to the CNS. Most patients with syncope during or immediately following swallowing have had structural abnormalities of the esophagus or the heart (diverticula, diffuse esophageal spasm, achalasia, and stricture). Cardiac conditions have included acute rheumatic carditis treated with digitalis, acute myocardial infarction, and a calcified mass over the aortic valve and septum. Bradyarrhythmias (sinus arrest or asystole, complete AV block, nodal or sinus bradycardia, and sinoatrial block) have been demonstrated during swallow syncope.

Airway stimulation (e.g., during endotracheal intubation or bronchoscopy) may also result in marked bradycardia resulting from similar mechanisms involving vagal afferent neural transmission to the CNS with subsequent vagal efferents leading to bradycardia and hypotension. A similar mechanism is probably operative in *cough syncope,* which consists of the very brief loss of consciousness after paroxysms of severe cough, described almost exclusively (> 90 per cent) in middle-aged men who drink ethanol, smoke, and have chronic lung disease. Coughing may produce very high intrathoracic pressure, with a sudden decrease in venous return and cardiac output and transmission of high intrathoracic pressure during cough to the subarachnoid space, which may reduce cerebral blood and lead to syncope. Alternatively, reflex syncope may be the predominant mechanism.

Rare case reports have associated cough syncope with Mobitz II or complete AV block, obstructive cardiomyopathy, hypersensitive carotid sinus syndrome, herniated-cerebellar tonsils, and severe bilateral cerebrovascular disease. A related syndrome, *sneeze syncope,* is probably due to similar mechanisms and has been associated with the Arnold-Chiari malformation. In the treatment of cough syncope due to underlying lung disease, smoking cessation is the most important factor, in addition to bronchodilators and cough suppressants.

CAROTID SINUS SYNCOPE. The carotid sinus baroreceptors consist of sensory nerve endings located in the internal carotid artery just above the bifurcation of the common carotid artery. Afferent impulses travel via the sinus nerve of Hering and join the glossopharyngeal nerve and perhaps cervical sympathetic and vagus nerves to enter the sensory nucleus of the vagus (solitary tract) and the vasomotor center. Efferent pathways include sympathetic adrenergic nerves to the heart, resistance and capacitance vessels, and cardiac vagus nerve.[12,13]

Three types of carotid sinus hypersensitivity are generally recognized.[12,13] *Cardioinhibitory carotid sinus hypersensitivity* is widely defined as cardiac asystole of 3 sec or more. The pure *vasodepressor type* is defined as a systolic blood pressure decline of 50 mm Hg or more (in the absence of significant bradycardia). A *mixed type* consists of a combination of cardioinhibitory and vasodepressor response. The prevalence of carotid sinus hypersensitivity in an asymptomatic population is reported to be 5 to 25 per cent, occurring primarily in older individuals (≥ 60 years); the condition is found more commonly in men. The cardioinhibitory variety accounts for 34 to 78 per cent and vasodepressor 5 to 10 per cent of cases of carotid sinus hypersensitivity.

Five to 20 per cent of individuals with abnormal carotid sensitivity suffer spontaneous fainting, termed *carotid sinus syncope.* Attacks may be precipitated by factors that exert pressure on the carotid sinus (e.g., tight collar, shaving, sudden turning), a history of which is obtained in only a quarter of patients with this syndrome. Syncope occurs predominantly in men, 70 per cent of whom are 50 years of age or older. The majority have coronary artery disease and hypertension. Other predisposing factors include neck pathology such as enlarged lymph nodes, tissue scars, carotid body tumors, parotid, thyroid, and head and neck tumors. Possible associations with digitalis, alpha-methyldopa, and propranolol have been reported. Abnormalities of sinus node function and atrioventricular conduction are often found in patients with carotid sinus hypersensitivity.

Survival in patients with carotid sinus hypersensitivity is similar to that in the general population and is largely related to underlying diseases. Survival appears to be unrelated to pacemaker therapy.[14] Prior studies had reported symptom recurrence in 20 to 25 per cent of untreated or medically treated patients with carotid sinus syndrome. However, syncope recurred in 57 per cent of those without pacemakers vs. 9 per cent of a paced group in a prospective study of patients with severe carotid sinus syndrome (i.e., patients with recurrent syncope, trauma, and reproduction of symptoms upon massage).[15]

GLOSSOPHARYNGEAL NEURALGIA. This is a severe unilateral paroxysmal pain in the oropharynx, tonsillar fossa, base of tongue, or ear precipitated by swallowing, chewing, or coughing. Occasionally, syncope and seizures occur during the attack, which in most instances is caused by asystole or bradycardia and rarely by a vasodepressor reaction. Seizures are consistent with hypoxemic convulsions. Neoplasms have been reported in one-sixth of the patients with syncope and consist of neck tumors or lymphoma with meningeal involvement. Trigeminal neuralgia has also been associated with syncope and seizures due to bradycardia and asystole or a vasodepressor reaction. Syncope is probably due to spread of afferent impulses from the trigger zone in the pharynx (conducted in the glossopharyngeal nerve) to the dorsal motor nucleus of the vagus, causing intense vagal stimulation. In the vasodepressor variety, inhibition of peripheral sympathetic activity is implicated.

HIGH-ALTITUDE SYNCOPE. A young healthy individual's recent arrival at moderate or very high altitudes can result in syncope without long-term adverse sequelae.[16] Possible mechanisms include reflex bradycardia, hyperventilation, and subsequent hypocapnia resulting in reflex cerebral vasoconstriction, which may decrease cerebral oxygen delivery. Mild volume depletion due to diuresis at high altitude or due to physical activity may lead to vasovagal syncope.

PSYCHIATRIC ILLNESSES. Stress and psychiatric illnesses probably cause syncope by precipitating vasovagal reactions. Patients with psychiatric syncope are generally young, are more often female, and have recurrent syncope but no organic heart disease.[17–19] Generalized anxiety disorder, panic disorder, and major depression account for the majority of psychiatric causes. Several epidemics of fainting described in young individuals have been attributed to transitory anxiety attacks in response to environmental stresses. Syncope constitutes a somatic complaint in up to 9 per cent of the patients with panic disorder. Major depression may lead to syncope through the common association with anxiety disorder, or syncope may be a somatic manifestation of depression, because medical patients with depression often present with nonspecific cardiopulmonary and other physical complaints indicating masked or atypical depression.

OTHER ENTITIES. Neurally mediated reflex mechanism is also implicated for syncope in association with exercise, especially syncope occurring immediately after exercise in individuals without structural heart disease.[20–22] An increase in catecholamines and force of ventricular contraction may stimulate the cardiac mechanoreceptors in the setting of mild volume depletion and shifts of blood flow to dissipate heat.

NEURALLY MEDIATED SYNCOPE. This may also occur with drugs that decrease venous return to the heart in an upright position. For example, nitrates lead to marked venous dilatation, decreased venous return, and diminished cardiac output, which normally results in tachycardia and increased cardiac inotropic state. However, in susceptible individuals, this may lead to stimulation of cardiac mechanoreceptors and syncope.[23] Syncope with aortic stenosis,[24] hypertrophic cardiomyopathy,[25] supraventricular tachycardias,[26] paroxysmal atrial fibrillation,[27] and that related to pacemakers[28] (i.e., pacemaker syndrome), appears to be neurally mediated.

Orthostatic Hypotension

When a person assumes upright posture, 500 to 700 ml of blood is pooled in the lower extremities and the splanchnic circulation. The consequent reduction in venous return to the heart results in decreased cardiac output and stimulation of aortic, carotid, and cardiopulmonary baroreceptors. This stimulation reflexly increases sympathetic outflow and inhibits parasympathetic activity. These adjustments lead to an increase in heart rate and vascular resistance to maintain systemic blood pressure upon standing upright.[29] Orthostatic hypotension results when a defect exists in regulation of systemic blood pressure in any element of this system, from the circulating volume to neural input to the vascular system.

Symptoms due to orthostatic hypotension include dizziness or light-headedness, blurring or loss of vision, a sense of profound weakness, and syncope. Loss of consciousness is generally brief, and there are no associated symptoms of autonomic hyperactivity. These symptoms are often worse on arising in the morning and may be especially prominent after meals or exercise.

Decreased intravascular volume and adverse effects of drugs are the most common causes of symptomatic orthostatic hypotension (Table 28–2).[29] Drugs cause syncope by leading to alterations of vascular volume or tone (e.g., antihypertensive agents, nitrates) or by causing an allergic or anaphylactic reaction. Drugs are responsible for 2 to 9 per cent of symptoms in patients presenting with syncope. Elderly patients are especially vulnerable to symptoms resulting from drugs and volume depletion because of reduced baroreceptor sensitivity, decreased cerebral blood flow, excessive renal sodium wasting, and an impaired thirst mechanism that develops with aging.[30]

Orthostatic hypotension is an important manifestation of diseases affecting the autonomic nervous system (Table 28–2).[31] *Idiopathic orthostatic hypotension* is a rare illness that affects men five times more frequently than women, and is often associated with other autonomic disturbances such as sphincter malfunction, impotence, impaired erection and ejaculation, and impaired sweating. Plasma norepinephrine levels are markedly reduced at rest and remain unchanged on standing, suggesting peripheral dysfunction. Shy-Drager syndrome is associated with autonomic failure and involvement of the corticospinal, extrapyramidal, and cerebellar tracts including a parkinson-like syndrome. This disease may also be associated with cholinergic dysfunction

TABLE 28–2 CAUSES OF ORTHOSTATIC HYPOTENSION

1. PRIMARY
- Pure autonomic failure (idiopathic orthostatic hypotension)
- Autonomic failure with multiple system atrophy (Shy-Drager syndrome)
- Autonomic failure with Parkinson's disease

2. SECONDARY
- General medical disorders: diabetes; amyloid; alcoholism
- Autoimmune disease: Guillain-Barré syndrome; mixed connective tissue disease; rheumatoid arthritis; Eaton-Lambert syndrome; systemic lupus erythematosus
- Carcinomatous autonomic neuropathy
- Metabolic disease: Vitamin B12-deficiency; porphyria; Fabry's disease; Tangier disease
- Hereditary sensory neuropathies, dominant or recessive
- Infections of the nervous system: syphilis; Chagas' disease; HIV infection; botulism; herpes zoster
- Central brain lesions: vascular lesion or tumors involving the hypothalamus and midbrain, for example craniopharyngioma; multiple sclerosis; Wernicke's encephalopathy
- Spinal cord lesions
- Familial dysautonomia
- Familial hyperbradykininism
- Renal failure
- Dopamine beta-hydroxylase deficiency
- Ageing

3. DRUGS
- Selective neurotoxic drugs; alcoholism
- Tranquilizers: phenothiazines; barbiturates
- Antidepressants: tricyclics; monoamine oxidase inhibitors
- Vasodilators: prazosin; hydralazine; calcium channel blockers
- Centrally acting hypotensive drugs: methyldopa; clonidine
- Adrenergic neuron blocking drugs: guanethidine
- Alpha-adrenergic blocking drugs: phenoxybenzamine; labetalol
- Ganglion-blocking drugs: hexamethonium; mecamylamine
- Angiotensin-converting enzyme inhibitors: captopril; enalapril; lisinopril

Adapted from Bannister, S. R. (ed.): Autonomic Failure. 2nd ed. Oxford, Oxford University Press, 1988, p. 8.

affecting the vagal, ocular, bladder, and sweat glands. Norepinephrine levels are normal at rest but remain unchanged on standing, suggesting an inability to stimulate normally functioning peripheral neurons.

Postprandial syncope can be a rare problem in the elderly due to hypotension after meals. Possible mechanism includes failure to maintain compensatory norepinephrine levels and cardioacceleratory responses. A systolic blood pressure decline of about 20 mm Hg after a meal has been reported in up to 36 per cent of elderly nursing home residents, occurring at 45 to 60 minutes in most patients.[32] This decline is often asymptomatic but rarely may lead to syncope and presyncope.

Neurological Disorders

These are infrequent causes of syncope.

CEREBROVASCULAR DISEASE. Approximately 6 per cent of ischemic strokes or transient ischemic attacks (TIAs) are associated with syncope. In 483 syncope patients seen in an emergency department, 7.7 per cent had TIAs.[33] All patients had concurrent neurological symptoms, most frequently vertigo, ataxia, and paresthesia. Almost all patients had vertebrobasilar TIAs.[33] Syncope is a rare manifestation of bilateral severe carotid artery disease. TIAs may result from atherosclerotic disease, inflammatory disorders (e.g., giant cell arteritis, systemic lupus erythematosus), aortic arch syndrome, dissection of extracranial arteries, cardiac diseases leading to emboli (e.g., rheumatic heart disease, myxoma), sickle cell disease, and anomalies of the cervical spine or cervical spondylosis. Syncope is also a manifestation of subclavian steal syndrome in which there is a stenosis of the subclavian artery and reversal of blood flow in the ipsilateral vertebral artery leading to vertebrobasilar ischemia.

MIGRAINES. A "faint sensation" is reported in 12 to 18 per cent of patients with migraine. Basilar artery migraine is a rare disorder affecting adolescents when syncope is associated with symptoms of brainstem ischemia. Localized brain stem ischemia due to spasm is the postulated mechanism. Migraine may result in syncope and orthostatic hypotension possibly because of hyper-responsiveness of dopamine receptors with inhibition of the vasomotor center. Migraines may also lead to a vasovagal reaction secondary to pain.

SEIZURE. Fewer than 2 per cent of patients presenting with syncope are diagnosed as having a seizure disorder as a cause of their loss of consciousness.[34,35] Atonic seizures or epileptic "drop attacks" are nonconvulsive seizures found most commonly with secondary generalized epilepsy or partial epilepsy affecting mesial frontal or central cortical regions. Sudden falls also occur with temporal lobe epilepsy.[36] *Temporal lobe syncope* is the term used for complex partial seizure when patients also have drop attacks resembling syncope.[37] Patients may have a brief loss of consciousness followed by partial responsiveness or confusion and may exhibit formed speech or reactive automatisms. Characteristically, an interictal electroencephalogram (EEG) shows temporal lobe epileptic abnormalities. Temporal lobe epilepsy has been rarely associated with bradyarrhythmias.[38]

Cardiac Syncope

Severe obstruction to cardiac output or rhythm disturbance can lead to syncope. Occasionally, obstructive lesions and arrhythmias coexist, and one disorder may accentuate the other.

OBSTRUCTION TO FLOW. This may be due to structural lesions of either the left or right side of the heart (Table 28–1). Exertional syncope is a common manifestation of all types of heart disease in which cardiac output is fixed and does not rise (or even falls) with exercise. Syncope occurs in up to 42 per cent of patients with severe aortic stenosis (see p. 1039), commonly with exercise.[24] The most likely mechanisms of exertional syncope in aortic stenosis, as in other entities that cause left ventricular outflow obstruction, are ventricular baroceptor-mediated hypotension and bradycardia. Exercise leads to a marked increase in left ventricular systolic pressure without a corresponding increase in aortic pressure. This results in excessive stimulation of left ventricular mechanoreceptors leading to inhibition of sympathetic and activation of parasympathetic tone through cardiac vagal afferent fibers.[24,39] Myocardial ischemia may be present during syncope (even in patients without coexistent coronary artery disease), suggesting ischemia as contributing to vasodepressor syncope or reduction in coronary artery perfusion due to hypotension and bradycardia.[39] Other rare potential causes of syncope include ventricular tachyarrhythmias, paroxysmal AV block, and atrial fibrillation with loss of "atrial kick." Syncope is prognostically important in aortic stenosis, with an average survival of 2 to 3 years after its onset in the absence of valve replacement.

Similar pathophysiological processes may be responsible for syncope in hypertrophic cardiomyopathy (see p. 1419).[25] Syncope is reported in as many as 30 per cent of patients with hypertrophic cardiomyopathy. Left ventricular outflow obstruction is dynamic and worsened by an increase in contractility, a decrease in chamber size, or a decrease in afterload and distending pressure. Thus, Valsalva maneuver, severe coughing paroxysm, or specific drugs (e.g., digitalis) may precipitate hypotension and syncope. Myocardial ischemia is frequently found with syncope.[40] Ventricular tachycardia is reported in approximately 25 per cent of adult patients with hypertrophic cardiomyopathy and is an important cause of syncope.[41] Predictors of syncope include age less than 30 years, left ventricular end-diastolic volume index less than 60 ml/m^2, and nonsustained ventricular tachycardia.[42] Extensive hypertrophy and ventricular tachycardia are associated with poorer prognosis.[43]

Effort syncope commonly occurs in pulmonary hypertension (up to 30 per cent in primary pulmonary hypertension [see p. 788]). The limitations to right ventricular outflow may lead to diminished capacity to increase cardiac output, which, in association with lowered peripheral resistance with exercise, may lead to hypotension and syncope. Exertional syncope may also occur with severe pulmonic stenosis on the basis of a similar mechanism (see p. 1059). Patients with congenital heart disease (e.g., tetralogy of Fallot, patent ductus arteriosus, and interventricular or interatrial septal defects) can experience syncope with effort or crying as a result of sudden reversal of a left-to-right shunt and a fall in arterial oxygen saturation.

Syncope, which may occasionally occur with exertion, is reported in 10 to 15 per cent of patients with pulmonary embolism and is more likely to occur with massive embolism (> 50 per cent obstruction of the pulmonary vascular bed) (Chap. 46). Massive pulmonary embolism results in acute right ventricular failure, which leads to increased right ventricular filling pressure and reduced stroke volume. Subsequent decreased cardiac output and hypotension may lead to loss of consciousness. Consciousness may be regained if the embolus migrates to a distal location in the pulmonary artery. Alternatively, activation of cardiopulmonary mechanoreceptors in the setting of increased force of ventricular contraction may be the cause of syncope.

Atrial myxomas may result in obstruction of the mitral or tricuspid valve leading to symptoms of cardiac failure and rarely syncope (see p. 1466). Syncope, dyspnea, and cardiac murmurs that change with body position are particularly indicative of myxoma. Mitral stenosis rarely leads to syncope; it may be due to severe obstruction to outflow, atrial fibrillation with rapid ventricular response, pulmonary hypertension, or a cerebral embolic event.

OTHER ORGANIC HEART DISEASE. Syncope may be the presenting symptom in 5 to 12 per cent of elderly patients with acute myocardial infarction (see p. 1199). Mechanisms responsible for syncope include (1) sudden pump failure producing hypotension and a decrease in perfusion of the brain, and (2) rhythm disturbance that may include ventricular tachycardia or bradyarrhythmias. Vasovagal reactions resulting from stimulation of left ventricular baroreceptors may occur during acute inferior infarction or ischemia involving the right coronary artery. Unstable angina and coronary artery spasm also have been rarely associated with syncope.

Syncope occurs in 5 per cent of patients with aortic dissection. Loss of consciousness may be due to stroke or related to rupture into the pericardial space, resulting in sudden cardiac tamponade.

ARRHYTHMIAS. Bradycardia leads to a prolonged ventricular filling period resulting in increased stroke volume to maintain cardiac output (see p. 449). Severe bradycardia may result in an inadequate compensatory increase in stroke volume and lead to syncope. Mild to moderate tachycardias increase cardiac output, whereas markedly fast rates lead to a decrease in diastolic filling and cardiac output resulting in hypotension and syncope. Supraventricular tachycardias and paroxysmal atrial fibrillation may activate cardiac mechanoreceptors because of diminished cardiac volume and vigorous ventricular contraction, leading to neurally mediated syncope.[26,27]

Sinus bradycardia may be from excessive vagal tone, decreased sympathetic tone, or sinus node disease. Sinus bradycardia in healthy young athletes is generally attributed to increased vagal tone and decreased sympathetic activity but rarely results in syncope. Sinus bradycardia also occurs with eye surgery, myxedema, intracranial and mediastinal tumors, and with use of many parasympathomimetic, sympatholytic, beta blocker, and other drugs. Conjunctival instillation of beta blockers may also cause symptomatic bradycardia.

Syncope is reported in 25 to 70 per cent of patients with sick sinus syndrome (see p. 648). This syndrome is characterized by disturbance of sinoatrial impulse formation or conduction. Electrocardiographic manifestations include sinus bradycardia, pauses, arrest, or exit block. Supraventricular tachycardia or atrial fibrillation may also occur in association with bradycardia or atrial fibrillation with slow ventricular response (bradycardia-tachycardia syndrome). Sick sinus syndrome may overlap with neurally mediated syndromes leading to recurrent syncope despite pacemaker therapy.[44]

Ventricular tachycardias generally occur in the setting of known organic heart disease. Severity of symptoms is related to the rate, duration, and myocardial pump function (see p. 679). Torsades de pointes and syncope occur in the setting of syndromes of congenital prolongation of Q-T interval (with or without deafness) as well as acquired long Q-T syndromes, which occur with drugs, electrolyte abnormalities, and CNS disorders (see p. 685). Antiarrhythmic drugs are the most common cause of torsades de pointes, occurring with quinidine (quinidine syncope), procainamide, disopyramide, flecainide, encainide, amiodarone, and satolol.

Other tachyarrhythmias that may cause syncope include atrial fibrillation or flutter with rapid ventricular response and AV nodal reentrant tachycardia (see p. 663). Syncope in Wolff-Parkinson-White syndrome may be related to rapid rate of reciprocating supraventricular tachycardia or to a rapid ventricular response over the accessory pathway during atrial fibrillation.[45] Syncope alone in Wolff-Parkinson-White syndrome may not predict risk of sudden death.[46,47]

Distribution of Causes of Syncope

There has been a wide variation in the proportion of patients diagnosed with various causes of syncope.[34,35,48–50] This is largely due to patient selection (differences ranging from emergency department to ICU patients) and lack of uniform criteria for assigning causes of syncope. The most common etiologies are vasovagal syncope (1 to 29 per cent), situational syncope (1 to 8 per cent), orthostatic hypotension (4 to 12 per cent), and drug-induced syncope (2 to 9 per cent). Organic cardiac diseases constitute 3 to 11 per cent and arrhythmias 5 to 30 per cent of causes of syncope. Each of the other causes is found in less than 5 per cent of patients. In studies in the 1980's, a cause of syncope was not diagnosed in 38 to 42 per cent. However, the proportion undiagnosed is probably substantially lower with wider use of event monitoring, tilt testing, electrophysiological studies, attention to psychiatric illnesses, and recognition that syncope in the elderly may be multifactorial. In a cardiology tertiary care referral center where patients underwent electrophysiological studies and tilt testing, a cause was not established in 26 per cent.[51]

Outcome in Syncope of Various Etiologies

The one-year mortality of patients with cardiac causes of syncope has been consistently high, ranging between 18 and 33 per cent.[34,35,49,50] These rates have been found to be higher than those in patients with a noncardiac cause (0 to 12 per cent) or in patients with unknown cause (6 per cent). The incidence of sudden death in patients with cardiac causes was also markedly higher as compared with the other two groups.[34,35] Even when adjustments for differences in comorbidity were made, cardiac syncope was still an independent predictor of mortality and sudden death. It is not known whether syncope predisposes to increased risk of mortality independent of underlying diseases. In the Framingham study, patients younger than age 60 experiencing syncope who did not have cardiovascular or neurological diseases had rates of mortality, sudden death, stroke, and myocardial infarction similar to patients without syncope.[52] In a study of patients with advanced heart failure, poor left ventricular function was associated with a high risk of sudden death regardless of the cause of syncope.[53,54] A comparative outcome study of unselected patients with and without syncope showed that underlying heart disease was associated with higher mortality.

There is an important difference in prognosis between cardiac syncope and neurally mediated or neurocardiogenic syncope. Neurocardiogenic syncope has excellent long-term prognosis, although recurrences are common and a major reason for seeking medical care. Similarly, syncope associated with psychiatric disease has no increased mortality but has one-year recurrence rates of 26 to 50 per cent.[17]

In patients presenting with syncope, the recurrence rate is 34 per cent over 3-year follow-up and it is lower in patients with cardiac causes as compared with the other groups, but not significantly so.[55] Although recurrences are associated with fractures and soft tissue injury in 12 per cent of patients, they do not predict an increased risk of mortality or sudden death.[55]

DIAGNOSTIC EVALUATION

The most important elements in the evaluation of syncope are (1) determining whether the patient has actually experienced syncope, (2) risk stratification, and (3) selective use of diagnostic tests to define the cause.

DETERMINING WHETHER THE PATIENT HAD SYNCOPE. A history from the patient and a witness, if present, is needed to separate syncope from other entities such as dizziness, vertigo, drop attacks, coma, and seizure. A particularly important issue is the distinction between syncope and seizure. Videometric analysis of patients with syncope has shown myoclonic activity in 90 per cent, predominantly consisting of multifocal arrhythmic jerks both in proximal and distal muscles.[56] Other findings include head turns, oral automatism, and visual and auditory hallucinations. Eyes remained open throughout syncope and upward deviation was common. Despite these findings, historical features are often sufficient to distinguish syncope from seizures. A comparison of seizures and syncope shows that seizures are associated with a blue face (or not pale), frothing at the mouth, tongue biting, disorientation, aching muscles, sleepiness after the event, and a duration of unconsciousness of more than 5 minutes. On the other hand, patients with syncope often report sweating or nausea before the event. The best discriminatory symptom is disorientation after the episode, which often signifies a seizure.[57] Tilt testing (see p. 870) may be useful to distinguish vasovagal syncope from seizure by provoking symptoms and hemodynamic changes with syncope that can be observed.[58]

RISK STRATIFICATION. This is important for initial management decisions such as admission to the hospital and the use of invasive testing such as electrophysiological studies. The issues include prediction of risk of sudden death and likelihood of cardiac syncope. In the assessment of risk, cause of syncope, presence of underlying cardiac disease, and abnormalities on electrocardiogram (ECG) are important.

Previous studies have consistently shown increased mortality and sudden death rates in patients with cardiac causes of syncope, thus identifying these patients as a high-risk subset. Examples include those with aortic stenosis, pulmonary hypertension, and arrhythmic syncope. Arrhythmias are primarily of concern in patients with heart disease or abnormal ECG. Thus, the presence of heart disease and certain abnormalities on ECG helps stratify patients into low- and high-risk groups. Patients with congestive heart failure, valvular heart disease, hypertrophic cardiomyopathy, and other types of organic heart disease constitute a high-risk group. Bundle branch block, old myocardial infarction, Wolff-Parkinson-White syndrome, and other evidence of AV block are also considered high-risk findings on ECG. If the presence or absence of heart disease cannot be determined clinically, specific tests such as echocardiogram, stress test, and ventricular function studies may be needed for risk stratification.

SELECTIVE USE OF DIAGNOSTIC TESTS. The evaluation of syncope is best approached by using the history and physical examination, ECG, and risk stratification to guide further diagnostic tests.

History, Physical Examination, and Baseline Laboratory Tests

A detailed account of syncope, the events leading to loss of consciousness, and symptoms following the episode is crucial to diagnosing specific entities. In diagnosing vasovagal syncope, precipitating factors, in conjunction with autonomic symptoms, can lead to diagnosis. Syncope during or immediately after micturition, cough, defecation, and swallowing is well described and easily diagnosed by history. Syncope associated with neurological symptoms of brain stem ischemia suggests transient ischemic attacks, basilar artery migraines, and subclavian steal syndrome. A detailed drug history may provide clues to possible drug-induced syncope. Table 28–3 shows other clinical presentations that may suggest specific entities.

Physical examination is used to diagnose specific entities and exclude others. Orthostatic hypotension, cardiovascular findings, and neurological examination are crucial in this regard. Orthostatic hypotension is generally defined as a decline of 20 mm Hg or more in systolic pressure upon assuming the upright position. However, this finding is reported in up to 24 per cent of the elderly and is frequently not associated with symptoms.[29] Thus, the clinical diagnosis of orthostatic hypotension should incorporate the presence of symptoms (e.g., dizziness and syncope) in association with a decrease in systolic blood pressure.

In the detection of orthostatic hypotension, supine blood pressure and heart rate should be measured after the patient has been recumbent for at least 5 minutes. Standing measurements should be obtained immediately and for at least 2 minutes. These measurements should be carried out to 10 minutes if there is a high suspicion of orthostatic hypotension without a drop in blood pressure having been

TABLE 28–3 CLINICAL FEATURES SUGGESTIVE OF SPECIFIC CAUSES

SYMPTOM OR FINDING	DIAGNOSTIC CONSIDERATION
After sudden unexpected pain, unpleasant sight, sound, or smell	Vasovagal syncope
During or immediately after micturition, cough, swallow, or defecation	Situational syncope
With neuralgia (glossopharyngeal or trigeminal)	Bradycardia or vasodepressor reaction
Upon standing	Orthostatic hypotension
Prolonged standing at attention	Vasovagal syncope
Well-trained athlete after exertion	Neurally mediated
Changing position (from sitting to lying, bending, turning over in bed)	Atrial myxoma, thrombus
Syncope with exertion	Aortic stenosis, pulmonary hypertension, pulmonary embolus, mitral stenosis, idiopathic hypertrophic subaortic stenosis, coronary artery disease, neurally-mediated
With head rotation, pressure on carotid sinus (as in tumors, shaving, tight collars)	Carotid sinus syncope
Associated with vertigo, dysarthria, diplopia, and other motor and sensory symptoms of brain stem ischemia	TIA, subclavian steal, basilar artery migraine
With arm exercise	Subclavian steal
Confusion after episode	Seizure

found earlier.[59] Sitting blood pressures are not reliable for detection of orthostatic hypotension.

Several cardiovascular findings are crucial diagnostically. Differences in the pulse intensity and blood pressure (generally over 20 mm Hg) in the two arms are suggestive of aortic dissection or subclavian steal syndrome. Special focus on cardiovascular examination for aortic stenosis, idiopathic hypertrophic subaortic stenosis, pulmonary hypertension, myxomas, and aortic dissection may uncover clues to these entities.

In those patients in whom the cause can be defined, the history and physical examination identify a potential cause in 49 to 85 per cent.[34,35,48–50] Furthermore, organic cardiac diseases causing syncope (e.g., aortic stenosis, idiopathic hypertrophic subaortic stenosis, pulmonary embolism), and neurological diseases (e.g., subclavian steal syndrome) can be strongly suspected by the history and physical examination. Testing for these diseases should be selective and based on findings of a careful history and physical examination. In one study, suggestive findings on history and physical examination were helpful in assigning the ultimate cause of syncope by directed testing in 8 per cent of additional patients.[34]

Initial laboratory blood tests rarely yield diagnostically helpful information. Hypoglycemia, hyponatremia, hypocalcemia, or renal failure is found in 2 to 3 per cent of patients, but most of these appear to result in seizures rather than syncope. These tests are often confirmatory of clinical suspicion of these laboratory abnormalities. Bleeding as a cause of syncope is generally diagnosed clinically and confirmed by a complete blood count or hemoccult tests.

Carotid Massage

The technique of carotid massage is not standardized. Commonly, massage is done in the supine position, and occasionally repeated in the sitting and standing positions if the vasodepressor variety is suspected and the test in the supine position is negative. Electrocardiographic and blood pressure monitoring is necessary. Mixed cardioinhibitory and vasodepressor response is diagnosed when carotid sinus massage is performed after cardioinhibitory response is abolished with atropine or atrioventricular sequential pacing. The duration of massage has varied from 5 sec to 40 sec,[12] but recent studies have used 6 to 10 sec.[14,15,60] Simultaneous bilateral massage should never be done. At least 15 seconds should be allowed to elapse between massage from one side to the other. Complications of carotid sinus massage include prolonged asystole, ventricular fibrillation, transient or permanent neurological deficit, and sudden death. Complication rates are not available but are considered extremely low; however, in patients with cerebrovascular disease the test should be done only if all other diagnostic modalities are exhausted and the pretest probability of carotid sinus syncope remains high.

Carotid sinus syncope is diagnosed in patients who are found to have carotid sinus hypersensitivity and have reproduction of spontaneous symptoms during carotid sinus massage. In the absence of symptom reproduction, carotid sinus syncope is likely when carotid sinus hypersensitivity is found and spontaneous episodes are related to activities that press or stretch the carotid sinus, or the patient has recurrent syncope with a negative workup.

Diagnostic Tests for Arrhythmias

Ascribing syncope to arrhythmias is often difficult because, in most patients, symptoms have already resolved by the time of testing; thus, a causal inference is often made on the basis of tests performed during asymptomatic periods. In diagnosing arrhythmias, every attempt should be made to attain symptomatic correlation. When this is not possible, uncertainty may remain regarding the cause of syncope because currently there are no validated criteria for attributing syncope to most arrhythmias by the use of electrocardiographic or electrophysiological abnormalities during asymptomatic periods.

ELECTROCARDIOGRAM. An abnormal ECG may be found in 50 per cent of patients presenting with syncope.[34] The most common abnormalities include bundle branch or bifascicular block, old myocardial infarction, and left ventricular hypertrophy. Arrhythmias as cause of syncope are assigned by ECG in 2 to 11 per cent of patients.[34,35,49,50] Exercise ECG (Chap. 5) can be used to evaluate syncope with exercise for the diagnosis of ischemia, exercise-induced tachyarrhythmias, or bradyarrhythmias after abrupt termination of exercise. However, the yield of this test for arrhythmias is very low.

Signal-averaged ECG, used for detection of low amplitude signals (late potentials) (see p. 583), has a sensitivity of 73 to 89 per cent and specificity of 89 to 100 per cent for prediction of inducible sustained ventricular tachycardia in patients with syncope.[61–63] Signal-averaged ECG has been used as a screening test in selecting patients for electrophysiological studies when ventricular tachycardia is the only concern. However, complete electrophysiological studies are generally needed to evaluate syncope when the decision is made to perform this test because abnormalities other than ventricular tachycardia (e.g., sinus node dysfunction, other conduction system disease, induced supraventricular tachycardia) as well as multiple abnormalities are often of concern.

PROLONGED ELECTROCARDIOGRAPHIC MONITORING. The central problem in attributing syncope to arrhythmias is that the vast majority of detected arrhythmias in syncope patients are brief and result in no symptoms.[64–67] On the other hand, arrhythmias are commonly reported in normal or ambulatory asymptomatic individuals, including sinus bradycardia, brief episodes of supraventricular tachycardia, and PACs or PVCs. Sinus pauses of more than 2 sec and brief runs of unsustained ventricular tachycardia (mostly less than 5 beat runs) are reported in up to 4 per cent of asymptomatic subjects. Mobitz II or complete AV block are very rare.

One method of assessing the impact of ambulatory monitoring in syncope is to determine the presence or absence of arrhythmias in patients who develop symptoms during monitoring. In studies that evaluated syncope or presyncope with approximately 12 hours of monitoring and reported on symptoms, only 4 per cent of patients had symptomatic correlation with arrhythmias.[67] In approximately 17 per cent of patients, symptoms were not associated with arrhythmias, thus potentially excluding rhythm disturbance as an etiology for syncope. In approximately 80 per cent of patients, no symptoms occurred but arrhythmias were often found. The causal relation between these arrhythmias and syncope therefore is uncertain. Furthermore, the finding of brief or no arrhythmias (without symptoms) on monitoring does not exclude arrhythmic syncope because of the episodic nature of arrhythmias. In patients with high pretest likelihood of arrhythmias, further evaluation for arrhythmias should be pursued by event monitoring or electrophysiological studies. Extending the duration of monitoring to 72 hours may increase the yield of brief arrhythmias detected (14.7 per cent during the first day, an additional 11.1 per cent the second day, and an additional 4.2 per cent the third day[65]), but not the yield for arrhythmias associated with symptoms.

Long-term monitoring (weeks to months) is possible with patient-activated intermittent loop recorders that can capture the rhythm during syncope after the patient has regained consciousness, because several minutes of retrograde electrocardiographic recording can be obtained. In one study of patients with multiple recurrences of syncope (median of 10 episodes), 7 of the 57 patients had an arrhythmia found with recurrent symptoms of which three were due to neurally mediated syncope.[68] Seven others had negative findings, therefore excluding arrhythmias as a cause of syncope. However, in 18 patients there were technical problems with use of the recorder that precluded a diagnosis. Thus, loop monitoring is most useful in patients with history of recurrent unexplained syncope because the probability of recurrence in these patients is higher, making it more likely that arrhythmias can be captured during an event.

ELECTROPHYSIOLOGICAL STUDIES (see p. 577). The indications for electrophysiological studies in patients with syncope have not been systematically defined, but they are more likely to be "positive" in patients with known heart disease, abnormal ventricular function, or abnormalities on the ECG or on ambulatory monitoring.[69–74] These tests are also more likely to be positive in patients with bundle branch block, identifying isolated conduction disease or ventricular tachyarrhythmias. Predictors of ventricular tachycardia by electrophysiological studies include organic heart disease, PVCs by ECG, and nonsustained ventricular tachycardia by Holter monitoring.[75] Sinus bradycardia, first-degree AV block, and bundle branch block by ECG predict bradyarrhythmic outcome.[75]

Predictors of a negative electrophysiological study in patients with syncope include the absence of heart disease, an ejection fraction over 40 per cent; normal ECG and Holter monitoring, absence of injury during syncope, and multiple or prolonged (> 5 minutes) episodes of syncope.[71] In studies of patients with syncope who have electrophysiological testing, the proportion of patients with positive findings has ranged between 18 and 75 per cent (mean of 60 per cent).[69] Approximately 35 per cent (range 0 to 80) had inducible ventricular tachycardia, 20 per cent (range 0 to 60) supraventricular tachycardia, 35 per cent (range 11 to 60) conduction disturbance (abnormal sinus node, atrioventricular node, or His-Purkinje function), and 10 per cent (range 0 to 24) other abnormalities (including hypervagotonia and carotid hypersensitivity).

Several issues need to be considered in using electrophysiological studies in the evaluation of syncope: First, induced arrhythmias presumed to be diagnostic should be associated with or capable of producing symptomatic hypotension. Second, the clinical significance of some of the electrophysiological abnormalities may be difficult to determine because of problems with sensitivity and specificity of several electrophysiological findings. For example, prolonged sinus node recovery time has a low sensitivity for diagnosis of sinus node dysfunction (18 to 69 per cent), but high specificity (88 to 100 per cent) when electrophysiological results are compared with ambulatory monitoring.[72,73] Tests for atrioventricular nodal conduction and refractoriness are also difficult to interpret and vary considerably with autonomic tone. A prolonged H-V interval and block between H and V with atrial pacing is a marker of significant conduction disease that may have resulted in bradyarrhythmias and syncope; however, cutpoints for the length of H-V interval have varied widely when syncope is attributed to conduction system disease (criteria have ranged from over 55 msec to over 100 msec).

Supraventricular tachycardia and atrial fibrillation or flutter may be occasionally initiated during electrophysiological studies, especially if aggressive induction procedures are used. The significance of these induced arrhythmias is uncertain unless they reproduce the patient's spontaneous symptoms.

Patients with structural heart disease have higher rates of inducible ventricular tachycardia as compared with those without cardiac disease (approximately 55 to 70 per cent vs. less than 20 per cent). The finding of *sustained monomorphic ventricular tachycardia* (see p. 679) has a high sensitivity and specificity for the presence of spontaneous ventricular tachycardia. However, induction of *polymorphic* or *nonsustained ventricular tachycardia* may frequently represent a nonspecific response to an aggressive ventricular stimulation protocol.

Third, the variations in the proportion of patients with positive findings on electrophysiological testing in syncope may be due to patient selection, testing methodology, and criteria for abnormal results. Patients have included those with single as well as multiple episodes and with many types of organic heart diseases as well as without heart disease. Testing variations include performance of left ventricular stimulation, use of isoproterenol, use of procainamide infusion during testing, and the number of extrastimuli for induction procedures.

In evaluation of outcomes, recurrence in follow-up is used as a measure of the effectiveness of testing with the assumption that treatment based on abnormal results leads to resolution of symptoms. In those who have normal studies, recurrence rates are 8 to 80 per cent with a mean of 35 per cent, while recurrence rates in those with abnormal testing are 0 to 32 per cent with a mean of 15 per cent over a mean length of follow-up of 11 to 36 months.[69] These data suggest potential outcome benefit for patients with an abnormal study. The interpretation of the rate of recurrence is, however, complicated because it may be caused by the side effects of drugs, noncompliance, inadequate treatment, or an incorrect initial diagnosis. Furthermore, recurrences are sporadic; thus, analysis of their rate over time may be difficult.

Mortality and incidence of sudden death in patients with positive findings are higher than in those with negative findings. For example, a 3-year sudden death rate of 48 per cent in patients with positive studies as compared with 9 per cent in those with negative studies has been found.[70] These differences are probably largely due to higher prevalence of cardiac comorbidity in patients with positive findings. These differences suggest that aggressive treatment of underlying heart disease should be pursued, in addition to the treatment of arrhythmia. A low rate of mortality and sudden death in patients with negative studies can also be reassuring because this defines a low-risk group of syncope patients.[76]

Upright Tilt Testing

Upright tilt testing refers to maintaining the patient in an upright position for a brief period to provoke vasovagal syncope. Upright tilt leads to pooling of blood in the lower limbs, resulting in decreased venous return (Fig. 28–2). Normal compensatory response to upright posture is reflex tachycardia, more forceful contraction of the ventricles, and vasoconstriction. However, in individuals susceptible to vasovagal syncope, this forceful ventricular contraction[76a] in the setting of a relatively empty ventricle, may activate the cardiac mechanoreceptors, triggering reflex hypotension and/or bradycardia. Catecholamine release (as may occur with anxiety, fear, and panic), by increasing ventricular contraction, may also activate the nerve endings responsible for triggering this reflex. Thus, catecholamines have been used to facilitate positive responses during upright tilt testing.[1,2]

Almost all tilt testing protocols employ tilt tables with footboard support. Saddle support is not used clinically because of poor specificity.[77] Testing is often performed in a fasting state and vasoactive drugs (e.g., calcium channel blockers, vasodilators, diuretics) are withheld before testing (approximately for 5 half-lives). The test should generally be performed in a quiet room, minimizing surrounding noise such as beepers and traffic. There should be ample lighting, and the temperature should be kept comfortably cool.

Monitoring of blood pressure during upright tilt testing has been done either noninvasively (e.g., with blood pressure cuff or digital plethysmography) or by invasive intraarterial blood pressure monitoring. Although concern has been voiced that invasive procedures may provoke vasova-

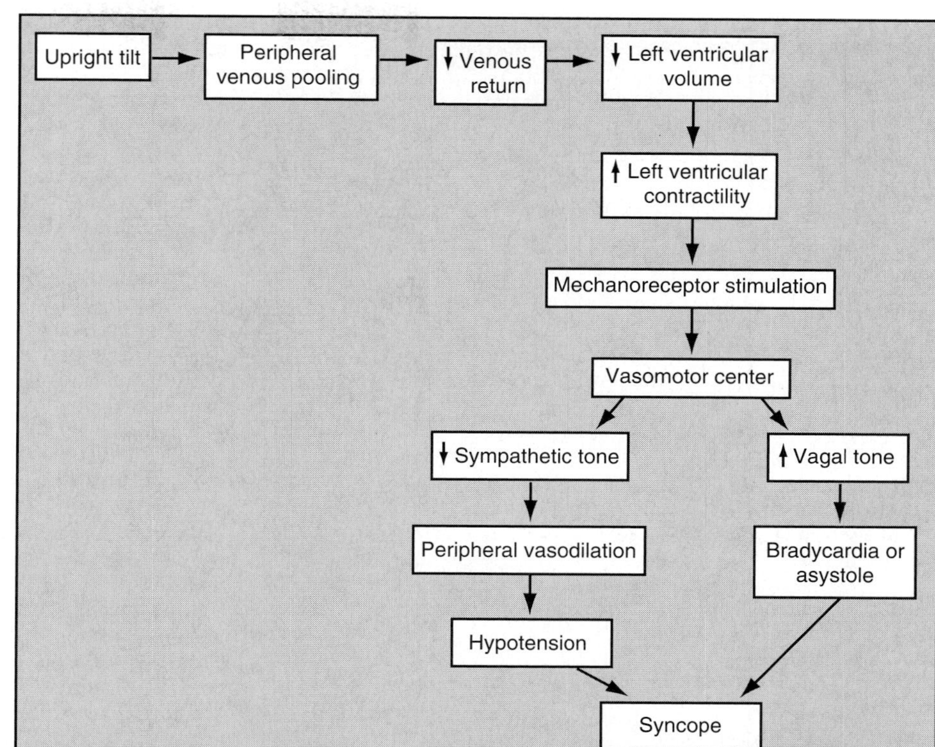

FIGURE 28–2. A pathophysiological mechanism for induction of vasovagal syncope during upright tilt testing.

gal reactions, the effect of monitoring has not been clearly established. Whenever possible, invasive monitoring should be avoided because of the provocation of vasovagal responses and increase in cost and complexity of testing.

The two general types of testing procedures are upright tilt testing alone (passive testing) and tilt testing in conjunction with a chemical agent. The vast majority of the reported studies employ passive testing[77–83] or use isoproterenol after a brief period of passive tilt testing.[51,84–93] Limited experiences with epinephrine,[94] edrophonium,[95] intravenous or sublingual nitroglycerin,[23] and esmolol tilt testing with esmolol withdrawal[96] are reported. These protocols cannot be recommended for general use because of limited data on their performance characteristics.

During passive tilt testing protocols, after baseline supine measurements of blood pressure and continuous monitoring of heart rate, patients are suddenly brought to an upright position. As shown in Table 28–4, most studies using passive testing protocols have employed a tilt angle of 60 degrees. Although protocols consisting of 60 minutes of testing have been studied, a total duration of 45 minutes is recommended because that time is two standard deviations away from mean time to positive responses (approximately 24 minutes).[77]

All testing protocols incorporating *isoproterenol* employ a passive phase of testing. The most common duration of this phase has been 10 to 15 minutes. If an endpoint of the study is not reached, the patient is generally brought to a supine position. Isoproterenol infusion is started while the patient is supine. The most common starting infusion rate is 1 μg/min; the most common duration of tilt testing with isoproterenol at each dose is 10 to 15 minutes. If patients do not develop an endpoint during this phase of testing, they are again brought to a supine position, isoproterenol infusion rate is increased, and patients are retilted for a similar duration of testing as during the initial dose of isoproterenol. This procedure is continued with increasing doses of isoproterenol until a positive response or another endpoint (e.g., maximum dosage, adverse effects, or development of severe tachycardia) is reached. The maximum dosage of isoproterenol used in reported studies is 3 to 5 μg/min. The endpoints of a positive response are syncope or presyncope in association with hypotension and/or bradycardia, although no standard definitions of hypotension or bradycardia are used across the studies.

POSITIVE RESPONSES IN PATIENTS WITH UNEXPLAINED SYNCOPE. In studies using passive upright tilt testing, 49 per cent (range 26 to 90 per cent) have had a positive response to tilt testing (Table 28–5), while in studies using isoproterenol, overall positive responses are approximately 64 per cent (range 39 to 87 per cent).[97] Approximately two-thirds of the positive responses occur during the isoproterenol phase. With either type of testing, about two-thirds of the responses appear to be cardioinhibitory (defined as bradycardia with or without associated hypotension), and the rest are pure vasodepressor reactions (defined as hypotension without significant bradycardia).

Higher angles and longer duration of testing are associated with higher positive responses to tilt testing.[97] The angle of testing during passive protocols has been 60 degrees, while with isoproterenol it predominantly has been 80 degrees, although studies have reported testing at 60, 70, and 90 degrees (Table 28–4). The duration of the passive phase of testing has also been variable, ranging from 5 to 60 minutes.[97] Additionally, the dosing of isoproterenol has also been variable, including bolus infusions starting at 2 μg as well as infusions based on body weight and heart rate increase (Table 28–4).[97] The maximum dosage of isoproterenol has also varied. The differences between positive responses on passive protocols and testing with isoproterenol appear to be due to differences in the angle and duration of testing. When studies of tilt testing with isoproterenol using 60 degree angles are compared with passive tilt testing at 60 degrees for 60 minutes, the positive responses are similar at 52 versus 54 per cent, respectively.[97]

SENSITIVITY AND SPECIFICITY. Sensitivity is determined by calculating the ratio of number of patients with positive tests over the number of patients who have the disease. The disease has to be diagnosed independently of the test by using a separate gold standard. In small studies of patients who have clinical vasovagal syncope, 67 to 83 per cent have had positive response, thus equalling the sensitivity of this test.[93,94] Specificity is defined as the propor-

TABLE 28–4 TILT TESTING PROTOCOLS

	PASSIVE (NO. OF STUDIES)	ISOPROTERENOL (NO. OF STUDIES)
Tilt Angle		
40°	1	—
60°	9	3
70°	—	1
80°	—	11
90°	—	1
Other*	1	—
Duration of Passive Tilt (in minutes)		
10	—	5
15	1	4
20	1	1
30	—	5
60	8	1
Other†	1	
Dose of Isoproterenol		
Starting dose		
1 μg/min		12
2 μg/min		1
0.02–0.04 μg/kg/min		1
2 μg‡		1
Other§		1
Increment in dose		
1 μg/min		10
2 μg/min		2
3 μg/min		1
0.05–0.1 μg/kg/min		1
2 μg‡		1
Other§		1
Highest		
3 μg/min		6
4 μg/min		1
5 μg/min		7
8 μg		1
0.05–0.1 μg/kg/min		1
Endpoints**		
Syncope	3	5
Syncope/Presyncope	2	3
Syncope or Presyncope in association with hypotension and/or bradycardia	4	8
Other	2††	6

* Endpoints were not specifically stated.
† 26 minutes.
‡ One study used bolus infusion starting only at 2 μg and increasing dose by 2 mg.
§ One study gave isoproterenol to elicit a 20 per cent increase in heart rate.
** 15°, 30°, 45° for 2 minutes, then 60° for 20 minutes.
†† Studies with isoproterenol report multiple other endpoints that are not mutually exclusive.
Adapted from Kapoor, W. N., et al.: Upright tilt testing in evaluating syncope: A comprehensive literature review. Am. J. Med. *97*:78, 1994.

tion of subjects without the disease or disorder who have a negative test. Specificity has generally been evaluated by performing upright tilt testing in subjects who have not had syncope previously. With passive tilt testing, specificity has been variable and has ranged between 0 and 100 per cent, although an overall rate is approximately 90 per cent.[97] The overall specificity of upright tilt testing with isoproterenol is approximately 75 per cent and range of 35 to 100 per cent.[97–99] Subjects of studies reporting poor specificity of tilt testing with isoproterenol were generally younger as compared with those reporting higher specificity.[97,98]

REPRODUCIBILITY. Reproducibility of upright tilt testing of 67 to 85 per cent has been adequate,[86,97,100–103] except for a recent study that showed remarkable lack of reproducibility.[104] In a study of 109 patients undergoing 2 consecutive days of passive testing, there was a 63 per cent rate of discordance between day 1 and day 2 of testing.[104] Of patients who had vasovagal syncope on day one, only 31 per cent had it on the second day.

TABLE 28–5 POSITIVE RESPONSES

	TOTAL SUBJECTS	NO. POSITIVE	% POSITIVE	POSITIVE RANGE
Passive tilt only	425	210	49	26–90
Isoproterenol tilt				
Passive phase	592	133	23	0–57
Isoproterenol phase	459	220	48	12–81
Overall	592	378*	64	39–87

* These 378 patients include 25 positive patients from one study that did not specify whether those patients were positive during the isoproterenol phase or the passive phase.
Adapted from Kapoor, W. N., et al.: Upright tilt testing in evaluating syncope: A comprehensive literature review. Am. J. Med. *97*:78, 1994.

Neurological Testing

Skull films, lumbar puncture, radionuclide brain scan, and cerebral angiography do not generally yield diagnostic information for a cause of syncope in the absence of clinical findings suggestive of a specific neurological process.[48] Studies of the EEG in patients with syncope have shown that an epileptiform abnormality was found in 1 per cent of patients; almost all of these were suspected clinically.[34,105] Treatment based on the EEG was initiated in 1 to 2 per cent of patients.[105] Head computed tomography (CT) scans are rarely useful to assign an etiology but are needed if a subdural hemorrhage due to head injury is suspected or in patients suspected to have a seizure as a cause of loss of consciousness.[34]

Specific tests of autonomic function are on occasion useful in defining further the nature of disease responsible for postural hypotension or when no clear reason for orthostasis is apparent.[31] These tests include cardiovascular responses to deep breathing, hyperventilation, stress (handgrip, noise, mental arithmetic, and cold pressor test), breath holding, and Valsalva maneuver. Protocols are also available for sweating and pupillary responses and pharmacological and biochemical testing of sympathetic and parasympathetic systems.[31] These tests are not recommended routinely because clinical data with a focus on autonomic symptoms, diseases causing orthostatic hypotension, and drugs frequently provide clues to the etiology of orthostatic hypotension, and there is often little need for additional diagnostic testing or for therapy selection.

Psychiatric Assessment

Psychiatric illnesses need to be considered as a cause of syncope, especially in young patients and those with multiple syncopal episodes who also have other nonspecific complaints. A high clinical suspicion for these disorders is needed because they are often not diagnosed in medical patients. Screening instruments for generalized anxiety disorder, panic attack and disorder, depression, and somatization disorder are recommended. A high rate of recurrence of syncope in these patients makes detection of these illnesses especially important.

Approach to Diagnostic Evaluation

As shown in Figure 28–3, history and physical examination are the starting points in the evaluation of the patient with syncope. Furthermore, the history and physical examination may reveal findings suggestive of specific entities as possible causes (e.g., findings of aortic stenosis or neurological signs and symptoms suggestive of a seizure disorder) that may require further noninvasive or invasive directed tests for establishing a diagnosis and initiating treatment.

An ECG is generally needed for the evaluation of patients with syncope, the cause of which is not evident from the history and physical examination. Although the diagnostic

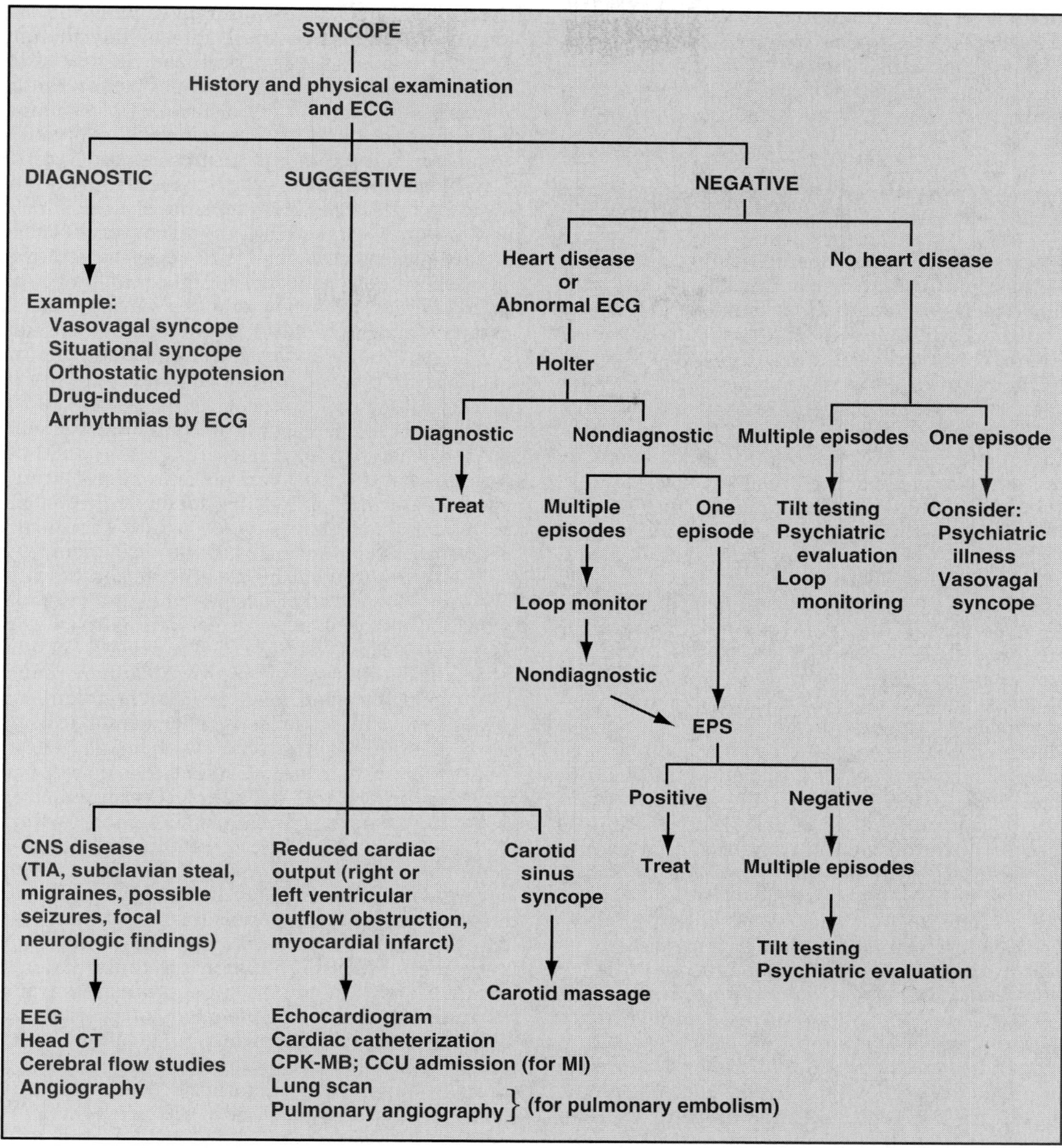

FIGURE 28–3. A flow diagram showing the approach to the evaluation of syncope.

yield of an ECG is low (e.g., for arrhythmias or suspicion of myocardial infarction), abnormalities can be treated quickly if found. Furthermore, patients with a normal ECG have a low likelihood of arrhythmias as a cause of syncope and are at low risk of sudden death. Thus, the ECG can offer both diagnostic and prognostic information which may have an important role in further evaluation and management.

In patients in whom a cause of syncope is not determined by the history, physical examination, and ECG, further testing can be approached by stratifying patients into those with and without heart disease and/or ECG abnormalities. If the presence or absence of heart disease cannot be determined clinically, specific tests such as echocardiogram, stress test, and ventricular function studies may be needed.

In patients with coronary artery disease, congestive heart failure, valvular heart disease, hypertrophic cardiomyopathy, or ECG abnormalities (e.g., bundle branch block or bifascicular block), prolonged ECG monitoring is the first step in evaluation. If prolonged monitoring is nondiagnostic, electrophysiological studies should be considered if symptoms are consistent with arrhythmic syncope. The findings of electrophysiological studies can form the basis for therapy. Patients with negative electrophysiological studies have a favorable prognosis, and thus empiric therapy with a pacemaker or antiarrhythmics is not justified. In patients with negative electrophysiological studies and recurrent unexplained syncope, upright tilt testing may help define neurally mediated syncope as a potential cause.

Younger patients (less than 60 years of age) with syncope and without heart disease have an excellent prognosis.[106] Furthermore, in patients with a normal ECG, the likelihood of arrhythmias is low, and prolonged electrocardiographic monitoring rarely leads to a specific diagnosis. The yield of electrophysiological studies in patients without heart disease is low. Thus, these studies are not justified in most patients. Many patients (especially those with recurrent syncope) probably have vasovagal syncope or psychiatric disorders that should be investigated. Although similar conclusions probably apply to older patients without heart disease, further studies are needed to better define the role of tests for detection of arrhythmias, especially for diagnosis of bradyarrhythmias.

Patients with recurrent syncope constitute a group in which management is difficult. Patients with multiple episodes (more than 5 in the last year) are less likely to have arrhythmias[71] and are more likely to have psychiatric illnesses.[17] The extent of initial evaluation of these patients is guided by the presence or absence of heart disease. In patients with frequent recurrent syncope in whom there is a high suspicion of arrhythmias, loop event recorders are especially valuable if a cause is not established by other means.

MANAGEMENT

Management issues include hospitalization decision, treatment selection, and patient instructions and education.

HOSPITAL ADMISSION. There are no studies evaluating the need for hospital admission in patients with syncope. Generally, patients are admitted if a rapid diagnostic evaluation is needed because of concerns about serious arrhythmias, sudden death, newly diagnosed serious cardiac disease (e.g., aortic stenosis, myocardial infarction), and new onset of seizure or stroke. Admission is also needed for treatment when etiology is clear (e.g., management of dehydration). In the large group of patients with unexplained syncope after initial history, physical examination, and ECG, risk stratification for arrhythmias and sudden death should guide the admission decision.

TREATMENT SELECTION. Because the treatment largely depends on the cause of syncope, a discussion of the treatment of all of the causes is beyond the scope of this review. General management issues and treatments of neurally mediated syncope that have recently received considerable attention will be reviewed.

Neurally Mediated Syncope. Patients may have a cluster of syncopal episodes at one time that may diminish or resolve spontaneously. Thus, the frequency and severity of events need to be considered when long-term therapy is started. Because of potential side effects, treatment should be reserved for patients with frequent or disabling symptoms. Because psychiatric illnesses probably lead to vasovagal reactions, screening for the psychiatric illnesses should be performed. Treatment of the psychiatric illness often will result in resolution of recurrent syncope.

Various drugs and pacemakers have been tried for patients with vasovagal syncope, and a decrease in recurrence of syncope or resolution of symptoms has been reported in almost every uncontrolled study. The most commonly used drugs are beta blockers (e.g., metoprolol 50 to 200 mg/day, atenolol 25 to 200 mg/day, and propranolol 40 to 160 mg/day),[97] which may inhibit the activation of cardiac mechanoreceptors by decreasing cardiac contractility. Anticholinergic drugs, such as transdermal scopolamine 1 patch every 2 to 3 days, have been tried,[97] particularly in patients with profound bradycardia during upright tilt testing. Disopyramide (200 to 600 mg/day) (see p. 609) has anticholinergic and negative inotropic effects that may inhibit activation of cardiac mechanoreceptors.[107,108] Measures to expand volume, such as increased salt intake, custom-fitted counterpressure support garments from ankle to waist, and fludrocortisone acetate (0.1 to 1 mg per day) are frequently used.[89,90,97] Potential side effects may include recumbent hypertension, hypokalemia, fluid retention, and congestive heart failure.

Theophylline (6 to 12 mg/kg/day) has been tried on occasion.[109] The mechanism of action of theophylline in the treatment of vasovagal syncope is not known; a blockade of effects of adenosine, which has vasodilatory effects, is postulated. Limited uncontrolled but favorable experiences are reported with serotonin reuptake inhibitors fluoxetine[110] and sertraline,[111] ephedrine,[112] etilephrine,[113] dihydroergotamine,[113] dextroamphetamine,[114] and pseudoephedrine.[115]

Finally, atrioventricular pacing has been utilized in patients with significant bradycardia in response to upright tilt testing.[116–118] Pacemakers may ameliorate symptoms but vasodepressor reactions still continue to occur. Even in patients with bradycardia and asystole as the major response to tilt testing, drug treatment is the therapy of choice. There is concern about the efficacy of any of the treatments for vasovagal syncope because one randomized trial showed no difference in recurrence of syncope between 15 treated (with a variety of drugs such as atenolol, dihydroergotamine, cafedrine) and 15 untreated patients.[113]

Orthostatic Hypotension. The initial approach to treatment of orthostatic hypotension is to ensure adequate salt and volume intake and to discontinue drugs that cause orthostatic hypotension. Patients with orthostatic hypotension should be advised to raise the head of the bed at night, to rise from bed or chair slowly, and to avoid prolonged standing. Compressive stockings applied up to thigh levels may help decrease venous pooling. Frequent small feedings may be helpful in patients with marked postprandial hypotension.

Pharmacological agents of potential benefit include fludrocortisone (0.1 to 1.0 mg/day), in conjunction with increased salt intake. Various adrenergic agents have been used, including ephedrine, phenylephrine, and others. A more detailed discussion of pharmacological treatment of orthostatic hypotension is found elsewhere.[31]

Elderly. Syncope in the elderly can be difficult to manage because elderly patients may have multiple chronic diseases and physiological impairments that predispose to syncope.[30] Thus, in the elderly, several seemingly mild abnormalities may contribute to a sudden reduction of cerebral blood flow and syncope. As an example, mild volume depletion with upper respiratory tract infection in an elderly patient with chronic renal insufficiency and systolic hypertension may be sufficient to cause syncope, whereas any one problem alone is not severe enough to cause loss of consciousness. The initial approach to the management of the elderly should be to search for a single condition as a cause of syncope. If a single condition is found (such as severe aortic stenosis, symptomatic bradycardia, or symptomatic orthostatic hypotension), treatment of that disease can be planned. However, a single disease as the cause of syncope is often not apparent. In these patients, inability to compensate for common situational stresses may be a factor in the setting of multiple medical problems, medications, and physiological impairments. A careful assessment of the effect of underlying pathological conditions and medications is important to determine whether multiple pathological processes could have led to syncope. Once these potential processes are identified, treatment should be directed to correcting these factors. As an example, consider an elderly patient presenting with syncope, who has taken enalapril 10 mg/day, has anemia (hemoglobin 9.0), mild orthostatic hypotension, and a recent upper respiratory tract infection. In this patient, if no other etiology of syncope is apparent on the basis of clinical findings and selective use of laboratory tests, volume repletion, treatment of anemia and adjustment or change of antihypertensive medication may help prevent further episodes of syncope.

PATIENT INSTRUCTIONS AND EDUCATION. Issues in patient education include instructions in prevention of syncope, non-pharmacologic treatment, and restriction of activities. Many patients with vasovagal syncope have precipitating factors or situations that should be identified and the patient instructed to avoid these situations. Common triggers include prolonged standing, venipuncture, large meals, and heat (such as hot baths or sunbathing). Additionally, fasting, lack of sleep, and alcohol intake may predispose to vasovagal syncope and should be avoided. Postexercise vasovagal syncope may occasionally be related to chronic inadequate salt and fluid replacement. Syncope may be prevented with the use of electrolyte-containing solutions and water in such instances. In other patients, exercise may have to be curtailed.

Patients with syncope should also be instructed to assume a supine position as soon as they develop premonitory symptoms. They should remain supine for 15 to 30 minutes. Patients with potential recurrences need to be instructed to avoid activities that may lead to serious injury to the patient or others. Activities such as swimming, mountain climbing, operating milling machines and saws, and other similar work should be curtailed or performed in the presence of a companion.

Although 84 per cent of states in the United States have specific regulations for driving restriction for seizures, only 26 states (52 per cent) have regulations that limit driving after an episode of loss of consciousness other than seizure (e.g., vasovagal syncope, arrhythmias, diabetic coma).[119] In nonseizure loss of consciousness, the average mandated duration of driving restriction is 4.3 months. In addition to adhering to state regulations on driving, the likelihood of recurrent episodes and the probability of treatment efficacy should be considered in restricting driving.[119,120]

REFERENCES

1. Benditt, D. G., Remole, S., Bailin, S., et al.: Tilt table testing for evaluation of neurally-mediated (cardioneurogenic) syncope: Rationale and proposed protocols. PACE *14*:1528, 1991.
2. Abboud, F. M.: Neurocardiogenic syncope. N. Engl. J. Med. *15*:1117, 1993.
3. Waxman, M. B., Cameron, D. A., and Wald, R. W.: Role of ventricular vagal afferents in the vasovagal reaction. J. Am. Coll. Cardiol. *21*:1138, 1993.
4. Scherrer, U., Vissing, S., Morgan, B. J., et al.: Vasovagal syncope after infusion of a vasodilator in a heart transplant recipient. N. Engl. J. Med. *32*:602, 1990.
5. Fitzpatrick, A. P., Banner, N., Cheng, A., et al.: Vasovagal reactions may occur after orthotopic heart transplantation. J. Am. Coll. Cardiol. *21*:1132, 1993.
6. Lightfoot, J. T., Rowe, S. A., and Fortney, S. M.: Occurrence of presyncope in subjects without ventricular innervation. Clin. Sci. *85*:695, 1993.
7. Moorita, H., Nishida, Y., Motochigawa, H., et al.: Opiate receptor-mediated decrease in renal nerve activity during hypotensive hemorrhage in conscious rabbits. Circ. Res. *63*:165, 1988.
8. Smite, M. L., Carlson, M. D., and Thames, M. D.: Naloxone does not prevent vasovagal syncope during simulated orthostatis in humans. J. Am. Nerv. *45*:1, 1993.
9. Schadt, J. C., and Ludbrook, J.: Hemodynamic and neurohumoral responses to acute hypovolemia in conscious mammals. Am. J. Physiol. (Heart Circ. Physiol. 29) *260*:H305, 1991.
10. Kapoor, W. N., Peterson, J., and Karpf, M.: Micturition syncope. JAMA *253*:796, 1985.
11. Kapoor, W. N., Peterson, J., and Karpf, M.: Defecation syncope. A symptom with multiple etiologies. Arch. Intern. Med. *146*:2377, 1986.
12. Strasberg, B., Sagie, A., Erdman, S., et al.: Carotid sinus hypersensivity and the carotid sinus syndrome. Prog. Cardiovasc. Dis. *5*:379, 1989.
13. Katritsis, D., Ward, D. E., and Camm, A. J.: Can we treat carotid sinus syndrome? PACE *14*:1367, 1991.
14. Brignole, M., Oddone, D., Cogorno, S., et al.: Long-term outcome in symptomatic carotid sinus hypersensitivity. Am. Heart J. *123*:687, 1992.
15. Brignole, M., Menozzi, C., Lolli, G., et al.: Long-term outcome of paced and nonpaced patients with severe carotid sinus syndrome. Am. J. Cardiol. *69*:1039, 1992.
16. Nicholas, R., O'Meara, P. D., and Calonge, N.: Is syncope related to moderate altitude exposure? JAMA *268*:904, 1992.
17. Kapoor, W. N., Fortunato, M., Hanusa, B. H., and Schulberg, H. C.: Psychiatric illnesses in patients with syncope. Am. J. Med. *99*:505, 1995.
18. Koenig, D., Linzer, M., Pontinenn, M., and Divine, G. W.: Syncope in young adults: evidence for a combined medical and psychiatric approach. J. Intern. Med. *232*:169, 1992.
19. Linzer, M., Felder, A., Hackel, A., et al.: Psychiatric syncope. Psychosom. Med. *31*:181, 1990.
20. Grubb, B. P., Temesy-Armos, P. N., Samoil, D., et al.: Tilt table testing in the evaluation and management of athletes with recurrent exercise-induced syncope. Med. Sci. Sports Exerc. *28*:24, 1993.
21. Osswald, S., Brooks, R., O'Nunain, S. S., et al.: Asystole after exercise in healthy persons. Ann. Intern. Med. *120*:1008, 1994.
22. Sneddon, J. F., Scalia, G., Ward, D. E., et al.: Exercise-induced vasodepressor syncope. Br. Heart J. *71*:554, 1994.
23. Raviele, A. N., Gasparini, G., DiPede, F., et al.: Nitroglycerine infusion during upright tilt: A new test for the diagnosis of vasovagal syncope. Am. Heart J. *127*:103, 1994.
24. Grech, E. D., and Ramsdale, D. R.: Exertional syncope in aortic stenosis. Am. Heart J. *121*:603, 1991.
25. Gilligan, D. M., Nihoyannopoulos, P., Chan, W. L., and Oakley, C. M.: Investigation of a hemodynamic basis for syncope in hypertrophic cardiomyopathy. Use of head-up tilt test. Circulation *85*:2140, 1992.
26. Leitch, J. W., Klein, G. J., Yee, R., et al.: Syncope associated with supraventricular tachycardia: An expression of tachycardia rate or vasomotor response? Circulation *85*:1064, 1992.
27. Brignole, M., Gianfranchi, L., Menozzi, C., et al.: Role of autonomic reflexes in syncope associated with paroxysmal atrial fibrillation. J. Am. Coll. Cardiol. *22*:1123, 1993.
28. Pavlovic, S. U., Kocovic, D., Djordjevic, M., et al.: The etiology of syncope in pacemaker patients. PACE *14*:2086, 1991.
29. Lipsitz, L.: Orthostatic hypotension in the elderly. N. Engl. J. Med. *321*:952, 1989.
30. Kapoor, W. N.: Syncope in the older person. J. Am. Geriatr. Soc. *42*:426, 1994.
31. Bannister, S. R. (ed.): Autonomic Failure: A Textbook of Clinical Disorders of the Autonomic Nervous System. 2nd ed. Oxford, Oxford Medical Publishers, 1988, pp. 1–20.
32. Vaitkevicius, P. V., Esserwein, D. M., Maynard, A. K., et al.: Frequency and importance of postprandial blood pressure reduction in elderly nursing-home patients. Ann. Intern. Med. *115*:865, 1991.
33. Davidson, E., Rotenbeg, Z., Fuchs, J., et al.: Transient ischemic attack–related syncope. Clin. Cardiol. *14*:141, 1991.
34. Kapoor, W.: Evaluation and outcome of patients with syncope. Medicine *69*:160, 1990.
35. Kapoor, W., Karpf, M., Wieand, S., et al.: A prospective evaluation and follow-up of patients with syncope. N. Engl. J. Med. *309*:197, 1983.
36. Gambardella, A., Reutens, D. C., Andermann, F., et al.: Late-onset drop attacks in temporal lobe epilepsy: A reevaluation of the concept of temporal lobe syncope. Neurology *44*:1074, 1994.
37. Jacome, D. E.: Temporal lobe syncope: Clinical variants. Clin. Electroencephal. *20*:58, 1989.
38. Constantin, L., Martins, J. B., Fincham, R. W., and Dagli, R. D.: Bradycardia and syncope as manifestations of partial epilepsy. J. Am. Coll. Cardiol. *15*:900, 1990.
39. Baltazar, R. F., Go, E. H., Benesh, S., and Mower, M. M.: Case report: Myocardial ischemia: an overlooked substrate in syncope of aortic stenosis. Am. J. Med. Sci. *303*:105, 1992.
40. Dilsizian, V., Bonow, R. O., Epstein, S. E., and Fananapazir, L.: Myocardial ischemia detected by thallium scintigraphy is frequently related to cardiac arrest and syncope in young patients with hypertrophic cardiomyopathy. J. Am. Coll. Cardiol. *22*:796, 1993.
41. Fananapazir, L., Tracy, C. M., Leon, M. B., et al.: Electrophysiologic abnormalities in patients with hypertrophic cardiomyopathy. Circulation *80*:1259, 1989.
42. Nienaber, C. A., Hiller, S., Spielmann, R. P., et al.: Syncope in hypertrophic cardiomyopathy: Multivariate analysis of prognostic determinants. J. Am. Coll. Cardiol. *15*:948, 1990.
43. Bradenburg, R. O.: Syncope and sudden death in hypertrophic cardiomyopathy. J. Am. Coll. Cardiol. *15*:962, 1990.
44. Sgarbossa, E. B., Pinski, S. L., Jaeger, F. J., et al.: Incidence and predictors of syncope in paced patients with sick sinus syndrome. PACE *15*:2055, 1992.
45. Paul, T., Guccione, P., and Garson, A.: Relationship of syncope in young patients with Wolff-Parkinson-White syndrome to rapid ventricular response during atrial fibrillation. Am. J. Cardiol. *65*:318, 1990.
46. Auricchio, A., Klein, H., Trappe, H., and Wenzlaff, P.: Lack of prognostic value of syncope in patients with Wolff-Parkinson-White syndrome. J. Am. Coll. Cardiol. *17*:152, 1991.
47. James, T. N.: Syncope and sudden death in the Wolff-Parkinson-White syndrome. J. Am. Coll. Cardiol. *17*:159, 1991.
48. Kapoor, W., Karpf, M., Maher, Y., et al.: Syncope of unknown origin: The need for a more cost-effective approach to its diagnostic evaluation. JAMA *247*:2687, 1982.
49. Silverstein, M. D., Singer, D. E., Mulley, A., et al.: Patients with syncope admitted to medical intensive care units. JAMA *248*:1185, 1982.
50. Martin, G. J., Adams, S. L., Martin, H. G., et al.: Prospective evaluation of syncope. Ann. Emerg. Med. *13*:499, 1984.
51. Sra, J. S., Anderson, A. J., Sheikh, S. H., et al.: Unexplained syncope evaluated by electrophysiologic studies and head-up tilt testing. Ann. Intern. Med. *114*:1013, 1991.
52. Savage, D. D., Corwin, L., McGee, D. L., et al.: Epidemiologic features of isolated syncope. The Framingham Study. Stroke *16*:626, 1985.
53. Middlekauff, H. R., Stevenson, W. G., and Sacon, L. A.: Prognosis after syncope: Impact of left ventricular function. Am. Heart J. *125*:121, 1993.
54. Middlekauff, H. R., Stevenson, W. G., Stevenson, L. W., and Saxon, L. A.: Syncope in advanced heart failure: High risk of sudden death regardless of origin of syncope. J. Am. Coll. Cardiol. *21*:110, 1993.
55. Kapoor, W., Peterson, J., Wieand, H. S., and Karpf, M.: Diagnostic and prognostic implications of recurrences in patients with syncope. Am. J. Med. *83*:700, 1987.
56. Lempert, T., Bauer, M., and Schmidt, D.: Syncope: A video metric analysis of 56 episodes of transient cerebral hypoxia. Ann. Neurol. *36*:233, 1994.
57. Hoefnagels, W. A. J., Padberg, G. W., Overweg, J., et al.: Syncope or seizure? The diagnostic value of the EEG and hyperventilation test in transient loss of consciousness. J. Neurol. *54*:953, 1991.
58. Grubb, B. P., Gerard, G., Roush, K., et al.: Differentiation of convulsive syncope and epilepsy with head-up tilt testing. Ann. Intern. Med. *115*:871, 1991.
59. Atkins, D., Hanusa, B., Sefcik, T., and Kapoor, W.: Syncope and orthostatic hypotension. Am. J. Med. *91*:179, 1991.
60. Kenny, R. A., and Traynor, G.: Carotid sinus syndrome: Clinical characteristics in elderly patients. Age Ageing *20*:449, 1991.
61. Winters, S. L., Stewart, D., and Gomes, J. A.: Signal averaging of the surface QRS complex predicts inducibility of ventricular tachycardia in

patients with syncope of unknown origin: A prospective study. J. Am. Coll. Cardiol. *10*(4):775, 1987.
62. Gang, E. S., Peter, T., Rosenthal, M. E., et al.: Detection of late potentials on the surface electrocardiogram in unexplained syncope. Am. J. Cardiol. *58*(10):14, 1986.
63. Steinberg, J. S., Prytowsky, E., Freedman, R. A., et al.: Use of the signal-averaged electrocardiogram for predicting inducible ventricular tachycardia in patients with unexplained syncope: Relation to clinical variables in a multivariate analysis. J. Am. Coll. Cardiol. *23*:99, 1994.
64. Gibson, T. C., and Heitzman, M. R.: Diagnostic efficacy of 24-hour electrocardiographic monitoring for syncope. Am. J. Cardiol. *53*:1013, 1984.
65. Bass, E. B., Curtiss, E. L., Arena, V. C., et al.: The duration of Holter monitoring in patients with syncope: Is 24 hours enough? Arch. Intern. Med. *150*:1073, 1990.
66. Kapoor, W., Cha, R., Peterson, J., et al.: Prolonged electrocardiographic monitoring in patients with syncope: The importance of frequent or repetitive ventricular ectopy. Am. J. Med. *82*:20, 1987.
67. DiMarco, J. P., and Philbrick, J. T.: Use of ambulatory electrocardiographic (Holter) monitoring. Ann. Intern. Med. *113*:53, 1990.
68. Linzer, M., Pritchett, E. L. C., Pontinenn, M., et al.: Incremental diagnostic yield of loop electrocardiographic recorders in unexplained syncope. Am. J. Cardiol. *66*:214, 1990.
69. Kapoor, W. N., Hammill, S. C., and Gersh, B. J.: Diagnosis and natural history of syncope and the role of invasive electrophysiologic testing. Am. J. Cardiol. *63*:730, 1989.
70. Bass, E. B., Elson, J. J., Fogoros, R. N., et al.: Long-term prognosis of patients undergoing electrophysiologic studies for syncope of unknown origin. Am. J. Cardiol. *62*:1186, 1988.
71. Klein, G. J., Gersh, B. J., and Yee, R.: Electrophysiological testing: The final court of appeal for the diagnosis of syncope? Circulation *92*:1332, 1995.
72. DiMarco, J. P.: Electrophysiologic studies in patients with unexplained syncope. Circulation *75*(Suppl III):140, 1987.
73. McAnulty, J. H.: Syncope of unknown origin: The role of electrophysiologic studies. Circulation *75*(Suppl III):144, 1987.
74. Moazes, F., Peter, T., Simonson, J., et al.: Syncope of unknown origin: clinical, noninvasive, and electrophysiologic determinants of arrhythmia induction and symptom recurrence during long-term follow-up. Am. Heart J. *121*:81, 1991.
75. Bachinsky, W. B., Linzer, M., Weld, L., and Estes, N. A. M.: Usefulness of clinical characteristics in predicting the outcome of electrophysiologic studies in unexplained syncope. Am. J. Cardiol. *69*:1044, 1992.
76. Kushner, J. A., Kou, W. H., Kadish, A. H., and Morady, F.: Natural history of patients with unexplained syncope and a nondiagnostic electrophysiologic study. J. Am. Coll. Cardiol. *14*:391, 1989.
76a. Yamanouchi, Y., Jaalouk, S., Shehadeh, A. A., et al.: Changes in left ventricular volume during head-up tilt in patients with vasovagal syncope. An echocardiographic study. Am. Heart J. *131*:73, 1996.
77. Fitzpatrick, A. P., Theodorakis, G., Vardas, P., and Sutton, R.: Methodology of head-up tilt testing in patients with unexplained syncope. J. Am. Coll. Cardiol. *17*:125, 1991.
78. Hackel, A., Linzer, M., Anderson, N., and Williams, R.: Cardiovascular and catecholamine responses to head-up tilt in the diagnosis of recurrent unexplained syncope in elderly patients. J. Am. Geriatr. Soc. *39*:663, 1991.
79. Kenny, R. A., Ingram, A., Bayliss, J., and Sutton, R.: Head-up tilt: A useful test for investigating unexplained syncope. Lancet *1*:1352, 1986.
80. Lerman-Sagie, T., Rechavia, E., Strasberg, B., et al.: Head-up tilt for the evaluation of syncope of unknown origin in children. J. Pediatr. *118*:676, 1991.
81. Raviele, A., Gasparini, G., DiPede, F., et al.: Usefulness of head-up tilt test in evaluating patients with syncope of unknown origin and negative electrophysiologic study. Am. J. Cardiol. *65*:1322, 1990.
82. Strasberg, B., Rechavia, E., Sagie, A., et al.: The head-up tilt table test in patients with syncope of unknown origin. Am. Heart J. *118*:923, 1989.
83. Abi-Samra, F., Maloney, J. D., Fouad-Tarazi, F. R., and Castle, L. W.: The usefulness of head-up tilt testing and hemodynamic investigations in the workup of syncope of unknown origin. PACE *11*:1202, 1988.
84. Almquist, A., Goldenberg, I. F., Milstein, S., et al.: Provocation of bradycardia and hypotension by isoproterenol and upright posture in patients with unexplained syncope. N. Engl. J. Med. *320*:346, 1989.
85. Chen, M. Y., Goldenberg, I. F., Milstein, S., et al.: Cardiac electrophysiologic and hemodynamic correlates of neurally mediated syncope. Am. J. Cardiol. *63*:66, 1989.
86. Chen, X. C., Chen, M. Y., Remole, S., et al.: Reproducibility of head-up tilt-table testing for eliciting susceptibility to neurally mediated syncope in patients without structural heart disease. Am. J. Cardiol. *69*:755, 1992.
87. Grubb, B. P., Temesy-Armos, P., Hahn, H., and Elliott, L.: Utility of upright tilt-table testing in the evaluation and management of syncope of unknown origin. Am. J. Med. *90*:6, 1991.
88. Grubb, B. P., Gerard, G., Roush, K., et al.: Cerebral vasoconstriction during head-upright tilt-induced vasovagal syncope. Circulation *84*:1157, 1991.
89. Grubb, B. P., Temesy-Armos, P., Moore, J., et al.: Head-upright tilt-table testing in evaluation and management of the malignant vasovagal syndrome. Am. J. Cardiol. *69*:904, 1992.
90. Grubb, B. P., Temesy-Armos, P., Moore, J., et al.: The use of head-upright tilt table testing in the evaluation and management of syncope in children and adolescents. PACE *15*:742, 1992.
91. Pongiglione, G., Fish, F. A., Strasburger, J. F., and Benson, D. W.: Heart rate and blood pressure response to upright tilt in young patients with unexplained syncope. J. Am. Coll. Cardiol. *16*:165, 1990.
92. Sheldon, R., and Killam, S.: Methodology of isoproterenol-tilt table testing in patients with syncope. J. Am. Coll. Cardiol. *19*:773, 1992.
93. Waxman, M. B., Yao, L., Cameron, D. A., et al.: Isoproterenol induction of vasodepressor-type reaction in vasodepressor-prone persons. Am. J. Cardiol. *63*:58, 1989.
94. Calkins, H., Kadish, A., Sousa, J., et al.: Comparison of responses to isoproterenol and epinephrine during head-up tilt in suspected vasodepressor syncope. Am. J. Cardiol. *67*:207, 1991.
95. Lurie, K. G., Dutton, J., Mangat, R., et al.: Evaluation of edrophonium as a provocative agent for vasovagal syncope during head-up tilt-table testing. Am. J. Cardiol. *72*:1286, 1993.
96. Ovadia, M., and Thoele, D.: Esmolol tilt testing with esmolol withdrawal for the evaluation of syncope in the young. Circulation *89*:228, 1994.
97. Kapoor, W. N., Smith, M., and Miller, N. L.: Upright tilt testing in evaluating syncope: a comprehensive literature review. Am. J. Med. *97*:78, 1994.
98. Kapoor, W. N., and Brant, N.: Evaluation of syncope by upright tilt testing with isoproterenol. Ann. Intern. Med. *116*:358, 1992.
99. Nwosu, E. A., Rahkoo, P. S., Hanson, P., and Grogan, E. W.: Hemodynamic and volumetric response of the normal left ventricle to upright tilt test. Am. Heart J. *128*:106, 1994.
100. Sheldon, R., Splawinski, J., and Killam, S.: Reproducibility of isoproterenol tilt table tests in patients with syncope. Am. J. Cardiol. *69*:1300, 1992.
101. Blanc, J. J., Mansourati, J., Maheu, B., et al.: Reproducibility of a positive passive upright tilt test at a seven-day interval in patients with syncope. Am. J. Cardiol. *72*:469, 1993.
102. Fish, F. A., Strasburger, J. F., and Benson, D. W.: Reproducibility of a symptomatic response to upright tilt in young patients with unexplained syncope. Am. J. Cardiol. *70*:605, 1992.
103. de Buitleir, M., Grogan, E. W., Picone, M., and Casteen, J. A.: Immediate reproducibility of the tilt-table test in adults with unexplained syncope. Am. J. Cardiol. *71*:304, 1993.
104. Brooks, R., Ruskin, J. N., Powell, A. C., et al.: Prospective evaluation of day-to-day reproducibility of upright tilt-table testing in unexplained syncope. Am. J. Cardiol. *71*:1289, 1993.
105. Davis, T. L., and Freemoon, F. R.: Electroencephalography should not be routine in the evaluation of syncope in adults. Arch. Intern. Med. *150*:2027, 1990.
106. Kapoor, W., Snustad, D., Peterson, J., et al.: Syncope in the elderly. Am. J. Med. *80*:419, 1986.
107. Kelly, P. A., Mann, D. E., Adler, S. W., et al.: Low-dose disopyramide often fails to prevent neurogenic syncope during head-up tilt testing. PACE *17*:573, 1994.
108. Morilo, C. A., Leith, J. W., Yee, R., and Klein, G. J.: A placebo-controlled trial of intravenous and oral disopyramide for prevention of neurally mediated syncope induced by head-up tilt. J. Am. Coll. Cardiol. *22*:1843, 1993.
109. Nelson, S. D., Stanley, M., Love, C. J., et al.: The autonomic and hemodynamic effects of oral theophylline in patients with vasodepressor syncope. Arch. Intern. Med. *151*(12):2425, 1991.
110. Grubb, B. P., Wolfe, D. A., Samoil, D., et al.: Usefulness of fluoxetine hydrochloride for prevention of resistant upright tilt induced syncope. PACE *16*:458, 1993.
111. Grubb, B. P., Samoil, D., Kosinski, D., et al.: Use of sertraline hydrochloride in the treatment of refractory neurocardiogenic syncope in children and adolescents. J. Am. Coll. Cardiol. *24*:490, 1994.
112. Janoski, D., Holt, D., Fredman, C., and Bjerregaard, P.: Efficacy of oral ephedrine sulfate in preventing neurocardiogenic syncope (abst). Circulation *84*:929, 1991.
113. Brignole, M., Menozzi, C., Gianfranchi, L., et al.: A controlled trial of acute and long-term medical therapy in tilt-induced neurally mediated syncope. Am. J. Cardiol. *70*:339, 1992.
114. Susmano, A., Volgman, A. S., and Buckingham, T. A.: Beneficial effects of dextro-amphetamine in the treatment of vasodepressor syncope. PACE *16*:1235, 1993.
115. Strieper, M. J., and Campbell, R. M.: Efficacy of alpha-adrenergic agonist therapy for prevention of pediatric neurocardiogenic syncope. J. Am. Coll. Cardiol. *22*:594, 1993.
116. Benditt, D. G., Petersen, M., Lurie, K. G., et al.: Cardiac pacing for prevention of recurrent vasovagal syncope. Ann. Intern. Med. *122*:204, 1995.
117. Petersen, M. E. V., Price, D., Williams, T., et al.: Short AV interval VDD Pacing does not prevent tilt induced vasovagal syncope in patients with cardioinhibitory vasovagal syndrome. PACE *17*:882, 1994.
118. Sra, J. S., Jazayeri, M. R., Avitall, B., et al.: Comparison of cardiac pacing with drug therapy in the treatment of neurocardiogenic (vasovagal) syncope with bradycardia or asystole. N. Engl. J. Med. *328*:1085, 1993.
119. Strickberger, S. A., Cantillon, C. O., and Friedman, P. L.: When should patients with lethal ventricular arrhythmia resume driving? An analysis of state regulations and physician practices. Ann. Intern. Med. *115*:560, 1991.
120. Decter, B. M., Goldner, B., and Cohen, T. J.: Vasovagal syncope as a cause of motor vehicle accidents. Am. Heart J. *127*:1619, 1994.

Index 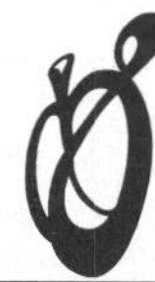

Note: Page numbers in *italics* indicate illustrations; those followed by t indicate tables. **Boldface page numbers** indicate main discussion. **Plate numbers** indicate color plates.

ISBN 0-7216-5664-1